## Section 8
## Problems of Ingestion, Digestion, Absorption, and Elimination



## Section 9
## Problems of Urinary Function



## Section 10
## Problems Related to Regulatory and Reproductive Mechanisms



## Section 11
## Problems Related to Movement and Coordination



## Section 12
## Nursing Care in Critical Care Settings



## Appendixes



Dig toxicity causes PVCs

# MEDICAL-SURGICAL NURSING

## Assessment and Management of Clinical Problems

10th Edition

# MEDICAL-SURGICAL NURSING

## Assessment and Management of Clinical Problems


**Sharon L. Lewis, RN, PhD, FAAN**
Professor Emerita, University of New Mexico, Albuquerque, New Mexico
Former Castella Distinguished Professor, School of Nursing, University of Texas Health Science Center at San Antonio, San Antonio, Texas
Developer and Consultant, Stress-Busting Program for Family Caregivers

**Linda Bucher, RN, PhD, CEN, CNE**
Emerita Professor, School of Nursing, University of Delaware, Newark, Delaware
Per Diem Staff Nurse, Emergency Department, Virtua Memorial Hospital, Mt. Holly, New Jersey

**Margaret McLean Heitkemper, RN, PhD, FAAN**
Professor and Chairperson, Biobehavioral Nursing and Health Systems, Elizabeth Sterling Soule Endowed Chair in Nursing, School of Nursing
Adjunct Professor, Division of Gastroenterology, School of Medicine, University of Washington, Seattle, Washington

**Mariann M. Harding, RN, PhD, CNE**
Associate Professor of Nursing, Kent State University at Tuscarawas, New Philadelphia, Ohio

*Section Editors*

**Jeffrey Kwong, DNP, MPH, ANP-BC, FAANP**
Associate Professor of Nursing at CUMC
Program Director, Adult-Gerontology Nurse Practitioner Program
Program Director, HIV Sub-Specialty
Program Director, Elder LGBT Interprofessional Collaborative Care Program (ELINC)
Program Director, Collaborative Access for LGBT Adults (CALA)
Columbia University School of Nursing
New York, New York

**Dottie Roberts, RN, EdD, MSN, MACI, OCNS-C, CMSRN, CNE**
Executive Director,
Orthopaedic Nurses Certification Board,
Chicago, Illinois;
Editor, "MEDSURG Nursing,"
Official Journal of the Academy of Medical-Surgical Nurses
Pitman, New Jersey


ELSEVIER

ELSEVIER

3251 Riverport Lane
St. Louis, Missouri 63043

MEDICAL-SURGICAL NURSING; ASSESSMENT AND MANAGEMENT OF CLINICAL PROBLEMS, 10TH EDITION

ISBN (single volume): 978-0-323-32852-4



**Notices**

Knowledge and best practice in this field are constantly changing. As new research and experience broaden our understanding, changes in research methods, professional practices, or medical treatment may become necessary.

Practitioners and researchers must always rely on their own experience and knowledge in evaluating and using any information, methods, compounds, or experiments described herein. In using such information or methods they should be mindful of their own safety and the safety of others, including parties for whom they have a professional responsibility.

With respect to any drug or pharmaceutical products identified, readers are advised to check the most current information provided (i) on procedures featured or (ii) by the manufacturer of each product to be administered, to verify the recommended dose or formula, the method and duration of administration, and contraindications. It is the responsibility of practitioners, relying on their own experience and knowledge of their patients, to make diagnoses, to determine dosages and the best treatment for each individual patient, and to take all appropriate safety precautions.

To the fullest extent of the law, neither the Publisher nor the authors, contributors, or editors, assume any liability for any injury and/or damage to persons or property as a matter of products liability, negligence or otherwise, or from any use or operation of any methods, products, instructions, or ideas contained in the material herein.

Herdman, T.H. & Kamitsuru, S. (Eds.). (2014). *NANDA International Nursing Diagnoses: Definitions & Classification, 2015-2017.* Oxford: Wiley Blackwell.

Previous editions copyrighted 2014, 2011, 2007, 2004, 2000, 1996, 1992, 1987, and 1983 by Mosby, Inc., an affiliate of Elsevier Inc.

**Library of Congress Cataloging-in-Publication Data**

Names: Lewis, Sharon Mantik, author.
Title: Medical-surgical nursing : assessment and management of clinical problems / Sharon L. Lewis [and five others].
Description: Tenth edition. | St. Louis, Missouri : Elsevier, Inc, [2017] | Includes bibliographical references and index.
Identifiers: LCCN 2016018182| ISBN 9780323328524 (v. 1 : hardcover : alk. paper) | ISBN 9780323355933 (v. 2 : hardcover : alk. paper)
Subjects: | MESH: Nursing Care | Nursing Assessment | Perioperative Nursing
Classification: LCC RT41 | NLM WY 100 | DDC 617/.0231—dc23 LC record available at https://lccn.loc.gov/2016018182

*Senior Content Strategist:* Jamie Blum
*Content Development Manager:* Jean Sims Fornango
*Content Development Specialist:* Jennifer Hermes, Melissa Rawe
*Publishing Services Manager:* Julie Eddy
*Senior Project Manager:* Mary G. Stueck
*Design Direction:* Ashley Miner, Renée Duenow

Printed in Canada

Last digit is the print number: 9 8 7 6 5 4 3

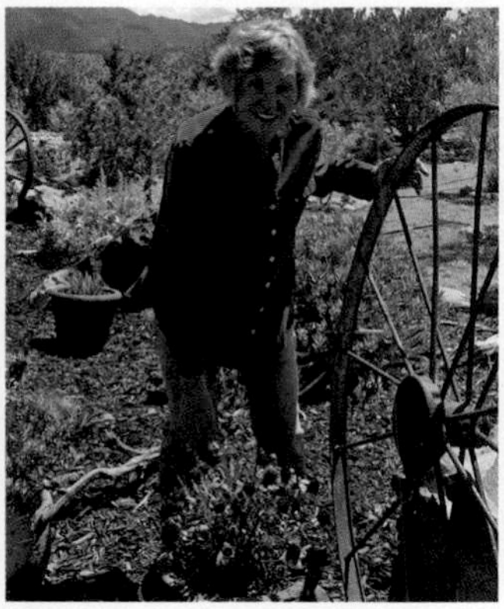

## SHARON L. LEWIS, RN, PhD, FAAN

Sharon Lewis received her Bachelor of Science in nursing from the University of Wisconsin–Madison, Master of Science in nursing with a minor in biological sciences from the University of Colorado–Denver, and PhD in immunology from the Department of Pathology at the University of New Mexico School of Medicine. She had a 2-year postdoctoral fellowship from the National Kidney Foundation. Her more than 45 years of teaching experience include inservice education and teaching in associate degree, baccalaureate, master's degree, and doctoral programs in Maryland, Illinois, Wisconsin, New Mexico, and Texas. Favorite teaching areas are pathophysiology, immunology, and family caregiving. She has been actively involved in clinical research for the past 35 years, investigating altered immune responses in various disorders and developing a stress management program for family caregivers. Her current primary professional responsibility is disseminating the Stress-Busting for Family Caregivers Program that she developed. Her free time is spent biking, landscaping, gardening, and being a grandmother.

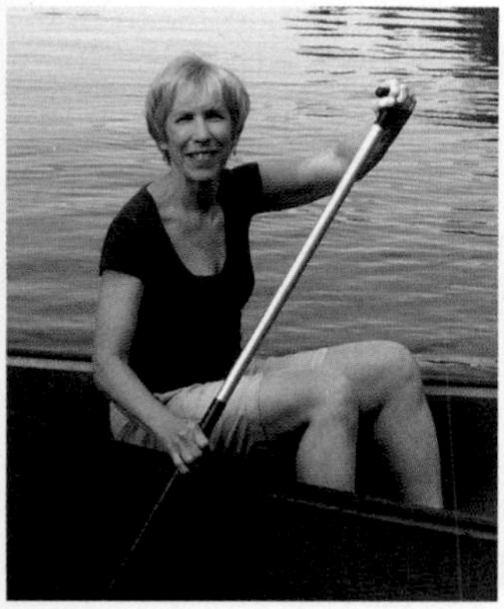

## LINDA BUCHER, RN, PhD, CEN, CNE

Linda Bucher is an Emerita Professor in the School of Nursing at the University of Delaware in Newark, Delaware. She received her Bachelor of Science in nursing from Thomas Jefferson University in Philadelphia, her Master of Science in adult health and illness from the University of Pennsylvania in Philadelphia, and her doctorate in nursing from Widener University in Chester, Pennsylvania. Her 40 years of nursing experience have spanned staff and patient education, acute and critical care nursing, and teaching in associate, baccalaureate, and graduate nursing programs in New Jersey, Pennsylvania, and Delaware. Her preferred teaching areas include emergency and cardiac nursing and evidence-based practice. She maintains her clinical practice by working as an emergency nurse, actively participates in the American Association of Critical Care Nurses, and volunteers as a postoperative nurse for Operation Smile. In her free time, she enjoys traveling and skiing with her family.

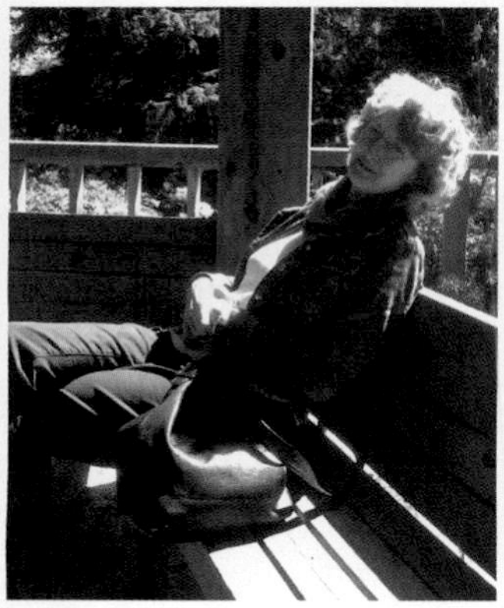

## MARGARET MCLEAN HEITKEMPER, RN, PhD, FAAN

Margaret Heitkemper is Professor and Chairperson, Department of Biobehavioral Nursing and Health Systems at the School of Nursing, and Adjunct Professor, Division of Gastroenterology at the School of Medicine at the University of Washington. She is also Director of the National Institutes of Health-National Institute for Nursing Research–funded Center for Research on Management of Sleep Disturbances at the University of Washington. In the fall of 2006, Dr. Heitkemper was appointed the Elizabeth Sterling Soule Endowed Chair in Nursing. Dr. Heitkemper received her Bachelor of Science in nursing from Seattle University, a Master of Nursing in gerontologic nursing from the University of Washington, and a doctorate in Physiology and Biophysics from the University of Illinois–Chicago. She has been on faculty at the University of Washington since 1981 and has been the recipient of three School of Nursing Excellence in Teaching awards and the University of Washington Distinguished Teaching Award. In addition, in 2002 she received the Distinguished Nutrition Support Nurse Award from the American Society for Parenteral and Enteral Nutrition (ASPEN), in 2003 the American Gastroenterological Association and Janssen Award for Clinical Research in Gastroenterology, and in 2005 she was the first recipient of the Pfizer and Friends of the National Institutes for Nursing Research Award for Research in Women's Health.

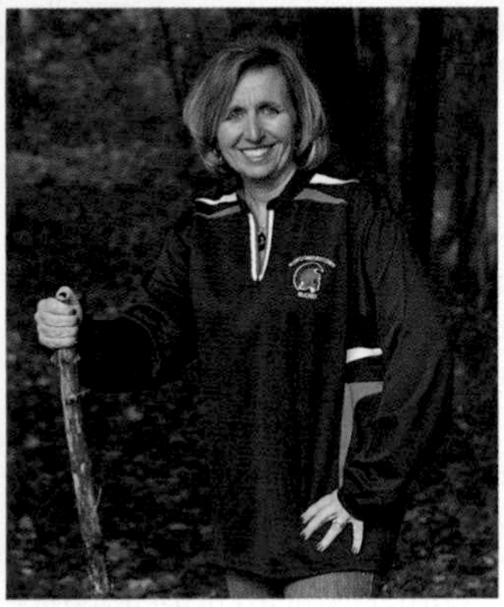

## MARIANN M. HARDING, RN, PhD, CNE

Mariann Harding is an Associate Professor of Nursing at Kent State University Tuscarawas, New Philadelphia, Ohio, where she has been on the faculty since 2005. She received her diploma in nursing from Mt. Carmel School of Nursing in Columbus, Ohio, her Bachelor of Science in nursing from Ohio University in Athens, Ohio, her Master of Science in Nursing as an adult nurse practitioner from the Catholic University of America in Washington D.C., and her doctorate in nursing from West Virginia University in Morgantown, West Virginia. Her 29 years of nursing experience has primarily been in critical care nursing, and teaching in licensed practical, associate, and baccalaureate nursing programs. She currently teaches medical-surgical nursing, health care policy, and evidence-based practice. Her research has focused on promoting student success and health promotion among individuals with gout and facing cancer. Free time is spent with her family or traveling, walking, and reading.

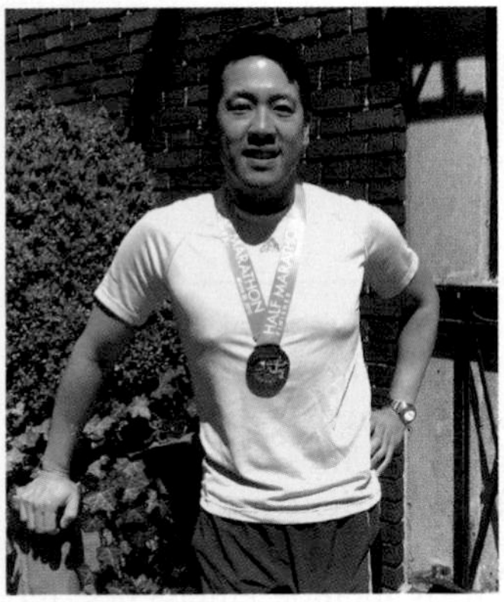

## JEFFREY KWONG, DNP, MPH, ANP-BC, FAANP

Jeffrey Kwong is an Associate Professor of Nursing at Columbia University School of Nursing where he also serves as Director of the Adult-Gerontology Nurse Practitioner Program. He has worked in the area of adult primary care with a special focus on HIV for over 20 years. He received his undergraduate degree from the University of California–Berkeley, his nurse practitioner degree from the University of California–San Francisco, and completed his doctoral training at the University of Colorado–Denver. He also has a Master's Degree in Public Health with a focus on Health Education and Behavioral Sciences from the University of California–Los Angeles and was appointed a Hartford Geriatric Interprofessional Scholar while completing his gerontology education at NYU. In addition to teaching, Dr. Kwong maintains a clinical practice at Gotham Medical Group in New York City. In 2015 he was inducted as a Fellow in the American Association of Nurse Practitioners.

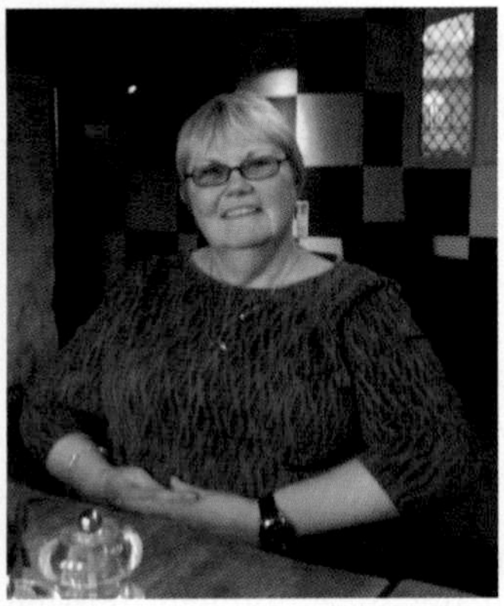

## DOTTIE ROBERTS, RN, EdD, MSN, MACI, OCNS-C, CMSRN, CNE

Dottie Roberts received her Bachelor of Science in nursing from Beth-El College of Nursing, Colorado Springs, Colorado, Master of Science in adult health nursing from Beth-El College of Nursing and Health Sciences, Master of Arts in curriculum and instruction from Colorado Christian University, Colorado Springs, Colorado, and EdD in healthcare education from Nova Southeastern University, Ft. Lauderdale, Florida. She has over 25 years of experience in medical-surgical and orthopaedic nursing, and holds certifications in both specialties. She has also taught in two baccalaureate programs in the Southeast and is certified as a nurse educator. For her dissertation, Dottie completed a phenomenological study on facilitation of critical-thinking skills by clinical faculty in a baccalaureate nursing program. She has been Executive Director of the Orthopaedic Nurses Certification Board since 2005 and editor of "MEDSURG Nursing," the official journal of the Academy of Medical-Surgical Nurses, since 2003. Her free time is spent traveling, reading, and cross-stitching.

**Richard B. Arbour, RN, MSN, CCRN, CNRN, CCNS, FAAN**
Clinical Faculty
School of Nursing
LaSalle University
Philadelphia, Pennsylvania

**Adena Bargad, RN, PhD, CNM**
Assistant Professor, Columbia University Medical Center
Director, Sub-Specialty Program in Women's Health
Columbia University School of Nursing
New York, New York

**Diana Taibi Buchanan, RN, PhD**
Associate Professor
Biobehavioral Nursing and Health Systems
University of Washington
Seattle, Washington

**Darcy Burbage, RN, MSN, AOCN, CBCN**
Survivorship Nurse Navigator
Helen F. Graham Cancer Center and Research Institute
Newark, Delaware

**Kim K. Choma, RN, DNP, WHNP**
Women's Health Nurse Practitioner–Training Consultant
NY/NJ AIDS Education and Training Centers (AETC)
New York, New York

**Susan Collazo, MSN, APN-CNP**
Thoracic Surgery
Northwestern Memorial Hospital
Chicago, Illinois

**Paula P. Cox-North, PhD, ARNP**
Clinical Assistant Professor
School of Nursing
University of Washington School of Nursing
Seattle, Washington

**Hazel A. Dennison, RN, DNP, APNc, CPHQ, CNE**
Director of Education Services
American Nephrology Nurses Association
Anthony J. Jannetti, Pub.
Pitman, New Jersey

**Jane K. Dickinson, RN, PhD, CDE**
Program Coordinator/Faculty
Diabetes Education and Management
Teachers College
Columbia University
New York, New York

**Rose Ann DiMaria-Ghalili, RN, PhD, CNSC**
Associate Professor of Nursing
College of Nursing and Health Professions
Drexel University
Philadelphia, Pennsylvania

**Mechele Fillman, RN, MSN**
Nursing Practitioner
Pain Management
Stanford Healthcare
Palo Alto, California

**Diana L. Gallagher, RN, MS, CWOCN, CFCN**
Clinical Nursing and Education
HealthMatters Consulting
Fayetteville, Arkansas

**Sherry A. Greenberg, RN, PhD, GNP-BC**
Coordinator, Advanced Practice Nursing: Geriatrics Program
Hartford Institute for Geriatric Nursing
New York University College of Nursing
New York, New York

**Angela DiSabatino Herman, RN, MS**
Manager, Cardiovascular Clinical Trials
Christiana Care Health Services
Newark, Delaware

**Christine R. Hoch, RN, MSN**
Nursing Instructor
University of Delaware
Newark, Delaware

**David M. Horner, CRNA, MS, APN**
CRNA Anesthesia
Marlton Hospital
Marlton, New Jersey

**Melissa L. Hutchinson, RN, MN, CCNS, CCRN**
Clinical Nurse Specialist
MICU/CCU
VA Puget Sound Health Care System
Seattle, Washington

**Katherine A. Kelly, RN, DNP, FNP-C, CEN**
Assistant Professor of Nursing
California State University
Sacramento, California

**Judy Knighton, RN, MScN**
Clinical Nurse Specialist—Burns
Ross Tilley Burn Centre
Sunnybrook Health Sciences Centre
Toronto, Ontario, Canada

**Nancy Kupper, RN, MSN**
Associate Professor of Nursing
Tarrant County College
Fort Worth, Texas

**Janet Lenart, RN, MN, MPH**
Senior Lecturer and Director for Online Education
University of Washington School of Nursing
Seattle, Washington

**Linda Littlejohns, RN, MSN, CNRN, FAAN**
Neuroscience Clinical Nursing Consultant
San Juan Capistrano, California

**Amy McKeever, PhD, CRNP, WHNP-BC**
Assistant Professor
College of Nursing
Villanova University
Villanova, Pennsylvania

**De Ann F. Mitchell, RN, PhD**
Director of Nursing
Tarrant County College
Fort Worth, Texas

**Carolyn Moffa, RN, MSN, FNP-C, CHFN**
Clinical Leader, Heart Failure Program
Christiana Care Health System
Newark, Delaware

**Eugene E. Mondor, RN, MN, CNCC(C)**
Clinical Nurse Educator—Adult Critical Care
Royal Alexandra Hospital
Edmonton, Alberta, Canada

**Janice A. Neil, RN, PhD**
Associate Professor and Chair
Undergraduate Nursing Science Junior Division
College of Nursing
East Carolina University
Greenville, North Carolina

**Suzanne Teresa Parsell, MSN, ANP-BC, CUNP**
Division of Endourology
University of Michigan
Ann Arbor, Michigan

**Madona Dawn Plueger, RN, MSN, ACNS-BC, CNRN**
Neuroscience Clinical Nurse Specialist
Barrow Neurological Institute
St. Joseph's Hospital and Medical Center
Phoenix, Arizona

**Carolee Polek, RN, PhD, AOCNS, BMTCN**
Associate Professor
School of Nursing
University of Delaware
Newark, Delaware

**Rosemary C. Polomano, RN, PhD, FAAN**
Professor of Pain Practice
Department of Biobehavioral Health Sciences
University of Pennsylvania School of Nursing;
Professor of Anesthesiology and Critical Care (Secondary)
University of Pennsylvania Perelman School of Medicine
Philadelphia, Pennsylvania

**Matthew C. Price, RN, MS, CNP, ONP-C, RNFA**
Manager, Orthopedic Advanced Practice Providers
Orthopedics
Riverside Methodist Hospital
Columbus, Ohio

**Susanne A. Quallich, RN, MSN, ANP-BC, NP-C, CUNP**
Andrology Nurse Practitioner
Urology
University of Michigan Health System
Ann Arbor, Michigan

**Kathleen A. Rich, RN, PhD, CCNS, CCRN-CSC, CNN**
Cardiovascular Clinical Specialist
Patient Care Services
IU Health La Porte Hospital
La Porte, Indiana

**Sandra Irene Rome, RN, MN, AOCN, CNS**
Clinical Nurse Specialist
Blood and Marrow Transplant Program
Cedars-Sinai Medical Center
Los Angeles, California

**Jennifer Saylor, RN, PhD, ACNS-BC**
Assistant Professor
School of Nursing
University of Delaware
Newark, Delaware

**Maureen A. Seckel, RN, MSN, APN, ACNS-BC, CCNS, CCRN**
Clinical Nurse Specialist
Medical Pulmonary Critical Care
Christiana Care Health System
Newark, Delaware

**Rose Shaffer, RN, MSN, ACNP-CS, CCRN**
Cardiology Nurse Practitioner
Thomas Jefferson University Hospital
Philadelphia, Pennsylvania

**Anita Jo Shoup, RN, MSN, CNOR**
Perioperative Clinical Nurse Specialist
Swedish Edmonds
Edmonds, Washington

**Cindy M. Sullivan, MN, ANP-C, CNRN**
Nurse Practitioner
Neurosurgery
Barrow Neurological Institute
Phoenix, Arizona

**Linda A. L. Upchurch, DNP, ANP-BC**
Assistant Professor
School of Nursing
Georgia Southern University
Statesboro, Georgia

**Deidre D. Wipke-Tevis, RN, PhD**
Associate Professor
PhD Program Director
MU Sinclair School of Nursing
University of Missouri
Columbia, Missouri

**Mary K. Wollan, RN, BAN, ONC**
Orthopaedic Nurse Educator
Excelen
Minneapolis, Minnesota

**Kathy H. Wu, MSN, ANP-BC**
Nurse Practitioner
Liver Transplant Center
New York Columbia Presbyterian Hospital
New York, New York

**Meg Zomorodi, RN, PhD, CNL**
Clinical Associate Professor
School of Nursing
University of North Carolina at Chapel Hill
Chapel Hill, North Carolina

**Michael E. Zychowicz, RN, DNP, ANP, ONP, FAAN, FAANP**
Associate Professor and Director, MSN Program
School of Nursing
Duke University
Durham, North Carolina

# REVIEWERS

**Karen S. Abate, PhD, FNP-BC**
Trenton, New Jersey

**Marian Altman, RN, MS, CNS-BC, ANP**
Richmond, Virginia

**Carol Annesser, RN, MSN, BC, CNE**
Toledo, Ohio

**Tara Back, RN, MSN**
St. Louis, Missouri

**Carolyn Baird, DNP, MBA, RN-BC, CARN-AP, CCDPD, FIAAN**
Canonsburg, Pennsylvania

**Adena Bargad, PhD, CNM**
New York, New York

**Janica Barnett, JD, AGPCNP-BC**
New York, New York

**Margaret Barton-Burke, RN, PhD, FAAN**
St. Louis, Missouri

**Vera Barton-Caro, RN, PhD, FNP-BC, CHFN**
Wheeling, West Virginia

**Cecilia M. Bidigare, RN, MSN, CNS-BC, CNE**
Dayton, Ohio

**Sonya H. Blevins, RN, DNP, CMSRN, CNE**
Greenville, South Carolina

**Donna C. Bond, RN, DNP, CCNS, AE-C, CTTS**
Roanoke, Virginia

**Marilyn Borkgren, APN, MS, CCNS**
Elk Grove Village, Illinois

**Elisabeth G. Bradley, MS, APN, ACNS-BC, AGPCNP-BC**
Newark, Delaware

**Marylee Bressie, RN, DNP, CCRN, CCNS, CEN**
Minneapolis, Minnesota

**Barbara Brunow, RN, MSN, MEd, CNS, CNE**
Sandusky, Ohio

**Diana Taibi Buchanan, RN, PhD**
Seattle, Washington

**Geraldine M. Budd, RN, PhD, FNP-BC, FAANP**
Harrisburg, Pennsylvania

**Darcy Burbage, RN, MSN, AOCN, CBCN**
Newark, Delaware

**Patricia Gable Burke, RN, BSN, CWOCN**
Cincinnati, Ohio

**Hope Bussenius, DNP, APRN, FNP-BC**
Atlanta, Georgia

**Judy Carlyle, RN, MNSc**
Nashville, Arkansas

**Kim K. Choma, RN, DNP, WHNP**
New York, New York

**Kim Clevenger, RN, EdD, BC**
Morehead, Kentucky

**Deborah Cline, RN, MS**
Reno, Nevada

**Susan Collazo, MSN, APN-CNP**
Chicago, Illinois

**Janie Corbitt, RN, MLS**
Milledgeville, Georgia

**Hazel A. Dennison, RN, DNP, APNc, CPHQ, CNE**
Pitman, New Jersey

**Jane K. Dickinson, RN, PhD, CDE**
New York, New York

**Vickie Lee Doscher, MSN, FNP-C, APRN**
Chesapeake, Virginia

**Deborah Ehlers, RN, MSN**
Yakima, Washington

**Susan J. Eisel, RN, MSEd**
Toledo, Ohio

**Rowena W. Elliott, RN, PhD, CNN, CNE, AGNP-C, FAAN**
Hattiesburg, Mississippi

**Dana R. Epstein, RN, PhD**
Tempe, Arizona

**Deborah Erickson, RN, PhD**
Peoria, Illinois

**Christine Espina, RN, DNP**
Seattle, Washington

**Cora Espina, RN, MN, ARNP, CWN**
Seattle, Washington

**Abimbola Farinde, PharmD, MS**
Orange Beach, Alabama

**Brian J. Fasolka, RN, MSN, CEN**
Philadelphia, Pennsylvania

**Marianne Ferrin, MSN, ACNP-BC**
Philadelphia, Pennysylvania

**Diana L. Gallagher, RN, MS, CWOCN, CFCN**
Fayetteville, Arkansas

**Karen Gilbert, RN, MSN, CNSC, CRNP**
Riverton, New Jersey

**Nelda S. Godfrey, RN, PhD, ACNS-BC, FAAN**
Kansas City, Kansas

**Roberta Goff, MSN Ed, RN-BC, ACNS-BC, ONC**
Traverse City, Michigan

**Regina Gonzalez-Lama, RN, MS**
Staten Island, New York

**Debra B. Gordon, RN-BC, DNP, ACNS-BC, FAAN**
Seattle, Washington

**Shari Gould, RN, MSN**
Victoria, Texas

**Sherry A. Greenberg, RN, PhD, GNP-BC**
New York, New York

**Kelly S. Grimshaw, RN, MSN, APRN, CCRN, CCTN**
New Haven, Connecticut

**Sharon Haas, RN, MSN, CDN**
Milwaukee, Wisconsin

**Debra Hagler, RN, PhD, ACNS-BC, CNE, CHSE, ANEF, FAAN**
Phoenix, Arizona

**Cynthia Hambach, RN, MSN, CCRN**
Philadelphia, Pennsylvania

**Janet L. Hannah, RN, CGRN**
Leesburg, Virginia

**Carla V. Hannon, MS, APRN, CCRN, CCNS**
New Haven, Connecticut

**Helene Harris, RN, MSN**
Temple, Texas

**Misty Hobart, RN, MSN, CNE**
Spokane, Washington

**Deena Hollingsworth, MSN, FNP-BC, CORLN**
Arlington, Virginia

**Michele M. Hughes, RN, MSN, ACNP, ONP-C**
Mechanicvsille, Virginia

**Melissa Hutchinson, RN, MN, CCNS, CCRN**
Seattle, Washington

**Stephanie Jackson, RN, MSN, AOCNS**
Los Angeles, California

**Suzanne Jed, MSN, FNP-BC**
Pretoria, South Africa

**Monica L. Johnson, RN, MSN, MBA-HCM, CMSRN, ONC, LNC**
New Orleans, Louisiana

**Jane Kaufman, MS, CRNP, ANP-BC**
Philadelphia, Pennsylvania

**Christina D. Keller, RN, MSN-Ed**
Radford, Virginia

**Lauren Kemph, RN, DNP, AGPCNP**
New York, New York

**Tracy H. Knoll, RN, MSN**
St. Louis, Missouri

**Regina Kukulski, RN, MSN, ACNS, BC, CNE**
Trenton, New Jersey

**Jane E. Lacovara, RN, MSN, CMSRN**
Tucson, Arizona

**Katherine A. Ladetto, RN, MSN, APRN, ANP-BC, GNP-BC**
Peabody, Massachusetts

**Susan C. Landis, RN, MN**
Seattle, Washington

**Marci Langenkamp, RN, MS**
Piqua, Ohio

**Patricia Lea, RN, DNP, CCRN**
Galveston, Texas

**Judith M. Lewis, DNP, APRN, CRNA**
Akron, Ohio

**Linda R. Lewis, MSN, RN-BC**
Scranton, Pennsylvania

**Rebecca Liebert, RN, MSN, FNP-C, ONP-C**
Tomah, Wisconsin

**Linda Littlejohns, RN, MSN, CNRN, FAAN**
San Juan Capistrano, California

**Anthony R. Lutz, RN, MSN, A-GNP-C**
Charlotte, North Carolina

**Carolyn Lyon, RN, MSN**
Roanoke, Virginia

**Angela M. Martinelli, RN, PhD, CNOR**
Fairfield, Connecticut

**Donna E. McCabe, DNP, APRN-BC, GNP**
New York, New York

**Molly McClelland, RN, PhD, ACNS-BC, CMSRN**
Detroit, Michigan

**Tara McMillan-Queen, RN, MSN, ANP, GNP**
Charlotte, North Carolina

**Molly McNett, RN, PhD, CNRN**
Cleveland, Ohio

**Karen Meneses, RN, PhD, FAAN**
Birmingham, Alabama

**Eugene E. Mondor, RN, MN, CNCC(C)**
Edmonton, Alberta, Canada

**Heidi E. Monroe, MSN, RN-BC, CPAN, CAPA**
Green Bay, Wisconsin

**Anna P. Moore, RN, MS**
Richmond, Virginia

**Kathy Morrison, RN, MSN, CNRN, SCRN**
Hershey, Pennsylvania

**Pamela K. Newland, RN, PhD, CMSRN**
St. Louis, Missouri

**Lorraine Nowakowski-Grier, MSN, APRN-BC, CDE**
Newark, Delaware

**Ellen Odell, DNP, ACNS-BC, CNE, APRN**
Siloam Springs, Arkansas

**Suzanne Teresa Parsell, MSN, ANP-BC, CUNP**
Ann Arbor, Michigan

**Jessica Pastor, MSN, DNP(c), ACNP-BC, SANE-A, TNCC**
Detroit and Troy, Michigan

**Rebecca Personett, RN, PhD, NEA-BC**
Gainesville and Dallas, Texas

**Madona Dawn Plueger, RN, MSN, ACNS-BC, CNRN**
Phoenix, Arizona

**Carolee Polek, RN, PhD, AOCNS, BMTCN**
Newark, Delaware

**Julia R. Popp, RN, MSN**
Toledo, Ohio

**Sarah Byram Poppe, MSN, ANP-BC**
Olympia, Washington

**Matthew C. Price, RN, MS, CNP, ONP-C, RNFA**
Columbus, Ohio

**Susanne A. Quallich, RN, MSN, ANP-BC, NP-C, CUNP**
Ann Arbor, Michigan

**Margaret R. Rateau, RN, PhD, CNE**
East Liverpool, Ohio

**Patricia S. Regojo, RN, MSN**
Philadelphia, Pennsylvania

**Courtney Reinisch, RN, DNP, APN-BC, DCC**
Newark, New Jersey

**Janet M. Riggs, RN, DrNP**
Philadelphia, Pennsylvania

**Julie Rogan, RN, MSN, ACCNS-AG, AOCNS, CCRN**
Philadelphia, Pennsylvania

**Diane Marie Rudolphi, RN, MS**
Newark, Delaware

**Diane Ryzner, MSN, APN, CNS, OCNS-C**
Arlington Heights, Illinois

**Susan A. Sandstrom, RN, MSN, BC, CNE**
Omaha, Nebraska

**Christine L. Savage, RN, PhD, CARN, FAAN**
Baltimore, Maryland

**Jennifer Saylor, RN, PhD, ACNS-BC**
Newark, Delaware

**Mary Scheid, RN, MSN, OCN, CBCN**
Greeley, Colorado

**Teresa J. Seright, RN, PhD, CCRN**
Bozeman, Montana

**Crystal Sheaves, RN, MSN, APRN, FNP-BC**
Charleston, West Virginia

**Crystal R. Sherman, DNP, CNP, FNP-BC, APHN-BC**
Portsmouth, Ohio

**Michelle Smeltzer, RN, MSN, DNPc, CEN**
East Norriton, Pennsylvania

**Matthew Soos, RN, BSN, BA, EMT**
Atlantic City, New Jersey

**Lisa Spruce, DNP, ACNS, ACNP, ANP, CNOR, CNS-CP**
Denver, Colorado

**Whitney Starr, MSN, FNP-BC**
Denver, Colorado

**Cynthia M. Steinwedel, RN, PhD, CNE**
Peoria, Illinois

**Laura A. Stokowski, RNC, MS**
Falls Church, Virginia

**Beth D. Strauss, RN, DNP, ACNS-BC**
Madison, Wisconsin

**Cindy M. Sullivan, MN, ANP-C, CNRN**
Phoenix, Arizona

**Joseph Tariman, RN, PhD, ANP-BC**
Chicago, Illinois

**Allison J. Terry, RN, PhD**
Montgomery, Alabama

**Tamekia L. Thomas, MSN, APN, PCCN, ACNS-BC**
Newark, Delaware

**Andrea H. Thurler, RN, DNP, FNP-BC**
Boston, Massachusetts

**Bonnie Tong, MSN, ACNP-BC**
New York, New York

**Mary Ellen Tresgallo, DNP, MPH, FNP-BC**
New York, New York

**Kathryn J. Trotter, DNP, CNM, FNP-C**
Durham, North Carolina

**Linda A. L. Upchurch, DNP, ANP-BC**
Statesboro, Georgia

**Olga Van Dyke, RN, MSN, CAGS**
Boston, Massachusetts

**Dawn M. Vanderhoef, PhD, DNP, PMHNP/CS-BC**
Nashville, Tennessee

**Deborah Kirk Walker, DNP, FNP-BC, NP-C, AOCN**
Birmingham, Alabama

**Colleen R. Walsh, RN, DNP, ONC, ONP-C, CNS, ACNP-BC**
Evansville, Indiana

**Daryle Wane, PhD, ARNP, FNP-BC**
New Port Richey, Florida

**Robert M. Welch, RN, MSN, FNP, CRNO**
Reno, Nevada

**Laura C. Williams, RN, MSN, CNS, ONC, CCNS**
Orlando, Florida

**Daniel Worrall, MSN, ANP-BC**
Boston, Massachusetts

**Kathy H. Wu, MSN, ANP-BC**
New York, New York

**Elsa Wuhrman, DNP, RN-BC, FNP, BC, DCC**
New York, New York

**Kenneth Wysocki, PhD, FNP-BC, FAANP**
Scottsdale, Arizona

**Linda H. Yoder, RN, PhD, AOCN, FAAN**
Austin, Texas

**Meg Zomorodi, RN, PhD, CNL**
Chapel Hill, North Carolina

**To the Profession of Nursing**
**and to the Important People in Our Lives**

**Sharon**
*My husband Peter and our grandchildren*
*Malia, Halle, Aidan, Cian, Layla, Ryker, and Archer*

**Linda**
*My nieces, Stefany and Jayme,*
*who so admirably reflect the ideals of the nursing profession*
*and my godchild, Liz, for her love of written words.*

**Margaret**
*My husband David, our daughters Elizabeth and Ellen,*
*and our grandsons Jaxon James and Axel*

**Mariann**
*My husband Jeff and our daughters Kate and Sarah*

**Jeff**
*To my mother, Virginia, whose dedication to the field of nursing*
*led me on this wonderful journey.*

**Dottie**
*My husband Steve and my children Megan, E.J., Jessica, and Matthew,*
*who have supported me through four college degrees and countless writing projects,*
*and to our grandsons Oscar and Stephen.*

The tenth edition of *Medical-Surgical Nursing: Assessment and Management of Clinical Problems* has been thoroughly revised to incorporate the most current medical-surgical nursing information in an easy-to-use format. More than just a textbook, this is a comprehensive resource containing essential information that students need to prepare for lectures, classroom activities, examinations, clinical assignments, and the safe, comprehensive care of patients. In addition to the readable writing style and full-color illustrations, the text and accompanying resources include many special features to help students learn key medical-surgical nursing content, including patient and caregiver teaching, gerontology, interprofessional care, cultural and ethnic considerations, patient safety, genetics, nutrition and drug therapy, evidence-based practice, and much more.

The comprehensive and timely content, special features, attractive layout, and student-friendly writing style combine to make this the number one medical-surgical nursing textbook used in more nursing schools than any other medical-surgical nursing textbook.

The strengths of the first nine editions have been retained, including the use of the nursing process as an organizational theme for nursing management. Numerous new features have been added to address some of the rapid changes in practice. Contributors have been selected for their expertise in specific content areas; one or more specialists in the subject area have thoroughly reviewed each chapter to increase accuracy. The editors have undertaken final rewriting and editing to achieve internal consistency. All efforts have been directed toward building on the strengths of the previous edition while preparing an even more effective new edition.

## ORGANIZATION

Content is organized into two major divisions. The first division, Section 1 (Chapters 1 through 10), discusses general concepts related to adult patients. The second division, Sections 2 through 12 (Chapters 11 through 68), presents nursing assessment and nursing management of medical-surgical problems.

The various body systems are grouped to reflect their interrelated functions. Each section is organized around two central themes: assessment and management. Chapters dealing with assessment of a body system include a discussion of the following:

1. A brief review of anatomy and physiology, focusing on information that will promote understanding of nursing care
2. Health history and noninvasive physical assessment skills to expand the knowledge base on which treatment decisions are made
3. Common diagnostic studies, expected results, and related nursing responsibilities to provide easily accessible information

Management chapters focus on the pathophysiology, clinical manifestations, diagnostic studies, interprofessional care, and nursing management of various diseases and disorders. The nursing management sections are organized into assessment, nursing diagnoses, planning, implementation, and evaluation. To emphasize the importance of patient care in various clinical settings, nursing implementation of all major health problems is organized by the following levels of care:

1. Health Promotion
2. Acute Care
3. Ambulatory Care

## CLASSIC FEATURES

- **Nursing management** is presented in a consistent and comprehensive format, with headings for Health Promotion, Acute Care, and Ambulatory Care. Over 60 nursing care plans on the Evolve website incorporate Nursing Interventions Classification (NIC) and Nursing Outcomes Classification (NOC) in a way that clearly shows the linkages among NIC, NOC, and nursing diagnoses, and applies them to nursing practice.
- **Cultural and ethnic health disparities** content and boxes in the text highlight risk factors and important issues related to the nursing care of various ethnic groups. A special Culturally Competent Care heading denotes cultural and ethnic content related to diseases and disorders. Chapter 2: Health Disparities and Culturally Competent Care discusses health status differences among groups of people related to access to care, economic aspects of health care, gender and cultural issues, and disease risk.
- **Interprofessional care** is highlighted in special Interprofessional Care sections in all management chapters and Interprofessional Care tables throughout the text.
- **Coverage on delegation and prioritization** includes the following:
  - Teamwork & Collaboration boxes highlight the nurse's role in working with members of the interprofessional team and also cover specific topics and skills related to delegation
  - Delegation and prioritization questions in case studies and Bridge to NCLEX Examination Questions
  - Nursing interventions throughout the text are listed in order of priority
  - Nursing diagnoses in the nursing care plans are listed in order of priority
- **Focused Assessment boxes** in all assessment chapters provide brief checklists that help students do a more practical "assessment on the run" or bedside approach to assessment. They can be used to evaluate the status of previously identified health problems and monitor for signs of new problems.
- **Safety Alert boxes** highlight important patient safety issues and focus on the National Patient Safety Goals.
- **Pathophysiology Maps** outline complex concepts related to diseases in flowchart format, making them easier to understand.
- **Patient and caregiver teaching** is an ongoing theme throughout the text. Chapter 4: Patient and Caregiver Teaching emphasizes the increasing importance and prevalence of patient management of chronic illnesses and conditions and the role of the caregiver in patient care.
- **Gerontology and chronic illness** are discussed in Chapter 5: Chronic Illness and Older Adults, and included throughout

the text under Gerontologic Considerations headings and in Gerontologic Differences in Assessment tables.

- **Nutrition** is highlighted throughout the book. Nutritional Therapy tables summarize nutritional interventions and promote healthy lifestyles in patients with various health problems.
- ***Healthy People* boxes** present health care goals as they relate to specific disorders such as diabetes and cancer.
- **Extensive drug therapy** content includes Drug Therapy tables and concise Drug Alerts highlighting important safety considerations for key drugs.
- **Genetics content** includes:
  - Genetics in Clinical Practice boxes that summarize the genetic basis, genetic testing, and clinical implications for genetic disorders that affect adults
  - A genetics chapter that focuses on practical application of nursing care as it relates to this important topic
  - Genetic Risk Alerts in the assessment chapters call attention to important genetic risks
  - Genetic Link headings in the management chapters highlight the specific genetic bases of many disorders
- **Gender Differences** boxes discuss how women and men are affected differently by conditions such as pain and hypertension.
- **Complementary & Alternative Therapies boxes** expand on this information and summarize what nurses need to know about therapies such as herbal remedies, acupuncture, and biofeedback.
- **Ethical/Legal Dilemmas boxes** promote critical thinking for timely and sensitive issues that nursing students may deal with in clinical practice—topics such as informed consent, advance directives, and confidentiality.
- **Emergency Management tables** outline the emergency treatment of health problems most likely to require emergency intervention.
- **Assessment Abnormalities tables** in assessment chapters alert the nurse to frequently encountered abnormalities and their possible etiologies.
- **Nursing Assessment tables** summarize the key subjective and objective data related to common diseases. Subjective data are organized by functional health patterns.
- **Health History tables** in assessment chapters present key questions to ask patients related to a specific disease or disorder.
- **Evidence-based practice** is covered throughout the book in Applying the Evidence boxes, Translating Research Into Practice boxes, and evidence-based practice-focused questions in the case studies.
- **Student-friendly pedagogy** includes the following:
  - Learning Outcomes and Key Terms at the beginning of each chapter help students identify the key content for that chapter.
  - Evolve website boxes at the end of each chapter alert students to supplemental online content and exercises, making it easy for students to facilitate online learning.
  - Bridge to NCLEX® Examination Questions at the end of each chapter are matched to the learning outcomes and help students learn the important points in the chapter. Answers are provided just below the questions for immediate feedback, and rationales are provided on the Evolve website.
  - Case Studies with photos bring patients to life. Management chapters have case studies at the end of the chapters. These cases help students learn how to prioritize care and manage patients in the clinical setting. Unfolding case studies are included in each assessment chapter and case studies that focus on managing care of multiple patients are included at the end of each section. Discussion questions with a focus on prioritization, delegation, and evidence-based practice are included in all case studies. Answer guidelines are provided on the Evolve website.
- A **glossary** of key terms and definitions is provided at the back of the text. An expanded version of the glossary with audio pronunciations is included on the Evolve website.

## NEW FEATURES

- **Check Your Practice boxes** challenge students to think critically, analyze patient assessment data, and implement the appropriate intervention. Scenarios and discussion questions are provided to promote active learning.
- **Becoming a Nurse Leader boxes** introduce students to concepts related to being a responsible team member and leader. They cover topics such as how nurses can build supportive relationships in the work environment, how to manage a team when providing care, dealing with a changing environment, and more.
- **Informatics boxes and content** in the Patient and Caregiver Teaching chapter reflect the current use and importance of technology as it relates to patient self-management.
- **Increased focus on developing critical thinking skills** is apparent in the Evidence-Based Practice boxes where students are engaged in discussing the implications of EBP findings for nursing practice. The unfolding case studies in assessment chapters also include additional discussion questions to facilitate critical thinking.
- **Increased focus on ambulatory and chronic care** addresses the increasing management of patients on an outpatient basis.
- **QSEN competencies** are highlighted in the core content, case studies, and nursing care plans.

## LEARNING SUPPLEMENTS FOR STUDENTS

- The handy **Clinical Companion** presents approximately 200 common medical-surgical conditions and procedures in a concise, alphabetical format for quick clinical reference. Designed for portability, this popular reference includes the essential, need-to-know information for treatments and procedures in which nurses play a major role. An attractive and functional four-color design highlights key information for quick, easy reference.
- An exceptionally thorough **Study Guide** contains over 500 pages of review material that reflect the content found in the book. It features a wide variety of clinically relevant exercises and activities, including NCLEX-format multiple choice and alternate format questions, case studies, anatomy review, critical thinking activities, and much more. It features an attractive four-color design and many alternate-item format questions to better prepare students for the NCLEX examination. An answer key is included to provide students with immediate feedback as they study.

- The **Evolve Student Resources** are available online at http://evolve.elsevier.com/Lewis/medsurg and include the following valuable learning aids organized by chapter:
  - Printable **Key Points** summaries for each chapter
  - 1000 NCLEX Examination **Review Questions**
  - **Answer Guidelines** to the case studies in the textbook
  - **Rationales for the Bridge to NCLEX® Examination Questions** in the textbook
  - 55 **Interactive Case Studies** with state-of-the-art animations and a variety of learning activities, which provide students with immediate feedback. Ten of the case studies are enhanced with photos and narration of the clinical scenarios.
  - Customizable **Nursing Care Plans**
  - **Conceptual Care Map Creator** and conceptual care maps for selected case studies in the textbook
  - **Audio glossary** of key terms, available as comprehensive alphabetical glossary and organized by chapter
  - **Stress-Busting Kit**
  - **Supporting Media**, including animations and audio clips
  - **Fluids and Electrolytes Tutorial**
  - **Content Updates**
- **Virtual Clinical Excursions (VCE)** is an exciting learning tool that brings learning to life in a "virtual" hospital setting. VCE simulates a realistic, yet safe, nursing environment where the routine and rigors of the average clinical rotation abound. Students can conduct a complete assessment of a patient and set priorities for care, collect data, analyze and interpret data, prepare and administer medications, and reach conclusions about complex problems. Each lesson has a textbook reading assignment and online activities based on "visiting" patients in the hospital. Instructors receive an implementation manual with directions for using VCE as a teaching tool.
- More than just words on a screen, **Elsevier eBooks** come with a wealth of built-in study tools and interactive functionality to help students better connect with the course material and their instructors. Plus, with the ability to fit an entire library of books on one portable device, students have the ability to study when, where, and how they want.

## TEACHING SUPPLEMENTS FOR INSTRUCTORS

- The **Evolve Instructor Resources** (available online at http://evolve.elsevier.com/Lewis/medsurg) remain the most comprehensive set of instructor's materials available, containing the following:
  - **TEACH for Nurses Lesson Plans** with electronic resources organized by chapter to help instructors develop and manage the course curriculum. This exciting resource includes:
    - Objectives
    - Teaching focus
    - Key terms
    - Nursing curriculum standards
    - Student and instructor chapter resource listings
    - Teaching strategies with learning activities and assessment methods tied to learning outcomes
    - **Case studies** with answer guidelines
  - The **Test Bank** features over 2000 NCLEX Examination test questions with text page references and answers coded for NCLEX Client Needs category, nursing process, and cognitive level. The test bank includes hundreds of prioritization, delegation, and multiple patient questions. All alternate item format questions are included. The ExamView software allows instructors to create new tests; edit, add, and delete test questions; sort questions by NCLEX category, cognitive level, nursing process step, and question type; and administer and grade online tests.
  - The **Image Collection** contains more than 800 full-color images from the text for use in lectures.
  - An extensive collection of **PowerPoint Presentations** includes over 125 different presentations focused on the most common diseases and disorders. The presentations have been thoroughly revised to include helpful instructor notes/teaching tips, unfolding case studies, new illustrations and photos not found in the book, new animations, and updated audience response questions for use with iClicker and other audience response systems.
  - Course management system.
  - Access to all student resources listed above.
- The **Simulation Learning System (SLS)** is an online toolkit that helps instructors and facilitators effectively incorporate medium- to high-fidelity simulation into their nursing curriculum. Detailed patient scenarios promote and enhance the clinical decision-making skills of students at all levels. The SLS provides detailed instructions for preparation and implementation of the simulation experience, debriefing questions that encourage critical thinking, and learning resources to reinforce student comprehension. Each scenario in the SLS complements the textbook content and helps bridge the gap between lecture and clinical. The SLS provides the perfect environment for students to practice what they are learning in the text for a true-to-life, hands-on learning experience.

## ACKNOWLEDGMENTS

The editors are especially grateful to many people at Elsevier who assisted with this major revision effort. In particular, we wish to thank the team of Jamie Blum, Jennifer Hermes, Mary Stueck, Julie Eddy, and Ashley Miner. In addition, we want to thank Becky Ramsaroop in marketing.

Special thanks and appreciation go to Peter Bonner who assisted with many details of manuscript preparation and review and photography for the book and interactive case studies.

We are particularly indebted to the faculty, nurses, and student nurses who have put their faith in our book to assist them on their path to excellence. The increasing use of this book throughout the United States, Canada, Australia, and other parts of the world has been gratifying. We appreciate the many users who have shared their comments and suggestions on the previous editions. All feedback is welcome.

We also wish to thank our contributors and reviewers for their assistance with the revision process. We sincerely hope that this book will assist both students and clinicians in practicing truly professional nursing.

*Sharon L. Lewis*
*Linda Bucher*
*Margaret McLean Heitkemper*
*Mariann M. Harding*
*Jeffrey Kwong*
*Dottie Roberts*

## TEST BANK

**Debra Hagler, RN, PhD, ACNS-BC, CNE, CHSE, ANEF, FAAN**
Clinical Professor
College of Nursing and Healthcare Innovation
Arizona State University
Phoenix, Arizona

## CASE STUDIES

### Interactive and Managing Care of Multiple Patients Case Studies

**Katherine A. Kelly, RN, DNP, FNP-C, CEN**
Assistant Professor of Nursing
California State University
Sacramento, California

**Sarah Barnes, RN, DNP**
Assistant Professor of Nursing
California State University
Sacramento, California

## POWERPOINT PRESENTATIONS

**Jane E. Oehme, RN, MS**
Associate Professor of Nursing
Pennsylvania College of Technology
Williamsport, Pennsylvania

**Michele A. Walczak, RN, MSN**
Associate Professor of Nursing
Pennsylvania College of Technology
Williamsport, Pennsylvania

## TEACH FOR NURSES

**Margaret R. Rateau, RN, PhD, CNE**
Assistant Professor of Nursing
Robert Morris University
Moon Township, Pennsylvania

## AUDIENCE RESPONSE QUESTIONS

**Jane E. Oehme, RN, MS**
Associate Professor of Nursing
Pennsylvania College of Technology
Williamsport, Pennsylvania

**Michele A. Walczak, RN, MSN**
Associate Professor of Nursing
Pennsylvania College of Technology
Williamsport, Pennsylvania

## NCLEX EXAMINATION REVIEW QUESTIONS

**Mary Boyce, RN, MSN, CCRN, CNE**
Mesa Community College
Mesa, Arizona

**Sarah Barnes, RN, DNP**
Assistant Professor of Nursing
California State University
Sacramento, California

**Leigh W. Moore, RN, MSN, CNOR, CNE**
Associate Professor of Nursing–ADN
Southside Virginia Community College
Alberta, Virginia

## STUDY GUIDE

**Susan A. Sandstrom, RN, MSN, BC, CNE**
Associate Professor in Nursing, Retired
College of Saint Mary
Omaha, Nebraska

## CLINICAL COMPANION

**Debra Hagler, RN, PhD, ACNS-BC, CNE, CHSE, ANEF, FAAN**
Clinical Professor
College of Nursing and Healthcare Innovation
Arizona State University
Phoenix, Arizona

## ETHICAL/LEGAL DILEMMAS BOXES

**Katherine K. Anselmi, JD, PhD, WHNP-BC**
Associate Clinical Professor
Assistant Dean of Accreditation/Regulatory Affairs and Online Innovation
College of Nursing and Health Professions
Drexel University
Philadelphia, Pennsylvania

**Vicki D. Lachman, RN, PhD, APRN, FAAN, NEA-BC**
President
V.L. Associates
Avalon, New Jersey

## EVIDENCE-BASED PRACTICE BOXES

**Shannon Ruff Dirksen, RN, PhD, FAAN**
Associate Professor
College of Nursing and Health Innovation
Arizona State University
Phoenix, Arizona

## NURSING CARE PLANS

**Collin Bowman-Woodall, RN, MS**
Assistant Professor
Samuel Merritt University
San Francisco Peninsula Learning Center
San Mateo, California

## BECOMING A NURSE LEADER BOXES

**Donna Jean Middaugh, RN, PhD**
Associate Dean for Academic Programs
College of Nursing
University of Arkansas for Medical Sciences
Little Rock, Arkansas

## GLOSSARY

**Cory Retherford, MSOM**
Former Research Assistant
University of Texas Health Science Center at San Antonio
San Antonio, Texas

## SPECIAL PROJECTS

**Peter Bonner, MS**
Former Professor and Research Statistician
New Mexico Highlands University
Las Vegas, New Mexico;
DSI
Placitas, New Mexico

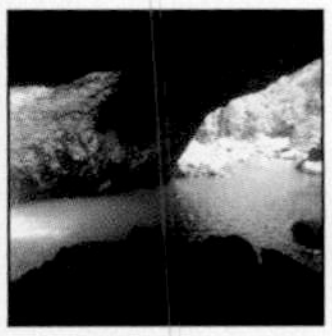

## Section 1
## Concepts in Nursing Practice



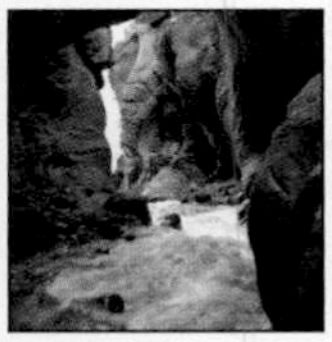

## Section 2
## Pathophysiologic Mechanisms of Disease



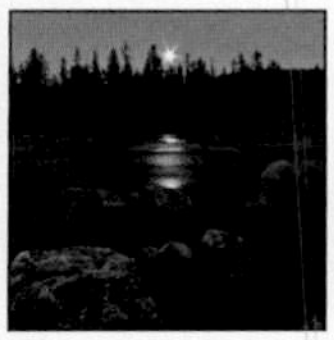

## Section 3
## Perioperative Care



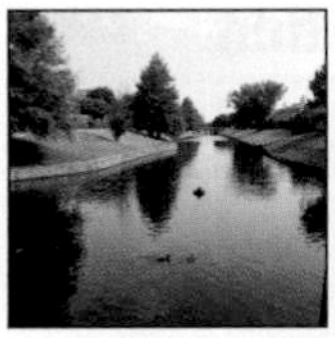

## Section 4
## Problems Related to Altered Sensory Input



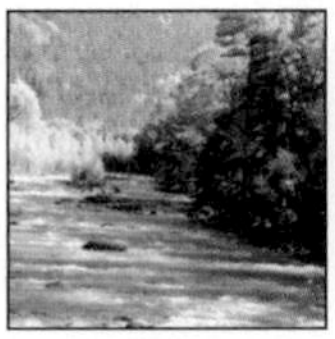

## Section 5
## Problems of Oxygenation: Ventilation



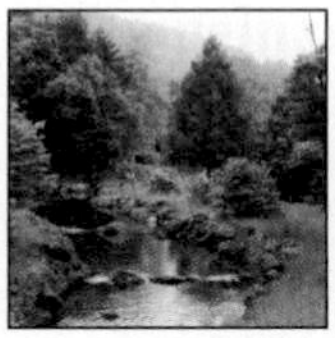

## Section 6
## Problems of Oxygenation: Transport



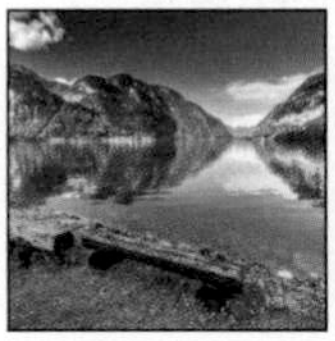

## Section 7
## Problems of Oxygenation: Perfusion

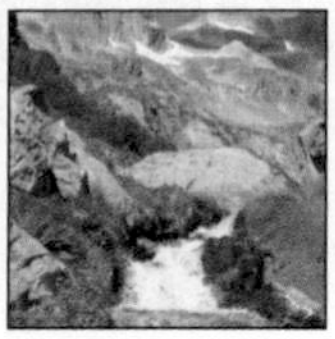

## Section 8
## Problems of Ingestion, Digestion, Absorption, and Elimination



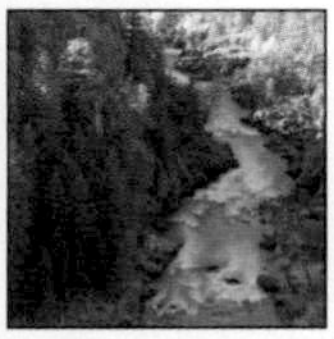

## Section 9
## Problems of Urinary Function



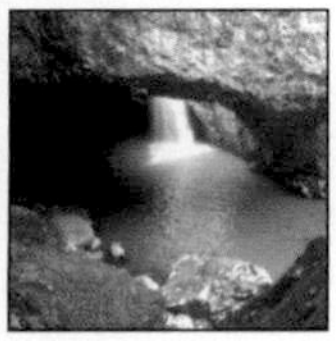

## Section 10
## Problems Related to Regulatory and Reproductive Mechanisms



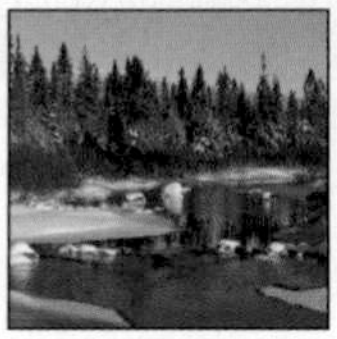

## Section 11
## Problems Related to Movement and Coordination



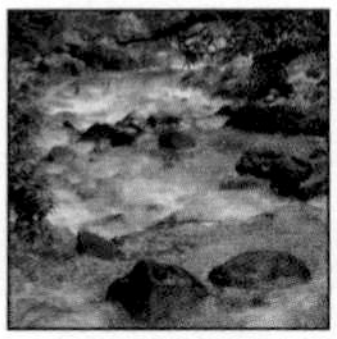

## Section 12
## Nursing Care in Critical Care Settings



## Appendixes

## ASSESSMENT ABNORMALITIES TABLES



## BECOMING A NURSE LEADER BOXES



## CASE STUDIES

### End-of-Chapter Case Studies



### Managing Care of Multiple Patients Case Studies



### Assessment Case Studies

## COMPLEMENTARY & ALTERNATIVE THERAPIES BOXES



## CULTURAL & ETHNIC HEALTH DISPARITIES BOXES



## DIAGNOSTIC STUDIES TABLES



## DRUG THERAPY TABLES

## EMERGENCY MANAGEMENT TABLES



## ETHICAL/LEGAL DILEMMAS BOXES



## EVIDENCE-BASED PRACTICE BOXES

### Applying the Evidence Boxes

### Translating Research Into Practice Boxes



## FOCUSED ASSESSMENT BOXES



## GENDER DIFFERENCES BOXES



## GENETICS IN CLINICAL PRACTICE BOXES



## GERONTOLOGIC ASSESSMENT DIFFERENCES TABLES

## HEALTH HISTORY TABLES



## *HEALTHY PEOPLE* BOXES



## INFORMATICS IN PRACTICE BOXES



## INTERPROFESSIONAL CARE TABLES

## NURSING ASSESSMENT TABLES



## NURSING MANAGEMENT TABLES



## NUTRITIONAL THERAPY TABLES

## PATIENT & CAREGIVER TEACHING TABLES



## TEAMWORK & COLLABORATION BOXES

# MEDICAL-SURGICAL NURSING

## Assessment and Management of Clinical Problems

SECTION 1

# Concepts in Nursing Practice

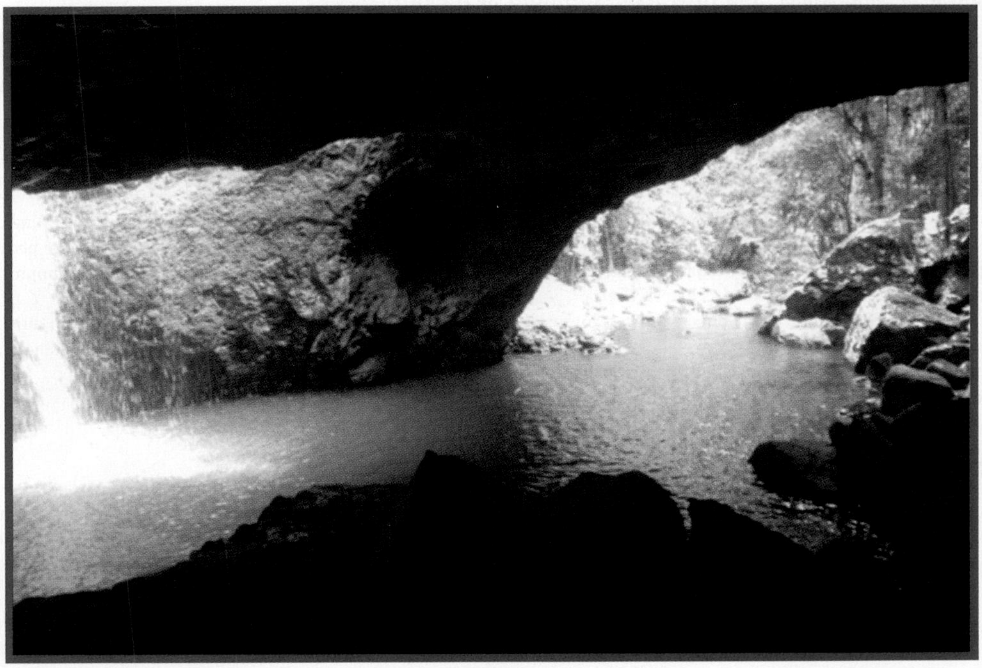

Peter Bonner

*Life is like the river, sometimes it sweeps you gently along and sometimes the rapids come out of nowhere.*
***Emma Smith***

# 1

# Professional Nursing Practice

*Mariann M. Harding*

*Knowledge has to be improved, challenged, and increased constantly, or it vanishes.*

***Peter Drucker***

http://evolve.elsevier.com/Lewis/medsurg/

## LEARNING OUTCOMES

1. Describe professional nursing practice in terms of domain, definitions, and recipients of care.
2. Compare the different scopes of practice available to professional nurses.
3. Analyze the effect of external influences on professional nursing practice.
4. Describe the role of critical thinking skills and use of the nursing process to provide patient-centered care.
5. Explain how standardized nursing terminologies for nursing diagnoses, patient outcomes, and nursing interventions can be used and linked.
6. Explore the role of the professional nurse in delegating care to licensed practical/vocational nurses and unlicensed assistive personnel.
7. Discuss the role of integrating safety and quality improvement processes into nursing practice.
8. Evaluate the role of informatics and technology in nursing practice.
9. Apply concepts of evidence-based practice to nursing practice.

## KEY TERMS

advanced practice registered nurse (APRN), p. 3
case management, p. 9
clinical pathways, p. 10
clinical reasoning, p. 9
critical thinking, p. 9
delegation, p. 11
electronic health records (EHRs), p. 14
evidence-based practice (EBP), p. 15
interprofessional team, p. 9
nursing, p. 3
nursing process, p. 5
nursing-sensitive patient outcome, p. 7
SBAR (Situation-Background-Assessment-Recommendation), p. 10
serious reportable event (SRE), p. 12
telehealth, p. 9

This chapter presents an overview of professional nursing practice, discussing the wide variety of roles and responsibilities that nurses fulfill to meet the health care needs of society.

## PROFESSIONAL NURSING PRACTICE

### Domain of Nursing Practice

Nursing practice today consists of a wide variety of roles and responsibilities necessary to meet society's health care needs. As a nurse, you are the frontline professional of health care (Fig. 1-1). You can practice in virtually all health care settings and communities. You have never been more important to health care than you are today. As a nurse, you (1) offer skilled care to those recuperating from illness or injury, (2) advocate for patients' rights, (3) teach patients to manage their health, (4) support patients and their caregivers at critical times, and (5) help them navigate the complex health care system. Although the majority of nurses work in acute care facilities, many nurses practice in long-term care, home care, primary and preventive care, ambulatory or outpatient clinics, and community health. Wherever you practice, recipients of your care include individuals, families, groups, or communities.

The American Nurses Association (ANA) states that the authority for the practice of nursing is based on a contract with society that acknowledges professional rights and responsibilities, as well as mechanisms for public accountability.[1] The knowledge and skills that make up nursing practice are derived from society's expectations and needs. Nursing practice continues to evolve according to society's health care needs and as knowledge and technology expand. This chapter introduces concepts and factors that affect professional nursing practice.

### Definitions of Nursing

Several well-known definitions of nursing indicate that the basic themes of health, illness, and caring have existed since Florence Nightingale described nursing. Following are two such examples:

- Nursing is putting the patient in the best condition for nature to act (Nightingale).[2]
- The nurse's unique function is to assist patients, sick or well, in the performance of those activities contributing to health or its recovery (or to peaceful death) that they would perform unaided if they had the necessary strength, will, or

Reviewed by Nelda S. Godfrey, PhD, RN, ACNS-BC, FAAN, Associate Dean and Clinical Professor, University of Kansas School of Nursing, Kansas City, Kansas; Laura A. Stokowski, RNC, MS, Inova Fairfax Hospital for Children, Falls Church, Virginia; and Dawn M. Vanderhoef, PhD, DNP, PMHNP/CS-BC, Assistant Professor, Vanderbilt University School of Nursing, Nashville, Tennessee.

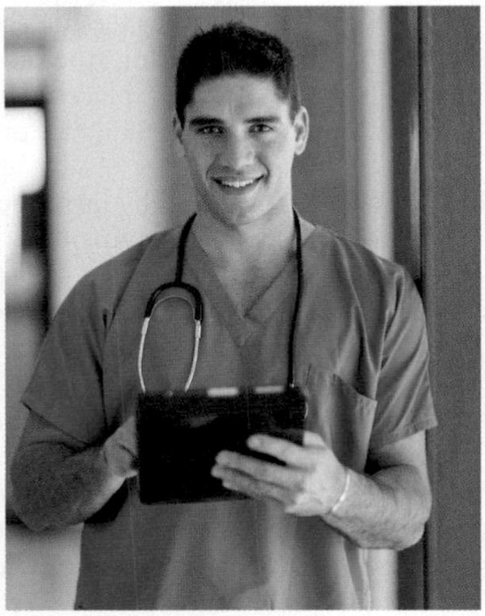

**FIG. 1-1** Nurses are frontline professionals of health care. (©Michael Jung/iStock/Thinkstock)

knowledge—and to do this in such a way as to help them gain independence as rapidly as possible (Henderson).[3]

In 1980 the ANA defined **nursing** as "the diagnosis and treatment of human responses to actual and potential health problems."[1] In this context, your care of a person with a fractured hip would focus on the patient's possible responses to impaired mobility, pain, and loss of independence.

The widely accepted ANA definition of nursing was reaffirmed in the 2010 edition of the ANA's *Nursing: A Social Policy Statement* to reflect the continuing evolution of nursing practice:

> ***Nursing*** *is the protection, promotion, and optimization of health and abilities, prevention of illness and injury, alleviation of suffering through the diagnosis and treatment of human response, and advocacy in the care of individuals, families, communities, and populations.*[1]

This definition reflects nurses' increasing role in promoting health and wellness and advocating for the recipients of their care.

## Nursing's View of Humanity

An individual has physiologic (or biophysical), psychologic (or emotional), sociocultural (or interpersonal), spiritual, and environmental components or dimensions. In this book, the individual is considered "a biopsychosocial spiritual being in constant interaction with a changing environment."[4] The individual is composed of dimensions that are interrelated and not separate entities. Thus a problem in one dimension may affect one or more of the other dimensions. A person's behavior is meaningful and oriented toward fulfilling needs, coping with stress, and developing one's self. However, at times a person requires help to meet these needs, cope successfully, or develop his or her unique potential.

## Scope of Nursing Practice

The essential core of nursing practice is to deliver holistic, patient-centered care. It includes assessment and evaluation, administering a variety of interventions, patient and family teaching, and being a member of the interprofessional health care team.

The extent that nurses engage in the scope of practice depends on their educational preparation, experience, and role and is guided by individual state laws. To enter into practice, a nurse must complete an accredited program and pass an examination verifying that the nurse has the knowledge necessary to provide safe care. Entry-level nurses with associate or baccalaureate degrees are prepared to function as generalists. At this level, nurses provide direct health care and focus on ensuring coordinated and comprehensive care to patients in a variety of settings. Nurses work collaboratively with other health care providers to manage the needs of individuals and groups.[5]

With experience and continued study, nurses may specialize in an area of practice. Certification is a formal way for nurses to obtain professional recognition for having expertise in a specialty area. A variety of nursing organizations offer certification in a number of nursing specialties.[6] Certification usually requires a certain amount of clinical experience and successful completion of an examination. Recertification usually requires ongoing clinical experience and continuing education. Common nursing specialties include cardiovascular care; critical care; women's health; nursing informatics; and geriatric, medical-surgical, perinatal, emergency, psychiatric/mental health, and community health nursing.

Additional formal education and experience can prepare nurses for advanced practice. An **advanced practice registered nurse (APRN)** is a nurse educated at the master's or doctoral level, with advanced education in pathophysiology, pharmacology, and health assessment and expertise in a specialized area of practice. APRNs include clinical nurse specialists, nurse practitioners, nurse midwives, and nurse anesthetists. APRNs play a vital role in the health care delivery system. In addition to managing and delivering direct patient care, APRNs have roles in leadership, quality improvement, evidence-based practice, and informatics.[5]

The doctor of nursing practice (DNP) degree is a practice-focused terminal nursing degree. By raising the educational preparation for APRNs to the doctoral level, nursing is moving in the same direction as other health professions that offer practice doctorates (e.g., pharmacy [PharmD], physical therapy [DPT]). Nurses with a research-focused doctorate (PhD) typically serve as faculty in schools of nursing, policy analysts, and researchers. However, they are being increasingly used in health care settings as clinical experts, researchers, and health care system executives.

# INFLUENCES ON PROFESSIONAL NURSING PRACTICE

## Complex Health Care Environments

**Expanding Knowledge and Technology.** Rapidly changing technology and dramatically expanding knowledge are adding to the complexity of health care environments. Advances in patient care technologies are transforming care delivery and extending patients' lives. Discoveries in genetics are changing the way we think about a number of diseases, such as cancer and heart disease. For example, genetic information guides breast cancer screening. If cancer is diagnosed, this information then allows for treatment and drug therapy based on the patient's genetic makeup. With advances in knowledge, ethical dilemmas and controversies arise regarding the use of new scientific knowledge and the disparities that exist in patients' access to technologically advanced health care. Throughout this book, expanding knowledge and technology's impact on nursing

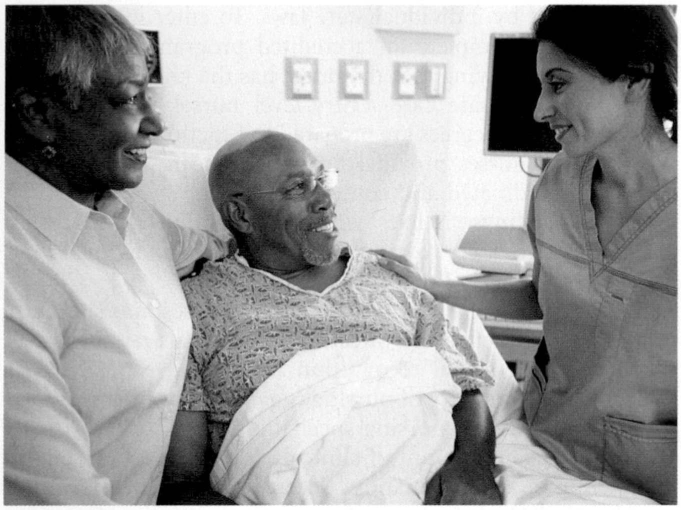

**FIG. 1-2** The patient, family, and nurse collaborate as part of coordinating high-quality care. (©monkebusinessimages/iStock/Thinkstock)

practice are highlighted in genetics, informatics, and ethical/legal boxes.

**Diverse Populations.** Patient populations are more diverse than ever. Americans are living longer, with the number of people with chronic illnesses and multiple comorbidities increasing. Unlike those who receive acute, episodic care, patients with chronic illnesses have complex needs. They see a variety of health care providers in various settings over an extended period. With care shifting from hospitals and nursing homes to managed care in the community, you need to be able to manage and coordinate care when patients are transitioning among different settings.

At the same time, you will be caring for a more culturally and ethnically diverse population. When delivering care, you must consider the patient's and caregiver's cultural beliefs and values. Immigrants, particularly undocumented immigrants, often lack the resources necessary to access health care. Inability to pay for health care is associated with a tendency to delay seeking care, resulting in illnesses that are more serious at the time of diagnosis. Boxes throughout this book emphasize the influence of such factors as gender, culture, and ethnicity on nursing practice.

**Consumerism.** Health care is a consumer-focused business, and patients today are more involved in their health care. They want more control over their health care and expect high-quality, coordinated, and financially reasonable care. Health information is readily available. Many patients are very knowledgeable about their health and seek information about health problems and health care from media and Internet sources. They gather information so that they can have a voice in making decisions about their health care. As a nurse, you must be able to help patients access, interpret, and use appropriate and valid health care information (Fig. 1-2).

## Health Care Systems

**Health Care Financing.** Many changes in health care systems that influence nursing care delivery are initiated by the government, employers, insurance companies, and regulating agencies in efforts to provide more cost-effective health care. Historically, the most notable event related to reimbursement was the establishment of prospective payment systems in the Medicare program. With this system, payment for hospital services for Medicare patients are based on flat fees determined by the diseases and problems treated during the admission. For example, if a patient had a total knee replacement, the hospital receives a set sum of money, such as $45,000 for the patient's care.

Other health care systems followed by introducing managed care systems that use prospective payment as a means of offering cost-effective health care delivery. In health maintenance organizations (HMOs) and preferred provider organizations (PPOs), charges are negotiated in advance of the delivery of care using predetermined reimbursement rates or capitation fees for medical care, hospitalization, and other health care services.

Now, quality and performance initiatives are driving further changes in health care financing. Value-based purchasing programs base reimbursement to health care providers on their performance on certain quality measures. These quality measures include clinical outcomes, patient safety, patient satisfaction, and the provider's adherence to evidence-based practice. Those who provide quality care at a lower cost may receive additional payments.

As part of value-based purchasing, payment for care can be withheld if a patient experiences events such as developing a pressure ulcer during a hospital stay or having something happen that is considered preventable (e.g., acquiring an injury after falling or having wrong site surgery).[7] This type of event is considered a *serious reportable event (SRE)*. SREs are discussed later in this chapter on p. 12.

**Health Policy.** Legislation has serious implications for health care delivery and nursing practice. The 2010 Patient Protection and Affordable Care Act (ACA) is the most important health care legislation since the creation of Medicare in 1965. The ACA's main goal is to increase access to health care. Other provisions affect how health care is delivered, expand wellness and preventive care, and promote quality and efficiency in the health care system.

The ACA encourages the creation of Accountable Care Organizations (ACOs). ACOs are groups of physicians, hospitals, and other health care providers who unite to coordinate care for Medicare patients. The goal of an ACO is to ensure that patients, especially the chronically ill, get the right care at the right time, while avoiding duplicate services and preventing errors.

The ACA supports nursing through funding for education and nurse-based clinics. The ACA has triggered changes throughout the health care system. As a nurse, you must take a leadership role in creating health care systems that provide safe, quality, patient-centered care. Becoming a Nurse Leader boxes throughout this book focus on developing leadership skills needed to fulfill this role.

## *Healthy People* Initiative

The U.S. government is active in establishing goals and objectives for improving health through the *Healthy People* initiative.[8] The vision of *Healthy People* is a society in which all people live long, healthy lives. The overarching goals of the *Healthy People 2020* initiative are presented in Table 1-1. You will play a significant role in the *Healthy People* agenda by emphasizing health promotion, health maintenance, and cost-effective care that is responsive to the needs of older adults, culturally diverse groups, and underserved populations. *Healthy People* boxes related to these goals are integrated throughout this book.

**TABLE 1-1 *Healthy People 2020***

**Overarching Goals**
- Attain high-quality, longer lives free of preventable disease, disability, injury, and premature death.
- Achieve health equity, eliminate disparities, and improve the health of all groups.
- Create social and physical environments that promote good health for all.
- Promote quality of life, healthy development, and healthy behaviors across all life stages.

Source: U.S. Department of Health and Human Services: *Healthy People 2020.* Retrieved from *www.healthypeople.gov.*

## Organizational Influences

**Professional Nursing Organizations.** The American Nurses Association is the primary professional nursing organization. There are numerous professional specialty organizations, such as the American Association of Critical-Care Nurses (AACN), Association of periOperative Registered Nurses (AORN), and Oncology Nursing Society (ONS). Professional organizations have numerous roles in promoting quality patient care and professional nursing practice. These roles include developing standards of practice and codes of ethics, supporting research, and lobbying for legislation and regulations. Major nursing organizations promote research into the causes of errors, develop strategies to prevent future errors, and address nursing issues that affect the nurse's ability to deliver patient care safely. Nurses join a professional organization to keep current in their practice and network with others who are interested in a particular practice area.

A program that supports nurses is the American Nurses Credentialing Center's Magnet Recognition Program. The Magnet program "recognizes health care organizations for quality patient care, nursing excellence and innovations in professional nursing practice."[9] Magnet designation demonstrates a high quality of nursing care and achievement of a positive practice environment for nurses. Nurses who work in Magnet facilities have low turnover and burnout rates and more opportunities for professional and personal growth. This leads to better patient outcomes and greater career satisfaction.

**Quality and Safety Education for Nurses (QSEN).** A number of high-profile reports over the past 15 years have highlighted problems with the quality of health care. One of these reports, *The Future of Nursing: Leading Change, Advancing Health* from the Health and Medicine Division (HMD) of the National Academy of Medicine (formerly called the Institute of Medicine), acknowledges the link between professional nursing practice and health care delivery. The report discusses how health care providers, including nurses, are not being adequately prepared to provide the highest quality care possible. It recommends making changes so that nurses will have the skills to advance health care and play leadership roles in a reformed health care system[10] (Table 1-2).

To address nursing's role in solving these problems, the Robert Wood Johnson Foundation funded the *Quality and Safety Education for Nurses (QSEN) Institute.* QSEN has made a major contribution to nursing by defining specific competencies that nurses need to have to practice safely and effectively in today's complex health care system. The remainder of this chapter describes each of the QSEN competencies and the knowledge, skills, and attitudes (KSAs) necessary in each of the six areas: (1) patient-centered care, (2) teamwork and collaboration, (3) safety, (4) quality improvement, (5) informatics, and (6) evidence-based practice[11] (Table 1-3).

**TABLE 1-2 Key Messages for the Future of Nursing**

- Nurses should practice to the full extent of their education and training.
- Nurses should achieve high education and training through an improved education system that promotes seamless academic progression.
- Nurses should be full partners with physicians and other health professionals in redesigning health care.
- Effective workforce planning and policy making require better data collection and information infrastructure.

Source: IOM (now HMD) Recommendations. Retrieved from *www.thefutureofnursing.org/recommendations.*

## PATIENT-CENTERED CARE

Nurses have long demonstrated that they truly deliver patient-centered care based on each patient's unique needs and understanding of the patient's preferences, values, and beliefs. Patient-centered care is interrelated with quality and safety. In the patient-centered care model, patients and caregivers seek and receive care from competent and knowledgeable health care professionals. In addition, patients and caregivers are involved in making decisions and coordinating care.

### Nursing Process

Nurses provide patient-centered care using an organizing framework called the *nursing process.* The **nursing process** is a problem-solving approach to the identification and treatment of patient problems that is the foundation of nursing practice. The nursing process framework provides a structure for the delivery of nursing care and the knowledge, judgments, and actions that nurses use to achieve best patient outcomes. Once started, the nursing process is continuous and cyclic.

The nursing process consists of five phases: assessment, diagnosis, planning, implementation, and evaluation (Fig. 1-3). There is a basic order to the nursing process, beginning with assessment. *Assessment* is the collection of subjective and objective patient information on which you will base your plan of care. *Nursing diagnosis* is the act of analyzing the assessment data and making a judgment about the nature of the data. It includes identifying and labeling human responses to actual or potential health problems or life processes. During *planning* the nursing diagnosis directs developing patient outcomes or goals and identifying nursing interventions to accomplish the outcomes. *Implementation* is the activation of the plan with the use of nursing interventions. *Evaluation* is a continual activity in the nursing process. Evaluation determines whether the patient outcomes have been met as a result of nursing interventions. If the outcomes were not met, a review of the steps of the process is necessary to determine why not. Revision may be needed in assessment (data collection), nursing diagnoses, planning (determining patient outcomes), or implementation (nursing interventions).

### Standardized Nursing Terminologies

The demands of the health care system challenge nursing to define its contribution to health care. The nursing profession can describe its unique role by answering questions such as: What do nurses do? How do they do it? How does it make a measurable difference in the health of those for whom they

**TABLE 1-3 QSEN Competencies**

| Competency | Knowledge, Skills, and Attitudes |
|---|---|
| **Patient-Centered Care**<br>Recognize the patient and caregiver as full partners in providing compassionate and coordinated care based on respect for patient's preferences, values, and needs | • Provide care with sensitivity and respect, taking into consideration the patient's perspectives, beliefs, and cultural background<br>• Assess level of comfort and treat appropriately<br>• Engage the patient in an active partnership that promotes health, well-being, and self-care management<br>• Facilitate patient's informed consent for care |
| **Teamwork and Collaboration**<br>Function effectively within nursing and interprofessional teams | • Value the expertise of each interprofessional member<br>• Initiate referrals when appropriate<br>• Follow communication practices that minimize risks associated with handoffs and transitions in care<br>• Participate in interprofessional rounds |
| **Safety**<br>Minimize risk of harm to patients and providers | • Follow recommendations from national safety campaigns<br>• Appropriately communicate observations or concerns related to hazards and errors<br>• Contribute to designing systems to improve safety |
| **Quality Improvement**<br>Use data to monitor the outcomes of care and to improve the quality and safety of health care systems | • Use quality measures to understand performance<br>• Identify gaps between local and best practices<br>• Participate in investigating the circumstances surrounding a sentinel event (never event) or serious reportable event (SRE) |
| **Informatics**<br>Use information and technology to communicate, manage knowledge, reduce errors, and support decision making | • Protect confidentiality of patient's protected health information<br>• Document appropriately in electronic health records<br>• Use communication technologies to coordinate patient care<br>• Respond correctly to clinical decision-making alerts |
| **Evidence-Based Practice**<br>Integrate best current evidence with clinical expertise and the patient/family preferences and values for delivery of optimal health care | • Read research, clinical practice guidelines, and evidence reports related to area of practice<br>• Base individual patient care plan on patient's values, clinical expertise, and evidence<br>• Continuously improve clinical practice based on new knowledge |

Source: QSEN Competencies. Retrieved from *http://qsen.org/competencies.*

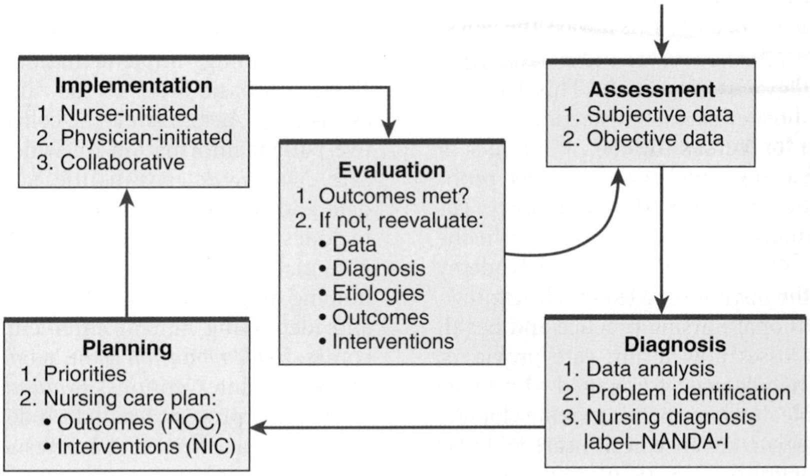


**FIG. 1-3** Nursing process.

care? How are nursing's contributions different from those of medicine?

In response to these questions, nursing uses standardized terminologies (also called *nomenclatures, classification systems,* and *taxonomies*) to clearly define and evaluate nursing care. This promotes continuity of patient care and provides data showing nursing's impact on patient outcomes. Instead of using a variety of words to describe the same patient problems and nursing interventions, nurses use a readily understood common language to improve communication.

Standardized terminologies help identify new knowledge and practice guidelines and are essential in exchanging information between different electronic records systems. For example, do the patient problems of pressure ulcer and skin breakdown mean the same thing? What nursing interventions prevent these problems? Does turning the patient every 2 hours mean the same thing as repositioning the patient every 2 hours? If the patient is turned or repositioned every 2 hours, what happens as a result? Does placing the patient on a pressure-relieving mattress or a standard mattress change the results? How are the results described? How do you know what works best?

Three of the most widely used nursing terminologies focus on specific phases of the nursing process: (1) NANDA International (NANDA-I): Nursing Diagnoses, Definitions, and Classification; (2) the Nursing Outcomes Classification (NOC); and (3) the Nursing Interventions Classification (NIC). Patients' responses or problems can be labeled using the nursing diagnoses classified and defined by NANDA-I.[12] Nursing-sensitive patient outcomes can be identified and evaluated by selecting appropriate NOC outcomes and nursing interventions, or treatments, can be selected and implemented from NIC.[13,14]

**NANDA-I Nursing Diagnoses.** NANDA-I is the nursing organization that develops and maintains the standard classification system for nursing diagnoses.[12] Nursing diagnoses provide the basis for selecting nursing interventions to achieve patient outcomes for which nursing is accountable. Delivering care based on accurately identified nursing diagnoses results in more effective and safer patient care. The NANDA-I list is continually evolving as new research results are available and nurses identify new human responses.

**Nursing Outcomes Classification (NOC).** Nursing Outcomes Classification (NOC) is a list of patient outcomes developed to evaluate the effects of interventions provided by nurses. A **nursing-sensitive patient outcome** is defined as an individual, family, or community state, behavior, or perception that is measured along a continuum in response to a nursing intervention(s).[13] The impact of your nursing practice on patient outcomes can be identified and measured when you choose a NOC outcome. Currently there are more than 490 outcomes. Each outcome has a designated code, definition, a set of indicators to use to evaluate patient status, and a five-point Likert scale for rating the outcome and indicators. A rating of a "5" is always the best possible score and "1" is always the worst possible score.

**Nursing Interventions Classification (NIC).** Nursing Interventions Classification (NIC) includes independent and collaborative interventions that you carry out, or direct others to carry out, on behalf of patients. An intervention is "any treatment, based upon clinical judgment and knowledge, which a nurse performs to enhance patient/client outcomes."[14] It includes treatments that you perform in all settings and includes direct and indirect care. NIC includes more than 550 interventions with a label name, a definition, and a set of activities for you to choose from to carry out the intervention.

A list of more than 550 interventions may seem overwhelming. You will soon discover those interventions that are often used in your particular specialty or with your patient population. When planning care for a patient, choose specific interventions that are appropriate for the patient based on the nursing diagnosis and desired patient outcomes. Each intervention has a list of activities, and you select the appropriate activities from the list to implement the intervention. NIC does not prescribe interventions for specific situations. You are responsible for making the important decision of when and which interventions to use for a specific patient and situation based on your knowledge of the patient and the patient's condition.

**NANDA-NOC-NIC Linkages.** NANDA, NOC, and NIC (NNN) linkages show how the three distinct nursing terminologies can be connected and used together when planning care for patients. Linkages may assist in determining a nursing diagnosis, projecting a desired outcome, and selecting interventions to achieve the desired outcome. Because each outcome or intervention has a coded number, the use of NNN facilitates electronic collection of standardized nursing data to evaluate the effectiveness of nursing care. Table 1-4 shows an example of an NNN linkage.

**TABLE 1-4 Example of NANDA-I–NOC–NIC Linkage**

**NANDA-I Nursing Diagnosis:** *Impaired skin integrity:* A state in which the individual has altered epidermis and/or dermis

| NANDA-I–Related Factors | NOC Outcomes | NIC Interventions |
|---|---|---|
| **Pressure** | Tissue integrity: skin and mucous membranes | Pressure management<br>Skin surveillance |
| **Nutritional deficit** | Nutritional status: food and fluid intake | Nutrition monitoring<br>Nutrition therapy |
| **Knowledge deficit** | Knowledge: illness care | Teaching: disease |

Source: *Nursing Diagnoses—Definitions and Classification 2015-2017.* © 2014, 1994-2014 by NANDA International. Used by arrangement with Blackwell Publishing Limited, a company of John Wiley & Sons, Inc.
*NANDA-I*, NANDA International; *NIC*, Nursing Interventions Classification; *NOC*, Nursing Outcomes Classification.

## Nursing Care Plans

In any clinical setting, you are responsible for providing an individualized plan of care that includes nursing diagnoses, outcomes, and interventions. In clinical practice, electronic care plans often follow a standard format that has been adapted to the specific setting. These plans are guides for routine nursing care. You individualize each to your patient's unique needs and problems.

In nursing education, the nursing process is often documented differently from clinical practice. The nursing process is frequently recorded in nursing care plans similar to those located on the website for this book *(http://evolve.elsevier.com/Lewis/medsurg)*. These nursing care plans are teaching and learning tools. You practice and learn the nursing process by collecting assessment data, identifying nursing diagnoses, and selecting patient outcomes and nursing interventions. You usually have to identify rationales for the selected interventions.

The nursing care plans associated with this book use NANDA-I–approved nursing diagnoses, listed in order of priority, with NOC outcomes and NIC interventions (NCP 1-1). When any of these care plans are used, you should individualize the plan for your specific patient. You must use critical thinking to continually evaluate the situation and revise the nursing diagnoses, outcomes, and interventions to fit each patient's unique care needs.

With *collaborative problems,* the nurse must monitor the patient to detect the onset or change in status of actual or potential complications.[15] Nurses use physician and nurse prescribed interventions to manage collaborative problems and prevent morbidity and mortality. During the diagnosis phase of the nursing process, you identify these risks in addition to nursing diagnoses. Identifying collaborative problems requires knowledge of pathophysiology and possible complications of medical treatment. Collaborative problem statements are usually written as "potential complication: ______" or "PC:

## NURSING CARE PLAN 1-1

***Patient With Heart Failure****

### Nursing Diagnosis

**Impaired gas exchange** *related to* increased preload and alveolar-capillary membrane changes *as evidenced by* abnormal $O_2$ saturation,, hypoxemia, dyspnea, tachypnea, tachycardia, restlessness, and patient's statement, "I am so short of breath"

### Patient Goal

Maintains adequate $O_2/CO_2$ exchange at the alveolar-capillary membrane to meet $O_2$ needs of the body

#### Outcomes (NOC)

**Respiratory Status: Gas Exchange**

- $O_2$ saturation _____
- Arterial pH _____
- $PaO_2$ _____
- $PaCO_2$ _____
- Chest x-ray findings _____

**Measurement Scale**
1 = Severe deviation from normal range
2 = Substantial deviation from normal range
3 = Moderate deviation from normal ranage
4 = Mild deviation from normal range
5 = No deviation from normal range

- Dyspnea with exertion _____
- Dyspnea at rest _____
- Restlessness _____
- Impaired cognition _____

**Measurement Scale**
1 = Severe
2 = Substantial
3 = Moderate
4 = Mild
5 = None

#### Interventions (NIC) and *Rationales*

**Respiratory Monitoring**

- Monitor pulse oximetry, respiratory rate, rhythm, depth, and effort of respirations *to evaluate changes in respiratory status.*
- Auscultate breath sounds, noting areas of decreased or absent ventilation and presence of adventitious sounds *to detect presence of pulmonary edema.*
- Monitor for increased restlessness, anxiety, and work of breathing *to detect increasing hypoxemia.*

**Oxygen Therapy**

- Administer supplemental $O_2$ or other noninvasive ventilator support (e.g., bilevel positive airway pressure [BiPAP]) as needed *to maintain adequate $O_2$ levels.*
- Monitor the $O_2$ liter flow rate and placement of $O_2$ delivery device *to ensure $O_2$ is adequately delivered.*
- Change $O_2$ delivery device from mask to nasal prongs during meals as tolerated *to sustain $O_2$ levels while eating.*
- Monitor the effectiveness of $O_2$ therapy *to identify hypoxemia and establish range of $O_2$ saturation.*

**Positioning**

- Position patient to alleviate dyspnea (e.g., semi-Fowler's position), as appropriate, *to improve ventilation by decreasing venous return to the heart and increasing thoracic capacity.*

*This example presents one nursing diagnosis for heart failure. The complete nursing care plan for heart failure is available on *http://evolve.elsevier.com/Lewis/medsurg.*

_____" without a "*related to*" statement. An example is PC: pulmonary embolism.

A *concept map* is another method of recording a nursing care plan. In a concept map the nursing process is recorded in a visual diagram of patient problems and interventions that illustrates the relationships among clinical data. Nurse educators use concept mapping to teach nursing process and care planning. There are various formats for concept maps.

*Conceptual care maps* blend a concept map and a nursing care plan. On a conceptual care map, assessment data used to identify the patient's primary health concern are centrally positioned. Diagnostic testing data, treatments, and medications surround the assessment data. Positioned below are nursing diagnoses that represent the patient's responses to the health state. Listed with each nursing diagnosis are the assessment data that support the nursing diagnosis, outcomes, nursing interventions with rationales, and evaluation. After completing the map, you draw connections between identified relationships and concepts. A conceptual care map creator is available online on the website for this book. For selected case studies at the end of the management chapters, related concept maps are available on the website at *http://evolve.elsevier.com/Lewis/medsurg.*

## Continuum of Patient Care

Nursing is a part of health care at all points along the patient care continuum. Depending on their health status, patients often move among a multitude of different health care settings. For example, a young man is in a trauma unit of an acute care hospital following a motor vehicle crash. After he is stabilized, he may be transferred to a general medical-surgical unit and then to an acute rehabilitation facility. After rehabilitation is complete, he is discharged home to continue with outpatient rehabilitation, with follow-up by home health care nurses and care in an ambulatory clinic.

Decisions regarding the most appropriate setting for obtaining health care frequently depend on the cost of care and the patient's health care insurance plan and personal finances. Although the hospital remains the mainstay for acute care interventions, community-based settings offer patients the opportunity to live or recover in settings that maximize their independence and preserve human dignity.

Community-based health care settings include ambulatory care, transitional care, and long-term care. *Transitional care* settings provide care in between the acute care and the home or long-term care setting. Patients may receive transitional care at an acute rehabilitation facility after head trauma or a spinal cord injury. *Long-term care* refers to the care of patients for a period greater than 30 days. It may be required for those who are severely developmentally disabled, who are mentally impaired, or who have physical deficits requiring continuous medical and nursing management (e.g., patients who are ventilator dependent or have Alzheimer's disease). Long-term care facilities include skilled nursing facilities, assisted living facilities, and residential care facilities.

With the Affordable Care Act, there is a new emphasis on care coordination when patients transition between care settings. *Transitions of care* refer to patients moving among health care practitioners, settings, and home as their condition and care needs change.[16] As a nurse, you are an essential part of care coordination by stressing actions that meet patient's needs and facilitate safe, quality care. Collaborating with other members of the interprofessional team is critical. A lack of communication can result in an ineffective care transition, leading to medication errors and higher hospital readmission rates. For example, you are a nurse in acute care admitting a long-term care patient who has been receiving propranolol 20 mg/5 mL twice a day. The admitting orders read "propranolol 20 mg/mL, give 5 mL twice a day."

### Delivery of Nursing Care

Nurses deliver patient-centered care in collaboration with the interprofessional health care team and within the framework of a care delivery model. A care delivery model outlines how responsibilities and authority are structured to accomplish patient care.[17] More positive care outcomes occur when the number and type of care providers match patient needs and there is a designated care coordinator.

In acute care settings, two basic models are used, team care and total patient care. *Team care* models involve a group of providers who work together to deliver care. A professional nurse is usually the team leader. As team leader, you manage and coordinate care with others, such as licensed practical/vocational nurses (LPNs/LVNs) and unlicensed assistive personnel (UAP). You have accountability for the quality of care delivered by team members during a work period. In total patient care models, you are responsible for planning and providing all care.

Other care models include case management and telehealth. **Case management** is "a collaborative process of assessment, planning, facilitation, care coordination, evaluation, and advocacy for options and services to meet an individual's and family's comprehensive health needs through communication and available resources to promote quality, cost-effective outcomes."[18] Although health care agencies implement case management in various ways, it involves managing the patient's care with other interprofessional team members across multiple care settings and levels of care.

A professional nurse often serves as the case manager. In this role, the nurse assesses the needs of patients and/or caregivers, coordinates services for them, makes referrals as appropriate, and evaluates the progress towards meeting care goals.

For example, a nurse case manager in an outpatient clinic has been working for 3 months with an older male patient who has multiple co-morbidities, including severe coronary artery disease, diabetes, and osteoarthritis. After he is scheduled for a coronary artery bypass, the nurse manager coordinates his care with other members of the interprofessional team. She arranges his preoperative appointments and informs the other team members so that all health care providers understand the patient's unique needs. After the patient has surgery, he develops a deep venous thrombosis in his leg. The case manager then works with the interprofessional team to evaluate the patient's discharge needs and determine whether rehabilitation or home health care are necessary for the patient. With the patient and caregiver, the team decides to discharge the patient to a rehabilitation facility. The case manager assists with the transition, again coordinating care so that the providers at the rehabilitation facility are aware of the patient's needs.

**Telehealth** nursing is using the nursing process to provide nursing care to patients through telecommunication technologies, including high-speed Internet, wireless, satellite, and video communications.[17] Among the many uses of telehealth are triaging patients, monitoring patients with chronic or critical conditions, helping patients manage symptoms, providing patient and caregiver education and emotional support, and providing follow-up care. Telehealth increases access to care. The nurse engaged in telehealth can assess the patient's health status, deliver interventions, and evaluate the outcomes of nursing care while separated geographically from the patient (Fig. 1-4).

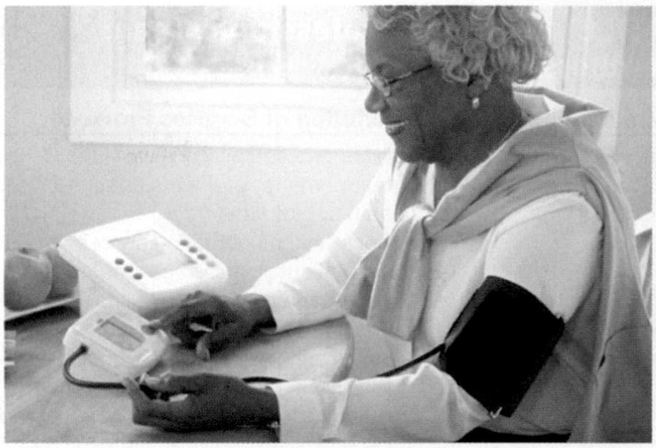

**FIG. 1-4** An older adult performing remote blood pressure monitoring. (From Cooper K, Gosnell K: *Foundations of nursing,* St Louis, 2015, Elsevier.)

### Critical Thinking

Complex health care environments require that you use critical thinking and clinical reasoning skills to make decisions that lead to the best patient outcomes. **Critical thinking**, your ability to focus your thinking to get the results you need in various situations, has been described as knowing how to learn, be creative, generate ideas, make decisions, and solve problems.[19]

Critical thinking is not memorizing a list of facts or the steps of a procedure. Instead, it is the ability to make judgments and solve problems by making sense of information. Learning and using critical thinking is a continual process that occurs inside and outside of the clinical setting.

**Clinical reasoning** is using critical thinking to examine and analyze patient care issues.[19] It involves understanding the medical and nursing implications of a patient's situation when making decisions regarding patient care. You use clinical reasoning when you identify a change in a patient's status, take into account the context and concerns of the patient and caregiver, and decide what to do about it.

Given the complexity of patient care today, nurses are required to learn and implement critical thinking and clinical reasoning skills long before they gain those skills through the experience of professional practice. Clinical experiences during nursing education provide opportunities for you to learn and make decisions about patient care. Various education models and techniques, including interactive case studies and simulation exercises, promote practice in critical thinking and clinical reasoning. Throughout this book, select boxes, case studies, and review questions promote your use of critical thinking and clinical reasoning skills.

## TEAMWORK AND COLLABORATION

### Interprofessional Team

To deliver high-quality care, you need to establish effective working relationships with members of the health care team. The **interprofessional team** is composed of providers from various disciplines, working together and sharing their expertise to provide individualized care. It may consist of physicians, nurses, pharmacists, occupational and physical therapists, social workers, and others (Table 1-5). To be competent in interprofessional practice, you must collaborate in many ways by exchanging knowledge, sharing responsibility for problem

**TABLE 1-5 Interprofessional Team Members**

| Team Member | Description of Services Provided |
|---|---|
| **Dentist** | Provides preventive and restorative treatments for problems affecting the teeth and mouth |
| **Dietitian** | Provides general nutrition services, including dietary consultation regarding health promotion or specialized diets |
| **Occupational therapist (OT)** | May assist patient with fine motor coordination, performance of activities of daily living, cognitive-perceptual skills, sensory testing, and the construction or use of assistive or adaptive equipment |
| **Pastoral care** | Offers spiritual support and guidance to patients and caregivers |
| **Pharmacist** | Prepares medications and infusion products |
| **Physical therapist (PT)** | Works with patients on improving strength and endurance, gait training, transfer training, and developing a patient education program |
| **Physician (medical doctor [MD])** | Practices medicine and treats illness and injury by prescribing medication, performing diagnostic tests and evaluations, performing surgery, and providing other medical services and advice |
| **Physician assistant** | Conducts physical exams, diagnoses and treats illnesses, and counsels on preventive health care in collaboration with a physician |
| **Respiratory therapist** | May assist with oxygen therapy in the home, provide specialized respiratory treatments, and instruct patient or caregiver regarding the proper use of respiratory equipment |
| **Social worker** | Assists patients with developing coping skills, meeting caregiver concerns, securing adequate financial resources or housing assistance, or making referrals to social service or volunteer agencies |
| **Speech pathologist** | Focuses on treatment of speech defects and disorders, especially through the use of physical exercises to strengthen muscles used in speech, speech drills, and audiovisual aids that develop new speech habits |

solving, and making patient care decisions. You may be responsible for coordinating care among the team members, participating in interprofessional team meetings or rounds, and initiating appropriate referrals when you need expertise in specialized areas to help the patient. To do so, you must be aware of the knowledge and skills of other team members and be able to communicate effectively with them.

To assist you in developing the competencies necessary to practice within an interprofessional clinical environment, you may participate in education activities with students from other disciplines. Throughout this book, teamwork and collaboration boxes, case studies, and review questions discuss the roles other professionals have in managing clinical problems.

## Coordinating Care

**Communication.** Effective communication is a key component of fostering teamwork and coordinating care. To provide safe, effective care, everyone involved in a patient's care should understand the patient's condition and his or her needs.

**TEAMWORK & COLLABORATION**

***Teamwork & Collaboration Boxes Throughout Book***



Unfortunately many issues result from a breakdown in communication. Miscommunication often occurs during transitions of care. One structured model used to improve communication is the **SBAR (Situation-Background-Assessment-Recommendation)** technique (Table 1-6). This technique provides a way to talk about a patient's condition among members of the health care team in a predictable, structured manner. Other ways to enhance communication during transitions include performing surgical time-outs, using a standard change-of-shift process, and conducting interprofessional rounds to identify risks and develop a plan for delivering care.

**Clinical Pathways.** **Clinical pathways** (critical paths, patient care protocols, care maps) are interprofessional care plans that specify care and desired outcomes during a specific time period for patients with a particular diagnosis or health condition. Think of a clinical pathway as a road map the patient and health care team should follow. As the patient progresses along the road, the patient should receive specific care and accomplish specific goals. If a patient's progress differs from the planned path, a variance has occurred. A negative variance occurs when specific goals are not met. The nurse usually identifies when a negative variance is present and works with the interprofessional team to create a plan to address the issue.[16]

The exact content and format of clinical pathways vary among agencies and settings. Each agency usually develops its own pathways based on evidence-based practice guidelines. Common components include assessment guidelines, laboratory and diagnostic testing, medications, activity, diet, and teaching. In

**TABLE 1-6 Guidelines for Communicating Using SBAR**

**Purpose:** SBAR is a model for effective transfer of information by providing a standardized structure for concise factual communications from nurse-to-nurse, nurse-to-physician, or nurse-to–other health professionals.
**Steps to Use:** Before speaking with a physician or other health care professional about a patient problem, assess the patient yourself, read the most recent physician progress and nursing notes, and have the patient's chart available.

| | |
|---|---|
| **S** Situation | • What is the situation you want to discuss? What is happening at the present time?<br>• Identify self, unit. State: I am calling about: *patient, room number.*<br>• Briefly state the problem: what it is, when it happened or started, and how severe it is. State: I have just assessed the patient and I am concerned about: *identify why you are concerned.* |
| **B** Background | • What is the background or circumstances leading up to the situation? State pertinent background information related to the situation that may include<br>• Admitting diagnosis and date of admission<br>• List of current medications, allergies, IV fluids<br>• Most recent vital signs<br>• Date and time of any laboratory testing and results of previous tests for comparison<br>• Synopsis of treatment to date<br>• Code status |
| **A** Assessment | • What do you think the problem is? What is your assessment of the situation? State what you think the problem is:<br>• Changes from prior assessments<br>• Patient condition unstable or worsening |
| **R** Recommendation/ Request | • What should we do to correct the problem? What is your recommendation or request? State your request.<br>• Specific treatments<br>• Tests needed<br>• Patient needs to be seen now |

Source: Institute for Health Care Improvement: SBAR technique for communication: a situational briefing model. Retrieved from *www.ihi.org/resources/Pages/Tools/SBARTechniqueforCommunicationASituationalBriefingModel.aspx.*

acute care, clinical pathways often describe which patient care components are required at specific times for each day of hospitalization. The case types selected for this type of pathway are usually those that are high volume or high risk and predictable, such as myocardial infarction and surgical procedures (e.g., joint replacements, cholecystectomies, cataract surgery).

**Delegation and Assignment.** As a registered nurse (RN), you will delegate nursing care and supervise others who are qualified to deliver care. **Delegation** is transferring authority to a competent individual for completing selected nursing tasks in a selected situation.[20] The delegation and assignment of nursing activities is a process that, when used appropriately, can result in safe, effective, and efficient patient care. Delegating can allow you more time to focus on complex patient care needs. Delegating care and supervising others will be one of your fundamental roles as a professional nurse.

Delegation typically involves tasks and procedures that licensed practical/vocational nurses (LPNs/LVNs) and unlicensed assistive personnel (UAP) perform. Nursing interventions that require independent nursing knowledge, skill, or judgment (e.g., initial assessment, determining nursing diagnoses, patient teaching, evaluating care) are your responsibility and cannot be delegated. State boards of nursing and agency policies identify activities that you can delegate to LPNs/LVNs and UAP. You need to use professional judgment to determine appropriate activities to delegate based on the patient's needs, the LPN/LVN's and UAP's education and training, and extent of supervision required. The most common delegated nursing actions occur during the implementation phase of the nursing process. For example, the nurse can delegate measuring oral intake and urine output to UAP, but the RN uses nursing judgment to decide if the intake and output are adequate.

The general guideline for LPN/LVN practice is that they can function independently in a stable, routine situation. However, they must work under the direct supervision of a professional nurse in acute, unstable situations when a patient's condition can rapidly change. In most states, LPNs/LVNs may administer medications, perform sterile procedures, and provide a wide variety of interventions planned by the RN. The procedure itself is not the issue in determining what can be delegated. Rather, the stability of the patient determines whether it is appropriate for an RN to delegate a procedure to an LPN/LVN. For example, the LPN/LVN can change a dressing on an abdominal surgical wound, but the RN should perform the initial dressing change and wound assessment.

UAPs hold many titles, including nurse aides, orderlies, nursing assistants, patient care assistants, or technicians. The activities UAPs perform typically include obtaining routine vital signs on stable patients, feeding and assisting patients at mealtimes, ambulating stable patients, and helping patients with bathing and hygiene.

Delegation can also occur among professional nurses. For example, if one RN has accountability for an outcome and asks another RN to perform a specific intervention related to that outcome, that is delegation. This type of delegation typically occurs when one RN leaves the unit/work area for a meal break.

*Assignment* is different from delegation in that assignment is the work each staff member is to accomplish during a given work period.[20] Staff members can only be assigned activities that are within their scope of practice. Therefore the term *assign* is used when you direct a person to do something that he or she is authorized to do. For example, you can assign an LPN/LVN to administer medications to a patient, because this is within the LPN/LVN's scope of practice. You cannot assign an LPN/LVN to a patient who needs an admission assessment, because an RN must perform the initial patient assessment.

Whether you delegate or are working with staff to whom you assign tasks, you are responsible for the patient's total care during your work period. You need to determine what patient care tasks must be accomplished during the given time period, identify who will accomplish them, and prioritize the order in which the tasks must be completed. You are responsible for supervising UAP or LPNs/LVNs. Clearly communicate what tasks must be done and provide necessary guidance. Since you are accountable for ensuring that delegated tasks are completed in a competent manner, evaluate the care given, follow-up as needed, and make sure no care was missed.

Delegation is a skill that is learned and you must practice to be proficient in managing patient care. You need to use critical thinking and professional judgment to ensure that the Five Rights of Nursing Delegation are implemented (Table 1-7). To

**TABLE 1-7 Five Rights of Delegation**

**The Five Rights of Delegation**

The registered nurse uses critical thinking and professional judgment to be sure that the delegation or assignment is:

1. The right task
2. Under the right circumstances
3. To the right person
4. With the right directions and communication
5. Under the right supervision and evaluation

| Rights of Delegation | Description | Questions to Ask |
|---|---|---|
| **Right Task** | One that can be delegated for a specific patient | Is it appropriate to delegate based on legal and agency factors? Has the person been trained and evaluated in performing the task? Is the person able and willing to do this specific task? |
| **Right Circumstances** | Appropriate patient setting, available resources, and considering relevant factors, including patient stability | What are the patient's needs right now? Is staffing such that the circumstances support delegation strategies? |
| **Right Person** | Right person is delegating the right task to the right person to be performed on right person | Is the prospective delegatee a willing and able employee? Are the patient needs a "fit" with the delegatee? |
| **Right Directions and Communication** | Clear, concise description of task, including its objective, limits, and expectations | Have you clearly communicated the task? With directions, limits, and expected outcomes? Does the delegatee know what and when to report? Does the delegatee understand what needs to be done? |
| **Right Supervision and Evaluation** | Appropriate monitoring, evaluation, intervention, and feedback | Do you know how and when you will interact about patient care with the delegatee? How often will you need to provide direct observation? Will you be able to give feedback to the staff member if needed? |

Source: Delegation Joint Statement NCSBN-ANA. Retrieved from *www.ncsbn.org/1625.htm.*

assist you, information on delegation is presented in teamwork and collaboration boxes and questions in case studies at the end of the management chapters.

## SAFETY

As the complexity of health care environments increases, patient safety is affected. It is estimated that between 210,000 and 440,000 patients each year suffer some type of harm that contributes to their death because of preventable medical errors.[21] A number of organizations are addressing this issue by providing safety goals for health care organizations and identifying safety competencies for health professionals. By implementing various procedures and systems to improve health care delivery to meet safety goals, health care systems are working to attain a culture of safety that minimizes the risk of harm to the patient.

### Serious Reportable Events

The National Quality Forum (NQF) uses the term **serious reportable event (SRE)**, also called a *"never" event,* to describe adverse events that are serious, largely preventable, and of concern to the public and health care providers.[22] These events include such things as a patient acquiring a stage III or greater pressure ulcer while hospitalized and death or disability from a fall or hypoglycemia.

To reduce the occurrence of these events, the NQF provides a list of effective *Safe Practices* that should be used in health care settings to improve the safety of care. You are implementing NQF practices when you perform a time-out prior to a surgical procedure, complete accurate medication records, and implement interventions to prevent catheter-associated urinary tract infections, pressure ulcers, and falls.

### National Patient Safety Goals

The Joint Commission (TJC), the accrediting agency for health care organizations, gathers and reports data on serious errors they call sentinel events. A *sentinel event* is a patient safety event not related to the patient's illness or underlying condition that reaches a patient and results in death, permanent harm, or severe temporary harm.[23] Events are "sentinel" because they signal the need for immediate investigation and response. Many sentinel events are also serious reportable events. If the patient undergoes a wrong-site or wrong-procedure surgery, experiences an assault in the health care setting or receives an incompatible blood product, the occurrence is both a sentinel event, reportable to TJC, and a serious reportable event, reportable to NQF.

To address specific patient safety concerns, TJC issues National Patient Safety Goals (NPSGs).[23] NPSGs promote patient safety by providing evidence-based solutions to common safety problems. The 2016 NPSGs are listed in Table 1-8.

The latest safety goal, focusing on improving the safety of clinical alarm systems, will greatly affect nursing. Patient monitoring systems provide important information. Alarms that work well improve patient safety and care by telling you when a patient requires your attention. However, so many alarms can go off that *alarm fatigue* occurs, and nurses can become desensitized to the sounds. By better managing alarms, alarm fatigue will be reduced and patient safety improved.

Because you have the greatest amount of interaction with patients, you play a key role in promoting safety. Many describe nurses as the patient's last line of defense. Every nurse has the responsibility to ensure the patient receives care in a manner that prevents errors and promotes patient safety. Throughout this book, safety alerts highlighting patient care issues and NPSGs will assist you in learning to apply safety principles.

## QUALITY IMPROVEMENT

Quality care is related to safety: the higher the culture of safety, the better the quality of care. Health care systems focused on

**TABLE 1-8 National Patient Safety Goals**

| Safety Goal | Examples |
|---|---|
| **Goal 1:** Identify patients correctly. | • Use at least two ways to identify patients (e.g., have them state full name and date of birth).<br>• Give the correct patient the correct blood with every blood transfusion. |
| **Goal 2:** Improve communication among the health care team. | • Quickly get critical test results to the right staff person. |
| **Goal 3:** Use medications safely. | • Label all medicines that are not already labeled. Discard any found unlabeled.<br>• Use appropriate precautions with patients who take anticoagulants.<br>• Find out what medications each patient is taking. Make certain that it is safe for the patient to take any new medicines with his or her current medicines.<br>• Give a list of the patient's medicines to the patient and his or her caregiver before they go home. Explain the list. |
| **Goal 6:** Use clinical alarm systems safely. | • Respond to alarms in a timely manner.<br>• Do not turn alarms off. |
| **Goal 7:** Prevent health care–associated infections. | • Use soap, water, and hand sanitizer before and after every patient contact.<br>• Use evidence-based practices to prevent infections related to central lines, indwelling urinary catheters, and multidrug-resistant organisms. |
| **Goal 15:** Identify the safety risks inherent in the agency's patient population. | • Assess patients at risk for suicide.<br>• Assess any risks for patients who are getting home oxygen therapy, such as fires. |
| **Universal Protocol (UP)**<br>Preprocedure verification<br>Mark procedure site<br>Performance of time-out | • Conduct a time-out before the start of any invasive or surgical procedure.<br>• Confirm correct patient, procedure, and site. |

Adapted from The Joint Commission (TJC): *2016 National patient safety goals,* Oakbrook Terrace, Ill. Retrieved from *www.jointcommission.org/assets/1/6/2016_NPSG_HAP_ER.pdf/.*

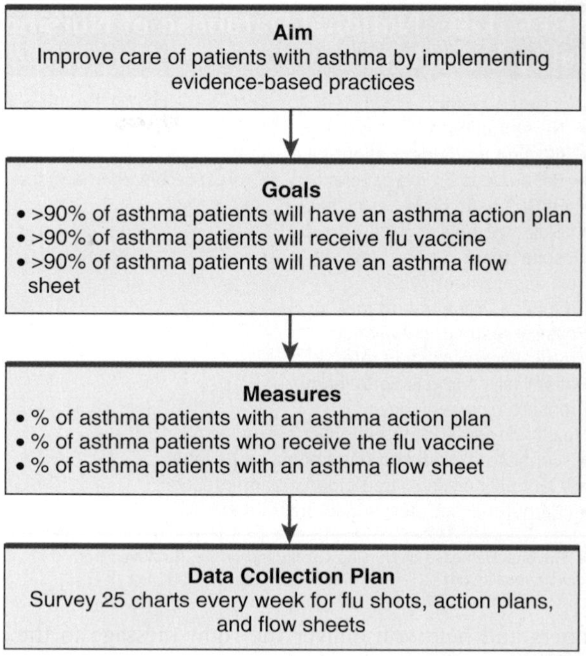


**FIG. 1-5** Quality improvement system. (Adapted from Courtlandt CD, Noonan L, Leonard GF: Model for improvement—part 1: A framework for health care quality, *Ped Clin North Am* 56:757, 2009.)

quality outcomes use practice standards and protocols based on best evidence while considering the patient's unique preferences and needs. Your role is to coordinate the complex aspects of patient care, including the care delivered by others, and identify and correct issues associated with poor quality and unsafe care.

Quality improvement (QI) programs involve systematic actions that monitor, assess, and improve health care quality. QI is an interprofessional team effort that is required by accrediting agencies. As part of professional nursing practice, you need to be able to collect data using QI tools, implement interventions to improve quality of care, and monitor patient outcomes. Several public and private groups focusing on improving health care quality have developed standard QI measures. These performance measures assess how well the health care team cares for a patient with a certain condition or receives a specific treatment. They describe what data must be collected and monitored. Fig 1-5 shows an example of a QI system for adult patients with asthma. In this example, you would monitor patient medical records to determine if the rate of flu vaccine administration exceeds 90%. You would share the results with the interprofessional team and, if the identified proficiency was not met, work as a team to implement measures to correct the deficiency.

### National Database of Nursing Quality Indicators

The National Database of Nursing Quality Indicators (NDNQI) provides data on nursing-sensitive measures to evaluate the impact of nursing care on patient outcomes. Patient outcomes are nursing sensitive if they improve with a greater quantity or quality of nursing care. NDNQI outcomes are unique because they identify how nursing workforce factors, including nurse staffing and skill mix, directly influence patient outcomes. NDNQI data show the incidence of falls and health care–associated pressure ulcers and infections decreases with adequate staffing and increased nurse education and satisfaction with the work environment. Table 1-9 lists the current NDNQI.

## INFORMATICS

Nursing is an information-intense profession. Advances in informatics and technology have changed the way nurses plan, deliver, document, and evaluate care. All nurses, regardless of their setting or role, use informatics and technology every day in practice. Informatics has changed how you obtain and review diagnostic information, make clinical decisions, communicate with patients and health care team members, document, and provide care.

Technology advances have increased the efficiency of nursing care, improving the work environment and the care nurses provide. Computers and mobile devices allow you to document at the time you deliver care and give you quick and easy access to information, including clinical decision-making tools, patient education materials, and references. Texting, video chat, and e-mail enhance communication among health care team

**TABLE 1-9 National Database of Nursing Quality Indicators**

- Workforce factors
  - Nurse turnover
  - Nursing hours per patient day
  - RN surveys on job satisfaction and practice environment scale
  - RN education and certification
  - Skill mix: RNs, LPNs/LVNs, UAP
- Hospital readmission rates
- Pain assessment cycle
- Peripheral IV infiltration rate
- Physical restraint prevalence
- Physical/sexual assault rate
- Patient falls and falls with injury
- Pressure ulcer incidence
- Health care–associated infections (HAI)
  - Ventilator-associated pneumonia and events
  - Central line-associated bloodstream infection
  - Catheter-associated urinary tract infection

Source: National Database of Nursing Quality Indicators. Retrieved from *www.nursingquality.org*.

members and help you deliver the right message to the right person at the right time.

Technology plays a key role in providing safe, quality patient care. Medication administration applications improve patient safety by flagging potential errors, such as look-alike and sound-alike medications and adverse drug interactions, before they can occur. Computerized provider order entry (CPOE) systems can eliminate errors caused by misreading or misinterpreting handwritten orders. Sensor technology can decrease the number of falls in high-risk patients. Care reminder systems provide cues that decrease the amount of missed nursing care.

Being able to use technology skills to communicate and access information is now an essential component of your professional nursing practice. You must be able to use word processing software, communicate by e-mail and book messaging, access appropriate information, and follow security and confidentiality rules. You need to demonstrate the skills to safely use patient care technologies and navigate electronic documentation systems.

*Protected health information (PHI)* is highly sensitive. *The Health Insurance Portability and Accountability Act (HIPAA)* is part of federal legislation that addresses actions for how PHI is used and disclosed. With the increased use of informatics and technology come new concerns on how to comply with HIPAA regulations and maintain a patient's privacy. New wireless technologies, increased use of e-mail and computer networking, and the ongoing threat of computer viruses increase the need for properly protecting a patient's privacy.

As a nurse, you have an obligation to ensure the privacy of your patient's health information. To do so, you need to understand your agency's policies regarding the use of technology. You need to know the rules regarding accessing patient records and releasing PHI, what to do if information is accidentally or intentionally released, and how to protect any passwords you use. If you are using social networking, you must be careful not to place any individually identifiable PHI online. Throughout this book, Informatics in Practice boxes offer suggestions on how to use informatics in your practice.

### Electronic Health Records

The largest use of informatics is **electronic health records (EHRs)**, also called *electronic medical records.* An EHR is a computerized record of patient information. It is shared among all health care team members involved in a patient's care and moves with the patient—to other providers and across care settings. The ideal EHR provides a single place for team members to review and update a patient's health record, document care given, and enter patient care orders, including medications, procedures, diets, and diagnostic and laboratory tests (Fig. 1-6). The EHR should contain a patient's medical history, diagnoses, medications, treatment plans, immunization dates, allergies, and test results.[24]

With the ACA, an increase in EHR use is under way. EHRs have the potential to reduce medical errors associated with traditional paper records and improve clinical decision making, patient safety, and quality of care. Unfortunately, several obstacles remain in the way of fully implementing EHRs. Systems are expensive and technologically complex, requiring a number of resources to implement and maintain. In addition, communication is still lacking among computer systems and software

**ETHICAL/LEGAL DILEMMAS**

***Social Networking: HIPAA Violation***

**Situation**

You log into a closed group on a social networking site and read a posting from a fellow nursing student. The posting describes in detail the complex care the student provided to an older patient in a local hospital the previous day. The student comments on how stressful the day was and asks for advice on how to deal with similar patients in the future.

**Ethical/Legal Points for Consideration**

- Protecting and maintaining patient privacy and confidentiality are basic obligations defined in the Code of Ethics for Nurses, which nurses and nursing students should uphold.[1]
- As outlined in the Health Insurance Portability and Accountability Act (HIPAA), a patient's private health information is any information that relates to the person's past, present, or future physical or mental health. This includes not only specific details such as a patient's name or picture but also information that gives enough details that someone may be able to identify that person.
- You may unintentionally breach privacy or confidentiality by posting patient information (diagnosis, condition, or situation) on a social networking site. Using privacy settings or being in a closed group does not guarantee the secrecy of posted information. Others can copy and share any post without your knowledge.
- Potential consequences for improperly using social networking vary based on the situation. These may include (1) disciplinary action by the state board of nursing, (2) being disciplined, suspended, or fired by an employer, (3) dismissal from a nursing program, and (4) civil and/or criminal charges.
- A student nurse who experienced a stressful day and is looking for advice and support from peers (e.g., "Today my patient died. I wanted to cry.") could share the experience by clearly limiting the posts to the student's personal perspective and not sharing any identifying information. This is one area in which it is safest to err on the side of caution to avoid the appearance of impropriety.

**Discussion Questions**

1. How would you deal with the situation involving the fellow nursing student or a nursing colleague?
2. How would you handle a situation in which you observed a staff member who violated HIPAA?

**Reference**

1. Code of Ethics for Nurses: Retrieved from *www.nursingworld.org/MainMenuCategories/EthicsStandards/Ethics-Position-Statements.*

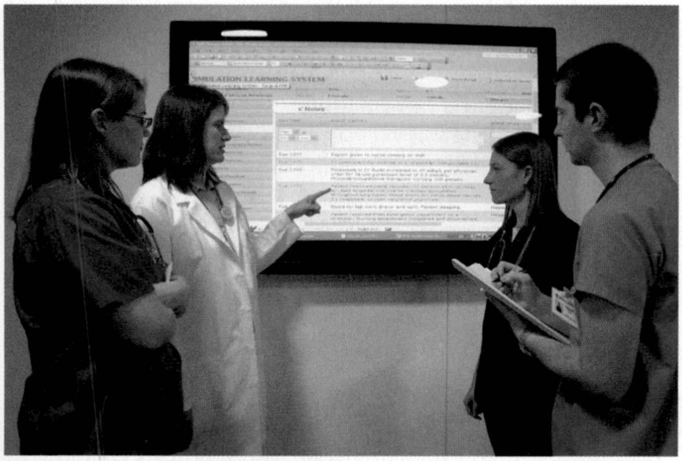

**FIG. 1-6** Members of the interprofessional team review a patient's electronic health record. (From Arnold EC, Boggs KU: *Interpersonal relationships*, St Louis, 2011, Mosby.)

applications in use. Finally, patients must be assured of their privacy and that information is only accessed by those with a right to know.

## EVIDENCE-BASED PRACTICE

Evidence-based practice (EBP) is a problem-solving approach to clinical decision making. Using the best available evidence (e.g., research findings, QI data), combined with your expertise and the patient's unique circumstances and preferences, leads to better clinical decisions and improved patient outcomes. EBP closes the gap between research and practice, providing more reliable and predictable care than that based on tradition, opinion, and trial and error.

EBP does not mean that you have to conduct a research study. Instead, EBP depends on you to take an active role in using the best available evidence when delivering care. You need to have an ongoing curiosity about what are the best nursing practices and routinely ask questions about your patient's care. Recognize when you need more information. When you base your practice on valid evidence, you are solving problems and supporting best patient outcomes.

### Steps of EBP Process

The EBP process has six steps (Table 1-10).

**Step 1.** Step 1 is asking a clinical question in the PICOT format. Developing the clinical question is the most important step in the EBP process.[25] A good clinical question sets the context for integrating evidence, clinical judgment, and patient preferences. In addition, the question guides the literature search for the best evidence to influence practice.

An example of a clinical question in PICOT format is, "In adult abdominal surgery patients (**P** = patients/population) is splinting with an elasticized abdominal binder (**I** = intervention) or a pillow (**C** = comparison) more effective in reducing pain associated with ambulation (**O** = outcome) on the first postoperative day (**T** = time period)?" A properly stated clinical question may not have all components of PICOT. Some only include four components. The (T) timing or (C) comparison components are not appropriate for every question. The (C) component of PICOT may include a comparison with a specific intervention, the usual standard of care, or no intervention at all.

**TABLE 1-10 Steps of Evidence-Based Practice (EBP) Process**

| |
|---|
| 1. Ask the clinical question using the **PICOT** format:<br>**P**atients/population<br>**I**ntervention<br>**C**omparison or comparison group<br>**O**utcome(s)<br>**T**ime (as applicable) |
| 2. Search for the best evidence based on the clinical question. |
| 3. Critically appraise and synthesize the evidence. |
| 4. Implement the evidence in practice. |
| 5. Evaluate the practice decision or change. |
| 6. Share the outcomes of the decision or change. |

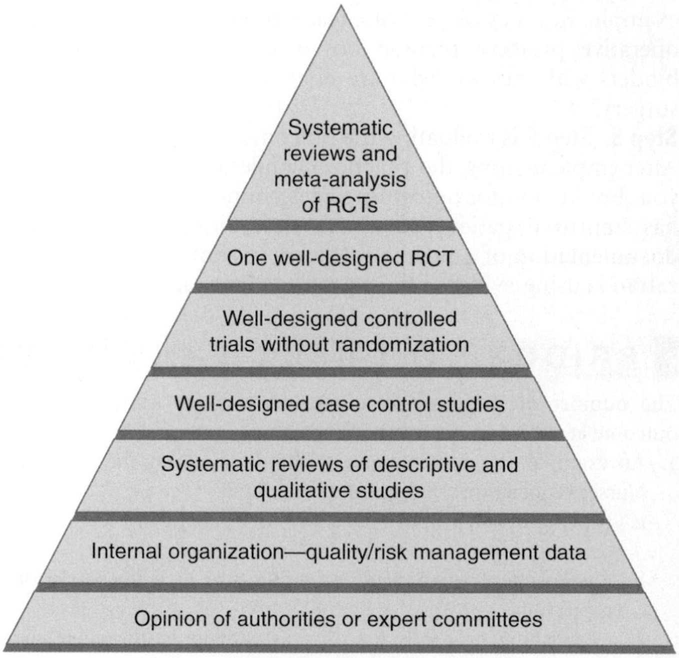


**FIG. 1-7** Hierarchy of evidence. (Modified from Guyatt G, Rennie D: *User's guide to the medical literature*, Chicago, 2002, American Medical Association; Harris RP, et al: Current methods of the U.S. Prevention Services Task Force: a review of the process. *Am J Prevent Med* 20:21, 2001; Melnyk BM, Fineout-Overholt E: *Evidence-based practice in nursing and healthcare: a guide to best practice*, ed 3, Philadelphia, 2014, Lippincott Williams & Wilkins.)

**Step 2.** Step 2 is searching for the best evidence that applies to the clinical question. Technology provides you with ready access to data. You can easily search a number of online resources and collect large amounts of clinical information and evidence. It is important to evaluate all data sources for their credibility and reliability. Not all evidence is equal. Figure 1-7 presents the hierarchy of evidence. As you go down the pyramid, the strength of the evidence becomes weaker. Systematic reviews and evidence-based clinical practice guidelines save time and effort in the EBP process. However, they are available for only a limited number of clinical topics and may not suit all types of clinical questions. When insufficient research exists to guide practice, recommendations from expert panels and authority figures may be the best evidence available.

**Step 3.** Step 3 is critically appraising and synthesizing evidence found in the search. A successful critical appraisal process focuses on three essential questions: (1) What are the results? (2) Are the results reliable and valid? and (3) Will the results help me in caring for my patients? You must determine the strength of the evidence and synthesize the findings related to the clinical question to conclude what is the best practice. For example, you find strong evidence supporting effectiveness of elasticized binders and pillows in reducing pain associated with ambulation. However, the binder appears to be more effective if the patient is obese or has had prior abdominal surgery.

**Step 4.** Step 4 involves implementing the evidence in practice. The decision to implement change is made by combining the evidence, clinical judgment, and the preferences and values of patients and caregivers. You may be part of an interprofessional team charged with implementing a practice change or applying evidence in a specific patient care situation. This may include developing clinical practice guidelines; policies and procedures; or new assessment, teaching, or documentation tools. For example, you may be part of a team implementing a new postoperative protocol focused on using elasticized abdominal binders with patients who are obese or had prior abdominal surgery.

**Step 5.** Step 5 is evaluating the outcome in the clinical setting. After implementing the practice change for a specific period, you should monitor outcomes to determine whether the change has improved patient outcomes. Accrediting bodies require documentation of outcome measures to show that the organization is using evidence to improve patient care.[25]

**Step 6.** Step 6 is sharing the results of the EBP change. If you do not share the outcomes of EBP, then other health care providers and patients cannot benefit from what you learned from your experience. Information is shared locally using unit- or hospital-based newsletters and posters and regionally and nationally through journal publications and presentations at conferences.

### Implementing EBP

To implement EBP, you must develop the skills to be able to seek and incorporate into practice scientific evidence that supports best patient outcomes. Throughout this book, two different types of EBP boxes are used to show how EBP is used in nursing practice. The Translating Research into Practice boxes provide initial answers to specific clinical questions. These boxes contain the clinical question, critical appraisal of the supportive evidence, implications for nursing practice, and the source of the evidence. Applying the Evidence boxes provide an opportunity for you to practice your critical thinking skills in applying EBP to patient scenarios. To assist you in identifying the use of evidence incorporated throughout this book, an asterisk (*) is used in the reference list at the end of each chapter to indicate evidence-based information for clinical practice.

## BRIDGE TO NCLEX EXAMINATION

The number of the question corresponds to the same-numbered outcome at the beginning of the chapter.

1. An example of a nursing activity that best reflects the American Nurses Association's definition of nursing is
   a. treating dysrhythmias that occur in a patient in the coronary care unit.
   b. diagnosing a patient with a feeding tube as being at risk for aspiration.
   c. establishing protocols for treating patients in the emergency department.
   d. providing antianxiety drugs for a patient who has disturbed sleep patterns.
2. A nurse working on the medical-surgical unit at an urban hospital would like to become certified in medical-surgical nursing. The nurse knows that this process would most likely require
   a. a bachelor's degree in nursing.
   b. formal education in advanced nursing practice.
   c. experience for a specific period in medical-surgical nursing.
   d. membership in a medical-surgical nursing specialty organization.
3. A nurse is providing care to a patient after right hip surgery. Within a pay-for-performance system, a critical role of the nurse is to
   a. ensure that care is provided using a minimal amount of supplies.
   b. discharge the patient at completion of the number of approved days of care.
   c. implement measures to decrease the risk of the patient acquiring an infection.
   d. assess the patient's ability to pay for health care services at the time of admission.
4. The nurse is assigned to care for a newly admitted patient. Number in order the steps for using the nursing process to prioritize care. (Number 1 is the first step, and number 5 is the last step.)
   ___ Evaluate whether the plan was effective.
   ___ Identify any health problems.
   ___ Collect patient information.
   ___ Carry out the plan.
   ___ Determine a plan of action.
5. The linkages among NANDA-I nursing diagnoses, NOC patient outcomes, and NIC nursing interventions can be used to
   a. evaluate patient outcomes.
   b. provide guides for planning care.
   c. predict the results of nursing care.
   d. shorten written care plans for individual patients.
6. The nurse is caring for a diabetic patient in the ambulatory surgical unit who has undergone debridement of an infected toe. Which task is appropriate for the nurse to delegate to unlicensed assistive personnel (UAP)?
   a. Check the patient's vital signs.
   b. Monitor the patient's pain level.
   c. Assess the patient's IV catheter site.
   d. Evaluate the patient's tibial and pedal pulses.
7. The nurse's role in addressing the National Patient Safety Goals established by The Joint Commission includes *(select all that apply)*
   a. answering monitoring alarms in a timely manner.
   b. using side rails and alarm systems as necessary to prevent patient falls.
   c. obtaining a complete, accurate list of the patient's medications on admission.
   d. memorizing and implementing all the rules published by The Joint Commission.
   e. encouraging patients to be actively involved in and question their own health care.

8. Advantages of using informatics in health care delivery are *(select all that apply)*
   **a.** reduced need for nurses in acute care.
   **b.** increased patient anonymity and confidentiality.
   **c.** the ability to achieve and maintain high standards of care.
   **d.** access to standard plans of care for many health problems.
   **e.** improved communication of the patient's health status to the health care team.
9. When using evidence-based practice, the nurse
   **a.** must use clinical practice guidelines developed by national health agencies.
   **b.** should use findings from randomized controlled trials to plan care for all patient problems.
   **c.** uses clinical decision making and judgment to determine what evidence is appropriate for a specific clinical situation.
   **d.** statistically analyzes the relationship of nursing interventions to patient outcomes to establish evidence for the most appropriate patient interventions.

1. b, 2. c, 3. c, 4. 5, 2, 1, 4, 3, 5. b, 6. a, 7. a, b, c, 8. c, d, e, 9. c.

For rationales to these answers and even more NCLEX review questions, visit *evolve.elsevier.com/Lewis/medsurg*

## EVOLVE WEBSITE

http://evolve.elsevier.com/Lewis/medsurg
**Review Questions (Online Only)**
**Key Points**
**Answer Key for Questions**
- Rationales for Bridge to NCLEX Examination Questions

**Conceptual Care Map Creator**
**Audio Glossary**
**Content Updates**

## REFERENCES

1. American Nurses Association: *Nursing: a social policy statement,* ed 3, Washington DC, 2010, The Association. (Classic)
2. Nightingale F: *Notes on nursing: what it is and what it is not* (facsimile edition), Philadelphia, 1946, Lippincott. (Classic)
3. Henderson V: *The nature of nursing,* New York, 1966, Macmillan. (Classic)
4. Roy S, Andrews H: *The Roy adaptation model,* ed 2, Stamford, Conn, 1999, Appleton & Lange. (Classic)
5. American Association of Colleges of Nursing: Essentials of baccalaureate education for professional nursing practice. Retrieved from *www.aacn.nche.edu.*
6. American Nurses Credentialing Center: Certification. Retrieved from *www.nursecredentialing.org/certification.aspx.*
7. Robert Wood Johnson Foundation: Achieving the potential of health care performance measures. Retrieved from *www.rwjf.org.*
8. US Department of Health and Human Services: *Healthy People 2020.* Retrieved from *www.healthypeople.gov.*
9. ANCC Magnet Recognition Program. Retrieved from *www.nursecredentialing.org/magnet.aspx.*
10. Committee on the Robert Wood Johnson Foundation Initiative on the Future of Nursing at the Institute of Medicine: *The future of nursing: leading change, advancing health,* Washington, DC, 2011, National Academies Press.
11. QSEN Institute. Retrieved from *http://qsen.org.*
12. NANDA International: Defining the knowledge of nursing. Retrieved from *www.nanda.org.*
13. Overview: Nursing Outcomes Classification (NOC). Retrieved from *www.nursing.uiowa.edu/cncce/nursing-outcomes-classification-overview.*
14. Overview: Nursing Interventions Classification (NIC). Retrieved from *www.nursing.uiowa.edu/cncce/nursing-interventions-classification-overview.*
15. Carpenito LJ: *Nursing care plans: transitional patient and family-centered care,* ed 6, Philadelphia, 2014, Lippincott Williams & Wilkins.
16. Transitions of care portal. Retrieved from *www.jointcommission.org/toc.aspx.*
17. Cherry B, Jacob SR: *Contemporary nursing practice,* ed 6, St Louis, 2013, Elsevier.
18. What is a case manager? Retrieved from *www.cmsa.org.*
19. Alfaro-LeFevre R: *Critical thinking, clinical reasoning, and clinical judgment,* ed 5, St Louis, 2013, Saunders.
20. Delegation. Retrieved from *www.ncsbn.org/1625.htm.*
21. James J: A new, evidence-based estimate of patient harms associated with hospital care, *Journal of Patient Safety* 9:122, 2013.
22. Safe practices for better healthcare. Retrieved from *www.qualityforum.org/Projects/Safe_Practices_2010.aspx.*
23. National Patient Safety Goals. Retrieved from *www.jointcommission.org/standards_information/npsgs.aspx.*
24. Benefits of EHRs. Retrieved from *www.healthit.gov/providers-professionals.*
25. Echevarria IM, Walker S: To make your case, start with a PICOT question, *Nursing* 44:18, 2014.

2

# Health Disparities and Culturally Competent Care

*Janet Lenart*

*No culture can live if it attempts to be exclusive.*

*Mahatma Gandhi*

http://evolve.elsevier.com/Lewis/medsurg/

## LEARNING OUTCOMES

1. Identify the key determinants of health and equity.
2. Describe the factors that contribute to health disparities and health equity.
3. Define the terms *culture, values, acculturation, ethnicity, race, stereotyping, ethnocentrism, cultural imposition, cultural competency,* and *culture-bound syndrome.*
4. Explain how culture and ethnicity may affect a person's physical and psychologic health.
5. Describe strategies for successfully communicating with a person who speaks a language that you do not understand.
6. Apply strategies for incorporating cultural information in the nursing process with all patients.
7. Describe the role of nursing in reducing health disparities.
8. Examine ways that your own cultural background may influence nursing care.

## KEY TERMS

acculturation, p. 22
cultural competence, p. 23
culture, p. 21
culture-bound syndromes, p. 29
determinants of health, p. 18
ethnicity, p. 19
ethnocentrism, p. 23
folk healers, p. 24
health disparities, p. 19
health equity, p. 19
health status, p. 18
lesbian, gay, bisexual, and transgender (LGBT), p. 21
place, p. 20
race, p. 19
sexuality, p. 21
stereotyping, p. 23
transcultural nursing, p. 23
values, p. 21

This chapter discusses health disparities and culture. Nurses play a key role in recognizing and reducing health disparities and providing culturally competent care.

## DETERMINANTS OF HEALTH

Why are there differences in the health status of people in America? How do these differences occur? The **determinants of health** are factors that (1) influence the health of individuals and groups and (2) help explain why some people experience poorer health than others.[1] Where people are born, grow up, live, work, and age helps determine their health status, behaviors, and care.

**Health status** describes the health of a person or a community.[2] Many measures make up the concept of health status. For individuals, this means the sum of their current health problems plus their coping resources (e.g., family, financial resources). For a community, health status is the combination of health measures for all individuals living in the community. Community health measures include birth and death rates, life expectancy, access to care, and morbidity and mortality rates related to disease and injury.

Factors in a person's social and physical environment, including personal relationships, workplace, housing, transportation, and neighborhood violence, contribute to health status.[1] For example, the risk of youth homicide is much higher in neighborhoods with gang activity and high crime rates. The physical environment in which one lives, works, and plays may expose a person to such risks as environmental hazards (workplace injuries), toxic agents (chemical spills, industrial pollution), unsafe traffic patterns (lack of sidewalks), or absence of fresh and healthy food choices.

An individual's behavior is influenced by his or her environment, education, and economic status. Behaviors such as tobacco and illicit drug use are strongly linked to a number of health conditions (e.g., lung cancer, liver disease). An individual's biologic makeup, such as genetics and family history of disease (e.g., heart disease), can increase the risk for specific diseases.

Reviewed by Christine Espina, RN, DNP, Nurse Planner and Continuing Education Specialist, University of Washington Continuing Nursing Education, Seattle, Washington; Shari Gould, RN, MSN, Associate Professor of Nursing, Victoria College, Victoria, Texas; and Ellen Odell, DNP, ACNS-BC, CNE, APRN, Director of Nursing, Associate Professor, Department of Nursing, John Brown University, Siloam Springs, Arkansas.

The availability of health care also contributes to an individual's health. The Affordable Care Act (ACA) reduced the number of uninsured Americans by 5.4 million in the first year of implementation. However, millions remain uninsured and have limited access to care, which will affect both individual and community health.[3]

## HEALTH DISPARITIES AND HEALTH EQUITY

**Health disparities** are differences in the incidence, prevalence, mortality rate, and burden of diseases that exist among specific population groups in the United States because of social, economic, or environmental disadvantages. Health disparities can affect population groups based on gender, age, ethnicity, socioeconomic status, education, geography, sexual orientation, disability, or special health care needs.[4] **Health equity** is achieved when every person has the opportunity to attain his or her health potential, and no one is disadvantaged.

### Factors and Conditions Leading to Health Disparities

Many factors and conditions can lead to the development of health disparities (Table 2-1). Awareness of these factors will assist you in providing optimal care for your patients.

#### ETHICAL/LEGAL DILEMMAS

***Health Disparities***

**Situation**

E.M., a 47-year-old Mexican American woman with type 2 diabetes mellitus, comes to the clinic to have her blood glucose measured. It has been 12 months since her last visit. At that time the nurse requested that she bring along her glucometer and strips to demonstrate how she checks her blood glucose because her glucose values were high at her previous visits.

When you check E.M.'s equipment and glucose strips, it is clear that the strips are for a different machine and they expired more than 2 years ago. When you inquire about the situation, E.M. explains that she cannot afford to come to the clinic or to buy new equipment and supplies to check her blood glucose level. During the day E.M. cares for her three grandchildren so her daughter can work. E.M. spends most of her income on food for her family, so little money is left over for her own health care.

**Ethical/Legal Points for Consideration**

- Ethnic minorities and other vulnerable or disadvantaged groups experience certain chronic illnesses at higher rates. Limited access to high-quality, accessible, and affordable health care services is clearly associated with an increased incidence of illness and complications, as well as a reduced life span.
- People with certain health problems such as diabetes may have difficulty obtaining health care insurance. These issues must be considered in the broader context of social justice.
- In many states the legal definition of the role of the professional nurse includes patient advocacy. Advocacy includes the obligation to provide adequate follow-up care for all patients, especially those who are experiencing health care disparities.
- When disparities are observed in an individual patient and family, as a nurse you must consider the possibilities of discrimination and abuse. Professional nurses are legally and ethically responsible for patient advocacy. When failure to fulfill this obligation results in harm to the patient, the nurse may incur legal liability.

**Discussion Questions**

1. How would you work with E.M. to help her obtain the necessary resources and knowledge to care for her diabetes?
2. What can you do to begin working on the problems of health disparities in your community?

**TABLE 2-1 Factors and Conditions Leading to Health Disparities**

| | |
|---|---|
| • Ethnicity and race | • Age |
| • Place | • Sexual orientation |
| • Income status | • Disability status |
| • Education | • Health care provider attitudes |
| • Occupation or unemployment | • Lack of health care services access |
| • Health literacy | • Language barrier |
| • Gender | |

**Ethnicity and Race.** The terms **ethnicity** and **race** are subjective and based on self-report. These terms are used interchangeably in conversation and cannot be defined by genetic markers. Social context and lived experiences influence people's decision about the ethnic and race category to which they identify or are assigned. For example, ethnic and race categories may differ on a person's birth certificate and death certificate.

People are asked to identify their own ethnicity and race for the purpose of health data collection (e.g., for birth and death certificates). Collection of health data based on self-reported ethnic and race categories is important for research, to inform policy, and to understand and eliminate disparities. For example, federal agencies are required to list a minimum of two ethnicities for people who self-identify as either *Hispanic or Latino* and *Not Hispanic or Latino.* A Hispanic or Latino is typically a person of Cuban, Mexican, Puerto Rican, South or Central American, or other Spanish descent, regardless of race.

In addition, federal agencies are required to list a minimum of five race categories: white, black or African American, American Indian or Alaska Native, Asian, and Native Hawaiian or other Pacific Islander. People are asked to identify their race using one or more categories. In this book the terms *ethnicity* and *race* are used interchangeably or together.

Despite dramatic improvements in treatments to prolong life and improve quality of life for most individuals, racial and ethnic minorities have benefited far less from these advances. Disparities are generally determined by comparing population groups. In the United States minority groups include Hispanics/Latinos 16.3%, African Americans 12.6%, Asian Americans 4.8%, Native Hawaiians and other Pacific Islanders 0.2%, Native Americans and Native Alaskans 0.9%, and two or more races 2.9% of the U.S. population.[5] The percentages for most of these groups are expected to increase in the coming decades.

Obesity and chronic illness rates for diabetes, hypertension, chronic obstructive pulmonary diseases, cancer, and stroke are higher among minority people. Racial, ethnic, and cultural differences exist in health services, treatments provided, and access to health care providers (HCPs). For example, African American men are less likely to be offered intervention procedures for cardiovascular disease and stroke. African American and Hispanic women are less likely to have mammography for breast cancer screening. Differences in access to screening and treatment exist even when minority groups are insured at the same level as whites. When patient groups are given the same care, the treatment outcomes are similar across racial and ethnic groups.[6]

Disease risk and outcomes are also influenced by race and ethnicity. For example, compared with U.S. white and African American populations, Native Americans have a higher incidence of stroke and are more likely to die as a consequence.[7] Cervical cancer mortality rates are higher in Hispanic and

## CULTURAL & ETHNIC HEALTH DISPARITIES

### *Cultural & Ethnic Health Disparities Boxes Throughout Book*

| Title | Chapter | Page |
|---|---|---|
| Alzheimer's Disease and Dementia | 59 | 1402 |
| Arthritis and Connective Tissue Disorders | 64 | 1525 |
| Brain Tumors | 56 | 1333 |
| Breast Cancer | 51 | 1218 |
| Cancer | 15 | 267 |
| Cancers of the Female Reproductive System | 53 | 1256 |
| Cancers of the Male Reproductive System | 54 | 1276 |
| Chronic Kidney Disease | 46 | 1076 |
| Colorectal Cancer | 42 | 954 |
| Coronary Artery Disease | 33 | 704 |
| Diabetes Mellitus | 48 | 1137 |
| Heart Failure | 34 | 738 |
| Hematologic Problems | 30 | 607 |
| Hypertension | 32 | 682 |
| Integumentary Problems | 23 | 410 |
| Liver, Pancreas, and Gallbladder Disorders | 43 | 986 |
| Lung Cancer | 27 | 514 |
| Obesity | 40 | 878 |
| Obstructive Pulmonary Diseases | 28 | 539 |
| Oral, Pharyngeal, and Esophageal Problems | 41 | 898 |
| Osteoporosis | 63 | 1511 |
| Sexually Transmitted Infections | 52 | 1228 |
| Stroke | 57 | 1347 |
| Tuberculosis | 27 | 506 |
| Urologic Disorders | 45 | 1034 |
| Visual and Auditory Problems | 21 | 368 |

African American women than in other American women. Numerous strategies are being developed to promote health equity and reduce disparities.

**Place.** Place refers to the geographic and environmental location where a person is born, grows, lives, works, and ages. Place affects the use of health services, health status, and health behaviors.

Approximately 25% of Americans live in nonurban or rural areas.[5] Three percent of Americans live in designated frontier counties. Differences in access to health care services among frontier, rural, and urban settings can create geographic health disparities. For example, rural populations and Native Americans living on reservations may need to travel long distances to receive health care. This can result in inadequate or less-frequent access to health care services. Some parts of the rural United States are considered "medically underserved" because of decreased numbers of health care providers per population.

People living in rural areas have higher rates of cancer, heart disease, diabetes, depression, and injury-related deaths than people living in urban areas. For example, in rural Appalachia the rates of lung, colon, cervical, and colorectal cancer are higher than the national average. Rural populations tend to be older than urban populations. Many rural areas have higher rates of obesity and chronic disease. The impact of social and physical environment on health choices can be illustrated by the problem of intimate partner violence in rural communities.[8] The decision to seek help is affected by geographic isolation, traditional gender roles, patriarchal attitudes, fear of lack of confidentiality, and economic factors that exist in some small rural communities.

Living in urban centers may also predispose a person to health disparities. Concerns about personal safety (e.g., clinics located in high-crime neighborhoods) can make patients reluctant to visit HCPs. At the same time, providers, such as home health nurses, working in high-risk areas may experience distress when they witness crime, drug use, or other illegal activities.

Among the most obvious health behaviors affected by place are physical activity and nutrition. Safe, walkable neighborhoods with playgrounds and sources of healthy foods promote physical activity and healthy eating. Social support and networks are related to health and coping with illness. Social networks are more likely to be found in communities where neighbors interact and rely on one another.

**Income, Education, and Occupation.** People of lower income, education, or occupational status experience worse health. In addition, they die at a younger age than those who are more affluent. Adults without a high school diploma or equivalent are three times more likely to die before age 65 than those with a college degree. Health care costs are one of the important factors that contribute to health disparities. Individuals who have no insurance, are underinsured, or lack financial resources to pay for treatment of diseases may forgo health care visits, screenings, and treatments. Patients who lack the knowledge and/or access to apply for government assistance programs (e.g., Medicaid) are also at risk. Hazardous work environments and high-risk occupations of laborers also increase health risk and contribute to higher rates of illness, injury, and death.

**Health Literacy.** *Health literacy* is defined as the degree to which individuals have the capacity to obtain, process, and understand basic health information and services needed to make appropriate health decisions. This includes the ability to (1) read, comprehend, and analyze information; (2) understand instructions; (3) weigh risks and benefits; and (4) ultimately make decisions and take action. The most recent national literacy survey reported that more than 40% and two thirds of people over age 60 have basic to below basic literacy skills, and another 5% are nonliterate in English.[9] Low health literacy is associated with more hospitalizations, greater use of emergency department care, decreased use of cancer screening and influenza vaccine, decreased ability to use medications correctly, and higher mortality rates among older adults.

On a daily basis, patients need to self-manage conditions such as diabetes and asthma. For example, patients with diabetes may not be able to maintain adequate blood glucose levels if they cannot read or understand the numbers on the home glucose monitoring system. The inability to read and understand medication labels can result in taking medications at the wrong time or in the wrong dose. Health literacy is discussed further in Chapter 4.

**Gender.** Health disparities exist between men and women. Adult women use health care services more than men. Women may not receive the same quality of care (Fig. 2-1). For example, women are less likely than men to receive procedures (e.g., coronary angiography) for cardiovascular disease.[10] When gender is combined with racial and ethnic differences, the disparities are even greater. (Gender Differences boxes are presented throughout this book, which highlight gender differences in disease risk, manifestations, and treatment.)

**Age.** Older adults are at risk for experiencing health disparities in the number of diagnostic tests performed and aggressiveness of treatments used. Biases toward older adults that affect their care, or ageism, are discussed in Chapter 5. Older women are less likely to be offered mammograms. Older people of low

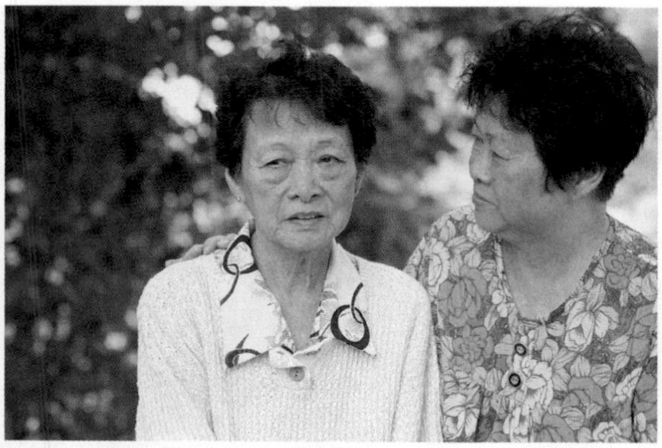

FIG. 2-1 Older Asian women are especially at risk for health disparities. (©szefei/iStock/Thinkstock)

socioeconomic status experience greater disability, more limitations in activities of daily living, and more frequent and rapid cognitive decline. Older adults who belong to minority groups are less likely than their white counterparts to receive screening for prostate and colorectal cancer.

**Sexual Orientation.** Sexuality is defined as a person's romantic, emotional, or sexual attraction to another person.

***Lesbian, Gay, Bisexual, and Transgender (LGBT).*** Lesbian, gay, bisexual, and transgender (LGBT) is a term that refers to the sexual orientation of these groups of people. LGBT individuals encompass all races and ethnicities, religions, and social classes. Being LGBT places an individual at risk for health disparities resulting from social, economic, or environmental disadvantages. Personal, family, and social acceptance of sexual orientation and gender identity affects the mental health and personal safety of LGBT individuals. Discrimination against LGBT people has been associated with high rates of psychiatric disorders, substance abuse, and suicide.[2]

Lesbian women are more likely to be obese when compared with their heterosexual counterparts. Lesbian and bisexual women have increased risk factors for cardiovascular disease.[11] Gay men have higher rates of human immunodeficiency virus and hepatitis infections than other groups. Gay men and lesbian women have higher smoking rates than heterosexuals.

Older LGBT individuals may face additional barriers to health because of isolation and a lack of social services and culturally competent providers.[2]

Understanding the cause of these disparities among LGBT individuals is essential to providing safe and high-quality care. One of the barriers to accessing high-quality health care by LGBT adults is the current lack of HCPs who are knowledgeable about their health needs. LGBT people may also experience fear of discrimination in health care settings.

Some health care settings are addressing the negative stereotypes that health care professionals may have, but of which they may not be aware. The Joint Commission (TJC) requires that patients be allowed the presence of a support individual of their choice. In addition, hospitals must adopt policies that bar discrimination based on factors such as sexual orientation and gender identification and expression.

**Health Care Provider Attitudes.** Certain behaviors and biases of the HCP can contribute to health disparities. Factors such as bias and prejudice can affect health care–seeking behavior in minority populations.[12] The health care system may also contribute to the problem of health disparities. For example, a clinic located in an area with a large population of Vietnamese

## HEALTHY PEOPLE

**Lesbian, Gay, Bisexual, and Transgender (LGBT) Individuals**

A *Healthy People 2020* goal is to improve the health, safety, and well-being of LGBT individuals.

- Efforts to improve LGBT health include the following:
  - Decreasing human immunodeficiency virus (HIV)/sexually transmitted infections (STI) with effective interventions
  - Implementing antibullying policies in schools
  - Creating advisory groups consisting of community representatives
  - Providing supportive social services to reduce suicide and homelessness risk among young people
  - Appropriately inquiring about and being supportive of a patient's sexual orientation to enhance the patient-provider interaction and patient's regular use of care
  - Providing health care professional students with access to LGBT patients to increase their knowledge of the health care needs of LGBT patients and ability to provide care to them
- Efforts to address health disparities among LGBT people include the following:
  - Expansion of domestic partner health insurance coverage
  - Establishment of LGBT health centers
  - Dissemination of effective HIV/STI interventions
  - Guarantee of appropriate health care screening

immigrants that does not provide interpreters or educational materials and financial forms in Vietnamese may limit these families' ability to understand how to access health care.

*Discrimination* and *bias* based on a patient's race, ethnicity, gender, age, body size, sexual orientation, or ability to pay are likely to result in less aggressive or negative treatment practices. Discrimination can result in the delay of a proper diagnosis due to assumptions made about the patient. Sometimes discrimination is difficult to identify, especially when it occurs at the institutional level.

Because an HCP's overt discriminatory behavior may not be immediately evident to the patient or yourself, it may be difficult to confront. Even well-intentioned providers who try to eliminate bias in their care can demonstrate their prior beliefs or prejudices through nonverbal communication. Many policies are in place to eliminate discrimination, but it still exists.[12]

## CULTURE

Culture is a way of life for a group of people. It includes the behaviors, beliefs, values, traditions, and symbols that the group accepts, generally without thinking about them. This way of life is passed along by communication and imitation from one generation to the next. You can also think of culture as cultivated behavior that is acquired through social learning. It is the totality of a person's learned, accumulated experience that is socially transmitted. The four classic characteristics of culture are described in Table 2-2.

Values are the sets of rules by which individuals, families, groups, and communities live. They are the principles and standards that serve as the basis for beliefs, attitudes, and behaviors. Although all cultures have values, the types and expressions of those values differ from one culture to another. These cultural values develop over time, guide decision making and actions, and may affect a person's self-esteem. Cultural values are often unconsciously developed early in life as a child learns about acceptable and unacceptable behaviors. The extent to which a person's cultural values are internalized influences that person's

**TABLE 2-2 Basic Characteristics of Culture**

- *Dynamic* and ever-changing
- *Not always shared* by all members of a cultural group
- *Adapted* to specific conditions such as environmental factors
- *Learned* through oral and written histories, as well as socialization

**TABLE 2-3 Cultural Characteristics of Different Ethnic Groups**

**Native American**
- Doing the honorable thing
- Folk healing
- Living in harmony with people and nature
- Respect for tribal elders and children
- Respect for all things living
- Returning what is taken from nature
- Spiritual guidance

**Hispanic/Latino**
- Cultural foods
- Folk healing
- Extended family valued
- Interdependence and collectivism
- Involvement of family in social activities
- Religion and spirituality highly valued
- Respect for elders and authority

**African American**
- Cultural foods
- Family networks
- Folk healing
- Importance of religion
- Interdependence within ethnic group
- Music and physical activities valued

**European American**
- Equal rights of genders
- Independence and freedom
- Individualistic and competitive
- Materialistic
- Self-reliance valued
- Youth and beauty valued

**Asian American**
- Cultural foods
- Family loyalty
- Folk healing
- Harmonious relationships
- Harmony and balance within body vital for preservation of life energy
- Respect for elders
- Respect for one's parents and ancestors

**Pacific Islander American**
- Collective concern and involvement
- Kinship alliance among nuclear and extended family
- Knowledge is collective; belongs to group, not individual
- Natural order and balanced relationships

Adapted from Andrews MM, Boyle JS: *Transcultural concepts in nursing care*, ed 6, Philadelphia, 2012, Lippincott Williams & Wilkins; and Giger JN, Davidhizar RE: *Transcultural nursing: assessment and intervention*, ed 6, St Louis, 2012, Mosby.

tendency toward judging other cultures, while usually using his or her own culture as the accepted standard. Table 2-3 provides some examples of cultural characteristics of different ethnic groups in the United States.[13]

Although individuals within a cultural group may have many similarities through their shared values, beliefs, and practices, there is also diversity within groups (Fig. 2-2). Each person is culturally unique. Such diversity may result from different perspectives and interpretations of situations. These differences may be based on age, gender, marital status, family structure, income, education level, religious views, and life experiences. Within any cultural group, there are smaller groups that may not hold all of the values of the dominant culture. These smaller cultural groups have experiences that differ from those of the dominant group. These differences may be related to ethnic background, residence, religion, occupation, health, age, gender, education, or other factors that unite the group. Members of a subculture share certain aspects of culture that are different from those of the overall cultural group. For example, among

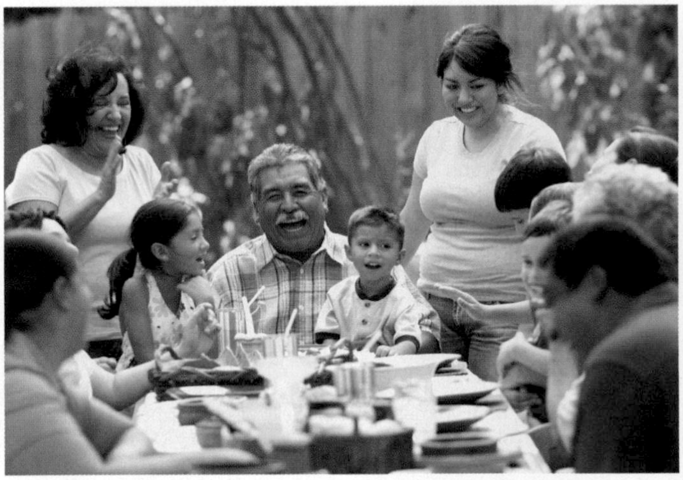

**FIG. 2-2** Members of this family share a common heritage. (©Jack Hollingsworth/Photodisc/Thinkstock)

Hispanics some seek professional health care immediately when symptoms appear, whereas other Hispanics rely first on folk healers. Other Hispanics first seek the opinion of family and friends before seeking formal health care.

*Cultural beliefs* about symptom tolerance and health care–seeking behavior can contribute to health disparities. Some cultures consider pain something to be endured or ignored, and as a result, the patient does not seek help. Some cultures may view diseases or problems fatalistically; that is, people see no reason to seek treatment because they believe it is unlikely to have any benefit. Some cultures view the signs and symptoms of an illness as "God's will" or as a punishment for some prior behavior.

Fatalism is higher in individuals with lower socioeconomic status. Fatalistic beliefs are associated with reduced cancer prevention activities such as exercising, not smoking, and following a healthy diet.[14] In some cultures it may not be acceptable to see an HCP who is not of the same gender or ethnic group. Such beliefs can result in delays in seeking health care or inadequate treatment.

**Acculturation** is the lifelong process of incorporating cultural aspects of the contexts in which a person grows, lives, works, and ages.[15] Acculturation is often bidirectional. In other words, the context also changes as it is influenced by a person's culture. Change may be in attitudes, behaviors, and values. For example, a sedentary person who loves to cook may change his or her attitude toward exercise when living with athletic roommates, who in turn also change as they begin to appreciate cooking. Behaviors change when an immigrant child learns the local language while also influencing the conduct of classmates. Last, a deeply held value such as self-sufficiency may change for a person exposed to a culture in which reliance on others dominates.

Newcomers may adopt both the strengths and limitations of the dominant culture. This is relevant when considering health behaviors of individuals and the quality of health care delivered by professionals. For example, an immigrant may be negatively influenced by a dominant cultural context in which unhealthy eating habits prevail.[16] As a new nurse, you may be negatively or positively influenced by the culture of care that is most prevalent in your workplace.

The result of acculturation for the individual may be new cultural variations in attitudes, behaviors, and values. All people participate in this process over their lives. People who move to a new cultural context are more aware of the acculturation experience than people who are not exposed to new experiences. Exposure to new cultural contexts increases the cultural competency of nurses.

**Stereotyping** refers to an overgeneralized viewpoint that members of a specific culture, race, or ethnic group are alike and share the same values and beliefs. This oversimplified approach does not take into account the individual differences that exist within a culture. Being a member of a particular cultural, ethnic, or racial group does not make the person an expert on other members of that same group. Such stereotyping can lead to false assumptions and affect a patient's care. For example, it would be inappropriate for you to assume that just because a nurse is Mexican American, he would know how a Mexican American patient's beliefs may affect that patient's health care practices. As another example, a young Mexican American nurse born and raised in a large city has experienced a different culture than the older patient who was born and raised in a rural area of Mexico.

**Ethnocentrism** refers to the belief that one's own culture and worldview are superior to those of others from different cultural, ethnic, or racial backgrounds. Comparing others' ways to your own can lead to seeing others as different or inferior. HCPs' ethnocentrism can result in poor communication, patient alienation, and potentially inadequate treatment. To avoid ethnocentrism, you need to remain open to a variety of perspectives and maintain a nonjudgmental view of the values, beliefs, and practices of others. Failure to do this can result in ethnic stereotyping or cultural imposition.

*Cultural imposition* occurs when one's own cultural beliefs and practices are imposed on another person or group of people. In health care it can result in disregarding or trivializing a patient's health care beliefs or practices. Cultural imposition may happen when an HCP is unaware of the patient's cultural beliefs and plans and implements care without taking them into account.[17]

*Cultural safety* describes care and advocacy for a person of another culture determined by that person or family. Care that is culturally safe prevents cultural imposition. Culturally safe practice requires cultural competency and action to ensure that cultural histories, experiences, and traditions of patients, their families, and communities are valued and shape health care approaches and policies.[18]

The term **transcultural nursing** was coined by Madeleine Leininger in the 1950s. Transcultural nursing is a specialty that focuses on the comparative study and analysis of cultures and subcultures. The goal of transcultural nursing is the discovery of culturally relevant facts that can guide the nurse in providing culturally appropriate care.[19]

## CULTURAL COMPETENCE

**Cultural competence** is the ability to understand, appreciate, and work with individuals from cultures other than your own. It involves an awareness and acceptance of cultural differences, self-awareness, knowledge of the patient's culture, and adaptation of skills to meet the patient's needs. The four components of cultural competence are (1) cultural awareness, (2) cultural knowledge, (3) cultural skill, and (4) cultural encounter[20] (Table 2-4).

Specific information is presented throughout this book to assist you in developing an awareness of cultural differences and learning assessment skills for different cultural groups. Table 2-7 (later in this chapter) presents a cultural assessment guide. It may be helpful to review general cultural characteristics associated with a cultural group when preparing to interview a patient. However, recognize that the patient may not identify with the assumed cultural group, and the provider's own biases and stereotypes may impact the patient and result in more patient-provider barriers.

Providing culturally competent care may increase patient satisfaction, reduce health disparities, increase patient safety,

**TABLE 2-4 How to Develop Cultural Competence**

| Description | Role of Nurse |
|---|---|
| **Cultural Awareness** | |
| • Ability to understand patients' unique cultural needs | • Identify your own cultural background, values, and beliefs, especially as related to health and health care.<br>• Examine your own cultural biases toward people whose cultures differ from your own culture. |
| **Cultural Knowledge** | |
| • Process of learning key aspects of a group's culture, especially as it relates to health and health care practices<br>• Patients are best source of information about their culture | • Learn basic general information about predominant cultural groups in your geographic area. Cultural pocket guides can be a good resource.<br>• Assess patients for presence or absence of cultural traits based on an understanding of generalizations about a cultural group.<br>• Do not make assumptions based on cultural background because the degree of acculturation varies among individuals.<br>• Read research studies that describe cultural differences.<br>• Read ethnic newspaper articles and books.<br>• View documentaries about cultural groups. |
| **Cultural Skill** | |
| • Ability to collect relevant cultural data<br>• Performance of a cultural assessment | • Be alert for unexpected responses with patients, especially as related to cultural issues.<br>• Become aware of cultural differences in predominant ethnic groups.<br>• Develop assessment skills to do a competent cultural assessment for any patient.*<br>• Learn assessment skills for different cultural groups, including cultural beliefs and practices. |
| **Cultural Encounter** | |
| • Direct cross-cultural interactions between people from culturally diverse backgrounds<br>• Extended contact with a cultural group to enhance understanding of its values and beliefs | • Create opportunities to interact with predominant cultural groups.<br>• Attend cultural events, such as religious ceremonies, significant life passage rituals, social events, and demonstrations of cultural practices.<br>• Visit markets and restaurants in ethnic neighborhoods.<br>• Explore ethnic neighborhoods, listen to different types of ethnic music, and learn games of various ethnic groups.<br>• Visit or volunteer at health fairs in local ethnic neighborhoods.<br>• Learn about prominent cultural beliefs and practices, and incorporate this knowledge into planning nursing care. |

*See Table 2-7 later in the chapter.

and prevent misunderstandings between you and your patients. It also involves integrating cultural practices into Western medicine. For example, before some diagnostic procedures and interventions, it is typical to have patients remove personal objects that are worn on the body. Ask patients whether they wear personal objects and the significance of their removal, since they may have cultural or spiritual significance. You also should know whether wearing these objects will compromise patient safety, test results, or outcomes of the intervention.

## CULTURAL DIVERSITY IN THE HEALTH CARE WORKPLACE

Poorer health outcomes for minorities are linked to the shortage of culturally and ethnically diverse HCPs, who have historically been underrepresented in the health professions. A diversity gap exists between the ethnic composition of the interprofessional health care team and the overall population in the United States (Fig. 2-3). For example, the diversity of nurses in the United States is increasing but still lags behind that of the overall population. African Americans, Hispanic/Latino Americans, and Native Americans make up more than 35% of the population but only 17% of the nation's nurses. Biased behaviors against nurses of diverse cultural and ethnic backgrounds by patients and health care professionals may contribute to their underrepresentation.

Cultural differences exist in how well patients believe they can communicate with their HCP. Communication issues include not understanding the HCP, feeling that they are not listened to, and having questions but not asking them. In the United States approximately 25% to 33% of minority patients have difficulty communicating with their HCP, compared with 16% of white patients. As increasing numbers of internationally educated nurses join the workforce, sufficient training and transitional support must be in place to ensure communication and quality of care.[21]

When HCPs from different cultures work together as members of the health care team, opportunities for miscommunication and conflict can occur. This is termed *cultural conflict.* The cultural origins of miscommunication and conflict in the workplace are often interconnected with cultural beliefs, values, and etiquette. Seeking clarification about misperceptions and misunderstandings is a communication strategy to foster effective teamwork among a multicultural health care team. To ensure the recruitment and retention of nurses from minority populations, all members of the health care team and leadership must create an environment that promotes effective cross-cultural communication and reduces bias and discrimination.

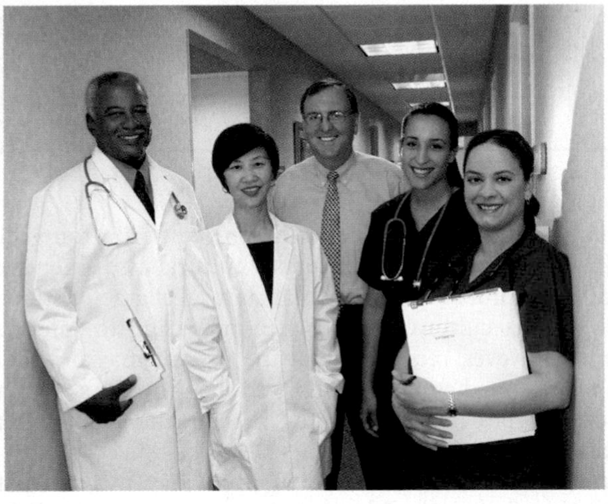

**FIG. 2-3** Interprofessional team working together in a multicultural health care environment. (©Thinkstock/Stockbyte/Thinkstock)

## CULTURAL FACTORS AFFECTING HEALTH AND HEALTH CARE

Many cultural factors affect the patient's health and health care. Several potential factors are presented in Table 2-5.

### Folk Healers and Traditions

Many cultures have **folk healers**, who are also known as *traditional healers.* Most folk healers speak the person's native language and cost less than conventional HCPs. Among the many folk healers found worldwide, Hispanics, particularly from regions in Mexico and Central and South America, may choose to use a *curandero* (or *curandera*), African Americans may visit a *hougan,* Native Americans may seek help from a medicine man or *shaman,* and Asian Americans may use folk healers such as a Chinese herbal therapist. In addition to folk healers, some cultures involve lay midwives (e.g., *parteras* for Hispanic women) in the care of pregnant women.

Folk medicine and traditions are forms of prevention and treatment that are culturally based and traditionally rely on oral transmission of healing techniques from one generation to the next. The patient may not use the term *folk medicine* but thinks of these as cultural home remedies or treatment practices. Folk medicine may be practiced in the home without the guidance of a folk healer. It is important to assess whether the patient is practicing traditional or folk healing.

Some traditions that are practiced as a rite of passage in some cultures can be considered harmful in the dominant culture in the United States. For example, female genital cutting is a tradition that is illegal in most countries yet still practiced in many countries in Africa and the Middle East. It results in physical and emotional trauma and may affect childbirth. Nurses have the opportunity to advocate for immigrant women who have experienced this trauma and to prevent return of young girls to their country of origin for the procedure.

### Spirituality and Religion

Spirituality and religion are aspects of culture that may affect a person's beliefs about health, illness, and end-of-life care. They may also play a role in nutrition and decisions related to health, wellness, and how to respond to or treat an illness.

*Spirituality* refers to a person's effort to find purpose and meaning in life. It is influenced by a person's unique life experiences and reflects one's personal understanding of life's mysteries. Spirituality relates to the soul or spirit more than to the body, and it may provide hope and strength for an individual during an illness.

*Religion* is a more formal and organized system of beliefs, including belief in or worship of God or gods. Religious beliefs include the cause, nature, and purpose of the universe and involve prayer and rituals. Religion is based on beliefs about life, death, good, and evil. You can use several interventions to meet a patient's religious and spiritual needs, including prayer, scripture reading, listening, and referral to a chaplain, rabbi, or priest.

Many patients find that rituals help them during times of illness. Rituals help a person make sense of life experiences and may take the form of prayer, meditation, or other rituals that

**TABLE 2-5 Cultural Factors Affecting Health and Health Care**

**Time Orientation**
- For some cultures it is more important to attend to a social role than to arrive on time for an appointment with HCP.
- Some cultures are future oriented; others are past or present oriented.

**Language and Communication**
- Patients may not speak English and may not be able to communicate with HCP.
- Even with interpreters, communication may be difficult.

**Economic Factors**
- Patients may not get health care because they cannot pay for it or because of the costs associated with travel for health care.
- Refugee or undocumented immigrant status may deter some patients from using the health care system.
- Immigrant women who are heads of households or single mothers may not seek health care for themselves because of child care costs.
- Patients may lack health insurance.

**Health Care System**
- Patients may not make or keep appointments because of the time lag between the onset of an illness and an available appointment.
- Hours of operation of health care facilities may not accommodate patients' need to work or use public transportation.
- Requirements to access some types of care may discourage some patients from taking the steps to qualify for health care or health care payment assistance.
- Some patients have a general distrust of HCPs and health care systems.
- Lack of ethnic-specific health care programs may deter some individuals from seeking health care.
- Transportation may be a problem for patients who have to travel long distances for health care.
- Adequate interpreter services may be unavailable.
- Patients may not have a primary HCP and may use emergency departments or urgent care centers for health care.
- Shortages of HCPs from specific ethnic groups may deter some people from seeking health care.
- Patients may lack knowledge about the availability of existing health care resources.
- Facility policies may not be culturally competent (e.g., hospital policy may limit the number of visitors, which is problematic for cultures that value having many family members present).

**Beliefs and Practices**
- Care provided in established health care programs may not be perceived as culturally relevant.
- Religious reasons, beliefs, or practices may affect a person's decision to seek (or not seek) health care.
- Patients may delay seeking health care because of fear or dependence on folk medicine and herbal remedies.
- Patients may stop treatment or discontinue visits for health care because the symptoms are no longer present, and they believe that further care is not required.
- Some patients associate hospitals and extended care facilities with death.
- The patient may have had a previous negative experience with culturally incompetent HCPs or discriminatory practices.
- Some people mistrust the majority population and institutions dominated by them.
- Some patients may feel apprehensive about unfamiliar diagnostic procedures and treatment options.

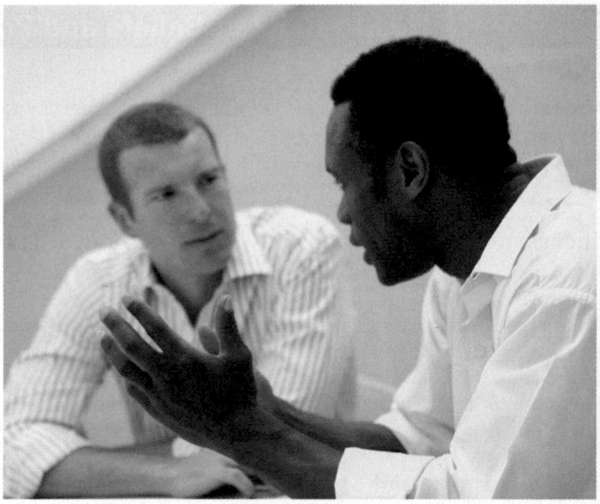

**FIG. 2-4** Co-workers from different cultures communicate with verbal and nonverbal cues. (©BananaStock/Thinkstock)

the patient may create. With appropriate training, you may include spiritual questions in the complete assessment of the patient and plan care based accordingly. (Table 9-5 has a spiritual assessment guide that may be used with patients.) Table 2-6 summarizes health-related beliefs and practices of selected religious groups.[19]

## Cross-Cultural Communication

*Communication* refers to an organized, patterned system of behavior that may be verbal or nonverbal (Fig. 2-4). *Verbal communication* includes not only one's language or dialect, but also voice tone, volume, timing, and ability to share thoughts and feelings. More than 45 million people in the United States speak a language other than English in their home, with Spanish being the most common. Hispanic people who do not speak English at home are less likely to receive a variety of health care services regardless of whether or not they are comfortable speaking English.

*Nonverbal communication* may take the form of writing, gestures, body movements, posture, facial expressions, and personal dress in some cultures. Nonverbal communication also includes eye contact, use of touch, body language, style of greeting, and spatial distancing. Eye contact varies greatly among cultural groups. Patients who are Asian, Arab, or Native American may avoid direct eye contact and consider it disrespectful or aggressive. Hispanic patients may expect you to look directly at them but may not return that direct gaze. Other variables to consider include the role of gender, age, acculturation, status, or position on what is considered appropriate eye contact. For example, Muslim-Arab women exhibit modesty when avoiding eye contact with men other than their husbands and when in public situations.

*Silence* has many meanings, and it is important to understand the meaning of silence for different cultural groups. Some people are comfortable with silence, whereas others become uncomfortable and may speak to decrease the amount of silent time. It is important to clarify what silence means in an interaction with a patient. Patients sometimes nod their head or say "yes" as if agreeing with you or to indicate they understand. Actually, they may be doing this because it is a culturally acceptable manner of showing respect, not because they understand or agree.

Many Native Americans are comfortable with silence and interpret silence as essential for thinking and carefully considering a response. In these interactions, silence shows respect

**TABLE 2-6 Health-Related Beliefs and Practices of Selected Religious Groups**

**Amish**
- Alcoholic beverages and drugs are prohibited unless prescribed by HCPs.
- Abortion, artificial insemination, and stem cell use are prohibited.
- Amish seldom purchase commercial health insurance.

**Catholicism**
- Many fast and abstain from meat and meat products on Ash Wednesday and the Fridays of Lent.
- Artificial contraception and direct abortion are prohibited. Indirect abortion (e.g., treatment of uterine cancer in a pregnant woman) may be morally justified.
- Sacrament of the Sick includes anointing of sick with oil, blessing by a priest, and communion (unleavened wafer made of flour and water).

**Church of Jesus Christ of Latter-Day Saints (Mormons)**
- Strict dietary code called Word of Wisdom prohibits all alcoholic beverages, hot drinks (nonherbal teas and coffee), tobacco, and illegal or recreational drugs.
- Fasting for 24-hour period occurs monthly on "Fast Sunday."
- During hospitalization or serious illness, an elder anoints the ill person with oil while a second elder seals the anointing with a prayer and blessing (laying on of hands).
- Abortion is prohibited except when the mother's life is in danger.

**Hinduism**
- Eating meat is prohibited because it involves harming a living creature.
- Cremation is most common form of body disposal, but fetuses or newborns are sometimes buried.

**Islam**
- Fasting during daytime hours occurs during a month-long period called Ramadan.
- Ritual cleansing with water before eating and before prayer is practiced.
- Eating pork or taking medicines with pork derivatives is prohibited.
- Drinking alcoholic beverages is prohibited.
- Artificial insemination is permissible only if from the husband to his own wife.

**Jehovah's Witness**
- Transfusions of blood in any form or agents in which blood is an ingredient are not acceptable. Blood volume expanders are acceptable if they are not derivatives of blood.
- Transplants that involve bodily mutilation are prohibited.
- Therapeutic and on-demand abortions are prohibited.
- Artificial insemination is prohibited for both donors and recipients.

**Judaism**
- Strictly observant Jews never eat pork, shellfish, or predatory fowl and never mix milk dishes and meat dishes in preparing foods. Fish with fins and scales are permissible.
- Certain foods and drink are designated as kosher, which means "proper." All animals must be ritually slaughtered.
- On the eighth day after birth, boys are circumcised in a ritual called Brit Milah, and girls are given a dedication ceremony involving prayers and blessings.
- Abortion is morally unacceptable except when the mother's life is in danger.
- Organized support system for the sick includes a visit from the rabbi. The rabbi may pray with the sick person alone or in a minyan, a group of 10 adults over age 13.
- If an autopsy is performed, all body parts must be returned for burial.

**Seventh-Day Adventism**
- Vegetarian diet encouraged.
- Nonvegetarian members refrain from eating foods derived from any animal having a cloven hoof that chews its cud (e.g., pigs, goats). Eating fish with fins and scales is acceptable, but consuming shellfish is prohibited.
- Consumption of alcoholic beverages is prohibited.
- Fasting is practiced and involves abstaining from food or liquids by healthy members of the church.

**Buddhism**
- Consumption of alcoholic beverages and illicit drugs is prohibited.
- Moderation in diet and avoidance of extremes are practiced.
- Central tenets are maintaining right views, intentions, speech, actions, livelihood, effort, mindfulness, and concentration.

Data from Andrews MM, Boyle JS: *Transcultural concepts in nursing care*, ed 6, Philadelphia, 2012, Lippincott Williams & Wilkins.

for the other person and demonstrates the importance of the remarks. In traditional Japanese and Chinese cultures, the speaker may stop talking and leave a period of silence for the listener to think about what has been said before continuing. Silence may be intended to show respect for the speaker's privacy, whereas in some cultures (e.g., French, Spanish, Russian) the person may interpret silence as meaning agreement. Asian Americans may use silence to demonstrate respect for elders, whereas African Americans may use silence as a response to what is perceived to be an inappropriate question.

Racism and microaggression affect communication. *Racism* is a belief that differences among the various racial/ethnic groups determine cultural or individual achievement. It usually involves the idea that one's own race/ethnicity is superior and has the right to dominate others or that a particular racial/ethnic group is inferior to the others.

*Microaggression* is social exchanges in which a person says or does something than can either intentionally or unintentionally belittle or alienate a person, especially someone of a different racial/ethnic group. It is imperative that nurses seek to understand racism and microaggression through education, self-awareness, and open dialogue with peers.[22]

## Family Roles and Relationships

Family roles differ from one culture to another (Fig. 2-5). It is important for you to determine who should be involved in communication and decision making related to health care. Some cultural groups emphasize interdependence rather than independence. In the United States many in the mainstream culture have strong beliefs related to autonomy. An individual is expected to sign consent forms when receiving health care. In other cultural groups a family member may be expected to make health care decisions. When you encounter a family that values interdependence over independence, the health care system may have difficulty adapting to how decisions are made. Treatment may have to be delayed while the patient waits for significant family members to arrive before giving consent for a procedure or treatment. In other instances the patient may make a decision that is best for the family despite adverse outcomes for the patient. Being aware of such values will better prepare you to advocate for the patient.

Some cultural differences relate to expectations of family members in providing care. In some cultures, family members expect to provide care for the patient even in the hospital. The patient may expect that the family, along with the HCPs, will provide all care. This view is the opposite of the predominant Western expectation that the patient will assume self-care as quickly as possible.

Ask about culturally relevant gender relationships. For example, in some cultures, such as many Arab groups, it is not appropriate for a man to be alone with a woman other than his wife. Nor is it appropriate for a woman other than a man's wife to provide physical care for him. The clinical implication of this cultural belief is that for many patients from Arab cultures, nurses cannot provide direct physical care for patients of the opposite gender. In some instances, procedures or treatments may be carried out for patients from the opposite gender but only if a third party is present.

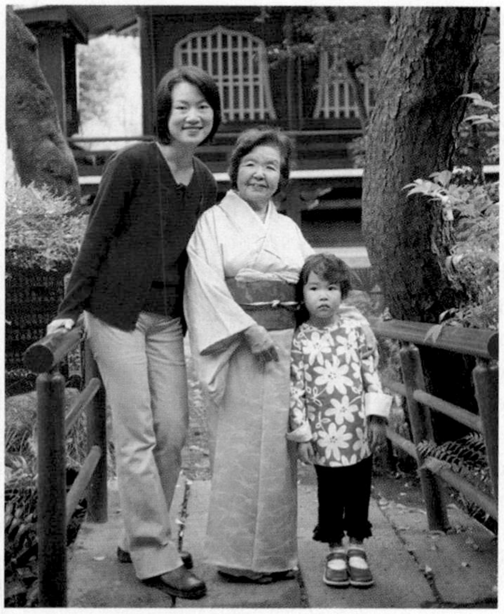

**FIG. 2-5** Family roles and relationships differ from one culture to another. (©Jupiterimages/Photos.com/Thinkstock)

### Personal Space

Personal space zones are the variable and subjective distance at which one person feels comfortable talking to another. A representative example of personal space zones for European Americans is shown in Fig. 2-6. Personal space distances vary from culture to culture, as well as within a culture. As a nurse, you often interact with patients in the intimate or personal distance, which may be uncomfortable for the patient.

Cultural groups have wide variations in their perception of appropriate distances. Whereas an American nurse of European descent may be comfortable with a certain distance, a person from a Hispanic or Middle Eastern background may believe that the distance is too far and will move closer, perhaps causing you to feel uncomfortable. If you then move away to a more comfortable distance, this may cause the other person to think that you are unfriendly, or the person may be offended. Personal space distance also varies within cultures.

### Touch

Physical contact with patients conveys various meanings depending on the culture. Performing a comprehensive assessment requires touching a patient. Many people of Asian and Hispanic heritage believe that touching a person's head is a sign of disrespect, especially because the head is believed to be the source of one's strength and/or soul. Numerous people in the world believe in the evil eye, or *mal ojo.* In this culture-bound syndrome, the illness—usually in a child or a woman—is believed to result from excessive admiration by another person. In some cultures the proper way to ward off the evil eye is to touch the area of admiration. For example, if the person admires

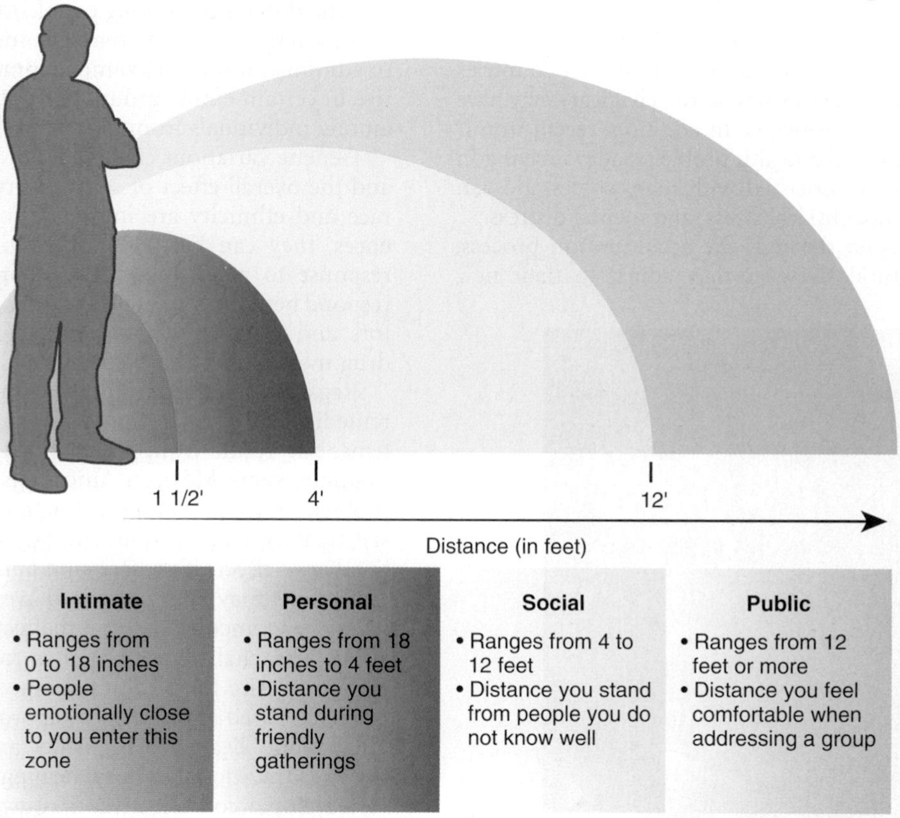


**FIG. 2-6** Personal space zones.

the hair, the top of the head may be touched. It is important for you to ask permission before touching anyone, particularly if it is necessary to touch the person's head.

### Nutrition

An important part of cultural practices is food, including both the foods that are eaten and rituals and practices associated with food. Muslims fast during the daytime during the Islamic month of Ramadan. Such practices may affect when and how medications are taken. Patients may be asked to make major changes in their diets because of health problems, or alternatively food may be used to cope with life changes such as homesickness. Specific foods may be considered essential to good health during pregnancy or other life stages. The HCP should take into account food-related cultural beliefs, practices, and habits when discussing nutrition with patients and planning their diets.

When individuals and families immigrate to an area that is very different from their country of origin, they may experience unfamiliar foods, food-storage systems, and food-buying habits. They also may come from countries that have limited food supplies because of poverty, wars, and poor sanitation. They may arrive with conditions such as malnutrition, diarrhea, and dental caries. Other problems may develop after the person arrives in the new country. For example, second-generation Hispanic immigrants have a greater chance of becoming overweight than their first-generation counterparts. The increase in weight is related to the degree of acculturation experienced by the immigrant.

### Immigrants and Immigration

Migration is driven by a number of conditions, such as overcrowding, natural disasters, geopolitical conflict, persecution, and economic forces. Because of these migrations, a rich diversity of cultures exists in many communities and countries today (Fig. 2-7).

Recent immigrants may be at risk for physical and mental health problems for many reasons. Conditions in their countries of origin (e.g., malnutrition, poor sanitation, civil war) may have resulted in chronic health problems. In addition, recent immigrants are at increased risk for health problems after arriving in a new area. Relocation is associated with many losses and can cause economic hardship, physical stress, and mental distress.

As new immigrants go through the acculturation process, many experience cultural stress as they adjust to their new environment, especially if they have left relatives behind or are unable to return to their home country. Older immigrants are especially affected by changes in role and social position. This may result in depression. Posttraumatic stress disorder is seen in immigrants who have survived wars and violence. Immigrants may face barriers to social acceptance, such as prejudice or discrimination, and experience a lack of ethnic and cultural resources. For some, it may mean loss of the social status that they experienced in their countries of origin.

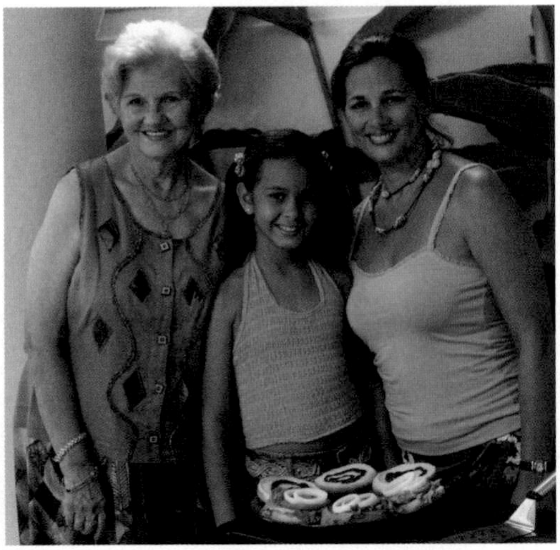

**FIG. 2-7** Recently arrived immigrants join a neighbor for a barbecue, a common American tradition. (©Jack Hollingsworth/Photodisc/Thinkstock)

Another potential problem is tuberculosis (TB). More than half of the TB cases in the United States occur in individuals born outside the country. Individuals who have recently immigrated from areas that have a high endemic rate of TB are more likely to have TB. Foreign-born Hispanics and Asians combined account for 48% of the nation's TB cases. The top five countries of the origin of foreign-born people with TB are Mexico, Philippines, Vietnam, India, and China. The *Refugee Health Guidelines* from the Centers for Disease Control and Prevention supports early identification and treatment.[23]

During the past 45 years, the migration pattern of North America has shifted. Whereas once most immigrants came from Europe, now most immigrants originate from Asia, Latin America, and Africa. Additionally, an increased number of first- and second-generation immigrants enter the United States after visiting friends and relatives. These individuals have a higher risk for malaria, typhoid fever, cholera, and hepatitis A than people born in the United States. Many immigrants lack health insurance and may primarily obtain their health care in emergency departments and urgent care clinics. Therefore nurses in all settings need to be aware of refugee health screening, treatment recommendations, and resources for access to health care and social services.

### Medications

Genetic differences among people from diverse ethnic or racial groups may explain differences in medication selection, dosage, or administration. For example, some medicines are more effective in certain ethnic groups than others. Side effects may vary among individuals from diverse backgrounds.

Genetic variations can affect how the body processes a drug and the overall effect of selected drugs on the body. Although race and ethnicity are imprecise indicators of genetic differences, they can be helpful in anticipating variations in the response to medications. For example, European Americans respond better to angiotensin-converting enzyme (ACE) inhibitors and β-blockers than African Americans. (Genetics and drug metabolism are discussed in Chapter 12.)

Regardless of their cultural origins, many people use cultural remedies and prescription drugs to treat their illnesses. Problems can result from interactions of these substances. For example, some Mexican Americans may treat gastrointestinal problems with preparations that contain lead. Individuals may self-treat their depression with St. John's wort, which can result in adverse effects if prescription antidepressants are also taken.

Patients may avoid standard Western medicine until herbs and other remedies become ineffective or the illness becomes acute. The challenge for you is to try to accommodate the patient's desire for traditional aspects of care while also using evidence-based approaches as appropriate and as acceptable to the patient. Evaluate the safety and appropriateness of the patient's traditional cultural healing therapies.

Develop a collaborative, trusting relationship with patients and encourage them to discuss their traditional approaches to healing. Seek out information on potential drug and herbal

**TABLE 2-7 Cultural Assessment**

*A cultural assessment should include the following:*
- Brief history of the cultural group with which person identifies
- Values orientation
- Cultural sanctions and restrictions
- Communication
- Health-related beliefs and practices
- Nutrition
- Socioeconomic considerations
- Organizations providing cultural support
- Educational background
- Religious affiliation
- Spiritual considerations

Adapted from Jarvis C: *Physical examination and health assessment*, ed 6, Philadelphia, 2012, Saunders.

product interaction from the pharmacist. Honor the patient's choices, if safe and effective, since this will enhance collaboration and may have a positive impact on health outcomes.

### Psychologic Factors

Symptoms are interpreted through a person's cultural norms and may vary from the recognized interpretations of Western medicine. All symptoms have meaning, and the meanings may vary from one culture to another. For example, the degree of depression following a cardiac diagnosis is mediated by cultural views. It is important to ask patients what their illness means to them, what they believe is the cause, and what they think is the best treatment (Table 2-7).

**Culture-bound syndromes** are illnesses or afflictions that are recognized only within a cultural group (Table 2-8). The symptoms, course of the illness, and people's reactions to the illness are limited to specific cultures. Culture-bound syndromes are expressed through psychologic or physical symptoms.

**TABLE 2-8 Culture-Bound Syndromes**

| Syndrome | Description |
|---|---|
| **Hispanics/Latinos** | |
| ***Bilis or Colera*** | Caused by strong anger or rage. Many Hispanic/Latino groups believe that anger results in excess bile that gets into the systemic circulation. Symptoms include acute nervous tension, headache, trembling, screaming, stomach disturbances, and, in severe cases, loss of consciousness. |
| ***Ataque de Nervios*** | Brought on by a stressful family event (e.g., death, divorce). Symptoms may include uncontrollable shouting, crying and trembling, and verbal or physical aggression. |
| ***Empacho*** | Condition described as food forming into a ball that clings to the stomach or intestines, causing pain and cramping. |
| ***Susto*** | Sometimes referred to as "fright sickness" or "soul loss." A traumatic anxiety-depressive state that may result from a frightening experience, such as a loud sound or some threat. Can cause anxiety, insomnia, listlessness, loss of appetite, and social withdrawal. One treatment is to have the affected person lie on the floor. The healer then sweeps indigenous herbs over the person's body while praying to release the evil wind. |
| **Native Americans** | |
| ***Ghost Sickness*** | Condition sometimes associated with witchcraft and a preoccupation with death. Symptoms include general weakness, loss of appetite, a feeling of suffocation, recurring nightmares, and a pervasive feeling of terror. |
| **Chinese** | |
| ***Shenjing Shuairuo*** | Characterized by physical and mental fatigue, headaches and other pains, dizziness, sleep disturbances, and concentration difficulties. |
| **African Americans** | |
| ***Brain Fag*** | Term describing brain "fatigue" caused by the challenges of school. Symptoms include difficulties concentrating, remembering, and thinking. |
| ***Thin Blood*** | Affects older adults, women, and children. Generally weakens an individual and increases susceptibility to illness. |
| **Caribbean and Southern United States** | |
| ***Falling Out*** | Characterized by a sudden collapse, which may sometimes be preceded by dizziness or "swimming" in the head. The person can hear but is unable to move. |
| **Cambodians** | |
| ***Koucharang or Kit Chroeun*** | Translates as "thinking too much," brought about by having witnessed or experienced a horrific trauma. Characterized by physical and emotional exhaustion, immobilization, and constant preoccupation with past suffering and loss. |
| **Koreans** | |
| ***Hwa-Byung*** | Ailment characterized by resentment that is brought about by bitterness and discontent. |

## NURSING MANAGEMENT: REDUCING HEALTH DISPARITIES AND INCREASING CULTURAL COMPETENCY

### Nurse's Self-Assessment

The first step in reducing health disparities and providing culturally competent care is for you to assess your own cultural background, values, and beliefs, especially those that are related to health and health care. Many tools are available to assist you with this process *(http://nccc.georgetown.edu)*.

Table 2-4 suggests ways for you to improve your cultural competence. This information can help you better understand patients and provide culturally competent care. It is important to understand that cultures evolve and change over time. Culturally competent care requires continual learning and self-reflection.[24] Many other important aspects of culture related to health care are included in the Culturally Competent Care sections throughout this book.

In today's increasingly multicultural environment, you will meet patients, families, significant others, and members of the health care team from many different cultures. You will find yourself in patient care situations that require an understanding of the patient's cultural beliefs and practices. Even when you provide care for patients from your own cultural background, you may be from a different subculture than the patient. For example, there are more than 550 federally recognized Native American tribes in the United States, so it would be inappropriate for you to assume that a Native American nurse can give culturally appropriate care to a Native American patient when they may be from different tribes. A white nurse from an urban upbringing may find cultural differences with a white patient from a rural community. Cultural competence is a lifelong process that involves self-reflection and continual learning.[24]

### Patient Assessment

HCPs play an important role in reducing health disparities. However, the causes of health disparities are not always easy to identify. Assess patients for their risk for reduced health care services because of limited access, inadequate resources, age, or low health literacy.

A cultural assessment should be included in the nursing process.[25] Table 2-7 lists important components of the assessment. Determine the patient's (1) health beliefs and health care practices; and (2) perspective of the meaning, cause, and preferred treatment of illness. Ask questions that you are comfortable with based on your own culture.

How can you be aware of the differences among ethnic groups? Using guides for cultural assessment will facilitate the nursing process when working with patients, families, or other groups who are from different cultures. Although guides can assist in this process, you need to be careful not to stereotype or assume that common cultural characteristics pertain to each individual patient. Use guides to explore the degree to which patients share commonalities with the traits generally attributed to their cultural group. You must be informed about traditional characteristics of cultural groups while recognizing that culture is constantly evolving and unique for each individual.

### Nursing Implementation

Although the issues associated with health disparities can seem overwhelming, a number of strategies are available to reduce and ultimately eliminate health disparities. Table 2-9 presents nursing interventions to reduce health disparities.

**Advocacy.** The solutions to reduce health disparities often rest with the policymakers. Economic issues often determine health care delivery. Access and public policy decisions determine who is eligible for federal and state health insurance coverage. You, along with the social worker, can help by identifying key resources in the community, including transportation services, reduced-fee screening programs, and appropriate federal and state offices for Medicaid and Medicare.

You can be an advocate in your health care setting by helping to create a community advisory group. Such a group can be very helpful when establishing health programs within a community. This can also increase the distribution of culturally sensitive information. Another powerful strategy is to increase the number of underrepresented populations in the health care professions (Fig. 2-8).

**Standardized Guidelines.** The use of standardized, evidence-based care guidelines can reduce disparities in diagnosis and treatments. For example, guidelines for the management of hypertension should be based on the patient's BP, symptoms, history, and laboratory values rather than other characteristics such as gender, age, or culture. Racial or cultural differences in outcomes are reduced when the guidelines are followed. In addition, recommendations related to cultural competency will guide you in your learning and practice.

The National Standards for Culturally and Linguistically Appropriate Services in Health Care (CLAS standards) are guidelines that improve the quality of health care. The CLAS standards provide practical guidance for care of people with limited English proficiency and of diverse cultural backgrounds.

**Communication.** Improving interpersonal skills is an important first step in reducing health disparities and providing culturally competent care. To show respect for the patient, take into account the patient's usual communication style. For instance, conduct a health history in an unhurried manner and in a way that is appropriate for the culture. In some cultures it is best to start with general rather than direct questions. For some cultures it is most effective to engage in "small talk," with the discussion including answers that may seem to be unrelated to the questions. If you appear to be "too busy," communication may be impaired.

When meeting patients or family members, introduce yourself and indicate how you would like them to address you—whether they should use first names; Mr., Ms., or Mrs.; or a title, such as nurse. Also ask the patient how he or she prefers to be addressed. This shows respect and will help you begin the relationship in a culturally appropriate manner.

If you need to gather personal information, it is important to understand the most effective approach to use. For instance,

**TABLE 2-9 Nursing Interventions to Reduce Health Disparities**

- Treat all patients equally.
- Be aware of your own biases or prejudices and work toward eliminating them.
- Learn about services and programs that focus on specific cultural/ethnic groups.
- Inform patients about health care services available for their specific cultural/ethnic group.
- Make sure the same standards of care are followed for all patients regardless of culture or ethnicity.
- Identify health care practices and cultural practices that are important to cultural and ethnic identity.
- Participate in research focused on understanding and improving care to culturally and ethnically diverse populations.
- Identify stereotypic attitudes toward a culture/ethnic group that may interfere with getting appropriate health care.
- Support patients of specific cultural/ethnic groups who are fearful about traveling outside the accepted neighborhood for health care services.
- Advocate for patients of specific cultural/ethnic groups to receive health care services that pay special attention to English-language limitations and cultural health practices.
- Learn advocacy and interpersonal strategies from leaders of specific cultural/ethnic groups. For example, African Americans may respond to themes such as "do it for your loved ones." Asian Americans may respond to fear of dependency themes.
- Ensure availability of culturally appropriate patient educational resources.

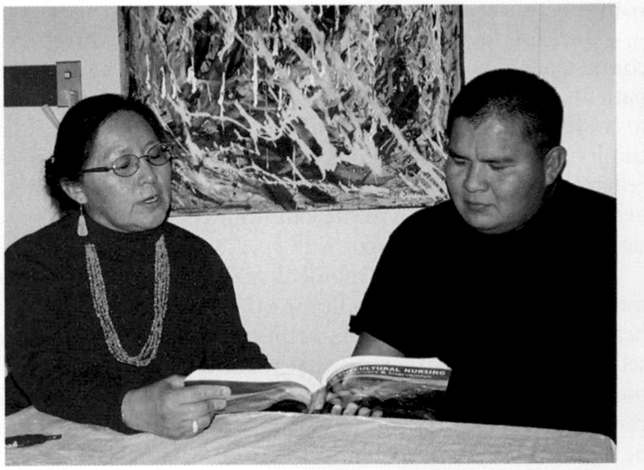

**FIG. 2-8** A Navajo nurse teaching a Navajo patient. (From Giger JN: *Transcultural nursing*, ed 6, St Louis, 2013, Mosby.)

**TABLE 2-10 Using a Medical Interpreter**

**Choosing an Interpreter**

- Use an agency interpreter if possible.
- Use a trained medical interpreter who knows how to interpret, has a health care background, understands patients' rights, and can help with advice about the cultural relevance or appropriateness of the health care plan and instructions.
- Use a family member only if necessary. Be aware of limitations if the family member does not understand medical terms, is younger or a different gender than the patient, or is not aware of the health care procedures or medical ethics.
- Interpreter should be able to do the following:
  - Interpret the patient's nonverbal as well as verbal communication.
  - Translate the message into understandable terms.
  - Act as a patient advocate to represent the patient's needs to the health care team.
  - Be culturally competent and understand how to provide teaching instructions.

**Strategies for Working With an Interpreter**

- If possible, have the interpreter meet with the patient ahead of time to establish rapport before the interpreting begins.
- Speak slowly.
- Maintain eye contact with the patient.
- Talk to the patient, not the interpreter.
- Use simple language with as few medical terms as possible.
- Speak one or two sentences at a time to allow for easier interpretation.
- Avoid raising your voice during the interaction.
- Obtain feedback to be certain the patient understands.
- Plan on taking twice as long to complete the interaction.

when talking with people from some cultural groups, it is imperative that you take time to establish trust and listen to the patient's responses to questions. There may be long silences as the person thinks about the question, showing respect by giving the question appropriate consideration before answering. Take time to listen and help establish trust.

Consider how the patient's age may impact his or her views and communication. For example, African American older adults with mental health concerns may struggle with shame, uncertainty, and lack of trust in the system.

Do not try to serve as an interpreter if your patient does not understand English, because this could lead to misunderstandings. Get the assistance of a person who is qualified to do medical interpretation when you cannot speak the patient's primary language (Table 2-10). Interpreters are available by phone anywhere in the United States through a fee-based service and should be used rather than a family member. Table 2-11 provides guidelines for communicating when no interpreter is available.

**TABLE 2-11 Communicating When No Interpreter Is Available**

1. Be polite and formal.
2. Pronounce name correctly. If unsure, ask about the correct pronunciation of the name. Use proper titles of respect, such as "Mr.," "Mrs.," "Ms.," "Dr." Greet the person using the last or complete name.
3. Gesture to yourself and say your name.
4. Offer a handshake or nod. Smile.
5. Proceed in an unhurried manner. Pay attention to any effort by the patient or family to communicate.
6. Speak in a low, moderate voice and avoid excessive hand gestures. Remember that there is a tendency to raise the volume and pitch of your voice when the listener appears not to understand. The listener may perceive that you are shouting or angry.
7. Use any words that you might know in the person's language. This indicates that you are aware of and respect his or her culture.
8. Use simple words such as "pain" instead of "discomfort." Avoid medical jargon, idioms, and slang. Avoid using contractions (e.g., don't, can't, won't). Use nouns repeatedly instead of pronouns. *Example:*
   Do not say: "He has been taking his medicine, hasn't he?"
   Do say: "Does Juan take medicine?"
9. Pantomime words and simple actions while you verbalize them.
10. Give instructions in the proper sequence. *Example:*
    Do not say: "Before you rinse the bottle, sterilize it."
    Do say: "First, wash the bottle. Second, rinse the bottle."
11. Discuss one topic at a time. Avoid using conjunctions. *Example:*
    Do not say: "Are you cold and in pain?"
    Do say: "Are you cold [while pantomiming]? Are you in pain?"
12. Validate whether the person understands by having him or her repeat instructions, demonstrate the procedure, or act out the meaning.
13. Write out several short sentences in English and determine the person's ability to read them.
14. Try a third language. Many Indochinese people speak French. Europeans often know two or more languages. Try Latin words or phrases. Use English words that have Latin roots (e.g., use precipitation instead of rain).
15. Ask the person's family and friends who could serve as an interpreter.
16. Use websites that translate words from one language to another. Some of them also have audio to help you know how to say the word correctly.
17. Obtain phrase books from a library or bookstore, make or purchase flash cards, contact hospitals for a list of interpreters, and use both a formal and an informal network to locate a suitable interpreter.

Source: Jarvis C: *Physical examination and health assessment*, ed 6, Philadelphia, 2012, Saunders.

**INFORMATICS IN PRACTICE**

***Use of Translation Applications***

- Communication barriers can negatively affect the type of care received by non–English-speaking patients.
- Use a language translation app to help you translate one language into another language.
- Some apps allow you to speak critical phrases and have the translation immediately spoken back to you or the patient in a natural human voice with the proper accent.
- Check the policy of the health care institution on the use of medical interpreters or translators, including the use of apps for translation.

A dictionary that translates from both your language and the patient's language (e.g., Spanish-English/English-Spanish dictionary) is useful. Patients may find it helpful if you have a list of questions and potential answers in several languages prepared by using these types of dictionaries. Many websites translate words and documents from one language into another (see Informatics in Practice box).

It is helpful to have resources for those cultural groups who frequently use the health care facility. This is especially beneficial when a qualified medical interpreter is not readily available and you need to learn important phrases in another language.

## CASE STUDY

### *Health Disparities*

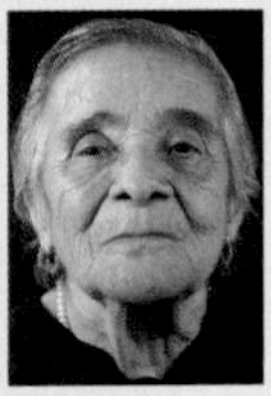

(©Luevanos/ iStock/ Thinkstock)

**Patient Profile**

M.S. is an 81-year-old woman who came to the United States from India 4 years ago with her son and daughter-in-law and their four children. She has a number of health problems, including coronary artery disease, hypertension, osteoarthritis in her right hip, and diabetes. Her daughter-in-law is the primary caregiver and frequently brings her to the urban community health clinic for a variety of health-related complaints. Recently M.S. has been experiencing memory problems.

The entire family comes to the health clinic with M.S. Because English is a second language (Hindustani is their first language) for all of the adult family members, the staff relies on the oldest granddaughter to interpret.

At this clinic visit, M.S. is complaining of shortness of breath. Through her granddaughter's interpretation, she tells the nurse that she is having trouble walking up the stairs in the apartment building. The nurse does the history and assessment, checks her blood glucose (which is within normal limits), and advises that she get more exercise. Given M.S.'s memory problems and limited English, the nurse does not complete a 24-hour dietary recall or counsel her or the family about diabetes management. M.S. is scheduled for an appointment with the cardiologist for an evaluation of her hypertension and heart disease. Two weeks later, when she is seen by the cardiologist, her shortness of breath is much worse and she is complaining of chest pain. She is hospitalized immediately.

Meanwhile, the clinic supervisor is completing a chart audit for the clinic's quality review program. She is reviewing M.S.'s chart and notices that, although she has been a patient in the clinic for 3 years, she has never received instructions on blood glucose monitoring or general diabetes management. The clinic has a nurse diabetes educator who teaches individual patients and groups of patients with diabetes. The clinic manager reviews these findings with the nurse and asks why she has not recommended that M.S. see the diabetes educator. The nurse states that with M.S.'s memory problems and the language barrier, she just assumed that M.S. and her family would not benefit from the consultation.

**Discussion Questions**

1. What type of health disparity has M.S. experienced?
2. What factors led to her not receiving the standard of care?
3. What additional assessment should have been done at the initial visit?

***Patient-Centered Care***

4. What strategies may have worked to enhance patient education?
5. How would you assess M.S.'s religious and spiritual needs?

***Quality Improvement***

6. If you were the clinic manager, how would you recommend that the nurse improve her practice?

Answers available at *http://evolve.elsevier.com/Lewis/medsurg.*

## BRIDGE TO NCLEX EXAMINATION

The number of the question corresponds to the same-numbered outcome at the beginning of the chapter.

1. What are the *leading* determinants of a patient's health (*select all that apply*)?
   - **a.** Genetics
   - **b.** Health behaviors
   - **c.** Family history of disease
   - **d.** Social and physical environment
   - **e.** Type and quality of medical care received
2. In identifying patients at the *greatest* risk for health disparities, the nurse would note that
   - **a.** patients who live in urban areas have readily available access to health care services.
   - **b.** cultural differences exist in patients' ability to communicate with their health care provider.
   - **c.** a patient receiving care from a health care provider of a different culture would have decreased quality of care.
   - **d.** men are more likely than women to have their cardiovascular disease symptoms ignored by their health care provider.
3. Forcing one's own cultural beliefs and practices on another person is an example of
   - **a.** stereotyping.
   - **b.** ethnocentrism.
   - **c.** cultural relativity.
   - **d.** cultural imposition.
4. Which statement *most* accurately describes cultural factors that may affect health?
   - **a.** Diabetes and cancer rates differ by cultural/ethnic groups.
   - **b.** Most patients find that religious rituals help them during times of illness.
   - **c.** There are limited ethnic variations in physiologic responses to medications.
   - **d.** Silence during a nurse-patient interaction usually means that the patient understands the instructions.
5. When communicating with a patient who speaks a language that the nurse does not understand, it is important to *first* attempt to
   - **a.** have a family member interpret.
   - **b.** use a trained medical interpreter.
   - **c.** use specific medical terminology so there will be no mistakes.
   - **d.** focus on the translation rather than nonverbal communication.
6. As part of the nursing process, cultural assessment is *best* accomplished by
   - **a.** judging the patient's cultural values based on observations.
   - **b.** using a cultural assessment guide as part of the nursing process.
   - **c.** seeking guidance from a nurse from the patient's cultural background.
   - **d.** relying on the nurse's previous experience with patients from that cultural group.

7. Nurses play an important role in reducing health disparities. An important mechanism to do this is to
   a. discourage use of evidence-based practice guidelines.
   b. insist that patients adhere to the *Healthy People 2020* guidelines.
   c. teach patients to use the Internet to find resources related to their health.
   d. engage in active listening and establish relationships with patients and families.

8. What is the *first* step in developing cultural competence?
   a. Create opportunities to interact with a variety of cultural groups.
   b. Examine the nurse's own cultural background, values, and beliefs about health and health care.
   c. Learn about a multitude of folk medicines and herbal substances that different cultures use for self-care.
   d. Learn assessment skills for different cultural groups, including cultural beliefs and practices and physical assessments.

1. a, b, d, 2. b, 3. d, 4. a, 5. b, 6. b, 7. d, 8. b.

For rationales to these answers and even more NCLEX review questions, visit *http://evolve.elsevier.com/Lewis/medsurg.*

## EVOLVE WEBSITE

http://evolve.elsevier.com/Lewis/medsurg
**Review Questions (Online Only)**
**Key Points**
**Answer Keys for Questions**
- Rationales for Bridge to NCLEX Examination Questions
- Answer Guidelines for Case Study on p. 32

**Conceptual Care Map Creator**
**Audio Glossary**
**Content Updates**

## REFERENCES


1. World Health Organization: Health impact assessment. Retrieved from *www.who.int.hia.en.*
2. Healthy People 2020: Social determinants of health. Retrieved from *www.healthypeople.gov/2020/topicsobjectives2020/overview.spx?topicid=39.*
3. Health Reform Monitoring Survey: Number of uninsured adults falls by 5.4 million since 2013. Retrieved from *http://hrms.urban.org/quicktakes/changeInUninsurance.html.*
4. Centers for Disease Control and Prevention: Chronic disease prevention and health promotion. Retrieved from *www.cdc.gov/chronicdisease/healthequity.*
5. US Census Bureau: Population estimates. Retrieved from *www.census.gov/prod/cen2010/briefs/c2010br-02.pdf.*
6. Cancer Facts & Figures for African Americans 2013-2014. Retrieved from *www.cancer.org/acs/groups/content/@epidemiologysurveilance/documents/document/acspc-036921.pdf.*
*7. Schieb LJ, Ayala C, Valderrama AL, et al: Trends and disparities in stroke mortality by region for American Indians and Alaska Natives, *Am J Public Health* 104(suppl 3):s359, 2014.
8. Edwards KM: Intimate partner violence and the rural-urban-suburban divide: myth or reality? A critical review of the literature, *Trauma Violence Abuse* 16:359, 2015.
9. The Joint Commission: What did the doctor say? Improving health literacy to protect patient safety. Retrieved from *www.jointcommission.org/assets/1/18/improving_health_literacy.pdf.*
10. Fabreau GI, Leung AA, Southern DA, et al: Sex, socioeconomic status, access to cardiac catheterization, and outcomes for acute coronary syndromes in the context of universal healthcare coverage, *Circ Cardiovasc Qual Outcomes* 7:540, 2014.
11. Farmer GW, Jabson JM, Bucholz KK, Bowen DJ: A population-based study of cardiovascular disease risk in sexual-minority women, *Am J Public Health* 103(10):1845, 2013.
*12. Blair I, Havranek E, Price D, et al: Assessment of biases against Latinos and African Americans among primary care providers and community members, *Am J Public Health* 103:92, 2013.
13. Giger JN, Davidhizar RE: *Transcultural nursing: assessment and intervention,* ed 6, St Louis, 2012, Mosby.
14. Harper FW, Nevedal A, Eggly S, et al: "It's up to you and God": understanding health behavior change in older African American survivors of colorectal cancer, *Transl Behav Med* 3:94, 2013.
15. Lopez-Class M, Castro FG, Ramirez AG: Conceptions of acculturation: a review and statement of critical issues, *Soc Sci Med* 72:1555, 2011.
*16. Ramírez A, Rutten L, Oh A, et al: Perceptions of cancer controllability and cancer risk knowledge: the moderating role of race, ethnicity, and acculturation, *J Cancer Educ* 28:254, 2013.
17. Melluish S: Globalization, culture and psychology, *Int Rev Psychiatry* 26:538, 2014.
18. Doutrich D, Arcus K, Dekker L, et al: Cultural safety in New Zealand and the United States. Looking at a way forward together, *J Transcult Nurs* 23:143, 2012.
19. Andrews MM, Boyle JS: *Transcultural concepts in nursing care,* ed 6, Philadelphia, 2012, Lippincott Williams & Wilkins.
20. Douglas MK, Pierce JU, Rosenkoetter M, et al: Standards of practice for culturally competent nursing care: 2011 update, *J Transcult Nurs* 22:317, 2011.
21. Sherwood G, Shaffer F: The role of internationally educated nurses in a quality, safe workforce, *Nurs Outlook* 62:46, 2014.
22. Hall J, Fields B: Continuing the conversation in nursing on race and racism, *Nurs Outlook* 61:164, 2013.
23. CDC: Implementation of new TB screening requirements for U.S.-bound immigrants and refugees—2007-2014. Retrieved from *www.cdc.gov/mmwr/preview/mmwrhtml/mm6311a3.htm.*
24. American Association of Colleges in Nursing: Cultural competency in baccalaureate nursing education. Retrieved from *www.aacn.nche.edu/education-resources/cultural-competency.*
25. Jarvis C: *Physical examination and health assessment,* ed 6, Philadelphia, 2012, Saunders.


*Evidence-based information for clinical practice.

3

# Health History and Physical Examination

*Jennifer Saylor*

*Believe in yourself and all that you are. Know that there is something inside you greater than any obstacle.*

***Christian D. Larson***

http://evolve.elsevier.com/Lewis/medsurg/

## LEARNING OUTCOMES

1. Explain the purpose, components, and techniques of a patient's health history and physical examination.
2. Obtain a nursing history using a functional health pattern format.
3. Select appropriate techniques of inspection, palpation, percussion, and auscultation for physical examination of a patient.
4. Differentiate among emergency, comprehensive, and focused types of assessment in terms of indications, purposes, and components.

## KEY TERMS

auscultation, p. 40
database, p. 34
functional health patterns, p. 35
inspection, p. 39
nursing history, p. 34
objective data, p. 35
palpation, p. 39
percussion, p. 39
subjective data, p. 35

During the assessment phase of the nursing process, you will obtain a patient's health history and perform a physical examination. The findings of your assessment (1) contribute to a database that identifies the patient's current and past health status and (2) provide a baseline against which future changes can be evaluated. The purpose of the nursing assessment is to enable you to make clinical judgments or nursing diagnoses about your patient's health status.[1] Assessment is the first step of the nursing process, but it is performed continually throughout the nursing process to validate nursing diagnoses, evaluate nursing interventions, and determine whether patient outcomes and goals have been met.

The language of assessment is complex, with many overlapping and confusing terms. In this text, *assessment* describes a hands-on data collection process, whereas a database identifies a specific list of information (data) to be collected.

## DATA COLLECTION

In the broadest sense, the **database** is all the health information about a patient. This includes the nursing history and physical examination, the medical history and physical examination, results of laboratory and diagnostic tests, and information contributed by other health care providers (HCPs). As a nurse, you and HCPs perform a patient history and a physical examination but use different formats and analyze the data based on each discipline's focus.

### Medical Focus

A *medical history* is designed to collect data to be used primarily by the HCP to determine risk for disease and diagnose medical conditions. The medical history is usually collected by a member of the health care team (e.g., physician, advanced practice nurse [APN], resident, physician's assistant, medical student). The HCP's physical examination and diagnostic tests aid in establishing medical diagnoses, effectiveness of previous treatments, and new treatment plan (if indicated). The information collected and reported by the HCP is also used by nurses and other members of the health care team (e.g., pharmacist, physical therapist, dietitian, social worker) based on the focus of their care. For example, the abnormal results of a neurologic examination by an APN may assist in the diagnosis of a stroke. You may use the same results of the neurologic examination to identify a nursing diagnosis of risk for falls. A physical therapist may also use this information to plan therapy involving range-of-motion exercises.

### Nursing Focus

The focus of nursing care is the diagnosis and treatment of human responses to actual or potential health problems or life processes. The information obtained from the **nursing history** and physical examination is used to determine the patient's strengths and responses to a health problem. For example, for the patient with a diagnosis of diabetes, the patient's responses

Reviewed by Karen S. Abate, PhD, FNP-BC, Family Nurse Practitioner/Nurse Educator, W. Cary School of Nursing, Thomas Edison State College, Trenton, New Jersey; Janie Corbitt, RN, MLS, Retired Instructor of Nursing, Milledgeville, Georgia; and Misty Hobart, RN, MSN, CNE, Department Chair, Nursing, Spokane Community College, Spokane, Washington.

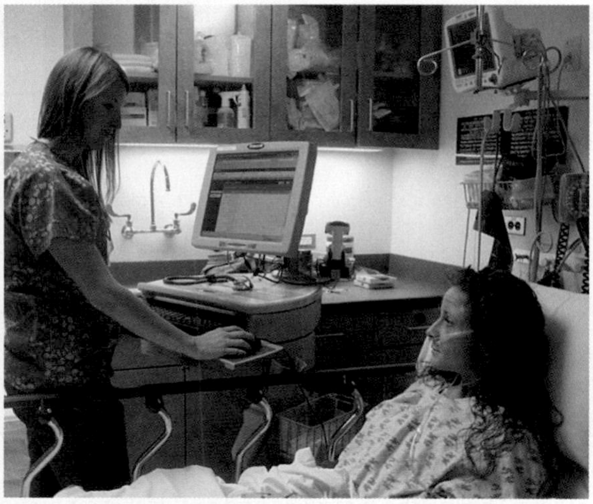

**FIG. 3-1** Obtaining and recording data from a nursing history and physical examination using a computer. (Courtesy Linda Bucher, RN, PhD, CEN, CNE, Staff Nurse, Virtua Memorial Hospital, Mt. Holly, N.J.)

may include anxiety or a lack of knowledge about self-management of the condition. This patient may also experience the physical response of fluid volume deficit because of the abnormal fluid loss caused by hyperglycemia. These human responses to the condition of diabetes are diagnosed and treated by nurses. During the nursing history interview and physical examination, you will obtain and record the data to support the identification of nursing diagnoses (Fig. 3-1).

## Types of Data

The database includes subjective and objective data. **Subjective data**, also known as *symptoms,* are collected by interviewing the patient and/or caregiver during the nursing history. This type of data includes information that can be described or verified only by the patient or caregiver. It is what the person tells you either spontaneously or in response to a direct question.

**Objective data**, also known as *signs,* are data that can be observed or measured. You obtain this type of data using inspection, palpation, percussion, and auscultation during the physical examination. Objective data are also acquired by diagnostic testing. Patients will often provide subjective data while you are performing the physical examination. You will also observe objective signs while interviewing the patient. All of the findings related to a specific problem, whether subjective or objective, are known as *clinical manifestations* of that problem.

## Interview Considerations

The purpose of the patient interview is to obtain a health history (i.e., subjective data) about the patient's past and present health state. Effective communication is a key factor in the interview process. Creating a climate of trust and respect is critical to establishing a therapeutic relationship.[2] You need to communicate acceptance of the patient as an individual by using an open, responsive, nonjudgmental approach. You communicate not only through language but also in your manner of dress, gestures, and body language. Modes of communication are learned through one's culture and influence: not only the words, gestures, and postures one uses but also the information that is shared with others (see discussion on culture in Chapter 2).

In addition to understanding the principles of effective communication, you have to develop a personal style of relating to patients. Although no single style fits all people, your wording of questions can increase the probability of eliciting the needed information. The ease of asking questions, particularly those related to sensitive areas such as sexual functioning, comes with training and experience.

The amount of time you need to complete a nursing history varies with the format used and your experience. The nursing history may be completed in one or several sessions, depending on the setting and patient. For example, you may have to plan several short sessions for an older adult patient with a low energy level to allow time for the patient to provide the needed information. You must also make a judgment about the amount of information collected on initial contact with the patient. In interviews with patients with chronic disease, patients in pain, and patients in emergency situations, ask only those questions that are pertinent to a specific problem. You can complete the health history interview at a more appropriate time.

Judge the reliability of the patient as a historian. An older adult may give a false impression about his or her mental status because of a prolonged response time or visual and hearing impairments. The complexity and long duration of health problems may make it hard for an older adult or a chronically ill younger patient to be an accurate historian.

It is important for you to determine the patient's priority concerns and expectations, since your priorities may be different from the patient's. For example, your priority may be to complete the health history, whereas the patient is interested only in relief from symptoms. Until the patient's priority need is met, you will probably be unsuccessful in obtaining complete and accurate data.

## Symptom Investigation

At any time during the assessment the patient may report a symptom such as pain, fatigue, or weakness. Symptoms experienced by the patient are not observed, so the symptom must be explored. Table 3-1 shows a mnemonic (PQRST) to help you remember the areas to explore if a symptom is reported. The information you receive may help determine the cause of the symptom. A common symptom that you will assess is pain (see Chapter 8). For example, if a patient states that he has "pain in his leg," you would assess and record the data using PQRST.

> Has right midcalf pain that usually occurs at work when climbing stairs after lunch (P). Pain is alleviated by stopping and resting for 2 to 3 minutes. Patient states he has been "eating a banana every day for extra potassium" but "it hasn't helped" (P). Pain is described as "stabbing" and is non-radiating (Q, R). Pain is so severe (rating 9 on 0-10 scale) that patient cannot continue activity (S). Onset is abrupt, occurring once or twice daily. It last occurred yesterday while cutting the lawn (T).

## Data Organization

Assessment data must be systematically obtained and organized so that you can readily analyze and make judgments about the patient's health status and any health problems. Some assessment forms are organized using body systems. Although helpful, these types of forms may be incomplete because they omit areas such as health promotion behaviors, sleep, coping, and values.

**Functional health patterns**, developed by Gordon,[3] provide the framework used throughout this book for obtaining a nursing history. This format includes an initial collection of important health information followed by assessment of 11

**TABLE 3-1 Investigation of Patient-Reported Symptom**

| | Factor | Questions for Patient and Caregiver | Record |
|---|---|---|---|
| P | Precipitating and Palliative | Were there any events that came before the symptom? What makes it better? Worse? What have you done for the symptom? Did this help? | Influence of physical and emotional activities. Patient's attempts to alleviate (or treat) the symptom. |
| Q | Quality | Tell me what the symptom feels like (e.g., aching, dull, pressure, burning, stabbing). | Patient's own words (e.g., "Like a pinch or stabbing feeling"). |
| R | Radiation | Where do you feel the symptom? Does it move to other areas? | Region of body. Local or radiating, superficial or deep. |
| S | Severity | On a scale of 0-10, with 0 meaning no pain and 10 being the worst pain you could imagine, what number would you give your symptom? | Pain rating number (e.g., 5/10). |
| T | Timing | When did the symptom start? Any particular time of day, week, month, or year? Has the symptom changed over time? Where are you and what are you doing when the symptom occurs? | Time of onset, duration, periodicity, and frequency. Course of symptoms. Where patient is and what patient is doing when the symptom occurs. |

## TEAMWORK & COLLABORATION
### *Assessment and Data Collection*

Ongoing data collection is expected of all members of the health care team. In acute care the initial (admission) nursing assessment must be completed by a registered nurse (RN) and within the timeframe determined by the agency.

**Role of Nursing Personnel**

***Role of Registered Nurse (RN)***

- On admission, complete a comprehensive assessment (Table 3-4).
- Obtain patient's health history by interviewing patient and/or caregiver.
- Perform physical examination using inspection, palpation, percussion, and auscultation as appropriate.
- Document findings from the health history and physical examination in the patient's record.
- Organize patient data into functional health patterns, if appropriate (Table 3-2).
- Develop and prioritize nursing diagnoses and collaborative problems for the patient.
- Throughout hospitalization, perform focused assessments based on patient's history or clinical manifestations (Table 3-7).

***Role of Licensed Practical/Vocational Nurse (LPN/LVN)***

- Collect and document specific patient data as delegated by the RN (after the RN has developed the plan of care based on the admission assessment).
- Perform focused assessment based on patient's history, clinical manifestations, or as instructed by the RN (Table 3-7).

***Role of Unlicensed Assistive Personnel (UAP)***

- Take and record vital signs, including oxygen saturation.
- Report abnormal findings to RN.
- Measure and document patient's height and weight, oral intake and output.
- Report patient's subjective complaints to RN.
- Per agency policy, perform point-of-care testing (e.g., glucose) and report findings to RN.

areas of health status or function (Table 3-2). Data organized in this format allow for the identification of areas of wellness (or positive function) as well as health problems.[2]

### Culturally Competent Care: Assessment

The process of obtaining a health history and performing a physical examination is an intimate experience for you and the patient. As noted earlier in the chapter, one's culture influences patterns of communication and what information is shared with others. During the interview and physical examination, be sensitive to issues of eye contact, space, modesty, and touching, as discussed in Chapter 2. Knowing the cultural norms related to male-female relationships is especially important during the physical examination. To avoid violating any culturally based practices, ask the patient about cultural values. Determine if the patient would like to have someone present during the history or physical examination or someone of the same gender to perform the history and physical examination.[1]

## NURSING HISTORY: SUBJECTIVE DATA

### Important Health Information

Important health information provides an overview of past and present medical conditions and treatments. Past health history, medications, allergies, and surgery or other treatments are included in this part of the history.

**Past Health History.** The past health history provides information about the patient's prior state of health. Ask the patient about major childhood and adult illnesses, injuries, hospitalizations, and surgeries. Specific questions are more effective than simply asking whether the patient has had any illness or health problems in the past. For example, asking "Do you have a history of diabetes?" elicits better information than asking "Do you have any chronic health problems?"

**Medications.** Ask the patient for specific details related to past and current medications, including prescription and illicit drugs, over-the-counter drugs, vitamins, herbs, and dietary supplements. Patients frequently do not consider herbs and dietary supplements as drugs. It is important to specifically ask about their use because they can interact adversely with existing or newly prescribed medications (Complementary & Alternative Therapies box).

Question older adult and chronically ill patients about medication routines. Polypharmacy, including medication costs and changes in absorption, metabolism, and elimination of drugs can pose serious potential problems for these patients.[4]

**Allergies.** Fully explore the patient's history of allergies to drugs, latex, contrast media, food, and the environment (e.g., pollen). Include a detailed description of any allergic reaction(s) reported by the patient.

**Surgery or Other Treatments.** Record all surgeries, along with the date of the event, reason for the surgery, and outcome. The outcome includes whether the problem was completely resolved or has residual effects. Be sure to ask about and record any blood products that the patient has received.

## TABLE 3-2 Health History

***Functional Health Pattern Format***

**Demographic Data**

Name, address, age, occupation, gender
Race, ethnicity, culture, spirituality

**Important Health Information**

Past health history
Medications, supplements
Allergies
Surgery or other treatments

**Health Perception–Health Management Pattern**

1. Reason for visit?
2. General state of health?
3. Most important things done to keep healthy? Testicular self-examination? Colorectal cancer, hypertension, and cardiac disease risk screening? Papanicolaou (Pap) test? Immunizations such as tetanus, pneumonia, hepatitis, and flu vaccines?
4. Who is your primary health care provider?
5. Health adherence problems?
6. Cause of illness? Action taken? Results?
7. Things important to you while here?
8. Family health history (e.g., cardiovascular disease, hypertension, cancer, diabetes, psychiatric illness, genetic disorders)?
9. Illness and injury risk factors (e.g., sexual abuse, intimate partner abuse, violence, use of tobacco or alcohol, substance abuse)?

**Nutritional-Metabolic Pattern**

1. Typical daily food intake (describe)? Supplements?
2. Typical daily fluid intake (describe)?
3. Weight loss or gain (amount, time span, intentional)?
4. Desired weight?
5. Appetite?
6. Food or eating: Discomfort? Diet restrictions?
7. Change in appetite with anxiety?
8. Heal well or poorly?
9. Skin problems: Lesions? Dryness?
10. Dentition: Dental problems? Well-fitting dentures?
11. Food preferences?
12. Food allergies?

**Elimination Pattern**

1. Bowel elimination pattern (describe): Frequency? Character? Discomfort? Laxatives? Enemas?
2. Urinary elimination pattern (describe): Frequency? Problem in control? Diuretics?
3. Any external devices?
4. Excess perspiration? Odor problems? Itching?

**Activity-Exercise Pattern**

1. Sufficient energy for desired or required activities?
2. Exercise pattern? Type? Regularity?
3. Spare time (leisure) activities?
4. Dyspnea? Chest pain? Palpitations? Stiffness? Aching? At rest? With activity?
5. Perceived ability for (rate Functional Level 0-III for each):
   Eating __ Cooking __ Grooming __
   Transfer (e.g., bed to chair) __ Toileting __
   Bathing __Dressing __ Shopping __ General mobility __

   *Functional Levels*
   Level 0: Full self-care
   Level I: Requires use of equipment or device
   Level II: Requires assistance or supervision from another person
   Level III: Is dependent and does not participate

**Sleep-Rest Pattern**

1. Generally rested and ready for daily activities after sleep?
2. Sleep onset problems? Aids (e.g., drugs, CPAP)? Dreams (nightmares)? Early awakening?
3. Usual sleep rituals?
4. Usual sleep pattern?

**Cognitive-Perceptual Pattern**

1. Hearing impairment? Hearing aids?
2. Vision? Wear glasses? Wear contact lens? Last checked?
3. Any change in taste? Any change in smell?
4. Any recent change in memory?
5. Easiest way to learn things?
6. Any discomfort? Pain (rating on scale of 0-10)? How managed?
7. Ability to communicate (e.g., primary language)?
8. Understanding of illness?
9. Understanding of treatments?

**Self-Perception–Self-Concept Pattern**

1. Self-description? Self-perception?
2. Effect of illness on self-image?

**Role-Relationship Pattern**

1. Live alone? Family/caregiver? Family structure?
2. Family problems?
3. Family problem solving?
4. Family dependence on you for things? How managing?
5. Family's and others' feelings about illness or hospitalization?*
6. Problems with children? Difficulty handling?*
7. Belong to social groups? Have close friends? Feel lonely (frequency)?
8. Work (school) satisfaction? Income sufficient for needs?*
9. Feel part of or isolated from neighborhood where living?

**Sexuality-Reproductive Pattern**

1. Any changes or problems in sexual relations?*
2. Effect of illness?
3. Use of contraceptives? Problems?
4. When menstruation started? Last menstrual period? Menstrual problems? Gravida? Para?†
5. Effect of present condition or treatment on sexuality?
6. Sexually transmitted infections?

**Coping–Stress Tolerance Pattern**

1. Tense a lot of the time? What helps? Use any drugs, alcohol?
2. Have someone to confide in? Available to you now?
3. Recent life changes?
4. Problem-solving techniques? Effective?

**Value-Belief Pattern**

1. Satisfied with life?
2. Religion important in your life?
3. Conflict between treatment and beliefs?

Modified from Gordon M: *Manual of nursing diagnosis*, ed 13, Boston, 2014, Jones & Bartlett.
*CPAP*, Continuous positive airway pressure.
*If appropriate.
†For women.

## COMPLEMENTARY & ALTERNATIVE THERAPIES

### *Assessment of Use of Herbs and Dietary Supplements*

**Why Assessment Is Important**

- Herbs and dietary supplements may have side effects or may interact adversely with prescription or OTC drugs.
- Patients at high risk for drug-herb interactions include those taking anticoagulant, antihypertensive, antidepressant, or immune-regulating therapy and patients undergoing anesthesia. Most herbs must be discontinued 2 to 3 weeks before surgery.
- Many patients do not tell health care providers (HCPs) that they are using herbs and dietary supplements. They may fear HCPs will disapprove of their use.
- Many herbal preparations contain a variety of ingredients. Ask the patient or caregiver to bring labeled containers to the health care site to determine the composition of the products.

**Nurse's Role**

- Patients typically share information about the use of herbs and dietary supplements with you if they are specifically asked.
- Create an accepting and nonjudgmental attitude when assessing use or interest in herbs or dietary supplements.
- Use open-ended questions such as, "What types of herbs, vitamins, or supplements do you take?" and "What effects have you noticed from using them?"
- Document the use of any herb(s) or dietary supplements in the patient record, including the name, amount, frequency of use, and any side effects.
- Inform patients of the following:
  - Risks and benefits associated with herbal use, including drug-herb interactions
  - Employees of health food stores are not licensed HCPs
  - Importance of carefully reading the labels of herbal therapies and dietary supplements and only taking the recommended amount
  - Moisture, sunlight, and heat may change the components of herbs
  - Many herbal therapies have side effects and these should be reported immediately to the HCP

## Functional Health Patterns

Assess the patient's functional health patterns to identify positive, dysfunctional, and potential dysfunctional health patterns. *Dysfunctional health patterns* result in nursing diagnoses, and *potential dysfunctional patterns* identify risk conditions for problems. In addition, you may identify patients with effective health function who express a desire for a higher level of wellness. Examples of possible questions to ask the patient related to the functional health patterns are presented in Table 3-2.

**Health Perception–Health Management Pattern.** Assessment of the health perception–health management functional health pattern focuses on the patient's perceived level of health and well-being and on personal practices for maintaining health. Ask the patient to describe his or her personal health and any concerns about it. Explore the patient's feelings of effectiveness at staying healthy by asking what helps and what hinders his or her well-being. Ask the patient to rate his or her health as excellent, good, fair, or poor. When possible, record this information in the patient's own words.

Next, ask about the type of HCP the patient uses. For example, if the patient is Native American, a medicine man may be considered the primary HCP. If the patient is of Hispanic origin, a *curandero* (Hispanic healer who uses folk medicine and herbs to treat patients) may be the primary HCP (see Chapter 2).

The questions for this pattern also seek to identify risk factors by obtaining a thorough family history (e.g., cardiac disease, cancer, genetic disorders), history of personal health habits (e.g., tobacco, alcohol, drug use), and history of exposure to environmental hazards (e.g., asbestos). If the patient is hospitalized, ask about the expectations for this experience. Have the patient describe his or her understanding of the current health problem, including its onset, course, and treatment. These questions obtain information about a patient's knowledge of the health problem and ability to use appropriate resources to manage the problem.

**Nutritional-Metabolic Pattern.** The processes of ingestion, digestion, absorption, and metabolism are assessed in this pattern. Obtain a 24-hour diet recall from the patient to evaluate the quantity and quality of foods and fluids consumed. If a problem is identified, ask the patient to keep a 3-day food diary for a more careful analysis of dietary intake. Assess the impact of psychologic factors such as depression, anxiety, stress, and self-concept on nutrition. Additionally, determine socioeconomic and cultural factors such as food budget, who prepares the meals, and food preferences. Determine whether the patient's present condition has interfered with eating and appetite by exploring any symptoms of nausea, intestinal gas, or pain. Food allergies should be differentiated from food intolerances, such as lactose or gluten intolerance.

**Elimination Pattern.** Assess bowel, bladder, and skin function in this pattern. Ask the patient about the frequency of bowel and bladder activity, including laxative and diuretic use. The skin is assessed in the elimination pattern in terms of its excretory function.

**Activity-Exercise Pattern.** Assess the patient's usual pattern of exercise, work activity, leisure, and recreation. Question the patient about his or her ability to perform activities of daily living and note any specific problems. Table 3-2 includes a scale for rating the functional levels of common activities.

**Sleep-Rest Pattern.** This pattern describes the patient's perception of his or her pattern of sleep, rest, and relaxation in a 24-hour period. This information can be elicited by asking, "Do you feel rested when you wake up?"

**Cognitive-Perceptual Pattern.** Assessing this pattern involves a description of all of the senses and cognitive functions. In addition, assess pain as a sensory perception in this pattern. (See Chapter 8 for details on pain assessment.) Ask the patient about any sensory deficits that affect the ability to perform activities of daily living. Record ways in which the patient compensates for any sensory-perceptual problems. To plan for patient teaching, ask the patient how he or she communicates best and what he or she understands about the illness and treatment plan. (See Chapter 4 for details on patient teaching.)

**Self-Perception–Self-Concept Pattern.** This pattern describes the patient's self-concept, which is critical in determining the way the person interacts with others. Included are attitudes about self, perception of personal abilities, body image, and general sense of worth. Ask the patient for a self-description and about how his or her health condition affects self-concept. Patients' expressions of hopelessness or loss of control frequently reflect an inability to care for oneself.

**Role-Relationship Pattern.** This pattern reveals the patient's roles and relationships, including major responsibilities. Ask the patient to describe family, social, and work roles and relationships and to rate his or her performance of the expected behaviors related to these. Determine whether patterns in these roles and relationships are satisfactory or whether strain is evident. Note the patient's feelings about how the present condition affects his or her roles and relationships.

**Sexuality-Reproductive Pattern.** This pattern describes satisfaction or dissatisfaction with personal sexuality and describes reproductive issues. Assessing this pattern is important because many illnesses, surgical procedures, and drugs affect sexual function. A patient's sexual and reproductive concerns may be expressed and teaching needs may be identified through information obtained in this pattern.

Obtaining information related to sexuality may be difficult for you. However, it is important to take a health history and screen for sexual function and dysfunction in a nonjudgmental way and provide information as appropriate, or refer the patient to a more experienced HCP.

**Coping–Stress Tolerance Pattern.** This pattern describes the patient's general coping pattern and the effectiveness of the coping mechanisms. Assessment of this pattern involves analyzing the specific stressors or problems that confront the patient, the patient's perception of the stressors, and the patient's response to the stressors. Document any major losses or stressors experienced by the patient in the previous year. Note strategies used by the patient to deal with stressors and relieve tension. Ask about individuals and groups that make up the patient's social support networks.

**Value-Belief Pattern.** This pattern describes the values, goals, and beliefs (including spiritual) that guide health-related choices. Document the patient's ethnic background and effects of culture and beliefs on health practices. Note and respect the patient's wishes about continuation of religious or spiritual practices and the use of religious articles.

## PHYSICAL EXAMINATION: OBJECTIVE DATA

### General Survey

After the nursing history, make a *general survey statement.* This is your general impression of a patient, including behavioral observations. This initial survey begins with your first encounter with the patient and continues during the health history interview.

Although you may include other data that seem pertinent, the major areas included in the general survey statement are (1) body features, (2) mental state, (3) speech, (4) body movements, (5) obvious physical signs, (6) nutritional status, and (7) behavior. Vital signs and body mass index (BMI) (calculated from height and weight [$kg/m^2$]) may be included. The following is a sample of a general survey statement:

> A.H. is a 34-year-old Hispanic woman, BP 130/84, P 88, R 18. No distinguishing body features. Alert but anxious. Speech rapid with trailing thoughts. Wringing hands and shuffling feet during interview. Skin flushed, hands clammy. Overweight relative to height (BMI = 28.3 $kg/m^2$). Sits with eyes downcast and shoulders slumped and avoids eye contact.

### Physical Examination

The *physical examination* is the systematic assessment of a patient's physical status. Throughout the physical examination, explore any positive findings using the same criteria used during the investigation of a symptom in the nursing history (Table 3-1). A *positive finding* indicates that the patient has or has had the particular problem or sign under discussion (e.g., if the patient with jaundice has an enlarged liver, it is a positive finding). Relevant information about this problem should then be gathered.

Negative findings may also be significant. A pertinent *negative finding* is the absence of a sign or symptom usually associated with a problem. For example, peripheral edema is common with advanced liver disease. If edema is not present in a patient with advanced liver disease, specifically note this as "no peripheral edema."

**Techniques.** Four major techniques are used in performing the physical examination: inspection, palpation, percussion, and auscultation. The techniques are usually performed in this sequence, except for the abdominal examination (inspection, auscultation, percussion, and palpation). Performing percussion and palpation of the abdomen before auscultation can alter bowel sounds and produce false findings. Not every assessment area requires the use of all four assessment techniques (e.g., musculoskeletal system requires only inspection and palpation).

***Inspection.*** Inspection is the visual examination of a part or region of the body to assess normal conditions or deviations. Inspection is more than just looking. This technique is deliberate, systematic, and focused. Compare what is seen with the known, generally visible characteristics of the body part that you are inspecting. For example, most 30-year-old men have hair on their legs. Absence of hair may indicate a vascular problem and the need for further investigation, or it may be normal for a patient of a particular ethnicity (e.g., Filipino men have little body hair). Always compare one side of the patient's body to the other to assess bilaterally for any abnormal findings.

***Palpation.*** Palpation is the examination of the body using touch. Using light and deep palpation can yield information related to masses, pulsations, organ enlargement, tenderness or pain, swelling, muscular spasm or rigidity, elasticity, vibration of voice sounds, crepitus, moisture, and texture. Different parts of the hand are more sensitive for specific assessments. For example, use the palmar surface (base of fingers) to feel vibrations, the dorsa (backs) of your hands and fingers to assess skin temperature, and tips of your fingers to palpate the abdomen[1] (Fig. 3-2).

***Percussion.*** Percussion is a technique that produces a sound and vibration to obtain information about the underlying

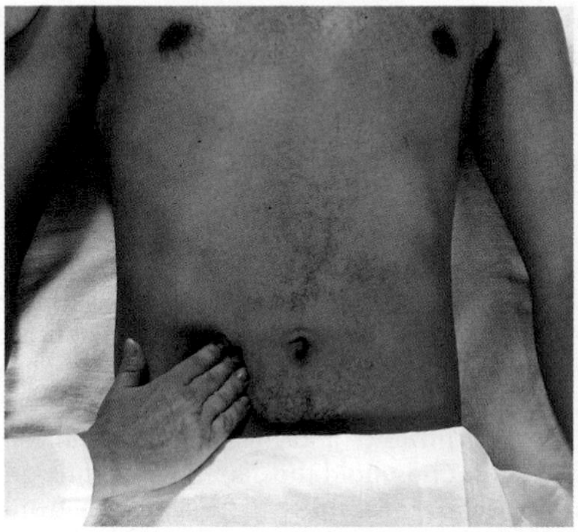

**FIG. 3-2** Palpation is the examination of the body using touch. (From Jarvis C: *Physical examination and health assessment,* ed 6, St Louis, 2012, Saunders.)

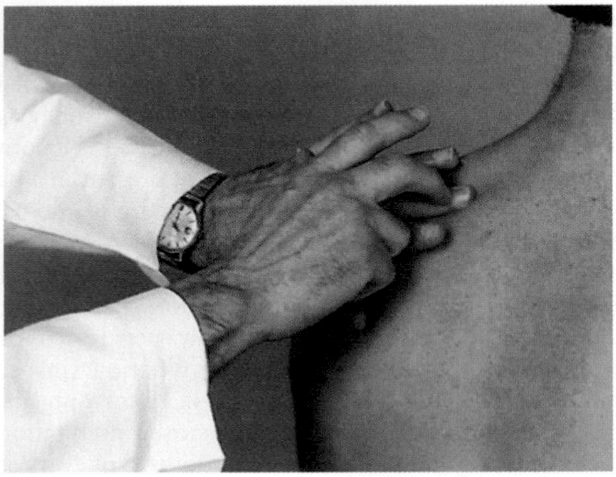

**FIG. 3-3** Percussion technique. Tapping the interphalangeal joint. Only the middle finger of the nondominant hand should be in contact with the skin surface. Normal percussion sounds: *resonant*—lung tissue; *tympany*—air-filled viscus (e.g., intestines); *dull*—dense organs (e.g., liver); *flat*—no air present (e.g., bone, muscle). (Modified from Seidel HM, Ball JW, Dains JE, et al: *Mosby's guide to physical examination*, ed 7, St Louis, 2011, Saunders.)

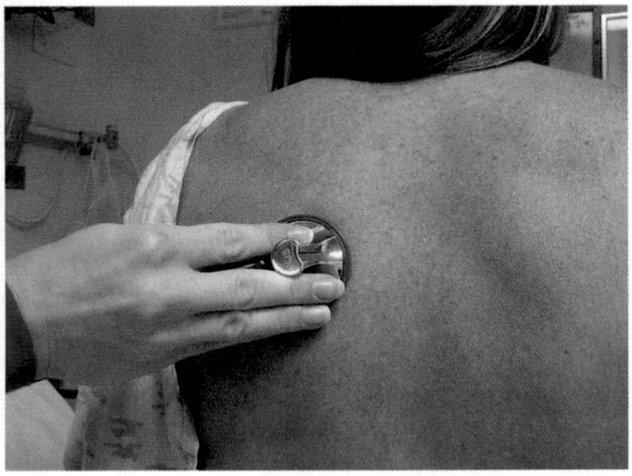

**FIG. 3-4** Auscultation is listening to sounds produced by the body to assess normal conditions and deviations from normal. (Courtesy Linda Bucher, RN, PhD, CEN, CNE, Staff Nurse, Virtua Memorial Hospital, Mt. Holly, N.J.)

area (Fig. 3-3). The sounds and vibrations are relative to the underlying structures. A change from an expected sound may indicate a problem (Fig. 3-3). For example, dullness in the right lower quadrant instead of the normal sound of tympany should be explored. (Specific percussion sounds of various body parts and regions are discussed in the appropriate assessment chapters.)

***Auscultation.*** Auscultation is listening to sounds produced by the body with a stethoscope to assess normal conditions and deviations from normal. This technique is particularly useful in evaluating sounds from the heart, lungs, abdomen, and vascular system. The bell of the stethoscope is more sensitive to low-pitched sounds (e.g., heart murmurs). The diaphragm of the stethoscope is more sensitive to high-pitched sounds (e.g., bowel sounds). Some stethoscopes have only a diaphragm, designed to transmit low- and high-pitched sounds. To listen for low-pitched sounds, hold the diaphragm lightly on the skin. For high-pitched sounds, press the diaphragm firmly on the skin[1] (Fig. 3-4). (Specific auscultatory sounds and techniques are discussed in the appropriate assessment chapters.)

**TABLE 3-3 Equipment for Physical Examination***

| | |
|---|---|
| • Alcohol swabs<br>• Blood pressure cuff<br>• Cotton balls<br>• Examining table or bed<br>• Eye chart (e.g., Snellen eye chart)<br>• Paper cup with water<br>• Patient gown<br>• Pocket flashlight | • Reflex hammer<br>• Stethoscope (with bell and diaphragm or a dual-purpose diaphragm; tubing 15-18 inches [38-46 cm])<br>• Tongue blades<br>• Watch (with second hand or digital) |

*These are examples of commonly used equipment; other equipment may be used depending on the situation.

**Equipment.** Collect the equipment needed for the physical examination before you begin (Table 3-3). This saves time and energy for you and the patient. (The uses of specific equipment are discussed in the appropriate assessment chapters.)

**Organization of Examination.** Perform the physical examination systematically and efficiently. Provide explanations to the patient as the examination proceeds and consider the patient's comfort, safety, and privacy. If you follow the same sequence every time, you are less likely to forget a procedure, a step in the sequence, or a portion of the body. Table 3-4 presents a comprehensive and organized physical examination outline.

Adaptations of the physical examination are often useful for the older adult patient, who may have age-related problems such as decreased mobility, limited energy, and perceptual changes.[5] An outline listing some of the useful adaptations is found in Table 3-5.

**Recording Physical Examination.** At the conclusion of the examination, record the normal and abnormal findings in the patient's record. See Table 3-6 for an example of how to record findings of a normal physical examination of a healthy adult. See Table 5-5 to locate age-related assessment findings in the book.

## TYPES OF ASSESSMENT

Various types of assessment are used to obtain information about a patient. These approaches can be divided into three types: emergency, comprehensive, and focused (Table 3-7). You need to decide what type of assessment to perform based on the clinical situation. Sometimes the health care agency provides guidelines, and other times it is a nursing judgment.

### Emergency Assessment

In an emergency or life-threatening situation an *emergency assessment* may be done. This involves a rapid history and examination of a patient while maintaining vital functions.

### Comprehensive Assessment

A *comprehensive assessment* includes a detailed health history and physical examination of all body systems. This is typically done on admission to the hospital or onset of care in a primary care setting.

### Focused Assessment

A *focused assessment* is an abbreviated health history and examination. It is used to evaluate the status of previously

## TABLE 3-4 Outline for Physical Examination

### 1. General Survey

*Observe general state of health (patient is seated).*

- Body features
- Mental state and level of orientation
- Speech
- Body movements
- Physical appearance
- Nutritional status
- Behavior

### 2. Vital Signs

*Record vital signs.*

- Blood pressure—both arms for comparison
- Apical/radial pulse
- Respiration
- Temperature
- Oxygen saturation

*Record height and weight; calculate body mass index (BMI).*

### 3. Integument

*Inspect and palpate skin for the following:*

- Color
- Integrity (e.g., lacerations, lesions, breakdown)
- Scars, tattoos, piercings
- Bruises, rash
- Edema
- Moisture
- Texture
- Temperature
- Turgor
- Vascularity

*Inspect and palpate nails for the following:*

- Color
- Lesions
- Size
- Shape
- Angle
- Capillary refill time

### 4. Head and Neck

*Inspect and palpate head for the following:*

- Shape and symmetry of skull
- Masses
- Tenderness
- Condition of hair and scalp
- Temporal arteries
- Temporomandibular joint
- Sensory (CN V, light touch, pain)
- Motor (CN VII, shows teeth, purses lips, raises eyebrows)
- Looks up, wrinkles forehead (CN VII)
- Raises shoulders against resistance (CN XI)

*Inspect and palpate (occasionally auscultate) neck for the following:*

- Skin (vascularity and visible pulsations)
- Symmetry
- Range of motion
- Pulses and bruits (carotid)
- Midline structure (trachea, thyroid gland, cartilage)
- Lymph nodes (preauricular, postauricular, occipital, mandibular, tonsillar, submental, anterior and posterior cervical, infraclavicular, supraclavicular)

*Test visual acuity.*

*Inspect and lightly palpate eyes/eyebrows for the following:*

- Position and movement of eyelids (CN VII)
- Visual fields (CN II)
- Extraocular movements (CN III, IV, VI)
- Cornea, sclera, conjunctiva
- Pupillary response (CN III)
- Red reflex*

*Inspect and palpate nose and sinuses for the following:*

- External nose: shape, blockage
- Internal nose: patency of nasal passages, shape, turbinates or polyps, discharge
- Frontal and maxillary sinuses

*Inspect and palpate ears for the following:*

- Placement
- Pinna
- Auditory acuity (whispered voice, ticking watch) (CN VIII)
- Mastoid process
- Auditory canal
- Tympanic membrane

*Inspect and palpate mouth for the following:*

- Lips (symmetry, lesions, color)
- Buccal mucosa (Stensen's and Wharton's ducts)
- Teeth (absence, state of repair, color)
- Gums (color, receding from teeth)
- Tongue for strength (asymmetry, ability to stick out tongue, side to side, fasciculations) (CN XII)
- Palates
- Tonsils and pillars
- Uvular elevation (CN IX)
- Posterior pharynx
- Gag reflex (CN IX and X)
- Jaw strength (CN V)
- Moisture
- Color
- Floor of mouth

### 5. Extremities

*Observe size and shape, symmetry and deformity, involuntary movements. Inspect and palpate arms, fingers, wrists, elbows, shoulders for the following:*

- Strength
- Range of motion
- Joint pain
- Swelling
- Pulses (radial, brachial)
- Sensation (light touch, pain, temperature)
- Test reflexes: triceps, biceps, brachioradialis

*Inspect and palpate legs for the following:*

- Strength
- Range of motion
- Joint pain
- Swelling, edema
- Hair distribution
- Sensation (light touch, pain, temperature)
- Pulses (dorsalis pedis, posterior tibialis)
- Test reflexes: patellar, Achilles, plantar

### 6. Posterior Thorax

*Inspect for muscular development, scoliosis, respiratory movement, approximation of AP diameter.*

- Palpate for symmetry of respiratory movement, tenderness of CVA, spinous processes, tumors or swelling, tactile fremitus
- Percuss for pulmonary resonance
- Auscultate for breath sounds
- Auscultate for egophony, bronchophony, and whispered pectoriloquy

### 7. Anterior Thorax

- Assess breasts for configuration, symmetry, dimpling of skin
- Assess nipples for rash, direction, inversion, retraction
- Inspect for apical impulse, other precordial pulsations
- Palpate the apical impulse and the precordium for thrills, lifts, heaves, tenderness
- Inspect neck for venous distention, pulsations, waves
- Palpate lymph nodes in the subclavian, axillary, and brachial areas
- Palpate breasts
- Auscultate for rate and rhythm; character of $S_1$ and $S_2$ in the aortic, pulmonic, Erb's point, tricuspid, mitral areas; bruits at carotid, epigastrium

*Continued*

## TABLE 3-4 Outline for Physical Examination—cont'd

**8. Abdomen**

- Inspect for scars, shape, symmetry, bulging, muscular position and condition of umbilicus, movements (respiratory, pulsations, presence of peristaltic waves)
- Auscultate for peristalsis (i.e., bowel sounds), bruits
- Percuss then palpate to confirm positive findings; check liver (size, tenderness), spleen, kidney (size, tenderness), urinary bladder (distention)
- Palpate femoral pulses, inguinofemoral nodes, and abdominal aorta

**9. Neurologic**

*Observe motor status.*

- Gait
- Toe walk
- Heel walk
- Drift

*Observe coordination:*

- Finger to nose
- Romberg sign
- Heel to opposite shin

*Observe the following:*

- Proprioception (position sense of great toe)

**10. Genitalia***

***Male External Genitalia***

- Inspect penis, noting hair distribution, prepuce, glans, urethral meatus, scars, ulcers, eruptions, structural alterations, discharge
- Inspect epidermis of perineum, rectum
- Inspect skin of scrotum; palpate for descended testes, masses, pain

***Female External Genitalia***

- Inspect hair distribution; mons pubis, labia (minora and majora); urethral meatus; Bartholin's, urethral, Skene's glands (may also be palpated, if indicated); introitus; any discharge
- Assess for presence of cystocele, prolapse
- Inspect perineum, rectum

*AP,* Anteroposterior; *CN,* cranial nerve; *CVA,* costovertebral angle.
*If the nurse has the appropriate education, additional techniques can be performed. A retinal reflex examination (red reflex) would be performed with the eye examination. Speculum and bimanual examination of women and the prostate gland examination of men would be performed after inspection of genitalia. Examination of the genitalia may require a second person to be present in the room.

## TABLE 3-5 Gerontologic Assessment Differences

### *Adaptations in Physical Assessment Techniques*

**General Approach**
Keep patient warm and comfortable because loss of subcutaneous fat decreases ability to stay warm. Adapt positioning to physical limitations. Avoid unnecessary changes in position. Perform as many activities as possible in the position of comfort for the patient.

**Skin**
Handle with care because of fragility and loss of subcutaneous fat.

**Head and Neck**
Provide a quiet environment free from distraction because of possible sensory impairments (e.g., decreased vision, hearing).

**Extremities**
Use gentle movements and reinforcement techniques. Avoid having patient hop on one foot or perform deep knee bends if patient has limited range of motion of the extremities, decreased reflexes, or diminished sense of balance.

**Thorax**
Adapt examination for changes related to decreased force of expiration, weakened cough reflex, and shortness of breath.

**Abdomen**
Use caution in palpating patient's liver because it is readily accessible because of a thinner, softer abdominal wall. The older adult patient may have diminished pain perception in the abdominal wall.

identified problems and monitor for signs and symptoms of new problems. It can be done when a specific problem (e.g., pneumonia) is identified. The patient's clinical manifestations should alert you to the appropriate focused assessment. For example, abdominal pain indicates the need for a focused assessment of the abdomen. Some problems require a focused assessment of more than one body system. A complaint of headache may indicate the need to do musculoskeletal, neurologic, and head and neck examinations. Examples of focused assessments for the various body systems can be found in each assessment chapter of this book.

## Using Assessment Approaches

Assessment in a hospital inpatient setting, particularly in acute care, is markedly different from assessment in other settings. Focused assessment of the hospitalized patient is frequent and performed by many different people. Such a team approach demands a high degree of consistency among different HCPs.

As you provide ongoing care for a patient, you will be constantly refining your mental image of the patient. As you gain experience, you will form a mental image of a patient's status from a few basic details, such as "85-year-old African American woman admitted for COPD exacerbation." Your picture of her becomes clearer as you receive a more complete verbal report, such as length of stay, laboratory results, physical findings, and vital signs. Next, perform your own assessment using a focused approach. During your assessment, you will confirm or revise the findings that you read in the medical record and what you heard from other HCPs.

Keep in mind that the process does not end once you have done your first assessment on a patient during your rounds. You will continue to gather information about all your patients throughout your shift. Everything that you learned previously about each patient is considered in the light of new information. For example, when you are doing a respiratory assessment on your patient with COPD, you hear crackles in her lungs. This finding should lead you to do a cardiovascular assessment because cardiac problems (e.g., heart failure) can also cause crackles. As you gain experience, the importance of new findings will be more obvious to you. Assessment case studies are integrated into all of the assessment chapters for this book to help you develop your assessment skills and knowledge.

Table 3-8 shows how you can perform different types of assessments based on a patient's progress through a given hospitalization. When a patient arrives at the emergency

## TABLE 3-6 Findings From a Physical Examination of a Healthy Adult

***Example***

**General Status**
Well-nourished, well-hydrated, well-developed white (woman) or (man) in NAD, appears stated age, speech clear and evenly paced; is alert and oriented ×3; cooperative, calm; BMI 23.8

**Skin**
Clear s̄ lesions, warm and dry, trunk warmer than extremities, normal skin turgor, no ↑ vascularity, no varicose veins

**Nails**
Well-groomed, round 160-degree angle s̄ lesions, nail beds pink, capillary refill <2 sec

**Hair**
Thick, brown, shiny, normal (male, female) distribution

**Head**
Normocephalic, nontender

**Eyes**
Visual fields intact on gross confrontation
Visual acuity: Right eye 20/20
Left eye 20/20
Both eyes 20/20
s̄ glasses
EOM: Intact on all gazes s̄ ptosis, nystagmus
Pupils: PERRLA, negative cover and uncover tests

**Ears**
Pinna intact, in proper alignment; external canal patent; small amount of cerumen present bilaterally; TMs intact; pearly gray LM, LR visible, not bulging; whisper heard at 3 ft bilaterally

**Nose**
Patent bilaterally; turbinates pink, no swelling
Sinuses nontender

**Mouth**
Moist and pink, soft and hard palates intact, uvula rises midline on "ahh," 24 teeth present and in good repair

**Throat**
Tonsils surgically removed, no redness

**Tongue**
Moist, pink, size appropriate for mouth, no lesions

**Neck**
Supple, s̄ masses, s̄ bruits, lymph nodes nonpalpable and nontender
Thyroid: Palpable, smooth, not enlarged
ROM: Full, intact strong
Trachea: Midline, nontender

**Breasts**
Soft, nonpendulous, s̄ venous pattern, s̄ dimpling, puckering
Nipples: s̄ inversion, point in same direction, areola dark and symmetric, no discharge, no masses, nontender

**Axilla**
Hair present, no lesions, no palpable lymph nodes

**Thorax and Lungs**
Respiratory rate 18, regular rhythm, oxygen saturation 98% on room air; AP < transverse diameter, no ↑ in tactile fremitus, no tenderness, lungs resonant throughout, diaphragmatic excursion 4 cm bilaterally, chest expansion symmetric, lung fields clear throughout

**Heart**
Rate 82, regular rate and rhythm; blood pressure: RA: 122/76, LA: 120/78; no lifts, heaves
Apical impulse: 5th ICS at MCL; no palpable thrills; $S_1$, $S_2$ louder, softer in appropriate locations; no $S_3$, $S_4$; no murmurs, rubs, clicks
Carotid, femoral, pedal, and radial pulses present; equal, 2+ bilaterally

**Abdomen**
No pulsations visible, rounded, positive bowel sounds in four quadrants, no bruits or CVA tenderness, no palpable masses

**Liver**
Lower border percussed at costal margin, smooth, nontender; approx. 9-cm span

**Spleen**
Nonpalpable, nontender

**Neurologic System**
Cranial nerves I-XII intact
Motor (drift, toe stand) intact
Coordination (FN, Romberg) intact
Reflexes: *See diagram*

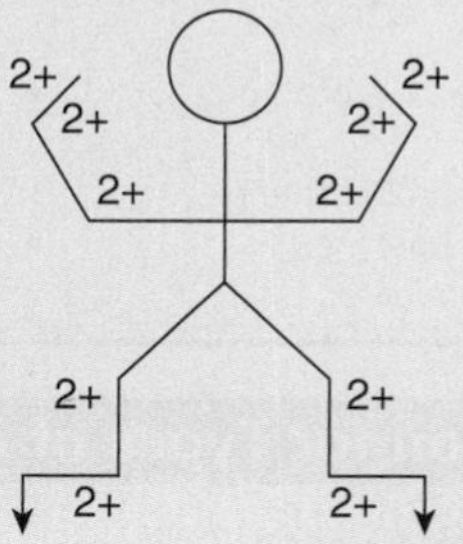


***Grading Scale***
0 No response
1+ Diminished
2+ Normal
3+ Increased
4+ Hyperactive
Sensation (touch, vibration, proprioception) normal bilaterally, upper and lower extremities

**Musculoskeletal System**
Well developed, no muscle wasting; s̄ crepitus, nodules, swelling; no scoliosis
ROM: Full and equal bilaterally, upper and lower extremities
Strength: Equal, strong 5/5 bilaterally, upper and lower extremities
Gait: Walks erect 2-foot steps, arms swinging at side s̄ staggering

*Continued*

**TABLE 3-6 Findings From a Physical Examination of a Healthy Adult Example—cont'd**

| Female Genitalia* | Male Genitalia* |
|---|---|
| External genitalia: No swelling, redness, tenderness in BUS; normal hair distribution, no cysts<br>Vagina: No lesions, discharge; bulging, pink<br>Cervix: Os closed; pink, no lesions, erosions, nontender<br>Uterus: Small, firm, nontender<br>Adnexa: No enlargement; nontender<br>Rectovaginal: Sphincter intact; confirms above findings | Normal male hair distribution, negative inguinal hernia<br>Penis: Urethral opening patent; no redness, swelling, discharge; no lesions, structural alterations<br>Scrotum: Testes descended; no redness, masses, tenderness<br>Rectal: No lesions, redness; sphincter intact; prostate small, nontender |

*AP,* Anterior-posterior; *BMI,* body mass index; *BUS,* Bartholin's gland, urethral meatus, Skene's duct; *CVA,* costovertebral angle; *EOM,* extraocular movements; *FN,* finger to nose; *ICS,* intercostal space; *LA,* left arm; *LM,* landmarks; *LR,* light reflex; *MCL,* midclavicular line; *NAD,* no acute distress; *PERRLA,* pupils equal, round, reactive to light and accommodation; *RA,* right arm; *ROM,* range of motion; $\bar{s}$, without; $S_1$, $S_2$, $S_3$, and $S_4$, heart sounds; *TM,* tympanic membrane.
*These data would be obtained from an examination of the genitalia if the nurse has the appropriate education.

**TABLE 3-7 Types of Assessment**

*The following describes types of assessment that you may use in various situations.*

| Description | When and Where Performed | Where to Find in Book |
|---|---|---|
| **Emergency**<br>• Limited to assessing life-threatening conditions (e.g., inhalation injuries, anaphylaxis, myocardial infarction, shock, stroke)<br>• Conducted to ensure survival. Focuses on elements in primary survey (e.g., airway, breathing, circulation, disability)<br>• After life-saving interventions are initiated, perform brief systematic assessment to identify any and all other injuries or problems | • Performed in any setting when signs or symptoms of a life-threatening condition appear (e.g., emergency department, critical care unit, surgical setting) | • Chapter 68, Table 68-3 and Table 68-5<br>• Emergency management tables throughout the book and listed in Table 68-1 |
| **Comprehensive**<br>• Detailed assessment of all body systems (head-to-toe assessment) | • Onset of care in primary or ambulatory care setting<br>• On admission to hospital, rehabilitation, or long-term care setting<br>• On initial home care visit | • Assessment chapters for each body system<br>• Outline for physical examination (Table 3-4)<br>• Findings for normal physical examination (Table 3-6) |
| **Focused**<br>• Abbreviated assessment that focuses on one or more body systems that are the focus of care<br>• Includes an assessment related to a specific problem (e.g., pneumonia, specific abnormal laboratory findings)<br>• Monitors for signs and symptoms of new problems | • Throughout hospital admission—at beginning of a shift and as needed throughout shift<br>• Revisit in ambulatory care setting or home care setting | • Focused assessment boxes in each assessment chapter<br>• Tables on nursing assessment of specific diseases throughout book |

**TABLE 3-8 Clinical Application for Types of Assessment**

*The following is an example of how various types of assessment would be used for a patient progressing from the emergency department to a clinical unit of a hospital.*

| Timeline | Type of Assessment |
|---|---|
| **Emergency Department**<br>Patient arrives in acute respiratory distress.<br>Problem is identified and critical interventions are performed.<br>Patient stabilizes. | • Perform emergency assessment (see Table 68-3).<br>• Conduct a focused assessment of the respiratory and related body systems (e.g., cardiovascular).<br>• May begin comprehensive assessment of all body systems. |
| **Clinical Unit**<br>Patient is admitted to a monitored clinical unit.<br>Beginning of each shift: reassess per orders and more frequently as determined by the nurse. | • Complete comprehensive assessment of all body systems within proper timeframe.<br>• Perform focused assessment of respiratory system and other related body systems per agency protocol.<br>• Perform focused assessment of appropriate body system(s) if new symptoms are reported. |

department with a life-threatening condition, you will perform an emergency assessment based on the elements of a primary survey (e.g., airway, breathing, circulation, disability) (see Table 68-3). Once the patient is stabilized, you can begin a focused assessment of the respiratory and related body systems. Once the patient is admitted, a comprehensive assessment of all body systems, whether or not they are involved in the current clinical problem, is obtained.

## PROBLEM IDENTIFICATION AND NURSING DIAGNOSES

After completing the history and physical examination, analyze the data to develop a list of nursing diagnoses and collaborative problems. See Chapter 1 for a description of the nursing process, including the identification of nursing diagnoses and collaborative problems.

## BRIDGE TO NCLEX EXAMINATION

The number of the question corresponds to the same-numbered outcome at the beginning of the chapter.

1. The patient health history and physical examination provide the nurse with information to primarily
   - **a.** diagnose a medical problem.
   - **b.** investigate a patient's signs and symptoms.
   - **c.** classify subjective and objective patient data.
   - **d.** identify nursing diagnoses and collaborative problems.
2. The nurse would place information about the patient's concern that his illness is threatening his job security in which functional health pattern?
   - **a.** Role-relationship
   - **b.** Cognitive-perceptual
   - **c.** Coping–stress tolerance
   - **d.** Health perception–health management
3. The nurse is preparing to examine a patient's abdomen. Identify the proper order of the steps in the assessment of the abdomen, using the numbers 1-4, with 1 = the first technique and 4 = the last technique:
   - ___ Inspection
   - ___ Palpation
   - ___ Percussion
   - ___ Auscultation
4. Which situation would require the nurse to obtain a focused assessment *(select all that apply)*?
   - **a.** A patient denies a current health problem.
   - **b.** A patient reports a new symptom during rounds.
   - **c.** A previously identified problem needs reassessment.
   - **d.** A baseline health maintenance examination is required.
   - **e.** An emergency problem is identified during physical examination.

1. d, 2. a, 3. 1, 4, 3, 2, 4. b, c.

For rationales to these answers and even more NCLEX review questions, visit *http://evolve.elsevier.com/Lewis/medsurg.*

## EVOLVE WEBSITE

http://evolve.elsevier.com/Lewis/medsurg

**Review Questions (Online Only)**

**Key Points**

**Answer Key for Questions**

- Rationales for Bridge to NCLEX Examination Questions

**Conceptual Care Map Creator**

**Audio Glossary**

**Content Updates**

## REFERENCES


1. Jarvis C: *Physical examination and health assessment*, ed 6, St Louis, 2012, Saunders.
2. Wilson S, Giddens J: *Health assessment for nursing practice*, ed 5, St Louis, 2013, Mosby.
3. Gordon M: *Manual of nursing diagnosis*, ed 13, Boston, 2014, Jones & Bartlett.
4. Lehne R: *Pharmacology for nursing care*, ed 8, St Louis, 2013, Mosby.
5. Eliopoulos C: *Gerontological nursing*, ed 8, Philadelphia, 2013, Lippincott Williams & Wilkins.

4

# Patient and Caregiver Teaching

*Linda Bucher*

*Tell me and I'll forget; show me and I may remember; involve me and I'll understand.*

***Chinese Proverb***

ⓔ http://evolve.elsevier.com/Lewis/medsurg/

## LEARNING OUTCOMES

1. Apply the teaching-learning process to diverse patient populations.
2. Apply strategies to manage challenges to nurse-teacher effectiveness.
3. Evaluate the role of the caregiver in patient teaching.
4. Relate the physical, psychologic, and sociocultural characteristics of the patient and caregiver to the teaching-learning process.
5. Prioritize patient teaching goals for diverse patients and caregivers.
6. Select appropriate teaching strategies for diverse patient populations and their caregivers.
7. Select appropriate methods to evaluate patient and caregiver teaching.

## KEY TERMS

caregivers, p. 49
health literacy, p. 52
learning, p. 47
learning needs, p. 53
motivational interviewing, p. 47
positive reinforcement, p. 53
self-efficacy, p. 48
teaching, p. 46
teaching plan, p. 46
teaching process, p. 51

This chapter describes the process of patient and caregiver teaching. In addition, it discusses the strategies and methods that contribute to successful teaching and learning experiences.

## ROLE OF PATIENT AND CAREGIVER TEACHING

Patient and caregiver (family member or significant other) teaching is an interactive and dynamic process that involves a change in a patient's knowledge, behavior, and/or attitude to maintain or improve health. You will find that teaching is one of your most challenging and rewarding roles. Teaching patients and caregivers is a key nursing intervention that makes a difference in their lives.

General goals of patient teaching include health promotion, disease prevention, management of illness, and appropriate selection and use of treatment options. In patients with acute and chronic health problems, teaching can prevent complications and promote recovery, self-care, and independence. The leading causes of death and disability in the United States are chronic diseases.[1] Whether patients adequately manage their health problems and maintain quality of life depends on what they learn about their conditions and what they choose to do with this knowledge. Patients who have the knowledge, skills, and desire to take responsibility for managing their health are less likely to be readmitted or visit the emergency department than patients who do not have this information or motivation.[2]

Teaching may occur wherever you work. Although agencies may employ advanced practice nurses and patient educators to establish and oversee patient teaching programs, you are always responsible for patient and caregiver teaching.[3] It is a responsibility that cannot be delegated to unlicensed assistive personnel (UAP).

Every interaction with a patient and a caregiver is a potential *teachable moment.* On any given day, more informal opportunities to teach will occur than formal opportunities. Take advantage of and document all of these moments. For example, when you teach a patient with asthma how to use a peak flow meter, you do not need a formal teaching plan. However, when your patient has a specific learning need about health promotion or management of a health problem, you should develop a teaching plan. A **teaching plan** includes (1) assessment of the patient's ability and readiness to learn, (2) identification of teaching needs, (3) development of learning goals with the patient, (4) implementation of the teaching, and (5) evaluation of the patient's learning.

## TEACHING-LEARNING PROCESS

Teaching is not just imparting information. **Teaching** is a process of deliberately arranging conditions to promote learning that results in a change in behavior.[4] Teaching can be a planned or informal experience. It uses a combination of methods such as instruction, counseling, and behavior modification.

Reviewed by Debra Hagler, RN, PhD, ACNS-BC, CNE, CHSE, ANEF, FAAN, Clinical Professor, Arizona State University, College of Nursing and Health Innovation, Phoenix, Arizona; Regina Kukulski, RN, MSN, ACNS, BC, CNE, Clinical Nurse Specialist Renal Services, Capital Health Regional Medical Center, Trenton, New Jersey; and Laura A. Stokowski, RNC, MS, Inova Fairfax Hospital for Children, Falls Church, Virginia.

**Learning** is acquiring knowledge and/or skills. It can result in a permanent change in a person.[4] Observation of this change is an indication that learning has occurred. Learning may also result in the potential or capability to change behavior. This is seen in a patient who understands the instruction and is fully informed but chooses not to change behavior. In this case, teaching gives the patient the capability to change behavior, but the decision to change is the patient's.

Although learning may occur without teaching, teaching helps to organize information and skills to make learning more efficient. In patient teaching the teaching-learning process involves the patient, the patient's caregiver(s), and you.

## Adult Learner

**Adult Learning Principles.** Understanding how and why adults learn is important for you to effectively teach patients and their caregivers. Many theories of adult learning have evolved from the work of Malcolm Knowles. He identified six principles of *andragogy* (adult learning) that are important for you to consider when teaching adults[5] (Table 4-1).

**Models to Promote Health.** When a change in health behaviors is recommended, patients and their caregivers may progress through a series of steps before they are willing or able to accept the change. Prochaska and Velicer proposed six stages of change in their *Transtheoretical Model of Health Behavior Change*[6] (Table 4-2). This model is frequently used to help patients stop smoking, manage diabetes, and lose weight.

**Motivational interviewing** *(www.motivationalinterview.org)* uses nonconfrontational interpersonal communication techniques to motivate patients to change behavior.[7] This strategy includes the use of any intervention that enhances the patient's motivation for change (Table 4-3). The techniques used in motivational interviewing are linked to the stages of change as identified by Prochaska and Velicer.

During the process of change, relapse and recycling through the stages are expected. Sometimes patients do not change behaviors or return to previous behaviors after a period of change. This may indicate that the interventions used did not consider the patient's stage of change.[8] Identify the patient's current stage of readiness for change and the stage to which the patient is moving. Patients who are in the early stages of change need and use different kinds of motivational support than patients at later stages of change.

For example, a patient who smokes cigarettes who is hospitalized is often in the *precontemplation* or *contemplation* stage of change. In the precontemplation stage, patients are not concerned about their substance use and are not considering changing their behavior. During this stage, help the patient increase awareness of risks and problems related to smoking and create doubt about the use of cigarettes. Ask the patient what he or she thinks could happen if the behavior is continued, provide evidence of the problem (e.g., x-ray changes), and share facts about the risks of smoking. Although patients may not be ready to change behavior while experiencing an acute health problem, the seeds of doubt are sown. In other cases, such as when a patient experiences a life-threatening condition (e.g., heart attack), there may be an immediate awareness of the problem and motivation to change.

**TABLE 4-1 Adult Learning Principles Applied to Patient and Caregiver Teaching**

| Principles | Teaching Implications for Nurse | Examples |
|---|---|---|
| Need to know | • Patients need to know why they should learn something, what they need to learn, and how it will benefit them.<br>• Ask the patient questions such as, "What do you think you need to learn about this topic?" | Your patient and his caregiver ask what they need to know about exercise guidelines after a heart attack. |
| Readiness to learn | • Readiness and motivation to learn are high when facing new tasks.<br>• Health crises provide opportunities for patients to learn and change behavior.<br>• Stress and anxiety may interfere with learning, thus requiring frequent reinforcement of content. | While recovering from a transient ischemic attack, your patient tells you that she is ready to learn about the changes she needs to take to reduce her risk for stroke. |
| Prior experiences | • Motivation is increased when patients already know something about the subject from past experiences.<br>• Identification of past knowledge and experiences can help find familiar ground to increase patients' confidence. | Your patient needs to begin injections of enoxaparin (Lovenox). She tells you that she gives her father insulin injections and is ready to learn how to administer this medication. |
| Motivation to learn | • Patients prefer to apply learning immediately.<br>• Long-term goals may have less appeal than short-term goals.<br>• Focus teaching on information that the patient views as being needed right now. | Your patient is scheduled to be discharged in the morning. Both she and her caregiver have received instruction on wound care and have watched the procedure. The caregiver tells you that he wants to perform the wound care today. |
| Orientation to learning | • Patients seek out various resources for specific learning and prefer to have choices.<br>• When the patient does not recognize the relevancy of the teaching, offer explanations of the value of the learning.<br>• Teaching should target the specific problem or circumstance. | Your patient, who is newly diagnosed with diabetes mellitus, tells you that he is worried about the diet changes he will need to make. Share several options with him to learn about diet changes (e.g., cooking classes, Web-based tutorials, mobile applications, individual sessions with the dietitian, brochures). |
| Self-concept | • Patients need control and self-direction (sense of autonomy) to maintain their sense of self-worth.<br>• Patients do not learn when they are treated like children and told what they must do. | Your patient has a temporary colostomy. She says she is not ready to look at the stoma. Work out a schedule with her for learning colostomy care that meets her need for control and prepares her for self-care. |

**TABLE 4-2 Stages of Change in Transtheoretical Model**

| Stage | Patient Behavior | Nursing Implications |
|---|---|---|
| **1. Precontemplation** | Is not considering a change. Is not ready to learn. | Provide support, increase awareness of condition. Describe benefits of change and risks of not changing. |
| **2. Contemplation** | Thinks about a change. May verbalize recognition of need to change. Says "I know I should," but identifies barriers. | Introduce what is involved in changing the behavior. Reinforce the stated need to change. |
| **3. Preparation** | Starts planning the change, gathers information, sets a date to initiate change, shares decision to change with others. | Reinforce the positive outcomes of change, provide information and encouragement, develop a plan, help set priorities, and identify sources of support. |
| **4. Action** | Begins to change behavior through practice. Tentative and may experience relapses. | Reinforce behavior with reward, encourage self-reward, discuss choices to help minimize relapses and regain focus. Help patient plan to deal with potential relapses. |
| **5. Maintenance** | Practices the behavior regularly. Able to sustain the change. | Continue to reinforce behavior. Provide additional teaching on the need to maintain change. |
| **6. Termination** | Change has become part of lifestyle. Behavior no longer considered a change. | Evaluate effectiveness of the new behavior. No further intervention needed. |

Adapted from Prochaska J, Velicer W: The transtheoretical model of health behavior change, *Am J Health Promot* 12:38, 1997. (Classic)

**TABLE 4-3 Key Aspects of Motivational Interviewing**

- Listen rather than tell.
- Adjust to, rather than oppose, patient resistance.
- Express empathy through reflective listening.
- Focus on the positive. Do not criticize the patient.
- Gently persuade with the understanding that change is up to the patient.
- Focus on the patient's strengths to support the hope needed to make changes.
- Avoid argument and direct confrontation, which can cause defensiveness and a power struggle.
- Help the patient recognize the "gap" between where he or she is and where he or she hopes to be.

A patient in the *contemplation* stage of change often experiences ambivalence. The patient understands that the behavior is a problem and that change is necessary. However, he or she believes that change is too difficult or that the pleasures of the behavior are worth the risks. This is seen in the patient who says, "I know that I have to stop smoking. This heart attack really scared me. I know I need to lose weight and start exercising, but I can't change everything all at once. Smoking helps me control my eating—I can't stop until I lose some weight." During this stage of change, help the patient consider the positive and negative aspects of his or her behavior (e.g., tobacco use), gently trying to tip the balance in favor of positive behavior. Helping the patient discover internal motivators in addition to those external motivators (e.g., second heart attack, lung disease) that push the patient toward change can move the patient from contemplating change to preparation and action. Throughout this process, emphasize the patient's personal choices and responsibilities for change.

As the patient moves from contemplation to *preparation,* a commitment to change is strengthened by helping the patient develop self-efficacy, which is the belief that one can succeed in a given situation. In this case it is the patient's belief that tobacco-use behaviors can be changed. Support even the smallest effort to change. Movement through action and maintenance stages of change requires continued support to increase the patient's involvement and participation in treatment. A comprehensive discussion of motivational interviewing is presented in the Treatment Improvement Protocols available at *www.ncbi.nlm.nih.gov/books/NBK14856.*

The resolution of acute health problems or discharge from the hospital often occurs before the patient moves to the preparation and action stages of change. As the patient develops readiness to change in the contemplative stage of change, continue to support him or her with referral to appropriate community and outpatient resources.

## Nurse as Teacher

### Required Competencies

***Knowledge of Subject Matter.*** Although it is impossible to be an expert in all subject areas, develop confidence as a teacher by becoming knowledgeable about the topic to be taught. For example, if you are teaching patients about the management of hypertension, you must be able to explain what hypertension is and why it is important to treat it. Also teach patients what they need to know about exercise, diet, and side effects of medications. Teach the patient and caregiver how to use BP equipment to monitor BP and to describe situations that must be reported to the HCP. Finally, provide the patient with additional resources, such as valid websites, brochures, and information about support organizations (e.g., American Heart Association).

Sometimes you will not be able to answer patients' or caregivers' questions. Clarify their questions to be sure of what they are asking. When you do not have the knowledge to answer the question, tell this to the patient and caregiver and seek help from co-workers, patient educators, and other reliable sources.

***Communication Skills.*** Patient teaching depends on effective communication between you and the patient or caregiver. Medical jargon is intimidating and frightening to most patients and their caregivers. Introduce medical words and define their meanings. Limit the use of acronyms (e.g., CABG for coronary artery bypass graft) and abbreviations (e.g., IV) when talking with patients. Have the patient and caregiver clarify their understanding of the disease process. Ask them to explain what they know in their own words. For example, if a patient is told that he has leukopenia, define this term in words that mean something to him. Explain that *leuko-* refers to a leukocyte, a white blood cell that fights infections; and that

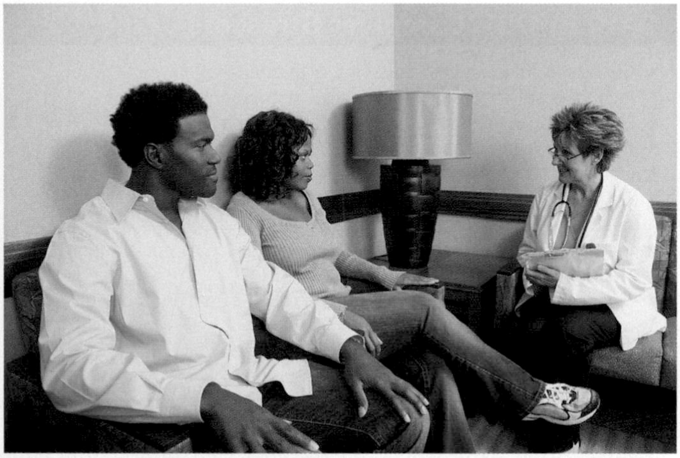

FIG. 4-1 Open, relaxed positioning of patient, spouse, and nurse at eye level promotes communication in teaching and learning. (©Jupiterimages/Photos.com/Thinkstock.)

*penia* refers to a shortage. To enhance learning, use a brief explanation such as, "You have a shortage of white blood cells, the cells that fight infection."

*Nonverbal communication* is critical when teaching. Nonverbal communication is often guided by cultural practices. For example, in Western culture, sitting in an open, relaxed position facing the patient with eyes at the same level delivers a positive nonverbal message (Fig. 4-1). In a hospital setting this may require raising the patient's bed or sitting in a chair at the bedside. Open body gestures communicate interest and a willingness to share. With patients from Eastern cultures, you may need to avoid direct eye contact and provide health information to a family spokesperson rather than directly to the patient.

Also develop the art of *active listening* by paying attention to what is said, observing the patient's nonverbal cues, and not interrupting. Nod in response to the patient's statements and restate what the patient is saying to help clarify communication.

*Empathy* is the courage to enter into the world of another in a manner that does not judge or correct but attempts to understand. Empathy means putting aside your own self and stepping into the patient's shoes. Active listening, combined with empathy, is a powerful way to communicate caring and prepare the patient to learn.

**Challenges to Nurse-Teacher Effectiveness.** Teaching patients and caregivers has many challenges, including (1) lack of time, (2) your own feelings as a teacher, (3) nurse-patient differences in learning goals, and (4) early discharge from the health care system.

*Lack of time* can be a barrier to effective teaching. For example, the patient's physical needs may compete for time that could be used for teaching. To make the most of limited time, it is critical to set learning priorities with the patient. Tell the patient at the beginning of the interaction how much time you can devote to the session. Some teaching should be delivered or reinforced during every contact with the patient or caregiver. For example, when giving medications, explain the purpose and side effects of each drug. Reinforcing small pieces of information over time is an effective teaching strategy, especially if information is new or complex.

Additional barriers are your *own feelings as a teacher* and insecurity about your own knowledge and skill. Teaching is a skill that takes time to master. Become familiar with the various resources for patient teaching that are available at your agency.

**TABLE 4-4 Assessment of Caregiver Needs**

*Ask caregivers the following questions:*

1. How are you coping with your caregiver role?
2. Do you have any difficulties performing your caregiver responsibilities?
3. How much support do you get from outside sources (e.g., other family members, friends)?
4. Are you aware of and do you use community resources (e.g., disease-specific professional organizations [such as Alzheimer's Association, American Heart Association], adult day care centers, church, synagogue)?
5. Do you know about resources that are available for respite (someone caring for your loved one while you have time to yourself)?
6. What kind of help or services do you need now and in the near future?
7. How can I or other health care providers help you in your caregiving role?

Consult with nurse educators or experienced co-workers for further help with developing your teaching skills.

Also, disagreements can arise among the patient, the caregiver, and you regarding the expectations or outcomes of teaching. Having realistic discussions about discharge plans, identifying timelines, and exploring home care options can emphasize the need for learning. For example, after a diagnosis of heart failure due to aortic valve insufficiency and subsequent emergent valve surgery, the patient and caregiver may reject teaching efforts until they realize and accept the seriousness of the patient's health problem.

Last, another important challenge to patient teaching relates to patients having early and quick discharges from the health care system. Shortened lengths of hospital stays have resulted in patients only having basic teaching plans implemented.

### Caregiver Support in the Teaching-Learning Process

The teaching and learning process is applicable to the caregiver as well as the patient. **Caregivers** are people who care for those who cannot care for themselves. Most common, caregivers are family members or significant others who (1) give or assist with direct patient care; (2) provide emotional, social, spiritual, and possibly financial support for the patient; and (3) manage and coordinate health care services.

Approximately one in four American adults provides care to someone on a daily basis. Caregivers are often categorized by their relationship to the patient. The most common types of caregivers are spouses, adult children, parents, grandparents, and life partners. Although older adult women are the most common family caregivers, other examples include husbands who care for wives with Alzheimer's disease, adult children who care for a parent with a stroke, grandparents who care for a grandchild with a developmental disorder, parents who care for an adult child with a spinal cord injury, and life partners who care for loved ones with a chronic illness.[9]

Identify the key caregiver(s) for the patient. Assess the caregiver's roles and relationships to the patient. The patient's health problem affects family roles and functions. Identify the needs of caregivers, whether it is in the acute care setting, during the transition to home, or in a home setting[10] (Table 4-4).

Consider cultural differences when assessing the caregiver. In some cultures a male family member may be the designated spokesperson. This person would receive and communicate information among family members and the patient. In planning for discharge to home, it is important to include caregivers who will actually provide the care for the patient, along with the family spokesperson (see Chapter 2 for more information on culturally competent care).

As much as possible, teach the caregiver along with the patient. Explain the goals of the teaching plan to both of them. Caregivers may need help to learn the physical and technical requirements of care, find resources for home care, locate equipment and supplies, and rearrange the home to accommodate the patient. Sources of support for the transition from hospital to home include community-based agencies, Medicare and Medicaid offices, and case managers at the hospital and insurance companies.

Patients and caregivers may have different teaching needs. For example, the first priority of an older patient with a diabetic leg ulcer may be to learn how to transfer from a bed to a chair in the least painful manner. On the other hand, the caregiver may be most concerned about learning the technique for dressing changes. Both the patient's and caregiver's learning needs are important. The patient and caregiver may also have differing or conflicting views of the illness and treatment options. Developing a successful teaching plan requires you to view the patient's needs within the context of the caregiver's needs. For instance, you may teach a patient with right-sided *paresis* (weakness) self-feeding techniques with special tools, but at a home visit you find the patient being fed by the caregiver. On questioning, the caregiver reveals that it is too hard to watch the patient struggle with feeding, it takes too long, and it is messy. As a result, the caregiver decides that it is easier to feed the patient. This is an example of a situation in which the patient and caregiver need additional discussion about the goals for self-care.

Finally, discuss the potential that support groups, family and friends, and community resources have for providing ongoing support. Support groups help by people sharing experiences and information, offering understanding and acceptance, and suggesting solutions to common problems and concerns. Encourage the caregiver to seek help from the social support system on matters such as housing, health coverage, finances, and respite care. *Respite care,* which is planned temporary care for the patient, includes adult day care, in-home care, and assisted living services.

**Caregiver Stress.** Caregiver responsibilities are usually taken on gradually with the progression of the patient's illness. As the caregiving responsibilities become more demanding, caregivers often realize that their lives have changed because of this experience. Overwhelmingly, caregivers want to continue their usual activities (e.g., work) despite the hardships they face in caring for acute and chronically ill patients.[11]

Prolonged periods of caregiving coupled with a patient's life-limiting illness can contribute to stress and burnout. Some common caregiver stressors are listed in Table 4-5. As caregiving progresses, stressors may change. For example, a caregiver may initially need only to adjust work schedules to accommodate a patient's health care appointments. Later, as the patient's condition worsens, the caregiver may have to reduce work hours, incurring financial hardships.

Caregiving is an experience for which most people are not prepared. It is common for caregivers to become physically, emotionally, and economically overwhelmed by the responsibilities and demands of caring for a loved one. The stress of caregiving may lead to emotional problems such as depression, anger, and resentment. Signs of caregiver stress include irritability, inability to concentrate, fatigue, and sleeplessness. The caregiver often experiences decreased social interactions and may be at risk for social isolation. Multiple commitments, fatigue, and, at times, the patient's socially inappropriate behaviors contribute to the caregiver's social isolation. Stress can progress to burnout and result in negligence and abuse of the patient by the caregiver. See Chapter 5 for information on elder mistreatment and abuse.

**TABLE 4-5 Caregiver Stressors**

- Change in roles and relationships within family unit
- Lack of respite or relief from caregiving responsibilities
- Need to juggle day-to-day activities, decisions, and caregiving
- Change in living conditions to accommodate family member
- Conflict in the family unit related to decisions about caregiving
- Other people's lack of understanding of the time and energy needed for caregiving
- Inability to meet personal self-care needs, such as socialization, sleep, eating, exercise, and rest
- Financial depletion of resources as a result of patient's or caregiver's inability to work
- Inadequate information or skills related to specific caregiving tasks such as bathing, drug administration, wound care

In the family system an illness experienced by one family member affects the entire family and alters family interactions. Often family members do not communicate with each other about the patient's needs, and this results in tension. Family conflicts regarding how patient care should be given can lead to disagreements and conflict within the family.

At the same time, many family members involved in caregiver activities also share rewards associated with this role. Positive aspects of caregiving include (1) knowing that their loved one is receiving good care (often in a home environment), (2) learning and mastering new skills, and (3) finding opportunities for intimacy. The tasks involved in caregiving often provide opportunities for family members to gain greater insights into each other and strengthen their relationships.

Encourage caregivers to take care of themselves. Suggest journaling or joining a support group to help them share feelings that may be difficult to express. Remind caregivers that getting regular exercise and sleep and eating balanced meals enhance their well-being. Encourage contact with others to provide emotional support. Finally, humor is important, and sometimes its use by caregivers can provide distraction and relieve stress-filled situations. See the Caregiving Resource Center at *www.aarp.org/home-family/caregiving* for additional information.

### Regulatory Mandates for Patient Teaching

Several important agencies have provided specific mandates related to teaching hospitalized patients. The Joint Commission's (TJC's) accreditation standards, National Patient Safety Goals,[12] and the American Hospital Association's Patient Care Partnership[13] clearly state that patients have a fundamental right to receive information about their care. This information includes their diagnosis, treatment, and prognosis in terms that they can reasonably be expected to understand. For example, this means that written materials must be appropriate for the patient's reading level. One program initiated by TJC, called Speak Up, was developed to encourage patients to become more involved and informed about their plan of care[14] (Table 4-6). Another program proposed by the National Patient Safety Foundation is called Ask Me 3.[15] A variety of resources that

### TABLE 4-6 The Joint Commission's Speak Up Initiative

**S**peak up if you have questions or concerns. If you still do not understand, ask again. It is your body and you have a right to know.
**P**ay attention to the care you get. Always make sure you are getting the right treatments and medicines by the right health care professionals. Do not assume anything.
**E**ducate yourself about your illness. Learn about the medical tests you get and your treatment plan.
**A**sk a trusted family member or friend to be your advocate (advisor or supporter).
**K**now what medicines you take and why you take them. Medicine errors are the most common health care mistakes.
**U**se a hospital, clinic, surgery center, or other type of health care organization that has been carefully checked out.
**P**articipate in all decisions about your treatment. You are the center of the health care team.

Source: The Joint Commission: To prevent health care errors, patients are urged to Speak Up (poster). Retrieved from *www.jointcommission.org/assets/1/18/SpeakUp_Poster.pdf.*

prompt patients to ask specific questions about their care are available as a part of these initiatives *(www.jointcommission.org/topics/speakup_brochures.aspx).*

## PROCESS OF PATIENT TEACHING

Many different approaches are used in the process of patient teaching. However, the approach used most frequently by nurses parallels the nursing process. The **teaching process** and the nursing process involve the development of a plan that includes assessment, setting of patient goals, implementation, and evaluation. The teaching process, like the nursing process, may not always flow in linear order, but the steps serve as checkpoints.

### Assessment

During the general nursing assessment, gather data to determine if the patient has learning needs. For example, what does the patient know about the health problem? How does he or she perceive the problem? If a learning need is identified, a more detailed assessment is needed, and that problem is addressed with the teaching plan. Assessment also includes the caregivers to determine their role and ability to care for the patient at home.[10] Key questions to use in the assessment are included in Table 4-7.

**Physical Factors.** The patient's age is a factor to consider in the teaching plan. Age affects the patient's experiences and rate of learning.[16] Some effects of increased age on learning may be obvious, but the inexperience of younger people can also affect learning. For example, a man in his twenties who has never thought about his own mortality may be unable to accept the long-term health implications of diabetes mellitus.

Sensory impairments (e.g., hearing or vision loss) decrease sensory input and can alter learning. Magnifying glasses, bright lighting, and materials printed in a large font may help the patient with impaired vision read teaching materials. People with hearing loss can be helped with hearing aids and teaching techniques that use more visual stimuli. Cognition may be affected by disorders of the nervous system (e.g., stroke, head trauma), and by other diseases (e.g., liver impairment, heart failure). Patients with alterations in cognition may have difficulty learning and may require greater caregiver involvement in the teaching process. Manual dexterity is needed to perform skills such as administration of injections or BP monitoring.

### TABLE 4-7 Assessment of Factors Affecting Patient Teaching

**Key Factors and Questions**

**Physical**
- What is the patient's age?
- Is the patient acutely ill?
- Is the patient fatigued or in pain?
- What is the primary diagnosis?
- Are there additional medical problems?
- What is the patient's current mental status?
- What is the patient's hearing ability? Visual ability? Motor ability?
- What drugs does the patient take that may affect learning?

**Psychologic**
- Does the patient appear anxious, afraid, depressed, defensive?
- Is the patient in a state of denial?
- What is the patient's level of motivation? Self-efficacy?

**Sociocultural**
- What are the patient's beliefs regarding his or her illness or treatment?
- Is proposed teaching consistent with the patient's cultural values?
- What is the patient's educational experience, reading ability, primary language?
- What is the patient's present or past occupation?
- How does the patient describe his or her financial status?
- What is the patient's living arrangement?
- Does the patient have family or close friends?

**Learner**
- What does the patient already know about his or her health problem?
- What does the patient think is most important to learn?
- What prior learning experiences could act as a frame of reference for current learning needs?
- Is the patient ready to learn? Change behavior?
- How does the patient learn best (e.g., reading, listening, looking at pictures, doing, playing games)?
- In what kind of environment does the patient learn best? Formal classroom? Computer/Web-based setting? Informal setting, such as home? Alone or in a group?
- In what way should the caregiver(s) be involved in patient teaching?

Problems performing manual skills may be resolved by using adaptive equipment.

Pain, fatigue, and certain drugs also influence the patient's ability to learn. No one can learn effectively when in pain. Provide teaching only after the patient's pain is controlled. A fatigued and weakened patient cannot learn effectively because of the inability to concentrate. Sleep disruption is common during hospitalization, and patients are frequently sleep deprived at the time of discharge. Drugs that cause central nervous system depression, such as opioids and sedatives, cause a general decrease in mental alertness and can affect the patient's ability to learn new information. Adjust the teaching plan to accommodate these factors by setting high-priority goals based on need-to-know information and realistic expectations. Patients often need a referral for follow-up so that teaching continues and learning is confirmed after discharge.

**Psychologic Factors.** Psychologic factors have a major influence on the patient's ability to learn. Anxiety and depression are common reactions to illness. Although mild anxiety increases the learner's perceptual and learning abilities, moderate or severe anxiety limits learning. Anxiety and depression can negatively affect the patient's motivation and readiness to learn. For instance, the patient newly diagnosed with diabetes mellitus who is depressed about the diagnosis may not listen or respond to instructions about glucose testing. Discussions with the patient about these concerns or referrals to an appropriate support group may help the patient to learn that management of diabetes is possible.

Patients also respond to the stress of illness with a variety of defense mechanisms, such as denial, rationalization, or even humor. A patient who denies having cancer will not be receptive to information related to treatment options. Similarly, a caregiver may have difficulty accepting a terminal diagnosis. A patient using rationalization will imagine any number of reasons for avoiding change or for rejecting teaching. For example, a patient with heart disease who does not want to change dietary habits will relate stories of people who have eaten bacon and eggs every day and lived to be 100. Some patients also use humor to filter reality or decrease anxiety. They may use laughter to escape from the experience of facing threatening situations. Humor in the teaching process is important and useful, but determine when humor is used excessively or inappropriately to avoid reality.

One important determinant of successful adoption of new behaviors is the patient's sense of self-efficacy. There is a strong relationship between self-efficacy and outcomes of illness management.[17] Self-efficacy increases when a person gains new skills in managing a threatening situation but decreases when the individual experiences repeated failure, especially early in the course of events. Plan easily achievable goals early in the teaching sessions. Proceed from simple to more complex content to create a feeling of success.

### Sociocultural Factors

***Health Literacy.*** *Literacy* is the ability to use printed and written information to function in society. The recent focus on the literacy rates of the U.S. population and their effects on health and health care have major implications for patient and caregiver teaching. The most recent national literacy survey reported that 43% of the general population and 66% of people older than 60 have basic to below basic literacy skills and another 5% are not literate in English.[18] Assessment of literacy is challenging, since patients rarely admit they have difficulty reading because of feelings of inadequacy and low self-esteem.[19]

Health literacy is the degree to which individuals have the capacity to obtain and understand basic health information needed to make appropriate health decisions.[12] Patients with limited literacy have trouble understanding and acting on health information, leading to *health illiteracy*. Even patients with higher general literacy can have low health literacy when trying to understand complex health information. Health illiteracy results in poor patient outcomes, nonadherence to treatment plans, limited self-management skills, and increased health disparities.[20]

Easy-to-use assessment tools are available to determine a patient's health literacy. The Single-Item Literacy Screener (SILS) uses one question to identify adults who need help with reading.[21] The question is, "How often do you need to have someone help you when you read instructions, pamphlets, or other written material from your doctor or pharmacy?"

Patient teaching materials should be written at the fifth-grade or lower reading level.[21] TJC has established that patient teaching should be tailored to the patient's literacy needs. For example, patients should be taught in their primary language.

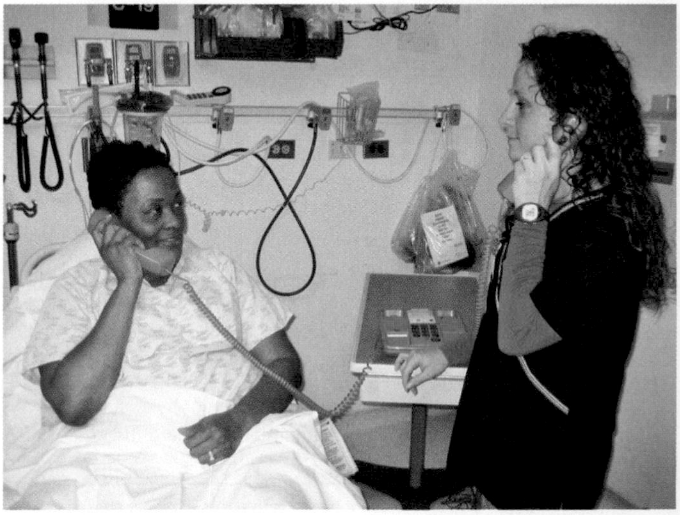

**FIG. 4-2** Nurse communicating with a non-English-speaking patient using a translation phone service. (Courtesy Linda Bucher, RN, PhD, CEN, CNE, Staff Nurse, Virtua Memorial Hospital, Mt. Holly, N.J.)

This is accomplished using medical interpreters (e.g., translators, sign language interpreters)[22] (Fig. 4-2). (Medical interpreters are discussed in Chapter 2 on p. 31.) Many patient teaching materials are currently available in languages other than English. Ideally, written materials should always be available in the patient's primary language.

***Cultural Considerations.*** Learning is influenced by the wider culture to which a patient belongs. Health practices, beliefs, and behavior are influenced by one's cultural traditions. These traditions, which can affect patient teaching, can be identified in a cultural assessment (see Table 2-7). TJC requires that patient teaching be tailored to the patient's cultural needs.[22] To prevent stereotyping patients, it is important to simply ask if there is a cultural group with which the patient identifies. Ask patients to describe their beliefs regarding health and illness.

One cultural element that specifically affects the teaching-learning process is a conflict between the patient's cultural beliefs and values and the behaviors promoted by the health care team. For example, a patient who values a trim figure can be taught to use diet and exercise to retain that figure while at the same time improving BP control. However, in another patient's culture, being heavier may be valued as a sign of financial success and sexuality. This patient may have more difficulty accepting the need for diet and exercise unless the importance of BP control is understood.

Assess the patient's use of cultural remedies and folk healers (see the Complementary & Alternative Therapies Box: Assessment of Use of Herbs & Dietary Supplements in Chapter 3, p. 38). Also consider the cultural remedies that may interfere with or are contraindicated by the treatment plan.

Last, it is important to know who has authority in the patient's culture. The patient may defer to the authority, such as an elder or a spiritual leader, for decisions. In this case, identify and work with the decision makers in the patient's cultural group. (See Chapter 2 for more information on cultural competence.)

***Socioeconomic Considerations.*** A variety of socioeconomic factors are considered when preparing to teach patients. Knowing the patient's present or past occupation may assist you in determining the vocabulary to use during teaching. For example, an auto mechanic may understand the volume

## EVIDENCE-BASED PRACTICE

### *Translating Research Into Practice*

**Does Culturally Appropriate Education Improve Diabetic Glycemic Control and Knowledge?**

***Clinical Question***

For adults with diabetes mellitus (P), what is the effect of culturally appropriate health education (I) versus usual care (C) on glycemic control and diabetes knowledge (O) in the short- and long-term (T)?

***Synthesis of Best Available Evidence***

- Systematic review of randomized controlled trials (RCTs) and quasi RCTs.
- 33 trials of patients ($n = 7453$) from ethnic minority groups with type 2 diabetes. Culturally appropriate interventions were any type of health education tailored for cultural needs of a minority group with type 2 diabetes. Glycemic control was measured by glycosylated hemoglobin A1C (A1C). Knowledge assessment varied across studies.
- A1C levels improved at 3, 6, 12, and 24 months after the intervention.
- Knowledge scores increased at 6 and 12 months after the intervention.

***Conclusion***

- Culturally appropriate education improved glycemic control and diabetes knowledge on a short- and long-term basis.

***Implications for Nursing Practice***

1. How would you modify diabetes education for someone from an ethnic minority group?
2. Why is it important for health care providers to provide culturally appropriate diabetes education?

***Reference for Evidence***

Attridge M, Creamer J, Ramsden M, et al: Culturally appropriate health education for people in ethnic minority groups with type 2 diabetes mellitus. Cochrane Database Syst Rev (9):CD006424, 2014.

*P*, Patient population of interest; *I*, intervention or area of interest; *C*, comparison of interest or comparison group; *O*, outcomes of interest; *T*, timing (see p. 15).

overload associated with heart failure as flooding an engine. An engineer may understand the principles of physics associated with gravity and pressures when discussing vascular problems.

Ask the patient about living arrangements. Whether the patient lives alone, with friends, or with family influences who is included in the teaching process. You may need to modify the teaching plan if the patient does not have access to electricity or phones. If the patient has unmet learning needs by the time of discharge, arrange for ongoing teaching after discharge.

**Learner Factors.** Finally, assess learner factors, including the patient's learning needs, readiness to learn, and learning style.

***Learning Needs.*** Learning needs are the new knowledge and skills that an individual must have to meet a goal. The assessment of learning needs determines what the patient already knows and any past experiences with health problems. Patients with long-standing health problems may have different learning needs from those patients with newly diagnosed health problems.

What patients should learn about managing an illness or what behaviors have to be changed to promote health may seem obvious to you. However, what you think is important may be different from what patients want to know. Remember that adults learn best when the teaching provides information that they view as being immediately needed (Table 4-1). Ask patients to prioritize what they see as the most critical information. Start by giving the patient a list of the recommended topics and then ask the patient to identify other topics not on the list. Having patients prioritize their own learning needs lets you begin with the patient's most important needs. If critical information needs to be taught, explain why the information is "need to know."

***Readiness to Learn.*** Readiness to learn and motivation depend on multiple factors, such as perceived need, attitudes, and beliefs. When teaching adults, identify what information the person values. Readiness to learn is increased if the patient perceives a need for information, has a belief that a behavior change has value, or perceives the learning activities as new and stimulating.[5]

Before implementing the teaching plan, determine where the patient is in the stages of change (Table 4-2). If the patient is in the precontemplation stage, provide support and increase the patient's awareness of the problem until the patient is ready to consider a change in behavior. Nurses in outpatient settings and home health care can continue to evaluate the patient's readiness to learn and implement the teaching plan as the patient moves through the stages of change. Reinforcement is a strong motivational factor for achieving a desired behavior and must be incorporated throughout the change process. Positive reinforcement involves rewarding the target behavior with positive feedback or other rewards to maintain the behavior.[6]

***Learning Style.*** Each person has a distinct style of learning. The three general learning styles are (1) *visual* (reading, pictures), (2) *auditory* (listening), and (3) *physical* (doing things). People often use more than one learning style to gain new knowledge or skills. To assess a patient's learning style, ask how the patient likes to learn and has learned in the past.[23] During assessment of the patient's learning style, identify the patient who does not read or who has limited health literacy. For example, the patient may tell you that he or she does not read much but likes to learn from television. In addition, assess the patient's *ehealth literacy*. This refers to the degree that patients use digital information (e.g., webinars, online health management tools) and communication technologies (e.g., online communication with HCP, online support groups) to improve their health[24] (Fig. 4-3). If possible, always use the patient's or caregiver's preferred learning style.

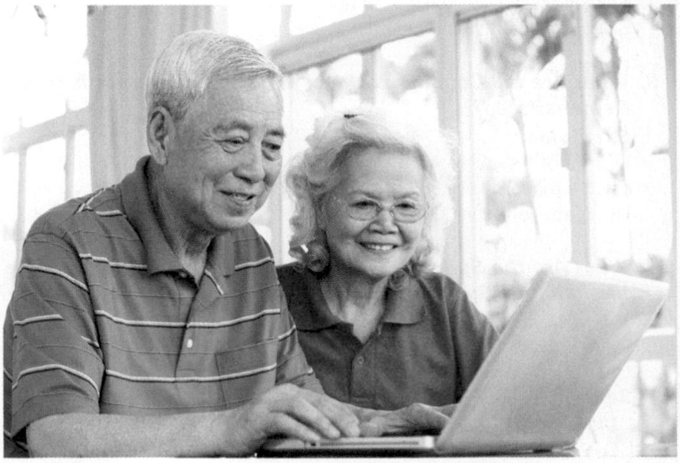

**FIG. 4-3** Older couple accessing the Web for health information. (©monkebusinessimages/iStock/Thinkstock.)

## Planning

Prioritize the patient's learning needs and agree on learning goals. If the patient's physical or psychologic condition interferes with his or her participation, involve the patient's caregiver(s) in the planning phase.

**Setting Goals.** It is important to have clear and measurable learning goals or outcomes (Table 4-8). Learning goals relate to the intended outcome of the learning process, guide the selection of teaching strategies, and help evaluate the patient's progress. Learning goals are parallel to patient outcomes in the nursing care plan (NCP). Most settings have standardized NCPs that contain preset goals and interventions for specific learning needs. You will modify these NCPs based on the patient's unique sociocultural and learner characteristics.

**Selecting Teaching Strategies.** Three factors that influence the selection of teaching strategies are (1) patient characteristics (e.g., learning style, educational background, culture, language skills), (2) subject matter, and (3) available resources. Table 4-9 provides a summary of the learner characteristics and recommended teaching approaches based on the generation of the patient or caregiver.[25,26]

Consider various teaching strategies (Table 4-10) when developing a teaching plan. Often, multiple strategies are used to improve learning (Fig. 4-4). Discussion is the most common type of interaction used in teaching patients and caregivers. Another type of group teaching involves *peer teaching*, as occurs in support groups. Patients dealing with common problems such as cancer, alcoholism, and eating disorders can benefit from peer teaching.

***Learning Materials.*** Use learning materials that are provided in multiple formats. Learn what resources are available in your agency and from support services and professional groups. The use of CDs/DVDs is helpful, particularly when teaching content

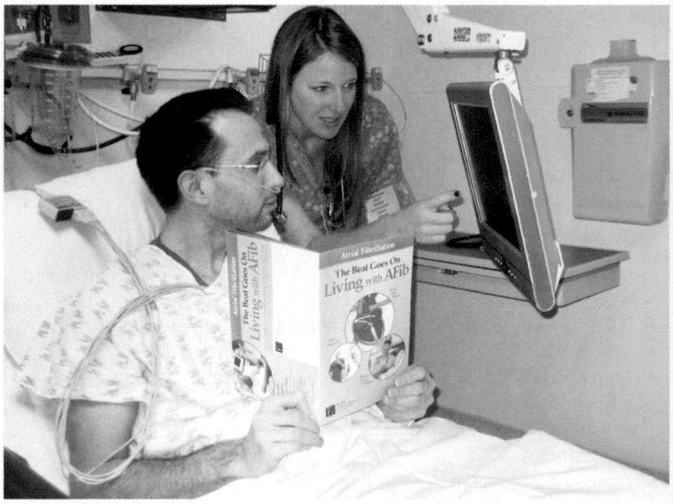

**FIG. 4-4** Effective teaching using a variety of strategies (written materials, computer-based patient education programs). (Courtesy Linda Bucher, RN, PhD, CEN, CNE, Staff Nurse, Virtua Memorial Hospital, Mt. Holly, N.J.)

### TABLE 4-8 Writing Learning Goals

**Elements of Learning Goals**

Learning goals (also called outcomes or objectives) are written statements that define exactly how patients demonstrate their mastery of the content. Goals address the following four questions:

1. ***Who Will Perform the Activity or Acquire the Desired Behavior?***
   ***Examples:***
   I (the patient) will
   I (the caregiver) will
   We (patient's family/caregivers) will
2. ***What Is the Actual Behavior That the Learner Will Exhibit to Demonstrate Mastery of the Goal?***
   ***Examples:***
   List the symptoms.
   Self-administer an insulin injection.
   Select from a hospital menu.
3. ***What Are the Conditions Under Which the Behavior Is to Be Demonstrated?***
   ***Examples:***
   In front of the nurse
   From a random list
   Using sterile technique
4. ***What Are the Specific Criteria That Will Be Used to Measure the Patient's Success, Such as Time and Degree of Accuracy?***
   ***Examples:***
   With 100% accuracy
   Over the next week
   Before discharge

**Verbs in Learning Goals**

| *Avoid vague, ambiguous verbs that are difficult to measure:* | *Use verbs that have precise descriptions with few interpretations:* |
|---|---|
| • Appreciate | • Identify |
| • Learn | • List |
| • Understand | • Describe |
| • Enjoy | • Demonstrate |
| • Feel | • Perform |
| • Value | • Select |

**Poorly and Well-Written Learning Goals**

| Example of Poorly Written Learning Goal | Examples of Well-Written Learning Goals |
|---|---|
| • The patient will understand the importance of managing his own colostomy.<br>*Analysis*: It is not clear how the patient will demonstrate that he "understands" the importance of managing his colostomy, when and to whom he will demonstrate this behavior, or what criteria will be used to determine whether the objective has been met. | • The patient will describe to the nurse the basic steps for changing the colostomy pouch and skin barrier by 2/14/17.<br>• Using correct technique, the patient will empty his colostomy pouch when one-third full.<br>• The patient's caregiver will perform colostomy care including changing the pouch and skin barrier.<br>• Given a list of signs and symptoms related to complications of a colostomy, the patient and caregiver will identify signs and symptoms to report to a health care provider before discharge.<br>*Analysis*: When learning goals are clear and specific and when they are documented in the patient's record, all members of the health care team can work together to accomplish the same outcomes. |

**TABLE 4-9 Learner Characteristics and Teaching Strategies by Generation**

| Birth Year | Learner Characteristics | Recommended Teaching Strategies |
|---|---|---|
| **Millennials (Generation Y, Yers, Nexters, Digital Natives)** | | |
| 1981-2000 | • Multitaskers<br>• Prefer interactive and virtual environments<br>• Technologically focused<br>• Require flexibility<br>• Short attention span<br>• Team players<br>• Prefer more structured learning compared to Xers<br>• Demand 24/7 access to learning | • Integrate technology and media in teaching (e.g., webinars, social networking sites, Avatars, Podcasts, Wii Fit).<br>• Discuss reliable websites.<br>• Consider health-related mobile applications.<br>• Download health information to smart phones, tablets, or similar devices.<br>• Consider group teaching. |
| **Generation X (Xers, Digital Natives)** | | |
| 1965-1980 | • Self-directed or self-paced learning<br>• Self-reliant<br>• Consumers of education<br>• Short attention span | • Integrate technology and media in teaching.<br>• Discuss reliable websites.<br>• Consider health-related mobile applications.<br>• Provide Web-based education materials.<br>• Provide education materials that are brief and easy to read.<br>• Encourage questions. |
| **Baby Boomers (Digital Immigrants)** | | |
| 1946-1964 | • Emphasis on self-knowledge<br>• Solve problems by action<br>• Acquisition of knowledge from authoritative sources<br>• Receptive to feedback<br>• Prefer text over graphics<br>• Process (step-by-step) oriented | • Assess ehealth literacy and consider strategies as appropriate.<br>• Consider lecture or lecture-discussion (e.g., PowerPoint presentation).<br>• Use patient education TV channels.<br>• Provide printed materials. |
| **Veterans (Traditionalists, Digital Immigrants)** | | |
| Born before 1946 | • Emphasis on rote learning<br>• Memorization of knowledge<br>• Follow rules | • Assess ehealth literacy and consider strategies as appropriate.<br>• Consider lecture or lecture-discussion.<br>• Use pictures and printed materials such as books. |

Compiled from Bradshaw M, Lowenstein A: *Innovative teaching strategies in nursing*, ed 6, Burlington, MA, 2014, Jones & Bartlett Learning; and United Nations Joint Staff Pension Fund: Traditionalists, baby boomers, generation X, generation Y (and generation Z) working together. Retrieved from *www.un.org/staffdevelopment/pdf/Designing%20Recruitment,%20Selection%20&%20Talent%20Management%20Model%20tailored%20to%20meet%20UNJSPF's%20Business%20Development%20Needs.pdf.*

that is mostly visual, such as the steps of a procedure (e.g., suctioning a tracheostomy). The health care agency's television system may also provide patient teaching programs (Fig. 4-4). A dedicated channel may be available and contain high-quality, professionally produced programs provided on demand or on a rotating schedule.

Printed materials continue to be used for teaching patients and caregivers and especially for those whose preferred learning style is reading. Many of these can be printed as needed for teaching (e.g., *www.kramesstaywell.com/home*). These materials are often used in combination with previously discussed teaching strategies. For instance, after a discussion on the effects of smoking on health, you may use material from the American Cancer Society to reinforce the information.

When writing teaching materials, use several techniques to keep the reading level at a fifth-grade level. These include the following: (1) place key information first using bold or italics; (2) use short, common words of one or two syllables; (3) define medical words in simple language if used; (4) keep sentences under 10 words if possible, and 15 at the most; (5) use pictures or drawings; and (6) use an active voice in the manner you would normally say something.[27] Whenever possible, evaluate written materials for readability level using word processing (e.g., Microsoft Word) or Web-based (e.g., *www.wordscount.info*) programs.

***Using Technology.*** Patients' use of the Internet and other digital technology (e.g., smart phones) to obtain health information and manage their health has steadily increased.[28] Patients can quickly do a Web search or open an application and have access to information about their disease, drugs, treatments, and surgeries (e.g., *www.hhs.gov/digitalstrategy/mobile/mobile-apps.html*). Your job is to help patients sift through the wide variety of information to decide if it is valid, reliable, and usable.[29] Understanding the principles of Web searching for health information and instructing patients in finding valid information are critical skills. The presence of Internet connections in many patient rooms (e.g., *www.getwellnetwork.com*) provides an opportunity for you to teach patients about their illness and how to use the Web to find related information.

Explore the use of digital technology by young and older patients and their caregivers. Factors that predict the use of the Web for health information (ehealth literacy) include access to high-speed connections, younger age, some college education, and confidence in using technology.[28] Patients who are chronically ill are more likely to seek health information on the Web.[30,31] Encourage patients to use websites established by the government, universities, or reputable health-related organizations (e.g., American Diabetes Association, American Heart Association, National Institutes of Health, U.S. Food and Drug Administration).

Although older adults are accessing the Web in greater numbers, many may not have the mental capacity, patience, or technical skills to successfully find health information.[32] Organizations dedicated to improving the quality of life for older adults promote the development of user-friendly websites (e.g., *www.nlm.nih.gov/pubs/checklist.pdf*) and publish guides to help older adults evaluate Web-based health information (e.g., *www.mlanet.org/resources/userguide.html*).

The quantity and complexity of digital health care technology available to patients and you will continue to increase.[33] *Telehealth*, a broad term that refers to the delivery of health-related services and information via telecommunications technologies, allows for (1) remote HCP-patient consultations *(telemedicine)*; (2) monitoring of vital signs, weight, heart rhythm, blood glucose, etc.; and (3) ongoing patient teaching[34] (see Fig. 34-7). Always educate yourself about these technologies and determine if any will be used when teaching patients.

## Implementation

During the implementation phase, use the planned teaching strategies to present information and teach new skills

**TABLE 4-10 Comparison of Teaching Strategies**

| Description | Advantages | Limitations |
|---|---|---|
| **Discussion ("Teach Back")** | | |
| • Purpose is to exchange points of view about a topic or to arrive at a decision or conclusion<br>• Can be done with patient, with patient and caregiver, or with group<br>• *Example:* Weight loss | • Allows for an active exchange of information and previous experiences among participants<br>• Good choice when patients have previous experience with subject and have information to share<br>• Nonthreatening format<br>• Can use peers (patients with common problems) to teach | • May require additional time depending on topic and number of participants |
| **Lecture-Discussion** | | |
| • Commonly used when group of patients and caregivers can benefit from basic information<br>• Lecture portion is short (i.e., 15-20 min)<br>• Discussion ("teach back") follows lecture<br>• *Example:* Basic principles of cardiac rehabilitation (e.g., exercise, nutrition) | • Combines short lecture to present basic information with time for discussion<br>• Provision of printed material related to lecture content is useful and recommended | • Need to limit number of lecture topics to three to five<br>• May require additional time depending on topic and number of participants |
| **Demonstration/Return Demonstration ("Show Back")** | | |
| • Purpose is to teach patient and caregiver to perform a skill<br>• Through return demonstration ("show back") can evaluate patient's ability to perform skill (Fig. 4-5)<br>• *Examples:* Dressing change, injection | • Provides for learning and practice of physical skills<br>• Dividing skill into series of smaller steps facilitates mastery and provides reinforcement | • May require additional time for practice needed to master skill<br>• Patients with limited manual dexterity may have difficulty |
| **Use of Teaching Resources** | | |
| • Audiovisual aids to supplement teaching<br>• Printed materials (e.g., brochures)<br>• CDs/DVDs<br>• Hospital-based TV (Fig. 4-4)<br>• Digital and communication technologies (e.g., mobile applications, Web-based patient education programs, game-based education, online support groups)<br>• Telehealth (see Fig. 34-7) | • Enhance the presentation through visual and/or auditory stimulation<br>• Best used in combination with other teaching strategies<br>• Use of digital and communication technologies for health information is the preferred choice for many<br>• Web access in patient rooms is standard in most health care agencies<br>• Health information can be provided and reinforced to patients remotely | • Materials must be previewed and evaluated (e.g., accuracy, completeness, reading level) before using<br>• Websites, games, applications, programs, etc. must be evaluated for validity of information<br>• May not be appropriate for all learners (e.g., lack of interest, decreased mental capacity)<br>• Finances (e.g., equipment purchase, Internet service) may be a limiting factor to using digital technology |

(Table 4-10). Incorporate verbal and nonverbal communication skills, active listening, and empathy into the process. Based on the assessment of the patient's physical, psychologic, sociocultural, and learner characteristics, determine how much the patient can participate. Whenever possible and appropriate, involve the patient's caregiver(s) in the teaching-learning process.

In implementing the teaching plan, remember the principles and characteristics of the adult learner. Reinforcement and reward are important, but be aware that phrases such as, "Aren't you doing well!" in a tone one would use with a child can be condescending to adult learners.

## Evaluation

Evaluation, the final step in the learning process, is a measure of the degree to which the patient has achieved the learning goals. Various evaluation techniques can be used (Table 4-11). Use techniques such as "teach back" and "show back" to determine the knowledge and skill levels of the patient and/or caregiver throughout the teaching and learning process[35] (Fig. 4-5). If certain goals are not reached, reassess the patient and revise the teaching plan accordingly.

The patient most likely had been administering insufficient insulin to himself for some time. The patient's vision had declined over the 20 years, and special equipment was now necessary for him to safely and correctly administer the insulin. The lesson here is that assumptions regarding a patient's

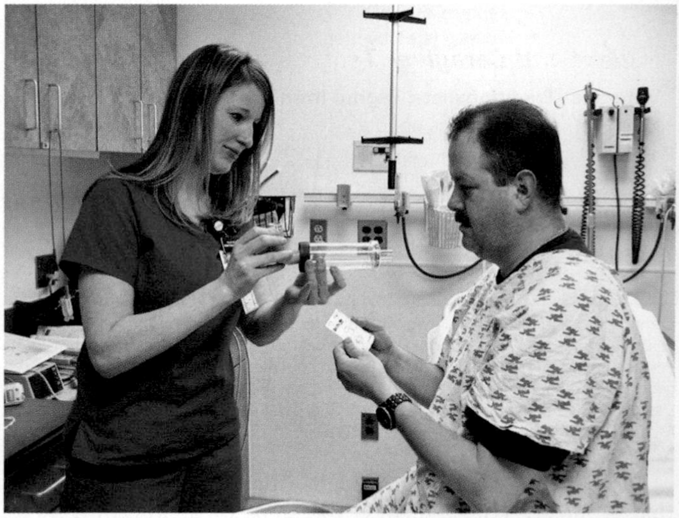

FIG. 4-5 Teaching using discussion ("teach back") and demonstration/return demonstration ("show back") increases successful learning by the patient. (Courtesy Linda Bucher, RN, PhD, CEN, CNE, Staff Nurse, Virtua Memorial Hospital, Mt. Holly, N.J.)

**TABLE 4-11 Evaluation of Patient and Caregiver Learning**

| Technique | Strategy and Examples |
|---|---|
| **Observe patient or caregiver directly.** | • Ask person to show you how to change the dressing.<br>• Return demonstration ("show back") determines whether<br>  • Skill has been mastered<br>  • Further instruction is needed<br>  • Patient and caregiver are ready for new or additional content |
| **Observe verbal and nonverbal cues.** | • Teaching may have to be delayed, further teaching is needed, or different strategy should be used if patient or caregiver<br>  • Asks you to repeat instructions<br>  • Loses eye contact<br>  • Begins to doze in chair or bed<br>  • Becomes restless or fidgety<br>  • Does not speak English |
| **Ask open-ended questions ("teach back").** | • Open-ended questions provide more information about understanding than close-ended questions, which require only a "yes" or "no."<br>• Ask questions such as<br>  • "How often do you need to change the dressing?"<br>  • "What will you do if you develop chest pain at home?" |
| **Talk with caregiver ("teach back").** | • Involve caregiver in the evaluation process.<br>• Ask questions such as<br>  • "What medications is she taking?"<br>  • "When does he use his oxygen?" |
| **Seek the patient's self-evaluation of progress.** | • Ask patient's opinion about his or her progress.<br>  • What evidence does the patient have that the goals are being met?<br>  • Is the patient ready to go forward with learning new material? |

## CHECK YOUR PRACTICE

Your patient is a 53-yr-old male with type 1 diabetes mellitus who entered the hospital with a blood glucose level of 550 mg/dL (30.53 mmol/L). He is now stable and soon will be discharged.

You prepare his insulin and plan to give him the syringe to let him do his own injection. Before you go to his room, your preceptor suggests that you observe his technique of preparing the insulin as well as the injection. You are puzzled by this comment because he has had diabetes for 32 years and should know how to do it.

When you go to his room, you ask him to prepare the insulin injection ("show back"). You notice that he filled the syringe with 30 units of insulin and 10 units of air, instead of 40 units of insulin. After correcting the dose and questioning the patient more fully ("teach back"), you wonder what happened because you thought he knew the correct dosage of insulin.

- What are possible reasons that he did not draw up the correct amount of insulin?

knowledge and skills are dangerous. Always evaluate past and new knowledge and skills.

Long-term evaluation of learning goals often requires follow-up after discharge. Provide a written schedule of visits and other appropriate referrals for the patient before he or she leaves the hospital or clinic. The patient's caregiver(s) also must be familiar with the follow-up plan so that everyone involved in the patient's long-term progress is on the same page.[36]

Documentation is an essential and required component throughout the entire teaching-learning process. Record everything from the assessment through plans for evaluation and follow-up. Because various members of the health care team use these records in different settings and for different reasons, the teaching goals, strategies, and evaluation results need to be clear, complete, and available to all members of the health care team.

## CASE STUDY

### *Patient and Caregiver Teaching*

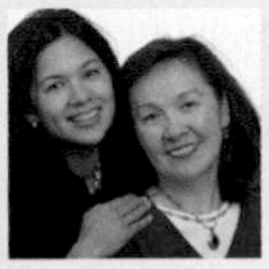

(©Thomas M Perkins/ Shutterstock)

**Patient Profile**

M.L., a 60-year-old Asian woman, is admitted to the hospital with a diagnosis of exacerbation of chronic obstructive pulmonary disease (COPD).

**Subjective Data**

- History of COPD for 10 years. Reports a chronic cough but denies any recent change in color of sputum. States "I stopped smoking last year, but my son-in-law smokes."
- Past medical history: gastroesophageal reflux disease; macular degeneration in right eye.
- Social history: widowed 5 years ago and since then has lived with daughter and son-in-law who work full time. Cares for two young grandchildren after school. English is M.L.'s second language.

**Objective Data**

***Physical Examination***

- Alert, cognitively intact, anxious, thin woman with dyspnea on minimal exertion. Speaking in short phases or sentences. States "I have no energy."
- Using oxygen via nasal cannula at 2 L/min
- Weight 100 lb, height 5 ft 2 in

***Diagnostic Studies***

- Chest x-ray negative for acute infection
- Arterial blood gases on room air: pH 7.35, $PaCO_2$ 47 mm Hg, $PaO_2$ 75 mm Hg, $HCO_3^-$ 30 mEq/L
- $O_2$ saturation (via pulse oximetry) during 6-minute walk test on room air = 83%
- Forced expiratory volume in 1 second of expiration ($FEV_1$) = 60% of predicted

**Interprofessional Care**

- Medications: bronchodilator therapy (inpatient nebulizer therapy, inhalers on discharge), oral corticosteroids
- Continuous home $O_2$ therapy: $O_2$ at 2 L/min via nasal cannula
- Pulmonary rehabilitation: inpatient and outpatient

**Discussion Questions**

1. ***Priority Decision:*** Given M.L.'s history, what are the priority learning needs?
2. ***Patient-Centered Care:*** What factors (e.g., sociocultural, physical, psychologic) may influence M.L.'s response to teaching?
3. ***Patient-Centered Care:*** What potential challenges might you expect when planning to teach M.L.? How would you manage them?
4. ***Priority Decision:*** Identify two priority nursing diagnoses. Develop a teaching plan for M.L. based on these nursing diagnoses.

Answers available at *http://evolve.elsevier.com/Lewis/medsurg.*

## BRIDGE TO NCLEX EXAMINATION

The number of the question corresponds to the same-numbered outcome at the beginning of the chapter.

1. Which technique is *most* appropriate when using motivational interviewing with a patient who tells you that he is ready to start a weight-loss program?
   - **a.** Confirm that the patient is serious about losing weight.
   - **b.** Insist that the patient consider an organized group weight-loss program.
   - **c.** Focus on the patient's strengths to support his optimism that he can successfully lose weight.
   - **d.** Ask a prescribed set of questions to increase the patient's awareness of his dietary behaviors.
2. Which is the *priority* patient teaching strategy when limited time is available?
   - **a.** Setting realistic goals that have high priority for the patient
   - **b.** Referring the patient to a nurse educator in private practice for teaching
   - **c.** Observing more experienced nurse-teachers to learn how to teach faster and more efficiently
   - **d.** Providing reading materials for the patient instead of discussing information the patient needs to learn
3. The nurse needs to include caregivers in patient teaching primarily because *(select all that apply)*
   - **a.** they provide all of the care for patients after discharge.
   - **b.** they might feel rejected if they are not included in the teaching.
   - **c.** patients have better outcomes when their caregivers are involved.
   - **d.** the patient may be too ill or too stressed to fully understand the teaching.
   - **e.** caregivers are responsible for the overall management of the patient's care.
4. Which patient characteristic enhances the teaching-learning process?
   - **a.** Moderate anxiety
   - **b.** High self-efficacy
   - **c.** Being in the precontemplative stage of change
   - **d.** Being able to laugh about the current health problem
5. What would be the *priority* teaching goal for a middle-aged Hispanic woman regarding methods to relieve symptoms of menopause?
   - **a.** Prevent the development of future disease.
   - **b.** Maintain the patient's current state of health.
   - **c.** Provide information on possible treatment options.
   - **d.** Change the patient's beliefs about herbal supplements.
6. A patient tells the nurse that she enjoys talking with others and sharing experiences but often falls asleep when reading. Which teaching strategy would be *most* effective with this patient?
   - **a.** Role playing
   - **b.** Group teaching
   - **c.** Lecture-discussion
   - **d.** Web-based programs
7. The nurse has taught a patient's wife (his primary caregiver) how to administer insulin to her husband. Evaluation of the nurse's teaching effectiveness before discharge would include
   - **a.** arranging for follow-up with a home care nurse.
   - **b.** monitoring the patient's glucose readings before discharge.
   - **c.** asking the caregiver to "show back" her ability to administer insulin.
   - **d.** asking the caregiver what she found helpful about the teaching experience.

1. c, 2. a, 3. c, d, 4. b, 5. c, 6. b, 7. c.

For rationales to these answers and even more NCLEX review questions, visit *http://evolve.elsevier.com/Lewis/medsurg*.

## EVOLVE WEBSITE

http://evolve.elsevier.com/Lewis/medsurg

**Review Questions (Online Only)**

**Key Points**

**Answer Keys for Questions**

- Rationales for Bridge to NCLEX Examination Questions
- Answer Guidelines for Case Study on p. 57

**Conceptual Care Map Creator**

**Audio Glossary**

**Content Updates**

## REFERENCES


1. Centers for Disease Control and Prevention: Chronic disease prevention and health promotion, Washington, DC, 2014. Retrieved from *www.cdc.gov/chronicdisease/overview/#sec1*.

*2. Mitchell S, Gardiner P, Sadikova E, et al: Patient activation and 30-day post-discharge hospital utilization, *J Gen Int Med* 29:349, 2014.

3. American Nurses Credentialing Center: Forces of magnetism: force 11: nurses as teachers, 2014. Retrieved from *www.nursecredentialing.org/ForcesofMagnetism.aspx#11*.

4. Redman BK: *The practice of patient education*, ed 10, St Louis, 2007, Mosby.

5. Knowles MS, Holton EF, Swanson RA: *The adult learner: the definitive classic in adult education and human resource development*, ed 7, St Louis, 2011, Mosby.

*6. Prochaska J, Velicer W: The transtheoretical model of health behavior change, *Am J Health Promot* 12:38, 1997. (Classic)

7. Rollnick S, Miller WR, Yahne CE: *Motivational interviewing in health care: helping patients change behavior*, New York, 2008, Guilford Press. (Classic)

*8. Miller WR: *Enhancing motivation for change in substance abuse treatment: Treatment Improvement Protocol (TIP) series 35, DHHS pub no (SMA) 99-3354*, Rockville, Md, 1999, US Department of Health and Human Services. Retrieved from *www.ncbi.nlm.nih.gov/books/NBK64967*. (Classic)

9. Feinberg L, Reinhard SC, Houser A, et al: Valuing the invaluable: 2011 update—the growing contributions and costs of family caregiving, AARP Public Policy Institute. Retrieved from *http://assets.aarp.org/rgcenter/ppi/ltc/i51-caregiving.pdf*.

10. Levine C: Supporting family caregivers: the hospital nurse's assessment of family caregiver needs, *Am J Nurs* 111:47, 2011.

11. Fowler C: Caring for the caregiver, *Nursing* 44:60, 2014.

12. The Joint Commission: 2014 Hospital national patient safety goals. Retrieved from *www.jointcommission.org/standards_information/npsgs.aspx*.

13. American Hospital Association: The patient care partnership. Retrieved from *www.aha.org/advocacy-issues/communicatingpts/pt-care-partnership.shtml*.

14. The Joint Commission: Speak up initiatives, 2014. Retrieved from *www.jointcommission.org/speakup.aspx*.

15. National Patient Safety Foundation: Ask me 3. Retrieved from *https://npsf.site-ym.com/default.asp?page=askme3*.

16. Geriatric Mental Health Foundation: Consumer/patient information. Retrieved from *www.gmhfonline.org/gmhf/consumer/factsheets/hlthage_mental.html.*
*17. Farrell K, Wicks MN, Martin JC: Chronic disease self-management improved with enhanced self-efficacy, *Clin Nurs Res* 13(4):289, 2004. (Classic)
18. The Joint Commission: What did the doctor say? Improving health literacy to protect patient safety, 2007. Retrieved from *www.jointcommission.org/assets/1/18/improving_health_literacy.pdf.*
19. Barclay L: Screening questions may help predict limited health literacy, *Ann Fam Med* 7:24, 2009.
20. U.S. Department of Health and Human Services, Office of Disease Prevention and Health Promotion: Quick guide to health literacy, fact sheet, health literacy and health outcomes. Retrieved from *www.health.gov/communication/literacy/quickguide/factsliteracy.htm.*
*21. Morris NS, MacLean CD, Chew LD, et al: The single item literacy screener: evaluation of a brief instrument to identify limited reading ability, *BMC Fam Pract* 7:21, 2006. (Classic)
22. Wilson-Stronks A, Lee KK, Cordero CL, et al: One size does not fit all: meeting the health care needs of diverse populations, Oakland Terrace, Ill, The Joint Commission. Retrieved from *www.jointcommission.org/assets/1/6/HLCOneSizeFinal.pdf.*
23. Inott T, Kennedy BB: Assessing learning styles: practical tips for patient education, *Nurs Clin North Am* 46:313, 2011.
24. Office of Disease Prevention and Health Promotion: What is e-health? Retrieved from *www.health.gov/communication/ehealth.*
25. Bradshaw M, Lowenstein A: *Innovative teaching strategies in nursing*, ed 6, Burlington, Mass, 2014, Jones & Bartlett Learning.
26. United Nations Joint Staff Pension Fund: Traditionalists, baby boomers, generation X, generation Y (and generation Z) working together. Retrieved from *www.un.org/staffdevelopment/pdf/Designing%20Recruitment,%20Selection%20&%20Talent%20Management%20Model%20tailored%20to%20meet%20UNJSPF's%20Business%20Development%20Needs.pdf.*
27. Medline Plus: How to write easy-to-read health materials, 2013. Retrieved from *www.nlm.nih.gov/medlineplus/etr.html.*
28. Pew Research Internet Project: Trends to watch. Retrieved from *www.pewinternet.org/2009/06/11/trends-to-watch.*
29. Wood F, Robson M, Thompson M, et al: Selecting the best type of mobile application for chronic disease self-management, *Comput Inform Nurs* 31:208, 2013.
*30. Stellefson M, Chaney B, Ochipa K, et al: YouTube as a source of chronic obstructive pulmonary disease patient education: a social media content analysis, *Chronic Resp Dis* 11:61, 2014.
*31. Lee S, Shin S: Effectiveness of virtual reality using video gaming technology in elderly adults with diabetes mellitus, *Diabetes Technol Ther* 15:489, 2013.
*32. Levy H, Janke AT, Langa KM: Health literacy and the digital divide among older Americans, *J Gen Intern Med* 30:384, 2015.
33. Trossman S: Back to the future? Telehealth services, tele-nursing are on the rise, *American Nurse* Sept/Oct:1, 2014.
34. GlobalMed: Telehealth, telecare, telemedicine…what's the difference? Retrieved from *www.globalmed.com/additional-resources/telehealth-telecare-and-telemedicine-whats-the-difference.php.*
35. Minnesota Health Literacy Partnership: Teach-back: what does your patient really understand? Retrieved from *healthliteracymn.org/sites/default/files/images/files/Teach-Back_program_guide_updated_011212.pdf.*
*36. Agency for Healthcare Research and Quality: Implementing re-engineered hospital discharges (Project RED): frequently asked questions, 2009. Retrieved from *www.ahrq.gov/news/kt/red/redfaq.htm.*

*Evidence-based information for clinical practice.

5

# Chronic Illness and Older Adults

*Sherry A. Greenberg*

*You don't stop laughing when you grow old, you grow old when you stop laughing.*

***George Bernard Shaw***

http://evolve.elsevier.com/Lewis/medsurg/

## LEARNING OUTCOMES

1. Describe the prevention and major causes of chronic illness.
2. Explain the characteristics of a chronic illness.
3. Describe the demographics of aging.
4. Define *ageism.*
5. Explain the needs of special populations of older adults.
6. Describe nursing interventions to assist older adults with chronic illnesses.
7. Describe common problems of older adults related to hospitalization and acute illness and the nurse's role in assisting them.
8. Differentiate among care alternatives to meet needs of older adults.
9. Describe the nurse's role in health promotion, disease prevention, and managing the special needs of older adults.

## KEY TERMS

ageism, p. 63
chronic illness, Table 5-1, p. 61
elder mistreatment (EM), p. 66
ethnogeriatric, p. 66
frail older adult, p. 63
gerontologic nursing, p. 69
Medicaid, p. 68
Medicare, p. 68
old-old adult, p. 63
young-old adult, p. 63

This chapter discusses issues related to chronic illness and aging. The population of older adults is growing rapidly. You need to consider their multiple, complex health care conditions and needs.

## CHRONIC ILLNESS

Illness can be categorized as either acute or chronic (Table 5-1). The U.S. health care system faces a growing burden of chronic illness as the population ages. Chronic illnesses account for 70% of all deaths in the United States. Chronic illness results in limitations in physical functioning, work productivity, and quality of life for nearly 1 out of 10 Americans. Older adults often live with more than one chronic illness, frequently up to six or more. A significant portion of U.S. health care dollars go toward the treatment of chronic illnesses.[1] The management of a chronic illness can greatly affect the lives of the patient, family, and caregiver. Table 5-2 presents the impact of some chronic illnesses.

In addition to people living longer, other societal changes have contributed to the increase in chronic illnesses. These include insufficient physical activity, lack of access to fresh fruits and vegetables, tobacco use, and alcohol consumption.[1]

### Trajectory of Chronic Illness

The individual with a chronic illness can move from a level of optimum functioning, with the illness well controlled, to a period of physical instability. Corbin and Strauss proposed a view of chronic illness as a trajectory (Fig. 5-1) with overlapping phases[2] (Table 5-3). This trajectory characterizes the common course of most chronic conditions. In addition, Corbin and Strauss identified the seven tasks of those who are chronically ill (Table 5-4). These tasks are discussed in the following sections.

**Preventing and Managing a Crisis.** Most chronic illnesses have the potential for an acute exacerbation of symptoms, which may result in further disability or death. Examples include the patient with heart disease who has another myocardial infarction or the patient with asthma who has a severe attack. A major task for the patient and caregiver is to learn to prevent or manage the crisis. First, the patient and caregiver need to understand the potential for the crisis to occur. Second, they need to know ways to prevent or modify the threat. This often involves adherence to a prescribed medical regimen. Patients also need to know the signs and symptoms of the onset of a crisis. Depending on the chronic illness, signs and symptoms may occur suddenly (e.g., bleeding in a patient with inflammatory bowel disease) or

Reviewed by Donna E. McCabe, DNP, APRN-BC, GNP, New York University, College of Nursing, New York, New York; and Lorraine Nowakowski-Grier, MSN, APRN, BC, CDE, Diabetes Nurse Practitioner, Christiana Care Health Services, Nursing Development & Education, Newark, Delaware.

**TABLE 5-1 Characteristics of Acute and Chronic Illness**

| Description | Characteristics |
|---|---|
| **Acute Illness** | |
| Diseases that have a rapid onset and short duration<br>*Examples:* colds, influenza, acute gastroenteritis | • Usually self-limiting<br>• Responds readily to treatment<br>• Complications infrequent<br>• After illness, return to previous level of functioning |
| **Chronic Illness** | |
| Diseases that are prolonged, do not resolve spontaneously, and are rarely cured completely<br>*Examples:* see Table 5-2 | • Permanent impairments or deviations from normal<br>• Irreversible pathologic changes<br>• Residual disability<br>• Special rehabilitation required<br>• Need for long-term medical and/or nursing management |

slowly (e.g., heart failure in a patient with untreated hypertension). It is important for the patient and caregiver to develop a plan to manage a crisis that is likely to occur.

**Carrying Out Prescribed Treatment Regimen.** Treatment regimens vary in degree of difficulty and the impact they have on the person's lifestyle. Treatment regimens may appear challenging or time consuming, such as changing a dressing multiple times a day or instituting a toileting program. However, they generally save time and prevent complications.

**Controlling Symptoms.** An important task for those with chronic illnesses is to learn to control symptoms so that desired activities may be continued. Some individuals redesign their lifestyle by learning to plan ahead, such as individuals with heart failure adjusting the time they take diuretics to avoid needing to rush to a bathroom if going out for the day. Independence in decision making is encouraged, but changes in treatment regimens should be done in collaboration with their health care provider (HCP) to avoid an exacerbation of the illness. Others may redesign their living space. Patients and their families and/or caregivers need to learn about the pattern of symptoms, such as typical onset, duration, and severity, so that lifestyle may be changed accordingly, while maintaining safety.

**Reordering Time.** People with chronic illness often report having too much or too little time. Treatment plans that require large amounts of time for the person, as well as caregivers, may necessitate changing schedules or eliminating other activities. For example, the patient with a new ileostomy needs to plan for increased time in the bathroom to change the drainage bag.

**Adjusting to Changes in the Course of Disease.** Some diseases, such as multiple sclerosis, have unpredictable courses that make planning activities difficult. Part of the individual's task is to develop a personal identity that includes the chronic illness and adjust to the lifestyle changes it necessitates. For example, an individual taking warfarin (Coumadin) due to a mechanical heart valve may need to avoid extreme physical sports that have a high potential for injury.

**Preventing Social Isolation.** Social isolation may occur with chronic illness because the individual chooses to withdraw from previous activities or because others withdraw from the chronically ill person. For example, a woman who has aphasia secondary to a stroke may be unwilling to go out in public because of embarrassment related to communication issues.

**TABLE 5-2 Impact of Chronic Illnesses**

| Chronic Illness | Impact | CONTENT IN BOOK Chapter | CONTENT IN BOOK Page |
|---|---|---|---|
| **Alzheimer's disease** | • Affects 5.4 million people<br>• Sixth leading cause of death | 59 | 1401 |
| **Arthritis** | • Affects 1 in 5 people<br>• One of most common chronic illnesses | 64 | 1517 |
| **Cancer** | • Second leading cause of death | 15 | 234 |
| **Chronic obstructive pulmonary disease** | • Affects many older adults<br>• Third leading cause of death | 28 | 557 |
| **Coronary artery disease** | • Affects about 17 million adults<br>• Leading cause of death | 33 | 702 |
| **Diabetes** | • Affects >29 million Americans<br>• 8.1 million do not know they have the disease<br>• Seventh leading cause of death | 48 | 1120 |
| **Heart failure** | • Most common reason older adults are hospitalized | 34 | 737 |
| **Obesity** | • Affects about 34% of adults<br>• Major contributor to other health problems | 40 | 874 |
| **Stroke** | • Affects about 7 million adults, 15%-30% disabled<br>• Leading cause of serious disability<br>• Fifth leading cause of death | 57 | 1345 |
| **HIV/AIDS** | • 50,000 new cases each year<br>• Affects >1 million Americans | 14 | 213 |

Data from Centers for Disease Control and Prevention: CDC's Chronic Disease Press Releases. Retrieved from *www.cdc.gov/chronicdisease/resources/press*, 2014.
*AIDS,* Acquired immunodeficiency syndrome; *HIV,* human immunodeficiency virus.

**Attempting to Normalize Interactions With Others.** Most individuals with chronic illness attempt to manage symptoms so that they can hide their disabilities or disfigurement. This may involve wearing a prosthesis or demonstrating that they can function the same as a person without a disability or chronic illness. An example of this is the woman with heart failure who stops walking to catch her breath but appears to be inspecting a plant or looking in a store window.

### Prevention of Chronic Illness

Chronic illnesses are often preventable. *Primary prevention* refers to measures such as nutritious diet, proper exercise, and immunizations that prevent the occurrence of a specific disease. Appropriate immunizations for older adults include influenza, pneumococcal, herpes zoster, tetanus/diphtheria/pertussis (Td/Tdap), and hepatitis A and B. *Secondary prevention* refers to actions aimed at early detection of disease that can lead

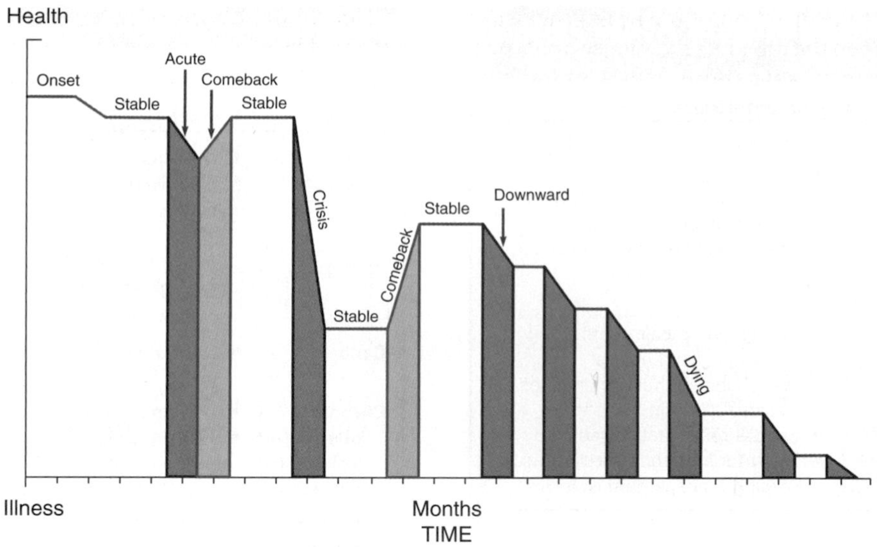


**FIG. 5-1** The Chronic Illness Trajectory is a theoretical model of chronic illness. The trajectory model of chronic illness recognizes that chronic illness will have many phases (Table 5-3). (From Woog P: *The chronic illness trajectory framework: the Corbin and Strauss nursing model,* New York, 1992, Springer.)

**TABLE 5-3 Chronic Illness Trajectory**

| Phases | Description |
|---|---|
| **Onset** | • Signs and symptoms are present.<br>• Disease diagnosed. |
| **Stable** | • Illness course and symptoms controlled by treatment regimen.<br>• Person maintains everyday activities. |
| **Acute** | • Active illness with severe and unrelieved symptoms or complications.<br>• Hospitalization may be required for management. |
| **Comeback** | • Gradual return to an acceptable way of life. |
| **Crisis** | • Life-threatening situation occurs.<br>• Emergency services are necessary. |
| **Unstable** | • Unable to keep symptoms or disease course under control.<br>• Life becomes disrupted while patient works to regain stability.<br>• Hospitalization not required. |
| **Downward** | • Gradual and progressive deterioration in physical or mental status.<br>• Accompanied by increasing disability and symptoms.<br>• Continuous alterations in everyday life activities. |
| **Dying** | • Patient has to relinquish everyday life interests and activities, let go, and die peacefully.<br>• Immediate weeks, days, hours preceding death. |

Source: Woog P: *The chronic illness trajectory framework: the Corbin and Strauss nursing model,* New York, 1992, Springer.

to interventions to prevent disease progression. *Tertiary prevention* refers to activities that limit disease progression such as rehabilitation.

## ❖ NURSING MANAGEMENT: CHRONIC ILLNESS

Diagnosis and treatment of the acute phase or acute exacerbations of a chronic illness sometimes take place in a hospital. Other phases of a chronic illness are regularly assessed and managed in an ambulatory care setting, at home, in an assisted living facility, or in a skilled nursing facility.

**TABLE 5-4 Seven Tasks of People With Chronic Illness**

1. Prevent and manage a crisis.
2. Carry out prescribed treatment regimen.
3. Control symptoms.
4. Reorder time.
5. Adjust to changes in course of disease.
6. Prevent social isolation.
7. Attempt to normalize interactions with others.

Source: Corbin JM, Strauss A: A nursing model for chronic illness management based upon the trajectory framework, *Sch Inq Nurs Pract* 5:155, 1991.

An assessment of health status, at least annually, includes an individual's level of daily functioning and his or her perception of relative health, function, and/or illness. Health assessment includes activities of daily living (ADLs), such as bathing, dressing, eating, toileting, and transferring. It also includes instrumental ADLs (IADLs), such as using a phone, shopping, preparing food, housekeeping, doing laundry, arranging transportation, taking medications, and handling finances.[3]

Because the majority of chronic illnesses are treated in an ambulatory care setting, it is increasingly important for patients and caregivers to understand and manage their own health. The term *self-management* refers to the individual's ability to manage his or her health, especially in response to living with a chronic illness. It refers to the ability to manage symptoms, medications and treatment regimen, physical and psychosocial consequences, and lifestyle changes.[4] Self-management is in conjunction with family and HCP.

You play an important role in the management of individuals with chronic illness. This includes conducting a comprehensive history and physical assessment, participating in interventions and plan of care, teaching the patient and caregiver regarding the treatment plan, implementing strategies for symptom management, and evaluating patient outcomes.

Family caregivers (e.g., spouses, partners, adult children) often have important roles in the life of the chronically ill person. The ideal situation is one in which family caregivers work together with the patient to manage the chronic condition(s). This collaboration begins under the direction of the health care team at the time of diagnosis. When the caregiver is a spouse or partner who is also older, he or she may have a chronic illness or multiple chronic conditions as well, which may complicate the coordination of care.[5] The stresses and needs of family caregivers are discussed in Chapter 4.

# OLDER ADULTS

## DEMOGRAPHICS OF AGING

The older adult population (those 65 years of age and older) continues to outpace the rest of the population. More than 41 million people, or 13% of the population, are age 65 or older.[6] Nearly one in five U.S. residents is expected to be 65 or older by 2030. The U.S. Census Bureau predicts life expectancy to continue to increase for both men and women. Those reaching 65 years have an average life expectancy of an additional 19.2 years, specifically 20.4 years for females and 17.8 years for males.[7] Whether this gender difference is due to differences in health behaviors (e.g., smoking, alcohol use) or occupation is not known.

### GENDER DIFFERENCES

#### *Older Adults*

**Men**

- More likely to be married and living with spouse or partner
- More likely to have health insurance
- Higher income after retirement
- Less likely to be involved in caregiving activities
- Generally have fewer chronic health conditions than women

**Women**

- More likely to live alone
- More likely to be widowed
- Less likely to have health insurance
- More likely to live in poverty
- Poverty rates highest among minority women
- More likely to lack formal work experience leading to lower income
- More likely to rely on Social Security as major source of income
- More likely to be caregiver of ill spouse or partner
- Have a higher incidence of chronic health conditions such as arthritis, hypertension, stroke, and diabetes

The fastest-growing segment of older Americans is people ages 85 or older. The increase in life span is due to declining infant mortality, new drug therapies, mechanical devices, and improved surgical interventions. In addition, greater emphasis on health promotion, disease prevention, and earlier detection as well as better care management has led to more Americans living past 85 years.

In the United States 13% of people over age 65 are of racial or ethnic minority populations, including 9% African Americans; 4% Asian/Pacific Islanders; and less than 1% American Indians, Eskimos, and Aleuts. People of Hispanic/Latino ethnicity (who may be of any race) represent 7% of the older population.[7] By 2030 the proportion of older adults who are people of racial or ethnic minority will increase 125% (Latinos 155%; African Americans 104%; American Indians, Eskimos, and Aleuts 116%; and Asian/Pacific Islanders 119%), while growth in the European-American population will increase by only 54%.[7]

Upcoming cohorts of older adults will likely have increased access to higher education, employment, technology, and resources than previous cohorts. According to the U.S. Census Bureau, the majority of the population 65 and older completed high school or higher education. Additionally, a quarter of the population 65 and older earned a bachelor's degree or higher.[8]

The terms **young-old adult** (65 to 74 years of age) and **old-old adult** (85 years of age and older) describe two groups of older adults with different characteristics and needs. Nearly 6% of individuals age 65 to 74 and 25% of those 85 and older live in nursing homes. The old-old adult is often a widowed, divorced, or single woman dependent on family for support or care. Many old-old adults have outlived children, spouses or partners, and siblings.

The **frail older adult** is usually over age 75 and has physical, cognitive, and/or mental conditions that may interfere with independently performing ADLs. (Frail older adults are discussed later in this chapter.)

## ATTITUDES TOWARD AGING

Who is old? The answer to this question often depends on the respondent's age and attitude. It is important to understand that aging is normal and is not related to pathology or disease. Age is established by a date in time and is influenced by many factors, including emotional and physical health, developmental stage, socioeconomic status, culture, and ethnicity.

As people age, they are exposed to new and different life experiences. The accumulation of these differences makes older adults more diverse than any other age group. As you assess older adults, consider and value their diversity and life history. Also assess their own perceptions of what it means to be an older adult. The majority of older adults report having good-to-excellent health despite having a chronic condition. However, older adults with poor health often report a higher perceived age and lower sense of well-being when compared with healthy older adults. Age is important, but it may not be the most relevant factor in determining appropriate care of an individual older adult.

Myths and stereotypes about aging are often supported by media reports of older adults who are "problematic." These commonly held misconceptions may lead to omissions or errors in assessment and unnecessary limitations or interventions. For example, if you think that all older people are rigid in their thinking, you may not present new ideas to a patient.[9]

**Ageism** is a negative attitude based on age. Ageism leads to discrimination and disparities in the care given to older adults. If you demonstrate negative attitudes, it may be because you fear your own aging process or you are not knowledgeable about aging and the health care needs of the older adult.

## BIOLOGIC AGING

From a biologic view, *aging* reflects the changes that occur over time. Biologic aging is a multifactorial process involving genetics, diet, and environment.[10] In part, biologic aging can be viewed as a balance of positive and negative factors (Fig. 5-2). Current research is directed at increasing the average life span and the quality of life of older adults. The hope is that new antiaging therapies will be developed to slow down or reverse age-related changes that result in chronic illness and disability.

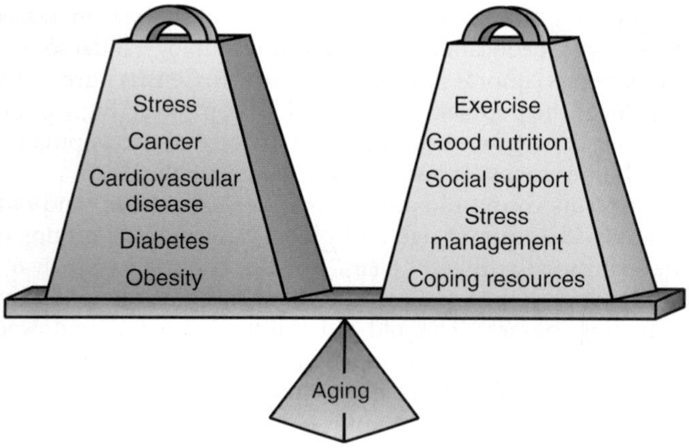


**FIG. 5-2** The aging process can be viewed as a balance between negative and positive factors.

## AGE-RELATED PHYSIOLOGIC CHANGES

Age-related changes affect every body system. These changes are normal and occur as people age. However, the age at which specific changes occur differs from person to person and within the same person. For instance, a person may have gray hair at age 45 but have relatively unwrinkled skin at age 80. In your role as a nurse, assess for age-related changes. Table 5-5 presents a list of tables in which specific age-related assessment findings can be found throughout the book.

**TABLE 5-5 Gerontologic Assessment Differences**

***Summary of Tables***

| Body System | Table Number | Page |
|---|---|---|
| Visual | 20-1 | 353 |
| Auditory | 20-7 | 361 |
| Integumentary | 22-1 | 397 |
| Respiratory | 25-4 | 459 |
| Hematologic | 29-3 | 593 |
| Cardiovascular | 31-1 | 663 |
| Gastrointestinal | 38-5 | 840 |
| Urinary | 44-2 | 1020 |
| Endocrine | 47-3 | 1108 |
| Reproductive | 50-3 | 1191 |
| Nervous | 55-2 | 1302 |
| Musculoskeletal | 61-1 | 1451 |

## SPECIAL OLDER ADULT POPULATIONS

### Chronically Ill Older Adults

Daily living with chronic illness is a reality for many older adults. The incidence of chronic illness triples after age 45. Most people 65 years of age and older have at least one chronic condition, and many have multiple conditions.[1] The most common chronic conditions in older adults are hypertension, heart failure, coronary artery disease, chronic obstructive pulmonary disease, cancer, diabetes, and osteoarthritis. Other common chronic conditions include Alzheimer's disease, vision and hearing deficits, osteoporosis, stroke, Parkinson's disease, and depression.

### Cognitively Impaired Older Adults

Most healthy older adults have no noticeable decline in cognitive abilities (Table 5-6). Older adults may have a mild decline in memory and may require more time to recall events or new information. This differs from cognitive impairment. New learning may be slower. Encourage older adults with memory loss to be evaluated by their HCP and to use memory aids, attempt recall in a calm and quiet environment, and actively engage in enhancing memory. Memory aids include clocks, calendars, notes, marked pillboxes, safety alarms on stoves, and identification necklaces or bracelets. Memory techniques include word association, mental imaging, and mnemonics.

Dementia, delirium, and depression are common and may co-exist in older adults. Declining physical health and acute illness are important factors that may influence cognition. For example, an older adult who undergoes surgery may demonstrate an acute change in mental status known as *delirium*.[11] Delirium superimposed on dementia may signify an acute or emergent condition such as heart failure. Hence, it is important to differentiate signs and symptoms of each. Cognitive impairment, delirium, dementia, and differentiation of each are discussed in Chapter 59.

**TABLE 5-6 Gerontologic Assessment Differences**

***Cognitive Function***

| Effect of Aging | Cognitive Function |
|---|---|
| Improves with aging | • Vocabulary and verbal reasoning<br>• Crystallized intelligence (ability to use skills, knowledge, and experience) |
| Declines during middle age | • Mental performance speed<br>• Synthesis of new information<br>• Fluid intelligence (ability to think logically and solve problems in new situations) |
| Declines during old age | • Short-term recall memory |
| Constant (no changes with aging) | • Long-term recall memory |

### Rural Older Adults

Five barriers to health care access for rural older adults are transportation, limited supply of health care workers and facilities, lack of quality health care, social isolation, and financial limitations. Particularly vulnerable are older adults of racial or ethnic minority living in rural areas, who have even less access to HCPs. In addition, older adults who live in rural areas may be less likely to engage in health-promoting activities.

When you work with older adults in rural areas, recognize lifestyle values and practices of rural life (Fig. 5-3). In planning care, be aware that transportation is the number one barrier to health care for rural older adults. Alternative service approaches such as computer-based Internet sources and chat rooms, DVDs, radio, community centers, and church social events may be used to promote healthy practices or to conduct health screening (Fig. 5-4).

The use of telehealth devices for monitoring patients in their home environments has enhanced the ability to provide care, including to those more isolated.[12] Innovative models of nursing practice must continue to be developed to assist the rural older adult. Older adults are increasingly using technology in their daily lives. Most older adults use the Internet and own a cell phone.[12]

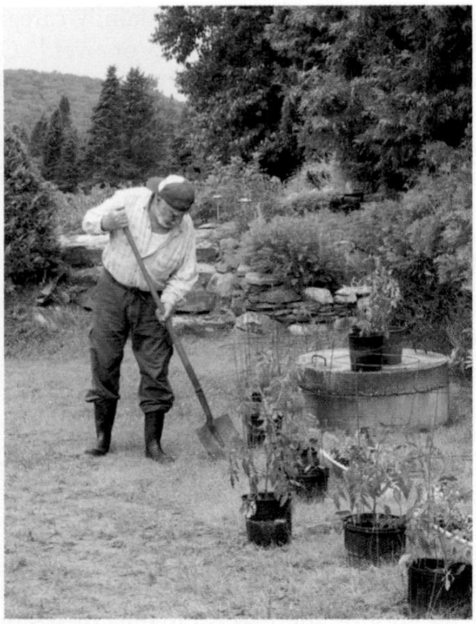

**FIG. 5-3** Older adults living in rural areas often enjoy outside activities, such as gardening. (©iStockphoto/Thinkstock.)

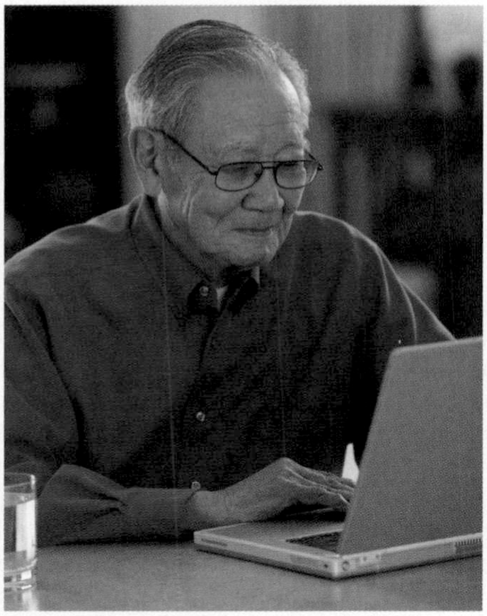

**FIG. 5-4** Older adults are using computers more frequently and accessing health care information on the Internet. (©iStockphoto/Thinkstock.)

## INFORMATICS IN PRACTICE

### *Older Adults and Internet Use*

- Thirty percent of older adults use the Internet to look for health information.
- Many adults over age 65 track their weight, diet, and exercise using apps.
- Older adults are more likely to accept as true what they read on the Internet. This is related to limited Internet experience and confusion from the large amounts of available information.
- Teach patients who use the Internet as a source of information how to assess the credibility of a website.
- Suggest the use of websites and apps that include senior-friendly design elements.

Source: *http://nihseniorhealth.gov/#.U4T10ruX3IA.emai.*

## Homeless Older Adults

The number of older adults who are homeless is increasing. Key factors associated with homelessness include (1) having a low income, (2) having reduced cognitive capacity, (3) living alone, and (4) living in a community that lacks affordable housing. Homeless older adults may be chronically homeless or recently homeless because of a crisis in either health, economic, or social status.

Mortality rates for homeless older adults are higher than for older adults who have housing. Older homeless adults are at higher risk for more health problems because many aging network services are not designed to reach out to homeless people. Older people who are homeless are less likely to use shelters or meal site services than younger homeless people. This may be due to fear of institutionalization. Care for homeless older adults requires an interprofessional approach (including nurses, physicians, social workers, clerical workers, and transporters) that links shelters with outreach, primary care clinics, Medicare and Medicaid offices, pharmacies, senior centers, and Area Agencies on Aging. Long-term care placement is often an alternative to homelessness, especially when the person is cognitively impaired.

## Frail Older Adults

*Frailty* is a common clinical syndrome seen in older adults. Clinical manifestations of frailty include older adults with three or more of the following criteria: (1) unintentional weight loss (greater than or equal to 10 pounds in a year); (2) self-reported exhaustion; (3) weakness (measured by grip strength); (4) slow walking speed; (5) low level of physical activity.[13] Risk factors include disability, multiple chronic conditions, and dementia. People are more likely to become frail if they smoke, have a history of depression or long-term medical health problems, or are underweight. The old-old population (85 years of age or older) is most at risk for frailty, although many in this age group remain healthy and robust.

Older frail adults experience declining function and decreasing daily energy. When stressful life events (e.g., death of a close friend) and daily strain (e.g., caring for an ill spouse) occur, frail older adults often show ineffective coping mechanisms and, as a result, may become ill. Common health problems of frail older adults include mobility limitations, sensory impairment, cognitive decline, and falls.

Frail older adults may tire easily; have little physical reserve; and are at risk for physical dependence and institutionalization. Frail older adults are especially at risk for malnutrition and dehydration, which are related to factors such as living alone, depression, and low income. Other factors, such as dementia, inadequate dental care, sensory deficits, fatigue, and limited mobility increase the risk of malnutrition and dehydration. Monitor frail older adults for adequate calorie, protein, iron, calcium, vitamin D, and fluid intake. A tool to assess the risk factors for poor nutritional status in older adults with or without evidence of frailty is presented in Table 5-7. Once an older adult's nutritional needs are identified, common interventions include home-delivered meals, dietary supplements, Supplemental Nutrition Assistance Program (SNAP),[14] dental referrals, and vitamin supplements. Because medications may affect appetite or interact with nutrients, perform a thorough medication review, including prescription drugs, over-the-counter (OTC) drugs, vitamins, minerals, supplements, as well as herbs and cultural remedies. Nutrition is discussed in Chapter 39.

**TABLE 5-7 SCALES: Nutritional Assessment of Older Adults**

*The acronym SCALES can remind you to assess important nutritional indicators:*

**S**adness, or mood change
**C**holesterol, high
**A**lbumin, low
**L**oss or gain of weight
**E**ating problems (e.g., mechanical problems such as impaired swallowing, poor dentition)
**S**hopping and food preparation problems

### Culturally Competent Care: Older Adults

The term ethnogeriatric describes the specialty area of providing culturally competent care to older adults.[15] As American society changes, ethnic institutions and neighborhoods may also change. For the older adult with strong ethnic and cultural roots, there may be a loss of friends who speak the "mother tongue," a loss of the religious institution that supports social ethnic activities, and a loss of stores that carry desired ethnic foods. This sense of loss is increased when children and others deny or ignore ethnic and cultural practices. Support for older adults of racial or ethnic minority is most frequently found in the family, religious practices, and isolated geographic or community ethnic clusters.

Ethnic populations of older adults face unique problems. Older adults may live in neighborhoods where physical security and personal safety related to crime may be a concern. Individuals who identify with particular ethnic groups often have disproportionately lower incomes and may not be able to afford Medicare deductibles or drugs needed to treat chronic illnesses. Older individuals from minority populations such as Hispanics use health care services less often when compared to nonminority groups.[15]

Assess each older adult's ethnic and cultural background. Assume that ethnicity and culture are important and of value to older adults and their families unless they tell you otherwise during an assessment. For you to be effective with the ethnic older adult, a sense of respect and clear communication are critical. Nursing interventions to assist in meeting the needs of ethnic populations[16] are described in Table 2-9. (Culturally competent care is discussed in Chapter 2.)

## SOCIAL SUPPORT FOR OLDER ADULTS

Social support for older adults occurs at three levels. First, family members are the primary and preferred providers of social support. Second, a semiformal level of support is found in clubs, religious (faith-based) organizations, neighborhoods, adult day care, and senior citizen centers. Third, older adults may be linked to formal systems of social welfare agencies, health facilities, and government support. Generally, you, as a nurse, are part of the formal support system.

### Family Caregivers

Many older adults require caregiving by family members. This includes those with multiple chronic conditions, those needing assistance with ADLs and IADLs, and older adults with dementia. Many family caregivers are caring for themselves, their aging parents, as well as their children and grandchildren. Caregiving contributes to stress or burden. Many family caregivers caring for older adults are themselves age 65 or over.[17] Older adults may take on the role of caregiver for someone in their family, usually their spouse or partner. Consider collaborating with a social worker if caregiver stress or strain is present and caregivers are in need of respite. The challenges of caregiving are discussed in Chapter 4 on p. 50.

### Elder Mistreatment

Elder mistreatment (EM) describes intentional acts of omission or commission by a caregiver or "trusted other" that cause harm or serious risk of harm to a vulnerable older adult. EM may occur in community (home or assisted living facility) or long-term care (institutional) settings.

Approximately 2% to 10% of community-dwelling older adults in the United States are abused, neglected, or exploited by trusted others.[18] The prevalence of EM in institutional settings is unknown, but it is thought to be widespread. Although EM rates are similar in women and men, the majority of victims are women because of the predominance of women in older age cohorts. Victims of EM have a mortality risk that is three times higher than that of non-mistreated peers. The higher mortality risk is not due to the abuse or neglect itself but rather may be due to stress-related illnesses associated with prolonged mistreatment.[18]

EM is a hidden problem. For every reported case in the community setting, more than five cases go unreported. Underreporting may be higher based on immigration status, ethnic background, or sexual orientation. Victims are unlikely to report mistreatment by "trusted others" because of isolation; impaired cognitive or physical function; feelings of shame, guilt, or self-blame; fear of reprisal; pressure from family members; fear of long-term care; or cultural norms. HCPs also underreport EM, possibly because of failure to suspect or recognize EM, perceived inability to successfully intervene, desire to avoid responsibility for further action, or ageism.

Family members are responsible for up to 90% of domestic EM.[18] Adult children who abuse, neglect, or exploit their parents are usually dependent on their parent(s) for housing and financial support, have a history of violence, are unemployed, and/or are disabled from substance abuse or mental illness. Abusive spouses or partners may either initiate intimate partner violence in older age or continue a lifelong pattern of abuse.

Many factors put community-dwelling older adults at risk for domestic EM. These include (1) physical or cognitive dysfunction that leads to an inability to perform ADLs (and therefore produces dependence on others for care), (2) any psychiatric diagnoses (especially dementia and depression), (3) alcohol abuse, and (4) decreased social support.[19] In long-term care settings the same factors that lead to institutionalization are risk factors for mistreatment by staff, visitors, and others. These include dependence on others for care because of physical or cognitive limitations.

Types of EM, characteristics, and manifestations are shown in Table 5-8. In institutional settings EM includes the types described in Table 5-8 but also includes failure to follow the plan of care, unauthorized use of physical or chemical restraints, overuse or underuse of medication, or isolation as punishment.

Follow your organization's protocols for EM screening and interventions. Perform a thorough history and physical examination that includes screening for mistreatment. It is important that you interview people alone because, if

**TABLE 5-8 Types of Elder Mistreatment**

| Characteristics | Manifestations |
|---|---|
| **Physical Abuse** | |
| Slapping, striking, restraining, incorrect positioning. Oversedation with medications. | Bruises, bilateral injuries (upper arms, ankles, wrists), repeated injuries in various stages of healing, burn marks, oversedation. Use of several emergency departments. |
| **Neglect** | |
| Failure or refusal to provide basic life needs, including food, water, medications, clothing, hygiene. Failure to provide physical aids such as dentures, eyeglasses, hearing aid. Failure to ensure safety. | Older adult's report of being neglected. Untreated or infected pressure ulcers on sacral area, heels. Loss of body weight. Laboratory values showing dehydration (e.g., ↑ Hct, ↑ serum sodium), malnutrition (↓ serum protein). Poor personal hygiene. Lack of adherence with medical treatment. |
| Failure to provide social stimulation. Leaving alone for long periods. Failure to provide companionship. | Depression, withdrawn behavior, agitation. Ambivalent attitude toward caregiver or family member. |
| **Psychologic Abuse** | |
| Berating verbally, harassment, intimidation, threats of punishment, or deprivation. Childlike treatment, isolation. | Depression, withdrawn behavior, agitation. Ambivalent attitude toward caregiver or family member. |
| **Sexual Abuse** | |
| Nonconsensual sexual contact, including touching inappropriately. Forced sexual contact. | Older adult's report of sexual abuse. Unexplained vaginal or anal bleeding, bruised breasts, unexplained STIs or genital infections. |
| **Financial Abuse** | |
| Denying access to personal resources, stealing money or possessions. Coercing to sign contracts or durable power of attorney. Making changes in will or trust. | Living situation below level of personal resources. Sudden change in personal finances, sudden transfer of assets. |
| **Violation of Personal Rights** | |
| Denying right to privacy or right to make decisions regarding health care or living environment. Forcible eviction. | Sudden inexplicable changes in living situation, confusion. |
| **Abandonment** | |
| Desertion of an older person by an individual who has assumed responsibility for providing care or by a person with physical custody. | Older adult's reports of being abandoned; desertion of an older adult at a hospital or skilled nursing facility, shopping center, or other public place. |

*Hct,* Hematocrit; *STIs,* sexually transmitted infections.

mistreatment is occurring, they may not disclose it in the presence of the person who accompanied them, especially if that person is the abuser. Be especially attentive to explanations about injuries that are not consistent with what you observe, contradictory explanations between the patient and the caregiver, or behavioral clues that suggest the patient is being threatened or intimidated. Additional nursing assessments and interventions are listed in Table 5-9. In most states, health care workers and others are mandated to report suspected or actual EM to Adult Protective Services (APS) and/or law enforcement. Know your legal responsibilities by checking the laws in your state.

### Self-Neglect

The majority of referrals made to APS are for self-neglect. Older adults who self-neglect are often unable to meet their basic needs and refuse help; have multiple, untreated medical or psychiatric conditions; and live alone and often in squalor. Older community-dwelling adults who self-neglect face a higher risk of mortality than peers who do not self-neglect.[20] Nursing interventions include assessment for possible self-neglect, referrals for long-term interprofessional case management, and referral to APS.

## SOCIAL SERVICES FOR OLDER ADULTS

A network of services supports older adults in the community and health care facilities. In the United States, most older adults are the beneficiaries of at least one social or governmental service. To understand the older adult's situation, learn about government structures that fund and regulate programs for older adults. The Administration on Aging (AoA), which is part of the Department of Health and Human Services, is the federal agency responsible for many older adult programs. Funding from the AoA is given to state and local Area Agencies on Aging (AAAs).

**TABLE 5-9 Nursing Assessment and Intervention**

***Elder Mistreatment***

*When elder mistreatment is suspected, it is important to do the following:*

- Screen for possible elder mistreatment, including domestic violence.
- Conduct a thorough history and head-to-toe physical assessment. Document your findings, including any statements made by the older adult or accompanying adult.
- If the older adult appears to be in immediate danger, develop and implement a safety plan in collaboration with the interprofessional team involved in the person's care.
- Identify, collect, and preserve physical evidence (e.g., dirty or bloody clothing, dressings, sheets).
- After obtaining consent, take photographs to document physical findings of suspected abuse or neglect. If possible and appropriate, do this before treating or bathing the alleged victim.
- If you suspect that mistreatment is occurring, report your findings to the appropriate state agency and/or law enforcement as mandated by the laws in your state.
- Initiate social work, forensic nursing, adult protective services, and other consultations as appropriate.

## MEDICARE AND MEDICAID

Medicare is a federally funded health insurance program for people ages 65 years or older, as well as for people under age 65 with certain disabilities and people of any age with end-stage renal disease (ESRD) requiring dialysis or a kidney transplant.

Medicare has four options for coverage: A, B, C, and D. Part A covers inpatient hospital care and partially covers skilled nursing facility care, hospice, and home health care. Part A coverage is "free" because workers support Medicare through payroll taxes. Medicare Part B partially covers outpatient care, physicians' or primary care providers' services, and home health care. It also covers some preventive services, such as mammograms. Medicare Part B is voluntary and has a monthly premium and an annual deductible before payment begins. Medicare Advantage Plans, sometimes called "Part C" or "MA Plans," are offered by private companies approved by Medicare to provide Part A and Part B benefits. Part D is available to Medicare enrollees and provides a prescription drug benefit. Members pay a yearly deductible, monthly premium, and copayment. People with lower incomes and limited assets may qualify for extra help to pay for prescriptions.

Medicare does not cover long-term care, custodial ADLs or IADLs care, dental care or dentures, hearing aids, or eyeglasses. (More information is available at *www.medicare.gov.*) Out-of-pocket expenditures for people on Medicare continue to rise. The costs increase with age, functional disabilities, number of chronic conditions, and number of hospitalizations.[21]

Medicaid is a state-administered, needs-based program to assist eligible low-income people, including Medicare beneficiaries, with certain medical expenses. Individuals who qualify for both Medicare and Medicaid are referred to as *dual-eligible.* Eligibility and coverage vary by state. For qualified Medicare beneficiaries, Medicaid pays Medicare premiums, deductibles, and co-insurance, as well as long-term care and home health expenses. In the United States the majority of long-term care is paid for by Medicaid or private pay. (More information is available at *www.medicaid.gov.*)

## CARE ALTERNATIVES FOR OLDER ADULTS

Older adults with special care needs include people who are homeless, in need of assistance with ADLs, cognitively impaired, homebound, or no longer able to live at home. Older adults may be served by adult day care, adult day health care, home health care, and long-term care. Continuing care retirement communities, congregate housing, and assisted living facilities are housing options for older adults.

### Adult Day Care and Adult Day Health Care

*Adult day care* centers provide social, recreational, and health-related services to individuals in a safe, community-based environment (Fig. 5-5). This includes daily supervision, social activities, opportunities for social interaction, and ADLs assistance for two major groups of adults: (1) those who are cognitively impaired and (2) those who have problems independently performing ADLs. Services offered in adult day care programs are individualized based on need. Programs designed for adults who are cognitively impaired offer therapeutic recreation, support for family, family counseling, and social involvement.

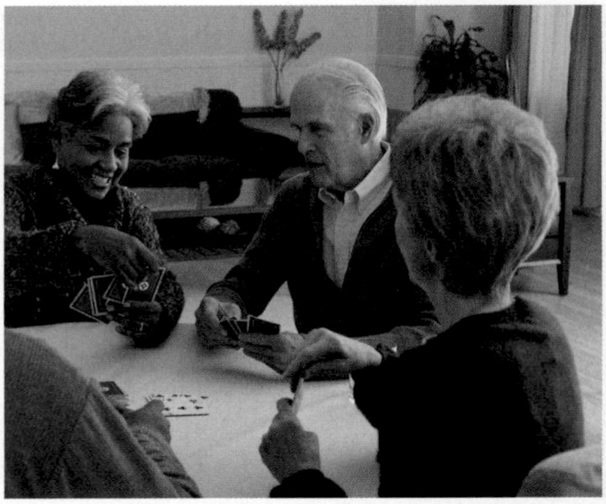

**FIG. 5-5** Senior centers offer places for older adults who live independently to meet and gather with friends. (©Jupiterimages/Comstock/Thinkstock.)

*Adult day health care* centers are similar to adult day care but are designed to meet the needs of older adults and people with disabilities who need a higher level of care. This might include health monitoring, therapeutic activities, one-on-one ADLs training, and personal services.

Adult day care centers and adult day health care centers may provide respite to allow continued employment for the caregiver and delay institutionalization of older adults. Centers are regulated, and standards are set by the state. Medicare does not cover costs. Adult day health care is tax deductible as dependent care. Appropriate placement in adult care programs that match participants' needs is important. You can assist caregivers and adults with self-care deficits by knowing the available centers in your area and assessing the needs of older adults and their families. You will then be in a position to assist older adults and their families in making good decisions about their care.

### Home Health Care

Home health care (HHC) can be a cost-effective care alternative for older adults who are homebound, have health needs that are intermittent or acute, and have supportive caregiver involvement. HHC is not an alternative for adults in need of 24-hour assistance with ADLs or continuous safety supervision. (Private duty care may be an alternative in these situations.) HHC services require physician orders and skilled nursing care for Medicare reimbursement. Unless these requirements are met, assistance by home health aides for ADLs management or assistance by a homemaker for IADLs management will not be paid by Medicare.

In addition to HHC, respite, and personal care, homemaker services are often sought by caregivers through organizations that provide nonmedical assistance. These services help older adults stay at home.

### Long-Term Care Facilities

Three factors appear to precipitate placement in a long-term care facility: (1) rapid patient deterioration, (2) caregiver inability to continue care because of stress and burnout, and (3) an alteration in or loss of the family support system. Progressive dementia, incontinence, or a major health event (e.g., stroke) can accelerate long-term care placement.

The conflicts and fears faced by older adults and their families make placement a difficult transition. Common caregiver

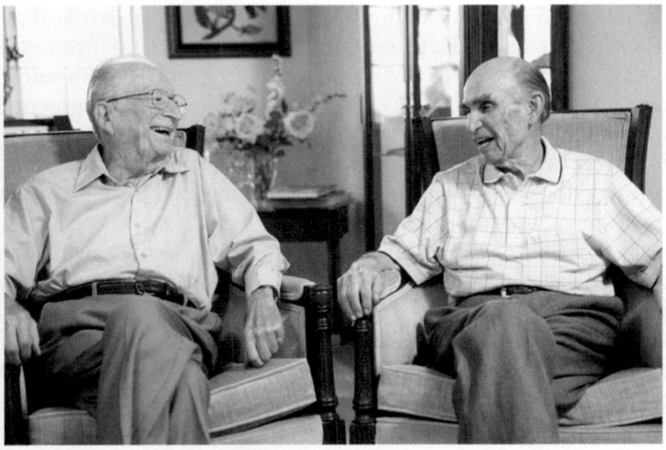

FIG. 5-6 Social interaction and acceptance are important for older adults. (©Hemera/Thinkstock.)

concerns include: (1) Will the older adult resist the admission process? (2) Will the level of care given by staff be insufficient? (3) Will the resident be lonely? and (4) Will nursing care be affordable?

The physical relocation of the older adult may lead to adverse health effects. *Relocation stress syndrome* is a nursing diagnosis that is associated with the disruption, confusion, and challenges that older adults face when moving from one environment to a new environment. Older adults may experience anxiety, depression, and disorientation. Appropriate interventions can reduce the effects of relocation. Whenever possible, involve older adults in the decision to move and fully inform them about the location. Caregivers can share information, pictures, or a video recording of the new location. Personnel at the institution can send a welcome message. On arrival, new residents can be greeted by staff members to provide orientation. To bridge the relocation, new residents can be "buddied" with seasoned residents (Fig. 5-6).

### Programs for All-Inclusive Care for the Elderly (PACE)

Programs for All-Inclusive Care for the Elderly (PACE) provide care for adults age 55 and older. PACE services include primary care including prescription medications and wound care; physical, occupational, recreational, and speech therapy; adult day care; dental; podiatry; social services; and home health care. Respite care, hospitalization, short-term rehabilitation, and long-term care are provided as needed.[22]

A person who has Medicaid will not have to pay a monthly premium for the long-term portion of the PACE benefit. A person who does not qualify for Medicaid but has Medicare will be charged a monthly premium to cover the long-term care portion.

## LEGAL AND ETHICAL ISSUES

Legal guidance and assistance is needed by many older adults. Legal issues include advance directives, estate planning, taxation issues, appeals for denied services (e.g., disability), financial decisions, or exploitation by strangers or "trusted others."

Advance directives are written statements of a person's wishes regarding medical care. A health care proxy may be appointed to make medical decisions in the event that a person is unable to make his or her own medical decisions. These documents allow individuals to more specifically direct their own care at end of life. Advance directives are discussed in detail in Chapter 9 and Table 9-6.

When working with older adults, you may find several ethical issues that influence practice, such as the assessment of older adults' ability to make decisions. Other ethical issues related to end-of-life care include decisions about resuscitation, treatment of infections, nutrition and hydration, and transfer to more intensive treatment units. These situations are often complex, especially during emotionally difficult times. You can assist the older adult, family, and other health care workers by (1) keeping current on the ethical issues, (2) acknowledging when an ethical dilemma is present, and (3) advocating for an institutional ethics committee to help provide guidance in the decision-making process and assist when differences of opinion occur.

## ❖ NURSING MANAGEMENT: OLDER ADULTS

**Gerontologic nursing** is the care of older adults based on the specialty body of knowledge of gerontology and nursing. These specialty nurses provide care for older adults using a whole-person (physical, psychologic, functional, developmental, socioeconomic, cultural) perspective. Care of older adults is complex and presents challenges that require skilled assessment and creative nursing interventions tailored to this population.

Diseases and conditions in older adults may be difficult to accurately assess and diagnose. Older adults may underreport symptoms and "treat" these symptoms by altering their functional status. For example, a woman having loss of feeling in her feet because of neuropathy may start using a walker to get around, while not reporting the symptom to her HCP. The older adult may attribute a new symptom to "aging" and ignore it. The older adult may eat less, sleep more, or "wait it out."

In older adults, disease symptoms are often atypical. For example, confusion may be a sign of an infection. Asymptomatic cardiac disease may be diagnosed when the patient is being treated for a urinary tract infection. Pathologic conditions with similar symptoms are often confused. For example, depression may be misdiagnosed and treated as dementia. The most common atypical illness presentations are "delirium" or "acute change in mental status" and change in functional status. A caregiver may say that their relative "is acting differently," "doesn't appear as him/herself," or is no longer participating in usual activities or self-care.

In older adults a *cascade disease pattern* may occur. For example, a person who experiences insomnia treats the condition with a sleeping medication, becomes lethargic and confused, falls, sustains a hip fracture, decreases activity and mobility, and subsequently develops pneumonia. You play a vital role in preventing this downward trajectory.

For older adults, the stress of an illness may lead to fear and anxiety. They may view health care personnel as helpful but perceive institutions as negative and potentially harmful places. Communicate a sense of concern and care by use of direct and simple statements, appropriate eye contact, direct touch, and gentle humor. These actions help the older adult relax in this stressful situation.

### ◆ Nursing Assessment

Prior to assessment, attend to the person's primary needs. For example, ensure that older adults are comfortable and ask if they need to use the bathroom. If older adults normally use eyeglasses and hearing aids, ask them to use these during the assessment. Place all assistive devices, such as walkers, within reach. Assess your patient's level of fatigue and pause the interview if necessary. Allow adequate time to offer information and time for the person to respond to questions. Interview both the older adult and his or her family or caregivers. This can be done separately, unless the patient is cognitively impaired or specifically requests the caregiver's presence. Although the health history may be lengthy, it is important to obtain. Review medical records and determine what information is most relevant or needs more detail.

The focus of a comprehensive geriatric assessment is to determine appropriate interventions to maintain and enhance the health, quality of life, function, and independence of older adults. Comprehensive geriatric assessment is interprofessional and, at a minimum, includes the medical history, functional assessment, medication review, cognitive and mood evaluation, social resources, physical examination, followed by recommended diagnostic tests. Comprehensive geriatric assessment is often conducted by an interprofessional geriatric assessment team. The interprofessional team minimally includes a staff nurse, an HCP such as a physician or adult-geriatric nurse practitioner, and a social worker. It may also include a physical and/or occupational therapist, dietitian, podiatrist, ophthalmologist, dentist, and pastoral care representative. After the assessment is complete, the interprofessional team meets with the patient and family to present the team's findings and recommendations.

Specific elements in a comprehensive nursing assessment include a thorough history, mood assessment, functional assessment including ADLs and IADLs, mental status evaluation, social-environmental assessment, and physical assessment. Evaluation of mental status is particularly important for older adults because these results often determine the potential for independent living. *SPICES,* an effective tool for obtaining assessment data in older adults, may be used as an initial nursing assessment when working in any setting (Fig. 5-7). Multiple evidence-based geriatric assessment tools and best practice approaches to nursing care for older adults are available from the *Try This* Series at the Hartford Institute for Geriatric Nursing (available at: *www.ConsultGeriRN.org/resources*).

A comprehensive geriatric assessment includes a fall risk (including fear of falling) and cause(s) of past falls. Individuals are at increased risk for falls if they have a history of falls or have a fear of falling. Many factors increase the risk of falls, including medications (including OTC ones), infection, electrolyte imbalance or other laboratory abnormalities, arthritis, changes in gait, balance, and mobility, neurologic impairment (e.g., stroke, Parkinson's disease), decreased muscle strength, and decreased visual acuity. Assess for symptoms of dizziness or lightheadedness upon standing. Other risk factors include environmental hazards, feet abnormalities, poor footwear, clutter, throw rugs, incorrect use of an assistive device such as a walker or cane, shiny or waxy floors, slippery floors, poor lighting, bed in an incorrect position such as too high, and uneven pavement.

Evaluation of the results of a comprehensive nursing assessment helps determine the service and potential long-term placement needs of older adults. Collect data regarding community resources that are needed to assist older adults and their caregivers in maintaining maximal functioning. The goal is to plan and implement actions that help older adults remain as functionally independent as possible and to promote their quality of life.

| Patient name: | Date: | |
|---|---|---|
| | EVIDENCE | |
| SPICES | Yes | No |
| **S**leep disorders | | |
| **P**roblems with eating or feeding | | |
| **I**ncontinence | | |
| **C**onfusion | | |
| **E**vidence of falls | | |
| **S**kin breakdown | | |

**FIG. 5-7** SPICES. (Adapted from Fulmer T: The geriatric nurse specialist role: a new model. *Nursing Management* 22:91, 1991. © Copyright Lippincott Williams & Wilkins, *http://lww.com.*)

## ◆ Planning

When setting goals with older adults, identify their strengths and abilities. Include caregivers in planning. Priority goals for older adults may include gaining a sense of control, feeling safe, and reducing stress.

## ◆ Nursing Implementation

When carrying out a plan of action for older adults, modify your approach and actions based on their physical, functional, and mental status. Small body size (common in older adults who meet frailty criteria) may necessitate the use of pediatric equipment (e.g., BP cuff). As with all patient groups, safety is a primary concern when caring for an older adult. Bone and joint changes often require transfer assistance, altered positioning, and use of gait belts and lift devices. Older adults with declining energy reserves may require additional time to complete tasks. A slower approach and the use of other adaptive equipment may be necessary. Cognitive impairment, if present, requires that you offer careful explanations and a calm approach to avoid producing anxiety and resistance in the older adult. Depression can result in apathy and poor cooperation with the treatment plan.

◆ **Health Promotion.** Health promotion and prevention of health problems for older adults focus on three areas: (1) increased participation in health promotion and disease prevention activities (Fig. 5-8), (2) reduction in diseases and health-related

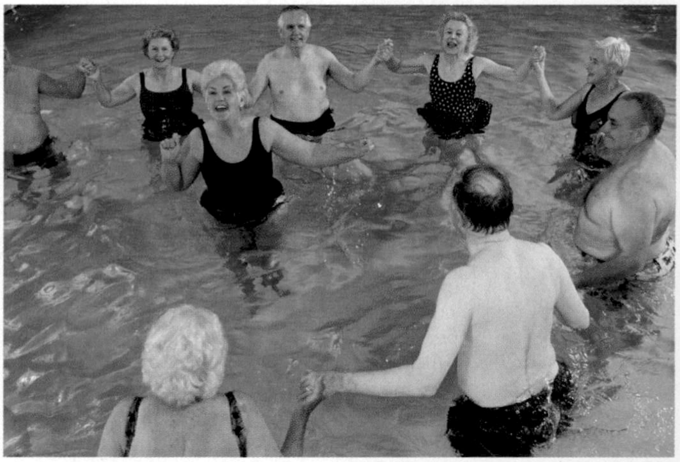

**FIG. 5-8** Water aerobics is an example of a health promotion activity for older adults. (©Purestock/Thinkstock.)

issues, and (3) increased use of services that reduce health hazards. Programs have been successfully developed for screening for chronic health conditions, tobacco cessation, geriatric foot care, vision and hearing screening, stress reduction, exercise programs, fall prevention programs, drug usage, crime prevention, elder mistreatment, and home safety assessment.[3,23] Teach older adults about the need for specific preventive services and available programs.

Health promotion and disease prevention should be included in nursing interventions and plans at any setting or level of care where nurses and older adults interact. You can use health promotion activities to increase personal responsibility for health and independent functioning. Teaching and reinforcement are important tools for you to use to enhance self-care practices by older adults. (Patient teaching is discussed in Chapter 4.)

◆ **Acute and Ambulatory Care.** The hospital may be the first point of contact for older adults with the health care system. Conditions that most commonly result in hospitalization include falls, dysrhythmias, heart failure, stroke, fluid and electrolyte imbalances (e.g., hyponatremia, dehydration), pneumonia, urosepsis, and hip fractures. Older adults are often hospitalized with multiple problems.

When older adults are being cared for in the acute care setting, both patients and caregivers need assistance with a variety of functions (Table 5-10). The outcome of hospitalization for older adults varies. Of particular concern are patients undergoing high-risk surgical procedures (e.g., hip replacement) and those who experience delirium while hospitalized.

◆ ***Care Transitions.*** The time of a care transition to another setting (e.g., acute care hospital to rehabilitation) is challenging for many older adults. While in the hospital, patients and caregivers are counseled on how to prepare for posthospital care. Those with multiple health conditions are particularly at high risk for rehospitalization.

Medicare regulations require a registered nurse, social worker, or qualified person to develop a care transition plan for patient discharge. Safe and effective care transitions are most likely to occur when interprofessional team members work together with the patient and family to coordinate care.

The Transitional Care Model (TCM) is an evidence-based, innovative approach to care coordination and management of the complex needs of older adults.[24] In this model a transitional care nurse delivers and coordinates care by nurses and other team members throughout potential and acute episodes of illness. Those most likely to benefit from transitional care nursing include those of older age and those with functional deficits, behavioral or psychiatric issues, multiple chronic conditions, a need for polypharmacy, a recent hospitalization, lack of a support system, low health literacy, and history of nonadherence to treatment.[24]

◆ ***Rehabilitation.*** The goal of rehabilitation is to help older adults adapt to or recover from disability or an acute functional decline. Rehabilitation may occur in acute inpatient rehabilitation, subacute rehabilitation, or long-term care settings. With proper training, assistive equipment, and attendant personal care, people with functional deficits may live independently. Older adults, primarily through Medicare reimbursement, can receive rehabilitative assistance through acute inpatient rehabilitation (limited days) and home health care programs (Fig. 5-9).

Older adults with chronic conditions, such as arthritis, have increased risk of functional decline. Decreased function or disabilities lead to increased self-care deficits, increased rates of institutionalization, decreased quality of life, and higher mortality rates.

Rehabilitation of older adults is influenced by several factors. First, preexisting conditions associated with decreased reaction time, visual acuity, fine motor ability, physical strength, and cognitive function affect the short- and long-term rehabilitation potential of older adults. Older adults may have anxiety, fear, or concern about falling. They may also be limited in the rehabilitation process by poor nutrition and financial issues. Encouragement, support, and acceptance from the interdisciplinary team members as well as their caregivers can assist older adults in remaining motivated for potentially physically challenging rehabilitation.

Second, older adults often lose function because of inactivity and immobility. This deconditioning can occur as a result of unstable acute medical conditions, lack of assistive devices, and a lack of motivation to stay fit. The effect of inactivity leads to "use it or lose it" consequences. Older adults can improve flexibility, strength, and aerobic capacity even into very old age. Passive and active range-of-motion exercises are used with all older adults to preserve muscle tone and strength and prevent deconditioning and subsequent functional decline.

### TABLE 5-10 Care of the Hospitalized Older Adult

*When an older adult is hospitalized, give special consideration to the following nursing interventions.*

- Identify older adults at risk for iatrogenesis (consequences of medical and/or surgical treatments).
- Consider discharge needs early in the hospital stay, especially assistance with ADLs, IADLs, and medications.
- Encourage the development and use of interprofessional teams, special care units, and individuals who focus on the special needs of older patients.
- Implement standard protocols to screen for at-risk conditions commonly present in the hospitalized older adult, such as urinary tract infection, falls, and delirium.
- Implement mobility programs to prevent functional decline such as *"The bed is not your friend."*
- Monitor for and prevent skin integrity changes.
- Focus on safety (e.g., prevention of falls).
- Advocate for referral of the patient to appropriate community-based services.

*ADLs,* Activities of daily living; *IADLs,* instrumental activities of daily living.

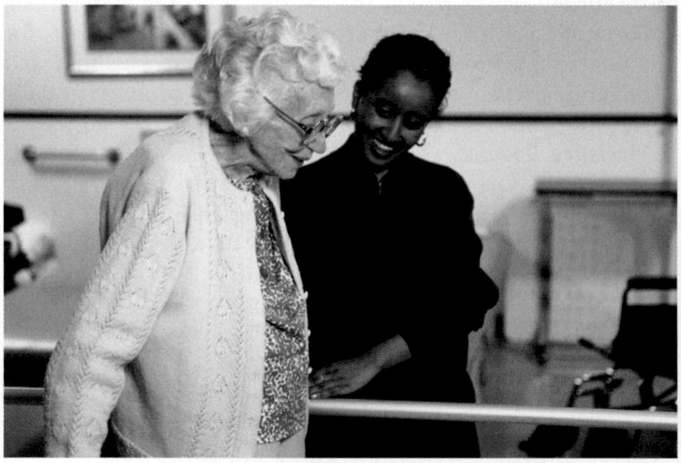

**FIG. 5-9** The nurse assists a patient in a geriatric rehabilitation facility. (©KeithBrofsky/Photodisc/Thinkstock.)

## EVIDENCE-BASED PRACTICE

### *Translating Research Into Practice*

**Can Tai Chi Help Cognitive Function in Older Adults?**

***Clinical Question***

In older adults (P), what is the effect of Tai Chi (I) on cognitive functioning (O)?

***Synthesis of Best Available Evidence***

- Systematic review of randomized controlled trials (RCTs), cross-sectional studies, and prospective randomized controlled and noncontrolled observational studies
- 20 studies of adults aged 60 years and older (*n* = 2553) in residential and community care settings with and without cognitive impairment. Intervention was Tai Chi lasting 20 to 60 minutes, 1 to 4 times per week, for up to 1 year. Most RCT control groups were stretching and toning, resistance and nonresistance exercise, and education. Outcomes of cognitive functioning were global cognition (dementia assessment), executive function (e.g., attention, memory), language, and learning.
- In cognitively healthy adults, Tai Chi had a positive effect on executive function with improvement maintained at 1 year. Global cognition, memory, learning, and fluency also improved.
- In cognitively impaired adults, Tai Chi had positive effects on global cognition and executive function.

***Conclusion***

- Tai Chi improved cognitive function, particularly in adults without significant cognitive impairment.

***Implications for Nursing Practice***

- How would you advise older adults who want information on activities that will help to maintain memory and ability to learn?
- How may the caregiver of a spouse or partner with dementia also benefit from engaging in Tai Chi?

***Reference for Evidence***

Wayne PM, Walsh JN, Taylor-Piliae RE, et al: Effect of Tai Chi on cognitive performance in older adults: systematic review and meta-analysis, *J Am Geriatr Soc* 62:25, 2014.

*P*, Patient population of interest; *I*, intervention or area of interest; *O*, outcomes of interest (see p. 15)

Last, the goal of rehabilitation is to strive for maximal function and physical capabilities considering the individual's current health and functional status. For example, on admission to an acute or long-term care facility and home health services, assess for fall risk as well as the person's fear of falling. Initiate appropriate fall prevention interventions and evaluate for ongoing risk. Conduct accurate and comprehensive foot and peripheral vascular assessments for all older adults, especially those with diabetes, and arrange appropriate follow-up care.

◆ ***Assistive Devices.*** Consider the use of assistive devices as interventions for older adults. Using appropriate assistive devices such as dentures, glasses, hearing aids, walkers, wheelchairs, adaptive utensils, elevated toilet seats, and skin protective devices can increase function. Include these tools and devices in the older adult's care plan when appropriate and provide instruction in the proper use of the devices. For example, using a cane appropriately may decrease fall risk.

Technology can assist with rehabilitation and living with functional impairments. For example, electronic monitoring equipment can be used to monitor heart rhythm and BP. Monitoring can also locate a person with dementia who has wandered away from home or a long-term care facility. Computerized assistive devices may help patients with speech difficulties following stroke, and small electronic devices can serve as memory aids.

◆ ***Safety.*** Safety is crucial in the health maintenance of older adults. When compared to younger adults, older adults are at higher risk for accidents due to normal sensory changes, slowed reaction time, decreased thermal and pain sensitivity, changes in gait and balance, and medication effects. Most accidents occur in or around the home. Falls, motor vehicle accidents, and fires are common causes of accidental death in older adults. Declining thermoregulation impairs the older person's ability to adapt to extremes in environmental temperatures. The bodies of older adults can neither conserve nor dissipate heat as efficiently as younger adults. Therefore both hypothermia and hyperthermia occur more readily. The older adult age-group accounts for the majority of deaths during severe cold spells and heat waves.

You can provide counsel regarding environmental changes, which may improve safety for older adults. Measures such as colored step strips, tub and toilet grab bars, and stairway handrails can be effective in "safety-proofing" the living spaces of older adults. Uncluttered floor space (e.g., removal of throw rugs), railings, and increased lighting and night-lights are some of the easiest and most practical adaptations. Social workers may help older adults implement these environmental changes. You can also advocate for home fire and security alarms.

Other interventions to decrease the risk of falling include exercise, physical therapy, and management of foot and footwear issues. Prevention of falls also includes encouraging the patient's use of glasses and hearing aid as ordered. Fear of falling can affect the older adults' decisions about the activities that they engage in and how active they remain.

Older adults who are new to inpatient or long-term care settings need a thorough orientation to the environment. Reassure the older adult that he or she is safe, and answer all questions and refer to interprofessional team members and specialists as needed. Foster orientation by displaying large-print clocks, avoiding complex or visually confusing wall designs, clearly designating doors and exits, and using simple bed and nurse or family-call controls. Provide diffuse lighting while avoiding glare.

◆ ***Medication Use.*** Medication use in older adults requires thorough and regular assessment, care planning, and evaluation. Nonadherence to medication regimens by older adults is common. Many older adults are unable to read prescription drug labels, and many are unable to understand the health information that is provided to them.

Age-related changes alter the pharmacodynamics and pharmacokinetics of drugs. Drug-drug, drug-nutrient, and drug-disease interactions influence the absorption, distribution, metabolism, and excretion of drugs. The most dramatic changes with aging are related to drug metabolism (Fig. 5-10). Hepatic blood flow decreases markedly with aging, and the enzymes largely responsible for drug metabolism are decreased as well. As a result, drug half-life is increased in older adults as compared with younger adults. This can lead to greater risk for drug toxicity and adverse drug events. Overall, by age 75 to 80, there is a 50% decline in the renal clearance of drugs. Older adults with altered renal function may need a lower dose and/or decreased frequency of administration of a drug excreted by the kidney. When drug level monitoring is available (e.g., digoxin [Lanoxin]), identify toxic levels by serum monitoring at regular

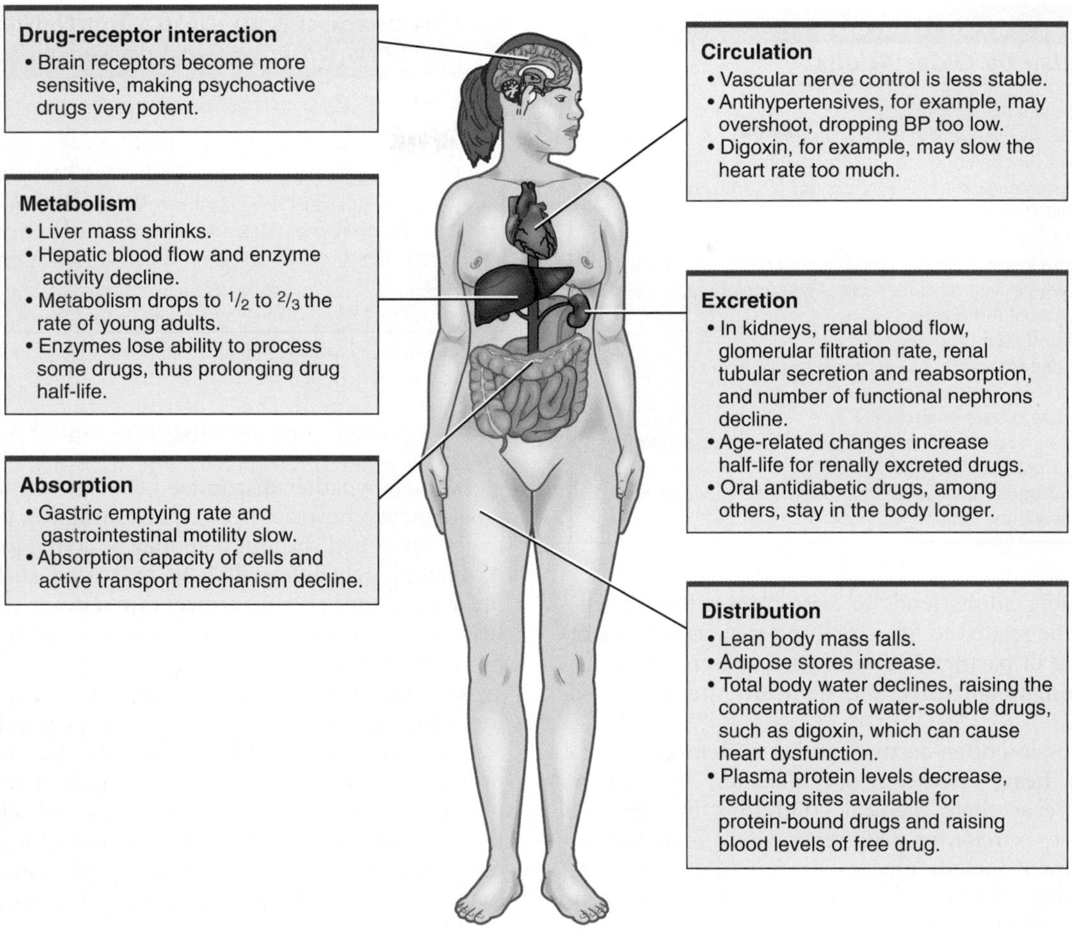


**FIG. 5-10** The effects of aging on drug metabolism.

**TABLE 5-11 Drug Therapy**

***Causes of Medication Errors by Older Adults***

- Decreased vision
- Forgetting to take drugs
- Use of nonprescription over-the-counter drugs
- Use of medications prescribed for someone else
- Lack of financial resources to obtain prescribed medication
- Failure to understand instructions or importance of drug treatment
- Refusal to take medication because of undesirable side effects

intervals, especially at change of dose and/or frequency of administration.

In addition to changes in the pharmacodynamics and pharmacokinetics of drugs, older adults may have difficulty managing medication regimens due to cognitive impairment, altered sensory perceptions, limited hand mobility or dexterity, and the high cost of many drugs. Common reasons for drug errors made by older adults are listed in Table 5-11.

*Polypharmacy* (the use of multiple medications by a person who has more than one health problem), overdose, and addiction to prescription drugs are major causes of illness in older adults.[25] Potential medication errors include the (1) administration of both brand and generic medications, (2) refilling medications too soon or too late (resulting in taking the medication incorrectly), and (3) drug-drug interactions. These errors can be prevented by having a pharmacist review the medication regimen regularly. Suggest the use of one pharmacy for filling all prescription medications.

The effects of medications in older adults with multiple health problems are particularly challenging to assess and manage. As one disease is treated, another may be affected. For example, the use of a drug such as oxybutynin (Ditropan), which is prescribed for overactive bladder, may cause confusion. To accurately assess medication knowledge and use, ask older adults to bring all medications (OTC drugs, prescription drugs, vitamins and supplements, laxatives, sleep aids, and herbal remedies) that they take regularly or occasionally to their health care appointment. You will then be able to accurately assess all medications that the patient is taking, including drugs that the person may have omitted or thought unimportant. The American Geriatrics Society (AGS) Beers Criteria are designed to reduce problems with medications in older adults.[25] Additional nursing interventions to assist older adults in following a safe medication routine are listed in Table 5-12.

***Depression.*** Depression is not a normal part of aging. However, it is often an underrecognized problem in older adults. Approximately 15% of older adults living in their homes have manifestations of depression. Rates of depressive symptoms in older adults in institutional settings are higher. The second highest rate of suicide occurs in those over 75.

Depression is associated with female gender, divorced or separated marital status, low socioeconomic status, poor social support, and a recent adverse and unexpected event.

**TABLE 5-12 Drug Therapy**

***Medication Use by Older Adults***

*When older adults are using medications, it is important to take the following measures to prevent medication errors.*

- Assess cognitive function and monitor for changes.
- Attempt to reduce medication use that is not essential by consulting the HCP and pharmacist.
- Assess ability to self-administer medication and overall medication use, including prescription drugs; over-the-counter drugs; antihistamines; cough syrups; vitamins, minerals, and supplements; sleep remedies; and herbal remedies.
- Assess alcohol and illicit drug use.
- Encourage the use of written or electronic medication-reminder systems.
- Encourage the use of one pharmacy.
- Work with HCPs and pharmacists to establish routine drug profiles on all older adult patients.
- Advocate, with drug companies and/or social work services, for low-income prescription support services.

Depression in older adults tends to arise from a loss of self-esteem and may be related to life situations, such as retirement or loss of a spouse or partner. Problems such as pain, insomnia, lethargy, agitation, weight loss, and dementia are associated with depression.

Late-life depression often occurs together with medical conditions, such as heart disease, stroke, diabetes, and cancer. Depression can exacerbate medical conditions by affecting adherence to diet, exercise, or drug regimens. It is important that your assessment include physical examination and interpretation of laboratory results for physical disorders that may have symptoms similar to those of depression (e.g., thyroid disorders, vitamin deficiencies).

Encourage older adults who exhibit depressive symptoms to seek treatment. Because older adults with depression may feel unworthy, withdrawn, and isolated, the support of the family or others in encouraging older adults to seek treatment is important. Assist older adult caregivers who exhibit depressive symptoms to seek medical attention, and assist them in securing respite services and support for their caregiving role. (Family caregiving is discussed in Chapter 4 on pp. 49 to 50.)

◆ ***Use of Restraints.*** *Physical restraints* are devices, materials, and equipment that physically prevent individuals from moving freely, such as walking, standing, lying, transferring, or sitting. *Chemical restraints* are drugs used to restrict the freedom or movement of a patient or in some cases to sedate a patient.

Before considering the use of any restraint, completely assess the perceived need for the restraint and document the assessment. Behavioral symptoms, such as crying and shouting, may arise from co-morbidities, pain, medication effects, unmet needs, and/or environmental factors. When behavioral manifestations are evident, ask the following questions to better understand the patient's behavior: Is the person able to verbalize what she or he needs and wants? People with dementia may respond by speaking, gesturing, nodding, or making eye contact. Questions that use "yes" or "no" answers are better than open-ended questions for gathering assessment information. Ask family, friends, or staff members from previous care settings about the patient's (1) history; (2) usual communication style and cues to indicate pain, fatigue, hunger, or a need to urinate or defecate; (3) abilities in ADLs; and (4) daily routines (e.g., "Is he often awake at night or an early riser?" "Does she prefer breakfast before dressing? Take an afternoon nap? Have a routine for dressing?").

**TABLE 5-13 Evaluating Nursing Care for Older Adults**

*Use the following questions to evaluate the effectiveness of care for older adults.*

- Is there an identifiable change in ADLs, IADLs, mental status, or signs and symptoms of the disease?
- Does the individual consider his or her health state to be improved?
- Does the individual think the plan is helpful?
- Do the individual and caregiver think the care is worth the time and cost?
- Can you document positive changes that support the interventions?

*ADLs,* Activities of daily living; *IADLs,* instrumental activities of daily living.

Evaluate whether disruptive behaviors signal unmet physiologic or psychosocial needs. For example, a patient who tries to get out of bed without help may be trying to reach the toilet. A toileting schedule will help to curtail such attempts and prevent incontinence. In critical care settings, patients emerging from sedation may be alarmed by an inability to speak or the presence of inserted tubes.

Restraints may be used only to ensure the person's safety or the safety of others. Physical and chemical restraints are a last resort in the care of older adults. The current standard is to provide safe care without using restraints of any form, whether physical or chemical. It is crucial to patient safety and prevention of falls that restraints not be used for this purpose. If physical or chemical restraints are used in acute, subacute, or long-term care settings, use of the least restrictive restraint is required. Restraints require an order from an HCP.

Carefully document restraint use and the behaviors that necessitate its perceived need. It is not appropriate to use restraints based on fall risk, avoidance of interference with medical devices, or perceived irritating behaviors, such as calling out. Frequent scheduled reviews of the ongoing necessity of the restraint are needed with consideration of discontinuation of the restraint. Long-term care regulations and The Joint Commission set standards for restraint usage. These include time limit, observation and care, use of least restrictive measures (e.g., mittens), and alternatives to the use of restraints. Restraint alternatives include low beds, body props, and electronic devices (such as bed and chair alarm signaling). Such approaches support the development of a "restraint-free," safe environment. Alternatives to restraints require vigilant, creative, and sensitive nursing care.

◆ ***Sleep.*** Adequacy of sleep is often a concern for older adults because of altered sleep patterns. Older people experience a marked decrease in deep sleep and are easily aroused. Many older adults report difficulty initiating sleep and maintaining prolonged sleep. They may state they feel "unrefreshed" after sleep. (Sleep problems of older adults are discussed in Chapter 7.)

## ◆ Evaluation

The evaluation phase of the nursing process is similar for all patients. The results of evaluation direct you to continue the plan of care or revise as indicated. When evaluating nursing care with older adults, focus on functional improvement and quality of life. Useful questions to consider when evaluating the plan of care for older adults are included in Table 5-13.

## CASE STUDY

### *Older Adults*

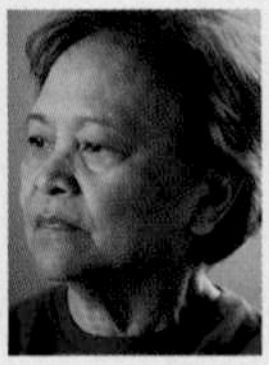

(©azndc/iStock/Thinkstock)

**Patient Profile**

C.L., a 73-year-old Taiwanese woman, was admitted through the emergency department with shortness of breath. She was diagnosed with community-acquired pneumonia. Her history also indicates she has chronic obstructive pulmonary disease (COPD), hypertension, diabetes, mild cognitive impairment, depression, macular degeneration, and significant hearing loss.

**Subjective Data**

- A stroke 5 years ago and has right-sided weakness
- A 100 pack-year history of tobacco use but quit smoking after her stroke
- Not seen primary care physician in 1 year
- In past year has had an unplanned weight loss of 15 pounds
- Spends her days either in bed or in a recliner watching television
- Shortness of breath for past 5 days

**Psychosocial Data**

- Came to the United States 15 years ago from Taiwan.
- Speaks Mandarin Chinese with limited English proficiency.
- Lives with her unemployed adult son who provides assistance with ADLs and IADLs.
- Has three daughters who live within a 2-hour drive.
- Limited financial resources but has Medicare and Medicaid benefits.
- Daughters raise concerns about their mother's care and safety at home, given their brother's history of anger issues and a gambling addiction.
- When daughters ask their brother about how he is caring for his mother, he says, "I'm doing the best I can. She refuses help. She refuses to go to the doctor. What do you want me to do? She's old. She's crazy. She's going to die anyway!"
- Daughters state their mother does not want to go to a nursing home.

**Objective Data**

***Physical Examination***

- Unwashed, matted hair, poor oral hygiene, overgrown toenails
- Two stage III sacral ulcers
- Unstageable right heel ulcer
- Multiple small bruises on her forearms and shins
- 5 × 10–cm bruise in the middle of her back

***Diagnostic Tests***

- Serum albumin 2.4 g/dL
- X-ray reveals consolidation in lower left and right lung lobes

**Discussion Questions**

1. What other information do you need to assess C.L.'s condition? How should questions regarding potential elder mistreatment be addressed?
2. Identify the stage(s) of Corbin and Strauss chronic illness trajectory that describe C.L.'s current status. Which stage(s) is the goal of your nursing care?
3. ***Patient-Centered Care:*** What is your assessment of C.L.'s ability to successfully complete these tasks? What will you include in your care planning to optimize her ability to complete these tasks?
4. ***Priority Decision:*** Based on your assessment of C.L., what are the priority nursing diagnoses? Are there collaborative problems?
5. ***Safety:*** To ensure C.L.'s safety, what nursing interventions are necessary during her hospitalization?
6. ***Teamwork and Collaboration:*** How would you use unlicensed assistive personnel (UAP) on the hospital unit to carry out the priorities that you identified in question 4?
7. ***Teamwork and Collaboration:*** What referrals may be indicated?
8. Define ageism, and explain how it may be manifested in this case.
9. What risk factors does C.L. have for development of frailty? Which of these factors are modifiable?
10. Based on your knowledge of care alternatives for older adults, what setting or settings may be appropriate for C.L. upon hospital discharge?
11. What risk factors does C.L. have for becoming a victim of elder mistreatment? List and provide the rationale for nursing interventions and legal and ethical responsibilities in this case.

Answers available at *http://evolve.elsevier.com/Lewis/medsurg.*

## BRIDGE TO NCLEX EXAMINATION

The number of the question corresponds to the same-numbered outcome at the beginning of the chapter.

1. Examples of primary prevention strategies include
   - **a.** colonoscopy at age 50.
   - **b.** avoidance of tobacco products.
   - **c.** teaching the importance of exercise to a patient with hypertension.
   - **d.** intake of a diet low in saturated fat in a patient with high cholesterol.
2. A characteristic of a chronic illness is that it *(select all that apply)*
   - **a.** has reversible pathologic changes.
   - **b.** has a consistent, predictable clinical course.
   - **c.** results in permanent deviation from normal.
   - **d.** is associated with many stable and unstable phases.
   - **e.** always starts with an acute illness and then progresses slowly.
3. Ageism is characterized by
   - **a.** denial of negative stereotypes regarding aging.
   - **b.** positive attitudes toward the elderly based on age.
   - **c.** negative attitudes toward the elderly based on age.
   - **d.** negative attitudes toward the elderly based on physical disability.
4. An ethnic older adult may feel a loss of self-worth when the nurse *(select all that apply)*
   - **a.** prohibits visits from a faith healer.
   - **b.** informs the patient about ethnic support services.
   - **c.** allows a patient to rely on ethnic health beliefs and practices.
   - **d.** emphasizes that a therapeutic diet does not allow ethnic foods.
   - **e.** uses a medical interpreter to provide explanations and teaching.
5. An important nursing action to help a chronically ill older adult is to
   - **a.** avoid discussing future lifestyle changes.
   - **b.** ensure the patient that the condition is stable.
   - **c.** treat the patient as a competent manager of the disease.
   - **d.** encourage the patient to "fight" the disease as long as possible.

6. Older adults who become ill are more likely than younger adults to
   a. complain about the symptoms of their problems.
   b. refuse to carry out lifestyle changes to promote recovery.
   c. seek medical attention because of limitations on their lifestyle.
   d. alter their daily living activities to accommodate new symptoms.
7. An appropriate care choice for an older adult who lives with an employed daughter but needs help with activities of daily living is
   a. adult day care.
   b. long-term care.
   c. a retirement center.
   d. an assisted living facility.
8. Nursing interventions directed at health promotion in the older adult are primarily focused on
   a. disease management.
   b. controlling symptoms of illness.
   c. teaching positive health behaviors.
   d. teaching regarding nutrition to enhance longevity.

1. b, 2. c, d, 3. c, 4. a, d, 5. c, 6. d, 7. a, 8. c.

For rationales to these answers and even more NCLEX review questions, visit *http://evolve.elsevier.com/Lewis/medsurg*.

## EVOLVE WEBSITE

http://evolve.elsevier.com/Lewis/medsurg

**Review Questions (Online Only)**

**Key Points**

**Answer Keys for Questions**

- Rationales for Bridge to NCLEX Examination Questions
- Answer Guidelines for Case Study on p. 75

**Conceptual Care Map Creator**

**Audio Glossary**

**Content Updates**

## REFERENCES


1. Centers for Disease Control and Prevention: Chronic diseases and health promotion, Retrieved from *www.cdc.gov/chronicdisease.*
2. Corbin JM, Strauss A: A nursing model for chronic illness management based upon the Trajectory Framework, *Sch Inq Nurs Pract* 5:155, 1991. (Classic)
3. Hartford Institute for Geriatric Nursing: Try This Series. Retrieved from *www.ConsultGeriRN.org/resources.*
4. Department of Health and Human Services. Self-management for health in chronic conditions. Retrieved from *www.grants.nih.gov/grants/guide/pa-files/PA-14-344.html.*

*5. Martinez-Marcos M, De la Cuesta-Benjumea C: Women's self management of chronic illnesses in the context of caregiving: a grounded theory study, *J Clin Nurs* 24:1557, 2015.

6. U.S. Census Bureau: Facts for features: Older Americans month: May 2014. Retrieved from *www.census.gov/newsroom/facts-for-features/2014/cb14-ff07.html.*
7. Administration on Aging: A profile of older Americans. Retrieved from *www.aoa.gov/Aging_Statistics/Profile/2012/docs/2012profile.pdf.*
8. Administration on Aging: Projected future growth of the older population. Retrieved from *www.aoa.acl.gov/Aging_Statistics/future_growth/future_growth.aspx.*
9. Scott G: Ageism is rife in health care, *Nurs Stan* 25:1, 2011.
10. Daniel M, Tollefsbol TO: Epigenetic linkage of aging, cancer and nutrition, *J Exp Biol* 218: 59, 2015.
11. Kim S, Brooks AK, Groban L: Preoperative assessment of the older surgical patient: honing in on geriatric syndromes, *Clin Interv Aging* 10:13, 2014.
12. Pew Research Internet Project. Older adults and technology use. Retrieved from *www.pewinternet.org/2014/04/03/older-adults-and-technology-use.*

*13. Xue QL: The frailty syndrome: definition and natural history, *Clin Geriatr Med* 27:1, 2011.

14. USDA Food and Nutrition Service. Supplemental Nutrition Assistance Program (SNAP). Retrieved from *www.fns.usda.gov/snap/snap-special-rules-elderly-or-disabled.*
15. Hardin SR: Ethnogeriatric in critical care, *Crit Care Nurs Clin North Am* 16:21, 2014.
16. Stanford Medicine, Geriatric Education Center. A national resource center in ethnogeriatrics. Retrieved from *http://sgec.stanford.edu.*
17. Administration on Aging Family Caregiver Alliance: Selected caregiver statistics. Retrieved from *www.caregiver.org/selected-caregiver-statistics.*
18. National Center for Elder Abuse. Retrieved from *www.ncea.aoa.gov/Library/Data.*
19. Preventing elder abuse and neglect in older adults: tools and tips. Retrieved from *www.ncea.aoa.gov/Library/Data.*

*20. Dong X: Self-neglect in an elderly community-dwelling U.S. Chinese population: findings from the population study of Chinese elderly in Chicago study, *J Am Geriatr Soc* 62:2391, 2014.

21. How much is enough? Out-of-pocket spending among Medicare beneficiaries: a chartbook. Retrieved from *www.kff.org/out+of+pocket.*
22. National PACE Association. Retrieved from *www.npaonline.org/website/article.asp.*
23. American Geriatrics Society. AGS/BGS Clinical practice guideline: prevention of falls in older persons. Retrieved from *www.americangeriatrics.org/health_care_professionals/clinical_practice/clinical_guidelines_recommendations/prevention_of_falls_summary_of_recommendations.*
24. Transitional care model: Essential elements. Retrieved from *www.transitionalcare.info/essential-elements.*
25. The American Geriatrics Society 2012 Beers criteria update expert panel for potentially inappropriate medication use in older adults, *J Am Geriatr Soc* 60:616, 2012.

*Evidence-based information for clinical practice.

6

# Stress and Stress Management

*Sharon L. Lewis, Peter N. Bonner*

*What is the triumph of the human spirit? It is the ability to rise above our problems and not only survive, but thrive in the face of adversity.*

**Brian Luke Seaward**

http://evolve.elsevier.com/Lewis/medsurg/

## LEARNING OUTCOMES

1. Differentiate between the terms *stressor* and *stress*.
2. Describe the role of the nervous and endocrine systems in the stress process.
3. Describe the effects of stress on the immune system.
4. Describe how stress affects the mind-body-spirit connection.
5. Discuss the effects of stress on health.
6. Explain the role of coping in managing stress.
7. Describe the coping and relaxation strategies that can be used by you, a patient, or caregiver experiencing stress.
8. Describe the nursing assessment and management of a patient experiencing stress.

## KEY TERMS

coping, p. 82
emotion-focused coping, p. 82
imagery, p. 84
massage, p. 85
meditation, p. 84
mind-body-spirit connection, p. 81
problem-focused coping, p. 82
psychoneuroimmunology (PNI), p. 80
relaxation breathing, p. 83
stress, p. 77
stressors, p. 77

High levels of stress are common among patients and their caregivers. How they deal with their stress is critical to their well-being. As a nurse, you have an important role in helping them manage stressful events.

Stress has a powerful effect on the mind and therefore a significant effect on one's health and well-being. This chapter focuses on how stress can affect the mind, body, and spirit and how a person can effectively cope with stress.

## WHAT IS STRESS?

**Stress** is the inability to cope with perceived (real or imagined) demands or threats to one's mental, emotional, or spiritual well-being.[1] What is perceived as stressful to one person may not be perceived as stressful to another. Individual responses to the same stressor vary greatly. *Perception* of the potential stressor influences the way an individual responds to that stressor (Fig. 6-1). This is demonstrated in the following examples.

- B.J., a 43-year-old woman, becomes depressed after a laparoscopic hysterectomy for fibroids. She is unwilling to participate in normal self-care activities. You are surprised by her response and think that this is fairly simple surgery and she should get on with her life. After further assessment, you discover that the removal of her uterus is a great psychologic stressor because she perceives it as a loss of her womanhood and femininity.
- K.R., a 52-year-old woman, has just been told by her physician of her new diagnosis of type 2 diabetes. After the physician's visit with her, you are prepared to provide emotional support. However, you are puzzled when she is smiling and breathing a sigh of relief. You think that this diagnosis should be stressful. However, K.R. tells you that she is so relieved because for weeks she has worried that her symptoms were related to cancer.

Many different events or factors can be **stressors**. They can be physiologic or emotional/psychologic (Fig. 6-1). The emotional/psychologic stressors can be positive or negative. For example, the birth of a baby is a positive stressor. Marital discord is a negative stressor.

### Is Stress Bad or Good?

We tend to think of stress as bad or a threat. Actually any event or situation that is out of the ordinary can be considered a stressor. Events that are normally considered happy or enjoyable (e.g., getting married, going on a vacation) are also stressors.

Stress can be helpful. A little stress can motivate you. Stress can actually inspire you to achieve a goal and become more confident or stronger physically.

Reviewed by Ellen Odell, DNP, ACNS-BC, CNE, APRN, Director of Nursing, Associate Professor, Department of Nursing, John Brown University, Siloam Springs, Arkansas; and Teresa J. Seright, RN, PhD, CCRN, Associate Teaching Professor, College of Nursing, Montana State University, Bozeman, Montana.

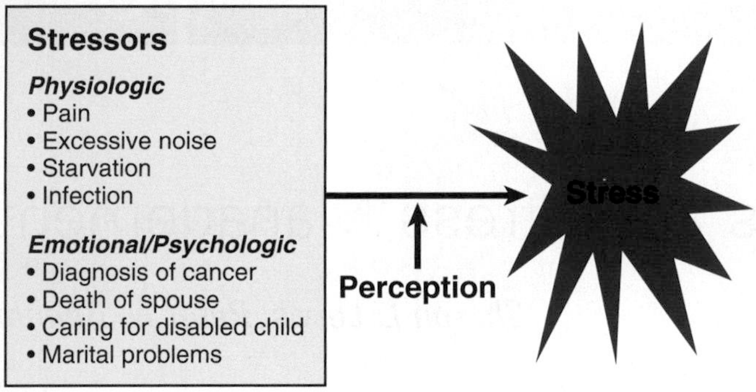


**FIG. 6-1** Stressors can be physiologic or emotional/psychologic. Your perception of these stressors will determine whether they cause stress. Events or circumstances become stressful when you perceive them to be.

The body does not differentiate between bad stress and good stress, or real or imaginary stress. It responds to the stressor with the same stress response. This stress response is the way our bodies react both physically and emotionally to any change, be it good, bad, real, or imagined.

For you as a nursing student, a test can be a stressful situation. A little bit of stress related to the upcoming test makes you study and become better prepared. If you are mildly stressed during the test, it may help your test performance as a little stress heightens your awareness and increases your mental acuity. However, if you are overly stressed, it causes mental blocks, lack of concentration, and inability to remember things.

Stress is a key for survival, but too much stress can be detrimental. That is why it is important for you and your patients to learn to cope more effectively with the stressors in life.

## Factors Affecting Response to Stress

Why do people respond so differently to stress? Why do some people cope better with stress than others? Interestingly, some individuals experience significant adverse life events but do not succumb to the effects of stress.

Differences in the responses to a stressor can be based on the duration of a stressor (acute or chronic) and intensity of a stressor (mild, moderate, or severe). For example, an individual dealing with the chronic stress of caring for a loved one may also be exposed to many acute stressors (e.g., car accident, influenza). Therefore the type, duration, and intensity of a stressor are important variables that can influence an individual's response (Fig. 6-2).

Factors that affect an individual's response to stress include internal and external influences (Table 6-1). These factors indicate the importance of using a holistic approach when assessing the impact of stress on a person. Four key personal characteristics that buffer the effects of stress are resilience, hardiness, attitude, and being optimistic.

*Resilience* is being resourceful and flexible and having good problem-solving skills. Individuals who possess a high degree of resilience are not as likely to perceive an event as stressful.

*Hardiness* is a combination of three characteristics: commitment, control, and openness to change. Together they provide the courage and motivation needed to turn stressful circumstances from potential calamities into opportunities for personal growth.[2]

*Attitude* can also influence the effect of stress on a person. People with positive attitudes view situations differently from those with negative attitudes. A person's attitude also influences how he or she manages stress. To some extent, positive emotional attitudes can prevent disease and prolong life.[3]

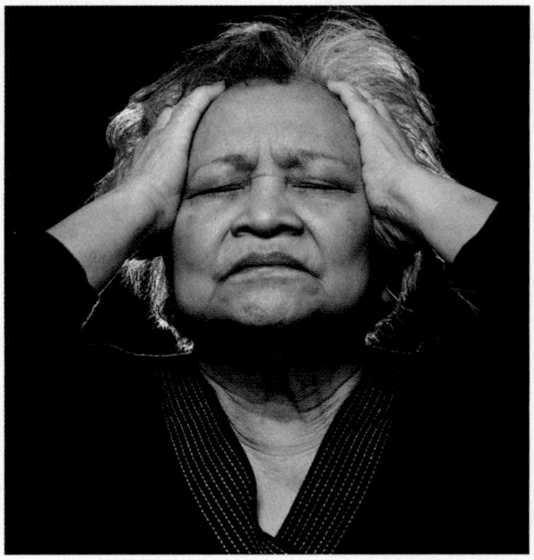

**FIG. 6-2** During stressful situations, the demands seem to exceed the resources. (©azndc/iStock/Thinkstock)

**TABLE 6-1 Factors Affecting Response to Stress**

| Internal | External |
|---|---|
| • Age | • Cultural and ethnic influences |
| • Health status | • Socioeconomic status |
| • Personality characteristics | • Social support |
| • Previous experience with stressors | • Religious or spiritual influences |
| • Genetic background | • Timing of stressors |
| • Resilience | • Number of stressors already experiencing |
| • Hardiness | |
| • Attitude | |
| • Optimistic outlook | |
| • Nutritional status | |
| • Sleep status | |

Being optimistic can help you cope more effectively with stress. Optimism also reduces a person's chances of developing stress-related illnesses. When optimistic people do become ill, they tend to recover more quickly. Pessimists are likely to deny the problem, distance themselves from the stressful event, focus on stressful feelings, or allow the stressor to interfere with achieving a goal. People with a more pessimistic attitude tend to report poorer health than people with optimistic attitudes.[3]

In addition to personal characteristics, external factors play an important role in one's ability to cope with stress. Being surrounded by a strong social support system and receiving positive support from friends and family have a large impact on an individual's ability to cope with stressors.

# PHYSIOLOGIC RESPONSE TO STRESS

The following section discusses the roles of the nervous, endocrine, and immune systems. These systems are interrelated, and that interrelationship is reflected in a person's physiologic response to stress (Fig. 6-3). Further, stress activation of these systems affects other body systems, such as the cardiovascular, respiratory, gastrointestinal, renal, and reproductive systems. A person's response to a stressor (real or imagined, and

PATHOPHYSIOLOGY MAP

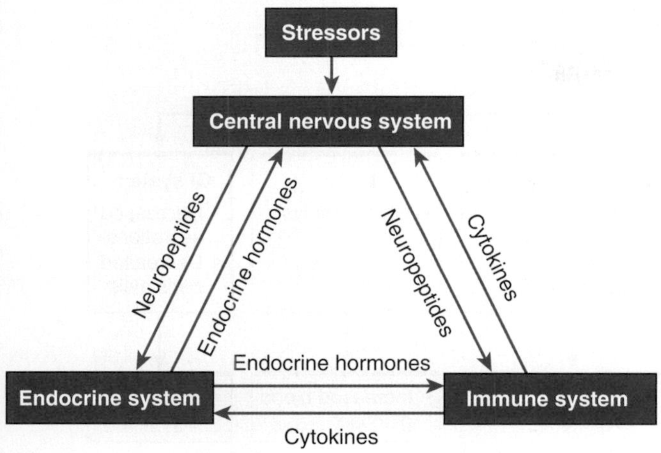


**FIG. 6-3** Neurochemical links among the nervous, endocrine, and immune systems. The communication among these three systems is bidirectional.

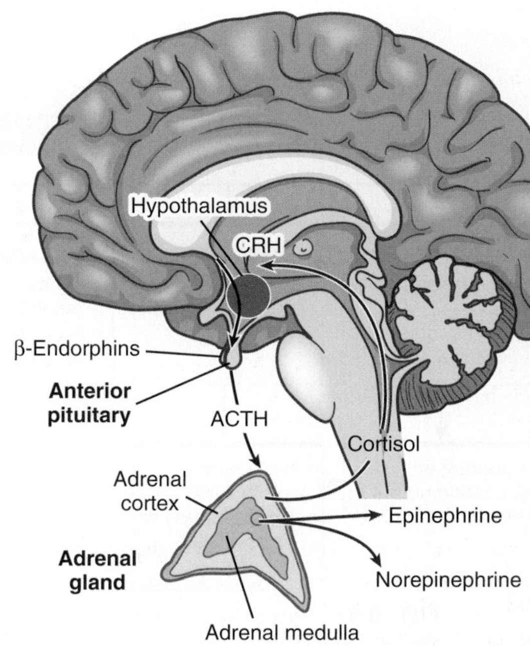


**FIG. 6-4** Hypothalamic-pituitary-adrenal axis. *ACTH,* Adrenocorticotropic hormone; *CRH,* corticotropin-releasing hormone.

physiologic or emotional/psychologic) determines the impact that stress will have on the body.

## Nervous System

**Cerebral Cortex.** The cerebral cortex evaluates the stressor in light of past experiences and future consequences. These functions are involved in the perception of a stressor.

**Limbic System.** The *limbic system* lies in the inner midportion of the brain near the base of the brain. The limbic system is an important mediator of emotions and behavior. When the limbic system is stimulated, emotions, feelings, and behaviors can occur that ensure survival and self-preservation.

**Reticular Formation.** The *reticular formation* is located between the lower end of the brainstem and thalamus. It contains the *reticular activating system* (RAS), which sends impulses contributing to alertness to the limbic system and cerebral cortex. When the RAS is stimulated, it increases its output of impulses, leading to wakefulness. Stress usually increases the degree of wakefulness and can lead to sleep disturbances.

**Hypothalamus.** The hypothalamus, which lies at the base of the brain just above the pituitary gland, has many functions that assist in adaptation to stress. Stress activates the limbic system, which in turn stimulates the hypothalamus. Because the hypothalamus secretes neuropeptides that regulate the release of hormones by the anterior pituitary, it is central to the connection between the nervous and endocrine systems in responding to stress (Fig. 6-4).

The hypothalamus plays a primary role in the stress response by regulating the function of both the sympathetic and parasympathetic branches of the autonomic nervous system. When an individual perceives a stressor, the hypothalamus sends signals that initiate both the nervous and endocrine responses to the stressor. It does this primarily by sending signals via nerve fibers to stimulate the sympathetic nervous system (SNS) and by releasing corticotropin-releasing hormone (CRH), which stimulates the pituitary to release adrenocorticotropic hormone (ACTH) (see Chapter 47).

## Endocrine System

Once the hypothalamus is activated in response to stress, the endocrine system becomes involved. The SNS stimulates the adrenal medulla to release epinephrine and norepinephrine (catecholamines). The effect of catecholamines and the activation of the SNS, including the response of the adrenal medulla, is referred to as the *sympathoadrenal response.* Epinephrine and norepinephrine prepare the body for the *fight-or-flight response* (Fig. 6-5).

Stress activates the hypothalamic-pituitary-adrenal (HPA) axis. In response to stress, the hypothalamus releases CRH, which stimulates the anterior pituitary to release proopiomelanocortin (POMC). Both ACTH (a hormone) and β-endorphin (a neuropeptide) are derived from POMC. Endorphins have analgesic-like effects and blunt pain perception during stress situations involving pain stimuli. ACTH, in turn, stimulates the adrenal cortex to synthesize and secrete corticosteroids (e.g., cortisol) and, to a lesser degree, aldosterone.

Corticosteroids are essential for the stress response. Cortisol produces a number of physiologic effects, such as increasing blood glucose levels, potentiating the action of catecholamines on blood vessels, and inhibiting the inflammatory response. Corticosteroids play an important role in "turning off" or blunting the stress response, which, if uncontrolled, can become self-destructive. This is shown by corticosteroids' ability to suppress the release of proinflammatory mediators, such as the cytokines tumor necrosis factor (TNF) and interleukin-1 (IL-1). The persistent release of such mediators is believed to initiate organ dysfunction in conditions such as sepsis. Thus corticosteroids act not only to support the body's adaptive response to a stressor but also to suppress an overzealous and potentially self-destructive response.

The stress response involves increases in (1) cardiac output (resulting from the increased heart rate and increased stroke volume), (2) blood glucose levels, (3) oxygen consumption, and (4) metabolic rate (Fig. 6-5). In addition, dilation of skeletal muscle blood vessels increases blood supply to the large muscles and provides for quick movement. Increased cerebral blood flow increases mental alertness. For example, in the case of stressful situations (e.g., blood loss from trauma), the increased

**PATHOPHYSIOLOGY MAP**

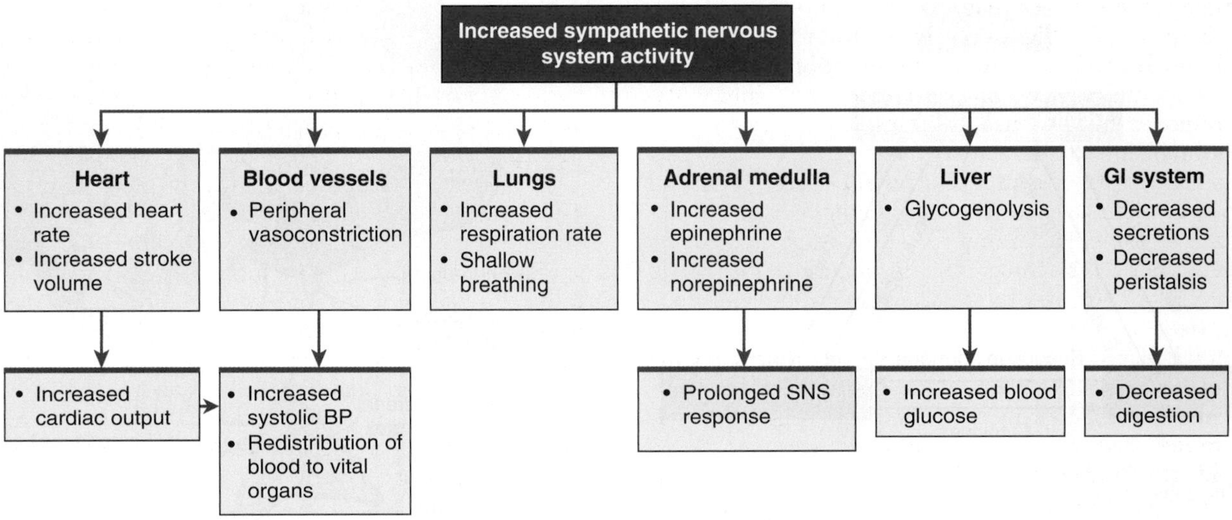


**FIG. 6-5** "Fight-or-flight" reaction. Alarm reaction responses resulting from increased sympathetic nervous system *(SNS)* activity.

blood volume (from increased extracellular fluid and the shunting of blood away from the gastrointestinal system) helps to maintain adequate circulation to vital organs.

## Summary of Stress Response

In summary, the fight-or-flight response is an important and necessary adaptive mechanism of the body to acute stress. This response to stressors is activated regardless of whether they are physiologic (e.g., acute pain) or emotional/psychologic (e.g., death of a child, loss of a home through fire, fear).

Acute stress leads to physiologic changes that are important to a person's survival. This is your "alarm system." It puts you on high alert. The acute stress response is a state of physiologic and psychologic arousal characterized by increased SNS activity that leads to increased heart and respiratory rate, increased BP, increased muscle tension, increased brain activity, and decreased skin temperature.

## Immune System

Stress also has an impact on the immune system. **Psychoneuroimmunology (PNI)** is an interdisciplinary science that studies the interactions among psychologic, neurologic, and immune responses.[4] Because the brain is connected to the immune system by neuroanatomic and neuroendocrine pathways, stressors have the potential to lead to alterations in immune function (Fig. 6-6).

Nerve fibers extend from the nervous system and synapse on cells and tissues of the immune system (i.e., spleen, lymph nodes). In turn, the cells of the immune system have receptors for many neuropeptides and hormones, which permit them to respond to nervous and neuroendocrine signals. As a result, the mediation of stress by the central nervous system leads to corresponding changes in immune cell activity.

Both acute and chronic stress can cause immunosuppression. Stress affects immune function by (1) decreasing the number and function of natural killer cells; (2) decreasing lymphocyte proliferation; (3) altering production of *cytokines* (soluble factors secreted by white blood cells and other cells, e.g., interferon, interleukins); and (4) decreasing phagocytosis

**PATHOPHYSIOLOGY MAP**

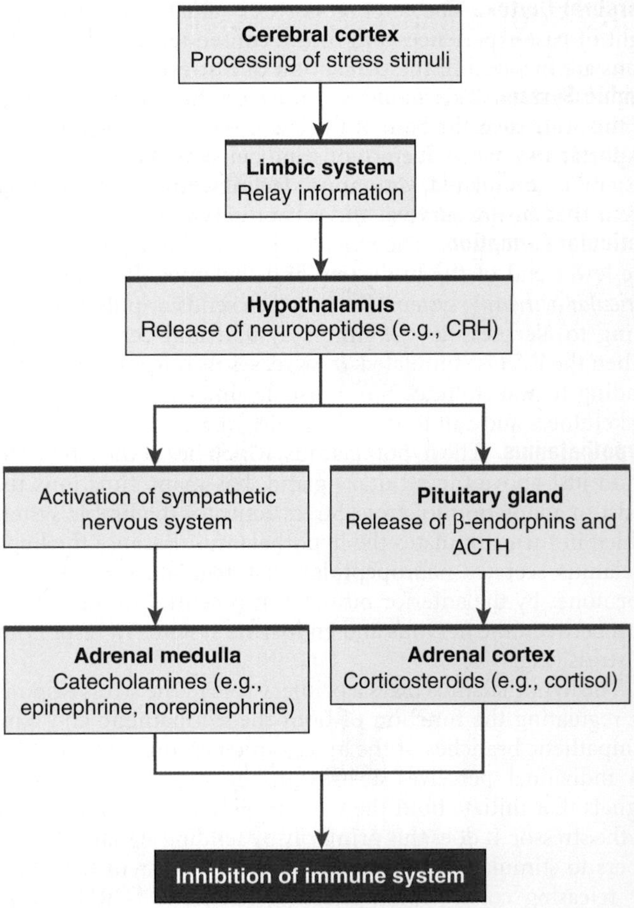


**FIG. 6-6** The cerebral cortex processes stressful stimuli and relays the information via the limbic system to the hypothalamus. Corticotropin-releasing hormone *(CRH)* stimulates the release of adrenocorticotropic hormone *(ACTH)* from the pituitary gland. ACTH stimulates the adrenal cortex to release corticosteroids. The sympathetic nervous system is also stimulated, resulting in the release of epinephrine and norepinephrine from the adrenal medulla. The end result is the inhibition of the immune system.

by neutrophils and monocytes.[4] (Natural killer cells, lymphocytes, and cytokines are discussed in Chapter 13.)

Importantly, the network that links the brain and immune system is bidirectional (Fig. 6-3). Signals from these systems travel back and forth, allowing for communication among these systems. Consequently, not only do emotions modify the immune response, but products of immune cells send signals back to the brain and alter its activity. Many of the communication signals sent from the immune system to the brain are mediated by cytokines, which are central to the coordination of the immune response. For example, IL-1 (a cytokine made by monocytes) acts on the temperature regulatory center of the hypothalamus and initiates the febrile response to infectious pathogens (see Fig. 11-4).

The central nervous system is capable of influencing the function of the immune system. Stress-induced immunosuppression may exacerbate or increase the risk of progression of immune-related diseases such as multiple sclerosis, asthma, rheumatoid arthritis, and cancer.[5]

Many questions about stress and the immune response remain unanswered. For example, it is not known how much stress (intensity or chronicity) is needed to cause changes or how much of an alteration in the immune system is necessary before disease susceptibility occurs.

## MIND-BODY-SPIRIT CONNECTION

The **mind-body-spirit connection** demonstrates the relationship and interconnectedness among the various parts that a person is made of: mind, body, and spirit (Fig. 6-7). All three parts are important in your life and in determining who you are. What goes on in your mind influences every part of the body. Your body and your mind are affected by how connected you feel to your spirit (soul). Spirit is the life force within you that gives life, energy, and power. You are a spiritual being with a mind that affects every aspect of your body.

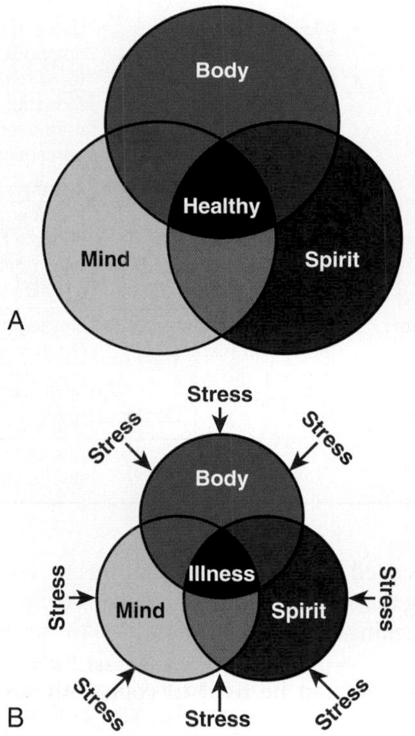


**FIG. 6-7** The connections among the mind, body, and spirit can lead to a person being healthy **(A)** or the effects of stress on the mind, body, and spirit connections can lead to illness **(B)**.

When your mind is healthy, your body can resist illness better. When your body is healthy, your feelings are more positive. When your spirit is renewed and energized, your mind is alert and your body feels good. The well-being of your spirit is linked to your mental, emotional, and physical health.

Stress has a powerful effect on your mind, body, and spirit. Therefore it has a significant effect on your health and well-being. Emotional thoughts and feelings can affect the body and spirit. Negative thoughts such as, "I am a terrible nurse … I cannot handle this one more day" can cause a physical response in your body (e.g., headaches, stomachaches), and it will make you feel down in your spirits; your life force feels sucked out. You can become physically ill.

Since the mind can affect the body and spirit, conscious use of the mind can effect positive changes in your body. Your mind is one of the most powerful weapons that you have to deal with and conquer stress.

How you deal with difficult situations or stressful times can greatly influence your overall well-being: your mind, body, and spirit. You have a choice in how you respond to a crisis or a difficult time. Even if the outcome of the situation is not what a person desired, one can emerge with a winning attitude. Sometimes you may feel that the world is against you and life is not fair. Or you can say, "This is rough, but I'm not going to let this get me down."

## EFFECTS OF STRESS ON HEALTH

As previously mentioned, the acute stress response is your alarm system and puts you on alert. However, your body was not meant to be on high alert all of the time. If stress is excessive or prolonged, these same "helpful" physiologic responses can lead to harm and disease. When a person sustains chronic, unrelieved stress, the body's defenses can no longer keep up with the demands. Therefore stress plays a role in the development and/or progression of diseases of adaptation, or stress-related illnesses (Table 6-2).

Stress is linked to leading causes of death, including cancer, accidents, and suicides. Stress can have effects on cognitive function, including poor concentration, memory problems, distressing dreams, sleep disturbances, and impaired decision making. Stress can also cause a wide variety of changes in behavior. These include people withdrawing from others, becoming quiet or unusually talkative, changing eating habits, drinking alcohol excessively, or becoming irritable.[5,6]

Long-term exposure to catecholamines resulting from excessive activation of the SNS may increase the risk of cardiovas-

**TABLE 6-2 Disorders With a Stress Component***

| | |
|---|---|
| • Depression | • Hypertension |
| • Dyspepsia | • Insomnia |
| • Eating disorders | • Irritable bowel syndrome |
| • Erectile dysfunction | • Low back pain |
| • Fatigue | • Menstrual irregularities |
| • Fibromyalgia | • Peptic ulcer disease |
| • Headaches | • Sexual dysfunction |

*List is not all inclusive.

cular diseases such as atherosclerosis and hypertension.[7] Other conditions that are precipitated or aggravated by stress include migraine headaches, irritable bowel syndrome, and peptic ulcers.[8,9] Control of metabolic conditions, such as diabetes mellitus, is also affected by stress. Behavioral interventions aimed at stress reduction and relaxation have helped manage these diseases in conjunction with standard medical therapy.[10]

Stressful life events can make a person more susceptible to infection. For example, psychologic stress may increase one's risk for developing the common cold. In a landmark study, healthy volunteers were inoculated intranasally with low doses of upper respiratory tract viruses. The subjects underwent psychologic testing to determine the occurrence of stressful events in their lives and their reactions to such stresses. The results showed that the rates of both viral infection and clinical colds increased with the degree of psychologic stress. In this study, social support buffered the harmful effects of stress.[11]

At the cellular level, stress may promote earlier onset of age-related diseases. There is a link between stress and telomere length. Telomeres are the protective end caps on chromosomes, and their diminishing size is an indication of age. Telomeres are highly susceptible to stress and depression. Telomeres are shorter in people who are stressed and depressed than in healthy people. Thus chronic stress can have a long-term effect on our overall health by changing our DNA and accelerating the rate at which our cells age.[12,13]

Chronic stress is a major contributor to chronic illness, which in turn is a major driver of escalating health care costs. It is critical that the entire health care community recognize the role of stress and unhealthy behaviors in causing and exacerbating chronic health conditions.

## COPING STRATEGIES

**Coping** is a person's efforts to manage stressors.[14] *Coping strategies* are what you do (your behaviors and actions) to help deal with stress. Coping can be either positive or negative. Positive coping includes activities such as exercise and spending time with friends and family. Healthy coping helps you handle your stressors so that they do not overwhelm you. Negative coping may include substance abuse and denial.

Unfortunately, some coping strategies actually make the stress worse. Sometimes coping strategies temporarily relieve the stress, but in the long run they actually increase the stress. For example, a person may really enjoy watching a favorite TV show as a form of coping. However, then it soon becomes a fixation on many soap operas and TV becomes an addiction and escape from dealing with the real stressors.

> You cannot always choose your destiny in life, but you can choose how you cope with it.
>
> **Norman Vincent Peale**

A variety of coping strategies can be used to cope with stress. Table 6-3 has examples of coping strategies that you can use in your life and teach to patients and caregivers. Coping strategies can be divided into two broad categories: emotion-focused coping and problem-focused coping. **Emotion-focused coping** involves managing the emotions that an individual feels when a stressful event occurs. Examples of emotion-focused coping include discussing feelings with a friend or taking a hot bath.

**TABLE 6-3 Coping Strategies**

| Strategy | Description | How to Implement |
|---|---|---|
| **Aromatherapy** | • Use of essential oils (fragrant molecules from plants) for inhalation or topical application<br>• Variety of essential oils including lavender, peppermint, rosemary, eucalyptus, sandalwood, etc. | • Place 5-8 drops in a full bath and agitate water before bathing.<br>• Place a few drops on a tissue or in diffuser or vaporizer. |
| **Art therapy** | • Allows a person to nonverbally express and communicate feelings, emotions, and thoughts<br>• Can reduce stress, promote relaxation, and help process experiences<br>• Based on the belief that the creative process is healing and life enhancing | • Close your eyes and draw a line on a piece of paper. Open your eyes. Continue to build on that line and draw whatever comes to mind.<br>• Get a piece of paper and doodle. Do not edit.<br>• Get a coloring book and crayons and just start coloring. |
| **Exercise** | • Any form of movement, especially aerobic movement<br>• Can be viewed as meditation in motion | • Walk, swim, garden, bicycle, dance, climb stairs, participate in group exercises. |
| **Humor** | • Can take the form of laughter, cartoons, funny movies, videos, riddles, comic books, and joke books | • Keep a "tickler" scrapbook with funny photos, cartoons, etc.<br>• Humor carts can be set up in many clinical settings to be used by patients and families. |
| **Journaling** | • Allows an individual to express self in writing<br>• Enhances personal development and awareness through self-reflection | • Use a journaling notebook or computer to write down thoughts, feelings, memories, and perceptions. |
| **Pet therapy (animal-assisted therapy)** (Fig. 6-8) | • Use of animals as a form of treatment<br>• Improves a patient's social, emotional, or cognitive functioning | • Pet therapist or family member or friend brings a pet with which patient can socialize. |
| **Social support** | • Relationships with family and friends<br>• Self-help groups and professional help | • Get together with family and friends on a regular basis.<br>• Join a support group that specifically helps to meet needs (e.g., grief support group). |

**Problem-focused coping** involves attempts to resolve the problems causing the stress. Setting priorities or collecting information and seeking advice are examples of problem-focused coping.

Both strategies can be used to cope with stressors, and a combination of these strategies can be used to cope with the same stressor. Table 6-4 provides examples of emotion- and problem-focused coping when applied to the same stressful situation. When a situation is unchangeable or uncontrollable,

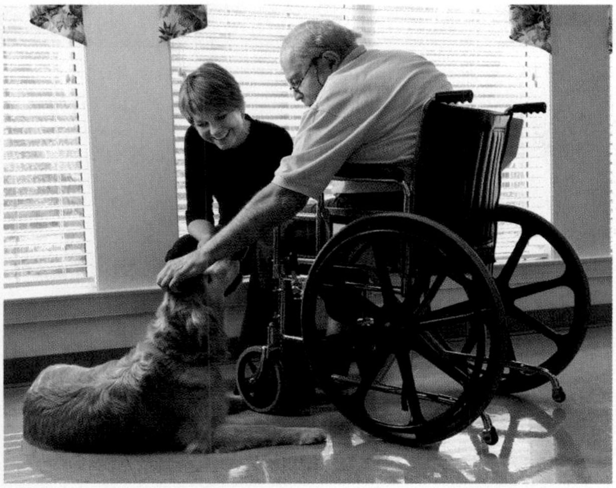

**FIG. 6-8** Pet therapy can be used in a variety of settings including rehabilitation. (©RonChappleStudios/Hemera/Thinkstock)

**TABLE 6-4 Problem- and Emotion-Focused Coping**

| Stressor | Problem-Focused Coping | Emotion-Focused Coping |
|---|---|---|
| Failing an examination | Obtaining a tutor | Going for a run |
| Being diagnosed with diabetes | Attending education classes about diabetes | Getting a massage |
| Receiving questionable mammogram results | Scheduling follow-up testing for ultrasound | Expressing feelings of anxiety to friends and nurse |

emotion-focused coping may predominate. The primary purpose of emotion-focused coping is to help decrease negative emotions and create a feeling of well-being. Although it may not seem to be working toward a solution, emotion-focused coping is a valid and appropriate way to deal with stressful situations.

If a problem can be changed or controlled, problem-focused coping is the most helpful coping strategy. Problem-focused coping strategies allow an individual to look at a challenge objectively, take action to address the problem, and thereby reduce the stress.

## RELAXATION STRATEGIES

The *relaxation response* is a state of physiologic and psychologic rest. It is the opposite of the stress response. The relaxation response is characterized by decreased SNS activity, which leads to decreased heart and respiratory rate, decreased BP, decreased muscle tension, decreased brain activity, and increased skin temperature.[15]

The relaxation response can be elicited through a variety of relaxation strategies (Table 6-5). Regular elicitation of the relaxation response has been proven to be an effective treatment for a wide range of stress-related disorders, including chronic pain, insomnia, and hypertension. Individuals who regularly engage in relaxation strategies are able to deal better with their stressors, increase their sense of control over stressors, and reduce their tension.[16]

**TABLE 6-5 Relaxation Strategies***

- Imagery
- Massage
- Meditation
- Muscle relaxation
- Music
- Qigong
- Relaxing breathing
- Tai Chi
- Yoga

*This list is not all inclusive. Further description of the most common ones are discussed in the text.

### COMPLEMENTARY & ALTERNATIVE THERAPIES

***Yoga***

Yoga is an ancient system of relaxation, exercise, and healing with origins in Indian philosophy. The goal of yoga is physical and mental well-being achieved through the use of stretching, postures, breathing practices, and meditation.

**Scientific Evidence**

Yoga can be used to treat hypertension and reduce stress and anxiety.

**Nursing Implications**

- Regardless of the type of yoga, deep abdominal relaxation breathing is a main component and helps one to focus on the inner self and promote the relaxation response.
- Yoga is often used to promote relaxation, decrease stress, improve flexibility, and enhance overall health.
- Yoga is generally considered safe. Some postures should not be used by patients with certain medical conditions or illnesses.

### Relaxation Breathing

The way one breathes affects every aspect of one's life. When a person is stressed, muscles tense and breathing becomes shallow and rapid. Therefore one of the simplest and most effective ways to stop the stress response is to breathe deeply and slowly. It is difficult to maintain tension when breathing in a slow, deep, and relaxed pattern.

**Relaxation** (abdominal) **breathing** can be performed while sitting, standing, or lying down. It is especially useful during a stressful or anxious situation to reduce stress. Relaxation breathing forms the basis for most relaxation strategies.

Before practicing relaxation breathing, it is important to assess one's normal breathing pattern (Table 6-6). Relaxation breathing, which involves the diaphragm, is natural for newborns and sleeping adults. It is a more efficient type of breathing. Chest breathing, which involves the upper chest and shoulders, is inefficient. This type of breathing is often used during times of anxiety and distress.

Relaxation breathing involves the primary use of the diaphragm and less use of the upper chest and shoulders to assist in each breath. In this type of breathing, the abdomen gently moves in and out during exhalation and inhalation. The breaths should be slow, steady, and deep.

One basic technique for relaxation breathing is as follows: (1) Inhale slowly and deeply, pushing the abdomen out. Think about breathing in peace. (2) Exhale slowly, letting the abdomen come in and all the muscles relax. Think about breathing out tension. (3) Repeat these deep breaths 10 times without interruption. As with any breathing exercise, if a light-headed feeling arises, stop for 30 seconds and then start again.

Other methods used to teach relaxation breathing are the 4 × 4 technique and relaxation sigh (Table 6-6). Breathing

**TABLE 6-6 Relaxation Breathing Techniques***

**Breathing Assessment**

1. Begin by placing one hand gently on your abdomen below your waistline.
2. Place the other hand on the center of your chest on the sternum.
3. Without changing the normal breathing pattern, take several breaths. During inhalation notice which hand rises the most.
4. When relaxation breathing is performed properly, the hand on the abdomen should rise more than the hand on the chest.

**4 × 4 Technique**

1. Sit up straight with your back flush to the support of the chair and your feet flat on the floor.
2. Rest your arms on your lap, thighs, or arms of the chair.
3. Take in a deep breath through your nose to a count of four (1 … 2 … 3 … 4).
4. Hold your breath to a count of four (1 … 2 … 3 … 4).
5. Release your breath through your mouth to a count of four (1 … 2 … 3 … 4).
6. Rest for a count of four (1 … 2 … 3 … 4).
7. Repeat the cycle four times.

**Relaxing Sigh**

1. Sit up straight with your back against the support of the chair and your feet flat on floor.
2. Inhale a natural breath and then sigh deeply. Let out a sound of relief as the air rushes out of your lungs.
3. Do not think about inhaling at the end of the sigh; just let the air come in naturally as you breathe deeply.
4. Repeat this sigh about 4 to 6 times very slowly.
5. You can repeat this exercise whenever you need it.

*Video demonstrations of these techniques are available in the Stress-Busting Kit for Nursing Students on the website for this book.

techniques are discussed in the Stress-Busting Kit for Nursing Students available on the website for this book.

Initially, relaxation breathing may feel unusual. With practice it becomes easier, and its relaxing benefits are soon obvious. You should personally learn to use relaxation breathing before teaching it to patients and their caregivers. Once learned, relaxation breathing can be easily taught to patients in a variety of settings, particularly when they are undergoing stressful and painful procedures.

## Meditation

**Meditation** is a practice of concentrated focus on a sound, object, visualization, the breath, or movement. The purpose of meditation is to increase awareness, reduce stress, promote relaxation, and enhance personal and spiritual growth.

Although meditation can be performed anywhere, it is best to practice meditation in a quiet place, free of distractions. Table 6-7 provides some basic guidelines on how to meditate. Meditation is often practiced while seated, and it is important to maintain a comfortable posture. Meditation can also be performed while walking and focusing on a single action such as the movement of the feet. In the beginning, individuals typically start with just 5 to 10 minutes of meditation at a time and often increase the time as the practice becomes more comfortable.

**Prayer.** Prayer can be a form of meditation. It is a spiritual communion with God or an object of worship. Many people find deep comfort in their faith. Religious services, conversations with clergy, and individual worship and prayer may help to alleviate a person's stress and give one a greater perspective, strength, and inspiration.

**TABLE 6-7 Guide to Meditation***

*You can teach yourself the basics of meditation by following a few simple steps:*

1. Find a quiet place.
2. Make sure there are no distractions.
3. Sit in a comfortable position.
4. Close your eyes.
5. Shut out the world so that your brain can stop processing information coming from your senses.
6. Pick a focus word, short phrase, song verse (melody), or prayer that is firmly rooted in your belief system, such as *one, peace, The Lord is my shepherd, Hail Mary full of grace,* or *shalom.*
7. Breathe slowly and practice relaxation breathing. Say your focus word, short phrase, song verse, or prayer silently to yourself as you exhale.
8. Say the word or phrase again and again.
9. Try saying the word or phrase silently to yourself with every exhalation. The monotony will help you focus.
10. Relax your muscles, progressing from your feet to your calves, thighs, abdomen, shoulders, head, and neck.
11. Do not be concerned when other thoughts come to mind. Just acknowledge them and return calmly to your word or phrase.
12. Continue for 10 to 20 minutes, but even 5 minutes can leave you feeling calm and refreshed. Rise slowly.
13. Practice once or twice daily.

*Meditation exercises are available in the Stress-Busting Kit for Nursing Students on the website for this book.

## Imagery

**Imagery** is the use of one's mind to generate images that have a calming effect on the body. It involves focusing the mind and incorporates all the senses to create physiologic and emotional changes. It is a simple relaxation technique that requires no equipment other than an active imagination. *Guided imagery* is a variation of imagery in which images are suggested by another person (either live or on a CD or in an MP3 file).

Imagery can be used in many clinical settings for stress reduction and pain relief. Benefits of imagery include anxiety reduction, decreased muscle tension, improved comfort during medical procedures, enhanced immune function, decreased recovery time after surgery, and reduction in sleeping problems.

You can use imagery in your own life or use guided imagery with your patients. One of the uses of imagery is to create a special place for a mental retreat. Table 6-8 describes the steps involved in creating a special place.

When imagery is performed, it is best to find a comfortable position. Take slow, deep breaths. Focus should involve all senses (sight, hearing, touch, smell). For example, one can use an image such as Fig. 6-9, engaging all the senses as one focuses on the image.

Imagery can also be used to specifically target a disease, problem, or stressor. Table 6-9 describes some suggestions for using imagery in specific diseases or disorders.

Imagery can also be used to enhance performance or process stressful or difficult tasks. For example, an athlete or musician can use imagery to achieve greater success. Imagery allows one to mentally rehearse the difficult or challenging situation. Imagery can help a fearful nurse start an IV line or perform a difficult procedure. It can also be used with a patient who is afraid to have a stressful or painful procedure performed (e.g., bone marrow biopsy).

**TABLE 6-8 Imagery: Creating Your Special Place***

1. Begin by closing your eyes and taking several slow, deep breaths.
2. Imagine a place where you feel completely comfortable and peaceful. It may be a real place or one you imagine: one from your past or some place you have always wanted to go.
3. Allow this special place to take form, slowly. As it takes form, look around to your left, to your right. Enjoy the scenery: the colors, the texture, the shapes.
4. Listen carefully to the sounds of your place. What do you hear?
5. Is there a gentle breeze or sunshine warming your face? Pick up or touch some favorite objects from your special place.
6. Take in a deep breath through your nose, and notice the rich smells around you. Perhaps your favorite flower is in bloom, or you smell the scents of the ocean.
7. Take another deep breath and relax. Enjoy the peace, comfort, and safety of your special place.
8. This is your special place. You relax and feel thankful that you are here, in your special place.
9. You can return to this place any time that you wish.

*Imagery exercises are available in the Stress-Busting Kit for Nursing Students on the website for this book.

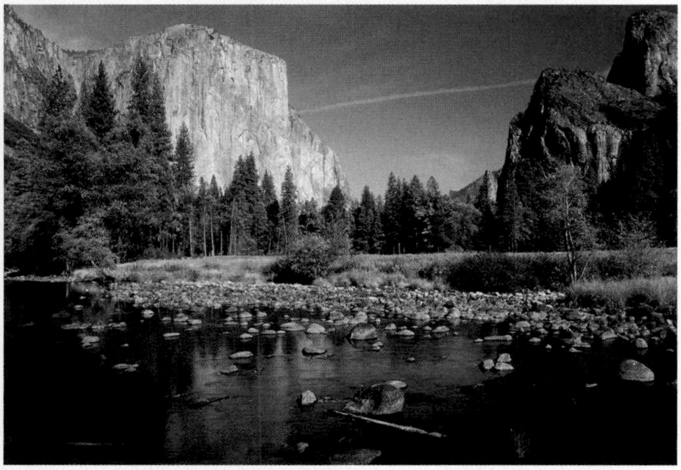

**FIG. 6-9** In imagery, special places are created involving all the senses, such as a place where one can hear rustling water, smell flowers, feel the wind, and see a colorful landscape. (©iStockphoto/Thinkstock)

## Music

*Music* can help achieve relaxation and bring about healthy changes in emotional or physical states. Listening to relaxing music can divert one's focus from a stressful situation.

Music has been used in many clinical settings. Music decreases anxiety and elicits the relaxation response. Music helps people with insomnia go to sleep. It can decrease muscle tension, pain sensation, and emotional stress.[17]

Music that contains approximately 60 to 80 beats/min is considered soothing. Low-pitched tones and music without words is recommended for relaxation. Mozart's music is a popular form of music used for relaxation. On the other hand, fast-tempo music can stimulate and uplift a person. Each person considers different types of music to be relaxing, so it is important to find music that best matches the person's needs and circumstance. To achieve optimal relaxation while listening to music, minimize all interruptions and assume a comfortable posture.

Music can be incorporated into clinical practice. It is noninvasive, safe, inexpensive, and easy to use. First, it is important to establish the purpose and benefit of using music with patients in a given clinical setting. Then assess each patient's interest and preference in music. Create a listening environment, encouraging the patient to find a comfortable position. Headphones or earphones and an MP3 or CD player can be used. Evaluate patients' response to the music, asking them how it sounds and how it makes them feel.

**TABLE 6-9 Examples of Imagery**

Imagery can be used to relieve stress and promote health and healing in conjunction with regular medical care. Special images can be created to alleviate symptoms or treat diseases or disorders. The image should be strong and vivid for the person, using many senses to create the image. Below are some examples that some people have found useful.

| Disease or Disorder | Images |
|---|---|
| **Infection** | • White blood cells with flashing red sirens arrest and imprison harmful germs. |
| **Cancer** | • Shark gobbles up cancer cells.<br>• Radiation or chemotherapy treatments enter the body like healing rays of light; they destroy cancer cells. |
| **Coronary artery disease** | • Water flows freely through a wide, open river. |
| **Weakened immune system** | • White blood cells rapidly multiply like millions of seeds bursting from a ripe seed pod. |
| **Asthma** | • Tiny elastic rubber bands that constrict the airways pop open. |
| **Depression** | • Troubles and feelings of sadness are attached to big colorful helium balloons and are floating off into a clear blue sky. |
| **Pain** | • Pain is washed away by a cool calm river flowing through the entire body. |

Adapted from Sobel DS, Ornstein R: *Healthy mind, healthy body,* New York, 1996, Patient Education Materials, Time Life.

## Massage

Massage includes a range of techniques that manipulate the soft tissues and joints of the body. Involving touch and movement, massage is typically delivered with the hands. It reduces muscle tension and positively affects mental and emotional states.

Massage is an important form of touch. It is also a form of caring, communication, and comfort. Your role related to massage differs from that of the registered massage therapist. Whereas massage therapists can provide more comprehensive massage therapies, as a nurse, you can use specific massage techniques as part of nursing care. For example, you can give a back massage to help promote sleep. For a bedridden patient, gentle massage can stimulate circulation and help prevent skin breakdown. A simple hand massage can be used to have a calming and relaxing effect, especially for patients who are anxious or agitated. During end-of-life care, hospice nurses may incorporate massage into their nursing care as the massaging touch can lessen pain and restlessness.

When you identify that massage may be useful, first assess the patient's preference regarding touch and massage. Consider cultural and social beliefs and discuss potential benefits with the patient. Family members can be taught to massage their loved one, providing a way for family members to participate in patient care. This can be therapeutic for the patient and family, even when the loved one is cognitively impaired or unresponsive.

> You may not be able to change the stressors in your life, but you can change your reaction or response to them.
>
> **Florence Nightingale**

## NURSING MANAGEMENT: STRESS

### Nursing Assessment

Patients and caregivers face many potential stressors that can have health consequences. Be aware of situations that are likely to result in stress and determine the patient's and caregiver's perception of these situations. In addition to the stressor itself, specific coping strategies have health consequences and therefore must be included in the assessment.

As a nurse, you are in a key position to (1) assess stress in patients and their caregivers, (2) assist them in identifying high-risk periods for stress, and (3) implement stress management strategies that can prevent the negative consequences of stress on their health (Fig. 6-10). Assess the number of stressors, duration of these stressors, and previous experience with similar demands. Assess the personal meaning attached to the stressful situation to provide useful insight for planning stress management strategies with the patient. Also consider the caregivers' responses to the stressors.

Be specific with your questions: Have you experienced this stressor before? How did you handle it? What worked well and what did not? Although the manifestations of stress may vary from person to person, assess the patient for the signs and symptoms of the stress response, including an increased heart rate and BP, hyperventilation, sweating, headache, musculoskeletal pain, gastrointestinal upset, loss of appetite, insomnia, and fatigue. In addition, the patient may exhibit some of the stress-related illnesses or diseases of adaptation (Table 6-2).

Behavioral manifestations may include an inability to concentrate, accident proneness, impaired speech, anxiety, crying, frustration, and irritability. Work-related responses to stress may include absenteeism or tardiness at work, decreased productivity, and job dissatisfaction. Cognitive responses include self-reports of an inability to make decisions and forgetfulness. Some of these responses may also be apparent to significant others.

Another major source of stress relates to the patient's illness, which often also causes stress for the caregiver and other family members. Assess what aspects of the illness are the most stressful for the patient and caregiver. These may include the patient's physical health, job responsibilities, finances, and children. This information is valuable because it helps you to understand the patient's perspective of the stressors. Knowledge of stressors, the feelings these stressors evoke, and the psychologic sequelae they can produce will assist you in identifying potential and actual sources of stress and their effect on the patient.

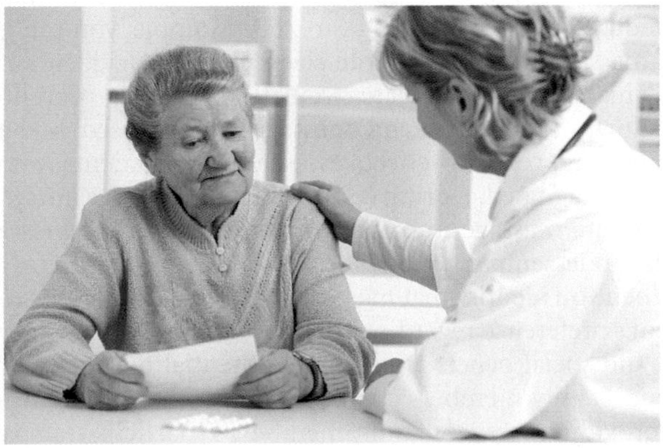

**FIG. 6-10** As a nurse, you have an important role in helping patients deal with stress. (©AlexRaths/iStock/Thinkstock)

### Nursing Implementation

The first step in managing stress is to become aware of its presence. This includes identifying what the stressors are and the person's response to them. Your role is to facilitate and enhance the patient's coping and adaptation. Nursing interventions depend on the severity of the stress experience. For example, a patient with multiple trauma expends energy in an attempt

## BECOMING A NURSE LEADER

### *Self-Care in Nursing*

**Situation**

You are a nursing student and becoming more anxious every day. You are constantly fatigued, have trouble sleeping, and are prone to muscle tension, headaches, and frequent gastrointestinal problems. In addition, you cannot concentrate or study, and you dread going to class and clinical. Seeing the pain and suffering of patients and family members is very stressful for you and causes you to feel hopeless. You are increasingly worried about being asked a question you cannot answer by physicians, nurses, and your instructors.

**Points for Consideration**

- Being an effective leader begins with taking care of yourself.
- Effective nurses remain honest with themselves and keep an open mind to getting help when they need it.
- Although nurses are taught to care for others, they often express reluctance to take the time required to care for themselves. Self-care can help practicing and student nurses cope with stressors and alleviate symptoms such as exhaustion, tension, and fatigue/burnout.[1]
- *Compassion fatigue* is identified as a unique form of burnout that affects individuals in caregiving roles. This may affect nurses when they personally experience the pain of their patients and families.[2]
- Be open to help. Don't feel ashamed or alone. Reach out for help by talking to your faculty, co-workers, or supervisor. Take advantage of student/employee health counseling.
- Keep work and home life separate. Easier said than done, but one of the key causes of compassion fatigue is losing sight of the boundaries between personal and work life.
- Some nursing school programs are incorporating self-care activities in their curriculums. These include discussions about self-care and stress management techniques (e.g., relaxation breathing, yoga, meditation, exercise, journaling) and seeing life as a blend and balance of teacher, healer, leader, and visionary.[2]

**Discussion Questions**

1. What are the first steps that you can take to decrease your stress and anxiety?
2. What self-care measures can you include in your daily life?
3. How can dealing with your own stressors help you to be a better nurse leader?

**References**

1. Blum CA: Practicing self-care for nurses: a nursing program initiative, *Online J Issues Nurs* 19(3), 2014. doi: 10.3912/OJIN.Vol19No03Man03.
2. Lombardo B, Eyre C: Compassion fatigue: a nurse's primer, *Online J Issues Nurs* 16(1):3, 2011. doi:10.3912/OJIN.Vol16No01Man03.

**TABLE 6-10 Personal Tips for Handling Stress**

- Do not try to be superhuman.
- Learn to "let go" of things that are outside of your control.
- Learn acceptance of yourself.
- Exercise regularly.
- Share your feelings.
- Keep a sense of humor; laugh often.
- Learn relaxation breathing.
- Use imagery.
- Meditate or pray.
- Get adequate sleep.
- Live a healthy lifestyle.
- Try to look at change as a positive challenge, not as a threat.
- Solve the little problems, since this can help you gain a feeling of control.
- Work to resolve conflicts with other people.
- If needed, get professional counseling.

**TABLE 6-11 How to Implement Stress Management in Practice**

1. Learn relaxation breathing. It is the easiest method of relaxation to use.
2. Practice teaching relaxation breathing with peers, then patients.
3. Pick coping strategies (Table 6-4) and relaxation strategies that are appropriate for your clinical area.
4. Practice using the strategy yourself. It becomes easier with time.
5. Take advantage of opportunities to teach coping and relaxation strategies to patients.
6. If you have setbacks, think about what went wrong. Do NOT quit!
7. Attend seminars and workshops on stress management to learn more.

to physically survive. As a nurse, your efforts are directed to life-supporting interventions and approaches aimed at reducing additional stressors for the patient. The patient with multiple trauma is much less likely to adapt or recover if faced with additional stressors such as sleep deprivation or an infection.

Coping strategies that are used should be helpful and not a source of additional stress for the patient. Coping strategies were previously discussed in this chapter.

You can assume a primary role in implementing stress management strategies. Some personal tips for handling stress are presented in Table 6-10. These tips will benefit you personally and enhance your own level of health and wellness. It is essential that you first care for yourself before you can help the patients who need your care. Once you have incorporated these strategies into your life, you can share them with patients and caregivers.

Ideas for how to incorporate stress management strategies into nursing practice are presented in Table 6-11. Although some may require additional training, many stress management strategies are within the scope of nursing practice. These include relaxation breathing, imagery, music, exercise, massage, meditation, art therapy, and journaling. (Additional resources are in the Stress-Busting Kit for Nursing Students on the website for this book.)

Most coping and relaxation strategies can be taught to patients in 10 to 15 minutes. Choose a coping or relaxation strategy to best suit the patient and situation. Give directions calmly and slowly in short, simple sentences.

Effective stress management provides an individual a sense of control of the stressful situation. As stress management practices are incorporated into daily activities, the individual is able to increase his or her confidence and self-reliance and limit the emotional response to the stressful circumstances. Having a sense of control can prevent the harmful effects of a stress response.

As a nurse, you are in an ideal situation to integrate stress management in clinical practice. You are also well equipped to develop and test the effectiveness of new approaches to manage stress and promote positive health outcomes. However, it is very important to recognize when the patient or caregiver needs to be referred to a professional with advanced training in counseling.

## CASE STUDY

### *Stress-Induced Complaints*

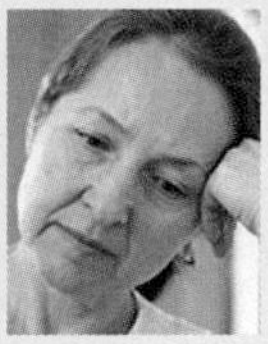

(©JackF/ iStock/ Thinkstock)

**Patient Profile**

K.F., a 48-year-old woman, recently moved to the United States from Romania with her two teenage children. She has no family in the country and was recently divorced. She has taken a job as a waitress in a hectic restaurant and works as a seamstress out of her home in the evenings.

She has developed some unusual symptoms and comes to see the nurse practitioner at a community clinic. Although she states that she was in good health when she left Romania, she now complains of fatigue, inability to sleep, and aches all over her body. Even when she is able to get some extra sleep, she still feels exhausted. Her co-worker told her she has fibromyalgia.

**Discussion Questions**

1. Consider K.F.'s situation and describe the stressors with which she is dealing. Describe the possible effects of these stressors on her health.
2. ***Priority Decision:*** What are the priority coping strategies that you should include in K.F.'s plan of care?
3. What limitations should be considered when discussing specific coping strategies?
4. ***Patient-Centered Care***: What cultural considerations should be included in the plan of care?

Answers available at *http://evolve.elsevier.com/Lewis/medsurg.*

## BRIDGE TO NCLEX EXAMINATION

The number of the question corresponds to the same-numbered outcome at the beginning of the chapter.

1. Determination of whether an event is a stressor is based on a person's
   a. tolerance.
   b. perception.
   c. adaptation.
   d. stubbornness.
2. The nurse would expect which finding in a patient as a result of the physiologic effect of stress on the reticular formation?
   a. An episode of diarrhea while awaiting painful dressing changes
   b. Refusal to communicate with nurses while awaiting a cardiac catheterization
   c. Inability to sleep the night before beginning to self-administer insulin injections
   d. Increased blood pressure, decreased urine output, and hyperglycemia after a car accident
3. The nurse uses knowledge of the effects of stress on the immune system by encouraging patients to
   a. sleep for 10 to 12 hours per day.
   b. avoid exposure to upper respiratory tract infections.
   c. receive regular immunizations when they are stressed.
   d. use emotion-focused rather than problem-focused coping strategies.
4. Which of the following examples reflects the relationship among the mind-body-spirit (*select all that apply*)?
   a. A 75-year-old man who enjoys doing crossword puzzles every day
   b. A 25-year-old man who has been successfully treated for testicular cancer
   c. A 55-year-old man who is impotent because of his prostate cancer surgery
   d. A 34-year-old woman who is angry because of her recent diagnosis of breast cancer
   e. A 65-year-old woman struggling with rehabilitation after having hip replacement surgery
5. The nurse recognizes that a person who experiences chronic stress could be at higher risk for (*select all that apply*)
   a. osteoporosis.
   b. fibromyalgia.
   c. colds and flu.
   d. high blood pressure.
   e. high serum cholesterol.
6. The nurse recognizes that a patient with newly diagnosed breast cancer is using an emotion-focused coping process when she
   a. joins a support group for women with breast cancer.
   b. considers the pros and cons of the various treatment options.
   c. delays treatment until her family can take a weekend trip together.
   d. tells the nurse that she has a good prognosis because the tumor is small.
7. During a stressful circumstance that is unchangeable, which type of coping strategy is the *most* effective?
   a. Avoidance
   b. Coping flexibility
   c. Emotion-focused coping
   d. Problem-focused coping
8. An appropriate nursing intervention for a hospitalized patient who states she cannot cope with her illness is
   a. controlling the environment to prevent sensory overload and promote sleep.
   b. encouraging the patient's family to offer emotional support by frequent visiting.
   c. arranging for the patient to phone family and friends to maintain emotional bonds.
   d. asking the patient to describe previous stressful situations and how she managed to resolve them.

1. b, 2. c, 3. b, 4. a, b, c, d, e, 5. b, c, d, 6. a, 7. c, 8. d.

For rationales to these answers and even more NCLEX review questions, visit *http://evolve.elsevier.com/Lewis/medsurg.*

## EVOLVE WEBSITE

http://evolve.elsevier.com/Lewis/medsurg
**Review Questions (Online Only)**
**Key Points**
**Answer Keys for Questions**
- Rationales for Bridge to NCLEX Examination Questions
- Answer Guidelines for Case Study on p. 87

**Conceptual Care Map Creator**
**Stress-Busting Kit for Nursing Students**
**Audio Glossary**
**Content Updates**

## REFERENCES


1. Seward BL: *Managing stress: principles and strategies for health and well-being*, ed 8, Burlington, Mass, 2014, Jones & Bartlett.
*2. Maddi SR: Hardiness: the courage to grow from stresses, *J Pos Psych* 1(3):160, 2006. (Classic)
3. Positive thinking: Stop negative self-talk to reduce stress. Retrieved from *www.mayoclinic.org/healthy-living/stress-management/in-depth/positive-thinking/art-20043950.*
4. Segerstrom S, editor: *The Oxford handbook of psychoneuroimmunology*, 2012.
5. American Institute of Stress. Retrieved from *http://www.stress.org.*
6. Chronic stress can damage brain structure and connectivity. Retrieved from *www.psychologytoday.com/blog/the-athletes-way/201402/chronic-stress-can-damage-brain-structure-and-connectivity.*
7. Stress and heart health. Retrieved from *www.heart.org/HEARTORG/Conditions/More/MyHeartandStrokeNews/Stress-and-Heart-Health_UCM_437370_Article.jsp.*
8. Feeling 'worn out'? Your heart may pay the price. Retrieved from *www.medicinenet.com/script/main/art.asp?articlekey=185327.*
9. Stress and migraines. Retrieved from *http://womenshealth.gov/publications/our-publications/fact-sheet/migraine.html.*
10. Feeling stressed? Stress relief might help your health. Retrieved from *http://newsinhealth.nih.gov/issue/Dec2014/Feature1.*
*11. Cohen S, Tyrrell DA, Smith AP: Psychological stress and susceptibility to the common cold, *N Engl J Med* 325:606, 1991. (Classic)
12. Mitchell C: Social disadvantage, genetic sensitivity and children's telomere length, *PNAS* 111:5944, 2014.
13. American Psychological Association: Stress in America: our health at risk. Retrieved from *www.apa.org/news/press/releases/stress.*
14. Lazarus R, Folkman S: *Stress, appraisal, and coping*, New York, 1984, Springer. (Classic)
15. Benson H: *The relaxation response*, New York, 1975, Avon. (Classic)
16. National Center for Complementary and Integrative Health. *https://nccih.nih.gov/health/stress/relaxation.htm.*
17. The power of music to reduce stress. Retrieved from *http://psychcentral.com/lib/the-power-of-music-to-reduce-stress/000930.*

*Evidence-based information for clinical practice.

# 7

# Sleep and Sleep Disorders

*Diana Taibi Buchanan*

*When you have a dream, you've got to grab it and never let go.*
*Carol Burnett*

http://evolve.elsevier.com/Lewis/medsurg/

## LEARNING OUTCOMES

1. Define sleep.
2. Describe the stages of sleep.
3. Explain the relationship of various diseases/disorders and sleep disorders.
4. Describe the etiology, clinical manifestations, and interprofessional and nursing management of insomnia.
5. Describe the etiology, clinical manifestations, interprofessional care, and nursing management of obstructive sleep apnea.
6. Describe the etiology, clinical manifestations, and interprofessional and nursing management of periodic limb movement disorder.
7. Describe clinical manifestations and interprofessional management of narcolepsy, parasomnias (including sleepwalking, sleep terrors, and nightmares), and circadian rhythm disorders.
8. Select appropriate strategies for managing sleep problems associated with shift work sleep disorder.

## KEY TERMS



## SLEEP

**Sleep** is a state in which an individual lacks conscious awareness of environmental surroundings but can be easily aroused. Sleep is distinct from unconscious states such as coma, in which the individual cannot be aroused. Sleep is a basic, dynamic, highly organized, and complex behavior that is essential for healthy functioning and survival. Over a life span of 80 years, an individual who sleeps 7 hours each night will spend approximately 24 years sleeping. Sleep influences both behavioral and physiologic functions, including memory, mood, hormone secretion, glucose metabolism, immune function, and body temperature.

Most adults require 7 to 8 hours of sleep within a 24-hour period.[1] Adequate sleep is defined as the amount of sleep one needs to be fully awake and alert the next day. *Insufficient sleep* refers to obtaining less than the recommended amount of sleep. *Fragmented sleep* refers to frequent arousals or actual awakenings that interrupt sleep continuity. *Nonrestorative sleep* refers to sleep that is of adequate duration but does not result in the individual feeling refreshed and alert the next day.

**Sleep disturbance** is a term used broadly to indicate conditions of poor sleep quality. Sleep disturbance may be related to external factors (e.g., noise, light), health-related factors (e.g., pain), or sleep disorders.

**Sleep disorders** refer to abnormalities unique to sleep. Sleep disorders discussed in this chapter include insomnia, obstructive sleep apnea syndrome, periodic limb movement disorder, circadian sleep disorders, narcolepsy, and parasomnias.

General sleep disturbances and sleep disorders can result in insufficient sleep. Many people get insufficient sleep because they simply do not allot enough time in bed to get adequate sleep. About 30% of Americans report getting less than 6 hours of sleep per night. An estimated 50 to 70 million people in the United States have a sleep disorder, and many are unaware that they have a problem[2] (Fig. 7-1).

Reviewed by Marylee Bressie, RN, DNP, CCRN, CCNS, CEN, Core Faculty/Nurse Planner, Department of Nursing, School of Public Service Leadership, Capella University, Minneapolis, Minnesota; Dana R. Epstein, RN, PhD, Chief, Nursing Research and Evidence-Based Practice Phoenix VA Health Care System, Phoenix, Arizona; and Teresa J. Seright, RN, PhD, CCRN, Associate Teaching Professor, College of Nursing, Montana State University, Bozeman, Montana.

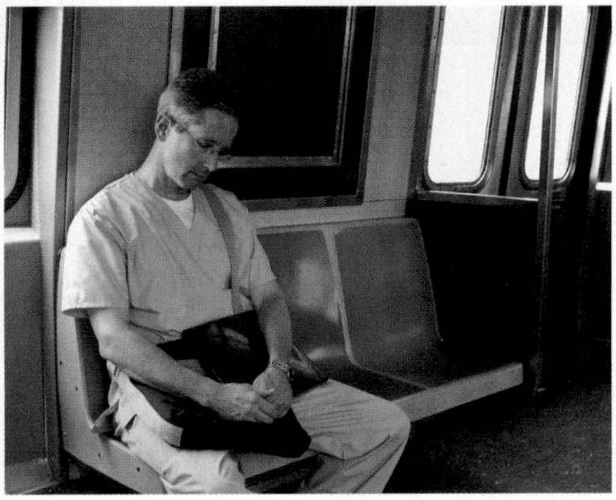

**FIG. 7-1** Sleep disorders are common in our society. (©Jupiterimages/Creatas/Thinkstock)

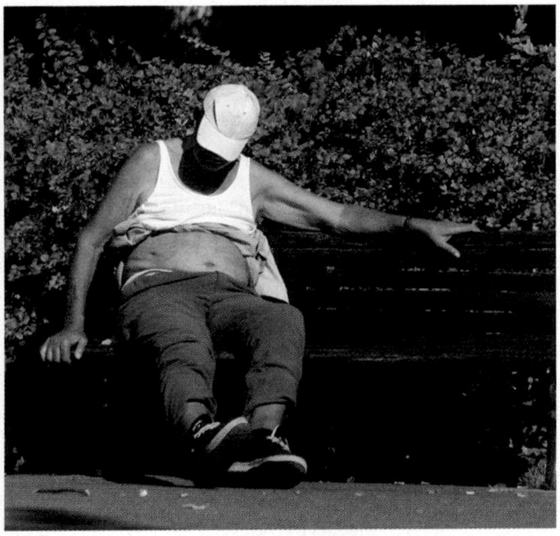

**FIG. 7-2** Excessive daytime sleepiness can occur in people with sleep disorders. (©iStockphoto/Thinkstock)

Untreated sleep disorders cause considerable health, safety, and economic consequences. Daytime sleepiness can be so severe that it interferes with work and social functioning (Fig. 7-2). People with chronic illnesses are at the greatest risk for sleep disturbances. Driving while drowsy is related to 100,000 accidents and 1500 traffic fatalities per year.[3] Each year, sleep disorders, sleep loss, and excessive daytime sleepiness cost the United States billions of dollars from the cost of health care, work-related accidents, and lost productivity.[2] Opportunities to address sleep problems are often missed because health care providers (HCPs) do not ask, and patients do not readily talk about them.

## PHYSIOLOGIC SLEEP MECHANISMS

### Sleep-Wake Cycle

The brain controls the cyclic changes between sleep and waking. Complex networks in the brainstem, hypothalamus, and thalamus interact to regulate the sleep and wake cycle.

**Wake Behavior.** **Wake behavior** is maintained by an integrated network of arousal systems from the brainstem and forebrain. A cluster of neuronal structures in the middle of the brainstem, called the *reticular activating system (RAS)*, is associated with generalized cortical activation and behavioral arousal. Various neurotransmitters (glutamate, acetylcholine, norepinephrine, dopamine, histamine, serotonin) promote wake behavior.[4]

People with Alzheimer's disease have a loss of cholinergic neurons in the forebrain, which results in sleep disturbances. People with Parkinson's disease have degeneration of dopamine neurons in the substantia nigra, leading to excessive daytime sleepiness. Histamine neurons in the hypothalamus stimulate cortical activation and wake behavior. The sedating properties of many over-the-counter (OTC) medications (e.g., diphenhydramine [Benadryl]) result from inhibiting histamine-related arousal systems.

*Orexin* (also called hypocretin) is a neuropeptide found in the hypothalamus. Orexin is involved in regulating the sleep-wake cycle and plays a role in keeping people awake.[5,6] Decreased levels of orexin or its receptors lead to difficulties staying awake, which is a syndrome called *narcolepsy*. (Narcolepsy is discussed later in this chapter on pp. 98-99.)

**Sleep Behavior.** An area in the hypothalamus just above the optic chiasm contains many sleep-promoting neurons. These neurons act to inhibit the RAS and promote sleep.[7] Sleep is stimulated by a variety of sleep-promoting neurotransmitters and peptides, including $\gamma$-aminobutyric acid (GABA), galanin, melatonin, adenosine, somatostatin, growth hormone–releasing hormone (GHRH), delta-sleep–inducing peptide, prostaglandins, and proinflammatory cytokines. When a person has an infection, proinflammatory cytokines (interleukin-1, tumor necrosis factor, interleukin-6) mediate symptoms such as sleepiness and lethargy. Peptides, such as cholecystokinin, released by the gastrointestinal tract after food ingestion, may mediate *postprandial sleepiness* (sleepiness after eating).

*Melatonin* is an endogenous hormone (from the amino acid tryptophan) produced by the pineal gland in the brain. Melatonin secretion is linked to the environmental light-dark cycle and its release signals the time for sleep. Under normal day-night conditions, melatonin is released in the evening as it gets dark. Light exposure at night can suppress melatonin secretion.[7]

**Circadian Rhythms.** Many biologic rhythms of behavior and physiology fluctuate within a 24-hour period. Because the **circadian** (*circa dian,* about a day) **rhythms** are controlled by internal clock mechanisms, they persist when people are placed in environments free of external time cues. The suprachiasmatic nucleus (SCN) in the hypothalamus is the master clock of the body. The 24-hour cycle of sleep and wake is synchronized to the environmental light and dark periods through specific light detectors in the retina. Pathways from the retina reach the SCN, and pathways from the SCN innervate brain regions controlling wake and sleep behavior.[7]

Light is the strongest time cue for the sleep-wake rhythm. Thus light can be used as a therapy to shift the timing of the sleep-wake rhythm. For example, bright light used early in the morning will cause the sleep-wake rhythm to move to an earlier time; bright light used in the evening will cause the sleep-wake rhythm to move to a later time.

### Sleep Architecture

*Sleep architecture* refers to the pattern of nighttime sleep recorded from physiologic measures of brain waves, eye movements, and muscle tone called *polysomnography* (PSG). Sleep consists of two basic states: *rapid eye movement (REM) sleep* and *non–rapid eye movement (NREM) sleep*. During sleep, the body cycles between NREM and REM sleep. Once asleep, a person goes through four to six NREM and REM sleep cycles, each cycle lasting 60 to 110 minutes.

**NREM Sleep.** In healthy adults the largest percentage of total sleep time, approximately 75% to 80%, is spent in NREM sleep. NREM sleep is subdivided into three stages:[8]

*Stage 1* occurs in the beginning of sleep, with slow eye movements, and is a transition phase from wakefulness to sleep. During this period the person can be easily awakened.

*Stage 2* encompasses most of the night's sleep. The heart rate slows down and body temperature drops. This stage is associated with specific electroencephalographic (EEG) wave forms that represent sleep-maintaining neural activity.

*Stage 3* is deep sleep or slow-wave sleep (SWS). This stage is associated with large EEG wave forms, called delta waves, which are used as a measure of sleep intensity. SWS sleep declines as people age such that most adults over 60 years of age have little NREM stage 3 sleep.

**REM Sleep.** REM sleep accounts for 20% to 25% of sleep. REM sleep follows NREM sleep in a sleep cycle. In this stage, brain waves resemble wakefulness and postural muscles are inhibited, leading to greatly reduced skeletal muscle tone. During REM sleep an individual cannot initiate muscle movement (e.g., cannot stand up). REM sleep is the period when the most vivid dreaming occurs.

## INSUFFICIENT SLEEP AND SLEEP DISTURBANCES

Insufficient sleep is associated with changes in body function (Fig. 7-3) and health problems (Table 7-1). Impaired cognitive function and impaired performance on simple behavioral tasks occur within 24 hours of sleep loss. The effects of sleep loss are cumulative.

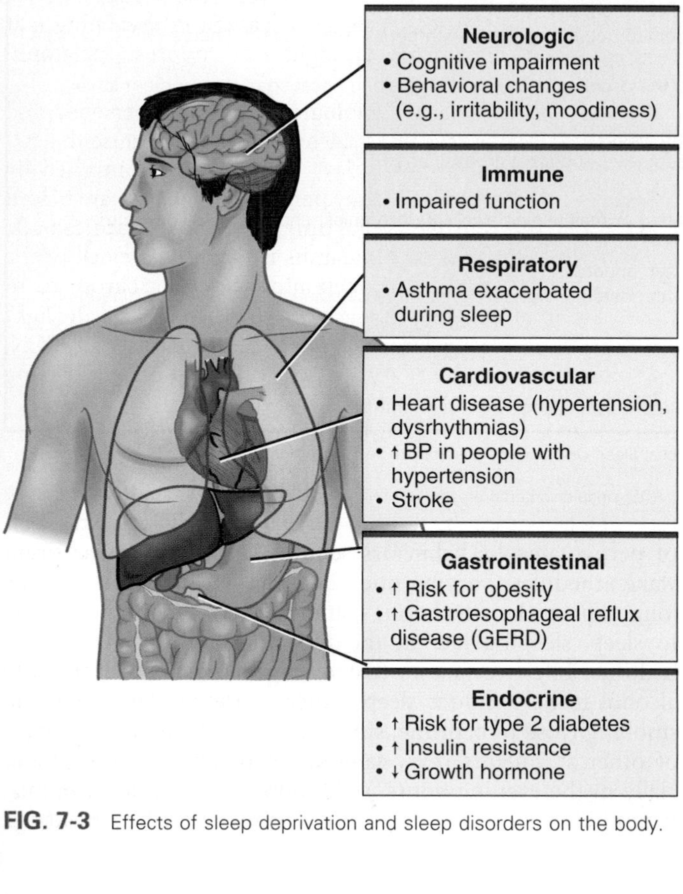


**FIG. 7-3** Effects of sleep deprivation and sleep disorders on the body.

Individuals who report less than 6 hours of sleep a night have a higher body mass index (BMI) and are more likely to be obese. The risk for developing glucose intolerance and diabetes is increased in individuals with a history of insufficient sleep. Chronic loss of sleep places older adults at risk for depression, impaired daytime functioning, social isolation, and overall reduction in quality of life. In patients with chronic illnesses, especially cardiovascular disease and stroke, insomnia and sleep-disordered breathing are associated with increased morbidity and mortality.[9]

### SLEEP DISTURBANCES IN THE HOSPITAL

Hospitalization, especially in the intensive care unit (ICU), is associated with decreased total sleep time and decreased SWS and REM sleep.[10] Because of the nature of a critical illness and its treatment, some degree of sleep loss may be inevitable for patients in ICUs. Preexisting sleep disorders may be aggravated or triggered in patients who are hospitalized.

In the hospital, environmental sleep-disruptive factors, psychoactive medications, and acute and critical illness all contribute to poor sleep. Patient symptoms, including pain, dyspnea, and nausea, can also contribute to sleep loss in the acutely ill patient. Medications commonly used in acutely and critically ill patients can further contribute to sleep loss. Hospitalized patients are also at risk for poor sleep because of circadian rhythm disruptions.

Hospital and ICU noise (e.g., staff paging system, ventilator alarms, bedside monitors, infusion alarms) and especially staff conversations near patients (e.g., in hallways) during both the day and night disturb sleep. Bright lights during the night also disrupt sleep and reduce melatonin levels. Patient care activities (e.g., dressing changes, blood draws, vital sign monitoring) disrupt sleep. Inactivity, boredom, and certain medications lead to napping during the day and evening that can affect nighttime sleep.

Decreased sleep duration and sleep loss increase the sensitivity and lower the tolerance to pain.[11] Adequate pain management may improve total sleep time, but medications commonly used to relieve pain, especially opioids, alter sleep and place an individual at risk for sleep-disordered breathing.

You have an important role in creating an environment conducive to sleep. This includes the scheduling of medications and procedures, including those performed by unlicensed assistive personnel (UAP). Reducing light and noise levels can promote opportunities for sleep. Hypnotic medications are often available on an as-needed basis.

## SLEEP DISORDERS

### INSOMNIA

The most common sleep disorder is insomnia, affecting one in three adults. **Insomnia** is characterized by difficulty falling asleep, difficulty staying asleep, waking up too early, or complaints of waking up feeling unrefreshed. The main complaint of people with insomnia is overall dissatisfaction with sleep quality and quantity.

*Acute insomnia* refers to difficulties falling or remaining asleep at least 3 nights per week for less than a month. *Chronic insomnia* is defined by the same symptoms and a daytime complaint (e.g., fatigue, poor concentration, interference with social

**TABLE 7-1 Relationship of Sleep Disturbances to Diseases and Disorders**

| Disease or Disorder | Sleep Disturbance |
|---|---|
| **Respiratory** | |
| **Asthma** | • Exacerbated during sleep |
| **Chronic obstructive pulmonary disease (COPD)** | • Associated with poor sleep quality, nocturnal oxygen desaturation, and coexisting sleep apnea |
| **Obstructive sleep apnea (OSA)** | • Linked with heart disease (hypertension, stroke, heart failure, coronary artery disease, dysrhythmias)<br>• Results in impaired glucose control similar to that which occurs in type 2 diabetes |
| **Renal** | |
| **End-stage renal disease (ESRD)** | • Disrupted nocturnal sleep with excessive daytime sleepiness<br>• Patients on dialysis have a high incidence of SDB and RLS, which are both significant predictors of mortality in these patients. |
| **Immune Disorders** | |
| **Human immunodeficiency virus (HIV)** | • Sleep disturbances and fatigue highly prevalent and associated with increased morbidity and mortality |
| **Endocrine** | |
| **Diabetes** | • Insufficient sleep linked to increased risk for type 2 diabetes<br>• Sleep deprivation in healthy people increases insulin resistance.<br>• Sleep duration and quality are predictors of HbA1C (A1C) levels, an important marker of blood glucose control. |
| **Musculoskeletal** | |
| **Arthritis** | • Increased rates of RLS and SDB<br>• Disease activity linked to sleep complaints |
| **Fibromyalgia** | • Co-morbid insomnia, especially complaint of nonrestorative sleep<br>• Increased rates of PLMD and RLS<br>• Lower levels of sleep-dependent hormones (growth hormone, prolactin) |
| **Systemic exertion intolerance disease (chronic fatigue syndrome)** | • Co-morbid insomnia<br>• Increased rates of SDB |
| **Cardiovascular (CV)** | • People with sleep apnea or sleep disorders are at increased risk for CV disorders, including hypertension, dysrhythmias, and coronary artery disease. |
| **Heart failure (HF)** | • Sleep disturbances (insomnia, PLMD, SDB) are common.<br>• Cheyne-Stokes breathing and central apnea are signs of HF exacerbation related to fluid overload. |
| **Hypertension** | • Inadequate sleep in people with hypertension can lead to further elevations in BP. |
| **Gastrointestinal** | |
| **Obesity** | • Association between short sleep duration and excess body weight. Short sleep duration may result in metabolic changes that are linked to obesity.<br>• Higher BMI in people who sleep <6 hours compared with people who sleep >8 hours<br>• Risk factor for SDB |
| **Gastroesophageal reflux disease (GERD)** | • Reflux of gastric contents into the esophagus occurs during sleep because of incompetent lower esophageal sphincter.<br>• Swallowing is depressed during sleep. |
| **Chronic liver disease** | • Associated with excessive sleepiness, nocturnal arousal, and RLS |
| **Neurologic** | |
| **Parkinson's disease** | • Associated with difficulty initiating or maintaining sleep, parasomnias, and excessive daytime sleepiness |
| **Alzheimer's disease** | • Many have SDB (frequently sleep apnea).<br>• Circadian rhythm alterations with nocturnal wandering, daytime sleepiness, and sleep disruption and awakening |
| **Pain (acute and chronic)** | • Decreased quantity and quality of sleep. Poor sleep can intensify pain. |
| **Cancer** | • Higher rates of insomnia<br>• Chemotherapy for cancer treatment associated with fragmented sleep and fatigue |

Source: National Center on Sleep Disorders and National Heart, Lung, and Blood Institute: National Sleep Disorders Research Plan: section 4, sleep and health. Retrieved from *www.cdc.gov/sleep/about_sleep/chronic_disease.htm.*
*BMI,* Body mass index; *PLMD,* periodic limb movement disorder; *RLS,* restless legs syndrome; *SDB,* sleep-disordered breathing.

or family activities) that persist for 3 months or longer. Chronic insomnia occurs in 10% to 15% of Americans and is more common in women than men. Insomnia is more common in people who are divorced, widowed, and separated than in those who are married. Insomnia is more prevalent in individuals with low socioeconomic status and less education.[3]

## Etiology and Pathophysiology

Behaviors, lifestyle, diet, physical and mental conditions, and medications contribute to insomnia. Insomnia is exacerbated or perpetuated by behaviors such as keeping irregular sleep-wake schedules (varying one's bedtime and rise time), taking long naps in the afternoon, spending more time in bed trying to sleep, sleeping late in the morning, and exercising near bedtime. Lifestyle factors that disrupt sleep include drinking alcohol to help induce sleep, which causes restless sleep, and smoking close to bedtime, since nicotine is a stimulant. Intake of other stimulants (e.g., caffeine, methamphetamine), especially in the evening hours, predisposes a person to insomnia. Insomnia is a common side effect of many medications (e.g., antidepressants, antihypertensives, corticosteroids, psychostimulants, analgesics).

Chronic insomnia often has no known medical or psychologic cause. Often individuals report that the onset occurred after a stressful life event (e.g., loss of loved one). In other cases, the onset of insomnia may be precipitated by psychiatric illnesses, medical conditions, medications, or substance abuse. Patients with psychiatric or medical conditions are more likely to have insomnia than individuals without these conditions. Once chronic insomnia manifests, symptoms are likely to persist over time.

### Clinical Manifestations

Manifestations of insomnia include one or more of the following symptoms: (1) difficulty falling asleep *(long sleep latency)*, (2) frequent awakenings *(fragmented sleep)*, (3) prolonged nighttime awakenings or awakening too early and not being able to fall back to sleep *(difficulty maintaining sleep)*, and (4) awakening feeling unrefreshed *(nonrestorative sleep)*. Daytime or functional consequences of insomnia include fatigue, having trouble concentrating at work or school, and having an altered mood. Behavioral manifestations of poor sleep include irritability, sleepiness during the day, forgetfulness, and attention and concentration problems.

### Diagnostic Studies

**Self-Report.** The diagnosis of insomnia is made based on subjective complaints and on an evaluation of a 1- or 2-week sleep diary completed by the patient. A diary or log usually includes the number and times of naps, times of going to bed, awakening and getting up, number of awakenings, as well as overall sleep quality.

In ambulatory care settings the evaluation of insomnia requires a comprehensive sleep history to establish the type of insomnia and to screen for possible psychiatric, medical, or other sleep disorders that would require specific treatment. Questionnaires, such as Pittsburgh Quality Sleep Index, Insomnia Severity Index, and Epworth Daytime Sleepiness, are commonly used to assess sleep quality and negative daytime symptoms related to insomnia.

**Actigraphy.** *Actigraphy* is a relatively noninvasive method of monitoring rest and activity cycles. An actigraph is a device that measures gross motor activity. It is worn on the wrist like a watch and is about the same size and shape. The unit continuously records the patient's movements, producing data that are downloaded to a computer and analyzed. Activity corresponds to time spent awake, and continuous inactivity corresponds to time spent asleep. Actigraphy is not necessary for diagnosing insomnia, but it is useful for confirming patient's sleep self-reports and monitoring the effects of treatments.

**Polysomnography.** A polysomnography (PSG) study is not required to establish a diagnosis of insomnia. A PSG study is done only if there are symptoms or signs of another sleep disorder, such as sleep-disordered breathing (discussed later in the chapter). In a PSG study, electrodes simultaneously record physiologic measures that define the main stages of sleep and wakefulness. These measures include (1) muscle tone recorded using an electromyogram (EMG), (2) eye movements recorded with an electro-oculogram (EOG), and (3) brain activity recorded through EEG. To determine additional characteristics of specific sleep disorders, other measures made during PSG include airflow at the nose and mouth, respiratory effort around the chest and abdomen, heart rate, noninvasive oxygen saturation, and EMG of the anterior tibialis muscles (used to detect periodic leg movements). Finally, a patient's gross body movements are monitored continuously by cameras and microphones.

### Interprofessional Care

Insomnia treatments are oriented toward symptom management (Table 7-2). A key to management is to change behaviors that perpetuate insomnia. The goal is to (1) prevent acute insomnia from becoming chronic and (2) treat chronic insomnia. An important first step is to provide teaching about sleep along with behavioral strategies. **Sleep hygiene** is a variety of different practices that are important to have normal, quality nighttime sleep and daytime alertness (Table 7-3). Patients often have some familiarity with sleep hygiene principles, but they may still benefit from coaching on how to use these principles effectively.

**Cognitive-Behavioral Therapy for Insomnia.** Although teaching about sleep hygiene practices is useful, individuals with chronic insomnia require more in-depth *cognitive-behavioral therapy for insomnia (CBT-I)*.[12] CBT-I is based on structured treatment plans that include cognitive and behavioral components.

**TABLE 7-2 Interprofessional Care**

***Insomnia***

| | |
|---|---|
| **Diagnostic Assessment**<br>***History***<br>• Self-report sleep log or diary<br>• Sleep assessment (Table 7-5)<br>• Pittsburgh Sleep Quality Index<br>• Insomnia Severity Index<br>• Epworth Sleepiness Scale | ***Drug Therapy*** (Table 7-4)<br>• Benzodiazepines<br>• Benzodiazepine-receptor–like agents<br>• Orexin-receptor antagonist<br>• Melatonin-receptor agonist<br>• Antidepressants<br>• Antihistamines |
| **Management**<br>***Nondrug Therapy***<br>• Sleep hygiene (Table 7-3)<br>• Cognitive behavioral therapies for insomnia (CBT-I) | ***Complementary and Alternative Therapy***<br>• Melatonin |

**TABLE 7-3 Patient Teaching**

***Sleep Hygiene***

*Include the following instructions when teaching a patient who has a sleep disturbance or disorder.*

- Do not go to bed unless you are sleepy.
- If you are not asleep after 20 minutes, get out of bed.
- Adopt a regular pattern in terms of bedtime and awakening.
- Begin rituals (e.g., warm bath, light snack, reading) that help you relax each night before bed.
- Get a full night's sleep on a regular basis.
- Make your bedroom quiet, dark, and a little bit cool.
- Do not read, write, eat, watch TV, talk on the phone, or use technologies such as smart phones and tablet computers in bed.
- Avoid caffeine, nicotine, and alcohol at least 4 to 6 hours before bedtime.
- Do not go to bed hungry, but don't eat a big meal near bedtime either.
- Avoid strenuous exercise within 6 hours of your bedtime.
- Avoid sleeping pills, or use them cautiously.
- Practice relaxation techniques (e.g., relaxation breathing) to help you cope with stress in your life (see Chapter 6).

Adapted from American Academy of Sleep Medicine: Healthy sleep habits, 2014. Retrieved from *www.sleepeducation.com/essentials-in-sleep/healthy-sleep-habits*.

**TABLE 7-4 Drug Therapy**

***Insomnia***

**Benzodiazepines**

- Diazepam (Valium)
- Flurazepam
- Lorazepam (Ativan)
- Quazepam
- Triazolam (Halcion)

**Benzodiazepine-Receptor–Like Agents**

- Zolpidem (Ambien, Ambien CR, Intermezzo, Edluar, ZolpiMist)
- Zaleplon (Sonata)
- Eszopiclone (Lunesta)

**Orexin-Receptor Antagonist**

- Suvorexant (Belsomra)

**Melatonin-Receptor Agonist**

- Ramelteon (Rozerem)

**Antidepressants**

- Amitriptyline
- Doxepin
- Trazodone

**Antihistamines**

- Diphenhydramine
- Doxylamine (Unisom)

The cognitive part of CBT-I may include stress management techniques (e.g., relaxation breathing, imagery) or cognitive strategies to address misconceptions about sleep. The specific approach used varies based on the patient's need. The behavioral part of CBT-I includes instructions to (1) limit the amount of time an individual can stay in bed, (2) maintain a scheduled time to get up in the morning, (3) go to bed only when feeling sleepy, and (4) get out of bed when unable to sleep. CBT-I also includes teaching about sleep hygiene practices (Table 7-3). CBT-I requires individuals to change behavior, which sometimes is difficult.

Although full CBT-I treatment should be delivered by qualified providers with training in this treatment, you can apply many of the principles to help patients. Encourage individuals with insomnia not to watch television or read in bed. Time in bed is limited to the actual time that the individual can sleep. Teach the person with insomnia to avoid naps and consumption of large meals, alcohol, and stimulants, especially a few hours before bedtime. Naps are less likely to affect nighttime sleep if they are limited to 15 to 20 minutes, once per day, and scheduled 7 to 9 hours after morning awakening. Regular exercise may enhance sleep quality but should not be performed within several hours of bedtime.

**Drug Therapy.** Most medications for insomnia work by producing sleepiness to promote the onset or maintenance of sleep. Medications are generally recommended for short-term treatment of insomnia. Medications that treat insomnia can cause next-day drowsiness and impair driving and other activities that require alertness. People can be impaired even when they feel fully awake. Hypnotic and anxiolytic medications are effective for improving sleep, but the benefits for improving daytime functioning are less certain.

Few studies have evaluated the use of hypnotics for chronic insomnia, and their use in older adults is controversial due to side effects and safety concerns, such as fall risk.[13] Many individuals with insomnia become accustomed to taking OTC or prescription medications to treat insomnia and risk becoming dependent on them, psychologically and physically. *Rebound insomnia* is common with abrupt withdrawal of some hypnotic medications. The daytime fatigue resulting from some medications can negatively influence the patient's efforts to use nondrug approaches.

Classes of medications used to treat insomnia include benzodiazepines, benzodiazepine-receptor agonists, orexin-receptor antagonist, melatonin-receptor agonist, antidepressants, and antihistamines (Table 7-4).

***Benzodiazepine Hypnotics.*** Benzodiazepines such as diazepam (Valium) activate the γ-aminobutyric acid (GABA) receptors to promote sleep. The prolonged half-life of some of these agents (e.g., flurazepam) can result in daytime sleepiness, amnesia, dizziness, and rebound insomnia. Tolerance to these agents develops, and there is a risk for dependence. The use of benzodiazepines should be limited to 2 to 3 weeks. All benzodiazepines have the potential for abuse. In addition, benzodiazepines interact with alcohol and other central nervous system (CNS) depressants. These agents are no longer recommended as first-line therapy for insomnia.

***Non-Benzodiazepine Hypnotics.*** Zolpidem (Ambien), zaleplon (Sonata), and eszopiclone (Lunesta) are the drugs of first choice for insomnia. Because they are benzodiazepine-receptor agonists, they work similarly to benzodiazepines. These drugs are effective and safe for use from 6 months to a year. Food has the potential to delay onset of action and should not be taken with these agents. These agents have short half-lives, making their duration of action short and reducing the risk of daytime sedation. The extended-release formulation of zolpidem (Ambien CR) is used for problems of sleep onset and sleep maintenance. A dissolvable tablet form of zolpidem (Edluar) and an oral spray formulation (ZolpiMist) may be useful for individuals who have difficulty swallowing pills or are on restricted oral fluid intake. Zolpidem tartrate (Intermezzo), a sublingual tablet, is used for patients with insomnia characterized by middle-of-the-night waking followed by difficulty returning to sleep.

***Orexin-Receptor Antagonist.*** Suvorexant (Belsomra) is the first approved orexin-receptor antagonist. It promotes sleep by blocking the effects of orexin. (Orexin is discussed on p. 90 earlier in this chapter.) Suvorexant should be taken no more than once per night, within 30 minutes of going to bed, with at least 7 hours remaining before the planned time of waking. The most common side effect is drowsiness.

***Melatonin-Receptor Agonist.*** Ramelteon (Rozerem) is a melatonin-receptor agonist. It has a rapid onset that is effective for sleep onset but a short duration of action. Ramelteon does not cause tolerance, but the drug is not always effective in improving sleep quality. Ramelteon is used for insomnia with sleep onset difficulty, not for sleep maintenance problems.

***Antidepressants.*** Certain atypical and tricyclic antidepressants are used as sleep aids due to their side effects of sedation. Trazodone, an atypical antidepressant, is one of the most common agents prescribed to treat insomnia, especially in older adults. The insomnia dose of antidepressants such as trazodone is much lower than the antidepressant dose. The administration of this drug to older adults is controversial. Daytime sleepiness is a common side effect. Tolerance can develop within a few weeks. Doxepin and amitriptyline are tricyclic antidepressants that may be used to treat insomnia. Doxepin improves sleep without next-day drowsiness in older and middle-aged adults with chronic primary insomnia.[14]

***Antihistamines.*** Many individuals with insomnia self-medicate with OTC sleep aids. Most OTC agents include diphenhydramine or doxylamine (Unisom). These drugs may also be constituents of "nighttime" pain medicines. Antihistamine agents are less effective than benzodiazepines, and tolerance develops quickly. In addition, antihistamines have anticholinergic side effects, including daytime sleepiness, impaired cognitive function, blurred vision, urinary retention, constipation, and risk of increased intraocular pressure. Agents with diphenhydramine are not intended for long-term use and should not be used by older adults.[15]

**Complementary and Alternative Therapy.** Many types of complementary and alternative therapies are used as sleep aids. As noted earlier in the chapter, melatonin is a hormone produced by the pineal gland (Complementary & Alternative Therapies box on below). Melatonin is effective for improving sleep disturbance associated with jet lag. It also helps night shift workers sleep during the daytime.[16] However, melatonin is not considered effective for improving nighttime sleep. Valerian is a herb that has been used for many years as a sleep aid and to relieve anxiety. Although valerian is safe, it is not effective in treating insomnia.[17] Additional sleep aids include white noise devices or relaxation strategies.

### COMPLEMENTARY & ALTERNATIVE THERAPIES

**Melatonin**

**Scientific Evidence**

Overall, the scientific evidence suggests the benefits of melatonin in people who take it for jet lag. The majority of scientific evidence suggests that it may decrease the time it takes to fall asleep (sleep latency).

**Nursing Implications**

- Regarded as safe in recommended doses for short-term use
- Avoid in patients using warfarin (Coumadin).
- Avoid in patients using central nervous system depressants.
- May cause a drop in BP. Caution is advised in patients taking drugs that may also lower BP.

Source: Based on a systematic review of scientific literature. Retrieved from *www.naturalstandard.com.*

## NURSING MANAGEMENT: INSOMNIA

### Nursing Assessment

As a nurse, you are in a key position to assess sleep problems in patients and their caregivers. Sleep assessment is important in helping patients identify personal habits and environmental factors that contribute to poor sleep. Family caregivers may experience sleep disruptions due to the necessity of providing care to patients in the home. These sleep disruptions can increase the burden of caregiving.

Self-report and objective data are used to assess sleep duration and quality. Many patients do not tell their HCP about their sleep problems. Make sure to ask patients about their sleep and problems with sleep. A sleep history includes characteristics of sleep such as sleep duration, the pattern of sleep, and daytime alertness (Table 7-5). Before using any questionnaire, assess the patient's cognitive function, reading level (if a paper form is used), and language ability. Also assess the diet. Question the patient about the intake of caffeine. Ask about alcohol consumption and whether it is used as a sleep aid. Although the sedative effects of alcohol hasten sleep onset, it suppresses REM sleep and increases awakenings later in the night.

Ask the patient about sleep aids. This includes OTC and prescription medications. Note the drug dose, frequency of use, and any side effects (e.g., daytime drowsiness, dry mouth). Many individuals also consume herbal or dietary supplements that they believe will improve sleep. Common supplements include valerian, melatonin, hops, lavender, passion flower, kava, and skullcap. Inform the patient that many of these products are sold as dietary supplements and do not have U.S. Food and Drug Administration (FDA) approval or regulatory oversight. The exact components and concentrations of herbs and supplements often are unknown, and patients may experience adverse effects. Certain agents such as kava are associated with liver toxicity.

### TABLE 7-5 Nursing Assessment

**Sleep**

*Use the following questions to do an initial assessment regarding sleep.*

1. What time do you normally go to bed at night? What time do you normally wake up in the morning?
2. Do you often have trouble falling asleep at night?
3. About how many times do you wake up at night?
4. If you do wake up during the night, do you usually have trouble falling back asleep?
5. Does your bed partner say or are you aware that you frequently snore, gasp for air, or stop breathing?
6. Does your bed partner say or are you aware that you kick or thrash about while asleep?
7. Are you aware that you ever walk, eat, punch, kick, or scream during sleep?
8. Are you sleepy or tired during much of the day?
9. Do you usually take one or more naps during the day?
10. Do you usually doze off without planning to during the day?
11. How much sleep do you need to feel alert and function well?
12. Are you currently taking any type of medication or other preparation to help you sleep?

Source: Bloom HG, Ahmed I, Alessi CA, et al: Evidence-based recommendations for the assessment and management of sleep disorders in older people, *J Am Geriatr Soc* 57:761, 2009.

Encourage individuals to keep a sleep diary for 1 to 2 weeks. In the diary have them record when they go to sleep, when they wake up, and how long they were awake during the night. The number and duration of naps should also be recorded.

The patient's medical history can also provide important information about factors that contribute to poor sleep. For example, a man with benign prostatic hyperplasia may report frequent awakenings during the night for voiding. Psychiatric problems (e.g., depression, anxiety, posttraumatic stress disorder [PTSD], drug abuse) are associated with sleep disturbances. Sleep disturbances often develop as a consequence or complication of a chronic or terminal condition (e.g., heart disease, dementia, cancer). Painful conditions such as arthritis may also contribute to nighttime awakenings.

Ask about work schedules and cross-country and international travel. Shift work contributes to reduced or poor-quality sleep. Work-related behaviors resulting from poor sleep may include poor performance, decreased productivity, and job absenteeism.

### Nursing Diagnoses

Nursing diagnoses related to sleep include insomnia, sleep deprivation, disturbed sleep pattern, and readiness for enhanced sleep.

### Nursing Implementation

Nursing interventions depend on the severity and duration of the sleep problem, as well as individual characteristics. Optimally, healthy adults should have 7 to 8 hours of sleep a night. Occasional difficulty getting to sleep or awakening during the night is not unusual. However, sleep disturbances longer than 1 month are problematic.

Although teaching about sleep hygiene practices (Table 7-3) is beneficial, individuals with chronic insomnia require more in-depth intervention using CBT-I strategies. An important component of sleep hygiene is reducing dietary intake of substances containing caffeine (Table 7-6). Caffeine has a half-life of about 6 hours, and possibly as long as 9 hours in older adults. Consuming caffeinated beverages after 12 noon should be avoided.

Suggest and implement changes in home and institutional environments to enhance sleep. Reducing light and noise levels enhances sleep. Awareness of time passing and watching the clock adds to anxieties about not falling asleep or returning to sleep. Keeping the bedroom dark and cool is conducive to good sleep.

Teach patients about sleeping medications. With the benzodiazepines, non-benzodiazepine hypnotics, and melatonin-receptor agonists, teach the patient to take the drug right before bedtime, be prepared to get a full night's sleep of at least 6 to 8 hours, and do not plan activities the next morning that require highly skilled psychomotor coordination. Advise patients not to take these medications with high-fat food (delays absorption), alcohol, or other CNS depressants. Patient follow-up regarding medications is important. Ask about daytime sleepiness, nightmares, and any difficulties in activities of daily living.

**TABLE 7-6 Caffeine Content of Foods and Beverages***

| Food or Beverage | Caffeine (mg) |
|---|---|
| Coffee, brewed (8 oz) | 95-200 |
| Coffee, instant (8 oz) | 27-173 |
| Coffee, decaffeinated | 2-12 |
| Tea, leaf or bag (8 oz) | 14-70 |
| Celestial Seasoning herbal tea, all varieties | 0 |
| Diet Coke (12 oz) | 23-47 |
| Coca-Cola (12 oz) | 23-35 |
| Dr. Pepper (12 oz) | 36-42 |
| Pepsi-Cola (12 oz) | 32-39 |
| Diet Pepsi-Cola (12 oz) | 27-37 |
| 7-Up, Sprite, or Diet 7-Up (12 oz) | 0 |
| A&W Root Beer (12 oz) | 0 |
| Red Bull (12 oz) | 75-80 |
| Mountain Dew (12 oz) | 42-55 |
| Ben & Jerry's no-fat coffee fudge frozen yogurt (1 cup) | 85 |
| Dannon coffee yogurt (8 oz) | 45 |
| Hershey's special dark chocolate bar (1.5 oz) | 31 |
| Hershey bar (milk chocolate) | 10 |
| Hot chocolate (8 oz) | 5 |

*List only includes selected foods and beverages.

## OBSTRUCTIVE SLEEP APNEA

The term **sleep-disordered breathing (SDB)** indicates abnormal respiratory patterns associated with sleep. These include snoring, apnea (temporary cessation of respiration), and hypopnea (temporary restriction of respiration without full cessation) with increased respiratory effort leading to frequent arousals. SDB results in frequent sleep disruptions and alterations in sleep architecture. Obstructive sleep apnea is the most commonly diagnosed SDB problem.

**Obstructive sleep apnea (OSA)**, also called *obstructive sleep apnea–hypopnea syndrome* (OSAHS), is characterized by partial or complete upper airway obstruction during sleep. *Apnea* is the cessation of respiratory airflow (90% or greater reduction) lasting longer than 10 seconds. *Hypopnea* is a condition characterized by shallow respirations (30% to 90% reduction in airflow).[8] Airflow obstruction in OSA occurs because of (1) narrowing of the air passages with relaxation of muscle tone during sleep and/or (2) the tongue and soft palate falling backward to partially or completely obstruct the pharynx (Fig. 7-4). Each obstruction may last from 10 to 90 seconds. During the apneic period the patient can experience *hypoxemia* (decreased $PaO_2$ or $SpO_2$) and *hypercapnia* (increased $PaCO_2$). These changes are ventilatory stimulants and cause brief arousals, but the patient may not fully awaken.

The patient has a generalized startle response, snorts, and gasps, which cause the tongue and soft palate to move forward and the airway to open. Apnea and arousal cycles occur repeatedly throughout the night. Apneic episodes occur most often during REM sleep, when airway muscle tone is lowest.

There is no single cause for OSA, but rather the condition is related to multiple factors that influence airway patency and the tone of airway musculature. Risk factors include obesity (BMI greater than 30 kg/m$^2$), age greater than 65 years, neck circumference greater than 17 inches, craniofacial abnormalities that affect the upper airway, and acromegaly (a pituitary disorder discussed in Chapter 49). Smokers are more likely to have OSA. OSA is more common in men than in women until after menopause, when the prevalence of the disorder is equal.[18] Women with OSA have higher mortality rates than men with OSA. OSA patients with excessive daytime sleepiness have increased mortality.

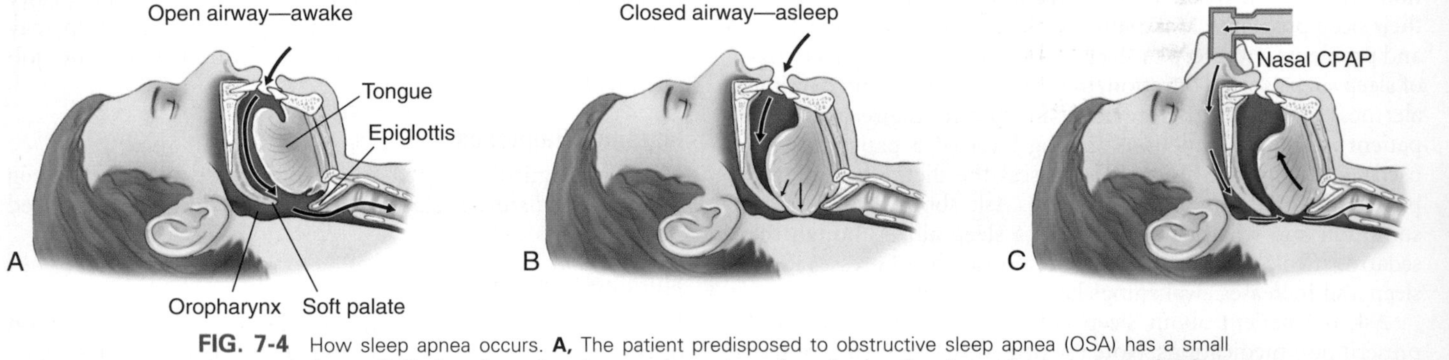


**FIG. 7-4** How sleep apnea occurs. **A,** The patient predisposed to obstructive sleep apnea (OSA) has a small pharyngeal airway. **B,** During sleep, the pharyngeal muscles relax, allowing the airway to close. Lack of airflow results in repeated apneic episodes. **C,** Continuous positive airway pressure *(CPAP)* splints the airway open, preventing airflow obstruction. (Modified from LaFleur Brooks M: *Exploring medical language: a student-directed approach,* ed 8, St Louis, 2012, Mosby.)

## INFORMATICS IN PRACTICE

### *Sleep Apnea Diagnosis and Monitoring*

- Home respiratory monitoring is a cost-effective alternative for diagnosing sleep-related breathing disorders that allows patients the convenience of sleeping in their own home.
- Home respiratory monitoring is used as part of a comprehensive sleep evaluation and in patients likely to have moderate to severe obstructive sleep apnea but without heart failure, obstructive lung disease, or neuromuscular disease.
- Home respiratory monitoring is used to monitor the effectiveness of non-CPAP therapies for patients with sleep-related breathing disorders.
- Wireless monitors can detect changes in vital signs and pulse oximetry, raising an alarm if values fall outside of set parameters.
- Your patient may benefit from telehealth to diagnose and monitor for sleep apnea in the home.

*CPAP,* Continuous positive airway pressure.

### Clinical Manifestations

Clinical manifestations of sleep apnea include frequent arousals during sleep, insomnia, excessive daytime sleepiness, and witnessed apneic episodes. The patient's bed partner may complain about the patient's loud snoring. Other symptoms include morning headaches (from hypercapnia or increased BP that causes vasodilation of cerebral blood vessels), personality changes, and irritability.

A major risk of OSA is cardiovascular complications. Apnea during sleep causes hypoxia, nocturnal arousals, and increased pressure in the thoracic cavity. These events can lead to negative physiologic consequences, including overactivation of the sympathetic nervous system, increased vascular resistance, and reduced oxygenation of the cardiac muscle. Long-term effects include hypertension, cardiac dysrhythmias, arteriosclerosis, heart failure, and cardiovascular-related mortality.[9]

Chronic sleep loss predisposes the person to diminished ability to concentrate, impaired memory, failure to accomplish daily tasks, and interpersonal difficulties. Men may experience impotence. Hypercapnia and arousals contribute to daytime sleepiness in people with OSA. Driving accidents may occur due to excessive daytime sleepiness. Family life and the patient's ability to maintain employment are often compromised. As a result, the patient may experience depression. Cessation of breathing reported by the bed partner is usually a source of great anxiety because of the fear that breathing may not resume.

### Diagnostic Studies

Assessment of the patient with OSA includes a thorough sleep and medical history. A common questionnaire used to screen for OSA is the STOP-BANG questionnaire,[18] which assesses for clinical manifestations highly suspicious of OSA.

Typically, OSA is diagnosed by PSG done in a clinical sleep laboratory. The patient's chest and abdominal movement, oral and nasal airflow, $SpO_2$, ocular movement, and heart rate and rhythm are monitored. In some instances, portable sleep studies are conducted in the home setting. Overnight pulse oximetry assessment may be done to determine whether nocturnal oxygen supplementation is indicated.

A diagnosis of sleep apnea requires documentation of apneic events or hypopneas of at least 10 seconds' duration. OSA is defined as more than 5 apnea/hypopnea events per hour accompanied by a 3% to 4% decrease in oxygen saturation. Severe apnea can be associated with apneic events of more than 30 to 50 per hour of sleep.[8]

## NURSING AND INTERPROFESSIONAL MANAGEMENT: SLEEP APNEA

### Conservative Treatment

Mild sleep apnea (5 to 10 apnea/hypopnea events per hour) may respond to simple measures. Conservative treatment at home begins with sleeping on one's side rather than on the back (called *positional therapy*), which reduces the effects of gravity on the airway. Elevating the head of the bed may eliminate OSA in some patients.

Medications that relax airway muscle tone often make OSA worse. Instruct the patient to avoid taking sedatives or consuming alcoholic beverages for 3 to 4 hours before sleep. Sleep medications often make OSA worse. Excessive weight worsens sleep apnea as the pressure of adipose tissue in the neck and on the chest restricts ventilation. Referral to a weight loss program may be indicated. Bariatric surgery may also reduce OSA.[19] Instruct the patient on the dangers of driving or using heavy equipment due to the profound sleepiness that is common in people with OSA. Insomnia is common in people with OSA, and they may need additional specific treatment for the insomnia (such as CBT-I).

Symptoms may resolve in up to half of patients with OSA who use a special mouth guard, also called an oral appliance, during sleep to prevent airflow obstruction. Oral appliances bring the mandible and tongue forward to enlarge the airway space, thereby preventing airway occlusion.[19] Some individuals find a support group beneficial, where they can express concerns and feelings and discuss strategies for resolving problems.

In patients with more severe symptoms (>15 apnea/hypopnea events/hour), *continuous positive airway pressure (CPAP)* by mask is the treatment of choice. With CPAP, the patient applies a nasal mask that is attached to a high-flow blower (Fig. 7-5). The blower is adjusted to maintain sufficient positive pressure (5 to 25 cm $H_2O$) in the airway during inspiration and expiration to prevent airway collapse.

Some patients cannot adjust to wearing a mask over the nose or mouth or to exhaling against the high pressure. A technologically more sophisticated therapy, bilevel positive airway pressure (BiPAP), can deliver a higher inspiration pressure and a lower

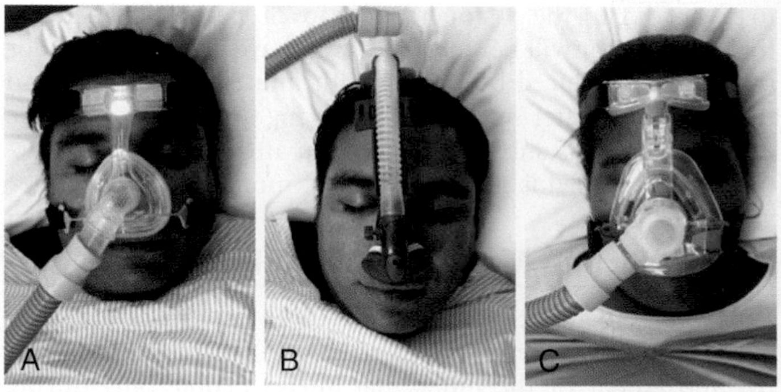


**FIG. 7-5** Examples of positive airway pressure devices for sleep apnea. **A,** Patient wearing a nasal mask and headgear (positive pressure only through nose). **B,** Patient wearing nasal pillows (positive pressure only through nose). **C,** Patient wearing a full face mask (positive pressure to nose and mouth). (From Goldman L, Schafer AI: *Goldman's Cecil medicine,* ed 24, Philadelphia, 2012, Saunders.)

pressure during expiration. With BiPAP, the apnea can be relieved with a lower mean pressure and may be better tolerated.

CPAP reduces apnea episodes, daytime sleepiness, and fatigue. It improves quality of life ratings and returns cognitive functioning to normal. Although CPAP is a highly effective treatment, patients have problems with adherence to using it on a daily basis.[19] Approximately two thirds of patients using CPAP report side effects such as nasal stuffiness.

First assess the patient's knowledge about OSA and CPAP, and involve the bed partner in teaching. Evaluate the patient for nasal resistance. To ensure successful adherence to CPAP treatment, patients need to be involved in the selection of the mask and device before the start of therapy.

When patients with a history of OSA are hospitalized, be aware that the administration of opioid analgesics and sedating medications (benzodiazepines, barbiturates, hypnotics) may worsen OSA symptoms by depressing respiration.[20] This will necessitate that the patient wear the CPAP or BiPAP when resting or sleeping. Many patients are able to use their own CPAP equipment, but hospital policy should be checked to be certain it can be used. Check with the HCP in charge of the patient's care to determine if a patient who uses home CPAP should continue this therapy in the hospital. If CPAP is ordered, you can encourage and assist with the patient's use of this therapy.

### ◆ Surgical Treatment

If other measures fail, OSA can be managed surgically. The goal of OSA surgery is to reduce collapsibility and increase patency of the upper airway, including oral, nasal, and pharyngeal passages. The two most common procedures are uvulopalatopharyngoplasty (UPPP or UP3) and genioglossal advancement and hyoid myotomy (GAHM). UPPP involves excision of the tonsillar pillars, uvula, and posterior soft palate to remove the obstructing tissue. GAHM involves advancing the attachment of the muscular part of the tongue on the mandible. When GAHM is performed, UPPP is generally done as well. Depending on the site of the obstruction, symptoms are relieved in up to 80% of patients. Radiofrequency ablation (RFA) of obstructive tissues alone or in combination with other surgical techniques is also used. RFA is the least invasive surgical intervention.

After surgery, complications of airway obstruction or hemorrhage occur most often in the immediate postoperative period. Patients can usually be discharged home within 1 day after the procedure. Before going home, teach the patient what to expect during the postoperative recovery period. Tell patients that their throat will be sore. They may have a foul breath odor that may be reduced by rinsing with diluted mouthwash and then salt water after several days. Snoring may persist until the inflammation has subsided. Follow-up after surgery is important. A repeat PSG is performed 3 to 4 months after surgery.

## PERIODIC LIMB MOVEMENT DISORDER

**Periodic limb movement disorder (PLMD)** is characterized by *periodic limb movements in sleep* (PLMS): involuntary, repetitive movement of the limbs that affects people only during sleep.[21] PLMD usually involves the legs and rarely involves the arms. Sometimes abdominal, oral, and nasal movement accompanies PLMD. Movements typically occur for 0.5 to 10 seconds, in intervals separated by 5 to 90 seconds. PLMD causes poor-quality sleep and excessive daytime sleepiness. The causes of PLMD are not fully understood, but iron deficiency and dopamine dysfunction in the CNS have been implicated.[21]

PLMS can occur with medical disorders (e.g., sleep apnea, narcolepsy) and certain medications. For a diagnosis of PLMD, the occurrence of PLMS must not be due to another disorder. PLMS affects many individuals with restless legs syndrome (RLS). (RLS is a disorder that is discussed in Chapter 58.)

PLMD is diagnosed using a detailed history from the patient and/or bed partner and doing PSG. PLMD is treated by medications aimed at reducing or eliminating the limb movements or the arousals. Clonazepam (Klonopin) (a benzodiazepine) is used to treat PLMD, although it likely helps patients by improving sleep quality rather than reducing limb movements. Other medications shown to be effective are valproic acid (Depakene), an antiseizure drug that reduces muscle activity, and selegiline (Eldepryl), a dopaminergic agent. Dopamine agonists (pramipexole [Mirapex] and ropinirole [Requip]) are recommended for RLS, but there is little research on their efficacy for PLMD. However, in common practice these drugs are prescribed to treat PLMD.

## CIRCADIAN RHYTHM DISORDERS

*Circadian rhythm disorders* can occur when the circadian time-keeping system loses synchrony with the environment. Lack of synchrony between the circadian time-keeping system and environment disrupts the sleep-wake cycle and affects the patient's ability to have quality sleep. The two common symptoms are insomnia and excessive sleepiness. Jet lag disorder and shift work sleep disorder (see Special Sleep Needs of Nurses section on p. 100) are the most common types of circadian rhythm disorders.[16]

**Jet lag disorder** occurs when a person travels across multiple time zones. One's body time is not synchronized with environmental time. Most individuals crossing at least three time zones experience jet lag. The number of time zones crossed affects the severity of symptoms and the time it takes to recover. Resynchronization of the body's clock occurs at a rate of about 1 hr/day when traveling eastward and 1.5 hr/day when traveling westward. Melatonin and exposure to daylight help to synchronize the body's rhythm.

Several strategies may help to reduce the risk of developing jet lag. Before travel the individual can start to get in harmony with the time schedule of the destination. When time at destination is brief (i.e., 2 days or less), keeping home-based sleep hours rather than adopting destination sleep hours may reduce sleepiness and jet lag symptoms.

## NARCOLEPSY

**Narcolepsy** is a chronic neurologic disorder caused by the brain's inability to regulate sleep-wake cycles normally. At various times throughout the day, people with narcolepsy experience uncontrollable urges to sleep. Patients with narcolepsy often go directly into REM sleep from wakefulness.[21] This does not occur in normal sleep and is a unique feature of narcolepsy. Patients with narcolepsy also experience fragmented and disturbed nighttime sleep. There are two types of narcolepsy: with cataplexy (type 1) and without cataplexy (type 2).[21] Cataplexy is a brief and sudden loss of skeletal muscle tone. It can manifest as a brief episode of muscle weakness or complete postural collapse and falling. Laughter, anger, or surprise often triggers episodes.

In both genders the onset of narcolepsy typically occurs in adolescence or early in the third decade. Head trauma, a sudden change in sleep-wake habits, and infection may trigger the onset of narcolepsy symptoms. The cause of narcolepsy remains unknown. It is associated with destruction of neurons that produce orexin. The resulting deficiency of orexin causes instability of wake and transitions from wake to sleep that occur unpredictably. The loss of neurons may be due to an autoimmune process.

Narcolepsy is diagnosed based on a history of sleepiness, PSG, and daytime *multiple sleep latency tests* (MSLTs).[21] For the MSLT, patients undergo an overnight PSG evaluation followed by four or five naps scheduled every 2 hours during the next day. Short sleep latencies and onset of REM sleep in more than two MSLTs are diagnostic signs of narcolepsy.

Narcolepsy cannot be cured. Management of narcolepsy is focused on symptom management (Table 7-3). Provide teaching about sleep and sleep hygiene. Advise the patient with narcolepsy to take three or more short (15-minute) naps throughout the day and to avoid large or heavy meals and alcohol. You can play a key role in ensuring patient safety by teaching safety behaviors and encouraging adherence to the prescribed medication regimen. Safety precautions, especially when driving, are critically important for patients with narcolepsy. The behavioral therapies for insomnia (discussed earlier in this chapter) are also used to address the sleep disturbances. Stimulants are used to counter daytime sleepiness.

Modafinil (Provigil), a nonamphetamine wake-promotion drug, is considered a first-line drug therapy. Sodium oxybate (Xyrem), a metabolite of GABA, is another wake-promoting medication that is used. High doses of selective serotonin reuptake inhibitors (SSRIs) (e.g., fluoxetine [Prozac], venlafaxine) may be prescribed for the management of cataplexy.

## PARASOMNIAS

**Parasomnias** are unusual and often undesirable behaviors that occur while falling asleep, transitioning between sleep stages, or arousing from sleep.[21] They are due to CNS activation and often involve complex behaviors. The parasomnia is generally goal directed, although the person is not aware or conscious of the act. Parasomnias may result in fragmented sleep and fatigue.

Sleepwalking and sleep terrors are arousal parasomnias that occur during NREM sleep. *Sleepwalking* behaviors can range from sitting up in bed, moving objects, and walking around the room to driving a car. During a sleepwalking event the individual may not speak and may have limited or no awareness of the event. On awakening, the individual does not remember the event. In the ICU, a parasomnia may be misinterpreted as ICU psychosis. Sedated ICU patients can exhibit manifestations of a parasomnia.

*Sleep terrors* (night terrors) are characterized by a sudden awakening from sleep along with a loud cry and signs of panic. The person has marked increases in heart rate and respiration and diaphoresis. Factors in the ICU such as sleep disruption and deprivation, fever, stress, and exposure to noise and light can contribute to sleep terrors.

*Nightmares* are a parasomnia characterized by recurrent awakening with recall of a frightful or disturbing dream. These normally occur during REM sleep during the final third of sleep. In critically ill patients nightmares are common and are most likely due to medications. Drug classes most likely to cause nightmares are sedative-hypnotics, β-adrenergic antagonists, dopamine agonists, and amphetamines.

### Gerontologic Considerations: Sleep

Older age is associated with overall shorter total sleep time, decreased sleep efficiency, and more awakenings (Fig. 7-6). A common misconception is that older people need less sleep than younger people. In fact, the amount of sleep needed as a person ages remains relatively constant. Other sleep disorders (e.g., sleep-disordered breathing) also increase with age and may manifest with symptoms of insomnia.[22]

Multiple factors impair older adults' ability to obtain quality sleep. Insomnia symptoms in older adults frequently occur with depression, cardiovascular disease, pain, and cognitive problems. Chronic conditions that are more common in older adults (COPD, diabetes, dementia, chronic pain, cancer) can affect sleep quality.[22] Medications used to treat these conditions can contribute to sleep problems. OTC medications also can lead to sleep disturbance. Cough and cold medications, especially those containing pseudoephedrine; caffeine-containing drugs; and drugs containing nicotine (e.g., nicotine gum, transdermal patches), are stimulants.

Awakening and getting out of bed during the night (e.g., to use the bathroom) increase the risk for falls. Older adults may use OTC medications or alcohol as a sleep aid. This practice can further increase the risk of falls at night. Chronic disturbed sleep in older adults can result in disorientation, delirium, impaired intellect, disturbed cognition, and increased risk of accidents and injury.

Because older adults may attribute their disturbed sleep to normal aging, they may fail to report symptoms of sleep disorders to their HCPs.[22] Use a sleeping assessment (Table 7-5) to detect sleep disturbances in older adults.

Sleep medications should be used with great caution in older adults. Diphenhydramine, alone or in combination with other drugs, is sedating with anticholinergic effects. Any OTC medication labeled "PM" probably has diphenhydramine and should be used cautiously by older adults. Metabolism of most hypnotic drugs decreases with aging. Older adults have increased sensitivity to hypnotic and sedative medications. Thus drug therapies for sleep disturbances are started at lower doses and monitored carefully. Whenever possible, long-acting benzodiazepines should be avoided. Older adults receiving

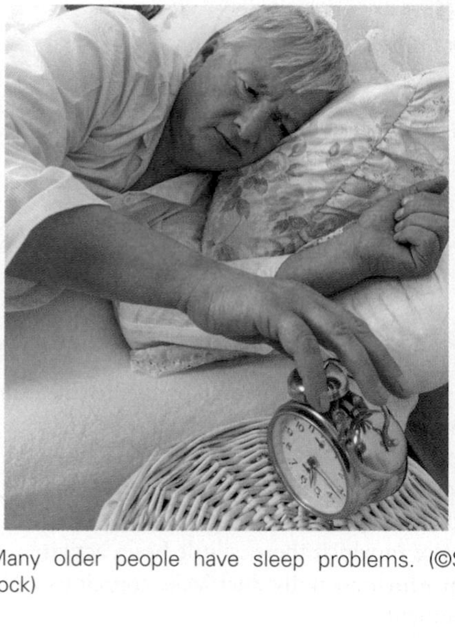

**FIG. 7-6** Many older people have sleep problems. (©Studio-Annika/iStock/Thinkstock)

benzodiazepines are at increased risk of daytime sedation, falls, and cognitive and psychomotor impairment.

## SPECIAL SLEEP NEEDS OF NURSES

Nursing is one of several professions that necessitates night shift and rotating shift schedules. In many settings, nurses are asked to or volunteer to work a variety of day and night shifts, often alternating and rotating them. Unfortunately, nurses who do shift work often report less job satisfaction and more job-related stress.[23] There is a higher incidence of driving errors in nurses doing shift work, especially those who work rotating shifts.[24]

Nurses on permanent night or rapidly rotating shifts are at increased risk of experiencing **shift work sleep disorder**, which is characterized by insomnia, sleepiness, and fatigue. Nurses on rotating shifts get the least amount of sleep. With repeated periods of inadequate sleep, the sleep debt grows. Chronic fatigue in nurses doing shift work poses challenges for the individual nurse's health and for patient safety.[23]

Shift work alters the synchrony between circadian rhythms and the environment, leading to sleep disruption. Nurses working the night shift are often too sleepy to be fully alert at work and too alert to sleep soundly the next day. Sustained alterations in circadian rhythms such as those imposed by rotating shift work have been linked to increased morbidity and mortality risks associated with cardiovascular problems. In addition, mood disorders such as anxiety are higher in nurses who work rotating shifts.

From a safety perspective, disturbed sleep and subsequent fatigue can result in errors and accidents for nurses as well as for their patients. Fatigue diminishes or distorts perceptual skills, judgment, and decision-making capabilities. Lack of sleep reduces the ability to cope and handle stress and may result in physical, mental, and emotional exhaustion.

The problem of sleep disruption is critically important to nursing. Several strategies may help reduce the distress associated with rotating shift work. These include brief periods of on-site napping. Maintaining a consistent sleep-wake schedule even on days off is optimum but perhaps unrealistic. For night shift work, scheduling the sleep period just before going to work increases alertness and vigilance, improves reaction times, and decreases accidents during night shift work. Nurses who have control over their work schedules appear to experience less sleep disruption than those whose schedule is imposed. As a nurse, you need to manage the impact of sleep disruption through the use of sleep hygiene practices.

## CASE STUDY

### *Insomnia*

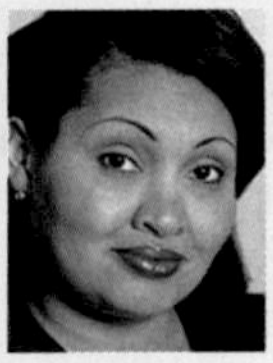

(©JackF/iStock/Thinkstock)

**Patient Profile**

G.P., a 49-year-old African American woman, is seen in the primary care clinic for complaints of chronic fatigue and disturbed sleep. She is postmenopausal based on self-report. In the past year, since the end of her periods, she has experienced daily hot flashes and sleep problems. She denies any other health problems. On a usual workday she drinks two cups of hot tea in the morning and one can of diet cola in the late afternoon. Currently she is taking OTC diphenhydramine for sleep. Her partner, who has accompanied her to the clinic, states that her snoring has gotten worse, and it is interfering with his sleep.

**Subjective Data**

- Reports hot flashes and nighttime sweating
- Reports daytime tiredness and fatigue
- States she has trouble getting to sleep and staying asleep

**Objective Data**

***Physical Examination***

- Laboratory evaluations within normal limits
- Height 5′6″
- Weight 180 lb

***Diagnostic Studies***

- Nighttime PSG study reveals episodes of obstructive sleep apnea

**Interprofessional Care**

- CPAP nightly
- Referred for weight reduction counseling
- Education about sleep hygiene

**Discussion Questions**

1. What are G.P.'s risk factors for sleep apnea?
2. How does CPAP work?
3. Based on the data above, what are the major health risks for G.P. from sleep apnea?
4. ***Patient-Centered Care:*** What specific sleep hygiene practices could G.P. use to improve the quality of her sleep?
5. ***Priority Decision:*** Based on your assessment of G.P., what are the priority nursing interventions for her?
6. ***Teamwork and Collaboration:*** For the interventions that you identified in the above question, which of the following personnel could be responsible for implementing them: RN, LPN, unlicensed assistive personnel (UAP)?
7. ***Priority Decision:*** Based on the assessment data provided, what are the priority nursing diagnoses?
8. ***Teamwork and Collaboration:*** What referrals may be indicated for G.P.?

Answers available at *http://evolve.elsevier.com/Lewis/medsurg.*

## BRIDGE TO NCLEX EXAMINATION

The number of the question corresponds to the same-numbered outcome at the beginning of the chapter.

1. Sleep is *best* described as a
   - **a.** loosely organized state similar to coma.
   - **b.** state in which pain sensitivity decreases.
   - **c.** quiet state in which there is little brain activity.
   - **d.** state in which an individual lacks conscious awareness of the environment.
2. Which statement(s) is/are true regarding rapid eye movement (REM) sleep (*select all that apply*)?
   - **a.** The EEG pattern is quiescent.
   - **b.** Muscle tone is greatly reduced.
   - **c.** It occurs only once in the night.
   - **d.** It is separated by distinct physiologic stages.
   - **e.** The most vivid dreaming occurs during this phase.

3. Insufficient sleep is associated with *(select all that apply)*
   a. increased body mass index.
   b. increased insulin resistance.
   c. impaired cognitive functioning.
   d. increased immune responsiveness.
   e. increased daytime body temperature.
4. When teaching the patient with primary insomnia about sleep hygiene, the nurse should emphasize
   a. the importance of daytime naps.
   b. the need to exercise before bedtime.
   c. the need for long-term use of hypnotics.
   d. avoiding caffeine-containing beverages 6-9 hours before bedtime.
5. While caring for a patient with a history of narcolepsy with cataplexy, the nurse can delegate which activity to the unlicensed assistive personnel (UAP)?
   a. Teaching about the timing of medications
   b. Walking the patient to and from the bathroom
   c. Developing a plan of care with a family member
   d. Planning an appropriate diet that avoids caffeine-containing foods
6. An overweight patient with sleep apnea would like to avoid using a nasal CPAP device if possible. To help him reach this goal, the nurse suggests that the patient
   a. lose excess weight.
   b. take a nap during the day.
   c. eat a high-protein snack at bedtime.
   d. use mild sedatives or alcohol at bedtime.
7. A patient on the surgical unit has a history of parasomnia (sleepwalking). What statement describes parasomnia?
   a. Hypnotic medications reduce the risk of sleepwalking.
   b. The patient is often unaware of the activity on awakening.
   c. The patient should be restrained at night to prevent personal harm.
   d. The potential for sleepwalking is reduced by exercise before sleep.
8. Strategies to reduce sleepiness during nighttime working include
   a. exercising before work.
   b. taking melatonin before working the night shift.
   c. sleeping for at least 2 hours immediately before work time.
   d. walking for 10 minutes every 4 hours during the night shift.

1. d, 2. b, e, 3. a, b, c, 4. d, 5. b, 6. a, 7. b, 8. c.

For rationales to these answers and even more NCLEX review questions, visit *http://evolve.elsevier.com/Lewis/medsurg.*

## EVOLVE WEBSITE

http://evolve.elsevier.com/Lewis/medsurg

**Review Questions (Online Only)**
**Key Points**
**Answer Keys for Questions**
- Rationales for Bridge to NCLEX Examination Questions
- Answer Guidelines for Case Study on p. 100

**Conceptual Care Map Creator**
**Audio Glossary**
**Content Updates**

## REFERENCES


1. National Heart, Lung, and Blood Institute: *How much sleep is enough?* Retrieved from *www.nhlbi.nih.gov/health/health-topics/topics/sdd/howmuch.html.*
2. Centers for Disease Control and Prevention: *Insufficient sleep is a public health epidemic.* Retrieved from *www.cdc.gov/features/dssleep/index.html#References.*
3. National Sleep Foundation: *Facts and stats.* Retrieved from *http://drowsydriving.org/about/facts-and-stats.*
4. Monti JM: The neurotransmitters of sleep and wake, a physiological reviews series, *Sleep Med Rev* 17:313, 2013.
5. de Lecea L, Huerta R: Hypocretin (orexin) regulation of sleep-to-wake transitions, *Front Pharmacol* 5:1, 2014.
6. National Sleep Foundation: *Orexin receptor antagonists: a new class of sleeping pill.* Retrieved from *http://sleepfoundation.org/sleep-news/orexin-receptor-antagonists-new-class-sleeping-pill.*
7. LeGates TA, Fernandez DC, Hattar S: Light as a central modulator of circadian rhythms, sleep and affect, *Nat Rev Neurosci* 15:443, 2014.
8. Iber C, Ancoli-Israel S, Chesson A, et al: *The American Academy of Sleep Medicine: The AASM manual for the scoring of sleep and associated events: rules, terminology and technical specifications,* 2007, Westchester, Ill.
9. Stopford E, Ravi K, Nayar V: The association of sleep disordered breathing with heart failure and other cardiovascular conditions, *Cardiol Res Pract* 2013:356280 (ISSN: 2090-8016), 2013.
10. Nesbitt L, Goode D: Nurses perceptions of sleep in the intensive care unit environment: a literature review, *Intensive Crit Care Nurs* 30:231, 2014.
11. Finan PH, Goodin BR, Smith MT: The association of sleep and pain: an update and a path forward, *J Pain* 14:1539, 2013.
12. Williams J, Roth A, Vatthauer K, et al: Cognitive behavioral treatment of insomnia, *Chest* 143:554, 2013.
*13. Tannenbaum C, Paquette A, Hilmer S, et al: A systematic review of amnestic and non-amnestic mild cognitive impairment induced by anticholinergic, antihistamine, GABAergic and opioid drugs, *Drugs Aging* 29:639, 2012.
*14. Yeung WF, Chung KF, Yung KP, et al: Doxepin for insomnia: a systematic review of randomized placebo-controlled trials, *Sleep Med Rev* 19:75, 2015.
15. Zisapel N: Drugs for insomnia, *Expert Opin Emerg Drugs* 17:299, 2012.
16. Zee PC, Attarian H, Videnovic A: Circadian rhythm abnormalities, *Continuum (Minneap Minn)* 19:132, 2013.
*17. Taibi DM, Landis CA, Petry H, et al: A systematic review of valerian as a sleep aid: safe but not effective, *Sleep Med Rev* 11:209, 2007.
*18. Chung F, Subramanyam R, Liao P, et al: High STOP-BANG score indicates a high probability of obstructive sleep apnoea, *Br J Anaesth* 108:768, 2012.
19. Freedman N: Improvements in current treatments and emerging therapies for adult obstructive sleep apnea, *F1000 Prime Rep* 6:1, 2014.
20. Ward CW: Safe use of opioids in individuals with obstructive sleep apnea, *Pain Manag Nurs* 16 (3):411, 2015.
21. American Academy of Sleep Medicine: *International classification of sleep disorders,* Darien, Ill, 2014, American Academy of Sleep Medicine.
22. Gooneratne NS, Vitiello MV: Sleep in older adults: normative changes, sleep disorders, and treatment options, *Clin Geriatr Med* 30:591, 2014.
*23. Matheson A, O'Brien L, Reid JA: The impact of shiftwork on health: a literature review, *J Clin Nurs* 23:3309, 2014.
*24. Ftouni S, Sletten TL, Howard M, et al: Objective and subjective measures of sleepiness, and their associations with on-road driving events in shift workers, *J Sleep Res* 22:58, 2013.

*Evidence-based information for clinical practice.

# 8

# Pain

*Rosemary C. Polomano, Mechele Fillman*

*It's not the load that breaks you down, it's the way you carry it.*

***Lou Holtz***

http://evolve.elsevier.com/Lewis/medsurg/

## LEARNING OUTCOMES

1. Define pain.
2. Describe the neural mechanisms of pain and pain modulation.
3. Differentiate between nociceptive and neuropathic types of pain.
4. Explain the physical and psychologic effects of unrelieved pain.
5. Interpret the subjective and objective data that are obtained from a comprehensive pain assessment.
6. Describe effective interprofessional pain management techniques.
7. Describe drug and nondrug methods of pain relief.
8. Explain your role and responsibility in pain management.
9. Discuss ethical and legal issues related to pain and pain management.
10. Evaluate the influence of one's own knowledge, beliefs, and attitudes about pain assessment and management.

## KEY TERMS

analgesic ceiling, p. 111
breakthrough pain (BTP), p. 108
central sensitization, p. 105
complex regional pain syndrome (CRPS), p. 107
equianalgesic dose, p. 117
modulation, p. 106
multimodal analgesia, p. 110
neuropathic pain, p. 106
nociception, p. 103
nociceptive pain, p. 104
pain, p. 102
patient-controlled analgesia (PCA), p. 120
patient-controlled epidural analgesia (PCEA), p. 120
peripheral sensitization, p. 104
transduction, p. 103
transmission, p. 104
trigger point, p. 121

**Pain** is a complex, multidimensional experience that can cause suffering and decreased quality of life. Pain is one of the major reasons that people seek health care. To effectively assess and manage patients with pain, you need to understand the physiologic and psychosocial dimensions of pain. This chapter presents evidence-based information to help you assess and safely manage pain in collaboration with other interprofessional team members.

## MAGNITUDE OF PAIN PROBLEM

Millions of people suffer from pain. Annually in the United States, at least 25 million people experience acute pain as a result of injury or surgery. Common chronic pain conditions such as arthritis, migraine headache, and back pain affect more than 100 million American adults.[1] Of the approximately 1.7 million people diagnosed with cancer each year, about 60% experience pain during treatment.[2] Despite the high prevalence and costs of acute and chronic pain, inadequate pain management occurs. Consequences of unrelieved acute pain are presented in Table 8-1.

## DEFINITIONS AND DIMENSIONS OF PAIN

In 1968 Margo McCaffery, a nurse and pioneer in pain management, defined **pain** as "whatever the person experiencing the pain says it is, existing whenever the person says it does."[3] The International Association for the Study of Pain (IASP) defines *pain* as "an unpleasant sensory and emotional experience associated with actual or potential tissue damage, or described in terms of such damage."[1]

These definitions emphasize the subjective nature of pain, in which the patient's self-report is the most valid means of assessment. Although understanding the patient's experience and relying on his or her self-report is essential, this view is problematic for many patients. For example, patients who are comatose or who suffer from dementia, patients who are mentally disabled or challenged, and patients with expressive aphasia

Reviewed by Marylee Bressie, RN, DNP, CCRN, CCNS, CEN, Core Faculty/Nurse Planner, Department of Nursing, School of Public Service Leadership, Capella University, Minneapolis, Minnesota; Debra B. Gordon, RN-BC, DNP, ACNS-BC, FAAN, Co-Director, Harborview Integrated Pain Care Program, Department of Anesthesiology and Pain Medicine, University of Washington, Seattle, Washington; and Elsa Wuhrman, DNP, RN-BC, FNP, BC, DCC, Nurse Practitioner and Assistant Professor of Nursing, Department of Anesthesiology/Acute Pain Services, Columbia University Medical Center, New York, New York.

**TABLE 8-1 Negative Consequences of Unrelieved Acute Pain**

| Response | Possible Consequences |
|---|---|
| **Endocrine and Metabolic** | |
| ↑ Adrenocorticotropic hormone (ACTH) | Weight loss (from ↑ catabolism) |
| ↑ Cortisol | ↑ Respiratory rate |
| ↑ Antidiuretic hormone (ADH) | ↑ Heart rate |
| ↑ Epinephrine and norepinephrine | Shock |
| ↑ Renin, ↑ aldosterone | Glucose intolerance |
| ↓ Insulin | Hyperglycemia |
| Gluconeogenesis | Fluid overload |
| Glycogenolysis | Hypertension |
| Muscle protein catabolism | Urinary retention, ↓ urine output |
| **Cardiovascular** | |
| ↑ Heart rate | Hypertension |
| ↑ Cardiac output | Unstable angina |
| ↑ Peripheral vascular resistance | Myocardial infarction |
| ↑ Myocardial oxygen consumption | Deep vein thrombosis |
| ↑ Coagulation | |
| **Respiratory** | |
| ↓ Tidal volume | Atelectasis |
| Hypoxemia | Pneumonia |
| ↓ Cough, sputum retention | |
| **Renal and Urologic** | |
| ↓ Urine output | Fluid imbalance |
| Urinary retention | Electrolyte disturbance |
| **Gastrointestinal** | |
| ↓ Gastric and intestinal motility | Constipation<br>Anorexia<br>Paralytic ileus |
| **Musculoskeletal** | |
| Muscle spasm | Immobility |
| Impaired muscle function | Weakness and fatigue |
| **Neurologic** | |
| Impaired cognitive function | Confusion<br>Impaired ability to think, reason, and make decisions |
| **Immunologic** | |
| ↓ Immune response | Infection |

**TABLE 8-2 Dimensions of Pain**

| Dimension | Description |
|---|---|
| **Physiologic** | • Genetic, anatomic, and physical determinants of pain influence how painful stimuli are processed, recognized, and described. |
| **Affective** | • Emotional responses to pain include anger, fear, depression, and anxiety.<br>• Negative emotions impair patient's quality of life. |
| **Cognitive** | • Beliefs, attitudes, memories, and meaning attributed to pain influence the ways in which a person responds to pain. |
| **Behavioral** | • Observable actions (e.g., grimacing, irritability, coping skills) are used to express or control pain.<br>• People unable to communicate may have behavioral changes (e.g., agitation, combativeness). |
| **Sociocultural** | • Age and gender influence nociceptive processes and responses to opioids.<br>• Families and caregivers influence patient's response to pain through their beliefs, behaviors, and support.<br>• Culture affects pain expression, medication use, and pain-related beliefs and coping methods. |

**GENDER DIFFERENCES**

***Pain***

**Men**

- Men are less likely to report pain than women.
- Men report more control over pain.
- Men are less likely than women to use alternative treatments for pain.

**Women**

- Women more frequently experience migraine headache, back pain, arthritis, fibromyalgia, irritable bowel syndrome, neuropathic pain, abdominal pain, and foot ache.
- Women are more likely to be diagnosed with a nonspecific, somatic disorder and less likely to receive analgesics for symptoms of chest and abdominal pain.

have varying abilities to report pain. In these instances, you must incorporate nonverbal information such as observed behaviors into your pain assessment.

The emotional distress of pain can cause *suffering,* which is the state of distress associated with loss. Suffering can result in a sense of insecurity, lack of control, and spiritual distress. It is important to assess the ways in which a person's spirituality influences and is influenced by pain.[4]

The meaning of the pain to the person is important. For example, a woman in labor may experience severe pain but can manage it without analgesics because for her it is associated with a joyful event. Moreover, she may feel control over her pain because of the training she received in prenatal classes and the knowledge that the pain is time-limited. In contrast, a woman with chronic, undefined musculoskeletal pain may be stressed by thoughts that her pain is "not real," is uncontrollable, or is caused by her own actions. Perceptions influence the ways in which a person responds to pain and must be incorporated into a comprehensive treatment plan.

Some people cope with pain by distracting themselves, whereas others convince themselves that the pain is permanent, untreatable, and overwhelming. People who believe that their pain is uncontrollable and overwhelming are more likely to have poor outcomes.[5] The biopsychosocial model of pain includes the physiologic, affective, cognitive, behavioral, and sociocultural dimensions of pain (Table 8-2).

Families and caregivers influence the patient's response to pain through their beliefs and behaviors. For example, families may discourage the patient from taking opioids because they have preconceived notions and fears that the patient may become addicted. Understanding these beliefs helps you address them through patient and family teaching.

## Pain Mechanisms

**Nociception** is the physiologic process by which information about tissue damage is communicated to the central nervous system (CNS). It involves four processes: (1) transduction, (2) transmission, (3) perception, and (4) modulation (Fig. 8-1).

**Transduction.** **Transduction** involves the conversion of a noxious mechanical, thermal, or chemical stimulus into an electrical signal called an action potential. Noxious (tissue-damaging) stimuli, including thermal (e.g., sunburn), mechanical (e.g.,

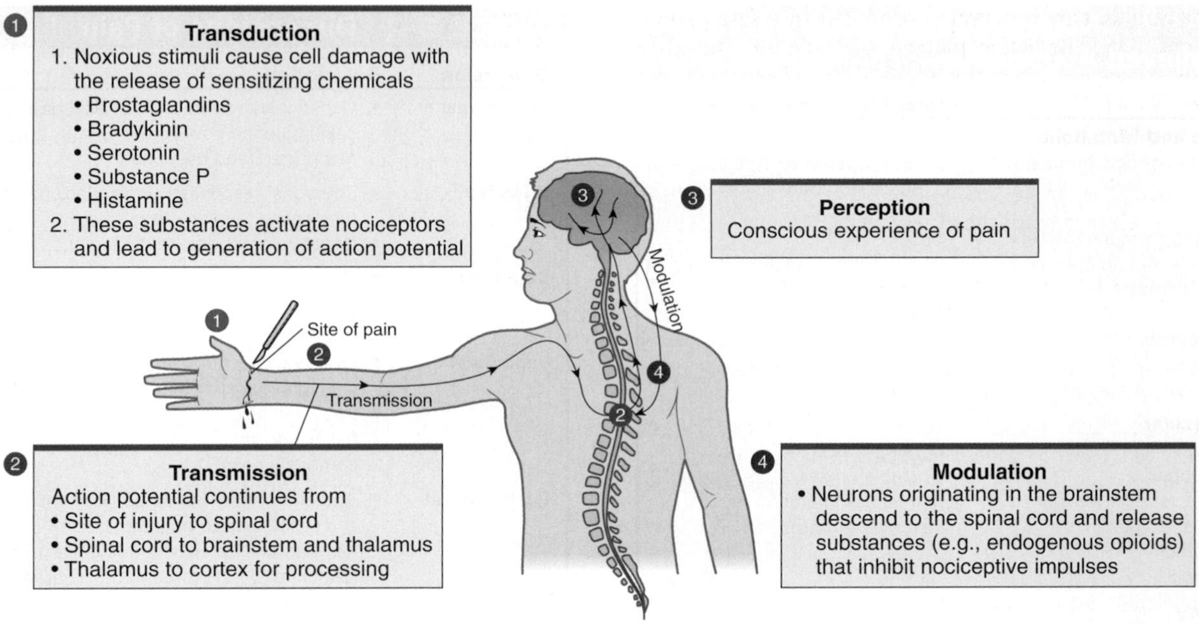


**FIG. 8-1** Nociceptive pain originates when the tissue is injured. *1,* Transduction occurs when there is release of chemical mediators. *2,* Transmission involves the conduct of the action potential from the periphery (injury site) to the spinal cord and then to the brainstem, thalamus, and cerebral cortex. *3,* Perception is the conscious awareness of pain. *4,* Modulation involves signals from the brain going back down the spinal cord to modify incoming impulses. (Developed by McCaffery M, Pasero C, Paice JA. Modified from McCaffery M, Pasero C: *Pain: clinical manual,* ed 2, St Louis, 1999, Mosby.)

surgical incision), or chemical (e.g., toxic substances) stimuli, cause the release of numerous chemicals such as substance P and adenosine triphosphate (ATP) into the damaged tissues. Other chemicals are released from mast cells (e.g., serotonin, histamine, prostaglandins) and macrophages (e.g., cytokines). These chemicals activate nociceptors, which are specialized receptors, or free nerve endings, that respond to painful stimuli. Activation of nociceptors results in an action potential that is carried from the nociceptors to the spinal cord primarily via small, rapidly conducting, myelinated A-delta fibers and slowly conducting unmyelinated C fibers.

In addition to stimulating nociceptors, inflammation and the subsequent release of chemical mediators lower nociceptor thresholds. As a result, nociceptors may fire in response to stimuli that previously were insufficient to elicit a response. They may also fire in response to non-noxious stimuli, such as light touch. This increased susceptibility to nociceptor activation is called **peripheral sensitization**. Leukotrienes, prostaglandins, cytokines, and substance P are involved in peripheral sensitization. Cyclooxygenase (COX), produced in the inflammatory response, also plays an important role in peripheral sensitization. A clinical example of this process is sunburn. This thermal injury causes inflammation that results in a sensation of pain when the affected skin is lightly touched. Peripheral sensitization amplifies signal transmission, which in turn contributes to central sensitization (discussed under Dorsal Horn Processing). The pain produced from activation of peripheral nociceptors is called **nociceptive pain** (described later in the chapter on p. 106).

Therapies that alter either the local environment or sensitivity of the peripheral nociceptors can prevent transduction and initiation of an action potential. Decreasing the effects of chemicals released at the periphery is the basis of several drug approaches to pain relief. For example, nonsteroidal antiinflammatory drugs (NSAIDs), such as ibuprofen (Advil), exert their analgesic effects by blocking the action of COX (see Fig. 11-2).

**Transmission.** **Transmission** is the process by which pain signals are relayed from the periphery to the spinal cord and then to the brain. Nerves that carry pain impulses from the periphery to the spinal cord are called *primary afferent fibers.* These include A-delta and C fibers, each of which is responsible for a different pain sensation. As previously mentioned, A-delta fibers conduct pain rapidly and are responsible for the initial, sharp pain that accompanies tissue injury. C fibers transmit painful stimuli more slowly and produce pain that is typically aching or throbbing. Primary afferent fibers terminate in the dorsal horn of the spinal cord. Activity in the dorsal horn integrates and modulates pain inputs from the periphery.

The propagation of pain impulses from the site of transduction to the brain is shown in Fig. 8-1. Three segments are involved in nociceptive signal transmission: (1) transmission along the peripheral nerve fibers to the spinal cord, (2) dorsal horn processing, and (3) transmission to the thalamus and cerebral cortex.

Drugs that stabilize the neuronal membrane act on peripheral sodium channels to inhibit propagation of nerve impulses. These medications include local anesthetics (e.g., injectable or topical lidocaine, bupivacaine [Sensorcaine]) and antiseizure drugs (e.g., gabapentin [Neurontin]).

***Transmission to Spinal Cord.*** The *first-order neuron* extends the entire distance from the periphery to the dorsal horn with no synapses. For example, an afferent fiber from the great toe travels from the toe through the fifth lumbar nerve root into the spinal cord; it is one cell. Once generated, an action potential travels all the way to the spinal cord unless it is blocked by a sodium channel inhibitor (e.g., local anesthetic) or disrupted by a lesion such as a dorsal root entry zone lesion.

The manner in which nerve fibers enter the spinal cord is central to the notion of spinal dermatomes. *Dermatomes* are areas on the skin that are innervated primarily by a single spinal cord segment. The distinctive pattern of the rash caused by herpes zoster (shingles) across the back and trunk is determined by dermatomes (see Fig. 23-7). Different dermatomes and their innervations are illustrated in Fig. 55-7.

***Dorsal Horn Processing.*** Once a nociceptive signal arrives in the spinal cord, it is processed within the dorsal horn. Neurotransmitters released from the afferent fiber bind to receptors on nearby cells. Some of these neurotransmitters (e.g., glutamate, substance P) produce activation, whereas others (e.g., γ-aminobutyric acid [GABA], serotonin) inhibit activation of nearby cells. In this area, exogenous and endogenous opioids (e.g., encephalin, β-endorphin) also play an important role by binding to opioid receptors and blocking the release of neurotransmitters, particularly substance P. They produce analgesic effects similar to those of exogenous opioids such as morphine. The neurons that project to the thalamus are called *second-order neurons.*

Increased sensitivity and hyperexcitability of neurons in the CNS is called **central sensitization**. Peripheral tissue damage or nerve injury can cause central sensitization, and continued nociceptive input from the periphery maintains it (Fig. 8-2). As a result of the increased excitability of CNS neurons, normal sensory inputs cause abnormal sensing and responses to painful and other stimuli. This explains why some people experience significant pain from touch or tactile stimulation in and around the areas of tissue or nerve injury. This is called *allodynia,* pain from a stimulus that is not typically painful. It also explains why some people experience *hyperalgesia,* an exaggerated or increased pain response to noxious stimuli.

With central sensitization, the central processing circuits are altered. In some cases, central sensitization can be long lasting due to multiple changes that occur in the periphery and CNS.[6]

With ongoing stimulation of slowly conducting unmyelinated C-fiber nociceptors, firing of specialized dorsal horn neurons gradually increases. These inputs can lead to the sprouting of wide dynamic range (WDR) neuron dendrites and the induction of glutamate-dependent *N*-methyl-D-aspartate (NMDA) receptors. This results in an increased capacity to transmit a broader range of stimuli-producing signals, which are then passed up the spinal cord and to the brain. This process is known as *windup.*[7]

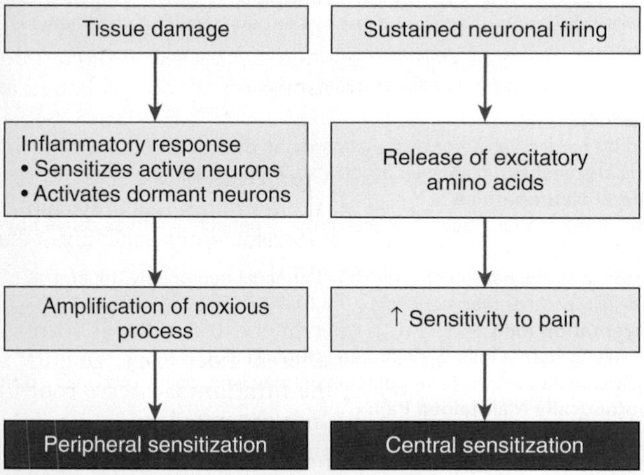


**FIG. 8-2** Sequence of mechanisms leading to peripheral and central sensitization. Increased susceptibility to nociceptor activation is called *peripheral sensitization.* Increased sensitivity and hyperexcitability of neurons in the CNS is called *central sensitization.*

Activation of NMDA receptors also plays a role in windup. NMDA receptor antagonists, such as ketamine (Ketalar), potentially interrupt or block mechanisms that lead to or sustain central sensitization. Windup is like central sensitization and hyperalgesia in that it occurs in response to C-fiber inputs. Windup is different, however, in that it can be short lasting, whereas central sensitization and hyperalgesia persist over time.

It is important for you to understand that acute, unrelieved pain leads to chronic pain through central sensitization. Even brief intervals of acute pain are capable of inducing long-term neuronal remodeling and sensitization *(plasticity),* chronic pain, and lasting psychologic distress.

*Neuroplasticity* refers to processes that allow neurons in the brain to compensate for injury and adjust their responses to new situations or changes in their environment.[8] Neuroplasticity contributes to adaptive mechanisms for reducing pain but also can result in maladaptive mechanisms that enhance pain sensitivity. Genetic variability among individuals may play an important role in changes that occur in the CNS as well as the response to different analgesic therapies to treat pain.[9] Understanding this phenomenon helps explain individual differences in response to pain and why some patients develop chronic pain conditions, whereas others do not.[10]

*Referred pain* must be considered when interpreting the location of pain reported by the person with an injury or a disease involving visceral organs. The location of a stimulus may be distant from the pain location reported by the patient (Fig. 8-3). For example, pain from liver disease is frequently located in the right upper abdominal quadrant but can also be referred to the anterior and posterior neck region, shoulder area, and posterior flank area. If referred pain is not considered when evaluating a pain location report, diagnostic tests and therapy could be misdirected.

***Transmission to Thalamus and Cortex.*** From the dorsal horn, nociceptive stimuli are communicated to the *third-order neuron,* primarily in the thalamus. Fibers of dorsal horn projection cells enter the brain through several pathways, including the spinothalamic tract and spinoreticular tract. Distinct thalamic nuclei

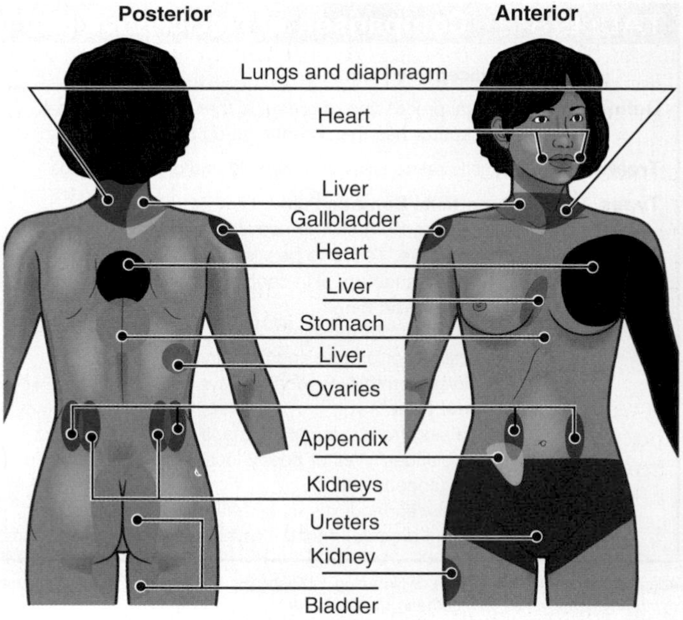


**FIG. 8-3** Typical areas of referred pain.

receive nociceptive input from the spinal cord and have projections to several regions in the cerebral cortex, where the perception of pain is presumed to occur.

Therapeutic approaches that target pain transmission include opioid analgesics that bind to opioid receptors on primary afferent and dorsal horn neurons. These agents mimic the inhibitory effects of endogenous opioids. Another medication, baclofen (Lioresal), inhibits pain transmission by binding to GABA receptors, thus mimicking the inhibitory effects of GABA.

**Perception.** *Perception* occurs when pain is recognized, defined, and assigned meaning by the individual experiencing the pain. In the brain, nociceptive input is perceived as pain. There is no single, precise location where pain perception occurs. Instead, pain perception involves several brain structures. For example, it is believed that the reticular activating system is responsible for warning the individual to attend to the pain stimulus; the somatosensory system is responsible for localization and characterization of pain; and the limbic system is responsible for the emotional and behavioral responses to pain. Cortical structures also are crucial to constructing the meaning of the pain.

Therefore behavioral strategies such as distraction and relaxation are effective pain-reducing therapies for many people. Meditation and imagery also affect pain perception. By directing attention away from the pain sensation, patients can reduce the sensory and affective components of pain.

**Modulation.** Modulation involves the activation of descending pathways that exert inhibitory or facilitatory effects on the transmission of pain (Fig. 8-1). Depending on the type and degree of modulation, nociceptive stimuli may or may not be perceived as pain. Modulation of pain signals can occur at the level of the periphery, spinal cord, brainstem, and cerebral cortex. Descending modulatory fibers release chemicals such as serotonin, norepinephrine, GABA, and endogenous opioids that can inhibit pain transmission.

Several antidepressants exert their effects through the modulatory systems. For example, tricyclic antidepressants (e.g., amitriptyline [Elavil]) and serotonin norepinephrine reuptake inhibitors (SNRIs) (e.g., venlafaxine [Effexor]) are used in the management of chronic noncancer and cancer pain. These agents interfere with the reuptake of serotonin and norepinephrine, thereby increasing their availability to inhibit noxious stimuli.

## CLASSIFICATION OF PAIN

Pain can be categorized in several ways. Most commonly, pain is categorized as nociceptive or neuropathic based on underlying pathology (Table 8-3). Another useful scheme is to classify pain as acute or chronic (Table 8-4).

### Nociceptive Pain

Nociceptive pain is caused by damage to somatic or visceral tissue. *Somatic pain* often is further categorized as superficial or deep. *Superficial pain* arises from skin, mucous membranes, and subcutaneous tissues. It is often described as sharp, burning, or prickly. *Deep pain* is often characterized as aching or throbbing and originates in bone, joint, muscle, or connective tissue.

*Visceral pain* comes from the activation of nociceptors in the internal organs and lining of the body cavities such as the thoracic and abdominal cavities. Visceral nociceptors respond to inflammation, stretching, and ischemia. Stretching of hollow viscera in the intestines and bladder that occurs from tumor involvement or obstruction can produce intense cramping pain. Examples of visceral nociceptive pain include pain from a surgical incision, pancreatitis, and inflammatory bowel disease.

### Neuropathic Pain

Neuropathic pain is caused by damage to peripheral nerves or structures in the CNS. While neuropathic pain is commonly associated with diabetic neuropathy and other neuropathic pain syndromes, approximately 8% of the general population has pain with neuropathic characteristics.[10] Typically described as numbing, hot, burning, shooting, stabbing, sharp, or electric shock–like, neuropathic pain can be sudden, intense, short lived, or lingering. Paroxysmal firing of injured nerves is

**TABLE 8-3 Comparison of Nociceptive and Neuropathic Pain**

| | Nociceptive Pain | Neuropathic Pain* |
|---|---|---|
| **Definition** | Normal processing of stimulus that damages normal tissue or has the potential to do so if prolonged | Abnormal processing of sensory input by the peripheral or central nervous system |
| **Treatment** | Usually responsive to nonopioid and/or opioid drugs | Treatment usually includes adjuvant analgesics. |
| **Types** | **Superficial Somatic Pain**<br>Pain arising from skin, mucous membranes, subcutaneous tissue. Tends to be well localized<br>*Examples:* sunburn, skin contusions<br>**Deep Somatic Pain**<br>Pain arising from muscles, fasciae, bones, tendons. Localized or diffuse and radiating<br>*Examples:* arthritis, tendonitis, myofascial pain<br>**Visceral Pain**<br>Pain arising from visceral organs, such as the GI tract and bladder. Well or poorly localized. Often referred to cutaneous sites<br>*Examples:* appendicitis, pancreatitis, cancer affecting internal organs, irritable bowel and bladder syndromes | **Central Pain**<br>Caused by primary lesion or dysfunction in the CNS<br>*Examples:* poststroke pain, pain associated with multiple sclerosis<br>**Peripheral Neuropathies**<br>Pain felt along the distribution of one or many peripheral nerves caused by damage to the nerve<br>*Examples:* diabetic neuropathy, alcohol-nutritional neuropathy, trigeminal neuralgia, postherpetic neuralgia<br>**Deafferentation Pain**<br>Pain resulting from a loss of or altered afferent input<br>*Examples:* phantom limb pain, postmastectomy pain, spinal cord injury pain<br>**Sympathetically Maintained Pain**<br>Pain that persists secondary to sympathetic nervous system activity<br>*Examples:* phantom limb pain, complex regional pain syndrome |

Adapted from National Institute of Neurological Disorders and Stroke: Complex regional pain syndrome fact sheet. Retrieved from *www.ninds.nih.gov/disorders/reflex_sympathetic_dystrophy/detail_reflex_sympathetic_dystrophy.htm.*

*CNS,* Central nervous system; *GI,* gastrointestinal.

*Note: Some types of neuropathic pain (e.g., postherpetic neuralgia) are caused by more than one neuropathologic mechanism.

**TABLE 8-4 Differences Between Acute and Chronic Pain**

| | Acute Pain | Chronic Pain |
|---|---|---|
| **Onset** | Sudden | Gradual or sudden |
| **Duration** | <3 mo or as long as it takes for normal healing to occur | >3 mo. May start as acute injury or event but continues past the normal time for recovery |
| **Severity** | Mild to severe | Mild to severe |
| **Cause of pain** | Generally can identify a precipitating event (e.g., illness, surgery) | May not be known. Original cause of pain may differ from mechanisms that maintain the pain. |
| **Course of pain** | Decreases over time and goes away as recovery occurs | Typically pain does not go away. Characterized by periods of increasing and decreasing pain |
| **Typical physical and behavioral manifestations** | Manifestations vary but can reflect sympathetic nervous system activation: • ↑ Heart rate, respiratory rate, BP • Diaphoresis, pallor • Anxiety, agitation, confusion • Urine retention | Predominantly behavioral manifestations: • Flat affect • ↓ Physical activity • Fatigue • Withdrawal from social interaction |
| **Usual goals of treatment** | Pain control with ability to participate in recovery activities. Minimize side effects of treatment | Pain control to the extent possible. Focus on enhancing function and quality of life. |

responsible for shooting and electric shock–like sensations. Common causes of neuropathic pain include trauma, inflammation, metabolic diseases (e.g., diabetes mellitus), alcoholism, infections of the nervous system (e.g., herpes zoster, human immunodeficiency virus), tumors, toxins, and neurologic diseases (e.g., multiple sclerosis). Examples of neuropathic pain conditions include phantom limb sensation, diabetic neuropathy, and trigeminal neuralgia. No single sign or symptom is diagnostic for neuropathic pain.

*Deafferentation pain* results from loss of or altered afferent input secondary to either peripheral nerve injury (e.g., amputation) or CNS damage, including a spinal cord injury. *Sympathetically maintained pain* is associated with dysregulation of the autonomic nervous system, and *central pain* is caused by CNS lesions or dysfunction. Painful peripheral polyneuropathies (pain felt along the distribution of multiple peripheral nerves) and painful mononeuropathies (pain felt along the distribution of a damaged nerve) arise from damage to peripheral nerves and generate pain that may be described as burning, paroxysmal, or shock-like. The patient may have associated positive or negative motor and sensory signs, including numbness, allodynia, or change in reflexes and motor strength.

One particularly debilitating type of neuropathic pain is **complex regional pain syndrome (CRPS)**. Typical features include dramatic changes in the color and temperature of the skin over the affected limb or body part, accompanied by intense burning pain, skin sensitivity, sweating, and swelling. CRPS type I is frequently triggered by tissue injury, surgery, or a vascular event such as stroke.[11] CRPS type II includes all these features in addition to a peripheral nerve lesion.

Neuropathic pain often is not well controlled by opioid analgesics alone. Treatment frequently necessitates a multimodal approach combining various adjuvant analgesics from different drug classes, including tricyclic antidepressants (e.g., amitriptyline [Elavil]), SNRIs (e.g., bupropion [Wellbutrin, Zyban]), antiseizure drugs (e.g., pregabalin [Lyrica]), transdermal lidocaine, and $\alpha_2$-adrenergic agonists (e.g., clonidine [Catapres]). NMDA receptor antagonists such as ketamine have shown promise in alleviating neuropathic pain refractory to other drugs.

### Acute and Chronic Pain

Acute pain and chronic pain differ in their cause, course, manifestations, and treatment (Table 8-4). Examples of *acute pain* include postoperative pain, labor pain, pain from trauma (e.g., lacerations, fractures, sprains), pain from infection (e.g., dysuria from cystitis), and pain from acute ischemia. For acute pain, treatment includes analgesics for symptom control and treatment of the underlying cause (e.g., splinting for a fracture, antibiotic therapy for an infection). Normally, acute pain diminishes over time as healing occurs. However, acute pain that persists can ultimately lead to disabling chronic pain states. For example, pain associated with herpes zoster subsides as the acute infection resolves, usually within a month. However, sometimes the pain persists and develops into a chronic pain state called *postherpetic neuralgia.* Because of the connection between inadequately treated acute pain and chronic pain, it is important to treat acute pain aggressively.

*Chronic pain,* or *persistent pain,* lasts for longer periods, often defined as longer than 3 months or past the time when an expected acute pain or acute injury should subside. The severity and functional impact of chronic pain often are disproportionate to objective findings because of changes in the nervous system not detectable with standard tests. Whereas acute pain functions as a signal, warning the person of potential or actual tissue damage, chronic pain does not appear to have an adaptive role. Chronic pain can be disabling and often is accompanied by anxiety and depression.

## PAIN ASSESSMENT

Assessment is an essential, although often overlooked, step in pain management. Regularly screen all patients for pain and, when present, perform a more thorough pain assessment. The key to accurate and effective pain assessment is to consider the principles of pain assessment (Table 8-5).

The goals of a nursing pain assessment are to (1) describe the patient's pain experience to identify and implement appropriate pain management techniques and (2) identify the patient's goal for therapy and resources for self-management.

### Elements of a Pain Assessment

Most components of a pain assessment involve direct interview or observation of the patient. Diagnostic studies and physical examination findings complete the initial assessment. Although the assessment differs according to the clinical setting, patient

**TABLE 8-5 Principles of Pain Assessment**

| Principles | Nursing Implications |
|---|---|
| **1.** Patients have the right to appropriate assessment and management of pain. | • Assess pain in *all* patients. |
| **2.** Pain is always subjective. | • Patient's self-report of pain is the single most reliable indicator of pain.<br>• Accept and respect this self-report unless there are clear reasons for doubt. |
| **3.** Physiologic and behavioral signs of pain (e.g., tachycardia, grimacing) are not reliable or specific for pain. | • Do not rely primarily on observations and objective signs of pain unless the patient is unable to self-report pain. |
| **4.** Pain is an unpleasant sensory and emotional experience. | • Address physical and psychologic aspects of pain when assessing pain. |
| **5.** Assessment approaches, including tools, must be appropriate for the patient population. | • Special considerations are needed for assessing pain in patients with difficulty communicating.<br>• Include family members in the assessment process (when appropriate). |
| **6.** Pain can exist even when no physical cause can be found. | • Do not attribute pain that does not have an identifiable cause to psychologic causes. |
| **7.** Different patients experience different levels of pain in response to comparable stimuli. | • A uniform pain threshold does not exist. |
| **8.** Patients with chronic pain may be more sensitive to pain and other stimuli. | • Pain tolerance varies among and within individuals depending on various factors (e.g., genetics, energy level, coping skills, prior experience with pain). |
| **9.** Unrelieved pain has adverse consequences. Acute pain that is not adequately controlled can result in physiologic changes that increase the likelihood of developing persistent pain. | • Encourage patients to report pain, especially patients who are reluctant to discuss pain, deny pain when it is probably present, or fail to follow through on prescribed treatments. |

population, and point of care (i.e., whether the assessment is part of an initial workup or a reassessment of pain following therapy), the evaluation of pain should always be multidimensional (Table 8-6).

Before beginning any assessment, recognize that patients may use words other than "pain." For example, older adults may deny that they have pain but respond positively when asked if they have soreness or aching. Document the specific words that the patient uses to describe pain. Then consistently ask the patient about pain using those words.

**Pain Pattern.** Assessing pain *onset* involves determining when the pain started. Patients with acute pain resulting from injury, acute illness, or treatment (e.g., surgery) typically know exactly when their pain began. Those with chronic pain may be less able to identify when the pain started. Establish the *duration* of the pain (how long it has lasted). This information helps to determine whether the pain is acute or chronic and assists in identifying the cause of the pain. For example, a patient with advanced cancer who also has chronic low back pain from spinal stenosis reports a sudden, severe pain in the back that began 2 days ago. Knowing the onset and duration can lead to a diagnostic workup that may reveal new metastatic disease in the spine.

Pain pattern also provides clues about the cause of the pain and directs its treatment. Many types of chronic pain (e.g., arthritis pain) can increase and decrease over time. A patient may have pain all the time (around-the-clock pain), as well as discrete periods of intermittent pain.

**Breakthrough pain (BTP)** is transient, moderate to severe pain that occurs in patients whose baseline persistent pain is otherwise mild to moderate and fairly well controlled. The average peak of BTP can be 3 to 5 minutes and can last up to 30 minutes or even longer. BTP can be either predictable or unpredictable, and patients can have one to many episodes per day. Several transmucosal fentanyl products are used specifically to treat BTP.

**TABLE 8-6 Nursing Assessment**

***Pain***

**Subjective Data**

***Important Health Information***

*Health history:* Pain history includes onset, location, intensity, quality, patterns, aggravating and alleviating factors, and expression of pain. Coping strategies. Past treatments and their effectiveness. Review of health care utilization related to the pain problem (e.g., emergency department visits, treatment at pain clinics, visits to primary HCPs and specialists)

*Medications:* Use of any prescription or over-the-counter, illicit, or herbal products for pain relief. Alcohol use

*Nondrug measures:* Use of therapies such as, but not limited to, massage, heat or ice, Reiki, aromatherapy, acupuncture, hypnosis, yoga, or meditation

***Functional Health Patterns***

*Health perception–health management:* Social and work history, mental health history, smoking history. Effects of pain on emotions, relationships, sleep, and activities. Interviews with family members. Records from psychologic/psychiatric treatment related to the pain

*Elimination:* Constipation related to opioid drug use, other medication use, or pain related to elimination

*Activity-exercise:* Fatigue, limitations in ability to perform ADLs (activities of daily living), IADLs (instrumental activities of daily living), and pain related to use of muscles

*Sexuality-reproductive:* Decreased libido

*Coping–stress tolerance:* Psychologic evaluation using standardized measures to examine coping style, depression, anxiety

**Objective Data**

*Physical examination,* including evaluation of functional limitations

*Psychosocial evaluation,* including mood

*End-of-dose failure* is pain that occurs before the expected duration of a specific analgesic. It should not be confused with BTP. Pain that occurs at the end of the duration of an analgesic often leads to a prolonged increase in the baseline persistent pain. For example, in a patient on transdermal fentanyl (Duragesic patches) the typical duration of action is 72 hours. An increase in pain after 48 hours on the drug would be characterized as end-of-dose failure. End-of-dose failure signals the need for changes in the dose or scheduling of the analgesic. Episodic, procedural, or *incident pain* is a transient increase in pain that is caused by a specific activity or event that precipitates pain. Examples include dressing changes, movement, position changes, and procedures such as catheterization.

**Location.** Determining the *location* of pain assists in identifying possible causes and treatment. Some patients may be able to specify the precise location(s) of their pain, whereas others may describe general areas or comment that they "hurt all over." The location of the pain may also be referred from its origin to another site (Fig. 8-3). For example, myocardial infarction can result in pain in the left shoulder. Pain may also radiate from its origin to another site. For example, angina pectoris can radiate from the chest to the jaw or down the left arm. This is referred to as radiating pain. *Sciatica* is pain that follows the course of the sciatic nerve. It may originate from joints or muscles around the back or from compression or damage to the sciatic nerve. The pain is projected along the course of the peripheral nerve, causing painful shooting sensations down the back of the thigh and inside of the leg to the foot.

Obtain information about the location of pain by asking the patient to (1) describe the site(s) of pain, (2) point to painful areas on the body, or (3) mark painful areas on a pain map. Because many patients have more than one site of pain, make certain that the patient describes every location.

**Intensity.** Assessing the severity, or *intensity,* of pain provides a reliable measure to determine the type of treatment and its effectiveness. Pain scales help the patient communicate pain intensity. Base your choice of a scale on the patient's developmental needs and cognitive status. Most adults can rate the intensity of their pain using a numeric rating scale (e.g., 0 = no pain, 10 = the worst pain), which is commonly used. A verbal descriptor scale (e.g., none, mild, moderate, severe) may be preferred for patients who wish to have word choices to quantify pain. For those oriented to vertical representations, the Pain Thermometer Scale is an option[12] (Fig. 8-4). Other visual pain measures such as the Wong-Baker FACES pain tool (*http://wongbakerfaces.org*) are useful for patients with cognitive or language barriers to describe their pain.[13] Pain assessment measures for cognitively impaired adults and nonverbal adults are addressed later in this chapter.

Although intensity is an important factor in determining analgesic approaches, do not dose patients with opioids solely based on reported pain scores.[14] Opioid "dosing by numbers" without taking into account a patient's sedation level and respiratory status can lead to unsafe practices and serious adverse events. Safer analgesic administration can be achieved by balancing an amount of pain relief with analgesic side effects and using a multimodal approach. (Multimodal approach is described later in this chapter.) Adjustments in therapy can be made to promote better pain control and minimize adverse outcomes.

**Quality.** The pain *quality* refers to the nature or characteristics of the pain. For example, patients often describe neuropathic

**Name** ____________________ **Date** __________

**Pain thermometer use**

This tool is excellent for patients whose cognitive deficits are moderate to severe, or who have difficulty communicating verbally. Ask the patient to circle words next to the thermometer or to mark the area on the thermometer to indicate the intensity of current pain.

**Pain thermometer scoring**

Document the words circled or those corresponding to the area of the thermometer the patient marks to identify level of pain intensity. Evaluate the change in pain descriptors selected by the patient over time to determine the effectiveness of pain treatments. Alternately, the words can be scored from 0 to 5 for recording purposes.

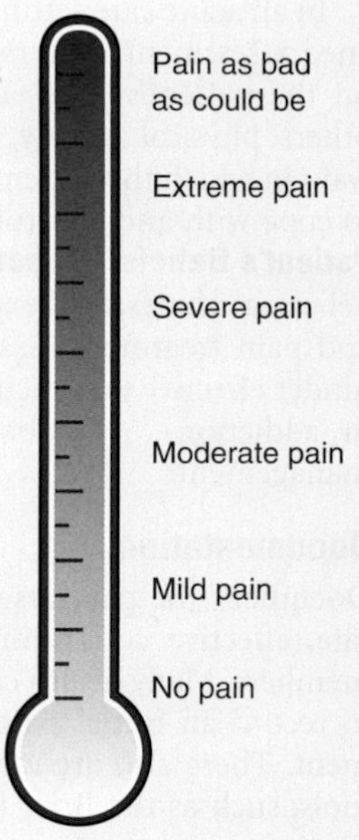


**FIG. 8-4** Pain thermometer scale. Ask the patient to circle words or point next to the thermometer or to mark or point to the area on the thermometer to indicate the intensity of pain. (Used with permission of Keela Herr, RN, PhD, AGSF, FAAN, University of Iowa.)

pain as burning, numbing, shooting, stabbing, electric shock–like, or itchy. Nociceptive pain may be described as sharp, aching, throbbing, dull, and cramping. Since the quality of pain relates to some degree to the classification of pain (e.g., neuropathic, nociceptive), these descriptors can help to guide treatment options that best address the specific mechanism of pain.

**Associated Symptoms.** *Associated symptoms* such as anxiety, fatigue, and depression may exacerbate or be exacerbated by pain. Patients with pain often report poor sleep and subsequent daytime sleepiness. Poor sleep can further increase pain perception. Ask about aggravating factors that increase pain as well as activities and situations that alleviate pain. For example, musculoskeletal pain may be increased or decreased with movement and ambulation. Resting or immobilizing a painful body part can decrease pain. Knowing what makes pain better or worse can help characterize the type of pain and be helpful in selecting treatments.

**Management Strategies.** As people experience and live with pain, they may cope differently and be more or less willing to try different strategies to manage it. Some strategies are successful, whereas others are not. To maximize the effectiveness of the pain treatment plan, ask patients what they are using now to control pain, what they have used in the past, and the outcomes of these methods. Strategies include prescription and nonprescription drugs and nondrug therapies, such as hot and cold applications, complementary and alternative therapies (e.g., acupuncture), and relaxation strategies (e.g., imagery). It is important to document both those that work and those that are ineffective.

**Impact of Pain.** Pain can have a profound influence on a patient's quality of life and functioning. Assess the effect of the pain on the patient's ability to sleep, enjoy life, interact with others, perform work and household duties, and engage in physical and social activities. Also assess the impact of pain on the patient's mood.

In an acute care setting, time limitations may dictate a shortened assessment. At a minimum, assess the effects of the pain on the patient's sleep and daily activities, relationships with others, physical activity, and emotional well-being. Include the ways in which the patient describes the pain and strategies used to cope with and control the pain.

**Patient's Beliefs, Expectations, and Goals.** Patient and family beliefs, attitudes, and expectations influence responses to pain and pain treatment. Assess for attitudes and beliefs that may hinder effective treatment (e.g., belief that opioid use will result in addiction). Ask about expectations and goals for pain management.

### Documentation

Document the pain assessment, since this is critical to ensure safe, effective communication among interprofessional team members. Many health care facilities have adopted specific tools to record an initial pain assessment, treatment, and reassessment. There also are many multidimensional pain assessment tools, such as the Brief Pain Inventory, the McGill Pain Questionnaire, and the Neuropathic Pain Scale.

### Reassessment

It is critical for you to reassess pain at appropriate intervals. The frequency and scope of reassessment are guided by factors such as pain severity, physical and psychosocial condition, type of intervention and risks of adverse effects, and institutional policy. For example, reassessment of a postoperative patient may be done frequently, such as at the time of peak effect for each analgesic dose. In a long-term care facility, residents with chronic pain are reassessed at least quarterly or with a change in condition or functional status.

## PAIN TREATMENT

### Basic Principles

All pain treatment plans are based on the following 10 principles and practice standards:

1. *Follow the principles of pain assessment* (Table 8-5). Remember that pain is a subjective experience. The patient is not only the best judge of his or her own pain but also the expert on the effectiveness of each pain treatment.
2. *Use a holistic approach to pain management.* The experience of pain affects all aspects of a person's life. Thus a holistic approach to assessment, treatment, and evaluation is required.
3. *Every patient deserves adequate pain management.* Many patient populations, including ethnic minorities, cognitively impaired adults, and people with past or current substance abuse, are at risk for inadequate pain management. Be aware of your own biases and ensure that all patients are treated respectfully.
4. *Base the treatment plan on the patient's goals.* Discuss with the patient realistic goals for pain relief during the initial pain assessment. Although goals can be described in terms of pain intensity (e.g., the desire for average pain to decrease from "8/10" to "3/10"), with chronic pain conditions functional goal setting should be encouraged (e.g., a goal of performing certain daily activities, such as socializing and recreational activities). Encourage functional activities for the patient with acute pain as well. For example, the pain must be at a level that allows the patient to use the incentive spirometer, get out of bed, and ambulate. Over time, reassess these goals and progress made toward meeting them. The patient, in collaboration with the interprofessional team, determines new goals. If the patient has unrealistic goals for therapy, such as wanting to be completely rid of all chronic arthritis pain or be completely pain free after a major surgery, work with the patient to establish a more realistic goal.
5. *Use both drug and nondrug therapies.* Although drugs are often considered the mainstay of therapy, incorporate self-care activities and nondrug therapies to increase the overall effectiveness of therapy and to allow for the reduction of drug dosages to minimize adverse drug effects.
6. *When appropriate, use a multimodal approach to analgesic therapy.* **Multimodal analgesia** employs the use of two or more classes of analgesic agents to take advantage of the various mechanisms of action. For acute, postoperative pain, a multimodal approach may include the use of an opioid (morphine), nonopioid (nonsteroidal antiinflammatory drug), and/or an antiseizure drug (e.g., gabapentin). Regional anesthesia and continuous peripheral neural blockade can be used with local anesthetics as part of multimodal regimens.[15] Factors such as age, type of surgery, risk for developing chronic pain, and co-existing conditions are all taken into account when designing a multimodal analgesic regimen. Multimodal analgesia is also used to treat chronic or persistent pain. Similar to the strategies for acute postoperative pain, the goal is to combine classes of analgesics for the maximum benefit of relieving pain with minimum doses to achieve relief and reduce adverse events from analgesics. Multimodal regimens achieve superior pain relief, enhance patient satisfaction, and decrease adverse effects of individual drugs.[16]
7. *Address pain using an interprofessional approach.* The expertise and perspectives of an interprofessional team are often necessary to provide effective assessment and therapies for patients with both acute and chronic pain. For hospitalized patients or those with complex acute or chronic pain issues, anesthesiology-based pain services may be available to manage patients with technology-supported pain care (e.g., patient-controlled analgesia or regional analgesia). Team members for these services can include pain management nurses, nurse practitioners, clinical nurse specialists, anesthesiologists, and clinical pharmacists. These teams also help to establish realistic goals with patients and families to facilitate recovery and discharge. Many outpatient pain management centers or clinics are available. Some provide comprehensive pain care and employ multiple providers including anesthesiologists, rehabilitation physicians, nurses, psychologists, physical and occupational therapists, and social workers. Services may focus on medication management, pain interventional therapies, psychologic counseling, cognitive and behavioral therapies, rehabilitative therapies (physical and occupational therapy), and social services. Specialized pain treatment centers may also offer more holistic therapies such as massage, music and art therapy, and acupuncture. Advise patients seeking specialized pain care from outpatient treatment centers to check about services that are provided.

**TABLE 8-7 Drug Therapy**
***Managing Side Effects of Pain Medications***

*Side effects can be managed in one or more of the following methods.*
- Decreasing the dose of analgesic by 10% to 15%
- Changing to a different medication in the same class
- Adding a drug to counteract the adverse effect of the analgesic (e.g., using a stool softener for patients experiencing opioid-induced constipation)
- Using an administration route that minimizes drug concentrations (e.g., intraspinal administration of opioids used to minimize high drug levels that produce sedation, nausea, and vomiting)

8. *Evaluate the effectiveness of all therapies to ensure that they are meeting the patient's goals.* Achievement of an effective treatment plan often requires trial and error. Adjustments in drug, dosage, or route are common to achieve maximal benefit while minimizing adverse effects. This trial-and-error process can become frustrating for the patient and caregivers. Reassure them that pain relief, if not pain cessation, is possible and that the interprofessional team will continue to work with them to achieve adequate pain relief.
9. *Prevent and/or manage medication side effects.* Side effects or adverse events are a major reason for treatment failure and nonadherence. Side effects are managed in one of several ways, as described in Table 8-7. You play a key role in monitoring for and treating side effects and in teaching patients and caregivers how to minimize these effects.
10. *Incorporate patient and caregiver teaching throughout assessment and treatment.* Content should include information about the causes of the pain, pain assessment methods, treatment goals and options, expectations of pain management, proper use of drugs, side effect management, and nondrug and self-help pain relief measures. Document the teaching and include evaluation of patient and caregiver comprehension.

## Drug Therapy for Pain

Pain medications generally are divided into three categories: nonopioids, opioids, and adjuvant drugs. Patient-centered treatment regimens may include medications from one or more of these groups. Mild pain often can be relieved using nonopioids alone. Moderate to severe pain usually requires an opioid. Certain types of pain, such as neuropathic pain, typically require adjuvant drug therapy alone or in combination with an opioid or another class of analgesics. Pain caused by cancer may be treated with chemotherapy or radiation therapy as well as pain medications.

**Nonopioids.** Nonopioid analgesics include acetaminophen, aspirin and other salicylates, and NSAIDs (Table 8-8). These agents are characterized by the following: (1) their analgesic properties have an **analgesic ceiling**; that is, increasing the dose beyond an upper limit provides no greater analgesia; (2) they do not produce tolerance or physical dependence; and (3) many are available without a prescription. To provide safe care, monitor over-the-counter (OTC) analgesic use to avoid serious problems related to drug interactions, side effects, and overdose.

Nonopioids are effective for mild to moderate pain. They are often used in conjunction with opioids because they allow for effective pain relief using lower opioid doses (thereby causing fewer opioid side effects). This phenomenon is called the *opioid-sparing effect.*

**TABLE 8-8 Drug Therapy**
***Selected Nonopioid Analgesics***

| Drug | Nursing Considerations |
|---|---|
| **Nonsalicylate** | |
| acetaminophen (Tylenol) | • Chronic overdose: liver toxicity<br>• Rectal suppository and injectable form (OFIRMEV) available. Sustained-release preparations available. Maximum daily dose of 3 g<br>• Oral doses of >3 g may cause hepatotoxicity.<br>• Acute overdose: acute liver failure<br>• Chronic overdose: liver toxicity<br>• Maximum daily IV dose should not exceed 4 g/day for adults ≥50 kg. |
| **Salicylates** | |
| aspirin | • Rectal suppository and sustained-release preparations available.<br>• Possibility of upper GI bleeding<br>• Used more commonly in low doses as a cardioprotective measure than for its analgesic properties |
| choline magnesium trisalicylate (Trilisate) | • Unlike aspirin and NSAIDs, does not increase bleeding time |
| **Nonsteroidal Antiinflammatory Drugs (NSAIDs)** | |
| ibuprofen (Advil) | • Use lowest effective dose for shortest possible duration.<br>• Increased risk of serious GI adverse events (bleeding, ulceration, perforation), especially in older adults<br>• May increase risk of serious cardiovascular thrombotic events, myocardial infarction, and stroke<br>• May increase risk of hypertension and renal insufficiency |
| naproxen (Naprosyn, Aleve) | • Use lowest effective dose for shortest possible duration.<br>• Increased risk of serious GI adverse events (bleeding, ulceration, perforation), especially in older adults<br>• Contraindicated for the treatment of perioperative pain in setting of coronary artery bypass graft (CABG) surgery |
| ketorolac | • Limit treatment to 5 days.<br>• May precipitate renal failure in dehydrated patients |
| diclofenac K (Cataflam) | • Use lowest effective dose for shortest possible duration.<br>• Available in oral, ophthalmic, topical preparations |
| celecoxib (Celebrex) | • Causes fewer GI side effects (e.g., bleeding) than other NSAIDs but risk still present. Is more costly than other NSAIDs<br>• May increase risk of serious cardiovascular thrombotic events, myocardial infarction, and stroke<br>• Risks may increase with duration of use, preexisting cardiovascular disease, or risk factors for cardiovascular disease. |

Aspirin is effective for mild pain, but its use is limited by its common side effects, including increased risk for bleeding, especially gastrointestinal (GI) bleeding. Other salicylates such as choline magnesium trisalicylate (Trilisate) cause fewer GI disturbances and bleeding abnormalities. Similar to aspirin, acetaminophen (Tylenol) has analgesic and antipyretic effects, but

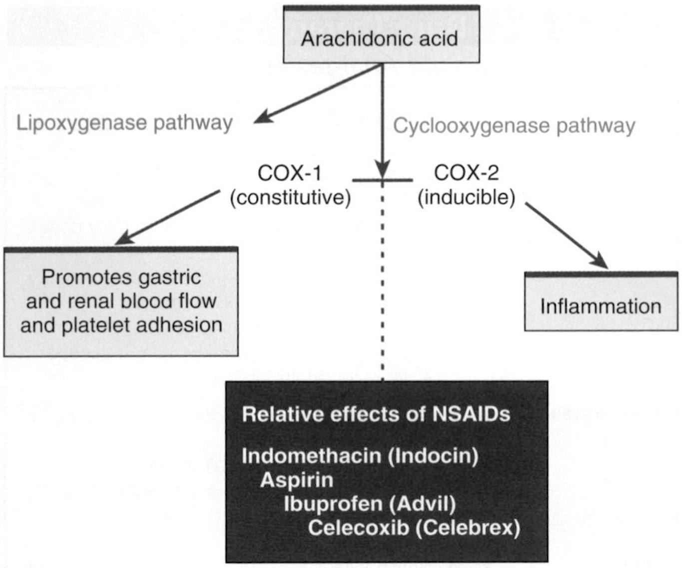


**FIG. 8-5** Arachidonic acid is oxidized by two different pathways: lipoxygenase and cyclooxygenase. The cyclooxygenase pathway leads to two forms of the enzyme cyclooxygenase: COX-1 and COX-2. COX-1 is known as *constitutive* (always present), and COX-2 is known as *inducible* (its expression varies markedly depending on the stimulus). Nonsteroidal antiinflammatory drugs (NSAIDs) differ in their actions, with some having more effects on COX-1 and others more on COX-2. Indomethacin acts primarily on COX-1, whereas ibuprofen is equipotent on COX-1 and COX-2. Celecoxib primarily inhibits COX-2.

unlike aspirin, it has no antiplatelet or antiinflammatory effects. Although acetaminophen is well tolerated, it is metabolized by the liver. Hepatotoxicity may result from chronic dosing of more than 3 g/day, acute overdose, or use by patients with severe preexisting liver disease.[17] The addition of acetaminophen to opioid therapy produces an opioid-sparing effect, lower pain scores, and fewer side effects, which is the reason for opioid-acetaminophen combinations such as Percocet. Acetaminophen is available for administration by parenteral route (OFIRMEV) administered over 15 minutes. IV acetaminophen is used for the treatment of acute mild to moderate pain and moderate to severe pain as an adjunct to opioid analgesics or part of a multimodal analgesic regimen. It has a short duration of action. The daily dose should not exceed 4 g/day.

NSAIDs represent a broad class of drugs with varying efficacy and side effects. All NSAIDs inhibit cyclooxygenase (COX), the enzyme that converts arachidonic acid into prostaglandins and related compounds. The enzyme has two forms: COX-1 and COX-2. COX-1 is found in almost all tissues and is responsible for several protective physiologic functions. In contrast, COX-2 is produced mainly at the sites of tissue injury, where it mediates inflammation (Fig. 8-5). Inhibition of COX-1 causes many of the untoward effects of NSAIDs, such as impairment of renal function, bleeding tendencies, GI irritation, and ulceration. Inhibition of COX-2 is associated with the therapeutic, antiinflammatory effects of NSAIDs. (Celecoxib [Celebrex] is a COX-2 inhibitor.) Older NSAIDs, such as ibuprofen, inhibit both forms of COX and are referred to as nonselective NSAIDs.

Patients vary greatly in their responses to a specific NSAID, so when one NSAID does not provide relief, another should be tried. NSAIDs are associated with many side effects, including GI problems ranging from dyspepsia to life-threatening ulceration and hemorrhage. NSAIDs can also cause cognitive impairment and hypersensitivity reactions with asthma-like symptoms.

Individuals at risk for NSAID-associated GI toxicity include those who have a recent history of peptic ulcer disease, patients who are older than 65, and those concurrently using corticosteroids or anticoagulants. If NSAIDs are used in patients at risk for GI bleeding, they should have concomitant therapy with misoprostol (Cytotec) or a proton pump inhibitor such as omeprazole (Prilosec). NSAIDs should not be administered concurrently with aspirin, since this increases the risk for GI bleeding.

**DRUG ALERT Nonsteroidal Antiinflammatory Drugs (NSAIDs)**
- NSAIDs (except aspirin) have been linked to a higher risk for cardiovascular events such as myocardial infarction, stroke, and heart failure.
- Patients who have just had heart surgery should not take NSAIDs.

**Opioids.** Opioids (Table 8-9) produce their effects by binding to receptors in the CNS. This results in (1) inhibition of the transmission of nociceptive input from the periphery to the spinal cord, (2) altered limbic system activity, and (3) activation of the descending inhibitory pathways that modulate transmission in the spinal cord. Thus opioids act on several nociceptive processes.

***Types of Opioids.*** Opioids are categorized according to their physiologic action (i.e., agonist, antagonist) and binding at specific opioid receptors (e.g., mu, kappa, delta). The most commonly administered subclass of opioids is the pure opioid agonists, or morphine-like opioids, which bind to mu receptors.

Opioid agonists are used for acute and chronic pain. Although nociceptive pain appears to be more responsive to opioids than neuropathic pain, opioids may be used to treat both types of pain. In the treatment of neuropathic pain, antineuropathic pain drugs such as antidepressants and antiseizure drugs are recommended as first-line agents. Pure opioid agonists include morphine, oxycodone (OxyContin), hydrocodone, codeine, methadone, hydromorphone (Dilaudid), oxymorphone (Opana), and levorphanol (Levo-Dromoran) (Table 8-9). These drugs are effective for moderate to severe pain because they are potent, theoretically have no analgesic ceiling, and can be administered via several routes. When opioids are prescribed for moderate pain, they are usually combined with a nonopioid analgesic such as acetaminophen (e.g., codeine plus acetaminophen [Tylenol #3], or hydrocodone plus acetaminophen or ibuprofen [Vicoprofen]). Addition of acetaminophen or NSAIDs limits the total daily dose that can be given.

**DRUG ALERT Morphine**
- Morphine may cause respiratory depression.
- If respirations are 12 or less breaths per minute, withhold medication and contact the HCP.

Methadone is a unique mu opioid receptor agonist, which is used primarily in the treatment of chronic pain but can be used for acute pain. It has a unique mechanism of action as an NMDA receptor antagonist, which is believed to produce analgesic effects independent of its action as an opioid.[18]

**DRUG ALERT Methadone (Dolophine)**
- Methadone may cause respiratory depression.
- Methadone can cause cardiac toxicity, specifically QT prolongation.

## TABLE 8-9 Drug Therapy

### *Opioid Analgesics*

| Drug | Routes of Administration | Nursing Considerations |
|---|---|---|
| **Mu Agonists** | | |
| morphine (MS Contin, Avinza, Kadian, Epimorph, Oramorph SR) | PO (short-acting and sustained-release forms), rectal, IV, subcutaneous, epidural, intrathecal, sublingual, intranasal | • Standard of comparison for opioid analgesics (Table 8-12 [later in chapter])<br>• Indicated for moderate to severe pain<br>• Can stimulate histamine release, leading to pruritus, with systemic administration<br>• Tablets for sustained-release preparations are to be swallowed whole, and must not be broken, chewed, dissolved, or crushed.<br>• Preparations for neuraxial* administration must be preservative free. |
| hydromorphone (Dilaudid) | PO (short-acting and long-acting forms), rectal, IV, subcutaneous, epidural, intrathecal | • Slightly shorter duration than morphine<br>• Indicated for moderate to severe pain<br>• Tablets for sustained-release preparations are to be swallowed whole, and must not be broken, chewed, dissolved, or crushed.<br>• Preparations for neuraxial* administration must be preservative free. |
| methadone (Dolophine) | PO, IV, IM | • High oral and rectal bioavailability<br>• Accumulates with repeated dosing<br>• Use with caution in older adults.<br>• Risk of QT interval prolongation |
| levorphanol (Levo-Dromoran) | PO, IV, IM, subcutaneous | • Accumulates with repeated dosing |
| fentanyl (Sublimaze [IV], Duragesic [transdermal], Actiq [transmucosal]), buccal tablet (Fentora), sublingual (Abstral), buccal soluble film (Onsolis), nasal spray (Lazanda) | IV, epidural, intrathecal, transmucosal, transdermal | • Immediate onset after IV route, 7-8 min after IM route, 5-15 min after transmucosal route, up to 6 hr after transdermal route<br>• For procedures, IV fentanyl often combined with benzodiazepines for analgesia and sedation<br>• Very potent; dosage is in micrograms (mcg).<br>• Transdermal fentanyl indicated only for chronic pain and should not be administered to opioid-naive patients. |
| oxymorphone (Opana, Opana ER, Numorphan) | IV, PO (short-acting and extended-release forms) | • Tablets for extended-release forms are to be swallowed whole and must not be broken, chewed, dissolved, or crushed.<br>• Use with caution in older and debilitated patients and patients with hepatic and renal impairment. |
| oxycodone (Roxicodone)<br>oxycodone extended-release (OxyContin)<br>oxycodone plus acetaminophen (Percocet)<br>oxycodone plus aspirin (Percodan)<br>oxycodone plus ibuprofen (Combunox)<br>oxycodone extended-release plus acetaminophen (Xartemis) | PO (short-acting and extended-release forms) | • Available as single entity and in combination with a nonopioid<br>• Can be used similarly to oral morphine for moderate to severe pain<br>• Often combined with a nonopioid for acute, moderate pain<br>• Extended-release indicated for chronic pain |
| oxycodone and naloxone extended release (Targiniq ER) | PO (extended release) | • Used for severe pain needing treatment around the clock<br>• Naloxone in drug blocks euphoric effects of oxycodone when crushed and snorted or crushed, dissolved, and injected.<br>• Makes it less liked by abusers than oxycodone alone |
| hydrocodone<br>(with acetaminophen [Norco])<br>(with bitartrate [Hysingla, Zohydro]) | PO (short acting and long-acting) | • Used for moderate or moderately severe pain<br>• Generally indicated for short-term management of acute pain (e.g., trauma, musculoskeletal) |
| codeine oral (with acetaminophen [Tylenol #3]), codeine injectable | PO, subcutaneous | • Associated with higher incidence of nausea and constipation than other mu agonists<br>• Many codeine preparations are combined with acetaminophen.<br>• 5%-10% of European Americans lack the enzyme to metabolize codeine to morphine. |
| tramadol (Ultram) | PO (short-acting and extended release) | • Dual mechanism of action: mu opioid agonist and blocks reuptake of norepinephrine and serotonin<br>• Used for moderate pain |
| tapentadol (Nucynta) | PO (short-acting and extended release) | • Dual mechanism of action: mu opioid agonist and blocks reuptake of norepinephrine and serotonin |

*Neuraxial anesthesia pertains to local anesthetics placed around the nerves of the central nervous system such as spinal and epidural anesthesia.

*Continued*

**TABLE 8-9 Drug Therapy**
***Opioid Analgesics—cont'd***

| Drug | Routes of Administration | Nursing Considerations |
|---|---|---|
| **Mixed Agonist-Antagonists** | | |
| pentazocine (Talwin)<br>pentazocine plus naloxone (Talwin NX) | Formulated in combination with acetaminophen, aspirin, ibuprofen<br>Abuse-deterrent preparation includes naloxone to discourage parenteral abuse | • May cause psychotomimetic effects (e.g., hallucinations) and may precipitate withdrawal in opioid-dependent patients<br>• Not recommended for treatment of chronic pain and rarely for acute pain |
| butorphanol | Available in a nasal spray and injectable form<br>Not available orally | • Psychotomimetic effects lower than with pentazocine<br>• May precipitate withdrawal in opioid-dependent patients<br>• Injectable used for acute pain<br>• Nasal spray indicated for migraine headaches |
| **Partial Agonists** | | |
| buprenorphine<br><br>buprenorphine plus naloxone sublingual (Suboxone) | Sublingual, injectable, implant | • Sublingual form should not be chewed or swallowed<br>• Lower abuse potential than morphine. Does not produce psychotomimetic effects<br>• May precipitate withdrawal in opioid-dependent patients. Not readily reversed by naloxone<br>• Buprenorphine plus naloxone used as a sublingual preparation to treat opioid dependence for easier withdrawal when necessary to taper from opioids |

Mixed agonist-antagonists (e.g., pentazocine [Talwin], butorphanol) bind as agonists on kappa receptors and as weak antagonists or partial agonists on mu receptors. Because of this difference in binding, mixed agonist-antagonists produce less respiratory depression than drugs that act only at mu receptors. These drugs cause more dysphoria and agitation. In addition, opioid agonist-antagonists have an analgesic ceiling and can precipitate withdrawal if used by a patient who is physically dependent on mu agonist drugs. Partial opioid agonists (e.g., buprenorphine [Buprenex]) can produce some pain relief but bind tightly to mu receptors and can block the effect of other drugs. Agonist-antagonists and partial agonists currently have limited clinical application in pain management.

***Dual-Mechanism Agents.*** Some analgesics have two distinct actions, or dual mechanisms. Tramadol (Ultram) is a weak mu agonist and inhibits the reuptake of norepinephrine and serotonin. It is effective in low back pain, osteoarthritis, fibromyalgia, diabetic peripheral neuropathic pain, polyneuropathy, and postherpetic neuralgia. The most common side effects are similar to those of other opioids, including nausea, constipation, dizziness, and sedation. As with other medications that increase serotonin and norepinephrine, avoid this drug in patients with a history of seizures because it lowers seizure threshold.

Tapentadol (Nucynta) is a centrally acting analgesic that works at mu receptors and inhibits norepinephrine reuptake. It is approved for management of moderate to severe acute pain. For chronic moderate to severe pain, an extended-release formula is available. The side effects are similar to those of conventional opioids, except that this drug is associated with less nausea and constipation.

***Opioids to Avoid.*** Some opioids should be avoided for pain relief because of limited efficacy and/or toxicities. Meperidine (Demerol) or pethidine is associated with neurotoxicity (e.g., seizures) caused by accumulation of its metabolite, normeperidine. Its use is limited for very short-term (i.e., less than 48 hours) treatment of acute pain when other opioid agonists are contraindicated.

**DRUG ALERT Meperidine (Demerol)**
The American Pain Society does not recommend the use of meperidine as an analgesic.

***Side Effects of Opioids.*** Common side effects of opioids include constipation, nausea and vomiting, sedation, respiratory depression, and pruritus. With continued use, many side effects diminish; the exception is constipation. Less common side effects include urinary retention, myoclonus, dizziness, confusion, and hallucinations. *Constipation* is the most common side effect of opioids. Left untreated, constipation may increase the individual's pain and can lead to fecal impaction and paralytic ileus.

Because tolerance to opioid-induced constipation does not develop, a bowel regimen should be initiated at the beginning of opioid therapy and continued for as long as the person takes opioids. Although dietary fiber, fluids, and exercise should be encouraged, these measures alone may not be sufficient. Most patients should use a gentle stimulant laxative (e.g., senna) plus a stool softener (e.g., docusate sodium [Colace]). Other agents (e.g., milk of magnesia, bisacodyl [Dulcolax], polyethylene glycol [MiraLAX], or lactulose [Constulose]) can be added if necessary. Methylnaltrexone (Relistor) and naloxegol (Movantik) are peripheral opioid receptor antagonists used for opioid-induced constipation when the response to traditional laxative and stool softener therapy is insufficient.

*Nausea* is often a problem in opioid-naive patients. The use of an antiemetic such as ondansetron (Zofran), metoclopramide (Reglan), transdermal scopolamine (Transderm Scōp), hydroxyzine (Vistaril), or a phenothiazine (e.g., prochlorperazine) can prevent or minimize nausea and vomiting until tolerance develops, usually within 1 week. Opioids delay gastric emptying (patient complains of gastric fullness), and this effect can be reduced by metoclopramide. If nausea and vomiting are severe and persistent, changing to a different opioid may be necessary.

*Sedation* is usually seen in opioid-naive patients being treated for acute pain. Regularly monitor patients receiving opioid analgesics for acute pain, especially in the first few days (e.g., after surgery). Be aware that the risk for unintended sedation in postoperative patients is greatest within 4 hours after leaving the postanesthesia care unit. Opioid-induced sedation resolves with the development of tolerance. Persistent sedation with chronic opioid use can be effectively treated with psychostimulants such as caffeine, dextroamphetamine (Dexedrine), methylphenidate (Ritalin), or the anticataleptic drug modafinil (Provigil).

The risk of *respiratory depression* is also higher in opioid-naive, hospitalized patients who are treated for acute pain. Clinically significant respiratory depression is rare in opioid-tolerant patients and when opioids are titrated to analgesic effect. Patients most at risk for respiratory depression include those who are age 65 or older, have a history of snoring or witnessed apneic episodes, report excessive daytime sleepiness, have underlying cardiac or lung disease, are obese (body mass index greater than 30 kg/m$^2$), have a history of smoking (more than 20 pack-years), or are receiving other CNS depressants (e.g., sedatives, benzodiazepines, antihistamines). For postoperative patients the greatest risk for opioid-related respiratory adverse events is within the first 24 hours after surgery. Clinically significant respiratory depression cannot occur in patients who are fully awake.

**CHECK YOUR PRACTICE**

A 74-yr-old male patient returned to the clinical unit following surgery for a hip replacement. You are having difficulty arousing him with either verbal or physical stimulation. His wife tells you to just let him sleep. His respiratory rate ranges from 8-10 breaths/min.
- What should you do?

Frequently monitor both the sedation level and respiratory rate in patients receiving opioid analgesics.[19] A sedation scale can be used for monitoring and providing appropriate interventions based on the level of sedation (Table 8-10).

**SAFETY ALERT Sedation and Respiratory Depression**
- If the number of patient's respirations falls below 8 or 10 breaths/minute and the sedation level is 3 or greater, you should vigorously stimulate the patient and try to keep the patient awake.
- If the patient becomes oversedated, administer oxygen.
- In this situation, the opioid dose should be reduced.

For patients who are excessively sedated or unresponsive, naloxone, an opioid antagonist that rapidly reverses the effects of opioids, can be administered. Naloxone can be given IV, subcutaneously, or intranasally. Evzio (handheld autoinjector containing naloxone) can be used by a caregiver or family member to treat a person known or suspected to have had an opioid overdose.

If the patient has been taking opioids regularly for more than a few days, use naloxone carefully because it can precipitate severe, agonizing pain; profound withdrawal symptoms; hypertension; and pulmonary edema. Because naloxone's half-life is shorter than that of most opioids, frequently monitor the patient.

*Pruritus* (itching) is another common side effect of opioids and occurs most frequently when opioids are administered via neuraxial (i.e., epidural, intrathecal) routes. Management of opioid-induced pruritus in non-cancer patients may include low-dose infusions of naloxone.

**TABLE 8-10 Pasero Opioid-Induced Sedation Scale (POSS) With Interventions**

| Level of Sedation | Nursing Intervention |
|---|---|
| **S** = Sleep, easy to arouse | • Acceptable<br>• No action necessary<br>• May increase opioid dose if needed |
| **1** Awake and alert | • Acceptable<br>• No action necessary<br>• May increase opioid dose if needed |
| **2** Slightly drowsy, easily aroused | • Acceptable<br>• No action necessary<br>• May increase opioid dose if needed |
| **3** Frequently drowsy, arousable, drifts off to sleep during conversation | • Unacceptable<br>• Monitor respiratory status and sedation level closely until sedation level is stable at less than 3 and respiratory status is satisfactory.<br>• Decrease opioid dose 25%-50% or notify HCP or anesthesiologist for orders.<br>• Consider administering a nonsedating, opioid-sparing nonopioid, such as acetaminophen or an NSAID, if not contraindicated. |
| **4** Somnolent, minimal or no response to verbal or physical stimulation | • Unacceptable<br>• Stop opioid<br>• Consider administering naloxone.<br>• Notify HCP or anesthesiologist.<br>• Monitor respiratory status and sedation level closely until sedation level is stable at less than 3 and respiratory status is satisfactory. |

Adapted from Pasero C: Assessment of sedation during opioid administration for pain management, *J PeriAnesthesia Nurs* 24:186, 2009.

A rare but concerning problem with long-term and even short-term use of high-dose opioids is *opioid-induced hyperalgesia* (OIH). OIH is a state of nociceptive sensitization caused by exposure to opioids. It is characterized by a paradoxic response in which patients actually become more sensitive to certain painful stimuli and report increased pain with opioid use. The exact mechanism is not clearly understood, but it may be due to neuroplasticity changes. This may explain why opioids tend to lose their effectiveness in certain patients over time.

**Adjuvant Analgesic Therapy.** Analgesic adjuvants are drugs that can be used alone or in conjunction with opioid and nonopioid analgesics (Table 8-11). Generally, these agents were developed for other purposes (e.g., antiseizure drugs, antidepressants) and found to be effective for treating pain.

***Corticosteroids.*** Corticosteroids include dexamethasone, prednisone, and methylprednisolone (Medrol). They are used for management of acute and chronic cancer pain, pain secondary to spinal cord compression, and inflammatory joint pain syndromes. Mechanisms of action may be related to the ability of corticosteroids to decrease edema and inflammation.

Corticosteroids have many side effects, especially when given chronically in high doses. These include hyperglycemia, fluid retention, dyspepsia and GI bleeding, impaired healing, muscle wasting, osteoporosis, adrenal suppression, and susceptibility to infection. Because they act through the same final pathway as NSAIDs, do not give corticosteroids at the same time as NSAIDs.

**TABLE 8-11 Drug Therapy**

***Adjuvant Drugs Used for Pain***

| Drug | Specific Indication | Nursing Considerations |
|---|---|---|
| **Corticosteroids** | Inflammation | • Avoid high doses for long-term use. |
| **Antidepressants** | | |
| ***Tricyclic Antidepressants*** | | |
| amitriptyline<br>doxepin<br>imipramine (Tofranil)<br>nortriptyline (Pamelor)<br>desipramine (Norpramin) | Neuropathic pain | • Side-effect profile differs for each agent and is often dose dependent.<br>• Common side effects include anticholinergic effects (e.g., dry mouth) and sedation.<br>• Monitor for anticholinergic side effects.<br>• Titrate slowly over days to weeks to reach optimal therapeutic doses. |
| ***Serotonin Norepinephrine Reuptake Inhibitor (SNRI) Antidepressants*** | | |
| venlafaxine<br>duloxetine (Cymbalta)<br>milnacipran (Savella) | Neuropathic pain<br>Multimodal therapy for acute pain (venlafaxine)<br>Fibromyalgia (duloxetine, milnacipran) | • Side effects vary with each agent.<br>• Decrease arousal and desire for sex |
| ***Other Antidepressants*** | | |
| bupropion (Wellbutrin) | Neuropathic pain<br>Headaches<br>Distinguished from TCAs and SNRIs as an inhibitor of norepinephrine and dopamine uptake | • Low risk of sexual dysfunction and sedation |
| **Antiseizure Drugs** | | |
| *First generation:*<br>carbamazepine (Tegretol)<br>phenytoin (Dilantin)<br>*Second generation:*<br>gabapentin (Neurontin)<br>pregabalin (Lyrica)<br>lamotrigine (Lamictal) | Neuropathic pain<br>Multimodal therapy for acute pain (gabapentin, pregabalin)<br>Fibromyalgia (pregabalin) | • Start with low doses, increase slowly.<br>• Side effects vary with each agent. |
| **GABA Receptor Agonist** | | |
| baclofen (Lioresal) | Neuropathic pain<br>Muscle spasms | • Monitor for weakness, urinary dysfunction.<br>• Avoid abrupt discontinuation because of CNS irritability. |
| **$\alpha_2$-Adrenergic Agonist** | | |
| clonidine (Duraclon)<br>tizanidine (Zanaflex) | Particularly useful for neuropathic pain when administered intrathecally | • Side effects include sedation, orthostatic hypotension, dry mouth.<br>• Often combined with anesthetics (e.g., bupivacaine [Sensorcaine]) |
| **Anesthetics: Oral or Systemic** | | |
| mexiletine | Diabetic neuropathy<br>Neuropathic pain | • Monitor for side effects: high incidence of nausea, dizziness, perioral numbness, paresthesias, tremor, seizures (at high doses), dysrhythmias, and myocardial depression.<br>• Avoid in patients with preexisting cardiac disease. |
| 5% lidocaine-impregnated transdermal patch (Lidoderm patch) | Postherpetic neuralgia | • Local skin reactions (e.g., change in color, colored spots, irritation, itching, rash, burning) occur at the site of application; typically mild. |
| **Anesthetics: Local** | | |
| lidocaine (L-M-X) | Topical local anesthetic cream applied to intact skin before venipuncture or lumbar puncture. Possibly effective for postherpetic neuralgia | • Apply bubble layer to intact skin, wait at least 20-30 min before wiping and performing painful procedure.<br>• Duration is approximately 60 min after wiped from skin.<br>• Available without prescription |
| lidocaine 2.5% + prilocaine 2.5% (topical EMLA [eutectic mixture of local anesthetics]) | Longer time to take effect than L-M-X | • Apply under an occlusive dressing (e.g., Tegaderm, DuoDerm) or on an anesthetic disk.<br>• Side effects include mild erythema, edema, skin blanching. |
| 5% lidocaine-impregnated transdermal patch (Lidoderm patch) | Postherpetic neuralgia | • Local skin reactions (e.g., change in color, colored spots, irritation, itching, rash, burning) occur at the site of application—typically mild. |
| capsaicin (active compound of chili peppers) | Pain associated with arthritis, postherpetic neuralgia, diabetic neuropathy | • Apply very sparingly onto affected area. Use gloves or wash hands with soap and water after application.<br>• Monitor for side effects: skin irritation (burning, stinging) at application site and cough when inhaled. |

Adapted from Pasero C, Polomano RC, McCaffery M, et al: Adjuvant analgesics. In Pasero C, McCaffery M, editors: *Pain: assessment and pharmacological management*, New York, 2011, Elsevier.

*CNS*, Central nervous system.

***Antidepressants.*** Tricyclic antidepressants (TCAs) enhance the descending inhibitory system by preventing the cellular reuptake of serotonin and norepinephrine. Higher levels of serotonin and norepinephrine in the synapse inhibit the transmission of nociceptive signals in the CNS. Other potential beneficial actions of TCAs include sodium channel modulation, $\alpha_1$-adrenergic antagonist effects, and a weak NMDA receptor modulation. They are effective for a variety of pain syndromes, especially neuropathic pain syndromes. However, side effects such as sedation, dry mouth, blurred vision, and weight gain limit their usefulness. Antidepressants that selectively inhibit reuptake of serotonin and norepinephrine (SNRIs) are effective for many neuropathic pain syndromes and have fewer side effects than the TCAs. These agents include venlafaxine, desvenlafaxine (Pristiq), milnacipran (Savella), and bupropion.

***Antiseizure Drugs.*** Antiseizure drugs affect peripheral nerves and the CNS in several ways, including sodium channel modulation, central calcium channel modulation, and changes in excitatory amino acids and other receptors. Agents such as gabapentin, lamotrigine, and pregabalin are valuable adjuvant agents in chronic pain therapy and are being used increasingly in the treatment of acute pain.

***GABA-Receptor Agonist.*** Baclofen, an agonist at GABA receptors, can interfere with the transmission of nociceptive impulses and is used for muscle spasms and neuropathic pain. It crosses the blood-brain barrier poorly and is much more effective for spasticity when delivered intrathecally.

***$\alpha_2$-Adrenergic Agonists.*** Clonidine and tizanidine (Zanaflex), the most widely used $\alpha_2$-adrenergic agonists, are thought to work on the central inhibitory $\alpha$-adrenergic receptors. These agents may also decrease norepinephrine release peripherally. They are used for chronic headache and neuropathic pain.

***Local Anesthetics.*** For acute pain from surgery or trauma, local anesthetics such as bupivacaine and ropivacaine can be administered epidurally by continuous infusion but also by intermittent or continuous infusion with regional nerve blocks. Topical applications of local anesthetics are used to interrupt transmission of pain signals to the brain. For example, 5% lidocaine patch (Lidoderm) is recommended as a first-line agent for the treatment of several types of neuropathic pain. In the treatment of chronic severe neuropathic pain that is refractory to other analgesics, oral therapy with mexiletine (Mexitil) may be tried. Systemic lidocaine administered in the form of an IV infusion is also sometimes used for neuropathic and postoperative visceral pain.

***Cannabinoids.*** Cannabinoid-derived medications show promise in the treatment of certain pain syndromes and symptoms. However, these preparations have sparked considerable controversy and confusion, mostly because cannabinoids are related to the cannabis plant, also known as marijuana. Synthetic cannabinoids (e.g., dronabinol [Marinol]) have been approved for medical use. Smoking marijuana or cannabis rapidly increases plasma levels of tetrahydrocannabinol (THC). The increase is dependent on composition of the marijuana cigarette and inhalation technique. As a result, this form of use is associated with variable pain relief. With commercially available oral preparations, the absorption and bioavailability are more reliable and predictable.

Cannabinoids exert their analgesic effects primarily through the cannabinoid-1 (CB1) and CB2 receptors. Activation of cannabinoid receptors modulates neurotransmission in the serotoninergic, dopaminergic, and glutamatergic systems, as well as other systems. Cannabinoids also enhance the endogenous opioid system. Other beneficial effects include alleviation of nausea and increased appetite. They may also have opioid-sparing effects, possibly reduce opioid tolerance, and even ameliorate symptoms of opioid withdrawal.[20]

### Administration

***Scheduling.*** Appropriate analgesic scheduling focuses on preventing or controlling pain, rather than providing analgesics only after the patient's pain has become severe. Premedicate a patient before procedures and activities that are expected to produce pain. Similarly, a patient with constant pain should receive analgesics around the clock rather than on an "as needed" (PRN) basis. These strategies control pain before it starts and usually result in lower analgesic requirements. Use fast-acting drugs for incident or breakthrough pain, whereas long-acting analgesics are more effective for constant pain. Examples of fast-acting and sustained-release analgesics are described later in this section.

***Titration.*** *Analgesic titration* is dose adjustment based on assessment of the adequacy of analgesic effect versus the side effects produced. The amount of analgesic needed to manage pain varies widely, and titration is an important strategy in addressing this variability. An analgesic can be titrated upward or downward, depending on the situation. For example, in a postoperative patient the dose of analgesic generally decreases over time as the acute pain resolves. On the other hand, opioids for chronic, severe cancer pain may be titrated upward many times over the course of therapy to maintain adequate pain control. The goal of titration is to use the smallest dose of analgesic that provides effective pain control with the fewest side effects.

***Equianalgesic Dosing.*** The term **equianalgesic dose** refers to a dose of one analgesic that is approximately equivalent in pain-relieving effects to a given dose of another analgesic (Table 8-12). This equivalence helps guide opioid dosing when changing routes or opioids when a particular drug is ineffective or causes intolerable side effects. Equianalgesic charts and conversion programs are widely available in clinical guidelines, in health care facility pain protocols, and on the Internet. They are useful tools, but you need to understand their limitations, since equianalgesic doses are estimates. To ensure safety, all changes

**TABLE 8-12 Opioid Equianalgesic Doses***

| | DOSE EQUAL TO PARENTERAL MORPHINE 10 MG | |
|---|---|---|
| **Drug** | **Oral (mg)** | **Parenteral (IM, IV, Subcutaneous) (mg)** |
| Morphine | 30 | 10 |
| Codeine | 200 | 120-130 |
| Fentanyl | NA | 0.1 (100 mcg) |
| Hydrocodone | 30 | NA |
| Hydromorphone | 7.5 | 1.5 |
| Levorphanol | 4 | 2 |
| Meperidine | 300 | 75 |
| Methadone† | | |
| Oxycodone | 15-30 | NA |
| Oxymorphone | NA | 1 |

*NA,* Not available.

*All equivalencies should be considered approximations. These amounts can be affected by many factors, including interpatient variability, type of pain, and tolerance. Monitor patients for effectiveness and adverse reactions and adjust the dose accordingly.

†The equianalgesic dose of methadone compared with other opioids varies widely in patients on chronic opioids (*www.aafp.org/afp/20050401/1353.html*).

in opioid therapy must be carefully monitored and adjusted for the individual patient.

***Administration Routes.*** Opioids and other analgesic agents can be delivered via many routes. This flexibility allows the HCP to (1) target a particular anatomic source of the pain, (2) achieve therapeutic blood levels rapidly when necessary, (3) avoid certain side effects through localized administration, and (4) provide analgesia when patients are unable to swallow. The following discussion highlights the uses and nursing considerations for analgesic agents delivered through a variety of routes.

**Oral.** Generally, oral administration is the route of choice for the person with a functioning GI system. Most pain medications are available in oral preparations, such as liquid and tablet. For opioids, larger oral doses are needed to achieve the equivalent analgesia of doses administered intramuscularly (IM) or IV (Table 8-12). For example, 10 mg of parenteral morphine is equivalent to approximately 30 mg of oral morphine. The reason larger doses are required is related to the *first-pass effect* of hepatic metabolism. This means that oral opioids are absorbed from the GI tract into the portal circulation and shunted to the liver. Partial metabolism in the liver occurs before the drug enters the systemic circulation and becomes available to peripheral receptors or can cross the blood-brain barrier and access CNS opioid receptors, which is necessary to produce analgesia. Oral opioids are as effective as parenteral opioids if the dose administered is large enough to compensate for the first-pass metabolism.

Many opioids are available in short-acting (immediate-release) and long-acting (sustained-release or extended-release) oral preparations. Immediate-release products are effective in providing rapid, short-term pain relief. Sustained- or extended-release preparations generally are administered every 8 to 12 hours, although some preparations (e.g., Kadian, Avinza, Exalgo) may be dosed every 24 hours.

**SAFETY ALERT Sustained- or Extended-Release Preparations**

- These should not be crushed, broken, dissolved, or chewed. These drugs are meant to be swallowed whole.
- If all of the medicine is released into a person at once, very serious side effects can occur, including death from overdose.

**Transmucosal and buccal routes.** Although morphine has historically been administered sublingually to people with cancer pain who have difficulty swallowing, little of the drug is actually absorbed from the sublingual tissue. Instead, most of the drug is dissolved in saliva and swallowed, making its absorption similar to oral morphine.

Several transmucosal fentanyl products are used for the treatment of breakthrough pain. These include (1) oral transmucosal fentanyl citrate (OTFC) (Actiq) with the fentanyl embedded in a flavored lozenge on a stick, which is absorbed by the buccal mucosa after being rubbed actively over it when administered as the lozenge (not sucked as a lollipop), (2) fentanyl buccal tablet (FBT) (Fentora) in the form of a buccal tablet that disintegrates, (3) fentanyl sublingual (Abstral), and (4) fentanyl buccal soluble film (Onsolis) for application to the buccal membrane. Transmucosal absorption allows the drug to enter the bloodstream and travel directly to the CNS. Pain relief typically occurs 5 to 7 minutes after administration. These formulations of fentanyl should only be used for patients who are already receiving and are tolerant to opioid therapy.[21]

An oromucosal spray delivery of cannabinoid extract (Sativex) is an adjunctive treatment for neuropathic pain and spasticity in patients with multiple sclerosis. It is not currently available in the United States.

**Intranasal route.** Intranasal administration allows delivery of medication to highly vascular mucosa and avoids the first-pass effect. Butorphanol is indicated for acute headache and other intense, recurrent types of pain. A transmucosal fentanyl nasal spray (Lazanda) is available for the treatment of breakthrough pain.

**Rectal.** The rectal route is often overlooked but is particularly useful when the patient cannot take an analgesic by mouth, such as those patients with severe nausea and vomiting. Analgesics that are available as rectal suppositories include hydromorphone, oxymorphone, morphine, and acetaminophen. If rectal preparations are not available, many oral formulations can be given rectally if the patient is unable to take medications by mouth.

**Transdermal route.** Fentanyl (Duragesic) is available as a transdermal patch system for application to intact, nonhairy skin. This delivery system is useful for the patient who cannot tolerate oral analgesic drugs. Absorption from the patch is slow, and it takes 12 to 17 hours to reach full effect with the first application. Therefore transdermal fentanyl is not suitable for rapid dose titration but can be effective if the patient's pain is stable, and the dose required to control it is known. Patches may have to be changed every 48 hours rather than the recommended 72 hours based on individual patient responses. Rashes caused by the adhesive of the patch may be reduced by preparing the skin 1 hour before placement with a weak corticosteroid cream. Biocclusive dressings are available if the patch keeps falling off because of sweating. A transdermal patient-controlled analgesia (PCA) system (iontophoretic transdermal system [ITS]) is available.

**DRUG ALERT Fentanyl Patches**

- Fentanyl patches (Duragesic) may cause death from overdose.
- Signs of overdose include trouble breathing or shallow respirations; tiredness, extreme sleepiness, or sedation; inability to think, talk, or walk normally; and faintness, dizziness, or confusion.

An important distinction should be made between transdermal patches designed for systemic drug delivery (e.g., Duragesic) and those for topical or local delivery (e.g., Lidoderm).

A 5% lidocaine-impregnated transdermal patch (Lidoderm patch) is used for postherpetic neuralgia. The patch is placed directly on the intact, nonhairy skin in the area of postherpetic pain and left in place for up to 12 hours. Topical local anesthetics are generally well tolerated and cause few systemic side effects, even with chronic use.

Creams and lotions containing 10% trolamine salicylate (Aspercreme, Myoflex Creme) are available for joint and muscle pain. This aspirin-like substance is absorbed locally. This route of administration avoids GI irritation but not the other side effects of high-dose salicylates. Topical diclofenac solution and a diclofenac patch (Flector) are effective for osteoarthritic pain of the knee.

Other topical analgesic agents, such as capsaicin (e.g., Zostrix) and lidocaine (L-M-X cream), also provide analgesia. Derived from red chili pepper, capsaicin acts on C-fiber heat receptors. If used three or four times a day for 4 to 6 weeks, it will cause the C nociceptor fibers to become inactive. The result is neuronal resistance to painful stimuli. Capsaicin is used to control pain associated with diabetic neuropathy, arthritis, and postherpetic neuralgia. L-M-X cream is useful for

## EVIDENCE-BASED PRACTICE

### *Translating Research Into Practice*

**What Is the Effect of Capsaicin on Chronic Neuropathic Pain?**

***Clinical Question***

For adults with chronic neuropathic pain (P), what is the effect of high-concentration capsaicin (I) versus placebo or usual care (C) on pain relief (O) for up to 12 weeks (T)?

***Synthesis of Best Available Evidence***

- Systematic review of randomized controlled trials (RCTs)
- Six trials ($n = 2073$) of participants with moderately intense postherpetic neuralgia or painful HIV-neuropathy lasting at least 3 months. Intervention was single application of high-concentration capsaicin patches to affected areas under carefully controlled conditions. The concentration of capsaicin (8%) was almost 100 times greater than conventional creams. Pain relief was expected to occur for approximately 12 weeks.
- About 1 in 8 patients with high-concentration capsaicin patch had significant pain relief. People with high pain relief reported improved sleep, fatigue, depression, and quality of life. Short-term local skin effects were erythema, burning, and pain at application site.

***Conclusion***

- High-concentration capsaicin patches may relieve chronic neuropathic pain.

***Implications for Nursing Practice***

1. What information would you provide a patient with intense chronic shingles pain who seeks your help when other therapies have failed?
2. What is your role as a member of the interprofessional pain management team for patients with constant, severe chronic pain?

***Reference for Evidence***

Derry S, Rice ASC, Cole P, et al: Topical capsaicin (high concentration) for chronic neuropathic pain in adults, *Cochrane Database Syst Rev* (2):CD007393, 2013.

*P*, Patient population of interest; *I*, intervention or area of interest; *C*, comparison of interest or comparison group; *O*, outcomes of interest; *T*, timing (see p. 15).

control of pain associated with venipunctures. Cover the targeted area of intact skin with a layer of L-M-X for at least 20 to 30 minutes before it is wiped off prior to beginning a painful procedure.

**Parenteral routes.** The parenteral routes include IV and subcutaneous administration. Single, repeated, or continuous dosing (IV or subcutaneous) is possible via parenteral routes. IV administration is the best route when immediate analgesia and rapid titration are necessary. Continuous IV infusions provide excellent steady-state analgesia through stable blood levels.

Onset of analgesia after subcutaneous administration is slow, and thus the subcutaneous route is rarely used for acute pain management. However, continuous subcutaneous infusions are effective for pain management at the end of life. This route is especially helpful for people with abnormal GI function and limited venous access.

The IM route is not recommended because injections cause significant pain and result in unreliable absorption. With chronic use, IM injections can result in abscesses and fibrosis.

**Intraspinal delivery.** Intraspinal or neuraxial opioid therapy involves inserting a catheter into the subarachnoid space

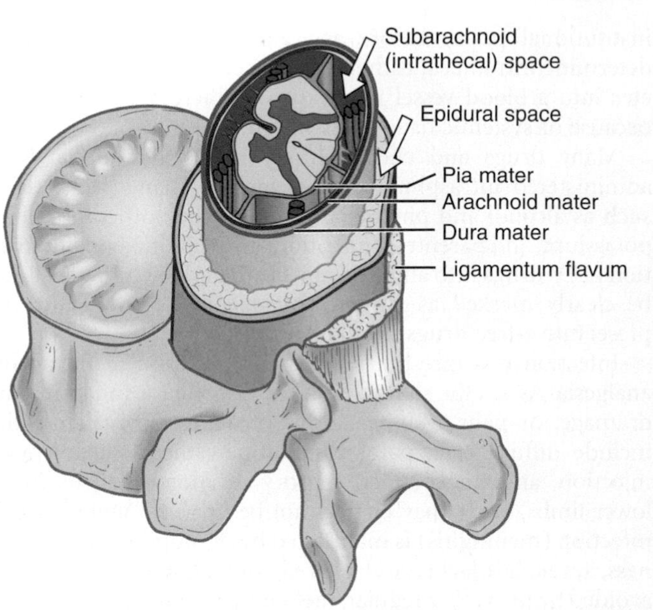


**FIG. 8-6** Spinal anatomy. The spinal cord extends from the foramen magnum to the first or second lumbar vertebral space. The subarachnoid space (intrathecal space) is filled with cerebrospinal fluid that continuously circulates and bathes the spinal cord. The epidural space is a potential space filled with blood vessels, fat, and a network of nerve extensions.

*(intrathecal delivery)* or the epidural space *(epidural delivery)* (Fig. 8-6). Analgesics are injected either by intermittent bolus doses or continuous infusion.

Percutaneously placed temporary catheters are used for short-term therapy (2 to 4 days), and surgically implanted catheters are used for long-term therapy. Although the lumbar region is the most common site of placement, epidural catheters may be placed at any point along the spinal column (cervical, thoracic, lumbar, or caudal). The tip of the epidural catheter is placed as close to the nerve supplying the painful dermatome as possible. For example, a thoracic catheter is placed for upper abdominal surgery, and a high lumbar catheter is used for lower abdominal surgery. Fluoroscopy is used to ensure correct placement of the catheter.

Intraspinally administered analgesics are highly potent because they are delivered close to the receptors in the spinal cord dorsal horn. Smaller doses of analgesics are needed than with other routes, including IV. For example, 1 mg of intrathecal morphine is approximately equivalent to 10 mg of epidural morphine, 100 mg of IV morphine, and 300 mg of oral morphine. Drugs that are delivered intraspinally include morphine, fentanyl, sufentanil (Sufenta), alfentanil (Alfenta), hydromorphone, ziconotide (Prialt) (a calcium channel receptor modulator for use in neuropathic pain syndromes), and clonidine. Nausea, itching, and urinary retention are common side effects of intraspinal opioids.

Complications of intraspinal analgesia include catheter displacement and migration, accidental infusions of neurotoxic agents, epidural hematomas, and infection. Clinical manifestations of catheter displacement or migration depend on catheter location and the drug being infused. A catheter that migrates out of the intrathecal or epidural space causes a decrease in pain relief with no improvement with additional boluses or increases in the infusion rate. If an epidural catheter migrates into the subarachnoid space, increased side effects become quickly apparent. Somnolence, confusion, and increased anesthesia (if the infusate contains an anesthetic) occur. Check with institutional policy before aspirating cerebrospinal fluid to determine intrathecal catheter placement. Migration of a catheter into a blood vessel may cause an increase in side effects because of systemic drug distribution.

Many drugs and chemicals are highly neurotoxic when administered intraspinally. These include many preservatives such as alcohol and phenol, antibiotics, chemotherapy agents, potassium, and parenteral nutrition. To avoid inadvertent injection of IV drugs into an intraspinal catheter, the catheter should be clearly marked as an intraspinal access device, and only preservative-free drugs should be injected.

Infection is a rare but serious complication of intraspinal analgesia. Assess the skin around the exit site for inflammation, drainage, or pain. Manifestations of an intraspinal infection include diffuse back pain, pain or paresthesia during bolus injection, and unexplained sensory or motor deficits in the lower limbs. Fever may or may not be present. Acute bacterial infection (meningitis) is manifested by photophobia, neck stiffness, fever, headache, and altered mental status. Infection is avoided by providing regular, meticulous wound care and using sterile technique when caring for the catheter and injecting drugs.

Long-term epidural catheters may be placed for terminal cancer patients or patients with certain pain syndromes that are unresponsive to other treatments. If a long-term indwelling epidural catheter is used, bacterial filters are recommended.

**Implantable pumps.** Intraspinal catheters can be surgically implanted for long-term pain relief. The surgical placement of an intrathecal catheter to a subcutaneously placed pump and reservoir allows for the delivery of drugs directly into the intrathecal space. The pump, which is normally placed in a pocket made in the subcutaneous tissue of the abdomen, may be programmable or fixed.

Changes are made by either reprogramming the pump or changing the mixture or concentration of drug in the reservoir. The pump is refilled every 30 to 90 days depending on flow rate, mixture, and reservoir size.

**Patient-controlled analgesia.** **Patient-controlled analgesia (PCA)** (demand analgesia) is a method that allows the patient to self-administer preset doses of an analgesic within a prescribed time period by activating an infusion pump. Routes of administration include oral, IV, epidural, inhaled, nasal, and transcutaneous. In acute care, PCA often refers to an electronically controlled infusion pump that delivers the medication by an IV or epidural route (**patient-controlled epidural analgesia [PCEA]**). PCEA often combines an opioid and local anesthetic. PCA can also be adapted for oral administration. With PCA/PCEA, a dose of opioid is delivered when the patient decides a dose is needed. PCA/PCEA uses an infusion system in which the patient pushes a button to receive a bolus infusion of an analgesic. PCA/PCEA is used widely for the management of acute pain, including postoperative pain and cancer pain.

Opioids, such as morphine and hydromorphone, are commonly administered via PCA therapy for acute and chronic pain. Sometimes IV PCA is administered with a continuous or background infusion called a *basal rate,* depending on the patient's opioid requirement. The addition of a basal rate in opioid-naive patients and those at risk for adverse respiratory outcomes (e.g., older age, obstructive sleep apnea, pulmonary disease) may lead to serious respiratory events. Basal rates are often used with epidural catheter pain management. Because the medication is delivered directly into the epidural space, the amount of opioid is 10 times less than is needed by IV route. This lessens the risk of respiratory depression but does not totally eliminate it.

Patient teaching is very important with the use of PCA/PCEA. Help the patient understand the mechanics of getting a drug dose and how to titrate the drug to achieve good pain relief. Teach the patient to self-administer the analgesic before pain is severe. Assure the patient that he or she cannot "overdose" because the pump is programmed to deliver a maximum number of doses per hour. Pressing the button after the maximum dose is administered will not result in additional analgesic. If the maximum doses are inadequate to relieve pain, the pump can be reprogrammed to increase the amount or frequency of dosing. In addition, you can give bolus doses if they are included in the HCP's orders. To make a smooth transition from infusion PCA to oral drugs, the patient should receive increasing doses of oral drug as the PCA analgesic is tapered.

Patient-controlled delivery systems are intended for use by the patient. An *authorized agent controlled analgesia (AACA)* is a method of delivery performed by a consistently available and competent individual for patients who are unable to independently activate PCA devices.[22] This authorized agent must be carefully selected, educated on the principles of PCA, and be capable of recognizing pain and the appropriate times to administer medication via the PCA device. Understand your institution's policies regarding PCA and AACA.

### Interventional Therapy

**Therapeutic Nerve Blocks.** Nerve blocks generally involve one-time or continuous infusion of local anesthetics into a particular area to produce pain relief. These techniques are also called *regional anesthesia.* Nerve blocks interrupt all afferent and efferent transmission to the area and thus are not specific to nociceptive pathways. They include local infiltration of anesthetics into a surgical area (e.g., chest incisions, inguinal hernia) and injection of anesthetic into a specific nerve (e.g., occipital or pudendal nerve) or nerve plexus (e.g., brachial or celiac plexus). Nerve blocks often are used during and after surgery to manage pain. For longer-term relief of chronic pain syndromes, local anesthetics can be administered via a continuous infusion.

Adverse effects of nerve blocks are similar to those for local anesthetics delivered via other systemic routes and include systemic toxicity resulting in dysrhythmias, confusion, nausea and vomiting, blurred vision, tinnitus, and metallic taste. Temporary nerve blocks affect motor function and sensation and typically last 2 to 24 hours, depending on the agent and the site of injection. Motor ability generally returns before sensation.

***Neuroablative Techniques.*** *Neuroablative interventions* are performed for severe pain that is unresponsive to all other therapies. Neuroablative techniques destroy nerves, thereby interrupting pain transmission. Destruction is by surgical resection or thermocoagulation, including radiofrequency coagulation. Neuroablative interventions that destroy the sensory division of a peripheral or spinal nerve are classified as *neurectomies, rhizotomies,* and *sympathectomies.* Neurosurgical procedures that ablate the lateral spinothalamic tract are classified as *cordotomies* if the tract is interrupted in the spinal cord, or *tractotomies* if the interruption is in the medulla or midbrain of the brainstem (Fig. 8-7). Cordotomy and tractotomy can be performed with the aid of local anesthesia by a percutaneous technique under fluoroscopy.

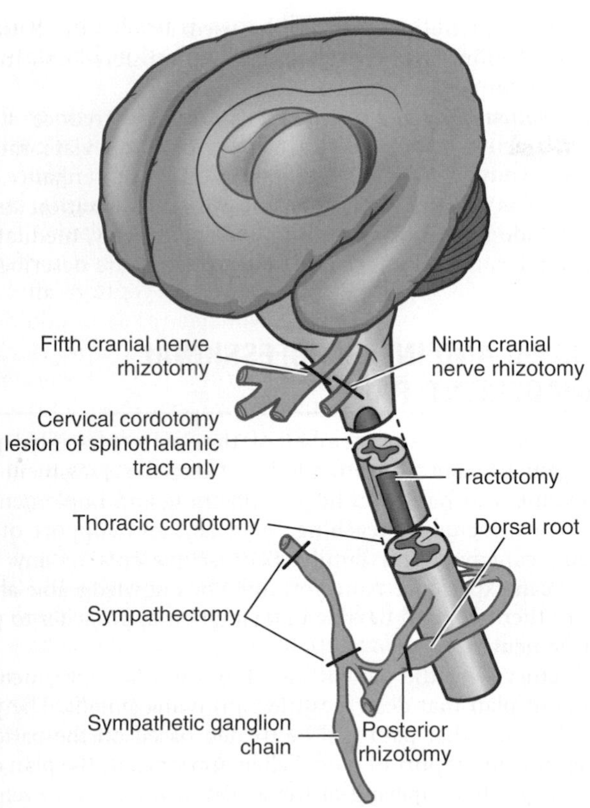


**FIG. 8-7** Sites of neurosurgical procedures for pain relief.

**TABLE 8-13 Nondrug Therapies for Pain**

| Physical Therapies | Cognitive Therapies |
|---|---|
| • Acupuncture<br>• Application of heat and cold (Table 8-14)<br>• Exercise<br>• Massage<br>• Transcutaneous electrical nerve stimulation (TENS) | • Distraction<br>• Hypnosis<br>• Imagery<br>• Relaxation strategies (see Chapter 6)<br>  • Relaxation breathing<br>  • Imagery<br>  • Meditation<br>  • Art therapy<br>  • Music therapy |

**Neuroaugmentation.** *Neuroaugmentation* involves electrical stimulation of the brain and spinal cord. Spinal cord stimulation (SCS) is performed much more often than brain stimulation. The most common use of SCS is for chronic back pain secondary to nerve damage that is unresponsive to other therapies. Other uses include complex regional pain syndrome (CRPS), spinal cord injury pain, and interstitial cystitis. Potential complications include those related to the surgery (bleeding and infection), migration of the generator (which usually is implanted in the subcutaneous tissues of the upper gluteal or pectoralis area), and nerve damage.

## Nondrug Therapies for Pain

Nondrug strategies play an important role in pain management (Table 8-13). They can reduce the dose of an analgesic required to relieve pain and thereby minimize side effects of drug therapy. Moreover, they increase the patient's sense of personal control about managing pain and increase coping skills. Some strategies are believed to alter ascending nociceptive input or stimulate descending pain modulation mechanisms (see the section on Perception on p. 106). These nondrug therapies are useful for both acute and chronic pain.

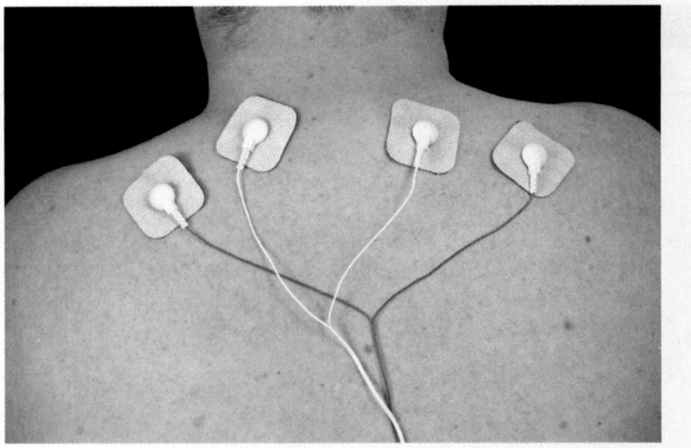

**FIG. 8-8** Transcutaneous electrical nerve stimulation (TENS) treatment being given for treatment of pain after shoulder surgery. (©Noel Moore/Hemera/Thinkstock)

### Physical Pain Relief Strategies

***Massage.*** Massage is useful for acute and chronic pain. Many different massage techniques exist, including moving the hands or fingers over the skin slowly or briskly with long strokes or in circles (superficial massage) or applying firm pressure to the skin to maintain contact while massaging the underlying tissues (deep massage). Another type is trigger point massage. A **trigger point** is a circumscribed hypersensitive area within a tight band of muscle. It is caused by acute or chronic muscle strain. It feels like a tight knot under the skin. Trigger point massage is performed by applying either strong, sustained digital pressure; deep massage; or gentler massage with ice followed by muscle heating. (Massage is discussed in Chapter 6.)

***Exercise.*** Exercise is an essential part of the treatment plan for patients with chronic pain, particularly those with musculoskeletal pain. Many patients become physically deconditioned as a result of their pain, which in turn leads to more pain. Exercise acts via many mechanisms to relieve pain. It enhances circulation and cardiovascular fitness, reduces edema, increases muscle strength and flexibility, and enhances physical and psychosocial functioning. Tailor an exercise program to the patient's physical needs and lifestyle. It may include aerobic exercise, stretching, and strengthening exercises. The program should be supervised by trained personnel (e.g., physical therapist).

***Transcutaneous Electrical Nerve Stimulation.*** *Transcutaneous electrical nerve stimulation* (TENS) involves the delivery of an electric current through electrodes applied to the skin surface over the painful region, at trigger points, or over a peripheral nerve. A TENS system consists of two or more electrodes connected by lead wires to a small, battery-operated stimulator (Fig. 8-8). Usually a physical therapist is responsible for administering TENS therapy, although nurses can be trained in the technique.

TENS may be used for acute pain, including postoperative pain and pain associated with physical trauma. The effects of TENS on chronic pain are less clear, but it may be effective in these cases.[23]

***Acupuncture.*** Acupuncture is a technique of Traditional Chinese Medicine in which very thin needles are inserted into the body at designated points. Acupuncture is used for many different kinds of pain.

**TABLE 8-14 Patient & Caregiver Teaching**
***Heat and Cold Therapy***

*Include the following instructions when teaching the patient and caregiver about superficial heat or cold techniques.*

**Heat Therapy**
- Do not use heat on an area that is being treated with radiation therapy, is bleeding, has decreased sensation, or has been injured in the past 24 hours.
- Do not use any menthol-containing products (e.g., Ben-Gay, Vicks, Icy Hot) with heat applications because this may cause burns.
- Cover the heat source with a towel or cloth before applying to the skin to prevent burns.

**Cold Therapy**
- Cover the cold source with a cloth or towel before applying to the skin to prevent tissue damage.
- Do not apply cold to areas that are being treated with radiation therapy, have open wounds, or have poor circulation.
- If it is not possible to apply the cold directly to the painful site, try applying it right above or below the painful site or on the opposite side of the body on the corresponding site (e.g., left elbow if the right elbow hurts).

***Heat Therapy.*** Heat therapy is the application of either moist or dry heat to the skin. Heat therapy can be either superficial or deep. Superficial heat can be applied using an electric heating pad (dry or moist), a hot pack, hot moist compresses, warm wax (paraffin), or a hot water bottle. To expose large areas of the body, patients can immerse themselves in a hot bath, shower, or whirlpool. Physical therapy departments provide deep-heat therapy through such techniques as short-wave diathermy, microwave diathermy, and ultrasound therapy. Patient and caregiver teaching regarding heat therapy is described in Table 8-14.

***Cold Therapy.*** Cold therapy involves the application of either moist or dry cold to the skin. Dry cold can be applied by means of an ice bag, moist cold by means of towels soaked in ice water, cold hydrocollator packs, or immersion in a bath or under running cold water. Icing with ice cubes or blocks of ice made to resemble Popsicles is another technique used for pain relief. Cold therapy is believed to be more effective than heat for a variety of painful conditions, including acute pain from trauma or surgery, acute flare-ups of arthritis, muscle spasms, and headache. Patient and caregiver teaching regarding cold therapy is described in Table 8-14.

**Cognitive Therapies.** Techniques to alter the affective, cognitive, and behavioral components of pain include a variety of cognitive strategies and behavioral approaches. For example, patients can identify and challenge negative pain-related thoughts and replace them with more positive coping thoughts. Some of these techniques require little training and often are adopted independently by the patient. For others, a trained therapist is necessary.

***Distraction.*** Distraction involves redirection of attention away from the pain and onto something else. It is a simple but powerful strategy to relieve pain. Distraction can be achieved by engaging the patient in any activity that can hold his or her attention (e.g., watching TV or a movie, conversing, listening to music). It is important to match the activity with the patient's energy level and ability to concentrate.

***Hypnosis.*** Hypnotherapy is a structured technique that enables a patient to achieve a state of heightened awareness and focused concentration that can be used to alter the patient's pain perception. Hypnosis should be administered and monitored only by specially trained clinicians.

***Relaxation Strategies.*** Relaxation strategies reduce stress, decrease acute anxiety, distract from pain, alleviate muscle tension, combat fatigue, facilitate sleep, and enhance the effectiveness of other pain relief measures.[24] Relaxation strategies include relaxation breathing, music, imagery, meditation, muscle relaxation, and art.[25] (These strategies are described in Chapter 6.)

## NURSING AND INTERPROFESSIONAL MANAGEMENT: PAIN

You are an important member of the interprofessional pain management team. You provide input into the assessment and reassessment of pain. You help in planning and implementing treatments, including teaching, advocacy, and support of the patient, caregiver, and family. Because patients in any care setting can experience pain, you must be knowledgeable about current therapies and flexible in trying new approaches to pain management.

Together with the patient, develop a written agreement or treatment plan that describes the pain management. The plan should ensure that pain will be treated based on the patient's perception and report of pain. When appropriate, the plan outlines the gradual tapering of the analgesic dose, with eventual substitution of parenteral analgesics with long-acting oral preparations, and possibly cessation of opioids.

Many nursing roles are described earlier in this chapter, including assessing pain, administering treatment, monitoring for side effects, and teaching patients and caregivers. However, the success of these actions depends on your ability to establish a trusting relationship with the patient and caregiver and to address their concerns regarding pain and its treatment.

### Effective Communication

Because pain is a subjective experience, patients need to feel confident that their reporting of pain will be believed and will not be perceived as "complaining." The patient and caregiver also need to know that you consider the pain significant and understand that pain may profoundly disrupt a person's life. Communicate concern and commit to helping the patient obtain pain relief and cope with any unrelieved pain. Support the patient and caregiver through the period of trial and error that may be necessary to implement an effective therapeutic plan. It also is important to clarify responsibilities in pain relief. Help the patient understand the role of the interprofessional team members, as well as the patient's roles and expectations.

In addition to addressing specific aspects of pain assessment and treatment, evaluate the impact that the pain has on the lives of the patient and caregiver. Table 8-15 addresses teaching needs of patients and caregivers related to pain management.

### Challenges to Effective Pain Management

Common challenges to effective pain management include misunderstandings about tolerance, physical dependence, and addiction. It is important for you to understand and be able to explain these concepts. Table 8-16 lists barriers to pain management and strategies to address them.

**Tolerance.** *Tolerance* occurs with chronic exposure to a variety of drugs. In the case of opioids, tolerance to analgesia is

**TABLE 8-15 Patient & Caregiver Teaching**

***Pain Management***

*Include the following information in the teaching plan for the patient with pain and caregiver.*

- Self-management techniques
- Realistic goals for pain control
- Negative consequences of unrelieved pain
- Need to maintain a record of pain level and effectiveness of treatment
- Treat pain with drugs and/or nondrug therapies before it becomes severe.
- Medication may stop working after it is taken for a period of time, and dosages may have to be adjusted.
- Potential side effects and complications associated with pain therapies can include nausea and vomiting, constipation, sedation and drowsiness, itching, urinary retention, and sweating.
- Need to report when pain is not relieved to tolerable levels

**TEAMWORK & COLLABORATION**

***Pain***

*Effective pain management should be a focus for all members of the nursing team.*

**Role of Nursing Personnel**

***Registered Nurse (RN)***

- Assess pain characteristics (pattern and onset, area or location, intensity, quality, associated symptoms, and management strategies).
- Develop treatment plan for patient's pain (including drug and nondrug therapies).
- Evaluate whether current treatment plan is effective.
- Teach patient and caregiver about treatment plan.
- Implement discharge teaching about pain management.

***Licensed Practical/Vocational Nurse (LPN/LVN)***

- Administer ordered pain medications (consider the state nurse practice act and agency policy, since LPNs may not be able to give medications by all routes).
- Assess patient's pain.

***Unlicensed Assistive Personnel (UAP)***

- Assist with screening for pain and notify RN if patient expresses pain.
- Take and report vital signs before and after pain medications are given.
- Note and report if patient is refusing to participate in ordered activities such as ambulation (since this may indicate inadequate pain management).

characterized by the need for an increased opioid dose to maintain the same degree of analgesia. Although the development of tolerance to side effects (except constipation) is more predictable, the incidence of clinically significant analgesic opioid tolerance in chronic pain patients is unknown, since dosage needs may increase as the disease (e.g., cancer) progresses. It is essential to assess for increased analgesic needs in patients on long-term therapy. The interprofessional team must evaluate and rule out other causes of increased analgesic needs, such as disease progression or infection.

If significant tolerance to opioids develops and it is believed that an opioid is losing its effectiveness, or intolerable side effects are associated with escalation of doses, the practice of *opioid rotation* may be considered. This involves switching from one opioid to another, assuming that the new opioid will be more effective at lower equianalgesic doses. However, very high opioid doses can result in opioid-induced hyperalgesia (OIH) rather than pain relief. This means that increases in the dose can lead to higher pain levels. (OIH is discussed on p. 115.)

◆ **Physical Dependence.** Like tolerance, physical dependence is a normal physiologic response to ongoing exposure to drugs. It is manifested by a withdrawal syndrome when the drug is abruptly decreased. Manifestations of opioid withdrawal are listed in Table 8-17. When opioids are no longer needed to provide pain relief, a tapering schedule should be used in conjunction with careful monitoring. A typical tapering schedule may involve reducing the dose by 20% to 50% per day. The goal is to reduce the amount of medication and at the same time minimize adverse and withdrawal effects.

◆ **Pseudoaddiction.** Inadequate treatment of pain can lead to a phenomenon called *pseudoaddiction*. This occurs when patients exhibit behaviors commonly associated with addiction (e.g., frequent requests for analgesic refills or higher dosages), but the behaviors resolve with adequate treatment of the patient's pain. These patients are often labeled as drug seeking, which can result in mistrust between the patient and HCP. This problem can be avoided by effective communication strategies and optimal pain management.

◆ **Addiction.** *Addiction* is a complex neurobiologic condition characterized by aberrant behaviors arising from a drive to obtain and take substances for reasons other than the prescribed therapeutic value (see Chapter 10). Tolerance and physical dependence are not indicators of addiction. Rather they are normal physiologic responses to chronic exposure to certain drugs, including opioids. Addiction rarely occurs in patients who receive opioids for pain control. If addiction is suspected, it must be investigated and diagnosed, if appropriate, but it should not be implied without evidence because this interferes with pain management. The hallmarks of addiction include (1) compulsive use, (2) loss of control of use, and (3) continued use despite risk of harm.

◆ **Risk Monitoring.** Several opioid risk assessments are available to help clinicians assess patient for abuse, misuse, and addiction. A controlled substance agreement for those at risk of addiction may be used. Addiction risk assessment tools such as the Opioid Risk Tool (*www.painmed.org/SOPResources/ClinicalTools*) and the Screener and Opioid Assessment for Patient Pain (*http://nhms.org/sites/default/files/Pdfs/SOAPP-14.pdf*) are available. Patient monitoring with urine drug screens and access to state prescription monitoring programs to track prescriptions are effective in detecting misuse of drugs. The risk of addiction should not prevent HCPs from using opioids to effectively treat moderate to severe acute and chronic pain.

## INSTITUTIONALIZING PAIN EDUCATION AND MANAGEMENT

Besides patient and caregiver barriers, other barriers to effective and safe pain management include inadequate HCP education and lack of institutional support. Traditionally, medical and nursing school curricula have spent little time teaching future physicians and nurses about pain and symptom management. The lack of emphasis on pain has contributed to inadequate training of HCPs.

Progress has been made in overcoming these barriers. Medical and nursing schools now devote more time to

**TABLE 8-16 Patient & Caregiver Teaching**
***Reducing Barriers to Pain Management***

*When teaching the patient and caregiver about pain management, discuss the following barriers.*

| Barrier | Nursing Considerations |
|---|---|
| **Fear of addiction** | • Explain that addiction is uncommon in patients taking opioids for pain. |
| **Fear of tolerance** | • Teach that tolerance is a normal physiologic response to chronic opioid therapy. If tolerance does develop, the drug may have to be changed (e.g., morphine in place of oxycodone).<br>• Teach that there is no absolute upper limit to pure opioid agonists (e.g., morphine). Dosages can be increased, and patient should not save drugs for when the pain is worse.<br>• Teach that tolerance develops more slowly to analgesic effects of opioids than to side effects (e.g., sedation, respiratory depression). Tolerance does not develop to constipation. Thus a regular bowel program should be started early. |
| **Concern about side effects** | • Teach methods to prevent and to treat common side effects.<br>• Emphasize that side effects such as sedation and nausea decrease with time.<br>• Explain that different drugs have unique side effects, and other pain drugs can be tried to reduce the specific side effect. |
| **Fear of injections** | • Explain that oral medicines are preferred.<br>• Emphasize that even if oral route becomes unusable, transdermal or indwelling parenteral routes can be used rather than injections. |
| **Desire to be "good" patient** | • Explain that patients are partners in their care and that partnership requires open communication by both patient and nurse.<br>• Emphasize to patients that they have a responsibility to keep you informed about their pain. |
| **Desire to be stoic** | • Explain that although stoicism is a valued behavior in many cultures, failure to report pain can result in undertreatment and severe, unrelieved pain. |
| **Forgetting to take analgesic** | • Provide and teach use of pill containers.<br>• Provide methods of record keeping for drug use.<br>• Recruit caregivers to assist with the analgesic regimen. |
| **Concern that pain indicates disease progression** | • Explain that increased pain or the need for analgesics may reflect tolerance.<br>• Emphasize that new pain may come from a non–life-threatening source (e.g., muscle spasm, urinary tract infection).<br>• Institute drug and nondrug strategies to reduce anxiety.<br>• Ensure that patient and caregivers have current, accurate, comprehensive information about the disease and prognosis.<br>• Provide psychologic support. |
| **Sense of fatalism** | • Explain that pain can be managed in most patients.<br>• Explain that most therapies require a period of trial and error.<br>• Emphasize that side effects can be managed. |
| **Ineffective medication** | • Teach that there are multiple options within each category of medication (e.g., opioids, NSAIDs), and another medication from the same category may provide better relief.<br>• Emphasize that finding the best treatment regimen often requires trial and error.<br>• Incorporate nondrug approaches in treatment plan. |

Adapted from Ersek M: Enhancing effective pain management by addressing patient barriers to analgesic use, *J Hospice Palliat Nurs* 1:87, 1999.
*NSAIDs,* Nonsteroidal antiinflammatory drugs.

**TABLE 8-17 Manifestations of Opioid Withdrawal Syndrome**

| | Early Response (6-12 Hr) | Late Response (48-72 Hr) |
|---|---|---|
| **Psychosocial** | • Anxiety | • Excitation |
| **Secretions** | • Lacrimation<br>• Rhinorrhea<br>• Diaphoresis | • Diarrhea |
| **Other** | • Yawning<br>• Piloerection<br>• Shaking, chills<br>• Dilated pupils<br>• Anorexia<br>• Tremor | • Restlessness<br>• Fever<br>• Nausea and vomiting<br>• Abdominal cramping pain<br>• Hypertension<br>• Tachycardia<br>• Insomnia |

addressing pain. Numerous professional organizations have published evidence-based guidelines for assessing and managing pain in many patient populations and clinical settings.

Institutional commitment and practices are changing clinical practice. One major step in institutionalizing pain management is the development and adoption of The Joint Commission (TJC) guideline on pain.[26] TJC is the accrediting body for most health care facilities (hospitals, nursing homes, and health care clinics). Under these standards, health care facilities are required to (1) recognize the patient's right to appropriate assessment and management of pain; (2) identify pain in patients during their initial assessment and as needed, during ongoing, periodic reassessments; (3) educate HCPs about pain assessment and management and ensure competency; and (4) educate patients and their families about pain management.

## ETHICAL ISSUES IN PAIN MANAGEMENT

### Fear of Hastening Death by Administering Analgesics

A common concern of health care professionals and caregivers is that providing a sufficient amount of drug to relieve pain will

## BECOMING A NURSE LEADER

### *Impaired Nurse*

#### Situation

You are a nurse on a very busy postsurgical cardiac care unit. Although Mr. Zeller is not your patient, you answer his call light while his nurse Bill is off the unit. Mr. Zeller is complaining of severe pain from his surgical site, stating he is not receiving relief from his pain medication. You check the medication administration record and notice that it is charted that he received morphine IV 30 minutes ago. You find this very strange and ask Bill about it when he returns from his break. Bill dismisses you and says that Mr. Zeller has a low pain tolerance. After you return from your break, Bill tells you that your patient Mrs. Zink is still complaining of severe pain, although he gave her morphine IV 15 minutes ago. While packing up to leave for the day, you notice Bill taking two syringes out of his pocket and throwing them in the hazardous waste container.

#### Points for Consideration

- As an advocate for the patient, nurses must be alert to and take appropriate action regarding any instances of incompetent, unethical, illegal, or impaired practice by any member of the health care team.[1]
- When nurses are aware of inappropriate or questionable practice in the provision or denial of health care, express your concern to the person carrying out the questionable practice.
- When the welfare of the patient is threatened, similar action should be directed to the responsible administrator and/or higher authority within the institution, or to an appropriate external authority.[1]
- About 1 in 10 nurses may be impaired or in recovery from alcohol or drug addiction. Nurses' overall pattern of dependency is unique because they have greater access to drugs in the workplace.[2]
- Nurses must educate themselves about the signs, symptoms, and behaviors that characterize substance abuse. It may be difficult to suspect a co-worker, and the fear of retaliation may keep some nurses from action. It is important to take steps to confront or notify the nurse manager of your suspicions.
- Do not allow yourself to be manipulated or fear confronting a nurse if patient safety is in jeopardy.[2]
- Substance-abusing nurses most likely will not seek treatment until confronted by peers, family, or nursing management, or if their job is in jeopardy. Those who do enter and complete structured treatment programs can be successful and reenter the profession of nursing.

#### Discussion Questions

1. Based on your suspicions of Bill, what action will you take first?
2. Do you have enough evidence to report Bill to your supervisor?
3. What responsibility do you have to Bill's patients?

#### References

1. American Nurses Association (ANA): Code of ethics for nurses with interpretive statements: Provision 3. Retrieved from *www.nursingworld.org/provision-3*.
2. Thomas CM, Siela D: The impaired nurse: would you know what to do if you suspected substance abuse? Retrieved from *www.americannursetoday.com/the-impaired-nurse-would-you-know-what-to-do-if-you-suspected-substance-abuse*.

hasten or precipitate death of a terminally ill person. However, there is no scientific evidence that opioids can hasten death, even among patients at the very end of life. Moreover, you have a moral obligation to provide comfort and pain relief at the end of life. Even if there is a concern about the possibility of hastening death, the rule of double effect provides ethical justification. This rule states that if an unwanted consequence (i.e., hastened death) occurs as a result of an action taken to achieve a moral good (i.e., pain relief), the action is justified if the nurse's intent is to relieve pain and not to hasten death.

### Requests for Assisted Suicide

Unrelieved pain is one of the reasons that patients make requests for assisted suicide. Aggressive and adequate pain management may decrease the number of such requests. Assisted suicide is a complex issue that extends beyond pain and pain management. Physician-assisted suicide is legal in some states (e.g., Oregon, Washington). To address the legal and ethical issues confronting nurses in this unique situation, the Oregon Nurses Association prepared a position paper on this topic.[27]

### Use of Placebos in Pain Assessment and Treatment

Placebos are still sometimes used to assess and treat pain. Using a placebo involves deceiving patients by making them believe that they are receiving an analgesic when in fact they are typically receiving an inert substance such as saline. The use of placebos to assess or treat pain is condemned by several professional organizations.

## Gerontologic Considerations: Pain

Persistent pain is a common problem in older adults and is often associated with physical disability and psychosocial problems. The prevalence of chronic pain among community-dwelling older adults exceeds 50%, and among older nursing home patients, it is approximately 80%. The most common painful conditions among older adults are musculoskeletal conditions such as osteoarthritis and low back pain. Chronic pain often results in depression, sleep disturbance, decreased mobility, increased health care utilization, and physical and social role dysfunction. Despite its high prevalence, pain in older adults is often inadequately assessed and treated.

Several barriers to pain assessment in the older patient exist. Older adults and their HCPs often believe that pain is a normal, inevitable part of aging and that nothing can be done to relieve the pain. Older adults may not report pain for fear of being a "burden" or a "complainer." They may fear taking opioids. In addition, older patients are more likely to use words such as "aching," "soreness," or "discomfort" rather than "pain." Be persistent in asking older adults about pain. Carry out the assessment in an unhurried, supportive manner.

Another barrier is the increased prevalence of cognitive, sensory-perceptual, and motor problems that interfere with a person's ability to process information and communicate. Examples include dementia and delirium, poststroke aphasia, and other communication barriers. Hearing and vision deficits may complicate assessment. Therefore pain assessment tools may have to be adapted for older adults. For example, it may be necessary to use a large-print pain intensity scale. Most older adults, even those with mild to moderate cognitive impairment, can use quantitative scales accurately and reliably.

In older patients with chronic pain, perform a thorough physical examination and history to identify causes of pain, possible therapies, and potential problems. Also assess for depression and functional impairments, because they are also common among older adults with pain.

Treatment of pain in older adults is complicated by several factors. First, older adults metabolize drugs more slowly than younger people and thus are at greater risk for higher blood levels and adverse effects. The adage "start low and go slow" must be applied to analgesic therapy in this age group. Second, the use of NSAIDs in older adults is associated with a high frequency of GI bleeding. Third, older adults often are taking many drugs for one or more chronic conditions. The addition of analgesics can result in dangerous drug interactions and increased side effects. Fourth, cognitive impairment and ataxia can be exacerbated by analgesics such as opioids, antidepressants, and antiseizure drugs. This requires that HCPs titrate drugs slowly and monitor carefully for side effects.

Treatment regimens for older adults must incorporate nondrug modalities. Exercise and patient teaching are important nondrug interventions for older adults with chronic pain. Also include family and caregivers in the treatment plan (Tables 8-15 and 8-16).

## MANAGING PAIN IN SPECIAL POPULATIONS

### Patients Unable to Self-Report Pain

Although the patient's self-report is the gold standard of pain assessment, many illnesses and conditions affect a patient's ability to report pain. These diagnoses and conditions include dementia and delirium. For these people, behavioral and physiologic changes may be the only indicators of pain. You must be astute at recognizing behavioral symptoms of pain.

A guide for assessing pain in nonverbal patients is presented in Table 8-18. Several scales have been developed to assess pain-related behaviors in nonverbal patients, particularly those with advanced dementia and the critically ill. Several pain assessment tools for people with dementia are available at the City of Hope Pain and Palliative Care Resource Center website *(http://prc.coh.org)*.

### Patients With Substance Abuse Problems

HCPs are often reluctant to administer opioids to patients at risk for addiction or those with substance-abuse disorders for fear of promoting or worsening addictions. However, there is no evidence that providing opioid analgesia to these patients in any way worsens their addictive disease. In fact, the stress of unrelieved pain may contribute to relapse in the recovering patient or increased drug use in the patient who is actively abusing drugs.

**TABLE 8-18 Assessing Pain in Nonverbal Patients**

*The following assessment techniques are recommended.*
- Obtain a self-report when possible.
- Never assume a nonverbal person is unable to communicate pain in some manner as blinking, writing, hand gestures, or nodding can be ways to express pain or the absence of pain.
- Investigate potential causes of pain.
- Observe patient behaviors that indicate pain (e.g., grimacing, frowning, rubbing a painful area, groaning, restlessness).
- Obtain surrogate reports of pain from professional and family caregivers.
- Try to use analgesics and reassess the patient to observe for a decrease in pain-related behaviors.

Modified from Herr K, Coyne PJ, McCaffery M, et al: Position statement from the American Society for Pain Management Nursing (ASPMN). Pain assessment in the patient unable to self-report: position statement with clinical practice recommendations, *Pain Manag Nurs* 12:230, 2011.

**CHECK YOUR PRACTICE**

A 36-yr-old male patient is recovering from abdominal surgery to remove his spleen after an automobile accident. He is a known drug user. You are taking care of him and he is very irritable because he is not getting enough pain medication. You are reluctant to give him his PRN morphine as you are afraid you will contribute to his addiction problem.
- What should you do?

Guidelines for pain management in patients with addictive disease have been established by the American Society for Pain Management Nursing (ASPMN). These guidelines reflect your role in a team approach in which patients with addictive disease and pain have the right to be treated with dignity, respect, and the same quality of pain assessment and management as all other patients.

If the patient acknowledges substance abuse, determine the types and amounts of drugs used. Avoid exposing the patient to the drug of abuse, and effective equianalgesic doses of other opioids may be determined if daily drug doses are known. If a history of drug abuse is unknown or if the patient does not acknowledge substance abuse, suspect abuse when normal doses of analgesics do not relieve the patient's pain.

Aggressive behavior patterns and signs of withdrawal may also occur. Withdrawal symptoms can exacerbate pain and lead to drug-seeking behavior or illicit drug use. Toxicology screens may be helpful in determining recently used drugs. Discussing these findings with the patient may help gain the patient's cooperation in pain control.

Severe pain should be treated with opioids and at much higher doses than those used with drug-naive patients. The use of a single opioid is preferred. Avoid using a mixed opioid agonist-antagonist such as butorphanol or a partial agonist such as buprenorphine because these drugs may precipitate withdrawal symptoms. Nonopioid and adjuvant analgesics and nondrug pain relief measures may also be used as appropriate. To maintain opioid blood levels and prevent withdrawal symptoms, provide analgesics around the clock. Use supplemental doses to treat breakthrough pain. IV or PCA infusions may be considered for acute pain management.

Pain management for people with addiction is challenging and requires an interprofessional team approach. When possible, the team includes pain management and addiction specialists. Team members need to be aware of their own attitudes about people with substance abuse problems, which may result in undertreatment of pain.

## CASE STUDY

### Pain

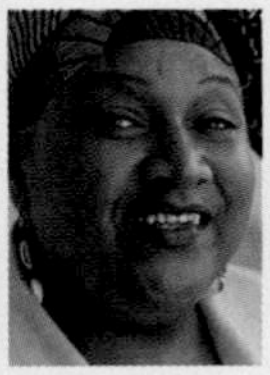

(©Ryan McVey/ Photodisc/ Thinkstock)

**Patient Profile**

K.C. is a 280-lb (127-kg) 68-year-old African American woman with diabetes who was admitted for an incision and drainage of a right abdominal abscess. She is being discharged on her second postoperative day. Her daughter will assist with dressing changes at home.

**Subjective Data**

- Lives alone
- Desires 0 pain but will accept 1 or 2 on a scale of 0 to 10
- Reports incision area pain as a 2 or 3 between dressing changes and as a 6 during dressing changes
- States sharp pain persists 1 to 2 hours after dressing change
- Reports pain between dressing changes controlled by two Percocet tablets
- Has history of fibromyalgia and is complaining of pain "everywhere"

**Objective Data**

- Requires qid dressing changes after discharge
- For discharge, Percocet (two tablets q4hr for pain PRN) is prescribed.

**Discussion Questions**

1. Describe the assessment data that are important for determining whether K.C. has adequate pain management.
2. How long should the daughter wait after the Percocet is given to begin the dressing change?
3. ***Patient-Centered Care:*** What additional pain therapies might you plan to help K.C. through the dressing change?
4. ***Priority Decision:*** What are the priority nursing interventions for K.C.?
5. ***Safety:*** What side effects might she experience because of her pain medication? How can these be safely managed?
6. ***Teamwork and Collaboration:*** To whom can you delegate teaching K.C. and her daughter the plan of care at home?
7. ***Priority Decision:*** Based on the data presented, what are the priority nursing diagnoses? Are there any collaborative problems?
8. ***Evidence-Based Practice:*** K.C.'s daughter asks you if any other strategies could be used to help decrease her mother's incisional pain and her overall fibromyalgia pain.

Answers available at *http://evolve.elsevier.com/Lewis/medsurg.*

## BRIDGE TO NCLEX EXAMINATION

The number of the question corresponds to the same-numbered outcome at the beginning of the chapter.

1. Pain is *best* described as
   **a.** a creation of a person's imagination.
   **b.** an unpleasant, subjective experience.
   **c.** a maladaptive response to a stimulus.
   **d.** a neurologic event resulting from activation of nociceptors.
2. A patient is receiving a PCA infusion after surgery to repair a hip fracture. She is sleeping soundly but awakens when the nurse speaks to her in a normal tone of voice. Her respirations are 8 breaths/minute. The *most* appropriate nursing action in this situation is to
   **a.** stop the PCA infusion.
   **b.** obtain an oxygen saturation level.
   **c.** continue to closely monitor the patient.
   **d.** administer naloxone and contact the physician.
3. Which words are *most* likely to be used to describe neuropathic pain *(select all that apply)*?
   **a.** Dull
   **b.** Mild
   **c.** Burning
   **d.** Shooting
   **e.** Shock-like
4. Unrelieved pain is
   **a.** expected after major surgery.
   **b.** expected in a person with cancer.
   **c.** dangerous and can lead to many physical and psychologic complications.
   **d.** an annoying sensation, but it is not as important as other physical care needs.
5. A cancer patient who reports ongoing, constant moderate pain with short periods of severe pain during dressing changes is
   **a.** probably exaggerating his pain.
   **b.** best treated by referral for surgical treatment of his pain.
   **c.** best treated by receiving a long-acting and a short-acting opioid.
   **d.** best treated by regularly scheduled short-acting opioids plus acetaminophen.
6. An example of distraction to provide pain relief is
   **a.** TENS.
   **b.** music.
   **c.** exercise.
   **d.** biofeedback.
7. Appropriate nonopioid analgesics for mild pain include *(select all that apply)*
   **a.** oxycodone.
   **b.** ibuprofen (Advil).
   **c.** lorazepam (Ativan).
   **d.** acetaminophen (Tylenol).
   **e.** codeine with acetaminophen (Tylenol #3).
8. An *important* nursing responsibility related to pain is to
   **a.** leave the patient alone to rest.
   **b.** help the patient appear to not be in pain.
   **c.** believe what the patient says about the pain.
   **d.** assume responsibility for eliminating the patient's pain.
9. Providing opioids to a dying patient who is experiencing moderate to severe pain
   **a.** may cause addiction.
   **b.** will probably be ineffective.
   **c.** is an appropriate nursing action.
   **d.** will likely hasten the person's death.

**10.** A nurse believes that patients with the same type of tissue injury should have the same amount of pain. This statement reflects
  **a.** a belief that will contribute to appropriate pain management.
  **b.** an accurate statement about pain mechanisms and an expected goal of pain therapy.
  **c.** a belief that will have no effect on the type of care provided to people in pain.
  **d.** a lack of knowledge about pain mechanisms, which is likely to contribute to poor pain management.

1. b, 2. c, 3. c, d, e, 4. c, 5. c, 6. b, 7. b, d, 8. c, 9. c, 10. d.

For rationales to these answers and even more NCLEX review questions, visit *http://evolve.elsevier.com/Lewis/medsurg.*

## EVOLVE WEBSITE

http://evolve.elsevier.com/Lewis/medsurg
**Review Questions (Online Only)**
**Key Points**
**Answer Keys for Questions**
- Rationales for Bridge to NCLEX Examination Questions
- Answer Guidelines for Case Study on p. 127

**Student Case Study**
- Patient With Pain

**Conceptual Care Map Creator**
**Audio Glossary**
**Content Updates**

## REFERENCES


1. Institute of Medicine Report from the Committee on Advancing Pain Research, Care, and Education: *Relieving pain in America: a blueprint for transforming prevention, care, education, and research*, Washington, DC, 2011, National Academies Press.
2. American Cancer Society. Retrieved from *http://www.cancer.org/research/survivaltreatmentresearch/palliative-care-research.*
3. McCaffery M: *Nursing practice theories related to cognition, bodily pain and man-environmental interactions*, Los Angeles, 1968, UCLA Students Store. (Classic)
4. Richardson P: Spirituality, religion and palliative care, *Ann Palliat Med* 3:150, 2014.
5. Sturgeon JA, Zautra AJ: Psychological resilience, pain catastrophizing, and positive emotions: perspectives on comprehensive modeling of individual pain adaptation, *Curr Pain Headache Rep* 17:317, 2013.
6. Mifflin KA, Kerr BJ: The transition from acute to chronic pain: understanding how different biological systems interact, *Can J Anaesth* 61:112, 2014.
7. Kerstman E, Ahn S, Battu S, et al: Neuropathic pain, *Handb Clin Neurol* 110:175, 2013.
8. Pelletier R, Higgins J, Bourbonnais D: Is neuroplasticity in the central nervous system the missing link to our understanding of chronic musculoskeletal disorders? *BMC Musculoskelet Disord* 12:25, 2015.
9. Mogil JS: Pain genetics: past, present and future, *Trends Genet* 28:258, 2012.

*10. van Hecke O, Austin SK, Khan RA, et al: Neuropathic pain in the general population: a systematic review of epidemiological studies, *Pain* 155:654, 2014.
*11. Bean DJ, Johnson MH, Kydd RR: The outcome of complex regional pain syndrome type 1: a systematic review, *J Pain* 15:677, 2014.
12. Herr K, Bjoro K, Decker S: Tools for assessment of pain in nonverbal older adults with dementia: a state-of-the-science review, *J Pain Symptom Manage* 31:170, 2006. (Classic)
13. Bashir MS, Khade A, Borkar P, et al: A comparative study between different pain rating scales in patients with osteoarthritis, *Indian J Physiol Pharmacol* 57:205, 2013.
*14. Gordon DB, Dahl J, Phillips P, et al: The use of "as-needed" range orders for opioid analgesic in the management of acute pain: a consensus statement of the American Society of Pain Management Nurses and the American Pain Society, *Pain Manag Nurs* 5:53, 2004. (Classic)
*15. de Leon-Casasola O: A review of the literature on multiple factors involved in postoperative pain course and duration, *Postgrad Med* 126:42, 2014.
16. Prabhakar A, Mancuso KF, Owen CP, et al: Perioperative analgesia outcomes and strategies, *Best Pract Res Clin Anesthesiol* 28:105, 2014.
*17. dela Cruz Ubaldo C, Hall NS, Le B: Postmarketing review of intravenous acetaminophen dosing based on Food and Drug Administration prescribing guidelines, *Pharmacotherapy* 34(Suppl 1):34S, 2014.
*18. Weimer MB, Chou R: Research gaps on methadone harms and comparative harms: findings from a review of the evidence for an American Pain Society and College on Problems of Drug Dependence clinical practice guideline, *J Pain* 15:366, 2014.
*19. Jungquist CR, Pasero C, Tripoli NM, et al: Instituting best practice for monitoring for opioid-induced advancing sedation in hospitalized patients, *Worldviews Evid Based Nurs* 11:350, 2014.
*20. Maguire DR, France CP: Impact of efficacy at the μ-opioid receptor on antinociceptive effects of combinations of μ-opioid receptor agonists and cannabinoid receptor agonists, *J Pharmacol Exp Ther* 35:383, 2014.
21. Simon SM, Schwartzberg LS: A review of rapid-onset opioids for breakthrough pain in patients with cancer, *J Opioid Manag* 10:207, 2014.
*22. Cooney MF, Czarnecki M, Dunwoody C, et al: American Society for Pain Management Nursing position statement with clinical practice guidelines: authorized agent controlled analgesia, *Pain Manag Nurs* 14:176, 2013.
23. Song JJ, Popescu A, Bell RL: Present and potential use of spinal cord stimulation to control chronic pain, *Pain Physician* 17:235, 2014.
*24. Shengelia R, Parker SJ, Ballin M, et al: Complementary therapies for osteoarthritis: are they effective? *Pain Manag Nurs* 14:e274, 2013.
*25. Crawford C, Lee C, Bingham J: Active Self-Care Therapies for Pain (PACT) Working Group: Sensory art therapies for the self-management of chronic pain symptoms, *Pain Med* 15(Suppl 1):S66, 2014.
26. The Joint Commission: Standard on pain assessment and management. Retrieved from *www.jointcommission.org.*
27. Oregon Nurses Association: ONA provides guidance on nurses' dilemma. Retrieved from *http://c.ymcdn.com/sites/www.oregonrn.org/resource/resmgr/imported/Assisted%20Suicide%20Adjusted.pdf.*

*Evidence-based information for clinical practice.

# Palliative Care at End of Life

*Linda A. L. Upchurch*

*You matter because you are you. You matter to the last moment of your life, and we will do all we can, not only to help you die peacefully, but also to live until you die.*

*Dame Cicely Saunders*

http://evolve.elsevier.com/Lewis/medsurg/

## LEARNING OUTCOMES

1. Discuss the purpose of palliative care.
2. Describe the purpose of and services provided by hospice.
3. Describe the physical and psychologic manifestations at the end of life.
4. Explain the process of grief and bereavement at the end of life.
5. Describe the nursing management of the dying patient.
6. Examine the cultural and spiritual issues related to end-of-life care.
7. Discuss vulnerable populations in end-of-life care.
8. Discuss ethical and legal issues in end-of-life care.
9. Explore the special needs of family caregivers in end-of-life care.
10. Discuss the special needs of the nurse who cares for dying patients and their families.

## KEY TERMS



## PALLIATIVE CARE

**Palliative care** is any form of care or treatment that focuses on reducing the severity of disease symptoms. The overall goals of palliative care are to (1) prevent and relieve suffering and (2) improve quality of life for patients with serious life-limiting illnesses[1] (Fig. 9-1). Specific goals of palliative care are listed in Table 9-1.

Ideally all patients receiving curative or restorative health care should receive palliative care at the same time. Palliative care extends into the period of end-of-life (EOL) care. Bereavement care follows the patient's death (Fig. 9-2).

Palliative care originated as EOL care in the 1960s. Initially this care focused on providing the relief of symptoms and emotional support to the patient, family, and significant others during the terminal phases of a serious life-limiting disease. Now that phase of palliative care is called palliative care at the end of life, which is the focus of this chapter.

The role of palliative care at the end of life is increasing in our current health care environment. Demographic changes in the population are increasing the demand for palliative care. For example, there are growing numbers of Baby Boomers turning 65. At the same time improvements in health care technology have led to longer life expectancies and an increased number of older adults. Older adults often have multiple chronic illnesses resulting in increased health care utilization.[2] Palliative care has been shown to (1) improve quality of life for those with chronic illness, (2) decrease the associated economic costs for their health care, and (3) alleviate the burden of caregivers for those with chronic and terminal illnesses.[3]

To optimize the benefits of palliative care, it should be initiated after a person receives a diagnosis of a life-limiting illness,

**TABLE 9-1 Goals of Palliative Care**

- Regard dying as a normal process.
- Provide relief from symptoms, including pain.
- Affirm life and neither hasten nor postpone death.
- Support holistic patient care and enhance quality of life.
- Offer support to patients to live as actively as possible until death.
- Offer support to the family during the patient's illness and in their own bereavement.

Adapted from World Health Organization: WHO definition of palliative care. Retrieved from *www.who.int/cancer/palliative/definition/en.*

Reviewed by Ellen Odell, DNP, ACNS-BC, CNE, APRN, Director of Nursing, Associate Professor, Department of Nursing, John Brown University, Siloam Springs, Arkansas; and Mary Ellen Tresgallo, DNP, MPH, FNP-BC, Assistant Professor of Nursing, Columbia University School of Nursing, New York, New York.

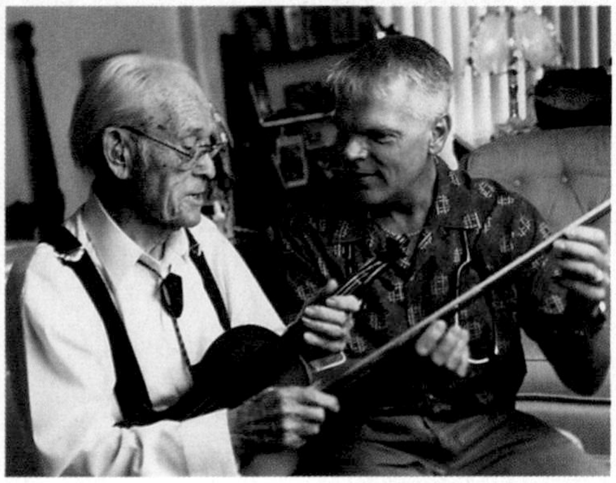

**FIG. 9-1** One goal of palliative care is to improve the quality of the patient's remaining life. (Courtesy Kathleen A. Pollard, RN, MSN, CHPN, Phoenix, Ariz.)

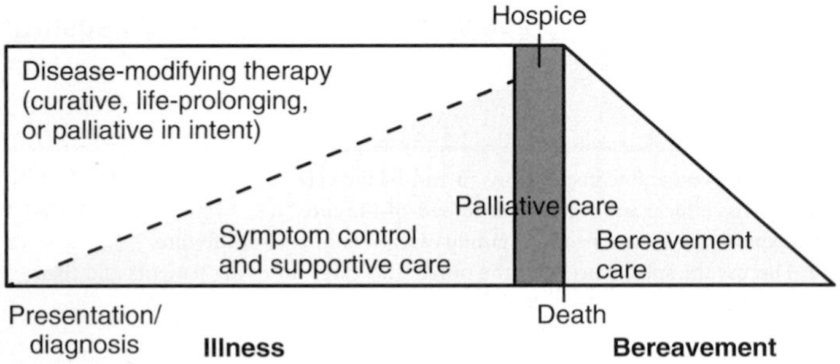


**FIG. 9-2** Continuum of care model showing integration of curative care, palliative and end-of-life/hospice care, and bereavement care. (Redrawn from Robert Wood Johnson Foundation: *The EPEC Project: Elements and models of end-of-life care*, 1999.)

such as cancer, heart failure, chronic obstructive pulmonary disease, dementia, or end-stage kidney disease. The palliative care team is an interprofessional collaboration involving physicians, nurses, social workers, pharmacists, chaplains, and other health care professionals. Communication among the patient, family, and interprofessional palliative team is important to provide optimal care. Patients may receive palliative care services in multiple settings, including the home, long-term and acute care, mental health facilities, rehabilitation centers, and prisons. Many institutions have established interprofessional palliative and hospice care teams.[1]

## HOSPICE CARE

Palliative care often includes hospice care before or at the end of life (Fig. 9-3). **Hospice** is not a place but a concept of care that provides compassion, concern, and support for persons in the last phases of a terminal disease (Fig. 9-4). The main goals of hospice care are to assist the patient to live fully as comfortable as possible and to die pain free and with dignity.[4] Hospice programs provide care with an emphasis on symptom management, advance care planning, spiritual care, and family support.

The major difference between palliative care and hospice care is that palliative care allows a person to simultaneously receive curative and palliative treatments. Hospice care is provided when the physician determines a person has 6 months or less to live, and that person or health care proxy decides to forgo curative treatments. Hospice is often underutilized, as many assume the person must be actively dying before hospice is necessary. On the contrary, it is important that the person be

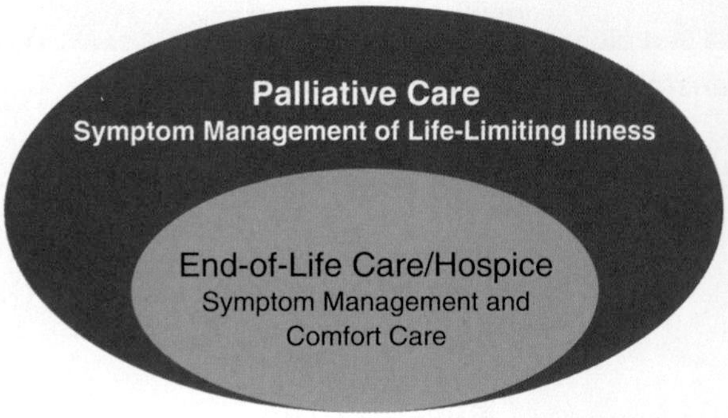


**FIG. 9-3** Relationship of palliative care and end-of-life care/hospice. (From Rosenberg M, Lamba S, Misra S: Palliative medicine and geriatric emergency care: challenges, opportunities, and basic principles, *Clin Geriatr Med* 29[1]:1, 2013.)

referred to hospice as soon as possible to facilitate palliation of physical, emotional, and spiritual distress so common at the end of life.

Approximately 1.5 million patients every year receive services through hospice programs. Almost half of the patients who die in the United States are under the care of a hospice program. More than three quarters of persons in hospice programs are over the age of 65 years, and the majority are white. The most common diagnoses are cancer and heart disease. Currently the median length of stay in a hospice program is 21 days.[4]

Hospice programs are organized under a variety of models. Some are hospital-based programs, others are part of existing home health care agencies, and others are freestanding or community-based programs. However, regardless of their organization, all hospice programs emphasize palliative rather than curative care, and quality rather than quantity of life.

Like palliative care, hospice care is provided in a variety of locations, including the home, inpatient settings, acute and long-term care facilities, and rehabilitation centers. Hospice services are available 24 hours a day, 7 days a week to provide help to patients and families in their homes. Inpatient hospice settings often have a relaxed and homelike atmosphere as much as possible (Fig. 9-5). Staff and volunteers are available for the patient and family.

A medically supervised interprofessional team and volunteers provide holistic hospice services. The hospice nurse plays a pivotal role in coordination of the hospice team.[5] Hospice nurses work with other interprofessional team members to provide care and support to the patient and family. Hospice

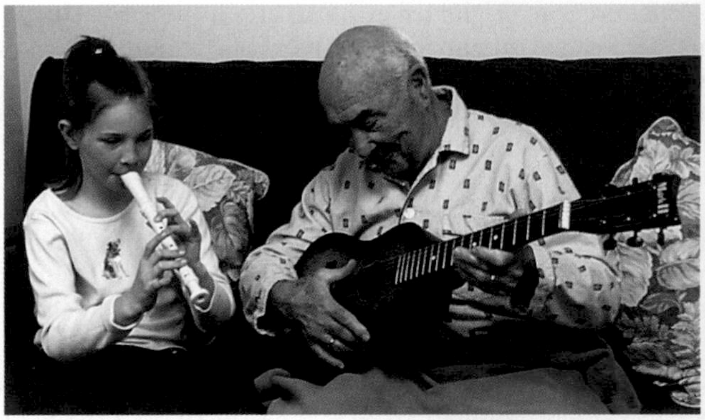

**FIG. 9-4** Hospice care is designed to provide compassion, concern, and support for the dying. (From Rick Brady, Riva, Md.)

## EVIDENCE-BASED PRACTICE

### *Translating Research Into Practice*

**Does Home Palliative Care Affect Odds of Dying at Home?**

***Clinical Question***

In adults with advanced disease (P) what is the effect of home palliative care (I) versus usual care (C) on odds of dying at home, caregiver outcomes, and cost-effectiveness (O)?

***Synthesis of Best Available Evidence***

- Systematic review of randomized controlled trials (RCTs), controlled clinical trials (CCTs), controlled before and after studies (CBAs), and interrupted time series (ITSs)
- 23 studies of family caregivers ($n = 4042$) and patients ($n = 37,561$) mainly with advanced cancer. Palliative care was specialized with home-based care teams for patients and/or family caregivers. Usual care included community, hospital, home health, and hospice care. Caregiver outcomes were (1) burden in last weeks of care and (2) grief after the patient's death.
- Although >50% of people worldwide prefer to die at home, less than 33% of all deaths take place at home.
- Specialized palliative home care almost doubled the odds of the patient's death occurring at home. There was no difference in caregiver grief when specialized care was compared to usual care from the time the patient died to 13 months later.
- Conflicting evidence exists if palliative home care reduces caregiver burden or is cost effective.

***Conclusions***

- Home palliative team care increases the likelihood of the patient dying at home compared to usual care.
- It is inconclusive if palliative home care is cost effective or affects caregiver outcomes.

***Implications for Nursing Practice***

1. How would you help patients who are undecided about palliative home care and yet desire to die at home?
2. What information would you provide caregivers who are concerned that palliative home care will result in greater grief related to the patient's death?

***Reference for Evidence***

Gomes B, Calanzani N, Curiale V, et al: Effectiveness and cost-effectiveness of home palliative care services for adults with advanced illness and their caregivers, *Cochrane Database Syst Rev* 6:CD007760, 2013.

*P*, Patient population of interest; *I*, intervention or area of interest; *C*, comparison of interest or comparison group; *O*, outcomes of interest; *T*, timing (see p. 15).

nurses are educated in pain control and symptom management, spiritual assessment, and assessment and management of family needs. To meet patient and family needs, the hospice nurse needs excellent teaching skills, compassion, flexibility, cultural competence, and adaptability.

The decision to begin hospice care is difficult for several reasons. Frequently patients, families, physicians, and other HCPs lack information about hospice care. Some cultural/ethnic groups may underutilize hospice because of lack of awareness of hospice services, desire to continue with potentially curative therapies, and concerns about lack of minority hospice workers.[6] Physicians may be reluctant to give referrals because they sometimes view a patient's decline as their personal failure. Some patients or family members see it as giving up.

It is important for you to consider potential barriers to hospice care in vulnerable populations. These may include veterans, homeless, immigrants, impoverished, disabled, or institutionalized persons. In these populations, besides the hospice team, you may need to collaborate with community partners to facilitate supportive services to meet everyday needs of the patient and family.[7]

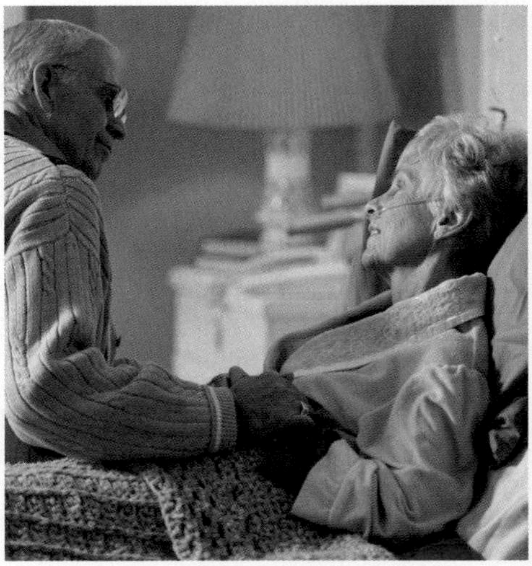

**FIG. 9-5** Inpatient hospice settings have been deinstitutionalized to make the atmosphere as relaxed and homelike as possible. (©Photodisc/Thinkstock)

Hospice services are covered by Medicare, Medicaid, and many private insurance agencies. Admission to a hospice program has two criteria. The first criterion is that the patient must desire the services and agree in writing that only hospice care (and not curative care) can be used to treat the terminal illness. Patients in hospice programs can withdraw from the program at any time (e.g., if their condition unexpectedly improves). Patients can receive care for other health problems that are not related to the terminal illness. However, those services may not be covered by the hospice, Medicare, Medicaid, or by the patient's insurance company.[8]

The second criterion is that the patient must be considered eligible for hospice. Medicare, Medicaid, and other insurers require that two physicians certify that the patient's prognosis is terminal, with less than 6 months to live. After this initial certification, only one physician (e.g., the hospice medical director) is needed to recertify the patient. It is important to realize that the physician who certified that a hospice patient is terminal does not "guarantee" death within 6 months. If a patient in hospice survives beyond 6 months, Medicare and other reimbursement organizations will continue to reimburse for more extended periods of treatment if the patient still meets enrollment criteria.

Occasionally, a patient's condition stabilizes, at which time the patient may be discharged from hospice care. This decision is made after review of the current treatment plan and input from members of the interprofessional hospice team.

## DEATH

**Death** occurs when all vital organs and body systems cease to function. It is the irreversible cessation of cardiovascular, respiratory, and brain function.

**Brain death** is an irreversible loss of all brain functions, including those of the brainstem. Brain death is a clinical diagnosis, and it occurs when the cerebral cortex stops functioning or is irreversibly destroyed.[9]

Since the development of technology that assists in supporting life, controversies have arisen over the exact definition of death. Questions and discussions have focused on whether brain death occurs when the whole brain (cortex and brainstem) ceases activity or when function of the cortex alone stops. The American Academy of Neurology developed the diagnostic criteria guidelines for clinical diagnosis of brain death. These criteria for brain death include coma or unresponsiveness, absence of brainstem reflexes, and apnea. Specific assessments by a physician are required to validate each of the criteria.[9]

Currently, legal and medical standards require that all brain function must cease for brain death to be pronounced and life support to be disconnected. Diagnosis of brain death is of particular importance when organ donation is an option. In some states and under specific circumstances, registered nurses are legally permitted to pronounce death. Policies and procedures may vary from state to state and among health care institutions.

## END-OF-LIFE CARE

**End of life** generally refers to the final phase of a patient's illness when death is imminent. The time from diagnosis of a terminal illness to death varies considerably, depending on the patient's diagnosis and extent of disease.

The Institute of Medicine defines *end of life* as the period during which an individual copes with declining health from a terminal illness or from the frailties associated with advanced age, even if death is not clearly imminent.[10] In some cases it is obvious to HCPs that the patient is at the end of life, but in other cases they may be uncertain if the end is close at hand. This uncertainty adds to the challenge of answering common questions the patient and family may ask, such as, "How much time is left?"

*End-of-life care* (EOL care) is the term used for issues and services related to death and dying. EOL care focuses on physical and psychosocial needs for the patient and family. The goals for EOL care are to (1) provide comfort and supportive care during the dying process, (2) improve the quality of the patient's remaining life, (3) help ensure a dignified death, and (4) provide emotional support to the family.

### Physical Manifestations at End of Life

As death approaches, metabolism is reduced and the body gradually slows down until all functions end. Respiratory changes are common at the end of life. Respirations may be rapid or slow, shallow, and irregular. Breath sounds may become wet and noisy, both audibly and on auscultation. Noisy, wet-sounding respirations, termed the **death rattle** or terminal secretions, are caused by mouth breathing and accumulation of mucus in the airways. **Cheyne-Stokes respiration** is a pattern of breathing characterized by alternating periods of apnea and deep, rapid breathing. When respirations cease, the heart stops beating within a few minutes. The physical manifestations of approaching death are listed in Table 9-2.

### Psychosocial Manifestations at End of Life

A variety of feelings and emotions can affect the dying patient and family at the end of life (Table 9-3). Most patients and families struggle with a terminal diagnosis and the realization that there is no cure. The patient and family may feel overwhelmed, fearful, powerless, and fatigued. The family's response

**TABLE 9-2 Physical Manifestations at End of Life**

| System | Manifestations |
|---|---|
| **Sensory system** | |
| Hearing | • Usually last sense to disappear |
| Touch | • Decreased sensation<br>• Decreased perception of pain and touch |
| Taste and smell | • Decreased with disease progression |
| Sight | • Blurring of vision<br>• Sinking and glazing of eyes<br>• Blink reflex absent<br>• Eyelids remain half-open |
| **Cardiovascular system** | • Increased heart rate; later slowing and weakening of pulse<br>• Irregular rhythm<br>• Decreased BP<br>• Delayed absorption of drugs administered IM or subcutaneously |
| **Respiratory system** | • Increased respiratory rate<br>• Cheyne-Stokes respiration (pattern of respiration characterized by alternating periods of apnea and deep, rapid breathing)<br>• Inability to cough or clear secretions resulting in grunting, gurgling, or noisy congested breathing (death rattle or terminal secretions)<br>• Irregular breathing, gradually slowing down to terminal gasps (may be described as guppy breathing) |
| **Urinary system** | • Gradual decrease in urine output<br>• Incontinence of urine<br>• Inability to urinate |
| **Gastrointestinal system** | • Slowing or cessation of GI function (may be enhanced by pain-relieving drugs)<br>• Accumulation of gas<br>• Distention and nausea<br>• Loss of sphincter control, producing incontinence<br>• Bowel movement before imminent death or at time of death |
| **Musculoskeletal system** | • Gradual loss of ability to move<br>• Sagging of jaw resulting from loss of facial muscle tone<br>• Difficulty speaking<br>• Swallowing becoming more difficult<br>• Difficulty maintaining body posture and alignment<br>• Loss of gag reflex<br>• Jerking seen in patients on high doses of opioids |
| **Integumentary system** | • Mottling on hands, feet, arms, and legs<br>• Cold, clammy skin<br>• Cyanosis of nose, nail beds, knees<br>• "Waxlike" skin when very near death |

**TABLE 9-3 Psychosocial Manifestations at End of Life**

| | |
|---|---|
| • Altered decision making | • Helplessness |
| • Anxiety about unfinished business | • Life review |
| • Decreased socialization | • Peacefulness |
| • Fear of loneliness | • Restlessness |
| • Fear of meaninglessness of one's life | • Saying goodbyes |
| • Fear of pain | • Unusual communication |
| | • Vision-like experiences |
| | • Withdrawal |

**TABLE 9-4 Kübler-Ross Model of Grief**

| Stage | What Person May Say | Characteristics |
|---|---|---|
| **Denial** | No, not me. It cannot be true. | Denies the loss has taken place and may withdraw. This response may last minutes to months. |
| **Anger** | Why me? | May be angry at the person who inflicted the hurt (even after death) or at the world for letting it happen. May be angry with self for letting an event (e.g., car accident) take place, even if nothing could have stopped it. |
| **Bargaining** | Yes me, but ... | May make bargains with God, asking, "If I do this, will you take away the loss?" |
| **Depression** | Yes me, and I am sad. | Feels numb, although anger and sadness may remain underneath |
| **Acceptance** | Yes me, but it is okay. | Anger, sadness, and mourning have tapered off. Accepts the reality of the loss |

Adapted from Kübler-Ross E: *On death and dying*, New York, 1969, Macmillan. (Classic)

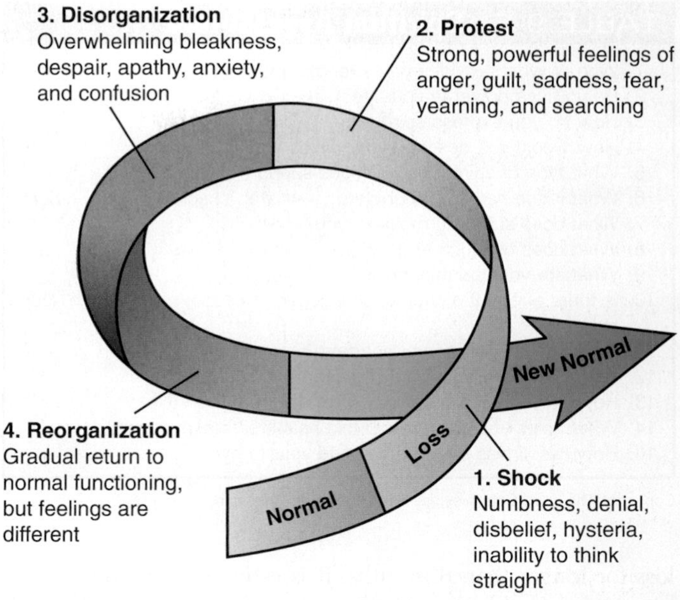


**FIG. 9-6** The grief wheel model begins with the normal state at the bottom. After a person goes through the grief process, eventually the grief will resolve. However, because of the loss, the normal state is not the same as before. The challenge is to accept the "new normal." (Adapted from Stress Free Living by Trevor Powell with permission from DK, a division of Penguin Random House LLC. Copyright © 2000 Dorling Kindersley Limited.)

depends in part on the type and length of the illness and their relationship with the person.

The patient's needs and wishes must be respected. Patients need time to think and express their feelings. Response time to questions may be sluggish because of fatigue, weakness, and confusion.

## Bereavement and Grief

Although the terms are often used interchangeably, *bereavement* refers to the state of loss, and *grief* refers to the reaction to loss. **Bereavement** is the period following the death of a loved one during which grief is experienced and mourning occurs. The time spent in bereavement depends on a number of factors, including how attached one was to the person who died and how much time was spent anticipating the loss.

**Grief** is a normal reaction to loss. Grief occurs in response to the real loss of a loved one and the loss of what might have been. Grief is dynamic and includes both psychologic and physiologic responses following a loss. Psychologic responses include anger, guilt, anxiety, sadness, depression, and despair. Physiologic reactions include sleeping problems, changes in appetite, physical problems, and illness.

Grief is a powerful emotional state that affects all aspects of a person's life. It is a complex and intense emotional experience. In the Kübler-Ross model of grief, there are five stages[11] (Table 9-4). Not every person experiences all the stages of grieving, and they are not always progressive. It is common to reach a stage and then go backward. For example, a person may have reached the stage of bargaining and then revert to the denial or anger stage.

Another model of grief is the grief wheel (Fig. 9-6). After a person experiences the loss, he or she feels *shock* (numbness, denial, inability to think straight). Next is the *protest* stage, in which a person experiences anger, guilt, sadness, fear, and searching. Then comes the *disorganization* stage, in which a person feels despair, apathy, anxiety, and confusion. The next stage is *reorganization*, in which a person gradually returns to normal functioning, but he or she feels different. The final stage is the *new normal*. Eventually the destabilization experienced in grief resolves and a normal state can begin. However, because of the loss, the normal state is not the same as before. The challenge is to accept the new normal. Trying to go back to the "old" normal (which is not there anymore) is what causes a great deal of anxiety and stress.

The manner in which a person grieves depends on factors such as the relationship with the person who has died (e.g., spouse, parent), physical and emotional coping resources, concurrent life stresses, cultural beliefs, and personality. Additional factors that affect the grief response include mental and physical health, economic resources, religious influences or spiritual beliefs, family relationships, social support, and time spent preparing for the death. Issues that occurred before the death (e.g., marital problems) may affect the grief response.[12]

The grief experience for the caregiver of the patient with a chronic illness often begins long before the actual death event. This is called *anticipatory grief*. Patients at the end of life can also experience anticipatory grief.

Working in a positive way through the grief process helps to adapt to the loss.[12] Grief that assists the person in accepting the reality of death is called *adaptive grief*, which is a healthy response. It may be associated with grieving before a death actually occurs or when the inevitability of the death is known. Indicators of adaptive grief include the ability to see some good resulting from the death and positive memories of the deceased person.

Dysfunctional reactions to loss can occur, and the physical and psychologic impact of the loved one's death may persist for years. *Prolonged grief disorder*, formerly called *complicated grief*, is a term used to describe prolonged and intense mourning. Prolonged grief disorder can include symptoms such as recurrent and severe distressing emotions and intrusive thoughts related to the loss of a loved one, self-neglect, and denial of the

**TABLE 9-5 Spiritual Assessment**

1. Who or what provides you strength and hope?
2. Do you use prayer in your life?
3. How do you express spirituality?
4. How would you describe your philosophy of life?
5. What type of spiritual or religious support do you desire?
6. What is the name of your clergy, minister, chaplain, pastor, rabbi?
7. What does suffering mean to you?
8. What does dying mean to you?
9. What are your spiritual goals?
10. Is there a role of a church, synagogue, mosque, or temple in your life?
11. Has belief in God been important in your life?
12. How does your faith help you cope with illness?
13. How do you keep going day after day?
14. What helps you get through this health care experience?
15. How has illness affected you and your family?



loss for longer than 6 months. It is estimated that one in five bereaved individuals experiences prolonged grief disorder. Those who experience prolonged grief disorder are at great risk for illness and may have work and social impairments.[13]

Bereavement and grief counseling are core components of patient- and family-centered palliative care. The goal of a bereavement program is to provide support and to assist survivors in the transition to a life without the deceased person. Incorporate grief support into the plan of care for the family and significant others during the patient's illness and after the death.

Priority interventions for grief must focus on providing an environment that allows the patient and family to express their feelings, such as anger, fear, and guilt. Discussion of feelings helps the patient and family work toward resolution of the grief process. Respect for the patient's privacy and need or desire to talk (or not to talk) is important. Honesty in answering questions and giving information is essential.

## Spiritual Needs

Assessment of spiritual needs in EOL care is a key consideration (Table 9-5). Spiritual needs do not necessarily equate to religion. **Spirituality** is defined as those beliefs, values, and practices that relate to the search for existential meaning and purpose. It may or may not include a belief in a higher power.[14] A person may not be part of a particular religion but have a deep spirituality. Many times at the end of life, patients question their beliefs about a higher power, their journey through life, religion, and an afterlife (Fig. 9-7). Some patients may choose to pursue a spiritual path. Some may not. Respect an individual's choice. Assess the patient's and family's preferences related to spiritual guidance or pastoral care services and make appropriate referrals.

Deep-seated spiritual beliefs may surface for some patients when they deal with their terminal diagnosis and related issues. Spiritual distress may occur.[15] Characteristics of spiritual distress include anger toward God or a higher being, change in behavior and mood, desire for spiritual assistance, or displaced anger toward clergy.

Spirituality has been associated with decreased despair in patients at the end of life. Some dying patients are secure in their faith about the future. It is common to observe patients relinquishing material possessions of life and focusing on values

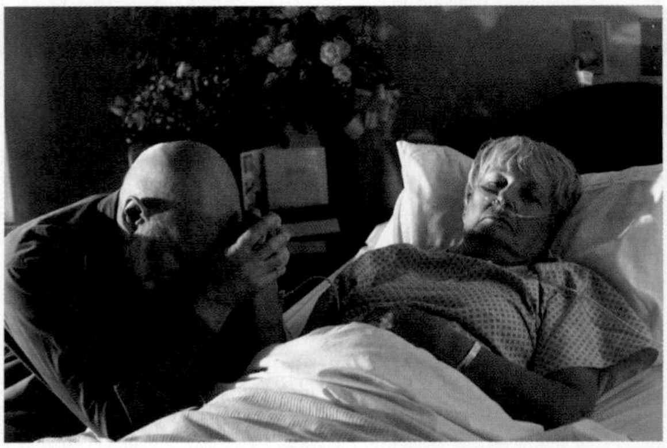

**FIG. 9-7** Spiritual needs are an important consideration in end-of-life care. (©Photodisc/Thinkstock)

that they believe will lead them on to another place. Many turn to religion because it may provide order to the world even in the presence of physical decline, social losses, suffering, and impending death. Religion may offer an existential meaning that offers a sense of peace and recognition of one's place in the broader cosmic context.[15]

## Culturally Competent Care: End of Life

Culture and ethnicity are important considerations for patients who are receiving palliative and EOL care and their families. Cultural beliefs affect a person's understanding of and reaction to death or loss. In some cultural/ethnic groups, death and dying are private matters shared only with significant others. Often feelings are repressed or internalized. People who believe in "toughing it out" or "being strong" may not express themselves when they are experiencing a loss. Some cultural groups, such as African Americans and Hispanic/Latinos, may easily express their feelings and emotions. Kinship tends to be strong in the Hispanic culture, and immediate and extended family provide support for one another. Expressing feelings of loss is encouraged and accepted easily.[16]

If palliative or hospice care is recommended, some cultural/ethnic groups are less likely to use these resources. For example, African Americans use hospice care less often because they value "toughness" in times of hardship. For Hispanics, often spouses and daughters are involved in decisions regarding palliative care and hospice.[16]

Consider patient attitudes toward death and suffering and preferences for information. The decision to use palliative care or hospice services may be perceived as "giving up" or receiving second-rate care. Such attitudes are best approached through clear, open discussions with the patient and family about the philosophy and services of palliative and hospice organizations. Culture and ethnicity affect decision making with regard to life support and withholding and withdrawing of treatments.[17] In some cultures, such as the Filipino American culture, it may be appropriate to first discuss a terminal diagnosis with the family before informing the patient.

Rituals associated with dying are part of all cultures.[16] In certain cultures the family may want to keep constant vigil in the room of a dying patient or in the waiting area. For example, some Jewish Americans believe that the spirit should not be alone when it leaves the body at the time of death. Therefore someone who is terminally ill should never be left alone. The

Jewish culture believes all body tissues must be buried with the individual. Once a death has occurred, some cultures, such as the Puerto Rican American culture, may want to kiss and touch the body to say goodbye. In the Islamic cultures the traditional rites of washing, shrouding, funeral prayers, and burial are done as soon as possible.

Families with non–English-speaking members are at risk for receiving less information about their family member's critical illness and prognosis.[18] Cultural variations also exist in symptom expression (e.g., pain expression) and use of health care services. Providing culturally competent care requires assessment of nonverbal cues such as grimaces, body position, and decreased or guarded movements. Issues related to pain assessment and management are discussed in Chapter 8.

Many differences exist among cultural beliefs and values in relation to death and dying. Your assessment of beliefs and preferences should be made on an individual basis to avoid stereotyping individuals with different cultural belief systems. This includes assessing and documenting the patient's cultural background, concerns, health practices, and attitudes about suffering. Early in the assessment, ask the patient and family to describe their desires for care before death and care of the body after death. Use open-ended questions related to the patient's perspectives on his or her illness and the patient's expectations of care. Use this assessment to guide the patient's plan of care and evaluation. You can also suggest or plan grief and bereavement counseling for the family. Accommodations must be made related to the patient's language, diet, and cultural beliefs and practices. When appropriate, access medical interpreter services so that the patient's wishes are known. (Culturally competent care is discussed in Chapter 2.)

## LEGAL AND ETHICAL ISSUES AFFECTING END-OF-LIFE CARE

Patients and families struggle with many decisions during the terminal illness and dying experience. Many people decide that the outcomes related to their care should be based on their own wishes and values. It is important to provide information to assist patients with these decisions. The decisions may involve the choice for (1) organ and tissue donations, (2) advance directives (e.g., medical power of attorney, living wills), (3) resuscitation, (4) mechanical ventilation, and (5) feeding tube placement.

*Decisional capacity* refers to the ability to consent or refuse care. It means that the individual has an understanding and appreciation of the information that is shared and has the capacity to engage in the reasoning process.

### Organ and Tissue Donation

Persons who are legally competent may choose organ donation. Any body part or the entire body may be donated. The decision to donate organs or to provide anatomic gifts may be made by a person before death or by immediate family after death. Family permission must be obtained at the time of donation.[19]

Some people carry donor cards. Some states allow organ donation to be marked on drivers' licenses. The names of agencies that handle organ donation vary by state and community. Common names for such an agency may be the organ bank, organ-sharing network, and organ-sharing alliance. Organ and tissue donations follow specific legal guidelines. Legal requirements and facility policies for organ or tissue donation must be followed. The physician must be notified immediately when organ donation is intended, because some tissues must be used within hours after death.

### Advance Care Planning and Advance Directives

*Advance care planning* is a process that involves having patients (1) think through their values and goals for treatment, (2) talk about their values and goals with others, and (3) document them. **Advance directives** are the written documents that provide information about the patient's wishes and his or her designated spokesperson (Table 9-6).

The first advance directive was known by laypersons as a *living will.* Most states have replaced the idea of living wills with *natural death acts,* which may include *directive to physicians* (DTPs), *durable power of attorney for health care* (DPAHC), *medical power of attorney* (MPOA), and *power of attorney for health care* (POAH). Under the natural death acts, an individual can tell the physician exactly what treatment is or is not desired. Each state has its own unique requirements. Keep in mind that patients often change their minds about desired treatments as their disease state progresses. Therefore it is important to reassess a patient's advance directives. For cognitively impaired older adults, consider the person's values and manner of life to make health care decisions consistent with decisions they made when they were cognitively intact.

Copies of state-specific forms can be obtained from local medical associations and on the Internet. However, a person may write his or her wishes without special forms. Verbal directives may be given to physicians with specific instructions in the presence of two witnesses. Based on this directive, the physician may use a Physician Order for Life-Sustaining Treatment (POLST) or Medical Order for Life-Sustaining Treatment (MOLST) to outline current treatment options that honor the person's desire for treatment (Table 9-6).

The person retains a copy of the order to be used in the case of any emergency in which the primary physician is not readily available for consultation. Attorneys and notaries may not be required in the development of these directives. If the person is not capable of communicating his or her wishes, the surrogate decision maker (most often family or significant other) determines the measures that will or will not be taken. In this case, the physician and nurse can discuss the options that are available with the family. Then it is important to document the family's decision. This is important because often nurses and other medical professionals do not know who can legally make EOL decisions for patients when they no longer have decisional capacity.

### Resuscitation

Cardiopulmonary resuscitation (CPR) has become common practice in health care. Patients who have respiratory or cardiac arrest are given CPR unless a *do-not-resuscitate (DNR) order* is given by the physician. A DNR order is a written medical order that documents a patient's wishes regarding resuscitation and, more important, the patient's desire to avoid CPR.[20]

The patient or family has the right to decide whether CPR will be used. It is no longer the sole decision of the physician. The American Nurses Association (ANA) supports the patient's right to self-determination and believes that nurses have a primary role in supporting the patient and family's decisions.[21]

**TABLE 9-6 Common Documents Used in End-of-Life Care**

| Document | Description | Special Considerations |
|---|---|---|
| **Advance directive** | General term used to describe documents that give instructions about future medical care and treatments and who should make the decisions in the event the person is unable to communicate | • Should comply with guidelines established by state of residence |
| **Allow Natural Death (AND)** | Written order acknowledging that comfort measures only are being provided to patient. Used in many palliative care and hospice settings to indicate that patient wants to die naturally with dignity and comfort | • In many settings may be used in conjunction with DNR terminology to ensure patient/family wishes for advance directives are followed (DNR/AND) |
| **Directive to physicians (DTP)** | Written document specifying the patient's wish to be allowed to die without heroic or extraordinary measures | • Indicates specific measures to be used or withheld |
| **Do not resuscitate (DNR)** | Written physician's order instructing HCPs not to attempt CPR. DNR order often requested by family | • Must indicate any specific measures to be used or withheld. Must be signed by a physician to be valid |
| **Power of attorney for health care (POAH)** | Term used by some states to describe a document used for listing the person(s) to make health care decisions should a patient become unable to make informed decisions for self | • May be the same as medical power of attorney<br>• Indicates specific measures to be used or withheld |
| **Living will** | Lay term used to describe any documents that give instructions about future medical care and treatments or the wish to be allowed to die without heroic or extraordinary measures should the patient be unable to communicate for self | • Must identify specific treatments that a person wants or does not want at end of life |
| **Medical power of attorney (MPOA)** | Term used by some states to describe a document used for listing the person(s) to make health care decisions should a patient become unable to make informed decisions for self | • May be the same as durable power of attorney for health care, health care proxy, or appointment of a health care agent or surrogate. Specifies measures to be used or withheld<br>• Person appointed may be called a health care agent, surrogate, attorney-in-fact, or proxy. |
| **Physician Order for Life-Sustaining Treatment (POLST) or Medical Order for Life-Sustaining Treatment (MOLST)** | A standardized physician order guided by the patient's medical condition and based upon personal preferences verbalized by patient or expressed in advance directive | • Only for those whose illness may limit life to less than 12 months<br>• Guides current treatments. Differs from advance directive, which guides future treatments<br>• Physician completes form based on discussion with patient or authorized representative, or in review of advance directive. Signed by physician, patient, or patient representative<br>• Printed on bright pink paper |

*CPR,* Cardiopulmonary resuscitation.

A physician's order should be written concerning the patient's or family's wishes for the use of CPR. Several different types of CPR decisions can be made. Complete and total heroic measures, which may include CPR, drugs, and mechanical ventilation, can be referred to as a *full code.* Some people choose variations of the full code. A *chemical code* involves the use of drugs for resuscitation without the use of CPR. A "no code," or a DNR order, allows the person to die with comfort measures only and without the interference of technology. Some states have implemented a form called *out-of-hospital DNR* for use by terminally ill patients who wish to have no heroic measures used to prolong life after they leave an acute care facility.[22]

*Allow Natural Death (AND)* is a term being used to replace "no code" or DNR. This term more accurately conveys what actually happens. It is also sometimes referred to as *"comfort measures only"* status, meaning that all comfort measures associated with pain control and symptom management are carried out, but the natural physiologic progression to death is not delayed or interrupted. The use of this type of language means that care is not withheld, but rather is supportive while allowing nature to take its course. It is meant to promote comfort and dignity at the end of life.

Withholding or withdrawing treatments must be included in an advance directive. The directive must clearly state what is to be done and what is not to be done. The ANA position statement states that the decision to withhold artificial nutrition and hydration should be made by the patient or surrogate together with the interprofessional team.[21] For patients who are no longer receiving artificial nutrition and hydration, it is important to continue to provide expert nursing care.

You need to be aware of legal issues and the patient's wishes. Advance directives and organ donor information should be located in the medical record and identified on the patient's record and/or the nursing care plan. All caregivers responsible for the patient need to know the patient's wishes. Additionally, you are responsible for becoming familiar with state, local, and agency procedures in EOL care documentation.

*Euthanasia* is the deliberate act of hastening death. The ANA statement on active euthanasia states that the nurse should not participate in active euthanasia, because such an act is in direct violation of the Code for Nurses, ethical traditions and goals of the profession, and its covenant with society.

*Physician-assisted suicide* is legal in some states. In this case, the physician provides the means and/or information about how the patient can commit suicide. As a nurse, you have an obligation to provide timely, humane, comprehensive, and compassionate EOL care. Euthanasia should not be confused with *palliative sedation,* which is the use of medications to intentionally produce sedation to relieve intractable symptoms and distress in a patient who is imminently dying.[5] The intent of palliative sedation is to relieve pain and suffering and not to shorten life or to hasten death, as is the case with euthanasia.

The use of opioids for symptom management at the end of life is often misunderstood and feared by patients, families, and HCPs. For this reason, many patients refuse to take the medications, which leads to physical and emotional suffering due to uncontrolled pain and symptoms. Your ethical obligation is to relieve suffering, which includes giving medications that have the potential of producing harm, such as with opioids. The *principle of double effect* refers to a principle that regards it morally permissible to give a medication that has the potential for harm if it is given with the intent of relieving pain and suffering and not intended to hasten death.[5]

As a nurse, your role is to teach the patient and family about addiction and tolerance to and dependence on medications. The person with terminal illness should not be concerned with addiction when the goal of treatment is comfort. Pain management is discussed in Chapter 8.

## NURSING MANAGEMENT: END OF LIFE

Nurses spend more time with patients near the end of life than any other health care professionals. Nursing care of terminally ill and dying patients is holistic and encompasses all psychosocial and physical needs. Respect, dignity, and comfort are important for the patient and family. Although there is no cure for the person's disease, the treatment plan still consists of assessment, planning, implementation, and evaluation. The main difference is that the focus of care is on the management of the symptoms of the disease, not necessarily the disease itself. Additionally, nurses who care for the dying need to recognize their own needs when dealing with grief and dying.

### Nursing Assessment

Assessment of the terminally ill or dying patient varies with the patient's condition. Be sensitive and do not impose repeated, unnecessary assessments on the dying patient. When possible, use health history data that are available in the medical record rather than tiring the patient with an interview.

Document the specific event or change that brought the patient into the health care setting. Record the patient's medical diagnoses, medication profile, and allergies.

If the patient is alert, do a brief review of the body systems. Assess for discomfort, pain, nausea, and dyspnea so that prompt interventions can be implemented using evidence-based tools for symptom assessment. These include numeric scales or visual analog scales for pain rating. In addition, evaluate and manage co-morbidities or acute episodes of problems such as diabetes mellitus or headache. Elicit information about the patient's abilities, food and fluid intake, patterns of sleep and rest, and response to the stress of terminal illness. Assess the patient's ability to cope with the diagnosis and prognosis of the illness. Also determine the family's capacity to manage the needed care and to cope with the illness and its consequences.

The physical assessment is abbreviated and focuses on changes that accompany terminal illness and the specific disease process.[23] The frequency of assessment depends on the patient's stability, but assessment is performed at least every 8 hours in the institutional setting. For patients cared for in their homes by hospice programs, assessment may occur weekly. As changes occur, assessment and documentation may have to be completed more frequently. If the patient is in the final hours of life, the physical assessment may be limited to essential data.

Key elements of a social assessment include determining the relationships and patterns of communication among the family. If multiple family members are present, listen to concerns from different members. Differences in expectations and interpersonal conflict can produce disruptions during the dying process and after the death of the loved one. Social assessment also includes evaluating the goals of the patient and family.

As death approaches, monitor the patient for multiple systems that often are failing during the EOL period. This requires vigilance and attention to physical changes that are often subtle. Neurologic assessment is especially important and

## ETHICAL/LEGAL DILEMMAS

### *End-of-Life Care*

**Situation**

A.P. is a terminally ill 50-year-old woman with metastatic breast cancer who has been hospitalized with severe bone pain. She moans at rest and verbalizes severe pain from any movement to reposition her. The present dose of IV morphine is not adequately controlling her pain. At the team conference the nurses discuss the need for more effective pain control but are concerned that additional pain medicine could hasten her death.

**Ethical/Legal Points for Consideration**

- Adequate pain relief is an important outcome for all patients, especially patients who are terminally ill.
- The *Code of Ethics for Nurses* addresses the responsibility of the nurse to relieve suffering and have conversations with patients and families about pain and symptom management.[1]
- The *principle of beneficence* means that care is provided to benefit patients. The goal of adequate pain control in the terminally ill to alleviate suffering is based on the *principle of nonmaleficence* (preventing or reducing harm to the patient). The secondary effect of hastening the patient's death is ethically justified and known as the *double effect*.
- Legally, the *standard of care* is used to define the nursing acts that are required for safe and competent nursing practice. When the actual nursing care falls below the standard of care, it is considered negligent and unsafe, and the nurse is at risk for being found incompetent.
- In a court of law, the standard of care in nursing is determined by nursing experts and evidence-based practices. The increasing use of technology to access the latest scientific findings is changing the standard of nursing care to a national, if not global, standard defined by research findings and nationally recognized expert testimony. Standards for providing expert nursing care and counseling at end of life are available.[1]
- In A.P.'s situation the standard of care is that the patient will experience pain relief. Failure of the nurse to act assertively to achieve pain relief for the patient and failure to effectively use resources to obtain that pain relief will be considered below the standard of care and unsafe and incompetent practice.

**Discussion Questions**

1. What types of discussions need to occur among the health care team, patient, and family as the terminally ill patient approaches this phase of care?
2. Distinguish between promotion of comfort and relief of pain in dying patients, and between assisted suicide and euthanasia.

**Reference**

1. Code of Ethics for Nurses: *www.nursingworld.org/MainMenuCategories/EthicsStandards/Ethics-Position-Statements.*

includes level of consciousness, presence of reflexes, and pupil responses. Evaluation of vital signs, skin color, and temperature indicates changes in circulation. Monitor and describe respiratory status, character and pattern of respirations, and characteristics of breath sounds. Monitor nutritional and fluid intake, urine output, and bowel function, since this provides assessment data for renal and gastrointestinal functioning. Assess skin condition on an ongoing basis, because skin becomes fragile and may easily break down.

In the last hours of life, assessments should be limited to only those that are needed to determine patient comfort. Assessment of pain and respiratory status may be the most important during this time. It may be more peaceful and comforting to the patient and family to refrain from overstimulation that may occur from certain types of assessments, such as measuring BP or checking for pupillary response. As death approaches, your efforts may be better spent providing emotional support to the patient and family rather than performing tasks that will have no impact on the patient's physical care.

## ◆ Planning

The patient and family need to be involved in planning and coordinating EOL care. In some cases, a family conference may be helpful to develop a coordinated plan of care.

Develop a comprehensive plan to support, teach, and evaluate patients and families. Nursing care goals during the last stages of life involve comfort and safety measures and care of the patient's emotional and physical needs. These goals may also include determining where the patient would like to die and whether this is possible. For example, the patient may want to die at home, but the family may object. Many factors contribute to the patient and family's decision. Interprofessional EOL care that includes the physician, social worker, chaplain, as well as other members of the palliative and/or hospice care team is important. Advocate for the patient so that his or her wishes are met as much as possible.

The last hours or days of the patient experiencing brain death (e.g., from trauma) are frequently spent in the ICU. Planning for EOL care may be particularly challenging in the ICU environment. At this time, some families are approached about organ donation. Consultation from palliative care specialists may help the family plan and cope with EOL issues.

## ◆ Nursing Implementation

Psychosocial care and physical care are interrelated for both the dying patient and family. Teaching them is an important part of EOL care. Families need ongoing information on the disease, the dying process, and any care that will be provided. They need information on how to cope with the many issues during this period of their lives. Denial and grieving may be barriers to learning and understanding at the end of life for both the patient and family.

◆ **Psychosocial Care.** As death approaches, respond appropriately to the patient's psychosocial manifestations at the end of life (Table 9-7).

◆ ***Anxiety and Depression.*** Patients often exhibit signs of anxiety and depression during the EOL period. Anxiety is an uneasy feeling whose cause is not easily identified. Anxiety is frequently related to fear.

Causes of anxiety and depression may include uncontrolled pain and dyspnea, psychosocial factors related to the disease process or impending death, altered physiologic states, and drugs used in high dosages. Encouragement, support, and teaching decrease some of the anxiety and depression. Management of anxiety and depression may include both medications and nonpharmacologic interventions. Relaxation strategies such as relaxation breathing, muscle relaxation, music, and imagery may be useful (see Chapter 6).

◆ ***Anger.*** Anger is a common and normal response to grief. A grieving person cannot be forced to accept the loss. The surviving family members may be angry with the dying loved one who is leaving them. Encourage the expression of feelings, but at the same time realize how difficult it is to come to terms with loss. As a nurse, you may be the target of the anger. You need to understand what is happening and not react on a personal level.

◆ ***Hopelessness and Powerlessness.*** Feelings of hopelessness and powerlessness are common during the EOL period. Encourage realistic hope within the limits of the situation. Allow the patient and family to deal with what is within their control, and help them to recognize what is beyond their control. When

**TABLE 9-7 Nursing Management**
***Psychosocial Care at End of Life***

| Characteristic | Nursing Management |
|---|---|
| **Withdrawal** | |
| Patient near death may seem withdrawn from the physical environment, maintaining the ability to hear but unable to respond. | Converse as though the patient were alert, using a soft voice and gentle touch. |
| **Unusual Communication** | |
| This may indicate that an unresolved issue is preventing the dying person from letting go. Patient may become restless and agitated or perform repetitive tasks (may also indicate terminal delirium). | Encourage the family to talk with and reassure the dying person. |
| **Vision-Like Experiences** | |
| Patient may talk to persons who are not there or see places and objects not visible. Vision-like experiences assist the dying person in coming to terms with meaning in life and transition from it. | Affirm the dying person's experience as a part of transition from this life. |
| **Saying Goodbyes** | |
| It is important for the patient and family to acknowledge their sadness, mutually forgive one another, and say goodbye. | Encourage the dying person and family to verbalize their feelings of sadness, loss, forgiveness and to touch, hug, cry.<br>Allow the patient and family privacy to express their feelings and comfort one another. |
| **Spiritual Needs** | |
| Patient or family may request spiritual support, such as the presence of a chaplain. | Assess spiritual needs. Allow patient to express his or her spiritual needs.<br>Encourage visit by appropriate spiritual care service provider, chaplain, or family member. |

possible, support the patient's involvement in decision making about care to foster a sense of control and autonomy.

***Fear.*** Fear is a typical feeling associated with dying. Four specific fears associated with dying are fear of pain, fear of shortness of breath, fear of loneliness and abandonment, and fear of meaninglessness.

**Fear of pain.** Many people assume that pain always accompanies death. Physiologically, there is no absolute indication that death is always painful. Psychologically, pain may occur based on the anxieties and separations related to dying. Terminally ill patients who do experience physical pain should have pain-relieving drugs available. Assure the patient and family that drugs will be given promptly when needed and that side effects of drugs can and will be managed. Reassessment of pain after medications are given is an important nursing action. Patients can participate in their own pain relief by discussing pain relief measures and their effects. Most patients want their pain relieved without the side effects of grogginess or sleepiness. Pain relief measures do not have to deprive the patient of the ability to interact with others.

**Fear of shortness of breath.** Respiratory distress and dyspnea are common near the end of life. The sensation of air hunger results in anxiety for the patient and family. Current therapies include opioids, bronchodilators, and oxygen, depending on the cause of the dyspnea. Anxiety-reducing agents (e.g., anxiolytics) may help produce relaxation.

**Fear of loneliness and abandonment.** Most terminally ill and dying people fear loneliness and do not want to be alone. Many dying patients are afraid that loved ones who are unable to cope with the patient's imminent death will abandon them. The simple presence of someone provides support and comfort (Fig. 9-8). Holding hands, touching, and listening are important nursing interventions. Providing companionship allows the dying person a sense of security.

**Fear of meaninglessness.** Fear of meaninglessness leads people to review their lives. They review their intentions during life, examining actions and expressing regrets about what might have been. *Life review* helps patients recognize the value of their lives. Assist patients and their families in identifying the positive qualities of the patient's life. Practical ways of helping may include looking at photo albums or collections of important mementos. Sharing thoughts and feelings may enhance spirituality and provide comfort for the patient at this time. Respect and accept the practices and rituals associated with the patient's life review while remaining nonjudgmental.[24]

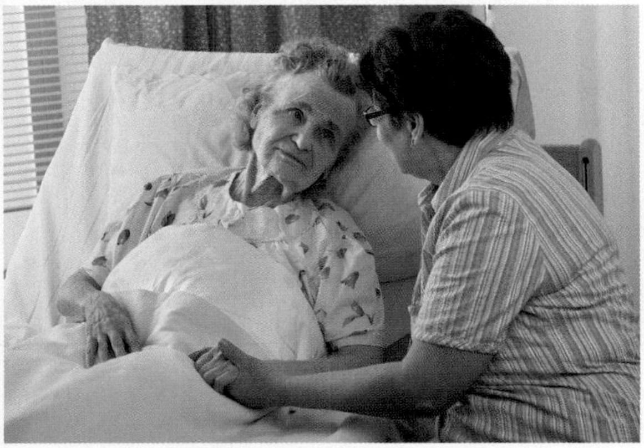

FIG. 9-8 Dying patients typically want someone whom they know and trust to stay with them. (©iStockphoto/Thinkstock)

***Communication.*** Communication among the interprofessional team, patient, and family is essential at the end of life. Empathy and active listening are essential components of communication in EOL care. *Empathy* is the identification with and understanding of another's situation, feelings, or motives. *Active listening* is paying attention to what is said, observing the patient's nonverbal cues, and not interrupting.

There may be silence. Frequently silence is related to the overwhelming feelings experienced at the end of life. Silence can also allow time to gather thoughts. Listening to the silence sends a message of acceptance and comfort. Communication also must be respectful of the patient's ethnic, cultural, and religious backgrounds.

Patients and family members may have difficulties expressing themselves emotionally. Allow time for them to express their feelings and thoughts. Make time to listen and interact in a sensitive way to enhance the relationship among you, the patient, and the family. A family conference is one way to create a more conducive environment for communication.

Prepare family members for changes in emotional and cognitive function that occur at the end of life. Unusual communication by the patient may take place at the end of life. The patient's speech may become confused, disoriented, or garbled. Patients may speak to or about family members or others who have predeceased them, give instructions to those who will survive them, or speak of projects yet to be completed. Active, careful listening allows for the identification of specific patterns in the dying person's communication and decreases the risk for inappropriate labeling of behaviors.

**Physical Care.** Nursing management related to physical care at the end of life focuses on symptom management and comfort rather than treatment for curing a disease or disorder (Table 9-8). The priority is meeting the patient's physiologic and safety needs. Physical care focuses on the needs for oxygen, nutrition, pain relief, mobility, elimination, and skin care. People who are dying deserve and require the same physical care as people who are expected to recover. If possible, it is important to discuss with the patient and family the goals of care before treatment begins. An advance directive should be completed so that the patient and family wishes are followed.

***Postmortem Care.*** After the patient is pronounced dead, prepare or delegate preparation of the patient's body for immediate viewing by the family with consideration for cultural customs and in accord with state law and agency policies and procedures. In some cultures and in some types of death, it may be important to allow the family to prepare or assist in caring for the patient's body. In general, close the patient's eyes, replace dentures, wash the body as needed (placing pads under the perineum to absorb urine and feces), and remove tubes and dressings (if appropriate). The patient's body is straightened, leaving the pillow to support the head and prevent pooling of blood and discoloration of the face.

Allow the family privacy and as much time as they need with the deceased person. When the death is unexpected or unanticipated, preparation of the patient's body for viewing or release to a funeral home depends on state law and agency policies and procedures. Never refer to the deceased person as "the body." Care of and discussion related to the person should continue to be respectful even after death.

## TABLE 9-8 Nursing Management

### *Physical Care at End of Life*

| Characteristic | Nursing Management |
|---|---|
| **Pain** | |
| • Pain may be a major symptom associated with terminal illness and the one most feared.<br>• Pain can be acute or chronic.<br>• Bone pain can be caused by metastases, fractures, arthritis, immobility.<br>• Physical and emotional stressors can aggravate pain. | • Assess pain thoroughly and regularly to determine the quality, intensity, location, and contributing and alleviating factors.<br>• Minimize possible irritants such as skin irritations from wetness, heat or cold, and pressure.<br>• Administer medications around the clock in a timely manner and on a regular basis to provide constant relief rather than waiting until the pain is unbearable and then trying to relieve it.<br>• Provide complementary and alternative therapies such as guided imagery, massage, and relaxation techniques as needed (see Chapter 6).<br>• Evaluate effectiveness of pain relief measures frequently to ensure that the patient is on a correct, adequate drug regimen.<br>• Do not delay or deny pain relief measures to a terminally ill patient. |
| **Delirium** | |
| • A state characterized by confusion, disorientation, restlessness, clouding of consciousness, incoherence, fear, anxiety, excitement, and often hallucinations<br>• May be misidentified as depression, psychosis, anger, or anxiety<br>• Use of opioids or corticosteroids as well as their withdrawal may cause delirium.<br>• Underlying disease process may contribute to delirium.<br>• Generally considered a reversible process | • Perform a thorough assessment for reversible causes of delirium, including pain, constipation, and urinary retention.<br>• Provide a room that is quiet, well lit, and familiar to reduce the effects of delirium.<br>• Reorient the dying person to person, place, and time with each encounter.<br>• Administer ordered benzodiazepines and sedatives as needed.<br>• Stay physically close to frightened patient. Reassure in a calm, soft voice with touch and slow strokes of the skin.<br>• Provide family with emotional support and encouragement in their efforts to cope with the behaviors associated with delirium. |
| **Anxiety/Restlessness** | |
| • May occur as death approaches and cerebral metabolism slows<br>• May occur with tachypnea, dyspnea, sweating | • Assess for previous anxiety disorder.<br>• Assess for spiritual distress and/or concerns related to death as causes of restlessness and agitation.<br>• Assess for urinary retention and stool impaction.<br>• Do not restrain.<br>• Use soothing music; slow, soft touch and voice.<br>• Limit the number of persons at the bedside. |
| **Dysphagia** | |
| • May occur because of extreme weakness and changes in level of consciousness<br>• Difficulty swallowing<br>• Aspiration of liquids and/or solids<br>• Drooling/inability to swallow secretions | • Identify the least invasive alternative routes of administration for drugs needed for symptom management.<br>• Suction orally as needed.<br>• Modify diet as tolerated/desired (soft, pureed, chopped meats).<br>• Hand feed small meals.<br>• Head elevated for meals and at least 30 minutes after<br>• If necessary use alternative (rectal, buccal, transdermal) medication routes.<br>• Discontinue nonessential medications.<br>• Discuss risk of aspiration. |
| **Weakness and Fatigue** | |
| • Expected at the end of life<br>• Metabolic demands related to disease process contribute to weakness and fatigue. | • Assess the patient's tolerance for activities.<br>• Time nursing interventions to conserve energy.<br>• Help the patient identify and complete valued or desired activities.<br>• Provide support as needed to maintain positions in bed or chair.<br>• Provide frequent rest periods. |
| **Dehydration** | |
| • May occur during the last days of life<br>• Hunger and thirst are rare in the last days of life.<br>• As the end of life approaches, patients tend to take in less food and fluid. | • Assess mucous membranes frequently for dryness, which can lead to discomfort.<br>• Maintain complete, regular oral care to provide for comfort and hydration of mucous membranes.<br>• Encourage consumption of ice chips and sips of fluids or use moist cloths to provide moisture to the mouth.<br>• Use moist cloths and swabs for unconscious patients to avoid aspiration.<br>• Apply lubricant to the lips and oral mucous membranes as needed.<br>• Do not force the patient to eat or drink.<br>• Teach family that hunger and thirst are rare in the last days of life.<br>• Reassure family that cessation of food and fluid intake is a natural part of the process of dying. |

## TABLE 9-8 Nursing Management

### *Physical Care at End of Life—cont'd*

| Characteristic | Nursing Management |
|---|---|
| **Dyspnea** | |
| • Subjective symptom<br>• Accompanied by fear of suffocation and anxiety<br>• Underlying disease process can exacerbate dyspnea.<br>• Coughing and expectorating secretions become difficult. | • Assess respiratory status regularly.<br>• Elevate the head and/or position patient on side to improve chest expansion.<br>• Use a fan or air conditioner to facilitate movement of cool air.<br>• Teach and encourage the use of pursed-lip breathing.<br>• Administer supplemental oxygen as ordered.<br>• Suction PRN to remove accumulation of mucus from the airways. Suction cautiously in the terminal phase.<br>• Administer expectorant as ordered. |
| **Myoclonus** | |
| • Mild to severe jerking or twitching sometimes associated with use of high dose of opioids.<br>• Patient may complain of involuntary twitching of extremities. | • Assess for initial onset, duration, and any discomfort or distress experienced by patient.<br>• If myoclonus is distressing or becoming more severe, discuss possible drug therapy modifications with the HCP.<br>• Changes in opioid medication may alleviate or decrease myoclonus. |
| **Skin Breakdown** | |
| • Skin integrity is difficult to maintain at the end of life.<br>• Immobility, urinary and bowel incontinence, dry skin, nutritional deficits, anemia, friction, and shearing forces lead to a high risk for skin breakdown.<br>• Disease and other processes may impair skin integrity.<br>• As death approaches, circulation to the extremities decreases and they become cool, mottled, and cyanotic. | • Assess skin for signs of breakdown.<br>• Implement protocols to prevent skin breakdown by controlling drainage and odor and keeping the skin and any wound areas clean.<br>• Perform wound assessments as needed.<br>• Follow appropriate nursing management protocol for dressing wounds.<br>• Follow appropriate nursing management protocol for a patient who is immobile, but consider realistic outcomes of skin integrity vs. maintenance of comfort.<br>• Follow appropriate nursing management to prevent skin irritations and breakdown from urinary and bowel incontinence.<br>• Use blankets to cover for warmth. Never apply heat.<br>• Prevent the effects of shearing forces. |
| **Bowel Patterns** | |
| • Constipation can be caused by immobility, use of opioid medications, depression, lack of fiber in the diet, and dehydration.<br>• Diarrhea may occur as muscles relax or from a fecal impaction related to the use of opioids and immobility. | • Assess bowel function.<br>• Assess for and remove fecal impactions.<br>• Encourage movement and physical activities as tolerated.<br>• Encourage fiber in the diet if appropriate.<br>• Encourage fluids if appropriate.<br>• Use suppositories, stool softeners, laxatives, or enemas if ordered.<br>• Assess for confusion, agitation, restlessness and pain, which may be signs of constipation. |
| **Urinary Incontinence** | |
| • May result from disease progression or changes in the level of consciousness.<br>• As death becomes imminent, the perineal muscles relax. | • Assess urinary function.<br>• Use absorbent pads for urinary incontinence.<br>• Follow appropriate nursing protocol for the consideration and use of indwelling or external catheters.<br>• Follow appropriate nursing management to prevent skin irritations and breakdown from urinary incontinence. |
| **Anorexia, Nausea, and Vomiting** | |
| • May be caused by complications of disease process<br>• Drugs contribute to nausea.<br>• Constipation, impaction, and bowel obstruction can cause anorexia, nausea, and vomiting. | • Assess the patient for complaints of nausea or vomiting.<br>• Assess possible contributing causes of nausea or vomiting.<br>• Have family provide the patient's favorite foods.<br>• Discuss modifications to the drug regimen with the HCP.<br>• Provide antiemetics before meals if ordered.<br>• Offer and provide frequent meals with small portions of favorite foods.<br>• Offer culturally appropriate foods.<br>• Provide frequent mouth care, especially after vomiting.<br>• Ensure uninterrupted mealtimes.<br>• If ordered, administer medications (e.g., megestrol, corticosteroids) to increase appetite.<br>• Teach family that appetite naturally decreases at end of life. |
| **Candidiasis** | |
| • White, cottage-cheese–like oral plaques<br>• Fungal overgrowth in the mouth due to chemotherapy and/or immunosuppression | • If ordered, administer oral antifungal nystatin.<br>• Clean dentures and other dental appliances to prevent reinfection.<br>• Provide oral hygiene and use soft toothbrush. |

## SPECIAL NEEDS OF CAREGIVERS AND NURSES IN END-OF-LIFE CARE

### Special Needs of Family Caregivers

Family caregivers are important in meeting the patient's physical and psychosocial needs. The role of caregivers includes working and communicating with the patient and other family members, supporting the patient's concerns, and helping the patient resolve any unfinished business. Families often face emotional, physical, and economic consequences as a result of caring for a family member who is dying. The caregiver's responsibilities do not end when the person is admitted to an acute care, inpatient hospice, or long-term care facility.

An understanding of the grieving process as it affects both the patient and family is important. Being present during a family member's dying process can be highly stressful. Recognize signs and behaviors among family members who may be at risk for abnormal grief reactions, and be prepared to intervene if necessary. Warning signs may include dependency and negative feelings about the dying person, inability to express feelings, sleep disturbances, a history of depression, difficult reactions to previous losses, perceived lack of social or family support, low self-esteem, multiple previous bereavements, alcoholism, or substance abuse. Caregivers with concurrent life crises (e.g., divorce) will be especially at risk.

Family caregivers and other family members need encouragement to continue their usual activities as much as possible. They need to discuss their activities and maintain some control over their lives. Inform caregivers about appropriate resources for support, including respite care. Resources such as community counseling and local support may assist some people in working through their grief.

Encourage caregivers to build a support system of extended family, friends, faith community, and clergy. The caregivers should have people to call on at any time to express any feelings they are experiencing. (The stressors and special needs of family caregivers are discussed in Chapter 4 on p. 50.)

### Special Needs of Nurses

Many nurses who care for dying patients do so because they are passionate about providing high-quality EOL care. Caring for patients and their families at the end of life is challenging and rewarding but also intense and emotionally charged.[24] A bond or connection may develop between you and the patient or family. Be aware of how grief personally affects you. When you provide care for terminally ill or dying patients, you are not immune to feelings of loss. It is common to feel helpless and powerless when dealing with death. Express feelings of sorrow, guilt, and frustration. It is important to recognize your own values, attitudes, and feelings about death.

Interventions are available that may help ease your physical and emotional stress. Be aware of what you can and cannot control. Recognizing personal feelings allows openness in exchanging feelings with the patient and family. Realizing that it is okay to cry with the patient or family during the end of life may be important for your well-being.

To meet your personal needs, focus on interventions that will help decrease your stress. Get involved in hobbies or other interests, schedule time for yourself, ensure time for sleep, maintain a peer support system, and develop a support system beyond the workplace.[25] Hospice agencies can help you cope through professionally assisted groups, informal discussion sessions, and flexible time schedules.

## CASE STUDY

### *Spiritual Distress at End of Life*

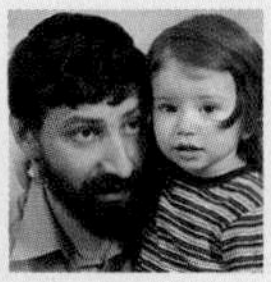

(©Mocker_bat/iStock/Thinkstock)

**Patient Profile**

G.M. is a 42-year-old Orthodox Jewish man. He is being visited by the hospice nurse for complaints of increasing abdominal pain, nausea, vomiting, lack of appetite, and constipation. He was diagnosed 6 months ago with pancreatic cancer that has metastasized to the liver and lungs. He quit work 1 month later. Two weeks ago he ended the drug trial he was on for 5 months and enrolled in hospice. Currently, he is taking oral opioids for pain, ondansetron (Zofran) PRN for nausea and vomiting, sertraline (Zoloft) for depression, and megestrol for appetite. His wife is worried that he will become addicted to the pain medication.

**Subjective Data**

- States that he is angry at God for giving him this illness
- Reports fatigue and lack of appetite
- Reports pain at 7 (0- to 10-point scale) not relieved by medication
- States he is worried about the loss of his health benefits and what will happen to his young family (including a son age 3) when he is gone

**Objective Data**

***Physical Examination***

- Underweight (20% less than ideal body weight for height)
- Skin is jaundiced
- Yellow sclera

**Interprofessional Care**

- Review pain medications for dosage adjustment.
- Hospice social worker to review medical benefits and disability application
- Ensure that advance directives are in place.
- Request a visit from his rabbi.

**Discussion Questions**

1. What are G.M.'s risk factors for spiritual distress?
2. Based on the data above, what are the major health problems for G.M.?
3. ***Patient-Centered Care:*** What specific palliative care needs does G.M. have?
4. ***Priority Decision:*** Based on the assessment data provided, what are the priority nursing diagnoses? Are there any collaborative problems?
5. ***Priority Decision:*** Based on your assessment of G.M., what are the priority nursing interventions for him?
6. ***Teamwork and Collaboration:*** For the interventions that you identified in the above question, which personnel could be responsible for implementing them: RN, LPN, unlicensed assistive personnel (UAP)?
7. ***Teamwork and Collaboration:*** What referrals may be indicated?

Answers available at *http://evolve.elsevier.com/Lewis/medsurg.*

## BRIDGE TO NCLEX EXAMINATION

The number of the question corresponds to the same-numbered outcome at the beginning of the chapter.

1. An 80-year-old female patient is receiving palliative care for heart failure. The *primary* purpose(s) of her receiving palliative care is (are) to (*select all that apply*)
   **a.** improve her quality of life.
   **b.** assess her coping ability with disease.
   **c.** have time to teach patient and family about disease.
   **d.** focus on reducing the severity of disease symptoms.
   **e.** provide care that the family is unwilling or unable to give.
2. The *primary* purpose of hospice is to
   **a.** allow patients to die at home.
   **b.** provide better quality of care than the family can.
   **c.** coordinate care for dying patients and their families.
   **d.** provide comfort and support for dying patients and their families.
3. A 67-year-old woman was recently diagnosed with inoperable pancreatic cancer. Before the diagnosis she was very active in her neighborhood association. Her husband is concerned because his wife is staying at home and missing her usual community activities. Which common EOL psychologic manifestation is she *most* likely demonstrating?
   **a.** Peacefulness
   **b.** Decreased socialization
   **c.** Decreased decision making
   **d.** Anxiety about unfinished business
4. For the past 5 years Tom has repeatedly asked his mother to donate his deceased father's belongings to charity, but his mother has refused. She sits in the bedroom closet, crying and talking to her long-dead husband. What type of grief is Tom's mother experiencing?
   **a.** Adaptive grief
   **b.** Disruptive grief
   **c.** Anticipatory grief
   **d.** Prolonged grief disorder
5. The home health nurse visits a 40-year-old patient with metastatic breast cancer who is receiving palliative care. The patient is experiencing pain at a level of 7 (0-10 point scale). In prioritizing activities for the visit, what should the nurse do *first*?
   **a.** Auscultate for breath sounds.
   **b.** Administer PRN pain medication.
   **c.** Check pressure points for skin breakdown.
   **d.** Ask family about patient's food and fluid intake.
6. While caring for his dying wife, the husband states that his wife is a devout Roman Catholic but he is a Baptist. Who is considered the *most* reliable source for spiritual preferences concerning EOL care for the dying wife?
   **a.** A priest
   **b.** Dying wife
   **c.** Hospice staff
   **d.** Husband of dying wife
7. A tearful patient tells the nurse that her brother (who is in prison) just received a diagnosis of terminal metastatic lung cancer. She is worried that her brother will die in pain and alone. What is the nurse's *best* response?
   **a.** "It's too bad that they don't have hospice services in prison."
   **b.** "I'm sure the prison will let him out if they know he is dying."
   **c.** "Maybe if he had not committed a crime, he wouldn't be in this situation."
   **d.** "Many prisons offer health care services, including hospice and palliative care."
8. The family attorney informed a patient's adult children and wife that the patient did not have an advance directive after he suffered a serious stroke. Who is responsible for making the decision about EOL measures when the patient cannot communicate his or her specific wishes?
   **a.** Notary and attorney
   **b.** Physician and family
   **c.** Wife and adult children
   **d.** Physician and nursing staff
9. The children caregivers of an older patient whose death is imminent have not left the bedside for the past 36 hours. In the nurse's assessment of the family, what findings indicate the potential for an abnormal grief reaction to occur *(select all that apply)*?
   **a.** Family cannot express their feelings to one another.
   **b.** Dying patient is becoming more restless and agitated.
   **c.** A family member is going through a difficult divorce.
   **d.** Family talks with and reassures the patient at frequent intervals.
   **e.** Siblings who were estranged from each other have now reunited.
10. A nurse has been working full time with terminally ill patients for 3 years. He has been experiencing irritability and mixed emotions when expressing sadness since four of his patients died on the same day. To optimize the quality of his nursing care, he should examine his own
    **a.** full-time work schedule.
    **b.** past feelings toward death.
    **c.** patterns for dealing with grief.
    **d.** demands for involvement in patient care.

1. a, d, 2. d, 3. b, 4. d, 5. b, 6. b, 7. d, 8. c, 9. a, c, 10. c.

For rationales to these answers and even more NCLEX review questions, visit *http://evolve.elsevier.com/Lewis/medsurg*.

## EVOLVE WEBSITE

http://evolve.elsevier.com/Lewis/medsurg

**Review Questions (Online Only)**

**Key Points**

**Answer Keys for Questions**

- Rationales for Bridge to NCLEX Examination Questions
- Answer Guidelines for Case Study on p. 142

**Student Case Study**

- Patient With Chronic Myelogenous Leukemia Including End-of-Life Care

**Conceptual Care Map Creator**

**Audio Glossary**

**Content Updates**

## REFERENCES


1. National Consensus Project for Quality Palliative Care: Clinical practice guidelines for quality palliative care, ed 3. Retrieved from *www.hpna.org/multimedia/NCP_Clinical_Practice_Guidelines_3rd_Edition.pdf.*
2. Centers for Disease Control and Prevention, U.S. Dept of Health and Human Services: The state of aging and health in America 2013. Retrieved from *www.cdc.gov/aging.*
3. Kelley AS, Deb P, Du Q, et al: Hospice enrollment saves money for Medicare and improves care quality across a number of different lengths-of-stay, *Health Aff* 32:552, 2013.
4. National Hospice and Palliative Care Organization: NHPCO facts and figures: hospice care in America. Alexandria, Va. Retrieved from *www.nhpco.org/sites/default/files/public/Statistics_Research/2014_Facts_Figures.pdf.*
5. Hospice and Palliative Nurses Association: HPNA position statements. Retrieved from *http://hpna.advancingexpertcare.org/education/position-statements.*
6. Johnson KS: Racial and ethnic disparities in palliative care, *J Palliat Med* 16:1329, 2013.
7. Olmsted CL, Johnson AM, Kaboli P, et al: Use of palliative care and hospice among surgical and medical specialties in the Veterans Health Administration, *JAMA Surg* 149:1169, 2014.
8. National Hospice and Palliative Care Organization: Palliative care costs and benefits. Retrieved from *www.caringinfo.org/i4a/pages/index.cfm?pageid=3297.*
9. Jackson J, Willmarth-Stec M, Shutter L: Update of clinical practice guidelines for brain death determination in an academic health center, *J Neurosci Nurs* 47:44, 2015.
10. Field M, Cassel C: *Approaching death: improving care at the end of life,* Washington, DC, 1997, National Academy Press. (Classic)
11. Kübler-Ross E: *On death and dying,* New York, 1969, Macmillan. (Classic).
12. National Cancer Institute: PDQ Grief, bereavement, and coping with loss, Bethesda, Md, 2014, National Cancer Institute. Retrieved from *http://cancer.gov/cancertopics/pdq/supportivecare/bereavement/HealthProfessional.*
13. Bryant RA, Kenny L, Joscelyne A, et al: Treating prolonged grief disorder: a randomized clinical trial, *JAMA Psychiatry* 71:1332, 2014.

*14. Skalla K, Ferrell B: Challenges in assessing spiritual distress in survivors of cancer, *Clin J Oncol Nurs* 19:99, 2015.

*15. Wilson KS, Korrke TE, Schettle S: Honoring Choices Minnesota: preliminary data from a community-wide advance care planning model, *J Am Geriatric Soc* 62:2420, 2014.

16. Rubin SS, Malkinson R, Witztum E: *Working with the bereaved: multiple lenses on loss and mourning,* Routledge Taylor and French, 2012, New York.

*17. LoPresti MA, Dement F, Gold HT: End-of-life care for people from ethnic minority groups: a systematic review, *Am J Hosp Palliat Care* 33(3):291, 2016.

*18. Leung D, Blastorah M, Nusdorfer L, et al: Nursing patients with chronic critical illness and their families: a qualitative study, *Nurs Crit Care* Feb 18, 2015. DOI: 10.1111/nicc.12154.

19. Stahler PA, Weese SE, Nygaard RM: Honoring patients' organ donation decisions when family conflict is present: experience from a single organ procurement organization, *J Trauma Acute Care Surg* 77:555, 2014.
20. Marcus B: Communicating patient DNR status using color-coded wristbands, *Am J Nurs* 115:11, 2015.
21. American Nurses Association: ANA position statements. Retrieved from *www.nursingworld.org/MainMenuCategories/EthicsStandards/Ethics-Position-Statements/etpain14426.pdf.*
22. Iowa Department of Public Health: Out of hospital DNR. Retrieved from *www.idph.state.ia.us/ems/dnr.asp.*

*23. Hui D, Dos Santos R, Chisholm G: Bedside clinical sign associated with impending death in patients with advanced cancer: preliminary findings of a prospective, longitudinal cohort study, *Cancer* 15:121, 2015.

24. Sliter MT, Sinclaire RR, Yuan Z, et al: Don't fear the reaper: trait death anxiety, mortality salience, and occupational health, *J Appl Psychol* 99:759, 2014.

*25. Wittenberg-Lyles E, Goldsmith J, Reno J: Perceived benefits and challenges of an oncology nurse support group, *Clin J Oncol Nurs* 18:E71, 2014.

*Evidence-based information for clinical practice.

10

# Substance Use Disorders

*Mariann M. Harding*

*No one is immune from addiction. It afflicts people of all ages, races, classes, and professions.*

**Patrick J. Kennedy**

http://evolve.elsevier.com/Lewis/medsurg/

## LEARNING OUTCOMES

1. Relate the effects of substance use to its resulting major health complications.
2. Differentiate among the effects of the use of stimulants, depressants, and cannabis.
3. Explain your role in promoting the cessation of smoking and tobacco use.
4. Summarize the nursing management and interprofessional care of patients who experience toxicity or withdrawal from stimulants and depressants.
5. Apply the Screening, Brief Intervention, and Referral to Treatment approach in clinical situations.
6. Describe the incidence and effects of substance use in the older adult.

## KEY TERMS

acute alcohol toxicity, p. 149
alcohol use disorder (AUD), p. 148
alcohol withdrawal syndrome (AWS), p. 150
binge drinking, p. 148
electronic cigarettes, p. 146
Screening, Brief Intervention, and Referral to Treatment (SBIRT), p. 153
substance use disorder (SUD), Table 10-1, p. 146
tobacco use disorder (TUD), p. 145

Substance use is a serious problem affecting society and the health care system. Substance-related disorders involve several types of substances, ranging from widely used and accepted tobacco and alcohol to illegal, brain-altering drugs such as heroin and cocaine. The *Diagnostic and Statistical Manual of Mental Disorders V (DSM-V)* outlines criteria used to identify the presence of substance use disorder (SUD)[1] (Table 10-1).

SUD is defined as mild, moderate, or severe based on the person's pattern of use and the functional impact of use on the person's daily life. Knowing the severity of substance use allows the health care team to tailor treatment according to a patient's needs. For example, a person who binge drinks may not have alcohol SUD but is at increased risk for it. On the other hand, a person who uses heroin or cocaine is likely to have severe SUD because these substances are highly addictive.

Many of the patients with substance use problems whom you will encounter are receiving care for problems associated with substance use. Almost every drug associated with SUD harms some tissue or organ. Substance use causes specific health problems, such as liver damage related to alcohol use or chronic obstructive pulmonary disease (COPD) related to smoking. Other health problems result from behaviors associated with substance use, such as malnutrition or trauma-related injuries from automobile accidents. Common health problems related to substance use are presented in Table 10-2.

This chapter focuses on the role of the medical-surgical nurse in identifying and managing the patient with SUD in the acute care setting. A hospitalized patient who uses substances can develop withdrawal when the use of the substance is abruptly stopped. You need to be able to recognize substance use and its effects on health problems and manage withdrawal. The health care setting provides an opportunity for screening and providing teaching regarding substance use and abuse. It is your responsibility to motivate the patient to change behavior and provide referrals to programs that provide treatment and rehabilitation. Failing to address a patient's substance use problem, thus enabling the behavior, is a breach of your professional responsibility.

## DRUGS ASSOCIATED WITH SUBSTANCE USE DISORDER

### NICOTINE

You are most likely to encounter people with **tobacco use disorder (TUD)**. People with TUD are dependent on the drug

Reviewed by Carolyn Baird, DNP, MBA, RN-BC, CARN-AP, CCDPD, FIAAN, Therapist, Counseling and Trauma Services, Canonsburg, Pennsylvania; Abimbola Farinde, PharmD, MS, Professor, Columbia Southern University, Orange Beach, Alabama; and Christine L. Savage, RN, PhD, CARN, FAAN, Professor and Chair, Community Public Health Johns Hopkins School of Nursing, Baltimore, Maryland.

**TABLE 10-1 Criteria for Substance Use Disorder**

The following criteria (clustered in four groups) can be used to identify substance use disorder (SUD). The severity of SUD can be classified as mild (2-3 criteria), moderate (4-5 criteria), or severe (6 or more criteria).

**Impaired Control**
- Taking more or for longer than intended
- Failing to quit using despite multiple times of trying to do so
- Spending a great deal of time obtaining, using, or recovering from use
- Craving the substance

**Social Impairment**
- Missing school, work, or other responsibilities due to use
- Continuing use despite problems caused or exacerbated by use
- Giving up or reducing important activities because of use

**Risky Use**
- Recurrent use in hazardous situations
- Continued use despite problems that are caused or worsened by use

**Pharmacologic Dependence**
- Physical tolerance to effects of the substance
- Presence of withdrawal symptoms when not using or using less

Source: American Psychiatric Association: *The diagnostic and statistical manual of mental disorders*, ed 5, Arlington, Va, 2013, The Association.

**TABLE 10-2 Health Problems Related to Substance Use**

| | Health Problems* |
|---|---|
| **Substance** | |
| **Cocaine** | • Cardiac dysrhythmias, myocardial ischemia and infarction<br>• Seizures, stroke<br>• Psychosis |
| **Amphetamines** | • Cardiac dysrhythmias, myocardial ischemia and infarction<br>• Liver, lung, kidney damage<br>• Mood disturbances, violent behavior, psychoses |
| **Sedative-hypnotics** | • Memory impairment<br>• Personality changes, depression |
| **Opioids** | • Sexual dysfunction<br>• Gastric ulcers<br>• Glomerulonephritis |
| **Inhalants** | • Cognitive and motor impairment<br>• Acute and chronic kidney injury |
| **Cannabis** | • Bronchitis, chronic cough<br>• Depression, anxiety, schizophrenia<br>• Memory impairment |
| **Behaviors** | |
| **Injecting drugs** | • Blood clots, phlebitis, skin infections<br>• Hepatitis B and C<br>• HIV/AIDS<br>• Other infections: endocarditis, tuberculosis, pneumonia, meningitis, tetanus, bone and joint infections, lung abscesses |
| **Snorting drugs** | • Nasal sores, septal necrosis or perforation<br>• Chronic sinusitis |
| **Risky sexual behavior** | • HIV/AIDS<br>• Hepatitis B and C<br>• Sexually transmitted infections |
| **Personal neglect** | • Malnutrition, impaired immunity<br>• Accidental injuries |

Adapted from National Institute on Drug Abuse: Medical consequence of drug abuse. Retrieved from *www.drugabuse.gov/related-topics/medical-consequences-drug-abuse*.
*Health problems related to substance use are discussed in the appropriate chapters throughout the text where they are identified as risk factors for these problems.

nicotine due to using tobacco products. A number of products contain nicotine, including smoked tobacco (cigarettes, cigars, pipes), smokeless tobacco (chew, snuff, dip), and some electronic cigarettes. Cigarette smoking is the main form of tobacco use in the United States.

### Effects of Use and Complications

Nicotine is a central nervous system stimulant. Within seconds of entering the body, nicotine reaches the brain, causing the release of adrenaline and creating feelings of a "high" or a "buzz." The effects last about 1 to 2 hours before withdrawal symptoms occur, leaving the person feeling tired, irritable, and anxious. The need to have the "high" or "buzz" feelings again makes the person crave more nicotine, leading to addiction.

Smoked tobacco is the most harmful method of nicotine use and injures nearly every organ in the body. Smoking alone accounts for 14 million major medical conditions affecting adults in the United States.[2] Smoking causes chronic lung disease, cardiovascular disease, and lung and other cancers and is a major factor in a variety of other conditions, including delayed wound healing and overall diminished health (Fig. 10-1).

Although those who use smokeless tobacco have less risk of lung disease, it is not without complications. Holding tobacco in the mouth is associated with periodontal disease and cancer of the mouth, cheek, tongue, throat, and esophagus. Smokeless tobacco produces the systemic effects of nicotine on the cardiovascular system, increasing the risk for cardiovascular disease.[3]

**Electronic cigarettes**, or e-cigs, have a similar look and feel as traditional cigarettes. These battery-operated devices turn nicotine and other chemicals, including propylene glycol and flavorings, into an aerosol. Emerging information indicates e-cigs are not harmless. This is a serious concern because the overall impact of their use on health remains uncertain. Potentially harmful chemicals have been found in some cartridges, including irritants, genotoxins, and carcinogens. E-cigs containing nicotine have the potential to increase the risk of cardiovascular and respiratory problems similar to traditional cigarettes.[4] Other problems, such as seizures and pneumonia, have been attributed to inhaling chemicals in the vapor. Although some believe substituting an e-cig for a traditional cigarette may aid in smoking cessation, no e-cigs are FDA approved. Do not recommend them as a smoking cessation aid.

## NURSING AND INTERPROFESSIONAL MANAGEMENT: TOBACCO USE DISORDER

### Tobacco Cessation

As a nurse, you have a professional responsibility to help people stop smoking or using tobacco. The Joint Commission mandates that every health professional is responsible for identifying tobacco users and providing them with information on ways to stop using tobacco. Patients who receive even brief advice and intervention from you are more likely to quit than those who receive no intervention.

With each patient encounter, encourage the patient to quit and offer specific smoking cessation interventions. The Agency for Healthcare Research and Quality has issued clinical practice guidelines for clinicians, including nurses, to use to motivate users to quit[5] (Tables 10-3 and 10-4). Use these brief clinical

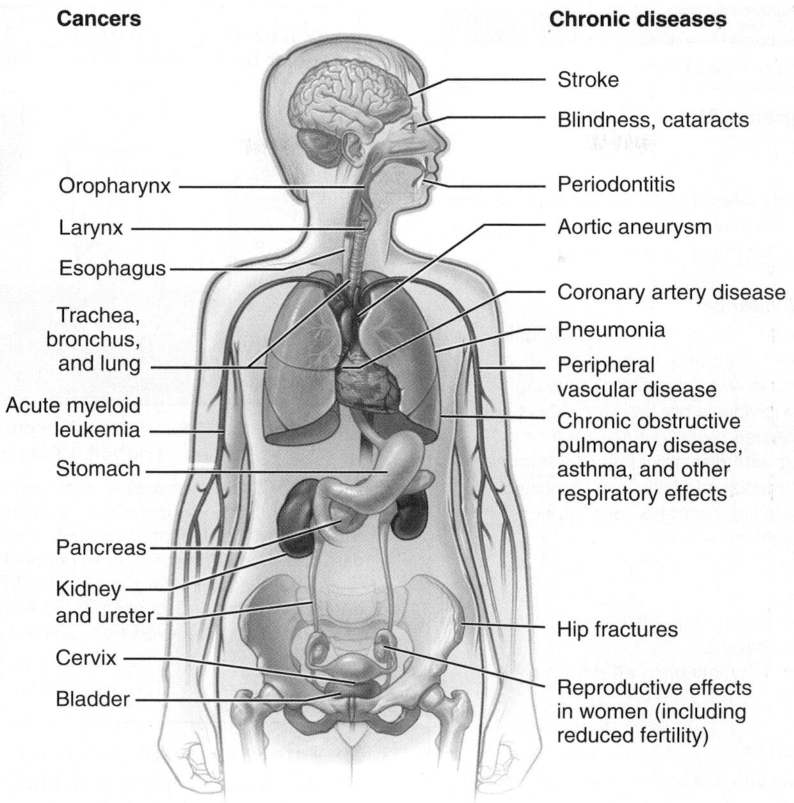


**FIG. 10-1** Health effects of smoking. (From Samet JM: Tobacco smoking, *Thorac Surg Clin* 23(2):103, 2013.)

### TABLE 10-3 Clinical Practice Guideline

***Treating Tobacco Use Disorder***

| The Five *A*s for Users Who Desire to Quit | The Five *R*s for Users Unwilling to Quit |
|---|---|
| 1. **Ask:** Identify all tobacco users at every contact.<br>2. **Advise:** Strongly urge all tobacco users to quit.<br>3. **Assess:** Determine willingness to make a quit attempt.<br>4. **Assist:** Develop a plan with the patient to help the patient quit (e.g., counseling, medication).<br>5. **Arrange:** Schedule follow-up contact. | 1. **Relevance:** Ask the patient to indicate why quitting is personally relevant (e.g., health).<br>2. **Risks:** Ask the patient to identify his or her potential risks/consequences of tobacco use.<br>3. **Rewards:** Ask the patient to identify potential benefits of stopping tobacco use.<br>4. **Roadblocks:** Ask patient to identify barriers or impediments to quitting.<br>5. **Repetition:** Repeat process every clinic visit. |

Source: Agency for Healthcare Research and Quality: *AHCPR supported clinical practice guideline: treating tobacco use and dependence: 2008 update,* Washington, DC, 2008, U.S. Public Health Service.

interventions, called the "5 *A*s," with each patient encounter. These interventions will help you identify tobacco users, encourage them to quit, determine their willingness to quit, assist them in quitting, and arrange for follow-up. A patient teaching guide (Table 10-5) expands on the fourth strategy, *Assist,* to help you aid the user willing to quit. If a tobacco user is unwilling to quit, using the "5 *R*s" may motivate the user to quit in the future.

A variety of smoking cessation products are available to help support users in quitting. These include prescription medicines as well as over-the-counter (OTC) products such as skin patches, lozenges, and gum. Nicotine replacement products are one type of smoking cessation product. These products reduce the craving and withdrawal symptoms associated with cessation by supplying the body with smaller amounts of nicotine (Table 10-6).

### TABLE 10-4 Inpatient Tobacco Cessation Interventions

*Take the following steps for every hospitalized patient.*

- Ask each patient on admission if he or she uses tobacco and document tobacco use status.
- For current tobacco users, list tobacco use status on the admission problem list and as a discharge diagnosis.
- Use counseling and medication to help all tobacco users maintain abstinence and to treat withdrawal symptoms.
- Provide advice and assistance on how to quit during hospitalization and remain abstinent after discharge.
- Arrange for follow-up regarding smoking status. Supportive contact should be provided for at least a month after discharge.

Source: Agency for Healthcare Research and Quality: *AHCPR supported clinical practice guideline: treating tobacco use and dependence: 2008 update,* Washington, DC, 2008, U.S. Public Health Service.

Because most health care facilities are tobacco-free environments, admitted patients who are addicted to nicotine may experience withdrawal symptoms since they are unable to smoke. These symptoms are the same as for the person who stops using tobacco "cold turkey." Offering nicotine replacement therapy to those who desire it will assist in controlling withdrawal symptoms during hospitalization and promote continued cessation after discharge.

Non-nicotine products also play a role in helping users quit. Varenicline (Chantix) is a drug used to aid smoking cessation. Varenicline is unique in that it has both agonist and antagonist actions. Its agonist activity at one subtype of nicotinic receptors

## EVIDENCE-BASED PRACTICE

### *Translating Research Into Practice*

**Do Tobacco Cessation Programs Affect Smoking Behavior?**

***Clinical Question***

In adults who regularly smoke cigarettes (P), do mass media tobacco cessation programs (I) versus no intervention (C) reduce smoking prevalence, cigarette consumption, quit attempts, and quit rates (O)?

***Synthesis of Best Available Evidence***

- Systematic review of randomized controlled trials (RCTs), quasi-RCTs, controlled trials, and interrupted time series
- 11 studies of state and community-wide programs; smoking prevalence generally >15,000 individuals per program. Mass media interventions were cessation-related messages focusing on smokers and motivation to quit with dissemination of information through television, radio, print media, and billboards. Smoking behavior outcomes were prevalence, cigarette consumption, attempts to quit, and quit or abstinence rates.

***Conclusions***

- Most studies suggested mass media programs have positive effects on individual smoking behaviors.
- Intensity and length of program may influence effectiveness of intervention.

***Implications for Nursing Practice***

1. What community resources can you use to help individuals who want to quit smoking?
2. How could you assist with a statewide program that seeks to reduce tobacco use?

***Reference for Evidence***

Bala M, Strzeszynski L, Topor-Madry R, et al: Mass media interventions for smoking cessation in adults, *Cochrane Database of Syst Rev* 6:CD004704, 2013.

*P*, Patient population of interest; *I*, intervention or area of interest; *C*, comparison of interest or comparison group; *O*, outcomes of interest; *T*, timing (see p. 15).

provides some nicotine effects to ease withdrawal symptoms. If the person does resume smoking, its antagonist action blocks the effects of nicotine at another subtype of nicotinic receptor, making smoking less enjoyable. Bupropion (Zyban), an antidepressant drug, reduces the urge to smoke, reduces some symptoms of withdrawal, and helps prevent weight gain associated with smoking cessation.

**DRUG ALERT Varenicline (Chantix) and Bupropion (Zyban)**

- Serious neuropsychiatric symptoms such as changes in behavior, hostility, agitation, depressed mood, suicidal thoughts and behavior, and attempted suicide can occur.
- Advise patients to stop taking these drugs and contact the HCP immediately if they experience any of these manifestations.

Along with using a smoking cessation product, users who wish to quit are more likely to succeed if they participate in a tobacco cessation program. You should be aware of community resources that assist users who are motivated to quit. Cessation programs may involve hypnosis, acupuncture, behavioral interventions, aversion therapy, group support programs, individual therapy, and self-help options. Many of these programs teach users to avoid high-risk situations for smoking relapse (e.g., those that promote cue-induced craving) and help them develop coping skills, such as cigarette refusal skills, assertiveness, alternative activities, and peer support systems.

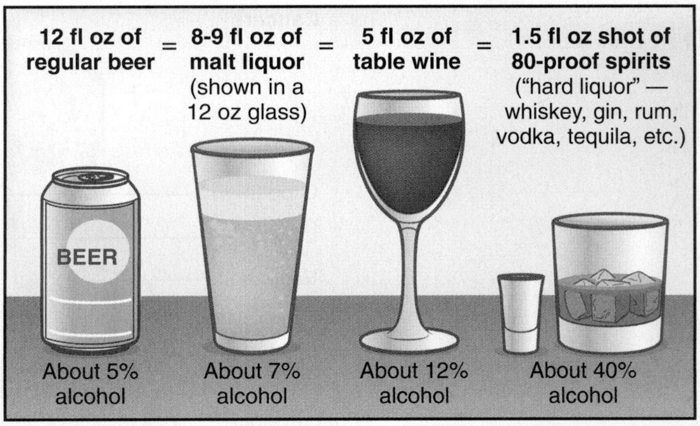


The percent of "pure" alcohol, expressed here as alcohol by volume (alc/vol), varies by beverage.

**FIG. 10-2** U.S. standard drink equivalents. The National Institute on Alcohol Abuse and Alcoholism (NIAAA) guidelines for alcohol use indicate that healthy men younger than 65 should consume no more than 14 standard drinks per week or 4 drinks per drinking occasion. Healthy, nonpregnant women and adults older than 65 should consume no more than 7 standard drinks per week or 3 drinks per drinking occasion. (From NIAAA: *What's a standard drink?* Retrieved from *www.niaaa.nih.gov.*)

## ALCOHOL

Sixty-five percent of Americans ages 18 and older consume alcohol. Most people use alcohol in moderation. *Risky drinking* is consuming alcohol in excess of established guidelines set forth by the National Institute on Alcohol Abuse and Alcoholism (Fig. 10-2). Risky drinking is associated with negative physical, emotional, and social consequences. **Alcohol use disorder (AUD)**, or alcoholism, affects about 7.2% of U.S. adults. A higher percent engage in periodic excess alcohol use. **Binge drinking** is alcohol use that brings blood alcohol concentration (BAC) levels over the legal limit for intoxication at least once per month.[6]

### Effects of Use and Complications

Alcohol affects almost all cells of the body. It changes levels of neurotransmitters in the central nervous system (CNS), affecting all areas and functions of the CNS. These include centers that control our impulses, mood, and behavior; coordinate motor activity; and promote respiratory and cardiac function. The immediate effects of alcohol depend on a person's susceptibility to alcohol and their BAC.

For the person who is not dependent on alcohol, the BAC is generally predictable of alcohol's effects. The relationship between BAC and behavior is different in a person who has developed tolerance to alcohol and its effects. The *tolerant person* is usually able to drink large amounts without obvious impairment and perform complex tasks without problems at BAC levels much higher than levels that would produce obvious impairment in the *nontolerant drinker*. Women have higher blood alcohol levels than men do after the same amount of alcohol intake.

Alcohol use has been linked to many health problems (Table 10-7), which frequently are the reason that people seek health care. Long-term alcohol use can lead to the development of high BP, heart disease, stroke, liver disease, and digestive problems. Short-term, excess alcohol use increases the risk of injury from motor vehicle crashes, falls, firearms, assault, drowning, and burns. A patient with AUD undergoing surgery has increased

**TABLE 10-5 Patient Teaching**

***Smoking and Tobacco Use Cessation***

*The following interventions are methods that work for quitting tobacco use. Tobacco users have the best chance of quitting if they use more than one method.*

**Develop a Quit Plan**

- Set a quit date, ideally within 2 weeks.
- Talk to your HCP about getting help to quit.
- Tell family, friends, and co-workers about quitting and request understanding and support.
- Anticipate withdrawal symptoms and challenges when quitting.
- Before quitting, avoid smoking in places where you spend a lot of time (work, car, home).
- Throw away all tobacco products from your home, car, and work.
- Have support options in place by your quit date.

**Use Approved Nicotine Replacement Systems**

- Use a nicotine replacement agent unless you are a pregnant or nursing woman (Table 10-6).
- Do not use other forms of tobacco when using nicotine replacement systems.

**Support and Encouragement**

- Joining a quit-tobacco support group will increase your chances of stopping permanently.
- If you get the urge for tobacco, call someone to help talk you out of it—preferably an ex-user.
- Be proud every time you reach a quit milestone and reward yourself.
- Do not be afraid to talk about how you feel while quitting, especially fears of not being able to quit for good. Ask your spouse or partner, friends, and co-workers to support you. Self-help materials, mobile phone applications, and hot lines are available:
  - American Lung Association: 800-586-4872; *www.lung.org*
  - American Cancer Society: 800-227-2345; *www.cancer.org*
  - National Cancer Institute: 800-784-8669; *www.smokefree.gov*

**Dealing With Urges to Use Tobacco**

- Identify situations that may cause you to want to smoke or use other tobacco, such as being around other smokers, being under time pressure, feeling sad or frustrated, and drinking alcohol.
- Avoid difficult situations while you are trying to quit. Try to lower your stress level.
- Exercise can help, such as walking, jogging, or bicycling.
- Distract yourself from thoughts of smoking and the urge to use tobacco by talking to someone, going to a movie, getting busy with a task, or having a game night with friends.
- Drink a lot of water.
- Keep your hands busy with a pen or toothpick.

**Avoiding Relapse**

Most relapses occur within the first 3 months after quitting. Do not be discouraged if you start using tobacco again. Remember, most people try several times before they finally quit. Explore different ways to break habits. You may have to deal with some of the following triggers that cause relapse.

- *Change your environment.* Get rid of cigarettes, tobacco (in any form), and ashtrays in your home, car, and place of work. Get rid of the smell of cigarettes in your car and home.
- *Alcohol.* Consider limiting or stopping alcohol use while you are quitting tobacco.
- *Other smokers at home.* Encourage housemates to quit with you. Work out a plan to cope with others who smoke, and avoid being around them.
- *Weight gain.* Tackle one problem at a time. Work on quitting tobacco first. You will not necessarily gain weight, and increased appetite is often temporary. Eat healthy and exercise.
- *Negative mood or depression.* If these symptoms persist, talk to your HCP. You may need treatment for depression.
- *Withdrawal symptoms.* Your body will go through many changes when you quit tobacco. You may have a dry mouth, cough, or scratchy throat, and you may feel irritable. The nicotine patch or gum may help with cravings (Table 10-6).
- *Focus on the benefits of quitting:*
  - Your BP and heart rate will lower almost immediately.
  - Your risk of a heart attack declines within 24 hours and the blood will become less likely to clot, making dangerous blood clots less likely.
  - Within a few weeks, you will be less short of breath, cough less, and have more energy. Your ability to smell and taste should improve.
  - Your immune system will be stronger, so you will be less likely to be sick.
  - Quitting will improve your night vision and help preserve your overall vision.

Adapted from National Cancer Institute: 18 ways smoking affects your health. Retrieved from *http://smokefree.gov/health-effects.*

readmission rates, increased in-hospital death rates, and longer length of stay.[7]

Complications may arise from the interaction of alcohol with commonly prescribed or OTC drugs. Drugs that interact with alcohol in an additive manner include antihypertensives, antihistamines, and antianginals. Alcohol taken with aspirin may cause or exacerbate GI bleeding. Alcohol taken with acetaminophen may increase the risk of liver damage. Taking an additional CNS depressant with alcohol can increase, or potentiate, the effect of both. An alcohol-dependent person may have cross-tolerance, requiring an increased dose of CNS depressants to achieve the desired effect.

## NURSING AND INTERPROFESSIONAL MANAGEMENT: ALCOHOL USE DISORDER

### Alcohol Toxicity

**Acute alcohol toxicity** occurs when a person has a high level of alcohol in his or her blood, generally after the ingestion of a large amount of alcohol. This leads to behavior changes and alcohol-induced CNS depression, resulting in respiratory and circulatory failure. Unconsciousness, coma, and possibly death can occur. Other common effects include hypokalemia, hypomagnesemia, and hypoglycemia.

Obtain as accurate a health history as possible and assess for injuries, diseases, and hypoglycemia. No antidote for alcohol is available. Implement supportive care measures to maintain airway, breathing, and circulation (the ABCs) until the alcohol metabolizes. Frequently monitor vital signs and level of consciousness. Treat alcohol-induced hypotension with IV fluids.

Patients with hypoglycemia may receive glucose-containing IV solutions. IV thiamine may be given before or with IV glucose solutions to prevent *Wernicke-Korsakoff syndrome,* which can cause seizures and brain damage.[8] Many patients have low serum magnesium levels and other signs of malnutrition, so HCPs frequently add multivitamins and magnesium to the IV fluids.

Agitation and anxiety are common. Stay with the patient as much as possible, orienting as necessary. Assess the patient for increasing belligerence and a potential for violence. Since the

**TABLE 10-6 Drug Therapy**

***Smoking Cessation****

| Agents | Common Side Effects | Considerations |
|---|---|---|
| **Nicotine Replacement Agents** | | |
| **Nicotine Gum (OTC)**<br>Nicorette 2 mg, 4 mg<br>• Use up to 12 wk<br>• Use 1 piece q1-2hr for 6 wk then q2-4hr for 3 wk<br>• Maximum dose: 24 pieces/day | Hiccups, mouth/jaw pain, mouth ulcers, indigestion, throat irritation, nausea | Specific 30-min chewing regimen with periods of holding the gum between cheek and teeth. Take only water 15 min before and during use. Difficult to use with dentures |
| **Nicotine Lozenge (OTC)**<br>Commit 2 mg, 4 mg<br>• Use 8-12 wk<br>• Use 1 lozenge q1-2hr tapering to 1 lozenge q4-8hr in 12 wk | Insomnia, nausea, sore throat, hiccups, cough, heartburn, headache, flatulence | Dissolves in mouth in 20 to 30 min. Do not chew or swallow. Avoid food and drink during use. Occasionally rotate around the mouth. |
| **Nicotine Patch (OTC)**<br>NicoDerm CQ, Habitrol, Nicotine transdermal system<br>• 18- or 24-hr doses<br>• Use ≥8 wk | Transient itching, burning, and redness at patch site. Insomnia, nausea, headache | Provides steady level of nicotine and is easy to use. Cannot be used by those with adhesive allergies. Rotate site to diminish skin irritation. |
| **Nicotine Nasal Spray**<br>Nicotrol NS<br>• 1-2 doses (2 sprays)/hr<br>• Use 3-6 mo | Nose and throat irritation, sneezing, rhinitis, headache, cough | Requires a prescription. Provides fastest nicotine delivery. Do not sniff or inhale while dosing. Tilt head back slightly for best results. |
| **Nicotine Inhaler**<br>Nicotrol nicotine inhalation system<br>• Use 1 cartridge q1-2hr<br>• Use 3-6 mo | Cough, mouth and throat irritation, headache, nausea, hiccups | Requires a prescription. Simulates smoking with mouthpiece and nicotine cartridge. May not be advisable for those with asthma or pulmonary disease |
| **Non-Nicotine Agents** | | |
| bupropion (Zyban)<br>• 150 mg/day for 3 days, then 150 mg bid<br>• Use 12 wk; can use up to 6 mo | Insomnia, dry mouth, irritability, rash, tremors, anorexia | Contraindicated with history of seizures or eating disorders. Promotes weight loss. First choice for smokers with depression |
| varenicline (Chantix)†<br>• 0.5 mg/day for 3 days, 0.5 mg bid for 4 days, then 1 mg bid<br>• Use 12 wk; additional 12 wk may be used in select patients | Nausea, sleep disturbances, constipation, flatulence, vomiting, headache | If taken concurrently with nicotine replacement therapy, incidence of nausea, headache, vomiting, dizziness, dyspepsia, and fatigue is increased, but nicotine pharmacokinetics not affected. |

*OTC nicotine replacement agents are also available in generic forms. Additional information and patient instructions are available from the American Lung Association at *www.lungusa.org*.

†See the Drug Alert for varenicline on p. 148.

patient is at risk for injury because of lack of coordination and impaired judgment, use protective measures.

### Alcohol Withdrawal Syndrome

**Alcohol withdrawal syndrome (AWS)** can develop in a hospitalized patient when the use of alcohol abruptly stops. The onset of AWS is variable depending on the quantity, frequency, pattern, and duration of alcohol use. The early signs usually develop within a few hours after the last drink. They peak after 24 to 48 hours and then disappear unless the withdrawal progresses to alcohol withdrawal delirium.

*Alcohol withdrawal delirium* is a serious complication that can occur from 2 to 3 days after the last drink and last 2 to 3 days. The greater the patient's dependence on alcohol, the greater the risk of alcohol withdrawal delirium. Death may result from hyperthermia, sepsis, aspiration pneumonia, or peripheral vascular collapse.[8]

Management begins with identifying at-risk people. Use a symptom assessment tool, such as the Clinical Institute Withdrawal Assessment of Alcohol Scale, Revised (CIWA-Ar), to determine treatment[8] (Table 10-8). Table 10-9 presents the clinical manifestations and suggested treatment for alcohol withdrawal. A nursing care plan (eNursing Care Plan 10-1) for a patient with AWS is available on the website at *http://evolve.elsevier.com/Lewis/medsurg*.

**CHECK YOUR PRACTICE**

A 34-yr-old male patient was admitted for multiple trauma following a car accident. His girlfriend tells you that he always drinks too much and she knew he would get in trouble someday.

- What signs and symptoms would alert you to the presence of alcohol withdrawal syndrome?
- What measures would you use to protect his safety?
- How would you involve members of the interprofessional team in planning patient care?

## USE OF OTHER SUBSTANCES

### STIMULANTS

Amphetamine-related stimulants are highly addictive substances. While the use of crack cocaine and methamphetamine is illegal, amphetamines have a role in treating narcolepsy and attention deficit disorder. While most people responsibly use prescribed stimulants, prescription stimulants are frequently misused. All stimulants increase cardiac activity and excite the CNS by increasing levels of norepinephrine, serotonin, and dopamine. People use these drugs to produce feelings of euphoria, increase alertness, and boost their energy. Health problems associated with using stimulants are presented in Table 10-2.

**TABLE 10-7 Effects of Chronic Alcohol Use**

| Body System | Effects |
|---|---|
| **Neurologic** | Alcoholic dementia, Wernicke-Korsakoff syndrome. Impaired cognitive function, psychomotor skills, abstract thinking, and memory. Depression, anxiety, attention deficit, labile moods, seizures, insomnia, peripheral neuropathy, chronic headache |
| **Immunologic** | Increased susceptibility to infections, depressed immune function |
| **Hematologic** | Bone marrow depression, anemia, leukopenia, thrombocytopenia, blood clotting abnormalities |
| **Musculoskeletal** | Myopathy, osteoporosis, gout |
| **Cardiac** | Hypertension, atrial fibrillation, cardiomyopathy, stroke, coronary artery disease, sudden cardiac death |
| **Hepatic** | Alcoholic hepatitis, cirrhosis, liver cancer |
| **Gastrointestinal** | Gastritis, gastroesophageal reflux disease (GERD), peptic ulcer, esophagitis, esophageal varices, gastrointestinal bleeding, pancreatitis, oropharyngeal cancer, colorectal cancer |
| **Nutrition** | Diabetes mellitus, anorexia, malnutrition, vitamin deficiencies (especially thiamine) |
| **Urinary** | Diuretic effect from inhibition of antidiuretic hormone |
| **Reproductive** | Breast cancer, testicular atrophy, decreased beard growth, decreased libido, decreased sperm count, gynecomastia |
| **Integumentary** | Palmar erythema, spider angiomas, rosacea, rhinophyma |

**TABLE 10-8 Clinical Institute Withdrawal Assessment of Alcohol Scale, Revised (CIWA-Ar)**

CIWA-Ar categories, with the range of scores in each category, are as follows:

| | | | |
|---|---|---|---|
| Agitation | 0-7 | Paroxysmal sweats | 0-7 |
| Anxiety | 0-7 | Tactile disturbances | 0-7 |
| Auditory disturbances | 0-7 | Tremor | 0-7 |
| Headache | 0-7 | Visual disturbances | 0-7 |
| Clouding of sensorium | 0-4 | | |

Source: University of Maryland School of Medicine. Available at *http://umem.org/files/uploads/1104212257_CIWA-Ar.pdf.*

## NURSING AND INTERPROFESSIONAL MANAGEMENT: STIMULANT USE

### Toxicity

Patients with stimulant toxicity present with *sympathetic overdrive* (increased stimulation of the sympathetic nervous system). The patient experiences restlessness, hypervigilance, agitated delirium, impaired judgment, and paranoia with psychotic symptoms. Physical effects include hypertension, tachycardia, fever, pupil dilation, seizures, confusion, and diaphoresis. Death may occur from stroke, dysrhythmias, or myocardial infarction.[1]

The emergency management depends on the clinical manifestations at the time of treatment (Table 10-10). A specific antidote for stimulant toxicity is not available. Supportive care measures include medications for agitation and cardiovascular symptoms.

### Withdrawal

Stimulant withdrawal is usually not an emergency. Abrupt cessation can lead to a "crash." The patient may be depressed and experience fatigue, prolonged sleep, vivid dreams, irritability, increased appetite, and disorientation. Craving for the stimulant drug is intense during the first hours to days of drug cessation and may continue for weeks. Supportive care includes maintaining a quiet environment and allowing the patient to sleep and eat as desired. If a patient has severe depression, initiate suicide precautions and refer for further treatment.

**TABLE 10-9 Manifestations and Treatment of Alcohol Withdrawal**

| Manifestations | Interprofessional Care |
|---|---|
| **Alcohol Withdrawal Syndrome** | |
| • Agitation<br>• Anxiety<br>• ↑ Heart rate<br>• ↑ BP<br>• Sweating<br>• Nausea<br>• Tremors<br>• Insomnia<br>• Hyperactivity | • Benzodiazepines (e.g., lorazepam [Ativan] or midazolam [Versed]) to prevent seizures and delirium<br>• Thiamine to prevent Wernicke-Korsakoff syndrome<br>• Multivitamins (e.g., folic acid, B vitamins)<br>• Magnesium sulfate to treat low serum magnesium<br>• IV glucose solution to treat hypoglycemia<br>• β-blockers (e.g., propranolol) or $\alpha_2$-agonists (e.g., clonidine) to stabilize VS<br>• Respiratory support |
| **Alcohol Withdrawal Delirium** | |
| • Disorientation<br>• Visual, tactile, or auditory hallucinations<br>• Seizures | • Continued use of benzodiazepines<br>• Carbamazepine (Tegretol) or valproate (Depakote) to treat seizures<br>• Antipsychotic agents (e.g., chlorpromazine [Thorazine], haloperidol [Haldol])<br>• Chlordiazepoxide (Librium) if psychosis persists after benzodiazepine administration |

**TABLE 10-10 Emergency Management**

***Stimulant Toxicity***

| Assessment Findings | Interventions |
|---|---|
| **Cardiovascular**<br>• Palpitations<br>• Tachycardia<br>• ↑ BP<br>• Dysrhythmias<br>• Myocardial ischemia or infarction<br>**Central Nervous System**<br>• Feeling of impending doom<br>• Euphoria<br>• Agitation<br>• Combativeness<br>• Seizures<br>• Hallucinations<br>• Confusion<br>• Paranoia<br>• Fever | • Ensure patent airway.<br>• Establish IV access and initiate fluid replacement as appropriate.<br>• Obtain a 12-lead ECG and initiate ECG monitoring.<br>• Treat ventricular dysrhythmias as appropriate with lidocaine, bretylium (Bretylol), or procainamide (Pronestyl).<br>• Hypertension and chest pain may require administration of nitroprusside (Nipride) or phentolamine (Regitine).<br>• Aspirin may be administered to lower the risk of myocardial infarction.<br>• Administer IV diazepam (Valium) or lorazepam (Ativan) for seizures.<br>• Administer IV antipsychotic drugs for psychosis and hallucinations.<br>• Monitor vital signs and level of consciousness.<br>• Initiate cooling measures for hyperthermia. |

## DEPRESSANTS

Commonly used depressants include sedative-hypnotics and opioids. Depressants have a rapid development of tolerance and dependence. Their use is also associated with medical emergencies involving toxicity and withdrawal. Deaths related to overdose are frequently caused by depressants and often from multiple depressants (e.g., opioids and benzodiazepines).[9] Excessive alcohol consumption is also common among those reporting high rates of depressant drug use.[9] Common health problems resulting from depressant use are listed in Table 10-2.

### Sedative-Hypnotics

Common sedative-hypnotic agents include barbiturates, benzodiazepines, and barbiturate-like drugs. Sedative-hypnotic drugs depress the CNS, causing sedation at low doses and sleep at high doses. Their use produces a euphoria and intoxication that resembles that of alcohol. Tolerance develops rapidly to the effects of these drugs, requiring higher doses to achieve euphoria. However, tolerance may not develop to the brainstem-depressant effects. As a result, an increased dose may trigger hypotension and respiratory depression, resulting in death.

### Opioids

The term *opioid* refers to a group of substances including opium, opium derivatives, and synthetic compounds. Individuals dependent on opioids include those who use illegal drugs sold on the street and those who misuse prescription opioids. Opioids act on opiate receptors and neurotransmitter systems in the CNS, causing sedation and analgesia. The person taking an opioid experiences euphoria, mood changes, mental clouding, drowsiness, and pain reduction. While this makes prescription opioids useful in treating a number of medical conditions, their pleasurable effects promote misuse. Misusing oxycodone (OxyContin) or acetaminophen plus hydrocodone can result in the same harmful consequences as abusing heroin.

## NURSING AND INTERPROFESSIONAL MANAGEMENT: DEPRESSANT USE

### Toxicity

Unintentional overdose frequently occurs with misuse of depressants, especially when used with alcohol or other drugs. The first priority of care is always the patient's ABCs. Depressant toxicity can cause death from CNS and respiratory depression. Continuous monitoring of neurologic status and supporting respiratory and cardiovascular function is critical until the patient is stable. The emergency management depends on the substance used and the clinical manifestations (Table 10-11).

**Sedative-Hypnotics.** On occasion, a patient with a benzodiazepine overdose may receive flumazenil, a specific benzodiazepine antagonist. Because flumazenil may have a shorter duration of action than some benzodiazepines, repeated doses may be needed until the benzodiazepine is metabolized. Place the patient on safety precautions, as flumazenil can cause seizures.

Since there are no antagonists for barbiturates or other sedative-hypnotic drugs, the patient who has overdosed on these agents receives treatment to promote drug elimination.[10]

**TABLE 10-11 Emergency Management**

***Depressant Toxicity***

| Assessment Findings | Interventions |
|---|---|
| • Aggressive behavior<br>• Agitation<br>• Confusion<br>• Lethargy<br>• Stupor<br>• Hallucinations<br>• Depression<br>• Slurred speech<br>• Pinpoint pupils<br>• Nystagmus<br>• Seizures<br>• Cold, clammy skin<br>• Rapid, weak pulse<br>• Slow or rapid shallow respirations<br>• Decreased $O_2$ saturation<br>• Hypotension<br>• Dysrhythmias<br>• ECG changes<br>• Cardiac or respiratory arrest | • Ensure patent airway.<br>• Anticipate intubation if respiratory distress evident.<br>• Establish IV access.<br>• Obtain temperature.<br>• Obtain 12-lead ECG and initiate continuous ECG monitoring.<br>• Obtain information about substance (name, route, when taken, amount).<br>• Obtain specific drug levels or comprehensive toxicology screen.<br>• Obtain a health history, including drug use and allergies.<br>• Administer antidotes as appropriate.<br>• Perform gastric lavage if necessary.<br>• Administer activated charcoal and cathartics as appropriate.<br>• Monitor vital signs, level of consciousness, and $O_2$ saturation. |

Dialysis is used to decrease the drug level and to prevent irreversible CNS effects and death. If the airway can be maintained, gastric lavage and activated charcoal are options.

**Opioids.** Opioid overdose can occur when a person deliberately misuses an illegal or prescription opioid, takes an opioid prescribed for someone else, takes an opioid in combination with other depressants, or inadvertently receives an incorrect opioid dose.[11] First-line treatment includes administering an opioid antagonist such as naloxone. Naloxone reverses respiratory depression, coma, and other manifestations of toxicity. Monitor the patient closely because naloxone has a shorter duration of action than most opioids. Repeated doses of naloxone may be required until the opioid is metabolized.

In some states, laws are making naloxone more widely available. This allows police, first responders, family members, and friends to administer naloxone in emergencies, thus reversing the effects of an overdose sooner. As a result, you may see more patients requiring postreversal care.

### Withdrawal

**Sedative-Hypnotics.** Withdrawal from sedative-hypnotics can be life threatening. The manifestations are nearly identical to those of alcohol withdrawal. Early, the patient may experience weakness, anxiety, insomnia, fever, orthostatic hypotension, and disorientation. Since the patient may experience delirium, seizures, and respiratory and cardiac arrest within 24 hours after the last dose, closely monitor the patient. Treatment consists of administering a long-acting benzodiazepine or phenobarbital in a tapered dose. IV diazepam is an option for severe manifestations. Supportive care includes implementing patient safety and comfort measures, frequently assessing neurologic status and vital signs, and providing reassurance and orientation.

**Opioids.** Opioid withdrawal symptoms depend on the opioid used, route of administration, and duration of use. It is usually not life threatening but can be extremely uncomfortable. Manifestations include intense drug craving, diaphoresis, GI distress, restlessness, fever, insomnia, watery eyes, tremors, muscle aches, runny nose, and altered mood.[1] With shorter-acting drugs, withdrawal occurs 6 to 8 hours after the last dose and peaks within 1 to 3 days. With longer-acting drugs, manifestations may not appear until 1 to 3 days after the last dose and peak in 4 to 6 days.

Treatment focuses on relieving symptoms and often requires medications. Substituting a long-acting opioid (e.g., methadone, buprenorphine) at low doses or $\alpha_2$-adrenergic agonists (e.g., clonidine [Catapres]) decreases withdrawal symptoms. Management includes GI medications (e.g., loperamide [Imodium], prochlorperazine [Compazine]), acetaminophen for muscle aches and fever, and benzodiazepines for acute anxiety and sleep disturbances.

## INHALANTS

Many products found in the home or workplace, such as markers, glues, and cleaning fluid, contain chemicals with psychoactive properties when they are inhaled. Many people do not consider these products as drugs. However, they are sometimes misused. Inhalants are rapidly absorbed and reach the CNS quickly. Most are depressants, and their effects are similar to alcohol, including slurred speech, lack of coordination, euphoria, and dizziness. The effects are relatively brief, lasting only 60 to 90 minutes. Long-term use can result in neurologic problems, including damage to parts of the brain that control cognition, movement, vision, and hearing (Table 10-2).

The patient with inhalant toxicity may experience dizziness, euphoria, disinhibition, nystagmus, slurred speech, and lethargy. The effects usually resolve within minutes to a few hours. Managing inhalant toxicity usually consists of providing supportive care. However, in some cases, users need emergency treatment for dysrhythmias, heart failure, or CNS hyperactivity (e.g., seizures). Using some inhalants (i.e., toluene) can result in nephrotoxicity; therefore monitor renal function. Withdrawal is rare as the duration of most inhaled substances is relatively short. Any manifestations that may occur require supportive care.

## CANNABIS

The use of cannabis, commonly referred to as marijuana or weed, continues to increase in the United States. The use patterns are similar to alcohol in that there is occasional use, misuse resulting in temporary problems, and the potential for SUD. The key ingredient in cannabis responsible for the psychoactive effects is tetrahydrocannabinol (THC). At low to moderate doses, THC produces effects similar to alcohol and other CNS depressants. These include euphoria, decreased inhibition, and impaired coordination. Long-term use is associated with a wide range of effects, particularly on cardiopulmonary and mental health[12] (Table 10-2).

The legalization of cannabis for medical and recreational use is controversial. While many states have legalized its use for specific medical reasons, legal sales for nonmedical use began for the first time in 2014.[12] THC-based medications, dronabinol (Marinol) and nabilone (Cesamet), are available to control nausea and vomiting resulting from cancer chemotherapy. Dronabinol is also used to stimulate the appetite in patients with acquired immunodeficiency syndrome (AIDS). Illegal synthetic THC derivatives (e.g., K2, Spice) contain varying amounts of different ingredients. The result is that these products have unpredictable effects and are more toxic. In some instances, death has occurred with a single use.

Patients with *acute marijuana toxicity* can present with acute psychotic episodes, especially if the patient used a synthetic derivative. Cannabis can induce tachycardia and hypertension, triggering dysrhythmias and myocardial infarction. Panic and flashbacks are managed by providing a quiet environment and reassuring the patient. Benzodiazepines provide symptom relief.

Withdrawal can occur in a hospitalized patient who heavily uses cannabis. The patient may experience irritability, anxiety, anorexia, chills, disturbed sleep, fever, and tremors.[1] These peak about 48 hours after cessation and last 3 to 4 days. No specific drug therapy is effective in treating withdrawal. Supportive care includes measures to ensure patient comfort, including analgesics and hydration.

## CAFFEINE

Caffeine is the most widely used psychoactive substance in the world. It is very weak when compared with the other stimulants. Most people use it to promote wakefulness. Other uses include facilitating motor activity and treating headaches. Its use is safe in most people. Recently, problems from high doses of caffeine have occurred in association with specialized drinks. A large caffeine intake can cause cardiac dysrhythmias, hypertension, disturbed sleep, seizures, and anxiety. Treatment consists of seizure control with benzodiazepines or phenobarbital and supportive care until the effects wear off. In a hospitalized patient, caffeine dependence can result in muscle pain or stiffness, drowsiness, irritability, and headaches after general anesthesia or during restrictions on usual caffeine intake.[1]

## ❖ NURSING MANAGEMENT: SUBSTANCE USE

### ◆ Nursing Assessment

You need to be able to determine if the patient uses substances in a way that places them at risk or if a SUD is present. Screening is a simple effective way to identify patients who need further assessment. The **Screening, Brief Intervention, and Referral to Treatment (SBIRT)** approach can be used (Fig. 10-3). SBIRT consists of three components: (1) screening

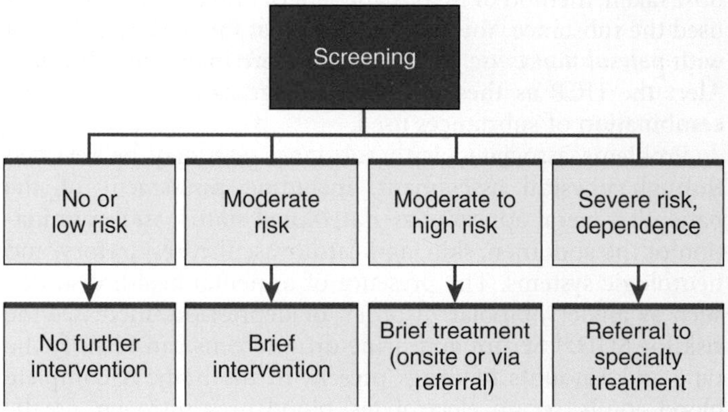


**FIG. 10-3** Screening, Brief Intervention, and Referral to Treatment Approach. (From Substance Abuse and Mental Health Services Administration [SAMHSA]: Systems-level implementation of screening, brief intervention, and referral to treatment. Technical Assistance Publication [TAP] Series 33. HHS Publication No. 13-4741. Rockville, Md, 2013, SAMHSA. Retrieved from *http://www.integration.samhsa.gov/SBIRT/tap33.pdf.*)

**TABLE 10-12 Brief Screening Tools for Substance Use**

**Single-Question Tests**

*Use one of the following questions to screen for the presence of alcohol, drug, or tobacco use.*
- How often in the past year have you had 5 (men) or 4 (women) or more drinks in a day?
- How many times in the past year have you used illegal drugs or prescription medications for nonmedical reasons?
- In the past year, how often have you used tobacco products?

**Two-Question Tests**

*Use the following two questions to screen for alcohol or drug use.*
- In the past year, have you ever drunk or used drugs more than you meant to?
- Have you felt you wanted or needed to cut down on your drinking or drug use in the past year?

Adapted from Strobbe S: Prevention and screening, brief intervention, and referral to treatment for substance use in primary care, *Prim Care Clin Office Pract* 41:185, 2014.

or assessing for substance use problems using standardized screening tools, (2) brief intervention or teaching patients about the consequences of substance use and abuse, and (3) referring those who screen positive for further treatment.[13]

The first step of SBIRT is using screening tools to identify those who may have problems with substance use. As a baseline, ask every patient about the use of all substances, including prescribed medications, OTC drugs, caffeine, tobacco, and recreational drugs. Use simple one- or two-question screening tests to detect alcohol, tobacco, and/or other substance use problems (Table 10-12). If a patient has a positive screen, follow up with a detailed assessment to identify specific problems. A screening tool for AUDIT, the Alcohol Use Disorders Identification Test, is shown in Table 10-13. A score of 8 points or more in men or 7 or more in women is considered problematic. Another useful tool is the Drug Abuse Screening Test (DAST-10), shown in Table 10-14.

If there is any indication of substance use, determine when the patient last used the substance. Knowing this information will let you know when to expect the onset of withdrawal and help you anticipate drug interactions. Assess for factors that influence the onset of withdrawal including the substance used, dose taken, method of intake, and length of time the patient has used the substance. You may discover that the patient is dealing with *polysubstance use*, or the use of more than one substance. Alert the HCP as these patients require care tailored to the combination of substances used.

Problems associated with substance use may be revealed through physical assessment, including assessment of the patient's general appearance, nutritional status, and examination of the abdomen, skin, and cardiovascular, respiratory, and neurologic systems. The presence of a mental health disorder, such as anxiety, bipolar disorder, or depression, increases the risk for SUD.[14] Serum and urine drug screens can identify the type and amounts of drugs present in the body. A complete blood count, serum electrolytes, blood urea nitrogen, creatinine, and liver function tests evaluate for electrolyte imbalances and cardiac, kidney, or liver dysfunction.

During your assessment, observe for patient behaviors such as denial, avoidance, underreporting or minimizing substance use, or provision of inaccurate information. Possible behaviors and physical manifestations suggesting substance use are listed in Table 10-15. However, these behaviors are not all inclusive.

**TABLE 10-13 Alcohol Use Disorders Identification Test (AUDIT)**

*Please answer each question by checking one of the circles in the second column.*

| Question | | Score |
|---|---|---|
| 1. How often do you have a drink containing alcohol? | ○ Never | (0) |
| | ○ Monthly or less | (1) |
| | ○ 2 to 4 times per month | (2) |
| | ○ 2 to 4 times per week | (3) |
| | ○ 4+ times per week | (4) |
| 2. How many drinks containing alcohol do you have on a typical day when you are drinking? | ○ 1 or 2 | (0) |
| | ○ 3 or 4 | (1) |
| | ○ 5 or 6 | (2) |
| | ○ 7 to 9 | (3) |
| | ○ 10 or more | (4) |
| 3. How often do you have six or more drinks on one occasion? | ○ Never | (0) |
| | ○ Less than monthly | (1) |
| | ○ Monthly | (2) |
| | ○ Weekly | (3) |
| | ○ Daily or almost daily | (4) |
| 4. How often during the last year have you found that you were not able to stop drinking once you had started? | ○ Never | (0) |
| | ○ Less than monthly | (1) |
| | ○ Monthly | (2) |
| | ○ Weekly | (3) |
| | ○ Daily or almost daily | (4) |
| 5. How often in the last year have you failed to do what was normally expected of you because you were drinking? | ○ Never | (0) |
| | ○ Less than monthly | (1) |
| | ○ Monthly | (2) |
| | ○ Weekly | (3) |
| | ○ Daily or almost daily | (4) |
| 6. How often during the last year have you needed a first drink in the morning to get yourself going after a heavy drinking session? | ○ Never | (0) |
| | ○ Less than monthly | (1) |
| | ○ Monthly | (2) |
| | ○ Weekly | (3) |
| | ○ Daily or almost daily | (4) |
| 7. How often during the last year have you had a feeling of guilt or remorse about drinking? | ○ Never | (0) |
| | ○ Less than monthly | (1) |
| | ○ Monthly | (2) |
| | ○ Weekly | (3) |
| | ○ Daily or almost daily | (4) |
| 8. How often during the last year have you been unable to remember what happened the night before because you had been drinking? | ○ Never | (0) |
| | ○ Less than monthly | (1) |
| | ○ Monthly | (2) |
| | ○ Weekly | (3) |
| | ○ Daily or almost daily | (4) |
| 9. Have you or someone else been injured as a result of your drinking? | ○ No | (0) |
| | ○ Yes, but not in the last year | (2) |
| | ○ Yes, during the last year | (4) |
| 10. Has a relative, friend, or other health worker been concerned about your drinking or suggested that you cut down? | ○ No | (0) |
| | ○ Yes, but not in the last year | (2) |
| | ○ Yes, during the last year | (4) |

Source: Babor TF, Higgins-Biddle JC, Saunders JB, Monteiro M: *The alcohol use disorders identification test*, ed 2, Geneva, Switzerland, 2001, WHO Press.
*Scoring for AUDIT:* Questions 1 through 8 are scored 0, 1, 2, 3, or 4. Questions 9 and 10 are scored 0, 2, or 4 only. The minimum score (nondrinkers) is 0 and the maximum possible score is 40. A score of 9 or more indicates hazardous or harmful alcohol consumption.

## ◆ Nursing Diagnoses

Nursing diagnoses for the patient with substance use disorder include, but are not limited to, the following:

**TABLE 10-14 Drug Abuse Screening Test (DAST-10)**

| *In the last 12 months:* | | |
|---|---|---|
| 1. Have you used drugs other than those required for medical reasons? | No | Yes |
| 2. Do you abuse more than one drug at a time? | No | Yes |
| 3. Are you always able to stop using drugs when you want to? | No | Yes |
| 4. Have you had "blackouts" or "flashbacks" as a result of drug use? | No | Yes |
| 5. Do you ever feel bad or guilty about your drug use? | No | Yes |
| 6. Does your spouse (or parents) ever complain about your involvement with drugs? | No | Yes |
| 7. Have you neglected your family because of your use of drugs? | No | Yes |
| 8. Have you engaged in illicit activities in order to obtain drugs? | No | Yes |
| 9. Have you ever experienced withdrawal symptoms or felt sick when you stopped taking drugs? | No | Yes |
| 10. Have you had medical problems as a result of your drug use? | No | Yes |



**TABLE 10-15 Manifestations Suggesting Substance Use**

- Fatigue
- Insomnia
- Headaches
- Seizure disorder
- Changes in mood
- Anorexia, weight loss
- Vague physical complaints
- Overuse of mouthwash or toiletries
- Appearing older than stated age, unkempt appearance
- Leisure activities that involve alcohol and/or other drugs
- Sexual dysfunction, decreased libido, erectile dysfunction
- Trauma secondary to falls, auto accidents, fights, or burns
- Driving while intoxicated (more than one citation suggests dependence)
- Failure of standard doses of sedatives to have a therapeutic effect
- Financial problems, including those related to spending for substances
- Defensive or evasive answers to questions about substance use and its importance in the person's life
- Problems in areas of life function (e.g., frequent job changes; marital conflict, separation, or divorce; work-related accidents, tardiness, absenteeism; legal problems; social isolation, estrangement from friends or family)

- Acute confusion *related to* toxicity or withdrawal
- Disturbed sensory perception *related to* toxicity or withdrawal
- Risk for injury *related to* altered mental status
- Ineffective health maintenance *related to* substance use

## Planning

The overall goals are that the patient with a substance use problem will (1) have normal physiologic functioning, (2) acknowledge a substance use problem, (3) explain the psychologic and physiologic effects of substance use, (4) abstain from substance use, and (5) cooperate with a proposed treatment plan.

## Nursing Implementation

**Health Promotion.** Your role in health promotion includes prevention and early detection of substance use. Prevention measures include abstinence from potentially harmful substances or limiting alcohol consumption. These measures decrease the risk of substance-related injury or illness.[14] You can help to prevent substance use problems by (1) teaching about the effects and negative outcomes of substance use and (2) providing support. Through early screening, you have the opportunity to prevent patients from becoming dependent on alcohol and other drugs. You can do this by initiating brief interventional techniques and helping them access appropriate care through referral to treatment if they exhibit risky behaviors or are already dependent.

**Acute Intervention.** The immediate result of overconsumption is acute toxicity or overdose. The patient may also present with trauma or injuries. The first priority of care is supporting the patient's ABCs, especially respiratory status. In addition to treating injuries, provide supportive care until detoxification can occur. Nursing care includes frequently assessing neurologic status and vital signs, administering IV fluids to prevent dehydration, orienting to time and place, and implementing patient safety measures.

Sometimes, uncertainty exists as to what substances are involved. If the patient used multiple substances, a complex clinical picture can result. For example, a patient presents with toxicity and the health care team does not know what substances are involved. Although blood and urine tests will help identify the substances, treatment is started while waiting for the test results. The patient in this situation would usually receive naloxone. If the substance used is a barbiturate or another CNS depressant, naloxone will not help the patient, but it will not hurt the patient either. If the patient does not respond to a total dose of 10 mg of naloxone, it is unlikely opioids are involved.

Once acute health issues are resolved, provide a brief intervention to teach patients about the consequences of substance use and support behavioral change. When patients have a substance use problem, it is critical to motivate the patient to engage in long-term treatment. You are in a unique position to facilitate behavior change. When a patient seeks care for health problems related to substance use or when hospitalization interferes with the usual pattern of use, the patient's awareness of a substance use problem is increased. Intervention at this time can promote behavior change. Take an active role in performing motivational interviewing and providing counseling aimed at cessation. (Motivational interviewing is discussed in Chapter 4.) Discuss the risks associated with substance use and provide feedback and advice. If the patient agrees, assist with referral to counseling or behavioral therapy.

## Gerontologic Considerations: Substance Use

Substance use in older adults is often difficult to recognize. Older adults do not fit the image of users. For example, older users are less likely to be involved in drug-related criminal activity and less likely to binge drink. They use different substances than younger users. The effects of alcohol and drug use can be mistaken for medical conditions common among older adults (e.g., insomnia, depression, hypertension, dementia). Therefore substance use problems may be attributed to another cause and not adequately treated (Fig. 10-4).

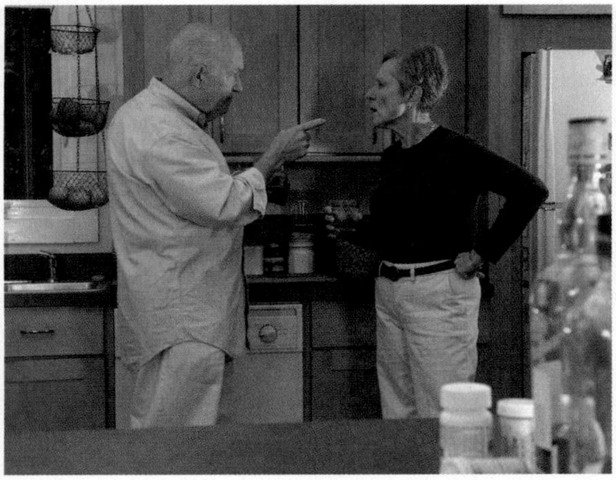

**FIG. 10-4** Older adults are often unaware of their substance use problems. (©Ned White/iStock/Thinkstock)

Because of the higher rate of co-existing medical problems, older adults are at greater risk for medical problems associated with substance use. Common problems include liver damage and cardiovascular, GI, and endocrine problems. Substance use may cause confusion, delirium, memory loss, and neuromuscular impairment. Physiologic changes may lead to toxicity at levels that may not have been a problem at a younger age. Withdrawal symptoms may be more severe than in younger individuals.

It is important to screen older adults for substance use. Family members are important sources of information. Other potential sources include friends, home health aides, meal delivery personnel, and staff members at senior citizen centers and long-term care facilities. It is important for you to discuss all drug and alcohol use with older adult patients, including OTC, herbal, and homeopathic drug use. Assess the patient's knowledge of currently used medications. Common screening questionnaires may not identify an older adult with a substance use problem. The Short Michigan Alcoholism Screening Test–Geriatric version (SMAST-G) is available as a short-form alcoholism-screening instrument for older adults *(http://consultgerirn.org)* and can identify those with a potential AUD.

Smoking and other tobacco use is an issue in older adults. Those who have been chronic smokers for decades may feel unable to stop or believe there is no benefit to stopping at an advanced age. However, smoking contributes to and exacerbates many chronic illnesses found in the older adult population. Smoking cessation at any age is beneficial. The information about smoking cessation discussed earlier is appropriate for helping older adults with smoking cessation (Tables 10-3 to 10-6).

Patient teaching for the older adult includes teaching about the desired effects, possible side effects, and appropriate use of prescribed and OTC drugs. When you suspect alcohol or substance use, refer the patient for treatment. It is a mistaken belief that older people have little to gain from alcohol and drug dependence treatment. The rewards of treatment can lead to greater quality and quantity of life for older adults.

## CASE STUDY

### *Substance Use Disorder*

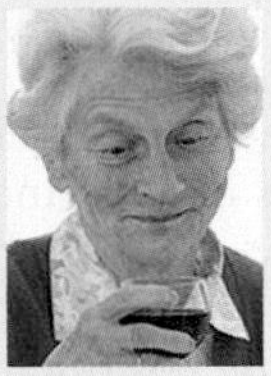

(©JPC-PROD/iStock/Thinkstock)

**Patient Profile**

C.M., a 78-year-old white woman, is admitted to the emergency department after falling and injuring her right hip. She has been widowed for 4 years and lives alone. Recently her best friend died. Her only family is a daughter who lives out of town. When contacted by phone, the daughter tells the nurse that her mother has appeared more disoriented and confused over the past few months when she has talked to her on the phone.

**Subjective Data**

- Is complaining of severe pain in her right hip
- Admits she had some wine in the late afternoon to stimulate her appetite
- Has experienced several falls in the past 2 months
- Reports that she fell after taking a sleeping pill prescribed by her physician because she does not sleep well
- Speech is hesitant and slurred
- Says she smokes about one-half pack of cigarettes a day

**Objective Data**

***Physical Examination***

- Oriented to person and place, but not time
- BP 162/94, pulse 92, respirations 24
- Severe pain and tenderness in the right hip region
- Tremors of hands

***Diagnostic Tests***

- X-ray reveals a subtrochanteric fracture of the right femur requiring surgical repair
- Blood alcohol concentration (BAC) 120 mg/dL (0.12 mg%)
- Complete blood count: hemoglobin 10.6 g/dL, hematocrit 33%

**Discussion Questions**

1. What other information is needed to assess C.M.'s condition?
2. How should you address questions regarding these areas?
3. What factors may contribute to C.M.'s substance use?
4. ***Priority Decision:*** Based on the assessment data presented, what are the priority nursing diagnoses? Are there any collaborative problems?
5. ***Priority Decision:*** What are the priority nursing interventions during C.M.'s preoperative period?
6. What possible complications and injury risks may become apparent during C.M.'s postoperative recovery?
7. ***Safety:*** To ensure C.M.'s safety, what nursing interventions are necessary after surgery?
8. ***Teamwork and Collaboration:*** How would you use the unlicensed assistive personnel (UAP) on the postoperative unit to carry out the interventions that you identified in question 5?
9. ***Teamwork and Collaboration:*** What referrals are indicated?

Answers available at *http://evolve.elsevier.com/Lewis/medsurg.*

## BRIDGE TO NCLEX EXAMINATION

The number of the question corresponds to the same-numbered outcome at the beginning of the chapter.

1. When admitting a patient, the nurse must assess the patient for substance use based on the knowledge that long-term use of addictive substances leads to
   - **a.** the development of coexisting psychiatric illnesses.
   - **b.** a higher risk for complications from underlying health problems.
   - **c.** potentiation of effects of similar drugs taken when the individual is drug free.
   - **d.** increased availability of dopamine, resulting in decreased sleep requirements.
2. The nurse would suspect cocaine toxicity in the patient who is experiencing
   - **a.** agitation, dysrhythmias, and seizures.
   - **b.** blurred vision, restlessness, and irritability.
   - **c.** diarrhea, nausea and vomiting, and confusion.
   - **d.** slow, shallow respirations; bradycardia; and hypotension.
3. The *most* appropriate nursing intervention for a patient who is being treated for an acute exacerbation of chronic obstructive pulmonary disease who is not interested in quitting smoking is to
   - **a.** accept the patient's decision and not intervene until the patient expresses a desire to quit.
   - **b.** realize that some smokers never quit, and trying to assist them increases the patient's frustration.
   - **c.** motivate the patient to quit by describing how continued smoking will worsen the breathing problems.
   - **d.** ask the patient to identify the risks and benefits of quitting and what barriers to quitting are present.
4. While caring for a patient who is experiencing alcohol withdrawal, the nurse should *(select all that apply)*
   - **a.** monitor neurologic status on a routine basis.
   - **b.** provide a quiet, nonstimulating, dimly lit environment.
   - **c.** pad the side rails and place suction equipment at the bedside.
   - **d.** orient the patient to environment and person with each contact.
   - **e.** administer antiseizure drugs and sedatives to relieve symptoms during withdrawal.
5. A patient admitted for scheduled surgery has a positive brief screening test result for an alcohol use disorder. Which initial action is *most* appropriate?
   - **a.** notify the health care provider.
   - **b.** complete a detailed alcohol use assessment.
   - **c.** initiate a referral to a specialty treatment center.
   - **d.** provide patient teaching on postoperative health risks.
6. Substance use problems in older adults are usually related to
   - **a.** use of drugs and alcohol as a social activity.
   - **b.** misuse of prescribed and over-the-counter drugs and alcohol.
   - **c.** continuing the use of illegal drugs initiated during middle age.
   - **d.** a pattern of binge drinking for weeks or months with periods of sobriety.

1. b, 2. a, 3. d, 4. a, c, d, e, 5. b, 6. b

For rationales to these answers and even more NCLEX review questions, visit *http://evolve.elsevier.com/Lewis/medsurg.*

## EVOLVE WEBSITE

http://evolve.elsevier.com/Lewis/medsurg

**Review Questions (Online Only)**

**Key Points**

**Answer Keys for Questions**

- Rationales for Bridge to NCLEX Examination Questions
- Answer Guidelines for Case Study on p. 156
- Answer Guidelines for Managing Care of Multiple Patients Case Study (Section 1) on p. 158

**Nursing Care Plan**

- eNursing Care Plan 10-1: Patient in Alcohol Withdrawal

**Conceptual Care Map Creator**

**Audio Glossary**

**Content Updates**

## REFERENCES


1. American Psychiatric Association: *The diagnostic and statistical manual of mental disorders*, ed 5, Arlington, Va, 2013, The Association.
2. CDC: Adult cigarette smoking in the U.S. Retrieved from *www.cdc.gov/tobacco/data_statistics/fact_sheets/adult_data/cig_smoking.*
3. CDC: Health effects of cigarette smoking. Retrieved from *www.cdc.gov/tobacco/data_statistics/fact_sheets/health_effects/effects_cig_smoking/#overview.*

*4. Hajek P, Etter J, Benowitz N, et al: Electronic cigarettes: review of use, content, safety, effects on smokers and potential for harm and benefit, *Addiction* 109:1801, 2014.

5. Agency for Healthcare Research and Quality: Treating tobacco use and dependence: 2008 update. Retrieved from *www.ahrq.gov/professionals/clinicians-providers/guidelines-recommendations/tobacco/index.html.*
6. Alcohol Facts and Statistics. Retrieved from *www.niaaa.nih.gov/alcohol-health/overview-alcohol-consumption/alcohol-facts-and-statistics.*
7. Miguel GM, Bejar-Prado L, Gili-Ortiz E, et al: Alcohol use disorders among surgical patients: Unplanned 30-days readmissions, length of hospital stay, excessive costs and mortality, *Drug Alc Dep* 137:55, 2014.
8. Patel G: The management of substance abuse in the critically ill, *Disease-a-Month* 60:429, 2014.
9. CDC: Prescription drug overdose in the United States. Retrieved from *www.cdc.gov/homeandrecreationalsafety/overdose/facts.html.*

*10. Mactier R, Laliberté M, Mardini J, et al: Extracorporeal treatment for barbiturate poisoning, *Am J of Kidney Dis* 64:347, 2014.

11. Substance Abuse and Mental Health Services Administration: *Opioid overdose prevention toolkit*, HHS Publication No. SMA 14-4742 2014, Rockville, Md, 2013, The Institute.
12. Durkin A: Legalization of marijuana for non-medical use, *J Psychosoc Nurs* 52:22, 2014.
13. SAMSA-HRSA Center for Integrated Health Solutions: SBIRT. Retrieved from *www.integration.samhsa.gov/clinical-practice/SBIRT.*
14. Strobbe S: Prevention and screening, brief intervention, and referral to treatment for substance use in primary care, *Prim Care Clin Office Pract* 41:185, 2014.


*Evidence-based information for clinical practice.

## CASE STUDY

### *Managing Care of Multiple Patients*

#### Introduction

You are assigned to care for the following five patients on a medical-surgical unit. Your team consists of yourself, a new LPN still on orientation, and a UAP (unlicensed assistive personnel).

#### Patients

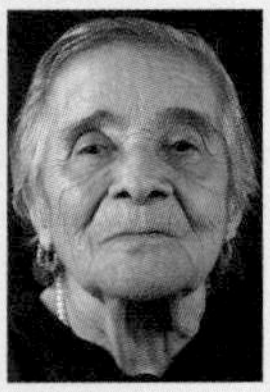

(©Luevanos/iStock/Thinkstock)

M.S. is an 81-yr-old woman who came to the United States from India 4 yr ago with her daughter, son-in-law, and their four children. She speaks minimal English, relying on her oldest granddaughter to translate. M.S., who has a history of diabetes mellitus, was admitted to the hospital yesterday with a diagnosis of heart failure.

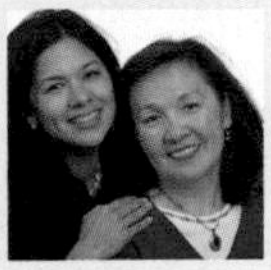

(©Thomas M Perkins/Shutterstock)

M.L. is a 60-yr-old Asian woman who was admitted to the hospital with a diagnosis of exacerbation of chronic obstructive pulmonary disease (COPD). She is receiving $O_2$ at 2 L/min via nasal cannula and her condition is currently stable.

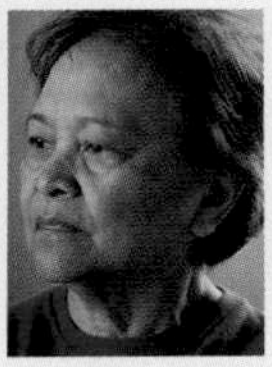

(©azndc/iStock/Thinkstock)

C.L. is a 73-yr-old Taiwanese woman who was brought to the ED by her son. Her chief complaint is shortness of breath. She has a history of COPD, hypertension, diabetes, and stroke. She was diagnosed with community-acquired pneumonia, which is being treated with IV antibiotics.

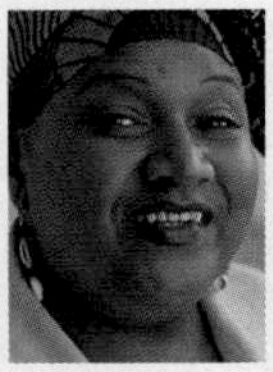

(©Ryan McVey/Photodisc/Thinkstock)

K.C. is a 280-lb (127-kg) 68-yr-old African American woman with diabetes who was admitted for an incision and drainage of a right abdominal abscess. She is being discharged on her second postoperative day. Her daughter will assist with dressing changes at home.

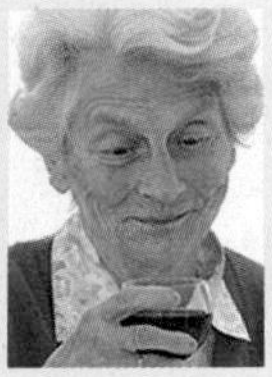

(©JPC-PROD/iStock/Thinkstock)

C.M. is a 78-yr-old white woman who was admitted from the ED after falling and fracturing her right hip. She is in Buck's traction and is scheduled to undergo surgical repair later this morning. She has a history of substance abuse and her blood alcohol content (BAC) was 120 mg/dL (0.12 mg%) on admission. The night nurse reports that she has been somewhat confused and restless overnight.

#### Discussion Questions

1. ***Priority Decision:*** After receiving report, which patient should you see first? Provide rationale.
2. **Teamwork and Collaboration:** Which morning task(s) could you delegate to the LPN *(select all that apply)*?
   a. Obtain a capillary blood glucose reading on K.C.
   b. Assess C.L.'s IV site for signs of phlebitis or infiltration.
   c. Access the hospital's available translation services for M.S.
   d. Provide discharge teaching on wound care for K.C. and her daughter.
   e. Titrate M.L.'s $O_2$ to obtain a pulse oximetry reading of 95% (as ordered by the health care provider).
3. ***Priority and Teamwork and Collaboration:*** When you and the LPN enter M.S.'s room, you find her sitting up in bed with labored respirations. Although you cannot understand what she is saying, you note that she is unable to say more than two words without stopping for a breath. Which *initial* action would be the *most* appropriate?
   a. Administer M.S.'s cardiac and respiratory medications and reassess her in 30 minutes.
   b. Ask the LPN to stay with M.S. while you go to the nurse's station to call her health care provider.
   c. Have the LPN find M.S.'s granddaughter so that she can translate what M.S. is trying to tell you.
   d. Ask the LPN to obtain an $O_2$ saturation and vital signs while you perform a respiratory assessment.

#### Case Study Progression

M.S.'s assessment reveals bibasilar crackles, 2+ dependent pitting edema, BP 175/84, pulse 116, RR 32, temp 36.8°C, and pulse oximetry 88% on room air. You administer $O_2$ at 4 L/min via nasal cannula and obtain an order from M.S.'s health care provider for furosemide 40 mg IV stat. After administering the diuretic, M.S.'s granddaughter arrives and you discuss her grandmother's condition. She tells you that her grandmother asked her to bring in potato chips and soda yesterday. She did not think her grandmother should be eating salt, but M.S. insisted that the dietitian said that she could eat them.

4. On further investigation, the dietitian tells you that an interpreter (translator) was not available when she saw M.S. yesterday. Because the dietitian did not understand what the patient was saying, she could not respond to any of her questions. She planned to visit M.S. today when the granddaughter is present. Being a culturally competent nurse, you realize that M.S. most likely interpreted the dietitian's silence as
   a. agreement with what A.Z. was asking.
   b. demonstrating a lack of respect for A.Z.'s wishes.
   c. a lack of understanding by the dietitian as to what she was asking.
   d. a need for the dietitian to get more information before answering her questions.
5. Which assessment findings may suggest elder mistreatment by C.L.'s son with whom she lives *(select all that apply)*?
   a. Two sacral ulcers
   b. Asking when her son is coming to visit
   c. Multiple small bruises on her forearms and shins
   d. Matted hair, poor oral hygiene, overgrown toenails
   e. C.L. becomes totally silent when her son comes to visit
6. Knowing that C.M.'s reported restlessness overnight may indicate acute alcohol withdrawal, you perform a more thorough assessment. Your assessment reveals a score of 11 on the Clinical Institute Withdrawal Assessment for Alcohol Scale. To prevent alcohol delirium, you plan to administer which medications per the health care provider's order *(select all that apply)*?
   a. IV thiamine
   b. morphine
   c. naloxone
   d. lorazepam (Ativan)
   e. haloperidol (Haldol)
7. ***Management Decision:*** The UAP informs you that the LPN is not following hospital protocol when caring for patients at risk for falling. What is your *most* appropriate action?
   a. Notify the unit manager as soon as possible.
   b. Ask the UAP to explain hospital protocol to the LPN.
   c. Write up the LPN's actions so they are included in her evaluation.
   d. Talk to the LPN about the importance of following hospital protocol to prevent injury in patients at risk for falling.

Answers available at *http://evolve.elsevier.com/Lewis/medsurg.*

# SECTION 2

# Pathophysiologic Mechanisms of Disease

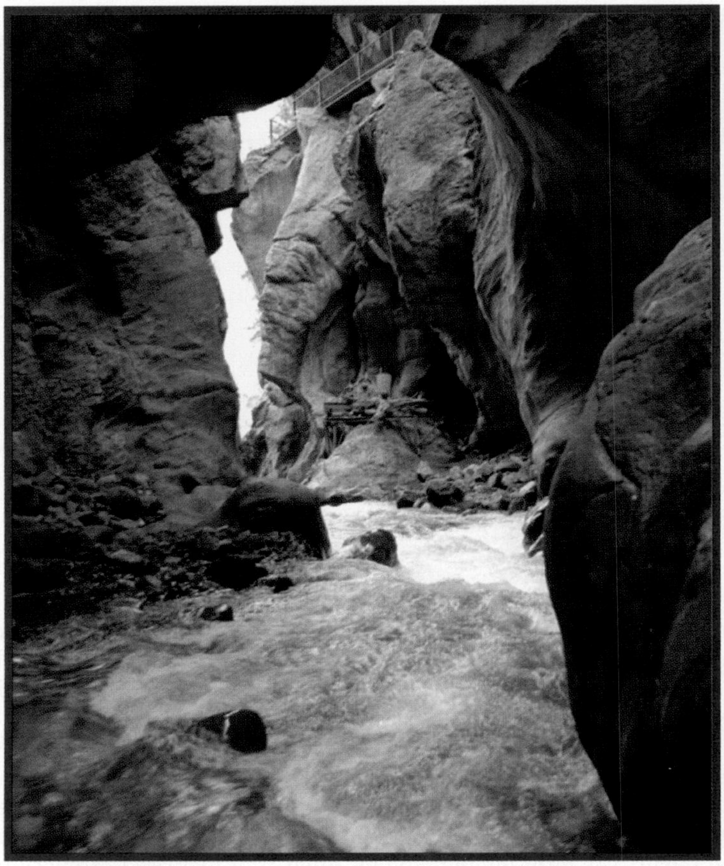

Peter Bonner

*May what I do flow from me like a river,*
*no forcing and no holding back,*
*the way it is with children.*

***Rainer Maria Rilke***

11

# Inflammation and Wound Healing

*Sharon L. Lewis*

*The most difficult thing is the decision to act, the rest is merely tenacity.*

*Amelia Earhart*

http://evolve.elsevier.com/Lewis/medsurg/

## LEARNING OUTCOMES

1. Describe the inflammatory response, including vascular and cellular responses and exudate formation.
2. Explain local and systemic manifestations of inflammation and their physiologic bases.
3. Describe the drug therapy, nutrition therapy, and nursing management of inflammation.
4. Differentiate among healing by primary, secondary, and tertiary intention.
5. Describe the factors that delay wound healing and common complications of wound healing.
6. Describe the nursing and interprofessional management of wound healing.
7. Explain the etiology and clinical manifestations of pressure ulcers.
8. Apply a patient risk assessment for pressure ulcers to measures used to prevent the development of pressure ulcers.
9. Discuss nursing and interprofessional management of a patient with pressure ulcers.

## KEY TERMS

**adhesions, Table 11-7, p. 167**
**dehiscence, Table 11-7, p. 167**
**evisceration, Table 11-7, p. 167**
**fibroblasts, p. 166**
**hypertrophic scars, Table 11-7, p. 167**
**inflammatory response, p. 160**
**pressure ulcer, p. 172**
**regeneration, p. 165**
**repair, p. 165**
**shearing force, p. 172**

This chapter focuses on inflammation and wound healing. Pressure ulcer prevention and treatment are also described.

## INFLAMMATORY RESPONSE

The **inflammatory response** is a sequential reaction to cell injury. It neutralizes and dilutes the inflammatory agent, removes necrotic materials, and establishes an environment suitable for healing and repair. The term *inflammation* is often but incorrectly used as a synonym for the term *infection.* Inflammation is always present with infection, but infection is not always present with inflammation. However, a person who is neutropenic may not be able to mount an inflammatory response. An infection involves invasion of tissues or cells by microorganisms such as bacteria, fungi, and viruses. In contrast, inflammation can also be caused by heat, radiation, trauma, chemicals, allergens, and an autoimmune reaction.

The mechanism of inflammation is basically the same regardless of the injuring agent. The intensity of the response depends on the extent and severity of injury and on the injured person's reactive capacity. The inflammatory response can be divided into a vascular response, cellular response, formation of exudate, and healing. Fig. 11-1 illustrates the vascular and cellular response to injury.

### Vascular Response

After cell injury, local arterioles briefly undergo transient vasoconstriction. After release of histamine and other chemicals by the injured cells, the vessels dilate. Chemical mediators cause increased capillary permeability and facilitate fluid movement from capillaries into tissue spaces. Initially composed of serous fluid, this inflammatory exudate later contains plasma proteins, primarily albumin. These proteins exert oncotic pressure that further draws fluid from blood vessels. Both vasodilation and increased capillary permeability are responsible for redness, heat, and swelling at the site of injury and the surrounding area.

As the plasma protein fibrinogen leaves the blood, it is activated to fibrin by the products of the injured cells. Fibrin strengthens a blood clot formed by platelets. In tissues, the clot functions to trap bacteria, prevent their spread, and serve as a framework for the healing process. Platelets release growth factors that start the healing process.

Reviewed by Marylee Bressie, RN, DNP, CCRN, CCNS, CEN, Core Faculty/Nurse Planner, Department of Nursing, School of Public Service Leadership, Capella University, Minneapolis, Minnesota; Diana L. Gallagher, RN, MS, CWOCN, CFCN, Clinical Nursing and Education, HealthMatters Consulting, Fayetteville, Arkansas; and Christina D. Keller, RN, MSN-Ed, Instructor, Clinical Simulation Center, Radford University, Radford, Virginia.

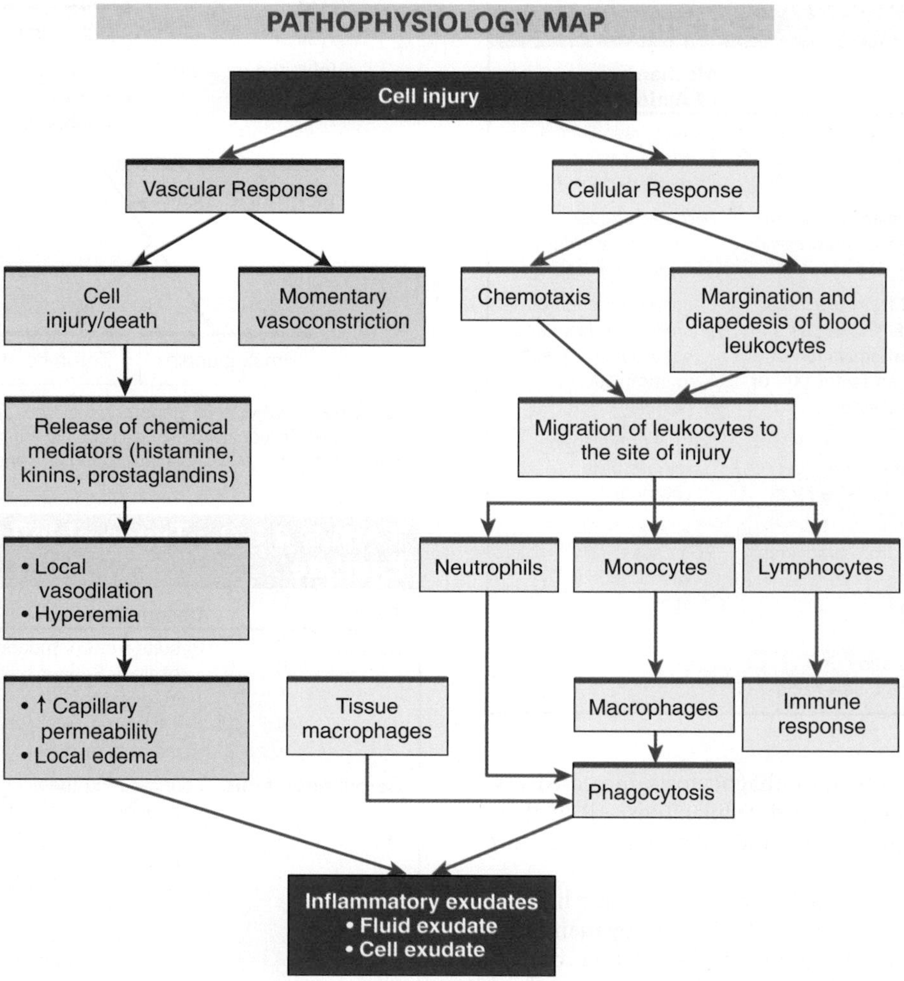


**FIG. 11-1** Vascular and cellular responses to tissue injury.

## Cellular Response

Neutrophils and monocytes move from circulation to the site of injury (Fig. 11-1). *Chemotaxis* is the directional migration of white blood cells (WBCs) to the site of injury, resulting in an accumulation of neutrophils and monocytes at the site.

**Neutrophils.** Neutrophils are the first leukocytes to arrive at the injury site (usually within 6 to 12 hours). They phagocytize (engulf) bacteria, other foreign material, and damaged cells. With their short life span (24 to 48 hours), dead neutrophils soon accumulate. In time a mixture of dead neutrophils, digested bacteria, and other cell debris accumulates as a creamy substance termed *pus.*

To keep up with the demand for neutrophils, the bone marrow releases more neutrophils into circulation. This results in an elevated WBC count, especially the neutrophil count. Sometimes the demand for neutrophils increases to the extent that the bone marrow releases immature forms of neutrophils *(bands)* into circulation. (Mature neutrophils are called *segmented neutrophils.*) The finding of increased numbers of band neutrophils in circulation is called a *shift to the left,* which is commonly found in patients with acute bacterial infections. (See Chapter 29 for a discussion of neutrophils.)

**Monocytes.** Monocytes are the second type of phagocytic cells that migrate from circulating blood. They usually arrive at the site within 3 to 7 days after the onset of inflammation. On entering the tissue spaces, monocytes transform into macrophages. Together with the tissue macrophages, these newly arrived macrophages assist in phagocytosis of the inflammatory debris. The macrophage role is important in cleaning the area before healing can occur. Macrophages have a long life span; they can multiply and may stay in the damaged tissues for weeks. These long-lived cells are important in orchestrating the healing process.

In cases in which particles are too large for a single macrophage, the macrophages accumulate and fuse to form a *multinucleated giant cell.* The giant cell is then encapsulated by collagen, leading to the formation of a granuloma. A classic example of this process occurs in tuberculosis of the lung. While the *Mycobacterium* bacillus is walled off, a chronic state of inflammation exists. The granuloma formed is a cavity of necrotic tissue.

**Lymphocytes.** Lymphocytes arrive later at the site of injury. Their primary role is related to humoral and cell-mediated immunity (see Chapter 13).

## Chemical Mediators

Mediators of the inflammatory response are presented in Table 11-1.

**Complement System.** The complement system is an enzyme cascade (C1 to C9) consisting of pathways to mediate inflammation and destroy invading pathogens. Major functions of the

**TABLE 11-1 Mediators of Inflammation**

| Mediator | Source | Mechanisms of Action |
|---|---|---|
| **Histamine** | Stored in granules of basophils, mast cells, platelets | Causes vasodilation and increased capillary permeability |
| **Serotonin** | Stored in platelets, mast cells, enterochromaffin cells of GI tract | Same as above. Stimulates smooth muscle contraction |
| **Kinins** (e.g., bradykinin) | Produced from precursor factor kininogen as a result of activation of Hageman factor (XII) of clotting system | Cause contraction of smooth muscle and vasodilation. Result in stimulation of pain |
| **Complement components** (C3a, C4a, C5a) | Anaphylatoxic agents generated from complement pathway activation | Stimulate histamine release and chemotaxis |
| **Prostaglandins** (PGs) **and leukotrienes** (LTs) | Produced from arachidonic acid (Fig. 11-2) | PGs cause vasodilation. LTs stimulate chemotaxis. |
| **Cytokines** | For information on cytokines, see Table 13-3 | |

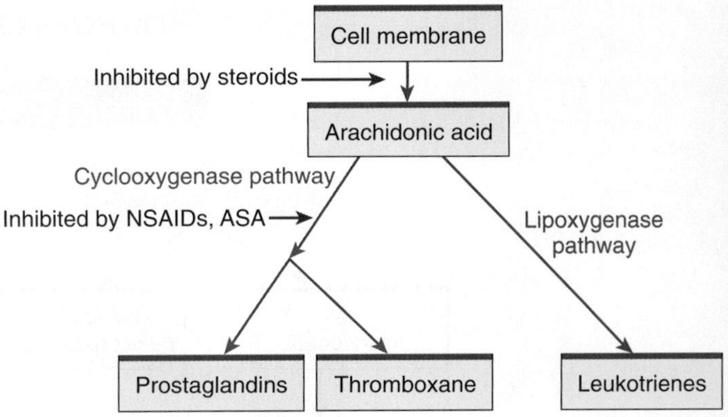


**FIG. 11-2** Pathway of generation of prostaglandins, thromboxane, and leukotrienes. Corticosteroids, nonsteroidal antiinflammatory drugs *(NSAIDs)*, and acetylsalicylic acid *(ASA)* act to inhibit various steps in this pathway.

complement system are enhanced phagocytosis, increased vascular permeability, chemotaxis, and cellular lysis. All of these activities are important mediators of the inflammatory response and healing.

Cell lysis occurs when the final components create holes in the cell membranes and cause targeted cell death by membrane rupture. In autoimmune disorders, healthy tissue can be damaged by complement activation and the resulting inflammatory response. Examples of this include rheumatoid arthritis and systemic lupus erythematosus.

**Prostaglandins and Leukotrienes.** When cells are activated by injury, the arachidonic acid in the cell membrane is rapidly converted to produce prostaglandins (PGs), thromboxane, and leukotrienes (Fig. 11-2). PGs are generally considered proinflammatory and are potent vasodilators contributing to increased blood flow and edema formation.

Some subtypes of PGs are formed when platelets are activated and can inhibit platelet and neutrophil aggregation. PGs also perform a significant role in sensitizing pain receptors to arousal by stimuli that would normally be painless. PGs have a pivotal role as pyrogens when stimulating the temperature-regulating area of the hypothalamus and producing a febrile response (see section on Fever on p. 163).

*Thromboxane* is a powerful vasoconstrictor and platelet-aggregating agent. It causes brief vasoconstriction and skin pallor at the injury site and promotes clot formation. It has a short half-life, and the pallor soon gives way to vasodilation and redness, which is caused by PGs and histamine.

*Leukotrienes* form the slow-reacting substance of anaphylaxis (SRS-A), which constricts smooth muscles of bronchi, causing narrowing of the airway, and increases capillary permeability, leading to airway edema.

## Exudate Formation

Exudate consists of fluid and leukocytes that move from the circulation to the site of injury. The nature and quantity of exudate depend on the type and severity of the injury and tissues involved (Table 11-2).

**TABLE 11-2 Types of Inflammatory Exudate**

| Type | Description | Examples |
|---|---|---|
| **Serous** | Results from outpouring of fluid. Seen in early stages of inflammation or when injury is mild | Skin blisters, pleural effusion |
| **Serosanguineous** | Found during the midpoint in healing after surgery or tissue injury<br>Composed of RBCs and serous fluid, which is semiclear pink and may have red streaks | Surgical drain fluid |
| **Fibrinous** | Occurs with increasing vascular permeability and fibrinogen leakage into interstitial spaces<br>Excessive amounts of fibrin that coats tissue surfaces may cause them to adhere. | Adhesions, gelatinous ribbons seen in surgical drain tubing<br>Frequently covers fluid-exuding wounds such as venous ulcers |
| **Hemorrhagic** | Results from rupture or necrosis of blood vessel walls | Hematoma, bleeding after surgery or tissue trauma |
| **Purulent (pus)** | Consists of WBCs, microorganisms (dead and alive), liquefied dead cells, and other debris | Furuncle (boil), abscess, cellulitis (diffuse inflammation in connective tissue) |
| **Catarrhal** | Found in tissues where cells produce mucus<br>Mucus production is accelerated by inflammatory response | Runny nose associated with upper respiratory tract infection |

## Clinical Manifestations

The *local manifestations* of inflammation include redness, heat, pain, swelling, and loss of function (Table 11-3 and Fig. 11-3).

**TABLE 11-3 Local Manifestations of Inflammation**

| Manifestations | Cause |
|---|---|
| **Redness** (rubor) | Hyperemia from vasodilation |
| **Heat** (calor) | Increased metabolism at inflammatory site |
| **Pain** (dolor) | Change in pH. Nerve stimulation by chemicals (e.g., histamine, prostaglandins). Pressure from fluid exudate |
| **Swelling** (tumor) | Fluid shift to interstitial spaces. Fluid exudate accumulation |
| **Loss of function** (functio laesa) | Swelling and pain |

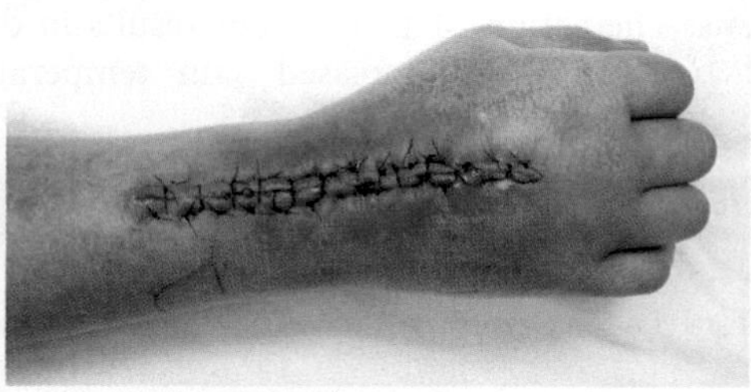

**FIG. 11-3** Inflammation secondary to postoperative deep wound infection following wrist surgery. (From Hayden RJ, Jebson PJL: Wrist arthrodesis, *Hand Clinics* 21[4]:631, 2005.)

*Systemic* manifestations of inflammation include an increased WBC count with a shift to the left, malaise, nausea and anorexia, increased pulse and respiratory rate, and fever.

Leukocytosis results from the increased release of WBCs from the bone marrow. Although the causes of other systemic manifestations are poorly understood, they may be related to complement activation and the release of *cytokines* (soluble factors secreted by WBCs and other types of cells that act as intercellular and intracellular messengers). Some of these cytokines (e.g., interleukins [ILs], tumor necrosis factor [TNF]) are important in causing the systemic manifestations of inflammation, as well as inducing fever. An increase in pulse and respiration follows the rise in metabolism as a result of an increase in body temperature. (Cytokines are discussed in Chapter 13.)

**Fever.** The onset of fever is triggered by the release of cytokines, which cause fever by initiating metabolic changes in the temperature-regulating center in the hypothalamus (Fig. 11-4). The synthesis of PGs is the most critical metabolic change. PGs act directly to increase the thermostatic set point. The hypothalamus then activates the autonomic nervous system to stimulate increased muscle tone and shivering and decreased perspiration and blood flow to the periphery. Epinephrine released from the adrenal medulla increases the metabolic rate. The net result is fever.

With the physiologic thermostat fixed at a higher-than-normal temperature, the rate of heat production is increased until the body temperature reaches the new set point. As the set point is raised, the hypothalamus signals an increase in heat production and conservation to raise the body temperature to the new level. At this point the individual feels chilled and shivers. The shivering response is the body's method of raising the body's temperature until the new set point is attained.[1] This seeming paradox is dramatic: the body is hot, yet an individual piles on blankets and may go to bed to get warm. When the

**PATHOPHYSIOLOGY MAP**

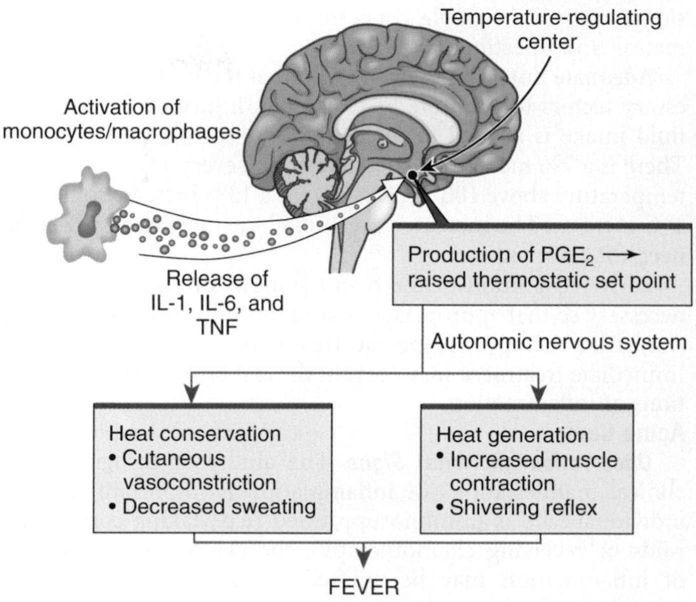


**FIG. 11-4** Production of fever. When monocytes/macrophages are activated, they secrete cytokines such as interleukin-1 *(IL-1)*, interleukin-6 *(IL-6)*, and tumor necrosis factor *(TNF)*, which reach the hypothalamic temperature-regulating center. These cytokines promote the synthesis and secretion of prostaglandin $E_2$ *($PGE_2$)* in the anterior hypothalamus. $PGE_2$ increases the thermostatic set point, and the autonomic nervous system is stimulated, resulting in shivering, muscle contraction, and peripheral vasoconstriction.

body temperature reaches the set point, the chills and warmth-seeking behavior cease.

The released cytokines and the fever that they trigger activate the body's defense mechanisms. Beneficial aspects of fever include increased killing of microorganisms, increased phagocytosis by neutrophils, and increased proliferation of T cells. Higher body temperatures may also enhance the activity of interferon, the body's natural virus-fighting substance (see Chapter 13).

### Types of Inflammation

The basic types of inflammation are acute, subacute, and chronic. In *acute inflammation*, the healing occurs in 2 to 3 weeks and usually leaves no residual damage. Neutrophils are the predominant cell type at the site of inflammation. A *subacute inflammation* has the features of the acute process but lasts longer. For example, infective endocarditis is a smoldering infection with acute inflammation, but it persists for weeks or months (see Chapter 36).

*Chronic inflammation* lasts for weeks, months, or even years. The injurious agent persists or repeatedly injures tissue. The predominant cell types present at the site of inflammation are lymphocytes and macrophages. Examples of chronic inflammation include rheumatoid arthritis and osteomyelitis. The prolongation and chronicity of any inflammation may be the result of an alteration in the immune response (e.g., autoimmune disease) and can lead to physical deterioration.

## ❖ NURSING AND INTERPROFESSIONAL MANAGEMENT: INFLAMMATION

### ◆ Nursing Implementation

◆ **Health Promotion.** The best management of inflammation is the prevention of infection, trauma, surgery, and contact with potentially harmful agents. This is not always possible. A simple mosquito bite causes an inflammatory response. Because occasional injury is inevitable, concerted efforts to minimize inflammation and infection are needed.

Adequate nutrition is essential so that the body has the necessary factors to promote healing when injury occurs. A high fluid intake is needed to replace fluid loss from perspiration. There is a 7% increase in metabolism for every 1° F increase in temperature above 100° F (37.8° C), or a 13% increase for every 1° C increase. The increased metabolic rate increases a patient's need for calories.

Early recognition of the manifestations of inflammation is necessary so that appropriate treatment can begin. This may be rest, drug therapy, or specific treatment of the injured site. Immediate treatment may prevent the extension and complications of inflammation.

### ◆ Acute Care

◆ ***Observation and Vital Signs.*** The ability to recognize the clinical manifestations of inflammation is important. In the individual who is immunosuppressed (e.g., taking corticosteroids or receiving chemotherapy), the classic manifestations of inflammation may be masked. In this individual, early symptoms of inflammation may be malaise or "just not feeling well."

Vital signs are important to note with any inflammation, especially when an infectious process is present. With infection, the temperature may rise, and pulse and respiration rates may increase.

◆ ***Fever.*** An important aspect of fever management is determining its cause. Although fever is usually regarded as harmful, an increase in body temperature is an important host defense mechanism. In the seventeenth century, Thomas Sydenham noted that "fever is a mighty engine which nature brings into the world for the conquest of her enemies."[2]

Steps are frequently taken to lower body temperature to relieve the anxiety of the patient and health care professionals. Because mild to moderate fever usually does little harm, imposes no great discomfort, and may benefit host defense mechanisms, antipyretic drugs are rarely essential to patient welfare. Moderate fevers (up to 103°F [39.4°C]) usually produce few problems in most patients. However, if the patient is very young or very old, is extremely uncomfortable, or has a significant medical problem (e.g., severe cardiopulmonary disease, brain injury), the use of antipyretics should be considered. Fever in the immunosuppressed patient should be treated immediately with antibiotic therapy because infections can rapidly progress to septicemia. (Neutropenia is discussed in Chapter 30 on pp. 632-633.)

Fever (especially if greater than 104° F [40° C]) can damage body cells, and delirium and seizures can occur. At temperatures greater than 105.8° F (41° C), regulation by the hypothalamic temperature control center becomes impaired. Damage can occur to many cells, including those in the brain.

Older adults have a blunted febrile response to infection. The body temperature may not rise to the level expected for a younger adult, or the rise may be delayed in its onset. The blunted response can delay diagnosis and treatment. By the time fever (as defined for younger adults) is present, the illness may be more severe. Patients who are taking nonsteroidal anti-inflammatory drugs (NSAIDs) on a regular basis (e.g., for treatment of rheumatoid arthritis) may also have a blunted febrile response.

Although sponge baths increase evaporative heat loss, they may not decrease the body temperature unless antipyretic drugs have been given to lower the set point. Otherwise, the body will initiate compensatory mechanisms (e.g., shivering) to restore body heat. The same principle applies to the use of cooling blankets, which are most effective in lowering body temperature when the set point has also been lowered.

A nursing care plan for the patient with a fever (eNursing Care Plan 11-1) is available on the website for this chapter.

◆ ***Drug Therapy.*** Drugs are used to decrease the inflammatory response and lower the body temperature (Table 11-4). Aspirin blocks PG synthesis in the hypothalamus and elsewhere in the body. Acetaminophen acts on the heat-regulating center in the hypothalamus. Some NSAIDs (e.g., ibuprofen [Motrin, Advil]) have antipyretic effects. Corticosteroids are antipyretic through the dual mechanisms of preventing cytokine production and PG synthesis. The action of these drugs results in dilation of superficial blood vessels, increased skin temperature, and sweating.

**CHECK YOUR PRACTICE**

A 76-yr-old female patient has acute osteomyelitis following a fractured femur. You are checking her temperature every 2 hours and giving acetaminophen when it is higher than 102° F. However, you notice that her temperature is greatly fluctuating from 96° F to 103° F.

- What should you do?

Antipyretics should be given around the clock to prevent acute swings in temperature. Chills may be evoked or perpetuated by the intermittent administration of antipyretics. These agents cause a sharp decrease in temperature. When the antipyretic wears off, the body may initiate a compensatory

**TABLE 11-4 Drug Therapy**

***Inflammation and Healing***

| Drug | Mechanism of Action |
|---|---|
| **Antipyretic Drugs** | |
| Salicylates (aspirin) | Inhibit synthesis of PGs (Fig. 11-2). Lower temperature by action on heat-regulating center in hypothalamus, resulting in peripheral vasodilation and heat loss |
| Acetaminophen (Tylenol) | Inhibits synthesis of PGs. Lowers temperature by action on heat-regulating center in hypothalamus |
| NSAIDs (e.g., ibuprofen [Advil]) | Inhibit synthesis of PGs |
| **Antiinflammatory Drugs** | |
| Salicylates (aspirin) | Inhibit synthesis of PGs, reduce capillary permeability |
| Corticosteroids (e.g., prednisone) | Interfere with tissue granulation, induce immunosuppressive effects (decreased synthesis of lymphocytes), prevent liberation of lysosomes |
| NSAIDs (e.g., ibuprofen, piroxicam [Feldene]) | Inhibit synthesis of PGs |
| **Vitamins** | |
| Vitamin A | Accelerates epithelialization |
| Vitamin B complex | Acts as coenzymes |
| Vitamin C | Assists in synthesis of collagen and new capillaries |
| Vitamin D | Facilitates calcium absorption |

*PGs,* Prostaglandins.

involuntary muscular contraction (i.e., chill) to raise the body temperature back up to its previous level. This unpleasant side effect of antipyretic drugs can be prevented by administering these agents regularly at 2- to 4-hour intervals.

Antihistamine drugs may also be used to inhibit the action of histamine. (Antihistamines are discussed in Chapters 13 and 26.)

◆ ***RICE.*** **R**est, **i**ce, **c**ompression, and **e**levation (RICE) is a key concept in treating soft tissue injuries and related inflammation.

◆ **Rest.** Rest helps the body use its nutrients and $O_2$ for the healing process. The repair process is facilitated by allowing fibrin and collagen to form across the wound edges with little disruption.

◆ **Cold and heat.** Cold application is usually appropriate at the time of the initial trauma to promote vasoconstriction and decrease swelling, pain, and congestion from increased metabolism in the area of inflammation. Heat may be used later (e.g., after 24 to 48 hours) to promote healing by increasing the circulation to the inflamed site and subsequent removal of debris. Heat is also used to localize the inflammatory agents. Warm, moist heat may help debride the wound site if necrotic material is present.

◆ **Compression and immobilization.** Compression counters the vasodilation effects and development of edema. Compression by direct pressure over a laceration occludes blood vessels and stops bleeding. Compression bandages provide support to injured joints that have tendons and muscles unable to provide support on their own. Assess distal pulses and capillary refill before and after application of compression to evaluate whether compression has compromised circulation (e.g., pale color of skin, loss of feeling).

Immobilization of the inflamed or injured area promotes healing by decreasing the tissues' metabolic needs. Immobilization with a cast or splint supports fractured bones and prevents further tissue injury from sharp bone fragments that could sever nerves or blood vessels (causing hemorrhage). As with compression, evaluate the patient's circulation after application and at regular intervals. Swelling can occur within the closed space of a cast and compromise circulation.

◆ **Elevation.** Elevating the injured extremity above the level of the heart reduces the edema at the inflammatory site by increasing venous and lymphatic return. Elevation also helps reduce pain associated with blood engorgement at the injury site. Elevation may be contraindicated in patients with significantly reduced arterial circulation.

## HEALING PROCESS

The final phase of the inflammatory response is healing. Healing includes two major components: regeneration and repair.

### Regeneration

**Regeneration** is the replacement of lost cells and tissues with cells of the same type. The ability of cells to regenerate depends on the cell type (Table 11-5).

### Repair

**Repair** is healing as a result of lost cells being replaced by connective tissue. Repair is the more common type of healing and usually results in scar formation. Repair is a more complex process than regeneration. Most injuries heal by connective tissue repair. Repair healing occurs by primary, secondary, or tertiary intention (Fig. 11-5).

**Primary Intention.** *Primary intention* healing takes place when wound margins are neatly approximated, as in a surgical incision or a paper cut. A continuum of processes is associated with primary healing (Table 11-6). These processes include three phases.

**TABLE 11-5 Regenerative Ability of Different Types of Tissues**

| Tissues | Cell Type | Description |
|---|---|---|
| Skin, lymphoid organs, bone marrow, and mucous membranes | Labile cells | Cells divide constantly. Injury to these organs is followed by rapid regeneration. |
| Liver, pancreas, kidney, and bone cells | Stable cells | Retain their ability to regenerate but do so only if the organ is injured. Regeneration is slow. |
| Neurons of the central nervous system (CNS) and skeletal and cardiac muscle cells | Permanent cells | Do not divide. Damage to CNS neurons or skeletal or heart muscle can lead to permanent loss. Healing of skeletal and cardiac muscle will occur by repair with scar tissue. If neurons in the CNS are destroyed, the tissue is generally replaced by glial cells. However, neurogenesis may occur from stem cells (see Chapter 55). |

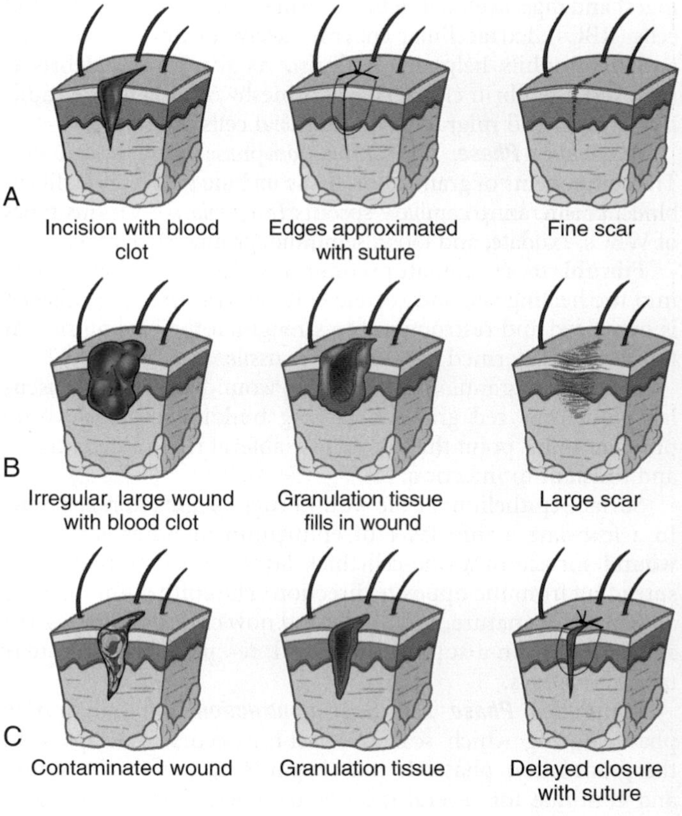


**FIG. 11-5** Types of wound healing. **A,** Primary intention. **B,** Secondary intention. **C,** Tertiary intention.

TABLE 11-6 **Phases in Primary Intention Healing**

| Phase | Duration | Description |
|---|---|---|
| Initial | 3 to 5 days | Approximation of incision edges. Migration of epithelial cells. Clot serving as meshwork for starting capillary growth |
| Granulation | 5 days to 4 wk | Migration of fibroblasts. Secretion of collagen. Abundance of capillary buds. Wound fragile |
| Maturation and scar contraction | 7 days to several months | Remodeling of collagen. Strengthening of scar |

***Initial Phase.*** In the *initial* (inflammatory) phase, the edges of the incision are first aligned and sutured (or stapled) in place. The incision area fills with blood from the cut blood vessels, blood clots form, and platelets release growth factors to begin the healing process. This forms a matrix for WBC migration. An acute inflammatory reaction occurs.

The area of injury is composed of fibrin clots, erythrocytes, neutrophils (dead and dying), and other debris. Macrophages ingest and digest cellular debris, fibrin fragments, and red blood cells (RBCs). Extracellular enzymes derived from macrophages and neutrophils help digest fibrin. As the wound debris is removed, the fibrin clot serves as a meshwork for future capillary growth and migration of epithelial cells.

***Granulation Phase.*** The *granulation* phase is the second step. The components of granulation tissue include proliferating fibroblasts; proliferating capillary sprouts *(angioblasts);* various types of WBCs; exudate; and loose, semifluid, ground substance.

**Fibroblasts** are immature connective tissue cells that migrate into the healing site and secrete collagen. In time, the collagen is organized and restructured to strengthen the healing site. At this stage it is termed *fibrous* or *scar tissue.*

During the granulation phase, the wound is pink and vascular. Numerous red granules (young budding capillaries) are present. At this point the wound is friable, at risk for dehiscence, and resistant to infection.

Surface epithelium at the wound edges begins to regenerate. In a few days a thin layer of epithelium migrates across the wound surface in a one-cell-thick layer until it contacts cells spreading from the opposite direction. The epithelium thickens and begins to mature, and the wound now closely resembles the adjacent skin. In a superficial wound, re-epithelialization may take 3 to 5 days.

***Maturation Phase and Scar Contraction.*** The *maturation* phase, during which scar contraction occurs, overlaps with the granulation phase. It may begin 7 days after the injury and continue for several months or years. This is the reason abdominal surgery discharge instructions limit lifting for up to 6 weeks.

Collagen fibers are further organized, and the remodeling process occurs. Fibroblasts disappear as the wound becomes stronger. The active movement of the myofibroblasts causes contraction of the healing area, helping to close the defect and bring the skin edges closer together. A mature scar is then formed. In contrast to granulation tissue, a mature scar is virtually avascular and pale. The scar may be more painful at this phase than in the granulation phase.

**Secondary Intention.** Wounds that occur from trauma, ulceration, and infection have large amounts of exudate and wide, irregular wound margins with extensive tissue loss. These wounds may have edges that cannot be *approximated* (brought together). The inflammatory reaction may be greater than in primary healing. This results in more debris, cells, and exudate. The debris may have to be cleaned away *(debrided)* before healing can take place.

The process of healing by secondary intention is essentially the same as healing by primary intention. The major differences are the greater defect and the gaping wound edges. Healing and granulation take place from the edges inward and from the bottom of the wound upward until the defect is filled. There is more granulation tissue, and the result is a much larger scar.

**Tertiary Intention.** *Tertiary intention* (delayed primary intention) healing occurs with delayed suturing of a wound in which two layers of granulation tissue are sutured together. This occurs when a contaminated wound is left open and sutured closed after the infection is controlled. It also occurs when a primary wound becomes infected, is opened, is allowed to granulate, and is then sutured. Tertiary intention usually results in a larger and deeper scar than primary or secondary intention.

### Wound Classification

A *wound* is a break or opening into the skin. Wounds often occur because of accidents or injuries. Types of wounds can range from minor scrapes to deep wounds involving bones, blood vessels, and nerves.

Identifying the etiology of a wound is essential to classifying the wound properly. Wounds can be classified by their cause (surgical or nonsurgical; acute or chronic) or depth of tissue affected (superficial, partial thickness, or full thickness). A *superficial wound* involves only the epidermis. *Partial-thickness* wounds extend into the dermis. *Full-thickness* wounds have the deepest layer of tissue destruction because they involve the subcutaneous tissue and sometimes even extend into the fascia and underlying structures such as the muscle, tendon, or bone (see Fig. 24-3).

A *skin tear* is a wound caused by shear, friction, and/or blunt force resulting in separation of skin layers. A skin tear can be partial thickness or full thickness. This type of wound is common, especially in older adults and critically or chronically ill adults.[3]

### Complications of Healing

Certain factors can interfere with wound healing and lead to complications (Table 11-7).

## NURSING AND INTERPROFESSIONAL MANAGEMENT: WOUND HEALING

### Nursing Assessment

The first step in wound care is to carefully assess and document the characteristics of the wound and surrounding area. This includes the location, size (longest length and widest width), depth, undermining and tunneling, wound margin (e.g., normal, macerated, erythema), and wound base (e.g., eschar, slough, exudate). Thoroughly assess the wound on admission (or first clinic visit) and on a regular basis thereafter. Deterioration in the wound requires you to assess and document changes more frequently.[4] Various methods exist for measuring wounds. One method is presented in Fig. 11-9.

**TABLE 11-7 Complications of Wound Healing**

**Adhesions**
- Bands of scar tissue that form between or around organs
- Adhesions may occur in the abdominal cavity or between the lungs and the pleura
- Adhesions in abdomen may cause an intestinal obstruction

**Contractions**
- Wound contraction is a normal part of healing
- Complications occur when excessive contraction results in deformity
- Shortening of muscle or scar tissue, especially over joints, results from excessive fibrous tissue formation (see Fig. 24-14)

**Dehiscence**
- Separation and disruption of previously joined wound edges (Fig. 11-6)
- Usually occurs when a primary healing site bursts open
- May be caused by the following:
  - Infection causing an inflammatory process
  - Granulation tissue not strong enough to withstand forces imposed on wound
  - Obesity placing individuals at high risk for dehiscence because adipose tissue has less blood supply and may slow healing
  - Pocket of fluid (seroma, hematoma) developing between tissue layers and preventing the edges of the wound from coming together

**Evisceration**
- Occurs when wound edges separate to the extent that intestines protrude through wound

**Excess Granulation Tissue ("Proud Flesh")**
- Excess granulation tissue may protrude above surface of healing wound
- If the granulation tissue is cauterized or cut off, healing continues in normal manner

**Fistula Formation**
- An abnormal passage between organs or a hollow organ and skin (abdominal or perianal fistula)

**Infection** (Fig. 11-3)
- ↑ Risk of infection when wound contains necrotic tissue or blood supply is ↓, patient's immune function is ↓ (e.g., from immunosuppressive drugs such as corticosteroids), undernutrition, multiple stressors, and hyperglycemia in diabetes

**Hemorrhage**
- Bleeding is normal immediately after tissue injury and ceases with clot formation
- Hemorrhage occurs as abnormal internal or external blood loss caused by suture failure, clotting abnormalities, dislodged clot, infection, or erosion of a blood vessel by a foreign object (tubing, drains) or infection process

**Hypertrophic Scars**
- Inappropriately large, raised red and hard scars (Fig. 11-7)
- Occur when an overabundance of collagen is produced during healing

**Keloid Formation**
- Great protrusion of scar tissue that extends beyond wound edges and may form tumor-like masses of scar tissue (Fig. 11-8)
- Permanent without any tendency to subside
- Patients often complain of tenderness, pain, and hyperparesthesia, especially in early stages
- Thought to be a hereditary condition occurring most often in dark-skinned people, particularly African Americans

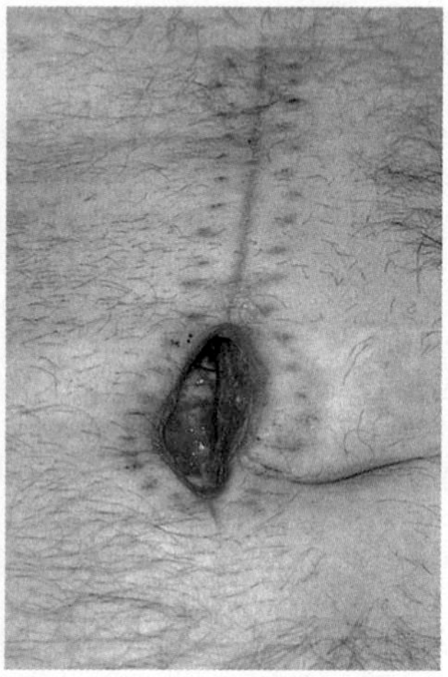

**FIG. 11-6** Dehiscence following a cholecystectomy. (From Bale S, Jones V: *Wound care nursing: a patient-centered approach,* ed 2, St Louis, 2006, Mosby.)

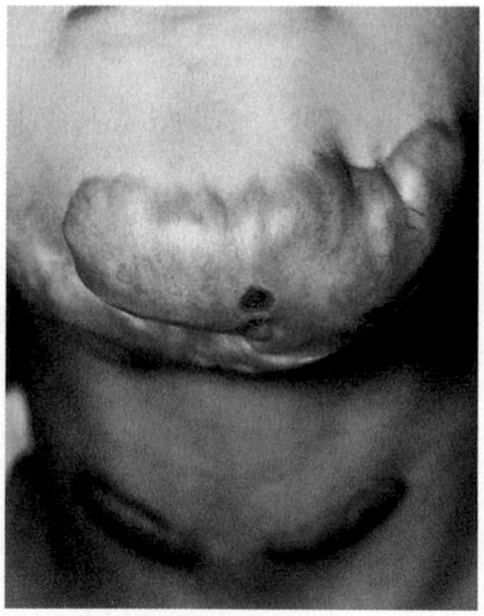

**FIG. 11-7** Hypertrophic scarring. (Reproduced with kind permission from Dr. C. Lawrence, Wound Healing Research Unit, Cardiff. In S Bale, V Jones, editors: *Wound care nursing: a patient-centered approach,* ed 2, St Louis, 2006, Mosby.)

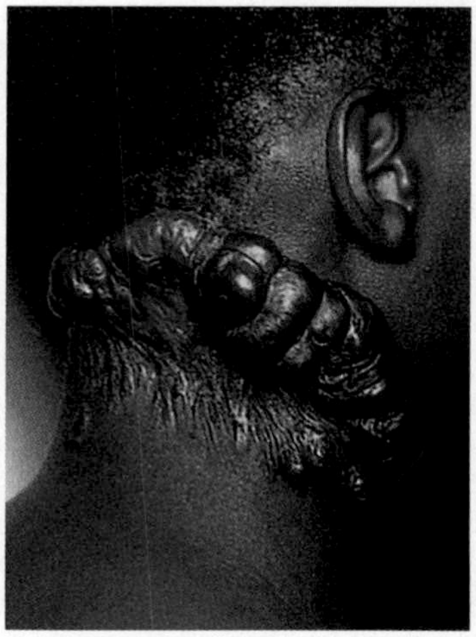

**FIG. 11-8** Keloid scarring. (Reproduced with kind permission from Dr. C. Lawrence, Wound Healing Research Unit, Cardiff. In Bale S, Jones V, editors: *Wound care nursing: a patient-centered approach,* ed 2, St Louis, 2006, Mosby.)

Record the consistency, color, and odor of any drainage and report if abnormal for the situation. *Staphylococcus* and *Pseudomonas* are common organisms that cause purulent, draining wounds.

In healthy people, wounds heal at a normal, predictable rate. Identify factors that may delay wound healing and contribute to chronic nonhealing wounds (Table 11-8).

*Chronic wounds* are those that do not heal within the normal time (approximately 3 months). If a wound fails to heal in a timely manner, assess and identify factors that may delay healing. Refer the patient to an HCP specializing in wound management. Time does not heal all wounds. While caring for patients during the healing process, you need to continually assess for complications (e.g., infection) associated with healing (Table 11-7).

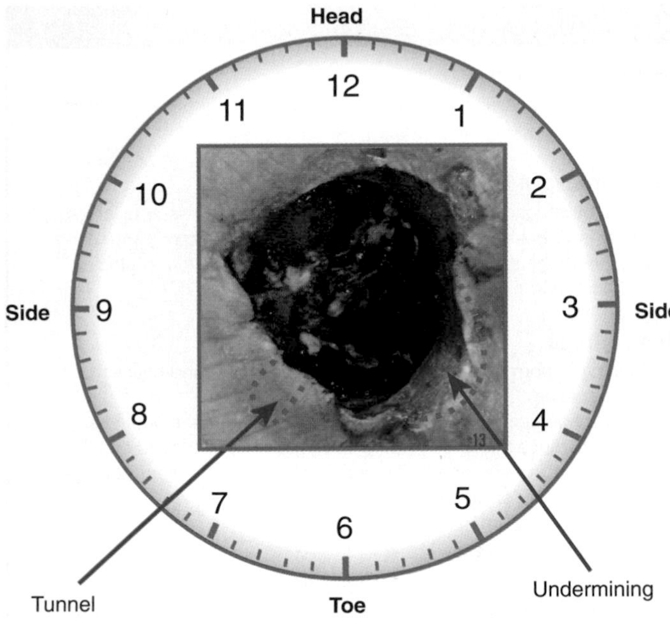


**FIG. 11-9** Wound measurements are made in centimeters. The first measurement is oriented from head to toe, the second is from side to side, and the third is the depth (if any). If there is any tunneling (when cotton-tipped applicator is placed in wound, there is movement) or undermining (when cotton-tipped applicator is placed in wound, there is a "lip" around the wound), this is charted in respect to a clock, with 12 o'clock being toward the patient's head. This wound would be charted as a full-thickness, red wound, 7 × 5 × 3 cm, with a 3-cm tunnel at 7 o'clock and 2 cm undermining from 3 o'clock to 5 o'clock. (Courtesy Robert B. Babiak, RN, BSN, CWOCN, San Antonio, Tex.)

## Nursing Implementation

The type of wound management and dressings required depend on the type, extent, and characteristics of the wound and the phase of healing. The purposes of wound management include (1) protecting a clean wound from trauma so that it can heal normally, (2) cleaning a wound to remove any dirt and debris from the wound bed, and (3) treating infection to prepare the wound for healing.

**Clean Wounds.** Superficial skin injuries may only need cleansing. Material used to close wounds include adhesive strips (e.g., Steri-Strips, butterflies), sutures (stitches), or tissue adhesives (fibrin sealants). Adhesive strips may be used instead of *sutures* in some injuries because they decrease *scarring,* and it is easier to care for them. Sutures are used to close wounds because suture material provides the mechanical support necessary to sustain closure. A wide variety of suturing materials are available. In contrast, tissue adhesives are a biologic adhesive that can be used by themselves or in conjunction with sutures or tape.

A dressing material that keeps the wound surface clean and slightly moist is optimal to promote epithelialization. For wounds that heal by primary intention, it is common to cover the wound or incision with a dry, sterile dressing that is removed as soon as the drainage stops or in 2 to 3 days. Medicated sprays that form a transparent film on the skin may be used for dressings on a clean incision or injury. Transparent film or adhesive semipermeable dressings (e.g., OpSite, Tegaderm) are occlusive dressings that are permeable to oxygen. The wound is then usually covered with a sterile dressing. Sometimes a surgeon will leave a surgical wound uncovered or remove the dressing within 48 hours after surgery.[5] (Examples of types of wound dressings are presented in Table 11-9.)

**TABLE 11-8 Factors Delaying Wound Healing**

| Factor | Effect on Wound Healing |
|---|---|
| **Nutritional deficiencies** | |
| • Vitamin C | Delays formation of collagen fibers and capillary development |
| • Protein | Decreases supply of amino acids for tissue repair |
| • Zinc | Impairs epithelialization |
| **Inadequate blood supply** | Decreases supply of nutrients to injured area, decreases removal of exudative debris, inhibits inflammatory response |
| **Corticosteroid drugs** | Impair phagocytosis by WBCs, inhibit fibroblast proliferation and function, depress formation of granulation tissue, inhibit wound contraction |
| **Infection** | Increases inflammatory response and tissue destruction |
| **Smoking** | Nicotine, a potent vasoconstrictor, impedes blood flow to healing areas |
| **Mechanical friction on wound** | Destroys granulation tissue, prevents apposition of wound edges |
| **Advanced age** | Slows collagen synthesis by fibroblasts, impairs circulation, requires longer time for epithelialization of skin, alters phagocytic and immune responses |
| **Obesity** | Decreases blood supply in fatty tissue |
| **Diabetes mellitus** | Decreases collagen synthesis, delays capillary growth, impairs phagocytosis (result of hyperglycemia), reduces supply of $O_2$ and nutrients secondary to vascular disease |
| **Poor general health** | Causes generalized absence of factors necessary to promote wound healing |
| **Anemia** | Supplies less $O_2$ at tissue level |

Clean wounds that are granulating and re-epithelializing should be kept slightly moist and protected from further trauma until they heal naturally.[6] Do not let a wound that has the potential to heal dry out. Dryness is an enemy of wound healing. "Airing out" a wound is a great mistake. Wounds need a moist environment to heal. Unnecessary manipulation during dressing changes may destroy new granulation tissue and break down fibrin formation.

Topical antimicrobials and antibactericidals (e.g., povidone-iodine [Betadine], Dakin's solution [sodium hypochlorite], hydrogen peroxide [$H_2O_2$], and chlorhexidine [Hibiclens]) should be used with caution in wound care because they can damage the new epithelium of healing tissue and delay healing. Therefore they should never be used in a clean granulating wound.

Sometimes drains are inserted into the wound to facilitate removal of fluid. The Jackson-Pratt drain is a suction drainage device consisting of a flexible plastic bulb connected to an internal plastic drainage tube (Fig. 11-10).

**Contaminated Wounds.** If the wound is contaminated, it must be converted into a clean wound before healing can occur normally. Debridement of a wound that has debris or dead tissue may be necessary. Absorption dressings can be used that absorb exudate and clean the wound surface. These dressings work by

TABLE 11-9 Types of Wound Dressings

| Type of Dressing | Description | Uses | Examples |
|---|---|---|---|
| **Gauze** | Made of woven or nonwoven material. Provide absorption of exudates. Most often combined with another kind of dressing | Can be used on almost any kind of wound. Cleansing, packing, and covering a variety of wounds | Numerous products available (e.g., Curity, Kerlix) |
| **Nonadherent** | Woven or nonwoven dressings. May be impregnated with saline, petrolatum, or antimicrobials. Minimally absorbent | Minor wounds or as a second dressing | Adaptic, Vaseline gauze, Xeroform |
| **Transparent films** | Generally composed of polyurethane. Transparency allows visualization of the wound. Minimally absorbent. Use with caution over superficial wounds. In fragile wounds (e.g., skin tears) can result in further tissue loss. In other wounds, can draw in moisture, increasing risk for infection | Dry, uninfected wounds or wounds with minimal drainage | Bioclusive, OpSite, Suresite, Tegaderm, Transeal |
| **Foams** | Film-coated gel or polyurethane. Able to hold large amounts of exudate. Some come with adhesive backings; others require gauze wrapping | Wounds with moderate to heavy drainage. Often used on new wounds | Allevyn, Cutimed, Hydrocell, Lyofoam, Mepilex, PolyMem |
| **Hydrocolloids** | Gelatin, pectin, or carboxymethylcellulose bonded to a film or sheet. Produce a flat occlusive dressing that forms a gel on wound surface. Occlusion does not interfere with wound healing. Support debridement and prevent secondary infections | Wounds with light to moderate drainage | Bursamed, Comfeel, DuoDerm, Primacol |
| **Hydrogels** | Available in gels, gel-covered gauze, or sheets. Donate moisture to a dry wound and maintain a moist environment. Can rehydrate wound tissue. Debridement because of moisturizing effects. Require a secondary dressing | Dry wounds. Wounds with minimal drainage. Necrotic wounds | Aquasite, Curasol, IntraSite, Purilon, Solosite |
| **Alginates** | Derived from seaweed or kelp. Form a nonsticky gel on contact with draining wound. Easy to use over irregular-shaped wounds. Generally require a secondary dressing | Wounds with moderate to heavy exudates (e.g., pressure ulcers, infected wounds) | AlgiSite, Kalginate, Melgisorb, Sorbsan |
| **Antimicrobials** | Wound covers that deliver agents such as silver and iodine, and polyhexamethylene biguanide (PHMB), which have antibacterial properties. Bacteria are not able to develop resistance to metals. Available as sponges, impregnated woven gauzes, film dressings, absorptive products, nylon fabric, nonadherent barriers, or a combination of materials | Partial- and full-thickness wounds, over surgical incisions, or around tracheostomies | Acticoat, Curity AMD, Iodoflex, SilverSorb, Silvercel |

For additional information, see *www.woundsource.com/product-category/dressings.*

drawing excess drainage from the wound surface. The amount of wound secretions determines the number of dressing changes.

In hydrocolloid dressings, such as DuoDerm, the inner part of these dressings interacts with the exudate, forming a hydrated gel over the wound. When the dressing is removed, the gel separates and stays over the wound. The wound must be cleansed gently to prevent damage to newly formed tissue. These types of dressings are designed to be left in place for up to 7 days or until leakage occurs around the dressing.

Dead tissue can be removed by debridement.[7] The debridement method used depends on the amount of debris and the condition of the wound tissue (Table 11-10).

**Negative-Pressure Wound Therapy.** Negative-pressure wound therapy (NPWT) is used to treat acute and chronic wounds. A vacuum source creates continuous or intermittent negative pressure inside the wound to remove fluid, exudates, and infectious materials to prepare the wound for healing and closure. NPWT systems consist of a vacuum pump, drainage tubing, a foam or gauze wound dressing, and an adhesive film dressing that covers and seals the wound.[8]

In this therapy, the wound is cleaned and a gauze or foam dressing is cut to the dimensions of the wound. A large occlusive dressing is applied and a small hole is made over the gauze or foam dressing where the tubing is attached (Fig. 11-11). The tubing is connected to a pump, which creates a negative pressure in the wound bed.

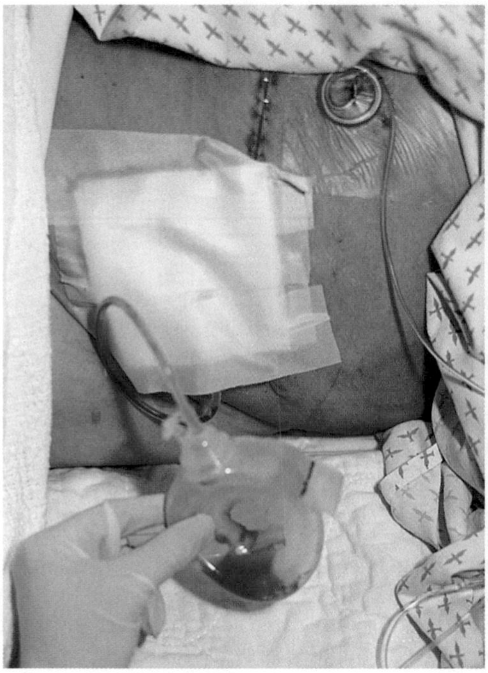

**FIG. 11-10** Jackson-Pratt drainage device. (From Perry AG, Potter PA, Elkin MK: *Nursing interventions and clinical skills,* ed 5, St Louis, 2012, Mosby.)

## TEAMWORK & COLLABORATION
### Wound Care

In general, wound care for complex or nonhealing wounds should be managed by the registered nurse (RN). State nurse practice acts vary in the wound care actions allowed by licensed practical/vocational nurses (LPNs/LVNs) and unlicensed assistive personnel (UAP).

**Role of Nursing Personnel**

***Registered Nurse (RN)***

- Assess patients for pressure ulcer risk and develop a plan of care to prevent the development of pressure ulcers.
- Assess patients for factors that may delay wound healing and develop a plan of care to address these factors.
- Assess and document initial wound appearance, including wound size, depth, color, and drainage.
- Plan nursing actions to assist with wound healing, including wound care, positioning, and nutritional interventions.
- Choose dressings and therapies for wound treatment (in conjunction with the HCP and/or wound care specialist).
- Implement wound care for complex or new wounds, including negative-pressure wound therapy and hyperbaric $O_2$ therapy.
- Evaluate whether wound care is effective in promoting wound healing.
- Provide teaching to patient and caregivers about home wound care and pressure ulcer prevention.

***Licensed Practical/Vocational Nurse (LPN/LVN)***

- Perform sterile dressing changes on acute and chronic wounds.
- Apply ordered topical antimicrobials and antibactericidals to wounds.
- Apply prescribed dressings or medications for wound debridement.
- Collect and record data about wound appearance.
- Reinforce teaching that was provided by the RN.

***Unlicensed Assistive Personnel (UAP)***

- Perform dressing changes for chronic wounds using clean technique (must consider state nurse practice act and agency policy).
- Empty wound drainage containers and document drainage on intake and output record.
- Report changes in wound appearance or drainage to RN.

**Role of Other Team Members**

***Dietitian***

- Assess and monitor patient's nutritional status.
- Establish an intervention together with the interprofessional team.
- Monitor patient's progress toward achieving the goals of care.

Although the exact mechanism for promoting healing is not known, it is thought that this therapy pulls excess fluid from the wound, reduces bacterial load, and encourages blood flow into the wound base.

Monitor the patient's serum protein levels and fluid and electrolyte balance because of losses from the wound. Additionally, monitor the patient's coagulation studies (platelet count, prothrombin time [PT], partial thromboplastin time [PTT]).

◆ **Hyperbaric Oxygen Therapy.** Hyperbaric $O_2$ therapy (HBOT) is the delivery of $O_2$ at increased atmospheric pressures. It can be given topically by creating a chamber around the injured limb. Alternatively it can be given systemically with the patient placed in an enclosed chamber, where 100% $O_2$ is administered at 1.5 to 3 times the normal atmospheric pressure.

**TABLE 11-10 Types of Debridement**

| Type | Description |
|---|---|
| **Surgical debridement** | • Quick method of debridement to prevent, control, or remove infection<br>• Used when large amounts of nonviable tissue are present<br>• Prepares wound bed for healing, skin grafting, or flaps |
| **Mechanical debridement** | • Two methods:<br>• *Wet-to-dry dressings,* in which open-mesh gauze is moistened with normal saline, lightly packed into wound surface, and outer layer allowed to dry. Wound debris adheres to dressing and then dressing is removed<br>• *Wound irrigation.* Make certain bacteria are not accidentally driven into wound with high irrigation pressure |
| **Autolytic debridement** | • Semiocclusive or occlusive dressings (Table 11-9) used to soften dry eschar by autolysis<br>• Assess area around wound for maceration when using these dressings |
| **Enzymatic debridement** | • Drugs applied topically to dissolve necrotic tissue and then covered with moist dressing (e.g., saline-moistened gauze)<br>• Examples of these drugs include collagenase (e.g., Santyl)<br>• Process can be slow, and thick eschar may have to be scored with scalpel |

HBOT allows $O_2$ to diffuse into the serum, rather than RBCs, and be transported to the tissues. By increasing the $O_2$ content in the serum, HBOT moves the $O_2$ past narrowed arteries and capillaries where RBCs cannot go.

In addition, elevated $O_2$ levels stimulate *angiogenesis* (production of new blood vessels), kill anaerobic bacteria, and increase the killing power of WBCs and certain antibiotics (e.g., fluoroquinolones, aminoglycosides). HBOT accelerates granulation tissue formation and wound healing.

The topical treatments can last 20 minutes twice daily or 4 to 6 hours daily. Most systemic treatments last from 90 to 120 minutes, and the number of treatments may vary from 10 to 60 depending on the condition being treated. The number of treatments is highly variable.

◆ **Drug Therapy.** Platelet-derived growth factor is released from the platelets and stimulates cell proliferation and migration. Becaplermin (Regranex), a recombinant human platelet–derived growth factor gel, actively stimulates wound healing. It is used to treat foot ulcers in patients with diabetes (see Chapter 48). Becaplermin should be used only when the wound is free of dead tissue and infection. It should not be used if cancer is suspected in the wound.

◆ **Nutritional Therapy.** Special nutritional measures facilitate wound healing. A high fluid intake is needed to replace fluid loss from perspiration and exudate formation. An increased metabolic rate intensifies water loss. Individuals at risk for wound healing problems are those with malabsorption problems (e.g., Crohn's disease, gastrointestinal [GI] surgery, liver disease), deficient intake or high energy demands (e.g., malignancy, major trauma or surgery, sepsis, fever), and diabetes.

Undernutrition puts a person at risk for poor healing. A diet high in protein, carbohydrate, and vitamins with moderate fat intake is necessary to promote healing. Protein is needed to

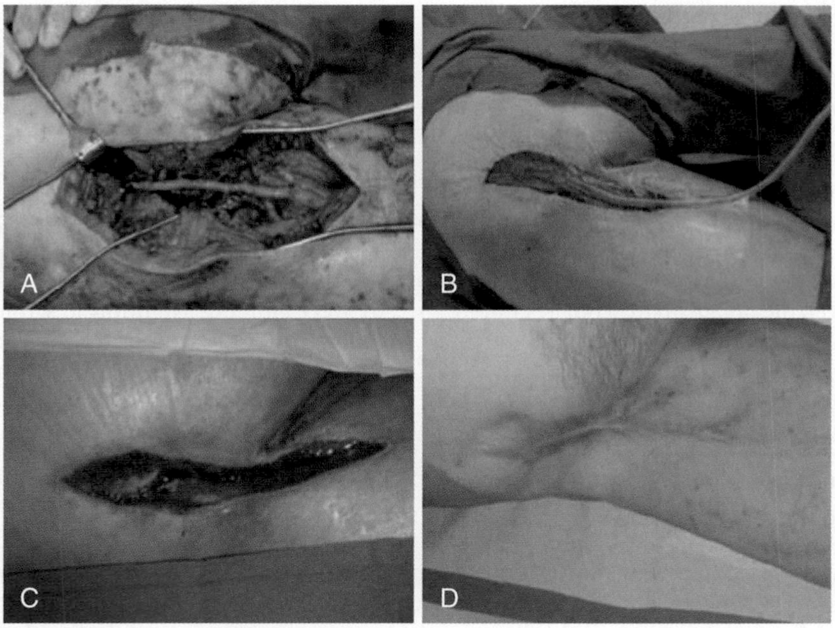


**FIG. 11-11** Negative-pressure wound therapy in woman with history of IV drug abuse. **A,** The completely destroyed femoral artery was reconstructed with a homograft. **B,** A black open-pore polyurethane foam was directly applied to the vascular reconstruction and negative pressure applied to wound. **C,** Wound site 16 days after surgery. **D,** Healed wound at 28 months without reinfection. (Source: Reprinted from Mayer D, Hasse B, Koelliker J, et al: Long-term results of vascular graft and artery preserving treatment with negative pressure wound therapy in Szilagyi grade III infections justify a paradigm shift, *Ann Surg* 254:754, 2011. Copyright Southeastern Surgical Congress.)

correct the negative nitrogen balance resulting from the increased metabolic rate. Protein is also necessary for synthesis of immune factors, leukocytes, fibroblasts, and collagen, which are the building blocks for healing. Carbohydrate is needed for the increased metabolic energy required in inflammation and healing. If there is a carbohydrate deficit, the body will break down protein for the needed energy. Fats are also a necessary component in the diet to help in the synthesis of fatty acids and triglycerides, which are part of the cellular membrane.[9]

Vitamin C is needed for capillary synthesis and collagen production by fibroblasts. The B-complex vitamins are necessary as coenzymes for many metabolic reactions. If a vitamin B deficiency develops, a disruption of protein, fat, and carbohydrate metabolism will occur. Vitamin A is also needed in healing because it aids in the process of epithelialization. It increases collagen synthesis and tensile strength of the healing wound.

If the patient is unable to eat, enteral feedings and supplements should be the first choice if the GI tract is functional. Parenteral nutrition is indicated when enteral feedings are contraindicated or not tolerated. (Enteral and parenteral nutrition is discussed in Chapter 39.)

◆ **Infection Prevention and Control.** You and the patient must scrupulously follow aseptic procedures, including handwashing, for keeping the wound free from infection. Do not allow the patient to touch a recently injured area. The patient's environment should be as free as possible from contamination from items introduced by roommates and visitors. Antibiotics may be administered prophylactically to some patients.

If an infection develops, a culture and sensitivity test should be done to determine the organism and the most effective antibiotic for that specific organism. The culture should be taken before the first dose of antibiotic is given. Cultures can be obtained by needle aspiration, tissue culture, or swab technique. Physicians obtain needle and tissue punch biopsy samples. As a nurse, you can obtain cultures using the swab technique.

Swab specimens can be obtained from wounds using Levine's technique, which involves rotating a culture swab over a cleansed 1-cm$^2$ area near the center of the wound. Use sufficient pressure to extract wound fluid from deep tissue layers. (A culture must be taken of the clean tissue because exudate and necrotic tissue will not provide an accurate sample.) When collecting samples, do not use cotton-tipped applicators.[10] The sample must be sent to the laboratory within 1 hour.

◆ **Psychologic Implications.** The patient may be distressed at the thought or sight of an incision or wound because of fear of scarring or disfigurement. Drainage and odor from a wound often cause increased alarm. The patient needs to understand the healing process and normal changes that occur as the wound heals.

When changing a dressing, avoid inappropriate facial expressions that may alert the patient to problems with the wound or raise doubts about your ability to care for it. Wrinkling your nose may convey disgust to the patient. Be careful not to focus on the wound to the extent that the patient is not treated as a total person.

◆ **Patient Teaching.** Because patients are being discharged earlier after surgery and many have surgery as outpatients, it is important that the patient and caregiver know how to care for the wound and perform dressing changes. Wound healing may not be complete for 4 to 6 weeks or longer. Emphasize the importance of adequate rest and good nutrition throughout this time. Physical and emotional stress should be minimal. Observing the wound for complications such as contractures, adhesions, and secondary infection is important. Teach the patient and caregiver the signs and symptoms of infection. Have them note changes in the wound color and amount of drainage. Teach the patient to notify the HCP of any signs of abnormal wound healing.

Drugs are often taken for a time after recovery from the acute infection. Review drug-specific side effects and adverse effects with the patient and caregiver, as well as methods to prevent side effects (e.g., taking with food or not). Teach the patient to contact the HCP if any of these effects occur. Inform the patient of the need to continue the drugs for the specified time. For example, a patient is instructed to take an antibiotic for 10 days but may stop taking the drug after 5 days because of decreased or absent symptoms. However, the organism may not be entirely eliminated, and it may also become resistant to the antibiotic if the drug is not continued.

## PRESSURE ULCERS

### Etiology and Pathophysiology

A **pressure ulcer** is localized injury to the skin and/or underlying tissue (usually over a bony prominence) as a result of pressure or pressure in combination with shear.[11] Pressure ulcers generally fall under the category of healing by secondary intention. The most common site for pressure ulcers is the sacrum, with heels being second.

Factors that influence the development of pressure ulcers include the amount of pressure (intensity), length of time the pressure is exerted on the skin (duration), and ability of the patient's tissue to tolerate the externally applied pressure. Other factors that contribute to pressure ulcer formation include **shearing force** (pressure exerted on the skin when it adheres to the bed and the skin layers slide in the direction of body movement [e.g., when pulling patient up in bed]) and *excessive moisture* (increases risk for skin breakdown).

Factors that put a patient at risk for the development of pressure ulcers are presented in Table 11-11. Individuals at risk include those who are older, incontinent, unable to reposition or unaware of the need to reposition (e.g., spinal cord injury), and bed- or wheelchair-bound.

### Clinical Manifestations

The clinical manifestations of pressure ulcers depend on the extent of the tissue involved. Pressure ulcers are staged or categorized based on the visible or palpable tissue in the ulcer bed. Table 11-12 illustrates the pressure ulcer stages based on the National Pressure Ulcer Advisory Panel (NPUAP) guidelines.[11]

If the pressure ulcer becomes infected, the patient may display signs of infection (e.g., leukocytosis, fever). In addition, the pressure ulcer may increase in size, odor, and drainage; have necrotic tissue; and be indurated, warm, and painful. Untreated ulcers may lead to *cellulitis* (spreading of inflammation to subcutaneous or connective tissue), chronic infection, sepsis, and possibly death. The most common complication of a pressure ulcer is recurrence. Therefore it is important to note the location of previously healed pressure ulcers on a patient's initial admission assessment.

**TABLE 11-11 Risk Factors for Pressure Ulcers**

| | |
|---|---|
| • Advanced age | • Incontinence |
| • Anemia | • Low diastolic blood pressure (<60 mm Hg) |
| • Contractures | • Mental deterioration |
| • Diabetes mellitus | • Neurologic disorders |
| • Elevated body temperature | • Obesity |
| • Friction (rubbing of surfaces together) | • Pain |
| • Immobility | • Prolonged surgery |
| • Impaired circulation | • Vascular disease |

## NURSING AND INTERPROFESSIONAL MANAGEMENT: PRESSURE ULCERS

In 1859 Florence Nightingale wrote, "If he has a bedsore, it's generally not the fault of the disease, but of the nursing."[12] Her comment emphasizes the critical role that nurses have in prevention and treatment of pressure ulcers.

**SAFETY ALERT Pressure Ulcers**
- Stage III or IV (full skin–thickness injury) pressure ulcer acquired after admission to a health care setting is considered a serious reportable event (SRE) (never event).[13] (SREs are discussed in Chapter 1.)

Nursing and interprofessional management are discussed together because the activities are interrelated. In addition to the nurse, other members of the health team, such as the wound care specialist, plastic surgeon, dietitian, physical therapist, and occupational therapist, can provide valuable input into the complex treatment necessary to prevent and treat pressure ulcers.

### Nursing Assessment

Assess patients for pressure ulcer risk initially on admission and at periodic intervals based on the patient's condition. Conduct a thorough head-to-toe assessment on admission to identify and document any pressure ulcers. Thereafter conduct periodic reassessment of the skin and wounds.

**SAFETY ALERT Assessing for Pressure Ulcers**
- In acute care, reassess patients for pressure ulcers every 24 hours.
- In long-term care, reassess residents weekly for the first 4 weeks after admission and then at least monthly or quarterly.
- In home care, reassess patients at every nurse visit.

To do a risk assessment, use a validated assessment tool such as the Braden Scale (available at *www.bradenscale.com*). Knowing the level of risk can help determine how aggressive preventive measures should be.

Identification of skin changes may be difficult in patients with dark skin. Table 11-13 presents techniques to help assess darker skin.

Subjective and objective data that should be obtained from a person with or at risk for a pressure ulcer are presented in Table 11-14.

### Nursing Diagnoses

Nursing diagnoses for the patient with a pressure ulcer may include, but are not limited to, the following:
- Impaired skin integrity *related to* mechanical factors and physical immobilization
- Impaired tissue integrity *related to* impaired circulation and imbalanced nutritional state

### Planning

The overall goals are that the patient with a pressure ulcer will (1) have no deterioration of the ulcer, (2) reduce or eliminate the factors that lead to pressure ulcers, (3) not develop an

## TABLE 11-12 Pressure Ulcer Stages/Categories

**Stage/Category I: Nonblanchable Erythema**

Intact skin with nonblanchable redness of a localized area usually over a bony prominence. Darkly pigmented skin may not have visible blanching. Its color may differ from the surrounding area. The area may be painful, firm, soft, warmer, or cooler as compared to adjacent tissue.

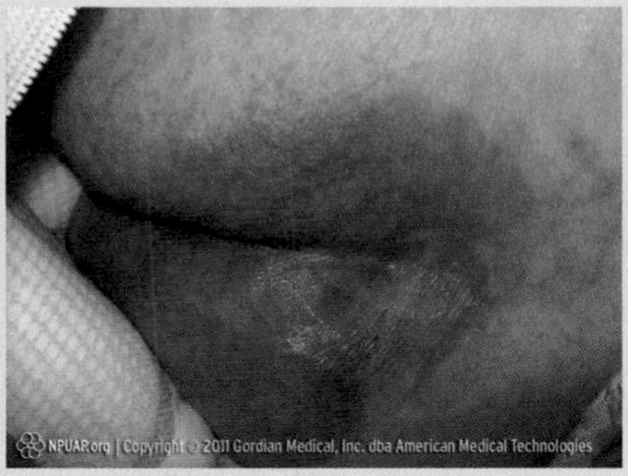


**Stage/Category II: Partial Thickness**

Partial-thickness loss of dermis presenting as a shallow open ulcer with a red-pink wound bed, without slough. May also present as an intact or open/ruptured serum-filled or serosanguineous-filled blister. Presents as a shiny or dry shallow ulcer without slough or bruising. (Bruising indicates deep tissue injury.)

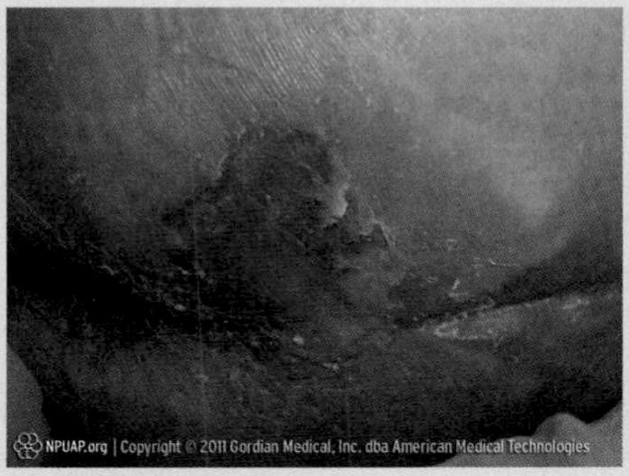


**Stage/Category III: Full-Thickness Skin Loss**

Full-thickness tissue loss. Subcutaneous fat may be visible but bone, tendon, or muscle are not exposed. Slough may be present but does not obscure depth of tissue loss. May include undermining and tunneling. The depth of a category/stage III pressure ulcer varies by anatomic location.

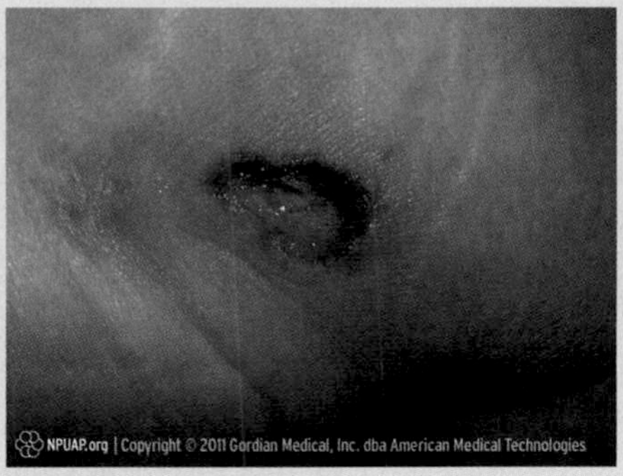


**Stage/Category IV: Full-Thickness Tissue Loss**

Full-thickness tissue loss with exposed bone, tendon, or muscle. Slough or eschar may be present. Often includes undermining and tunneling. Depth of pressure ulcer varies by anatomic location. Ulcers can extend into muscle and/or supporting structures (e.g., fascia, tendon, or joint capsule) making osteomyelitis or osteitis likely to occur. Exposed bone/muscle is visible or directly palpable.

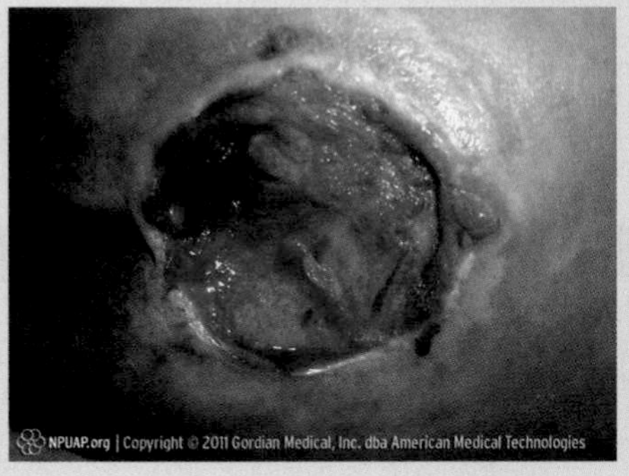


**Unstageable/Unclassified: Full-Thickness Skin or Tissue Loss (Depth Unknown)**

Full-thickness tissue loss in which actual depth of ulcer is completely obscured by slough (yellow, tan, gray, green, or brown) and/or eschar (tan, brown, or black) in wound bed. Until enough slough and/or eschar are removed to expose the base of wound, the true depth cannot be determined; but it will be either a stage III or stage IV. Stable (dry, adherent, intact without erythema, or fluctuance) eschar on the heels serves as "the body's natural (biologic) cover" and should not be removed.

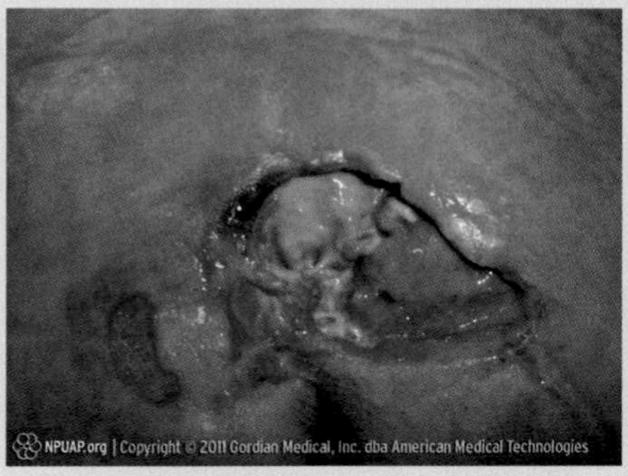


**Suspected Deep Tissue Injury (Depth Unknown)**

Purple or maroon localized area of discolored intact skin or blood-filled blister due to damage of underlying soft tissue from pressure and/or shear. The area may be preceded by tissue that is painful, firm, mushy, boggy, warmer, or cooler as compared to adjacent tissue. Deep tissue injury may be difficult to detect in individuals with dark skin tones. Evolution may include a thin blister over a dark wound bed. The wound may further evolve and become covered by thin eschar. Evolution may be rapid, exposing additional layers of tissue even with optimal treatment.

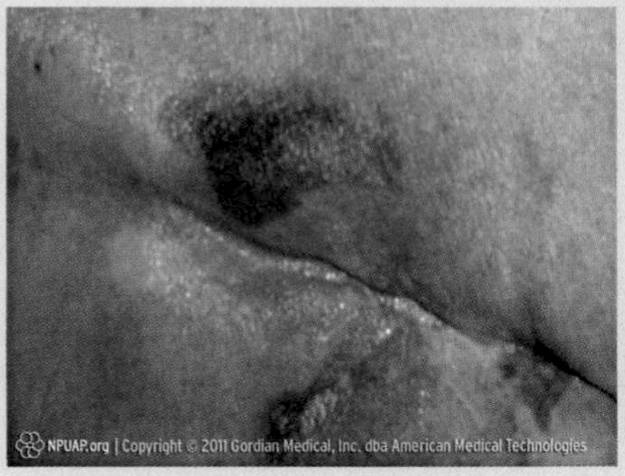


Photos used with permission of the National Pressure Ulcer Advisory Panel.

**TABLE 11-13 Assessing Patients With Dark Skin**

- Look for changes in skin color, such as skin that is darker (purplish, brownish, bluish) than surrounding skin.
- Use natural or halogen light source to accurately assess the skin color. Fluorescent light casts blue color, which can make skin assessment difficult.
- Assess the area for the skin temperature using your hand. The area may feel initially warm, then cooler.
- Touch the skin to feel its consistency. Boggy or edematous feel may indicate a stage I pressure ulcer.
- Ask the patient if he or she has any pain or itchy sensation.

**TABLE 11-14 Nursing Assessment**

***Pressure Ulcers***

**Subjective Data**

***Important Health Information***

*Past health history:* Stroke, spinal cord injury; prolonged bed rest or immobility; circulatory impairment; poor nutrition; altered level of consciousness; prior history of pressure ulcer; immunologic abnormalities; advanced age; diabetes; anemia; trauma

*Medications:* Use of opioids, hypnotics, systemic corticosteroids

*Surgery or other treatments:* Recent surgery

***Functional Health Patterns***

*Nutritional-metabolic:* Obesity, emaciation; decreased fluid, calorie, or protein intake; vitamin or mineral deficiencies; clinically significant malnutrition as indicated by low serum albumin, decreased total lymphocyte count, and decreased body weight (15% less than ideal body weight)

*Elimination:* Incontinence of urine, feces, or both

*Activity-exercise:* Weakness, debilitation, inability to turn and position body; contractures

*Cognitive-perceptual:* Pain or altered cutaneous sensation in pressure ulcer area; decreased awareness of pressure on body areas; capacity to follow treatment plan

**Objective Data**

***General***

Fever

**Integumentary**

Diaphoresis, edema, and discoloration, especially over bony areas such as sacrum, hips, elbows, heels, knees, ankles, shoulders, and ear rims, progressing to increased tissue damage characteristic of ulcer stages*

***Possible Diagnostic Findings***

Leukocytosis, positive cultures for microorganisms from pressure ulcer

*Table 11-12.

infection in the pressure ulcer, (4) have healing of pressure ulcers, and (5) have no recurrence.

## ◆ Nursing Implementation

◆ **Health Promotion.** A primary nursing responsibility is the (1) identification of patients at risk for developing pressure ulcers (Tables 11-11 and 11-14) and (2) implementation of pressure ulcer prevention strategies for those who are at risk. Prevention remains the best treatment for pressure ulcers. Implementing evidence-based pressure ulcer prevention programs can reduce the occurrence of health care–acquired pressure ulcers.[14,15]

**EVIDENCE-BASED PRACTICE**

***Applying the Evidence***

**Repositioning and Pressure Ulcers**

You are doing discharge planning with L.H., an obese 76-year-old woman with a history of diabetes, hypertension, and macular degeneration. L.H. has spent most of her time while hospitalized in a bed or wheelchair and now has a stage I pressure ulcer on her sacrum. You explain the importance of pressure ulcer care with her son, who is her primary caregiver.

***Making Clinical Decisions***

***Best Available Evidence.*** Repositioning is the primary method of reducing the risk for pressure ulcers. Pressure-reducing devices (e.g., foam dressings, foam mattress, padded commode, wheelchair seats) may also be used but should not be a substitute for repositioning.

***Clinician Expertise.*** You know that patients with pressure ulcers or at risk for pressure ulcers should be repositioned frequently. The frequency of repositioning is individualized based on patient need and risk. (It is no longer every 2 hours for every patient.)

***Caregiver Preferences and Values.*** L.H.'s caregiver states he will reposition his mother during the day and instruct the home health care aide to reposition her frequently at night.

***Implications for Nursing Practice***

1. In addition to repositioning, what information is important to discuss with L.H.'s son to prevent further skin breakdown?
2. What are the risk factors for L.H. to develop new pressure ulcers?
3. What is important for the home health care nurse to monitor on her visits to L.H. related to pressure ulcers and healing?

***Reference for Evidence***

National Pressure Ulcer Advisory Panel. Retrieved from *www.npuap.org/wp-content/uploads/2014/08/Updated-10-16-14-Quick-Reference-Guide-DIGITAL-NPUAP-EPUAP-PPPIA-16Oct2014.pdf.*

**! SAFETY ALERT Preventing Pressure Ulcers**

- Use devices to reduce pressure and shearing force (e.g., low-air-loss mattresses, foam mattresses, wheelchair cushions, padded commode seats, boots [foam, air], lift sheets) as appropriate. These devices do not replace the need for frequent repositioning.
- Reposition patients frequently to prevent pressure ulcers.

In the past, the "standard" was to turn and reposition patients every 2 hours. However, this "policy" is not evidence based. Time schedules and frequency should be individualized based on risk factors, patient's overall condition, and type of mattress and support surface. For example, some high-risk patients may need to be turned and repositioned every hour, whereas others at lower risk may need to be turned and repositioned only every 3 to 4 hours.[6,11]

◆ **Acute Care.** Care of a patient with a pressure ulcer requires local care of the wound and support measures of the whole person, such as adequate nutrition, pain management, control of other medical conditions, and pressure relief. Both conservative and surgical strategies are used in the treatment of pressure ulcers, depending on the stage and condition of the ulcer.

Once a pressure ulcer has developed, initiate interventions based on the ulcer characteristics (e.g., stage, size, location, amount of exudate, type of wound, presence of infection or pain) and the patient's general status (e.g., nutritional state, age, cardiovascular status, level of mobility). Carefully document the size of the pressure ulcer. A wound-measuring card or tape can be used to note the ulcer's maximum length and width in centimeters. To find the depth of the ulcer, take a sterile cotton-tipped applicator and soak it with saline. Gently place it into the deepest part of the ulcer, and then measure the length of the portion of the applicator that probed the ulcer. Documentation of the healing wound can be done using several available pressure ulcer healing tools such as the NPUAP Pressure Ulcer Scale for Healing (PUSH) tool (available at *www.npuap.org/wp-content/uploads/2012/03/push3.pdf*).

Some agencies require that pictures of the pressure ulcer be taken initially and at regular intervals during the course of treatment. The Informatics box has suggestions for digital imaging.

## INFORMATICS IN PRACTICE

### *Digital Images*

To monitor wound progress, use digital photography. For the best images:

- Include a ruler with date, length, width, and depth of the wound in each photo.
- Position the patient the same way for each photo.
- Take the photo from the same angle each time. Pointing perpendicularly at the wound is best.
- Use natural light, without flash, whenever possible.
- Show the wound on a solid background, avoiding shiny underpads.
- Avoid patient identifiers such as jewelry, tattoos, or visible family members.

Local care of the pressure ulcer may involve debridement, wound cleaning, application of a dressing, and relief of pressure. It is important to select the appropriate pressure-relieving technique (e.g., pad, overlay, mattress, specialty bed) to relieve pressure and keep the patient off of the pressure ulcer. Whenever possible, do not turn the patient onto a body surface that is still reddened. Massage is contraindicated in the presence of acute inflammation and where there is the possibility of damaged blood vessels or fragile skin.

Sliding down in bed causes shear. Encourage patients to reposition themselves by lifting rather than sliding and to use a trapeze if indicated. Lift sheets may be used to move patients up in bed or to transfer them.

A pressure ulcer that has necrotic tissue or eschar (except for dry, stable necrotic feet or heels) must have the tissue removed by surgical, mechanical, enzymatic, or autolytic debridement methods. Once the pressure ulcer has been successfully debrided and has a clean granulating base, the goal is to provide an appropriate wound environment that supports moist wound healing and prevents disruption of the newly formed granulation tissue. Reconstruction of the pressure ulcer site by surgical repair, including skin grafting, skin flaps, musculocutaneous flaps, or free flaps, may be necessary.

Clean pressure ulcers with noncytotoxic solutions (e.g., normal saline) that do not kill or damage cells, especially fibroblasts. Solutions such as Dakin's solution (sodium hypochlorite solution), acetic acid, povidone-iodine, and hydrogen peroxide are cytotoxic. Therefore they should not be used to clean pressure ulcers. It is also important to use enough irrigation pressure to adequately clean the pressure ulcer (4 to 15 psi) without causing trauma or damage to the wound. To obtain this pressure, use a 30-mL syringe and a 19-gauge needle.

After the pressure ulcer has been cleansed, cover it with an appropriate dressing. Keep a pressure ulcer slightly moist, rather than dry, to enhance re-epithelialization. Some factors to consider when selecting a dressing are maintenance of a moist environment, prevention of the wound from drying out, ability to absorb the wound drainage, location of the wound, amount of caregiver time required to change the dressing, cost of the dressing, presence of infection, clean versus sterile dressings, and care delivery setting. Never use a wet-to-dry dressing on a clean granulating pressure ulcer. This type of dressing should be used only for mechanical debridement of a wound that has necrotic or sloughing tissue. (Dressings are discussed in Table 11-9.)

Stages II through IV pressure ulcers are considered contaminated or colonized with bacteria. Remember that in people who have chronic wounds or are immunocompromised, the clinical signs and symptoms of infection (purulent exudate, odor, erythema, warmth, tenderness, edema, pain, fever, and elevated WBC count) may not be present even though the pressure ulcer is infected.

The maintenance of adequate nutrition is an important nursing responsibility for the patient with a pressure ulcer. Often the patient is debilitated and has a poor appetite secondary to inactivity. Oral feedings must be adequate in calories, protein, fluids, vitamins, and minerals to meet the patient's nutritional requirements. The caloric intake needed to correct and maintain nutritional balance may be 30 to 35 calories/kg/day and 1.25 to 1.50 g of protein/kg/day.

Enteral feedings can be used to supplement the oral feedings. When oral and enteral feedings are inadequate, parenteral nutrition consisting of amino acid and glucose solutions is used. (Parenteral and enteral nutrition are discussed in Chapter 39.)

◆ **Ambulatory Care.** Pressure ulcers affect the quality of life of patients and their caregivers. Because pressure ulcers commonly recur, teaching prevention techniques to the patient and caregiver is extremely important (Table 11-15). A sixth-grade–level version of the patient guide to pressure ulcer prevention is available for use in patient teaching *(www.npuap.org/PU_Prev_Points.pdf)*.

The caregiver needs to know the etiology of pressure ulcers, prevention techniques, early signs, nutritional support, and

## TABLE 11-15 Patient & Caregiver Teaching

### *Pressure Ulcer*

*When teaching the patient and caregiver to prevent and care for pressure ulcers, do the following.*

1. Identify and explain risk factors and etiology of pressure ulcers to patient and caregiver.
2. Assess all at-risk patients at time of first hospital and/or home visit or whenever the patient's condition changes. Thereafter assess at regular intervals based on care setting (every 24 hours for acute care or every visit in home care).
3. Teach the caregiver techniques for incontinence. If incontinence occurs, cleanse skin at time of soiling and use absorbent pads or briefs.
4. Demonstrate correct positioning to decrease risk of skin breakdown. Instruct caregiver to reposition a bed-bound patient at least every 2 hours, a chair-bound patient every hour. NEVER position the patient directly on the pressure ulcer.
5. Assess resources (i.e., caregiver's availability and skill, finances, equipment) of patients requiring pressure ulcer care at home. When selecting ulcer care dressing, consider cost and amount of caregiver time required.
6. Teach patient and/or caregiver to place clean dressings over sterile dressings using "no touch" technique when changing dressings. Instruct caregiver on disposal of contaminated dressings.
7. Teach patient and caregiver to inspect skin daily. Tell them to report any significant changes to the HCP.
8. Teach patient and caregiver the importance of good nutrition to enhance ulcer healing.
9. Evaluate program effectiveness.

care techniques for actual pressure ulcers. Because the patient with a pressure ulcer often requires extensive care for other health problems, it is important that the nurse support the caregiver with the added responsibility for pressure ulcer treatment. eNursing Care Plan 11-2 (available on the website for this chapter) outlines the care for the patient with a pressure ulcer.

### ◆ Evaluation

The expected outcomes are that the patient with a pressure ulcer will have

- Healing of pressure ulcer(s)
- Intact skin with no further breakdown

## CASE STUDY

### Inflammation and Infection

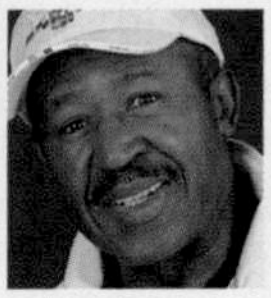

(©iStockphoto/ Thinkstock)

**Patient Profile**

G.N., a 65-year-old African American man, was admitted to the hospital emergency department with partial-thickness burns that involved his face, neck, and upper trunk. He also had a lacerated right leg. His injuries occurred about 36 hours earlier when he fell out of a tree onto his gas grill (which was lit) while trimming tree branches.

**Subjective Data**

- Complains of slightly hoarse voice and irritated throat
- States that he tried to treat himself because he does not have health insurance
- Has been coughing up sooty sputum
- Complains of severe pain in left hip

**Objective Data**

***Physical Examination***

- Leg wound is gaping and has drainage: temperature 101.1°F (38.4°C)
- X-rays reveal a fractured right tibia and fractured left hip

***Laboratory Studies***

- WBC count 26,400/μL ($26.4 \times 10^9$/L) with 80% neutrophils (10% bands)

**Interprofessional Care**

- Surgery is performed to repair the left hip.

**Discussion Questions**

1. What clinical manifestations of inflammation did G.N. exhibit, and what are their pathophysiologic mechanisms?
2. What type of exudate formation did he develop?
3. What is the basis for the development of the temperature?
4. What is the significance of his WBC count and differential?
5. Because his wound was gaping, primary tissue healing was not possible. How would you expect healing to take place? What complications could he develop?
6. What risk factors does G.N. have to develop a pressure ulcer?
7. ***Priority Decision:*** Based on the assessment data provided, what are the priority nursing diagnoses? Are there any collaborative problems?
8. ***Teamwork and Collaboration:*** What nursing activities related to wound care can be delegated to unlicensed assistive personnel (UAP)?
9. ***Quality Improvement:*** What outcomes would indicate that interprofessional care was effective?

Answers available at *http://evolve.elsevier.com/Lewis/medsurg.*

## BRIDGE TO NCLEX EXAMINATION

The number of the question corresponds to the same-numbered outcome at the beginning of the chapter.

1. A patient 1 day postoperative after abdominal surgery has incisional pain, 99.5°F temperature, slight erythema at the incision margins, and 30 mL serosanguineous drainage in the Jackson-Pratt drain. Based on this assessment, what conclusion would the nurse make?
   **a.** The abdominal incision shows signs of an infection.
   **b.** The patient is having a normal inflammatory response.
   **c.** The abdominal incision shows signs of impending dehiscence.
   **d.** The patient's physician must be notified about her condition.
2. The nurse assessing a patient with a chronic leg wound finds local signs of erythema and the patient complains of pain at the wound site. What would the nurse anticipate being ordered to assess the patient's systemic response?
   **a.** Serum protein analysis
   **b.** WBC count and differential
   **c.** Punch biopsy of center of wound
   **d.** Culture and sensitivity of the wound
3. A patient in the unit has a 103.7°F temperature. Which intervention would be *most* effective in restoring normal body temperature?
   **a.** Use a cooling blanket while the patient is febrile.
   **b.** Administer antipyretics on an around-the-clock schedule.
   **c.** Provide increased fluids and have the UAP give sponge baths.
   **d.** Give prescribed antibiotics and provide warm blankets for comfort.
4. A nurse is caring for a patient who has a pressure ulcer that is treated with debridement, irrigations, and moist gauze dressings. How should the nurse anticipate healing to occur?
   **a.** Tertiary intention
   **b.** Secondary intention
   **c.** Regeneration of cells
   **d.** Remodeling of tissues
5. A nurse is caring for a patient with diabetes who is scheduled for amputation of his necrotic left great toe. The patient's WBC count is $15.0 \times 10^6$/μL, and he has coolness of the lower extremities, weighs 75 lb more than his ideal body weight, and smokes two packs of cigarettes per day. Which *priority* nursing diagnosis addresses the primary factor affecting the patient's ability to heal?
   **a.** Imbalanced nutrition: obesity *related to* high-fat foods
   **b.** Impaired tissue integrity *related to* decreased blood flow secondary to diabetes and smoking
   **c.** Ineffective peripheral tissue perfusion *related to* narrowed blood vessels secondary to diabetes and smoking
   **d.** Ineffective individual coping *related to* indifference and denial of the long-term effects of diabetes and smoking
6. Which one of the orders should a nurse question in the plan of care for an elderly immobile stroke patient with a stage III pressure ulcer?
   **a.** Pack the ulcer with foam dressing.
   **b.** Turn and position the patient every hour.
   **c.** Clean the ulcer every shift with Dakin's solution.
   **d.** Assess for pain and medicate before dressing change.

7. An 85-year-old patient is assessed to have a score of 16 on the Braden Scale. Based on this information, how should the nurse plan for this patient's care?
   a. Implement a 1-hr turning schedule with skin assessment.
   b. Place DuoDerm on the patient's sacrum to prevent breakdown.
   c. Elevate the head of bed to 90 degrees when the patient is supine.
   d. Continue with weekly skin assessments with no special precautions.
8. A 65-year-old stroke patient with limited mobility has a purple area of suspected deep tissue injury on the left greater trochanter. Which nursing diagnoses are *most* appropriate (*select all that apply*)?
   a. Acute pain *related to* tissue damage and inflammation
   b. Impaired skin integrity *related to* immobility and decreased sensation
   c. Impaired tissue integrity *related to* inadequate circulation secondary to pressure
   d. Risk for infection *related to* loss of tissue integrity and undernutrition secondary to stroke
   e. Ineffective peripheral tissue perfusion *related* to arteriosclerosis and loss of blood supply to affected area
9. An 82-year-old man is being cared for at home by his family. A pressure ulcer on his right buttock measures 1 × 2 × 0.8 cm in depth, and pink subcutaneous tissue is completely visible on the wound bed. Which stage would the nurse document on the wound assessment form?
   a. Stage I
   b. Stage II
   c. Stage III
   d. Stage IV

1. b, 2. b, 3. b, 4. b, 5. b, 6. c, 7. a, 8. b, c, 9. c

For rationales to these answers and even more NCLEX review questions, visit *http://evolve.elsevier.com/Lewis/medsurg.*

## EVOLVE WEBSITE

http://evolve.elsevier.com/Lewis/medsurg

**Review Questions (Online Only)**

**Key Points**

**Answer Keys for Questions**

- Rationales for Bridge to NCLEX Examination Questions
- Answer Guidelines for Case Study on p. 176

**Student Case Study**

- Patient With Pressure Ulcers

**Nursing Care Plans**

- eNursing Care Plan 11-1: Patient With a Fever
- eNursing Care Plan 11-2: Patient With a Pressure Ulcer

**Conceptual Care Map Creator**

**Audio Glossary**

**Content Updates**

## REFERENCES


1. Knowlton MC: Nurses know how to manage fever, but what about shivering? *Nursing* 43:49, 2013.
2. Atkins E: Fever: its history, cause, and function, *Yale J Biol Med* 55:283, 1982. (Classic)
3. LeBlanc K, Baranoski S: Skin tears: Best practices for care and prevention, *Nursing* 44:36, 2014.
4. Bergevin RC: Assessing wounds in palliative care, *Nursing* 44(8):67, 2014.

*5. Lisy K: Early vs. delayed removal of dressings covering surgical wounds, *AJN* 114:23, 2014.

*6. Ayello EA, Baranoski S: Wound care prevention, *Nursing* 44:32, 2014.

*7. Wilcox JR, Carter MJ, Covington S: Frequency of debridements and time to heal: a retrospective cohort study of 312,744 wounds, *JAMA Dermatol* 149(9):1050, 2013.

8. Negative pressure wound therapy: use with care. Retrieved from *www.fda.gov/MedicalDevices/Safety/AlertsandNotices/TipsandArticleson DeviceSafety/ucm225038.htm.*
9. Posthauer ME: Nutrition: fuel for pressure ulcer prevention and healing, *Nursing* 44:67, 2014.
10. Huddleston Cross H: Obtaining a wound swab culture specimen, *Nursing* 44:68, 2014.

*11. National Pressure Ulcer Advisory Panel. Retrieved from *www.npuap.org.*

12. Nightingale F: *Notes on nursing*, Philadelphia, 1859, Lippincott. (Classic)
13. Nelson M, Harris R: Pressure ulcer alert! *Nursing* 43:64, 2013.

*14. Roe E, Williams DL: Using evidence-based practice to prevent hospital-acquired pressure ulcers and promote wound healing, *AJN* 114:61, 2014.

*15. Paul R, McCutcheon SP, Tregarthen JP, et al: Sustaining pressure ulcer best practices in high-volume cardiac care unit, *AJN* 114:34, 2014.


*Evidence-based information for clinical practice.

# 12

# Genetics and Genomics

*Sharon L. Lewis*

*You inherit your environment just as much as your genes.*

***Johnny Rich***

ⓔ http://evolve.elsevier.com/Lewis/medsurg/

## LEARNING OUTCOMES

1. Differentiate the common terms related to genetics and genetic disorders: autosomal, carrier, heterozygous, homozygous, mutation, recessive, and X-linked gene.
2. Differentiate between the two common causes of genetic mutations.
3. Compare and contrast the three most common inheritance patterns of genetic disorders.
4. Describe the most common classifications of genetic disorders.
5. Explore the complex ethical and social implications of genetic testing.
6. Analyze the role of pharmacogenomics and pharmacogenetics in developing personalized drug therapy.
7. Discuss your role in assisting the patient and family in dealing with genetic issues.

## KEY TERMS

epigenetics, p. 183
genetics, p. 178
genomics, p. 178
hereditary, Table 12-1, p. 179
heterozygous, Table 12-1, p. 179
homozygous, Table 12-1, p. 179
mutation, Table 12-1, p. 179
pharmacogenetics, p. 186
pharmacogenomics, p. 186

## GENETICS AND GENOMICS

In the 1860s an Austrian monk named Gregor Mendel, while experimenting with pea plants, discovered how traits are transmitted from parents to offspring. This discovery laid the foundation for modern **genetics**, the study of genes and their role in inheritance. Genetics determines the way that certain traits or conditions are passed down from one generation to another.

**Genomics** is the study of all of a person's genes (the *genome*), including interactions of these genes with each other and with the person's environment. (Common terms used in genetics and genomics are defined in Table 12-1.) Genomics includes the study of complex diseases such as heart disease, asthma, diabetes mellitus, and cancer, because these diseases are typically caused by a combination of genetic and environmental factors rather than by a single gene.

A person's genes can have a profound impact on health and disease. More than 4000 diseases are thought to be related to altered genes. Genomic factors play a role in 9 of the 10 leading causes of death in the United States, including heart disease, cancer, diabetes, stroke, and Alzheimer's disease.[1]

Genomics may help us understand why some people who eat healthy diets and exercise regularly still die at a young age of cancer, whereas some people eat unhealthy diets and never exercise and yet live to an old age.

The identification of a genetic basis for many human diseases has the potential to strongly influence the care of patients at risk for or diagnosed with a disease that has a genetic link. You need to know the basic principles of genetics, be familiar with the impact that genetics and genomics have on health and disease, and be prepared to assist the patient and family with genetic issues.

### Basic Principles of Genetics

**Genes.** *Genes* are the basic units of heredity. There are more than 22,000 genes in each person's genetic makeup, or *genome.* Genes encode (carry the instructions) for proteins that direct the activities of cells and functions of the body. Genes control how a cell functions, including how quickly it grows, how often it divides, and how long it lives. To control these functions, genes produce proteins that perform specific tasks and act as messengers for the cell. Therefore it is essential that each gene have the correct instructions or "code" for making its protein so that the protein can perform the proper function for the cell.

Genes are arranged in a specific linear formation along a chromosome (Fig. 12-1). Each gene has a specific location on a chromosome, termed a *locus.* An *allele* is one of two or more alternative forms of a gene that occupy corresponding loci on *homologous chromosomes* (a pair of chromosomes having corresponding deoxyribonucleic acid [DNA] sequences, with one

Reviewed by Judy Carlyle, RN, MNSc, Faculty/Clinical Liaison, Arkansas Rural Nursing Education Consortium (ARNEC), Nashville, Arkansas; Laura A. Stokowski, RNC, MS, Inova Fairfax Hospital for Children, Falls Church, Virginia; and Kenneth Wysocki, PhD, FNP-BC, FAANP, Family Nurse Practitioner, Asthma and Genetics Researcher, Clinical Services, Matrix Medical Network, Scottsdale, Arizona.

## TABLE 12-1 Glossary of Genetic and Genomic Terms

| Term | Definition |
|---|---|
| **Allele** | An alternative form of a gene. Each person receives two alleles of a gene, one from each biologic parent. Different alleles produce variations in inherited traits such as eye color and blood type. |
| **Autosome** | Any chromosome that is not a sex chromosome. Humans have 22 pairs of autosomes. |
| **Carrier** | Individual who carries a copy of a mutated gene for a recessive disorder. |
| **Chromosome** | A compact structure containing DNA and proteins present in nearly all cells of the body. Normally each cell has 46 chromosomes in 23 pairs. Each biologic parent contributes one of each pair of chromosomes. |
| **Codominance** | Two dominant versions of a trait that are both expressed in the same individual (e.g., AB blood type). |
| **Congenital disorder** | Condition present at birth. |
| **Dominant allele** | Gene that is expressed in the phenotype of a heterozygous individual. |
| **Familial disorder** | Condition that affects more than one person in a family. |
| **Gene** | The basic unit of heredity information located on a specific part of a chromosome. Genes direct cells to make proteins and guide almost every aspect of operation and repair of cells. |
| **Genetic risk factor** | A change in a gene that increases a person's risk of developing a disease. |
| **Genetics** | Study of genes and their role in inheritance. |
| **Genome** | All the DNA contained in an individual. |
| **Genome-wide association study (GWAS)** | A study approach that involves scanning complete sets of DNA (genomes) of many individuals to find genetic variations associated with a particular disease. |
| **Genomics** | Study of how genes interact and influence people's biologic and physical characteristics. |
| **Genotype** | Genetic identity of an individual. This identity does not show as outward characteristics. |
| **Hereditary** | Transmission of a disease, condition, or trait from parent to children. |
| **Heterozygous** | Having two different alleles for one given gene, one inherited from each parent. |
| **Homozygous** | Having two identical alleles for one given gene, one inherited from each parent. |
| **Locus** | Position of a gene on a chromosome. |
| **Mutation** | A change in DNA or a gene. Sometimes these changes are passed from parent to children. |
| **Oncogene** | Gene that is able to initiate and contribute to the conversion of normal cells to cancer cells. |
| **Pedigree** | Family tree that contains the genetic characteristics and disorders of that particular family. |
| **Pharmacogenetics** | Study of variability of responses to drugs related to variations in single genes. |
| **Pharmacogenomics** | Study of variability of responses to drugs related to variations in and interactions of multiple genes. |
| **Phenotype** | Observable traits or characteristics of an individual (e.g., hair color). |
| **Protooncogene** | Normal cellular genes that are important regulators of normal cellular processes. Mutations can activate them to become oncogenes. |
| **Recessive allele** | Allele that has no noticeable effect on the phenotype in a heterozygous individual. |
| **Trait** | Physical characteristic that one inherits, such as hair or eye color. |
| **X-linked gene** | Gene located on the X chromosome. In general, sex-linked disorders are only seen in males. |

coming from the mother and the other from the father). Each allele codes for a specific inherited characteristic.

When there are two different alleles, the allele that is fully expressed is the *dominant allele.* The other allele that lacks the ability to express itself in the presence of a dominant allele is the *recessive allele.* Physical traits expressed by an individual are termed the *phenotype,* and the actual genetic makeup of the individual is termed the *genotype.*

**Chromosomes.** *Chromosomes* are contained in the nucleus of a cell and occur in pairs. Humans have 23 pairs of chromosomes; 22 of the 23 pairs of chromosomes are *homologous* and are termed *autosomes.* Autosomes are the same in both males and females. The sex chromosomes make up the twenty-third pair of chromosomes. A female has two X chromosomes, and a male has one X and one Y chromosome. One chromosome of each pair is inherited from the mother and one from the father. One half of each child's chromosomes (and therefore the genetic makeup) comes from his or her father and one half from his or her mother.

**DNA.** Genes are made up of a nucleic acid called *deoxyribonucleic acid* (DNA). DNA stores genetic information and encodes the instructions for synthesizing specific proteins needed to maintain life. DNA also dictates the rate at which proteins are made. Every somatic cell in a person's body has the same DNA.

The information in DNA is stored as a code made up of four nitrogenous bases: adenine (A), guanine (G), cytosine (C), and thymine (T). Human DNA consists of about 3 billion bases, and more than 99% of those bases are the same in all people. The order (or sequence) of these bases determines the information for building and maintaining an organism. This is similar to the way letters of the alphabet are used to create words and sentences.

DNA bases pair up with each other, A with T and C with G, to form units called *base pairs.* Each base is also attached to a sugar molecule and a phosphate molecule (Fig. 12-2). Together, a base, sugar, and phosphate are called a *nucleotide.* Nucleotides are arranged in two long strands that form a spiral called a *double helix.* The structure of the double helix is somewhat like

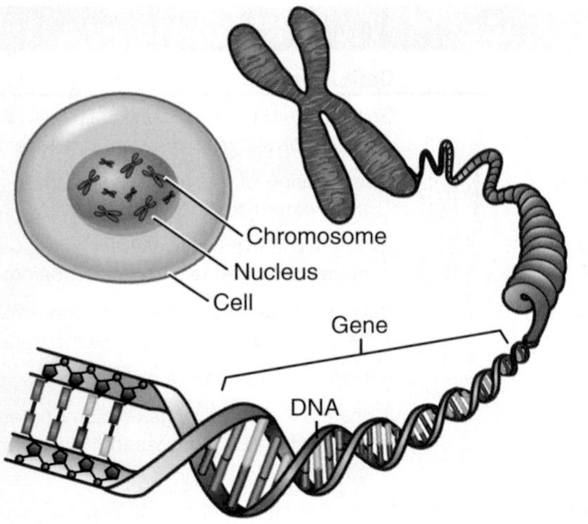


**FIG. 12-1** The long, stringy DNA that makes up genes is spooled within chromosomes inside the nucleus of a cell. (Note that a gene would actually be a much longer stretch of DNA than what is shown here.) (Adapted from *The New Genetics,* National Institute of General Medical Science, National Institutes of Health, U.S. Department of Health and Human Services.)

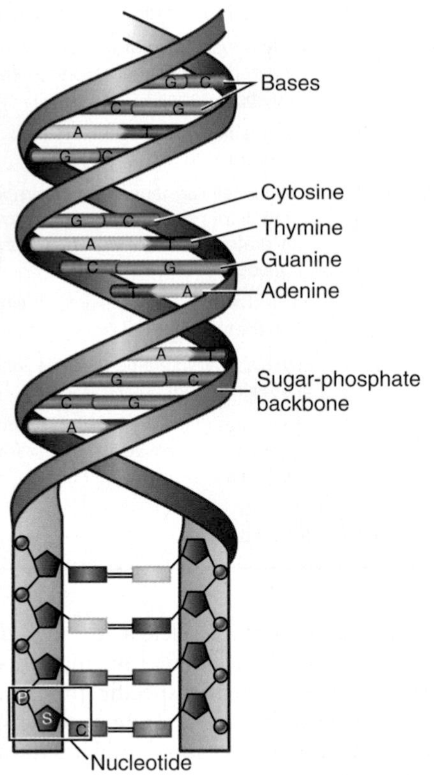


**FIG. 12-2** DNA consists of two long, twisted chains made up of nucleotides. Each nucleotide contains one base, one phosphate molecule *(P),* and the sugar molecule deoxyribose *(S).* The bases in DNA nucleotides are adenine *(A),* thymine *(T),* cytosine *(C),* and guanine *(G).* (Adapted from *The New Genetics.* National Institute of General Medical Science, National Institutes of Health, U.S. Department of Health and Human Services.)

a ladder, with the base pairs forming the ladder's rungs and the sugar and phosphate molecules forming the ladder's vertical sidepieces.

DNA can *replicate* (make copies of itself). Each strand of DNA in the double helix can serve as a pattern for duplicating the sequence of bases. When cells divide, each new cell must have an exact copy of the DNA that was in the parent (original) cell.

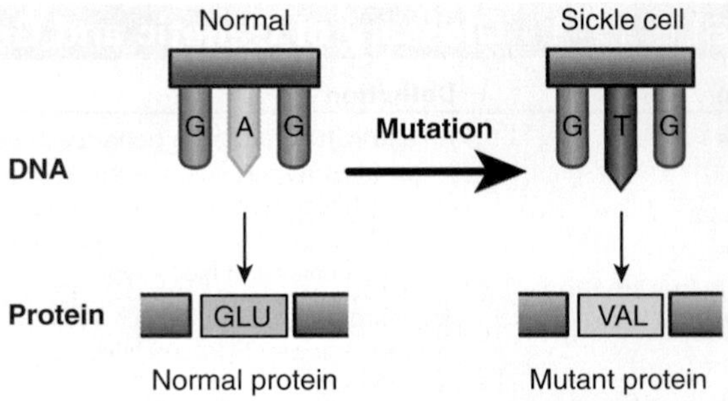


**FIG. 12-3** In sickle cell disease a single gene mutation leads to mutant (incorrect) protein. The substitution of valine *(VAL)* for glutamic acid on the β-globin chain of hemoglobin produces abnormal hemoglobin, hemoglobin S *(Hb S).* In response to low $O_2$ levels, the erythrocytes with Hb S stiffen and elongate, taking on a sickle shape (see Fig. 30-3).

If the chromosomes in one of your cells were uncoiled and placed end to end, the DNA would be about 6 feet long. If all of the DNA in your body were connected, it would stretch about 67 billion miles.[2]

**RNA.** *Ribonucleic acid* (RNA) is similar to DNA but with some significant differences. Like DNA, RNA contains the nitrogenous bases adenine, guanine, and cytosine. However, RNA lacks the nitrogenous base thymine and instead contains uracil. RNA is single stranded and contains ribose instead of deoxyribose sugar. RNA transfers the genetic information obtained from DNA to the proper location for protein synthesis.

**Protein Synthesis.** Protein synthesis, or the making of proteins, occurs in two steps: *transcription* and *translation.* Transcription is the process by which messenger RNA (mRNA) is synthesized from single-stranded DNA. The mRNA becomes attached to a ribosome, where translation occurs. At this point another specialized type of RNA, transfer RNA (tRNA), arranges the amino acids in the correct sequence to assemble the protein. Once the protein is completed, it is released from the ribosome and is able to perform its specific function in the cell.

**Mitosis.** *Mitosis* is a type of cell division that results in the formation of genetically identical daughter cells. Before cell division, the chromosomes duplicate, and each new cell (called daughter cells) receives an exact replica of the chromosomes from the original cell (called the parent cell).

**Meiosis.** *Meiosis* occurs only in sexual reproductive cells. In meiosis the number of chromosomes is reduced, resulting in half of the usual number of chromosomes. Therefore oocytes and sperm contain only a single copy of each chromosome, whereas all other body cells contain duplicates of each chromosome.

## Genetic Mutations

A *mutation* is any change in the usual DNA sequence. Subtle variations in DNA are called *polymorphisms* (meaning many forms). Many of these *gene* polymorphisms account for slight variations among people such as hair and eye color. However, some gene variations may result in disease or an increased risk for disease. These gene variations or changes are referred to as *mutations.*

A genetic mutation is like a spelling error in a gene's sequence. For example, in people with sickle cell disease, a substitution of a single base (adenine is replaced by thymine) in a single gene (β-globin gene) causes the disease (Fig. 12-3). Mutations range in size from a single DNA base (building block) to a large segment of a chromosome.

The change in gene structure may alter the type and/or amount of protein produced. The protein may not work at all, or it may work incorrectly. In some cases, genetic mutations do not have an obvious effect on the people who have them.

**Types of Mutations.** Genetic mutations occur in two ways. They can be inherited from a parent (germline mutation) or acquired (somatic mutation) during a person's lifetime.

*Germline mutations* are passed from parent to child. These mutations are present in the oocyte and sperm cells. This type of mutation is present throughout a person's life in virtually every cell in the body.

*Acquired (somatic) mutations* occur in the DNA of a cell at some time during a person's life. An acquired mutation is passed on to all cells that develop from that single cell. These mutations in somatic cells cannot be passed on to the next generation. Acquired mutations can occur if (1) a mistake is made as DNA replicates during cell division or (2) environmental factors alter the DNA.

Mutations can occur when a cell is dividing. Considering that 3 billion base pairs are replicated in each cell division, DNA replication is very accurate. However, during replication occasionally mistakes such as deletions, insertions, or duplication of DNA material can occur. Although DNA repair enzymes can correct replication errors, mistakes can go uncorrected.

In addition to cell division, DNA damage can also occur from environmental factors. For example, ultraviolet (UV) radiation can cause DNA damage, leading to skin cancer. Toxins in cigarettes can lead to lung cancer. Many chemotherapy drugs used to treat cancer target the DNA of cancer cells and healthy cells. In the process, these drugs increase a person's risk of developing secondary cancers (see Chapter 15).

Cells have built-in mechanisms that catch and repair most of the changes that occur during DNA replication or from environmental damage. However, as we age, our DNA repair does not work as effectively and we accumulate changes in our DNA.

## Inheritance Patterns

Genetic disorders can be categorized into autosomal dominant, autosomal recessive, or X-linked (sex-linked) recessive disorders (Table 12-2). If the mutant gene is located on an autosome, the genetic disorder is called *autosomal.* If the mutant gene is on the X chromosome, the genetic disorder is called *X-linked.*

*Family pedigrees* for autosomal recessive and dominant disorders and X-linked recessive disorders are shown in Figs. 12-4 and 12-5.

*Autosomal dominant disorders* are caused by a mutation of a single gene pair (heterozygous) on a chromosome. A dominant allele prevails over a normal allele. Autosomal dominant disorders show variable expression. *Variable expression* means that the symptoms expressed by the individuals with the mutated gene vary from person to person even though they have the same mutated gene. Although autosomal dominant disorders have a high probability of occurring in families, sometimes these disorders cause a new mutation or skip a generation. This is termed *incomplete penetrance.*

*Autosomal recessive disorders* are caused by mutations of two gene pairs (homozygous) on a chromosome. A person who inherits one copy of the recessive allele does not develop the

**TABLE 12-2 Comparison of Genetic Disorders**

| Characteristics | Examples |
|---|---|
| **Autosomal Dominant** | |
| • Males and females are affected* equally.<br>• More common than recessive disorders and usually less severe.<br>• Affected individuals show variable expression.<br>• Affected individuals may have an affected parent.<br>• Children of a heterozygous (affected) parent have a 50% chance of being affected.<br>• Individuals are affected in successive generations. | • Breast and ovarian cancer related to *BRCA* genes<br>• Familial hypercholesterolemia<br>• Hereditary nonpolyposis colorectal cancer<br>• Huntington's disease<br>• Neurofibromatosis<br>• Marfan's syndrome |
| **Autosomal Recessive** | |
| • Males and females are affected equally.<br>• Heterozygotes are carriers and usually asymptomatic.<br>• Affected individuals may have unaffected† parents who are heterozygous for trait.<br>• Children of two heterozygous parents have 25% chance of being affected and 50% chance of being carriers (Fig. 12-9).<br>• Frequently there is no family history of disease. | • Cystic fibrosis<br>• Phenylketonuria<br>• Sickle cell disease<br>• Tay-Sachs disease<br>• Thalassemia |
| **X-Linked Recessive** | |
| • Most affected individuals have unaffected parents.<br>• Affected individuals are usually males.<br>• Daughters of affected male are carriers.<br>• Sons of affected male are unaffected (unless mother is a carrier). | • Duchenne muscular dystrophy<br>• Hemophilia<br>• Wiskott-Aldrich syndrome |

*Have the disease.
†Do not have the disease.

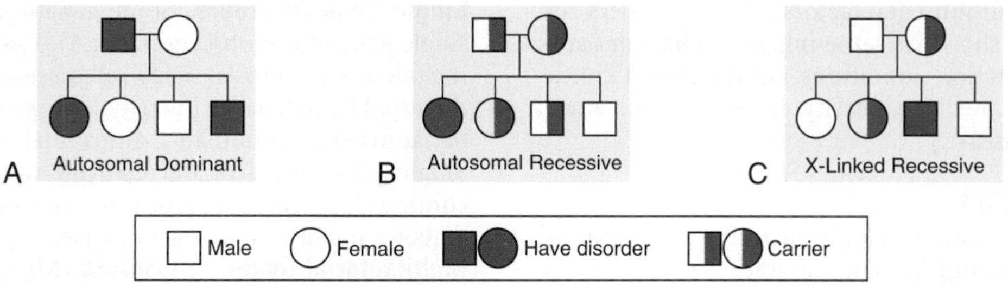


**FIG. 12-4** Examples of family pedigrees showing inheritance of **(A)** autosomal dominant, **(B)** autosomal recessive, and **(C)** X-linked recessive disorders.

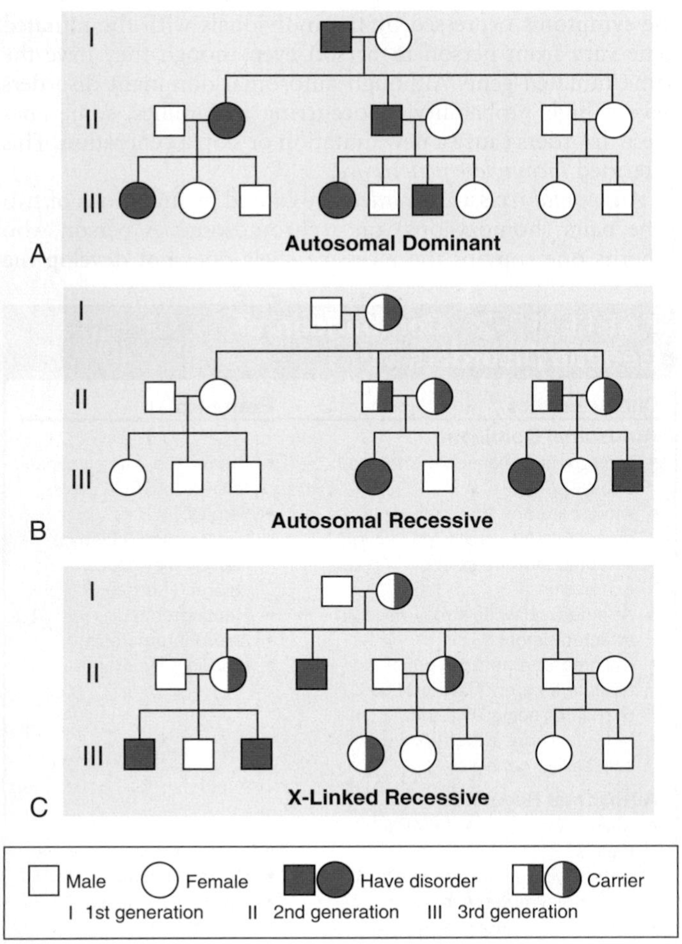


**FIG. 12-5** Family pedigrees showing three generations. **A,** Family pedigree suggestive of an autosomal dominant disorder. **B,** Family pedigree suggestive of an autosomal recessive disorder. **C,** Family pedigree suggestive of an X-linked recessive disorder.

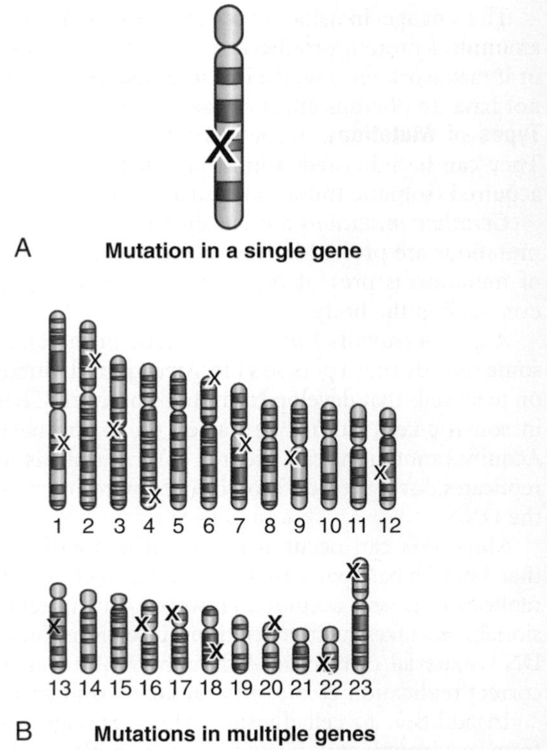


**FIG. 12-6** **A,** Genetic disorders can be caused by a mutation in a single gene (e.g., sickle cell disease, cystic fibrosis, hemophilia). **B,** Most genetic disorders are multifactorial genetic disorders caused by a combination of mutations in multiple genes, often interacting with environmental factors. Examples include cancer, diabetes mellitus, obesity, and hypertension.

disease because the normal allele predominates.[3] However, this person is a *carrier.*

*X-linked recessive disorders* are caused by a mutation on the X chromosome. Usually only men are affected by this disorder because women who carry the mutated gene on one X chromosome have another X chromosome to compensate for the mutation. However, women who carry the mutated gene can transmit it to their offspring. It is possible for women to have X-linked recessive disorders, and this can occur when an affected male mates with an unaffected female carrier. This points to the importance of testing the carrier status of the female partner of affected males. *X-linked dominant disorders* do exist, but they are rare.

*Multifactorial inherited conditions* are caused by a combination of genetic and environmental factors. These disorders run in families but do not show the same inherited characteristics as the single gene mutation conditions. Multifactorial conditions include diabetes mellitus, obesity, hypertension, cancer, and coronary artery disease.

### Human Genome Project

The Human Genome Project (HGP), which was completed in 2003, mapped the entire human genome.[4] Analysis of the data will continue for many years. The knowledge gained through the HGP will (1) help improve the diagnosis of diseases, (2) allow for earlier detection of genetic predisposition to diseases, and (3) play a critical role in determining risk assessment for genetic-related diseases. In addition, the results of the HGP assist in matching organ donors with transplant recipients.

## GENETIC DISORDERS

A *genetic disorder* is caused in whole or in part by an alteration in the DNA sequence. As discussed in the section on genetic mutations (pp. 180-181), genetic disorders can be inherited (person born with altered genetic code) or they can be acquired (e.g., replication errors, damage to DNA from toxins).[5] Genetic disorders can be caused by (1) a mutation in one gene (single gene disorder); (2) mutations in multiple genes (multifactorial inheritance disorder), which are often related to environmental factors; or (3) damage to chromosomes (changes in the number or structure of chromosomes).

### Classification of Genetic Disorders

**Single Gene Disorders.** Some genetic disorders result from a single gene mutation (Fig. 12-6, *A*). Examples of these diseases include cystic fibrosis, sickle cell disease, and polycystic kidney disease. The pattern of inheritance for single gene disorders can be autosomal dominant, autosomal recessive, or X-linked. Single gene disorders are relatively rare compared with more commonly occurring multifactorial genetic disorders such as diabetes mellitus and heart disease.

**Multifactorial Genetic Disorders.** Multifactorial genetic disorders are complex diseases that result from small inherited variations in genes, often acting together with environmental factors

(Fig. 12-6, *B*). Heart disease, diabetes, and most cancers are examples of such disorders.

Although many common diseases are usually caused by inheritance of mutations in multiple genes, such diseases can also be caused by rare hereditary mutations in a single gene. In these cases, genetic mutations that cause or strongly predispose a person to these diseases run in a family. These mutations can significantly increase each family member's risk of developing the disease. One example is breast cancer, in which inheritance of a mutated *BRCA1* or *BRCA2* gene confers significant risk of developing the disease.

***Epigenetics.*** Environmental factors can alter the way our genes are expressed (i.e., which genes are "switched" on or off). Epigenetics is the study of the chemical modification of specific genes or gene-associated proteins of an organism. Epigenetic modifications can define how the information in genes is expressed and used by cells. Genetic and environmental factors interact to influence a person's predisposition to different diseases. The expression of genes can be affected both positively and negatively by environmental factors, such as exercise, diet, chemicals, toxins, or smoking.

Identical twins, who have the same genetic makeup, do not always develop the same diseases or at the same rate. Twins share the same genes but their environments become more different as they age. This unique aspect of twins makes them an excellent model for understanding how genes and the environment contribute to certain traits, especially complex behaviors and diseases.[6]

**Chromosome Disorders.** *Chromosome disorders* are caused by structural changes within chromosomes or by an excess or deficiency of the genes that are located on chromosomes. For example, Down syndrome is caused by an extra copy of chromosome 21 (called trisomy 21), so there are three copies of this chromosome instead of two. In Down syndrome there is no individual abnormal gene on the chromosome.

Chronic myelocytic leukemia can be caused by a chromosomal translocation, in which portions of two chromosomes (chromosomes 9 and 22) are exchanged. This translocation is called the *Philadelphia chromosome*.

Throughout the book, genetic disorders are highlighted in Genetics in Clinical Practice boxes, Genetic Risk Alert boxes (in the assessment chapters), and Genetic Links content (in the management chapters).

## GENETIC TESTING

Genetic testing includes any procedure done to analyze chromosomes, genes, or any gene product that can determine whether a mutation or predisposition to a condition exists. Genetic tests have been developed for more than 2000 diseases. A person's blood, skin, hair, or saliva can be used to obtain samples for genetic testing. Tissues and cells can also be obtained prenatally.

Genetic testing has been very useful in health care (Table 12-3). Most tests assess single genes and are used to diagnose genetic disorders such as cystic fibrosis or Duchenne muscular dystrophy.[7] Some genetic tests look at rare inherited mutations of otherwise protective genes, such as *BRCA1* and *BRCA2*, which are responsible for some types of hereditary breast and ovarian cancers.[8]

The results of these tests are used in diagnosing an illness or risk for a disorder and provide the basis for appropriate treatments. Other genetic tests identify people at high risk for conditions that may be preventable. For example, monitoring for and removing polyps or the entire colon in those inheriting a gene for familial adenomatous polyposis (FAP) have saved many lives.[8] (FAP is discussed in Chapter 42 on p. 953.)

Genetic testing of individuals may raise ethical and social issues. People considering genetic testing should be aware that test results in their medical records may not be kept private. However, the Genetic Information Nondiscrimination Act (GINA) protects people from discrimination by employers and health insurance companies.

If an individual has genetic testing, it may uncover information that may also affect a family member who was not tested. These individuals are frequently not a part of the decision-making process to undergo testing. Similarly, if a whole family is tested, the results may indicate that the biologic relationship is not what the family believed it to be. Some tests are used to help guide HCPs' recommendations for treatment in consultation with the patient (e.g., *BRCA* testing). Other tests allow families to make the decision about not having children with diseases (e.g., cystic fibrosis) or identify people at high risk for conditions that may be prevented by monitoring or having prophylactic surgery (e.g., familial adenomatous polyposis [FAP]).

Currently, many genetic tests are available from testing laboratories. In most cases, insurance companies will not cover the cost of genetic testing. For more information about genetic testing, see *www.cdc.gov/genomics/gtesting/index.htm.*

### Interpreting Genetic Test Results

The results of genetic tests are not always straightforward, which often makes them challenging to interpret and explain. When interpreting test results, HCPs need to consider a person's medical history and family history and the type of genetic test that was done.

A *positive test* result means that the laboratory found a change in a particular gene, chromosome, or protein that was being tested. Depending on the purpose of the test, this result may confirm a diagnosis (e.g., Huntington's disease), indicate

**GENETICS IN CLINICAL PRACTICE**

***Genetics in Clinical Practice Boxes Throughout Book***

**TABLE 12-3 Use of Genetic Tests***

| Type of Test | Description | Examples |
|---|---|---|
| **Diagnostic testing** | • Used to diagnose, rule out, or confirm a specific genetic or chromosomal condition<br>• Used to confirm findings when patient's signs and symptoms suggest a genetic disorder<br>• Can be performed at any time during a person's life but is not available for all genes or all genetic conditions | • Cystic fibrosis<br>• Sickle cell disease<br>• Polycystic kidney disease<br>• Hemophilia<br>• Familial hypercholesterolemia |
| **Carrier screening** | • Can be used to identify unaffected individuals who carry one copy of a gene<br>• Offered to individuals who have a family history of a genetic disorder and to people in ethnic groups with an increased risk of specific genetic conditions<br>• If both parents are tested, the test can provide information about a couple's risk of having a child with a genetic condition | • Cystic fibrosis<br>• Sickle cell disease<br>• Hemophilia |
| **Preimplantation genetic diagnosis (PGD)** | • Fertilized embryos tested before implantation and pregnancy<br>• Allows embryos free of particular disorders to be placed into the uterus<br>• Embryos that test positive for genetic disorders can be destroyed | • For individuals known to have or be a carrier for a genetic mutation (e.g., Huntington's disease) |
| **Prenatal diagnostic testing** | • Fluid obtained from amniocentesis or tissue from chorionic villus used to obtain fetal cells. Can also obtain fetal samples from mother's blood<br>• Used to detect changes in genes or chromosomes of fetus before birth<br>• Type of testing offered to couples with an increased risk of having a baby with a genetic or chromosomal disorder<br>• Can decrease a couple's uncertainty or help them decide whether to terminate the pregnancy | • Down syndrome<br>• Other genetic alterations in fetuses |
| **Newborn screening** | • Most widespread use of genetic testing<br>• Early intervention to treat these disorders can eliminate or reduce symptoms that may otherwise cause a lifetime of disability | • Phenylketonuria<br>• Congenital hypothyroidism<br>• Cystic fibrosis |
| **Presymptomatic testing** | • Used to detect genetic mutations associated with disorders that appear later in life<br>• Can be helpful to people who have a family member with a genetic disorder but who have no features of the disorder themselves at the time of testing<br>• Results can provide information about a person's risk of developing a specific disorder and help with making decisions about treatment | • Huntington's disease<br>• Adult polycystic kidney disease<br>• Hemochromatosis<br>• Familial adenomatous polyposis<br>• Hereditary nonpolyposis colorectal cancer syndrome |
| **Predictive testing** | • Can identify mutations that increase a person's risk of developing disorders<br>• If results are positive, person can have prophylactic measures (e.g., mastectomy, oophorectomy) to prevent development of cancer | • Breast cancer<br>• Ovarian cancer |
| **Forensic testing** | • Done to identify an individual for legal purposes | • Identify crime or victims in catastrophic situations<br>• Rule out or implicate a crime suspect |
| **Parental testing** | • Establish biologic relationships between people | • Paternity testing |
| **Pharmacogenomic testing** | • Identifies genetic variations that influence a person's response to drugs<br>• Results provide information to help select drug therapy that is best for the person | • Warfarin (Coumadin) dose |

*The laboratory performing the tests must, by law, keep your personal information and test results confidential.

## GENETICS IN CLINICAL PRACTICE

### *Genetic Information Nondiscrimination Act (GINA)*

**What Is GINA?**

The Genetic Information Nondiscrimination Act (GINA) prohibits discrimination in health care coverage and employment based on genetic information

**Why Was GINA Needed?**

- Decreases concerns about discrimination that might prevent people from getting genetic tests
- Enables people to take part in research studies without fear that their DNA information may be used against them in the workplace or prevent them from getting health insurance

**What Is a Genetic Test?**

- An analysis of human genes (DNA, RNA), chromosomes, proteins, or metabolites that detects genotypes, mutations, or chromosomal changes

**What Is Genetic Information?**

- Any information about a person's genetic tests, family members' genetic tests, and family history of a genetic disease or disorder
- Referral of a person or family for, or use of, genetic services and participation in clinical research that involves genetic services

**What Does GINA Do?**

- Prevents health insurers from denying health insurance coverage, adjusting premiums, and discriminating against a person based solely on his or her genetic or family history information
- Prevents health insurers from requesting that a person have a genetic test
- Prohibits most employers from using genetic information for hiring, firing, or promotion decisions, and for any decisions regarding terms of employment
- GINA's health coverage nondiscrimination protection does not extend to life insurance, disability insurance, and long-term care insurance

**For more information see**

- *www.genome.gov/Pages/PolicyEthics/GeneticDiscrimination/GINAInfoDoc.pdf*
- Frequently Asked Questions about GINA at *www.dnapolicy.org/gina/faqs.html*

that a person is a carrier of a particular genetic mutation (e.g., cystic fibrosis), identify an increased risk of developing a disease (e.g., breast cancer), or suggest a need for further testing. A positive result of a predictive or presymptomatic genetic test usually cannot establish the absolute risk of developing a disorder. In addition, a positive test cannot predict the course or severity of a condition.

In some situations, it is difficult to interpret a positive result because some people who have the genetic mutation being tested never develop the disease. For example, having the *apolipoprotein E-4 (Apo E-4)* allele increases the risk of developing Alzheimer's disease. However, many people who test positive for *Apo E-4* never develop Alzheimer's disease (see Chapter 59).

A *negative test* result means that the laboratory did not find an altered form of the gene, chromosome, or protein under consideration. This result can indicate that a person is not affected by a particular disorder, is not a carrier of a specific genetic mutation, or does not have an increased risk of developing a certain disease. However, it is possible that the test missed a disease-causing genetic alteration, since many tests cannot detect all the genetic changes that cause a particular disorder. Further testing may be required to confirm a negative result.

### Direct-to-Consumer Genetic Tests

Direct-to-consumer genetic tests (at-home testing) are marketed directly to people (consumers) via television, print advertisements, or the Internet. The test kit is mailed to the person instead of being ordered through an HCP's office. The test typically involves collecting a DNA sample at home, often by swabbing the inside of the cheek, and mailing the sample back to the laboratory. In some cases, the person must visit a health clinic to have blood drawn.

Consumers are notified of their results by mail or over the telephone, or the results are posted online. In some cases a genetic counselor or other HCP is available to explain the results and answer questions. The cost of genetic testing can range from under $100 to more than $2,000, depending on the nature and complexity of the test. The cost increases if more than one test is necessary or if multiple family members must be tested to obtain a meaningful result.

Direct-to-consumer genetic tests have significant risks and limitations. People may want their genetic information, but they may not understand what it means. Consumers are vulnerable to being misled by the results of unproven or invalid tests. Without guidance from an HCP, they may make important decisions about disease treatment or prevention based on inaccurate, incomplete, or misunderstood information about their health. Consumers may also experience an invasion of genetic privacy if testing companies use their genetic information in an unauthorized way.

If your patients are considering using these kinds of genetic tests, let them know that they first need to discuss the issue with their HCP or a genetic counselor. Patient teaching related to genetic testing is presented in Table 12-4.

### ETHICAL/LEGAL DILEMMAS
#### *Genetic Testing*

**Situation**

A 30-year-old woman informs you that she is 3 months pregnant. She has two children with her current husband. This pregnancy was unplanned, and her youngest child has cystic fibrosis (CF). She expresses concern regarding the possibility of having another child with CF. She mentions that she would like to have genetic testing on her fetus. Her husband asks you what the likelihood is of having another child with CF.

**Ethical/Legal Points for Consideration**

- With genetic testing, the patient and her family can find out whether their child will have CF. The woman and her husband can then make an informed decision.
- Genetic counseling is recommended before and after obtaining genetic testing because of the complexity of the information and the emotional issues involved with implications and options.
- Knowing that CF is an autosomal recessive condition, you can use Punnett squares (Fig. 12-9) or a family pedigree (Figs. 12-4 and 12-5) to show the woman and her husband the probability of having another child with CF.
- Be mindful of the privacy and confidentiality of genetic information and the potential conflict between one person's right to privacy and another person's right to information.

**Discussion Questions**

1. What information would you give the patient and her husband regarding genetic testing in order for them to make an informed decision?
2. What options are available for this couple?
3. How would you assist this couple as they are considering terminating the pregnancy if the results of the genetic testing reveal that the fetus will have CF?

### TABLE 12-4 Patient & Family Teaching
#### *Genetic Testing*

**Genetic Counselors**

- Individuals who are considering genetic testing should meet with a genetic counselor who is specially trained in medical genetics and counseling.
- Counseling is advised to help you understand the purpose of genetic testing, considerations before testing, and the emotional and medical impact of the test results.
- Genetic counseling can help you understand the pros and cons of genetic testing before making a decision to undergo a genetic test.

**General Information**

*The following includes some important general information about genetic testing.*

- Genetic testing can be expensive and may not be included in your medical insurance policy.
- Genetic testing may determine whether you are predisposed to developing an inherited disease.
- A particular genetic test will only tell you whether there is a specific genetic variant or mutation. Positive tests do not mean you will develop that disease or disorder. Neither can the results tell you when you will develop the disease.
- If a genetic test demonstrates a genetic predisposition to an inherited disorder, the news can be depressing.
- Knowledge of a genetic predisposition to a disease may give you the motivation to take preventive measures (e.g., taking drugs for familial hypercholesterolemia) or make lifestyle changes to lower the risk of a disease (e.g., exercising to decrease the risk of type 2 diabetes).
- If a genetic test reveals a strongly negative result, you probably will not develop that disease.
- If a genetic test reveals you are at risk for a specific genetic disorder, there is the possibility that other family members may also be at risk.
- If a genetic test reveals you are at risk for developing an inherited disease, whether you decide to share that information with family members is a personal and an ethical decision that you will have to make.
- Genetic testing may provide important information that you can use when making decisions about having children.

### Genetic Technology

**DNA Fingerprinting.** DNA (genetic) fingerprinting begins by extracting DNA from the cells in a sample of blood, saliva, semen, or other appropriate fluid or tissue. *Polymerase chain reaction (PCR)* is a quick, easy method to provide unlimited copies of a DNA or RNA sequence using only a small amount of sample. PCR involves the artificial replication of a DNA or RNA sequence. The DNA or RNA strands can be separated to form new templates that are used for replication.

PCR is a key element in *genetic fingerprinting.* It is an essential technique to finding mutations in genes. It is also used extensively in forensic medicine to identify DNA of criminal suspects by using samples from blood, hair, saliva, and semen. PCR has also been used in paternity testing and finding evidence to free wrongly incarcerated prisoners. PCR can also be used as a confirmatory test in HIV testing. This is especially important when an infant of a mother who is HIV-antibody positive also tests HIV positive. In this situation, it is not known whether the antibodies from the infant's blood are from the baby or the mother. PCR techniques can be used on the baby's lymphocytes to determine whether the baby is infected with HIV.

**DNA Microarray (DNA Chip).** Although all of a person's somatic cells contain identical genetic material, the same genes are not active in every cell. Studying which genes are active and which are inactive in different cell types helps to understand (1) how these cells function normally and (2) how they are affected when various genes do not perform properly.

Gene expression profiling uses a technology called *DNA microarrays* (DNA chips). This technology is used to measure the expression levels of large numbers of genes simultaneously or to genotype multiple regions of a genome. The chips are laid out by robots that can position DNA fragments so precisely that more than 20,000 of them can fit on one microscope slide.

Then fluorescent-tagged molecules are washed over the DNA fragments. Some molecules (with green fluorescent tags) bind to their complementary sequence. These molecules can be identified because they glow under fluorescent light when scanned using automated equipment. Complete patterns of gene activity can be captured with this technology.

### Genome-Wide Association Study (GWAS)

*Genome-wide association study (GWAS)* is an approach that involves rapidly scanning complete sets of DNA, or genomes, of many individuals to find genetic variations associated with the development or progression of a particular disease.

Until recently, researchers looked at single genes and the proteins that they encode. With GWAS, researchers study large numbers of genes and proteins, including how they act and interact. This provides a more complete picture of what goes on in a person. After the genetic associations are identified, researchers may be able to learn how to stop or jump-start genes on demand, change the course of a disease, or prevent it from ever happening. GWAS is particularly useful in finding genetic variations that contribute to multifactorial inherited disorders such as asthma, cancer, diabetes, and heart disease.

To carry out a GWAS, researchers use two groups of participants: people with the disease being studied and similar people without the disease. Each person's complete set of DNA, or genome, is then purified from the blood or cells, placed on tiny chips, and scanned on automated laboratory machines. The machines quickly survey each participant's genome for strategically selected markers of genetic variation.

If certain genetic variations are found to be significantly more common in people with the disease compared to people without the disease, the variations are said to be "associated" with the disease. The associated genetic variations can serve as powerful pointers to the region of the human genome where the disease-causing problem resides.

The potential impact of GWAS is substantial, since it lays the groundwork for personalized medicine, in which the current one-size-fits-all approach to health care gives way to more customized strategies. Tools such as GWAS can provide patients with individualized information about their risks of developing certain diseases. The information will help health care professionals tailor prevention programs to each person's unique genetic makeup.

## PHARMACOGENOMICS AND PHARMACOGENETICS

Patients vary widely in their response to drugs. Although the reasons for this are complex, genetic factors may account for a large percentage of patient variability in response to individual drugs. **Pharmacogenomics** is the study of genomic variation associated with drug responses.

Pharmacogenomics examines the entire genome and allows for the identification of variations in multiple genes affecting the drug response. **Pharmacogenetics** is the study of genetic variability of drug responses related to variations in single genes.

These two terms are frequently used interchangeably in describing the relationship between pharmacology and genetic variability in determining an individual's response to drugs. However, pharmacogenetics has a much narrower focus.[9]

Pharmacogenetic and pharmacogenomic studies can potentially lead to drugs that can be tailor-made or adapted to each person's particular genetic makeup. This makes it possible to have personalized medicine by choosing the right drug and the right dose for the right person.[9,10] Table 12-5 has examples of pharmacogenetics.

One important area of study has been focused on the cytochrome P450 (CYP450) family of major enzymes, which are important in drug metabolism. Alterations in the *CYP450* gene can affect how the liver breaks down certain drugs, such as warfarin (Coumadin). People with a less active form of the enzyme (who metabolize the drug slowly) may get too much of the drug, whereas people with a more active form of the enzyme (who metabolize the drug quickly) may get too little of the drug. Too much warfarin can lead to internal bleeding, whereas too little warfarin may still allow blood clots to form. Pharmacogenomic testing can assist HCPs in prescribing the right amount of a medicine based on a patient's particular genetic makeup (Fig. 12-7).

Currently a genetic test for identifying *CYP450* polymorphisms is available. In addition to maximizing the safety and effectiveness of drugs, this type of genetic testing can lead to individualized drug therapy.

HCPs are starting to use pharmacogenomic information to prescribe drugs, but at this time such tests are routine for only a few diseases or disorders (examples are presented in Table 12-5). However, given the field's rapid growth, pharmacogenomics may soon lead to personalized medicine and individualized drug therapy to manage heart disease, cancer, asthma, depression, and many other common diseases.

**TABLE 12-5 Examples of Pharmacogenetics**

| Drug | Role of Pharmacogenetics |
|---|---|
| **trastuzumab (Herceptin)** | • In breast cancer, drug only works for women whose tumors have genes that lead to the overproduction of a protein called HER-2.<br>• Drug is a monoclonal antibody to HER-2. After the antibody attaches to the antigen, it kills the cells.<br>• Genetic testing provides information on which patients are good candidates for treatment with drug.<br>• Drug does not work for patients whose tumor genes do not express HER-2. |
| **crizotinib (Xalkori)** | • Drug used to treat patients with late-stage (locally advanced or metastatic), non–small cell lung cancers (NSCLC) who express the abnormal anaplastic lymphoma kinase *(ALK)* gene.<br>• *ALK* gene abnormality causes cancer development and growth.<br>• Crizotinib works by blocking certain proteins called *kinases,* including the protein produced by the abnormal *ALK* gene.<br>• Drug was approved for use with a companion genetic diagnostic test that determines whether a patient with NSCLC has the abnormal *ALK* gene. |
| **vemurafenib (Zelboraf)** | • Approved for patients with late-stage (metastatic) or unresectable melanoma.<br>• Indicated for the treatment of patients with melanoma whose tumors express a gene mutation called *BRAF V600E.*<br>• To be considered for treatment, patients must first have genetic testing to determine whether melanoma cells have the *BRAF V600E* mutation. |
| **warfarin (Coumadin)** (Fig. 12-7) | • Genetic variants in the genes *VKORC1* and cytochrome P450 2C9 *(CYP2C9)* have a significant impact on people's sensitivity to warfarin (Fig. 12-7)<br>• Individuals with particular variations in these genes require a lower warfarin dose to maintain therapeutic levels of anticoagulation.<br>• Individuals with other variations require higher doses.<br>• Together these genetic variations explain about 50% of the required dose difference between individuals.<br>• Testing for patient's *CYP2C9* and *VKORC1* genotype information can assist in selecting the starting dose. |
| **abacavir (Ziagen)** | • Some people are at greater risk for serious allergic reactions when first starting treatment with this drug.<br>• Genetic testing for *HLA-B*5701* before taking the drug can identify people who carry a genetic marker that is associated with life-threatening hypersensitivity reactions. |
| **clopidogrel (Plavix)** | • For clopidogrel to work, cytochrome P450 enzymes in the liver (particularly CYP2C19) must convert the drug to its active form.<br>• About 2% to 14% of the population are poor metabolizers of the drug, and these patients may not receive the full benefits of the drug.<br>• Genetic tests are available to identify genetic differences in CYP2C19 function. |

## GENE THERAPY

Gene therapy is an experimental technique that uses genes to treat or prevent disease. Gene therapy is an approach to treating potentially lethal and disabling diseases that are caused by single gene deficiencies. With specialized techniques, gene expression can be manipulated to correct the problem in the particular patient, although the correction will not be passed along to offspring of that person. Approaches to gene therapy include the following:[11]

- Replacing a mutated gene that causes disease with a healthy copy of the gene
- Inactivating, or "knocking out," a mutated gene that is functioning improperly
- Introducing a new gene into the body to help fight a disease

A gene that is inserted directly into a cell usually does not function. A carrier molecule called a *vector* must be used to deliver the therapeutic gene to the patient's target cells. Currently, the most common vector is a virus that has been genetically altered to carry normal human DNA. The vector can be injected or given IV directly into specific tissue. The vector unloads its genetic material containing the therapeutic human gene into the target cell. If the treatment is successful, the new gene will make a functional protein and restore the target cell to a normal state. A diagram of gene therapy is depicted in Fig. 12-8.

Although gene therapy is a promising treatment option for a number of diseases (including inherited disorders, some types of cancer, and certain viral infections), the technique remains risky and is still under study to make sure that it will be safe and effective. Gene therapy is currently only being tested for the treatment of diseases that have no other cure.[11]

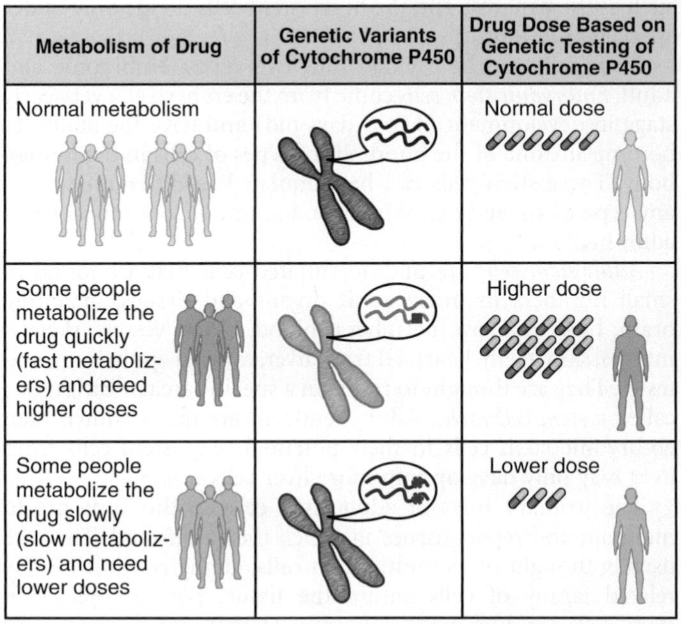


**FIG. 12-7** Individuals respond differently to the drug warfarin (Coumadin). The diversity of responses is partially due to genetic variants in one of the cytochrome *P450* genes.

## STEM CELL THERAPY

Stem cells are the subject of much discussion because they may offer treatment for many diseases. The use of stem cells may allow for the regeneration of lost tissue and restoration of function in various diseases.

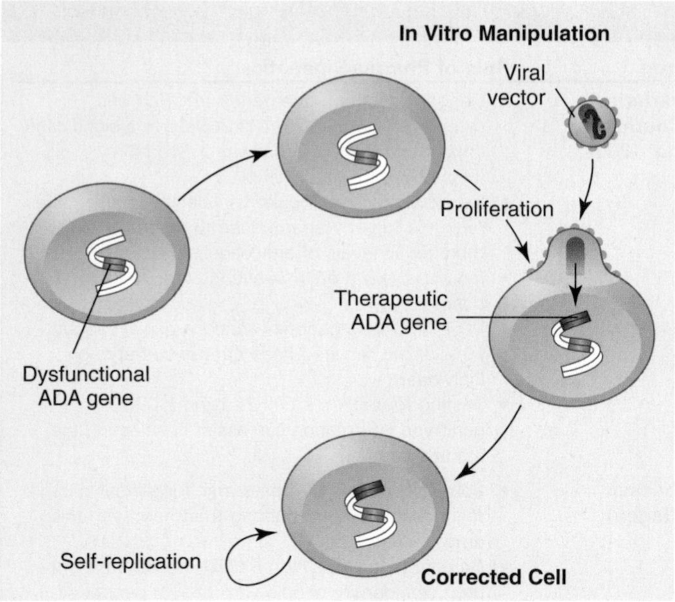


**FIG. 12-8** Gene therapy for adenosine deaminase *(ADA)* deficiency attempts to correct this immunodeficiency state. The viral vector containing the therapeutic ADA gene is inserted into the patient's lymphocytes. These cells can then make the ADA enzyme.

*Stem cells* are unspecialized cells in the body that have the ability to (1) remain in their unspecialized state and divide or (2) differentiate and develop into specialized cells such as a brain cell or a muscle cell. In some body organs such as the gastrointestinal (GI) tract and bone marrow, stem cells divide to repair and replace damaged or old tissues. In other organs such as the pancreas and the heart, stem cells divide only under special conditions.

Stem cells can be divided into two types: embryonic and adult. *Embryonic stem cells* come from the embryo at a very early stage in development (4 to 5 days old) and have the ability to become any one of the hundreds of types of cells in the human body. These stem cells can be stimulated to differentiate into any type of tissue (e.g., skin, liver, kidney, blood) found in an adult human.

*Adult stem cells* are undifferentiated cells that are found in small numbers in many adult organs and tissues, including brain, bone marrow, peripheral blood, blood vessels, skeletal muscle, skin, teeth, heart, GI tract, liver, ovarian epithelium, and testes. They are thought to reside in a specific area of each tissue called a *stem cell niche.* Adult stem cells are more limited than embryonic stem cells in their potential (e.g., stem cells from liver may only develop into more liver cells).

The primary roles of adult stem cells in the body are to maintain and repair tissues in which they are found. They are usually thought of as multipotent cells, giving rise to a closely related family of cells within the tissue. For example, skin stem cells produce new skin cells. Hematopoietic stem cells found within the bone marrow are capable of forming all of the various blood cells. These cells are prolific by design and are already being used for bone marrow transplants (see Chapter 15).

Medical researchers are investigating the use of stem cells to repair or replace damaged body tissues, similar to whole organ transplants. Currently not enough donated organs are available to meet the demand for transplants. In organ transplants, when tissues from a donor are placed into a patient's body, the patient's immune system may react and reject the donated tissue as "foreign." However, using stem cells presents less risk of this immune rejection, and the therapy may be more successful.

In addition, stem cells could be directed to differentiate into specific cell types. They would then become a renewable source of replacement cells and tissues to treat conditions such as Alzheimer's disease, spinal cord injury, stroke, burns, heart disease, diabetes, osteoarthritis, and rheumatoid arthritis. It may become possible to generate healthy heart muscle cells in the laboratory and then transplant those cells into patients with chronic heart disease. Whether these cells can generate heart muscle cells or stimulate the growth of new blood vessels is under investigation.[12]

## ❖ NURSING MANAGEMENT: GENETICS AND GENOMICS

You must be knowledgeable about the fundamentals of genetics and genomics.[13,14] By understanding the profound influence that genetics has on health and illness, you can assist the patient and family in making critical decisions related to genetic issues, such as genetic testing. You also must collaborate with the health care team to involve a genetic nurse or a genetic counselor.

A genetic nurse is a licensed professional nurse with special education and training in genetics. Nurses with *GCN* after their names are baccalaureate-prepared licensed registered nurses who have received specialty credentialing as a Genetic Clinical Nurse (GCN). Nurses with *APNG* after their names are licensed registered nurses with a master's degree who have received specialty credentialing as an Advanced Practice Nurse in Genetics (APNG).

As a basic professional nurse, you should be an advocate for patients and families by facilitating access to genetics resources. In addition, you must provide or reinforce accurate information pertaining to genetics or a genetic disease or concern. This information should be tailored to the patient based on culture, religion, knowledge level, literacy, and preferred language.[15]

You can identify and assess inheritance patterns and explain them to the patient and family through the use of family pedigrees (see Figs. 12-4 and 12-5) and Punnett squares (Fig. 12-9). Maintain the patient's confidentiality and respect the patient's values and beliefs because genetic information may have major health and social implications.

Genetic testing may raise many psychologic and emotional issues. Knowledge of carrier status of a genetic disorder may influence a person's decisions for a career, marriage, and childbearing. It may also affect significant others in grappling with serious life and health care issues. For example, how should a wife deal with a husband who has tested positive for Huntington's disease and shows early signs of cognitive impairment but does not yet show any other neurologic manifestations of the disease? Should their children be tested for the disease? A 43-year-old woman who has a family history of breast cancer and is now diagnosed with breast cancer wants to know if she and her two teenage daughters should have *BRCA* testing. What do you tell her?

Furthermore, there are ethical concerns. Who should know the results of a genetic test? Who should protect the privacy of individuals' test results and prevent individuals from possible

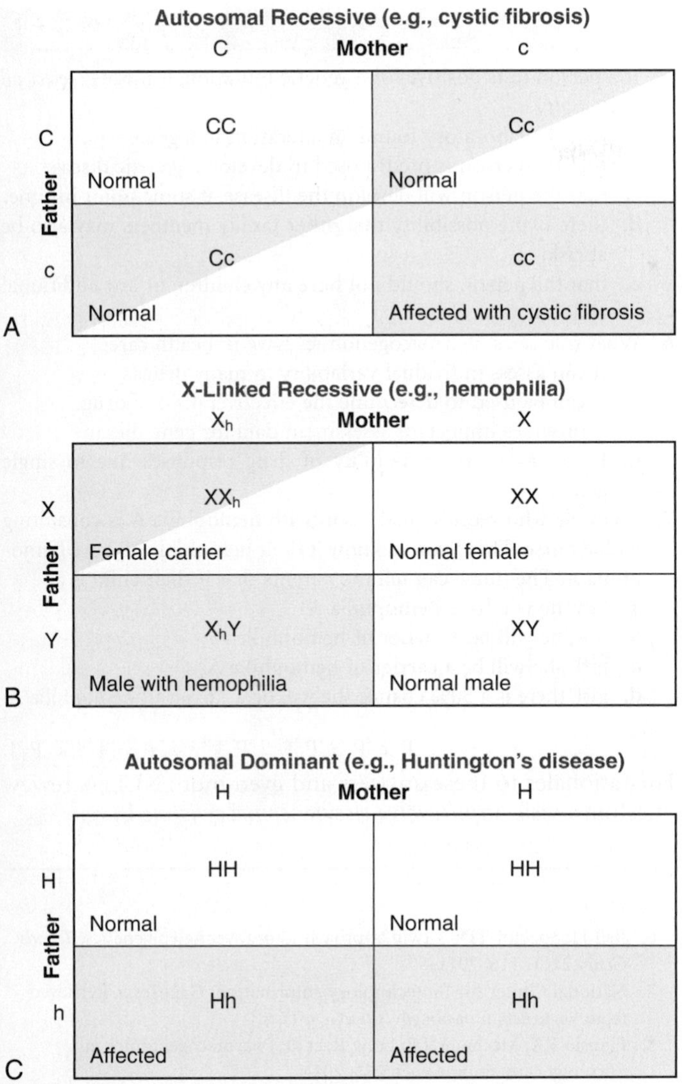


**FIG. 12-9** Punnett squares illustrate inheritance possibilities. **A,** If the mother and father are both carriers for cystic fibrosis, there is a 25% chance that offspring will have cystic fibrosis. **B,** If the mother is a carrier for the hemophilia gene and the father has a normal genotype, there is a 50% chance that any male offspring will have hemophilia. There is a 50% chance that any female offspring will be a carrier. **C,** If the mother has a normal genotype and the father has Huntington's disease, there is a 50% chance that offspring will have the disease.

discrimination? Genetic information should not be misused to label individuals or particular ethnic groups. Close attention must be paid to better understand the psychosocial needs of individuals and societal responses and health care policy related to genetic testing.

People may be reluctant to share or disclose information about family history or genetic test results. They fear they are vulnerable to discrimination based on their DNA. Inform your patients about the Genetic Information Nondiscrimination Act (GINA), which protects them from discrimination by employers and health care insurance companies (see Genetics in Clinical Practice Box on p. 184).

## ◆ Nursing Assessment: Family History

Family history is one of the strongest influences on a person's risk of developing genetic-related disorders such as heart disease, stroke, diabetes, or cancer. The family history is a free genetic test. Even though a person cannot change his or her genetic makeup, knowing the family history can help in the prevention or early diagnosis and treatment of a disorder. For example, it is important to monitor cholesterol levels in a person with a family history of familial hypercholesterolemia.

The key features of a family history that may increase a person's risk for genetic-related diseases are

- Disease in more than one close relative
- Disease that does not usually affect a certain gender (e.g., breast cancer in a male)
- Diseases that occur at an earlier age than expected (e.g., myocardial infarction before age 35)
- Certain combinations of diseases within a family (e.g., breast and ovarian cancer, heart disease and diabetes)

If a family has one or more of these features, the family history may hold important clues about a person's risk for a genetic disease. People with a family history of disease may have the most to gain from lifestyle changes and screening tests. People cannot change their genes, but they can change unhealthy behaviors (e.g., smoking, poor eating habits). They can also get screening tests to detect diseases and disease risk factors (e.g., elevated cholesterol, hypertension) that can be treated.

Genetic Risk Alert boxes in the assessment chapters in this book highlight a patient's risks related to genetic diseases and disorders. Use the information in these boxes when obtaining a nursing history.

Family health history is a written or graphic record of the diseases and health conditions present in one's family (see Chapter 3). A useful family health history shows three generations of a person's biologic relatives, the age of diagnosis of a disease, and the age and cause of death of deceased family members. A family health history is a useful tool for understanding health risks and preventing disease in individuals and their close relatives.

Talk with your own family members about your family's health history. Record this information and update it periodically so that you and your family members will have organized and accurate information ready to share with your HCP. Family health history information may help HCPs determine which tests and screenings are recommended to help you and your family know your health risk.

To help individuals collect and organize their family history information, the Centers for Disease Control and Prevention (CDC) has collaborated with the U.S. Surgeon General and other federal agencies to develop a Web-based tool called *My Family Health Portrait (https://familyhistory.hhs.gov/fhh-web/home.action).*

## BRIDGE TO NCLEX EXAMINATION

The number of the question corresponds to the same-numbered outcome at the beginning of the chapter.

1. If a person is heterozygous for a given gene, it means that the person
   - **a.** is a carrier for a genetic disorder.
   - **b.** is affected by the genetic disorder.
   - **c.** has two identical alleles for the gene.
   - **d.** has two different alleles for the gene.
2. Common causes of genetic mutations include *(select all that apply)*
   - **a.** DNA damage from toxins.
   - **b.** DNA damage from UV radiation.
   - **c.** inheritance of altered genes from father.
   - **d.** inheritance of altered genes from mother.
   - **e.** inheritance of somatic mutations from either parent.
3. A father who has an X-linked recessive disorder and a wife with a normal genotype will
   - **a.** pass the carrier state to his male children.
   - **b.** pass the carrier state to all of his children.
   - **c.** pass the carrier state to his female children.
   - **d.** not pass on the genetic mutation to any of his children.
4. What characterizes multifactorial genetic disorders?
   - **a.** Genetic testing available for most disorders
   - **b.** Commonly caused by single gene alterations
   - **c.** Many family members report having the disorder
   - **d.** Caused by complex interactions of genetic and environmental factors
5. If a person tests positive for a genetic mutation, it means *(select all that apply)*
   - **a.** that the laboratory found an alteration in a gene.
   - **b.** that the person is predisposed to develop a genetic disease.
   - **c.** that the person will develop the disease at some point in time.
   - **d.** there is the possibility that other family members may also be at risk.
   - **e.** that the person should not have any children or any additional children.
6. What role does pharmacogenomics have in health care?
   - **a.** It can assess individual variability to many drugs.
   - **b.** It can be used to determine the effectiveness of a drug.
   - **c.** It provides important assessment data for gene therapy.
   - **d.** It can assess the variability of drug responses due to single genes.
7. A couple who recently had a son with hemophilia A is consulting with a nurse. They want to know if their next child will have hemophilia A. The nurse can tell the parents that if their child is a
   - **a.** boy, he will have hemophilia A.
   - **b.** boy, he will be a carrier of hemophilia A.
   - **c.** girl, she will be a carrier of hemophilia A.
   - **d.** girl, there is a 50% chance she will be a carrier of hemophilia A.

1. d, 2. a, b, c, d, 3. c, 4. d, 5. a, d, 6. b, 7. d

For rationales to these answers and even more NCLEX review questions, visit *http://evolve.elsevier.com/Lewis/medsurg.*

## EVOLVE WEBSITE

http://evolve.elsevier.com/Lewis/medsurg

**Review Questions (Online Only)**

**Key Points**

**Answer Key for Questions**

- Rationales for Bridge to NCLEX Examination Questions

**Conceptual Care Map Creator**

**Audio Glossary**

**Content Updates**

## REFERENCES


1. US Department of Health and Human Services: Genomics. Retrieved from *www.healthypeople.gov.*
2. The New Genetics, National Institute of General Medical Sciences, National Institutes of Health, US Department of Health and Human Services. Retrieved from *http://publications.nigms.nih.gov/thenewgenetics.*
3. Nakano S, Tluczek A: Genomic breakthroughs in the diagnosis and treatment of cystic fibrosis, *AJN* 114:36, 2014.
4. US Department of Energy: Human Genome Project information. Retrieved from *www.ornl.gov.*
5. Genes and diseases. Retrieved from *www.ncbi.nlm.nih.gov/books/NBK22183.*
6. Bell JT, Spector TD: A twin approach to unraveling epigenetics, *Trends Genet* 27(3):116, 2011.
7. National Center for Biotechnology Information: GeneTests. Retrieved from *www.ncbi.nlm.nih.gov/sites/GeneTests.*
8. Filipski KK, Mechanic LE, Long R, et al: Pharmacogenomics in oncology care, *Front Genet* 5:73, 2014.

*9. Knisely MR, Carpenter JS, Von Ah D: Pharmacogenonics in the nursing literature: an integrative review, *Nursing Outlook* 62(4):285, 2014.

10. Cheek DJ: What you need to know about pharmacogenomics, *Nursing* 43:44, 2013.
11. Gene therapy. Retrieved from *http://ghr.nlm.nih.gov/handbook/therapy/genetherapy.*
12. National Institutes of Health: Stem cell basics. Retrieved from *stemcells.nih.gov.*
13. Genetic Science Learning Center, University of Utah: Learning genetics. Retrieved from *http://learn.genetics.utah.edu.*
14. *Journal of Nursing Scholarship* Genomics Webinar Series (2013). Retrieved from *www.genome.gov/27552312#al-2.*

*15. International Society of Nurses in Genetics: *Position statements: genetic counseling for vulnerable populations: the role of nursing.* Retrieved from *www.isong.org.*

*Evidence-based information for clinical practice.

13

# Altered Immune Responses and Transplantation

*Sharon L. Lewis*

*Happiness is not something readymade. It comes from your own actions.*

*Dalai Lama*

http://evolve.elsevier.com/Lewis/medsurg/

## LEARNING OUTCOMES

1. Describe the functions and components of the immune system.
2. Compare and contrast humoral and cell-mediated immunity, including lymphocytes involved, types of reactions, and effects on antigens.
3. Characterize the five types of immunoglobulins.
4. Differentiate among the four types of hypersensitivity reactions in terms of immunologic mechanisms and resulting alterations.
5. Identify the clinical manifestations and emergency management of a systemic anaphylactic reaction.
6. Describe the assessment and interprofessional care of a patient with chronic allergies.
7. Explain the relationship between the human leukocyte antigen system and certain diseases.
8. Describe the etiologic factors, clinical manifestations, and treatment modalities of autoimmune diseases.
9. Describe the etiologic factors and categories of immunodeficiency disorders.
10. Differentiate among the types of rejections following transplantation.
11. Identify the types and side effects of immunosuppressive therapy.

## KEY TERMS

**anergy**, p. 196
**antigen**, p. 191
**autoimmunity**, p. 204
**cell-mediated immunity**, p. 196
**cytokines**, p. 194
**human leukocyte antigen (HLA)**, p. 206
**humoral immunity**, p. 195
**hypersensitivity reactions**, p. 197
**immunocompetence**, p. 196
**immunodeficiency**, p. 205
**immunosuppressive therapy**, p. 209

This chapter discusses the normal immune response and the altered immune responses of hypersensitivity (including allergies), autoimmunity, and immunodeficiency. Histocompatibility, organ transplantation, and immunosuppressive therapy are also presented.

## NORMAL IMMUNE RESPONSE

*Immunity* is the body's ability to resist disease. Immune responses serve the following three functions:

1. *Defense:* The body protects against invasions by microorganisms and prevents the development of infection by attacking foreign antigens and pathogens.
2. *Homeostasis:* Damaged cellular substances are digested and removed. Through this mechanism, the body's different cell types remain uniform and unchanged.
3. *Surveillance:* Mutations continually arise in the body but are normally recognized as foreign cells and destroyed.

### Antigens

An **antigen** is a substance that elicits an immune response. Most antigens are composed of protein. However, other substances such as large polysaccharides, lipoproteins, and nucleic acids can act as antigens. All of the body's cells have antigens on their surface that are unique to that person and enable the body to recognize itself. The immune system normally becomes "tolerant" to the body's own molecules. Therefore it is nonresponsive to "self" antigens.

### Types of Immunity

Immunity is classified as innate or acquired.

**Innate Immunity.** *Innate immunity* is present at birth, and its primary role is first-line defense against pathogens. This type of immunity involves a nonspecific response, and neutrophils and monocytes are the primary white blood cells (WBCs) involved. Innate immunity is not antigen specific, so it can respond within minutes to an invading microorganism without prior exposure to that organism.

Reviewed by Kelly S. Grimshaw, RN, MSN, APRN, CCRN, CCTN, Acute Care Nurse Practitioner, Transplant Department, Yale New Haven Hospital, New Haven, Connecticut; and Allison J. Terry, RN, PhD, Associate Professor of Nursing, Assistant Dean of Clinical Practice, School of Nursing, Auburn University Montgomery, Montgomery, Alabama.

TABLE 13-1 **Types of Acquired Specific Immunity**

| Type | Natural | Artificial |
|---|---|---|
| **Active** | Natural contact with antigen through actual infection (e.g., chickenpox, measles, mumps) | Immunization with antigen (e.g., vaccines for chickenpox, measles, mumps) |
| **Passive** | Transplacental and colostrum transfer from mother to child (e.g., maternal immunoglobulins passed to baby) | Injection of serum with antibodies from one person (e.g., injection of hepatitis B immune globulin) to another person who does not have antibodies |

**Acquired Immunity.** *Acquired immunity* is the development of immunity, either actively or passively (Table 13-1).

***Active Acquired Immunity.*** *Active acquired immunity* results from the invasion of the body by foreign substances such as microorganisms and subsequent development of antibodies and sensitized lymphocytes. With each reinvasion of the microorganisms, the body responds more rapidly and vigorously to fight off the invader. Active acquired immunity may result naturally from a disease or artificially through immunization. Because antibodies are synthesized, immunity takes time to develop but is long lasting.

***Passive Acquired Immunity.*** *Passive acquired immunity* implies that the host receives antibodies to an antigen rather than synthesizing them. This may take place naturally through the transfer of immunoglobulins across the placental membrane from mother to fetus. Artificial passive acquired immunity occurs through injection with gamma globulin (serum antibodies). The benefit of this immunity is its immediate effect. Unfortunately, passive immunity is short lived because the person does not synthesize the antibodies and consequently does not retain memory cells for the antigen.

## Lymphoid Organs

The lymphoid system is composed of central (or primary) and peripheral lymphoid organs. The *central lymphoid organs* are the thymus gland and bone marrow. The *peripheral lymphoid organs* are the lymph nodes; tonsils; spleen; and gut-, genital-, bronchial-, and skin-associated lymphoid tissues (Fig. 13-1).

Lymphocytes are produced in the bone marrow and eventually migrate to the peripheral organs. The thymus is involved in the differentiation and maturation of T lymphocytes and is therefore essential for a cell-mediated immune response. During childhood the thymus is large. It shrinks with age, and in the older person the thymus is a collection of lymphocytes and connective tissue.

When antigens are introduced into the body, they may be carried by the bloodstream or lymph channels to regional lymph nodes. The antigens interact with B and T lymphocytes and macrophages in the lymph nodes. The two important functions of lymph nodes are (1) filtration of foreign material brought to the site and (2) circulation of lymphocytes.

The tonsils are an example of lymphoid tissue. The spleen, a peripheral lymph organ, is important as the primary site for filtering foreign antigens from the blood. Lymphoid tissue is found in the submucosa of the gastrointestinal (GI) (gut-associated), genitourinary (genital-associated), and respiratory (bronchial-associated) tracts. This tissue protects the body from external microorganisms.

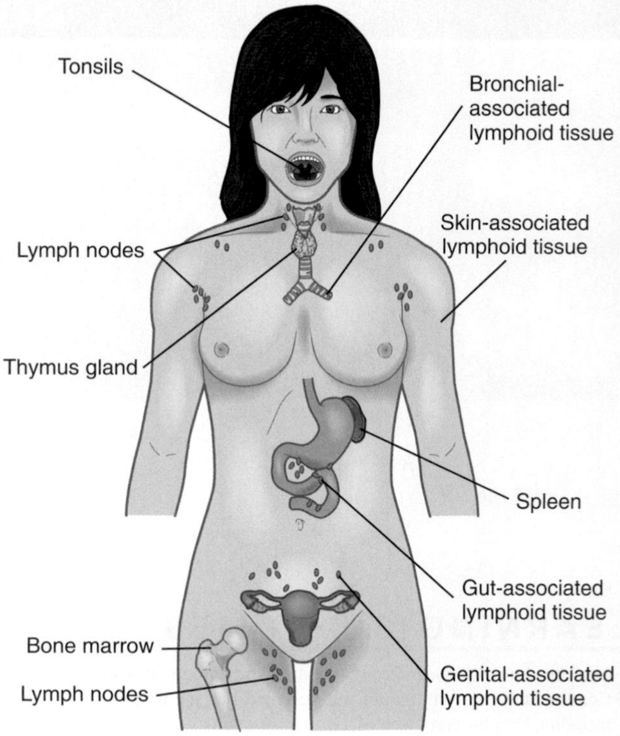

**FIG. 13-1** Organs of the immune system.

The skin-associated lymph tissue consists primarily of lymphocytes and Langerhans' cells (type of dendritic cell) found in the epidermis of skin. When Langerhans' cells are depleted, the skin cannot initiate an immune response. Therefore a delayed hypersensitivity reaction (as determined by skin testing with injected antigens) does not occur.

## Cells Involved in Immune Response

**Mononuclear Phagocytes.** The *mononuclear phagocyte system* includes monocytes in the blood and macrophages found throughout the body. Mononuclear phagocytes have a critical role in the immune system. They are responsible for capturing, processing, and presenting the antigen to the lymphocytes. This stimulates a humoral or cell-mediated immune response. Capturing is accomplished through phagocytosis. The macrophage-bound antigen, which is highly immunogenic, is presented to circulating T or B lymphocytes and thus triggers an immune response (Fig. 13-2).

**Lymphocytes.** Lymphocytes are produced in the bone marrow (Fig. 13-3). They then differentiate into B and T lymphocytes.

***B Lymphocytes.*** In the early research on *B lymphocytes* (bursa-equivalent lymphocytes) in birds, it was discovered that they mature under the influence of the bursa of Fabricius, hence the name *B cells.* However, this lymphoid organ does not exist in humans. The bursa-equivalent tissue in humans is the bone marrow. B cells differentiate into *plasma cells* when activated. Plasma cells produce antibodies (immunoglobulins) (Table 13-2).

***T Lymphocytes.*** Cells that migrate from the bone marrow to the thymus differentiate into *T lymphocytes* (thymus-dependent cells). The thymus secretes hormones, including thymosin, that stimulate the maturation and differentiation of T lymphocytes.

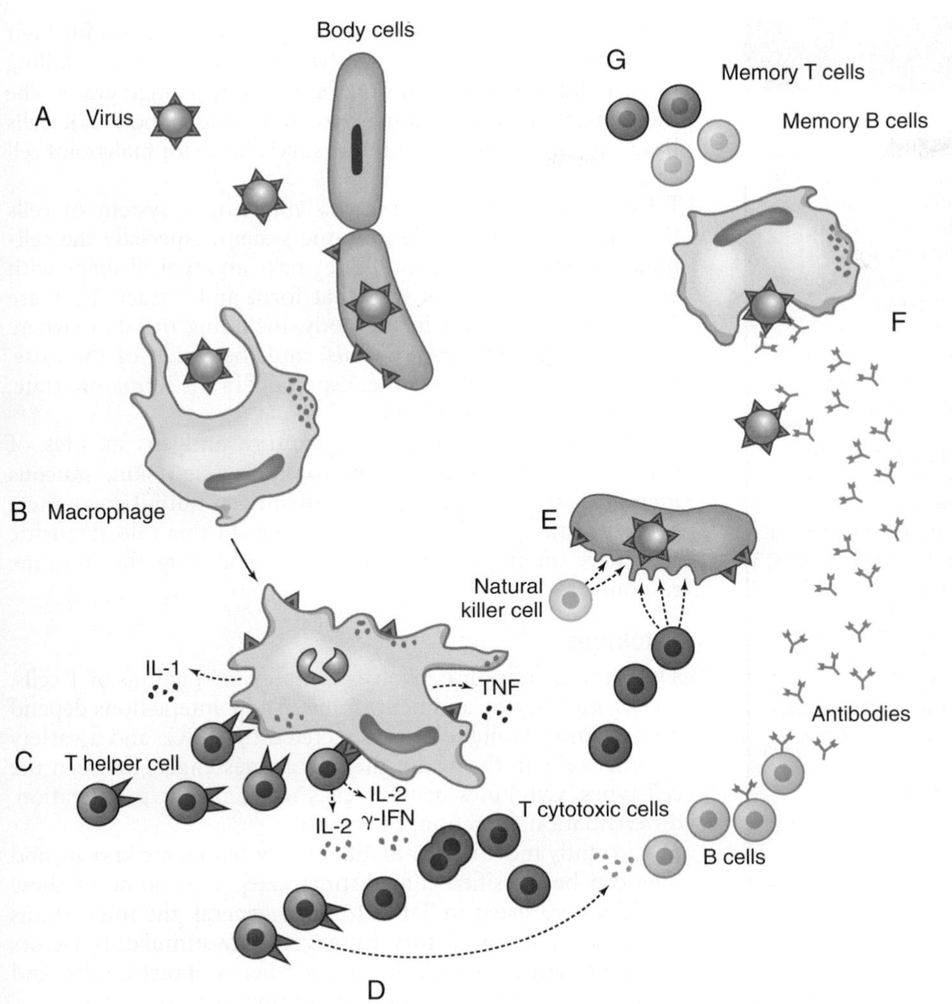


**FIG. 13-2** The immune response to a virus. **A,** A virus invades the body through a break in the skin or another portal of entry. The virus must make its way inside a cell to replicate itself. **B,** A macrophage recognizes the antigens on the surface of the virus. The macrophage digests the virus and displays pieces of the virus (antigens) on its surface. **C,** T helper cell recognizes the antigen displayed and binds to the macrophage. This binding stimulates the production of cytokines (interleukin-1 *[IL-1]* and tumor necrosis factor *[TNF]*) by the macrophage and interleukin-2 *(IL-2)* and γ-interferon *(γ-IFN)* by the T cell. These cytokines are intracellular messengers that provide communication among the cells. **D,** IL-2 instructs other T helper cells and T cytotoxic cells to proliferate (multiply). T helper cells release cytokines, causing B cells to multiply and produce antibodies. **E,** T cytotoxic cells and natural killer cells destroy infected body cells. **F,** The antibodies bind to the virus and mark it for macrophage destruction. **G,** Memory B and T cells remain behind to respond quickly if the same virus attacks again.

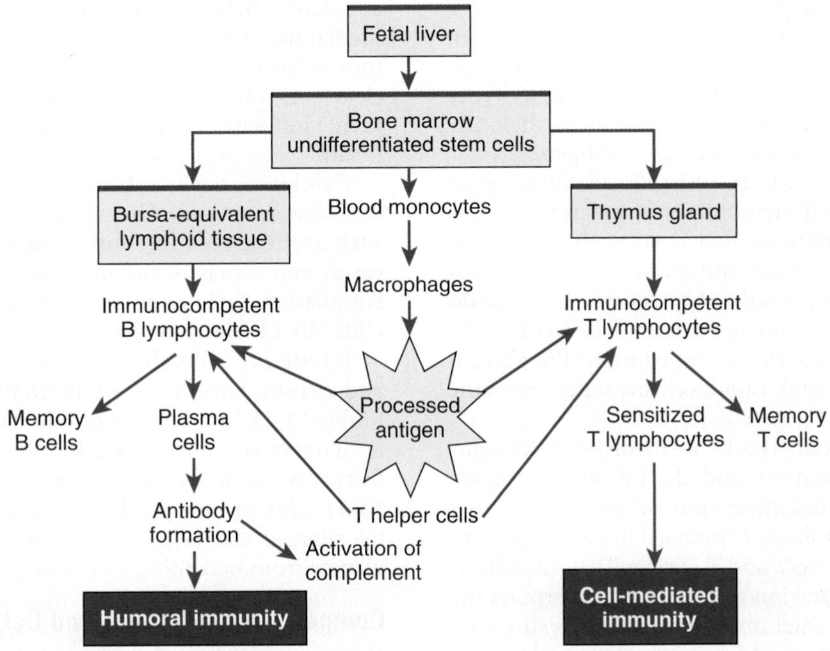


**FIG. 13-3** Relationships and functions of macrophages, B lymphocytes, and T lymphocytes in an immune response.

TABLE 13-2 **Characteristics of Immunoglobulins**

| Class | Serum Concentration | Location | Characteristics |
|---|---|---|---|
| **IgG** | 76% | Plasma, interstitial fluid | Is only immunoglobulin that crosses placenta<br>Is responsible for secondary immune response |
| **IgA** | 15% | Body secretions, including tears, saliva, breast milk, colostrum | Lines mucous membranes and protects body surfaces |
| **IgM** | 8% | Plasma | Is responsible for primary immune response<br>Forms antibodies to ABO blood antigens |
| **IgD** | 1% | Plasma | Is present on lymphocyte surface<br>Assists in the differentiation of B lymphocytes |
| **IgE** | 0.002% | Plasma, interstitial fluids | Causes symptoms of allergic reactions<br>Fixes to mast cells and basophils<br>Assists in defense against parasitic infections |

T cells make up 70% to 80% of the circulating lymphocytes and are primarily responsible for immunity to intracellular viruses, tumor cells, and fungi. T cells live from a few months to the life span of an individual and account for long-term immunity.

T lymphocytes can be categorized into T cytotoxic and T helper cells. Antigenic characteristics of WBCs have now been classified using monoclonal antibodies. These antigens are classified as *clusters of differentiation,* or *CD antigens.* Many types of WBCs, especially lymphocytes, are referred to by their CD designations. All mature T cells have the CD3 antigen.

**T cytotoxic cells.** T cytotoxic (CD8) cells are involved in attacking antigens on the cell membrane of foreign pathogens and releasing cytolytic substances that destroy the pathogen. These cells have antigen specificity and are sensitized by exposure to the antigen. Much like B cells, some sensitized T cells do not attack the antigen but remain as memory T cells. As in the humoral immune response, a second exposure to the antigen results in a more intense and rapid cell-mediated immune response.

**T helper cells.** T helper (CD4) cells are involved in the regulation of cell-mediated immunity and the humoral antibody response. T helper cells differentiate into subsets of cells that produce distinct types of cytokines (discussed in a later section). These subsets are called $T_H1$ cells and $T_H2$ cells. $T_H1$ cells stimulate phagocyte-mediated ingestion and killing of microbes, the key component of cell-mediated immunity. $T_H2$ cells stimulate eosinophil-mediated immunity, which is effective against parasites and is involved in allergic responses.

***Natural Killer Cells.*** Natural killer (NK) cells are also involved in cell-mediated immunity. These cells are not T or B cells but are large lymphocytes with numerous granules in the cytoplasm. NK cells do not require prior sensitization for their generation. These cells are involved in recognition and killing of virus-infected cells, tumor cells, and transplanted grafts. The mechanism of recognition is not fully understood. NK cells have a significant role in immune surveillance for malignant cell changes.

**T Dendritic Cells.** *Dendritic cells* make up a system of cells that are important to the immune system, especially the cell-mediated immune response. They have an atypical shape with extensive dendritic processes that form and retract. They are found in many places in the body, including the skin (where they are called *Langerhans' cells*) and the lining of the nose, lungs, stomach, and intestine. Especially in the immature state, they are found in the blood.[1]

They function primarily to capture antigens at sites of contact with the external environment (e.g., skin, mucous membranes) and then transport an antigen until it encounters a T cell with specificity for the antigen. In this role, dendritic cells have an important function in activating the immune response.

## Cytokines

The immune response involves complex interactions of T cells, B cells, monocytes, and neutrophils. These interactions depend on **cytokines** (soluble factors secreted by WBCs and a variety of other cells in the body) that act as messengers between the cell types. Cytokines instruct cells to alter their proliferation, differentiation, secretion, or activity.

Currently more than 100 different cytokines are known, and they can be classified into distinct categories. Some of these cytokines are listed in Table 13-3. In general, the interleukins act as immunomodulatory factors, colony-stimulating factors act as growth-regulating factors for hematopoietic cells, and interferons are antiviral and immunomodulatory.

The net effect of an inflammatory response is determined by a balance between proinflammatory and antiinflammatory mediators. Sometimes cytokines are classified as proinflammatory or antiinflammatory (Table 13-3). However, it is not that clear-cut, since many other factors (e.g., target cells, environment) influence the inflammatory response to a given injury or insult.

Cytokines have a beneficial role in hematopoiesis and immune function. They can also have detrimental effects such as those seen in chronic inflammation, autoimmune diseases, and sepsis. Cytokines such as erythropoietin, colony-stimulating factors, interferons, and interleukin-2 are used clinically (Table 13-4).

Interferon helps the body's natural defenses attack tumors and viruses. Three types of interferon have now been identified (Table 13-3). Interferon is not directly antiviral but produces an antiviral effect in cells by reacting with them and inducing the formation of a second protein termed *antiviral protein* (Fig. 13-4). This protein mediates the antiviral action of interferon by altering the cell's protein synthesis and preventing new viruses from becoming assembled.

## Comparison of Humoral and Cell-Mediated Immunity

Humans need both humoral and cell-mediated immunity to remain healthy. Each type of immunity has unique properties, different methods of action, and reactions against particular antigens. Table 13-5 compares humoral and cell-mediated immunity.

TABLE 13-3 **Types and Functions of Cytokines**

| Type | Primary Functions |
|---|---|
| **Interleukins (ILs)** | |
| IL-1 | Proinflammatory mediator. Promotes proliferation of B cells. Activates T cells, NK cells, and macrophages |
| IL-2 | Activates T cells, NK cells, and macrophages. Stimulates release of other cytokines (α-IFN, TNF, IL-1, IL-6) |
| IL-3 | Hematopoietic growth factor for hematopoietic precursor cells |
| IL-4 | Antiinflammatory mediator. B cell growth and differentiation. Induces differentiation into $T_H2$ cells. Stimulates growth of mast cells |
| IL-5 | B cell growth and differentiation. Promotes growth and differentiation of eosinophils |
| IL-6 | Proinflammatory mediator. T- and B-cell growth factor, promotes differentiation of B cells into plasma cells and stimulates antibody secretion. Induces fever. Synergistic effects with IL-1 and TNF |
| **Interferons (IFNs)** | |
| α-IFN<br>β-IFN | Inhibit viral replication, activate NK cells and macrophages, antiproliferative effects on tumor cells |
| γ-IFN | Proinflammatory mediator. Activates macrophages, neutrophils, and NK cells. Promotes B cell differentiation. Inhibits viral replication |
| **Tumor Necrosis Factor (TNF)** | Proinflammatory mediator. Activates macrophages and granulocytes. Promotes immune and inflammatory responses. Kills tumor cells. Responsible for weight loss associated with chronic inflammation and cancer |
| **Colony-Stimulating Factors (CSFs)** | |
| Granulocyte colony-stimulating factor (G-CSF) | Stimulates proliferation and differentiation of neutrophils, enhances functional activity of mature PMNs |
| Granulocyte-macrophage colony-stimulating factor (GM-CSF) | Stimulates proliferation and differentiation of PMNs and monocytes |
| Macrophage colony-stimulating factor (M-CSF) | Promotes proliferation, differentiation, and activation of monocytes and macrophages |
| **Erythropoietin** | Stimulates erythroid progenitor cells in bone marrow to produce red blood cells |

*NK*, Natural killer; *PMNs*, polymorphonuclear neutrophils.

TABLE 13-4 **Clinical Uses of Cytokines**

| Cytokine | Clinical Uses |
|---|---|
| **α-Interferon** (Roferon-A, Intron A) | Hairy cell leukemia, chronic myelogenous leukemia, malignant melanoma, renal cell carcinoma, ovarian cancer, multiple myeloma, Kaposi sarcoma, hepatitis B and C |
| **β-Interferon** (Betaseron, Avonex, Rebif) | Multiple sclerosis |
| **Colony-Stimulating Factors** | |
| ***G-CSF*** | |
| • filgrastim (Neupogen)<br>• pegfilgrastim (Neulasta) | Chemotherapy-induced neutropenia |
| ***GM-CSF*** | |
| • sargramostim (Leukine) | Neutropenia, myeloid recovery after bone marrow transplantation |
| **Soluble TNF Receptor** | |
| etanercept (Enbrel) | Rheumatoid arthritis |
| **Interleukin-2** | |
| aldesleukin (Proleukin) | Metastatic renal cell carcinoma, metastatic melanoma |
| **Interleukin 11** (platelet growth factor) | |
| oprelvekin (Neumega) | Thrombocytopenia related to chemotherapy |
| **Erythropoietin** | |
| epoetin alfa (Epogen, Procrit)<br>darbepoetin alfa (Aranesp) | Anemia related to chronic kidney disease, cancer, and chemotherapy |
| **IL-1 Receptor Antagonist** | |
| anakinra (Kineret) | Rheumatoid arthritis |

*G-CSF*, Granulocyte colony-stimulating factor; *GM-CSF*, granulocyte-macrophage colony-stimulating factor; *IL*, interleukin; *TNF*, tumor necrosis factor.

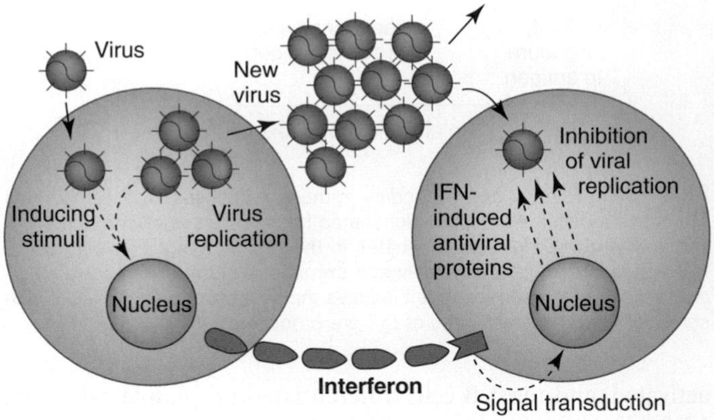


**FIG. 13-4** Mechanism of action of interferon (IFN). When a virus attacks a cell, the cell begins to synthesize viral DNA and interferon. Interferon serves as an intercellular messenger and induces the production of antiviral proteins. Then the virus is not able to replicate in the cell.

**Humoral Immunity.** Humoral immunity consists of antibody-mediated immunity. The term *humoral* comes from the Greek word *humor*, which means body fluid. Since antibodies are produced by plasma cells (differentiated B cells) and found in plasma, the term *humoral immunity* is used. Production of antibodies is an essential component in a humoral immune response. Each of the five classes of immunoglobulins (Igs) (IgG, IgA, IgM, IgG, IgE) has specific characteristics (Table 13-2).

When a pathogen (especially bacteria) enters the body, it may encounter a B cell that is specific for antigens located on that bacterial cell wall. In addition, a monocyte or macrophage may phagocytize the bacteria and present its antigens to a B cell. The B cell recognizes the antigen because it has receptors on its cell surface specific for that antigen. When the antigen comes in contact with the cell surface receptor, the B cell becomes

**TABLE 13-5 Comparison of Humoral and Cell-Mediated Immunity**

| Characteristics | Humoral Immunity | Cell-Mediated Immunity |
|---|---|---|
| **Cells involved** | B lymphocytes | T lymphocytes, macrophages |
| **Products** | Antibodies | Sensitized T cells, cytokines |
| **Memory cells** | Present | Present |
| **Protection** | Bacteria<br>Viruses (extracellular)<br>Respiratory and GI pathogens | Fungus<br>Viruses (intracellular)<br>Chronic infectious agents<br>Tumor cells |
| **Examples** | Anaphylactic shock<br>Atopic diseases<br>Transfusion reaction<br>Bacterial infections | Tuberculosis<br>Fungal infections<br>Contact dermatitis<br>Graft rejection<br>Destruction of cancer cells |

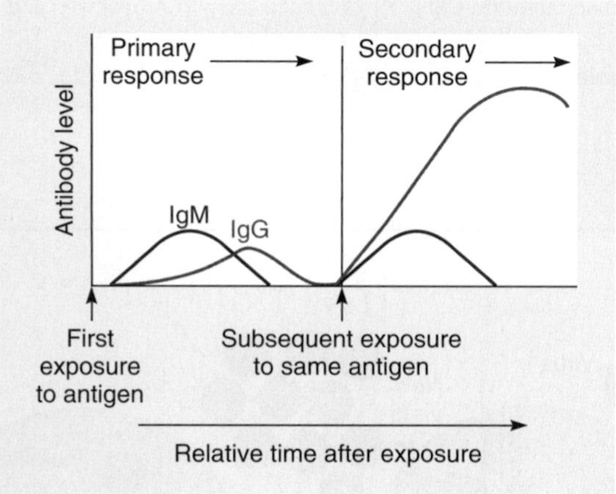


**FIG. 13-5** Primary and secondary immune responses. The introduction of antigen induces a response dominated by two classes of immunoglobulins, IgM and IgG. IgM predominates in the primary response, with some IgG appearing later. After the host's immune system is primed, another challenge with the same antigen induces the secondary response, in which some IgM and large amounts of IgG are produced.

activated, and most B cells differentiate into plasma cells (Fig. 13-3). The mature plasma cell secretes immunoglobulins. Some stimulated B cells remain as memory cells.

The primary immune response becomes evident 4 to 8 days after the initial exposure to the antigen (Fig. 13-5). IgM is the first type of antibody formed. Because of the large size of the IgM molecule, this immunoglobulin is confined to the intravascular space. As the immune response progresses, IgG is produced, and it can move from intravascular to extravascular spaces.

When the individual is exposed to the antigen the second time, a secondary antibody response occurs. This response occurs faster (1 to 3 days), is stronger, and lasts for a longer time than a primary response. Memory cells account for the memory of the first exposure to the antigen and the more rapid production of antibodies. IgG is the primary antibody found in a secondary immune response.

IgG crosses the placental membrane and provides the newborn with passive acquired immunity for at least 3 months. Infants may also get some passive immunity from IgA in breast milk and colostrum.

**TABLE 13-6 Gerontologic Assessment Differences**

***Effects of Aging on the Immune System***

- Thymic involution
- ↓ Cell-mediated immunity
- ↓ Delayed hypersensitivity reaction
- ↓ IL-1 and IL-2 synthesis
- ↓ Expression of IL-2 receptors
- ↓ Proliferative response of T and B cells
- ↓ Primary and secondary antibody responses
- ↑ Autoantibodies

*IL,* Interleukin.

**Cell-Mediated Immunity.** Immune responses that are initiated through specific antigen recognition by T cells are termed cell-mediated immunity. Several cell types and factors are involved in cell-mediated immunity. The cell types involved include T cells, macrophages, and NK cells. Cell-mediated immunity is of primary importance in (1) immunity against pathogens that survive inside of cells, including viruses and some bacteria (e.g., mycobacteria); (2) fungal infections; (3) rejection of transplanted tissues; (4) contact hypersensitivity reactions; and (5) tumor immunity.

### Gerontologic Considerations: Effects of Aging on the Immune System

With advancing age, there is a decline in the function of the immune response (Table 13-6). The primary clinical evidence of *immunosenescence* is the high incidence of malignancies in older adults. Older people are also more susceptible to infections (e.g., influenza, pneumonia) from pathogens that they were relatively immunocompetent against earlier in life. Bacterial pneumonia is the leading cause of death from infections in older adults. The antibody response to immunizations (e.g., flu vaccine) in older adults is considerably lower than in younger adults.[2]

The bone marrow remains relatively unaffected by increasing age. Immunoglobulin levels decrease with age and therefore lead to a suppressed humoral immune response in older adults. *Thymic involution* (shrinking) occurs with aging, along with decreased numbers of T cells. These changes in the thymus gland are a primary cause of immunosenescence. Both T and B cells show deficiencies in activation, transit time through the cell cycle, and subsequent differentiation. However, the most significant alterations involve T cells. As thymic output of T cells diminishes, the differentiation of T cells increases. Consequently, there is an accumulation of memory cells rather than new precursor cells responsive to previously unencountered antigens.

The delayed hypersensitivity reaction, as determined by skin testing with injected antigens, is frequently decreased or absent in older adults. This altered response reflects anergy (an immunodeficient condition characterized by lack of or diminished reaction to an antigen or a group of antigens).

## ALTERED IMMUNE RESPONSE

Immunocompetence exists when the body's immune system can identify and inactivate or destroy foreign substances. When the immune system is incompetent or underresponsive, severe infections, immunodeficiency diseases, and malignancies may occur.

**TABLE 13-7 Types of Hypersensitivity Reactions**

| Type I: IgE-Mediated | Type II: Cytotoxic | Type III: Immune-Complex | Type IV: Delayed Hypersensitivity |
|---|---|---|---|
| **Antigen** | | | |
| Pollen, food, drugs, dust | Cell surface of RBCs<br>Cell basement membrane | Extracellular fungal, viral, bacterial | Intracellular or extracellular |
| **Antibody Involved** | | | |
| IgE | IgG, IgM | IgG, IgM | None |
| **Complement Involved** | | | |
| No | Yes | Yes | No |
| **Mediators of Injury** | | | |
| Histamine<br>Mast cells<br>Leukotrienes<br>Prostaglandins | Complement lysis<br>Macrophages in tissues | Neutrophils<br>Complement lysis<br>Monocytes, macrophages<br>Lysosomal enzymes | Cytokines<br>T cytotoxic cells |
| **Examples** | | | |
| Allergic rhinitis<br>Asthma<br>Atopic dermatitis<br>Urticaria<br>Angioedema | Transfusion reaction<br>Goodpasture syndrome<br>Immune thrombocytopenic purpura<br>Graves' disease | Systemic lupus erythematosus<br>Rheumatoid arthritis<br>Acute glomerulonephritis | Contact dermatitis (e.g., to poison ivy) |
| **Skin Test** | | | |
| Wheal and flare | None | Erythema and edema in 3-8 hr | Erythema and edema in 24-48 hr (e.g., TB test) |

When the immune system overreacts, hypersensitivity disorders such as allergies and autoimmune diseases may develop.

## Hypersensitivity Reactions

Sometimes the immune response is overreactive against foreign antigens or reacts against its own tissue, resulting in tissue damage. These responses are termed **hypersensitivity reactions**. *Autoimmune diseases,* a type of hypersensitivity response, occur when the body fails to recognize self-proteins and reacts against self-antigens.

Hypersensitivity reactions can be classified according to the source of the antigen, time sequence (immediate or delayed), or immunologic mechanisms causing the injury. Four types of hypersensitivity reactions exist (Table 13-7). Types I, II, and III are immediate and are examples of humoral immunity. Type IV is a delayed hypersensitivity reaction and is related to cell-mediated immunity.

**Type I: IgE-Mediated Reactions.** *Anaphylactic reactions* are type I reactions that occur only in susceptible people who are highly sensitized to specific allergens. IgE antibodies, produced in response to the allergen, have a characteristic property of attaching to mast cells and basophils (Fig. 13-6; see Fig. 28-2). Within these cells are granules containing potent chemical mediators (histamine, serotonin, leukotrienes, eosinophil chemotactic factor of anaphylaxis [ECF-A], kinins, and bradykinin). (Chemical mediators of inflammation are discussed in Chapter 11 and Table 11-1.)

On the first exposure to the allergen, IgE antibodies are produced and bind to mast cells and basophils. On any subsequent exposures, the allergen links with the IgE bound to mast cells or basophils and triggers degranulation of the cells and the release of chemical mediators from the granules. In this process, the mediators that are released attack target tissues, causing clinical symptoms of an allergic response. These effects include smooth muscle contraction, increased vascular permeability, vasodilation, hypotension, increased secretion of mucus, and itching. Fortunately, the mediators are short acting and their effects are reversible. (The mediators are listed in Table 13-8.)

**TABLE 13-8 Mediators of Allergic Response***

- Anaphylatoxins (C3a, C4a, C5a from complement activation)
- Histamine
- Kinins
- Leukotrienes†
- Platelet-activating factor
- Prostaglandins
- Serotonin

*Mediators of inflammation and their mechanism of action are presented in Table 11-1.
†See Chapter 11, Fig. 11-2.

A genetic predisposition to the development of allergic diseases exists. The capacity to become sensitized to an allergen, rather than the specific allergic disorder, appears to be the inherited trait. For example, a father with asthma may have a son who has allergic rhinitis.

The clinical manifestations of an anaphylactic reaction depend on whether the mediators remain local or become systemic, or whether they affect particular organs. When the mediators remain localized, a cutaneous response termed the *wheal-and-flare reaction* occurs. This reaction is characterized by a pale wheal containing edematous fluid surrounded by a red flare from the hyperemia. The reaction occurs in minutes or hours and is usually not dangerous. A classic example of a wheal-and-flare reaction is the mosquito bite. The wheal-and-flare reaction serves a diagnostic purpose as a means of demonstrating allergic reactions to specific allergens during skin tests.

Common allergic reactions include anaphylaxis and atopic reactions.

***Anaphylaxis.*** *Anaphylaxis* can occur when mediators are released systemically (e.g., after injection of a drug, after an insect sting). The reaction occurs within minutes and can be life threatening because of bronchial constriction and subsequent airway obstruction and vascular collapse. The target organs affected are seen in Fig. 13-7. Initial symptoms include

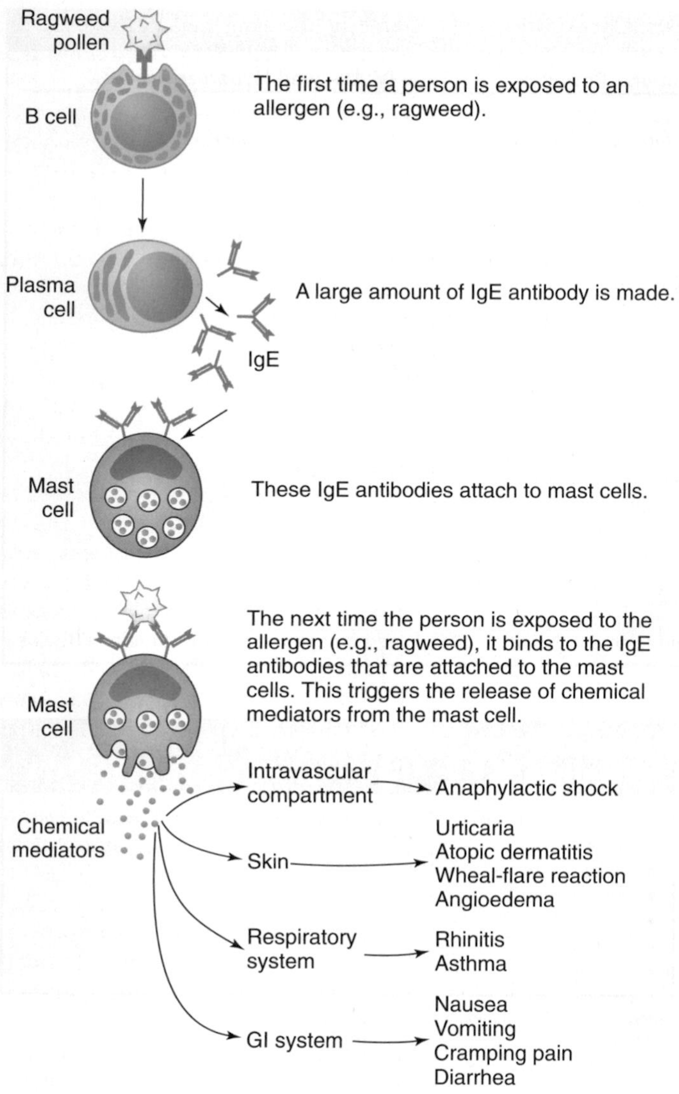


**FIG. 13-6** Steps in a type I allergic reaction.

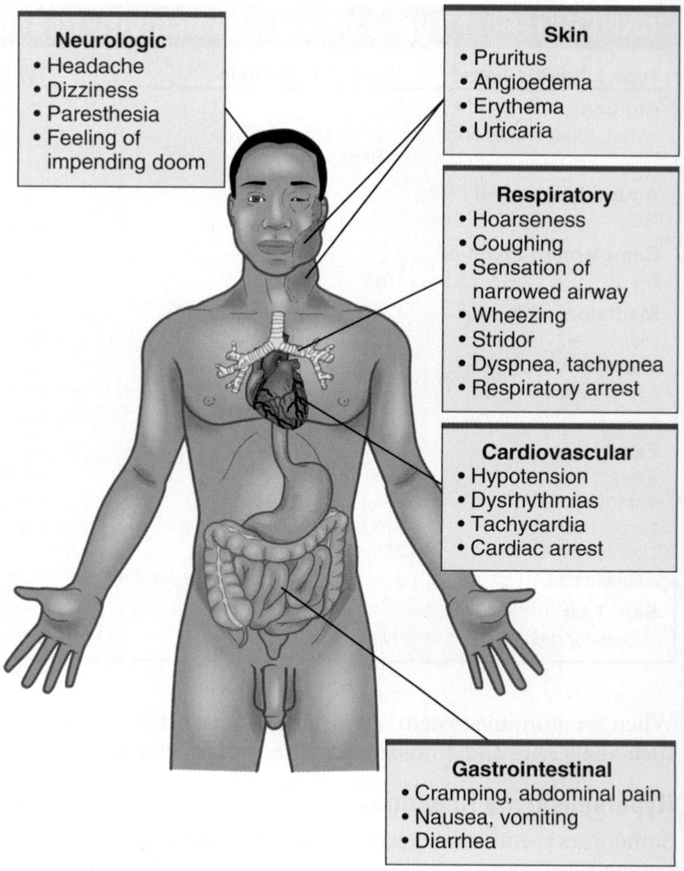


**FIG. 13-7** Clinical manifestations of a systemic anaphylactic reaction.

edema and itching at the site of exposure to the allergen. Shock can occur rapidly and is manifested by rapid, weak pulse; hypotension; dilated pupils; dyspnea; and possibly cyanosis. This is compounded by bronchial edema and angioedema. Death will occur if emergency treatment is not initiated. Some of the important allergens that can cause anaphylactic shock in hypersensitive people are listed in Table 13-9. Drugs are the leading cause of anaphylaxis-related deaths.[3]

***Atopic Reactions.*** An estimated 20% of the population is *atopic,* having an inherited tendency to become sensitive to environmental allergens. The atopic diseases that can result are allergic rhinitis, asthma, atopic dermatitis, urticaria, and angioedema.

*Allergic rhinitis,* or hay fever, is the most common type I hypersensitivity reaction. It may occur year-round (perennial allergic rhinitis), or it may be seasonal (seasonal allergic rhinitis). Airborne substances such as pollens, dust, and molds are the primary causes of allergic rhinitis. Perennial allergic rhinitis may be caused by dust, molds, and animal dander. Seasonal allergic rhinitis is commonly caused by pollens from trees, weeds, or grasses. The target areas affected are the conjunctiva of the eyes and the mucosa of the upper respiratory tract. Symptoms include nasal discharge; sneezing; lacrimation; mucosal swelling with airway obstruction; and pruritus around the eyes, nose, throat, and mouth. (Treatment of allergic rhinitis is discussed in Chapter 26 on p. 478.)

Many patients with *asthma* have an allergic component to their disease. These patients frequently have a history of atopic disorders (e.g., infantile eczema, allergic rhinitis, food intolerances). Inflammatory mediators produce bronchial smooth muscle constriction, excessive secretion of viscoid mucus, edema of the mucous membranes of the bronchi, and decreased

**TABLE 13-9 Allergens Causing Anaphylactic Shock**

| | |
|---|---|
| **Drugs**<br>• Aspirin<br>• Cephalosporins<br>• Chemotherapy drugs<br>• Insulins<br>• Local anesthetics<br>• Nonsteroidal antiinflammatory drugs<br>• Penicillins<br>• Sulfonamides<br>• Tetracycline | **Treatment Measures**<br>• Allergenic extracts used in immunotherapy<br>• Blood products (whole blood and components)<br>• Iodine-contrast media for CT scan or other radiologic procedures |
| **Foods**<br>• Eggs, milk, nuts, peanuts, shellfish, fish, chocolate, strawberries | **Insect Venoms**<br>• Wasps, hornets, yellow jackets, bumblebees, ants<br>**Animal Sera**<br>• Diphtheria antitoxin<br>• Rabies antitoxin<br>• Snake venom antitoxin<br>• Tetanus antitoxin |

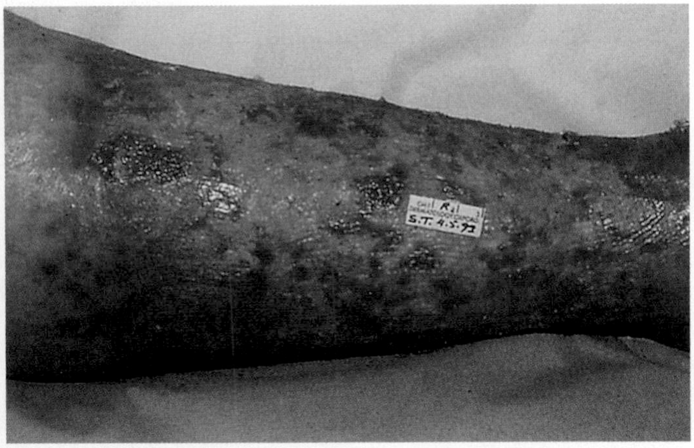

**FIG. 13-8** Atopic dermatitis of the lower leg. (From Morison MJ: *Nursing management of chronic wounds,* Edinburgh, 2001, Mosby.)

lung compliance. Because of these physiologic alterations, patients manifest dyspnea, wheezing, coughing, tightness in the chest, and thick sputum. (Pathophysiology and management of asthma are discussed in Chapter 28.)

*Atopic dermatitis* is a chronic, inherited skin disorder characterized by exacerbations and remissions. It is caused by several environmental allergens that are difficult to identify. Although patients with atopic dermatitis have elevated IgE levels and positive skin tests, the histopathologic features do not represent the typical, localized wheal-and-flare type I reactions. The skin lesions are more generalized and involve vasodilation of blood vessels, resulting in interstitial edema with vesicle formation (Fig. 13-8). (Dermatitis is discussed in Chapter 23.)

*Urticaria (hives)* is a cutaneous reaction against systemic allergens occurring in atopic people. It is characterized by transient wheals (pink, raised, edematous, pruritic areas) that vary in size and shape and may occur all over the body. Urticaria develops rapidly after exposure to an allergen and may last minutes or hours. Histamine causes localized vasodilation (erythema), transudation of fluid (wheal), and flaring. Flaring is due to dilated blood vessels on the edge of the wheal. Histamine is responsible for the pruritus associated with the lesions. (Urticaria is discussed in Chapter 23.)

*Angioedema* is a localized cutaneous lesion similar to urticaria but involving deeper layers of the skin and submucosa. The principal areas of involvement include the eyelids, lips, tongue, larynx, hands, feet, GI tract, and genitalia. Swelling usually begins in the face and then progresses to the airways and other parts of the body. Dilation and engorgement of the capillaries secondary to the release of histamine cause the diffuse swelling. Welts are not apparent as in urticaria. The outer skin appears normal or has a reddish hue. The lesions may burn, sting, or itch and can cause acute abdominal pain if in the GI tract. The swelling may occur suddenly or over several hours and usually lasts for 24 hours.

**Type II: Cytotoxic and Cytolytic Reactions.** Cytotoxic and cytolytic reactions are type II hypersensitivity reactions involving the direct binding of IgG or IgM antibodies to an antigen on the cell surface. Antigen-antibody complexes activate the complement system, which mediates the reaction. Cellular tissue is destroyed in one of two ways: (1) activation of the complement system resulting in cytolysis or (2) enhanced phagocytosis.

Target cells frequently destroyed in type II reactions are erythrocytes, platelets, and leukocytes. The tissue damage usually occurs rapidly. Some of the antigens involved are the ABO blood group, Rh factor, and drugs. Pathophysiologic disorders characteristic of type II reactions include ABO incompatibility transfusion reaction, Rh incompatibility transfusion reaction, autoimmune and drug-related hemolytic anemias, leukopenias, thrombocytopenias, erythroblastosis fetalis (hemolytic disease of the newborn), and Goodpasture syndrome.

***Hemolytic Transfusion Reactions.*** A classic type II reaction occurs when a recipient receives ABO-incompatible blood from a donor. Naturally acquired antibodies to antigens of the ABO blood group are in the recipient's serum but are not present on the erythrocyte membranes (see Table 29-8). For example, a person with type A blood has anti-B antibodies, a person with type B blood has anti-A antibodies, a person with type AB blood has no antibodies, and a person with type O blood has anti-A and anti-B antibodies.

If the recipient is transfused with incompatible blood, antibodies immediately coat the foreign erythrocytes, causing *agglutination* (clumping). The clumping of cells blocks small blood vessels in the body, uses existing clotting factors, and depletes them, leading to bleeding. Within hours, neutrophils and macrophages phagocytize the agglutinated cells. The complement system is activated and cell lysis occurs, which causes the release of hemoglobin into the urine and plasma. Acute kidney injury can result from the hemoglobinuria. (Blood transfusions are discussed in Chapter 30.)

***Goodpasture Syndrome.*** *Goodpasture syndrome* is a disorder involving the lungs and kidneys. An antibody-mediated autoimmune reaction occurs involving the glomerular and alveolar basement membranes. The circulating antibodies combine with tissue antigen to activate the complement system, which causes deposits of IgG to form along the cell basement membranes of the lungs or kidneys. This reaction may result in pulmonary hemorrhage and glomerulonephritis. (Goodpasture syndrome is discussed in Chapter 45.)

**Type III: Immune-Complex Reactions.** Tissue damage in immune-complex reactions, which are type III reactions, occurs secondary to antigen-antibody complexes. Soluble antigens combine with immunoglobulins of the IgG and IgM classes to form complexes that are too small to be effectively removed by the mononuclear phagocyte system. Therefore the complexes deposit in tissue or small blood vessels. They cause activation of the complement system and release of chemotactic factors that lead to inflammation and destruction of the involved tissue.

Type III reactions may be local or systemic and immediate or delayed. The clinical manifestations depend on the number of complexes and the location in the body. Common sites for deposit are the kidneys, skin, joints, blood vessels, and lungs. Severe type III reactions are associated with autoimmune disorders such as systemic lupus erythematosus, acute glomerulonephritis, and rheumatoid arthritis. (Systemic lupus erythematosus and rheumatoid arthritis are discussed in Chapter 64, and acute glomerulonephritis is discussed in Chapter 45.)

**Type IV: Delayed Hypersensitivity Reactions.** A *delayed hypersensitivity reaction*—a type IV reaction—is a *cell-mediated immune response.* Although cell-mediated responses are usually protective mechanisms, tissue damage occurs in delayed hypersensitivity reactions.

The tissue damage in a type IV reaction does not occur in the presence of antibodies or complement. Rather, sensitized T cells attack antigens or release cytokines. Some of these cytokines attract macrophages into the area. The macrophages and

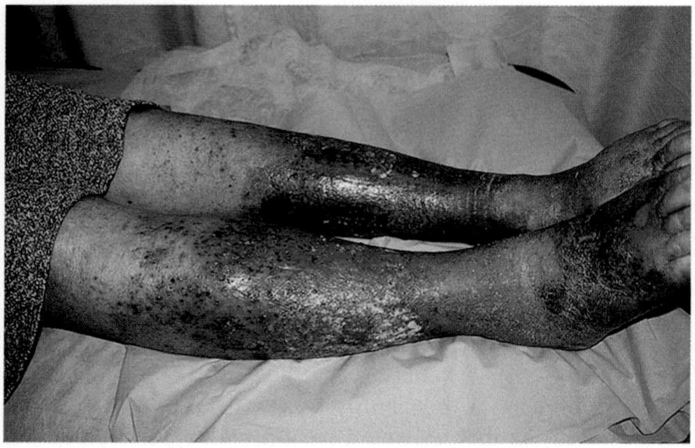

**FIG. 13-9** Contact dermatitis to rubber. (From Morison MJ: *Nursing management of chronic wounds*, Edinburgh, 2001, Mosby.)

enzymes released by them are responsible for most of the tissue destruction. In the delayed hypersensitivity reaction, it takes 24 to 48 hours for a response to occur.

Clinical examples of a delayed hypersensitivity reaction include contact dermatitis (Fig. 13-9); hypersensitivity reactions to bacterial, fungal, and viral infections; and transplant rejections. Some drug sensitivity reactions also fit this category.

***Contact Dermatitis.*** *Allergic contact dermatitis* is an example of a delayed hypersensitivity reaction involving the skin. The reaction occurs when the skin is exposed to substances that easily penetrate the skin to combine with epidermal proteins. The substance then becomes antigenic. Over a period of 7 to 14 days, memory cells form to the antigen. On subsequent exposure to the substance, a sensitized person develops eczematous skin lesions within 48 hours. The most common potentially antigenic substances are metal compounds (e.g., those containing nickel or mercury); rubber compounds; poison ivy, poison oak, and poison sumac; cosmetics; and some dyes.

In acute contact dermatitis, the skin lesions appear erythematous and edematous and are covered with papules, vesicles, and bullae. The involved area is pruritic but may also burn or sting. When contact dermatitis becomes chronic, the lesions resemble atopic dermatitis because they are thickened, scaly, and lichenified. The main difference between contact dermatitis and atopic dermatitis is that contact dermatitis is localized and restricted to the area exposed to the allergens, whereas atopic dermatitis is usually widespread.

***Microbial Hypersensitivity Reactions.*** The classic example of a microbial cell-mediated immune reaction is the body's defense against the tubercle bacillus. Tuberculosis results from invasion of lung tissue by the highly resistant tubercle bacillus. The organism itself does not directly damage the lung tissue. However, antigenic material released from the tubercle bacilli reacts with T cells, initiating a cell-mediated immune response. The resulting response causes extensive caseous necrosis of the lung.

After the initial cell-mediated reaction, memory cells persist, so subsequent contact with the tubercle bacillus or an extract of purified protein from the organism causes a delayed hypersensitivity reaction. This is the basis for the purified protein derivative (PPD) tuberculosis skin test, which is read 48 to 72 hours after the PPD is injected intradermally. (Tuberculosis is discussed in Chapter 27.)

## ALLERGIC DISORDERS

### Assessment

For a thorough assessment of a patient with allergies, perform a comprehensive patient history, physical examination, diagnostic workup, and skin testing for allergens. Obtain information from the patient about family allergies, past and present allergies, and social and environmental factors.

Family history, including information about atopic reactions in relatives, is especially important in identifying at-risk patients. Note past and present allergies. In addition to identifying the allergen, also obtain information about the clinical manifestations and course of allergic reaction. The time of year when an allergic reaction occurs can be a clue to a seasonal allergen. Also obtain information about any over-the-counter or prescription medications used to treat the allergies.

Social and environmental factors, especially the physical environment, are important. Ask about pets, trees and plants on the property, pollutants in the air, floor coverings, houseplants, and cooling and heating systems in the home and workplace. In addition, a daily or weekly food diary with a description of any untoward reactions is important.[4] Of particular interest is a screening for any reaction to medication. Finally, ask about the patient's lifestyle and stress level in connection with the allergic symptoms.

Do a comprehensive head-to-toe physical examination, with particular attention focused on the site of the allergic manifestations. Obtain a comprehensive assessment that includes subjective and objective data (Table 13-10).

### Diagnostic Studies

Many specialized immunologic techniques can be performed to detect abnormalities of lymphocytes, eosinophils, and immunoglobulins. A complete blood count (CBC) with WBC differential is done, with an absolute lymphocyte count and eosinophil count. Immunodeficiency is diagnosed if the lymphocyte count is below 1200/μL ($1.2 \times 10^9$/L). T cell and B cell quantification is used to diagnose specific immunodeficiency syndromes. The eosinophil count is elevated in type I hypersensitivity reactions involving IgE. The serum IgE level is also generally elevated in type I hypersensitivity reactions and serves as a diagnostic indicator of atopic diseases.

Sputum and nasal and bronchial secretions may also be tested for the presence of eosinophils. If asthma is suspected, pulmonary function tests (especially for forced expiratory volume) are helpful.

Skin testing for allergens is the preferred method, but in some cases blood testing may be ordered. Allergy blood testing is recommended if a person (1) is using a drug that interferes with skin test results (e.g., antihistamines, corticosteroids) and cannot stop taking it for a few days, (2) cannot tolerate the many needle scratches required for skin testing, or (3) has a skin disorder (e.g., severe eczema, dermatitis, psoriasis).

**Skin Tests.** Skin testing is used to identify the specific allergens that are causing the allergy symptoms. With the use of empiric allergy medications as the treatment of choice for most allergic rhinitis, it has become common practice to omit skin testing for specific allergens in these patients. However, diagnosing an allergy to a specific antigen enables the patient to avoid an allergen and makes him or her a candidate for immunotherapy. Unfortunately, skin testing cannot be done on patients who cannot stop taking drugs that suppress the histamine response or patients with food allergies.

**TABLE 13-10 Nursing Assessment**

***Allergies***

**Subjective Data**

***Important Health Information***

*Past health history:* Recurrent respiratory problems, seasonal exacerbations. Unusual reactions to insect bites or stings; past and present allergies

*Medications:* Unusual reactions to any medications; use of over-the-counter drugs or medications for allergies

***Functional Health Patterns***

*Health perception–health management:* Family history of allergies; malaise

*Nutritional-metabolic:* Food intolerances, vomiting

*Elimination:* Abdominal cramps, diarrhea

*Activity-exercise:* Fatigue; hoarseness, cough, dyspnea

*Cognitive-perceptual:* Itching, burning, stinging of eyes, nose, throat, or skin; chest tightness

*Role-relationship:* Altered home and work environment, presence of pets

**Objective Data**

***Integumentary***

Rashes, including urticaria, wheal and flare, papules, vesicles, bullae; dryness, scaliness, scratches, irritation

***Eyes, Ears, Nose, and Throat***

*Eyes:* Conjunctivitis; lacrimation; rubbing or excessive blinking; dark circles under the eyes ("allergic shiner")

*Ears:* Diminished hearing; immobile or scarred tympanic membranes; recurrent ear infections

*Nose:* Nasal polyps, nasal voice, nose twitching, itchy nose, rhinitis; pale, boggy mucous membranes; sniffling, repeated sneezing; swollen nasal passages; recurrent, unexplained nosebleeds; crease across the bridge of nose ("allergic salute")

*Throat:* Continual throat clearing; swollen lips or tongue; red throat; palpable neck lymph nodes

***Respiratory***

Wheezing, stridor; thick sputum

***Possible Diagnostic Findings***

Eosinophilia of serum, sputum, or nasal and bronchial secretions; ↑ serum IgE levels; positive skin tests; abnormal chest and sinus x-rays

***Procedure.*** Skin testing may be done by three different methods: (1) a scratch or prick test, (2) an intradermal test, or (3) a patch test. The areas of the body usually used in skin testing are the arms and back. Allergen extracts are applied to the skin in rows with a corresponding control site opposite the test site. Saline or another diluent is applied to the control site. In the *scratch test* a drop of allergen is placed on the skin, and then a pricking device is used so that the allergen can enter the skin. In the *intradermal test* the allergen extract is injected under the skin, similar to a PPD test for TB. In the *patch test* an allergen is applied to a patch that is placed on the skin (see Fig. 22-10).

***Results.*** In the scratch and intradermal tests the reaction occurs in 5 to 10 minutes. In the patch test the patches must be worn for 48 to 72 hours. If the person is hypersensitive to the allergen, a positive reaction will occur within minutes after insertion in the skin and may last for 8 to 12 hours. A positive reaction is manifested by a local wheal-and-flare response.

The size of the positive reaction does not always correlate with the severity of allergy symptoms. False-positive and false-negative results may occur. Negative results from skin testing do not necessarily mean the person does not have an allergic disorder, and positive results do not necessarily mean that the allergen was causing the clinical manifestations. Positive results imply that the person is sensitized to that allergen. Therefore correlating skin test results with the patient's history is important.

***Precautions.*** A highly sensitive person is always at risk for developing an anaphylactic reaction to skin tests. Therefore a patient should never be left alone during the testing period. Sometimes skin testing is completely contraindicated and blood allergy testing is used. If a severe reaction does occur with a skin test, the extract is immediately removed and antiinflammatory topical cream is applied to the site. For intradermal testing, the arm is used so that a tourniquet can be applied during a severe reaction. A subcutaneous injection of epinephrine may also be necessary.

## Interprofessional Care

After an allergic disorder is diagnosed, treatment is aimed at reducing exposure to the offending allergen, treating the symptoms, and, if necessary, desensitizing the person through immunotherapy.

**Anaphylaxis.** Anaphylactic reactions occur suddenly in hypersensitive patients after exposure to the offending allergen. They may occur after parenteral injection of drugs (especially antibiotics) or blood products, and after insect stings. The cardinal principle in management is speed in (1) recognition of signs and symptoms of an anaphylactic reaction, (2) maintenance of a patent airway, (3) prevention of spread of the allergen by using a tourniquet, (4) administration of drugs, and (5) treatment for shock. Table 13-11 summarizes the emergency treatment of anaphylactic shock.

Severe cases of anaphylaxis may result in hypovolemic shock because of the loss of intravascular fluid into interstitial spaces that occurs secondary to increased capillary permeability.[5] Peripheral vasoconstriction and stimulation of the sympathetic nervous system occur to compensate for the fluid shift. However, unless shock is treated early, the body will no longer be able to compensate, and irreversible tissue damage will occur, leading to death. (Hypovolemic shock is discussed in Chapter 66.)

All health care workers must be prepared for the rare but life-threatening anaphylactic reaction, which requires immediate medical and nursing interventions. It is extremely important to list all of a patient's allergies on the chart, nursing care plan, and medication record.[6]

**Chronic Allergies.** Most allergic reactions are chronic and are characterized by remissions and exacerbations of symptoms. Treatment focuses on identification and control of allergens, relief of symptoms through drug therapy, and hyposensitization of a patient to an offending allergen.

***Allergen Recognition and Control.*** You play an important role in helping the patient make lifestyle adjustments so that there is minimal exposure to offending allergens. Reinforce that, even with drug therapy and immunotherapy, the patient will never be totally desensitized or completely symptom free. Help the patient initiate various preventive measures to control the allergic symptoms.

Of primary importance is the need to identify the offending allergen. Sometimes this is done through skin testing. In the case of food allergies an elimination diet is sometimes valuable. If an allergic reaction occurs, all foods eaten shortly before the

**TABLE 13-11 Emergency Management**

***Anaphylactic Shock***

**Etiology**

- Injection of, inhalation of, ingestion of, or topical exposure to substance that produces profound allergic response (Table 13-9 for more complete listing).

**Assessment Findings**

Fig. 13-7.

**Interventions**

***Initial***

- Ensure patent airway. Intubation if evidence of impending obstruction.
- Remove insect stinger if present.
- Establish IV access.
- Epinephrine (1 mg/mL preparation): Give 0.3-0.5 mg IM preferably in the mid-outer thigh. Can repeat every 5-15 min.*
- Administer high-flow $O_2$ (8-10 L/min) via face mask. Can give up to 100% as needed.
- Nebulized albuterol (Proventil) for bronchospasm resistant to epinephrine.
- Diphenhydramine (Benadryl) IV for urticaria and itching.
- Corticosteroids: methylprednisolone (Solu-Medrol) IV.

***Hypotension***

- Place recumbent and elevate legs.
- IV normal saline rapid bolus of 1-2 L.
- Maintain BP with fluids, volume expanders, vasopressors (e.g., dopamine [Intropin]).

***Ongoing Monitoring***

- Monitor vital signs, respiratory effort, $O_2$ saturation, level of consciousness, cardiac rhythm, and urine output.
- Anticipate intubation with severe respiratory distress.
- Anticipate cricothyrotomy or tracheostomy with severe laryngeal edema.

*Patients receiving β-blockers may be resistant to treatment with epinephrine and can develop refractory hypotension and bradycardia. Glucagon should be administered in this setting because it has inotropic and chronotropic effects that are not mediated through β-receptors.

reaction should be eliminated and gradually reintroduced one at a time until the offending food is detected.

Many allergic reactions, especially asthma and urticaria, may be aggravated by fatigue and emotional stress. Assist the patient in planning a stress management program. Relaxation techniques can be practiced when the patient comes for frequent immunotherapy treatments.

Sometimes control of allergic symptoms requires environmental control, including changing an occupation, moving to a different climate, or giving up a favorite pet. In the case of airborne allergens, sleeping in an air-conditioned room, damp dusting daily, covering mattresses and pillows with hypoallergenic covers, and wearing a mask outdoors may be helpful.

If the allergen is a drug, instruct the patient to avoid the drug. The patient also has the responsibility to make his or her allergies well known to all health care providers. The patient should wear a Medic Alert bracelet listing the particular drug allergy and have the offending drug listed on all medical and dental records.

For a patient allergic to insect stings, commercial bee-sting kits containing preinjectable epinephrine and a tourniquet are available. Instruct the patient and family about the technique of applying the tourniquet and self-injecting the subcutaneous epinephrine. This patient also should wear a Medic Alert bracelet and carry a bee-sting kit whenever going outdoors.

**Drug Therapy.** The major categories of drugs used for symptomatic relief of chronic allergic disorders include antihistamines, sympathomimetic/decongestant drugs, corticosteroids, antipruritic drugs, and mast cell–stabilizing drugs. Many of these drugs can be obtained over the counter and are often misused by patients.

***Antihistamines.*** Antihistamines are the best drugs for treatment of allergic rhinitis and urticaria (see Chapter 26, Table 26-2). They are less effective for severe allergic reactions. They act by competing with histamine for $H_1$-receptor sites and thus blocking the effect of histamine. Best results are achieved if they are taken as soon as allergy symptoms appear. Antihistamines can be used effectively to treat edema and pruritus but are relatively ineffective in preventing bronchoconstriction. With seasonal rhinitis, antihistamines should be taken during peak pollen seasons. (Antihistamines are discussed in Chapter 26.)

***Sympathomimetic/Decongestant Drugs.*** The major sympathomimetic drug is epinephrine (Adrenalin), which is the drug of choice to treat an anaphylactic reaction. Epinephrine is produced by the adrenal medulla and stimulates α- and β-adrenergic receptors. Stimulation of the α-adrenergic receptors causes vasoconstriction of peripheral blood vessels. β-Receptor stimulation relaxes bronchial smooth muscles. Epinephrine also acts directly on mast cells to stabilize them against further degranulation. The action of epinephrine lasts only a few minutes. For the treatment of anaphylaxis, the drug must be given parenterally (IM, IV).

Several specific, minor sympathomimetic drugs differ from epinephrine because they can be taken orally or nasally and last for several hours. Included in this category are phenylephrine (Neo-Synephrine) and pseudoephedrine (Sudafed). The minor sympathomimetic drugs are used primarily to treat allergic rhinitis.

***Corticosteroids.*** Nasal corticosteroid sprays are effective in relieving the symptoms of allergic rhinitis (see Chapter 26 and Table 26-2). Occasionally patients have such severe manifestations of allergies that they are truly incapacitated. In these situations, a brief course of oral corticosteroids can be used.

***Antipruritic Drugs.*** Topically applied antipruritic drugs are most effective when the skin is not broken. These drugs protect the skin and provide relief from itching. Common over-the-counter drugs include calamine lotion, coal tar solutions, and camphor. Menthol and phenol may be added to other lotions to produce an antipruritic effect. Some more potent drugs that require a prescription include methdilazine (Tacaryl) and trimeprazine (Temaril).

***Mast Cell–Stabilizing Drugs.*** Cromolyn (NasalCrom) is a mast cell–stabilizing agent that inhibits the release of histamines, leukotrienes, and other agents from the mast cell after antigen-IgE interaction. It is available as an inhalant nebulizer solution or a nasal spray. Cromolyn is used in the management of allergic rhinitis (see Chapter 27).

***Leukotriene Receptor Antagonists.*** Leukotriene receptor antagonists (LTRAs) block leukotriene, one of the major mediators of the allergic inflammatory process (see Table 26-2). These medications can be taken orally. They may be used in the treatment of allergic rhinitis and asthma.

**Immunotherapy.** Immunotherapy is the recommended treatment for control of allergic symptoms when the allergen cannot be avoided and drug therapy is not effective. Relatively few patients with allergies have symptoms so intolerable that they require allergy immunotherapy. (In individuals with anaphylactic reactions to insect venom, immunotherapy is definitely indicated.)

Immunotherapy involves administration of small titers of an allergen extract in increasing strengths until hyposensitivity to the specific allergen is achieved. For best results, teach the patient to avoid the offending allergen whenever possible because complete desensitization is impossible. Unfortunately, not all allergy-related conditions respond to immunotherapy. Food allergies cannot be safely treated with this therapy, and eczema may worsen with immunotherapy.

***Mechanism of Action.*** The IgE level is elevated in atopic individuals. When IgE combines with an allergen in a hypersensitive person, a reaction occurs, releasing histamine in various body tissues. Allergens more readily combine with IgG than with other immunoglobulins. Therefore immunotherapy involves injecting allergen extracts that will stimulate increased IgG levels. The goal of long-term immunotherapy is to keep "blocking" IgG levels high. By increasing the IgG levels, the IgE is blocked from binding to the allergen. Thus mast cell degranulation is prevented. In addition, allergen-specific T suppressor cells develop in individuals receiving immunotherapy.

***Method of Administration.*** The allergens included in immunotherapy are chosen based on the results of skin testing with a panel of allergens.

**Subcutaneous immunotherapy.** *Subcutaneous immunotherapy (SCIT)* involves the subcutaneous injection of titrated amounts of allergen extracts biweekly or weekly. The dose is small at first and is increased slowly until a maintenance dosage is reached. Generally it takes 1 to 2 years of immunotherapy to reach the maximal therapeutic effect. Therapy may be continued for about 5 years. After that, discontinuing therapy is considered. In many patients a decrease in symptoms is sustained after the treatment is discontinued. For patients with severe allergies or sensitivity to insect stings, maintenance therapy is continued indefinitely. Best results are achieved when immunotherapy is administered throughout the year.

**Sublingual immunotherapy.** *Sublingual immunotherapy (SLIT)* involves allergen extracts taken under the tongue. SLIT has been used in Europe for decades. Recently the first sublingual products have become available in the United States. These include a five-grass pollen tablet (Oralair), a single grass pollen tablet (Grastek), and a ragweed pollen tablet (Ragwitek).[7]

SLIT is self-administered (usually daily) by patients at home, although the initial dose is usually given under medical supervision. Some patients experience local application site reactions (e.g., oral pruritus, throat irritation, tongue swelling), but systemic allergic reactions are markedly fewer than SCIT. Local reactions subside in many patients within a few days to a week.

SLIT has the advantage of being a convenient, self-administered oral therapy. Its primary disadvantage is that it requires the patient to be consistently compliant with therapy.[8]

## NURSING MANAGEMENT: IMMUNOTHERAPY

You will often be the person responsible for administering SCIT. Always anticipate adverse reactions, especially when using a new-strength dose, after a previous reaction, or after a missed dose. Early manifestations of a systemic reaction include pruritus, urticaria, sneezing, laryngeal edema, and hypotension. Emergency measures for anaphylactic shock should be initiated immediately. Describe a local reaction according to the degree of redness and swelling at the injection site. If the area is greater than the size of a quarter in an adult, report the reaction to the HCP so that the allergen dosage may be decreased.

Immunotherapy always carries the risk of a severe anaphylactic reaction. Therefore an HCP, emergency equipment, and essential drugs should be available whenever injections are given.

Record keeping must be accurate and can be invaluable in preventing an adverse reaction to the allergen extract. Before giving an injection, check the patient's name against the name on the vial. Next, determine the vial strength, amount of last dose, date of last dose, and any reaction information.

Always administer the allergen extract in an extremity away from a joint so that a tourniquet can be applied for a severe reaction. Rotate the site for each injection. Aspirate for blood before giving an injection to ensure that the allergen extract is not injected into a blood vessel. An injection directly into the bloodstream can potentiate an anaphylactic reaction. After giving the injection, carefully observe the patient for 20 to 30 minutes, since systemic reactions are most likely to occur immediately. However, warn the patient that a delayed reaction can occur as long as 24 hours later.

### Latex Allergies

Allergies to latex products have become an increasing problem, affecting patients and health care professionals. The increase in allergic reactions has coincided with the sharp increase in glove use. The more frequent and prolonged the exposure to latex, the greater the likelihood of developing a latex allergy.[9]

In addition to gloves, many latex-containing products are used in health care, such as blood pressure cuffs, stethoscopes, tourniquets, IV tubing, syringes, electrode pads, $O_2$ masks, tracheal tubes, colostomy and ileostomy pouches, urinary catheters, anesthetic masks, and adhesive tape. Latex proteins can become aerosolized through powder on gloves and can result in serious reactions when inhaled by sensitized individuals. It is recommended that all health care facilities use powder-free gloves to avoid respiratory exposure to latex proteins.[10]

**Types of Latex Allergies.** Two types of latex allergies can occur: type IV allergic contact dermatitis and type I allergic reactions. *Type IV contact dermatitis* is caused by the chemicals used in the manufacturing process of latex gloves. It is a delayed reaction that occurs within 6 to 48 hours. Typically the person first has dryness, pruritus, fissuring, and cracking of the skin, followed by redness, swelling, and crusting at 24 to 48 hours. Chronic exposure can lead to lichenification, scaling, and hyperpigmentation. The dermatitis may extend beyond the area of physical contact with the allergen.

A *type I allergic reaction* is a response to the natural rubber latex proteins and occurs within minutes of contact with the proteins. The manifestations of these allergic reactions can vary from skin redness, urticaria, rhinitis, conjunctivitis, or asthma to full-blown anaphylactic shock. Systemic reactions to latex may result from exposure to latex protein via various routes, including the skin, mucous membranes, inhalation, and blood.

**Latex-Food Syndrome.** Because some proteins in rubber are similar to food proteins, some foods may cause an allergic reaction in people who are allergic to latex. This is called *latex-food syndrome*. The most common of these foods are banana, avocado, chestnut, kiwi, tomato, water chestnut, guava, hazelnut, potato, peach, grape, and apricot. Most people with latex allergy have a positive allergy test to at least one related food.

## ❖ NURSING AND INTERPROFESSIONAL MANAGEMENT: LATEX ALLERGIES

Identifying patients and health care workers sensitive to latex is crucial to prevent adverse reactions. Obtain a thorough health history and history of any allergies, especially for patients with any complaints of latex contact symptoms. Not all latex-sensitive individuals can be identified, even with a careful and thorough history. The greatest risk factor is long-term multiple exposures to latex products (e.g., health care personnel, individuals who have had multiple surgeries, rubber industry workers). Additional risk factors include a patient history of allergic rhinitis, asthma, and allergies to certain foods (listed earlier).

Use latex precaution protocols for those patients identified as having a positive latex allergy test or a history of signs and symptoms related to latex exposure. Many health care facilities have created latex-free product carts that can be used for patients with latex allergies. The National Institute for Occupational Safety and Health (NIOSH) has published recommendations for preventing allergic reactions to latex in the workplace (Table 13-12).

Because of the potential for severe symptoms of food allergy, teach patients to avoid those foods. Other recommendations for people with latex and food allergies include wearing a Medic Alert bracelet or necklace and carrying an injectable epinephrine pen.

### Multiple Chemical Sensitivity

*Multiple chemical sensitivity (MCS)* is a subjective illness marked by recurrent, vague, nonspecific symptoms attributed to low levels of chemical, biologic, or physical agents.

Commonly accused substances include smoke, pesticides, plastics, synthetic fabrics, scented products, petroleum products, and paint fumes. Women between the ages of 30 and 50 are more likely to develop the symptoms. MCS is a controversial diagnosis and is not recognized as an illness by the American Medical Association or other authorities.[11]

The symptoms that people report are wide-ranging and not specific. They include headache, fatigue, dizziness, nausea, congestion, itching, sneezing, sore throat, chest pain, breathing problems, muscle pain or stiffness, skin rash, diarrhea, bloating, gas, confusion, difficulty concentrating, memory problems, and mood changes. These symptoms are usually subjective, and there is no evidence of a pathologic condition or physiologic dysfunction.

Diagnosis is usually made based on a patient's health history. There is no established test to diagnose MCS. The most effective treatment for MCS is to avoid the chemicals that may trigger the symptoms and create a chemical-free and odor-free home and workplace.

Psychotherapy is recommended as a primary option. In patients who are unwilling to undergo psychotherapy but willing to accept medications, antidepressants including selective serotonin reuptake inhibitors (SSRIs) (e.g., citalopram [Celexa]), have been used for treatment. Drugs for anxiety and sleep have also been used.

**TABLE 13-12 Guidelines for Preventing Allergic Latex Reactions**

- Use nonlatex gloves for activities that are not likely to involve contact with infectious materials (e.g., food preparation, housekeeping).
- Appropriate barrier protection is needed when handling infectious materials. If you choose latex gloves, use powder-free gloves with reduced protein content.
- When wearing latex gloves, do not use oil-based hand creams or lotions.
- Frequently clean work areas that are contaminated with latex-containing dust (e.g., carpets, ventilation ducts).
- Learn to recognize the symptoms of latex allergy: skin rash; hives; flushing; itching; nasal, eye, or sinus symptoms; asthma; and shock.
- If symptoms of latex allergy develop, avoid direct contact with latex gloves and products.
- Wear a Medic Alert bracelet and carry an epinephrine pen (e.g., EpiPen).

Source: National Institute for Occupational Safety and Health (NIOSH) (*www.cdc.gov/niosh*).

## AUTOIMMUNITY

**Autoimmunity** is an immune response against self in which the immune system no longer differentiates self from nonself. For some unknown reason, immune cells that are normally unresponsive (tolerant to self-antigens) are activated. In autoimmunity, autoantibodies and autosensitized T cells cause pathophysiologic tissue damage.

The cause of autoimmune diseases is still unknown. Age is thought to play some role because the number of circulating autoantibodies increases in people over age 50. However, the principal factors in the development of autoimmunity are (1) the inheritance of susceptibility genes, which may contribute to the failure of self-tolerance; and (2) initiation of autoreactivity by triggers, such as infections, which may activate self-reactive lymphocytes.

Autoimmune diseases tend to cluster, so that a given person may have more than one autoimmune disease (e.g., rheumatoid arthritis, Addison's disease), or the same or related autoimmune diseases may be found in other members of the same family. This observation has led to the concept of genetic predisposition to autoimmune disease. Most of the genetic research in this area correlates certain human leukocyte antigen (HLA) types with an autoimmune condition. (HLAs and disease association are discussed later in this chapter on p. 207.)

Even in a genetically predisposed person, some trigger is required for the initiation of autoreactivity. This may include infectious agents such as a virus. Viral infections can cause an alteration of cells or tissues that are not normally antigenic. The virally induced changes can make the cells or tissues antigenic. Viruses may be involved in the development of diseases such as type 1 diabetes mellitus. Rheumatic fever and rheumatic heart disease are autoimmune responses triggered by streptococcal infection and mediated by antibodies against group A $\beta$-hemolytic streptococci that cross-react with heart muscles and valves and synovial membranes.

Drugs can also be precipitating factors in autoimmune disease. Hemolytic anemia can result from methyldopa (Aldomet) administration. Procainamide (Pronestyl) can induce the formation of antinuclear antibodies and cause a lupus-like syndrome.

Gender and hormones also have a role in autoimmune disease. More women than men have autoimmune disease. During pregnancy, many autoimmune diseases get better. After delivery, the woman with an autoimmune disease frequently has an exacerbation.

### Autoimmune Diseases

Generally, autoimmune diseases are grouped according to organ-specific and systemic diseases (Table 13-13). Systemic lupus erythematosus (SLE) is a classic example of a systemic autoimmune disease characterized by damage to multiple organs. The cause is unknown, but there appears to be a loss of self-tolerance for the body's own DNA antigens.

In SLE, tissue injury appears to be the result of the formation of antinuclear antibodies. For some reason (possibly a viral infection), the cell membrane is damaged and deoxyribonucleic acid (DNA) is released into the systemic circulation, where it is viewed as nonself. This DNA is normally sequestered inside the nucleus of cells. On release into the circulation, the DNA antigen reacts with an antibody. Some antibodies are involved in immune complex formation, and others may cause damage directly. Once the complexes are deposited, the complement system is activated and further damages the tissue, especially the renal glomerulus. (SLE is discussed in Chapter 64.)

### Apheresis

Apheresis has been effectively used to treat autoimmune diseases and other diseases and disorders. *Apheresis* is a procedure to separate components of the blood followed by the removal of one or more of these components. Compound words are often used to describe any particular apheresis procedure, depending on the blood components being collected. *Plateletpheresis* is the removal of platelets, usually for collection from normal individuals to infuse into patients with low platelet counts (e.g., patients taking chemotherapy who develop thrombocytopenia). *Leukocytapheresis* is a general term indicating the removal of WBCs and is used in chronic myelogenous leukemia to remove high numbers of leukemic cells.

Apheresis is also used in hematopoietic stem cell transplantation to collect stem cells from peripheral blood. These stem cells can then be used to repopulate a person's bone marrow after high-dose chemotherapy (see section on hematopoietic stem cell transplants in Chapter 15).

**Plasmapheresis.** *Plasmapheresis* is the removal of plasma containing components causing or thought to cause disease. It can also be used to obtain plasma from healthy donors to administer to patients as replacement therapy.

When plasma is removed, it is replaced by substitute fluids such as saline, fresh-frozen plasma, or albumin. Thus the term *plasma exchange* more accurately describes this procedure.

Plasmapheresis has been used to treat autoimmune diseases such as SLE, glomerulonephritis, Goodpasture syndrome, myasthenia gravis, thrombocytopenic purpura, rheumatoid arthritis, and Guillain-Barré syndrome. Many disorders for which plasmapheresis is used are characterized by circulating autoantibodies (usually of the IgG class) and antigen-antibody complexes. The rationale for performing therapeutic plasmapheresis in autoimmune disorders is to remove pathologic substances present in plasma. Immunosuppressive therapy has been used to prevent recovery of IgG production, and plasmapheresis has been used to prevent antibody rebound.

In addition to removing antibodies and antigen-antibody complexes, plasmapheresis may also remove inflammatory mediators (e.g., complement) that are responsible for tissue damage. In the treatment of SLE, plasmapheresis is usually reserved for the patient having an acute attack who is unresponsive to conventional therapy.

Plasmapheresis involves the removal of whole blood through an IV device, and then the blood circulates through the apheresis machine. Inside the machine the blood is divided into plasma and its cellular components by centrifugation or membrane filtration. The plasma is generally replaced with normal saline, lactated Ringer's solution, fresh-frozen plasma, plasma protein fractions, or albumin. When blood is manually removed, only 500 mL can be taken at one time. However, with the use of apheresis procedures, more than 4 L of plasma can be pheresed in 2 to 3 hours.

As with administration of other blood products, be aware of side effects associated with plasmapheresis. The most common complications are hypotension and citrate toxicity. Hypotension is usually the result of a vasovagal reaction or transient volume changes. Citrate is used as an anticoagulant and may cause hypocalcemia, which may manifest as headache, paresthesias, and dizziness.

**TABLE 13-13 Examples of Autoimmune Diseases***

| | |
|---|---|
| **Systemic Diseases** | ***Endocrine System*** |
| • Rheumatoid arthritis | • Addison's disease |
| • Scleroderma (systemic sclerosis) | • Graves' disease |
| • Systemic lupus erythematosus | • Hypothyroidism |
| | • Thyroiditis |
| | • Type 1 diabetes mellitus |
| **Organ-Specific Diseases** | |
| ***Blood*** | ***Gastrointestinal System*** |
| • Autoimmune hemolytic anemia | • Celiac disease |
| • Hemochromatosis | • Inflammatory bowel disease |
| • Immune thrombocytopenic purpura (ITP) | • Pernicious anemia |
| ***Central Nervous System*** | ***Kidney*** |
| • Guillain-Barré syndrome | • Glomerulonephritis |
| • Multiple sclerosis | • Goodpasture syndrome |
| ***Muscle*** | ***Liver*** |
| • Myasthenia gravis | • Autoimmune hepatitis |
| | • Primary biliary cirrhosis |
| ***Heart*** | ***Eye*** |
| • Rheumatic fever | • Uveitis |

*These diseases are discussed in various chapters throughout the book.

## IMMUNODEFICIENCY DISORDERS

When the immune system does not adequately protect the body, **immunodeficiency** exists. Immunodeficiency disorders involve an impairment of one or more immune mechanisms, which include (1) phagocytosis, (2) humoral response, (3) cell-mediated response, (4) complement, and (5) a combined humoral and cell-mediated deficiency. Immunodeficiency disorders are *primary* if the immune cells are improperly developed or absent and *secondary* if the deficiency is caused by illnesses or treatment. Primary immunodeficiency disorders are rare and often serious, whereas secondary disorders are more common and less severe.

### Primary Immunodeficiency Disorders

The basic categories of primary immunodeficiency disorders are (1) phagocytic defects, (2) B cell deficiency, (3) T cell deficiency, and (4) a combined B cell and T cell deficiency (Table 13-14).

### Secondary Immunodeficiency Disorders

Some of the important factors that may cause secondary immunodeficiency disorders are listed in Table 13-15. Drug-induced immunosuppression is the most common. Immunosuppressive therapy is prescribed for patients to treat autoimmune disorders and to prevent transplant rejection. In addition, immunosuppression is a serious side effect of drugs used in cancer chemotherapy. Generalized leukopenia often results, leading to a decreased humoral and cell-mediated response. Therefore secondary infections are common in immunosuppressed patients.

Malnutrition alters cell-mediated immune responses. When protein is deficient over a prolonged period, the thymus gland atrophies and lymphoid tissue decreases. In addition, an increased susceptibility to infections always exists.

Hodgkin's lymphoma greatly impairs the cell-mediated immune response, and patients may die from severe viral or fungal infections. (Hodgkin's lymphoma is discussed in Chapter 30.) Viruses, especially rubella, may cause immunodeficiency by direct cytotoxic damage to lymphoid cells. Systemic infections can place such a demand on the immune system that resistance to a secondary or subsequent infection is impaired.

Radiation can destroy lymphocytes either directly or through depletion of stem cells. As the radiation dose is increased, more bone marrow atrophies, leading to severe pancytopenia and suppression of immune function. Splenectomy in children is especially dangerous and may lead to septicemia simply from respiratory tract infections.

Stress may alter the immune response. This response involves interrelationships among the nervous, endocrine, and immune systems (see Chapter 6).

**TABLE 13-14 Primary Immunodeficiency Disorders**

| Disorder | Affected Cells | Genetic Basis |
|---|---|---|
| Chronic granulomatous disease | PMNs, monocytes | X-linked |
| Job syndrome | PMNs, monocytes | — |
| Bruton's X-linked agammaglobulinemia | B | X-linked |
| Common variable hypogammaglobulinemia | B | — |
| Selective IgA, IgM, or IgG deficiency | B | Some X-linked |
| DiGeorge syndrome (thymic hypoplasia) | T | — |
| Severe combined immunodeficiency disease | Stem, B, T | X-linked or autosomal recessive |
| Ataxia-telangiectasia | B, T | Autosomal recessive |
| Wiskott-Aldrich syndrome | B, T | X-linked |
| Graft-versus-host disease | B, T | — |

*PMNs,* Polymorphonuclear neutrophils.

**TABLE 13-15 Causes of Secondary Immunodeficiency**

**Drug-Induced Immunodeficiency**
- Chemotherapy drugs
- Corticosteroids

**Age**
- Infants
- Older adults

**Malnutrition**
- Dietary deficiency
- Cachexia

**Therapies**
- Radiation
- Surgery
- Anesthesia

**Diseases or Disorders**
- Acquired immunodeficiency syndrome (AIDS)
- Cirrhosis
- Chronic kidney disease
- Diabetes mellitus
- Hodgkin's lymphoma
- Malignancies
- Systemic lupus erythematosus
- Burns
- Trauma
- Severe infection

**Stress**
- Chronic stress
- Trauma (physical or emotional)

## HUMAN LEUKOCYTE ANTIGEN SYSTEM

The antigens responsible for rejection of genetically unlike tissues are called the *major histocompatibility antigens.* These antigens are products of histocompatibility genes. In humans, they are called the **human leukocyte antigen (HLA)** system. The genes for the HLA antigens are linked and occur together on the sixth chromosome. HLAs are present on all nucleated cells and platelets. The HLA system is primarily used in matching organs and tissues for transplantation.

An important characteristic of HLA genes is that they are highly *polymorphic* (variable). Each HLA locus can have many different possible alleles, and thus many combinations exist. Each person has two alleles for each locus, one inherited from each parent. Both alleles of a locus are expressed independently (i.e., they are codominant). The proteins encoded by certain genes are known as *antigens.*

The entire set of A, B, C, D, and DR genes (the HLA genes) located on one chromosome is termed a *haplotype.* A complete set is inherited as a unit (haplotype). One haplotype is inherited from each parent (Fig. 13-10). This means that a person has HLA genes that are one-half identical to those of each parent. The HLA genes of one person have a 25% chance of being identical to the HLA genes of a sibling.

In organ transplantation A, B, and DR are primarily used for compatibility matching. The specific allele at each locus is identified by a number. For example, a person could have an HLA of A2, A6, B7, B27, DR4, and DR7. Currently more than 8000 HLA alleles have been identified for the various HLA genes.

### Human Leukocyte Antigen and Disease Associations

The early interest in HLAs was stimulated by the role of HLAs in matching donors and recipients of organ transplants. Since that time, the interest in the association between HLAs and disease has grown.

A number of diseases show significant associations with specific HLA alleles. People who have these alleles are much more likely to develop the associated disease than those who do not have the allele. However, the possession of a particular HLA allele does not mean that the person will necessarily develop the associated disease—only that the relative risk is greater than in the general population.

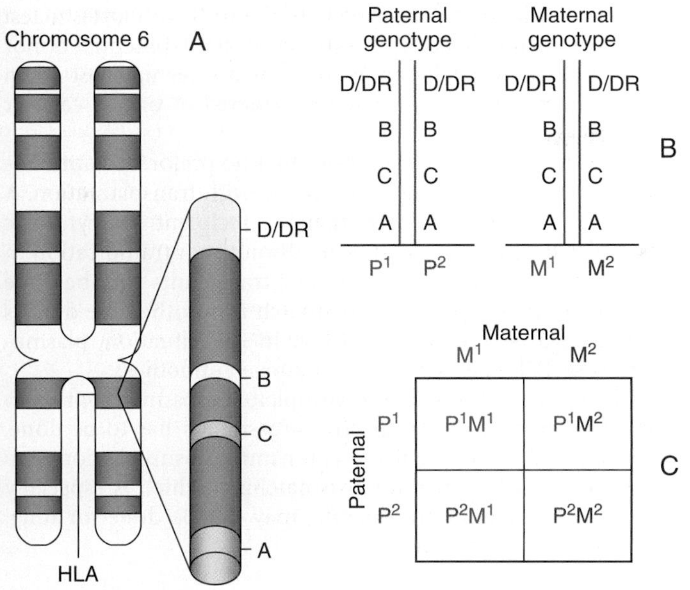


**FIG. 13-10** Patterns of human leukocyte antigen (HLA) inheritance. **A,** HLA genes are located on chromosome 6. **B,** The two haplotypes of the father are labeled $P^1$ and $P^2$, and the haplotypes of the mother are labeled $M^1$ and $M^2$. Each child inherits two haplotypes, one from each parent. **C,** Therefore only four combinations—$P^1M^1$, $P^1M^2$, $P^2M^1$, and $P^2M^2$—are possible, and 25% of the offspring will have identical HLA haplotypes.

Most of the HLA-associated diseases are classified as autoimmune disorders. Examples of HLA types and disease associations include (1) HLA-B27 and ankylosing spondylitis, (2) HLA-DR2 and HLA-DR3 and SLE, (3) HLA-DR3 and HLA-DR4 and diabetes mellitus, and (4) HLA-DR2 and narcolepsy.

The discovery of HLA associations with certain diseases is a major breakthrough in understanding the genetic bases of these diseases. It is now known that at least part of the genetic bases of HLA-associated diseases lies in the HLA region, but the actual mechanisms involved in these associations are still unknown. However, most individuals who inherit a specific HLA type (e.g., HLA-DR3) that is associated with a disease will never develop that disease.

Currently the association between HLAs and certain diseases is of minimal practical clinical importance. Nevertheless, there is promise for the development of clinical applications in the future. For example, with certain autoimmune diseases, it may be possible to identify members of a family at greatest risk for developing the same or a related autoimmune disease. These people would need close medical supervision, implementation of preventive measures (if possible), and early diagnosis and treatment to prevent chronic complications.

## ORGAN TRANSPLANTATION

Transplantation success has improved with advances in surgical technique, advances in histocompatibility testing, and more effective immunosuppressant drugs. Common tissue transplants include corneas, skin, bone marrow, heart valves, bone, and connective tissues (Fig. 13-11). Cornea transplants can prevent or correct blindness. Skin grafts are used in managing burn patients. Bone marrow is donated to help patients with leukemias and other malignancies.

Transplanted organs currently come from many different body systems. These organs include the heart, lung, liver, kidney, pancreas, and intestine. Multiple organs can be transplanted together, such as kidney and pancreas, kidney and liver, kidney and heart, or the complete intestinal tract. For example, many patients with diabetes who receive a pancreas transplant also receive a kidney transplant because the diabetes has not only impaired the pancreas but also led to renal failure.

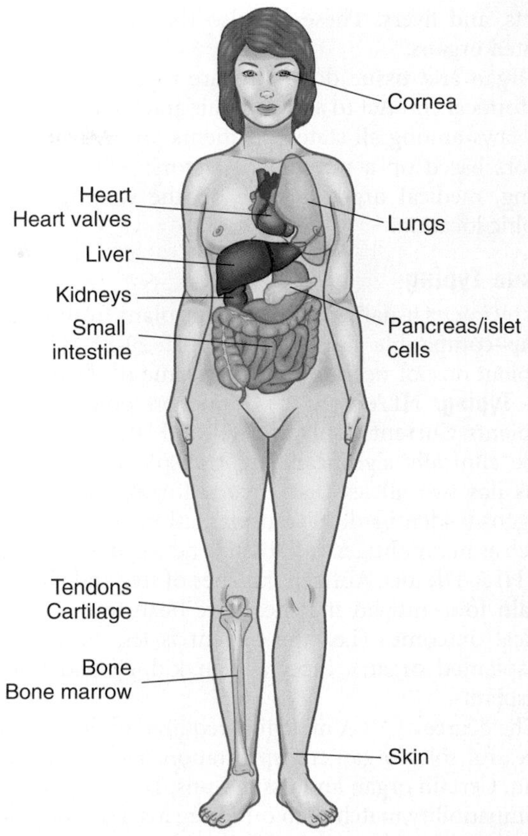


**FIG. 13-11** Tissues and organs that can be transplanted.

Some organs can be transplanted in parts or segments instead of transplanting an entire organ. Liver and lung lobes (rather than the whole organ) may be transplanted, or an intestine may be used in segments, thus allowing for one person's organ donation to benefit many recipients. This technique also enables living donors to donate part of an organ (or one of their organs in the case of kidneys).

Organ donations are taken from two sources: deceased (cadaver) and living donors. Most organs and tissues currently come from deceased donors. However, because of the shortage of organs from deceased donors, the use of related and living unrelated donor organs is increasing.

Individuals can make a decision to become a donor when they sign a donor card, the back of their driver's license, or a donor registry (depending on the state) and indicate their wish to donate organs. However, on their death or imminent death, the person's legal next of kin may need to consent to the donation regardless of whether the donor card is signed. Legal requirements and the facility's policy for a donor's legal next of kin to consent regardless of whether the donor card is signed vary from state to state and from facility to facility.

Currently more than 123,000 people are on the organ procurement and transplantation network's national waiting list, which is maintained by the United Network for Organ Sharing (UNOS). However, fewer than 30,000 people receive transplants annually. The organs in highest demand are kidneys, hearts, and livers. These are also the most commonly transplanted organs.[12]

Organ and tissue donations are regulated by the Uniform Anatomical Gift Act to allow for fair and consistent transplantation laws among all states.[13] Patients are matched to available donors based on a number of factors: ABO blood and HLA typing, medical urgency, time on the waiting list, and geographic location.

## Tissue Typing

The recipient usually receives a transplant from an ABO blood group–compatible donor (see Table 29-8). The donor and recipient do not need to share the same Rh factor.

**HLA Typing.** HLA typing is done on potential donors and recipients. Currently only the A, B, and DR antigens are thought to be clinically significant for transplantation. Because each locus has two alleles that encode for antigens, a total of six antigens is identified. In transplantation an attempt is made to match as many antigens as possible between the HLA-A, HLA-B, and HLA-DR loci. Antigen matches of five and six antigens and certain four-antigen matches have been found to have better clinical outcomes (i.e., the patient is less likely to reject the transplanted organ), especially in kidney and bone marrow transplants.

The degree of HLA matching required or deemed suitable for successful solid organ transplantation depends on the type of organ. Certain organ and tissue transplants require a closer histocompatibility match than other organs. For example, a cornea transplant can be accepted by nearly any individual because corneas are avascular and therefore no antibodies reach the cornea to cause rejection. In kidney and bone marrow transplantation, HLA matching is very important, since these transplants are at high risk for graft rejection. On the other hand, for liver transplants, HLA mismatches have little impact on graft survival. Heart and lung transplants fall somewhere in between, but minimizing HLA mismatches significantly improves survival. In addition, for liver, lung, and heart transplants, few donors are available, and it is difficult to get good HLA matches.

Transporting and storing donated organs can take time. The "best" match may live many miles from the "ideal" recipient. The need to have the "best" matches has to be balanced against the time it takes to harvest and transport a donated organ and then transplant it.

**Panel of Reactive Antibodies.** A *panel of reactive antibodies (PRA)* indicates the recipient's sensitivity to various HLAs before receiving a transplant. To detect preformed antibodies to HLA, the recipient's serum is mixed with a randomly selected panel of donor lymphocytes to determine reactivity. The potential recipient may have been exposed to HLA antigens by means of previous blood transfusions, pregnancy, or a previous organ transplant.

PRA allows for the determination of whether a recipient is of high or low reactivity to potential donors. The results for the PRA are calculated in percentages. A high PRA indicates that the person has a large number of cytotoxic antibodies and is highly sensitized, which means there is a poor chance of finding a crossmatch-negative donor. In patients awaiting transplantation, a PRA panel is usually done on a regular basis. In highly sensitized patients (high PRA), plasmapheresis and IV immunoglobulin (IVIG) can be used to lower the number of antibodies.

**Crossmatch.** A crossmatch is done to determine the existence of antibodies against the potential donor. A crossmatch uses serum from the recipient mixed with donor lymphocytes to test for any preformed anti-HLA antibodies to the potential donor organ. The crossmatch can be used as a screening test when possible living donors are being considered or once a cadaver donor is selected.

A negative crossmatch indicates that no preformed antibodies are present and it is safe to proceed with transplantation. A positive crossmatch indicates that the recipient has cytotoxic antibodies to the donor and is an absolute contraindication in living donor transplants. Live donor transplants may be done for patients with a positive crossmatch if no other live donors (with a negative crossmatch) exist. In this situation, plasmapheresis or IVIG can be done to remove antibodies.

It is not always possible to complete a crossmatch prior to transplantation. If a retrospective crossmatch has to be done, the results will have implications for immunosuppression protocols after the transplant. Crossmatching, which is especially important for kidney transplants, may not be done for lung, liver, and heart transplants.

## Transplant Rejection

Rejection is one of the major problems following organ transplantation. Rejection of organs occurs as a normal immune response to foreign tissue. The rejection can be prevented by using immunosuppression therapy, performing ABO and HLA matching, and ensuring that the crossmatch is negative. Unfortunately, many different HLAs exist, and a perfect match is nearly impossible unless the tissue is from oneself, an identical twin, or in some cases a sibling. Rejection can be hyperacute, acute, or chronic. Prevention, early diagnosis, and treatment of rejection are essential for long-term graft function.

**Hyperacute Rejection.** *Hyperacute rejection* occurs within 24 hours after transplantation because the blood vessels are rapidly destroyed. It occurs because the person had preexisting antibodies against the transplanted tissue or organ. There is no treatment for hyperacute rejection, and the transplanted organ is removed. Fortunately hyperacute rejection is a rare event because the final testing just before transplant usually determines whether the recipient is sensitized to any of the donor HLAs.

**Acute Rejection.** *Acute rejection* most commonly manifests in the first 6 months after transplantation. This type of rejection is usually a cell-mediated immune response by the recipient's lymphocytes, which have been activated against the donated (foreign) tissue or organ (Fig. 13-12). In addition to cell-mediated rejection, another type of acute rejection occurs when the recipient develops antibodies to the transplanted organ (humoral rejection).

It is not uncommon to have at least one rejection episode, especially with organs from deceased donors. These episodes are usually reversible with additional immunosuppressive therapy, which may include increased corticosteroid doses or polyclonal or monoclonal antibodies. Unfortunately, immunosuppressants increase the risk for infection. To combat acute rejection, all patients with transplants require long-term use of immunosuppressants, putting them at a high risk for infection, especially in the first few months after transplant when the immunosuppressive doses are highest.

**Chronic Rejection.** *Chronic rejection* is a process that occurs over months or years and is irreversible. Chronic rejection can occur for unknown reasons or from repeated episodes of acute rejection. The transplanted organ is infiltrated with large numbers of T and B cells characteristic of an ongoing,

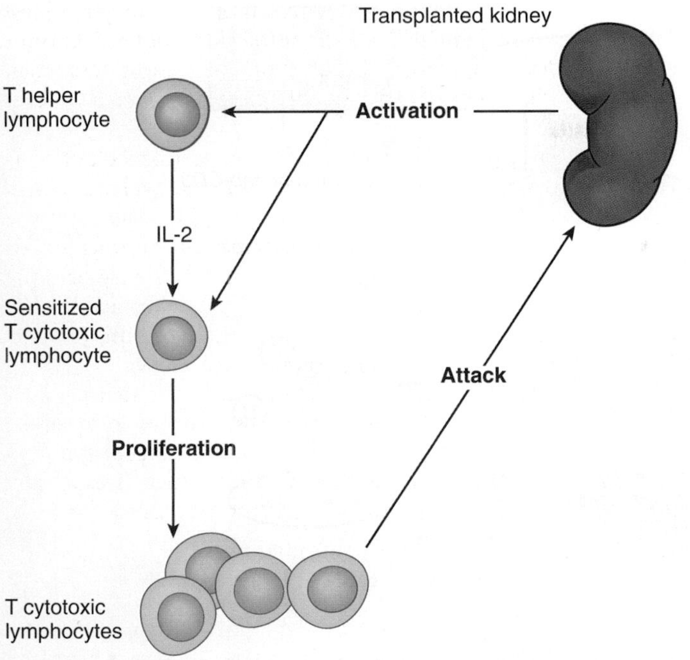


**FIG. 13-12** Mechanism of action of T cytotoxic lymphocyte activation and attack of transplanted tissue. The transplanted organ (e.g., kidney) is recognized as foreign and activates the immune system. T helper cells are activated to produce interleukin-2 *(IL-2),* and T cytotoxic lymphocytes are sensitized. After the T cytotoxic cells proliferate, they attack the transplanted organ.

low-grade, immune-mediated injury. Chronic rejection results in fibrosis and scarring. In heart transplants it manifests as accelerated coronary artery disease. In lung transplants it manifests as bronchiolitis obliterans. In liver transplants it is characterized by loss of bile ducts. In kidney transplants it manifests as fibrosis and glomerulopathy.

There is no definitive therapy for this type of rejection. Treatment is primarily supportive. This type of rejection is difficult to manage and is not associated with the optimistic prognosis of acute rejection.

## Immunosuppressive Therapy

**Immunosuppressive therapy** requires a lifelong balance between rejection and infection. On one hand, the immune response must be suppressed to prevent rejection of the transplanted organ. On the other hand, an adequate immune response must be maintained to prevent overwhelming infection and the development of malignancies.[14]

Many of the drugs used to achieve immunosuppression have significant side effects. Because transplant recipients must take immunosuppressants for life, the risk of toxicity continues for the rest of their lives.

Immunosuppressant drugs are listed in Table 13-16. With the use of a combination of agents that work during different phases of the immune response (Fig. 13-13), lower doses of each drug can be given to produce effective immunosuppression while minimizing side effects.

The major immunosuppressive agents are (1) calcineurin inhibitors, including cyclosporine (Sandimmune, Neoral, Gengraf) and tacrolimus (Prograf); (2) corticosteroids (prednisone, methylprednisolone [Solu-Medrol] IV); (3) mycophenolate mofetil (CellCept, Myfortic); and (4) sirolimus (Rapamune). Azathioprine (Imuran) and cyclophosphamide (Cytoxan) can also be used. Muromonab-CD3 (Orthoclone OKT3) and either horse antithymocyte globulin (Atgam) or rabbit antithymocycte globulin (ATG) are IV medications used for short periods to prevent early rejection or reverse acute rejection.

Immunosuppression protocols are highly variable among transplant centers, with different combinations of medications being used. Most patients are initially on triple therapy. The standard triple therapy usually includes a calcineurin inhibitor, a corticosteroid, and mycophenolate mofetil.

The doses of immunosuppressant drugs are reduced over time after the transplant. Patients taking corticosteroids may be weaned off after a few years. The trend in many transplant centers is to use immunosuppression protocols that do not contain corticosteroids because of their many side effects.

**Calcineurin Inhibitors.** This group of drugs, including tacrolimus and cyclosporine, is the foundation of most immunosuppression regimens. As the most effective immunosuppressants, these drugs prevent a cell-mediated attack against the transplanted organ (Fig. 13-13). These drugs do not cause bone marrow suppression or alterations of the normal inflammatory response. They are generally used in combination with corticosteroids, mycophenolate mofetil, and sirolimus. Tacrolimus is the most widely used calcineurin inhibitor. Cyclosporine is being used less frequently.

Many of the side effects of calcineurin inhibitors are dose related. These drugs are potentially nephrotoxic. Drug levels are monitored closely to prevent toxicity.

**DRUG ALERT Tacrolimus and Cyclosporine**
- A substance in grapefruit and grapefruit juice prevents metabolism of these drugs.
- Consuming grapefruit or grapefruit juice while using these drugs could increase their toxicity.

**Mycophenolate Mofetil.** Mycophenolate mofetil inhibits purine synthesis with suppressive effects on T and B cells. The major limitation of this drug is its GI toxicities, including nausea, vomiting, and diarrhea. In many cases the side effects can be diminished by lowering the dose or giving smaller doses more frequently.

**DRUG ALERT Mycophenolate Mofetil**
- When given IV, it must be reconstituted in $D_5W$ and no other solution.
- Do not give as IV bolus. Administer over 2 or more hours.

**Sirolimus.** Sirolimus is an immunosuppressive agent that suppresses T cell activation and proliferation. It is used in combination with corticosteroids, cyclosporine, and/or tacrolimus.

**Monoclonal Antibodies.** Monoclonal antibodies are used for preventing and treating acute rejection episodes. Muromonab-CD3 was the first of these monoclonal antibodies to be used in clinical transplantation. It is a mouse monoclonal antibody that binds with the CD3 antigen found on the surface of human thymocytes and mature T cells. It interferes with the function of T cells, the pivotal cells involved in rejection. It is administered via IV bolus. All T cells are affected, rather than just the subset active in graft rejection. Within minutes after the initial infusion of muromonab-CD3, the number of circulating T cells decreases significantly.

A flu-like syndrome occurs during the first few days of treatment because of cytokine release. Side effects include fever, rigors, headache, myalgias, and various GI disturbances. To reduce the expected side effects of muromonab-CD3, give patients acetaminophen (Tylenol), diphenhydramine

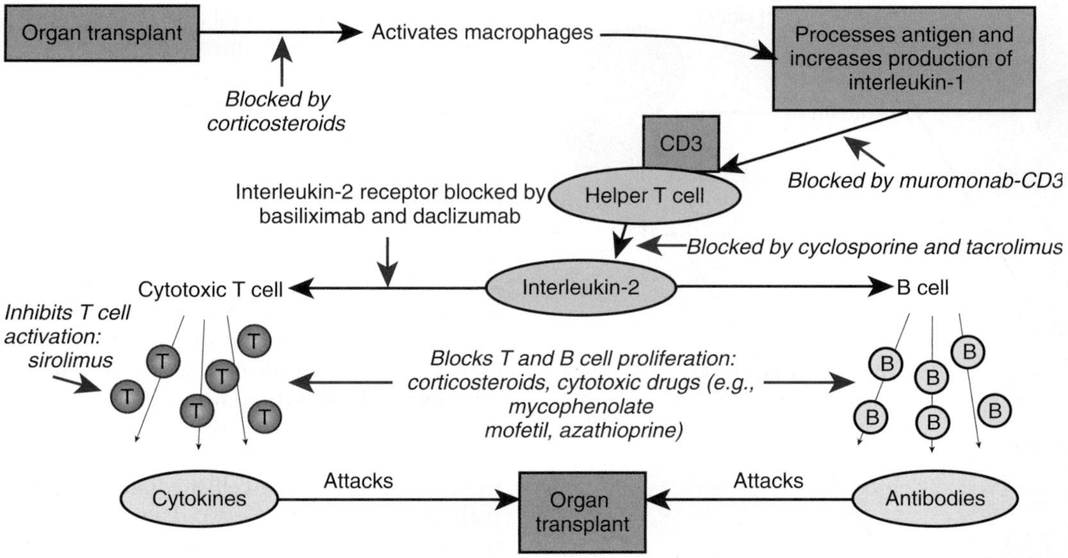


**FIG. 13-13** Sites of action for immunosuppressive agents. (Adapted from McKenry L, Tessier E, Hogan M: *Mosby's pharmacology in nursing,* St Louis, 2006, Mosby.)

(Benadryl), and IV methylprednisolone before administering the dose.

Newer-generation monoclonal antibodies are a hybrid of mouse and human antibodies and have fewer side effects than muromonab-CD3 because they have been "humanized." These include daclizumab (Zenapax) and basiliximab (Simulect), which target the IL-2 receptor and impair lymphocyte proliferation. Another monoclonal antibody is alemtuzumab (Campath), which targets the CD52 antigen found on T and B cells, monocytes, and macrophages. It can cause prolonged T cell depletion.

**Polyclonal Antibodies.** Polyclonal antibodies to T cells include horse antithymocyte globulin (Atgam) and rabbit antithymocycte globulin (Thymoglobulin, ATG). These agents are derived by injecting animals (rabbit or horse) with human lymphoid cells, then harvesting and purifying the resultant antibody. They have been commonly used for induction immunosuppression and treatment of acute rejection.

Allergic reactions to the foreign proteins from the host animal, manifested by fever, arthralgias, and tachycardia, are common but usually not severe enough to preclude use. These side effects can be decreased by administering the preparation slowly, over 4 to 6 hours, and premedicating patients with acetaminophen, diphenhydramine, and methylprednisolone. The main toxicities of polyclonal antibodies are leukopenia and thrombocytopenia caused by antibody contaminants that are not completely removed during preparation of the antibodies.

## GRAFT-VERSUS-HOST DISEASE

*Graft-versus-host disease (GVHD)* occurs when an immunoincompetent (immunodeficient) patient receives immunocompetent cells. A GVHD response is most commonly seen in hematopoietic stem cell transplants. In most transplantation situations, the biggest concern is the patient's (host's) rejection of the organ or transplant. However, in GVHD disease, the graft (donated tissue) rejects the host (recipient) tissue.[15]

The GVHD response may begin 7 to 30 days after transplantation. Once the reaction is started, little can be done to modify its course. The exact mechanism involved in this reaction is not completely understood. However, it involves donor T cells attacking and destroying vulnerable host (recipient) cells.

The target organs for the GVHD phenomenon are the skin, liver, and GI tract. The skin disease may be a maculopapular rash, which may be pruritic or painful. It initially involves the palms and soles of the feet but can progress to a generalized erythema with bullous formation and desquamation (shedding of the outer layer of skin). The liver disease may range from mild jaundice with elevated liver enzymes to hepatic coma. The GI manifestations may include mild to severe diarrhea, severe abdominal pain, GI bleeding, and malabsorption.

The biggest problem with GVHD is infection, with different types of infections seen in different periods. Bacterial and fungal infections predominate immediately after transplantation when granulocytopenia exists. The development of interstitial pneumonitis is the primary concern later in the course of the disease.

There is no adequate treatment of GVHD once it is established. Although corticosteroids are often used, they enhance the susceptibility to infection. The use of immunosuppressive agents (e.g., methotrexate, cyclosporine) has been most effective as a preventive rather than a treatment measure. Radiation of blood products before they are administered is another measure to prevent T cell replication.

## TABLE 13-16 Drug Therapy

### *Immunosuppressive Therapy*

| Agent | Route | Mechanism of Action | Side Effects |
|---|---|---|---|
| **Corticosteroids** | | | |
| prednisone, methylprednisolone (Solu-Medrol) | PO, IV | Suppress inflammatory response. Inhibit cytokine production (IL-1, IL-6, TNF) and T cell activation and proliferation | Peptic ulcers, hypertension, osteoporosis, $Na^+$ and $H_2O$ retention, muscle weakness, easy bruising, delayed healing, hyperglycemia, ↑ risk for infection |
| **Calcineurin Inhibitors** | | | |
| cyclosporine (Sandimmune, Neoral, Gengraf) | PO, IV | Acts on T helper cells to prevent production and release of IL-2. Inhibits proliferation of T and B cells | Nephrotoxicity, ↑ risk for infection, neurotoxicity (tremors, seizures), hepatotoxicity, lymphoma, hypertension, tremors, hirsutism, leukopenia, gingival hyperplasia |
| tacrolimus (Prograf) | PO, IV | Same as cyclosporine but more effective | Same as cyclosporine |
| **Cytotoxic (Antiproliferative) Drugs** | | | |
| mycophenolate mofetil (CellCept, Myfortic) | PO, IV | Inhibits purine synthesis. Suppresses proliferation of T and B cells | Diarrhea, nausea and vomiting, neutropenia, thrombocytopenia, ↑ risk for infection, ↑ incidence of malignancies |
| azathioprine (Imuran) | PO, IV | Inhibits purine synthesis. Suppresses proliferation of T and B cells | Bone marrow suppression (neutropenia, anemia, thrombocytopenia) |
| cyclophosphamide (Cytoxan, Neosar) | PO, IV | Cross-links DNA, leading to cell injury and death. Results in decrease in number and activity of T and B cells | Neutropenia, hemorrhagic cystitis |
| sirolimus (Rapamune) | PO | Binds to mechanistic target of rapamycin (mTOR), thereby suppressing T cell activation and proliferation | ↑ Risk for infection, leukopenia, anemia, thrombocytopenia, hyperlipidemia, hypercholesterolemia, arthralgias, diarrhea. ↑ incidence of malignancies |
| everolimus (Zortress) | PO | Same as above | Peripheral edema, constipation, hypertension, nausea, anemia, urinary tract infection, hyperlipidemia |
| **Monoclonal Antibodies** | | | |
| muromonab-CD3 (Orthoclone OKT3) | IV push | Monoclonal antibody that binds to CD3 receptors on T cells, causing cell lysis. Inhibits function of T cells | Fever, chills, dyspnea, chest pain, nausea and vomiting<br>Anaphylactic reactions include pulmonary edema, cardiac or respiratory arrest. |
| daclizumab (Zenapax) | IV | Monoclonal antibody that targets IL-2 receptor and inhibits T cell activation and proliferation | Can cause acute hypersensitivity reaction, including anaphylaxis |
| basiliximab (Simulect) | IV | Same as daclizumab | Same as daclizumab |
| alemtuzumab (Campath) | IV | Monoclonal antibody that targets the CD52 antigen on T and B cells, monocytes, and macrophages. Causes prolonged T cell depletion | Fever, chills, dyspnea, chest pain, nausea and vomiting. Neutropenia, anemia, thrombocytopenia<br>Increased risk of opportunistic infections |
| **Polyclonal Antibodies** | | | |
| Horse antithymocyte globulin (Atgam)<br>Rabbit antithymocyte globulin (Thymoglobulin, ATG) | IV | Prepared by immunizing horse or rabbit with human thymocytes or T cells. Polyclonal antibodies directed against T cells, thus depleting them | Fever, chills, dyspnea, myalgia, chest pain, nausea and vomiting, anaphylaxis, leukopenia, thrombocytopenia, rash, ↑ risk for infection |
| **Other** | | | |
| belatacept (Nulojix) | IV | Prevents the activation of T cells | Anemia, diarrhea, constipation, urinary tract infection, peripheral edema |

*IL,* Interleukin; *TNF,* tumor necrosis factor.

## BRIDGE TO NCLEX EXAMINATION

The number of the question corresponds to the same-numbered outcome at the beginning of the chapter.

1. The function of monocytes in immunity is related to their ability to
   **a.** stimulate the production of T and B lymphocytes.
   **b.** produce antibodies on exposure to foreign substances.
   **c.** bind antigens and stimulate natural killer cell activation.
   **d.** capture antigens by phagocytosis and present them to lymphocytes.
2. One function of cell-mediated immunity is
   **a.** formation of antibodies.
   **b.** activation of the complement system.
   **c.** surveillance for malignant cell changes.
   **d.** opsonization of antigens to allow phagocytosis by neutrophils.
3. The reason newborns are protected for the first 6 months of life from bacterial infections is because of the maternal transmission of
   **a.** IgG.
   **b.** IgA.
   **c.** IgM.
   **d.** IgE.
4. In a type I hypersensitivity reaction the primary immunologic disorder appears to be
   **a.** binding of IgG to an antigen on a cell surface.
   **b.** deposit of antigen-antibody complexes in small vessels.
   **c.** release of cytokines used to interact with specific antigens.
   **d.** release of chemical mediators from IgE-bound mast cells and basophils.

5. The nurse is alerted to possible anaphylactic shock immediately after a patient has received IM penicillin by the development of
   **a.** edema and itching at the injection site.
   **b.** sneezing and itching of the nose and eyes.
   **c.** a wheal-and-flare reaction at the injection site.
   **d.** chest tightness and production of thick sputum.
6. The nurse advises a friend who asks him to administer his allergy shots that
   **a.** it is illegal for nurses to administer injections outside of a medical setting.
   **b.** he is qualified to do it if the friend has epinephrine in an injectable syringe provided with his extract.
   **c.** avoiding the allergens is a more effective way of controlling allergies, and allergy shots are not usually effective.
   **d.** immunotherapy should only be administered in a setting where emergency equipment and drugs are available.
7. Association between HLA antigens and diseases is *most* commonly found in what disease conditions?
   **a.** Malignancies
   **b.** Infectious diseases
   **c.** Neurologic diseases
   **d.** Autoimmune disorders
8. A patient is undergoing plasmapheresis for treatment of systemic lupus erythematosus. The nurse explains that plasmapheresis is used in her treatment to
   **a.** remove T lymphocytes in her blood that are producing antinuclear antibodies.
   **b.** remove normal particles in her blood that are being damaged by autoantibodies.
   **c.** exchange her plasma that contains antinuclear antibodies with a substitute fluid.
   **d.** replace viral-damaged cellular components of her blood with replacement whole blood.
9. The *most* common cause of secondary immunodeficiencies is
   **a.** drugs.
   **b.** stress.
   **c.** malnutrition.
   **d.** human immunodeficiency virus.
10. What accurately describes rejection following transplantation?
    **a.** Hyperacute rejection can be treated with OKT3.
    **b.** Acute rejection can be treated with sirolimus or tacrolimus.
    **c.** Chronic rejection can be treated with tacrolimus or cyclosporine.
    **d.** Hyperacute reaction can usually be avoided if crossmatching is done before the transplantation.
11. In a person having an acute rejection of a transplanted kidney, what would help the nurse understand the course of events *(select all that apply)*?
    **a.** A new transplant should be considered.
    **b.** Acute rejection can be treated with OKT3.
    **c.** Acute rejection usually leads to chronic rejection.
    **d.** Corticosteroids are the most successful drugs used to treat acute rejection.
    **e.** Acute rejection is common after a transplant and can be treated with drug therapy.

1. d, 2. c, 3. a, 4. d, 5. a, 6. d, 7. d, 8. c, 9. a, 10. d, 11. b, e

For rationales to these answers and even more NCLEX review questions, visit *http://evolve.elsevier.com/Lewis/medsurg.*

## EVOLVE WEBSITE

http://evolve.elsevier.com/Lewis/medsurg

**Review Questions (Online Only)**

**Key Points**

**Answer Key for Questions**

- Rationales for Bridge to NCLEX Examination Questions

**Conceptual Care Map Creator**

**Audio Glossary**

**Supporting Media**

- Animations
  - Antibodies and Antigens
  - Vaccination

**Content Updates**

## REFERENCES


1. Sparber F: Langerhans cells: an update, *J Dtsch Dermatol Ges* 12(12):1107, 2014.
2. Pritz T, Weinberger B, Grubeck-Loebenstein B: The aging bone marrow and its impact on immune responses in old age, *Immunol Lett* 162(1 Pt B): 310, 2014.
3. Moore LE, Kemp AM, Kemp SF: Recognition, treatment, and prevention of anaphylaxis, *Immunol Allergy Clin North Am* 35(2):363, 2015.
4. Simmons S: Taking the bite out of food allergies, *Nursing* 44(12):44, 2014.
5. Vacca VM, McMahon-Bowen E: Anaphylaxis, *Nursing* 43(11):16, 2013.
6. Yunker NS, Wagner BJ: A pharmacologic review of anaphylaxis, *Plast Surg Nurs* 34(4):183, 2014.
7. Lee S, Nolte H, Benninger MS: Clinical considerations in the use of sublingual immunotherapy for allergic rhinitis, *Am J Rhinol Allergy* 29(2):106, 2015.
8. Compalati E, Braido F, Walter Canonica G: Sublingual immunotherapy: recent advances, *Allergol Int* 62(4):415, 2013.
9. Latex allergies. Retrieved from *www.webmd.com/allergies/latex-allergies.*
10. Preventing allergic reactions to natural rubber latex in the workplace. Retrieved from *http://www.cdc.gov/niosh/docs/97-135/pdfs/97-135.pdf.*
11. Multiple chemical sensitivity. Retrieved from *www.webmd.com/allergies/multiple-chemical-sensitivity.*
12. United Network of Organ Sharing (UNOS). Retrieved from *www.unos.org.*
13. Uniform Anatomical Gift Act. Retrieved from *http://uniformlaws.org/Act.aspx?title=Anatomical%20Gift%20Act.*
14. Immunosuppression. Retrieved from *http://emedicine.medscape.com/article/432316-overview.*
15. Flowers ME, Martin PJ: How we treat chronic graft-versus-host disease, *Blood* 125(4):606, 2015.

14

# Infection and Human Immunodeficiency Virus Infection

Jeffrey Kwong

*Do not allow the pain of loss to stop the process of living.*

*Trent Thomas*

http://evolve.elsevier.com/Lewis/medsurg/

## LEARNING OUTCOMES

1. Evaluate the impact of emerging and reemerging infections on health care.
2. Identify appropriate interventions to reduce health care-associated infections (HAIs).
3. Explain the ways human immunodeficiency virus (HIV) is transmitted and factors that affect transmission.
4. Describe the pathophysiology of HIV infection.
5. Chart the spectrum of untreated HIV infection.
6. Identify the diagnostic criteria for acquired immunodeficiency syndrome (AIDS).
7. Describe methods used to test for HIV infection.
8. Discuss the interprofessional management of HIV infection.
9. Summarize the characteristics of opportunistic diseases associated with AIDS.
10. Describe the potential complications associated with long-term treatment of HIV infection.
11. Compare and contrast HIV prevention methods.
12. Describe the nursing management of HIV-infected patients and HIV-at-risk patients.

## KEY TERMS

acquired immunodeficiency syndrome (AIDS), p. 221
antiretroviral therapy (ART), p. 219
emerging infection, p. 215
health care–associated infections (HAIs), p. 217
human immunodeficiency virus (HIV), p. 218
opportunistic diseases, p. 219
postexposure prophylaxis (PEP), p. 226
preexposure prophylaxis (PrEP) p. 223
reverse transcriptase, p. 219
standard precautions, p. 218
transmission-based precautions, p. 218
viral load, p. 220
window period, p. 222

This chapter presents a brief overview of emerging and health care–associated infections (HAIs). In addition, this chapter provides a comprehensive discussion of human immunodeficiency virus (HIV) infection, focusing on transmission, pathophysiology, interprofessional care, and nursing management.

## INFECTIONS

Infections, such as lower respiratory tract infections, malaria, HIV, and tuberculosis (TB), are responsible for a significant number of deaths worldwide. Infection occurs when a *pathogen* (a microorganism that causes disease) invades the body, begins to multiply, and produces disease, usually causing harm to the host. The signs and symptoms of infection are a result of specific pathogen activity, which triggers inflammation and other immune responses.

Infections can be categorized as localized, disseminated, or systemic. A *localized* infection is limited to a small area. A *disseminated* infection has spread to areas of the body beyond the initial site of infection. *Systemic* infections have spread extensively throughout the body, often via the blood.

### TYPES OF PATHOGENS

The many different kinds of pathogens can be classified into several groups, including bacteria, viruses, fungi, protozoa, and prions. *Bacteria* are one-celled organisms that are common throughout nature. Many bacteria are normal flora. They live harmoniously in or on the human body without causing disease under normal circumstances. Normal flora protect the human body by preventing the overgrowth of other microorganisms. For example, *Escherichia coli* is a bacteria that is part of the normal flora in the large intestine.

Bacteria cause disease in two ways: by entering the body and growing inside human cells (e.g., TB) or by secreting toxins that damage cells (e.g., *Staphylococcus aureus*). Bacteria are divided into categories based on the shape of their cells. *Cocci*, such as streptococci and staphylococci, are round. *Bacilli* are rod shaped

Reviewed by Suzanne Jed, MSN, FNP-BC, Senior Clinical Technical Advisor, International Training and Education Center for Health (I-TECH) South Africa, University of Washington, Pretoria, South Africa; Allison J. Terry, RN, PhD, Associate Professor of Nursing, Assistant Dean of Clinical Practice, School of Nursing, Auburn University Montgomery, Montgomery, Alabama; and Daniel Worrall, MSN, ANP-BC, Nurse Practitioner, Massachusetts General Hospital, Boston, Massachusetts.

**TABLE 14-1 Disease-Causing Bacteria**

| Bacteria | Diseases Caused |
|---|---|
| *Chlamydia trachomatis* | Chlamydia, lymphogranuloma venereum |
| Clostridia | |
| • *Clostridium botulinum* | Food poisoning with progressive muscle paralysis |
| • *Clostridium tetani* | Tetanus (lockjaw) |
| *Corynebacterium diphtheriae* | Diphtheria |
| *Escherichia coli* | Urinary tract infections, peritonitis, hemolytic-uremic syndrome |
| Haemophilus | |
| • *Haemophilus influenzae* | Nasopharyngitis, meningitis, pneumonia |
| • *Haemophilus pertussis* | Pertussis (whooping cough) |
| *Helicobacter pylori* | Peptic ulcers, gastritis |
| *Klebsiella-Enterobacter* organisms | Urinary tract infections, peritonitis, pneumonia |
| *Legionella pneumophila* | Pneumonia (Legionnaires' disease) |
| Mycobacteria | |
| • *Mycobacterium leprae* | Hansen's disease (leprosy) |
| • *Mycobacterium tuberculosis* | Tuberculosis |
| Neisseriae | |
| • *Neisseria gonorrhoeae* | Gonorrhea, pelvic inflammatory disease, proctitis |
| • *Neisseria meningitidis* | Meningococcemia, meningitis |
| *Proteus* species | Urinary tract infections, peritonitis |
| *Pseudomonas aeruginosa* | Urinary tract infections, meningitis |
| Salmonella | |
| • *Salmonella typhi* | Typhoid fever |
| • Other *Salmonella* organisms | Food poisoning, gastroenteritis |
| *Shigella* | Shigellosis; diarrhea, abdominal pain, and fever (dysentery) |
| *Staphylococcus aureus* | Skin infections, pneumonia, urinary tract infections, acute osteomyelitis, toxic shock syndrome |
| Streptococci | |
| • *Streptococcus faecalis* | Genitourinary infection, infection of surgical wounds |
| • *Streptococcus pneumoniae* | Pneumococcal pneumonia |
| • *Streptococcus pyogenes* (group A β-hemolytic streptococci) | Pharyngitis, scarlet fever, rheumatic fever, acute glomerulonephritis, erysipelas, pneumonia |
| • *S. pyogenes* (group B β-hemolytic streptococci) | Urinary tract infections |
| • *Streptococcus viridans* | Bacterial endocarditis |
| *Treponema pallidum* | Syphilis |

**TABLE 14-2 Disease-Causing Viruses**

| Virus | Diseases Caused |
|---|---|
| Adenoviruses | Upper respiratory tract infection, pneumonia |
| Arbovirus | Syndrome of fever, malaise, headache, myalgia; aseptic meningitis; encephalitis |
| Coronavirus | Upper respiratory tract infection |
| Coxsackieviruses A and B | Upper respiratory tract infection, gastroenteritis, acute myocarditis, aseptic meningitis |
| Ebola | Hemorrhagic fever |
| Echoviruses | Upper respiratory tract infection, gastroenteritis, aseptic meningitis |
| Hepatitis A, B, C | Viral hepatitis |
| Herpesviruses | |
| • Cytomegalovirus (CMV) | Gastroenteritis; pneumonia and retinal damage in immunosuppressed individuals, infectious mononucleosis-like syndrome |
| • Epstein-Barr | Mononucleosis, Burkitt's lymphoma (possibly) |
| • Herpes simplex type 1 | Herpes labialis ("fever blisters"), genital herpes infection |
| • Herpes simplex type 2 | Genital herpes infection |
| • Varicella-zoster | Chickenpox, shingles |
| Human immunodeficiency virus (HIV) | HIV infection, AIDS |
| Influenza A and B | Upper respiratory tract infection, H1N1 (swine) flu, H5N1 avian (bird) flu |
| Mumps | Parotitis, orchitis in postpubertal males |
| Papillomavirus | Genital warts, cervical and anal cancer |
| Parainfluenza 1-4 | Upper respiratory tract infection |
| Parvovirus | Gastroenteritis |
| Poliovirus | Poliomyelitis |
| Pox viruses | Smallpox, Molluscum contagiosum |
| Reoviruses 1, 2, 3 | Upper respiratory tract infection |
| Respiratory syncytial virus | Gastroenteritis, respiratory tract infection |
| Rhabdovirus | Rabies |
| Rhinovirus | Upper respiratory tract infection, pneumonia |
| Rotaviruses | Gastroenteritis |
| Rubella | German measles |
| Rubeola | Measles |
| West Nile virus | Flu-like symptoms, meningitis, encephalitis |

and include tetanus and TB. *Curved rods* include *Vibrio* bacteria, one of which causes cholera. *Spirochetes* are spiral shaped and include the organisms that cause leprosy and syphilis. Table 14-1 lists common bacteria that cause disease.

*Viruses,* unlike bacteria, do not have a cellular structure. They are simple infectious particles that consist of a small amount of genetic material (either ribonucleic acid [RNA] or deoxyribonucleic acid [DNA]) and a protein envelope. Viruses can reproduce only after releasing their genetic material into the cell of another living organism. Examples of diseases caused by viruses are presented in Table 14-2.

*Fungi* are organisms similar to plants, but they lack chlorophyll. *Mycosis* is any disease caused by a fungus. Pathogenic fungi cause infections that are usually localized but can become disseminated in an immunocompromised person. Tinea pedis (athlete's foot) and tinea corporis (ringworm) are two common mycotic infections. Some fungi are normal flora in the body, but when overgrowth occurs, disease can result. Overgrowth of *Candida albicans,* for example, can cause candidiasis in the mouth (thrush), esophagus, intestines, and vagina. Other fungi and their respective mycotic infections are listed in Table 14-3.

*Protozoa* are single-cell, animal-like microorganisms. Protozoa normally live in soil and bodies of water. When introduced into the human body, they can cause infection. Amoebic dysentery and giardiasis are caused by protozoal parasites. Malaria is caused by a sporozoa called *Plasmodium malariae.*

*Prions* are infectious particles that contain abnormally shaped proteins. Not all prions cause disease, but those that do

TABLE 14-3 **Disease-Causing Fungi**

| Fungi | Diseases Caused | Organs Affected |
|---|---|---|
| *Aspergillus fumigatus* | Aspergillosis | Lungs* |
| | Otomycosis | Ears |
| *Blastomyces dermatitidis* | Blastomycosis | Lungs, various organs |
| *Candida albicans* | Candidiasis | Intestines |
| | Vaginitis | Vagina |
| | Thrush | Skin,† mouth |
| *Coccidioides immitis* | Coccidioidomycosis | Lungs* |
| *Pneumocystis jiroveci* | Pneumocystis pneumonia (PCP) | Lungs* |
| *Sporothrix schenckii* | Sporotrichosis | Skin, lymph vessels |
| *Trichophyton* | Tinea pedis | Skin† |
| *Microsporum* | Tinea capitis | Skin† |
| *Epidermophyton* | Tinea corporis | Skin† |

*See Table 27-14: Fungal Infections of the Lung.
†See Table 23-7: Common Fungal Infections of the Skin.

typically affect the nervous system. They can cause a group of illnesses called *transmissible spongiform encephalopathies (TSEs)*. Examples of TSEs are Creutzfeldt-Jakob disease and bovine spongiform encephalopathy in cattle (also known as mad cow disease).

## EMERGING INFECTIONS

An **emerging infection** is an infectious disease that has recently increased in incidence or that threatens to increase in the immediate future.[1] Examples of emerging infections are described in Table 14-4. Emerging infectious diseases can originate from unknown sources or from contact with animals, changes in known diseases, or biologic warfare. For example, severe acute respiratory syndrome (SARS) and the West Nile virus come from animal sources. Others emerged when a previously treatable organism (e.g., *S. aureus*) developed resistance to antibiotics.

The battle against infection is not new, but modern technologies have changed the rules of the game. Global travel, population density, encroachment into new environments, misuse of antibiotics, and bioterrorism have increased the risk for widespread distribution of emerging infections.

Additionally, some diseases thought to be under control, such as TB, measles, and pertussis, have reemerged.[2] Newer infections have also been identified, such as Middle Eastern Respiratory Syndrome (MERS), SARS, Ebola virus, Chikungunya (a self-limiting viral illness causing flu-like symptoms seen in Africa, Asia, and more recently the Caribbean), and influenza A (H1N1) virus.

Studies in *zoonosis* (science of transmission of diseases from animals to humans) have shown that many known infectious diseases come from animal and insect vectors. The SARS outbreak in China in 2003, for instance, was linked to the civet cat, a small carnivorous mammal found throughout much of Asia and Africa. (SARS is discussed in Chapter 67.)

West Nile virus is carried and transmitted by mosquitoes. Mosquitoes acquire the virus as they draw blood from infected animals and people. The virus does not cause illness in the mosquito but can be transferred to uninfected animals and humans as the mosquito continues to feed. Bird deaths are an early warning sign of a West Nile virus outbreak, which can spread quickly if action is not taken in a timely manner. (West Nile virus is discussed in Chapter 56.)

TABLE 14-4 **Emerging Infections**

| Microorganism | Related Disease |
|---|---|
| **Bacteria** | |
| *Borrelia burgdorferi* | Lyme disease |
| *Campylobacter jejuni* | Diarrhea |
| *Escherichia coli* O157:H7 | Hemorrhagic colitis, hemolytic-uremic syndrome |
| *Helicobacter pylori* | Peptic ulcer disease |
| *Legionella pneumophila* | Pneumonia (Legionnaires' disease) |
| *Vibrio cholerae* 0139 | New strain associated with epidemic cholera |
| **Virus** | |
| Chikungunya | Fever, muscle aches, rash |
| Ebola virus | Ebola hemorrhagic fever |
| H1N1 | H1N1 (swine) flu |
| Hantavirus | Hemorrhagic fever associated with severe pulmonary syndrome |
| Hepatitis C virus | Parenterally transmitted hepatitis |
| Hepatitis E virus | Enterically transmitted hepatitis |
| Human immunodeficiency virus (HIV) | HIV infection and AIDS |
| Human herpesvirus 6 (HHV-6) | Roseola subitum |
| Human herpesvirus 8 (HHV-8) | Associated with Kaposi sarcoma in immunosuppressed patients, including people with HIV infection |
| West Nile virus | West Nile fever |
| Zika virus | Fever, rash, muscle aches; possible microcephaly in children born to infected mothers |
| **Parasite** | |
| *Cryptosporidium parvum* | Acute and chronic diarrhea |

Influenza viruses are examples of how disease can spread between animals and humans. Variants of influenza A viruses were responsible for influenza epidemics. These include the 2009 influenza A (H1N1) outbreak that was traced back to pigs, hence the name *swine flu*. In 1997 and 2003 outbreaks of the influenza A (H5N1) strain of avian flu resulted from transmission of influenza virus from chickens to humans.

Ebola virus has presented an ongoing challenge to public health since it was first seen in 1976. In 2014, rates of Ebola increased significantly in East Africa, and the first cases of Ebola were seen in the United States. These initial cases were primarily from travelers or medical aid workers who were working in Africa. Ebola virus can cause severe hemorrhagic fever and is usually lethal. Therapeutic and preventive measures are limited. The natural reservoir and path of transmission are unknown, which makes it impossible to effectively combat Ebola virus and the disease it causes.

### Reemerging Infections

Advances in the development of medications and vaccines has led to the near eradication of some infections (e.g., smallpox, polio), but infective agents can reemerge under the right conditions. Table 14-5 presents some diseases that have shown resurgence in recent decades.[3] For example, there have been outbreaks and the resurgence of vaccine-preventable infections such as measles and pertussis in recent years. This is in part due to people not receiving recommended preventive vaccines.

International travel has created a new obstacle for the local eradication of diseases. For example, measles is no longer

**TABLE 14-5 Reemerging Infections**

| Microorganism | Infection | Description |
|---|---|---|
| **Bacteria** | | |
| *Corynebacterium diphtheriae* | Diphtheria | Localized infection of mucous membranes or skin |
| *Bordetella pertussis* | Pertussis | Acute, highly contagious respiratory disease characterized by loud whooping inspiration. Also known as whooping cough |
| *Mycobacterium tuberculosis* | Tuberculosis | Chronic infection transmitted by inhalation of infected droplets (see Chapter 27) |
| **Virus** | | |
| Dengue viruses (flaviviruses) | Dengue fever | Acute infection transmitted by mosquitoes and occurring mainly in tropical and subtropical regions |
| Rubeola | Measles | Fever, malaise, cough, and maculopapular rash |
| **Parasite** | | |
| *Giardia* | Giardiasis | Diarrheal illness that usually originates in water contaminated with fecal matter. Also known as traveler's diarrhea |

**TABLE 14-6 Common Antibiotic-Resistant Organisms and Treatment**

| Bacteria | Resistant to | Preferred Treatment |
|---|---|---|
| *Staphylococcus aureus* | methicillin* | vancomycin |
| *Staphylococcus epidermidis* | methicillin* | vancomycin |
| *Enterococcus faecalis* | vancomycin<br>streptomycin<br>gentamicin | penicillin G or ampicillin |
| *Enterococcus faecium* | vancomycin<br>streptomycin<br>gentamicin | penicillin G or ampicillin |
| *Streptococcus pneumoniae* | penicillin G | ceftriaxone (Rocephin)<br>cefotaxime (Claforan) |
| *Klebsiella pneumoniae* | Third-generation cephalosporins (e.g., ceftazidime [Ceptaz, Fortaz]) | imipenem and cilastatin (Primaxin)<br>meropenem (Merrem IV) |
| *Neisseria gonorrheae* | Third-generation cephalosporins (e.g., cefixime and ceftriaxone) | gemifloxacin/ gentamicin plus azithromycin |

*This drug is no longer available in the United States.

considered endemic in the United States but remains a leading cause of death in developing countries. Domestic outbreaks have typically occurred in areas with low vaccination rates. Some cases have been found in people who have recently traveled to measles-endemic areas outside the United States.[4]

### Antimicrobial-Resistant Organisms

*Resistance* occurs when pathogenic organisms change in ways that decrease the ability of a drug (or a family of drugs) to treat disease.[5] Microorganisms can become resistant to classic treatments (e.g., penicillin) as well as to newer antibiotics and antiviral agents. Microorganisms are highly adaptable. They have evolved genetic and biochemical mechanisms to defend against antimicrobials. Genetic mechanisms include mutation and acquisition of new DNA or RNA. Biochemically, bacteria can resist antibiotics by producing enzymes that destroy or inactivate the drugs. Drug target sites are then altered so that the antibiotic cannot bind to or enter the bacteria. If the drug cannot enter the cell, it cannot kill the bacteria. Table 14-6 describes common antibiotic-resistant bacteria.

Methicillin-resistant *S. aureus* (MRSA), vancomycin-resistant enterococci (VRE), vancomycin-resistant *S. aureus* (VRSA), carbapenem-resistant enterobacteriaceae (CRE), and penicillin-resistant *Streptococcus pneumoniae* are examples of emerging strains of antibiotic-resistant organisms. These drug-resistant bacteria were initially seen primarily in health care settings but are becoming more prevalent in the community. For example, MRSA, a form of *S. aureus* that does not respond to methicillin- or penicillin-based therapies, was initially considered a health care–associated infection (HA-MRSA). However, a variant strain of MRSA that is primarily acquired in the community (community-acquired MRSA [CA-MRSA]) has emerged. This strain of MRSA is more *virulent* (able to cause disease or infection) compared with HA-MRSA.[6] CA-MRSA has been known to cause rapidly forming skin infections and systemic diseases, including pneumonia and sepsis. Rates of CA-MRSA infections appear to be on the rise. Conversely, there has been a reduction in HA-MRSA with the use of strict infection control measures in health care settings.

VRE is another antibiotic-resistant bacteria that has become a concern for patients and health care workers. VRE is more virulent than MRSA and can remain viable on environmental surfaces for weeks. Although antibiotic-resistant bacteria can infect anyone, patients who are hospitalized and those with a suppressed immune system are more likely to be exposed to these bacteria and to develop infection.

HCPs have contributed to the development of drug-resistant microorganisms by (1) administering antibiotics for viral infections, (2) succumbing to pressures from patients to prescribe unnecessary antibiotic therapy, (3) using inadequate drug regimens to treat infections, or (4) using broad-spectrum or combination agents for infections that should be treated with first-line medications.

Patients can also contribute to resistance development by (1) skipping doses, (2) not taking antibiotics for the full duration of prescribed therapy, or (3) saving unused antibiotics "in case I need them later." In addition, limited resources and access to medications make it difficult for some patients to get adequate treatment for infections. Teaching patients and their families the proper use of antibiotics (Table 14-7) is crucial to treatment success and prevention of drug-resistant pathogens. The Centers for Disease Control and Prevention (CDC), the Infectious Diseases Society of America (IDSA), and many health care organizations have been campaigning for greater vigilance in minimizing the misuse of antibiotics in reaction to this growing concern.

Although antibiotics are a class of drugs that are typically thought of when discussing drug-resistant organisms, any organism (virus, fungi, or parasite) can develop drug resistance to agents typically used to treat them. Hence, the term *antimicrobial resistance* is now used to describe the phenomena of resistance across different classes of organisms.

**TABLE 14-7 Patient & Caregiver Teaching**

***Decrease Risk for Antibiotic-Resistant Infection***

*Include the following instructions when teaching patients or their caregivers how to decrease the risk for antibiotic-resistant infection.*

**1. Do Not Take Antibiotics to Prevent Illness (unless prescribed)**

- Doing this increases your risk for developing resistant infection
- Exceptions include taking antibiotics as prescribed before certain surgeries and dental work or in the presence of immune dysfunction

**2. Wash Your Hands Frequently**

Hand washing is the single most important thing you can do to prevent infection.

**3. Follow Directions When Taking Antibiotics**

- Not taking your antibiotic as prescribed or skipping doses can allow antibiotic-resistant bacteria to develop.

**4. Do Not Request an Antibiotic for Flu or Colds**

- If your HCP says that you do not need an antibiotic, chances are you do not.
- Antibiotics are effective against bacterial infections but not viruses, which cause colds and flu.

**5. Finish Your Antibiotic**

- Do not stop taking your antibiotic when you feel better.
- If you stop taking your antibiotic early, the hardiest bacteria survive and multiply.
- Eventually you could develop an infection resistant to many antibiotics. You should never have leftover antibiotics.

**6. Do Not Take Leftover Antibiotics**

- Do not save unfinished antibiotics for later use or borrow leftover drugs from family or friends.
- This is dangerous because (1) the leftover antibiotic may not be appropriate for you, (2) your illness may not be a bacterial infection, (3) old antibiotics can lose their effectiveness and in some cases can even be fatal, and (4) there will not be enough doses in a leftover bottle to provide full treatment.

## HEALTH CARE–ASSOCIATED INFECTIONS

**Health care–associated infections (HAIs)** are infections that are acquired as a result of exposure to microorganisms in a health care setting.[7] Approximately 722,000 HAIs occur annually, and nearly 1 out of every 25 hospitalized patients has at least one HAI. Improvements in infection control have resulted in fewer infections in recent years.[8,9] In recent years there were decreases in several of the major types of HAIs, including central line–associated bloodstream infections, surgical site infections, *Clostridium difficile* infections, and methicillin-resistant *S. aureus* bacteremia. Surgical and immunocompromised patients are at highest risk. Any organism can cause HAIs, but certain bacteria, including *E. coli, S. aureus, Enterobacter aerogenes,* and various types of streptococci, are the more common culprits. Some bacteria that do not normally cause disease can cause infections in high-risk patients as a result of illness or treatment of illness.

Approximately one third of HAIs are preventable. HCPs often transmit HAIs from patient to patient through direct contact. First lines of defense to prevent the spread of HAIs include hand washing (or using an alcohol-based hand sanitizer) before and after patient contact or procedures, appropriate use of protective equipment such as gloves, and decontamination of equipment used for patient care.[10] Isolated infections can also be caused when bacteria that normally stay in one area of the body are introduced into another area. Therefore care must be taken to change gloves and wash hands when moving from one task to another, even when working with the same patient. Guidelines on reducing and controlling the spread of disease in health care settings, especially of antimicrobial-resistant organisms, have been developed and are implemented in most institutions[11,12] (Table 14-8). Nurses and all HCPs have the responsibility of using appropriate measures, including transmission-based precautions, to help protect patients from HAIs.

**TABLE 14-8 OSHA Requirements for Personal Protective Equipment**

*The following equipment is used to minimize exposure to blood-borne pathogens.*

| Equipment | Indications for Use |
|---|---|
| **Gloves** | • Must be used when the employee can reasonably anticipate having contact with blood or other potentially infectious materials, when performing vascular access procedures, and when handling or touching contaminated items or surfaces<br>• Gloves must be replaced if torn, punctured, or contaminated or their ability to function as a barrier is compromised. |
| **Clothing (gowns, aprons, caps, boots)** | • Must be used when occupational exposure is anticipated<br>• The type and characteristics depend on the task and degree of exposure anticipated. |
| **Face protection (mask and glasses with solid side shields or a chin-length face shield)** | • Must be used when splashes, sprays, spatters, or droplets of blood or other potentially infectious materials pose a hazard to the eyes, nose, or mouth |

Source: Occupational Safety and Health Administration: Bloodborne pathogens and needlestick prevention. Retrieved from *www.osha.gov/SLTC/bloodbornepathogens.*
NOTE: Employers must provide, make accessible, and require the use of personal protective equipment (PPE) at no cost to the employee. PPE also must be provided in appropriate sizes. Hypoallergenic gloves or similar alternatives must be made available to employees who have an allergic sensitivity to gloves.
*OSHA,* Occupational Safety and Health Administration.

### Gerontologic Considerations: Infections in Older Adults

For older adults, the rate of HAIs is two or three times higher than for younger patients. Individuals in long-term care facilities are at special risk for HAI. Age-related changes (e.g., impaired immune function, co-morbidities such as diabetes, physical disabilities) can contribute to higher infection rates in older adults.[13]

Infections common in older adults include pneumonia, urinary tract infections, skin infections, and TB. Urinary tract infections are more common in older adults who reside in long-term care facilities. Patients with indwelling catheters are at particular risk.

Infections in older adults often have atypical manifestations, such as cognitive and behavioral changes, before the emergence of fever, pain, or alterations in laboratory values. Do not rely on the presence of fever to indicate infection in older adults, because many have lower core body temperatures and decreased immune responses. Suspicion of disease should typically begin

**CHECK YOUR PRACTICE**

You are working in a long-term care facility and one of your residents, a 76-yr-old man who is recovering from a stroke, seems very confused today. You discuss your concerns with the unlicensed assistive personnel (UAP), explaining that he seemed so alert yesterday and you wonder if he may have an infection, such as pneumonia or a urinary tract infection. The UAP says, "I just took his temperature and it is normal so I don't think he has an infection."

- How should you follow up with this resident and UAP?

if a patient demonstrates changes in the ability to perform daily activities or in cognitive function. In addition, underlying diseases, increased frequency of drug reactions, and institutionalization can complicate the management of an older adult with infection.

## INFECTION PREVENTION AND CONTROL

### Occupational Safety and Health Administration (OSHA) Guidelines

OSHA is a federal agency that protects workers from injury and illness in places of employment and supports activities that minimize or eliminate exposure to infectious materials in the workplace. OSHA mandates that any employer whose employees could be exposed to potentially infectious materials implement standard policies and procedures for protection of those employees. Employees must be provided with appropriate personal protective equipment (PPE) and safety equipment.[11] These include gloves, gowns, facial protection, and disposal systems for sharps (Table 14-8). Appropriate PPE varies depending on the situation, and you need to use sound judgment when deciding when and how to use protective equipment.

### Infection Precautions

If a patient is admitted with or develops an infection that is considered a risk to others, infection precautions may need to be implemented. The CDC has established guidelines with two levels of precautions: (1) **standard precautions**, designed for the care of all patients in hospitals and health care facilities and (2) **transmission-based precautions**, designed for specific diseases.[11] The purpose of these precautions is to prevent the transmission of organisms from patients to HCPs, from HCPs to patients, from patients to other patients, and from health care personnel and patients to people outside of the hospital (Table 14-9).

The *standard precautions* system applies to (1) blood; (2) all body fluids, secretions, and excretions; (3) non-intact skin; and (4) mucous membranes. Standard precautions are designed to reduce the risk of transmission of microorganisms in hospitals. Standard precautions should be applied to *all* patients regardless of diagnosis or presumed infection status. The CDC's standard precautions incorporate all of the OSHA blood-borne pathogens standard requirements.

*Transmission-based precautions* are used for patients known to be or suspected of being infected with highly transmissible or epidemiologically important pathogens that require additional precautions to interrupt transmission and prevent infection. Transmission-based precautions include airborne precautions, droplet precautions, and contact precautions. *Airborne precautions* are used if the organism can cause infection over long distances when suspended in the air (e.g., TB, rubeola).

**TABLE 14-9 Types of Isolation Precautions Used in Health Care Settings**

| Type | Examples |
|---|---|
| **Standard Precautions** | |
| • Used for care of all patients, regardless of their diagnosis or presumed infection status | Includes the use of hand washing and appropriate personal protective equipment |
| **Transmission-Based Precautions** | |
| • Recommended to provide additional precautions beyond standard precautions to prevent transmission of pathogens<br>• Can be used for patients known or suspected to be infected or colonized with pathogens that can be transmitted by airborne or droplet transmission, or by contact with dry skin or contaminated surfaces<br>• These precautions should be used in addition to standard precautions. | **Airborne Precautions:** Used for infections spread in small particles in the air such as chickenpox (varicella), measles, and tuberculosis (TB)<br>**Droplet Precautions:** Used for infections spread in large droplets by coughing, talking, or sneezing such as influenza and bacterial meningitis<br>**Contact Precautions:** Used for infections spread by skin-to-skin contact or contact with other surfaces such as *C. difficile*, MRSA, and VRE |

*Droplet precautions* are used to minimize contact with pathogens that are spread through the air at close contact and that affect the respiratory system or mucous membranes (e.g., influenza, pertussis). *Contact precautions* are used to minimize the spread of pathogens that are acquired from direct or indirect contact, especially multidrug-resistant organisms (e.g., MRSA, VRE, CRE). Transmission-based precautions may be combined for diseases that have multiple routes of transmission. Whether used alone or in combination, transmission-based precautions should always be used in conjunction with standard precautions.

## HUMAN IMMUNODEFICIENCY VIRUS INFECTION

**Human immunodeficiency virus (HIV)** is a retrovirus that causes immunosuppression. People with HIV are more susceptible to infections that are normally controlled through immune responses. The term *HIV disease* is used interchangeably with HIV infection. With advances in treatment, HIV is managed as a chronic disease, since people with the disease are living longer.

More than 1 million people are currently living with HIV in the United States, with approximately 50,000 new infections occurring each year.[14] With the availability of effective HIV treatment, there has been a dramatic drop in the number of deaths attributable to HIV.

In North America HIV is most prevalent among men who have sex with men (MSM). However, increasing numbers of new HIV infections are occurring in women, people of color, people who live in poverty, and young adults.

### Transmission of HIV

HIV can be transmitted through contact with infected blood, semen, vaginal secretions, or breast milk. HIV transmission occurs through sexual intercourse with an infected partner; exposure to HIV-infected blood or blood products; and perinatal transmission during pregnancy, at delivery, or through breastfeeding. HIV is not spread casually.[15] The virus cannot be transmitted through hugging, dry kissing, shaking hands, sharing eating utensils, using toilet seats, or casual encounters in any setting. It is not spread by tears, saliva, urine, emesis, sputum, feces, sweat, respiratory droplets, or enteric routes. Health care personnel have a low risk of acquiring HIV at work, even after a needle-stick injury.[16]

**Sexual Transmission.** The most common mode of HIV transmission is unprotected sexual contact with an HIV-infected partner. Sexual activity involves contact with semen, vaginal secretions, and/or blood, all of which have lymphocytes that may contain HIV. During any form of sexual intercourse (anal, vaginal, or oral), the risk of infection is greater for the partner who receives the semen, although infection can also be transmitted to the inserting partner. This occurs because the receiver has prolonged contact with infected fluids, and it helps explain why it is easier to infect women than men during heterosexual intercourse. Sexual activities that cause trauma to local tissues can increase the risk of transmission. In addition, genital lesions from other sexually transmitted infections (e.g., herpes, syphilis) significantly increase the likelihood of transmission.

**Contact With Blood and Blood Products.** HIV can be transmitted from exposure to blood when sharing drug-using paraphernalia. Needles, syringes, straws, and other equipment may be contaminated with HIV or other blood-borne organisms, and sharing this equipment can result in disease transmission.

Routine screening of blood donors to identify at-risk individuals and testing donated blood for the presence of HIV have improved the safety of the blood supply. In countries that routinely test donated blood, HIV infection as a result of blood transfusions or hemophilia clotting factors is unlikely.

Puncture wounds are the most common means of work-related HIV transmission. The risk of infection after a needle-stick exposure to HIV-infected blood is 0.3% to 0.4% (or 3 or 4 out of 1000).[16] The risk is higher if the exposure involves blood from a patient with a high level of circulating HIV, a deep puncture wound, a needle with a hollow bore and visible blood, or a device used for venous or arterial access. Splash exposures of blood on skin with an open lesion present some risk, but it is much lower than from a puncture wound.

**Perinatal Transmission.** Perinatal transmission from an HIV-infected mother to her infant can occur during pregnancy, delivery, or breastfeeding. On average, 25% of infants born to women with untreated HIV infection are born with HIV. Fortunately, the risk of transmission can be reduced to less than 2% in settings in which pregnant women are routinely tested for HIV infection and, if found to be infected, treated with **antiretroviral therapy (ART)**, a combination of medication used to control and suppress HIV replication.[17,18]

## Pathophysiology

HIV is an RNA virus. RNA viruses are called *retroviruses* because they replicate in a "backward" manner (going from RNA to DNA). Like all viruses, HIV cannot replicate unless it is inside a living cell.[19] The *CD4⁺ T cell (CD4 cell)*, a type of lymphocyte, is the target cell for HIV. HIV enters the CD4⁺ T cell by binding to protein receptors on the outside of the cell (Fig. 14-1). This process is known as *fusion* (Fig. 14-2).

Once HIV is attached and fused with the CD4⁺ T cell, HIV RNA enters the CD4⁺ T cell. This triggers the release of **reverse transcriptase**, an enzyme that transforms HIV RNA into a single strand of DNA. This strand copies itself, becoming

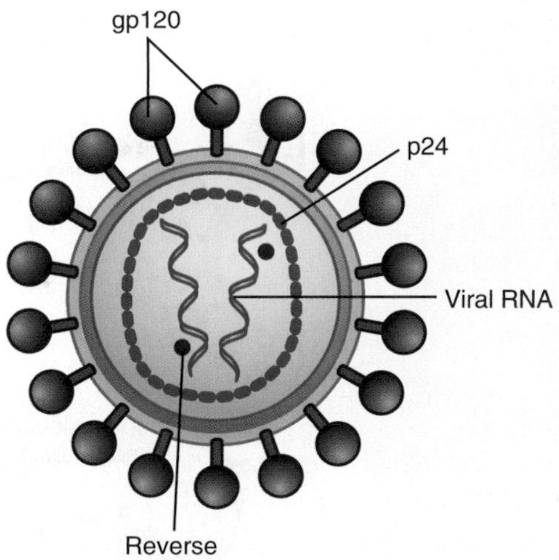


**FIG. 14-1** HIV is surrounded by an envelope made up of proteins (including gp120) and contains a core of viral RNA and proteins.

double-stranded viral DNA. Another enzyme, called *integrase*, allows the newly formed double-stranded DNA to integrate itself into the host's genetic structure. This action has two consequences: (1) because all genetic material is replicated during cell division, all daughter cells are also infected and (2) viral DNA in the genome directs the cell to make new HIV.

*Protease*, another enzyme involved in the replication process, cleaves the newly formed strands of HIV genetic material into smaller pieces. New HIV virions are then formed and released. The CD4⁺ T cell is then destroyed after the HIV virions are released.[19]

HIV destroys about 1 billion CD4⁺ T cells every day. For many years the body can produce new CD4⁺ T cells to replace the destroyed cells. However, over time the ability of HIV to destroy CD4⁺ T cells exceeds the body's ability to replace the cells. The decline in the CD4⁺ T cell count impairs immune function. Generally, the immune system remains healthy with more than 500 CD4⁺ T cells/μL. Immune problems begin to occur when the count drops below 500 CD4⁺ T cells/μL. Severe problems develop with fewer than 200 CD4⁺ T cells/μL.

With HIV, a point is eventually reached where so many CD4⁺ T cells have been destroyed that not enough are left to regulate immune responses (Fig. 14-3). This allows **opportunistic diseases** (infections and cancers that occur in immunosuppressed patients) to develop. Opportunistic diseases are the main cause of disease, disability, and death in patients with HIV infection.

### Clinical Manifestations and Complications

The typical course of untreated HIV infection follows the pattern shown in Fig. 14-4. It is important to remember that (1) disease progression is highly individualized, (2) treatment can significantly alter this pattern, and (3) an individual's prognosis is unpredictable.

**Acute Infection.** Approximately 2 to 4 weeks after someone becomes newly infected with HIV, individuals typically experience *acute HIV infection*, a period when people can have a mononucleosis-like syndrome of fever, swollen lymph nodes, sore throat, headache, malaise, nausea, muscle and joint pain, diarrhea, and/or a diffuse rash. Some people also develop neurologic complications, such as aseptic meningitis, peripheral neuropathy, facial palsy, or Guillain-Barré syndrome.[20] During

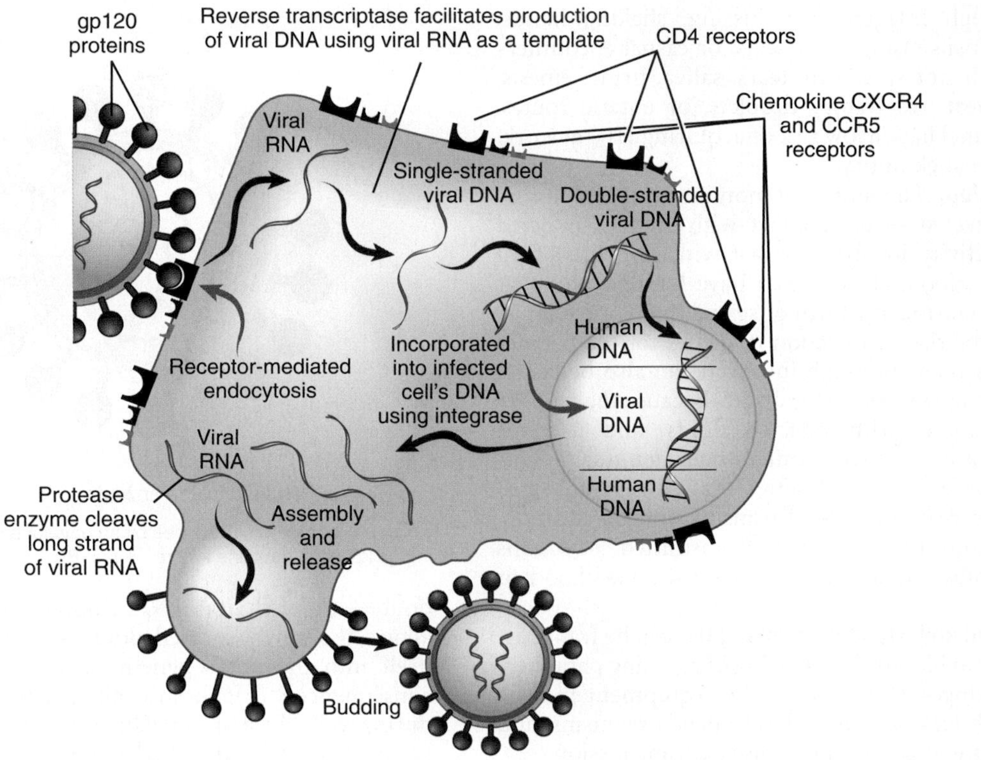


**FIG. 14-2** HIV has gp120 glycoproteins that attach to CD4 and chemokine CXCR4 and CCR5 receptors on the surface of CD4⁺ T cells. Viral RNA then enters the cell, produces viral DNA in the presence of reverse transcriptase, and incorporates itself into the cellular genome in the presence of integrase, causing permanent cellular infection and the production of new virions. New viral RNA develops initially in long strands that are cut in the presence of protease and leave the cell through a budding process that ultimately contributes to cellular destruction.

this time a high **viral load** (the amount of HIV circulating in the blood) is noted, and $CD4^+$ T cell counts fall temporarily but quickly return to baseline or near-baseline levels (Fig. 14-3). Many people, including HCPs, mistake acute HIV symptoms for a bad case of the flu. Individuals are most infectious during the acute infection stage because of the high amounts of circulating HIV.

### Chronic HIV Infection

***Asymptomatic Infection.*** The interval between initial HIV infection and a diagnosis of AIDS is about 10 years in untreated infection. During the first several years after initial infection, individuals are typically asymptomatic and have no symptoms or relatively limited signs of infection.

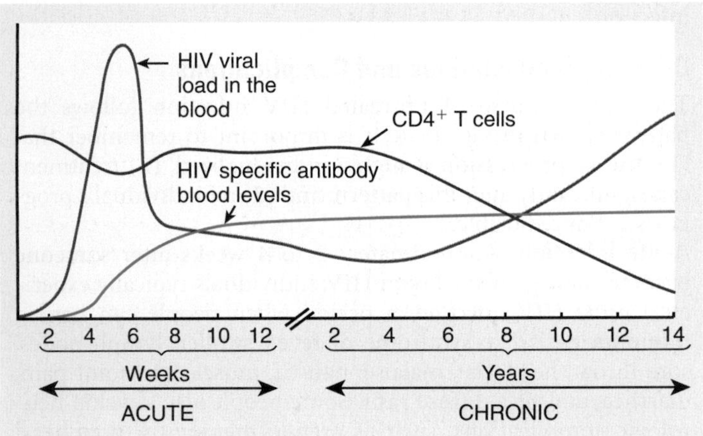


**FIG. 14-3** Viral load in the blood in relationship to number of $CD4^+$ T cells over the spectrum of untreated HIV infection.

Because most of the symptoms during early infection are vague and nonspecific for HIV, people may not be aware that they are infected. During this time, infected people continue their usual activities, which may include high-risk sexual and drug-using behaviors. This is a public health problem because infected individuals can transmit HIV to others even though they have no symptoms.[20] Personal health is also affected because people who do not know that they are infected have little reason to seek treatment and are less likely to make

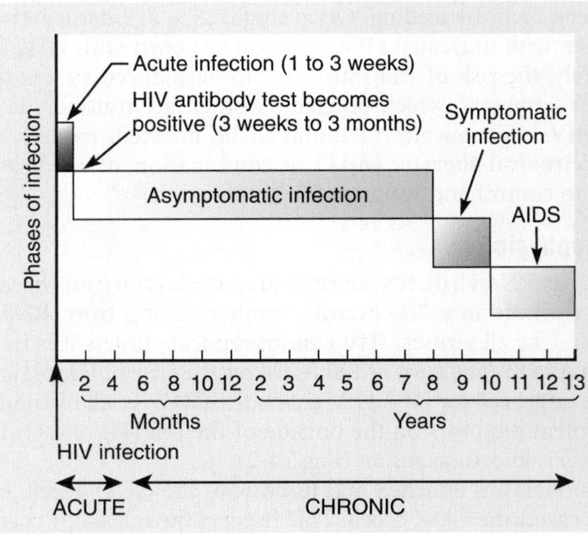


**FIG. 14-4** Timeline for the spectrum of untreated HIV infection. The timeline represents the course of untreated illness from the time of infection to clinical manifestations of disease.

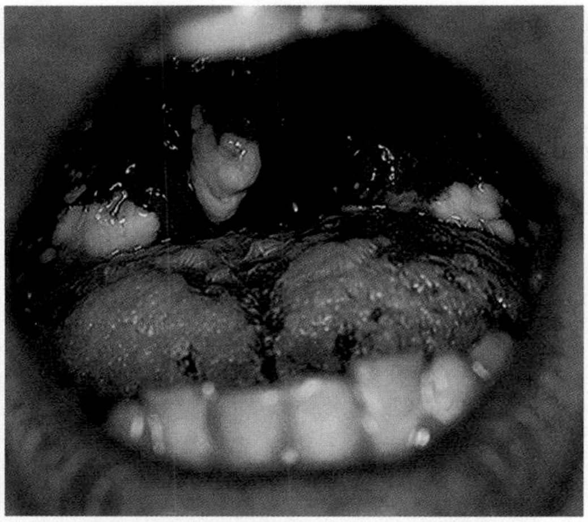

**FIG. 14-5** Oral thrush involving hard and soft palate. (From Emond R, Welsby P, Rowland H: *Colour atlas of infectious diseases,* ed 4, Edinburgh, 2003, Mosby.)

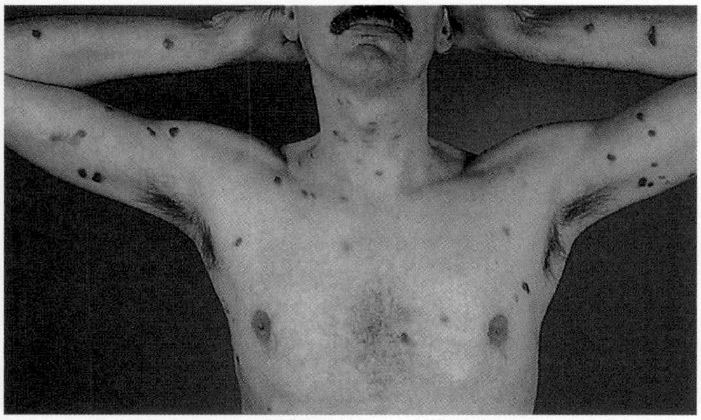

**FIG. 14-6** Kaposi sarcoma (KS). The malignant vascular lesions of KS can appear anywhere on the skin surface or on internal organs. Lesions vary in size from pinpoint to large and may appear in a variety of shades. (From Friedman-Kien AE: *Color atlas of AIDS,* Philadelphia, 1989, Saunders.)

behavior changes that could improve the quality and length of their lives.

***Symptomatic Infection.*** As the $CD4^+$ T cell count declines closer to 200 cells/μL and the viral load increases, HIV advances to a more active stage. Symptoms such as persistent fever, frequent night sweats, chronic diarrhea, recurrent headaches, and severe fatigue may develop.

One of the more common infections associated with this phase of HIV infection is oropharyngeal candidiasis (thrush) (Fig. 14-5). *Candida* organisms rarely cause problems in healthy adults but are more common in HIV-infected people. Other infections that can occur at this time include shingles (caused by the varicella-zoster virus); persistent vaginal candidal infections; outbreaks of oral or genital herpes; bacterial infections; and Kaposi sarcoma (KS), which is caused by human herpesvirus 8 (Fig. 14-6). *Oral hairy leukoplakia,* an Epstein-Barr virus infection that causes painless, white, raised lesions on the lateral aspect of the tongue (Fig. 14-7), is another indicator of disease progression.

***AIDS.*** A diagnosis of **acquired immunodeficiency syndrome (AIDS)** is made when an HIV-infected patient meets criteria established by the CDC.[21] These criteria occur when the immune system becomes severely compromised (Table 14-10). Opportunistic diseases generally do not occur in the presence of a functioning immune system. Many infections, a variety of

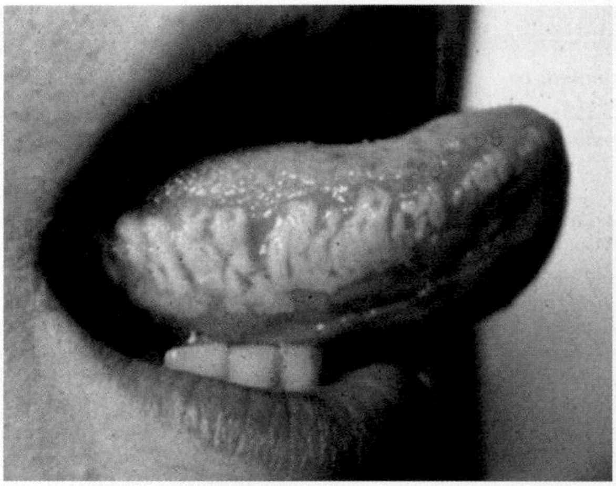

**FIG. 14-7** Oral hairy leukoplakia on the lateral aspect of the tongue. (Set of slides published in 1992 by Jon Fuller, MD, and Howard Libman, MD, at Boston University School of Medicine, Boston.)

**TABLE 14-10 Diagnostic Criteria for AIDS**

AIDS is diagnosed when an individual with HIV develops at least one of the following conditions:

1. $CD4^+$ T cell count drops below 200 cells/μL.
2. One of the following opportunistic infections (OIs):
   - *Fungal:* candidiasis of bronchi, trachea, lungs, or esophagus; *Pneumocystis jiroveci* pneumonia (PCP); disseminated or extrapulmonary coccidioidomycosis; disseminated or extrapulmonary histoplasmosis
   - *Viral:* cytomegalovirus (CMV) disease other than liver, spleen, or nodes; CMV retinitis (with loss of vision); herpes simplex with chronic ulcer(s) or bronchitis, pneumonitis, or esophagitis; progressive multifocal leukoencephalopathy (PML); extrapulmonary cryptococcosis
   - *Protozoal:* toxoplasmosis of the brain, chronic intestinal isosporiasis, chronic intestinal cryptosporidiosis
   - *Bacterial: Mycobacterium tuberculosis* (any site); any disseminated or extrapulmonary mycobacteria, including *Mycobacterium avium* complex (MAC) or *Mycobacterium kansasii;* recurrent pneumonia; recurrent *Salmonella* septicemia
3. One of the following opportunistic cancers:
   - Invasive cervical cancer
   - Kaposi sarcoma (KS)
   - Burkitt's lymphoma
   - Immunoblastic lymphoma
   - Primary lymphoma of the brain
4. Wasting syndrome. *Wasting* is defined as a loss of 10% or more of ideal body mass.

Modified from Centers for Disease Control and Prevention: 1993 Revised classification system for HIV infection and expanded surveillance case definition for AIDS among adolescents and adults, 1993. Retrieved from *www.cdc.gov/mmwr/preview/mmwrhtml/rr5710a1.htm?s_cid=rr5710a1_e*.

malignancies, wasting, and HIV-related cognitive changes can occur in patients with immune impairment (Table 14-11). Organisms that do not cause severe disease in people with functioning immune systems can cause debilitating, disseminated, and life-threatening infections during this stage. Several opportunistic diseases may occur at the same time, compounding the difficulties of diagnosis and treatment. Advances in HIV treatment have decreased the occurrence of opportunistic diseases.

## Diagnostic Studies

**Diagnosis of HIV Infection.** Diagnosis of HIV infection is made by testing for HIV antibodies and/or antigens in the blood.[22] HIV screening tests detect HIV-specific antibodies or antigens,

### TABLE 14-11 Common Opportunistic Diseases Associated With HIV Infection

| Organism or Disease | Clinical Manifestations |
|---|---|
| ***Candida albicans*** | Thrush (Fig. 14-5), esophagitis, vaginitis. Whitish yellow patches in mouth, esophagus, GI tract, vagina |
| ***Coccidioides immitis*** | Pneumonia and fever, weight loss, cough |
| **CNS lymphoma** | Cognitive dysfunction, motor impairment, aphasia, seizures, personality changes, headache |
| ***Cryptococcus neoformans*** | Meningitis, cognitive impairment, motor dysfunction, fever, seizures, headache |
| ***Cryptosporidium muris*** | Gastroenteritis, watery diarrhea, abdominal pain, weight loss |
| **Cytomegalovirus (CMV)** | *Retinitis:* retinal lesions, blurred vision, loss of vision<br>*Esophagitis, stomatitis:* difficulty swallowing, colitis or gastritis: bloody diarrhea, pain, weight loss<br>*Pneumonitis:* respiratory symptoms.<br>*Neurologic disease:* CNS manifestations |
| **Hepatitis B virus (HBV)** | Jaundice, fatigue, abdominal pain, loss of appetite, nausea, vomiting, joint pain. Some have no signs or symptoms |
| **Hepatitis C virus (HCV)** | Jaundice, fatigue, abdominal pain, loss of appetite, nausea, vomiting, dark urine. Many have no signs or symptoms. |
| **Herpes simplex** | *HSV-1 (type 1):* orolabial and mucocutaneous vesicular and ulcerative lesions. Keratitis, visual disturbances, encephalitis, CNS manifestations<br>*HSV-2 (type 2):* genital and perianal vesicular and ulcerative lesions |
| ***Histoplasma capsulatum*** | *Pneumonia:* fever, cough, weight loss<br>*Meningitis:* CNS manifestations, disseminated disease |
| **JC papovavirus** | Progressive multifocal leukoencephalopathy (PML), CNS manifestations, mental and motor declines |
| **Kaposi sarcoma (KS)** caused by human herpesvirus 8 (HHV-8) | Vascular lesions on the skin (Fig. 14-6), mucous membranes, and viscera with wide range of presentation: firm, flat, raised, or nodular; pinpoint to several cm in size; hyperpigmented, multicentric. Can cause lymphedema and disfigurement, particularly when confluent. Usually not serious unless occurring in the respiratory or gastrointestinal system |
| ***Mycobacterium avium* complex (MAC)** | Gastroenteritis, watery diarrhea, weight loss |
| ***Mycobacterium tuberculosis* (MTB, TB)** | Respiratory and disseminated disease. Productive cough, fever, night sweats, weight loss |
| ***Pneumocystis jiroveci* pneumonia (PCP)** | Pneumonia, nonproductive cough, hypoxemia, progressive shortness of breath, fever, night sweats, fatigue |
| ***Toxoplasma gondii*** | Encephalitis, cognitive dysfunction, motor impairment, fever, altered mental status, headache, seizures, sensory abnormalities |
| **Varicella-zoster virus (VZV)** | *Shingles:* erythematous maculopapular rash along dermatomal planes, pain, pruritus<br>*Ocular:* progressive outer retinal necrosis (PORN) |

but typically it takes several weeks after initial infection before evidence of HIV can be detected on a screening test (Fig. 14-3). This delay is known as the **window period**. HIV screening tests can be performed using blood or saliva. Combination antibody and antigen tests (also known as fourth-generation tests) are able to detect HIV earlier than previous versions of HIV screening tests. The fourth-generation test decreases the window period to within 3 weeks following infection (Table 14-12).

**Laboratory Studies in HIV Infection.** Two laboratory tests are used for monitoring HIV progression: $CD4^+$ T cell count and viral load. The $CD4^+$ T cell count provides a marker of immune function. As the disease progresses, the number of $CD4^+$ T cells usually decreases (Fig. 14-3). The normal range for $CD4^+$ T cells is 800 to 1200 cells/μL. Laboratory tests that measure viral levels provide an assessment of disease progression. The lower the viral load, the less active the disease. In HIV, viral loads are reported as real numbers (e.g., 1260 copies/μL). The goal of treatment is to suppress the viral load to the lowest level possible, which is below the level of detection on a commercial assay. This is often referred to as "undetectable." "Undetectable" does *not* mean that the virus has been eliminated from the body or that the individual can no longer transmit HIV to others. Rather, it refers to the fact that the amount of circulating HIV in the blood is below the level of detection of the test.

Abnormal blood test results are common in HIV infection and may be caused by HIV, opportunistic diseases, or complications of therapy. Decreased white blood cell (WBC) counts,

### TABLE 14-12 HIV Testing

#### *HIV-Antibody/Antigen Testing (Fourth-Generation Testing)*

A highly sensitive test detects antibodies and antigens associated with HIV. Blood samples that are negative for HIV infection are reported as negative. The new fourth-generation testing algorithm includes confirmatory testing with HIV viral load testing for any indeterminate results.

- If the patient has a negative fourth-generation test, but reports recent risky behaviors, encourage retesting in 4 to 6 weeks. Individuals at ongoing risk should be assessed or counseled for risk reduction interventions including preexposure prophylaxis (PrEP).
- If the results are positive and consistent with HIV infection, assist the patient in getting appropriate counseling, support, and follow-up HIV primary care.

**Rapid HIV-Antibody Testing**

1. Rapid testing is strongly recommended by the Centers for Disease Control and Prevention. Results are highly accurate, and it can be done in a variety of settings (mobile health units, HCPs' offices, or even in the privacy of an individual's home). Results are typically available within 20 minutes.
2. In-home HIV test kits are available. Testing is done on saliva.
3. Rapid tests are screening tests for antibodies, not for antigen.
4. Negative rapid tests should be followed by a risk assessment to determine the need for repeat tests.
5. Positive rapid tests can be disclosed to the patient but must be confirmed with a standard HIV assay. This step necessitates a blood draw and a return appointment to get results.

especially below-normal numbers of lymphocytes (lymphopenia) and neutrophils (neutropenia), are often seen. Low platelet counts (thrombocytopenia) may be caused by HIV, antiplatelet antibodies, or drug therapy. Anemia is associated with the chronic disease process and with adverse effects of ART. Altered liver function, caused by HIV infection, drug therapy, or co-infection with a hepatitis virus, is common. Early identification of co-infection with hepatitis B virus (HBV) or hepatitis C virus (HCV) is extremely important because these infections have a more serious course in patients with HIV, may ultimately limit options for ART, and can cause liver-related morbidity and mortality.[23]

Resistance tests can determine if a patient's HIV is resistant to drugs used for ART. *Genotype* and *phenotype* assays are used to help HCPs know which medications can be used to control a patient's infection. These tests are similar to culture and sensitivity testing used for antibiotic selection.

## Interprofessional Care

Interprofessional care of the HIV-infected patient focuses on (1) monitoring HIV disease progression and immune function, (2) initiating and monitoring ART, (3) preventing the development of opportunistic diseases, (4) detecting and treating opportunistic diseases, (5) managing symptoms, (6) preventing or decreasing complications of treatment, and (7) preventing further transmission of HIV. To accomplish these goals, ongoing assessment, clinician-patient interactions, and patient teaching and support are required.

The initial patient visit provides an opportunity to gather baseline data and to start establishing rapport. A complete history and physical examination, including an immunization history and psychosocial and dietary evaluations, should be conducted. Findings from the history, assessment, and laboratory tests help to determine patient needs. This is also a good time to complete the case reports required by the state health department. Patient teaching about the spectrum of HIV disease, treatment, prevention of transmission to others, improvements in health, and family planning can be initiated at this meeting. Use patient input to develop a plan of care and determine the need for referrals. Remember that a newly diagnosed patient may not be able to retain or understand information. Be prepared to repeat and clarify information over the course of several months.

**Drug Therapy for HIV Infection.** The goals of drug therapy in HIV infection are to (1) decrease the viral load, (2) maintain or increase $CD4^+$ T cell counts, (3) prevent HIV-related symptoms and opportunistic diseases, (4) delay disease progression, and (5) prevent HIV transmission. HIV cannot be cured, but ART can delay disease progression by decreasing viral replication.[24] When taken consistently and correctly, ART can reduce viral loads by 90% to 99%, which makes adherence to treatment regimens extremely important.

Drugs used to treat HIV work at various points in the HIV replication cycle (Table 14-13). The major advantage of using drugs from different classes is that combination therapy can inhibit viral replication in several different ways, making it more difficult for the virus to recover and decreasing the likelihood of drug resistance. A major problem with most drugs used in ART is that resistance develops rapidly when they are used alone *(monotherapy)* or taken in inadequate doses. For that reason, combinations of three or more drugs should be used.

**! SAFETY ALERT Interaction of ART With Other Drugs**

- Many ARTs have interactions with other commonly used drugs and herbal therapies (e.g., St. John's wort).
- Significant interactions with ARTs also occur with over-the-counter drugs, including antacids, proton pump inhibitors, and certain supplements.
- Be sure to ask patients about prescribed and over-the-counter drugs as well as herbal products and supplements.

**Drug Therapy for Opportunistic Diseases.** Management of HIV is complicated by the many opportunistic diseases that can develop as the immune system deteriorates (Table 14-11). Prevention is the preferred approach to opportunistic diseases. A number of opportunistic diseases associated with HIV can be delayed or prevented with adequate ART, vaccines (including hepatitis B, influenza, and pneumococcal), and disease-specific prevention measures.[25] Although it is usually not possible to eradicate opportunistic diseases once they occur, prophylactic medications can significantly decrease morbidity and mortality rates. Advances in the prevention, diagnosis, and treatment of opportunistic diseases have contributed significantly to increased life expectancy.

**Preventing Transmission of HIV.** Preexposure prophylaxis (PrEP) is a comprehensive HIV prevention strategy to reduce the risk of sexually acquired HIV infection in adults at high risk.[26] PrEP should be used in conjunction with other proven prevention interventions such as condoms, risk reduction counseling, and regular HIV testing.

Tenofovir in combination with emtricitabine, also known as Truvada, is used to reduce the risk of HIV infection in uninfected individuals who are at significant risk of acquiring HIV. Tenofovir/emtricitabine is also currently used in combination with other antiretroviral agents for the treatment of HIV-infected people.

# NURSING MANAGEMENT: HIV INFECTION

## Nursing Assessment

Nursing assessment of individuals not known to be infected with HIV should focus on behaviors that put the person at risk for HIV and other sexually transmitted and blood-borne infections. Assess patients for risky behaviors on a regular basis. Do not assume that someone is without risk because he or she is too old, too young, heterosexual, or married.

Help individuals assess risk by asking some basic questions: (1) Have you ever had a blood transfusion or used clotting factors? If so, was it before 1985? (2) Have you ever shared drug-using equipment with another person? (3) Have you ever had a sexual experience in which your penis, vagina, rectum, or mouth came into contact with another person's penis, vagina, rectum, or mouth? (4) Have you ever had a sexually transmitted infection? (5) Have you ever had sexual contact with someone known to have HIV? These questions provide the minimum information needed to initiate a risk assessment. Follow up a positive response to any of these questions with an in-depth exploration of issues related to the identified risk.

Specific assessments are needed for an individual who has been diagnosed with HIV infection. Subjective and objective data that should be obtained are presented in Table 14-14. Repeated nursing assessments over time are essential because people's circumstances change. Early recognition and treatment can slow the progression of HIV infection and prevent new

TABLE 14-13 **Drug Therapy**

***HIV Infection***

| Drug Classification | Mechanism of Action | Examples |
|---|---|---|
| **Entry Inhibitors** | Prevent binding of HIV to cells, thus preventing entry of HIV into cells where replication would occur | enfuvirtide (Fuzeon)<br>maraviroc (Selzentry) |
| **Reverse Transcriptase Inhibitors** | | |
| ***Nucleoside Reverse Transcriptase Inhibitors (NRTIs)*** | Insert a piece of DNA into the developing HIV DNA chain, blocking further development of the chain and leaving the production of the new strand of HIV DNA incomplete | zidovudine (AZT, ZDV, Retrovir)<br>didanosine (ddI, Videx, Videx-EC [time-released])<br>stavudine (d4T, Zerit)<br>lamivudine (3TC, Epivir)<br>abacavir (Ziagen)<br>emtricitabine (FTC, Emtriva) |
| ***Nonnucleoside Reverse Transcriptase Inhibitors (NNRTIs)*** | Inhibit the action of reverse transcriptase | nevirapine (Viramune XR)<br>delavirdine (Rescriptor)<br>efavirenz (Sustiva)<br>etravirine (Intelence)<br>rilpivirine (Edurant) |
| ***Nucleotide Reverse Transcriptase Inhibitor (NtRTI)*** | Combines with reverse transcriptase enzyme to block the process needed to convert HIV RNA into HIV DNA | tenofovir (Viread) |
| **Integrase Inhibitors** | Bind with integrase enzyme and prevent HIV from incorporating its genetic material into the host cell | raltegravir (Isentress)<br>elvitegravir (Vitekta)†<br>dolutegravir (Tivicay) |
| **Protease Inhibitors (PIs)** | Prevent the protease enzyme from cutting HIV proteins into the proper lengths needed to allow viable virions to assemble and bud out from the cell membrane | saquinavir (Fortovase, Invirase)<br>indinavir (Crixivan)<br>ritonavir (Norvir)‡<br>nelfinavir (Viracept)<br>atazanavir (Reyataz)<br>fosamprenavir (Lexiva)<br>tipranavir (Aptivus)<br>darunavir (Prezista)<br>lopinavir + ritonavir (Kaletra) |
| **Fixed-Dose Combination Products** | More than one drug combined into a single tablet. Drugs may be from the same or different classes. | Atripla (tenofovir DF + emtricitabine + efavirenz)<br>Combivir (lamivudine + zidovudine)<br>Complera (tenofovir DF + emtricitabine + rilpivirine)<br>Odefsky (tenofovir AF + emtricitabine + rilpivirine)<br>Epzicom (abacavir + lamivudine)<br>Triumeq (abacavir + lamivudine + dolutegravir)<br>Trizivir (abacavir + lamivudine + zidovudine)<br>Truvada (tenofovir DF + emtricitabine)<br>Descovy (tenofovir AF + emtricitabine)<br>Stribild (tenofovir DF + emtricitabine + elvitegravir + cobicistat§)<br>Genvoya (tenofovir AF + emtricitabine + elvitegravir + cobicistat§)<br>Evotaz (atazanavir + cobicistat§)<br>Prezcobix (darunavir + cobicistat§) |

*AF,* Alafenamide. *DF,* disoproxil fumarate.
†Vitekta must be administered with a boosted HIV protease inhibitor. Elvitegravir in other fixed dose combinations can be given with either a protease inhibitor or cobicistat.
‡Most often used in low doses with other PIs to boost effect.
§Cobicistat is a pharmacologic booster that enhances the potency of some HIV antiretrovirals. It has no direct effects against HIV.

infections. A complete history and thorough systems review can help identify and address problems in a timely manner.

## ◆ Planning

Nursing interventions can help the patient to (1) adhere to drug regimens; (2) adopt a healthy lifestyle that includes avoiding exposure to other sexually transmitted infections and blood-borne diseases; (3) protect others from HIV; (4) maintain or develop healthy and supportive relationships; (5) maintain activities and productivity; (6) explore spiritual issues; (7) come to terms with issues related to disease, disability, and death; and (8) cope with symptoms caused by HIV and its treatments.

## ◆ Nursing Implementation

The complexity of HIV disease is related to its chronic nature. As with most chronic and infectious diseases, primary prevention and health promotion are the most effective health care strategies. When prevention fails, disease results. Table 14-15 presents a summary of nursing goals, assessments, and interventions throughout the course of HIV infection.

◆ **Health Promotion.** Even with recent successes in HIV treatment, prevention remains a critical component to control the epidemic. In addition, health promotion encourages early detection of the disease so that, if primary prevention has failed, early intervention can be initiated.

◆ ***Prevention of HIV Infection.*** HIV infection is preventable. Avoiding or modifying risky behaviors is the most effective prevention tool. Nursing interventions to prevent disease transmission are based on an assessment of the individual's risk behaviors. Provide culturally sensitive, language-appropriate, and age-specific teaching and behavior change counseling. Nurses who are comfortable with and know how to talk about

## TABLE 14-14 Nursing Assessment

### *HIV-Infected Patient*

**Subjective Data**

***Important Health Information***

*Past health history:* Route of infection. Hepatitis, other sexually transmitted infections, tuberculosis. Frequent viral, fungal, and/or bacterial infections

*Medications:* Use of immunosuppressive drugs

***Functional Health Patterns***

*Health perception–health management:* Perception of illness. Alcohol and drug use. Malaise

*Nutritional-metabolic:* Weight loss, anorexia, nausea, vomiting. Lesions, bleeding, or ulcerations of lips, mouth, gums, tongue, or throat. Sensitivity to acidic, salty, or spicy foods. Difficulty swallowing, abdominal cramping. Skin rashes, lesions, or color changes

*Elimination:* Persistent diarrhea, change in character of stools. Painful urination, low back pain

*Activity-exercise:* Chronic fatigue, muscle weakness, difficulty walking. Cough, shortness of breath

*Sleep-rest:* Insomnia, night sweats, fatigue

*Cognitive-perceptual:* Headaches, stiff neck, chest pain, rectal pain, retrosternal pain. Blurred vision, photophobia, diplopia, loss of vision. Hearing impairment. Confusion, forgetfulness, attention deficit, changes in mental status, memory loss, personality changes Paresthesias, hypersensitivity in feet, pruritus

*Role-relationship:* Support system(s), career or job, financial resources

*Sexuality-reproductive:* Lesions on genitalia or anus (internal or external), pruritus or burning in vagina, penis, or anus. Painful sexual intercourse, rectal pain or bleeding, changes in menstruation, vaginal or penile discharge. Use of birth control measures, pregnancies, desire for future children

*Coping–stress tolerance:* Stress levels, previous losses, coping patterns, self-concept; social withdrawal

**Objective Data**

***General***

Lethargy, persistent fever, lymphadenopathy, peripheral wasting, fat deposits in truncal areas and upper back

***Eyes***

Presence of exudates, retinal lesions or hemorrhage, papilledema

***Integumentary***

Decreased skin turgor, dry skin, diaphoresis. Pallor, cyanosis. Lesions, eruptions, discolorations, bruises of skin or mucous membranes. Vaginal or perianal excoriation. Alopecia. Delayed wound healing

***Respiratory***

Tachypnea, dyspnea, intercostal retractions. Crackles, wheezing, productive or nonproductive cough

***Cardiovascular***

Pericardial friction rub, murmur, bradycardia, tachycardia.

***Gastrointestinal***

Mouth lesions, including blisters (HSV), white-gray patches (*Candida* infection), painless white lesions on lateral aspect of the tongue (hairy leukoplakia), discolorations (KS). Gingivitis, tooth decay or loosening. Redness or white patchy lesions of throat. Vomiting, diarrhea, incontinence, rectal lesions, hyperactive bowel sounds, abdominal masses, hepatosplenomegaly

***Musculoskeletal***

Muscle wasting, weakness

***Neurologic***

Ataxia, tremors, lack of coordination. Sensory loss, slurred speech, aphasia. Memory loss, peripheral neuropathy, apathy, agitation, depression, inappropriate behavior. Decreasing levels of consciousness, seizures, paralysis, coma

***Reproductive***

Genital lesions or discharge, abdominal tenderness secondary to pelvic inflammatory disease (PID)

***Possible Diagnostic Findings***

Positive HIV antibody/antigen assay. Detectable viral load. ↓ $CD4^+$ T cell count, ↓ WBC count, lymphopenia, anemia, thrombocytopenia. Electrolyte imbalances, abnormal liver function tests. ↑ cholesterol, triglycerides, and blood glucose

*HSV,* Herpes simplex virus; *KS,* Kaposi sarcoma; *WBC,* white blood cell.

sensitive topics such as sexuality and drug use are best prepared to provide prevention education.

A wide variety of activities can reduce the risk of HIV infection.[27] Individuals choose the methods that best fit their needs and circumstances. Prevention techniques can be divided into *safe sexual activities* (those that eliminate risk) and *risk-reducing sexual activities* (those that decrease, but do not eliminate, risk).

The goal is to develop safer, healthier, and less risky behaviors. The more consistently and correctly prevention methods are used, the more effective they are in preventing HIV infection. It is also a good idea to use a combination of prevention methods (e.g., using condoms and decreasing the number of sex partners) to increase the prevention effect.

**Decreasing risks related to sexual intercourse.** *Safe sexual activities* eliminate the risk of exposure to HIV in semen and vaginal secretions. Abstaining from all sexual activity is an effective way to accomplish this goal, but there are safe options for those who cannot or do not wish to abstain. Limiting sexual behavior to activities in which the mouth, penis, vagina, or rectum does not come into contact with a partner's mouth, penis, vagina, or rectum eliminates contact with blood, semen, or vaginal secretions. Safe activities include masturbation, mutual masturbation ("hand job"), and other activities that meet the "no contact" requirements. *Insertive sex* between partners who are not infected with HIV and not at risk of becoming infected with HIV is also considered safe.

*Risk-reducing sexual activities* decrease the risk of contact with HIV through the use of barriers. Barriers should be used when engaging in insertive sexual activity (oral, vaginal, or anal) with a partner who has HIV or whose HIV status is not known. The most commonly used barrier is the male condom. Male condoms can be used for protection during anal, vaginal, and oral intercourse. Female condoms provide an alternative to male condoms. Squares of latex (known as dental dams) can be used as a barrier during oral sexual activity.

**Decreasing risks related to drug use.** Drug use, including alcohol and tobacco, can cause immunosuppression, poor nutrition, and a host of psychosocial problems. However, drug use does not cause HIV infection. The major risk for HIV related to using drugs involves sharing equipment or having

## ETHICAL/LEGAL DILEMMAS

### *Individual vs. Public Health Protection*

**Situation**

A nurse in a community clinic is having a follow-up visit with V.T., a 38-year-old woman, who was found to have HIV during her annual examination 2 weeks ago. During the visit, V.T. discloses that she has been verbally and physically abused by her partner. V.T. also indicates that she had not yet told her partner about the HIV diagnosis because she is afraid that he will hurt her. She has not used any protection during sex with him since she learned of her test results because she suspects he infected her.

**Ethical/Legal Points for Consideration**

- You face a conflict between preventing further harm to V.T. (possible increase in intimate partner violence), providing care to her partner (his need for an HIV test, diagnosis, and treatment), and protecting the public health (potential spread of HIV infection to her partner or from her partner to others in the community). Patient teaching and support are essential because your primary obligation is to the patient.
- Because relevant law varies from state to state, your first step is to be familiar with your state law concerning mandated reporting for domestic partner abuse and infectious diseases.
- Laws regarding protection of privacy in HIV testing are federal and apply everywhere.
- In many states, reporting domestic abuse is mandatory only when the abuse is actually witnessed by the reporter or when the immediate effects of the abuse (e.g., wounds, contusions, broken bones) are witnessed.[1]
- You should be familiar with crisis counseling services for V.T. and offer her the following advice: collect and stash a set of car keys or taxi money in a safe place, keep a bag packed and hidden or even stored in a locker somewhere accessible, develop a code phrase to use with a friend or family member to call for help, keep a cell phone charged, and have money hidden in a safe place.

**Discussion Questions**

1. Within the parameters of your state's requirements for reportable conditions, how can you protect the patient's confidentiality to prevent further intimate partner violence?
2. What services are offered by your state to notify a partner without disclosing the source patient's name? How would V.T. access those services in your state?
3. How can you protect the partner from possible infection while also protecting V.T. from further violence?
4. How can you best address the issue of intimate partner violence? What resources would V.T. have in your community?
5. Discuss the benefits of universal, voluntary testing in light of V.T.'s case.

**Reference**

1. National Coalition Against Domestic Violence: *www.ncadv.com.*

unsafe sexual experiences while under the influence of drugs. Basic risk reduction rules are (1) do not use drugs; (2) if you use drugs, do not share equipment; and (3) do not have sexual intercourse when under the influence of any drug (including alcohol) that impairs decision making.[28]

The safest method is to abstain from drugs, but this may not be a viable option for users who are not prepared to quit or have no access to drug treatment services. The risk of HIV for these individuals can be eliminated if they do not share equipment. Injecting equipment ("works") includes needles, syringes, cookers (spoons or bottle caps used to mix the drug), cotton, and rinse water. Equipment used to snort (straws) or smoke (pipes) drugs can also be contaminated with blood and should not be shared.

## HEALTHY PEOPLE

### *Prevention and Early Detection of HIV*

- Increase safer sexual practices, including condom use.
- Decrease equipment sharing among IV drug users.
- Increase clinician skills to assess for risk factors for HIV infection, recommend HIV testing, and provide counseling for behavior change.
- Make voluntary HIV testing a routine part of health care.
- Increase access to new HIV testing technologies, especially rapid testing.
- Increase access to HIV testing facilities in traditional health care settings, as well as in alternative sites such as drug and alcohol treatment facilities and community-based organizations.
- Increase risk assessment and individualized behavior change messages to people with HIV to prevent new infections.
- Decrease perinatal HIV infection by offering voluntary HIV testing as a part of routine prenatal care.
- Provide counseling and appropriate HIV therapy to those who are infected.

Access to sterile equipment is an important risk elimination tactic. Some communities have needle and syringe exchange programs (NSEPs) that provide sterile equipment in exchange for used equipment. Opposition to these programs is related to the fear that access to injecting supplies will increase drug use. However, studies have shown that, in communities with NSEPs, drug use does not increase, rates of HIV and other blood-borne infections are controlled, and an overall cost benefit results.[29] Cleaning equipment before use can also reduce risk by decreasing the chance of blood contact.

In addition, providing support for patients with substance use and referring individuals to professionals who can assist patients manage the psychologic aspects of substance use is important. Other self-help programs (e.g., Narcotics Anonymous, Alcoholics Anonymous) may also be beneficial.

◆ **Decreasing risks of perinatal transmission.** The best way to prevent HIV infection in infants is to prevent HIV infection in women. Women who are already infected with HIV should be asked about their reproductive desires. Those who choose not to have children need to have family planning methods discussed in detail. Should they become pregnant, abortion may be desired and should be discussed in conjunction with other options, including the possibility of maintaining the pregnancy and using ART to decrease the risk of transmission.

If HIV-infected pregnant women are appropriately treated during pregnancy, the rate of perinatal transmission can be decreased from 25% to less than 2%. ART has significantly decreased the risk for infants born to HIV-infected women, and more of these women are now becoming mothers. The current standard of care is for all women who are pregnant or contemplating pregnancy to be counseled about HIV, routinely offered access to voluntary HIV-antibody testing, and, if infected, offered optimal ART.[24,30]

◆ **Decreasing risks at work.** The risk of infection from occupational exposure to HIV is small but real. OSHA requires employers to protect workers from exposure to blood and other potentially infectious materials (Table 14-8). Precautions and safety devices decrease the risk of direct contact with blood and body fluids. Should exposure to HIV-infected fluids occur, **postexposure prophylaxis (PEP)** with combination ART can significantly decrease the risk of infection.[16] The need for timely treatment and counseling makes it even more critical for nurses to report all blood exposures.

TABLE 14-15 **Nursing Interventions in HIV Infection**

| Nursing Care and Goals | Assessment | Interventions |
|---|---|---|
| **Health Promotion** | | |
| 1. Prevent HIV infection. | *Risk factors:* What behaviors or social, physical, emotional, pathogenic, or immune factors place the patient at risk? | • Education, including knowledge, attitudes, and behaviors, with emphasis on risk reduction to the following:<br>• *General population:* Cover general information<br>• *Pregnant women:* General information and information specific to HIV infection and pregnancy<br>• *Individual patient:* Specific to assessed need<br>• Empower patients to take control of prevention measures. |
| 2. Detect HIV infection early. | Does the patient need to be tested for HIV? | • Provide HIV antibody/antigen testing with appropriate counseling. |
| **Acute Care** | | |
| 1. Promote health and limit disability. | *Physical health:* Is the patient experiencing problems?<br>*Mental health:* How is the patient coping?<br>*Resources:* Does the patient have family or social support? Is the patient accessing community services? Is money or insurance a problem? Does the patient have access to spiritual support as desired? | • Provide case management or refer to interprofessional team, including social work.<br>• Teach regarding HIV, the spectrum of infection, options for care, signs and symptoms to report, treatment options, immune enhancement, risk reduction, and ways to adhere to treatment regimens.<br>• Establish long-term, trusting relationship with patient, family, and significant others.<br>• Provide emotional and spiritual support.<br>• Develop resources for legal needs: discrimination prevention, wills and advance directives, child care wishes.<br>• Empower the patient to identify needs, direct care, and seek services. |
| 2. Manage problems caused by HIV infection. | *Physical health:* Has the patient experienced acute exacerbation of problems related to immunodeficiency, opportunistic disease, or risk factors (e.g., substance use)?<br>*Mental health status:* Has the patient's ability to cope with psychosocial issues deteriorated? | • Provide care during acute exacerbations: recognition of life-threatening developments, life support, rapid intervention with treatments and drugs, comfort, and hygiene needs.<br>• Support patient and family during crisis.<br>• Assist the patient with mental health issues and provide referral to mental health specialist as needed. |
| **Ambulatory Care** | | |
| 1. Maximize quality of life. | *Physical health:* Are new symptoms developing? Is the patient experiencing drug side effects or interactions? | • Continue case management.<br>• Teach about changing treatment options and continued adherence.<br>• Empower patient to continue to direct care and to make desires known to family members and significant others. |
| 2. Resolve life and death issues. | *Mental health:* How is the patient coping? What adjustments have been made?<br>*Finances:* Can the patient maintain health care and basic standards of living?<br>*Family, social, and community support:* Are these available? Is the patient using support in an effective manner? Do family or significant others need teaching, encouragement, or stress relief?<br>*Spirituality issues:* Does the patient desire support from a religious organization or spiritual counselor? What assistance does the patient desire? | • Continue physical care for chronic disease process: treatments, drugs, comfort, and hygiene needs.<br>• Encourage health promotion measures (as above).<br>• Refer the patient to resources to support finances.<br>• Support patient and family or significant others in a trusting relationship.<br>• Assist with end-of-life issues: resuscitation orders, comfort measures, funeral plans, estate planning, child care, etc.<br>• Assess desires and refer to resources that will assist in meeting identified spiritual needs. |

***HIV Testing.*** An estimated 14% of people living with HIV in the United States are not aware that they are infected. People who do not know they are infected are more likely to transmit the infection to others. Current guidelines recommend universal, voluntary testing as part of routine medical care.[31,32] The goal is to normalize the test, decrease the stigma related to HIV testing, find hidden cases, get infected individuals into care, and prevent new cases of infection.

## Acute Care

***Early Intervention.*** Early intervention after detection of HIV infection can promote health and limit disability. The nursing assessment in HIV disease should focus on early detection of symptoms, opportunistic diseases, and psychosocial problems (Table 14-15).

**Initial response to diagnosis of HIV.** Reactions to an HIV diagnosis are similar to the reactions of people who are diagnosed with any life-threatening, debilitating, or chronic illness. These reactions include anxiety, panic, fear, depression, denial, hopelessness, anger, and guilt.[33] Unfortunately, all these emotions are overlaid with the stigma and discrimination that continue to pervade societal reactions to HIV. Many of these reactions are also seen in the patient's family members, friends, and caregivers. As time passes, patients and their loved ones will be confronted with complex treatment decisions; feelings of loss, anger, powerlessness, depression, and grief; social isolation; the possibility of death; and/or thoughts of suicide.

**Antiretroviral therapy.** ART can significantly slow the progression of HIV. However, treatment regimens can be complex,

## EVIDENCE-BASED PRACTICE

### Applying the Evidence

**Condom Use and HIV**

As a nurse in an HIV clinic, you are counseling M.J., a 27-year-old gay man, and his partner. M.J. is on antiretroviral therapy. His viral load is very low and his CD4⁺ T cell count is normal. He tells you that since the medications are working, he and his partner (who is not infected with HIV) are considering not using condoms in the future.

***Making Clinical Decisions***

***Best Available Evidence.*** One of the best ways to prevent HIV transmission from an infected person to an uninfected person is by using condoms.

***Clinician Expertise.*** You know that risk-reducing sexual activities in this situation include the continued use of condoms. However, you also know that although a very low viral load decreases the risk of HIV transmission, a partner may become infected.

***Patient Preferences and Values.*** M.J. tells you that he and his partner are in a committed relationship, have no other partners, and do not like using condoms.

***Implications for Practice***

1. What information would you discuss with M.J. related to HIV transmission, viral load, and the risks of unprotected sexual activity?
2. What measures besides condom use would you discuss with M.J. to reduce the risk of HIV transmission?

***References for Evidence***

Centers for Disease Control and Prevention: HIV prevention in the United States-proven HIV prevention methods. Retrieved from *www.cdc.gov/nchhstp/newsroom/HIVFactSheets/Prevention.*

Centers for Disease Control and Prevention: Condom fact sheet in brief. Retrieved from *www.cdc.gov/condomeffectiveness/brief.html.*

the drugs have side effects, ART does not work for everyone, and it is expensive. These factors can contribute to problems with adherence to treatment, a dangerous situation because of the high risk of developing drug resistance.

## CHECK YOUR PRACTICE

You are working in an outpatient HIV clinic and one of the patients, a 34-yr-old single mother with HIV infection, tells you, "I've been feeling well lately, and I've been so busy taking care of my 2-year-old son, so I have not been taking my HIV meds."

- How would you respond to this patient?

As a nurse, you are often the person who works most closely with patients who are trying to cope with the issues of dealing with the diagnosis and treatment of HIV. Table 14-16 provides a guide to providing patient and caregiver teaching on HIV treatment and initial follow up.

Interventions include teaching about (1) advantages and disadvantages of new treatments, (2) dangers of poor adherence to therapeutic regimens, (3) how and when to take each drug, (4) drug interactions to avoid, and (5) side effects that must be reported to the HCP.

Clinical guidelines provide information on initial drug regimens.[24] However, one of the most important considerations for initiating therapy is patient readiness for treatment. *Adherence* to ART is a critical component of successful drug therapy for people with HIV infection. Nurses are uniquely prepared to provide assistance with adherence to the drug regimen (Table 14-17). Taking drugs as prescribed (right dose and time) is important for all drug therapy, but with HIV infection, missing even a few doses can lead to drug resistance. Patients can be helped to adhere to difficult treatment regimens with electronic reminders, beepers, timers on pillboxes, and calendars. Group support and individual counseling can also help, but the best approach is to learn about the patient's life and assist with problem solving related to taking medications within the confines of that life.

## TABLE 14-16 Patient & Caregiver Teaching

### Antiretroviral Drugs

*Resistance to antiretroviral drugs is a major problem in treating HIV infection. Include the following instructions when teaching the patient and/or caregiver to decrease the risk of developing resistance.*

1. Discuss options with your HCP to find the best regimen for you. Your provider should order at least three different antiretroviral drugs from at least two different drug groups.
2. Know the drugs you are taking and how to take them (some have to be taken with food, some must be taken on an empty stomach, some cannot be taken together). If you do not understand, ask. Have your nurse write the instructions clearly for you.
3. Take the full dose prescribed, and take it on schedule. If you cannot take the drug because of side effects or other problems, report it to your HCP immediately.
4. Take all of your medications as prescribed. Do not quit taking one drug while continuing the others. If you cannot tolerate even one of your drugs, talk to your HCP, who will recommend a way to deal with the side effects or a new set of drugs.
5. Many antiretroviral drugs interact with other drugs, including a number of common drugs you can buy without a prescription. Be sure your HCP and pharmacist know all of the drugs that you are taking, and do not take any new drugs without checking for possible interactions.
6. The goals of antiretroviral therapy are to decrease the amount of virus in your blood (your viral load) and to keep your CD4⁺ T cell count high. The best results reduce your viral load below detectable levels and keep your CD4⁺ T cell count high. Most HCPs do routine laboratory work every 3 to 6 months whether you are taking antiretroviral agents or not.
7. Two to 4 weeks after you start on drug therapy (or change your therapy), your HCP will test your viral load to find out how the drugs are working.
   - Your viral load is reported in absolute numbers. All you need to know is that you want to see the viral load drop.
   - Your CD4⁺ T cell count is reported in absolute numbers or percentages. It is best for your CD4⁺ T cell count to be above 500 to 600 cells/μL. If reported in percentages, you would like your CD4⁺ T cell value to be above 14%.
8. An undetectable viral load means that the amount of virus is extremely low and HIV cannot be found in the blood using current testing technology. It does not mean that the virus is gone because the virus can be in lymph nodes and organs that blood tests cannot detect. It also does not mean that you are no longer able to transmit HIV to others. You will need to continue protecting all of your sexual and drug-using partners from HIV.

◆ **Delaying disease progression.** HIV disease progression may be delayed by promoting a healthy immune system, whether the patient chooses to take ART or not. Useful interventions for HIV-infected patients include (1) getting nutritional support to maintain lean body mass and ensure appropriate levels of vitamins and micronutrients; (2) moderating or eliminating alcohol, tobacco, and drug use; (3) keeping up to date with recommended vaccines; (4) getting adequate rest and exercise; (5) reducing stress; (6) avoiding exposure to new infectious agents; (7)

**TABLE 14-17 Patient & Caregiver Teaching**

***Improving Adherence to Antiretroviral Therapy***

*The following are strategies that you can use to improve a patient's adherence to using antiretroviral therapy:*

1. Determine whether the patient understands the importance of adherence and is ready to start therapy.
2. Provide teaching on medication dosing.
3. Review potential side effects of drugs.
4. Assure the patient that side effects can be treated. If not, medication regimens can be changed.
5. Use teaching and memory aids, including pictures, pillboxes, and calendars.
6. Engage family and friends in the teaching process. Solicit their support to help the patient take treatment.
7. Simplify regimens, dosing, and food requirements as much as possible.
8. Use a team of nurses, HCPs, pharmacists, case managers, and mental health and peer counselors to support the patient.
9. Help the patient integrate the medication regimen into his or her typical life activities and work schedules.

Modified from Centers for Disease Control and Prevention: Guidelines for the use of antiretroviral agents in HIV-1-infected adults and adolescents, 2015. Retrieved from *http://aidsinfo.nih.gov.*

**INFORMATICS IN PRACTICE**

***Use of Internet and Mobile Devices to Manage HIV***

- The Internet offers resources and support for patients that can assist them in coping with their illness and educate them about signs and symptoms of serious illness.
- By monitoring their health and quickly spotting warning signs of serious illnesses, patients are able to alert their HCPs and receive earlier treatment.
- These systems can help the patient manage antiretroviral therapy by sending medication reminders by text or e-mail.

accessing counseling; (8) getting involved in support groups and community activities; and (9) developing a consistent relationship with HCPs, including attendance at regular appointments.

Teach patients to recognize symptoms that may indicate disease progression and/or drug side effects so that prompt medical care can be initiated. Table 14-18 provides an overview of symptoms that patients should report.

◆ ***Acute Exacerbations.*** Chronic diseases are characterized by acute exacerbations of recurring problems. This is especially true in HIV disease in which infections, cancers, debility, and psychosocial or economic issues may interact to overwhelm the patient's ability to cope. Nursing care becomes more complex as the patient's immune system deteriorates and new problems arise to compound existing difficulties. When opportunistic diseases or difficult treatment side effects develop, symptom management, teaching, and emotional support are needed.

Nursing care can help prevent the many opportunistic diseases associated with HIV infection. The best way to prevent opportunistic disease is to ensure that the patient is adhering to an effective ART regimen and, if appropriate, taking prophylactic medications for opportunistic infections. Should an opportunistic disease occur, nursing care is an essential part of helping the patient adhere to medications and providing supportive care specific to the opportunistic disease. For example, if the patient has *Pneumocystis jiroveci* pneumonia (PCP)

**TABLE 14-18 Patient & Caregiver Teaching**

***Signs and Symptoms HIV-Infected Patients Need to Report***

*Teach the patient with HIV infection and the caregiver to report the following signs and symptoms.*

**Report Immediately**

- Any change in level of consciousness: lethargic, hard to arouse, unable to be aroused, unresponsive, unconscious
- Headache accompanied by nausea and vomiting, changes in vision, changes in ability to perform coordinated activities, or after any head trauma
- Vision changes: blurry or black areas in vision field, new floaters, double vision
- Persistent shortness of breath related to activity and not relieved by a short rest period
- Nausea and vomiting accompanied by abdominal pain
- Vomiting blood
- Dehydration: unable to eat or drink because of nausea, diarrhea, or mouth lesions; severe diarrhea or vomiting; dizziness when standing
- Yellow discoloration of the skin
- Any bleeding from the rectum that is not related to hemorrhoids or trauma (e.g., from anal sexual intercourse)
- Pain in the flank with fever and inability to urinate for more than 6 hr
- Blood in the urine
- New onset of weakness in any part of the body, new onset of numbness that is not obviously related to pressure, new onset of difficulty speaking
- Chest pain not obviously related to cough
- Seizures
- New rash accompanied by fever
- New oral lesions accompanied by fever
- Severe depression, anxiety, hallucinations, delusions, or thoughts of causing danger to self or others

**Report the Following Signs and Symptoms Within 24 Hours**

- New or different headache; constant headache not relieved by over-the-counter medication
- Headache accompanied by fever, nasal congestion, or cough
- Burning, itching, or discharge from the eyes
- New or productive cough
- Vomiting 2 or 3 times a day
- Vomiting accompanied by fever
- New, significant, or watery diarrhea (more than 6 times a day)
- Painful urination, bloody urine, urethral discharge
- Significant new rash (widespread; painful; or following a path down the leg or arm, around the chest, or on the face)
- Difficulty eating or drinking because of mouth lesions
- Vaginal discharge, pain, or itching

(Fig. 14-8), nursing interventions can ensure adequate oxygenation. If the patient has cryptococcal meningitis, an important nursing concern is maintaining a safe environment for a confused patient.

◆ **Ambulatory Care.** HIV infection has no cure, continues for life, causes physical disability, and contributes to impaired health. In many cases it can lead to death. HIV infection affects the entire range of a person's life from physical health to social, emotional, economic, and spiritual well-being.

◆ ***Stigma of HIV.*** HIV-infected patients share problems experienced by all individuals with chronic diseases, but these problems are exacerbated by negative social attitudes and beliefs surrounding HIV.[34] HIV-infected people may be thought to lack

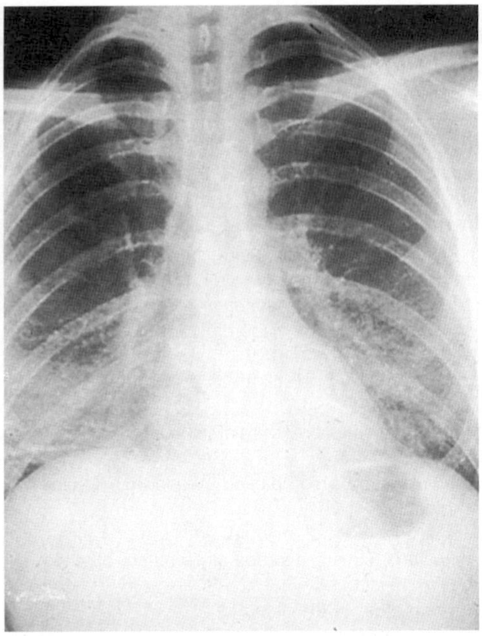

**FIG. 14-8** Chest x-ray showing interstitial infiltrates as the result of *Pneumocystis jiroveci* pneumonia. (From the Centers for Disease Control and Prevention. Courtesy Jonathan W.M. Gold, MD, New York.)

control over urges to have sex or use drugs. Some people conclude that people with HIV brought the disease upon themselves and deserve to be sick. Behaviors associated with HIV infection are viewed by some as immoral (e.g., homosexuality, promiscuity) and are sometimes illegal (e.g., using drugs, sex work). The fact that infected individuals can transmit HIV to others creates fear, which leads to stigma and discrimination in all facets of life.

In the United States, HIV-infected people have lost jobs, homes, and insurance, although these forms of discrimination are prohibited by the Americans with Disabilities Act (ADA). HIV-related stigma is a global problem that is often more severe for women. Discrimination can lead to social isolation, dependence, frustration, low self-image, loss of control, and economic pressures.

◆ ***Disease and Drug Side Effects.*** Physical problems related to HIV or its treatment can interfere with the patient's ability to maintain a desired lifestyle. HIV-infected patients frequently experience anxiety, fear, depression, diarrhea, peripheral neuropathy, pain, nausea, vomiting, and fatigue. Nursing interventions for these symptoms are similar to what they would be for the patient who does not have HIV infection. For example, nursing management of diarrhea includes helping patients collect specimens, recommending dietary changes, encouraging fluid and electrolyte replacement, instructing the patient about skin care, and managing skin breakdown around the perianal area. Nursing approaches for fatigue in HIV include teaching patients to assess fatigue patterns; determine contributing factors; set activity priorities; conserve energy; schedule rest periods; exercise regularly; and avoid substances such as caffeine, nicotine, alcohol, and other drugs that may disturb sleep.

Some HIV-infected patients, especially those who have been infected and on ART for a long time, may develop a set of metabolic disorders. These include (1) lipodystrophy (changes in body shape caused by a redistribution of fat in the abdomen, upper back, and breasts along with fat loss in the arms, legs, and face) (Fig. 14-9); (2) hyperlipidemia (elevated triglycerides, elevated low-density lipoproteins, and decreased high-density lipoproteins); (3) insulin resistance (4) hyperglycemia; (5) bone

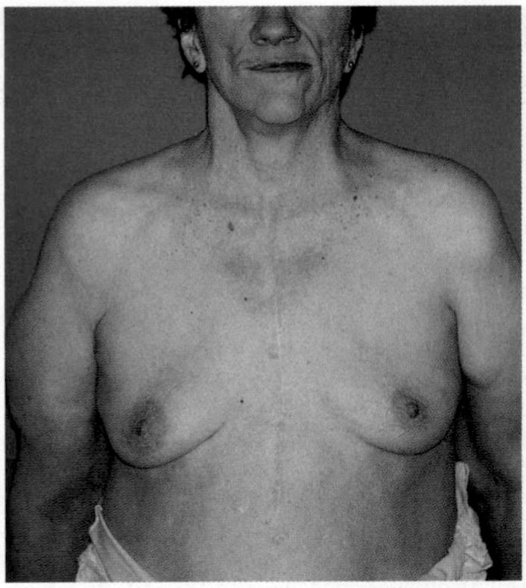

**FIG. 14-9** Lipodystrophy manifestations. (From James WD, Berger T, Elston D: *Andrews' diseases of the skin: clinical dermatology,* ed 11, St Louis, 2011, Saunders.)

disease (osteoporosis, osteopenia, avascular necrosis); (6) lactic acidosis; (7) renal disease; and (8) cardiovascular disease.[35,36]

It is still not clear why these disorders develop, but it is probably a combination of factors such as long-term infection with HIV, side effects of ART, genetic predisposition, and chronic stress. Management of metabolic disorders focuses on detecting problems early, dealing with symptoms, and helping the patient cope with emerging problems and changes to treatment regimens. It is important to recognize and treat these problems early, especially because cardiovascular disease and lactic acidosis are potentially fatal complications.

A frequent first intervention is to change ART medications because some drugs are more often associated with these disorders. Lipid abnormalities are generally treated with lipid-lowering drugs (see Table 33-5), dietary changes, and exercise. Insulin resistance is treated with hypoglycemic drugs and weight loss. Bone disease may be improved with exercise, dietary changes, and calcium and vitamin D supplements.

◆ ***End-of-Life Care.*** Despite new developments in the treatment of HIV infection, many patients eventually experience disease progression, disability, and death. Sometimes these occur because treatments do not work for the patient. Sometimes the patient's HIV becomes resistant to all available drug therapies. In addition, ART is now allowing people living with HIV to live longer and to develop diseases of aging, such as cardiovascular and endocrine problems that lead to death.

Nursing care during the terminal phase of any disease should focus on keeping the patient comfortable, facilitating emotional and spiritual acceptance of the finite nature of life, helping the patient's significant others deal with grief and loss, and maintaining a safe environment.[37] As a nurse, you are the pivotal care provider during this phase of illness, whether at home, through hospice, or in a health care facility. (End-of-life care is discussed in Chapter 9.)

## ◆ Evaluation

The expected outcomes are that the patient at risk for HIV infection will

- Analyze personal risk factors
- Develop and implement a personal plan to decrease risks
- Get tested for HIV

The expected outcomes are that the patient with HIV infection will

- Describe basic aspects of the effects of HIV on the immune system
- Compare and contrast various treatment options for HIV disease
- Work with a team of HCPs to achieve optimal health
- Prevent transmission of HIV to others

## Gerontologic Considerations: HIV Infection

The number of older adults who have HIV disease is increasing because (1) HIV treatment has been effective in reducing the number of deaths from HIV-related opportunistic infections and (2) people 60 and older are being infected at increasing rates. The number of people over the age of 60 living with HIV is expected to grow.

Remember that older people living with HIV are susceptible to the same diseases as non-HIV-infected older people. These include heart disease, cancer, diabetes, bone disease, arthritis, hypertension, kidney disease, and cognitive impairment. However, people with HIV infection may experience these diseases at an earlier age (compared with non-HIV-infected people) and may be at higher risk of co-morbidities related to the medications used to treat HIV.[38] For example, some of the HIV medications are associated with increased lipids and altered insulin metabolism. Focusing nursing care on early identification of these complications, and assisting patients in reducing their risk for heart disease, diabetes, or other chronic disease, are critical aspects of caring for the older HIV patient.

Another consideration with the aging HIV population is the impact of polypharmacy (taking multiple medications to treat a variety of conditions). In general, older adults are often prescribed multiple medications to manage various chronic diseases. Some of these medications may interact with or be potentiated by HIV medications. Therefore careful monitoring and assessment of possible drug interactions is important when providing care to this population.

Older adults may be ashamed and hesitate to tell anyone that they have an HIV infection. This may make it difficult for them to get the appropriate health care and support. As a nurse, you need to recognize that HIV is a chronic disease that will affect an increasing number of older adults and be prepared to help the older person who is living with HIV infection.

### CHECK YOUR PRACTICE

You are receiving report on a newly admitted patient to the rehabilitation unit. He is a 68-yr-old male patient who had a hip replacement 3 days ago. The nurse giving the report casually mentions, "Oh, by the way, he has AIDS. Can you believe that an old man like that has HIV?"

- How would you respond?

## CASE STUDY

### *HIV Infection*

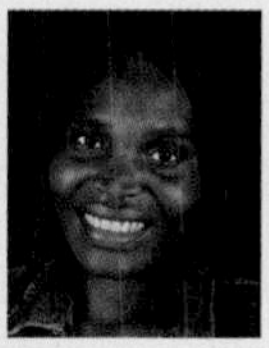

(©iStockphoto/Thinkstock)

**Patient Profile**

J.N., a 35-year-old African American woman, was admitted to the hospital in respiratory distress. AIDS and *Pneumocystis jiroveci* pneumonia (PCP) were both diagnosed 2 days ago.

**Subjective Data**

- Seen by an HCP 6 years ago for pain behind the sternum and difficulty swallowing, diagnosed as esophageal candidiasis; positive HIV-antibody test at that time
- Has consistently refused ART because, "We can't afford it"
- Married to Jim, a former IV drug user, for 15 years until his recent death from AIDS-related complications
- Has two children, ages 8 and 10; neither has been tested for HIV infection
- Experiences fatigue and frequent oral and vaginal candidiasis outbreaks
- Expresses concern about the welfare of her children, who are at home with her sister, and says, "Maybe I should take better care of myself for them"

**Objective Data**

***Physical Examination***

- 5 ft 6 in tall, 100 lb, temperature 100.4° F (38° C), $O_2$ saturation 92% on 3 L of $O_2$ via nasal cannula

***Laboratory Studies***

- CD4$^+$ T cell count 185 cells/µL
- Viral load 55,328 copies/µL
- Hematocrit 30%

**Interprofessional Care**

- Trimethoprim/sulfamethoxazole
- Combination antiretroviral therapy: tenofovir and emtricitabine (Truvada), with darunavir and cobicistat (Prezcobix)

**Discussion Questions**

1. Why did J.N.'s initial medical problem (esophageal candidiasis) lead to an HIV test?
2. Why was trimethoprim/sulfamethoxazole ordered, and what are its common side effects?
3. What diagnostic criteria for AIDS are present in J.N.?
4. Is there a potential advantage to J.N.'s refusal to take antiretroviral drugs in the past? If so, why or why not?
5. ***Priority Decision:*** What priority teaching needs should be covered before J.N. is discharged from the hospital to return home? What referrals must be made?
6. How can J.N. be helped to adhere to her medication schedule?
7. ***Priority Decision:*** What are the priority nursing interventions? What plans must be made for continued nursing care after discharge?
8. ***Evidence-Based Practice:*** J.N. asks you if her kids should be tested. She is afraid of what the results may be. How should you respond?
9. ***Teamwork and Collaboration:*** Women often put their children's welfare first. What barriers could this cause for J.N.'s treatment? How could an interprofessional team assist in addressing these issues?
10. ***Safety:*** The nurse needs to start an IV for fluid replacement on J.N. Before inserting the IV what type of personal protective equipment is recommended for this situation?

Answers available at *http://evolve.elsevier.com/Lewis/medsurg.*

## BRIDGE TO NCLEX EXAMINATION

The number of the question corresponds to the same-numbered outcome at the beginning of the chapter.

1. Emerging and reemerging infections affect health care by *(select all that apply)*
   a. reevaluating vaccine practices.
   b. revealing antimicrobial resistance.
   c. limiting antibiotics to those with life-threatening infection.
   d. challenging researchers to discover new antimicrobial therapies.
2. Which types(s) of isolation precautions is (are) appropriate for a patient with tuberculosis (*select all that apply*)?
   a. contact precautions
   b. droplet precautions
   c. airborne precautions
   d. standard precautions
   e. neutropenic precautions
3. Transmission of HIV from an infected individual to another most commonly occurs as a result of
   a. unprotected anal or vaginal sexual intercourse.
   b. low levels of virus in the blood and high levels of CD4$^+$ T cells.
   c. transmission from mother to infant during labor and delivery and breastfeeding.
   d. sharing of drug-using equipment, including needles, syringes, pipes, and straws.
4. During HIV infection
   a. reverse transcriptase helps HIV fuse with the CD4$^+$ T cell.
   b. HIV RNA uses the CD4$^+$ T cell's mitochondria to replicate.
   c. the immune system is impaired predominantly by the eventual widespread destruction of CD4$^+$ T cells.
   d. a long period of dormancy develops during which HIV cannot be found in the blood and there is little viral replication.
5. Which statements accurately describe HIV infection (*select all that apply*)?
   a. Untreated HIV infection has a predictable pattern of progression.
   b. Late chronic HIV infection is called acquired immunodeficiency syndrome (AIDS).
   c. Untreated HIV infection can remain in the early chronic stage for a decade or more.
   d. Untreated HIV infection usually remains in the early chronic stage for 1 year or less.
   e. Opportunistic diseases occur more often when the CD4$^+$ T cell count is high and the viral load is low.
6. A diagnosis of AIDS is made when an HIV-infected patient has
   a. a CD4$^+$ T cell count below 200/μL.
   b. a high level of HIV in the blood and saliva.
   c. lipodystrophy with metabolic abnormalities.
   d. oral hairy leukoplakia, an infection caused by Epstein-Barr virus.
7. Screening for HIV infection generally involves
   a. detecting CD8$^+$ cytotoxic T cells in saliva.
   b. laboratory analysis of saliva to detect CD4$^+$ T cells.
   c. analysis of lymph tissues for the presence of HIV RNA.
   d. laboratory analysis of blood to detect HIV antigen or antibody.
8. HIV antiretroviral drugs are used to
   a. cure acute HIV infection.
   b. decrease viral RNA levels.
   c. treat opportunistic diseases.
   d. decrease pain and symptoms in terminal disease.
9. Opportunistic diseases in HIV infection
   a. are usually benign.
   b. are generally slow to develop and progress.
   c. occur in the presence of immunosuppression.
   d. are curable with appropriate drug interventions.
10. Which statement(s) about metabolic side effects of ART is (are) true (*select all that apply*)?
    a. These are annoying symptoms that are ultimately harmless.
    b. ART-related body changes include fat redistribution and peripheral wasting.
    c. Lipid abnormalities include increases in triglycerides and decreases in high-density cholesterol.
    d. Insulin resistance and hyperlipidemia can be treated with drugs to control glucose and cholesterol.
    e. Compared to uninfected people, insulin resistance and hyperlipidemia are more difficult to treat in HIV-infected patients.
11. Which strategy can the nurse teach the patient to eliminate the risk of HIV transmission?
    a. Using sterile equipment to inject drugs
    b. Cleaning equipment used to inject drugs
    c. Taking lamivudine (Epivir) during pregnancy
    d. Using latex or polyurethane barriers to cover genitalia during sexual contact
12. What is the *most* appropriate nursing intervention to help an HIV-infected patient adhere to a treatment regimen?
    a. "Set up" a drug pillbox for the patient every week.
    b. Give the patient a video and a brochure to view and read at home.
    c. Tell the patient that the side effects of the drugs are bad but that they go away after a while.
    d. Assess the patient's routines and find adherence cues that fit into the patient's life circumstances.

1. a, b, d; 2. c, d; 3. a; 4. c; 5. a, b, c; 6. a; 7. d; 8. b; 9. c; 10. b, c, d; 11. a; 12. d

For rationales to these answers and even more NCLEX review questions, visit *http://evolve.elsevier.com/Lewis/medsurg*.

## EVOLVE WEBSITE

http://evolve.elsevier.com/Lewis/medsurg

**Review Questions (Online Only)**
**Key Points**
**Answer Keys for Questions**
- Rationales for Bridge to NCLEX Examination Questions
- Answer Guidelines for Case Study on p. 231

**Student Case Study**
- Patient With Human Immunodeficiency Virus (HIV) Infection and Acquired Immunodeficiency Syndrome (AIDS)

**Conceptual Care Map Creator**
**Audio Glossary**
**Content Updates**

## REFERENCES

1. Centers for Disease Control and Prevention: Emerging infectious diseases. Retrieved from *http://wwwnc.cdc.gov/eid*.
2. Centers for Disease Control and Prevention: The reemergence of vaccine-preventable diseases—exploring the public health successes and challenges, 2015. Retrieved from *www.cdc.gov*.

3. Khabbaz RF, Moseley RR, Steiner RJ, et al: Challenges of infectious diseases in the USA, *Lancet* 384:53, 2014.
4. Clemons NS, Gastanaduy PA, Fiebelkorn AP, et al: Measles—United States, January 4–April 2, 2015, *MMWR* 64:373, 2015.
5. Infectious Disease Society of America: Antimicrobial resistance. Retrieved from *www.idsociety.org/topic_antimicrobial_resistance.*
6. Velez R, VanGraafeiland B, Sloand E: Using clinical guidelines and clinical acumen to manage community-acquired methicillin-resistant *Staphylococcus aureus* infection, *J Nurse Pract* 11:124, 2015.
7. Centers for Disease Control and Prevention: Healthcare-associated infections. Retrieved from *www.cdc.gov/HAI.*
8. Centers for Disease Control and Prevention: Healthcare-associated infections: Data and statistics. Retrieved from *www.cdc.gov/HAI/surveillance/index.html.*
9. US Department of Health and Human Services Agency for Healthcare Research & Quality: Healthcare-associated infections. Retrieved from *www.ahrq.gov.*
10. Centers for Disease Control and Prevention: Top CDC recommendations to prevent healthcare-associated infections. Retrieved from *www.cdc.gov/HAI.*
11. Centers for Disease Control and Prevention: Guidelines for isolation precautions: preventing transmission of infectious agents in healthcare settings, 2007. Retrieved from *www.cdc.gov/hicpac.*
12. Society of Healthcare Epidemiology of America: Compendium of strategies to prevent healthcare-associated infection in acute care hospitals—2014 update. Retrieved from *www.shea-online.org/View/ArticleId/289/Compendium-of-Strategies-to-Prevent-Healthcare-Associated-Infections-in-Acute-Care-Hospitals-2014-Up.aspx.*
13. High K: Evaluation of infection in the older adult. Retrieved from *www.uptodate.com.*
14. Centers for Disease Control and Prevention: HIV surveillance report: diagnosis of HIV infection in the United States and dependent areas, 2013. Retrieved from *www.cdc.gov/hiv/statistics/basics.*
15. US Department of Health and Human Services. HIV/AIDS basics. Retrieved from *www.aids.gov/hiv-aids-basics.*
*16. Kuhar DT, Henderson DK, Struble KA, et al: Updated US public health service guidelines for the management of occupational exposures to human immunodeficiency virus and recommendations for postexposure prophylaxis, *Infect Control Hosp Epidemiol* 34:875, 2013.
17. World Health Organization. Mother-to-child transmission of HIV. Retrieved from *www.who.int/hiv/topics/mtct/en.*
18. Centers for Disease Control and Prevention: US Public Health Service Task Force recommendations for use of antiretroviral drugs in pregnant HIV-1–infected women for maternal health and interventions to reduce perinatal HIV transmission in the United States—July 31, 2012. Retrieved from *www.aidsinfo.nih.gov.*
19. US Department of Health and Human Services. The HIV life cycle. Retrieved from *http://aidsinfo.nih.gov/education-materials/fact-sheets/19/73/the-hiv-life-cycle.*
20. Smith MK, Rutstein SE, Powers KA, et al: The detection and management of early HIV infection: a clinical and public health emergency, *J Acquir Immune Defic Syndr* 63:S187, 2013.
21. US Department of Health and Human Services. The stages of HIV infection. Retrieved from *http://aidsinfo.nih.gov/education-materials/fact-sheets/19/46/the-stages-of-hiv-infection.*
22. Branson BM, Owen SM, Weslowski LG, et al: Laboratory testing for the diagnosis of HIV infection: updated recommendations, 2014. Retrieved from *http://stacks.cdc.gov/view/cdc/23447.*
23. Kang W, Tong HI, Sun Y, et al: Hepatitis C virus infection in patients with HIV-1 infection: epidemiology, natural history and management, *Expert Rev Gastroenterol Hepatol* 8:247, 2014.
*24. Panel on Antiretroviral Guidelines for Adults and Adolescents. Guidelines for the use of antiretroviral agents in HIV-1–infected adults and adolescents, 2015. Retrieved from *http://aidsinfo.nih.gov/guidelines/html/1/adult-and-adolescent-treatment-guidelines/0.*
25. Panel on Opportunistic Infections in HIV-infected Adults and Adolescents. Guidelines for the prevention and treatment of opportunistic infections in HIV-infected adults and adolescents, 2015. Retrieved from *www.aidsinfo.nih.gov.*
*26. Smith DK, Koenig LJ, Martin M, et al: Preexposure prophylaxis for the prevention of HIV infection – 2014: a clinical practice guideline. Retrieved from *http://stacks.cdc.gov/view/cdc/23109.*
27. Centers for Disease Control and Prevention, Health Resources and Services Administration, National Institutes of Health, American Academy of HIV Medicine, Association of Nurses in AIDS Care, the National Minority AIDS Council, and Urban Coalition for HIV/AIDS Prevention Services: Recommendations for HIV prevention with adults and adolescents with HIV in the United States, 2014. Retrieved from *http://stacks.cdc.gov/view/cdc/26062.*
28. US Department of Health and Human Services. Substance abuse/use. Retrieved from *www.aids.gov/hiv-aids-basics/prevention/reduce-your-risk/substance-abuse-use.*
29. Shoptaw S: HIV prevention for people who use substances: evidence-based strategies, *J Food Drug Anal* 21:S91, 2013.
*30. Panel on Treatment of HIV-infected Pregnant Women and Prevention of Perinatal Transmission. Recommendations for use of antiretroviral drugs in pregnant HIV-1-infected women for maternal health and interventions to reduce perinatal HIV transmission in the United States. Retrieved from *http://aidsinfo.nih.gov/guidelines/html/3/perinatal-guidelines/0#.*
31. Centers for Disease Control and Prevention: Revised guidelines for HIV testing of adults, adolescents, and pregnant women in health-care settings—September 22, 2006. (Classic) Retrieved from *www.aidsinfo.nih.gov.*
32. US Preventive Services Task Force. Human immunodeficiency virus (HIV) infection: screening, 2013. Retrieved from *www.uspreventiveservicestaskforce.org/Page/Topic/recommendation-summary/human-immunodeficiency-virus-hiv-infection-screening.*
33. US Department of Health and Human Services. Just diagnosed: next steps after testing positive for HIV. Retrieved from *http://aidsinfo.nih.gov/education-materials/fact-sheets/21/65/just-diagnosed–next-steps-after-testing-positive-for-hiv.*
34. French H, Greeff M, Watson MJ, et al: HIV stigma and disclosure experiences of people living with HIV in an urban and a rural setting, *AIDS Care* 8:1042, 2015.
35. Hemkens LG, Bucher HC: HIV infection and cardiovascular disease, *Eur Heart J* 35:1373, 2014.
36. Bociaga-Jasik M, Goralska J, Razny U, et al: Impact of antiretroviral therapy on selected metabolic disorders-pilot study, *Adv Clin Exp Med* 23:539, 2014.
37. Kirton C, Krakowski A, Witt Sherman D: Palliative care in HIV/AIDS. In Matzo M, editor: *Palliative care nursing: quality care to the end of life*, ed 4, New York, 2015, Springer.
*38. The HIV and Aging Consensus Project. Recommended treatment strategies for clinicians managing older patients with HIV. Retrieved from *http://hiv-age.org.*

*Evidence-based information for clinical practice.

# 15

# Cancer

*Carolee Polek*

*Every tomorrow has two handles. We can take hold of it by the handle of anxiety or by the handle of faith.*

***Author Unknown***

http://evolve.elsevier.com/Lewis/medsurg/

## LEARNING OUTCOMES

1. Describe the prevalence, incidence, survival, and mortality rates of cancer in the United States.
2. Describe the processes involved in the biology of cancer.
3. Differentiate among the three stages of cancer development.
4. Describe the role of the immune system related to cancer.
5. Discuss the role of the nurse in the prevention, detection, and diagnosis of cancer.
6. Explain the use of surgery, chemotherapy, radiation therapy, immunotherapy, targeted therapy, and hormone therapy in the treatment of cancer.
7. Identify the classifications of chemotherapy agents and methods of administration.
8. Differentiate between teletherapy (external beam radiation) and brachytherapy (internal radiation).
9. Describe the effects of radiation therapy and chemotherapy on normal tissues.
10. Identify the types and effects of immunotherapy and targeted therapy.
11. Describe the nursing management of patients receiving chemotherapy, radiation therapy, immunotherapy, and targeted therapy.
12. Describe nutritional therapy for patients with cancer.
13. Identify the complications associated with advanced cancer.
14. Describe support interventions for cancer patients, cancer survivors, and their caregivers.

## KEY TERMS

**bone marrow transplantation** (BMT), p. 259
**brachytherapy**, p. 250
**cancer**, p. 234
**carcinogens**, p. 237
**carcinoma in situ** (CIS), p. 241
**chemotherapy**, p. 245
**hematopoietic stem cell transplantation** (HSCT), p. 259
**histologic grading**, p. 241
**immunologic surveillance**, p. 239
**immunotherapy**, p. 257
**malignant neoplasms**, p. 240
**metastasis**, p. 238
**nadir**, p. 253
**oncogenes**, p. 236
**peripheral stem cell transplantation** (PSCT), p. 259
**protooncogenes**, p. 236
**radiation**, p. 249
**staging**, p. 241
**targeted therapy**, p. 257
**teletherapy**, p. 250
**tumor angiogenesis**, p. 238
**vesicants**, p. 246

**Cancer** is a group of diseases characterized by uncontrolled and unregulated growth of cells. Although cancer is often considered a disease of aging, with the majority of cases diagnosed in those over age 55 years, it occurs in people of all ages. An estimated 1,658,370 people in the United States are diagnosed annually with invasive carcinoma (excluding basal and squamous cell skin cancers).[1]

Overall both the incidence and mortality rate of cancer have been declining.[2] The incidences of many cancers, such as colorectal, lung, breast, and oropharyngeal cancers, have declined largely as a result of preventive efforts. However, the incidence of other types of cancers, such as kidney, thyroid, pancreas, liver, uterus, skin melanoma, multiple myeloma, and non-Hodgkin's lymphoma, has been increasing.[3]

Overall cancer incidence is higher in men than women. Gender differences in incidence and in death rates for specific cancers are presented in Tables 15-1 and 15-2 and the Gender Differences box.

Although mortality rates from all cancers combined are on the decline, cancer is still the second most common cause of

Reviewed by Margaret Barton-Burke, RN, PhD, FAAN, Mary Ann Lee Professor of Oncology Nursing, College of Nursing, University of Missouri–St Louis, St. Louis, Missouri; Stephanie Jackson, RN, MSN, AOCNS, Oncology Clinical Nurse Specialist, Hematology/Stem Cell Transplant, UCLA Medical Center, Los Angeles, California; Laura A. Stokowski, RNC, MS, Inova Fairfax Hospital for Children, Falls Church, Virginia; Joseph Tariman, RN, PhD, ANP-BC, Assistant Professor, School of Nursing, De Paul University, Chicago, Illinois; Deborah Kirk Walker, DNP, FNP-BC, NP-C, AOCN, Assistant Professor/Nurse Practitioner, Coordinator of Dual Adult—Gerontology Primary Care and Oncology Nurse Practitioner Specialty Track, Acute, Chronic, and Continuing Care Department, University of Alabama at Birmingham School of Nursing, Birmingham, Alabama; and Linda H. Yoder, RN, PhD, AOCN, FAAN, Associate Professor and Director, Nursing Administration and Healthcare Systems Management, Robert Wood Johnson Executive Nurse Alumna, Luci Baines Johnson Fellow in Nursing, The University of Texas at Austin School of Nursing, Austin, Texas.

**TABLE 15-1 Cancer Incidence by Site and Gender***

| MALE Type | % | FEMALE Type | % |
|---|---|---|---|
| Prostate | 26 | Breast | 29 |
| Lung | 14 | Lung | 13 |
| Colon/rectum | 8 | Colon/rectum | 8 |
| Urinary bladder | 7 | Uterus | 7 |
| Non-Hodgkin's lymphoma | 5 | Thyroid | 6 |
| Kidney and renal pelvis | 5 | Non-Hodgkin's lymphoma | 4 |
| Oral cavity and pharynx | 4 | Melanoma | 4 |
| Leukemia | 4 | Pancreas | 3 |

Source: American Cancer Society: *Cancer facts & figures 2015,* Atlanta, 2015, American Cancer Society.
*Numbers are estimates excluding basal and squamous cell skin cancers and carcinoma in situ.

**TABLE 15-2 Cancer Deaths by Site and Gender**

| MALE Type | % | FEMALE Type | % |
|---|---|---|---|
| Lung and bronchus | 28 | Lung and bronchus | 26 |
| Prostate | 9 | Breast | 15 |
| Colon/rectum | 8 | Colon/rectum | 9 |
| Pancreas | 7 | Pancreas | 7 |
| Liver and intrahepatic bile ducts | 5 | Ovary | 5 |
| | | Leukemia | 4 |
| Leukemia | 5 | Uterus | 4 |
| Esophagus | 4 | Non-Hodgkin's lymphoma | 3 |
| Urinary bladder | 4 | Liver and intrahepatic bile ducts | 3 |
| Non-Hodgkin's lymphoma | 4 | Brain and other nervous system | 2 |
| Kidney and renal pelvis | 3 | | |

Source: American Cancer Society: *Cancer facts & figures 2015,* Atlanta, 2015, American Cancer Society.

## GENDER DIFFERENCES

***Cancer***

**Men**
- More men than women die from cancer-related deaths each year.
- Mortality rate from lung cancer is higher in men than in women.
- Cancer with the highest incidence among men is prostate cancer.
- Men are more likely to develop liver cancer than women.
- Head and neck cancer occurs more frequently in men than in women.

**Women**
- Cancer with the highest death rate among women is lung cancer.
- Cancer with the highest incidence among women is breast cancer.
- Thyroid cancer is more prevalent in women than in men.
- Women are less likely to have colon cancer screenings than men.

death in the United States (heart disease is the most common). However, in people 40 to 79 years of age, cancer is the leading cause of death. Annually about 589,400 Americans are expected to die as a result of cancer, which is more than 1600 people per day.[1,2]

Considerable progress has been made in controlling cancer for long periods. More than 14.5 million Americans are alive today who have a history of cancer. This statistic represents Americans living with cancer, including those who are disease free, in remission, or undergoing treatment.[2] (Cancer survivors are discussed in this chapter on pp. 266-267).

Statistics are helpful in describing the scope of cancer as a public health problem, but they cannot describe the combined physiologic, psychologic, and social impact of cancer on individual patients, their caregivers, and families. Considerable apprehension is associated with a cancer diagnosis, proportionately more than with other chronic diseases such as heart disease. Despite advances in treatment and care, a great deal of anxiety and fear continue to be associated with a diagnosis of cancer. Education of health care professionals and the public is essential to promote realistic attitudes about cancer and cancer treatment.

You are in a strategic position to lead efforts at changing attitudes about cancer. Furthermore, you can also (1) assist individuals in decreasing their risk of cancer development, (2) increase rates of cancer screening, (3) help patients comply with cancer management regimens, and (4) support patients and their families as they cope with the effects of cancer and related treatment. You need to be knowledgeable about specific types of cancer, treatment options, management of side effects of therapy, and supportive therapies for cancer.

## BIOLOGY OF CANCER

Two major dysfunctions in the process of cancer development are defective cell proliferation (growth) and defective cell differentiation.

### Defect in Cell Proliferation

Normally, most tissues contain a population of undifferentiated cells known as stem cells. These stem cells ultimately differentiate and become mature, functioning cells of that tissue and only that tissue.

Cell proliferation originates in the stem cell and begins when the stem cell enters the cell cycle (Fig. 15-1). The time from when a cell enters the cell cycle to when the cell divides into two identical cells is called the *generation time of the cell.* A mature cell continues to function until it degenerates and dies.

All of the body's cells are controlled by an intracellular mechanism that determines when cell proliferation is necessary. Under normal conditions, a state of dynamic equilibrium is constantly maintained (i.e., cell proliferation equals cell degeneration or death). Normally the process of cell division and proliferation is activated only in the presence of cell degeneration or death *(apoptosis).* Cell proliferation also occurs if the body has a physiologic need for more cells. For example, a normal increase in white blood cell (WBC) count occurs in the presence of infection.

Another mechanism for proliferation control in normal cells is *contact inhibition.* Normal cells respect the boundaries and territory of the cells surrounding them. They will not invade a territory that is not their own. The neighboring cells are thought to inhibit cell growth through the physical contact of the surrounding cell membranes. Cancer cells grown in tissue culture are characterized by loss of contact inhibition. These cells have no regard for cell boundaries and grow on top of one another and also on top of or between normal cells.

The rate of normal cell proliferation (from the time of cell birth to the time of cell death) differs in each body tissue. In some tissues, such as bone marrow, hair follicles, and epithelial lining of the gastrointestinal (GI) tract, the rate of cell proliferation is rapid. In other tissues, such as myocardium and cartilage, cell proliferation does not occur or is slow.

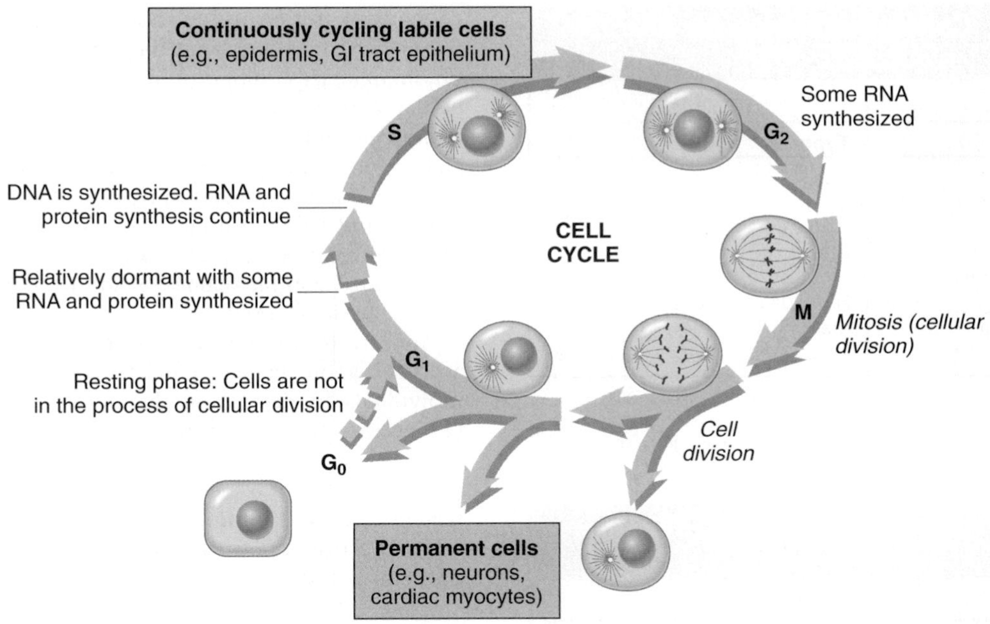


**FIG. 15-1** Cell life cycle and metabolic activity. Generation time is the period from *M* phase to *M* phase. Cells not in the cycle but capable of division are in the resting phase *($G_0$)*. (Adapted from Kumar V, Abbas AK, Fausto N, et al: *Robbins and Cotran pathologic basis of disease,* ed 8, Philadelphia, 2010, Saunders.)

Cancer cells proliferate at the same rate as the normal cells of the tissue from which they arise. However, cancer cells respond differently than normal cells to the intracellular signals that regulate the state of dynamic equilibrium. The difference is that proliferation of the cancer cells is indiscriminate and continuous. Sometimes they produce more than two cells at the time of mitosis. In this way, there is continuous growth of a tumor mass: $1 \times 2 \times 4 \times 8 \times 15$ and so on. This is termed the *pyramid effect.* The time required for a tumor mass to double in size is known as its *doubling time.*

## Defect in Cell Differentiation

*Cell differentiation* is normally an orderly process that progresses from a state of immaturity to a state of maturity. Because all body cells are derived from the fertilized ova, all cells have the potential to perform all body functions. As cells differentiate, this potential is repressed, and the mature cell is capable of performing only specific functions. With cell differentiation, there is a stable and orderly phasing out of cell potential. Under normal conditions, the differentiated cell is stable and will not *dedifferentiate* (i.e., revert to a previous undifferentiated state).

### Genetic Link

Cancer involves the malfunction of genes that control differentiation and proliferation. Two types of normal genes that can be affected by mutation are *protooncogenes* and *tumor suppressor genes.* **Protooncogenes** are normal cell genes that are important regulators of normal cell processes. Protooncogenes promote growth, whereas tumor suppressor genes suppress growth. Mutations that alter the expression of protooncogenes can activate them to function as **oncogenes** (tumor-inducing genes).

The protooncogene has been described as the genetic lock that keeps the cell in its mature functioning state. When this lock is "unlocked," as may occur through exposure to *carcinogens* (agents that cause cancer) or oncogenic viruses, genetic alterations and mutations occur. The abilities and properties that the cell had in fetal development are again expressed. Oncogenes can change a normal cell to a malignant one. This cell regains a fetal appearance and function. For example, some cancer cells produce new proteins, such as those characteristic of the embryonic and fetal periods of life. These proteins, located on the cell membrane, include carcinoembryonic antigen (CEA) and α-fetoprotein (AFP). They can be detected in human blood by laboratory studies (see Role of the Immune System later in this chapter). Other cancer cells, such as small cell carcinoma of the lung, produce hormones (see Complications of Cancer later in this chapter on pp. 261-267) that are ordinarily produced by cells arising from the same embryonic cells as the tumor cells.[4]

*Tumor suppressor genes* function to regulate cell growth. They prevent cells from going through the cell cycle. Mutations that alter tumor suppressor genes make them inactive, resulting in a loss of their tumor-suppressing action. Examples of tumor suppressor genes are *BRCA1* and *BRCA2.* Alterations in these genes increase a person's risk for breast and ovarian cancer. Another tumor suppressor gene is the *APC* gene. Alterations in this gene increase a person's risk for familial adenomatous polyposis, which is a precursor for colorectal cancer (see Chapter 42). Mutations in the *p53* tumor suppressor gene have been found in many cancers, including bladder, breast, colorectal, esophageal, liver, lung, and ovarian cancers.

## Development of Cancer

The following is a theoretical model of the development of cancer. The cause and development of each type of cancer are likely to be multifactorial. A common misbelief is that the development of cancer is a rapid, haphazard event. However, cancer is usually an orderly process that occurs over time and has several stages: initiation, promotion, and progression (Fig. 15-2).

**Initiation.** Cancer cells arise from normal cells as a result of changes in genes. The first stage, *initiation,* involves a mutation in the cell's genetic structure. A *mutation* is any change in the usual DNA sequence.

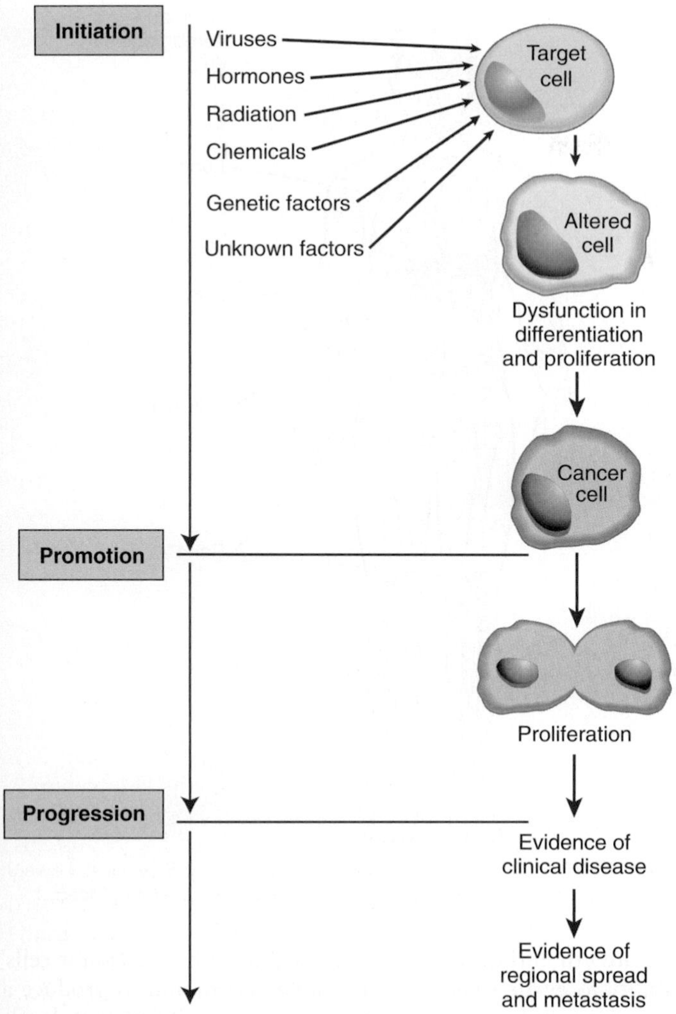


**FIG. 15-2** Process of cancer development.

## Genetic Link

Gene mutations can occur in two different ways: *inherited* from a parent (passed from one generation to the next) or *acquired* during a person's lifetime. (Mutations are discussed in Chapter 12.)

About 5% to 10% of all cancers or the predisposition to the cancer is inherited from one's parents.[5] These genetic alterations lead to a high risk of developing a specific type of cancer. However, most cancers do not result from inherited genes but are acquired from damage to genes occurring during one's lifetime. An acquired mutation is passed on to all cells that develop from that single cell. The damaged cell may die or repair itself. However, if cell death or repair does not occur before cell division, the cell will replicate into daughter cells, each with the same genetic alteration.

***Carcinogens.*** Many carcinogens (cancer-causing agents capable of producing cell alterations) are detoxified by protective enzymes and are harmlessly excreted. If this protective mechanism fails, carcinogens can enter the cell's nucleus and alter deoxyribonucleic acid (DNA). Carcinogens may be chemical, radiation, or viral.

**Chemical carcinogens.** Chemicals were identified as cancer-causing agents in the latter part of the eighteenth century when Percival Pott noted that chimney sweeps had a higher incidence of cancer of the scrotum associated with exposure to soot residue in chimneys. As the years passed, many chemical agents have been identified as carcinogens (e.g., benzene, arsenic, formaldehyde). People exposed to certain chemicals over time have a greater incidence of certain cancers than others. The long latency period from the time of exposure to the development of cancer makes it difficult to identify cancer-causing chemicals.

**Radiation.** Radiation can cause cancer in almost any body tissue. When cells are exposed to a source of radiation, damage occurs to DNA. Certain malignancies have been correlated with radiation as a carcinogenic agent:

- Leukemia, lymphoma, thyroid cancer, and other cancers increased in incidence in the general population of Hiroshima and Nagasaki after the atomic bomb explosions.
- A higher incidence of bone cancer occurs in people exposed to radiation in certain occupations, such as radiologists, radiation chemists, and uranium miners.

Ultraviolet (UV) radiation has long been associated with melanoma and squamous and basal cell carcinoma of the skin. Sunlight is the main source of UV exposure giving off UVA and UVB rays. Skin cancer is the most common type of cancer among whites in the United States. Of great concern is the increase in the incidence of melanoma. Although the cause of melanoma is probably multifactorial, UV radiation secondary to sunlight exposure is linked to the development of melanoma. UV radiation from tanning beds can cause skin cancer (melanoma, basal cell and squamous cell carcinoma).[6]

**Viral carcinogens.** Certain DNA and ribonucleic acid (RNA) viruses, termed *oncogenic,* can transform the cells they infect and induce malignant transformation. Viruses have been identified as causative agents of cancer in animals and humans. Burkitt's lymphoma is associated with Epstein-Barr virus (EBV).[7] People with acquired immunodeficiency syndrome (AIDS), which is caused by human immunodeficiency virus (HIV), have a high incidence of Kaposi sarcoma (see Chapter 14). Other viruses that have been linked to the development of cancer include hepatitis B virus, which is associated with hepatocellular carcinoma; and human papillomavirus (HPV), which is believed to induce lesions that progress to squamous cell carcinomas, such as cervical, anal, and head and neck cancers.

**Promotion.** A single alteration of the genetic structure of the cell is not sufficient to result in cancer. However, the odds of cancer development are increased with the presence of promoting agents. *Promotion,* the second stage in the development of cancer, is characterized by the reversible proliferation of the altered cells. An increase in the altered cell population further increases the likelihood of additional mutations.

An important distinction between initiation and promotion is that the activity of promoters is reversible. This is a key concept in cancer prevention. Promoting factors include such agents as dietary fat, obesity, cigarette smoking, and alcohol consumption. Changing a person's lifestyle to modify these risk factors can reduce the chance of cancer development. Approximately one third of cancer-related deaths in the United States are related to tobacco use, unhealthy diet, physical inactivity, and obesity.[1]

Several promoting agents have activity against specific types of body tissues. Therefore these agents tend to promote specific kinds of cancer. For example, cigarette smoke is a promoting agent in bronchogenic carcinoma and, in conjunction with alcohol intake, promotes esophageal and bladder cancers.

Some carcinogens, termed *complete carcinogens*, are capable of both initiating and promoting the development of cancer. Cigarette smoke is an example of a complete carcinogen capable of initiating and promoting cancer.

A period of time, ranging from 1 to 40 years, elapses between the initial genetic alteration and the actual clinical evidence of cancer. This period, called the *latent* period, includes both the initiation and promotion stages in the natural history of cancer. The variation in the length of time that elapses before the cancer becomes clinically evident is associated with the mitotic rate of the tissue of origin and environmental factors. In most cancers, the process of developing cancer is years or even decades in length.

For the disease process to become clinically evident, the cells must reach a critical mass. A tumor that is 1.0 cm (0.4 inch) (the size usually detectable by palpation) contains 1 billion cancer cells. A 0.5-cm tumor is the smallest that can be detected by current diagnostic measures, such as MRI.

**Progression.** *Progression* is the final stage in the natural history of a cancer. This stage is characterized by increased growth rate of the tumor, increased invasiveness, and **metastasis** (spread of the cancer to a distant site). Certain cancers seem to have an affinity for a particular tissue or organ as a site of metastasis (e.g., colon cancer often spreads to the liver). Other cancers (e.g., melanoma) are unpredictable in their pattern of metastasis. The most frequent sites of metastasis are lungs, liver, bone, brain, and adrenal glands (Fig. 15-3).

Metastasis is a multistep process beginning with the rapid growth of the primary tumor (Fig. 15-4). As the tumor increases in size, development of its own blood supply is critical to its survival and growth. The process of the formation of blood vessels within the tumor itself is termed **tumor angiogenesis** and is facilitated by tumor angiogenesis factors produced by the cancer cells.

Tumor cells are able to detach from the primary tumor, invade the tissue surrounding the tumor, and penetrate the walls of lymph or vascular vessels for metastasis to a distant site. Once free from the primary tumor, metastatic tumor cells frequently travel to distant organ sites via hematogenous or lymphatic routes.

*Hematogenous metastasis* involves several steps beginning with primary tumor cells penetrating blood vessels. These tumor cells then enter the circulation, travel through the body, and adhere to and penetrate small blood vessels of distant organs. Most tumor cells do not survive this process and are destroyed by mechanical mechanisms (e.g., turbulence of blood flow) and cells of the immune system. However, the formation of a combination of tumor cells, platelets, and fibrin deposits may protect some tumor cells from destruction in blood vessels.

In the lymphatic system, tumor cells may be "trapped" in the first lymph node confronted and likely to spread from a tumor. This lymph node is referred to as the *sentinel lymph node.* A biopsy can be done of the sentinel node to help determine the extent of the cancer. The procedure is less extensive requiring the removal of fewer lymph nodes. The tumor cells may bypass regional lymph nodes and travel to more distant lymph nodes, a phenomenon termed *skip metastasis.* This phenomenon is exhibited in malignancies such as esophageal cancers. Tumor cells that do survive the process of metastasis must create an environment in the distant organ site that is conducive to their growth and development.

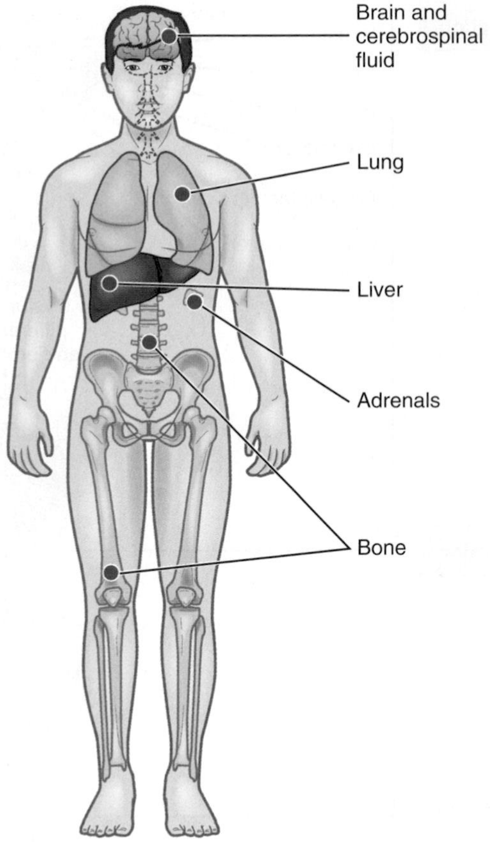


**FIG. 15-3** Main sites of metastasis. (Adapted from Stevens A, Lowe J: *Pathology: an illustrated review in colour,* ed 2, London, 2000, Mosby.)

Growth and development are facilitated by the tumor cells' ability to evade cells of the immune system and to produce a vascular supply within the metastatic site similar to that developed in the primary tumor site. Vascularization is critical to the supply of nutrients to the metastatic tumor and to the removal of waste products. Vascularization of the metastatic site is also facilitated by tumor angiogenesis factors produced by the cancer cells.

## Role of the Immune System

This section is limited to a discussion of the role of the immune system in the recognition and destruction of tumor cells. (For a detailed discussion of immune system function, see Chapter 13.)

The immune system has the potential to distinguish cells that are normal (self) from abnormal (nonself) cells. For example, cells of transplanted organs can be recognized by the immune system as *nonself* and thus elicit an immune response. This response can ultimately result in the rejection of the organ. Similarly, cancer cells can be perceived as nonself and elicit an immune response resulting in their rejection and destruction. However, unlike transplanted cells, cancer cells arise from normal human cells and, although they are mutated and thus different, the immune response that is mounted against cancer cells may be inadequate to effectively kill them.

Cancer cells may display altered cell-surface antigens as a result of malignant transformation. These antigens are termed *tumor-associated antigens (TAAs)* (Fig. 15-5). It is believed that one of the functions of the immune system is to respond to TAAs. The immune system's response to antigens of the

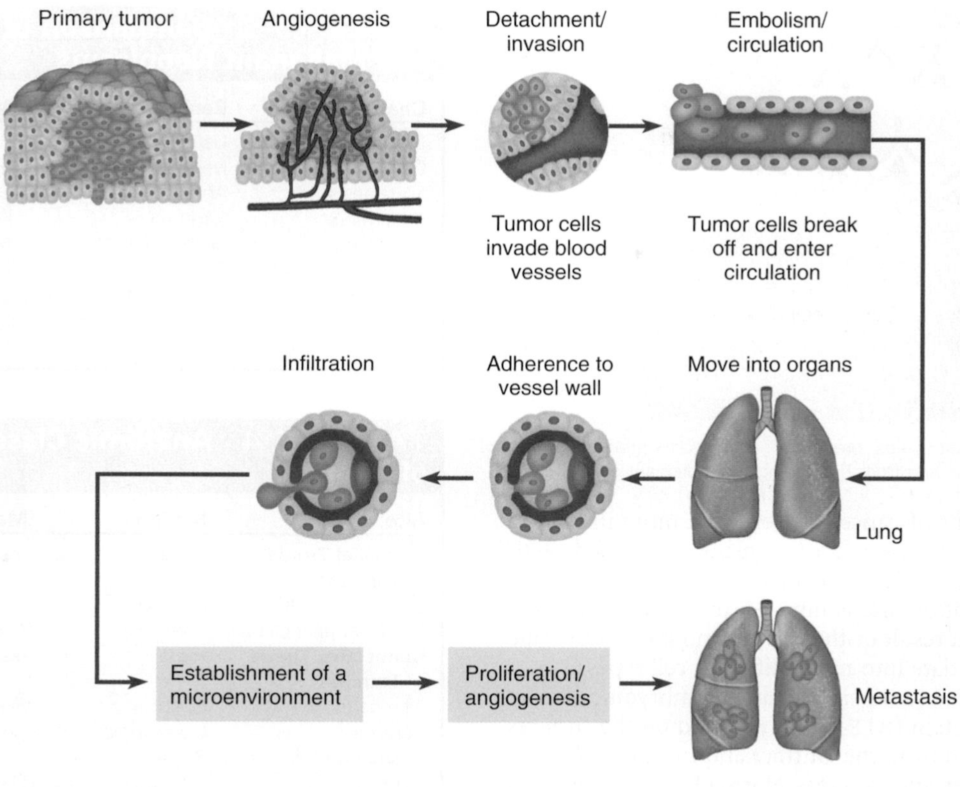


**FIG. 15-4** The pathogenesis of cancer metastasis. To produce metastases, tumor cells must detach from the primary tumor and enter the circulation, survive in the circulation to rest in the capillary bed, adhere to capillary basement membrane, gain entrance into the organ parenchyma, respond to growth factors, proliferate and induce angiogenesis, and evade host defenses. (Adapted from Fidler IT: The pathogenesis of cancer metastasis: the "seed and soil" hypothesis revisited, *Nat Rev Cancer* 3(6):453, 2003.)

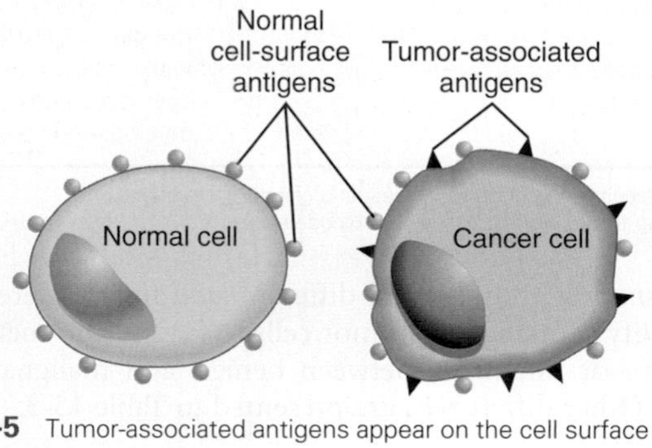


**FIG. 15-5** Tumor-associated antigens appear on the cell surface of malignant cells.

malignant cells is termed **immunologic surveillance**. In this process, lymphocytes continuously check cell-surface antigens and detect and destroy cells with abnormal or altered antigenic determinants. Under most circumstances, immune surveillance prevents these transformed cells from developing into clinically detectable tumors.

Immune response to malignant cells involves cytotoxic T cells, natural killer (NK) cells, macrophages, and B cells. *Cytotoxic T cells* play a dominant role in resisting tumor growth. These cells are capable of killing tumor cells. T cells are also important in the production of cytokines (e.g., interleukin-2 [IL-2] and γ-interferon), which stimulate T cells, NK cells, B cells, and macrophages.

*Natural killer (NK) cells* are able to directly lyse tumor cells spontaneously without any prior sensitization. These cells are stimulated by γ-interferon and IL-2 (released from T cells), resulting in increased cytotoxic activity.

*Monocytes* and *macrophages* have several important roles in tumor immunity. Macrophages can be activated by γ-interferon (produced by T cells) to become nonspecifically lytic for tumor cells. Macrophages also secrete cytokines, including interleukin-1 (IL-1), tumor necrosis factor (TNF), and colony-stimulating factors (CSFs). The release of IL-1, coupled with the presentation of the processed antigen, stimulates T cell activation and production. α-Interferon augments the killing ability of NK cells. TNF causes hemorrhagic necrosis of tumors and exerts cytocidal or cytostatic actions against tumor cells. CSFs regulate the production of various blood cells in the bone marrow and stimulate the function of various WBCs.

*B cells* can produce specific antibodies that bind to tumor cells. These antibodies are often detectable in the patient's serum and saliva.

**Escape Mechanisms From Immunologic Surveillance.** The process by which cancer cells evade the immune system is termed *immunologic escape*. Possible mechanisms by which cancer cells can escape immunologic surveillance include (1) suppression of factors that stimulate T cells to react to cancer cells; (2) weak surface antigens allowing cancer cells to "sneak through" immunologic surveillance; (3) development of tolerance of the immune system to some tumor antigens; (4) suppression of the immune response by products secreted by cancer cells; (5) induction of suppressor T cells by the tumor; and (6) blocking antibodies that bind TAAs, thus preventing their recognition by T cells (Fig. 15-6).

**Oncofetal Antigens and Tumor Markers.** *Oncofetal antigens* are a type of tumor antigen. They are found on the surfaces and the inside of cancer cells and fetal cells. These antigens are an

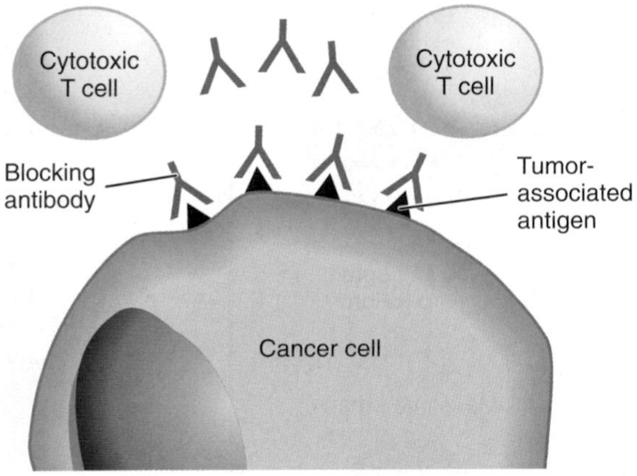


**FIG. 15-6** Blocking antibodies prevent T cells from interacting with tumor-associated antigens and from destroying the malignant cell.

expression of the shift of cancerous cells to a more immature metabolic pathway, an expression usually associated with embryonic or fetal periods of life. The reappearance of fetal antigens in malignant disease is not well understood, but it is believed to occur as a result of the cell regaining its embryonic capability to differentiate into many different cell types.

Examples of oncofetal antigens are carcinoembryonic antigen (CEA) and α-fetoprotein (AFP). CEA is found on the surfaces of cancer cells derived from the GI tract and from normal cells from the fetal gut, liver, and pancreas. Normally, CEA disappears during the last 3 months of fetal life. CEA was originally isolated from colorectal cancer cells. However, elevated CEA levels have also been found in nonmalignant conditions (e.g., cirrhosis of the liver, ulcerative colitis, heavy smoking).

These oncofetal antigens can be used as *tumor markers* that may be clinically useful to monitor the effect of therapy and indicate tumor recurrence. However, oncofetal antigens are not 100% specific for tumor recurrence. Tumor markers are affected by various factors that must be accounted for when reviewing these results. For example, the persistence of elevated preoperative CEA titers after surgery indicates that the tumor is not completely removed. A rise in CEA levels after chemotherapy or radiation therapy may indicate recurrence or spread of the cancer and may be affected by chronic lung or liver disease and smoking.

AFP is produced by malignant liver cells and fetal liver cells. AFP levels have also been found to be elevated in some cases of testicular carcinoma, viral hepatitis, and nonmalignant liver disorders. AFP has diagnostic value in primary cancer of the liver (hepatocellular cancer), but it is also produced when metastatic liver growth occurs. The detection of AFP is of value in tumor detection and determination of tumor progression.

Other examples of oncofetal antigens are CA-125 (found in ovarian carcinoma), CA-19-9 (found in pancreatic and gallbladder cancer), prostate-specific antigen (PSA) (found in prostate cancer), and CA-15-3 and CA-27-29 (found in breast cancer). Molecular markers for specific tumors include kRAS (expression of oncogene in colon cancer), epidermal growth factor receptor (EGFR) often overexpressed in lung cancer, and human epidermal growth factor receptor-2 (HER-2) expression in breast cancer.

## BENIGN VERSUS MALIGNANT NEOPLASMS

Tumors can be classified as benign or malignant. In general, *benign neoplasms* are well differentiated, and **malignant neoplasms** range from well differentiated to undifferentiated. The ability of malignant tumor cells to invade and metastasize is the major difference between benign and malignant neoplasms. Other differences are presented in Table 15-3.

**TABLE 15-3 Comparison of Benign and Malignant Neoplasms**

| Characteristic | Benign | Malignant |
|---|---|---|
| Encapsulated | Usually | Rarely |
| Differentiated | Normally | Poorly |
| Metastasis | Absent | Capable |
| Recurrence | Rare | Possible |
| Vascularity | Slight | Moderate to marked |
| Mode of growth | Expansive | Infiltrative and expansive |
| Cell characteristics | Fairly normal, similar to parent cells | Cells abnormal, become more unlike parent cells |

**TABLE 15-4 Anatomic Classification of Tumors**

| Site | Benign | Malignant |
|---|---|---|
| **Epithelial Tissue Tumors*** | **-oma** | **-carcinoma** |
| Surface epithelium | Papilloma | Carcinoma |
| Glandular epithelium | Adenoma | Adenocarcinoma |
| **Connective Tissue Tumors†** | **-oma** | **-sarcoma** |
| Fibrous tissue | Fibroma | Fibrosarcoma |
| Cartilage | Chondroma | Chondrosarcoma |
| Striated muscle | Rhabdomyoma | Rhabdomyosarcoma |
| Bone | Osteoma | Osteosarcoma |
| **Nervous Tissue Tumors** | **-oma** | **-oma** |
| Meninges | Meningioma | Meningeal sarcoma |
| Nerve cells | Ganglioneuroma | Neuroblastoma |
| **Hematopoietic Tissue Tumors** | | |
| Lymphoid tissue | — | Hodgkin's lymphoma, non-Hodgkin's lymphoma |
| Plasma cells | — | Multiple myeloma |
| Bone marrow | — | Lymphocytic and myelogenous leukemia |

*Body surfaces, lining of body cavities, and glandular structures.
†Supporting tissue, fibrotic tissue, and blood vessels.

## CLASSIFICATION OF CANCER

Tumors can be classified according to anatomic site, histology (grading), and extent of disease (staging). Tumor classification systems provide a standardized way to (1) communicate the status of the cancer to all members of the interprofessional care team, (2) assist in determining the most effective treatment plan, (3) evaluate the treatment plan, (4) predict prognosis, and (5) compare like groups for statistical purposes.

### Anatomic Site Classification

In the *anatomic classification* of tumors, the tumor is identified by the tissue of origin, anatomic site, and behavior of the tumor (i.e., benign or malignant) (Table 15-4). *Carcinomas* originate from embryonal *ectoderm* (skin and glands) and *endoderm* (mucous membrane linings of the respiratory tract, GI tract, and genitourinary [GU] tract). *Sarcomas* originate from embryonal *mesoderm* (connective tissue, muscle, bone, and fat).

Lymphomas and leukemias originate from the hematopoietic system.

### Histologic Classification

In **histologic grading** of tumors, the appearance of cells and degree of differentiation are evaluated pathologically. For many tumor types, four grades are used to evaluate abnormal cells based on the degree to which the cells resemble the tissue of origin. Tumors that are poorly differentiated (undifferentiated) have a poorer prognosis than those that are closer in appearance to the normal tissue of origin (well differentiated):

*Grade I:* Cells differ slightly from normal cells (mild dysplasia) and are well differentiated (low grade).
*Grade II:* Cells are more abnormal (moderate dysplasia) and moderately differentiated (intermediate grade).
*Grade III:* Cells are very abnormal (severe dysplasia) and poorly differentiated (high grade).
*Grade IV:* Cells are immature and primitive *(anaplasia)* and undifferentiated; cell of origin is difficult to determine (high grade).
*Grade X:* Grade cannot be assessed.

### Extent of Disease Classification

Classifying the extent and spread of disease is termed **staging**. This classification system is based on the anatomic extent of disease rather than on cell appearance. Although there are similarities in the staging of various cancers, there are many differences for specific types of cancer.

**Clinical Staging.** The clinical staging classification system determines the anatomic extent of the malignant disease process by stages:

*Stage 0:* cancer in situ
*Stage I:* tumor limited to the tissue of origin; localized tumor growth
*Stage II:* limited local spread
*Stage III:* extensive local and regional spread
*Stage IV:* metastasis

Clinical staging has been used as a basis for staging a variety of tumor types, including cancer of the cervix (see Table 53-13) and Hodgkin's lymphoma (see Fig. 30-14). Other malignant diseases (e.g., leukemia) do not use this staging approach.

**TNM Classification System.** The *TNM classification system* (Table 15-5) is used to determine the anatomic extent of the disease involvement according to three parameters: tumor size and invasiveness (T), presence or absence of regional spread to the lymph nodes (N), and metastasis to distant organ sites (M). (Examples of the TNM classification system can be found in Tables 27-17 and 51-6.) TNM staging cannot be applied to all malignancies. For example, leukemias are not solid tumors and therefore cannot be staged using these guidelines.

**Carcinoma in situ (CIS)** refers to a neoplasm whose cells are localized and show no tendency to invade or metastasize to other tissues. CIS has its own designation in the system ($T_{is}$) because it has all the histologic characteristics of cancer except invasion—a primary feature of the TNM staging system.

Staging of the disease can be performed initially and at several evaluation points. Clinical staging is done at the completion of the diagnostic workup to guide effective treatment selection. Examples of diagnostic studies that may be performed to assess for extent of disease include radiologic studies, such as bone and liver scans; ultrasonography; and computed tomography (CT), MRI, and positron emission tomography (PET) scans.

*Surgical staging* refers to the extent of the disease as determined by surgical excision, exploration, and/or lymph node sampling. For example, a laparotomy and a splenectomy may be performed in staging of Hodgkin's lymphoma. During a staging laparotomy, lymph node biopsies may be done, and margins of any masses may be marked with metal clips for use during radiation therapy. However, exploratory surgical staging is being used less frequently as noninvasive diagnostic technology becomes increasingly sophisticated.

After the extent of the disease is determined, the stage classification is not changed. The original description of the extent of the tumor remains part of the record. If additional treatment is needed, or if treatment fails, retreatment staging is done to determine the extent of the disease process before retreatment. "Restaging" classification (rTNM) is differentiated from the stage at diagnosis, since the clinical significance may be different.

In addition to tumor classification systems, other rating scales can be used to describe and document the status of patients with cancer at the time of diagnosis, treatment, and retreatment and at each follow-up examination. For example, the Karnofsky Performance Scale[8] and Katz Index of Independence in Activities of Daily Living[9] describe patient's functional performance.

**TABLE 15-5 TNM Classification System**

| | |
|---|---|
| **Primary Tumor (T)** | |
| $T_0$ | No evidence of primary tumor |
| $T_{is}$ | Carcinoma in situ |
| $T_{1-4}$ | Ascending degrees of increase in tumor size and involvement |
| $T_x$ | Tumor cannot be measured or found |
| **Regional Lymph Nodes (N)** | |
| $N_0$ | No evidence of disease in lymph nodes |
| $N_{1-4}$ | Ascending degrees of nodal involvement |
| $N_x$ | Regional lymph nodes unable to be assessed clinically |
| **Distant Metastases (M)** | |
| $M_0$ | No evidence of distant metastases |
| $M_{1-4}$ | Ascending degrees of metastatic involvement, including distant nodes |
| $M_x$ | Cannot be determined |

NOTE: For examples of TNM classification system applied to diseases, see Fig. 30-14 and Table 27-17.

## PREVENTION AND EARLY DETECTION OF CANCER

The war on cancer will not be won with drugs or radiation therapy. A stronger emphasis on prevention is needed.[10] As a nurse, you have an essential role in the prevention and early detection of cancer. Eliminating risk factors reduces the incidence of cancer. For example, rates of smoking-related cancers (e.g., lung and head and neck cancers) have declined following reduction in smoking rates.[1]

Early detection and prompt treatment are responsible for increased survival rates in patients with cancer. Colonoscopy is important in reducing colon cancer mortality both by early detection of colon cancers and by prevention (e.g., excision of adenomatous polyps).

Teach patients and the public about cancer prevention and early detection, including the following:

**TABLE 15-6 Seven Warning Signs of Cancer**

| |
|---|
| **C**hange in bowel or bladder habits |
| **A** sore that does not heal |
| **U**nusual bleeding or discharge from any body orifice |
| **T**hickening or a lump in the breast or elsewhere |
| **I** ndigestion or difficulty in swallowing |
| **O**bvious change in a wart or mole |
| **N**agging cough or hoarseness |

- Reduce or avoid exposure to known or suspected carcinogens and cancer-promoting agents, including cigarette smoke, tanning beds, and sun exposure.
- Eat a balanced diet that includes vegetables and fresh fruits (see Fig. 39-1 and Table 39-1), whole grains, and adequate amounts of fiber. Reduce dietary fat and preservatives, including smoked and salt-cured meats containing high nitrite concentrations.
- Limit alcohol intake.
- Participate in regular exercise (i.e., 30 minutes or more of moderate physical activity five times weekly).
- Maintain a healthy weight.
- Obtain adequate, consistent periods of rest (at least 6 to 8 hours per night).
- Eliminate, reduce, or change the perception of stressors and enhance the ability to effectively cope with stressors (see Chapter 6).
- Have a regular physical examination that includes a health history. Be familiar with your own family history and your risk factors for cancer.
- Learn and follow the American Cancer Society's recommended cancer screening guidelines for breast, colon, cervical, and prostate cancer.[11]
- Learn and practice self-examination (e.g., breast or testicular self-examination).
- Know the seven warning signs of cancer, and inform the health care provider if they are present (Table 15-6). (These actually detect fairly advanced disease.)
- Seek immediate medical care if you notice a change in what is normal for you and if cancer is suspected.

The goals of public education are to (1) motivate people to recognize and modify behaviors that may negatively affect health and (2) encourage awareness of and participation in health-promoting behaviors. When you teach about cancer, try to minimize the fear that surrounds the diagnosis.

## Diagnosis of Cancer

When a patient has a possible diagnosis of cancer, it is a stressful time for the patient and family. Patients may undergo several days to weeks of diagnostic studies. During this time, fear of the unknown may be more stressful than the actual diagnosis of cancer. Patients may also be overwhelmed or confused by the need for multiple diagnostic studies and consultations. Help to coordinate care between multiple specialists and explain the purpose of required tests and any special preparation needed for them.

Some facilities have comprehensive oncology teams and services that are all housed in the same building to help coordinate care among the cancer specialists. These centers consolidate appointments to make the experience convenient and comfortable for the patients and their families.

While patients are waiting for the results of diagnostic studies, be available to actively listen to their concerns. Their anxiety may arise from myths and misconceptions about cancer (e.g., cancer is a "death sentence," cancer treatment is worse than the illness). Correcting those misconceptions can help to minimize their anxiety.

Learn to recognize your own discomfort during difficult conversations. Avoid communication patterns that may hinder exploration of feelings and meaning, such as providing false reassurances (e.g., "It's probably nothing"), redirecting the discussion (e.g., "Let's discuss that later"), generalizing (e.g., "Everyone feels this way"), and using overly technical language as a means of distancing yourself from the patient. These self-protective strategies deny patients the opportunity to share the meaning of their experience. In addition, they can jeopardize your ability to build a trusting relationship with your patients.

During this time of high anxiety, the patient may need repeated explanations of the diagnostic workup. Include as much information as needed by the patient and family. Give clear, understandable explanations and reinforce them as needed. Written information is helpful for reinforcement of verbal information.

A diagnostic plan for the person suspected of having cancer includes the health history (including a history of present illness), identification of risk factors, the physical examination, and specific diagnostic studies. For many people, cancer is initially diagnosed after the findings of an abnormal screening test (e.g., mass on mammogram). For others, they are alerted to the presence of cancer by a presenting symptom or cluster of symptoms (e.g., cough and hemoptysis, anorexia and weight loss).

Concentrate on risk factors for cancer such as family or personal history of cancer, exposure to or use of known carcinogens (e.g., cigarette smoking, occupational pollutants or chemicals, radiation exposure), diseases characterized by chronic inflammation or immunosuppression (e.g., ulcerative colitis), and drug ingestion (e.g., hormone therapy, previous anticancer therapies). Also assess factors that may warrant additional supportive care during therapy, including alcohol or recreational drug use, living situation, social support, and coping strategies for perceived stressors.

Diagnostic studies depend on the suspected primary or metastatic site(s) of the cancer. (Specific procedures as they relate to each body system are discussed in the respective assessment chapters.) Examples of diagnostic studies include the following:

- Cytology studies (e.g., Papanicolaou [Pap] test, bronchial washings)
- Tissue biopsy
- Chest x-ray
- Complete blood count, chemistry profile

### HEALTHY PEOPLE

***Prevention and Early Detection of Cancer***

- Limit alcohol use.
- Get regular physical activity.
- Maintain a normal body weight.
- Obtain regular colorectal screenings.
- Avoid cigarette smoking and other tobacco use.
- Get regular mammography screening and Pap tests.
- Use sunscreen with a sun protection factor of 15 or higher.
- Practice healthy dietary habits, such as reducing fat consumption, avoiding processed meats, and increasing fruit and vegetable consumption.

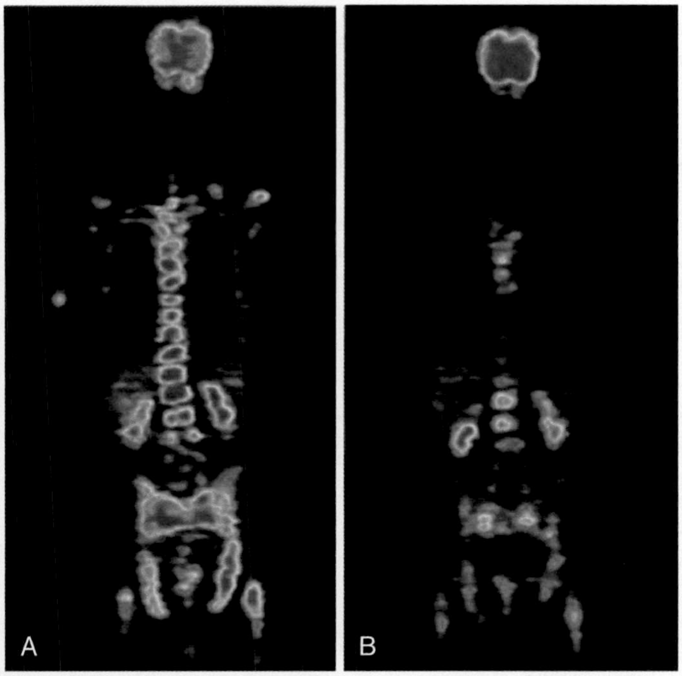


**FIG. 15-7** Positron emission tomography (PET) scan before treatment **(A)** indicating metastasis throughout the body. PET scan after treatment **(B)** indicates the effects of therapy. More radioactive material accumulates in areas that have higher levels of activity. This often corresponds to areas of disease and shows up as brighter spots on the PET scan. (From Shimizu N, Masuda H, Yamanaka H, et al: Fluorodeoxyglucose positron emission tomography scan of prostate cancer bone metastases with flare reaction after endocrine therapy, *J Urol* 151[2]:609, 1999.)

- Liver function studies (e.g., aspartate aminotransferase [AST])
- Endoscopic examination: upper GI, sigmoidoscopy, or colonoscopy (including guaiac test for occult blood)
- Radiographic studies (e.g., mammography, ultrasound, CT scan, MRI)
- Radioisotope scans (e.g., bone, lung, liver, brain)
- PET scan (Fig. 15-7)
- Tumor markers (e.g., CEA, AFP, PSA, CA-125)
- Genetic markers (e.g., *BRCA1, BRCA2*)
- Molecular receptor status (e.g., estrogen and progesterone receptors)
- Bone marrow examination (if a hematolymphoid malignancy is suspected or to document metastatic disease)

**Biopsy.** A *biopsy* is the removal of a tissue sample for pathologic analysis. Various methods are used to obtain a biopsy depending on the location and size of the suspected tumor. *Percutaneous biopsy* is commonly performed for tissue that can be safely reached through the skin. *Endoscopic biopsy* may be used for lung or other intraluminal lesions (esophageal, colon, bladder). When a tumor is not easily accessible, a *surgical procedure* (laparotomy, thoracotomy, craniotomy) is often necessary to obtain a piece of the tumor tissue. Many radiographic techniques may be used in conjunction with the biopsy procedure (e.g., CT, MRI, ultrasound-guided biopsy, stereotactic biopsy, fluoroscopic-assisted biopsy) to improve tissue localization.

Various types and sizes of biopsy needles are available and are selected according to the type of tissue to be sampled. *Fine-needle aspiration* (FNA) may be accomplished with a small-gauge aspiration needle that provides cells from the mass for cytologic examination. *Large-core biopsy* cutting needles deliver an actual piece of tissue (core) that can be analyzed with the advantage of preserving the histologic architecture of the tissue specimen. *Excisional biopsy* involves the surgical removal of the entire lesion, lymph node, nodule, or mass. Therefore it is therapeutic as well as diagnostic. If an excisional biopsy is not feasible, an *incisional biopsy* (partial excision) may be performed with a scalpel or dermal punch.

Pathologic evaluation of a tissue sample is the only definitive means to diagnose cancer. The pathologist examines the tissue to determine (1) whether it is benign or malignant, (2) the anatomic tissue from which the tumor arises *(histology),* and (3) the degree of cell differentiation *(histologic grade).* Other information that can be obtained includes the extent of malignant involvement (size of tumor and depth), evidence of invasiveness (extracapsular, lymphatic), adequacy of surgical excision (positive or negative surgical margin status), nuclear grade (mitotic rate), and special staining techniques that may provide insight into responsiveness of the tumor to treatment or disease behavior (receptor status, tumor markers).

## INTERPROFESSIONAL CARE

### Treatment Goals

The goals of cancer treatment are cure, control, and palliation (Fig. 15-8). Primary factors that determine what therapy is used are the tumor histology and staging outcomes. Other important factors are the patient's physiologic status (e.g., presence of co-morbid illnesses), psychologic status, and personal desires (e.g., active treatment versus palliation of symptoms).

These factors influence (1) the modalities chosen for treatment (i.e., surgery, radiation therapy, chemotherapy, immunotherapy, targeted therapy, hormone therapy), (2) how therapies are sequenced, and (3) the length of time the treatment is prescribed. Each type of therapy can be used alone or in any combination during initial treatment or as maintenance therapy, as well as in retreatment if the disease does not respond or recurs after remission.

For many cancers, two or more of the treatment modalities (known as *multimodality therapy* or *combined modality therapy*) are used to achieve the goal of cure or control for a long time. Multimodality therapy has the benefit of being more effective (because it takes advantage of more than one mechanism of action), but often at the expense of greater toxicity.

**Cure.** When caring for the patient and family with cancer, know the treatment goals to appropriately communicate with, teach, and support the patient. When *cure* is the goal, treatment is expected to have the greatest chance of disease eradication. Curative cancer therapy differs according to the particular cancer being treated and may involve local therapies (i.e., surgery or radiation) alone or in combination, with or without periods of adjunctive systemic therapy (i.e., chemotherapy).

For example, basal cell carcinoma of the skin is usually cured by surgical removal of the lesion and/or several weeks of radiation therapy. In the treatment plan for acute promyelocytic leukemia (which has curative potential), several chemotherapy drugs are given on a scheduled basis over many months to several years. Testicular cancer can be cured with a combination of surgery, chemotherapy, and radiation.

Although there is no benchmark that ensures "cure" for most cancers, in general the risk for recurrent disease is highest after treatment completion and gradually decreases the longer the

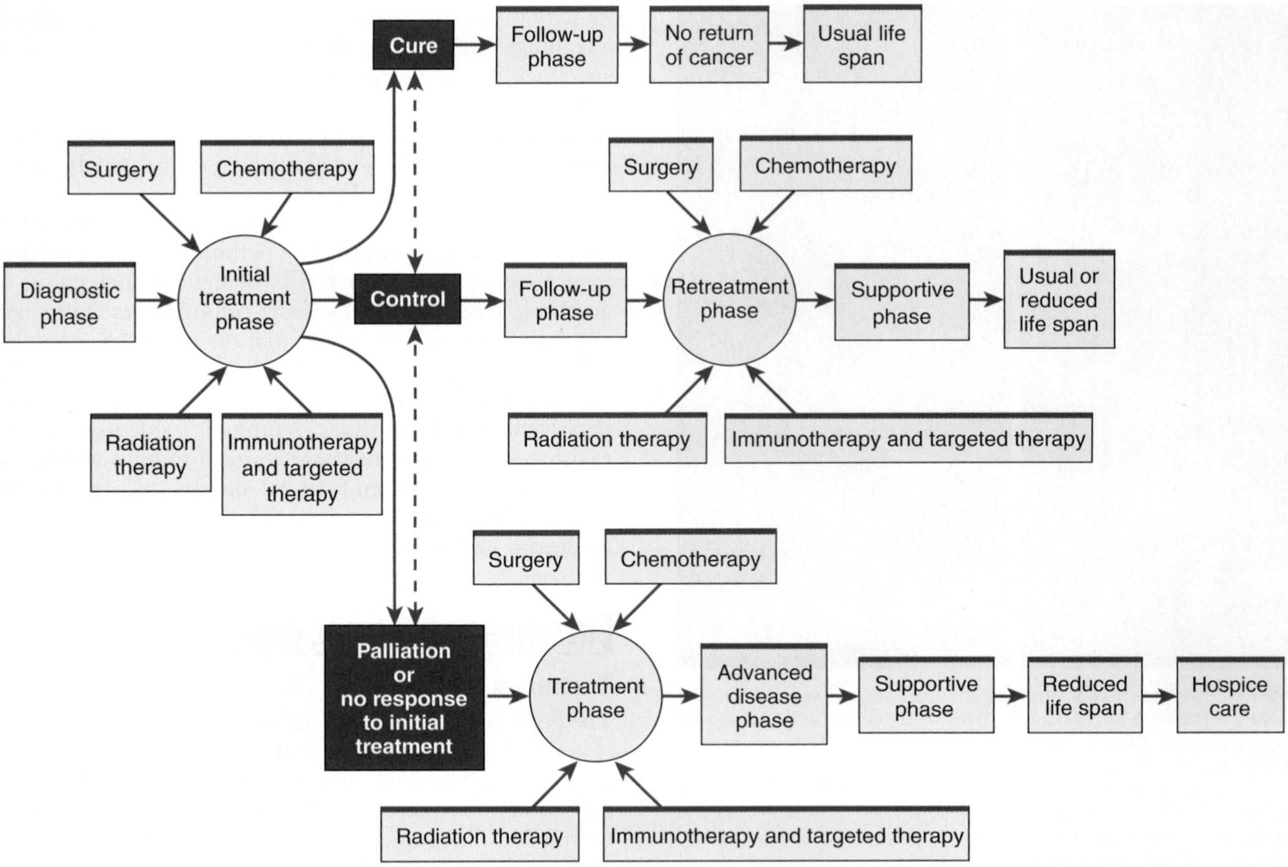


**FIG. 15-8** Goals of cancer treatment.

patient remains disease free following treatment. Cancers with a higher mitotic rate (e.g., testicular cancer) are more likely to recur than cancers with slower mitotic rates (e.g., postmenopausal breast cancer). Therefore the timeframe to consider a person "cured" may differ according to the tumor and its characteristics.

**Control.** *Control* is the goal of the treatment plan for many cancers that cannot be completely eradicated but are responsive to anticancer therapies. As with other chronic illnesses (e.g., diabetes mellitus, heart failure), cancer can be controlled for long periods with therapy. Examples include multiple myeloma and chronic lymphocytic leukemia (see Chapter 30). Patients may undergo an initial course of treatment followed by maintenance therapy for as long as the disease is responding. Patients are monitored closely for early signs and symptoms of disease recurrence or progression and the cumulative effects of therapy. Evidence of tumor resistance (such as disease progression) may warrant changing to an alternative therapy.

**Palliation.** *Palliation* is the treatment goal when relief or control of symptoms and the maintenance of a satisfactory quality of life are the primary objectives. Palliative care and treatment are not mutually exclusive and can take place concurrently. An example of treatment in which palliation is the primary goal includes using radiation therapy or chemotherapy to reduce tumor size and relieve subsequent symptoms such as the pain of bone metastasis.

## Personalized Cancer Medicine

An emerging trend in cancer care is *personalized medicine,* in which the patient's genetic information is used to guide (customize) decisions made about prevention, diagnosis, and treatment of cancer. Many of the diagnostic studies (tumor markers, genetic markers, molecular receptor status) are useful in determining treatment options for patients with cancer.

Before personalized medicine, most patients with a specific type and stage of cancer received the same treatment. However, some treatments worked well for some patients and not as well for others. With increasing research, it was found that genetic differences in people and their tumors explained many of these different responses to treatment. By performing more genetic tests and analysis, treatments can now be personalized.[12]

Targeted therapy (see Table 15-13 later in this chapter) targets a cancer's specific genes or proteins that contribute to cancer growth and survival. Treatment with a targeted therapy depends on assessing whether the tumor has the specific target. This is usually done by testing a sample of the tumor obtained through a biopsy.

*Pharmacogenomics* and *pharmacogenetics* is the study of genomic variation associated with drug responses.[13,14] Examples of how the results of genetic testing can be applied to the use of cancer drugs are presented in Table 12-5. For example, vemurafenib (Zelboraf) is used to treat patients with metastatic melanoma. However, it is indicated only for the treatment of patients with melanoma whose tumors express a gene mutation called *BRAF V600E.*

Despite the promises of personalized cancer treatments, not all types of cancer have personalized treatment options. Genetic testing of the patient and tumor sample may be costly and time consuming, and many insurance plans may not cover the costs

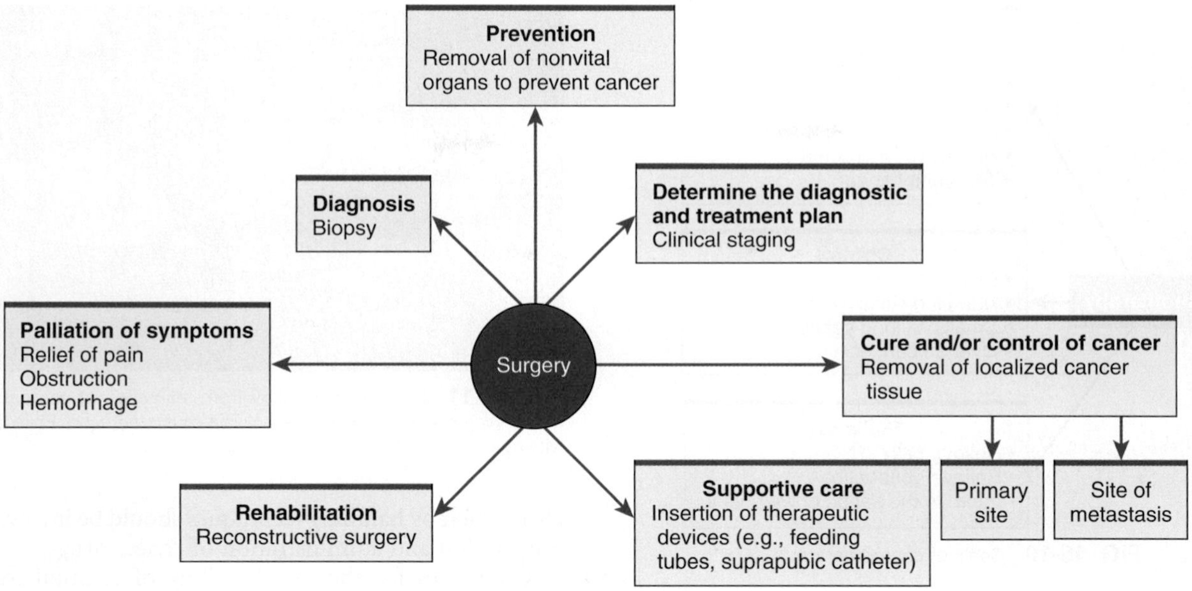


**FIG. 15-9** Role of surgery in the treatment of cancer.

of these tests. Some personalized treatments, such as targeted treatments, can also be expensive.[12]

## SURGICAL THERAPY

Surgery is the oldest form of cancer treatment. The treatment of choice for many years was to remove the cancer and as much of the surrounding normal tissue as possible. What this approach did not fully consider was the ability of cancer cells to travel from the original tumor site to other locations, making surgical cure possible only when the tumor was localized and relatively small. Today surgery is used to meet a variety of goals (Fig. 15-9), and the trend is toward less radical surgeries.

### Prevention

Surgical intervention can be used to eliminate or reduce the risk of cancer development. Prophylactic removal of nonvital organs has been successful in reducing the incidence of some cancers. For example, patients who have adenomatous familial polyposis may benefit from a total colostomy to prevent colorectal cancer (see Chapter 42). Individuals who have genetic mutations of *BRCA1* or *BRCA2* and have a strong family history of early-onset breast cancer may consider having a prophylactic mastectomy (see Chapter 51).

### Cure or Control

When the goal is cure or control, the objective is to remove all or as much resectable tumor as possible while sparing normal tissue. Examples of surgical procedures used for cure or control of cancer include radical neck dissection, mastectomy, orchiectomy, thyroidectomy, nephrectomy, hysterectomy, and/or oophorectomy.

A *debulking* or *cytoreductive procedure* may be used if the tumor cannot be completely removed (e.g., a tumor attached to a vital organ). When this occurs, as much tumor as possible is removed and the patient is given chemotherapy and/or radiation therapy. This type of surgical procedure can make chemotherapy or radiation therapy more effective, since the tumor mass is reduced before treatment is initiated. Other times, a patient may need to receive *neoadjuvant* (treatment before surgery) chemotherapy and/or radiation therapy to reduce tumor burden and improve the surgical outcome.

### Supportive and Palliative Care

When cure or control of cancer is no longer possible, the focus shifts to supportive care and palliation of symptoms. Surgical procedures may be used to provide supportive care that maximizes bodily function or facilitates cancer treatment. Examples of supportive surgical procedures include the following:

- Insertion of feeding tube to maintain nutrition during head and neck cancer treatment
- Placement of central venous access devices to deliver chemotherapy agents
- Prophylactic surgical fixation of bones at risk for pathologic fracture

Effects of treatment or symptoms from metastatic cancer may necessitate surgical intervention for palliation. Examples include (1) debulking of tumor to relieve pain or pressure, (2) colostomy for the relief of a bowel obstruction (see Chapter 42), and (3) laminectomy for the relief of a spinal cord compression (see Chapter 60).

## CHEMOTHERAPY

**Chemotherapy** (antineoplastic therapy) is the use of chemicals as a systemic therapy for cancer. In the 1940s nitrogen mustard, a chemical warfare agent used in World Wars I and II, was used in the treatment of lymphoma and acute leukemia. In the 1970s chemotherapy was established as an effective treatment modality for cancer. Chemotherapy is now a mainstay of cancer treatment for most solid tumors and hematologic malignancies (e.g., leukemias, lymphomas). Chemotherapy can offer cure for some cancers, control other cancers for long periods, and in some instances offer palliative relief of symptoms when cure or control is no longer possible (Fig. 15-10).

### Effect on Cells

The goal of chemotherapy is to eliminate or reduce the number of cancer cells in the primary tumor and metastatic tumor site(s). All cells (cancer cells and normal cells) enter the cell

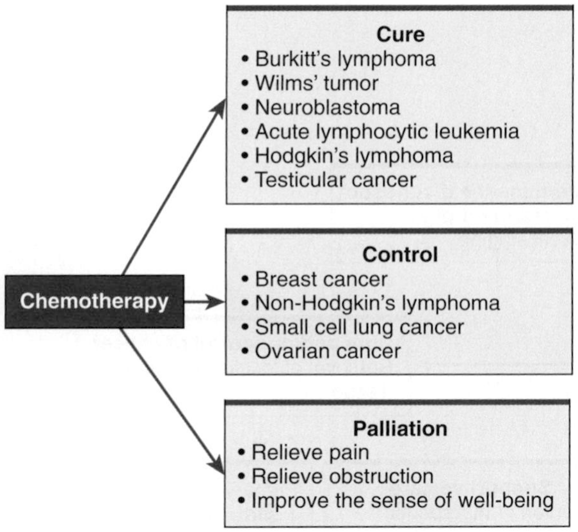


**FIG. 15-10** Goals of chemotherapy.

cycle for replication and proliferation (Fig. 15-1). The effects of the chemotherapy drugs are described in relation to the cell cycle.

The two major categories of chemotherapy drugs are cell cycle phase–nonspecific and cell cycle phase–specific drugs. *Cell cycle phase–nonspecific chemotherapy drugs* have their effect on the cells during all phases of the cell cycle, including the process of cell replication and proliferation and the resting phase ($G_0$). *Cell cycle phase–specific chemotherapy drugs* exert their most significant effects during specific phases of the cell cycle (i.e., when cells are in the process of cell replication or proliferation during $G_1$, S, $G_2$, or M). Cell cycle phase–specific and cell cycle phase–nonspecific agents are often administered in combination to maximize effectiveness by using agents that function by differing mechanisms and throughout the cell cycle.

When cancer first begins to develop, most of the cells are actively dividing. As the tumor increases in size, more cells become inactive and convert to a resting state ($G_0$). Because most chemotherapy agents are most effective against dividing cells, cells can escape death by staying in the $G_0$ phase. A major challenge is to overcome the effect of resistant resting and noncycling cells.

## Classification of Chemotherapy Drugs

Chemotherapy drugs are classified in general groups according to their molecular structure and mechanisms of action (Table 15-7). Each drug in a particular classification has many similarities. However, there are major differences in how the drugs work and the unique side effects associated with drugs in each class.

## Preparation of Chemotherapy

It is important to know the specific guidelines for administration of chemotherapy drugs. In addition, it is important to understand that drugs may pose an occupational hazard to health care professionals who do not follow safe handling guidelines. A person preparing, transporting, or administering chemotherapy may absorb the drug through inhalation of particles when reconstituting a powder and through skin contact from exposure to droplets or powder from oral agents. There may also be some risk in handling the body fluids and excretions of people receiving chemotherapy immediately after administration for 48 hours. Only those personnel specifically trained in chemotherapy handling techniques should be involved with the preparation and administration of cancer drugs.

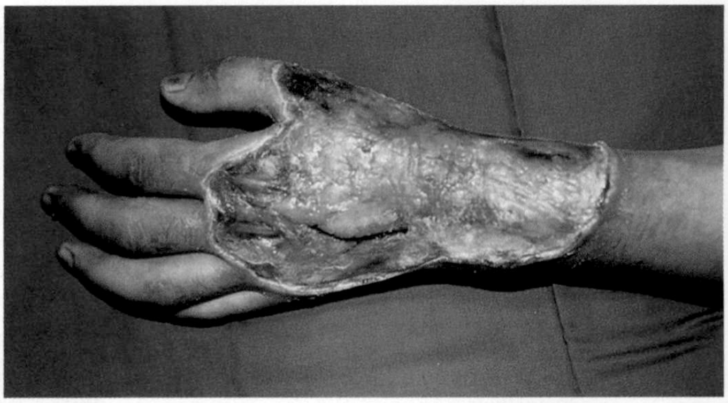

**FIG. 15-11** Extravasation injury from infiltration of chemotherapy drug. (From Weinzweig N, Weinzweig J: *The mutilated hand,* Philadelphia, 2005, Mosby.)

Guidelines for the safe handling of chemotherapy agents have been developed by the National Institute for Occupational Safety and Health (OSHA)[15] and the Oncology Nursing Society (ONS).[16]

## Methods of Administration

Chemotherapy can be administered by multiple routes (Table 15-8). With advances in drug formulation techniques, more oral chemotherapy agents are available. With oral agents, the patient will need to be taught about storage and side effects.

The IV route is the most common method of administering chemotherapy. Major concerns associated with the IV administration of antineoplastic drugs include venous access difficulties, device- or catheter-related infection, and *extravasation* (infiltration of drugs into tissues surrounding the infusion site) causing local tissue damage (Fig. 15-11).

Many chemotherapy drugs are either irritants or vesicants. *Irritants* will damage the intima of the vein, causing phlebitis and sclerosis and limiting future peripheral venous access but will not cause tissue damage if infiltrated. However, **vesicants**, if inadvertently infiltrated into the skin, may cause severe local tissue breakdown and necrosis. It is extremely important to monitor for and promptly recognize symptoms associated with extravasation of a vesicant and to take immediate action if it occurs. To minimize the associated physical discomforts, emotional distress, and risks of infection and infiltration, IV chemotherapy can be administered by a *central venous access device* (CVAD). CVADs are placed in large blood vessels and permit frequent, continuous, or intermittent administration of chemotherapy, immunotherapy, and targeted therapy, and other products, thus avoiding multiple venipunctures for vascular access. (CVADs are discussed in Chapter 16.)

## Regional Chemotherapy Administration

Regional treatment with chemotherapy involves delivery of the drug directly to the tumor site. The advantage of this method is that higher concentrations of the drug can be delivered to the tumor with reduced systemic toxicity. Several regional delivery methods have been developed, including intraarterial, intraperitoneal, intrathecal or intraventricular, and intravesical bladder chemotherapy.

**Intraarterial Chemotherapy.** Intraarterial chemotherapy delivers the drug to the tumor via the arteries supplying the tumor. This method has been used for the treatment of osteogenic

**TABLE 15-7 Drug Therapy**

***Chemotherapy***

| Mechanisms of Action | Examples |
|---|---|
| **Alkylating Agents** | |
| ***Cell Cycle Phase–Nonspecific Agents*** | |
| Damage DNA by causing breaks in the double-stranded helix. If repair does not occur, cells will die immediately (cytocidal) or when they attempt to divide (cytostatic). | bendamustine (Treanda), busulfan (Myleran), chlorambucil (Leukeran), cyclophosphamide, dacarbazine (DTIC-Dome), ifosfamide (Ifex), mechlorethamine (Mustargen), melphalan (Alkeran), temozolomide (Temodar), thiotepa |
| **Nitrosoureas** | |
| ***Cell Cycle Phase–Nonspecific Agents*** | |
| Like alkylating agents, break DNA helix, interfering with DNA replication. Cross blood-brain barrier. | carmustine (BiCNU, Gliadel), lomustine (Gleostine), streptozocin (Zanosar) |
| **Platinum Drugs** | |
| ***Cell Cycle Phase–Nonspecific Agents*** | |
| Bind to DNA and RNA, miscoding information and/or inhibiting DNA replication, and cells die. | carboplatin, cisplatin (Platinol-AQ), oxaliplatin (Eloxatin) |
| **Antimetabolites** | |
| ***Cell Cycle Phase–Specific Agents*** | |
| Mimic naturally occurring substances, thus interfering with enzyme function or DNA synthesis. Primarily act during S phase. Purine and pyrimidine are building blocks of nucleic acids needed for DNA and RNA synthesis | |
| • Interfere with purine metabolism | cladribine, clofarabine (Clolar), fludarabine, mercaptopurine (Purixan), nelarabine (Arranon), pentostatin (Nipent), thioguanine |
| • Interfere with pyrimidine metabolism | capecitabine (Xeloda); cytarabine (ara-C [Cytosar-U, DepoCyt]), floxuridine, 5-fluorouracil (5-FU), gemcitabine (Gemzar) |
| • Interfere with folic acid metabolism | methotrexate (Trexall), pemetrexed (Alimta) |
| • Interfere with DNA synthesis | hydroxyurea (Hydrea, Droxia) |
| **Antitumor Antibiotics** | |
| ***Cell Cycle Phase–Nonspecific Agents*** | |
| Bind directly to DNA, thus inhibiting the synthesis of DNA and interfering with transcription of RNA. | bleomycin, dactinomycin (Cosmegen), daunorubicin (Cerubidine, DaunoXome), doxorubicin (Doxil), epirubicin (Ellence), idarubicin, mitomycin, mitoxantrone, valrubicin (Valstar) |
| **Mitotic Inhibitors** | |
| ***Cell Cycle Phase–Specific Agents*** | |
| **Taxanes** | |
| Antimicrotubule agents that interfere with mitosis. Act during the late $G_2$ phase and mitosis to stabilize microtubules, thus inhibiting cell division. | albumin-bound paclitaxel (Abraxane), docetaxel (Taxotere), paclitaxel (Taxol) |
| **Vinca Alkaloids** | |
| Act in M phase to inhibit mitosis. | vinblastine, vincristine, vinorelbine (Navelbine) |
| **Others** | |
| Microtubular inhibitors. | estramustine (Emcyt), ixabepilone (Ixempra), eribulin (Halaven) |
| **Topoisomerase Inhibitors** | |
| ***Cell Cycle Phase–Specific Agents*** | |
| Inhibit topoisomerases (normal enzymes) that function to make reversible breaks and repairs in DNA that allow for flexibility of DNA in replication. | etoposide, irinotecan (Camptosar), teniposide (Vumon), topotecan (Hycamtin) |
| **Miscellaneous** | |
| Enzyme derived from the yeast Erwinia used to deplete the supply of asparagine (amino acid) for leukemic cells that are dependent on an exogenous source of this amino acid. Inhibits protein synthesis. | Erwinia asparaginase, L-asparaginase (Elspar) |
| Causes changes in DNA in leukemia cells and leads to cell death. | arsenic trioxide (Trisenox) |
| Suppresses mitosis. Appears to alter DNA, RNA, and protein. | procarbazine (Matulane) |

NOTE: Many of these drugs are irritants or vesicants that require special attention during administration to avoid extravasation. It is important to know this information about a drug before administering it.

sarcoma; cancers of the head and neck, bladder, and cervix; melanoma; primary liver cancer; and metastatic liver disease. One method of intraarterial drug delivery involves the surgical placement of a catheter that is subsequently connected to an external infusion pump or an implanted infusion pump for infusion of the chemotherapy agent.

**Intraperitoneal Chemotherapy.** Intraperitoneal chemotherapy involves the delivery of chemotherapy to the peritoneal cavity for treatment of peritoneal metastases from primary colorectal and ovarian cancers and malignant ascites. Temporary Silastic catheters (Tenckhoff, Hickman, and Groshong) are percutaneously or surgically placed into the peritoneal cavity for short-term administration of chemotherapy. Alternatively, an implanted port can be used to administer chemotherapy intraperitoneally. Chemotherapy is generally infused into the peritoneum in 1 to 2 L of fluid and allowed to *dwell* in the peritoneum for 1 to 4 hours. After the *dwell time,* the fluid is drained from the peritoneum.

**TABLE 15-8 Drug Therapy**

***Methods of Chemotherapy Administration***

| Method | Examples |
|---|---|
| Oral | cyclophosphamide, capecitabine (Xeloda), temozolomide (Temodar) |
| Intramuscular | bleomycin |
| Intravenous | doxorubicin, vincristine, cisplatin, 5-fluorouracil (5-FU), paclitaxel (Taxol) |
| Intracavitary (pleural, peritoneal) | Radioisotopes, alkylating agents, methotrexate |
| Intrathecal | methotrexate (preservative free), cytarabine |
| Intraarterial | dacarbazine, 5-FU, methotrexate |
| Perfusion | Alkylating agents |
| Subcutaneous | cytarabine, bortezomib |
| Topical | 5-FU cream |

**TABLE 15-9 Cells With Rapid Rate of Proliferation**

| Cells | Generation Time | Effect of Cell Destruction |
|---|---|---|
| Bone marrow stem cell | 6-24 hr | Myelosuppression (infection, bleeding, anemia) |
| Neutrophils | 12 hr | Leukopenia, infection |
| Epithelial cells lining the gastrointestinal tract | 12-24 hr | Anorexia, mucositis (including stomatitis, esophagitis), nausea and vomiting, diarrhea |
| Cells of the hair follicle | 24 hr | Alopecia |
| Ova or testes | 24-36 hr | Reproductive dysfunction |

**Intrathecal or Intraventricular Chemotherapy.** Cancers that metastasize to the central nervous system (CNS) are difficult to treat because the blood-brain barrier often prevents distribution of chemotherapy to this area. One method used to treat metastasis to the CNS is intrathecal chemotherapy. This method involves a lumbar puncture and injection of chemotherapy into the subarachnoid space. To reduce the need for repeated lumbar punctures, patients may have an Ommaya reservoir inserted. An Ommaya reservoir is a Silastic, dome-shaped disk with an extension catheter that is surgically implanted through the cranium into a lateral ventricle.

**Intravesical Bladder Chemotherapy.** *Intravesical bladder chemotherapy* involves instillation of chemotherapy into the bladder. The chemotherapy agent is instilled into the bladder via a urinary catheter and retained for 1 to 3 hours.

### Effects of Chemotherapy on Normal Tissues

Chemotherapy agents cannot selectively distinguish between normal cells and cancer cells. Chemotherapy-induced side effects are the result of the destruction of normal cells, especially those that are rapidly proliferating such as those in the bone marrow, lining of the GI system, and integumentary system (skin, hair, and nails) (Table 15-9). The general and drug-specific adverse effects of these drugs are classified as acute, delayed, or chronic.

*Acute toxicity* occurs during and immediately after drug administration and includes anaphylactic and hypersensitivity reactions, extravasation or a flare reaction, anticipatory nausea and vomiting, and cardiac dysrhythmias.

*Delayed effects* are numerous and include delayed nausea and vomiting, mucositis, alopecia, skin rashes, bone marrow suppression, altered bowel function (diarrhea or constipation), and a variety of cumulative neurotoxicities.

*Chronic toxicities* involve damage to organs such as the heart, liver, kidneys, and lungs. Chronic toxicities can be either long-term effects that develop during or immediately after treatment and persist or late effects that are absent during treatment and manifest later.

Some side effects fall into more than one category. For example, nausea and vomiting can be both acute and delayed.

### Treatment Plan

Although single-drug chemotherapy is sometimes prescribed, the more common modality is combining agents in multidrug regimens. This approach to treatment targets more than one signaling pathway and has proven to be more effective in managing most cancers. The regimens with multiple agents involve drugs with different mechanisms of action and varying toxicity profiles. However, when chemotherapy agents are used in combination, patients can experience an increase in toxicities.

Drug regimens are selected based on evidence supporting their use in specific cancers. Sometimes they are customized to meet the needs of an individual patient. Chemotherapy is most effective when the tumor burden is low, therapy is not interrupted, and the patient receives the intended dose. The dose of each drug is based on the individual's body weight and height using the body surface area calculation.

Mutation of cancer cells within the tumor can result in cells that are resistant to chemotherapy. With the use of multiple drugs that work at different places in the cell cycle, cancer cells can be more effectively killed. Thus mutation and resistance of cancer cells can be prevented.

**INFORMATICS IN PRACTICE**

***Managing Cancer Patients' Symptoms***

- Patients arriving at some clinics are handed a tablet computer. While in the waiting room or chemotherapy infusion unit, with the touch of a finger they select the symptoms that they are experiencing.
- HCPs can review the information and provide care aimed at managing the patient's specific symptoms.
- After the visit, the notes are stored in the patient's electronic health record. This system can assist with quality of care by determining if standards of care were followed.

## RADIATION THERAPY

Along with surgery, radiation therapy is one of the oldest methods of cancer treatment. It was first used by Emil Grubbe (a medical student) to treat an ulcerating breast cancer in 1896 (although the patient responded locally, she died later of metastatic disease). The observation that radiation exposure caused tissue damage led scientists to explore the use of radiation to treat tumors. The hypothesized association was that if radiation exposure resulted in the destruction of highly mitotic skin cells, it could be used in a controlled way to prevent the continued growth of cancer cells.

It was not until the 1960s that sophisticated equipment and treatment planning facilitated the delivery of adequate radiation doses to tumors and tolerable doses to normal tissues. Today many cancer patients receive radiation therapy at some point in their treatment.

### Effects of Radiation

**Radiation** is energy that is emitted from a source and travels through space or some material. Delivery of high-energy beams, when absorbed into tissue, produces ionization of atomic particles. The energy in ionizing radiation acts to break the chemical bonds in DNA. The DNA is damaged, resulting in cell death.

Different types of ionizing radiation are used to treat cancer, including *electromagnetic radiation* (i.e., x-rays, gamma rays) and *particulate radiation* (alpha particles, electrons, neutrons, protons). High-energy x-rays (photons) are generated by an electric machine, such as a linear accelerator.

Technologic advances have expanded and refined the sources and methods of delivering radiation therapy, thus offering more accurate and less invasive radiation treatment options. Most radiation centers in the United States currently use megavoltage linear accelerator technology. Larger radiation facilities may offer a combination of machines that permit expanded options for patients at one treatment site.

### Principles of Radiobiology

As the radiation beam passes through the treatment field, energy is deposited. *Low-energy beams* (such as electrons) expend energy quickly on impact with matter. Therefore they penetrate only a short distance. (They are clinically useful in treating superficial skin lesions.) *High-energy beams* (such as photons) have greater depth of penetration, not attaining full intensity until they reach a certain depth. Therefore they are suitable for delivering optimal doses to internal targets while sparing the skin.

Technically, all cancer cells could be killed with radiation given in high enough doses. However, to avoid serious toxicity and long-term complications of treatment, radiation to surrounding healthy tissue must be limited to the *maximal tolerated dose* for that specific tissue. Advances in planning and in delivery technology (such as *intensity-modulated radiation therapy [IMRT]* and *image-guided radiation therapy [IGRT]*) have greatly improved the ability to deliver maximal doses to the target volume while sparing critical structures (e.g., spinal cord, carotid arteries, optic chiasm) as much as possible.

Historically, the radiation dose was expressed in units called *rads* (radiation absorbed doses). Current nomenclature is *gray* (Gy) or centigray (cGy). A *centigray* is equivalent to 1 rad, and 100 centigray equals 1 gray. Once the total dose to be delivered is determined, that dose is divided into daily *fractions.* Doses between 180 and 200 cGy/day are considered *standard fractionation,* typically delivered once a day Monday through Friday for a period of 2 to 8 weeks (depending on the desired total dose).

Certain cancers are more susceptible to the effects of radiation than others (Table 15-10). In responsive tumors (such as lymphomas), even a large tumor burden is affected by radiation therapy. In less responsive tumors, a large tumor burden may result in a slower and perhaps incomplete response. Localized prostate cancer responds very slowly to radiation (several months after treatment is completed).

**TABLE 15-10 Tumor Radiosensitivity***

| | |
|---|---|
| **High Radiosensitivity** | **Mild Radiosensitivity** |
| • Ovarian dysgerminoma<br>• Testicular seminoma<br>• Hodgkin's lymphoma<br>• Non-Hodgkin's lymphoma<br>• Wilms' tumor<br>• Neuroblastoma | • Soft tissue sarcomas (e.g., chondrosarcoma)<br>• Gastric adenocarcinoma<br>• Renal adenocarcinoma<br>• Colon adenocarcinoma |
| **Moderate Radiosensitivity** | **Poor Radiosensitivity** |
| • Oropharyngeal carcinoma<br>• Esophageal carcinoma<br>• Breast adenocarcinoma<br>• Uterine and cervical carcinoma<br>• Prostate carcinoma<br>• Bladder carcinoma | • Osteosarcoma<br>• Malignant melanoma<br>• Malignant glioma<br>• Testicular nonseminoma |

*Radiosensitivity is the relative susceptibility of cells and tissues to the effects of radiation.

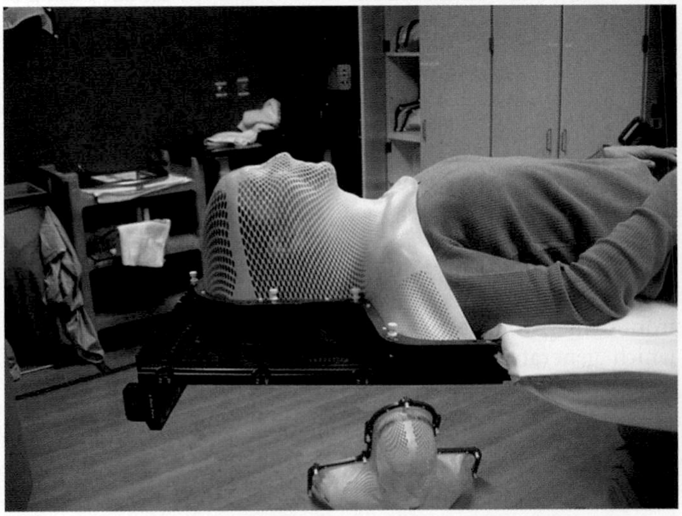

**FIG. 15-12** Immobilization device. A head holder and an immobilization mask may be used to ensure accurate positioning for daily treatment of head and neck cancer. (Courtesy Jormain Cady, Virginia Mason Medical Center, Seattle, Wash.)

### Simulation and Treatment Planning

*Simulation* is a process by which the radiation treatment fields are defined, filmed, and marked out on the skin. The radiation oncologist specifies the dose and volume of area to be treated. Treatment volumes include the (1) *gross target v*olume (GTV), which is the gross extent of the tumor identified by examination or imaging; (2) the *clinical target* volume (CTV), which is the GTV plus additional margin to encompass any potential microscopic or subclinical disease; and (3) the *planning target volume* (PTV), which is the GTV/CTV plus additional margin to allow for organ motion or variance in daily set-up position.

During the simulation, the patient is positioned on a simulator, which is a diagnostic x-ray machine that re-creates the actions of the linear accelerator and the radiation fields are marked on the patient's skin. Immobilization devices (e.g., casts, bite blocks, thermoplastic face masks) are typically used to help the patient maintain a stable position (Fig. 15-12).

The target is defined using a variety of possible imaging techniques (e.g., x-rays; CT, MRI, PET scans), physical examination, and surgical reports. Small tattoos may be placed to ensure the patient position is precisely reproduced on a daily basis.

### Treatment

Radiation is used to treat a carefully defined area of the body. Since radiation only has an effect on tissues within the treatment field, it is not appropriate as the primary treatment for systemic disease. However, radiation may be used by itself, in combination with chemotherapy or surgery to treat primary tumors, or for palliation of metastatic lesions.

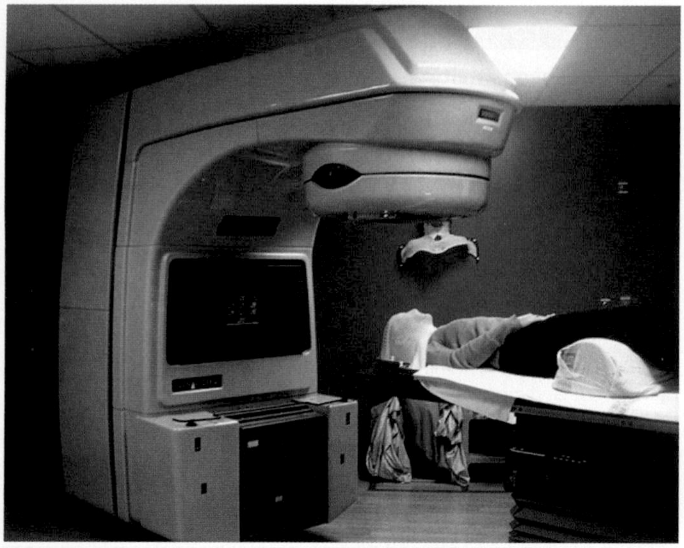

**FIG. 15-13** Linear accelerator. Varian Clinac EX linear accelerator with multiple photon and electron energies available for use according to the treatment plan. Patient is positioned on radiation treatment table for treatment of head and neck cancer. (Courtesy Jormain Cady, Virginia Mason Medical Center, Seattle, Wash.)

**External Radiation.** Radiation can be delivered externally (known as *teletherapy* or *external beam radiation therapy*) or internally *(brachytherapy)*. **Teletherapy** *(external beam radiation)* is the most common form of radiation treatment delivery. With this technique, the patient is exposed to radiation from a megavoltage treatment machine. A linear accelerator, which generates ionizing radiation from electricity and can have multiple energies, is the most commonly used machine for delivering external beam radiation (Fig. 15-13). *Gamma knife technology* (used to deliver highly accurate stereotactic treatment to a localized treatment volume) uses a cobalt source.

**Internal Radiation.** Radiation can also be delivered as **brachytherapy**, which means "close" or internal radiation treatment. It consists of the implantation or insertion of radioactive materials directly into the tumor (interstitial) or in close proximity to the tumor (intracavitary or intraluminal). This allows for direct delivery of radiation to the target with minimal exposure to surrounding healthy tissues. (In external radiation, the beam has to pass through external tissues to reach the internal target.) Brachytherapy is commonly used in combination with external radiation as a supplemental "boost" treatment, but may also be used as primary or adjuvant therapy.

Sources of radiation for brachytherapy include temporary sealed sources such as iridium-192 and cesium-137 and permanent sealed sources such as iodine-125, gold-198, and palladium-103. These are supplied in the form of seeds or ribbons. With a temporary implant, the source may be placed into a special catheter or metal tube that has been inserted into the tumor area. It is left in place until the prescribed dose of radiation has been reached in the calculated number of hours.

Brachytherapy may be delivered as high-dose-rate (HDR) treatment (i.e., several doses administered at varying intervals over a few minutes each time) or low-dose-rate (LDR) treatment (i.e., continuous treatment over several hours or days). A remote "afterloading" technique (i.e., the source is inserted after the applicator is in place) is designed to enhance physician and patient safety and is used for HDR brachytherapy with iridium-192. These methods are commonly used for head and neck, lung, breast, and gynecologic cancers.

Permanent implants, such as for prostate brachytherapy, involve the insertion of radioactive seeds directly into the tumor tissue, where they remain permanently. As interstitial seeds used for treatment emit low energies with limited tissue penetration, patients are not considered radioactive. However, some initial radiation precautions may be recommended because of a small risk of seed dislodgement. Over time, the isotopes that are used decay and are no longer radioactive. The timeframe for side effects induced by treatment can be predicted based on the rate of decay for the specific isotope used.

Radiopharmaceutical therapy employs unsealed liquid radioactive sources that are administered orally as a drink, such as iodine-131 for thyroid cancer, or IV as with yttrium-90 given for refractory lymphomas or samarium-153 used to treat bone metastases.

Caring for the person undergoing brachytherapy or receiving radiopharmaceuticals requires that you be aware that the patient is emitting radioactivity. Patients with temporary implants are radioactive only while the source is in place. In patients with permanent implants, because the sources have short half-lives and are weak emitters, the radioactive exposure to the outside and to others is low. These patients may be discharged with minimal precautions.

The principles of *ALARA (as low as reasonably achievable)* and *time, distance,* and *shielding* are vital to health care professional safety when caring for the person with a source of internal radiation. Organize care to limit the time spent in direct contact with the patient. To minimize anxiety and confusion, tell the patient the reason for time and distance limitations before the procedure.

The radiation safety officer will indicate how much time at a specific distance can be spent with the patient. This is determined by the dose delivered by the implant. Because the source is nonpenetrating, small differences in distance are critical. Only care that must be delivered near the source, such as checking placement of the implant, is performed in close proximity. Use shielding, if available, and do not deliver care without wearing a film badge (dosimeter) indicating cumulative radiation exposure. Do not share the film badge, do not wear it anywhere but at work, and return it according to the agency's protocol.

## NURSING MANAGEMENT: CHEMOTHERAPY AND RADIATION THERAPY

You have an important role in helping patients deal with the side effects of chemotherapy and radiation therapy. Before initiating teaching, assess the patient's ability to process information. Customize teaching to meet the patient's and family's learning needs.[17,18]

Common side effects of chemotherapy and radiation are presented in Table 15-11. Bone marrow suppression, fatigue, GI disturbances, integumentary and mucosal reactions, and pulmonary and reproductive effects are discussed in this section.

### Nursing Implementation

**Bone Marrow Suppression.** Myelosuppression is one of the most common effects of chemotherapy and, to a lesser extent,

**TABLE 15-11 Nursing Management of Problems Caused by Chemotherapy and Radiation Therapy**

| Etiology | Nursing Management |
|---|---|
| **Gastrointestinal System** | |
| ***Stomatitis, Mucositis, Esophagitis*** | |
| Epithelial cells are destroyed by chemotherapy or radiation treatment when located in field (e.g., head and neck, stomach, esophagus).<br>Inflammation and ulceration occur due to rapid cell destruction. | • Assess oral mucosa daily and teach patient to do this.<br>• Encourage nutritional supplements (e.g., Ensure, Carnation Instant Breakfast) if intake decreasing.<br>• Be aware that eating, swallowing, and talking may be difficult (may require analgesics).<br>• Instruct in avoidance of irritating spicy or acidic foods or too hot or too cold food (extremes in temperature).<br>• Instruct on how to select moist, bland, and softer foods.<br>• Encourage patient to keep oral cavity clean and moist by performing frequent oral rinses with saline or salt and soda solution.<br>• Encourage patient to use artificial saliva to manage dryness (radiation).<br>• Discourage use of irritants such as tobacco and alcohol.<br>• Apply topical anesthetics (e.g., viscous lidocaine, oxethazaine). |
| ***Nausea and Vomiting*** | |
| Release of intracellular breakdown products stimulates vomiting center in brain.<br>Drugs also stimulate vomiting center in brain (see Fig. 41-1).<br>GI lining destroyed with radiation and chemotherapy. | • Encourage patient to eat and drink when not nauseated.<br>• Administer antiemetics prophylactically before chemotherapy and also on as-needed basis.<br>• Instruct patient to take antiemetics on a scheduled basis for 2-3 days after highly emetogenic chemotherapy.<br>• Use diversional activities (if appropriate). |
| ***Anorexia*** | |
| Release of TNF and IL-1 from macrophages has appetite-suppressant effect.<br>Therapy-induced GI effects (mucositis, nausea and vomiting, bowel disturbances) and anxiety reduce appetite. | • Monitor weight.<br>• Encourage patient to eat small, frequent meals of high-protein, high-calorie foods.<br>• Gently encourage patient to eat, but avoid nagging.<br>• Recommend keeping a food diary to track daily calories and fluids.<br>• Serve food in pleasant environment. |
| ***Diarrhea*** | |
| From denuding of epithelial lining of intestines.<br>Side effect of chemotherapy.<br>Follows radiation to abdomen, pelvis, lumbosacral areas. | • Give antidiarrheal drugs as needed.<br>• Encourage low-fiber, low-residue diet.<br>• Encourage fluid intake of at least 3 L/day. |
| ***Constipation*** | |
| Decreased intestinal motility is related to autonomic nervous system dysfunction.<br>Caused by neurotoxic effects of plant alkaloids (vincristine, vinblastine). | • Instruct patient to take stool softeners as needed, eat high-fiber foods, and increase fluid intake.<br>• Instruct patient to increase activity (e.g., walking) if tolerated. |
| ***Hepatotoxicity*** | |
| Toxic effects from chemotherapy drugs (usually transient and resolve when drug is stopped). | • Monitor liver function tests. |
| **Hematologic System** | |
| ***Anemia*** | |
| Bone marrow depressed secondary to therapy.<br>Malignant infiltration of bone marrow by cancer. | • Monitor hemoglobin and hematocrit levels.<br>• Administer iron supplements and erythropoietin.<br>• Encourage intake of foods that promote RBC production (see Table 30-5). |
| ***Leukopenia*** | |
| Depression of bone marrow secondary to chemotherapy or radiation therapy.<br>Infection most frequent cause of morbidity and death in cancer patients.<br>Respiratory and genitourinary system usual sites of infection. | • Monitor WBC count, especially neutrophils.<br>• Tell patient to report temperature elevation and any other manifestations of infection.<br>• Teach patient to avoid large crowds and people with infections.<br>• Administer WBC growth factors (Table 15-15).<br>• For patient teaching, see Table 30-23. |
| ***Thrombocytopenia*** | |
| Bone marrow depressed secondary to chemotherapy.<br>Malignant infiltration of bone marrow crowds out normal marrow.<br>Spontaneous bleeding can occur with platelet counts ≤20,000/μL. | • Observe for signs of bleeding (e.g., petechiae, ecchymosis).<br>• Monitor platelet counts.<br>• For patient teaching, see Table 30-15. |
| **Integumentary System** | |
| ***Alopecia*** | |
| Destruction of hair follicles by chemotherapy or radiation to scalp.<br>Hair loss usually is temporary with chemotherapy, but usually permanent in response to radiation. | • Suggest ways to cope with hair loss (e.g., hair pieces, scarves, wigs).<br>• Cut long hair before therapy.<br>• Avoid excessive shampooing, brushing, and combing of hair.<br>• Avoid use of electric hair dryers, curlers, and curling rods.<br>• Discuss impact of hair loss on self-image. |
| ***Radiation Skin Changes (dry to moist desquamation)*** | |
| Radiation damages skin. | • See Table 15-12 for patient management details. |

*IL-1,* Interleukin-1; *TNF,* tumor necrosis factor.

*Continued*

**TABLE 15-11 Nursing Management of Problems Caused by Chemotherapy and Radiation Therapy—cont'd**

| Etiology | Nursing Management |
|---|---|
| **Integumentary System—cont'd**<br>***Chemotherapy-Induced Skin Changes*** | |
| Hyperpigmentation.<br>Telangiectasia.<br>Photosensitivity.<br>Acneiform eruptions.<br>Acral erythema. | • Alert patient to potential skin changes.<br>• Encourage patient to avoid sun exposure.<br>• Implement symptomatic management as needed depending on specific skin effect (e.g., application of lotions, benzoyl peroxide for acne, corticosteroid creams). |
| **Genitourinary Tract**<br>***Hemorrhagic Cystitis*** | |
| Cells lining bladder are destroyed by chemotherapy (e.g., cyclophosphamide, ifosfamide).<br>Side effect of radiation when located in treatment field. | • Encourage increased fluid intake 24-72 hr after treatment as tolerated.<br>• Monitor manifestations such as urgency, frequency, and hematuria.<br>• Administer cytoprotectant agent (mesna [Mesnex]) and hydration.<br>• Administer supportive care agents to manage symptoms (e.g., flavoxate [Urispas]). |
| ***Reproductive Dysfunction*** | |
| Cells of testes or ova are damaged by therapy. | • Discuss possibility with patients before treatment initiation.<br>• Offer opportunity for sperm and ova banking before treatment for patients of childbearing age. |
| ***Nephrotoxicity*** | |
| Direct renal cell damage from exposure to nephrotoxic agents (cisplatin and high-dose methotrexate).<br>Precipitation of metabolites of cell breakdown (tumor lysis syndrome [TLS]). | • Monitor BUN and serum creatinine levels.<br>• Avoid potentiating drugs.<br>• Alkalinize the urine by adding sodium bicarbonate to IV infusion and administer allopurinol (Zyloprim) or rasburicase for TLS prevention. |
| **Nervous System**<br>***Intracranial Pressure*** | |
| May result from radiation edema in central nervous system. | • Monitor neurologic status.<br>• May be controlled with corticosteroids. |
| ***Peripheral Neuropathy*** | |
| Paresthesias, areflexia, skeletal muscle weakness, and smooth muscle dysfunction can occur as a side effect of plant alkaloids, taxanes, and cisplatin. | • Monitor for these manifestations in patients on these drugs.<br>• Consider temporary chemotherapy dose interruption or reduction until symptoms improve.<br>• Antiseizure drugs (e.g., gabapentin [Neurontin]) may be considered. |
| ***Cognitive Changes ("chemo brain")*** | |
| Occur during and after treatment (especially with chemotherapy).<br>Difficulties in concentration, memory lapses, trouble remembering details, taking longer to finish tasks.<br>May happen quickly and last a short time. Sometimes people have mild long-term effects. | • Teach patients to do the following:<br>  • Use detailed daily planner.<br>  • Get enough sleep and rest.<br>  • Exercise brain (learn something new, do word puzzles).<br>  • Focus on one thing (no multitasking). |
| **Respiratory System**<br>***Pneumonitis*** | |
| Radiation pneumonitis develops 2-3 mo after start of treatment.<br>After 6-12 mo, fibrosis occurs and is evident on x-ray.<br>Side effect of some chemotherapy drugs. | • Monitor for dry, hacking cough; fever; and exertional dyspnea. |
| **Cardiovascular System**<br>***Pericarditis and Myocarditis*** | |
| Inflammation secondary to radiation injury.<br>Complication when chest wall is irradiated. May occur up to 1 yr after treatment.<br>Side effect of some chemotherapy drugs. | • Monitor for clinical manifestations of these disorders (e.g., dyspnea). |
| ***Cardiotoxicity*** | |
| Some chemotherapy drugs (e.g., anthracyclines, taxanes) can cause ECG changes and rapidly progressive heart failure. | • Monitor heart with ECG and cardiac ejection fractions.<br>• Drug therapy may need to be modified for symptoms or deteriorating cardiac function studies. |
| **Biochemical**<br>***Hyperuricemia*** | |
| Increased uric acid levels due to chemotherapy-induced cell destruction.<br>Can cause secondary gout and obstructive uropathy. | • Monitor uric acid levels.<br>• Allopurinol may be given as a prophylactic measure.<br>• Encourage increased fluid intake. |
| **Psychoemotional**<br>***Fatigue*** | |
| Anabolic processes result in accumulation of metabolites from cell breakdown. | • Assess for reversible causes of fatigue, and address them as indicated.<br>• Reassure patient that fatigue is a common side effect of therapy.<br>• Encourage patient to rest when fatigued, to maintain usual lifestyle patterns as much as possible, and to pace activities in accordance with energy level.<br>• Encourage moderate exercise as tolerated. |

*BUN*, Blood urea nitrogen; *ECG*, electrocardiogram.

it can also occur with radiation. Treatment-induced reductions in blood cell production can result in life-threatening and distressing effects, including infection, hemorrhage, and overwhelming fatigue. The major difference in manifestations between radiation therapy and chemotherapy is that with radiation (a local therapy), only bone marrow within the treatment field is affected, whereas chemotherapy (a systemic therapy) affects bone marrow function throughout the body. Therefore effects are more profound with chemotherapy and when the two therapies are combined.

In general, the onset of bone marrow suppression is related to the life span of the type of blood cell. WBCs (especially neutrophils) are affected most acutely (within 1 to 2 weeks), platelets in 2 to 3 weeks, and red blood cells (RBCs), with a longer life span of 120 days, at a later time. The severity of myelosuppression depends on the chemotherapy drugs used, dosages of drugs, and the specific radiation treatment field. Radiation to large marrow-containing regions of the body produces the most clinically significant myelosuppression. In the adult, most of the active marrow is in the pelvis or thoracic and lumbar vertebrae.

Monitor the complete blood count, particularly the neutrophil, platelet, and RBC counts, in patients receiving chemotherapy or radiation. Typically patients experience the lowest blood cell counts (called the **nadir**) between 7 and 10 days after initiation of therapy. However, the exact onset depends on the particular drug regimen.

*Neutropenia* is more common in patients receiving chemotherapy than radiation therapy. Neutropenia is a serious risk factor for life-threatening infection and sepsis. Significant neutropenia will prompt treatment delay or modification (i.e., lower dosages). Take every possible measure to prevent infections in these patients. Hand hygiene is the mainstay of patient protection. Patients and their contacts (including hospital staff) should follow hand-washing guidelines.

Monitor temperature routinely. Any sign of infection should be treated promptly, since fever in the setting of neutropenia is a medical emergency. WBC growth factors (i.e., filgrastim [Neupogen], pegfilgrastim [Neulasta]) are routinely used to reduce the duration of chemotherapy-induced neutropenia. They are also used as a prophylactic measure to prevent neutropenia when highly myelosuppressive chemotherapy drugs are used.[19] (Neutropenia is discussed in Chapter 30; see also the patient teaching guide in Table 30-23 and eNursing Care Plan 30-3 on the website for that chapter.)

*Thrombocytopenia* can result in spontaneous bleeding or major hemorrhage. Avoid invasive procedures and advise patients to avoid activities that place them at risk for injury or bleeding (including excessive straining). Risk of serious bleeding is generally not apparent until the platelet count falls below 50,000/μL. Platelet transfusions may be necessary and are usually administered when platelet counts fall below 20,000/μL. (Thrombocytopenia is discussed in Chapter 30; see also the patient teaching guide in Table 30-15 and eNursing Care Plan 30-2 on the website for that chapter.)

*Anemia* is common in patients undergoing either radiation therapy or chemotherapy. It generally has a later onset (about 3 to 4 months after treatment initiation). For patients with low hemoglobin levels, RBC growth factors (i.e., darbepoetin [Aranesp], epoetin [Procrit]) may be given according to clinical guidelines for use. In extreme circumstances (i.e., symptomatic anemia), RBC transfusions may also be indicated. However, in general, RBC transfusions should be avoided. (Hematopoietic growth factors are discussed later in this chapter and presented in Table 15-15.)

◆ **Fatigue.** *Fatigue* is the persistent subjective sense of tiredness associated with cancer and its treatment that interferes with usual day-to-day functioning. Fatigue is a nearly universal symptom affecting most patients with cancer. It is commonly reported by patients as the most distressful of treatment-related side effects. Furthermore, it may persist long after treatment has ended.

Anemia is one cause of fatigue. Other causes may be related to the (1) accumulation of toxic substances that are left in the body after cells are killed by cancer treatment, (2) need for extra energy to repair and heal body tissue damaged by treatment, and (3) lack of sleep caused by some chemotherapy drugs.

Assess for reversible causes of fatigue, such as anemia, hypothyroidism, depression, anxiety, insomnia, dehydration, or infection.

Help patients recognize that fatigue is a common side effect of therapy, and encourage energy conservation strategies. Help individuals identify days or times during the day when they typically feel better, and encourage them to remain more active during that time period.

Resting before activity and having others assist with work or home management may be necessary. Ignoring the fatigue or overstressing the body when fatigue is tolerable may lead to an increase in symptoms. However, maintaining exercise and activity within tolerable limits is often helpful in managing fatigue. Walking programs are a way for most patients to keep active without overtaxing themselves. Remaining active helps to improve mood and avoid the debilitating cycle of fatigue-depression-fatigue that can occur in patients with cancer. Guidelines for the evaluation and management of cancer-related fatigue are available.[20]

◆ **Gastrointestinal Effects.** The cells of the mucosal lining of the GI tract are highly proliferative, with epithelial cells being replaced every 2 to 6 days. The intestinal mucosa is one of the most sensitive tissues to radiation and chemotherapy. The etiology of GI reactions is related to a variety of mechanisms, including (1) the release of serotonin from the GI tract, which then stimulates the chemoreceptor trigger zone (CTZ) and the vomiting center in the brain and (2) cell death and resulting damage to GI mucosa. Additionally, radiation to treatment fields that contain GI structures (i.e., abdominopelvic, lumbosacral, and lower thoracic areas) and selected chemotherapy agents produce direct injury to GI epithelial cells. These injuries result in a variety of GI effects, including nausea and vomiting, diarrhea, mucositis, and anorexia. These problems can significantly affect the patient's hydration and nutritional status and sense of well-being.

◆ ***Nausea and Vomiting.*** Nausea and vomiting are common sequelae of chemotherapy and, in some instances, radiation therapy. Vomiting may occur within 1 hour of chemotherapy administration or a few hours after radiation therapy to the chest or abdomen and may persist for 24 hours or more. Several antiemetic drugs are available (see Table 41-1).

Metoclopramide (Reglan), prochlorperazine, serotonin (5-$HT_3$) receptor antagonists (ondansetron [Zofran], granisetron [Kytril], dolasetron [Anzemet], and palonosetron [Aloxi]), and dexamethasone have been used to decrease nausea and vomiting caused by chemotherapy. Aprepitant (Emend) and rolapitant (Varubi), substance P/neurokinin-1 receptor antagonists, are effective in preventing nausea and vomiting on the day of chemotherapy, as well as for delayed symptoms. Akynzeo is a fixed combination of two drugs: palonosetron and netupitant (a substance P/neurokinin-1 receptor antagonist).

Patients may also develop *anticipatory nausea and vomiting* if they experience poorly controlled nausea and vomiting after chemotherapy administration. In this phenomenon, encountering the cues even without receiving treatment may precipitate nausea and vomiting. Aggressive emesis control, including the prophylactic administration of antiemetic and antianxiety medication 1 hour before treatment, is recommended. The patient may find that eating a light meal of nonirritating food before treatment is also helpful.

*Delayed nausea and vomiting* can develop 24 hours to a week after treatment. Assess patients who are experiencing nausea and vomiting for signs and symptoms of dehydration and metabolic alkalosis. Nausea and vomiting can be successfully managed with antiemetic regimens, dietary modification, and other nondrug interventions (e.g., relaxation breathing).

◆ ***Diarrhea.*** Diarrhea is a reaction of the bowel mucosa to radiation and certain chemotherapy drugs. It is characterized by an increase in frequency and liquidity of stool. The small bowel is extremely sensitive and does not tolerate significant radiation doses. With pelvic radiation, patients may be treated with a full bladder to move the small bowel out of the treatment field. Both radiation- and chemotherapy-induced diarrhea are best managed with diet modification, antidiarrheals, antimotility agents, and antispasmodics (see Table 42-2).

Recommend a diet low in fiber and residue before treatment with chemotherapy known to cause diarrhea. This includes limiting foods that are high in roughage (e.g., fresh fruits, vegetables, seeds, nuts) (see Table 42-7). To prevent diarrhea, other foods to avoid include fried, fatty, or highly seasoned foods and other foods that are gas producing. Bowel mucosal injury from radiation may also result in temporary lactose intolerance. Therefore avoiding milk products is helpful for some patients during and immediately after treatment.

Depending on the severity of the diarrhea, hydration and electrolyte supplementation are also recommended. Lukewarm sitz baths may alleviate discomfort and cleanse the rectal area if significant rectal irritation has developed. The rectal area must be kept clean and dry to maintain skin integrity. You should visually inspect the perianal area for evidence of skin breakdown. Systemic analgesia may be used for the painful skin irritations that may develop. Note the number, volume, consistency, and character of stools per day. Teach patients to maintain a diary or log to record episodes and aggravating and alleviating factors.

◆ ***Mucositis.*** Mucositis (irritation, inflammation, and/or ulceration of the mucosa) is a common complication in almost all patients receiving radiation to the head and neck and in many patients receiving certain antineoplastic agents. Similar to the bowel mucosa, the mucosal linings of the oral cavity, oropharynx, and esophagus are extremely sensitive to the effects of radiation and chemotherapy.

Certain factors can compound the problem. For example, patients undergoing head and neck radiation may face the additional challenge of radiation-induced parotid gland dysfunction. This may result in decreased salivary flow, causing acute or chronic *xerostomia* (dry mouth). Dryness or thick saliva compromises the protective salivary functions of assisting with cleansing teeth, moistening food, and swallowing. Meticulous oral care during and for a long time after treatment reduces the risk of cavities related to the radiation, which may develop as a result of diminished saliva. Advise patients to continue regular dental follow-up every 6 months and to use fluoride supplements as recommended by their dentist. Saliva substitutes may be offered to patients with xerostomia, although many patients find that drinking small amounts of water frequently has a similar effect.

*Dysgeusia* (taste loss) may develop during therapy, and by the end of treatment, patients often report that all food has lost its flavor. Ultimately, nutritional status may be compromised. *Dysphagia* (difficulty swallowing), which characterizes pharyngeal and/or esophageal involvement, further impedes eating. Patients may report feeling that they have a "lump" as they swallow and that "foods get stuck." *Odynophagia* (painful swallowing) caused by oropharyngeal or esophageal irritation and ulceration may require the use of analgesics before meals.

Oral assessment and meticulous intervention to keep the oral cavity moist, clean, and free of debris are essential to prevent infection and to facilitate nutritional intake. Implementing standard oral care protocols that address prevention and management of mucositis facilitates routine assessment, patient and family teaching, and intervention.

Routinely assess the oral cavity, mucous membranes, characteristics of saliva, and ability to swallow. Having a dentist perform all necessary dental work before the initiation of treatment is also recommended. Teach the patient to self-examine the oral cavity as well as how to perform oral care (proper tooth brushing with a soft-bristle toothbrush, flossing, and use of fluoride trays to prevent caries). Oral care should be performed at least before and after each meal, at bedtime, and as needed through the day. A saline solution of 1 tsp of salt in 1 L of water is an effective cleansing agent. One tsp of sodium bicarbonate may be added to the oral care solution to decrease odor, alleviate pain, and dissolve mucin.

Mucositis or pain in the throat can be alleviated by systemic and/or topical analgesics and antibiotics if infection is present. Monitor and get prompt treatment for oral candidiasis (which often occurs with mucositis). Frequent cleansing with saline and water and topical application of anesthetic gels directly to the lesions are standard care.

◆ ***Anorexia.*** Anorexia (loss of appetite) is a common occurrence in patients with cancer. It is a side effect of the cancer itself as well as of cancer treatment. Anorexia may be related to an inflamed mouth or esophagus, which creates difficulty chewing or swallowing, or to emotions such as anxiety or depression. It is important to have a dietitian involved in patient care before cancer treatment begins.

Patients experiencing nausea and vomiting, bowel disturbances, mucositis, and taste alterations typically have little desire to eat. Although it is highly individual, anorexia seems to peak at about 4 weeks of treatment and to resolve more quickly than fatigue when treatment ends.

Monitor the patient with anorexia during and after treatment to ensure that weight loss does not become excessive. Also observe for dehydration. Small, frequent meals of high-protein, high-calorie foods are better tolerated than large meals. Nutritional supplements can be helpful as well. Enteral or parenteral nutrition may be indicated if the patient is severely malnourished, if symptoms are expected to interfere with nutrition for a time, or if the bowel is being rested. Monitor for and manage

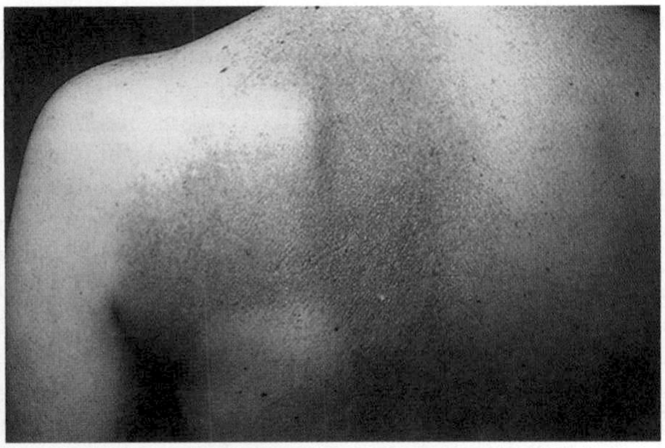

**FIG. 15-14** Dry desquamation.

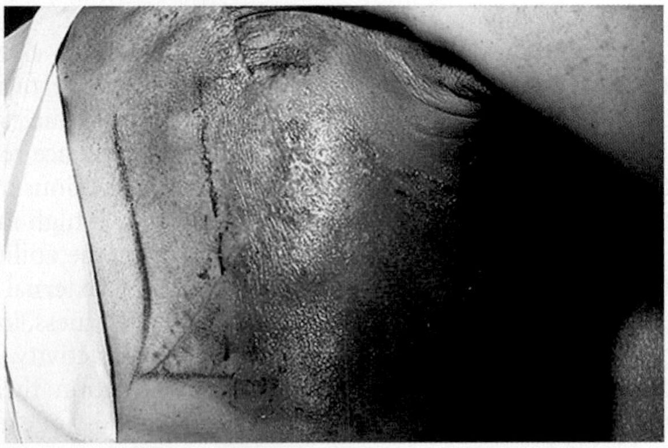

**FIG. 15-15** Wet desquamation.

other symptoms that may interfere with appetite (e.g., nausea, vomiting, pain, depression).

◆ **Skin Reactions**

◆ ***Radiation Skin Changes.*** With radiation therapy, skin effects are local, occurring only in the treatment field. Radiation-induced skin changes can be acute or chronic depending on the area irradiated, dosage, and technique. The skin-sparing ability of modern radiation equipment limits the severity of these reactions.

Erythema may develop 1 to 24 hours after a single treatment but generally occurs progressively as the treatment dose accumulates. Erythema is an acute response followed by dry desquamation (Fig. 15-14). If the rate of cell sloughing is faster than the ability of the new epidermal cells to replace dead cells, a wet desquamation occurs with exposure of the dermis and weeping of serous fluid (Fig. 15-15). Skin reactions are particularly evident in areas of skinfolds or where skin is subjected to pressure, such as behind the ear; in gluteal folds; or on the perineum, breast, collar line, and bony prominences.

Although skin care protocols vary among institutions, basic skin care principles apply. The goal is to prevent infection and facilitate wound healing. Protect radiated skin from temperature extremes. Do not use heating pads, ice packs, and hot water bottles in the treatment field. Avoid constricting garments, rubbing, harsh chemicals, and deodorants, since they may traumatize the skin. Dry reactions are uncomfortable and result in pruritus. Lubricate dry skin with a nonirritating lotion emollient that contains no metal, alcohol, perfume, or additives, since these can be irritating. Calendula ointment and topical hyaluronic acid cream are effective for the management of radiation dermatitis. Aloe vera gel is also used, especially for prevention of skin problems.

Wet desquamation of tissues generally produces pain, drainage, and increased risk of infection. Skin care to manage most desquamation includes keeping tissues clean with normal saline compresses or modified Burow's solution soaks. Then protect the skin from further damage with moisture vapor–permeable dressings or Vaseline petrolatum gauze. Because protocols vary widely, the guidelines presented in Table 15-12 should be verified with your institution's radiation oncology department before using.

◆ ***Chemotherapy Skin Changes.*** Chemotherapy produces a wide range of skin toxicities. These can range from mild erythema and hyperpigmentation to more distressing effects such as acral erythema and *erythrodysesthesia syndrome* (also called palmar-plantar erythrodysesthesia or hand-foot syndrome).

Erythrodysesthesia syndrome can cause mild symptoms of redness and tingling of the palms of the hands and soles of the feet. It may also cause severe symptoms of painful moist desquamation, ulceration, blistering, and pain.

### TABLE 15-12 Patient & Caregiver Teaching
#### *Radiation Skin Reactions*

*Include the following instructions when teaching the patient and caregiver to clean and protect the skin in a radiation treatment area.*

1. Gently cleanse the skin in the treatment field using a mild soap (Ivory, Dove), tepid water, a soft cloth, and a gentle patting motion. Rinse thoroughly and pat dry.
2. Apply nonmedicated, nonperfumed, moisturizing lotion or cream, such as calendula ointment, aloe gel, Aquaphor, or Biafine cream, to alleviate dry skin. Some substances must be gently cleansed from the treatment field before each treatment and reapplied. Over-the-counter hydrocortisone cream 1% may reduce itching.
3. Rinse the area with saline solution. Expose the area to air as often as possible. If copious drainage is present, use astringent compresses (such as Domeboro solution) and nonadhesive absorbent dressings (they must be changed as soon as they become wet). Observe the area daily for signs of infection.
4. Avoid wearing tight-fitting clothing such as brassieres and belts over the treatment field.
5. Avoid wearing harsh fabrics, such as wool and corduroy. A lightweight cotton garment is best. If possible, expose the treatment field to air.
6. Use gentle detergents such as Dreft and Ivory Snow to wash clothing that will come in contact with the treatment field.
7. Avoid direct exposure to the sun. If the treatment field is in an area that is exposed to the sun, wear protective clothing such as a wide-brimmed hat when out in the sun and apply sunscreen lotion.
8. Avoid all sources of excessive heat (hot water bottles, heating pads, sunlamps) on the treatment field.
9. Avoid exposing the treatment field to cold temperatures (ice bags or cold weather).
10. Avoid swimming in saltwater or in chlorinated pools during the time of treatment.
11. Avoid the use of potential irritants (e.g., perfumes, powders, or cosmetics) on the skin in the treatment field; review use of other topical medications or lotions with your health care provider during treatment. Also avoid tape, dressings, and adhesive bandages unless permitted by the radiation therapist. Avoid shaving the hair in the treatment field.
12. Continue to protect sensitive skin after the treatment is completed. Do the following:
    - Avoid direct exposure to the sun. A sunscreen agent and protective clothing must be worn if the potential of exposure to the sun is present.
    - Use an electric razor if shaving is necessary in the treatment field.

*Alopecia* is an easily recognizable effect of cancer therapy. It is frequently associated with varying degrees of emotional distress. Hair loss associated with radiation is local, whereas chemotherapy affects hair throughout the body. The degree and duration of hair loss experienced by patients depend on the type and dose of the chemotherapy agent.

Alopecia caused by the administration of chemotherapy agents is usually reversible. Usually the hair does not grow back until 3 to 4 weeks after the drugs are discontinued. Often the new hair has a different color and texture than the hair that was lost.

Patients experience a range of emotions at the prospect of losing their hair and when hair loss actually occurs. These may include anger, grief, embarrassment, or fear. Hair loss is a visible reminder of their cancer and the challenges of treatment. For some people, the loss of hair is one of the most stressful events experienced during the course of treatment. The American Cancer Society's "Look Good, Feel Better" program is an excellent support and resource for people experiencing not just hair loss but body image changes in general.

◆ **Pulmonary Effects.** Both chemotherapy and radiation have the potential to produce pulmonary tissue damage that is irreversible and progressive. Distinguishing between the complications of treatment and those related to disease is challenging. The effects of radiation on the lung include both acute and late reactions. Immediate pulmonary effects of radiation can be alarming to patients because they may mimic symptoms (e.g., cough, dyspnea) that precipitated the cancer diagnosis.

*Pneumonitis* is a delayed acute inflammatory reaction that may occur within 1 to 3 months after completion of thoracic radiation. This reaction is often asymptomatic, although an increase in cough, fever, and night sweats may occur. Some patients may develop pulmonary fibrosis (with or without prior pneumonitis), which is a late effect of therapy.

The most common pulmonary toxicities associated with chemotherapy include pulmonary edema (noncardiogenic) related to capillary leak syndrome or fluid retention, hypersensitivity pneumonitis, interstitial fibrosis, and pneumonitis produced by an inflammatory reaction or destruction of alveolar-capillary endothelium.

◆ **Cardiovascular Effects.** Radiation to the thorax can damage the pericardium, myocardium, valves, and coronary blood vessels. The pericardium is most commonly involved, with pericardial effusion or pericarditis the key problems. Patients with preexisting coronary artery disease are especially vulnerable.

Anthracyclines (e.g., doxorubicin [Adriamycin], daunorubicin) cause cardiotoxicity. Acute cardiotoxicities may cause electrocardiographic (ECG) abnormalities and late effects cause left ventricular dysfunction and heart failure. Baseline and periodic echocardiograms to monitor left ventricular function during treatment are usually done.

◆ **Cognitive Effects.** Cognitive effects can happen at any time during cancer, especially after treatment. This alteration in mental function, commonly described by patients as mental cloudiness or fog, is commonly called *chemo brain*.[21,22] Patients can experience thinking and memory problems. Although the brain will usually recover over time, the effects can last a short time or last for years. The effects can be so severe that patients may be unable to be involved in any activities that require mental effort such as school, work, or social activities.

◆ **Reproductive Effects.** Reproductive dysfunction secondary to radiation and chemotherapy varies according to the radiation treatment field and dosage, the particular chemotherapy agent and dose, and host factors (e.g., age). Treatment can cause temporary or permanent gonadal failure. Reproductive effects occur most often when reproductive organs are included in the radiation treatment field and when alkylating agents are used.

The testes are highly sensitive to radiation and should be protected with a testicular shield whenever possible. Pretreatment status may be a significant factor because a low sperm count and loss of motility are seen in individuals with testicular cancer and Hodgkin's lymphoma before any therapy is begun. Combined modality treatment or prior chemotherapy with alkylating agents enhances and prolongs the effects of radiation on the testes. When radiation is used alone with conventional doses and appropriate shielding, testicular recovery often occurs. Compromise of reproductive function in men may also result from erectile dysfunction after pelvic radiation.

The radiation dose that induces ovarian failure changes with age. Unlike the testes, there is no way to repair ovarian function. When radiation therapy is given, the ovaries are shielded whenever possible. Other factors that influence reproductive or sexual functioning in women include reactions in the cervix and endometrium. These tissues withstand a high radiation dose with minimal sequelae, accounting for the ability to treat endometrial and cervical cancer with high external and brachytherapy doses. Acute reactions such as tenderness, irritation, and loss of lubrication compromise sexual activity. Late effects of combined internal and external radiation therapy include vaginal shortening related to fibrosis and loss of elasticity and lubrication.

The patient and her or his partner require information about the expected effects of treatment relative to reproductive and sexual issues. Fertility preservation should be addressed prior to the start of any cancer treatment. Pretreatment harvesting of sperm, ova, or ovarian tissue may be considered.[23]

Potential infertility can be a significant consequence for the individual, and counseling may be indicated. However, in no case should the patient think that conception is not possible during treatment. Specific suggestions to manage side effects that have an impact on sexual functioning include using a water-soluble vaginal lubricant and routinely using a vaginal dilator after pelvic irradiation. Encourage discussion of issues related to reproduction and sexuality, offer specific suggestions, and make referrals for ongoing counseling when indicated.

## LATE EFFECTS OF RADIATION AND CHEMOTHERAPY

Cancer survivors are achieving long-term remission and survival with advancements in treatment modalities. However, these forms of therapy (especially radiation therapy and chemotherapy) may produce long-term sequelae termed *late effects* that occur months to years after cessation of therapy.[24,25] Every body system can be affected to some extent by radiation therapy or chemotherapy.

Acute radiation effects generally manifest as transient inflammatory changes in highly proliferative cells (e.g., epithelial tissues). In contrast, late radiation effects occur most commonly in post-mitotic cells (e.g., liver, kidney, lung, heart, muscle, bone, and connective tissues). Once they occur, the late effects may be progressive and generally are permanent. Examples range from skin telangiectasias to strictures, fistulas, or radiation necrosis.

Alteration of the lymphatic channels (e.g., axillary lymph node dissection) may contribute to lymphedema.

Long-term effects of chemotherapy include cardiac toxicity, cataracts, arthralgias, endocrine alterations, renal insufficiency, hepatitis, osteoporosis, neurocognitive dysfunction, or other effects depending on the agents. The additive effects of multiagent chemotherapy before, during, or after a course of radiation therapy can significantly increase the resulting late effects.

The cancer survivor may also be at risk for secondary malignancies, including leukemia, angiosarcoma, and skin cancer. Patients treated with alkylating agents and those treated with high-dose radiation have an increased risk. The potential risk for developing a secondary malignancy does not contraindicate the use of cancer treatment.

## IMMUNOTHERAPY AND TARGETED THERAPY

**Immunotherapy** uses the immune system, the body's main defense against infection and disease, to fight cancer. Some types of immunotherapy are called *biologic therapy*. Immunotherapy can (1) boost or manipulate the immune system and create an environment that is not conducive for cancer cells to grow or (2) attack cancer cells directly. Various types of immunotherapy include cytokines, vaccines, and monoclonal antibodies (Table 15-13). Monoclonal antibodies (drugs ending in -mab) are the most successful immunotherapy. Antibodies are proteins produced by the immune system that bind to a target antigen on the cell surface. Because each antibody is specific to an antigen, that mechanism is used to develop specific drugs to treat cancer. Many of the monoclonal antibodies are targeted therapies.

**Targeted therapy** interferes with cancer growth by targeting specific cell receptors and pathways that are important in tumor growth.[26,27] Targeted therapies work at sites that are on the cell surface, at the intracellular level, or in the extracellular domain (Fig. 15-16 and Table 15-13). Targeted therapies are more selective for specific molecular targets than chemotherapy drugs. Thus they act on specific targets that are associated with cancer. In comparison, chemotherapy acts on all rapidly dividing normal and cancer cells. A major advantage of targeted therapy (compared with chemotherapy) is that it does less damage to normal cells.

As more oncogene targets are identified, additional agents are being developed that target specific oncogenes. Targeted therapies provide for use of personalized therapy based on the biology of an individual's tumor. Examples of some targeted therapies are discussed in the next few paragraphs.

A major class of targeted therapy is tyrosine kinase inhibitors (Table 15-13). Tyrosine kinases are enzymes responsible for the activation of many proteins by signal transduction cascades. EGFR is a transmembrane molecule that works through activation of intracellular tyrosine kinase (TK). Overexpression of EGFR is associated with unregulated cell growth and a poor prognosis. Drugs that inhibit EGFR suppress cell proliferation and promote *apoptosis* (programmed cell death).

EGFRs belong to the same receptor family as human epidermal growth factor receptor-2 (HER-2), the target for trastuzumab (Herceptin), which is a drug primarily used to treat breast cancer. HER-2 is overexpressed in certain cancers (especially breast cancers) and is associated with more aggressive disease and decreased survival. Trastuzumab is a monoclonal antibody (MoAb) that binds to HER-2 and is given IV to inhibit the growth of breast cancer cells that overexpress the HER-2 protein. Lapatinib (Tykerb) is an oral agent used for breast cancer that overexpresses HER-2.

Chronic myeloid leukemia (CML) cells make an abnormal active enzyme called BCR-ABL tyrosine kinase. Drugs (e.g., imatinib [Gleevec]) that inhibit this enzyme suppress proliferation of CML cells and promote apoptosis.

*Angiogenesis inhibitors* work by preventing the mechanisms and pathways necessary for vascularization of tumors. Bevacizumab (Avastin), a recombinant human MoAb, binds with vascular endothelial growth factor (VEGF), a compound that stimulates blood vessel growth. When bevacizumab binds with VEGF, it prevents VEGF from binding with its receptors on vascular endothelial cells and promoting new vessel formation. As a result, further tumor growth is inhibited.

*Proteasomes* are intracellular multienzyme complexes that degrade proteins. In cancer cells, proteasome inhibitors (e.g., bortezomib [Velcade]) promote accumulation of proteins that leads to cell death.

Cancer cells can become resistant to targeted therapies. This can occur because the (1) target changes through mutation and the therapy no longer interacts with it and (2) tumor finds a new growth pathway and no longer depends on the target. Because of the possibility of resistance, targeted therapies work best in combination or in combination with a chemotherapy drug.

### Side Effects of Immunotherapy and Targeted Therapy

The administration of one type of immunotherapy usually induces the endogenous release of other agents. The release and action of these agents result in systemic immune and inflammatory responses. The toxicities and side effects of these agents are related to dose and schedule.

Common side effects include constitutional flu-like symptoms, including headache, fever, chills, myalgias, fatigue, malaise, weakness, photosensitivity, anorexia, and nausea. With interferon therapy, these flu-like symptoms almost invariably appear, but their severity generally decreases over time. Acetaminophen administered every 4 hours, as prescribed, often reduces the severity of the flu-like syndrome. The patient is commonly premedicated with acetaminophen in an attempt to prevent or decrease the intensity of these symptoms. In addition, large amounts of fluids help decrease the symptoms.

Tachycardia and orthostatic hypotension are also commonly reported. IL-2 and MoAbs can cause *capillary leak syndrome,* which can result in pulmonary edema. Other toxic and side effects may involve the CNS, renal and hepatic systems, and cardiovascular system. These effects are found particularly with interferons and IL-2.

A wide range of neurologic deficits has been observed with interferon and IL-2 therapy. The nature and extent of these problems are not yet completely understood. However, these problems are understandably frightening to the patient and family, who must be taught to observe for neurologic problems (e.g., confusion, memory loss, difficulty making decisions, insomnia), report their occurrence, and institute appropriate safety and support measures.

MoAbs are administered by infusion. Patients may experience infusion-related symptoms, which can include fever, chills, urticaria, mucosal congestion, nausea, diarrhea, and myalgias.

Skin rashes are common in patients receiving EGFR inhibitors and manifest generally as erythema and acneiform-like

**TABLE 15-13 Drug Therapy**

***Immunotherapy and Targeted Therapy****

| Mechanism of Action | Examples |
|---|---|
| **Cytokines** (see Table 13-4) | |
| Inhibits DNA and protein synthesis. Suppresses cell proliferation. Increases cytotoxic effects of natural killer (NK) cells | α-interferon (Intron A) |
| Stimulates proliferation of T and B cells<br>Activates NK cells | interleukin-2 (aldesleukin [Proleukin]) |
| **Vaccines** | |
| Live attenuated strain of *Mycobacterium bovis* induces immune response. Used intravesically to treat bladder cancer (see Chapter 45) | BCG vaccine |
| Vaccine against prostate cancer that stimulates the immune system against the cancer (see Chapter 54) | sipuleucel-T (Provenge) |
| **Kinase Inhibitors** | |
| ***EGFR Tyrosine Kinase (TK) Inhibitors*** | |
| Inhibit epidermal growth factor receptor (EGFR) TK | cetuximab (Erbitux)<br>erlotinib (Tarceva)<br>gefitinib (Iressa)<br>panitumumab (Vectibix) |
| Inhibit EGFR-TK and binds HER-2 | lapatinib (Tykerb) |
| ***BCR-ABL Tyrosine Kinase Inhibitors*** | |
| Inhibit BCR-ABL TK. Primarily used in chronic myeloid leukemia | bosutinib (Bosulif)<br>dasatinib (Sprycel)<br>imatinib (Gleevec)<br>nilotinib (Tasigna) |
| ***Multi-Tyrosine Kinase Inhibitors*** | |
| Inhibit multiple TKs | axitinib (Inlyta)<br>cabozantinib (Cometriq)<br>pazopanib (Votrient)<br>regorafenib (Stivarga)<br>sorafenib (Nexavar)<br>sunitinib (Sutent)<br>vandetanib (Caprelsa) |
| ***Anaplastic Lymphoma Kinase (ALK) Inhibitors*** | |
| Inhibit anaplastic lymphoma kinase (ALK) | ceritinib (Zykadia)<br>crizotinib (Xalkori) |
| ***BRAF and MEK Kinase Inhibitors*** | |
| Inhibit BRAF and MEK enzymes | dabrafenib (Tafinlar)<br>trametinib (Mekinist)<br>vemurafenib (Zelboraf)<br>cobimetinib (Cotellic) |
| ***mTOR Kinase Inhibitors*** | |
| Inhibits a specific protein known as the mechanistic target of rapamycin (mTOR) | everolimus (Afinitor)<br>temsirolimus (Torisel) |
| **Human Epidermal Growth Factor Receptor-2 (HER-2)** | |
| Monoclonal antibody to HER-2 that attaches to the antigen. It is taken into the cells and eventually kills them | pertuzumab (Perjeta)<br>trastuzumab (Herceptin) |
| Trastuzumab connected to a chemotherapy drug called DM1 | ado-trastuzumab emtansine (Kadcyla) |
| **CD20 Monoclonal Antibodies** | |
| Binds CD20 antigen, causing cytotoxicity and radiation injury | ibritumomab tiuxetan/yttrium-90 (Zevalin) |
| Binds CD20 antigen, causing cytotoxicity | ofatumumab (Arzerra)<br>rituximab (Rituxan) |
| **CD52 Monoclonal Antibody** | |
| Binds CD52 antigen (found on T and B cells, monocytes, NK cells, neutrophils) | alemtuzumab (Campath) |
| **Angiogenesis Inhibitors** | |
| Binds vascular endothelial growth factor (VEGF), thereby inhibiting angiogenesis | bevacizumab (Avastin)<br>pazopanib (Votrient)<br>ramucirumab (Cyramza) |
| **Proteasome Inhibitors** | |
| Inhibits proteasome activity, which functions to regulate cell growth | bortezomib (Velcade)<br>carfilzomib (Kyprolis) |
| **Immunomodulatory Drugs (IMiDs)** | |
| Inhibit production of TNF, IL-6, and VEGF (which leads to its antiangiogenic effects). Stimulates T and NK cells and increases γ-interferon and IL-2 production | apremilast (Otezla)<br>lenalidomide (Revlimid)<br>pomalidomide (Pomalyst)<br>thalidomide (Thalomid) |
| **Programmed Death Receptor (PD)-1 Blockers** | |
| Blocks PD-1, a protein on T cells that normally helps keep these cells from attacking other cells. Thus boosts immune response against cancer cells | nivolumab (Opdivo)<br>pembrolizumab (Keytruda) |

*BRAF*, B-Raf; *HER-2*, human epidermal growth factor receptor 2; *IL*, interleukin; *TNF*, tumor necrosis factor.
*This list is not all inclusive.

rash that can cover a large part of the upper body. Angiogenesis inhibitors can cause problems of arterial thrombi, hemorrhage, hypertension, impaired wound healing, and proteinuria. Other toxicities of MoAbs include hepatotoxicity, bone marrow depression, and CNS effects.

## ❖ NURSING MANAGEMENT: IMMUNOTHERAPY AND TARGETED THERAPY

Some problems experienced by the patient receiving immunotherapy and targeted therapy are different from those observed with more traditional forms of cancer therapy. These effects occur more acutely and are dose limited (i.e., effects resolve when the agent is discontinued). Patients may be hesitant to inform the HCP of intolerable side effects. Some patients may be afraid to discuss side effects because they may think that the drug will be stopped. Or they decide to discontinue the drug because of side effects. Assess and evaluate the patient's side effects and tolerance. Appropriate proactive nursing care can prevent these problems because you are in a position to intervene.

Capillary leak syndrome and pulmonary edema are problems that require critical care nursing. Bone marrow depression is generally more transient and less severe than that observed with chemotherapy. Fatigue associated with immunotherapy and targeted therapy can be so severe that it constitutes a dose-limiting toxicity. As these agents are increasingly combined with chemotherapy, the spectrum of therapy-related effects expands.

Nursing interventions for flu-like syndrome include the administration of acetaminophen before treatment and every 4

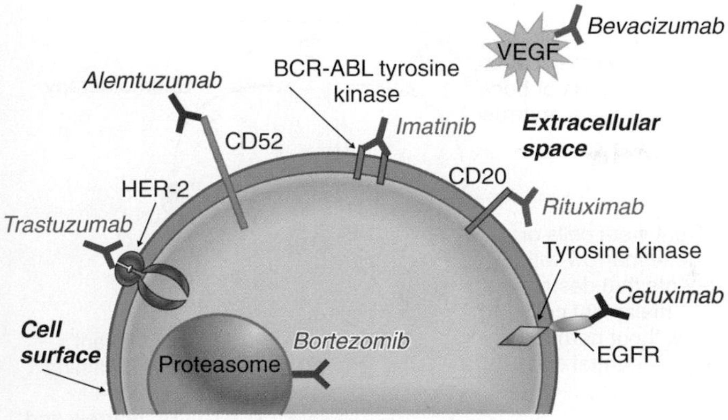


FIG. 15-16 Sites of action of targeted therapy. Examples of targeted therapy drugs that work at the specific site of action are indicated in colored, italicized font. *EGFR,* Epidermal growth factor receptor; *HER-2,* human epidermal growth factor receptor-2; *VEGF,* vascular endothelial growth factor.

hours after treatment. IV meperidine (Demerol) has been used to control the severe chills or rigors associated with some agents. Other nursing measures include monitoring vital signs and temperature, planning for periods of rest for the patient, assisting with activities of daily living (ADLs), and monitoring for adequate oral intake.

## HORMONE THERAPY

Hormones are substances that are produced in endocrine glands and function as chemical messengers in the body. The hormones estrogen and progesterone can enhance the growth of some breast cancers, and androgen (testosterone) can enhance the growth of some prostrate cancers. When given as a cancer treatment, drugs (hormone therapy) can block the effects of the hormone and stop the growth of cancer cells (Table 15-14).

Corticosteroids are used in combination with many drug regimens for cancer. They are antiinflammatory agents that reduce swelling and inflammation, which may be contributing to cancer pain. They are used with other drugs, such as ondansetron and aprepitant, to control and prevent nausea and vomiting caused by chemotherapy.

In addition to drug manipulation of hormones, surgical interventions (oophorectomy, castration) can be used to remove the effects of the hormone on cancer growth.

## HEMATOPOIETIC GROWTH FACTORS

Hematopoietic growth factors are used to support cancer patients through the treatment of the disease (Table 15-15). Colony-stimulating factors (CSFs) are a family of glycoproteins produced by various cells. CSFs stimulate production, maturation, regulation, and activation of cells of the hematologic system. The name of the CSF is based on the specific cell line it affects (Table 15-15).

Erythropoiesis-stimulating agents (ESAs) should be used only when treating anemia specifically caused by chemotherapy. ESA use is avoided in patients receiving chemotherapy with the intent to cure the disease. Use of these agents has raised safety concerns because they can cause potential harms (thromboembolic events, shorter survival) and increase the risk for death and for serious cardiovascular events when administered to achieve a target hemoglobin of greater than 12 g/dL. Therefore

### TABLE 15-14 Drug Therapy

***Hormone Therapy***

| | |
|---|---|
| **Corticosteroids** | |
| Disrupt the cell membrane and inhibit synthesis of protein. Decrease circulating lymphocytes, inhibit mitosis, depress immune system, increase sense of well-being. | cortisone, dexamethasone, hydrocortisone (Cortef), methylprednisolone (Medrol), prednisone |
| **Estrogen Receptor Blockers** | |
| Selectively attach to estrogen receptors, blocking estrogen from binding. Inhibits tumor growth. | fulvestrant (Faslodex), tamoxifen, toremifene (Fareston) |
| **Estrogen Receptor Modulator** | |
| Produces both estrogen-agonistic effects on bone and estrogen-antagonistic effects on breast tissue. | raloxifene (Evista) |
| **Aromatase Inhibitors** | |
| Inhibit aromatase, thus preventing the production of estrogen. | anastrozole (Arimidex), exemestane (Aromasin), letrozole (Femara) |
| **Estrogens** | |
| Interfere with effect of testosterone. | estradiol, estramustine (Emcyt), estrogen (Menest) |
| **Androgen Receptor Blockers** | |
| Selectively attach to androgen receptors, blocking androgen from binding, Inhibits tumor growth. | flutamide, bicalutamide (Casodex), enzalutamide (Xtandi) |

the lowest dose should be used that will gradually increase hemoglobin to the lowest level sufficient to avoid the need for blood transfusion. Monitor the hemoglobin level regularly.

## HEMATOPOIETIC STEM CELL TRANSPLANTATION

**Bone marrow transplantation** (BMT) and **peripheral stem cell transplantation** (PSCT) are effective, lifesaving procedures for the treatment of a number of malignant and nonmalignant diseases (Table 15-16). BMT and PSCT allow for the safe use of very high doses of chemotherapy agents and/or radiation therapy in patients whose tumors have developed resistance (refractory) or failed to respond to standard doses of chemotherapy and radiation. Although these procedures are lifesaving, patients may have long-term or delayed complications that can affect their quality of life.

This therapeutic approach was typically referred to as BMT because the bone marrow was the original source of stem cells when the procedure was first developed. However, advances in harvesting and cryopreservation technologies have opened new pathways to the collection of stem cells from the peripheral blood.[28] Consequently, the terminology has changed, and the procedure is now referred to as **hematopoietic stem cell transplantation** (HSCT). Overall cure rates are steadily increasing. Even when cure is not achieved, transplantation can result in a period of remission.

The approach in HSCT is to eradicate diseased tumor cells and/or clear the bone marrow of its components to make way for engraftment of the transplanted, healthy stem cells. This is accomplished by administering higher than usual dosages of chemotherapy with or without radiation therapy. Life-threatening consequences associated with pancytopenia and

**TABLE 15-15 Drug Therapy**

***Hematopoietic Growth Factors Used in Cancer Treatment***

| Growth Factor | Drug Name | Indications | Side Effects |
|---|---|---|---|
| **Granulocyte-macrophage colony-stimulating factor (GM-CSF)** | sargramostim (Leukine) | Myeloid cell recovery after bone marrow transplantation | Nausea, vomiting, diarrhea, fever, chills, myalgia, headache, fatigue |
| **Granulocyte colony-stimulating factor (G-CSF)** | filgrastim (Neupogen)<br>pegfilgrastim (Neulasta)<br>tbo-filgrastim (Granix)<br>filgrastim-sndz (Zarxio) | Chemotherapy-induced neutropenia | Bone pain, nausea, vomiting |
| **Erythropoietin** | epoetin α (Epogen, Procrit) | Anemia of chronic cancer | Hypertension, thrombosis, headache |
| | darbepoetin α (Aranesp) | Anemia related to chemotherapy | Hypertension, thrombosis, headache |
| **Interleukin-11 (platelet growth factor)** | oprelvekin (Neumega) | Thrombocytopenia related to chemotherapy | Fluid retention, peripheral edema, dyspnea, tachycardia, nausea, mouth sores |

**TABLE 15-16 Indications for Hematopoietic Stem Cell Transplantation**

| Malignant Diseases | Nonmalignant Diseases |
|---|---|
| • Acute and chronic myelogenous leukemia | • Aplastic anemia |
| • Acute and chronic lymphocytic leukemia | • Chronic granulomatous disease |
| • Hodgkin's lymphoma | • Fanconi's anemia |
| • Multiple myeloma | • Hematologic diseases |
| • Myelodysplastic syndrome | • Immunodeficiency diseases |
| • Non-Hodgkin's lymphoma | • Severe combined immunodeficiency disease (SCID) |
| | • Sickle cell disease (severe) |
| | • Thalassemia |
| | • Wiskott-Aldrich syndrome |

other adverse effects can result from this procedure. After chemotherapy and radiation therapy are completed, healthy stem cells are infused. These healthy stem cells "rescue" the damaged bone marrow through subsequent proliferation and differentiation of the donated stem cells in the recipient.

HSCT is an intensive procedure with many risks. Some patients die from treatment-related complications or from recurrence of the original disease. Because it is a highly toxic therapy, the patient must weigh the significant risks of treatment-related death or treatment failure (relapse) against the hope of cure.

## Types of Hematopoietic Stem Cell Transplants

HSCTs are categorized as allogeneic, syngeneic, or autologous. The sources of stem cells include the bone marrow, peripheral circulating blood, and umbilical cord blood. In *allogeneic transplantation,* stem cells are acquired from a donor (graft) who, through human leukocyte antigen (HLA) tissue typing, has been determined to be HLA matched to the recipient (host). HLA typing involves testing WBCs to identify genetically inherited antigens common to both donor and recipient that are important in compatibility of transplanted tissue. (HLA tissue typing is discussed in Chapter 13.) The donor is often a family member but may be an unrelated donor found through a national or international bone marrow registry (e.g., National Marrow Donor Program). These are known as MUD (matched unrelated donor) transplants. Increased risks and toxicities may be associated with an unrelated allogeneic transplant. Common indications for allogeneic transplant are certain leukemias, multiple myeloma, and lymphoma.

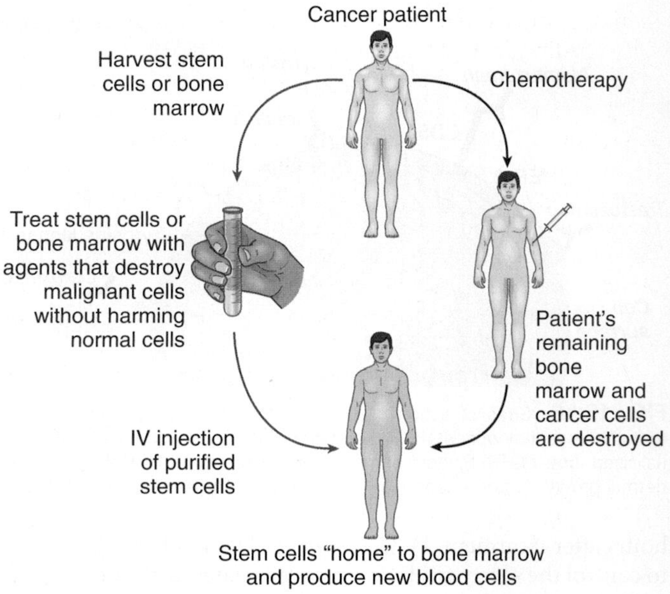


**FIG. 15-17** Autologous stem cell transplant.

*Syngeneic transplantation* is a type of allogeneic transplant that involves obtaining stem cells from one identical twin and infusing them into the other. Identical twins have identical HLA types and are a perfect match

In *autologous transplantation,* patients receive their own stem cells back after *myeloablative* (destroying bone marrow) chemotherapy (Fig. 15-17). The aim of this approach is purely "rescue." It enables patients to receive intensive chemotherapy and/or radiation by supporting them with their previously harvested stem cells until their marrow generates blood cells again on its own. Restoration usually takes about 4 to 6 weeks. Autologous transplants are typically used to treat hematologic malignancies if there is no suitable donor or the patient cannot undergo allogeneic transplantation.

The newer, nonmyeloablative or reduced intensity transplant uses lower doses of radiation or chemotherapy that result in less toxicity and myelosuppression. HSCT continues to be investigated in the management of some solid tumors refractory to treatment.

## Procedures

**Harvest Procedures.** Hematopoietic stem cells are *harvested* from a donor (for allogeneic transplantation) or from the recipient (for autologous transplantation) via two different methods. In one type of procedure, used for harvesting stem cells residing in bone marrow (as the process was originally developed), the procedure is performed in the operating room using general or spinal anesthesia. Multiple bone marrow aspirations (usually from the iliac crest, but sometimes from the sternum) are carried out to obtain stem cells. The entire bone marrow harvest procedure takes about 1 to 2 hours, and the patient can be discharged after recovery. Postharvest, the donor may experience pain at the collection site that lasts up to 7 days and can be treated with mild analgesics. The donor's body will replenish the removed bone marrow in a few weeks.

In the other type of procedure, peripheral stem cell transplants are obtained from the peripheral blood in an outpatient procedure. It is done using cell separator equipment that automatically separates the stem cells from the blood circulating through the machine and returns the remaining blood components to the donor. The process averages about 2 to 4 hours but can sometimes take longer depending on donor factors and the quality of the venous access. Often it takes more than one procedure to obtain enough stem cells. Because the blood has fewer stem cells than the bone marrow, "mobilization" of stem cells from the bone marrow into the peripheral blood can be accomplished using chemotherapy and/or hematopoietic growth factors.

To increase stem cell production for collection, common growth factors that are used are granulocyte-macrophage colony-stimulating factor (GM-CSF) and granulocyte colony-stimulating factor (G-CSF) (Table 15-15). When patients are given growth factors for mobilization, stem cells are harvested after 4 or 5 days of growth factor injections.

Harvested marrow is processed to strain out bone fragments (this is not necessary with peripheral collections). The marrow or peripherally collected stem cells are then bagged with preservative for cryopreservation and storage until they are needed, or they are used immediately. Since it is coming from the patient, autologous stem cells are sometimes treated (purged) to remove undetected cancer cells. Many different pharmacologic, immunologic, physical, and chemical agents have been used for this purpose.

Umbilical cord blood is also rich in hematopoietic stem cells, and successful allogeneic transplants have been performed using this source. Cord blood can be HLA-typed and cryopreserved. A disadvantage of cord blood is the possibility of insufficient numbers of stem cells to permit transplant to adults. Considerable research is currently ongoing to define the optimal application of this technology.

**Preparative Regimens and Stem Cell Infusions.** Patients receive myeloablative dosages of chemotherapy with or without adjunctive radiation to treat the underlying disease. Total-body irradiation (TBI) can be used for immunosuppression or to treat the disease. These preparative therapies are known as the *conditioning regimen.*

Stem cell infusions are administered IV, and can be injected via the slow bolus method or infused much like a blood transfusion (using tubing without a filter). The infused stem cells reconstitute the bone marrow elements, "rescuing" the recipient's hematopoietic system. Usually 2 to 4 weeks are required for the transplanted marrow to start producing hematopoietic blood cells. During this period, when the patient has pancytopenia, the patient must be protected from exposure to infectious agents and supported with electrolyte supplements, nutrition, and blood component transfusions (as needed) to maintain adequate levels of circulating RBCs and platelets.

**Complications.** Bacterial, viral, and fungal infections are common after HSCT, so prophylactic therapies are used to reduce their incidence. A potentially serious complication of allogeneic transplant is graft-versus-host disease. This occurs when the T cells from the donated marrow (graft) recognize the recipient (host) as foreign and begin to attack certain organs such as the skin, liver, and GI tract. (Graft-versus-host disease is discussed in Chapter 13.)

The occurrence and severity of posttransplant complications also depend on the drugs used (some are more toxic than others) and the stem cell source. Because stem cells in the peripheral blood are more mature than those harvested from the marrow, the hematologic recovery period in PSCT is shorter, and fewer, less severe complications are seen.

### GENE THERAPY

*Gene therapy* is an experimental therapy that involves introducing genetic material into a person's cells to fight disease. At this time, the use of gene therapy is investigational. (Gene therapy is discussed in Chapter 12.)

## COMPLICATIONS OF CANCER

The patient may develop complications related to the continual growth of the cancer into normal tissue or to the side effects of treatment.

### NUTRITIONAL PROBLEMS

#### Malnutrition

The patient with cancer may experience protein and calorie malnutrition characterized by fat and muscle depletion. (Assessment of malnutrition is discussed in Chapter 39.)

Soft, nonirritating high-protein and high-calorie foods should be eaten throughout the day. Foods suggested for increasing the protein intake are presented in Table 15-17. High-calorie foods that provide energy and minimize weight loss are presented in Table 15-18. (A sample high-calorie, high-protein diet is presented in Table 39-10.)

Teach the patient to avoid extremes of temperature, tobacco, alcohol, spicy or rough foods, and other irritants. Encourage nutritional supplements (e.g., Ensure) as an adjunct to meals and fluid intake. Weigh the patient at least twice each week to monitor for weight loss.

Suggest a referral for individualized nutritional counseling to the patient or HCP as soon as a 5% weight loss is noted or if the patient has the potential for protein and calorie malnutrition. Monitor albumin and prealbumin levels. Once a 10-lb (4.5-kg) weight loss occurs, it may be difficult to maintain the patient's nutritional status.

Teach the patient to use nutritional supplements in place of milk when cooking or baking. Foods to which nutritional supplements can be easily added include scrambled eggs, pudding, custard, mashed potatoes, cereal, and cream sauces. Packages of instant breakfast can be used as indicated or sprinkled on cereals, desserts, and casseroles.

Families are an integral part of the health care team. As symptom severity increases, the family's role in helping the patient eat becomes increasingly critical.

**TABLE 15-17 Nutritional Therapy**

***Protein Foods With High Biologic Value***

**Milk**

- Whole milk: 1 cup = 9 g protein.
- Double-strength milk (1 quart of whole milk plus 1 cup of dried skim milk blended and chilled): 1 cup = 14 g protein.
- Milk shake (1 cup of ice cream plus 1 cup of milk): 15 g protein, 415 cal.
- Use evaporated milk, double-strength milk, or half-and-half to make casseroles, hot cereals, sauces, gravies, puddings, milk shakes, and soups.
- Yogurt (regular and frozen): check labels and purchase brand with highest protein content: 1 cup = 10 g protein

**Eggs**

- Egg: 6 g protein.
- Eggnog: 1 cup = 15.5 g protein.
- Add eggs to salads, casseroles, and sauces. Deviled eggs are especially well tolerated.
- Desserts that contain eggs include angel food cake, sponge cake, custard, and cheesecake.

**Cheese**

- Cottage: ½ cup = 15 g protein.
- American: 1 slice = 3 g protein.
- Cheddar: 1 slice = 6 g protein.
- Cream: 1 Tbsp = 1 g protein.
- Use cheese in a sandwich or as a snack.
- Add cheese to salads, casseroles, sauces, and baked potatoes.
- Cheese spread with crackers is a wholesome snack that can be made and stored in the refrigerator for easy accessibility.
- Advise patient that cheese can be constipating.

**Meat, Poultry, Fish**

- Pork: 3 oz = approx. 19 g protein.
- Chicken: ½ breast = approx. 26 g protein.
- Fish: 3 oz = approx. 30 g protein.
- Tuna fish: 6½ oz = approx. 44.5 g protein.
- Add meat, poultry, and fish to salads, casseroles, and sandwiches.
- Add strained and junior baby meats to soups and casseroles.
- Cocktail wieners and deviled ham on crackers are wholesome snacks. These snacks can be made and stored in the refrigerator for easy accessibility.

If the malnutrition cannot be treated with dietary intake, it may be necessary to use enteral or parenteral nutrition. (Enteral and parenteral nutrition are discussed in Chapter 39.)

### Altered Taste Sensation (Dysgeusia)

Cancer cells may release substances that stimulate the bitter taste buds. The patient may also experience an alteration in the sweet, sour, and salty taste sensations. Meat may taste bitter or bland. The physiologic basis of these varied taste alterations is unknown.

Teach patients with altered taste problems to avoid foods that they dislike. Frequently the patient may feel compelled to eat certain foods that are believed to be beneficial. Tell the patient to experiment with spices and other seasoning agents in an attempt to mask the taste alterations. Lemon juice, onion, mint, basil, and fruit juice marinades may improve the taste of certain meats and fish. Ham may enhance the taste of vegetables. Increasing the amount of spice or seasoning agent is usually not an effective way to enhance the taste.

**TABLE 15-18 Nutritional Therapy**

***High-Calorie Foods***

| | | | |
|---|---|---|---|
| Mayonnaise | 1 Tbsp | = | 101 cal |
| Butter or margarine | 1 tsp | = | 35 cal |
| Sour cream | 1 Tbsp | = | 72 cal |
| Peanut butter | 1 Tbsp | = | 94 cal |
| Whipped cream | 1 Tbsp | = | 53 cal |
| Corn oil | 1 Tbsp | = | 119 cal |
| Jelly | 1 Tbsp | = | 49 cal |
| Ice cream | 1 cup | = | 256 cal |
| Honey | 1 Tbsp | = | 64 cal |

### Cancer Cachexia

*Cancer cachexia* (wasting syndrome) is a complex, multifactorial syndrome characterized by anorexia and/or unintended loss of weight and appetite. It is accompanied by generalized tissue wasting, skeletal muscle atrophy, immune dysfunction, and metabolic abnormalities. The weight loss cannot be reversed nutritionally.

Cancer patients can suffer from cachexia, especially those with upper gastrointestinal and pancreatic cancers. As cancer progresses, cachexia can affect many cancer patients, and is associated with increased morbidity.[29]

The best management of cancer cachexia is to effectively treat the cancer. Unfortunately, this is not a realistic goal for patients with advanced cancer. A second option is to increase nutritional intake, but this does not completely reverse the wasting associated with cachexia. A third option is to use megestrol acetate (Megace), a synthetic form of the hormone progesterone, which stimulates appetite in patients with cachexia.

## INFECTION

Infection is a primary cause of death in the patient with cancer. The usual sites of infection include the lungs, GU system, mouth, rectum, peritoneal cavity, and blood (septicemia). Infection occurs as a result of the ulceration and necrosis caused by the tumor, compression of vital organs by the tumor, and neutropenia caused by the disease process or the cancer treatment.

Instruct patients at risk for neutropenia to call their HCP if they have a temperature of 100.4° F (38° C) or greater. Assessment most often includes signs and symptoms of fever, determination of possible etiology (e.g., sinuses, mucous membranes, respiratory, GI, urinary, sites of any tubes or lines), and complete blood count.

Many patients are neutropenic when an infection develops. In these individuals, infection may cause significant morbidity and may be rapidly fatal if not treated promptly. The classic manifestations of infection are often subtle or absent in a patient with neutropenia and a depressed immune system. (Neutropenia was discussed earlier in this chapter on p. 253 and is also discussed in Chapter 30.)

## ONCOLOGIC EMERGENCIES

*Oncologic emergencies* are life-threatening emergencies that can occur as a result of cancer or cancer treatment. These emergencies can be obstructive, metabolic, or infiltrative (Table 15-19).

TABLE 15-19 **Oncologic Emergencies**

| Description | Manifestations | Management |
|---|---|---|
| **Obstructive Emergencies** | | |
| ***Superior Vena Cava Syndrome (SVCS)*** | | |
| • Results from obstruction of superior vena cava by tumor or thrombosis.<br>• Common causes are lung cancer, non-Hodgkin's lymphoma, and metastatic breast cancer.<br>• Presence of central venous catheter and previous mediastinal radiation increase risk of development. | • Facial edema, periorbital edema.<br>• Distention of veins of head, neck, and chest (Fig. 15-18).<br>• Headache, seizures.<br>• Mediastinal mass on chest x-ray. | • Considered a serious medical problem.<br>• Radiation therapy to site of obstruction.<br>• Chemotherapy for tumors more sensitive to this therapy. |
| ***Spinal Cord Compression*** | | |
| • Neurologic emergency caused by cancer in epidural space of spinal cord.<br>• Common causes are breast, lung, prostate, GI, and renal cancers and melanomas.<br>• Lymphomas can also invade epidural space. | • Intense, localized, and persistent back pain accompanied by vertebral tenderness.<br>• Motor weakness, sensory paresthesia and loss.<br>• Autonomic dysfunction (e.g., change in bowel or bladder function). | • Radiation therapy and corticosteroids.<br>• Surgical decompressive laminectomy.<br>• Activity limitations and pain management. |
| ***Third Space Syndrome*** | | |
| • Shifting of fluid from vascular space to interstitial space.<br>• Occurs secondary to extensive surgical procedures, immunotherapy, or septic shock. | • Signs of hypovolemia: hypotension, tachycardia, low central venous pressure, decreased urine output. | • Fluid, electrolyte, and plasma protein replacement.<br>• During recovery hypervolemia can occur, resulting in hypertension, elevated central venous pressure, weight gain, and shortness of breath. |
| **Metabolic Emergencies** | | |
| ***Syndrome of Inappropriate Antidiuretic Hormone (SIADH)*** | | |
| • Tumor cells can produce abnormal or sustained production of antidiuretic hormone (ADH).<br>• Many chemotherapy agents may also contribute to ectopic ADH production or potentiate ADH effects. | • Water retention and hyponatremia (hypotonic hyponatremia) (see Chapter 49).<br>• Weight gain without edema, weakness, anorexia, nausea, vomiting, personality changes, seizures, oliguria, decrease in reflexes, and coma. | • Treat underlying malignancy.<br>• Take measures to correct sodium-water imbalance, including fluid restriction, oral salt tablets or isotonic (0.9%) saline administration, and IV 3% sodium chloride solution (severe cases).<br>• Furosemide (Lasix) used in initial phases.<br>• Monitor sodium level because correcting SIADH rapidly may result in seizures or death. |
| ***Hypercalcemia*** | | |
| • Occurs in metastatic disease of bone or multiple myeloma, or when a parathyroid hormone–like substance is secreted by cancer cells.<br>• Immobility and dehydration can contribute to or exacerbate hypercalcemia. | • Serum calcium in excess of 12 mg/dL (3 mmol/L) often produces symptoms.<br>• Apathy, depression, fatigue, muscle weakness, ECG changes, polyuria and nocturia, anorexia, nausea, and vomiting.<br>• High calcium elevations can be life threatening.<br>• Chronic hypercalcemia can result in nephrocalcinosis and irreversible renal failure. | • Treat primary disease.<br>• Hydration (3 L/day) and bisphosphonate therapy.<br>• Diuretics (particularly loop diuretics) used to prevent heart failure or edema.<br>• Infusion of bisphosphonate zoledronate (Zometa) or pamidronate (Aredia). |
| ***Tumor Lysis Syndrome (TLS)*** | | |
| • Metabolic complication characterized by rapid release of intracellular components in response to chemotherapy and radiation therapy (less commonly).<br>• Massive cell destruction releases intracellular components (potassium, phosphate, DNA, RNA) that are metabolized to uric acid by liver. | • *Hallmark signs*: hyperuricemia, hyperphosphatemia, hyperkalemia, hypocalcemia.<br>• Weakness, muscle cramps, diarrhea, nausea, and vomiting.<br>• Occurs within first 24 to 48 hr after initiation of chemotherapy.<br>• May persist for about 5 to 7 days.<br>• Metabolic abnormalities and concentrated uric acid (which crystallizes in distal tubules of kidneys) can lead to acute kidney injury. | • Identify patients at risk.<br>• Increase urine production using hydration therapy.<br>• Decrease uric acid concentrations using allopurinol.<br>• Use IV sodium bicarbonate to counter effects of acidic properties that are released. |
| **Infiltrative Emergencies** | | |
| ***Cardiac Tamponade*** | | |
| • Fluid accumulation in pericardium.<br>• Caused by constriction of pericardium by tumor or pericarditis secondary to radiation therapy to the chest. | • Heavy feeling over chest, shortness of breath, tachycardia, cough, dysphagia, hiccups, hoarseness.<br>• Nausea, vomiting, excessive perspiration.<br>• Decreased level of consciousness, distant or muted heart sounds.<br>• Extreme anxiety. | • Decrease fluid around heart using (1) surgery to create a pericardial window or an (2) indwelling pericardial catheter.<br>• Administer $O_2$ therapy, IV hydration, and vasopressor therapy. |
| ***Carotid Artery Rupture*** | | |
| • Invasion of arterial wall by tumor or erosion following surgery or radiation therapy.<br>• Occurs most frequently in patients with head and neck cancer. | • Bleeding: ranges from minor oozing to spurting of blood in the case of a "blowout" of artery. | • Administer IV fluids and blood products.<br>• Surgery: ligation of carotid artery above and below rupture site and reduction of local tumor. |

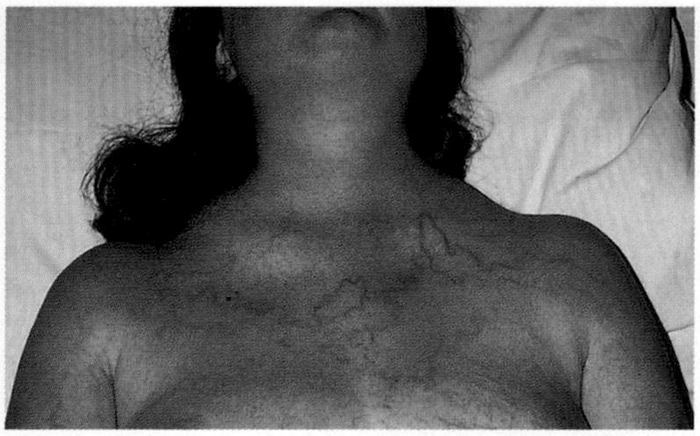

**FIG. 15-18** Superior vena caval obstruction in bronchial carcinoma. Note the swelling of the face and neck and the development of collateral circulation in the veins. (From Forbes CD, Jackson WF: *Colour atlas and text of clinical medicine,* ed 3, London, 2003, Mosby.)

### Obstructive Emergencies

*Obstructive emergencies* are primarily caused by tumor obstruction of an organ or blood vessel. Obstructive emergencies include superior vena cava syndrome (Fig. 15-18), spinal cord compression syndrome, third space syndrome, and intestinal obstruction.

### Metabolic Emergencies

*Metabolic emergencies* are caused by the production of ectopic hormones directly from the tumor or are secondary to metabolic alterations caused by the tumor or by cancer treatment. Ectopic hormones arise from tissues that do not normally produce these hormones. Cancer cells return to a more embryonic form, thus allowing the cells' stored potential to become evident.

Metabolic emergencies include syndrome of inappropriate antidiuretic hormone secretion, hypercalcemia, tumor lysis syndrome, septic shock (discussed in Chapter 66), and disseminated intravascular coagulation (discussed in Chapter 30).

### Infiltrative Emergencies

*Infiltrative emergencies* occur when malignant tumors infiltrate major organs or secondary to cancer therapy. The most common infiltrative emergencies are cardiac tamponade and carotid artery rupture.

## CANCER PAIN

Moderate to severe pain occurs in approximately 50% of patients who are receiving active treatment for their cancer and in 80% to 90% of patients with advanced cancer.[30] What is concerning is that these statistics have not changed in the past 30 years. Undertreatment of cancer pain is common and causes needless suffering, decreases quality of life, and increases the burden on family caregivers.

### Pain Assessment

Inadequate pain assessment is the single greatest barrier to effective pain management. Data such as vital signs and patient behaviors are not reliable indicators of pain, especially longstanding, chronic pain. It is important to distinguish between persistent and episodic, positional, or breakthrough pain. Therefore it is essential that a comprehensive pain assessment include a detailed history to elicit the following characteristics of pain: quality, location, intensity, duration, and precipitating and alleviating factors. Differentiating between types of pain (e.g., visceral, bone, neuropathic) is important in developing an effective pain management plan.

Assess pain on an ongoing basis to determine the effectiveness of the treatment plan. Obtain data and document at regular intervals the location and intensity of the pain, what it feels like, and how it is relieved. Assess change in pain (e.g., a significant change in the intensity, character, worsening, or location of pain) to determine the cause (e.g., progression of disease).

Always believe the patient report and accept it as the primary source of assessment data. Table 15-20 presents assessment questions that may facilitate data collection.

**TABLE 15-20 Pain Assessment in Cancer Patients**

| Characteristic | Questions to Ask |
|---|---|
| **Location** | • Where is the pain?<br>• Is the pain in more than one place? Is the pain in a new location?<br>• Does location of pain correlate with known diagnosis? |
| **Intensity** | • How bad is the pain?<br>• Rate the pain on a scale of 0 to 10. (See Chapter 8 for rating scales.) |
| **Quality** | • What does the pain feel like—sharp, dull, burning, shooting, aching, or other? (See Chapter 8 for descriptors.) |
| **Pattern** | • Has the pain changed?<br>• Is the pain getting better, worse, or unchanged?<br>• What makes the pain better or worse? |
| **Relief measures** | • What do you do to control your pain?<br>• Do you use medications?<br>• Do the relief measures help much? How much? |

### Pain Management

Pain management for the cancer patient must address both persistent and breakthrough components of pain if they are present. Adjuvant therapies need to be developed specific to the type or nature of the pain. In addition, teach patients how to keep a pain management diary.[30]

Drug therapy, including nonsteroidal antiinflammatory drugs, opioids, and adjuvant pain medications, should be used and selected based on the character and/or cause of the pain. Opioids normally are prescribed for the treatment of moderate to severe cancer pain. Analgesic medications (e.g., morphine, fentanyl) should be given on a regular schedule (around the clock) with additional doses available as needed for breakthrough pain. In general, oral administration of the medication is preferred, but other routes (e.g., transdermal, transmucosal) are also available.

It is critical for you to pay attention to common side effects of pain medications (e.g., constipation) to ensure the patient's well-being and adherence with the pain management program. Nonsteroidal antiinflammatories (e.g., ibuprofen) often serve as helpful adjuncts to opioid therapy, particularly for bone pain. Other adjuvant therapies, such as antidepressant and antiseizure drugs, may be beneficial in neuropathic pain, which is often resistant to opioids.

Radiopharmaceuticals (e.g., samarium-153) may benefit patients with diffuse bone pain (particularly if no further chemotherapy is planned). Patients may experience an initial pain *flare* after administration. Nerve blocks or epidural or intrathecal analgesia may also be used to treat patients with unrelieved pain or to minimize the requirements for opioids.

Remember that with opioid drugs (e.g., morphine) the appropriate dosage is whatever is necessary to control the pain with the fewest side effects. Fear of addiction is not warranted. However, it must be addressed as part of patient teaching, since it is a significant barrier for patients and nurses in appropriate pain management. In addition, you need to assess the patient for possible risk factors for opioid misuse/abuse.

Discuss the goals of analgesic therapy with patients, especially those requiring large or chronic doses of opioids. Treatment plans should be developed that balance analgesia and side effects to maintain optimal functional status.

Patient teaching should clarify myths and misconceptions and reassure patients and family caregivers that cancer pain can be effectively relieved. Furthermore, addiction and tolerance are not problems associated with effective cancer pain management. Nondrug interventions, including relaxation therapy and imagery, can be effectively used to manage pain (see Chapter 6). Additional strategies to relieve pain are discussed in Chapter 8.

## COPING WITH CANCER AND TREATMENT

You have a key role in assisting patients in coping with the psychosocial issues associated with cancer and cancer treatment. The patient may experience a variety of concerns, including fears of dependency, loss of control, family and relationship stress, financial burden, and fear of death. Anxiety and fear may be experienced throughout the cancer continuum, including at diagnosis, during or after treatment, and in association with long-term follow-up.

Repetitive office visits or hospitalizations, continuing medications, and frequent laboratory testing force the individual to confront the cancer on a daily basis. Treatment-related uncertainties and fears are often most evident at the beginning of therapy. However, anxiety and fear may be present throughout treatment, and when therapy is completed (e.g., fear of recurrence, less available support).

Adaptation and coping with a cancer diagnosis may be influenced by a variety of patient factors, including demographics, prior coping skills and strategies, social support, and religious and spiritual beliefs (Table 15-21). You are in a key position to assess the patient's and family's responses and support positive coping strategies. To facilitate the development of effective coping and to support the patient and family during the various stages of cancer, you should do the following:

- Be available and continue to be available, especially during difficult times.
- Exhibit a caring attitude.
- Listen actively to fears and concerns.
- Help provide relief from distressing symptoms.
- Provide essential information regarding cancer and cancer care that is accurate and establishes realistic expectations about what the patient will experience.
- Maintain a relationship based on trust and confidence. Be open, honest, and caring in the approach.
- Use touch to exhibit caring. A squeeze of the hand or a hug may at times be more effective than words.
- Assist the patient in setting realistic, reachable short-term and long-term goals.
- Assist the patient in maintaining usual lifestyle patterns.

**TABLE 15-21 Factors Affecting How Patients Cope With Cancer**

| Factor | Description |
|---|---|
| **Ability to cope with stressful events in the past** | How patients coped with previous stressful events (e.g., loss of job, major disappointment, significant traumatic event) affects how they cope with diagnosis of cancer. |
| **Availability of significant others** | Patients who have effective support systems cope more effectively than those who do not. |
| **Ability to express feelings and concerns** | Patients who express feelings and needs and ask for help cope more effectively than those who internalize feelings and needs. |
| **Age at the time of diagnosis** | Age determines coping strategies to a great degree. For example, a young mother with cancer may have concerns that differ from those of a 70-yr-old woman with cancer. |
| **Extent of disease** | Cure or control of the disease process is usually easier to cope with than the reality of terminal illness. |
| **Disruption of body image** | Disruption of the body image (e.g., radical neck dissection, alopecia, mastectomy) may intensify the psychologic impact of cancer. |
| **Presence of symptoms** | Symptoms such as fatigue, nausea, diarrhea, and pain may intensify the psychologic impact of cancer. |
| **Past experience with cancer** | Negative experiences with cancer (personal or in others) influence perceptions about the current situation. |
| **Attitude associated with the cancer** | Patients who feel in control and have a positive attitude about cancer and cancer treatment cope better with the diagnosis and treatment of cancer than those who feel hopeless, helpless, and out of control. |

- Maintain hope, which is the key to effective cancer care. Hope varies, depending on the patient's status—hope that the symptoms are not serious, hope that the treatment is curative, hope for independence, hope for relief of pain, hope for a longer life, hope to achieve meaningful goals, or hope for a peaceful death. Hope provides control over what is occurring and is the basis of a positive attitude toward cancer and cancer care.

Tell patients that they will be followed and reassure them that support is ongoing. Provide information and support to help minimize the negative impact of cancer therapy on a person's quality of life. Patient teaching and symptom management help patients to self-manage their illness (e.g., adjusting treatment schedules to permit patients to work when possible, making referrals to support groups). Collaborate with the oncology nurse navigators who serve as the liaison between the patient and members of the interprofessional care team.

Arrange for patients to meet with individuals who have successfully completed therapy as this can increase their hopefulness and confidence. In addition, make regular supportive telephone contacts between office visits and assist with planning for transportation, nutrition, and emotional support.

Do not forget the caregiver and other family members. They need education and support throughout the trajectory of diagnosis, treatment, and follow-up.[31] Patients and caregivers may benefit from a variety of psychosocial interventions, such as supportive listening, stress management techniques, individual or group counseling, and cognitive-behavioral therapy. Assess

## ETHICAL/LEGAL DILEMMAS

***Medical Futility***

**Situation**

D.M., a 65-year-old Asian woman, has breast cancer with metastasis to the liver and bone. The family asks you why their mother is not receiving chemotherapy. In addition, they want to make sure that she will be resuscitated should her heart stop. They are aware of her diagnosis and that she may have only a few months to live. In morning rounds you were told that D.M. does not want any treatment that would prolong her life.

**Ethical/Legal Points for Consideration**

- Although court decisions have varied, legally there is substantial consensus concerning the right to privacy (a constitutional right), right to informed consent and refusal of treatment, and rights pertaining to end-of-life decision making. The *Code of Ethics for Nurses* addresses the key components in the informed consent process that nurses must address.[1]
- A patient who is an adult and is competent (defined as capable of understanding and interpreting information, making choices, and communicating those choices) solely retains the right to make personal health care decisions.
- The Patient Self-Determination Act requires that the patient be asked on admission whether he or she has an advance directive. If available, it is placed in the medical record. If the patient does not have an advance directive, it must be documented.
- The National POLST Paradigm is an approach to end-of-life planning that emphasizes patients' wishes about the care they receive. The POLST Paradigm is an approach to end-of-life planning emphasizing the medical orders and includes coverage regardless of location (e.g., hospital, home, assisted living).[2]
- Often families have difficulty accepting the finality of a terminal diagnosis.
- Sometimes family members have conflicting interests (e.g., finances, property, inheritance rights) that influence their decision-making abilities.

**Discussion Questions**

1. How can you help D.M. communicate her wishes to her family?
2. How can you and the interprofessional care team assist the family in planning end-of-life care that incorporates the wishes of their mother?
3. What are the cultural issues in D.M.'s case?

**References**

1. Code of Ethics for Nurses. *www.nursingworld.org/MainMenuCategories/EthicsStandards/Ethics-Position-Statements.*
2. Physician Orders for Life Sustaining Treatment (POLST) Paradigm: *www.polst.org.*

the psychosocial concerns and emotional responses of patients, caregivers, and families so you can connect patients with appropriate supportive care resources. Use the available resources in the community such as the American Cancer Society, Cancer Lifeline, churches, and other community resources.

### Gerontologic Considerations: Cancer

Cancer is usually a disease of aging with 78% of cancers occurring in people 55 years or older.[1] The cancer mortality rate is exceedingly high in older adults, with 70% of all deaths due to cancer occurring in those over age 65. This is especially important since the normal life span is increasing and the proportion of the population who are older than 65 years is increasing.

Clinical manifestations of cancer in older adults may be mistakenly attributed to age-related changes and ignored by the person.[32] Older adults are particularly vulnerable to the complications of both cancer and cancer therapy. This is due to their decline in physiologic functioning, social and emotional resources, and cognitive function.

The older adult's functional status should be taken into consideration when developing a treatment plan. Age alone is not a good predictor of tolerance or response to treatment. Advances in the treatment of cancer are making cancer therapies beneficial to an increasing number of older adults, including patients with suboptimal health.

Assess the patient at the time of diagnosis to identify important issues that may affect decisions about treatment options. Issues to assess include projected life expectancy, estimate of morbidity from cancer, co-morbidities that would affect treatment, and patient decision-making capacity and wishes.

Some important questions to consider when an older person is diagnosed with cancer include the following: Will the treatment provide more benefits than harm? Will he or she be able to tolerate the treatment safely? Is there need to optimize other co-morbidities or nutritional or functional status before starting treatment? What are the patient's preferences and wishes?

## CANCER SURVIVORSHIP

Although the overall incidence and death rate from cancer has decreased, the number of cancer survivors continues to increase. It is estimated that there are currently more than 14.5 million cancer survivors in the United States. Some of these individuals are cancer free, whereas others still have evidence of cancer and may be undergoing treatment. The increase in survivorship is attributed to the aging and growth of the population as well as improvements in early detection and treatment. Survival statistics vary greatly by the type and stage of cancer.[1,33]

The rapid increase in cancer survivors has been accompanied by a greater awareness of the long-term health and quality-of-life issues that a cancer diagnosis imposes. Cancer survivors experience a variety of long-term and late sequelae following treatment (discussed earlier in this chapter on pp. 256-257). You need to be aware of the long-term late effects of the various treatments so that you can teach patients and their caregivers.

The impact of cancer and its treatment confers greater risk of non–cancer-related death and co-morbidities (e.g., heart disease, diabetes, metabolic syndrome, endocrine dysfunction, osteoporosis) among cancer survivors. Furthermore, cancer survivors may continue to experience symptoms or functional impairment related to treatment for years after treatment.

The impact of a cancer diagnosis can affect many aspects of a patient's life, with cancer survivors commonly reporting financial, vocational, marital, and spiritual concerns long after treatment is over. Psychosocial/emotional issues can play a profound role in a patient's life after cancer, with issues related to living in uncertainty being frequently encountered.

Some patients may wish to return to their normal lives as soon as possible, and they may fail to attend scheduled follow-up appointments. Other survivors may become cancer advocates or active members of a cancer support group. Still others may allow their lives to revolve around the cancer and may even resist giving up the illness role.

Tips to help cancer survivors are presented in Table 15-22. Connecting cancer survivors to online support and resources is a strategy to enhance positive health outcomes[34,35] (Table 15-23).

## TABLE 15-22 Patient Teaching

### *Cancer Survivors*

*You can help cancer survivors by doing the following:*

1. Provide all cancer patients with a treatment summary and care plan outlining treatment exposures, risk of late effects, preventive care recommendations, and follow-up surveillance plan after completion of treatment.
   - Care plans should clearly identify all members of the interprofessional team and their responsibilities for follow-up care.
   - Include referrals to appropriate supportive care and community resources that would benefit the patient in recovery or ongoing care.
2. Coordinate care among the oncology team, primary HCP, and other specialists.
3. Teach HCPs about the needs of cancer survivors, including long-term effects of cancer and cancer treatments.
4. Teach cancer survivors to look for and report any ongoing symptoms resulting from treatment, including late effects of radiation therapy and chemotherapy.
5. Promote healthy behaviors:
   - *Prevention:* good nutrition, exercise, smoking avoidance, maintenance of proper weight, cardiac risk reduction, bone health.
   - *Early detection:* routine health screenings (e.g., breast, colon), cholesterol, diabetes, osteoporosis screening as recommended.
6. Encourage cancer survivors to have regular follow-up examinations with their HCP.
7. Assess for psychoemotional, financial, health insurance, or vocational problems related to cancer. Assist patients in getting appropriate help if necessary.

## TABLE 15-23 Resources for Cancer Survivors

| Organization | Purpose |
|---|---|
| **ACS Cancer Survivors Network** | Provides survivorship information and resources and online forum for connecting with others affected by cancer. *(www.cancer.org/cancersurvivorsnetwork)* |
| **CancerCare** | Provides a variety of free support services delivered by professional oncology social workers for patients and anyone else affected by cancer. *(www.cancercare.org)* |
| **Cancer.Net** | American Society of Clinical Oncology (ASCO) patient support site that includes extensive information and resources for cancer survivors. *(www.cancer.net)* |
| **National Cancer Institute Office of Cancer Survivorship** | Supports research into the short- and long-term physical, social, emotional, and economic effects of cancer survivorship. Offers educational and support resources for cancer survivors, caregivers, and advocates. *(www.cancercontrol.cancer.gov/ocs/)* |
| **National Coalition for Cancer Survivorship** | Advocates for quality cancer care. Seeks to empower and educate patients and advocates on issues that affect the quality of life of cancer survivors. *(www.canceradvocacy.org)* |

## Culturally Competent Care: Cancer

Cancer incidence and death rates are disproportionately higher in African Americans than in whites and other minority groups (see Cultural & Ethnic Health Disparities box). Although overall racial disparities in cancer death rates have been declining, death rates continue to be higher among African Americans than whites. In addition, African Americans are more likely to have later stage disease at the time of diagnosis than whites.[1]

Differences in survival rates from cancer are attributed primarily to a combination of factors, including poverty, difficult access to and poorer quality of health care, more co-morbid conditions, and differences in tumor biology. Disparities in cancer care exist throughout the continuum from cancer prevention and screening to end-of-life care and survivorship. The disparity in prevention and screening results in cancer being in advanced stages at the time of diagnosis.[1,2]

### CULTURAL & ETHNIC HEALTH DISPARITIES

#### *Cancer*

- Cancer incidence and death rates for men are highest among African Americans, followed by whites, Hispanics, and Asians/Pacific Islanders.
- Cancer incidence rates for women are highest among whites, followed by African Americans, Hispanics, and Asians/Pacific Islanders.
- However, cancer death rates for women are highest among African Americans, followed by whites, Hispanics, and Asians/Pacific Islanders.

Culturally competent care in oncology is needed to meet the needs of diverse groups. Culturally competent care involves awareness of personal background, how culture affects care delivery, and how to adapt to meet cultural needs. Nurses need to actively seek to understand cultural differences to meet the individualized needs. (Culture is discussed in Chapter 2 and culturally competent care related to specific cancers is presented in the chapters where the cancer is discussed.)

## BRIDGE TO NCLEX EXAMINATION

The number of the question corresponds to the same-numbered outcome at the beginning of the chapter.

1. Trends in the incidence and death rates of cancer include the fact that
   a. lung cancer is the most common type of cancer in men.
   b. a higher percentage of women than men have lung cancer.
   c. breast cancer is the leading cause of cancer deaths in women.
   d. African Americans have a higher death rate from cancer than whites.
2. What features of cancer cells distinguish them from normal cells *(select all that apply)*?
   a. Cells lack contact inhibition.
   b. Oncogenes maintain normal cell expression.
   c. Cells return to a previous undifferentiated state.
   d. Proliferation occurs when there is a need for more cells.
   e. New proteins characteristic of embryonic stage emerge on cell membrane.

3. A characteristic of the stage of progression in the development of cancer is
   a. oncogenic viral transformation of target cells.
   b. a reversible steady growth facilitated by carcinogens.
   c. a period of latency before clinical detection of cancer.
   d. proliferation of cancer cells despite host control mechanisms.
4. The primary protective role of the immune system related to malignant cells is
   a. surveillance for cells with tumor-associated antigens.
   b. binding with free antigen released by malignant cells.
   c. production of blocking factors that immobilize cancer cells.
   d. reacting to a new set of antigenic determinants on cancer cells.
5. The nurse is caring for a 59-year-old woman who had surgery 1 day ago for removal of a malignant abdominal mass. The patient is awaiting the pathology report. She is tearful and says that she is scared to die. The *most* effective nursing intervention at this point is to use this opportunity to
   a. motivate change in an unhealthy lifestyle.
   b. teach her about the seven warning signs of cancer.
   c. instruct her about healthy stress relief and coping practices.
   d. let her communicate about the meaning of this experience.
6. The goals of cancer treatment are based on the principle that
   a. surgery is the single most effective treatment for cancer.
   b. initial treatment is always directed toward cure of the cancer.
   c. a combination of treatment modalities is effective for controlling many cancers.
   d. although cancer cure is rare, quality of life can be increased with treatment modalities.
7. The *most* effective method of administering a chemotherapy agent that is a vesicant is to
   a. give it orally.
   b. give it intraarterially.
   c. use an Ommaya reservoir.
   d. use a central venous access device.
8. The nurse explains to a patient undergoing brachytherapy of the cervix that she
   a. must undergo simulation to locate the treatment area.
   b. requires the use of radioactive precautions during nursing care.
   c. may experience desquamation of the skin on the abdomen and upper legs.
   d. requires shielding of the ovaries during treatment to prevent ovarian damage.
9. A patient on chemotherapy and radiation for head and neck cancer has a WBC count of $1.9 \times 10^3/\mu L$, hemoglobin of 10.8 g/dL, and a platelet count of $99 \times 10^3/\mu L$. Based on the CBC results, what is the *most* serious clinical finding?
   a. Cough, rhinitis, and sore throat
   b. Fatigue, nausea, and skin redness at site of radiation
   c. Temperature of 101.9° F, fatigue, and shortness of breath
   d. Skin redness at site of radiation, headache, and constipation
10. To prevent fever and shivering during an infusion of rituximab (Rituxan), the nurse should premedicate the patient with
    a. aspirin.
    b. acetaminophen.
    c. sodium bicarbonate.
    d. meperidine (Demerol).
11. The nurse counsels the patient receiving radiation therapy or chemotherapy that
    a. effective birth control methods should be used for the rest of the patient's life.
    b. if nausea and vomiting occur during treatment, the treatment plan will be modified.
    c. after successful treatment, a return to the person's previous functional level can be expected.
    d. the cycle of fatigue-depression-fatigue that may occur during treatment may be reduced by restricting activity.
12. A patient on chemotherapy for 10 weeks started at a weight of 121 lb. She now weighs 118 lb and has no sense of taste. Which nursing intervention would be a *priority*?
    a. Advise the patient to eat foods that are fatty, fried, or high in calories.
    b. Discuss with the physician the need for parenteral or enteral feedings.
    c. Advise the patient to drink a nutritional supplement beverage at least three times a day.
    d. Advise the patient to experiment with spices and seasonings to enhance the flavor of food.
13. A 70-year-old male patient has multiple myeloma. His wife calls to report that he sleeps most of the day, is confused when awake, and complains of nausea and constipation. Which complication of cancer is this *most* likely caused by?
    a. Hypercalcemia
    b. Tumor lysis syndrome
    c. Spinal cord compression
    d. Superior vena cava syndrome
14. A patient has recently been diagnosed with early stages of breast cancer. What is *most* appropriate for the nurse to focus on?
    a. Maintaining the patient's hope
    b. Preparing a will and advance directives
    c. Discussing replacement child care for the patient's children
    d. Discussing the patient's past experiences with her grandmother's cancer

1. d, 2. a, c, e, 3. d, 4. a, 5. d, 6. c, 7. d, 8. b, 9. c, 10. b, 11. c, 12. d, 13. a, 14. a

For rationales to these answers and even more NCLEX review questions, visit *http://evolve.elsevier.com/Lewis/medsurg.*

## EVOLVE WEBSITE

http://evolve.elsevier.com/Lewis/medsurg
**Review Questions (Online Only)**
**Key Points**
**Answer Keys for Questions**
- Rationales for Bridge to NCLEX Examination Questions

**Conceptual Care Map Creator**
**Supporting Media**
- Animations
  - Chemotherapy
  - Radiation Therapy

**Audio Glossary**
**Content Updates**

## REFERENCES

1. American Cancer Society: *Cancer facts & figures 2015,* Atlanta, 2015, American Cancer Society.
2. Siegel RL, Miller KD, Jemal A: Cancer statistics 2015, *CA Cancer J Clin* 65:5, 2015.
3. National Cancer Institute, NIH, DHHS: Cancer trends progress report, Bethesda, Md, March 2015. Retrieved from *http://progressreport.cancer.gov.*

4. Vockley JG, Niederhuber JE: Diagnosis and treatment of cancer using genomics, *BMJ* 350:h1832, 2015.
5. Ariga H: Common mechanisms of onset of cancer and neurodegenerative diseases, *Biol Pharm Bull* 38(6):795, 2015.
6. Cancer Prevention and Control, Centers for Disease Control and Prevention: Skin cancer. Retrieved from *www.cdc.gov/cancer/skin/index.htm.*
7. Casulo C, Friedberg J: Treating Burkitt lymphoma in adults, *Curr Hematol Malig Rep* 10(3):266, 2015.
8. Karnofsky Performance Scale. Retrieved from *www.pennmedicine.org/homecare/hcp/elig_worksheets/Karnofsky-Performance-Status.pdf.*
9. Katz Index of Independence in Activities of Daily Living. Retrieved from *http://consultgerirn.org/uploads/File/trythis/try_this_2.pdf.*
10. Stewart BW, Wild P: World cancer report. World Health Organization.

*11. American Cancer Society: Cancer screening guidelines. Retrieved from *www.cancer.org/healthy/findcancerearly/cancerscreeningguidelines/american-cancer-society-guidelines-for-the-early-detection-of-cancer.*

12. American Society of Clinical Oncology (ASCO): What is personalized cancer medicine? Retrieved from *www.cancer.net/navigating-cancer-care/how-cancer-treated/personalized-and-targeted-therapies/what-personalized-cancer-medicine.*
13. Low SK, Takahashi A, Mushiroda T, et al: Genome-wide association study: a useful tool to identify common genetic variants associated with drug toxicity and efficacy in cancer pharmacogenomics, *Clin Cancer Res* 20(10):2541, 2014.
14. McLeod HL: Cancer pharmacogenomics: early promise, but concerted effort needed, *Science* 339(6127):1563, 2013.
15. National Institute for Occupational Safety and Health: Safe handling of chemotherapy agents. Retrieved from *www.cdc.gov/niosh/topics/antineoplastic.*
16. Polovich M, Olsen M, LeFebvre K: *Chemotherapy and biotherapy guidelines and recommendations for practice*, ed 4, Pittsburgh, 2014, Oncology Nursing Society.

*17. Tariman JD, Doorenbos A, Schepp KG, et al: Information needs priorities in patients diagnosed with cancer: a systematic review, *J Adv Pract Oncol* 2014(5):115, 2014.

18. Matsuyama RK, Kuhn LA, Molisani A, et al: Cancer patients' information needs the first nine months after diagnosis, *Patient Educ Couns* 90(1):96, 2013.

*19. Mhaskar R, Clark OA, Lyman G, et al: Colony-stimulating factors for chemotherapy-induced febrile neutropenia, *Cochrane Database Syst Rev* 10:CD003039, 2014.

20. National Cancer Institute: Guidelines for the evaluation and management of cancer-related fatigue. Retrieved from *www.cancer.gov/cancertopics/pdq/supportivecare/fatigue/HealthProfessional/page4.*
21. Kaiser J, Bledowski C, Dietrich J: Neural correlates of chemotherapy-related cognitive impairment, *Cortex* 54C:33, 2014.
22. American Cancer Society: Chemo brain. Retrieved from *www.cancer.org/treatment/treatmentsandsideeffects/physicalsideeffects/chemotherapyeffects/chemo-brain.*
23. Wright CI, Coad J, Morgan S, et al: "Just in case": the fertility information needs of teenagers and young adults with cancer, *Eur J Cancer Care (Engl)* 23(2):189, 2014.
24. A[illegible] SH, Kremer LC, Sklar C: Approaches to reduce the long-term b[illegible]-related complications in survivors of childhood c[illegible] *Book* 35:196, 2015.

*25. S[illegible] al: Are we ready to predict late e[illegible] of clinically useful prediction models, *Eur J Cancer* 51(6):758, 2015.

26. American Cancer Society: How does targeted cancer therapy work? Retrieved from *www.cancer.org/treatment/treatmentsandsideeffects/treatmenttypes/targetedtherapy/targeted-therapy-how-work.*
27. National Cancer Institute: What are targeted cancer therapies? Retrieved from *www.cancer.gov/about-cancer/treatment/types/targeted-therapies/targeted-therapies-fact-sheet#q4.*
28. Ozkan MC, Sahin F, Saydam G: Peripheral blood stem cell mobilization from healthy donors, *Transfus Apher Sci* 53:13, 2015.
29. Aoyagi T, Terracina KP, Raza A, et al: Cancer cachexia, mechanism and treatment, *World J Gastrointest Oncol* 7(4):17, 2015.
30. National Council of Cancer Nurses' guidelines for management of adult cancer pain. Retrieved from *www.nccn.org/professionals/physician_gls/pdf/pain.pdf.*
31. Longacre ML: Cancer caregivers information needs and resource preferences, *J Cancer Educ* 28(2):297, 2013.
32. National Institute on Aging: Global health and aging. Retrieved from *www.nia.nih.gov/research/publication/global-health-and-aging/living-longer.*
33. DeSantis CE, Lin CC, Mariotto AB, et al:. Cancer treatment and survivorship statistics, 2014, *CA Cancer J Clin* 64(4):252, 2014.
34. Warren E, Footman K, Tinelli M, et al: Do cancer-specific websites meet patient's information needs? *Patient Educ Couns* 95(1):126, 2014.
35. Shea-Budgell MA, Kostaras X, Myhill KP, et al: Information needs and sources of information for patients during cancer follow-up, *Curr Oncol* 21(4):165, 2014.


*Evidence-based information for clinical practice.

16

# Fluid, Electrolyte, and Acid-Base Imbalances

*Mariann M. Harding*

*Water is the driving force in nature.*

***Leonardo da Vinci***

http://evolve.elsevier.com/Lewis/medsurg/

## LEARNING OUTCOMES

1. Describe the composition of the major body fluid compartments.
2. Define processes involved in the regulation of movement of water and electrolytes between the body fluid compartments.
3. Describe the etiology, laboratory diagnostic findings, clinical manifestations, and nursing and interprofessional management of the following disorders:
   a. Extracellular fluid volume imbalances: fluid volume deficit and fluid volume excess
   b. Sodium imbalances: hypernatremia and hyponatremia
   c. Potassium imbalances: hyperkalemia and hypokalemia
   d. Magnesium imbalances: hypermagnesemia and hypomagnesemia
   e. Calcium imbalances: hypercalcemia and hypocalcemia
   f. Phosphate imbalances: hyperphosphatemia and hypophosphatemia
4. Identify the processes involved in maintaining acid-base balance.
5. Discuss the etiology, laboratory diagnostic findings, clinical manifestations, and nursing and interprofessional management of the following acid-base imbalances: metabolic acidosis, metabolic alkalosis, respiratory acidosis, and respiratory alkalosis.
6. Describe the composition of and indications for common IV fluid solutions.
7. Discuss the types and nursing management of commonly used central venous access devices.

## KEY TERMS

acidosis, p. 287
active transport, p. 272
alkalosis, p. 287
anions, p. 271
buffers, p. 287
cations, p. 271
central venous access devices (CVADs), p. 294
electrolytes, p. 271
fluid spacing, p. 274
hydrostatic pressure, p. 273
hypertonic, p. 273
hypotonic, p. 273
isotonic, p. 273
oncotic pressure, p. 273
osmolality, p. 272
osmosis, p. 272
osmotic pressure, p. 272

## HOMEOSTASIS

Body fluids and electrolytes play an important role in maintaining *homeostasis,* the body's stable internal environment. Body fluids are in constant motion transporting nutrients, electrolytes, and oxygen to cells and carrying waste products away from cells. The body uses a number of adaptive responses to keep the composition and volume of fluids and electrolytes within narrow limits to maintain homeostasis and promote health.

Many diseases and their treatments affect fluid and electrolyte balance. For example, a patient with metastatic colon cancer may develop hypercalcemia because of bone destruction from tumor invasion. Chemotherapy used to treat the cancer may result in nausea and vomiting and, subsequently, dehydration and acid-base imbalances. When correcting dehydration with IV fluids, the patient requires close monitoring to prevent fluid overload.

It is important to anticipate the potential for fluid and electrolyte imbalances associated with certain disorders and medical therapies, recognize the signs and symptoms of imbalances, and intervene with the appropriate action. This chapter describes the (1) normal control of fluids, electrolytes, and acid-base balance; (2) conditions that disrupt homeostasis and resulting manifestations; and (3) actions that the health care provider and you can take to manage fluid, electrolyte, and acid-base imbalances and restore homeostasis.

## WATER CONTENT OF THE BODY

The body is composed primarily of water. It accounts for about 50% to 60% of body weight in the adult. Water content varies with body mass, gender, and age (Fig. 16-1). Lean body mass has a higher percentage of water, while adipose tissue has a lesser percentage of water. So, the more fat present in the body, the less the total water content. Women generally have a lower percentage of body water because they tend to have less lean body mass than men. Older adults also tend to have less lean body mass, resulting in a lower percentage of body water when compared to younger adults. In older adults, body water content

Reviewed by Helene Harris, RN, MSN, Clinical Educator, Central Texas Veterans Healthcare System, Temple, Texas; Ellen Odell, DNP, ACNS-BC, CNE, APRN, Director of Nursing, Associate Professor, Department of Nursing, John Brown University, Siloam Springs, Arkansas; and Daryle Wane, PhD, ARNP, FNP-BC, RN to BSN Coordinator, Professor of Nursing, Department of Health Occupations, Pasco-Hernando State College, New Port Richey, Florida.

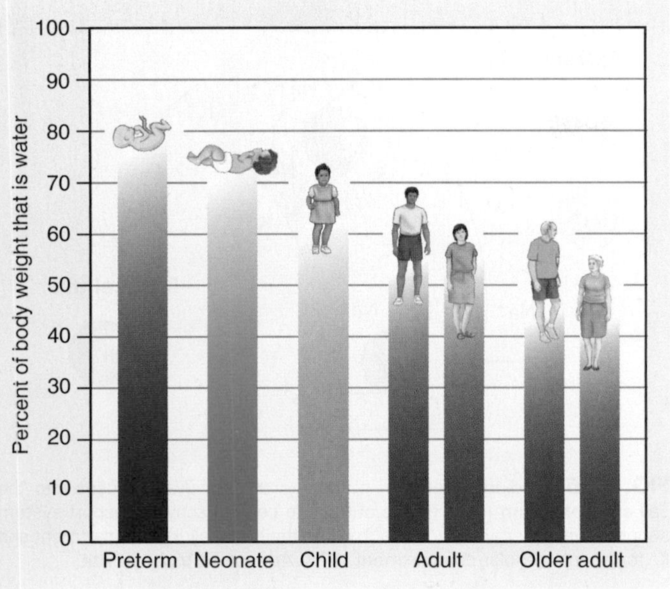


**FIG. 16-1** Body water over the life span.

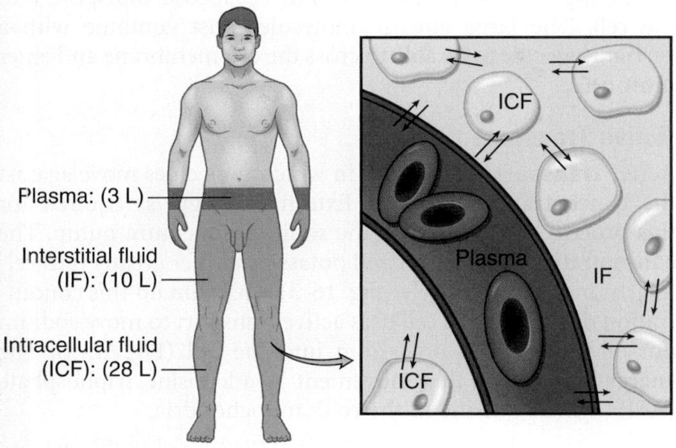


**FIG. 16-2** Relative volumes of three body fluids. Values represent fluid distribution in a young male adult.

averages 45% to 50% of body weight. This places them at a higher risk for fluid-related problems than young adults.

## Body Fluid Compartments

The two fluid compartments in the body are the *intracellular space* (inside the cells) and the *extracellular space* (outside the cells) (Fig. 16-2). About two thirds of the body water is located within cells and is termed *intracellular fluid* (ICF). ICF makes up about 40% of body weight of an adult. This means a 70-kg young man would have about 42 L of water, with about 28 L of that water located within his cells.

The fluid in the extracellular space is *extracellular fluid* (ECF). The two main compartments containing ECF are the *interstitial fluid,* or the fluid in the spaces between cells, and the intravascular fluid or *plasma,* the liquid part of blood. Other ECF compartments include lymph and *transcellular fluids.* Transcellular fluids include cerebrospinal fluid; fluid in the gastrointestinal (GI) tract and joint spaces; and pleural, peritoneal, intraocular, and pericardial fluid. ECF makes up about one third of the body water; this amounts to about 14 L in a 70-kg man. About one third of ECF is in the intravascular space as plasma (3 L in a 70-kg man), and two thirds is in the interstitial space (10 L in a 70-kg man). The fluid in the transcellular spaces totals about 1 L at any given time.

## Calculation of Fluid Gain or Loss

One liter of water weighs 2.2 lb (1 kg). Body weight change, especially sudden change, is an excellent indicator of overall fluid volume loss or gain. For example, if a patient drinks 240 mL (8 oz) of fluid, weight gain will be 0.5 lb (0.23 kg). A patient receiving diuretic therapy who loses 4.4 lb (2 kg) in 24 hours has experienced a fluid loss of about 2 L. An adult patient who is fasting may lose 1 to 2 lb/day. A weight loss exceeding this is likely due to loss of body fluid.

# ELECTROLYTES

**Electrolytes** are substances whose molecules dissociate, or split, into ions when placed in water. *Ions* are electrically charged particles. **Cations** are positively charged ions. Examples include sodium ($Na^+$), potassium ($K^+$), calcium ($Ca^{2+}$), and magnesium ($Mg^{2+}$) ions. **Anions** are negatively charged ions. Examples include bicarbonate ($HCO_3^-$), chloride ($Cl^-$), and phosphate ($PO_4^{3-}$) ions. Most proteins bear a negative charge and are thus anions.

## Measurement of Electrolytes

The concentration of electrolytes in body fluids is expressed in milliequivalents (mEq) per liter. Since electrolytes are active chemicals, it is useful to express their concentration according to their chemical activity, or the number of electrolytes able to combine chemically. Ions combine milliequivalent for milliequivalent. For example, 1 mEq (1 mmol) of sodium combines with 1 mEq (1 mmol) of chloride.

## Electrolyte Composition of Fluid Compartments

Electrolyte composition varies between ECF and ICF. The overall concentration of electrolytes is nearly the same in the two compartments. However, concentrations of specific ions differ greatly (Fig. 16-3). In ECF the main cation is sodium, with small amounts of potassium, calcium, and magnesium. The primary ECF anion is chloride, with small amounts of bicarbonate, sulfate, and phosphate anions.

In ICF the most prevalent cation is potassium, with small amounts of magnesium and sodium. The prevalent ICF anion is phosphate, with some protein and a small amount of bicarbonate. See Table 16-1 for normal serum electrolyte values.

# MECHANISMS CONTROLLING FLUID AND ELECTROLYTE MOVEMENT

The movement of electrolytes and water between ICF and ECF to maintain homeostasis involves many different processes, including simple diffusion, facilitated diffusion, and active transport. Water moves as driven by two forces: hydrostatic pressure and osmotic pressure.

## Diffusion

*Diffusion* is the movement of molecules from an area of high concentration to low concentration (Fig. 16-4). Net movement of molecules stops when the concentrations are equal in both areas. It occurs in liquids, gases, and solids. Simple diffusion requires no external energy.

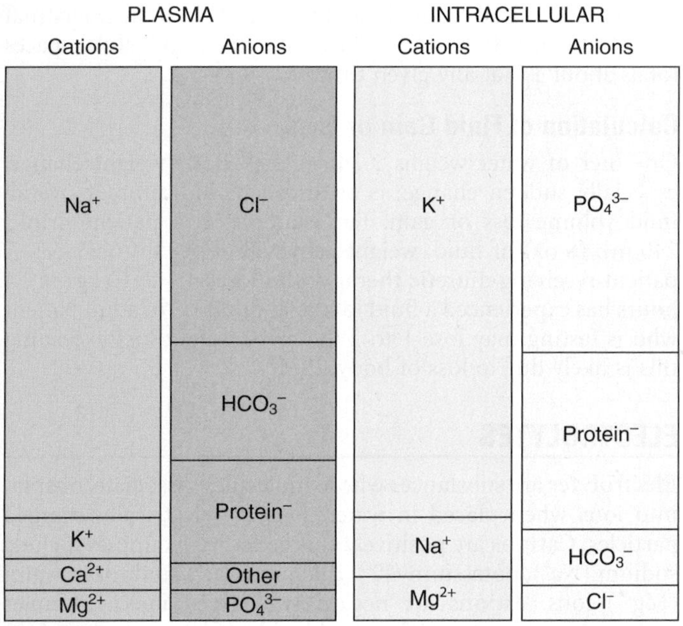


**FIG. 16-3** The relative concentrations of the major cations and anions in the intracellular space and the plasma.

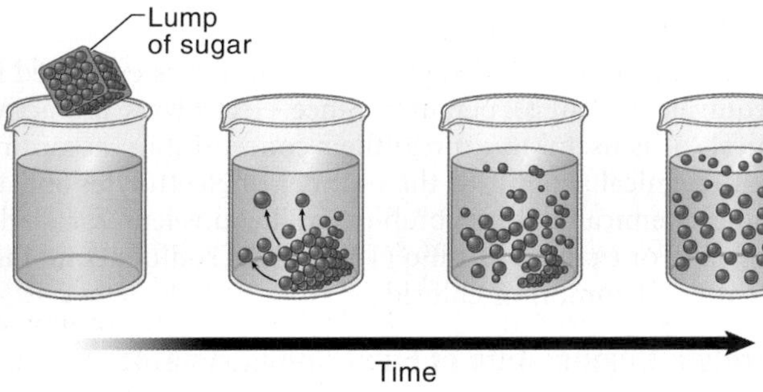


**FIG. 16-4** Diffusion is the movement of molecules from an area of high concentration to an area of low concentration. Eventually the sugar molecules are evenly distributed.

**TABLE 16-1 Normal Serum Electrolyte Values**

| Electrolyte | Reference Interval |
|---|---|
| **Anions** | |
| Bicarbonate ($HCO_3^-$) | 22-26 mEq/L (22-26 mmol/L) |
| Chloride ($Cl^-$) | 96-106 mEq/L (96-106 mmol/L) |
| Phosphate ($PO_4^{3-}$)* | 2.4-4.4 mg/dL (0.78-1.42 mmol/L) |
| **Cations** | |
| Potassium ($K^+$) | 3.5-5.0 mEq/L (3.5-5.0 mmol/L) |
| Magnesium ($Mg^{2+}$) | 1.5-2.5 mEq/L (0.75-1.25 mmol/L) |
| Sodium ($Na^+$) | 135-145 mEq/L (135-145 mmol/L) |
| Calcium ($Ca^{2+}$) (total) | 8.6-10.2 mg/dL (2.15-2.55 mmol/L) |
| Calcium (ionized) | 4.6-5.3 mg/dL (1.16-1.32 mmol/L) |

*The majority of the phosphorus (P) in the body is found as phosphate ($PO_4^{3-}$). The terms are used interchangeably in this text.

## Facilitated Diffusion

*Facilitated diffusion* involves the use of a protein carrier in the cell membrane. The protein carrier combines with a molecule, especially one too large to pass easily through the cell membrane, and assists in moving the molecule across the membrane from an area of high to low concentration. Like simple diffusion, facilitated diffusion is passive and requires no energy. An example of facilitated diffusion is glucose transport into the cell. The large glucose molecule must combine with a carrier molecule to be able to cross the cell membrane and enter most cells.

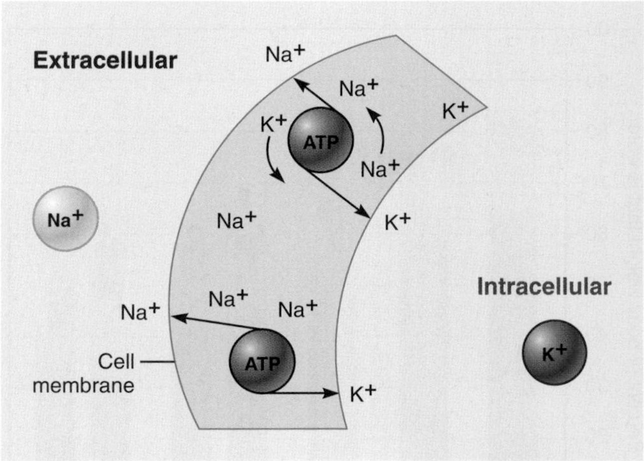


**FIG. 16-5** Sodium-potassium pump. As sodium *($Na^+$)* diffuses into the cell and potassium *($K^+$)* diffuses out of the cell, an active transport system supplied with energy delivers $Na^+$ back to the extracellular compartment and $K^+$ to the intracellular compartment. *ATP,* Adenosine triphosphate.

## Active Transport

**Active transport** is a process in which molecules move against the concentration gradient. External energy is required for this process. An example is the sodium-potassium pump. The concentrations of sodium and potassium differ greatly intracellularly and extracellularly (Fig. 16-3). To maintain this concentration difference, the cell uses active transport to move sodium out of the cell and potassium into the cell (Fig. 16-5). The energy source for this movement is adenosine triphosphate (ATP), which is made in the cell's mitochondria.

## Osmosis

**Osmosis** is the movement of water "down" a concentration gradient, that is, from a region of low solute concentration to one of high solute concentration, across a semipermeable membrane. Osmosis requires no outside energy sources. It stops when the concentration differences disappear or when hydrostatic pressure builds and opposes any further movement of water. Imagine a chamber with two compartments separated by a semipermeable membrane, one that allows only the movement of water (Fig. 16-6). If you add albumin to one side, water will move from the less concentrated side (has more water) to the more concentrated side of the chamber water (has less water) until the concentrations are equal.

Whenever dissolved substances are contained in a space with a semipermeable membrane, they can pull water into the space by osmosis. The concentration of the solution determines the strength of the osmotic pull. The higher the concentration, the greater a solution's pull, or **osmotic pressure.** Osmotic pressure is measured in milliosmoles (mOsm). It may be expressed as either fluid osmolarity or fluid osmolality. Although you will often see the terms *osmolarity* and *osmolality* used interchangeably, they are different measurements. *Osmolarity* measures the total milliosmoles per liter of solution, or the concentration of molecules per volume of solution (mOsm/L). **Osmolality**

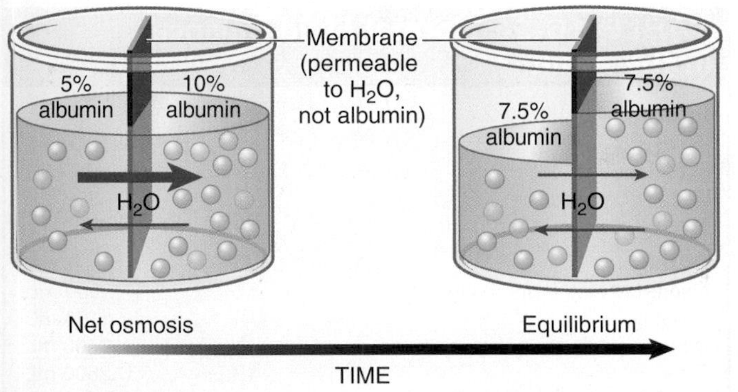


**FIG. 16-6** Osmosis is the process of water movement through a semipermeable membrane from an area of low solute concentration to an area of high solute concentration.

measures the number of milliosmoles per kilogram of water, or the concentration of molecules per weight of water. Osmolality is the preferred measure to evaluate the concentration of plasma, urine, and body fluids.[1]

**Measurement of Osmolality.** Osmolality is nearly the same in the various body fluid spaces. Therefore measuring or estimating plasma osmolality is a useful way to assess the state of the body's water balance. Calculate the plasma osmolality using the following formula.[2]

$$\text{Plasma osmolality} = (2 \times \text{Na}) + \left(\frac{\text{BUN}}{2.8}\right) + \left(\frac{\text{Glucose}}{18}\right)$$

Normal plasma osmolality is between 280 and 295 mOsm/kg. A value greater than 295 mOsm/kg indicates that the concentration of solute is too great or the water content is too little. This condition is termed *water deficit.* A value less than 275 mOsm/kg indicates too little solute for the amount of water or too much water for the amount of solute. This condition is termed *water excess.* Both conditions are clinically significant.

Osmolality of urine can range from 100 to 1300 mOsm/kg. Urine osmolality depends on fluid intake, the amount of antidiuretic hormone (ADH) in circulation, and the renal response to ADH.

**Osmotic Movement of Fluids.** The osmolality of the fluid surrounding cells affects them. Fluids with the same osmolality as the cell interior are termed **isotonic**. Normally, ECF and ICF are isotonic to one another, so no net movement of water occurs.

Changes in the osmolality of ECF alter the volume of cells. Solutions in which the solutes are less concentrated than in the cells are termed **hypotonic** (hypoosmolar). If a cell is surrounded by hypotonic fluid, water moves into the cell, causing it to swell and possibly to burst. Fluids with solutes more concentrated than in cells, or an increased osmolality, are termed **hypertonic** (hyperosmolar). If hypertonic fluid surrounds a cell, water leaves the cell to dilute ECF; the cell shrinks and may eventually die (Fig. 16-7).

### Hydrostatic Pressure

**Hydrostatic pressure** is the force of fluid in a compartment pushing against a cell membrane or vessel wall. In the blood vessels, hydrostatic pressure is the BP generated by the contraction of the heart. Hydrostatic pressure in the vascular system gradually decreases as the blood moves through the arteries until it is about 30 mm Hg in the capillary bed. At the capillary level, hydrostatic pressure is the major force that pushes water out of the vascular system and into the interstitial space.

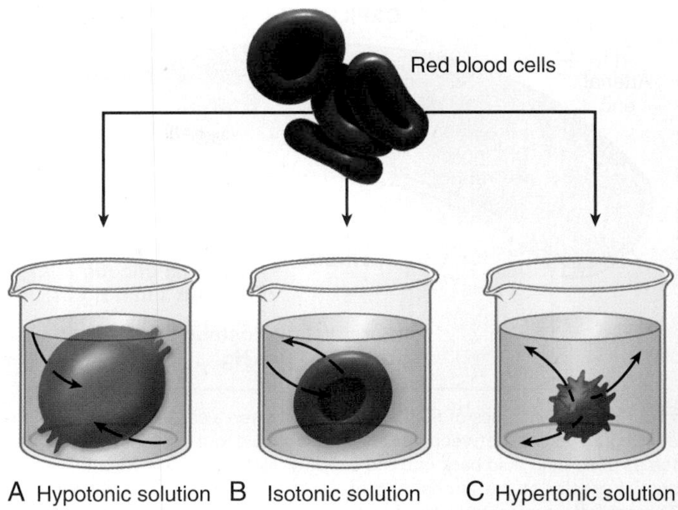


**FIG. 16-7** Effects of water status on red blood cells. **A,** Hypotonic solution ($H_2O$ excess) results in cellular swelling. **B,** Isotonic solution (normal $H_2O$ balance) results in no change. **C,** Hypertonic solution ($H_2O$ deficit) results in cellular shrinking.

### Oncotic Pressure

**Oncotic pressure** (colloidal osmotic pressure) is the osmotic pressure caused by plasma colloids in solution. The major colloids in the vascular system contributing to osmotic pressure are proteins, such as albumin. Plasma has substantial amounts of protein, while the interstitial space has very little. The plasma protein molecules attract water, pulling fluid from the tissue space to the vascular space. Under normal conditions, plasma oncotic pressure is about 25 mm Hg. The small amount of protein found in the interstitial space exerts an oncotic pressure of about 1 mm Hg.

## FLUID MOVEMENT IN CAPILLARIES

As plasma flows through the capillary bed, four factors determine if fluid moves out of the capillary and into the interstitial space or if fluid moves back into the capillary from the interstitial space. The amount and direction of movement are determined by the interaction of (1) capillary hydrostatic pressure, (2) plasma oncotic pressure, (3) interstitial hydrostatic pressure, and (4) interstitial oncotic pressure.

Capillary hydrostatic pressure and interstitial oncotic pressure move water out of the capillaries. Plasma oncotic pressure and interstitial hydrostatic pressure move fluid into the capillaries. At the arterial end of the capillary, capillary hydrostatic pressure exceeds plasma oncotic pressure, and fluid moves into the interstitial space. At the venous end of the capillary, the capillary hydrostatic pressure is lower than plasma oncotic pressure, drawing fluid back into the capillary by the oncotic pressure created by plasma proteins (Fig. 16-8).

### Fluid Shifts

If capillary or interstitial pressures change, fluid may abnormally shift from one compartment to another, resulting in edema or dehydration.

**Shifts of Plasma to Interstitial Fluid.** *Edema,* an accumulation of fluid in the interstitial space, occurs if venous hydrostatic

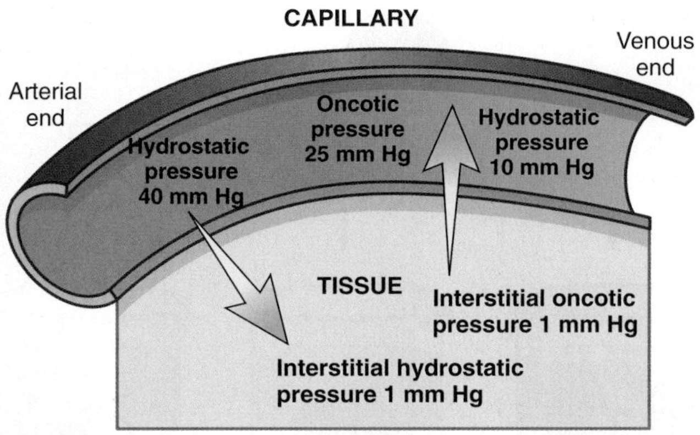


**FIG. 16-8** Dynamics of fluid exchange between a capillary and tissue. An equilibrium exists between forces filtering fluid out of the capillary and forces absorbing fluid back into the capillary. Note that the hydrostatic pressure is greater at the arterial end of the capillary than at the venous end. The net effect of pressures at the arterial end of the capillary causes a movement of fluid into the tissue. At the venous end of the capillary, there is net movement of fluid back into the capillary.

pressure rises, plasma oncotic pressure decreases, or interstitial oncotic pressure rises. Edema may also develop if an obstruction of lymphatic outflow causes decreased removal of interstitial fluid.

***Elevation of Venous Hydrostatic Pressure.*** Increasing the pressure at the venous end of the capillary inhibits fluid movement back into the capillary, which results in edema. Causes of increased venous pressure include fluid overload, heart failure, liver failure, obstruction of venous return to the heart (e.g., tourniquets, restrictive clothing, venous thrombosis), and venous insufficiency (e.g., varicose veins).

***Decrease in Plasma Oncotic Pressure.*** Fluid remains in the interstitial space if the plasma oncotic pressure is too low to draw fluid back into the capillary. Low plasma protein content decreases oncotic pressure. This can result from excessive protein loss (renal disorders), deficient protein synthesis (liver disease), and deficient protein intake (malnutrition).

***Elevation of Interstitial Oncotic Pressure.*** Trauma, burns, and inflammation can damage capillary walls and allow plasma proteins to accumulate in the interstitial space. This increases interstitial oncotic pressure, draws fluid into the interstitial space, and holds it there.

**Shifts of Interstitial Fluid to Plasma.** An increase in the plasma osmotic or oncotic pressure draws fluid into the plasma from the interstitial space. This could happen with administration of colloids, dextran, mannitol, or hypertonic solutions. Increasing the tissue hydrostatic pressure is another way of causing a shift of fluid into plasma. Wearing elastic compression gradient stockings or hose to decrease peripheral edema is a therapeutic application of this effect.

## FLUID SPACING

**Fluid spacing** is a term used to describe the distribution of body water. *First spacing* describes the normal distribution of fluid in ICF and ECF compartments. *Second spacing* refers to an abnormal accumulation of interstitial fluid (i.e., edema). *Third spacing* occurs when excess fluid collects in the nonfunctional area between cells. This fluid is trapped where it is difficult or impossible for it to move back into the cells or blood vessels. Third spacing occurs with ascites; fluid leaking into the abdominal cavity with peritonitis or pancreatitis; and edema associated with burns, trauma, or sepsis.

**TABLE 16-2 Normal Fluid Balance in the Adult**

| | |
|---|---|
| **Intake** | |
| Fluids | 1200 mL |
| Solid food | 1000 mL |
| Water from oxidation | 300 mL |
| Total | 2500 mL |
| **Output** | |
| Insensible loss (skin and lungs) | 900 mL |
| In feces | 100 mL |
| Urine | 1500 mL |
| Total | 2500 mL |

## REGULATION OF WATER BALANCE

A number of factors are involved in maintaining the finely tuned balance among water intake, use, and excretion. For proper fluid balance, an average healthy adult requires a daily water intake between 2000 and 3000 mL (Table 16-2). This amount replaces what is lost from the body in urinary output and insensible losses. Oral fluid intake accounts for most of the water intake. Water intake also includes water from food metabolism and water present in solid foods.

*Insensible water loss,* which is invisible vaporization from the lungs and skin, assists in regulating body temperature. Accelerated body metabolism, which occurs with increased body temperature and exercise, increases the amount of water lost and may result in the need for additional water replacement.

Do not confuse water loss through the skin with the vaporization of water excreted by sweat glands. Insensible perspiration causes only water loss. Excessive sweating *(sensible perspiration)* caused by exercise, fever, or high environmental temperatures may lead to large losses of water and electrolytes.

### Hypothalamic-Pituitary Regulation

Water ingestion equals water loss in the individual who has free access to water, intact thirst and ADH mechanism, and normally functioning kidneys. A body fluid deficit or increase in plasma osmolality activates osmoreceptors in the hypothalamus, which stimulate thirst and the release of ADH from the posterior pituitary gland. ADH acts on the distal tubules and collecting ducts in the kidney by making them more permeable to water. The result is increased water reabsorption from the tubular filtrate into the blood and decreased excretion in the urine. Because ADH is only able to regulate how much water the body holds onto, an intact thirst mechanism is our main protection against developing dehydration or hyperosmolality. Thirst causes us to increase the amount of water we drink. Together these result in increased free water in the body, decreasing plasma osmolality and restoring fluid volume.

Many factors influence ADH secretion and thirst. Decreased BP, nausea, pain, hypoglycemia, and hypoxemia stimulate ADH release. In the postoperative patient, the stress response to surgery and receiving analgesics and anesthesia cause ADH release and decreased osmolality. The unconscious or cognitively impaired patient is at increased risk for fluid deficit and hyperosmolality because of an inability to express thirst and act on it. A dry mouth will cause a person to drink, even when there is no body water deficit.

### Renal Regulation

The primary function of the kidneys is to regulate fluid and electrolyte balance by adjusting urine volume and the excretion of most electrolytes (see Chapter 44). The kidneys filter the total plasma volume many times each day. In the average adult, the kidneys reabsorb 99% of this filtrate, producing around 1.5 L of urine per day. Under the influence of ADH, aldosterone, and other hormones, selective reabsorption and secretion of water and electrolytes in the renal tubules results in urine that is greatly different in composition and concentration from plasma. This process helps maintain normal plasma osmolality, electrolyte balance, blood volume, and acid-base balance.

With severely impaired renal function, the kidneys cannot maintain fluid and electrolyte balance. This condition results in edema, potassium and phosphorus retention, acidosis, and other electrolyte imbalances (see Chapter 46).

### Adrenal Cortical Regulation

Glucocorticoids and mineralocorticoids secreted by the adrenal cortex help regulate water and electrolyte balance. The glucocorticoids (e.g., cortisol) primarily have an antiinflammatory effect and increase serum glucose levels, while the mineralocorticoids (e.g., aldosterone) enhance sodium retention and potassium excretion (Fig. 16-9). When sodium is reabsorbed, water follows because of osmotic changes.

Aldosterone is a mineralocorticoid with strong sodium-retaining and potassium-excreting capabilities. Decreased renal perfusion or decreased sodium in the distal portion of the renal tubule activates the renin-angiotensin-aldosterone system (RAAS), resulting in aldosterone secretion. In addition to the RAAS, increased serum potassium, decreased serum sodium, and adrenocorticotropic hormone (ACTH) stimulate aldosterone secretion. Aldosterone increases sodium and water reabsorption in the renal distal tubules, decreasing plasma osmolality and restoring fluid volume.

Cortisol is the most abundant glucocorticoid. In large doses, cortisol has both glucocorticoid (glucose-elevating and antiinflammatory) and mineralocorticoid (sodium-retention) effects. Normally cortisol secretion is in a diurnal or circadian pattern. Increased cortisol secretion occurs in response to physical and psychologic stress. This affects many body functions, including fluid and electrolyte balance (Fig. 16-10).

### Cardiac Regulation

Natriuretic peptides, including atrial natriuretic peptide (ANP) and b-type natriuretic peptide (BNP), are hormones produced by cardiomyocytes. They are produced in response to increased atrial pressure (increased volume, such as occurs in heart failure) and high serum sodium levels. They are natural antagonists to the RAAS and suppress secretion of aldosterone, renin, and ADH, and the action of angiotensin II. In the renal tubules, peptides promote excretion of sodium and water, decreasing blood volume and BP.

### Gastrointestinal Regulation

In addition to oral intake, the GI tract normally secretes around 8000 mL of digestive fluids each day. The GI tract normally reabsorbs most of this fluid, with only a small amount eliminated in feces. This is why diarrhea and vomiting, which prevent GI reabsorption of secreted fluid, can lead to significant fluid and electrolyte loss.

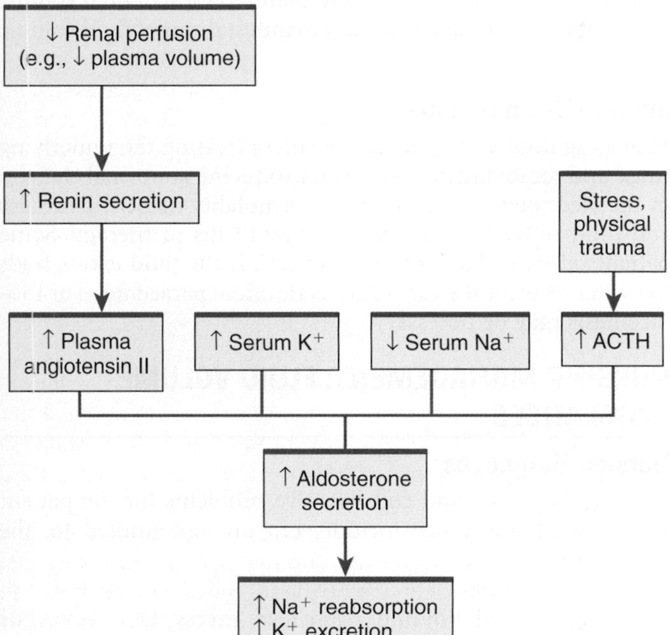


**FIG. 16-9** Factors affecting aldosterone secretion. *ACTH,* Adrenocorticotropic hormone.

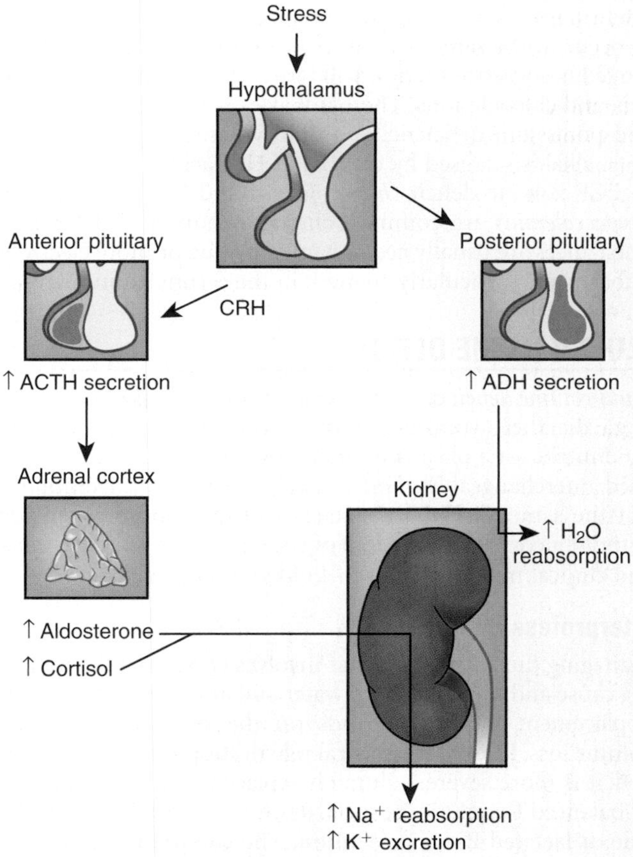


**FIG. 16-10** Effects of stress on fluid and electrolyte balance. *ACTH,* Adrenocorticotropic hormone; *ADH,* antidiuretic hormone; *CRH,* corticotropin-releasing hormone.

### Gerontologic Considerations: Fluid and Electrolytes

The older adult experiences normal physiologic changes that increase susceptibility to fluid and electrolyte imbalances. Structural changes to the kidneys and a decrease in the renal blood flow lead to decreased glomerular filtration rate and loss of the ability to concentrate urine and conserve water. Hormonal changes include a decrease in renin and aldosterone and an increase in ADH and ANP. The loss of subcutaneous tissue and thinning of the dermis lead to increased moisture lost through the skin and an inability to respond quickly to heat or cold.

Do not automatically attribute older patients' fluid and electrolyte problems to the natural processes of aging. Throughout this chapter are suggestions for adapting your assessment and nursing interventions when caring for the older adult.

## FLUID VOLUME IMBALANCES

Fluid and electrolyte imbalances occur to some degree in most patients with a major illness or injury because illness disrupts normal homeostatic mechanisms. Illness or disease directly causes some fluid and electrolyte imbalances (e.g., burns, heart failure). Other times therapeutic measures (e.g., colonoscopy preparation, diuretics) cause or contribute to imbalances. Perioperative patients are at risk for developing fluid and electrolyte imbalances because of fluid restrictions, blood or fluid loss, and the stress of surgery.

Fluid and electrolyte imbalances are commonly classified as *deficits* or *excesses.* Although each imbalance is discussed separately in this chapter, it is common for more than one imbalance to occur in the same patient. For example, a patient with prolonged nasogastric suction will lose sodium, potassium, hydrogen, and chloride ions. These imbalances may result in sodium and potassium deficiencies, a fluid volume deficit, and metabolic alkalosis caused by the loss of HCl acid.

ECF volume deficit *(hypovolemia)* and ECF volume excess *(hypervolemia)* are common clinical conditions. ECF volume imbalances are usually accompanied by one or more electrolyte imbalances, particularly changes in the serum sodium level.

## FLUID VOLUME DEFICIT

*Fluid volume deficit* can occur with abnormal loss of body fluids (e.g., diarrhea, vomiting, hemorrhage, polyuria), inadequate fluid intake, or a plasma to interstitial fluid shift. Though often used interchangeably, *fluid volume deficit* and *dehydration* are not the same. *Dehydration* refers to loss of pure water alone without a corresponding loss of sodium. Table 16-3 lists causes and clinical manifestations of fluid volume deficit.

### Interprofessional Care

Managing fluid volume deficit involves correcting the underlying cause and replacing both water and any needed electrolytes. Replacement therapy depends on the severity and type of volume loss. In mild losses, oral rehydration may be used. If the deficit is more severe, volume is replaced with blood products or balanced IV solutions, such as isotonic (0.9%) sodium chloride or lactated Ringer's solution. The choice of fluid depends on the cause and patient's electrolyte status. For rapid volume replacement, 0.9% sodium chloride is preferred. Blood is administered when volume loss is due to blood loss.

**TABLE 16-3 Extracellular Fluid Imbalances: Causes and Manifestations**

| ECF Volume Deficit | ECF Volume Excess |
|---|---|
| **Causes** | |
| • ↑ Insensible water loss or perspiration (high fever, heatstroke)<br>• Diabetes insipidus<br>• Osmotic diuresis<br>• Hemorrhage<br>• GI losses: vomiting, NG suction, diarrhea, fistula drainage<br>• Overuse of diuretics<br>• Inadequate fluid intake<br>• Third-space fluid shifts: burns, pancreatitis | • Excessive isotonic or hypotonic IV fluids<br>• Heart failure<br>• Renal failure<br>• Primary polydipsia<br>• SIADH<br>• Cushing syndrome<br>• Long-term use of corticosteroids |
| **Manifestations** | |
| • Restlessness, drowsiness, lethargy, confusion<br>• Thirst, dry mucous membranes<br>• Cold clammy skin<br>• Decreased skin turgor, ↓ capillary refill<br>• Postural hypotension, ↑ pulse, ↓ CVP<br>• ↓ Urine output, concentrated urine<br>• ↑ Respiratory rate<br>• Weakness, dizziness<br>• Weight loss<br>• Seizures, coma | • Headache, confusion, lethargy<br>• Peripheral edema<br>• Jugular venous distention<br>• S3 heart sound<br>• Bounding pulse, ↑ BP, ↑ CVP<br>• Polyuria (with normal renal function)<br>• Dyspnea, crackles, pulmonary edema<br>• Muscle spasms<br>• Weight gain<br>• Seizures, coma |

*CVP,* Central venous pressure; *ECF,* extracellular fluid; *SIADH,* syndrome of inappropriate antidiuretic hormone.

## FLUID VOLUME EXCESS

Fluid volume excess may result from excess intake of fluids, abnormal retention of fluids (e.g., heart failure, renal failure), or a shift of fluid from interstitial fluid into plasma fluid. Weight gain is the most consistent manifestation of fluid volume excess. Table 16-3 lists causes and manifestations of fluid volume excess.

### Interprofessional Care

Managing fluid volume excess involves treating the underlying cause and removing fluid without producing abnormal changes in the electrolyte composition or osmolality of ECF. Diuretics and fluid restriction are the primary forms of therapy. Some patients also need sodium restrictions. If the fluid excess leads to ascites or pleural effusion, an abdominal paracentesis or thoracentesis may be necessary.

## NURSING MANAGEMENT: FLUID VOLUME IMBALANCES

### Nursing Diagnoses

Nursing diagnoses and collaborative problems for the patient with a fluid imbalance include, but are not limited to, the following:

*ECF volume deficit:*

- Deficient fluid volume *related to* excess ECF losses or decreased fluid intake
- Decreased cardiac output *related to* excess ECF losses or decreased fluid intake

- Risk for impaired oral mucous membrane *related to* fluid volume deficit
- Potential complication: hypovolemic shock

*ECF volume excess:*

- Excess fluid volume *related to* increased water and/or sodium retention
- Impaired gas exchange *related to* water retention leading to pulmonary edema
- Risk for impaired skin integrity *related to* edema
- Activity intolerance *related to* increased water retention, fatigue, and weakness
- Disturbed body image *related to* altered body appearance secondary to edema
- Potential complications: pulmonary edema, ascites

## Nursing Implementation

**Daily Weights.** Daily weights are the most accurate measure of volume status. An increase of 1 kg (2.2 lb) is equal to 1000 mL (1 L) of fluid retention, provided the person has maintained usual dietary intake or has not been on NPO status. Obtain the weight under standardized conditions. Weigh the patient at the same time every day, wearing the same garments and on the same carefully calibrated scale. Remove excess bedding and empty all drainage bags before the weighing. If items are present that are not there every day, such as bulky dressings or tubes, note this along with the weight.

**Intake and Output.** Intake and output records provide valuable information about fluid and electrolyte problems. An accurately recorded intake and output will identify sources of excessive intake or fluid losses. Intake should include oral, IV, and tube feedings and retained irrigants. Output includes urine, excess perspiration, wound or tube drainage, vomitus, and diarrhea. Estimate fluid loss from wounds and perspiration. Note the amount and color of the urine and measure the urine specific gravity. Readings greater than 1.025 indicate concentrated urine, while readings less than 1.010 indicate dilute urine.

**Laboratory Findings.** Monitor laboratory results when available and calculate the serum osmolality. The patient with a fluid volume deficit often has increased BUN, sodium, and hematocrit levels with increased plasma and urine osmolality. With fluid volume excess, the patient will have decreased BUN, sodium, and hematocrit levels with decreased plasma and urine osmolality.

**Cardiovascular Care.** Monitor vital signs and perform a thorough cardiovascular assessment as needed. Changes in BP, central venous pressure, pulse force, and jugular venous distention reflect ECF volume imbalances. In fluid volume excess, the pulse is full, bounding, and not easily obliterated. Increased volume causes distended neck veins (jugular venous distention), increased central venous pressure, and high BP. Auscultate heart sounds, being alert for the presence of an S3.

In mild to moderate fluid volume deficit, sympathetic nervous system compensation increases the heart rate and results in peripheral vasoconstriction in an effort to maintain BP within normal limits. Pulses may be weak and thready. Assess for orthostatic changes. A change in position from lying to sitting or standing may elicit a decrease in BP or a further increase in the heart rate (orthostatic hypotension). In more severe deficits, hypotension may be present.

**Respiratory Care.** Monitor pulse oximetry and auscultate lung sounds as needed. ECF excess can result in pulmonary congestion and pulmonary edema, as increased hydrostatic pressure in the pulmonary vessels forces fluid into the alveoli. The patient will experience shortness of breath and moist crackles on auscultation. The patient with ECF deficit will demonstrate an increased respiratory rate because of decreased tissue perfusion and resultant hypoxia. Administer oxygen as ordered.

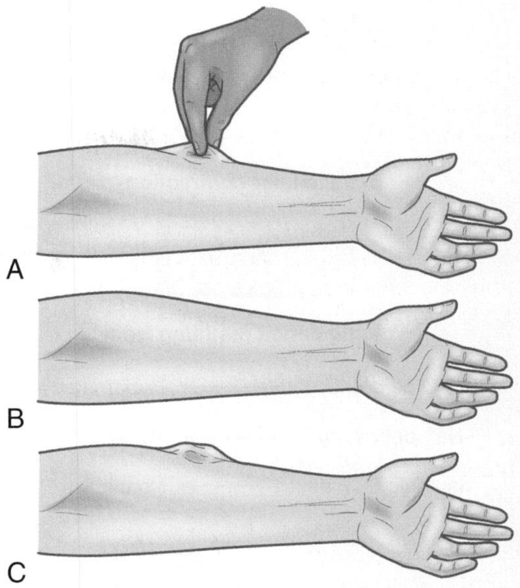


**FIG. 16-11** Assessment of skin turgor. **A** and **B,** When normal skin is pinched, it resumes shape in seconds. **C,** If the skin remains wrinkled for 20 to 30 seconds, the patient has poor skin turgor.

**Patient Safety.** The patient with fluid volume deficit is at risk for falls because of orthostatic hypotension, muscle weakness, and changes in level of consciousness. Assess level of consciousness, gait, and muscle strength. Implement fall precautions. If orthostatic hypotension is present, teach the patient to change positions slowly when rising from a bed or chair. Place alarm monitors on patients who are confused and try to get out of bed without assistance.

**Skin Care.** Examine the skin for turgor and mobility. Normally a fold of skin, when pinched, will readily move and, on release, rapidly return to its former position. In ECF volume deficit, skin turgor is diminished, and there is a lag in the pinched skinfold's return to its original state (referred to as *tenting*). Skin areas over the sternum, abdomen, and anterior forearm are the usual sites for evaluation of tissue turgor (Fig. 16-11). In older people, decreased skin turgor is less predictive of fluid deficit because of the loss of tissue elasticity.[3]

In mild fluid deficits, the skin may appear warm, dry, and wrinkled. These signs may be difficult to evaluate in the older adult because the patient's skin may be normally dry, wrinkled, and nonelastic. In more severe deficits, the skin may be cool and moist if there is vasoconstriction to compensate for the decreased fluid volume. Oral mucous membranes will be dry, the tongue may be furrowed, and the individual often complains of thirst. Routine oral care is critical for the comfort of a patient who is dehydrated or on a fluid restriction.

Edematous skin may feel cool because of fluid accumulation and a decrease in blood flow secondary to the pressure of the fluid. The fluid can stretch the skin, causing it to feel taut and hard. Assess edema by pressing with a thumb or forefinger over the edematous area. A grading scale is used to standardize the description if an indentation (ranging from 1+ [slight edema; 2-mm indentation] to 4+ [pitting edema; 8-mm indentation]) remains when pressure is released. Evaluate for edema in areas

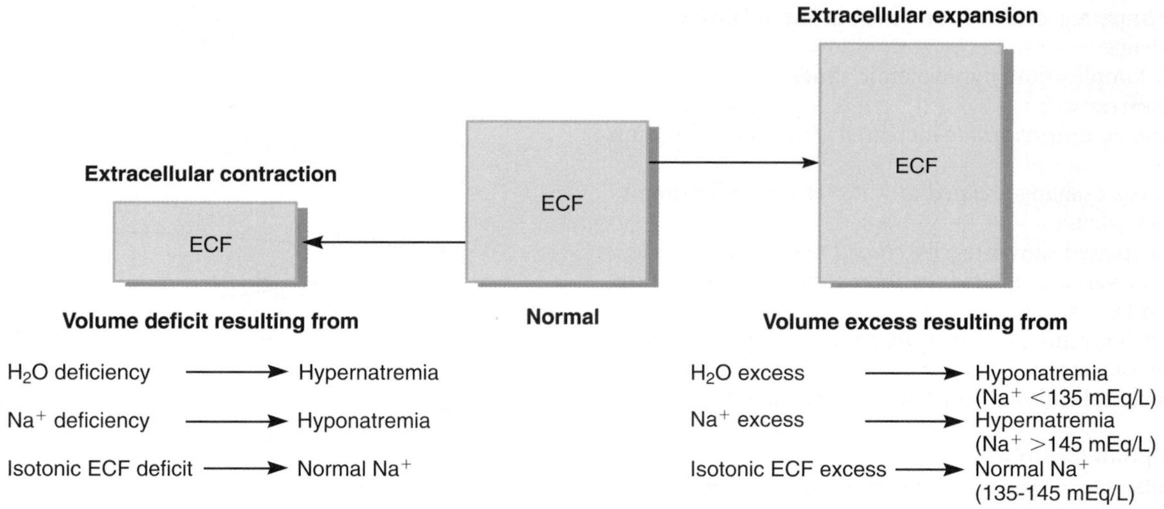


**FIG. 16-12** Differential assessment of extracellular fluid (ECF) volume.

where soft tissues overlie a bone, particularly the tibia, fibula, and sacrum.

Good skin care is important. Protect tissues from extremes of heat and cold, prolonged pressure, and trauma. Frequent skin care and changes in position will prevent skin breakdown. Elevate edematous extremities to promote venous return and fluid reabsorption. Dehydrated skin needs frequent care without the use of soap. Applying moisturizing creams or oils increases moisture retention and stimulates circulation.

◆ **Fluid Therapy.** Administer IV fluids as ordered. Carefully monitor the rates of infusion of IV fluid solutions, especially when large volumes of fluid are being given. This is especially true in patients with cardiac, renal, or neurologic problems.

In the presence of fluid volume deficit, you can use several interventions to maintain adequate oral intake. Assess the patient's ability to obtain adequate fluids independently, express thirst, and swallow effectively. Fluids should be easily accessible. Provide a variety of fluids that the patient likes. Serve fluids at a temperature preferred by the patient. Offer fluids every 1 to 2 hours and at select times, such as when administering medications. Remind the patient to finish all drinks.

If the patient is choosing to limit intake to decrease nocturia or incontinence, make it easier for the patient to reach the toilet when needed.[3] Assist those with physical limitations, such as arthritis, to open and hold containers. Involve the dietitian, speech therapist, or occupation therapist for help with patients with dysphagia or physical limitations.

## SODIUM IMBALANCES

Sodium, the main cation of ECF, plays a major role in maintaining the concentration and volume of ECF and influencing water distribution between ECF and ICF. Sodium has an important role in the generation and transmission of nerve impulses, muscle contractility, and regulation of acid-base balance.

The serum sodium level reflects the ratio of sodium to water, not necessarily the amount of sodium in the body. Changes in the serum sodium level can reflect a primary water imbalance, primary sodium imbalance, or combination of the two. Sodium imbalances are typically associated with imbalances in ECF volume (Figs. 16-12 and 16-13). Because sodium is the primary determinant of ECF osmolality, sodium imbalances are typically associated with parallel changes in osmolality.

The GI tract absorbs sodium from foods. Typically, daily intake of sodium far exceeds the body's daily requirements. Sodium leaves the body through urine, sweat, and feces. The

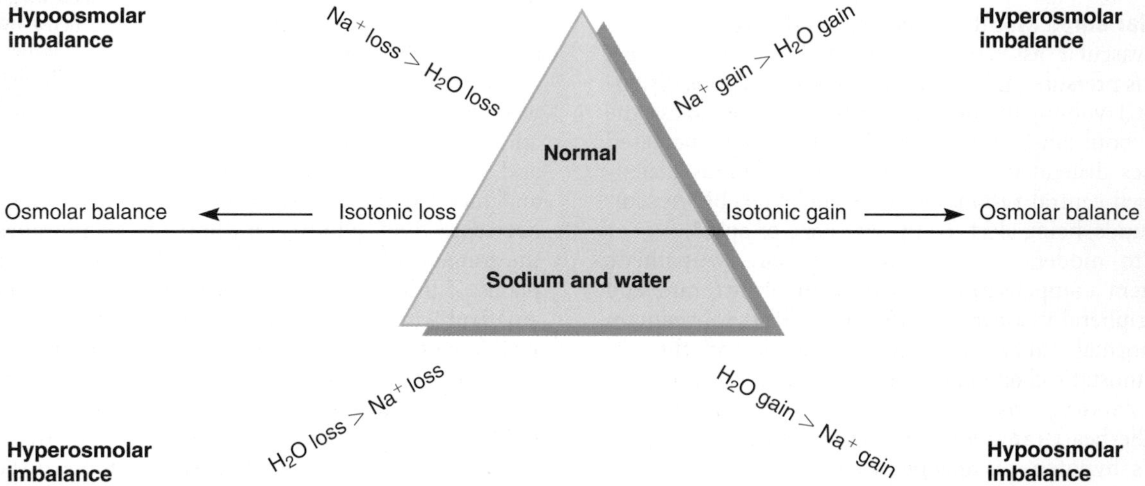


**FIG. 16-13** Isotonic gains and losses affect mainly the extracellular fluid (ECF) compartment with little or no water movement into the cells. Hypertonic imbalances cause water to move from inside the cell into ECF to dilute the concentrated sodium, causing cell shrinkage. Hypotonic imbalances cause water to move into the cell, causing cell swelling.

kidneys primarily regulate sodium balance. The kidneys control ECF sodium concentration by excreting or retaining water under the influence of ADH. Aldosterone plays a smaller role in sodium regulation by promoting sodium reabsorption from the renal tubules.

## HYPERNATREMIA

*Hypernatremia* (elevated serum sodium) may occur with inadequate water intake, excess water loss or, rarely, sodium gain. Because sodium is the major determinant of ECF osmolality, hypernatremia causes hyperosmolality. ECF hyperosmolality causes water to move out of the cells to restore equilibrium, leading to cellular dehydration. As discussed earlier, the primary protection against the development of hyperosmolality is thirst. Hypernatremia is not a problem in an alert person who has access to water, can sense thirst, and is able to swallow. Hypernatremia secondary to water deficiency is often the result of an impaired level of consciousness or an inability to obtain fluids.

Several clinical states can produce hypernatremia from water loss (Table 16-4). A deficiency in the synthesis or release of ADH from the posterior pituitary gland (central diabetes insipidus) or a decrease in kidney responsiveness to ADH (nephrogenic diabetes insipidus) can result in profound diuresis, producing a water deficit and hypernatremia. Hyperosmolality with osmotic diuresis can result from hyperglycemia associated with uncontrolled diabetes mellitus or administering concentrated hyperosmolar tube feedings.

Excess sodium intake with inadequate water intake can also lead to hypernatremia. Examples of sodium gain include IV administration of hypertonic saline or sodium bicarbonate, use of sodium-containing drugs, excessive oral intake of sodium (e.g., ingestion of seawater), and *primary aldosteronism* (hypersecretion of aldosterone) caused by a tumor of the adrenal glands.

### Clinical Manifestations

The manifestations of hypernatremia are primarily the result of water shifting out of cells into ECF with resultant dehydration and shrinkage of cells (Table 16-4). Dehydration of brain cells results in alterations in mental status, ranging from agitation, restlessness, confusion, and lethargy to coma.[3] If there is any accompanying ECF volume deficit, manifestations such as postural hypotension, tachycardia, and weakness occur.

**TABLE 16-4 Sodium Imbalances: Causes and Manifestations**

| Hypernatremia ($Na^+$ >145 mEq/L [mmol/L]) | Hyponatremia ($Na^+$ <135 mEq/L [mmol/L]) |
|---|---|
| **Causes** | |
| ***Excessive Sodium Intake*** | ***Excessive Sodium Loss*** |
| • IV fluids: hypertonic NaCl, excessive isotonic NaCl, IV sodium bicarbonate<br>• Hypertonic tube feedings without water supplements<br>• Near-drowning in salt water | • *GI losses:* diarrhea, vomiting, fistulas, NG suction<br>• *Renal losses:* diuretics, adrenal insufficiency, $Na^+$ wasting renal disease<br>• *Skin losses:* burns, wound drainage |
| ***Inadequate Water Intake*** | ***Inadequate Sodium Intake*** |
| • Unconscious or cognitively impaired individuals | • Fasting diets |
| ***Excessive Water Loss (↑ sodium concentration)*** | ***Excessive Water Gain (↓ sodium concentration)*** |
| • ↑ Insensible water loss (high fever, heatstroke, prolonged hyperventilation)<br>• Osmotic diuretic therapy<br>• Diarrhea | • Excessive hypotonic IV fluids<br>• Primary polydipsia |
| ***Diseases*** | ***Diseases*** |
| • Diabetes insipidus<br>• Primary hyperaldosteronism<br>• Cushing syndrome<br>• Uncontrolled diabetes mellitus | • SIADH<br>• Heart failure<br>• Primary hypoaldosteronism<br>• Cirrhosis |
| **Manifestations** | |
| ***Hypernatremia With Decreased ECF Volume*** | ***Hyponatremia With Decreased ECF Volume*** |
| • Restlessness, agitation, lethargy, seizures, coma<br>• Intense thirst, dry swollen tongue, sticky mucous membranes<br>• Postural hypotension, ↓ CVP, weight loss, ↑ pulse<br>• Weakness, muscle cramps | • Irritability, apprehension, confusion, dizziness, personality changes, tremors, seizures, coma<br>• Dry mucous membranes<br>• Postural hypotension, ↓ CVP, ↓ jugular venous filling, ↑ pulse, thready pulse<br>• Cold and clammy skin |
| ***Hypernatremia With Normal or Increased ECF Volume*** | ***Hyponatremia With Normal or Increased ECF Volume*** |
| • Restlessness, agitation, twitching, seizures, coma<br>• Intense thirst, flushed skin<br>• Weight gain, peripheral and pulmonary edema, ↑ BP, ↑ CVP | • Headache, apathy, confusion, muscle spasms, seizures, coma<br>• Nausea, vomiting, diarrhea, abdominal cramps<br>• Weight gain, ↑ BP, ↑ CVP |

*CVP,* Central venous pressure; *ECF,* extracellular fluid; *SIADH,* syndrome of inappropriate antidiuretic hormone.

## NURSING AND INTERPROFESSIONAL MANAGEMENT: HYPERNATREMIA

### Nursing Diagnoses

Nursing diagnoses and collaborative problems for the patient with hypernatremia include, but are not limited to, the following:

- Risk for electrolyte imbalance *related to* inadequate water intake, excess sodium intake and/or water loss injury *related to* altered sensorium and seizures
- Risk for fluid volume deficit *related to* inadequate water intake and/or water loss
- Risk for injury *related to* altered sensorium and seizures
- Potential complications: seizures and coma

### Nursing Implementation

Managing hypernatremia depends on the underlying cause and the patient's volume status. In primary water deficit, fluid replacement is provided either orally or IV with isotonic such as 0.9% sodium chloride.[2] If the problem is sodium excess, expect diluting the high sodium concentration with sodium-free IV fluids, such as 5% dextrose in water, and promoting sodium excretion with diuretics. Dietary sodium intake is often restricted. If the patient has an altered sensorium or is having seizures, initiate seizure precautions.

Monitor serum sodium levels, serum osmolality, and the patient's response to therapy. The serum sodium level should not decrease by more than 8 to 15 mEq/L in an 8-hour period.[2] Quickly reducing levels can cause a rapid shift of water back into the cells, resulting in cerebral edema and neurologic complications. This risk is greatest in the patient who developed hypernatremia over several days or longer.

## HYPONATREMIA

*Hyponatremia* (low serum sodium) may result from a loss of sodium-containing fluids, water excess in relation to the amount of sodium (dilutional hyponatremia), or a combination of both (Table 16-4). Hyponatremia is usually associated with ECF hypoosmolality from the excess water. To restore balance, fluid shifts out of the ECF and into the cells, leading to cellular edema.

Common causes of hyponatremia from loss of sodium-rich body fluids include draining wounds, diarrhea, vomiting, and primary adrenal insufficiency. Inappropriate use of sodium-free or hypotonic IV fluids causes hyponatremia from water excess. This may occur in patients after surgery or major trauma or administering fluids to patients with renal failure. Patients with psychiatric disorders may have an excessive water intake. Syndrome of inappropriate antidiuretic hormone secretion (SIADH) results in dilutional hyponatremia caused by abnormal retention of water. See Chapter 49 for a discussion of the causes of SIADH.

### Clinical Manifestations

The manifestations of hyponatremia are due to cellular swelling and first appear in the central nervous system (CNS). Mild hyponatremia has minor, nonspecific neurologic symptoms including headache, irritability, and difficulty concentrating. More severe hyponatremia can cause confusion, vomiting, seizures, and even coma. If hyponatremia is severe and develops rapidly, irreversible neurologic damage or death from brain herniation can occur.[4]

## ◆ NURSING AND INTERPROFESSIONAL MANAGEMENT: HYPONATREMIA

### ◆ Nursing Diagnoses

Nursing diagnoses and collaborative problems for the patient with hyponatremia include, but are not limited to, the following:

- Risk for electrolyte imbalance *related to* excess sodium loss and/or excess water intake or retention
- Risk for injury *related to* altered sensorium and decreased level of consciousness
- Risk for acute confusion *related to* electrolyte imbalance
- Potential complication: severe neurologic changes

### ◆ Nursing Implementation

Managing hyponatremia from fluid loss includes replacing fluid using isotonic sodium-containing solutions, encouraging oral intake, and withholding all diuretics.[2] In mild hyponatremia caused by water excess, fluid restriction is often the only treatment. The aim of the restriction is 500 mL less than the previous 24-hour urine output.[4] Loop diuretics and demeclocycline may be given. If hyponatremia is acute or more serious, small amounts of IV hypertonic saline solution (3% sodium chloride) can restore the serum sodium level while the body is returning to a normal water balance.

Vasopressor receptor antagonists (drugs that block the activity of ADH), are used to treat patients who cannot tolerate fluid restrictions or have more severe symptoms.[4] These drugs include conivaptan (Vaprisol) and tolvaptan (Samsca). Conivaptan is given IV to hospitalized patients with severe hyponatremia from water excess. Tolvaptan is an oral preparation used to treat hyponatremia from heart failure and SIADH.

Monitor serum sodium levels and the patient's response to therapy to avoid rapid or overcorrection. The level should not increase by more than 8 to 12 mEq/L in the first 24 hours.[4] Quickly increasing levels of sodium can cause osmotic demyelination syndrome with permanent damage to nerve cells in the brain. An accurate urine output record is essential. The patient may need a urinary catheter placed if unable to assist with monitoring output. If the patient has an altered sensorium or is having seizures, initiate seizure precautions.

## POTASSIUM IMBALANCES

Potassium is the major ICF cation, with 98% of the body potassium being intracellular. For example, potassium concentration within muscle cells is around 140 mEq/L; potassium concentration in ECF is 3.5 to 5.0 mEq/L. The sodium-potassium pump in cell membranes maintains this concentration difference by pumping potassium into the cell and sodium out. Insulin helps by stimulating the sodium-potassium pump.

Because the ratio of ECF potassium to ICF potassium is the major factor in the resting membrane potential of nerve and muscle cells, neuromuscular and cardiac function are often affected by potassium imbalances. Potassium is involved with regulating intracellular osmolality and promoting cellular growth. It is required for glycogen to be deposited in muscle and liver cells. Potassium also plays a role in acid-base balance (discussed in the section on Acid-Base Regulation later in this chapter).

Diet is the source of potassium. The typical Western diet contains roughly 50 to 100 mEq of potassium daily, mainly from protein-rich foods and many fruits and vegetables. Many salt substitutes used in low-sodium diets contain substantial potassium. Patients may receive potassium from parenteral sources, including IV fluids; transfusions of stored, hemolyzed blood; and medications (e.g., potassium penicillin).

The kidneys are the primary route for potassium loss, eliminating about 90% of the daily potassium intake. Potassium excretion depends on the serum potassium level, urine output, and renal function. When serum potassium is high, urine potassium excretion increases and when serum levels are low, excretion decreases. Large urine output can cause excess potassium loss. Impaired kidney function can cause potassium retention. There is an inverse relationship between sodium and potassium reabsorption in the kidneys. Factors that cause sodium retention (e.g., low blood volume, hyponatremia, aldosterone secretion) cause potassium excretion.

## HYPERKALEMIA

*Hyperkalemia* (high serum potassium) may result from impaired renal excretion, a shift of potassium from ICF to ECF, a massive intake of potassium, or a combination of these factors (Table 16-5). The most common cause of hyperkalemia is renal failure. Adrenal insufficiency with a subsequent aldosterone deficiency leads to potassium retention. Factors that cause potassium to move from ICF to ECF include acidosis, massive cell destruction (as in burn or crush injury, tumor lysis, severe infections), and intense exercise. In metabolic acidosis, potassium ions shift

**TABLE 16-5 Potassium Imbalances: Causes and Manifestations**

| Hyperkalemia ($K^+$ >5.0 mEq/L [mmol/L]) | Hypokalemia ($K^+$ <3.5 mEq/L [mmol/L]) |
|---|---|
| **Causes** | |
| ***Excess Potassium Intake*** | ***Potassium Loss*** |
| • Excessive or rapid parenteral administration<br>• Potassium-containing drugs (e.g., potassium penicillin)<br>• Potassium-containing salt substitute | • *GI losses:* diarrhea, vomiting, fistulas, NG suction, ileostomy drainage<br>• *Renal losses:* diuretics, hyperaldosteronism, magnesium depletion<br>• *Skin losses:* diaphoresis<br>• Dialysis |
| ***Shift of Potassium Out of Cells*** | ***Shift of Potassium Into Cells*** |
| • Acidosis<br>• Tissue catabolism (e.g., fever, crush injury, sepsis, burns)<br>• Intense exercise<br>• Tumor lysis syndrome | • Increased insulin release (e.g., IV dextrose load)<br>• Insulin therapy (e.g., with diabetic ketoacidosis)<br>• Alkalosis<br>• ↑ Epinephrine (e.g., stress) |
| ***Failure to Eliminate Potassium*** | ***Lack of Potassium Intake*** |
| • Renal disease<br>• Adrenal insufficiency<br>• *Medications:* Angiotensin II receptor blockers, ACE inhibitors, heparin, potassium-sparing diuretics, NSAIDs | • Starvation<br>• Diet low in potassium<br>• Failure to include potassium in parenteral fluids if NPO |
| **Clinical Manifestations** | |
| • Fatigue, irritability<br>• Muscle weakness, cramps<br>• Loss of muscle tone<br>• Paresthesias, decreased reflexes<br>• Abdominal cramping, diarrhea, vomiting<br>• Confusion<br>• Irregular pulse<br>• Tetany | • Fatigue<br>• Muscle weakness, leg cramps<br>• Soft, flabby muscles<br>• Paresthesias, decreased reflexes<br>• Constipation, nausea, paralytic ileus<br>• Shallow respirations<br>• Weak, irregular pulse<br>• Hyperglycemia |
| ***ECG Changes*** | ***ECG Changes*** |
| • Tall, peaked T wave<br>• Prolonged PR interval<br>• ST segment depression<br>• Widening QRS<br>• Loss of P wave<br>• Ventricular fibrillation<br>• Ventricular standstill | • Flattened T wave<br>• Presence of U wave<br>• ST segment depression<br>• Prolonged QRS<br>• Peaked P wave<br>• Ventricular dysrhythmias<br>• First- and second-degree heart block |

*ACE,* Angiotensin-converting enzyme.

from ICF to ECF in exchange for hydrogen ions moving into the cell.

Digoxin-like drugs and β-adrenergic blockers (e.g., propranolol) can impair entry of potassium into cells, resulting in a higher ECF potassium concentration. Several drugs, such as heparin, potassium-sparing diuretics, angiotensin II receptor blockers (e.g., losartan), and angiotensin-converting enzyme (ACE) inhibitors (e.g., lisinopril), can contribute to hyperkalemia by reducing the kidney's ability to excrete potassium.[5]

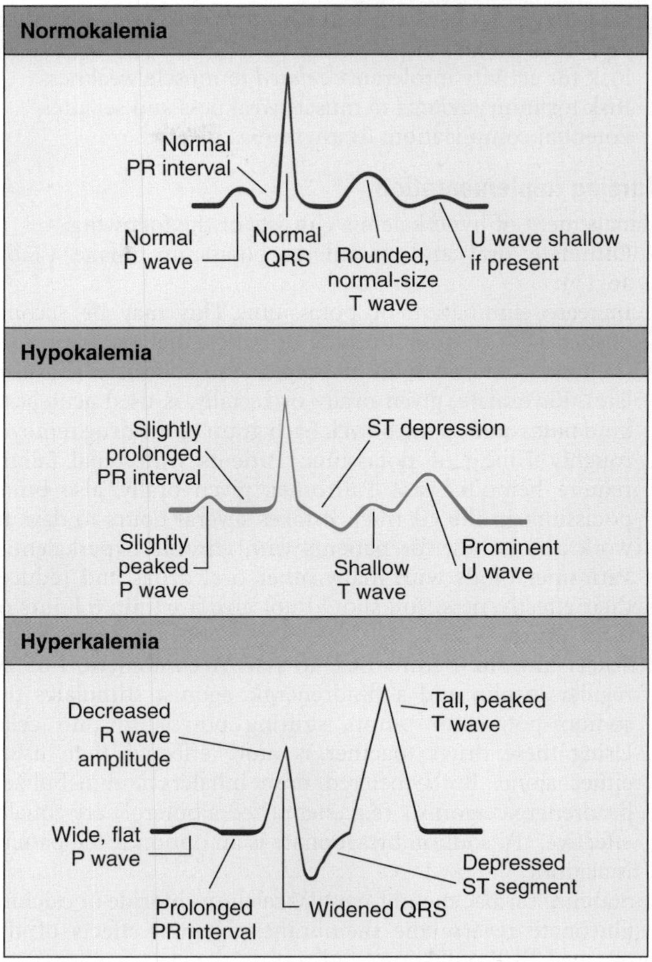


**FIG. 16-14** ECG changes associated with alterations in potassium status.

### Clinical Manifestations

The increased potassium concentration outside the cell changes the normal ECF and ICF ratio, resulting in increased cell excitability and changes in impulse transmission to the nerves and muscles. The most clinically significant problems are the disturbances in cardiac conduction. The initial finding is tall, peaked T waves. As potassium increases, cardiac depolarization decreases, leading to loss of P waves, a prolonged PR interval, ST segment depression, and widening QRS complex (Fig. 16-14). Heart block, ventricular fibrillation, or cardiac standstill may occur. Elevated potassium may cause failure to capture in a patient who has a pacemaker.[6]

The patient may experience fatigue, confusion, tetany, muscle cramps, paresthesias, and weakness. As potassium increases, loss of muscle tone and weakness or paralysis of other skeletal muscles, including the respiratory muscles can occur, leading to respiratory arrest. Abdominal cramping, vomiting, and diarrhea occur from hyperactivity of gastrointestinal smooth muscles.

## ❖ NURSING AND INTERPROFESSIONAL MANAGEMENT: HYPERKALEMIA

### ◆ Nursing Diagnoses

Nursing diagnoses and collaborative problems for the patient with hyperkalemia include, but are not limited to, the following.

- Risk for electrolyte imbalance *related to* excessive retention or cellular release of potassium
- Risk for activity intolerance *related to* muscle weakness
- Risk for injury *related to* muscle weakness and seizures
- Potential complication: dysrhythmias

### ◆ Nursing Implementation

Management of hyperkalemia consists of the following:

1. Eliminate oral and parenteral potassium intake (Table 46-11).
2. Increase elimination of potassium. This may be accomplished with loop or thiazide diuretics, dialysis, patiromer (Veltassa), and/or sodium polystyrene sulfonate (Kayexalate). Kayexalate, given orally or rectally, is used acutely to bind potassium in the bowel. Each gram of the drug removes roughly 1 mEq of potassium. Patients with renal failure require hemodialysis.[6] Patiromer, given orally, also binds potassium in the GI tract. It takes several hours to days to work and is best for patients with chronic hyperkalemia. Patiromer binds with many other oral drugs and reduces their effectiveness. You should not give it within 6 hours of other drugs.
3. Force potassium from ECF to ICF. A combination of IV regular insulin and a β-adrenergic agonist stimulates the sodium-potassium pump, shifting potassium into cells. Using these drugs together is more effective than using either alone. Both metered dose inhalers and nebulized β-adrenergic agonists (e.g., nebulized albuterol) are equally effective.[5] IV sodium bicarbonate is an option if the patient is acidotic.
4. Stabilize cardiac membranes. IV calcium chloride or calcium gluconate reverse the membrane potential effects of the elevated ECF potassium and restore the electrical gradient. This protects the patient from life-threatening dysrhythmias.[6]

When the potassium elevation is mild and the kidneys are functioning, it may be sufficient to (1) withhold potassium from the diet and IV sources and (2) increase renal potassium elimination by administering fluids and loop or thiazide diuretics. Patients with severe hyperkalemia or symptomatic patients should receive one of the treatments to force potassium into cells.

Provide continuous ECG monitoring of all patients with clinically significant hyperkalemia to detect dysrhythmias and monitor the effects of therapy. The patient experiencing dangerous cardiac dysrhythmias should receive IV calcium immediately. Monitor BP because rapidly administering calcium can cause hypotension. When administering insulin, monitor for hypoglycemia and give glucose as needed.

## HYPOKALEMIA

Hypokalemia (low serum potassium) can result from an increased loss of potassium, an increased shift of potassium from ECF to ICF, or rarely from deficient dietary potassium intake. The most common causes of hypokalemia are abnormal losses from either the kidneys or GI tract. GI tract losses are associated with diarrhea, laxative misuse, vomiting, and ileostomy drainage. Renal losses occur when a patient is diuresing or has a low magnesium level. Low plasma magnesium levels stimulate renin and aldosterone release, resulting in potassium excretion.

Among the factors causing potassium to move from ECF to ICF are insulin therapy, especially in conjunction with diabetic ketoacidosis, and β-adrenergic stimulation (catecholamine release in stress, coronary ischemia). Alkalosis can cause a shift of potassium into cells in exchange for hydrogen, lowering potassium in ECF and causing symptomatic hypokalemia.

### Clinical Manifestations

Hypokalemia alters the resting membrane potential, resulting in hyperpolarization (an increased negative charge within the cell) and impaired muscle contraction. Therefore the manifestations of hypokalemia involve changes in cardiac and muscle function (Table 16-5).

The most serious clinical problems are cardiac changes, including impaired repolarization, resulting in a flattened T wave, depressed ST segment, and the presence of a U wave. The P waves peak and the QRS complex is prolonged (Fig. 16-14). There is an increased incidence of heart block and potentially lethal ventricular dysrhythmias.

As with hyperkalemia, skeletal muscle weakness and paresthesias may occur. Severe hypokalemia can cause paralysis. This usually involves the extremities but can involve the respiratory muscles, leading to shallow respirations and respiratory arrest. Alterations in smooth muscle function may lead to decreased GI motility (e.g., constipation, paralytic ileus). Finally, hypokalemia impairs insulin secretion, leading to glucose intolerance and hyperglycemia.

## ❖ NURSING AND INTERPROFESSIONAL MANAGEMENT: HYPOKALEMIA

### ◆ Nursing Diagnoses

Nursing diagnoses and collaborative problems for the patient with hypokalemia include, but are not limited to, the following:

- Risk for electrolyte imbalance *related to* excess potassium loss
- Risk for activity intolerance *related to* muscle weakness
- Risk for injury *related to* muscle weakness and hyporeflexia
- Potential complication: dysrhythmias

### ◆ Nursing Implementation

Managing hypokalemia consists of oral or IV potassium chloride (KCl) supplements and increased dietary intake of potassium. Consuming potassium-rich foods can usually correct mild hypokalemia. Clinically significant hypokalemia requires administering oral or IV KCl.

**! SAFETY ALERT Administering IV KCl**

- IV KCl must always be diluted and never given in concentrated amounts.
- Never give KCl via IV push or as a bolus.
- Invert IV bags containing KCl several times to ensure even distribution in the bag.
- Do not add KCl to a hanging IV bag to prevent giving a bolus dose.

IV KCl infusion rates should not exceed 10 mEq/hr unless the patient is in a critical care setting with continuous ECG monitoring and central line access for administration.[5] IV KCl must be given by infusion pump to ensure correct administration rate. Because KCl is irritating to the vein, assess IV sites at least hourly for phlebitis and infiltration. Infiltration can cause necrosis and sloughing of the surrounding tissue.

**TABLE 16-6 Patient & Caregiver Teaching**

***Prevention of Hypokalemia***

*Include the following instructions when teaching at-risk patients how to prevent hypokalemia:*

1. For all patients at risk:
   - Report the signs and symptoms of hypokalemia (Table 16-5) to the HCP.
   - Have serum potassium levels checked regularly.
   - Regularly include foods high in potassium in your diet (see Table 46-11).
   - Consume alcohol in moderation only.
   - Avoid consuming large amounts of licorice.
2. For patients taking oral potassium supplements:
   - Take the medication as prescribed to prevent overdosing.
   - Take the supplement with a full glass of water. Do not crush or chew tablets.

Patients who are critically ill and those at risk for hypokalemia should have continuous ECG monitoring to detect cardiac changes. Monitor serum potassium levels and urine output as appropriate.

**CHECK YOUR PRACTICE**

You are taking care of a 78-yr-old female patient with heart failure. She is taking furosemide (Lasix) and digitalis.

- What should you be alert for in a patient who takes both of these drugs?

KCl is usually given only if the urine output is at least 0.5 mL/kg of body weight per hour. Because patients on digoxin therapy have an increased risk of toxicity if their serum potassium level is low, monitor the patient for digitalis toxicity.

Teach patients ways to prevent hypokalemia (Table 16-6). Patients at risk for hypokalemia should have regular serum potassium levels monitored. Teach the patient taking digitalis to report signs and symptoms of digoxin toxicity immediately to the HCP.

## CALCIUM IMBALANCES

Calcium is necessary for many metabolic processes. It is the major cation in bones and teeth. Calcium plays a role in blood clotting, transmission of nerve impulses, myocardial contractions, and muscle contractions. The source of calcium is dietary intake. Calcium absorption requires the active form of vitamin D. Vitamin D is obtained from foods or made in the skin by the action of sunlight on cholesterol.

The total body content of calcium is about 1200 g. The bones contain 99% of the body's calcium; the remainder is in plasma and body cells. Of the calcium in plasma, 50% is bound to plasma proteins, primarily albumin; 40% is in a free or ionized form, and the remainder is found bound with phosphate, citrate, or carbonate. The ionized or free calcium is biologically active. The serum pH influences how much calcium is ionized or bound to albumin. A decreased plasma pH (acidosis) decreases calcium binding to albumin, leading to more ionized calcium. An increased plasma pH (alkalosis) increases calcium binding, leading to decreased ionized calcium.

Serum calcium levels reflect the total level of all forms of plasma calcium. Serum albumin levels affect the interpretation of total calcium levels. Total calcium values increase or decrease directly with serum albumin levels. Ionized calcium levels are measured using special laboratory techniques or calculated using a formula. Albumin levels do not affect ionized calcium levels.

Parathyroid hormone (PTH) and calcitonin regulate calcium levels. Since the bones serve as a readily available store of calcium, the body is usually able to maintain normal serum calcium levels by regulating the movement of calcium into or out of the bone. Low serum calcium levels stimulate the parathyroid glands to produce and release PTH. PTH increases bone resorption (movement of calcium out of bones), increases GI absorption of calcium, and increases renal tubule reabsorption of calcium. High serum calcium levels stimulate the release of calcitonin from the thyroid gland. Calcitonin has the opposite effect of PTH. It lowers the serum calcium level by increasing calcium deposition into bone, increasing renal calcium excretion, and decreasing GI absorption.

### HYPERCALCEMIA

*Hypercalcemia* (high serum calcium) is caused by hyperparathyroidism in about two thirds of persons. Malignancies, especially from hematologic, breast, and lung cancers, cause the remaining third. Malignancies lead to hypercalcemia through bone destruction from tumor invasion or tumor secretion of parathyroid-related proteins, which stimulate calcium release from bones.[7] More rare causes include thiazide diuretic use, prolonged immobilization, and increased calcium intake (e.g., use of calcium-containing antacids).

Excess calcium acts like a sedative, leading to reduced excitability of muscles and nerves. Neurologic manifestations begin with fatigue, lethargy, weakness, and confusion and progress to hallucinations, seizures, and coma. Disturbances in cardiac conduction can lead to dysrhythmias, including heart block and ventricular tachycardia. Table 16-7 lists the causes and manifestations of hypercalcemia.

### NURSING AND INTERPROFESSIONAL MANAGEMENT: HYPERCALCEMIA

#### Nursing Diagnoses

Nursing diagnoses and collaborative problems for the patient with hypercalcemia include, but are not limited to, the following:

- Risk for electrolyte imbalance *related to* excessive bone destruction
- Risk for activity intolerance *related to* generalized muscle weakness
- Risk for injury *related to* neuromuscular and sensorium changes
- Potential complication: dysrhythmias

#### Nursing Implementation

Management depends on the degree of hypercalcemia, patient's condition, and the underlying cause. Patients with mild hypercalcemia should stop any medications related to hypercalcemia, start a diet low in calcium, increase weight-bearing activity, and maintain adequate hydration. The patient must drink 3000 to 4000 mL of fluid daily to promote the renal excretion of calcium and decrease the chance of kidney stone formation. Fluids that promote urine acidity (cranberry or prune juice) will help to prevent formation of stones.

Managing severe hypercalcemia includes administering saline, a bisphosphonate, and calcitonin. Begin with hydrating

**TABLE 16-7 Calcium Imbalances: Causes and Manifestations**

| Hypercalcemia ($Ca^{2+}$ >10.2 mg/dL [2.55 mmol/L]) | Hypocalcemia ($Ca^{2+}$ <8.6 mg/dL [2.15 mmol/L]) |
|---|---|
| **Causes** | |
| ***Increased Total Calcium*** | ***Decreased Total Calcium*** |
| • Hyperparathyroidism | • Primary hypoparathyroidism |
| • Hematologic malignancy | • Renal insufficiency |
| • Malignancies with bone metastasis | • Acute pancreatitis |
| • Prolonged immobilization | • Elevated phosphorus |
| • Vitamin A or D overdose | • Vitamin D deficiency, malnutrition |
| • Paget's disease | • Magnesium deficiency |
| • Adrenal insufficiency | • Bisphosphonates |
| • Thyrotoxicosis | • Tumor lysis syndrome |
| • Thiazide diuretics | • Loop diuretics |
| • Milk-alkali syndrome | • Chronic alcoholism |
| • Calcium-containing antacids | • Diarrhea |
| • *Mycobacterium* infection | • ↓ Serum albumin |
| ***Increased Ionized Calcium*** | ***Decreased Ionized Calcium*** |
| • Acidosis | • Alkalosis |
| | • Excess administration of citrated blood |
| **Manifestations** | |
| • Lethargy, weakness, fatigue | • Weakness, fatigue |
| • Decreased memory | • Depression, irritability, confusion |
| • Depressed reflexes | • Hyperreflexia, muscle cramps |
| • ↑ BP | • ↓ BP |
| • Confusion, psychosis | • Numbness and tingling in extremities and region around mouth |
| • Anorexia, nausea, vomiting | • Chvostek's sign |
| • Bone pain, fractures | • Trousseau's sign |
| • Polyuria, dehydration | • Laryngeal and bronchial spasms |
| • Nephrolithiasis | • Tetany, seizures |
| • Seizures, coma | |
| ***ECG Changes*** | ***ECG Changes*** |
| • Shortened ST segment | • Elongation of ST segment |
| • Shortened QT interval | • Prolonged QT interval |
| • Ventricular dysrhythmias | • Ventricular tachycardia |
| • Increased digitalis effect | |

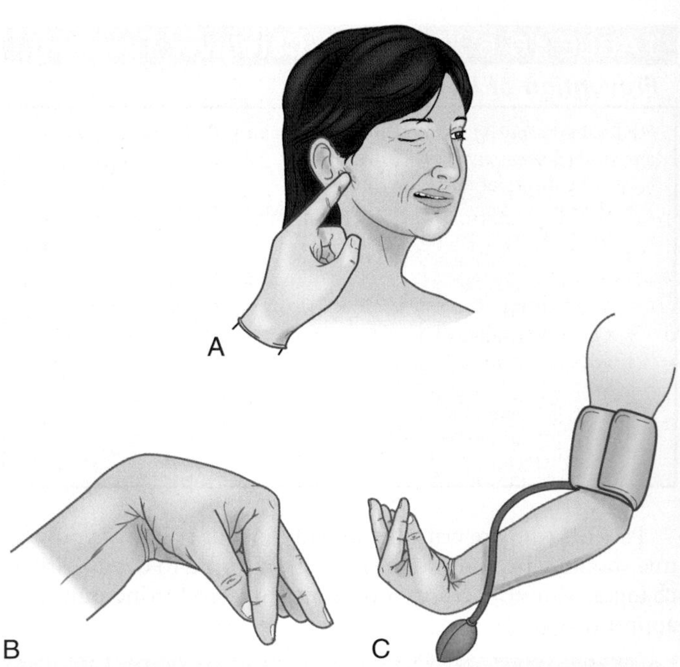


**FIG. 16-15** Tests for hypocalcemia. **A,** Chvostek's sign is contraction of facial muscles in response to a light tap over the facial nerve in front of the ear. **B,** Trousseau's sign is a carpal spasm induced by **C,** inflating a BP cuff above the systolic pressure for a few minutes.

the patient with IV isotonic saline to maintain a urine output of 100 to 150 mL per hour.[8] IV saline therapy requires careful monitoring. Fluid overload can occur in patients who cannot excrete the excess sodium because of impaired renal function. Bisphosphonates (e.g., pamidronate, zoledronic acid) are the most effective agents in treating hypercalcemia, particularly when caused by a malignancy.[7] They interfere with the activity of osteoclasts, cells that break down bone. Because it takes 2 to 4 days for bisphosphonates to achieve maximum effect, patients receive IM or SC calcitonin for an immediate effect. Calcitonin rapidly increases renal calcium excretion. However, therapy is only effective for a few days and may cause tachycardia. Dialysis is an option in life-threatening situations.

## HYPOCALCEMIA

*Hypocalcemia* (low serum calcium) can result from any condition associated with PTH deficiency. This may occur with surgical removal of a portion of or injury to the parathyroid glands during thyroid or neck surgery or with neck radiation. The patient who receives multiple blood transfusions can become hypocalcemic because the citrate used to anticoagulate the blood binds with calcium, decreasing ionized calcium levels. Sudden alkalosis may result in symptomatic hypocalcemia despite a normal total serum calcium level. The high pH increases calcium binding to protein, decreasing the amount of ionized calcium. Table 16-7 lists causes and manifestations of hypocalcemia.

Low ionized calcium levels decrease the threshold for activating the sodium channels that cause cell membrane depolarization. This results in increased nerve excitability and sustained muscle contraction, or *tetany.* Clinical signs of tetany include Chvostek's sign and Trousseau's sign. *Chvostek's sign* is contraction of facial muscles in response to a tap over the facial nerve in front of the ear (Fig. 16-15, *A*). *Trousseau's sign* refers to carpal spasms induced by inflating a BP cuff on the arm (Fig. 16-15, *B* and *C*). When the cuff is inflated above the systolic pressure, carpal spasms occur within 3 minutes if hypocalcemia is present. Other manifestations of tetany are laryngeal stridor, dysphagia, paresthesia, and numbness and tingling around the mouth or in the extremities. Cardiac effects of hypocalcemia include decreased cardiac contractility and ECG changes. A prolonged QT interval may develop into ventricular tachycardia.

## NURSING AND INTERPROFESSIONAL MANAGEMENT: HYPOCALCEMIA

### Nursing Diagnoses

Nursing diagnoses and collaborative problems for the patient with hypocalcemia include, but are not limited to, the following:

- Risk for electrolyte imbalance *related to* decreased PTH level
- Ineffective breathing pattern *related to* laryngospasm
- Acute pain *related to* sustained muscle contractions
- Risk for injury *related to* tetany and seizures
- Potential complications: fracture, respiratory arrest

### Nursing Implementation

Managing hypocalcemia depends on the underlying cause and the presence of symptoms. Treating mild or asymptomatic hypocalcemia involves a diet high in calcium-rich foods and calcium and vitamin D supplementation. Symptomatic hypocalcemia is treated with IV calcium gluconate.[9] Measures to promote $CO_2$ retention, such as breathing into a paper bag or sedating the patient, can control muscle spasm and other symptoms of tetany until the calcium level is corrected. Patients taking loop diuretics may need to change to thiazide diuretics to decrease urinary calcium excretion. Closely observe any patient who had thyroid or neck surgery in the immediate postoperative period for manifestations of hypocalcemia because of the proximity of the surgery to the parathyroid glands. Adequately treat pain and anxiety because hyperventilation-induced respiratory alkalosis can precipitate hypocalcemic symptoms.

## PHOSPHATE IMBALANCES

Phosphorus is the primary anion in ICF and the second most abundant element in the body after calcium. Most phosphorus is in bones and teeth as calcium phosphate. The remaining phosphorus is metabolically active and essential to the function of muscle, red blood cells, and the nervous system. It is involved in the acid-base buffering system; the mitochondrial formation of ATP; cellular uptake and use of glucose; and carbohydrate, protein, and fat metabolism.

PTH maintains serum phosphorus levels and balance. Proper phosphate balance requires adequate renal functioning because the kidneys are the major route of phosphate excretion. When the phosphate level in the glomerular filtrate falls below normal or PTH levels are low, the kidneys reabsorb additional phosphorus. A reciprocal relationship exists between phosphorus and calcium. This means a low serum calcium level stimulates the release of PTH, decreasing reabsorption of phosphorus and lowering phosphorus levels.

## HYPERPHOSPHATEMIA

*Hyperphosphatemia* (high serum phosphate) is common in patients with acute kidney injury or chronic kidney disease, which alters the kidney's ability to excrete phosphate. Other causes include excess phosphate intake from the use of phosphate-containing laxatives or enemas or a shift of phosphate from ICF to ECF. This may occur in patients with tumor lysis syndrome or rhabdomyolysis. Hypoparathyroidism and Vitamin D intoxication cause increased kidney phosphate reabsorption. Table 16-8 summarizes causes and clinical manifestations of hyperphosphatemia.

Hyperphosphatemia is often asymptomatic unless calcium binds with phosphate, leading to manifestations of hypocalcemia.[8] These manifestations include tetany, muscle cramps, paresthesias, and seizures. Long term, increased phosphate levels result in the development of calcified deposits outside of the bones. These calcium deposits can be found in soft tissues such as joints, arteries, skin, corneas, and kidneys and produce organ dysfunction, notably renal failure.

Managing hyperphosphatemia involves identifying and treating the underlying cause. Intake of foods and fluids high in phosphorus (e.g., dairy products) should be restricted. Oral phosphate-binding agents (e.g., calcium carbonate) limit intestinal phosphate absorption and increase phosphate secretion in the intestine. With severe hyperphosphatemia, hemodialysis may be used to rapidly decrease levels. Volume expansion and forced diuresis with a loop diuretic may increase phosphate excretion. If hypocalcemia is present, institute measures to correct calcium levels. See Chapter 46 for more information regarding treating hyperphosphatemia associated with kidney disease.

**TABLE 16-8 Phosphate Imbalances: Causes and Manifestations**

| Hyperphosphatemia ($PO_4^{3-}$ >4.4 mg/dL [1.42 mmol/L]) | Hypophosphatemia ($PO_4^{3-}$ <2.4 mg/dL [0.78 mmol/L]) |
|---|---|
| **Causes** | |
| • Renal failure<br>• Phosphate enemas (e.g., Fleet Enema)<br>• Excessive ingestion (e.g., phosphate-containing laxatives)<br>• Rhabdomyolysis<br>• Tumor lysis syndrome<br>• Thyrotoxicosis<br>• Hypoparathyroidism<br>• Sickle cell anemia, hemolytic anemia<br>• Hyperthermia | • Malabsorption syndromes<br>• Chronic diarrhea<br>• Malnutrition, vitamin D deficiency<br>• Parenteral nutrition<br>• Chronic alcoholism<br>• Phosphate-binding antacids<br>• Diabetic ketoacidosis<br>• Hyperparathyroidism<br>• Refeeding syndrome<br>• Respiratory alkalosis |
| **Manifestations** | |
| • Hypocalcemia<br>• Numbness and tingling in extremities and region around mouth<br>• Hyperreflexia, muscle cramps<br>• Tetany, seizures<br>• Calcium-phosphate precipitates in skin, soft tissue, cornea, viscera, blood vessels | • CNS depression (confusion, coma)<br>• Muscle weakness, including respiratory muscle weakness<br>• Polyneuropathy, seizures<br>• Cardiac problems (dysrhythmias, heart failure)<br>• Osteomalacia, rickets<br>• Rhabdomyolysis |

## HYPOPHOSPHATEMIA

Hypophosphatemia (low serum phosphate) can result from decreased intestinal absorption, increased urinary excretion, or from ECF to ICF shifts. Malabsorption, diarrhea, and phosphate-binding antacids lead to decreased absorption. Phosphate shifts occur in respiratory alkalosis, treatment of diabetic ketoacidosis, and refeeding syndrome (reinstitution of nutrition to patients who are severely malnourished). Hypophosphatemia may occur in those who are malnourished or receive parenteral nutrition with inadequate phosphorus replacement. Table 16-8 lists causes and clinical manifestations of hypophosphatemia.

Most of the manifestations of hypophosphatemia result from impaired cellular energy and $O_2$ delivery due to low levels of cellular ATP and 2,3-diphosphoglycerate (2,3-DPG), an enzyme in RBCs that facilitates $O_2$ delivery to the tissues. Mild to moderate hypophosphatemia is often asymptomatic. Severe hypophosphatemia may be fatal because of decreased cellular function. Acute manifestations include CNS depression, muscle weakness and pain, respiratory failure, and heart failure. Chronic hypophosphatemia alters bone metabolism, resulting in rickets and osteomalacia.

Managing mild phosphorus deficiency involves increasing oral intake with dairy products or phosphate supplements. Dairy products are better tolerated because phosphate supplements are often associated with adverse GI effects.[10] Symptomatic hypophosphatemia can be fatal and usually requires IV administration of sodium phosphate or potassium phosphate.[8] Frequent monitoring is necessary during IV therapy as complications include hypocalcemia, hyperkalemia, hypotension, and dysrhythmias.

## MAGNESIUM IMBALANCES

Magnesium, the second most abundant intracellular cation, plays an important role in essential cellular processes. It is a cofactor in many enzyme systems, including those responsible for carbohydrate metabolism, DNA and protein synthesis, blood glucose control, and BP regulation. Magnesium is required for the production and use of adenosine triphosphate (ATP), the energy source for the sodium-potassium pump. Muscle contraction and relaxation, normal neurologic function, and neurotransmitter release depend on magnesium.

About 50% to 60% of the body's magnesium is stored in muscle and bone; 30% is in cells. Only 1% is in ECF. The intestines and kidneys regulate magnesium levels. GI absorption increases when magnesium levels are low. The kidney regulates serum magnesium by controlling the amount of magnesium reabsorbed in the ascending loop of Henle and distal tubules.[8]

### HYPERMAGNESEMIA

*Hypermagnesemia* (high serum magnesium level) usually occurs only with increased magnesium intake accompanied by renal insufficiency or failure. A patient with chronic kidney disease who ingests products containing magnesium (e.g., Maalox, milk of magnesia) will have a problem with excess magnesium. Magnesium excess could develop in a pregnant woman receiving magnesium sulfate for the treatment of eclampsia or in patients taking laxatives and antacids that contain magnesium. Table 16-9 lists the causes and manifestations of hypermagnesemia.

Excess magnesium inhibits acetylcholine release at the myoneural junction and calcium movement into cells, impairing nerve and muscle function. Initial manifestations include hypotension, facial flushing, lethargy, urinary retention, nausea, and vomiting. As the serum magnesium level increases, deep tendon reflexes are lost, followed by muscle paralysis and coma. Respiratory and cardiac arrest can occur.

**TABLE 16-9 Magnesium Imbalances: Causes and Manifestations**

| Hypermagnesemia ($Mg^+$ >2.5 mEq/L [1.25 mmol/L]) | Hypomagnesemia ($Mg^+$ <1.5 mEq/L [0.75 mmol/L]) |
|---|---|
| **Causes** | |
| • Renal failure | • GI tract fluid losses (e.g., diarrhea, NG suction) |
| • IV administration of magnesium, especially for treatment of eclampsia | • Chronic alcoholism |
| • Tumor lysis syndrome | • Malabsorption syndromes |
| • Hypothyroidism | • Prolonged malnutrition |
| • Metastatic bone disease | • ↑ Urine output |
| • Adrenal insufficiency | • Hyperglycemia |
| • Antacids, laxatives | • Proton pump inhibitor therapy |
| **Manifestations** | |
| • Lethargy, drowsiness | • Confusion |
| • Muscle weakness | • Muscle cramps |
| • Urinary retention | • Tremors, seizures |
| • Nausea, vomiting | • Vertigo |
| • Diminished deep tendon reflexes | • Hyperactive deep tendon reflexes |
| • Flushed, warm skin, especially facial | • Chvostek's and Trousseau's signs |
| • ↓ Pulse, ↓ BP | • ↑ Pulse, ↑ BP, dysrhythmias |

Management begins with avoiding magnesium-containing drugs and limiting diet intake of magnesium-containing foods (e.g., green vegetables, nuts, bananas, oranges, peanut butter, chocolate). If renal function is adequate, increased fluids and diuretics promote urinary excretion. In the patient with impaired renal function, dialysis is required. If hypermagnesemia is symptomatic, giving IV calcium gluconate will oppose the effects of the excess magnesium on cardiac muscle.

### HYPOMAGNESEMIA

*Hypomagnesemia* (low serum magnesium level) occurs in patients with limited magnesium intake or increased gastrointestinal or renal losses. Causes of hypomagnesemia from insufficient food intake include prolonged fasting or starvation and chronic alcoholism. Another potential cause is prolonged parenteral nutrition without magnesium supplementation. Fluid loss from the GI tract, inflammatory bowel disease, and proton pump inhibitors interfere with magnesium absorption. Many diuretics and osmotic diuresis from high glucose levels may cause magnesium loss through increased urinary excretion.[11] Table 16-9 lists the causes and manifestations of hypomagnesemia.

Clinically, hypomagnesemia resembles hypocalcemia. Neuromuscular manifestations are common, such as muscle cramps, tremors, hyperactive deep tendon reflexes, Chvostek's sign, and Trousseau's sign. Neurologic manifestations include confusion, vertigo, and seizures.

Magnesium deficiency can lead to cardiac dysrhythmias, such as torsades de pointes and ventricular fibrillation. Hypomagnesemia is associated with digitalis toxicity.

Managing hypomagnesemia depends on the underlying cause and the patient's symptoms. Mild magnesium deficiencies involve oral supplements and increased dietary intake of foods high in magnesium. If hypomagnesemia is severe or if hypocalcemia is present, IV magnesium (e.g., magnesium sulfate) is given. Monitor vital signs and use an infusion pump, since rapid administration can lead to hypotension and cardiac or respiratory arrest.

## ACID-BASE IMBALANCES

The body normally maintains a steady balance between the acids continually produced during normal metabolism and the bases that neutralize and promote the excretion of the acids. Because these acids alter the body's internal environment, their regulation is necessary to maintain homeostasis and acid-base balance. Many health problems may lead to acid-base imbalances. Patients with diabetes mellitus, chronic obstructive pulmonary disease, and kidney disease frequently develop acid-base imbalances.

Remember that an acid-base imbalance is not a disease but a symptom of an underlying health problem. Always consider the possibility of acid-base imbalance in patients with serious illnesses.

### pH AND HYDROGEN ION CONCENTRATION

The acidity or alkalinity of a solution depends on its hydrogen ion ($H^+$) concentration. An increase in $H^+$ concentration leads

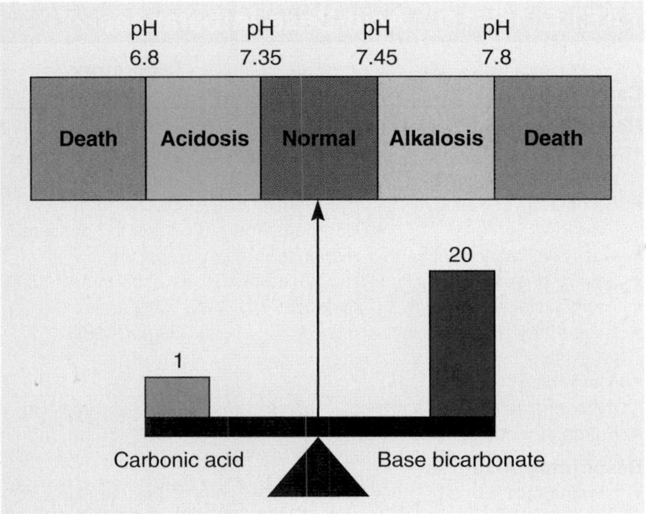


**FIG. 16-16** The normal range of plasma pH is 7.35 to 7.45. A normal pH is maintained by a ratio of 1 part carbonic acid to 20 parts bicarbonate.

to acidity; a decrease leads to alkalinity. $H^+$ concentration is usually expressed as a negative logarithm (symbolized as *pH*). The use of the negative logarithm means that the lower the pH, the higher the $H^+$ concentration. In contrast to a pH of 7, a pH of 8 represents a 10-fold decrease in $H^+$ concentration.

The pH of a chemical solution may range from 1 to 14. A solution with a pH of 7 is considered neutral. An acid solution has a pH less than 7, and an alkaline solution has a pH greater than 7. Blood is slightly alkaline and has a normal arterial pH of 7.35 to 7.45. Medically, if the pH drops below 7.35, a person has **acidosis**. If the blood pH is greater than 7.45, the person has **alkalosis** (Fig. 16-16).

## ACID-BASE REGULATION

The body uses three mechanisms to regulate acid-base balance and maintain the pH between 7.35 and 7.45. These are the buffer systems, respiratory system, and renal system. Each mechanism reacts at different speeds. Buffers are the fastest, reacting immediately. The respiratory system responds in minutes and reaches maximum effectiveness in hours. The renal response occurs hours to days after a change in pH, but the kidneys can maintain balance indefinitely in patients with chronic imbalances.

### Buffer System

Buffering is the primary regulator of acid-base balance. **Buffers** act chemically to change strong acids into weaker ones or bind them to neutralize them. This minimizes the effect of acids on blood pH until their excretion from the body. Buffers can only maintain pH when the respiratory and renal systems function adequately.

All body fluids contain buffers. The major buffer system in ECF is carbonic acid–bicarbonate. Other buffers include phosphate, protein, and hemoglobin. The cell can act as a buffer by shifting $H^+$ in and out of the cell. When ECF levels of $H^+$ are increased, $H^+$ enters the cell in exchange for potassium. This may result in hyperkalemia. Conversely, with decreased $H^+$ levels, $H^+$ enters plasma in exchange for potassium. This is why alkalosis can cause hypokalemia.

A buffer consists of a weak acid, which releases $H^+$ when fluid is too alkaline, or a base and its salt, which takes up $H^+$ when fluid is too acidic. The carbonic acid–bicarbonate ($H_2CO_3$/$HCO_3^-$) buffer system neutralizes hydrochloric (HCl) acid in the following manner:

$$\underset{\text{Strong acid}}{HCl} + \underset{\text{Strong base}}{Na_2CO_3} \rightarrow \underset{\text{Salt}}{NaCl} + \underset{\text{Weak acid}}{H_2CO_3}$$

In this way, combining a strong acid with a strong base prevents the acid from making a large decrease in pH. The carbonic acid is broken down to $H_2O$ and $CO_2$. The lungs excrete $CO_2$, either combined with insensible $H_2O$ as carbonic acid, or alone as $CO_2$.

The phosphate, protein, and hemoglobin buffer systems act in the same way as the bicarbonate system. The main components of the phosphate system are monohydrogen phosphate ($HPO_4^{2-}$) and dihydrogen phosphate ($H_2PO_4^-$). A phosphate, combined with sodium, can neutralize a strong acid such as HCl, by forming sodium chloride (NaCl) and sodium biphosphate ($NaH_2PO_4$), a weak acid. If a strong base, such as sodium hydroxide (NaOH), is present, sodium biphosphate ($NaH_2PO_4$) neutralizes it to a weaker base ($Na_2HPO_4$) and $H_2O$.

Intracellular and extracellular proteins can act as acids or bases. Because the chemical structure of amino acids has an acid (the carboxyl group [COOH]) and a base (amine), they can accept $H^+$ if pH decreases or release $H^+$ if fluid is too alkaline. Some amino acids have basic radicals ($NH_3OH$ [ammonium hydroxide]), which can dissociate into $NH_3^+$ (ammonia) and $OH^-$ (hydroxide). The $OH^-$ can combine with $H^+$ to form $H_2O$.

Hemoglobin is able to bind with both $H^+$, forming a weak acid, and $CO_2$, forming carbaminohemoglobin ($HbCO_2$). $HbCO_2$ dissociates in the lungs, releasing $CO_2$ for exhalation. Because $H^+$ can only combine with hemoglobin that has released its oxygen, hemoglobin less saturated with oxygen (venous blood) is a better buffer than saturated hemoglobin (arterial blood). Hemoglobin also assists in controlling pH by shifting chloride in and out of RBCs in exchange for bicarbonate.

The buffer system maintains a 20:1 ratio between $HCO_3^-$ and carbonic acid in ECF. The body's ability to maintain this ratio is important in controlling pH. For example, excess carbonic acid increases the ratio and decreases pH, resulting in acidosis. In response, the body can increase $HCO_3^-$ levels to keep the ratio 20:1 and maintain the pH near normal, a state called *compensation*. For example, a ratio of 40:2 would be present in compensated acid-base balance.

### Respiratory System

The lungs help maintain a normal pH by excreting $CO_2$ and water, which are by-products of cellular metabolism. When released into the circulation, $CO_2$ enters RBCs and combines with $H_2O$ to form $H_2CO_3$. This carbonic acid dissociates into $H^+$ and $HCO_3^-$. Hemoglobin buffers the free $H^+$, and the $HCO_3^-$ diffuses into the plasma. This process is reversed in the pulmonary capillaries, forming $CO_2$ that is then excreted by the lungs. The overall reversible reaction is expressed in the following manner:

$$CO_2 + H_2O \rightarrow H_2CO_3 \rightarrow H_3 + HCO_3^-$$

The amount of $CO_2$ in the blood directly relates to carbonic acid concentration and subsequently to $H^+$ concentration. With increased respirations, more $CO_2$ is expelled and less remains in the blood. This leads to less carbonic acid and less $H^+$. With decreased respirations, more $CO_2$ remains in the blood. This leads to increased carbonic acid and more $H^+$.

The respiratory center in the medulla in the brainstem controls the rate of excretion of $CO_2$. If increased amounts of $CO_2$ or $H^+$ are present, the respiratory center stimulates an increased rate and depth of breathing to "blow off" $CO_2$ through hyperventilation. If the center senses low $H^+$ or $CO_2$ levels, respirations are inhibited and $CO_2$ retained. If a respiratory problem (e.g., respiratory failure) is the cause of an acid-base imbalance, the respiratory system loses ability to correct a pH alteration. The older adult has an impaired compensatory ability because of decreased respiratory function.

### Renal System

Under normal conditions, the body depends on the kidneys to reabsorb and conserve all of the $HCO_3^-$ they filter and excrete a portion of the acid produced by cellular metabolism. The three mechanisms of acid elimination are (1) secretion of small amounts of free hydrogen into the renal tubule, (2) combination of $H^+$ with ammonia ($NH_3$) to form ammonium ($NH_4^+$), and (3) excretion of weak acids.

The kidneys normally excrete acidic urine (average pH is 6). As a compensatory mechanism, the pH of the urine can decrease to 4 or increase to 8. To compensate for acidosis, the kidneys can reabsorb additional $HCO_3^-$ and eliminate excess $H^+$. This increases the blood pH and decreases the urine pH. If the renal system is the cause of an acid-base imbalance (e.g., renal failure), it loses the ability to correct a pH alteration. In the older adult, the kidneys are less able to compensate for acid load.

## ALTERATIONS IN ACID-BASE BALANCE

An acid-base imbalance results when there is an alteration in the ratio of 20:1 between base and acid content. This occurs when a disease or process alters one side of the ratio (e.g., $CO_2$ retention in pulmonary disease) and the compensatory processes that maintain the other side of the ratio (e.g., increased renal $HCO_3^-$ reabsorption) either fail or are inadequate. The compensatory process may be inadequate because either the pathophysiologic process is overwhelming or there is insufficient time for the compensatory process to work.

Acid-base imbalances are classified as respiratory or metabolic. *Respiratory imbalances* result from the retention or an excess of $CO_2$ altering carbonic acid concentrations. *Metabolic imbalances* affect the base $HCO_3^-$. Acidosis occurs with an increase in carbonic acid (respiratory acidosis) or a decrease in $HCO_3^-$ (metabolic acidosis). Alkalosis occurs with a decrease in carbonic acid (respiratory alkalosis) or an increase in $HCO_3^-$ (metabolic alkalosis). Imbalances are further classified as acute or chronic. Chronic imbalances allow greater time for compensatory changes.

### Respiratory Acidosis

*Respiratory acidosis* (carbonic acid excess) occurs whenever the person hypoventilates (Table 16-10). Hypoventilation leads to a buildup of $CO_2$, resulting in an accumulation of carbonic acid in the blood. Carbonic acid dissociates, releasing $H^+$ and decreasing pH. If $CO_2$ is not eliminated from the blood, acidosis results from the accumulation of carbonic acid (Fig. 16-17, *A*).

During acute respiratory acidosis, the renal compensatory mechanisms begin to operate within 24 hours. The kidneys conserve $HCO_3^-$ and secrete increased concentrations of $H^+$ into the urine. Until the renal mechanisms have an effect, the serum $HCO_3^-$ level will usually be normal, and then it will increase.

**TABLE 16-10 Acid-Base Imbalances**

| Causes | Pathophysiology | Laboratory Findings |
|---|---|---|
| **Respiratory Acidosis** | | |
| • Chronic respiratory disease (e.g., COPD)<br>• Barbiturate or sedative overdose<br>• Chest wall abnormality<br>• Severe pneumonia<br>• Atelectasis<br>• Respiratory muscle weakness<br>• Mechanical hypoventilation<br>• Pulmonary edema | • ↑ $CO_2$ retention from hypoventilation<br>• Compensatory response is ↑ $HCO_3^-$ retention by kidney | ↓ Plasma pH<br>↑ $PaCO_2$<br>$HCO_3^-$ normal (uncompensated)<br>↑ $HCO_3^-$ (compensated)<br><br>*Sample ABG*<br>Uncompensated:<br>pH 7.31<br>$PaCO_2$ 54 mm Hg<br>$HCO_3^-$ 25 mEq/L |
| **Respiratory Alkalosis** | | |
| • Hyperventilation (e.g., hypoxia, anxiety, fear, pain, exercise, fever)<br>• Stimulated respiratory center (e.g., septicemia, stroke, meningitis, encephalitis, brain injury, salicylate poisoning)<br>• Liver failure<br>• Mechanical hyperventilation | • ↑ $CO_2$ excretion from hyperventilation<br>• Compensatory response is ↑ $HCO_3^-$ excretion by kidney | ↑ Plasma pH<br>↓ $PaCO_2$<br>$HCO_3^-$ normal (uncompensated)<br>↓ $HCO_3^-$ (compensated)<br><br>*Sample ABG*<br>Uncompensated:<br>pH 7.52<br>$PaCO_2$ 27 mm Hg<br>$HCO_3^-$ 24 mEq/L |
| **Metabolic Acidosis** | | |
| • Diabetic ketoacidosis<br>• Lactic acidosis<br>• Starvation<br>• Diarrhea<br>• Renal tubular acidosis<br>• Renal failure<br>• Gastrointestinal fistulas<br>• Shock | • Gain of fixed acid, inability to excrete acid or loss of base<br>• Compensatory response is ↑ $CO_2$ excretion by lungs | ↓ Plasma pH<br>$PaCO_2$ normal (uncompensated)<br>↓ $PaCO_2$ (compensated)<br>↓ $HCO_3^-$<br><br>*Sample ABG*<br>Uncompensated:<br>pH 7.29<br>$PaCO_2$ 38 mm Hg<br>$HCO_3^-$ 18 mEq/L |
| **Metabolic Alkalosis** | | |
| • Vomiting<br>• Nasogastric suctioning<br>• Diuretic therapy<br>• Hypokalemia<br>• Excess $NaHCO_3$ intake<br>• Mineralocorticoid use | • Loss of strong acid or gain of base<br>• Compensatory response is ↑ $CO_2$ retention by lungs | ↑ Plasma pH<br>$PaCO_2$ normal (uncompensated)<br>↑ $PaCO_2$ (compensated)<br>↑ $HCO_3^-$<br><br>*Sample ABG*<br>Uncompensated:<br>pH 7.50<br>$PaCO_2$ 40 mm Hg<br>$HCO_3^-$ 34 mEq/L |

*ABG*, Arterial blood gas.

### Respiratory Alkalosis

*Respiratory alkalosis* (carbonic acid deficit) occurs with hyperventilation, or an increase in respiratory rate or volume (Table 16-10). The primary cause of respiratory alkalosis is hypoxemia from acute pulmonary disorders (e.g., pneumonia, pulmonary embolus). Hyperventilation can occur as a physiologic response

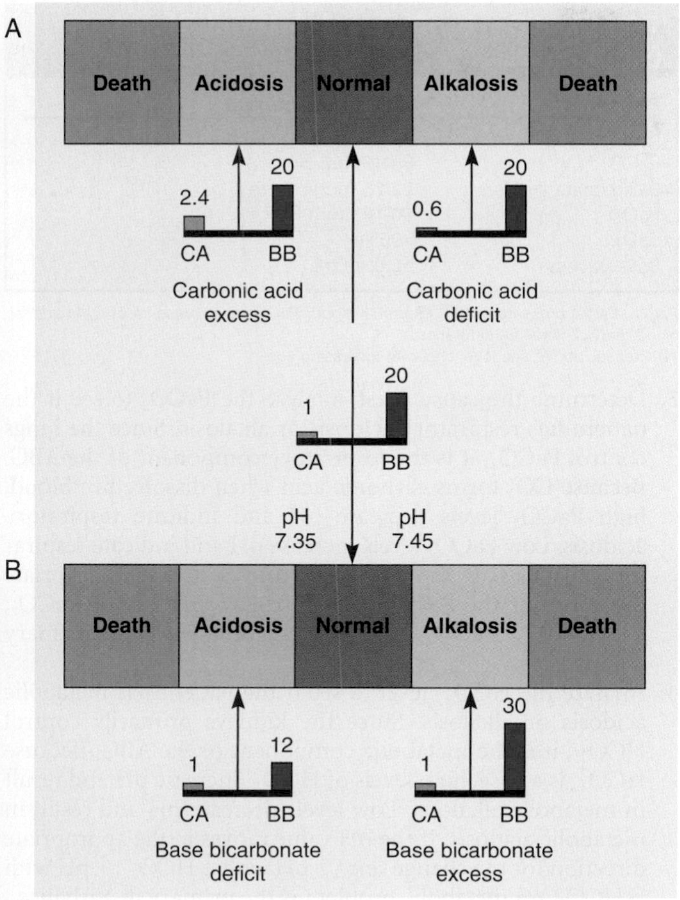


**FIG. 16-17** Kinds of acid-base imbalances. **A,** Respiratory imbalances caused by carbonic acid (*CA*) excess and carbonic acid deficit. **B,** Metabolic imbalances caused by base bicarbonate (*BB*) deficit and base bicarbonate excess.

to metabolic acidosis and increased metabolic demands (e.g., fever). Pain, anxiety, and some CNS disorders can increase respirations without a physiologic need. The decrease in the arterial $CO_2$ level leads to decreased carbonic acid concentration in the blood and an increased pH (Fig. 16-17, *A*).

Compensated respiratory alkalosis is rare. In acute respiratory alkalosis, aggressive treatment of the cause of hypoxemia is essential and usually does not allow time for compensation to occur. Some buffering may occur with shifting of $HCO_3^-$ into cells in exchange for chloride ions ($Cl^-$). In chronic respiratory alkalosis that occurs with pulmonary fibrosis or CNS disorders, compensation may include renal excretion of $HCO_3^-$.

### Metabolic Acidosis

*Metabolic acidosis* (base bicarbonate deficit) occurs when an acid other than carbonic acid accumulates in the body or when bicarbonate is lost in body fluids (Table 16-10 and Fig. 16-17, *B*). Ketoacid accumulation in diabetic ketoacidosis and lactic acid accumulation with shock are examples of acid accumulation. Severe diarrhea results in loss of $HCO_3^-$. In renal disease, the kidneys lose their ability to reabsorb $HCO_3^-$ and secrete $H^+$. To compensate for metabolic acidosis, the kidneys attempt to excrete additional acid and the lungs increase $CO_2$ excretion. The patient often develops *Kussmaul respirations* (deep, rapid breathing).

If metabolic acidosis is present, calculating the anion gap will help determine the source of the acidosis. The *anion gap* is the difference between the measured serum cations and anions in ECF. Calculate the anion gap using the following formula:

$$\text{Anion gap} = Na^+ - (HCO_3^- + Cl^-)$$

A normal anion gap is 8 to 12 mmol/L. The anion gap increases in metabolic acidosis associated with acid gain (e.g., lactic acidosis, diabetic ketoacidosis) but is normal in metabolic acidosis caused by bicarbonate loss (e.g., diarrhea).

### Metabolic Alkalosis

*Metabolic alkalosis* (base bicarbonate excess) occurs when a loss of acid (e.g., from prolonged vomiting or gastric suction) or a gain in $HCO_3^-$ (e.g., from ingestion of baking soda) occurs (Table 16-10 and Fig. 16-17, *B*). Renal excretion of $HCO_3^-$ occurs in response to metabolic alkalosis. The lung's compensatory response is limited. The respiratory rate decreases in order to increase plasma $CO_2$. However, once hypoxemia occurs or plasma $CO_2$ reaches a certain level, stimulation of chemoreceptors increases respirations.

### Mixed Acid-Base Disorders

A mixed acid-base disorder occurs when two or more disorders are present at the same time. The pH depends on the type, severity, and acuity of each disorder involved and any compensatory mechanisms at work. Respiratory acidosis combined with metabolic alkalosis (e.g., a patient with atelectasis and NG suction) may result in a near-normal pH, whereas respiratory acidosis combined with metabolic acidosis causes a greater decrease in pH than either disorder alone. An example of a mixed acidosis is a patient in severe shock with poor perfusion and hypoventilation. Mixed alkalosis can occur in a patient hyperventilating because of postoperative pain and losing acid secondary to NG suctioning.

## CLINICAL MANIFESTATIONS OF ACID-BASE IMBALANCES

Clinical manifestations of acidosis and alkalosis are summarized in Tables 16-11 and 16-12. In both respiratory and metabolic acidosis, the CNS is depressed. Headache, lethargy, weakness, and confusion develop, leading eventually to coma and death. Compensatory mechanisms also produce specific clinical manifestations. For example, the deep, rapid respirations of a patient with metabolic acidosis occur with respiratory compensation.

In both types of alkalosis, symptoms usually result from an accompanying electrolyte abnormality rather than the alkalosis. Hypocalcemia occurs due to increased calcium binding with albumin, lowering the amount of ionized, active calcium. Therefore, muscle cramping, tingling and numbness of the fingers, and tetany occur. Once $HCO_3^-$ levels are higher than 50 mEq/L, patients may develop seizures, hypoventilation, and coma.[12]

### Blood Gas Values

Arterial blood gas (ABG) values provide objective information about a patient's acid-base status, the underlying cause of an imbalance, and the body's ability to regulate pH. Knowing the patient's clinical situation and the extent of renal and respiratory compensation allows you to identify acid-base disorders and the patient's ability to compensate. Blood gas analysis also

**TABLE 16-11 Manifestations of Acidosis**

| Respiratory (↑ $PaCO_2$) | Metabolic (↓ $HCO_3^-$) |
|---|---|
| **Neurologic** | |
| Lethargy | Lethargy |
| Confusion | Confusion |
| Dizziness | Dizziness |
| Headache | Headache |
| Coma | Coma |
| **Cardiovascular** | |
| ↓ BP | ↓ BP |
| Ventricular fibrillation (related to hyperkalemia from compensation) | Dysrhythmias (related to hyperkalemia from compensation) |
| Warm, flushed skin | Cold, clammy skin |
| **Gastrointestinal** | |
| No significant findings | Nausea, vomiting, diarrhea, abdominal pain |
| **Neuromuscular** | |
| Seizures | Muscle weakness |
| **Respiratory** | |
| Hypoventilation with hypoxia | Deep, rapid respirations |

**TABLE 16-12 Manifestations of Alkalosis**

| Respiratory (↓ $PaCO_2$) | Metabolic (↑ $HCO_3^-$) |
|---|---|
| **Neurologic** | |
| Dizziness | Irritability |
| Light-headedness | Lethargy |
| Confusion | Confusion |
| Headache | Headache |
| **Cardiovascular** | |
| Tachycardia | Tachycardia |
| Dysrhythmias (related to hypokalemia from compensation) | Dysrhythmias (related to hypokalemia from compensation) |
| **Gastrointestinal** | |
| Nausea, vomiting, diarrhea | Nausea, vomiting |
| Epigastric pain | Anorexia |
| **Neuromuscular** | |
| Tetany | Tetany |
| Numbness | Tremors |
| Tingling of extremities | Tingling of fingers and toes |
| Hyperreflexia | Muscle cramps, hypertonic muscles |
| Seizures | Seizures |
| **Respiratory** | |
| Hyperventilation (lungs are unable to compensate if there is a respiratory problem) | Hypoventilation (compensatory action by lungs) |

shows the partial pressure of arterial $O_2$ ($PaO_2$) and $O_2$ saturation. These values help you evaluate the patient's overall oxygenation status and identify hypoxemia.

To interpret the results of an ABG, perform the following six steps:

1. Look at each of the values. If the pH is between 7.35 and 7.45, and the $CO_2$, $HCO_3^-$, and $PaO_2$ are within normal limits, the ABGs are normal. If any value is out of normal, then continue.
2. Determine if the pH is acidotic or alkalotic. Values less than 7.35 are acidotic and values greater than 7.45 are alkalotic. A normal pH may indicate normal acid-base status, compensation is occurring, or a mixed disorder is present.

**TABLE 16-13 Normal Arterial Blood Gas Values**

| Parameter | Reference Interval |
|---|---|
| pH | 7.35-7.45 |
| $PaCO_2$ | 35-45 mm Hg |
| Bicarbonate ($HCO_3^-$) | 22-26 mEq/L (mmol/L) |
| $PaO_2$† | 80-100 mm Hg |
| $SaO_2$ | >95% |
| Base excess | ±2.0 mEq/L |

*$PaCO_2$*, Partial pressure of $CO_2$ in arterial blood; *$PaO_2$*, partial pressure of $O_2$ in arterial blood; *$SaO_2$*, arterial $O_2$ saturation.
†Decreases above sea level and with increasing age.

3. Determine the cause. First, analyze the $PaCO_2$ to see if the patient has respiratory acidosis or alkalosis. Since the lungs control $PaCO_2$, it is the respiratory component of the ABG. Because $CO_2$ forms carbonic acid when dissolved in blood, high $PaCO_2$ levels decrease pH and indicate respiratory acidosis. Low $PaCO_2$ levels increase pH and indicate respiratory alkalosis. If the pH value moves in the appropriate direction for the $PaCO_2$ change (e.g., ↓ pH with ↑ $PaCO_2$; ↑ pH with ↓ $PaCO_2$), a respiratory problem is the primary disturbance.
4. Analyze the $HCO_3^-$ level to see if the patient has metabolic acidosis or alkalosis. Since the kidneys primarily control $HCO_3^-$, it is the metabolic component of the ABG. Because $HCO_3^-$ is a base, high levels of $HCO_3^-$ increase pH and result in metabolic alkalosis. Low levels decrease pH and result in metabolic acidosis. If the pH value moves in the appropriate direction for the change (e.g., ↓ pH with ↓ $HCO_3^-$; ↑ pH with ↑ $HCO_3^-$), a metabolic problem is the primary disturbance.
5. Determine if the patient is compensating or a mixed disorder is present. Look at the component ($CO_2$ or $HCO_3^-$) that is not the cause of the primary disturbance. If the component that does not match the pH is moving in the opposite direction, the body is attempting to compensate. For example, if the pH is slightly acidotic (7.33), the $CO_2$ is high (55 mm Hg), and the $HCO_3^-$ is high (36 mEq/L), the $CO_2$ is the parameter that matches the acidotic pH. The patient's underlying acid-base imbalance is respiratory acidosis. The $HCO_3^-$ level is alkalotic. Since this is in the opposite direction of respiratory acidosis, compensation is occurring. If both parameters match the pH, consider the possibility that a combined respiratory or metabolic acidosis or alkalosis is present. For example, if the pH is acidotic (7.28), the $CO_2$ is high (55 mm Hg), and the $HCO_3^-$ is low (16 mEq/L), the patient's underlying acid-base imbalance is combined respiratory-metabolic acidosis.
6. Assess the $PaO_2$ and $O_2$ saturation. If these values are abnormal, hypoxemia is present.

Table 16-13 lists normal blood gas values. Table 16-14 explains how to analyze ABG results. The laboratory findings section of Table 16-10 provides ABG findings of the four major acid-base disturbances. Table 16-15 shows *ROME*, a quick memory device for understanding acid-base imbalances. See Chapter 25 for further discussion of ABGs.

## ASSESSMENT OF FLUID, ELECTROLYTE, AND ACID-BASE IMBALANCES

Assessing patients for fluid, electrolyte, and acid-base imbalances is an important part of your nursing practice. In addition

**TABLE 16-14 Arterial Blood Gas (ABG) Analysis**

| ABG Values | Analysis |
|---|---|
| pH 7.30<br>$PaCO_2$ 30 mm Hg<br>$HCO_3^-$ 16 mEq/L<br>$PaO_2$ 95 mm Hg on room air | 1. The pH, $PaCO_2$, and $HCO_3^-$ are abnormal. pH <7.35 indicates acidosis.<br>2. $PaCO_2$ is low, indicating respiratory alkalosis.<br>3. $HCO_3^-$ is low, indicating metabolic acidosis.<br>4. $HCO_3^-$ matches the pH, indicating metabolic acidosis is the primary problem.<br>5. The $CO_2$ is moving in the opposite direction, indicating the lungs are attempting to compensate for the metabolic acidosis.<br>6. $PaO_2$ is normal and does not indicate hypoxemia. |

**Interpretation**

This ABG is interpreted as metabolic acidosis with partial compensation.

**TABLE 16-15 ROME: Memory Device for Acid-Base Imbalances**

For acid-base imbalances a quick memory device (mnemonic) can be used.

In ***Respiratory*** conditions, the pH and the $PaCO_2$ go in ***Opposite*** directions.

- In respiratory alkalosis, the pH is ↑ and the $PaCO_2$ is ↓.
- In respiratory acidosis, the pH is ↓ and the $PaCO_2$ is ↑.

In ***Metabolic*** conditions, the pH and the $HCO_3^-$ go in the same direction (***Equal***). The $PaCO_2$ may also go in the same direction.

- In metabolic alkalosis, pH and $HCO_3^-$ are ↑ and the $PaCO_2$ is ↑ or normal.
- In metabolic acidosis, pH and $HCO_3^-$ are ↓ and the $PaCO_2$ is ↓ or normal.

| | | | |
|---|---|---|---|
| **Respiratory** | | **pH** | **$PaCO_2$** |
| **O**pposite | Acidosis | ↓ | ↑ |
| | Alkalosis | ↑ | ↓ |
| **Metabolic** | | **pH** | **$HCO_3^-$** |
| **E**quivalent | Acidosis | ↓ | ↓ |
| | Alkalosis | ↑ | ↑ |

to assessing for the clinical manifestations presented earlier in this chapter, obtain subjective and objective data from any patient with suspected fluid, electrolyte, or acid-base imbalances as discussed below.

## Subjective Data

### Important Health Information

***Past Health History.*** Question the patient about any history of problems involving the kidneys, heart, GI system, or lungs that could affect the present fluid, electrolyte, and acid-base balance. Obtain information about specific diseases such as diabetes mellitus, diabetes insipidus, chronic obstructive pulmonary disease, renal failure, ulcerative colitis, and Crohn's disease. Ask the patient about any prior fluid, electrolyte, or acid-base disorders.

***Medications.*** Assess the patient's current and past use of medications. The ingredients in many drugs, especially over-the-counter drugs, are often hidden sources of sodium, potassium, calcium, magnesium, and other electrolytes. Many prescription drugs, including diuretics, corticosteroids, and electrolyte supplements, can cause fluid and electrolyte imbalances.

***Surgery or Other Treatments.*** Ask the patient about past or present renal dialysis, kidney surgery, or bowel surgery resulting in a temporary or permanent external collecting system such as an ileostomy.

### Functional Health Patterns

***Health Perception–Health Management Pattern.*** If the patient is currently experiencing a problem related to fluid, electrolyte, and acid-base balance, obtain a careful description of the illness, including onset, course, and treatment. Question the patient about any recent changes in body weight.

***Nutritional-Metabolic Pattern.*** Ask the patient about diet and any special dietary practices. Weight reduction diets, fad diets, or any eating disorders, such as anorexia or bulimia, can lead to fluid and electrolyte problems. If the patient is on a special diet, such as low sodium or high potassium, assess the ability to adhere to the dietary prescription.

***Elimination Pattern.*** Make note of the patient's usual bowel and bladder habits. Carefully document any deviations from the expected elimination pattern, such as diarrhea, oliguria, polyuria, or incontinence.

***Activity-Exercise Pattern.*** Ask about the patient's exercise pattern and any complaints of excessive perspiration. Determine if the patient is exposed to extremely high temperatures during leisure or work activity. Ask the patient what he or she does to replace fluid and electrolytes lost through excessive perspiration. Assess the patient's activity level to determine any functional problems that could lead to lack of ability to obtain food or fluids.

***Cognitive-Perceptual Pattern.*** Ask about any changes in sensations, such as numbness, tingling, or muscle weakness, which could indicate a fluid and electrolyte problem. Ask the patient and caregiver if there have been any changes in mentation or alertness, such as confusion, memory impairment, or lethargy.

## Objective Data

**Physical Examination.** A complete physical examination is needed because fluid, electrolyte, and acid-base balance affects all body systems. As you assess each system, check for manifestations that you would expect with an imbalance. Common abnormal assessment findings of major body systems offer clues to possible imbalances (Table 16-16).

**Laboratory Values.** Assessing serum electrolyte values is a good starting point for evaluating fluid and electrolyte balance (Table 16-1). Serum electrolytes can also provide important information about a patient's acid-base balance. Changes in the serum $HCO_3^-$ (often reported as total $CO_2$ or $CO_2$ content on an electrolyte panel) indicate metabolic acidosis (low $HCO_3^-$ level) or alkalosis (high $HCO_3^-$ level).

**! SAFETY ALERT Managing Critical Test Results**

- Promptly report critical laboratory values to the HCP.
- Assess the patient and initiate appropriate actions (e.g., ECG monitoring).

Remember serum electrolyte values often provide limited information. They reflect the concentration of that electrolyte in ECF but not necessarily in ICF. For example, most potassium is found in the cells. Changes in serum potassium values may be the result of a true deficit or excess of potassium or reflect the movement of potassium into or out of the cell during acid-base imbalances. An abnormal serum sodium level may reflect a sodium problem or, more likely, a water problem.

Other useful laboratory tests include serum and urine osmolality, serum glucose, blood urea nitrogen, serum creatinine, venous blood gas sampling, urine specific gravity, and urine electrolytes.

**TABLE 16-16 Assessment Abnormalities**

***Fluid and Electrolyte Imbalances***

| Finding | Possible Etiology |
|---|---|
| **Skin** | |
| Poor skin turgor | Fluid volume deficit |
| Cold, clammy skin | Fluid volume deficit, $Na^+$ deficit |
| Pitting edema | Fluid volume excess |
| Flushed, dry skin | $Na^+$ excess, $Mg^{2+}$ excess |
| **Pulse** | |
| Bounding pulse | Fluid volume excess |
| Rapid, weak, thready pulse | Fluid volume deficit |
| Weak, irregular, rapid pulse | Severe $K^+$ deficit, $Mg^{2+}$ deficit |
| Weak, irregular, slow pulse | Severe $K^+$ excess, $Mg^{2+}$ excess |
| **Blood Pressure** | |
| Hypotension | Fluid volume deficit, $Ca^{2+}$ deficit, $Mg^{2+}$ excess |
| Hypertension | Fluid volume excess, $Ca^{2+}$ excess, $Mg^{2+}$ deficit |
| **Respirations** | |
| Rapid respirations | Fluid volume deficit |
| Shortness of breath | Fluid volume excess |
| Moist crackles | Fluid volume excess |
| Restricted airway | $Ca^{2+}$ deficit, $PO_4^{3-}$ excess |
| **Skeletal Muscles** | |
| Muscle cramping | $K^+$ excess , $Ca^{2+}$ deficit, $PO_4^{3-}$ excess, $Mg^{2+}$ deficit |
| Muscle weakness | $K^+$ excess, $K^+$ deficit, $Ca^{2+}$ excess, $PO_4^{3-}$ deficit, $Mg^{2+}$ excess |
| Trousseau's sign | $Ca^{2+}$ deficit, $Mg^{2+}$ deficit, $PO_4^{3-}$ excess |
| Chvostek's sign | $Ca^{2+}$ deficit, $Mg^{2+}$ deficit, $PO_4^{3-}$ excess |
| **Neurologic** | |
| Tremors, seizures | $Na^+$ excess, $K^+$ excess, $Ca^{2+}$ deficit, $PO_4^{3-}$ excess, $Mg^{2+}$ deficit |
| Irritability | $Na^+$ deficit, $K^+$ excess, $Ca^{2+}$ deficit, $PO_4^{3-}$ excess |
| Fatigue | Fluid volume deficit, $K^+$ deficit, $Ca^{2+}$ excess |
| Confusion | Fluid volume excess, $Na^+$ deficit, $K^+$ excess, $K^+$ deficit, $Ca^{2+}$ excess, $Mg^{2+}$ excess, $Mg^{2+}$ deficit, $PO_4^{3-}$ deficit |
| Decreased level of consciousness | Fluid volume deficit, fluid volume excess, $Na^+$ excess, $Na^+$ deficit, $PO_4^{3-}$ deficit |

## ORAL FLUID AND ELECTROLYTE REPLACEMENT

In all cases of fluid, electrolyte, and acid-base imbalances, the primary treatment involves correcting the underlying cause. Oral rehydration solutions containing water, potassium, sodium, and glucose may be used to correct mild fluid and electrolyte deficits. Glucose not only provides calories, but also promotes sodium and water absorption in the small intestine. Commercial oral rehydration solutions are now available for home use. Cola drinks are avoided because they do not contain adequate electrolyte replacement and the sugar content may lead to osmotic diuresis.

## IV FLUID AND ELECTROLYTE REPLACEMENT

IV fluid and electrolyte therapy is necessary to treat many different fluid and electrolyte imbalances. Many patients need maintenance IV fluid therapy when they cannot take oral fluids (e.g., during and after surgery). Other patients need corrective or replacement therapy for losses that are ongoing or have already occurred. The amount and type of solution is determined by the normal daily maintenance requirements and by imbalances identified by laboratory results. IV replacement solutions are classified by their concentration or tonicity (Table 16-17). Tonicity is an important factor in determining the appropriate solution to correct imbalances.

### Solutions

**Hypotonic.** A hypotonic solution has more water than electrolytes, with an osmolality of less than 250 mOsm/kg.[13] Infusing a hypotonic solution dilutes ECF, lowering serum osmolality. Osmosis then produces a movement of water from ECF to interstitial spaces and cells, causing cells to swell. After achieving equilibrium, ICF and ECF have the same osmolality. Hypotonic solutions (e.g., 0.45% NaCl) are useful in treating patients with hypernatremia and are a good maintenance fluid because normal daily losses are hypotonic. They are not good for replacement because they can deplete ECF and lower BP. Because hypotonic solutions have the potential to cause cellular swelling, monitor patients for changes in mentation that may indicate cerebral edema.[13]

Although 5% dextrose in water is technically an isotonic solution, the dextrose quickly metabolizes. The net result is the administration of hypotonic free water with equal expansion of ECF and ICF. One liter of a 5% dextrose solution provides 50 g of dextrose, or 170 calories. While this amount of dextrose is not enough to meet caloric requirements, it helps prevent ketosis associated with starvation.

**Isotonic.** An isotonic solution has a similar concentration of water and electrolytes to plasma, with an osmolality of 250 to 375 mOsm/L.[13] Because of the similarity, administering an isotonic solution expands only ECF, and the fluid does not move into cells. This makes isotonic solutions the ideal fluid replacement for patients with ECF volume deficits. Examples of isotonic solutions include 0.9% NaCl and lactated Ringer's solution.

Isotonic saline (0.9% NaCl) or *normal saline* has a sodium concentration (154 mEq/L) somewhat higher than that of plasma (135 to 145 mEq/L) and a chloride concentration (154 mEq/L) significantly higher than the plasma chloride level (96 to 106 mEq/L). Therefore excessive administration of isotonic saline has the potential to increase sodium and chloride levels. Isotonic saline is used when a patient has experienced both fluid and sodium losses (e.g., diarrhea, vomiting). It is the fluid of choice for replacement.[13]

Lactated Ringer's solution contains sodium, potassium, chloride, calcium, and lactate (the precursor of bicarbonate) in about the same concentrations as ECF. This makes it the ideal fluid in certain situations, such as surgery, burns, or GI fluid losses. Patients with liver dysfunction, hyperkalemia, and severe hypovolemia should not receive lactated Ringer's because they have a decreased ability to convert lactate to bicarbonate.

**Hypertonic.** A hypertonic solution initially raises the osmolality of ECF and expands volume. The higher osmotic pressure draws water out of the cells into ECF. It is useful in the treatment of hyponatremia and trauma patients with head injury. Hypertonic solutions require frequent monitoring of BP, lung sounds, and serum sodium levels because of the risk for intravascular fluid volume excess.

Although concentrated dextrose and water solutions (10% dextrose or greater) are hypertonic solutions, once the dextrose

TABLE 16-17 **Commonly Used Crystalloid Solutions**

| Solution | Tonicity | mOsm/kg | Contents | Indications and Considerations |
|---|---|---|---|---|
| **Dextrose in Water** | | | | |
| 5% | Isotonic, but physiologically hypotonic | 278 | 50 g/L dextrose | • Contains free water only, no electrolytes<br>• Provides 170 cal/L<br>• Used to replace water losses and treat hypernatremia |
| 10% | Hypertonic | 556 | 100 g/L dextrose | • Contains free water only, no electrolytes<br>• Provides 340 cal/L<br>• Used with parenteral nutrition |
| **Saline** | | | | |
| 0.45% | Hypotonic | 154 | 77 mEq/L $Na^+$<br>77 mEq/L $Cl^-$ | • Contains free water, $Na^+$ and $Cl^-$, no calories<br>• Used to treat hypernatremia and uncontrolled hyperglycemia<br>• Used as a maintenance solution |
| 0.9% | Isotonic | 308 | 154 mEq/L $Na^+$<br>154 mEq/L $Cl^-$ | • Contains $Na^+$ and $Cl^-$ in excess of plasma levels<br>• Does not contain free water or calories<br>• Used to expand intravascular volume and replace extracellular fluid losses<br>• Only solution that may be administered with blood products<br>• May cause volume overload in patients with cardiac or renal disease |
| 3.0% | Hypertonic | 1026 | 513 mEq/L $Na^+$<br>513 mEq/L $Cl^-$ | • Contains $Na^+$ and $Cl^-$ in excess of plasma levels<br>• Used to treat symptomatic hyponatremia and trauma patients with head injury<br>• Administer slowly because it may cause volume overload and pulmonary edema |
| **Dextrose in Saline** | | | | |
| 5% in 0.25% | Isotonic | 355 | 50 g/L dextrose<br>34 mEq/L $Na^+$<br>34 mEq/L $Cl^-$ | • Provides $Na^+$, $Cl^-$, and free water<br>• Used to replace hypotonic losses and treat hypernatremia<br>• Provides 170 cal/L |
| 5% in 0.45% | Hypertonic | 432 | 50 g/L dextrose<br>77 mEq/L $Na^+$<br>77 mEq/L $Cl^-$ | • Provides $Na^+$, $Cl^-$, and free water<br>• Used as a maintenance solution |
| 5% in 0.9% | Hypertonic | 586 | 50 g/L dextrose<br>154 mEq/L $Na^+$<br>154 mEq/L $Cl^-$ | • Contains $Na^+$ and $Cl^-$ in excess of plasma levels<br>• Used to treat metabolic alkalosis and volume deficits in patients with hyponatremia |
| **Multiple Electrolyte Solutions** | | | | |
| Ringer's solution | Isotonic | 309 | 147 mEq/L $Na^+$<br>156 mEq/L $Cl^-$<br>4 mEq/L $K^+$<br>4 mEq/L $Ca^{2+}$ | • Similar in composition to plasma except that it has excess $Cl^-$, no $Mg^{2+}$, no $HCO_3^-$<br>• Does not provide free water or calories<br>• Used to expand the intravascular volume and replace extracellular fluid losses |
| Lactated Ringer's (Hartmann's) solution | Isotonic | 273 | 130 mEq/L $Na^+$<br>109 mEq/L $Cl^-$<br>4 mEq/L $K^+$<br>3 mEq/L $Ca^{2+}$<br>28 mmol/L lactate | • Similar in composition to normal plasma except does not contain $Mg^{2+}$<br>• Does not provide free water or calories<br>• Used to treat hypovolemia, burns, and GI fluid losses<br>• Cannot be used in patients with alkalosis or lactic acidosis |

is metabolized, the net result is the administration of water. This free water ultimately expands ECF and ICF. The primary use of these solutions is providing calories as part of parenteral nutrition (see Chapter 39). You may administer solutions containing 10% dextrose or less through a peripheral line. You must use a central line to administer solutions with dextrose concentrations greater than 10%.

**IV Additives.** Additives in basic IV solutions replace specific losses. KCl, $CaCl_2$, $MgSO_4$, and $HCO_3^-$ are common additives. The use of each was described earlier in the discussion of the specific electrolyte deficiencies. Many premixed IV solutions containing specific additives are available. Using these solutions reduces error as the solution contains the correct amount of the electrolyte in the proper volume and type of IV solution.

**Colloids.** Colloids solutions contain large molecules that increase oncotic pressure and pull fluid into the blood vessels. Because this action restores blood volume, colloids are also called volume expanders or plasma expanders. Colloids include human plasma products (albumin, fresh frozen plasma, blood) and semisynthetics (dextran, starches).

Albumin is available in 5% and 25% solutions. The 5% solution has an albumin concentration similar to plasma and results in plasma volume expansion equal to the volume infused. This makes the 5% concentration ideal for treating hypovolemic patients. In contrast, 25% albumin solution is hypertonic and draws fluid from the interstitial space. This makes it useful in treating patients with burns, hepatic failure, and ascites.

Dextrans are synthetic complex sugar solutions. There are two types: low-molecular-weight dextran (dextran 40) and high-molecular-weight dextran (dextran 70). Because dextran metabolizes slowly, it remains in the vascular system for a prolonged period. It pulls additional fluid into the intravascular space, expanding it by more volume than what is infused. Hydroxylethyl starches (e.g., Hespan) are synthetic colloids that work similarly to dextran to expand plasma volume.

Colloids can lead to circulatory overload because they pull fluid into ECF. Monitor vital signs and urine output frequently and assess for signs and symptoms of fluid volume excess. All colloids affect blood coagulation, with dextran and starches having the strongest anticoagulation effect. Monitor coagulation times and implement any necessary precautions. Fatal anaphylactic reactions have occurred with Hespan and dextran. Monitor the patient closely for a hypersensitivity reaction and discontinue an infusion immediately if a reaction occurs.

If the patient has lost blood, whole blood or packed RBCs are necessary. Packed RBCs have the advantage of giving the patient primarily RBCs rather than RBCs and fluid volume. Although packed RBCs have a decreased plasma volume, they increase the oncotic pressure and pull fluid into the intravascular space. The use of whole blood, with its additional fluid volume, may cause circulatory overload, particularly in patients who are susceptible to complications from excess circulating volume (e.g., heart failure). To prevent fluid volume excess, loop diuretics may be administered with blood and colloids. See Chapter 30 for more information on the administration of blood and blood products.

## TEAMWORK & COLLABORATION

### *IV Therapy*

Although many states permit licensed practical nurses (LPNs) to administer IV fluids and drugs, the registered nurse (RN) should administer IV fluids or medications to unstable or critically ill patients.

**Role of Nursing Personnel**

***Registered Nurse (RN)***

- Assess patient for clinical manifestations of fluid and electrolyte disturbances.
- Determine if ordered IV therapies are appropriate.
- Choose and insert appropriate IV catheters and infusion devices.
- Administer IV fluids and medications to unstable and critically ill patients.
- Evaluate patient for clinical manifestations of fluid overload or hypovolemia and initiate appropriate changes in IV fluids.
- Evaluate if IV therapies are addressing patient's fluid and electrolyte needs.

***Licensed Practical/Vocational Nurse (LPN/LVN)***

- Administer IV fluids and medications to stable patients (consider state nurse practice act and agency policy).
- Adjust IV flow rate for stable patients according to HCP orders (consider state nurse practice act and agency policy).
- Insert IV catheters (consider state nurse practice act and agency policy).
- Monitor for clinical manifestations of adverse reactions to IV fluids or medications.

***Unlicensed Assistive Personnel (UAP)***

- Measure and record oral intake and output.
- Report swelling or redness at IV site or patient complaints of discomfort at IV site to RN.

**Role of Other Team Members**

***Pharmacist***

- Determine appropriateness of IV therapies and need for dose adjustments.
- Prepare IV infusions and medications.
- Screen for potential problems, such as compatibility issues.
- Monitor response to therapy.

## CENTRAL VENOUS ACCESS DEVICES

**Central venous access devices (CVADs)** are catheters placed in large blood vessels (e.g., subclavian vein, jugular vein) of people who require frequent or special access to the vascular system. There are three main types of CVADs: centrally inserted catheters, peripherally inserted central catheters (PICCs), and implanted ports.

Advantages of CVADs include immediate access to the central venous system, a reduced need for multiple venipunctures, and decreased risk of extravasation injury. CVADs permit frequent, continuous, rapid, or intermittent administration of fluids and medications. They allow for the administration of drugs that are potential *vesicants* (agents that can cause tissue damage), blood and blood products, and parenteral nutrition. CVADs can provide a means to perform hemodynamic monitoring and obtain venous blood samples. They are useful with patients who have limited peripheral vascular access or who have a projected need for long-term vascular access. CVADs can also be used for injections of radiopaque contrast media. Table 16-18 provides examples of conditions where CVADs are used.

The major disadvantages of CVADs are an increased risk of systemic infection and the invasiveness of the procedure. Extravasation (leakage of fluid) can still occur if there is displacement of or damage to the device.

### Centrally Inserted Catheters

The tip of centrally inserted catheters (also called central venous catheters [CVCs]) rests in the distal end of the superior vena cava near its junction with the right atrium (Fig. 16-18). The other end of the catheter exits through a separate incision on the chest or abdominal wall. *Nontunneled catheters* are usually placed in the subclavian or internal jugular vein, more rarely in the femoral vein. They are best for patients with short-term needs in an acute care setting. *Surgically placed tunneled catheters* (e.g., Hickman) are suitable for long-term needs. Tunneling of the catheter through subcutaneous tissue and the synthetic cuff used to anchor the catheter provide stability and decrease infection risk. After the site heals, the catheter does not require a dressing, making it easier for the patient to maintain the site at home.

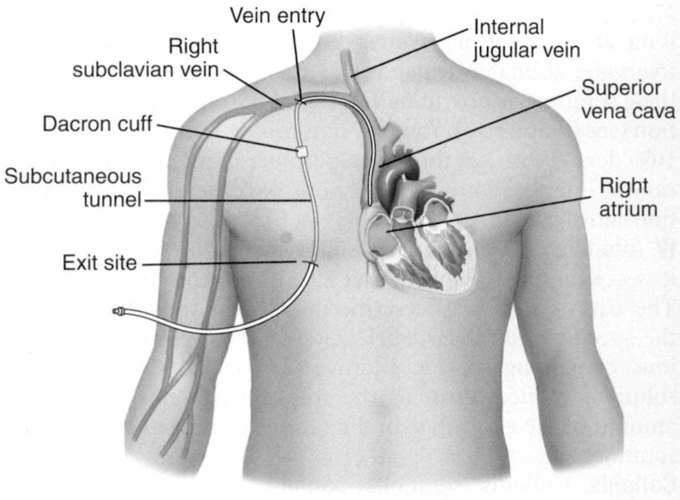


**FIG. 16-18** Tunneled central venous catheter. Note tip of the catheter in the superior vena cava.

**TABLE 16-18 Indications for Central Venous Access Devices (CVADs)***

| Condition | Indications for Use |
|---|---|
| **Medication administration** | |
| • Cancer | • Chemotherapy, infusion of irritating or vesicant medications |
| • Infection | • Long-term administration of antibiotics |
| • Pain | • Long-term administration of pain medication |
| • Drugs at risk for causing phlebitis | • Epoprostenol (Flolan)<br>• Calcium chloride<br>• Potassium chloride<br>• Amiodarone (Cordarone) |
| **Nutritional replacement** | • Infusion of parenteral nutrition<br>• Infusion of high percentage dextrose solutions |
| **Blood samples** | • Multiple blood draws for diagnostic tests over time |
| **Blood transfusions** | • Infusion of blood or blood products |
| **Renal failure** | • Perform hemodialysis (especially on an acute basis) or continuous renal replacement therapy |
| **Shock, burns** | • Infusion of high volumes of fluid and electrolyte replacement |
| **Hemodynamic monitoring** | • Used to measure central venous pressure to assess fluid balance |
| **Heart failure** | • Perform ultrafiltration |
| **Autoimmune disorders** | • Perform plasmapheresis |

*This list is not all-inclusive, and these are examples only.

CVCs are available with single-, double-, triple-, or quad-lumens. Multi-lumen catheters are useful in the critically ill patient because each lumen can be simultaneously used to provide a different therapy. For example, incompatible drugs infuse in separate lumens without mixing while a third lumen provides access for blood sampling.

### Peripherally Inserted Central Catheters

Peripherally inserted central catheters (PICCs) are central venous catheters inserted into a vein in the arm. The basilic vein is preferred because of its large diameter (Fig. 16-19). The cephalic, median cubital, or brachial veins are other options. Single-, double-, or triple-lumens are available; double lumens are preferred, because they allow for simultaneous uses. PICCs are used with patients who need vascular access for 1 week to 6 months, but they can be in place for longer periods.

Advantages of a PICC over a CVC are lower infection rate, fewer insertion-related complications, decreased cost, and ability to insert at the bedside or in an outpatient area. PICCs, however, are associated with an increased risk of deep vein thrombosis and phlebitis (Table 16-19). If phlebitis occurs, it usually happens within 7 to 10 days after insertion. Do not use the arm with the PICC to obtain a BP reading or draw blood. When the BP cuff is inflated, the PICC can touch the vein wall, increasing the risk of vein damage and thrombosis.

### Implanted Infusion Ports

An implanted infusion port consists of a surgically implanted central venous catheter connected to a reservoir or port (Fig. 16-20, *A*). The catheter tip lies in the desired vein. The port lies in a surgically created subcutaneous pocket on the upper chest or arm. It consists of a titanium or plastic reservoir covered with a self-sealing silicone septum. You access the port by using a special noncoring needle with a deflected tip. This prevents damage to the septum that could make the port useless (Fig. 16-20, *B*).

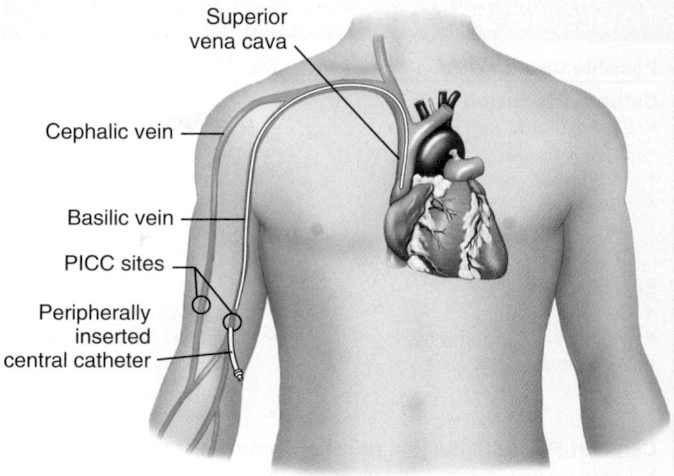


**FIG. 16-19** Peripherally inserted central catheter (PICC) can be inserted using the basilic or cephalic vein.

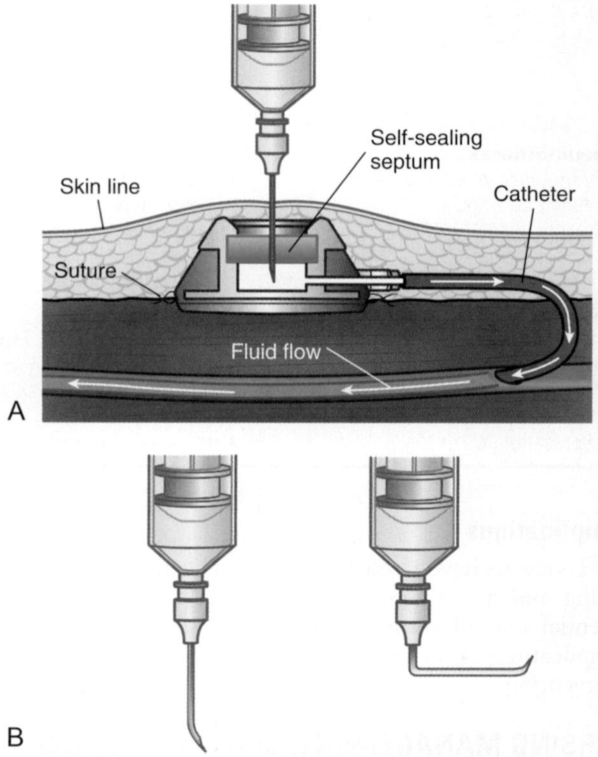


**FIG. 16-20** **A,** Cross section of implantable port displaying access of the port with the Huber-point needle. Note the deflected point of the Huber-point needle, which prevents coring of the port's septum. **B,** Two Huber-point needles used to enter the implanted port. The 90-degree needle is used for top-entry ports for continuous infusion.

Drugs are placed in the reservoir either by a direct injection or through injection into an established IV line. The reservoir then slowly releases the medicine into the bloodstream. Implanted ports are good for long-term therapy and have a low risk of infection. The hidden port offers the patient cosmetic advantages and overall has less maintenance than other types of CVADs. Monitor accessed ports for infiltration that can occur if the needle is not in place or dislodges.

**TABLE 16-19 Complications of Central Venous Access Devices (CVADs)**

| Possible Cause | Manifestations | Management |
|---|---|---|
| **Catheter Occlusion** | | |
| • Clamped or kinked catheter<br>• Tip against wall of vessel<br>• Thrombosis<br>• Precipitate buildup in lumen | • Sluggish infusion or aspiration<br>• Inability to infuse and/or aspirate | • Instruct patient to change position, raise arm, and cough.<br>• Assess for and alleviate clamping or kinking.<br>• Flush with normal saline using a 10-mL syringe. Do not force flush.<br>• Perform fluoroscopy to determine cause and site.<br>• Instill anticoagulant or thrombolytic agent. |
| **Embolism** | | |
| • Catheter breaking<br>• Dislodgment of thrombus<br>• Entry of air into circulation | • Chest pain<br>• Respiratory distress (dyspnea, tachypnea, hypoxia, cyanosis)<br>• Hypotension<br>• Tachycardia | • Administer $O_2$.<br>• Clamp catheter.<br>• Place patient on left side with head down (air emboli).<br>• Notify physician. |
| **Catheter-Related Infection (local or systemic)** | | |
| • Contamination during insertion or use<br>• Migration of organisms along catheter<br>• Immunosuppressed patient | • *Local:* redness, tenderness, purulent drainage, warmth, edema<br>• *Systemic:* fever, chills, malaise | ***Local***<br>• Culture drainage from site.<br>• Apply warm, moist compresses.<br>• Remove catheter if indicated.<br>***Systemic***<br>• Take blood cultures.<br>• Give antibiotic therapy.<br>• Give antipyretic therapy.<br>• Remove catheter if indicated. |
| **Pneumothorax** | | |
| • Perforation of visceral pleura during insertion | • Decreased or absent breath sounds<br>• Respiratory distress (cyanosis, dyspnea, tachypnea)<br>• Chest pain<br>• Distended unilateral chest | • Administer $O_2$.<br>• Position in semi-Fowler's position.<br>• Prepare for chest tube insertion. |
| **Catheter Migration** | | |
| • Improper suturing<br>• Insertion site trauma<br>• Changes in intrathoracic pressure<br>• Forceful catheter flushing<br>• Spontaneous | • Sluggish infusion or aspiration<br>• Edema of chest or neck during infusion<br>• Patient complaint of gurgling sound in ear<br>• Dysrhythmias<br>• Increased external catheter length | • Perform fluoroscopy to verify position.<br>• Assist with removal and new CVAD placement. |

### Complications

CVADs always have a potential for complications. Careful monitoring and assessment may assist in early identification of potential complications. Table 16-19 lists common possible complications, potential causes, clinical manifestations, and interventions.

## ❖ NURSING MANAGEMENT: CENTRAL VENOUS ACCESS DEVICES

Nursing management of CVADs includes assessment, dressing changes and cleansing, injection cap changes, and maintenance of catheter patency. The exact frequency and procedures for these requirements vary by type of CVAD and institution, so it is important to follow your specific institution's policies and procedures. The following section discusses some general guidelines.

Catheter and insertion site assessment includes inspecting the site for redness, edema, warmth, drainage, and tenderness or pain. Observing the catheter for misplacement or slippage is important. Perform a comprehensive pain assessment, particularly noting any complaints of chest or neck discomfort, arm pain, or pain at the insertion site. Do not use a newly placed CVAD until the tip position is verified with a chest x-ray.

Before manipulating a catheter for any reason, perform hand hygiene. Perform dressing changes and cleanse the catheter insertion site using strict sterile technique. Typical dressings include transparent semipermeable dressings or gauze and tape. If the site is bleeding, a gauze dressing may be preferable. Otherwise, transparent dressings are preferred. They allow observation of the site without having to remove the dressing. Transparent dressings may be left in place for up to 1 week. Change any dressing immediately if it becomes damp, loose, or soiled.

Cleanse the skin around the catheter insertion site according to institution policy. A chlorhexidine-based preparation is the cleansing agent of choice. Its effects last longer than either povidone-iodine or isopropyl alcohol, offering improved killing of bacteria.[14] When using chlorhexidine, cleansing the skin with friction is critical to preventing infection. When applying a new dressing, allow the area to air dry completely. Secure the lumen ports to the skin above the dressing site. Document the date and time of the dressing change and initial the dressing.

Disinfect catheter hubs, needleless connectors, and injection ports before accessing the catheter. Use an alcoholic chlorhexidine preparation, 70% alcohol, or povidone-iodine. Change injection caps at regular intervals according to institution policy or if they have damage from excessive punctures. Use strict sterile technique. Teach the patient to turn the head to the opposite side of the CVAD insertion site during cap change. If you cannot clamp the catheter, instruct the patient to lie flat in bed and perform the Valsalva maneuver whenever the catheter is open to air to prevent an air embolism.

Flushing is one of the most effective ways to maintain catheter patency. It also keeps incompatible drugs or fluids from mixing. Use a normal saline solution in a syringe that has a barrel capacity of 10 mL or more to avoid excess pressure on the catheter. If you feel resistance, do not apply force. This could result in a ruptured catheter or create an embolism if a thrombus is present. Because of the risk of contamination and infection, prefilled syringes or single-dose vials are preferred over multiple-dose vials. If you are not using a positive-pressure valve cap, clamp any unused lines after flushing.

Use the push-pause technique when flushing all catheters. Push-pause creates turbulence within the catheter lumen, promoting the removal of debris that adheres to the catheter lumen and decreasing the chance of occlusion. This technique involves injecting saline with a rapid alternating push-pause motion, instilling 1 to 2 mL with each push on the syringe plunger. If you are using a negative-pressure cap or neutral pressure cap, clamp the catheter while maintaining positive pressure while instilling the last 1 mL of saline. This prevents reflux of blood back into the catheter. If a positive-pressure valve cap is present, it works to prevent the reflux of blood and resultant catheter lumen occlusion. Remove the syringe before clamping the catheter to allow the positive pressure valve to work correctly.

### Removal of CVADs

Removing a CVAD is done according to institution policy and the nurse's scope of practice. In many agencies, nurses with demonstrated competency can remove PICCs and nontunneled central venous catheters. The procedure involves removing any sutures and then gently withdrawing the catheter. Instruct the patient to perform the Valsalva maneuver as the last 5 to 10 cm of the catheter is withdrawn. Immediately apply pressure to the site with sterile gauze to prevent air from entering and to control bleeding. Inspect the catheter tip to determine that it is intact. After bleeding has stopped, apply an antiseptic ointment and sterile dressing to the site.

## CASE STUDY

### *Fluid and Electrolyte Imbalance*

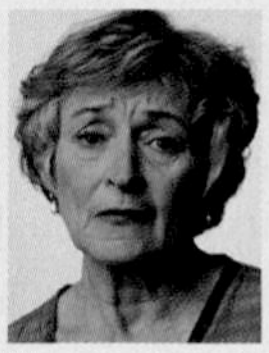

(©Kevin Peterson/ Photodisc/ Thinkstock)

**Patient Profile**

S.S., a 63-year-old white woman with acute lymphocytic leukemia, has been receiving chemotherapy on an outpatient basis. She completed her third treatment 5 days ago and has been experiencing nausea and vomiting for 2 days despite using ondansetron (Zofran). S.S.'s daughter brings her to the hospital, where she is admitted to the medical unit. As the admitting nurse, you perform a thorough assessment.

**Subjective Data**

- Complains of lethargy, weakness, dizziness, and dry mouth
- States she has been too nauseated to eat or drink anything for 2 days

**Objective Data**

- Heart rate 110 beats/min, pulse thready
- BP 100/65
- Weight loss of 5 lb since she received her chemotherapy treatment 5 days ago
- Dry oral mucous membranes

**Discussion Questions**

1. Based on her clinical manifestations, what fluid imbalance does S.S. have?
2. What additional assessment data should you obtain?
3. What are her risk factors for fluid and electrolyte imbalances?
4. You draw blood for a serum chemistry evaluation. What electrolyte imbalances are likely and why?
5. S.S. is at risk for which acid-base imbalance? Describe the changes that would occur in S.S.'s ABGs with this acid-base imbalance. How would the body compensate?
6. ***Teamwork and Collaboration:*** What is the interprofessional team's priority at this time for S.S.?
7. The physician orders dextrose 5% in 0.45% saline to infuse at 100 mL/hr. What type of solution is this, and how will it help S.S.'s fluid imbalance?
8. ***Priority Decision:*** What are the priority nursing interventions for S.S.?
9. ***Evidence-Based Practice:*** S.S. has a double-lumen PICC in her left arm. One lumen is connected to the IV infusion; the other is unused. What is the recommended practice for maintaining the patency of the unused lumen?
10. ***Quality Improvement:*** What outcomes will indicate that interprofessional care was effective?

Answers available at *http://evolve.elsevier.com/Lewis/medsurg.*

## BRIDGE TO NCLEX EXAMINATION

The number of the question corresponds to the same-numbered outcome at the beginning of the chapter.

1. During the postoperative care of a 76-year-old patient, the nurse monitors the patient's intake and output carefully, knowing that the patient is at risk for fluid and electrolyte imbalances primarily because
   - **a.** older adults have an impaired thirst mechanism and need reminding to drink fluids.
   - **b.** water accounts for a greater percentage of body weight in the older adult than in younger adults.
   - **c.** older adults are more likely than younger adults to lose extracellular fluid during surgical procedures.
   - **d.** small losses of fluid are significant because body fluids account for 45% to 50% of body weight in older adults.

2. During administration of a hypertonic IV solution, the mechanism involved in equalizing the fluid concentration between ECF and the cells is
   - **a.** osmosis.
   - **b.** diffusion.
   - **c.** active transport.
   - **d.** facilitated diffusion.

3a. An older woman was admitted to the medical unit with GI bleeding and fluid volume deficit. Clinical manifestations of this problem are (*select all that apply*)
   - **a.** weight loss.
   - **b.** dry oral mucosa.
   - **c.** full bounding pulse.
   - **d.** engorged neck veins.
   - **e.** decreased central venous pressure.

**3b.** The nursing care for a patient with hyponatremia and fluid volume excess includes
- **a.** fluid restriction.
- **b.** administration of hypotonic IV fluids.
- **c.** administration of a cation-exchange resin.
- **d.** placement of an indwelling urinary catheter.

**3c.** The nurse should be alert for which manifestations in a patient receiving a loop diuretic?
- **a.** Restlessness and agitation
- **b.** Paresthesias and irritability
- **c.** Weak, irregular pulse and poor muscle tone
- **d.** Increased blood pressure and muscle spasms

**3d.** Which patient is at *greatest* risk for developing hypermagnesemia?
- **a.** 83-year-old man with lung cancer and hypertension
- **b.** 65-year-old woman with hypertension taking β-adrenergic blockers
- **c.** 42-year-old woman with systemic lupus erythematosus and renal failure
- **d.** 50-year-old man with benign prostatic hyperplasia and a urinary tract infection

**3e.** It is important for the nurse to assess for which clinical manifestation(s) in a patient who has just undergone a total thyroidectomy (*select all that apply*)?
- **a.** Confusion
- **b.** Weight gain
- **c.** Depressed reflexes
- **d.** Circumoral numbness
- **e.** Positive Chvostek's sign

**3f.** The nurse expects the long-term treatment of a patient with hyperphosphatemia secondary to renal failure will include
- **a.** fluid restriction.
- **b.** calcium supplements.
- **c.** magnesium supplements.
- **d.** increased intake of dairy products.

**4.** The lungs act as an acid-base buffer by
- **a.** increasing respiratory rate and depth when $CO_2$ levels in the blood are high, reducing acid load.
- **b.** increasing respiratory rate and depth when $CO_2$ levels in the blood are low, reducing base load.
- **c.** decreasing respiratory rate and depth when $CO_2$ levels in the blood are high, reducing acid load.
- **d.** decreasing respiratory rate and depth when $CO_2$ levels in the blood are low, increasing acid load.

**5.** A patient has the following arterial blood gas results: pH 7.52, $PaCO_2$ 30 mm Hg, $HCO_3^-$ 24 mEq/L. The nurse determines that these results indicate
- **a.** metabolic acidosis.
- **b.** metabolic alkalosis.
- **c.** respiratory acidosis.
- **d.** respiratory alkalosis.

**6.** The typical fluid replacement for the patient with a fluid volume deficit is
- **a.** dextran.
- **b.** 0.45% saline.
- **c.** lactated Ringer's.
- **d.** 5% dextrose in 0.45% saline.

**7.** The nurse is unable to flush a central venous access device and suspects occlusion. The *best* nursing intervention would be to
- **a.** apply warm moist compresses to the insertion site.
- **b.** attempt to force 10 mL of normal saline into the device.
- **c.** place the patient on the left side with head-down position.
- **d.** instruct the patient to change positions, raise arm, and cough.

1. d, 2. a, 3a. a, b, e, 3b. a, 3c. c, 3d. c, 3e. a, d, e, 3f. b, 4. a, 5. d, 6. c, 7. d

For rationales to these answers and even more NCLEX review questions, visit *http://evolve.elsevier.com/Lewis/medsurg.*

## EVOLVE WEBSITE

*http://evolve.elsevier.com/Lewis/medsurg*

**Review Questions (Online Only)**

**Key Points**

**Answer Keys for Questions**
- Answer Guidelines for Case Study on p. 297
- Rationales for Bridge to NCLEX Examination Questions
- Answer Guidelines for Managing Care of Multiple Patients Case Study (Section 2) on p. 299

**Student Case Study**
- Patient With Hyponatremia/Fluid Volume Imbalance

**Conceptual Care Map Creator**

**Audio Glossary**

**Fluids and Electrolytes Tutorial**

**Content Updates**

## REFERENCES

1. McCance K, Huether SE: *Pathophysiology: the biologic basis for disease in adults and children*, ed 7, St Louis, 2014, Mosby.
2. Harring TR, Deal NS, Kuo DC: Disorders of sodium and water balance, *Emerg Med Clin N Am* 32:379, 2014.
3. Hooper L, Bunn D, Jimoh FO, Fairweather-Tait SJ: Water-loss dehydration and ageing, *Mech Ageing Dev* 136:50, 2014.
*4. Verbalis JG, Goldsmith SR, Greenberg A, et al: Diagnosis, evaluation, and treatment of hyponatremia: expert panel recommendations, *Am J Med* 126:S1, 2013.
5. Medford-Davis L, Rafique Z: Derangements of potassium, *Emerg Med Clin North Am* 32:329, 2014.
6. Crawford AH: Hyperkalemia: recognition and management of a critical electrolyte disturbance, *J Infus Nurs* 37:167, 2014.
7. Reagan P, Pani A, Rosner MH: Approach to the diagnosis and treatment of hypercalcemia in a patient with malignancy, *Am J Kidney Dis* 63:141, 2014.
8. Chang WT, Radin B, McCurdy MT: Calcium, magnesium, and phosphate abnormalities in the emergency department, *Emerg Med Clin North Am* 31:349, 2014.
9. Kelly A, Levine MA: Hypocalcemia in the critically ill patient, *J Int Care Med* 28:166, 2013.
10. Patel R, Taylor A, Pile T: Management of hypophosphataemia, *Br J Hosp Med* 74:C66, 2013.
11. Demssie Y, Patel L, Kumar M, Syed A: Hypomagnesemia: clinical relevance and management, *Br J Hosp Med* 75:39, 2014.
12. Soifer JT, Hyung TK: Approach to metabolic alkalosis, *Emerg Med Clin North Am* 32:453, 2014.
*13. Davison D, Rajit KB, Goldstein SL, Chawla LS: Fluid management in adults: core curriculum 2014, *Am J Kidney Dis* 63:700, 2014.
*14. Marschall J, Mermel LA, Fakih M, et al: Strategies to prevent central line–associated bloodstream infections in acute care hospitals: 2014 update, *Strategies* 35:753, 2014.

*Evidence-based information for clinical practice.

## CASE STUDY

### *Managing Care of Multiple Patients*

You and another RN are assigned to care for the following three patients in the intensive care unit (ICU). There is also a UAP (unlicensed assistive personnel) on duty.

#### Patients

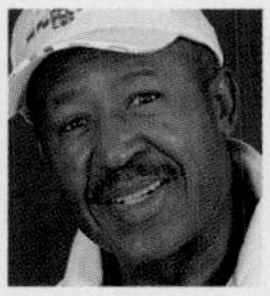
(©Stockphoto/ Thinkstock)

G.N., a 65-yr-old African American man, was admitted to the ICU after falling out of a tree onto a lit gas grill. He has partial-thickness burns on his face, neck, and upper trunk. He has undergone surgical repair of right tibia and left hip fractures as well as debridement of a severely lacerated right leg. His voice is slightly hoarse and he is coughing up sooty sputum. He is receiving $O_2$ at 4 L/min via nasal cannula, and his $O_2$ saturation is 93%. His WBC count is 26,400/μL (26.4 × $10^9$/L) with 80% neutrophils (10% bands).

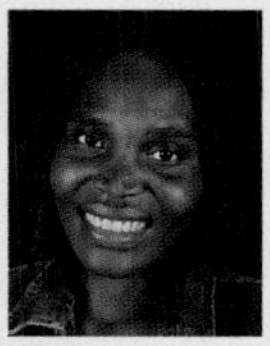
(©Stockphoto/ Thinkstock)

J.N., a 35-yr-old African American woman, was transferred to the ICU from the clinical unit last evening with acute respiratory failure. She was diagnosed 2 days ago with AIDS and *Pneumocystis jiroveci* pneumonia (PCP). Prior to this hospital admission she had consistently refused antiretroviral therapy (ART) because she could not afford it. She was started on oral trimethoprim/sulfamethoxazole (Bactrim) and combination antiretroviral therapy. However, her respiratory distress worsened and she was transferred to the ICU for intubation and mechanical ventilation. She is now receiving IV Bactrim.

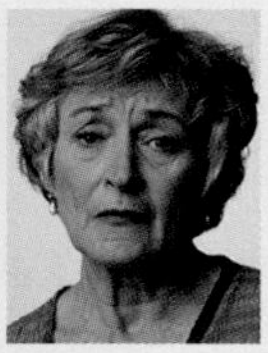
(© Kevin Peterson/ Photodisc/ Thinkstock)

S.S., a 63-yr-old white woman with acute lymphocytic leukemia, has been receiving chemotherapy on an outpatient basis. She completed her third treatment 5 days ago and has been experiencing nausea and vomiting for 2 days despite using ondansetron (Zofran). She was initially admitted to the clinical unit but was transferred to the ICU for close monitoring after becoming severely hypotensive overnight. Her most recent blood pressure was 98/50, HR 82 and regular, $O_2$ saturation 95% on 2L via nasal cannula, RR 22 and regular.

#### Discussion Questions

1. ***Priority Decision:*** After receiving report, which patient should you see first? Provide rationale.
2. ***Teamwork and Collaboration:*** Which morning tasks should you delegate to the UAP *(select all that apply)*?
   a. Take blood pressure readings on S.S.
   b. Perform respiratory assessment on G.N.
   c. Document strict intake and output on S.S.
   d. Provide oral care around the endotracheal tube for J.N.
   e. Titrate S.S.'s IV infusion rate based on her blood pressure reading.
3. ***Priority and Teamwork and Collaboration:*** When you enter J.N.'s room, the ventilator alarms are going off. The UAP had just finished providing oral care and she tells you that J.N. has become increasingly agitated within the last 5 minutes. Which *initial* action would be *most* appropriate?
   a. Suction J.N.'s endotracheal tube.
   b. Have the UAP stay with J.N. while you obtain IV sedation for her.
   c. Ask the UAP to describe exactly what she did when she was performing oral care.
   d. Assess the ventilator to identify what alarm is going off and to make sure all connections are secure.

#### Case Study Progression

J.N.'s ventilator tubing became disconnected. You quickly reconnect her tubing, and as she settles down her oxygenation improves. You ask the UAP to obtain vital signs on all your patients while you begin a more thorough assessment of J.N.

4. During your assessment of J.N., you note gray-white patches on the inside of her mouth. You recognize these as *most* likely caused by
   a. *Candida albicans.*
   b. poor oral hygiene.
   c. *Coccidioides immitis.*
   d. irritation from recent mouth care.
5. G.N.'s family asks you why surgery was performed on his leg wound. Your response is based on the knowledge that debridement *(select all that apply)*
   a. is used to remove infected tissue.
   b. is used to remove nonviable tissue.
   c. prepares the wound bed for healing.
   d. can only be accomplished in surgery.
   e. is necessary in any burn wound involving the skin.
6. S.S.'s morning laboratory results reveal a serum potassium level of 2.8 mEq/L. You notify the health care provider and obtain an order for IV potassium. During infusion of the potassium replacement, you prioritize assessment of S.S.'s
   a. bowel function.
   b. cardiac rhythm.
   c. muscle strength.
   d. level of consciousness.
7. ***Management Decision:*** While sitting at the computer charting your patients' morning assessments, you overhear the UAP telling a nursing student that J.N. deserves what she got because HIV is God's way of punishing those who sin. Your *most* appropriate response would be to
   a. report the UAP's actions to your supervisor.
   b. ask the UAP to keep her opinions to herself.
   c. ignore the conversation because it does not affect patient care.
   d. talk to the UAP and student about keeping personal feelings separate from patient care.

Answers available at *http://evolve.elsevier.com/Lewis/medsurg.*

# SECTION 3

# Perioperative Care

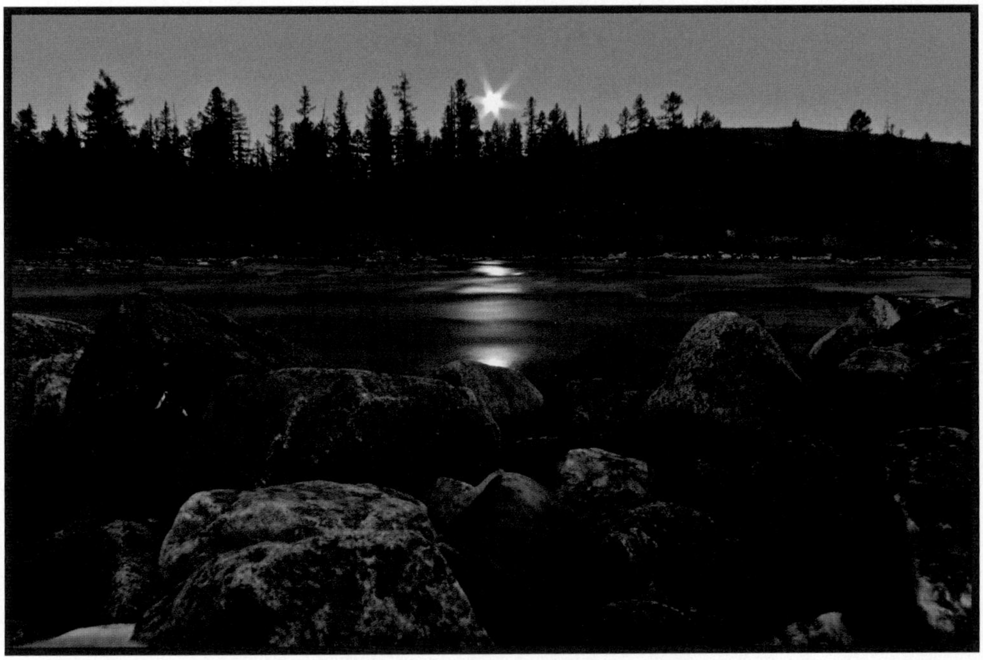

Thinkstock

*I choose to listen to the river for a while, thinking river thoughts, before joining the night and the stars.*

***Edward Abbey***

17

# Preoperative Care

*Janice A. Neil*

*The oldest and strongest emotion of mankind is fear, and the oldest and strongest kind of fear is fear of the unknown.*

***H.P. Lovecraft***

http://evolve.elsevier.com/Lewis/medsurg/

## LEARNING OUTCOMES

1. Differentiate the common purposes and settings of surgery.
2. Apply knowledge of the purpose and components of a preoperative nursing assessment.
3. Interpret the significance of data related to the preoperative patient's health status and operative risk.
4. Analyze the components and purpose of the patient's informed consent for surgery.
5. Examine the nursing role in the physical, psychologic, and educational preparation of the surgical patient.
6. Prioritize the nursing responsibilities related to day-of-surgery preparation for the surgical patient.
7. Differentiate the purposes and types of common preoperative medications.
8. Apply knowledge of the special considerations of preoperative preparation for the older adult surgical patient.

## KEY TERMS

ambulatory surgery, p. 302
elective surgery, p. 301
emergency surgery, p. 301
informed consent, p. 309
same-day admission, p. 301
surgery, p. 301

Preparation of patients for surgery is an important nursing role. This chapter discusses preoperative care that is applicable to all surgical patients regardless of where the surgery is performed. Preparation measures for specific surgical procedures (e.g., abdominal, thoracic, or orthopedic surgery) are discussed in appropriate chapters of this text.

**Surgery** is the art and science of treating diseases, injuries, and deformities by operation and instrumentation. The surgical experience involves an interprofessional team, including the patient, surgeon, anesthesia care provider (ACP), nurse, and other health care team members. Surgery may be performed for any of the following purposes:

- *Diagnosis:* Determination of the presence and extent of a pathologic condition (e.g., lymph node biopsy, bronchoscopy)
- *Cure:* Elimination or repair of a pathologic condition (e.g., removal of ruptured appendix or benign ovarian cyst)
- *Palliation:* Alleviation of symptoms without cure (e.g., cutting a nerve root [rhizotomy] to remove symptoms of pain, creating a colostomy to bypass an inoperable bowel obstruction)
- *Prevention* (e.g., removal of a mole before it becomes malignant, removal of the colon in a patient with familial polyposis to prevent cancer)
- *Cosmetic improvement* (e.g., repairing a burn scar, breast reconstruction after a mastectomy)
- *Exploration:* Surgical examination to determine the nature or extent of a disease (e.g., laparotomy). With the advent of advanced diagnostic tests, exploration is less common because many problems can be identified noninvasively.

Specific suffixes are commonly used in combination with a body part or organ in naming surgical procedures (Table 17-1).

## SURGICAL SETTINGS

Surgery may be a carefully planned event (**elective surgery**) or may arise with unexpected urgency (**emergency surgery**). Both elective and emergency surgeries are performed in a variety of settings. The setting where a surgical procedure may be safely performed is influenced by the type of surgery, potential complications, and the patient's health status. (Specific surgeries are described in chapters throughout the text in discussions of interventions for specific problems.)

For inpatient surgery, patients who are going to be admitted to the hospital are usually admitted on the day of surgery (**same-day admission**). Patients who are in the hospital before surgery are usually there because of acute or chronic medical conditions.

Reviewed by Janie Corbitt, RN, MLS, Retired Instructor of Nursing, Milledgeville, Georgia; Shari Gould, RN, MSN, Associate Professor of Nursing, Victoria College, Victoria, Texas; and Lisa Spruce, DNP, ACNS, ACNP, ANP, CNOR, CNS-CP, Director of Evidence-Based Perioperative Practice, Association of periOperative Registered Nurses, Denver, Colorado.

**TABLE 17-1 Suffixes Describing Surgical Procedures**

| Suffix | Meaning | Example |
|---|---|---|
| -ectomy | Excision or removal of | Appendectomy |
| -lysis | Destruction of | Electrolysis |
| -orrhaphy | Repair or suture of | Herniorrhaphy |
| -oscopy | Looking into | Endoscopy |
| -ostomy | Creation of opening into | Colostomy |
| -otomy | Cutting into or incision of | Tracheotomy |
| -plasty | Repair or reconstruction of | Mammoplasty |

The majority of surgical procedures are performed as **ambulatory surgery** (also called *same-day* or *outpatient surgery*). Many of these surgeries use minimally invasive techniques (e.g., laparoscopic techniques). Ambulatory surgery may be conducted in endoscopy clinics, physicians' offices, freestanding surgical clinics, and outpatient surgery units in hospitals. These procedures can be performed using general, regional, or local anesthetic and require less than a 24-hour stay postoperatively. Many patients go home with a caregiver within hours of surgery.

Ambulatory surgery is often preferred by patients and health care providers (HCPs). Generally, it requires fewer laboratory tests and preoperative and postoperative drugs and reduces the patient's risk for health care–associated infections. Patients like the convenience of recovering at home, HCPs prefer the flexibility in scheduling, and the cost is usually less for the patient and the insurer.

You play an essential role in preparing the patient for surgery, caring for the patient during surgery, and aiding the patient's recovery after surgery. To perform these functions effectively, first know the nature of the disorder requiring surgery and any co-morbidities. Second, identify the individual patient's response to the stress of surgery. Third, know the results of appropriate preoperative diagnostic tests. Last, identify potential risks and complications associated with the surgical procedure and any co-morbidities that should be included in the plan of care. The nurse caring for the patient preoperatively is likely to be different from the nurse in the operating room (OR), postanesthesia care unit (PACU), surgical intensive care unit (SICU), or surgical unit. Thus communication and documentation of important preoperative assessment findings are essential for quality care.

## PATIENT INTERVIEW

One of the most important nursing actions is the preoperative interview. The nurse who works in the physician's office, ambulatory surgery center, or hospital may do the interview.

The preoperative interview can occur in advance or on the day of surgery. The primary purposes of the patient interview are to (1) obtain the patient's health information, including drug and food allergies; (2) provide and clarify information about the planned surgery, including anesthesia; and (3) assess the patient's emotional state and readiness for surgery, including his or her expectations about the surgical outcomes. The interview also provides the patient and caregiver an opportunity to ask questions about surgery, anesthesia, and postoperative care. Often patients ask about taking their routine drugs, such as insulin, anticoagulants, or heart medications, and if they will experience pain. By being aware of the patient's and caregiver's needs, you can provide the information and support needed during the perioperative period.

## NURSING ASSESSMENT OF PREOPERATIVE PATIENT

The overall goal of the preoperative assessment is to identify risk factors and plan care to ensure patient safety throughout the surgical experience. To achieve this, you will need to do the following:

- Establish baseline data for comparison in the intraoperative and postoperative period.
- Determine the patient's psychologic status to reinforce the use of coping strategies during the surgical experience.
- Determine physiologic factors directly or indirectly related to the surgical procedure that may contribute to operative risk factors.
- Participate in the identification and documentation of the surgical site according to agency protocol.
- Identify prescription drugs, over-the-counter drugs, and herbs taken by the patient that may result in drug interactions affecting the surgical outcome.
- Review the results of all preoperative diagnostic studies in the patient's record, and share this information with the appropriate HCPs.
- Identify cultural and ethnic factors that may affect the surgical experience.
- Determine if the patient received adequate information from the surgeon to make an informed decision to have surgery and that the consent form is signed and witnessed.

### Subjective Data

**Psychosocial Assessment.** Surgery is a stressful event, even when the procedure is minor. The psychologic and physiologic reactions to surgery may elicit the stress response (e.g., elevated BP and heart rate). The stress response enables the body to meet the demands in the perioperative period. If stressors or the responses to the stressors are excessive, the stress response can be magnified and may affect recovery. Many factors influence the patient's reaction to stress, including age, past experiences with illness and pain, current health, and socioeconomic status.

The use of common language and avoidance of medical jargon are essential. Use words and language that are familiar to the patient to help the patient understand the surgery. Familiar language also helps reduce preoperative anxiety.

Your role in psychologically preparing the patient for surgery is to assess the patient for potential or actual stressors that could negatively affect surgery (Table 17-2). Communicate all concerns to the appropriate surgical team member, especially if the concern requires intervention later in the surgical experience. Because many patients are admitted directly into the preoperative area from their homes, you must be skilled in assessing important psychologic factors in a short time. The most common psychologic factors are anxiety, fear, and hope.

***Anxiety.*** Most people are anxious when facing surgery because of the unknown. This is normal and is an inborn survival mechanism. However, if the anxiety level is high, cognition, decision making, and coping abilities can be reduced.

Anxiety can arise from lack of knowledge. This can range from not knowing what to expect to uncertainty about the outcome and may result from past experiences or stories heard through friends or the media. You can decrease some anxiety

**TABLE 17-2 Psychosocial Assessment of Preoperative Patient**

**Situational Changes**
- Define current degree of personal control, decision making, and independence.
- Determine the presence of hope and anticipation of positive results.
- Consider the impact of surgery and hospitalization and possible effects on lifestyle.
- Identify support systems, including family, other caregivers, group and institutional structures, and religious and spiritual groups.

**Concerns With the Unknown**
- Identify specific areas and degree of anxiety and fears related to the surgery (e.g., pain).
- Identify expectations of surgery, changes in current health status, effects on daily living, and sexual activity (if appropriate).

**Concerns With Body Image**
- Identify current roles or relationships and view of self.
- Determine perceived or potential changes in roles or relationships and their impact on body image.

**Past Experiences**
- Review previous surgical experiences, hospitalizations, and treatments.
- Determine responses to those experiences (positive and/or negative).
- Identify current perceptions of surgical procedure in relation to the above and information from others (e.g., a friend's view of a personal surgical experience).

**Knowledge Deficit**
- Identify the amount and type of preoperative information the patient wants.
- Assess understanding of surgical procedure, including preparation, care, interventions, preoperative activities, restrictions, and expected outcomes.
- Identify the accuracy of information the patient has received from others, including health care team, family, friends, and media.

for the patient by providing information about what to expect. This is often done through classes or Web-based or audiovisual teaching materials before surgery. Inform the surgeon if the patient requires any additional information or if anxiety is excessive.

Patients may experience anxiety when surgery is in conflict with their religious or cultural beliefs. In particular, identify, record, and communicate patient decisions regarding the possibility of blood transfusions. For example, Jehovah's Witnesses may choose to refuse blood or blood products.[1]

***Common Fears.*** Patients fear surgery for a number of reasons. The most common fear is the risk of death or permanent disability resulting from surgery. Sometimes the fear comes after hearing or reading about the risks during the informed consent process. Other fears are related to pain, change in body image, or results of diagnostic procedures.

*Fear of death* can be extremely harmful. Notify the HCP if the patient has a strong fear of death. A patient's strong fear of impending death may prompt the HCP to delay the surgery because the emotional state influences the stress response and thus the surgical outcome.

*Fear of pain and discomfort* during and after surgery is common. If the fear is extreme, notify the ACP or the surgeon. Reassure the patient that drugs are available for anesthesia and analgesia during surgery. For pain after surgery, tell patients to ask for pain medication before pain becomes severe. Teach the patient how to use a pain intensity scale (e.g., 0 to 10, FACES). (Pain scales are explained in Chapter 8.)

Drugs may also be given that provide an amnesic effect so that the patient will not remember what occurs during surgery. Tell the patient that this effect assists in decreasing anxiety after surgery.

*Fear of mutilation* or *alteration in body image* can occur whether the surgery is radical, such as amputation, or minor, such as a breast biopsy. Even a small scar on the body can upset some, and others fear keloid development (overgrowth of a scar). Listen to and assess the patient's concern about this fear with an accepting attitude.

*Fear of anesthesia* may arise from the unknown, personal experience, or tales of others' bad experiences. These concerns can also result from information about the risks of anesthesia (e.g., brain damage, paralysis). Many patients fear losing control while under anesthesia. If these fears are identified, inform the ACP immediately so that he or she can talk further with the patient.

*Fear of disruption of life functioning* may be present in varying degrees. It can range from fear of permanent disability to concern about not being able to engage in activities of daily living for a few weeks. Concerns about loss of role function, separation from family, and how the family will manage may be revealed. Financial concerns may be related to an anticipated loss of income or the costs of surgery.

If you identify any of these fears, a consult with the patient's caregiver, a social worker, a spiritual advisor, or a psychologist

**EVIDENCE-BASED PRACTICE**

***Applying the Evidence***

**Music and Preoperative Anxiety**

You are taking care of D.G., a 74-year-old woman scheduled for aortic valve replacement surgery. She was admitted early this morning to the preoperative unit. Unfortunately, an emergency surgery has resulted in at least a 4-hour delay of her surgery. You note that she is currently experiencing a high level of anxiety.

***Making Clinical Decisions***

***Best Available Evidence.*** Music intervention in the preoperative period, including listening to pre-recorded music or individually tailored music administered by a trained therapist, may be effective in reducing anxiety.

***Clinician Expertise.*** Anxiety can increase BP and pulse rate and may lengthen postoperative recovery. Excessive anxiety in a patient can even result in surgery being cancelled. Nonpharmacologic methods of reducing preoperative anxiety, such as listening to music, may help patients reduce their anxiety.

***Patient Preference and Values.*** D.G. tells you that she is not able to relax and would like "a strong pill" to reduce her anxiety. D.G.'s family mentioned to you earlier that she enjoys listening to classical music at home.

***Implications for Practice***

1. What information would you share with D.G. related to the use of drugs to reduce her anxiety?
2. How would you respond to D.G. when she asks how music could possibly help in reducing her anxiety?

***Reference for Evidence***

Bradt J, Dileo C, Shim M: Music interventions for preoperative anxiety, *Cochrane Database Syst Rev* 6:CD006908, 2013.

## CHECK YOUR PRACTICE

Your 19-year-old male patient is in the holding area. He is scheduled for an orchiectomy for testicular cancer. He is visibly sweating and agitated. When you ask him how he is doing, he responds, "I am scared. Wouldn't you be?"

- What can you do to reduce his fear?

may be appropriate. Financial advisors at the hospital may be able to provide information about financial support.

***Hope.*** Although many psychologic factors related to surgery seem to be negative, hope is a positive attribute.[2] Hope may be the patient's strongest method of coping. To deny or minimize hope may negate the positive mental attitude necessary for a quick and full recovery. Some surgeries are hopefully anticipated. These can be the surgeries that repair (e.g., plastic surgery for burn scars), rebuild (e.g., total joint replacement to reduce pain and improve function), or save and extend life (e.g., repair of aneurysm, organ transplant). Assess and support the presence of hope and the patient's anticipation of positive results.

**Past Health History.** Ask the patient about any previous health problems and surgeries. Determine if the patient understands the need for surgery. For example, the patient scheduled for a total knee replacement may indicate that increasing pain and immobility are the reasons for the surgery.

Document the reason for any past hospitalizations, including previous surgeries and the dates. Also identify any problems with previous surgeries. For example, the patient may have experienced a wound infection or a reaction to a drug.

Ask women about their menstrual and obstetric history. This includes the date of their last menstrual period, the number of pregnancies, and any history of cesarean section.

When obtaining a family health history, ask the patient and caregiver about any inherited traits, since they may contribute to the surgical outcome. Record any family history of heart and endocrine diseases. For example, if a patient reports a parent with hypertension, sudden cardiac death, or myocardial infarction, this should alert you to the possibility that the patient may have a similar predisposition or condition. Also obtain information about the patient's family history of adverse reactions to or problems with anesthesia. For example, malignant hyperthermia has a genetic predisposition. Measures to decrease complications associated with this condition can be taken. (For further information on malignant hyperthermia, see Chapter 18.)

**Medications.** Document all current medication use, including over-the-counter drugs and herbs. In many ambulatory surgery centers, patients are asked to bring their medications with them when reporting for surgery. This helps to accurately assess and document the name and dosage of medications.

The interaction of the patient's current drugs and anesthetics can increase or decrease the desired physiologic effect of anesthetics. Consider the effects of opioids and prescribed drugs for chronic health conditions (e.g., heart disease, hypertension, depression, seizure disorder, diabetes). For example, certain antidepressants can potentiate the effect of opioids, agents that can be used for anesthesia. Antihypertensive drugs may predispose the patient to shock from the combined effect of the drug and the vasodilator effect of some anesthetic agents. Insulin or oral hypoglycemic drugs may require adjustments during the perioperative period because of increased body metabolism, decreased oral intake, stress, and anesthesia. Antiplatelet drugs (e.g., aspirin, clopidogrel [Plavix]) and nonsteroidal antiinflammatory drugs (NSAIDs) inhibit platelet aggregation and may contribute to postoperative bleeding.

Surgeons may instruct patients to withhold these drugs before surgery. Specific timeframes for withholding drugs depend on the drug and the patient. Patients on long-term anticoagulation therapy (e.g., warfarin [Coumadin], rivaroxaban [Xarelto], dabigatran [Pradaxa], apixaban [Eliquis]) present a unique challenge. The options for these patients include (1) continuing therapy, (2) withholding therapy for a time before and after surgery, or (3) withholding the therapy and starting subcutaneous or IV heparin therapy during the perioperative period. The management strategy selected is determined by patient history and the nature of the surgery.[3]

Ask about the use of herbs and dietary supplements because their use is so common. Many patients do not think to include supplements in their list of medications. They believe that herbal and dietary supplements are "natural" and do not pose a surgical risk.[4] (See the Complementary & Alternative Therapies box in Chapter 3 on p. 38 on how to assess for the use of herbal supplements.) Excessive use of vitamins and herbs can cause harmful effects in patients undergoing surgery. In patients taking anticoagulants or antiplatelets, herbal supplements can produce excessive postoperative bleeding that may require a return to the OR.[5] The effects of specific herbs that are of concern during the perioperative period are listed in the Complementary & Alternative Therapies box.

## COMPLEMENTARY & ALTERNATIVE THERAPIES

### *Herbal Products and Surgery*

The following can be used as a guide for patient teaching:

- Notify your HCP of all vitamins, herbs, and dietary supplements that you are taking.
- Avoid astragalus and ginseng, since they can increase BP before and during surgery.
- Avoid garlic, vitamin E, ginkgo, and fish oils because they can increase bleeding.
- Avoid kava and valerian because they can cause excess sedation.
- In general, discontinue all herbs 2 to 3 weeks before any surgical procedure. Consult your HCP for specific instructions.

**Helpful Herbs and Vitamins**

- Arnica is a homeopathic remedy useful in soft tissue healing.
- Multivitamins can be taken until the day before surgery. Taking them on the day of surgery on an empty stomach may contribute to nausea and vomiting after surgery.

Also ask the patient about any recreational drug use. The substances most likely to be used include tobacco, alcohol, opioids, marijuana, cocaine, and amphetamines. Ask questions about the use of these substances in a frank manner. Stress that recreational drug use may affect the type and amount of anesthesia that will be needed. When patients become aware of the potential interactions of these substances with anesthetics, most patients respond honestly about using them.

Chronic alcohol use can place the patient at risk because of lung, gastrointestinal, or liver damage. When liver function is decreased, metabolism of anesthetic agents is prolonged, nutritional status is altered, and the potential for postoperative complications is increased. Alcohol withdrawal can also occur during lengthy surgery or in the postoperative period. Although this can be a life-threatening event, it can be avoided with appropriate planning and management (see Chapter 10).

Record and share all findings of the drug history with the perioperative health care team. The ACP will determine the appropriate schedule and dose of the patient's routine drugs before and after surgery. Ensure that all of the patient's drugs are identified, implement any changes in the medication plan, and monitor the patient for potential interactions and complications.

**Allergies.** Ask the patient about drug intolerances and drug allergies. Drug intolerance usually results in side effects that are unpleasant for the patient but are not life threatening. These effects can include nausea, constipation, diarrhea, or *idiosyncratic* (opposite than expected) reactions. A true drug allergy produces hives and/or an anaphylactic reaction, causing cardiopulmonary compromise (e.g., hypotension, tachycardia, bronchospasm). Being aware of drug intolerances and drug allergies aids the health care team to maintain patient comfort and safety.

Record all drug intolerances and allergies and, if appropriate, place an allergy identification band on the patient on the day of surgery.

**SAFETY ALERT Allergies**

- Some local anesthetic agents contain bisulfite preservatives.
- Notify the ACP if the patient reports an allergy to sulfur-containing drugs.

Also inquire about nondrug allergies, specifically food and environmental (e.g., latex, pollen, animals) allergies. The patient with a history of any allergic reactions has a greater potential for hypersensitivity reactions to drugs given during anesthesia. Patients need to be screened specifically for latex allergies by gathering data in the following areas:

- Risk factors
- Contact dermatitis
- Contact urticaria (e.g., hives)
- Aerosol reactions
- History of reactions that suggest an allergy to latex

Risk factors for latex allergy include long-term, multiple exposures to latex products, such as those experienced by health care and rubber industry workers. Additional risk factors include a history of hay fever, asthma, and allergies to certain foods (e.g., eggs, avocados, bananas, chestnuts, potatoes, peaches).[6] (Latex allergies are discussed in Chapter 13.)

**Review of Systems.** The last component of the patient history is the body systems review. Ask specific questions to confirm the presence or absence of any diseases. Current health problems can alert you to areas that should be more closely examined in the preoperative physical examination. The combined review of systems and patient history provide essential data to determine the specific preoperative tests that need to be ordered.

***Cardiovascular System.*** Evaluate cardiovascular (CV) function to determine preexisting disease or problems (e.g., coronary artery disease, prosthetic heart valve). In reviewing the CV system, you may find a history of hypertension, angina, dysrhythmias, heart failure, or myocardial infarction. Inquire about the patient's current treatment for any CV condition (e.g., drugs) and the level of functioning. A cardiology consult is often required before surgery if the patient has a significant CV history (e.g., recent myocardial infarction [MI], valvular heart disease, implantable cardioverter-defibrillator).

If indicated, a 12-lead electrocardiogram (ECG) and coagulation studies should be ordered, and the results should be on the chart before surgery. The CV assessment provides data on what other measures have to be done. For example, the patient who is on diuretic therapy needs to have a serum potassium level drawn preoperatively. If the patient has a history of hypertension, the ACP may give vasoactive drugs to maintain adequate BP during surgery. If the patient has a prosthetic heart valve, antibiotic prophylaxis may be needed before surgery to decrease the risk of infective endocarditis (see Chapter 36).

Postoperative venous thromboembolism (VTE), a condition that includes deep vein thrombosis and pulmonary embolism, is a concern for any surgical patient. Patients at high risk for VTE include those with a history of previous thrombosis, blood-clotting disorders, cancer, varicosities, obesity, tobacco use, heart failure, or chronic obstructive pulmonary disease (COPD).[7] People are also at risk for developing a VTE because of immobility and positioning during the operative procedure. Antiembolism stockings or sequential compression devices (SCDs) may be applied in the preoperative holding area.

***Respiratory System.*** Ask the patient about any recent or chronic respiratory disease or infections. Elective surgery may be postponed if the person has an upper respiratory tract infection. Upper airway infections increase the risk of bronchospasm, laryngospasm, decreased $O_2$ saturation, and problems with respiratory secretions. Also report a patient's history of dyspnea at rest or with exertion, coughing (dry or productive), or hemoptysis (coughing blood) to the ACP and surgeon.

If a patient has a history of asthma, ask about the use of inhaled or oral corticosteroids and bronchodilators, as well as the frequency and triggers of asthma attacks. The patient with a history of COPD is at high risk for postoperative pulmonary complications, including hypoxemia and atelectasis.

Gather information about the patient's tobacco use. The patient should be encouraged to stop smoking at least 6 weeks preoperatively by the HCP, as smoking increases the risk for pulmonary complications during and after surgery. Report conditions likely to affect respiratory function such as sleep apnea, obesity, and spinal, chest, and airway deformities. For example, patients may be asked to bring their sleep apnea devices with them to the hospital or surgical center. Depending on the patient's history and physical examination, baseline pulmonary function tests and arterial blood gases may be ordered preoperatively.

***Neurologic System.*** Preoperative evaluation of neurologic functioning includes assessing the patient's ability to respond to questions, follow commands, and maintain orderly thought patterns. Alterations in the patient's hearing and vision may affect responses and the ability to follow directions throughout the perioperative assessment and evaluation. Record the patient's ability to pay attention, concentrate, and respond appropriately to establish a preoperative baseline for postoperative comparison.

If you note deficits in cognitive function, determine the extent of the problems and whether they can be corrected before surgery. If the problems cannot be corrected, it is important to involve a legal guardian or person with durable power of attorney for health care to assist the patient and provide informed consent for surgery.

Preoperative assessment of the older person's baseline cognitive function is especially crucial for intraoperative and postoperative evaluation. The older adult may have intact mental abilities preoperatively but is more prone to adverse outcomes during and after surgery than the younger adult. This is due to the additional stressors of the surgical procedure, dehydration, hypothermia, and anesthesia and adjunctive drugs. These factors may contribute to the development of *emergence delirium,* a condition that may be falsely labeled as senility or dementia. Thus preoperative findings are critical for postoperative comparison.

In the review of the neurologic system, inquire about any history of strokes, transient ischemic attacks, or spinal cord injury. Also ask about neurologic diseases, such as myasthenia gravis, Parkinson's disease, and multiple sclerosis, and any treatments used.

***Genitourinary System.*** Assess for a history of renal or urinary tract diseases, such as chronic kidney disease or repeated urinary tract infections. Record the present disease state and current treatment of the disease. Renal dysfunction is associated with a number of alterations, including fluid and electrolyte imbalances, coagulopathies, increased risk for infection, and impaired wound healing. Because many drugs are metabolized and excreted by the kidneys, a decrease in renal function can lead to an altered response to drugs and unpredictable drug elimination. Renal function tests (e.g., serum creatinine, blood urea nitrogen [BUN]) are commonly ordered preoperatively.

Record and share with the perioperative team if the patient has problems voiding (e.g., incontinence, hesitancy). Older male patients may have an enlarged prostate that can interfere with the insertion of a bladder catheter or impair voiding in the postoperative period.

For a woman of childbearing age, determine if she is pregnant or thinks she could be pregnant. Most agencies require a pregnancy test for all women of childbearing age before surgery.[8] Immediately inform the surgeon if the patient states that she may be pregnant, since maternal and fetal exposure to anesthetics during the first trimester should be avoided.

***Hepatic System.*** The liver is involved in glucose homeostasis, fat metabolism, protein synthesis, drug and hormone metabolism, and bilirubin formation and excretion. The liver detoxifies many anesthetics and adjunctive drugs. The patient with hepatic dysfunction may have an increased perioperative risk for clotting abnormalities and adverse responses to drugs. Consider the presence of liver disease if there is a history of jaundice, hepatitis, alcohol abuse, or obesity.

***Integumentary System.*** Ask about a history of skin problems. Assess the current condition of the skin, especially at the incision site, for rashes, breakdown, or other dermatologic conditions. A patient with a history of pressure ulcers may require extra padding during surgery. Skin problems can affect postoperative healing.

Body art such as tattoos and piercings are increasingly common. When possible, select pigment-free areas for injections, IV sites, and laboratory draws.

***Musculoskeletal System.*** Note any musculoskeletal and mobility problems, especially in the older adult. If the patient has arthritis, identify all affected joints. Mobility restrictions may influence intraoperative and postoperative positioning and ambulation. Spinal anesthesia may be difficult if the patient cannot flex the lumbar spine adequately to allow easy needle insertion. If the neck is affected, intubation and airway management may be difficult. Any mobility aids (e.g., cane, walker) should be brought with the patient on the day of surgery.

***Endocrine System.*** The patient with diabetes mellitus is especially at risk for adverse effects of anesthesia and surgery. Hypoglycemia, hyperglycemia, delayed wound healing, and infection are common complications of diabetes during the perioperative period. Clarify with the patient's surgeon or ACP whether the patient should take the usual dose of insulin or oral hypoglycemic agents on the day of surgery. ACPs may vary the usual insulin dose based on the patient's current status and history of glucose control. Regardless of the preoperative insulin or oral hypoglycemic orders, measure serum or capillary glucose levels the morning of surgery to establish baseline levels. Assess the patient's glucose levels regularly and, if necessary, manage according to agency protocol.

Determine if the patient has a history of thyroid dysfunction. Hyperthyroidism or hypothyroidism can place the patient at surgical risk because of alterations in metabolic rate. If the patient takes a thyroid replacement drug, check with the ACP about administration of the drug on the day of surgery. If the patient has a history of thyroid dysfunction, laboratory tests may be ordered to determine current levels of thyroid function.

The patient with Addison's disease also requires special consideration during surgery. Addisonian crisis or shock can occur if a patient abruptly stops taking replacement corticosteroids, and the stress of surgery may require additional IV corticosteroid therapy[9] (see Chapter 49).

***Immune System.*** If the patient has a history of a compromised immune system or takes immunosuppressive drugs, record it. Corticosteroids used in immunosuppressive doses may be tapered before surgery. Impairment of the immune system can lead to delayed wound healing and increased risk for postoperative infections.[10] If the patient has an acute infection (e.g., upper respiratory tract infection, sinusitis, influenza), elective surgery is often cancelled. Patients with active chronic infections such as hepatitis B or C, acquired immunodeficiency syndrome, or tuberculosis may have surgery if indicated. However, when preparing the patient for surgery, remember to take infection control precautions for the protection of the patient and staff.[11] (Infection control guidelines are discussed in Chapter 14.)

***Fluid and Electrolyte Status.*** Ask the patient about any recent conditions that increase the risk for fluid and electrolyte imbalances, such as vomiting, diarrhea, or preoperative bowel preps. For example, surgery may be planned for a patient with cholecystitis who has been vomiting for several days. Also identify drugs that alter fluid and electrolyte status, such as diuretics. Serum electrolyte levels are often assessed before surgery. Many patients may have restricted fluids for some time before surgery. If the surgery is delayed, they could develop dehydration. A patient with or at risk for dehydration may need additional fluids and electrolytes before or during surgery.

Although a preoperative fluid balance history should be completed for all patients, it is especially critical for older adults. Their reduced adaptive capacity leaves a narrow margin of safety between overhydration and underhydration.

***Nutritional Status.*** Nutritional deficits include overnutrition and undernutrition, both of which require considerable time to correct. However, knowing that a patient has a nutritional deficit can help the health care team provide more individualized care. For example, if the patient is thin, provide more padding than usual (pressure points on all patients are protected routinely) on the OR table. Notify the team if a patient is severely obese (body mass index [BMI] greater than 40 $kg/m^2$) to allow time to obtain special equipment needed for the patient's care (e.g., longer instruments for abdominal surgery).

Obesity stresses the cardiac and pulmonary systems and makes access to the surgical site and anesthesia administration more difficult.[12] It predisposes the patient to wound dehiscence, wound infection, and incisional herniation postoperatively. Adipose tissue is less vascular than other types of tissue. In addition, the patient may be slower to recover from anesthesia because inhalation agents are absorbed and stored by adipose tissue, thus leaving the body more slowly. (See Chapter 40 for special needs of obese patients undergoing surgery.)

Nutritional deficiencies impair the ability to recover from surgery. Remember that the obese patient and the very thin patient can also be protein and vitamin deficient. If the nutritional problem is severe, surgery may be postponed. Protein and vitamins A, C, and B complex deficiencies are particularly significant because these substances are essential for wound healing.[13]

**TABLE 17-3 American Society of Anesthesiologists' Physical Classification System**

| Rating | Definition |
|---|---|
| P1 | Normal healthy person |
| P2 | Patient with mild systemic disease |
| P3 | Patient with severe systemic disease |
| P4 | Patient with severe systemic disease that is a constant threat to life |
| P5 | Moribund patient who is not expected to survive without surgery |
| P6 | Declared brain-dead patient whose organs are being removed for donor purposes |

Source: American Society of Anesthesiologists: ASA physical status classification system, 2014. Retrieved from *www.asahq.org/clinical/physicalstatus.htm*.
NOTE: Patients selected for surgery in ambulatory or outpatient settings generally have ratings of P1, P2, or P3.

Supplemental nutrition may be given during the perioperative period to patients who are malnourished. The older adult is often at risk for malnutrition and fluid volume deficits.[8]

Identify patients who consume large quantities of coffee or caffeinated soft drinks. In many cases, withholding caffeinated beverages preoperatively or for some time postoperatively can lead to severe withdrawal headaches.[14] Caffeine withdrawal headaches can be confused with spinal headaches if the preoperative data are not recorded. Giving caffeinated beverages postoperatively, when possible, may prevent these headaches.

## Objective Data

**Physical Examination.** The Joint Commission requires that all patients admitted to the OR have a documented history and physical examination (H&P) in their chart.[15] This may be done in advance of surgery or on the day of surgery. It may be performed by any qualified person, including advanced practice nurses, physicians, physician assistants, or ACPs. Findings from the patient's H&P will enable the ACP to assign the patient a physical status rating for anesthesia administration (Table 17-3). This rating is an indicator of the patient's perioperative risk and may influence perioperative decisions.

In addition to the health assessment, also complete a physical examination of the patient before surgery (Table 17-4). Review

**TABLE 17-4 Health Assessment and Physical Examination of Preoperative Patient***

**Cardiovascular System**
- Identify acute or chronic problems. Note presence of angina, hypertension, heart failure, recent myocardial infarction, renal disease, diabetes.
- Identify any drugs (e.g., aspirin) or herbs (e.g., ginkgo) that may affect coagulation.
- Identify patients with prosthetic heart valves, pacemakers, or implantable cardioverter-defibrillators.
- Assess for edema (including dependent areas), noting location and severity.
- Inspect neck veins for distention.
- Obtain bilateral baseline BPs.
- Assess capillary refill and pulses (bilaterally when appropriate) for rate, rhythm, and quality: apical, radial, and pedal.

**Respiratory System**
- Identify acute or chronic problems. Note presence of infection, chronic obstructive pulmonary disease, or asthma. Note use of CPAP machine.
- Assess tobacco history, including date/time of last cigarette and number of pack-years.
- Determine baseline $O_2$ saturation and respiratory rate and rhythm.
- Observe for cough, dyspnea, and use of accessory muscles of respiration.
- Auscultate lungs for normal and adventitious breath sounds.

**Neurologic System**
- Determine orientation to person, place, and time.
- Assess baseline mental status. Note presence of confusion, disorderly thinking, or inability to follow commands.
- Identify past history of strokes, transient ischemic attacks, or neurologic diseases (e.g., Parkinson's disease, multiple sclerosis).

**Genitourinary System**
- Identify any infection or preexisting disease.
- Determine ability to void.
- Note color, amount, and characteristics of urine (if appropriate).
- Determine pregnancy status (if appropriate).

**Hepatic System**
- Review past history of substance abuse, especially alcohol and IV drug use.
- Inspect skin color and sclera of eyes for any signs of jaundice.

**Integumentary System**
- Determine skin status. Note any current or previous skin disorders (e.g., pressure ulcers, eczema, bruising).
- Inspect skin for rashes, boils, or infection, especially around the planned surgical site.
- Inspect mucous membranes and skin turgor for signs of dehydration.
- Assess skin moisture and temperature.

**Musculoskeletal System**
- Examine skin around bone pressure points.
- Assess for limitations in joint range of motion and muscle strength.
- Assess for joint or muscle pain.
- Assess mobility, gait, and balance.

**Gastrointestinal System**
- Determine patterns of food and fluid intake and any recent changes in weight.
- Determine usual pattern of bowel movements, including date of last bowel movement.
- Assess for presence of dentures and bridges (loose dentures or teeth may be dislodged during intubation).
- Weigh patient.
- Auscultate abdomen for presence of bowel sounds.

**Immune System**
- Identify any immunodeficiency or autoimmune disorders.
- Assess for use of corticosteroids or other immunosuppressant drugs.

**Laboratory and Diagnostic Studies**
- Review results of all laboratory and diagnostic studies completed preoperatively (see Table 17-5).

*CPAP*, Continuous positive airway pressure.
*See specific body system chapters for more detailed assessments and related laboratory studies.

**TABLE 17-5 Common Preoperative Diagnostic Studies**

| Test | Assessment |
|---|---|
| **ABGs, pulse oximetry** | Respiratory and metabolic function, oxygenation status |
| **Blood glucose** | Metabolic status, diabetes |
| **Blood urea nitrogen, creatinine** | Renal function |
| **Chest x-ray** | Pulmonary disorders, cardiac enlargement, heart failure |
| **CBC: RBCs, Hgb, Hct, WBCs** | Anemia, immune status, infection |
| **Electrocardiogram** | Cardiac disease, dysrhythmias |
| **Electrolytes** | Metabolic status, renal function, diuretic side effects |
| **hCG** | Pregnancy status |
| **Liver function tests** | Liver status |
| **PT, PTT, INR, platelet count** | Coagulation status |
| **Pulmonary function studies** | Pulmonary status |
| **Serum albumin** | Nutritional status |
| **Type and crossmatch** | Blood available for replacement (elective surgery patients may have own blood available) |
| **Urinalysis** | Renal status, hydration, urinary tract infection |

*CBC,* Complete blood count; *hCG,* human chorionic gonadotropin; *Hct,* hematocrit; *Hgb,* hemoglobin; *INR,* international normalized ratio; *PT,* prothrombin time; *PTT,* partial thromboplastin time.

the documentation already present in the patient's chart, including the H&P, to better proceed with your examination. Record all findings and share any relevant findings immediately with the surgeon or ACP.

**Diagnostic Studies.** Obtain and assess the results of diagnostic studies ordered preoperatively (Table 17-5). For example, if the patient is taking an antiplatelet drug (e.g., aspirin), a coagulation profile is ordered; if the patient is on diuretic therapy, a potassium level is assessed; if the patient is of childbearing age, a pregnancy test is done; or if the patient is taking drugs for dysrhythmias, a preoperative ECG is obtained. Blood glucose is monitored for patients with diabetes. In many settings, tests for methicillin-resistant *Staphylococcus aureus* are done preoperatively. Patients with positive results are prescribed antibiotics for several days before surgery.[16]

Ideally, preoperative tests are ordered based on the patient's H&P. However, many agencies and insurers have protocols for preoperative tests, which may not include all those in Table 17-5. In addition, the preoperative tests may be done days before surgery. Ensure that all laboratory and diagnostic reports are in the patient's chart. Missing reports may result in a delay or cancellation of the surgery.

## NURSING MANAGEMENT: PREOPERATIVE PATIENT

Preoperative nursing interventions are derived from the nursing assessment and must reflect each patient's specific needs. Physical preparations are determined by the pending surgery and routines of the surgery setting. Preoperative teaching may be minimal or extensive. The Association of periOperative Registered Nurses (AORN) provides standards and recommended practices to guide nursing interventions in all perioperative settings.[7]

### Preoperative Teaching

The patient has a right to know what to expect and how to participate effectively during the surgical experience. Preoperative teaching increases patient satisfaction and can reduce postoperative fear, anxiety, and stress.[17] Teaching may also decrease the development of complications, length of hospitalization, and recovery time after discharge.

In most surgical settings, patients often arrive only a short time before surgery is scheduled. Preoperative teaching for these patients is generally done in the surgeon's office or a preadmission surgical clinic and reinforced on the day of surgery. After ambulatory surgery the patient usually goes home several hours after recovery, depending on the patient's progress and procedure-specific needs. Teaching must include information that focuses on the patient's safety. Provide written materials for patients and caregivers to use for review and reinforcement at home. Discharge teaching is required for all patients[18] and is discussed in Chapter 19.

When doing preoperative teaching, find a balance between explaining so much that the patient is overwhelmed and telling so little that the patient is unprepared. If you observe and listen carefully to the patient, you can usually determine how much information is enough. Remember that anxiety and fear may limit learning ability. Also assess what the patient wants to know and give priority to those concerns.

Generally, preoperative teaching includes three types of information: sensory, process, and procedural. Different patients, with varying cultures, backgrounds, and experience, may want different types of information. See Table 4-7 for factors affecting patient teaching.

With *sensory information,* patients find out what they will see, hear, smell, and feel during the surgery. For example, you may tell them that the OR will be cold, but they can ask for a warm blanket; the lights in the OR are bright; or many unfamiliar sounds and specific smells will be present.

Patients wanting *process information* may not want specific details but just the general flow of what is going to happen. This information would include the patient's transfer to the holding area, visits by the nurse and the ACP before transfer to the OR, and waking up in the PACU.

With *procedural information,* patients desire details that are more specific. For example, this information would include that an IV line will be started while the patient is in the holding area and the surgeon will mark the operative area with an indelible marker to verify the surgical site.[7]

Share the preoperative teaching given to the patient with the nurses providing postoperative care to evaluate learning and avoid duplication of teaching. Because the time for teaching is limited, the team approach is often used. For example, teaching may be started in the outpatient setting. Your responsibility is to assess the patient's understanding of this teaching and fill in the gaps at this point in the surgical process.

Record all teaching in the patient's chart. A guide for preoperative patient and caregiver teaching is presented in Table 17-6. See Chapter 4 for additional information on patient and caregiver teaching.

**General Surgery Information.** Unless contraindicated (e.g., after craniotomy, tonsillectomy), all patients should receive instruction about deep breathing, coughing, and early ambulation postoperatively. This is essential because patients may not want to do these activities postoperatively unless they know the reason for them and practice them preoperatively. Tell patients

**TABLE 17-6 Patient & Caregiver Teaching**

***Preoperative Preparation***

*Include the following information in the preoperative teaching plan for the patient and caregiver.*

**Sensory Information**

- Preoperative holding area may be noisy.
- Drugs and cleaning solutions may be odorous.
- Operating room (OR) can be cold. Forced air warming devices may be used. Warm blankets are also available and can be requested.
- Talking may be heard in OR but may be distorted because of masks. Ask questions if something is not understood.
- OR bed will be narrow. A safety strap will be applied over the thighs.
- Lights in the OR may be bright.
- Monitoring machines may be heard (e.g., beeping noises) when awake.

**Procedural Information**

- What to bring and what type of clothing to wear to the surgery center
- Any changes in time of surgery.
- Fluid and food restrictions.
- Physical preparation required (e.g., shower, bowel, or skin preparation).
- Purpose of frequent vital signs assessment.
- Pain control and other comfort measures.
- Why turning, deep breathing, and coughing postoperatively are important. Practice sessions must be done preoperatively.
- Insertion of IV lines.
- Procedure for anesthesia administration.
- Expect surgical site to be marked with indelible ink or marker.

**Process Information**

***Information About General Flow of Surgery***

- Admission area.
- Preoperative holding area, OR, and postanesthesia care unit (PACU).
- Caregivers can usually stay in preoperative holding area until surgery.
- Caregivers will be able to see patient after discharge from the PACU or possibly in PACU once the patient is awake.
- Identification of any technology that may be present on awakening, such as monitors, central lines, sequential compression devices.

***Where Caregivers Can Wait During Surgery***

- Encourage caregivers to ask questions and express any concerns.
- OR staff will update caregivers during surgery and when surgery is completed.
- Surgeon will usually talk with caregivers after surgery.

and caregivers if tubes, drains, monitoring devices, or special equipment will be used after surgery. Explain that these devices help you to safely care for the patient. Examples of individualized teaching may include how to use incentive spirometers or postoperative patient-controlled analgesia pumps. Patients should have a clear understanding of how to rate their pain and how their pain will be managed.[19] (See Chapter 8 for additional information on pain.)

The patient should also receive accurate surgery-specific information. For example, a patient having a total joint replacement may have an immobilizer after surgery, or a patient having heart surgery should be told about waking up in the intensive care unit.

◆ **Ambulatory Surgery Information.** The ambulatory surgery patient or the patient admitted to the hospital the day of surgery needs to receive information before admission. Some ambulatory surgical centers telephone the patients several days before the procedure to obtain health information, give instructions, and answer questions. Each center has policies and procedures that direct this communication in a timely manner.

In addition to specifics on the procedure, patients need information on day-of-surgery events such as arrival time, registration, parking, what to wear, what to bring, and the need to have a responsible adult present for transportation home after surgery.

Traditionally, patients having elective surgery are told to have nothing by mouth (NPO) starting at midnight on the night before surgery. Evidence-based guidelines published by the American Society of Anesthesiologists are less strict[20] (Table 17-7). Restriction of fluids and food is designed to reduce the risk of pulmonary aspiration and postoperative nausea and vomiting. Protocols may vary for patients having local anesthesia or surgery scheduled late in the day. Follow the NPO protocol of each surgical setting. The patient who has not followed the NPO instructions may have surgery delayed or cancelled. It is critical that the patient understands the reason for and follows all restrictions.

**TABLE 17-7 Preoperative Fasting Recommendations***

| Liquid and Food Intake | Minimum Fasting Period (Hr) |
|---|---|
| Clear liquids (e.g., water, clear tea, black coffee, carbonated beverages, fruit juice without pulp) | 2 |
| Breast milk | 4 |
| Nonhuman milk, including infant formula | 6 |
| Light meal (e.g., toast and clear liquids) | 6 |
| Regular meal (may include fried or fatty food, meat) | 8 or more |

Source: Practice guidelines for preoperative fasting and the use of pharmacologic agents to reduce the risk of pulmonary aspiration: application to healthy patients undergoing elective procedures: an updated report by the American Society of Anesthesiologists Task Force on Preoperative Fasting. Retrieved from *http://anesthesiology.pubs.asahq.org/Article.aspx?articleid=1933410.*

*For healthy patients of all ages undergoing elective surgery (excluding women in labor).

## ◆ Legal Preparation for Surgery

Legal preparation for surgery consists of checking that all required forms have been correctly signed and are present in the patient's chart, and that the patient and caregiver clearly understand what is going to happen. Standard consent forms include those for the surgical procedure and blood transfusions. Other forms may include advance directives and durable power of attorney for health care (see Chapter 9).

◆ **Consent for Surgery.** Before nonemergency surgery can be legally performed, the patient must voluntarily sign an informed consent form in the presence of a witness. **Informed consent** is an active, shared decision-making process between the HCP and recipient of care. Three conditions must be met for consent to be valid. First, there must be *adequate disclosure* of the (1) diagnosis; (2) nature and purpose of the proposed treatment; (3) risks and consequences of the proposed treatment; (4) probability of a successful outcome; (5) availability, benefits, and risks of alternative treatments; and (6) prognosis if treatment is not instituted. Second, the patient must demonstrate clear *understanding* of the information being provided before receiving sedating preoperative drugs. If a patient is sedated prior to signing the consent, surgery may be cancelled or delayed. Third, the recipient of care must *give consent voluntarily.* The patient must not be persuaded or coerced in any way by anyone to undergo the procedure.[21]

The surgeon is ultimately responsible for obtaining the patient's consent for surgical treatment. You may be asked to witness the patient's signature on the consent form. At this time, you must be a patient advocate, verifying that the patient understands the information in the consent and the implications of consent, and that consent for surgery is truly voluntary. If the patient is unclear about the surgical plans, contact the surgeon about the patient's need for additional information. The patient should also be aware that consent, even when signed, can be withdrawn at any time.

If the patient is a minor, unconscious, or mentally incompetent to sign the permit, a legally appointed representative or responsible family member may give written permission. An *emancipated minor* is one who is younger than the legal age of consent but is recognized as having the legal capacity to provide consent.[19] Procedures for obtaining consent vary among states and agencies. Follow specifics required by your state's nurse practice act and agency policies that apply to an individual situation.

## ETHICAL/LEGAL DILEMMAS

### *Informed Consent*

**Situation**

J.S., a 72-year-old woman, is waiting in the preoperative holding area. You are discussing her impending surgery when you realize that this competent adult does not fully understand her surgery and was not informed of the alternatives to this surgery. Although she has previously signed a consent form, your assessment is that she was not fully informed about her treatment options or does not recall them.

**Ethical/Legal Points for Consideration**

- Informed consent requires that patients have complete information about the proposed treatment, as well as alternative treatments, risks and benefits of each treatment option, and possible consequences of the surgical procedure. The person (usually the surgeon) performing the procedure usually has this responsibility.
- An opportunity to have questions answered about the various treatment options and their possible outcomes is also an important element of informed consent.
- A patient can revoke the consent at any time, even at the very last minute. It is essential that you report any circumstance that suggests that the patient does not understand the information or is revoking the informed consent to the person who obtained the consent.
- In most states, the registered nurse's legal role is to witness the signing of the document. This means that as a nurse, you attest to the fact that the patient's signature was valid.

**Discussion Questions**

1. What do you think you should do next?
2. What is your role as a patient advocate in the informed consent process?
3. What should you do if the patient states that she does not want to know about the surgical procedure or alternatives to surgery?

A true medical emergency may override the need to obtain consent.[19] When immediate medical treatment is needed to preserve life or prevent serious impairment to life or limb and the patient is incapable of giving consent, the next of kin may give consent. If reaching the next of kin is not possible, the HCP may begin treatment without written consent. A note is written in the chart documenting the medical necessity of the procedure. In the case of an emergency in which consent cannot be obtained, you will usually need to complete an event report because it is an occurrence that is inconsistent with routine agency practices.

## ◆ Day-of-Surgery Preparation

◆ **Nursing Role.** Day-of-surgery preparation varies a great deal depending on whether the patient is an inpatient or an ambulatory surgical patient. Your responsibilities immediately before surgery include final preoperative teaching, assessment, and communication of pertinent findings. In addition, ensure that all preoperative orders are done and that the chart is complete and accompanies the patient to the OR. It is especially important to verify the presence of a signed informed consent, results of laboratory and diagnostic studies, an H&P, a record of any consultations, baseline vital signs, proper skin preparation, and completed nursing notes. In addition, the surgical site is identified and marked with an indelible marker by the surgeon and documented to indicate that the patient agrees.[7]

Hospitals often require that a patient wear a hospital gown with no underclothes. Surgical centers may allow the patient to wear underwear, depending on the procedure to be performed. The patient should remove any cosmetics, since observation of skin color is important. Nail polish and artificial nails should be removed so that capillary refill and pulse oximetry can be assessed. Place an identification band on the patient and, if applicable, an allergy band (Fig. 17-1). Return all patient valuables to a caregiver or secure according to agency policy. All prostheses, including dentures, contact lenses, and glasses, are generally removed to prevent loss or damage. If electrocautery devices will be used during surgery, jewelry in piercings must be removed as a safety measure. Hearing aids should be left in place to allow the patient to better follow instructions. Return glasses to the patient as soon as possible after surgery.

Encourage the patient to void before preoperative drugs are given and before transfer to the OR. An empty bladder prevents involuntary elimination under anesthesia and reduces the risk of urinary retention during the early postoperative recovery.

Many preoperative drugs interfere with balance and increase the risk for a fall during ambulation. Carefully assess each patient for responses to preoperative drugs and adjust the plan of care accordingly.

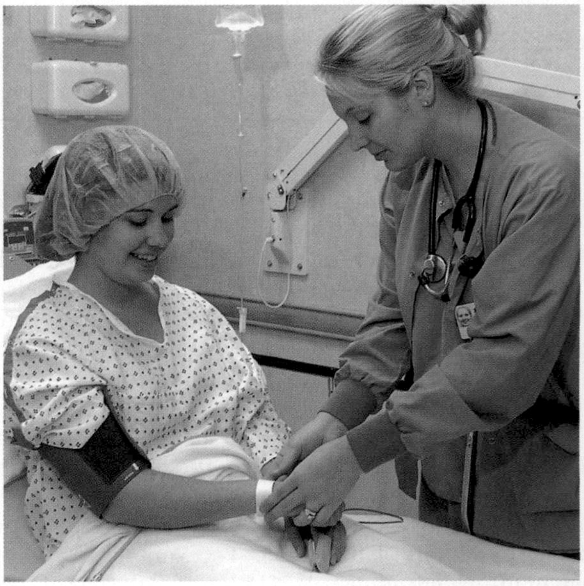

**FIG. 17-1** The nurse performs a safety check by verifying that the patient has an identification band (wristband) as part of the preoperative preparations before she goes to surgery. (Courtesy Susan R. Volk, RN, MSN, CCRN, CPAN, Staff Development Specialist, Christiana Care Health System, Newark, Del.)

## CHECK YOUR PRACTICE

You are caring for an older female patient who received a dose of alprazolam (Xanax) for preoperative anxiety. One hour later, she requests to use the bathroom. You ask her if she can walk and she replies "yes." When assisting her to stand, she becomes dizzy and almost falls. You return her to bed.

- Instead of trying to help this patient ambulate to the bathroom, what should have you done?

**Preoperative Medications.** Preoperative medications are used for a variety of reasons (Table 17-8). A patient may receive a single drug or a combination of drugs. Benzodiazepines are used for their sedative and amnesic properties. Anticholinergics are sometimes given to reduce secretions. Opioids may be given to decrease pain and intraoperative anesthetic requirements. Antiemetics may be given to decrease nausea and vomiting.

Other drugs that may be given preoperatively include antibiotics, eyedrops, and routine prescription drugs. Antibiotics may be given throughout the perioperative period for patients with a history of prosthetic heart valve to prevent infective endocarditis and for patients with previous joint replacement. Antibiotics may also be ordered for the patient undergoing surgery where wound contamination is a potential risk (e.g., gastrointestinal surgery). Antibiotics are most often given IV and are usually started preoperatively (e.g., 30 to 60 minutes before the surgical incision).

## INFORMATICS IN PRACTICE

### *Computer-Based Timing for Antibiotic Administration*

- A patient who receives the appropriate preoperative antibiotic has a decreased risk of a health care–associated infection.
- Using a computer to time the administration of preoperative antibiotics can decrease the incidence of wound infections.
- Computer-based timing systems assist with quality of care by tracking patient outcomes.
- You can look at the time patients received antibiotics and compare the rate of wound infections for those who did and did not receive timely treatment.

β-Adrenergic blockers (β-blockers) are sometimes used in people with known hypertension or coronary artery disease to control BP or reduce the chances of MI and cardiac arrest.[22] People with diabetes are also carefully monitored and may receive insulin in the preoperative period.[19] Eyedrops are often ordered and given preoperatively for the patient undergoing cataract and other eye surgery. Many times the patient will require multiple sets of eyedrops given at 5-minute intervals. It is important to give these drugs as ordered and on time to adequately prepare the eye for surgery.

Drugs that patients routinely take may or may not be used on the day of surgery. To aid patient teaching and remove confusion about which drugs should be taken, carefully check written preoperative orders and clarify the orders with the surgeon and/or ACP if there is any question.

Preoperative drugs may be ordered by mouth (PO), IV, or subcutaneously. Provide PO drugs with a small sip of water 60 to 90 minutes before the patient goes to the OR unless otherwise ordered. Subcutaneous injections (e.g., insulin) and IV drugs are usually given to the patient after arrival in the preoperative holding area or OR. Inform the patient about the expected effects of the drugs (e.g., drowsiness).

## TABLE 17-8 Drug Therapy

### *Commonly Used Preoperative Medications*

| Class | Drug | Purpose |
|---|---|---|
| **Antibiotics** | cefazolin (Ancef) | Prevent postoperative infection |
| **Anticholinergics** | atropine<br>glycopyrrolate (Robinul)<br>scopolamine (Transderm-Scop) | ↓ Oral and respiratory secretions<br>Prevent nausea and vomiting<br>Provide sedation |
| **Antidiabetics** | insulin (Humulin R) | Stabilize blood glucose |
| **Antiemetics** | metoclopramide (Reglan)<br>ondansetron (Zofran) | ↑ Gastric emptying<br>Prevent nausea and vomiting |
| **Benzodiazepines** | midazolam<br>diazepam (Valium)<br>lorazepam (Ativan) | ↓ Anxiety, induce sedation, amnesic effects |
| **β-Blockers** | labetalol | Manage hypertension |
| **Histamine ($H_2$)-receptor antagonists** | famotidine (Pepcid)<br>ranitidine (Zantac) | ↓ HCl acid secretion, ↑ pH, ↓ gastric volume |
| **Opioids** | morphine (Duramorph)<br>fentanyl (Sublimaze) | Relieve pain during preoperative procedures |

**SAFETY ALERT Preoperative Checklist**

- Use a preoperative checklist (Table 17-9) to ensure that all preoperative preparations have been completed.
- This is especially important to do before the patient is given any sedating drugs.

## Transportation to Operating Room

For inpatients, transport staff move the patient by stretcher to the OR. Assist the patient in moving from the bed to the stretcher, raise the side rails, and ensure that the completed chart and any ordered preoperative equipment (e.g., SCDs) goes with the patient. In many agencies the caregiver may go with the patient to the holding area.

In an ambulatory surgical center the patient may be transported to the OR by stretcher or wheelchair. If no sedatives have been given, the patient may even walk accompanied to the OR. In all cases it is important to ensure patient safety during transport. Record the method of transportation and the person who transports the patient to the OR. Provide the hand-off communication to the nurse receiving the patient. This allows each of you to ensure that all pertinent information regarding the patient has been shared.[23] To avoid adverse events related to miscommunication, AORN recommends the use of the Situation-Background-Assessment-Recommendation (SBAR) model for the hand-off process in this setting[19] (see Table 1-6).

Show the caregiver where to wait for the patient during surgery. Many hospitals have a surgical waiting room where OR staff communicate the patient's status to the caregiver(s) and notify them when the surgery is complete. The surgeon also can locate the caregiver in this room after surgery to discuss the outcome. Some hospitals provide pagers to caregivers so that they may eat or do errands during the surgery.

## Culturally Competent Care: Preoperative Patient

Include cultural considerations when assessing and implementing care for the patient's preoperative needs. For example, culture often determines one's expression of pain, family expectations, and ability to verbally express needs. One's culture may

**TABLE 17-9 Preoperative Checklist**

| Preoperative Data | Initials |
|---|---|
| Height ____ Weight ____ | |
| Isolation Y or N Type ____ | |
| Allergies noted on chart Y or N | |
| Vital signs (baseline) T ____ P ____ R ____ BP ____ Pulse Ox ____ | |
| **Chart Review** | |
| H&P on chart | |
| H&P within 30 days? Y or N | |
| Signed and witnessed informed consent form on chart Y or N | |
| Signed consent for blood administration Y or NA | |
| Blood type and crossmatch Y or NA | |
| **Diagnostic Results** | |
| Hgb/Hct ____/____ NA | |
| PT/INR/PTT ____/____/____ NA | |
| CXR ____ NA | |
| ECG ____ NA<br>hCG ____ Negative ____ Positive ____NA | |
| Other labs: | |
| **Final Chart Review** | |
| Additional forms attached: | |

| Day of Surgery | Initials |
|---|---|
| Surgical site marked Y or NA | |
| ID band on patient Y or N | |
| Allergy band on patient Y or NA | |
| Vital signs Time ________<br>T ____ P ____ R ____ BP ____ Pulse Ox ____ | |
| **Procedures** | |
| NPO since ____ | |
| Capillary blood glucose Time ____ Result: ____ NA | |
| Voided/catheter Time ____ | |
| Preoperative drugs given Time ____ NA | |
| Preoperative antibiotics given Time ____ NA | |
| Preoperative skin prep Y or NA<br>Shower____ Scrub____ Clip____ | |
| Makeup, nail polish, false fingernails, and false eyelashes removed Y or NA | |
| Hospital gown applied Y or NA | |
| **Valuables** | |
| Dentures Y or N | |
| Wig or hairpiece Y or N | |
| Eyeglasses Y or N | |
| Contact lenses Y or N | |
| Hearing aid Y or N | |
| Prosthesis Y or N | |
| Jewelry Y or N Piercings with jewelry Y or N | |
| Clothing Y or N | |
| Disposition of valuables: Hearing aid in place Y or NA | |

Time to OR ________________ Date ________________
Transported to OR by ________________
Final check by ________________ RN ________________

require that the family be included in any decision making. For example, many older Hispanic women may defer to their family for the decision whether or not to have surgery. Respect these decisions. If the patient or caregiver does not speak English, it is mandated that a qualified interpreter or translator communication system be used.[24] (Culturally competent care is discussed in Chapter 2.)

## Gerontologic Considerations: Preoperative Patient

Many surgical procedures are done on patients older than 65 years of age. Surgery on older adults requires careful evaluation.[25] Frequently performed procedures in older adults include cataract extraction, coronary and vascular procedures, prostate surgery, herniorrhaphy, cholecystectomy, and joint repair or replacement.

Be particularly alert when assessing and caring for the older adult surgical patient. An event that has little effect on a younger adult may be overwhelming to the older patient. Emotional reactions to impending surgery and hospitalization often intensify in the older adult. Hospitalization may represent a physical decline and loss of health, mobility, and independence. The older adult may view the hospital as a place to die or as a stepping-stone to a nursing home. Help to decrease anxieties and fears while maintaining the self-esteem of the older adult during the surgical experience.

The risks associated with anesthesia and surgery increase in the older patient. In general, the older the patient, the greater the risk of complications after surgery. In planning care, consider the patient's physiologic status, not only the chronologic age. The surgical risk in the older adult relates to normal physiologic aging and changes that compromise organ function, reduce reserve capacity, and limit the body's ability to adapt to stress. This decreased ability to cope with stress, often compounded by the burden of one or more chronic illnesses, and the surgery itself increase the risk of complications.[25]

When preparing the older adult for surgery, obtain a detailed H&P. Preoperative laboratory tests, an ECG, and a chest x-ray are important in planning the choice and type of anesthesia. The patient's primary HCP is usually not the surgeon, and frequently several HCPs are involved in the patient's care.

Older adults may have some sensory deficits. Vision and hearing may be reduced, and bright lights may bother those with eye problems. Thought processes and cognitive abilities may be slowed or impaired. Assess and record baseline sensory and cognitive function. Physical reactions are often slowed as a result of mobility and balance problems. All these changes may require more time for the older adult to complete preoperative testing and understand preoperative instructions. These changes also require attention to promote patient safety and prevent injury. (See Chapter 5 for more discussion about older adults.)

When older adults live in a long-term care or assisted living facility, you may need to coordinate transportation from these facilities so that timely arrival allows for surgery preparation. A legal representative of the patient must be present to provide consent for surgery if the patient cannot sign for himself or herself.

Finally, determine the presence of or need for caregiver support for the older adult undergoing surgery. With the increase in outpatient surgical procedures and shorter postoperative length of stays, caregiver support is critical in the continuity of care for this population.

## CASE STUDY

### *Preoperative Patient*

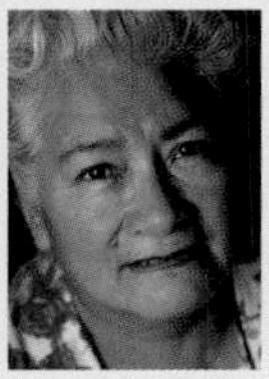

(©Ryan McVay/ Photodisc/ Thinkstock)

**Patient Profile**

F.D., a 72-year-old Hispanic retired librarian, is admitted to the hospital with compromised circulation of the right lower leg and a necrotic right foot. She has diabetes and takes insulin to maintain appropriate blood glucose levels. She has been NPO since midnight. It is now 10 AM on the morning of the surgery.

**Subjective Data**

- History of type 2 diabetes for 30 years; states, "My blood sugar is hard to control" and "I just started taking insulin"
- History of hypertension
- History of stage 2 chronic kidney disease
- History of peripheral vascular disease
- History of macular degeneration in right eye; reports poor vision
- Surgical history: cesarean section at age 30, cholecystectomy at age 65; reports poor wound healing after last surgery
- States her Social Security checks barely cover her living expenses
- States she often runs out of her drugs and cannot always afford to refill them right away
- Reports chronic burning pain in both legs and has trouble sleeping at night
- Lives alone but has family who want her to move in with them after surgery
- Uses herbs to control blood glucose levels and frequently skips her insulin

**Objective Data**

***Physical Examination***

- Alert, cognitively intact, anxious, older woman with complaints of numbness and lack of feeling in right leg
- Weight 190 lb, height 5 ft 3 in
- BP 180/94, pulse 84 and slightly irregular
- Wears glasses for close work and reading

***Diagnostic Studies***

- Admission serum blood glucose level 272 mg/dL (15.2 mmol/L), glycosylated hemoglobin (Hb A1C) 14%
- Morning capillary blood glucose level 198 mg/dL (11 mmol/L)
- Doppler pulses for right lower leg weak, absent in right foot
- Doppler pulses in left lower leg present, weak in left foot
- Serum creatinine 2.0 mg/dL (176 mmol/L)

**Interprofessional Care**

- Scheduled for a below-the-knee amputation of the right leg at 1 PM today

**Discussion Questions**

1. What factors may influence F.D.'s response to hospitalization and surgery?
2. ***Priority Decision:*** Given F.D.'s history, what priority preoperative nursing assessments would you want to complete and why?
3. What potential perioperative complications may you expect for F.D.?
4. ***Priority Decision:*** What priority topics would you include in F.D.'s preoperative teaching plan?
5. ***Priority Decision:*** Based on the assessment data presented, identify the priority nursing diagnoses and related interventions. Are there any collaborative problems?
6. ***Teamwork and Collaboration:*** Identify appropriate preoperative interventions that must be completed and could be delegated to unlicensed assistive personnel (UAP).
7. ***Safety:*** To ensure F.D.'s safety, what preoperative nursing interventions are essential?
8. ***Evidence-Based Practice:*** F.D. asks you why she received insulin this morning when she has not eaten anything since midnight. How would you respond to her?

Answers available at *http://evolve.elsevier.com/Lewis/medsurg.*

## BRIDGE TO NCLEX EXAMINATION

The number of the question corresponds to the same-numbered outcome at the beginning of the chapter.

1. An overweight patient (BMI 28.1 kg/m$^2$) is scheduled for a laparoscopic cholecystectomy at an outpatient surgery setting. The nurse knows that
   **a.** surgery will involve multiple small incisions.
   **b.** this setting is not appropriate for this procedure.
   **c.** surgery will involve removing a portion of the liver.
   **d.** the patient will need special preparation because of obesity
2. The patient tells the nurse in the preoperative setting that she has noticed she has a reaction when wearing rubber gloves. What is the *most* appropriate intervention?
   **a.** Notify the surgeon so that the case can be cancelled.
   **b.** Ask additional questions to assess for a possible latex allergy.
   **c.** Notify the OR staff immediately so that latex-free supplies can be used.
   **d.** No intervention is needed because the patient's rubber sensitivity has no bearing on surgery.
3. A 59-year-old man scheduled for a herniorrhaphy in 2 days reports that he takes ginkgo daily. What is the *priority* intervention?
   **a.** Inform the surgeon, since the procedure may have to be rescheduled.
   **b.** Notify the anesthesia care provider, since this herb interferes with anesthetics.
   **c.** Ask the patient if he has noticed any side effects from taking this herbal supplement.
   **d.** Tell the patient to continue to take the herbal supplement up to the day before surgery.
4. A 17-year-old patient with a leg fracture who is scheduled for surgery is an emancipated minor. She has a statement from the court for verification. Which intervention is *most* appropriate?
   **a.** Witness the permit after consent is obtained by the surgeon.
   **b.** Call a parent or legal guardian to sign the permit, since the patient is under 18.
   **c.** Obtain verbal consent, since written consent is not necessary for emancipated minors.
   **d.** Investigate your state's nurse practice act related to emancipated minors and informed consent.

5. A *priority* nursing intervention to assist a preoperative patient in coping with fear of postoperative pain would be to
   a. inform the patient that pain medication will be available.
   b. teach the patient to use guided imagery to help manage pain.
   c. describe the type of pain expected with the patient's particular surgery.
   d. explain the pain management plan, including the use of a pain rating scale.
6. A patient is scheduled for surgery requiring general anesthesia at an ambulatory surgical center. The nurse asks him when he ate last. He replies that he had a light breakfast a couple of hours before coming to the surgery center. What should the nurse do *first*?
   a. Tell the patient to come back tomorrow, since he ate a meal.
   b. Proceed with the preoperative checklist, including site identification.
   c. Notify the anesthesia care provider of when and what the patient last ate.
   d. Have the patient void before administering any preoperative medications.
7. A patient who normally takes 40 units of glargine insulin (long acting) at bedtime asks the nurse what to do about her dose the night before surgery. The *best* response would be to have her
   a. skip her insulin altogether the night before surgery.
   b. get instructions from her surgeon or HCP on any insulin adjustments.
   c. take her usual dose at bedtime and eat a light breakfast in the morning.
   d. eat a moderate meal before bedtime and then take half her usual insulin dose.
8. Preoperative considerations for older adults include (*select all that apply*)
   a. using only large-print educational materials.
   b. speaking louder for patients with hearing aids.
   c. recognizing that sensory deficits may be present.
   d. providing warm blankets to prevent hypothermia.
   e. teaching important information early in the morning.

1. a, 2. b, 3. a, 4. a, 5. d, 6. c, 7. b, 8. c, d

For rationales to these answers and even more NCLEX review questions, visit *http://evolve.elsevier.com/Lewis/medsurg*.

## EVOLVE WEBSITE

http://evolve.elsevier.com/Lewis/medsurg

**Review Questions (Online Only)**

**Key Points**

**Answer Keys for Review Questions**

- Rationales for Bridge to NCLEX Examination Questions
- Answer Guidelines for Case Study on p. 313

**Conceptual Care Map Creator**

**Audio Glossary**

**Content Updates**

## REFERENCES


1. Jehovah's Witness Official Website: Why don't Jehovah's Witnesses accept blood transfusions? Retrieved from *www.jw.org/en/jehovahs-witnesses/faq/jehovahs-witnesses-why-no-blood-transfusions/#?insight[search_id]=b9ef370f-ef34-4500-a973-7cbe6fe12c54&insight[search_result_index]=2.*
2. Seyedfatemi N, Rafii F, Rezaer M, et al: Comfort and hope in the preanesthesia stage in patients undergoing surgery, *J Perianesth Nurs* 29:213, 2014.
3. Tran H, Joseph J, Young L, et al: New oral anticoagulants: a practical guide on prescription, laboratory testing and peri-procedural/bleeding management, *Intern Med J* 44:525, 2014.
4. Society of Gastroenterology Nurses and Associates: Patient safety issues with use of herbal supplements. Retrieved from *www.sgna.org/issues/sedationfactsorg/patientcare_safety/herbalsupplements.aspx.*
5. Erian M, McLaren G: Be wary of "natural" therapy in gynecological surgery, *Int J Womens Health* 5:345, 2013.
6. American College of Allergy, Asthma, and Immunology: Latex allergy. Retrieved from *www.acaai.org/ALLERGIST/ALLERGIES/TYPES/LATEX-ALLERGY/Pages/default.aspx.*

*7. Association of periOperative Registered Nurses: *Guidelines for perioperative practice*, Denver, 2015, The Association.

8. Hepner DL: The role of testing in the preoperative evaluation, *Cleve Clin J Med* 76:s22, 2009.
9. Yalamarthi S: Perioperative steroids in surgical patients. Retrieved from *www.hmjanaesthesia.4t.com/periopsteroid.htm.*
10. Neil JA: Perioperative care of the immunocompromised patient, *AORN J* 85:544, 2007.
11. Neil JA: Perioperative care of the patient with tuberculosis, *AORN J* 88:942, 2008.
12. Neil JA: Perioperative care of the bariatric revision surgery patient, *AORN J* 97:210, 2013.
13. Evans DC, Martindale RG, Kiraly LN, et al: Nutrition optimization prior to surgery, *Nutr Clin Prac* 29:10, 2014.
14. Lack L, Johannson K: Caffeine withdrawal: cost or benefit? *Sleep Med* 14:e53, 2013.
15. Department of Health and Human Services: CMS manual. Retrieved from *www.cms.gov/Regulations-and-Guidance/Guidance/Transmittals/downloads/R71SOMA.pdf.*
16. Marimuthu K, Harbarth S: Screening for methicillin-resistant *Staphylococcus aureus* ... all doors closed? *Curr Opin Infect Dis* 27:356, 2014.

*17. Ping G: Preoperative education interventions to reduce anxiety and improve recovery among cardiac surgery patients: a review of randomised controlled trials, *J Clin Nurs* 24:34, 2014.

18. American Hospital Association: The patient care partnership: understanding expectations, rights and responsibilities. Retrieved from *www.aha.org/content/00-10/pcp_english_030730.pdf.*
19. Rothrock JC, editor: *Alexander's care of the patient in surgery*, ed 15, St Louis, 2015, Mosby.

*20. American Society of Anesthesiologists Committee: Practice guidelines for preoperative fasting and the use of pharmacologic agents to reduce the risk of pulmonary aspiration: application to healthy patients undergoing elective procedures: an updated report by the American Society of Anesthesiologists Committee on Standards and Practice Parameters, *Anesthesiology* 114:3, 2011.

21. American College of Surgeons: Informed consent. Retrieved from *www2.facs.org/public_info/operation/consent.html.*
22. Sear JW: Perioperative renin-angiotensin blockade: to continue or discontinue, that is the question! *Anesth Analg* 118:909, 2014.
23. Association of periOperative Registered Nurses: Patient hand off tool kit. Retrieved from *www.aorn.org/PracticeResources/ToolKits/PatientHandOffToolKit.*
24. Wilson-Stronks A, Lee KK, Cordero CL, et al: One size does not fit all: meeting the health care needs of diverse populations, Washington, DC, 2008, The Joint Commission. Retrieved from *www.jointcommission.org/assets/1/6/HLCOneSizeFinal.pdf.*

*25. Chow WB, Ko CY, Rosenthal RA, et al: American College of Surgeons NSQIP®/AGS best practice guidelines: optimal preoperative assessment of the geriatric surgical patient. Retrieved from *http://site.acsnsqip.org/wp-content/uploads/2011/12/ACS-NSQIP-AGS-Geriatric-2012-Guidelines.pdf.*


*Evidence-based information for clinical practice.

18

# Intraoperative Care

*Anita Jo Shoup, David M. Horner**

*Do not go where the path may lead, go instead where there is no path and leave a trail.*

**Ralph Waldo Emerson**

http://evolve.elsevier.com/Lewis/medsurg/

## LEARNING OUTCOMES

1. Differentiate the purposes of the various areas of the surgery department and the proper attire for each area.
2. Differentiate the roles and responsibilities of the interprofessional surgical team members.
3. Prioritize needs of patients undergoing surgery.
4. Analyze the role of the perioperative nurse in the management of patients undergoing surgery.
5. Apply basic principles of aseptic technique used in the operating room.
6. Evaluate the importance of safety in the operating room related to patients, equipment, and anesthesia.
7. Differentiate among the various anesthesia techniques and commonly used anesthesia drugs.

## KEY TERMS

**anesthesia care provider (ACP), p. 318**
**anesthesiology, p. 318**
**epidural block, p. 326**
**general anesthesia, p. 322**
**local anesthesia, p. 324**
**malignant hyperthermia (MH), p. 327**
**nurse anesthetist, p. 318**
**regional anesthesia, p. 324**
**spinal anesthesia, p. 325**

Historically, surgery took place in the traditional environment of the hospital operating room (OR). Now, the majority of surgical procedures are done as ambulatory surgery (outpatient surgery). In addition, the use of *minimally invasive surgery* (MIS) is rapidly increasing. More procedures use endoscopes and other advanced technology (e.g., robotics). Incisions are smaller, blood loss is reduced, postoperative pain is decreased, recovery time is shorter, and patients are discharged sooner. This chapter discusses the intraoperative care that is applicable to all surgical patients regardless of where or how the surgery is performed.

## PHYSICAL ENVIRONMENT OF THE OPERATING ROOM

### Department Layout

The *surgical suite* is a controlled environment designed to minimize the spread of pathogens and allow a smooth flow of patients, staff, and equipment needed to provide safe patient care. The suite is divided into three distinct areas: unrestricted, semirestricted, and restricted areas. The *unrestricted area* is where people in street clothes can interact with those in surgical attire. These areas typically include the points of entry for patients (e.g., holding area), staff (e.g., locker rooms), and information (e.g., nursing station or control desk). The *semirestricted area* includes the surrounding support areas and corridors. Only authorized staff are allowed access to the semirestricted areas. All staff in the semirestricted area must wear surgical attire and cover all head and facial hair. In the *restricted area* masks are required to supplement surgical attire.[1] The restricted area can include the OR, scrub sink area, and sterile core.

In addition, the physical layout is designed to reduce cross-contamination. The flow of clean and sterile supplies and equipment is separated from contaminated supplies, equipment, and waste by space, time, and traffic patterns. Staff members move supplies from clean areas, such as the sterile core, through the OR for surgery, and on to the surrounding areas, such as the instrument decontamination area.

### Holding Area

The *holding area,* frequently called the *preoperative holding area,* is a special waiting area inside of or next to the surgical suite. The size can range from a centralized area to handle numerous patients to a small designated area immediately outside the actual room scheduled for the surgical procedure. In the holding area you will identify and assess the patient before transferring him or her to the OR.

The *Surgical Care Improvement Project* (SCIP) is a national quality partnership of organizations focused on improving

*Contributed section on anesthesia content.

Reviewed by Judith M. Lewis, DNP, APRN, CRNA, Co-Chief Nurse Anesthetist, Akron's Children's Hospital, Akron, Ohio; Angela M. Martinelli, RN, PhD, CNOR, Clinical Professor, College of Nursing, Sacred Heart University, Fairfield, Connecticut; Crystal R. Sherman, DNP, CNP, FNP-BC, APHN-BC, Assistant Professor of Nursing, Shawnee State University, Portsmouth, Ohio; and Olga Van Dyke, RN, MSN, CAGS, Assistant Professor, School of Nursing, Massachusetts College of Pharmacy and Health Sciences, Boston, Massachusetts.

surgical care by significantly reducing the number of complications from surgery.[2] Several SCIP measures may be completed in the holding area, such as drug administration, patient warming, and application of sequential compression devices (SCDs). Many minor procedures (e.g., inserting IV catheters) can also be performed here.

The National Patient Safety Goals (NPSGs) require a preprocedure verification process, including the verification of relevant documentation (e.g., history and physical examination, signed consent forms, nursing and preanesthesia assessment).[3] In addition, any required blood products, implants, devices, and special equipment must be available. Further, the results of any diagnostic studies (e.g., x-rays, biopsy reports) must be included. In addition, the NPSGs require that the surgeon mark the procedure site. If possible, the marking should be done with the patient's involvement.[3]

In some settings, another area for holding is identified as the *admission, observation, and discharge* (AOD) area. This area is designed to allow early morning admission for outpatient surgery, same-day admission, and inpatient holding before surgery. In this area you can assess preoperative information, observe the patient before and after surgery, and allow sufficient recovery time before the patient is discharged to either the home or an inpatient room. The AOD area is important in the patient's stay throughout outpatient surgery and prevents unnecessary overnight stays in the inpatient setting.

Separation from caregivers just before surgery can produce anxiety for the patient. This anxiety can be reduced when the caregiver is permitted to wait with the patient in the holding area until the patient is transferred to the OR.

### Operating Room

The traditional surgical environment, or OR, is a unique setting separate from other clinical units. It is controlled geographically, environmentally, and aseptically, and it is restricted in terms of the flow of staff (Fig. 18-1). It is preferred to have the OR next to the postanesthesia care unit (PACU) and the surgical intensive care unit. This allows for quick transport of the postoperative patient and close proximity to anesthesia staff if complications arise.

Several methods are used to prevent the transmission of infection. Filters and controlled airflow in the ventilating systems provide dust control. Positive air pressure in the rooms prevents air from entering the OR from the halls and corridors. Ultraviolet (UV) lighting may be used because UV radiation reduces the number of microorganisms in the air. Dust-collecting surfaces such as open shelves and tables are omitted. Materials that are resistant to the corroding effects of strong disinfectants are used.

Overall safety and comfort are aided by the use of OR furniture that is adjustable, easy to clean, and easy to move. All equipment is checked frequently to ensure proper functioning and electrical safety. The lighting is designed to provide a low- to high-intensity range for a precise view of the surgical site (Fig. 18-2). A communication system provides a means for the delivery of routine and emergency messages.[4]

## SURGICAL TEAM

### Registered Nurse

The *perioperative nurse* is a registered nurse (RN) who implements the patient's plan of care during the perioperative period.

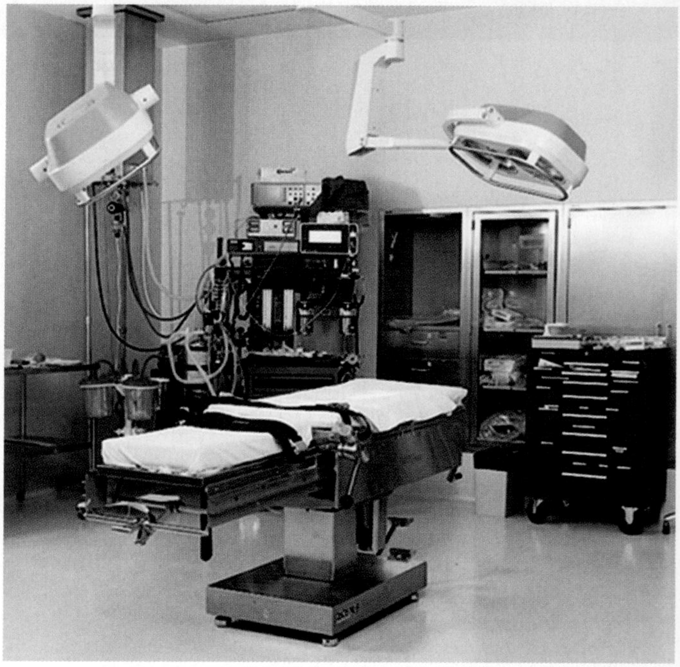

**FIG. 18-1** Typical operating room. (Courtesy Greg McVicar.)

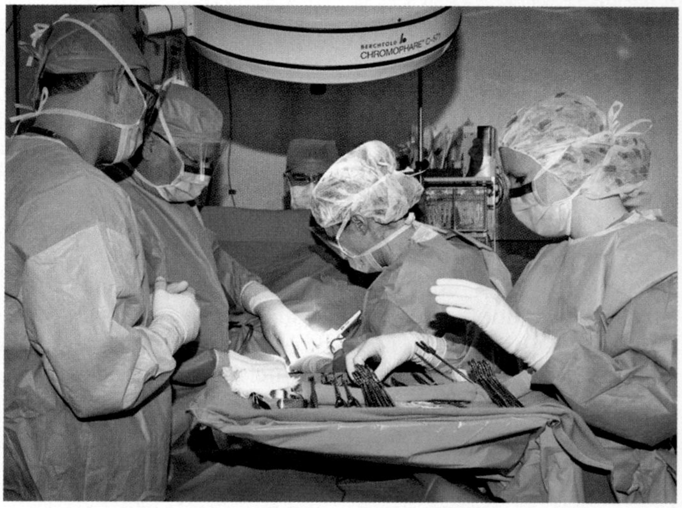


**FIG. 18-2** The complexity of surgery requires maintaining asepsis. (Courtesy Swedish Edmonds Hospital, Edmonds, Wash. Photograph by Amy Wesley.)

Through close collaboration with the other members of the surgical team, you prepare the OR for patients before they arrive. You are usually the first member of the surgical team who meets the patient. You are the patient's advocate throughout the intraoperative experience. This includes (1) maintaining the patient's safety, privacy, dignity, and confidentiality; (2) communicating with the patient; and (3) providing physical care.

Assess the patient to determine any additional needs or tasks to complete before surgery. Provide physical and emotional comfort for the patient and teaching regarding the upcoming surgery for the patient and caregivers. In addition, work with the patient's caregivers, keeping them informed and answering questions. This is particularly important in day-surgery settings, where caregivers must assume greater responsibility for preoperative and postoperative care.

In the perioperative role, you assume functions that involve either sterile or unsterile activities (Table 18-1). When you

**TABLE 18-1 Intraoperative Nursing Activities**

| |
|---|
| **Circulating, Nonsterile Activities** |
| • Reviews anatomy, physiology, and surgical procedure |
| • Assists in preparing room, ensuring that supplies and equipment are available, in working order, and sterile (if required) |
| • Maintains aseptic technique in all required activities |
| • Monitors practices of aseptic technique in self and others |
| • Checks mechanical and electrical equipment and environmental factors |
| • Conducts a preprocedure verification process |
| • Assesses patient's physical and emotional status |
| • Confirms and implements ordered SCIP measures |
| • Plans and coordinates intraoperative nursing care |
| • Checks chart and relates pertinent data to team members |
| • Helps with the application of monitoring devices and insertion of invasive lines and other devices |
| • Assists with and ensures patient safety in transferring and positioning patient |
| • Assists with induction of anesthesia |
| • Monitors draping procedure |
| • Participates in surgical time-out |
| • Records intraoperative care |
| • Prepares, records, labels, and sends blood, pathology, and any anatomic specimens to proper locations |
| • Measures blood, urine output, and other fluid loss |
| • Confirms, dispenses, and records drugs used, including local anesthetics |
| • Coordinates all intraoperative activities with team members and other staff and departments |
| • Maintains accurate count of sponges, needles, instruments, and medical devices that could be retained in the patient |
| • Goes with patient to PACU |
| • Gives hand-off report to PACU nurse with information relevant to care of patient |
| **Scrubbed, Sterile Activities** |
| • Reviews anatomy, physiology, and surgical procedure |
| • Assists in preparing the operating room |
| • Completes surgical hand antisepsis and gowns and gloves self and other members of surgical team |
| • Prepares instrument table and arranges sterile equipment for functional use |
| • Assists with draping procedure |
| • Participates in surgical time-out procedure |
| • Passes instruments to surgeon and assistants by anticipating their needs |
| • Maintains accurate count of sponges, needles, instruments, and medical devices that could be retained in the patient |
| • Monitors practices of aseptic technique in self and others |
| • Keeps track of irrigation solutions used for calculation of blood loss |
| • Accepts, verifies, and reports drugs used by surgeon and/or ACP, including local anesthetics |

*ACP*, Anesthesia care provider; *PACU*, postanesthesia care unit; *SCIP*, Surgical Care Improvement Project.

serve in the role of *scrub nurse*, you follow the designated surgical hand antisepsis procedure, are gowned and gloved in sterile attire, and remain in the sterile field (Fig. 18-2). When you serve in the role of *circulating nurse*, you remain in the unsterile field and so you are not gowned and gloved in sterile attire.

Ongoing assessment of the patient is essential because the patient's condition may change quickly. You respond to these changes and revise the plan of care as needed. Examples of nursing activities that characterize each phase surrounding the surgical experience are presented in Table 18-2.

As patients move through the surgical experience, they are cared for by many team members. Chances for error arise whenever clinical information is shared among these members.[5] The Joint Commission requires that all health care providers use a standardized approach to hand-off communication. The perioperative RN ensures that a complete and accurate hand-off using a consistent format, such as SBAR (see Table 1-6), occurs every time patient care is transferred to another professional. Examples of such transfers include change of shift, surgeon to nurse, and OR nurse to postanesthesia nurse.

You have the opportunity to become a certified perioperative nurse (CNOR). Nursing certification is an objective measure (written test) that validates that a nurse has the essential knowledge needed to provide perioperative nursing care.[6]

### Licensed Practical/Vocational Nurse and Surgical Technologist

Depending on your state nurse practice act, the role of the circulating or scrub nurse may be filled by a licensed practical/vocational nurse or a surgical technologist. Surgical technologists may attend an associate degree program, a vocational training program, or a hospital or military training program. The Association of Surgical Technologists sets the standards for education, provides continuing education opportunities, and offers certification for surgical technologists.[7]

If the circulating nurse is not an RN, the licensed practical/vocational nurse or surgical technologist must have access to an RN at all times. You are responsible for supervising the licensed practical/vocational nurse or surgical technologist in the performance of all delegated nursing tasks.[8]

### Surgeon and Assistant

The *surgeon* is the physician who performs the surgical procedure. The surgeon is primarily responsible for the following:

- Preoperative medical history and physical assessment, including need for surgical intervention, choice of surgical procedure, management of preoperative testing, and discussion of the risks of and alternatives to surgical intervention
- Patient safety and management in the OR
- Postoperative management of the patient

The *surgeon's assistant* can be a physician who functions in an assisting role during the surgical procedure. The assistant usually holds retractors to expose surgical areas and assists with hemostasis and suturing. In some instances, especially in educational settings, the assistant may perform some portions of the surgery under the surgeon's direct supervision. In many institutions the surgeon's assistant is a registered nurse first assistant or a physician's assistant (PA) who functions under the physician's direct supervision.

### Registered Nurse First Assistant

The *registered nurse first assistant* (RNFA) works in collaboration with the surgeon to produce an optimal surgical outcome for the patient. The Association of periOperative Registered Nurses (AORN) position statement on RNFAs states that the perioperative nurse must have formal education for this role and works collaboratively with the surgeon, patient, and surgical team by preparing and using instruments, providing exposure to the surgical site, handling tissue, assisting with hemostasis, and suturing.[9] RNFA education programs provide RNs with the education necessary to assume this expanded role. The RNFA can also obtain certification.

**TABLE 18-2 Perioperative Nursing Activities***

| BEFORE SURGERY | DURING SURGERY | AFTER SURGERY |
|---|---|---|
| **Assessment and Planning** | **Implementation** | **Evaluation** |
| **Home, Clinic, Holding Area**<br>• Initiates preoperative assessment<br>• Plans teaching appropriate to patient's needs<br>• Involves caregiver<br>**Surgical Unit**<br>• Completes preoperative assessment<br>• Coordinates patient teaching with staff<br>• Develops a plan of care that reflects patient's level of function and ability<br>• Safely gives ordered drugs<br>**Surgical Suite**<br>• Conducts preprocedure verification<br>• Assesses patient's level of consciousness, skin integrity, mobility, emotional status, and functional limitations<br>• Reviews chart<br>• Ensures all supplies and equipment needed are available, functioning, and sterile, if appropriate | **Safety Maintenance**<br>• Ensures integrity of sterile field<br>• Ensures that sponge, needle, instrument, and medical device counts are correct<br>• Positions patient to ensure correct alignment, exposure of surgical site, and prevention of injury<br>• Prevents chemical injury from prepping solutions, drugs, etc.<br>• Ensures safe use of electrical equipment<br>• Safely gives ordered drugs<br>**Monitoring Physical Status**<br>• Monitors and reports changes in patient's vital signs<br>• Monitors blood loss and urine output<br>**Monitoring Psychologic Status**<br>• Provides emotional support to patient<br>• Ensures patient's right to privacy is maintained<br>• Communicates patient's emotional status to health care team | **Postanesthesia, Discharge Area**<br>• Determines patient's response to surgical intervention<br>• Monitors ABCs, vital signs, level of consciousness<br>• Safely gives ordered drugs<br>**Clinical Unit**<br>• Evaluates effectiveness of nursing care in OR using patient outcome criteria<br>• Determines patient's level of satisfaction with care given during perioperative period<br>• Assesses patient's psychologic status<br>• Assists with discharge planning<br>**Home, Clinic**<br>• Seeks patient's perception of surgery in terms of effects of anesthetic agents, impact on body image, immobilization<br>• Determines caregiver's perceptions of surgery |

*ABCs,* Airway, breathing, circulation.
*List of activities is not all-inclusive.

### Anesthesia Care Provider

The **anesthesia care provider (ACP)** is a person who administers anesthesia and can be an anesthesiologist, nurse anesthetist, or anesthesiologist assistant (AA). ACPs are responsible for giving anesthetic agents to provide a temporary state of depressed or loss of consciousness, relieve pain, and manage vital life functions (e.g., breathing, BP during surgery). After surgery, they provide care during recovery.[10]

**Anesthesiology** is a specialty within the practice of medicine that focuses on the following:

- Medically managing patients who are rendered unconscious or insensible to pain and emotional stress during surgical and other medical procedures
- Protecting functions and vital organs under the stress of anesthetic, surgical, or other medical procedures
- Managing pain
- Managing cardiopulmonary resuscitation
- Managing problems in pulmonary care
- Managing critically ill patients in special care units

A **nurse anesthetist** is a master's-prepared RN who has graduated from an accredited nurse anesthesia program and completed a national certification examination to become a certified registered nurse anesthetist (CRNA).

The CRNA scope of practice includes the following[11]:

- Performing and documenting a preanesthetic assessment and evaluation
- Developing and implementing a plan for delivering anesthesia
- Selecting and starting the planned anesthetic technique
- Selecting, obtaining, and administering the anesthesia, adjuvant drugs, and fluids
- Selecting, applying, and inserting appropriate noninvasive and invasive monitoring devices
- Managing a patient's airway and pulmonary status
- Managing emergence and recovery from anesthesia
- Releasing or discharging patients from a PACU
- Ordering, starting, or modifying pain relief therapy
- Responding to emergency situations by providing airway management, and giving emergency fluids and drugs
- Assuming additional responsibilities within the expertise of the individual

An AA is a master's-prepared health professional who serves under the direction of an anesthesiologist. The AA has graduated from an accredited program and completed a national certification examination. AAs participate in all types of anesthesia, including giving drugs, obtaining vascular access, applying and interpreting monitors, establishing and maintaining airways, and assisting with preoperative assessments.

## NURSING MANAGEMENT: PATIENT BEFORE SURGERY

The preoperative assessment of the surgical patient provides baseline data for intraoperative and postoperative care and is used to plan the intraoperative care. Preoperative care of the patient is discussed in Chapter 17.

### Psychosocial Assessment

Knowing about the activities that occur when a patient is moved into the surgical suite allows you to provide explanations and reassurances, especially to the anxious patient. You can usually answer general questions regarding surgery or anesthesia, such as, "When will I go to sleep?" "Who will be in the room?" "When will my surgeon arrive?" "How much of my body will be exposed?" "Will I be cold?" "When will I wake up?" Specific questions relating to details of the surgical procedure and anesthesia may be referred to the surgeon or ACP. For patients who do not speak English, a qualified interpreter must be used (see Table 2-10).

### Physical Assessment

Perform a thorough physical assessment during the preoperative preparation of the patient (see Chapter 17).

## Chart Review

Required chart data vary with agencies, patient conditions, and surgical procedures. Because ambulatory surgery centers tend to have a healthier patient population, fewer tests may be needed. Examples of data that are obtained during the preoperative assessment are found in Tables 17-2 and 17-4. This information provides an understanding of past and present history, current health status, and potential for infection and other complications.

## Admitting the Patient

Agency policy guides the protocol to be followed when admitting the patient to the holding area and OR. A general routine includes initial greeting, proper identification, and offer of human contact and warmth. A preprocedure verification process is conducted before the start of surgery. In some agencies this takes place in the holding area; in others it takes place in the OR itself.

The admitting procedure is continued with reassessment of the patient and with time allowed for last-minute questions. Complete the chart review for the previously mentioned data and note any abnormalities or changes. Question the patient concerning valuables, prostheses, and last intake of food and fluid. Confirm that the correct preoperative drugs were given (if ordered). Provide a pillow or adjust the patient's position if requested. Most hospitals require the patient's hair to be covered just before transfer to the OR suite to reduce potential shedding. Specific SCIP measures may include (1) a prophylactic antibiotic started within 30 to 60 minutes before the surgical incision and (2) application of a warming blanket and SCDs.

Complementary and alternative therapies such as therapeutic touch, aromatherapy, music therapy, guided imagery, and even movies may be used for surgical patients (see the Complementary & Alternative Therapies box). These therapies may decrease anxiety, promote relaxation, reduce pain, and facilitate the healing process.[12] In some agencies these therapies are started before the patient is admitted to the OR. In others, such as ambulatory settings, they may be started after the patient arrives in the holding area.

**CHECK YOUR PRACTICE**

Your patient has arrived in the holding area. As you review the chart, you realize that the consent for blood has not been signed. You also know that the patient has Alzheimer's disease and is not mentally competent to give consent.

- How would you proceed?

**COMPLEMENTARY & ALTERNATIVE THERAPIES**

***Music Therapy***

Music is an ancient healing tool recognized in the writings of Plato.

**Scientific Evidence**

Strong scientific evidence for use in reducing stress and anxiety and enhancing mood.*

**Nursing Implications**

- To be effective, the music selected must be appropriate for the situation. Music can have many different physiologic effects.
- Listening to calming music can result in slower, deeper breathing and a decrease in heart rate and BP. Both of these indicate relaxation.
- Music with a faster pace can energize a person and promote mental alertness.
- Music therapy is safe in combination with other treatment approaches.

*Based on a systematic review of scientific literature. Retrieved from *www.naturalstandard.com.*

# NURSING MANAGEMENT: PATIENT DURING SURGERY

Whether surgery is only minutes long or lasts several hours, the circulating nurse is responsible for implementing the intraoperative plan of care. Patient care in the perioperative setting is dynamic and depends on the knowledge, skills, and judgment of the perioperative RN.[4] One of the critical duties of the circulating nurse is to serve as the patient's advocate. While each member of the perioperative team is focused on their specific activities, the circulating nurse focuses on the patient as a whole. This involves ongoing assessment, reassessment, and adjustment of the care plan so that the patient achieves a level of wellness equal to or improved from the preoperative level.

## Room Preparation

Before transferring the patient into the OR, prepare the room to ensure privacy, prevention of infection, and safety. Individualization of this preparation is essential to achieve the expected patient outcomes.

**CHECK YOUR PRACTICE**

You are assigned to observe in the OR. A severely obese patient is admitted to the holding area. The circulating nurse tells you that the unique needs of each patient must be addressed for a safe surgical experience.

- What special considerations are needed for this patient?

When a patient is severely obese, special equipment is needed to safely transfer the patient to and from the OR table. Extra staff may also be needed for the positioning of the patient for the procedure. During surgery, special equipment (e.g., extra-long instrumentation) may be used.

Surgical attire (pants and shirts, masks, protective eyewear, and caps or hoods) is worn by all people entering the OR (Fig. 18-3). All electrical and mechanical equipment is checked for proper functioning. Aseptic technique is practiced as each surgical item is opened and placed on the instrument table. Sponges, needles, instruments, and small medical devices (e.g., surgical clip cartridges, universal adapters) are counted according to strict processes to ensure accurate retrieval at the end of the procedure. Any retained surgical supplies, devices, or instruments are sentinel events (never events) or serious reportable events that can result in negative outcomes for the patient.[1,4] (Sentinel events and serious reportable events are discussed in Chapter 1.)

During room preparation and the surgical procedure, the scrub person performs surgical hand antisepsis, dons sterile gown and gloves, and touches only those items in the sterile field. The circulating nurse remains in the unsterile field and performs those activities that permit touching all unsterile items and the patient. This coordinated effort allows for smooth functioning throughout the procedure.

## Transferring Patient

Once the patient's identity has been confirmed and the OR has been prepared, the patient is moved into the room for the surgery. Each time a patient is transferred from one bed to another, the wheels of the stretcher must be locked. A sufficient number of staff members using ergonomic tools for safe patient handling and movement should be available to lift, guide, and

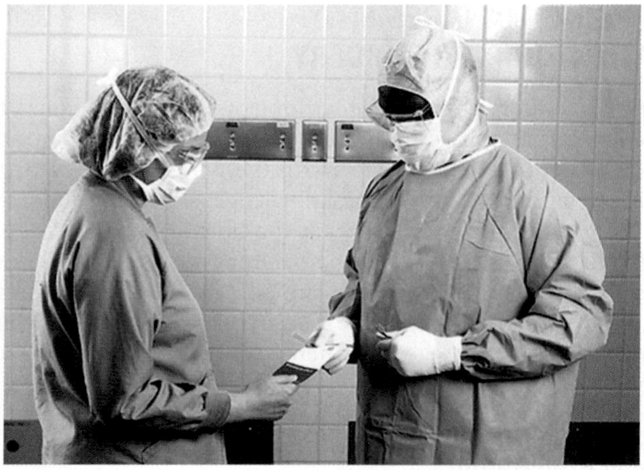

**FIG. 18-3** Surgical attire is worn by all people entering the operating room.

prevent accidental falling or injury to self, other staff, or the patient. Once the patient is on the OR bed, place safety straps snugly across the patient's thighs. At this time the monitor leads (e.g., ECG leads), BP cuff, and pulse oximeter are usually applied and an IV catheter is inserted if it was not done in the holding area.

## ◆ Scrubbing, Gowning, and Gloving

Surgical hand antisepsis is required of all sterile members of the surgical team (scrub nurse, surgeon, and assistant). When the procedure of scrubbing is the chosen method for surgical hand antisepsis (often for the first case of the day), your fingers and hands should be scrubbed first with progression to the forearms and elbows. The hands should be held away from surgical attire and higher than the elbows at all times to prevent contamination from clothing or detergent suds and water from draining from the unclean area above the elbows to the clean and previously scrubbed areas of the hands and fingers.

Waterless, alcohol-based agents are replacing soap and water in many agencies. When using an alcohol-based surgical handscrub product, prewash hands and forearms with soap and dry completely before applying the alcohol-based product. After application of the alcohol-based product, rub hands and forearms thoroughly until dry before donning sterile gloves.[1,4]

Once surgical hand antisepsis is completed, the team members enter the OR to put on surgical gowns and two pairs of gloves to protect patients and themselves from the transmission of microorganisms.[1,4] Because the gowns and gloves are sterile, those who have scrubbed can manipulate and organize all sterile items for use during the procedure.

## ◆ Basic Aseptic Technique

Aseptic technique is practiced in the OR to prevent infection. This is implemented through the creation and maintenance of a sterile field (Fig. 18-4). The center of the sterile field is the site of the surgical incision. Items used in the sterile field, including surgical instruments and equipment, have been sterilized by appropriate sterilization methods.

Team members must understand specific principles to practice aseptic technique (Table 18-3). Unless these principles are followed, the patient's safety is compromised and the potential for postoperative infection is increased.[1,4]

In addition to following the principles of aseptic technique, the surgical team is responsible for following the guidelines established by the U.S. Occupational Safety and Health Administration (OSHA) and the AORN to protect the patient and the team from exposure to blood-borne pathogens.[13] These guidelines emphasize (1) standard and transmission-based precautions; (2) engineering and work practice controls; and (3) the use of personal protective equipment such as gloves, gowns, caps, face shields, masks, and protective eyewear. This is especially important in the OR because of the high potential for exposure to blood-borne pathogens.

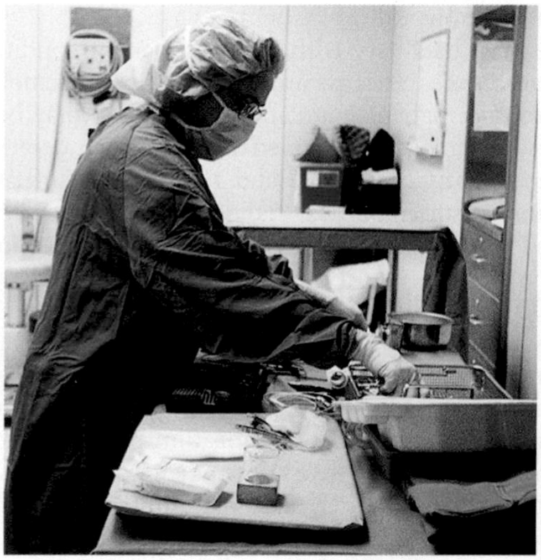

**FIG. 18-4** A sterile field is created before surgery. (Courtesy The Methodist Hospital, Houston, Tex. Photograph by Donna Dahms, RN, CNOR.)

### TABLE 18-3 Principles of Aseptic Technique in Operating Room

- All materials that enter the sterile field must be sterile.
- If a sterile item comes in contact with an unsterile item, it is contaminated.
- Contaminated items are removed immediately from the sterile field. If the unsterile item is small (e.g., unopened suture), once it is removed, the area is marked off (i.e., covered with a sterile drape). If the entire field is contaminated, it should be set up again with all new materials.
- The surgical team working in the operative field must wear sterile gowns and gloves. Once dressed for procedure, they must recognize that the only parts of the gown considered sterile are the front from chest to table level and sleeves to 2 inches above elbow.
- A wide margin of safety must be maintained between sterile and unsterile fields.
- Tables are considered sterile only at tabletop level. Items extending beneath this level are considered contaminated.
- The edges of a sterile package are considered contaminated once the package has been opened. If a sterile package (e.g., package of sutures) is placed on the sterile field, that entire package remains sterile even when opened.
- Microorganisms travel on airborne particles and will enter the sterile field with excessive air movements and currents.
- Microorganisms travel by capillary action through moist fabrics, resulting in contamination.
- Microorganisms harbor on the patient's and team members' hair, skin, and respiratory tracts and must be confined by appropriate attire.

## ◆ Assisting Anesthesia Care Provider

While you check the OR to complete the final preparations, the ACP prepares the patient for the administration of the anesthetic. You need to understand the effects of the anesthetic agents and know the location of all emergency drugs and equipment.

If you are the circulating nurse, you may be involved in placing monitoring devices to be used during the surgical procedure (e.g., ECG leads). If the patient is to have general anesthesia, remain at the patient's side to ensure safety and assist the ACP. These responsibilities may include measuring BP and assisting in the maintenance of the patient's airway. During the surgical procedure, you also provide a vital communication link for the ACP to other departments, such as the laboratory or blood bank.

## ◆ Safety Considerations

All surgical procedures, regardless of where they take place, can put the patient at risk for injury. These injuries can be infections, physical trauma from positioning or equipment used, or physiologic effects of surgery itself. Be alert to all safety issues, since the patient in the OR is often compromised from the effects of anesthesia.

Fire in the OR can have devastating consequences for the patient. Fortunately, surgical fires can be prevented with awareness of the hazards and emphasis on safe practices.[14] Care must be taken to correctly place the grounding pad and all electrosurgical equipment to prevent injury from burns or fire (Fig. 18-5). The electrosurgery plume of smoke contains toxic gas and vapors, bio-aerosols, and viruses as well as additional hazardous chemical compounds. These airborne contaminants can cause problems with visibility of the surgical site and tissue irritation and have mutagenic and carcinogenic potential.[1] Smoke evacuators may be used to minimize this exposure.

The *Universal Protocol,* one of the NPSGs, is followed to prevent wrong site, wrong procedure, and wrong surgery.[15] A patient safety checklist for ORs is the cornerstone of a major focus to make surgery safer. The use of the World Health Organization (WHO) Surgical Safety Checklist has improved

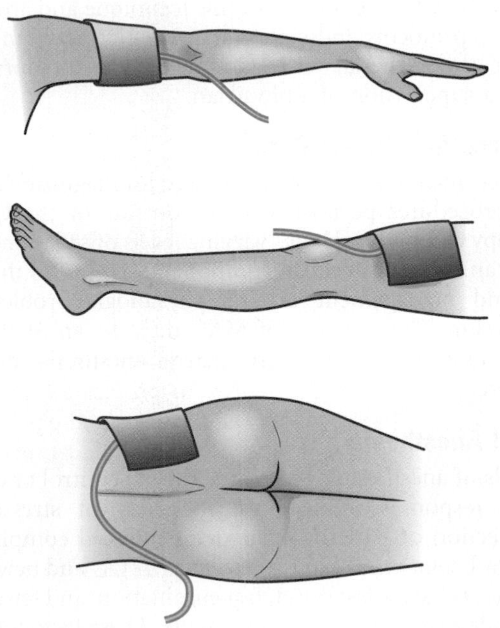

**FIG. 18-5** When an electrosurgical unit is used, the patient must be properly grounded to prevent unintended injury. A well-vascularized muscle mass is an optimal site. Safety can be compromised by excessive hair, adipose tissue, bony prominences, fluid (edema), adhesive failure, and scar tissue. (Courtesy Covidien, Mansfield, Mass.)

compliance with standards and decreased complications from surgery.[16]

Similarly, the AORN has developed a position statement regarding correct site surgery and guidelines for implementing the Universal Protocol.[17] All members of the surgical team stop what they are doing during a *surgical time-out* just before the procedure starts to verify patient identification, surgical procedure, and surgical site. In addition, OR staff complete a fire risk assessment (per agency protocol) to identify and reduce the potential for an OR fire.

**! SAFETY ALERT Surgical Time-Out**

- Before the induction of anesthesia, ask the patient to confirm name, birthdate, surgical procedure and site, and consent.
- Wrong surgical procedure and surgery performed on the wrong body part or wrong patient are *sentinel events (never events)* or *serious reportable events* (described in Chapter 1).

## ◆ Positioning Patient

Positioning the patient is a critical part of every procedure and usually follows administration of the anesthetic. The ACP indicates when to begin the positioning. The patient's position should allow for accessibility to the operative site, administration and monitoring of anesthetic agents, and maintenance of the patient's airway. When positioning for the surgical procedure, take care to (1) provide correct musculoskeletal alignment; (2) prevent undue pressure on nerves, skin over bony prominences, earlobes, and eyes; (3) provide for adequate thoracic excursion; (4) prevent occlusion of arteries and veins; (5) provide modesty in exposure; and (6) recognize and respect individual needs such as previously assessed aches, pains, or deformities. It is your responsibility to secure the extremities, provide adequate padding and support, and obtain sufficient physical or mechanical help to avoid unnecessary straining of self or patient.

The patient may be placed in various positions, including supine, prone, lateral, lithotomy, or sitting. The supine is the most common position used. It is suited for surgery involving the abdomen, heart, and breast. The prone position allows easy access for back surgery (e.g., laminectomy). The lithotomy position is used for some types of pelvic organ surgery (e.g., vaginal hysterectomy).

Whatever position is needed for the procedure, take great care to prevent injury to the patient. Because anesthesia blocks the sensory nerve impulses, the patient will not feel pain, discomfort, or stress being placed on nerves, muscles, bones, and skin. Improper positioning could potentially result in muscle strain, joint damage, pressure ulcers, nerve damage, and other untoward effects.

Pressure ulcers are costly and debilitating complications of surgery. They are also considered preventable events.[18] Hypoperfusion of tissue under pressure in an immobile patient plays a major role in the development of pressure ulcers in the OR. A primary safety consideration for positioning is the redistribution of pressure, especially at the patient's bony prominences.

General anesthesia causes peripheral vessels to dilate. Position changes affect where the pooling of blood occurs. If the head of the OR bed is raised, the lower torso will have increased blood volume and the upper torso may become compromised. Hypovolemia and cardiovascular disease can further compromise the patient's status. Consequently, the entire surgical team carefully plans and implements the patient's positioning and then closely monitors the patient throughout the surgical procedure.

### Preventing Hypothermia

Research has shown a relationship between unintended hypothermia and impaired wound healing, adverse cardiac events, altered drug metabolism, and coagulopathies.[19] To prevent hypothermia, the surgical team needs to closely monitor the patient's temperature. A thermal warming blanket and warm IV fluids may be used to maintain the patient's normal body temperature.

### Preparing Surgical Site

The purpose of skin preparation, or "prepping," is to reduce the number of microorganisms available to migrate to the surgical wound. The task of prepping is completed intraoperatively by the circulating nurse, surgeon, or surgical assistant.

The skin is prepared by mechanically scrubbing or cleansing around the surgical site with an antimicrobial agent identified as one that reduces microorganisms on intact skin, contains a nonirritating antimicrobial agent, has broad-spectrum activity, is fast acting and persistent, and is nonallergenic to the patient. A liberal area is scrubbed in a circular motion. The principle of scrubbing from the clean area (site of the incision) to the dirty area (distal to the incision) is observed at all times.

Antiseptic agents used for skin preparation may contain alcohol and be flammable. Skin injury can occur if these agents are allowed to pool under the patient. Care must be taken to ensure that these agents are properly confined and allowed to fully dry. After the skin is prepped and the fumes are allowed to dispel to reduce the risk of fire, the sterile members of the surgical team drape the area. Only the site to be incised is left exposed.

## NURSING MANAGEMENT: PATIENT AFTER SURGERY

Through constant observation of the surgical process, the ACP anticipates the end of the surgical procedure. Appropriate types and doses of anesthetic agents are used so that their effects will be minimal at the end of the surgical procedure. This also allows greater physiologic control of the patient during the transfer to the PACU.

The patient's response to your care is evaluated based on outcome criteria established during the development of the patient's plan of care. These outcome criteria are published as the *Perioperative Nursing Data Set (PNDS)* by AORN. The PNDS reflects standards and recommended practices related to the delivery of nursing care in any perioperative setting.[20]

The ACP and you or another member of the surgical team go with the patient to the PACU. A hand-off of the patient that includes his or her status and the procedure performed is communicated to the nurse receiving the patient in the PACU to promote safe, ongoing care.

# ANESTHESIA

The American Society of Anesthesiologists (ASA) defines anesthesia according to the effect that it has on the patient's sensorium and pain perception. These definitions include minimal sedation (e.g., anxiolysis), moderate sedation/analgesia, deep sedation/analgesia, and general anesthesia. The art and science of providing anesthesia continues to evolve. For example, noninvasive electroencephalogram-based technology allows ACPs to track the level of patient awareness (i.e., *awareness monitoring*) during surgery and adjust anesthesia as needed.

The anesthetic technique and agents are selected by the ACP in collaboration with the surgeon and patient. The ACP has ultimate responsibility for the choice of anesthesia. Factors contributing to the decision include the patient's current physical and mental status, age, allergy and pain history, expertise of the ACP, and factors relating to the operative procedure (e.g., length, site, discharge plans). An absolute contraindication to any anesthetic technique or agent is patient refusal.

The ACP obtains anesthesia consent, writes orders for preoperative and postoperative drugs, and assigns the patient an anesthesia classification. The ASA physical status classification system is based on the patient's physiologic status with no regard to the surgical procedure to be performed. A scale of P1 to P6 is used, with a rating of P6 reserved for a brain-dead patient undergoing organ harvest (see Table 17-3). An intraoperative complication is more likely to develop with a higher classification number.

Other designations can be added to the ASA status (e.g., "E" to designate an "emergent" procedure). ASA physical status is dynamic and represents the patient's status immediately before surgery. For example, a healthy 26-year-old adult who is severely injured in an automobile collision may be classified as ASA P5E because life-threatening injuries require emergent surgery.

## ANESTHESIA TECHNIQUES

Types of anesthesia techniques include moderate to deep sedation, monitored anesthesia care (MAC), general anesthesia, and local and regional anesthesia[21] (Table 18-4).

### Moderate to Deep Sedation

*Moderate to deep sedation* is used for procedures performed outside of the OR (e.g., reduction of dislocated joints in the emergency department) and does not require the presence of an ACP. RNs who are trained in this technique and are allowed by agency protocols and state nurse practice acts can provide this type of anesthesia.[22] It is administered by the nurse under the direct supervision of a physician.

### Monitored Anesthesia Care

*Monitored anesthesia care (MAC)* is used for diagnostic or therapeutic procedures performed in or outside of the OR (e.g., endoscopy clinic). It includes varying levels of sedation, analgesia, and anxiolysis. A critical component of MAC is the assessment and management of any physiologic problems that may develop. The provider of MAC must be an ACP, since it may be necessary to change to general anesthesia during the procedure.

### General Anesthesia

The goals of anesthesiology include the (1) control of excessive biologic responses induced by a variety of stressors and (2) protection of patients from stress-induced complications. To this end, *total intravenous anesthesia (TIVA)* and newer inhalation agents have a fast onset, fast elimination, and fewer undesirable side effects than previous agents. These factors facilitate early discharge from the PACU and ambulatory surgery centers.

**General anesthesia** is the technique of choice for patients who are having surgical procedures that are of significant duration, require skeletal muscle relaxation, require uncomfortable

**TABLE 18-4 Anesthesia Techniques and Effects**

| Technique | Patient Effects |
|---|---|
| **Moderate to deep sedation (formerly called *conscious sedation*)** | • Sedative, anxiolytic, and/or analgesic drugs used<br>• Does not include use of inhalation agents<br>• Patients responsive and breathe without assistance<br>• Not expected to induce levels of sedation that would impair patients' ability to protect their airway<br>• Most often used for minor therapeutic procedures (e.g., realignment of a fracture in the emergency department) |
| **Monitored anesthesia care (MAC)** | • Sedative, anxiolytic, and/or analgesic drugs used<br>• Does not usually involve inhalation agents<br>• Patients less responsive and may require airway management<br>• Provides maximum flexibility to match sedation level to patient needs and procedural requirements<br>• Often used in conjunction with regional or local anesthesia<br>• Often used for minor therapeutic and diagnostic procedures (e.g., eye surgery, colonoscopy) |
| **General anesthesia** | • Loss of sensation with loss of consciousness<br>• Combination of hypnosis, analgesia, and amnesia<br>• Usually involves use of inhalation agents<br>• Skeletal muscle relaxation<br>• Elimination of coughing, gagging, vomiting, and sympathetic nervous system responsiveness<br>• Requires advanced airway management |
| **Local anesthesia** | • Loss of sensation without loss of consciousness<br>• Induced topically or via infiltration, intracutaneously, or subcutaneously<br>• Topical applications may be aerosolized or nebulized |
| **Regional anesthesia** | • Loss of sensation to a region of body without loss of consciousness<br>• Involves blocking a specific nerve or group of nerves with administration of a local anesthetic<br>• Includes spinal, caudal, and epidural anesthesia and IV and peripheral nerve blocks (e.g., interscalene, axillary, infraclavicular or supraclavicular, popliteal, femoral, sciatic) |

Source: American Society of Anesthesiologists: *Distinguishing monitored anesthesia care ("MAC") from moderate sedation/analgesia (conscious sedation),* Schaumburg, Ill, 2013, The Society.

operative positions because of the location of the incision site, or require control of ventilation. Additional reasons for general anesthesia include patient refusal of local or regional techniques, contraindications to other techniques, and uncooperative patients. Patients may be uncooperative due to intoxication, emotional lability, head injury, impaired cognition, or inability to remain immobile for any length of time. Phases of general anesthesia are presented in Table 18-5.

General anesthesia may be induced by IV or inhalation, and maintained by either one or a combination of the two (Table 18-6). A *balanced technique,* using adjunctive drugs to complement the induction, is the most common approach used for general anesthesia.

**IV Agents.** All routine general anesthetics begin with an IV induction agent, whether it is a hypnotic, an anxiolytic, or a dissociative agent. When used during the initial period of anesthesia, these agents induce a pleasant sleep with a rapid onset of action that patients find desirable. A single dose lasts only a few minutes, which is long enough for a laryngeal mask airway (LMA) or an endotracheal (ET) tube to be placed. Once this is done, the ACP uses the selected inhalation and IV agent(s).

Recent advances in IV hypnotics (e.g., dexmedetomidine [Precedex]) and opioids (e.g., remifentanil [Ultiva]) have led to the more frequent use of TIVA. However, the patient may still require advanced airway management (e.g., LMA, ET tube) and will receive oxygen/air mixtures via this route.

**Inhalation Agents.** Inhalation agents are the cornerstone of general anesthesia. They may be volatile liquids or gases. Volatile liquids are given through a specially designed vaporizer after being mixed with oxygen as a carrier gas. This gas mixture is then delivered to the patient via the anesthesia circuit. Waste gases are removed using negative evacuation pressure venting to the outside of the agency.

Inhalation agents enter the body through the alveoli in the lungs. Ease of administration and rapid excretion by ventilation make them desirable agents. One undesirable trait is the irritating effect some inhalation agents (e.g., desflurane [Suprane]) have on the respiratory tract. Possible complications include coughing, laryngospasm, and increased secretions.[23]

Once the patient has been induced with an IV agent, the choice for delivering inhalation agents is usually through an ET tube or LMA. The ET tube permits control of ventilation and protects the airway from aspiration. LMAs are currently an important option for patients with difficult airways, but they do not provide access to the trachea or airway protection with the same certainty as ETs. Complications of ET tube or LMA include those associated primarily with insertion and removal. These include failure to intubate, damage to teeth and lips, laryngospasm, laryngeal edema, postoperative sore throat, and hoarseness caused by injury or irritation of the vocal cords or surrounding tissues.

**Adjuncts to General Anesthesia.** The administration of general anesthesia is rarely limited to one agent. Drugs added to an inhalation anesthetic (other than an IV induction drug) are termed *adjuncts.* These drugs are added to the anesthetic regimen specifically to achieve unconsciousness, analgesia, amnesia, muscle relaxation, or autonomic nervous system control. Adjuncts include opioids, benzodiazepines, neuromuscular blocking agents (muscle relaxants), and antiemetics (Table 18-7). It is important to know that these drugs are often given in combination and may have synergistic or antagonistic effects. You may observe deeper levels of sedation or more drug-related side effects beyond those seen with inhalation anesthetics alone. If needed, drugs are available to reverse the effects of some of these adjuncts.

**Dissociative Anesthesia.** *Dissociative anesthesia* interrupts associative brain pathways while blocking sensory pathways. The patient may appear catatonic, is amnesic, and experiences profound analgesia that lasts into the postoperative period. Ketamine (Ketalar) (given IV or IM) is a common dissociative anesthetic. It is a potent analgesic and amnesic. Ketamine is used in asthmatic patients undergoing surgery because it promotes bronchodilation and in trauma patients requiring surgery because it increases heart rate and helps maintain cardiac output. Because ketamine is a phenylcyclohexyl piperidine (PCP) derivative, the drug may cause hallucinations and nightmares, greatly limiting its usefulness. Concurrent use of midazolam (Versed) can reduce or eliminate hallucinations associated with ketamine.

**TABLE 18-5 Phases of General Anesthesia**

| Preinduction | Induction | Maintenance | Emergence |
|---|---|---|---|
| **Description** | | | |
| • Period starting with initiation of IV or arterial access, application of monitors (e.g., ECG), administration of preoperative drugs | • Initiation of drugs that make patient unconscious<br>• Airway secured with airway assist devices | • Period during which surgical procedure is performed<br>• Patient remains in an unconscious state with measures to ensure airway safety | • Period when surgical procedure is completed<br>• Patient is prepared for return to consciousness and removal of airway assist devices |
| **Role of Anesthesia Care Provider** | | | |
| • Determine final anesthetic care plan<br>• Insert and monitor IV or arterial access<br>• Confirm antibiotic prophylaxis<br>• Give drugs for anxiety, aspiration prophylaxis | • Give appropriate drugs<br>• Secure airway<br>• Position patient appropriately for surgical procedure | • Monitor patient's physiologic status<br>• Give drugs and titrate fluids as appropriate | • Reverse residual neuromuscular blocking agents<br>• Assess for return of all protective reflexes<br>• Remove airway assist devices<br>• Assess pain |
| **Role of Perioperative Nurse** | | | |
| • Complete preoperative assessment<br>• Check and confirm signed informed consent<br>• Complete surgical time-out. | • Assist with application of monitors (noninvasive and invasive)<br>• Assist with airway management | • Adjust patient position as necessary<br>• Monitor patient safety | • Assist in placement of dressing<br>• Protect patient during return of reflexes<br>• Prepare patient to move to postanesthesia care unit |
| **Classes of Drugs Used** (Tables 17-8, 18-6, and 18-7) | | | |
| • Benzodiazepines<br>• Opioids<br>• Antibiotics<br>• Aspiration prophylaxis:<br>  • $H_2$ receptor blockers (e.g., ranitidine [Zantac])<br>  • Gastric motility agents (e.g., metoclopramide [Reglan])<br>  • Anticholinergics (e.g., scopolamine [Transderm-Scōp]) | • Benzodiazepines<br>• Opioids<br>• Barbiturates<br>• Hypnotics<br>• Volatile gases | • Benzodiazepines<br>• Opioids<br>• Barbiturates<br>• Hypnotics<br>• Volatile gases<br>• Neuromuscular blocking agents | • Reversal agents (PRN):<br>  • Anticholinesterases (e.g., neostigmine)<br>  • Opioid antagonists (e.g., naloxone)<br>  • Benzodiazepine antagonists (e.g., flumazenil)<br>  • Neuromuscular block reversal of rocuronium [Zemuron] and vecuronium [Norcuron] (e.g., sugammadex [Bridon])<br>• Supplemental opioids (PRN)<br>• Antiemetics (PRN) |

Provide a quiet, unhurried environment in the PACU for all patients receiving dissociative anesthesia.[24]

## Local and Regional Anesthesia

**Local anesthesia** interrupts the generation of nerve impulses by altering the flow of sodium into nerve cells. The result is autonomic nervous system blockade, anesthesia, and skeletal muscle flaccidity or paralysis. Local anesthetics are topical, ophthalmic, nebulized, or injectable. A local anesthetic, such as lidocaine (Xylocaine), is applied to a specific area of the body by the surgeon or ACP and does not require sedation or loss of consciousness.

**Regional anesthesia** (or block) using a local anesthetic is always injected. It involves a central nerve (e.g., spinal) or group of nerves (e.g., plexus) that innervate a site remote to the point of injection. Administration of a local or regional anesthetic may involve concurrent use of MAC or moderate to deep sedation (Table 18-4), either preinjection or intraoperatively. Regional blocks are used as preoperative analgesia, intraoperatively to manage surgical pain, and postoperatively to control pain. Indwelling catheters that deliver local anesthetic via a pump to the surgical site may be implanted before the patient emerges from anesthesia to provide continuous pain relief up to 72 hours postoperatively.

Advantages of local and regional anesthesia include rapid recovery and discharge with continued postoperative analgesia without any accompanying cognitive dysfunction. Local and regional anesthesia can be safely used in patients who have co-morbidities that would preclude the use of general anesthesia.

Disadvantages of local and regional anesthesia include the potential for technical difficulties; discomfort at the injection site; and the risk of inadvertent vascular injection leading to refractory hypotension, dysrhythmias, and possible seizures. Another disadvantage is the inability to precisely match the agent's duration of action to the duration of the surgical procedure.

In ambulatory or outpatient procedures, you may assist the ACP in the administration of a peripheral or regional block. Consequently, you must be familiar with the drugs, including the methods of administration and adverse and toxic effects. Initial assessment of the patient should include detailed questioning of the patient's history with the use of local anesthetics and any adverse events associated with their use by the patient or blood relatives.

Many patients report "allergies" to local anesthetics. Although true allergies to local anesthetics occur, they are rare. Allergies are likely to be a result of additives or preservatives in the preparation. Moreover, some local anesthetics are combined with epinephrine to provide localized vasoconstriction. This decreases absorption and extends the action of the agent. However, if the local anesthetic is absorbed in the tissues or inadvertently injected IV and enters the general circulation, the patient may experience tachycardia, hypertension, and a general perception of panic.

**Methods of Administration.** Local anesthetics are injected at the surgical site, nebulized, or applied topically. Topical applications of creams, ointments, aerosols, and liquids are standard methods of administration. The drug is applied directly to the skin, mucous membranes, or open surface. Eutectic mixture of

TABLE 18-6 **Drug Therapy**

***General Anesthesia***

| Drugs | Advantages | Disadvantages | Nursing Interventions |
|---|---|---|---|
| **IV Agents** | | | |
| ***Barbiturates*** | | | |
| methohexital (Brevital) | Rapid induction, duration of action <5 min. | Adverse cardiac effects (e.g., myocardial depression), hypotension, respiratory depression, excitation, involuntary movement. | Usually have minimal postoperative effects because of short duration of action. Increased incidence of postoperative nausea in patients with barbiturate sensitivity, histamine-triggered nausea, vomiting. |
| ***Nonbarbiturate Hypnotics*** | | | |
| etomidate (Amidate) | Produces little change in cardiovascular dynamics. Useful for hemodynamically unstable patients. Only minor respiratory depression. No histamine release. | Associated with adverse effects of myoclonia, nausea and vomiting, hiccups, and adrenocortical inhibition. | Observe for transient skeletal muscle movements (myoclonia), nausea and vomiting, hiccups, hypotension, hypoglycemia. |
| propofol (Diprivan) | Ideal for short outpatient procedures because of rapid onset of action, metabolic clearance. May be used for induction and maintenance of anesthesia. | May cause bradycardia and other dysrhythmias, hypotension, apnea, transient phlebitis, nausea and vomiting, hiccups. May cause hypertriglyceridemia. | Monitor for postoperative hypotension, bradycardia. Monitor serum triglycerides q24hr when sedated >24 hr. |
| **Inhalation Agents** | | | |
| ***Volatile Liquids*** | | | |
| isoflurane (Forane)<br>desflurane (Suprane)<br>sevoflurane (Ultane) | All cause skeletal muscle relaxation.<br>*isoflurane:* No increase in ventricular irritability. Does not cause liver or renal toxicity. Resistant to metabolic breakdown.<br>*desflurane:* Fastest onset and emergence, widely used in ambulatory settings. Least postoperative cognitive dysfunction. Potential airway irritant.<br>*sevoflurane:* Predictable effects on cardiovascular and respiratory systems, rapid acting. Preferred for inhalation induction as nonirritating to respiratory tract. | All cause respiratory depression, hypotension, myocardial depression.<br>*isoflurane and desflurane:* May be unsuitable for patients with coronary artery disease.<br>*sevoflurane:* May be associated with emergence delirium (see Chapter 19). Atypical seizure-like activity has been reported. | Assess and treat pain during early anesthesia recovery. Assess for adverse reactions such as cardiopulmonary depression with hypotension and prolonged respiratory depression. Monitor for nausea and vomiting. |
| ***Gaseous Agents*** | | | |
| nitrous oxide | Potentiates volatile agents, thus speeding induction and reducing total dosage and side effects. Good analgesic potency. Produces little or no toxicity at therapeutic concentrations. | Weak anesthetic, rarely used alone. Must be given with $O_2$ to prevent hypoxemia. Avoid in patients with strong history of nausea and vomiting. | Avoid in patients with bone marrow depression. |
| **Dissociative Anesthetic** | | | |
| ketamine (Ketalar) | Can be given IV or IM. Potent analgesic and amnesic. | May cause hallucinations and nightmares, increased intracranial and intraocular pressure, ↑ heart rate, ↑ BP. | Anticipate administration of a benzodiazepine if agitation and hallucinations occur. Calm, quiet environment is essential in postoperative care. |

local anesthetics (EMLA cream, a combination of prilocaine and lidocaine) is an example of a cream applied to the site 30 to 60 minutes before the procedure for analgesia. The success of injected local anesthetics may be limited by prolonged duration of procedure or infection at the injection site, thus interfering with drug absorption.

When a patient is prepared for regional anesthesia, airway equipment, emergency drugs, and a cardiac monitor/defibrillator should be immediately available to provide advanced airway and cardiopulmonary support if necessary. Inadvertent IV injection of the agent or excessive absorption of bupivacaine (Sensorcaine), in particular, may lead to cardiac depression, severe dysrhythmias, or cardiac arrest.[25]

Examples of common regional nerve blocks include brachial plexus block; IV regional anesthesia (IVRA) or Bier block anesthesia; and femoral, axillary, cervical, sciatic, ankle, and retrobulbar blocks. For IVRA or Bier block, the patient has a double-cuff tourniquet applied as a safety measure. You can aid the success of regional anesthesia by assisting in patient positioning, monitoring vital signs during block delivery, administering oxygen therapy, and using supporting devices (at the direction of the ACP) that contribute to the anesthesia (e.g., ultrasound imaging, nerve stimulator, tourniquets).

***Spinal and Epidural Anesthesia.*** Spinal anesthesia and epidural anesthesia are also types of regional anesthesia. **Spinal anesthesia** involves the injection of a local anesthetic into the cerebrospinal fluid in the subarachnoid space, usually below the level of L2 (Fig. 18-6, *A*). The local anesthetic mixes with cerebrospinal fluid. Depending on the extent of its spread, various levels of anesthesia are achieved. Because the local anesthetic is given directly into the cerebrospinal fluid, a spinal anesthetic produces an autonomic, sensory, and motor blockade. Patients experience vasodilation and may become hypotensive as a result of the autonomic block. They feel no pain as a result of the

**TABLE 18-7 Drug Therapy**

***Adjuncts to General Anesthesia***

| Agents | Uses During Anesthesia | Adverse Effects | Nursing Interventions |
|---|---|---|---|
| **Opioids** | | | |
| fentanyl (Sublimaze)<br>sufentanil (Sufenta)<br>morphine sulfate<br>hydromorphone (Dilaudid)<br>alfentanil (Alfenta)<br>remifentanil (Ultiva)<br>methadone (Dolophine) | Induce and maintain anesthesia, reduce stimuli from sensory nerve endings, provide analgesia during surgery and recovery in PACU. | Respiratory depression, stimulation of vomiting center, possible bradycardia and peripheral vasodilation (when combined with anesthetics). High incidence of pruritus in both regional and IV administration. | • Assess respiratory rate and rhythm, monitor pulse oximetry, protect airway in anticipation of vomiting.<br>• Use standing orders for antipruritics and antiemetics.<br>• Reverse opioid-induced respiratory depression with naloxone (Narcan). If used, reversal of analgesic effects also occurs. |
| **Benzodiazepines** | | | |
| midazolam (Versed)<br>diazepam (Valium)<br>lorazepam (Ativan) | Reduce anxiety preoperatively and postoperatively, induce and maintain anesthesia, induce amnesia, treat emergence delirium.<br>Supplement sedation in local and regional anesthesia and MAC. | Synergistic effect with opioids, increasing potential for respiratory depression. Hypotension and tachycardia. Prolonged sedation or confusion. | • Monitor level of consciousness. Assess for respiratory depression, hypotension, and tachycardia.<br>• Reverse severe benzodiazepine-induced respiratory depression with flumazenil (Romazicon). |
| **Neuromuscular Blocking Agents** | | | |
| *Depolarizing agent:*<br>succinylcholine (Anectine)<br><br>*Nondepolarizing agents:*<br>pancuronium<br>rocuronium<br>atracurium<br>cisatracurium (Nimbex) | Facilitate endotracheal intubation, promote skeletal muscle relaxation (paralysis) to enhance access to surgical sites.<br>Effects of nondepolarizing agents are usually reversed toward end of surgery by administration of anticholinesterase agents (e.g., neostigmine, pyridostigmine). | Apnea related to paralysis of respiratory muscles. Duration of action of nondepolarizing agents may be longer than surgery. Reversal agents may not completely eliminate effects. Confusion and nausea. Recurrence of muscle weakness with correction of hypothermia. | • If intubated, monitor return of muscle strength, level of consciousness, and ventilation.<br>• Maintain patent airway. Monitor respiratory rate and rhythm until patient able to cough and return to previous levels of muscle strength. Ensure availability of nondepolarizing reversal agents (e.g., neostigmine [Prostigmin]) and emergency respiratory support equipment.<br>• Monitor temperature and levels of muscle strength with temperature changes. |
| **Antiemetics** | | | |
| ondansetron (Zofran)<br>dolasetron (Anzemet)<br>granisetron (Kytril)<br>metoclopramide (Reglan)<br>prochlorperazine<br>promethazine<br>scopolamine (Transderm-Scōp) | Counteract emetic effects of inhalation agents and opioids. Prophylactic prevention of nausea and vomiting related to histamine release, vagal stimulation, vestibular disturbance, surgical procedure (e.g., abdominal and laparoscopic procedures). | Headache, dizziness, IV irritation, dysrhythmias, dysphoria, dystonia, dry mouth, central nervous system sedation. | • Monitor heart rhythm, cardiopulmonary status, level of central nervous system excitation or sedation, ability to move limbs, presence of nausea or vomiting. |
| **Miscellaneous** | | | |
| dexmedetomidine (Precedex) | Induces and maintains sedation in nonintubated patients prior to and/ or during surgical procedures. | Hypotension, bradycardia, sinus arrest, transient hypertension during administration of loading dose. | • Monitor heart rate and rhythm, and BP for possible side effects. |
| dexamethasone | Counteracts emetic effects of inhalation agents and opioids (off-label use).* | Insomnia, nervousness, abdominal distention. | • Monitor for possible side effects. |

*MAC,* Monitored anesthesia care; *PACU,* postanesthesia care unit.
*For an explanation of off-label drug use, see *www.cancer.org/docroot/ETO/content/ETO_1_2x_Off-Label_Drug_Use.asp.*

sensory block. They cannot move as a result of the motor block. The duration of action of the spinal anesthetic depends on the drug selected and the dose given. A spinal anesthetic may be used for procedures involving the extremities (e.g., joint replacements) and lower gastrointestinal, prostate, and gynecologic surgeries.[23]

An **epidural block** involves injection of a local anesthetic into the epidural space via a thoracic or lumbar approach (Fig. 18-6, *B*). The anesthetic agent does not enter the cerebrospinal fluid but binds to nerve roots as they enter and exit the spinal cord. With the use of a low concentration of local anesthetic, sensory pathways are blocked but motor fibers remain intact. In higher doses, sensory and motor fibers are blocked. Epidural anesthesia may be used as the sole anesthetic for a surgical procedure. In addition, a catheter may be placed to allow for intraoperative use and continued analgesia in the postoperative period (Fig. 18-6, *C*). For postoperative analgesia, lower doses of epidurally administered local anesthetic, usually in combination with an opioid, are used. Epidural anesthesia is commonly used for analgesia, or in combination with MAC or general anesthesia, in obstetrics, vascular procedures involving the lower extremities, lung resections, and renal and midabdominal surgeries. The desirable effects of vasodilation and analgesia contribute to better surgical outcomes.

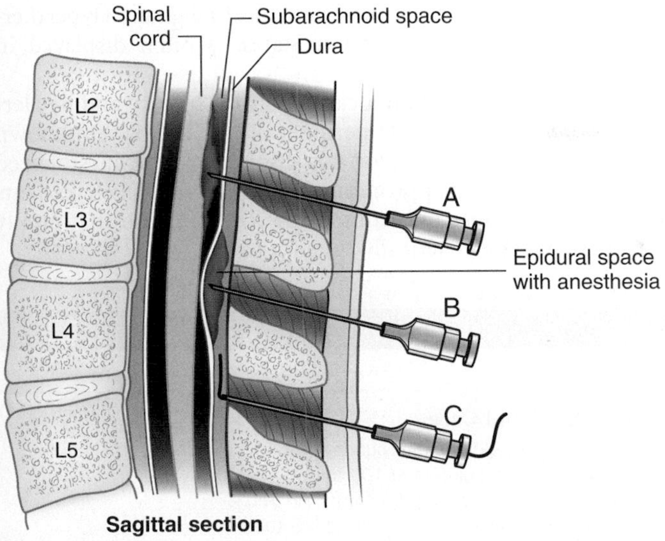


**FIG. 18-6** Location of needle point and injected anesthetic relative to dura and spinal cord. **A,** Spinal anesthesia. **B,** Single-injection epidural. **C,** Epidural catheter. (Interspaces most commonly used are L2-3, L4-5, L3-4.)

When spinal or epidural anesthesia is used, the patient can remain fully conscious, receive MAC, or choose general anesthesia. The onset of spinal anesthesia is more rapid than that of epidural anesthesia. Spinal and epidural anesthesia may be extended in duration using indwelling catheters, thus allowing for additional doses of anesthetic.

When spinal or epidural anesthesia is used, closely observe the patient for manifestations of autonomic nervous system blockade. These include hypotension, bradycardia, nausea, and vomiting. There is less autonomic nervous system blockade with epidural anesthesia than with spinal anesthesia. Should "too high" a block be achieved, the patient may experience tingling in the arms and hands or inadequate breathing and apnea.[23] Other complications of spinal or epidural anesthesia include postdural puncture headache, back pain, isolated nerve injury, and meningitis.

### Gerontologic Considerations: Patient During Surgery

Although anesthetic agents have become safer and more predictable, the aging process affects the pharmacokinetics of drugs, specifically the absorption, distribution, and metabolism of medications. This results in alterations in the onset, peak, and duration of drugs independent of the route of administration. Because of this, anesthetic drugs should be carefully titrated when given to older adults. Physiologic changes in aging may alter the patient's response not only to the anesthetic but also to blood and fluid loss and replacement, hypothermia, pain, and tolerance of the surgical procedure and positioning. Carefully monitor the older adult's response to all anesthetic agents. Assess the postoperative recovery from these agents before the patient is transferred out of the PACU.

Some older adults may have difficulty communicating and following directions as a result of alterations in hearing or vision. These factors increase the need for clear and concise communication in the OR, especially when preoperative sedation is combined with already existing sensory deficits. Because of decreased ability to perceive discomfort or pressure on vulnerable areas and a loss of skin elasticity, the older adult's skin is at risk for injury from tape, electrodes, warming and cooling blankets, and certain types of dressings. In addition, pooling of solutions used to prepare the skin in dependent areas can quickly create skin burns or abrasions.

The care and vigilance of the entire surgical team are needed in preparing and positioning the older patient. The older adult often has osteoporosis and/or osteoarthritis. Misalignment, pressure, or other insults to arthritic joints that may be desensitized from administration of an anesthetic may create long-term injury and disability. Older adults are also at a greater risk of perioperative hypothermia. Consider the use of a variety of warming devices and carefully monitor them if used.

## CATASTROPHIC EVENTS IN THE OPERATING ROOM

Unanticipated intraoperative events occasionally occur. Although some may be anticipated (e.g., cardiac arrest in an unstable patient, massive blood loss during trauma surgery), others may occur without warning, demanding immediate intervention by all members of the OR team. Two such events are anaphylactic reactions and malignant hyperthermia.

### Anaphylactic Reactions

*Anaphylaxis* is the most severe form of an allergic reaction, manifesting with life-threatening pulmonary and circulatory complications. The initial clinical manifestations of anaphylaxis may be masked by anesthesia. ACPs give a variety of drugs to patients, such as anesthetics, antibiotics, blood products, and plasma expanders. Because any parenterally administered material can stimulate an allergic response, vigilance and rapid intervention are essential. An anaphylactic reaction causes hypotension, tachycardia, bronchospasm, and possibly pulmonary edema. Anesthetic agents, antibiotics, and latex are responsible for many perioperative allergic reactions. (Anaphylaxis is discussed in Chapter 13.)

*Latex allergy* has become a particular concern in the perioperative setting, given the use of gloves, catheters, and many other devices containing natural rubber latex. Reactions to natural rubber latex range from urticaria to anaphylaxis with symptoms appearing immediately or at some time during the surgical procedure. Latex allergy protocols should be set up in each agency to provide a latex-safe environment for susceptible individuals.[26] (Latex allergies are discussed in Chapter 13.)

### Malignant Hyperthermia

**Malignant hyperthermia (MH)** is a rare disorder characterized by hyperthermia with rigidity of skeletal muscles that can result in death. It occurs in susceptible people when they are exposed to certain anesthetic agents. Succinylcholine (Anectine), especially when given with volatile inhalation agents, appears to be the primary trigger of the disorder. Other factors, such as stress, trauma, and heat, also have been implicated. When MH does occur, it is usually during general anesthesia, but it may manifest in the recovery period as well.[27]

MH is an autosomal dominant trait but is variable in its genetic manifestation, so predictions based on family history are important but not reliable. (Autosomal dominant disorders are discussed in Chapter 12.) The fundamental defect is hypermetabolism of skeletal muscle resulting from altered control of intracellular calcium. This leads to muscle contracture, hyperthermia, hypoxemia, lactic acidosis, and hemodynamic and cardiac alterations.

Tachycardia, tachypnea, hypercarbia, and ventricular dysrhythmias are generally seen but are nonspecific to MH. MH is generally diagnosed after all other causes of the hypermetabolism are ruled out. The rise in body temperature is not an early sign of MH. Unless promptly detected and treated, MH can result in cardiac arrest and death. The definitive treatment of MH is prompt administration of dantrolene (Dantrium). Dantrolene slows metabolism, reduces muscle contraction, and mediates the catabolic processes associated with MH.[25] A treatment protocol, available from the Malignant Hyperthermia Association of the United States, is often displayed in the OR.[28]

To prevent MH, obtain a careful family history and be alert to the development of MH perioperatively. The patient known or suspected to be at risk for this disorder can be anesthetized with minimal risks if appropriate precautions are taken. Patients with MH should be informed of the condition so that family members may be genetically tested.

## CASE STUDY

### *Intraoperative Patient*

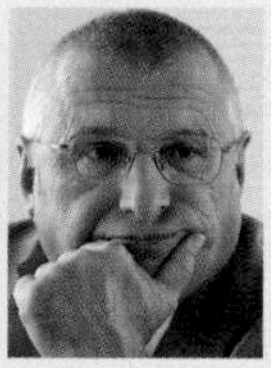

(©shironosov/ iStock/ Thinkstock)

**Patient Profile**

G.S., a 63-year-old retired accountant, was admitted to the hospital for severe pain from acute cholecystitis. G.S.'s medical history includes hypertension and type 2 diabetes. His pain has been managed with hydromorphone (Dilaudid) using patient-controlled analgesia. His intractable nausea and vomiting required the placement of a nasogastric (NG) tube. He is scheduled for a laparoscopic cholecystectomy. The surgery will be performed under general anesthesia.

**Subjective Data**

- G.S. is awake and able to identify himself, his birth date, surgical procedure, and surgical site
- States pain is controlled and rates it a 4 on a 0 to 10 scale on arrival to the holding area

**Objective Data**

- Admitted to the holding area with an NG tube in place and one peripheral IV catheter
- Capillary blood glucose 1 hour ago was 125 mg/dL
- Oxygen saturation 96% on room air

**Interprofessional Care**

- Vital signs per holding area routine
- 0.9 normal saline solution at 100 mL/hr
- Titrate $O_2$ therapy to keep $O_2$ saturation >90%
- Provide low, intermittent suction to NG tube

**Discussion Questions**

1. What are the potential intraoperative problems that you may expect with G.S.?
2. ***Priority Decision:*** What priority nursing interventions would be appropriate to prevent these complications from occurring?
3. ***Teamwork and Collaboration:*** What are the interprofessional team's priorities for G.S.?
4. ***Evidence-Based Practice:*** G.S. tells you that he is cold in spite of a blanket in place. Why is it important that G.S. remains warm?
5. ***Safety:*** Identify two areas of risk for injury to G.S. What actions can be taken to ensure patient safety?

Answers available at *http://evolve.elsevier.com/Lewis/medsurg.*

## BRIDGE TO NCLEX EXAMINATION

The number of the question corresponds to the same-numbered outcome at the beginning of the chapter.

1. Proper attire for the semirestricted area of the surgery department is
   - **a.** street clothing.
   - **b.** surgical attire and head cover.
   - **c.** surgical attire, head cover, and mask.
   - **d.** street clothing with the addition of shoe covers.
2. Activities that the nurse might perform in the role of a scrub nurse during surgery include (*select all that apply*)
   - **a.** checking electrical equipment.
   - **b.** preparing the instrument table.
   - **c.** passing instruments to the surgeon and assistants.
   - **d.** coordinating activities occurring in the operating room.
   - **e.** maintaining accurate counts of sponges, needles, and instruments.
3. The nurse is caring for a patient undergoing surgery for a knee replacement. What is critical to the patient's safety during the procedure (*select all that apply*)?
   - **a.** Universal protocol is followed.
   - **b.** The ACP is an anesthesiologist.
   - **c.** The patient has adequate health insurance.
   - **d.** The patient's family is in the surgery waiting area.
   - **e.** The patient's allergies are conveyed to the surgical team.
4. The nurse's *primary* responsibility for the care of the patient undergoing surgery is
   - **a.** developing an individualized plan of nursing care for the patient.
   - **b.** carrying out specific tasks related to surgical policies and procedures.
   - **c.** ensuring that the patient has been assessed for safe administration of anesthesia.
   - **d.** performing a preoperative history and physical assessment to identify patient needs.
5. When scrubbing at the scrub sink, the nurse should
   - **a.** scrub from elbows to hands.
   - **b.** scrub without mechanical friction.
   - **c.** scrub for a minimum of 10 minutes.
   - **d.** hold the hands higher than the elbows.
6. When positioning a patient in preparation for surgery, the nurse understands that injury to the patient is *most* likely to occur as a result of
   - **a.** incorrect musculoskeletal alignment.
   - **b.** loss of perception of pain or pressure.
   - **c.** pooling of blood in peripheral vessels.
   - **d.** disregarding the patient's need for modesty.

7. IV induction for general anesthesia is the method of choice for *most* patients because
   a. the patient is not intubated.
   b. the agents are nonexplosive.
   c. induction is rapid and pleasant.
   d. emergence is longer but with fewer complications.

1. b, 2. b, c, e, 3. a, e, 4. a, 5. d, 6. a, 7. c

For rationales to these answers and even more NCLEX review questions, visit *http://evolve.elsevier.com/Lewis/medsurg.*

## EVOLVE WEBSITE

http://evolve.elsevier.com/Lewis/medsurg

**Review Questions (Online Only)**
**Key Points**
**Answer Keys for Questions**
- Rationales for Bridge to NCLEX Examination Questions
- Answer Guidelines for Case Study on p. 328

**Conceptual Care Map Creator**
**Audio Glossary**
**Content Updates**

## REFERENCES


*1. Association of periOperative Registered Nurses: *Perioperative standards and recommended practices*, Denver, 2012, The Association.
2. The Joint Commission: Surgical care improvement project, 2014. Retrieved from *www.jointcommission.org/surgical_care_improvement_project.*
3. The Joint Commission: Hospital national patient safety goals. Retrieved from *www.jointcommission.org/assets/1/6/2015_NPSG_HAP.pdf.*
4. Rothrock JC: *Alexander's care of the patient in surgery*, ed 15, St Louis, 2015, Mosby.
5. Agency for Healthcare Research and Quality: Patient safety network. Retrieved from *http://psnet.ahrq.gov/primer.aspx?primerID=9.*
6. Competency and Credentialing Institute: CNOR certification, 2014. Retrieved from *www.cc-institute.org/cnor/aboutabout.*
7. Association of Surgical Technologists: About the profession, 2014. Retrieved from *www.ast.org/AboutUs/About_AST.*
8. Association of periOperative Registered Nurses: AORN position statement on allied health care providers and support personnel in the perioperative practice setting, 2011. Retrieved from *www.aorn.org/TwoColumnInsert.aspx?id=21939&terms=POSITION%20STATEMENTS.*
9. Association of periOperative Registered Nurses: AORN position statement on RN first assistants, 2013. Retrieved from *www.aorn.org/TwoColumnInsert.aspx?id=21939&terms=POSITION%20STATEMENTS.*
10. American Society of Anesthesiologists: Anesthesia fast facts, 2014. Retrieved from *www.asahq.org/For-the-Public-and-Media/Press-Room/Anesthesia-Fast-Facts.aspxaspx.*
11. American Association of Nurse Anesthetists: Qualifications and capabilities of the certified Registered Nurse anesthetist, 2014. Retrieved from *www.aana.com/ceandeducation/becomeacrna/Pages/Qualifications-and-Capabilities-of-the-Certified-Registered-Nurse-Anesthetist-.aspx.*
*12. Jiménez-Jiménez M, García-Escalona A, Martín-López A, et al: Intraoperative stress and anxiety reduction with music therapy: a controlled randomized clinical trial of efficacy and safety, *J Vasc Nurs* 31:101, 2013.
13. Occupational Safety and Health Administration: Occupational safety and health standards, toxic and hazardous substances: bloodborne pathogens, 29 CFR §1910.1030 2012. Retrieved from *www.osha.gov/pls/oshaweb/owadisp.show_document?p_table=STANDARDS&p_id=10051.*
14. ECRI Institute: Surgical fire prevention. Retrieved from *www.ecri.org/Accident_Investigation/Pages/Surgical-Fire-Prevention.aspx.*
15. The Joint Commission: Universal protocol, 2014. Retrieved from *www.jointcommission.orghttp://www.jointcommission.org/standards_information/up.aspx..*
*16. Collins SJ, Newhouse R, Porter J, Talsma A: Effectiveness of the surgical safety checklist in correcting errors: a literature review applying Reason's Swiss cheese model, *AORN J* 100:65, 2014.
17. Association of periOperative Registered Nurses: Preventing wrong-patient, wrong-site, wrong-procedure events. Retrieved from *www.aorn.org/Clinical_Practicehttps://www.aorn.org/TwoColumnInsert.aspx.*
*18. Lumbley J, Ali S, Tchokouani L: Retrospective review of predisposing factors for intraoperative pressure ulcer development, *J Clin Anesth* 26:368, 2014.
*19. Leeds I, Wick E, Melton GB: Does close temperature regulation affect surgical site infection rates? *Adv Surg* 48:65, 2014.
20. Association of periOperative Registered Nurses: *Perioperative nursing data set: the perioperative nursing vocabulary*, ed 3, Denver, 2011, The Association.
21. American Society of Anesthesiologists: *Distinguishing monitored anesthesia care ("MAC") from moderate sedation/analgesia (conscious sedation)*, Schaumburg, Ill, 2013, The Society.
22. American Association of Nurse Anesthetists: Registered nurses engaged in the administration of sedation and analgesia, 2013. Retrieved from *www.aana.com/resources2/professionalpractice/Documents/PPM%20Consid%204.2%20RNs%20Engaged%20in%20Sedation%20Analgesia.pdf*
23. Naglehout JJ, Plaus KL, editors: *Nurse anesthesia*, ed 5, St Louis, 2014, Saunders.
24. Skidmore-Roth L: *Mosby's 2015 nursing drug reference*, ed 28, St Louis, 2015, Mosby.
25. Morrell RC: Intralipid might save lives as a rescue from bupivacaine toxicity, 2007. Retrieved from *www.apsf.org/newsletters/html/2007/summer/03_intralipid.htm.*
26. Shoup AJ: Latex allergy. In Watson DS, editor: *Perioperative safety*, St Louis, 2011, Mosby.
27. Seifert P, Wahr J, Pace M, et al: Crisis management of malignant hyperthermia in the OR, *AORN J* 100:189, 2014.
28. Malignant Hyperthermia Association of the United States: Emergency treatment for an acute MH event. Retrieved from *www.mhaus.org/healthcare-professionals/managing-a-crisis.*


*Evidence-based information for clinical practice.

# Postoperative Care

*Christine R. Hoch*

*You may have to fight a battle more than once to win it.*

***Margaret Thatcher***

ⓔ http://evolve.elsevier.com/Lewis/medsurg/

## LEARNING OUTCOMES

1. Prioritize nursing responsibilities related to managing patients in the postanesthesia care unit (PACU).
2. Prioritize nursing responsibilities related to maintaining patient safety and preventing postoperative complications in the PACU and clinical unit.
3. Apply data from the initial nursing assessment to the management of the patient after transfer from the PACU to the clinical unit.
4. Select appropriate nursing interventions to manage potential problems during the postoperative period.
5. Differentiate discharge criteria from Phase I and Phase II postanesthesia care.

## KEY TERMS

airway obstruction, p. 332
atelectasis, p. 334
delayed emergence, p. 338
emergence delirium, p. 338
fast-tracking, p. 331
patient-controlled analgesia (PCA), p. 340
postoperative ileus (POI), p. 341
rapid postanesthesia care unit progression (RPP), p. 331

The postoperative period begins immediately after surgery and continues until the patient is discharged from medical care. This chapter focuses on the common features of postoperative nursing. Specific surgical procedures and the related postoperative care are discussed in the appropriate chapters of this text.

## POSTOPERATIVE CARE OF SURGICAL PATIENT

The patient's immediate recovery period is managed in a *postanesthesia care unit* (*PACU*), which is located adjacent to the operating room (OR). This location limits transportation of the patient immediately after surgery and provides ready access to anesthesia and OR staff. During the three phases of postanesthesia care, different levels of care are provided depending on the patient's needs[1] (Table 19-1).

**TABLE 19-1 Phases of Postanesthesia Care**

**Phase I**

- Care during the immediate postanesthesia period
- ECG and more intense monitoring (e.g., arterial BP monitoring, mechanical ventilation)

*Goal:* Prepare patient for transfer to Phase II level of care, an inpatient unit, or intensive care setting

**Phase II**

- Ambulatory surgery patients
- Fast-tracking (i.e., patients who have bypassed Phase I level of care)

*Goal:* Prepare patient for transfer to extended observation, home, or extended care facility

**Extended Observation**

- Extended care or observation after transfer/discharge from Phase I or Phase II levels of care

*Goal:* Prepare patient for self-care

**Blended Levels of Care**

- Various levels of care offered in the same environment

Source: American Society of PeriAnesthesia Nurses: 2015-2017 *Perianesthesia nursing standards, practice recommendations and interpretive statements,* Cherry Hill, NJ, 2015, The Society.

### Postanesthesia Care Unit Admission

The patient's initial admission to the PACU is a joint effort among the anesthesia care provider (ACP), OR nurse, and PACU nurse. This collaborative effort fosters a smooth transfer of care to the PACU and helps determine the phase to which the patient is assigned.

**PACU Progression.** How patients move through the phases of care in the PACU is determined by their condition. If a patient assigned to Phase I care on admission to the PACU is stable and recovering well, the patient may rapidly progress through Phase

Reviewed by Diane Marie Rudolphi, RN, MS, Continuing Non-Tenure Track Nursing Faculty, University of Delaware, Newark, Delaware; and Lisa Spruce, DNP, ACNS, ACNP, ANP, CNOR, CNS-CP, Director of Evidence-Based Perioperative Practice, Association of periOperative Registered Nurses, Denver, Colorado.

**TABLE 19-2 PACU Hand-Off Report**

**General Information**
- Patient name and age
- Surgeon and ACP
- Surgical procedure
- Presence of tubes, drains, catheters, and IV lines
- Type of anesthesia (e.g., general, regional, monitored anesthesia care)
- Use of any reversal agents
- Airway status (artificial airway and/or interventions to maintain adequate oxygenation)
- Pain management interventions
- NPO status and postoperative orders to be started

**Patient History**
- Indication for surgery
- Medical history, medications, allergies
- Preoperative or baseline vital signs, laboratory and diagnostic findings
- Level of consciousness, orientation
- Specific patient characteristics (e.g., hearing loss, vision impairment, mobility limitations)
- Patient preferences (e.g., cultural, personal beliefs/restrictions)
- Patient emotional status on arrival to OR

**Intraoperative Management**
- Anesthetic agents
- Other drugs received preoperatively or intraoperatively
- Last dose of opioid administration/pain management plan
- Total fluid replacements, including blood transfusions
- Total fluid losses (e.g., blood, nasogastric drainage)
- Urine output

**Intraoperative Course**
- Unexpected anesthetic events or reactions
- Unexpected surgical events
- Most recent vital signs and monitoring trends
- Results of intraoperative laboratory tests and x-rays

*ACP*, Anesthesia care provider; *PACU*, postanesthesia care unit.

I to either Phase II care or an inpatient unit. This accelerated progress is called **rapid postanesthesia care unit progression (RPP)**. Another accelerated system of care is **fast-tracking**, which involves admitting ambulatory surgery patients directly to Phase II care.[1] Although both RPP and fast-tracking can potentially result in time and cost savings, the patient's safety is the primary determining factor of where and at what level postoperative care is provided.

**Phase I Initial Assessment.** On admission of the patient to the PACU, the ACP gives you a postanesthesia hand-off report (Table 19-2). Hand-off reports should be standardized and interactive allowing for questions and clarification of information.[2] The ACP should remain in the PACU until you accept responsibility for the nursing care of the patient. The goals of PACU care are to maintain patient safety during recovery from anesthesia, identify actual and potential patient problems that may occur as a result of anesthesia and surgery, and to intervene appropriately. Potential problems in the postoperative period are identified in Fig. 19-1. Table 19-3 identifies key components of a PACU assessment.

Begin your initial assessment with an evaluation of the patient's airway, breathing, and circulation (ABC) status. Oxygenation and ventilation can be affected by residual neuromuscular blockade, use of opioids, and patient characteristics such as sleep-disordered breathing (e.g., central or obstructive sleep apnea [OSA], abnormal airway anatomy). Identify signs of inadequate oxygenation and ventilation (Table 19-4). Any evidence of respiratory distress requires prompt intervention.

Pulse oximetry monitoring provides a noninvasive means of assessing oxygenation and can provide an early warning of hypoxemia. *Transcutaneous carbon dioxide ($PtcCO_2$) and end-tidal $CO_2$ ($PetCO_2$) (capnography) monitoring* are used to detect respiratory depression in high-risk patients.[3] Volumetric capnography and acoustic respiratory rate monitoring have also demonstrated benefit in early identification of postoperative respiratory distress.[4] (Pulse oximetry, capnography, $PtcCO_2$, and $PetCO_2$ are discussed in Chapter 25.)

**TABLE 19-3 Initial PACU Assessment**

**Airway**
- Patency
- Oral or nasal airway
- Laryngeal mask airway
- Endotracheal tube with ventilator settings

**Breathing**
- Respiratory rate and quality
- Auscultated breath sounds
- Pulse oximetry
- Capnography or other technology supported monitoring if indicated
- Supplemental $O_2$

**Circulation**
- ECG monitoring: rate and rhythm
- BP: noninvasive or arterial line
- Hemodynamic pressure readings (if applicable)
- Temperature
- Capillary refill
- Color, temperature, moisture of skin
- Apical and peripheral pulses

**Genitourinary**
- Urine output

**Neurologic**
- Level of consciousness
- Orientation
- Sensory and motor status
- Pupil size and reaction

**Gastrointestinal**
- Nausea, vomiting
- Intake (fluids, irrigations)
- Output (vomitus)
- Bowel sounds

**Surgical Site**
- Dressings and visible incisions
- Drains: type, patency, and drainage
- IV assessment: location and condition of sites, solutions infusing

**Pain**
- Incision
- Other

**Patient Safety Needs**
- Patient position
- Fall risk assessment

**TABLE 19-4 Signs of Inadequate Oxygenation**

**Central Nervous System**
- Restlessness
- Agitation
- Confusion
- Muscle twitching
- Seizures
- Coma

**Respiratory System**
- Increased to absent respiratory effort
- Use of accessory muscles
- Abnormal breath sounds
- Abnormal arterial blood gases

**Cardiovascular System**
- Hypertension
- Hypotension
- Tachycardia
- Bradycardia
- Dysrhythmias
- Delayed capillary refill
- Weak peripheral pulses
- Decreased $O_2$ saturation

**Integumentary System**
- Flushed, cool, or moist skin
- Cyanosis

**Renal System**
- Urine output <0.5 mL/kg/hr

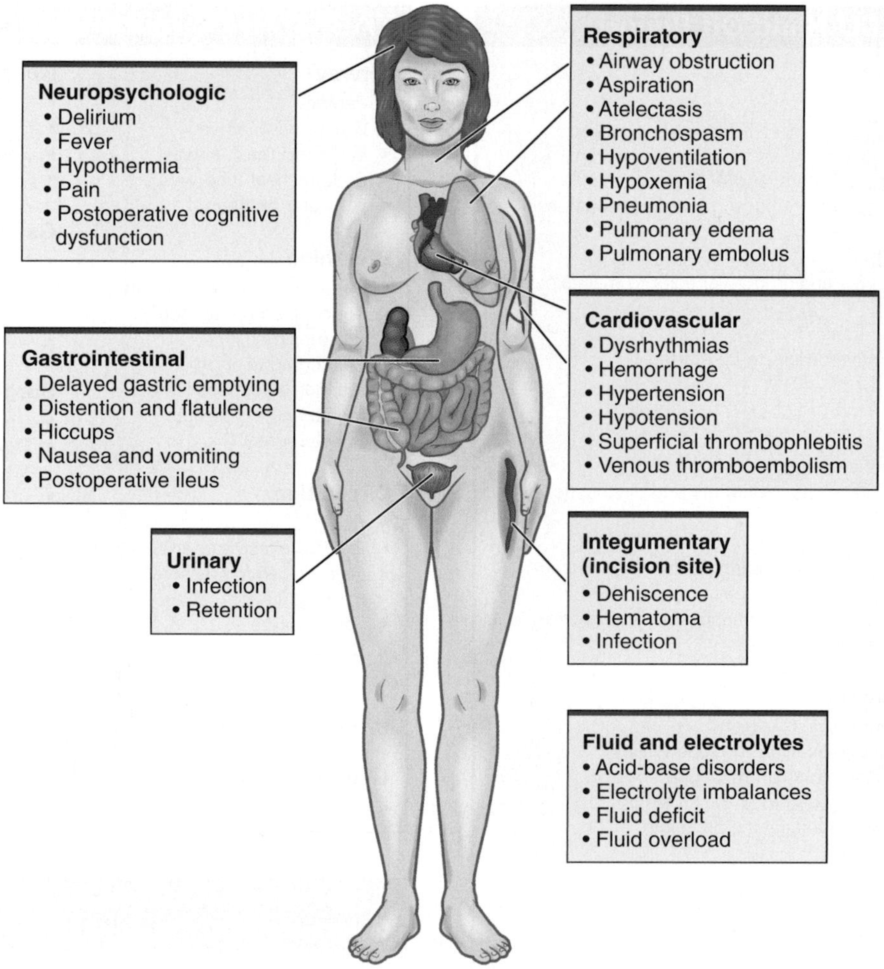


**FIG. 19-1** Potential problems in the postoperative period.

Note and assess changes in ECG findings from the preoperative baseline. Measure the BP and compare it with baseline readings. Invasive monitoring (e.g., arterial BP) is started if needed. Also assess body temperature, peripheral pulses, capillary refill, and skin condition (e.g., color, moisture). Any signs of inadequate tissue perfusion require prompt intervention.

Focus the initial neurologic assessment on level of consciousness; orientation; sensory and motor status; and size, equality, and reactivity of the pupils. The patient may be awake, drowsy but arousable, or asleep. Because hearing is the first sense to return in the unconscious patient, explain all activities to the patient from the moment of admission to the PACU. If the patient received a regional anesthetic (e.g., spinal, epidural), sensory and motor blockade may still be present, and you should check a dermatome level (see Fig. 55-7). (Dermatomes are also discussed in Chapter 8.) During recovery from regional anesthesia, sensory and motor function returns from the extremities to the site where the anesthetic was given. Therefore the areas near the site of injections are the last to recover.

Assess the urinary system by measuring intake and output and determining fluid balance. Intraoperative fluid totals are part of the anesthesia report. Note the presence of all IV lines; all irrigation solutions and infusions; and all output devices, including catheters and wound drains. Assess the surgical site, noting the condition of any dressings and the type and amount of any drainage. Implement postoperative orders related to incision care.

Nursing management of select problems is discussed in the following pages and can be applied to patients in both the PACU and clinical unit.

## RESPIRATORY PROBLEMS

### Etiology

**PACU.** In the immediate postanesthesia period the most common causes of airway compromise include obstruction, hypoxemia, and hypoventilation (Table 19-5). Patients at high risk include those who (1) have had general anesthesia; (2) are older than 55 years of age; (3) have a history of tobacco use; (4) have preexisting lung disease and/or sleep-disordered breathing; (5) are obese; (6) have co-morbidities (e.g., renal disease, diabetes, hypertension); or (7) have undergone airway, thoracic, or abdominal surgery. However, respiratory problems may occur with any patient who has been anesthetized. The greatest risk for respiratory distress occurs in the first 24 hours following surgery.[5]

**Airway obstruction** is commonly caused by blockage of the airway by the patient's tongue (Fig. 19-2). The base of the tongue falls backward against the soft palate and occludes the pharynx. It is most pronounced in the supine position and in the patient who is extremely sleepy after surgery.

*Hypoxemia*, a partial pressure of arterial oxygen ($PaO_2$) less than 60 mm Hg, is characterized by a variety of nonspecific clinical signs and symptoms, ranging from agitation to

TABLE 19-5 **Postoperative Respiratory Complications**

| Complications | Mechanisms | Manifestations | Interventions |
|---|---|---|---|
| **Airway Obstruction** | | | |
| Tongue falling back | Muscular flaccidity associated with ↓ consciousness and muscle relaxants | Use of accessory muscles<br>Snoring respirations<br>↓ Air movement | • Patient stimulation<br>• Head tilt, jaw thrust (Fig. 19-2)<br>• Artificial airway |
| Retained thick secretions | Secretion stimulation by anesthetic agents<br>Dehydration of secretions | Noisy respirations<br>Coarse crackles | • Suctioning<br>• Deep breathing and coughing<br>• IV hydration<br>• Chest PT |
| Laryngospasm | Irritation from endotracheal tube, anesthetic gases, or gastric aspiration<br>Most likely to occur after removal of endotracheal tube | Inspiratory stridor (crowing respirations)<br>Sternal retraction<br>Acute respiratory distress | • $O_2$ therapy<br>• Positive pressure ventilation<br>• IV muscle relaxant<br>• Lidocaine<br>• Corticosteroids |
| Laryngeal edema | Allergic drug reaction<br>Mechanical irritation from intubation<br>Fluid overload | Similar to laryngospasm | • $O_2$ therapy<br>• Antihistamines<br>• Corticosteroids<br>• Sedatives<br>• Possible intubation |
| **Hypoxemia** | | | |
| Atelectasis | Bronchial obstruction caused by retained secretions or ↓ lung volumes | ↓ Breath sounds<br>↓ $O_2$ saturation | • Humidified $O_2$ therapy<br>• Deep breathing<br>• Incentive spirometry<br>• Early mobilization |
| Pulmonary edema | Fluid overload<br>↑ Hydrostatic pressure<br>↓ Interstitial pressure<br>↑ Capillary permeability | ↓ $O_2$ saturation<br>Crackles<br>Infiltrates on chest x-ray | • $O_2$ therapy<br>• Diuretics<br>• Fluid restriction |
| Pulmonary embolism | Thrombus dislodged from peripheral venous system and lodged in pulmonary arterial system | Acute tachypnea<br>Dyspnea<br>Tachycardia<br>Hypotension<br>↓ $O_2$ saturation<br>Bronchospasm | • $O_2$ therapy<br>• Cardiopulmonary support<br>• Anticoagulant therapy |
| Aspiration | Inhalation of gastric contents into lungs | Unexplained tachypnea<br>Bronchospasm<br>↓ $O_2$ saturation<br>Atelectasis<br>Interstitial edema<br>Alveolar hemorrhage<br>Respiratory failure | • $O_2$ therapy<br>• Cardiopulmonary support<br>• Antibiotics |
| Bronchospasm | ↑ Smooth muscle tone with closure of small airways | Wheezing<br>Dyspnea<br>Tachypnea<br>↓ $O_2$ saturation | • $O_2$ therapy<br>• Bronchodilators |
| **Hypoventilation** | | | |
| Depression of central respiratory drive | Medullary depression from anesthetics, opioids, sedatives | Shallow respirations<br>↓ Respiratory rate, apnea<br>↓ $PaO_2$<br>↑ $PaCO_2$ | • Initiate capnography or other technology supported respiratory monitoring<br>• Stimulation<br>• Reversal of opioids or benzodiazepines<br>• Mechanical ventilation |
| Poor respiratory muscle tone | Neuromuscular blockade<br>Neuromuscular disease | As above | • Reversal of paralysis<br>• Mechanical ventilation |
| Mechanical restriction | Tight casts, dressings, abdominal binders<br>Positioning and obesity preventing lung expansion | As above | • Elevate head of bed<br>• Repositioning<br>• Loosen dressings |
| Pain | Shallow breathing to prevent incisional pain | ↑ Respiratory rate<br>Hypotension<br>Hypertension<br>↓ $PaCO_2$<br>↓ $PaO_2$<br>Complaints of pain<br>Guarding behavior | • Opioid analgesic drug therapy<br>• Nonsteroidal antiinflammatory drug therapy<br>• Complementary and alternative therapies (e.g., music, imagery) |

*$PaCO_2$*, Partial pressure of arterial carbon dioxide; *$PaO_2$*, partial pressure of arterial oxygen.

## TEAMWORK & COLLABORATION

### Caring for the Postoperative Patient

In the PACU, patients require frequent assessment and intervention by RNs. On the clinical units, the RN is responsible for assessment, development of an individualized plan of care, implementation and evaluation of the plan of care, and discharge teaching. Much of the care can be delegated to LPNs/LVNs and UAP. Respiratory and physical therapy may also have a role in the patient's care, depending on the type of surgery and the patient's past medical history.

| PACU | Clinical Unit |
|---|---|
| **Role of Nursing Personnel** | |
| ***Registered Nurse (RN)*** | |
| • Assess patient's initial airway, breathing, and circulation status.<br>• Evaluate for the return to consciousness, ability to maintain airway and breathing.<br>• Provide ongoing assessments for postoperative problems (e.g., airway obstruction, hypoventilation, hypotension or hypertension, dysrhythmias, emergence delirium).<br>• Evaluate patient's readiness to be transferred to clinical unit or be discharged from ambulatory surgery.<br>• Provide hand-off report about patient status when transferring patient to RN on clinical unit.<br>• Provide discharge teaching for patient and caregiver after ambulatory surgery. | • Assess patient on initial admission to clinical unit.<br>• Assess for postoperative complications (e.g., atelectasis, hemodynamic instability, cognitive dysfunction, pain, fluid and electrolyte imbalance, fever or hypothermia, nausea and vomiting, urinary retention, wound infection).<br>• Develop and implement an individualized plan of care based on identification of patient risk factors and potential complications.<br>• Develop and implement individualized patient and caregiver education, including discharge teaching. |
| ***Licensed Practical/Vocational Nurse (LPN/LVN)*** | |
| • Administer and titrate $O_2$ based on agency protocols.<br>• Give analgesics and IV fluids (consider state nurse practice act and agency policy). | • Titrate $O_2$ administration according to prescribed parameters.<br>• Monitor pain level and give prescribed analgesics.<br>• Give medications (consider state nurse practice act and agency policy for medications).<br>• Provide wound care, including dressing changes.<br>• Use bladder ultrasound to check for urinary retention.<br>• Insert catheter as prescribed for urinary retention. |
| ***Unlicensed Assistive Personnel (UAP)*** | |
| • Assist with positioning of patients in the lateral recovery position.<br>• Obtain vital signs, pulse oximetry and capillary blood glucose levels (per agency policy). Report abnormal levels to RN.<br>• Assist patient with elimination needs.<br>• Assist in transfer of patient to clinical unit. | • Record oral intake and output.<br>• Assist patient with deep breathing and coughing exercises.<br>• Report complaints of pain to RN or LPN/LVN.<br>• Reposition and ambulate patients as instructed.<br>• Provide hygiene, including oral care.<br>• Assist with nutrition and elimination needs. |
| **Role of Other Team Members** | |
| ***Respiratory Therapist*** | |
| • Provide respiratory care modalities that support patient recovery from anesthesia (e.g., $O_2$ therapy, nebulizer treatments, pulmonary drainage procedures, mechanical ventilation, and airway support).<br>• Institute extubation protocols.<br>• Monitor pulse oximetry, capnography, or other technology-assisted means of assessing hypoxemia or hypoventilation.<br>• Assist with $O_2$ and/or ventilation management during patient transport.<br>• Perform arterial blood gas sampling in the absence of an arterial line. | • Institute rapid intubation protocols if necessary in the absence of ACP.<br>• Provide respiratory care modalities (e.g., $O_2$ therapy, nebulizer treatments, pulmonary drainage procedures).<br>• Assist with $O_2$ and/or ventilation support during patient transport.<br>• Monitor pulse oximetry and capnography and titrate $O_2$ as needed.<br>• Perform arterial blood gas sampling as needed. |
| ***Physical Therapist*** | |
| • Perform initial assessment to ascertain normal functioning level if surgery was emergent.<br>• Support patient motion and joint mobility. | • Support patient motion and joint mobility.<br>• Support patient return to baseline functional mobility following surgery.<br>• Support nursing staff on best measures for joint positioning, transferring from bed to chair, and/or ambulation. |

somnolence, hypertension to hypotension, and tachycardia to bradycardia. Pulse oximetry will indicate low $O_2$ saturation (less than 90%).

The most common cause of postoperative hypoxemia is atelectasis. **Atelectasis** (alveolar collapse) may be the result of bronchial obstruction caused by retained secretions, decreased respiratory excursion, or general anesthesia. Atelectasis occurs when mucus blocks bronchioles or when the amount of alveolar surfactant (substance that holds the alveoli open) is reduced (Fig. 19-3). As air becomes trapped beyond the plug and is eventually absorbed, the alveoli collapse. Atelectasis may affect a portion of or an entire lobe of the lungs.

Other causes of hypoxemia include pulmonary edema, pulmonary embolism (PE), aspiration, and bronchospasm. *Pulmonary edema* is caused by an accumulation of fluid in the alveoli. It may be the result of fluid overload, heart failure, prolonged airway obstruction, sepsis, or aspiration.

*Aspiration* of gastric contents into the lungs is a potentially serious emergency. Gastric aspiration may also cause laryngospasm, infection, and pulmonary edema. Because of the serious consequences of aspiration of gastric fluids, prevention is the goal.

*Bronchospasm* is the result of an increase in bronchial smooth muscle tone with resultant closure of small airways. Airway edema develops, causing secretions to build up in the airway. The patient will have wheezing, dyspnea, use of accessory muscles, hypoxemia, and tachypnea. Bronchospasm may be due to aspiration, endotracheal intubation, pharyngeal suctioning, or an allergic response. (Allergic responses are discussed in Chapter 13.) Bronchospasm

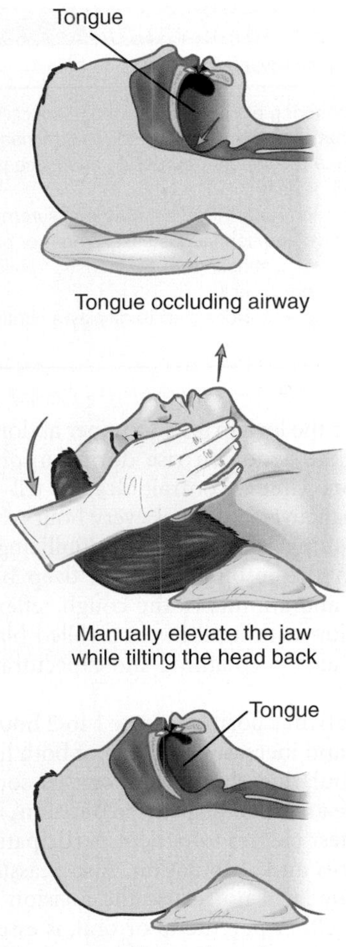


**FIG. 19-2** Etiology and relief of airway obstruction.

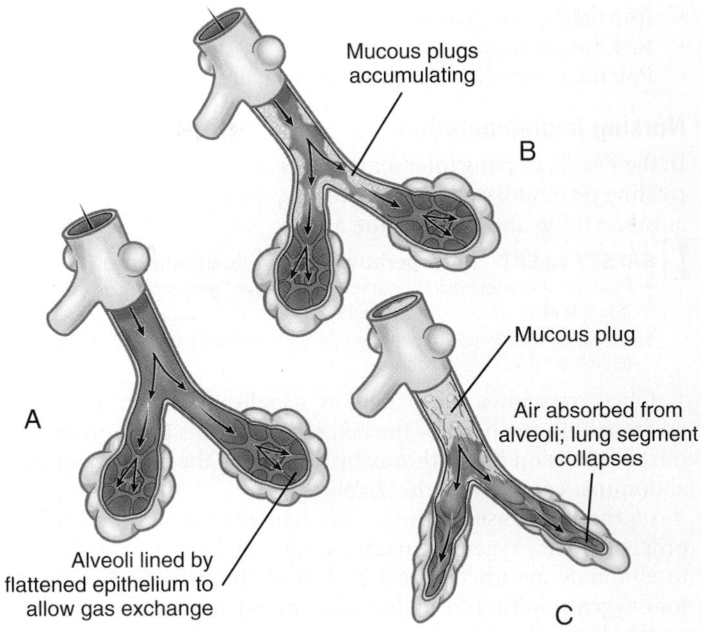


**FIG. 19-3** Postoperative atelectasis. **A,** Normal bronchiole and alveoli. **B,** Mucous plug in bronchiole. **C,** Collapse of alveoli resulting from atelectasis after absorption of air.

may occur in any patient but is seen more frequently in patients with asthma and chronic obstructive pulmonary disease (COPD).

*Hypoventilation,* a common complication in the PACU, is characterized by a decreased respiratory rate or effort, hypoxemia, and an increasing partial pressure of arterial carbon dioxide ($PaCO_2$) (*hypercapnia*). Hypoventilation may result from depression of the central respiratory drive (secondary to anesthesia or use of opioids), poor respiratory muscle tone (secondary to neuromuscular blockade or disease), or a combination of both.

**SAFETY ALERT Hypoventilation**
- Always monitor for respiratory depression when giving opioids.
- Use a sedation assessment scale (e.g., Richmond Agitation and Sedation Scale) to assess for levels of sedation and promote patient safety when giving opioids in the PACU.

Richmond Agitation Scale available at *www.icudelirium.org/docs/RASS.pdf.*

**Clinical Unit.** Common causes of respiratory problems for postoperative patients in the clinical unit are atelectasis and pneumonia, especially in patients with co-morbidities (e.g., OSA, COPD, heart failure)[6,7] and following abdominal and thoracic surgery. The postoperative development of mucous plugs and decreased surfactant production is directly related to hypoventilation, immobility and bed rest, ineffective coughing, and history of tobacco use. Increased bronchial secretions occur when the respiratory passages have been irritated by heavy smoking; acute or chronic pulmonary infection or disease; and the drying of mucous membranes that occurs with intubation, inhalation anesthesia, and dehydration. Without intervention, atelectasis can progress to pneumonia.

## NURSING MANAGEMENT: RESPIRATORY PROBLEMS

### Nursing Assessment

For an adequate respiratory assessment, evaluate airway patency; chest symmetry; and depth, rate, and character of respirations. Observe the chest wall for symmetry of movement. Impaired ventilation may first be seen as slowed breathing or reduced chest and abdominal movement during breathing. Also assess for the use of abdominal or accessory muscles, which may indicate respiratory distress. Auscultate breath sounds, since decreased or absent breath sounds are found when airflow is diminished or obstructed. Patients with poor respiratory effort, noisy respirations, or other signs of respiratory distress should be aroused immediately and instructed to take deep breaths.

Regular monitoring of vital signs, including pulse oximetry, capnography or other technology-supported monitoring (e.g., acoustic monitoring), and a thorough respiratory assessment permit you to recognize early signs of respiratory problems. Manifestations of hypoxemia include tachypnea, gasping, anxiety, restlessness, confusion, and a rapid or thready pulse.

Note and record the characteristics of sputum or mucus. Mucus from the trachea and throat is normally colorless and thin in consistency. Sputum from the lungs and bronchi is normally thick with a pale yellow tinge. Changes in sputum (e.g., color) may indicate a respiratory infection.

### Nursing Diagnoses

Nursing diagnoses and collaborative problems related to respiratory problems include, but are not limited to, the following:
- Ineffective airway clearance *related to* ineffective cough, obstruction, pain
- Ineffective breathing pattern *related to* anesthetic agents, pain, use of opioids

- Impaired gas exchange *related to* hypoventilation
- Risk for aspiration
- Potential complications: pneumonia, atelectasis

### ◆ Nursing Implementation

In the PACU, nursing interventions are aimed at preventing and treating respiratory problems. Proper positioning of the patient aids breathing and protects the airway.

**SAFETY ALERT Postoperative Patient Positioning**

- Position the unconscious patient in a lateral "recovery" position (Fig. 19-4).
- This position keeps the airway open and reduces the risk of aspiration if vomiting occurs.

Once conscious, the patient is usually placed in a supine position with the head of the bed elevated. This position maximizes expansion of the thorax by decreasing the pressure of the abdominal contents on the diaphragm.

$O_2$ therapy is used if the patient had general anesthesia or if ordered. Give oxygen via nasal cannula or face mask. $O_2$ helps to eliminate anesthetic gases and meet the increased demand for oxygen resulting from decreased blood volume or increased metabolism.

Deep breathing is encouraged to aid gas exchange and promote the return to consciousness. Once the patient is more awake, deep breathing, coughing, and use of an incentive spirometer help prevent alveolar collapse and move respiratory secretions to larger airway passages for expectoration. One technique, known as *sustained maximal inspiration,* requires the patient to inhale as deeply as possible and, at the peak of inspiration, hold the breath for a few seconds, and then exhale. This should be followed by a second deep breath and cough.

The use of an incentive spirometer helps by giving visual feedback of respiratory effort (Fig. 19-5). Diaphragmatic or abdominal breathing involves inhaling slowly and deeply through the nose, holding the breath for a few seconds, and then exhaling slowly and completely through the mouth. Place the patient's hands lightly over the lower ribs and upper abdomen so that the patient can feel the abdomen rise during inspiration and fall during expiration. Unless contraindicated, tell the patient to perform these maneuvers 10 times every hour while awake.

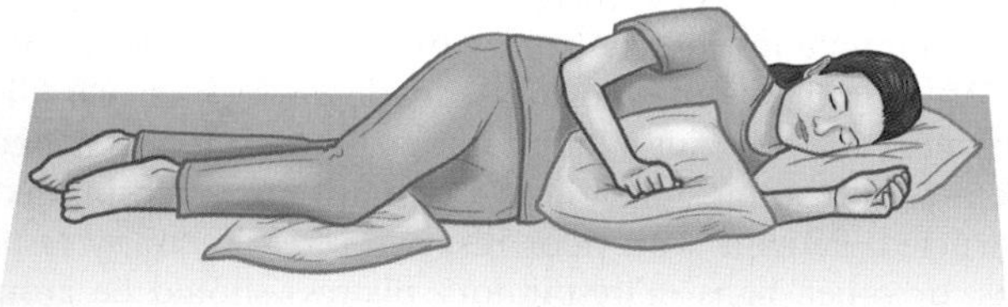

**FIG. 19-4** Position of patient during recovery from general anesthesia.

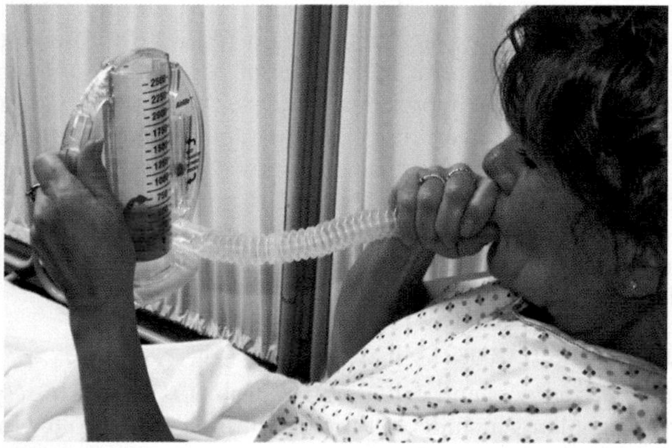

**FIG. 19-5** Proper use of an incentive spirometer. (Courtesy Christine R. Hoch, MSN, RN, ACNS-BC, Nursing Instructor, University of Delaware, Newark, Del.)

**INFORMATICS IN PRACTICE**

***Respiratory Monitoring***

- Continuous monitoring of respiratory rate is especially important for postoperative patients receiving PCA for pain management, as opioids can cause respiratory depression and place patients at risk of serious injury or death.
- Acoustic Respiration Rate (RRa) is a new measurement that allows for the noninvasive and continuous assessment of patients' breathing. RRa uses a sensor with an acoustic transducer that is applied to the patient's neck.
- The respiratory signal is processed to display a continuous respiration rate.

Source: *www.masimo.com/rra*

Effective coughing is essential in mobilizing secretions. If secretions are in the respiratory tract, deep breathing often moves them up and stimulates the cough reflex. Splinting an abdominal incision with a pillow or a rolled blanket supports the incision and aids in coughing and expectorating secretions (Fig. 19-6).

Change the patient's position every 1 to 2 hours to allow full chest expansion and increase perfusion of both lungs. Sitting in a chair and ambulating should be done as soon as ordered. Provide adequate and regular pain medication. Incisional pain often is the greatest barrier to patient participation in effective breathing exercises and ambulation. Also reassure the patient that these activities will not cause the incision to open. Adequate hydration, either parenteral or oral, is essential to maintain the integrity of mucous membranes and to keep secretions thin and loose for easy expectoration.

Other nursing interventions appropriate for specific respiratory problems are detailed in Table 19-5. A nursing care plan for the postoperative patient (eNursing Care Plan 19-1) is available on the website for this chapter.

## CARDIOVASCULAR PROBLEMS

### Etiology

**PACU.** In the immediate postanesthesia period the most common cardiovascular problems include hypotension, hypertension, and

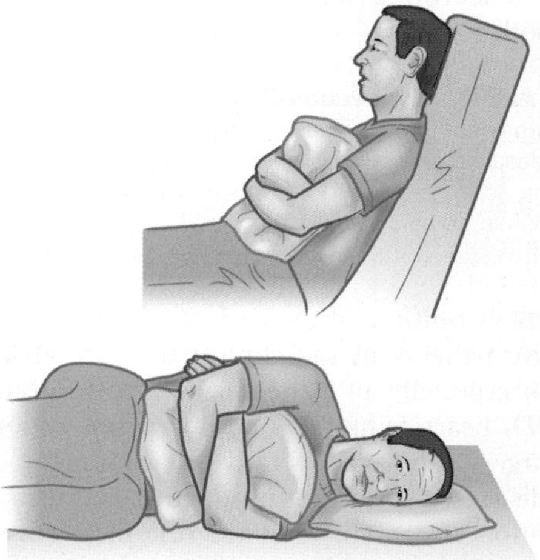

**FIG. 19-6** Techniques for splinting incision when coughing.

dysrhythmias. Patients at greatest risk for alterations in cardiovascular function include those with alterations in respiratory function, those with a history of cardiovascular disease, older adults, the debilitated, and the critically ill.

*Hypotension* is evidenced by signs of hypoperfusion to the vital organs, especially the brain, heart, and kidneys. Clinical signs of disorientation, loss of consciousness, chest pain, and oliguria reflect hypoperfusion, hypoxemia, and the loss of physiologic compensation. Intervention must be timely to prevent the devastating complications of cardiac ischemia or infarction, cerebral ischemia, renal ischemia, and bowel infarction.

The most common cause of hypotension in the PACU is fluid and blood loss, which may lead to hypovolemic shock. Hemorrhage is always a risk of surgery. Marked blood loss is possible when cauterization or sutures fail. Hemorrhage most often occurs internally, requiring assessment for changes in level of consciousness and vital signs. If changes are detected, treatment is directed toward restoring circulating volume. If there is no response to fluid administration, heart dysfunction should be considered the cause of hypotension.

Primary heart dysfunction, as may occur in myocardial infarction, cardiac tamponade, or pulmonary embolism, results in an acute drop in cardiac output. Secondary heart dysfunction occurs as a result of the negative *chronotropic* (rate of heart contraction) and negative *inotropic* (force of heart contraction) effects of drugs, such as β-adrenergic blockers, digoxin, or opioids. Other causes of hypotension include decreased systemic vascular resistance, dysrhythmias, and measurement errors (e.g., taking BP with an incorrectly sized cuff).

*Hypertension,* a common finding in the PACU, is most frequently the result of sympathetic nervous system stimulation that may be the result of pain, anxiety, bladder distention, or respiratory distress. Hypertension may also be the result of hypothermia and preexisting hypertension.

In the PACU, *dysrhythmias* are caused by hypoxemia, hypercapnia, electrolyte and acid-base imbalances, circulatory instability, and preexisting heart disease. Hypothermia, pain, surgical stress, and many anesthetic agents can also cause dysrhythmias.

**Clinical Unit.** In the clinical unit, postoperative fluid and electrolyte imbalances are contributing factors to heart problems. Such imbalances may result from a combination of the body's normal response to the stress of surgery, excessive fluid losses, and improper IV fluid replacement. The body's fluid status directly affects cardiac output.

Fluid retention during postoperative days 1 to 3 can result from the stress response, which maintains both blood volume and BP. Fluid retention is caused by the secretion and release of two hormones by the pituitary—antidiuretic hormone (ADH) and adrenocorticotropic hormone (ACTH)—and activation of the renin-angiotensin-aldosterone system (RAAS). ADH release leads to increased water reabsorption and decreased urine output, increasing blood volume. ACTH stimulates the adrenal cortex to secrete cortisol and, to a lesser degree, aldosterone (see Figs. 16-9 and 16-10). Fluid losses resulting from surgery decrease kidney perfusion, stimulating the RAAS and causing marked release of aldosterone (see Chapter 16). Both mechanisms that increase aldosterone lead to significant sodium and fluid retention, thus increasing blood volume.

Fluid overload may occur during this period of fluid retention when IV fluids are infused too rapidly, when chronic (e.g., heart, kidney) disease exists, or when the patient is an older adult. Fluid deficits from untreated preoperative dehydration, intraoperative blood losses, or slow or inadequate fluid replacement can lead to decreases in cardiac output and tissue perfusion. Postoperative losses from vomiting, bleeding, wound drainage, or suctioning can also contribute to fluid deficits.

*Hypokalemia* can be a consequence of urinary and gastrointestinal (GI) tract losses. Low serum potassium levels directly affect the contractility of the heart and may contribute to decreases in cardiac output and tissue perfusion. Potassium replacement, usually 40 mEq/day, should not be given until renal function is assessed. A urine output of at least 0.5 mL/kg/hr is generally considered indicative of adequate renal function.

Cardiovascular status is also affected by the state of tissue perfusion or blood flow. The stress response contributes to an increase in clotting tendencies by increasing platelet production. In addition, general anesthesia causes peripheral vasodilation, which may contribute to damage of the vascular lining.

A *venous thromboembolism* (VTE) may form in leg veins as a result of inactivity, body position, and pressure, all of which lead to venous stasis and decreased perfusion. VTE is especially common in older adults, obese individuals, immobilized patients, and patients with a history of PE. It is a potentially life-threatening complication, because it may lead to PE and infarction. Suspect PE in any patient with tachypnea, dyspnea, and tachycardia, particularly when the patient is already receiving $O_2$ therapy. Other manifestations may include agitation, chest pain, hypotension, hemoptysis, dysrhythmias, and heart failure. Superficial thrombophlebitis is an uncomfortable but less serious complication that may develop in a leg vein as a result of venous stasis or in the arm veins as a result of irritation from IV catheters or solutions. (PE and VTE are discussed in Chapters 27 and 37, respectively.)

*Syncope* (fainting) may indicate decreased cardiac output, fluid deficits, or defects in cerebral perfusion. Syncope frequently occurs as a result of postural hypotension when the patient ambulates. It is more common in the older adult or in the patient who has been immobile for long periods. Normally when the patient stands up quickly, the arterial baroreceptors respond to the accompanying fall in BP with sympathetic nervous system stimulation. This produces vasoconstriction and thereby maintains BP. These sympathetic and vasomotor functions may be diminished in the older adult and the immobile or postanesthesia patient.

## NURSING MANAGEMENT: CARDIOVASCULAR PROBLEMS

### Nursing Assessment

The most important aspect of the cardiovascular assessment is frequent monitoring of vital signs. They are usually monitored every 15 minutes in Phase I, or more often until stabilized, and then less frequently in Phase II. Compare postoperative vital signs with pre- and intraoperative findings to determine when the signs are returning to baseline. Notify the ACP or surgeon if any of the following occurs:

- Systolic BP <90 mm Hg or >160 mm Hg
- Pulse rate <60 beats/minute or >120 beats/minute
- Pulse pressure (difference between systolic and diastolic BP) narrows
- BP trends gradually decrease or increase over several consecutive readings
- Change in heart rhythm

Hypotension accompanied by a normal pulse and warm, dry, pink skin usually represents the residual vasodilating effects of anesthesia and suggests only a need for continued observation. Hypotension accompanied by a rapid or weak pulse and cold, clammy, pale skin may indicate impending hypovolemic shock and requires immediate treatment.

ECG monitoring is recommended for patients who have a history of heart disease and for all older patients who have undergone major surgery, regardless of whether they have heart problems. Assess the apical-radial pulse carefully, and report any deficits or irregularities. Assess peripheral pulses and skin color, temperature, and moisture to gain valuable information about tissue perfusion.

### ◆ Nursing Diagnoses

Nursing diagnoses and collaborative problems related to cardiovascular problems include, but are not limited to, the following:

- Decreased cardiac output *related to* hypovolemia, dysrhythmias
- Ineffective peripheral tissue perfusion *related to* prolonged immobility, venous stasis
- Risk for imbalanced fluid volume
- Risk for impaired cardiovascular function
- Potential complications: hypovolemic shock, venous thromboembolism

### ◆ Nursing Implementation

◆ **PACU.** Begin treatment of hypotension with $O_2$ therapy to promote oxygenation of hypoperfused organs. Inspect the surgical incision to determine if excessive bleeding is the cause of volume loss. Because the most common cause of hypotension is fluid loss, give IV fluid boluses to normalize BP. Primary heart dysfunction may require drug intervention. Peripheral vasodilation and hypotension may require vasoconstrictive agents to increase systemic vascular resistance.

Treatment of hypertension centers on removing the cause of sympathetic nervous system stimulation. Treatment may include the use of analgesics, assistance in voiding, and correction of respiratory problems. Rewarming corrects hypothermia-induced hypertension. If the patient has preexisting hypertension or has undergone heart or vascular surgery, drug therapy to reduce BP is usually needed.

Because the majority of dysrhythmias seen in the PACU have identifiable causes, treatment is directed toward removing the cause. Correction of these physiologic alterations usually corrects the dysrhythmias. In the event of life-threatening dysrhythmias (e.g., ventricular tachycardia), follow the agency's protocol for advanced cardiac life support.

◆ **Clinical Unit.** Maintain an accurate intake and output record, monitor laboratory findings (e.g., electrolytes, hematocrit), and manage IV therapy during the postoperative period. Ongoing assessment of the potential complications associated with IV therapy (e.g., extravasation; redness, pain at the site) is essential.

Early ambulation is the most significant general nursing measure to prevent postoperative complications. The exercise associated with walking (1) increases muscle tone; (2) stimulates circulation, which prevents venous stasis and VTE, and speeds wound healing; and (3) increases vital capacity and maintains normal respiratory function. Progression to ambulation can be achieved by first raising the head of the patient's bed for 1 to 2 minutes and then assisting the patient to sit, with legs dangling, while monitoring the pulse rate. If no changes or complaints are noted, start ambulation with ongoing monitoring of the pulse. If changes in the pulse are noted or dizziness occurs, sit the patient in a nearby chair. The patient should remain in this location until the BP and pulse are stable. Then help the patient back to the bed. If dizziness occurs, it is often frightening for the patient and you. Injury can result from a fall, so take measures to ensure patient and staff safety.

**CHECK YOUR PRACTICE**

You are caring for an older, obese male patient who is 1 day post colon resection with activity orders for moving out of the bed to a chair. While he is in bed, you help him to a sitting position with his legs dangling. He tells you that he feels dizzy. You take his BP and it is 108/64 and his pulse is 124.

- What should you do?

## NEUROLOGIC AND PSYCHOLOGIC PROBLEMS

### Etiology

**PACU.** Postoperatively, **emergence delirium** is a short-term neurologic alteration manifested by behaviors such as restlessness, agitation, disorientation, thrashing, and shouting. This condition may be caused by hypoxia, anesthetic agents, bladder distention, postoperative pain, long duration of preoperative fasting, residual neuromuscular blockade, or the presence of an endotracheal tube.[8] If delirium occurs, first suspect hypoxia.

**Delayed emergence** may also be a problem postoperatively. The most common cause of delayed emergence is prolonged drug action, particularly of opioids, sedatives, residual neuromuscular blockade, and inhalation anesthetics. It is not usually due to neurologic injury. Delayed emergence is associated with longer PACU and hospital length of stay.[8]

**Clinical Unit.** Two types of postoperative cognitive impairments seen in surgical patients are *postoperative cognitive dysfunction* (POCD) and *delirium.* POCD is a decline in the patient's cognitive function (e.g., memory, ability to concentrate) for weeks or months after surgery. POCD is seen primarily in the older surgical patient. Preexisting cognitive impairment, age, duration of anesthesia, intraoperative complications, and postoperative infections are related to the development of POCD. Any changes in mental status should be quickly and thoroughly investigated, as the causes may be life threatening.

Postoperative delirium is more common in the older patient, but it can occur in patients of any age. Delirium may be the result of severe postoperative pain, fluid and electrolyte imbalances, hypoxemia, drug effects, sleep deprivation, and sensory deprivation or overload. It is characterized by cognitive dysfunction, varying levels of consciousness, altered psychomotor activity, and a disturbed sleep/wake cycle. (Delirium is discussed in Chapter 59.)

Anxiety and depression may also occur in postoperative patients. Patients may experience depressive symptoms and delirium at the same time. This increases the likelihood of postoperative complications.[9] Any patient may have these responses as part of grieving for lost body parts or functions or for loss of independence during recovery and rehabilitation.

*Alcohol withdrawal delirium* results from alcohol withdrawal in a postoperative patient. It is characterized by restlessness, insomnia and nightmares, irritability, and auditory or visual hallucinations. Chapter 10 discusses the identification and management of alcohol withdrawal delirium.

## NURSING MANAGEMENT: NEUROLOGIC AND PSYCHOLOGIC PROBLEMS

### Nursing Assessment

Assess the patient's level of consciousness, orientation, memory, and ability to follow commands. Determine the size, reactivity, and equality of the pupils. Also assess the patient's sleep/wake cycle and sensory and motor status. If the neurologic status is altered, try to determine possible causes. If the patient was mentally alert before surgery and becomes cognitively impaired postoperatively, you should suspect delirium or POCD.

### Nursing Diagnoses

Nursing diagnoses related to neurologic or psychologic problems include, but are not limited to, the following:

- Acute confusion *related to* hypoxia, postoperative cognitive dysfunction, delirium
- Anxiety *related to* change in health status, hospital environment
- Disturbed body image *related to* loss of body part(s), function
- Disturbed sleep pattern *related to* pain, hospital environment

### Nursing Implementation

**PACU.** The most common cause of postoperative agitation in the PACU is hypoxemia. As a result, focus your attention on evaluating respiratory function. Once you have ruled out hypoxemia or other known causes of postoperative delirium, sedation may be beneficial in controlling the agitation. Because the most common cause of delayed emergence is prolonged drug action, delays in awakening usually spontaneously resolve with time. If necessary, benzodiazepines and opioids may be reversed with drug antagonists.

Until the patient is awake and able to communicate effectively, be a patient advocate and maintain patient safety at all times. This includes monitoring physiologic status, having the side rails up and the call bell available, securing equipment (e.g., IV lines, artificial airways), using two unique patient identifiers before giving drugs or completing treatments, and verifying allergies.

**Clinical Unit.** To prevent or manage postoperative delirium or POCD, address factors that are known to contribute to the condition. Maintain normal physiologic function by achieving fluid and electrolyte balance, adequate nutrition and sleep, pain management, proper bowel and bladder function, and early mobilization. To help orient the patient, use specific aids, such as clocks, calendars, and photos.

To prevent or limit psychologic problems, provide adequate support for the patient. This includes listening to and talking with the patient, offering explanations and reassurance, and encouraging the presence and assistance of the patient's caregiver(s). Evaluate the patient's behavior to distinguish a normal reaction to a stressful situation from one that is becoming abnormal or excessive. The recognition of alcohol withdrawal delirium presents a particular challenge. Record and report any unusual or disturbed behavior so that a diagnosis can be made and treatment started.

## PAIN AND DISCOMFORT

### Etiology

Despite the availability of pain-relieving drugs and techniques, pain remains a common problem and a significant fear for patients. Postoperative pain is caused by the interaction of a number of physiologic and psychologic factors. The skin and underlying tissues have been traumatized by the incision and retraction during surgery. In addition, there may be reflex muscle spasms around the incision. Anxiety and fear, sometimes related to the anticipation of pain, create tension and further increase muscle tone and spasm. Positioning during surgery or the use of internal devices such as an endotracheal tube or catheters may also cause discomfort. The effort and movement associated with deep breathing, coughing, and ambulating may aggravate pain by creating tension on the incision area. Other sources of discomfort include nausea and vomiting, environmental noises, noxious odors, and shivering.

When the internal viscera are cut, no pain is felt. However, pressure in the internal viscera causes pain. Therefore deep visceral pain may signal a complication such as intestinal distention, bleeding, or abscess formation. Pain also increases the risk of atelectasis and impaired respiratory function.

## NURSING MANAGEMENT: PAIN

### Nursing Assessment

The patient's self-report is the single most reliable indicator of pain. Pain scales such as a numeric or FACES pain scale can assist with assessing the severity or intensity of pain. (Pain scales are discussed in Chapter 8.) Assess pain levels at rest and during activities. Since verbalization of pain is not always possible in the PACU, observe the patient for other indications of pain (e.g., restlessness, grimacing, changes in vital signs). You should expect that patients will experience incisional pain, especially with movement, and with certain procedures (e.g., removal of drains).

Assessment of patients from different cultures or who do not speak English may be challenging. Take extra time to explore the pain experience with these patients. (Chapter 2 discusses the use of an interpreter.) Adapt care as needed to meet the patient's unique needs and expectations for pain control.

Assess the patient on arrival to the PACU and at frequent intervals. Identifying the location of the pain is important. Incisional pain is to be expected, but other causes of pain, such as a full bladder, may also be present. Always involve patients in the assessment and management of their pain.

### Nursing Diagnoses

Nursing diagnoses for the patient experiencing pain include, but are not limited to, the following:

- Acute pain *related to* inflammation or injury in surgical area
- Chronic pain *related to* preexisting conditions (e.g., arthritis)

### Nursing Implementation

A plan for pain control that includes behavioral modalities and control of anxiety is developed preoperatively. Adjustments to or continuation of drugs used to treat any chronic pain is also evaluated in the preoperative phase of care. During this time, patients are taught to report pain and how it will be managed postoperatively. Pain management plans should be shared during the hand-off report.

Postoperative pain control techniques include the use of single modalities (e.g., opioid drugs, patient-controlled analgesia [PCA], regional analgesic [local anesthetic infiltration]) and multimodal analgesia. *Multimodal analgesia,* or the use of two or more analgesics with different mechanisms of action (e.g., opioid and a nonsteroidal antiinflammatory drug [NSAID]), is recommended when possible to achieve better pain relief with fewer or less severe side effects.[10] These drugs may be given via the same or different routes. The choice of modalities should be procedure and patient specific.

Orders for pain medication and other comfort measures are often written on an as-needed (PRN) basis. Time the administration of analgesics to ensure that they are in effect during activities that may be painful, such as walking. Although opioid analgesics are often essential for the postoperative patient's comfort, there are undesirable side effects. The most common include constipation, nausea and vomiting, respiratory and cough depression, and hypotension.

Before giving any analgesic, first assess the patient's pain, including location, quality, and intensity; vital signs; and level of consciousness. Treat incisional pain as ordered. If the patient reports chest or leg pain, analgesics may mask a complication (e.g., VTE). If it is gas pain, opioids can aggravate it. If the analgesic either fails to relieve the pain or makes the patient lethargic or somnolent, notify the health care provider (HCP) and request a change in the order.

**Patient-controlled analgesia (PCA)** is a method of pain management that allows the self-administration of predetermined doses of analgesia by the patient. The goals of PCA are to provide immediate analgesia and maintain an acceptable level of pain control. A continuous infusion in addition to patient-administered bolus doses may also be ordered especially in opioid tolerant patients.[10] Continuous infusions allow for a steady blood level of analgesia with the additional patient doses used prior to anticipated painful events (e.g., walking, deep breathing, and coughing) or for breakthough pain. The route of delivery may be IV, oral, epidural, or transdermal. The transdermal route is designed for short-term pain management and may offer advantages over the IV route (e.g., needleless, low infection risk, decreased drug errors associated with pump malfunction or inaccurate programming). Some advantages of PCA are early ambulation, better pain management than with PRN analgesia, and greater patient satisfaction. (PCA is discussed in Chapter 8.)

**CHECK YOUR PRACTICE**

Although PCA is infusing as ordered, your postoperative patient reports ongoing pain that is rated 8 on a 0 to 10 scale.

- What steps would you take next to manage this patient's pain more effectively?

*Epidural analgesia* is the infusion of opioid analgesics through a catheter placed into the epidural space surrounding the spinal cord. The goal of epidural analgesia is delivery of the drug directly to opiate receptors in the spinal cord. Administration methods include intermittent bolus dosing, continuous infusion, and patient-controlled epidural analgesia. This technique results in a constant circulating level and a reduced total dose of medication. The use of epidural analgesia for postoperative pain is increasing.

*Perineural local anesthesia*, the infiltration of a nonopioid drug into the surgical site, is another method of managing postoperative pain. A disposable or mechanical infusion pump delivers the local anesthetic via a catheter directly to the surgical incision site. A single dose of bupivacaine liposome injectable suspension (Exparel) provides pain relief with reduced opioid needs for up to 72 hours.

The acute pain of surgery almost always requires the use of analgesics. However, nondrug approaches such as repositioning, massage, and distraction can enhance pain management. Complementary and alternative therapies such as music therapy, guided imagery, relaxation exercises, and aromatherapy are effective adjuncts in pain management.

Organizational approaches have also demonstrated a reduction in postoperative pain intensity with decreases in side effects associated with the use of analgesia. These approaches include the use of procedure-specific, multimodal pain management guidelines with titration of analgesia based on specific patient needs.[10,11]

**SAFETY ALERT Patient-Controlled Analgesia (PCA)**

- Carefully check the HCP's order for PCA and properly program the pump to deliver the ordered dose of analgesic (e.g., continuous rate, bolus dose, maximum dose).
- A patient's death or serious injury associated with a drug error (e.g., wrong drug, wrong dose, wrong patient, wrong rate) is a serious reportable event (never event) or sentinel event. (See Chapter 1 for discussion of these events.)

## ALTERATIONS IN TEMPERATURE

### Etiology

The patient's temperature in the postoperative period provides valuable information (Table 19-6).

**Hypothermia.** Perioperative *hypothermia* is a core body temperature less than 96.8° F (36° C). Hypothermia occurs when heat loss exceeds heat production. Heat loss may occur due to skin exposure by the surgical procedure, use of cold irrigants and skin preparations, as well as unwarmed inhaled gases. Although all patients are at risk for hypothermia, patients with low preoperative core body temperatures, systolic BP less than 140 mm Hg, older patients, female patients, and patients who receive epidural or spinal anesthesia are at a higher risk of developing hypothermia postoperatively.[12] Long surgical procedures and prolonged anesthetic administration lead to redistribution of body heat from the core to the periphery. This places the patient at an increased risk for hypothermia.

Hypothermia can affect the patient's perception of the perioperative experience. The complications associated with hypothermia can include vasoconstriction with resultant hypertension, compromised immune function, bleeding, untoward cardiac events, surgical site infection (SSI), altered drug metabolism, and postoperative pain and shivering. Shivering can increase resting energy expenditure and $O_2$ consumption up to 500%, which can lead to hypoxemia and myocardial ischemia (angina). Shivering can also increase carbon dioxide production, contribute to increased heart rate, BP, and intracranial pressure, as well as significantly affect the patient's comfort level.

**Fever.** Fever may occur at any time during the postoperative period (Table 19-6). Wound infection, particularly from aerobic

**TABLE 19-6 Postoperative Temperature Changes**

| Time After Surgery | Temperature | Possible Causes |
|---|---|---|
| Up to 12 hr | Hypothermia: ≤96.8° F (36° C) | Effects of anesthesia, body heat loss during surgical procedure |
| First 48 hr (postop days 1 and 2) | Mild elevation: ≤100.4° F (38° C) | Inflammatory response to surgical stress |
| | Moderate elevation: >100.4° F (38° C) | Lung congestion, dehydration |
| After first 48 hr (postop day 3 and later) | Elevation >100° F (37.8° C) | Infection (e.g., wound, urinary, respiratory) |

organisms, is often accompanied by a fever that spikes in the afternoon or evening and returns to near-normal levels in the morning. The respiratory tract may be infected secondary to stasis of secretions in areas of atelectasis. The urinary tract may be infected secondary to catheterization. Superficial thrombophlebitis may occur at the IV site. VTE in the leg veins may produce a temperature elevation.

Surgical patients who take antibiotics for a period of time are at risk for *Clostridium difficile* infections. Manifestations of *C. difficile* may include fever, diarrhea, and abdominal pain.

Intermittent high fever accompanied by shaking chills and diaphoresis suggests septicemia. This may occur at any time during the postoperative period because microorganisms may have been introduced into the bloodstream during surgery, especially in GI or genitourinary (GU) procedures. Septicemia may also occur later from a wound or urinary tract infection.

*Malignant hyperthermia* (MH) causes a rapid rise in core body temperature to 105° F (40.5° C) or higher and severe muscle contractions after receiving general anesthesia. Additional signs of MH include tachycardia, hypercarbia, metabolic and respiratory acidosis, myoglobinuria, and elevated creatine kinase levels. MH is a life-threatening complication. While most cases of MH occur during general anesthesia, the 1-hour period immediately following surgery (e.g., in the PACU) is also a critical time.[13]

## NURSING MANAGEMENT: ALTERED TEMPERATURE

### Nursing Assessment

Record the patient's temperature on arrival to the PACU and every hour if the patient remains normothermic. Temperature may be taken orally, temporally, or via the tympanic membrane. Use the same route of measuring temperature during the patient's stay in the PACU. If the patient is hypothermic, measure the temperature every 15 minutes until normothermia is reached. Unintended hypothermia is an independent risk factor for surgical site infections (SSIs). Perioperative temperature management remains a quality measure by the Surgical Care Improvement Project (SCIP), a national partnership of organizations whose goal is to reduce SSIs.[14]

Risk factors for hypothermia or MH should be communicated to all members of the perioperative team. Supplies recommended by the Malignant Hyperthermia Association of the United States should be readily available to manage MH. Assess the color and temperature of the skin. Observe the patient for early signs of inflammation and infection that may precede a fever so that any complications can be treated in a timely manner.

### Nursing Diagnoses

Nursing diagnoses related to an altered temperature include, but are not limited to, the following:

- Hypothermia *related to* long surgical procedures, prolonged use of anesthetics
- Hyperthermia *related to* hypermetabolic state, infection
- Risk for imbalanced body temperature
- Risk for perioperative hypothermia

### Nursing Implementation

*Passive warming measures* include the use of warmed cotton blankets, socks, and reflective blankets and limiting skin exposure. *Active warming measures* involve the application of external warming devices, including forced air warmers; heated water mattresses; radiant warmers; heated, humidified $O_2$; and warmed IV fluids. When using any external warming device, record body temperature and the patient's comfort level at 15-minute intervals. In addition, take care to prevent skin injuries.

$O_2$ therapy via nasal prongs or mask is used to treat the increased demand for $O_2$ caused by shivering. Shivering can be treated with opioids (e.g., meperidine [Demerol]). Treatment for MH includes the administration of dantrolene (Dantrium) with the onset of symptoms in addition to measures to cool the patient (e.g., ice packs, cold IV solutions). Acid-base imbalances should also be corrected to reverse signs of MH.

Meticulous asepsis is required with wound and IV site care. Airway clearance is encouraged with deep breathing, coughing, and the use of the incentive spirometer. If fever develops, chest x-rays may be taken and antipyretic drugs given. Depending on the suspected cause of the fever, obtain cultures of the wound, sputum, urine, or blood. If a bacterial infection is the source of the fever, antibiotics are started as soon as cultures have been obtained. If the fever rises above 103° F (39.4° C), body-cooling measures may be used.

## GASTROINTESTINAL PROBLEMS

### Etiology

*Postoperative nausea and vomiting* (PONV) are the most common complications affecting as many as 80% of high-risk patients. Risk factors include younger age (less than 50 years of age), gender (female), history of motion sickness or previous PONV, nonsmoking status, action of anesthetics or opioids, and duration and type of surgery.[15] Delayed gastric emptying and slowed peristalsis that result from handling of the bowel during abdominal surgery also contribute to PONV, as does starting oral intake too soon after surgery.

*Constipation* may also occur postoperatively and can be due to anesthetics used during surgery that may paralyze the intestine; immobility; alterations in diet and fluid intake pre- and postoperatively; and the use of opioids for pain relief. Opioids contribute to constipation by decreasing peristalsis and slowing fecal transport through the intestinal tract. Opioids may also decrease a patient's urge to defecate. (Constipation is discussed in Chapter 42).

**Postoperative ileus (POI)**, or the temporary impairment of gastric and bowel motility after surgery, results from the handling or reconstruction of the intestine during surgery and limited dietary intake before and after surgery. After abdominal surgery, motility in the large intestine may be reduced for 3 to 5 days, although motility in the small intestine resumes within several hours following surgery. Although POI is expected following abdominal surgery, it may occur following non-abdominal surgery.

Risk factors for POI include the use of opioids, immobility, older age, previous abdominal surgery, and early postoperative feeding. Use of opioid analgesia may prolong the duration of POI. Abdominal cramps, increasing abdominal distention, complaints of constipation or vomiting, and dehydration often accompany POI.

*Hiccups (singultus)* are intermittent spasms of the diaphragm caused by irritation of the phrenic nerve, which innervates the diaphragm. The phrenic nerve may be irritated postoperatively by gastric distention, intestinal obstruction, intraabdominal bleeding, and a subphrenic abscess. Indirect irritation of the phrenic nerve may be produced by acid-base and electrolyte imbalances. Reflex irritation may come from drinking hot or cold liquids or from the presence of a nasogastric (NG) tube. Hiccups usually last a short time and stop spontaneously.

## NURSING MANAGEMENT: GASTROINTESTINAL PROBLEMS

### Nursing Assessment

Ask the patient about feelings of nausea. If nausea is present, assess the severity using a verbal descriptor or numerical scale. If vomiting occurs, determine the quantity, characteristics, and color of the vomitus. Assess the abdomen for distention and presence of bowel sounds. Because bowel sounds are frequently absent or diminished in the immediate postoperative period, auscultate all four quadrants to determine the presence, frequency, and characteristics of the sounds. The return of normal bowel motility is usually accompanied by the passage of gas or stool and the patient's ability to tolerate oral intake without complaints of nausea or vomiting.

### Nursing Diagnoses

Nursing diagnoses and collaborative problems related to GI problems include, but are not limited to, the following:

- Nausea *related to* anesthetic agents, manipulation of abdominal contents
- Imbalanced nutrition: less than body requirements *related to* vomiting, decreased appetite, decreased peristalsis
- Constipation *related to* anesthetics, opioid analgesics, immobility, and dietary changes
- Risk for imbalanced fluid volume
- Risk for electrolyte imbalance
- Potential complications: POI, hiccups

### Nursing Implementation

In the PACU when the patient is NPO, IV fluids are given to maintain fluid and electrolyte balance. Begin oral fluids as ordered and tolerated. Depending on the type of the surgery, the patient may begin oral intake as soon as the gag reflex returns. When oral intake is allowed, offer clear liquids first and continue the IV fluids, usually at a reduced rate. If oral intake is well tolerated, the IV fluids are stopped.

Be alert to prevent aspiration if the patient vomits while still sleepy from anesthesia. Position the patient in the lateral recovery position and have suction equipment available. Interventions for PONV include verifying hydration status and BP and giving appropriate antiemetic or prokinetic drugs (see Chapter 41, Table 41-1). Consider complementary and alternative therapy interventions for PONV (e.g., imagery, music, aromatherapy, acupressure).

Constipation may be prevented using bowel protocols that include the use of a stool softener and laxative. Assess the patient regularly to detect the return of peristalsis. Encourage the patient to expel gas. Gas pains, which tend to become pronounced on the second or third postoperative day, may be relieved by ambulation and frequent repositioning. Positioning the patient on the right side permits gas to rise along the transverse colon and aids its release. Bisacodyl (Dulcolax) suppositories may be ordered to stimulate colonic peristalsis and expulsion of gas and stool. Resuming a normal diet after bowel sounds have returned also aids the return of normal peristalsis.

The goal of treatment for POI is the relief of associated symptoms and return of normal gastrointestinal function. Management includes bowel rest or the withholding of solid foods with a gradual reintroduction of food starting with clear liquids. Diet is advanced to solid food with an ongoing assessment of tolerance to oral intake.

An NG tube may be needed to decompress the stomach to prevent nausea, vomiting, and abdominal distention. Oral care is critical for comfort and stimulation of salivary glands when the patient is NPO or has an NG tube. Chewing gum has been studied as a treatment strategy for POI in select populations. Chewing gum mimics the act of eating, which is thought to stimulate gastric and bowel motility. This adjunctive intervention has been found to decrease the time for passage of flatus and stool for patients who undergo abdominal surgery.[16]

## URINARY PROBLEMS

### Etiology

Low urine output (800 to 1500 mL) in the first 24 hours after surgery may be expected, regardless of fluid intake. This low output is caused by increased aldosterone and ADH secretion resulting from the stress of surgery; fluid restriction before surgery; and fluid loss through surgery, drainage, and diaphoresis. By the second or third day, after fluid has been mobilized and the immediate stress reaction subsides, the patient will begin to have increasing urine output.

Acute urinary retention can occur in the postoperative period for a variety of reasons. Anesthesia depresses the nervous system, including the micturition reflex arc and the higher centers that influence it. This allows the bladder to fill more completely than normal before the urge to void is felt. Anesthesia also impedes voluntary micturition. Anticholinergic and opioid drugs may also interfere with the ability to initiate voiding or to empty the bladder completely.

Urinary retention is more likely to occur after lower abdominal or pelvic surgery because spasms or guarding of the abdominal and pelvic muscles interferes with their normal function in micturition. Pain may alter perception and interfere with the patient's awareness of bladder filling. Voiding ability is probably impaired to the greatest extent by immobility and bed rest. The supine position reduces the ability to relax the perineal muscles and external sphincter.

*Oliguria* (diminished output of urine) can be a sign of renal failure and is a less common, although more serious, problem after surgery. It may result from renal ischemia caused by inadequate renal perfusion.

## NURSING MANAGEMENT: URINARY PROBLEMS

### Nursing Assessment

Examine the urine for both quantity and quality. Note the color, amount, and odor of the urine. Assess indwelling catheters for patency. Urine output should be at least 0.5 mL/kg/hr. To decrease the risk of catheter-associated urinary tract infection (CAUTI), remove the catheter as soon as possible or within 24 hours, unless there is a reason to continue its use. Most patients void within 6 to 8 hours after surgery. If no voiding occurs, scan or percuss the suprapubic area for signs of bladder fullness or distention.

### Nursing Diagnoses

Nursing diagnoses and collaborative problems related to urinary problems include, but are not limited to, the following:

- Urinary retention *related to* anesthetic agents, pain
- Potential complication: acute kidney injury, CAUTI

### Nursing Implementation

You can aid voiding by normal positioning of the patient—sitting for women and standing for men. Reassure the patient regarding the ability to void. Helpful techniques include providing privacy, running water, offering water for the patient to drink, or pouring warm water over the perineum. Walking, preferably to the bathroom, and the use of a bedside commode are additional helpful measures to assist in voiding.

The surgeon often leaves an order to catheterize the patient in 6 to 8 hours if voiding has not occurred. Because of the possibility of CAUTI, first try to confirm that the bladder is actually full. Consider fluid intake during and after surgery and determine bladder fullness (e.g., discomfort when the bladder is palpated). Scan the bladder with a portable ultrasound to assess volume of urine in the bladder and avoid unnecessary catheterization. If catheterization is required, a straight catheterization (as compared to an indwelling catheter) is preferred to limit the risk of CAUTI.

## INTEGUMENTARY PROBLEMS

### Etiology

Surgery generally involves an incision through the skin and underlying tissues, disrupting the protective skin barrier. One of the greatest risks during the perioperative period is *surgical site infection (SSI)*. SSIs continue to be the most common health care–acquired infection and have been associated with prolonged hospitalizations, increased cost of care, and poor patient outcomes.[17] Wound healing is therefore a major concern during the postoperative period. The majority of SSIs are preventable with evidence-based strategies to prevent them (e.g., selection, timing, and duration of prophylactic antibiotics, surgical site skin preparation including hair removal, perioperative blood glucose management). Adherence to these strategies is known to reduce the incidence of SSIs and is a major goal of the SCIP initiative.

Wound infection may result from contamination of the wound from three major sources: (1) exogenous flora present in the environment and on the skin, (2) oral flora, and (3) intestinal flora. The incidence of wound sepsis is higher in patients who are malnourished, immunosuppressed, or older, or who have had a long hospital stay or a lengthy surgical procedure (more than 3 hours). Patients needing bowel surgery, particularly after a traumatic injury, are at high risk. Infection may involve the entire incision and may extend downward through deeper tissues. An abscess may form locally, or it may spread throughout entire body cavities, as in peritonitis.

Evidence of wound infection usually does not become apparent before the third to fifth postoperative day. Local manifestations include redness, swelling, and increasing pain and tenderness at the site. Systemic manifestations are fever and leukocytosis.

An accumulation of fluid in a wound may create pressure, impair circulation and wound healing, and predispose the patient to infection. To allow for drainage, the surgeon may place a drain in the incision or make a stab wound adjacent to the incision. These drains may be made of soft rubber and drain into a dressing, or they may be firm catheters attached to a Hemovac or other source of gentle suction.

An adequate nutritional state is essential for wound healing. The patient who is well nourished preoperatively can tolerate the postoperative delay in nutritional intake for several days. However, the patient with preexisting nutritional deficits that occur with chronic diseases (e.g., diabetes, ulcerative colitis, alcoholism) is more prone to problems of wound healing. The patient who cannot meet postoperative nutritional needs may be given enteral or parenteral nutrition to promote healing.

## NURSING MANAGEMENT: SURGICAL WOUNDS

### Nursing Assessment

Nursing assessment of the wound and dressing requires knowledge of the type of wound, the drains inserted, and expected drainage related to the specific type of surgery. Immediately postoperatively, check the wound every 15 to 30 minutes or as ordered. A small amount of serous drainage is common from any type of wound. If a drain is in place, a moderate to large amount of drainage may be expected. For example, an abdominal incision with an accompanying drain is expected to have a moderate amount of serosanguineous drainage in the first 24 hours. In contrast, an inguinal herniorrhaphy should have only minimal serous drainage during the postoperative period.

In general, drainage is expected to change from sanguineous (red) to serosanguineous (pink) to serous (clear yellow). The drainage should decrease over hours or days, depending on the type of surgery. Wound infection may be accompanied by purulent drainage. *Wound dehiscence* (separation and disruption of previously joined wound edges) may be preceded by a sudden discharge of brown, pink, or clear drainage. (Wound dehiscence is discussed in Chapter 11.)

### Nursing Diagnoses

Nursing diagnoses related to surgical wounds include, but are not limited to, the following:

- Impaired skin integrity *related to* surgical incision
- Risk for infection: SSI

### Nursing Implementation

When drainage appears on the dressing, record the type, amount, color, and odor of drainage. Expected drainage from tubes is outlined in Table 19-7. Also assess the effect of position changes on drainage. Notify the surgeon of any excessive or abnormal drainage or significant changes in vital signs.

The incision may be covered with a dressing immediately after surgery. Many surgeons prefer to change the first postoperative dressing. If the initial operative dressing is saturated, follow agency policy to determine whether you may change the dressing or simply reinforce it. Skin graft dressings may stay in place for 3 to 5 days to avoid disturbing the graft site and promote graft acceptance. These dressings may be changed by specially trained nurses. (Skin grafts are discussed in Chapter 23.)

When a dressing is changed, note the number and type of drains present and avoid dislodging the drains. Inspect the incision site carefully. The area around the sutures may be slightly reddened and swollen, which is an expected inflammatory response. However, the skin around the incision should be of normal color and temperature. If the wound is healing by primary intention, has little or no drainage, or has no drains in place, a single-layer dressing or no dressing is sufficient. A multilayer dressing is used when drains are in place, when moderate to heavy drainage is occurring, or when healing occurs other than by primary intention. (Wound healing and care are discussed in Chapter 11.)

**TABLE 19-7 Output From Tubes, Drains, and Catheters**

| Substance | Daily Amount | Color | Odor | Consistency |
|---|---|---|---|---|
| **Indwelling Catheter** | | | | |
| Urine | 800-1500 mL for first 24 hr<br>Minimum expected output: 0.5 mL/kg/hr | Clear, yellow | Ammonia | Watery |
| **Nasogastric Tube or Gastrostomy Tube** | | | | |
| Gastric contents | <1500 mL/day | Pale, yellow-green<br>Bloody after GI surgery | Sour | Watery |
| **Open Drains (e.g., Penrose)** | | | | |
| Wound drainage | Varies with procedure<br>May decrease over hours or days | Varies with procedure<br>Initially may be sanguineous or serosanguineous, changing to serous | Same as wound dressing<br>Foul odor may indicate infection | Thin, watery |
| **Closed Suction Drains (e.g., Hemovac, Jackson-Pratt)** | | | | |
| Wound drainage | Varies with procedure<br>May decrease over hours or days | Varies with procedure<br>Initially may be sanguineous or serosanguineous, changing to serous | Little to no odor<br>Foul odor may indicate infection | Thin, watery |
| **T-Tube** | | | | |
| Bile | 500 mL | Bright yellow to dark green | Acid | Thick |
| **Mediastinal Chest Tube** | | | | |
| Wound drainage post cardiothoracic surgery | Varies with procedure<br>Should decrease over several hours postoperatively | Sanguineous or serosanguineous | N/A | Thin |
| **Pleural Chest Tube** | | | | |
| Fluid that has collected in the pleural space | Varies with procedure<br>Decreases over hours or days<br>>100 mL/hr is considered excessive | Varies with indication for insertion and fluid collected in the pleural spaces | N/A | Varies with indication for insertion |

**TABLE 19-8 Surgery Discharge Criteria**

**PACU Discharge Criteria (Phase I)**

- Patient awake, easily arousable (or baseline)
- Vital signs at baseline or stable
- No excess bleeding or drainage
- No respiratory depression
- $O_2$ saturation >90%
- Pain controlled or acceptable
- Nausea and vomiting controlled
- Report given

**Ambulatory Surgery Discharge Criteria (Phase II or Extended Observation)**

- All PACU discharge criteria (Phase I) met
- No IV opioid drugs for last 30 min
- Voided if appropriate to surgical procedure or orders
- Able to ambulate if not contraindicated
- Responsible adult present to accompany and drive patient home
- Written discharge instructions given and patient and caregiver understanding confirmed

## DISCHARGE FROM THE PACU

The choice of discharge site is based on patient acuity, access to follow-up care, and the potential for postoperative complications. The decision to discharge the patient from the PACU is based on written discharge criteria approved by the agency's anesthesiology and medical staff[1] (Table 19-8). Standardized scoring systems (e.g., *Modified Aldrete Scoring System*) are often used to determine the patient's general condition and readiness for discharge from the PACU.

### Discharge to Clinical Unit

Before discharging the patient from the PACU to the clinical unit, provide a hand-off report about the patient to the receiving nurse. The report summarizes the operative and postanesthesia period. It should also include information as to where the patient's caregivers are waiting. Nurse-to-nurse communication must be accurate and allow for questions. The use of a standardized communication tool, such as SBAR (*Situation-Background-Assessment-Recommendation*), provides a complete report and enhances a safe transfer of the patient from PACU to the clinical unit (Table 19-9). (Hand-off communication is discussed in Chapter 1, and SBAR is presented in Table 1-6.)

As the nurse who receives the patient on the clinical unit, assist the PACU transport staff to safely move the patient from the stretcher to the bed. Take care to protect IV lines, drains, and traction devices. Obtain vital signs and compare the patient status with the report provided by the PACU nurse. After this, perform a more focused assessment and initiate postoperative orders and nursing care as appropriate (Table 19-10).

## AMBULATORY SURGERY

### Phase II and Extended Observation

Advances in minimally invasive and noninvasive procedures, anesthesia, and analgesia have resulted in an increase in ambulatory surgical procedures. Ambulatory surgery patients include those patients receiving Phase II and extended observation postoperative care (Table 19-1). PONV and pain are significant problems after ambulatory surgery. These can lead to delirium, prolonged PACU stay, delayed discharge, readmission, delayed resumption of usual activities, and decreased patient satisfaction.

### Ambulatory Surgery Discharge

The patient leaving an ambulatory surgery setting must be mobile and alert to provide a degree of self-care when discharged to home (Table 19-8). PONV and pain must be controlled. Overall, the patient must be stable and near the level of preoperative functioning for discharge from the unit. At discharge, provide teaching for the patient and caregiver

**TABLE 19-9 Postoperative SBAR Hand-Off Communication**

**Situation**

Patient transferring to Room # __________ Date __________
Surgeon __________ Anesthesia __________
Procedure __________
Surgical site(s) __________

**Background**

Allergies __________
Medications received in PACU __________
IV site/fluids __________
Dressings and/or drains __________
Operative comments __________

**Assessment**

PACU vital signs T ____ P ____ RR ____ BP ____ $O_2$ Sat ____
$O_2$ source __________ $FIO_2$ __________
Pain rating at discharge __________
Method of pain management __________
Last dose of pain medication __________
Nausea/vomiting at discharge __________
Intake __________ Output __________
Recovery comments __________

**Recommendations**

Equipment needed __________
Physician orders to be completed __________
Other notes __________
Transferring RN __________ Phone # for questions __________
Receiving RN __________

Modified from Sandlin D: Improving patient safety by implementing a standardized and consistent approach to hand-off communication, *J Perianesth Nurs* 22:290, 2007.

**TABLE 19-10 Nursing Assessment**

***Care of Patient on Admission to Clinical Unit***

1. Record time of patient's return to unit and assess airway, breathing, and circulation.
2. Obtain baseline vital signs, including $O_2$ saturation.
3. Assess neurologic status, including level of consciousness and movement of extremities.
4. Assess level of pain:
   - Last dose and type of pain control
   - Current pain rating
5. Assess wound, dressing, and drainage tubes:
   - Type and amount of drainage
   - Tubing connected to gravity or suction drainage (per orders)
6. Assess color, temperature, and appearance of skin.
7. Assess urinary status:
   - Time of voiding
   - Presence of catheter, patency, and total output
   - Bladder distention or urge to void
8. Position for airway maintenance, comfort, and safety (bed in low position, side rails up).
9. Check IV infusion:
   - Type of solution
   - Amount of fluid remaining
   - Patency and flow rate
   - Condition of insertion site and size of catheter
10. Position call bell within reach, and orient patient to use of call bell.
11. Assess for any nausea or vomiting.
    - Availability of emesis basin and tissues
12. Determine emotional state and provide support as needed.
13. Check for presence of caregiver.
    - Patient and caregiver oriented to immediate environment
14. Check and carry out postoperative orders.

specific to the type of anesthesia and surgery, and reinforce with written instructions. The patient may not drive and must be accompanied by an adult at the time of discharge. A follow-up evaluation of the patient's status is made by telephone, and any specific questions and concerns are addressed.

Carefully assess the patient's readiness for discharge and home care needs. Determine availability of caregivers (e.g., family, friends) and access to (1) a pharmacy for prescriptions, (2) a phone in the case of an emergency, and (3) follow-up care.

Discuss the patient's expectations regarding activity and assistance needed after discharge. The patient and caregiver must be included in discharge planning and provided with the information and support to make informed decisions about ongoing care.

**INFORMATICS IN PRACTICE**

***Discharge Teaching***

- When discharging a patient who requires a complex dressing change and the written instructions are not adequate, consider using a video. This may be available on the hospital's television system or the Internet (e.g., YouTube). You could also take a series of pictures that show how to perform the procedure.
- If using a video from the Internet, check it to ensure that the procedure is properly performed.
- The patient and caregiver can view the video or pictures at home as a reference when performing the procedure.

### Planning for Discharge and Follow-up Care

Preparation for the patient's discharge is an ongoing process that begins during the preoperative phase. The informed patient is prepared as events unfold and gradually assumes more responsibility for self-care during the postoperative period. As discharge approaches, be sure that the patient and caregiver(s) have the following information:

- Symptoms to be reported (e.g., fever, increased incisional drainage, unrelieved incisional pain, discomfort in other parts of the body)
- When and how to take prescribed drugs and possible side effects
- Care of incision and any dressings, including bathing recommendations
- Activities allowed and prohibited. When various activities can be resumed safely (e.g., driving, return to work, sexual intercourse, leisure activities)
- Dietary restrictions or modifications
- Where and when to return for follow-up appointment
- Answers to any individual questions or concerns

Common reasons patients seek help after discharge include unrelieved pain, need for advice about drugs, and wound issues (e.g., drainage). Attention to complete discharge instructions may prevent needless distress for the patient and caregiver. Standardized, preprinted discharge instructions that are surgery specific and easy to read ensure that information is complete.

Record the discharge teaching in the chart. For the patient, the postoperative phase of care continues and extends into the recuperative period. Assessment and evaluation of the patient after discharge may be done with a follow-up call or by a visit from a home health nurse.

Increasingly, patients are being discharged from the hospital with many care needs. They may be transferred to transitional care facilities, to long-term care facilities, or directly to their homes. When discharged directly to home, the patient is expected to continue self-care, with assistance from caregivers or home health care personnel (e.g., nurses, physical therapists). The care may include dressing changes, wound care, catheter or drain care, home antibiotics, or continued physical therapy. Working together with the discharge planner or case manager, ensure the patient's safe transition from hospital-based care to community- or home-based care.

### Gerontologic Considerations: Postoperative Patient

The older postoperative patient deserves special consideration. The older adult has decreased respiratory function, including decreased ability to cough and decreased thoracic compliance. These alterations lead to an increase in the work of breathing and a decreased ability to eliminate drugs. Carefully monitor reactions to anesthetic drugs. Pneumonia is a common postoperative complication in older adults.

Vascular function in the older adult is altered due to atherosclerosis and decreased elasticity in the blood vessels. Cardiac function is often compromised, and compensatory responses to changes in BP and volume are limited. Circulating blood volume is decreased, and hypertension is common. Cardiovascular status must be closely monitored throughout surgery and the postoperative period.

Drug toxicity is a potential problem in the older adult. Renal perfusion in the older adult normally decreases, along with a reduced ability to remove drugs that are excreted by the kidneys. Decreased liver function also leads to reduced drug metabolism and increased drug activity. Carefully assess renal and liver function in the postoperative phase to prevent drug overdose and toxicity.

Observing for changes in mental status is an important part of postoperative care in older adults. Factors such as age, history of alcohol abuse, poor baseline cognition, hypoxia, metabolic imbalances, hypotension, and polypharmacy can contribute to postoperative delirium. Anesthetics, especially anticholinergic drugs and benzodiazepines, also increase the risk for delirium. Despite knowledge of risk factors, postoperative delirium in older adults is poorly understood.

Pain control in the older patient is challenging because of possible preexisting cognitive deficits, impaired communication, and physiologic changes that affect how drugs are metabolized. Older patients may hesitate to ask for pain medication because they believe that pain should be tolerated because it is an inevitable result of surgery. Some older patients may be nervous about using PCA machines.

Thoroughly assess pain in a surgical patient who does not report any pain. Encourage the use of analgesics, and explain to the patient and caregiver that untreated pain has a negative effect on recovery.

## CASE STUDY

### *Postoperative Patient*

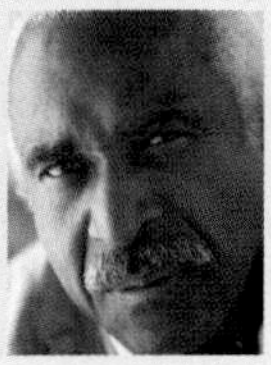

(©BananaStock/ BananaStock/ Thinkstock)

#### Patient Profile

E.G., a 74-year-old, African American, retired college professor, has just undergone surgery for a fractured hip. He fell off a ladder while painting his house. E.G.'s medical history includes type 2 diabetes and COPD. The surgery, performed while the patient was under general anesthesia, lasted 3 hours.

#### Subjective Data

- Active walker in his home community
- Smokes 1 pack of cigarettes per day × 58 years
- Always had problems sleeping
- Difficulty hearing, wears hearing aid
- Upset with injury and its impact on life
- Is a widower and has no relatives nearby or friends to assist with care
- Reports pain is 8 on a 0 to 10 scale on arrival to PACU

#### Objective Data

- Admitted to PACU with abduction pillow between his legs, one peripheral IV catheter, a self-suction drain from the hip dressing, an indwelling urinary catheter
- $O_2$ saturation 91% on 40% $O_2$ face mask

#### Interprofessional Care

##### *Postoperative Orders*

- Vital signs per PACU routine
- Capillary blood glucose level on arrival and every 4 hours. Call for blood glucose level <70 mg/dL or >250 mg/dL. Follow agency guidelines for management of hypoglycemia.
- 0.45 normal saline at 100 mL/hr
- Morphine via patient-controlled analgesia 1 mg q10min (20 mg max in 4 hr) for pain
- Advance diet as tolerated
- Incentive spirometry q1hr × 10 while awake
- $O_2$ therapy to keep $O_2$ saturation >90%
- Respiratory: Albuterol 2.5 mg via nebulizer every 4 hours PRN for wheezing
- Neurovascular checks q1hr × 4 hr
- Empty and measure self-suction drain every shift
- Strict intake and output

#### Discussion Questions

1. What are the potential postanesthesia problems that you may expect with E.G.?
2. ***Priority Decision:*** What priority nursing interventions would be appropriate to prevent these problems from occurring?
3. ***Teamwork and Collaboration:*** Which of these interventions could you delegate to unlicensed assistive personnel (UAP)?
4. What factors may predispose E.G. to the following problems: atelectasis, infection, pulmonary embolism, nausea and vomiting?
5. How can you determine when E.G. is sufficiently recovered from general anesthesia to be discharged to the clinical unit?
6. What potential postoperative problems on the clinical unit might you expect?
7. What are risk factors for this patient developing postoperative delirium? What are the signs and symptoms of delirium?
8. Why is drug toxicity a potential problem for E.G.?
9. ***Priority Decision:*** Based on the assessment data presented, identify two priority nursing diagnoses. Are there any collaborative problems?
10. ***Evidence-Based Practice:*** E.G. tells you he doesn't want the "catheter" to be removed because he doesn't want anyone to help him to the bathroom. How would you respond to this request?
11. ***Patient-Centered Care:*** What teaching will you provide so that E.G. can successfully self-manage his care?
12. ***Teamwork and Collaboration:*** What referrals may be indicated based on E.G.'s medical history?
13. ***Safety:*** Identify two areas of risk for injury to E.G. What actions can be taken to ensure patient safety?
14. ***Quality Improvement:*** What outcomes would indicate that interprofessional care with respiratory therapy was effective?

Answers available at *http://evolve.elsevier.com/Lewis/medsurg.*

## BRIDGE TO NCLEX EXAMINATION

The number of the question corresponds to the same-numbered outcome at the beginning of the chapter.

1. When a patient is admitted to the PACU, what are the *priority* interventions the nurse performs?
   - **a.** Assess the surgical site, noting presence and character of drainage.
   - **b.** Assess the amount of urine output and the presence of bladder distention.
   - **c.** Assess for airway patency and quality of respirations and obtain vital signs.
   - **d.** Review results of intraoperative laboratory values and medications received.
2. A patient is admitted to the PACU after major abdominal surgery. During the initial assessment the patient tells the nurse he thinks he is going to "throw up." A *priority* nursing intervention is to
   - **a.** increase the rate of the IV fluids.
   - **b.** obtain vital signs, including $O_2$ saturation.
   - **c.** position patient in lateral recovery position.
   - **d.** administer antiemetic medication as ordered.
3. After admission of the postoperative patient to the clinical unit, which assessment data require the *most* immediate attention?
   - **a.** $O_2$ saturation of 85%
   - **b.** Respiratory rate of 13/min
   - **c.** Temperature of 100.4° F (38° C)
   - **d.** Blood pressure of 90/60 mm Hg
4. A 70-kg postoperative patient has an average urine output of 25 mL/hr during the first 8 hours. The *priority* nursing intervention(s) given this assessment would be to
   - **a.** perform a straight catheterization to measure the amount of urine in the bladder.
   - **b.** notify the physician and anticipate obtaining blood work to evaluate renal function.
   - **c.** continue to monitor the patient because this is a normal finding during this time period.
   - **d.** evaluate the patient's fluid volume status since surgery and obtain a bladder ultrasound.
5. Discharge criteria for the Phase II patient include (*select all that apply*)
   - **a.** no nausea or vomiting.
   - **b.** ability to drive self home.
   - **c.** no respiratory depression.
   - **d.** written discharge instructions understood.
   - **e.** opioid pain medication given 45 minutes ago.

1. c, 2. c, 3. a, 4. d, 5. c, d, e

For rationales to these answers and even more NCLEX review questions, visit *http://evolve.elsevier.com/Lewis/medsurg.*

## EVOLVE WEBSITE

http://evolve.elsevier.com/Lewis/medsurg

**Review Questions (Online Only)**

**Key Points**

**Answer Keys for Questions**

- Rationales for Bridge to NCLEX Examination Questions
- Answer Guidelines for Case Study on p. 346
- Answer Guidelines for Managing Care of Multiple Patients Case Study (Section 3) on p. 348

**Student Case Study**

- Patient Undergoing Surgery

**Nursing Care Plan**

- eNursing Care Plan 19-1: Postoperative Patient

**Conceptual Care Map Creator**

**Audio Glossary**

**Content Updates**

## REFERENCES


*1. American Society of PeriAnesthesia Nurses: *2015-2017 Perianesthesia nursing standards, practice recommendations and interpretive statements*, Cherry Hill, NJ, 2015, The Society.

2. Joint Commission Center for Transforming Healthcare: Hand-off communications, 2014. Retrieved from *www.centerfortransforminghealthcare.org/projects/detail.aspx?Project=1.*

3. Tusman G, Groisman I, Fiolo FE, et al: Noninvasive monitoring of lung recruitment maneuvers in morbidly obese patients: the role of pulse oximetry and volumetric capnography, *Anesth Analg* 118:137, 2014.

*4. Atkins JH, Mandel JE: Performance of Masimo rainbow acoustic monitoring for tracking changing respiratory rates under laryngeal mask airway general anesthesia for surgical procedures in the operating room: a prospective observational study, *Anesth Analg* 119:1307, 2014.

*5. ASPAN US PR Strategic Work Team: The APSAN prevention of unwanted sedation in the adult patient. Evidence-based practice recommendation, *J Perianesth Nurs* 29:344, 2014.

*6. American Society of Anesthesiologists: Practice guidelines for the perioperative management of patients with obstructive sleep apnea: an updated report by the American Society of Anesthesiologists Task Force on perioperative management of patients with obstructive sleep apnea, *Anesthesiology* 120:268, 2014.

*7. Maile MD, Engoren MC, Trempor KK, et al: Worsening preoperative heart failure is associated with mortality and noncardiac complications, but not myocardial infarction after noncardiac surgery: a retrospective cohort study, *Anesth Analg* 119:522, 2014.

8. Xara D, Acacio S, Mendoca J, et al: Inadequate emergence after anesthesia: emergence delirium and hypoactive emergence in the postanesthesia care unit, *J Clin Anesth* 25:439, 2013.

*9. Radinovic KS, Markovic-Denic L, Dubljanin-Raspopovic E, et al: Effect of the overlap syndrome of depressive symptoms and delirium on outcomes in elderly adults with hip fracture: a prospective cohort study, *J Am Geriatr Soc* 62:1640, 2014.

10. Chou R, Gordon DB, de Leon-Casasola OA, et al: Management of postoperative pain: A clinical practice guideline from the American Pain Society, the American Society of Regional Anesthesia and Pain Medicine, and the American Society of Anesthesiologists' Committee on Regional Anesthesia, Executive Committee, and Administrative Council, *J Pain* 17:131, 2016.

*11. Usichenko TI, Rottenbacher I, Kohlmann T, et al: Implementation of the quality management system improves postoperative pain treatment: a prospective pre-/post-interventional questionnaire study, *Br J Anaesth* 110:87, 2013.

*12. Hooper VD, Chard R, Clifford T, et al: ASPAN's evidence-based clinical practice guideline for the promotion of perioperative normothermia, ed 2, *J Perianesth Nurs* 25:346, 2010.

13. Larach MG, Brandom BW, Allen GC, et al: Malignant hyperthermia deaths related to inadequate temperature monitoring, 2007-2012: a report from the North American malignant hyperthermia registry of

the malignant hyperthermia association of the United States, *Anesth Analg* 119:1359, 2014.

14. The Joint Commission: Specifications manual for national hospital inpatient quality measures. Retrieved from *http://www.jointcommission.org/specifications_manual_for_national_hospital_inpatient_quality_measures.aspx.*

*15. Gan TJ, Diemunsch P, Habib AS, et al: Consensus guidelines for the management of postoperative nausea and vomiting, *Anesth Analgesia* 118:85, 2014.

16. Wronski S: Chew on this: reducing postoperative ileus with chewing gum, *Nursing* 44:19, 2014.

17. Magill SS, Hellinger W, Cohen J, et al: Prevalence of healthcare-associated infections in acute care hospitals in Jacksonville, Florida, *Infect Control Hosp Epidemiol* 33:283, 2012.

*Evidence-based information for clinical practice.

## CASE STUDY

### *Managing Care of Multiple Patients*

You have been called into work at 10:00 AM to cover patients for a nurse who had a family emergency. You take over care for the following three patients on a surgical unit. You have one UAP available who is assigned to help you and two other RNs.

#### Patients

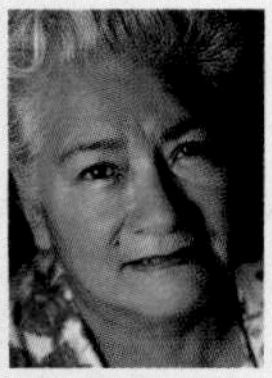

(©Ryan McVay/ Photodisc/ Thinkstock)

F.D., a 72-yr-old woman, was admitted to the hospital with compromised circulation of the right lower leg and a necrotic right foot as a complication of her diabetes. She is scheduled for a below-the-knee amputation of the right leg at 1:00 PM today. She has been NPO since midnight. Her morning capillary blood glucose level was 198 mg/dL. She received 4 units of regular insulin at 8 AM. She has an IV of normal saline infusing at 125 mL/hr.

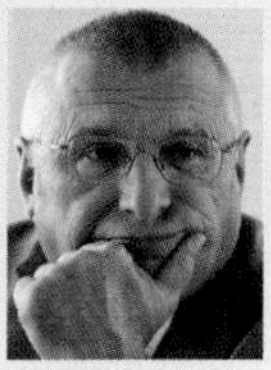

(©shironosov/ iStock/ Thinkstock)

G.S., a 63-yr-old male, was admitted to the hospital for severe pain and intractable vomiting from acute cholecystitis. G.S.'s medical history includes hypertension and type 2 diabetes. He had a laparoscopic cholecystectomy yesterday. His capillary blood glucose 1 hour ago was 135 mg/dL.

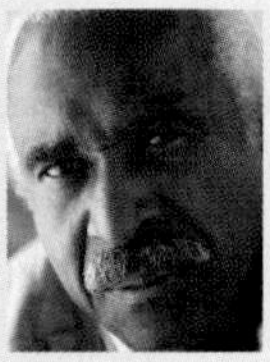

(©BananaStock/ BananaStock/ Thinkstock)

E.G., a 74-yr-old man, underwent surgery for a fractured hip yesterday. He is currently receiving dextrose 5% in 0.45 normal saline at 100 mL/hr, morphine via patient-controlled analgesia at 1 mg q10min (20 mg max in 4 hr) for pain, heparin 5000 units subcutaneously every 12 hours, and $O_2$ to keep $O_2$ saturation >93%. He has a self-suction drain in place at the surgical site. He has good respiratory effort when using his incentive spirometer.

#### Discussion Questions

1. ***Priority Decision:*** After receiving report, which patient should you see first? Provide a rationale for your decision.
2. ***Teamwork and Collaboration:*** Which tasks should you delegate to the UAP? *(select all that apply)*
   a. Explain discharge instructions to G.S.
   b. Obtain noon vital signs on E.G. and F.D.
   c. Obtain capillary blood glucose levels on F.D. and G.S.
   d. Confirm E.G.'s understanding of how to use the PCA pump.
   e. Remind E.G. and G.S. to use their incentive spirometers every hour.
3. ***Priority Decision and Teamwork and Collaboration:*** When you enter F.D.'s room, you find her somewhat withdrawn and lethargic. Her face is cool and slightly clammy. What initial action would be most appropriate?
   a. Give 1 ampule of $D_{50}$ IV stat.
   b. Increase F.D.'s IV rate to 150 mL/hour.
   c. Obtain a stat capillary blood glucose level.
   d. Ask the UAP to give F.D. a glass of orange juice.

#### Case Study Progression

F.D.'s capillary blood glucose reading was 64 mg/dL. You notify her HCP and administer 1 ampule of $D_{50}$ IV dextrose as ordered. You also change her IV infusion to $D_5$ ½NS. You check her capillary blood glucose within 15 minutes and then monitor her blood glucose levels on an hourly basis.

4. A preoperative checklist for F.D. is used to ensure completion of *(select all that apply)*
   a. removal of nail polish and jewelry.
   b. signed and witnessed informed consent.
   c. patient understanding of sensory information.
   d. identification of surgical site with surgical skin marker.
   e. notification of family of where to wait for the surgeon postoperatively.
5. F.D. tells you that she is afraid they may amputate the wrong leg. She tells you she has read stories of that happening at other hospitals. Your *best* response to F.D. would be to
   a. ask her if she would like a sedative to calm her fears.
   b. reassure her that it has never happened in this hospital.
   c. explain the "time-out" procedure for preventing such errors.
   d. offer to go to the operating room with her to ensure the correct leg is amputated.
6. ***Priority Decision:*** The charge nurse on the unit reports that E.G.'s aPTT (activated partial thromboplastin time) is 84 seconds. Upon assessing him, the nurse notes that the dressing on his hip is saturated with serosanguinous drainage. The next dose of heparin is due at 2100 this evening; the last dose was at 0900 this morning. The patient's blood pressure is 92/54 with a heart rate of 110 bpm. Respiratory rate is 30 breaths/minute and $O_2$ saturation is 98% on 2 L of $O_2$. The nursing *priority* for this patient would be to
   a. notify physical therapy that the patient's session today will have to be postponed until tomorrow.
   b. notify the previous RN that a medication error may have occurred with the patient's heparin dose at 0900.
   c. send an order to the laboratory for stat CBC and type and screen for 4 units of packed red blood cells.
   d. notify the health care provider of the laboratory result and anticipate orders for reversal agent such as protamine.
7. ***Management Decision:*** When providing discharge instructions to G.S., he tells you that the UAP told him that he could do whatever activity he was comfortable doing—to let pain guide his progress. Your *initial* reaction to this statement should be to
   a. ask the UAP to clarify what was said to G.S.
   b. report the UAP's actions to the nurse manager.
   c. teach G.S. about the reason for activity restrictions.
   d. clarify the discharge instructions with the health care provider.

Answers available at *http://evolve.elsevier.com/Lewis/medsurg.*

# SECTION 4

# Problems Related to Altered Sensory Input

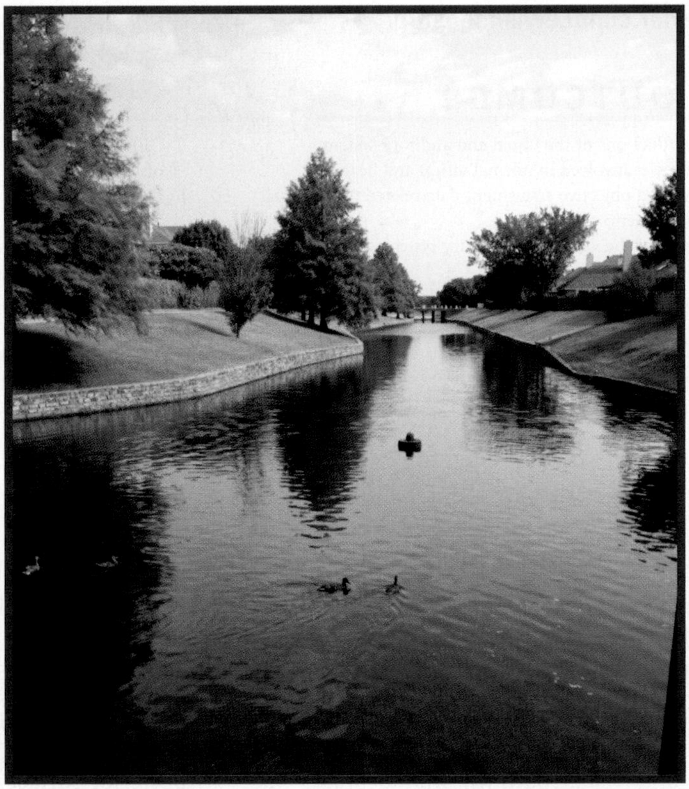

*Rivers know this.*
*There is no hurry.*
*We will get there someday.*

***Winnie the Pooh***

Peter Bonner

20

# Assessment of Visual and Auditory Systems

*Sharon L. Lewis*

*The most pathetic person in the world is someone who has sight, but has no vision.*

*Helen Keller*

http://evolve.elsevier.com/Lewis/medsurg/

## LEARNING OUTCOMES

1. Describe the structures and functions of the visual and auditory systems.
2. Explain the physiologic processes involved in normal vision and hearing.
3. Obtain significant subjective and objective assessment data related to the visual and auditory systems from a patient.
4. Perform a physical assessment of the visual and auditory systems using the appropriate techniques.
5. Differentiate normal from common abnormal findings of a physical assessment of the visual and auditory systems.
6. Link the age-related changes in the visual and auditory systems to differences in assessment findings.
7. Describe the purpose, significance of results, and nursing responsibilities related to diagnostic studies of the visual and auditory systems.

## KEY TERMS

astigmatism, p. 351
conjunctiva, p. 352
hyperopia, p. 351
lens, p. 352
myopia, p. 351
nystagmus, p. 361
presbycusis, p. 361
presbyopia, p. 351
refraction, p. 351
retina, p. 352
sclera, p. 352
tinnitus, p. 361
vertigo, p. 361

## VISUAL SYSTEM

## STRUCTURES AND FUNCTIONS OF VISUAL SYSTEM

The visual system consists of the external tissues and structures surrounding the eye, external and internal structures of the eye, refractive media, and visual pathway in the brain. The external structures are the eyebrows, eyelids, eyelashes, lacrimal system, conjunctiva, cornea, sclera, and extraocular muscles. The internal structures are the iris, lens, ciliary body, choroid, and retina. The entire visual system is important for visual function. Light reflected from an object in the field of vision passes through the transparent structures of the eye and, in doing so, is *refracted* (bent) so that a clear image can fall on the retina. From the retina, the visual stimuli travel through the visual pathway to the occipital cortex, where they are perceived as an image.

### Structures and Functions of Vision

**Eyeball.** The eyeball, or globe, is composed of three layers (Fig. 20-1). The tough outer layer is composed of the sclera and transparent cornea. The middle layer consists of the uveal tract (iris, choroid, and ciliary body), and the innermost layer is the retina. The *anterior cavity* is divided into the anterior and posterior chambers. The anterior chamber lies between the iris and posterior surface of the cornea, and the posterior chamber lies between the anterior surface of the lens and posterior surface of the iris. The *posterior cavity* lies in the large space behind the lens and in front of the retina.

**Refractive Media.** For light to reach the retina, it must pass through a number of structures: the cornea, aqueous humor, lens, and vitreous. All these structures must remain clear for light to reach the retina and stimulate the photoreceptor cells. The transparent cornea is the first structure through which light passes. It is responsible for the majority of light refraction necessary for clear vision.

*Acknowledgment:* We would like to acknowledge the contributions of Sarah Smith, RN, MA, CRNO, COT, Nurse Manager, Department of Ophthalmology, University of Iowa Health Care, Iowa City, Iowa, to this chapter over the past six editions of the book.
Reviewed by Hope Bussenius, DNP, APRN, FNP-BC, Clinical Assistant Professor, Nell Hodgson Woodruff School of Nursing, Emory University, Atlanta, Georgia; Deborah Ehlers, RN, MSN, Director of Nursing and Administrator of The Eye Center, Yakima, Washington; Deena Hollingsworth, MSN, FNP-BC, CORLN, Family Nurse Practitioner, ENT Specialists of Northern Virginia, Arlington, Virginia; Michelle Smeltzer, RN, MSN, DNPc, CEN, Clinical Education Specialist, Emergency Department, Einstein Medical Center Montgomery, East Norriton, Pennsylvania; Allison J. Terry, RN, PhD, Associate Professor of Nursing, Assistant Dean of Clinical Practice, School of Nursing, Auburn University Montgomery, Montgomery, Alabama; and Robert M. Welch, RN, MSN, FNP, CRNO, Family Nurse Practitioner, Nevada Retina Associates, Reno, Nevada.

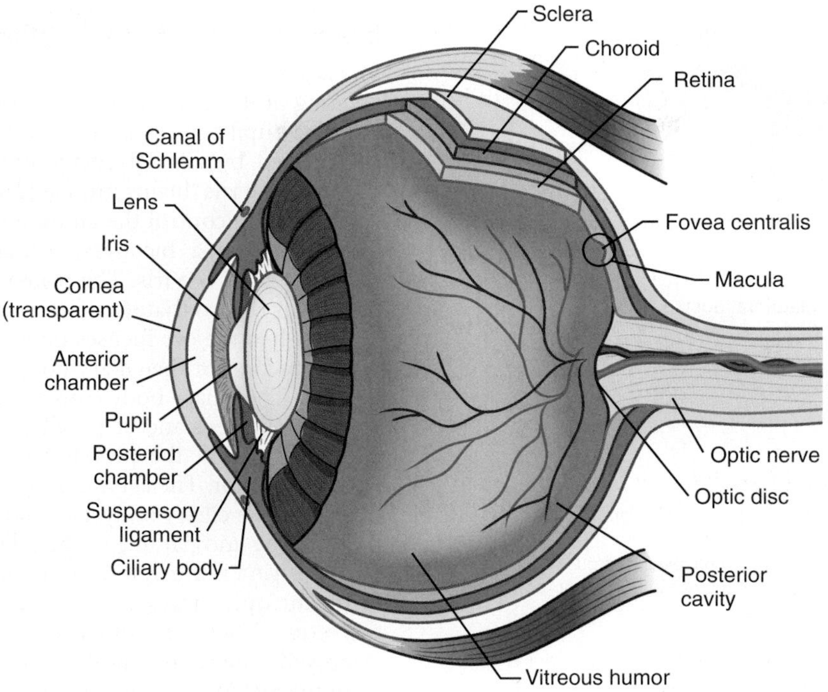


**FIG. 20-1** The human eye. (Modified from Patton KT, Thibodeau GA: *Anatomy and physiology,* ed 8, St Louis, 2013, Mosby.)

*Aqueous humor,* a clear watery fluid, fills the anterior and posterior chambers of the anterior cavity of the eye. Aqueous humor is produced from capillary blood in the ciliary body. It is drained away by the scleral veins *(canal of Schlemm),* which enter the circulation of the body. The aqueous humor bathes and nourishes the lens and endothelium of the cornea. Excess production or decreased outflow can elevate intraocular pressure above the normal 10 to 21 mm Hg, a condition termed *glaucoma.*

The lens is a biconvex structure located behind the iris and supported in place by small fibers collectively called the *suspensory ligament* (also called *zonule*). The ligament is a "scaffolding," a series of microscopic wire-like threads that connect the lens to the ciliary body. The primary function of the lens is to bend light rays, allowing the rays to fall onto the retina. The lens shape is modified by action of the ciliary body as part of *accommodation,* a process that allows a person to focus. An example of accommodation is the ability to focus on near objects, such as when reading. Anything altering the clarity of the lens affects light transmission.

*Vitreous humor* is a transparent gel-like substance that fills the posterior cavity (Fig. 20-1). Light passing through the vitreous may be blocked by any nontransparent substance within the vitreous. The effect on vision varies, depending on the amount, type, and location of the substance blocking the light.

**Refractive Errors.** **Refraction** is the eye's ability to bend light rays so that they fall on the retina. In the normal eye, parallel light rays are focused through the lens into a sharp image on the retina. When the light does not focus properly, it is called a *refractive error.*

The individual with **myopia** (nearsightedness) can see near objects clearly, but objects in the distance are blurred. The individual with **hyperopia** (farsightedness) can see distant objects clearly, but close objects are blurred. **Astigmatism** is an uneven curvature of the cornea, which results in visual distortion.

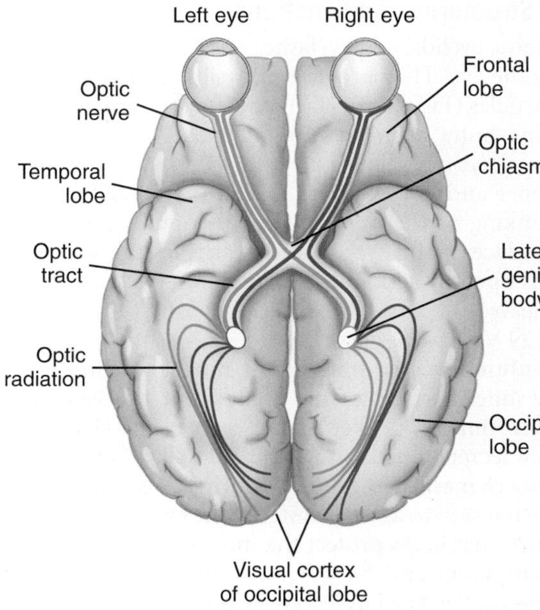


**FIG. 20-2** The visual pathway. Fibers from the nasal portion of each retina cross over to the opposite side of the optic chiasma, terminating in the lateral geniculate body of the opposite side. Location of a lesion in the visual pathway determines the resulting visual defect.

**Presbyopia** is a loss of accommodation, causing an inability to focus on near objects. Manifestations of presbyopia appear around age 40.

**Visual Pathways.** Once the image travels through the refractive media, it is focused on the retina (Fig. 20-2). From the retina, the impulses travel through the optic nerve to the optic chiasm, where the nasal fibers of each eye cross over to the other side. Fibers from the left field of both eyes form the left optic tract and travel to the left occipital cortex. The fibers from the right field of both eyes form the right optic tract and travel to the

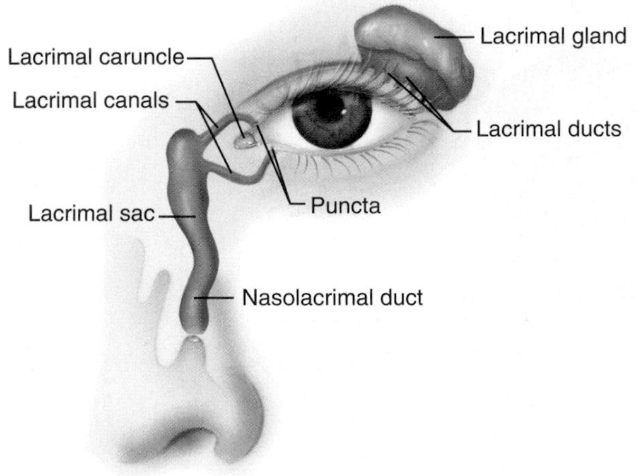


**FIG. 20-3** External eye and lacrimal apparatus. Tears produced in the lacrimal gland pass over the surface of the eye and enter the lacrimal canal. From there the tears are carried through the nasolacrimal duct to the nasal cavity. (Modified from Patton KT, Thibodeau GA: *Anatomy and physiology*, ed 8, St Louis, 2013, Mosby.)

right occipital cortex. This arrangement of the nerve fibers in the visual pathways allows determination of the anatomic location of abnormalities.

### External Structures and Functions

The eyebrows, eyelids, and eyelashes serve an important role in protecting the eye. They provide a physical barrier to dust and foreign particles (Fig. 20-3). The eye is further protected by the surrounding bony orbit and by fat pads located below and behind the *globe*, or eyeball.

The upper and lower eyelids join at the medial and lateral canthi. Blinking of the upper eyelid distributes tears over the anterior surface of the eyeball and nourishes the surface cells. The eyelids open by action of the cranial nerve (CN) III (oculomotor nerve) and close through the action of muscles innervated by CN VII (facial nerve).

The **conjunctiva** is a transparent mucous membrane that covers the inner surfaces of the eyelids and also extends over the sclera, forming a "pocket" under each eyelid. Glands in the conjunctiva secrete mucus and tears. The **sclera** is composed of collagen fibers meshed together to form an opaque structure commonly referred to as the "white" of the eye. The sclera forms a tough shell that helps protect the intraocular structures.

The transparent and avascular cornea allows light to enter the eye (Fig. 20-1). The curved cornea refracts (bends) incoming light rays to help focus them on the retina. The cornea consists of six layers: epithelium, Bowman's layer, stroma, Descemet's membrane, Dua's layer, and endothelium.[1] The lacrimal system consists of the lacrimal gland and ducts, lacrimal canals and puncta, lacrimal sac, and nasolacrimal duct (Fig. 20-3). In addition to the lacrimal gland, other glands provide secretions to make up the mucous, aqueous, and lipid layers of the tear film. The tear film moistens the eye and provides oxygen to the cornea.

Each eye is moved by three pairs of extraocular muscles: (1) superior and inferior rectus muscles, (2) medial and lateral rectus muscles, and (3) superior and inferior oblique muscles. Neuromuscular coordination produces simultaneous movement of the eyes in the same direction.

### Internal Structures and Functions

The iris provides the color of the eye. The iris has a small round opening in its center, the *pupil*, which allows light to enter the eye. The pupil constricts via action of the iris sphincter muscle (innervated by CN III [oculomotor nerve]) and dilates via action of the iris dilator muscle (innervated by CN V [trigeminal nerve]) to control the amount of light that enters the eye.

The **lens** is a biconvex, avascular, transparent structure located behind the iris. The primary function of the lens is to bend light rays so that they focus on the retina. *Accommodation* occurs when the eye focuses on a near object and is facilitated by contraction of the ciliary body, which changes the shape of the lens. The ciliary body consists of the ciliary muscles, which surround the lens and lie parallel to the sclera. The ciliary processes lie behind the peripheral part of the iris and secrete aqueous humor. The *choroid* is a highly vascular structure that nourishes the ciliary body, iris, and outer portion of the retina. It lies inside and parallel to the sclera (Fig. 20-1).

The **retina** is the innermost layer of the eye that extends and forms the optic nerve. Neurons make up the major portion of the retina. Therefore retinal cells are unable to regenerate if destroyed. The retina lines the inside of the eyeball, extending from the area of the optic nerve to the ciliary body (Fig. 20-1). It is responsible for converting images into a form that the brain can understand and process as vision.

The retina is composed of two types of photoreceptor cells: rods and cones. Rods provide vision in dim or darkened environments, and cones are receptive to colors in bright environments. The central region of the retina is called the *macula*, a 6-mm diameter area that is responsible for the central visual field. The *fovea centralis*, located at the center of the macula, is composed only of densely packed cones. This area of the retina provides the sharpest visual acuity, which is necessary for activities in which visual detail is of primary importance, such as reading and driving.[2]

### Gerontologic Considerations: Effects of Aging on Visual System

Every structure of the visual system is subject to changes as the individual ages. Whereas many of these changes are relatively benign, others may result in severely compromised visual acuity in the older adult. The psychosocial impact of poor vision or blindness can be highly significant. Age-related changes in the visual system and differences in assessment findings are presented in Table 20-1.

## ASSESSMENT OF VISUAL SYSTEM

Assessment of the visual system may be as simple as determining a patient's visual acuity or as complex as collecting complete subjective and objective data pertinent to the visual system. To perform an appropriate visual evaluation, determine which parts of the data collection are important for each patient.

### Subjective Data

#### Important Health Information

***Past Health History.*** Obtain information about the patient's past health history, including the ocular and nonocular history. Question the patient specifically about systemic diseases, such as diabetes, hypertension, cancer, rheumatoid arthritis, syphilis and other sexually transmitted infections (STIs), acquired

## TABLE 20-1 Gerontologic Assessment Differences

### Visual System

| Changes | Differences in Assessment Findings |
|---|---|
| **Eyebrows and Eyelashes** | |
| Loss of pigment in hair | Graying of eyebrows, eyelashes |
| **Eyelids** | |
| Loss of orbital fat, decreased muscle tone | Entropion, ectropion, mild ptosis |
| Tissue atrophy, prolapse of fat into eyelid tissue | Blepharodermachalasis (excessive upper lid skin) |
| **Conjunctiva** | |
| Tissue damage related to chronic exposure to ultraviolet light or to other chronic environmental exposure | Pinguecula (small yellowish spot usually on medial aspect of conjunctiva) |
| **Sclera** | |
| Lipid deposition | Scleral color yellowish as opposed to bluish |
| **Cornea** | |
| Cholesterol deposits in peripheral cornea | Arcus senilis (milky white-gray ring encircling periphery of cornea) (Fig. 20-4) |
| Tissue damage related to chronic exposure | Pterygium (thickened, triangular bit of pale tissue that extends from inner canthus of eye to nasal border of cornea) |
| Decrease in water content, atrophy of nerve fibers | Decreased corneal sensitivity and corneal reflex |
| Epithelial changes | Loss of corneal luster |
| Accumulation of lipid deposits | Blurring of vision |
| **Lacrimal Apparatus** | |
| Decreased tear secretion | Dryness |
| Malposition of eyelid resulting in tears overflowing lid margins instead of draining through puncta | Tearing, irritated eyes |
| **Iris** | |
| Increased rigidity of iris | Decreased pupil size |
| Dilator muscle atrophy or weakness | Slower recovery of pupil size after light stimulation |
| Loss of pigment | Change of iris color |
| Ciliary muscle becoming smaller, stiffer | Decrease in near vision and accommodation |
| **Lens** | |
| Biochemical changes in lens proteins, oxidative damage, chronic exposure to ultraviolet light | Cataracts |
| Increased rigidity of lens | Presbyopia |
| Opacities in lens (may also be related to opacities in cornea and vitreous) | Complaints of glare, night vision impaired |
| Accumulation of yellow substances | Yellow color of lens |
| **Retina** | |
| Retinal vascular changes related to atherosclerosis and hypertension | Narrowed, pale, straighter arterioles. Acute branching |
| Decrease in number of cones | Changes in color perception, especially blue and violet |
| Loss of photoreceptor cells, retinal pigment, epithelial cells, and melanin | Decreased visual acuity |
| Age-related macular degeneration as a result of vascular changes | Loss of central vision, presence of drusen, atrophy of macular retinal pigment |
| **Vitreous** | |
| Liquefaction and detachment of vitreous | Increased complaints of "floaters" |

## CASE STUDY

### Patient Introduction

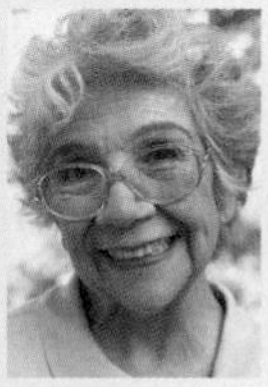

(©Jack Hollingsworth/ Photodisc/ Thinkstock)

F.M. is an 81-year-old Hispanic woman who comes to the emergency department with complaints of visual disturbances. F.M. states that her vision "looks like everything is covered with a spider web." She also reports seeing periodic light flashes and small white spots "floating" in the air.

**Discussion Questions**

1. What are the possible causes of F.M.'s visual disturbances?
2. Is her condition stable or an emergency?

You will learn more about F.M. and her condition as you read through this assessment chapter.

(See p. 356 for more information on F.M.)

Answers available at *http://evolve.elsevier.com/Lewis/medsurg.*

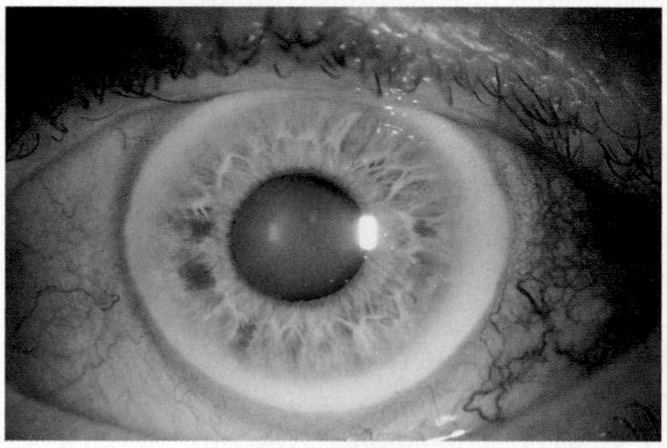

**FIG. 20-4** Arcus senilis, or age-related degeneration of the cornea. (From Kanski JJ: *Clinical ophthalmology: a synopsis,* ed 2, New York, 2009, Butterworth-Heinemann.)

immunodeficiency syndrome (AIDS), muscular dystrophy, myasthenia gravis, multiple sclerosis, inflammatory bowel disease, and hypothyroidism or hyperthyroidism. Many of these diseases have ocular manifestations. It is particularly important to determine whether the patient has any history of cardiac or pulmonary disease because β-adrenergic blockers (β blockers) are often used to treat glaucoma. These medications can slow heart rate, decrease BP, and exacerbate asthma or chronic obstructive pulmonary disease (COPD).

Obtain a history of tests for visual acuity, including the date of the last examination and change in glasses or contact lenses. Ask the patient about a history of strabismus, amblyopia, cataracts, retinal detachment, refractive surgery, or glaucoma. Note any trauma to the eye, its treatment, and sequelae.

The patient's nonocular history can be significant in assessing or treating the ophthalmic condition. Ask the patient about previous surgeries, treatments, or trauma related to the head.

## TABLE 20-2 Health History

### *Visual System*

**Health Perception–Health Management**
- Describe the change in your vision. Describe how this affects your daily life.
- Do you wear protective eyewear (sunglasses, safety goggles, hats)?*
- Do you wear contact lenses? If so, how do you take care of them?
- If you use eyedrops, how do you instill them?
- Do you have any allergies that cause eye symptoms?*
- Do you have a family history of cataracts, glaucoma, or macular degeneration?*

**Nutritional-Metabolic**
- Do you take any nutritional supplements?*
- Does your visual problem affect your ability to obtain and prepare food?*

**Elimination**
- Do you have to strain to void or defecate?*

**Activity-Exercise**
- Are your activities limited in any way by your eye problem?*
- Do you participate in any leisure activities that have the potential for eye injury?*

**Sleep-Rest**
- Is your vision affected by the amount of sleep you get?*
- Does your eye problem affect your sleeping patterns?*

**Cognitive-Perceptual**
- Does your eye problem affect your ability to read?*
- Do you have any eye pain?* Do you have any eye itching, burning, or foreign body sensation?*

**Self-Perception–Self-Concept**
- How does your eye problem make you feel about yourself?

**Role-Relationship**
- Do you have any problems at work or home because of your eyes?*
- Have you made any changes in your social activities because of your eyes?*

**Sexuality-Reproductive**
- Has your eye problem caused a change in your sex life?*
- For women: Are you pregnant? Do you use birth control pills?*
- For men: Do you use any erectile dysfunction drugs? Any vision problems with their use?*

**Coping–Stress Tolerance**
- Do you feel able to cope with your eye problem?*
- How do you feel that your eye problem has affected your life, and how do you cope with these changes?*

**Value-Belief**
- Do you have any conflicts about the treatment of your eye problem?*

*If yes, describe.

***Medications.*** If a patient takes medication, obtain a complete list, including dosage and frequency of over-the-counter (OTC) medicines, eye drops, and herbal therapies or dietary supplements. Many patients do not think of these as "real" drugs and may not mention their use unless specifically questioned. However, many of these drugs have ocular effects. For example, many cold preparations contain a form of epinephrine (e.g., pseudoephedrine) that can dilate the pupil. Note the use of any antihistamine or decongestant, since these drugs can cause ocular dryness. In addition, specifically ask whether the patient uses any prescription drugs such as corticosteroids, thyroid medications, or agents such as oral hypoglycemics and insulin to lower blood glucose levels. Long-term use of corticosteroid preparations can contribute to the development of glaucoma or cataracts.[3] Also note whether the patient is taking any β blockers, since these can be potentiated by the β blockers used to treat glaucoma.

***Surgery or Other Treatments.*** Note any surgical procedures related to the eye or brain. Brain surgery and the subsequent swelling can cause pressure on the optic nerve or tract, resulting in visual alterations. Also document any laser procedures on the eye. The effect of any eye surgery or laser treatment on visual acuity is important information to obtain.

**Functional Health Patterns.** Ocular problems do not always affect the patient's visual acuity. For example, patients with blepharitis or diabetic retinopathy may not have noticeable visual deficits. The focus of the functional health pattern assessment depends on the presence or absence of vision loss and whether the loss is permanent or temporary. Table 20-2 lists suggested health history questions related to the functional health patterns.

***Health Perception–Health Management Pattern.*** Patient characteristics such as gender, ethnicity, and age are important in assessing ophthalmic conditions. Men are more likely than women to have color blindness. The leading cause of blindness among African Americans is glaucoma.[4] Older individuals are also at greater risk for glaucoma.

The ophthalmic patient in a clinic or office setting is often seeking routine eye care or a change in the prescription of eyewear. However, the patient may have some underlying concerns that he or she does not mention or even recognize. Ask the patient, "Why are you here today?"

The patient's visual health can affect activities at home or at work. It is important to know how the patient perceives the current health problem. As outlined in Table 20-2, guide the patient in describing the current problem. Assess the patient's ability to accomplish necessary self-care, especially any eye care related to the patient's ophthalmic problem.

The patient may not recognize the importance of eye-safety practices, such as wearing protective eyewear during potentially hazardous activities or avoiding noxious fumes and other eye irritants. Obtain information about the use of sunglasses in bright light. Prolonged exposure to ultraviolet (UV) light can affect the retina. Ask about night driving habits and any problems encountered. Today, millions of people wear contact lenses, but many do not care for them properly. The type of contact lenses used and the patient's wearing and care habits may provide information for teaching.

Obtain information about allergies. Allergies often cause eye symptoms such as itching, burning, watering, drainage, and blurred vision.

Hereditary systemic diseases (e.g., sickle cell anemia) can significantly affect ocular health. In addition, many refractive errors and other eye problems are hereditary. Specifically, ask whether the patient has a family history of diseases such as arteriosclerosis, diabetes, thyroid disease, hypertension, arthritis, or cancer. In addition, determine whether the patient has a family history of ocular problems such as cataracts, tumors, glaucoma, refractive errors (especially myopia and hyperopia), or retinal degenerative conditions (e.g., macular degeneration, retinal detachment).

### GENETIC RISK ALERT

**Glaucoma**

- Certain types of glaucoma have a strong genetic link. Many different glaucoma genes have been discovered.
- People with a family history of glaucoma have a much greater risk of developing it.

**Age-Related Macular Degeneration (AMD)**

- Some cases of AMD have a genetic link. Multiple genes may be associated with AMD.

***Nutritional-Metabolic Pattern.*** High doses of vitamins containing antioxidants (vitamins C and E and beta-carotene) may be important to ocular health. Some patients with AMD may benefit from supplements of these vitamins.

***Elimination Pattern.*** Straining to defecate (Valsalva maneuver) can raise the intraocular pressure. After patients have eye surgery, many surgeons do not want them to strain. Assess the patient's usual pattern of elimination and determine whether there is the potential for constipation in the patient who has had ophthalmic surgical procedures.

***Activity-Exercise Pattern.*** The patient's usual level of activity or exercise may be affected by reduced vision, symptoms accompanying an ocular problem, or activity restrictions after a surgical procedure. Inquire about leisure activities during which the patient may incur an ocular injury. For example, gardening, woodworking, and other craft activities can result in corneal or conjunctival foreign bodies or even penetrating injuries of the globe. Sports activities such as racquetball, baseball, and tennis carry risks for blunt trauma to the eyes. Protection goggles should be worn for these sports.

***Sleep-Rest Pattern.*** In the otherwise healthy person, lack of sleep may cause ocular irritation, especially if the patient wears contact lenses. Normal sleep patterns may be disrupted in the patient with painful eye problems such as corneal abrasions.

***Cognitive-Perceptual Pattern.*** The entire assessment of the ophthalmic patient focuses on the sense of sight but does not overlook other cognitive or perceptual problems. For example, the functional ability of a patient with a visual deficit will be further compromised if the patient also has hearing problems. The patient who cannot see to read has increased difficulty following postoperative instructions if he or she also has trouble hearing or remembering verbal instructions. Eye pain is always an important symptom to assess. If eye pain is present, question the patient about treatment and response.

***Self-Perception–Self-Concept Pattern.*** The loss of independence that can follow a partial or complete loss of vision, even if the condition is temporary, can have devastating effects on the patient's self-concept. Carefully evaluate the potential effect of vision loss on the patient's self-image. For instance, disabling glare from a cataract may prevent nighttime driving. In today's highly mobile society, the loss of the ability to drive can represent a significant loss of independence and self-esteem.

***Role-Relationship Pattern.*** Ocular problems can negatively affect the patient's ability to maintain the necessary or desired roles and responsibilities in the home, work, and social environments. For example, AMD may decrease visual acuity so that the patient can no longer adequately function at work. Many occupations place workers in conditions in which eye injury may occur. For example, factory workers may be at risk from flying metal debris. Eye-safety practices, such as the use of goggles or safety glasses, are now a legal requirement in the workplace. The patient with diabetes may not be able to see well enough to self-administer insulin. This patient may resent dependence on a family member who takes over this function. Sensitively inquire if the ocular problem has affected the patient's preferred roles and responsibilities.

***Sexuality-Reproductive Pattern.*** The patient with severe vision loss may develop such a poor self-image that the ability to be sexually intimate is lost. Assure the patient that low vision or blindness does not affect a person's ability to be sexually expressive. Often touch is more important than vision.

***Coping–Stress Tolerance Pattern.*** The patient with temporary or permanent visual problems may experience emotional stress. Assess the patient's coping strategies and availability of support systems.

***Value-Belief Pattern.*** Be sensitive to each patient's individual values and spiritual beliefs, since these may guide the patient's decisions regarding ophthalmic care. It can be difficult to understand why a patient refuses treatment that has potential benefit or wants treatment that may have limited potential benefit.

## Objective Data

**Physical Examination.** Physical examination of the visual system includes inspecting the ocular structures and determining the status of their respective functions. Physiologic functional assessment includes (1) determining the patient's visual acuity, ability to judge closeness and distance, and extraocular muscle (EOM) function; (2) evaluating visual fields; (3) observing pupil function; and (4) measuring the intraocular pressure. Assessment of ocular structures should include examining the ocular adnexa, external eye, and internal structures. Some structures, such as the retina, blood vessels, and optic disc, must be assessed with an ophthalmoscope.

Assessment of the visual system may include all of the components discussed in the following sections, or it may be as brief as measuring the patient's visual acuity. Assess what is appropriate and necessary for the specific patient. Many of the following assessments are within your scope of practice, but some require special training.

Normal physical assessment of the visual system is outlined in Table 20-3. Age-related visual changes and differences in assessment findings are listed in Table 20-1. Assessment techniques related to vision are summarized in Table 20-4, and assessment abnormalities are listed in Table 20-5 on p. 357.

A *focused assessment* is used to evaluate the status of previously identified visual problems and to monitor for signs of new problems (see Table 3-7). A focused assessment of the visual system is presented in the box on p. 356.

***Initial Observation.*** Your initial observation of the patient can provide information that will help focus the assessment. When first encountering the patient, you may observe that the patient is dressed in clothing with unusual color combinations. This may indicate a color-vision deficit. Also note an unusual head position. The patient with diplopia may hold the head in a skewed position in an attempt to see a single image. The patient with a corneal abrasion or photophobia will cover the eyes with the hands to try to block out room light. Make a crude estimate of depth perception by extending a hand for the patient to shake.

## CASE STUDY
### *Subjective Data*

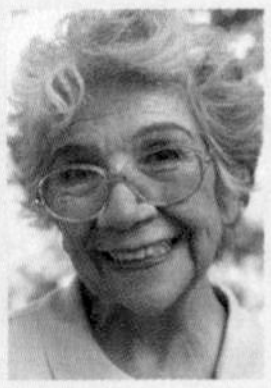

(©Jack Hollingsworth/ Photodisc/ Thinkstock)

A focused subjective assessment of F.M. revealed the following information:

- ***PMH:*** Extraocular extraction of cataract on R eye with implantation of intraocular lens 2 mo ago. Type 2 diabetes mellitus, hypothyroidism, and hypertension.
- ***Medications:*** Glyburide (DiaBeta) 5 mg/day, levothyroxine (Synthroid) 100 mcg/day, metoprolol (Lopressor) 50 mg PO daily.
- ***Health Perception–Health Management:*** States she was compliant with postoperative antibiotic and corticosteroid eyedrops and with office follow-up with eye surgeon. Recovery from surgery was uneventful, and eyedrops were discontinued 2 wk ago. Does not have allergies. Had excellent eyesight until today.
- ***Elimination:*** Has had difficulty moving bowels with increased straining. Trying prune juice to help.
- ***Activity-Exercise:*** Walks in the mall at least ½ mile three times a week. No resistance or isotonic exercises.
- ***Cognitive-Perceptual:*** Denies eye pain, itching, or tearing. Having difficulty reading.
- ***Coping–Stress Tolerance:*** Afraid she is having a stroke.

**Discussion Questions**

1. What type of assessment would be most appropriate for F.M.: comprehensive, focused, or emergency?
2. What assessment questions will you ask her?
3. How will you individualize the assessment based on her age, ethnic/cultural background, and condition?
4. Which subjective assessment findings are of most concern to you?
5. Based on the subjective assessment findings, what type of physical assessment should be performed?

You will learn more about the physical assessment of the visual system in the next section.

(See p. 359 for more information on F.M.)

Answers available at *http://evolve.elsevier.com/Lewis/medsurg.*

## FOCUSED ASSESSMENT
### *Visual System*

*Use this checklist to make sure the key assessment steps have been done.*

**Subjective**

*Ask the patient about any of the following and note responses.*

| | | |
|---|---|---|
| Changes in vision (e.g., acuity, blurred) | Y | N |
| Eye redness, itching, discomfort | Y | N |
| Drainage from eyes | Y | N |

**Objective: Physical Examination**

***Inspect***

| | |
|---|---|
| Eyes for any discoloration or drainage | ✓ |
| Conjunctiva and sclera for color and vascularity | ✓ |
| Lens for clarity | ✓ |
| Eyelid for ptosis | ✓ |

***Assess***

| | |
|---|---|
| Vision based on patient looking at nurse or Snellen chart | ✓ |
| Extraocular movements | ✓ |
| Peripheral vision | ✓ |
| PERRLA | ✓ |

*PERRLA,* Pupils equal, round, reactive to light and accommodation.

## TABLE 20-3 Normal Physical Assessment of Visual System

- Visual acuity 20/20 OU. No diplopia.
- External eye structures symmetric and without lesions or deformities.
- Lacrimal apparatus nontender and without drainage.
- Conjunctiva clear. Sclera white.
- PERRLA.
- Lens clear.
- EOMI.
- Optic disc margins sharp.
- Retinal vessels without AV nicking, with no hemorrhages or spots.

*EOMI,* Extraocular movements intact; *OU,* both eyes; *PERRLA,* pupils equal, round, reactive to light and accommodation.

## TABLE 20-4 Nursing Assessment
### *Assessment Techniques: Visual System*

| Description | Purpose |
|---|---|
| **Visual Acuity Testing** | |
| Patient reads from Snellen chart at 20 ft (distance vision test) or Jaeger chart at 14 in (near vision test). Examiner notes smallest print patient can read on each chart. | Determines distance and near visual acuity |
| **Confrontation Visual Field Test** | |
| Patient faces examiner, covers one eye, fixates on examiner's face, and counts number of fingers that examiner brings into patient's field of vision. | Determines if patient has a full field of vision, without obvious scotomas |
| **Pupil Function Testing** | |
| Examiner shines light into patient's pupil and observes pupillary response. Each pupil is examined independently. Examiner also checks for consensual and accommodative response. | Determines if patient has normal pupillary response |
| **Intraocular Pressure Testing: Tonometry** | |
| Covered end of probe is gently touched several times to anesthetized corneal surface. Examiner records several readings to obtain a mean intraocular pressure. | Measures intraocular pressure (normal pressure is 10-21 mm Hg) |
| **Ophthalmoscopy** | |
| Examiner holds ophthalmoscope close to patient's eye, shining light into back of eye and looking through aperture on ophthalmoscope. Examiner adjusts dial to select one of lenses in ophthalmoscope that produces desired amount of magnification to inspect retina. | Provides magnified view of retina and optic nerve head (Fig. 20-5) |
| **Color Vision Testing** | |
| In the Ishihara test, a patient identifies numbers or paths formed by pattern of dots in series of color plates. | Determines ability to distinguish colors |
| **Keratometry** | |
| Examiner aligns projection and notes readings of corneal curvature. | Measures corneal curvature. Often done before fitting contact lenses, before refractive surgery, or after corneal transplantation |

## TABLE 20-5 Assessment Abnormalities

### *Visual System*

| Finding | Description | Possible Etiology and Significance |
|---|---|---|
| **Subjective Data** | | |
| Pain | Foreign body sensation | Superficial corneal erosion or abrasion. Can result from contact lens wear or trauma. Conjunctival or corneal foreign body |
| | Severe, deep, throbbing | Anterior uveitis, acute glaucoma, infection. Acute glaucoma also associated with nausea, vomiting |
| Photophobia | Persistent abnormal intolerance to light | Inflammation or infection of cornea or anterior uveal tract (iris and ciliary body) |
| Blurred vision | Gradual or sudden inability to see clearly | Refractive errors, corneal opacities, cataracts, migraine aura, retinal changes (detachment, macular degeneration) |
| Spots, floaters | Patient describes seeing spots, "spider webs," "curtain," or floaters within the field of vision | Most common cause is vitreous liquefaction (benign phenomenon). Other possible causes include hemorrhage into the vitreous humor, retinal holes or tears. |
| Dryness | Discomfort, sandy, gritty, irritation, or burning | Decreased tear formation or changes in tear composition because of aging or various systemic diseases |
| Diplopia | Double vision | Abnormalities of extraocular muscle action related to muscle or cranial nerve pathologic condition |
| **Objective Data** | | |
| ***Eyelids*** | | |
| Allergic reactions | Redness, excessive tearing, and itching of lid margins | Many possible allergens. Associated eye trauma can occur from rubbing itchy eyelids. |
| Hordeolum (sty) | Small, superficial white nodule along lid margin | Infection of sebaceous gland of eyelid. Causative organism is usually bacterial (most commonly *Staphylococcus aureus*). |
| Blepharitis | Redness, swelling, and crusting along lid margins | Bacterial invasion of lid margins. Often chronic |
| Ptosis | Drooping of upper lid margin, unilateral or bilateral | Mechanical causes as a result of eyelid tumors or excess skin. Myasthenia gravis |
| Entropion | Inward turning of upper or lower lid margin, unilateral or bilateral | Congenital causes resulting in development abnormalities |
| Ectropion | Outward turning of lower lid margin | Mechanical causes as a result of eyelid tumors, herniated orbital fat, or extravasation of fluid |
| ***Conjunctiva*** | | |
| Conjunctivitis | Redness, swelling of conjunctiva. May be itchy | Bacterial or viral infection. May be allergic response or inflammatory response to chemical exposure |
| Subconjunctival hemorrhage | Appearance of blood spot on sclera. May be small or can affect entire sclera | Conjunctival blood vessels rupture, leaking blood into the subconjunctival space. |
| ***Cornea*** | | |
| Corneal abrasion | Localized painful disruption of the epithelial layer of cornea. Can be visualized with fluorescein dye | Trauma. Overwear or improper fit of contact lenses |
| ***Globe*** | | |
| Exophthalmos | Protrusion of globe beyond its normal position within bony orbit. Sclera often visible above iris when eyelids are open | Intraocular or periorbital tumors. Hyperthyroidism |
| ***Pupil*** | | |
| Anisocoria | Pupils unequal (constricted) | Central nervous system disorders. Slight difference in pupil size is normal in some people. |
| Abnormal response to light or accommodation | Pupils respond asymmetrically or abnormally to light stimulus or accommodation. | Central nervous system disorders, general anesthesia |
| ***Extraocular Muscles*** | | |
| Strabismus | Deviation of eye position in one or more directions | Overaction or underaction of one or more extraocular muscles |
| ***Lens*** | | |
| Cataract | Opacification of lens. Pupil can appear cloudy or white when opacity is visible behind pupil opening. | Aging, trauma, diabetes, long-term systemic corticosteroid therapy |
| ***Visual Field Defect*** | | |
| Peripheral | Partial or complete loss of peripheral vision | Glaucoma. Interruption of visual pathway (e.g., tumor). Migraine headache |
| Central | Loss of central vision | Macular disease |

During the initial observation, observe the patient's overall facial and ophthalmic appearance. The eyes should be symmetric and normally placed on the face. The globes should not have a bulging or sunken appearance.

***Assessing Functional Status***

**Visual acuity.** Always record the patient's visual acuity for medical and legal reasons. When doing a physical examination of the eyes, assess the right eye first and then the left eye. Document the patient's visual acuity before the patient receives any ophthalmic care.

To assess visual acuity, position the person on a mark exactly 20 ft (6 m) from the Snellen eye chart. If the person wears glasses or contacts, leave them on. Cover one eye at a time during the test. Ask the person to read down the lines of the chart to the smallest line of letters possible. Record the result using the numeric fraction at the end of the last successful line read. Indicate whether any letters were missed and if corrective lenses were worn (e.g., "Right eye, 20/30-2, with contacts"). Next ask the patient to cover the other eye, and repeat the process. Normal visual acuity is 20/20. The first number indicates the distance the person is standing or sitting from the chart; the second number gives the distance at which a normal eye can read the particular line. *Legal blindness* is defined as the best-corrected vision in the better eye of 20/200 or less.

If the patient reports near vision difficulty or is 40 years of age or older, you would also use a hand-held vision screener with varying print sizes (e.g., a Jaeger chart). Hold the card at 14 in (35 cm) from the eye in good light to assess near vision. Examine each eye separately with glasses on. A normal result is "14/14" in each eye, read without hesitancy and without the patient moving the card.

Hand motion or light perception may be used for distance vision assessment if a specific vision chart for distance assessment is not available. If you must assess near visual acuity without access to a Jaeger eye chart, an accurate assessment is still possible using newsprint or the label on a container. Record the acuity as "reads newspaper headline at X inches."

**Extraocular muscle functions.** Observe the corneal light reflex to evaluate for weakness or imbalance of the extraocular muscles (EOM). In a darkened room, ask the patient to look straight ahead while shining a penlight directly on the cornea. The light reflection should be located in the center of both corneas as the patient faces the light source.

To assess eye movement, hold a finger or an object within 10 to 12 inches of the patient's nose. Ask the patient to follow with eyes only the movement of the object or finger in the six cardinal positions of gaze. This test can indicate weakness or paralysis in the EOM and cranial nerves (oculomotor nerve [CN III], trochlear nerve [CN IV], and abducens nerve [CN VI]).[5]

**Pupil function and intraocular pressure.** Pupil function is determined by inspecting the pupils and their reactions to light. The normal finding is commonly abbreviated as PERRL (pupils are equal [in size], round, and reactive to light). To test for accommodation, ask the person to focus on a distant object. This process dilates the eyes. Then have the person shift the focus to a near object (e.g., your finger held about 3 inches from the person's nose). A normal response is constriction of the eyes and convergence (inward movement of both eyes toward each other). When accommodation is assessed in addition to the pupillary light reflex, a normal response is *PERRLA* (pupils are equal, round, and reactive to light and accommodation).

In a small percentage of the population, the pupils are unequal in size (*anisocoria*). The pupils should react to light directly (pupil constricts when a light shines into the eye) and consensually (pupil constricts when a light shines into the opposite eye).

Intraocular pressure (Table 20-4) can be measured by a variety of methods, including tonometry. Normal intraocular pressure ranges from 10 to 21 mm Hg.

***Assessing Structures.*** The visual system structures are assessed primarily by inspection. The visual system is unique because not only the external structures but also many of the internal structures can be directly inspected. The iris, lens, vitreous, retina, and optic nerve can be visualized directly through the clear cornea and pupil opening.

This direct inspection requires special observation equipment, such as the slit lamp microscope and ophthalmoscope. This equipment permits examination of the conjunctiva, sclera, cornea, anterior chamber, iris, lens, vitreous, and retina under magnification. The *ophthalmoscope* is a hand-held instrument with a light source and magnifying lenses that is held close to the patient's eye to visualize the posterior part of the eye. Little pain or discomfort is associated with these examinations.

**Eyebrows, eyelashes, and eyelids.** All structures should be present and symmetric, without deformities, redness, or swelling. Eyelashes extend outward from the lid margins. In normal closing, the upper and lower eyelid margins just touch. The lacrimal puncta should be open and positioned properly against the globe.

**Conjunctiva and sclera.** The conjunctiva and sclera can easily be examined at the same time. Evaluate the color, smoothness, and presence of lesions or foreign bodies. The conjunctiva covering the sclera is normally clear, with fine blood vessels visible. These blood vessels are more common in the periphery.

The sclera is normally white, but it may take on a yellowish hue in the older adult because of lipid deposition. A pale blue cast caused by scleral thinning can also be normal in older adults. A slight yellow cast may also be found in some dark-skinned people, such as African Americans and Native Americans.

**Cornea.** The cornea should be clear, transparent, and shiny. The iris should appear flat and not bulge toward the cornea. The area between the cornea and iris should be clear, with no blood or purulent material visible in the anterior chamber.

**Iris.** Both irides should be of similar color and shape. However, a color difference between the irides occurs normally in a small portion of the population.

**Retina and optic nerve.** An ophthalmoscope is used to magnify the retina and optic nerves and bring them into crisp focus (Fig. 20-5). Examine the optic nerve or disc for size, color, and abnormalities. The optic disc is creamy yellow with distinct margins. A central depression in the disc, called the *physiologic cup*, may be seen. This area is the exit site for the optic nerve. The cup should be less than one half the diameter of the disc. Normally, no hemorrhages or exudates are present in the fundus (retinal background). Careful inspection of the fundus can reveal retinal holes, tears, detachments, or lesions. Small hemorrhages can be associated with diabetes or hypertension and can appear in various shapes, such as dots or flames. Finally, examine the macula for shape and appearance. This area of high reflectivity is devoid of any blood vessels.

Important information about the vascular system and central nervous system (CNS) can be obtained through direct

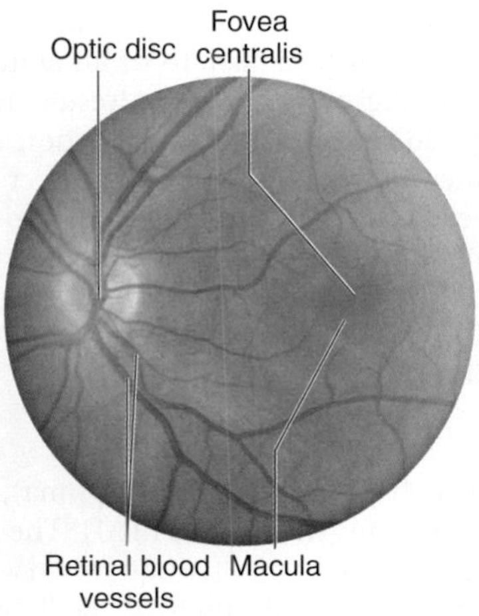


**FIG. 20-5** Magnified view of retina through the ophthalmoscope. (From Newell FW: *Ophthalmology: principles and concepts*, ed 7, St Louis, 1992, Mosby.)

visualization with an ophthalmoscope. Skilled use of this instrument requires practice.

### Special Assessment Techniques

***Color Vision.*** Testing the patient's ability to distinguish colors can be an important part of the overall assessment because some occupations may require accurate color discrimination. The Ishihara color test determines the patient's ability to distinguish a pattern of color in a series of color plates.[6]

***Stereopsis.*** Stereoscopic vision allows a patient to see objects in three dimensions. Any event that causes a patient to have monocular vision (e.g., enucleation, patching) results in the loss of stereoscopic vision. Without stereopsis, the individual's ability to judge distances or the height of a step is impaired. This disability can have serious consequences if the patient trips over a step when walking or follows too closely behind another vehicle when driving.

## CASE STUDY

### *Objective Data: Physical Examination*

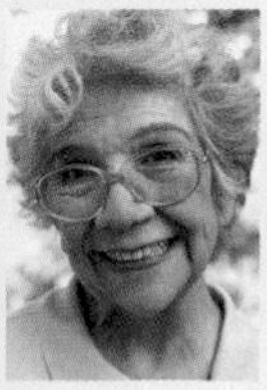

(©Jack Hollingsworth/ Photodisc/ Thinkstock)

Physical examination findings of F.M. were as follows:

- PERRL. No abnormalities noted on visual examination of external eye structures. EOM intact and symmetric.

**Discussion Questions**

1. What should be included in the physical assessment? For what would you be looking?
2. What diagnostic studies might you expect to be ordered?

As you continue to read this chapter, consider diagnostic studies that you would anticipate being performed for F.M.

Answers available at *http://evolve.elsevier.com/Lewis/medsurg.*

## DIAGNOSTIC STUDIES OF VISUAL SYSTEM

Diagnostic studies of the visual system provide important information in monitoring the patient's condition and planning appropriate interventions. These studies are considered objective data. Table 20-6 presents common diagnostic studies of the visual system.

**TABLE 20-6 Diagnostic Studies**

***Visual System***

| Study | Description, Purpose, and Nursing Responsibility* |
|---|---|
| **Refractometry** | Measure of refractive error. Patient sits looking through apertures at Snellen acuity chart and lenses are changed. Patient chooses lenses that make acuity sharpest. Dilation of eyes may help visualize retina and optic nerves. Procedure is painless.<br>Pupil dilation, which may last 3-4 hr, makes it difficult to focus on near objects. |
| **Ultrasonography** | *A-scan* determines the right power of a lens implant before cataract surgery.<br>*B-scan* used to diagnose ocular pathologic conditions such as intraocular foreign bodies or tumors, vitreous opacities, retinal detachments |
| **Fluorescein Angiography** | Fluorescein injected IV into peripheral vein followed by serial photographs (over 10-min period) of retina through dilated pupils<br>Provides diagnostic information about flow of blood through retinal vessels<br>If extravasation occurs, fluorescein is toxic to tissue. Tell patient that dye can sometimes cause transient nausea or vomiting. Yellow-orange discoloration of urine and skin may occur. |
| **Amsler Grid Test** | Self-administered test using a hand-held card printed with a grid of lines (similar to graph paper) (Fig. 20-6). Using one eye at a time, patient fixates on center dot and records any abnormalities of grid lines, such as wavy, missing, or distorted areas. Used to monitor macular problems |
| **Perimetry (Visual Field) Testing** | Can detect alterations in central and peripheral vision, which may be caused by various conditions such as glaucoma, stroke, brain tumors, or other neurologic deficits. Person sits and looks inside a bowl-shaped instrument called a *perimeter.* While staring at the center of bowl, a light flashes and the person presses a button each time flash is seen. A computer records the results, and a printout shows if there are areas where flashes of light are not seen. |

*Patient teaching regarding the purpose and method of testing is a nursing responsibility for all diagnostic procedures.

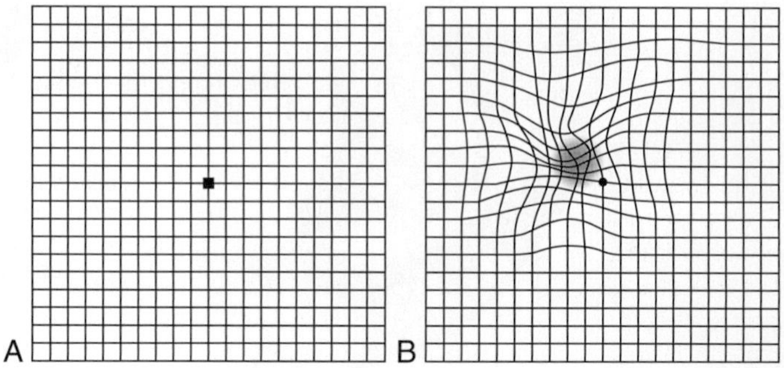


**FIG. 20-6** Amsler grid. **A,** Normal grid. **B,** Abnormal grid as seen by person with macular degeneration.

## CASE STUDY

### *Objective Data: Diagnostic Studies*

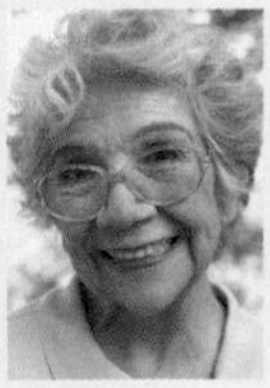

(©Jack Hollingsworth/ Photodisc/ Thinkstock)

The health care provider performs an ophthalmoscopic examination on F.M. and identifies a partial retinal detachment. This diagnosis is confirmed via ultrasonography.

**Discussion Questions**

1. Are these the diagnostic studies that you expected to be ordered?
2. Which diagnostic study results are of most concern to you?

Answers available at *http://evolve.elsevier.com/Lewis/medsurg.*

# AUDITORY SYSTEM

## STRUCTURES AND FUNCTIONS OF AUDITORY SYSTEM

The auditory system is composed of the peripheral auditory system and central auditory system. The peripheral auditory system includes the structures of the ear itself: external, middle, and inner ear (Fig. 20-7). This system is concerned with the reception and perception of sound. The inner ear functions in hearing and balance.

The central auditory system integrates and assigns meaning to what is heard. This system includes the vestibulocochlear nerve (CN VIII) and auditory cortex of the brain. The brain and its pathways transmit and process sound and sensations that maintain a person's equilibrium.

The role of the external and middle portion of the ear is to conduct and amplify sound waves from the environment. This portion of sound conduction is termed *air conduction.* Problems in these two parts of the ear may cause *conductive hearing loss,* resulting in a decrease in sound intensity and/or a distortion in sound.[7]

Disturbances in equilibrium can impair coordination, balance, and orientation. Damage to or an abnormality of the inner ear or along the nerve pathways results in *sensorineural hearing loss.* In addition to causing distortion or faintness of sound, sensorineural hearing loss may affect the ability to understand speech or cause complete hearing loss. Impairment within the auditory pathways of the brain causes *central hearing loss.* This type of hearing loss causes difficulty in understanding the meaning of words that are heard. (Types of hearing loss are discussed in Chapter 21 on pp. 387-388.)

### External Ear

The external ear consists of the *auricle* (pinna), external auditory canal, and tympanic membrane (TM). The auricle is composed of cartilage and connective tissue covered with epithelium, which also lines the external auditory canal (Fig. 20-7). The external auditory canal is a slightly S-shaped tube about 1 inch (2.5 cm) in length in the adult. The lining of the proximal one third of the canal contains fine hairs (cilia), sebaceous (oil) glands, and ceruminous (wax) glands. The oil and wax lubricate the ear canal, keep it free from debris, and kill bacteria. The distal two thirds of the canal is lined with thin epithelium over the bone and is very sensitive.

The function of the external ear and canal is to collect and transmit sound waves to the *tympanic membrane* (eardrum). This shiny, translucent, pearl-gray membrane is composed of epithelial cells, connective tissue, and mucous membrane. It serves as a partition and an instrument of sound transmission between the external auditory canal and middle ear.

### Middle Ear

The middle ear cavity is an air space located in the temporal bone. Mucous membrane lines the middle ear and is continuous from the nasal pharynx via the eustachian (auditory) tube. The eustachian tube equalizes atmospheric air pressure between the middle ear and throat and allows the tympanic membrane to move freely. It is normally closed and opened with the movement of the jaw, usually during yawning and swallowing.

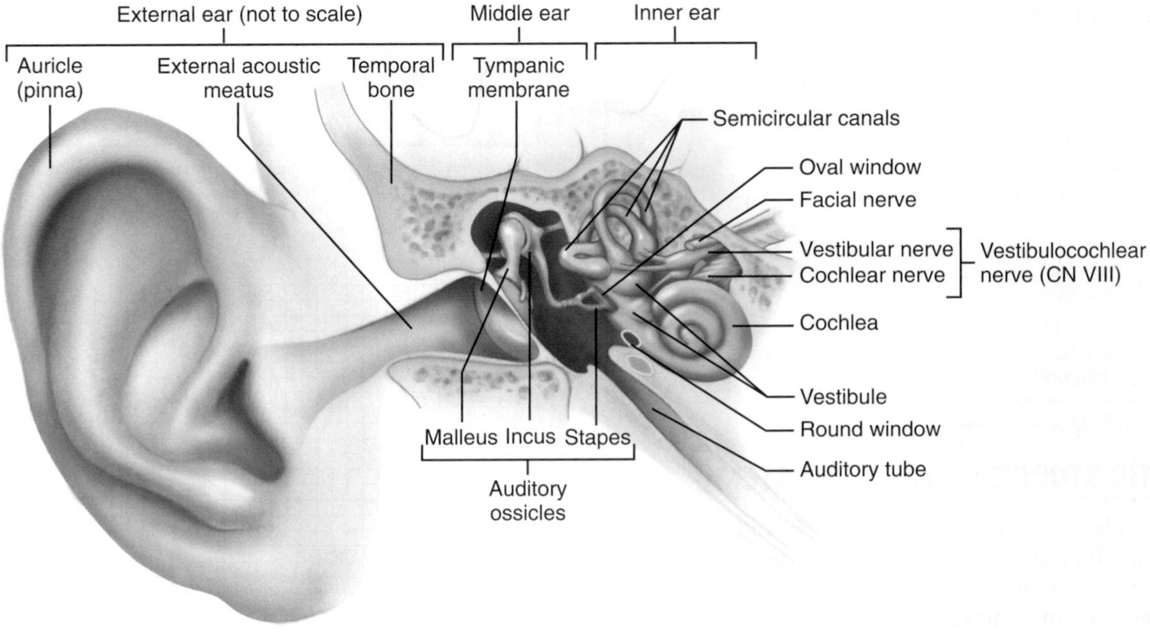


**FIG. 20-7** External, middle, and inner ear. (Modified from Patton KT, Thibodeau GA: *Anatomy and physiology,* ed 8, St Louis, 2013, Mosby.)

Blockage of this tube can occur with allergies, nasopharyngeal infections, or enlarged adenoids. When the eustachian tube remains open, it is referred to as *patulous*. When this occurs, a person can hear one's own voice (autophony).

The middle ear contains the three smallest bones in the body: *malleus, incus,* and *stapes* (ossicles). Vibrations of the TM cause the ossicles to move and transmit sound waves to the oval window. The superior part of the middle ear is called the *epitympanum,* or the attic. It also communicates with air cells within the mastoid bone. The mastoid is the posterior part of the temporal bone. The facial nerve (CN VII) traverses above the oval window of the middle ear. The thin, bony covering of the facial nerve can become damaged by chronic ear infection, skull fracture, or trauma during ear surgery. Problems may occur related to voluntary facial movements, eyelid closure, and taste discrimination. Permanent damage to the facial nerve can also result.

### Inner Ear

The inner ear is composed of a bony labyrinth (maze) surrounding a membrane. Perilymphatic fluid lies between the bone and membrane. The fluid inside the membrane is called *endolymph.* The inner ear contains the functional organs for hearing and balance. The receptor organ for hearing is the *cochlea,* which is a coiled structure. It contains the *organ of Corti,* whose tiny hair cells respond to stimulation of selected portions of the basilar membrane according to pitch. This stimulus is converted into an electrochemical impulse and then transmitted by the acoustic portion of the vestibulocochlear nerve (CN VIII) to the temporal lobe of the brain to process and interpret the sound.

Three semicircular canals and the vestibule make up the organ of balance, the membranous labyrinth, which is housed within the bony labyrinth. The membranous labyrinth is filled with endolymphatic fluid, and the bony labyrinth is filled with perilymphatic fluid. Nervous stimuli are communicated by the vestibular portion of CN VIII. Debris such as loose crystals of calcium or excessive pressure within the lymphatic fluid can produce disorders such as benign paroxysmal positional vertigo (BPPV). (BPPV is discussed in Chapter 21.)

**Transmission of Sound.** Sound waves travel by air (air conduction) and are picked up by the auricles and auditory canal. Sound waves strike the TM, causing it to vibrate. The central area of the TM is connected to the malleus, which also starts to vibrate. The malleus transmits the vibration to the incus and then the stapes. As the stapes moves back and forth, it pushes the membrane of the oval window in and out. Movement of the oval window produces waves in the perilymph.

Once sound waves are transmitted to the liquid medium of the inner ear, the vibration is picked up by the tiny sensory hair cells of the cochlea, which initiate nerve impulses. These impulses are carried by nerve fibers to the main branch of the acoustic portion of CN VIII and then to the brain.

The bones of the skull can also transmit sound directly to the inner ear (bone conduction). (Tuning fork tests are discussed in Table 20-11.)

### Gerontologic Considerations: Effects of Aging on Auditory System

Approximately 20% of American adults report some degree of hearing loss, with aging being the primary cause.[8] **Presbycusis**, or hearing loss due to aging, can result from a variety of sources. Noise exposure, systemic diseases, poor nutrition, ototoxic drugs, and pollution exposure over the life span can damage the delicate hair cells of the organ of Corti or atrophy lymph-producing cells. Sound transmission is also diminished by calcification of the ossicles. The loss associated with presbycusis is usually greater for high-pitched sounds. Accumulation of dry cerumen (earwax) in the external canal can also interfere with the transmission of sound. **Tinnitus**, or ringing in the ears, may accompany the hearing loss that results from the aging process. As the average life span increases, the number of people with hearing loss will also increase. Prevention and early identification of problems ensure a more active and healthy aging population.

Age-related changes in the auditory system and differences in assessment findings are presented in Table 20-7.

## ASSESSMENT OF AUDITORY SYSTEM

Assessment of the auditory system should include assessment of hearing and equilibrium because the auditory and *vestibular* (balance) systems are closely related. It is often difficult to separate symptoms related to these two systems. Help the patient describe symptoms and problems to differentiate the source of the problems. Health history questions to ask a patient with an auditory problem are listed in Table 20-8.

Problems with balance may manifest as vertigo or nystagmus. **Vertigo** is a sense that the person or objects around the person are moving or spinning and is usually stimulated by movement of the head. *Dizziness* is a sensation of being off-balance that occurs when standing or walking. **Nystagmus** is an abnormal eye movement that may be observed as a twitching of the eyeball or described by the patient as a blurring of vision with head or eye movement.

Initially try to categorize symptoms related to balance and separate them from symptoms related to hearing loss or

**TABLE 20-7 Gerontologic Assessment Differences**

***Auditory System***

| Changes | Differences in Assessment Findings |
|---|---|
| **External Ear** | |
| Increased production of and drier cerumen | Impacted cerumen, potential hearing loss |
| Increased hair growth | Visible hair, especially in men |
| Loss of elasticity in cartilage | Collapsed ear canal |
| **Middle Ear** | |
| Atrophic changes of tympanic membrane | Conductive hearing loss |
| **Inner Ear** | |
| Hair cell degeneration, neuron degeneration in auditory nerve and central pathways, reduced blood supply to cochlea, calcification of ossicles | Presbycusis, diminished sensitivity to high-pitched sounds, impaired speech reception, tinnitus |
| Less effective vestibular apparatus in semicircular canals | Alterations in balance and body orientation |
| **Brain** | |
| Decline in ability to filter out unwanted and unnecessary sound | Difficulty hearing in a noisy environment, heightened sensitivity to loud sounds |

tinnitus. The symptoms can be combined later in the assessment to help make the diagnosis and plan for the patient.

## Subjective Data

### Important Health Information

***Past Health History.*** Many problems related to the ear may result from childhood illnesses or problems of adjacent organs. Consequently, a careful assessment of past health problems is important.

Ask the patient about previous problems regarding the ears, especially during childhood. Record the (1) frequency of acute middle ear infections (otitis media); (2) surgical procedures (e.g., myringotomy); (3) perforations of the eardrum; (4) drainage; and (5) history of mumps, measles, or scarlet fever. Congenital hearing loss can result from infectious diseases (e.g., rubella, influenza, syphilis), teratogenic medications, or hypoxia in the first trimester of pregnancy. Document head injury because it may result in hearing loss. Information about food and environmental allergies is important because they can cause the eustachian tube to become edematous and prevent aeration of the middle ear.

Record symptoms such as vertigo, tinnitus, and hearing loss in the patient's words. Guide the description by asking for specific details of the sensations and situations that may cause them or make them worse. Information regarding family members with hearing loss and type of hearing loss is important. Some congenital hearing loss is hereditary. The age of onset of presbycusis also follows a familial pattern.

***Medications.*** Obtain information about present or past medications that are ototoxic (cause damage to CN VIII) and can produce hearing loss, tinnitus, and vertigo. The amount and frequency of aspirin use are important because tinnitus can result from high aspirin intake. Aminoglycosides and many other antibiotics, salicylates, antimalarial agents, chemotherapy drugs, diuretics, and nonsteroidal antiinflammatory drugs (NSAIDs) are groups of drugs that are potentially ototoxic. Monitor for hearing and balance problems in patients receiving these drugs. Many drugs produce hearing loss that may be reversible if treatment is stopped.

***Surgery or Other Treatments.*** Document previous hospitalizations for ear surgery, including myringotomy (ventilation holes placed in the TM with or without tubes), tympanoplasty (surgical repair of TM), tonsillectomy, and adenoidectomy (removal of tonsils and adenoids). Record the use of and satisfaction with a hearing aid. Also note any problems with impacted cerumen.

**Functional Health Patterns.** Hearing and balance problems can affect all aspects of a person's life. To assess the impact of hearing loss, ask health history questions based on a functional health patterns approach (Table 20-8).

### TABLE 20-8 Health History

***Auditory System***

**Health Perception–Health Management**

***Hearing***

- Have you had a change in your hearing?* If yes, how does this change affect your daily life?
- Do you use any devices to improve your hearing (e.g., hearing aid, special volume control, headphones for television or stereo)?*
- How do you protect your hearing?
- Do you have any allergies that result in ear problems?*

***Equilibrium***

- When did the dizziness or spinning sensation first occur?
- Does this sensation occur when you first stand up, when you are lying down, or both?
- Have you ever fallen because of the dizziness?*
- Can you drive or walk alone? If no, elaborate.
- Are there any times of the day when your symptoms are worse?*

***Tinnitus***

- How long have you experienced ringing in your ears? Has it changed?* Describe the ringing (e.g., buzzing, ringing, roaring). Do you also have a feeling of fullness or pressure?*
- When does it bother you the most?
- What things have you tried that help or have not helped?
- What medications are you taking?

**Nutritional-Metabolic**

- Do you notice any differences in symptoms with changes in diet?*
- Does your ear problem cause nausea that interferes with your food intake?*
- Does chewing or swallowing cause you any ear discomfort?*

**Elimination**

- Does straining during a bowel movement cause ear pain?*

**Activity-Exercise**

- Do you need help with certain activities (e.g., lifting, bending, climbing stairs, driving, speaking) because of symptoms?*

**Sleep-Rest**

- Is your sleep disturbed by noises or ringing in the ears or by a sensation of spinning?*

**Cognitive-Perceptual**

- Do you experience ear pain?* What relieves the pain? What makes it worse? Does the pain affect your hearing or balance?
- Have you noticed any problem with communicating or understanding what people are saying?*

**Self-Perception–Self-Concept**

- Have changes in your hearing affected how you feel about yourself or your feeling of independence?*

**Role-Relationship**

- What effect has your ear problem had on your work, family, or social life?
- Are you able to recognize the effects of your ear problems on your life?*

**Sexuality-Reproductive**

- Has your ear problem caused a change in your sex life?*

**Coping–Stress Tolerance**

- Do you consider your ear problem a source of stress?*
- How do you cope when you are experiencing symptoms?

**Value-Belief**

- Do you have a conflict between what your health care provider would like you to do and what you believe you should do?

*If yes, describe.

***Health Perception–Health Management Pattern.*** Note the onset of hearing loss, whether sudden or gradual, and who noted the onset (e.g., patient, family, significant others). Gradual hearing losses are most often noted by those who communicate with the patient. Sudden losses and those exacerbated by some other condition are most often reported by the patient.

Assess the patient for personal measures used to preserve hearing. The use of protective ear covers or earplugs is good practice for people in high-noise environments. Document if the patient is a swimmer and the frequency and duration of swimming and use of ear protection. Note the type of water (pool, lake, or ocean) in which the swimming takes place to help identify contact with contaminated water. Assess for the placement of any item in the ear, including hearing aids, which can cause trauma to the canal and TM.

***Nutritional-Metabolic Pattern.*** Alcohol, sodium, and dietary supplements affect the amount of endolymph in the inner ear system. Patients with Ménière's disease may notice some improvement in their symptoms with alcohol restriction and a low-sodium diet. Note changes in symptoms with food intake. Question the patient about any ear pain (otalgia) or discomfort associated with chewing or swallowing that may decrease nutritional intake. This situation is often associated with a problem in the middle ear.

Assessment of clenching or grinding of the teeth helps differentiate problems of the ear from referred pain of the temporomandibular joint (TMJ). Ask about dental problems and dentures.

***Elimination Pattern.*** Elimination patterns are mainly of interest in the patient with perilymph fistula and after surgical procedures. Frequent constipation or straining with bowel or bladder elimination may interfere with healing or repair of a perilymph fistula. After middle ear surgery (stapedectomy) the patient needs to prevent increased intracranial (and consequent inner ear) pressure associated with straining during bowel movements. Stool softeners may be ordered postoperatively for the patient who reports chronic problems with constipation.

***Activity-Exercise Pattern.*** A review of the patient's activity-exercise pattern is essential when assessing for equilibrium problems. Question the patient specifically about the onset, duration, and frequency of symptoms. Identify activities that relieve or worsen symptoms and how they relate to the time of the day. For example, patients with Ménière's disease are less able to compensate for environmental input as the day progresses.

***Sleep-Rest Pattern.*** Ask the patient with chronic tinnitus about sleep problems. Find out if the patient has tried any techniques to modify the tinnitus (e.g., having fan on, using white noise devices). Also assess for snoring because it can be caused by swelling or hypertrophy of tissue in the nasopharynx. This excessive tissue can impair the functioning of the eustachian tube and cause the sensation of ear fullness or pain.

***Cognitive-Perceptual Pattern.*** Pain is associated with some ear problems, particularly those involving the middle ear and auditory canal. If pain is present, ask the patient to describe the pain, presence of drainage *(otorrhea)*, history of teeth grinding, and the treatments used for relief. Note the effect on the pain level when the auricle is moved or the tragus is palpated.

Note the patient's ability to pay attention and follow directions. Problems with these tasks may be an early indicator of hearing loss. The patient may not recognize a gradual hearing loss. Ask significant others if they have noted any change in the patient's hearing.

***Self-Perception–Self-Concept Pattern.*** Ask the patient to describe how the ear problem has affected his or her personal life and feelings about himself or herself. Hearing loss and chronic vertigo are particularly distressing for the patient. Hearing loss can result in embarrassing social situations that affect the patient's self-concept. Sensitively question the patient about such situations.

At times the patient with chronic vertigo may be accused of acting intoxicated. Clarify the symptom history with the patient and consider an evaluation with a hearing specialist.

***Role-Relationship Pattern.*** Question the patient about the effect that the ear problem has had on family life, work responsibilities, and social relationships. Hearing loss can result in strained family relations and misunderstandings.

Also ask about employment or contact with environments that have excessive noise levels, such as work with jet engines and machinery and electronically amplified music. Document the use of preventive devices worn in noisy environments. Many jobs rely on the ability to hear accurately and respond appropriately. If a hearing loss is present, gather detailed information on the effect this has on the patient's job.

The unpredictability of vertigo attacks can have devastating effects on all aspects of a patient's life. Ordinary activities such as driving or cooking and work that requires balance all have an element of danger. Assess the effect of the vertigo on the patient's many roles and responsibilities.

***Sexuality-Reproductive Pattern.*** Determine whether hearing loss or vertigo has interfered with the establishment of a satisfactory sex life. Although intimacy does not depend on the ability to hear, a hearing loss could interfere with establishing or maintaining a relationship.

***Coping–Stress Tolerance Pattern.*** Ask the patient about his or her usual coping style, stress management strategies, and available support. If the patient seems unable to manage the situation, outside intervention may be required. Denial is a common response to a hearing problem and should be assessed.

***Value-Belief Pattern.*** Question the patient about any conflicts produced by the problem or treatment related to values or beliefs. Every effort should be made to resolve the problem so that the patient does not experience additional stress. Ask about the use of home remedies such as hot oil in the ear.

## Objective Data

**Physical Examination.** During the interview to obtain a health history, obtain objective data regarding the patient's ability to hear. Note clues such as posturing of the head and appropriateness of responses. Does the patient ask to have certain words repeated? Does the patient intently watch the examiner but miss comments when *not* looking at the examiner? Is the patient lip reading? Record these significant observations. This is also important because the patient is often unaware of hearing loss or does not admit to changes in hearing until moderate losses have occurred.

A normal assessment of the auditory system is listed in Table 20-9. Age-related changes of the auditory system and differences in assessment findings are listed in Table 20-7.

A *focused assessment* is used to evaluate the status of previously identified auditory problems and to monitor for signs of new problems (see Table 3-7). A focused assessment of the auditory system is presented in the box on p. 364.

**TABLE 20-9 Normal Physical Assessment of Auditory System**

- Ears symmetric in location and shape
- Auricles and tragus nontender, without lesions
- Canal clear, tympanic membrane intact, landmarks and light reflex intact
- Able to hear low whisper at 30 cm. Weber test results, no lateralization. Rinne test results AC > BC

*AC*, Air conduction; *BC*, bone conduction.

## FOCUSED ASSESSMENT

### *Auditory System*

*Use this checklist to make sure the key assessment steps have been done.*

**Subjective**

*Ask the patient about any of the following and note responses.*

| | | |
|---|---|---|
| Changes in hearing | Y | N |
| Ear pain | Y | N |
| Ear drainage | Y | N |

**Objective: Physical Examination**

***Inspect***

| | |
|---|---|
| Alignment and position of ears on head | ✓ |
| Size, shape, symmetry, color, and skin intactness | ✓ |
| External auditory meatus for discharge or lesions | ✓ |

***Assess***

| | |
|---|---|
| Hearing based on ability to respond to conversation, respond to a whisper, or hear a ticking watch | ✓ |

***External Ear.*** Inspect and palpate the external ear before examining the external canal and tympanum. Observe the auricle, preauricular area, and mastoid area for symmetry, color of skin, swelling, redness, and lesions. Then palpate the auricle and mastoid areas for tenderness and nodules. Grasping the auricle or pressing on the tragus may elicit pain, especially if the external ear or canal is inflamed.

***External Auditory Canal and Tympanum.*** Before inserting an otoscope, inspect the canal opening for patency, palpate the tragus, and gently move the auricle to check for discomfort. Select a speculum slightly smaller than the size of the ear canal. Tip the patient's head to the opposite shoulder. Grasp the top of the auricle and gently pull up and backward to straighten the canal. Hold the otoscope while stabilizing it with your fingers on the patient's cheek, and then insert it slowly. A pneumatic otoscope creates negative pressure to pull at the TM and is helpful in confirming TM retraction or fluid behind the membrane. A tight seal of the speculum is essential during this step of the examination. Observe the canal for size and shape and the color, amount, and type of cerumen. Be careful when clearing the canal of cerumen. Damage can occur to the middle ear if the TM is perforated.

Inspect the TM for color, fluid behind the membrane, landmarks, contour, and intactness (Fig. 20-8). The TM is normally pearl gray, white, or pink; shiny; and translucent. The handle (manubrium) of the malleus and its short process (umbo) should be visible through the membrane. The position and dome (concave) shape of the TM cause the light from the otoscope to reflect back in a cone shape with crisp edges. If the TM is bulging or retracted, the edges of the light reflex will be fuzzy (diffuse) and may spread over the TM. The middle and inner ear cannot be examined with the otoscope because of the TM.

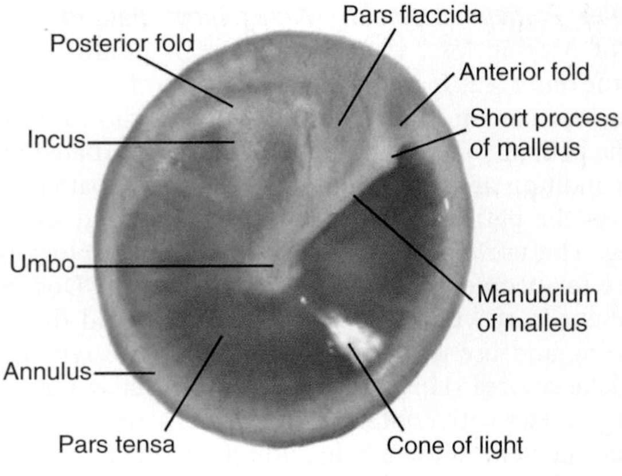


**FIG. 20-8** Normal tympanic membrane. (Jarvis C: *Physical examination and health assessment*, ed 7, St Louis, 2015, Elsevier.)

Table 20-10 summarizes assessment abnormalities of the auditory system.

## DIAGNOSTIC STUDIES OF AUDITORY SYSTEM

Table 20-11 describes diagnostic studies commonly used to assess the auditory system.

### Audiometry

Audiometry is beneficial as a screening test for hearing acuity and as a diagnostic test to determine the degree and type of hearing loss. The most common test performed by the audiologist is pure-tone audiometry.[9] The audiometer produces pure tones at varying intensities to which the patient can respond. Sound is characterized by the number of vibrations or cycles that occur each second. Hertz (Hz) is the unit of measurement used to classify the frequency of a tone. The higher the frequency is, the higher the pitch.

Hearing loss can affect certain sound frequencies. The specific pattern produced on the audiogram by these losses can assist in the diagnosis of the type of hearing loss. The intensity or strength of a sound wave is expressed in terms of decibels (dB), ranging from 0 to 110 dB. The intensity of a sound required to make any frequency barely audible to the average normal ear is 0 dB. Threshold refers to the signal level at which pure tones are detected (pure-tone thresholds) or the signal level at which the patient correctly hears 50% of the signals (speech detection thresholds).

Normal speech is approximately 40 to 65 dB; a soft whisper is 20 dB. Normally, a child and a young adult can hear frequencies from about 16 to 20,000 Hz, but hearing is most sensitive between 500 and 4000 Hz. This is similar to the frequencies of normal speech. A 40- to 45-dB loss in these frequencies causes moderate difficulty in hearing normal speech. A hearing aid may be helpful because it makes sound information louder but not clearer. A hearing aid may not be helpful to the patient who has problems with discrimination of sounds or sound information because the consonants are still not heard enough to make speech understandable.

### Specialized Tests

More sophisticated tests are available to determine the cause of certain hearing losses (Table 20-11). CT scan and MRI are used to diagnose the site of a lesion, such as a tumor of the auditory nerve.

## TABLE 20-10 Assessment Abnormalities

### *Auditory System*

| Finding | Description | Possible Etiology and Significance |
|---|---|---|
| **External Ear and Canal** | | |
| **Sebaceous cyst behind ear** | Usually within skin, possible presence of black dot (opening to sebaceous gland) | Removal or incision and drainage if painful |
| **Tophi** | Hard nodules in the helix or antihelix consisting of uric acid crystals | Associated with gout, metabolic disorder. Further diagnosis needed |
| **Impacted cerumen** | Wax that has not normally been excreted from the ear. No visualization of eardrum | Decreased hearing possible, pain, sensation of fullness in auditory canal, removal necessary before otoscopic examination |
| **Discharge in canal** | Infection of external ear, usually painful | Swimmer's ear, infection of external ear. Possibly caused by ruptured eardrum and otitis media |
| **Swelling of pinna, pain** | Infection of glands of skin, hematoma caused by trauma | Aspiration (for hematoma) |
| **Scaling or lesions** | Change in usual appearance of skin | Seborrheic dermatitis, actinic keratosis, basal or squamous cell carcinoma |
| **Exostosis** | Bony growth extending into canal causing narrowing of canal | Possible interference with visualization of tympanum. Usually asymptomatic |
| **Tympanum** | | |
| **Retracted eardrum** | Appearance of shorter, more horizontal malleus. Absent or bent cone of light | Vacuum in middle ear, blockage of eustachian tube, negative pressure in middle ear |
| **Hairline fluid level, yellow-amber bubbles above fluid level** | Caused by transudate of blood and serum, meniscus of fluid producing hairline appearance | Serous otitis media |
| **Bulging red or blue eardrum, lack of landmarks** | Fluid-filled middle ear, pus, blood | Acute otitis media, perforation possible |
| **Perforation of eardrum** (Fig. 20-8) | Previous perforations of the eardrum that have failed to heal. Thin, transparent layer of epithelium surrounding eardrum | Chronic otitis media, mastoiditis, drainage |
| **Recruitment** | Perception that sounds are getting too loud too fast | Sensorineural hearing loss. Hearing aid difficult to use |

## TABLE 20-11 Diagnostic Studies

### *Auditory System*

| Study | Description, Purpose, and Nursing Responsibility* |
|---|---|
| **Auditory** | |
| **Audiometry** | *Pure-tone audiometry* quantifies hearing loss. Sounds are presented through earphones in soundproof room. Patient responds when sound is heard. Response is recorded on an audiogram. Purpose is to determine patient's hearing range in terms of decibels (dB) and Hertz (Hz) for diagnosing hearing loss. Tinnitus can cause inconsistent results.<br>*Speech audiometry* includes speech reception threshold (measure of intensity at which speech is recognized) and word recognition score (ability to discriminate among various speech sounds). |
| **Auditory evoked potential (AEP)** | Procedure is similar to electroencephalogram (see Chapter 55 and Table 55-7). Electrodes are attached to patient in a darkened room. Electrodes are placed typically at vertex, mastoid process, or earlobes and forehead. A computer is used to isolate auditory from other electrical activity of brain. |
| **Electrocochleography** | Test records electrical activity in cochlea and auditory nerve. Electrode placed on or through the eardrum. Used to assess and monitor patients with dizziness. |
| **Auditory brainstem response (ABR)** | Study measures electrical peaks along auditory pathway of inner ear to brain and provides diagnostic information related to acoustic neuromas, brainstem problems, and stroke. |
| **Tympanometry** | Used to check middle ear and mobility of eardrum. A probe is placed snugly into external ear canal, and positive and negative pressures are then applied. Measurements are made of movement of eardrum. |
| **Tuning Fork Tests** | |
| **Weber test** | Stem of vibrating tuning fork is placed on midline of skull or forehead. Patient asked to indicate where the sound is heard best. In normal auditory function, the patient perceives a midline tone and the sound is heard equally in both ears. If a patient has conductive hearing loss in one ear, the sound will be heard louder (lateralizes) in that ear. If sensorineural loss is present, the sound is louder (lateralizes) in the normal (unaffected) ear. |
| **Rinne test** | Hearing by bone conduction (BC) and air conduction (AC) is compared. Stem of vibrating tuning fork held against mastoid bone (for BC of sound) and time noted. When the sound is no longer perceived behind the ear (BC of sound), time is noted once again and the still-vibrating fork is moved close to the pinna (AC of sound).<br>Have the patient report when the sound next to the ear canal (AC) is no longer heard and note time. Normally, the sound is heard twice as long in front of the ear as it is on the bone.<br>With conductive hearing loss, the relationship is reversed; BC is longer than AC. With sensorineural hearing loss, both AC and BC are reduced, but AC remains longer. |

*Continued*

**TABLE 20-11 Diagnostic Studies**
***Auditory System—cont'd***

| Study | Description, Purpose, and Nursing Responsibility* |
|---|---|
| **Vestibular Tests** | |
| **Electronystagmography (ENG)** | Used to diagnose diseases of vestibular system such as dizziness and balance disorders. Electrodes are placed near patient's eyes, and movement of eyes (nystagmus) is recorded on graph during specific eye movements and when ear is irrigated. Caloric test may be part of testing to measure responses to warm and cold water circulated into the ear canal. Instruct patient to eat light meal before test to avoid nausea. Observe patient for vomiting. Ensure patient safety. |
| **Posturography** | Balance test that can isolate one semicircular canal from others to determine site of lesion. Test is done in a boxlike device in which floor moves in response to a correction in balance by patient. Inform patient that test may be uncomfortable. Test can be discontinued at any time at patient's request. |
| **Rotary chair testing** | Evaluates peripheral vestibular system. Patient is seated in a chair driven by a motor under computer control. Test is usually done in the dark. Instruct patient to eat light meal before test to avoid nausea. Observe patient for vomiting. Ensure patient safety. |

*Patient teaching regarding the purpose and method of testing is a nursing responsibility for all diagnostic procedures.

## BRIDGE TO NCLEX EXAMINATION

The number of the question corresponds to the same-numbered outcome at the beginning of the chapter.

1. In a patient who has a hemorrhage in the posterior cavity of the eye, the nurse knows that blood is accumulating
   **a.** in the aqueous humor.
   **b.** between the lens and retina.
   **c.** between the cornea and lens.
   **d.** in the space between the iris and lens.
2. Increased intraocular pressure may occur as a result of
   **a.** edema of the corneal stroma.
   **b.** dilation of the retinal arterioles.
   **c.** blockage of the lacrimal canals and ducts.
   **d.** increased production of aqueous humor by the ciliary process.
3. Question patients using eye drops to treat their glaucoma about
   **a.** use of corrective lenses.
   **b.** their usual sleep pattern.
   **c.** a history of heart or lung disease.
   **d.** sensitivity to opioids or depressants.
4. Always assess the patient with an ophthalmic problem for
   **a.** visual acuity.
   **b.** pupillary reactions.
   **c.** intraocular pressure.
   **d.** confrontation visual fields.
5. During an assessment of hearing, the nurse would expect that a normal finding would be
   **a.** absent cone of light.
   **b.** bluish purple tympanic membrane.
   **c.** midline tone heard equally in both ears.
   **d.** fluid level at hairline in the tympanum.
6. Age-related changes in the auditory system commonly include *(select all that apply)*
   **a.** drier cerumen.
   **b.** tinnitus in both ears.
   **c.** auditory nerve degeneration.
   **d.** atrophy of the tympanic membrane.
   **e.** greater ability to hear high-pitched sounds.
7. Before injecting fluorescein for angiography, it is important for the nurse to *(select all that apply)*
   **a.** obtain an emesis basin.
   **b.** ask if the patient is fatigued.
   **c.** administer a topical anesthetic.
   **d.** inform patient that skin may turn yellow.
   **e.** assess for allergies to iodine-based contrast media.

1. b, 2. d, 3. c, 4. a, 5. c, 6. a, c, d, 7. a, d

For rationales to these answers and even more NCLEX review questions, visit *http://evolve.elsevier.com/Lewis/medsurg.*

## EVOLVE WEBSITE

http://evolve.elsevier.com/Lewis/medsurg
**Review Questions (Online Only)**
**Key Points**
**Answer Keys for Questions**
- Rationales for Bridge to NCLEX Examination Questions
- Answer Guidelines for Case Study on pp. 353, 356, 359, and 360

**Conceptual Care Map Creator**
**Audio Glossary**
**Supporting Media**
- Animation
  - Weber Test

**Content Updates**

## REFERENCES


1. Dua HS, Fara LA, Said DG, et al: Human corneal anatomy redefined: a novel pre-Descmet's layer (Dua's layer), *Ophthalmology* 120(9):1778, 2013.
2. Thibodeau G, Patton K: *Structure and function of the body*, ed 14, St Louis, 2012, Mosby.
3. *Saunders nursing drug handbook 2015*, St Louis, 2015, Saunders.
4. American Foundation for the Blind: AFB senior site. Retrieved from *www.afb.org*.
5. Goldman L, Schafer A, editors: *Goldman's Cecil medicine*, ed 25, St Louis, 2016, Saunders.
6. Rakel R, Rakel D, editors: *Textbook of family medicine*, ed 9, St Louis, 2015, Saunders.
7. National Institute on Deafness and Other Communication Disorders: Quick statistics. Retrieved from *www.nidcd.nih.gov/health/statistics/Pages/quick.aspx*.
8. Hearing Loss Association of America. Retrieved from *http://hearingloss.org*.
9. Bope E, Kellerman R, editors: *Conn's current therapy 2015*, St Louis, 2015, Saunders.

21

# Visual and Auditory Problems

*Sharon L. Lewis*

*It is only with the heart that one can see rightly; what is essential is invisible to the eye.*

***Antoine de Saint-Exupery***

http://evolve.elsevier.com/Lewis/medsurg/

## LEARNING OUTCOMES

1. Compare and contrast the types of refractive errors and appropriate corrections.
2. Describe the etiology and nursing and interprofessional management of extraocular disorders.
3. Explain the pathophysiology, clinical manifestations, interprofessional care, and nursing management of the patient with intraocular disorders.
4. Discuss the nursing measures that promote the health of the eyes and ears.
5. Discuss the general preoperative and postoperative care of patients undergoing surgery of the eye or ear.
6. Summarize the action and uses of drug therapy for treating problems of the eyes and ears.
7. Explain the pathophysiology, clinical manifestations, and nursing and interprofessional management of common ear problems.
8. Compare the causes, management, and rehabilitative potential of conductive and sensorineural hearing loss.
9. Explain the use, care, and patient teaching related to assistive devices for eye and ear problems.
10. Describe the common causes and assistive measures for severe visual impairment and deafness.
11. Describe the measures used to assist the patient in adapting psychologically to decreased vision and hearing.

## KEY TERMS

acoustic neuroma, p. 387
age-related macular degeneration (AMD), p. 378
astigmatism, p. 368
benign paroxysmal positional vertigo (BPPV), p. 386
cataract, p. 373
conjunctivitis, p. 371
enucleation, p. 382
external otitis, p. 383
glaucoma, p. 379
hordeolum, p. 370
hyperopia, p. 368
keratitis, p. 372
Ménière's disease, p. 386
myopia, p. 367
otosclerosis, p. 385
presbycusis, p. 391
presbyopia, p. 368
refractive error, p. 367
retinal detachment, p. 376
retinopathy, p. 376
strabismus, p. 373

The chapter describes visual and auditory problems, with an emphasis on their pathophysiology, clinical manifestations, interprofessional care, and nursing management. Assistive devices for visual and hearing impairment are also discussed.

## VISUAL PROBLEMS

### REFRACTIVE ERRORS

The most common visual problem is **refractive error**. This defect prevents light rays from converging into a single focus on the retina. Defects are a result of irregularities of the corneal curvature, focusing power of the lens, or length of the eye. The major symptom is blurred vision. In some cases, the patient may also complain of ocular discomfort, eyestrain, or headaches. Most refractive errors can be corrected by the use of lenses in the form of eyeglasses or contact lenses, refractive eye laser surgery, or surgical implantation of an artificial lens.

**Myopia** (nearsightedness) is an inability to accommodate for objects at a distance. It causes light rays to be focused in front of the retina. Myopia may occur because of excessive light refraction by the cornea or lens or because of an abnormally long eye. Myopia is the most common refractive error, with approximately 25% of Americans having this disorder.

*Acknowledgment*: We would like to acknowledge the contributions of Sarah Smith, RN, MA, CRNO, COT, Nurse Manager, Department of Ophthalmology, University of Iowa Health Care, Iowa City, Iowa, to this chapter over the past six editions of the book.
Reviewed by Marylee Bressie, RN, DNP, CCRN, CCNS, CEN, Core Faculty/Nurse Planner, Department of Nursing, School of Public Service Leadership, Capella University, Minneapolis, Minnesota; Hope Bussenius, DNP, APRN, FNP-BC, Clinical Assistant Professor, Nell Hodgson Woodruff School of Nursing, Emory University, Atlanta, Georgia; Deborah Ehlers, RN, MSN, Director of Nursing and Administrator of The Eye Center, Yakima, Washington; Deena Hollingsworth, MSN, FNP-BC, CORLN, Family Nurse Practitioner, ENT Specialists of Northern Virginia, Arlington, Virginia; Michelle Smeltzer, RN, MSN, DNPc, CEN, Clinical Education Specialist, Emergency Department, Einstein Medical Center Montgomery, East Norriton, Pennsylvania; and Robert M. Welch, RN, MSN, FNP, CRNO, Family Nurse Practitioner, Nevada Retina Associates, Reno, Nevada.

**Hyperopia** (farsightedness) is an inability to accommodate for near objects. It causes the light rays to focus behind the retina and requires the patient to use accommodation to focus the light rays on the retina for near objects. This type of refractive error occurs when the cornea or lens does not have adequate focusing power or when the eyeball is too short.

**Presbyopia** is the loss of accommodation associated with age. This condition generally appears at about age 40. As the eye ages, the lens becomes larger, firmer, and less elastic. These changes, which progress with aging, result in an inability to focus on near objects.

**Astigmatism** is caused by an irregular corneal curvature. This irregularity causes the incoming light rays to be bent unequally. Consequently, the light rays do not come to a single point of focus on the retina. Astigmatism can occur in conjunction with any of the other refractive errors.

*Aphakia* is the absence of the lens. Rarely, the lens may be absent congenitally, or it may be removed during cataract surgery. A lens that is traumatically injured is removed and replaced with an intraocular lens (IOL) implant. The absence of the lens generally results in a significant refractive error. Without the focusing ability of the lens, images are projected behind the retina.

### Nonsurgical Corrections

**Corrective Glasses.** Myopia, hyperopia, presbyopia, and astigmatism can be modified by using the appropriate corrective lenses. Glasses for presbyopia are often called "reading glasses" because they are usually only worn for close work. The presbyopic correction may also be combined with a correction for another refractive error, such as myopia or astigmatism. In these combined glasses, the presbyopic correction is in the lower portion of the spectacle lens. A traditional bifocal or trifocal has visible lines. However, most lenses today that correct vision at various distances do not have visible lines. The prescription varies throughout the lens, allowing distance focusing in the top two thirds and near focus in the bottom one third of the lens.

**Contact Lenses.** Contact lenses are another way to correct refractive errors. Contact lenses are made from various plastic and silicone substances that are highly permeable to oxygen and have a high water content. These features allow for increased wearing time with greater comfort. If the oxygen supply to the cornea is decreased, it becomes swollen, visual acuity decreases, and the patient experiences severe discomfort.

In general, you need to know whether the patient wears contact lenses, the pattern of wear (daily versus extended), and care practices. Shining a light obliquely on the eyeball can help visualize a contact lens. Contact lenses are associated with microbial keratitis, a severe sight-threatening complication. Risk factors for keratitis include poor hand cleaning, poor lens case hygiene, and inadequate lens cleaning. Teach the patient the importance of following recommended cleaning practices and reporting redness, sensitivity, vision problems, and pain to the eye care professional. Instruct the patient to remove contact lenses immediately if any of these problems occur.

### Surgical Therapy

Surgical procedures are designed to eliminate or reduce the need for eyeglasses or contact lenses and correct refractive errors by changing the focus of the eye. Surgical management for refractive errors includes laser surgery and IOL implantation.

**Laser.** *Laser-assisted in situ keratomileusis* (LASIK) may be considered for patients with low to moderately high amounts of myopia or hyperopia, with or without astigmatism.[1] The procedure first involves using a laser or surgical blade to create a flap in the cornea. The flap is folded back, exposing the middle section (stroma) of the cornea. Pulses from a computer-controlled laser vaporize a part of the stroma. The flap is then repositioned, adhering on its own without sutures in a few minutes.[2]

*Photorefractive keratectomy* (PRK) is indicated for low to moderate amounts of myopia or hyperopia, with or without astigmatism and is a good option for a patient with insufficient corneal thickness for a LASIK flap. In PRK only the epithelium is removed, and the laser sculpts the cornea to correct the refractive error. *Laser-assisted subepithelial keratomileusis* (LASEK) is similar to PRK, except that the epithelium is replaced after surgery.

**Implant.** *Refractive intraocular lens* (refractive IOL) implantation is an option for patients with a high degree of myopia or hyperopia. Like cataract surgery, it involves removal of the patient's natural lens and implantation of an IOL, which is a small plastic lens to correct a patient's refractive error. Accommodating IOLs correct both myopia and presbyopia.

*Phakic intraocular lenses* (phakic IOLs) are sometimes referred to as *implantable contact lenses.* They are implanted into the eye without removing the eye's natural lens. They are used for patients with high degrees of myopia or hyperopia. Unlike refractive IOLs, the phakic IOL is placed in front of the eye's natural lens. Leaving the natural lens in the eye preserves the eye's ability to focus for reading vision.

**CULTURAL & ETHNIC HEALTH DISPARITIES**

***Visual and Auditory Problems***

- Whites have a higher incidence of hearing impairment than African Americans or Asian Americans.
- Glaucoma has an increased incidence and severity among African Americans compared with whites.
- Hispanic Americans have an increased incidence of diabetic retinopathy.
- Native Americans have an increased incidence of otitis media when compared with whites.
- Whites have a higher incidence of macular degeneration than Hispanics, African Americans, and Asian Americans.

## VISUAL IMPAIRMENT

Visual impairment describes vision that cannot be fully corrected by corrective lenses, medical treatment, or surgery. The term *visual impairment* includes conditions ranging from low vision to the absence of any sight at all (total blindness).[3] Many terms are used when people refer to visual impairment, including:

- *Low vision* is a term used to describe impaired vision that cannot be improved by conventional eyeglasses, contact lenses, medications, or surgery in which some good usable vision remains.
- *Severe visual impairment* describes visual impairment in people who are unable to read ordinary newsprint even with correction. People with a severe visual impairment may or may not be legally blind.
- *Legal blindness* refers to central visual acuity of 20/200 or less in the better eye with correction, or a peripheral visual field of 20 degrees or less.

Almost all blindness in the United States is the result of common eye diseases, including cataracts, glaucoma, age-related macular degeneration, and diabetic retinopathy.

## NURSING MANAGEMENT: VISUAL IMPAIRMENT

### Nursing Assessment

It is important to assess how long the patient has had a visual impairment, since recent loss of vision has different implications for nursing care. Determine how the patient's visual impairment affects normal functioning. Question the patient about the level of difficulty involved in doing certain tasks. For example, ask how much difficulty the patient has when reading a newspaper, writing a check, moving from one room to the next, or viewing television. Other questions can help determine the personal meaning that the patient attaches to the visual impairment. Ask how the vision loss has affected specific aspects of the patient's life, whether the patient has lost a job, or what activities the patient does not engage in because of the visual impairment.

Determine the patient's emotional reactions, coping strategies, and support systems. The patient may attach many negative meanings to the impairment because of societal views of blindness. For example, the patient may view the impairment as punishment or view himself or herself as useless and burdensome.

### Planning

The overall goals are that the patient with impaired vision will (1) make a successful adjustment to the impairment, (2) verbalize feelings related to the loss, (3) identify personal strengths and support systems, and (4) use appropriate coping strategies. If the patient has been functioning at an appropriate or acceptable level, the goal is to maintain the current level of function.

### Nursing Implementation

**Health Promotion.** Encourage the patient with preventable causes of further visual impairment to seek appropriate health care. For example, the patient with vision loss from glaucoma may prevent further visual impairment by complying with prescribed therapies and ophthalmic evaluations.

**Acute Care.** Provide emotional support and direct care to the patient with recent visual impairment. Allow the patient to express fear, anger, and grief. Help the patient identify appropriate coping strategies. The family is intimately involved in the experiences that occur with vision loss. With the patient's knowledge and permission, include family members in discussions and encourage them to express their concerns.

Many people are uncomfortable around an individual with visual impairment because they are not sure what behaviors are appropriate. Being sensitive to the patient's feelings without being overly worried or smothering the patient's independence is vital in creating a therapeutic nursing presence. Always communicate in a normal conversational tone and manner with the patient, and address the patient, not the caregiver. Common courtesy dictates introducing oneself and any other people who approach patients with visual impairment. It is also important to say good-bye when leaving the presence of the visually impaired person. Making eye contact with the patient accomplishes several objectives. It ensures that you are speaking while facing the patient so that the patient has no difficulty hearing. Your head position validates that you are attentive to the patient. In addition, establishing eye contact ensures that you can observe the patient's facial expressions and reactions.

Assist the patient using a *sighted-guide technique.* Stand slightly in front and to one side of the patient, and offer an elbow for the patient to hold. Serve as the sighted guide, walking slightly ahead of the patient with the patient holding the back of your arm. As you walk, describe the environment to help orient the patient. For example, "We're going through an open doorway and approaching two steps down." Help the patient sit by placing one of his or her hands on the seat of the chair.

**Ambulatory Care.** In working with the patient who is visually impaired, remember that a person classified as legally blind may have some useful vision. Rehabilitation after partial or total loss of vision can foster independence, self-esteem, and productivity. Know what services and devices are available for the patients with visual impairments, and make appropriate referrals. For the legally blind patient the primary resource for services is the state agency for rehabilitation of the blind. Legally blind individuals are often eligible for federal and state assistance and income tax benefits. A list of agencies that serve the partially sighted or blind patient is available from the American Foundation for the Blind *(www.afb.org).*

Braille or audio books for reading and a cane or guide dog for ambulation are examples of vision substitution techniques. These are usually most appropriate for the patient with no functional vision. For most patients who have some remaining vision, vision enhancement techniques can provide help in learning to ambulate, read printed material, and accomplish activities of daily living (ADLs).

***Optical Devices for Vision Enhancement.*** A wide range of newer technologies are available to assist people with low vision. These devices include desktop video magnification/closed circuit units, electronic hand-held magnifiers, text-to-speech scanners (material read aloud to you), E-readers, and computer tablets (material read aloud, magnification, image zooming, brighter screen, voice recognition). Many of these devices require some training by an assistive technology professional. Encourage patients to practice with the technologic device to ensure they can use it successfully.

***Nonoptical Methods for Vision Enhancement.*** *Approach magnification* is a simple way to enhance the patient's residual vision. Recommend that the patient sit closer to the television or hold books closer to the eyes. Contrast enhancement techniques include watching television in black and white, using a black felt-tip marker, and using contrasting colors (e.g., a red stripe at the edge of steps or curbs). Increased lighting can be provided by halogen lamps, direct sunlight, or gooseneck lamps that can be aimed directly at the reading material or other near objects. Large type is often helpful, especially in conjunction with other optical or nonoptical vision enhancements.

***Non–24-Hour Sleep-Wake Disorder.*** A common problem that can occur in blind people (especially those who are totally blind) is *non–24-hour sleep-wake disorder (Non-24).* It is a circadian rhythm sleep disorder in which an individual's biologic clock fails to synchronize to a 24-hour day.[4] (Sleep and sleep disorders are discussed in Chapter 7.) It is caused by lack of light input to the circadian clock.

People with this disorder have difficulty falling asleep or staying asleep at night. During the day they may have an uncontrollable urge to sleep. This disorder can result in severe sleep issues including insomnia, excessive sleepiness, changing patterns of when a person sleeps, and social and work consequences.

Melatonin is used to shift the circadian clock earlier (an advance) or later (a delay). Tasimelteon (Hetlioz), a melatonin receptor agonist, can also be used for treatment. It works by targeting receptors in the brain that control the timing of the sleep-wake cycle.

### ◆ Evaluation

The overall expected outcomes are that the patient with visual impairment will

- Follow treatment plan to prevent further loss of vision
- Be able to use adaptive coping strategies
- Not experience low self-esteem or a decrease in social interactions
- Function safely within her or his own environment

#### HEALTHY PEOPLE

***Health Impact of Responsible Eye Care***

- Regular hand washing prevents the spread of disease from one eye to the other.
- Seeking appropriate health care can lead to early detection of disease and prevent further loss of vision in patients with certain types of partial vision loss.
- Wearing sunglasses and practicing proper nutrition may help prevent cataract development and age-related macular degeneration.
- Wearing eye protection during potentially hazardous work, hobby, and sport activities reduces the risk of eye injuries.

### Gerontologic Considerations: Visual Impairment

The older adult is at an increased risk for vision loss caused by eye disease.[5] This older person may have other deficits, such as cognitive impairment or limited mobility, that further affect the ability to function in usual ways. Societal devaluation of the older adults may compound the self-esteem or isolation issues associated with the older patient's visual impairment. Financial resources may be inadequate to meet the increased demands of vision services or assistive devices.

The older patient may become increasingly confused or disoriented when visually compromised. The combination of decreased vision and confusion increases the risk of falls, which have potentially serious consequences for the older adult. Decreased vision may compromise the older patient's ability to function, resulting in concerns about maintaining independence and a diminished self-image. Decreased manual dexterity may make the instillation of prescribed eye drops difficult for some older adults. Those with low vision are more likely to make medication errors that are potentially dangerous, such as taking too much insulin or mistaking one drug for another.

## EYE TRAUMA

Although the eyes are well protected by the bony orbit and fat pads, everyday activities can result in ocular trauma. The most common ocular injuries in the United States occur in the home due to gardening, power tool use, and home repair work. Sport- and work-related injuries are additional causes of eye trauma.[6]

Table 21-1 outlines emergency management of the patient with an eye injury. A *Morgan lens* may be used to provide continuous irrigation of an injured eye. It consists of a sterile plastic device resembling a contact lens that floats over the eye (never physically touches it) and allows copious irrigation of the eye. The device is connected to tubing that delivers irrigating solution. The Morgan lens provides relief for chemical or thermal burns and removes nonembedded foreign materials in the eye.

#### CHECK YOUR PRACTICE

You are working in your garden when your neighbor comes running into your yard. She is screaming and waving her arms. Her husband was using a chain saw to cut down a tree when a piece of wood chip flew into his eye. When you go to your neighbor's yard, the husband is on the ground crying in pain and you assess that the wood chip is embedded in his eye.

- What should you do next?

Trauma is often a preventable cause of visual impairment. Many eye injuries could be prevented by wearing protective eyewear. Your role in individual and community education is extremely important in reducing the incidence of ocular trauma.

# EXTRAOCULAR DISORDERS

## INFLAMMATION AND INFECTION

One of the most common eye conditions is inflammation or infection of the external eye. Many external irritants or microorganisms can affect the eye, conjunctiva, and avascular cornea.

An external **hordeolum** (commonly called a *sty*) is an infection of the sebaceous glands in the lid margin (Fig. 21-1). The most common bacterial infective agent is *Staphylococcus aureus.* A red, swollen, circumscribed, and acutely tender area develops rapidly. Instruct the patient to apply warm, moist compresses at least four times a day until it improves. This may be the only treatment necessary. If it tends to recur, teach the patient to perform lid scrubs daily. In addition, appropriate antibiotic ointments or drops may be indicated.

A *chalazion* is a chronic inflammatory granuloma of the meibomian (sebaceous) glands in the lid. It may evolve from a hordeolum or occur in response to the material released into the lid when a blocked gland ruptures. The chalazion usually appears on the upper lid as a swollen, tender, reddened area that may be painful. Initial treatment is similar to that for a hordeolum. If warm, moist compresses are ineffective in promoting spontaneous drainage, the ophthalmologist may drain the lesion (this is normally an office procedure) or inject the lesion with corticosteroids.

*Blepharitis* is a common chronic bilateral inflammation of the lid margins. The lids are red rimmed with many scales or

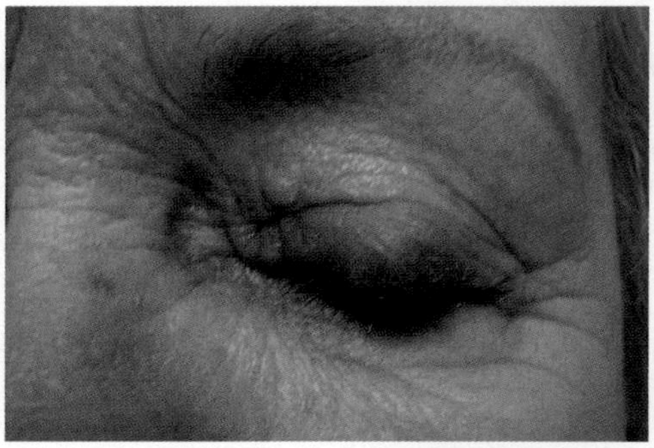

**FIG. 21-1** Hordeolum (sty) on the upper eyelid caused by staphylococcal infection. (Courtesy Cory J. Bosanko, OD, FAAO, Eye Centers of Tennessee, Crossville, Tenn.)

**TABLE 21-1 Emergency Management**

***Eye Injury***

| Etiology | Assessment Findings | Interventions |
|---|---|---|
| **Trauma**<br>• Blunt (e.g., fist)<br>• Penetrating (e.g., glass, metal, or wood fragments. Knife, stick, or other object)<br>**Chemical Burn**<br>• Alkaline<br>• Acid<br>**Thermal Burn**<br>• Direct burn from hot surface<br>• Indirect burn from UV light (e.g., welding torch, looking directly at sun)<br>**Foreign Bodies**<br>• Glass<br>• Metal<br>• Wood<br>• Plastic<br>• Ceramics | • Pain<br>• Photophobia<br>• Redness—diffuse or localized<br>• Swelling<br>• Ecchymosis<br>• Tearing<br>• Blood in the anterior chamber<br>• Absent eye movements<br>• Fluid drainage from eye (e.g., blood, CSF, aqueous humor)<br>• Abnormal or decreased vision<br>• Visible foreign body<br>• Prolapsed globe<br>• Abnormal intraocular pressure<br>• Visual field defect | **Initial**<br>• Determine mechanism of injury.<br>• Ensure airway, breathing, and circulation.<br>• Assess for other injuries.<br>• Assess for chemical exposure.<br>• Begin ocular irrigation *immediately* in case of chemical exposure. Do not stop until emergency personnel arrive to continue irrigation. Use sterile saline or water if saline is unavailable.<br>• Assess visual acuity.<br>• Do not put pressure on the eye.<br>• Instruct patient not to blow nose.<br>• Do not attempt to treat the injury (except as noted above for chemical exposure).<br>• Stabilize foreign objects.<br>• Cover the eye(s) with dry, sterile patches and a protective shield.<br>• Do not give the patient food or fluids.<br>• Elevate head of bed 45 degrees.<br>• Do not put medication or solutions in the eye unless ordered by physician.<br>• Administer analgesia as appropriate.<br>**Ongoing Monitoring**<br>• Reassure the patient.<br>• Monitor pain.<br>• Anticipate surgical repair for penetrating injury, globe rupture, or globe avulsion. |

*CSF*, Cerebrospinal fluid; *UV*, ultraviolet.

crusts on the lid margins and lashes. The patient may primarily complain of itching but may also experience burning, irritation, and photophobia. Conjunctivitis may occur simultaneously.

If blepharitis is caused by a staphylococcal infection, an appropriate ophthalmic antibiotic ointment must be used. Often blepharitis is caused by both staphylococcal and seborrheal microorganisms, and the treatment must be more vigorous to avoid hordeolum, *keratitis* (inflammation of the cornea), and other eye infections. Emphasize thorough cleaning practices of the skin and scalp. Gentle cleansing of the lid margins with baby shampoo can effectively soften and remove crusting.

## Conjunctivitis

**Conjunctivitis** is an infection or inflammation of the conjunctiva. These infections may be caused by bacteria or viruses.[7] Conjunctival inflammation may result from exposure to allergens or chemical irritants. The tarsal conjunctiva (lining the interior surface of the lids) may become inflamed as a result of a chronic foreign body in the eye, such as a contact lens. Careful hand washing and use of individual or disposable towels help prevent spreading the condition.

**Bacterial Infections.** Acute bacterial conjunctivitis *(pinkeye)* is a common infection. Although it occurs in every age group, epidemics are common among children. *S. aureus* is the most common cause. The patient with bacterial conjunctivitis may complain of discomfort, pruritus, redness, and a mucopurulent drainage. Although it typically occurs initially in one eye, it generally spreads to the unaffected eye. It is usually self-limiting, but treatment with antibiotic drops (e.g., besifloxacin [Besivance]) shortens the course of the disorder. Teach patients the importance of hand washing and avoiding contact with an infected person.

**Viral Infections.** Conjunctival infections may be caused by many different viruses. The patient with viral conjunctivitis may complain of tearing, foreign body sensation, redness, and mild photophobia. This condition is usually mild and self-limiting. However, it can be severe, with increased discomfort and subconjunctival hemorrhaging. Adenovirus conjunctivitis may be contracted in contaminated swimming pools and through direct contact with an infected patient. Treatment is usually palliative. If the patient is severely symptomatic, topical corticosteroids can provide temporary relief.

**Chlamydial Infections.** *Trachoma* is a chronic conjunctivitis caused by *Chlamydia trachomatis* (serotypes A through C). It is a major cause of blindness worldwide. This preventable eye disease is transmitted mainly by the hands and by flies. Adult inclusion conjunctivitis (AIC) is caused by *C. trachomatis* (serotypes D through K). AIC is becoming more prevalent in the United States because of the increase in sexually transmitted chlamydial infection.[8]

Manifestations of both trachoma and AIC are mucopurulent ocular discharge, irritation, redness, and lid swelling. For unknown reasons, AIC does not carry the long-term consequences of trachoma. AIC also differs from trachoma in that it is common in economically developed countries, whereas trachoma is most commonly seen in underdeveloped countries. Antibiotic therapy is usually effective for trachoma and AIC.

Although antibiotic treatment may be successful, patients with AIC have a high risk of concurrent chlamydial genital infection, as well as other sexually transmitted infections.

**Allergic Conjunctivitis.** Conjunctivitis caused by exposure to an allergen can be mild and transitory, or it can be severe enough to cause significant swelling, sometimes ballooning the conjunctiva beyond the eyelids. The defining symptom of allergic conjunctivitis is itching. The patient may also complain of burning, redness, and tearing. In addition to pollens, the patient may develop allergic conjunctivitis in response to animal dander, ocular solutions, and medications. Instruct the patient to avoid the allergen if it is known. Artificial tears can be effective in diluting the allergen and washing it from the eye. Effective topical medications include antihistamines and corticosteroids.

## Keratitis

**Keratitis** is an inflammation or infection of the cornea that is caused by a variety of microorganisms or by other factors. The condition may involve the conjunctiva and/or the cornea. When it involves both, the disorder is termed *keratoconjunctivitis.*

**Bacterial Infections.** The cornea can become infected by a variety of bacteria. Topical antibiotics are generally effective, but eradicating the infection may require subconjunctival antibiotic injection or, in severe cases, IV antibiotics. Risk factors include mechanical or chemical corneal epithelial damage, contact lens wear, nutritional deficiencies, immunosuppressed states, and contaminated products (e.g., lens care solutions and cases, topical medications, cosmetics).

**Viral Infections.** Herpes simplex virus (HSV) keratitis is the most frequently occurring infectious cause of corneal blindness in the Western hemisphere. It is a growing problem, especially with immunosuppressed patients. The corneal ulcer has a characteristic dendritic (tree-branching) appearance. Pain and photophobia are common.

Antiviral treatments include trifluridine drops (Viroptic), oral acyclovir (Zovirax), and topical vidarabine (Vira-A) ointment. Therapy may also involve corneal debridement. Topical corticosteroids are usually contraindicated because they contribute to a longer course and possible deeper ulceration of the cornea.

The varicella-zoster virus (VZV) causes both chickenpox and herpes zoster ophthalmicus (HZO). HZO may occur by reactivation of an endogenous infection that has persisted in a latent form after an earlier attack of varicella or by contact with a patient with chickenpox or herpes zoster. It occurs most frequently in the older adult and in the immunosuppressed patient. Care of the patient with acute HZO may include analgesics for pain, topical corticosteroids to reduce inflammation, antiviral agents such as acyclovir to reduce viral replication, mydriatic agents to dilate the pupil and relieve pain, and topical antibiotics to combat secondary infection. The patient may apply warm compresses and povidone-iodine gel to the affected skin (gel should not be applied near the eye).

*Epidemic keratoconjunctivitis* (EKC) is the most serious ocular adenoviral disease. EKC is spread by direct contact, including sexual activity. In the medical setting, contaminated hands and instruments can be the source of spread. The patient may complain of tearing, redness, photophobia, and foreign body sensation. In most patients the disease involves only one eye. Treatment is primarily palliative and includes ice packs and dark glasses. In severe cases therapy can include mild topical corticosteroids to temporarily relieve symptoms and topical antibiotic ointment. Teach the patient the importance of good hygiene practices to avoid spreading the disease.

**Other Causes of Keratitis.** Keratitis may also be caused by fungi (most commonly *Aspergillus, Candida,* and *Fusarium* species), especially in the case of ocular trauma in an outdoor setting where fungi are prevalent in the soil and moist organic matter.

*Acanthamoeba* keratitis is caused by a parasite that is associated with contact lens wear, probably as a result of contaminated lens care solutions or cases. Homemade saline solution is particularly susceptible to *Acanthamoeba* contamination. Instruct the patient who wears contact lenses about good lens care practices. Medical treatment of *Acanthamoeba* keratitis is difficult, since the organism is resistant to most drugs. Antifungal agents (e.g., ketoconazole [Nizoral] and polyhexamethylene biguanide [PHMB]) may be used. If antimicrobial therapy fails, the patient may require a corneal transplant.

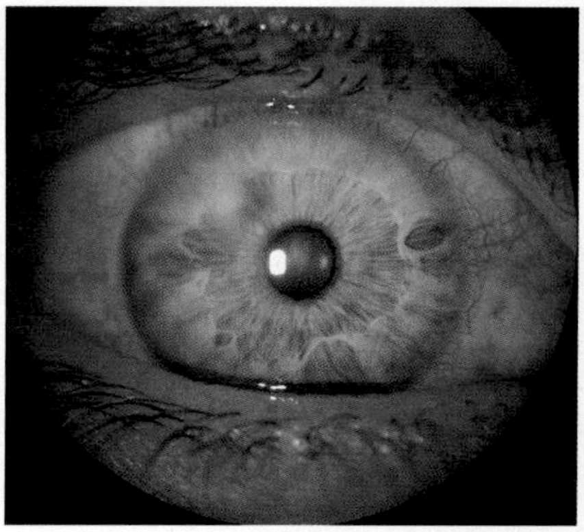

**FIG. 21-2** Corneal ulcer. Infection associated with poor contact lens care. (Courtesy Cory J. Bosanko, OD, FAAO, Eye Centers of Tennessee, Crossville, Tenn.)

Exposure keratitis occurs when the patient cannot adequately close the eyelids. The patient with *exophthalmos* (protruding eyeball) from thyroid eye disease or masses posterior to the globe is susceptible to exposure keratitis.

**Corneal Ulcer.** Tissue loss caused by infection of the cornea produces a *corneal ulcer* (infectious keratitis) (Fig. 21-2). The infection can be due to bacteria, viruses, or fungi. Corneal ulcers are often painful, and patients may feel as if there is a foreign body in their eye. Other symptoms can include tearing, purulent or watery discharge, redness, and photophobia. Treatment is generally aggressive to avoid permanent loss of vision. Antibiotic, antiviral, or antifungal eye drops may be prescribed as frequently as every hour night and day for the first 24 hours. An untreated corneal ulcer can result in corneal scarring and perforation (hole in the cornea). A corneal transplant may be indicated.

## ❖ NURSING MANAGEMENT: INFLAMMATION AND INFECTION

Assess ocular changes, such as edema, redness, decreased visual acuity, feelings that a foreign body is present, or discomfort. Document the findings in the patient's record. Also consider the psychosocial aspects of the patient's condition, especially when vision is impaired.

Careful asepsis and frequent, thorough hand washing are essential to prevent spreading organisms from one eye to the other, to other patients, to family members, and to health care professionals. Teach the patient and family about avoiding sources of ocular irritation or infection and responding appropriately if an ocular problem occurs. Inform the patient about appropriate use and care of lenses and lens care products. The patient with infective disorders that may have a sexual mode of transmission needs specific information about those disorders.

Apply warm or cool compresses if indicated for the patient's condition. Darkening the room and providing an appropriate analgesic are other comfort measures. If the patient's visual acuity is decreased, modify the patient's environment or activities for safety.

The patient may require eye drops as frequently as every hour. If the patient receives two or more different drops, stagger the eye drops to promote maximum absorption. For example, if two different eye drops are ordered hourly, administer one drop on the hour and one drop on the half hour (unless otherwise prescribed). The patient who needs frequent eye drop administration may experience sleep deprivation.

The patient's primary need is for information about required care and how to accomplish that care. Also instruct the patient and caregiver about the proper techniques for medication administration. If the patient's vision is compromised, suggest alternative ways to accomplish necessary daily activities and self-care. Inform the patient who wears contact lenses and develops infections to discard all opened or used lens care products and cosmetics to decrease the risk of reinfection from contaminated products (a common problem and a probable source of infection for many patients).

## DRY EYE DISORDERS

*Keratoconjunctivitis sicca* (dry eyes) is a common complaint, particularly of older adults and individuals with certain systemic diseases such as scleroderma and systemic lupus erythematosus. Patients with dry eyes complain of irritation or "sand in my eye" and that the sensation typically worsens through the day. This condition is caused by a decrease in the quality or quantity of the tear film, and treatment is directed at the underlying cause.

With decreased tear secretion, the patient may use artificial tears or ointments. Restasis (cyclosporine ophthalmic emulsion) helps to increase the eyes' natural ability to produce tears. In severe cases, closure of the lacrimal puncta may be necessary. Patients with dry eyes associated with dry mouth may have Sjögren's syndrome (see Chapter 64).

## STRABISMUS

**Strabismus** is a condition in which the patient cannot consistently focus two eyes simultaneously on the same object. One eye may deviate in *(esotropia)*, out *(exotropia)*, up *(hypertropia)*, or down *(hypotropia)*. Strabismus in the adult may be caused by thyroid disease, neuromuscular problems of the eye muscles, retinal detachment repair, or cerebral lesions. In the adult the primary complaint with strabismus is double vision.

## CORNEAL DISORDERS

### Corneal Scars

The cornea is an optically transparent tissue that allows light rays to enter the eye and focus on the retina, thus producing a visual image. Any wound (trauma, infection) to the cornea can cause it to become scarred and opacified, thus decreasing the normal transparency. The treatment for corneal scars is a corneal transplant.

### Keratoconus

*Keratoconus* is a noninflammatory, usually bilateral disease that has a familial tendency. Keratoconus usually appears during adolescence and slowly progresses between ages 20 and 60 years. The anterior cornea thins and protrudes forward, taking on a cone shape. The only symptom is blurred vision. The astigmatism may be corrected with glasses or rigid contact lenses.

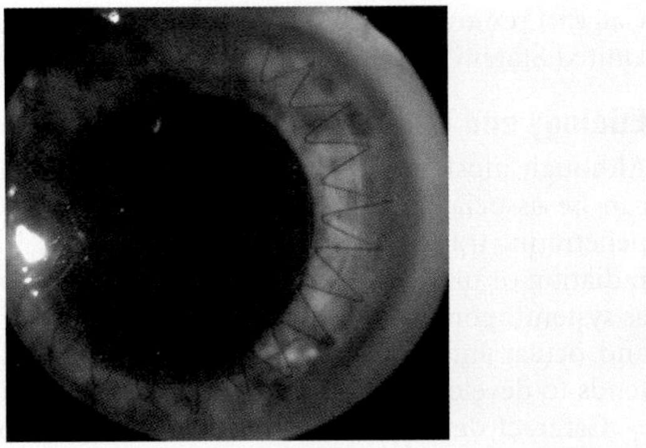

**FIG. 21-3** Sutures on a donated cornea after penetrating keratoplasty (corneal transplant). (Courtesy Cory J. Bosanko, OD, FAAO, Eye Centers of Tennessee, Crossville, Tenn.)

Intacs inserts are two clear plastic lenses surgically inserted on the cornea perimeter to reduce astigmatism and myopia. Intacs are generally used to delay the need for a corneal transplant when contact lenses or glasses no longer help a patient achieve adequate vision.

In keratoconus the cornea can perforate as central corneal thinning progresses. In advanced cases, a corneal transplant is indicated before the cornea perforates.

**Corneal Transplant.** Indications for corneal transplants (keratoplasty) are corneal scarring and keratoconus. Types of corneal transplants include penetrating (full thickness) corneal transplant and lamellar corneal transplant.

*Penetrating (full thickness) cornea transplant* involves transplanting all the layers of the cornea using a donor cornea. In this procedure, the ophthalmic surgeon removes the full thickness of the patient's cornea and replaces it with a donor cornea that is sutured into place (Fig. 21-3). Vision may not be restored for up to 12 months.

During a *lamellar cornea transplant*, only some layers of the cornea are replaced with the transplant. This can include the deepest layer, called the *endothelium* (posterior lamellar cornea transplant). Commonly performed versions of this procedure include Descemet's stripping endothelial keratoplasty (DSEK) or Descemet's membrane endothelial keratoplasty (DMEK). Lamellar transplants may be more appropriate than full penetrating transplants when the disease process is limited to only a portion of the cornea.

Approximately 40,000 corneal transplants are performed in the United States each year. The surgery is one of the fastest and safest of all tissue or organ transplant surgeries.[9] The time between the donor's death and the removal of the tissue should be as short as possible. The eye banks test donors for human immunodeficiency virus (HIV) and hepatitis B and C. The tissue is preserved in a special nutritive solution. Improved methods of tissue procurement and preservation, postoperative topical corticosteroids, and careful follow-up have decreased graft rejection. Matching the blood type of the donor and recipient may also improve the success rate.

# INTRAOCULAR DISORDERS

## CATARACT

A **cataract** is an opacity within the lens. The patient may have a cataract in one or both eyes. If cataracts are present in both eyes, one may affect the patient's vision more than the other.

Cataract removal is the most common surgical procedure in the United States.[10]

## Etiology and Pathophysiology

Although most cataracts are age related *(senile cataracts),* they can be associated with other factors. These include blunt or penetrating trauma, congenital factors such as maternal rubella, radiation or ultraviolet (UV) light exposure, certain drugs such as systemic corticosteroids or long-term topical corticosteroids, and ocular inflammation. The patient with diabetes mellitus tends to develop cataracts at a younger age.

Cataract development is mediated by a number of factors. In senile cataract formation altered metabolic processes within the lens cause an accumulation of water and alterations in the lens fiber structure. These changes affect lens transparency, causing vision changes.

## Clinical Manifestations and Diagnostic Studies

The patient with cataracts may complain of a decrease in vision, abnormal color perception, and glare. Glare is due to light scatter caused by the lens opacities, and it may be significantly worse at night when the pupil dilates. The visual decline is gradual, but the rate of cataract development varies from patient to patient.

Diagnosis is based on decreased visual acuity or other complaints of visual dysfunction. The opacity is directly observable by ophthalmoscopic or slit lamp microscopic examination. A totally opaque lens creates the appearance of a white pupil. Table 21-2 lists other diagnostic studies that may be helpful in evaluation of a cataract.

## Interprofessional Care

The presence of a cataract does not necessarily indicate a need for surgery. For many patients the diagnosis is made long before they actually decide to have surgery. Nonsurgical therapy may postpone the need for surgery. Interprofessional care for cataracts is presented in Table 21-2.

**TABLE 21-2 Interprofessional Care**

***Cataract***

| Diagnostic Assessment / Management | Acute Care: Surgical Therapy |
|---|---|
| **Diagnostic Assessment**<br>• History and physical examination<br>• Visual acuity measurement<br>• Ophthalmoscopy (direct and indirect)<br>• Slit lamp microscopy<br>• Glare testing, potential acuity testing in selected patients<br>• Keratometry and A-scan ultrasound (if surgery is planned)<br>• Other tests (e.g., visual field perimetry) to determine cause of visual loss<br><br>**Management**<br>***Nonsurgical***<br>• Change in glasses prescription<br>• Strong reading glasses or magnifiers<br>• Increased lighting<br>• Lifestyle adjustment | ***Preoperative***<br>• Mydriatic, cycloplegic agents<br>• Nonsteroidal antiinflammatory drugs<br>• Topical antibiotics<br>• Antianxiety medications<br><br>***Surgery***<br>• Removal of lens<br>• Phacoemulsification<br>• Extracapsular extraction<br>• Correction of surgical aphakia<br>• Intraocular lens implantation (most frequent type of correction)<br>• Contact lenses<br><br>***Postoperative***<br>• Topical antibiotic<br>• Topical corticosteroid or other antiinflammatory agent<br>• Mild analgesia if necessary<br>• Eye patch or shield and activity as prescribed by patient's surgeon |

**Nonsurgical Therapy.** Currently, no treatment is available to "cure" cataracts other than surgical removal. Often changing the patient's eyewear prescription can improve visual acuity, at least temporarily. Other visual aids, such as strong reading glasses or magnifiers of some type, may help the patient with near vision. Increasing the amount of light to read or accomplish other near-vision tasks is another useful measure. The patient may be willing to adjust his or her lifestyle to adjust to visual decline. For example, if glare makes it difficult to drive at night, a patient may elect to drive only during daylight hours or to have a family member drive at night. Sometimes informing and reassuring the patient about the disease process makes the patient comfortable about choosing nonsurgical measures, at least temporarily.

**Surgical Therapy.** When palliative measures no longer provide an acceptable level of visual function, the patient is an appropriate candidate for surgery. The patient's occupational needs and lifestyle changes are also factors affecting the decision to have surgery. In some instances, factors other than the patient's visual needs may influence the need for surgery. Lens-induced problems such as increased intraocular pressure (IOP) may require lens removal. Opacities may prevent the ophthalmologist from obtaining a clear view of the retina in the patient with diabetic retinopathy or other sight-threatening pathologic conditions. In those cases, the cataract may be removed to allow visualization of the retina and adequate management of the problem.

***Preoperative Phase.*** The patient's preoperative preparation should include an appropriate history and physical examination. Because almost all patients have local anesthesia, many physicians and surgical facilities do not require an extensive preoperative physical assessment. However, most patients with cataracts are older adults who may have several medical problems that should be evaluated and controlled before surgery. Almost all patients with cataracts are admitted to a surgical facility on an outpatient basis. The patient is normally admitted several hours before surgery to allow time for preoperative procedures.

The patient receives dilating drops and a nonsteroidal antiinflammatory eye drop to reduce inflammation (depends on ophthalmologist's preference). One type of drug used for dilation is a *mydriatic,* an α-adrenergic agonist that produces pupillary dilation by contraction of the iris dilator muscle. Another type of drug is a *cycloplegic,* an anticholinergic agent that produces paralysis of accommodation (cycloplegia) by blocking the effect of acetylcholine on the ciliary body muscles. Cycloplegics (tropicamide [Mydriacyl, Tropicacyl]) produce pupillary dilation (mydriasis) by blocking the effect of acetylcholine on the iris sphincter muscle. The patient may receive preoperative antianxiety medication.

**DRUG ALERT Cycloplegics and Mydriatics**
- Instruct patient to wear dark glasses to minimize photophobia.
- Monitor for signs of systemic toxicity (e.g., tachycardia, central nervous system [CNS] effects).

***Intraoperative Phase.*** Cataract extraction is an intraocular procedure using an operating microscope. The most common form of cataract surgery is *phacoemulsification.* In this procedure, a very small incision is made in the surface of the eye in or near the cornea. A thin ultrasound probe is inserted into the

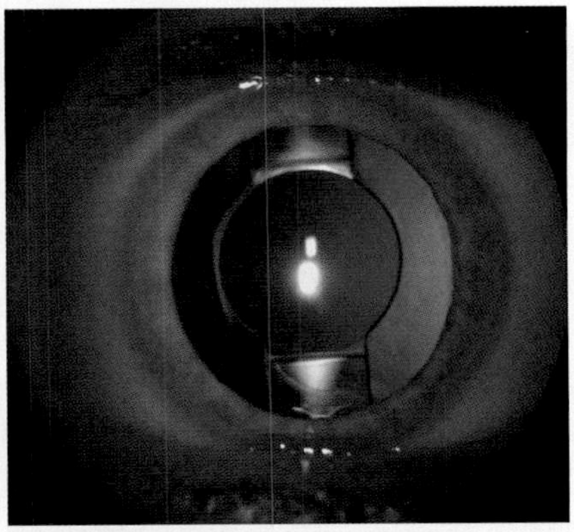

FIG. 21-4 Intraocular lens implant after cataract surgery. (Courtesy Cory J. Bosanko, OD, FAAO, Eye Centers of Tennessee, Crossville, Tenn.)

eye and ultrasonic vibrations are used to dissolve (phacoemulsify) the clouded lens into fragments. These pieces are then suctioned out through the same ultrasound probe. The small incisions are self-sealing and usually do not require sutures.

An *extracapsular cataract extraction procedure* is used mainly for very advanced cataracts where the lens is too dense to dissolve into fragments. This technique requires a larger incision so that the cataract can be removed in one piece without being fragmented inside the eye. This surgical technique requires sutures to close the larger wound, and visual recovery is often slower.

Almost all patients have an IOL implanted at the time of cataract extraction surgery (Fig. 21-4). The lens of choice is a posterior chamber lens that is implanted in the capsular bag behind the iris. At the end of the procedure, additional medications such as antibiotics and corticosteroids may be administered.

***Postoperative Phase.*** Unless complications occur, the patient is usually ready to go home as soon as the effects of sedative agents have worn off. Postoperative medications usually include antibiotic drops to prevent infection and corticosteroid drops to decrease the postoperative inflammatory response. Recommendations for postoperative activity restrictions and nighttime eye shielding vary based on the ophthalmologist's preference. Many still prefer that the patient avoid activities that increase the IOP, such as bending or stooping, coughing, or lifting.

During each postoperative examination the ophthalmologist measures the patient's visual acuity, checks anterior chamber depth, assesses corneal clarity, and measures intraocular pressure (IOP). Even on the operative day the patient's uncorrected visual acuity in the operative eye may be good. However, it is not unusual or indicative of any problem if the patient's visual acuity is reduced immediately after surgery.

The postoperative eye drops are gradually reduced in frequency and finally discontinued when the eye has healed. Multifocal IOL can correct for both near and far vision. Regardless of the type of IOL used, patients may still need glasses or contact lenses to achieve their best visual acuity.

## ❖ NURSING MANAGEMENT: CATARACTS

### ◆ Nursing Assessment

Assess the patient's distance and near visual acuity. If the patient is going to have surgery, especially note the visual acuity in the patient's unoperated eye. Use this information to determine how visually compromised the patient may be while the operative eye is healing. In addition, assess the psychosocial impact of the patient's visual disability and the level of knowledge regarding the disease process and therapeutic options. Postoperatively, assess the patient's level of comfort and ability to follow the postoperative regimen.

### ◆ Nursing Diagnoses

Nursing diagnoses for the patient with a cataract include, but are not limited to, the following:

- Self-care deficits *related to* visual deficit
- Anxiety *related to* lack of knowledge about the surgical and postoperative experience

### ◆ Planning

Preoperatively, the overall goals are that the patient with a cataract will (1) make informed decisions regarding therapeutic options and (2) experience minimal anxiety. Postoperatively, the overall goals are that the patient with a cataract will (1) understand and comply with postoperative therapy, (2) maintain an acceptable level of physical and emotional comfort, and (3) remain free of infection and other complications.

### ◆ Nursing Implementation

◆ **Health Promotion.** There are no proven measures to prevent cataract development. However, it is probably wise (and certainly does no harm) to suggest that the patient wear sunglasses, avoid extraneous or unnecessary radiation, and maintain appropriate intake of antioxidant vitamins (e.g., vitamins C and E) and good nutrition. Also provide information about vision enhancement techniques for the patient who chooses not to have surgery.

◆ **Acute Care.** Preoperatively, the patient with cataracts needs accurate information about the disease process and treatment options, especially because cataract surgery is considered an elective procedure. Be available to give the patient and family information to help them make an informed decision about appropriate treatment. For the patient who elects to have surgery, provide information, support, and reassurance about the surgical and postoperative experience to reduce or alleviate anxiety.

Photophobia is common when administering pupil dilation medications. Therefore decreasing the room lighting is helpful. These medications produce transient stinging and burning. Table 21-3 outlines patient and caregiver teaching after eye surgery.

If a patch is used, inform patients that they will not have depth perception until the patch is removed. This necessitates special considerations to avoid falls or other injuries. The patient with significant visual impairment in the unoperated eye requires more assistance while the operative eye is patched. Some patients may require 1 or 2 weeks for the visual acuity in the operated eye to reach an adequate level for most visual needs. These patients also need some special assistance until the vision improves.

After cataract surgery the patient usually experiences little or no pain but may have some scratchiness or blurriness in the operative eye. Mild analgesics are usually sufficient to relieve any pain. If the pain is intense, the patient should notify the surgeon because this may indicate hemorrhage, infection, or increased IOP. Also instruct the patient to notify the surgeon if there is increased or purulent drainage, increased redness, or any decrease in visual acuity. A nursing care plan for the patient

**TABLE 21-3 Patient & Caregiver Teaching**
***After Eye Surgery***

*Include the following information in the teaching plan for the patient and caregiver after eye surgery.*

- Proper hygiene and eye care techniques to ensure that medications, dressings, and/or surgical wound is not contaminated during eye care
- Signs and symptoms of infection and when and how to report these to allow for early recognition and treatment of possible infection
- Importance of complying with postoperative restrictions on head positioning, bending, coughing, and Valsalva maneuver to optimize visual outcomes and prevent increased intraocular pressure
- How to instill eye medications using aseptic techniques and adherence with prescribed eye medication routine to prevent infection
- How to monitor pain, take pain medication, and report pain not relieved by medication
- Importance of continued follow-up as recommended to maximize potential visual outcomes

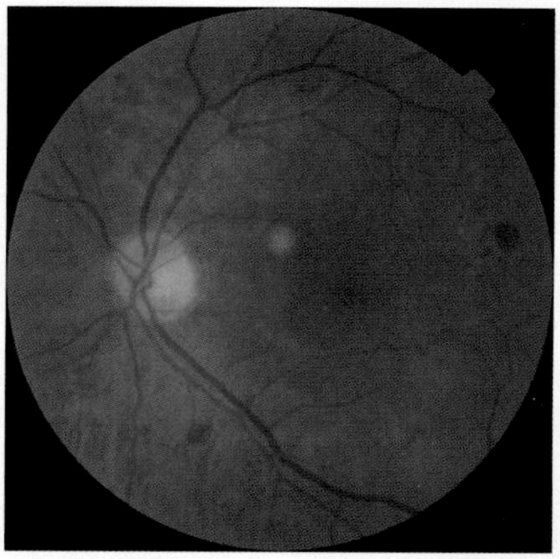

**FIG. 21-5** Diabetic retinopathy. Intraretinal dot or blot hemorrhages. (Courtesy Cory J. Bosanko, OD, FAAO, Eye Centers of Tennessee, Crossville, Tenn.)

after eye surgery (eNursing Care Plan 21-1) is available on the website for this chapter.

◆ **Ambulatory Care.** Patients with cataracts who have surgery remain in the surgical facility for only a few hours. The patient and caregiver are responsible for almost all postoperative care. Give them written and verbal instructions before discharge, including information about postoperative eye care, activity restrictions, medications, follow-up visit schedule, and signs and symptoms of possible complications. Include the patient's caregiver in the instructions because some patients may have difficulty with self-care activities, especially if the vision in the unoperated eye is poor. Provide an opportunity for the patient and caregiver to perform return demonstrations of any self-care activities.

Most patients experience little visual impairment after surgery. IOL implants provide immediate visual rehabilitation, and many patients achieve a usable level of visual acuity within a few days after surgery.

A few patients may have significant visual impairment postoperatively. These include patients who do not have an IOL implanted at the time of surgery, those who require several weeks to achieve a usable level of visual acuity following surgery, or those with poor vision in their unoperated eye. For those patients the time between surgery and receiving glasses or contacts can be a period of significant visual disability. Suggest ways the patient and caregiver can modify activities and the environment to maintain an adequate level of safe functioning. Suggestions may include getting assistance with steps, removing area rugs and other potential obstacles, preparing meals for freezing before surgery, or obtaining audio books for diversion until visual acuity improves.

### ◆ Evaluation

The overall expected outcomes are that the patient following cataract surgery will

- Have improved vision
- Be better able to take care of self
- Have minimal to no pain
- Be optimistic about expected outcomes

### Gerontologic Considerations: Cataracts

Most patients with cataracts are older. When the older patient is visually impaired, even temporarily, the patient may experience a loss of independence, lack of control over her or his life, and a significant change in self-perception. Societal devaluation of the older individual complicates these experiences. The older patient often needs emotional support and encouragement, as well as specific suggestions to allow a maximum level of independent function. Assure the older patient that cataract surgery can be accomplished safely and comfortably with minimal sedation.

## RETINOPATHY

**Retinopathy** is a process of microvascular damage to the retina. It can develop slowly or rapidly and lead to blurred vision and progressive vision loss. Retinopathy occurs most often in adults with diabetes mellitus or hypertension.

*Diabetic retinopathy* is a common complication of diabetes mellitus, especially in patients with long-standing uncontrolled diabetes.[11] *Nonproliferative retinopathy* is the most common form of diabetic retinopathy and is characterized by capillary microaneurysms, retinal swelling, and hard exudates. Macular edema represents a worsening of the retinopathy as plasma leaks from macular blood vessels. As capillary walls weaken, they can rupture, leading to intraretinal "dot or blot" hemorrhaging (Fig. 21-5). A severe loss in central vision can result. As the disease advances, *proliferative retinopathy* may occur. New blood vessels grow, but they are abnormal, fragile, and predisposed to leak, thus causing severe vision loss. (Diagnosis and treatment of diabetic retinopathy are discussed in Chapter 48.)

*Hypertensive retinopathy* is caused by high BP creating blockages in retinal blood vessels. (Hypertension is discussed in Chapter 32.) These changes may not initially affect a person's vision. On a routine eye examination, retinal hemorrhages, anoxic cotton-wool spots, and macular swelling can be noted. Sustained, severe hypertension can cause sudden visual loss from swelling of the optic disc and nerve *(papilledema)*. Treatment, which may be an emergency, focuses on lowering the BP. Normal vision is restored in most patients with treatment of the underlying cause of the hypertension.

## RETINAL DETACHMENT

A **retinal detachment** is a separation of the sensory retina and the underlying pigment epithelium, with fluid accumulation between the two layers. In the patient with no other risk factors who has had a retinal detachment in one eye, the risk of detachment in the second eye is as high as 25%.[12] Almost all patients with an untreated, symptomatic retinal detachment become blind in the involved eye.

### Etiology and Pathophysiology

Retinal detachment has many causes, the most common of which is a retinal break. *Retinal breaks* are an interruption in the full thickness of the retinal tissue, and they can be classified as tears or holes. *Retinal holes* are atrophic retinal breaks that occur spontaneously. *Retinal tears* can occur as the vitreous humor shrinks during aging and pulls on the retina. The retina tears when the traction force exceeds the strength of the retina. Once the retina has a break, liquid vitreous can enter the subretinal space between the sensory layer and the retinal pigment epithelium layer, causing a *rhegmatogenous* retinal detachment. Risk factors for retinal detachment are listed in Table 21-4.

### Clinical Manifestations and Diagnostic Studies

Patients with a detaching retina describe symptoms that include *photopsia* (light flashes); floaters; and a "cobweb," "hairnet," or ring in the field of vision. Once the retina has detached, the patient describes a painless loss of peripheral or central vision, "like a curtain" coming across the field of vision.

The area of visual loss corresponds inversely to the area of detachment. For example, if the retinal detachment involves the superior retina, the defect is seen in the inferior visual field. If the detachment is small or develops slowly, the patient may not be aware of a visual problem.

Visual acuity measurements should be the first diagnostic procedure with any complaint of vision loss (Table 21-5). The retinal detachment can be directly visualized using direct and indirect ophthalmoscopy or slit lamp microscopy in conjunction with a special lens to view the far periphery of the retina.

**TABLE 21-4 Risk Factors for Retinal Detachment**

- Increasing age
- Severe myopia
- Eye trauma
- Cataract surgery
- Family or personal history of retinal detachment

Source: National Eye Institute, National Institutes of Health: Retinal detachment. Retrieved from *www.nei.nih.gov/health/retinaldetach*.

**TABLE 21-5 Interprofessional Care**
***Retinal Detachment***

|  |  |
|---|---|
| **Diagnostic Assessment**<br>• History and physical examination<br>• Visual acuity measurement<br>• Ophthalmoscopy (direct and indirect)<br>• Slit lamp microscopy<br>• Ultrasound if cornea, lens, or vitreous is hazy or opaque | ***Surgery***<br>• Laser photocoagulation<br>• Cryopexy<br>• Scleral buckling procedure<br>• Vitrectomy<br>• Intravitreal bubble |
| **Management**<br>***Preoperative***<br>• Mydriatic, cycloplegic agents<br>• Photocoagulation of retinal break that has not progressed to detachment | ***Postoperative***<br>• Topical antibiotic<br>• Topical corticosteroid<br>• Analgesia<br>• Mydriatics<br>• Positioning and activity as prescribed by patient's surgeon |

Ultrasound may be useful in identifying a retinal detachment if the retina cannot be directly visualized (e.g., when the cornea, lens, or vitreous is hazy or opaque).

### Interprofessional Care

Some retinal breaks are not likely to progress to detachment. In these situations the ophthalmologist simply monitors the patient, giving precise information about the warning signs and symptoms of impending detachment and instructing the patient to seek immediate evaluation if any of those signs or symptoms is recognized. The ophthalmologist usually refers the patient with a detachment to a retinal specialist. Treatment objectives are to seal any retinal breaks and relieve inward traction on the retina. Several techniques are used to accomplish these objectives.

#### Surgical Therapy

***Laser Photocoagulation and Cryopexy.*** These techniques seal retinal breaks by creating an inflammatory reaction that causes a chorioretinal adhesion or scar. *Laser photocoagulation* involves using an intense, precisely focused light beam to create an inflammatory reaction. The light is directed at the area of the retinal break. *Cryopexy* involves freezing (cryotherapy) the retinal break by placing a probe on the ocular surface at the location of the break. The probe is activated with compressed nitrous oxide gas that temporarily freezes the break. The freeze thaw reaction creates scarring in the area that will seal the break.

For retinal breaks accompanied by significant detachment, the retinal specialist may use photocoagulation or cryopexy intraoperatively in conjunction with scleral buckling. Tears or holes without accompanying retinal detachment may be treated prophylactically with laser photocoagulation or cryopexy if there is a high risk of progression to a retinal detachment. When used alone, laser photocoagulation or cryopexy therapy is an outpatient procedure that usually requires only topical anesthesia. The patient may experience minimal adverse symptoms during or after the procedure.

***Scleral Buckling.*** *Scleral buckling* is an extraocular surgical procedure that involves indenting the globe so that the pigment epithelium, choroid, and sclera move toward the detached retina. The retinal surgeon sutures a silicone implant against the sclera, causing the sclera to buckle inward. The surgeon may place an encircling band over the implant if there are multiple retinal breaks, if suspected breaks cannot be located, or if there is widespread inward traction on the retina (Fig. 21-6). If present, subretinal fluid may be drained by inserting a small-gauge needle to facilitate contact between the retina and buckled sclera. Scleral buckling is usually done as an outpatient procedure.

***Intraocular Procedures.*** In addition to the extraocular procedures described, retinal surgeons may also use one or more intraocular procedures in treating some retinal detachments. *Pneumatic retinopexy* is the intravitreal injection of a gas to form a temporary bubble in the vitreous that closes retinal breaks and provides apposition of the separated retinal layers. Because the intravitreal bubble is temporary, this technique is combined with laser photocoagulation or cryopexy. The patient with an intravitreal bubble must position the head so that the bubble is in contact with the retinal break. The patient may need to maintain this position as much as possible for up to several weeks.

*Vitrectomy* (surgical removal of the vitreous) may be used to relieve traction on the retina, especially when the traction results from proliferative diabetic retinopathy. Vitrectomy may

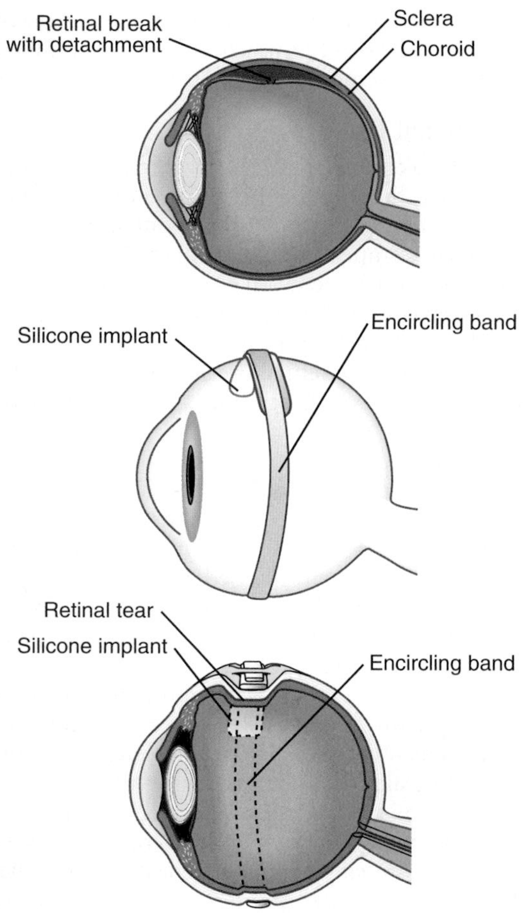


**FIG. 21-6** Retinal break with detachment and surgical repair by scleral buckling technique.

be combined with scleral buckling to provide a dual effect in relieving traction.

***Postoperative Considerations.*** Visual prognosis varies, depending on the extent, length, and area of detachment. Postoperatively the patient may be on bed rest and may require special positioning to maintain proper position of an intravitreal bubble. The patient may need multiple topical medications, including antibiotics, antiinflammatory agents, or dilating agents. The level of activity restriction after retinal detachment surgery varies greatly. Verify the prescribed level of activity with each patient's surgeon, and help the patient plan for any necessary assistance related to activity restrictions.

In most cases, retinal detachment is an urgent situation, and the patient is suddenly confronted with the need for surgery. The patient needs emotional support, especially during the immediate preoperative period when preparations for surgery can lead to additional anxiety. When the patient experiences postoperative pain, administer prescribed pain medications and teach the patient to take the medication as necessary after discharge. The patient may go home within a few hours of surgery or may remain in the hospital for several days, depending on the surgeon and type of repair.

Discharge planning and teaching are important and should begin as early as possible because the patient does not remain hospitalized long. Patient and caregiver teaching after eye surgery is discussed in Table 21-5. Because the patient is at increased risk for retinal detachment in the other eye, teach the patient the signs and symptoms of retinal detachment. Also promote the use of proper protective eyewear to help avoid ocular damage related to trauma.

## AGE-RELATED MACULAR DEGENERATION

**Age-related macular degeneration** (AMD) is the most common cause of irreversible central vision loss in people over age 60 in the United States. AMD is divided into two forms: dry (nonexudative) and wet (exudative). People with *dry AMD,* which is the more common form (90% of all cases), often notice that close vision tasks are becoming more difficult. In this form of AMD the macular cells start to atrophy, leading to a slowly progressive and painless vision loss.

*Wet AMD* is the more severe form. Wet AMD accounts for the majority of the cases of AMD-related blindness. Wet AMD has a more rapid onset of vision loss and is characterized by the development of abnormal blood vessels in or near the macula. Patients with wet AMD had dry AMD first.

### Etiology and Pathophysiology

AMD is related to retinal aging. Genetic factors also play a major role, and family history is a major risk factor for AMD.[13] Increased risk factors for AMD include white ethnicity, family history of AMD, chronic inflammation conditions, smoking, and hypertension.

Nutritional factors may play a role in the progression of AMD. A dietary supplement of vitamin C, vitamin E, lutein, zeaxanthin, and zinc decreases the progression of advanced AMD but has no effect on people with minimal AMD or those with no evidence of AMD. Eating lots of dark green, leafy vegetables containing lutein (e.g., kale and spinach) may help reduce the risk of AMD (*www.nei.nih.gov/health/maculardegen/armd_facts.asp*).

The dry form of AMD starts with the abnormal accumulation of yellowish extracellular deposits called *drusen* in the retinal pigment epithelium. Over time atrophy and degeneration of macular cells occur. Wet AMD is characterized by the growth of new blood vessels in an abnormal location in the retinal epithelium. As the new blood vessels grow, they leak fluid and can bleed, causing scar tissue to gradually form. Acute vision loss may occur from either the dry or wet forms of AMD.

### Clinical Manifestations and Diagnostic Studies

The patient may complain of blurred and darkened vision, *scotomas* (blind spots in the visual field), and *metamorphopsia* (distortion of vision). If patients have only one eye affected, they may not notice early changes in their vision. In addition to visual acuity measurement, the primary diagnostic procedure is ophthalmoscopy. The examiner looks for drusen and other fundus changes associated with AMD. The Amsler grid test may help define the involved area, and it provides a baseline for future comparison (see Fig. 20-6). Fundus photography and IV angiography with fluorescein and/or indocyanine green dyes may help to further determine the extent and type of AMD. Retinal anatomy can also be analyzed using optical coherence tomography (OCT) or scanning laser ophthalmoscopy.

### Interprofessional Care

Visual prognosis varies greatly for people with AMD. Limited treatment options for patients with wet AMD include several medications that are injected directly into the vitreous cavity. Ranibizumab (Lucentis), bevacizumab (Avastin), aflibercept

(Eylea), and pegaptanib (Macugen) are selective inhibitors of endothelial growth factor, thus helping to slow vision loss in wet AMD. Side effects can include blurred vision, eye irritation, eye pain, and photosensitivity. Injections are given at 4- to 6-week intervals, depending on treatment response. Disease stability is determined by OCT, which allows the physician to identify pathology in the macula. The findings determine the need for continued intravitreal injections.

*Photodynamic therapy* (PDT) uses verteporfin (Visudyne) IV and a "cold" laser to excite the dye. The PDT procedure is used in wet AMD and damages the abnormal blood vessels in wet AMD. Verteporfin is a photosensitizing drug that becomes active when exposed to the low-level laser light wave. Until the drug is completely excreted by the body, it can be activated by exposure to sunlight or other high-intensity light such as halogen. Therefore caution patients to avoid direct exposure to sunlight and other intense forms of light for 5 days after treatment. After receiving therapy, patients must be completely covered because any exposure of the skin to sunlight could activate the drug in that area, resulting in a chemical burn.

People at risk for developing advanced AMD should consider supplements of vitamins and minerals (in consultation with their HCP). The cessation of smoking may also help in halting the progression of dry AMD to a more advanced stage.

Many patients with low-vision assistive devices can continue reading and retain a license to drive during the daytime and at lowered speeds. The permanent loss of central vision has significant psychosocial implications for nursing care. Management of the patient with visual impairment is discussed on p. 369 and is appropriate for the patient with AMD. Avoid giving the impression that "nothing can be done" about the problem when caring for the patient with AMD. Although therapy may not recover lost vision, much can be done to augment the remaining vision.

## GLAUCOMA

**Glaucoma** is a group of disorders characterized by increased IOP and the consequences of elevated pressure, optic nerve atrophy, and peripheral visual field loss. Glaucoma is the second leading cause of permanent blindness in the United States and the leading cause of blindness among African Americans.[14] Many people with glaucoma are unaware of their condition. The incidence of glaucoma increases with age. Blindness from glaucoma is largely preventable with early detection and appropriate treatment. Genetic factors have been identified in some types of glaucoma.[13]

### Etiology and Pathophysiology

A proper balance between the rate of aqueous production (referred to as *inflow*) and the rate of aqueous reabsorption (referred to as *outflow*) is essential to maintain the IOP within normal limits. The place where the outflow occurs is called the *angle* because it is the angle where the iris meets the cornea. When the rate of inflow is greater than the rate of outflow, IOP can increase above the normal limits. If IOP remains elevated, permanent vision loss may occur.

*Primary open-angle glaucoma* (POAG) is the most common type of glaucoma. In POAG the outflow of aqueous humor is decreased in the trabecular meshwork. The drainage channels become clogged, like a clogged kitchen sink. Damage to the optic nerve can then result.

*Primary angle-closure glaucoma* (PACG) is due to a reduction in the outflow of aqueous humor that results from angle closure. Usually this is caused by the lens bulging forward as a result of the aging process. Angle closure may also occur as a result of pupil dilation in the patient with anatomically narrow angles. An acute attack may be precipitated by situations in which the pupil remains partially dilated long enough to cause an acute and significant rise in the IOP. This may occur because of drug-induced mydriasis, emotional excitement, or darkness. Drug-induced mydriasis may occur not only from topical ophthalmic preparations but also from many systemic medications (both prescription and over-the-counter [OTC] drugs). Check drug records and documentation before administering medications to the patient with angle-closure glaucoma, and instruct the patient not to take any mydriatic medications.

### Clinical Manifestations

POAG develops slowly and without symptoms of pain or pressure. The patient usually does not notice the gradual visual field loss until peripheral vision has been severely compromised. Eventually the patient with untreated glaucoma has "tunnel vision," in which only a small center field can be seen and all peripheral vision is absent.

Acute angle-closure glaucoma causes definite symptoms, including sudden, excruciating pain in or around the eye. This is often accompanied by nausea and vomiting. Visual symptoms include seeing colored halos around lights, blurred vision, and ocular redness.

Manifestations of subacute or chronic angle-closure glaucoma appear more gradually. The patient who has had a previous, unrecognized episode of subacute angle-closure glaucoma may report a history of blurred vision, seeing colored halos around lights, ocular redness, or eye or brow pain.

### Diagnostic Studies

IOP is usually elevated in glaucoma (normal is 10 to 21 mm Hg). In the patient with elevated pressures, the ophthalmologist usually repeats the measurements over time to verify the elevation. In open-angle glaucoma, IOP is usually between 22 and 32 mm Hg. In acute angle-closure glaucoma, IOP may be more than 50 mm Hg.

In open-angle glaucoma, slit lamp microscopy reveals a normal angle. In angle-closure glaucoma the examiner may note a markedly narrow or flat anterior chamber angle, an edematous cornea, a fixed and moderately dilated pupil, and ciliary injection (hyperemia of the ciliary blood vessels produces a red color).

Measures of peripheral and central vision provide additional diagnostic information. Whereas central acuity may remain 20/20 even in the presence of severe peripheral visual field loss, visual field perimetry may reveal subtle changes in the peripheral vision early in the disease process, long before actual scotomas develop. In acute angle-closure glaucoma, central visual acuity is reduced if the patient has corneal edema, and the visual fields may be markedly decreased. As glaucoma progresses, *optic disc cupping* may be one of the first signs of chronic open-angle glaucoma. The optic disc becomes wider, deeper, and paler (light gray or white), which is visible with direct or indirect ophthalmoscopy (Fig. 21-7).

### Interprofessional Care

The primary focus of glaucoma therapy is to keep the IOP low enough to prevent the patient from developing optic nerve

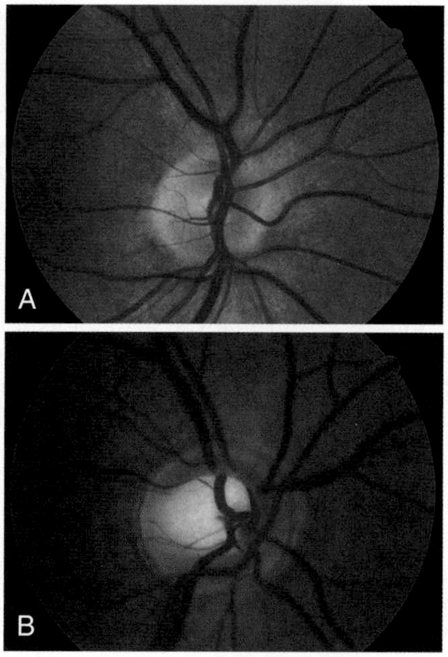

FIG. 21-7 **A,** In the normal eye the optic cup is pink with little cupping. **B,** In glaucoma the optic cup is bleached and optic cupping is present. (Note the appearance of the retinal vessels, which travel over the edge of the optic cup and appear to dip into it.)

**TABLE 21-6 Interprofessional Care**

***Glaucoma***

| | |
|---|---|
| **Diagnostic Assessment**<br>• History and physical examination<br>• Visual acuity measurement<br>• Tonometry<br>• Ophthalmoscopy (direct and indirect)<br>• Slit lamp microscopy<br>• Gonioscopy<br>• Visual field perimetry<br><br>**Management**<br>***Chronic Open-Angle Glaucoma***<br>*Drug Therapy* (Table 21-7)<br>• β-Adrenergic blockers<br>• α-Adrenergic agonists<br>• Cholinergic agents (miotics)<br>• Carbonic anhydrase inhibitors | *Surgical Therapy*<br>• Argon laser trabeculoplasty (ALT)<br>• Trabeculectomy with or without filtering implant<br><br>***Acute Angle-Closure Glaucoma***<br>• Topical cholinergic agent<br>• Hyperosmotic agent<br>• Laser peripheral iridotomy<br>• Surgical iridectomy |

damage. Therapy varies with the type of glaucoma. The diagnostic and interprofessional care of glaucoma is summarized in Table 21-6.

**Chronic Open-Angle Glaucoma.** Initial treatment in chronic open-angle glaucoma is with drugs (Table 21-7). The patient must understand that continued treatment and supervision are necessary because the drugs control, but do not cure, glaucoma.

*Argon laser trabeculoplasty* (ALT) is a noninvasive option to lower IOP when medications are not successful or when the patient either cannot or will not use the drug therapy as recommended. ALT is an outpatient procedure that requires only topical anesthetic. The laser stimulates scarring and contraction of the trabecular meshwork, which opens the outflow channels. ALT reduces IOP most of the time. The patient uses topical corticosteroids for 3 to 5 days after the procedure. The most common postoperative complication is an acute rise in IOP. The ophthalmologist examines the patient 1 week and again at 4 to 6 weeks after surgery.

Filtration surgery, also called a *trabeculectomy,* may be indicated if medical management and laser therapy are not successful.

**Acute Angle-Closure Glaucoma.** Acute angle-closure glaucoma is an ocular emergency that requires immediate intervention. Miotics (Table 21-7) and oral or IV hyperosmotic agents, including glycerin liquid (Ophthalgan), isosorbide solution (Ismotic), and mannitol solution (Osmitrol), are usually successful in immediately lowering the IOP. A laser peripheral iridotomy or surgical iridectomy is necessary for long-term treatment and prevention of subsequent episodes. These procedures allow the aqueous humor to flow through a newly created opening in the iris and into normal outflow channels. One of these procedures may also be performed on the other eye as a precaution because many patients often experience an acute attack in the other eye.

**DRUG ALERT Miotics**
- Warn patients about decreased visual acuity, especially in dim light.

## NURSING MANAGEMENT: GLAUCOMA

### Nursing Assessment

Because glaucoma is a chronic condition requiring long-term management, assess the patient's ability to understand and adhere to the rationale and regimen of the prescribed therapy. In addition, assess the patient's psychologic reaction to the diagnosis of a potentially sight-threatening chronic disorder. Include the patient's caregiver in the assessment process because the chronic nature of this disorder affects the family in many ways. Some families may become the primary care providers, such as eye drop administration, if the patient is unwilling or unable to accomplish these self-care activities.

### Nursing Diagnoses

Nursing diagnoses for the patient with glaucoma include, but are not limited to, the following:

- Risk for injury *related to* visual acuity deficits
- Self-care deficits *related to* visual acuity deficits
- Acute pain *related to* pathophysiologic process and surgical correction
- Noncompliance *related to* the inconvenience and side effects of glaucoma medications

### Planning

The overall goals are that the patient with glaucoma will (1) have no progression of visual impairment, (2) understand the disease process and rationale for therapy, (3) comply with all aspects of therapy (including medication administration and follow-up care), and (4) have no postoperative complications.

### Nursing Implementation

**Health Promotion.** Loss of vision as a result of glaucoma is a preventable problem. Teach the patient and caregiver about the risk of glaucoma and that it increases with age. Stress the importance of early detection and treatment in preventing visual impairment. A comprehensive ophthalmic examination is important in identifying people with glaucoma or those at risk of developing glaucoma. The current recommendation is for an ophthalmologic examination every 2 to 4 years for people between ages 40 and

## TABLE 21-7 Drug Therapy

### *Acute and Chronic Glaucoma*

| Drug | Action | Side Effects | Nursing Considerations |
|---|---|---|---|
| **β-Adrenergic Blockers** | | | |
| betaxolol (Betoptic) | $\beta_1$ cardioselective blocker. ↓ IOP, ↓ aqueous humor production | Transient discomfort. Systemic reactions rarely reported but include bradycardia, heart block, pulmonary distress, headache, depression | Topical drugs. Minimal effect on pulmonary and cardiovascular parameters. Contraindicated in patient with bradycardia, cardiogenic shock, or overt cardiac failure. Systemic absorption can have additive effect with systemic $\beta_1$-blocking agents. |
| levobunolol (Betagan)<br>timolol maleate (Timoptic, Istalol) | $\beta_1$ and $\beta_2$ noncardioselective blockers. ↓ IOP, ↓ aqueous humor production | Transient ocular discomfort, blurred vision, photophobia, bradycardia, decreased BP, bronchospasm, headache, depression | Topical drops. Same as betaxolol. These noncardioselective $\beta_2$-blockers are also contraindicated in patients with asthma or COPD. |
| **α-Adrenergic Agonists** | | | |
| dipivefrin (Propine) | α- and β-adrenergic agonist. Converted to epinephrine inside the eye. ↓ aqueous humor production, enhances outflow facility | Ocular discomfort and redness, tachycardia, hypertension | Topical drops. Contraindicated in patient with narrow-angle glaucoma. Teach punctal occlusion if patient at risk of systemic reactions. |
| epinephrine | Same as dipivefrin | Same as dipivefrin, but can be more pronounced | Topical drops. Same as dipivefrin |
| apraclonidine (Iopidine)<br>brimonidine | α-Adrenergic agonists. ↓ aqueous humor production | Ocular redness. Irregular heart rate | Topical drops. Used to control or prevent acute postlaser IOP rise (used before and immediately after ALT and iridotomy, Nd:YAG laser capsulotomy). Teach patient at risk of systemic reactions to occlude puncta. |
| latanoprost (Xalatan)<br>travoprost<br>bimatoprost (Lumigan) | Prostaglandin F analogs | Increased brown iris pigmentation, ocular discomfort and redness, dryness, itching, and foreign body sensation | Topical drops. Teach patient to not exceed 1 drop per evening. Have patient remove contact lens 15 min before instilling. |
| **Cholinergic Agents (Miotics)** | | | |
| carbachol (Miostat, Isopto Carbachol) | Parasympathomimetic. Stimulates iris sphincter contraction, causing miosis and opening of trabecular meshwork, facilitating aqueous outflow. Also partially inhibits cholinesterase | Transient ocular discomfort, headache, blurred vision, decreased adaptation to the dark, syncope, salivation, dysrhythmias, vomiting, diarrhea, hypotension | Topical drops. Caution patient about ↓ visual acuity caused by miosis, particularly in dim light. |
| pilocarpine (Isopto Carpine, Pilocar) | Parasympathomimetic. Stimulates iris sphincter contraction, causing miosis and opening of trabecular meshwork, facilitating aqueous humor outflow | Same as carbachol | Topical drops. Same as carbachol |
| **Carbonic Anhydrase Inhibitors** | | | |
| ***Systemic*** | | | |
| acetazolamide (Diamox)<br>dichlorphenamide (Daranide)<br>methazolamide | ↓ Aqueous humor production | Paresthesias, especially "tingling" in extremities. Hearing dysfunction or tinnitus. Loss of appetite, taste alteration, GI disturbances. Drowsiness, confusion | Oral nonbacteriostatic sulfonamides. Anaphylaxis and other sulfa-type allergic reactions may occur in patient allergic to sulfa. Diuretic effect can ↓ electrolyte levels. Should not be given to patient on high-dose aspirin therapy |
| ***Topical*** | | | |
| brinzolamide (Azopt)<br>dorzolamide (Trusopt) | — | Transient stinging, blurred vision, redness | Same as above |

*ALT,* Argon laser trabeculoplasty; *IOP,* intraocular pressure.

64 years, and every 1 to 2 years for people age 65 years or older. African Americans in every age category should have examinations more often because of the increased incidence and more aggressive course of glaucoma in these individuals.[13]

◆ **Acute Care.** Acute nursing interventions are directed primarily toward the patient with acute angle-closure glaucoma and the surgical patient. The patient with acute angle-closure glaucoma requires immediate medication to lower the IOP. It must be administered in a timely and appropriate manner according to the ophthalmologist's prescription. Most surgical procedures for glaucoma are outpatient procedures. The patient needs postoperative instructions and may require nursing measures to relieve discomfort related to the procedure. Patient and caregiver teaching after eye surgery is discussed in Table 21-3.

◆ **Ambulatory Care.** Because of the chronic nature of glaucoma, remind the patient to follow the therapeutic regimen and follow-up recommendations prescribed by the ophthalmologist. Provide accurate information about the disease process and treatment options, including the rationale underlying each option. In addition, the patient needs information about the purpose, frequency, and technique for administration of antiglaucoma drugs. Encourage adherence by helping the patient identify the most convenient and appropriate times for medication administration or advocating a change in therapy if the patient reports unacceptable side effects.

### ◆ Evaluation

The overall expected outcomes are that the patient with glaucoma will

- Have no further loss of vision
- Adhere to the recommended therapy
- Safely function within own environment
- Obtain relief from pain associated with the disease and surgery

### Gerontologic Considerations: Glaucoma

Many older patients with glaucoma have systemic illnesses or take systemic medications that may affect their therapy. In particular, the patient using a β-adrenergic blocking glaucoma agent may experience an additive effect if a systemic β-adrenergic blocking drug is also being taken. All β-adrenergic blocking glaucoma agents are contraindicated in the patient with bradycardia, heart block greater than first-degree heart block, cardiogenic shock, and overt cardiac failure. The noncardioselective β-adrenergic blocking glaucoma agents are also contraindicated in the patient with chronic obstructive pulmonary disease (COPD) or asthma. The hyperosmolar agents may precipitate heart failure or pulmonary edema in the susceptible patient. The older patient on high-dose aspirin therapy for rheumatoid arthritis should not take carbonic anhydrase inhibitors. The α-adrenergic agonists can cause tachycardia or hypertension, which may have serious consequences in the older patient. Teach the older patient to occlude the puncta to limit the systemic absorption of glaucoma medications.

## INTRAOCULAR INFLAMMATION AND INFECTION

The term *uveitis* is used to describe inflammation of the uveal tract, retina, vitreous body, or optic nerve. This inflammation may be caused by bacteria, viruses, fungi, or parasites. *Cytomegalovirus retinitis* (CMV retinitis) is an opportunistic infection that occurs in patients with acquired immunodeficiency syndrome (AIDS) and in other immunosuppressed patients. The etiology of sterile intraocular inflammation includes autoimmune disorders, AIDS, malignancies, or those disorders associated with systemic diseases such as inflammatory bowel disease. Pain and photophobia are common symptoms.

*Endophthalmitis* is an extensive intraocular inflammation of the vitreous cavity. Bacteria, viruses, fungi, or parasites can induce this serious inflammatory response. The mechanism of infection may be endogenous, in which the infecting agent arrives at the eye through the bloodstream, or exogenous, in which the infecting agent is introduced through a surgical wound or a penetrating injury. Although rare, endophthalmitis is a devastating complication of intraocular surgery or penetrating ocular injury. It can lead to irreversible blindness within hours or days. Manifestations include ocular pain, photophobia, decreased visual acuity, headaches, reddened and swollen conjunctiva, and corneal edema.

Treatment of intraocular inflammation depends on the underlying cause. Intraocular infections require antimicrobial agents, which may be delivered topically, subconjunctivally, intravitreally, systemically, or in some combination. Sterile inflammatory responses require antiinflammatory medications such as corticosteroids. The patient with intraocular inflammation is usually uncomfortable and may be noticeably anxious and frightened. Provide accurate information and emotional support to the patient and family. In severe cases, enucleation may be necessary. When the patient has lost visual function or even the entire eye, the patient will grieve the loss. Your role includes helping the patient through the grieving process.

## OCULAR TUMORS

Benign and malignant tumors can occur in many areas of the eye, including the conjunctiva, retina, and orbit.[15] Malignancies of the eyelid include basal cell and squamous cell carcinomas (see Chapter 23).

*Uveal melanoma* is a cancerous neoplasm of the iris, choroid, or ciliary body. It is more frequently found in light-skinned people over age 60 with chronic UV exposure. Genetic factors may also increase a person's risk.[16] Uveal melanoma can arise from preexisting nevi in the eye. Tumors may be asymptomatic or associated with vision loss depending on their size and location and presence of hemorrhage and retinal detachment. As with other cancers, cancer stage and cell type are important variables in the patient's prognosis. Diagnostic testing may include ultrasound, MRI, and fine-needle aspiration biopsy. Uveal melanoma commonly appears as a dome-shaped, well-circumscribed, solid brown to golden pigment in the iris, choroid, or ciliary body (Fig. 21-8). Many patients do not lose their eye, and some may experience good vision after treatment in the affected eye.

Depending on the status of the involved eye, treatment options can include enucleation, radiation therapy (brachytherapy), external beam radiation, transpupillary photocoagulation, eye wall resection, and exenteration.

## ENUCLEATION

**Enucleation** is the removal of the eye. The primary indication for enucleation is a blind, painful eye. This may result from glaucoma, infection, or trauma. Enucleation may also be indicated in ocular malignancies. The surgical procedure includes severing the extraocular muscles close to their insertion on the globe, inserting an implant to maintain the intraorbital anatomy, and suturing the ends of the extraocular muscles over the

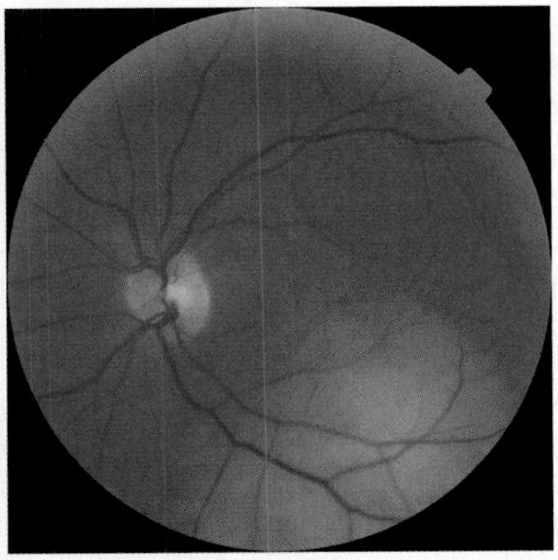

**FIG. 21-8** Uveal melanoma. A large tumor in the choroid, the most common location in the eye for melanoma. (Courtesy Cory J. Bosanko, OD, FAAO, Eye Centers of Tennessee, Crossville, Tenn.)

implant. The conjunctiva covers the joined muscles, and a clear conformer is placed over the conjunctiva until the permanent prosthesis is fitted. A pressure dressing helps prevent postoperative bleeding.

Postoperatively, observe the patient for signs of complications, including excessive bleeding or swelling, increased pain, displacement of the implant, or temperature elevation. Patient teaching should include the instillation of topical ointments or drops and wound cleansing. Instruct the patient in the method of inserting the conformer into the socket in case it falls out. The patient is often devastated by the loss of an eye, even when enucleation occurs after a lengthy period of painful blindness. Recognize and validate the patient's emotional response and provide support to the patient and family.

Approximately 6 weeks after surgery the wound is sufficiently healed for the permanent prosthesis. The prosthesis is fitted by an ocularist and designed to match the remaining eye. Teach the patient how to remove, cleanse, and insert the prosthesis. Special polishing is required periodically to remove dried protein secretions.

## OCULAR MANIFESTATIONS OF SYSTEMIC DISEASES

Many systemic diseases have significant ocular manifestations. Ocular signs and symptoms may be the first finding or complaint in the patient with a systemic disease. One example is the patient with undiagnosed diabetes who seeks ophthalmic care for blurred vision. A careful history and examination of the patient can reveal that the underlying cause of the blurred vision is lens swelling caused by hyperglycemia. Another example is the patient who seeks care for a conjunctival lesion. The ophthalmologist may be the first health care professional to make the diagnosis of AIDS based on the presence of a conjunctival Kaposi sarcoma (KS).

# AUDITORY PROBLEMS: EXTERNAL EAR AND CANAL

## TRAUMA

Trauma to the external ear can cause injury to the subcutaneous tissue that may result in a hematoma. If the hematoma is not aspirated, inflammation of the membranes of the ear cartilage (perichondritis) can result. Blows to the ear can also cause conductive hearing loss if the ossicles in the middle ear are damaged or the tympanic membrane (TM) is perforated. Head trauma that injures the temporal lobe of the cerebral cortex can impair the ability to understand the meaning of sounds.

## EXTERNAL OTITIS

The skin of the external ear and canal is subject to the same problems as skin anywhere on the body. **External otitis** involves inflammation or infection of the epithelium of the auricle and ear canal. Swimming may alter the flora of the external canal because of chemicals and contaminated water. This can result in an infection often referred to as "swimmer's ear." Trauma from picking the ear or using sharp objects (e.g., hairpins) frequently causes the initial break in the skin. Piercing of cartilage in the upper part of the auricle also places the patient at higher risk for infection.

Infections and skin conditions may cause external otitis. Bacteria or fungi may be the cause. *Pseudomonas aeruginosa* is the most common bacterial cause. Fungi, especially *Candida albicans* and *Aspergillus,* thrive in warm, moist climates. The warm, dark environment of the ear canal provides a good growth medium for microorganisms.

*Malignant external otitis* is a serious infection caused by *P. aeruginosa.* It occurs mainly in older patients with diabetes. The infection, which can spread from the external ear to the parotid gland and temporal bone (osteomyelitis), is usually treated with antibiotics.

Ear pain *(otalgia)* is one of the first signs of external otitis. Even in mild cases, the patient may experience significant discomfort with chewing, moving the auricle, or pressing on the tragus. Swelling of the ear canal can muffle hearing. There may be serosanguineous (blood-tinged fluid) or purulent (white to green thick fluid) drainage. Fever occurs when the infection spreads to surrounding tissue.

## ❖ NURSING AND INTERPROFESSIONAL MANAGEMENT: EXTERNAL OTITIS

Diagnosis of external otitis is made by otoscopic examination of the ear canal. Care must be taken to avoid pain when pulling on the pinna to straighten out the canal or when inserting the otoscope speculum. The eardrum may be difficult to see due to swelling in the canal. Culture and sensitivity studies of the drainage may be done. Moist heat, mild analgesics, and topical anesthetic drops usually control the pain. Topical treatments may include antibiotics for infection and corticosteroids for inflammation. If the surrounding tissue is involved, systemic antibiotics are prescribed. Improvement should occur in 48 hours, but the patient needs to adhere to the prescribed therapy for 7 to 14 days for complete resolution.

Hands should be washed before and after administration of otic drops (eardrops). The drops should be administered at room temperature. Cold drops can cause vertigo due to stimulation of the semicircular canals, and heated drops can burn the tympanum. The tip of the dropper should not touch the ear during administration to prevent contamination of the entire bottle of drops. The ear is positioned so that the drops can run into the canal. The patient should maintain this position for 2 minutes to allow the drops to spread. Sometimes the drops are placed onto a wick of cotton that is placed in the canal. Instruct the patient not to push the cotton farther into the ear. Careful

**TABLE 21-8 Patient & Caregiver Teaching**

***Prevention of External Otitis***

*Include the following instructions when teaching the patient and caregiver.*

1. Do not put anything in your ear canal unless requested by your health care provider.
2. Report itching if it becomes a problem.
3. Earwax is normal.
   - It lubricates and protects the canal.
   - Report chronic excessive cerumen if it impairs your hearing.
4. Keep your ears as dry as possible.
   - Use earplugs if you are prone to swimmer's ear.
   - Turn your head to each side for 30 seconds at a time to help water run out of the ears.
   - Do not dry with cotton-tipped applicators.
   - A hair dryer set to low and held at least 6 in from the ear can speed water evaporation.

handling and disposal of material saturated with drainage are important. Instruct the patient on methods to reduce the risk of external otitis (Table 21-8).

## CERUMEN AND FOREIGN BODIES IN EXTERNAL EAR CANAL

Impacted cerumen (earwax) can cause discomfort and decreased hearing. In the older person the cerumen becomes dense and drier. The hair in the ear becomes thicker and coarser, entrapping the hard, dry cerumen in the canal. Symptoms of cerumen impaction include hearing loss, otalgia, tinnitus, and vertigo.

Management of impacted cerumen involves irrigation of the canal with body-temperature solutions to soften the cerumen. Special syringes can be used and vary from a simple bulb syringe to special irrigating equipment. Place the patient in a sitting position with an emesis basin under the ear. Pull the auricle up and back, and direct the flow of solution above or below the impaction. It is important that the ear canal not be completely occluded with the syringe tip. If irrigation does not remove the wax, mild lubricant drops may be used to soften the earwax. Severe impactions may need to be removed by the HCP.

Attempts to remove a foreign object from the ear may result in pushing it farther into the canal. Vegetable matter in the ear tends to swell and may create a secondary inflammation, making removal more difficult. Mineral oil or lidocaine drops can be used to kill an insect before removal with microscope guidance. Removal of impacted objects should be performed by an HCP.

Ears should be cleaned with a washcloth and finger. Cotton-tipped applicators should be avoided. Penetration of the middle ear by a cotton-tipped applicator can cause serious injury to the TM and ossicles. The use of cotton-tipped applicators can also cause cerumen to become impacted against the TM and impair hearing.

## MALIGNANCY OF EXTERNAL EAR

Skin cancers are the only common malignancies of the ear. Rough sandpaper-like changes to the upper border of the auricle are premalignant lesions (actinic keratoses) associated with chronic sun exposure. They are often treated with liquid nitrogen. Malignancies in the external ear canal include basal cell carcinoma in the pinna and squamous cell carcinoma in the ear canal. If left untreated, they can invade underlying tissue. Teach the patient about the dangers of sun exposure and the importance of using hats and sunscreen when outdoors.

# MIDDLE EAR AND MASTOID

## OTITIS MEDIA

### Acute Otitis Media

*Acute otitis media* is an infection of the tympanum, ossicles, and space of the middle ear. Swelling of the auditory tube from colds or allergies can trap bacteria, causing a middle ear infection. Pressure from the inflammation pushes on the TM, causing it to become red, bulging, and painful. Acute otitis media is usually a childhood disease because in children the auditory tube that normally drains fluid and mucus from the middle ear is shorter and narrower and its position is flatter than in adults. Infection can be due to viruses or bacteria. Pain, fever, malaise, and reduced hearing are signs and symptoms of infection. Referred pain from the temporomandibular joint, teeth, gums, sinuses, or throat may also cause ear pain.

Antibiotics are used if an infection is present. Surgical intervention is generally reserved for the patient who does not respond to medical treatment. A *myringotomy* involves an incision in the tympanum to release the increased pressure and exudate from the middle ear. A tympanostomy tube may be placed for short- or long-term use. Prompt treatment of an episode of acute otitis media generally prevents spontaneous perforation of the TM. If allergies are a causative factor, antihistamines may also be prescribed.

### Otitis Media With Effusion

*Otitis media with effusion* is an inflammation of the middle ear with a collection of fluid in the middle ear space. The fluid may be thin, mucoid, or purulent. If the auditory tube does not open and allow equalization of atmospheric pressure, negative pressure within the middle ear pulls fluid from surrounding tissues. This problem commonly follows upper respiratory tract or chronic sinus infections, barotrauma (caused by pressure change), or otitis media.

Complaints include a feeling of fullness of the ear, a "plugged" feeling or popping, and decreased hearing. The patient does not experience pain, fever, or discharge from the ear. It is common to have otitis media with effusion for weeks to months after an episode of acute otitis media. It usually resolves without treatment but may recur.

### Chronic Otitis Media and Mastoiditis

Repeated attacks of otitis media may lead to chronic otitis media, especially in adults who have a history of recurrent otitis media in childhood. Because the mucous membrane of the middle ear is continuous with the air cells of the mastoid bone, both can be involved in the chronic infectious process.

*Chronic otitis media* is characterized by a purulent exudate and inflammation that can involve the ossicles, auditory tube, and mastoid bone. It is often painless. Hearing loss, nausea, and episodes of dizziness can occur. Hearing loss is a complication from inflammatory destruction of the ossicles, a TM perforation, or accumulation of fluid in the middle ear space. A mass of epithelial cells and cholesterol in the middle ear *(cholesteatoma)* may also develop. The cholesteatoma enlarges and can

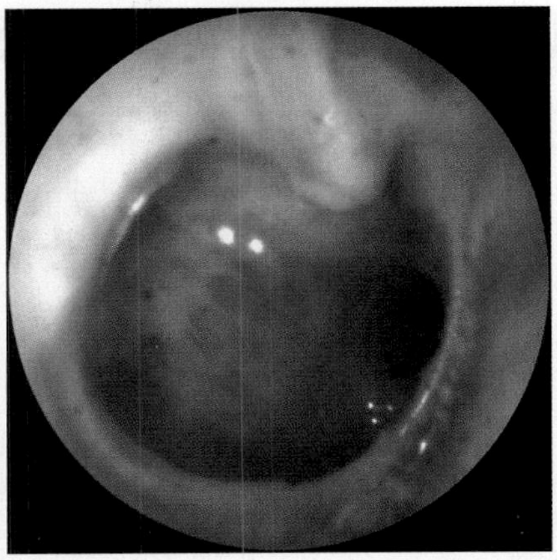

FIG. 21-9 Perforation of the tympanic membrane (TM). (From Flint P, Haughey B, Lund V, Niparko JK, editors: *Cummings otolaryngology: head and neck surgery,* ed 5, St Louis, 2010, Mosby.)

**TABLE 21-9 Interprofessional Care**

***Chronic Otitis Media***

| Diagnostic Assessment | Management |
|---|---|
| • History and physical examination<br>• Otoscopic examination<br>• Culture and sensitivity of middle ear drainage<br>• Mastoid x-ray | • Ear irrigations<br>• Otic, oral, or parenteral antibiotics<br>• Analgesics<br>• Antiemetics<br>• Surgery<br>  • Tympanoplasty<br>  • Mastoidectomy |

destroy the adjacent bones. Unless removed surgically, it can cause extensive damage to the ossicles and impair hearing.

Otoscopic examination of the TM may reveal changes in color and mobility or a perforation (Fig. 21-9). Culture and sensitivity tests of the drainage are necessary to identify the organisms involved so that appropriate antibiotic therapy can be prescribed. The audiogram may demonstrate a hearing loss as great as 50 to 60 dB if the ossicles have been damaged or separated. Sinus x-rays, MRI, or a CT scan of the temporal bone is done to assess for bone destruction and the presence of a mass.

## NURSING AND INTERPROFESSIONAL MANAGEMENT: CHRONIC OTITIS MEDIA

The goals of treatment are to clear the middle ear of infection, repair any perforations, and preserve hearing (Table 21-9). Otic and systemic (oral and IV) antibiotic therapy is started based on the culture and sensitivity results. In many cases of chronic otitis media, antibiotic resistance is present. The patient may need to undergo frequent evacuation of drainage and debris in an outpatient setting.

Often chronic TM perforations do not heal with conservative treatment, and surgery is necessary. *Tympanoplasty (myringoplasty)* involves reconstruction of the TM and/or the ossicles. A *mastoidectomy* is often performed with a tympanoplasty to remove infected portions of the mastoid bone. Removal of tissue stops at the middle ear structures that appear capable of conducting sound. Sudden pressure changes in the ear and postoperative infections can disrupt the surgical repair during the healing phase or cause facial nerve paralysis.

**TABLE 21-10 Interprofessional Care**

***Otosclerosis***

| Diagnostic Assessment | Management |
|---|---|
| • History and physical examination<br>• Otoscopic examination<br>• Rinne test<br>• Weber test<br>• Audiometry<br>• Tympanometry | • Hearing aid<br>• Surgery (stapedectomy or stapes prosthesis)<br>• Drug therapy<br>  • Sodium fluoride with vitamin D<br>  • Calcium carbonate |

Impaired hearing is expected during the postoperative period if there is packing in the ear. A cotton ball dressing is used for the incision made through the external auditory canal (endaural). Instruct the patient to change the cotton packing as needed. If a postauricular (behind the ear) incision is used and a drain is in place, place a dressing over the mastoid area. A small gauze pad is cut to fit behind the ear, and soft dressing material is applied over the ear to prevent the outer circular head dressing from placing pressure on the auricle. Monitor the tightness of the dressing to prevent tissue necrosis and assess the amount and type of drainage. Keep the suture line dry.

## OTOSCLEROSIS

Otosclerosis is a hereditary autosomal dominant disease. It is the most common cause of hearing loss in young adults. Spongy bone develops from the bony labyrinth, preventing movement of the footplate of the stapes in the oval window. This reduces the transmission of vibrations to the inner ear fluids and results in conductive hearing loss. Although otosclerosis is typically bilateral, one ear may show faster progression of hearing loss. The patient is often unaware of the problem until the loss becomes so severe that communication is difficult.

Otoscopic examination may reveal a reddish blush of the tympanum (Schwartz's sign) caused by the vascular and bony changes within the middle ear. Tuning fork tests (e.g., Rinne) and an audiogram demonstrate good hearing by bone conduction but poor hearing by air conduction (air-bone gap). (These diagnostic tests are discussed in Table 20-11). Usually a difference of at least 20 to 25 dB between air and bone conduction levels of hearing is seen in otosclerosis.

The hearing loss associated with otosclerosis may be stabilized by the oral administration of sodium fluoride with vitamin D and calcium carbonate. These medications retard bone resorption and encourage the calcification of bony lesions. Amplification of sound by a hearing aid can be effective because the inner ear function is normal.

Interprofessional care of otosclerosis is presented in Table 21-10. Microdrill or laser surgical treatment involves opening the footplate (stapedotomy) or replacing the stapes with a metal or Teflon substitute (prosthesis). These procedures are usually performed with the patient under conscious sedation. The ear with poorer hearing is repaired first, and the other ear may be operated on within a year. Immediately after surgery the patient often reports a significant improvement in hearing in the operative ear. Because of the accumulation of blood and fluid in the middle ear during the postoperative period, the hearing level decreases initially, but it improves gradually with healing.

Nursing management of the patient undergoing surgery to correct otosclerosis is similar to that for the patient having a tympanoplasty. Use Gelfoam on the incision flap to limit bleeding. Place a cotton ball in the ear canal, and cover the ear with a small dressing. The patient may experience dizziness, nausea, and vomiting as a result of stimulation of the labyrinth during surgery. Some patients demonstrate nystagmus because of disturbance of the perilymph fluid. The patient should take care to avoid sudden movements that may bring on or exacerbate vertigo. Actions that increase inner ear pressure, such as coughing, sneezing, lifting, bending, and straining during bowel movements, should be avoided.

## INNER EAR PROBLEMS

Three manifestations that indicate disease of the inner ear are vertigo, sensorineural hearing loss, and tinnitus. Symptoms of vertigo arise from the vestibular labyrinth, whereas hearing loss and tinnitus arise from the auditory labyrinth. There is an overlap between manifestations of inner ear problems and CNS disorders.

**TABLE 21-11 Interprofessional Care**

***Ménière's Disease***

**Diagnostic Assessment**
- History and physical examination
- Audiometric studies (including speech discrimination, tone decay)
- Vestibular tests (including caloric test, positional test)
- Electronystagmography
- Neurologic examination
- Glycerol test

**Management**

***Acute Care***

*Drug Therapy*
- Sedatives
- Benzodiazepines
- Anticholinergics
- Antihistamines
- Antiemetics

*Surgical Therapy*
- Endolymphatic sac decompression
- Endolymphatic shunt
- Vestibular nerve section
- Labyrinthectomy

***Ambulatory Care***
- Diuretics
- Antihistamines
- Calcium channel blockers
- Sedatives
- Hydrops diet: restriction of sodium, caffeine, nicotine, alcohol, and foods with monosodium glutamate (MSG)

### MÉNIÈRE'S DISEASE

**Ménière's disease** (endolymphatic hydrops) is characterized by symptoms caused by inner ear disease, including episodic vertigo, tinnitus, fluctuating sensorineural hearing loss, and aural fullness. The patient experiences significant disability because of sudden, severe attacks of vertigo with nausea, vomiting, sweating, and pallor. Symptoms usually begin between 30 and 60 years of age.[17]

The cause of the disease is unknown, but it results in an excessive accumulation of endolymph in the membranous labyrinth. The volume of endolymph increases until the membranous labyrinth ruptures. Attacks may be preceded by a sense of fullness in the ear, increasing tinnitus, and muffled hearing. The patient may experience the feeling of being pulled to the ground ("drop attacks"). Some patients report that they feel like they are whirling in space. Attacks may last hours or days and may occur several times a year. The clinical course of the disease is highly variable.

### NURSING AND INTERPROFESSIONAL MANAGEMENT: MÉNIÈRE'S DISEASE

Interprofessional care of Ménière's disease (Table 21-11) includes diagnostic tests to rule out other causes of the symptoms, including CNS disease. Results that suggest Ménière's disease include a mild, low-frequency sensorineural hearing loss on audiogram and abnormalities with vestibular tests. A glycerol test may aid in diagnosis. An oral dose of glycerol is given, followed by serial audiograms over 3 hours. Improvement in hearing or speech discrimination supports a diagnosis of Ménière's disease. The improvement is attributed to the osmotic effect of glycerol that pulls fluid from the inner ear.

During the acute attack, antihistamines (e.g., diphenhydramine), anticholinergics (e.g., atropine), and benzodiazepines (e.g., lorazepam [Ativan]) can be used to decrease the abnormal sensation and lessen nausea and vomiting. Acute vertigo is treated symptomatically with bed rest, sedation, and antiemetics (e.g., prochlorperazine) or antivertigo drugs (e.g., meclizine [Antivert]) for motion sickness. The patient requires reassurance and counseling that the condition is not life threatening. Management between attacks may include diuretics, antihistamines, calcium channel blockers, and a low-sodium diet. Diazepam (Valium), meclizine, and fentanyl with droperidol may be used to reduce the vertigo. Over time, most patients respond to the prescribed medications but must learn to live with the unpredictability of the attacks and the loss of hearing.

Frequent and incapacitating attacks are indications for surgical intervention. Decompression of the endolymphatic sac and shunting are performed to reduce the pressure on the cochlear hair cells and to prevent further damage and hearing loss. If relief is not achieved, vestibular nerve section (cutting the nerve) may be performed. When involvement is unilateral, surgical ablation of the labyrinth, resulting in loss of the vestibular and hearing cochlear function, is performed. Some patients with severe attacks of vertigo have shown improvement with the injection of gentamicin through the TM. This results in inner ear damage and a reduction in endolymph production.

Plan nursing interventions to minimize vertigo and provide for patient safety. During an acute attack keep the patient in a quiet, darkened room in a comfortable position. Teach the patient to avoid sudden head movements or position changes. Fluorescent or flickering lights or a television may exacerbate symptoms and should be avoided. Make an emesis basin available because vomiting is common. To minimize the risk of falling, keep the side rails up and the bed in a low position when the patient is in bed. Instruct the patient to call for assistance when getting out of bed. Medications and fluids are administered parenterally, and intake and output are monitored. When the attack subsides, assist the patient with ambulation because unsteadiness may remain.

### BENIGN PAROXYSMAL POSITIONAL VERTIGO

**Benign paroxysmal positional vertigo (BPPV)** is a common cause of vertigo. Approximately 50% of the cases of vertigo may be due to BPPV. In BBPV, free-floating debris in the semicircular canal causes vertigo with specific head movements, such as getting out of bed, rolling over in bed, and sitting up from lying down. The debris ("ear rocks") is composed of small crystals of calcium carbonate that derive from the utricle in the inner ear. The utricle may be injured by head trauma, infection, or degeneration from the aging process. However, for many patients, a cause cannot be found.

Symptoms of BPPV include nystagmus, vertigo, lightheadedness, loss of balance, and nausea. There is no hearing loss, and symptoms tend to be intermittent. The symptoms of BPPV may be confused with those of Ménière's disease. Diagnosis is based on the results of auditory and vestibular tests.

Although BPPV is bothersome, it is rarely serious unless a person falls. The Epley maneuver, or canalith repositioning procedure, is effective in providing symptom relief for many patients. In this maneuver, the ear debris is moved from areas in the inner ear that cause symptoms and repositioned into less sensitive areas where they do not cause these problems. The Epley maneuver does not address the actual presence of debris but rather changes their location. A trained HCP can instruct the patient how to perform the maneuver.

## ACOUSTIC NEUROMA

An acoustic neuroma is a unilateral benign tumor that occurs where the vestibulocochlear nerve (cranial nerve [CN] VIII) enters the internal auditory canal. Early diagnosis is important because the tumor can compress the trigeminal and facial nerves and arteries within the internal auditory canal. Symptoms usually begin between 40 and 60 years of age.

Early symptoms are associated with CN VIII compression and destruction. They include unilateral, progressive, sensorineural hearing loss; reduced touch sensation in the posterior ear canal; unilateral tinnitus; and mild, intermittent vertigo. Diagnostic tests include neurologic, audiometric, and vestibular tests; CT scans; and MRI.

Surgery to remove small tumors generally preserves hearing and vestibular function. Large tumors (larger than 3 cm) and the surgery required to remove them can leave the patient with permanent hearing loss and facial paralysis. Stereotactic radiosurgery may slow tumor growth and preserve the facial nerve. Instruct the patient to report any clear, colorless discharge from the nose. This may be cerebrospinal fluid (CSF), which increases the risk of infection. Teach the importance of follow-up care after surgery to monitor hearing and for recurrence of the tumor.

## HEARING LOSS AND DEAFNESS

Hearing disorders are a common cause of disability in the United States. Nearly half of the people who need assistance with hearing disorders are 65 years of age or older. With the aging of the population, the incidence of hearing loss is increasing.[18] Causes of hearing loss are shown in Fig. 21-10.

### Types of Hearing Loss

**Conductive Hearing Loss.** *Conductive hearing loss* occurs when conditions in the outer or middle ear impair the transmission of sound through air to the inner ear. A common cause is otitis media with effusion. Other causes are impacted cerumen, perforation of the TM, otosclerosis, and narrowing of the external auditory canal.

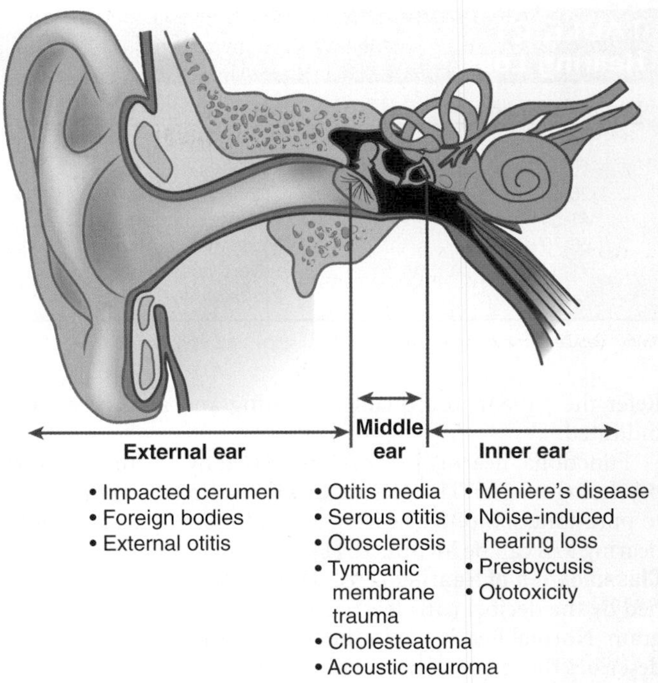


**FIG. 21-10** Causes of hearing loss.

The audiogram demonstrates better hearing through bone than through air (air-bone gap). The patient often speaks softly because hearing his or her own voice (which is conducted by bone) seems loud. This patient hears better in a noisy environment. The first step is to identify and treat the cause if possible. If correction of the cause is not possible, a hearing aid may help if the loss is greater than 40 to 50 dB.

**Sensorineural Hearing Loss.** *Sensorineural hearing loss* is caused by impairment of function of the inner ear or the vestibulocochlear nerve (CN VIII). Congenital and hereditary factors, noise trauma over time, aging (presbycusis), Ménière's disease, and ototoxicity can cause sensorineural hearing loss. Ototoxic drugs include aspirin, nonsteroidal antiinflammatory drugs, antibiotics (aminoglycosides, erythromycin, vancomycin), loop diuretics, and chemotherapy drugs (e.g., vincristine [Oncovin], cisplatin [Platinol]).

Systemic infections, such as Paget's disease of the bone, immune diseases, diabetes mellitus, bacterial meningitis, and trauma, are associated with this type of hearing loss. The main problems are the ability to hear sound but not to understand speech, and the lack of understanding of the problem by others. The ability to hear high-pitched sounds (including consonants) diminishes. Sounds become muffled and difficult to understand. An audiogram demonstrates a loss in decibel levels of the 4000-Hz range and eventually the 2000-Hz range. A hearing aid may help some patients, but it only makes sounds and speech louder, not clearer.

**Mixed Hearing Loss.** Mixed hearing loss occurs due to a combination of conductive and sensorineural causes. Careful evaluation is needed if corrective surgery for conductive loss is planned because the sensorineural component of the hearing loss will still remain.

**Central and Functional Hearing Loss.** Central hearing loss involves an inability to interpret sound, including speech, because of a problem in the brain (CNS). A careful history is helpful because there are usually cases of deafness in the family.

**TABLE 21-12 Classification of Hearing Loss**

| Decibel (dB) Loss | Meaning |
|---|---|
| 0-15 | Normal hearing |
| 16-25 | Slight hearing loss |
| 26-40 | Mild impairment |
| 41-55 | Moderate impairment |
| 56-70 | Moderately severe impairment |
| 71-90 | Severe impairment |
| >90 | Profound deafness* |

*Most people in this category have been deaf since birth (congenitally deaf).

Refer the patient to a qualified hearing and speech service if indicated.

Functional hearing loss may be caused by an emotional or a psychologic factor. The patient does not seem to hear or respond to pure-tone subjective hearing tests, but no physical reason for hearing loss can be identified. Psychologic counseling may help.

**Classification of Hearing Loss.** Hearing loss can also be classified by the decibel (dB) level or loss as recorded on the audiogram. Normal hearing is in the 0- to 15-dB range. Table 21-12 describes the levels of hearing loss.

### Clinical Manifestations

Common early signs of hearing loss are answering questions inappropriately, not responding when not looking at the speaker, asking others to speak up, and showing irritability with others who do not speak up. Other behaviors that suggest hearing loss include straining to hear, cupping the hand around the ear, reading lips, and an increased sensitivity to slight increases in noise level. Often the patient is unaware of minimal hearing loss. Family and friends who get tired of repeating or talking loudly are often the first to notice the hearing loss. Pressure exerted by significant others is a significant factor in whether the patient seeks help for hearing impairment.

*Sudden hearing loss*, commonly known as sudden deafness, occurs as an unexplained, rapid loss of hearing (usually in one ear) either at once or over several days. It is a medical emergency, and the patient should see an HCP immediately.[19]

Deafness is often called the "unseen handicap" because the difficulty in communication with a deaf person is not realized until you initiate a conversation with that person. You need to thoroughly validate the deaf person's understanding of health teaching. Descriptive visual aids can be helpful. If the significantly hearing-impaired individual uses sign language to communicate, the Americans with Disabilities Act requires providing an interpreter when significant information is presented such as for patient consent or discharge teaching.[20]

Interference in communication and interaction with others can be the source of many problems for the patient and caregiver. Often the patient refuses to admit or may be unaware of impaired hearing. Irritability is common because the patient must concentrate so hard to understand speech. The loss of clarity of speech in the patient with sensorineural hearing loss is most frustrating. The patient may hear what is said but not understand it. Withdrawal, suspicion, loss of self-esteem, and insecurity are commonly associated with advancing hearing loss.[21]

**Tinnitus and Hearing Loss.** *Tinnitus* is the perception of *sound* in the ears where no external source is present. It is "ringing in the ears" or "head noise" (see *www.ata.org*). Tinnitus is sometimes the first symptom of hearing loss, especially in older people. It may be soft or loud, high pitched or low pitched.

Tinnitus and hearing loss are directly related. Both are caused by inner ear nerve damage. The main difference between tinnitus and hearing loss is the extent of the damage (since tinnitus can still be heard).

Although the most common cause of tinnitus is noise, it can also be a side effect of medications (see discussion on drugs causing sensorineural hearing loss on p. 387). More than 200 drugs are known to cause tinnitus.

**CHECK YOUR PRACTICE**

Your newly assigned 68-yr-old female patient is being discharged today following a hip replacement. Before going to her room, you prepared the materials and information for her discharge. You sit down by her bed and start talking with her. She shakes her head and says, "No, no." You are perplexed until she flashes a bracelet that says *I am deaf.*

- How will you proceed?

## NURSING AND INTERPROFESSIONAL MANAGEMENT: HEARING LOSS AND DEAFNESS

### Health Promotion

**Environmental Noise Control.** Noise is the most preventable cause of hearing loss. (Fig. 21-11 lists the levels of environmental noise generated by common indoor and outdoor sounds.) Sudden severe loud noise (acoustic trauma) and chronic exposure to loud noise (noise-induced hearing loss) can damage hearing. Acoustic trauma causes hearing loss by destroying the hair cells of the organ of Corti. Sensorineural hearing loss as a result of increased and prolonged environmental noise, such as amplified sound, is occurring in young adults at an increasing rate. Amplified music (e.g., on iPods or MP3 players) should not exceed 50% of maximum volume. Ear protection should be worn when firing a gun and during other recreational pursuits with high noise levels. Health teaching regarding avoidance of continued exposure to noise levels greater than 70 dB is essential.

In work environments known to have high noise levels (more than 85 dB), ear protection should be worn. Occupational Safety and Health Administration (OSHA) standards require ear protection for workers in environments where the noise levels consistently exceed 85 dB. Periodic audiometric screening should be part of the health maintenance policies of industry. This provides baseline data on hearing to measure subsequent hearing loss.

Employees should participate in hearing conservation programs in work environments. Such programs should include noise exposure analysis, provision for control of noise exposure (hearing protectors), measurements of hearing, and employee-employer notification and education. Young adults should be encouraged to keep amplified music at a reasonable level and limit their exposure time. Hearing loss caused by noise is not reversible.

**HEALTHY PEOPLE**

***Health Impact of Wearing Ear Protection***

- Ear protection should be worn during all recreational and work activities involving high noise levels.
- Ear protection can greatly reduce the damage to the ear from loud noise.
- Periodic audiometric screening is important to detect hearing loss before it progresses.

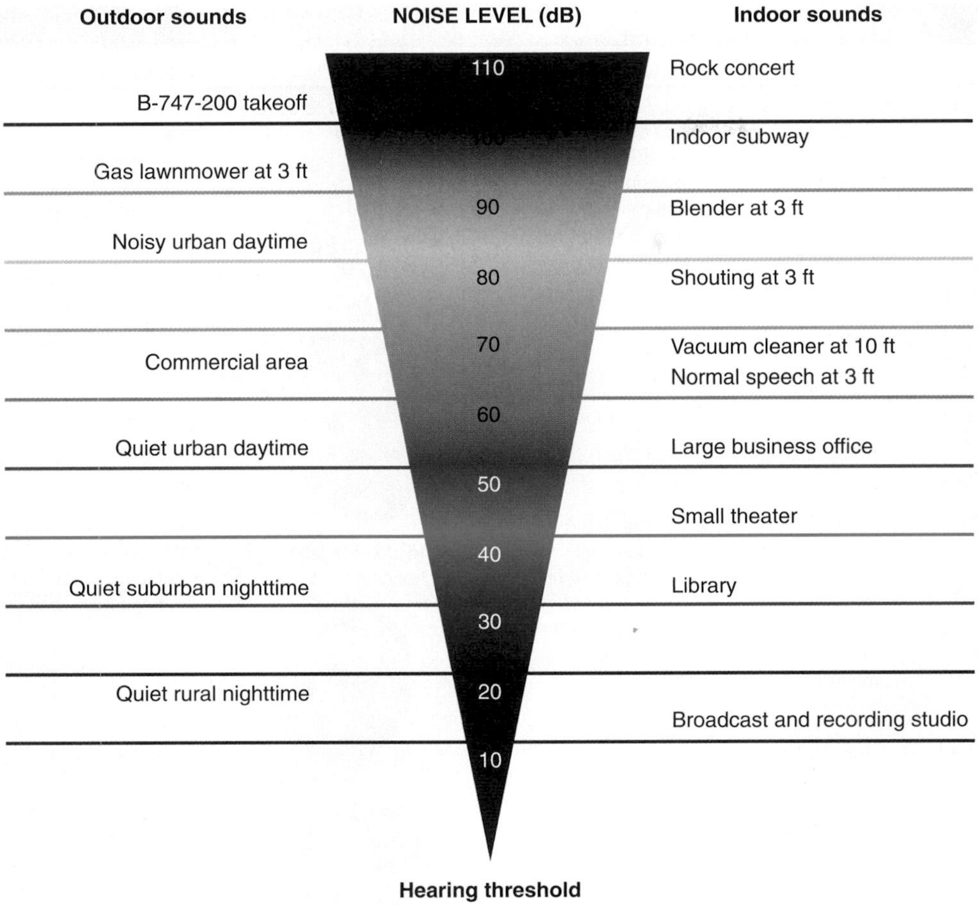


**FIG. 21-11** Range of common environmental sounds.

**Immunizations.** Various viruses can cause deafness as a result of fetal damage and malformations affecting the ear. Promote childhood and adult immunizations, including the measles, mumps, and rubella (MMR) vaccine. Rubella infection during the first 8 weeks of pregnancy is associated with a high incidence of congenital rubella syndrome, which causes sensorineural deafness. Women of childbearing age should be tested for antibodies to these viral diseases. Women should avoid pregnancy for at least 3 months after being immunized. Immunization must be delayed if the woman is pregnant. Women who are susceptible to rubella can be vaccinated safely during the postpartum period.

**Ototoxic Substances.** Drugs commonly associated with ototoxicity include salicylates, loop diuretics, chemotherapy drugs, and antibiotics. Chemicals used in industry (e.g., toluene, carbon disulfide, mercury) may damage the inner ear. The patient who is receiving ototoxic drugs or is exposed to ototoxic chemicals should be monitored for signs and symptoms associated with ototoxicity, including tinnitus, diminished hearing, and changes in equilibrium. If these symptoms develop, immediate withdrawal of the drug may prevent further damage and may cause the symptoms to disappear.

## Assistive Devices and Techniques

**Hearing Aids.** The patient with a suspected hearing loss should have a hearing assessment by a qualified audiologist. If a hearing aid is indicated, it should be fitted by an audiologist or a speech and hearing specialist. Many types of hearing aids are available, each with advantages and disadvantages (Table 21-13). The conventional hearing aid serves as a simple amplifier. For the patient with bilateral hearing impairment, binaural hearing aids provide the best sound lateralization and speech discrimination.

The goal of hearing aid therapy is improved hearing with consistent use. Patients who are motivated and optimistic about using a hearing aid are more successful users. Determine the patient's readiness for hearing aid therapy, including acknowledgment of a hearing problem, the patient's feelings about wearing a hearing aid, the degree to which the hearing loss affects life, and any difficulties the patient has manipulating small objects such as putting a battery in a hearing aid.

Initially, use of the hearing aid should be restricted to quiet situations in the home. The patient must first adjust to voices (including the patient's own voice) and household sounds. The patient should also experiment by increasing and decreasing the volume as situations require. As the patient adjusts to the increase in sounds and background noise, he or she can progress to situations where several people will be talking simultaneously. Next, the environment can be expanded to the outdoors and then a shopping mall or grocery store. Adjustment to different environments occurs gradually, depending on the individual patient.

When the hearing aid is not being worn, it should be placed in a dry, cool area where it will not be inadvertently damaged or lost. The battery should be disconnected or removed when not in use. A standard hearing aid battery lasts anywhere from 3 to 22 days, depending on the hearing aid type, battery type and capacity, and the amount of hearing aid use. Battery life

**TABLE 21-13 Types of Hearing Aids**

| Type | Advantages | Disadvantages |
|---|---|---|
| **Completely in the canal** (mild to moderate hearing loss) 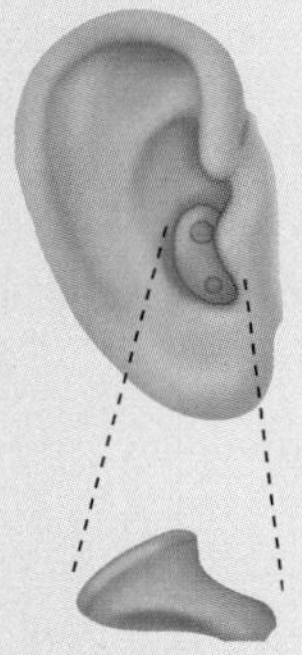 | Smallest and least visible aid. Protected from sounds such as wind noise. | Costly. No space for add-ons such as directional microphones or volume controls. Small, short-lived batteries. |
| **In the canal** (mild to severe hearing loss) 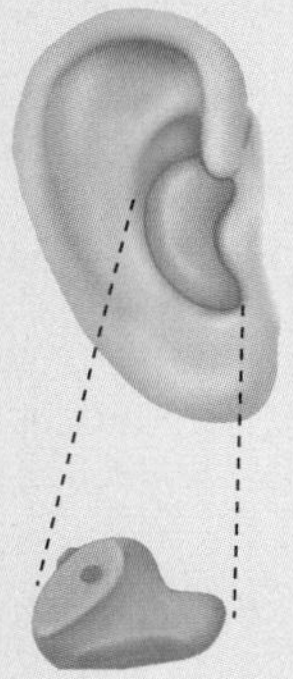 | More powerful than aids completely in the canal. Has adjustable features such as noise reduction. | Small size of aid with its additional features may be difficult to operate for patients with visual loss or arthritis. |
| **In the ear** (mild to severe hearing loss) 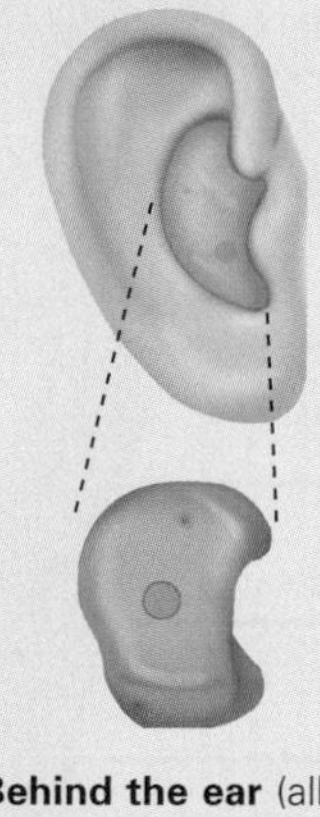 | Powerful amplification. Inserts and adjusts easily. Longer-lasting batteries. | Visible. May pick up wind noise readily. |
| **Behind the ear** (all types of hearing loss) 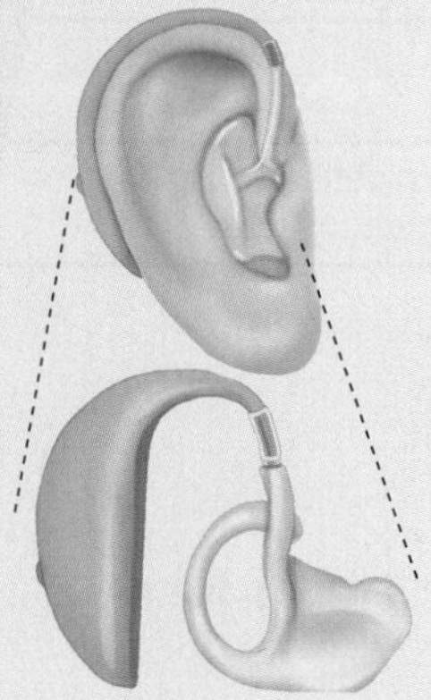 | Most powerful aid. Adjusts easily. Longest battery life. | Largest, most visible aid. Newer models may be smaller and less obvious. |

averages 1 week (depends on hearing aid, battery, and amount of use), and patients should be advised to purchase only a month's supply at a time. Ear molds should be cleaned weekly or as needed. Toothpicks or pipe cleaners may be used to clear a clogged ear tip.

An *implantable hearing device* or aid is available to patients who cannot or will not use traditional hearing aids or cochlear implants. Implanted hearing devices amplify sound and transmit the sound vibrations through the ear. The device does not have external components that are visible. There are two types of implantable hearing devices: fully implantable and partially implantable. The fully implantable devices are surgically placed and nothing is visible externally. Partially implanted devices have an internal device that is implanted surgically but have an external device that is worn behind or in the ear.

**Speech Reading.** *Speech reading,* commonly called *lip reading,* can be helpful in increasing communication. It allows for approximately 40% understanding of the spoken word. The patient is able to use visual cues associated with speech, such as gestures and facial expression, to help clarify the spoken message. In speech reading, many words look alike to the patient (e.g., rabbit, woman). Help the patient by using and teaching verbal and nonverbal communication techniques as described in Table 21-14.

**Sign Language.** *Sign language* is used as a form of communication for people with profound hearing impairment. It involves gestures and facial features such as eyebrow motion and lip-mouth movements. Sign language is not universal. American Sign Language (ASL) is used in the United States and the English-speaking parts of Canada.

**Cochlear Implant.** The *cochlear implant* is used as a hearing device for people with severe to profound sensorineural hearing

**TABLE 21-14 Communication With Patients With Hearing Impairment**

**Nonverbal Aids**

- Draw attention with hand movements.
- Have speaker's face in good light.
- Avoid covering mouth or face with hands.
- Avoid chewing, eating, smoking while talking.
- Maintain eye contact.
- Avoid distracting environments.
- Avoid careless expression that the patient may misinterpret.
- Use touch.
- Move close to better ear.
- Avoid light behind speaker.

**Verbal Aids**

- Speak normally and slowly.
- Do not overexaggerate facial expressions.
- Do not overenunciate.
- Use simple sentences.
- Rephrase sentence. Use different words.
- Write name or difficult words.
- Do not shout.
- Speak in normal voice directly into better ear.

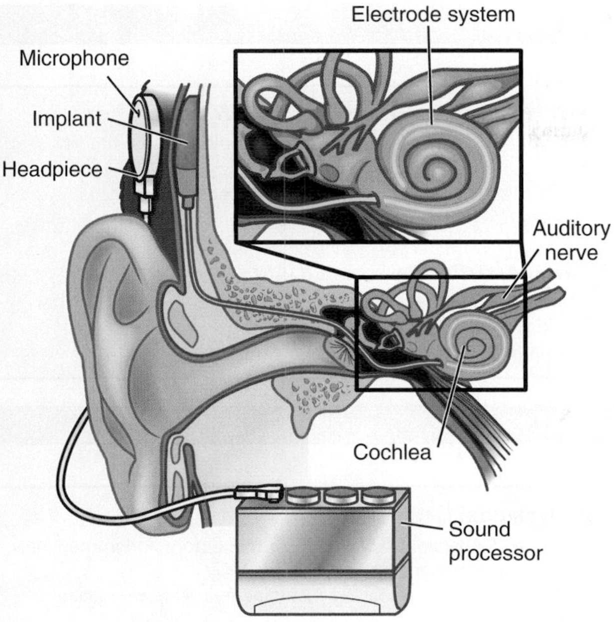


**FIG. 21-12** Cochlear implant.

loss in one or both ears.[22] The ideal candidate is one who has become deaf after acquiring speech and language. The system consists of an external microphone placed behind the ear, a speech processor and a transmitter implanted under the skin that change sounds into electrical impulses, and a group of electrodes placed within the cochlea that stimulate the auditory nerves in the ear (Fig. 21-12). Cochlear implants send information that covers the entire range of sound frequencies. The cochlear implant electrodes are inserted as far as possible into the cochlea to send both high- and low-frequency information. For patients with conductive and mixed hearing loss, the cochlear Baha system may be surgically implanted. The system works through direct bone conduction and integrates with the skull bone over time.

Extensive training and rehabilitation are essential to receive maximum benefit from these implants. The positive aspects of a cochlear implant include providing sound to the person who heard none, improving lip-reading ability, monitoring the loudness of the person's own speech, improving the sense of security, and decreasing feelings of isolation.

**Assistive Listening Devices.** Numerous devices are now available to assist the hearing-impaired person. Direct amplification devices, amplified telephone receivers, alerting systems that flash when activated by sound, an infrared system for amplifying the sound of the television, and a combination FM receiver and hearing aid are all devices that you can explore based on patient needs. People with profound deafness may be assisted by text-telephone alerting systems that flash when activated by sound, closed captioning on television, and a specially trained dog. The dogs are trained to alert their owners to specific sounds within the environment, thus increasing the person's safety and independence.

**TABLE 21-15 Classification of Presbycusis**

| Type | Hearing Change and Prognosis |
|---|---|
| **Sensory** | |
| Atrophy of auditory nerve. Loss of sensory hair cells | Loss of high-pitched sounds. Little effect on speech understanding. Good response to sound amplification |
| **Neural** | |
| Degenerative changes in cochlea and spinal ganglion | Loss of speech discrimination. Amplification alone not sufficient |
| **Metabolic** | |
| Atrophy of blood vessels in wall of cochlea with interruption of essential nutrient supply | Uniform loss for all frequencies accompanied by recruitment.* Good response to hearing aid |
| **Cochlear** | |
| Stiffening of basilar membrane, which interferes with sound transmission in the cochlea | Hearing loss increases from low to high frequencies. Speech discrimination affected with higher-frequency losses. Helped by appropriate forms of amplification |

*Abnormally rapid increase in loudness as sound intensity increases.

## Gerontologic Considerations: Hearing Loss

**Presbycusis**, hearing loss associated with aging, includes the loss of peripheral auditory sensitivity, a decline in word recognition ability, and associated psychologic and communication issues. Because consonants (high-frequency sounds) are the letters by which spoken words are recognized, the older person with presbycusis has a diminished ability to understand the spoken word. Vowels are heard, but some consonants fall into the high-frequency range and cannot be differentiated. This may lead to confusion and embarrassment because of the difference in what was said and what was heard.[23]

The cause of presbycusis is related to degenerative changes in the inner ear. Noise exposure is thought to be a common factor. Table 21-15 describes the classification of specific causes and associated hearing changes of presbycusis. Often a person may have more than one type of presbycusis. The prognosis for hearing depends on the cause of the loss. Sound amplification with the appropriate device is often helpful in improving the understanding of speech. In other situations, an audiologic rehabilitation program can be valuable.

The older adult is often reluctant to use a hearing aid for sound amplification. Reasons cited most often include cost, appearance, insufficient knowledge about hearing aids, amplification of competing noise, and unrealistic expectations. Most hearing aids and batteries are small, and neuromuscular changes such as stiff fingers, enlarged joints, and decreased sensory perception often make the care and handling of a hearing aid difficult and frustrating for an older person. Some older adults may also tend to accept their losses as part of getting older and believe there is no need for improvement.

## TEAMWORK & COLLABORATION

### *Corrective Lenses and Hearing Aids*

**Role of Nursing Personnel**

***Registered Nurse (RN)***
- Assess patient vision and hearing with and without corrective devices.
- Teach patient about the use of and care for corrective lenses and hearing aids.
- Evaluate whether corrective lenses or hearing aids are effective in maintaining or improving vision or hearing.
- Evaluate for problems that may occur with contact lenses (e.g., conjunctivitis) or with hearing aids (e.g., external ear irritation).

***Licensed Practical/Vocational Nurse (LPN/LVN)***
- Perform Snellen and/or Jaeger testing as delegated by the RN (consider state nurse practice act and agency policy).
- Monitor for adverse effects of contact lenses (e.g., redness, complaints of irritation) and report these to the RN.

***Unlicensed Assistive Personnel (UAP)***
- Clean corrective lenses with ordered solutions.
- Help patients with hearing aid placement.
- Clean and replace batteries in hearing aids.

## CASE STUDY

### *Glaucoma and Diabetic Retinopathy*

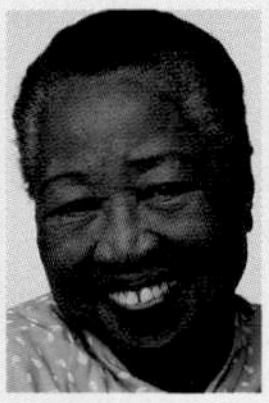
(©Kevin Peterson/ Stockbyte/ Thinkstock)

**Patient Profile**

J.K. is a 68-year-old African American woman who has been diagnosed with osteoarthritis and type 2 diabetes mellitus for the past 15 years. She now has diabetic retinopathy. She returns to the eye clinic with her daughter for continued care of primary open-angle glaucoma (POAG) and reexamination for changes in diabetic retinopathy. Her current medical regimen for POAG includes topical timolol maleate 0.5% extended (Timoptic-XE) once daily OU and latanoprost (Xalatan) 0.005% OU at bedtime. At her last examination it was noted that she had microaneurysms and hard exudates of the retina.

**Subjective Data**
- She can no longer read the newspaper and reports that medication labels are difficult to read.
- States she is not always successful in getting the eye drops instilled because her hands are gnarled and painful from osteoarthritis.

**Objective Data**
- Distant and near visual acuity are stable at 20/60 (OD) and 20/50 (OS). This is a reduction from 20/40 (OU) at her last visit.
- Intraocular pressures are stable at 20 mm Hg (OU). There is a new scotoma on visual field testing in the OS.
- Fluorescein angiography reveals diabetic macular edema OU.

**Interprofessional Care**
- Brimonidine (Alphagan) 0.15% (OS) 15 min before and immediately after argon laser trabeculoplasty (ALT)
- Argon laser (OU) to seal leaking microaneurysms from macular edema
- Check intraocular pressure (IOP) 1 hr after ALT
- Continue previous glaucoma drop regimen
- Follow-up examination for glaucoma in 2 wk for possible ALT (OD)
- Follow-up examination for diabetic macular edema in 8 wk

**Discussion Questions**
1. Explain the etiology of the new scotoma.
2. Why may ALT be an appropriate therapy for J.K.?
3. What is the purpose of the eye drops before and immediately after ALT?
4. ***Patient-Centered Care:*** What are the priority topics that should be discussed in discharge teaching with J.K.?
5. What is the etiology of the vision loss from diabetic retinopathy?
6. ***Priority Decision:*** What are the priority nursing interventions for J.K.?
7. ***Priority Decision:*** Based on the assessment data, what are the priority nursing diagnoses? Are there any collaborative problems?
8. ***Evidence-Based Practice:*** J.K. wants to know if her glaucoma is related to her diabetes. How would you respond to her question?

Answers available at *http://evolve.elsevier.com/Lewis/medsurg*.

## BRIDGE TO NCLEX EXAMINATION

The number of the question corresponds to the same-numbered outcome at the beginning of the chapter.

1. Presbyopia occurs in older individuals because
   **a.** the eyeball elongates.
   **b.** the lens becomes inflexible.
   **c.** the corneal curvature becomes irregular.
   **d.** light rays are focusing in front of the retina.
2. The *most* important intervention for the patient with epidemic keratoconjunctivitis is
   **a.** cleansing the affected area with baby shampoo.
   **b.** monitoring spread of infection to the opposing eye.
   **c.** regular instillation of artificial tears to the affected eye.
   **d.** teaching the patient and family members good hygiene techniques.
3. Inflammation and infection of the eye
   **a.** are caused by irritants and microorganisms.
   **b.** have a higher incidence in sexually active patients.
   **c.** are chronic problems that result in a loss of vision.
   **d.** are frequently treated with cold compresses and antibiotics.
4. Which patient behaviors would the nurse promote for healthy eyes and ears *(select all that apply)*?
   **a.** Wearing protective sunglasses when bicycling
   **b.** Supplemental intake of B vitamins and magnesium
   **c.** Playing amplified music at 75% of maximum volume
   **d.** Patient notifying the health care provider of tinnitus while on antibiotics
   **e.** A woman avoiding pregnancy for 4 weeks after receiving MMR immunization
5. What should be included in the postoperative teaching of the patient who has undergone cataract surgery *(select all that apply)*?
   **a.** Eye discomfort is often relieved with mild analgesics.
   **b.** A decline in visual acuity is common for the first week.
   **c.** Stay on bed rest and limit activity for the first few days.
   **d.** Notify surgeon if an increase in redness or drainage occurs.
   **e.** Nighttime eye shielding and activity restrictions are essential to prevent eyestrain.

6. What should be included in the nursing plan for a patient who needs to administer antibiotic eardrops?
   a. Cool the drops so that they decrease swelling in the canal.
   b. Avoid placing a cotton wick to assist in administering the drops.
   c. Be careful to avoid touching the tip of the dropper bottle to the ear.
   d. Keep the head tilted 5 to 7 minutes after administration of the drops.
7. What is *important* for the nurse to include in the postoperative care of the patient following tympanoplasty?
   a. Check the gag reflex.
   b. Encourage independence.
   c. Avoid changing the cotton padding.
   d. Instruct patient to refrain from forceful nose blowing.
8. The patient who has a conductive hearing loss
   a. hears better in a noisy environment.
   b. hears sound but does not understand speech.
   c. often speaks loudly because his or her own voice seems low.
   d. experiences clearer sound with a hearing aid if the loss is less than 30 dB.
9. Instruct the patient who is newly fitted with bilateral hearing aids to *(select all that apply)*
   a. replace the batteries monthly.
   b. clean the ear molds weekly or as needed.
   c. clean ears with cotton-tipped applicators daily.
   d. disconnect or remove the batteries when not in use.
   e. initially restrict usage to quiet listening in the home.
10. Which strategies would *best* assist the nurse in communicating with a patient who has a hearing loss *(select all that apply)*?
    a. Overenunciate speech.
    b. Speak normally and slowly.
    c. Exaggerate facial expressions.
    d. Raise the voice to a higher pitch.
    e. Write out names or difficult words.
11. Patients with permanent visual impairment
    a. feel most comfortable with other visually impaired people.
    b. may feel threatened when others make eye contact during a conversation.
    c. usually need others to speak louder so that they can communicate appropriately.
    d. may experience the same grieving process that is associated with other losses.

1. b, 2. d, 3. a, 4. a, 5. a, d, 6. c, 7. d, 8. a, 9. b, d, e, 10. b, e, 11. d

For rationales to these answers and even more NCLEX review questions, visit *http://evolve.elsevier.com/Lewis/medsurg.*

## EVOLVE WEBSITE

http://evolve.elsevier.com/Lewis/medsurg

**Review Questions (Online Only)**

**Key Points**

**Answer Keys for Review Questions**

- Rationales for Bridge to NCLEX Examination Questions
- Answer Guidelines for Case Study on p. 392

**Student Case Study**

- Patient Undergoing Cataract Surgery

**eNursing Care Plan**

- eNursing Care Plan 21-1: Patient After Eye Surgery

**Conceptual Care Map Creator**

**Audio Glossary**

**Supporting Media**

- Animations
  - Cataract Removal
  - LASIK
  - Myringotomy
  - Scleral Buckling

**Content Updates**

## REFERENCES


1. Sutton G, Lawless M, Hodge C: Laser in situ keratomileusis in 2012: a review, *Clin Exp Optom* 97(1):18, 2014.
2. FDA: Lasik. Retrieved from *www.fda.gov/MedicalDevices/ProductsandMedicalProcedures/SurgeryandLifeSupport/LASIK/default.htm.*
3. American Foundation for the Blind: Aging and vision fact sheet. Retrieved from *www.afb.org/info/programs-and-services/public-policy-center/directconnect-newsletter/new-learning-opportunity-from-afb-finding-the-numbers-we-need/1235.*
4. National Sleep Foundation: Non-24. Retrieved from *https://sleepfoundation.org/non-24/content/non-24.*
5. Akpek EK, Smith RA: Overview of age-related ocular conditions, *Am J Manag Care* 19(5 Suppl):S67, 2013.
6. Lin A, Confait C, Ahmad M, et al: Severe ocular trauma in the emergency room, *J Miss State Med Assoc* 55(6):176, 2014.
7. Durning MV: Conjunctivitis, *Nursing* 43:39, 2013.

*8. Lockwood C, Stern C: Interventions for the treatment of trachoma: an overview of Cochrane systematic reviews, *Int J Nurs Pract* 20(6):709, 2014.

*9. Güell JL, El Husseiny MA, Manero F, et al: Historical review and update of surgical treatment for corneal endothelial diseases, *Ophthalmol Ther* 3(1-2):1, 2014.

10. National Eye Institute: Facts about cataracts. Retrieved from *www.nei.nih.gov/health/cataract/cataract_facts.*
11. Nentwich MM, Ulbig MW: Diabetic retinopathy—ocular complications of diabetes mellitus, *World J Diabetes* 6(3):489, 2015.
12. Steel D: Retinal detachment, *BMJ Clin Evid* 3;2014. pii: 0710.
13. Mackey DA, Hewitt AW: Genome-wide association study success in ophthalmology, *Curr Opin Ophthalmol* 25(5):386, 2014.
14. Glaucoma Research Foundation: African Americans and glaucoma. Retrieved from *www.glaucoma.org/glaucoma/african-americans-and-glaucoma.php.*
15. American Cancer Society: Eye cancer. Retrieved from *www.cancer.org/cancer/eyecancer.*
16. Nielsen M, Dogrusöz M, Bleeker JC, et al: The genetic basis of uveal melanoma, *J Fr Ophthalmol* 38(6):516, 2015.

*17. Tassinari M, Mandrioli D, Gaggioli N, et al: Ménière's disease treatment: a patient-centered systematic review, *Audiol Neurootol* 20(3):153, 2015.

18. Hearing Loss Association of America: *http://hearingloss.org.*
19. Sudden deafness. Retrieved from *www.nidcd.nih.gov/health/hearing/pages/sudden.aspx.*
20. American Disabilities Act. Retrieved from *www.ada.gov/pubs/ada.htm.*
21. Shuler GK, Mistler LA, Torrey K, et al: Bridging communication gaps with the deaf, *Nursing* 43:24, 2013.
22. National Institute on Deafness and Other Communication Disorders: Cochlear implants. Retrieved from *www.nidcd.nih.gov.*
23. Öberg M: Hearing care for older adults: beyond the audiology clinic, *Am J Audiol* 2015 Apr 7. doi:10.1044/2015_AJA-14-0077. [Epub ahead of print]


*Evidence-based information for clinical practice.

# 22

# Assessment of Integumentary System

*Diana L. Gallagher*

*Nobody grows old merely by living a number of years. We grow old by deserting our ideals. Years may wrinkle the skin, but to give up enthusiasm wrinkles the soul.*

***Samuel Ullman***

http://evolve.elsevier.com/Lewis/medsurg/

## LEARNING OUTCOMES

1. Describe the structures and functions of the integumentary system.
2. Link the age-related changes in the integumentary system to differences in assessment findings.
3. Obtain significant subjective and objective data related to the integumentary system from a patient.
4. Describe specific assessments to be made during the physical examination of the skin and appendages.
5. Compare and contrast the critical components for describing primary and secondary lesions.
6. Perform a physical assessment of the integumentary system using appropriate techniques.
7. Specify the structural and assessment differences in light- and dark-skinned persons.
8. Differentiate normal from common abnormal findings of a physical assessment of the integumentary system.
9. Describe the purpose, significance of results, and nursing responsibilities related to diagnostic studies of the integumentary system.

## KEY TERMS

alopecia, Table 22-8, p. 403
dermis, p. 395
epidermis, p. 394
erythema, Table 22-8, p. 403
hirsutism, Table 22-8, p. 403
intertriginous, p. 399
keloid, p. 403
keratinocytes, p. 394
melanocytes, p. 395
mole (nevus), Table 22-8, p. 403
pruritus, p. 399
sebaceous glands, p. 396

The integumentary system is the largest organ of the body. It is composed of the skin, hair, nails, and certain glands. The skin has two major layers: epidermis (outer layer) and dermis (inner layer). The subcutaneous tissue (layer) lies under the dermis (Fig. 22-1). The skin is as complex as any organ, but unlike the others, it is readily visible. Being able to see and touch the skin helps you assess your patients. You can see abnormalities, understand their significance, and intervene early.

## STRUCTURES AND FUNCTIONS OF SKIN AND APPENDAGES

### Structures

**Epidermis.** The epidermis, the outer layer of the skin, is relatively thin, ranging from 0.05 mm on the eyelids to 0.1 mm on the soles.[1] There are no lymphatic or vascular structures in the epidermis. It is supported by passive circulation from the dermis.

The epidermis can be divided into five distinct but interrelated layers. Two of the layers are the stratum corneum (the surface layer) and the stratum germinativum (deepest, basal layer) (Fig. 22-1).

The major cells in the epidermis are the keratinocytes (90%) and melanocytes (5%). The remaining cells are Langerhans' cells and Merkel cells.

Keratinocytes are synthesized from epidermal cells in the basal layer. Initially they are undifferentiated and shaped like columns. As they mature (keratinize), they move to the surface, where they flatten and die to form the outer skin layer (stratum corneum). Keratinocytes produce a fibrous protein, keratin, which is vital to the skin's protective barrier function. The upward movement of keratinocytes from the basal layer to the outermost levels of the stratum corneum takes about 14 days. The keratinocytes remain there for another 14 days, allowing the epidermis to regenerate every 28 days. (Each month you have a new layer of skin.)

Many skin problems result from changes in this cell cycle. If dead cells slough off too rapidly, the skin appears thin and eroded. If new cells form faster than old cells are shed, the skin becomes scaly and thickened. Failure of the epidermis to

Reviewed by Patricia Gable Burke, RN, BSN, CWOCN, Patient Educator Wound, Ostomy, Continence Care, Bethesda North Hospital, Cincinnati, Ohio; Kim Clevenger, RN, EdD, BC, Associate Professor of Nursing, BSN Program Coordinator, Morehead State University, Morehead, Kentucky; and Allison J. Terry, RN, PhD, Associate Professor of Nursing, Assistant Dean of Clinical Practice, School of Nursing, Auburn University Montgomery, Montgomery, Alabama.

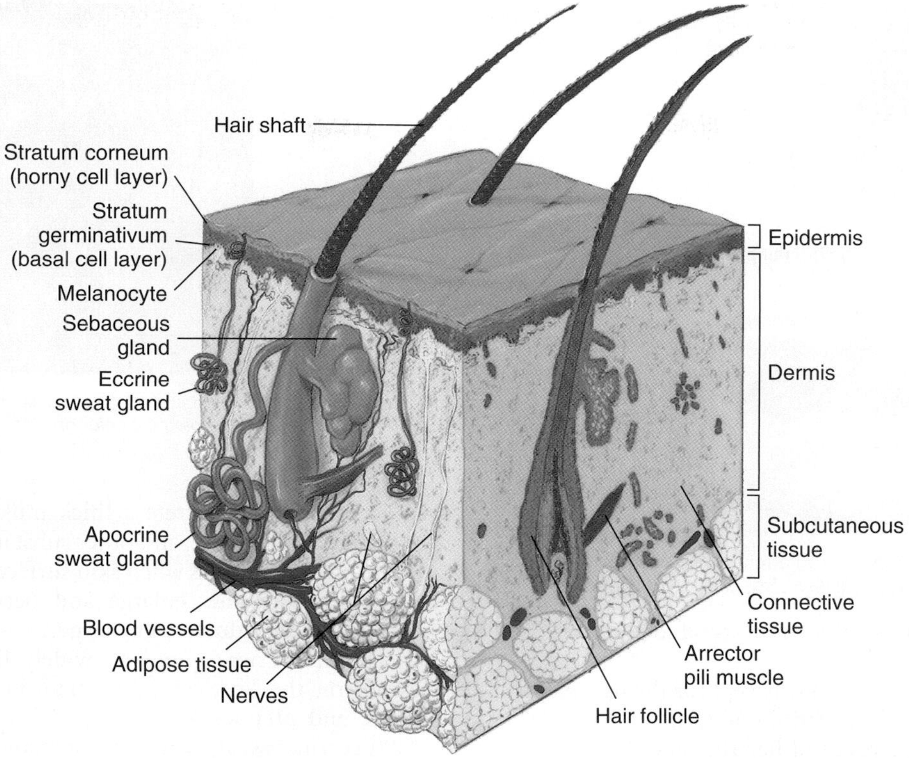


**FIG. 22-1** Microscopic view of the skin in longitudinal section. (From Jarvis C: *Physical examination and health assessment,* ed 6, St Louis, 2012, Saunders.)

function normally occurs with skin cancer and psoriasis (discussed in Chapter 23).

**Melanocytes** are also found in the deep, basal layer. They contain melanin, a pigment that gives color to the skin and hair and protects the body from damaging ultraviolet (UV) sunlight. Sunlight and hormones stimulate the melanosome (within the melanocyte) to increase the production of melanin. People of all races have similar numbers of melanocytes. In darker skin, the melanosomes are larger and more numerous, thus producing more melanin.[1] This increased melanin forms a natural sun shield for dark skin and results in a decreased incidence of skin cancer in these persons. The distribution of melanocytes varies from one area of the body to another. For example, the face has more melanocytes than the abdomen.

*Langerhans' cells* are a type of dendritic cell (discussed in Chapter 13 on p. 194). They are immunocompetent cells that are essential to recognize antigens. When they are depleted, the skin cannot initiate an immune response. The Langerhans' cells in bioengineered skin grafts have been removed to prevent graft rejection. In skin diseases such as psoriasis and sarcoidosis, there are decreased numbers of Langerhans' cells.

*Merkel cells* are touch receptors found in the epidermis and involved in the sensation of light touch. They are used when feeling the texture of an object and determining what it is. High concentrations of Merkel cells are found in the fingertips and also in the lips, but they are also present in areas of hairy skin.[2]

The basement membrane zone is between the epidermis and dermis. This structure provides for the (1) exchange of fluids between the epidermis and dermis and (2) structural support for the epidermis. The basement membrane also helps to secure the two layers together. Inflammation and separation of the epidermal and dermal layers result in the blisters seen with problems such as burns, full-thickness wounds, and mechanical trauma.

**Dermis.** The **dermis** is the connective tissue below the epidermis. Dermal thickness ranges from 0.3 mm on the eyelid to 3.0 mm on the back.[3] The dermis is very vascular, containing many blood vessels. It also contains nerves, lymphatic vessels, hair follicles, sebaceous glands, and specialized cells such as mast cells and macrophages that protect the body from external stimuli.

The dermis is made of three types of connective tissue: collagen, elastic fibers, and reticular fibers. Collagen forms the greatest part of the dermis. It is responsible for the skin's mechanical strength. The primary cell type in the dermis is the *fibroblast,* which produces collagen and elastin. Collagen is critical in wound healing.

The dermis has two layers: upper thin papillary layer and a deeper, thicker reticular layer. The papillary layer is arranged haphazardly in ridges, or papillae, which extend into the outer epidermal layer. These elevated surface ridges form fingerprints and footprints. The reticular layer forms the bulk of the dermis. It is made up of thick collagen bundles arranged perpendicular to the skin's surface.

**Subcutaneous Tissue.** The subcutaneous tissue lies below the dermis. It is made of loose connective tissue and fat cells that provide insulation, cushioning, temperature regulation, and energy storage. The subcutaneous tissue attaches the skin to underlying tissues, such as muscle and bone. The distribution pattern of subcutaneous tissue varies with gender, heredity, age, and nutritional status.

**Skin Appendages.** *Skin appendages* include the hair, nails, and glands (sebaceous, apocrine, and eccrine). These appendages are epidermal extensions that have their roots in the dermis. These structures receive nutrients, electrolytes, and fluids from the dermis. Hair and nails form from specialized keratin.

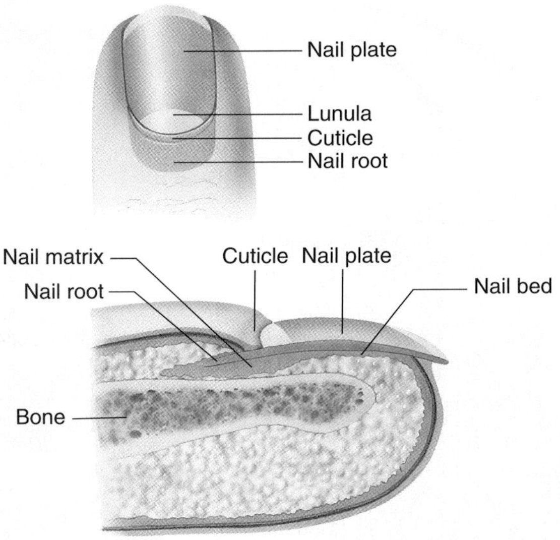


**FIG. 22-2** Structure of a nail. (From Patton KT, Thibodeau GA, Douglas M: *Essentials of anatomy and physiology,* St Louis, 2012, Mosby.)

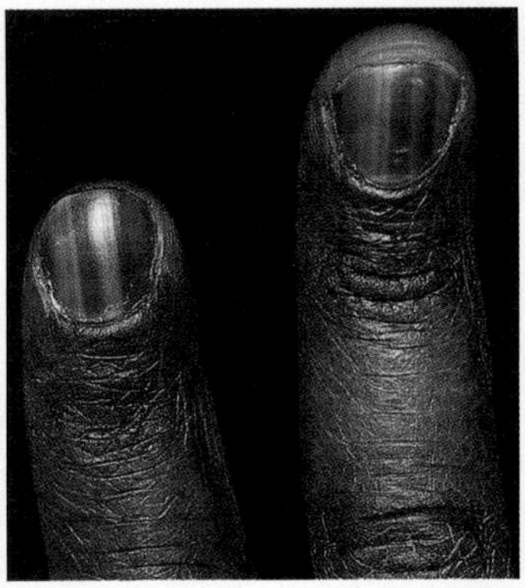

**FIG. 22-3** Pigmented nail bed normally seen with dark skin color. (From Habif TP: *Clinical dermatology: a color guide to diagnosis and therapy,* ed 5, St Louis, 2011, Mosby.)

Systemic diseases can affect the condition and health of both hair and nails.

Hair grows on most of the body except for the lips, palms of the hands, interdigital spaces, portions of the genitalia, and soles of the feet. Hair color is a result of heredity and determined by the type and amount of melanin in the hair shaft. Hair grows approximately 1 cm per month. People lose an average of 25 to 100 hairs each day.[1] When lost hair is not replaced, baldness, or *alopecia,* results.

Fingernails and toenails are made of heavily keratinized cells. The part of the nail that you can see is the nail body. The rest is the nail root. A fold of skin hides most of the nail root. The cuticle borders this skin fold. Nail growth begins in the nail root. The portion of the nail root you can see is the *lunula.* This white, crescent-shaped area is the site of mitosis and nail growth (Fig. 22-2). Under the nail is an area of epidermis called the *nail bed.* The nail bed contains many blood vessels. Fingernails grow at a rate of 0.7 to 0.84 mm per week, with toenail growth 30% to 50% slower.[4] A lost fingernail usually regenerates in 3 to 6 months, while a lost toenail may require 12 months or longer to regenerate. Nail growth varies based on a person's age and health. Nails grow faster in men and in warm weather. Nail color ranges from pink to yellow or brown depending on skin color. Color and texture variations in the nails may represent normal or abnormal conditions. Pigmented longitudinal bands *(melanonychia striata)* occur in the nail bed in approximately 90% or more of people with dark skin[2] (Fig. 22-3).

Two major types of glands are associated with the skin: sebaceous and sweat (apocrine and eccrine) glands. **Sebaceous glands** secrete *sebum,* which is emptied into the hair follicles. Sebum waterproofs and lubricates the skin and promotes the absorption of fat-soluble substances. Sebum is somewhat bacteriostatic and fungistatic. These glands depend on sex hormones, particularly testosterone, to regulate sebum secretion and production. Actual production varies depending on age, sex, and testosterone and estrogen levels. Sebaceous glands are present on all areas of the skin except the palms and soles and dorsum of the feet. These glands are most abundant on the face, scalp, upper chest, and back.

The *apocrine sweat glands* are located in the axillae, breast areolae, umbilical and anogenital areas, external auditory canals, and eyelids. They secrete a thick milky substance containing protein, carbohydrate, and other substances.[5] The secretions are odorless. Odor occurs when skin surface bacteria alter the secretions. These glands enlarge and become active at puberty because of reproductive hormones.

The *eccrine sweat glands* are widely distributed over the body, except on the lips, ear canals, nail beds, labia minora, glans penis, and prepuce. One square inch of skin contains about 3000 eccrine sweat glands. Their main function is to cool the body by evaporation, excrete waste products, and moisturize surface cells. Sweat is a transparent watery solution composed of salts, ammonia, urea, and other wastes. In extreme situations, the body can produce 2 to 4 L of sweat per hour or up to 12 liters in 24 hours. Heat, certain mental stimuli, and ingestion of hot, spicy foods stimulate sweat secretion.

## Functions of Integumentary System

The skin's primary function is to protect the underlying body tissues by serving as a barrier to the external environment. The skin acts as a barrier against invasion by bacteria and viruses and prevents excessive water loss. The fat in the subcutaneous layer insulates the body and provides protection from trauma. Melanin screens and absorbs ultraviolet radiation.

The skin with its nerve endings and special receptors provides sensory perception for environmental stimuli. These highly specialized nerve endings supply information to the brain related to pain, heat and cold, touch, pressure, and vibration.

The skin controls heat regulation by responding to changes in internal and external temperature with vasoconstriction or vasodilation. The skin's excretory function and heat regulation are related. Between 600 and 900 mL of water is lost daily through insensible water loss (invisible vaporization from the lungs and skin), which assists in regulating body temperature. Sebum and sweat lubricate the skin surface. Endogenous synthesis of vitamin D, which is critical to calcium and phosphorus balance, occurs in the epidermis. Vitamin D is synthesized by the action of UV light on vitamin D precursors in epidermal cells.

The skin is a delivery system for drugs. An increasing number of systemic drugs are effectively delivered via patches or creams applied directly to the skin.

## Gerontologic Considerations: Effects of Aging on Integumentary System

Many skin changes are associated with aging. Depending on a person's view of themselves, the normal, visible effects of aging

## TABLE 22-1 Gerontologic Assessment Differences

### *Integumentary System*

| Changes | Differences in Assessment Findings |
|---|---|
| **Skin** | |
| Decreased subcutaneous fat, muscle laxity, degeneration of elastic fibers, collagen stiffening | Increased wrinkling, sagging breasts and abdomen, redundant flesh around eyes, slowness of skin to flatten when pinched (tenting) |
| Decreased extracellular water, surface lipids, and sebaceous gland activity | Dry, flaking skin with possible signs of excoriation caused by scratching |
| Decreased activity of apocrine and sebaceous glands | Dry skin with minimal to no perspiration, skin color uneven |
| Increased capillary fragility and permeability | Bruising |
| Increased focal melanocytes in basal layer with pigment accumulation | Solar lentigines on face and back of hands |
| Diminished blood supply | Decrease in rosy appearance of skin and mucous membranes. Skin cool to touch. Diminished awareness of pain, touch, temperature, peripheral vibration |
| Decreased proliferative capacity | Diminished rate of wound healing |
| Decreased immunocompetence | Increase in neoplasms |
| **Hair** | |
| Decreased melanin and melanocytes | Gray or white hair |
| Decreased oil | Dry, coarse hair. Scaly scalp |
| Decreased density of hair | Thinning and loss of hair |
| Cumulative androgen effect; decreasing estrogen levels | Facial hirsutism, baldness |
| **Nails** | |
| Decreased peripheral blood supply | Thick, brittle nails with diminished growth |
| Increased keratin | Longitudinal ridging |
| Decreased circulation | Prolonged return of blood to nails on blanching |

on the skin and hair may have a profound psychologic effect. Having a youthful look may affect a person's self-image. The appearance of the signs of aging can be a threat to self-concept. Other changes in skin structure related to normal changes with aging can pose serious risk. Age-related changes of the integumentary system and differences in assessment findings are listed in Table 22-1.

Chronic UV exposure is the major contributor to the photoaging and wrinkling of skin.[6] Sun damage to the skin is cumulative (Fig. 22-4). The wrinkling of sun-exposed areas such as the face and hands is more marked than that of a sun-shielded area, such as the buttocks. Poor nutrition, with decreased intake of protein, calories, and vitamins, contributes to skin aging. Collagen fibers stiffen, elastic fibers degenerate, and the amount of subcutaneous tissue decreases. These changes, with the added effects of gravity, lead to wrinkling.

The junction between the dermis and epidermis flattens. This causes the two layers to lose their tight bond. Skin tears and other trauma become common as the epidermis slides separately from the dermis. Fewer free fatty acids in the epidermis results in dry, scaly, itchy skin. Dryness, combined with trauma caused by scratching, increases the risk of fissures (cracks) in the skin and secondary infections. Decreased subcutaneous fat

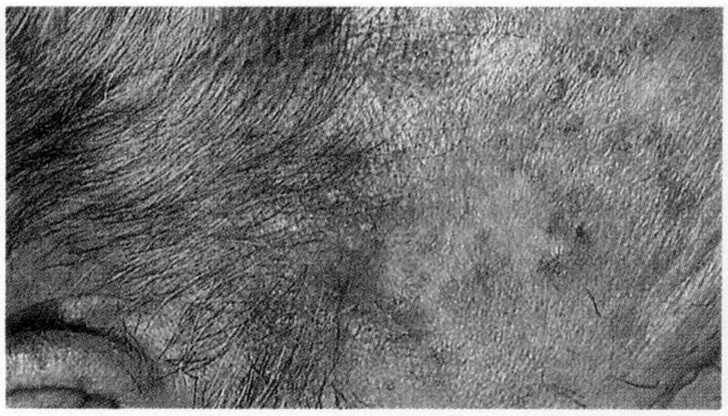

**FIG. 22-4** Photoaging. Irregular pigmentation and keratoses occur on sun-damaged skin on forehead. (From Gawkrodger D, Ardern-Jones MR: *Dermatology,* ed 5, Edinburgh, 2012, Churchill Livingstone.)

## TABLE 22-2 Normal Physical Assessment of Integumentary System

| | |
|---|---|
| **Skin** | • Evenly pigmented. No petechiae, purpura, lesions, or excoriations<br>• Warm, good turgor |
| **Nails** | • Pink, oval, adhere to nail bed with 160-degree angle |
| **Hair** | • Shiny and full; amount and distribution appropriate for age and gender<br>• No flaking of scalp, forehead, or pinna |

increases the risk of traumatic injury, hypothermia, and skin shearing, which may lead to pressure ulcers.

Fewer melanocytes are present, and with decreased levels of melanin, hair color fades. Hormonal and vitamin deficiencies can cause dry, thin hair and alopecia. The growth rate of the hair and nails decreases because of atrophy. The nail plate thins, and nails become brittle and more prone to splitting and yellowing. Nails, especially the toenails, may thicken with age. With aging, the apocrine and eccrine sweat glands atrophy, causing dry skin and decreased body odor.

Benign neoplasms related to the aging process can occur. These growths include seborrheic keratoses, vascular lesions such as cherry angiomas, and skin tags. *Actinic keratoses* appear on areas of chronic sun exposure, especially in the person who has a fair complexion and light eyes (blue, green, or hazel). These premalignant cutaneous lesions place a person at increased risk for squamous cell and basal cell carcinomas. A photoaged person is more susceptible to skin cancers because UV exposure decreases the capacity to repair cellular damage. Chronic UV exposure from tanning beds causes the same damage as UV from the sun.

## ASSESSMENT OF INTEGUMENTARY SYSTEM

The general skin assessment begins with your initial contact with the patient and continues throughout the examination. As you are meeting your patient for the first time, take a moment to note the overall condition of their skin and hair. Specific areas of the skin are assessed during the examination of other body systems, unless the chief complaint is a dermatologic problem. Record a general statement about the skin's physical condition (Table 22-2). In addition, ask the health history questions presented in Table 22-3 when a skin problem is noted.

### Subjective Data

People with skin problems may have complaints that you are not able to readily observe. A thorough health history yields information about possible causes and the effect of the problem on the person's life.

## TABLE 22-3 Health History

### *Integumentary System*

**Health Perception–Health Management**
- Describe your daily hygiene practices.
- What skin products are you currently using?
- Describe any current skin condition, including onset, course, and treatment (if any).

**Nutritional-Metabolic**
- Describe any changes in the condition of your skin, hair, nails, and mucous membranes.
- Have you noticed any recent changes in the way sores or wounds heal?*
- Have you had any weight loss or dietary changes, including supplemental vitamins and minerals?*

**Elimination**
- Have you noticed recent changes in your skin related to excessive sweating, dryness, or swelling?*

**Activity-Exercise**
- Do your leisure or work activities involve the use of any chemicals that are irritating to your skin?*
- Do you do anything to protect yourself from the sun?*

**Sleep-Rest**
- Does your skin condition keep you awake or awaken you after you have fallen asleep?*

**Cognitive-Perceptual**
- Do you have any unusual sensations of heat, cold, or touch?*
- Do you have any pain associated with your skin condition?*
- Do you have any joint pain?*

**Self-Perception–Self-Concept**
- How does your skin condition make you feel about yourself?

**Role-Relationship**
- Has your skin condition changed your relationships with others?*
- Have you changed your lifestyle because of your skin condition?*

**Sexuality-Reproductive**
- Has your skin condition changed your intimate relationships with others?*
- Has your birth control method (if used) caused a skin problem?*

**Coping–Stress Tolerance**
- Are you aware of any situation or stressor that changes your skin condition?*
- Do you think that stress plays a role in your skin condition?*
- How do you handle stress?

**Value-Belief**
- Are there any cultural beliefs that influence your thinking or feelings about your skin condition?*
- Are there any treatment options that you would be opposed to using?

*If yes, describe.

## CASE STUDY

### *Patient Introduction*

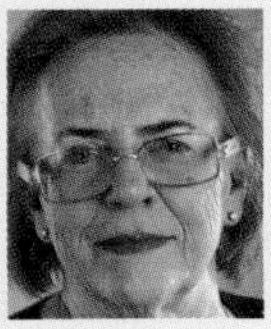

(©iStockphoto/Thinkstock)

D.A. is a 74-year-old woman who comes to the medical clinic with concerns related to various "spots" on her face. She says they have been there for a while and she thought they were just "age spots" but got concerned after her friend was diagnosed with a malignant melanoma.

**Discussion Questions**

1. What type of assessment should you perform: comprehensive, focused, or emergency?
2. What are the possible causes of D.A.'s facial lesions?
3. What questions would you ask D.A. to determine the possible causes?

You will learn more about D.A. and her condition as you read through this assessment chapter.

(See p. 400 for more information on D.A.)

Answers available at *http://evolve.elsevier.com/Lewis/medsurg.*

### Important Health Information

***Past Health History.*** Past health history reveals previous trauma, surgery, or disease that involves the skin. Many diseases have dermatologic manifestations (Table 22-4). Determine if the patient has noticed any problems such as jaundice (liver disease), delayed wound healing (diabetes mellitus), cyanosis (respiratory disorder), or pallor (anemia). Obtain specific information related to food sensitivities, pet or drug allergies, and skin reactions to insect bites and stings. Note any history of chronic or unprotected exposure to UV light, including tanning bed use and radiation treatments.

***Medications.*** A thorough medication history is important. Ask the patient about skin-related problems that occurred because of taking prescription or over-the-counter (OTC) medications. Many vitamins, hormones, antibiotics, corticosteroids, and antimetabolites have side effects that are manifested in the skin. Document the use of medications specifically used to treat a primary skin problem, such as acne, or a secondary skin problem, such as itching. Record the drug's name, length of use, method of application, and effectiveness.

***Surgery or Other Treatments.*** Determine if any surgical procedures, including cosmetic surgery, were done on the skin. Record any previous biopsy results. Note any treatments specific for a skin problem (e.g., phototherapy) or for a health problem (e.g., radiation therapy). Document any treatments undergone primarily for cosmetic purposes, such as tanning booth use, laser resurfacing, or cosmetic "peels."

### Functional Health Patterns

***Health Perception–Health Management Pattern.*** Question the patient about health practices, such as self-care habits related to daily hygiene. Document the frequency of use and sun protection factor (SPF) of sunscreen products. Assess the use of personal care products (e.g., shampoos, moisturizing agents, cosmetics), including brand name, quantity, and frequency. Record a description of any current skin problem, including onset, symptoms, course, and treatment. Note any medications used for treating hair loss.

Obtain information about the family history of any skin diseases, including congenital and familial diseases (e.g., alopecia, psoriasis) and systemic diseases with dermatologic manifestations (e.g., diabetes, thyroid disease, cardiovascular diseases, immune disorders). Note any family and personal history of skin cancer, particularly melanoma.

**TABLE 22-4 Diseases With Dermatologic Manifestations**

| Systemic Problem | Dermatologic Manifestations |
|---|---|
| **Endocrine** | |
| Hyperthyroidism | Increased sweating, warm skin with persistent flush, thin nails, alopecia. Fine, soft hair |
| Hypothyroidism | Cold, dry, pale to yellow skin. Generalized nonpitting edema. Dry, coarse, brittle hair. Brittle, slow-growing nails |
| Glucocorticoid excess (Cushing syndrome) | Atrophy, striae, epidermal thinning, telangiectasia, acne. Decreased subcutaneous fat over extremities. Thin, loose dermis. Impaired wound healing. Increased vascular fragility. Mild hirsutism. Excessive collection of fat over clavicles, back of neck, abdomen, and face |
| Addison's disease | Loss of body hair (especially axillary), generalized hyperpigmentation (accentuated in folds) |
| Androgen excess | Enlarged facial pores, male sex characteristics, acne, acceleration of coarse hair growth |
| Androgen deficiency | Development of sparse hair. Marked reduction in sebum production |
| Hypoparathyroidism | Opaque, brittle nails with transverse ridges. Coarse, sparse hair with patchy alopecia |
| Hyperpituitarism (acromegaly) | Coarsened skin, deepened lines. Increased oiliness and sweating, acne. Increased number of nevi, hyperpigmentation; hypertrichosis (excess hair growth) |
| Diabetes mellitus | Erythematous plaques of shins, delayed wound healing, neuropathy, acanthosis nigricans (velvety, dark skin on the neck and in skin folds) |
| **Reproductive Organs** | |
| Primary syphilis | Chancre |
| Secondary syphilis | Generalized skin lesions, alopecia |
| Tertiary syphilis | Gummas |
| Paget's disease | Eczematous patch of nipple and areola |
| **Gastrointestinal** | |
| Inflammatory bowel disease | Mouth ulcers, erythema nodosum |
| Liver disease and biliary tract obstruction | Jaundice, itching, pigmentary abnormalities, alterations in nails and hair, spider angiomas, telangiectasia |
| Deficiency of essential fatty acids | Scaly skin |
| Malabsorption syndrome | Acquired ichthyosis (dry, scaly skin) |
| Cystic fibrosis | Abnormal sweat gland function |
| **Musculoskeletal and Connective Tissue** | |
| Systemic lupus erythematosus | Discoid lesions, maculopapular semiconfluent rash (butterfly rash), alopecia, mouth ulcers |
| Scleroderma | Leathery hardening and stiffness of skin |
| Dermatomyositis | Edema; purplish-red upper eyelids; scaly, macular erythema over knuckles |
| **Metabolic** | |
| Vitamin $B_1$ (thiamine) deficiency | Edema, redness of soles of feet |
| Vitamin $B_2$ (riboflavin) deficiency | Red fissures at corner of mouth, glossitis |
| Nicotinic acid (niacin) deficiency | Redness of exposed areas of skin of hand or foot, face, or neck; infected dermatitis |
| Vitamin C deficiency | Petechiae, purpura, bleeding gums |
| **Immune** | |
| Hodgkin's lymphoma | Pruritus, sensitive skin |
| Non-Hodgkin's lymphoma | Papules, nodules, plaques, pruritus |
| HIV infection | Kaposi sarcoma, eosinophilic folliculitis |
| **Cardiovascular** | |
| Rheumatic heart disease | Petechiae, urticaria, nodules, erythema |
| Thromboangiitis obliterans (Buerger's disease) | Pallor or cyanosis, gangrene, ulceration |
| Peripheral vascular disease | Loss of hair on hands and feet. Delayed capillary filling. Dependent rubor (redness), pain |
| Venous ulcers | Leathery, brownish skin on lower leg; pruritus, concave lesion with edema. Scar tissue with healing |
| **Respiratory** | |
| Inadequate oxygenation due to respiratory disease | Cyanosis |
| **Hematologic** | |
| Anemia | Pallor, hyperpigmentation, pale mucous membranes, hair loss, nail dystrophy |
| Clotting disorders | Purpura, petechiae, ecchymosis |
| **Renal** | |
| Chronic kidney disease | Dry skin, pruritus, uremic frost, pallor, bruises |
| **Neurologic** | |
| Chronic sensory polyneuropathies | Trophic changes in skin resulting from sensory denervation, pressure ulcers, |
| Spinal cord trauma | anesthesia, paresthesias |

**GENETIC RISK ALERT**

- The primary risk factor leading to skin cancer and melanoma is environmental exposure to UV radiation. UV radiation damages DNA, causing an error in the genetic code and resulting in abnormal skin cells.[6]
- Inherited genetic factors can increase the risk for skin cancer. A person has an increased risk for developing melanoma if he or she has a first-degree relative (e.g., parent, full sibling) who had a melanoma.
- The risk for skin cancer is increased in people who have a fair complexion (light-colored skin that easily freckles, red or blond hair, and blue or light-colored eyes).

***Nutritional-Metabolic Pattern.*** Question the patient about any changes in the condition of skin, hair, nails, and mucous membranes and whether they are related to dietary changes. A diet history reveals the adequacy of nutrients essential to healthy skin such as vitamins A, D, E, and C; dietary fat; and protein. Note any food allergies that cause a skin reaction. Ask obese patients if they have areas of chafing or a rash in **intertriginous** areas, where skin surfaces overlap and rub on each other (e.g., below the breasts, axillae, and groin). Note any excessive or absent sweating. Question the patient about poor or delayed wound healing.

***Elimination Pattern.*** Ask the patient about conditions of the skin such as dehydration, edema, and **pruritus** (itching), which can indicate alterations in fluid balance. If urinary or fecal incontinence is a problem, determine the condition of the skin in the anal and perineal areas.

***Activity-Exercise Pattern.*** Obtain information about environmental hazards in relation to hobbies and recreational activities, including exposure to known carcinogens, chemical irritants, and allergens. Ask the patient if any changes occur in the skin during exercise or other activities.

***Sleep-Rest Pattern.*** Question the patient about disturbances in sleep patterns caused by a skin condition. For example, pruritus can be distressing and cause major alterations in normal sleep patterns. Poor sleep and resulting tiredness are often reflected in a patient's face by dark circles under the eyes and a decreased firmness in the facial skin.

***Cognitive-Perceptual Pattern.*** Determine the patient's perception of the sensations of heat, cold, pain, and touch. Note any discomfort associated with a skin condition, especially when observed in intact skin, or any complaints of unusual skin sensations. Patients with neuropathy may describe numbness, tingling, or crawling sensations in their arms or legs. Assess and record any joint pain. Assess the mobility of the joints, since the patient's skin condition may cause alterations in mobility.

***Self-Perception–Self-Concept Pattern.*** Assess any feelings related to the patient's skin condition such as sadness, anxiety, despair, or altered body image. These feelings can occur with classic signs of aging or visible skin problems such as acne, rosacea, and psoriasis, which alter physical appearance.

***Role-Relationship Pattern.*** Determine how the patient's skin condition affects relationships with family members, peers, and work associates. In addition, question the patient regarding the effect of environmental factors on the skin such as occupational exposure to irritants, sun, and unusually cold or unhygienic conditions. Contact dermatitis caused by allergens and irritants is a common problem associated with occupation.

***Sexuality-Reproductive Pattern.*** Tactfully question and assess the effect of the patient's skin condition on sexual activity. In particular, note the reproductive status of the female patient relative to possible therapeutic interventions. For example, isotretinoin (Accutane), used to treat acne, and topical fluorouracil (Efudex, Fluoroplex), used to treat actinic keratoses, are teratogenic drugs that may cause abnormal fetal development. Pregnant women or women who could become pregnant should not use them.

***Coping–Stress Tolerance Pattern.*** Assess and question the patient about the role that stress may play in creating or exacerbating the skin condition. Ask the patient what coping strategies are used to manage the skin condition.

***Value-Belief Pattern.*** Ask about cultural or religious beliefs that could influence the patient's self-image as related to the skin condition. Assess values and beliefs that may influence or limit the choice of treatment options.

## Objective Data

**Physical Examination.** A physical examination of the skin begins with a systematic, general inspection and then a more specific assessment of problem areas. A normal range of differences exists in the skin, hair, and nails. Your assessment should note normal skin changes related to age, genetic factors, and environmental exposures from other changes. Look for changes in the color of the skin, turgor, temperature, dryness, thickness, and vascularity. General principles when assessing the skin are as follows:

- Have a private examination room of moderate temperature with good lighting; a room with exposure to daylight is preferred.
- Ensure that the patient is comfortable and in a dressing gown that allows easy access to all skin areas.
- Be systematic and proceed from head to toe.

### CASE STUDY

### *Subjective Data*

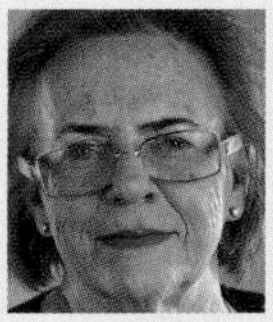

(©iStockphoto/ Thinkstock)

A focused subjective assessment of D.A. reveals the following:

- ***PMH:*** Negative except for an appendectomy at age 16.
- ***Medications:*** None at present. NKA.
- ***Health Perception–Health Management:*** Currently washes her face with a skin cleanser in the morning and nighttime. After cleansing, she applies a moisturizer with SPF 15. She has used these facial products for the past 3 years since she first started noticing small age spots appearing. Before that, she just used soap and water.
- ***Nutritional:*** D.A. reports that her skin seems to be drier as she ages but otherwise no changes besides the "age spots" or "whatever they are." Denies any changes in the way cuts or sores heal. No weight loss. Does not take any supplemental vitamins or minerals.
- ***Elimination:*** Although skin is a little dry, D.A. does not perceive it to be excessively dry. Denies excessive sweating or any swelling.
- ***Activity-Exercise:*** Loves to garden and go for walks outdoors. Reports a history of frequent, sometimes severe, sunburns as a child. No use of sunscreen growing up but does remember her mother making her wear T-shirts over her bathing suits to help prevent sunburn. Has used sunscreen for the past 20 years when outdoors. Reapplies as needed.
- ***Cognitive-Perceptual:*** Denies any pain or discomfort associated with skin lesions.
- ***Coping–Stress Tolerance:*** Fearful that she might have skin cancer.

**Discussion Questions**

1. Which subjective assessment findings are of most concern to you?
2. What should be included in the physical assessment? What specific characteristics of the skin lesions would you be looking for?

You will learn more about the physical examination of the skin in the next section.

(See p. 404 for more information on D.A.)

Answers available at *http://evolve.elsevier.com/Lewis/medsurg.*

- Compare symmetric parts.
- Perform a general inspection and then a lesion-specific examination.
- Use the metric system when taking measurements.
- Use appropriate terminology and nomenclature when reporting or documenting.

Photographs are useful when accurate findings are needed. Follow clinical agency protocol regarding obtaining a patient's consent to photograph skin lesions for inclusion in the medical record.

***Inspection.*** Inspect the skin for general color and pigmentation, vascularity, bruising, and lesions or discolorations. The critical factor in assessment of skin color is change. A skin color that is normal for a particular patient can be a sign of a pathologic condition in another patient. The skin color depends on the amount of melanin (brown), carotene (yellow), oxyhemoglobin (red), and reduced hemoglobin (bluish red) present at a particular time. The most reliable areas to assess erythema, cyanosis, pallor, and jaundice are the areas of least pigmentation, such as the sclera, conjunctivae, nail beds, lips, and buccal mucosa. The true skin color is best observed in photo-protected areas such as the buttocks. Activity, sun (UV) exposure, emotions, cigarette smoking, and edema, as well as respiratory, renal, cardiovascular, and hepatic disorders, can all directly affect skin color.

In your general inspection, note the presence of body art such as piercings and tattoos. The nose, ears, eyebrows, lips, navel, and nipples are common sites of piercing. Examine tattoos and needle-track marks and note the location and characteristics of the surrounding skin area. Tattoo pigments deposited in the skin may cause itching, pain, and sensitivity for several weeks after the tattoo is placed.

Examine the skin for possible problems related to vascularity, including bruising and vascular and purpuric lesions such as *angioma* (benign tumor of blood or lymph vessels), *petechiae* (tiny, flat, purplish red pinpoint lesions on skin), *ecchymosis* (bruise larger than petechiae), or *purpura* (purple colored spots and patches characterized by ecchymosis or other small hemorrhages). Note the reaction to direct pressure on the lesion. If a lesion blanches on direct pressure and then refills, the redness is due to dilated blood vessels. If the discoloration remains, it is the result of subcutaneous or intradermal bleeding or a nonvascular lesion. Note any pattern of bruising such as discoloration in the shape of the hand or fingers or bruises at different stages of resolution. These may indicate other health problems or abuse and require further investigation.

Record the color, size, height, distribution, location, and shape of any lesions. Lesions may be primary or secondary lesions. *Primary skin lesions* develop on previously unaltered skin. The common characteristics of primary skin lesions are shown in Table 22-5. *Secondary skin lesions* are lesions that change with time or occur because of factors such as scratching or infection. Secondary skin lesions are shown in Table 22-6.

Skin lesions are usually described in terms related to the lesions' configuration (solitary or pattern in relation to other lesions) and distribution (arrangement of lesions over an area of skin) (Table 22-7). Note any unusual odors. Skin sites with lesions, such as rashes, may be colonized with yeast or bacteria, which can be associated with distinctive odors in intertriginous areas (Fig. 22-5).

Inspect all body hair. Note the distribution, texture, and quantity of hair. Changes in the normal distribution of body hair and growth may indicate an endocrine or vascular disorder. Carefully inspect the nails, including nail shape, thickness, curvature, and surface. Note any grooves, pitting, ridges, or detachment from nail bed. Changes in nail smoothness or thickness can occur with anemia, psoriasis, thyroid problems, decreased vascular circulation, and some infections.

***Palpation.*** Palpate the skin to obtain information about temperature, turgor, moisture, and texture. Use the back of your hand to gauge skin temperature. The skin should be warm, not hot. Skin temperature increases when blood flow to the dermis is increased. A localized temperature increase occurs with burns and local inflammation. A generalized increase occurs when a person has a fever. A decreased body temperature may occur when shock or other circulatory problems, chilling, or infection are present.

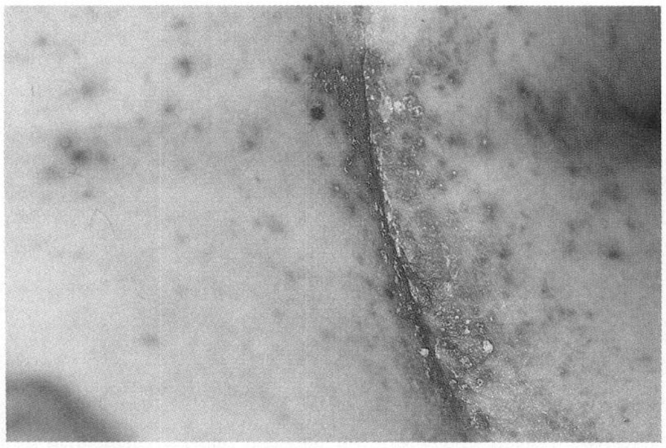

**FIG. 22-5** Intertrigo. Rash in body folds with *Candida* infection. (From Graham-Brown R, Bourke J, Cunliffe T: *Dermatology: fundamentals of practice,* Edinburgh, 2008, Mosby Ltd.)

*Turgor* refers to the elasticity of the skin. Assess turgor by gently pinching an area of skin under the clavicle or on the back of the hand. Skin with good turgor should move easily when lifted and immediately return to its original position when released. In patients with dehydration and aging, a loss of turgor occurs and can cause tenting of the skin.

Skin moisture (dampness or dryness of the skin) increases in intertriginous areas and with high humidity. Skin moisture

**TABLE 22-5 Primary Skin Lesions**

| Lesion | Description |
|---|---|
| **Macule** 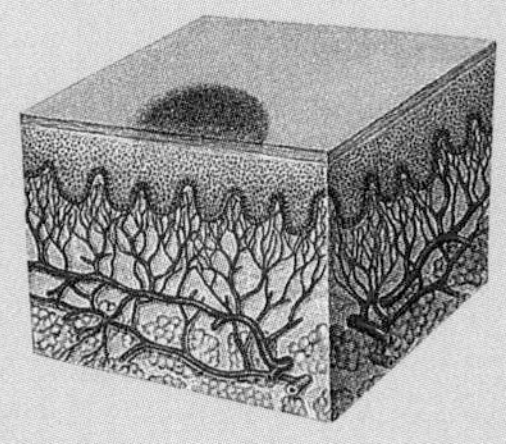 | Circumscribed, flat area with a change in skin color. <0.5 cm in diameter. If lesion >0.5 cm, it is a *patch.* *Examples:* freckles, petechiae, measles, flat mole (nevus), café-au-lait spots, vitiligo (complete depigmentation) |
| **Papule** 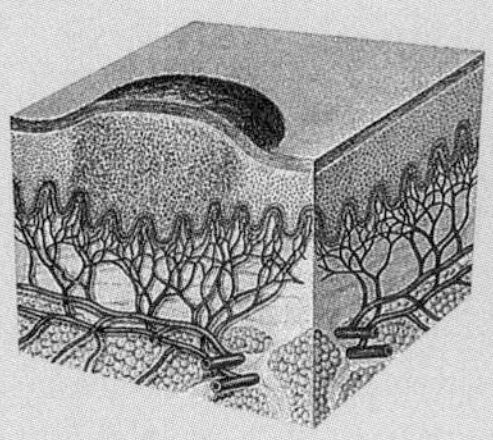 | Elevated, solid lesion. <0.5 cm in diameter. If lesion is >0.5 cm in diameter, it is a *nodule.* *Examples:* wart (verruca), elevated moles, lipoma, basal cell carcinoma |
| **Vesicle** 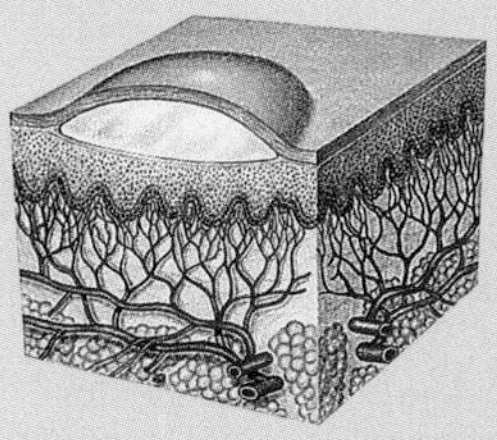 | Circumscribed, superficial collection of serous fluid. <0.5 cm in diameter *Examples:* varicella (chickenpox), herpes zoster (shingles), second-degree burn |
| **Plaque** 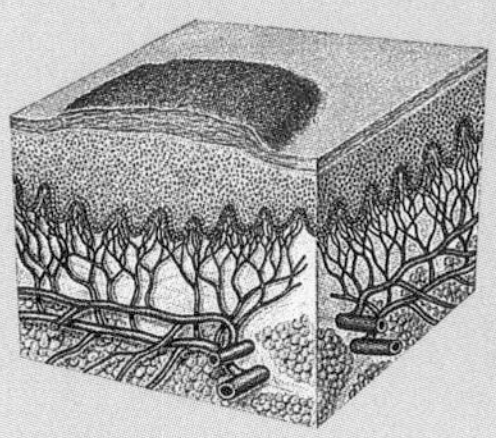 | Circumscribed, elevated, superficial, solid lesion. >0.5 cm in diameter *Examples:* psoriasis, seborrheic and actinic keratoses |
| **Wheal** 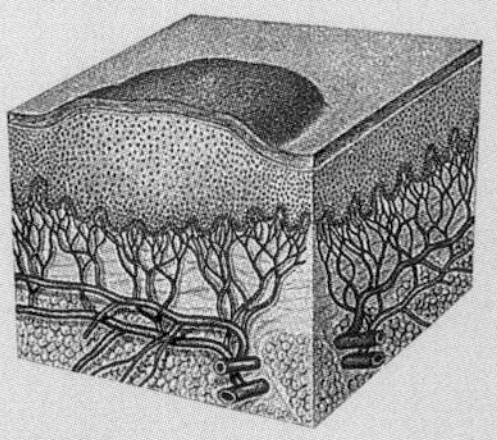 | Firm, edematous, irregularly shaped area. Diameter variable *Examples:* insect bite, urticaria |
| **Pustule** 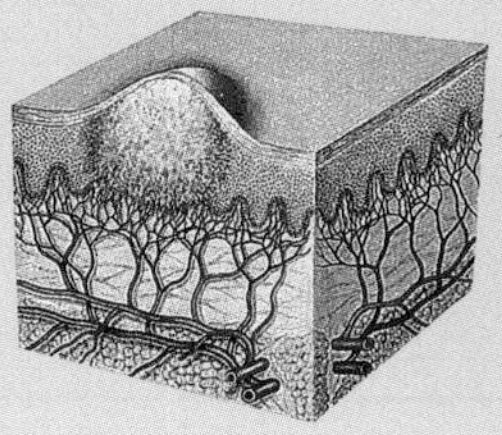 | Elevated, superficial lesion filled with purulent fluid *Examples:* acne, impetigo |

varies with environmental temperature, muscular activity, body weight, and body temperature. The skin should be intact with no flaking, scaling, or cracking. Skin generally becomes drier with increasing age.

*Texture* refers to the fineness or coarseness of the skin. The skin should feel smooth and firm with the surface evenly thin in most areas. Thickened callus areas are normal on the soles and palms and relate to weight bearing. Increased skin thickness is often work related and the result of excessive pressure. Excessive calluses on the soles of patients with neuropathy or diabetes predispose them to developing lesions.

Use a *focused assessment* to evaluate the status of previously identified skin problems and to monitor for signs of new problems. A focused assessment of the skin is presented in the box below. Assessment abnormalities of the skin are described in Table 22-8.

### Assessment of Dark Skin

The structures of dark skin are no different from those of lighter skin, but they are often more difficult to assess (Table 22-9). Color is easiest to assess in areas where the epidermis is thin and pigmentation is not influenced by sun exposure, such as

**TABLE 22-6 Secondary Skin Lesions**

| Lesion | Description |
| --- | --- |
| **Fissure** 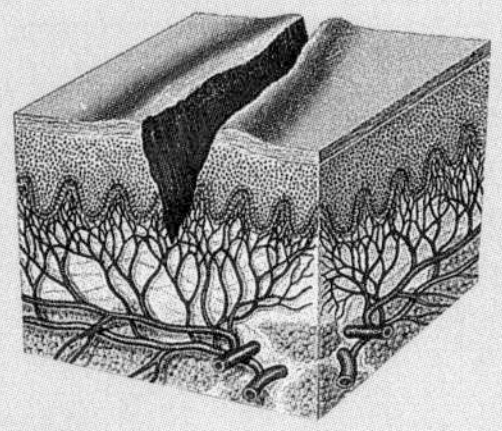 | Linear crack or break from the epidermis to the dermis. Dry or moist *Examples:* athlete's foot, cracks at corner of the mouth |
| **Scale** 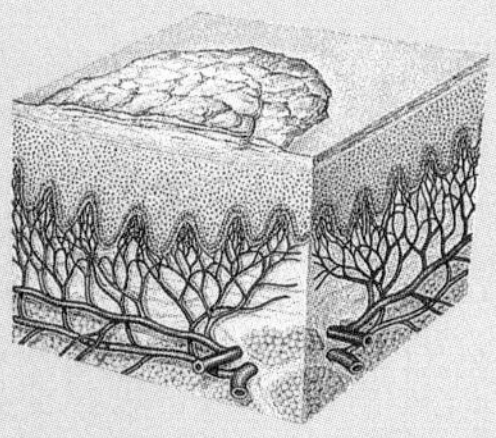 | Excess, dead epidermal cells produced by abnormal keratinization and shedding *Examples:* flaking of skin after a drug reaction or sunburn |
| **Scar** 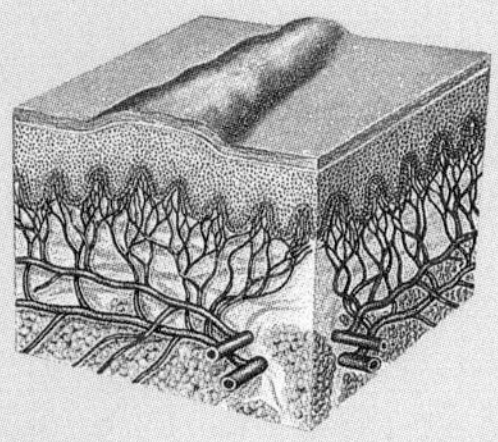 | Abnormal formation of connective tissue that replaces normal skin *Examples:* surgical incision, healed wound |
| **Ulcer** 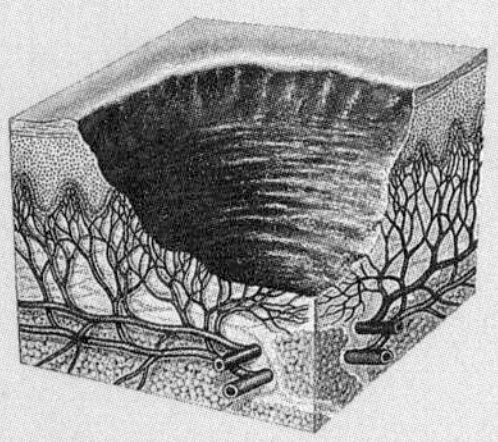 | Loss of the epidermis, extending into the dermis. Crater-like, irregular shape *Examples:* pressure ulcer, chancre |
| **Atrophy** 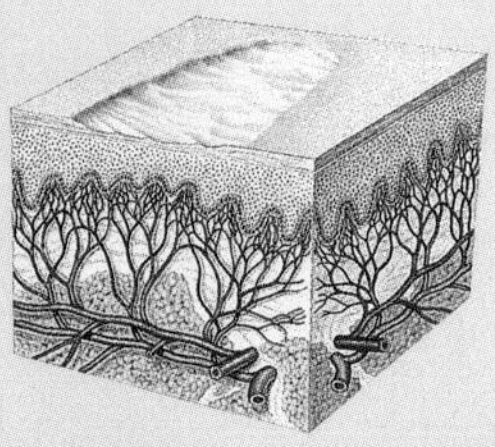 | Depression in skin resulting from thinning of the epidermis or dermis *Examples:* aged skin, striae |
| **Excoriation** 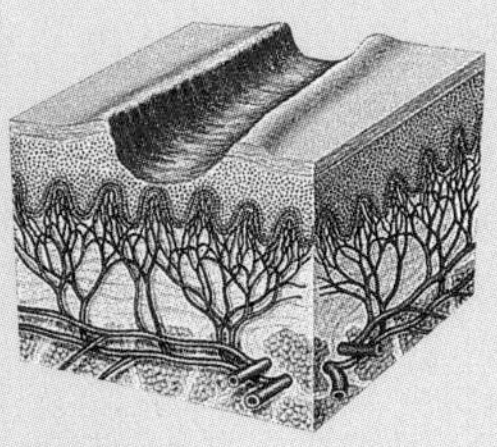 | Area in which epidermis is missing, exposing the dermis *Examples:* abrasion, scratch |

**FOCUSED ASSESSMENT**

***Integumentary System***

*Use this checklist to make sure the key assessment steps have been done.*

**Subjective**

*Ask the patient about any of the following and note responses.*

| | | |
| --- | --- | --- |
| Hair loss (unusual or rapid) | Y | N |
| Changes in skin (e.g., lesions, bruising) | Y | N |
| Nail discoloration | Y | N |

**Objective: Diagnostic**

*Check the following for results and critical values.*

| | |
| --- | --- |
| Biopsy results | ✓ |
| Albumin | ✓ |

**Objective: Physical Examination**

***Inspect***

| | |
| --- | --- |
| Skin for color, integrity, scars, lesions, signs of breakdown | ✓ |
| Facial and body hair for distribution, color, quantity, hygiene | ✓ |
| Nails for shape, contour, color, thickness, cleanliness | ✓ |
| Dressings if present | ✓ |

***Palpate***

| | |
| --- | --- |
| Skin for temperature, texture, moisture, thickness, turgor, mobility | ✓ |

**TABLE 22-7 Lesion Distribution Terminology**

| Term | Description |
| --- | --- |
| **Annular** | Circular, begins in center and spreads to periphery (e.g., tinea corporis [ringworm]) |
| **Asymmetric** | Unilateral distribution |
| **Confluent** | Merging together (e.g., urticaria [hives]) |
| **Discrete** | Distinct individual lesions that remain separate (e.g., acne) |
| **Gyrate** | Twisted, coiled spiral, snakelike |
| **Grouped** | Clusters of lesions (e.g., vesicles of contact dermatitis) |
| **Localized** | Limited areas of involvement that are clearly defined (confined to one area) |
| **Polycyclic** | Annular lesions grow together (e.g., psoriasis) |
| **Solitary** | Single lesion |
| **Symmetric** | Bilateral distribution |
| **Zosteriform** | Linear arrangement along a dermatome area (e.g., herpes zoster) |

## TABLE 22-8 Assessment Abnormalities

### *Integumentary System*

| Finding | Description | Possible Etiology and Significance |
|---|---|---|
| **Alopecia** | Loss of hair (localized or general) | Heredity, friction, rubbing, traction, trauma, stress, infection, inflammation, chemotherapy, pregnancy, emotional shock, tinea capitis, immunologic factors |
| **Angioma** | Tumor consisting of blood or lymph vessels | Normal increase in incidence with aging, liver disease, pregnancy, varicose veins |
| **Carotenemia (carotenosis)** | Yellow discoloration of skin, no yellowing of sclerae, most noticeable on palms and soles | Vegetables containing carotene (e.g., carrots, squash), hypothyroidism |
| **Comedo (acne lesion)** | Enlarged hair follicle plugged with sebum, bacteria, and skin cells; can be open (blackhead) or closed (whitehead) | Heredity, certain drugs, hormonal changes with puberty and pregnancy |
| **Cyanosis** | Slightly bluish gray or dark purple discoloration of the skin and mucous membranes caused by excessive amounts of reduced hemoglobin in capillaries | Cardiorespiratory problems, vasoconstriction, asphyxiation, anemia, leukemia, and malignancies |
| **Cyst** | Sac containing fluid or semisolid material | Obstruction of a duct or gland, parasitic infection |
| **Ecchymosis** | Large, bruise-like lesion caused by collection of extravascular blood in dermis and subcutaneous tissue | Trauma, bleeding disorders |
| **Erythema** | Redness occurring in patches of variable size and shape | Heat, certain drugs, alcohol, ultraviolet rays, any problem that causes dilation of blood vessels in the skin |
| **Hematoma** | Extravasation of blood of sufficient size to cause visible swelling | Trauma, bleeding disorders |
| **Hirsutism** | Male distribution of hair in women | Abnormality of ovaries or adrenal glands, decrease in estrogen level, familial trait |
| **Hypopigmentation** | Loss of pigmentation resulting in lighter patches than the normal skin | Chemical agents, nutritional factors, burns, inflammation, infection |
| **Intertrigo** | Dermatitis of overlying surfaces of the skin | Moisture, irritation, obesity; may be complicated by *Candida* infection (Fig. 22-5) |
| **Jaundice** | Yellow (in white patients) or yellowish brown (in African Americans) discoloration of the skin, best observed in the sclera, secondary to increased bilirubin in the blood | Liver disease, red blood cell hemolysis, pancreatic cancer, common bile duct obstruction |
| **Keloid** | Hypertrophied scar beyond wound margins (Fig. 22-6) | Predisposition more common in African Americans |
| **Lichenification** | Thickening of the skin with accentuated normal skin markings | Repeated scratching, rubbing, and irritation usually as a result of pruritus or neurosis |
| **Mole (nevus)** | Benign overgrowth of melanocytes | Defects of development; excessive numbers and large, irregular moles; often familial |
| **Petechiae** | Pinpoint, discrete deposits of blood <1-2 mm in the extravascular tissues and visible through the skin or mucous membrane | Inflammation, marked vasodilation, blood vessel trauma, blood dyscrasia that results in bleeding tendencies (e.g., thrombocytopenia) |
| **Telangiectasia** | Visibly dilated, superficial, cutaneous small blood vessels, commonly found on face and thighs | Aging, acne, sun exposure, alcohol, liver failure, corticosteroids, radiation, certain systemic diseases, skin tumors |
| **Tenting** | Failure of skin to return immediately to normal position after gentle pinching | Aging, dehydration, cachexia |
| **Varicosity** | Increased prominence of superficial veins | Interruption of venous return (e.g., from tumor, incompetent valves, inflammation), commonly found on lower legs with aging |
| **Vitiligo** | Complete absence of melanin (pigment) resulting in chalky white patch (Fig. 22-7) | Autoimmune, familial, thyroid disease |

the lips, mucous membranes, nail beds, and protected areas (e.g., buttocks). Palmar and plantar surfaces are lighter than other skin areas in darker-skinned persons. Rashes are often more difficult to observe and may have to be palpated. Wrinkling is less apparent in those with dark skin.

Persons with dark skin are predisposed to certain skin and hair conditions. **Keloid** is an overgrowth of collagenous tissue at the site of a skin injury (e.g., ear piercing) (Fig. 22-6). *Vitiligo* is total loss of pigment in the affected area (Fig. 22-7). In *dermatosis papulosa nigra,* the person has small, pigmented wart-like papules, commonly on the face. *Nevus of Ota* is a slate-gray or blue-gray birthmark located on the forehead and face around the eye area. It may also involve the sclera (Fig. 22-8). *Traction alopecia* may be the result of trauma from hair rollers or from tight braiding of the hair (Fig. 22-9). The hair loss may be temporary or permanent. *Pseudofolliculitis* is an inflammatory response to ingrown hairs that occurs after shaving too closely

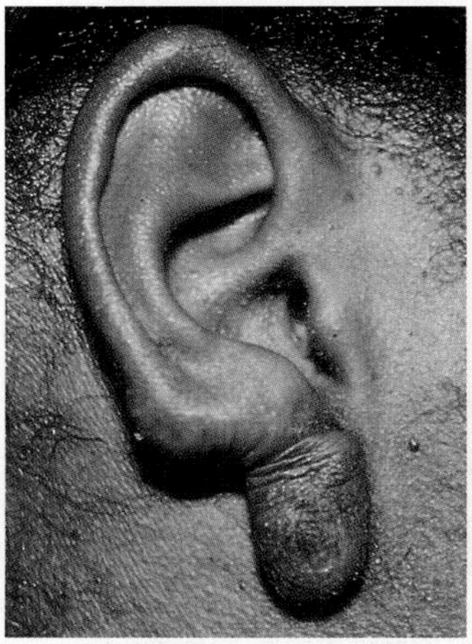

**FIG. 22-6** Keloid. Hypertrophic scarring after skin injury, which is more common in dark-skinned persons. (From Habif TP: *Clinical dermatology: a color guide to diagnosis and therapy,* ed 5, St Louis, 2011, Mosby.)

## TABLE 22-9 Nursing Assessment

### *Assessment Variations in Light- and Dark-Skinned Persons*

| Light Skin | Dark Skin |
|---|---|
| **Cyanosis** | |
| Grayish blue tone, especially in nail beds, earlobes, lips, mucous membranes, palms, and soles | Ashen or gray color most easily seen in the conjunctiva of the eye, mucous membranes, and nail beds |
| **Ecchymosis** | |
| Dark red, purple, yellow, or green color, depending on age of bruise | Purple to brownish black. Difficult to see unless occurring in an area of light pigmentation |
| **Erythema** | |
| Reddish tone, possibly accompanied by increased skin temperature secondary to localized inflammation | Deeper brown or purple skin tone with evidence of increased skin temperature secondary to inflammation |
| **Jaundice** | |
| Yellowish color of skin, sclera, fingernails, palms, and oral mucosa | Yellowish green color most obviously seen in sclera of eye (do not confuse with yellow eye pigmentation, which may be evident in dark-skinned patients), palms, and soles |
| **Pallor** | |
| Pale skin color that may appear white or ashen; also evident on lips, nail beds, and mucous membranes | Lack of underlying red tone in brown or black skin. In light-skinned African Americans, yellowish brown skin. In dark-skinned African Americans, ashen or gray skin |
| **Petechiae** | |
| Lesions appearing as small, reddish purple pinpoints, best observed on abdomen and buttocks | Difficult to see. May be evident in the buccal mucosa of the mouth or conjunctiva of the eye |
| **Rash** | |
| May be visualized and felt with light palpation | Not easily visualized, but may be felt with light palpation |
| **Scar** | |
| Generally heals, showing narrow scar line | Higher incidence of keloid development, resulting in a thickened, raised scar (Table 22-6) |

## CASE STUDY

### *Objective Data: Physical Examination*

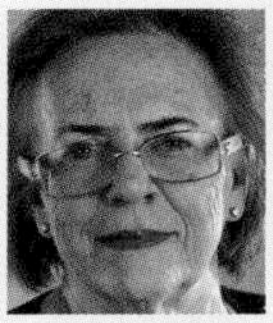

(©iStockphoto/Thinkstock)

- Physical examination findings of D.A.'s skin are as follows:
  - Complexion fair. Wrinkles around eyes, above upper lip, and on sides of cheeks bilaterally. Normal skin temperature and turgor.
  - Lesions: on upper right forehead measuring 2 × 3 mm; on left forehead near hairline measuring 1 × 2 mm; and on left lower cheek measuring 2 × 2.5 mm.

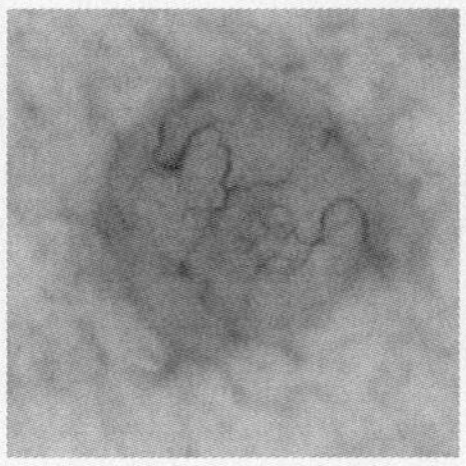

Cheek lesion. (From Bolognia JL, Schaffer JV, Duncan KO, et al: *Dermatology essentials,* Philadelphia, 2014, Saunders.)

- The lesions are slightly erythematous but do not blanch when direct pressure is applied. Borders distinct. The lesions on the forehead have minimal elevation noted on palpation. The lesion on the cheek is slightly elevated.
- No other skin lesions noted on rest of body.

**Discussion Questions**

1. Which physical assessment findings are of most concern to you?
2. Based upon the subjective and objective assessment data presented so far, what would be three priority nursing diagnoses?
3. What diagnostic studies do you think may be ordered for D.A.?

You will learn more about diagnostic studies related to the skin in the next section.

(See p. 406 for more information on D.A.)

Answers available at *http://evolve.elsevier.com/Lewis/medsurg.*

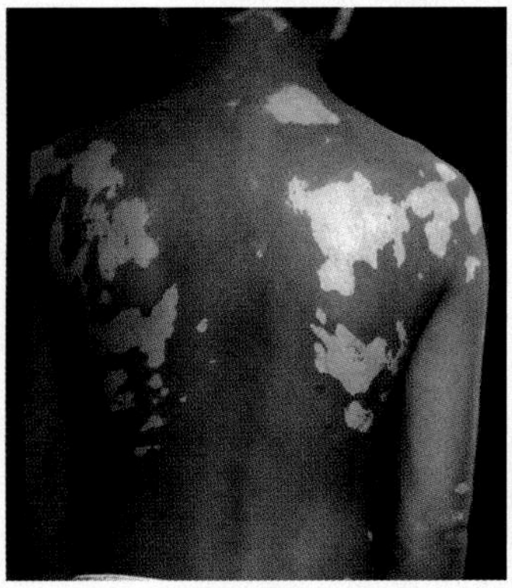

**FIG. 22-7** Vitiligo. Total loss of pigment in the affected area. (From Graham-Brown R, Bourke J, Cunliffe T: *Dermatology: fundamentals of practice,* Edinburgh, 2008, Mosby Ltd.)

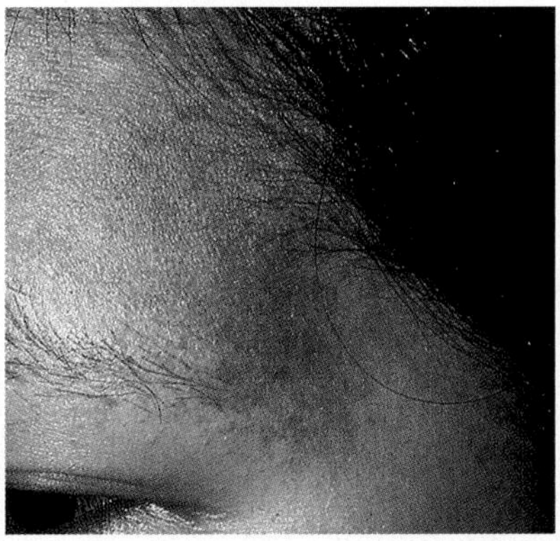

**FIG. 22-8** Nevus of Ota. Flat gray to blue pigmentation in the upper trigeminal area, which is more common in dark-skinned persons. (From Gawkrodger D, Ardern-Jones MR: *Dermatology,* ed 5, Edinburgh, 2012, Churchill Livingstone.)

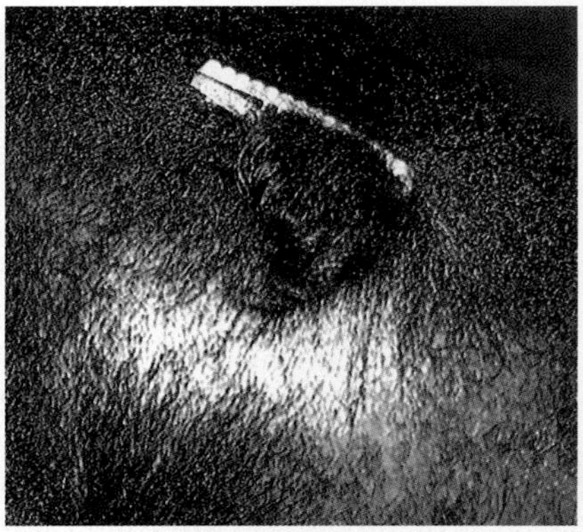

**FIG. 22-9** Traction alopecia. Hair loss in scalp because of prolonged tension from hair rollers, braiding, or straightening combs. (From Hurwitz S: *Clinical pediatric dermatology: a textbook of skin disorders of childhood and adolescence,* ed 2, Philadelphia, 1993, Saunders.)

in the beard area. The ingrown hairs result in pustules and papules.

Because of the darkness of the skin in some people, color may not be a reliable indicator of systemic conditions (e.g., flushed skin with fever). Cyanosis may be difficult to determine because a normal bluish hue occurs in dark-skinned people. Dark skin rarely shows a blanch response, making it more difficult to identify pressure ulcers.

## DIAGNOSTIC STUDIES OF INTEGUMENTARY SYSTEM

Table 22-10 presents diagnostic studies commonly used for the integumentary system. The main diagnostic techniques related to skin problems are inspection of an individual lesion and a careful history related to the problem. If a definitive diagnosis cannot be made by these techniques, additional tests may be indicated, such as *dermatoscopy* (examination of the skin through a lighted instrument with optical magnification).[7]

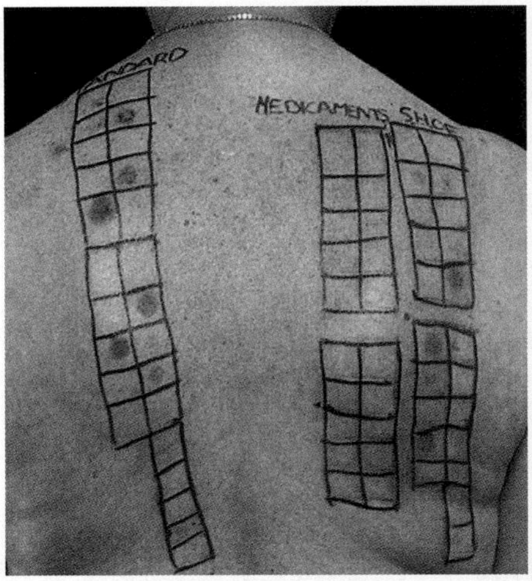


**FIG. 22-10** Patch test. Results from an application of possible allergens to the skin shows positive reactions in the sites labeled "standard" and "shoe." (From Graham-Brown R, Bourke J, Cunliffe T: *Dermatology: fundamentals of practice*, Edinburgh, 2008, Mosby Ltd.)

**TABLE 22-10 Diagnostic Studies**
***Integumentary System***

| Study | Description and Purpose | Nursing Responsibility |
|---|---|---|
| **Biopsy** | | |
| **Punch** | Special punch biopsy instrument of appropriate size used. Instrument rotated to appropriate level to include dermis and some fat. Suturing may or may not be done. Provides full-thickness skin for diagnostic purposes | *Before:* Verify that consent form is signed (if needed). *During:* Assist with site preparation, anesthesia, procedure, and hemostasis. Properly identify specimen. *After:* Apply dressing, give postprocedure instructions to patient. |
| **Excisional** | Used when good cosmetic results and/or entire lesion removal desired. Skin closed with subcutaneous and skin sutures | Same as above |
| **Incisional** | Wedge-shaped incision made in lesion too large for excisional biopsy. Useful when larger specimen than shave or punch biopsy is needed | Same as above |
| **Shave** | Single-edged razor blade used to shave off superficial lesions or small sample of a large lesion. Provides thin specimen for diagnostic purposes | Same as above |
| **Microscopic Tests** | | |
| **Potassium hydroxide (KOH)** | Hair, scales, or nails examined for superficial fungal infection. Specimen put on glass slide and 10%-20% concentration of KOH added | *Before:* Instruct patient regarding purpose of test. *During:* Prepare slide. |
| **Tzanck test (Wright's and Giemsa's stain)** | Fluid and cells from vesicles examined. Used to diagnose herpes infections. Specimen put on slide, stained, and examined microscopically | *Before:* Inform patient of purpose of test. *During:* Use sterile technique for collection of fluid. |
| **Culture** | Test identifies fungal, bacterial, and viral organisms. For *fungi,* scraping or swab of skin performed. For *bacteria,* material obtained from intact pustules, bullae, or abscesses. For *viruses,* vesicle or bulla and exudate taken from base of lesion | *Before:* Instruct patient regarding purpose and procedure. *During:* Properly identify specimen. Follow instructions for storing specimen if not immediately sent to laboratory. |
| **Mineral oil slides** | To check for infestations, scrapings are placed on slide with mineral oil and viewed microscopically. | *Before:* Instruct patient about purpose of test. *During:* Prepare slide. |
| **Immunofluorescent studies** | Some skin diseases have specific, abnormal antibody proteins that can be identified by fluorescent studies. Both skin tissue and serum can be examined. | *Before:* Inform patient about purpose of test. *During:* Assist in obtaining specimen. For punch biopsy, place specimen in special fixative (e.g., Michel's) and not formalin. |
| **Miscellaneous** | | |
| **Wood's lamp (black light)** | Examination of skin with long-wave ultraviolet light causes specific substances to fluoresce (e.g., *Pseudomonas* fungal, infections, vitiligo). | *Before:* Explain purpose of examination. Inform patient it is not painful. *During:* Darken room. |
| **Patch test** (Fig. 22-10) | Used to assess for allergic dermatitis and photoallergic reactions. Application of allergens to the patient's skin (usually on the back) for 48 hr. Test sites examined 48 hr later for a reaction, characterized by the presence of erythema, papules, vesicles, or all of these. Additional readings beyond 48 hr may be done. | *Before:* Explain purpose and procedure to patient. *After:* Instruct patient that patches are left in place for 48 hr, during which time it is important not to wash the area or play vigorous sport because if the adhesive tapes peel off the process will have to be repeated. The patches should not be exposed to sunlight or other sources of ultraviolet (UV) light. |

Biopsy is one of the most common diagnostic tests used to evaluate a skin lesion. A biopsy is indicated when a malignancy is suspected or a specific diagnosis is questionable. Techniques include punch, incisional, excisional, and shave biopsies. The method used depends on factors such as the site of the biopsy, cosmetic result desired, and type of tissue needed.

Other diagnostic procedures include stains and cultures for fungal, bacterial, and viral infections. Direct immunofluorescence is a special diagnostic technique used on biopsy specimens and may be indicated in certain conditions such as bullous diseases and systemic lupus erythematosus. Indirect immunofluorescence is performed on a sample of blood.

## CASE STUDY

### *Objective Data: Diagnostic Studies*

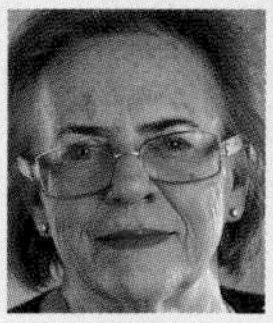
(©iStockphoto/Thinkstock)

The HCP examines the lesion via dermatoscopy and uses a Wood's lamp to rule out a fungal infection. The HCP suspects basal cell carcinoma.

**Discussion Questions**

1. Are these the diagnostic tests you expected the HCP to perform?
2. What, if any, additional diagnostic studies would you anticipate being ordered for D.A.?
3. What are the interprofessional team's priorities for D.A. at this time?

Answers available at *http://evolve.elsevier.com/Lewis/medsurg.*

## BRIDGE TO NCLEX EXAMINATION

The number of the question corresponds to the same-numbered outcome at the beginning of the chapter.

1. The primary function of the skin is
   - **a.** insulation.
   - **b.** protection.
   - **c.** sensation.
   - **d.** absorption.
2. Age-related changes in the hair and nails include *(select all that apply)*
   - **a.** oily scalp.
   - **b.** scaly scalp.
   - **c.** thinner nails.
   - **d.** thicker, brittle nails.
   - **e.** longitudinal nail ridging.
3. When assessing the nutritional-metabolic pattern in relation to the skin, the nurse questions the patient regarding
   - **a.** joint pain.
   - **b.** the use of moisturizing shampoo.
   - **c.** recent changes in wound healing.
   - **d.** self-care habits related to daily hygiene.
4. During the physical examination of a patient's skin, the nurse would
   - **a.** use a flashlight in a poorly lit room.
   - **b.** note cool, moist skin as a normal finding.
   - **c.** pinch up a fold of skin to assess for turgor.
   - **d.** perform a lesion-specific examination first and then a general inspection.
5. The nurse assessed the patient's skin lesions as firm, edematous, irregularly shaped with a variable diameter. They would be called
   - **a.** wheals.
   - **b.** papules.
   - **c.** pustules.
   - **d.** plaques.
6. To assess the skin for temperature and moisture, the *most* appropriate technique for the nurse to use is
   - **a.** palpation.
   - **b.** inspection.
   - **c.** percussion.
   - **d.** auscultation.
7. Persons with dark skin are more likely to develop
   - **a.** keloids.
   - **b.** wrinkles.
   - **c.** skin rashes.
   - **d.** skin cancer.
8. On inspection of a patient's dark skin, the nurse notes a blue-gray birthmark on the forehead and eye area. This assessment finding is called
   - **a.** vitiligo.
   - **b.** intertrigo.
   - **c.** Nevus of Ota.
   - **d.** telangiectasia.
9. Diagnostic testing is recommended for skin lesions when
   - **a.** a health history cannot be obtained.
   - **b.** a more definitive diagnosis is needed.
   - **c.** percussion reveals an abnormal finding.
   - **d.** treatment with prescribed medication has failed.

1. b, 2. b, d, e, 3. c, 4. c, 5. a, 6. a, 7. a, 8. c, 9. b

For rationales to these answers and even more NCLEX review questions, visit *http://evolve.elsevier.com/Lewis/medsurg.*

## EVOLVE WEBSITE

http://evolve.elsevier.com/Lewis/medsurg

**Review Questions (Online Only)**
**Key Points**
**Answer Keys for Questions**
- Rationales for Bridge to NCLEX Examination Questions
- Answer Guidelines for Case Study on pp. 398, 400, 404, and 406

**Conceptual Care Map Creator**
**Audio Glossary**
**Content Updates**

## REFERENCES


1. Marks JG, Miller JJ: *Principles of dermatology*, ed 5, St Louis, 2013, Mosby.
2. Bryant R, Nix D: *Acute and chronic wounds: current management concepts*, ed 4, St Louis, 2012, Elsevier. (Classic)
3. Habif TP: *Clinical dermatology*, ed 5, St Louis, 2011, Mosby. (Classic)
4. Patton KT, Thibodeau GA: *Anatomy and physiology*, ed 8, St Louis, 2013, Mosby.
5. Ball JW, Dains JE, Flynn JA, et al: *Seidel's guide to physical examination*, ed 8, St Louis, 2014, Mosby.
6. Han A, Chien AL, Kang S: Photoaging, *Dermatol Clin* 32:291, 2014.
7. Marchetti MA, Marghoob AA: Dermoscopy, *CMAJ* 186:1167, 2014.

# 23

# Integumentary Problems

*Diana L. Gallagher*

*I am tired of all this nonsense about beauty being skin deep. That is deep enough. What do you want, an adorable pancreas?*

*Jean Kerr*

http://evolve.elsevier.com/Lewis/medsurg/

## LEARNING OUTCOMES

1. Specify health promotion practices related to the integumentary system.
2. Explain the etiology, clinical manifestations, and nursing and interprofessional management of malignant dermatologic disorders.
3. Explain the etiology, clinical manifestations, and nursing and interprofessional management of bacterial, viral, and fungal infections of the integument.
4. Describe the etiology, clinical manifestations, and nursing and interprofessional management of infestations and insect bites.
5. Explain the etiology, clinical manifestations, and nursing and interprofessional management of allergic dermatologic disorders.
6. Explain the etiology, clinical manifestations, and nursing and interprofessional management related to benign dermatologic disorders.
7. Select appropriate nursing interventions to manage the patient with a dermatologic disorder.
8. Summarize the psychologic effects of chronic dermatologic conditions.
9. Explain the indications and nursing management related to common cosmetic procedures and skin grafts.

## KEY TERMS

acne vulgaris, Table 23-10, p. 419
actinic keratosis, p. 411
basal cell carcinoma (BCC), p. 411
cellulitis, Table 23-5, p. 414
cryosurgery, p. 422
curettage, p. 422
dysplastic nevi (DN), p. 413
herpes zoster, Table 23-6, p. 415
impetigo, Table 23-5, p. 414
lichenification, p. 424
malignant melanoma, p. 411
psoriasis, p. 417
squamous cell carcinoma (SCC), p. 411
sun protection factor (SPF), p. 408

This chapter discusses health promotion of the skin, common dermatologic conditions, and malignant skin neoplasms. An emphasis is placed on the nursing management of patients with dermatologic conditions.

## HEALTH PROMOTION

Health promotion practices related to the skin often parallel practices for general good health. The skin reflects both physical and psychologic well-being. Specific health promotion activities appropriate to good skin health include avoiding environmental hazards, attention to hygiene, good nutrition, adequate hydration, skin self-exam, and periodic professional exams for areas that are difficult to see.

### Environmental Hazards

**Sun Exposure.** Exposure to the sun comes with serious risk. Sun exposure results in permanent sun damage. The damage caused by ultraviolet (UV) rays is cumulative. It results in degenerative changes in the dermis, premature aging (e.g., loss of elasticity, thinning, wrinkling, abnormal dryness), and an impaired immune response. Prolonged and repeated sun exposure is a major factor in precancerous and cancerous lesions. Other problems directly associated with sun exposure include actinic keratosis, basal cell carcinoma, squamous cell carcinoma, and malignant melanoma.

Specific wavelengths (Table 23-1) have different effects on the skin. Sunlight is composed of visible light and UV light. There are two types of UV light: UVA and UVB. UVA light is responsible for tanning, UVB for sunburn. Both types can damage the skin, increase the risk of skin cancer, and accelerate the aging of skin. Tanning is the skin's response to injury. It is caused by the increased production of melanin. When sun exposure is excessive, the skin's turnover time becomes shortened, which can result in peeling. Fair-skinned persons and those with light-colored eyes should be especially cautious about excess sun exposure. They have less melanin and thus less natural protection.

Reviewed by Patricia Gable Burke, RN, BSN, CWOCN, Patient Educator Wound, Ostomy, Continence Care, Bethesda North Hospital, Cincinnati, Ohio; Kim Clevenger, RN, EdD, BC, Associate Professor of Nursing, BSN Program Coordinator, Morehead State University, Morehead, Kentucky; and Allison J. Terry RN, PhD, Associate Professor of Nursing, Assistant Dean of Clinical Practice, School of Nursing, Auburn University Montgomery, Montgomery, Alabama.

**TABLE 23-1 Wavelengths of Sun and Effects on Skin**

| Wavelength | Effect |
|---|---|
| **Long** (ultraviolet A [UVA]) | Can produce elastic tissue damage and actinic skin damage. Contributes to formation of skin cancer. |
| **Middle** (ultraviolet B [UVB]) | Causes sunburn and cumulative effect of sun damage. Major factor in development of skin cancer. |
| **Short** (ultraviolet C [UVC]) | Does not reach earth, since it is blocked by atmosphere. |

Other factors that increase the possibility of sunburn include being at a high altitude, being in snow (reflects 80% of the sun's rays), or being in or near water. Warn people of the dangers of tanning booths and sun lamps, which emit UVA. Tanning booths increase the risk of sunburn, cataracts, and skin cancer.[1]

Your patient teaching should include information on sun protection. People often do not understand the serious risks of sun exposure. Education is important. Teach patients sun safety guidelines, including sun avoidance, wearing protective clothing, and using appropriate sunscreen. Avoiding exposure to the midday sun and using protective clothing and sunscreens beginning early in life can prevent the formation of skin cancer later in life.

Teach the patient ways to avoid the damaging effects of the sun. This includes wearing sunglasses, a large-brimmed hat, and a darker-colored, long-sleeved shirt of a tightly woven fabric or carrying an umbrella. The greatest risk is between the hours of 10:00 AM and 2:00 PM, regardless of the latitude. This is when 80% of UV rays occur. Even on overcast days, serious sunburn can occur because up to 80% of the sun's UV rays can penetrate the clouds.

## EVIDENCE-BASED PRACTICE

### *Applying the Evidence*

**Tanning Booths and Skin Cancer**

You are a nurse working in a dermatology clinic. D.F., a 30-year-old female with fair skin (blonde hair and blue eyes), is completing her health history before a skin screening examination. She says she regularly visits an indoor tanning salon every other week. She tells you that being tan makes her feel "more healthy and attractive."

***Making Clinical Decisions***

***Best Available Evidence.*** There is a strong link between exposure to UV from indoor tanning booth use and increased risk of skin cancer and melanoma.

***Clinician Expertise.*** You note that D.F. has the following skin cancer risk factors: fair skin, blue eyes, frequent use of tanning booths.

***Patient Preferences and Values.*** After listening, D.F. tells you that she will consider reducing the frequency of her visits, going only when she has an important event to attend.

***Implications for Nursing Practice***

1. How would you respond to D.F., given the information that she has provided to you?
2. What resources can help address her view that a "tan looks healthy"?
3. What sun safe precautions should she take when outdoors to prevent skin cancer?

***Reference for Evidence***

Wehner M, Chren M, Nameth D, et al: International prevalence of indoor tanning: a systematic review and meta-analysis, *JAMA Dermatol* 150:390, 2014.

**TABLE 23-2 Drug Therapy**

***Drugs That May Cause Photosensitivity***

| Categories | Examples |
|---|---|
| **Antidepressants** | amitriptyline, doxepin, venlafaxine |
| **Antidysrhythmics** | quinidine, amiodarone (Cordarone) |
| **Antihistamines** | diphenhydramine, chlorpheniramine, clemastine, cetirizine (Zyrtec) |
| **Antimicrobials** | tetracycline, sulfamethoxazole, azithromycin (Zithromax), ciprofloxacin (Cipro) |
| **Antifungals** | griseofulvin, ketoconazole |
| **Antipsychotics** | chlorpromazine, haloperidol |
| **Chemotherapy** | methotrexate, dacarbazine (DTIC), 5-fluorouracil (5-FU) |
| **Diuretics** | furosemide (Lasix), hydrochlorothiazide |
| **Hypoglycemics** | tolbutamide, glipizide (Glucotrol), glyburide |
| **Nonsteroidal antiinflammatory drugs** | diclofenac (Voltaren), piroxicam (Feldene), sulindac |

Sunscreens can filter both UVA and UVB wavelengths. The two types of topical sunscreens are chemical and physical. Chemical sunscreens are light creams or lotions designed to absorb or filter UV light, resulting in decreased UV light penetration. Physical sunscreens are thick, opaque, heavy creams that reflect UV radiation. Regular sunscreen use decreases the risk of developing melanoma.

The U.S. Food and Drug Administration (FDA) rates sunscreen products on their **sun protection factor (SPF)**. The SPF measures the effectiveness of a sunscreen in filtering and absorbing UV radiation. All sunscreen labels in the United States must state which rays they protect against. Products labeled with "broad spectrum" block both UVA and UVB.[2] Sunscreens with broad spectrum labeling must have an SPF of at least 15. Sunscreens with an SPF of 15 or more filter 92% of the UVB rays and make sunburn unlikely when applied appropriately.

People need to select the sunscreen most appropriate for their needs. Para-aminobenzoic acid (PABA) and PABA esters, cinnamates, salicylates, and methyl anthranilate block UVB rays. Many sunscreen products no longer contain PABA because it stains clothing and can cause allergic reactions, including contact dermatitis. Avobenzone (Parsol) blocks UVA rays and has been added to some sunscreens. Benzophenones block both UVA and UVB rays.

The general recommendation is that everyone should use daily sunscreen with a minimum SPF of 15. Teach patients to look for the term *broad spectrum* on sunscreen packaging. Patients who have a history of skin cancer or problems with sun sensitivity should use a product with an SPF of at least 30. Sunscreens should be applied 20 to 30 minutes before going outdoors, even in cloudy weather. The SPF value of all sunscreens decreases with time. Sunscreen must be reapplied every 2 hours in a sufficient amount. One ounce per total body application is recommended. The ears, toes, and lips also need sunscreen. Sunscreens are not "waterproof" and must be reapplied immediately after swimming.

Certain medications potentiate the sun's effects, even with brief exposure. Drug categories that contain common photosensitizing medications are listed in Table 23-2. Be aware

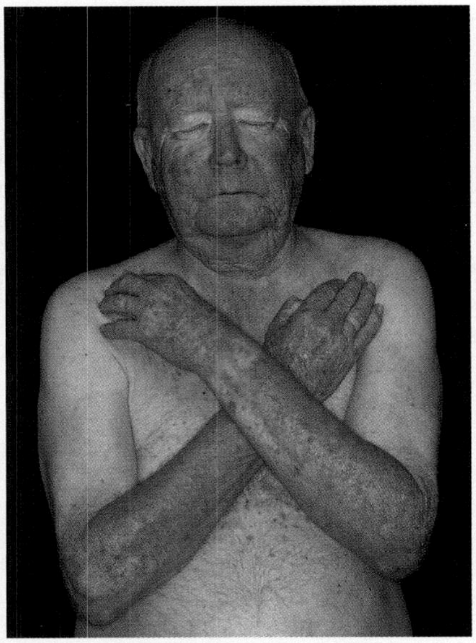

**FIG. 23-1** Intense eruption in areas exposed to sunlight after patient started on hydrochlorothiazide. (From Habif TP: *Clinical dermatology: a color guide to diagnosis and therapy,* ed 5, St Louis, 2011, Mosby.)

that many drugs are included in these categories. Assess the photosensitivity of each individual drug. The chemicals in these medications absorb light when exposed to natural sunlight and release energy that harms cells and tissues. The clinical manifestations of drug-induced photosensitivity (Fig. 23-1) are similar to those of exaggerated sunburn. These include swelling, erythema, vesicles, and papular, plaquelike lesions. Teach patients who are taking these drugs about their photosensitizing effect and the need to protect the skin from photosensitivity reactions by using sunscreen products.

**Irritants and Allergens.** Patients can seek treatment for irritant or allergic dermatitis, which are two types of contact dermatitis. *Irritant contact dermatitis* results from direct chemical injury to the skin. *Allergic contact dermatitis* is an antigen-specific, type IV delayed hypersensitivity response. This response requires sensitization and occurs only in those who are predisposed to react to a particular antigen (see Chapter 13).

Teach patients to avoid known irritants (e.g., ammonia, harsh detergents). Skin patch testing (application of allergens) can sometimes help determine the most likely sensitizing agent. Sometimes the HCP is the first to detect a contact allergy to various metals or medical products, such as gloves (latex) and adhesives in wound or ostomy products. Medications used to treat a variety of conditions may contain fragrances and preservatives that can cause dermatologic reactions.

**Radiation.** Although most radiology departments are extremely cautious in protecting both themselves and their patients from the effects of excessive radiation, it is important for you to help the patient make decisions about radiologic procedures. X-rays are valuable in both diagnosis and therapy. They can cause serious side effects to the skin, including erythema, dry and moist desquamation, edema, and changes in pigmentation.

## Rest and Sleep

Sleep is restorative to the skin. Pruritic skin diseases often interfere with sleep. Therefore helping patients obtain high-quality sleep is an important health-promotion consideration. Adequate rest increases the patient's ability to tolerate itching, thereby decreasing skin damage from the resultant scratching.

## Exercise

Exercise increases circulation and dilates the blood vessels. In addition to the healthy glow produced by exercise, the psychologic effects can improve one's appearance and mental outlook. However, caution must be used to prevent overexposure to heat, cold, and sun during outdoor exercise.

## Hygiene

The patient's skin type, lifestyle, culture, age, and gender influence hygienic practices. The normal acidity of the skin and perspiration protect against bacterial overgrowth. Most soaps are alkaline and neutralize the skin surface, leading to a loss of protection. Using mild, moisturizing soaps and lipid-free cleansers, and avoiding hot water and vigorous scrubbing can noticeably decrease local skin irritation and inflammation. Skin piercings in which jewelry has been inserted can be cared for with antibacterial soaps that do not contain sulfites.

In general, skin and hair must be washed often enough to remove excess oil and excretions and to prevent odor. Older persons should avoid harsh soaps and shampoos and frequent bathing because of the dryness of their skin and scalp. Moisturizers used immediately after a bath or shower (while the skin is still damp) seal in the moisture.

## Nutrition

A well-balanced diet adequate in all food groups can produce healthy skin, hair, and nails. Important elements of skin nutrition include the following:

- *Vitamin A:* Essential for maintenance of normal cell structure, specifically epithelial cells. It is necessary for normal wound healing. The absence of vitamin A causes dryness of the conjunctiva and poor wound healing.
- *Vitamin B complex:* Essential for complex metabolic functions. Deficiencies of niacin and pyridoxine ($B_6$) manifest as dermatologic symptoms such as erythema, bullae, and seborrhea-like lesions.
- *Vitamin C (ascorbic acid):* Essential for connective tissue formation and normal wound healing. Absence of vitamin C causes symptoms of scurvy, including petechiae, bleeding gums, and purpura.
- *Vitamin $D_3$ (cholecalciferol):* Essential for bone health. It is produced naturally by cutaneous photosynthesis after UVB exposure. A deficiency manifests as bone and muscle weakness and pain.
- *Vitamin K:* Essential for synthesizing blood clotting factors. A deficiency can lead to bruising.
- *Protein:* Necessary in amounts adequate for cell growth and maintenance and normal wound healing. A deficiency can lead to decreased wound healing.

Obesity has adverse effects on the skin. The increase in subcutaneous fat can lead to stretching and overheating (see Chapter 40). Overheating secondary to the greater insulation provided by fat causes increased sweating, which inflames and dries the skin. Obesity is a risk factor for poor wound healing and is associated with developing type 2 diabetes mellitus. Increased skin folds contribute to skin problems. Skin in these intertriginous (skin on skin) areas is predisposed to skin tags *(acrochordons),* and candidiasis (yeast), intertrigo (bacteria, fungi, yeast), and erythrasma (bacteria) infections.

### Self-Treatment

Determine if the patient is aware of the dangers of ignoring a skin problem, self-diagnosis, and treatment. The increasing variety of OTC skin preparations can be confusing.

In your general instructions to the patient, stress the duration of the treatment and the need to follow package directions. Skin problems may be slow to produce symptoms and slow to resolve. Tell the patient to follow package directions when using OTC drugs. If the package insert says its use should not exceed 7 days, patients should heed this warning. Teach the patient to stop self-care and seek the help of a HCP if any systemic signs of inflammation or extensions of the skin problem (e.g., an increasing number of lesions, increased erythema, increased swelling) develop.

## SKIN CANCER

Skin cancer is the most commonly diagnosed cancer.[3] Skin cancers are either nonmelanoma or melanoma. The fact that skin lesions are so visible increases the likelihood of early detection and diagnosis. Early detection and treatment can often lead to a highly favorable prognosis.

Teach patients to self-examine their skin at least on a monthly basis. The cornerstone of skin self-examination is the ABCDE rule.[4] Examine skin lesions for ***A**symmetry,* ***B**order* irregularity, ***C**olor* change and variation, ***D**iameter* of 6 mm or more, and ***E**volving* in appearance (Fig. 23-2). Emphasize that a persistent skin lesion that does not heal and lesions once flat and now raised, once small and recently growing, or changing in appearance are warning signs. These lesions must be examined by an HCP.

### Risk Factors

Risk factors for skin cancer include having fair skin, blond or red hair, light eye color, history of chronic sun exposure, family or personal history of skin cancer, and indoor tanning.[5] The Fitzpatrick Classification of Skin Type can assist you in determining a skin complexion and how likely a person is to get skin cancer (Table 23-3).

Because of genetic markers, people of Celtic ancestry (fair skin, blue eyes, red or fair hair, an inability to tan) are at a higher risk for squamous cell carcinoma. Environmental factors that increase the risk of skin cancer include living near the equator, outdoor occupations, and frequent outdoor recreational activities. Using indoor tanning booths and outdoor sunbathing are controllable risk factors for skin cancer. Patients treated with oral methoxsalen (psoralen) and psoralen plus ultraviolet A radiation (PUVA) may be at greater risk for melanoma.

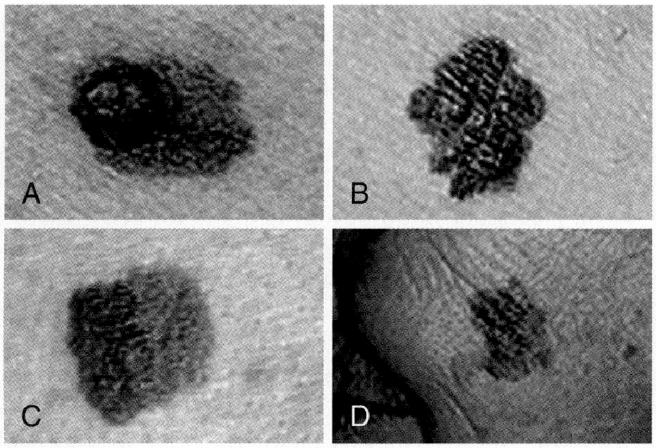


**FIG. 23-2** The ABCDEs of melanoma. **A,** Asymmetry: one half unlike the other half. **B,** Border irregularity: edges are ragged, notched, or blurred. **C,** Color: varied pigmentation; shades of tan, brown, and black. **D,** Diameter: greater than 6 mm (diameter of a pencil eraser). **E,** (not pictured) Evolving; changing appearance (change in shape, size, color, or other characteristic is noted over time). (From The Skin Cancer Foundation, New York, N.Y.)

**CULTURAL & ETHNIC HEALTH DISPARITIES**

***Integumentary Problems***

- African Americans and Hispanics have a lower incidence of skin cancer than whites.
- In the United States, rates of BCC and SCC are increasing among Hispanic and Asian women.
- Melanoma can occur in dark-skinned persons but often goes unrecognized until the advanced stages.
- When darker skin heals after injury or inflammation, it tends to be hypopigmented or hyperpigmented.
- African Americans and Asians are more likely to develop a keloid at the site of an injury.

Dark-skinned persons are less susceptible to skin cancer because of their increased melanin, which acts like a sunscreen. However, there is still a risk and a need to wear sunscreen. They often have melanomas on areas with less melanin, such as the palms, soles, mucous membranes, and under the nails. Since it is common for people with dark skin to have pigmented, longitudinal bands on their nails, assess and follow any nail discoloration.

## NONMELANOMA SKIN CANCER

Nonmelanoma skin cancers (basal cell and squamous cell carcinomas) are the most common forms of skin cancer. More than 3.5 million new cases are diagnosed each year.[3] Nonmelanoma skin cancers do not develop from melanocytes. They develop in the basement membrane of the skin. Although there are few deaths from nonmelanoma skin cancer, they have the potential for severe local destruction, permanent disfigurement, and disability.

Nonmelanoma skin cancers usually develop in sun-exposed areas, such as the face, head, neck, back of the hands, and arms. The most common causative factor is sun exposure. There are some differences between basal and squamous cell cancers. Squamous cell cancers usually occur on the head and neck where there is the highest degree of UV radiation. Basal cell

**TABLE 23-3 Fitzpatrick Classification of Skin Type**

| Skin Type | Skin Color | Characteristics |
|---|---|---|
| I | White, freckles, very fair. Red or blond hair. Blue eyes | Always burns, never tans |
| II | White, fair. Red or blond hair. Blue, hazel, or green eyes | Usually burns, tans with difficulty |
| III | Cream white, fair. Any eye or hair color | Sometimes mild burn, gradually tan |
| IV | Brown, typical Mediterranean skin | Rarely burns, tans with ease |
| V | Dark brown, Middle Eastern skin types | Very rarely burns, tans very easily |
| VI | Black | Never burns, tans very easily |

cancers do not follow that pattern and may occur in sun-protected areas.

### Actinic Keratosis

Actinic keratosis, also known as *solar keratosis,* consists of hyperkeratotic papules and plaques on sun-exposed areas. Actinic keratoses are premalignant skin lesions that affect nearly all of the older white population. These are the most common of all precancerous skin lesions. The clinical appearance of actinic keratoses can be highly varied. The typical lesion is an irregularly shaped, flat, slightly erythematous papule with indistinct borders and an overlying hard keratotic scale or horn (Table 23-4). Actinic keratoses may spontaneously resolve when exposure to sunlight is reduced. Sun exposure is a key factor. They are often first noticed in the summer.

Because actinic keratosis is impossible to differentiate from squamous cell carcinoma, treatment should be aggressive. Nonsurgical procedures are the first-line treatment (Table 23-4). Any lesion that persists should be evaluated for a possible biopsy.

### Basal Cell Carcinoma

Basal cell carcinoma (BCC) is a locally invasive malignancy arising from epidermal basal cells. It is the most common type of skin cancer but the least deadly. BCC usually occurs in middle-aged to older adults. It commonly develops at the site of earlier trauma, such as scarring, thermal burns, and injuries.[6]

Clinical manifestations are described in Table 23-4. Some BCC are pigmented, with curled borders and an opaque appearance. They may be hard to distinguish from melanoma. A tissue biopsy is needed to confirm the diagnosis. BCC rarely metastasize (Fig. 23-3). However, if BCC is left untreated, massive tissue destruction may result.

Treatment depends on the tumor location and histologic type, history of recurrence, and patient characteristics (Table 23-4). Location and size are important factors in determining the best treatment.

### Squamous Cell Carcinoma

Squamous cell carcinoma (SCC) is a malignant neoplasm of keratinizing epidermal cells. It frequently occurs on sun-exposed skin at the base of an actinic keratosis or another lesion. SCC is less common than BCC. It can be highly aggressive, has the potential to metastasize, and may lead to death if not treated early and correctly. Pipe, cigar, and cigarette smoking contribute to the formation of SCC on the mouth and lips. Immunosuppression leads to a dramatic increase in the incidence of SCC. Renal transplant recipients have a 253-fold increase in the risk of SCC.[6] The clinical manifestations of SCC are described in Table 23-4. A biopsy should always be performed when a lesion is suspected to be SCC.

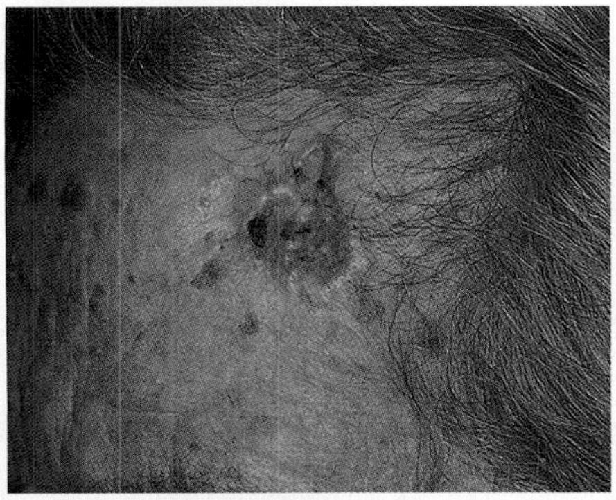

**FIG. 23-3** Basal cell carcinoma. Rolled, well-defined border and central erosion. (From Swartz MH: *Textbook of physical diagnosis: history and examination,* ed 6, Philadelphia, 2010, Saunders.)

## MALIGNANT MELANOMA

Malignant melanoma is a tumor arising in melanocytes, the cells producing melanin. Melanoma causes the majority of skin cancer deaths. More than 132,000 new cases are diagnosed every year worldwide.[3] The incidence of melanoma in whites has tripled in the last 40 years. Non-whites have a decreased incidence of melanoma, but they often have more advanced disease at initial diagnosis and a higher mortality rate than whites.[7] Melanoma can occur in the eyes, ears, gastrointestinal tract, leptomeninges, and oral and genital mucous membranes. When it begins in the skin, it is called *cutaneous melanoma.* Melanoma has the ability to metastasize to any organ, including the brain and heart.

Although the exact cause of melanoma is unknown, a combination of environmental and genetic factors is involved. UV radiation from the sun is the main cause of melanomas, but artificial sources of UV radiation, such as sunlamps and tanning booths, play a role. UV radiation damages the deoxyribonucleic acid (DNA) in skin cells, causing "misspellings" (mutations) in their genetic code. This alters the cells. Although anyone can develop melanoma, the risk is greatest for people who have red or blond hair, blue or light-colored eyes, and light-colored skin that freckles easily. These people have less melanin and thus less protection from UV radiation. The use of immunosuppressive drugs and a history of dysplastic nevi also increase a person's risk.

A person may have a genetic predisposition toward getting melanoma. Between 5% and 10% of people with melanoma have a first-degree relative (e.g., parent, full sibling) who had melanoma. This risk increases significantly if multiple relatives have a history of melanoma. Mutated genes have been identified in some families who have a high familial incidence of melanoma.

### Clinical Manifestations

About one fourth of melanomas occur in existing nevi or moles; about 20% occur in dysplastic nevi (Table 23-4). Melanoma frequently occurs on the lower legs and backs in women and on the trunk, head, and neck in men. Because most melanoma cells continue to produce melanin, melanoma tumors are often dark brown or black. Patients should consult their HCP immediately if their moles or lesions show any of the clinical signs (ABCDEs) of melanoma (Fig. 23-2). Any sudden or progressive change or increase in the ABCDE rule must be evaluated.

### Interprofessional Care

One of the initial steps in correctly diagnosing a suspicious lesion is dermoscopic examination. Dermoscopes use magnification to see patterns and structures not visible with the naked eye. Handheld screening devices (e.g., MelaFind) can assist the HCP in determining if a lesion without the obvious ABCDE signs should be biopsied. Biopsy is a critical tool for identifying a lesion. All suspicious lesions should be biopsied using an excisional biopsy technique. They should not be shave-biopsied, shave-excised, or electrocauterized. These techniques fail to provide an accurate measurement of depth.

The most important prognostic factor is tumor thickness at the time of diagnosis. Two methods to determine thickness are currently in use. The *Breslow measurement* indicates the depth of the tumor in millimeters (Fig. 23-4). The *Clark level* indicates the depth of invasion of the tumor; the higher the number, the deeper the melanoma.

Treatment depends on the site of the original tumor, stage of the cancer, and patient's age and general health. The staging

**TABLE 23-4 Premalignant and Malignant Conditions of the Skin**

| Etiology and Pathophysiology | Clinical Manifestations | Treatment and Prognosis |
|---|---|---|
| **Actinic Keratosis** | | |
| • Actinic (sun) damage<br>• Premalignant skin lesions<br>• Common in older whites | • Flat or elevated, dry, hyperkeratotic scaly papule. Often multiple<br>• Possibly flat, rough, or verrucous (wartlike)<br>• Rough adherent scale on red base, which returns when removed<br>• Often on erythematous sun-exposed area<br>• Increase in number with age | • Cryosurgery. Topical application of 5-FU, imiquimod (Aldara) or diclofenac (Solaraze), chemical peels, laser resurfacing, photodynamic therapy (PDT, with 5-aminolevulinic acid [5-ALA] or methyl aminolevulinate [MAL] followed by light irradiation)<br>• Recurrence possible even with adequate treatment |
| **Atypical or Dysplastic Nevi** | | |
| • Morphologically between common acquired nevi and melanoma<br>• May be precursor of malignant melanoma | • Often >5 mm. Irregular border, possibly notched. Frequently multiple<br>• Variegated color of tan, brown, black, red, or pink within single mole<br>• Presence of at least one flat portion, often at edge of mole<br>• Most common site on back, but possible in uncommon mole sites such as scalp or buttocks (Fig. 23-5) | • Increased risk for melanoma<br>• Careful monitoring of persons suspected of familial tendency to melanoma or dysplastic nevi<br>• Excisional biopsy for suspicious lesions |
| **Basal Cell Carcinoma** | | |
| • Change in basal cells. No maturation or normal keratinization<br>• Continuing division of basal cells and formation of enlarging mass<br>• Related to excessive sun exposure, genetic skin type, x-ray radiation, scars, and some types of nevi | *Nodular and ulcerative:*<br>• Small, slowly enlarging papule<br>• Borders semitranslucent or "pearly" with overlying telangiectasia<br>• Erosion, ulceration, and depression of center<br>• Normal skin markings lost (Fig. 23-3)<br>*Superficial:*<br>• Erythematous, pearly, sharply defined, barely elevated plaques | • Surgical excision, electrodessication and curettage, cryosurgery, radiation therapy, topical or systemic chemotherapy, and photodynamic therapy<br>• 90% cure rate with primary lesions<br>• Slow-growing tumor that invades local tissue. Metastasis rare<br>• 5-FU and imiquimod for superficial lesions, photodynamic therapy for small lesions, vismodegib (Erivedge) or sonidegib (Odomzo) for metastatic or recurrent locally invasive lesions |
| **Squamous Cell Carcinoma** | | |
| • Frequent occurrence on previously damaged skin (e.g., from sun, radiation, scar)<br>• Malignant tumor of squamous cell of epidermis. Invasion of dermis, surrounding skin | • Most common on sun-exposed areas such as face and hands<br>• *Superficial:* Thin, scaly erythematous plaque without invasion into the dermis<br>• *Early:* Firm nodules with indistinct borders, scaling, and ulceration<br>• *Late:* Covering of lesion with scale or horn from keratinization, ulceration | • Surgical excision, cryosurgery, radiation therapy, chemotherapy, electrosurgery<br>• Untreated lesion may metastasize to regional lymph nodes and distant organs.<br>• 13-*cis*-retinoic acid and interferon alfa-2A for metastatic lesions<br>• High cure rate with early detection and treatment |
| **Malignant Melanoma** | | |
| • Neoplastic growth of melanocytes anywhere on skin, eyes, or mucous membranes<br>• Classification according to major histologic mode of spread<br>• Potential invasion and widespread metastases | • Irregular color, surface, and border Variegated color, including red, white, blue, black, gray, brown<br>• Flat or elevated. Eroded or ulcerated<br>• Often <1 cm in size<br>• Most common sites in males are back, then chest. In females are legs, then back (Fig. 23-2) | • Surgical excision and possible sentinel lymph node evaluation<br>• Possible use of adjuvant therapy after surgery if lesion >1.5 mm in depth<br>• Correlation between survival rate and depth of invasion<br>• Poor prognosis unless diagnosed and treated early<br>• Spreading by local extension, regional lymphatic vessels, and bloodstream |
| **Cutaneous T-Cell Lymphoma** | | |
| • Origins in skin. Localized chronic, slowly progressing disease<br>• Possibly related to environmental toxins and chemical exposure<br>• Mycosis fungoides (MF) is most common form.<br>• Sézary syndrome is an advanced form of MF.<br>• Prevalence twice as high in men as in women | • Classic presentation involves 3 stages: patch (early), plaque, and tumor (advanced).<br>• History of persistent macular eruption followed by gradual appearance of indurated erythematous plaques on trunk that appears similar to psoriasis<br>• Pruritus, lymphadenopathy | • Treatment usually controls symptoms but is not curative. UVB, PUVA, corticosteroids, topical nitrogen mustard, radiation therapy in patch and plaque stage of disease<br>• Interferon, systemic chemotherapy, extracorporeal photopheresis, romidepsin (Istodax) for progressive disease<br>• Bexarotene (Targretin), denileukin diftitox (Ontak), and vorinostat (Zolinza) for advanced disease<br>• Disease course is unpredictable. 10% will have progressive disease. |

*5-FU,* Fluorouracil; *PUVA,* psoralen ultraviolet A; *UVB,* ultraviolet B.

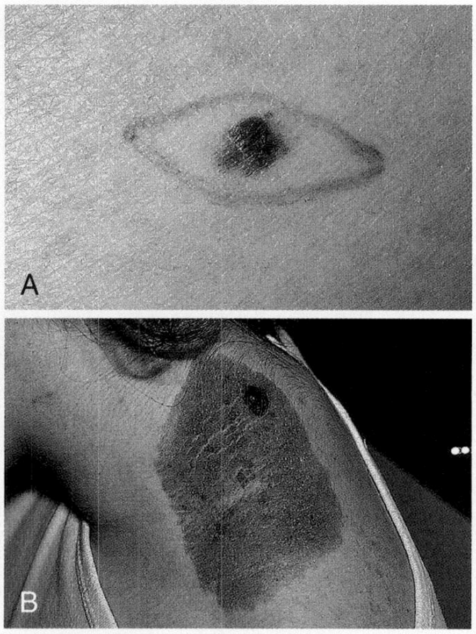

FIG. 23-4 Breslow measurement of tumor thickness. **A,** Thin (0.08-mm) superficial spreading melanoma, good prognosis. **B,** Thick nodular melanoma with lymph node involvement, poor prognosis. (From Gawkrodger D, Ardern-Jones MR: *Dermatology,* ed 5, Edinburgh, 2012, Churchill Livingstone.)

of melanoma (stages 0 to IV) is based on tumor size (thickness), nodal involvement, and metastasis. In stage 0 the melanoma is confined to one place (in situ) in the epidermis. Melanoma is nearly 100% curable by excision if diagnosed at stage 0. The 5-year survival rate depends on sentinel node biopsy results, which indicate if metastasis has occurred. The presence of metastasis in the sentinel lymph node is the most important prognostic factor for recurrence.[6]

The initial treatment of malignant melanoma is wide surgical excision. Melanoma that has spread to the lymph nodes or nearby sites usually requires additional (adjuvant) therapy such as chemotherapy, immunotherapy, targeted therapy, and/or radiation therapy. Chemotherapy includes dacarbazine (DTIC) and temozolomide (Temodar). Adding combinations of cisplatin, carmustine, carboplatin (Paraplatin), or vincristine improves response rate.

Immunotherapy can include cytokines (α-interferon, interleukin-2), PD-1 inhibitors, and CTLA-4 inhibitors. PD-1 inhibitors include nivolumab (Opdivo) and pembrolizumab (Keytruda). These drugs block PD-1, a protein on T cells that normally keeps these cells from attacking other cells in the body. By blocking PD-1, these drugs boost the immune response against melanoma cells. Ipilimumab (Yervoy), a CTLA-4 inhibitor, also boosts the immune system, but it has a different target. It blocks CTLA-4, a protein that normally helps keep T cells in check. By blocking the action of CTLA-4, ipilimumab boosts the immune response against melanoma cells.[8]

Targeted therapy for melanoma includes BRAF and MEK inhibitors. About half of all melanomas have mutations in the *BRAF* gene, which makes an altered BRAF protein that signals melanoma cells to proliferate. Vemurafenib (Zelboraf), dabrafenib (Tafinlar), and cobimetinib (Cotellic) are BRAF inhibitor drugs that attack the BRAF protein directly.

The *MEK* gene is involved in the activation of the BRAF pathway. Therefore a MEK inhibitor drug, trametinib (Mekinist), can be used to treat melanomas with *BRAF* gene changes.

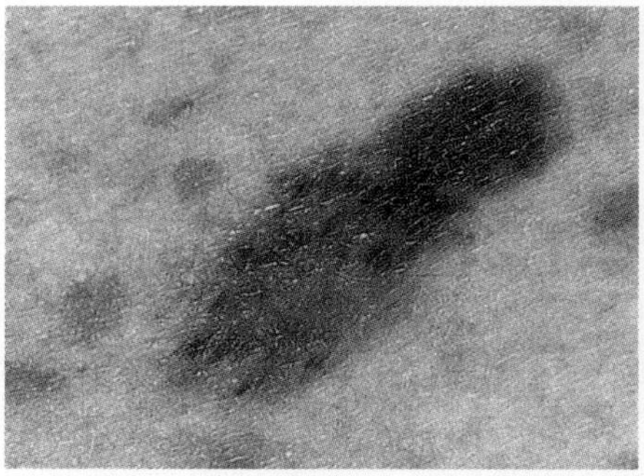

FIG. 23-5 Dysplastic nevus. Irregular border and color. (From Graham-Brown R, Bourke J, Cunliffe T: *Dermatology: fundamentals of practice,* Edinburgh, 2008, Mosby Ltd.)

### Atypical or Dysplastic Nevus

An abnormal nevus pattern called *dysplastic nevus syndrome* identifies a person at increased risk of melanoma. Approximately 2% to 8% of the white population have moles classified as atypical or dysplastic nevi. **Dysplastic nevi (DN)**, or atypical moles, are nevi that are larger than usual (greater than 5 mm across) with irregular borders and various shades of color (Fig. 23-5). These nevi may have the same ABCDE characteristics as melanoma, but they are less pronounced. A difference between DN and common nevi is that DN do not appear until a person is nearing puberty and continue to develop beyond the fourth decade. The average number of normal nevi in adults is about 40. Those with DN may have more than 100 normal-appearing nevi.

Obtain a detailed family history related to melanoma and DN. The risk of developing melanoma doubles with the presence of one DN, and having multiple DN increases the risk up to 12-fold.

**CHECK YOUR PRACTICE**

You are working in a dermatology clinic, and your assigned patient is a 78-yr-old white man. He is worried about his many "brown" spots on his face and arms. He tells you that they probably developed because he worked outside in construction most of his life.

- How do you distinguish among an age spot (lentigo), normal mole, and malignant melanoma?
- What risk factors would you assess for in a patient with a suspected cancerous lesion?

## SKIN INFECTIONS AND INFESTATIONS

### Bacterial Infections

The skin provides an ideal environment for bacterial growth with an abundant supply of nutrients, water, and warm temperature. Bacterial infection occurs when the balance between the host and microorganisms is altered. This can occur as a primary infection after a break in the skin. It can occur as a secondary infection in already damaged skin or as a sign of a systemic disease (Table 23-5). *Staphylococcus aureus* and group A β-hemolytic streptococci are the major types of bacteria responsible for primary and secondary skin infections. Streptococci cause impetigo, erysipelas, cellulitis, and lymphangitis. *S. aureus* causes impetigo, folliculitis, cellulitis, and furuncles (Fig. 23-6).

Healthy persons can develop bacterial skin infections. Predisposing factors such as moisture, obesity, atopic dermatitis,

**TABLE 23-5 Common Bacterial Infections of the Skin**

| Etiology and Pathophysiology | Clinical Manifestations | Treatment and Prognosis |
|---|---|---|
| **Impetigo**<br>• Group A β-hemolytic streptococci, staphylococci, or combination of both<br>• Associated with poor hygiene<br>• Primary or secondary infection. Contagious | • Vesiculopustular lesions that develop thick, honey-colored crust surrounded by erythema<br>• Pruritic<br>• Most common on face as primary infection | *Topical:*<br>• Wound care with warm saline or aluminum acetate soaks followed by soap-and-water removal of crusts and application of topical antibiotic cream or ointment (mupirocin [Bactroban], retapamulin [Altabax])<br>• Meticulous hygiene essential<br>*Systemic:*<br>• Systemic antibiotics (e.g., cephalosporins, amoxicillin, clindamycin) for widespread infections or systemic manifestations |
| **Folliculitis**<br>• Usually staphylococci<br>• Present in areas subjected to friction, moisture, rubbing, or oil<br>• Increased incidence in patients with diabetes mellitus | • Small pustule at hair follicle opening with minimal erythema<br>• Development of crusting<br>• Most common on scalp, beard, extremities in men<br>• Tender to touch | • Antistaphylococcal soap (e.g., Hibiclens, Lever 2000, Dial) and water cleansing<br>• Topical antibiotics (e.g., mupirocin)<br>• Warm compresses of water or aluminum acetate solution<br>• Usually heals without scarring<br>• If lesions extensive and deep, possible scarring, loss of involved hair follicles, and treatment with systemic antibiotics |
| **Furuncle**<br>• Deep infection with staphylococci around hair follicle<br>• Often associated with severe acne or seborrheic dermatitis | • Tender erythematous area around hair follicle that is painful<br>• Draining pus and core of necrotic debris on rupture<br>• Most common on face, back of neck, axillae, breasts, buttocks, perineum, thighs | • Incision and drainage (possibly with packing), antibiotics, meticulous care of involved skin, frequent application of warm, moist compresses |
| **Furunculosis**<br>• Increased incidence in patients who are obese, diabetic, chronically ill, or regularly exposed to moisture, pressure | • Lesions as above<br>• Malaise, regional adenopathy, elevated body temperature | *Topical:*<br>• Incision and drainage of painful nodules<br>• Warm, moist compresses to erythematous plaques<br>• Measures to reduce surface staphylococci include antimicrobial cream to nares, armpits, and groin and antiseptic to entire skin.<br>• Meticulous personal hygiene<br>*Systemic:*<br>• Systemic antibiotic effective against MRSA pending culture and sensitivity results<br>• Often recurrent with scarring |
| **Carbuncle**<br>• Multiple, interconnecting furuncles | • Many pustules appearing in erythematous area<br>• Most common at nape of neck | • Treatment same as for furuncles<br>• Often recurrent despite production of antibodies<br>• Heal slowly with scar formation |
| **Cellulitis**<br>• Inflammation of subcutaneous tissues<br>• Possibly secondary complication or primary infection<br>• Often following break in skin<br>• *Staphylococcus aureus* and streptococci usual causative agents<br>• Deep inflammation of subcutaneous tissue from enzymes produced by bacteria | • Hot, tender, erythematous, and edematous area with diffuse borders<br>• Chills, malaise, and fever (Fig. 23-6) | *Topical:*<br>• Moist heat, immobilization, and elevation<br>*Systemic:*<br>• Systemic antibiotic therapy<br>• Hospitalization if severe for IV antibiotic therapy (dalbavancin [Dalvance], vancomycin, linezolid [Zyvox], ceftaroline fosamil [Teflaro], daptomycin [Cubicin])<br>• Progression to gangrene possible if untreated |
| **Erysipelas**<br>• Superficial cellulitis primarily involving the dermis<br>• Group A β-hemolytic streptococci | • Red, hot, sharply demarcated plaque that is indurated and painful<br>• Bacteremia possible<br>• Most common on face and extremities<br>• Toxic signs: fever, ↑ WBC count, headache, malaise | • Systemic antibiotics, usually penicillin<br>• Hospitalization often required |

*MRSA,* Methicillin-resistant *S. aureus.*

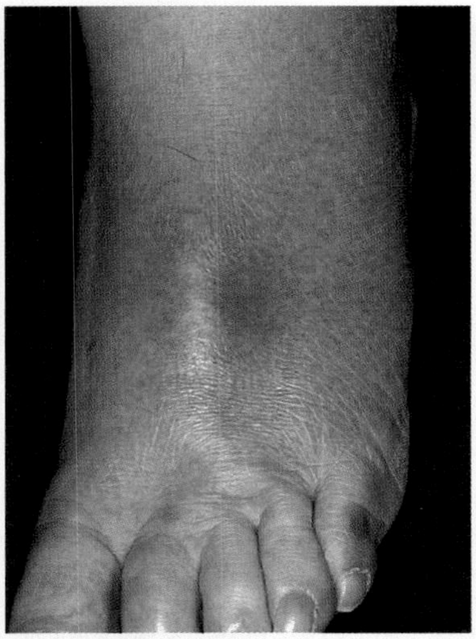

**FIG. 23-6** Cellulitis with characteristic erythema, tenderness, and edema. (From Habif TP: *Clinical dermatology: a color guide to diagnosis and therapy,* ed 5, St Louis, 2011, Mosby.)

systemic corticosteroids and antibiotics, and chronic disease such as diabetes mellitus increase the likelihood of infection. Good hygiene practices and general good health inhibit bacterial infections. If an infection is present, the resulting drainage is infectious. Good skin hygiene and infection control practices are necessary to prevent the spread of the infection.

### Viral Infections

Similar to viral infections anywhere in the body, viral infections of the skin are difficult to treat. When a virus infects a cell, a skin lesion may develop. Lesions can also result from an inflammatory response to viral infections. Herpes simplex, herpes zoster (Fig. 23-7), and warts (Fig. 23-8) are the most common viral infections affecting the skin (Table 23-6).

### Infestations and Insect Bites

The possibilities for exposure to *infestations* (harboring insects or worms) and insect bites are numerous (Table 23-7). In many instances, an allergy to the venom plays a major role in the reaction. In other cases, the clinical manifestations are a

**TABLE 23-6 Common Viral Infections of the Skin**

| Etiology and Pathophysiology | Clinical Manifestations | Treatment and Prognosis |
|---|---|---|
| **Herpes Simplex Virus (HSV) Types 1 and 2** | | |
| • Oral or genital HSV infections serotyped as either HSV-1 or HSV-2<br>• Both are recurrent lifelong viral infections.<br>• Exacerbated by sunlight, trauma, menses, stress, and systemic infection<br>• Contagious to those not previously infected<br>• Transmitted by respiratory droplets or virus-containing fluid (e.g., saliva, cervical secretions)<br>• Infection in one area readily transmitted to another site by contact | *First episode:*<br>• Symptoms occurring 2 days to 2 weeks after contact<br>• Painful local reaction<br>• Single or grouped vesicles on erythematous base<br>• Systemic symptoms (e.g., fever, malaise) possible or no symptoms possible<br>*Recurrent:*<br>• Recurrence in similar spot<br>• Characteristic grouped vesicles on erythematous base | • Symptomatic<br>• Soothing, moist compresses. White petroleum to lesions<br>• Scarring not usual result<br>• Antiviral agents such as acyclovir (Zovirax), famciclovir (Famvir), and valacyclovir (Valtrex)<br>• Vaccine not currently available for HSV-1 or HSV-2 |
| **Herpes Zoster (Shingles)** | | |
| • Activation of the varicella-zoster virus<br>• Incidence increases with age.<br>• Potentially contagious to anyone who has not had varicella or who is immunosuppressed | • Linear distribution along a dermatome of grouped vesicles and pustules on erythematous base resembling chickenpox (Fig. 23-7)<br>• Usually unilateral on trunk, face, and lumbosacral areas<br>• Burning, pain, and neuralgia preceding outbreak<br>• Mild to severe pain during outbreak | • Symptomatic<br>*Topical:*<br>• Wet compresses, silver sulfadiazine (Silvadene) to ruptured vesicles<br>*Systemic:*<br>• Antiviral agents (e.g., acyclovir, famciclovir, valacyclovir) within 72 hr to prevent postherpetic neuralgia<br>• Analgesia. Mild sedation at bedtime<br>• Gabapentin (Neurontin) to treat postherpetic neuralgia<br>• Usually heals without complications, but scarring and postherpetic neuralgia possible<br>• Vaccine (Zostavax) to prevent shingles for adults ≥50 yr |
| **Verruca Vulgaris** | | |
| • Caused by human papillomavirus (HPV)<br>• Spontaneous disappearance in 1-2 yr possible<br>• Mildly contagious by autoinoculation<br>• Specific response dependent on body part affected<br>• Prevalence greater in youth and immunosuppressed | • Circumscribed, hypertrophic, flesh-colored papule limited to epidermis<br>• Painful on lateral compression | • Multiple treatments, including surgery using blunt dissection with scissors or curette<br>• Liquid nitrogen therapy<br>• Blistering agent (cantharidin)<br>• Keratolytic agent (salicylic acid)<br>• $CO_2$ laser destruction |
| **Plantar Warts** | | |
| • Caused by HPV | • Wart on bottom surface of foot, growing inward because of pressure of walking or standing (Fig. 23-8)<br>• Painful when pressure applied<br>• Interrupted skin markings<br>• Cone shaped with black dots (thrombosed vessels) when wart removed | • Topical immunotherapy (imiquimod), cryosurgery, salicylic acid, duct tape |

**TABLE 23-7 Common Infestations and Insect Bites**

| Etiology and Pathophysiology | Clinical Manifestations | Treatment and Prognosis |
|---|---|---|
| **Bees and Wasps** | | |
| *Hymenoptera* species | • Intense, burning, local pain<br>• Swelling and itching<br>• Severe hypersensitivity possibly leading to anaphylaxis | • Cool compresses<br>• Local application of antipruritic lotion<br>• Antihistamines if indicated<br>• Usually uneventful recovery |
| **Bedbugs** | | |
| • *Cimicidae* species<br>• Feeding periodic, usually at night<br>• Present in furniture, walls during day | • Wheal surrounded by vivid flare<br>• Firm urticaria transforming into persistent lesion<br>• Severe pruritus<br>• Often grouped in threes appearing on uncovered parts of body | • Bedbug controlled by chlorocyclohexane<br>• Lesions usually require no treatment<br>• Severe itching possibly requires use of antihistamines or topical corticosteroids |
| **Pediculosis (Head Lice, Body Lice, Pubic Lice)** | | |
| • *Pediculus humanus* var. capitis, *Pediculus humanus* var. corporis, *Phthirus pubis*<br>• Obligate parasites that suck blood, leave excrement and eggs on skin and hair, live in seams of clothing (if body lice) and in hair as nits. Transmission of pubic lice often by sexual contact | • Minute, red, noninflammatory<br>• Points flush with skin. Progression to papular wheal-like lesions<br>• Pruritus<br>• Secondary excoriation, especially parallel linear excoriations in intrascapular region<br>• Nits and eggs are firmly attached to hair shaft in head and body. | • γ-Benzene hexachloride or pyrethrins to treat various parts of body<br>• Spinosad (Natroba) topical suspension 0.9% to treat scalp and hair<br>• Close contacts (e.g., bed partners and playmates) should be screened and treated.<br>• Do not share head gear. |
| **Scabies** | | |
| • *Sarcoptes scabiei*<br>• Mite penetrates stratum corneum, deposits eggs.<br>• Allergic reaction to eggs, feces, mite parts<br>• Transmission by direct physical contact, only occasionally by shared personal items<br>• Rarely seen in dark-skinned people | • Severe itching, especially at night, usually not on face<br>• Presence of burrows, especially in interdigital webs, flexor surface of wrists, genitalia, and anterior axillary folds<br>• Erythematous papules (may be crusted), possible vesiculation, interdigital web crusting | • 5% permethrin topical lotion, one overnight application with second application 1 wk later, may yield 95% eradication.<br>• Treat all family members, treat environment with plastic covering for 5 days, launder all clothes and linen with bleach.<br>• Treat sexual partner.<br>• Antibiotics if secondary infections present<br>• Possible residual pruritus up to 4 wk after treatment<br>• Recurrence possible if inadequately treated |
| **Ticks** | | |
| • *Borrelia burgdorferi* (spirochete transmitted by ticks in certain areas) causes Lyme disease.<br>• Endemic areas include Northeast, Mid-Atlantic states, parts of Midwest and West (see Chapter 64). | • Spreading, ringlike rash 3-4 wk after bite (see Fig. 64-7)<br>• Rash commonly in groin, buttocks, axillae, trunk, and upper arms and legs<br>• Warm, itchy, or painful rash<br>• Flu-like symptoms<br>• Cardiac, arthritic, and neurologic manifestations possible<br>• Unreliable laboratory test | • Oral antibiotics, such as doxycycline, tetracycline<br>• IV antibiotics for arthritic, neurologic, and cardiac symptoms<br>• Rest and healthy diet<br>• Most patients recover. |

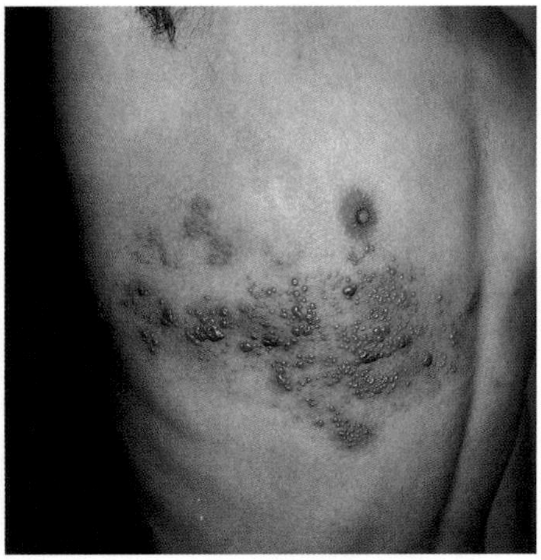

**FIG. 23-7** Herpes zoster (shingles) on the anterior chest, classic dermatomal distribution. (From James WD, Berger T, Elston DMD: *Andrews' diseases of the skin,* ed 11, Philadelphia, 2011, Saunders.)

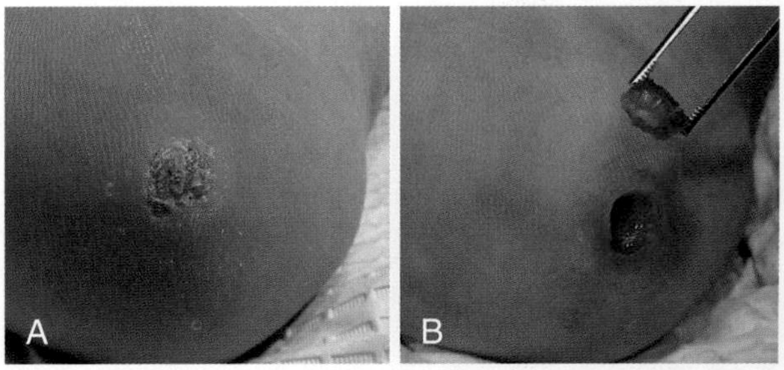


**FIG. 23-8** Plantar wart. **A,** Keratotic lesion. **B,** After excision. (From Swartz MH: *Textbook of physical diagnosis: history and examination,* ed 6, Philadelphia, 2010, Saunders.)

reaction to the eggs, feces, or body parts of the invading organism. Some people react with a severe hypersensitivity (anaphylaxis), which can be life threatening. (Anaphylaxis is discussed in Chapter 13.)

Preventing insect bites by avoidance or using repellents is somewhat effective. Meticulous hygiene related to personal articles, clothing, bedding, and examination and care of pets, as well as careful selection of sexual partners, can reduce the incidence of infestations. Prompt, routine skin inspection is necessary in geographic areas where there is a risk of tick bite. (Lyme disease, which is caused by a tick, is discussed in Chapter 64.)

### Fungal Infections

Because of the large number of fungi that are present everywhere, exposure to some pathologic varieties may occur. Skin, hair, and nails can become infected with fungi, including candidiasis and tinea unguium (Fig. 23-9). Common fungal infections of the skin are presented in Table 23-8. Most infections are relatively harmless in healthy adults, but they can be embarrassing and distressing to the patient.

The microscopic examination of the scraping of suspicious scaly skin lesions in 10% to 20% potassium hydroxide (KOH) is an inexpensive diagnostic measure to determine the presence of a fungus. The appearance of microscopic hyphae (threadlike structures) is indicative of a fungal infection.

## ALLERGIC DERMATOLOGIC PROBLEMS

Dermatologic problems associated with allergies and hypersensitivity reactions may present a challenge to the clinician (Table 23-9). (The pathophysiology related to allergic and contact dermatitis is discussed in Chapter 13.) A careful family history and discussion of exposure to possible offending agents can provide valuable data. Patch testing is used to help to determine possible causative agents (see Fig. 22-10). The best treatment of allergic dermatitis is avoidance of the causative agent. The extreme pruritus and its potential for chronicity make it a frustrating problem for you and the patient, especially if the offending agent cannot be identified.

## BENIGN DERMATOLOGIC PROBLEMS

Although the list of benign dermatoses is extensive, some of the most commonly seen and distressing problems include acne vulgaris (Fig. 23-10), psoriasis, and seborrheic keratoses. Benign problems are summarized in Table 23-10.

**Psoriasis** is an autoimmune disease. Men and women develop psoriasis at equal rates. It occurs in all racial groups, but at varying rates. About 1.3% of African Americans have psoriasis, compared to 2.5% of whites.[9] It usually develops in persons between 15 and 35 years old. One third of people with psoriasis have at least one relative with the disease.

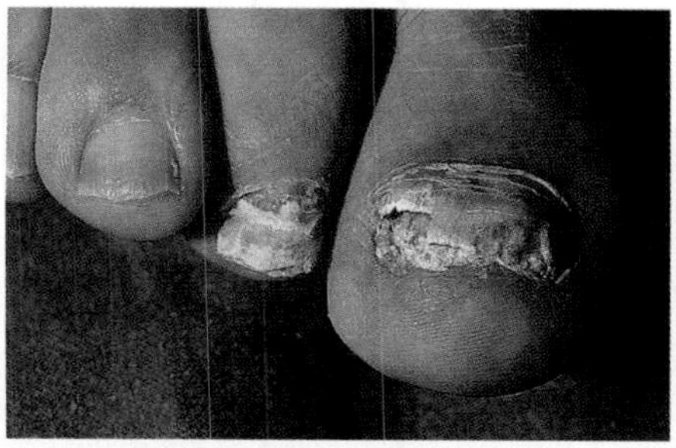

**FIG. 23-9** Tinea unguium (onychomycosis). Fungal infection of toenails. Crumbly, discolored, and thickened nails. (From Gawkrodger D, Ardern-Jones MR: *Dermatology,* ed 5, Edinburgh, 2012, Churchill Livingstone.)

Diagnosis is often based on the skin's appearance (Fig. 23-11). Lesions are distinctive and appear as red, scaling papules that merge to form plaques. The affected area is normally rounded, with adherent silver scales that bleed easily when removed.

While most people have mild disease, many with severe disease often have a weakened immune system, diabetes mellitus, depression, and cardiovascular disease. Psoriatic arthritis affects 10% to 30% of all persons with psoriasis. (Psoriatic arthritis is discussed in Chapter 64.) The chronicity of psoriasis can be severe and disabling. People withdraw from social contacts because of visible lesions, and quality of life can diminish.

**DRUG ALERT Isotretinoin (Accutane)**
- Used to treat acne (Table 23-10)
- Can cause serious damage to fetus
- Contraindicated in women who are pregnant or want to become pregnant while on the drug
- Blood donation prohibited for those taking the drug and for 1 month after treatment ends
- Linked to liver function test abnormalities

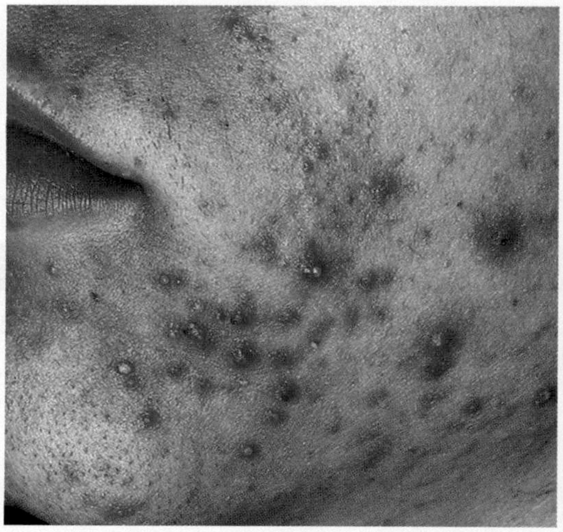

**FIG. 23-10** Acne vulgaris. Papules and pustules. (From James WD, Berger T, Elston DMD: *Andrews' diseases of the skin,* ed 11, Philadelphia, 2011, Saunders.)

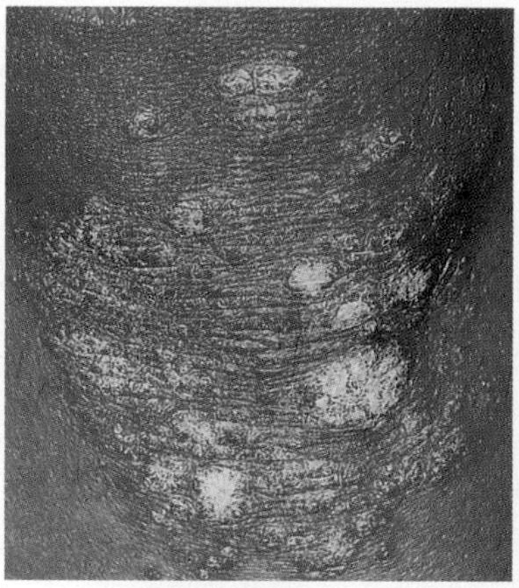

**FIG. 23-11** Psoriasis. Characteristic inflammation and scaling. (From Habif TP: *Clinical dermatology: a color guide to diagnosis and therapy,* ed 5, St Louis, 2011, Mosby.)

**TABLE 23-8 Common Fungal Infections of the Skin**

| Etiology and Pathophysiology | Clinical Manifestations | Treatment and Prognosis |
|---|---|---|
| **Candidiasis**<br>• Caused by *Candida albicans*<br>• Also known as *moniliasis*<br>• 50% of adults symptom-free carriers<br>• Appears in warm, moist areas such as groin area, oral mucosa, and submammary folds<br>• Immunosuppression (e.g., from HIV infection, chemotherapy, radiation, and organ transplantation) allows yeast to become pathogenic. | *Mouth:* White, cheesy plaque, resembles milk curds<br>*Vagina:* Vaginitis with red, edematous, painful vaginal wall, white patches. Vaginal discharge. Pruritus. Pain on urination and intercourse<br>*Skin:* Diffuse papular erythematous rash with pinpoint satellite lesions around edges of affected area | • Azole antifungals (e.g., fluconazole, ketoconazole) or other specific medication such as vaginal suppository or oral lozenge<br>• Sexual abstinence or use of condom<br>• Skin hygiene to keep area clean and dry<br>• Powder is effective on nonmucosal surfaces of skin to prevent recurrence. |
| **Tinea Corporis**<br>• Various dermatophytes, commonly referred to as *ringworm* | • Typical annular (ringlike) scaly appearance, well-defined margins<br>• Erythematous | • Cool compresses<br>• Topical antifungals for isolated patches. Creams or solutions of miconazole, ketoconazole, clotrimazole, butenafine |
| **Tinea Cruris**<br>• Various dermatophytes<br>• Commonly referred to as *jock itch* | • Well-defined scaly plaque in groin area<br>• Does not affect mucous membranes | • Topical antifungal cream or solution |
| **Tinea Pedis**<br>• Various dermatophytes<br>• Commonly referred to as *athlete's foot* | • Interdigital scaling and maceration<br>• Scaly plantar surfaces sometimes with erythema and blistering<br>• May be pruritic. Possibly painful | • Topical antifungal cream, gel, solution, spray, or powder |
| **Tinea Unguium (Onychomycosis)**<br>• Various dermatophytes<br>• Incidence increases with age. | • Only few nails on one hand may be affected. Toenails more commonly affected<br>• Scaliness under distal nail plate<br>• Brittle, thickened, broken, or crumbling nails with yellowish discoloration (Fig. 23-9) | • Oral antifungal (terbinafine [Lamisil], itraconazole [Sporanox])<br>• Topical antifungal cream or solution (minimal effectiveness) if unable to tolerate systemic treatment<br>• Thinning of toenails if needed<br>• Nail avulsion (removal) is an option. |

**TABLE 23-9 Common Allergic Conditions of the Skin**

| Etiology and Pathophysiology | Clinical Manifestations | Treatment and Prognosis |
|---|---|---|
| **Allergic Contact Dermatitis**<br>• Type IV delayed hypersensitivity response (see Chapter 13)<br>• Absorbed agent acts as antigen.<br>• Sensitization occurs after one or more exposures.<br>• Appearance of lesions 2-7 days after contact with allergen | • Red papules and plaques<br>• Sharply circumscribed with occasional vesicles (see Fig. 13-9)<br>• Usually pruritic<br>• Area of dermatitis frequently takes shape of causative agent (e.g., metal allergy and bandlike dermatitis on ring finger). | • Topical or oral corticosteroids, antihistamines<br>• Skin lubrication<br>• Elimination of contact allergen<br>• Avoidance of irritating affected area<br>• Systemic corticosteroids if sensitivity severe |
| **Urticaria**<br>• Usually allergic phenomenon<br>• Erythema and edema in upper dermis resulting from a local increase in permeability of capillaries (usually from histamine release) | • Spontaneously occurring, raised or irregularly shaped wheals, varying size, usually multiple<br>• A single lesion usually resolves in 24 hr.<br>• Can occur anywhere on the body | • Removal of triggering agent, if known<br>• Oral antihistamine therapy<br>• Possibly systemic corticosteroids |
| **Drug Reaction**<br>• May be caused by any drug that acts as antigen and causes hypersensitivity reaction<br>• Certain drugs (e.g., penicillin) more likely to cause reactions<br>• Not all reactions are allergic, some are intolerance (e.g., gastric upset). | • Rash of any morphology<br>• Often red, macular and papular, semiconfluent, generalized rash with abrupt onset<br>• Appearance as late as 14 days after cessation of drug. Possibly pruritic<br>• Some reactions may be life threatening requiring immediate and intensive care. | • Withdrawal of drug if possible<br>• Antihistamines, topical or systemic corticosteroids may be necessary depending on severity of symptoms. |
| **Atopic Dermatitis**<br>• Type 1 hypersensitivity response (see Chapter 13)<br>• Genetically influenced, chronic, relapsing disease<br>• Exaggerated by a skin response to environmental allergens<br>• Associated with allergic rhinitis and asthma | • Multiple presentations, including acute, subacute, and chronic stages. All are pruritic.<br>• *Acute stage:* Bright erythema, oozing vesicles, with extreme pruritus (see Fig. 13-8)<br>• *Subacute stage:* Scaly, light red to red-brown plaques<br>• *Chronic stage:* Thickened skin with accentuation of skin markings (lichenification), possible hypopigmentation, or hyperpigmentation. Dry skin. Common in antecubital and popliteal space | • Lubrication of dry skin<br>• Topical immunomodulators (pimecrolimus [Elidel], tacrolimus [Protopic])<br>• Reduction of stress reduces flares<br>• Corticosteroids, phototherapy for severe inflammation and pruritus<br>• Antibiotics for secondary infection as needed |

## TABLE 23-10 Common Benign Conditions of the Skin

| Etiology and Pathophysiology | Clinical Manifestations | Treatment and Prognosis |
|---|---|---|
| **Acne Vulgaris** | | |
| • Inflammatory disorder of sebaceous glands<br>• More common in teenagers but possible development and persistence in adulthood<br>• Flare can occur with use of corticosteroids and androgen-dominant birth control pills and before menses. | • Noninflammatory lesions, including open comedones (blackheads) and closed comedones (whiteheads)<br>• Inflammatory lesions, including papules and pustules<br>• Most common on face, neck, and upper back (Fig. 23-10) | *Topical:*<br>• Mechanical removal of multiple lesions with comedo extractor<br>• Topical benzoyl peroxide, retinoids, or antimicrobials (clindamycin, erythromycin)<br>*Systemic:*<br>• Systemic antibiotics<br>• Use of isotretinoin (Accutane) for severe nodulocystic acne to possibly provide lasting remission. Pregnancy tests, monitor liver function, cholesterol, triglycerides, and for depression<br>• Aim of treatment to suppress new lesions and minimize scarring<br>• Spontaneous remission possible<br>• Often improvement with exposure to sun<br>• May last many years |
| **Nevi (Moles)** | | |
| Grouping of normal cells derived from melanocyte-like precursor cells | • Hyperpigmented areas that vary in form and color<br>• Flat, slightly elevated, verrucoid, polypoid, dome-shaped, sessile, or papillomatous<br>• Preservation of normal skin markings<br>• Hair growth possible | • No treatment necessary except for cosmetic reasons<br>• Skin biopsy for suspicious nevi |
| **Psoriasis** | | |
| • Autoimmune chronic dermatitis that involves excessively rapid turnover of epidermal cells<br>• Family predisposition<br>• Usually develops before age 40 | • Sharply demarcated silvery scaling plaques on reddish colored skin commonly on the scalp, elbows, knees, palms, soles, and fingernails (Fig. 23-11)<br>• Itching, burning, pain<br>• Localized or general, intermittent or continuous<br>• Symptoms vary in intensity from mild to severe. | Goal to reduce inflammation and suppress rapid turnover of epidermal cells. No cure, but control is possible<br>*Topical treatments:*<br>• Corticosteroids, tar, salicylic acid, calcipotriene, anthralin<br>• Intralesional injection of corticosteroids for chronic plaques<br>*Systemic treatments:*<br>• Natural or artificial UVB. PUVA (UVA with topical or systemic photosensitizer (psoralen)<br>• Antimetabolite (methotrexate), PDE-4 inhibitor (apremilast [Otezla]), retinoid (acitretin), immunosuppressant (cyclosporine), biologic therapy (adalimumab [Humira], etanercept [Enbrel], infliximab [Remicade], ustekinumab [Stelara], certolizumab pegol [Cimzia], secukinumab [Cosentyx], golimumab [Simponi]), and ixekizumab (Taltz) for moderate to severe plaque disease |
| **Seborrheic Keratoses** | | |
| • Benign, familial, exact etiology unknown<br>• Usually occur after age 40, increase in number with age | • Irregularly round or oval, often verrucous papules or plaques<br>• Well-defined shape, appearance of being stuck on<br>• Increase in pigmentation with time<br>• Usually multiple and possibly itchy | • Removal by curettage or cryosurgery for cosmetic reasons or to eliminate source of irritation<br>• Biopsy if unable to distinguish from melanoma |
| **Acrochordons (Skin Tags)** | | |
| • Common after midlife<br>• Appearance on neck, axillae, and upper trunk secondary to mechanical friction or redundant skin (associated with obesity) | • Small, skin-colored, soft, pedunculated papules<br>• May become irritated | • No treatment medically necessary<br>• Surgical removal when needed<br>• Usually just snipping without anesthesia |
| **Lipoma** | | |
| • Benign tumor of adipose tissue, often encapsulated<br>• Most common in 40- to 60-yr-old age group | • Rubbery, compressible, round mass of adipose tissue<br>• Single or multiple<br>• Variable in size, possibly extremely large<br>• Most common on trunk, back of neck, and forearms | • Usually no treatment<br>• Biopsy to differentiate from liposarcoma<br>• Excision usual treatment (when indicated) |
| **Lentigo** | | |
| • Increased number of normal melanocytes in basal layer of epidermis related to sun exposure and aging<br>• Also called "liver spots" or "age spots" | • Hyperpigmented, brown to black macule or patch (flat lesion) on sun-exposed areas | • Evaluate carefully for progression.<br>• Treatment only for cosmetic purposes: liquid nitrogen, laser resurfacing<br>• May recur<br>• Biopsy when suspicious of melanoma. |

*PUVA,* Psoralen ultraviolet A; *UVA,* ultraviolet A; *UVB,* ultraviolet B.

## INTERPROFESSIONAL CARE: DERMATOLOGIC PROBLEMS

### Diagnostic Studies

A careful history is of prime importance in diagnosing skin problems. The HCP must be skilled at detecting any evidence that could lead to the cause of many different skin diseases and conditions. After a careful history and physical examination, inspect individual lesions. The history, physical examination, and appropriate diagnostic test results guide therapy.

### Interprofessional Therapy

Many different treatment methods are used in dermatology. Advances in this field have brought relief to many previously chronic, untreatable conditions. Many of the specific therapeutic treatments require specialized equipment and are usually reserved for use by a dermatologist.

**Phototherapy.** Ultraviolet light (UVL) of different wavelengths may be used to treat many dermatologic conditions, including psoriasis, cutaneous T-cell lymphoma, atopic dermatitis, vitiligo, and pruritus. Light sources available include broadband UVB, narrowband UVB, and long-wave UV (UVA1). One form of phototherapy involves the use of psoralen plus UVA light (PUVA). Psoralen is a photosensitizing drug given to patients for a prescribed amount of time before exposure to UVA.

Treatments are generally given two to four times a week. Side effects of oral psoralen include nausea and vomiting, sunburn, and persistent pruritus. Perform frequent skin assessments on all patients receiving phototherapy, since erythema is a side effect of treatment. Topical corticosteroids may reduce painful erythema. Use psoralen with extreme caution in patients with liver or renal disease because slower metabolism and excretion can lead to prolonged photosensitivity.

Since there is risk with any UV exposure, discuss the risks and benefits with the patient prior to initiating phototherapy. Caution patients about the potential hazards of using photosensitizing chemicals and further exposure to UV rays from sunlight or artificial UVL during therapy. Because the lens of the eye absorbs psoralen, patients receiving PUVA need prescription protective eyewear that blocks 100% of UVL. Using the eyewear prevents cataract formation. Instruct patients to use the eyewear for 24 hours after taking the medication when outdoors or near a bright window because UVA penetrates glass. Ongoing monitoring is essential because of the immunosuppressive effects of PUVA, including an increased risk of SCC, BCC, and melanoma.

**CHECK YOUR PRACTICE**

You are working in a dermatology clinic preparing a 64-yr-old woman for phototherapy to treat multiple actinic keratoses on her nose and both cheeks. She says the first lesion appeared a few years ago. She then got worried about all of the time she spent in her garden without sunscreen. She thought the lesions were just "age spots" and was unconcerned until a few started to grow and periodically bleed.

- Prior to therapy, what teaching will you do to get her ready for the procedure and to take care of herself after the procedure?

Photodynamic therapy is a special type of phototherapy used to treat actinic keratosis and some malignant skin tumors. This therapy uses a photosensitizing agent in a different way than other phototherapy treatments. The patient receives the photosensitizing agent IV or topically, depending on the area treated. Time is allowed for the drug to be absorbed by the target cells. Light is then applied to the area, causing the drug to react with oxygen. This starts a reaction that kills the cells.[10]

**TABLE 23-11 Skin Conditions Treated by Laser**

| | |
|---|---|
| • Acne scars | • Psoriasis |
| • Hair removal | • Resurfacing of skin |
| • Hemangiomas | • Rosacea |
| • Leg veins | • Skin lesions |
| • Pigment discoloration in epidermis | • Tattoo removal |
| • Pigmented nevi | • Vascular lesions |
| • Port wine stain | • Wrinkles |

**Radiation Therapy.** The use of radiation therapy to treat BCC, SCC, and malignant melanoma varies greatly according to local practice and availability. Radiation may be given to reduce tumor size or as palliative treatment. One advantage of radiation therapy is minimal damage to surrounding tissue. This is of prime consideration in locations such as the nose, eyelids, and canthal areas. Radiation therapy is particularly effective for the older adult or debilitated patient who cannot tolerate even a minor surgical procedure.

Radiation therapy usually requires multiple visits to a radiology department. It can produce permanent hair loss *(alopecia)* of the irradiated areas. Other adverse effects, depending on anatomic location and dose of radiation delivered, include telangiectasia, atrophy, hyperpigmentation, depigmentation, ulceration, hearing loss, ocular damage, atrophy, and mucositis. Careful shielding is necessary to prevent ocular lens damage if the irradiated area is around the eyes. (Radiation therapy is discussed in Chapter 15.)

Total-body skin irradiation (body is bombarded with high-energy electrons) is one treatment for cutaneous T-cell lymphoma. Treatment follows a lengthy course and causes premature aging of the skin. Patients experience varying degrees of permanent alopecia and radiation dermatitis with a transient loss of sweat gland function.

**Laser Technology.** Laser treatment is expanding rapidly as an efficient surgical tool for many types of dermatologic problems (Table 23-11). Depending on the type of laser and the wavelength, lasers serve a wide variety of functions. Lasers are able to produce measurable, repeatable, consistent zones of tissue damage. They can cut, coagulate, and vaporize tissue to some degree. Laser light does not accumulate in body cells and cannot cause cumulative cellular changes or damage. With less damage to surrounding tissue, there is a decreased risk of scarring.

The surgical use of laser energy requires a focusing device to produce a small, high-density spot of energy. Several types of lasers are available. The $CO_2$ laser, the most common, has numerous applications as a vaporizing and cutting tool for most tissues. The argon laser emits light that is primarily absorbed by hemoglobin. It helps in the treatment of vascular and other pigmented lesions. Other, less common lasers include copper and gold vapors and neodymium:yttrium-aluminum-garnet (Nd:YAG). Written policies and procedures should cover laser safety and be reviewed by all personnel working with laser equipment.

### Drug Therapy

***Antibiotics.*** A number of topical and systemic antibiotics are used to treat dermatologic problems. Sometimes topical and systemic antibiotics are used concurrently. Common OTC topical antibiotics include bacitracin-neomycin-polymyxin (Neosporin), bacitracin, and polymyxin B. Many HCPs do not recommend Neosporin because of the risk of allergic contact dermatitis. Prescription topical antibiotics include mupirocin (for superficial *Staphylococcus* infections such as impetigo), gentamicin (used for *Staphylococcus* and most gram-negative organisms), and erythromycin (used for gram-positive cocci [staphylococci and streptococci] and gram-negative cocci and bacilli). Topical erythromycin and clindamycin (Cleocin solutions or gels) are used in the treatment of acne vulgaris. Topical metronidazole is used to treat rosacea and bacterial vaginosis. Many popular systemic antibiotics are not used topically because of the danger of allergic contact dermatitis.

If there are manifestations of systemic infection, a systemic antibiotic is used. Frequently used drugs include penicillin, minocycline, erythromycin, tetracycline, and for severe infections, vancomycin. These drugs are particularly useful for acne vulgaris and bacterial infections, such as erysipelas, cellulitis, carbuncles, and severe infected eczema. Teach patients drug-specific instructions on the proper technique of taking or applying antibiotics.

***Corticosteroids.*** Corticosteroids are effective in treating a wide variety of dermatologic conditions. They can be used topically, intralesionally, or systemically. Topical corticosteroids have local antiinflammatory and antipruritic effects. Since corticosteroids may alter the clinical manifestations, attempt to diagnose a skin problem before applying a corticosteroid preparation. Accurate and adequate topical therapy is often the key to a successful outcome. Once a sufficient amount of medication is dispensed, limits should be set on the duration and frequency of application.

The potency of a particular preparation depends on the concentration of active drug. With prolonged use, more potent corticosteroid formulations can cause adrenal suppression, especially if a large surface area is covered and occlusive dressings are used. Over time, high-potency corticosteroids may produce side effects, including skin atrophy resulting from impaired cell mitosis, capillary fragility, and susceptibility to bruising. In general, dermal and epidermal atrophy does not occur until a corticosteroid has been used for 2 to 3 weeks. If drug use is discontinued at the first sign of atrophy, recovery usually occurs in several weeks. Rosacea eruptions and severe exacerbations of acne vulgaris may also occur. Rebound dermatitis is common when therapy is stopped. Tapering the use of high-potency topical corticosteroids when improvement is noted reduces the risk.

Low-potency corticosteroids such as hydrocortisone act more slowly but can be used for a longer time without producing serious side effects. Low-potency corticosteroids are safe to use on the face and intertriginous areas, such as the axillae and groin.

The most potent delivery system for a topical corticosteroid is an ointment form. Apply creams and ointments in thin layers and slowly massage into the site 1 to 3 times a day.

Intralesional corticosteroids are injected directly into or just beneath the lesion. This method provides a reservoir of medication with an effect lasting several weeks to months. Intralesional injection is common in the treatment of psoriasis, alopecia areata (patchy hair loss), cystic acne, hypertrophic scars, and keloids. Triamcinolone acetonide (Kenalog) is the most common drug used for intralesional injection.

Systemic corticosteroids can have remarkable results in the treatment of skin conditions. However, they often have undesirable systemic effects (see Chapter 49). Corticosteroids can be given as short-term therapy for acute conditions such as contact dermatitis caused by poison ivy. Long-term corticosteroid therapy for dermatologic conditions is reserved for severe disease such as bullous (blistering) disorders.

***Antihistamines.*** Oral antihistamines are helpful in treating urticaria, angioedema, and pruritus that can occur in problems such as atopic dermatitis, allergic dermatitis, and other allergic cutaneous reactions. Several different antihistamines may be tried before the satisfactory therapeutic effect is achieved. Antihistamines may have sedative effects. Sedating antihistamines, such as hydroxyzine and diphenhydramine, are often preferred for pruritic conditions because the tranquilizing and sedative effects offer symptomatic relief. Warn the patient about sedative effects, a problem when driving or operating heavy machinery. Antihistamines, such as loratadine (Claritin), fexofenadine (Allegra), and cetirizine (Zyrtec), bind to peripheral histamine receptors, providing antihistamine action without sedation. They are not effective for controlling pruritus. All antihistamines should be used with caution in older adults because of their long half-life and anticholinergic effects.

***Topical Fluorouracil.*** Fluorouracil (5-FU) is a topical cytotoxic agent with selective toxicity for sun-damaged cells. It is used to treat premalignant (especially actinic keratosis) and some malignant skin diseases. Because systemic absorption of the drug is minimal, systemic side effects are not a problem. Patient compliance is a consideration in the use of 5-FU. The medication produces erythema and pruritus within 3 to 5 days. Painful, eroded areas over the damaged skin occur within 1 to 3 weeks, depending on skin thickness at the site. Low-potency topical corticosteroids are often applied 20 minutes after 5-FU to reduce erythema and pruritus and increase patient adherence with therapy. 5-FU is available in four strengths (0.5%, 1%, 2%, and 5%). Treatment must continue with applications 1 (only in the 0.5% strength) or 2 times a day for 2 to 4 weeks. Healing may take up to 4 weeks after medication is stopped.[11]

Because 5-FU is a photosensitizing drug, instruct the patient to avoid sunlight during treatment. Teach patients about the effect of the medication. Tell them they will look worse before they look better. Adherence depends on thoroughness of your instruction, which should include a written handout. After treatment, skin should be smooth and free of actinic keratosis. Actinic keratosis may recur in treated areas, and multiple courses of therapy may be necessary over the years for those with severely sun-damaged skin.

***Immunomodulators.*** Topical immunomodulators, such as pimecrolimus (Elidel) and tacrolimus (Protopic), are used to treat atopic dermatitis. They work by suppressing an overreactive immune system. The side effects are minimal and may include a transient burning or feeling of heat at the application site. An increased risk of skin cancer and precancerous lesions may be associated with these drugs.

Another topical immunomodulator, imiquimod (Aldara), acts to stimulate the production of $\alpha$-interferon and other cytokines to enhance cell-mediated immunity. It boosts the immune response only where applied and is safe for transplant patients. Imiquimod is used for external genital warts, actinic keratoses, and superficial BCC. Most patients using this cream experience skin reactions, including redness, swelling, blistering, excoriations, peeling, itching, and burning. Dosing varies depending on the type of lesion treated and the strength of medication prescribed.[11]

### Diagnostic and Surgical Therapy

**Skin Scraping.** Scraping with a scalpel blade is done to obtain a sample of surface cells (stratum corneum) for microscopic inspection and diagnosis. The most common tests of skin scrapings are mineral oil examination for scabies and 10% to 20% potassium hydroxide (KOH) for fungus.

**Electrodessication and Electrocoagulation.** Electrical energy can be converted to heat with the tip of an electrode. The heat burns and destroys tissue. The major uses of this type of therapy are coagulation of bleeding vessels to obtain hemostasis and destruction of small *telangiectasias* (dilation of groups of superficial capillaries and venules). *Electrodessication* usually involves more superficial destruction, and a monopolar electrode is used. *Electrocoagulation* uses a dipolar electrode. It has a deeper effect, with better hemostasis but an increased possibility of scarring. While minor electrosurgery on patients with a pacemaker poses minimal risk, both pacemakers and internal defibrillators can be affected by the electrical energy being used.

**Curettage.** Curettage is the removal and scooping away of tissue using an instrument called a *curette.* A curette looks like a small spoon with very sharp edges. Although a curette is not usually strong enough to cut normal skin, it can remove many types of small, soft skin tumors and superficial lesions, such as warts, actinic keratoses, seborrheic keratosis, and small BCC and SCC. The area to be curetted is anesthetized before the procedure. The lesion is removed, and then the skin is cauterized. The removed tissue is usually biopsied. A dressing may be applied, and you will need to teach the patient wound care. A small scar and hypopigmentation can result.

**Punch Biopsy.** Punch biopsy is a common procedure used to obtain a tissue sample for histologic study or to remove small lesions (Fig. 23-12). The procedure is simple. The biopsy area is marked and then anesthetized so that the anesthetizing agent will not obscure the landmarks. The HCP rotates the punch into the skin and removes a small cylinder of skin. Hemostasis is achieved with pressure or absorbable gelatin (Gelfoam) packing. Sites of 4 mm or larger are usually closed with sutures. Punch biopsies are not done below the knee if other sites are available. Circulatory changes can make evaluation of the tissue sample more difficult.

**Cryosurgery.** Cryosurgery is the use of subfreezing temperatures to destroy epidermal lesions. Cryosurgery is a useful treatment for common benign, precancerous conditions, including common and genital warts, cutaneous tags, thin seborrheic keratoses, lentigines, actinic keratoses, BCC, and SCC. Topical liquid nitrogen (−196° F) is the agent most commonly used for cryosurgery.[12] The mechanism of injury involves direct cellular freezing and vascular stasis (stoppage or slowdown in the flow of blood), which develops after thawing. Intracellular ice formation causes the cell to rupture during thaw, leading to cell death and necrosis of the treated tissue.

Liquid nitrogen is applied topically (directly onto the lesion) with a direct spray or a cotton-tipped applicator. Tell patients that they will feel a stinging cold sensation. The lesion first becomes swollen and red, and it may blister. A scab forms and falls off in 1 to 3 weeks. The skin lesion sloughs along with the scab. Growth of new skin follows.

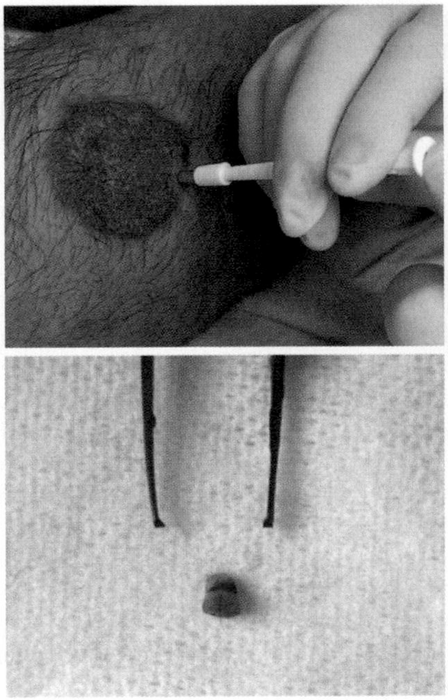



**FIG. 23-12** Punch biopsy. **A,** Removal of skin for diagnostic purposes. **B,** Specimen obtained. (From Graham-Brown R, Bourke J, Cunliffe T: *Dermatology: fundamentals of practice,* Edinburgh, 2008, Mosby Ltd.)

The low temperature of liquid nitrogen can easily destroy melanocytes, leaving an area of hypopigmentation resembling a scar. The size of an affected area to be treated may limit the use of cryotherapy. The disadvantages of this treatment are the lack of a tissue specimen for histologic confirmation of cell type before destruction and the potential for destruction of adjacent healthy tissue.

**Excision.** Excision is an option if the lesion involves the dermis. Complete closure of the excised area usually results in a good cosmetic result.

A specific type of excision is *Mohs surgery,* which is a microscopically controlled removal of a skin malignancy. In this procedure, the HCP removes tissue sections in thin horizontal layers. All of the specimen's margins are examined to determine whether any malignant cells remain (Fig. 23-13). Any residual tumor not removed by the first surgical excision is removed in serial excisions performed the same day. Benefits of Mohs surgery are preserving normal tissue, producing the smallest possible wound, and completely removing the cancer before surgical closure. Although this can become a lengthy procedure, it is done in an outpatient setting using local anesthesia.

## NURSING MANAGEMENT: DERMATOLOGIC PROBLEMS

### Ambulatory Care

Dermatologic conditions are not usually the primary reason for hospitalization. Nevertheless, many hospitalized patients have skin problems that need nursing intervention and patient education. Nursing interventions related to skin conditions fall into broad categories. They are applicable to many problems in both inpatient and outpatient settings. A nursing care plan for the patient with chronic skin lesions (eNursing Care Plan 23-1) is available on the website for this chapter.

**Wet Compresses.** For superficial skin problems that involve inflammation, itching, and infection, wet compresses are

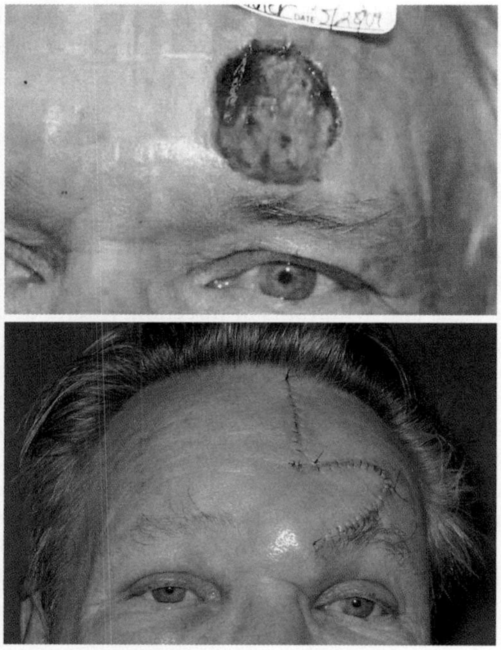

FIG. 23-13 **A,** Removal of melanoma by Mohs surgery. **B,** After plastic surgery using a skin flap to repair defect. (Courtesy Peter Bonner, Placitas, N. Mex.)

commonly used. They are appropriate for damaged, oozing skin. Wet compresses are an excellent way to remove crusts and scabs that are adhering to the wound surface. Wet compresses provide comfort and treatment of conditions such as poison ivy, insect bites, and skin infections.

It is important to understand how to do a wet compress (dressing) correctly. Unless there is a concern about water quality, tap water at room temperature is the best choice. If drinkable water is not available, filtered, bottled, or sterile water may be used. Depending on the problem, additives may be used. Antibacterial solutions may contain aluminum acetate (Domeboro powder), silver nitrate, or acetic acid. Concentrations are critical when additives are used. For example, the desired concentration for acetic acid (vinegar) for a compress is 1% to 2.5%. Kitchen vinegar is 5% and must be diluted. Either white or brown vinegar using ½ cup diluted in 1 pint of water will yield a 1% concentration. Wet compresses should be tepid. However, when an antiinflammatory effect is desired, the wet dressing should be cool.

The material you select for wet compresses should be four to eight layers thick and slightly larger than the area that you are treating. Use gauze or any clean material (e.g., thin cotton sheeting, thermal underwear, tube socks). Ingenuity is sometimes required when covering odd-shaped body parts. Do not use gauze sponges with fillers (abdominal pads), because they will retain too much solution, and fibers can be left in the wound if the skin is open. Place the prescribed compress material into fresh solution and squeeze out excess water. Your goal is a wet compress—not simply damp and not dripping.

Wet compresses are applied continuously or intermittently. When used continuously, use new solution as needed. Do not add additional solution. This can alter the concentration and damage the skin. Depending on the desired effect, intermittent compresses are placed for 10 to 30 minutes, 2 to 4 times a day. Careful monitoring of the skin is important. If the skin appears *macerated* (softens and turns white), discontinue the dressings for 2 to 3 days. Change and wash daily any material used repeatedly throughout the day. Protect the patient from discomfort and chilling. A water-resistant pad will help protect the mattress, linens, and furniture.

**TABLE 23-12 Drug Therapy**
***Common Bases for Topical Medications***

| Agent | Therapeutic Considerations |
|---|---|
| **Powder** | Promotion of dryness. Lubricates skinfold areas to prevent irritation. Base for antifungal preparations. Protect patient from inhaling. |
| **Lotion** | Emulsions of water, alcohol, and/or oil. Cooling and drying. Some leave residual powder film after evaporation of water. Useful in subacute pruritic eruptions |
| **Cream** | Emulsions of oil and water. Most common base for topical medications. Lubrication and protection |
| **Ointment** | Oil with differing amounts of water added in suspension. Lubrication and prevention of dehydration. Petrolatum most common |
| **Paste** | Mixture of powder and ointment, used when drying effect necessary because moisture is absorbed |
| **Gel** | Nongreasy combination of propylene glycol and water. May contain alcohol |

◆ **Baths.** Baths are an appropriate intervention when large areas of the body need treatment. Baths may be relaxing and will help decrease itching. Agents such as colloidal oatmeal (Aveeno) and sodium bicarbonate can be added directly to bath water. Fill the tub with tepid water to cover the affected areas. Depending on the severity of the problem and the patient's discomfort, have the patient soak for 15 to 20 minutes 3 or 4 times a day. Stress to the patient not to rub the skin dry with a towel but gently pat to prevent increased irritation and inflammation. Avoid adding oils as their use increases the risk of falls. To sustain the hydrating effect, apply cream, ointment emollients (moisturizers), or other prescribed topical agents after the bath. This helps seal the moisture in the hydrated cells and increases the absorption of any topical medications.

◆ **Topical Medications.** Topical medications are commonly used to treat cutaneous problems. The effectiveness of topical therapy depends on which base the medication is prepared in. Table 23-12 summarizes the common agents used as bases for topical preparations and their therapeutic considerations. The base selected depends on the properties needed.

Creams are very versatile and most commonly prescribed. They are a mix of organic oils, water, and usually a preservative. Ointments are primarily organic oils with little or no water. Many are preservative free. They are more lubricating than creams and offer enhanced potency of the active ingredient. They may be too occlusive for conditions with high levels of exudate or in body creases. Gels work well on the scalp, where other compounds may mat the hair and for acute exudative conditions such as poison ivy. Lotions can be a mix of water, alcohols, and/or oils. They are also appropriate for the scalp but may cause stinging and drying when used in skin folds. Pastes are a compound of 50% or more powder in an ointment base. They are good for protecting the skin but are messy. A limited number of foams are available.

Apply topical medications as directed. Proper administration will yield best results, maintain consistency, and avoid waste. Some are very costly. As a general rule, topical medication should be applied in a thin film to clean skin and spread evenly in a downward motion in the direction of hair growth. Thick creams will spread easier if the skin is still damp. If a secondary dressing is going to be used, you can apply the medication directly onto a dressing. Teach the patient and caregiver proper dosing, application technique, anticipated results, and common reactions.

Occlusion with a plastic wrap is an effective way of increasing the absorption of topical corticosteroids or simple emollients. The plastic wrap traps perspiration against the outer layer of the epidermis. Applying preparations to moist skin increases absorption 10-fold. Use tape or stretch wraps to keep the plastic wrap in place. For conditions on the feet or lower legs, socks can be worn over the plastic wrap. Wraps applied multiple times daily are kept in place for 2 to 8 hours. Some patients choose to use the occlusion technique at bedtime. Recommend occlusion with discretion. It is not appropriate in areas prone to infection, such as skin creases.

- **Control of Pruritus.** *Pruritus* (itching) can be caused by dry skin, almost any physical or chemical stimulus to the skin (such as drugs or insects), and any scaling skin disorder. The itch sensation is carried by the same nonmyelinated nerve fibers as pain and temperature. The patient will have pain rather than an itch if the epidermis is damaged or absent.

The itch/scratch cycle must be broken to prevent excoriation and lichenification. Control of pruritus is important because it is difficult to diagnose an excoriated and inflamed lesion. Certain circumstances make itching worse. Have the patient avoid anything that causes vasodilation, such as heat or rubbing. Dryness of the skin lowers the itch threshold and increases the itch sensation.

Teach the patient ways to help break the itch/scratch cycle. A cool environment may cause vasoconstriction and decrease itching. Hydration, wet compresses, and moisturizers (including antipruritic lotions) are normally helpful. Apply wet compresses for 30 to 60 minutes, pat the skin dry, and apply a lubricant or medication. Topical and injectable corticosteroids are occasionally ordered. Topically applied menthol, camphor, or phenol numb the itch receptors. Systemic antihistamines may provide relief. The principal side effect of most antihistamines is sedation. This may be desirable because pruritus is often worse at night and can interfere with sleep.

**Lichenification** is a thickening of epidermis with exaggerated markings resembling a washboard. It is caused by chronic scratching or rubbing of the skin. Lichenification is often associated with atopic dermatoses and other pruritic conditions. Although any area of the body may be affected, the hands, forearms, shins, and nape of the neck are common sites. Itching may become habitual. The persistent scratching can cause excoriations. Treating the cause of the itching is the key to preventing lichenification.

- **Prevention of Spread.** Although most skin problems are not contagious, infection control precautions indicate wearing gloves when working with any open wounds or lesions with drainage. Not all infected drainage is purulent. Careful hand washing and properly disposing of soiled dressings are the best means of preventing the spread of infections or infestations. The most common contagious lesions include impetigo, streptococcal infections, staphylococcal infections (e.g., methicillin-resistant *S. aureus* [MRSA]), fungal infections, primary chancre, scabies, and pediculosis.
- **Prevention of Secondary Infections.** Open skin lesions are susceptible to invasion by other viral, bacterial, or fungal organisms. Meticulous hygiene, hand washing, and dressing changes are important to minimize the potential for secondary infections. Warn the patient about scratching lesions, which can cause excoriations and create a portal of entry for pathogens. Trim the patient's nails short to minimize trauma from scratching.
- **Specific Skin Care.** You are often in a position to teach patients skin care after simple dermatologic surgical procedures, such as skin biopsy, excision, and cryosurgery. In general, your instructions should include dressing changes, use of topical antibiotics, and the signs and symptoms of infection. After a dermatologic procedure, any oozing wound should be cleansed with a saline solution twice daily or as ordered by the HCP. Potable (safe, drinking water) is a safe alternative in some situations. Antibiotic or plain petrolatum ointment may be applied with a secondary dressing that is both absorbent and nonadherent.

Wounds that are kept moist and covered heal more rapidly and with less scarring. The initial crust that forms should be left undisturbed as a protective coating for the damaged skin beneath it. Healing crusts that have been moisturized and protected will separate naturally from healed epidermis.

A sutured wound may be covered with a variety of dressings. Sutures are generally removed in 4 to 14 days, depending on the placement site. Sometimes alternating sutures are removed after the third day. Incision lines may require daily cleansing, usually with plain water. If necessary, a topical antibiotic is applied and the wound either is covered with a dry dressing or left open to air. The patient may experience some swelling and discomfort in the first 24 hours. Intermittent application of cold (ice packs) over the surgical dressing may reduce edema. Mild analgesics such as acetaminophen or a nonsteroidal antiinflammatory medication should control discomfort. Teach the patient how to differentiate normal inflammation from an infection. A slight red border during the first few days after a procedure is normal inflammation. Redness that persists longer than a week or extends beyond a 1 cm border, a fever above 101° F, increased pain, pronounced swelling, and purulent drainage are all signs and symptoms of a possible infection. If these occur, they should be promptly reported to the HCP.

- **Psychologic Effects of Chronic Dermatologic Problems.** Emotional stress can occur for persons who suffer from chronic skin problems such as psoriasis, atopic dermatitis, or acne. The sequelae of chronic skin problems could result in social and employment problems with subsequent financial implications, a poor self-image, problems with sexuality, and increasing and progressive frustration. The usual lack of systemic illness coupled with the visibility of the skin lesions often presents a real problem to the patient.

Help the patient comply with the prescribed regimen. Allow the patient to verbalize the "Why me?" question, even though there is no ready answer. Refer the patient to dermatology support groups. Many are listed on the American Academy of Dermatology website *(www.aad.org)*. These groups are extremely helpful for patient support and accurate education materials.

The location of lesions and scars is the determining factor with respect to its cosmetic implications. Facial scars are the most damaging psychologically because they are so visible. Creative use of cosmetics can do much to mask lesions and scarring. Consider individual sensitivity to product ingredients when selecting cosmetics. Oil-free, hypoallergenic cosmetics are available and may be beneficial for the allergic patient.

## TEAMWORK & COLLABORATION

### *Skin Care*

**Role of Nursing Personnel**

***Registered Nurse (RN)***

- Assess patient's skin for acute and chronic integumentary problems.
- Assess patient's risk factors for integumentary problems.
- Document skin condition and risk factor assessment, and develop a plan of care.
- Determine whether patient is taking drugs that increase photosensitivity.
- Teach about risks associated with sun exposure and methods for decreasing exposure to the sun.
- Teach about therapies used for integumentary disorders, including dressings, baths, and oral or topical medications used on an outpatient basis.
- Evaluate treatment for effectiveness and any adverse effects.

***Licensed Practical/Vocational Nurse (LPN/LVN)***

- Administer prescribed therapies such as dressings and oral or topical medications.
- Monitor the skin for changes in appearance or texture that may indicate worsening of integumentary problem or adverse reactions to treatment.
- Reinforce teaching done by the RN.

***Unlicensed Assistive Personnel (UAP)***

- Assist patient with bathing.
- Apply wet dressings to skin or add medications (such as oilated oatmeal) to patient baths (consider state nurse practice act and agency policy).
- Report changes in skin appearance or patient complaints of discomfort to the RN.

Rehabilitative cosmetics are available to help camouflage and deemphasize such lesions as *vitiligo* (loss of pigmentation), *melasma* (tan to brown patches on the face), or healed postoperative wound sites. These commercially available products are opaque, smudge resistant, and water resistant.

## COSMETIC PROCEDURES

A vast array of cosmetic procedures is available, including chemical peels, toxin injections, fillers, laser surgery, breast enlargement and reduction (see Chapter 51), face-lift, eyelid-lift, and liposuction. Common cosmetic topical procedures are presented in Table 23-13. Other types of cosmetic procedures include the injection of botulinum toxin (Botox), deoxycholic acid (Kybella), calcium hydroxylapatite (Radiesse), collagen (Zyplast), and hyaluronic acid fillers (e.g., Restylane, Perlane, Juvéderm). Transitory side effects may occur, such as mild redness, pain, swelling, and bruising. Uncommon side effects from cosmetic procedures include allergic reaction, infection, or lumps at the injection sites; undercorrection or overcorrection of wrinkles; and reactivation of human papillomavirus (HPV). Tell the patient that he or she will need to repeat the procedure at prescribed intervals to maintain the desired appearance.

The reasons for undergoing these procedures are as varied as the techniques. The most common reason that people suffer the discomfort and financial expense (most are not covered by health insurance) of a cosmetic procedure is to improve their body image. If they feel better about themselves after having cosmetic procedures, they often act more confident and self-assured. Often social position and economic considerations are part of the decision. Increased longevity provides a larger population to whom cosmetic procedures are especially appealing.

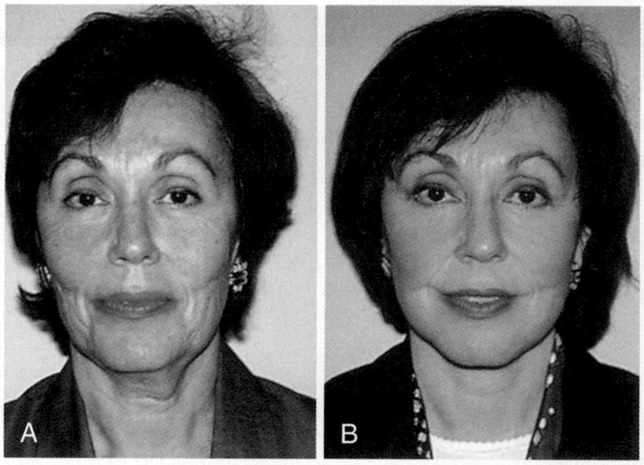


**FIG. 23-14** Face-lift. **A,** Preoperative. **B,** Postoperative. (From Pastorek N, Bustillo A: Deep plane face-lift, *Facial Plast Surg Clin North Am* 13:433-449, 2005.)

Regardless of the patient's reasons for seeking cosmetic procedures, maintain a supportive, nonjudgmental attitude about these procedures. If the patient wishes to change or enhance a body feature perceived as unattractive and has realistic expectations about the outcome, you should support this decision.

### Elective Surgery

**Laser Surgery.** Laser surgery is used to treat congenital and acquired vascular lesions (cherry angiomas, spider leg veins, hemangiomas, port wine stains, and tattoo removal) and for skin resurfacing and hair removal. Lasers can reduce scarring and fine wrinkles around the lips or eyes and remove facial lesions (Table 23-11). Swelling, redness, and bruising are common after treatment. The treated areas usually are kept moist with ointment or occlusive dressings for the first few days. The patient must protect treated skin from the sun.

**Face-Lift.** A face-lift *(rhytidectomy)* is the lifting and repositioning of the lower two thirds of the face and neck to improve appearance (Fig. 23-14). Indications for this procedure include the following:

- Redundant soft tissue or scarring resulting from disease (e.g., acne scarring)
- Asymmetric redundancy of soft tissues (e.g., facial palsy)
- Redundant soft tissue resulting from trauma
- Preauricular lesions
- Redundant soft tissues resulting from *solar elastosis* (sagging of the skin from sun damage), changes in body weight, and the effects of gravity
- Restoration of body image

The surgical approach and lines of incisions vary according to the desired correction and the position of the hairline. Eyelid-lifts *(blepharoplasty)* can remove redundant tissue and possibly improve the field of vision. Preventing hematoma formation is the most important postoperative consideration. Ice packs are usually applied for the first 24 to 48 hours to reduce swelling and decrease the possibility of hematoma formation. Usually the pain is minimal. Antibiotics are used at the surgeon's discretion. Complications can occur if the person smokes or is involved in vigorous exercise.

**TABLE 23-13 Common Cosmetic Topical Procedures**

| Tretinoin (Retin-A, Renova) | Chemical Peels (e.g., Beta Hydroxy Acid, Jessner's Peel, TCA) | Microdermabrasion | α-Hydroxy Acids (e.g., Glycolic Acid, Lactic Acid) |
|---|---|---|---|
| **Indications** | | | |
| Improves appearance of photodamaged skin, especially fine wrinkling. Reduces actinic keratoses | Improves appearance of photodamaged skin, acne scarring, actinic and seborrheic keratoses | Smoothes appearance of photodamaged and wrinkled skin, acne scarring | Smoothes appearance of photodamaged and wrinkled skin, acne scarring |
| **Description** | | | |
| Initially applied every 2 to 3 days. Treatment stopped if severe inflammation occurs. Maximum response in 8-12 mo | Solution applied in varying amounts to the skin, causing a controlled burn with a loss of melanin. | Epidermis and top dermal layer removed by applying aluminum oxide or baking soda crystals. Re-epithelialization of abraded surface then occurs. | Low concentrations (<10%) in many skin care products consumers can apply to the skin. Higher concentrations (50%-70%) applied only by an HCP |
| **Side Effects** | | | |
| Erythema, swelling, flaking, pigmentation changes. Teratogenic. Increases phototoxicity if taking other photosensitive drugs | Moderate swelling and crusting for 1 wk. Redness for 6-8 wk. Pink tone possible for several mo. Photosensitivity | Light pink tone that resolves within 24 hr. Photosensitivity | Photosensitivity, slight irritation at lower concentrations, severe redness, oozing, and flaking skin possible with higher concentrations |
| **Patient Teaching** | | | |
| Apply at night since preparation is inactivated by light. Apply emollients, use sunscreen, use sun avoidance measures, avoid using abrasive or drying facial cleansers for severe sensitivity (e.g., excess irritation). | Use sunscreen. Avoid sun for 6 mo to prevent hyperpigmentation. | Generous application of emollients and sunscreen | Use sunscreen and sun avoidance measures. |

**Liposuction.** Liposuction is a technique for removing subcutaneous fat to improve facial and body contours. Although not a substitute for diet and exercise, it can be successful in removing areas of fat from virtually any body area that is resistant to other techniques.

Liposuction is relatively free of complications. Possible contraindications include the use of anticoagulants, uncontrolled hypertension, diabetes mellitus, and poor cardiovascular status. Persons under 40 years of age with good skin elasticity are the best candidates. However, patients over 40 can be treated successfully.

The procedure is usually done on an outpatient basis under local anesthesia. One or more sessions may be necessary, depending on the size of the area to be treated. The HCP inserts a blunt-tipped cannula through a small incision and pushes into the fat to break it loose from the fibrous stroma. Multiple repeated thrusts disrupt the fat and create tunnels. The loosened fat is removed with a powerful suction. Afterwards, firm pressure is applied to the wounds and compression garments are worn for 3 to 4 weeks.[13] Bandaging also helps to contour the skin. It may take several months for the results to be evident.

## NURSING MANAGEMENT: COSMETIC SURGERY

Many cosmetic surgical procedures are done in well-equipped day-surgery units or in dermatologist or plastic surgeon in-office surgery suites.

### Preoperative Management

A major preoperative consideration relates to informed consent and realistic expectations of what cosmetic surgery can accomplish. Although the HCP should provide this information, reinforce it and answer questions and concerns. For instance, a face-lift has little or no effect on deep wrinkling of the forehead and temples, deep nasolabial grooves, or vertical lip wrinkles. Before-and-after treatment photographs of similar cases are often useful in helping the patient to set realistic expectations.

Your teaching plan should include the timeframe for healing. Explain the oozing, crusting stage of an abrasive procedure so the patient can plan time off from work if necessary. Since wound healing may not be complete for 1 year, the patient should not anticipate complete results immediately. The final result is affected by the patient's age, general state of health, and skin type and the extent (severity) of the condition being treated. Efforts should be made to correct or control any existing health problem before the procedure.

### Postoperative Management

Most cosmetic procedures are not extremely painful. Usually mild analgesics are sufficient to keep the patient comfortable. Although infection is not a common problem after cosmetic surgery, assess the sites for signs of infection. Teach the patient signs and symptoms of infection with instructions to report them immediately so that appropriate antibiotic intervention can be started.

If the surgery involved an alteration in the skin's circulation, as in a face-lift, carefully monitor for adequate circulation. Warm, pink skin that blanches on pressure indicates that adequate circulation is present in the surgical area. Supportive, compressive dressings and ice packs may be necessary early in the postoperative period.

## SKIN GRAFTS

### Uses

Skin grafts may be necessary to protect underlying structures or to reconstruct areas for cosmetic or functional purposes.

They may be used to facilitate rapid closure and minimize complications. Ideally, wounds heal by primary intention. However, large wounds, surgically created wounds, trauma, and chronic wounds can result in extensive tissue destruction, making healing by primary intention impossible. In these cases, skin grafting may be necessary to close the defect. Improved surgical techniques make it possible to graft skin, bone, cartilage, fat, fascia, muscles, and nerves. For cosmetically pleasing results, the color, thickness, texture, and hair-growing nature of skin used for grafting should match the recipient site. (See Chapter 24 for a discussion of skin grafting for patients with burn injuries.)

## Types

The two types of traditional skin grafts are free grafts and skin flaps. Free grafts are further classified according to the method of providing a blood supply to the grafted skin. One method is to transfer the graft (epidermis and part or all of the dermis) to the recipient site from the donor site. The *autograft* (from the patient's own body) or *isograft* (from an identical twin) revascularizes and becomes fixed to the new site. The other method of free skin grafting is by *reconstructive microsurgery.* With the use of an operating microscope, circulation is established immediately in the graft by anastomosis of the blood vessels from the skin flap to the vessels in the recipient site.

Skin flaps involve moving a section of skin and subcutaneous tissue from one part of the body to another without terminating the vascular attachment *(pedicle).* Skin flaps are used to cover wounds with a poor vascular bed, provide padding when needed, and cover wounds over cartilage and bone. The patient may need intermediate flap placement if the recipient site is far removed from the donor site. For instance, a skin flap from the thigh to the head would require an intermediate graft. The flap is advanced to the recipient site when circulation is well established at the intermediate site. The patient's needs and the type of defect determine the type of flap and the route of transfer.

Soft tissue expansion is a technique for providing skin (1) for resurfacing of a defect, such as a burn scar; (2) for removal of a disfiguring mark (e.g., a tattoo); or (3) as a preliminary step in breast reconstruction. A subcutaneous tissue expander of an appropriate size and shape is placed under the skin, usually as an outpatient procedure. Weekly expansion with saline solution can be done in a health care setting or by the patient at home. This expansion procedure is repeated until the skin reaches the size needed for the repair. This may take from several weeks to 3 to 4 months. Once sufficient skin is available, the old incision is opened, the expander is removed, and the soft tissue is ready to be used as an advancement flap. The tissue expander next to a defect retains the primary tissue characteristics such as color and texture.

Newer engineered skin substitutes (e.g., Apligraf, Dermagraft, Integra, Alloderm) are gaining popularity. There are a number available and each offers its own benefits. Some are two-layered membranes with both dermal and epidermal components. Others are only one layer. The skin is engineered from neonatal foreskins and cadavers. Because the tissue is engineered, Langerhans' cells are removed, reducing the risk of rejection.[14] Engineered skin grafts have an extended shelf life. Some are cryopreserved, others shipped overnight as they are needed. Advantages include ready availability, the avoidance of a donor site, application in outpatient settings, minimal scarring, and less pain.

## CASE STUDY

### *Malignant Melanoma and Dysplastic Nevi*

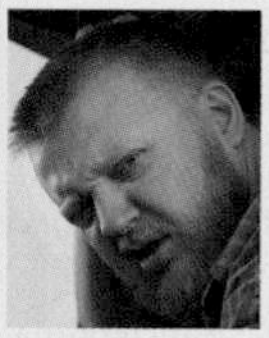

(©Dimedrol68/ iStock/ Thinkstock)

**Patient Profile**

G.L. is a 44-year-old white, fair-skinned man who is a long-distance truck driver. In his leisure time, he enjoys swimming. He comes to the clinic for evaluation of a changing lesion on his left arm.

**Subjective Data**

- History of a basal cell carcinoma (BCC) on his left ear in the last 4 years
- Father treated for metastatic malignant melanoma in the last 2 years
- First noted the lesion 5 months ago when it started changing size
- Anxious the lesion might have spread and require extensive, disfiguring surgery

**Objective Data**

***Physical Examination***

- Has a 4-mm lesion, dark brown, scalloped with vaguely defined borders
- Four dysplastic nevi found on back

***Diagnostic Studies***

- Excisional biopsy confirmed malignant melanoma.
- Sentinel node biopsy results were negative.
- Diagnostic tests indicate melanoma stage I.

**Discussion Questions**

1. What risk factors for malignant melanoma does he have?
2. What are the usual clinical manifestations associated with malignant melanoma?
3. What is the prognosis for a patient with this stage of malignant melanoma?
4. What treatment options are available for him?
5. ***Priority Decision:*** Based on the assessment data presented, what are the priority nursing diagnoses? Are there any collaborative problems?
6. ***Patient-Centered Care:*** How would you help G.L. deal with his anxiety over the treatment outcomes?
7. ***Priority Decision:*** What is the priority of care for G.L.?
8. ***Safety:*** What would you include in his patient teaching plan to address future sun exposure?
9. ***Teamwork and Collaboration:*** Which of the following nursing personnel should be responsible for teaching G.L.: RN, LPN/LVN, or UAP?
10. ***Evidence-Based Practice:*** G.L. wants to know whether regularly applying sunscreen will reduce his risk for developing a second melanoma. How would you reply?

Answers available at *http://evolve.elsevier.com/Lewis/medsurg.*

## BRIDGE TO NCLEX EXAMINATION

The number of the question corresponds to the same-numbered outcome at the beginning of the chapter.

1. Which safe sun practices would the nurse include in the teaching plan for a patient who has photosensitivity *(select all that apply)*?
   - **a.** Wear protective clothing.
   - **b.** Apply sunscreen liberally and often.
   - **c.** Emphasize the short-term use of a tanning booth.
   - **d.** Avoid exposure to the sun, especially during midday.
   - **e.** Wear any sunscreen as long as it is purchased at a drugstore.
2. When teaching a patient with malignant melanoma about this disorder, the nurse recognizes that the patient's prognosis is *most* dependent on
   - **a.** the thickness of the lesion.
   - **b.** the degree of asymmetry in the lesion.
   - **c.** the amount of ulceration in the lesion.
   - **d.** how much the lesion has spread superficially.
3. The nurse determines that a patient with a diagnosis of which disorder is *most* at risk for spreading the disease?
   - **a.** Tinea pedis
   - **b.** Impetigo on the face
   - **c.** Candidiasis of the nails
   - **d.** Psoriasis on the palms and soles
4. A mother and her two children have been diagnosed with pediculosis corporis at a health care center. An appropriate measure in treating this condition is
   - **a.** applying pyrethrins to the body.
   - **b.** topical application of griseofulvin.
   - **c.** moist compresses applied frequently.
   - **d.** administration of systemic antibiotics.
5. A common site for the lesions associated with atopic dermatitis is the
   - **a.** buttocks.
   - **b.** temporal area.
   - **c.** antecubital space.
   - **d.** plantar surface of the feet.
6. During the assessment of a patient, you note an area of red, sharply defined plaques covered with silvery scales that are mildly itchy on the patient's knees and elbows. You recognize this finding as
   - **a.** lentigo.
   - **b.** psoriasis.
   - **c.** actinic keratosis.
   - **d.** seborrheic keratosis.
7. In teaching a patient who is using topical corticosteroids to treat acute dermatitis, the nurse should tell the patient that *(select all that apply)*
   - **a.** the cream form is the most efficient system of delivery.
   - **b.** short-term use of topical corticosteroids usually does not cause systemic side effects.
   - **c.** apply creams and ointments with a glove in small amounts to prevent further infection.
   - **d.** abruptly discontinuing the use of topical corticosteroids may cause a reappearance of the dermatitis.
   - **e.** systemic side effects may be experienced from topical corticosteroids if the person is malnourished.
8. A patient with acne vulgaris tells the nurse that she has quit her job as a receptionist because she believes her facial appearance is unattractive to customers. The nursing diagnosis that *best* describes this patient response is
   - **a.** ineffective coping related to lack of social support.
   - **b.** impaired skin integrity related to presence of lesions.
   - **c.** anxiety related to lack of knowledge of the disease process.
   - **d.** social isolation related to decreased activities secondary to fear of rejection.
9. Important patient teaching after a chemical peel includes
   - **a.** avoidance of sun exposure.
   - **b.** application of firm bandages.
   - **c.** limitation of vigorous exercise.
   - **d.** use of moist heat to relieve discomfort.

1. a, b, d; 2. a; 3. b; 4. a; 5. c; 6. b; 7. b, d; 8. d; 9. a

For rationales to these answers and even more NCLEX review questions, visit *http://evolve.elsevier.com/Lewis/medsurg.*

## EVOLVE WEBSITE

http://evolve.elsevier.com/Lewis/medsurg

**Review Questions (Online Only)**

**Key Points**

**Answer Keys for Questions**

- Rationales for Bridge to NCLEX Examination Questions
- Answer Guidelines for Case Study on p. 427

**Nursing Care Plan**

- eNursing Care Plan 23-1: Patient With Chronic Skin Lesions

**Conceptual Care Map Creator**

**Audio Glossary**

**Supporting Media**

- Animation
  - Mohs Surgery

**Content Updates**

## REFERENCES


1. Centers for Disease Control: Indoor tanning is not safe. Retrieved from *www.cdc.gov/cancer/skin/basic_info/indoor_tanning.htm.*
2. US Food and Drug Administration: Sunscreen drug products for over-the-counter human use. Retrieved from *www.fda.gov/drugs/guidancecomplianceregulatoryinformation/guidances/ucm330694.htm.*
3. American Cancer Society: Skin cancer facts. Retrieved from *www.cancer.org/cancer/cancercauses/sunanduvexposure/skin-cancer-facts.*
4. Tsao H, Olazagasti J, Cordoro KM, et al: Early detection of melanoma: reviewing the ABCDEs, *J Am Acad Dermatol* 72:717, 2015.
5. CDC: What are the risk factors for skin cancer? Retrieved from *www.cdc.gov/cancer/skin/basic_info/risk_factors.htm.*
6. Habif TP: *Clinical dermatology*, ed 5, St Louis, 2011, Elsevier. (Classic)
7. Stubblefield J, Kelly B: Melanoma in Non-Caucasian populations, *Surg Clin N Am* 94:1115, 2014.

*8. Kim DW, Trinh VA, Hwu WJ: Ipilimumab in the treatment of advanced melanoma, *Expert Opin Biol Ther* 14:1709, 2014.

9. National Psoriasis Foundation: About psoriasis. Retrieved from *www.psoriasis/org/about.*
10. Rkein AM, Ozog DM: Photodynamic therapy, *Dermatol Clin* 32:415, 2014.

*11. Micali G, Lacarrubba F, Nasca MR, et al: Topical pharmacotherapy for skin cancer, *J Am Acad Derm* 70:979, 2014.

12. Marks JG, Miller JJ: *Principles of dermatology*, ed 5, St Louis, 2013, Elsevier.
13. Afrooz PN, Pozner JN, DiBernado BE: Noninvasive and minimally invasive techniques in body contouring, *Clin Plastic Surg* 41:789, 2014.
14. Nathoo R, Howe N, Cohen G: Skin substitutes: An overview of the key players in wound management, *J Clin Aesthet Derm* 7:44, 2014.

*Evidence-based information for clinical practice.

24

# Burns

*Judy Knighton*

*With the new day comes new strength and new thoughts.*

***Eleanor Roosevelt***

http://evolve.elsevier.com/Lewis/medsurg/

## LEARNING OUTCOMES

1. Relate the causes of burns to the prevention strategies for burn injuries.
2. Differentiate between partial-thickness and full-thickness burns.
3. Apply tools used to determine the severity of burns.
4. Compare the pathophysiology, clinical manifestations, complications, and interprofessional care throughout the three burn phases.
5. Compare the fluid and electrolyte shifts during the emergent and acute burn phases.
6. Differentiate the nutritional needs of the burn patient throughout the three burn phases.
7. Compare the various burn wound care techniques and surgical options for partial-thickness and full-thickness burn wounds.
8. Prioritize nursing interventions in the management of the burn patient's physiologic and psychosocial needs.
9. Examine the various physiologic and psychosocial aspects of burn rehabilitation.
10. Design a plan of care to prepare the burn patient and caregiver for discharge.

## KEY TERMS

burn, p. 429
carboxyhemoglobin, p. 430
chemical burns, p. 429
contracture, p. 446
cultured epithelial autograft (CEA), p. 445
debridement, p. 439
electrical burns, p. 431
escharotomy, p. 437
excision and grafting, p. 444
full-thickness burns, p. 432
partial-thickness burns, p. 432
smoke and inhalation injuries, p. 430
thermal burns, p. 429

The focus of this chapter is the care of patients who have experienced a burn. A **burn** is an injury to the tissues of the body caused by heat, chemicals, electric current, or radiation. The resulting effects are influenced by the temperature of the burning agent, duration of contact time, and type of tissue that is injured.

An estimated 450,000 Americans seek medical care each year for burns.[1] Approximately 40,000 people are hospitalized, one half of whom requires care in specialized burn centers. About 3400 Americans die annually as a direct result of their injuries. The highest fatality rates occur in children ages 4 years and younger and adults over age 65. Around the world, nearly 11 million people need medical attention annually for burn injuries, and about 265,000 die.[2]

Although burn incidence has decreased over the past 20 years, burn injuries still occur too frequently and mainly to those at a lower socioeconomic level and with histories of substance abuse and mental health illness. Most burn incidents are preventable. The focus of burn prevention has shifted from blaming individuals and changing behaviors to making legislative changes and collecting global burn data to address the unique prevention needs of low- and middle-income countries.[3]

Coordinated national programs in developed countries have focused on child-resistant lighters, nonflammable children's clothing, tap water anti-scald devices, stricter building codes, hardwired smoke detectors and alarms, and fire sprinklers. As a nurse, you can advocate for and teach about burn risk–reduction strategies in the home and at work (Tables 24-1 and 24-2).

## TYPES OF BURN INJURY

### Thermal Burns

**Thermal burns**, caused by flame, flash, scald, or contact with hot objects, are the most common type of burn injury (Fig. 24-1). The severity of the injury depends on the temperature of the burning agent and duration of contact time. Scald injuries can occur in the bathroom or while cooking. Flash, flame, or contact burns can occur while cooking, smoking, burning leaves in the backyard, or using gasoline or hot oil.

### Chemical Burns

**Chemical burns** are the result of contact with acids, alkalis, and organic compounds. In addition to tissue damage, eyes can be

Reviewed by Cecilia M. Bidigare, RN, MSN, CNS-BC, CNE, Associate Professor of Nursing, Sinclair Community College, Dayton, Ohio; Patricia S. Regojo, RN, MSN, Nurse Manager, Burn Intensive Care Unit and Thoracic Surgery Unit, Temple University Hospital, Philadelphia, Pennsylvania; and Olga Van Dyke, RN, MSN, CAGS, Assistant Professor, School of Nursing, Massachusetts College of Pharmacy and Health Sciences, Boston, Massachusetts.

injured if they are splashed with the chemical. Acids are found in the home and at work and include hydrochloric, oxalic, and hydrofluoric acid. Alkali burns can be more difficult to manage than acid burns, since alkalis adhere to tissue, causing protein hydrolysis and liquefaction. Alkalis are found in cement, oven and drain cleaners, and heavy industrial cleansers.[4] Organic compounds, including phenols (chemical disinfectants) and petroleum products (creosote and gasoline), produce contact burns and systemic toxicity.

**TABLE 24-1 Sources of Burn Injury***

**Home Hazards**

***Kitchen and Bathroom***
- Microwaved food
- Steam, hot grease or liquids from cooking
- Hot water heaters set at 140°F (60°C) or higher

***General Household***
- Heat lamps
- Fireplaces (e.g., gas, wood)
- Open space heaters
- Radiators (e.g., home, automobile)
- Outdoor grills (e.g., propane, charcoal)
- Frayed or defective wiring
- Multiple extension cords per outlet
- Flammables (e.g., starter fluid, gasoline, kerosene)
- Carelessness with cigarettes, matches, candles

**Occupational Hazards**
- Tar
- Cement
- Chemicals
- Hot metals
- Steam pipes
- Combustible fuels
- Fertilizers, pesticides
- Electricity from power lines
- Sparks from live electric sources

*List is not all-inclusive.

**TABLE 24-2 Strategies to Reduce Burn Injury**

**Flame or Contact**
- Never smoke in bed.
- Use "child-resistant" lighters.
- Hold regular home fire exit drills.
- Never leave hot oil unattended while cooking.
- Never use gasoline or other flammable liquids to start a fire.
- Never leave candles unattended or near open windows or curtains.
- Consider a flame-retardant smoking apron for older or "at-risk" people.
- Exercise caution when microwaving food and beverages as they can get very hot.

**Scald**
- Use "anti-scald" devices with showerhead or faucet fixtures.
- Lower hot water temperature to the "lowest point" or 120°F (49°C).
- After running bath water, check temperature with back of hand or bath thermometer.
- Supervise bathing with small children, older adults, or anyone with impaired physical movement, physical sensation, or judgment.

**Inhalation**
- Install smoke and carbon monoxide detectors and change batteries annually (if appropriate).

**Chemical**
- Store chemicals safely in approved containers and label clearly.
- Ensure safety of workers handling chemicals (education, protective eyewear, gloves, masks, clothing).

**Electrical**
- Avoid or repair frayed wiring.
- Avoid outdoor activities during electrical (i.e., lightning) storms.
- Ensure electrical power source is shut off before beginning repairs.
- Wear protective eyewear and gloves when making electrical repairs.

## Smoke and Inhalation Injury

Smoke and inhalation injuries from breathing noxious chemicals or hot air can cause damage to the respiratory tract. Three types of smoke and inhalation injuries can occur: metabolic asphyxiation, upper airway injury, and lower airway injury. Smoke inhalation injuries are a major predictor of mortality in burn patients. Rapid initial and ongoing assessment is critical. Airway compromise and pulmonary edema can develop over the first 12 to 48 hours.[5]

**Metabolic Asphyxiation.** The majority of deaths at a fire scene are the result of inhaling certain smoke elements, primarily carbon monoxide (CO) or hydrogen cyanide. Oxygen delivery to or consumption by tissues is impaired. The result is hypoxia and, ultimately, death when carboxyhemoglobin (i.e., hemoglobin combined with CO) blood levels are greater than 20%. CO and hydrogen cyanide poisoning may occur in the absence of burn injury to the skin.

**Upper Airway Injury.** Upper airway injury results from an inhalation injury to the mouth, oropharynx, and/or larynx. The injury may be caused by thermal burns or the inhalation of hot

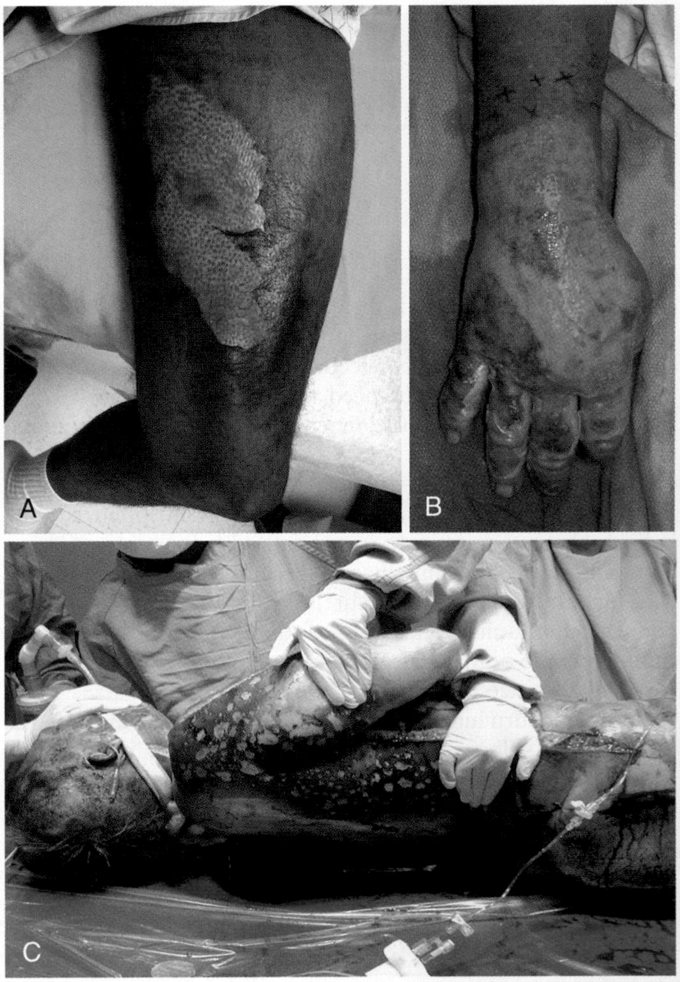


**FIG. 24-1** Types of burn injury. **A,** Superficial, partial-thickness scald burn to thigh. **B,** Deep, partial-thickness flame burn to hand. **C,** Full-thickness flame burn to posterior chest and arm. (Courtesy Judy Knighton, Toronto, Canada.)

**TABLE 24-3 Manifestations of Lung Injury Associated With Burns**

| Upper Airway | Lower Airway |
|---|---|
| • Blisters, edema<br>• Hoarseness<br>• Difficulty swallowing<br>• Copious secretions<br>• Stridor<br>• Substernal and intercostal retractions<br>• Total airway obstruction | • High degree of suspicion if patient was trapped in a fire in an enclosed space or clothing caught fire<br>• Presence of facial burns or singed nasal or facial hair<br>• Dyspnea<br>• Carbonaceous sputum<br>• Wheezing<br>• Hoarseness<br>• Altered mental status |

air, steam, or smoke. Mucosal burns of the oropharynx and larynx are manifested by redness, blistering, and edema (Table 24-3). The swelling can be massive and the onset rapid. Flame burns to the neck and chest may make breathing more difficult because of the burn eschar, which becomes tight and constricting from the underlying edema. Swelling from scald burns to the face and neck can also be lethal, as can external pressure from edema pressing on the airway. Mechanical obstruction can occur quickly, presenting a true airway emergency.

**Lower Airway Injury.** An inhalation injury to the trachea, bronchioles, and alveoli is usually caused by breathing in toxic chemicals or smoke. Tissue damage is related to the duration of exposure to toxic fumes or smoke. Clinical manifestations of lower airway lung injury are presented in Table 24-3. Carefully assess the patient for facial burns, singed nasal hair, hoarseness, painful swallowing, darkened oral and nasal membranes, carbonaceous sputum, history of being burned in an enclosed space, and clothing burns around the neck and chest. Pulmonary edema may not appear until 12 to 48 hours after the burn, and then it may manifest as acute respiratory distress syndrome (ARDS) (see Chapter 67).

### Electrical Burns

**Electrical burns** result from intense heat generated from an electric current. Direct damage to nerves and vessels, causing tissue anoxia and death, can also occur. The severity of the electrical injury depends on the amount of voltage, tissue resistance, current pathways, surface area in contact with the current, and length of time that the current flow was sustained (Fig. 24-2). Tissue densities offer various amounts of resistance to electric current. For example, fat and bone offer the most resistance, whereas nerves and blood vessels offer the least resistance. Current that passes through vital organs (e.g., brain, heart, kidneys) produces more life-threatening sequelae than that which passes through other tissues. In addition, electric sparks may ignite the patient's clothing, causing a flash injury.

As with inhalation injury, perform a rapid assessment of the patient with an electrical injury. Transfer to a burn center is indicated. The severity of an electrical injury can be difficult to determine, since most of the damage is below the skin (known as the *iceberg effect*). Determination of electric current contact points and history of the injury may help reveal the likely path of the current and potential areas of injury. Contact with electric current can cause muscle contractions strong enough to fracture the long bones and vertebrae. Another reason to suspect long bone or spinal fractures is a fall resulting from the electrical injury. For this reason, consider all patients with electrical

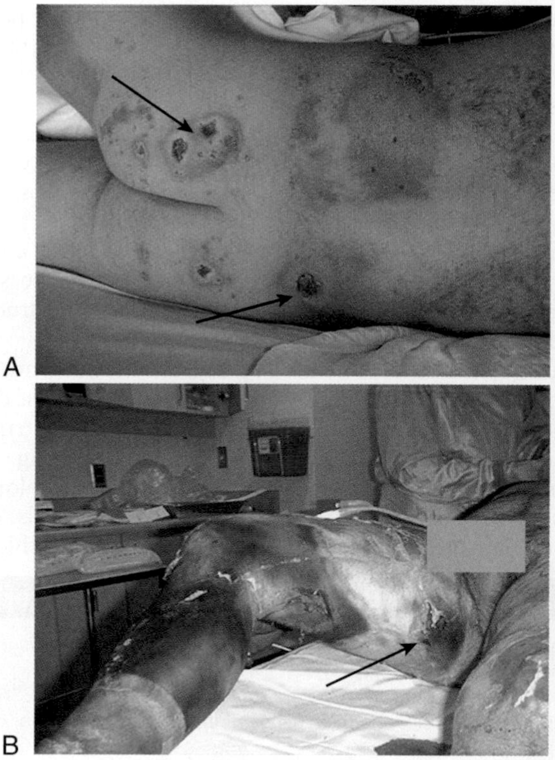

**FIG. 24-2** Electrical injury produces heat coagulation of blood supply and contact area as electric current passes through the skin. **A,** Back and buttock *(arrows)*. **B,** Leg *(arrow)*. (Courtesy Judy Knighton, Toronto, Canada.)

burns at risk for a cervical spine injury. Use cervical spine immobilization during transport and subsequent diagnostic testing until injury is ruled out.

Electrical injury puts the patient at risk for dysrhythmias or cardiac arrest, severe metabolic acidosis, and myoglobinuria.[6] The electric shock can cause immediate heart standstill or ventricular fibrillation. Delayed dysrhythmias or arrest can also occur without warning during the first 24 hours after injury. Myoglobin from injured muscle and hemoglobin from damaged red blood cells (RBCs) are released into the circulation whenever massive muscle and blood vessel damage occurs. The released myoglobin travels to the kidneys and can block the renal tubules. This can result in acute tubular necrosis (ATN) and acute kidney injury (see Chapter 46).

### Cold Thermal Injury

Cold thermal injury, or frostbite, is discussed in Chapter 68.

## CLASSIFICATION OF BURN INJURY

The treatment of burns is related to the severity of the injury.[7] Severity is determined by (1) depth of burn, (2) extent of burn calculated in percent of total body surface area (TBSA), (3) location of burn, and (4) patient risk factors (e.g., age, past medical history). The American Burn Association (ABA) uses referral criteria to determine which burn injuries should be treated in burn centers (Table 24-4). The majority of patients with minor burn injuries can be managed in community hospitals.[8]

### Depth of Burn

Burn injury involves the destruction of the integumentary system. The skin is divided into three layers: epidermis, dermis, and subcutaneous tissue (Fig. 24-3). The *epidermis,* or nonvascular protective outer layer of the skin, is approximately as thick as a sheet of paper. (The structure and function of the skin are discussed in Chapter 22.)

The *dermis,* which lies below the epidermis, is approximately 30 to 45 times thicker than the epidermis. The dermis contains connective tissues with blood vessels, hair follicles, nerve endings, sweat glands, and sebaceous glands.

Under the dermis lies the *subcutaneous tissue,* which contains major vascular networks, fat, nerves, and lymphatics. The subcutaneous tissue acts as a heat insulator for underlying structures, including muscles, tendons, bones, and internal organs.

Burns continue to be defined by degrees: first, second, third, and fourth degree. The ABA recommends a more precise definition and classifies burns according to depth of skin destruction: **partial-thickness burns** and **full-thickness burns** (Fig. 24-3). Skin-reproducing (re-epithelializing) cells are located along the shafts of the hair follicles, sweat glands, and oil glands. If significant damage occurs to the dermis (i.e., a full-thickness burn), not enough skin cells remain to regenerate new skin. A permanent, alternative source of skin must be found. Table 24-5 compares the various burn classifications according to the depth of injury.

**TABLE 24-4 Burn Center Referral Criteria**

*Burn injuries that should be referred to a burn center include the following:*

1. Partial-thickness burns >10% of total body surface area (TBSA)
2. Burns that involve the face, hands, feet, genitalia, perineum, or major joints
3. Third-degree burns in any age group
4. Electrical burns, including lightning injury
5. Chemical burns
6. Inhalation injury
7. Burn injury in patients with preexisting medical disorders that could complicate management, prolong recovery, or affect mortality risk (e.g., heart or kidney disease, diabetes)
8. Any patients with burns and concomitant trauma (e.g., fractures) in which the burn injury poses the greatest risk of morbidity or mortality. In such cases, if the trauma poses the greater immediate risk, the patient may be initially stabilized in a trauma center before being transferred to a burn center. The HCP will need to use his or her judgment, in consultation with the regional medical control plan and triage protocols.
9. Burn injury in children in hospitals without qualified personnel or equipment needed to care for them
10. Burn injury in patients who will require special social, emotional, or long-term rehabilitative intervention

Source: American Burn Association: Guidelines for the operation of burn centers. Retrieved from *http://www.ameriburn.org/Chapter14.pdf.*

## Extent of Burn

Two commonly used tools for determining the TBSA affected or the extent of a burn wound are the *Lund-Browder chart* (Fig. 24-4, *A*) and the *Rule of Nines* (Fig. 24-4, *B*). (First-degree burns, equivalent to a sunburn, are not included when calculating TBSA.) The Lund-Browder chart is considered more accurate because it considers the patient's age in proportion to relative body-area size. The Rule of Nines is often used for initial assessment of a burn patient because it is easy to remember. For irregular- or odd-shaped burns, the patient's hand (including the fingers) is approximately 1% TBSA. The *Sage Burn Diagram* is a free, web-based tool for estimating TBSA burned (*www.sagediagram.com*). There are also mobile applications (e.g., uBurn, Mersey Burns) available to estimate the percentage of burn and fluid resuscitation needs.[9]

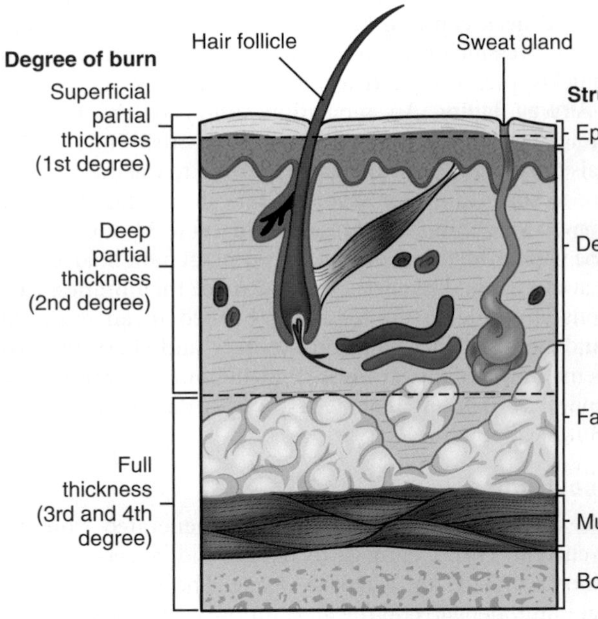


**FIG. 24-3** Cross section of skin indicating the depth of burn and structures involved.

**TABLE 24-5 Classification of Burn Injury Depth**

| Classification | Appearance | Possible Cause | Structures Involved |
|---|---|---|---|
| **Partial-Thickness Skin Destruction** | | | |
| **Superficial (first-degree) burn** | Erythema, blanching on pressure, pain and mild swelling, no vesicles or blisters (although after 24 hr skin may blister and peel) | Superficial sunburn<br>Quick heat flash | Superficial epidermal damage with hyperemia. Tactile and pain sensation intact |
| **Deep (second-degree) burn** | Fluid-filled vesicles that are red, shiny, wet (if vesicles have ruptured). Severe pain caused by nerve injury. Mild to moderate edema | Flame<br>Flash<br>Scald<br>Contact burns<br>Chemicals<br>Tar, cement<br>Electric current | Epidermis and dermis involved to varying depths. Skin elements, from which epithelial regeneration occurs, remain viable. |
| **Full-Thickness Skin Destruction** | | | |
| **Third- and fourth-degree burns** | Dry, waxy white, leathery, or hard skin. Visible thrombosed vessels. Insensitivity to pain because of nerve destruction. Possible involvement of muscles, tendons, and bones | Flame<br>Scald<br>Chemical<br>Tar, cement<br>Electric current | All skin elements and local nerve endings destroyed. Coagulation necrosis present. Surgical intervention required for healing |

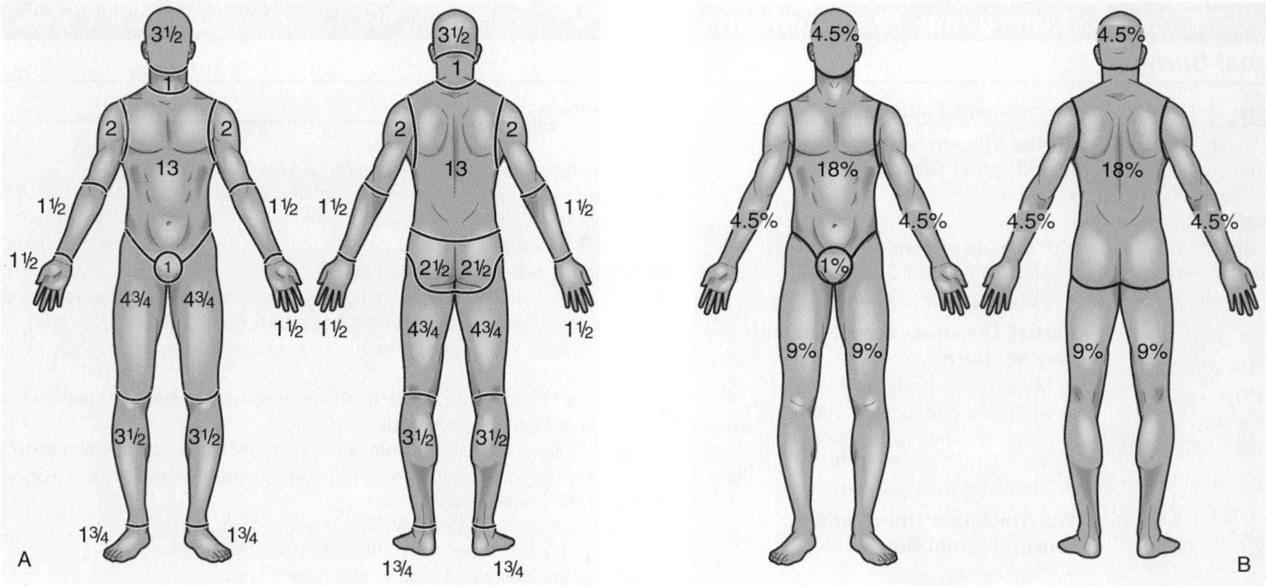


FIG. 24-4 A, Lund-Browder chart. By convention, areas of partial-thickness injury are colored in blue and areas of full-thickness injury in red. Superficial partial-thickness burns are not calculated. B, Rule of Nines chart.

### Location of Burn

The severity of the burn injury is also determined by the location of the burn. Burns to the face and neck and circumferential burns to the chest or back may interfere with breathing as a result of mechanical obstruction from edema or leathery, devitalized burn tissue *(eschar)*. These burns may also indicate possible smoke or inhalation injury.

Burns to the hands, feet, joints, and eyes are of concern because they make self-care difficult and may jeopardize future function. Burns to the hands and feet are challenging to manage because of superficial vascular and nerve supply systems that must be protected while the burn wounds are healing.

Burns of the ears and nose are at risk for infection as the skin is very thin and the underlying skeleton is frequently exposed. Burns to the buttocks or perineum are at high risk for infection from urine or feces contamination. Circumferential burns to the extremities can cause circulation problems distal to the burn, with possible nerve damage to the affected extremity. Patients may also develop compartment syndrome (see Chapter 62) from direct heat damage to the muscles, swelling, and/or preburn vascular problems.

### Patient Risk Factors

Any patient with preexisting heart, lung, or kidney disease has a poorer prognosis for recovery because of the increased demands placed on the body by a burn injury. The patient with diabetes or peripheral vascular disease is at high risk for poor healing, especially with foot and leg burns.[10] General physical weakness from any chronic disease, including alcoholism, drug abuse, or malnutrition, makes it challenging for the patient to fully recover from a burn injury. In addition, the burn patient who has also sustained fractures, head injuries, or other trauma has a more difficult recovery.

## PREHOSPITAL AND EMERGENCY CARE

At the scene of the injury, priority is given to removing the person from the source of the burn and stopping the burning process. Rescuers must also protect themselves from being injured. In the case of electrical and chemical injuries, initial care involves removal of the patient from contact with the electrical or chemical source.

Small thermal burns (10% or less of TBSA) should be covered with a clean, cool, tap water–dampened towel for the patient's comfort and protection until medical care is available. Cooling of the injured area (if small) within 1 minute helps minimize the depth of the injury. If the burn is large (greater than 10% TBSA) or an electrical or inhalation burn is suspected and the patient is unresponsive, first focus your attention on CAB:

- *Circulation:* Check for presence of pulses and elevate the burned limb(s) above the heart to decrease pain and swelling.
- *Airway:* Check for patency, soot around nares and on the tongue, singed nasal hair, darkened oral or nasal membranes.
- *Breathing:* Check for adequacy of ventilation.

If the patient is responsive, your priorities would follow the order of the ABCs: airway, breathing, and circulation.

To prevent hypothermia, cool large burns for no more than 10 minutes. Do not immerse the burned body part in cool water because it may cause extensive heat loss. Never cover a burn with ice, since this can cause hypothermia and vasoconstriction of blood vessels, thus further reducing blood flow to the injury. Gently remove as much burned clothing as possible to prevent further tissue damage. Leave adherent clothing in place until the patient is transferred to a hospital. Wrap the patient in a dry, clean sheet or blanket to prevent further contamination of the wound and to provide warmth.

Chemical burns are best treated by quickly removing any chemical particles or powder from the skin. Remove all clothing containing the chemical because the burning process continues while the chemical is in contact with the skin. Flush the affected area with copious amounts of water to irrigate the skin anywhere from 20 minutes to 2 hours postexposure. Tap water is acceptable for flushing eyes exposed to chemicals. Tissue destruction may continue for up to 72 hours after contact with some chemicals.

Watch patients with inhalation injuries closely for signs of respiratory distress. These patients need to be treated quickly and efficiently if they are to survive. If CO poisoning is suspected, treat the patient with 100% humidified $O_2$. Patients who have both body burns and an inhalation injury must be transferred to the nearest burn center.

**TABLE 24-6 Emergency Management**

***Thermal Burns***

| Etiology | Assessment Findings | Interventions |
|---|---|---|
| • Hot liquids or solids<br>• Flash flame<br>• Open flame<br>• Steam<br>• Hot surface<br>• Ultraviolet rays | **Partial-Thickness (superficial; first-degree) Burn**<br>• Redness<br>• Pain<br>• Moderate to severe tenderness<br>• Minimal edema<br>• Blanching with pressure<br>**Partial-Thickness (deep; second-degree) Burn**<br>• Moist blebs, blisters<br>• Mottled white, pink to cherry-red<br>• Hypersensitive to touch or air<br>• Moderate to severe pain<br>• Blanching with pressure<br>**Full-Thickness (third- and fourth-degree) Burns**<br>• Dry, leathery eschar<br>• Waxy white, dark brown, or charred appearance<br>• Strong burn odor<br>• Impaired sensation when touched<br>• Absence of pain with severe pain in surrounding tissues<br>• Lack of blanching with pressure | **Initial**<br>• If unresponsive, assess circulation, airway, and breathing.<br>• If responsive, monitor airway, breathing, and circulation.<br>• Stabilize cervical spine.<br>• Assess for inhalation injury.<br>• Provide supplemental $O_2$ as needed.<br>• Anticipate endotracheal intubation and mechanical ventilation with circumferential full-thickness burns to the neck and chest or large TBSA burn.<br>• Monitor vital signs, level of consciousness, respiratory status, $O_2$ saturation, and heart rhythm.<br>• Remove nonadherent clothing, shoes, watches, jewelry, glasses or contact lenses (if face was exposed).<br>• Cover any concurrent thermal burns with dry dressings or clean sheet.<br>• Establish IV access with two large-bore catheters if burn >15% TBSA.<br>• Begin fluid replacement.<br>• Insert indwelling urinary catheter if burn >15% TBSA.<br>• Elevate burned limbs above heart to decrease edema.<br>• Give IV analgesia and assess effectiveness frequently.<br>• Identify and treat other associated injuries (e.g., fractures, head injury).<br>**Ongoing Monitoring**<br>• Monitor airway, breathing, and circulation.<br>• Monitor vital signs, $O_2$ saturation, heart rhythm, and level of consciousness.<br>• Monitor pain level.<br>• Monitor urine output. |

*TBSA,* Total body surface area.

Always remember that the burn patient may also have sustained other injuries that could take priority over the burn itself. Persons involved in the prehospital phase of burn care must fully share the circumstances of the injury to emergency department (ED) staff. This is especially important if the patient was trapped in a closed space, exposed to hazardous chemicals or electricity, or suffered a possible traumatic injury (e.g., fall).

Prehospital and emergency care are presented in tables that describe thermal burns (Table 24-6), inhalation injury (Table 24-7), electrical burns (Table 24-8), and chemical burns (Table 24-9).

## PHASES OF BURN MANAGEMENT

Burn management can be organized chronologically into three phases: emergent (resuscitative), acute (wound healing), and rehabilitative (restorative). Overlap in care does exist. For example, the emergent phase begins at the time of the burn injury, and care often begins prehospital or in the ED. Wound care is the primary focus of the acute phase, but wound care also takes place in both the emergent and rehabilitation phases. Planning for rehabilitation begins on the day of the burn injury or admission to the burn center. Formal rehabilitation begins as soon as functional assessments can be performed.

## EMERGENT PHASE

The *emergent (resuscitative) phase* is the time required to resolve the immediate, life-threatening problems resulting from the burn injury.[11] This phase usually lasts up to 72 hours from the time the burn occurred. The primary concerns are the onset of hypovolemic shock and edema formation. The emergent phase ends when fluid mobilization and diuresis begin.

### Pathophysiology

**Fluid and Electrolyte Shifts.** The greatest initial threat to a patient with a major burn is hypovolemic shock (Fig. 24-5). It is caused by a massive shift of fluids out of the blood vessels as a result of increased capillary permeability and can begin as early as 20 minutes postburn. As the capillary walls become more permeable, water, sodium, and plasma proteins (especially albumin) move into the interstitial spaces and other surrounding tissue. The colloidal osmotic pressure decreases with progressive loss of protein from the vascular space. This results in more fluid shifting out of the vascular space into the interstitial spaces (Fig. 24-6).

Fluid also moves to areas that normally have minimal to no fluid, a phenomenon termed *third spacing.* Examples of third spacing in burn injury are exudate and blister formation, as well as edema in unburned areas.

Other sources of fluid loss are insensible losses by evaporation from large, denuded body surfaces and the lungs. The normal insensible loss of 30 to 50 mL/hr is increased in the severely burned patient. The net result of the fluid shifts and losses is termed *intravascular volume depletion.* Clinical signs of hypovolemic shock are decreased BP and increased heart rate. If hypovolemic shock is not corrected, refractory shock and death may result. (Shock is discussed in Chapter 66.)

The circulatory system is also affected by the hemolysis of RBCs from circulating factors (e.g., oxygen free radicals) released at the time of the burn, as well as by the direct insult of the burn injury. Thrombosis in the capillaries of burned tissue causes an additional loss of circulating RBCs. An elevated hematocrit is commonly caused by hemoconcentration due to fluid loss. After fluid balance is restored, the hematocrit levels drop.

Major electrolyte shifts of sodium and potassium also occur during this phase. A potassium shift develops first because

## TABLE 24-7 Emergency Management

### *Inhalation Injury*

| Etiology | Assessment Findings | Interventions |
|---|---|---|
| • Exposure of respiratory tract to intense heat or flames<br>• Inhalation of noxious chemicals, smoke, or CO | • History of being trapped in an enclosed space, being in an explosion, or having clothing catch fire<br>• Rapid, shallow respirations<br>• Increasing hoarseness<br>• Coughing<br>• Singed nasal or facial hair<br>• Darkened oral or nasal membranes<br>• Smoky breath<br>• Carbonaceous sputum<br>• Productive cough with black, gray, or bloody sputum<br>• Irritation of upper airways or burning pain in throat or chest<br>• Difficulty swallowing<br>• Cherry-red skin color (CO levels >20%)<br>• Restlessness, anxiety<br>• Altered mental status, including confusion, coma<br>• Decreased $O_2$ saturation<br>• Dysrhythmias | **Initial**<br>• If unresponsive, assess circulation, airway, and breathing.<br>• If responsive, monitor airway, breathing, and circulation.<br>• Stabilize cervical spine.<br>• Assess for concurrent thermal burn.<br>• Provide 100% humidified $O_2$.<br>• Anticipate endotracheal intubation and mechanical ventilation with significant inhalation injury.<br>• Monitor vital signs, level of consciousness, $O_2$ saturation, and heart rhythm.<br>• Remove nonadherent clothing, jewelry, glasses, or contact lenses (if face was exposed).<br>• Establish IV access with two large-bore catheters if burn >15% TBSA.<br>• Begin fluid replacement.<br>• Insert indwelling urinary catheter if burn >15% TBSA.<br>• Elevate burned limb(s) above heart to decrease edema.<br>• Obtain arterial blood gas, carboxyhemoglobin levels, and chest x-ray.<br>• Give IV analgesia and assess effectiveness frequently.<br>• Identify and treat other associated injuries (e.g., fractures, pneumothorax, head injury).<br>• Cover concurrent burned areas with dry dressings or clean sheet.<br>• Anticipate need for fiberoptic bronchoscopy or intubation.<br>**Ongoing Monitoring**<br>• Monitor airway, breathing, and circulation.<br>• Monitor vital signs, $O_2$ saturation, heart rhythm, and level of consciousness.<br>• Monitor pain level.<br>• Monitor urine output. |

*CO,* Carbon monoxide; *TBSA,* total body surface area.

## TABLE 24-8 Emergency Management

### *Electrical Burns*

| Etiology | Assessment Findings | Interventions |
|---|---|---|
| • Electric wires<br>• Utility wires<br>• Lightning<br>• Defibrillator | • Leathery, white, or charred skin<br>• Burn odor<br>• Loss of consciousness<br>• Impaired touch sensation<br>• Minimal or absent pain<br>• Dysrhythmias<br>• Cardiac arrest<br>• Location of contact points<br>• Diminished peripheral circulation in injured extremity<br>• Thermal burns if clothing ignites<br>• Fractures or dislocations from force of current<br>• Head or neck injury if fall occurred<br>• Depth and extent of wound difficult to visualize. Assume injury greater than what is seen. | **Initial**<br>• Remove patient from electrical source while protecting rescuer.<br>• If unresponsive, assess circulation, airway, and breathing.<br>• If responsive, monitor airway, breathing, and circulation.<br>• Stabilize cervical spine.<br>• Provide supplemental $O_2$ as needed.<br>• Monitor vital signs, heart rhythm, level of consciousness, respiratory status, and $O_2$ saturation.<br>• Check pulses distal to burns.<br>• Remove nonadherent clothing, shoes, watches, jewelry, glasses or contact lenses (if face was exposed).<br>• Cover burned areas with dry dressings or clean sheet.<br>• Establish IV access with two large-bore catheters if burn >15% TBSA.<br>• Begin fluid replacement.<br>• Obtain arterial blood gas to assess acid-base balance.<br>• Insert indwelling urinary catheter if burn >15% TBSA.<br>• Elevate burned limb(s) above heart to decrease edema.<br>• Give IV analgesia and assess effectiveness frequently.<br>• Identify and treat other associated injuries (e.g., fractures, head injury, thermal burns).<br>**Ongoing Monitoring**<br>• Monitor airway, breathing, and circulation.<br>• Monitor vital signs, $O_2$ saturation, heart rhythm, level of consciousness, and neurovascular status of injured limbs.<br>• Monitor pain level.<br>• Monitor urine output.<br>• Monitor urine for development of myoglobinuria secondary to muscle breakdown and hemoglobinuria secondary to RBC breakdown.<br>• Anticipate possible administration of $NaHCO_3$ to alkalinize the urine and maintain serum pH >6.0. |

*$NaHCO_3$,* Sodium bicarbonate; *TBSA,* total body surface area.

## TABLE 24-9 Emergency Management

***Chemical Burns***

| Etiology | Assessment Findings | Interventions |
| --- | --- | --- |
| • Acids<br>• Alkalis<br>• Organic compounds | • Burning<br>• Redness, swelling of injured tissue<br>• Degeneration of exposed tissue<br>• Discoloration of injured skin<br>• Localized pain<br>• Edema of surrounding tissue<br>• Tissue destruction continuing for up to 72 hr<br>• Respiratory distress if chemical inhaled<br>• Decreased muscle coordination (if organophosphate)<br>• Paralysis | **Initial**<br>• If unresponsive, assess circulation, airway, and breathing before decontamination procedures.<br>• If responsive, monitor airway, breathing, and circulation.<br>• Stabilize cervical spine.<br>• Provide supplemental $O_2$ as needed.<br>• Brush dry chemical from skin before irrigation.<br>• Remove nonadherent clothing, shoes, watches, jewelry, glasses or contact lenses (if face was exposed).<br>• Flush chemical from wound and surrounding area with copious amounts of saline solution or water.<br>• For chemical burn of the eye(s), flush from inner to outer corner of eye with water or lactated Ringer's (if available).<br>• Cover burned areas with dry dressings or clean sheet.<br>• Establish IV access with two large-bore catheters if burn >15% TBSA.<br>• Begin fluid replacement.<br>• Insert indwelling urinary catheter if burn >15% TBSA.<br>• Elevate burned limb(s) above heart to decrease edema.<br>• Give IV analgesia and assess effectiveness frequently.<br>• Contact poison control center for assistance.<br>**Ongoing Monitoring**<br>• Monitor airway if exposed to chemicals.<br>• Monitor pain level.<br>• Monitor urine output.<br>• Consider possibility of systemic impact of identified chemical, and monitor and treat accordingly.<br>• Monitor pH of eye if exposed to chemicals. |

*TBSA,* Total body surface area.

**PATHOPHYSIOLOGY MAP**

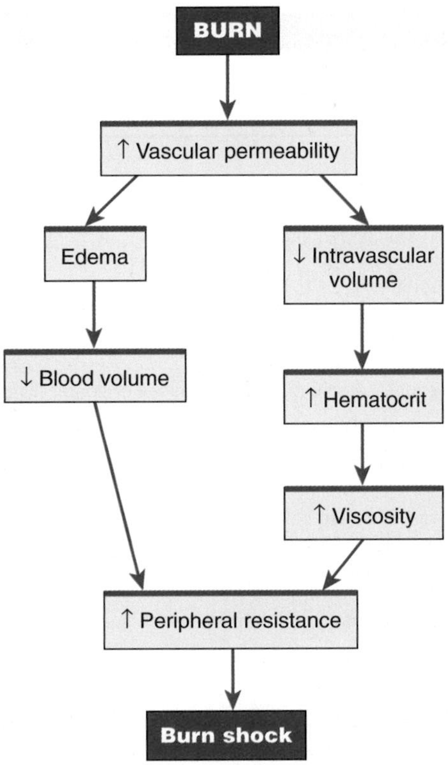


**FIG. 24-5** At the time of major burn injury, there is increased capillary permeability. All fluid components of the blood begin to leak into the interstitium, causing edema and a decreased blood volume. Hematocrit increases, and the blood becomes more viscous. The combination of decreased blood volume and increased viscosity produces increased peripheral resistance. Burn shock, a type of hypovolemic shock, rapidly ensues and, if not corrected, can result in death.

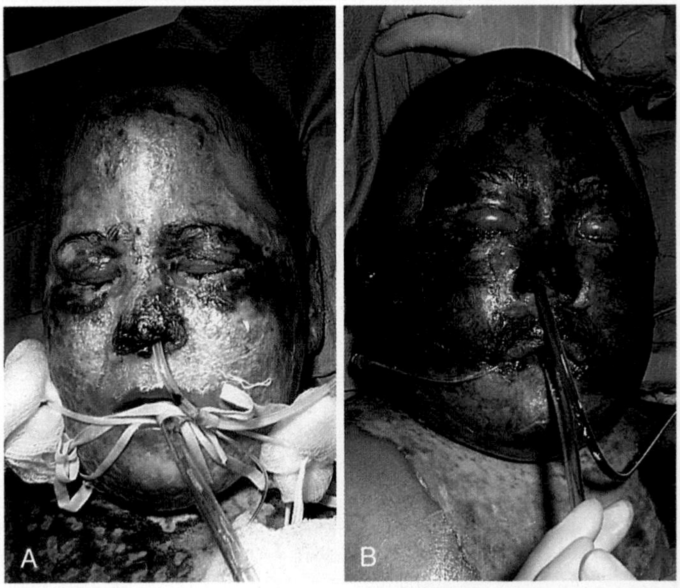


**FIG. 24-6** **A,** Facial edema before fluid resuscitation. **B,** Facial edema after 24 hours. (Courtesy Judy Knighton, Toronto, Canada.)

injured cells and hemolyzed RBCs release potassium into the circulation. Sodium rapidly moves to the interstitial spaces and remains there until edema formation ends (Fig. 24-7).

Toward the end of the emergent phase, capillary membrane permeability is restored if fluid replacement is adequate. Fluid loss and edema formation end. Interstitial fluid gradually returns to the vascular space (Fig. 24-7). Diuresis occurs, and the urine has a low specific gravity.

**Inflammation and Healing.** Burn injury to tissues and vessels causes coagulation necrosis. Neutrophils and monocytes accumulate at the site of injury. Fibroblasts and newly formed collagen fibrils appear and begin wound repair within the first 6

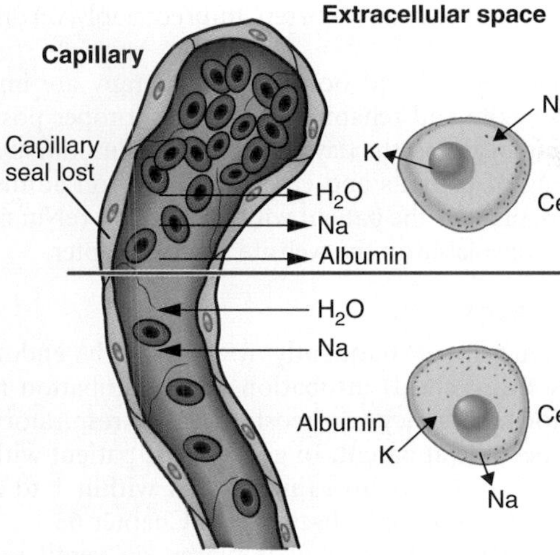


FIG. 24-7 The effects of burn shock are shown above the blue line. As the capillary seal is lost, interstitial edema develops. The cellular integrity is also altered, with sodium *(Na)* moving into the cell in abnormal amounts and potassium *(K)* leaving the cell. The shifts after the resolution of burn shock are shown below the blue line. The water and sodium move back into the circulating volume through the capillary. The albumin remains in the interstitium. Potassium is transported into the cell and sodium is transported out as the cellular integrity returns.

to 12 hours after injury. (The inflammatory response is discussed in Chapter 11.)

**Immunologic Changes.** The body's immune system is challenged when a burn injury occurs. The skin barrier to invading organisms is destroyed, bone marrow depression occurs, and circulating levels of immunoglobulins are decreased. Defects occur in the function of white blood cells (WBCs). The inflammatory cytokine cascade, triggered by tissue damage, impairs the function of lymphocytes, monocytes, and neutrophils. Thus the patient is at a greater risk for infection.

## Clinical Manifestations

The patient with severe burns is likely to be in shock from hypovolemia. Often the areas of full-thickness and deep partial-thickness burns are at first painless because the nerve endings have been destroyed. Superficial to moderate partial-thickness burns are very painful. Blisters, filled with fluid and protein, are common in partial-thickness burns. The patient with a larger burn area may develop a paralytic ileus, with absent or decreased bowel sounds. Shivering may occur as a result of chilling that is caused by heat loss, anxiety, or pain.

The patient may be alert and able to answer questions shortly after admission or until he or she is intubated (if there is respiratory compromise). Patients are often frightened and need your calm reassurances. Give simple explanations of what to expect as you provide care. Unconsciousness or altered mental status in a burn patient usually results from hypoxia associated with smoke inhalation. Other possibilities include head trauma, substance abuse, or excessive amounts of sedation or pain medication.

## Complications

The three major organ systems most susceptible to complications during the emergent phase of burn injury are the cardiovascular, respiratory, and urinary systems.

**Cardiovascular System.** Cardiovascular system complications include dysrhythmias and hypovolemic shock, which, if untreated, may progress to refractory shock. Circulation to the extremities

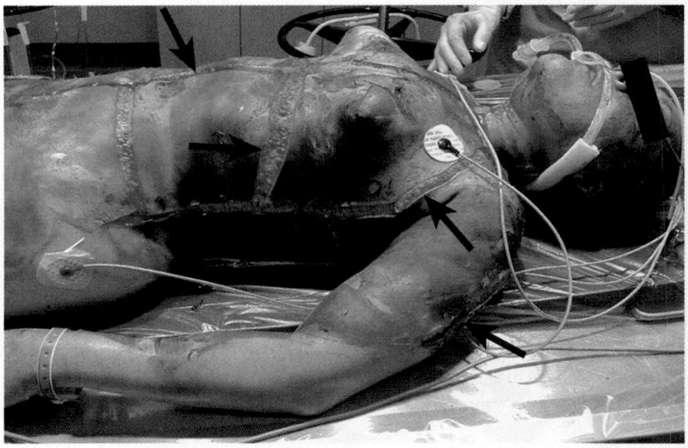

FIG. 24-8 Escharotomies of the anterior and lateral chest and arm (indicated by *arrows*). (Courtesy Judy Knighton, Toronto, Canada.)

can be severely impaired by deep circumferential burns and subsequent edema formation, which act like a tourniquet. If untreated, ischemia, paresthesias, and necrosis can occur. An **escharotomy** (an incision through the full-thickness eschar) is frequently done after transfer to a burn center to restore circulation to compromised extremities (Fig. 24-8).

Initially, blood viscosity increases because of the fluid loss. Microcirculation is impaired because of the damage to skin structures that contain small capillary systems. These two events result in a phenomenon termed *sludging*. Sludging is corrected by adequate fluid replacement.

Burn patients are at an increased risk for venous thromboembolism (VTE) if one or more of the following conditions are present: advanced age, obesity, extensive or lower-extremity burns, concomitant lower-extremity trauma, and prolonged immobility. VTE prophylaxis with anticoagulant drugs should be started, unless contraindicated.[12]

**Respiratory System.** The respiratory system is vulnerable to two types of injury: (1) upper airway burns and (2) lower airway injury (Table 24-3). Upper airway distress may occur with or without smoke inhalation, and airway injury at either level may occur in the absence of burn injury to the skin. (Smoke and inhalation injuries are discussed earlier in this chapter on pp. 430-431.)

The patient may need a fiberoptic bronchoscopy and carboxyhemoglobin blood levels to confirm a suspected inhalation injury. Look in the prehospital and ED notes to see if the patient was exposed to smoke or fumes. Examine any sputum for carbon. Watch for signs of respiratory distress, such as increased agitation, anxiety, restlessness, or a change in the rate or character of the patient's breathing, since symptoms may not be present immediately.

In general, there is no correlation between the percentage TBSA burn (% TBSA) and the severity of inhalation injury. In a patient with inhalation injury, a chest x-ray may appear normal on admission, but changes usually occur over the next 24 to 48 hours. Arterial blood gas (ABG) values may also be within the normal range on admission and change over time.

**Other Cardiopulmonary Problems.** Patients with preexisting heart disease (e.g., myocardial infarction) or lung disease (e.g., chronic obstructive pulmonary disease [COPD]) are at an increased risk for complications. If fluid replacement is too vigorous, watch for early signs of heart failure or pulmonary edema. Invasive measures (e.g., hemodynamic monitoring) may be necessary to monitor fluid resuscitation.

Patients with preexisting lung disease are more likely to develop a respiratory infection. Pneumonia, a common complication of major burns, is the leading cause of death in patients with an inhalation injury.

**Urinary System.** The most common complication of the urinary system in the emergent phase is ATN. If your patient becomes hypovolemic, blood flow to the kidneys is decreased, causing renal ischemia. If this continues, acute kidney injury may develop.

With full-thickness and major electrical burns, myoglobin (from muscle cell breakdown) and hemoglobin (from RBC breakdown) are released into the bloodstream and block renal tubules. Carefully monitor the adequacy of fluid replacement because this can reverse the obstruction of the tubules.

## NURSING AND INTERPROFESSIONAL MANAGEMENT: EMERGENT PHASE

In the emergent phase the patient's survival depends on rapid and thorough assessment and appropriate interventions.[13] Usually the health care provider (HCP) and you make an initial assessment of the depth and extent of the burn and coordinate the actions of others on the health care team. In a community hospital, determine whether the patient requires inpatient or outpatient care. In the case of inpatient care, decide whether the patient remains in the hospital or should be transferred to a burn center (Table 24-4). Care predominantly focuses on airway management, fluid therapy, and wound care (Table 24-10). Patients often improve and worsen, unpredictably, on an almost daily basis.

Although physical and occupational therapy are important in both the acute and rehabilitation phases, proper positioning and splinting begin on the day of admission. Emotional support and teaching of patients and caregivers begin on admission. A nursing care plan for the patient with burn injury (eNursing Care Plan 24-1) is available on the website for this chapter.

### Airway Management

Airway management frequently involves early endotracheal (preferably orotracheal) intubation. Early intubation removes the need for emergency tracheostomy after respiratory problems have become apparent. In general, the patient with burns to the face and neck requires intubation within 1 to 2 hours after injury. (Intubation is discussed in Chapter 65.)

After intubation the patient is placed on ventilatory support, with the oxygen concentration based on ABG values.

### INFORMATICS IN PRACTICE

***Staff Training Using Gaming***

1. Preparing burn center staff for a mass casualty incident involving burn victims is essential.
2. Interactive, video game–based training modules simulate real-life emergency events surrounding a mass casualty burn incident.
3. Critical skills for triage and initial resuscitation (emergent phase) for multiple victims can be practiced.

### TABLE 24-10 Interprofessional Care

***Burn Injury***

| Emergent Phase | Acute Phase | Rehabilitation Phase |
|---|---|---|
| **Fluid Therapy** (Table 24-11)<br>• Assess fluid needs.<br>• Begin IV fluid replacement.<br>• Insert indwelling urinary catheter.<br>• Monitor urine output.<br>**Wound Care**<br>• Start daily shower and wound care.<br>• Debride as necessary.<br>• Assess extent and depth of burns.<br>• Administer tetanus toxoid or tetanus antitoxin.<br>**Pain and Anxiety**<br>• Assess and manage pain and anxiety.<br>**Physical and Occupational Therapy**<br>• Place patient in position that prevents contracture formation and reduces edema.<br>• Assess need for splints.<br>**Nutritional Therapy**<br>• Assess nutritional needs and begin feeding patient by most appropriate route as soon as possible.<br>**Respiratory Therapy**<br>• Assess oxygenation needs.<br>• Provide supplemental $O_2$ as needed.<br>• Intubate if necessary.<br>• Monitor respiratory status.<br>**Psychosocial Care**<br>• Provide support to patient and caregiver during initial crisis phase. | **Fluid Therapy**<br>• Continue to replace fluids, depending on patient's clinical response.<br>**Wound Care**<br>• Continue daily shower and wound care.<br>• Continue debridement (if necessary).<br>• Assess wound daily and adjust dressing protocols as necessary.<br>• Observe for complications (e.g., infection).<br>**Early Excision and Grafting**<br>• Provide temporary allografts.<br>• Provide permanent autografts.<br>• Care for donor sites.<br>**Pain and Anxiety**<br>• Continue to assess for and treat pain and anxiety.<br>**Physical and Occupational Therapy**<br>• Begin daily therapy program for maintenance of range of motion.<br>• Assess need for splints and anticontracture positioning.<br>• Encourage and assist patient with self-care as possible.<br>**Nutritional Therapy**<br>• Continue to assess diet to support wound healing.<br>**Respiratory Therapy**<br>• Continue to assess oxygenation needs.<br>• Continue to monitor respiratory status.<br>• Monitor for signs of complications (e.g., pneumonia).<br>**Psychosocial Care**<br>• Provide ongoing support, counseling, and teaching to patient and caregiver about physical and emotional aspects of care and recovery.<br>• Begin to anticipate discharge needs.<br>**Drug Therapy** (Table 24-13)<br>• Assess need for drugs (e.g., antibiotics).<br>• Continue to monitor effectiveness and adjust dosage as needed. | • Continue to counsel and teach patient and caregiver about wound care.<br>• Continue to encourage and assist patient in resuming self-care.<br>• Continue to prevent or minimize contractures and assess likelihood for scarring (surgery, physical and occupational therapy, splinting, pressure garments).<br>• Discuss possible reconstructive surgery.<br>• Prepare for discharge home or transfer to rehabilitation hospital.<br>• Discuss possible need for home care nursing. |

Extubation may be indicated when the edema resolves, usually 3 to 6 days after burn injury, unless severe inhalation injury exists. Escharotomies of the chest may be needed to relieve respiratory distress secondary to circumferential, full-thickness burns of the neck and chest (Fig. 24-8).

Within 6 to 12 hours after injury in which smoke inhalation is suspected, a fiberoptic bronchoscopy should be done to assess the lower airway. When intubation is not done, treatment of inhalation injury includes giving 100% humidified $O_2$. Place the patient in a high Fowler's position, unless contraindicated (e.g., spinal injury), and encourage deep breathing and coughing every hour. Reposition the patient every 1 to 2 hours. Provide suctioning and chest physiotherapy (as ordered).

If severe respiratory distress (e.g., hoarseness, shortness of breath) develops, intubation and mechanical ventilation are started. Positive end-expiratory pressure (PEEP) may be used to prevent collapse of the alveoli and progressive respiratory failure (see Chapters 65 and 67). Bronchodilators may be given to treat severe bronchospasm. CO poisoning is treated by administering 100% $O_2$ until carboxyhemoglobin levels return to normal.

**SAFETY ALERT Pulse CO Oximetry Monitoring**

- Standard pulse oximetry ($SpO_2$) does not distinguish oxyhemoglobin from carboxyhemoglobin. A patient with CO poisoning will have normal $SpO_2$ readings in spite of elevated carboxyhemoglobin levels.
- For patients with suspected or confirmed CO poisoning, use a pulse CO oximetry (SpCO) device.[14]

## Fluid Therapy

Obtaining IV access is critical for fluid resuscitation and drug administration. At least two large-bore IVs must be in place for patients with burns that are 15% TBSA or more. It is critical to obtain IV access that can handle large volumes of fluid. For patients with burns greater than 30% TBSA, consider a central line for fluid and drug administration and blood sampling (central lines are discussed in Chapter 16). An arterial line is often placed if frequent ABGs or invasive BP monitoring is needed.

Assess the extent of the burn wound using a standardized tool (Fig. 24-4). Then use a standardized formula to estimate the patient's fluid resuscitation needs. Fluid replacement is achieved with crystalloid solutions (usually lactated Ringer's), colloids (albumin), or a combination of the two. IV saline is usually started during the prehospital phase.

The Parkland (Baxter) formula for fluid replacement is the most common formula used (Table 24-11 or *www.mdcalc.com/parkland-formula-for-burns*). Remember that all formulas are estimates. Fluids are titrated based on the patient's response (e.g., hourly urine output, vital signs). Patients with an electrical injury have greater than normal fluid needs. They generally require an osmotic diuretic (mannitol [Osmitrol]) to increase their urine output and overcome high levels of hemoglobin and myoglobin in the urine. Too much fluid and overestimation of TBSA contribute to over-resuscitation of fluids or "fluid creep."[15] For the first 24 hours, the recommendation is 2 to 4 mL lactated Ringer's/kg/%TBSA burned.

Colloidal solutions (e.g., 5% albumin) may also be given. However, administration is recommended after the first 12 to 24 hours postburn when capillary permeability returns to normal or near normal. After this time, the plasma remains in the vascular space and expands the circulating volume. The replacement volume is calculated based on the patient's body weight and TBSA burned (e.g., 0.3 to 0.5 mL/kg/%TBSA burned).

**TABLE 24-11 Fluid Resuscitation**

**Parkland (Baxter) Formula***

4 mL lactated Ringer's solution per kilogram (kg) of body weight per percent of total body surface area (% TBSA) burned = Total fluid requirements for first 24 hr after burn

**Application**

½ of total in first 8 hr
¼ of total in second 8 hr
¼ of total in third 8 hr

**Example**

For a 70-kg patient with a 50% TBSA burn:

$$4\ \text{mL} \times 70\ \text{kg} \times 50\ (\%\text{TBSA})\ \text{burned} = 14{,}000\ \text{mL in 24 hr}$$

½ of total in first 8 hr = 7000 mL (875 mL/hr)
¼ of total in second 8 hr = 3500 mL (437 mL/hr)
¼ of total in third 8 hr = 3500 mL (437 mL/hr)

*Formulas are guidelines. Fluid is given at a rate to produce 0.5-1.0 mL/kg/hr of urine output. The American Burn Association Consensus Fluid Resuscitation Formula has suggested 2-4 mL lactated Ringer's solution per kg of body weight per %TBSA burned = total fluid requirements for first 24 hr after burn. This strategy avoids over-resuscitation of fluids or "fluid creep."

Assess for the adequacy of fluid resuscitation hourly using clinical parameters. Urine output, the most commonly used parameter, and cardiac parameters are defined as follows.

- *Urine output:* 0.5 to 1 mL/kg/hr; 75 to 100 mL/hr for electrical burn patient with evidence of hemoglobinuria or myoglobinuria.
- *Cardiac parameters:* Mean arterial pressure (MAP) greater than 65 mm Hg, systolic BP greater than 90 mm Hg, heart rate less than 120 beats/minute. MAP and BP are best measured by an arterial line. Manual BP measurement is often invalid because of edema and vasoconstriction.

**CHECK YOUR PRACTICE**

You are assigned to a new male burn patient who weighs 72 kg and has 45% TBSA burn.

- What rate (mL/hr) should fluids be infused over the second 8 hours of fluid resuscitation for him?

## Wound Care

Once a patent airway, effective circulation, and adequate fluid replacement have been achieved, priority is given to care of the burn wound. Partial-thickness burn wounds appear pink to cherry-red and are wet and shiny with serous exudate. These wounds may or may not have intact blisters; are painful when touched; and have only minor, localized sensation because nerve endings may have been destroyed in the burned dermis.

You and unlicensed assistive personnel (UAP) can perform cleansing and gentle debridement (using scissors and forceps) on a shower cart (Fig. 24-9), in a regular shower, or on a patient's bed or stretcher. Extensive, surgical debridement is done in the operating room (OR) (Fig. 24-10). During **debridement**, necrotic skin is removed. Releasing escharotomies and fasciotomies are done in the emergent phase, usually in burn centers by burn physicians.

Patients find the first wound care to be both physically and mentally demanding. Provide emotional support and begin to build trust during this activity. A once-daily shower and dressing change in the morning, with an evening dressing change in

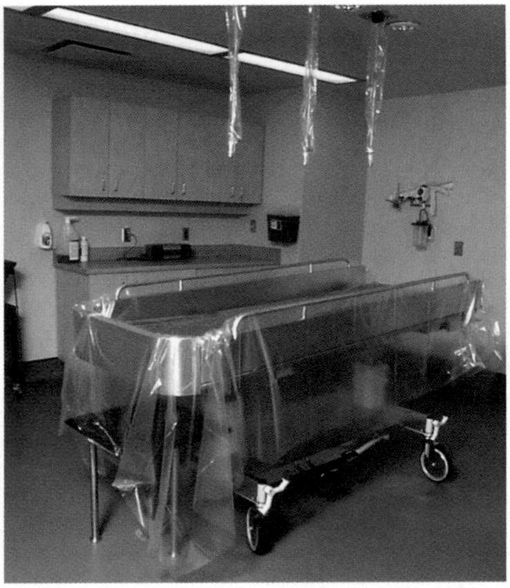

FIG. 24-9 Shower cart. Showering presents an opportunity for wound care and physical therapy. (Courtesy Judy Knighton, Toronto, Canada.)

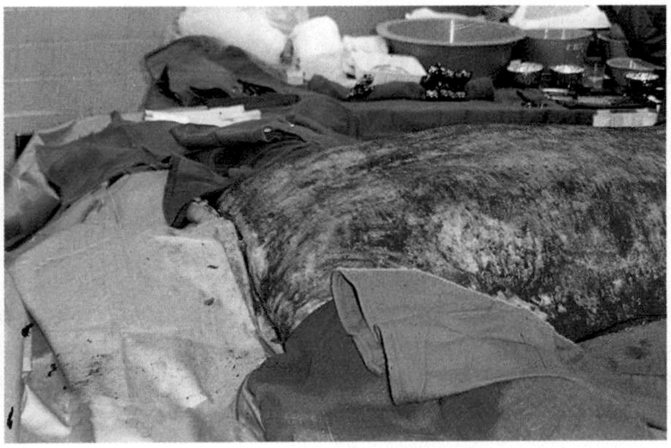

FIG. 24-10 Surgical debridement of full-thickness burns is necessary to prepare the wound for grafting. (Courtesy Judy Knighton, Toronto, Canada.)

the patient's room, are part of the routine in many burn centers. Others opt to shower the patient on admission and then perform all other dressing changes in the patient's room. Some of the newer antimicrobial dressings can be left in place from 3 to 14 days, thereby reducing the frequency of dressing changes.

Infection can cause further tissue injury and possible sepsis.[16] The source of infection in burn wounds is likely the patient's own flora, mostly from the skin and respiratory and gastrointestinal (GI) systems. Preventing cross-contamination from one patient to another is a priority.

Two approaches to burn wound treatment are (1) the open method and (2) the use of multiple dressing changes (closed method). In the *open method* the patient's burn is covered with a topical antimicrobial and has no dressing over the wound. This approach is usually limited to the care of facial burns. In the *multiple dressing change,* or *closed method,* sterile gauze dressings are impregnated with or laid over a topical antimicrobial (Fig. 24-11). These dressings are changed anywhere from every 12 to 24 hours to once every 14 days (depending on the product). Most burn centers support the concept of moist wound healing and use dressings to cover the burned areas, with the exception of facial burns.

When the patient's open burn wounds are exposed, always wear personal protective equipment (PPE) (e.g., disposable hats, masks, gowns, gloves). When removing contaminated dressings and washing the wound, use nonsterile, disposable gloves. Use sterile gloves when applying ointments and sterile dressings. In addition, prevent shivering by keeping the room warm (approximately 85°F [29.4°C]). Before leaving one patient, remove your PPE. Don new PPE before you treat another patient. Thoroughly wash your hands both before and after patient contact to prevent cross-contamination.

Permanent skin coverage is the primary goal for burn wound care. There is rarely enough unburned skin in the major (greater than 50% TBSA) burn patient for immediate skin grafting. In this situation, temporary wound closure methods are needed. *Allograft (homograft) skin* (from skin donor cadavers) is used, along with newer biosynthetic options. Treatment approaches vary among burn centers (Table 24-12).

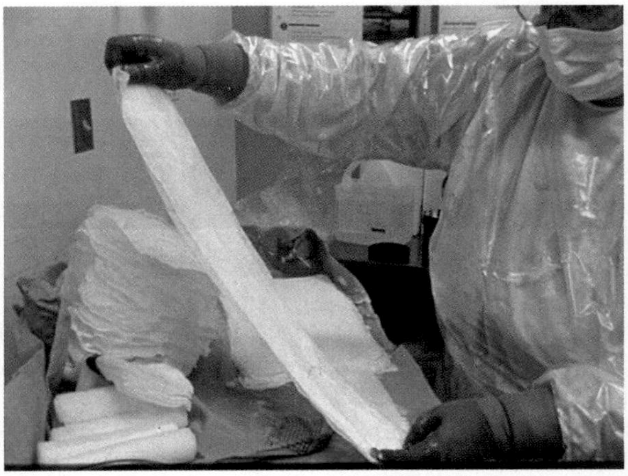

FIG. 24-11 Application of silver sulfadiazine cream to saline-moistened gauze. (Courtesy Judy Knighton, Toronto, Canada.)

**TABLE 24-12 Skin Grafts Used for Burn Injury**

| Graft Type | Source and Description | Coverage |
|---|---|---|
| Xenograft (or heterograft) (different species) | Porcine skin | Temporary (3 days to 2 wk) |
| Allograft (or homograft) (same species) | Cadaveric skin | Temporary (3 days to 2 wk) |
| Autograft | Patient's own skin | Permanent |
| Cultured epithelial autograft (CEA)–Epicel | Patient's own skin cell cultures | Permanent |
| Biobrane | Semipermeable silicone membrane bonded to nylon fabric | Temporary (10-21 days) |
| Integra | Biodegradable dermal layer made of bovine collagen and glycosaminoglycan bonded to silicone membrane | Permanent |
| AlloDerm | Acellular dermal matrix derived from donated human skin | Permanent |
| OrCel | Donated neonatal foreskin fibroblasts and keratinocytes in bovine collagen sponge | Permanent |
| Apligraf | Donated neonatal foreskin fibroblasts and keratinocytes in bovine collagen gel | Permanent |
| Matriderm | Bovine collagen and elastin matrix | Permanent |

## Other Care Measures

Certain parts of the body (e.g., face, eyes, hands, arms, ears, perineum) need vigilant nursing care. The face is highly vascular and can become very swollen. It is often covered with ointments and gauze but not wrapped to limit pressure on delicate facial structures. An ophthalmology exam should occur soon after admission for all patients with facial burns. Periorbital edema can prevent eye opening and is often frightening for the patient. Always check that the patient's eyelashes are not turned inward towards the eyeball. Provide assurance that the swelling is not permanent. Instill methylcellulose drops or artificial tears into the eyes for moisture and additional comfort. Apply antibiotic eye ointment for corneal burns or edema as ordered.

Ears should be kept free from pressure because of their poor vascularization and tendency to become infected. Do not use pillows for the patient with ear burns. The pressure on the cartilage may cause chondritis. Further, the ear may stick to the pillowcase, causing pain and bleeding. Raise your patient's head using a rolled towel placed under the shoulders, being careful to avoid pressure necrosis. Follow the same strategy for the patient with neck burns to hyperextend the neck and prevent neck contracture.

Extend your patient's burned hands and arms and raise them on pillows or plastic-covered foam wedges to reduce edema. Ask the physical therapist and the HCP if splints should be applied to burned hands and feet to keep them in positions of function. Remove the splints often and inspect the skin and bony prominences to avoid areas of pressure from inappropriate or prolonged application.

Keep your patient's perineum as clean and dry as possible after each voiding or bowel movement. In addition to monitoring hourly urine outputs, an indwelling catheter prevents urine contamination of the perineal area. Regular once- or twice-daily perineal care, in the presence or absence of a perineal burn wound, is essential. Assess the need for an indwelling urinary catheter on a daily basis. Remove when no longer needed to limit the risk of a urinary tract infection. If your patient has frequent, loose stools, consider using a fecal diversion device.

Perform necessary laboratory tests to monitor fluid and electrolyte balance. Draw ABGs, as necessary, to assess adequacy of ventilation and oxygenation in patients with suspected or confirmed inhalation or electrical injury.

Work with the physical therapist to perform range-of-motion (ROM) exercises during dressing changes and throughout the day. Movement aids the shift of the leaked fluid back into the vascular bed. Active and passive exercise of body parts also maintains function, prevents skin and joint contractures, and reassures the patient that movement is still possible.

## Drug Therapy

**Analgesics and Sedatives.** Promote the use of analgesics for the patient's comfort. Early in the postburn period, IV pain medications should be given because (1) onset of action is fastest with this route; (2) oral drugs have a slower onset of action and are not as effective when GI function is slowed or impaired because of shock or paralytic ileus; and (3) IM injections are not absorbed well in burned or edematous areas, causing pooling of drugs in the tissues. Consequently, when fluid mobilization starts, the patient could be inadvertently overdosed from the interstitial accumulation of previous IM drugs.

Common drugs used for pain control are listed in Table 24-13. Initially, opioids are the drug of choice for pain control.

**TABLE 24-13 Drug Therapy**
***Burns***

| Drugs | Purpose |
|---|---|
| **Analgesics** | |
| morphine (Avinza) | Relieve pain |
| sustained-release morphine (MS Contin) | |
| hydromorphone (Dilaudid) | |
| sustained-release hydromorphone (Dilaudid CR) | |
| fentanyl (Sublimaze) | |
| oxycodone and acetaminophen (Percocet) | |
| methadone (Dolophine) | |
| Nonsteroidal antiinflammatory (e.g., ketorolac) | |
| Adjuvant analgesics (e.g., gabapentin [Neurontin]) | |
| **Sedatives/Hypnotics** | |
| lorazepam (Ativan) | Reduce anxiety |
| midazolam | Provide short-acting amnesic effects |
| zolpidem (Ambien) | Promote sleep |
| **Antidepressants** | |
| sertraline (Zoloft) | Reduce depression, improve mood |
| citalopram (Celexa) | |
| **Anticoagulants** | |
| enoxaparin (Lovenox) | Prevent venous thromboembolism |
| heparin | |
| **Nutritional Support** | |
| Vitamins A, C, E, and multivitamins | Promote wound healing |
| Minerals: zinc, iron (ferrous sulfate) | Promote cell integrity and hemoglobin formation |
| **Gastrointestinal Support** | |
| ranitidine (Zantac) | Decrease stomach acid and risk of Curling's ulcer |
| esomeprazole (Nexium) | |
| calcium carbonate and magnesium carbonate (Mylanta) | Neutralize stomach acid |
| aluminum hydroxide and magnesium hydroxide (Maalox) | |
| nystatin | Prevent overgrowth of *Candida albicans* in oral mucosa |

When given appropriately, these drugs should provide adequate pain relief. Evaluate the pain management plan often, since the patient's needs may change and tolerance to drugs may develop over time. Remember that the patient's pain level may not directly correlate with the extent and depth of burn. Analgesic needs vary from one patient to another. Consider a multimodal approach to pain control. Sedatives/hypnotics and antidepressants can also be given with analgesics to control the anxiety, insomnia, or depression that patients may experience (Table 24-13).

**Tetanus Immunization.** Tetanus toxoid is given routinely to all burn patients because of the likelihood of anaerobic burn wound contamination. If the patient has not received an active immunization within 10 years before the burn injury, tetanus immunoglobulin should be considered. (Tetanus immunization is discussed in Table 68-6.)

**Antimicrobial Agents.** After the wound is cleansed, topical antimicrobial agents may be applied (Fig. 24-11) and covered with a light dressing. Systemic antibiotics are not routinely used to control burn wound flora because the burn eschar has little or no blood supply, and consequently little antibiotic is delivered to the wound. In addition, the routine use of systemic antibiotics increases the chance of developing multidrug-resistant organisms.

Some topical burn agents penetrate the eschar and inhibit bacterial invasion of the wound. Silver-impregnated dressings can be left in place from 3 to 14 days, depending on the patient's clinical situation and the particular product. Silver sulfadiazine (Silvadene) and mafenide acetate (Sulfamylon) creams are also used.[17]

**SAFETY ALERT Drug Allergy Check**

- Check the patient for any allergies to sulfa, since many burn antimicrobial creams contain sulfa.

Sepsis remains a primary cause of death in the patient with major burns and may lead to multiple organ dysfunction syndrome (see Chapter 66). Systemic antibiotic therapy is started when the diagnosis of sepsis is made or when some other source of infection is identified (e.g., pneumonia).

Fungal infections may develop in the patient's mucous membranes (mouth and genitalia) as a result of systemic antibiotic therapy and low resistance. The offending organism is usually *Candida albicans.* Oral infection is treated with nystatin (Mycostatin) mouthwash. When a normal diet is resumed, yogurt or *Lactobacillus* (Lactinex) may be given to reintroduce the normal intestinal flora that was destroyed by antibiotic therapy.

◆ **Venous Thromboembolism Prophylaxis.** Burn patients are at risk for VTE. If there are no contraindications, it is recommended that low-molecular-weight heparin (enoxaparin) or low-dose unfractionated heparin be started as soon as it is considered safe. For burn patients who have a high bleeding risk, VTE prophylaxis with sequential compression devices and/or graduated compression stockings are used until the bleeding risk decreases and heparin can be started (Table 24-13). (VTE prophylaxis is discussed in Chapter 37.)

### ◆ Nutritional Therapy

Once fluid replacement needs have been addressed, nutrition takes priority in the initial emergent phase. Early and aggressive nutritional support within several hours of the burn injury can decrease complications and mortality, optimize burn wound healing, and minimize the negative effects of hypermetabolism and catabolism.[18] Nonintubated patients with a burn of less than 20% TBSA will usually be able to eat enough to meet their nutritional needs.

Intubated patients and those with larger burns require additional support. Enteral feedings have almost entirely replaced parenteral feeding. Early enteral feeding, usually with smaller-bore tubes, preserves GI function, increases intestinal blood flow, and promotes optimal conditions for wound healing. In general, begin the feedings slowly at a rate of 20 to 40 mL/hr and increase to the goal rate within 24 to 48 hours. If a large nasogastric tube is used, gastric residuals should be checked to rule out delayed gastric emptying. Assess bowel sounds every 8 hours.

A *hypermetabolic state* proportional to the size of the wound occurs after a major burn injury. Resting metabolic expenditure may be increased by 50% to 100% above normal in patients with major burns. Core temperature is elevated. Catecholamines, which stimulate catabolism and heat production, are increased. Massive catabolism can occur and is characterized by protein breakdown and increased gluconeogenesis.

Failure to supply adequate calories and protein leads to malnutrition and delayed healing. Calorie-containing nutritional supplements are often given to meet the caloric needs. Protein powder can also be added to food and liquids. Supplemental vitamins may be started in the emergent phase, with iron supplements often given in the acute phase[19] (Table 24-13).

## ACUTE PHASE

The *acute phase* of burn care begins with the mobilization of extracellular fluid and subsequent diuresis. It concludes when partial-thickness wounds are healed or full-thickness burns are covered by skin grafts. This may take weeks or months.

### Pathophysiology

A healing burn injury causes many pathophysiologic changes in the body. Diuresis from fluid mobilization occurs, and the patient is less edematous. Bowel sounds return. The depth of the burn wounds may be more apparent as they "declare" themselves as partial or full thickness. The patient may now become more aware of the enormity of his or her situation and will benefit from emotional support and information.

Some healing begins as WBCs surround the burn wound and phagocytosis occurs. Necrotic tissue begins to slough. Fibroblasts lay down matrices of the collagen precursors that eventually form granulation tissue. A partial-thickness burn will heal, from both the wound edges and the dermal bed below, if kept free from infection and *desiccation* (dryness). However, full-thickness burn wounds, unless extremely small, must have the burn eschar surgically removed (excised) and skin grafts applied in order to heal. In some cases, healing time and length of hospitalization are decreased by early excision and grafting.

### Clinical Manifestations

Partial-thickness wounds form eschar, which begins separating fairly soon after injury. Once the eschar is removed, re-epithelialization begins at the wound margins and appears as red or pink scar tissue. Epithelial buds, from the hair follicles and glands in the dermal bed, eventually close the wound. Healing is spontaneous and usually occurs within 10 to 21 days.

Margins of full-thickness eschar take longer to separate. As a result, full-thickness burn wounds require surgical debridement and skin grafting to heal.

### Laboratory Values

Because the body is attempting to reestablish fluid and electrolyte balance in the initial acute phase, it is important to follow serum electrolyte levels closely.

**Sodium.** *Hyponatremia* can develop from excessive GI suction and diarrhea. Manifestations of hyponatremia include weakness, dizziness, muscle cramps, fatigue, headache, tachycardia, and confusion. The patient may also develop a *dilutional hyponatremia* called *water intoxication* from excess water intake. To avoid this condition, offer the patient fluids other than water, such as juice or nutritional supplements, to drink.

*Hypernatremia* may be seen after successful fluid resuscitation if large amounts of hypertonic solutions were used. Hypernatremia may also be caused by tube feedings or inappropriate fluid administration. Manifestations of hypernatremia include thirst; dried, furry tongue; lethargy; confusion; and possibly seizures. Sodium restrictions may be applied to IV fluids and enteral or oral feedings until levels return to safe limits.

**Potassium.** *Hyperkalemia* may occur if the patient has renal failure, adrenocortical insufficiency, or massive deep muscle injury (e.g., electrical burn) with large amounts of potassium released from damaged cells. Heart dysrhythmias and arrest can occur with elevated potassium levels. Check for muscle weakness, cramping, and paralysis.

*Hypokalemia* occurs with vomiting, diarrhea, prolonged GI suction, and IV therapy without potassium supplementation. Potassium is also lost through the patient's burn wounds. Signs and symptoms of hypokalemia include fatigue, muscle weakness, leg cramps, heart dysrhythmias, paresthesias, and decreased reflexes (see Chapter 16).

## Complications

**Infection.** A burn injury destroys the body's first line of defense, the skin. The burn wound is now colonized with the person's own organisms that were on the skin before the burn. If the levels of bacteria between the eschar and viable wound bed rise to greater than $10^5$ per gram of tissue, the patient has a burn wound infection. Localized inflammation, induration, and sometimes suppuration can be seen at the burn wound margins. Partial-thickness burns can change to full-thickness wounds when these bacteria invade viable, unburned tissue. Wound infections may be treated with systemic antibiotics based on wound culture and sensitivity results.

Watch for signs and symptoms, including hypothermia or hyperthermia, increased heart and respiratory rate, decreased BP, and decreased urine output. The patient may have mild confusion, chills, malaise, and loss of appetite. The WBC count usually is between 10,000/μL ($10 \times 10^9$/L) and 20,000/μL ($20 \times 10^9$/L). The WBCs have functional defects and the patient is immunosuppressed for many months after the burn injury.

The causative organisms of sepsis are usually gram-negative bacteria (e.g., *Pseudomonas, Proteus*), putting the patient at further risk for septic shock. When sepsis is suspected, immediately obtain cultures from all possible sources, including the burn wound, blood, urine, sputum, oropharynx and perineal regions, and IV site. Treatment immediately begins with antibiotics. When the culture and sensitivity results are known, the antibiotic in use may be continued or changed based on the results. At this stage the patient's condition is considered critical, and close monitoring of vital signs and mental status is needed.

**Cardiovascular and Respiratory Systems.** The same cardiovascular and respiratory system complications present in the emergent phase may continue into the acute phase of care. In addition, new problems might arise, requiring timely intervention.

**Neurologic System.** Neurologically, the patient probably has no physical symptoms, unless severe hypoxia from respiratory injuries or complications from electrical injuries occur. Probable causes of neurologic complications include electrolyte imbalance, stress, cerebral edema, sepsis, sleep disturbances, and the use of analgesics and antianxiety drugs. However, some patients may demonstrate certain behaviors that are not completely understood.

The patient may become extremely disoriented, may withdraw or become combative, and may have hallucinations and frequent nightmare-like episodes. Delirium is more acute at night and occurs more often in the older patient. Start appropriate nursing interventions to prevent delirium and use a screening tool to diagnose delirium (see Table 59-18). Orient and reassure your patient if he or she is confused or agitated. This state is usually transient, lasting from a day or two to several weeks, but complications and sequelae can last for years and be serious.

**Musculoskeletal System.** The musculoskeletal system is particularly prone to complications during the acute phase, and the involvement of both the physical and occupational therapist is vitally important. As the burns begin to heal and scar tissue forms, the skin is less supple and pliant. ROM may be limited, and skin and joint contractures can occur. Because of pain, the patient prefers a flexed position for comfort. Have the patient stretch and move the burned body parts as much as possible. Consult with the physical or occupational therapist about proper positioning and splinting to prevent or reduce contracture formation.

**Gastrointestinal System.** The GI system may also experience complications during this phase. Paralytic ileus can be caused by sepsis. Diarrhea may result from the use of enteral feedings or antibiotics. Constipation can occur as a side effect of opioids, decreased mobility, and a low-fiber diet. *Curling's ulcer* is a type of gastroduodenal ulcer characterized by diffuse superficial lesions (including mucosal erosion). It is caused by a generalized stress response to decreased blood flow to the GI tract. The patient has increased gastric acid secretion.

Aim to prevent Curling's ulcer by feeding the patient as soon as possible after the burn injury. Antacids, $H_2$-histamine blockers (e.g., ranitidine [Zantac]), and proton pump inhibitors (e.g., esomeprazole [Nexium]) are used prophylactically to neutralize stomach acids and inhibit histamine and the secretion of hydrochloric acid (Table 24-13). Patients with major burns may also have occult blood in their stools during the acute phase and require close monitoring for bleeding.

**Endocrine System.** Watch for transient increases in the patient's blood glucose levels as a result of stress-mediated cortisol and catecholamine release. There is an increased mobilization of glycogen stores and gluconeogenesis. Subsequently, glucose is produced, along with an increase in insulin production. However, insulin's effectiveness is decreased because of relative insulin insensitivity. This results in an elevated blood glucose level. Hyperglycemia may also be caused by the increased caloric intake necessary to meet some patients' metabolic requirements. When this occurs, treat with IV or subcutaneous insulin, not decreased feeding. Check blood glucose levels and give insulin as ordered. Point-of-care testing of glucose can be done, but serum glucose testing is more accurate. As the patient's metabolic demands are met and less stress is placed on the entire system, this stress-induced condition is reversed.

# ◆ NURSING AND INTERPROFESSIONAL MANAGEMENT: ACUTE PHASE

The major therapeutic interventions in the acute phase are (1) wound care, (2) excision and grafting, (3) pain management, (4) physical and occupational therapy, and (5) nutritional therapy.

## ◆ Wound Care

The goals of wound care are to (1) prevent infection by cleansing and debriding the area of necrotic tissue that would promote bacterial growth and (2) promote wound re-epithelialization and/or successful skin grafting.

Wound care consists of ongoing observation, assessment, cleansing, debridement, and dressing reapplication. Nonsurgical debridement, dressing changes, topical antimicrobial therapy, graft care, and donor site care are performed as often as necessary, depending on the topical cream or dressing ordered. Enzymatic debriding agents made of natural ingredients, such as collagen, may be used for *enzymatic debridement* of burn wounds, which speeds up the removal of dead tissue from the healthy wound bed.

Cleanse wounds with soap and water or normal saline-moistened gauze to gently remove the old antimicrobial agent and any loose necrotic tissue, scabs, or dried blood. During the debridement phase, cover the wound with topical antimicrobial creams (e.g., silver sulfadiazine) or silver-impregnated dressings. When the partial-thickness burn wounds have been fully debrided, a protective, coarse or fine-meshed, greasy-based (paraffin or petroleum) gauze dressing is applied to protect the re-epithelializing keratinocytes as they resurface and close the open wound bed.

If grafting is necessary, protect the skin graft (discussed later) with the same greasy gauze dressings next to the graft, followed by saline-moistened middle dressing, and dry gauze outer dressings. With facial grafts the unmeshed sheet graft is left open, so it is possible for *blebs* (serosanguineous exudate) to form between the graft and recipient bed. Blebs prevent the graft from permanently attaching to the wound bed. The evacuation of blebs is best performed by aspiration with a tuberculin syringe and only by those trained in this specialized skill. (Dressings are discussed in Table 11-9.)

## Excision and Grafting

Management of full-thickness burn wounds involves early removal (surgical excision) of the necrotic tissue followed by application of split-thickness autograft skin.[20] This approach has improved the management and survival rate of burn patients. In the past, patients with major burns had low rates of survival because healing and wound coverage took so long that the patient usually died of sepsis or malnutrition.

Many patients, especially those with major burns, are taken to the OR for wound excision on day 1 or 2 (emergent phase). The wounds are covered with a biologic dressing or allograft for temporary coverage until permanent grafting can occur (Table 24-12).

During the procedure of **excision and grafting**, devitalized tissue (eschar) is excised down to the subcutaneous tissue or fascia, depending on the degree of injury. Surgical excision can result in massive blood loss. To decrease surgical blood loss, topical application of epinephrine or thrombin, injection of saline and epinephrine, application of extremity tourniquets, or application of a new fibrin sealant (Artiss) is used.

Once hemostasis has been achieved, a graft is then placed on clean, viable tissue to achieve good adherence. Whenever possible, the freshly excised wound is covered with *autograft* (the person's own) skin (Table 24-12). Recently, fibrin sealant has been used to attach skin grafts to the wound bed. Grafts can also be stapled or sutured into place (Fig. 24-12, *A*). Negative pressure wound therapy dressings are often placed on top of skin grafts to optimize adherence of the graft to the excised wound bed.[21] A temporary allograft can be used to test the suitability of the recipient site to accept a graft. The allograft is then removed several days later in the OR and an autograft applied.

With early excision, function is restored and scar tissue formation is minimized. Clots between the graft and wound keep the graft from adhering to the wound. Outer occlusive dressings apply just enough pressure to promote adherence of the graft to the wound bed and help control bleeding. Protect the grafted area from shearing, friction, and pressure. Facial, neck, and hand burns require skilled nursing care to identify and manage clots quickly for the best functional and esthetic outcomes.

Donor skin is taken from the patient for grafting by means of a *dermatome*, which removes a thin (14/1000 to 16/1000 inch) split-thickness layer of skin from an unburned site (Fig. 24-12, *B*). The donor skin can be meshed (usually ratio of 1.5 : 1) to allow for greater wound coverage, or it may be applied as an unmeshed sheet for a better cosmetic result when grafting the face, neck, and hands. The donor site now becomes a new open wound.

The goals of donor site care are to promote rapid, moist wound healing; decrease pain at the site; and prevent infection.

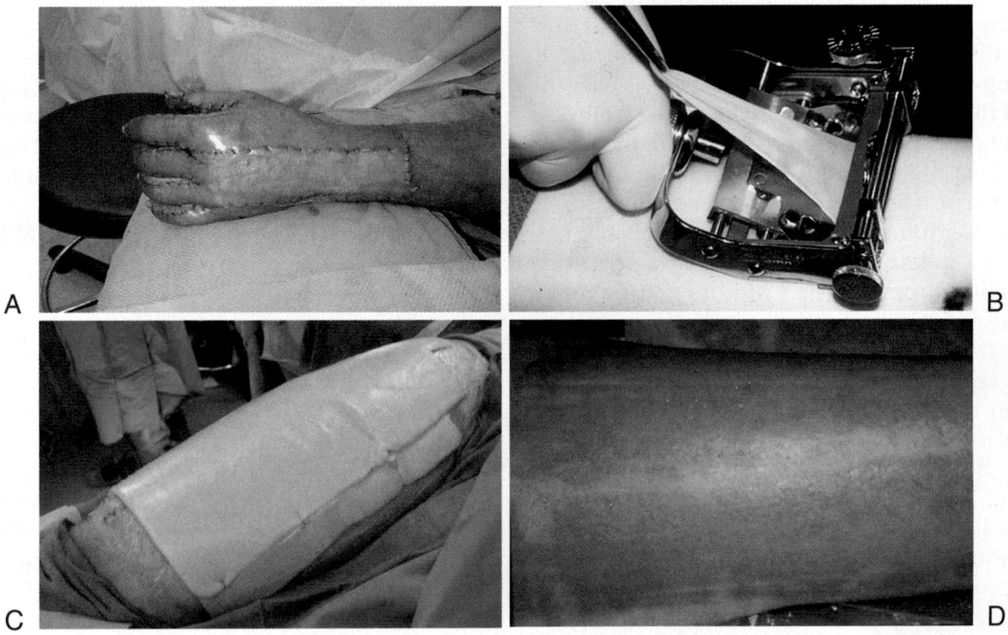


**FIG. 24-12** **A,** Freshly applied split-thickness sheet skin graft to the hand. **B,** Split-thickness skin graft is harvested from a patient's thigh using a dermatome. **C,** Donor site is covered with a hydrophilic foam dressing after harvesting. **D,** Healed donor site. (Courtesy Judy Knighton, Toronto, Canada.)

The choices of dressings for donor sites include transparent dressings (e.g., OpSite), xenograft, silver sulfadiazine, silver-impregnated dressings, calcium alginate, and hydrophilic foam dressings (Fig. 24-12, *C*). Nursing care of the donor site is specific to the dressing selected. Several of the newer dressings decrease healing time, which allows earlier reharvesting of skin at the same site. The average healing time for a donor site is 10 to 14 days (Fig. 24-12, *D*).

**Cultured Epithelial Autografts.** In the patient with large body burns, only a limited amount of unburned skin may be available as donor sites for grafting, and some of that skin may not be suitable for harvesting. Cultured epithelial autograft (CEA) is a method of getting permanent skin from a person with limited skin available for harvesting. CEA is grown from biopsies obtained from the patient's unburned skin. This procedure is performed in suitable patients in some burn centers as soon as possible. The specimens are sent to a commercial laboratory, where the biopsied keratinocytes are grown in a culture medium containing epidermal growth factor. After approximately 18 to 25 days, the keratinocytes have expanded up to 10,000 times and form sheets that can be used as skin grafts. The cultured skin is returned to the burn center, where it is placed on the patient's excised burn wounds (Fig. 24-13, *A*). CEA grafts generally form a seamless, smooth replacement skin tissue (Fig. 24-13, *B*). Problems related to CEA include a poor graft take because of thin epidermal skin, graft loss during healing, infection, and contracture development.

**Artificial Skin.** Artificial skin can replace all functions of the skin and consists of both dermal and epidermal elements.[22] The Integra artificial skin dermal regeneration template is an example of a skin replacement system. As with CEA, it is indicated for use in the treatment of life-threatening, full-thickness or deep partial-thickness burn wounds when a conventional autograft is not available or advisable, as in older or high anesthetic-risk patients. It has also been successfully used in reconstructive burn surgery procedures. It must be applied within a few days postburn for greatest success.

Integra artificial skin has a bilayer membrane composed of acellular dermis and silicone. The wound is excised, the bilayer membrane is placed dermal layer down, and the wound is wrapped with dressings in the OR. The dermal layer functions as a biodegradable template that induces organized regeneration of new dermis by the body. The silicone layer remains intact for 3 weeks as the dermal layer degrades and epidermal autografts become available. At this point, the silicone is removed during a second surgical procedure and replaced by the patient's own epidermal autografts. Some burn centers use CEA as the source of the epidermis.

Another dermal replacement is AlloDerm, a cryopreserved allogenic dermis. Human allograft dermis, harvested from cadavers, is decellularized to make it immunogenic and then freeze-dried. Once thawed, AlloDerm is rehydrated with ultra-thin epidermal autografts immediately before placement on a freshly excised wound.

## Pain Management

Many aspects of burn care cause pain. However, patients will experience acceptable levels of relative comfort if they receive adequate analgesia. To provide effective pain management, you must understand both the physiologic and psychologic aspects of pain. (Pain management is discussed in Chapter 8.)

Burn patients experience two kinds of pain: (1) *continuous, background pain* that might be present throughout the day and night; and (2) *treatment-induced pain* associated with dressing changes, ambulation, and rehabilitation activities. The first line of pain treatment is drugs (Table 24-13). With background pain, a continuous IV infusion of an opioid (e.g., hydromorphone [Dilaudid]) provides a steady, therapeutic level of the drug. If an IV infusion is not ordered, slow-release, twice-a-day opioids (e.g., morphine [MS Contin]) are used.

Breakthrough doses of analgesia must be available regardless of the regimen selected. Anxiolytics, which can enhance analgesics, are also indicated and include lorazepam (Ativan) and midazolam. Adjuvant analgesics, such as gabapentin (Neurontin) and pregabalin (Lyrica), also enhance opioids. The use of these drugs can help reduce the opioid dosage and undesirable side effects.

For treatment-induced pain, premedicate with an analgesic and possibly an anxiolytic via the IV or oral route. For patients with an IV, a short-acting analgesic is often used.

Elimination of all pain is difficult, and most patients will accept a "tolerable" level of discomfort. Some pain can be managed using

### CHECK YOUR PRACTICE

Your patient with a burn injury is ordered fentanyl (Sublimaze) before a dressing change. The patient has multiple IV lines and you are not sure which line to use to insert the drug. You know that mixing up IV lines can lead to serious drug errors.

- How would you determine which IV line to use to give the drug?

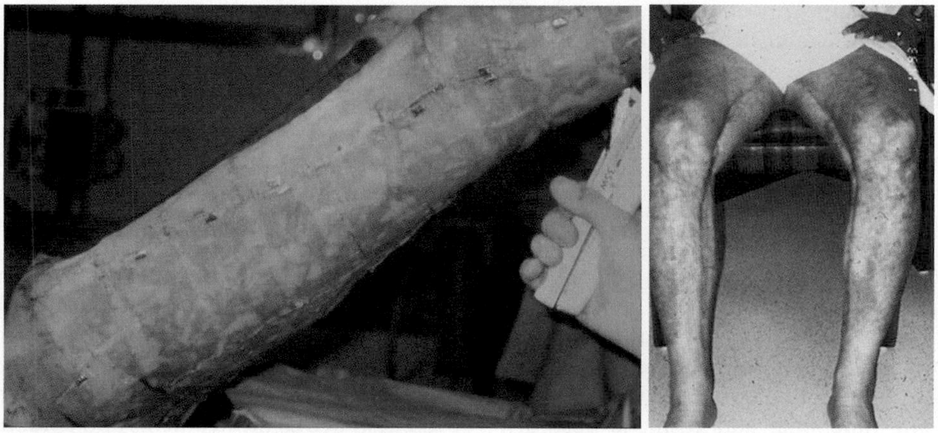

A B

**FIG. 24-13** Patient with cultured epithelial autograft (CEA). **A,** Intraoperative application of CEA. **B,** Appearance of healed CEA.

nondrug strategies. Relaxation breathing, guided imagery, hypnosis, biofeedback, computerized gaming, and music therapy can also help patients cope with pain[23] (see Chapters 6 and 8).

Remember, the more control the patient has in managing pain, the more successful the chosen strategies will be. Active participation in asking for time-outs and scheduling treatments and rest periods can help the patient manage feelings of anticipatory pain. Patient-controlled analgesia (PCA) is used in some burn centers, with varying degrees of success. (PCA is discussed in Chapter 8.)

### ◆ Physical and Occupational Therapy

Continuous physical therapy throughout burn recovery is imperative if the patient is to regain and maintain muscle strength and optimal joint function. A good time for exercise is during and after wound cleansing, when the skin is softer and bulky dressings are removed. Passive and active ROM should be performed on all joints. Ensure that the patient with neck burns continues to sleep without pillows or with the head hanging slightly over the top of the mattress to encourage hyperextension.

Maintain the occupational therapy schedule for wearing custom-fitted splints, which are designed to keep joints in functional position. Check the splints often to ensure an optimal fit, with no undue pressure that may lead to skin breakdown or nerve damage.

### ◆ Nutritional Therapy

The goal of nutritional therapy during the acute burn phase is to provide adequate calories and protein to promote healing. When the wounds are still open, the burn patient is in a hypermetabolic and highly catabolic state.

The patient may benefit from an antioxidant protocol, which includes selenium, vitamin E, acetylcysteine, ascorbic acid, zinc, and a multivitamin. Meeting daily caloric requirements is crucial and should start within the first 1 to 2 days postburn. The daily estimated caloric needs must be regularly calculated by a dietitian and readjusted as the patient's condition changes (e.g., wound healing improves, sepsis develops). Monitor laboratory values (e.g., albumin, prealbumin, total protein, transferrin) on a regular basis.

If the patient is mechanically ventilated or unable to eat enough calories by mouth, a small-bore feeding tube is placed and enteral feedings are started. When the patient is extubated, contact the speech pathologist for a swallowing assessment before an oral diet is started. Encourage the patient to eat high-protein, high-carbohydrate foods to meet caloric goals. Ask caregivers to bring in favorite foods from home. Appetite is usually reduced, and you will need to reinforce whatever steps are taken to achieve adequate intake. Ideally, weight loss should not be more than 10% of preburn weight. Record the patient's daily caloric intake using calorie count sheets, which are reviewed by the dietitian. Weigh your patient weekly to evaluate progress.

## REHABILITATION PHASE

The formal *rehabilitation phase* begins when the patient's wounds have healed and he or she is engaging in some level of self-care. This may happen as early as 2 weeks or as long as 7 to 8 months after a major burn injury. Goals for the patient now are to (1) work toward resuming a functional role in society and (2) rehabilitate from any functional and cosmetic postburn reconstructive surgery that may be necessary.[24]

### Pathophysiologic Changes and Clinical Manifestations

Burn wounds heal either by spontaneous re-epithelialization or by skin grafting. Layers of keratinocytes begin rebuilding the tissue structure destroyed by the burn injury. Collagen fibers, present in the new scar tissue, assist with healing and add strength to weakened areas. The new skin appears flat and pink. In about 4 to 6 weeks, the area becomes raised and hyperemic. If adequate ROM is not started, the new tissue will shorten, causing a **contracture**. Mature healing is reached in about 12 months when suppleness has returned, and the pink or red color has faded to a slightly lighter hue than the surrounding unburned tissue.

Tell patients who have more heavily pigmented skin that it will take longer for it to regain its color because many of the melanocytes have been destroyed. Frequently, the skin does not regain its original color. Provide teaching and emotional support to assist the patient with grieving about these changes to his or her body. Cosmetic camouflage, the implantation of pigment within the skin, can help even out unequal skin tones and improve the patient's overall appearance and self-image.

Scarring has two characteristics: discoloration and contour. The discoloration of scars fades somewhat with time. However, scar tissue tends to develop altered contours; that is, it is no longer flat or slightly raised but becomes elevated and enlarged above the original burned area. Some burn care providers believe that pressure can eventually help keep a scar flat. Gentle pressure is maintained on the healed burn with custom-fitted pressure garments and clear, thermoplastic face masks. Pressure garments and masks should never be worn over unhealed wounds. Once a wearing schedule has been set, they are removed only for short periods while bathing. Pressure garments are worn up to 24 hours a day for as long as 12 to 18 months.

The patient typically reports discomfort from itching where healing is occurring. Teach your patient about the application of water-based moisturizers and selective, short-term use of oral antihistamines (e.g., hydroxyzine [Atarax]) to help reduce the itching. Massage oil, silicone gel sheeting (e.g., Biodermis), gabapentin, and injectable corticosteroids also may help.[25]

As "old" epithelium is replaced by new cells, flaking occurs. The newly formed skin is extremely sensitive to trauma. Blisters and skin tears are likely to develop from slight pressure or friction. Additionally, these newly healed areas can be hypersensitive or hyposensitive to cold, heat, and touch. Grafted areas are more likely to be hyposensitive until peripheral nerve regeneration occurs. Teach your patients to protect healed burn areas from direct sunlight for about 3 months to prevent hyperpigmentation and sunburn injury. Tell them to always wear sunscreen when outside.

### Complications

The most common complications during the rehabilitation phase are skin and joint contractures and hypertrophic scarring.[26] A *joint contracture* (an abnormal condition of a joint characterized by flexion and fixation) develops as a result of the shortening of scar tissue in the flexor tissues of a joint. Areas that are most susceptible to skin and joint contractures include the anterior and lateral neck areas, axillae, antecubital fossae, fingers, groin areas, popliteal fossae, knees, and ankles (Fig. 24-14). Some areas encompass major joints. Not only does the skin over these areas develop contractures, but the underlying tissues, such as the ligaments and tendons, also have a tendency to shorten during the healing process.

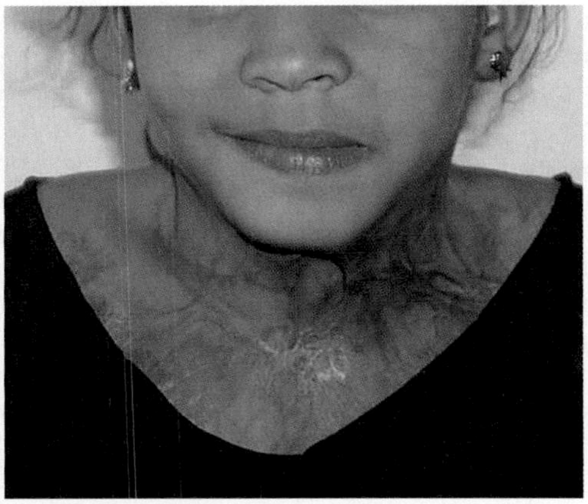

**FIG. 24-14** Neck contracture. (Courtesy Linda Bucher, RN, PhD, CEN, CNE, Staff Nurse, Virtua Memorial Hospital, Mt. Holly, N.J.)

Carefully watch the patient for these potential problems. Encourage proper positioning, splinting, and exercise to minimize this complication. Tell the patient to continue with these strategies until the skin matures at around 1 year posthealing. Rehabilitative therapy is aimed at the extension of body parts because the flexors are stronger than the extensors. Burned legs may first be wrapped with elastic (e.g., tensor, Ace) bandages to assist with circulation to leg-graft and donor sites before ambulation. Burned arms can be wrapped with a layer of tubular elastic gauze (e.g., Tubigrip). This interim pressure prevents blister formation, promotes venous return, and decreases pain and itchiness. Once the skin is completely healed and less fragile, custom-fitted pressure garments replace the elastic bandages and tubular gauze.

## NURSING AND INTERPROFESSIONAL MANAGEMENT: REHABILITATION PHASE

During the rehabilitation phase, encourage both the patient and caregiver to participate in care. Since the patient may go home with unhealed wounds, teach your patient and caregiver the skills for wound care. Before discharge, have the patient or caregiver return demonstrate (show-back) the proper dressing change. In addition, make sure the patient or caregiver knows when to contact the burn team (e.g., signs of infection, increased pain) and the need to keep outpatient visits to ensure good wound healing.

If needed, arrange home care nursing to assist with care. The newly discharged patient will need to know how to gently remove the dressings in the shower, once daily, if a nonadherent, greasy gauze dressing is used or twice daily, if a topical, antimicrobial cream is ordered. Teach that showering, not bathing, with mild soap and warm water keeps the wounds clean.

Give advice on scar management, moisturizing, and sun protection. Suggest using water-based creams that penetrate into the dermis (e.g., Vaseline Intensive Rescue) on healed areas to keep the skin supple and moisturized. This will decrease itching and flaking. Occasionally antihistamines are used at bedtime if itching persists.

Base ongoing pain management and nutritional needs on individual patient status. Continue to encourage the patient to perform the physical and occupational therapy routines. Suggest computerized gaming devices for breaks from the exercise routines.[27] Encourage and reassure the patient to maintain morale, particularly once the patient realizes that recovery can be slow. Rehabilitation may have to be a primary focus for at least the next 6 to 12 months.

Postburn reconstructive surgery is frequently required after a major burn. The need for further surgery is reviewed at the outpatient burn clinic appointments after discharge.

### Gerontologic Considerations: Burns

The older patient presents many challenges for the burn team. The normal aging process puts the patient at risk for injury because of unsteady gait, limited eyesight, and diminished hearing. As people age, skin becomes drier and more wrinkled. Older adults have thinning of the dermal layer, a loss of elastic fibers, a reduction in subcutaneous adipose tissue, and a decrease in vascularity. As a result, the thinner dermis, with reduced blood flow, sustains deeper burns with poorer rates of healing.

Once injured, the older adult has more complications in the emergent and acute phases of burn resuscitation because of preexisting co-morbidities. For example, older patients with diabetes, heart failure, or COPD have morbidity and mortality rates exceeding those of healthy, younger patients. In older patients, pneumonia is a frequent complication, burn wounds and donor sites take longer to heal, and surgical procedures are not well tolerated. Weaning from a ventilator can be a challenge. Although usually self-limiting, delirium, if it develops, may be distressing. It usually takes longer for these patients to rehabilitate to the point where they can safely return home. For some, a return home to independent living may not be possible. As the population ages, developing strategies to prevent burn injuries in older adults is a priority.

## EMOTIONAL/PSYCHOLOGIC NEEDS OF PATIENTS AND CAREGIVERS

Patients and caregivers have many emotional/psychologic needs during the often lengthy, unpredictable, and complex course of care.[28] You have an important supportive and counseling role as patients struggle to get their lives back on track.

To manage the enormous range of emotional responses that the burn patient may exhibit, assess the circumstances of the burn (e.g., cause, people involved), family relationships, and previous coping experiences with stressful stimuli. At any time the patient may experience a variety of emotions such as fear, anxiety, anger, guilt, and depression (Table 24-14).

Burn survivors frequently experience thoughts and feelings that are frightening and disturbing, such as guilt about the burn incident, reliving the burn experience, fear of dying, concern about future therapy and surgery, frustrations with ongoing discomfort and treatment, and hopelessness about the future. During recovery, as more independence is expected from the patient, new fears may occur: "Can I really do this?" "Am I a desirable person?" "How can I go outside looking like this?" These challenges confront patients throughout their recovery and often for years to come.

A person's self-esteem may be adversely affected by a burn injury. Some individuals may fear the loss of relationships because of perceived or actual physical disfigurement. In a society that values physical beauty, alterations in body image can result in psychologic distress.

Open and frequent communication among the patient, caregivers, close friends, and burn team members is essential. Because of the tremendous psychologic impact of a burn injury, be particularly sensitive to the patient's emotions and concerns. Encourage the patient to discuss fears regarding loss of life as

**TABLE 24-14 Emotional Responses of Burn Patients***

| Emotion | Possible Verbal Expression |
|---|---|
| **Fear** | • Will I die?<br>• What will happen next?<br>• Will I be disfigured?<br>• Will my family and friends still love me? |
| **Anxiety** | • I feel out of control.<br>• What's going to happen to me?<br>• When will I look normal again? |
| **Anger** | • Why did this happen to me?<br>• The nurses enjoy hurting me.<br>• I hope the person who did this to me dies. |
| **Guilt** | • If only I'd been more careful<br>• I'm being punished because I did something wrong. |
| **Hopefulness** | • What do I need to do to survive this injury emotionally and return to my life/family/friends?<br>• What am I meant to learn from this injury? |
| **Depression** | • It's no use going on like this.<br>• I don't care what happens to me.<br>• I wish people would leave me alone. |

*List is not all-inclusive.

he or she once knew it, loss of function, temporary or permanent deformity and disfigurement, return to work and home life, and financial burdens resulting from a long and costly hospitalization and rehabilitation.[29]

Encourage appropriate independence and an eventual return to preburn activities, such as school or work. Peer counseling and informal interactions with other burn survivors may bring comfort and help to restore confidence.[30] Reassure patients that their feelings, during this period of adjustment, are a normal reaction to an extraordinary life event. Their frustration and impatience are to be expected as they work to establish a new life. Assist patients in adapting to a realistic, yet positive appraisal of their particular situation, emphasizing what they *can* do instead of what they *cannot* do.

Caregivers may share some or all of these challenges and feelings. At times, they may feel helpless or too exhausted to assist their loved one. Continued support from trusted and familiar burn team members is essential. Helping caregivers assist with aspects of the patient's care helps them to reconnect with their loved one and eases the transition home. Many burn survivors and their caregivers remark on the powerful learning experience of the burn and a renewed appreciation of life, despite the ongoing challenges of a prolonged recovery. You must acknowledge that their feelings are real and common. Most burn survivors speak of a real satisfaction with their postburn life and are more empowered as time goes on.

It is important to address individual spiritual and cultural needs because both have a role in treatment decisions and recovery. Pastoral care may be a helpful resource for the patient and caregiver. The need for support, information, and family involvement may vary among cultures. Identify what is important to your patient and caregiver, and communicate that information in the patient's plan of care. Encourage the burn care team to remain culturally aware of and sensitive to the individual patient's and caregiver's cultural needs.

The difficult issue of sexuality must be met with honesty.[31] Physical appearance is altered in the patient who has sustained a major burn. Acceptance of any changes is difficult at first for the patient and significant other. The nature of skin injury in itself can cause modifications in processing sexual stimuli. Touch is an important part of sexuality, and immature scar tissue may make the sensation of touch unpleasant or may dull it. This may only be transient, but the patient and partner need to know that it is normal and receive anticipatory guidance from the burn team to avoid undue emotional strain.

A significant number of burn survivors have preexisting mental health or substance abuse issues, any of which may have contributed to the burn incident. The stress of the burn injury can precipitate a psychologic crisis. Assessment by a psychiatrist who can prescribe appropriate drugs, if needed, and begin counseling is often helpful. Early psychiatric intervention is essential if the patient has been previously treated for a psychiatric illness or if the injury was a suicide attempt. The diagnosis of posttraumatic stress disorder is made in a number of burn patients. However, it has been noted that distress and trauma symptoms can act as a catalyst for positive posttraumatic growth. Coping styles and social support appear to assist in these positive changes postburn.[32]

Psychologic care typically begins in the hospital, but links to community resources must be made before discharge to ensure continuity of treatment. A referral to a psychiatrist, psychologist, psychiatric advanced practice nurse (APN), mental health counselor, or social worker should be discussed if concerns are raised at burn clinic follow-up.

Caregiver and patient support groups may be beneficial in meeting the patient's and caregiver's emotional needs at any phase of the recovery process. Speaking with others who have experienced burn trauma can be beneficial, both in terms of confirming that the patient's feelings are normal and in sharing helpful advice. The Phoenix Society *(www.phoenix-society.org)* is an international, highly respected burn survivors' support group. For many years the society has offered valuable support and resources (e.g., annual World Burn Congress conference) to burn survivors, caregivers, and burn team staff.

## SPECIAL NEEDS OF NURSES

Warm, trusting, and mutually satisfying relationships frequently develop between burn patients and nursing staff, not only during hospitalization but also during the long-term rehabilitation period. Sometimes the bond can be so strong that the patient has difficulty separating from the hospital and staff. The frequency and intensity of family contact can be rewarding as well as draining to you. You may find it difficult to cope with the deformities caused by the burn injury, odors, unpleasant sight of the wound, and reality of the pain that accompanies the burn and its treatment. Do not hesitate to seek help from co-workers, a manager, or the employee assistance program should you feel the need.

In time, you will come to know that the specialized burn care you provide makes a critical difference in helping patients not only survive but also cope with and triumph over an intense and complex injury.

Ongoing support services or critical incident stress debriefings led by a psychiatrist, psychologist, psychiatric APN, or social worker may also be helpful. Peer support groups (e.g., ABA, International Society for Burn Injuries) can serve a similar purpose by helping you cope with difficult feelings experienced when caring for burn patients. Because burn nursing is physically, psychologically, and intellectually demanding, it has many challenges and inherent rewards.[33] Attention to your own self-care is important to maintain a positive attitude and healthy work-life balance. Time with family and friends and rest and relaxation at home are essential parts of self-care and a balanced life with purpose and meaning.

## CASE STUDY

### Burn Injury

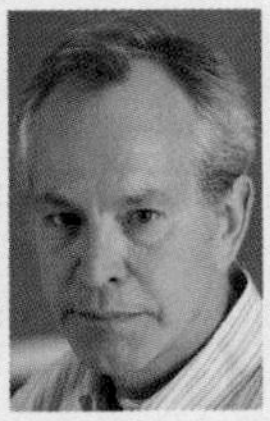

(©Comstock/ Thinkstock)

**Patient Profile**

G.M., a 52-year-old married white man, arrives at the emergency department with burns to his face, neck, chest, right arm and hand, and right foot. He was burning brush on his farm when the fire went out of control. He has an 18-gauge IV with NSS running at 100 mL/hr, and he is receiving 100% humidified $O_2$ by mask.

**Subjective Data**

- Complains of blurry vision and trouble swallowing
- States his burns are painful and that he is scared
- States he is a "diabetic" and has "high blood pressure"

**Objective Data**

***Physical Examination***

- Is awake, alert, and oriented, but in some distress
- Eyes are red, irritated
- Voice is hoarse; nasal hair is singed
- Face is reddened with blisters noted on the nose and forehead
- Right arm, right hand, anterior chest, neck, and right foot have shiny, bright red, wet wounds
- Is shivering

**Discussion Questions**

1. ***Priority Decision:*** What are the priorities of care in the prehospital setting and emergency department? How should his airway, breathing, and circulation be managed?
2. ***Priority Decision:*** What factors place G.M. at high risk for an inhalation injury? What priority interventions can be anticipated?
3. ***Patient-Centered Care:*** What pain medications might be considered to relieve his pain?
4. Which of the criteria for burn center referral does G.M. meet for admission to the hospital burn unit?
5. What metabolic disturbances would be expected soon after G.M.'s admission? Explain the physiologic basis for these changes.
6. How might G.M.'s co-morbidities affect his burn care and rehabilitation?
7. ***Patient-Centered Care:*** What measures should be taken to support G.M.'s caregivers?
8. ***Priority Decision:*** Based on the assessment data presented, what are the priority nursing diagnoses? Identify any collaborative problems.
9. ***Evidence-Based Practice:*** What are the most effective wound care strategies to manage G.M.'s burn wounds?
10. ***Patient-Centered Care:*** Prior to discharge what teaching should be provided to G.M. and his family so they can successfully manage his care at home?
11. ***Safety:*** To ensure G.M.'s safety at home, what interventions are necessary prior to discharge?
12. ***Quality Improvement:*** What outcomes will indicate that interprofessional care was effective?

Answers available at *http://evolve.elsevier.com/Lewis/medsurg.*

## BRIDGE TO NCLEX EXAMINATION

The number of the question corresponds to the same-numbered outcome at the beginning of the chapter.

1. Knowing the most common causes of household fires, which prevention strategy would the nurse focus on when teaching about fire safety?
   - **a.** Set hot water temperature at 140° F.
   - **b.** Use only hardwired smoke detectors.
   - **c.** Encourage regular home fire exit drills.
   - **d.** Never permit older adults to cook unattended.
2. The injury that is *least* likely to result in a full-thickness burn is
   - **a.** sunburn.
   - **b.** scald injury.
   - **c.** chemical burn.
   - **d.** electrical injury.
3. When assessing a patient with a partial-thickness burn, the nurse would expect to find *(select all that apply)*
   - **a.** blisters.
   - **b.** exposed fascia.
   - **c.** exposed muscles.
   - **d.** intact nerve endings.
   - **e.** red, shiny, wet appearance.
4. A patient is admitted to the burn center with burns to his head, neck, and anterior and posterior chest after an explosion in his garage. On assessment, the nurse auscultates wheezes throughout the lung fields. On reassessment, the wheezes are gone and the breath sounds are greatly diminished. Which action is the *most* appropriate for the nurse to take *next*?
   - **a.** Encourage the patient to cough and auscultate the lungs again.
   - **b.** Obtain vital signs, oxygen saturation, and a STAT arterial blood gas.
   - **c.** Document the findings and continue to monitor the patient's breathing.
   - **d.** Anticipate the need for endotracheal intubation and notify the physician.
5. Fluid and electrolyte shifts that occur during the early emergent phase of a burn injury include
   - **a.** adherence of albumin to vascular walls.
   - **b.** movement of potassium into the vascular space.
   - **c.** sequestering of sodium and water in interstitial fluid.
   - **d.** hemolysis of red blood cells from large volumes of rapidly administered fluid.
6. To maintain a positive nitrogen balance in a major burn, the patient must
   - **a.** eat a high-protein, high-carbohydrate diet.
   - **b.** increase normal caloric intake by about three times.
   - **c.** eat at least 1500 calories/day in small, frequent meals.
   - **d.** eat a gluten-free diet for the chemical effect on nitrogen balance.
7. A patient has 25% TBSA burn from a car fire. His wounds have been debrided and covered with a silver-impregnated dressing. The nurse's *priority* intervention for wound care would be to
   - **a.** reapply a new dressing without disturbing the wound bed.
   - **b.** observe the wound for signs of infection during dressing changes.
   - **c.** apply cool compresses for pain relief in between dressing changes.
   - **d.** wash the wound aggressively with soap and water three times a day.

**8.** Pain management for the burn patient is *most* effective when *(select all that apply)*
  **a.** a pain rating tool is used to monitor the patient's level of pain.
  **b.** painful dressing changes are delayed until the patient's pain is completely relieved.
  **c.** the patient is informed about and has some control over the management of the pain.
  **d.** a multimodal approach is used (e.g., sustained-release and short-acting opioids, NSAIDs, adjuvant analgesics).
  **e.** nonpharmacologic therapies (e.g., music therapy, distraction) replace opioids in the rehabilitation phase of a burn injury.

**9.** A therapeutic measure used to prevent hypertrophic scarring during the rehabilitation phase of burn recovery is
  **a.** applying pressure garments.
  **b.** repositioning the patient every 2 hours.
  **c.** performing active ROM at least every 4 hours.
  **d.** massaging the new tissue with water-based moisturizers.

**10.** A patient is recovering from second- and third-degree burns over 30% of his body and the burn care team is planning for discharge. The *first* action the nurse should take when meeting with the patient would be to
  **a.** arrange a return-to-clinic appointment and prescription for pain medications.
  **b.** teach the patient and the caregiver proper wound care to be performed at home.
  **c.** review the patient's current health care status and readiness for discharge to home.
  **d.** give the patient written information and websites for information for burn survivors.

1. c, 2. a, 3. a, d, e, 4. d, 5. c, 6. a, 7. b, 8. a, c, d, 9. a, 10. c

For rationales to these answers and even more NCLEX review questions, visit *http://evolve.elsevier.com/Lewis/medsurg.*

## EVOLVE WEBSITE

http://evolve.elsevier.com/Lewis/medsurg

**Review Questions (Online Only)**

**Key Points**

**Answer Keys for Questions**
- Rationales for Bridge to NCLEX Examination Questions
- Answer Guidelines for Case Study on p. 449
- Answer Guidelines for Managing Care of Multiple Patients Case Study (Section 4) on p. 451

**Student Case Study**
- Patient With Burns

**Nursing Care Plan**
- eNursing Care Plan 24-1: Patient With a Thermal Burn Injury

**Conceptual Care Map Creator**

**Audio Glossary**

**Content Updates**

## REFERENCES


1. American Burn Association: Burn incidence and treatment in the US: 2013 fact sheet. Retrieved from *www.ameriburn.org/resources?factsheet.php.*
2. WHO International: Burns fact sheet number 365, updated April 2014. Retrieved from *www.Who.int/mediacentrefactsheets/fs365/en.*
3. Peck M: Epidemiology and prevention of burns throughout the world. In Jeschke MG, Kamolz L-P, Sjoberg F, et al, editors: *Handbook of burns: acute burn care,* vol 1, Wein, Austria, 2012, Springer-Verlag.
4. Summers A: Treating cement burns in the emergency department, *Emerg Nurse* 20:30, 2013.
5. Jeschke MG: Critical care of burn victims including inhalation injury. In Jeschke MG, Kamolz L-P, Shahrokhi S, editors: *Burn care and treatment: a practical guide,* Wein, Austria, 2013, Springer-Verlag.

*6. Saracogli A, Kuzucuoglu T, Yakupoglu S, et al: Prognostic factors in electrical burns: a review of 101 patients, *Burns* 40:702, 2014.

7. Burn injury. Retrieved from *www.burninjury.org.*
8. Payne S, Cole E: Treatment of acute burn blisters in unscheduled care settings, *Emerg Nurse* 20:32, 2012.

*9. Morris R, Javed M, Bodger O, et al: A comparison of two smartphone applications and the validation of smartphone applications as tools for fluid calculation for burns resuscitation, *Burns* 40:826, 2014.

10. Somerset A, Coffee R, Jones L, et al: The impact of prediabetes on glycemic control and clinical outcomes post-burn injury, *J Burn Care Res* 35:5, 2014.
11. Rice PL, Orgill DP: Emergency care of moderate and severe thermal burns in adults, 2014. Retrieved from *www.uptodate.com.*
12. Faraklas I, Ghanem M, Brown A, et al: Evaluation of an enoxaparin dosing calculator using burn size and weight, *J Burn Care Res* 34:621, 2013.
13. Culleiton AL, Simko LM: Caring for patients with burn injuries, *Nursing* 43:27, 2013.

*14. Hampson NB, Piantadosi CA, Thom SR, et al: Practice recommendations in the diagnosis, management, and prevention of carbon monoxide poisoning, *Am J Resp Crit Care Med* 186:1095, 2012.

15. Fahlstrom K, Boyle C, Makic MBF: Implementation of a nurse-driven burn resuscitation protocol: a quality improvement project, *Crit Care Nurse* 33:25, 2013.
16. Shahrokhi S: Infections in burns. In Jeschke MG, Kamolz L-P, Shahrokhi S, editors: *Burn care and treatment: a practical guide,* Germany, 2014, Springer Wien.

*17. Scheckter CC, VanVliet MM, Krishnan NM, et al: Cost effectiveness comparison between topical silver sulfadiazine and enclosed silver dressings for partial-thickness burn treatment, *J Burn Care Res* 35:284, 2014.

18. Jeschke MG: Nutrition of the burn patient and treatment of the hypermetabolic response. In Jeschke MG, Kamolz L-P, Shahrokhi S, editors: *Burn care and treatment: a practical guide,* Germany, 2014, Springer Wien.

*19. Nordlund MJ, Pham TN, Gibran NS: Micronutrients after burn injury: a review, *J Burn Care Res* 35:121, 2014.

20. Kamolz L-P: Acute burn surgery. In Jeschke MG, Kamolz L-P, Shahrokhi S, editors: *Burn care and treatment: a practical guide,* Germany, 2014, Springer Wien.

*21. Waltzman JT, Bell DE: Vacuum-assisted closure device as a split-thickness skin graft bolster in the burn population, *J Burn Care Res* 35:e338, 2014.

22. Jeschke MG, Finerty CC, Shahrokhi S, et al: Wound coverage technologies in burn care: novel technologies, *J Burn Care Res* 34:612, 2013.

*23. Jeffs D, Dorman D, Brown S, et al: Effect of virtual reality on adolescent pain during burn wound care, *J Burn Care Res* 35:39, 2014.

*24. Stergiou-Kita M, Grigorovich A, Gomez M: Development of an interprofessional clinical practice guideline for vocational evaluation following severe burn, *Burns* 40:1149, 2014.

*25. Carrougher GJ, Martinez EM, McMullen KS, et al: Pruritus in adult burn survivors: post-burn prevalence and risk factors associated with increased intensity, *J Burn Care Res* 34:94, 2013.

*26. Godleski M, Oeffling A, Bruflat AK, et al: Treating burn-associated joint contracture: results of an inpatient rehabilitation stretching protocol, *J Burn Care Res* 34:420, 2013.

27. Perry IS, Carbullido C, Kowada J, et al: Keeping up with video game technology: objective analysis of XBox Kinect™ and PlayStation 3 Move™ for use in burn rehabilitation, *Burns* 40:852, 2014.
28. Kornhaber R, Wilson A, Abu-Kumar MZ, et al: Coming to terms with it all: adult burn survivors' "lived experience" of acknowledgement and acceptance, *Burns* 40:589, 2014.

*29. Stavrou D, Weissman O, Tessone A, et al: Health-related quality of life in burn patients: a review of the literature, *Burns* 40:788, 2014.

*30. Tolley JS, Foroushani PS: What do we know about one-to-one peer support for adults with a burn injury? A scoping review, *J Burn Care Res* 35:233, 2014.
*31. Goncalves N, Melo A, Caltran MP, et al: Sexuality in burn victims: an integrative literature review, *Burns* 40:552, 2014.
32. Baillie SE, Sellwood W, Wisely JA: Post-traumatic growth in adults following a burn, *Burns* 40:1089, 2014.
*33. Leggatt JM, Wassa K, Sinacore JM, et al: A pilot study examining moral distress in nurses working in one United States burn center, *J Burn Care Res* 34:521, 2013.

*Evidence-based information for clinical practice.

## CASE STUDY

### *Managing Care of Multiple Patients*

#### Introduction

You are working the day shift on a medical-surgical unit and have been assigned to care for the following five patients. You have one UAP who is assigned to work with you. There are 15 other patients on the unit being cared for by an additional 3 RNs and 3 UAP.

#### Patients

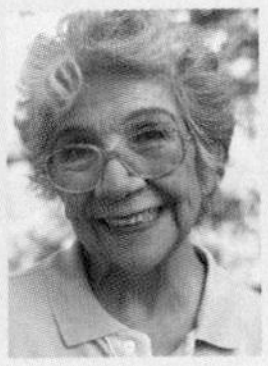

(©Jack Hollingsworth/ Photodisc/ Thinkstock)

F.M., an 81-yr-old Hispanic woman, had pneumatic retinopexy surgery yesterday to repair a partial detached retina. She has a history of type 2 diabetes, hypothyroidism, and hypertension. She is scheduled to be discharged today, but the night nurse is concerned because her BP is elevated at 150/94 mm Hg.

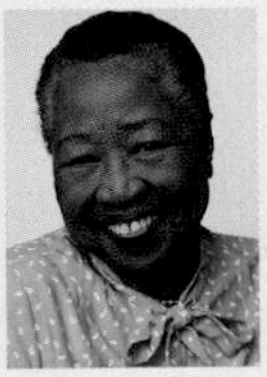

(©Kevin Peterson/ Stockbyte/ Thinkstock)

J.K., a 68-yr-old African American woman with osteoarthritis and type 2 diabetes mellitus for the past 15 years, now has diabetic retinopathy. She had argon laser therapy to her right eye yesterday to seal leaking microaneurysms from macular edema. She was admitted with uncontrolled postoperative hyperglycemia.

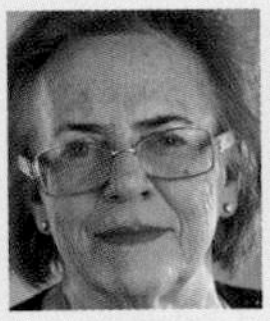

(©Stockphoto/ Thinkstock)

D.A., a 74-yr-old woman, is admitted to the hospital with complaints of chest tightness and shortness of breath. Her past medical history is negative except for a recent diagnosis of basal cell carcinoma (BCC) on her face. She was scheduled to have the BCC surgically removed tomorrow. The health care provider suspects D.A.'s symptoms are caused by anxiety but first needs to rule out any coronary artery disease before surgery.

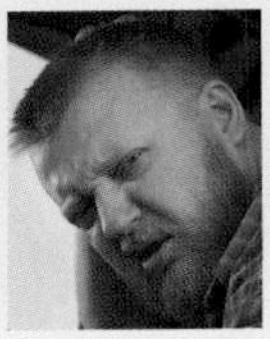

(©Dimedrol68/ iStock/ Thinkstock)

G.L., a 51-yr-old white man, just arrived for admission. He is scheduled for surgical removal of malignant melanoma lesions on his face at 1200. He is worried that the surgery will be disfiguring.

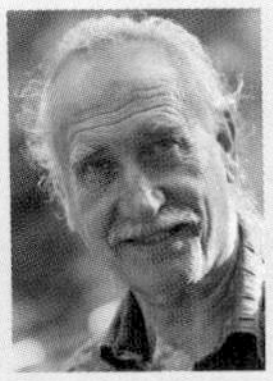

(©Stockphoto/ Thinkstock)

D.B., a 74-yr-old white man, was admitted 3 hours ago from the ED with partial thickness burns on his chest and arms (estimated to be 6% TBSA). He was burning leaves and branches using gasoline. The pile exploded and his clothes caught fire.

#### Discussion Questions

1. ***Priority Decision:*** After receiving report, which patient should you see first? Provide rationale.
2. ***Teamwork and Collaboration:*** Which tasks could you delegate to the UAP *(select all that apply)*?
   a. Obtain vital signs on F.M.
   b. Take a blood pressure reading on D.B.
   c. Perform an admission assessment on G.L.
   d. Explain planned diagnostic testing to D.A.
   e. Obtain a capillary blood glucose reading on J.K.
3. ***Priority Decision and Teamwork and Collaboration:*** When you enter D.B.'s room, he tells you he is not feeling well. He says he has a headache and his legs are "cramping up." He is also somewhat confused as he is unaware that he is in the hospital. What initial action would be *most* appropriate?
   a. Administer acetaminophen for headache relief.
   b. Have the UAP obtain a stat capillary blood glucose reading.
   c. Notify D.B.'s health care provider of his altered level of consciousness.
   d. Ask the UAP to obtain vital signs on D.B. while you look at his most recent lab work.

#### Case Study Progression

D.B.'s vital signs are BP 154/88 mm Hg, heart rate is 112 bpm, respirations are 18 breaths/min, and temperature is 98°F (36.8°C). His most recent lab work reveals a serum sodium level of 128 mEq/L (128 mmol/L). You notify his health care provider, who orders a normal saline IV to infuse at 100 mL/hr.

4. D.B. complains of thirst and asks for something to drink. Which fluid would be appropriate to give him *(select all that apply)*?
   a. Gatorade
   b. Tap water
   c. Cola soda
   d. Apple juice
   e. Orange juice
5. In addition to teaching F.M. how to administer postoperative eye drops, you will also explain
   a. position and activity restrictions.
   b. how to change the dressing on her eye.
   c. the necessity for restricting fluid intake.
   d. that protective eyewear will no longer be required.
6. When giving report to your UAP regarding your assigned patients, you are asked by the UAP if there is a significant difference between D.A. and G.L.'s skin cancers. You reply based on knowledge that
   a. basal cell carcinoma is the most deadly form of skin cancer.
   b. malignant melanoma typically appears as red, rough patches on the skin.
   c. basal cell carcinoma typically presents during the second and third decades of life.
   d. melanoma has the ability to metastasize to any organ, including the brain and heart.
7. ***Management Decision:*** Another RN offers to help you by providing care for F.M. Which observed action by the RN would require your immediate intervention?
   a. The RN assists F.M. to lie flat on her back.
   b. The RN gives F.M. oral medication for pain.
   c. The RN assures F.M. that retinal reattachment is usually successful.
   d. The RN explains to F.M. that she is at risk for detachment in the other eye.

Answers available at *http://evolve.elsevier.com/Lewis/medsurg*.
*TBSA*, Total body surface area.

# SECTION 5

# Problems of Oxygenation: Ventilation

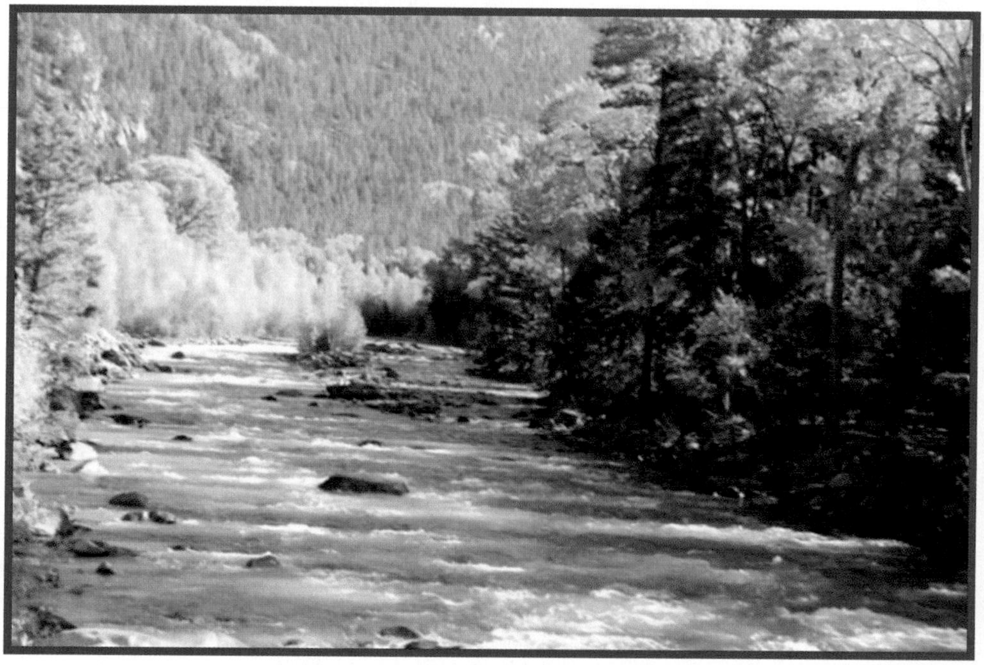

Peter Bonner

*The mark of a successful man is one that has spent an entire day on the bank of a river without feeling guilty about it.*

***Chinese Philosopher***

# 25

# Assessment of Respiratory System

*Eugene E. Mondor*

*For breath is life, and if you breathe well you will live long on earth.*

***Sanskrit Proverb***

http://evolve.elsevier.com/Lewis/medsurg/

## LEARNING OUTCOMES

1. Differentiate among the structures and functions of the upper respiratory tract, lower respiratory tract, and chest wall.
2. Describe the process that initiates and controls inspiration and expiration.
3. Describe the process of oxygenation and ventilation within the lungs.
4. Identify the respiratory defense mechanisms.
5. Describe the significance of arterial blood gas values in relation to respiratory function.
6. Relate the signs and symptoms of inadequate oxygenation to physical assessment findings.
7. Link the age-related changes of the respiratory system to the differences in assessment findings.
8. Obtain significant subjective and objective assessment data related to the respiratory system from a patient.
9. Perform a physical assessment of the respiratory system using the appropriate techniques.
10. Differentiate normal from common abnormal findings in a physical assessment of the respiratory system.
11. Describe the purpose, significance of results, and nursing responsibilities related to diagnostic studies of the respiratory system.

## KEY TERMS

adventitious breath sounds, p. 466
chemoreceptor, p. 458
compliance, p. 456
crackles, Table 25-8, p. 468
dyspnea, p. 456
elastic recoil, p. 456
fremitus, p. 464
mechanical receptors, p. 458
oxygenation, p. 456
pleural friction rub, Table 25-8, p. 468
resistance, p. 456
surfactant, p. 455
tidal volume (VT), p. 454
ventilation, p. 456
wheezes, Table 25-8, p. 468

## STRUCTURES AND FUNCTIONS OF RESPIRATORY SYSTEM

The primary purpose of the respiratory system is gas exchange. This involves the transfer of $O_2$ and $CO_2$ between the atmosphere and blood. The respiratory system is divided into two parts: upper respiratory tract and lower respiratory tract (Fig. 25-1).

### Upper Respiratory Tract

The *upper respiratory tract* includes the nose, mouth, pharynx, epiglottis, larynx, and trachea. Air enters into the respiratory tract through the nose. The nose is made of bone and cartilage and is divided into two nares by the nasal septum. The inside of the nose is shaped into three passages by projections called *turbinates.* The turbinates increase the surface area of the nasal mucosa, which warms and moistens the air as it enters the nose. The internal nose opens directly into the sinuses. The nasal cavity connects with the pharynx, a tubular passageway that is subdivided into three parts: the *nasopharynx, oropharynx,* and *laryngopharynx.*

The nose functions to protect the lower airway by warming and humidifying air and filtering small particles before air enters the lungs. Olfactory nerve endings, located in the roof of the nose, are responsible for the sense of smell.

Air moves through the oropharynx to the laryngopharynx. It then travels through the epiglottis to the larynx before moving into the trachea. The *epiglottis* is a small flap located behind the tongue that closes over the larynx during swallowing. This prevents solids and liquids from entering the lungs. The vocal cords are located in the larynx. Air passes through the glottis (the opening between the vocal cords) and into the trachea. The trachea is a cylindrical tube about 5 in (10 to 12 cm) long and 1 in (1.5 to 2.5 cm) in diameter. U-shaped cartilages keep the trachea open but allow the adjacent esophagus to expand for swallowing. The trachea bifurcates into the right and left mainstem bronchi at a point called the *carina.* The carina is located at the level of the manubriosternal junction, also called the

Reviewed by Donna C. Bond, RN, DNP, CCNS, AE-C, CTTS, Pulmonary Clinical Nurse Specialist, Carilion Clinic, Roanoke, Virginia; Deborah Cline, RN, MS, Nursing Faculty, Carrington College, Reno, Nevada; and Cynthia M. Steinwedel, RN, PhD, CNE, Assistant Professor, Department of Nursing, Bradley University, Peoria, Illinois.

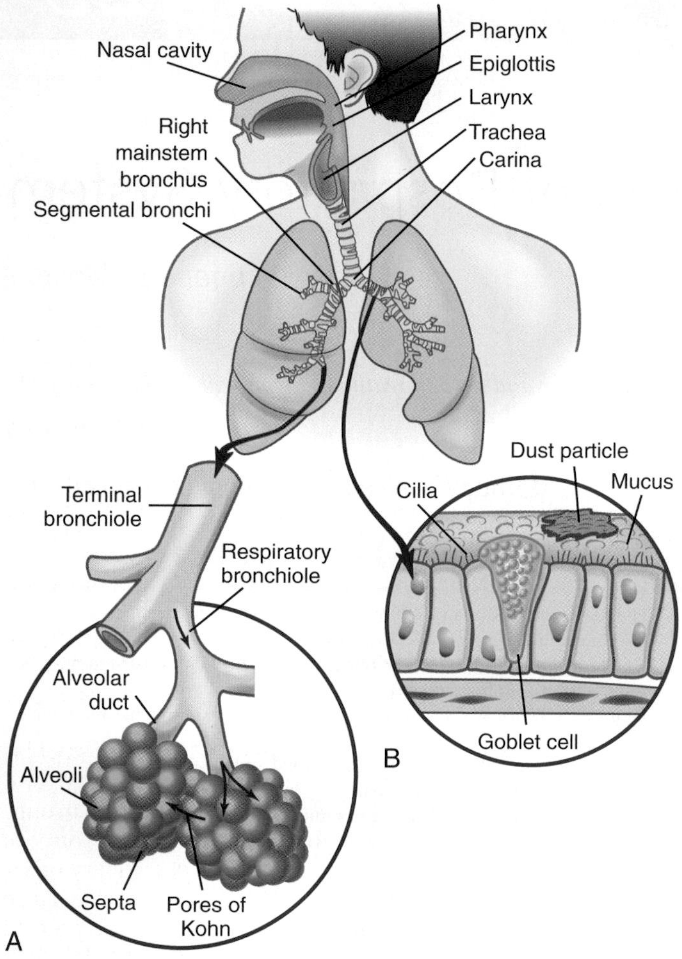


**FIG. 25-1** Structures of the respiratory tract. **A,** Pulmonary functional unit. **B,** Ciliated mucous membrane. (Redrawn from Price SA, Wilson LM: *Pathophysiology: clinical concepts of disease processes,* ed 6, St Louis, 2003, Mosby.)

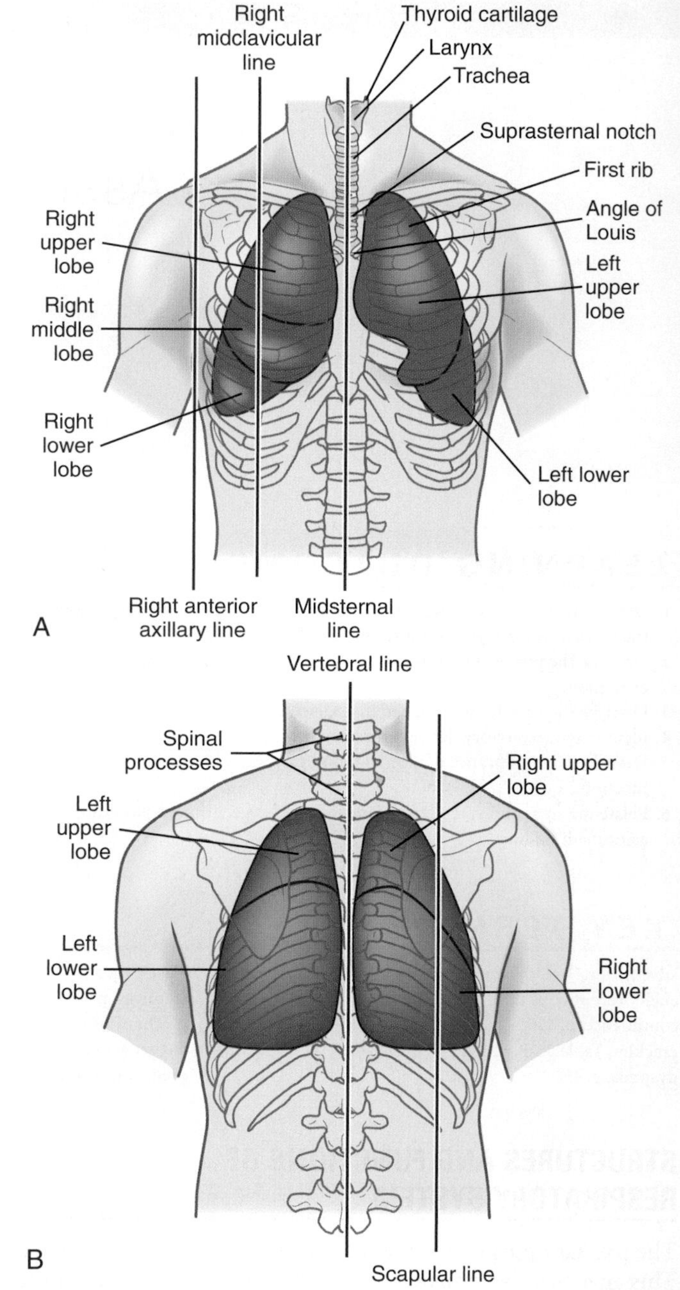


**FIG. 25-2** Landmarks and structures of the chest wall. **A,** Anterior view. **B,** Posterior view. (Redrawn from Thompson JM, McFarland GK, Hirsch JE, Tucker SM: *Mosby's clinical nursing,* ed 5, St Louis, 2002, Mosby.)

*angle of Louis.* The carina is highly sensitive, and stimulation of this area during suctioning causes vigorous coughing.[1]

## Lower Respiratory Tract

Once air passes the carina, it is in the lower respiratory tract. The *lower respiratory tract* consists of the bronchi, bronchioles, alveolar ducts, and alveoli. With the exception of the right and left mainstem bronchi, all lower airway structures are located inside the lungs. The right lung is divided into three lobes (upper, middle, and lower) and the left lung into two lobes (upper and lower) (Fig. 25-2). The structures of the chest wall (ribs, pleura, muscles of respiration) are also important for respiration.

The mainstem bronchi, pulmonary vessels, and nerves enter the lungs through a slit called the *hilus.* The right mainstem bronchus is shorter, wider, and straighter than the left mainstem bronchus. For this reason, aspiration is more likely to occur in the right lung than in the left lung.

The mainstem bronchi subdivide several times to form the lobar, segmental, and subsegmental bronchi. Further divisions form the bronchioles. The most distant bronchioles are called the respiratory bronchioles. Beyond these lie the alveolar ducts and alveoli (Fig. 25-3). The bronchioles are encircled by smooth muscles that constrict and dilate in response to various stimuli. The terms *bronchoconstriction* and *bronchodilation* refer to a decrease or increase in the diameter of the airways caused by contraction or relaxation of these muscles.

The trachea and bronchi act as a pathway to conduct gases to and from the alveoli. The trachea plus the bronchi are called *anatomic dead space* (VD).The air filling this space does not participate in gas exchange. In adults a normal **tidal volume (VT)**, or volume of air exchanged with each breath, is about 500 mL (in a 150-lb man). Of each 500 mL inhaled, about 150 mL is VD.

After moving through the VD, air reaches the respiratory bronchioles and alveoli (Fig. 25-4). *Alveoli* are small sacs in the lungs that are the primary site of gas exchange for $O_2$ and $CO_2$. The adult lung has over 300 million alveoli, each 0.3 mm in diameter. The alveoli are interconnected by pores of Kohn,[1,2]

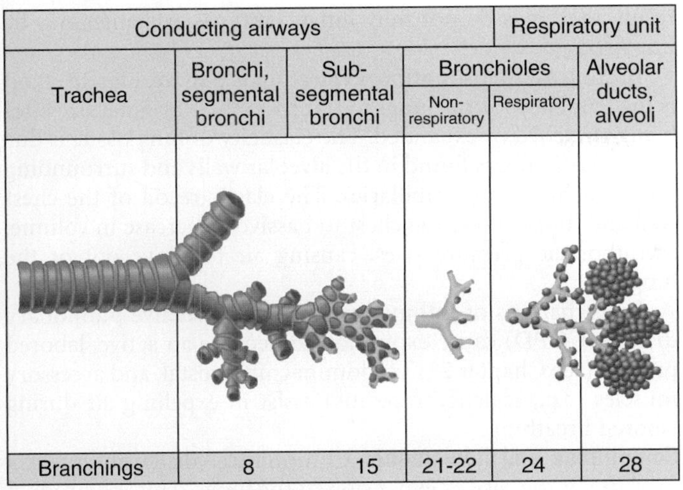


FIG. 25-3 Structures of lower airways. (Redrawn from Thompson JM, McFarland GK, Hirsch JE, Tucker SM: *Mosby's clinical nursing,* ed 5, St Louis, 2002, Mosby.)

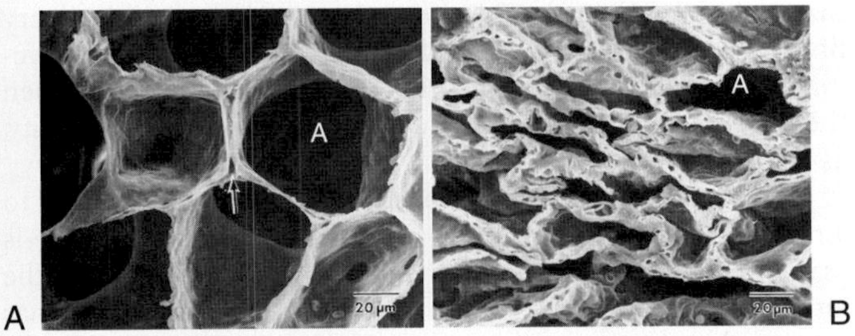


FIG. 25-4 Scanning electron micrograph of lung parenchyma. **A,** Alveoli *(A)* and alveolar-capillary membrane *(arrow).* **B,** Effects of atelectasis. Alveoli *(A)* are partially or totally collapsed. (*A,* From Dantzker DR, Bone RC, George RB, editors: *Pulmonary and critical care medicine,* vol 1, St Louis, 1993, Mosby. *B,* From Albertine KH, Williams MC, Hyde DM: Anatomy of the lungs. In RJ Mason, VC Broaddus, JF Murray, et al, editors: *Murray and Nadel's textbook of respiratory medicine,* ed 4, Philadelphia, 2005, Saunders.)

which allow movement of air from alveolus to alveolus (Fig. 25-1). Deep breathing promotes air movement through these pores and assists in moving mucus out of the respiratory bronchioles. Bacteria can also move through these pores, spreading infection to previously uninfected areas. Alveoli have a total volume of about 2500 mL and a surface area for gas exchange that is about the size of a tennis court.

Gases are exchanged at the alveolar-capillary membrane, where the alveoli come in contact with pulmonary capillaries (Fig. 25-5). In conditions such as pulmonary edema, excess fluid fills the interstitial space and alveoli, markedly reducing gas exchange.

**Surfactant.** Because alveoli are unstable, they have a natural tendency to collapse. Alveolar cells secrete surfactant. **Surfactant** is a lipoprotein that lowers the surface tension in the alveoli.[3] It reduces the amount of pressure needed to inflate the alveoli and makes them less likely to collapse. Normally, each person takes a slightly larger breath, termed a *sigh,* after every five or six breaths. This sigh stretches the alveoli and promotes surfactant secretion.

When not enough surfactant is present, the alveoli collapse. The term *atelectasis* refers to collapsed, airless alveoli (Fig. 25-4, *B*). The postoperative patient is at risk for atelectasis because of

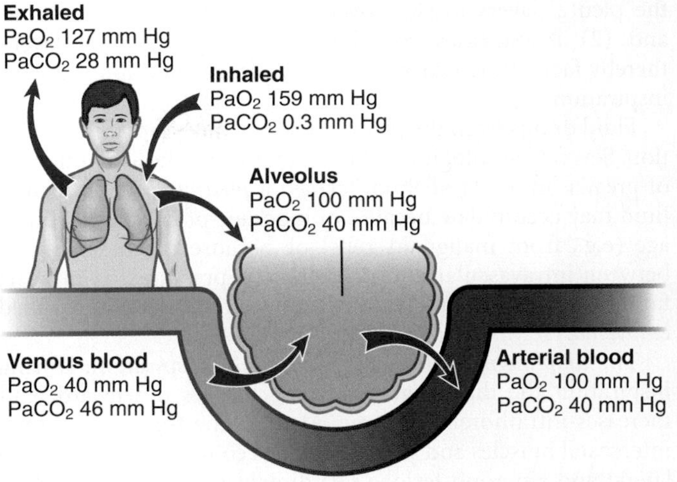


FIG. 25-5 Partial pressure of respiratory gases in normal respiration. The pressures are shown in inhaled and exhaled air from the lungs and at the level of the alveoli and pulmonary venous and arterial blood vessels.

the effects of anesthesia and restricted breathing with pain (see Chapter 19). In acute respiratory distress syndrome (ARDS), lack of surfactant contributes to widespread atelectasis (see Chapter 67).

**Blood Supply.** The lungs have two different types of circulation: pulmonary and bronchial. The pulmonary circulation provides the lungs with blood that participates in gas exchange. The pulmonary artery receives deoxygenated blood from the right ventricle of the heart and delivers it to pulmonary capillaries that lie directly alongside the alveoli. $O_2$–$CO_2$ exchange occurs at this point. The pulmonary veins return oxygenated blood to the left atrium, which then delivers it to the left ventricle. This oxygenated blood is pumped by the left ventricle into the aorta, which supplies the arteries of the systemic circulation. Venous blood is collected from capillary networks of the body and returned to the right atrium by way of the superior and inferior vena cava.

The *bronchial circulation* starts with the bronchial arteries, which arise from the thoracic aorta. The bronchial circulation provides $O_2$ to the bronchi and other pulmonary tissues. Deoxygenated blood returns from the bronchial circulation through the azygos vein into the superior vena cava.

## Chest Wall

The chest wall is shaped, supported, and protected by 24 ribs (12 on each side). The ribs and sternum protect the lungs and the heart from injury and are called the *thoracic cage.* The *mediastinum* is the space in the middle of the thoracic cavity. It contains many major organs of the chest, including the heart, aorta, and esophagus. The mediastinum physically separates the right and left lungs into two separate compartments.

The chest cavity is lined with a membrane called the *parietal pleura,* and the lungs are lined with a membrane called the *visceral pleura.* The parietal and visceral pleurae join to form a closed, double-walled sac. The visceral pleura does not have any sensory pain fibers or nerve endings, whereas the parietal pleura does have sensory pain fibers. Therefore irritation and inflammation of the parietal pleura causes pain with each breath.

The space between the pleural layers is called the *intrapleural space.* Normally this space contains 20 to 25 mL of fluid. This fluid serves two purposes: (1) it provides lubrication, allowing the pleural layers to slide over each other during breathing; and (2) it increases cohesion between the pleural layers, thereby facilitating expansion of the pleurae and lungs during inspiration.

Fluid drains from the pleural space by the lymphatic circulation. Several pathologic conditions may cause the accumulation of greater amounts of fluid, termed a *pleural effusion.* Pleural fluid may accumulate because of blockage of lymphatic drainage (e.g., from malignant cells) or because of an imbalance between intravascular and oncotic fluid pressures, as in heart failure. Purulent pleural fluid with bacterial infection is called *empyema.*

The *diaphragm* is the major muscle of respiration. During inspiration the diaphragm contracts, moves downward, and increases intrathoracic volume. At the same time the external intercostal muscles and scalene muscles contract, increasing the lateral and anteroposterior (AP) dimension of the chest. This causes the size of the thoracic cavity to increase and intrathoracic pressure to decrease, so air is pulled into the lungs.

The diaphragm is made up of two hemidiaphragms, each innervated by the right and left phrenic nerves. The phrenic nerves arise from the spinal cord between C3 and C5, the third and fifth cervical vertebrae. Injury to the phrenic nerve results in hemidiaphragm paralysis on the side of the injury. Complete spinal cord injuries above the level of C3 result in total diaphragm paralysis and dependence on a mechanical ventilator.

## Physiology of Respiration

**Oxygenation.** Oxygenation refers to the process of obtaining $O_2$ from the atmospheric air and making it available to the organs and tissues of the body. The lungs' ability to oxygenate arterial blood adequately is assessed by clinical assessment of the patient (Table 25-2), partial pressure of $O_2$ in arterial blood ($PaO_2$), and arterial $O_2$ saturation ($SaO_2$).

$O_2$ is carried in the blood in two forms: dissolved $O_2$ and hemoglobin-bound $O_2$. The $PaO_2$ represents the amount of $O_2$ dissolved in the plasma and is expressed in millimeters of mercury (mm Hg). The $SaO_2$ is the amount of $O_2$ bound to hemoglobin in comparison with the amount of $O_2$ the hemoglobin can carry. The $SaO_2$ is expressed as a percentage. For example, if the $SaO_2$ is 90%, this means that 90% of the hemoglobin attachments for $O_2$ have $O_2$ bound to them.

$O_2$ and $CO_2$ move back and forth across the alveolar-capillary membrane by diffusion. The overall direction of movement is from the area of higher concentration to the area of lower concentration. Thus $O_2$ moves from alveolar gas (atmospheric air) into the arterial blood and $CO_2$ from the arterial blood into the alveolar gas. Diffusion continues until equilibrium is reached.

**Ventilation.** Ventilation involves *inspiration,* or inhalation (movement of air into the lungs), and *expiration,* or exhalation (movement of air out of the lungs). Air moves in and out of the lungs because intrathoracic pressure changes in relation to pressure at the airway opening. Contraction of the diaphragm and intercostal and scalene muscles increases chest dimensions, thereby decreasing intrathoracic pressure. Gas flows from an area of higher pressure (atmospheric) to one of lower pressure (intrathoracic). When dyspnea (shortness of breath) occurs, neck and shoulder muscles can assist the effort. Some conditions (e.g., phrenic nerve paralysis, rib fractures, neuromuscular disease) may limit diaphragm or chest wall movement and cause the patient to breathe with smaller tidal volumes. As a result, the lungs do not fully inflate, and gas exchange may be impaired.

In contrast to inspiration, expiration is passive. Elastic recoil is the tendency for the lungs to return to their original size after being stretched or expanded. The elasticity of lung tissue is due to the elastin fibers found in the alveolar walls and surrounding the bronchioles and capillaries. The elastic recoil of the chest wall and lungs allows the chest to passively decrease in volume. Intrathoracic pressure rises, causing air to move out of the lungs.

Exacerbations of asthma or chronic obstructive pulmonary disease (COPD) cause expiration to become an active, labored process (see Chapter 28). Abdominal, intercostal, and accessory muscles (e.g., scalene, trapezius) assist in expelling air during labored breathing.

**Compliance and Resistance.** Compliance (distensibility) is a measure of the ease of expansion of the lungs. This is a product of the elasticity of the lungs and elastic recoil of the chest wall.[4] When compliance is decreased, the lungs are more difficult to inflate. Examples include conditions that increase fluid in the lungs (e.g., pulmonary edema, ARDS, pneumonia), conditions that make lung tissue less elastic or distensible (e.g., pulmonary fibrosis, sarcoidosis), and conditions that restrict lung movement (e.g., pleural effusion). Compliance is increased when there is destruction of alveolar walls and loss of tissue elasticity, as in COPD.

On the other hand, resistance refers to any impediment to airflow during inspiration and expiration. Airway resistance is primarily affected by changes in the diameter (size) of the airways. For example, a patient with an acute asthma attack has narrowed airways, resulting in increased resistance. Smaller-size airways make it more difficult for patients to get air into their lungs. The presence of secretions in the bronchi also increases resistance. The administration of bronchodilators decreases resistance by increasing the diameter of the bronchi, facilitating air entry into the lungs.

Changes in either compliance and/or resistance have the ability to seriously affect both oxygenation and ventilation of the patient.

**Arterial Blood Gases.** Two methods are used to assess the efficiency of gas transfer in the lung and tissue oxygenation: (1) analysis of *arterial blood gases* (ABGs) and (2) pulse oximetry. ABGs are measured to determine oxygenation status and acid-base balance. ABG analysis includes measurement of the $PaO_2$, $PaCO_2$ (the partial pressure of $CO_2$ in arterial blood), acidity (pH), bicarbonate ($HCO_3^-$), and $SaO_2$. Normal values for ABGs are given in Table 25-1.

Blood for ABG analysis can be obtained by arterial puncture or from an arterial catheter, which is usually in the radial or femoral artery. Both techniques allow only intermittent analysis. Continuous intraarterial blood gas monitoring is also possible via a fiberoptic sensor or an $O_2$ electrode inserted into an arterial catheter. An arterial catheter permits ABG sampling without repeated arterial punctures.

The normal $PaO_2$ decreases with advancing age. It also varies in relation to the distance above sea level. At higher altitudes the barometric pressure is lower, resulting in a lower inspired $O_2$ pressure and a lower $PaO_2$ (Table 25-1).

**Mixed Venous Blood Gases.** For the patient with a normal or near-normal cardiac status, assessment of $PaO_2$ or $SaO_2$ is usually sufficient to determine the level of oxygenation. The patient with impaired cardiac output or hemodynamic

### TABLE 25-1 Normal Arterial and Venous Blood Gas Values*

| | ARTERIAL BLOOD GASES | | VENOUS BLOOD GASES | |
|---|---|---|---|---|
| Laboratory Value | Sea Level BP 760 mm Hg | 1 Mile Above Sea Level BP 629 mm Hg | Mixed Venous Blood Gases | |
| pH | 7.35-7.45 | 7.35-7.45 | pH | 7.32-7.43 |
| $PaO_2$† | 80-100 mm Hg | 65-75 mm Hg | $PvO_2$ | 38-42 mm Hg |
| $SaO_2$† | >95%‡ | >95%‡ | $SvO_2$ | 60%-80%‡ |
| $PaCO_2$ | 35-45 mm Hg | 35-45 mm Hg | $PvCO_2$ | 38-55 mm Hg |
| $HCO_3^-$ | 22-26 mEq/L (mmol/L) | 22-26 mEq/L (mmol/L) | $HCO_3^-$ | 22-26 mEq/L (mmol/L) |

*BP*, Barometric pressure; *$HCO_3^-$*, bicarbonate; *$PaO_2$*, partial pressure of $O_2$ in arterial blood; *$PaCO_2$*, partial pressure of arterial $CO_2$; *$PvCO_2$*, partial pressure of $CO_2$ in venous blood; *$PvO_2$*, partial pressure of $O_2$ in venous blood; *$SaO_2$*, arterial $O_2$ saturation; *$SvO_2$*, venous $O_2$ saturation.
$HCO_3^-$, BE (base excess), and $SaO_2$ are all calculated values unless identified as "measured."
*Assumes patient is ≤60 yr of age and breathing room air.
†Values decrease with age.
‡The same normal values apply when $SpO_2$ and $SvO_2$ are obtained by oximetry.

instability (e.g., altered level of consciousness, alterations in heart rate and rhythm, low BP) may have inadequate tissue $O_2$ delivery or abnormal $O_2$ consumption.

The amount of $O_2$ delivered to the tissues or consumed can be calculated. A catheter positioned in the pulmonary artery, termed a *pulmonary artery (PA) catheter,* is used for mixed venous sampling (see Chapter 65). Blood drawn from a PA catheter is termed a *mixed venous blood gas* ($SvO_2$) sample because it consists of venous blood that has returned to the right side of the heart from all parts of the body and "mixes" in the right ventricle. Normal $SvO_2$ is 60% to 80%. Other normal mixed venous values are given in Table 25-1.

$SvO_2$ can be monitored intermittently by obtaining a blood sample from the PA catheter. A decrease in $SvO_2$ suggests that less $O_2$ is being delivered to the tissues or that more $O_2$ is being consumed. Changes in $SvO_2$ provide an early warning of a change in cardiac output or tissue $O_2$ delivery.

**Oximetry.** Arterial $O_2$ saturation can be monitored noninvasively and continuously using a *pulse oximetry* probe on the finger, toe, ear, or bridge of the nose. The abbreviation $SpO_2$ is used to indicate the $O_2$ saturation of hemoglobin as measured by pulse oximetry.[5] $SpO_2$ and heart rate are displayed on the monitor as digital readings. Normal $SpO_2$ values are 94% to 99%.

$SpO_2$ is assessed with each routine vital sign check in many inpatient areas. Oximetry is also used during exercise testing and when adjusting flow rates during long-term $O_2$ therapy. Pulse oximetry is particularly valuable in intensive care and perioperative situations, in which sedation or decreased consciousness may mask hypoxia (Table 25-2). Changes in $SpO_2$ can be detected quickly and treated immediately (Table 25-3).

Values obtained by pulse oximetry are less accurate if the $SpO_2$ is less than 70%. At this level the oximeter may display a value that is ±4% of the actual value. For example, if the $SpO_2$ reading is 70%, the actual value can range from 66% to 74%. Pulse oximetry is also inaccurate if hemoglobin variants (e.g., carboxyhemoglobin, methemoglobin) are present. Other factors that can alter the accuracy of pulse oximetry include motion, low perfusion, anemia, cold extremities, bright fluorescent lights, intravascular dyes, thick acrylic nails, and dark skin color. If there is doubt about the accuracy of the $SpO_2$ reading, obtain an ABG analysis to verify the results.

**$CO_2$ Monitoring.** $CO_2$ can be monitored using transcutaneous $CO_2$ ($PtcCO_2$) and end-tidal $CO_2$ ($PetCO_2$) capnography. Transcutaneous measurement of $CO_2$ is a noninvasive method of estimating arterial pressure of $CO_2$ ($PaCO_2$) using an electrode placed on the skin.

### TABLE 25-2 Manifestations of Inadequate Oxygenation

| | ONSET | |
|---|---|---|
| Manifestations | Early | Late |
| **Central Nervous System** | | |
| Unexplained apprehension | X | |
| Unexplained restlessness or irritability | X | |
| Unexplained confusion or lethargy | X | X |
| Combativeness | | X |
| Coma | | X |
| **Respiratory** | | |
| Tachypnea | X | |
| Dyspnea on exertion | X | |
| Dyspnea at rest | | X |
| Use of accessory muscles | | X |
| Retraction of interspaces on inspiration | | X |
| Pause for breath between sentences, words | | X |
| **Cardiovascular** | | |
| Tachycardia | X | |
| Mild hypertension | X | |
| Dysrhythmias | X | X |
| Hypotension | | X |
| Cyanosis | | X |
| Cool, clammy skin | | X |
| **Other** | | |
| Diaphoresis | X | X |
| Decreased urine output | X | X |
| Unexplained fatigue | X | X |

$PetCO_2$ is the noninvasive measurement of alveolar $CO_2$ during exhalation when $CO_2$ concentration is at its peak. It is used to monitor and assess trends in the patient's ventilatory status. Expired gases are sampled from the patient's airway and are analyzed by a $CO_2$ sensor that uses infrared light to measure exhaled $CO_2$.[6] The sensor may be attached to an adaptor on the endotracheal tube or the tracheostomy tube. A nasal cannula with a sidestream capnometer can be used in patients without an artificial airway. Capnography is usually presented as a graph of expiratory $CO_2$ plotted against time.

In the past, capnography was used mainly intraoperatively, postoperatively, and in critical care units. Today's monitors are portable and practical for use in emergency departments and on inpatient units.

Measurement of $O_2$ saturation (oximetry) is primarily used to assess for hypoxia. $CO_2$ monitoring assesses for hypercapnia. The use of both measures together is important in determining the patient's oxygenation and ventilatory status.

**TABLE 25-3 Normal and Critical Values for $PaO_2$ and $SpO_2$**

| $PaO_2$ (mm Hg) | $SpO_2$ (%) | Significance | Manifestations | Management |
|---|---|---|---|---|
| 80-100 | ≥94 | Normal value | Asymptomatic | • Routine assessment of patient |
| 60-79 | 90 | Mild hypoxemia | Restlessness, tachycardia, dysrhythmias, dyspnea, hypertension | • Assess patient condition as necessary<br>• Supplemental $O_2$ may be required |
| 40-59 | 88 | Moderate hypoxemia | Confusion, lethargy, dysrhythmias, hypotension, respiratory distress, accessory muscle use | • $O_2$ required<br>• Escalate level of care. Obtain critical care consult<br>• Monitor frequently for sudden deterioration in condition |
| <40 | 75 | Severe hypoxemia | Cyanosis, coma, respiratory and/or cardiac arrest possible | • High $FIO_2$, intubation, mechanical ventilation<br>• Continuous patient assessment and evaluation |

## Control of Respiration

The respiratory center in the medulla (located in the brainstem) responds to chemical and mechanical signals. Impulses are sent from the medulla to the respiratory muscles through the spinal cord and phrenic nerves.

**Chemoreceptors.** A chemoreceptor is a receptor that responds to a change in the chemical composition ($PaCO_2$ and pH) of the fluid around it. Central chemoreceptors are located in the medulla and respond to changes in the hydrogen ion ($H^+$) concentration. An increase in the $H^+$ concentration *(acidosis)* causes the medulla to increase the respiratory rate and tidal volume ($V_T$). A decrease in $H^+$ concentration *(alkalosis)* has the opposite effect. Changes in $PaCO_2$ regulate ventilation primarily by their effect on the pH of the cerebrospinal fluid. When the $PaCO_2$ level is increased, more $CO_2$ is available to combine with $H_2O$ and form carbonic acid ($H_2CO_3$). This lowers the cerebrospinal fluid pH and stimulates an increase in respiratory rate. The opposite process occurs with a decrease in $PaCO_2$ level.

Peripheral chemoreceptors are located in the carotid bodies at the bifurcation of the common carotid arteries and in the aortic bodies above and below the aortic arch. The peripheral chemoreceptors respond to decreases in $PaO_2$ and pH and to increases in $PaCO_2$. These changes also stimulate the respiratory center.

In a healthy person an increase in $PaCO_2$ or a decrease in pH causes an immediate increase in the respiratory rate. The $PaCO_2$ does not vary more than about 3 mm Hg if lung function is normal. Conditions such as COPD alter lung function and may result in chronically elevated $PaCO_2$ levels. In these instances, the patient is relatively insensitive to further increases in $PaCO_2$ as a stimulus to breathe and may be maintaining ventilation largely because of a hypoxic drive from the peripheral chemoreceptors (see Chapter 28).

**Mechanical Receptors.** Mechanical receptors (juxtacapillary and irritant) are located in the lungs, upper airways, chest wall, and diaphragm. They are stimulated by a variety of physiologic factors, such as irritants, muscle stretching, and alveolar wall distortion. Signals from the stretch receptors aid in the control of respiration. As the lungs inflate, pulmonary stretch receptors activate the inspiratory center to inhibit further lung expansion. This is termed the *Hering-Breuer reflex,* and it prevents overdistention of the lungs. Impulses from the mechanical sensors are sent through the vagus nerve to the brain. The stimulation of juxtacapillary receptors causes the rapid respiration (tachypnea) seen in pulmonary edema. These receptors are stimulated by fluid entering the pulmonary interstitial space.

## Respiratory Defense Mechanisms

Respiratory defense mechanisms are efficient in protecting the lungs from inhaled particles, microorganisms, and toxic gases. The defense mechanisms include the filtration of air, mucociliary clearance system, cough reflex, reflex bronchoconstriction, and alveolar macrophages.

**Filtration of Air.** Nasal hairs filter inspired air. In addition, the abrupt changes in direction of airflow that occur as air moves through the nasopharynx and larynx increase air turbulence. This causes particles and bacteria to contact the mucosa lining these structures. Most large particles (greater than 5 μm) are less dangerous because they are removed in the nasopharynx or bronchi and do not reach the alveoli.

The velocity of airflow slows greatly after it passes the larynx, facilitating the deposition of smaller particles (1 to 5 μm). They settle out the way that sand does in a river, a process termed *sedimentation.* Particles less than 1 μm in size are too small to settle in this manner and are deposited in the alveoli. An example of small particles that can build up is coal dust, which can lead to pneumoconiosis (see Chapter 27).

**Mucociliary Clearance System.** Below the larynx, the movement of mucus is accomplished by the mucociliary clearance system, commonly referred to as the *mucociliary escalator.* This term is used to indicate the relationship between the secretion of mucus and the ciliary activity. Mucus is continuously secreted at a rate of about 100 mL/day by goblet cells and submucosal glands. It forms a mucous blanket that contains the impacted particles and debris from distal lung areas (Fig. 25-1). The small amount of mucus normally secreted is swallowed without being noticed. Secretory immunoglobulin A (IgA) in the mucus helps protect against bacteria and viruses.

Cilia cover the airways from the level of the trachea to the respiratory bronchioles (Fig. 25-1). Each ciliated cell contains approximately 200 cilia, which beat rhythmically about 1000 times per minute in the large airways, moving mucus toward the mouth. The ciliary beat is slower further down the tracheobronchial tree. As a consequence, particles that penetrate more deeply into the airways are removed less rapidly. Ciliary action is impaired by dehydration, smoking, inhalation of high $O_2$ concentrations, infection, and ingestion of drugs such as atropine, anesthetics, alcohol, or cocaine. Patients with COPD and cystic fibrosis have repeated lower respiratory tract infections. In these conditions cilia are often destroyed, resulting in impaired secretion clearance, a chronic productive cough, and chronic colonization by bacteria, which leads to frequent respiratory tract infections.

**Cough Reflex.** The cough is a protective reflex action that clears the airway by a high-pressure, high-velocity flow of air. It is a backup for mucociliary clearance, especially when this clearance mechanism is overwhelmed or ineffective. Coughing is only effective in removing secretions above the subsegmental level (large or main airways). Secretions below this level must be moved upward by the mucociliary mechanism before they can be removed by coughing.

**Reflex Bronchoconstriction.** *Reflex bronchoconstriction* is another defense mechanism. In response to the inhalation of large amounts of irritating substances (e.g., dusts, aerosols), the bronchi constrict in an effort to prevent entry of the irritants. A person with hyperreactive airways, such as a person with asthma, may experience bronchoconstriction after inhalation of triggers such as cold air, perfume, or other strong odors.

**Alveolar Macrophages.** Because ciliated cells are not found below the level of the respiratory bronchioles, the primary defense mechanism at the alveolar level is alveolar macrophages. *Alveolar macrophages* rapidly phagocytize inhaled foreign particles such as bacteria. The debris is moved to the level of the bronchioles for removal by the cilia or removed from the lungs by the lymphatic system. Particles (e.g., coal dust, silica) that cannot be adequately phagocytized tend to remain in the lungs for indefinite periods and can stimulate inflammatory responses (see Chapter 27). Because alveolar macrophage activity is impaired by cigarette smoke, the smoker who is employed in an occupation with heavy dust exposure (e.g., mining, foundries) is at an especially high risk for lung disease.

### Gerontologic Considerations: Effects of Aging on Respiratory System

Age-related changes in the respiratory system can be divided into alterations in structure, defense mechanisms, and respiratory control (Table 25-4). Structural changes include calcification of the costal cartilages, which can interfere with chest expansion. The outward curvature of the spine is marked, especially with osteoporosis, and the lumbar curve flattens. Therefore the chest may appear barrel shaped, and the older person may need to use accessory muscles to breathe. Respiratory muscle strength progressively declines after age 50. Overall, the lungs in the older adult are harder to inflate.

Within the lung, the number of functional alveoli decreases, and they become less elastic. Small airways in the lung bases close earlier in expiration. As a consequence, more inspired air is distributed to the lung apices and ventilation is less well matched to perfusion, lowering the $PaO_2$. Therefore older adults have less tolerance for exertion, and dyspnea can occur if their activity exceeds their normal exercise.

In older adults *respiratory defense mechanisms* are less effective because of a decline in both cell-mediated and humoral immunity (ability to produce antibodies). The alveolar macrophages are less effective at phagocytosis. An older patient has a less forceful cough and fewer and less functional cilia. Mucous membranes tend to be drier. Retained mucus predisposes the older adult to respiratory tract infections. Formation of secretory IgA, an important defense mechanism, is diminished. Swallowing is slower because of transit time in the pharyngeal area, and there is reduced sensation in the pharynx. If the older adult patient has a superimposed neurologic condition (e.g., stroke), aspiration is more likely.

*Respiratory control* is also altered as a result of the aging process, resulting in a more gradual response to changes in blood $O_2$ or $CO_2$ level. The $PaO_2$ may drop to a slightly lower than normal level, and the $PaCO_2$ may rise to a slightly higher than normal level before the respiratory rate changes.

The extent of these changes in people of the same age varies greatly. The older adult who has a significant smoking history, is obese, and has a chronic illness is at greatest risk of adverse outcomes.

**TABLE 25-4 Gerontologic Assessment Differences**

***Respiratory System***

| Changes | Differences in Assessment Findings |
|---|---|
| **Structures** | |
| Chest wall stiffening<br>Costal cartilage calcification<br>↑ Anteroposterior diameter<br>↓ Elastic recoil<br>↓ Chest wall compliance<br>↓ Functioning alveoli<br>↓ Respiratory muscle strength | Barrel chest appearance, kyphotic posture, ↓ chest wall movement, ↓ deep breathing<br>Mucus thickened<br>↓ Vital capacity, ↑ residual volume, ↑ functional residual capacity<br>Diminished breath sounds, particularly at lung bases<br>↓ $PaO_2$ and $SaO_2$, normal pH and $PaCO_2$ |
| **Defense Mechanisms** | |
| ↓ Cell-mediated immunity<br>↓ Specific antibodies<br>↓ Cilia function<br>↓ Cough force<br>↓ Alveolar macrophage function<br>↓ Sensation in pharynx | ↓ Cough effectiveness, ↓ secretion clearance<br>↑ Risk of upper respiratory aspiration, infection, influenza, pneumonia<br>Respiratory infections may be more severe and last longer |
| **Respiratory Control** | |
| ↓ Response to hypoxemia<br>↓ Response to hypercapnia | Slight ↓ in $PaO_2$ and ↑ in $PaCO_2$ before respiratory rate changes<br>↓ Ability to maintain acid-base balance<br>Significant hypoxemia or hypercapnia may develop from relatively small incidents<br>Retained secretions, excessive sedation, or positioning that impairs chest expansion may substantially alter $PaO_2$ or $SpO_2$ values |

## ASSESSMENT OF RESPIRATORY SYSTEM

Determining a patient's needs related to the respiratory system requires an accurate health history and a thorough physical examination.[7] A respiratory assessment can be done as part of a comprehensive physical examination or as a focused respiratory examination. Use judgment in determining whether all or part of the history and physical examination will be completed based on the patient's problems and degree of respiratory distress. If respiratory distress is severe, only obtain pertinent information and defer a thorough assessment until the patient's condition stabilizes.

### Subjective Data

#### Important Health Information

***Past Health History.*** It is important to determine the frequency of upper respiratory problems (e.g., colds, sore throats, sinus problems, allergies) and whether seasonal changes have an effect on these problems. Question the patient with allergies about possible precipitating factors or triggers such as medications, pollen, smoke, mold, or pet exposure. Document the characteristics and severity of the allergic reaction such as runny nose, wheezing, scratchy throat, or chest tightness. Inquire about a past history of lower respiratory problems, such as asthma, COPD, pneumonia, and tuberculosis (TB). Also determine the frequency of asthma exacerbations and triggers, if

## CASE STUDY

### Patient Introduction

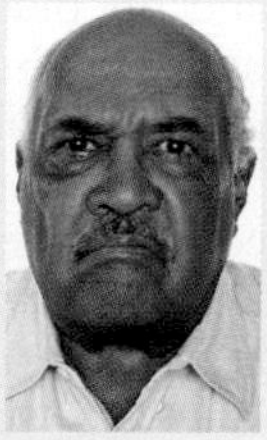

(©Fuse/ Thinkstock)

F.T. is a 70-year-old African American man who comes to the emergency department (ED) complaining of increased shortness of breath. He states that he started using his albuterol inhaler every 4 hours a few days ago, but it does not seem to be helping. He has been having trouble sleeping or doing any activity because of his shortness of breath.

**Discussion Questions**

1. What are the possible causes of F.T.'s shortness of breath?
2. Does F.T. require urgent admission to the hospital or is his condition stable and he can be seen by an HCP in a few hours?

You will learn more about F.T. and his condition as you read through this assessment chapter.

(See p. 463 for more information on F.T.)

Answers available at *http://evolve.elsevier.com/Lewis/medsurg.*

known. Because respiratory symptoms are often manifestations of problems that involve other body systems, it is important to ask about a history of additional health problems. For example, the patient with cardiac dysfunction may experience dyspnea (shortness of breath) as a consequence of heart failure. The patient with human immunodeficiency virus (HIV) infection may experience frequent respiratory tract infections because immune function is compromised.

***Medications.*** Take a thorough medication history, including both prescription and over-the-counter medications. Ask about the reason for taking the medication, its name, the dose and frequency, length of time taken, its effect, and any side effects. Assess for overuse of short-term bronchodilators as a key indicator of symptom control, since this information will help guide management. Inquire about the use of an angiotensin-converting enzyme (ACE) inhibitor, since cough is a relatively common side effect of this class of drugs. Encourage the patient to bring her or his medication bottles and any inhalers to each visit with an HCP.

If the patient is using $O_2$ for a breathing problem, document the fraction of inspired $O_2$ concentration ($FIO_2$), flow rate (liters per minute), method of administration, number of hours used per day, and effectiveness of the therapy. Assess safety practices, including the patient's cognitive and physical ability related to using $O_2$ and any metered-dose inhalers.

***Surgery or Other Treatments.*** Determine if the patient has been hospitalized for a respiratory problem. Note the dates, therapy (including surgery), and current status of the problem. Determine if the patient has ever been intubated because of a respiratory problem. Ask about the use of and response to respiratory treatments such as a nebulizer, humidifier, airway clearance modalities (see Chapter 28), high-frequency chest wall oscillation, postural drainage, and percussion.

**Functional Health Patterns.** Health history questions to ask a patient with a respiratory problem are presented in Table 25-5.

***Health Perception–Health Management Pattern.*** Ask the patient if there has been a perceived change in health status within the last several days, months, or years. In COPD, lung function declines slowly over many years. The patient may not notice this decline because activity is altered to accommodate reduced exercise tolerance. If an upper respiratory tract infection is superimposed on a chronic problem, dyspnea and decreased exercise tolerance may occur very quickly. In asthma, symptoms may occur or worsen during exercise, in the presence of mold, or following changes in temperature or air pollution.

Explore and document common manifestations of respiratory problems (e.g., cough, dyspnea). Also describe the course of the patient's illness, including when it began, type of symptoms, and factors that alleviate or aggravate these symptoms. Because of the chronic nature of respiratory problems, the patient may relate a change in symptoms rather than the onset of new symptoms when describing the present illness. Carefully document any changes because they often suggest the cause of illness. For example, increased shortness of breath or increased purulence of sputum may suggest an acute exacerbation of COPD.

If a cough is present, evaluate its quality. For example, a loose-sounding cough indicates secretions; a dry, hacking cough indicates airway irritation or obstruction; a harsh, barky cough suggests upper airway obstruction from inhibited vocal cord movement related to subglottic edema. Assess whether the cough is strong enough to clear secretions, and note whether it is productive or nonproductive of secretions. Determine if a cough is acute or chronic (longer than 3 weeks in duration) or if it first began with an upper respiratory tract infection. The pattern and etiology of the cough are determined by asking questions such as the following: What has been the pattern of coughing? Has it been regular or paroxysmal (i.e., sudden, periodic onset), or related to a time of day, the weather, certain activities, talking, or deep breathing? Any change over time? Do you clear your throat a lot? What have you tried to alleviate the coughing? Did you try any prescription or over-the-counter drugs?

If the patient has a productive cough, evaluate the following characteristics of sputum: amount, color, consistency, and odor. Quantify the amount of sputum in teaspoons, tablespoons, or cups per day. Note any recent increases or decreases in the amount. The normal color is clear or slightly whitish. If a patient is a cigarette smoker, the sputum is usually clear to gray with occasional specks of brown. The patient with COPD may exhibit clear, whitish, or slightly yellow sputum, especially in the morning on rising. If the patient reports any change from baseline color, suspect pulmonary complications. Note any changes in consistency of sputum to thick, thin, or frothy and pink tinged. These changes may indicate dehydration, postnasal drip or sinus drainage, or possible pulmonary edema. Normally sputum should be odorless. A foul odor or exceptionally bad breath or taste in the mouth suggests an infectious process. Ask the patient if sputum production has increased or decreased with a change in position (e.g., increased with lying down) or activity.

When assessing mucus, determine if the patient has a history of spitting or coughing up blood *(hemoptysis)*. Hemoptysis can range from a slight streaking of blood in the mucus to massive coughing up of blood, in which the patient loses more than 600 mL of blood in a 24-hour period. Massive hemoptysis is an immediate medical emergency.

Frequently the patient cannot differentiate between hemoptysis and *hematemesis* (vomiting blood). Hemoptysis can be found with a variety of conditions such as pneumonia, TB, lung cancer, and severe bronchiectasis.

Assess for a history of any difficulty breathing. For example, *wheezes* are musical sounds that can be audible. Wheezing indicates some degree of airway obstruction, such as asthma, foreign body aspiration, and emphysema. Assess for any history of family exposure to *Mycobacterium tuberculosis.*

## TABLE 25-5 Health History

### *Respiratory System*

**Health Perception–Health Management**
- Describe your daily activities. Have breathing problems prevented you from doing activities that you used to be able to do?* Are your breathing problems better, worse, or about the same compared with 6 months ago?
- How do your breathing problems affect your self-care abilities?
- Have you ever smoked? Do you smoke now? If so, what have you smoked? Cigarettes? Cigars? Pipes? Electronic cigarettes?
- If yes, how many cigarettes each day and for how long? Are you interested in stopping smoking? Are there aids we can tell you about that would assist your quitting? Would you be willing to come back for a visit so that we can explore your quitting? If you stopped smoking, did you do so because of your health?* How did you stop?
- Have you ever used chewing tobacco?
- Have you ever smoked street drugs?*
- Do you get the flu shot yearly? When was your last flu shot? Have you had a Pneumovax vaccination?
- What equipment helps you manage your respiratory problems? How often do you use it? Does it help? Cause problems?
- Do you feel that your respiratory problem is getting better or worse?

**Nutritional-Metabolic**
- Have you recently lost weight because of difficulty eating related to your respiratory problem? How much weight have you lost? Have you lost this weight voluntarily?
- Do any particular foods affect your breathing?* Sputum production?*

**Elimination**
- Does your breathing problem make it difficult for you to get to the toilet?*
- Are you inactive because of shortness of breath to the point that it causes incontinence?* Constipation?*

**Activity-Exercise**
- Are you ever short of breath during exercise?* At rest?*
- Do you get too short of breath to do the things you want to do?*
- Is your home one story? Two stories? How many steps from the street to your door?
- Can you walk up a flight of steps without stopping?
- Are you able to maintain your typical activities of daily living? If not, what are you able to do independently? What do you need help with? What have you had to give up?
- What do you do when you get short of breath? Does this help? How long does it take you to recover after you have been short of breath?

**Sleep-Rest**
- Do breathing problems cause you to wake up during the night?*
- Can you lie flat at night? If not, how many pillows do you use?
- Do you need to sleep upright in a chair?*
- Are you or your partner aware of any snoring?
- Do you awaken in the morning feeling rested?
- Do you ever wake up in the morning with a headache?*
- Do you fall asleep easily during the day?*

**Cognitive-Perceptual**
- Do you have any pain associated with breathing?* On a scale from 0 to 10, with 0 being "no pain" and 10 being "the worst pain you can imagine," where would you rate your pain? Does it hurt more on inspiration?* Expiration?* Or both?*
- If you are experiencing pain with breathing, describe the pain.
- Has the pain gotten better, worse, or stayed about the same over the past 6 months?
- Do you ever feel restless, irritable, or confused without a reason?*
- Do you have difficulty remembering things?*

**Self-Perception–Self-Concept**
- Describe how your respiratory problems have changed your life.
- If you use $O_2$, do you ever go out without bringing it with you? How often does this occur? Why?

**Role-Relationship**
- Has your respiratory problem caused any difficulties in your work, family, or social relationships?*

**Sexuality-Reproductive**
- Has your respiratory problem caused a change in your sexual activity?*
- Have you and your partner talked about ways to minimize your breathing problems during sexual activity?

**Coping–Stress Tolerance**
- On a daily/weekly basis, how often do you leave your home?
- Do you feel under any stress right now?
- Does stress have an effect on your breathing?*
- Do you notice if your emotions have any effect on your respiratory problems?
- Are you aware of any respiratory support groups in your area?

**Value-Belief**
- What do you think causes/has caused your respiratory problem(s)?
- How are you feeling right now?
- Do you think the things you have been told to do for your respiratory problems really help? If not, why?
- What are you looking for/expecting from the HCP today, in terms of your breathing problem(s)?

*If answer "yes" to any of the above questions, ask patient to describe.

## GENETIC RISK ALERT

- Respiratory problems that have a strong genetic link include cystic fibrosis, COPD resulting from $\alpha_1$-antitrypsin deficiency, and asthma.
- If people have a family history of these respiratory problems, they have a much greater risk of developing them.
- Although cigarette smoking is a major risk factor for COPD, only a minority of cigarette smokers develop symptomatic disease. The risk for COPD related to cigarette smoking is genetically related.
- Determine if there is a family history of any of these respiratory problems that may have genetic or familial tendencies.

Smoking is the most important risk factor for COPD and lung cancer. Ask about cigarette use, and find out about the use of any tobacco products, including cigars, pipes, chewing tobacco, electronic cigarettes (e-cigarettes), and hookah (instrument for vaporizing and smoking flavored tobacco). Also find out about exposure to secondhand smoke. Determine if the patient has tried to quit using tobacco products, including using prescription, over-the-counter, and herbal remedies.

Discuss current and past smoking habits. Quantify smoking habits in *pack-years.* This is done by multiplying the number of packs smoked per day by the number of years smoked. For example, a person who smoked 1 pack per day for 15 years has a 15 pack-year history.

Assess if the patient received immunizations for influenza (flu) and pneumococcal pneumonia. Influenza vaccine should be administered yearly in the fall. Recommendations for pneumococcal vaccines are presented in Table 27-5.

Ask where the patient has lived and traveled. Risk factors for TB include prior residence in China, India, Africa, the former Soviet Republics, Latin America, or any developing country. Other TB risk factors include exposure to people with high rates of TB transmission such as the homeless, injection drug users, and people with HIV infection. Risk factors for fungal infections of the lung include individuals who may be exposed to bird and rodent feces and/or live or travel in the Southwest (coccidioidomycosis) and the Mississippi River Valley (histoplasmosis).

Ask the patient about the use of equipment to manage respiratory symptoms (e.g., home $O_2$ therapy equipment, inhalers, devices for sleep apnea). Question the patient about the type of equipment used, cleaning of the device, frequency of use, its effect, and any side effects. Have patients demonstrate the use of their inhalers. Many patients do not know how to use these devices correctly (see Chapter 28).

***Nutritional-Metabolic Pattern.*** Weight loss is a symptom of many respiratory diseases. Determine if weight loss was intentional and, if not, if food intake is altered by anorexia (from medications), fatigue (from hypoxemia, increased work of breathing), or feeling full quickly (from lung hyperinflation). Anorexia, weight loss, and chronic malnutrition are common in patients with COPD, lung cancer, TB, and chronic severe infection (bronchiectasis). Also note fluid intake. Dehydration can cause mucus to thicken and obstruct the airway. Rapid weight gain from fluid retention may decrease pulmonary gas exchange.

***Elimination Pattern.*** Healthy elimination habits depend on the ability to reach a toilet when necessary. Activity intolerance secondary to dyspnea could result in incontinence. Dyspnea can also be the cause of limited mobility, which can cause constipation. Question the patient with dyspnea about incontinence and constipation. People with a chronic cough, especially women, may be troubled with urinary incontinence during paroxysms of coughing.

***Activity-Exercise Pattern.*** Determine if the patient's activity is limited by dyspnea at rest or during exercise. Also note whether the patient's residence (e.g., number of steps, levels) poses a problem that increases social isolation. Record and objectively measure the degree of the patient's dyspnea. For example, can the patient walk up one flight of stairs without stopping because of dyspnea? Is dyspnea that is associated with an activity better, worse, or about the same in the last few months? Determine if the patient has difficulty breathing in a certain position, or if relief of dyspnea can be obtained by assuming a different position (e.g., tripod position in COPD).

Discuss whether the patient is able to carry out activities of daily living without dyspnea or other respiratory symptoms. If unable, document the amount and type of care needed. Immobility and sedentary habits can be risk factors for hypoventilation leading to atelectasis or pneumonia.

***Sleep-Rest Pattern.*** Determine if the patient wakes up because of pulmonary problems. The patient with asthma or COPD may awaken at night with chest tightness, wheezing, or coughing. This suggests a need for adjunct therapy or other medication changes. The patient with cardiovascular disease (e.g., heart failure) may sleep with the head elevated on several pillows to avoid respiratory problems brought on by lying flat *(orthopnea)*. Excessive weight interferes with normal ventilation and may cause sleep apnea (see Chapter 7). Extremely obese individuals may hypoventilate while awake or asleep, and weight loss can improve respiratory function. Manifestations of sleep apnea include snoring, insomnia, abrupt awakenings, daytime drowsiness, and early morning headaches. Night sweats may be a manifestation of TB.

***Cognitive-Perceptual Pattern.*** Because hypoxia can cause neurologic symptoms, ask the patient about apprehension, restlessness, irritability, and memory changes, which can indicate inadequate cerebral oxygenation (Table 25-2). Hypoxemia interferes with the ability to learn and retain information. For this reason, teaching may be more effective if the caregiver is present during teaching sessions to provide reinforcement at a later date.

Assess the patient's cognitive ability to cooperate with treatment. Failure or inability to participate in needed therapy may result in exacerbation of respiratory problems.

Inquire about any discomfort or pain with breathing. Explore a complaint of chest pain carefully to rule out cardiac involvement. Problems such as pleurisy, fractured ribs, and costochondritis cause chest pain. Careful assessment of the patient experiencing pain with breathing, such as onset, exact location of the pain, and factors that make the pain with breathing better or worse can help establish an accurate diagnosis.

***Self-Perception–Self-Concept Pattern.*** Dyspnea limits activity, impairs ability to fulfill normal roles, and often alters self-esteem. A patient may be reluctant to appear in public with a highly visible nasal cannula and $O_2$ equipment. Discuss with the patient his or her personal body image. A barrel chest, clubbed fingers, pursed-lip breathing, and frequent expectoration of sputum or throat clearing can be embarrassing and can lead to social isolation. Referral to a support group or pulmonary rehabilitation program may be beneficial in developing a support system and coping strategies.

***Role-Relationship Pattern.*** Acute and chronic respiratory problems can seriously affect performance in work or other activities. Discuss the impact of medications, $O_2$ therapy, and special routines (e.g., pulmonary hygiene for cystic fibrosis) on the patient's family, job, and social life.

Document the nature of the patient's work and frequency and intensity of exposure to fumes, toxins, asbestos, coal, fibers, or silica. Inquire whether symptoms are worse in specific situations (e.g., home versus work environments). Investigate any patient-specific allergens, such as dust or fumes, that could be present in the work environment. Hobbies such as woodworking (sawdust) or pottery (silica) and exposure to animals (allergies) may also cause respiratory problems. Because of hyperreactive airways, exposure to fumes, smoke, and other chemicals may trigger an attack in the patient with asthma.

***Sexuality-Reproductive Pattern.*** Most patients can continue to have satisfactory sexual relationships despite marked physical limitations. In a tactful manner, determine whether breathing difficulties have caused alterations in sexual activity. If so, provide teaching about positions that decrease dyspnea during sexual activity and alternative strategies for sexual fulfillment. Many patients need to perform good pulmonary hygiene (bronchodilators, coughing, and deep breathing) before intimacy. This is similar to what they would do before strenuous physical activity. They may need to use $O_2$ therapy equipment during intercourse.

***Coping–Stress Tolerance Pattern.*** Dyspnea causes anxiety, and anxiety exacerbates dyspnea. The result is a vicious cycle—the patient avoids activities that cause dyspnea, becoming more

## CASE STUDY

### Subjective Data

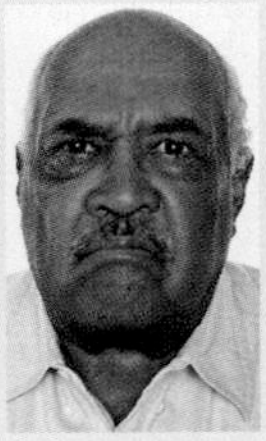
(©Fuse/ Thinkstock)

A focused subjective assessment of F.T. revealed the following information:

***PMH:*** COPD, hypertension, and benign prostatic hyperplasia. No history of allergies.

***Medications:*** metoprolol (Lopressor) 50 mg/day PO, furosemide (Lasix) 20 mg PO daily, finasteride (Proscar) 5 mg/day PO, Advair inhaler (fluticasone and salmeterol) 2 puffs bid, and albuterol inhaler 2 puffs q4hr PRN. Does not use $O_2$ at home.

***Health Perception–Health Management:*** F.T. states he usually manages his COPD well with the Advair inhaler and occasional use of albuterol inhaler PRN. He thinks he caught a cold from his granddaughter last week. Increasing difficulty breathing, even with albuterol. Has a history of 30 pack-years of smoking, quitting 5 years ago.

***Nutritional-Metabolic Pattern:*** Not eating, drinking very little over past 2 to 3 days.

***Activity-Exercise:*** At present, cannot walk 100 feet without feeling short of breath, nor walk up one flight of stairs without stopping to catch his breath.

***Sleep-Rest:*** Difficulty sleeping at present. Last night he slept upright in his recliner.

***Cognitive-Perceptual:*** Denies any pain associated with shortness of breath. Feels slightly irritable because of lack of sleep.

***Coping–Stress Tolerance:*** Denies any stress or emotional disturbance.

**Discussion Questions**

1. What type of assessment would be most appropriate for F.T.: comprehensive, focused, or emergency?
2. From the information provided by F.T., what other information would you ask him about his condition (time permitting)?
3. How will you individualize the assessment based on his current physiologic condition?
4. What considerations will you make based on his age? Ethnic/cultural background?
5. Of the information provided, which subjective assessment findings are of most concern to you?
6. F.T. cannot use his inhaler appropriately while he is talking with you. Is this an appropriate time to teach him about the proper use of his inhaler?
7. What should be included in the physical assessment? What do you think will be the priorities in your physical assessment?

You will learn about the physical assessment of the respiratory system in the next section.

(See p. 464 for more information on F.T.)

Answers available at *http://evolve.elsevier.com/Lewis/medsurg.*

deconditioned and more dyspneic. The outcome is often physical and social isolation. Assess how often the patient leaves home and interacts with others. Referral to a support group or pulmonary rehabilitation program may be beneficial.

The chronic nature of many respiratory problems such as COPD and asthma can cause prolonged stress. Inquire about the patient's coping strategies to manage this stress.

***Value-Belief Pattern.*** Determine the patient's adherence to the management regimen. Explore reasons for lack of adherence, including conflict with cultural beliefs, financial constraints (e.g., costs of prescriptions), or failure to understand benefit. Including the patient and caregiver in the planning of care can improve adherence.

## Objective Data

**Physical Examination.** Vital signs, including temperature, pulse, respirations, BP, and $SpO_2$ are important data to collect before examination of the respiratory system.

***Nose.*** Inspect the nose for patency, inflammation, deformities, symmetry, and discharge. Check each naris for air patency with respiration while the other naris is briefly occluded. Tilt the patient's head backward and push the tip of the nose upward gently. With a nasal speculum and a good light, inspect the interior of the nose. The mucous membrane should be pink and moist, with no evidence of edema (bogginess), exudate, or bleeding. Inspect the nasal septum for deviation, perforations, and bleeding. Some septal deviation is normal in an adult. Inspect the turbinates for polyps, which are abnormal, finger-like projections of swollen nasal mucosa. Polyps may result from long-term irritation of the mucosa (e.g., from allergies). Assess any discharge for color and consistency. Purulent and malodorous discharge could indicate the presence of a foreign body. Watery discharge could be secondary to allergies or from cerebrospinal fluid. Bloody discharge could be from trauma or dryness. Thick mucosal discharge could indicate infection.

***Mouth and Pharynx.*** Using a good light source, inspect the interior of the mouth for color, lesions, masses, gum retraction, bleeding, and poor dentition. Inspect the tongue for symmetry and lesions. Observe the pharynx by pressing a tongue blade against the middle of the back of the tongue. If the oropharynx is tight, have the patient yawn, since this usually allows more structures to be visible. The pharynx should be smooth and moist, with no evidence of exudate, ulcerations, swelling, or postnasal drip. Note the color, symmetry, and any enlargement of the tonsils. Stimulate the gag reflex by placing a tongue blade along the side of the pharynx behind the tonsil. A normal response (gagging) indicates that cranial nerves IX (glossopharyngeal) and X (vagus) are intact and that the airway is protected.[8]

***Neck.*** Inspect the neck for symmetry and tender or swollen areas. Palpate the lymph nodes while the patient is sitting erect with the neck slightly flexed. Progression of palpation is from the nodes around the ears, to the nodes at the base of the skull, and then to those located under the angles of the mandible to the midline. The patient may have small, mobile, nontender nodes *(shotty nodes)*, which are not a sign of a pathologic condition. Tender, hard, or fixed nodes indicate disease. Describe the location and characteristics of any palpable nodes.

***Thorax and Lungs.*** Picture imaginary lines on the chest to help identify abnormalities (Fig. 25-2). Describe abnormalities in terms of their location relative to these lines (e.g., 2 cm from the right midclavicular line).

Chest examination is best performed in a well-lit, warm room with measures taken to ensure the patient's privacy. The patient's chest is exposed. Perform all physical assessment maneuvers (inspection, palpation, percussion, auscultation) on either the anterior or the posterior chest first rather than moving from anterior to posterior or vice versa with each maneuver. It is best to begin on the posterior chest, particularly with female patients, since more information can be obtained without interference from the breast tissue. In addition, if the patient tires or you are interrupted, baseline data with the most information will have been obtained from examining the posterior of the chest.

**Inspection.** When inspecting the *anterior chest,* have the patient sit upright, or, position the patient supine with the head of the bed elevated to thirty degrees (semi-Fowler's position). The patient may need to lean forward for support on the bedside table to facilitate breathing.

First, observe the patient's appearance and note any evidence of respiratory distress, such as tachypnea or use of accessory muscles. Next, determine the shape and symmetry of the chest. Chest movement should be equal on both sides, and the anterior-posterior (AP) diameter should be less than the side-to-side or transverse diameter. Normal AP ratio is 1:2. An increase in AP diameter (e.g., barrel chest) may be due to normal aging or result from lung hyperinflation. Observe for abnormalities in the sternum (e.g., *pectus carinatum* [a prominent protrusion of the sternum] and *pectus excavatum* [an indentation of the lower sternum above the xiphoid process]).

Next observe the respiratory rate, depth, and rhythm. The normal adult respiratory rate is 12 to 20 breaths/minute. Inspiration (I) should take half as long as expiration (E) (I:E ratio = 1:2). Observe for abnormal breathing patterns, such as *Kussmaul* (rapid, deep breathing), *Cheyne-Stokes* (abnormal respirations characterized by alternating periods of apnea and deep, rapid breathing), or *Biot's* (irregular breathing with apnea every four to five cycles) respirations.

Skin color provides clues to respiratory status. Cyanosis, a late sign of hypoxemia, is best observed in light-skinned patients as a bluish tinge to the mucous membranes, lips, and palms of the hands. In dark-skinned individuals, cyanosis may be reflected as a gray or white discoloration in the conjunctivae or around the mouth. Causes of cyanosis include hypoxemia or decreased cardiac output. Inspect the fingers for evidence of long-standing hypoxemia known as *clubbing* (an increase in the angle between the base of the nail and the fingernail to 180 degrees or more, usually accompanied by an increase in the depth, bulk, and sponginess of the end of the finger).

When inspecting the *posterior chest,* ask the patient to lean forward with arms folded. This position moves the scapulae away from the spine, exposing more of the area to be examined. The same sequence of observations that was done on the anterior part of the chest is performed on the posterior part. In addition, any spinal curvature is noted. Spinal curvatures that affect breathing include kyphosis, scoliosis, and kyphoscoliosis.

**Palpation.** Determine tracheal position by gently placing the index fingers on either side of the trachea just above the suprasternal notch and gently pressing backward. Normal tracheal position is midline; deviation to the left or right is abnormal. Tracheal deviation occurs away from the side of a tension pneumothorax or a neck mass, but toward the side of a pneumonectomy or lobar atelectasis.

Symmetry of chest expansion and extent of movement are determined at the level of the diaphragm. Place your hands over the lower anterior chest wall along the costal margin and move them inward until the thumbs meet at midline. Ask the patient to breathe deeply. Observe the movement of the thumbs away from each other. Normal expansion is 1 in (2.5 cm). Hand placement on the posterior side of the chest is at the level of the tenth rib. Move the thumbs until they meet over the spine (Fig. 25-6). Check expansion anteriorly or posteriorly, but it is not necessary to check both.

Normal chest movement is equal. Unequal expansion occurs when air entry is limited by conditions involving the lung (e.g., atelectasis, pneumothorax) or the chest wall (e.g., incisional pain). Equal but diminished expansion occurs in conditions that produce a hyperinflated or barrel chest or in neuromuscular diseases (e.g., amyotrophic lateral sclerosis, spinal cord lesions). Movement may be absent or unequal over a pleural effusion, an atelectasis, or a pneumothorax.

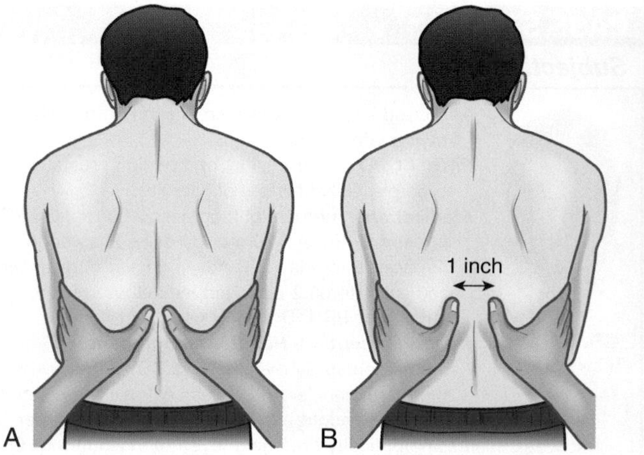


**FIG. 25-6** Estimation of thoracic expansion. **A,** Exhalation. **B,** Maximal inhalation.

## CASE STUDY

### *Objective Data: Physical Examination*

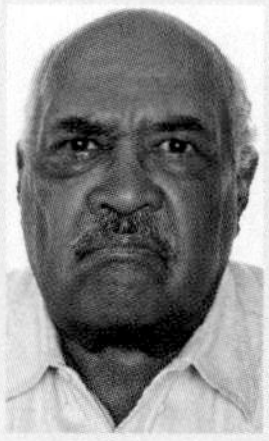

(©Fuse/Thinkstock)

Physical examination findings of F.T. are as follows:

Temperature: 38°C (100.4°F), apical pulse 110, respiratory rate 30 (regular, shallow, slightly labored), BP 170/90. $O_2$ saturation ($SpO_2$) 87% on room air. Patient sitting on edge of bed with arms resting on bedside table. Skin color normal for race with no signs of cyanosis. Slight use of accessory muscles in neck and shoulders noted. Trachea midline. Chest expansion equal. Prolonged expiration. No clubbing noted. Lungs: adequate air entry at apices bilaterally with fine crackles; decreased air entry to both bases with coarse crackles. Slight expiratory wheeze heard throughout all lung fields. F.T. has a moist, productive cough with yellow-tinged sputum.

**Discussion Questions**

1. What physical assessment findings are of most concern to you?
2. Based upon the subjective and objective assessment data presented so far, what would be three priority nursing diagnoses?
3. Identify three interventions that may be considered immediately post-assessment?
4. Can any of your priority interventions be delegated to unlicensed assistive personnel (UAP)?
5. With this additional physical assessment information, what diagnostic studies would you now anticipate being ordered for F.T.?

You will learn more about diagnostic studies of the respiratory system in the next section.

(See p. 473 for more information on F.T.)

Answers available at *http://evolve.elsevier.com/Lewis/medsurg.*

**Fremitus** is the vibration of the chest wall produced by vocalization. Tactile fremitus can be felt by placing the palmar surface of the hands against the patient's chest with the fingers hyperextended. Ask the patient to repeat a phrase such as "boy-oh-boy" in a deeper, louder-than-normal voice. Move your hands from side to side at the same time from top to bottom on the patient's chest (Fig. 25-7). Palpate all areas of the chest and compare vibrations from similar areas. Tactile fremitus is most intense adjacent to the sternum and between the scapulae because these areas are closest to the major bronchi. Fremitus is less intense farther away from these areas.

Note any increase, decrease, or absence of fremitus. Increased fremitus occurs when the lung becomes filled with fluid or is

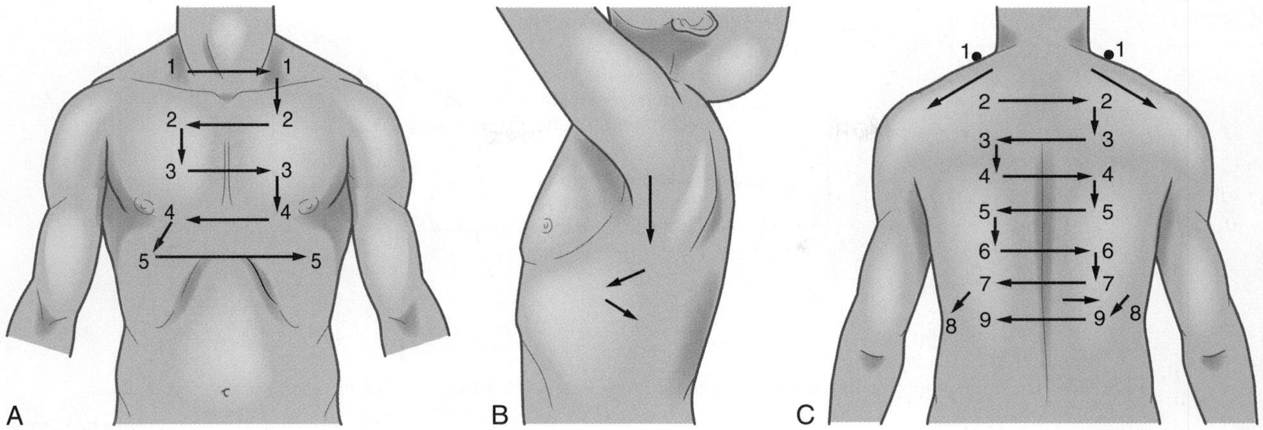


**FIG. 25-7** Sequence for examination of the chest. **A,** Anterior sequence. **B,** Lateral sequence. **C,** Posterior sequence. For palpation, place the palms of the hands in the position designated as *"1"* on the right and left sides of the chest. Compare the intensity of vibrations. Continue for all positions in each sequence. For percussion, tap the chest at each designated position, moving downward from side to side. Compare percussion sounds at all positions. For auscultation, place the stethoscope at each position and listen to at least one complete inspiratory and expiratory cycle. Keep in mind that, with a female patient, the breast tissue will modify the completeness of the anterior examination.

**TABLE 25-6 Percussion Sounds**

| Sound | Description |
|---|---|
| **Resonance** | Low-pitched sound heard over normal lungs |
| **Hyperresonance** | Loud, lower-pitched sound than normal resonance heard over hyperinflated lungs, such as in chronic obstructive pulmonary disease and acute asthma |
| **Tympany** | Drum-like, loud, empty quality sound heard over pneumothorax |
| **Dull** | Sound with medium-intensity, pitch and duration heard over areas of "mixed" solid and lung tissue, such as top area of liver, partially consolidated lung tissue (pneumonia), or fluid-filled pleural space |
| **Flat** | Soft, high-pitched sound of short duration heard over very dense tissue where air is not present, such as posterior chest below level of diaphragm |

denser. As the patient's voice moves through a dense tissue or fluid, you can feel that the vibration is increased. This is found in pneumonia, in lung tumors, with thick bronchial secretions, and above a pleural effusion (the lung is compressed upward). Fremitus is decreased if the hand is farther from the lung (e.g., pleural effusion) or the lung is hyperinflated (e.g., barrel chest). Absent fremitus may be noted with pneumothorax or atelectasis. The anterior of the chest is more difficult to palpate for fremitus because of the large muscles and breast tissue.

**Percussion.** Percussion is performed to assess the density or aeration of the lungs. Percussion sounds are described in Table 25-6. (The technique for percussion is described in Chapter 3 and Fig. 3-3.)

The anterior chest is usually percussed with the patient in a semi-sitting or supine position. Starting above the clavicles, percuss downward, interspace by interspace (Fig. 25-7). The area over lung tissue should be resonant, with the exception of the area of cardiac dullness (Fig. 25-8). For percussion of the posterior chest, have the patient sit leaning forward with arms folded. The posterior chest should be resonant over lung tissue to the level of the diaphragm (Fig. 25-9).

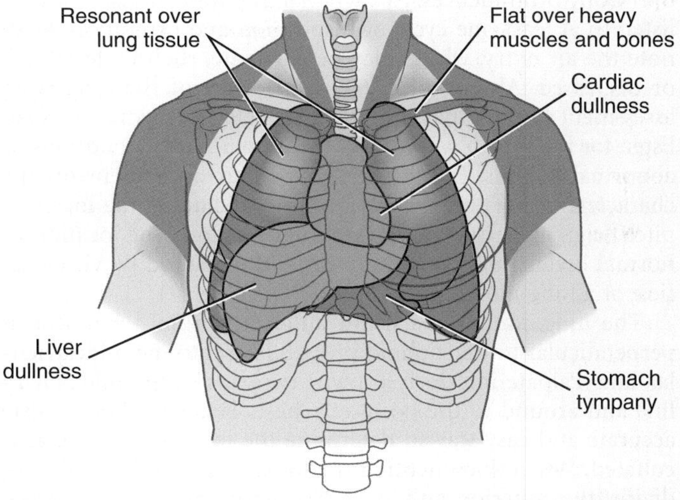


**FIG. 25-8** Diagram of percussion areas and sounds on the anterior side of the chest. (Redrawn from Thompson JM, McFarland GK, Hirsch JE, Tucker SM: *Mosby's clinical nursing,* ed 5, St Louis, 2002, Mosby.)

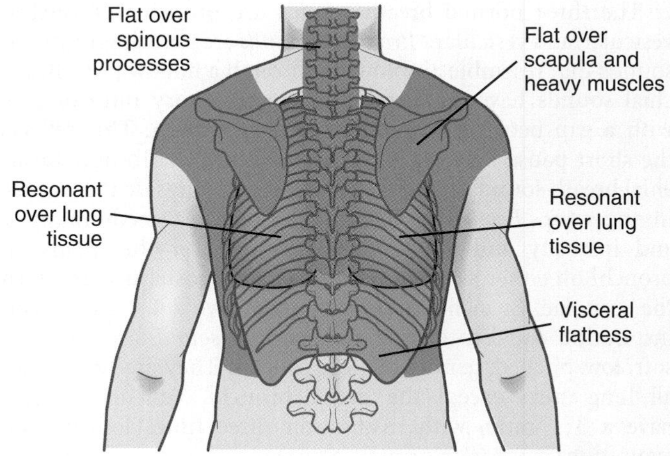


**FIG. 25-9** Diagram of percussion areas and sounds on the posterior side of the chest. Percussion proceeds from the lung apices to the lung bases while comparing sounds in opposite areas of the chest. (Redrawn from Thompson JM, McFarland GK, Hirsch JE, Tucker SM: *Mosby's clinical nursing,* ed 5, St Louis, 2002, Mosby.)

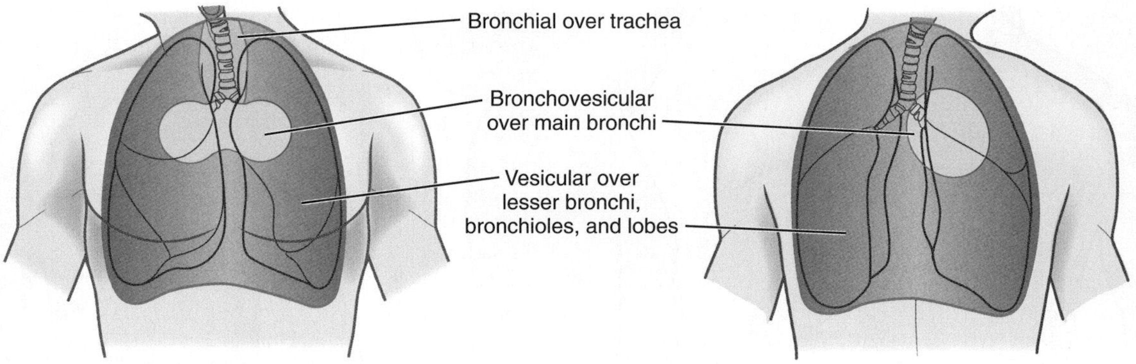


**FIG. 25-10** Normal auscultatory sounds. (Redrawn from Beare PG, Myers JL: *Adult health nursing,* ed 3, St Louis, 1998, Mosby.)

**Auscultation.** During chest auscultation, instruct the patient to breathe slowly and a little more deeply than normal through the mouth. Auscultation should proceed from the lung apices to the bases, comparing opposite areas of the chest, unless the patient is in respiratory distress or will tire easily; if so, start at the bases (Fig. 25-7). Place the stethoscope over lung tissue, not over bony prominences. At each placement of the stethoscope, listen to at least one cycle of inspiration and expiration. First, note the air entry, which may be adequate, slightly decreased, or decreased. Absent air entry in any part of the lung is an assessment finding that should be reported immediately. Next, listen for the breath sound, and the presence of adventitious or abnormal sounds. Specifically focus your assessment on the characteristics of the abnormal sound, including the location, pitch (e.g., high, low), and duration of sound. The location of normal breath sounds is more easily understood by visualization of a lung model (Fig. 25-10).

The lung sounds are heard anteriorly from a line drawn perpendicular to the xiphoid process lateral to the midclavicular line. Palpate inferiorly (down) two ribs in the midaxillary line and around to the posterior chest. This gives you a fairly accurate and easy way to determine the lung fields to be auscultated. When documenting the location of the lung sounds, divide the anterior and posterior lung into thirds (upper, middle, and lower) and note, for example, "crackles posterior right lower lung field." You are not expected to define which lobe of the lung has particular lung sounds.

The three normal breath sounds are bronchial, bronchovesicular, and vesicular.[9] *Bronchial sounds* are loud, high-pitched sounds that resemble air blowing through a hollow pipe. Bronchial sounds have an inspiratory to expiratory ratio of 2:3, with a gap between inspiration and expiration. This reflects the short pause between the respiratory cycles. To hear bronchial breath sounds, place the stethoscope alongside the trachea in the neck. *Bronchovesicular sounds* have a medium pitch and intensity and are heard anteriorly over the mainstem bronchi on either side of the sternum and posteriorly between the scapulae. Bronchovesicular sounds have a 1:1 ratio, with inspiration equal to expiration. *Vesicular sounds* are relatively soft, low-pitched, gentle, rustling sounds. They are heard over all lung areas except the major bronchi. Vesicular sounds have a 3:1 ratio, with inspiration three times longer than expiration.

A variety of terms have been used inconsistently over time to describe breath sounds.[10] Rales are now referred to as *crackles,* and rhonchi are referred to as *wheezes.* Breath sounds are categorized into two main categories: normal and abnormal (adventitious).[11] **Adventitious breath sounds** include fine crackles, coarse crackles, wheezes, stridor, and pleural friction rub (Table 25-8).

A record of the normal physical assessment of the respiratory system is shown in Table 25-7. Assessment abnormalities of the thorax and lungs are presented in Table 25-8. Chest examination findings in common pulmonary problems are presented in Table 25-9. Age-related changes in the respiratory system and assessment findings are presented in Table 25-4.

A *focused assessment* is used to evaluate the status of previously identified respiratory problems and to monitor for signs of new problems (see Chapter 3, Table 3-7). A focused assessment of the respiratory system is presented in the box on this page.

## FOCUSED ASSESSMENT

### *Respiratory System*

*Use this checklist to make sure the key assessment steps have been done.*

**Subjective**

*Ask the patient about any of the following and note responses.*

| | | |
|---|---|---|
| Shortness of breath | Y | N |
| Wheezing | Y | N |
| Sputum production (color, quantity) | Y | N |
| Pain with breathing | Y | N |
| Cough | Y | N |

**Objective: Diagnostic**

*Check the following diagnostic tests for critical values.*

| | |
|---|---|
| Arterial blood gases | ✓ |
| Chest x-ray | ✓ |
| Hct, Hgb | ✓ |

**Objective: Physical Examination**

***Observe***

| | |
|---|---|
| Respirations: Rate, quality, and pattern | ✓ |

***Inspect***

| | |
|---|---|
| Skin and nails for integrity and color | ✓ |
| Neck for position of trachea | ✓ |
| Shape, symmetry, and movement of chest wall | ✓ |

***Palpate***

| | |
|---|---|
| Chest and back for masses | ✓ |

***Auscultate***

| | |
|---|---|
| Lung (breath) sounds | ✓ |

*Hct,* Hematocrit; *Hgb,* hemoglobin.

## DIAGNOSTIC STUDIES OF RESPIRATORY SYSTEM

Numerous diagnostic studies are available to assess the respiratory system. Table 25-10 identifies the most common studies, and select studies are described in more detail below.

### Sputum Studies

Sputum samples can be obtained by expectoration, tracheal suction, or bronchoscopy (discussed later). When the patient is unable to expectorate spontaneously, sputum may also be collected by inhalation of an irritating aerosol, usually hypertonic saline. This is called *sputum induction*. The specimens may be examined for culture and sensitivity to identify an infecting organism (e.g., *Mycobacterium, Pneumocystis jiroveci*) or to confirm a diagnosis (e.g., malignant cells). Regardless of whether specimen tests are ordered, observe the sputum for color, volume, viscosity, and presence or absence of blood.

### Skin Tests

Skin tests may be performed to test for allergic reactions (see Chapter 13) or exposure to TB bacilli or fungi. Skin tests involve the intradermal injection of an antigen. A positive result on a TB skin test indicates that the patient has been exposed to the antigen. It does not indicate that TB is currently present. A negative result indicates either no exposure or a depression of cell-mediated immunity such as occurs in HIV infection (Table 25-11 for interpreting responses to tuberculin skin testing).

Nursing responsibilities are similar for all skin tests. First, to prevent a false-negative reaction, be certain that the injection is intradermal and not subcutaneous. After the injection, circle the site(s) and instruct the patient not to remove the marks. When charting administration of the antigen, draw a diagram of the forearm and hand and label the injection site. The diagram is especially helpful when more than one test is administered.

When reading test results, use a good light. If an induration is present, use a marking pen to indicate the periphery on all four sides of the induration. As the pen touches the raised area, make a mark. Then determine the diameter of the induration in millimeters. Reddened, flat areas are not measured.

### Endoscopy

**Bronchoscopy.** *Bronchoscopy* is a procedure in which the bronchi are visualized through a fiberoptic tube (Fig. 25-11). Bronchoscopy may be used for diagnostic purposes to obtain biopsy specimens and assess results of treatment. Bronchoscopy is also

**TABLE 25-7 Normal Physical Assessment of the Respiratory System**

| | |
|---|---|
| **Nose** | • Symmetric with no deformities<br>• Nasal mucosa pink, moist with no edema, exudate, blood, or polyps<br>• Nasal septum straight (slight nasal deviation possible). Nares patent bilaterally |
| **Oral mucosa** | • Light pink, moist, no exudate or ulcerations |
| **Pharynx** | • Smooth, moist, and pink |
| **Neck** | • Trachea midline |
| **Chest** | • AP (anteroposterior to lateral) diameter 1:2<br>• Respirations nonlabored at 12-20 breaths/min<br>• Breath sounds vesicular without crackles or wheezes<br>• Excursion equal bilaterally with no increase in tactile fremitus |

**TABLE 25-8 Assessment Abnormalities**

***Respiratory System***

| Finding | Description | Possible Etiology and Significance* |
|---|---|---|
| **Inspection** | | |
| Pursed-lip breathing | Exhalation through mouth with lips pursed together to slow exhalation. | COPD, asthma. Suggests ↑ breathlessness<br>Strategy taught to slow expiration, ↓ dyspnea |
| Tripod position. Inability to lie flat | Leaning forward with arms and elbows supported on overbed table. | COPD, asthma exacerbation, pulmonary edema<br>Indicates moderate to severe respiratory distress |
| Accessory muscle use. Intercostal retractions | Neck and shoulder muscles used to assist breathing; muscles between ribs pull in during inspiration. | COPD, asthma exacerbation, secretion retention<br>Indicates severe respiratory distress/failure, hypoxemia |
| Splinting | Voluntary ↓ in tidal volume to ↓ pain on chest expansion | Thoracic or abdominal incision, chest trauma, pleurisy |
| ↑ AP diameter | AP chest diameter equal to lateral. Slope of ribs more horizontal (90 degrees) to spine | COPD, asthma, cystic fibrosis, lung hyperinflation, advanced age |
| Tachypnea | Rate >20 breaths/min | Fever, anxiety, hypoxemia, restrictive lung disease<br>Magnitude of ↑ above normal rate reflects increased work of breathing. |
| Kussmaul respirations | Regular, rapid, and deep respirations | Metabolic acidosis. Increases $CO_2$ excretion |
| Cyanosis | Bluish color of skin best seen in lips and on the palpebral conjunctiva (inside the lower eyelid) | Reflects 5-6 g of hemoglobin not bound with $O_2$. ↓ $O_2$ transfer in lungs, ↓ cardiac output. Nonspecific, unreliable indicator |
| Finger clubbing | ↑ Depth, bulk, sponginess of distal portion of finger | Chronic hypoxemia, cystic fibrosis, lung cancer, bronchiectasis |
| Abdominal paradox | Inward (rather than normal outward) movement of abdomen during inspiration | Inefficient and ineffective breathing pattern. Nonspecific indicator of severe respiratory distress |
| **Palpation** | | |
| Tracheal deviation | Leftward or rightward movement of trachea from normal midline position | Nonspecific indicator of change in position of mediastinal structures. Medical emergency if caused by tension pneumothorax (trachea deviates to side opposite collapsed lung) |

*Continued*

## TABLE 25-8 Assessment Abnormalities

### *Respiratory System—cont'd*

| Finding | Description | Possible Etiology and Significance* |
|---|---|---|
| **Palpation—cont'd** | | |
| Altered tactile fremitus | Increase or decrease in vibrations | ↑ In pneumonia, pulmonary edema. ↓ in pleural effusion, lung hyperinflation. Absent in pneumothorax, atelectasis |
| Altered chest movement | Unequal or equal but diminished movement of two sides of chest with inspiration | Unequal movement caused by atelectasis, pneumothorax, pleural effusion, splinting. Equal but diminished movement caused by barrel chest, restrictive disease, neuromuscular disease |
| **Percussion** | | |
| Hyperresonance | Loud, lower-pitched sound over areas that normally produce a resonant sound | Lung hyperinflation (COPD), lung collapse (pneumothorax), air trapping (asthma) |
| Dullness | Medium-pitched sound over areas that normally produce a resonant sound | ↑ Density (pneumonia, large atelectasis), ↑ fluid in pleural space (pleural effusion) |
| **Auscultation** | | |
| Fine crackles | Series of short-duration, discontinuous, high-pitched sounds heard just before the end of inspiration. Result of rapid equalization of gas pressure when collapsed alveoli or terminal bronchioles suddenly snap open. Similar sound to that made by rolling hair between fingers | Interstitial edema (early pulmonary edema), alveolar filling (pneumonia), loss of lung volume (atelectasis), early phase of heart failure, idiopathic pulmonary fibrosis |
| Coarse crackles | Series of long-duration, discontinuous, low-pitched sounds caused by air passing through airway intermittently occluded by mucus, unstable bronchial wall. Evident on inspiration and, at times, expiration. Similar sound to blowing through straw under water. Increase in bubbling quality with more fluid | Excessive fluid within the lungs, heart failure, pulmonary edema, pneumonia with severe congestion, COPD |
| Wheezes | Continuous high-pitched squeaking or musical sound caused by rapid vibration of bronchial walls. First evident on expiration but possibly evident on inspiration as obstruction of airway increases. Possibly audible without stethoscope | Bronchospasm (caused by asthma), airway obstruction (caused by foreign body, tumor), COPD |
| Stridor | Continuous musical or crowing sound of constant pitch. Result of partial obstruction of larynx or trachea | Croup, epiglottitis, vocal cord edema after extubation, foreign body |
| Absent breath sounds | No sound evident over entire lung or area of lung | Pneumothorax, pleural effusion, mainstem bronchi obstruction, large atelectasis, pneumonectomy, lobectomy |
| Pleural friction rub | Creaking or grating sound from roughened, inflamed pleural surfaces rubbing together. Evident during inspiration, expiration, or both and no change with coughing. Often uncomfortable, especially on deep inspiration | Pleurisy, pneumonia, pulmonary infarct |
| Bronchophony, whispered pectoriloquy | Spoken or whispered syllable more distinct than normal on auscultation | Pneumonia. |
| Egophony | Spoken "E" similar to "A" on auscultation because of altered transmission of voice sounds | Pneumonia, pleural effusion |

*Limited to common etiologic factors. (Further discussion of conditions listed may be found in Chapters 26 through 28.)

## TABLE 25-9 Chest Examination Findings in Respiratory Problems

| Problem | Inspection | Palpation | Percussion | Auscultation |
|---|---|---|---|---|
| **Chronic obstructive pulmonary disease** | Barrel chest, cyanosis, tripod position, use of accessory muscles | ↓ Movement | Hyperresonant or dull if consolidation | Crackles, wheezes, distant breath sounds |
| **Asthma** | | | | |
| Exacerbation | Prolonged expiration, tripod position, pursed lips | ↓ Movement | Hyperresonance | Wheezes, ↓ breath sounds ominous sign (severely diminished air movement) |
| No exacerbation | Normal | Normal | Normal | Normal |
| **Pneumonia** | Tachypnea, use of accessory muscles, duskiness or cyanosis | ↑ Fremitus over affected area | Dull over affected areas | *Early:* Bronchial sounds<br>*Later:* Fine and/or coarse crackles, egophony, whispered pectoriloquy |
| **Atelectasis** | No change unless involves entire segment, lobe | If small, no change<br>If large, ↓ movement, ↓ fremitus | Dull over affected area | Fine crackles (may disappear with deep breaths)<br>Absent sounds if large |
| **Pulmonary edema** | Tachypnea, labored respirations, cyanosis, blood-tinged sputum | ↓ Movement or normal movement | Dull or normal depending on amount of fluid | Fine or coarse crackles |
| **Pleural effusion** | Tachypnea, use of accessory muscles | ↑ Movement<br>↑ Fremitus above effusion<br>Absent fremitus over effusion | Dull | Diminished or absent over effusion, egophony above effusion |
| **Pulmonary fibrosis** | Tachypnea | ↓ Movement | Normal | Crackles or sounds like Velcro being pulled apart |

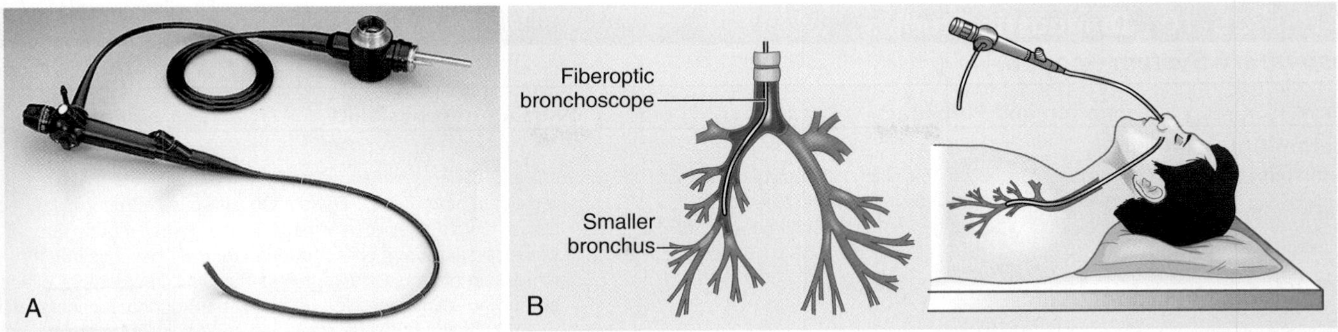


**FIG. 25-11** Fiberoptic bronchoscope. **A,** The transbronchoscopic balloon-tipped catheter and the flexible fiberoptic bronchoscope. **B,** The catheter is introduced into a small airway and the balloon inflated with 1.5 to 2 mL of air to occlude the airway. Bronchoalveolar lavage is performed by injecting and withdrawing 30-mL aliquots of sterile saline solution, gently aspirating after each instillation. Specimens are sent to the laboratory for analysis. *(A, Courtesy Olympus America Inc, Melville, N.Y.)*

## TABLE 25-10 Diagnostic Studies
### *Respiratory System*

| Study | Description and Purpose | Nursing Responsibility |
|---|---|---|
| **Blood Studies** | | |
| **Hemoglobin** | Test reflects amount of hemoglobin available for combination with $O_2$. Venous blood sample obtained.<br>*Male:* 13.2-17.3 g/dL (132-173 g/L)<br>*Female:* 11.7-16.0 g/dL (117-160 g/L) | *Before:* Explain procedure and its purpose. |
| **Hematocrit** | Test reflects ratio of RBCs to plasma. Increased hematocrit (polycythemia) found in chronic hypoxemia. Venous blood sample obtained.<br>*Male:* 39%-50% (0.39-0.50)<br>*Female:* 35%-47% (0.35-0.47) | *Before:* Explain procedure and its purpose. |
| **Arterial blood gases (ABGs)** | Arterial blood is obtained through puncture of radial or femoral artery or through arterial catheter. Performed to assess acid-base balance, oxygenation/ventilation status, need for and/or change in $O_2$ therapy, or change in ventilator settings.* | *Before:* Indicate whether patient is using $O_2$ (flow rate in L/min). Avoid change in $O_2$ therapy or interventions (e.g., suctioning, position change) for 15 min before obtaining sample.<br>*During:* Assist with positioning (e.g., palm up, wrist slightly hyperextended if radial artery is used). Collect blood in heparinized syringe. To ensure accurate results, expel all air bubbles.<br>*After:* Apply pressure to radial artery for at least 5 min after specimen is obtained to prevent hematoma at the arterial puncture site. Send sample to lab promptly for analysis. |
| **$O_2$ Monitoring** | | |
| **Oximetry** | Monitors arterial or venous $O_2$ saturation. Probe attaches to finger, toe, earlobe, bridge of the nose for $SpO_2$ monitoring or is contained in a pulmonary artery catheter for $SvO_2$ monitoring. Oximetry is used for intermittent or continuous monitoring and exercise testing.<br>*Normal $SpO_2$:* 94%-99%; *normal $SvO_2$:* 60%-80%. | *During:* Apply probe. When interpreting $SpO_2$ and $SvO_2$ values, first assess patient status and presence of factors that can alter accuracy of pulse oximeter reading. For $SpO_2$ these include motion, low perfusion, cold extremities, bright lights, acrylic nails, dark skin color, carbon monoxide, and anemia. For $SvO_2$, these include change in $O_2$ delivery or $O_2$ consumption. |
| **$CO_2$ Monitoring** | | |
| **End-tidal $CO_2$ ($PetCO_2$) (capnography)** | Assesses the level of $CO_2$ in exhaled air. Graphically displays partial pressure of $CO_2$<br>Expired gases are sampled from patient's airway and analyzed by a $CO_2$ sensor that uses infrared light to measure exhaled $CO_2$. Sensor may be attached to an adaptor on endotracheal or tracheostomy tube. A nasal cannula with a sidestream capnometer can be used in patients without an artificial airway.<br>Can be used as a diagnostic measure to detect lung disease and for monitoring patients.<br>Normal difference between $PaCO_2$ and $PetCO_2$ is 2-5 mm Hg ($PaCO_2$: 35-45 mm Hg; $PetCO_2$: 37-50 mm Hg). | *Before:* Teach patient and caregiver about purpose of capnography monitoring, emphasizing the benefit of continuous monitoring.<br>*During:* Make sure that sensor is properly attached. Record and document data per institution policy. |
| **Sputum Studies** | | |
| **Culture and sensitivity** | Purpose is to diagnose bacterial infection, select antibiotic, and evaluate treatment. Sputum specimen is collected in a sterile container. Takes 48-72 hr for results. | *Before:* Instruct patient on how to produce a good specimen (see Gram stain in this table). If patient cannot produce specimen, bronchoscopy may be used (Fig. 25-11).<br>*After:* Send specimen to laboratory promptly for analysis. |

*For reference intervals, see Table 25-1.

*Continued*

**TABLE 25-10 Diagnostic Studies**

***Respiratory System—cont'd***

| Study | Description and Purpose | Nursing Responsibility |
|---|---|---|
| **Sputum Studies—cont'd** | | |
| **Gram stain** | Staining of sputum permits classification of bacteria into gram-negative and gram-positive types. Results guide therapy until culture and sensitivity results are obtained. | *Before:* Instruct patient to expectorate sputum into container after coughing deeply. *During:* Obtain sputum (mucoidlike), not saliva. Obtain specimen in early morning after mouth care because secretions collect during night. If unsuccessful, try increasing oral fluid intake unless fluids are restricted. Collect sputum in sterile container (sputum trap) during suctioning via endotracheal tube or by aspirating secretions from the trachea. *After:* Send specimen to laboratory promptly for analysis. |
| **Acid-fast bacteria (AFB) smear and culture** | Two different tests used to assess sputum for acid-fast bacilli (e.g., *Mycobacterium tuberculosis*). In AFB smear (a rapid test), sputum sample spread thinly on glass slide, treated with a fluorochrome stain, and examined under a microscope for AFB. Culture for AFB may take up to 6 wk. | *Before:* Instruct patient how to produce a good specimen (see Gram stain in this table). *After:* Send specimen to laboratory promptly for analysis. |
| **Cytology** | Determines presence of abnormal cells that may indicate malignant condition. Single sputum specimen is collected in special container with fixative solution. | *Before:* Instruct patient on how to produce a good specimen (see Gram stain in this table). If patient cannot produce specimen, bronchoscopy may be used (Fig. 25-11). *After:* Send specimen to laboratory promptly for analysis. |
| **Radiology** | | |
| **Chest x-ray** | Used to screen, diagnose, and evaluate changes in respiratory system. Most common views are anteroposterior (AP) and lateral. | *Before:* Instruct patient to undress to waist, put on gown, and remove any metal between neck and waist. |
| **Computed tomography (CT) scan** | Performed for diagnosis of suspicious lesions difficult to assess (e.g., mediastinum, hilum, pleura) by conventional x-ray. Common types are helical or spiral CT (contrast medium is usually used) and high-resolution CT scan (contrast medium is not used). Spiral CT used to diagnose a pulmonary embolism. | Same as for chest x-ray. Contrast medium may be given IV. *Before:* Before contrast medium used evaluate BUN and serum creatinine to assess renal function. Assess if patient is allergic to shellfish (iodine), since the contrast is iodine based. Be sure the patient is well hydrated before and after procedure (to excrete contrast). *During:* Warn patient that contrast injection may cause a feeling of being warm and flushed. Instruct patient to lie still on a hard table and that scanner will revolve around body with clicking noises. |
| **Magnetic resonance imaging (MRI)** | Used for in-depth diagnosis of lesions difficult to assess by CT scan (e.g., lung apex) and for differentiating vascular from nonvascular structures. | Same as for chest x-ray and CT scan, except contrast medium is not iodine based. *Before:* Explain MRI unit will be close to patient's body. If patient has claustrophobia, provide relaxation suggestions to help cope. Patient must remove all metal (e.g., jewelry, watch) before test. Patients with pacemakers and implantable cardioverter-defibrillators may not be able to have MRI. |
| **Ventilation-perfusion (V/Q) scan** | Used to assess ventilation and perfusion of lungs. IV radioisotope given to assess perfusion. For the ventilation portion, patient inhales a radioactive gas (xenon or krypton) that outlines alveoli. Normal scans show homogeneous radioactivity. Diminished or absent radioactivity suggests lack of perfusion or airflow. Ventilation without perfusion suggests a pulmonary embolus. | Same as for chest x-ray. No precautions needed afterward because the gas and isotope transmit radioactivity for only a brief interval. Not useful for patients in critical care who are intubated and mechanically ventilated. |
| **Pulmonary angiogram** | Used to visualize pulmonary vasculature and locate obstruction or pathologic conditions (e.g., pulmonary embolus). Contrast medium is injected through a catheter threaded into pulmonary artery or right side of heart. Series of x-rays are taken after contrast medium is injected into pulmonary artery. Chest CT is replacing angiography, since it is less invasive. | Same as for chest x-ray. (See CT scan in this table for contrast media precautions.) *After:* Check pressure dressing site after procedure. Monitor BP, pulse, and circulation distal to injection site. Report and record significant changes. |
| **Positron emission tomography (PET) scan** | Used to distinguish benign from malignant pulmonary nodules. Because malignant lung cells have an increased uptake of glucose, the PET scan, which uses an IV radioactive glucose preparation, can demonstrate increased uptake of glucose in malignant lung cells. | *Before:* Patient is NPO at least 4-6 hr preprocedure. Check the blood glucose levels as high levels may interfere with test. *After:* Encourage fluids to excrete radioactive substance. |
| **Endoscopy** | | |
| **Bronchoscopy** (Fig. 25-11) | Flexible fiberoptic scope is used for diagnosis, biopsy, specimen collection, or assessment of changes. It may also be done to suction mucous plugs, lavage lungs, or remove foreign objects. | *Before:* Obtain signed consent. Instruct patient to be NPO for 6-12 hr before the test. Give sedative (as ordered). *After:* Keep patient NPO until gag reflex returns. Monitor for recovery from sedation. Blood-tinged mucus is not abnormal. If biopsy was done, monitor for hemorrhage and pneumothorax. |

TABLE 25-10 **Diagnostic Studies**
***Respiratory System—cont'd***

| Study | Description and Purpose | Nursing Responsibility |
|---|---|---|
| **Mediastinoscopy** | Scope is inserted through a small incision in suprasternal notch and advanced into mediastinum to inspect and biopsy lymph nodes. Used to diagnose lung cancer, non-Hodgkin's lymphoma, granulomatous infections, and sarcoidosis. | *Before:* Obtain signed consent. Prepare patient for surgical intervention. Performed in OR using a general anesthetic<br>*After:* Monitor as for bronchoscopy. |
| **Lung Biopsy** | Specimens may be obtained by transbronchial or percutaneous biopsy or via transthoracic needle aspiration (TTNA), video-assisted thoracoscopic surgery (VATS), or open lung biopsy. Transbronchial biopsy and VATS can be performed in the bronchoscopy suite. TTNA is done under CT guidance in radiology department. Open lung is performed in the OR. VATS can also be done in the OR. These tests are used to obtain specimens for laboratory analysis. | *Before:* Obtain signed consent. Same as bronchoscopy if procedure done with bronchoscope, and same as thoracotomy if open lung biopsy done<br>*After TTNA:* Check breath sounds q4hr for 24 hr and report any respiratory distress. Check incision site for bleeding. A chest x-ray should be done after TTNA or transbronchial biopsy to check for pneumothorax.<br>*After VATS:* A chest tube may be placed postprocedure until lung has reexpanded. Monitor breath sounds to follow chest reexpansion. Encourage deep breathing for lung reinflation. |
| **Thoracentesis** (Fig. 25-13) | Used to obtain specimen of pleural fluid for diagnosis, remove pleural fluid, or instill medication. Chest x-ray is always obtained after procedure to check for pneumothorax. | *Before:* Explain procedure to patient and obtain signed consent before procedure.<br>*During:* Usually performed in patient's room. Position patient upright with elbows on an overbed table and feet supported. Instruct patient not to talk or cough during procedure.<br>*After:* Observe for signs of hypoxia and pneumothorax, and verify breath sounds in all fields. Encourage deep breaths to expand lungs. Send labeled specimens to laboratory promptly for analysis. |
| **Pulmonary Function Tests** | Used to evaluate lung function. Involves use of spirometer to assess air movement as patient performs prescribed respiratory maneuvers.† | *Before:* Avoid scheduling immediately after mealtime. Avoid administration of inhaled bronchodilator 6 hr before procedure. Explain procedure to patient. Assess for respiratory distress.<br>*During:* Assess for respiratory distress.<br>*After:* Assess for respiratory distress. Provide rest after procedure. |
| **Exercise Testing** | Used in diagnosis and determining exercise capacity. A *complete test* involves walking on a treadmill while expired $O_2$ and $CO_2$, respiratory rate, heart rate, and heart rhythm are monitored. In a *modified test* (desaturation test) only $SpO_2$ is monitored. | *Before:* Instruct patient to wear comfortable shoes.<br>*During:* Encourage patient to hold handlebars on treadmill and walk as quickly as possible. |
| **6-Min walk test** | Used to measure functional capacity and response to treatment in patients with heart or lung disease. Pulse oximetry is usually monitored during walk. Distance walked is measured and used to monitor progression of disease or improvement after rehabilitation. | *During:* Patient is instructed by a trained practitioner to walk as far as possible during 6 min, stopping when short of breath and continuing when able. Continually assess and observe patient tolerance to test. |

†For reference intervals, see Tables 25-12 and 25-13.

used for treatment (e.g., to remove mucous plugs or foreign bodies). Laser therapy, electrocautery, cryotherapy, and stents may be placed through a bronchoscope to achieve patency of an airway that has been completely or partially obstructed by tumors.

Bronchoscopy can be performed in an outpatient procedure room, in a surgical suite, or at the bedside in the intensive care unit or on a medical-surgical unit, with the patient lying down or seated. The bronchoscope may be inserted through either the nose or the mouth. Depending upon the approach, after the nasopharynx or oropharynx are anesthetized with local anesthetic spray, the bronchoscope is coated with water-soluble lubricant and inserted down into the airways. Small amounts (30 mL) of sterile saline may be injected through the scope and withdrawn and examined for cells, a technique termed *bronchoalveolar lavage* (BAL). On mechanically ventilated patients in ICU, bronchoscopy can be done through the endotracheal tube.

## Lung Biopsy

Lung biopsy may be done (1) transbronchially, (2) percutaneously or via transthoracic needle aspiration (TTNA), (3) by video-assisted thoracic surgery (VATS), or (4) as an open lung biopsy. The purpose of a lung biopsy is to obtain tissue, cells, or secretions for evaluation. Transbronchial lung biopsy involves passing a forceps or needle through the bronchoscope for a specimen (Fig. 25-12). Specimens can be cultured or examined for malignant cells. A combination of transbronchial lung biopsy and BAL is used to differentiate infection and rejection in lung transplant recipients.

The procedure for percutaneous or TTNA involves inserting a needle through the chest wall, usually under CT guidance. Because of the risk of a pneumothorax, a chest x-ray is ordered after TTNA.

In VATS a rigid scope with a lens is passed through a trocar placed into the pleura via one or two small incisions in the intercostal muscles. The physician views the lesions on a monitor directly via the scope, and biopsy specimens can be taken. A chest tube is kept in place until the lung expands. Lesions in the pleura or peripheral lung are biopsied via VATS. VATS is much less invasive than open lung biopsy and is the procedure of choice when appropriate.

**TABLE 25-11 Interpreting Responses to Tuberculin Skin Testing**

| Types of Responses | Consider Positive in the Following Groups |
|---|---|
| **Positive Reactions** | |
| ≥5-mm induration | • HIV-infected people<br>• People who had recent contact with a person with TB disease<br>• People with fibrotic lesions on chest x-ray consistent with prior TB<br>• Patients with organ transplants<br>• People who are immunosuppressed (e.g., taking the equivalent of ≥15 mg/day of prednisone for ≥1 mo) |
| ≥10-mm induration | • Recent immigrants (<5 yr) from high-prevalence countries<br>• Injecting drug users<br>• Residents and employees of high-risk congregate settings<br>• Mycobacteriology laboratory personnel<br>• People with clinical conditions (e.g., diabetes mellitus, end-stage kidney disease) that place them at high risk |
| ≥15-mm induration | • Any person (including those with no known risk factors for TB) |
| **False Reactions** | **Possible Causes** |
| False-negative reactions (do not react even though infected) | • Anergy, immunosuppression<br>• Recent TB infection (within 8-10 wk of exposure)<br>• Overwhelming TB infection<br>• Very old TB infection (many years)<br>• Recent live virus vaccination (e.g., measles, chickenpox) |
| False-positive reactions (react even though not infected) | • Nontuberculous mycobacteria (e.g., *Mycobacterium avium-intracellulare* [MAI] or *Mycobacterium avium* complex [MAC])<br>• Previous BCG vaccine |

Source: Centers for Disease Control and Prevention: Tuberculosis (TB) fact sheet: tuberculin skin testing. Retrieved from *www.cdc.gov/tb/publications/factsheets/testing/skintesting.htm.*

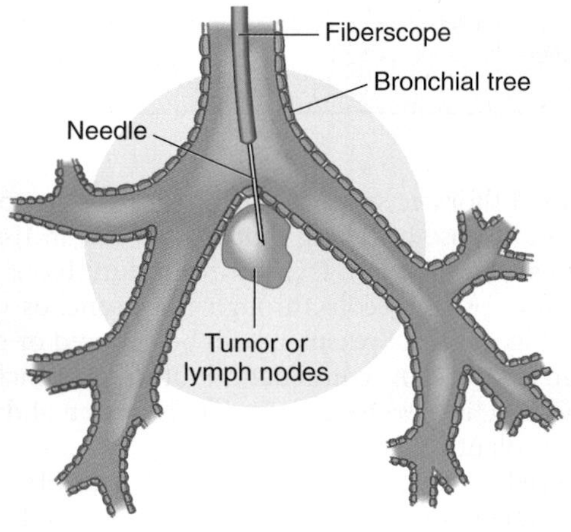


**FIG. 25-12** Transbronchial biopsy needle penetrating the bronchial wall and entering a mass of subcarinal lymph nodes or tumor. (Redrawn from Du Bois RM, Clarke SW: *Fiberoptic bronchoscopy in diagnosis and management,* Orlando, 1987, Grune & Stratton.)

Open lung biopsy is used when pulmonary disease cannot be diagnosed by other procedures. The patient is anesthetized, the chest is opened with a thoracotomy incision, and a biopsy specimen is obtained. Nursing care for the procedure is the same as after thoracotomy (see Chapter 27).

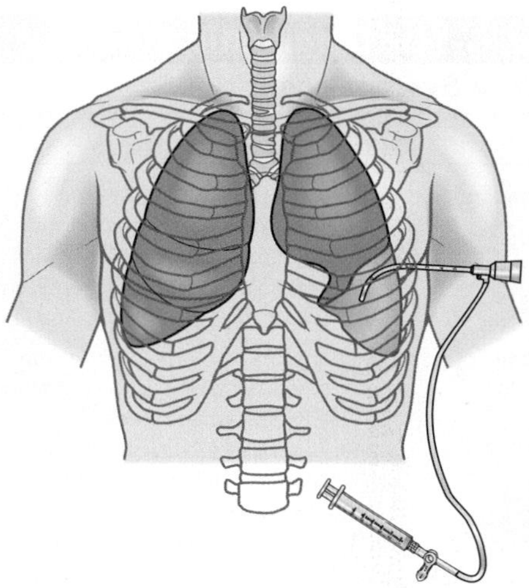

**FIG. 25-13** Thoracentesis. A catheter is positioned in the pleural space to remove accumulated fluid.

## Thoracentesis

*Thoracentesis* is the insertion of a large-bore needle through the chest wall into the pleural space to obtain specimens for diagnostic evaluation, remove pleural fluid, or instill medication (Fig. 25-13). The patient is positioned sitting upright with elbows on an overbed table and feet supported. The skin is cleansed and a local anesthetic (lidocaine) is injected subcutaneously. A chest tube may be inserted to permit further drainage of fluid.

## Pulmonary Function Tests

*Pulmonary function tests* (PFTs) measure lung volumes and airflow. The results of PFTs are used to diagnose pulmonary disease, monitor disease progression, evaluate disability, and assess response to bronchodilators. Airflow measurement is administered by trained personnel using a spirometer. The patient inserts a mouthpiece, takes as deep a breath as possible, and exhales as hard, fast, and for as long as possible. Verbal coaching is given to ensure that the patient continues blowing out until exhalation is complete.

The computer calculates the patient's percentage of predicted values, that is, how well the performance compares with an average based on age, gender, race, and height.[12] Normal values are approximately 80% to 120% of the predicted value. Normal values for PFTs are shown in Tables 25-12 and 25-13.

Spirometry may be ordered before and after the administration of a bronchodilator to determine the patient's response. This may help document reversibility of airway obstruction (e.g., asthma). A positive response to the bronchodilator is greater than 200 mL increase or greater than 12% increase between preadministration and postadministration values.

Home spirometry may be used to monitor lung function in people with asthma, cystic fibrosis, or COPD, as well as before and after lung transplantation or other thoracic surgeries. A peak flow meter is the instrument used at home. It is a hand-held device through which one blows forcefully and quickly after taking a deep breath. Spirometry changes at home can warn of early lung transplant rejection or infection. Data from a peak flow meter provide important feedback to patients with asthma so that they can learn to modify activities and medications in response to changes in peak expiratory flow rates (see Chapter 28).

More specific pulmonary function parameters can be directly assessed at the bedside in the high-acuity or critical care unit to determine the need for or liberation (weaning and extubation) from mechanical ventilation (see Table 65-13).

### TABLE 25-12 Lung Volumes and Capacities

| Parameter | Definitions | Normal Value* |
|---|---|---|
| **Volumes** | | |
| **Tidal volume (VT)** | Volume of air inhaled and exhaled with each breath. Only a small proportion of total capacity of lungs | 0.5 L |
| **Expiratory reserve volume (ERV)** | Additional air that can be forcefully exhaled after normal exhalation is complete | 1.0 L |
| **Residual volume (RV)** | Amount of air remaining in lungs after forced expiration. Air available in lungs for gas exchange between breaths | 1.5 L |
| **Inspiratory reserve volume (IRV)** | Maximum volume of air that can be inhaled forcefully after normal inhalation | 3.0 L |
| **Capacities** | | |
| **Total lung capacity (TLC)** | Maximum volume of air that lungs can contain (TLC = IRV + VT + ERV + RV) | 6.0 L |
| **Functional residual capacity (FRC)** | Volume of air remaining in lungs at end of normal exhalation (FRC = ERV + RV). Increase or decrease possible with lung disease | 2.5 L |
| **Vital capacity (VC)** | Maximum volume of air that can be exhaled after maximum inspiration (VC = IRV + VT + ERV). Higher VC for men (generally) | 4.5 L |
| **Inspiratory capacity (IC)** | Maximum volume of air that can be inhaled after normal expiration (IC = VT + IRV) | 3.5 L |

*Normal values vary with patient's height, weight, age, race, and gender.

### TABLE 25-13 Pulmonary Function Airflow

| Measure | Description | Normal Value* |
|---|---|---|
| **Forced vital capacity (FVC)** | Amount of air that can be quickly and forcefully exhaled after maximum inspiration | >80% of predicted |
| **Forced expiratory volume in first second of expiration ($FEV_1$)** | Amount of air exhaled in first second of FVC. Grades severity of airway obstruction | >80% of predicted |
| **$FEV_1$/FVC ratio** | Dividing value for $FEV_1$ by value for FVC. Useful in differentiating obstructive and restrictive pulmonary dysfunction | *Age <50:* ≥75% of predicted *Age ≥50:* ≥70% of predicted |
| **Forced midexpiratory flow rate ($FEF_{25\%-75\%}$)** | Measurement of airflow rate in middle half of forced expiration. Early indicator of disease of small airways | *Age <50:* ≥75% of predicted *Age ≥50:* ≥70% of predicted |
| **Maximal voluntary ventilation (MVV)** | Deep breathing as rapidly as possible for specified period. Fairly nonspecific test that gives information about exercise capacity. Used in conjunction with exercise stress test | About 170 L/min |
| **Peak expiratory flow rate (PEFR)** | Maximum airflow rate during forced expiration. Aids in monitoring bronchoconstriction in asthma. Can be measured with peak flow meter | Up to 600 L/min |

*Normal values vary with patient's height, age, race, and gender.

## CASE STUDY

### *Objective Data: Diagnostic Studies*

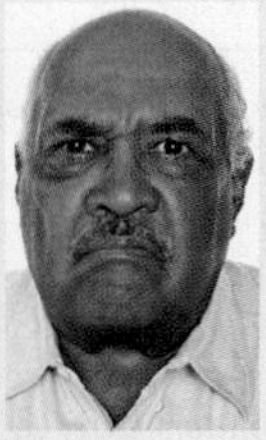

(©Fuse/ Thinkstock)

The HCP orders the following diagnostic studies for F.T.:

- CBC, basic metabolic panel (electrolytes, BUN, creatinine)
- ABGs
- Chest x-ray
- Sputum for culture and sensitivity

The ABGs indicate a compensated respiratory alkalosis with hypoxemia. The WBC is 17,350/µL, potassium 2.9 mEq/L, and chest x-ray shows bilateral consolidation to both lower lobes. F.T. is admitted to the cardiopulmonary medical-surgical nursing unit.

**Discussion Questions**

1. Are these the diagnostic studies that you expected to be ordered?
2. Of the diagnostic test results, is anything abnormal?
3. Of the diagnostic test results, which ones are of most concern to you?
4. What do you think is the pathophysiologic cause of F.T.'s problems?
5. F.T. asks you what he could have done differently to prevent this problem from happening. What will you tell him?
6. F.T. will be admitted to the hospital. What patient teaching can you do with F.T. as he is waiting to be admitted?
7. What is the interprofessional team's top priority for F.T. at this time?
8. What patient outcomes would indicate that the interprofessional team was effective?

You will learn more about the upper and lower respiratory problems and chronic obstructive pulmonary disease (COPD) in the next three chapters.

Answers available at *http://evolve.elsevier.com/Lewis/medsurg.*

## BRIDGE TO NCLEX EXAMINATION

The number of the question corresponds to the same-numbered learning outcome identified at the beginning of this chapter.

1. To promote the release of surfactant, the nurse encourages the patient to
   **a.** take deep breaths.
   **b.** cough five times per hour to prevent alveolar collapse.
   **c.** decrease fluid intake to reduce fluid accumulation in the alveoli.
   **d.** sit with head of bed elevated to promote air movement through the pores of Kohn.
2. A patient with a respiratory condition asks, "How does air get into my lungs?" The nurse bases her answer on knowledge that air moves into the lungs because of
   **a.** increased $CO_2$ and decreased $O_2$ in the blood.
   **b.** contraction of the accessory abdominal muscles.
   **c.** stimulation of the respiratory muscles by the chemoreceptors.
   **d.** decrease in intrathoracic pressure relative to pressure at the airway.

3. The nurse can *best* determine adequate arterial oxygenation of the blood by assessing
   a. heart rate.
   b. hemoglobin level.
   c. arterial oxygen partial pressure.
   d. arterial carbon dioxide partial pressure.
4. When teaching a patient about the *most* important respiratory defense mechanism distal to the respiratory bronchioles, which topic would the nurse discuss?
   a. Alveolar macrophages
   b. Impaction of particles
   c. Reflex bronchoconstriction
   d. Mucociliary clearance mechanism
5. A student nurse asks the RN what can be measured by arterial blood gas (ABG). The RN tells the student that the ABG can measure *(select all that apply)*
   a. acid-base balance.
   b. oxygenation status.
   c. acidity of the blood.
   d. bicarbonate ($HCO_3^-$) in arterial blood.
   e. overall balance of electrolytes in arterial blood.
6. To detect early signs or symptoms of inadequate oxygenation, the nurse would examine the patient for
   a. dyspnea and hypotension.
   b. apprehension and restlessness.
   c. cyanosis and cool, clammy skin.
   d. increased urine output and diaphoresis.
7. During the respiratory assessment of an older adult, the nurse would expect to find *(select all that apply)*
   a. a vigorous reflex cough.
   b. increased chest expansion.
   c. increased residual volume.
   d. diminished lung sounds at base of lungs.
   e. increased anteroposterior (AP) chest diameter.
8. When assessing activity-exercise patterns related to respiratory health, the nurse inquires about
   a. dyspnea during rest or exercise.
   b. recent weight loss or weight gain.
   c. ability to sleep through the entire night.
   d. willingness to wear $O_2$ equipment in public.
9. When auscultating the chest of an older patient in respiratory distress, it is *best* to
   a. begin listening at the apices.
   b. begin listening at the lung bases.
   c. begin listening on the anterior chest.
   d. Ask the patient to breathe through the nose with the mouth closed.
10. Which assessment finding of the respiratory system does the nurse interpret as abnormal?
    a. Inspiratory chest expansion of 1 inch
    b. Symmetric chest expansion and contraction
    c. Resonance (to percussion) over the lung bases
    d. Bronchial breath sounds in the lower lung fields
11. The nurse is preparing the patient for a diagnostic procedure to remove pleural fluid for analysis. The nurse would prepare the patient for which test?
    a. Thoracentesis
    b. Bronchoscopy
    c. Pulmonary angiography
    d. Sputum culture and sensitivity

1. a, 2. d, 3. c, 4. a, 5. a, b, c, d, 6. b, 7. c, d, e, 8. a, 9. b, 10. d, 11. a

For rationales to these answers and even more NCLEX review questions, visit *http://evolve.elsevier.com/Lewis/medsurg.*

## EVOLVE WEBSITE

http://evolve.elsevier.com/Lewis/medsurg

**Review Questions (Online Only)**

**Key Points**

**Answer Keys for Questions**

- Rationales for Bridge to NCLEX Examination Questions
- Answer Guidelines for Case Study on pp. 460, 463, 464, and 473

**Conceptual Care Map Creator**

**Audio Glossary**

**Supporting Media**

- Animations
  - Inhalation
  - Oxygenation
  - Pulse Oximetry
  - Respiration Cycle
  - Respiratory System Overview
- Audio
  - Bronchial Breath Sounds
  - Bronchovesicular Breath Sounds
  - High-Pitched Crackles
  - High-Pitched Wheeze
  - Low-Pitched Crackles
  - Low-Pitched Wheeze
  - Pleural Friction Rub
  - Stridor
  - Vesicular Breath Sounds

**Content Updates**

## REFERENCES


1. McCance KL, Huether SE: *Pathophysiology: the biological basis for disease in adults and children*, ed 7, St Louis, 2014, Mosby.
2. Urden LD, Stacy KM, Lough ME: *Critical care nursing: diagnosis and management*, ed 7, St Louis, 2013, Mosby.
3. Patton KT, Thibodeau GA. *The human body in health and disease*, ed 6, St Louis, 2014, Mosby.
4. Heuer AJ, Scanlan CL: *Wilkins' clinical assessment in respiratory care*, ed 7, St Louis, 2014, Mosby.
5. Mechem CC: Pulse oximetry. Retrieved from *www.uptodate.com/contents/pulse-oximetry.*
6. Press CD: End tidal capnography. Retrieved from *http://emedicine.medscape.com/article/2116444.*
7. Jarvis C: *Physical examination and health assessment*, ed 7, St Louis, 2015, Elsevier.
8. Ball JW, Dains JE, Flynn JA, et al: *Seidel's guide to physical examination*, ed 8, St Louis, 2015, Saunders.
9. Bohadana A, Izbicki G, Kraman SS: Fundamentals of lung auscultation, *NEJM* 370:744, 2014.
10. Mikami R, Murao M, Cugell DW, et al: International symposium on lung sounds: Synopsis of proceedings, *Chest* 2:342, 1987. (Classic)
11. Stahlheber CL: Breath sound assessment. Retrieved from *http://emedicine.medscape.com/article/1894146.*
12. Dancer R, Thickett D: Pulmonary function tests, *Medicine* 40:186, 2012.

# 26

# Upper Respiratory Problems

*Eugene E. Mondor*

*When you own your breath, nobody can steal your peace.*

**Author unknown**

http://evolve.elsevier.com/Lewis/medsurg/

## LEARNING OUTCOMES

1. Describe the clinical manifestations and nursing and interprofessional management of problems of the nose.
2. Discuss the clinical manifestations and nursing and interprofessional management of problems of the paranasal sinuses.
3. Describe the clinical manifestations and nursing and interprofessional management of problems of the pharynx and larynx.
4. Discuss the nursing and interprofessional management of the patient who requires a tracheostomy.
5. Identify the steps involved in performing tracheostomy care and suctioning an airway.
6. Describe the risk factors for and clinical manifestations of head and neck cancer.
7. Discuss the nursing and interprofessional management of patients requiring surgery for head and neck cancer.
8. Explain essential components of discharge teaching for the patient going home with a permanent tracheostomy after total laryngectomy for cancer.

## KEY TERMS

allergic rhinitis, p. 477
decannulation, p. 490
deviated septum, p. 475
epistaxis, p. 476
nasal polyps, p. 483
rhinoplasty, p. 476
sinusitis, p. 482
tracheostomy, p. 485

Disorders of the upper respiratory system, including nose, sinuses, pharynx, and larynx, are presented in this chapter. Nursing management of patients with a tracheostomy or requiring surgery for head and neck cancer is also discussed.

## PROBLEMS OF NOSE AND PARANASAL SINUSES

### DEVIATED SEPTUM

**Deviated septum** is a deflection of the normally straight nasal septum. Although up to 80% of adults may have septa that are slightly off center, the diagnosis of deviated septum is generally reserved for those whose septa are severely shifted.[1] Trauma to the nose, either at birth or later in life, is the most common cause of deviated septum.[2] Deviation of the septum from midline can interfere with both airflow and sinus drainage through the narrowed passageway.

Symptoms vary depending on the degree of deviation. Minor septal deviations may be asymptomatic. Manifestations of severe septal deviation include obstruction to nasal breathing, nasal congestion, frequent sinus infections, nosebleeds *(epistaxis)*, and facial pain.

The diagnosis of deviated septum is made by an HCP during physical examination with a nasal speculum. Medical management of minor septal deviation is focused on symptom control of nasal inflammation and congestion using saline rinses and decongestants to clear nasal passages. For severe septal deviation, a nasal septoplasty, performed under local or general anesthetic, reconstructs and properly aligns the deviated septum.

### NASAL FRACTURE

*Nasal fracture* is the most common facial fracture and the third most common fracture of any bone.[3] Fracture of the nose most often occurs as a result of blunt trauma, including fights, automobile accidents, falls, and sports injuries. Complications associated with nasal fractures include airway obstruction, epistaxis, meningeal tears causing cerebrospinal fluid (CSF) leakage, septal hematoma, and cosmetic deformity. Many cases of facial trauma can be prevented by using protective sports equipment and protecting against falls.

There is no standardized classification system for nasal fractures. Most nasal fractures, however, can be classified as simple or complex. *Simple fractures* may be unilateral or bilateral and

Reviewed by Donna C. Bond, RN, DNP, CCNS, AE-C, CTTS, Pulmonary Clinical Nurse Specialist, Carilion Clinic, Roanoke, Virginia; Marylee Bressie, RN, DNP, CCRN, CCNS, CEN, Core Faculty/Nurse Planner, Department of Nursing, School of Public Service Leadership, Capella University, Minneapolis, Minnesota; Deborah Cline, RN, MS, Nursing Faculty, Carrington College, Reno, Nevada; and Cynthia M. Steinwedel, RN, PhD, CNE, Assistant Professor, Department of Nursing, Bradley University, Peoria, Illinois.

typically produce little or no displacement. Powerful frontal blows can cause *complex fractures,* which may also involve subsequent damage to adjacent facial structures such as the teeth or eyes. Patients with complex nasal fractures should be evaluated for possible injury to the cervical spine and orbital or mandibular fractures.[4]

Diagnosis of a nasal fracture is based on the health history and physical examination. Clinical manifestations suggestive of a nasal fracture include localized pain, crepitus on palpation, swelling, difficulty breathing out of the nostrils, epistaxis, ecchymosis, and cosmetic deformity. Although facial deformity with a nasal fracture is common, often epistaxis may be the only initial manifestation of a nasal fracture.

On inspection, assess the patient's ability to breathe through each side of the nose and note the presence of edema, bleeding, or hematoma. Ecchymosis may be under one or both eyes. Ecchymosis involving both eyes is often termed *raccoon eyes* and may suggest a basilar skull fracture (see Chapter 56). Inspect the nose internally for evidence of septal deviation, hemorrhage, or clear drainage.

Clear, pink-tinged, or persistent drainage after control of epistaxis suggests a possible CSF leak. Checking this fluid for glucose at the bedside to help confirm the presence of CSF is highly unreliable and influenced by many factors. If possible, send a specimen to the laboratory to determine the fluid type. Goals of nursing management are to maintain the airway, reduce edema and pain, prevent complications, and provide emotional support.

The best way to maintain the airway is to keep the patient sitting upright. Apply ice to the face and nose in 10- to 20-minute intervals to help reduce edema and bleeding. Administer analgesia as ordered to control pain. Acetaminophen is preferred over nonsteroidal antiinflammatory drugs (NSAIDs) or acetylsalicylic acid (ASA; aspirin) for the first 48 hours to avoid prolonging clotting time and increasing the risk for bleeding. Nasal stuffiness may be relieved with nasal decongestants, saline nasal sprays, and a humidifier. The patient should avoid hot showers and alcohol for the first 48 hours to prevent an increase in swelling. Encourage the patient to quit or decrease smoking to facilitate tissue healing.

When a fracture is confirmed, the goals are to realign the fracture using closed or open reduction.[5] Simple fractures are often reduced with manual manipulation. With complex nasal fractures, considerable swelling of soft tissues occurs, and it may be necessary to wait to repair the fracture until after the edema subsides, which may be 5 to 10 days.

Septoplasty and rhinoplasty are surgical options. These procedures provide an adequate airway and function of the nose, and help to reestablish a person's cosmetic appearance. The presence of septal hematoma increases the patient's risk for infection, which may necessitate drainage and antibiotic therapy.

## RHINOPLASTY

**Rhinoplasty**, surgical reconstruction of the nose, is performed to improve airway function (when trauma or developmental deformities result in nasal obstruction) or for cosmetic reasons. When caring for rhinoplasty patients before surgery, assess the patient's expectations of the surgery. Actual or perceived alterations in body image (e.g., deformed or enlarged nose) can affect self-esteem and interactions with others. Computerized photographs can be used to show the patient's appearance after the surgery. These images can help patients decide whether to undergo rhinoplasty.

Rhinoplasty is often performed as an outpatient procedure using regional or general anesthesia. Nasal tissue is added or removed, and the nose may be lengthened or shortened. Plastic implants are sometimes used to reshape the nose. Incisions are typically inside the nose and hidden. Sonic rhinoplasty incorporates the use of an ultrasonic device to gently aspirate bone, enabling a refined cosmetic result.[6]

After surgery, nasal packing may be inserted in some patients to apply pressure and prevent bleeding or septal hematoma formation. An external plastic splint protects and supports the new shape of the nose during the healing process. If present, nasal packing is usually removed 1 or 2 days after surgery. The splint may be left in place for approximately 1 to 2 weeks.

## ❖ NURSING MANAGEMENT: NASAL SURGERY

Before surgery, instruct patients to notify the HCP about any medications that they take at home. Aspirin-containing drugs and NSAIDs may have to be discontinued for 5 days to 2 weeks preoperatively to reduce the risk of bleeding. Encourage smoking cessation to promote postoperative wound healing. During the immediate postoperative period, nursing interventions include maintenance of the airway; assessment of respiratory status; pain management; and observation of the surgical site for bleeding, infection, and edema.

Teaching is important because the patient must be able to detect complications at home. The patient typically experiences temporary edema and ecchymosis. Cold compresses and elevation of the head can help minimize swelling and discomfort. Teach about activity restrictions aimed at preventing bleeding and injury (no nose blowing, swimming, heavy lifting, strenuous exercise). Subtle swelling may be slow to resolve, delaying the achievement of a full cosmetic result for up to 1 year.

## EPISTAXIS

**Epistaxis** (nosebleed) most often occurs in adults over age 50. Epistaxis can be caused by trauma, hypertension, low humidity, upper respiratory tract infections, allergies, sinusitis, foreign bodies, chemical irritants (such as street drugs), overuse of decongestant nasal sprays, facial or nasal surgery, anatomic malformation, and tumors.[7] Conditions that prolong bleeding time or alter platelet counts will predispose the patient to epistaxis. Bleeding time may be prolonged if the patient takes aspirin, NSAIDs, warfarin, or other anticoagulant drugs.

Approximately 90% of nosebleeds occur in the anterior portion of the nasal cavity and are easily visualized. Anterior bleeding can be self-treated and usually stops spontaneously. Posterior bleeding may require medical treatment.

Posterior bleeding occurs more commonly with older adults secondary to other health problems (e.g., hypertension). Since posterior nosebleeds occur closer to the throat, it is often difficult to determine how much blood loss has occurred.

## ❖ NURSING AND INTERPROFESSIONAL MANAGEMENT: EPISTAXIS

Use simple first aid measures to control epistaxis including (1) calm the patient; (2) place the patient in a sitting position, leaning slightly forward with head tilted forward; and (3) apply direct pressure by squeezing the entire soft lower portion of the nose (nostrils) together for 5 to 15 minutes. If bleeding does not stop within 15 minutes, seek medical assistance.

Medical management involves attempting to identify the location of the bleed. For anterior bleeds, a pledget (nasal tampon) impregnated with anesthetic solution (lidocaine) and/or vasoconstrictive agents such as epinephrine may be placed into the nasal cavity. Alternatively, absorbable materials such as oxidized cellulose (surgical), gelatin foam (Gelfoam), or a gelatin-thrombin combination (Floseal) may be used. Packing for anterior bleeds can remain in place for 48 to 72 hours. Silver nitrate may also be used to chemically cauterize an identified bleeding point. Thermal cauterization is reserved for more severe bleeding and may require the use of local or general anesthesia.[8]

It may be much more difficult to identify the location of a posterior bleed. Posterior bleeds often require packing. Packing with compressed nasal sponges (e.g., Merocel) or epistaxis balloons (e.g., Rapid Rhino) is preferred over the use of traditional Vaseline ribbon gauze because of the ease of placement. Packing is inserted into the nares and advanced along the floor of the nasal cavity. The sponge expands with moisture to fill the nasal cavity and tamponade bleeding. The epistaxis balloon is inflated with air to achieve the same pressure effect (Fig. 26-1). In the absence of a specific nasal device, a size 10F, 12F, or 14F Foley catheter with a 30 mL balloon may be used. A nasal sling (folded 2 × 2-inch gauze pad) may be gently taped under the nares to absorb drainage. If packing fails to stop the bleeding, arterial embolization may be required.

Nasal sponges, packing, and balloons may impair respiratory status. Closely monitor the level of consciousness, heart rate and rhythm, respiratory rate, $O_2$ saturation using pulse oximetry ($SpO_2$), and observe for any signs of difficulty breathing or swallowing. Because of the risk of complications, all patients with posterior packing should be admitted to a monitored unit for close observation.

Nasal packing is painful because sufficient pressure must be applied to stop the bleeding. Nasal packing predisposes patients to infection from bacteria (e.g., *Staphylococcus aureus*) present in the nasal cavity. The patient should receive a mild opioid analgesic for pain (e.g., acetaminophen with codeine). Antibiotics effective against staphylococci may be prescribed.

Nasal packing may be left in place for 2 to 3 days. Before removal, medicate the patient for pain because this procedure is uncomfortable. After removal, cleanse the nares gently and lubricate them with water-soluble jelly.

Before discharge teach the patient and caregiver about home care. Teach the patient to use saline nasal spray and/or a humidifier, sneeze with the mouth open, and avoid the use of aspirin-containing products or NSAIDs. Instruct the patient to avoid vigorous nose blowing, engaging in strenuous activity, lifting, and straining for 4 to 6 weeks.

## ALLERGIC RHINITIS

**Allergic rhinitis** is inflammation of the nasal mucosa in response to a specific allergen. Allergic rhinitis can be classified according to the causative allergen (seasonal or perennial) or the frequency of symptoms (episodic, intermittent, or persistent). *Episodic* refers to symptoms related to sporadic exposure to allergens not typically encountered in the patient's normal environment, such as exposure to animal dander when visiting another person's home. *Intermittent* means that the symptoms are present less than 4 days a week or less than 4 weeks per year. *Persistent* means that symptoms are present more than 4 days a week and for more than 4 weeks per year.

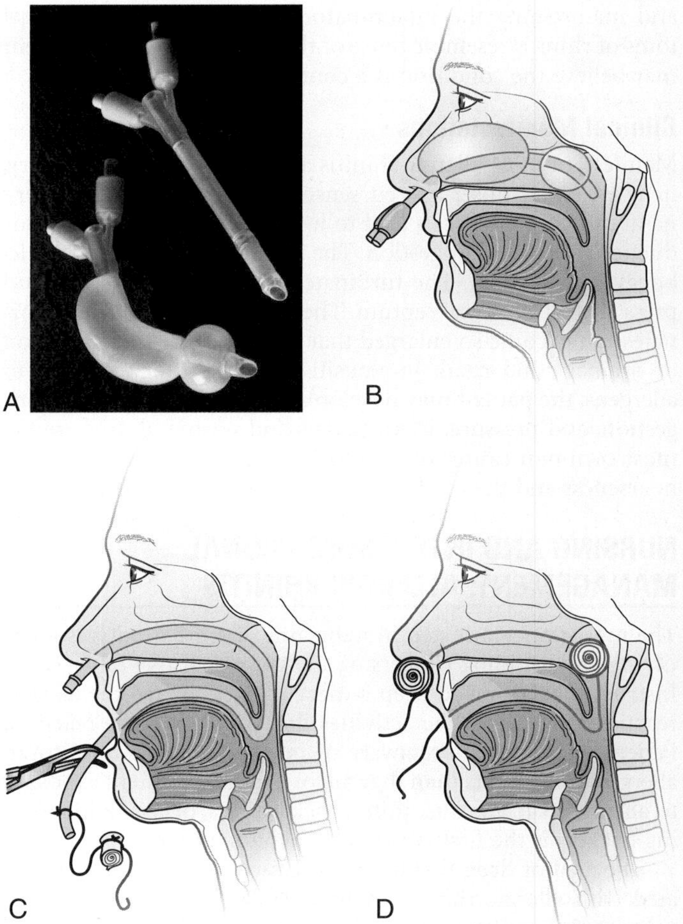


**FIG. 26-1** **A,** Epistaxis balloon. The balloon is inflated after insertion. (Courtesy Boston Medical, Westborough, Mass.) **B,** Epistaxis balloon in proper position in nares. (From Roberts JR, Hedges JR: *Clinical procedures in emergency medicine,* ed 5, Philadelphia, 2009, Saunders.) **C,** Method for placing posterior nasal pack. Catheter is passed through the bleeding side of the nose and pulled out through the mouth with a hemostat. Strings are tied to the catheter, and the pack is pulled up behind the soft palate and into the nasopharynx. **D,** Nasal pack in position in the posterior nasopharynx. Dental roll at the nose helps maintain correct position.

*Seasonal rhinitis* usually occurs in the spring and fall, and is caused by allergy to pollens from trees, flowers, grasses, or weeds. The typical attack lasts for several weeks during times when pollen counts are high; then it disappears and recurs at the same time the following year. *Perennial rhinitis* occurs year round from exposure to environmental allergens, such as animal dander, dust mites, cockroaches, fungi, and molds. Both seasonal and perennial rhinitis can be classified as episodic, intermittent, or persistent, depending on the duration and frequency of symptoms.

Sensitization to an allergen occurs with initial allergen exposure, which results in the production of antigen-specific immunoglobulin E (IgE) (see Fig. 13-6). After exposure, mast cells and basophils release histamine, cytokines, prostaglandins, and leukotrienes, which cause the early symptoms of sneezing, itching, rhinorrhea, and congestion.[9] Four to 8 hours after exposure, inflammatory cells infiltrate the nasal tissues, causing and maintaining the inflammatory response. Because symptoms of rhinitis resemble those of the common cold, the patient may believe the condition is a continuous or repeated cold.

### Clinical Manifestations

Manifestations of allergic rhinitis are initially sneezing; watery, itchy eyes and nose; altered sense of smell; and thin, watery nasal discharge that can lead to a more sustained mucus production and nasal congestion. The nasal turbinates appear pale, boggy, and swollen. The turbinates may fill the air space and press against the nasal septum. The posterior ends of the turbinates can become so enlarged that they obstruct sinus aeration or drainage and result in sinusitis. With chronic exposure to allergens, the patient may develop a headache, stuffy nose, congestion, and pressure. Nasal polyps and postnasal drip are the most common causes of cough. The patient may complain of hoarseness and the recurrent need to clear the throat.

## ❖ NURSING AND INTERPROFESSIONAL MANAGEMENT: ALLERGIC RHINITIS

The most important step in managing allergic rhinitis is identifying and avoiding triggers of allergic reactions (Table 26-1). Instruct the patient to keep a diary of times when the allergic reaction occurs and the activities that precipitate the reaction. Patients are often more aware of intermittent exposure to an allergen such as pets than they are of a more persistent exposure to allergens such as dust mites, cockroaches, or mold. Identifying triggers is the first step toward avoiding them.

The goal of drug therapy is to reduce inflammation associated with allergic rhinitis, reduce nasal symptoms, minimize associated complications, and maximize quality of life. Nasal corticosteroid sprays are the first line and most effective treatment for allergic rhinitis.[10] Appropriate oral medication options include $H_1$-antihistamines, decongestants, and leukotriene receptor antagonists (LTRAs). Intranasal medications include antihistamines, anticholinergics, corticosteroids, cromolyn, and decongestants[11] (Table 26-2).

Second-generation antihistamines are preferred over first-generation antihistamines because of their nonsedating effects. Remind patients who are taking antihistamines to have adequate fluid intake to reduce adverse symptoms. Nasal corticosteroid sprays are used to decrease inflammation locally with little absorption in the systemic circulation. Therefore systemic side effects are rare. If symptoms are not relieved with monotherapy, a two-drug combination (such as an oral $H_1$-antihistamine and an intranasal corticosteroid) may be helpful.

**DRUG ALERT Antihistamines**

- First-generation antihistamines (e.g., chlorpheniramine [Chlor-Trimeton]) can cause drowsiness and sedation.
- Warn patients that operating machinery and driving may be dangerous because of the sedative effect.

**DRUG ALERT Pseudoephedrine (Sudafed)**

- Large doses may produce tachycardia and palpitations, especially in patients with cardiac disease.
- Overdose in those over 60 years of age may result in central nervous system depression, seizures, and hallucinations.

Immunotherapy (allergy shots) may be used when a specific, unavoidable allergen is identified and drugs are not tolerated or are ineffective in controlling symptoms. Immunotherapy involves controlled exposure to small amounts of the known allergen through frequent (at least weekly) injections with the goal of decreasing sensitivity. Sublingual or intranasal administration of allergen immunotherapy may be appropriate for selected patients. (Immunotherapy is discussed in Chapter 13.)

**TABLE 26-1 Patient & Caregiver Teaching**

***Avoiding Allergens in Allergic Rhinitis***

Include the following instructions when teaching a patient or caregiver about allergic rhinitis.

| What to Avoid | Specific Approaches |
|---|---|
| **House dust** | • Focus on the bedroom. Remove carpeting. Limit furniture.<br>• Put the pillows, mattress, and springs in airtight vinyl bags or containers.<br>• Limit clothing in the bedroom to items used frequently. Place clothing in airtight, zipper-sealed vinyl clothes bags.<br>• Install an air filter. Close the air conditioning vent into room. Use blinds rather than draperies. |
| **House dust mites** | • Wash bedding in hot water (130° F [54° C]).<br>• Wear a mask when vacuuming. Install a filter on the outlet port of vacuum cleaner.<br>• Avoid sleeping or lying on upholstered furniture.<br>• Keep house temperature and conditions cool and dry. |
| **Pet allergens** | • Remove pets from interior of home.<br>• Clean living area thoroughly.<br>• Do not expect instant relief. Symptoms usually do not improve significantly for 2 months after pet removal. |
| **Mold spores** | • The three *D*s that promote growth of mold spores are darkness, dampness, and drafts.<br>• Ventilate closed rooms and open doors. Consider adding windows to dark rooms. Consider keeping a small light on in closets.<br>• Basement light with a timer that provides light several hours a day may decrease mold growth.<br>• Avoid places where humidity is high (e.g., basements, clothes hampers, greenhouses, barns). Dehumidifiers are rarely helpful. |
| **Pollens** | • Stay inside with closed doors and windows during high-pollen season.<br>• Install an air conditioner with a good air filter. Wash filters weekly during high-pollen season.<br>• Put the car air conditioner on "recirculate" when driving.<br>• Avoid having plants, especially in the bedroom. |
| **Smoke** | • Presence of a smoker will sabotage the best of all possible symptom reduction programs. |

## ACUTE VIRAL RHINITIS

*Acute viral rhinitis* (common cold or acute coryza) is an infection of the upper respiratory tract that can be caused by more than 200 different viruses. The majority of colds, caused by rhinoviruses, are mild and self-limiting. Other viruses, such as coxsackieviruses and adenoviruses, can cause a more severe illness. Acute viral rhinitis is the most prevalent infectious disease, with the average adult contracting one to three colds per year.

The virus is spread by airborne droplets emitted by the infected person while breathing, talking, sneezing, or coughing. Because the virus can survive on inanimate objects for up to 3 days, transmission can also occur by direct hand contact. Frequency of the infection increases in the winter months when

## TABLE 26-2 Drug Therapy

### *Rhinitis and Sinusitis*

| Drug | Mechanism of Action | Side Effects | Nursing Actions |
|---|---|---|---|
| **Corticosteroids** | | | |
| ***Nasal Spray***<br>beclomethasone<br>budesonide (Rhinocort)<br>ciclesonide (Omnaris)<br>flunisolide<br>fluticasone (Flonase)<br>fluticasone furoate (Veramyst)<br>mometasone (Nasonex)<br>triamcinolone | Inhibits inflammatory response of allergic rhinitis. At recommended dose, systemic side effects are unlikely because of low systemic absorption. Systemic effects may occur with higher than recommended doses. | Mild transient nasal burning and stinging, mucosal drying.<br>In rare instances, localized fungal infection with *Candida albicans.* | • Instruct patient to use on regular basis and not PRN.<br>• Instruct patient to clear nasal passages before use.<br>• Reinforce that spray acts to decrease inflammation and it may take several days or weeks to achieve maximum effects.<br>• Discontinue use if nasal infection develops. |
| **Mast Cell Stabilizer** | | | |
| ***Nasal Spray***<br>cromolyn spray | Suppresses release of histamine and other inflammatory mediators from mast cells. | Minimal side effects. Occasional burning or nasal irritation. | • Reinforce that spray prevents symptoms.<br>• Begin 2 wk before pollen season starts and use throughout pollen season.<br>• If isolated allergy, such as cat, use prophylactically before exposure to allergen. |
| **Leukotriene Receptor Antagonists (LTRAs) and Inhibitors** | | | |
| ***Antagonists***<br>zafirlukast (Accolate)<br>montelukast (Singulair)<br>***Inhibitors***<br>zileuton (Zyflo) | Suppress leukotriene activity, thereby inhibiting airway edema, bronchoconstriction, mucus production, and inflammation (see Fig. 11-2). | Generally well tolerated<br>May cause headaches, dizziness, rash, altered liver function tests, GI disturbances<br>*Zafirlukast and zileuton:* Monitor PT levels and theophylline levels if patient is taking warfarin or theophylline. | • Monitor liver function tests periodically while on therapy. Discontinue if elevated.<br>• Administer on empty stomach.<br>• Do not discontinue therapy without consulting HCP.<br>• Not to be used for acute attacks. |
| **Anticholinergic** | | | |
| ***Nasal Spray***<br>ipratropium bromide (Atrovent) | Blocks nasal cholinergic receptors, reducing nasal secretions in the common cold and nonallergic rhinitis. | Nasal dryness and irritation may occur. Does not cause systemic side effects. | • Need to prime pump with seven actuations before initial use<br>• May reduce the need for other rhinitis medications. |
| **Antihistamines** | | | |
| ***First-Generation Agents (Oral)***<br>brompheniramine<br>chlorpheniramine (Chlor-Trimeton)<br>clemastine<br>dexchlorpheniramine<br>diphenhydramine<br>levocetirizine (Xyzal) | Bind with $H_1$ receptors on target cells, blocking histamine binding. Relieve acute symptoms of allergic response (itching, sneezing, rhinorrhea). | Cross blood-brain barrier, frequently causing sedation and somnolence.<br>Can also cause paradoxic stimulation (restlessness, nervousness, insomnia).<br>Anticholinergic side effects (e.g., palpitations, dry mouth, constipation, urinary hesitancy). | • Warn patient that operating machinery and driving may be dangerous because of sedative effect.<br>• Teach patient to report palpitations, change in heart rate, change in bowel or bladder habits.<br>• Instruct patient not to use alcohol with antihistamines because of additive depressant effect.<br>• Rapid onset of action, no drug tolerance with prolonged use. |
| ***Second-Generation Agents (Oral)***<br>loratadine (Claritin)<br>cetirizine (Zyrtec)<br>fexofenadine (Allegra)<br>desloratadine (Clarinex)<br>levocetirizine (Xyzal) | Same as above. | Limited affinity for brain $H_1$ receptors. Cause minimal sedation, few effects on psychomotor activities or bladder function. | • Teach patient to expect few, if any, side effects.<br>• More expensive than traditional antihistamines<br>• Rapid onset of action, no drug tolerance with prolonged use. |
| ***Second-Generation Agents (Intranasal)***<br>azelastine (Astelin)<br>olopatadine (Patanase) | Same as above. | Headache, bitter taste, somnolence, nasal irritation. | • Longer use increases risk of rebound vasodilation, which can increase congestion. |
| **Decongestants** | | | |
| ***Oral***<br>pseudoephedrine (Sudafed) | Stimulates adrenergic receptors on blood vessels, promotes vasoconstriction, reduces nasal congestion. | CNS stimulation, causing insomnia, excitation, headache, irritability, increased blood and ocular pressure, dysuria, palpitations, tachycardia. | • Advise patient of adverse reactions.<br>• Advise that some preparations are contraindicated for patients with cardiovascular disease, hypertension, diabetes, glaucoma, benign prostatic hyperplasia, hepatic and renal disease. |
| ***Topical (Nasal Spray)***<br>oxymetazoline<br>phenylephrine | Same as above. | Same as above, plus rebound nasal congestion. | • Teach patient that these drugs should not be used for >3 days or >3-4 times/day. |

*PT,* Prothrombin time.

*Continued*

TABLE 26-2 **Drug Therapy**

***Rhinitis and Sinusitis—cont'd***

| Drug | Mechanism of Action | Side Effects | Nursing Actions |
|---|---|---|---|
| **Combination Cold Medications** | | | |
| Zutripro oral solution (hydrocodone, chlorpheniramine, and pseudoephedrine)<br>Rezira oral solution (hydrocodone and pseudoephedrine) | Hydrocodone suppresses cough. Mechanism of action of chlorpheniramine and pseudoephedrine discussed above. | See individual drugs above. | • Avoid in patients with head injury or increased intracranial pressure.<br>• Use with caution in patients with acute abdominal conditions. |

people stay indoors and overcrowding is more common. Other factors that increase susceptibility include fatigue, physical and emotional stress, allergies that affect the nose and throat, and compromised immune status. Exercise may reduce the number of upper respiratory tract infections.

Symptoms of acute viral rhinitis typically begin 2 or 3 days after infection and may include runny nose, watery eyes, nasal congestion, sneezing, cough, sore throat, fever, headache, and fatigue. Symptoms may last 2 to 14 days, with typical recovery in 7 to 10 days.

**COMPLEMENTARY & ALTERNATIVE THERAPIES**

***Echinacea***

**Scientific Evidence**

- Echinacea may have some benefit in reducing the incidence and duration of the common cold.
- However, there is conflicting evidence on its use in prevention and treatment of upper respiratory tract infections.

**Nursing Implications**

- Echinacea is considered safe when used on a short-term basis in recommended doses.
- Patients with asthma or allergies to plants in the daisy family (including ragweed, mums, marigolds, and daisies) are more likely to have allergic reactions.
- It may interfere with drugs that suppress the immune system and those that are metabolized by the liver.
- Caution is advised for patients with autoimmune disorders using this herb.

Source: *www.nlm.nih.gov/medlineplus/druginfo/natural/981.html.*

## NURSING AND INTERPROFESSIONAL MANAGEMENT: ACUTE VIRAL RHINITIS

Interventions are directed at relieving symptoms. Rest, oral fluids, antipyretics, and analgesics are recommended. Warm salt water gargles, ice chips, lozenges, or sprays may help alleviate a sore throat. Petroleum jelly soothes a raw nose. Saline nasal spray reduces nasal congestion. Antihistamine and decongestant therapy reduces postnasal drip and significantly decreases the severity of cough, nasal obstruction, and nasal discharge. Caution patients to use intranasal decongestant sprays for no more than 3 days to prevent rebound congestion from occurring. Cough suppressants, such as dextromethorphan, and expectorants, such as guaifenesin, may be used.

Complications of acute viral rhinitis include pharyngitis, sinusitis, otitis media, tonsillitis, and lung infections. Unless complications are present, antibiotic therapy is not indicated. Antibiotics have no effect on viruses. If symptoms remain for 10 to 14 days with no improvement, an HCP should be consulted.

Teach the patient to recognize the manifestations of secondary bacterial infection, such as a temperature higher than 103° F (39.4° C); tender, swollen glands; severe sinus or ear pain; or significantly worsening symptoms. Green, purulent nasal drainage during the later stages of a cold is not uncommon and is not always indicative of bacterial infection. In the patient with pulmonary disease, signs of infection often include a change in consistency, color, or volume of the sputum. Because infection can progress rapidly, teach the patient with chronic respiratory disease to immediately report sputum changes, increased shortness of breath, and chest tightness.

During the cold season, advise patients with a chronic illness or a compromised immune system to avoid crowded situations and other individuals who have obvious cold symptoms. Frequent hand washing and avoiding hand-to-face contact can help prevent direct spread.

## INFLUENZA

*Influenza* (flu) is a highly contagious respiratory illness that causes significant morbidity and mortality. Millions of Americans (about 5% to 20% of U.S. population) contract influenza each year. The flu season begins in September and continues through April of each year, peaking anywhere from November to March. More than 225,000 people are hospitalized each year for flu-related complications.[12] On average, influenza is responsible for 20,000 deaths annually. Vaccination of high-risk groups can prevent many of these deaths.

### Etiology and Pathophysiology

Influenza viruses are classified into three serotypes (A, B, and C), but only A and B cause significant illness in humans. Influenza A is subtyped based on the presence of two surface proteins: hemagglutinin (H) and neuraminidase (N). The H antigens enable the virus to enter the cell, and the N antigens facilitate cell-to-cell transmission. As a result, influenza A viruses are named according to their H and N type (e.g., H3N2).

Influenza A is the most common and most virulent flu virus and can infect a variety of animals as well as humans. More than 100 types of influenza A are found in birds (avian flu), pigs (swine flu), horses, seals, and dogs. The virus mutates (changes) to allow it to infect different species. When a new viral strain reaches humans, people do not have immunity, and the virus can spread quickly around the globe, causing a *pandemic.* For example, type A H1N1 influenza (swine flu) emerged in 2009 and had never been seen in humans before. A worldwide pandemic resulted. Pandemics can also be triggered by the reemergence of a viral strain that has not circulated for many years. *Epidemics* are more localized outbreaks, usually occurring yearly, caused by variants of already circulating strains.

Influenza B and C viruses are not divided into subtypes and only infect humans. Outbreaks of influenza B can also cause regional epidemics, but the disease it produces is generally milder than that caused by influenza A. Influenza C causes mild illness and does not cause epidemics or pandemics.

Every flu season is different. Several different strains of influenza viruses exist, and the viruses are able to mutate over time; this explains the need for annual vaccination. Fewer cases of influenza result when a minor change in the virus occurs because most persons have partial immunity.

Influenza is transmitted from animals to humans by direct or indirect contact with infected animals (e.g., animal feces). Influenza is communicable between humans primarily through infected droplets and inhalation of aerosolized particles and to a lesser extent through direct contact with contaminated surfaces. The virus has an incubation period of 1 to 4 days, with peak transmission risk starting approximately 1 day before onset of symptoms and continuing for 5 to 7 days after a person first becomes sick.[13]

### Clinical Manifestations

For some patients, it may be difficult to distinguish between the common cold and flu (Table 26-3). The onset of flu is typically abrupt, with systemic symptoms of chills, fever, and generalized myalgia, often accompanied by a headache, cough, sore throat, and fatigue. Physical examination findings are usually minimal, with normal assessment on chest auscultation. In uncomplicated cases, symptoms often subside within 7 days. Dyspnea and diffuse crackles are signs of pulmonary complications. Some patients, particularly older adults, experience weakness or lethargy that may persist for weeks.

Common complications of influenza include pneumonia (which can be either primary influenza [viral] pneumonia or secondary bacterial pneumonia) and ear or sinus infections. The patient who develops secondary bacterial pneumonia usually experiences gradual improvement of influenza symptoms, then worsening cough and purulent sputum. Treatment with antibiotics is usually effective if started early. Older adults are particularly prone to dehydration.

### Diagnostic Studies

Influenza is commonly diagnosed based on the patient's health history, clinical findings, and the knowledge of other cases of influenza in the community.

Viral cultures are considered the "gold standard" for diagnosing influenza. However, they can take up to 3 to 10 days for results. Viral cultures may be obtained from a throat swab, nasopharyngeal swab, expectorated sputum, ET tube sample, or bronchoscopy (bronchial wash).[14] A viral culture has the advantage of identifying which virus (A, B, or another respiratory virus) and which strains of virus are present. These data are used in the formulation of the following season's flu vaccine.

Rapid flu tests can help in the diagnosis by detecting the virus in nasal secretions. Depending on the method, the test may be completed in the HCP's office in less than 30 minutes or be sent to a laboratory, with results available the same day. The test can help differentiate influenza from other viral and bacterial infections with similar manifestations that may be serious and must be treated differently. Rapid flu tests are best used within the first 48 hours of the onset of symptoms to help diagnose influenza and determine whether antiviral drugs are a treatment option.[15] The main disadvantages of the rapid flu test are that it will miss some cases or occasionally be positive when a person does not actually have the flu.

**TABLE 26-3 Comparison of Common Cold and Influenza**

| Manifestations and Treatment | Common Cold (Viral Rhinitis) | Influenza |
|---|---|---|
| **Symptom onset** | Appear gradually | Abrupt onset. Within 3 to 6 hr |
| **Fever** | Rare | Characteristically high 102-104° F (38.9-40° C]). Lasts 3-4 days |
| **Headache** | Uncommon | Common (can be severe) |
| **General aches and pains** | Slight | Usual. Often severe |
| **Fatigue and weakness** | Sometimes. Usually mild | Usual. Starts early and can last up to 2-3 wk |
| **Exhaustion** | Uncommon | Usual at beginning of illness |
| **Stuffy nose** | Common | Sometimes |
| **Sneezing** | Common | Sometimes |
| **Sore throat** | Common | Sometimes |
| **Chest discomfort, cough** | Common. Mild to moderate hacking cough | Common |
| **Complications** | Sinus congestion. Earache | Bronchitis, pneumonia, acute respiratory failure. Can be life-threatening |
| **Prevention** | Hand washing. Avoid close contact with anyone who has a cold | Hand washing. Annual vaccination. Antiviral drugs. Avoid close contact with anyone who has the flu |
| **Treatment** | Temporary relief of symptoms: rest, hydration, decongestants, acetaminophen or ibuprofen for headache, aches, and pains | Antiviral drugs if given within 24-48 hr of onset. Rest, hydration, acetaminophen or ibuprofen for headache, aches, and pains |

Adapted from Johnson K: Is it a cold or the flu? Retrieved from *www.webmd.com/cold-and-flu/is-it-a-cold-or-flu.*

## ❖ NURSING AND INTERPROFESSIONAL MANAGEMENT: INFLUENZA

The most effective strategy for managing influenza is prevention. Two types of flu vaccines are available: inactivated and live attenuated (Table 26-4). Administration of the flu vaccine results in the production of antibodies against the viruses contained in the vaccine.

The influenza vaccine is changed on a yearly basis, depending on the virus strains identified by the Centers for Disease Control and Prevention (CDC) as being most likely to cause illness in the upcoming flu season. The best time to receive the vaccine is in September (before flu exposure) because it takes 2 weeks for full protection to occur. However, the vaccine can be administered at any time during the flu season.

**TABLE 26-4 Types of Influenza Immunization**

| Trivalent Inactivated Influenza Vaccine (TIV) | Live Attenuated Influenza Vaccine (LSIV) |
|---|---|
| Given by injection | Given by nasal spray |
| Approved for use in people ≥6 mo of age | Approved for healthy people ages 2-49 yr |
| Can be used in people at increased risk:<br>• People of any age with chronic medical conditions<br>• Residents of nursing homes and long-term care facilities<br>• People who are immunocompromised<br>• Pregnant women | Should NOT be used in:<br>• Children <2 yr or adults >50 yr<br>• Pregnant women<br>• People with known immunodeficiency<br>• Children or adolescents receiving aspirin or other salicylates<br>• People who have medical conditions that place them at increased risk for complications from influenza (chronic cardiovascular, pulmonary, or neurologic diseases; diabetes mellitus; renal or hepatic dysfunction; hemoglobinopathies)<br>• HCPs of high-risk patients because of risk of viral transmission from vaccine (should not care for high-risk patients for 7 days after vaccination) |
| Most common side effects are injection site reactions, such as pain, redness, and swelling | Most common side effects are runny nose and nasal congestion in all ages, fever in children ages 2-6 yr old and sore throat in adults |

**SAFETY ALERT Influenza Vaccination**

- Advocate for vaccination of all people older than 6 months of age, but especially for those at high risk (e.g., health care workers, residents of long-term care facilities).
- Give high priority to groups, such as health care workers, who can transmit influenza to high-risk persons.

Vaccination of healthy people decreases the incidence and risk of transmitting influenza to those who have less ability to cope with the effects of this illness. Despite obvious benefits, many persons are reluctant to be vaccinated. Current vaccines are highly purified, and reactions are extremely rare. Soreness at the injection site is usually the most frequently reported adverse effect. Contraindications are a history of severe allergic reactions to previous flu vaccine. Patients with anaphylactic hypersensitivity to eggs should discuss the vaccine with their HCP, as alternatives for vaccinating patients with egg allergies are now available.

The primary nursing goals in influenza are relief of symptoms and prevention of secondary infection. Unless the patient with influenza is at high risk or complications develop, only supportive therapy is necessary. Rest, hydration, analgesics, and antipyretics can provide symptom relief. Older adults and those with a chronic illness may require hospitalization.

To treat influenza, three antiviral medications are used: zanamivir (Relenza), oseltamivir (Tamiflu), and peramivir (Rapivab).[16] Zanamivir is administered using an inhaler, oseltamivir is available as an oral capsule, and peramivir is given IV.

These antiviral drugs are neuraminidase inhibitors that prevent the virus from being released and spreading to other cells. These drugs shorten the duration of influenza symptoms and reduce the risk of complications. Treatment should be initiated as soon as possible in patients who are hospitalized with influenza, have severe or complicated illness, or are at high risk for complications. For maximum benefit in the treatment of influenza, therapy should begin within 2 days of the onset of symptoms, but it can be started later (based on clinical judgment).

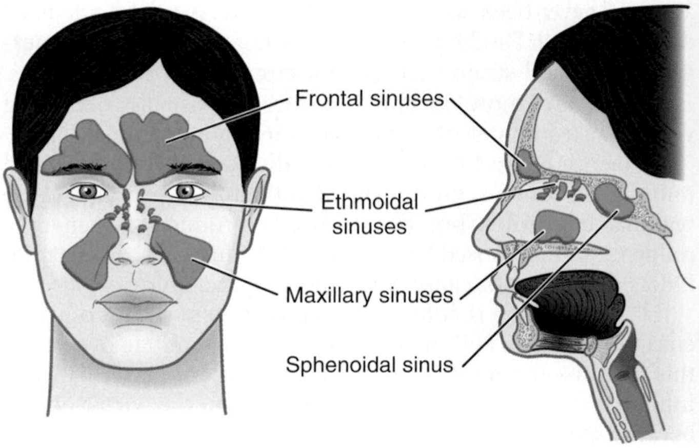


**FIG. 26-2** Location of the sinuses.

**COMPLEMENTARY & ALTERNATIVE THERAPIES**

***Zinc***

**Scientific Evidence**

- Zinc is available in two forms: oral zinc (e.g., lozenges, tablets, syrup) and intranasal zinc (e.g., swabs, gels).
- When administered within 24 hr of onset of symptoms, zinc reduces the duration and severity of cold symptoms.
- When zinc supplementation is taken in low doses for at least 5 mo, the incidence of colds is reduced.

**Nursing Implications**

- Intranasal zinc has been linked to a severe side effect (irreversible loss of the sense of smell) and should not be used.
- Zinc is regarded as relatively safe when taken at recommended doses.
- Zinc lozenges are more apt to cause adverse effects (bad taste, nausea) than syrup or tablets.
- Oral zinc should not be taken with foods that will reduce its absorption, such as caffeine and dairy products.
- Zinc may interact with drugs, including antibiotics and penicillamine.

Source: *https://nccih.nih.gov/health/tips/flucold.htm.*

## SINUSITIS

**Sinusitis** affects one out of every seven adults. It develops when inflammation or hypertrophy (swelling) of the mucosa blocks the openings (ostia) in the sinuses, through which mucus drains into the nose (Fig. 26-2). *Rhinosinusitis,* which may accompany sinusitis, is concurrent inflammation or infection of the nasal mucosa. Obstruction of mucus drainage can also be caused by nasal polyps, foreign bodies, deviated septa, or tumors. The secretions that accumulate behind the blocked ostia provide a rich medium for growth of bacteria, viruses, and fungi, all of which may cause infection.

Viral sinusitis typically follows an upper respiratory tract infection in which the virus penetrates the mucous membrane and decreases ciliary function. Viral infections usually resolve without treatment in less than 14 days. If symptoms worsen after 3 to 5 days or persist for longer than 10 days, a secondary bacterial infection may be present. Only 5% to 10% of patients with viral sinusitis develop a bacterial infection requiring antibiotic therapy.

*Streptococcus pneumoniae, Haemophilus influenzae,* and *Moraxella catarrhalis* are the most common causes of bacterial sinusitis. Fungal sinusitis is uncommon, usually occurring in patients who are debilitated or immunocompromised.

Sinusitis can be classified as acute, subacute, or chronic.[17] *Acute sinusitis* typically begins within 1 week of an upper respiratory tract infection and lasts less than 4 weeks. *Subacute sinusitis* is present when symptoms progress over 4 to 8 weeks. *Chronic sinusitis* (lasting longer than 8 weeks) is a persistent infection usually associated with allergies and nasal polyps. Chronic sinusitis generally results from repeated episodes of acute sinusitis that result in irreversible loss of the normal ciliated epithelium lining the sinus cavity.

### Clinical Manifestations

Acute sinusitis causes significant pain over the affected sinus, purulent nasal drainage, nasal obstruction, congestion, fever, and malaise. The patient may appear acutely ill. Assessment involves inspection of the nasal mucosa and palpation of the sinus pressure points for pain. Findings that indicate acute sinusitis include edematous mucosa, discolored purulent nasal drainage, enlarged turbinates, tenderness over the involved frontal and/or maxillary sinuses, and *halitosis* (bad breath). Recurrent headaches that change in intensity with position changes or when secretions drain are not uncommon.

Chronic sinusitis is difficult to diagnose because symptoms are often nonspecific. The patient is rarely febrile. The patient may experience facial or dental pain, nasal congestion, and increased drainage, but severe pain and purulent drainage are often absent. Some symptoms mimic those seen with allergies. X-rays or CT scan of the sinuses may help confirm the diagnosis. CT scans may show the sinuses to be filled with fluid or a thickened mucous membrane. Nasal endoscopy with a flexible scope may be used to examine the sinuses, obtain a specimen for culture, and restore normal drainage.

As many as 50% of patients with moderate to severe asthma have chronic sinusitis. The exact link between these diseases is unclear. Postnasal drip associated with sinusitis may trigger asthma by stimulating bronchoconstriction. Gastroesophageal reflux disease (GERD) and smoking may increase the risk of a person with asthma developing sinusitis. Appropriate treatment of sinusitis often causes a reduction in asthma symptoms.

## NURSING AND INTERPROFESSIONAL MANAGEMENT: SINUSITIS

If allergies are the precipitating cause of sinusitis, instruct the patient about ways to reduce sinus inflammation and infection, including environmental control of allergens and appropriate drug therapy (see allergic rhinitis presented earlier in this chapter).

Initial treatment for acute sinusitis focuses on symptom relief. Medications include oral or topical decongestants to promote drainage, intranasal corticosteroids to decrease inflammation, analgesics to relieve pain, and saline nasal spray to relieve congestion. A clinical response to treatment should be observed within 72 hours.[18] Instruct patients using topical decongestants to use the medication for no longer than 4 to 5 days to prevent rebound congestion caused by vasodilation.

**TABLE 26-5 Patient & Caregiver Teaching**

***Acute or Chronic Sinusitis***

*Include the following instructions when teaching the patient and caregiver about management of sinusitis.*

1. Get plenty of rest to help body fight infection and promote recovery.
2. Keep well hydrated by drinking six to eight glasses of water to loosen secretions.
3. Take hot showers twice daily. Use a steam inhaler (15-min vaporization of boiled water), bedside humidifier, or nasal saline spray to promote secretion drainage.
4. Apply warm, damp towels around nose, cheeks, and eyes to ease facial pain.
5. Sleep with head elevated to help sinuses drain and reduce congestion.
6. Report a temperature of 100.4° F (38° C) or higher, which indicates infection.
7. Follow prescribed medication regimen:
   - Take analgesics to relieve pain.
   - Take decongestants/expectorants to relieve swelling.
   - Take antibiotics (as prescribed) for infection. Be sure to take entire prescription and report continued symptoms or a change in symptoms.
   - Administer nasal sprays correctly.
8. Perform nasal saline washes once or twice a day to wash sinuses.
9. Do not smoke, and avoid exposure to smoke. Smoke is an irritant and will worsen symptoms.
10. If allergies predispose to sinusitis, follow instructions regarding environmental control, drug therapy, and immunotherapy to reduce the inflammation and prevent sinus infection.

Saline irrigation of the nasal cavity can be used to rinse nasal passages, facilitate drainage, and decrease inflammation. Saline nasal spray is available over the counter.

If symptoms worsen or persist for longer than 1 week, antibiotic therapy may be prescribed. Amoxicillin is the first-line drug of choice and is continued for 10 to 14 days to prevent the formation of antibiotic-resistant organisms.[19] If symptoms do not resolve, the antibiotic should be changed to a fluoroquinolone or broader-spectrum cephalosporin antibiotic.

With chronic sinusitis, mixed bacterial flora is often present and infections are difficult to eliminate. Broad-spectrum antibiotics may be used for 4 to 6 weeks. Patient and caregiver teaching for acute and chronic sinusitis is presented in Table 26-5.

Medical therapy may not relieve the symptoms of some patients with persistent, recurrent, or chronic sinus illnesses. They may require nasal endoscopic surgery to relieve blockage caused by hypertrophy or septal deviation. This is usually performed as an outpatient procedure using local anesthesia. Propel, a self-expanding implant, can be placed directly in the sinus during surgery. Propel helps to maintain postoperative patency to the sinus cavity and provide localized corticosteroid delivery directly to the sinus lining before dissolving after 30 days.

## OBSTRUCTION OF NOSE AND SINUSES

### Nasal Polyps

**Nasal polyps** are soft, painless, benign (noncancerous) growths that form slowly in response to repeated inflammation of the sinus or nasal mucosa. They are most common in adults over age 40 and are twice as likely to occur in men than women.[20]

Polyps, which appear as chronic yellow, gray, or pink semitransparent projections in the naris, can exceed the size of a grape.

Small polyps are typically asymptomatic. Clinical manifestations of larger polyps include nasal obstruction, nasal discharge (usually clear mucus), and speech distortion. Topical and systemic corticosteroids are the primary medical therapy used to shrink nasal polyps. Endoscopic or laser surgery can remove nasal polyps, but recurrence is common.

### Foreign Bodies

A variety of foreign bodies may potentially lodge in the upper respiratory tract of adults, but these are rare occurrences. Some of these situations may be the result of trauma or found in patients with mental illness. Foreign bodies may be inorganic or organic. Inorganic foreign bodies may cause no symptoms and be incidentally discovered on routine examination. Organic foreign bodies may produce a local inflammatory reaction and nasal discharge, which may become purulent and foul smelling if the object remains in the nasal cavity for an extended time. Foreign bodies can also cause pain, difficulty breathing, and nasal bleeding.

Foreign bodies should be removed from the nose through the route of entry. Sneezing or blowing the nose with the opposite nostril closed may be effective in removing the foreign object. Avoid irrigating the nose or pushing the object backward, since either could cause aspiration and airway obstruction. If sneezing or blowing the nose does not remove the object, an HCP should be consulted.

# PROBLEMS OF PHARYNX

## ACUTE PHARYNGITIS

*Acute pharyngitis* is an acute inflammation of the pharyngeal walls. It may include the tonsils, palate, and uvula. It can be caused by a viral, bacterial, or fungal infection. Viral pharyngitis accounts for approximately 90% of cases. Bacterial pharyngitis ("strep throat") usually results from group A β-hemolytic streptococci and accounts for 5% to 10% of cases.[21]

Fungal pharyngitis, such as candidiasis, can develop with the prolonged use of antibiotics or inhaled corticosteroids. It can also occur in immunosuppressed patients, especially those with human immunodeficiency virus (HIV) infection. Other causes of pharyngitis include dry air, smoking, GERD, allergy and postnasal drip, endotracheal (ET) intubation, chemicals, and cancer.

### Clinical Manifestations

Symptoms of acute pharyngitis range in severity from a "scratchy" throat to pain so severe that swallowing is difficult. Because both viral and streptococcal infections appear as a red and edematous pharynx (with or without patchy exudates), it may be difficult to distinguish between the two types.

Four classic manifestations present in bacterial pharyngitis include fever greater than 100.4° F (38° C), anterior cervical lymph node enlargement, tonsillar or pharyngeal exudate, and the absence of cough.[22] However, appearance is not always diagnostic. When two or three of the above criteria are present, a rapid antigen detection test and/or a throat culture is done to establish the cause and direct appropriate management. White, irregular patches on the oropharynx suggest fungal infection with *Candida albicans.*

## ❖ NURSING AND INTERPROFESSIONAL MANAGEMENT: ACUTE PHARYNGITIS

The goals of nursing management are infection control, symptom relief, and prevention of secondary complications. For viral pharyngitis, antibiotics are not recommended. Instruct patients to use ibuprofen or acetaminophen for pain relief. Encourage the patient to increase fluid intake.

For symptom relief, instruct the patient to gargle with warm salt water ( ½ tsp of salt in 8 oz of water); drink warm or cold liquids; and suck on popsicles, hard candies, or throat lozenges. Cool, bland liquids and gelatin will not irritate the pharynx; citrus juices are often irritating. Encourage the patient to use a cool mist vaporizer or humidifier.

For bacterial pharyngitis caused by group A β-hemolytic streptococci, penicillin is the drug of choice. This antibiotic must be taken several times a day for a full 10 days to prevent complications such as rheumatic fever. For patients allergic to penicillin, erythromycin or clindamycin may be appropriate substitutes.[23] Other antibiotics (amoxicillin, azithromycin [Zithromax], cephalosporins) may also be used. Most people with streptococcal infections are contagious until they have been on antibiotics for 24 to 48 hours. Repeat throat cultures after antibiotic therapy are not required.

*Candida* infections are treated with nystatin, an antifungal antibiotic. Instruct patients to swish the preparation in their mouths for as long as possible before swallowing it. Treatment should continue until symptoms are gone. Patients taking inhaled corticosteroids are at risk for infection with *Candida* organisms. Thoroughly rinsing the mouth with water after using corticosteroids can prevent this infection.

## PERITONSILLAR ABSCESS

*Peritonsillar abscess* is a complication of tonsillitis and is most often caused by group A β-hemolytic streptococci. The abscess causes pain, swelling, and blockage of the throat (when severe), threatening airway patency. The patient also experiences a high fever, chills, leukocytosis, difficulty swallowing, and a muffled voice. Treatment consists of IV antibiotic therapy and needle aspiration or incision and drainage of the abscess. In some cases an emergency tonsillectomy is performed, or an elective tonsillectomy is scheduled after the infection has subsided.

# PROBLEMS OF TRACHEA AND LARYNX

## AIRWAY OBSTRUCTION

Acute airway obstruction is a medical emergency. Airway obstruction can be caused by aspiration of food or a foreign body, allergic reactions, edema and inflammation caused by infections or burns, peritonsillar or retropharyngeal abscesses, malignancy, laryngeal or tracheal stenosis, and trauma.

Airway obstruction may be partial or complete. Clinical presentation of an airway obstruction often depends on the cause of the obstruction and/or location of the blockage due to an aspirated object such as food.[24] For example, objects lodged within the larynx may produce voice hoarseness or complete airway obstruction. Tracheal obstruction may produce wheezing, whereas objects lodged within the lower respiratory system (e.g., bronchus) may produce a cough or decreased air entry on the affected side.

Manifestations include choking, stridor, use of accessory muscles, suprasternal and intercostal retractions, flaring nostrils, wheezing, restlessness, tachycardia, cyanosis, and change in level of consciousness. Prompt assessment and treatment are essential because partial obstruction may quickly progress to complete obstruction. Complete airway obstruction can result in permanent brain damage or death if not corrected within 3 to 5 minutes.

Your immediate priority is to ensure the patient has a patent airway. Interventions to reestablish a patent airway include the obstructed airway (Heimlich) maneuver (see Appendix A), cricothyroidotomy, ET intubation, and tracheostomy. Unexplained partial airway obstruction or recurrent symptoms indicate the need for additional tests, such as a chest x-ray, laryngoscopy, and rigid bronchoscopy.

## TRACHEOSTOMY

A **tracheostomy** is a surgically created stoma (opening) in the anterior portion of the trachea (Fig. 26-3, *A*). A tracheostomy may be undertaken to (1) establish a patent airway, (2) bypass an upper airway obstruction, (3) facilitate removal of secretions, (4) permit long-term mechanical ventilation, and (5) facilitate weaning from mechanical ventilation.[25]

The tracheostomy tube is shorter in length and slightly wider in diameter than an ET tube, thereby making it easier to keep the tube clean and facilitate better oral and bronchial hygiene. With the use of a tracheostomy (compared to an ET tube), patient comfort may be increased, because no tube is present in the mouth. There is also less risk of long-term damage to vocal cords.

A variety of tracheostomy tubes are available to meet individual patient needs (Table 26-6). All tracheostomy tubes contain a faceplate, or *flange,* which rests on the neck. In addition, all tracheostomy tubes come with an *obturator,* which is used to help insert the tube. Tracheostomy tubes have an *outer cannula* (which keeps the airway patent), and an *inner cannula* (which can be disposable or nondisposable and removed for cleaning) (Fig. 26-3).

*Cuffed* and *uncuffed* tracheostomy tubes are available. A tracheostomy tube with an inflated cuff (balloon) is most commonly used, particularly if the patient needs mechanical ventilation or is at risk of aspiration. The cuff, inflated via the *balloon inflation port* on the tracheostomy tube, helps keep the tracheostomy tube in place. Cuffless tubes are primarily used for the patient with a long-term tracheostomy, making eating and talking possible.

The outer and/or inner cannula may be *fenestrated* or *nonfenestrated.* A *fenestrated tube* has an opening (a hole) on the surface of the tube. A fenestrated tube allows the patient to breathe spontaneously. For example, with the use of a cuffed, fenestrated tracheostomy tube, when the cuff is deflated and the inner cannula removed, air can pass from the lungs up through the opening in the tracheostomy tube through the vocal cords and larynx, into the upper airway, and out the mouth and nose. This permits the patient to speak with the tracheostomy tube in place. When the cuff is reinflated and the inner cannula reinserted, air is prevented from passing from the lungs through the vocal cords.

Most patients who require mechanical ventilation are initially managed with an ET tube, which can be quickly inserted in an emergency. (The care of the patient with an ET tube is discussed in Chapter 65.) When swelling, trauma, or upper airway obstruction prevents ET intubation, an emergent *surgical tracheostomy* is required.

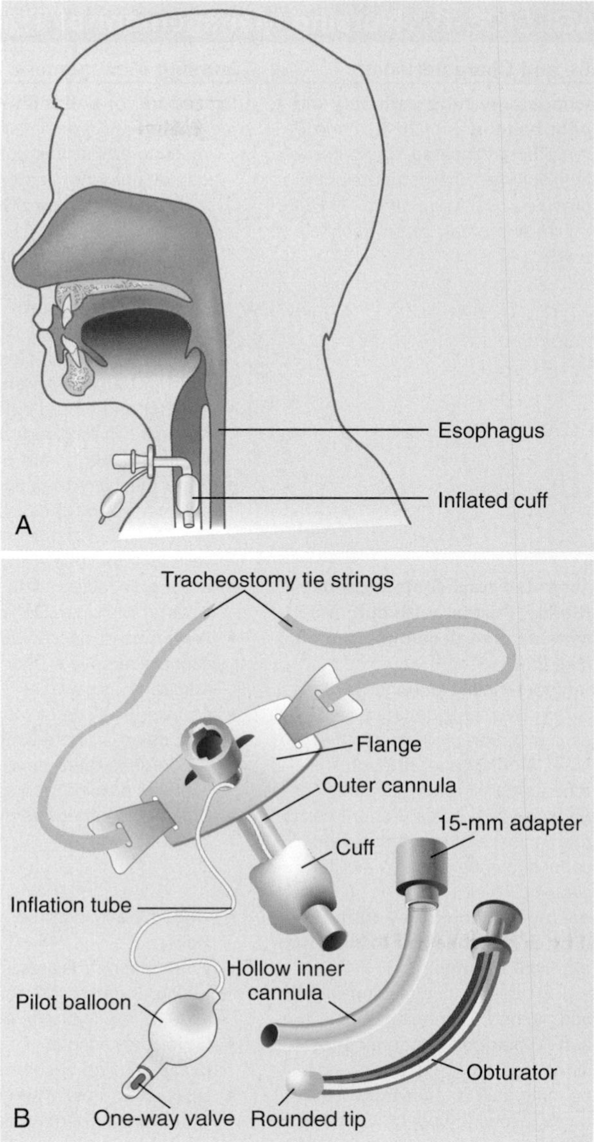


**FIG. 26-3** Tracheostomy tube. **A,** Tracheostomy tube inserted in airway with inflated cuff. (See Table 26-6 and eNursing Care Plan 26-1 [on the website for this chapter] for related nursing management.) **B,** Parts of a tracheostomy tube.

Most surgical tracheostomies are performed in the operating room using general anesthesia. These may be undertaken electively on patients who are already intubated but require prolonged mechanical ventilation. A vertical incision is made on the anterior portion of the trachea. The tracheostomy tube is inserted, the incision is sutured, and a sterile dressing is applied.

A newer surgical technique is the *percutaneous tracheostomy.* Using local anesthesia, sedation, and under video-assisted guidance, a needle is placed into the middle of the trachea. A dilator is placed over the top of the needle. The opening is progressively made larger (with increasingly larger dilators) until the hole is big enough for insertion of the tracheostomy tube. Percutaneous tracheostomy approaches have less risk of bleeding and fewer postoperative complications.[26]

**TABLE 26-6 Nursing Management of Tracheostomies**

| Tube and Characteristics | Nursing Management |
|---|---|
| **Tracheostomy tube with cuff and pilot balloon** (Fig. 26-3, *A* and *B*)<br>When properly inflated, low-pressure, high-volume cuff distributes cuff pressure over large area, minimizing pressure on tracheal wall. | **Procedure for cuff inflation**<br>• *Mechanically ventilated patient:* Inflate the cuff using *minimal occlusion volume (MOV) technique* by slowly injecting air into the cuff until no leak (sound) is heard at peak inspiratory pressure (end of ventilator inspiration) when a stethoscope is placed over the trachea. An alternative approach, termed *minimal leak technique* (MLT), involves inflating the cuff to minimal occlusion pressure and then withdrawing 0.1 mL of air.<br>• *Spontaneously breathing patient:* Inflate cuff using MOV by slowly injecting air into the cuff until no sound is heard after deep breath or during inhalation with bag-valve-mask. If using MLT, remove 0.1 mL of air while maintaining seal. MLT should not be used if there is risk of aspiration.<br>• *Immediately after cuff inflation (both groups):* Verify pressure is within accepted range (20 to 25 cm $H_2O$) with a manometer. Record cuff pressure and volume of air used for cuff inflation in chart.<br>**Care of patients with an inflated cuff**<br>• Monitor and record cuff pressure q8hr. Cuff pressure should be 20 to 25 cm $H_2O$ to allow adequate tracheal capillary perfusion. If needed, remove or add air to the pilot tubing using a syringe and stopcock. Afterward, verify cuff pressure is within accepted range with manometer.<br>• Report inability to keep the cuff inflated or need to use progressively larger volumes of air to keep cuff inflated. Potential causes include tracheal dilation at the cuff site or a crack or slow leak in the housing of the one-way inflation valve. If the leak is due to tracheal dilation, the physician may intubate the patient with a larger tube. |
| **Fenestrated tracheostomy tube (Shiley, Portex) with cuff, inner cannula, and decannulation plug** (Fig. 26-6)<br>When nonfenestrated inner cannula is removed, cuff deflated, and decannulation plug inserted, air flows around tube, through fenestration in outer cannula, and up over vocal cords. Patient can then speak. A fenestrated inner cannula can be used to facilitate cleaning. | • If possible, assess risk of aspiration before removing inner cannula. A speech pathologist may be able to assist if available. Deflate cuff. Note coughing.<br>• ***Never*** insert decannulation plug in tracheostomy tube until cuff is deflated and nonfenestrated inner cannula removed. Prior insertion will prevent patient from breathing (no air inflow). This may precipitate a respiratory arrest.<br>• Assess for signs of respiratory distress when a fenestrated cannula is first used. If this occurs, remove the cap, insert a nonfenestrated inner cannula, and reinflate the cuff.<br>• A nonfenestrated inner cannula must be used to suction patient to prevent tracheal damage from suction catheter passing through fenestrated openings.<br>• Cuff management as described above. |
| **Speaking tracheostomy tube (Portex, National) with cuff, two external tubings**<br>Has two tubings, one leading to cuff and second to opening above the cuff. When port is connected to air source, air flows out of opening and up over the vocal cords, allowing speech with cuff inflated. | • Once tube is inserted, wait 2 days before use so that the stoma can close around the tube and prevent leaks.<br>• When patient desires to speak, connect port to compressed air (or $O_2$). Be certain to identify correct tubing. If gas enters the cuff, it will overinflate and rupture, requiring an emergency tube change. Use lowest flow (typically 4-6 L/min) that results in speech. High flows dehydrate mucosa.<br>• Cover port adapter. This will cause the air to flow upward. Instruct patient to speak in short sentences because voice becomes a whisper with long sentences.<br>• Disconnect flow when patient does not want to speak to prevent mucosal dehydration.<br>• Cuff management as described above. |
| **Tracheostomy tube (Bivona Fome-Cuf) with foam-filled cuff**<br>Cuff is filled with plastic foam. Before insertion, cuff is deflated. After insertion, cuff is allowed to fill passively with air. Pilot tubing is not capped, and no cuff pressure monitoring is required. | • Before insertion, withdraw all air from the cuff using a 20-mL syringe. Cap pilot balloon tubing to prevent reentry of air. After tracheostomy is inserted, remove cap from pilot tubing, allowing cuff to passively reinflate.<br>• Do not inject air into tubing or cap pilot balloon tubing while it is in patient. Air will flow in and out in response to pressure changes (head turning). Place tag on tubing to alert staff not to cap or inflate cuff.<br>• Deflate cuff daily via pilot balloon to evaluate integrity of cuff. Also assess ability to easily deflate cuff. Difficulty deflating cuff indicates a need for tube change. If aspirate returns with air, cuff is no longer intact.<br>• Tube can be used for up to 1 mo in patients on home mechanical ventilation.<br>• Good choice for patients who require inflated cuff at home, since teaching about cuff pressure is simplified. |

The choice of tracheostomy often depends on the surgeon's personal preference. Both surgical and percutaneous tracheostomies may also be performed at the patient's bedside in the emergency department or ICU.

## ❖ NURSING MANAGEMENT: TRACHEOSTOMY

### ◆ Acute Care

Before the tracheostomy procedure (and time permitting), explain the purpose of the procedure to both the patient and caregiver. If the patient is having the tracheostomy in the operating room, follow all hospital policies and procedures for preparing the patient for surgery. (Care of the preoperative patient is discussed in Chapter 17.)

If the procedure is being done at the patient's bedside, ensure all appropriate personnel, including respiratory therapy, have been notified. Emergency resuscitation equipment, including a bag-valve-mask (BVM), should be readily available.

Record vital signs, including heart rate, respiratory rate and rhythm, BP, and $SpO_2$. Ensure an existing IV line is patent and that bedside suction is working. Help assemble and set up all necessary equipment. Position the patient supine. Administer

**TABLE 26-7 Complications of Tracheostomy**

*Closely monitor patients with a tracheostomy for the following potential complications:*

- Air leak
- Airway obstruction
- Altered body image
- Aspiration
- Bleeding
- Fistula formation
- Impaired cough
- Infection: wound or respiratory tract
- Subcutaneous emphysema
- Tracheal necrosis
- Tracheal stenosis
- Tube displacement

analgesia and sedation as ordered by the surgeon, and monitor patient response to analgesia and/or sedatives. Observe patient's tolerance to the procedure.

If you are asked to help during the procedure, ensure you place the obturator inside the outer cannula with its rounded tip protruding from the end of the tube to ease insertion. After insertion, immediately remove the obturator so that air can flow through the tube. Keep the obturator in an easily accessible place at the bedside so that it can be used quickly in case of accidental decannulation (removal of the tracheostomy).

Immediately after the procedure, the cuff (balloon) is inflated. The patient's chest is auscultated for air entry. Air entry should be heard in all lung fields. When placement is confirmed, the ET tube (if present) is removed. The tracheostomy tube is sutured and secured in place with cotton tracheostomy ties, tracheostomy tapes, or Velcro straps.

Many different complications can occur as a result of tracheostomy (Table 26-7). You must be aware of them, especially airway obstruction, bleeding, and infection.

Monitor and record the patient's heart rate, respiratory rate, BP, and $SpO_2$. $SpO_2$ readings should remain stable. Note and record the mechanical ventilator settings, including mode, $FIO_2$, and positive end expiratory pressure (PEEP). Observe the amount of blood at the tracheostomy insertion site. Notify the surgeon or most appropriate personnel if the bleeding persists. A chest x-ray should be taken after the procedure. (Care of the patient receiving mechanical ventilation is discussed in Chapter 65.)

Considerable variation in practice exists with regard to the care of a patient with a new tracheostomy. In some centers, it is a shared responsibility between nursing and respiratory therapy. You need to be familiar with your hospital's policies and procedures. The following discussion highlights general guidelines when caring for a patient with a tracheostomy in the first few days after the procedure.

The tracheostomy site must be assessed every shift (at a minimum). Observe the site for any redness, inflammation, edema, ulceration, or signs of infection. Clean around the stoma with normal saline. Apply a sterile pre-cut dressing around the tracheostomy tube site at least once per shift or more frequently based upon your nursing assessment.

Because an inflated cuff exerts pressure on the tracheal mucosa, it is important to inflate the cuff with the minimum volume of air required to obtain an airway seal. Cuff inflation pressure can be measured with a hand-held cuff manometer. The pressure should be monitored at least every 8 hours. Cuff inflation pressure should not exceed 20 to 25 cm $H_2O$ because higher pressures may compress tracheal capillaries, limit blood flow, and predispose the patient to tracheal necrosis. The minimal leak technique (MLT) and the minimal occlusion volume (MOV) are two commonly used methods to inflate the tracheostomy cuff (Table 26-6). Routine cuff deflation is no longer recommended.[27]

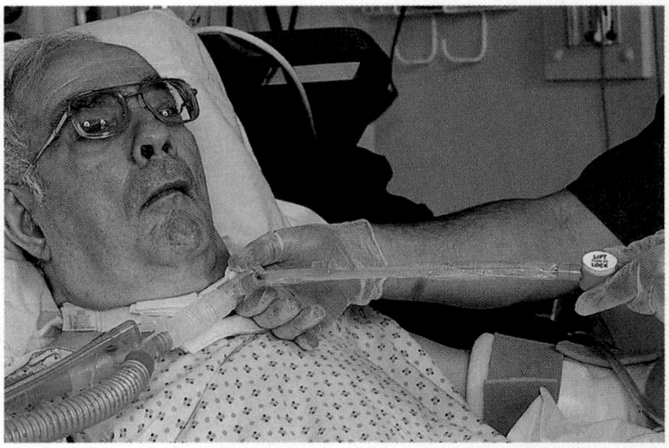

**FIG. 26-4** Suctioning tracheostomy with closed system suction catheter. (From Potter PA, Perry AG: *Basic nursing: essentials for practice,* ed 7, St Louis, 2011, Mosby.)

Suction the airway via the tracheostomy tube as needed (Fig. 26-4 and Table 26-8). Try to avoid suctioning through the newly created tracheostomy in the first few hours after the procedure, as this may aggravate discomfort and promote bleeding. Initially, patients should receive humidified air to compensate for the loss of the upper airway to warm and moisturize secretions. Humidification is essential to prevent retention of tenacious secretions and formation of mucous plugs.

If the inner cannula is disposable, replace as per manufacturer and institutional guidelines. If nondisposable, clean the inner cannula at least every shift. Cleaning removes mucus from the inside of the tube to prevent airway obstruction (Table 26-9).

Change the tracheostomy tapes after the first 24 hours and then as required (Fig. 26-5 and Table 26-9). A two-person technique, one person to stabilize the tracheostomy and one to change the tapes, is best practice to ensure that the tracheostomy does not become accidentally dislodged during the procedure. At the end of the procedure, place two fingers underneath the tapes to ensure they are not too tight around the neck.

When turning and repositioning the patient, take care not to dislodge the tracheostomy tube. Because tube replacement is difficult, several precautions are required, including (1) keep a replacement tube of equal or smaller size at the bedside, readily available for emergency reinsertion; (2) do not change tracheostomy tapes for at least 24 hours after the insertion procedure; and (3) if necessary, an HCP performs the first tube change usually no sooner than 7 days after the tracheostomy.

**CHECK YOUR PRACTICE**

You are caring for a patient who had a surgically created tracheostomy 6 hours ago. While suctioning the patient, he coughs and the tracheostomy tube is dislodged.

- What should you do?

If the tube is accidentally dislodged, immediately call for help. While waiting for the HCP, a respiratory therapist, or other designated individual to arrive, several options may be used (depending on nursing scope of practice and hospital policies and procedures). One option is to quickly obtain a hemostat to spread the opening where the tube was displaced. Insert the obturator in the replacement (spare) tracheostomy tube,

## TABLE 26-8 Suctioning a Tracheostomy

1. Assess the need for suctioning hourly. Indications include visible coughing, coarse crackles or wheezes over large airways, moist cough, increase in peak inspiratory pressure on mechanical ventilator, and restlessness or agitation. May be accompanied by decrease in $SpO_2$. Do not suction routinely.
2. If suctioning is indicated, explain procedure to patient.
3. Collect necessary sterile equipment: suction catheter (no larger than half the lumen of the tracheostomy tube), gloves, sterile water, cup, and drape. If a closed tracheal suction system is used, the catheter is enclosed in a plastic sleeve and reused (Fig. 26-4). No additional equipment is needed.
4. Check suction source and regulator. Adjust suction pressure to no greater than 125 mm Hg pressure with tubing occluded.
5. Assess heart rate and rhythm and $SpO_2$ to provide baseline for detecting change during suctioning.
6. Wash hands and put on personal protective equipment (eye goggles).
7. Use sterile technique to open package, fill cup with sterile water, put on sterile gloves, and connect catheter to suction tubing. Designate one hand as contaminated for (1) connecting and disconnecting the tubing at the suction catheter, (2) using the manual resuscitation bag (MRB), and (3) operating the suction control. Suction sterile water through the catheter to test the system.
8. Provide preoxygenation for a minimum of 30 seconds by (1) adjusting ventilator to deliver 100% $O_2$; or (2) using a reservoir-equipped bag-valve-mask connected to 100% $O_2$. The method chosen depends on whether the patient is attached to a mechanical ventilator or has a tracheostomy tube in place but is spontaneously breathing and receiving supplemental $O_2$. The patient who has had a tracheostomy for an extended period and is not acutely ill may be able to tolerate suctioning without use of an MRB or the ventilator.
9. Gently insert catheter *without suction* to minimize the amount of $O_2$ removed from the lungs. Insert the catheter to the point where the patient coughs. Do NOT insert the catheter until you meet resistance (this is the carina, and repeated trauma with suction catheter can promote bleeding). Apply suction as you slowly begin to withdraw the catheter.
10. Continuous suction should be applied for no more than 10 to 15 seconds.
11. Discontinue suctioning and immediately remove the suction catheter from the patient's trachea if heart rate decreases from baseline by 20 beats/min, increases from baseline by 40 beats/min, a dysrhythmia occurs, or $SpO_2$ decreases to less than 90%. A vagal response may have occurred.
12. After each suction pass, wait at least 30 seconds before suctioning again. Always hyperoxygenate for at least 30 sec (via mechanical ventilator or MRB with 5-6 breaths) in between each suctioning pass.
13. Repeat procedure until airway is clear. Limit insertions of suction catheter to as few as possible. If airway is not clear after three suction passes, allow the patient to rest before additional suctioning.
14. Return $O_2$ concentration to prior setting.
15. Rinse catheter. If using the in-line suction catheter (via mechanical ventilation), ensure that normal saline used to flush out the suction catheter does not enter the patient's airway. For disposable suction catheters, dispose of catheter by wrapping it around fingers of gloved hand and pulling glove over catheter. Discard equipment in proper waste container.
16. Suction the oropharynx or use mouth suction.
17. Reassess heart rate and rhythm and $SpO_2$. Auscultate to assess changes in lung sounds. Record time, amount, and character of secretions and patient response to suctioning.

lubricate with saline, and insert the tube into the stoma. Once the tube is inserted, remove the obturator immediately so that air can flow through the tube.

Another option is to insert a suction catheter to allow passage of air and to serve as a guide for insertion. Thread the tracheostomy tube over the catheter and remove the suction catheter.

If the tube cannot be replaced, immediately and quickly assess the patient's level of respiratory distress and position the patient in semi-Fowler's position to alleviate dyspnea until assistance arrives. Severe dyspnea may progress to respiratory arrest. If respiratory arrest occurs, cover the stoma with a sterile dressing and ventilate the patient with the BVM over the nose

## TABLE 26-9 Tracheostomy Care

*The following are general guidelines for basic tracheostomy care. Become familiar with the specific policies and/or procedures in your institution.*

1. Explain procedure to patient.
2. Use tracheostomy care kit or collect necessary sterile equipment (e.g., suction catheter, gloves, water basin, drape, tracheostomy ties, tube brush or pipe cleaners, 4 × 4-inch gauze pads, sterile water or normal saline, and tracheostomy dressing [optional]). NOTE: Clean rather than sterile technique is used at home.
3. Position patient in semi-Fowler's position.
4. Assemble needed materials on bedside table next to patient.
5. Wash hands. Put on personal protective equipment (goggles and clean gloves).
6. Auscultate chest sounds. If wheezes or coarse crackles are present, suction the patient if unable to cough up secretions (Table 26-8). Remove soiled dressing and clean gloves.
7. Open sterile equipment, pour sterile $H_2O$ or normal saline into two compartments of sterile container or two basins, and put on sterile gloves. NOTE: Hydrogen peroxide (3%) is no longer recommended unless an infection is present. If it is used, rinse the inner cannula and skin with sterile $H_2O$ or normal saline afterward to prevent trauma to tissue.
8. Unlock and remove inner cannula, if present. Many tracheostomy tubes do not have inner cannulas. Care for these tubes includes all steps except for inner cannula care.
9. If disposable inner cannula is used, replace with new cannula. If a nondisposable cannula is used:
   - Immerse inner cannula in sterile solution and clean inside and outside of cannula using tube brush or pipe cleaners.
   - Rinse cannula in sterile solution. Remove from solution and shake to dry.
   - Insert inner cannula into outer cannula with the curved part downward, and lock in place.
10. Remove dried secretions from stoma using 4 × 4-inch gauze pad soaked in sterile water or saline. Gently pat area around the stoma dry. Be sure to clean under the tracheostomy flange (faceplate), using cotton swabs to reach this area.
11. Change tracheostomy tapes. Use two-person change technique or secure new tapes to flanges before removing the old ones. Tie tracheostomy tapes securely with room for two fingers between tapes and skin (Fig. 26-5). To prevent accidental tube removal, secure the tracheostomy tube by gently applying pressure to the flange of the tube during the tape changes. *Do not change tracheostomy tapes for 24 hours after the tracheostomy procedure.*
13. As an alternative, some patients prefer tracheostomy tapes made of Velcro, which are easier to adjust.
14. If drainage is excessive, place dressing around tube (Fig. 26-5). A pre-cut tracheostomy dressing or unlined gauze should be used. Do not cut the gauze because threads may be inhaled or wrap around the tracheostomy tube. Change the dressing as required. Wet dressings promote infection and stoma irritation.
15. Repeat care three times/day and as needed.

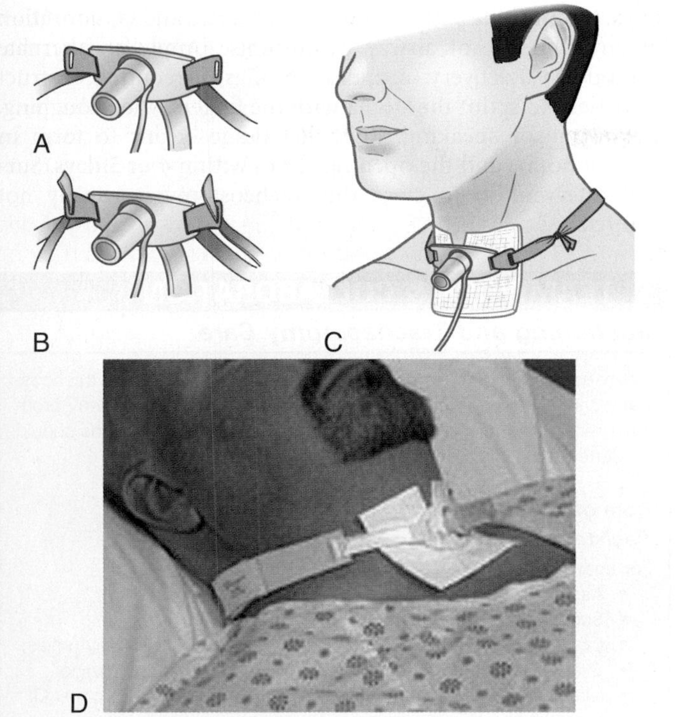


FIG. 26-5 Changing tracheostomy tapes. **A,** A slit is cut about 1 inch (2.5 cm) from the end. The slit end is put into the opening of the cannula. **B,** A loop is made with the other end of the tape. **C,** The tapes are tied together with a double knot on the side of the neck. **D,** A Velcro tracheostomy tube holder can be used instead of twill ties to make tracheostomy tube stabilization more secure. (*D,* Courtesy Dale Medical Products, Inc, Plainville, Mass.)

and mouth. If a patient has had a total laryngectomy, there will be complete separation between the upper airway and trachea. Ventilate this patient through the tracheostomy stoma.

## Chronic Care

Some patients will never be able to be weaned from mechanical ventilation and will require a tracheostomy for life. Care of the patient with a long-term tracheostomy includes all of the same care as patients with a new tracheostomy, including observing the tracheostomy site, cleaning the inner cannula, suctioning, and changing tracheostomy tapes.

The tracheostomy tube should be changed approximately 1 month after the first tube change and monthly thereafter. When a tracheostomy has been in place for several months, the healed tract should be well formed. Changing the tracheostomy tube may be undertaken for two main reasons. First, it permits assessment of the stoma and cleaning of the tube. The patient may be taught to change the tube at home using a clean technique. Second, exchanging the tracheostomy tube for one of a different size (smaller internal diameter) will increase airway resistance and work of breathing for the patient. This will strengthen the respiratory muscles and help promote weaning from mechanical ventilation.

## Swallowing Dysfunction

The patient with a tracheostomy who cannot protect the airway from aspiration requires an inflated cuff. However, an inflated cuff may result in swallowing dysfunction by interfering with the normal function of muscles used to swallow.

For long-term tracheostomy patients, it is important to evaluate the patient's swallowing ability and risk for aspiration.

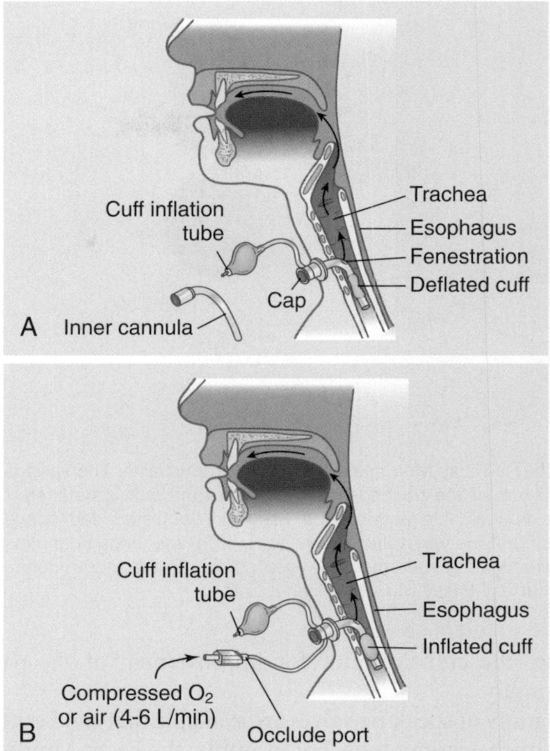


FIG. 26-6 Speaking tracheostomy tubes. **A,** Fenestrated tracheostomy tube with cuff deflated, inner cannula removed, and tracheostomy tube capped to allow air to pass over the vocal cords. **B,** Speaking tracheostomy tube. One tube is used for cuff inflation. The second tube is connected to a source of compressed air or $O_2$. When the port on the second tube is occluded, air flows up over the vocal cords, allowing speech with an inflated cuff. (See Table 26-6 and eNursing Care Plan 26-1 for related nursing management.)

Assessment of the patient's ability to swallow is most often done by a speech therapist. The patient is evaluated for aspiration and/or microaspiration using different consistencies of thickened fluids and under videofluoroscopy or with a fiberoptic endoscopy. If the patient is able to swallow without aspiration when the cuff is deflated, the cuff may be left deflated or a cuffless tube substituted. At this time, patients may also be permitted varying levels of thickened fluids and soft foods.

## Speech With a Tracheostomy Tube

A number of techniques promote speech in the patient with a tracheostomy. When the patient initially requires attachment to a mechanical ventilator, provide the patient with a paper and pencil, a white board, or Magic Slate. A communication board with pictures of common needs is convenient for patients who may speak other languages. A visual alphabet for spelling words is useful for patients who are weak or have difficulty writing.

The spontaneously breathing patient may be able to talk with a tracheostomy. Several options are available depending upon the type of tracheostomy. For example, if it has been determined that the patient is at low risk for aspiration, (1) remove the inner cannula (if nonfenestrated), (2) deflate the cuff, and (3) place the decannulation cap in the tube (Fig. 26-6).

When the tracheostomy cuff is deflated, exhaled air is allowed to flow upward over the vocal cords. When a fenestrated cannula is first used, frequently assess the patient for signs of respiratory distress. If the patient is not able to tolerate the procedure, remove the cap, insert a nonfenestrated inner cannula, and

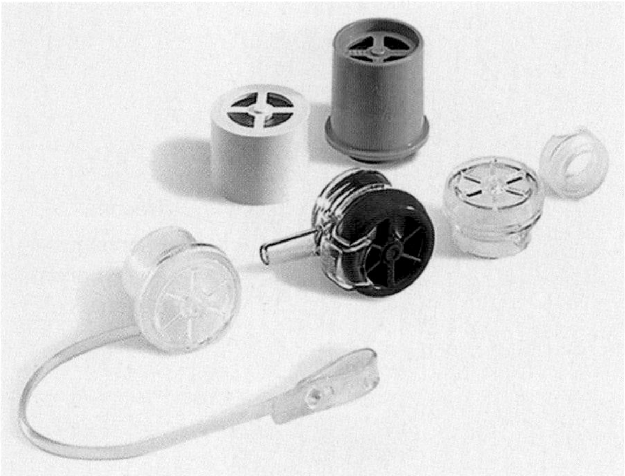

**FIG. 26-7** Passy-Muir speaking tracheostomy valve. The valve is placed over the hub of the tracheostomy tube after the cuff is deflated. Multiple options are available and can be used for ventilated and nonventilated patients. The one-way valve allows air to enter the lungs during inspiration and redirects air upward over the vocal cords into the mouth during expiration. (Courtesy Passy-Muir, Inc, Irvine, Calif.)

reinflate the cuff. Monitor for improvement of the patient's condition.

A variety of speaking valves are available that can be attached to the tracheostomy tube. For example, the Passy-Muir valve is a simple device that attaches to the hub of the tracheostomy tube (Fig. 26-7). With the cuff deflated, the valve redirects air flow through the vocal cords. On inspiration, the valve on the device opens, allowing the patient to inhale. When the patient exhales, the valve closes, air flows upward around the tracheostomy, and through the vocal cords. The patient exhales through the nose and mouth instead of through the tracheostomy, allowing speech. The patient may initially only be able to tolerate short periods of use until he or she becomes accustomed to exhaling through the mouth. Remove the valve immediately if there are any signs and symptoms of respiratory distress. Advocating for the use of alternative speaking devices may help improve self-care and increase self-esteem for the patient with a tracheostomy.

### ◆ Decannulation

Removal of the tracheostomy from the trachea is known as **decannulation**. Removal is possible when the primary condition for which the patient initially received a tracheostomy has been resolved. In addition, the patient needs to (1) be hemodynamically stable; (2) have a stable, intact respiratory drive; and (3) be able to adequately exchange air and expectorate secretions.

Immediately prior to decannulation, explain to the patient what will occur. Monitor and record the vital signs. Suction the patient prior to decannulation through the tracheostomy. Clear the mouth of any oral secretions. Loosen and/or cut the tracheostomy tapes, and remove any visible sutures holding the tracheostomy in place. Most importantly, ensure that the tracheostomy cuff is deflated. Pull the tracheostomy tube outwards in one smooth motion. Stop if you meet any resistance and notify the appropriate personnel.

Once the tracheostomy tube is removed, post-decannulation care involves application of a sterile occlusive dressing and monitoring the site for bleeding. The dressing must be changed if it gets soiled or wet. If necessary, close the stoma with tape strips. Monitor the patient's respiratory status and $O_2$ saturation for any evidence of airway compromise. Apply an alternate method of $O_2$ delivery (e.g., nasal prongs) if required. Instruct the patient to splint the stoma with the fingers when coughing, swallowing, or speaking. Epithelial tissue begins to form in 24 to 48 hours, and the opening closes within 4 or 5 days. Surgical intervention to close the tracheostomy is usually not required.

### TEAMWORK & COLLABORATION
#### *Suctioning and Tracheostomy Care*

Licensed practical nurses (LPNs) may do suctioning and give tracheostomy care to stable patients. In patients who have acute airway problems requiring an ET or tracheostomy tube, these interventions should be done by the registered nurse (RN).

**Role of Nursing Personnel**

***Registered Nurse (RN)***

For unstable patients:
- Assess for the need for suctioning.
- Suction the ET or tracheostomy tube.
- Evaluate for adverse effects of suctioning such as dysrhythmias.
- Evaluate whether patient status is improved after suctioning.
- Maintain appropriate cuff inflation pressure at 20 to 25 cm $H_2O$, or use minimal leak technique to maintain cuff pressure.
- Assess tracheostomy and any retention sutures for evidence of complications (e.g., infection).
- Replace the tracheostomy tube after accidental dislodgment.
- Ventilate the patient with a bag-valve-mask device after accidental tracheostomy dislodgment if needed.
- Assess swallowing ability and risk for aspiration.
- Develop plan to avoid aspiration in a patient with a tracheostomy.
- Teach patient and caregiver about home tracheostomy care.

***Licensed Practical/Vocational Nurse (LPN/LVN)***

For stable patients:
- Determine the need for suctioning.
- Suction the tracheostomy.
- Evaluate whether patient status is improved after suctioning.
- Provide tracheostomy care using sterile technique.

***Unlicensed Assistive Personnel (UAP)***
- Provide oral care to patient with a tracheostomy.
- Suction patient's oropharynx (after being trained and evaluated in this procedure).
- Report increased need for oropharyngeal suctioning to the RN.

**Role of Other Team Members**

***Respiratory Therapist***
- Ensures proper equipment is available for suctioning and tracheotomy care
- Has similar role to that of RN (see above)

## LARYNGEAL POLYPS

*Laryngeal polyps* develop on the vocal cords from vocal abuse (e.g., excessive talking, singing) or irritation (e.g., intubation, cigarette smoking). The most common symptom is hoarseness. Polyps are treated conservatively with voice rest and adequate hydration. Surgical removal may be indicated for large polyps, which may cause dysphagia, dyspnea, and stridor. Polyps are usually benign but may be removed because they can become malignant.

## HEAD AND NECK CANCER

Head and neck cancer is classified according to the area where it occurs. These cancers may involve the nasal cavity and paranasal sinuses, nasopharynx, oropharynx, larynx, oral cavity, and/or salivary gland. (Cancer of the oral cavity is discussed in Chapter 41.) Most head and neck cancers arise from squamous cells that line the mucosal surfaces of the head and neck.

More than 52,000 new cases of head and neck cancer are diagnosed each year in the United States. Eighty-five percent of head and neck cancers are caused by tobacco (including smokeless tobacco). Excessive alcohol consumption is also a major risk factor. Head and neck cancer most frequently occurs in people over age 50 and twice as often in men (compared to women). Head and neck cancers in patients younger than 50 years are often associated with human papillomavirus (HPV) infection. Other risk factors include sun exposure, radiation therapy to the head and neck, exposure to asbestos and other industrial carcinogens, and poor oral hygiene.[28]

Unfortunately, most people have locally advanced disease at the time of diagnosis. Disability from both the disease and subsequent treatment is significant because of the potential loss of voice, adverse effects from chemotherapy and/or radiation, disfigurement, and social concerns.

### Clinical Manifestations

Early clinical manifestations of head and neck cancer vary with the location of the tumor. For example, cancer of the oral cavity may initially be seen as a white or red patch in the mouth, an ulcer that does not heal, or a change in the fit of dentures. Some patients experience what feels like a lump in the throat or a change in the quality of the voice. Hoarseness that lasts more than 2 weeks may be a symptom of early laryngeal cancer.

Other clinical manifestations may include a sore throat that does not get better with treatment, a unilateral sore throat or otalgia (ear pain), swelling or lumps in the neck, and coughing up blood. Unintentional weight loss and difficulty with chewing, swallowing, moving the tongue or jaw, and breathing are typically late symptoms. A partially or fully obstructed airway is also often a late manifestation of head and neck cancer.

### Diagnostic Studies

Early detection is key to patient survival. Physical assessment involves thoroughly examining the oral cavity, including the area under the tongue and dentures, with a flashlight. There may be thickening of the normally soft and pliable oral mucosa. Inspect the floor of the mouth and tongue, and bimanually palpate the lymph nodes in the neck. *Leukoplakia* (white patch) or *erythroplakia* (fiery red patch) may be found. Both leukoplakia and carcinoma in situ (localized to a defined area) may precede invasive carcinoma by many years.

If lesions are suspected, the upper airways may be examined using indirect pharyngoscopy and laryngoscopy (which involves using a laryngeal mirror). The larynx and vocal cords are visually inspected for lesions and tissue mobility. Typically, multiple biopsy specimens are obtained to help determine the extent of the disease. A CT scan or MRI may be performed to detect local and regional spread. Positron emission tomography (PET) scanning is also used in diagnosis. (Interprofessional care of head and neck cancer is presented in Table 26-10.)

**TABLE 26-10 Interprofessional Care**

***Head and Neck Cancer***

| Diagnostic Assessment | Management |
|---|---|
| • History and physical examination<br>• Indirect pharyngoscopy and laryngoscopy<br>• Endoscopy<br>• Biopsy<br>• Chest x-ray<br>• Barium swallow | • Surgery<br>  • Vocal cord stripping<br>  • Laser surgery<br>  • Cordectomy<br>  • Partial or total laryngectomy<br>  • Pharyngectomy<br>  • Lymph node removal with neck dissection<br>  • Tracheostomy<br>  • Reconstructive procedures<br>• Radiation therapy<br>• Chemotherapy<br>• Targeted therapy<br>• Physical therapy<br>• Occupational therapy<br>• Speech therapy |

### Staging of Head and Neck Cancer

Head and neck cancer is staged based on the size of the tumor (T), number and location of involved lymph nodes (N), and extent of metastasis (M). This is referred to as *TNM staging*.[29] TNM staging classifies head and neck cancers as Stage 0 (carcinoma in situ) through Stage IV (spread to distant organs and tissues). (TNM staging is discussed in Chapter 15 on p. 241.)

### Interprofessional Care

The choice of treatment for head and neck cancer is based on many factors, including the location of tumor, TNM stage, patient's age and overall general health, urgency of treatment, cosmetic and functional considerations (e.g., ability to talk, swallow, and chew), and patient choice. Treatment options may include surgery, radiation therapy, chemotherapy, targeted therapy, or any combination of these modalities.[30]

**Surgical Therapy.** Surgery is often the first-line treatment option for head and neck cancers. Some patients may be treated with surgery alone. For other patients, combining surgery with radiation therapy and/or chemotherapy may be appropriate. Depending on the location and stage of cancer, the following surgical procedures may be done:

- *Vocal cord stripping:* Removal of outer layers of tissue on the vocal cords. This approach may be used for a biopsy or to treat some stage 0 cancers confined to the vocal cords. Vocal cord stripping rarely affects speech.
- *Laser surgery:* An endoscope with a laser is inserted down the throat and the tumor can be vaporized or removed.
- *Cordectomy:* Part or all of the vocal cords are removed. Patients may experience changes in speech. Removing part of a vocal cord may lead to a hoarse voice. If both vocal cords are removed, speech will no longer be possible.
- *Partial or total laryngectomy:* A surgical procedure in which part or all of the larynx is removed. For the patient with a total laryngectomy, airflow in and out of the lungs will be altered as a result of surgery and normal voice production will not be possible (Fig. 26-8).
- *Pharyngectomy:* Part or all of the throat is removed.
- *Tracheostomy:* A tracheostomy is done to create an alternate pathway for breathing by creating a stoma in the trachea. (Tracheostomy was previously discussed on pp. 485-490.)

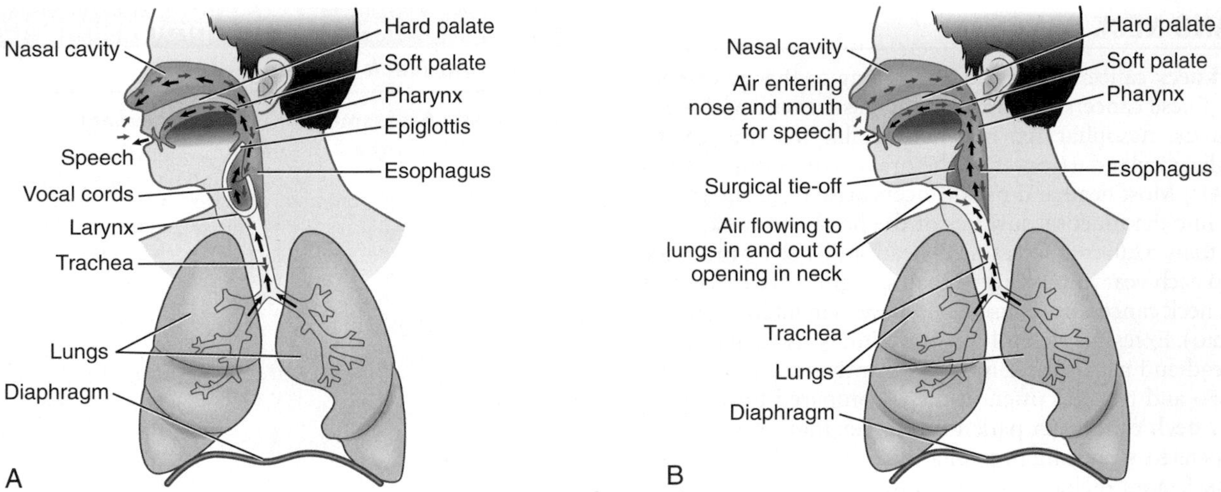


**FIG. 26-8** **A,** Normal airflow in and out of the lungs. **B,** Airflow in and out of the lungs after total laryngectomy.

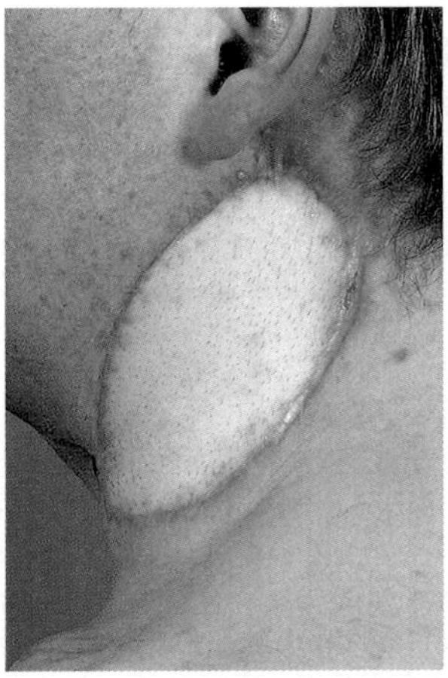

**FIG. 26-9** Reconstructive surgery involving skin grafts and skin flaps may be needed after a radical neck dissection. (From Eggers G, Flechtenmacher C, Kurzen J, Hassfeld S: Infiltrating basal cell carcinoma of the neck 34 years after irradiation of an haemangioma in early childhood. A case-report, *J Craniomaxillofac Surg* 33:199, 2005.)

- *Lymph node removal:* Head and neck cancer sometimes spreads to the lymph nodes. The amount of tissue and number of lymph nodes that are removed depend on how far the cancer has spread.
- *Neck dissection surgery:* Three main types include:
  - *Radical neck dissection:* All the tissue on the side of the neck from the mandible to the clavicle is removed. The muscle, nerve, salivary gland, and major blood vessels in this area are removed.
  - *Modified radical neck dissection:* This is the most common type of neck dissection. All lymph nodes are removed. Less neck tissue is taken out than in radical dissection. This surgery may also spare the nerves in the neck and, sometimes, the blood vessels or muscle.
  - *Selective neck dissection:* If cancer has not spread far, fewer lymph nodes have to be removed. The muscle, nerve, and blood vessels in the neck may also be saved.

Following extensive surgery to remove head and neck cancer, reconstructive operations can help restore both the structure and function of the affected areas (Fig. 26-9).

**Radiation Therapy.** Radiation therapy can be delivered by either external-beam therapy or internal implants (brachytherapy). Brachytherapy is a concentrated and localized method of delivering radiation that involves placing a radioactive source into or near the tumor. The goal is to deliver high doses of radiation to the target area while limiting exposure of surrounding tissues. Thin, hollow, plastic needles are inserted into the tumor area, and radioactive seeds are placed in the needles. The seeds emit continuous radiation. (Radiation therapy and brachytherapy are discussed in Chapter 15.)

Radiation therapy is often preferred for patients with early head and neck cancer because it offers the patient good results with voice preservation. Some patients refuse surgical intervention for advanced lesions because of the extent of the procedure and potential risks involved. In this situation, radiation therapy is used as the sole treatment or in combination with chemotherapy. Other patients may opt for surgery and a combination of either radiation and/or chemotherapy treatments.

**Chemotherapy and Targeted Therapy.** Chemotherapy is used in combination with radiation therapy for patients with stage III or IV cancers. Chemotherapy agents include cisplatin, methotrexate, 5-fluorouracil (5-FU), docetaxel (Taxotere), ifosfamide (Ifex), and bleomycin.

Cetuximab (Erbitux), a targeted therapy, is used with chemotherapy to treat patients with late-stage head and neck cancer. The drug targets epidermal growth factor receptor (EGFR), a specific protein within cancer cells, and stops the cells from growing. (Targeted therapy is discussed in Chapter 15 and Table 15-13.)

**Nutritional Therapy.** Many patients with head and neck cancer are malnourished even before treatment begins. Treatment modalities increase the risk of malnutrition. For example, after radical neck surgery the patient may be unable to take in nutrients orally because of swelling, the location of sutures, or difficulty with swallowing. Side effects from chemotherapy and radiation therapy can impair the patient's ability to maintain adequate nutrition. Painful oral mucositis frequently leads to breaks in treatment if the patient is relying solely on oral intake for nutrition.

A thorough nutritional assessment and prophylactic placement of a gastrostomy tube in high-risk patients are vital to maintaining adequate nutrition. Enteral nutrition may be started before initiation of treatment to obtain and maintain optimal nutritional status needed for tissue repair. (Enteral nutrition is described in Chapter 39.) Observe for tolerance of the feedings and adjust the amount, time, and formula if nausea, vomiting, diarrhea, or distention occurs. Instruct the patient and caregiver about the tube feedings.

Patients who are not candidates for or who refuse tube feedings need to be monitored closely for weight loss. Antiemetics or analgesics may be given before meals to reduce nausea and mouth pain. Bland foods are easier for patients to tolerate. Patients can increase caloric intake by adding dry milk to foods during preparation, selecting foods high in calories, and using oral supplements. It is helpful to add mild sauces and gravies to food, which adds calories and moistens food so that it is more easily swallowed. Elevate the head of the bed while the patient is eating.

Anticipate swallowing problems when the patient resumes eating after surgery. The type and degree of difficulty varies depending on the surgical procedure. Videofluoroscopic swallowing studies may be used to evaluate the safety of the patient's swallowing. When the patient can successfully swallow with low or no risk of aspiration, small amounts of thickened liquids or pureed foods may be given with the patient in high Fowler's position. Avoid thin, watery fluids because they are difficult to swallow and increase the risk of aspiration. Closely observe for choking. Suctioning may be necessary to prevent aspiration.

**Physical Therapy.** After surgery for head and neck cancer, the physical therapist will help teach the patient how to use the upper extremities to assist with support and movement of the head. In the immediate postoperative period, the patient should begin an exercise program to maintain strength and movement in the shoulders and neck. Without exercise, the patient will be left with a "frozen" shoulder and limited range of neck motion. The patient should continue his or her exercise program after discharge to prevent future functional disabilities.

**Speech Therapy.** Preoperatively a speech therapist should meet with the patient and caregiver to discuss any effect that surgery will have on the voice and potential voice restoration options. The International Association of Laryngectomees, an association of laryngectomy patients, focuses on helping patients reestablish speech. Local groups, called "Lost Chord" or "New Voice" Clubs, often provide volunteers to visit the patient preoperatively.

There are three major approaches used to restore oral communication: (1) electrolarynx, (2) tracheoesophageal puncture (TEP) voice restoration, and (3) esophageal speech. An *electrolarynx* is a hand-held, battery-powered device that creates speech with the use of sound waves (Fig. 26-10, *A*). This option allows for speech immediately after surgery, is easy to learn, and requires little maintenance. The primary disadvantage of the electrolarynx is the mechanical sound quality, which many patients find unacceptable.

In *transesophageal puncture (TEP)* a fistula is created in the tracheoesophageal wall that diverts pulmonary air across the pharyngoesophageal mucosa for phonation when the tracheostoma is occluded. A one-way valve prosthesis is placed in the tract. The valve prevents aspiration of food or saliva from the esophagus into the tracheostomy. To speak, the patient manually blocks the stoma with the finger. Air moves from the lungs, through the prosthesis, into the esophagus, and out the mouth. Speech is produced by the air vibrating against the esophagus and is formed into words by moving the tongue and lips. A commonly used voice prosthesis is the Blom-Singer prosthesis (Fig. 26-10, *B*). TEP offers the best speech quality with the highest patient satisfaction.

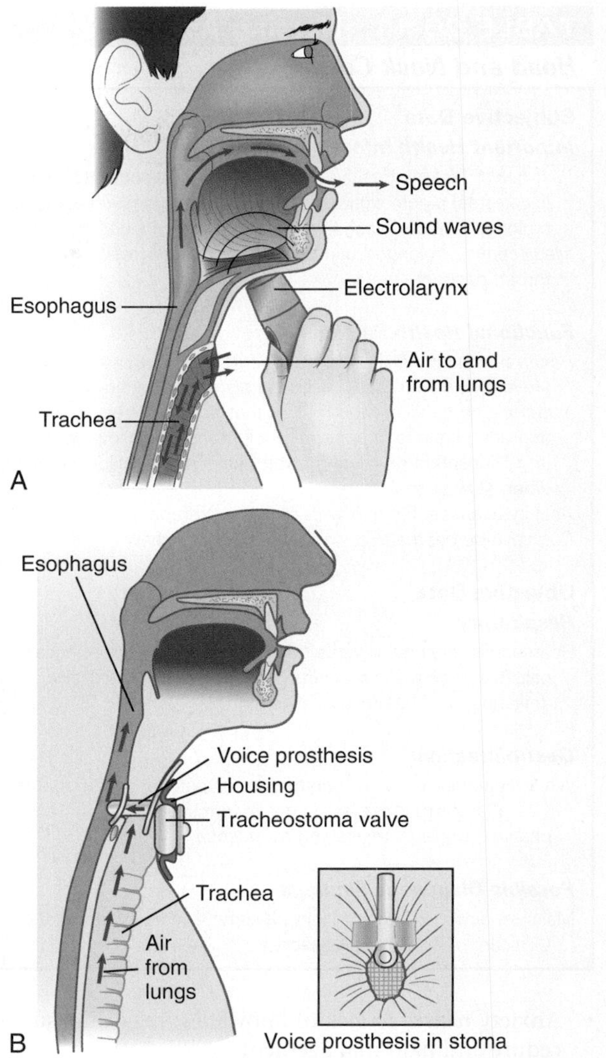


**FIG. 26-10** **A,** The sound waves created by the electrolarynx allow the person to speak. **B,** The Blom-Singer voice prosthesis and valve.

*Esophageal speech* production depends upon air that is introduced into the esophagus and is then expelled past the pharyngoesophageal segment, the vibratory source for sound production. The primary disadvantages of developing esophageal speech are the length of time required to learn the technique and the reduction in voice quality.

## ❖ NURSING MANAGEMENT: HEAD AND NECK CANCER

### ◆ Nursing Assessment

Table 26-11 presents subjective and objective data to obtain from a person with head and neck cancer.

### ◆ Nursing Diagnoses

Nursing diagnoses for the patient with head and neck cancer include, but are not limited to, the following:

- Ineffective airway clearance *related to* presence of artificial airway and excessive mucus
- Risk for aspiration *related to* presence of tracheostomy tube and impaired swallowing

**TABLE 26-11 Nursing Assessment**
***Head and Neck Cancer***

**Subjective Data**
***Important Health Information***
*Past health history:* Positive family history; prolonged tobacco use (cigarettes, pipes, cigars, chewing tobacco, smokeless tobacco); prolonged, heavy alcohol use; poor intake of fruits and vegetables
*Medications:* Prolonged use of over-the-counter medication for sore throat, decongestants

***Functional Health Patterns***
*Health perception–health management:* Does not participate in preventive health measures, long history of alcohol and tobacco use
*Nutritional-metabolic:* Mouth ulcer that does not heal, change in fit of dentures, change in appetite, weight loss, swallowing difficulty (e.g., sensation of lump in throat, pain with swallowing, aspiration when swallowing)
*Activity-exercise:* Fatigue with minimal exertion
*Cognitive-perceptual:* Sore throat, pain on swallowing, referred ear pain

**Objective Data**
***Respiratory***
Hoarseness, change in voice quality, chronic laryngitis, nasal voice, palpable neck mass and lymph nodes (tender, hard, fixed), tracheal deviation; dyspnea, stridor (late sign)

***Gastrointestinal***
White (leukoplakia) or red (erythroplakia) patches inside mouth, ulceration of mucosa, asymmetric tongue, exudate in mouth or pharynx, mass or thickening of mucosa

***Possible Diagnostic Findings***
Mass on direct or indirect laryngoscopy; tumor on soft tissue x-ray, CT scan, or MRI; positive biopsy

- Anxiety *related to* lack of knowledge regarding surgical procedure and pain management
- Acute pain *related to* tissue injury from surgery
- Impaired verbal communication *related to* removal of vocal cords

Additional information on nursing diagnoses for the patient with head and neck cancer is presented in eNursing Care Plan 26-2 on the website for this chapter.

## ◆ Planning

The overall goals are that the patient will have (1) a patent airway, (2) no spread of cancer, (3) no complications related to therapy, (4) adequate nutritional intake, (5) minimal to no pain, (6) the ability to communicate, and (7) an acceptable body image.

## ◆ Nursing Implementation

◆ **Health Promotion.** Most head and neck cancer can be prevented. The development of head and neck cancer is closely related to personal habits, primarily tobacco use and excessive alcohol ingestion. Poor oral hygiene and HPV infection are also risk factors for head and neck cancer.

Include information about risk factors in health teaching. Encourage good oral hygiene. Teach patients about safe sex practices to prevent HPV infection (e.g., use condoms for every sex act, be in a monogamous relationship, choose a partner who has had no or few previous partners). If cancer has been diagnosed, tobacco and alcohol cessation is still important. The likelihood of a cure, by any treatment modality, for a patient with head and neck cancer who continues to smoke and ingest alcoholic beverages is decreased. Additionally, the risk of a second primary cancer is significantly increased. Give patients information about smoking cessation programs and techniques for success. If necessary, refer to an alcohol treatment program. (Smoking cessation and treatment of alcohol abuse are discussed in Chapter 10.)

◆ **Acute Care.** Teach the patient and caregiver about the type of treatment to be performed and care required. Help prepare them to deal with the psychologic impact of the diagnosis of cancer, alteration of physical appearance, possible need for enteral feedings, and potential for altered methods of communication because of the loss of a voice.

The care plan should include assessment of the patient's support system. The patient may not have someone to provide assistance after discharge, may be unemployed, or may have a job that cannot be continued.

◆ ***Surgical Therapy.*** Preoperatively assess the patient's physical and psychosocial needs. Physical preparation is the same as for any major surgery, with an emphasis on oral hygiene. Assess knowledge and understanding of the planned surgical procedure, and clarify information as needed. Include the caregiver in preoperative teaching.

Tailor teaching to the planned surgical procedure. For example, include information about expected changes in speech following a laryngectomy. Magic Slates, alphabet boards, writing materials, pictorial guides, or hand signals are useful methods for communicating. Programmable speech-generating devices allow use of recorded messages that are matched with a graphic representing each message. Integration of this technology into patient care enhances the patient's ability to communicate basic needs postoperatively.

**INFORMATICS IN PRACTICE**
***Communication Devices for Patient With Laryngectomy***

- Assisting with communication will improve a patient's quality of life after a laryngectomy.
- Use an iPad or iPhone and download a text-to-speech application. These applications allow the patient to type in text, and then a computer voice says the text aloud.
- You can also teach the patient how to use a keyboard-based communication program. The patient types on a traditional keyboard and generates speech that is transmitted through hand-held speakers.

Immediately after surgery, focus your nursing care on airway management, wound care, nutrition, communication, and psychosocial issues related to body image changes. Maintenance of a patent airway is essential. The inflammation in the surgical area may compress the trachea. Keep the patient in a semi-Fowler's position to decrease edema and limit tension on the suture lines. The patient with a laryngectomy requires frequent suctioning via the tracheostomy tube. (Care of a patient with a tracheostomy was discussed earlier in this chapter on pp. 486-490.) Secretions typically change in amount and consistency over time. The patient may initially have copious blood-tinged secretions that diminish and thicken. Maintain adequate fluid intake (IV, enteral, and oral when allowed) and humidification of inspired gases to keep secretions liquid and mucous membranes moist. Encourage deep breathing and coughing.

Administer analgesic drugs as needed for pain control. Because patients may not be able to speak, have them nonverbally rate their pain (e.g., visual pain scale such as FACES) to help assess the effectiveness of the medication. (Pain management is discussed in Chapter 8.)

Monitor vital signs frequently because of the risk of hemorrhage. Many of the structures in the head and neck area are very vascular.

Pressure dressings, packing, or drainage tubes may be used for wound management, depending on the type of surgical procedure. Do not change the dressing unless you have a specific order from the surgeon. If skin flaps are used, dressings are typically not used. This allows better visualization of the flap and avoids excessive pressure on tissue (Fig. 26-9). Skin flaps must initially be checked hourly for color and any change in size or edema. Doppler ultrasound may be used to determine the presence of a pulse, depending upon the location of the skin flap. Hemovac, Jackson-Pratt, and Penrose are some of the drainage tubes that may be used.

Drainage may initially be bloody, then serosanguineous, and gradually decrease in volume over 24 hours. Monitor patency of drainage tubes every 4 hours to ensure proper functioning. If the tubing becomes obstructed, fluid will accumulate under the skin flap and predispose the patient to formation of hematomas or seromas, impair wound healing, and increase the risk for infection. After drainage tubes are removed, closely monitor the area to detect any swelling. Closely monitor incision sites for signs of infection.

The patient may have a nasogastric tube inserted during surgery to remove gastric contents via intermittent suction for the first 24 to 48 hours until peristalsis returns. Because the nasogastric tube lies close to internal incision lines, do not manipulate or move the tube. When bowel sounds return, enteral feedings may be started slowly and advanced to meet nutritional needs.

◆ ***Radiation Therapy.*** Dry mouth *(xerostomia)*, a frequent and annoying problem, typically begins within a few weeks of treatment. The patient's saliva decreases in volume and becomes thick. The change may be temporary or permanent. Pilocarpine hydrochloride (Salagen) is often effective in increasing saliva production.

**CHECK YOUR PRACTICE**

Your 64-yr-old male patient with oral cancer has been receiving radiation therapy for 3 weeks. He has developed xerostomia and oral mucositis. He asks if you have any suggestions to help relieve his symptoms.

- How would you respond?

Once patients are permitted to have foods or fluids by mouth, they can get symptom relief by increasing fluid intake, chewing sugarless gum or sugarless candy, using nonalcoholic mouth rinses (baking soda or glycerin solutions), and using artificial saliva. Instruct patients to always carry a water bottle with them. Fluoride gels or treatments can help prevent dental deterioration caused by xerostomia.

Oral mucositis can cause irritation, ulceration, and pain. Instruct the patient on oral care basics, including the use of a soft toothbrush and regular flossing. Empty fluoride gel trays, along with bite blocks, athletic mouth guards, or gauze pads, can be worn during radiation treatments. This prevents radiation scatter to the tongue and cheek from metal work in the mouth. Warm bland rinses such as those with salt and baking soda four to six times daily may be helpful. Sucking on ice chips can also help with the pain. Patients should avoid commercial mouthwashes and hot, spicy, or acidic foods because they are irritating.

Skin over the irradiated area often becomes reddened and sensitive to touch. Instruct patients to use only prescribed lotions and skin products while undergoing radiation therapy and to not use any lotions within 2 hours before treatment. (Skin care for patients having radiation therapy is discussed in Chapter 15.)

Fatigue is a common side effect of radiation therapy as well as chemotherapy. Encourage patients to walk 15 to 30 minutes each day, since regular exercise can give them more energy. Instruct patients to do activities that are most important to them and to rest during periods of low energy. Identify support systems and encourage patients to ask for help.

◆ ***Stoma Care.*** Should the patient have a stoma created as a result of surgery, instruct the patient before discharge in the proper care of the stoma. The patient should wash the area around the stoma daily with a moist cloth. A nasal wash spray (e.g., Alkalol) can be used every 1 to 2 hours to keep the stoma moist and prevent crusting. Dried secretions can be removed with tweezers. If a laryngectomy tube is in place, the patient must remove the entire tube at least daily and clean it in the same manner as a tracheostomy tube. The inner cannula may have to be removed and cleaned more frequently. A scarf or loose shirt can be used to hide the stoma.

The patient should cover the stoma when coughing (because mucus may be expectorated) and during any activity (e.g., shaving, applying makeup) that may lead to inhalation of foreign materials. Because water can easily enter the stoma, the patient should wear a plastic collar when taking a shower. Swimming is contraindicated. Initially, humidification is administered via a mechanical ventilation or, after extubation, with a tracheostomy mask. After discharge, the patient can use a bedside humidifier.

◆ ***Psychosocial Needs.*** Psychosocial care of the patient with head and neck cancer is very important. Issues concerning depression, change in body image, and sexuality are very common. Although changes are discussed before surgery, the patient may not be psychologically prepared for the extent of these changes.

Depression may occur for many reasons: inability to speak because of surgical procedure and/or presence of ET or tracheostomy tube, altered physical appearance due to the surgery and edema, loss of independence and reliance upon others, and feelings of helplessness and hopelessness. Depression may also be related to concern about the prognosis.

Allow the patient and caregiver to express their feelings and emotions, verbally or nonverbally. Convey acceptance to help patients regain positive feelings about their body image and self-concept. Encourage participation in support groups. Information about available groups can be obtained through the local branch of the American Cancer Society. A psychiatric referral may be appropriate for the patient who is experiencing prolonged or severe depression.

Surgery and foreign attachments such as tracheostomy and gastrostomy tubes may dramatically affect body image. Xerostomia and fatigue can physically affect sexuality. It may be difficult for the patient to talk about sexual problems because of the alteration in communication. Assist the patient and partner by allowing them to talk about their sexuality, and how surgery and treatment may affect their relationship. Helping the patient see that sexuality involves much more than appearance may relieve some anxiety.

◆ **Ambulatory Care.** The patient may be discharged with a tracheostomy and a nasogastric or gastrostomy feeding tube. Some patients initially need home health care to evaluate the patient's or caregiver's ability to perform self-care activities. The patient and caregiver need to learn how to manage tubes and whom to call if there are problems. Provide pictorial instructions for tracheostomy care, suctioning, stoma and skin care, and enteral feeding as appropriate. Encouraging the patient to participate in self-care is an important part of rehabilitation.

Inform the patient about the importance of wearing a Medic Alert bracelet or other identification that alerts emergency personnel of the possible alterations in breathing status as a result of surgery. Because the patient no longer breathes through the nose, the ability to smell smoke and food is often lost. Advise the patient to install smoke and carbon monoxide detectors in the home. Encourage preparation of food that is colorful, attractive, and nutritious because taste may also be diminished secondary to the loss of smell and radiation therapy.

The patient can resume exercise, recreation, and sexual activity when able. Most patients can return to work 1 to 2 months after surgery. However, many never return to full-time employment. The changes that follow a total laryngectomy can be upsetting. Loss of speech, loss of the ability to taste and smell, inability to produce audible sounds (including laughing and weeping), and the presence of a permanent tracheal stoma that produces undesirable mucus are often overwhelming to the patient. Although changes are discussed before surgery, the patient may not be prepared for the extent of these changes. If the patient has a significant other, this person's reaction to the patient's altered appearance is important. Acceptance by another person can promote an improved self-image.

## ◆ Evaluation

Expected outcomes for the patient with head and neck cancer who is treated surgically are that the patient will

- Demonstrate effective coughing and secretion clearance
- Demonstrate the ability to swallow oral foods without aspiration
- Report satisfaction with pain relief
- Use written and nonverbal techniques to effectively communicate with others

Other outcomes for the patient with head and neck cancer who is treated surgically are addressed in eNursing Care Plans 26-1 and 26-2 on the website for this chapter.

## CASE STUDY

### *Laryngeal Cancer*

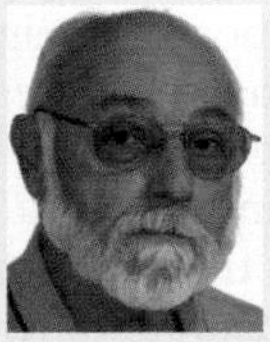

(©iStockphoto/ Thinkstock)

**Patient Profile**

M.R., a 60-yr-old baker, was admitted to the hospital for influenza. He explained to his HCP that he has also experienced "a cough that just won't go away," some pain and difficulty swallowing, and "a sore throat that really hasn't gotten better" over the past year. His wife passed away 6 years ago. He has three children; one daughter lives in the same city. He has a history of hypertension, smoking, alcohol use, and type 2 diabetes mellitus.

**Subjective Data**

- States that his symptoms worsened in the past 3 months
- Has used various cough and cold remedies over the past 6 months to relieve symptoms without relief
- Has lost weight because of decrease in appetite and difficulty swallowing
- Has smoked three packs of cigarettes a day for 40 yr
- Consumes 4 to 6 cans of beer a day

**Objective Data**

***Physical Examination***

- *Vital signs:* Temperature 102.4° F (39.1° C), heart rate 99 beats/minute (pulse strong, regular), respiratory rate 24 breaths/minute (short, shallow, slightly labored), BP 176/84 (cuff), $SpO_2$ 87% on room air
- *Inspection:* Awake and alert, appears gray, malnourished, dehydrated. Small, irregular white patches on the sides of oral cavity
- *Palpation:* Enlarged cervical nodes bilaterally (nontender)
- *Auscultation:* Adequate and clear air entry to upper lung fields; slightly decreased air entry to bases with occasional fine crackles on expiration

***Diagnostic Studies***

- Chest x-ray: Lung fields clear
- Laryngoscopy: Mass in subglottic area (requires further evaluation)
- CT scan: Subglottic lesion with lymph node involvement
- Diagnosis: Laryngeal cancer

**Interprofessional Care**

- *Surgery:* Suggests a total laryngectomy
- *Oncology:* Suggests radiation and chemotherapy postoperatively
- *ICU:* Preoperative consult (ICU admission for 24 hours postoperatively)
- *Gastroenterology:* Percutaneous gastrostomy tube preoperatively for enteral tube feeding
- *Dietary:* Explain nutritional options with/without ET tube/ tracheostomy.
- *Physical therapy:* Visit pre-surgery to explain postoperative exercise routine.
- *Social worker:* Determine social supports available postoperatively.

**Discussion Questions**

1. What information in the assessment suggests that M.R. is at risk for cancer of the larynx?
2. ***Priority Decision:*** What are your priority teaching strategies for M.R. before and after total laryngectomy?
3. How would you explain the gastrostomy tube to M.R.?
4. Discuss methods that can be used to facilitate communication in the postoperative period.
5. Is there anything in his history that may affect wound healing after surgery?
6. ***Priority Decision:*** In the recovery room, M.R.'s heart rate is 138 (tachycardia), BP is 84/32, and $SpO_2$ is 91%. What are your priority nursing interventions?
7. ***Teamwork and Collaboration:*** M.R. is discharged from the ICU after 24 hours. What information would you want to know from the ICU nurse who has just transported M.R. to the clinical unit?

**Progression of Case**

M.R. is awake and alert. Vital signs are stable. BP 168/94. Large surgical dressing on neck with three Jackson-Pratt drains. Tracheostomy tube in place. Receiving $O_2$ via tracheal mask. Tube feeding @ 60 mL/hour via gastrostomy tube. Voiding independently. M.R. nonverbally indicating to you that he "wants to get out of bed."

8. ***Priority Decision:*** Based on the assessment data presented, what are your priority nursing diagnoses? Are there any collaborative problems?
9. ***Teamwork and Collaboration:*** M.R. has a tracheostomy. What role can unlicensed assistive personnel (UAP) have in relation to the tracheostomy?
10. ***Evidence-Based Practice:*** How could you best meet M.R.'s communication needs during the first few postoperative days?
11. Shortly after transfer to the clinical unit, M.R. is tearful and is staring at the wall. What should you do?
12. ***Patient-Centered Care:*** What teaching is required to help this patient assume self-care after his surgery? What precautions should the patient take because of his stoma?

Answers available at *http://evolve.elsevier.com/Lewis/medsurg.*

## BRIDGE TO NCLEX EXAMINATION

The number of the question corresponds to the same-numbered outcome at the beginning of the chapter.

1. A patient was seen in the clinic for an episode of epistaxis, which was controlled by placement of anterior nasal packing. During discharge teaching, the nurse instructs the patient to
   **a.** use aspirin for pain relief.
   **b.** remove the packing later that day.
   **c.** skip the next dose of antihypertensive medication.
   **d.** avoid vigorous nose blowing and strenuous activity.
2. A patient with allergic rhinitis reports severe nasal congestion; sneezing; and watery, itchy eyes and nose at various times of the year. To teach the patient to control these symptoms, the nurse advises the patient to
   **a.** avoid all intranasal sprays and oral antihistamines.
   **b.** limit the usage of nasal decongestant spray to 10 days.
   **c.** use oral decongestants at bedtime to prevent symptoms during the night.
   **d.** keep a diary of when the allergic reaction occurs and what precipitates it.
3. A patient is seen at the clinic with fever, muscle aches, sore throat with yellowish exudate, and headache. The nurse anticipates that the interprofessional management will include *(select all that apply)*
   **a.** antiviral agents to treat influenza.
   **b.** treatment with antibiotics starting ASAP.
   **c.** a throat culture or rapid strep antigen test.
   **d.** supportive care, including cool, bland liquids.
   **e.** comprehensive history to determine possible etiology.
4. The *best* method for determining the risk of aspiration in a patient with a tracheostomy is to
   **a.** consult a speech therapist for swallowing assessment.
   **b.** have the patient drink plain water and assess for coughing.
   **c.** assess for change of sputum color 48 hours after patient drinks small amount of blue dye.
   **d.** suction above the cuff after the patient eats or drinks to determine presence of food in trachea.
5. Which nursing action would be of *highest priority* when suctioning a patient with a tracheostomy?
   **a.** Auscultating lung sounds after suctioning is complete
   **b.** Providing a means of communication for the patient during the procedure
   **c.** Assessing the patient's oxygenation saturation before, during, and after suctioning
   **d.** Administering pain and/or antianxiety medication 30 minutes before suctioning
6. When planning health care teaching to prevent or detect early head and neck cancer, which people would be the *priority* to target *(select all that apply)*?
   **a.** 65-year-old man who has used chewing tobacco most of his life
   **b.** 45-year-old rancher who uses snuff to stay awake while driving his herds of cattle
   **c.** 21-year-old college student who drinks beer on weekends with his fraternity brothers
   **d.** 78-year-old woman who has been drinking hard liquor since her husband died 15 years ago
   **e.** 22-year-old woman who has been diagnosed with human papilloma virus (HPV) of the cervix
7. While in the recovery room, a patient with a total laryngectomy is suctioned and has bloody mucus with some clots. Which nursing interventions would apply?
   **a.** Notify the physician immediately.
   **b.** Place the patient in the prone position to facilitate drainage.
   **c.** Instill 3 mL of normal saline into the tracheostomy tube to loosen secretions.
   **d.** Continue your assessment of the patient, including $O_2$ saturation, respiratory rate, and breath sounds.
8. Appropriate discharge teaching for the patient with a permanent tracheostomy after a total laryngectomy for cancer would include *(select all that apply)*
   **a.** encouraging regular exercise such as swimming.
   **b.** washing around the stoma daily with a moist washcloth.
   **c.** encouraging participation in postlaryngectomy support group.
   **d.** providing pictures and "hands-on" instruction for tracheostomy care.
   **e.** teaching how to hold breath and trying to gag to promote swallowing reflex.

1. d, 2. d, 3. c, d, e, 4. a, 5. c, 6. a, b, d, e, 7. d, 8. b, c, d

For rationales to these answers and even more NCLEX review questions, visit *http://evolve.elsevier.com/Lewis/medsurg.*

## EVOLVE WEBSITE

http://evolve.elsevier.com/Lewis/medsurg

**Review Questions (Online Only)**

**Key Points**

**Answer Keys for Questions**
- Rationales for Bridge to NCLEX Examination Questions
- Answer Guidelines for Case Study on p. 496

**Student Case Study**
- Patient With Head and Neck Cancer/Laryngectomy With Tracheostomy

**Nursing Care Plans**
- eNursing Care Plan 26-1: Patient With a Tracheostomy
- eNursing Care Plan 26-2: Patient Having Total Laryngectomy and/or Radical Neck Surgery

**Conceptual Care Map Creator**

**Supporting Media**
- Animation
  - Tracheotomy

**Audio Glossary**

**Content Updates**

## REFERENCES


1. American Academy of Otolaryngology–Head and Neck Surgery: Deviated septum. Retrieved from *www.entnet.org/content/deviated-septum.*
2. Patton KT, Thibodeau GA: *Human body in health and disease*, ed 6, St Louis, 2014, Elsevier Mosby.
3. Becker DG: Nasal and septal fractures. Retrieved from *http://emedicine.medscape.com/article/878595-overview#a03.*

4. Urden LD, Stacy KM, Lough ME: *Critical care nursing: diagnosis and management*, ed 7, St Louis, 2014, Mosby.
5. Haraldson SJ: Nasal fracture treatment and management. Retrieved from: *http://emedicine.medscape.com/article/84829-treatment*.
6. Pribitkin EA, Lavasani LS, Shindle C et al: Sonic rhinoplasty: Sculpting with the ultrasound bone aspirator. In Schiffman MA, Di Giuseppe A, editors: *Advanced aesthetic rhinoplasty: art, science, and new clinical techniques*, New York, 2013, Springer.
7. Fried MP: Epistaxis. Retrieved from *www.merckmanuals.com*.
8. Newson L: Nosebleed (epistaxis). Retrieved from *www.patient.co.uk/doctor/nosebleed-epistaxis-pro*.
9. deSchazo RD, Kemp SF: Patient information: allergic rhinitis (seasonal allergies). Retrieved from *www.uptodate.com/contents/allergic-rhinitis-seasonal-allergies-beyond-the-basics*.
10. Henochowicz SI: Allergic rhinitis. Retrieved from *www.nlm.nih.gov/medlineplus/ency/article/000813.htm*.
11. Sheikh J: Allergic rhinitis medication summary. Retrieved from *http://emedicine.medscape.com/article/134825-medication#1*.
12. New York Department of Health: Influenza (flu) fact sheet. Retrieved from *www.health.ny.gov/diseases/communicable/influenza/fact_sheet.htm*.
13. Centers for Disease Control and Prevention: Key facts about influenza (flu) & flu vaccine. Retrieved from *www.cdc.gov/flu/keyfacts.htm*.
14. Blanco EM: Diagnostic influenza tests. Retrieved from *http://emedicine.medscape.com/article/2053517-overview#aw2aab6b2*.
15. Centers for Disease Control and Prevention: Rapid Diagnostic Testing for Influenza: Information for Health Care Professionals. Retrieved from *www.cdc.gov/flu/professionals/diagnosis/rapidclin.htm*.
16. U.S. Food and Drug Administration (FDA): Influenza (Flu) Antiviral Drugs and Related Information. Retrieved from *www.fda.gov/Drugs/DrugSafety/InformationbyDrugClass/ucm100228.htm*.
17. Nazario B: Sinus infection: An overview of sinusitis. Retrieved from *www.webmd.com/allergies/sinusitis-and-sinus-infection*.
18. Kaplan A: Canadian guidelines for acute bacterial rhinosinusitis, *Canadian Family Physician* 60:227, 2014.
19. Hwang PH, Patel ZM: Acute sinusitis and rhinosinusitis in adults: treatment. Retrieved from *www.uptodate.com/contents/acute-sinusitis-and-rhinosinusitis-in-adults-treatment*.
20. Seidu L: Nasal polyps. Retrieved from *www.webmd.com/allergies/guide/nasal-polyps-symptoms-and-treatments*.
21. Carrillo-Marquez MA: Bacterial pharyngitis. Retrieved from *http://emedicine.medscape.com/article/225243-overview*.
22. Acerra JR: Pharyngitis clinical presentation. Retrieved from *http://emedicine.medscape.com/article/764304-clinical*.
23. Chow AW, Doron S: Evaluation of acute pharyngitis in adults. Retrieved from *www.uptodate.com/contents/evaluation-of-acute-pharyngitis-in-adults#H1*.
24. Murray AD: Foreign bodies of the airway. Retrieved from *http://emedicine.medscape.com/article/872498-overview*.
25. Morris L, Whitmer A, McIntosh E: Tracheostomy care and complications in the intensive care unit, *Critical Care Nurse* 33:18, 2013.
26. Batuwitage B, Webber S, Glossop A: Percutaneous tracheostomy. Continuing Education in Anesthesia, Critical Care, and Pain. Retrieved from *http://ceaccp.oxfordjournals.org/content/early/2014/01/02/bjaceaccp.mkt068.full.pdf+html*.
27. Agency for Clinical Innovation: Care of adult patients in acute care facilities with tracheostomy – clinical practice guidelines. Retrieved from *www.aci.health.nsw.gov.au/__data/assets/pdf_file/0005/181454/ACI_Tracheostomy_CPG.pdf*.
28. American Cancer Society: Retrieved from *www.cancer.org/research/cancerfactsstatistics/cancerfactsfigures2015/index*.
29. American Society of Clinical Oncology: Stages of cancer. Retrieved from *www.cancer.net/navigating-cancer-care/diagnosing-cancer/stages-cancer*.
30. American Society of Clinical Oncology: Head and neck cancer: treatment options. Retrieved from *www.cancer.net/cancer-types/head-and-neck-cancer/treatment-options*.

27

# Lower Respiratory Problems

*Eugene E. Mondor*

*What oxygen is to the lungs, such is hope to the meaning of life.*

**Emil Brunner**

http://evolve.elsevier.com/Lewis/medsurg/

## LEARNING OUTCOMES

1. Compare and contrast the clinical manifestations and nursing and interprofessional management of patients with acute bronchitis and pertussis.
2. Differentiate among the types of pneumonia and their etiology.
3. Describe the pathophysiology, clinical manifestations, diagnostic studies, interprofessional care, and nursing management of patients with pneumonia.
4. Describe the pathogenesis, classification, clinical manifestations, complications, diagnostic abnormalities, interprofessional care, and nursing management of patients with tuberculosis.
5. Describe the causes, clinical manifestations, and nursing and interprofessional management of patients with pulmonary fungal infections.
6. Explain the pathophysiology, clinical manifestations, and nursing and interprofessional management of a patient with a lung abscess.
7. Identify the causative factors, clinical manifestations, and nursing and interprofessional management of patients with environmental lung diseases.
8. Describe the etiology, risk factors, pathophysiology, clinical manifestations, interprofessional care, and nursing management of lung cancer.
9. Compare and contrast the pathophysiology, clinical manifestations, and nursing and interprofessional management of pneumothorax, fractured ribs, and flail chest.
10. Describe the purpose, function, and nursing responsibilities related to chest tubes and various chest drainage systems.
11. Explain the types of chest surgery and appropriate preoperative and postoperative care.
12. Describe the etiology, clinical manifestations, and nursing and interprofessional management of patients with restrictive lung disorders such as pleural effusion, pleurisy, and atelectasis.
13. Describe the pathophysiology, clinical manifestations, and nursing and interprofessional management of pulmonary embolism, pulmonary hypertension, and cor pulmonale.
14. Discuss the use of lung transplantation as a treatment for pulmonary disorders, emphasizing nursing and interprofessional management of the postoperative lung transplant patient.

## KEY TERMS

**acute bronchitis, p. 499**
**community-acquired pneumonia (CAP), p. 501**
**cor pulmonale, p. 533**
**empyema, p. 527**
**flail chest, p. 521**
**hemothorax, p. 520**
**hospital-acquired pneumonia (HAP), p. 501**
**lung abscess, p. 512**
**pertussis, p. 500**
**pleural effusion, p. 527**
**pleurisy (pleuritis), p. 528**
**pneumoconiosis, p. 513**
**pneumonia, p. 500**
**pneumothorax, p. 519**
**pulmonary edema, p. 529**
**pulmonary embolism (PE), p. 529**
**pulmonary hypertension, p. 531**
**tension pneumothorax, p. 520**
**thoracentesis, p. 527**
**thoracotomy, p. 524**
**tuberculosis (TB), p. 506**

A variety of problems affect the lower respiratory system. Lung diseases that are characterized primarily by an obstructive disorder, such as asthma, chronic obstructive pulmonary disease (COPD), and cystic fibrosis, are discussed in Chapter 28. This chapter discusses other lower respiratory tract diseases, including infectious, oncologic, traumatic, restrictive, and vascular disorders.

## LOWER RESPIRATORY TRACT INFECTIONS

Lower respiratory tract infection is both a common and serious occurrence. It is responsible for thousands of clinic and emergency department visits and hospital admissions each year. In the United States, pneumonia and influenza are responsible for more than 56,000 deaths annually.[1,2]

## ACUTE BRONCHITIS

**Acute bronchitis** is a self-limiting inflammation of the bronchi in the lower respiratory tract and a common reason for seeking medical care. Most acute bronchial infections are caused by viruses. Air pollution, dust, inhalation of chemicals, smoking, chronic sinusitis, and asthma are other triggers of acute bronchitis.

Reviewed by Donna C. Bond, RN, DNP, CCNS, AE-C, CTTS, Pulmonary Clinical Nurse Specialist, Carilion Clinic, Roanoke, Virginia; Marylee Bressie, RN, DNP, CCRN, CCNS, CEN, Core Faculty/Nurse Planner, School of Public Service Leadership, Capella University, Minneapolis, Minnesota; Deborah Cline, RN, MS, Nursing Faculty, Carrington College, Reno, Nevada; and Cynthia M. Steinwedel, RN, PhD, CNE, Assistant Professor, Department of Nursing, Bradley University, Peoria, Illinois; and Beth D. Strauss, RN, DNP, ACNS-BC, Associate Professor, Edgewood College, Henry Predolin School of Nursing, Madison, Wisconsin.

## HEALTHY PEOPLE

### *Prevention of Respiratory Diseases*

- Avoid cigarette smoking and exposure to environmental smoke.
- Wash hands frequently to prevent and avoid spreading infections.
- Avoid exposure to allergens, indoor pollutants, and ambient air pollutants.
- Get a pneumococcal vaccine and yearly flu vaccine as directed by HCP.
- Wear proper personal protective equipment when working in an occupation with prolonged exposure to dust, fumes, or gases.

Cough, which is the most common symptom, lasts for up to 3 weeks. Clear, mucoid secretions are often present, although some patients produce purulent sputum. The presence of colored (e.g., green) sputum is not a reliable indicator of bacterial infection. Associated symptoms may include headache, fever, malaise, hoarseness, myalgias, dyspnea, and chest pain.

Diagnosis of acute bronchitis is based on clinical assessment. Assessment may reveal normal breath sounds or crackles or wheezes, usually on expiration and with exertion. *Consolidation* (occurs when fluid accumulates in the lungs), suggestive of pneumonia, is absent with bronchitis. Chest x-rays would be normal and are therefore not indicated unless pneumonia is suspected. (Chronic bronchitis is discussed in Chapter 28.)

The goal in acute bronchitis is to relieve symptoms and prevent pneumonia. Treatment is supportive, including cough suppressants, encouraging oral fluid intake, and using a humidifier. $\beta_2$-agonist (bronchodilator) inhalers are useful for patients with wheezes. Generally antibiotics are not prescribed for treating a viral infection, as they may cause side effects and promote antibiotic resistance. However, antibiotics may be prescribed for patients with underlying chronic conditions and who have a prolonged infection associated with systemic symptoms.

Patients should be encouraged not to smoke, avoid secondhand smoke, and to frequently wash their hands. If the acute bronchitis is due to an influenza virus, treatment with antiviral drugs, either zanamivir (Relenza) or oseltamivir (Tamiflu), can be started. These drugs should be initiated within 48 hours of the onset of symptoms.

## PERTUSSIS

**Pertussis** is a highly contagious infection of the respiratory tract caused by a gram-negative bacillus, *Bordetella pertussis*. The bacteria attach to the cilia of the respiratory tract and release toxins that damage the cilia, causing inflammation and swelling. The incidence of pertussis has been steadily increasing in the United States since the 1980s, with the largest increase noted in adults. It is thought that immunity resulting from childhood vaccination with DPT (diphtheria, pertussis, tetanus) may diminish over time, allowing a milder (but still contagious) infection. The Centers for Disease Control and Prevention (CDC) currently recommends that all adults age 19 years and older who have not received a dose of Tdap (tetanus, diphtheria, and pertussis) receive a one-time vaccination as soon as possible.[3]

Clinical manifestations of pertussis occur in stages. The first (catarrhal) stage, occurring within the first 2 weeks of infection, manifests as a mild upper respiratory tract infection (URI) with a low-grade or no fever, runny nose, watery eyes, and mild, nonproductive cough. The second (paroxysmal) stage, from the second to tenth week of infection, is characterized by paroxysms of cough. The final (convalescent) stage lasts 2 to 3 weeks and is characterized by less severe cough and weakness.

The hallmark characteristic of pertussis is uncontrollable, violent coughing. Inspiration after each cough produces the typical "whooping" sound as the patient tries to breathe in air against an obstructed glottis. The "whoop" is often not present in teens and adults (especially those who have been vaccinated). Like acute bronchitis, the coughing is more frequent at night. Vomiting may also occur with the coughing. Unlike bronchitis, the cough with pertussis may last from 6 to 10 weeks.

The primary treatment for pertussis is antibiotics, usually macrolides (erythromycin, azithromycin [Zithromax]), to minimize symptoms and prevent spread of the disease. The patient is infectious from the beginning of the catarrhal stage through the third week after onset of symptoms or until 5 days after antibiotic therapy has been initiated. Cough suppressants and antihistamines should not be used, since they are ineffective and may induce coughing episodes. Corticosteroids and bronchodilators are also not useful.

## PNEUMONIA

**Pneumonia** is an acute infection of the lung parenchyma. Until 1936, pneumonia was the leading cause of death in the United States.[4] The discovery of sulfa drugs and penicillin was pivotal in the treatment of pneumonia. Since that time, remarkable progress has been made in the development of antibiotics to treat pneumonia. However, despite newer antimicrobial agents, pneumonia is still associated with significant morbidity and mortality rates. The CDC reports that pneumonia and influenza are the eighth leading cause of death in the United States.[5]

### Etiology

Normally, the airway distal to the larynx is protected from infection by various defense mechanisms. Mechanisms that create a mechanical barrier to microorganisms entering the tracheobronchial tree include air filtration, epiglottis closure over the trachea, cough reflex, mucociliary escalator mechanism, and reflex bronchoconstriction (see Chapter 25). Immune defense mechanisms include secretion of immunoglobulins A and G and alveolar macrophages.

Pneumonia is more likely to occur when defense mechanisms become incompetent or are overwhelmed by the virulence or quantity of infectious agents. Decreased consciousness weakens the cough and epiglottal reflexes, which may allow aspiration of oropharyngeal contents into the lungs. Tracheal intubation bypasses normal filtration processes and interferes with the cough reflex and mucociliary escalator mechanism. Air pollution, cigarette smoking, viral URIs, and normal changes that occur with aging can also impair the mucociliary mechanism. Chronic diseases can suppress the immune system's ability to inhibit bacterial growth. The risk factors for pneumonia are listed in Table 27-1.

Organisms that cause pneumonia reach the lung by three ways:

1. *Aspiration* of normal flora from the nasopharynx or oropharynx. Many organisms that cause pneumonia are normal inhabitants of the pharynx in healthy adults.
2. *Inhalation* of microbes present in the air. Examples include *Mycoplasma pneumoniae* and fungal pneumonias.
3. *Hematogenous spread* from a primary infection elsewhere in the body. Examples are streptococci and *Staphylococcus aureus* from infective endocarditis.

### TABLE 27-1 Risk Factors for Pneumonia

- Abdominal or thoracic surgery
- Age >65 yr
- Air pollution
- Altered consciousness: alcoholism, head injury, seizures, anesthesia, drug overdose, stroke
- Bed rest and prolonged immobility
- Chronic diseases: chronic lung and liver disease, diabetes mellitus, heart disease, cancer, chronic kidney disease
- Debilitating illness
- Exposure to bats, birds, rabbits, farm animals
- Immunosuppressive disease and/or therapy (corticosteroids, cancer chemotherapy, human immunodeficiency virus [HIV] infection, immunosuppressive therapy after organ transplant)
- Inhalation or aspiration of noxious substances
- Intestinal and gastric feedings via nasogastric or nasointestinal tubes
- IV drug use
- Malnutrition
- Recent antibiotic therapy
- Resident of a long-term care facility
- Smoking
- Tracheal intubation (endotracheal intubation, tracheostomy)
- Upper respiratory tract infection

### TABLE 27-2 Organisms Causing Pneumonia

| Community-Acquired Pneumonia | Hospital-Acquired Pneumonia |
|---|---|
| *Streptococcus pneumoniae** | *Pseudomonas aeruginosa*† |
| *Mycoplasma pneumoniae* | *Escherichia coli*† |
| *Haemophilus influenzae* | *Klebsiella pneumoniae*† |
| Respiratory viruses | *Acinetobacter* species† |
| *Chlamydophila pneumoniae* | *Haemophilus influenzae* |
| *Chlamydophila psittaci* | *Staphylococcus aureus* |
| *Coxiella burnettii* | *Streptococcus pneumoniae* |
| *Legionella pneumophila* | *Proteus* species |
| Oral anaerobes | *Enterobacter* species |
| *Moraxella catarrhalis* | Oral anaerobes |
| *Staphylococcus aureus* | |
| *Pseudomonas aeruginosa* | |
| Enteric aerobic gram-negative bacteria (e.g., *Klebsiella* species) | |
| Fungi | |
| *Mycobacterium tuberculosis* | |

*Most common cause of community-acquired pneumonia (CAP).
†Most common causes of hospital-acquired pneumonia (HAP).

## Types of Pneumonia

Bacteria, viruses, *Mycoplasma* organisms, fungi, parasites, and chemicals are potential causes of pneumonia. Although pneumonia can be classified many different ways (e.g., according to the causative organism), the most widely recognized and clinically effective way is to classify pneumonia as *community-acquired* or *hospital-acquired* pneumonia. Classifying pneumonia is important because of the differences in the likely causative organisms (Table 27-2) and the selection of appropriate antimicrobial therapy.

**Community-Acquired Pneumonia.** Community-acquired pneumonia (CAP) is an acute infection of the lung occurring in patients who have not been hospitalized or resided in a long-term care facility within 14 days of the onset of symptoms. The decision to treat the patient at home or admit him or her to the hospital is based on several factors such as the patient's age, vital signs, mental status, presence of co-morbid conditions, and current physiologic condition. Clinicians can use tools such as the CURB-65 scale (Table 27-3) to supplement clinical judgment.

### TABLE 27-3 Assessing Pneumonia Using CURB-65

**The CURB-65 scale** may be used as a supplement to clinical judgment to determine the severity of pneumonia and if patients need to be hospitalized.

**Identifying the Level of Risk**

**Patients receive 1 point for each of the following indicators:**

- **C:** Confusion (compared to baseline)
- **U:** BUN >20 mg/dL
- **R:** Respiratory rate ≥30 breaths/min
- **B:** Systolic blood pressure <90 mm Hg or diastolic blood pressure ≤60 mm Hg
- **65:** ≥Age 65 yr

**Scoring and Decision Making**

| Score | Decision |
|---|---|
| **0** | Treat at home |
| **1-2** | Consider hospital admission |
| **3 or more** | Hospital admission |
| **4-5** | Consider admission to intensive care unit |

Source: Lim WS, van der Eerden MM, Laing R, et al: Defining community acquired pneumonia severity on presentation to hospital: an international derivation and validation study, *Thorax* 58(5):377, 2003.

Empiric antibiotic therapy should be started as soon as possible. *Empiric antibiotic therapy,* the initiation of treatment before a definitive diagnosis or causative agent is confirmed, should be started as soon as CAP is suspected. Empiric antibiotic administration is based on experience and knowledge of drugs known to be effective for the most likely causative agent.

**Hospital-Acquired Pneumonia.** Hospital-acquired pneumonia (HAP), also known as *nosocomial pneumonia,* is a pneumonia in a nonintubated patient that begins 48 hours or longer after admission to hospital and was not present at the time of admission. *Ventilator-associated pneumonia* (VAP), also a type of HAP, refers to pneumonia that occurs more than 48 hours after endotracheal intubation.[6] (VAP is discussed in Chapter 65.) Once the diagnosis of HAP or VAP is made, treatment of pneumonia is initiated based on known risk factors, early versus late onset, and probable organism. Antibiotic therapy can be adjusted once the results of sputum cultures identify the exact pathogen. Both HAP and VAP are associated with longer hospital stays, increased associated costs, sicker patients, and increased risk of morbidity and mortality.

A major problem in treating pneumonia today is the development of multidrug-resistant (MDR) organisms. Primary culprits include methicillin-resistant *Staphylococcus aureus* and gram-negative bacilli. Risk factors for development of MDR pneumonia include advanced age, immunosuppression, history of antibiotic use, and prolonged mechanical ventilation. Antibiotic susceptibility tests can identify MDR organisms. The virulence of these organisms can severely limit the available and appropriate antimicrobial therapy. MDR organisms also increase the morbidity and mortality risks associated with pneumonia. (Chapter 14 discusses MDR organisms.)

**Aspiration Pneumonia.** *Aspiration pneumonia* results from the abnormal entry of material from the mouth or stomach into the trachea and lungs. Conditions that increase the risk of aspiration include decreased level of consciousness (e.g., seizure, anesthesia, head injury, stroke, alcohol intake), difficulty swallowing, and insertion of nasogastric tubes with or without tube feeding. With loss of consciousness, the gag and cough reflexes are depressed, and aspiration is more likely to occur.

The aspirated material (food, water, vomitus, or oropharyngeal secretions) triggers an inflammatory response. The most common form of aspiration pneumonia is a primary bacterial infection. Typically, more than one organism is identified on sputum culture, including aerobes and anaerobes, since they both make up the flora of the oropharynx.

Until cultures are completed and results obtained, initial antibiotic therapy is based on an assessment of probable causative organism, severity of illness, patient factors (e.g., malnutrition, current use of antibiotic therapy), and ability to treat common community-acquired organisms. For patients who aspirate in hospitals, appropriate antibiotics should include coverage for both gram-negative organisms and MRSA. In contrast, aspiration of acidic gastric contents causes *chemical (noninfectious) pneumonitis,* which may not require antibiotic therapy. However, secondary bacterial infection can occur 48 to 72 hours later.

**Necrotizing Pneumonia.** *Necrotizing pneumonia* is a rare complication of bacterial lung infection. It is characterized by liquefaction and, in some situations, cavitation of lung tissue. This often occurs as a result of community-acquired pneumonia (CAP). Although the exact pathophysiologic mechanisms involved are controversial, causative organisms include *Staphylococcus, Klebsiella,* and *Streptococcus.* Lung abscesses commonly occur. Signs and symptoms of necrotizing pneumonia include immediate respiratory insufficiency and/or failure, leukopenia, and bleeding into the airways.[7] Treatment often includes long-term antibiotic therapy and possible surgery.

**Opportunistic Pneumonia.** *Opportunistic pneumonia* is inflammation and infection of the lower respiratory tract in immunocompromised patients. Individuals at risk for opportunistic pneumonia include those with altered immune responses. This can include people with severe protein-calorie malnutrition or immunodeficiencies (e.g., human immunodeficiency virus [HIV] infection) and those receiving radiation therapy, chemotherapy, and any immunosuppressive therapy, including long-term corticosteroid therapy. In addition to the risk of bacterial and viral pneumonia, the immunocompromised person may develop an infection from microorganisms that do not normally cause disease, such as *Pneumocystis jiroveci* (formerly *carinii*) and cytomegalovirus (CMV).

*P. jiroveci* pneumonia (PJP) rarely occurs in the healthy individual but is the most common form of pneumonia in people with HIV disease. The onset is slow and subtle with symptoms of fever, tachypnea, tachycardia, dyspnea, nonproductive cough, and hypoxemia. The chest x-ray usually shows diffuse bilateral infiltrates. In widespread disease, the lungs have massive consolidation. PJP can be life-threatening, causing acute respiratory failure and death. Infection can also spread to other organs, including the liver, bone marrow, lymph nodes, spleen, and thyroid. Bacterial and viral pneumonias must first be ruled out because of the vague presentation of PJP. Although the causative agent is fungal, PJP does not respond to antifungal agents. Treatment consists of a course of trimethoprim/sulfamethoxazole (Bactrim, Septra) either IV or orally depending on the severity of disease and the patient's response.

CMV, a herpesvirus, can cause viral pneumonia. Most CMV infections are asymptomatic or mild, but severe disease can

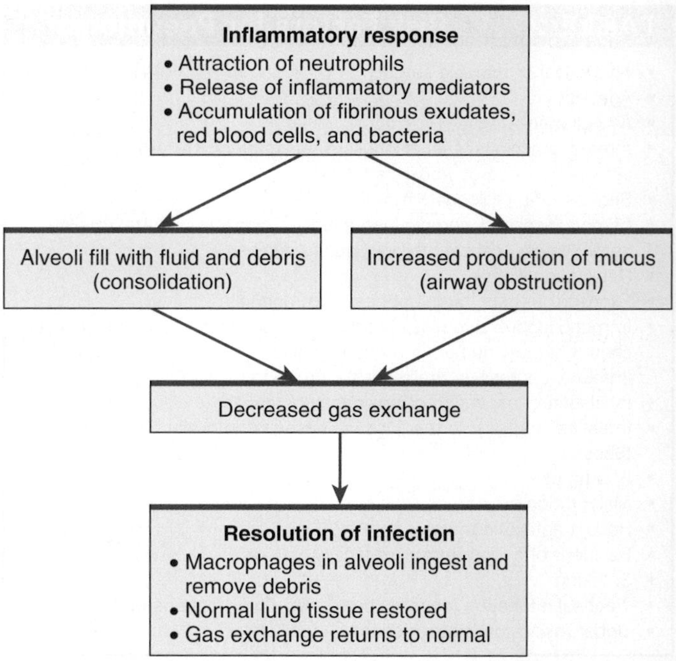


**FIG. 27-1** Pathophysiologic course of pneumonia.

occur in people with an impaired immune response. CMV is the most common life-threatening infectious complication after hematopoietic stem cell transplantation.[8] Antiviral medications (e.g., ganciclovir [Cytovene], foscarnet [Foscavir], cidofovir) and high-dose immunoglobulin are used for treatment.

## Pathophysiology

Specific pathophysiologic changes related to pneumonia vary according to the offending organism, but the majority of organisms trigger an inflammatory response in the lungs (Fig. 27-1). Inflammation, characterized by an increase in blood flow and vascular permeability, activates neutrophils to engulf and kill the offending organisms. As a result, the inflammatory process attracts more neutrophils, edema of the airways occurs, and fluid leaks from the capillaries and tissues into alveoli. Normal $O_2$ transport is affected, leading to clinical manifestations of hypoxia (e.g., tachypnea, dyspnea, tachycardia). *Consolidation,* a feature typical of bacterial pneumonia, occurs when the normally air-filled alveoli become filled with fluid and debris. Mucus production also increases, which can potentially obstruct airflow and impair gas exchange even further. Over time and with appropriate antibiotic therapy, macrophages lyse and process the debris, lung tissue is allowed to recover, and gas exchange returns to normal. Resolution and healing occur if there are no complications.

## Clinical Manifestations

The most common presenting symptoms of pneumonia are cough, fever, chills, dyspnea, tachypnea, and pleuritic chest pain. The cough may or may not be productive. Sputum may appear green, yellow, or even rust colored (bloody). Viral pneumonia may initially be seen as influenza, with respiratory symptoms appearing and/or worsening 12 to 36 hours after onset.

The older or debilitated patient may not have classic symptoms of pneumonia. Confusion or stupor (possibly related to hypoxia) may be the only finding. Hypothermia, rather than fever, may also be noted with the older patient. Nonspecific clinical manifestations include diaphoresis, anorexia, fatigue, myalgias, and headache.

On physical examination, fine or coarse crackles may be auscultated over the affected region. If consolidation is present, bronchial breath sounds, egophony (a change in the sound of the voice of the patient), and increased fremitus (vibration of the chest wall produced by vocalization) may be noted. Patients with pleural effusion may exhibit dullness to percussion over the affected area.

## Complications

Complications develop more frequently in older individuals and those with underlying chronic diseases. Potential complications include the following:

- *Atelectasis* (collapsed, airless alveoli) of one or part of one lobe may occur. These areas may clear with effective deep breathing and coughing.
- *Pleurisy* (inflammation of the pleura) may occur.
- *Pleural effusion* (fluid in the pleural space) can occur. In most cases, the effusion is sterile and is reabsorbed in 1 to 2 weeks. Occasionally, effusions require aspiration by thoracentesis.
- *Bacteremia* (bacterial infection in the blood) is more likely to occur in infections with *Streptococcus pneumoniae* and *Haemophilus influenzae.*
- *Pneumothorax* can occur when air collects in the pleural space, causing the lungs to collapse.
- *Meningitis* can be caused by *Streptococcus pneumoniae.* The patient with pneumonia who is disoriented, confused, or drowsy may have a lumbar puncture to evaluate the possibility of meningitis.
- *Acute respiratory failure* is one of the leading causes of death in patients with severe pneumonia. Failure occurs when pneumonia damages the lungs' ability to facilitate the exchange of $O_2$ and $CO_2$ across the alveolar-capillary membrane.
- *Sepsis/septic shock* can occur when bacteria within alveoli enter the bloodstream. Severe sepsis can lead to shock and multisystem organ dysfunction syndrome (MODS) (see Chapter 66).

*Lung abscess* is not a common complication of pneumonia. However, it may occur with pneumonia caused by *S. aureus* and gram-negative organisms. *Empyema,* the accumulation of purulent exudate in the pleural cavity, occurs in less than 5% of cases and requires antibiotic therapy and drainage of the exudate by a chest tube or open surgical drainage.[9] Pleurisy, pleural effusion, atelectasis, lung abscess, and pneumothorax are discussed later in this chapter.

## Diagnostic Studies

The common diagnostic measures for pneumonia are presented in Table 27-4. History, physical examination, and chest x-ray often provide enough clinical information to make decisions about early treatment. Chest x-ray often shows a typical pattern characteristic of the infecting organism and is important in the diagnosis of pneumonia. X-ray may also show pleural effusions. A thoracentesis and/or bronchoscopy with washings may be used to obtain fluid samples from patients not responding to initial therapy.

Ideally, a sputum specimen for culture and Gram stain to identify the organism are obtained before beginning antibiotic therapy. However, antibiotic administration should not be delayed if a specimen cannot be readily obtained. Delays in antibiotic therapy can increase the risk of morbidity and mortality. Blood cultures are done for patients who are seriously ill. Arterial blood gases (ABGs) may be obtained to assess for hypoxemia (partial pressure of $O_2$ in arterial blood [$PaO_2$] less than 80 mm Hg), hypercapnia (partial pressure of carbon dioxide in arterial blood [$PaCO_2$] greater than 45 mm Hg), and acidosis (pH <7.35). Leukocytosis occurs in the majority of patients with bacterial pneumonia; the white blood cell (WBC) count is usually greater than 15,000/μL ($15 \times 10^9$/L) with the presence of bands (immature neutrophils).

The use of biologic markers of infection to guide clinical decisions for treatment of pneumonia is under investigation. Serum levels of C-reactive protein (CRP) and procalcitonin are currently being explored as possible sources of information to help guide clinicians in distinguishing pneumonia from other types of cardiac and respiratory failure.[10-12]

**TABLE 27-4 Interprofessional Care**
***Pneumonia***

| Diagnostic Assessment | Management |
|---|---|
| • History and physical examination<br>• Chest x-ray<br>• Gram stain of sputum<br>• Sputum culture and sensitivity test<br>• Pulse oximetry or ABGs (if indicated)<br>• Complete blood count, WBC differential, and routine blood chemistries (if indicated)<br>• Blood cultures (if indicated) | • Increased fluid intake (at least 3 L/day)<br>• Balance between activity and rest<br>• $O_2$ therapy (if indicated)<br><br>***Drug Therapy***<br>• Appropriate antibiotic therapy (Table 27-6)<br>• Antipyretics<br>• Analgesics |

## Interprofessional Care

Pneumococcal vaccine is used to prevent *Streptococcus pneumoniae* (Table 27-5). Prompt treatment with the appropriate antibiotic is essential. Antibiotics are highly effective for both bacterial and mycoplasma pneumonia. In uncomplicated cases, the patient responds to drug therapy within 48 to 72 hours. Indications of improvement include decreased temperature, improved breathing, and reduced chest discomfort. Abnormal physical findings can last more than 7 days. A repeat chest x-ray may be obtained in 6 to 8 weeks to assess for resolution.

In addition to antibiotic therapy, supportive measures are individualized to the patient's needs. These may include $O_2$ therapy to treat hypoxemia, analgesics to relieve chest pain, and antipyretics (e.g., aspirin, acetaminophen) for elevated temperature. Although cough suppressants, mucolytics, bronchodilators, and corticosteroids are often prescribed as adjunctive therapy, the use of these drugs is controversial. However, they may be prescribed for patients with underlying chronic conditions.

Individualize rest and activity to each patient's tolerance. Benefits of mobility include improved diaphragm movement and chest expansion, mobilization of secretions, and prevention of venous stasis.

Currently, no definitive treatment exists for the majority of viral pneumonias. As identified earlier, care is generally supportive. In most circumstances, viral pneumonia is self-limiting and will often resolve in 3 to 4 days. Antiviral therapy may be used to treat pneumonia caused by influenza (e.g., oseltamivir, zanamivir) and a few other viruses (e.g., acyclovir [Zovirax] for herpes simplex virus).[13]

**Drug Therapy.** Once the pneumonia is classified, the HCP selects empiric therapy on the likely infecting organism (Table 27-2). Table 27-6 presents the drug therapy for bacterial CAP.

For all types of pneumonia, empiric antibiotic therapy is based on whether the patient has risk factors for MDR organisms. The prevalence and resistance patterns of MDR pathogens vary among localities and institutions. Therefore the antibiotic regimen must be adapted to local patterns of antibiotic resistance. Multiple regimens exist, but all should initially include antibiotics that are effective against both resistant gram-negative and resistant gram-positive organisms.

Clinical improvement usually occurs in 3 to 5 days. Patients who deteriorate or fail to respond to therapy require aggressive reevaluation to assess for noninfectious etiologies, complications, coexisting infectious processes, or pneumonia caused by a drug-resistant pathogen.

IV antibiotic therapy should be switched to oral therapy as soon as the patient is hemodynamically stable, is improving clinically, is able to ingest oral medication, and has a functioning gastrointestinal tract. Stable patients do not need to be observed in the hospital and can be discharged to home on oral antibiotics. Total treatment time for patients with CAP should be a minimum of 5 days, and the patient should be afebrile for 48 to 72 hours before stopping treatment. However, you need to emphasize the importance of completing the full course of antibiotic treatment. Longer treatment time may be needed if initial therapy was not active against the identified pathogen or complications occur.

**TABLE 27-5 Pneumococcal Vaccines**

| Vaccine* | Recommendations for Use |
|---|---|
| **Pneumococcal conjugate vaccine (PCV13, Prevnar 13)†** | • All children <5 yr<br>• All adults ≥65 yr<br>• Anyone 2-64 yr old with certain medical conditions (e.g., sickle cell disease, asplenia, immunodeficiencies, HIV infection, chronic renal failure, leukemia, generalized malignancy, long-term immunosuppressive therapy, cerebrospinal fluid leaks, cochlear implant[s]) |
| **Pneumococcal polysaccharide vaccine (PPSV23, Pneumovax 23)†** | • All adults ≥65 yr<br>• Anyone 2-64 yr old with certain long-term health problems (e.g., heart disease, lung disease, diabetes mellitus, alcoholism, cirrhosis, sickle cell disease, leaks of cerebrospinal fluid, cochlear implant)<br>• Anyone 2-64 yr with a disease or condition that weakens the immune system or taking drugs that lowers body's resistance to infection (e.g., HIV infection; lymphoma or leukemia; kidney failure; damaged or no spleen; multiple myeloma; receiving immunosuppressive chemotherapy, radiation therapy, or long-term corticosteroids; after organ or bone marrow transplantation)<br>• Adults 19-64 yr who smoke cigarettes or have asthma |

*For additional details on scheduling of pneumococcal vaccinations, see *www.cdc.gov/mmwr/preview/mmwrhtml/mm6434a4.htm?s_cid=mm6434a4_w*.
†As their names imply, PCV13 and Prevnar 13 protect against 13 types of pneumococcal bacteria, and PPSV23 and Pneumovax 23 protect against 23 types of pneumococcal bacteria. The vaccinations have different mechanisms of action.

**Nutritional Therapy.** Hydration is important in the supportive treatment of pneumonia to prevent dehydration and to thin and loosen secretions. Individualize and carefully monitor fluid intake. If the patient is an older adult, has heart failure, or has a known preexisting respiratory condition, IV administration of fluids and electrolytes may be necessary.

**TABLE 27-6 Drug Therapy**

***Bacterial Community-Acquired Pneumonia***

| Patient Variable | Treatment Options |
|---|---|
| **Outpatient** | |
| **Previously healthy** | |
| No recent antibiotic therapy in past 3 mo and no risk for drug-resistant *Staphylococcus pneumoniae* (DRSP) | Macrolide OR doxycycline |
| **Co-morbidities** (e.g., COPD; diabetes; chronic heart, liver, lung, or renal disease; malignancy; use of antibiotics in past 3 mo) | Respiratory fluoroquinolone<br>OR<br>β-Lactam plus macrolide (doxycycline may be substituted for macrolide) |
| **Regions with ≥25% macrolide-resistant *S. pneumoniae*** | Respiratory fluoroquinolone<br>OR<br>β-Lactam plus macrolide |
| **Inpatient** | |
| **Medical unit** | Respiratory fluoroquinolone<br>OR<br>β-Lactam plus macrolide |
| **ICU** | β-Lactam plus either azithromycin or respiratory fluoroquinolone |
| **Special conditions** | |
| • *Pseudomonas* infection | Antipneumococcal, antipseudomonal β-lactam plus either ciprofloxacin or levofloxacin<br>OR<br>Antipneumococcal, antipseudomonal β-lactam plus aminoglycoside and azithromycin<br>OR<br>Antipneumococcal, antipseudomonal β-lactam plus an aminoglycoside and an antipneumococcal fluoroquinolone |
| • *Pseudomonas* infection but patient has penicillin allergy | Substitute aztreonam for the above β-lactam |
| • Community-acquired methicillin-resistant *Staphylococcus aureus* (CA-MRSA) | Add vancomycin or linezolid (Zyvox) |
| **Types of Antibiotics** | |
| **Macrolides** | erythromycin, azithromycin (Zithromax), clarithromycin (Biaxin) |
| **Fluoroquinolones** | moxifloxacin (Avelox, Vigamox), levofloxacin (Levaquin), gemifloxacin (Factive) |
| **β-Lactams** | High-dose amoxicillin, amoxicillin/clavulanate (Augmentin), cefpodoxime, ceftriaxone (Rocephin), cefuroxime (Ceftin) |
| **Antipneumococcal, antipseudomonal β-lactams** | imipenem/cilastatin (Primaxin), meropenem (Merrem), cefepime (Maxipime), piperacillin/tazobactam (Zosyn) |

Source: Adapted from the Infectious Diseases Society of America Practice Guidelines for CAP. Retrieved from *www.idsociety.org/Organ_System/#CommunityAcquiredPneumoniaCAP*. For updated guidelines, check website.

Weight loss may occur in patients with pneumonia because of increased metabolic needs and difficulty eating due to nonspecific abdominal complaints or shortness of breath. Small, frequent meals are easier for dyspneic patients to tolerate. Offer foods high in calories and nutrients.

## NURSING MANAGEMENT: PNEUMONIA

### Nursing Assessment

Table 27-7 presents subjective and objective data to obtain from a patient with pneumonia.

### Nursing Diagnoses

Nursing diagnoses for the patient with pneumonia may include, but are not limited to, the following:

- Impaired gas exchange *related to* fluid and exudate accumulation within the alveoli and surrounding lung tissue
- Ineffective breathing pattern *related to* inflammation and chest discomfort
- Acute pain (chest) *related to* inflammation and ineffective pain management and/or comfort measures
- Activity intolerance *related to* chest discomfort, inflammation, shortness of breath, generalized weakness

Additional information on nursing diagnoses for the patient with pneumonia is presented in eNursing Care Plan 27-1 on the website for this chapter.

**TABLE 27-7 Nursing Assessment**

***Pneumonia***

**Subjective Data**

***Important Health Information***

*Past health history:* Lung cancer, COPD, diabetes mellitus, chronic debilitating disease, malnutrition, altered consciousness, immunosuppression, exposure to chemical toxins, dust, or allergens

*Medications:* Antibiotics, corticosteroids, chemotherapy, or any immunosuppressants

*Surgery or other treatments:* Recent abdominal or thoracic surgery, splenectomy, endotracheal intubation, or any surgery with general anesthesia. Tube feedings

***Functional Health Patterns***

*Health perception–health management:* Cigarette smoking, alcoholism; recent upper respiratory tract infection, malaise

*Nutritional-metabolic:* Anorexia, nausea, vomiting. Chills

*Activity-exercise:* Prolonged bed rest or immobility. Fatigue, weakness. Dyspnea, cough (productive or nonproductive). Nasal congestion

*Cognitive-perceptual:* Pain with breathing, chest pain, sore throat, headache, abdominal pain, muscle aches

**Objective Data**

***General***

Fever, restlessness or lethargy. Splinting of affected area

***Respiratory***

Tachypnea, pharyngitis, asymmetric chest movements or retraction, decreased excursion, nasal flaring. Use of accessory muscles (neck, abdomen). Crackles, friction rub on auscultation, dullness on percussion over consolidated areas, increased tactile fremitus on palpation. Pink, rusty, purulent, green, yellow, or white sputum (amount may be scant to copious)

***Cardiovascular***

Tachycardia

***Neurologic***

Changes in mental status, ranging from confusion to delirium

***Possible Diagnostic Findings***

Leukocytosis. Abnormal ABGs with ↓ or normal $PaO_2$, ↓ or normal $PaCO_2$, and ↑ or normal pH initially, and later ↓ $PaO_2$, ↑ $PaCO_2$, and ↓ pH. Positive sputum on Gram stain and culture. Patchy or diffuse infiltrates, abscesses, pleural effusion, or pneumothorax on chest x-ray

### Planning

The overall goals are that the patient with pneumonia will have (1) clear breath sounds, (2) normal breathing patterns, (3) no signs of hypoxia, (4) normal chest x-ray, (5) normal white blood cell (WBC) count, and (6) absence of complications related to pneumonia.

### Nursing Implementation

**Health Promotion.** To reduce the risk of pneumonia, teach individuals to practice good health habits, such as frequent hand washing, proper nutrition, adequate rest, regular exercise, and coughing or sneezing into the elbow rather than hands. Avoidance of cigarette smoke is one of the most important health-promoting behaviors. If possible, avoid exposure to people with URIs. If a URI occurs, it requires prompt attention with supportive measures (e.g., rest, fluids). If symptoms persist for longer than 7 days, the person should seek medical care. Encourage those at risk for pneumonia (e.g., chronically ill, older adult) to obtain both influenza and pneumococcal vaccines (Table 27-5). Identifying patients at risk (Table 27-1) and taking measures to prevent pneumonia are priority interventions.

In the acute care setting, place the patient with altered consciousness in positions (e.g., side-lying, upright) that will prevent or minimize the risk of aspiration. Turn and reposition the patient at least every 2 hours to facilitate adequate lung expansion and mobilization of secretions. Encourage and assist with ambulation and positioning into a chair. In the ICU, strict adherence to all aspects of the ventilator bundle (see Table 67-8), a group of interventions aimed at reducing the risk of VAP, has been shown to significantly reduce VAP.

For the patient who has difficulty swallowing and needs assistance in eating, drinking, and taking medication to prevent aspiration, elevate the patient's head-of-bed to at least 30 degrees and have the patient sit up for all meals. Assess for a gag reflex before giving food or fluids. Patients who have orogastric or nasogastric tubes are at risk for aspiration pneumonia (see Chapter 39). Although feeding tubes are small, any interruption in the integrity of the lower esophageal sphincter can allow reflux of gastric contents. To prevent aspiration, elevate the head of the bed to at least 30 degrees and monitor gastric residual volumes (see Table 39-12).

Patients with impaired mobility from any cause need assistance with turning and moving as well as encouragement to breathe deeply at frequent intervals. Observe the patient's skin and all pressure points for any evidence of redness or breakdown, especially the sacrum and coccyx. Early mobilization, the use of an incentive spirometer, and twice-daily oral hygiene with chlorhexidine swabs have been shown to significantly reduce the incidence of pneumonia in postoperative patients.[14] Treat pain to a comfort level that permits the patient to deep breathe and cough but yet remain awake and alert and achieve optimum mobility.

Practice strict medical asepsis and adherence to infection control guidelines to reduce the incidence of health care–associated infection (HAI). Staff and visitors should wash their hands on entering and leaving the patient's room. Staff must wash or use sanitizing hand gel before and after providing care and on removing gloves. Use strict sterile aseptic technique when suctioning the patient's trachea, and use caution when handling ventilator circuits, tracheostomy tubing, and nebulizer circuits that can become contaminated from patient secretions. Avoid inappropriate use of antibiotics to prevent the development of drug-resistant organisms.

◆ **Acute Care.** Although many patients with pneumonia are treated on an outpatient basis, the nursing care plan for a patient with pneumonia (see eNursing Care Plan 27-1) applies to both individuals at home and in-hospital patients. Essential nursing care for patients with pneumonia includes monitoring physical assessment parameters, providing treatment, and monitoring the patient's response to treatment. Along with physical assessment (including pulse oximetry monitoring), prompt collection of specimens and initiation of antibiotics are critical. $O_2$ therapy, hydration, nutritional support, breathing exercises, early ambulation, and therapeutic positioning are part of nursing management. Collaborate with respiratory therapists for assistance in monitoring the patient's condition and with physical therapy for postural drainage and chest percussion.

◆ **Ambulatory Care.** Teach the patient about the importance of taking every dose of the prescribed antibiotic, any drug-drug and food-drug interactions for the prescribed antibiotic, and the need for adequate rest to facilitate recovery. Instruct the patient to drink plenty of liquids (at least 6 to 10 glasses/day, unless contraindicated) and to avoid alcohol and smoking. A cool mist humidifier or warm bath may help the patient breathe easier. Tell patients that it may be several weeks before their usual vigor and sense of well-being return. Explain that a follow-up chest x-ray may be done in 6 to 8 weeks to evaluate resolution of pneumonia. A prolonged period of convalescence may be necessary for the older adult or chronically ill patient.

Teaching should also include information about available influenza and pneumococcal vaccines. Patients can receive the pneumococcal vaccine and influenza vaccine at the same time but not in the exact same location, and the vaccines cannot be mixed into one injection.

### ◆ Evaluation

The expected outcomes are that the patient with pneumonia will have

- Effective respiratory rate, rhythm, and depth of respirations
- Lungs clear to auscultation

Additional information on expected outcomes for the patient with pneumonia is presented in eNursing Care Plan 27-1 available on the website for this chapter.

## TUBERCULOSIS

**Tuberculosis (TB)** is an infectious disease caused by *Mycobacterium tuberculosis.* It usually involves the lungs, but any organ can be infected, including brain, kidneys, and bones. The CDC reports that more than 2 billion people (one third of the world's population) are infected with TB. It is the leading cause of mortality in patients with HIV infection. The incidence of TB worldwide declined until the mid-1980s when HIV disease emerged. The major factors contributing to the resurgence of TB were (1) high rates of TB among patients with HIV infection and (2) the emergence of MDR strains of *M. tuberculosis.* Although the prevalence of TB has increased in Europe, it has steadily declined in the United States since reaching a resurgence peak in 1992.[15]

TB occurs disproportionately in the poor, underserved, and minorities. People most at risk include the homeless, residents of inner-city neighborhoods, foreign-born people, those living or working in institutions (long-term care facilities, prisons, shelters, hospitals), IV injecting drug users, poor people, and those with poor access to health care. Immunosuppression from any etiology (e.g., HIV infection, malignancy, long-term corticosteroid use) increases the risk of active TB infection.

### CULTURAL & ETHNIC HEALTH DISPARITIES

#### *Tuberculosis*

- Of the reported tuberculosis (TB) cases in the United States, most occur in racial and ethnic minorities.
- Asians have the highest TB rate of any ethnic group in the United States. Native Hawaiian and other Pacific Islanders have the second-highest TB rate.
- Of all the TB cases in the United States, 65% occur in foreign-born people. This rate is 13 times higher than in U.S.-born people.
- The percentage of foreign-born people with multidrug-resistant TB has increased from 31% in 1993 to 90% in 2013.

Source: Centers for Disease Control and Prevention: Trends in tuberculosis—United States 2013. Retrieved from *www.cdc.gov/tb/statistics/reports/2013/pdf/report2013.pdf.*

Once a strain of *M. tuberculosis* develops resistance to two of the most potent first-line antituberculous drugs (e.g., isoniazid [INH], rifampin [Rifadin]), it is defined as *multidrug-resistant tuberculosis* (MDR-TB).[16] Extensively drug-resistant TB (XDR-TB) occurs when the organism is also resistant to any of the fluoroquinolones plus any injectable antibiotic agent. Resistance results from several problems, including incorrect prescribing, lack of public health case management, and patient nonadherence to the prescribed regimen.

### Etiology and Pathophysiology

*M. tuberculosis* is a gram-positive, acid-fast bacillus (AFB) that is usually spread from person to person via airborne particles expectorated when breathing, talking, singing, sneezing, and coughing. A process of evaporation leaves small droplet nuclei, 1 to 5 μm in size, suspended in the air for minutes to hours. These bacteria are then inhaled by another person. TB is not highly infectious, as transmission usually requires close, frequent, or prolonged exposure. The disease cannot be spread by touching, sharing food utensils, kissing, or any other type of physical contact.

Factors that influence the likelihood of transmission include the (1) number of organisms expelled into the air, (2) concentration of organisms (small spaces with limited ventilation would mean higher concentration), (3) length of time of exposure, and (4) immune system of the exposed person. Once inhaled, these small particles lodge in bronchioles and alveoli. A local inflammatory reaction occurs, and the focus of infection is established. This is called the *Ghon lesion* or *focus,* which represents a calcified TB granuloma, the hallmark of a primary TB infection. The formation of a granuloma is a defense mechanism aimed at walling off the infection and preventing further spread. Replication of the bacillus is inhibited and the infection is stopped.

Most immunocompetent adults infected with TB are able to completely kill the mycobacteria. Some people contain the mycobacteria in a nonreplicating dormant state. Of these individuals, 5% to 10% develop active TB infection when the bacteria begin to multiply months or years later. *M. tuberculosis* is aerophilic ($O_2$ loving) and thus has an affinity for the lungs. However, the infection can spread via the lymphatic system and find favorable environments for growth in other organs, including the cerebral cortex, spine, epiphyses of the bone, and adrenal glands.

## Classification

Several systems can be used to classify TB. The American Thoracic Society classifies TB based on development of the disease (Table 27-8). TB can also be classified according to (1) its presentation (primary, latent, or reactivated) and (2) whether it is pulmonary or extrapulmonary.

*Primary TB infection* occurs when the bacteria are inhaled and initiate an inflammatory reaction. The majority of people mount effective immune responses to encapsulate these organisms for the rest of their lives, preventing primary infection from progressing to disease.

*Latent TB infection* (LTBI) occurs in a person who does not have active TB disease (Table 27-9). People with LTBI have a positive skin test but are asymptomatic (Table 27-9). These individuals cannot transmit the TB bacteria to others but can develop active TB disease at some point. Immunosuppression, diabetes mellitus, poor nutrition, aging, pregnancy, stress, and chronic disease can precipitate the reactivation of LTBI. Consequently, treatment of LTBI is important (discussed later in this chapter).

If the initial immune response is not adequate, the body cannot contain the organisms. As a result, the bacteria replicate and *active TB disease* results. When active disease develops within the first 2 years of infection, it is termed *primary TB*. Individuals co-infected with HIV are at greatest risk for developing active TB. Post-primary TB, or *reactivation TB*, is defined as TB disease occurring 2 or more years after the initial infection. If the site of TB is pulmonary or laryngeal, the individual is considered infectious and can transmit the disease to others.

## Clinical Manifestations

Symptoms of pulmonary TB usually do not develop until 2 to 3 weeks after infection or reactivation. The characteristic pulmonary manifestation is an initial dry cough that frequently becomes productive with mucoid or mucopurulent sputum. Active TB disease may initially manifest with constitutional symptoms such as fatigue, malaise, anorexia, unexplained weight loss, low-grade fevers, and night sweats. Dyspnea is a late symptom that may signify considerable pulmonary disease or a pleural effusion. Hemoptysis, which occurs in less than 10% of patients with TB, is also a late symptom.

Sometimes TB has a more acute, sudden presentation. The patient may have a high fever, chills, generalized flu-like symptoms, pleuritic pain, and a productive cough. Auscultation of the lungs may be normal or reveal crackles, and/or adventitious (such as bronchial) breath sounds.

Immunosuppressed (e.g., HIV-infected) people and older adults are less likely to have fever and other signs of an infection. In patients with HIV, classic manifestations of TB such as fever, cough, and weight loss may be wrongly attributed to *P. jiroveci* pneumonia (PJP) or other HIV-associated opportunistic diseases. Clinical manifestations of respiratory problems in patients with HIV must be carefully investigated to determine the cause. A change in cognitive function may be the only initial presenting sign of TB in an older person.

The clinical manifestations of extrapulmonary TB depend on the organs infected. For example, renal TB can cause dysuria and hematuria. Bone and joint TB may cause severe pain.

**TABLE 27-8 Classification of Tuberculosis**

| Class | Exposure or Infection | Description |
|---|---|---|
| 0 | No TB exposure | No TB exposure, not infected (no history of exposure, negative tuberculin skin test) |
| 1 | TB exposure, no infection | TB exposure, no evidence of infection (history of exposure, negative tuberculin skin test) |
| 2 | Latent TB infection, no disease | TB infection without disease (significant reaction to tuberculin skin test, negative bacteriologic studies, no x-ray findings compatible with TB, no clinical evidence of TB) |
| 3 | TB, clinically active | TB infection with clinically active disease (positive bacteriologic studies or both a significant reaction to tuberculin skin test and clinical or x-ray evidence of current disease) |
| 4 | TB, but not clinically active | No current disease (history of previous episode of TB or abnormal, stable x-ray findings in a person with a significant reaction to tuberculin skin test. Negative bacteriologic studies if done. No clinical or x-ray evidence of current disease) |
| 5 | TB suspect | TB suspect (diagnosis pending). Individual should not be in this classification for >3 mo |

Source: American Thoracic Society.

**TABLE 27-9 Latent Tuberculosis Infection (LTBI) Compared to TB Disease**

| Latent TB Infection (LTBI) | TB Disease |
|---|---|
| Has no symptoms | Has symptoms that may include the following:<br>• Bad cough that lasts ≥3 wk<br>• Pain in the chest<br>• Coughing up blood or sputum<br>• Weakness or fatigue<br>• Weight loss<br>• No appetite<br>• Chills<br>• Fever<br>• Sweating at night |
| Does not feel sick | Usually feels sick |
| Cannot spread TB bacteria to others | May spread TB bacteria to others |
| Usually has a skin test or blood test result indicating TB infection | Usually has a skin test or blood test result indicating TB infection |
| Has a normal chest x-ray and a negative sputum smear | May have an abnormal chest x-ray or positive sputum smear or culture |
| Needs treatment for latent TB infection to prevent active TB disease | Needs treatment for active TB disease |

Source: Centers for Disease Control and Prevention: Latent tuberculosis infection: a guide for primary health care providers (2013). Retrieved from *www.cdc.gov/tb/publications/ltbi/pdf/TargetedLTBI.pdf*.

Headaches, vomiting, and lymphadenopathy may be present with TB meningitis.

### Complications

Appropriately treated pulmonary TB typically heals without complications, except for scarring and residual cavitation within the lung. Significant pulmonary damage, although rare, can occur in patients who are poorly treated or who do not respond to TB treatment.

*Miliary TB* is the widespread dissemination of the mycobacterium. The bacteria are spread via the bloodstream to several distant organs. The infection is characterized by a large amount of TB bacilli and may be fatal if left untreated. It can occur as a result of primary disease or reactivation of latent infection. Clinical manifestations of miliary TB slowly progress over a period of days, weeks, or even months. Symptoms vary depending on the organs that are affected. Fever, cough, and lymphadenopathy are present. Hepatomegaly and splenomegaly may also occur.

*Pleural TB,* a specific type of extrapulmonary TB, can result from either primary disease or reactivation of a latent infection. Chest pain, fever, cough, and presence of a unilateral pleural effusion are common. A pleural effusion is caused by bacteria in the pleural space, which trigger an inflammatory reaction and a pleural exudate of protein-rich fluid. Empyema is less common than effusion but may occur from large numbers of tubercular organisms in the pleural space. Diagnosis is confirmed by AFB cultures and a pleural biopsy.

Because TB can infect organs throughout the body, various acute and long-term complications can result. TB in the spine (Pott's disease) can lead to destruction of the intervertebral disc and adjacent vertebrae. Central nervous system TB can cause severe bacterial meningitis. Abdominal TB can lead to peritonitis, especially in HIV-positive patients. The kidneys, adrenal glands, lymph nodes, and urogenital tract may also be affected.

### Diagnostic Studies

**Tuberculin Skin Test.** The tuberculin skin test (TST) (Mantoux test) using purified protein derivative (PPD) is the standard method to screen people for *M. tuberculosis*. The test is administered by injecting 0.1 mL of PPD intradermally on the ventral surface of the forearm. The test is read by inspection and palpation 48 to 72 hours later for the presence or absence of induration. Induration, a palpable, raised, hardened area or swelling (not redness) at the injection site means the person has been exposed to TB and has developed antibodies.[17] (Antibody formation occurs 2 to 12 weeks after initial exposure to the bacteria.) The indurated area (if present) is measured and recorded in millimeters. Based on the size of the induration and the risk factors, an interpretation is made according to standards for determining a positive test reaction. Because the immunocompromised patient may have a decreased response to TST, smaller induration reactions (5 mm or larger) are considered positive. (See Table 25-11 for guidelines in interpreting responses to the TST.)

Some people who were previously infected with TB may have a waning immune response to the TST, resulting in a false negative result. However, repeating the TST may stimulate (boost) the body's ability to react to tuberculin in future tests. A positive reaction to a subsequent test could then be misinterpreted as a new infection, rather than the result of the boosted reaction to an old infection. To prevent misinterpretation in future testing, a two-step testing process is recommended for initial testing for health care workers (who get repeated testing) and for individuals who have a decreased response to allergens. A previously negative two-step TST ensures that any future positive results can be accurately interpreted as being caused by a new infection.

**Interferon-γ Release Assays.** Interferon-γ (INF-gamma) release assays (IGRAs) provide another screening tool for TB. IGRAs are blood tests that detect INF-gamma release from T cells in response to *Mycobacterium tuberculosis.* Examples of IGRAs include QuantiFERON-TB test and the T-SPOT.TB test. Test results are available in a few hours.

IGRAs offer several advantages over the TST in that they require only one patient visit, are not subject to reader bias, have no booster phenomenon, and are not affected by prior bacillus Calmette-Guérin (BCG) vaccination. The cost of an IGRA is substantially higher than the TST. Current guidelines suggest that both tests are viable options and that selection should be based on context and reasons for testing. Neither IGRAs nor TST can distinguish between LTBI and active TB infection. LTBI can only be diagnosed by excluding active TB.

**Chest X-ray.** Although the findings on chest x-ray examination are important, it is not possible to make a diagnosis of TB solely on chest x-ray findings. The chest x-ray may appear normal in a patient with TB. Findings suggestive of TB include upper lobe infiltrates, cavitary infiltrates, lymph node involvement, and pleural and/or pericardial effusion. Other diseases, such as sarcoidosis, can mimic the appearance of TB.

**Bacteriologic Studies.** Three consecutive sputum specimens obtained on different days are sent for smear and culture. The initial testing involves a microscopic examination of stained sputum smears for AFB. However, the definitive diagnosis of TB requires the demonstration of tubercle bacilli bacteriologically by sputum culture, which can take up to 8 weeks. Treatment is warranted pending the culture results for patients in whom clinical suspicion of TB is high. Samples for other suspected TB sites can be collected from gastric washings, cerebrospinal fluid (CSF), or fluid from an effusion or abscess.

### Interprofessional Care

Most patients with TB are treated on an outpatient basis (Table 27-10). Many people can continue to work and maintain their lifestyles with few changes. Patients with sputum smear–positive TB are generally considered infectious for the first 2 weeks after starting treatment. Advise these patients to restrict visitors and avoid travel on public transportation and trips to public places. Remind them of the importance of good handwashing and oral hygiene. Hospitalization may be needed for the severely ill or debilitated. The mainstay of TB treatment is drug therapy

**TABLE 27-10 Interprofessional Care**

***Pulmonary Tuberculosis***

| Diagnostic Assessment | Management |
|---|---|
| • History and physical examination<br>• Tuberculin skin test (TST)<br>• QuantiFERON-TB test<br>• Chest x-ray<br>• Bacteriologic studies<br>• Sputum smear for acid-fast bacilli (AFB)<br>• Sputum culture | • Long-term treatment with antimicrobial drugs (Tables 27-11 and 27-12)<br>• Follow-up AFB smears, cultures, and chest x-rays<br>• Follow-up care involving community health care workers and social workers |

TABLE 27-11 **Drug Therapy**

***Tuberculosis (TB)***

| Drug | Side Effects* |
|---|---|
| isoniazid | Hepatitis, asymptomatic elevation of aminotransferases (ALT, AST)<br>Monitor liver function tests monthly |
| rifampin (Rifadin) | Hepatitis, thrombocytopenia, orange discoloration of bodily fluids (sputum, urine, sweat, tears) |
| pyrazinamide | Hepatitis, arthralgias, hyperuricemia |
| ethambutol (Myambutol) | Ocular toxicity (decreased red-green color discrimination)<br>Monitor visual acuity and color discrimination regularly |
| rifabutin (Mycobutin) | Hepatitis, thrombocytopenia, neutropenia, orange discoloration of bodily fluids (sputum, urine, sweat, tears) |
| rifapentine (Priftin) | Similar to those of rifampin |
| streptomycin | Ototoxicity, neurotoxicity, nephrotoxicity |
| bedaquiline (Sirturo) | Dysrhythmias |
| aminoglycosides | Ototoxicity, nephrotoxicity |
| • capreomycin (Capastat)<br>• amikacin | Used in selected cases for treatment of resistant strains |
| fluoroquinolones | GI disturbance, neurologic effects (dizziness, headache), rash |
| • levofloxacin (Levaquin)<br>• moxifloxacin (Avelox, Vigamox) | Used in drug-resistant TB |

*ALT,* Alanine transaminase; *AST,* aspartate aminotransferase.
*Only common side effects are listed.

TABLE 27-12 **Drug Therapy**

***Tuberculosis Disease Regimens***

| Initial Phase | Continuation Phase |
|---|---|
| **Option 1** | |
| 4-drug regimen consisting of isoniazid, rifampin, pyrazinamide, ethambutol<br>Given daily for 56 doses (8 wk) OR 5 days/wk DOT for 40 doses (8 wk) | isoniazid, rifampin daily for 126 doses (18 wk) OR 5 days/wk DOT for 90 doses (18 wk) |
| **Option 2** | |
| 4-drug regimen consisting of isoniazid, rifampin, pyrazinamide, ethambutol<br>Given daily for 14 doses (2 wk), followed by twice weekly for 12 doses (6 wk) OR 5 days/wk DOT for 10 doses (2 wk), then twice weekly for 12 doses (6 wk) | isoniazid, rifampin twice weekly for 36 doses (18 wk) OR once weekly for 18 doses (18 wk) |
| **Option 3** | |
| 4-drug regimen consisting of isoniazid, rifampin, pyrazinamide, ethambutol<br>Given three times weekly for 24 doses (8 wk) | isoniazid, rifampin three times weekly for 54 doses (18 wk) |
| **Option 4** | |
| 3-drug regimen consisting of isoniazid, rifampin, ethambutol<br>Given daily for 56 doses (8 wk) OR 5 days/wk DOT for 40 doses (8 wk) | isoniazid, rifampin daily for 217 doses (31 wk) OR 5 days/wk DOT for 155 doses (31 wk) OR twice weekly for 62 doses (31 wk) |

*DOT,* Directly observed therapy.
Source: American Thoracic Society, Centers for Disease Control and Prevention, and Infectious Diseases Society of America: Treatment of tuberculosis. Retrieved from *www.cdc.gov/mmwr/PDF/rr/rr5211.pdf.*

(Table 27-11). Promoting and monitoring adherence are critical for treatment to be successful.

### Drug Therapy

***Active TB Disease.*** Because of the growing prevalence of MDR-TB, it is important to manage the patient with active TB aggressively. Drug therapy is divided into two phases: initial and continuation (Table 27-12). In most circumstances the treatment regimen for patients with previously untreated TB consists of a 2-month initial phase with four drugs (isoniazid, rifampin, pyrazinamide, and ethambutol). If drug susceptibility test results indicate that the bacteria are susceptible to all drugs, ethambutol may be discontinued. If pyrazinamide cannot be included in the initial phase (because of liver disease, pregnancy, etc.), the remaining three drugs are used for the initial phase.

**DRUG ALERT Isoniazid**
- Alcohol may increase hepatotoxicity of the drug.
- Instruct patient to avoid drinking alcohol during treatment.
- Monitor for signs of hepatitis before and while taking drug.

If the patient develops a toxic reaction to the primary drugs, other drugs can be used, including rifabutin and rifapentine (Priftin). Treatment for drug-resistant TB is guided by sensitivity testing. MDR-TB therapy typically includes a fluoroquinolone and an injectable antibiotic (Table 27-11). Bedaquiline (Sirturo), a relatively new drug, is used in combination with other drugs to treat MDR-TB. It works by inhibiting an enzyme needed for *M. tuberculosis* to replicate.

*Directly observed therapy* (DOT) involves providing the antituberculosis drugs directly to patients and watching as they swallow the medications. To ensure adherence, it is the preferred strategy for all patients with TB, especially for those at risk for nonadherence.[18] Nonadherence is a major factor in the emergence of multidrug resistance and treatment failures. Many individuals do not adhere to the treatment program in spite of understanding the disease process and value of treatment. DOT is an expensive but essential public health measure. The risk for reactivation of TB and MDR-TB is increased in patients who do not complete the full course of therapy. In many areas, the public health nurse administers DOT at a clinic site.

When DOT is not used, fixed-dose combination drugs may enhance adherence. Combinations of isoniazid and rifampin (Rifamate) and of isoniazid, rifampin, and pyrazinamide (Rifater) are available to simplify therapy. The therapy for people with HIV follows the same therapy options outlined in Table 27-12. However, alternative regimens that include once-weekly isoniazid plus rifapentine continuation dosing in any HIV-infected patient and twice-weekly isoniazid plus rifampin or rifabutin should not be used if $CD4^+$ counts are less than 100/μL. HCPs must also be alert for possible drug interactions between antiretrovirals (used to treat HIV) and rifamycins.

Teaching patients about the adverse effects of these drugs and when to seek prompt medical attention is critical. The major side effect of isoniazid, rifampin, and pyrazinamide is nonviral hepatitis. Baseline liver function tests (LFTs) are done at the start of treatment and monitored closely (e.g., every 2 to 4 weeks), if results are abnormal.

***Latent Tuberculosis Infection.*** In people with LTBI, drug therapy helps prevent a TB infection from developing into active TB disease. Because a person with LTBI has fewer bacteria, treatment is much easier. Usually only one drug is needed. Drug therapy regimens for LTBI are presented in Table 27-13.

**TABLE 27-13 Drug Therapy**

***Latent Tuberculosis Infection Regimens***

| Drugs | Duration | Interval | Minimum Doses |
|---|---|---|---|
| isoniazid | 9 mo | Daily | 270 |
| | | Twice weekly* | 76 |
| isoniazid | 6 mo | Daily | 180 |
| | | Twice weekly* | 52 |
| isoniazid and rifapentine | 3 mo | Once weekly* | 12 |
| rifampin | 4 mo | Daily | 120 |

Source: Centers for Disease Control and Prevention: Latent tuberculosis infection: a guide for primary health care providers (2013). Retrieved from *www.cdc.gov/tb/publications/ltbi/pdf/TargetedLTBI.pdf*
*Use directly observed therapy (DOT).

## ETHICAL/LEGAL DILEMMAS

***Patient Adherence***

**Situation**

A health clinic at a homeless shelter discovers that F.C., a 64-yr-old male with tuberculosis (TB), has not been taking his prescribed medication. He tells you that it is hard for him to get to the clinic to obtain the medication, much less to keep on a schedule. You are concerned not only about this patient but also about the risks for the other people at the shelter, in the park, and at the meal sites.

**Ethical/Legal Points for Consideration**

- Adherence is a complex issue involving a person's culture and values, perceived risk of disease, availability of resources, access to treatment, and perceived consequences of available choices.
- Advocacy for the patient and the community obliges you to involve other members of the health care team, such as social services, to assist in obtaining the necessary resources or support for the patient to complete a course of treatment.
- Some cities and states have instituted a stepwise legal process for managing nonadherent TB patients.[1]
- Legally the constitutionally granted right to control one's own body may be limited by the state and federal obligation to protect public health and safety. Most of these laws have provisions for the protection of constitutional rights such as right to counsel, right to least restrictive alternative in terms of confinement setting, and right to prompt judicial review.
- The federal government and many states have provisions for quarantine, detention, and treatment. With the threats of bioterrorism and the globalization of exposure to highly lethal infectious diseases, it seems unlikely that the government's power to detain will be removed.

**Discussion Questions**

1. What alternatives of care can be offered to F.C.?
2. Under what circumstances are HCPs justified in overriding a patient's autonomy or decision making?

**Reference**

1. Guidelines for the Civil Detention of Persistently Non-Adherent Tuberculosis Patients in California. Retrieved from *http://ctca.org/fileLibrary/file_50.pdf.*

The standard treatment regimen for LTBI is 9 months of daily isoniazid. It is an effective and inexpensive drug that the patient can take orally. The 9-month regimen is more effective, but adherence issues may make a 6-month regimen preferable. For HIV patients and those with fibrotic lesions on chest x-ray, isoniazid is given for 9 months. An alternative 3-month regimen of isoniazid and rifapentine may be used for otherwise healthy patients who are not presumed to be infected with drug-resistant bacilli. Four-month therapy with rifampin may be indicated if the patient is resistant to isoniazid. Because of severe liver injury and deaths, the CDC does not recommend the combination of rifampin and pyrazinamide for treatment of LTBI.[19]

## EVIDENCE-BASED PRACTICE

***Applying the Evidence***

**Adherence to Tuberculosis Treatment Program**

You are a nurse working in an outpatient health clinic with C.J., a 42-year-old male diagnosed 3 months ago with active tuberculosis (TB). You notice C.J. frequently misses or is late for his clinic appointments. He tells you he forgets when his appointments are scheduled and asks if he needs to continue with his visits because he is feeling much better.

***Making Clinical Decisions***

***Best Available Evidence.*** TB clinic attendance and treatment completion rates are higher when patients receive pre-appointment reminder phone calls or letters. When appointments are missed, phone calls, letters, or home visits re-engage patients, resulting in improved clinic attendance and treatment completion.

***Clinician Expertise.*** You know patients may stop attending clinics and taking their medications when feeling well again, which can lead to treatment failure and multidrug resistance.

***Patient Preferences and Values.*** C.J. tells you that he has a busy lifestyle and that he does not remember his appointment dates or consider them important since he is feeling better.

***Implications for Nursing Practice***

1. What information would you provide C.J. regarding the importance of his clinic visits?
2. Your clinic indicates interest in starting a reminder system for clinic appointments. How will you support these efforts, and what system will you recommend?
3. How will you determine if C.J. is adhering to the recommended drug treatment program?

***Reference for Evidence***

Liu Q, Abba K, Alejandria MM, et al: Reminder systems to improve patient adherence to tuberculosis clinic appointments for diagnosis and treatment, *Cochrane Database Syst Rev* 11:CD006594, 2014.

***Bacille-Calmette-Guerin Vaccine.*** Bacille-Calmette-Guerin (BCG) vaccine is a live, attenuated strain of *Mycobacterium bovis.* The vaccine is given to infants in parts of the world with a high prevalence of TB. In the United States it is typically not recommended because of the low risk of infection, the vaccine's variable effectiveness against adult pulmonary TB, and potential interference with TB skin test reactivity. The BCG vaccination can result in a false-positive TST. IGRA results are not affected. The BCG vaccine should be considered only for select individuals who meet specific criteria (e.g., health care workers who are continually exposed to patients with MDR-TB and when infection control precautions are not successful).

## NURSING MANAGEMENT: TUBERCULOSIS

### Nursing Assessment

Ask the patient about a previous history of TB, chronic illness, or any immunosuppressive medications. Obtain a social and occupational history to determine risk factors for transmission of TB. Assess the patient for productive cough, night sweats, temperature elevation, weight loss, pleuritic chest pain, and abnormal lung sounds. If the patient has a productive cough, early morning is the ideal time to collect sputum specimens for an AFB smear.

### Nursing Diagnoses

Nursing diagnoses for the patient with TB may include, but are not limited to, the following:

- Ineffective breathing pattern *related to* decreased lung capacity
- Ineffective airway clearance *related to* increased secretions, fatigue, and decreased lung capacity
- Risk for infection (spread of infection to others) *related to* cough and sputum production, lack of knowledge of disease process, and social/economic circumstances
- Noncompliance and ineffective health management *related to* lack of knowledge of disease process, lack of motivation, long-term nature of treatment, and lack of resources

### Planning

The overall goals are that the patient with TB will (1) comply with the therapeutic regimen, (2) have no recurrence of disease, (3) have normal pulmonary function, and (4) take appropriate measures to prevent the spread of the disease.

### Nursing Implementation

**Health Promotion.** The ultimate goal is to eradicate TB worldwide. Screening programs in known risk groups are of value in detecting individuals with TB. Treatment of LTBI reduces the number of TB carriers in the community. The person with a positive TST should have a chest x-ray to assess for active TB disease. Individuals with a diagnosis of TB must be reported to the public health authorities for identification and assessment of contacts and risk to the community.

Programs to address the social determinants of TB are necessary to decrease transmission of TB. Reducing HIV infection, poverty, overcrowded living conditions, malnutrition, smoking, and drug and alcohol abuse can help minimize TB infection rates. Improving access to health care and education is also important.

**Acute Care.** Patients admitted to the emergency department or directly to the nursing unit with respiratory symptoms should be assessed for the possibility of TB. Those strongly suspected of having TB should (1) be placed on airborne isolation; (2) receive a medical workup, including chest x-ray, sputum smear, and culture; and (3) receive appropriate drug therapy. Airborne infection isolation is indicated for the patient with pulmonary or laryngeal TB until the patient is noninfectious. *Airborne infection isolation* refers to isolation of patients infected with organisms spread by the airborne route. It requires a single-occupancy room with negative pressure and airflow of 6 to 12 exchanges per hour.

High-efficiency particulate air (HEPA) masks are worn whenever entering the patient's room. These masks are highly effective at protecting from small particles 5 μm or less in diameter. Because there are many different types of HEPA masks currently available, health care professionals should be "fit tested" each time a different brand or model of mask is used to ensure proper mask size. Otherwise, the CDC recommends that yearly mask "fit testing" is acceptable.[20] To be effective, the mask must be molded to fit tightly around the nose and mouth.

Teach patients to cover the nose and mouth with paper tissues every time they cough, sneeze, or produce sputum. The tissues should be thrown into a paper bag and disposed of with the trash or flushed down the toilet. Emphasize careful hand washing after handling sputum and soiled tissues. If patients need to be out of the negative-pressure room, they must wear a standard isolation mask to prevent exposure to others. Minimize prolonged visitation to other parts of the hospital.

Identify and screen close contacts of the person with TB. Anyone testing positive for TB infection will undergo further evaluation and needs to be treated for either LTBI or active TB disease.

**Ambulatory Care.** Patients who respond clinically are discharged home (even with positive cultures) if their household contacts have already been exposed and the patient is not posing a risk to others. A sputum specimen for AFB smear and culture should be obtained at a minimum of monthly intervals until two consecutive specimens are negative on culture. More frequent AFB smears may be useful to assess the early response to treatment and provide an indication of infectiousness. Negative cultures are needed to declare the patient not infectious.

Teach the patient how to minimize exposure to close contacts and household members. Homes should be well ventilated, especially the areas where the infected person spends a lot of time. While still infectious, the patient should sleep alone, spend as much time as possible outdoors, and minimize time in congregate settings or on public transportation.

Teach the patient and caregiver about adherence with the prescribed regimen. This is important, since most treatment failures occur because the patient neglects to take the drug, discontinues it prematurely, or takes it irregularly. Strategies to improve adherence to drug therapy include teaching and counseling, reminder systems, incentives or rewards, contracts, and DOT.

Notification of the public health department is required. The public health nurse is responsible for follow-up on household contacts and assessment of the patient for adherence. If adherence is an issue, the public health agency may be responsible for DOT. Most individuals can be considered adequately treated when the therapy regimen has been completed and there is evidence of negative cultures, clinical improvement, and improvement on chest x-ray.

Because about 5% of individuals experience relapses, teach the patient to recognize the symptoms that indicate recurrence of TB. If these symptoms occur, the patient should seek immediate medical attention. Instruct the patient about certain factors that could reactivate TB, such as immunosuppressive therapy, malignancy, and prolonged debilitating illness. If the patient experiences any of these events, the HCP must be told so that TB can be closely monitored for reactivation. In some situations it is necessary to put the patient on anti-TB therapy. Because smoking is associated with poor outcomes in TB, patients should be encouraged to quit. Provide patients with teaching and resources to help them stop smoking.

### Evaluation

**Evaluation.** The expected outcomes are that the patient with TB will have

- Resolution of the disease
- Normal pulmonary function
- Absence of any complications
- No further transmission of TB

## ATYPICAL MYCOBACTERIA

There are more than 30 varieties of acid-fast mycobacteria that do not cause TB but can cause pulmonary disease, lymphadenitis,

**TABLE 27-14 Fungal Infections of the Lung**

| Infection | Organism |
|---|---|
| **Endemic Fungal Infections** | |
| Histoplasmosis | *Histoplasma capsulatum* |
| Coccidioidomycosis | *Coccidioides immitis* |
| Blastomycosis | *Blastomyces dermatitidis* |
| **Opportunistic Fungal Infections** | |
| Candidiasis | *Candida albicans* |
| Aspergillosis | *Aspergillus niger* or *Aspergillus fumigatus* |
| Cryptococcosis | *Cryptococcus neoformans* |

skin or soft tissue disease, or disseminated disease. Pulmonary disease is indistinguishable from TB clinically and radiologically but can be differentiated by bacteriologic culture. Atypical mycobacteria are not airborne and not transmitted by droplets. They can be found in tap water, soil, bird feces, and house dust.

*Mycobacterium avium* complex (MAC), found in aerosols generated from baths, hot spas, and swimming pools, is one cause of atypical mycobacteria pulmonary infection. Only a small number of people exposed to the organism actually develop MAC lung disease. People who are immunosuppressed (e.g., HIV/AIDS) or have chronic pulmonary disease are most susceptible. Treatment is similar to that for TB.

## PULMONARY FUNGAL INFECTIONS

Pulmonary fungal pneumonia is an infectious process in the lungs caused by endemic (native and common) or opportunistic fungi (Table 27-14). *Endemic* fungal pathogens cause infection in healthy people and in immunocompromised people in certain geographic locations in the United States. For example, *Coccidioides*, which causes coccidioidomycosis, is a fungus found in the soil of dry, low-rainfall areas.[21] It is endemic in many areas of the southwestern United States. *Opportunistic* fungal infections occur in immunocompromised patients (e.g., those being treated with corticosteroids, chemotherapy, and immunosuppressive drugs) and in patients with HIV and cystic fibrosis. These infections can be very serious.

Fungal infections are acquired by inhalation of spores. These infections are not transmitted from person to person, and the patient does not have to be placed in isolation. The clinical manifestations are similar to those of bacterial pneumonia. Skin testing, serology, and biopsy methods assist in identifying the infecting organism.

Amphotericin B remains the standard therapy for treating serious systemic fungal infections. It must be given IV to achieve adequate blood and tissue levels because the GI tract does not absorb it well. Less serious infections can be treated with oral antifungals such as ketoconazole (Nizoral), fluconazole (Diflucan), voriconazole (Vfend), and itraconazole (Sporanox). Effectiveness of therapy can be monitored with fungal serology titers.

## LUNG ABSCESS

### Etiology and Pathophysiology

A **lung abscess** is necrosis of lung tissue typically resulting from bacteria aspirated from the oral cavity in patients with periodontal disease. Because oral secretions can contain large amounts of bacteria, even small amounts *(microaspiration)* can cause infection. The abscess usually develops slowly, beginning with an enlarging area of infection that becomes necrotic and eventually forms a cavity filled with purulent material. Lung abscesses can also result from IV drug use, malignancy, pulmonary emboli, TB, and various parasitic and fungal diseases. Abscesses usually contain more than one type of microbe, most commonly reflecting the anaerobic flora of the mouth.

The area of the lung most often affected due to aspiration is the posterior segment of the upper lobes. The abscess may erode into the bronchial system, causing the production of foul-smelling or sour-tasting sputum. It may grow toward the pleura and cause pleuritic pain. Multiple small abscesses, sometimes referred to as *necrotizing pneumonia,* can occur within the lung.

### Clinical Manifestations and Complications

Clinical manifestations usually occur slowly over a period of weeks to months, especially if anaerobic organisms are the primary cause. Symptoms of abscess caused by aerobic bacteria develop more acutely and resemble bacterial pneumonia. The most common manifestation is cough-producing purulent sputum (often dark brown) that is foul smelling and foul tasting. Hemoptysis is common, especially when an abscess ruptures into a bronchus. Other common manifestations are fever, chills, prostration, night sweats, pleuritic pain, dyspnea, anorexia, and weight loss.

Physical examination of the lungs indicates dullness to percussion and decreased breath sounds on auscultation over the involved segment of lung. Bronchial breath sounds may be transmitted to the periphery if the communicating bronchus becomes patent and the segment begins to drain. Crackles may also be present in the later stages as the abscess drains.

The infection can also spread via the bloodstream and produce a number of other possible complications. Pulmonary abscess, bronchopleural fistula, bronchiectasis, and empyema from perforation of the abscess into the pleural cavity, have been reported.

### Diagnostic Studies

A chest x-ray is often the only test needed for diagnosis of lung abscess. The presence of a solitary cavitary lesion with an air-fluid level and local infiltrate can confirm the diagnosis. CT scanning may be helpful if the cavitation is not clear on chest x-ray. As long as there is drainage via the bronchus, sputum will contain the microorganisms that are present in the abscess. However, expectorated sputum samples are contaminated with oral flora, making it difficult to determine the offending organisms.

Bronchoscopy may be used to (1) avoid oropharyngeal contamination, (2) collect a specimen if drainage is delayed, or (3) investigate if there is a possibility of an underlying malignancy. Pleural fluid and blood cultures may be useful to identify the offending organisms. Although nonspecific, an elevated neutrophil count from a complete blood count (CBC) may indicate an infectious process.

## ❖ NURSING AND INTERPROFESSIONAL MANAGEMENT: LUNG ABSCESS

Monitor the patient's vital signs, level of consciousness, and respiratory status for any signs of hypoxia. Note any cyanosis or clubbing of the fingers. Administer $O_2$ as needed. IV antibiotic therapy should be started as soon as possible. Clindamycin is first-line therapy. Parenteral antibiotics are switched to oral antibiotics once the patient shows clinical and x-ray evidence of improvement.

Because of the need for prolonged antibiotic therapy, the patient must be aware of the importance of continuing the medication for the prescribed period. To avoid the risk of a secondary or worsening infection, all antibiotics should be taken, as directed, for the entire prescribed period. Sometimes the patient is asked to return periodically during the course of antibiotic therapy for repeat cultures and sensitivity tests to ensure that the infecting organism is not becoming resistant to the antibiotic. When antibiotic therapy is completed, the patient is reevaluated.

Teach the patient how to cough effectively (see Table 28-23). Chest physiotherapy and postural drainage are not recommended because they may facilitate movement of microorganisms into other bronchi, extending infection. Rest, good nutrition, and adequate fluid intake are supportive measures to facilitate recovery. If dentition is poor and dental hygiene is not adequate, encourage the patient to obtain dental care. Consider collaboration with the social worker to evaluate available options for dental care if the patient has limited resources.

Percutaneous drainage of the abscess may be necessary if the patient does not adequately respond to antibiotic treatment. A small catheter, guided by CT or ultrasound, may be placed to drain the abscess. Surgery is rarely indicated but occasionally necessary when reinfection of a large cavitary lesion occurs or to establish a diagnosis when there is evidence of an underlying problem such as a neoplasm. The usual procedure in such cases is a lobectomy. A pneumonectomy may be necessary for multiple abscesses.

## ENVIRONMENTAL LUNG DISEASES

Environmental or occupational lung diseases result from inhaled dust or chemicals. The extent of lung damage is influenced by the toxicity of the inhaled substance, amount and duration of exposure, and individual susceptibility. Environmentally induced lung disease includes pneumoconiosis, chemical pneumonitis, and hypersensitivity pneumonitis.

**Pneumoconiosis** is a general term for a group of lung diseases caused by inhalation and retention of mineral or metal dust particles. The literal meaning of *pneumoconiosis* is "dust in the lungs." These diseases are classified according to the origin of the dust (e.g., silicosis, asbestosis, berylliosis). Coal worker's pneumoconiosis (CWP), also known as *black lung,* is caused by inhalation of large amounts of coal dust, an occupational hazard for underground coal miners. The inhaled substance is ingested by macrophages, which releases substances that cause cell injury and death. Fibrosis occurs as a result of tissue repair after inflammation. Breathing problems become evident after many years of repeated exposure, resulting in diffuse *pulmonary fibrosis* (excess connective tissue).

*Chemical pneumonitis* results from exposures to toxic chemical fumes. Acutely, there is diffuse lung injury characterized as pulmonary edema. Chronically, the clinical picture is that of *bronchiolitis obliterans* (obstruction of the bronchioles due to inflammation and fibrosis), which is usually associated with a normal chest x-ray or one that shows hyperinflation. An example is silo filler's disease.

*Hypersensitivity pneumonitis,* or extrinsic allergic alveolitis, is a form of parenchymal lung disease seen when an individual inhales antigens to which he or she is allergic. Examples include bird fancier's lung and farmer's lung.

Asbestos is a group of minerals composed of microscopic fibers. For many years, asbestos was primarily used for insulation and to help fireproof buildings. When disturbed, asbestos releases tiny filament particles into the air. Once inhaled, the tiny fibers become deposited within the lung. Asbestosis is chronic inflammation of the lung, and people with repeated exposure are at a greater risk of disease. Lung cancer, either squamous cell carcinoma or adenocarcinoma, is the most frequent cancer associated with asbestos exposure. There is a minimum lapse of 15 to 19 years between first exposure and development of lung cancer. Mesothelioma, both pleural and peritoneal, is associated with asbestos exposure.

### Clinical Manifestations

Symptoms of many environmental lung diseases may not occur until at least 10 to 15 years after the initial exposure to the inhaled irritant. Clinical manifestations common to all pneumoconioses include dyspnea, cough, wheezing, and weight loss. Pulmonary function studies often show reduced vital capacity. A chest x-ray often reveals lung involvement specific to the primary problem. CT scans have been useful in detecting early lung involvement.

Cor pulmonale, a condition in which the right side of the heart fails, is a late complication, especially in conditions characterized by diffuse pulmonary fibrosis. COPD is the most common complication of environmental lung disease. Other associated disorders include lung cancer, mesothelioma, and TB. Manifestations of these complications are often the reason the patient seeks health care.

Signs of acute hypersensitivity pneumonitis occur 4 to 6 hours after exposure and include chills, fever, cough, shortness of breath, and malaise. Symptoms of chronic hypersensitivity pneumonitis include cough, anorexia, and weight loss. Acute pulmonary edema may occur after exposure to chemical fumes.

### Interprofessional Care

The best approach to management of environmental lung diseases is to prevent or decrease environmental and occupational exposure. Teach the public about the risk and the appropriate protective equipment. Using well-designed, effective ventilation systems and wearing masks are appropriate for some occupations and household activities. Inhalation of smoke by nonsmokers has led to regulations requiring a smoke-free workplace. Periodic inspections and monitoring of workplaces by agencies such as the Occupational Safety and Health Administration (OSHA) and the National Institute for Occupational Safety and Health (NIOSH) reinforce employers' obligations to provide a safe work environment. NIOSH is responsible for workplace safety and health regulations in the United States.

Early diagnosis is essential to halting the disease process. Strategies are directed toward preventing disease progression and improving or controlling respiratory symptoms. Strategies include $O_2$ therapy, inhaled bronchodilators, percussion therapy, and pulmonary rehabilitation. Patients should also be immunized against pneumococcal pneumonia and influenza. Discontinuation of exposure to the offending inhalant and smoking cessation may or may not be effective in stopping disease progression.

## LUNG CANCER

*Lung cancer* is the leading cause of cancer-related deaths in the United States.[22] Lung cancer accounts for 28% of all cancer deaths, more than those caused by breast, prostate, and colon cancer combined. Annually about 221,000 new cases of lung cancer are diagnosed and 158,000 Americans die. Although lung cancer is associated with a high mortality and low cure rate, advances in medical treatment are improving the response to treatment.[23]

## Etiology

Smoking is responsible for 80% to 90% of all lung cancers.[23] Tobacco smoke contains 60 carcinogens in addition to substances (carbon monoxide, nicotine) that interfere with normal cell development. Exposure to tobacco smoke causes changes in the bronchial epithelium, which usually returns to normal when smoking is discontinued. The risk of lung cancer gradually decreases with smoking cessation, reaching that of nonsmokers within 10 to 15 years of quitting.

The risk of developing lung cancer is directly related to total exposure to tobacco smoke, measured by total number of cigarettes smoked in a lifetime, age of smoking onset, depth of inhalation, tar and nicotine content, and the use of unfiltered cigarettes. Both smokers and nonsmokers can develop lung cancer. Sidestream smoke (smoke from burning cigarettes, cigars) contains the same carcinogens found in mainstream smoke (smoke inhaled and exhaled by the smoker). This exposure to secondhand smoke creates a health risk for nonsmoking adults and children.

Other common causes of lung cancer include high levels of pollution, radiation (especially radon exposure), and asbestos. Heavy or prolonged exposure to industrial agents such as ionizing radiation, coal dust, nickel, uranium, chromium, formaldehyde, and arsenic can also increase the risk of lung cancer, especially in smokers.[24]

Marked variations exist in a person's propensity to develop lung cancer. Differences in lung cancer incidence, risk factors, and survival exist between men and women (see Gender Differences box). Genetic, hormonal, and molecular influences may contribute to these differences.

## Pathophysiology

Most primary lung tumors are believed to arise from mutated epithelial cells. The development of mutations, which are caused by carcinogens, is also influenced by various genetic factors. Once underway, tumor development is promoted by epidermal growth factor. These cells grow slowly, taking 8 to 10 years for a tumor to reach 1 cm in size, the smallest lesion detectable on x-ray. Lung cancers occur primarily in the segmental bronchi or beyond and usually occur in the upper lobes of the lungs (Figs. 27-2 and 27-3).

Primary lung cancers are categorized into two broad subtypes (Table 27-15): non–lung cancer (NSCLC) (80%) and small cell lung cancer (SCLC) (20%).[25] Lung cancers metastasize primarily by direct extension and via the blood and lymph system. The common sites for metastasis are the lymph nodes, liver, brain, bones, and adrenal glands.

**Paraneoplastic Syndrome.** Lung cancers can cause *paraneoplastic syndrome.* Paraneoplastic syndrome may be caused by hormones, cytokines, or enzymes (secreted by tumor cells) or by

### GENDER DIFFERENCES
**Lung Cancer**

**Men**
- More men than women are diagnosed with lung cancer.
- More men than women die from lung cancer.
- Male smokers are 10 times more likely to develop lung cancer than nonsmokers.
- Men with lung cancer have a worse prognosis than women.
- Lung cancer incidence and deaths are decreasing in men.

**Women**
- Lung cancer incidence and deaths are increasing in women.
- Women develop lung cancer after fewer years of smoking than men do.
- Women develop lung cancer at a younger age than men.
- Nonsmoking women are at greater risk of developing lung cancer than men.
- Women with lung cancer live, on the average, 12 months longer than men.

### CULTURAL & ETHNIC HEALTH DISPARITIES
**Lung Cancer**

**African Americans**
- Have the highest incidence of lung cancer
- Are more likely to die from lung cancer than any other ethnic group
- Have a higher rate of lung cancer among men than in other ethnic groups

**Whites**
- Have the second-highest death rate from lung cancer
- Have a higher rate of lung cancer among women than in other ethnic groups

**Asian/Pacific Islanders and Hispanics**
- Have the lowest rates of lung cancer in both men and women

**Other**
- Regional variations among ethnic groups may be due to smoking prevalence, exposure to cancer-causing substances, and other factors.
- Cigarette consumption has decreased dramatically in developed countries such as the United States and Canada.
- Cigarette smoking is increasing in developing countries (e.g., nations in Africa, Asia, Latin America).

Source: Centers for Disease Control and Prevention: Racial/ethnic disparities and geographic differences in lung cancer incidence—38 states and the District of Columbia, 1998-2006. Retrieved from *www.cdc.gov/mmwr/PDF/wk/mm5944.pdf.*

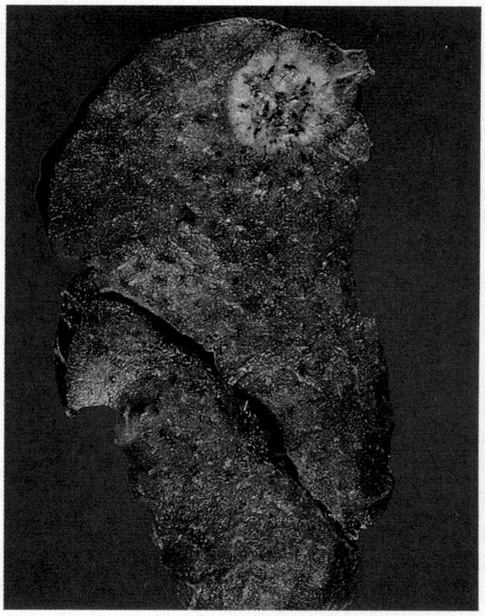

**FIG. 27-2** Lung cancer (peripheral adenocarcinoma). The tumor shows prominent black pigmentation, suggestive of having evolved from anthracosis (coal dust in the lungs). (From Damjanov I, Linder J: *Anderson's pathology,* ed 10, St Louis, 1996, Mosby.)

**TABLE 27-15 Types of Primary Lung Cancer**

| Type | Growth Rate | Characteristics | Response to Therapy |
|---|---|---|---|
| **Non–Small Cell Lung Cancer (NSCLC)** | | | |
| **Squamous cell carcinoma** | Slow | • Accounts for 20%-30% of lung cancers<br>• Centrally located, producing early symptoms of nonproductive cough and hemoptysis<br>• Does not have a strong tendency to metastasize | • Surgical resection may be attempted.<br>• Adjuvant chemotherapy and radiation<br>• Depending on the staging, life expectancy is better than for small cell lung cancer. |
| **Adenocarcinoma** | Moderate | • Accounts for 30%-40% of lung cancers<br>• Most common lung cancer in people who have not smoked<br>• Peripherally located<br>• Often has no clinical manifestations until widespread metastasis is present | • Surgical resection may be attempted depending on staging.<br>• Does not respond well to chemotherapy |
| **Large cell (undifferentiated) carcinoma** | Rapid | • Accounts for 10% of lung cancers<br>• Composed of large cells that are anaplastic and often arise in bronchi<br>• Is highly metastatic via lymphatics and blood | • Surgery is not usually attempted because of high rate of metastases.<br>• Tumor may be radiosensitive but often recurs. |
| **Small Cell Lung Cancer (SCLC)** | | | |
| **Small cell carcinoma** | Very rapid | • Accounts for about 20% of lung cancers<br>• Most malignant form of lung cancer<br>• Spreads early via lymphatics and bloodstream<br>• Frequent metastasis to brain<br>• Associated with endocrine disturbances | • Chemotherapy mainstay of treatment but overall poor prognosis<br>• Radiation is used as adjuvant therapy and palliative measure. |

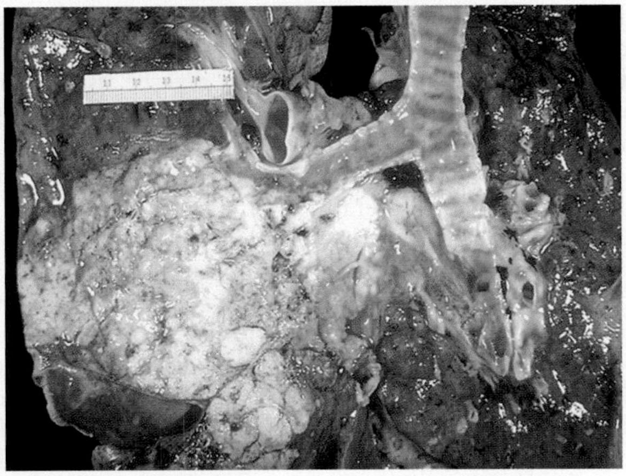

**FIG. 27-3** Lung carcinoma. The gray-white tumor tissue is infiltrating the lung. Histologically this tumor is identified as a squamous cell carcinoma. (From Kumar V, Abbas AK, Aster JC, Fausto N: *Robbins and Cotran pathologic basis of disease*, ed 8, Philadelphia, 2010, Saunders.)

antibodies (produced by the body in response to the tumor) that destroy healthy cells. Sometimes the symptoms of paraneoplastic syndrome manifest even before the malignancy is diagnosed.

Examples of paraneoplastic syndrome include hypercalcemia, syndrome of inappropriate antidiuretic hormone secretion (SIADH), adrenal hypersecretion, polycythemia, and Cushing syndrome. SCLCs are most often associated with the paraneoplastic syndrome. These conditions may stabilize with treatment of the underlying neoplasm. (These effects of paraneoplastic syndrome are discussed in the section on metabolic emergencies in Chapter 15 on pp. 264.)

## Clinical Manifestations

The clinical manifestations of lung cancer are usually nonspecific and appear late in the disease process. Symptoms may be masked by a chronic cough attributed to smoking or smoking-related lung disease. Manifestations depend on the type of primary lung cancer, its location, and metastatic spread. Lung cancer frequently manifests as a lobar pneumonia that does not respond to treatment.

One of the most common symptoms of lung cancer, and often the one reported first, is a persistent cough. Blood-tinged sputum may be produced because of bleeding caused by the cancer. The patient may complain of dyspnea or wheezing. Chest pain, if present, may be localized or unilateral, ranging from mild to severe.

Later manifestations include nonspecific systemic symptoms such as anorexia, fatigue, weight loss, and nausea and vomiting. Hoarseness may be present as a result of laryngeal nerve involvement. Unilateral paralysis of the diaphragm, dysphagia, and superior vena cava obstruction may occur because of intrathoracic spread of the malignancy. Sometimes there are palpable lymph nodes in the neck or axillae. Mediastinal involvement may lead to pericardial effusion, cardiac tamponade, and dysrhythmias.

## Diagnostic Studies

A chest x-ray is the initial diagnostic test used for patients with suspected lung cancer. The x-ray may initially be normal or identify a lung mass or infiltrate. Evidence of metastasis to the ribs or vertebrae and a pleural effusion may also be seen on chest x-ray. CT scanning is used to further evaluate the lung mass. CT scans can identify the location and extent of masses in the chest, any mediastinal involvement, and lymph node enlargement.

Sputum cytologic studies can identify malignant cells, but sputum samples are rarely used in diagnosing lung cancer because malignant cells are not always present in the sputum. Biopsy is required for a definitive diagnosis. Cells for biopsy can be obtained by CT-guided needle aspiration, bronchoscopy, mediastinoscopy, or video-assisted thoracoscopic surgery (VATS). If a thoracentesis is performed to relieve a pleural effusion, the fluid is also analyzed for malignant cells.

Accurate assessment of lung cancer is critical for staging and determining appropriate treatment. Bone scans and CT scans of the brain, pelvis, and abdomen are used to determine if metastatic disease is present. A complete history and physical examination, CBC with differential, chemistry panel, liver function tests, renal function tests, and pulmonary function tests are necessary. MRI and/or positron emission tomography (PET)

**TABLE 27-16 Interprofessional Care**
***Lung Cancer***

| Diagnostic Assessment | Management |
|---|---|
| • History and physical examination | • Surgery |
| • Chest x-ray | • Radiation therapy |
| • Bronchoscopy | • Chemotherapy |
| • Cytologic study of bronchial washings or pleural space fluid | • Targeted therapy and immunotherapy |
| • CT scan, MRI | • Prophylactic cranial radiation |
| • Positron emission tomography (PET) | • Bronchoscopic laser therapy |
| • Mediastinoscopy | • Photodynamic therapy |
| • Video-assisted thoracoscopic surgery (VATS) | • Airway stenting |
| • Transbronchial or percutaneous fine-needle aspiration | • Radiofrequency ablation |

**TABLE 27-17 Staging of Non–Small Cell Lung Cancer**

| Stages | | Characteristics |
|---|---|---|
| I | | Tumor is small and localized to lung. No lymph node involvement |
| | A | Tumor <3 cm |
| | B | Tumor 3-5 cm and invading surrounding local areas. |
| II | | Increased tumor size, some lymph node involvement |
| | A | Tumor 3-5 cm with invasion of lymph nodes on same side of chest OR<br>Tumor 5-7 cm without lymph node involvement |
| | B | Tumor 5-7 cm involving the bronchus and lymph nodes on same side of chest and tissue of other local organs OR<br>Tumor >7 cm without lymph node involvement |
| III | | Increased spread of tumor |
| | A | Tumor spread to the nearby structures (chest wall, pleura, pericardium) and regional lymph nodes |
| | B | Extensive tumor involving heart, trachea, esophagus, mediastinum, malignant pleural effusion, contralateral lymph nodes, scalene or supraclavicular lymph nodes |
| IV | | Distant metastasis |

may also be used to evaluate and stage lung cancer. Table 27-16 summarizes the diagnostic assessment of lung cancer.

**Staging.** Staging of NSCLC is performed according to the TNM staging system (see Table 15-5). Under the TNM system, the tumor is grouped into four stages with A or B subtypes. A simplified version of staging of NSCLC is presented in Table 27-17. Patients with stages I, II, and IIIA disease may be surgical candidates. However, stage IIIB or IV disease is usually inoperable and has a poor prognosis.

Staging of SCLC by TNM has not been useful because this cancer is aggressive and is always considered systemic. The stages of SCLC are *limited* and *extensive*. *Limited* means that the tumor is confined to one side of the chest and regional lymph nodes. *Extensive* SCLC means that the cancer extends beyond the limited stage. Most patients with SCLC have extensive disease at time of diagnosis.

**Screening for Lung Cancer.** Screening for high-risk patients is recommended by the U.S. Preventive Services Task Force (USPSTF).[26] Recommendations include annual screening for lung cancer in adults ages 55 to 80 with a history of smoking (30-pack year smoking history or currently smoke) or quit smoking but less than 15 years ago. Screening is done using low-dose CT. These guidelines have been endorsed by several other groups, including the American Cancer Society.[27]

## Interprofessional Care

**Surgical Therapy.** Surgical resection is the treatment of choice in NSCLC stages I to IIIA without mediastinal involvement, since resection provides the best chance for a cure. Factors that affect survival include the size of the primary tumor and co-morbidities. For other NSCLC stages, patients may require surgery in conjunction with radiation therapy, chemotherapy, and targeted therapy. Many NSCLCs are not resectable at the time of diagnosis.

Surgical procedures that may be performed include pneumonectomy (removal of one entire lung), lobectomy (removal of one or more lobes of the lung), or segmental or wedge resection procedures. VATS may be used to treat lung cancers near the outside of the lung. Surgery is generally not indicated for SCLC because of its rapid growth and dissemination at the time of diagnosis.

When the tumor is considered operable, the patient's cardiopulmonary status must be evaluated to determine the ability to have surgery. Pulmonary function studies, ABGs, and an anesthesia consult are often completed preoperatively to assess the patient's cardiopulmonary status.

**Radiation Therapy.** Radiation therapy may be used as treatment for both NSCLC and SCLC. Radiation therapy may be given as curative therapy, palliative therapy (to relieve symptoms), or adjuvant therapy in combination with surgery, chemotherapy, or targeted therapy.

Radiation therapy may be used as primary therapy in the individual who is unable to tolerate surgical resection because of co-morbidities. Radiation therapy also relieves symptoms of dyspnea and hemoptysis resulting from bronchial obstructive tumors and treats superior vena cava syndrome. It can also be used to treat pain that is caused by metastatic bone lesions or cerebral metastasis. Sometimes radiation is used preoperatively to reduce the tumor mass before surgical resection. Complications of radiation therapy include esophagitis, skin irritation, nausea and vomiting, anorexia, and radiation pneumonitis (see Chapter 15).

***Stereotactic Body Radiotherapy.*** Stereotactic body radiotherapy (SBRT), also called *stereotactic surgery* or *radiosurgery,* is a new lung cancer treatment. It is a type of radiation therapy that uses high doses of radiation delivered accurately to tumors outside the CNS. SBRT uses special positioning procedures and radiology techniques so that a higher dose of radiation can be delivered to the tumor and only a small part of the healthy lung is exposed. Therapy is given over 1 to 3 days. SBRT provides an option for patients with early stage lung cancers who are not surgical candidates for other medical reasons.

**Chemotherapy.** Chemotherapy is the primary treatment for SCLC. In NSCLC, chemotherapy may be used in the treatment of nonresectable tumors or as adjuvant therapy to surgery. A variety of chemotherapy drugs and multidrug regimens (i.e., protocols) are used. Chemotherapy for lung cancer typically consists of combinations of two or more of the following drugs: etoposide, carboplatin, cisplatin, paclitaxel (Taxol), vinorelbine (Navelbine), cyclophosphamide, ifosfamide (Ifex), docetaxel (Taxotere), gemcitabine (Gemzar), and pemetrexed (Alimta).

**Targeted Therapy.** Targeted therapy uses drugs that block the growth of molecules involved in specific aspects of tumor growth (see Chapter 15). Because this type of therapy inhibits growth rather than directly killing cancer cells, targeted therapy may be less toxic than chemotherapy. One type of targeted therapy for patients with NSCLC inhibits tyrosine kinase, an enzyme associated with speeding up molecular reactions. Tyrosine kinase inhibitors, which block signals for growth in the cancer cells, include cetuximab (Erbitux), erlotinib (Tarceva), afatinib (Gilotrif), gefitinib (Iressa), osimertinib (Tagrisso), and necitumumab (Portrazza).

Another type of kinase inhibitor is used to treat patients with NSCLC who have an abnormal anaplastic lymphoma kinase *(ALK)* gene. Drugs in this class include crizotinib (Xalkori) and ceritinib (Zykadia). These drugs directly inhibit the kinase protein produced by the *ALK* gene that is responsible for cancer development and growth.

Another type of targeted therapy used to treat lung cancer inhibits the growth of new blood vessels (angiogenesis) by targeting vascular endothelial growth factor. Bevacizumab (Avastin) is an angiogenesis inhibitor.

**Immunotherapy.** Nivolumab (Opdivo) and pembrolizumab (Keytruda) are drugs that target PD-1, a protein on T cells that normally helps keep these cells from attacking other cells in the body. By blocking PD-1, these drugs boost the immune response against cancer cells. This can shrink some tumors or slow their growth. Nivolumab and pembrolizumab can be used in people with metastatic NSCLC whose cancer has progressed after other treatments and with tumors that express PD-1.

**Other Therapies**

***Prophylactic Cranial Radiation.*** Patients with SCLC have early metastases, especially to the central nervous system. Most chemotherapy does not penetrate the blood-brain barrier. Therefore after successful systemic treatment, the patient is at risk for cerebral metastases. Prophylactic radiation has been shown to decrease the incidence of cerebral metastases and improve the survival rate in patients with limited SCLC.[28]

***Bronchoscopic Laser Therapy.*** Bronchoscopic laser therapy makes it possible to remove obstructing bronchial lesions. The laser's thermal energy is transmitted to the target tissue. It is a safe and effective treatment of endobronchial obstructions from tumors. Symptoms of airway obstruction are relieved as a result of thermal necrosis and shrinkage of the tumor. The procedure may be repeated as needed.

***Photodynamic Therapy.*** Photodynamic therapy (PDT) is a form of treatment for early stage lung cancers that uses a combination of a drug and a specific type of light. Cancer cells are killed when the drug, known as a photosynthesizer, is exposed to a specific wavelength of light. Porfimer (Photofrin) is the most commonly used photosynthesizer. It is injected IV and selectively concentrates in tumor cells in the esophagus and outer layers of the airways. After a set time (usually 48 hours), the tumor is exposed to laser light via bronchoscopy, activating the drug and causing cell death. Necrotic tissue is removed with bronchoscopy a few days later. This process can also be repeated as required. PDT can also affect nutrient delivery to cancer cells and stimulate the immune system to attack the cancer cells.

***Airway Stenting.*** Stents are used alone or in combination with other techniques for relief of dyspnea, cough, or respiratory insufficiency. The advantage of an airway stent is that it supports the airway wall against collapse or external compression and can delay extension of tumor into the airway lumen.

***Radiofrequency Ablation.*** Radiofrequency ablation therapy is used to treat small NSCLC lung tumors that are near the outer edge of the lungs. This therapy is an alternative to surgery in patients who cannot or elect not to have surgery. A thin, needle-like probe is inserted through the skin into the tumor. CT scans are used to guide placement. An electric current is then passed through the probe, which heats and destroys tumor cells. Local anesthesia is used for this outpatient procedure.

## ❖ NURSING MANAGEMENT: LUNG CANCER

### ◆ Nursing Assessment

It is important to determine the patient and caregiver's understanding of diagnostic tests (those completed as well as those planned), the diagnosis or potential diagnosis, the treatment options, and the prognosis. At the same time, assess the patient's level of anxiety and support provided by the patient's significant others. Subjective and objective data that should be obtained from a patient with lung cancer are presented in Table 27-18.

### ◆ Nursing Diagnoses

Nursing diagnoses for the patient with lung cancer may include, but are not limited to, the following:

- Ineffective airway clearance *related to* increased tracheobronchial secretions and presence of tumor
- Ineffective breathing pattern *related to* decreased lung capacity and presence of space-occupying lesion
- Impaired gas exchange *related to* tumor obstructing airflow
- Anxiety *related to* lack of knowledge of diagnosis or unknown prognosis and treatments
- Grieving *related to* new cancer diagnosis, lack of knowledge about the disease process, and therapeutic regimen

### ◆ Planning

The overall goals are that the patient with lung cancer will have (1) effective breathing patterns, (2) adequate airway clearance, (3) adequate oxygenation of tissues, (4) minimal to no discomfort, and (5) a realistic attitude about treatment and prognosis.

### ◆ Nursing Implementation

◆ **Health Promotion.** The best way to halt the epidemic of lung cancer is to prevent people from smoking, help smokers stop smoking, and decrease exposure to environmental pollutants. Because most smokers start in the teenage years, prevention of teen smoking has the most significant role in reducing the incidence of lung cancer. A wealth of material is available to the smoker who is interested in smoking cessation. (Smoking cessation is discussed in Chapter 10.)

Modeling healthy behavior by not smoking, promoting smoking cessation programs, and actively supporting education and policy changes related to smoking are important nursing activities. Many changes have occurred as a result of the recognition that passive smoke is a health hazard. Laws prohibit smoking in most public places and limit public smoking to designated areas. Most hospital environments are now completely smoke free, prohibiting smoking by employees and patients. A new trend is for hospitals to refuse employment to anyone testing positive for nicotine. This includes not only smokers but also nonsmokers who are routinely exposed to secondhand smoke.

◆ **Acute Care.** Care of the patient with lung cancer initially involves support and reassurance during the diagnostic evaluation. It is important to recognize the multiple stressors that

**TABLE 27-18 Nursing Assessment**
***Lung Cancer***

**Subjective Data**
***Important Health Information***
*Past health history:* Exposure to secondhand smoke, airborne carcinogens (e.g., asbestos, radon, hydrocarbons), or other pollutants. Urban living environment. Chronic lung disease (e.g., TB, COPD, bronchiectasis)
*Medications:* Cough medicines or other respiratory medications

***Functional Health Patterns***
*Health perception–health management:* Smoking history, including amount per day and number of years. Family history of lung cancer. Frequent respiratory tract infections
*Nutritional-metabolic:* Anorexia, nausea, vomiting, dysphagia (late). Weight loss. Chills
*Activity-exercise:* Fatigue. Persistent cough (productive or nonproductive). Dyspnea at rest or with exertion, hemoptysis (late symptom)
*Cognitive-perceptual:* Chest pain or tightness, shoulder and arm pain, headache, bone pain (late symptom)

**Objective Data**
***General***
Fever, neck and axillary lymphadenopathy, paraneoplastic syndrome (e.g., syndrome of inappropriate ADH secretion)

***Integumentary***
Jaundice (liver metastasis). Edema of neck and face (superior vena cava syndrome), digital clubbing

***Respiratory***
Wheezing, hoarseness, stridor, unilateral diaphragm paralysis, pleural effusions (late signs)

***Cardiovascular***
Pericardial effusion, cardiac tamponade, dysrhythmias (late signs)

***Neurologic***
Confusion, disorientation, unsteady gait (brain metastasis)

***Musculoskeletal***
Pathologic fractures, muscle wasting (late)

***Possible Diagnostic Findings***
Observance of lesion on chest x-ray, CT scan, or PET scan. MRI findings of vertebral, spinal cord, or mediastinal invasion. Positive sputum or bronchial washings for cytologic studies. Positive fiberoptic bronchoscopy and biopsy findings

*ADH,* Antidiuretic hormone.

occur when someone is diagnosed with lung cancer. The stress response is a normal and adaptive response but can become detrimental when stress is overwhelming and intense. Patients suffer the stress of their symptoms, including dyspnea and cough. Diagnostic and therapeutic procedures provide additional stress by placing patients in unfamiliar environments with unusual and perhaps painful results. Emotional stressors include the knowledge of the high mortality rate of lung cancer and the causal effect of cigarette smoking. Worries about role performance and ability to care for their family while undergoing cancer treatment provide further stress. Carefully assess each individual, since he or she will experience unique stressors. The insight gained will help the patient and caregiver cope with the stress of the illness and treatment.

Care of the patient undergoing thoracic surgery is discussed later in this chapter on pp. 524-527. Care of the patient undergoing radiation therapy and chemotherapy is discussed in Chapter 15. Individualized care depends on the plan for treatment. Assessment and intervention in symptom management are pivotal, as is teaching the patient to recognize signs and symptoms that may indicate progression or recurrence of disease. Provide patient comfort, teach methods to reduce pain, monitor for side effects of prescribed medications, foster appropriate coping strategies for both the patient and caregiver, assess smoking cessation readiness, and help patient access resources to deal with the illness.

◆ **Ambulatory Care.** Teach signs and symptoms to report, such as hemoptysis, dysphagia, chest pain, and hoarseness.

**CHECK YOUR PRACTICE**

You are doing discharge teaching with a 72-yr-old woman who had a lobectomy for NSCLC. She tells you, "I'm not going to give up smoking my cigarettes because I am just going to die anyhow. I might as well enjoy smoking while I still can."
- How would you respond?

Counseling patients on smoking cessation and prevention is essential in decreasing morbidity and mortality risks associated with lung cancer. Encourage the patient and family to provide a smoke-free environment. This may include smoking cessation for multiple family members. If the treatment plan includes home $O_2$, the teaching plan must include the safe use of $O_2$.

For many individuals who have lung cancer, little can be done to significantly prolong their lives. Radiation therapy and chemotherapy can provide palliative relief from distressing symptoms. Constant pain may become a major problem. (Measures used to relieve pain are discussed in Chapter 8. Care of the patient with cancer is discussed in Chapter 15.) The palliative care team should be involved as the patient and family move toward the end of life (see Chapter 9). The team can provide information about disability, financial planning, and community resources for end-of-life care such as hospice and home care.

## ◆ Evaluation

The expected outcomes are that the patient with lung cancer will
- Have adequate breathing patterns
- Have adequate oxygenation
- Experience minimal to no pain
- Convey feelings openly and honestly, with a realistic attitude about prognosis

## OTHER TYPES OF LUNG TUMORS

SCLC and NSCLC account for 95% of lung tumors. The other 5% include the following:
- *Hamartomas,* the most common benign tumor, is a slow-growing congenital tumor composed of fibrous tissue, fat, and blood vessels.
- *Mucous gland adenoma* is a benign tumor arising in the bronchi that consists of columnar cystic spaces.
- *Mesotheliomas* are either malignant or benign and originate from the visceral pleura. Malignant mesotheliomas are associated with exposure to asbestos. Benign mesotheliomas are localized lesions.

Secondary metastases from other malignancies can occur. Malignant cells from another part of the body reach the lungs via the pulmonary capillaries or the lymphatic network. The primary malignancies that spread to the lungs often originate in the GI or genitourinary tract and in the breast. General symptoms of lung metastases are chest pain and nonproductive cough.

## CHEST TRAUMA AND THORACIC INJURIES

Traumatic injuries to the chest contribute to the majority of all traumatic deaths. Thoracic injuries range from simple rib fractures to complex life-threatening rupture of organs. The mechanisms of injuries causing chest trauma are separated into two categories: blunt trauma and penetrating trauma.

*Blunt trauma* occurs when the chest strikes or is struck by an object. The impact can cause shearing and compression of thoracic structures. The external injury may appear minor, but internally the organs may have severe injuries. Rib and sternal fractures can lacerate lung tissue. In a high-velocity impact, shearing forces can result in laceration or tearing of the aorta. Compression of the chest may result in contusion, crush injury, and organ rupture.

*Penetrating trauma* is an injury in which a foreign object impales or passes through the body tissues, creating an open wound. Examples include knife wounds, gunshot wounds, and injuries with other sharp objects. Emergency care of the patient with a chest injury is presented in Table 27-19. The most common thoracic emergencies and their management are described in Table 27-20.

## PNEUMOTHORAX

A **pneumothorax** is caused by air entering the pleural cavity. Normally, negative (subatmospheric) pressure exists between the visceral pleura (surrounding the lung) and parietal pleura (lining the thoracic cavity), known as the *pleural space.* The pleural space contains a few milliliters of lubricating fluid to reduce friction when the tissues move. When air enters this space, the change to positive pressure causes a partial or complete lung collapse (Fig. 27-4). As the volume of air in the pleural space increases, the lung volume decreases. This condition should be suspected after any trauma to the chest wall.

If a pneumothorax is small, mild tachycardia and dyspnea may be the only manifestations. If the pneumothorax occupies a large area, respiratory distress may be present, including shallow, rapid respirations; dyspnea; air hunger; and $O_2$ desaturation. On auscultation, no breath sounds are detected over the affected area. A chest x-ray shows air or fluid in the pleural space and reduction in lung volume.

### Types of Pneumothorax

**Spontaneous Pneumothorax.** A spontaneous pneumothorax typically occurs due to the rupture of small blebs (air-filled sacs) located on the surface of the lung. These blebs can occur in healthy, young individuals or as a result of lung disease such

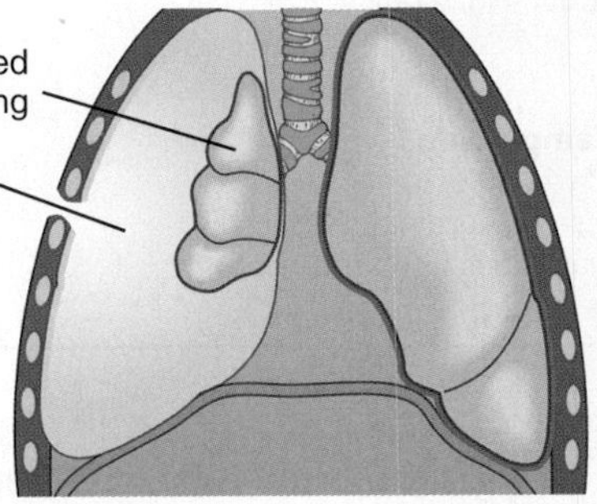


**FIG. 27-4** Open pneumothorax resulting from collapse of lung due to disruption of chest wall and outside air entering.

### TABLE 27-19 Emergency Management

**Chest Trauma**

| Etiology | Assessment Findings | Interventions |
|---|---|---|
| **Blunt**<br>• Motor vehicle accident<br>• Pedestrian accident<br>• Fall<br>• Assault with blunt object<br>• Crush injury<br>• Explosion<br>**Penetrating**<br>• Knife<br>• Gunshot<br>• Stick<br>• Arrow<br>• Other missiles | **Respiratory**<br>• Dyspnea, respiratory distress<br>• Cough with or without hemoptysis<br>• Cyanosis of mouth, face, nail beds, mucous membranes<br>• Tracheal deviation<br>• Audible air escaping from chest wound<br>• Decreased breath sounds on side of injury<br>• Decreased $O_2$ saturation<br>• Frothy secretions<br>**Cardiovascular**<br>• Rapid, thready pulse<br>• Decreased BP<br>• Narrowed pulse pressure<br>• Asymmetric BP values in arms<br>• Distended neck veins<br>• Muffled heart sounds<br>• Chest pain<br>• Dysrhythmias<br>**Surface Findings**<br>• Bruising<br>• Abrasions<br>• Open chest wound<br>• Asymmetric chest movement<br>• Subcutaneous emphysema | **Initial**<br>• If unresponsive, assess circulation, airway, and breathing.<br>• If responsive, monitor airway, breathing, and circulation.<br>• Administer high-flow $O_2$ to keep $SpO_2$ >90%.<br>• Establish IV access with two large-bore catheters. Begin fluid resuscitation as appropriate.<br>• Remove clothing to assess injury.<br>• Cover sucking chest wound with nonporous dressing taped on three sides.<br>• Stabilize impaled objects with bulky dressings. *Do not remove object.*<br>• Assess for other significant injuries and treat appropriately.<br>• Place patient in a semi-Fowler's position if breathing is easier *after* cervical spine injury has been ruled out.<br>• Administer small amounts of analgesia as necessary for pain and to help with breathing.<br>• Prepare for emergency needle decompression if tension pneumothorax or cardiac tamponade present.<br>**Ongoing Monitoring**<br>• Monitor vital signs, level of consciousness, $O_2$ saturation, cardiac rhythm, respiratory status, and urine output.<br>• Anticipate intubation for respiratory distress.<br>• Release dressing if tension pneumothorax develops after sucking chest wound is covered. |

**TABLE 27-20 Emergency Management**

***Thoracic Injuries***

| Injury and Description | Manifestations | Intervention |
|---|---|---|
| **Pneumothorax** Air in pleural space (Fig. 27-4). | Dyspnea, decreased movement of involved chest wall, diminished or absent breath sounds on the affected side, hyperresonance to percussion | Chest tube insertion with chest drainage system. |
| **Hemothorax** Blood in the pleural space, may or may not occur in conjunction with pneumothorax. | Dyspnea, diminished or absent breath sounds, dullness to percussion, decreased Hgb, shock depending on blood volume lost | Chest tube insertion with chest drainage system. Autotransfusion of collected blood, treatment of hypovolemia as necessary. |
| **Tension Pneumothorax** Air in pleural space that does not escape Increased air in the pleural space shifts organs and increases intrathoracic pressure (Fig. 27-5). | Cyanosis, air hunger, extreme agitation, tracheal deviation away from affected side, subcutaneous emphysema, neck vein distention, hyperresonance to percussion | Medical emergency: needle decompression followed by chest tube insertion with chest drainage system. |
| **Flail Chest** Fracture of two or more adjacent ribs in two or more places with loss of chest wall stability (Fig. 27-6). | Paradoxical movement of chest wall, respiratory distress. May be associated hemothorax, pneumothorax, pulmonary contusion | $O_2$ as needed to maintain $O_2$ saturation, analgesia. Stabilize flail segment with positive pressure ventilation (intubation and mechanical ventilation). Treat associated injuries. Surgical fixation. |
| **Cardiac Tamponade** Blood rapidly collects in pericardial sac, compresses myocardium because pericardium does not stretch, and prevents ventricles from filling. | Muffled, distant heart sounds, hypotension, neck vein distention, increased central venous pressure | Medical emergency: pericardiocentesis with surgical repair as appropriate. |

as COPD, asthma, cystic fibrosis, and pneumonia. Smoking increases the risk for bleb formation. Other risk factors include being tall and thin, male gender, family history, and previous spontaneous pneumothorax.

**Iatrogenic Pneumothorax.** *Iatrogenic pneumothorax* can occur due to laceration or puncture of the lung during medical procedures. For example, transthoracic needle aspiration, subclavian catheter insertion, pleural biopsy, and transbronchial lung biopsy all have the potential to injure the lung. Barotrauma from excessive ventilatory pressure during manual or mechanical ventilation can rupture alveoli or bronchioles. Esophageal procedures may also be involved in the development of a pneumothorax. Tearing during insertion of a gastric tube can allow air from the esophagus to enter the mediastinum and pleural space.

**Tension Pneumothorax.** Tension pneumothorax occurs when air enters the pleural space but cannot escape. The continued accumulation of air in the pleural space causes increasingly elevated intrapleural pressures. This results in compression of the lung on the affected side and pressure on the heart and great vessels, pushing them away from the affected side (Fig. 27-5). The mediastinum shifts toward the unaffected side, compressing the "good" lung, which further compromises oxygenation. As the pressure increases, venous return is decreased and cardiac output falls.

Tension pneumothorax may result from either an open or a closed pneumothorax. In an open chest wound, a flap may act as a one-way valve. Thus air can enter on inspiration but cannot escape. Tension pneumothorax can occur with mechanical ventilation and resuscitative efforts. It can also occur if chest tubes are clamped or become blocked in a patient with a pneumothorax. Unclamping the tube or relieving the obstruction may correct this situation.

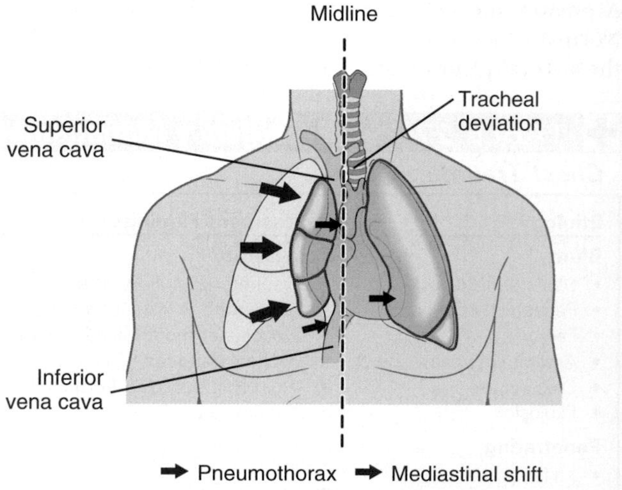


**FIG. 27-5** Tension pneumothorax. As pleural pressure on the affected side increases, mediastinal displacement ensues with resultant respiratory and cardiovascular compromise. Tracheal deviation is an external (but late) manifestation of the mediastinal shift.

Tension pneumothorax is a medical emergency, with both the respiratory and cardiovascular systems affected. Manifestations include dyspnea, marked tachycardia, tracheal deviation, decreased or absent breath sounds on the affected side, neck vein distention, cyanosis, and profuse diaphoresis. If the tension in the pleural space is not relieved, the patient is likely to die from inadequate cardiac output or severe hypoxemia.

**Hemothorax.** Hemothorax is an accumulation of blood in the pleural space resulting from injury to the chest wall, diaphragm, lung, blood vessels, or mediastinum.[29] When it occurs with pneumothorax, it is called a *hemopneumothorax*. The patient with a traumatic hemothorax requires immediate insertion of a chest tube for evacuation of the blood, which can be recovered and reinfused for a short time after the injury. (Autotransfusion is discussed in Chapter 30.)

**Chylothorax.** *Chylothorax* is the presence of lymphatic fluid in the pleural space. The thoracic duct is disrupted either traumatically or from a malignancy, and the lymphatic fluid fills the pleural space.[30] This milky white fluid is high in lipids. Normal lymphatic flow through the thoracic duct is 1500 to 2500 mL/day. This amount can be increased up to tenfold after ingestion of fats. Some cases heal with conservative treatment (chest drainage, bowel rest, and dietary modifications). Octreotide has been used with some success to reduce the flow of lymphatic fluid. Surgery (thoracic duct ligation) and pleurodesis (the artificial production of adhesions between the parietal and visceral pleura) may be considered for refractory cases.

### Interprofessional Care

Treatment of a pneumothorax depends on its severity and the underlying cause. If the patient is stable and has minimal air and/or fluid accumulated in the intrapleural space, no treatment may be necessary, since the condition may resolve spontaneously.

Pneumothorax can be classified as *open* (air entering through an opening in the chest wall) or *closed* (no external wound). Penetrating trauma allows air to enter the pleural space through an opening in the chest wall (Fig. 27-4). Examples include stab or gunshot wounds and surgical thoracotomy. A penetrating chest wound may be referred to as a *sucking chest wound,* since air enters the pleural space through the chest wall during inspiration.

Emergency treatment consists of covering the wound with an occlusive dressing that is secured on three sides (vent dressing). During inspiration, as negative pressure is created in the chest, the dressing pulls against the wound, preventing air from entering the pleural space. During expiration, as the pressure rises in the pleural space, the dressing is pushed out and air escapes through the wound and from under the dressing. If the object that caused the open chest wound is still in place, do not remove it until an HCP is present. Stabilize the impaled object with a bulky dressing.

The most definitive and common treatment of pneumothorax and hemothorax is to insert a chest tube and connect it to water-seal drainage. Repeated spontaneous pneumothorax may have to be treated surgically by a partial pleurectomy, stapling, or pleurodesis to promote adherence of the pleurae to one another. Tension pneumothorax is a medical emergency, requiring urgent needle decompression followed by chest tube insertion to water-seal drainage.

## FRACTURED RIBS

Rib fractures are the most common type of chest injury resulting from blunt trauma. Ribs 5 through 9 are most frequently fractured because they are the least protected by chest muscles. If the fractured rib is splintered or displaced, it may damage the pleura, lungs, and other internal organs.

Clinical manifestations of fractured ribs include pain at the site of injury, especially during inspiration and with coughing. The patient splints the affected area and takes shallow breaths to try to decrease the pain. Atelectasis and pneumonia may develop because of decreased chest wall movement and retained secretions.

The goal of treatment is to decrease pain so that the patient can breathe adequately and clear secretions. Strapping the chest with tape or using a thoracic binder is not recommended, since it limits chest expansion and predisposes the individual to atelectasis. Nonsteroidal antiinflammatory drugs (NSAIDs), opioids, and thoracic nerve blocks can be used to reduce pain and aid with deep breathing and coughing. Patient teaching should emphasize deep breathing, coughing, incentive spirometry, and appropriate use of pain medications.

## FLAIL CHEST

**Flail chest** results from the fracture of several consecutive ribs, in two or more separate places, causing an unstable segment (Fig. 27-6). It can also be caused by fracture of the sternum and several consecutive ribs. The resultant instability of the chest wall causes paradoxical movement during breathing. The affected (flail) area moves in the opposite direction with respect to the intact portion of the chest. During inspiration, the affected portion is sucked in, and during expiration, it bulges out. This paradoxical chest movement not only prevents adequate ventilation but also increases the work of breathing. The underlying lung may have a pulmonary contusion aggravating hypoxemia.

A flail chest is usually apparent on visual examination. The patient manifests rapid, shallow respirations and tachycardia. The patient moves air poorly, and movement of the thorax is asymmetric and uncoordinated. The patient may

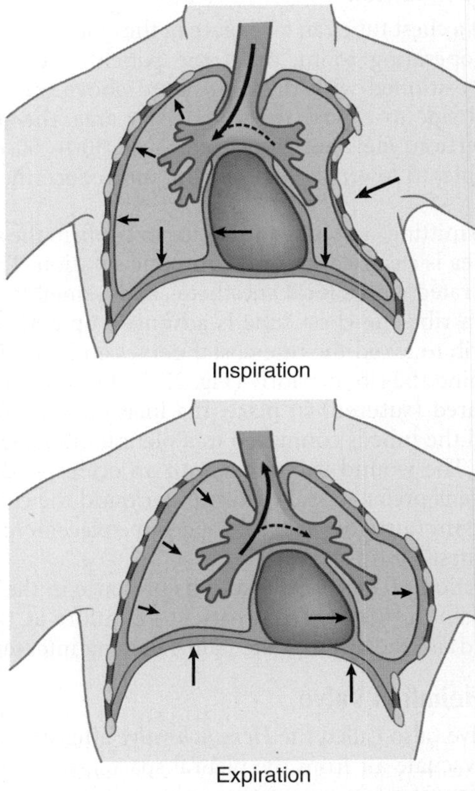


FIG. 27-6 Flail chest produces paradoxical respiration. On inspiration, the flail section moves inward with mediastinal shift to the uninjured side. On expiration, the flail section bulges outward with mediastinal shift to the injured side.

also attempt to splint the chest to assist with breathing. Observation of abnormal thoracic cavity movement, palpation for crepitus near the rib fractures, and chest x-ray all assist in the diagnosis.

Initial therapy consists of ensuring adequate ventilation and supplemental $O_2$ therapy. The goal is to facilitate lung expansion and ensure adequate oxygenation. Analgesia is necessary to help promote adequate respiration. Although many patients can be managed without mechanical ventilation, intubation and ventilation may be necessary. Surgical fixation of the flail segment may be done. The lung parenchyma and fractured ribs heal with time. Some patients continue to experience intercostal pain after the flail chest has resolved.

## CHEST TUBES AND PLEURAL DRAINAGE

If enough fluid or air accumulates in the pleural space, the negative pressure becomes positive and the lungs collapse. As a result, chest tubes are inserted to drain the pleural space, reestablish negative pressure, and allow for proper lung expansion. Tubes may also be inserted in the mediastinal space to drain air and fluid postoperatively.

Chest tubes are approximately 20 inches (51 cm) long and vary in size from 12F to 40F. The size inserted is determined by the patient's condition. Large (36F to 40F) tubes are used to drain blood, medium (24F to 36F) tubes are used to drain fluid, and small (12F to 24F) tubes are used to drain air. Pigtail tubes are very small (10F to 14F) tubes with a curly end designed to keep them in place. They are a safe and effective alternative to larger-bore chest tubes for treatment of pneumothorax.

### Chest Tube Insertion

Insertion of a chest tube can take place in the emergency department, the operating room, or at the patient's bedside. The patient is positioned with the arm raised above the head on the affected side to expose the midaxillary area, the standard site for insertion. Elevate the patient's head 30 to 60 degrees, when possible, to lower the diaphragm and reduce the risk of injury.

Time permitting, a chest x-ray is used to confirm the affected side. The area is cleansed with an antiseptic solution. The chest wall is infiltrated with a local anesthetic, and a small incision is made over a rib. The chest tube is advanced up and over the top of the rib to avoid the intercostal nerves and blood vessels that are behind the rib inferiorly (Fig. 27-7). Once inserted, the tube is secured (sutured) in place, the incision is closed with sutures, and the tube is connected to a pleural drainage system (Fig. 27-8). The wound is covered with an occlusive dressing. Most clinicians prefer to seal the wound around the chest tube with petroleum (airtight) gauze. Proper tube placement is confirmed by chest x-ray.

The insertion of a chest tube and its presence in the pleural space are painful. Monitor the patient's comfort at frequent intervals and use the appropriate pain-relieving interventions.

### Flutter or Heimlich Valve

A flutter valve (also called the *Heimlich valve* after its inventor) is used to evacuate air from the pleural space (Fig. 27-9). This device consists of a one-way rubber valve within a rigid plastic tube. It is attached to the external end of the chest tube. During inspiration, when pressure in the chest is greater than atmospheric pressure, the valve opens. During expiration, when intrathoracic pressure is less than atmospheric pressure, the valve closes.

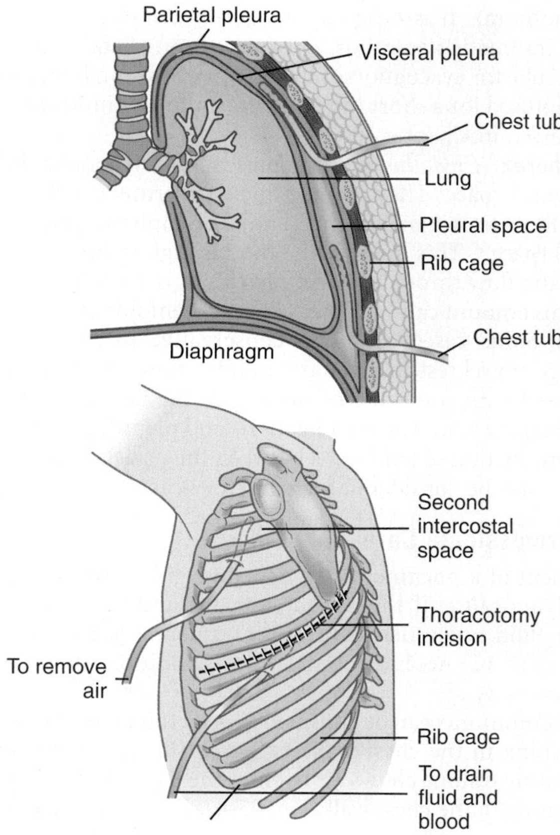


**FIG. 27-7** Placement of chest tubes.

The flutter valve can be used for small to moderate-sized pneumothorax. It also allows for patient mobility, since the smaller drainage bag can be hidden under the clothes while the patient ambulates. Drainage bags attached to the flutter valve must have a vent to the atmosphere to prevent a potential tension pneumothorax. This can be accomplished by simply cutting a small slit in the top of any drainage bag that does not have a built-in vent. Patients may go home with a flutter valve in place.

### Pleural Drainage

Insertion of a chest tube often requires attachment to a drainage device or chamber to collect fluid, air, and/or blood from the thoracic cavity. Several different disposable chest drainage units are currently available, but common to all drainage units are three basic compartments (Fig. 27-8).

The *first compartment,* or collection chamber, receives fluid and air from the pleural or mediastinal space. The drained fluid stays in this chamber while expelled air vents to the second compartment. The *second compartment,* the water-seal chamber, contains 2 cm of water, which acts as a one-way valve. Incoming air enters from the collection chamber and bubbles up through the water. The water prevents backflow of air into the patient. Brisk bubbling of air often occurs in this chamber when a pneumothorax is initially evacuated. Intermittent bubbling during exhalation, coughing, or sneezing (when the patient's intrathoracic pressure is increased) may be observed as long as there is air in the pleural space. Eventually, as the air leak resolves and the lung becomes more fully expanded, bubbling ceases.

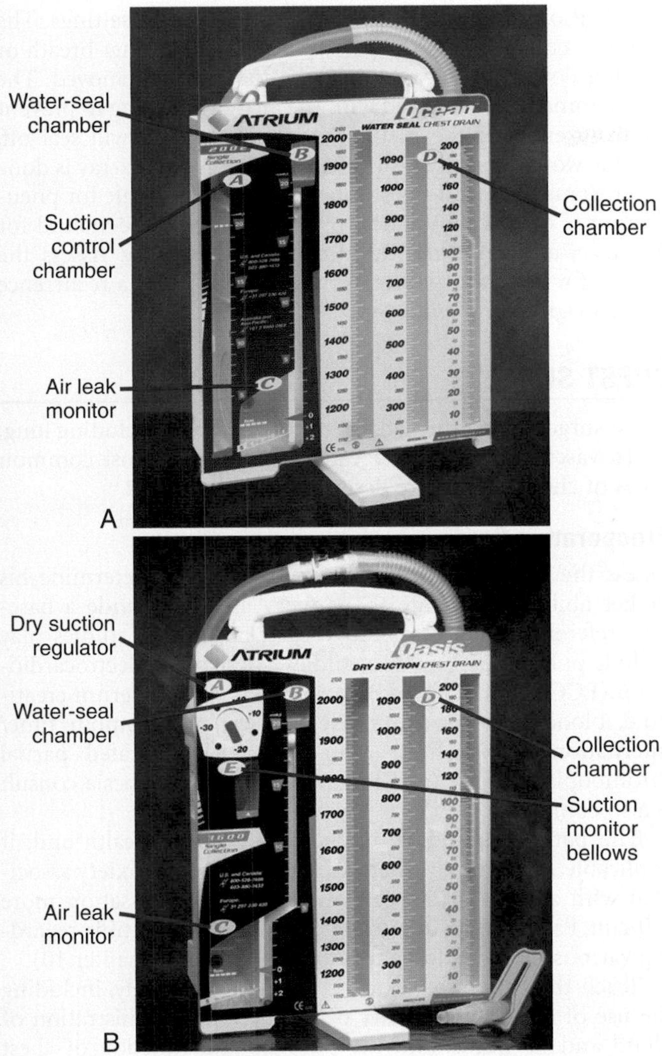


**FIG. 27-8** Chest drainage unit. Both units have three chambers: (1) collection chamber; (2) water-seal chamber; and (3) suction control chamber. Suction control chamber requires a connection to a wall suction source that is dialed up higher than the prescribed suction for the suction to work. **A,** Water suction. This unit uses water in the suction control chamber to control the wall suction pressure. **B,** Dry suction. This unit controls wall suction by using a regulator control dial. (From Atrium Medical Corporation, Hudson, N.H.)

Normal fluctuation of the water within the water-seal chamber is called *tidaling*. This up and down movement of water in concert with respiration reflects intrapleural pressure changes during inspiration and expiration. Investigate any sudden cessation of tidaling, since this may signify an occluded chest tube. Gradual reduction and eventual cessation of tidaling are expected as the lung reexpands.

The *third compartment,* the suction control chamber, applies suction to the chest drainage system. There are two main types of suction control: water and dry. The water suction control chamber uses a column of water to control the amount of suction from the wall regulator. The chamber is typically filled with 20 cm of water. When the negative pressure generated by the suction source exceeds the set 20 cm, air from the atmosphere enters the chamber through a vent on top of the chest drainage unit and the air bubbles up through the water, causing a suction-breaker effect. As a result, excess pressure is relieved.

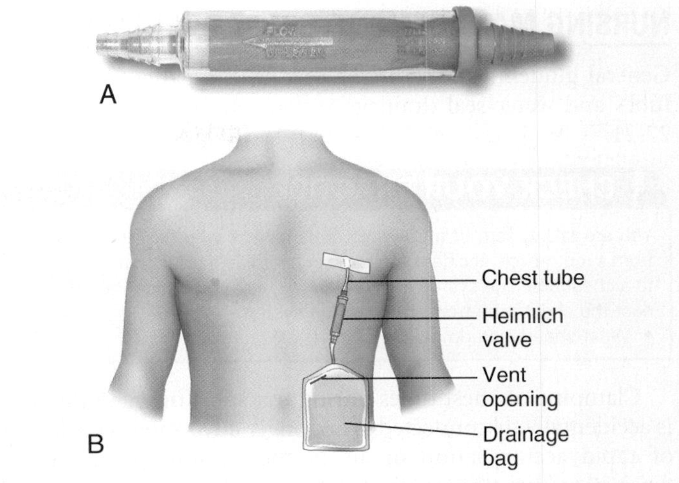


**FIG. 27-9** **A,** Heimlich chest drain valve is a specially designed flutter valve that is used in place of a chest drainage unit for small uncomplicated pneumothorax with little or no drainage and no need for suction. The valve allows for escape of air but prevents the reentry of air into the pleural space. (*A,* Courtesy and © Copyright Becton, Dickinson and Company.) **B,** Placement of valve between chest tube and vented drainage bag, which can be worn under a person's clothes.

The amount of suction applied is regulated by the amount of water in this chamber and not by the amount of suction applied to the system. An increase in suction does not result in an increase in negative pressure to the system because any excess suction merely draws in air through the vent on top of the third chamber. The suction pressure is usually ordered to be −20 cm $H_2O$, although higher pressures (−40 cm $H_2O$) are sometimes necessary to evacuate the pleural space; lower pressure (−10 cm $H_2O$) may be used for frail and older patients at risk for tissue damage with higher pressures.

To initiate suction, adjust (increase) the vacuum source until gentle bubbling is present in the third chamber. Excessive bubbling does not increase the amount of suction but does increase the rate of evaporation of the water and the amount of noise made by the device.

The dry suction chest drainage system contains no water. It has a visual alert that indicates if the suction is working. It uses either a restrictive device or a regulator to dial the desired negative pressure; this is internal in the chest drainage system. To increase the suction pressures, turn the dial on the drainage system. Increasing the vacuum source does not increase the pressure. When decreasing suction, depress the manual vent to reduce excess vacuum to the lower prescribed level.

A variety of commercially disposable plastic chest drainage systems are available. Manufacturers include directions for set-up and use with each unit. Atrium Medical Corporation offers online educational videos of the principles of chest drainage and products at *www.atriummed.com/Products/Chest_Drains/education.asp.*

## INFORMATICS IN PRACTICE

### *Chest Drainage System*

- You find yourself in a situation in which you need to set up a chest drainage system. You have not done this since simulation lab in nursing school.
- On the Internet, find a procedure manual or watch a video or podcast on this procedure.

## NURSING MANAGEMENT: CHEST DRAINAGE

General guidelines for nursing care of the patient with chest tubes and water-seal drainage systems are presented in Table 27-21.

**CHECK YOUR PRACTICE**

You are taking care of a 26-yr-old male patient who has chest injuries from a motorcycle accident. He has a chest tube in place that is attached to a chest drainage system. While turning him, you accidentally disconnect the chest tube from the drainage system.

- What should you do next?

Clamping of chest tubes during transport or when the tube is accidentally disconnected is no longer advocated. The danger of rapid accumulation of air in the pleural space, causing tension pneumothorax, is far greater than that of a small amount of atmospheric air that enters the pleural space. If a chest tube becomes disconnected, the immediate priority is to reestablish the water-seal system. In some hospitals, when disconnection occurs, the chest tube is immersed in sterile water (about 2 cm) until the system can be reestablished. It is important to know the unit protocol, individual clinical situation (whether an air leak exists), and HCP preference before any chest tube clamping occurs.

Chest tubes may be momentarily clamped to change the drainage apparatus or to check for air leaks. Appearance of a new air leak warrants assessment of the drainage system to identify whether the air leak is coming from the patient or the system. Once again, you are encouraged to become familiar with the policies and procedures of their workplace regarding specific clinical situations and circumstances when chest tubes may be clamped.

Closely monitor the patient for complications associated with chest tube placement and drainage. If volumes from 1 to 1.5 L of fluid and/or blood are removed rapidly, reexpansion pulmonary edema or severe, symptomatic hypotension can occur. Subcutaneous emphysema can occur from air leaking into the tissue surrounding the chest tube insertion site. A "crackling" sensation will be felt when palpating the skin. A small amount of subcutaneous air is harmless and will be reabsorbed. However, severe subcutaneous emphysema can cause drastic swelling of the head and neck with potential airway compromise.

Meticulous sterile technique during dressing changes can reduce the incidence of infected sites. Nursing care and patient teaching can minimize the risk of atelectasis and shoulder stiffness. Encourage coughing, deep breathing, incentive spirometer use, and range-of-motion exercises. Monitor integrity of the chest tube system. Monitor the color and amount of drainage hourly in the first few hours post-chest tube insertion. Drainage greater than 200 mL in the first hour, development of subcutaneous emphysema, or any signs and symptoms of respiratory distress should be reported to the appropriate HCP at once.

### Chest Tube Removal

The chest tubes are removed when the lungs are reexpanded and fluid drainage has ceased or is minimal. In some centers, suction is discontinued and the chest drain is on gravity drainage for 24 hours before the tube is removed. Give the patient pain medication about 30 to 60 minutes before tube removal.

Gather dressing supplies and petroleum jelly dressing. Explain the procedure to the patient. The tube is removed by the HCP or an advanced practice nurse in most settings. The suture is cut, and with the patient holding his or her breath or bearing down (Valsalva maneuver), the tube is removed. The site is immediately covered with the airtight dressing to prevent air from entering the pleural space. The pleura will seal off, and the wound usually heals in a few days. A chest x-ray is done 30 to 60 minutes post-chest tube removal to evaluate for pneumothorax or reaccumulation of fluid. Observe the wound for drainage, and reinforce the dressing if necessary. Assess the patient for respiratory distress, which may signify a recurrence of the original problem.

## CHEST SURGERY

Chest surgery is performed for various reasons, including lung, heart, vascular, and esophageal disorders. The most common types of chest surgery are described in Table 27-22.

### Preoperative Care

Assess the patient's cardiopulmonary status to determine his or her ability to tolerate the surgery and to provide a baseline reference for postoperative care. Diagnostic studies may include pulmonary function studies, chest x-ray, electrocardiogram (ECG), ABGs, blood urea nitrogen (BUN), serum creatinine, blood glucose, serum electrolytes, prothrombin time/international normalized ratio (PT/INR), activated partial thromboplastin time (aPTT), and CBC. An anesthesia consult is also completed.

The patient should be in the best possible health and, if applicable, stop smoking before elective surgery. Anxiety associated with anticipated surgery makes smoking cessation more difficult. Provide encouragement, support, and teaching regarding various methods to help stop smoking (see Chapter 10).

Teach the patient what to expect postoperatively, including the use of $O_2$, the possibility of intubation, administration of blood and IV fluids, and the purpose and function of chest tubes. Reassure the patient that adequate medication will be used to reduce pain. Explain how to use patient-controlled analgesia (PCA), if planned. Preoperative teaching should always include exercises for effective deep breathing and use of incentive spirometry. If the patient practices these techniques before surgery, they will be easier to perform postoperatively. Show the patient how to splint the incision with a pillow to facilitate deep breathing. Teach and have the patient provide a return demonstration of range-of-motion exercises on the surgical side (similar to those for the mastectomy patient [see Fig. 51-9]).

The thought of losing part of a vital organ is frequently frightening. Reassure the patient that the lungs have a large degree of functional reserve. Even after the removal of one lung, enough lung tissue is left to maintain adequate oxygenation. Be available to answer the patient and caregiver's questions. Answer questions openly and honestly. Try to facilitate the expression of concerns, feelings, and questions. (General preoperative care and teaching are discussed in Chapter 17.)

### Surgical Procedures

**Thoracotomy.** A thoracotomy is a surgical incision into the chest to gain access to the heart, lungs, esophagus, thoracic aorta, or anterior spine. Two common approaches to a thoracotomy are the median sternotomy and lateral thoracotomy. The median sternotomy involves splitting the sternum and is primarily used for surgery involving the heart. The lateral

## TABLE 27-21 Chest Tubes and Water-Seal Drainage

### Set-Up and Insertion

1. Make sure patient is aware of the procedure and informed consent is obtained.
2. Gather equipment.
   - Thoracotomy tray
   - Chest drainage unit (CDU)
   - Chest tube
   - Bottle of sterile water
   - 1% lidocaine
   - Suction tubing and collection container
   - Occlusive dressing
3. Prepare CDU.
   - *Wet suction:* add sterile water to 2-cm mark in water-seal chamber and to 20-cm mark (or as ordered) in suction control chamber.
   - *Dry suction:* add sterile water to the fill line of the air leak meter. Attach suction tubing and increase suction until the bellows-like float moves across the display window.
4. Position and support the patient to minimize movement during procedure.

### Drainage System

1. Keep all tubing loosely coiled below chest level. Tubing should drop straight from bed or chair to drainage unit. Do not let it be compressed.
2. Keep all connections between chest tubes, drainage tubing, and the drainage collector tight, and tape at connections.
3. Observe for air fluctuations (tidaling) and bubbling in the water-seal chamber.
   - If tidaling (rising with inspiration and falling with expiration in the spontaneously breathing patient) is not observed, the drainage system is blocked, the lungs are reexpanded, or the system is attached to suction.
   - If bubbling increases, there may be an air leak in the drainage system or a leak from the patient (bronchopleural leak).
4. If the chest tube is connected to suction, disconnect from wall suction to check for tidaling.
5. Suspect a system leak when bubbling is continuous.
   - Retape tubing connections.
   - Ensure that dressing is air occlusive.
   - If leak persists, briefly clamp the chest tube at the patient's chest. If the leak stops, then the air is coming from the patient.*
   - If the air leak persists, briefly and methodically move the clamps down the tubing away from the patient until the air leak stops. The leak will then be present between the last two clamp points. If the air leak persists all the way to the drainage unit, replace the unit.*
6. High fluid levels in the water seal indicate residual negative pressure.
   - The chest system may have to be vented by using the high-negativity release valve available on the drainage system to release residual pressure from the system.
   - Do not lower water-seal column when wall suction is not operating or when patient is on gravity drainage.

### Patient's Clinical Status

1. Monitor the patient's clinical status. Assess vital signs, lung sounds, and pain.
2. Assess for manifestations of reaccumulation of air and fluid in the chest (↓ or absent breath sounds), significant bleeding (>100 mL/hr), chest drainage site infection (drainage, erythema, fever, ↑ WBC), or poor wound healing. Notify HCP for management plan.
3. Evaluate for subcutaneous emphysema at chest tube site.
4. Encourage the patient to breathe deeply periodically to facilitate lung expansion and encourage range-of-motion exercises to the shoulder on the affected side. Encourage use of incentive spirometry every hour while awake to prevent atelectasis or pneumonia.

### Chest Drainage

1. Never elevate the drainage system to the level of the patient's chest because this will cause fluid to drain back into the lungs. Secure the unit to the drainage stand. Change the unit if the collection chamber is full. Do not try to empty it.
2. Mark the time of measurement and the fluid level on the drainage unit according to the unit standards. Report any change in the quantity or characteristics of drainage (e.g., clear yellow to bloody) to the HCP and record the change. Notify HCP if >100 mL/hr drainage.
3. Check the position of the chest drainage container. If the drainage system is overturned and the water seal is disrupted, return it to an upright position and encourage the patient to take a few deep breaths, followed by forced exhalations and cough maneuvers.
4. If the drainage system breaks, place the distal end of the chest tubing connection in a sterile water container at a 2-cm level as an emergency water seal.
5. Milking or stripping chest tubes is no longer recommended, since these practices can dangerously increase intrapleural pressures and damage lung tissues. Position tubing so that drainage flows freely to negate need for milking or stripping.

### Monitoring Wet Vs. Dry Suction Chest Drainage Systems

***Suction Control Chamber in Wet Suction System***

1. Keep the suction control chamber at the appropriate water level by adding sterile water as needed to replace water lost to evaporation.
2. Keep the cover over the suction control chamber in place to prevent more rapid evaporation of water and to decrease the noise of the bubbling.
3. After filling the suction control chamber to the ordered suction amount (generally 20 cm $H_2O$ suction), connect the suction tubing to the wall suction.
4. Dial the wall suction regulator until continuous gentle bubbling is seen in the suction control chamber (generally 80-120 mm Hg). Vigorous bubbling is not necessary and will increase the rate of evaporation.
5. If no bubbling is seen in the suction control chamber, (1) there is no suction, (2) suction is not high enough, or (3) the pleural air leak is so large that suction is not high enough to evacuate it.

***Suction Control Chamber in Dry Suction System***
*(see manufacturer's directions)*

1. After connecting patient to system, turn the dial on the chest drainage system to amount ordered (generally −20 cm $H_2O$ pressure), connect suction tubing to wall suction source, and increase the suction until the float appears in the window of the CDU.
2. If ordered to decrease suction, turn the dial down, depress the high-negativity vent, and assess for a rise in the water level of the water-seal chamber.

### Chest Tube Dressings

1. Change dressing according to unit protocol and HCP preference.
2. Remove old dressing carefully. Assess the site for any evidence of inflammation or infection and culture site as indicated.
3. Cleanse the site according to protocol, maintaining strict sterile asepsis.
4. Redress with occlusive dressing. Some HCPs prefer the use of petroleum gauze dressing around the tube to prevent air leak. Date the dressing and document dressing change.

*As per institutional policy and procedures.

**TABLE 27-22 Chest Surgeries**

| Type | Description | Indications |
|---|---|---|
| **Lobectomy**<br>Removal of one lobe of lung | • Most common lung surgery<br>• Need chest tubes postoperatively<br>• Lung tissue expands to fill up space left by resected lobe | Lung cancer, bronchiectasis, TB, emphysematous bullae, benign lung tumors, fungal infections |
| **Pneumonectomy**<br>Removal of entire lung | • Done only when lobectomy or segmental resection will not remove all diseased lung<br>• May have chest tube postoperatively<br>• Fluid will gradually fill space where lung has been removed<br>• Position patient on operative side to facilitate expansion of remaining lung | Lung cancer (most common) |
| **Segmental Resection**<br>Removal of one or more lung segments | • Done to remove bronchovascular lung segment<br>• Need chest tubes postoperatively<br>• Remaining lung tissue expands to fill space<br>• Indicated for a patient unable to handle more extensive surgery | Lung cancer, bronchiectasis |
| **Wedge Resection**<br>Removal of small, localized lesion that occupies only part of a segment | • Most conservative approach<br>• Need chest tubes postoperatively<br>• Done to remove small peripheral nodules or for patients unable to handle more extensive surgery | Lung biopsy, excision of small nodules |
| **Decortication**<br>Removal or stripping of thick, fibrous membrane from visceral pleura | • Need chest tubes postoperatively | Empyema or other inflammatory process unresponsive to conservative management |
| **Exploratory Thoracotomy**<br>Incision into thorax to look for injured or bleeding tissues | • Need chest tubes postoperatively | Chest trauma |
| **Thoracotomy (Not Involving Lungs)**<br>Incision into thorax for surgery on other organs | • Postoperative care related to thoracotomy and primary reason for surgical procedure<br>• Need chest tubes postoperatively | Hiatal hernia repair, open heart surgery, esophageal surgery, tracheal resection, thoracic aorta repair |
| **Video-Assisted Thoracoscopic Surgery (VATS)**<br>Video-assisted technique with a rigid scope with a distal lens inserted into pleura and image shown on a monitor screen | • Allows surgeon to manipulate instruments passed into pleural space through separate small intercostal incisions<br>• VATS done under general anesthesia in operating room<br>• May require chest tube postoperatively | Procedures performed using VATS include lung biopsy, lobectomy, resection of nodules, repair of fistulas |
| **Lung Volume Reduction Surgery (LVRS)**<br>**Open surgical procedure** | • Involves reducing lung volume by multiple wedge excisions or VATS<br>• Removes most diseased lung tissue | Advanced bullous emphysema, $\alpha_1$-antitrypsin emphysema |
| **Bronchoscopic procedure** | • Used to place one-way valves in airways leading to the diseased parts of the lung<br>• Valves let air out, but not in, thus collapsing a certain segment of lungs | |

thoracotomy incision can be done using a posterolateral or anterolateral incision. The *posterolateral incision* is used for most surgeries involving the lung. The incision is made from front to back at the level of the fourth, fifth, or sixth intercostal space. Strong mechanical retractors are used to separate the ribs and gain access to the lung. The *anterolateral incision* is made in the fourth or fifth intercostal space from the sternal border to the midaxillary line. This procedure is commonly used for surgery or trauma victims, mediastinal operations, and wedge resections of the upper and middle lobes of the lung.

**Video-Assisted Thoracic Surgery.** *Video-assisted thoracoscopic surgery* (VATS) is a widely used, minimally invasive surgical approach. It provides a real-time two-dimensional video image of the inside of the chest cavity. It is used for diagnosis and treatment of diseases of the pleura, pulmonary masses and nodules, mediastinal masses, and interstitial lung disease. Through incisions just large enough to insert the instruments, the surgeon can inspect the chest cavity, biopsy suspicious areas, obtain samples of fluids for analysis, and remove tissue. VATS is increasingly being used for patients with thoracic trauma. The surgeon can examine, diagnose, and manage intrathoracic injuries in both blunt and penetrating trauma, including injuries to the diaphragm. A chest tube is placed in the pleural space through one or more of the incisions at the end of the procedure, secured with sutures, and connected to a drainage unit in the usual manner.

The advantages of VATS include less discomfort, faster return to normal activity level, reduced length of hospital stay, lower postoperative morbidity risk, and fewer complications.[31] Patients who have marginal respiratory reserve or are too debilitated to tolerate an open thoracotomy approach may benefit from the VATS procedure.

#### Postoperative Care

The thoracotomy incision is the most painful surgical incision for patients and one of the most difficult for medical-surgical nurses to manage. Postoperative pain after a thoracotomy is typically intense because respiratory muscles are cut during surgery. For most chest surgeries, chest tubes are placed in the pleural space to allow for lung reexpansion. In a pneumonectomy, chest tubes may or may not be placed in the space from which the lung was removed. Adequate pain management is a priority to prevent respiratory compromise. The use of PCA, epidural infusions, and intercostal nerve blocks enables patients to breathe deeply, cough, and move the arm and shoulder on the operative side.

Nursing care priorities in the postoperative period include assessment of respiratory function, including observation of respiratory rate and effort, sputum volume and color, breath sounds, and chest tube function and drainage. Daily chest x-rays are often ordered. Assessment of pain, monitoring of temperature, and observation of the surgical site are similar to care provided for other postoperative patients (see Chapter 19). Care after thoracotomy is presented in eNursing Care Plan 27-2 (available on the website for this chapter).

## RESTRICTIVE RESPIRATORY DISORDERS

Disorders that impair the ability of the chest wall and diaphragm to move with respiration are called *restrictive respiratory disorders.* There are two categories: *extrapulmonary conditions,* in which the lung tissue is normal, and *intrapulmonary conditions,* in which the cause is the lung or pleura. Examples of extrapulmonary conditions that alter respirations are listed in Table 27-23. These disorders are further described in their respective chapters.

Examples of intrapulmonary causes are listed in Table 27-24. Lung damage can be caused by inflammation and scarring of lung tissue (interstitial lung disease), air spaces (pneumonitis), or pleura (empyema).

Pulmonary function tests are the best means of differentiating between restrictive and obstructive respiratory disorders. The hallmark characteristic of a restrictive lung disorder is a reduced total lung capacity (TLC), whereas the hallmark characteristic of an obstructive disorder is reduced forced expiratory volume ($FEV_1$). Mixed obstructive and restrictive disorders sometimes occur together. For example, a patient may have both asthma (an obstructive problem) and pulmonary fibrosis (a restrictive problem).

**TABLE 27-23 Extrapulmonary Causes of Restrictive Lung Disease**

| Central Nervous System | Chest Wall |
|---|---|
| • Head injury, CNS lesion (e.g., tumor, stroke)<br>• Opioid and barbiturate use | • Chest wall trauma (e.g., flail chest, fractured rib)<br>• Obesity-hypoventilation syndrome (Pickwickian syndrome)<br>• Kyphoscoliosis |
| **Neuromuscular System** | |
| • Spinal cord injury<br>• Guillain-Barré syndrome<br>• Amyotrophic lateral sclerosis<br>• Myasthenia gravis<br>• Muscular dystrophy | |

## PLEURAL EFFUSION

### Types

The pleural space normally contains 5 to 15 mL of fluid that acts as a lubricant between the chest wall (parietal pleura) and lungs (visceral pleura). **Pleural effusion** is an abnormal collection of fluid in this space. It is not a disease but rather an indication of disease. A balance between hydrostatic pressure, oncotic pressure, and capillary membrane permeability governs movement of fluid in and out of the pleural space. Fluid accumulation can be a result of increased pulmonary capillary pressure, decreased oncotic pressure, increased pleural membrane permeability, or obstruction of lymphatic flow.

Pleural effusion is classified as transudative or exudative according to the protein content. A *transudate* occurs primarily in noninflammatory conditions and is an accumulation of protein-poor, cell-poor fluid. Transudative pleural effusions are clear, pale yellow, and caused by (1) increased hydrostatic pressure found in heart failure or (2) decreased oncotic pressure (from hypoalbuminemia) found in chronic liver or renal disease. An *exudative effusion* results from increased capillary permeability characteristic of an inflammatory reaction. It is most commonly associated with infections and malignancies.

An **empyema** is the collection of purulent fluid in the pleural space. It is caused by conditions such as pneumonia, TB, lung abscess, and infection of surgical wounds of the chest. Therapeutic treatment options for empyema include appropriate antibiotic therapy (necessary to eradicate the causative organism), percutaneous drainage, tube thoracostomy, VATS, intrapleural fibrinolytic therapy (instilled via the chest tube) to dissolve fibrous adhesions, decortication, and open window thoracostomy.

### Clinical Manifestations

Common clinical manifestations of pleural effusion are dyspnea; cough; and occasional sharp, nonradiating chest pain that is worse on inhalation. Physical examination of the chest may indicate decreased movement of the chest on the affected side, dullness to percussion, and diminished breath sounds over the affected area. A chest x-ray and CT reveal the volume and location of the effusion. Indication of a possible empyema include the manifestations of pleural effusion as well as fever, night sweats, cough, and weight loss.

### Thoracentesis

**Thoracentesis** is aspiration of intrapleural fluid for diagnostic and therapeutic purposes. For a thoracentesis, the patient may sit on the edge of a bed and lean forward over a bedside table. A chest x-ray or ultrasound images are used to determine the optimal puncture site. The skin is cleansed with an antiseptic solution and injected with a local anesthetic. The thoracentesis

**TABLE 27-24 Intrapulmonary Causes of Restrictive Lung Disease**

| Pleural Disorders | Parenchymal Disorders |
|---|---|
| • Pleural effusion<br>• Pleurisy (pleuritis)<br>• Pneumothorax | • Acute respiratory distress syndrome (ARDS)<br>• Atelectasis<br>• Interstitial lung diseases<br>• Pneumonia |

needle is inserted into the intercostal space (see Fig. 25-13). Fluid is aspirated with a syringe, or tubing is connected to the needle to allow fluid to drain into a sterile container. After the fluid is removed, the needle is withdrawn, and a bandage is applied over the insertion site.

Usually only 1000 to 1200 mL of pleural fluid is removed at one time. Rapid removal of a large volume can result in hypotension, hypoxemia, or reexpansion pulmonary edema. A chest x-ray may be done after the procedure to assess for possible complications such as pneumothorax. During and after the procedure, monitor vital signs and pulse oximetry, and observe the patient for any manifestations of respiratory distress.

### Interprofessional Care

The management of pleural effusions is to treat the underlying cause. For example, adequate treatment of heart failure with diuretics and sodium restriction may result in a decreased incidence of pleural effusion. The treatment of pleural effusions secondary to malignant disease represents a more difficult problem. These types of pleural effusions are frequently recurrent and reaccumulate quickly after thoracentesis.

*Chemical pleurodesis* is performed to obliterate the pleural space and prevent reaccumulation of effusion fluid in both malignant and nonmalignant pleural effusions. This procedure first requires chest tube drainage of the effusion. Once the fluid is drained, a chemical slurry is instilled into the pleural space. Talc is the most effective agent for pleurodesis. Other agents such as doxycycline and bleomycin can also be used. The chest tube is clamped for 8 hours while the patient is turned in different positions to allow the chemical to contact the entire pleural space. After 8 hours the chest tube is unclamped and attached to a drainage unit. Fever and chest pain are the most common side effects associated with pleurodesis. Chest tubes are left in place until fluid drainage is less than 150 mL/day and no air leaks are noted.

## PLEURISY

**Pleurisy (pleuritis)** is an inflammation of the pleura. Inflammation can be caused by infectious diseases, neoplasms, autoimmune disorders, chest trauma, GI disease, and certain medications. The inflammation usually subsides with adequate treatment of the primary disease. The pain of pleurisy is typically abrupt, sharp in onset, and aggravated by inspiration. The patient's breathing is shallow and rapid to avoid unnecessary movement of the pleura and chest wall. A pleural friction rub may occur, which is the sound heard over areas where inflamed visceral pleura and parietal pleura rub over one another during inspiration. This sound, like a squeaking door, is usually loudest at peak inspiration but may be heard during exhalation as well.

Treatment of pleurisy is aimed at treating the underlying disease and providing pain relief. NSAIDs or analgesics and lying on or splinting the affected side may provide some relief. Teach the patient to splint the rib cage when coughing. If the pain is severe, intercostal nerve blocks may be considered.

## ATELECTASIS

*Atelectasis* is a lung condition characterized by collapsed, airless alveoli. There may be diminished or absent breath sounds and dullness to percussion over the affected area. The most common cause of atelectasis is obstruction of the small airways with secretions. This is common in bedridden patients and in postoperative abdominal and thoracic surgery patients. Normally the pores of Kohn (see Fig. 25-1) provide collateral passage of air from one alveolus to another. Deep inspiration is necessary to open the pores effectively. For this reason, deep-breathing exercises, coughing, incentive spirometry, and early mobility are important to prevent atelectasis and treat the patient at risk. (The prevention and treatment of atelectasis are discussed in Chapter 19.)

# INTERSTITIAL LUNG DISEASES

*Interstitial lung disease* (ILD), also called *diffuse parenchymal lung disease,* refers to more than 200 lung disorders in which the tissue between the air sacs of the lungs (the interstitium) is affected by inflammation or scarring (fibrosis).[32] ILDs can be caused by inhalation of occupational and environmental toxins, certain medications, radiation therapy, connective tissue disorders, malignancy, and infection. Treatment is aimed at reducing exposure to the causative agent and/or treating the underlying disease process. Although scarring is irreversible, treatment with corticosteroids and immunosuppressant drugs can minimize progression. A lung transplant may be an option for some patients.

Most of the ILDs are extremely rare. Many times the cause of ILD is unknown. The most common ILDs of unknown etiology are idiopathic pulmonary fibrosis and sarcoidosis.

## IDIOPATHIC PULMONARY FIBROSIS

*Idiopathic pulmonary fibrosis* (IPF) is a chronic, progressive disorder characterized by chronic inflammation and formation of scar tissue in the connective tissue. Risk factors for IPF include a history of cigarette smoking and exposure to wood and metal dust. IPF affects more men than women and typically first appears between the ages of 50 and 70 years. There is no known cure for IPF.

Clinical manifestations of IPF include exertional dyspnea; dry, nonproductive cough; clubbing of the fingers; and inspiratory crackles. Fatigue, weakness, anorexia, and weight loss may occur as the disease progresses. Chest x-ray findings are generally nonspecific. Pulmonary function tests may be abnormal with evidence of restriction (reduced vital capacity) and impaired gas exchange. Open lung biopsy using VATS often helps to confirm the pathology and is considered the "gold standard" for diagnosis.

The clinical course of IPF is variable and the prognosis is poor, with a 5-year survival rate of 30% to 50% after diagnosis. Many people diagnosed with IPF are initially treated with a corticosteroid (prednisone), sometimes in combination with other drugs that suppress the immune system (e.g., methotrexate, cyclosporine). Kinase inhibitor drugs, which block multiple pathways that are involved in scarring, include nintedanib (Ofev) and pirfenidone (Esbriet).

$O_2$ therapy and pulmonary rehabilitation should be prescribed for all patients. Lung transplantation may be an option for those who meet the criteria.[33] (Lung transplantation is discussed later in this chapter on p. 533.)

## SARCOIDOSIS

*Sarcoidosis* is a chronic, multisystem granulomatous disease of unknown cause that primarily affects the lungs. The disease may also involve the skin, eyes, liver, kidney, heart, and lymph nodes. African Americans and those with a family history of sarcoidosis are at higher risk for developing sarcoidosis.

Signs and symptoms vary depending on what organs are affected. Pulmonary symptoms include dyspnea, cough, and chest pain. Many patients do not have symptoms.

The disease is staged and treatment decisions are based on pulmonary function and progression of the disease. Some patients have a spontaneous remission. Treatment is aimed at suppression of the inflammatory response. Patients are followed every 3 to 6 months with pulmonary function tests, chest x-ray, and CT scan to monitor disease progression.

# VASCULAR LUNG DISORDERS

## PULMONARY EDEMA

**Pulmonary edema** is an abnormal accumulation of fluid in the alveoli and interstitial spaces of the lungs. It is a complication of various heart and lung diseases (Table 27-25). In severe circumstances, pulmonary edema can be a life-threatening medical emergency.

The most common cause of pulmonary edema is left-sided heart failure. (Pathophysiology, clinical manifestations, and management of pulmonary edema are described in Chapter 34.)

## PULMONARY EMBOLISM

### Etiology and Pathophysiology

**Pulmonary embolism (PE)** is the blockage of one or more pulmonary arteries by a thrombus, fat or air embolus, or tumor tissue. The word *embolus* derives from a Greek word meaning "plug" or "stopper." *Emboli* are mobile clots that generally do not stop moving until they lodge at a narrowed part of the circulatory system. A pulmonary embolus consists of material that gains access to the venous system and then to the pulmonary circulation. The embolus travels with blood flow through ever-smaller blood vessels until it lodges and obstructs perfusion of the alveoli (Fig. 27-10). The lower lobes of the lung are most commonly affected. Approximately 10% of patients with massive PE die within the first hour. Treatment with anticoagulants significantly reduces mortality.

Most pulmonary emboli arise from deep vein thrombosis (DVT) in the deep veins of the legs. *Venous thromboembolism* (VTE) is the preferred term to describe the spectrum of pathologic conditions from DVT to PE (see Table 37-7). Other sites of origin of PE include femoral or iliac veins, right side of the heart (atrial fibrillation), and pelvic veins (especially after surgery or childbirth). Upper extremity DVT occasionally occurs in the presence of central venous catheters or arterial lines. These cases may resolve with the removal of the catheter. A *saddle embolus* refers to a large thrombus lodged at an arterial bifurcation.

In addition to dislodged thrombi, less common causes of PE include fat emboli (from fractured long bones), air emboli (from improperly administered IV therapy), bacterial vegetation on heart valves, amniotic fluid, and tumors. Risk factors for PE include immobility or reduced mobility, surgery within the last 3 months (especially pelvic and lower extremity surgery), history of DVT, malignancy, obesity, oral contraceptives, hormone therapy, cigarette smoking, prolonged air travel, heart failure, pregnancy, and clotting disorders.

### Clinical Manifestations

The signs and symptoms of PE are varied and nonspecific, making diagnosis difficult. Clinical manifestations depend on the size and extent of emboli. Small emboli may go undetected or produce vague, transient symptoms. Symptoms may begin slowly or suddenly. Dyspnea is the most common presenting symptom, occurring in 85% of patients with PE. A mild to moderate hypoxemia may be observed. Other manifestations may include tachypnea, cough, chest pain, hemoptysis, crackles, wheezing, fever, accentuation of the pulmonic heart sound, tachycardia, and syncope. Massive emboli may produce a sudden change in mental status, hypotension, and feelings of impending doom.

### Complications

Complications of pulmonary emboli include pulmonary infarction and pulmonary hypertension. *Pulmonary infarction* (death of lung tissue) is most likely when the following factors are present: (1) occlusion of a large or medium-sized pulmonary vessel (more than 2 mm in diameter), (2) insufficient collateral blood flow from the bronchial circulation, or (3) preexisting lung disease. Infarction results in alveolar necrosis and hemorrhage. Occasionally the necrotic tissue becomes infected, and an abscess may develop. Concomitant pleural effusion is frequent.

*Pulmonary hypertension* results from hypoxemia or from involvement of more than 50% of the area of the normal pulmonary bed. As a single event, an embolus rarely causes pulmonary hypertension. Recurrent pulmonary emboli gradually cause a reduction in the capillary bed and eventual pulmonary hypertension. Dilation and hypertrophy of the right

**TABLE 27-25 Causes of Pulmonary Edema**

- Heart failure
- Overhydration with IV fluids
- Hypoalbuminemia: nephrotic syndrome, hepatic disease, nutritional disorders
- Altered capillary permeability of lungs: inhaled toxins, inflammation (e.g., pneumonia), severe hypoxia, near-drowning
- Malignancies of the lymph system (e.g., non-Hodgkin's lymphoma)
- $O_2$ toxicity
- Acute respiratory distress syndrome (ARDS)
- Unknown causes: neurogenic condition, opioid overdose, reexpansion pulmonary edema, high altitude

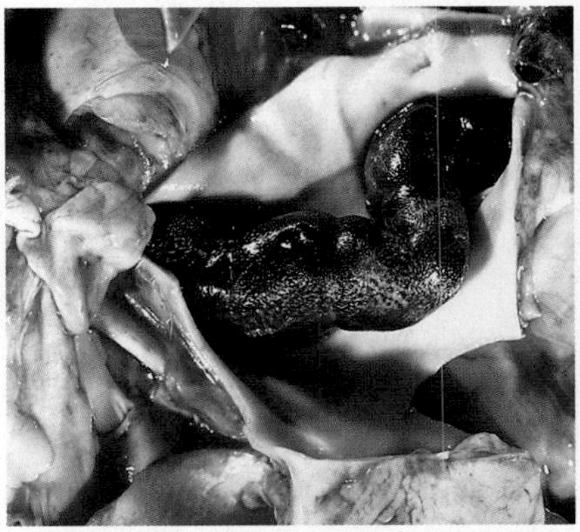

**FIG. 27-10** Large embolus from the femoral vein lying in the main left and right pulmonary arteries. (From the teaching collection of the Department of Pathology, University of Texas Southwestern Medical School, Dallas, Tex. In Kumar V, Abbas AK, Aster JC, Fausto N, editors: *Robbins and Cotran pathologic basis of disease,* ed 8, Philadelphia, 2010, Saunders.)

ventricle can develop secondary to pulmonary hypertension. Depending on the degree of pulmonary hypertension and its rate of development, outcomes can vary, with some patients dying within months of the diagnosis and others living for decades.

## Diagnostic Studies

*D-dimer* is a laboratory test that measures the amount of cross-linked fibrin fragments. These fragments are the result of clot degradation and are rarely found in healthy individuals. The disadvantage of D-dimer testing is that it is neither specific (many other conditions cause elevation) nor sensitive, because up to 50% of patients with small pulmonary emboli have normal results. Patients with suspected PE and an elevated D-dimer level but normal venous ultrasound may need a spiral CT or lung scan.

A *spiral (helical) CT scan* (also known as CT angiography or CTA) is the most frequently used test to diagnose PE (Table 27-26). An IV injection of contrast media is required to view the pulmonary blood vessels. The scanner continuously rotates around the patient while obtaining views (slices) of the pulmonary vasculature. This allows visualization of all anatomic regions of the lungs. Computer software reconstructs the data to provide a three-dimensional picture and assist in emboli visualization.

If a patient cannot have contrast media, a ventilation-perfusion (V/Q) scan is done. The V/Q scan has two components and is most accurate when both are performed:

1. *Perfusion scanning* involves IV injection of a radioisotope. A scanning device images the pulmonary circulation.
2. *Ventilation scanning* involves inhalation of a radioactive gas such as xenon. Scanning reflects the distribution of gas through the lung. The ventilation component requires the patient's cooperation and may be impossible to perform in the critically ill patient, particularly if the patient is intubated.

Pulmonary angiography is the most sensitive and specific test for PE. However, it is an expensive and invasive procedure that involves insertion of a catheter through the antecubital or femoral vein, advancement of the catheter to the pulmonary artery, and injection of contrast medium. The accessibility and accuracy of the spiral CT have greatly diminished the need for pulmonary angiography.

ABG analysis is important but not diagnostic. The $PaO_2$ may be low because of inadequate oxygenation secondary to occluded pulmonary vasculature preventing matching of perfusion to ventilation. The pH is often normal unless respiratory alkalosis develops as a result of prolonged hyperventilation or to compensate for lactic acidosis caused by shock. Abnormal findings are usually identified on the chest x-ray (atelectasis, pleural effusion) and the ECG (ST segment and T wave changes), but they are not diagnostic for PE. Serum troponin levels and b-type natriuretic peptide (BNP) levels are frequently elevated but not diagnostic.

### TABLE 27-26 Interprofessional Care

***Acute Pulmonary Embolism***

| Diagnostic Assessment | Management |
|---|---|
| • History and physical examination<br>• Chest x-ray<br>• Continuous ECG monitoring<br>• ABGs<br>• Spiral (helical) CT scan<br>• Ventilation-perfusion (V/Q) lung scan<br>• D-dimer level<br>• Troponin level, BNP level<br>• Pulmonary angiography | • Supplemental $O_2$, intubation if necessary<br>• Monitor aPTT and INR levels<br>• Balance activity and rest<br>• Inferior vena cava filter<br>• Pulmonary embolectomy in life-threatening situation<br><br>***Drug Therapy***<br>• Fibrinolytic agent<br>• Unfractionated heparin IV<br>• Low-molecular-weight heparin (e.g., enoxaparin [Lovenox])<br>• Warfarin (Coumadin) for long-term therapy<br>• Opioids for pain relief |

*ABGs,* Arterial blood gases; *aPTT,* activated partial thromboplastin time; *BNP,* b-type natriuretic peptide; *INR,* international normalized ratio.

## Interprofessional Care

Prevention of PE begins with prevention of DVT. DVT prophylaxis includes the use of sequential compression devices, early ambulation, and anticoagulant medications.

To reduce mortality risk, treatment is begun as soon as PE is suspected (Table 27-26). The objectives are to (1) prevent further growth or extension of thrombi in the lower extremities, (2) prevent embolization from the upper or lower extremities to the pulmonary vascular system, and (3) provide cardiopulmonary support if indicated.

Supportive therapy for the patient's cardiopulmonary status varies according to the severity of the PE. $O_2$ can be given via mask or cannula, and the concentration of $FIO_2$ is determined by ABG analysis. In some situations, endotracheal intubation and mechanical ventilation are necessary to maintain adequate oxygenation. Respiratory measures such as turning, coughing, deep breathing, and incentive spirometry are important to help prevent or treat atelectasis. If manifestations of shock are present, IV fluids are administered followed by vasopressor agents as needed to support perfusion (see Chapter 66). If heart failure is present, diuretics are used (see Chapter 34). Pain resulting from pleural irritation or reduced coronary blood flow is treated with opioids.

**Drug Therapy.** Immediate anticoagulation is required for patients with PE. Subcutaneous administration of low-molecular-weight heparin (LMWH) (e.g., enoxaparin [Lovenox]) or fondaparinux has been found to be safer and more effective than use of unfractionated heparin.[34] It is the recommended treatment for patients with acute PE, administered once daily. Advantages of LMWH over unfractionated heparin include greater bioavailability, subcutaneous administration, and longer duration of therapeutic effect; furthermore, monitoring the aPTT is not necessary or useful with LMWH. Unfractionated IV heparin can be as effective but is more difficult to titrate to therapeutic levels.

Warfarin (Coumadin), an oral anticoagulant, should also be initiated at the time of diagnosis.[34] Warfarin should be administered for at least 3 months and then reevaluated. Alternatives to warfarin include apixaban (Eliquis), dabigitran (Pradaxa), and edoxaban (Savaysa). Anticoagulant therapy may be contraindicated if the patient has complicating factors such as blood dyscrasias, hepatic dysfunction causing alterations in the clotting, overt bleeding, a history of hemorrhagic stroke, or heparin-induced thrombocytopenia (HIT).

Although not common, some HCPs use direct thrombin inhibitors (see Table 37-10) in the treatment of PE. Similarly, fibrinolytic agents, such as tissue plasminogen activator (tPA) or alteplase (Activase), may help dissolve the pulmonary embolus and the source of the thrombus in the pelvis or deep leg veins, thereby decreasing the likelihood of recurrent emboli. Fibrinolytic therapy is discussed in Chapter 33.

**Surgical Therapy.** Hemodynamically unstable patients with massive PE in whom thrombolytic therapy is contraindicated may be candidates for immediate pulmonary embolectomy. Embolectomy, removal of emboli to help decrease right ventricular afterload, can be achieved via a vascular (catheter) or surgical approach. Surgical outcomes have improved in recent years, in part due to rapid diagnosis and enhanced surgical procedures, with mortality rates decreasing from 30% to 19%.[35]

To prevent further emboli, an inferior vena cava (IVC) filter may be the treatment of choice in patients who remain at high risk and patients for whom anticoagulation is contraindicated. This device, inserted percutaneously via the femoral vein, is placed at the level of the diaphragm in the inferior vena cava. Once inserted, the filter expands and prevents migration of large clots into the pulmonary system. Complications associated with this device are rare but include misplacement, migration, and perforation.

## NURSING MANAGEMENT: PULMONARY EMBOLISM

### Nursing Implementation

Nursing measures aimed at prevention of PE are similar to those for prophylaxis of VTE (see Chapter 37, pp. 818-819).

The prognosis of a patient with PE is good if therapy is promptly instituted. Keep the patient on bed rest in a semi-Fowler's position to facilitate breathing. Administer $O_2$ therapy as ordered. Assess the patient's cardiopulmonary status with careful monitoring of vital signs, cardiac rhythm, pulse oximetry, ABGs, and lung sounds. Maintain an IV line for medications and fluid therapy. Monitor laboratory results to ensure therapeutic ranges of INR (for warfarin) and aPTT (for IV heparin). Monitor the patient for complications of anticoagulant and fibrinolytic therapy (e.g., bleeding, hematomas, bruising). Provide appropriate interventions related to immobility and fall precautions, once the patient is permitted out of bed.

The patient is usually anxious because of pain, inability to breathe, and fear of death. Carefully explain the situation, the medications, and provide emotional support and reassurance to help relieve the patient's anxiety.

Patient teaching regarding long-term anticoagulant therapy is critical. Anticoagulant therapy continues for at least 3 months. Patients with recurrent emboli may be treated indefinitely with anticoagulants. INR levels are drawn at intervals and warfarin dosage is adjusted. Some patients are monitored by nurses in an anticoagulation clinic.

Long-term management of PE is similar to that for the patient with VTE (see discussion of VTE in Chapter 37 on pp. 818-819). Discharge planning is aimed at preventing worsening of the condition and avoiding complications and recurrence. Reinforce the need for the patient to return to the HCP for regular follow-up examinations.

### Evaluation

The expected outcomes are that the patient who has a PE will have

- Adequate tissue perfusion and respiratory function
- Adequate cardiac output
- Increased level of comfort
- Prevention of further recurrence of PE

## PULMONARY HYPERTENSION

**Pulmonary hypertension** is characterized by elevated pulmonary artery pressure resulting from an increase in resistance to blood flow through the pulmonary circulation. Normally the pulmonary circulation is characterized by low resistance and low pressure. In pulmonary hypertension the pulmonary pressures are elevated with the mean pulmonary artery pressure greater than 25 mm Hg at rest (normal is 12 to 16 mm Hg) or greater than 30 mm Hg with exercise.

The World Health Organization (WHO) has identified five categories (groups) of pulmonary hypertension. Each group is based on etiology of the disorder.

*Group 1:* Pulmonary arterial hypertension attributable to medication, specific diseases, genetic (inherited) link, or idiopathic

*Group 2:* Related to left-sided heart failure

*Group 3:* Related to the lungs and hypoxemia

*Group 4:* Related to the cardiovascular system and thromboembolic occlusion

*Group 5:* Multifactorial (and often unclear) origins with hematologic or metabolic involvement

The disease commonly manifests with shortness of breath and fatigue. Pulmonary hypertension can occur as a primary disease *(idiopathic pulmonary arterial hypertension)* or as a secondary complication of a respiratory, cardiac, autoimmune, hepatic, or connective tissue disorder *(secondary pulmonary arterial hypertension).*

## IDIOPATHIC PULMONARY ARTERIAL HYPERTENSION

*Idiopathic pulmonary arterial hypertension* (IPAH) is pulmonary hypertension that occurs without an apparent cause. (It was previously known as *primary pulmonary hypertension* [PPH].) If untreated, this disorder can be rapidly progressive, causing right-sided heart failure and death within a few years. Although new drug therapy has greatly improved survival, the disease remains incurable.

### Etiology and Pathophysiology

The etiology of IPAH is unknown. It has been associated with connective tissue diseases, cirrhosis, and HIV, but the exact relationship between these disorders and IPAH remains unclear. Similarly, the pathophysiology of IPAH is poorly understood. It has been suggested that some type of insult (e.g., hormonal, mechanical) to the pulmonary endothelium may occur, causing a cascade of events leading to vascular scarring, endothelial dysfunction, and smooth muscle proliferation (Fig. 27-11). IPAH affects females more than males.

### Clinical Manifestations and Diagnostic Studies

Classic symptoms of pulmonary hypertension are dyspnea on exertion and fatigue. Exertional chest pain, dizziness, and syncope are other symptoms. These symptoms are related to the inability of cardiac output to increase in response to increased $O_2$ demand. Abnormal heart sounds may also be auscultated, including an S3. Eventually, as the disease progresses, dyspnea occurs at rest. Pulmonary hypertension increases the workload of the right ventricle and causes right ventricular hypertrophy (a condition called *cor pulmonale*) and eventually heart failure.

Right-sided cardiac catheterization is the definitive test to diagnose any type of pulmonary hypertension. In addition to providing an accurate measurement of pulmonary artery pressures, it also determines cardiac output and pulmonary vascular resistance. Confirmation of IPAH requires a thorough workup to exclude conditions that may cause secondary pulmonary hypertension. Diagnostic evaluation often includes ECG, chest x-ray, pulmonary function tests, echocardiogram, and CT scan.

The mean time between onset of symptoms and the diagnosis is about 2 years. By the time patients become symptomatic, the disease is already in the advanced stages and the pulmonary artery pressure is two to three times normal.

**PATHOPHYSIOLOGY MAP**

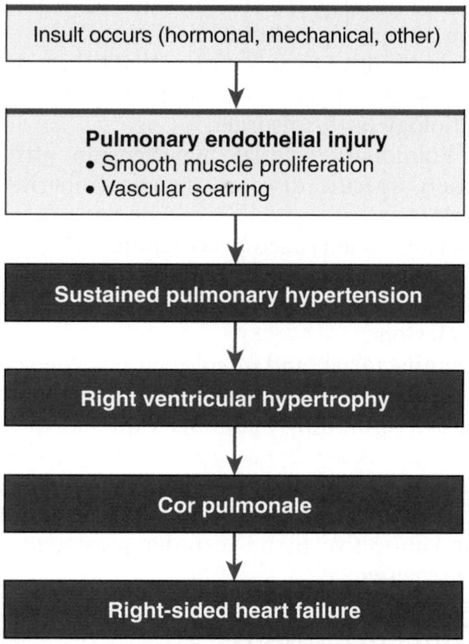


**FIG. 27-11** Pathogenesis of pulmonary hypertension and cor pulmonale.

## ❖ NURSING AND INTERPROFESSIONAL MANAGEMENT: PULMONARY HYPERTENSION

Early recognition of pulmonary hypertension is essential to interrupt the vicious cycle responsible for progression of the disease. Encourage patients to report unexplained shortness of breath, syncope, chest discomfort, and edema of the feet and ankles to their primary care provider.[36]

Although IPAH has no cure, treatment can relieve symptoms, improve quality of life, and prolong life. Drug therapy consists of several drug classifications that promote vasodilation of the pulmonary blood vessels, reduce right ventricular overload, and reverse remodeling (Table 27-27). Diuretics are used to manage peripheral edema. The use of anticoagulants is also beneficial in pulmonary complications related to thrombus formation. Because hypoxia is a potent pulmonary vasoconstrictor, low-flow $O_2$ provides symptomatic relief. The goal is to keep $O_2$ saturation 90% or greater.

Surgical interventions for pulmonary hypertension include atrial septostomy (AS) and lung transplantation. AS is a palliative procedure that involves the creation of an intraatrial right-to-left shunt to decompress the right ventricle. It is used for a select group of patients awaiting lung transplantation.

**TABLE 27-27 Drug Therapy**
***Pulmonary Hypertension***

| Drug | Mechanism of Action | Considerations |
|---|---|---|
| **Calcium Channel Blockers** | | |
| nifedipine (Adalat CC, Procardia)<br>diltiazem (Cardizem, Cardizem LA, Cartia XT, Tiazac) | • Act on vascular smooth muscle, causing dilation<br>• Lower pulmonary artery pressure | • Can only be used in patients who do not have right-sided heart failure<br>• Used at high doses in comparison to other uses of calcium channel blockers |
| **Phosphodiesterase (Type 5) Enzyme Inhibitors** | | |
| sildenafil (Revatio)<br>tadalafil (Adcirca) | • Promote selective smooth muscle relaxation in lung vasculature | • Given orally<br>• Contraindicated in patients taking nitroglycerin, since may cause refractory hypotension |
| **Vasodilators (Parenteral)** | | |
| epoprostenol (Flolan, Veletri)<br>treprostinil (Remodulin)<br>adenosine (Adenocard) | • Prostacyclin analog<br>• Promote pulmonary vasodilation and reduce pulmonary vascular resistance | • Given IV to patients who do not respond to calcium channel blockers or have New York Heart Association (NYHA) class III or IV right-sided heart failure<br>• Given by continuous IV (central line) or continuous subcutaneous route. Half-life of epoprostenol is short. Potential clinical deterioration from abrupt withdrawal if infusion disrupted |
| **Vasodilators (Inhaled)** | | |
| iloprost (Ventavis)<br>treprostinil (inhaled) (Tyvaso) | Synthetic analogs of prostacyclin ($PGI_2$)<br>Dilate systemic and pulmonary arterial vasculature | • Indicated for patients with NYHA class III or IV heart failure<br>• Administered 6-9 times a day using a disk inserted into a nebulizer<br>• Can cause orthostatic hypotension. Do not give to patients with systolic BP <85 mm Hg. |
| **Endothelin Receptor Antagonists** | | |
| bosentan (Tracleer)<br>ambrisentan (Letairis)<br>macitentan (Opsumit) | • Binds to endothelin-1 receptors and blocks the constriction of pulmonary arteries<br>• Promote relaxation of pulmonary arteries and decrease pulmonary artery pressure | • Given orally<br>• Indicated for patients with NYHA class II to IV symptoms<br>• Hepatotoxic<br>• Monitor liver function tests monthly. |

Lung transplantation is indicated for those patients who do not respond to drug therapy and progress to severe right-sided heart failure. Recurrence of the disease has not been reported in individuals who have undergone transplantation.

## SECONDARY PULMONARY ARTERIAL HYPERTENSION

*Secondary pulmonary arterial hypertension* (SPAH) occurs when a primary disease causes a chronic increase in pulmonary artery pressures. SPAH can develop as a result of parenchymal lung disease, left ventricular dysfunction, intracardiac shunts, chronic pulmonary thromboembolism, or systemic connective tissue disease. The specific primary disease pathology can result in anatomic or vascular changes causing the pulmonary hypertension.

The symptoms can reflect the underlying disease, but some are directly attributable to SPAH, including dyspnea, fatigue, lethargy, and chest pain. The initial physical findings can include right ventricular hypertrophy and signs of right ventricular failure (increased pulmonic heart sound, right-sided fourth heart sound, peripheral edema, and hepatomegaly).

Diagnosis of SPAH is similar to that of IPAH. Treatment of SPAH consists mainly of treating the underlying primary disorder. When irreversible pulmonary vascular damage has occurred, therapies used for IPAH are initiated. A pulmonary thromboendarterectomy (PTE) may offer a cure for patients with chronic pulmonary hypertension caused by thromboembolism. It is a technically demanding procedure and is performed only at selected centers.

## COR PULMONALE

**Cor pulmonale** is enlargement of the right ventricle caused by a primary disorder of the respiratory system. Pulmonary hypertension is usually a preexisting condition in cor pulmonale. Cor pulmonale may be present with or without overt cardiac failure. The most common cause of cor pulmonale is COPD. Almost any disorder that affects the respiratory system can cause cor pulmonale. Fig. 27-11 outlines the etiology and pathogenesis of pulmonary hypertension and cor pulmonale.

### Clinical Manifestations and Diagnostic Studies

Clinical manifestations are subtle and often masked by the symptoms of the pulmonary condition. Common symptoms include exertional dyspnea, tachypnea, cough, and fatigue. Physical signs include evidence of right ventricular hypertrophy on ECG and an increase in intensity of the second heart sound. Chronic hypoxemia leads to polycythemia and increased total blood volume and viscosity of the blood. Polycythemia is often present in cor pulmonale secondary to COPD.

If heart failure accompanies cor pulmonale, additional manifestations such as peripheral edema, weight gain, distended neck veins, full, bounding pulse, and enlarged liver may also be found. (Heart failure is discussed in Chapter 34.) Various laboratory tests and imaging studies are used to confirm the diagnosis of cor pulmonale (Table 27-28).

## NURSING AND INTERPROFESSIONAL MANAGEMENT: COR PULMONALE

Early identification of cor pulmonale is essential before changes to the heart occur that may be irreversible. The primary management of cor pulmonale is difficult but often directed at investigating the cause and treating the underlying pulmonary problem (Table 27-28).

Long-term $O_2$ therapy, the mainstay of treatment to correct the hypoxemia, reduces vasoconstriction and pulmonary hypertension. All other strategies must be individualized for each patient but are often directed at treating pulmonary hypertension that can lead to cor pulmonale. If fluid, electrolyte, and acid-base imbalances are present, they must be corrected. Diuretics may help decrease the plasma volume and reduce the workload on the heart but must be used with extreme caution. In some cases, decreases in fluid volume from diuresis can worsen cardiac function. Bronchodilator therapy is indicated if the underlying respiratory problem is due to an obstructive disorder.

Other treatments may include vasodilator therapy, calcium channel blockers, anticoagulants, digitalis, and phlebotomy, all of which have varying degrees of success. Chronic management of cor pulmonale resulting from COPD is similar to that described for COPD (see Chapter 28).

**TABLE 27-28 Interprofessional Care**

***Cor Pulmonale***

| Diagnostic Assessment | Management |
|---|---|
| • History and physical examination | • $O_2$ therapy |
| • ABGs, $SpO_2$ | • Low-sodium diet |
| • Serum and urine electrolytes | |
| • b-Type natriuretic peptide (BNP) | ***Drug Therapy*** |
| • ECG | • Bronchodilators |
| • Chest x-ray | • Diuretics |
| • Echocardiography | • Vasodilators (if indicated) |
| • CT scan | • Calcium channel blockers (if indicated) |
| • MRI | |
| • Cardiac catheterization | • Inotropic agents |

**TABLE 27-29 Indications for Lung Transplantation***

- Chronic obstructive pulmonary disease
- Idiopathic pulmonary fibrosis
- Cystic fibrosis
- Idiopathic pulmonary arterial hypertension
- $\alpha_1$-Antitrypsin deficiency

*These are the most common indications.

## LUNG TRANSPLANTATION

*Lung transplantation* has become an important mode of therapy for patients with end-stage lung disease. The limiting factor for this therapy is the availability of donors. A variety of pulmonary disorders are potentially treatable with lung transplantation (Table 27-29). Improved patient selection criteria, technical advances, and better methods of immunosuppression have resulted in improved survival rates.

### Preoperative Care

Patients being considered for lung transplantation need to undergo extensive evaluation. Absolute contraindications for lung transplant include malignancy within past 2 years (some types of skin cancer are excluded), chronic active hepatitis B or C, HIV, untreatable advanced dysfunction of another major organ system (e.g., liver or renal failure), current smoker, poor nutritional status, poor rehabilitation potential, and significant psychosocial problems. The patient and family must be able to cope with a complex postoperative regimen (e.g., strict adherence to immunosuppressive therapy, continuous monitoring for early signs of infection, prompt reporting of manifestations of infection). Many transplant centers require preoperative outpatient pulmonary rehabilitation to maximize physical conditioning.

In the United States, the United Network for Organ Sharing (UNOS) is a private, non-profit organization that works with the federal government to manage organ transplantation. UNOS designates recipients of donor lungs based on a lung allocation score (LAS). The LAS helps to prioritize waiting list recipients based on the urgency of need and expected post-transplant survival expectations.

Patients who are accepted as transplant candidates must carry a pager with them at all times in case a donor organ becomes available. These patients must be prepared to move to the location of their chosen transplant center at a moment's notice. Such patients may be encouraged to limit their travel within a certain geographic region to facilitate rapid transportation to a transplant center.

## Surgical Procedure

Four types of transplant procedures are available: single-lung transplantation, bilateral lung transplantation, heart-lung transplantation, and transplantation of lobes from a living-related donor.

*Single-lung transplantation* involves a thoracotomy incision on the side of the chest. The opposite lung is ventilated while the diseased lung is excised, and the donor lung implanted. Three anastomoses are done: bronchus, pulmonary artery, and pulmonary veins. In *bilateral lung transplantation,* the incision is made across the sternum and the donor lungs are implanted separately. A median sternotomy incision is used for a *heart-lung transplant* procedure. *Lobar transplantation* from living donors is reserved for candidates who urgently need transplantation and are unlikely to survive until a donor becomes available. The majority of these transplant recipients are patients with cystic fibrosis, and their parents or relatives are donors. Once anastomosis is complete, the lung is gently reinflated, perfusion is reestablished, chest tubes are inserted, and the surgical incision is closed.

## Postoperative Care

Early postoperative care often includes admission to ICU and provision of ventilatory support, fluid and hemodynamic management, immunosuppression, nutritional support, detection of early rejection, and prevention or treatment of infection. Once hemodynamic stability has been achieved, the patient is often transferred to a high acuity observation or surgical unit. Maintenance of accurate fluid balance is vital in the postoperative phase.

Lung transplant recipients are at high risk for multiple complications after surgery. Noninfectious issues may include VTE, diaphragmatic dysfunction, and malignancy. Infectious complications may be caused by bacteria, viruses, fungi, or protozoa. Infections are the leading cause of death at all time points after lung transplant. Bacterial bronchitis and pneumonia are the most common infections, but cytomegalovirus (CMV), fungi, viruses, and mycobacteria are also etiologic factors.

Immunosuppressive therapy usually includes a three-drug regimen of tacrolimus, mycophenolate mofetil (CellCept), and prednisone. (The mechanisms of action of these drugs are discussed in Table 13-16 and Fig. 13-13.) Drug levels are monitored on a regular basis. Lung transplant recipients usually receive higher levels of immunosuppressive therapy than other organ recipients.

Acute rejection is fairly common in lung transplantation, typically occurring in the first 5 to 10 days after surgery. Low-grade fever, fatigue, dyspnea, dry cough, and $O_2$ desaturation are possible signs of rejection. Accurate diagnosis of rejection is by transtracheal biopsy. Treatment consists of high doses of IV corticosteroids administered for 3 days, followed by high doses of oral prednisone. In patients with persistent or recurrent acute rejection, antilymphocyte therapy may be useful.

*Bronchiolitis obliterans* (BOS) is a manifestation of chronic rejection in lung transplant patients. BOS is characterized by airflow obstruction that progresses over time. The onset is often subacute, with gradual development of exertional dyspnea, nonproductive cough, wheezing, and/or low-grade fever. Airway obstruction is not responsive to bronchodilators and corticosteroid therapy. Although not proven effective, additional immunosuppressive agents may be used in the treatment of chronic rejection. Because acute rejection is a major risk factor for BOS, prevention of acute rejection is key to decreasing the incidence of chronic rejection.

Before discharge, the patient needs to be able to perform self-care activities, including medication management and activities of daily living, and to accurately identify when to call the transplant team. Patients should be instructed on pulmonary clearance measures, including aerosolized bronchodilators, chest physiotherapy, and deep-breathing and coughing techniques, to help minimize any potential complication. Home spirometry is useful in monitoring trends in lung function. Teach patients to keep medication logs, laboratory results, and spirometry records. Patients are placed in an outpatient rehabilitation program to improve physical endurance.

After discharge, the transplant team follows patients for transplant-related issues. Patients return to their primary care team for health maintenance and routine illnesses. As transplant procedures become more frequent, transplant patients will return to hospitals for other routine procedures. Coordination of care between the transplant team, primary care team, and inpatient teams is essential for ongoing successful management of these patients. (Organ transplantation, histocompatibility, rejection, and immunosuppressive therapy are discussed in Chapter 13.)

## CASE STUDY

### *Pneumonia and Lung Cancer*

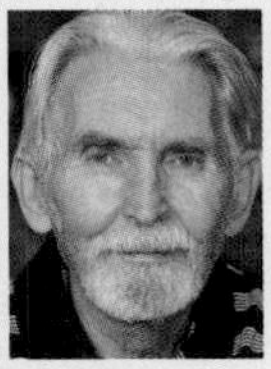

(©iStockphoto/ Thinkstock)

**Patient Profile**

J.H. is a 52-year-old white man who comes to the emergency department complaining of shortness of breath. He has not seen an HCP for many years.

**Subjective Data**

- Has a 38 pack-year history of cigarette smoking
- States he has always been slender but has had 25-lb weight loss despite a normal appetite in the past few months
- Admits to a "smoker's cough" for the past 2 to 3 years; recently coughing up blood
- Is married and the father of three adult children

**Objective Data**

***Physical Examination***

- Thin, pale man, looking older than stated age
- Height 6 ft (182.9 cm); weight 135 lb (61.2 kg)
- Intermittently confused and anxious with rapid shallow respirations
- Vital signs: temperature 102.6° F (39.2° C), heart rate 120, respiratory rate 36
- Chest wall has limited excursion on right side; auscultation of left side reveals coarse crackles but clear with cough; right side has diminished breath sounds

**Diagnostic Studies**

- Arterial blood gases: pH 7.51, $PaO_2$ 58 mm Hg, $PaCO_2$ 30 mm Hg, $HCO_3^-$ 22 mEq/L, $O_2$ saturation 84% (room air)
- Chest x-ray: consolidation of the right lung, especially in the base with possible mass in the area of right bronchus; pleural effusion on the right side
- Bronchoscopy with biopsy of mass: small cell lung carcinoma

**Interprofessional Care**

- Diagnosis: pneumonia with small cell lung cancer
- Follow-up with patient and family to consider treatment options

**Discussion Questions**

1. How would you classify J.H.'s pneumonia? Why is this important?
2. What is your analysis of J.H.'s arterial blood gas results?
3. ***Priority Decision:*** Based on the assessment data presented, what are the priority nursing diagnoses? Are there any collaborative problems?
4. ***Priority Decision:*** What are the priority nursing interventions for J.H.?
5. ***Teamwork and Collaboration:*** Identify activities that can be delegated to unlicensed assistive personnel (UAP).
6. ***Patient-Centered Care:*** You are planning a meeting with J.H. and his family to discuss their needs. The physician tells you that J.H. is terminally ill. Who will you include in this meeting?
7. ***Evidence-Based Practice:*** J.H.'s children tell you that they are worried they will get lung cancer, since their father has it and they grew up around his secondhand smoke. They want to know what kind of screening is available for them. How will you respond?
8. What is the goal if radiation therapy is used for J.H.?
9. ***Patient-Centered Care:*** What issues should be addressed in your teaching of J.H. and his wife as you prepare him for discharge and care at home?

Answers available at *http://evolve.elsevier.com/Lewis/medsurg.*

## BRIDGE TO NCLEX EXAMINATION

The number of the question corresponds to the same-numbered outcome at the beginning of the chapter.

1. When caring for a patient with acute bronchitis, the nurse will *prioritize*
   - **a.** auscultating lung sounds.
   - **b.** encouraging fluid restriction.
   - **c.** administering antibiotic therapy.
   - **d.** teaching the patient to avoid cough suppressants.
2. For which patients with pneumonia would the nurse suspect aspiration as the likely cause of pneumonia *(select all that apply)*?
   - **a.** Patient with seizures
   - **b.** Patient with head injury
   - **c.** Patient who had thoracic surgery
   - **d.** Patient who had a myocardial infarction
   - **e.** Patient who is receiving nasogastric tube feeding
3. An appropriate nursing intervention for a patient with pneumonia with the nursing diagnosis of ineffective airway clearance related to thick secretions and fatigue would be to
   - **a.** perform postural drainage every hour.
   - **b.** provide analgesics as ordered to promote patient comfort.
   - **c.** administer $O_2$ as prescribed to maintain optimal $O_2$ levels.
   - **d.** teach the patient how to cough effectively to bring secretions to the mouth.
4. A patient with TB has been admitted to the hospital and is placed in an airborne infection isolation room. What should the patient be taught *(select all that apply)*?
   - **a.** Expect routine TST to evaluate infection.
   - **b.** Visitors will not be allowed while in airborne isolation.
   - **c.** Take all medications for full length of time to prevent multidrug-resistant TB.
   - **d.** Wear a standard isolation mask if leaving the airborne infection isolation room.
   - **e.** Maintain precautions in airborne infection isolation room by coughing into a paper tissue.
5. A patient has been receiving high-dose corticosteroids and broad-spectrum antibiotics for treatment secondary to a traumatic injury and infection. The nurse plans care for the patient knowing that the patient is most susceptible to
   - **a.** candidiasis.
   - **b.** aspergillosis.
   - **c.** histoplasmosis.
   - **d.** coccidioidomycosis.
6. When caring for a patient with a lung abscess, what is the nurse's *priority* intervention?
   - **a.** Postural drainage
   - **b.** Antibiotic administration
   - **c.** Obtaining a sputum specimen
   - **d.** Patient teaching regarding home care

7. The emergency department nurse is caring for patients exposed to a chlorine leak from a local factory. The nurse would closely monitor these patients for
   a. pulmonary edema.
   b. anaphylactic shock.
   c. respiratory alkalosis.
   d. acute tubular necrosis.
8. The nurse receives an order for a patient with lung cancer to receive influenza vaccine and pneumococcal vaccines. The nurse will
   a. call the health care provider to question the order.
   b. administer both vaccines at the same time in different arms.
   c. administer the flu shot and tell the patient to come back 1 week later to receive the pneumococcal vaccine.
   d. administer the pneumococcal vaccine and suggest FluMist (nasal vaccine) instead of the influenza injection.
9. The nurse identifies a flail chest in a trauma patient when
   a. multiple rib fractures are determined by x-ray.
   b. a tracheal deviation to the unaffected side is present.
   c. paradoxical chest movement occurs during respiration.
   d. there is decreased movement of the involved chest wall.
10. The nurse notes tidaling of the water level in the tube submerged in the water-seal chamber in a patient with closed chest tube drainage. The nurse should
   a. continue to monitor the patient.
   b. check all connections for a leak in the system.
   c. lower the drainage collector further from the chest.
   d. clamp the tubing at progressively distal points away from the patient until the tidaling stops.
11. Following a pneumonectomy, an appropriate nursing intervention is
   a. monitoring chest tube drainage and functioning.
   b. positioning the patient on the unaffected side or back.
   c. doing range-of-motion exercises on the affected upper limb.
   d. auscultating frequently for lung sounds on the affected side.
12. A *priority* nursing intervention for a patient who has just undergone a chemical pleurodesis for recurrent pleural effusion is
   a. administering ordered analgesia.
   b. monitoring chest tube drainage.
   c. sending pleural fluid for laboratory analysis.
   d. monitoring the patient's level of consciousness.
13. When planning care for a patient at risk for pulmonary embolism, the nurse *prioritizes*
   a. maintaining the patient on bed rest.
   b. using sequential compression devices.
   c. encouraging the patient to cough and deep breathe.
   d. teaching the patient how to use the incentive spirometer.
14. Which statement(s) describe(s) the management of a patient following lung transplantation *(select all that apply)*?
   a. High doses of $O_2$ are administered around the clock.
   b. The use of a home spirometer will help to monitor lung function.
   c. Immunosuppressant therapy usually involves a three-drug regimen.
   d. Most patients experience an acute rejection episode in the first 2 days.
   e. The lung is biopsied using a transtracheal method if rejection is suspected.

1. a, 2. a, b, e, 3. d, 4. c, d, e, 5. a, 6. b, 7. a, 8. b, 9. c, 10. a, 11. c,
12. a, 13. b, 14. b, c, e

For rationales to these answers and even more NCLEX review questions, visit *http://evolve.elsevier.com/Lewis/medsurg.*

## EVOLVE WEBSITE

http://evolve.elsevier.com/Lewis/medsurg

**Review Questions (Online Only)**

**Key Points**

**Answer Keys for Questions**

- Rationales for Bridge to NCLEX Examination Questions
- Answer Guidelines for Case Study on p. 355

**Student Case Studies**

- Patient With Lung Cancer
- Patient With Pulmonary Embolism and Respiratory Failure

**Nursing Care Plans**

- eNursing Care Plan 27-1: Patient With Pneumonia
- eNursing Care Plan 27-2: Patient After Thoracotomy

**Conceptual Care Map Creator**

**Audio Glossary**

**Content Updates**

## REFERENCES


1. Centers for Disease Control and Prevention: Pneumonia deaths. Retrieved from *www.cdc.gov/nchs/fastats/pneumonia.htm.*
2. Centers for Disease Control and Prevention: Influenza deaths. Retrieved from *www.cdc.gov/nchs/fastats/flu.htm.*
3. Centers for Disease Control and Prevention: Pertussis (whooping cough): causes and transmission. Retrieved from *www.cdc.gov/pertussis/about/causes-transmission.html.*
4. American Lung Association: Influenza and pneumonia. Retrieved from *www.lung.org/assets/documents/publications/solddc-chapters/i-p.pdf.*
5. Centers for Disease Control and Prevention: Leading causes of death. Retrieved from *www.cdc.gov/nchs/fastats/leading-causes-of-death.htm.*
6. Kalanuria AA, Zai W, Mirski M: Ventilator-associated pneumonia in the ICU, *Crit Care* 18:208, 2014.
7. Löffler B, Niemann S, Ehrhardt C, et al: Pathogenesis of *Staphylococcus aureus* necrotizing pneumonia, *Expert Rev Anti Infect Ther* 11:1041, 2013.
8. Elborai Y: Management of cytomegalovirus (CMV) in hematopoietic stem cell transplant (HSCT), *J Pediatr Neonatal Care* 1:23, 2014.
9. Burgos J, Falcó V, Pahissa A: The increasing incidence of empyema, *Curr Opin Pulmonary Med* 19:350, 2013.
10. van Vugt SF, Broekhuizen BD, Lammens C, et al: Use of serum C reactive protein and procalcitonin concentrations in addition to symptoms and signs to predict pneumonia in patients presenting to primary care with acute cough: diagnostic study, *Br Med J* 346:f2450, 2013.

*11. Niu WY, Wan YG, Li MY, et al: The diagnostic value of serum procalcitonin, IL-10 and C-reactive protein in community-acquired pneumonia and tuberculosis, *Eur Rev Med Pharmacol Sci* 17:3329, 2013.

12. Joseph GG: Prognostic value of serum procalcitonin and C-reactive protein levels in critically ill patients who developed ventilator-associated pneumonia, *Ann Thorac Med* 10:137, 2015.
13. U.S. Food and Drug Administration: Influenza (flu) antiviral drugs and related information. Retrieved from *www.fda.gov/Drugs/DrugSafety/InformationbyDrugClass/ucm100228.htm#AntiviralMedications.*

*14. Keyt H, Faverio P, Restrepo MI: Prevention of ventilator-associated pneumonia in the intensive care unit: a review of clinically relevant recent advancements, *Indian J Med Res* 139:814, 2014.
15. Centers for Disease Control and Prevention: TB incidence in the United States, 1953-2013. Retrieved from *www.cdc.gov/tb/statistics/tbcases.htm.*
16. World Health Organization. Multidrug-resistant tuberculosis (MDR-TB): 2013 update. Retrieved from *www.who.int/tb/challenges/mdr/mdr_tb_factsheet.pdf?ua=1.*
17. Centers for Disease Control and Prevention: Tuberculosis (TB) fact sheets: skin testing. Retrieved from *www.cdc.gov/tb/publications/factsheets/testing/skintesting.htm.*
18. Joseph MR, Thomas RA, Nair S, et al: Directly observed treatment short course for tuberculosis. What happens to them in the long term? *Indian J Tuberc* 62:29, 2015.
19. Centers for Disease Control and Prevention: Tuberculosis (TB): treatment for latent TB infection. Retrieved from *www.cdc.gov/tb/topic/treatment/ltbi.htm.*
20. Centers for Disease Control and Prevention: The national personal protective technology laboratory (NPPTL): respirator trusted-source information. Section 3: Ancillary respirator information. Retrieved from *www.cdc.gov/niosh/npptl/topics/respirators/disp_part/RespSource3fittest.html#fith.*
21. Centers for Disease Control and Prevention: Fungal diseases: Valley fever (coccidioidomycosis). Retrieved from *www.cdc.gov/fungal/diseases/coccidioidomycosis.*
22. Centers for Disease Control and Prevention: Lung cancer. Retrieved from *www.cdc.gov/cancer/lung.*
23. American Lung Association: Lung cancer fact sheet. Retrieved from *www.lung.org/lung-disease/lung-cancer/resources/facts-figures/lung-cancer-fact-sheet.html.*
24. American Lung Association: Causes of cancer. Retrieved from *www.lung.org/associations/states/colorado/lung-disease/lung-cancer.html.*
25. Lung Cancer.Org: Lung cancer 101-Types and staging of lung cancer. Retrieved from *www.lungcancer.org/find_information/publications/163-lung_cancer_101/268-types_and_staging.*
*26. Blackmon SH, Feinglass SR: The United States Preventive Services Task Force Recommendations for Lung Cancer Screening, *Thorac Surg Clin* 25(2):199, 2015.
*27. Smith RA, Manassaram-Baptiste D, Brooks D, et al: Cancer screening in the United States, 2014: a review of current American Cancer Society guidelines and current issues in cancer screening, *CA Cancer J Clin* 64:30, 2014.
*28. Zhang W, Jiang W, Luan L, et al: Prophylactic cranial irradiation for patients with small-cell lung cancer: a systematic review of the literature with meta-analysis, *BMC Cancer* 14:793, 2014.
29. Mancini MC: Hemothorax. Retrieved from *emedicine.medscape.com/article/2047916-overview.*
30. Adams SD: Chylothorax. Retrieved from *emedicine.medscape.com/article/172527-overview.*
31. Hennon MW, Demmy TL: Video-assisted thoracoscopic surgery (VATS) for locally advanced lung cancer. Retrieved from *www.annalscts.com/article/view/476/608.*
32. British Lung Foundation: What is interstitial lung disease? Retrieved from *www.blf.org.uk/Page/What-is-interstitial-lung-disease.*
*33. Kistler KD, Nalysnyk L, Rotella P, et al: Lung transplantation in idiopathic pulmonary fibrosis: a systematic review of the literature, *BMC Pulm Med* 14:139, 2014.
*34. Guyatt GH, Akl EA, Crowther M, et al for the American College of Chest Physicians Antithrombotic Therapy and Prevention of Thrombosis Panel: Executive summary: Antithrombotic therapy and prevention of thrombosis, 9th ed: American College of Chest Physicians evidence-based clinical practice guidelines, *Chest* 141 (2 Suppl):7S, 2012.
35. Weinberg I, Jaff MR: Treating large pulmonary emboli: Do the guidelines guide us? *Curr Opin Pulmonary Med* 19:413, 2013.
36. Healthline Networks, Inc: The symptoms of pulmonary arterial hypertension. Retrieved from *www.healthline.com/health-slideshow/symptoms-pulmonary-arterial-hypertension#9.*

*Evidence-based information for clinical practice.

28

# Obstructive Pulmonary Diseases

*Susan Collazo*

*A nation that destroys its soils destroys itself. Forests are the lungs of our land, purifying the air and giving fresh strength to our people.*

**Franklin D. Roosevelt**

http://evolve.elsevier.com/Lewis/medsurg/

## LEARNING OUTCOMES

1. Describe the etiology, pathophysiology, clinical manifestations, and interprofessional care of asthma.
2. Describe the nursing management of the patient with asthma.
3. Describe the etiology, pathophysiology, clinical manifestations, and interprofessional care of the patient with chronic obstructive pulmonary disease (COPD).
4. Describe the effects of cigarette smoking on the lungs.
5. Identify the indications for $O_2$ therapy, methods of delivery, and complications of $O_2$ administration.
6. Explain the nursing management of the patient with COPD.
7. Describe the pathophysiology, clinical manifestations, interprofessional care, and nursing management of the patient with cystic fibrosis.
8. Describe the pathophysiology, clinical manifestations, interprofessional care, and nursing management of the patient with bronchiectasis.

## KEY TERMS

$\alpha_1$-antitrypsin (AAT) deficiency, p. 558
asthma, p. 539
bronchiectasis, p. 580
chest physiotherapy (CPT), p. 569
chronic bronchitis, p. 557
chronic obstructive pulmonary disease (COPD), p. 557
cor pulmonale, p. 560
cystic fibrosis (CF), p. 576
emphysema, p. 557
$O_2$ toxicity, p. 565
postural drainage, p. 570
pursed-lip breathing (PLB), p. 569

Imagine needing to consciously think about every breath that you take for minutes, hours, or even days. Many individuals with obstructive lung disease have this experience.

Approximately 31.5 million adult Americans are living with asthma or chronic obstructive pulmonary disease (COPD).[1,2]

Obstructive pulmonary disease, the most common chronic lung disease, is characterized by increased resistance to airflow as a result of airway obstruction or airway narrowing. Types of obstructive lung diseases include asthma, COPD, cystic fibrosis (CF), and bronchiectasis. *Asthma* is a lung disease that causes inflammation with variable episodes of airflow obstruction, but it is usually reversible. *COPD* is an obstructive pulmonary disease with progressive limitation in airflow that is not fully reversible. The patient with asthma has variations in airflow over time, usually with normal lung function between exacerbations. In contrast, the limitation in expiratory airflow in the patient with COPD is generally more constant. The pathophysiology of asthma and the response to therapy differ from those associated with COPD. However, the patient with a diagnosis of obstructive pulmonary disease may have features of both asthma and COPD. Patients with asthma who have less responsive reversible airflow obstruction are difficult to distinguish from COPD patients.

*Cystic fibrosis,* another form of obstructive pulmonary disease, is a genetic disorder. It produces airway obstruction because of changes in exocrine glandular secretions, resulting in increased mucus production.

*Bronchiectasis* is an obstructive disease characterized by dilated bronchioles, making it difficult to clear secretions. It most frequently results from untreated or poorly treated pulmonary infections, immune system problems, or genetic factors.

*Acknowledgment:* We would like to acknowledge the contributions of Jane Kaufman, MS, CRNP, ANP-BC, Advanced Senior Lecturer, University of Pennsylvania School of Nursing, Philadelphia, Pennsylvania, to this chapter over the past four editions of the book.
Reviewed by Marilyn Borkgren, APN, MS, CCNS, Pulmonary APN, Suburban Lung Associates, Elk Grove Village, Illinois; Kim Clevenger, RN, EdD, BC, Associate Professor of Nursing, BSN Program Coordinator, Morehead State University, Morehead, Kentucky; Deborah Cline, RN, MS, Nursing Faculty, Carrington College, Reno, Nevada; Marianne Ferrin, MSN, ACNP-BC, Coordinator Penn Lung Center, Adult Cystic Fibrosis Program, Philadelphia, Pennsylvania; Jane Kaufman, MS, CRNP, ANP-BC, Advanced Senior Lecturer, University of Pennsylvania School of Nursing, Philadelphia, Pennsylvania; Eugene E. Mondor, RN, MN, CNCC(C), Clinical Nurse Educator–Adult Critical Care, Royal Alexandra Hospital, Edmonton, Alberta, Canada; Cynthia M. Steinwedel, RN, PhD, CNE, Assistant Professor, Department of Nursing, Bradley University, Peoria, Illinois; and Kenneth Wysocki, PhD, FNP-BC, FAANP, Family Nurse Practitioner, Asthma and Genetics Researcher, Clinical Services, Matrix Medical Network, Scottsdale, Arizona.

## GENDER DIFFERENCES

### Asthma

**Men**
- Before puberty, more boys are affected than girls.

**Women**
- After puberty and into adulthood, more women are affected than men.
- Women who are admitted to the emergency department are more likely to need hospitalization than men.
- Death rate from asthma is greater in women than in men.

## CULTURAL & ETHNIC HEALTH DISPARITIES

### Obstructive Pulmonary Diseases

**Asthma**
- Asthma prevalence rates are more than 38% higher among African Americans than whites.
- Puerto Ricans have higher asthma prevalence rates and age-adjusted death rates than all other racial and ethnic subgroups.
- Female African Americans have the highest mortality rates from asthma among all ethnic/gender groups.

**Chronic Obstructive Pulmonary Disease (COPD)**
- Whites have the highest incidence of COPD despite higher rates of smoking among other ethnic groups.
- Hispanics have lower death rates related to COPD than other ethnic groups.

**Cystic Fibrosis**
- Whites have the highest incidence of cystic fibrosis.
- Cystic fibrosis is uncommon among African Americans, Hispanics, and Asian Americans.

## ASTHMA

**Asthma** is a heterogenous disease characterized by a combination of clinical manifestations along with reversible expiratory airflow limitation or bronchial hyperresponsiveness. The variability of signs and symptoms can include episodes of wheezing, breathlessness, chest tightness, and cough, particularly at night or in the early morning. These episodes are associated with widespread but variable airflow obstruction that is usually reversible, either spontaneously or with treatment. The clinical course of asthma is unpredictable, ranging from periods of adequate control to exacerbations with poor control of symptoms.[3]

Asthma affects an estimated 18.8 million adult Americans. Among adults, women are 62% more likely to have asthma than men. Asthma is a public health concern, with more than 14.2 million lost workdays in adults. However, the good news is that after a long period of an increasing incidence of asthma, the mortality and use of health care services for asthma are continuing to plateau and/or decrease. Despite the decline in the number of deaths from asthma over the past 10 years, more than 3300 people yearly still die from asthma.[1]

### Risk Factors for Asthma and Triggers of Asthma Attacks

Risk factors for asthma and triggers of asthma attacks can be related to the patient (e.g., genetic factors) or the environment (e.g., pollen) (Table 28-1). Male gender is a risk factor for asthma in children, but not adults. Obesity is also a risk factor for asthma.[4] Other factors and triggers are discussed in this section.

**TABLE 28-1 Triggers of Asthma Attacks**

**Allergen Inhalation**
- Animal dander (e.g., cats, mice, guinea pigs)
- Cockroaches
- House dust mite
- Molds
- Pollens

**Air Pollutants**
- Aerosol sprays
- Cigarette smoke
- Exhaust fumes
- Oxidants
- Perfumes
- Sulfur dioxides

**Viral or Bacterial Infection**
- Sinusitis, allergic rhinitis
- Viral upper respiratory tract infection

**Drugs**
- β-Adrenergic blockers
- Aspirin
- Nonsteroidal antiinflammatory drugs

**Occupational Exposure**
- Agriculture, farming
- Industrial chemicals and plastics
- Laundry detergents
- Metal salts
- Paints, solvents
- Pharmaceutical agents
- Wood and vegetable dusts

**Food Additives**
- Beer, wine, dried fruit, shrimp, processed potatoes
- Monosodium glutamate
- Sulfites (bisulfites and metabisulfites)
- Tartrazine

**Other Factors**
- Exercise and cold, dry air
- Gastroesophageal reflux disease (GERD)
- Hormones, menses
- Stress

**Genetics.** Asthma has a component that is inherited, but the genetics are complex. Numerous genes may be involved in the development of asthma and a person's response to various asthma medications.[3,4] *Atopy,* the genetic predisposition to develop an allergic (immunoglobulin E [IgE]–mediated) response to common allergens, is a major risk factor for asthma.

**Immune Response.** The *hygiene hypothesis* suggests that a newborn baby's immune system must be conditioned so that it will function properly during infancy and the rest of life. People who have a lower incidence of asthma are exposed to certain infections early in life, use few antibiotics, are exposed to other children (e.g., siblings, day care), or live in rural settings or with pets. People for whom these factors are not present in childhood have a higher incidence of asthma.[3]

**Allergens.** Indoor and outdoor allergens, such as cockroaches, furry animals, fungi, pollen, and molds, can trigger asthma attacks. However, their role in the actual development of asthma is not as clear.[3,4]

**Exercise.** Asthma that is induced or exacerbated during physical exertion is called *exercise-induced asthma* (EIA) or *exercise-induced bronchospasm* (EIB). Typically, EIB occurs after vigorous exercise, not during it (e.g., jogging, aerobics, walking briskly, climbing stairs). Symptoms of EIA are pronounced during activities where there is exposure to cold, dry air. For example, swimming in an indoor heated pool is less likely to produce symptoms than downhill skiing. Airway obstruction may occur due to changes in the airway mucosa caused by hyperventilation during exercise, with either cooling or rewarming of air and capillary leakage in the airway wall.

**Air Pollutants.** Various air pollutants, such as cigarette or wood smoke or vehicle exhaust, can trigger asthma attacks. In heavily industrialized or densely populated areas, climatic conditions often lead to concentrated pollution in the atmosphere, especially with thermal inversions and stagnant air masses. Ozone alert days are regularly noted on the news reports, and patients should minimize outdoor activity during these times. Cigarette smoking is associated with an accelerated decline of lung functioning in a person with asthma, increases the severity of the disease, may cause the patient to be less responsive to treatment, and reduces the chance of the asthma being controlled. Despite the relationship of pollutants in triggering asthma attacks, the role of outdoor air pollution as a cause of asthma development remains controversial.[4]

**Occupational Factors.** *Occupational asthma* is the most common occupational respiratory disorder, with up to 15% of new asthma cases arising from job-related exposures to more than 300 agents.[4,5] Irritants cause a change in the responsiveness of the airways. However, the development of symptoms from this alteration may not occur until the patient has had months to years of exposure. Occupations with a high risk of occupational asthma include agricultural worker, baker, hospital worker, plastics manufacturer, and beautician. Characteristically people with occupational asthma give a history of arriving at work feeling well but gradually develop symptoms by the end of the day.

**Respiratory Tract Infections.** Respiratory tract infections (i.e., viral and not bacterial) are often the major precipitating factor of an acute asthma attack. Acute infection can increase airway narrowing and airway hyperresponsiveness. Viral-induced alterations of epithelial cells, increased inflammatory cell accumulation, edema of airway walls, and exposure of airway nerve endings contribute to altered airway function. These alterations in airway function may exacerbate asthma.

**Nose and Sinus Problems.** Most patients with asthma have a history of allergic rhinitis. Treatment of allergic rhinitis usually improves the symptoms of asthma. Additional information on the relationship of rhinitis and asthma can be found at *www.whiar.org*.

Acute and chronic sinusitis, especially allergic rhinosinusitis, may worsen asthma. Some patients with asthma have chronic sinus problems that cause inflammation of the mucous membranes. Sinusitis must be treated and large nasal polyps removed for an asthma patient to have good control. (Sinusitis is discussed in Chapter 26.)

**Drugs and Food Additives.** Sensitivity to specific drugs may occur in some people, especially those with nasal polyps and sinusitis. Some people with asthma have what is termed the *asthma triad:* nasal polyps, asthma, and sensitivity to aspirin and nonsteroidal antiinflammatory drugs (NSAIDs). Salicylic acid can be found in many over-the-counter (OTC) drugs and some foods, beverages, and flavorings. Some asthmatics who use aspirin or NSAIDs (e.g., ibuprofen [Motrin]) develop wheezing within 2 hours. In addition, there is usually profound rhinorrhea, congestion, tearing, and even angioedema. Avoidance of aspirin and NSAIDs is required. However, patients with aspirin sensitivity under the care of an allergist can be desensitized by daily administration of the drug.

β-Adrenergic blockers in oral form (e.g., metoprolol [Toprol XL]) or topical eye drops (e.g., timolol [Timoptic]) may trigger asthma because they can cause bronchospasm. Angiotensin-converting enzyme (ACE) inhibitors (e.g., lisinopril [Prinivil]) may produce cough in susceptible individuals, thus making asthma symptoms worse.

Other agents that may precipitate asthma in the susceptible patient are tartrazine (yellow dye no. 5, found in many foods) and sulfiting agents widely used in the food and pharmaceutical industries as preservatives and sanitizing agents. Sulfiting agents are commonly found in fruits, beer, and wine and used extensively in salad bars to protect vegetables from oxidation. Asthma exacerbations can occur after the use of sulfite-containing preservatives found in topical ophthalmic solutions, IV corticosteroids, and some inhaled bronchodilator solutions.

Food allergies triggering asthma reactions in adults are rare. Avoidance diets are not recommended until an allergy has been demonstrated, usually by oral challenges performed by a specialized HCP provider, such as an allergist.

**Gastroesophageal Reflux Disease.** Gastroesophageal reflux disease (GERD) is more common in people with asthma than in the general population. GERD may worsen asthma symptoms because reflux may trigger bronchoconstriction and cause aspiration. Asthma medications may worsen GERD symptoms. $\beta_2$-Agonists (especially given orally), which are used to treat asthma, relax the lower esophageal sphincter, thus allowing stomach contents to reflux into the esophagus and possibly be aspirated into the lungs. Effective treatment for GERD in an asthma patient can improve nocturnal asthma control, quality of life, and possibly exacerbations in these patients.[4,6] (GERD is discussed in Chapter 41.)

**Psychologic Factors.** Asthma is not a psychosomatic disease. However, many people with asthma report that symptoms worsen with stress. Certainly psychologic factors cause bronchoconstriction via stimulation of the cholinergic reflex pathways. Extreme emotional expressions (e.g., crying, laughing, anger, fear) can lead to hyperventilation and hypocapnia, which can cause airway narrowing.[4]

An asthma attack caused by any triggering event can produce panic, stress, and anxiety. However, it varies from patient to patient and in the same patient from episode to episode.

## Pathophysiology

The primary pathophysiologic process in asthma is persistent but variable inflammation of the airways. The airflow is limited because the inflammation results in bronchoconstriction, airway hyperresponsiveness (hyperreactivity), and edema of the airways. Exposure to allergens or irritants initiates the inflammatory cascade (Fig. 28-1). A variety of inflammatory cells are involved, including mast cells, macrophages, eosinophils, neutrophils, T and B lymphocytes, and epithelial cells of the airways.

As the inflammatory process begins, mast cells (found beneath the basement membrane of the bronchial wall) degranulate and release multiple inflammatory mediators (Fig. 28-2). IgE antibodies are linked to mast cells, and the allergen cross-links the IgE. Then inflammatory mediators such as leukotrienes, histamine, cytokines, prostaglandins, and nitric oxide are released. Some inflammatory mediators have effects on the (1) blood vessels, causing vasodilation and increasing capillary permeability (runny nose), (2) nerve cells causing itching, (3) smooth muscle cells causing bronchial spasms and airway narrowing, and (4) goblet cells causing mucus production (Fig. 28-3). This whole process is sometimes referred to as the *early-phase response* in asthma. Clinically it can occur within 30 to 60 minutes after exposure to an allergen or irritant.

Symptoms can recur 4 to 6 hours after the early response because of the influx of many inflammatory cells, which are set in motion by the initial response. At this later time the patient may develop symptoms again or worsening of symptoms. This

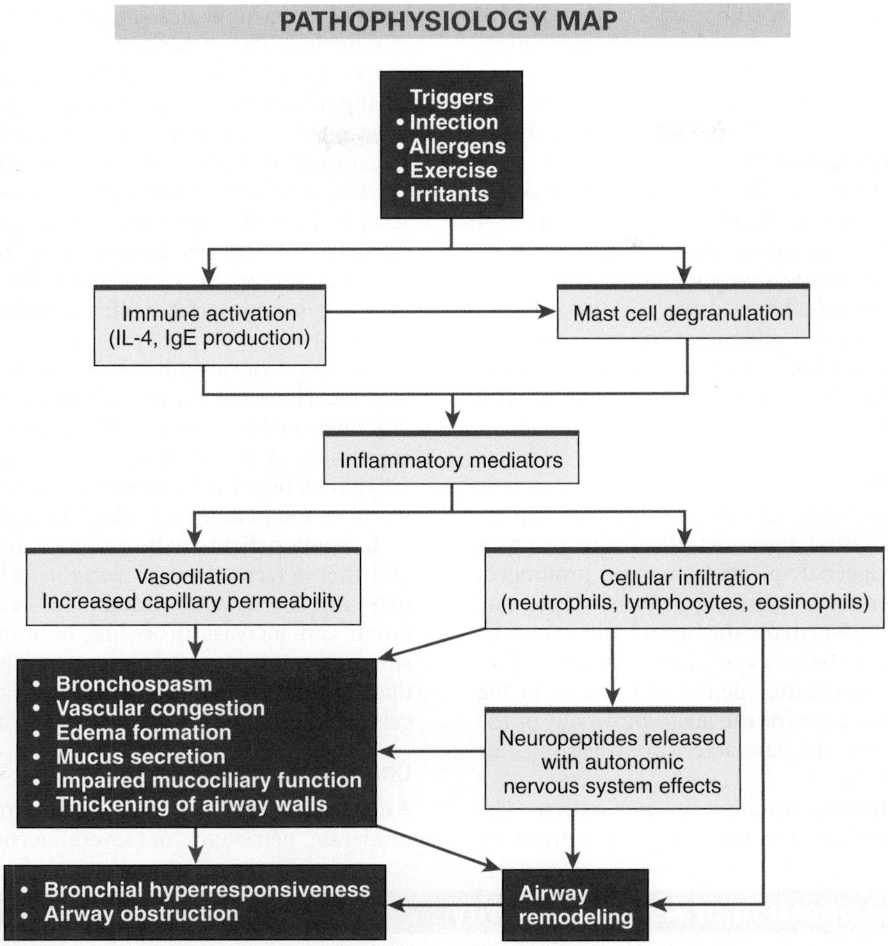


**FIG. 28-1** Pathophysiology of asthma. *IL,* Interleukin. (Adapted from McCance KL, Huether SE, editors: *Pathophysiology: the biologic basis for disease in adults and children,* ed 6, St Louis, 2010, Mosby.)

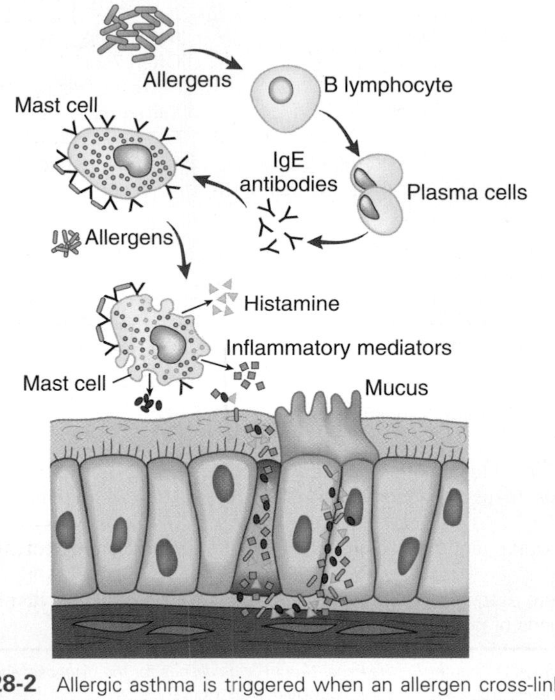


**FIG. 28-2** Allergic asthma is triggered when an allergen cross-links IgE receptors on mast cells, which are then activated to release histamine and other inflammatory mediators (early-phase response). A late-phase response may occur due to further inflammation.

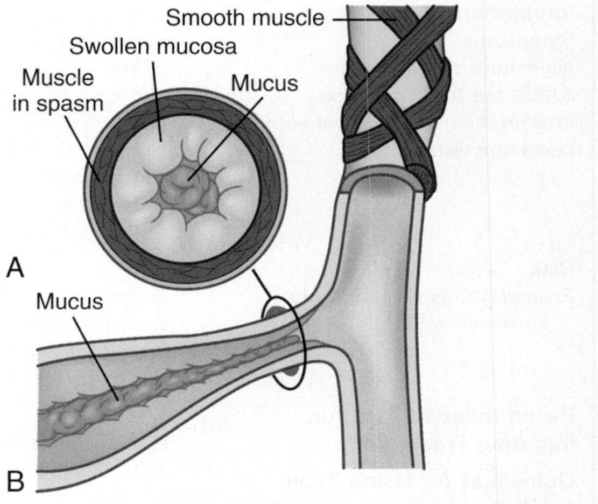


**FIG. 28-3** Factors causing obstruction (especially expiratory obstruction) in asthma. **A,** Cross section of a bronchiole occluded by muscle spasm, swollen mucosa, and mucus in the lumen. **B,** Longitudinal section of a bronchiole. (Redrawn from Price SA, Wilson LM: *Pathophysiology: clinical concepts of disease processes,* ed 6, St Louis, 2003, Mosby.)

is called the *late-phase response*, which occurs in about 50% of individuals with asthma. In this late-phase response, more inflammatory cells are recruited and activated, with continuing inflammation of the airways. Thus bronchoconstriction with symptoms persists for 24 hours or more. Corticosteroids are effective in treating this inflammation.

Chronic inflammation may result in structural changes in the bronchial wall known as *remodeling*. A progressive loss of lung function occurs that is not prevented or fully reversed by therapy. The changes in structure may include fibrosis of the subepithelium, smooth muscle hypertrophy of the airways, mucus hypersecretion, continued inflammation, and *angiogenesis* (proliferation of new blood vessels). Remodeling is thought to explain why some individuals have persistent asthma and limited response to therapy.[3,4]

## Clinical Manifestations

The characteristic clinical manifestations of asthma are wheezing, cough, dyspnea, and chest tightness after exposure to a precipitating factor or trigger. Expiration may be prolonged. Instead of a normal inspiratory-expiratory ratio of 1 : 2, it may be prolonged to 1 : 3 or 1 : 4. Normally the bronchioles constrict during expiration. However, the airways become narrower than usual as a result of bronchospasm, edema, and mucus in the bronchioles. Thus it takes longer for the air to move out of the bronchioles. This produces the characteristic wheezing, air trapping, and hyperinflation.

Asthma signs and symptoms can differ for each patient. The most common manifestations include cough, shortness of breath (dyspnea), wheezing, chest tightness, and variable airflow obstruction. The presence of any of these (usually in combination) can indicate that an asthma episode or attack is occurring. Changes have taken place to trigger the airways, and airflow is obstructed. A cough, either dry or productive, may be present specifically at night and early morning or after laughing or playing sports. Symptoms are variable both in frequency and severity in each individual asthma patient at any time. The frequency of nocturnal awakenings due to cough, wheezing, or dyspnea is used as an indicator for the severity of asthma. Symptoms can interfere with the patient's ADLs as they increase in severity.

The physical examination in people with asthma is often normal. The most common finding is expiratory wheezing on auscultation but may be absent or only heard during forced expiration. A runny nose, swollen nasal passages, and nasal polyps can be present. An examination of the patient's skin may reveal eczema and hives, which have been linked to asthma.

In some patients with asthma, cough is the only symptom, and this is termed *cough variant asthma*. The bronchospasm may not be severe enough to cause airflow obstruction, but it can increase bronchial tone and cause irritation with stimulation of the cough receptors. The cough may be nonproductive or with secretions, which may be thick, tenacious, white, gelatinous mucus, which makes their removal difficult.

## Classification of Asthma

Asthma can be classified as intermittent, mild persistent, moderate persistent, or severe persistent (Table 28-2). The

**TABLE 28-2 Classification of Asthma Severity**

| | ASTHMA SEVERITY | | | |
|---|---|---|---|---|
| | | PERSISTENT | | |
| **Components of Severity** | **Intermittent** | **Mild** | **Moderate** | **Severe** |
| **Impairment** | | | | |
| **Symptoms** | ≤2 days/wk | >2 days/wk, not daily | Daily | Continuous |
| **Nighttime awakenings** | ≤2/mo | 3-4/mo | >1/wk, not nightly | Often 7/wk |
| **SABA use for symptoms** | ≤2 days/wk | >2 days/wk, not daily | Daily | Several times per day |
| **Interference with normal activity** | None | Minor limitation | Some limitation | Extremely limited |
| **Lung function*** | Normal $FEV_1$ between exacerbations<br>$FEV_1$ >80%<br>$FEV_1$/FVC normal | $FEV_1$ >80% predicted<br>$FEV_1$/FVC normal | $FEV_1$ 60%-80% predicted<br>$FEV_1$/FVC reduced by 5% | $FEV_1$ <60% predicted<br>$FEV_1$/FVC reduced by 5% |
| **Risk** | | | | |
| **Exacerbations requiring oral corticosteroids** | 0-1/yr | ≥2/yr even in the absence of impairment. | | |
| | Consider severity and interval since last exacerbation. → | | | |
| | Frequency and severity may fluctuate over time. → | | | |
| | Relative annual risk of exacerbation may be related to $FEV_1$. → | | | |
| **Recommended Step for Initiating Treatment** | Step 1 | Step 2 | Step 3† | Step 4 or 5† |
| | Reevaluate asthma control in 2-6 wk and adjust therapy accordingly. | | | |

**Guidelines for Using Table**
- Patients should be assigned to the most severe step in which any feature occurs. Clinical features for individual patients may overlap across steps. Determine level of severity by assessment of both impairment and risk. Assess impairment by patient's recall of previous 2- to 4-wk spirometry results.
- An individual's classification should change over time as treatment is initiated. After treatment, the focus switches to the level of control, not the classification of severity.
- Patients at any level of severity of chronic asthma can have mild, moderate, or severe exacerbations of asthma. Some patients with intermittent asthma experience severe and life-threatening exacerbations separated by long periods of normal lung function and no symptoms.

Source: Adapted from National Asthma Education and Prevention Program, National Heart, Lung, and Blood Institute: *Expert Panel Report 3: guidelines for the diagnosis and management of asthma*, NIH pub no 08-4051, Bethesda, Md, 2007, National Institutes of Health. Retrieved from *www.nhlbi.nih.gov/guidelines*.
*$FEV_1$*, Forced expiratory volume in 1 sec; *FVC*, forced vital capacity; *SABA*, short-acting $\beta_2$-adrenergic agonist.
*Percent predicted values for $FEV_1$ or ratio of $FEV_1$/FVC. Normal $FEV_1$/FVC: 8-19 yr, 85%; 20-39 yr, 80%; 40-59 yr, 75%; 60-80 yr, 70%.
†Consider short-term corticosteroid therapy.

classification system is used to determine the treatment. Patients may move to different asthma classifications over the course of their disease.

## Complications

Asthma exacerbations may occur and are classified as mild, moderate, severe, or life-threatening. Asthma is characterized by an unpredictable and variable course, with a person's asthma attacks ranging from seemingly minor interferences in breathing to life-threatening episodes. Depending on an individual's response, asthma can rapidly progress from normal breathing to acute severe or life-threatening asthma.

An attack of asthma may have an abrupt onset, but usually symptoms occur more gradually. Attacks may last for a few minutes to several hours. Between attacks, the patient may be asymptomatic with normal or near-normal spirometry, depending on the severity of disease. However, in some people, compromised pulmonary function (indicated by abnormal spirometry results) may lead to a state of continuous symptoms and chronic debilitation characterized by irreversible airway disease. Acute exacerbations of asthma are discussed in Table 28-7 later in this chapter in the section on Interprofessional Care on p. 546.

## Diagnostic Studies

Underdiagnosis of asthma is common. A detailed history is important to determine if a person has had similar attacks, which are often precipitated by a known trigger. (Triggers are discussed on pp. 539-540.) Because wheezing and cough are seen with a variety of disorders (e.g., COPD, GERD, vocal cord dysfunction, heart failure), it is important to determine if asthma is the cause of these problems. (A comparison of asthma and COPD is presented in Table 28-3.)

Numerous tests that are used to diagnose asthma are presented in Table 28-4. In general, the HCP should consider the diagnosis of asthma if various indicators (i.e., clinical manifestations, health history, peak flow variability or spirometry) are positive.

The peak expiratory flow rate (PEFR) measured by the peak flow meter (at home or in a health care setting) is an aid to diagnose and monitor asthma. However, PEFR measurements are not interchangeable with other lung measurements of lung function (e.g., forced expiratory volume in 1 second [$FEV_1$]). Since types of peak flow meters vary, PEFR should be compared with the patient's own previous best measurements using their own meter.

Spirometry (measured in a health care setting) is usually normal between asthma attacks if the patient has no other underlying pulmonary disease. However, the patient with asthma may show an obstructive pattern including a decrease in forced vital capacity (FVC), $FEV_1$, PEFR, and $FEV_1$ to FVC ratio ($FEV_1$/FVC). (The normal values for spirometry and pulmonary function tests are discussed in Table 25-13 and Chapter 25.)

When spirometry is scheduled, ask the patient to stop taking any bronchodilator medications for 6 to 12 hours before the tests. Spirometry can be done before and after the administration of a bronchodilator to determine the degree of the response. This may help determine reversibility of airway obstruction, which is critical information for diagnosing asthma. A positive response to the bronchodilator is an increase of more than 200 mL and an increase of more than 12% between preadministration and postadministration values.

### TABLE 28-3 Comparison of Asthma and COPD*

| | Asthma | COPD |
|---|---|---|
| **Clinical Features** | | |
| Age | Usually <40 yr (onset). | Usually 40-50 yr (onset). |
| Smoking history | Not causal. | Often long history (>10-20 pack-years). |
| Health and family history | Presence of allergy, rhinitis, eczema. Family history of asthma. | Infrequent allergies. May have exposure to environmental pollutants. With $\alpha_1$-antitrypsin deficiency, family history of lung or liver disease without smoking history. |
| Clinical symptoms | Intermittent, vary day to day, worse at night or early morning. | Slowly progressive and persistent. |
| Dyspnea | Absent except in exacerbations or poor control. | Dyspnea during exercise. |
| Sputum | Infrequent. | Often. |
| Disease course | Stable (with exacerbations). | Progressive worsening (with exacerbations). |
| **Diagnostic Study Results** | | |
| ABGs | Normal between or during exacerbations. | Between exacerbations in advanced COPD<br>• Often low-normal pH and $PaO_2$<br>• High-normal $PaCO_2$ with high $HCO_3^-$ (compensated respiratory acidosis) |
| pH | ↑ Early in exacerbation, then ↓ if prolonged or severe exacerbation. | N→↓ |
| $PaO_2$ | ↓ | N→↓ |
| $PaCO_2$ | ↓ Early in exacerbation, then ↑ if prolonged or severe exacerbation. | N→↑ |
| Chest x-ray | May reveal hyperinflation. | Hyperinflation. May have cardiac enlargement, flattened diaphragm. |
| Lung volumes | Often normalizes. | Never normalizes. |
| • Total lung capacity | Increased. | Increased. |
| • Residual volume | Increased. | Increased. |
| • $FEV_1$ | Decreased or normal. | Decreased. |
| • $FEV_1$/FVC | Normal to decreased. | Decreased (<70%). |

*ABGs*, Arterial blood gases; *$FEV_1$*, forced expiratory volume in 1 sec; *FVC*, forced vital capacity.
*Individuals may have features of both asthma and COPD.

Some patients with symptoms of asthma have normal lung function. During an exacerbation of asthma, lung function parameters fall from their baseline levels.

An elevated serum eosinophil count and elevated serum IgE levels are highly suggestive of *atopy* (genetic predisposition to develop an allergic response), which may be a risk factor for asthma. Allergy skin testing may be of some value to determine sensitivity to specific allergens. However, a positive skin test does not necessarily mean that the allergen is causing the asthma attack. On the other hand, a negative allergy test does not mean that the asthma is not allergy related. (Allergy testing is discussed in Chapter 13.)

A chest x-ray in an asymptomatic patient with asthma is usually normal but can tell if something else (i.e., pneumonia, foreign body in the airway) could be causing symptoms similar to asthma. A routine chest x-ray in a patient with asthma is usually not done unless additional manifestations are present such as fever, chills, or upper airway stridor.

**TABLE 28-4 Interprofessional Care**

***Asthma***

**Diagnostic Assessment**

- History and physical examination
- Spirometry, including response to bronchodilator therapy
- Peak expiratory flow rate (PEFR)
- Chest x-ray
- Measurement of oximetry
- Allergy skin testing (if indicated)
- Blood level of eosinophils and IgE (if indicated)

**Management**

***Intermittent or Persistent Asthma***

- Identification and avoidance or elimination of triggers
- Patient and caregiver teaching
- Drug therapy (Tables 28-6 and 28-8 and Fig. 28-4)
- Asthma action plan (Fig. 28-8)
- Desensitization (immunotherapy) if indicated
- Assess for control (e.g., Asthma Control Test [ACT])*

***Acute Exacerbations*** *(Table 28-7)*

- $SaO_2$ monitoring
- ABGs
- Inhaled $\beta_2$-adrenergic agonists
- Inhaled anticholinergics
- $O_2$ by nasal cannula or mask
- IV or oral corticosteroids
- IV fluids
- IV magnesium
- Intubation and assisted ventilation

*ABGs,* Arterial blood gases; *IgE,* immunoglobulin E; *$SaO_2$,* $O_2$ saturation.
*See *www.asthmacontroltest.com.*

### Interprofessional Care

The goal of asthma treatment is to achieve and maintain control of the disease. Once the patient is diagnosed, guidelines provide direction on classification of asthma severity (Table 28-2) and which medications (based on steps 1 through 6) the patient requires (Table 28-5 and Fig. 28-4). The current guidelines focus on (1) assessing the severity of the disease at diagnosis and initial treatment and then (2) monitoring periodically to control the disease.[3,4]

At the initial diagnosis, a patient may have severe asthma and require steps 4 through 6 asthma medication. After treatment, the patient's level of control is assessed (i.e., well controlled, not well controlled, or very poorly controlled; Table 28-5). The HCP steps down the medication as the patient achieves control of the symptoms or steps it up if the symptoms worsen. Achieving rapid control of the symptoms is the goal to return the patient to his or her daily functioning at the best possible level (Fig. 28-4).

Validated questionnaires (e.g., Asthma Control Test [ACT] available at *www.asthmacontroltest.com*) can be used to assess quality-of-life issues in asthma patients. The level of control is determined by the patient's current peak flow or $FEV_1$. In addition, any exacerbations or adverse effects of treatment will determine the level of control.

**Intermittent and Persistent Asthma.** The classification of severity of asthma at initial diagnosis helps determine which types of drugs are best suited to control the asthma symptoms (Tables 28-2 and 28-5). Patients in all classifications of asthma require a short-term (rescue or reliever) medication. Short-acting $\beta_2$-adrenergic agonists (SABAs) (e.g., albuterol [ProAir HFA, Proventil HFA, Ventolin HFA]) are the most effective class of drugs used as rescue or reliever medications. Patients with persistent asthma must also be on a long-term or controller medication (Table 28-6). Inhaled corticosteroids (ICSs) (e.g., fluticasone [Flovent Diskus or HFA]) are the most effective class of drugs to treat the inflammation. (See later section on drug therapy in this chapter.)

**TABLE 28-5 Components of Asthma Control**

| | CLASSIFICATION OF ASTHMA CONTROL | | |
|---|---|---|---|
| **Components of Control** | **Well Controlled** | **Not Well Controlled** | **Very Poorly Controlled** |
| **Impairment** | | | |
| **Symptoms** | ≤2 days/wk | >2 days/wk | Throughout the day |
| **Nighttime awakenings** | ≤2/mo | 1-3/wk | ≥4/wk |
| **Interference with normal activity** | None | Some limitation | Extremely limited |
| **SABA use** | ≤2 days/wk | >2 days/wk | Several times/day |
| **$FEV_1$ or peak flow** | >80% predicted/personal best | 60%-80% predicted/personal best | <60% predicted/personal best |
| **Risk** | | | |
| **Exacerbations requiring oral corticosteroids** | 0-1/yr | ≥2/yr | ≥2/yr |
| **Progressive loss of lung function** | Consider severity and interval since last exacerbation. → | | |
| **Treatment-related adverse effects** | Evaluation requires long-term follow-up. → Can vary in intensity from none to very troublesome and worrisome. Level of intensity does not correlate to specific levels of control but should be considered in the overall assessment of risk. → | | |
| **Recommended Action for Treatment** (Based on assessment of control) | • Maintain current step.<br>• Regular follow-up every 1-6 mo to maintain control<br>• Consider step down if well controlled for at least 3 mo. | • Step up one step.<br>• Reevaluate in 2-6 wk.<br>• For side effects, consider alternative treatment options. | • Consider oral corticosteroids.<br>• Step up one or two steps and reevaluate in 2 wk.<br>• For side effects, consider alternative treatment options. |

Source: Adapted from National Asthma Education and Prevention Program, National Heart, Lung, and Blood Institute: *Expert Panel Report 3: guidelines for the diagnosis and management of asthma,* NIH pub no 08-4051, Bethesda, Md, 2007, National Institutes of Health. Retrieved from *www.nhlbi.nih.gov/guidelines.*
*$FEV_1$,* Forced expiratory volume in 1 sec; *SABA,* short-acting $\beta_2$-adrenergic agonist.

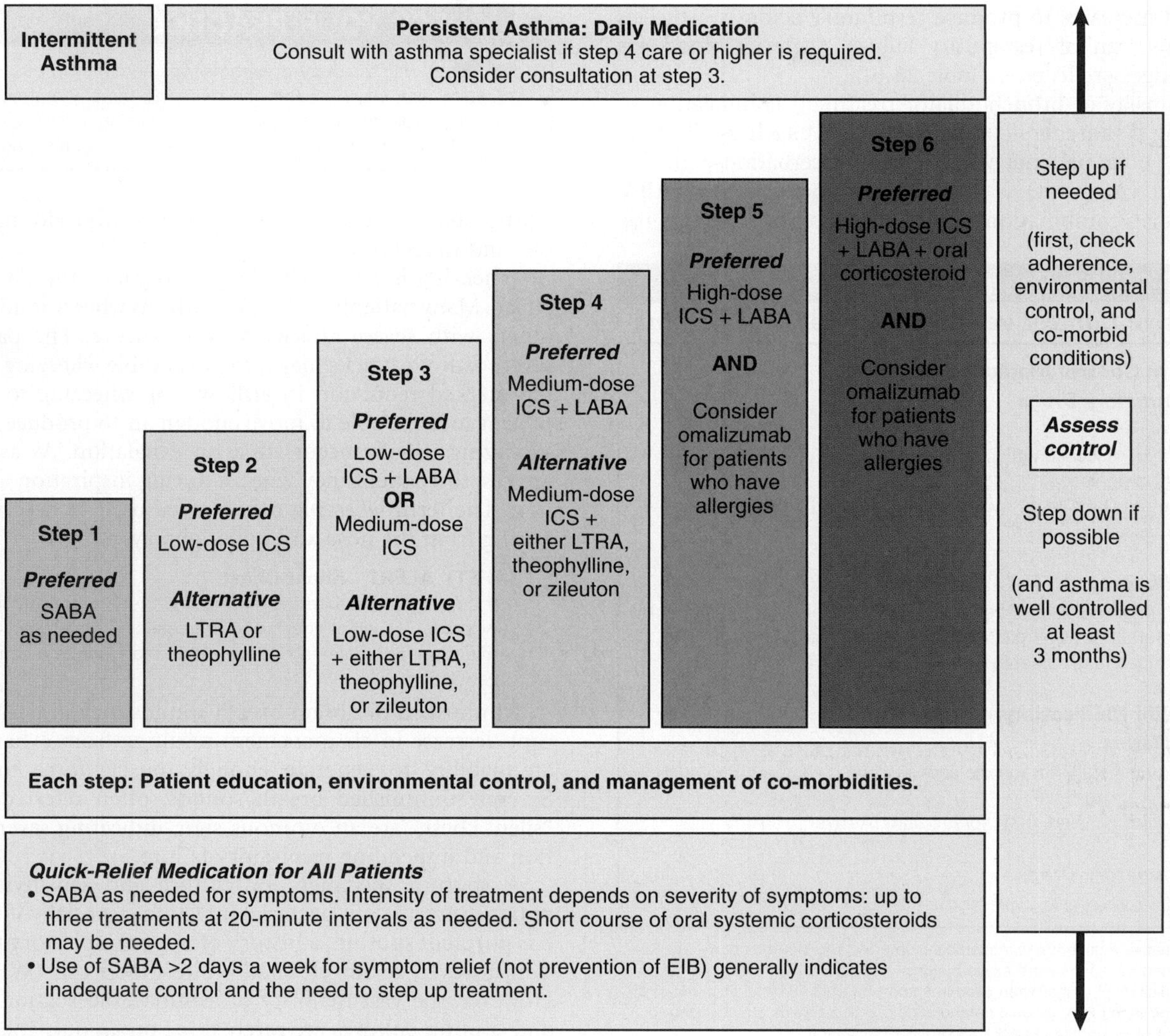


*EIB*, Exercise-induced bronchospasm; *ICS*, inhaled corticosteroid; *LABA*, long-acting inhaled $\beta_2$-agonist; *LTRA*, leukotriene receptor antagonist; *SABA*, short-acting inhaled $\beta_2$-agonist.

**FIG. 28-4** Drug therapy: stepwise approach for managing asthma. (Modified from *Expert Panel Report 3: Guidelines for the Diagnosis and Management of Asthma.* Bethesda, Md, 2007, National Asthma Education and Prevention Program, National Heart, Lung, and Blood Institute.)

**Acute Asthma Exacerbations.** Acute asthma exacerbations can be classified as mild, moderate, severe, or life-threatening (Table 28-7). During an acute attack, the person sits forward to maximize the diaphragmatic movement with prominent wheezing, a respiratory rate higher than 30 breaths/minute, and pulse greater than 120 beats/minute. Accessory muscles in the neck are straining to lift the chest wall, and the patient is often agitated (from hypoxemia). Percussion of the lungs indicates hyperresonance. Auscultation of the lungs indicates inspiratory or expiratory wheezing. As the episode resolves, coughing produces thick, stringy mucus.

If a patient has wheezing and acute distress, it is not feasible to obtain a detailed health history (although a family member may supply some pertinent information). Continuous monitoring of the patient is critical. During an acute attack of asthma, bedside PEFR may be used to monitor airflow obstruction. Serial PEFR results, oximetry, and measurement of ABGs provide information about the severity of the attack and the response to therapy. These objective measures more reliably indicate the severity of the exacerbation than symptoms do. A few patients perceive asthma symptoms poorly and may have a significant decrease in lung function without any change in symptoms. Obtaining a PEFR during a severe asthma attack is usually not possible. However, if it can be obtained, and it is less than 200 L/min, it indicates severe obstruction in all but very small adults.

Management of the patient with acute exacerbations focuses on correcting hypoxemia and improving ventilation. $O_2$ monitoring should be continuous with pulse oximetry. Supplemental $O_2$ is given by nasal cannula or mask to achieve a $PaO_2$ of at least 60 mm Hg or $O_2$ saturation greater than 90%.

Hyperventilation occurs during an asthma attack as lung receptors respond to increased lung volume from trapped air and airflow limitation. Decreased perfusion and ventilation of the alveoli and increased alveolar gas pressure lead to ventilation-perfusion abnormalities in the lungs. The patient is hypoxemic early on with decreased $PaCO_2$ and increased pH (respiratory alkalosis) because he or she is hyperventilating. As the airflow limitation worsens with air trapping, the patient works much harder to breathe. The $PaCO_2$ normalizes as the patient tires, and then it increases to produce respiratory acidosis, which is an ominous sign of respiratory failure. (Arterial blood gas [ABG] changes are listed in Table 28-3.)

The mainstay of bronchodilator treatment is inhalation of short-acting $\beta_2$-adrenergic agonists (SABAs) such as albuterol (Table 28-2). In patients with severe exacerbations, inhaled ipratropium (Atrovent) is used in conjunction with SABA. Combivent is a combination of both ipratropium and albuterol.

## TABLE 28-6 Drug Therapy

### *Long-Term Control versus Quick Relief of Asthma*

**Long-Term Control Medications**

***Antiinflammatory Drugs***

Corticosteroids
- Inhaled (e.g., fluticasone [Flovent Diskus or HFA])
- Oral (e.g., prednisone)

Leukotriene modifiers (e.g., montelukast [Singulair])
Anti-IgE (omalizumab [Xolair])

***Bronchodilators***

Long-acting inhaled $\beta_2$-adrenergic agonists (e.g., salmeterol [Serevent])
Long-acting oral $\beta_2$-adrenergic agonists (e.g., albuterol [VoSpire ER])
Methylxanthines (e.g., theophylline [Theo-24])

**Quick-Relief Medications**

***Bronchodilators***

Short-acting inhaled $\beta_2$-adrenergic agonists (e.g., albuterol [Proventil HFA])
Anticholinergics (inhaled) (e.g., ipratropium [Atrovent HFA])*

***Antiinflammatory Drugs***

Corticosteroids (systemic) (e.g., prednisone)†

*Used as alternative if patient has intolerable side effects to albuterol or in emergency department for severe exacerbations.
†Considered quick-relief drugs when used in a short burst (3-10 days) at the start of therapy or during a period of gradual deterioration. Corticosteroids are not used for immediate relief of an ongoing attack.

## CHECK YOUR PRACTICE

Your patient with a history of asthma was admitted to the ED in acute respiratory distress. He has been receiving therapy and seems to be responding. You notice he is no longer wheezing.
- Should you consider this finding an indication that he is doing better?

Corticosteroids are used for patients who do not initially respond to SABA alone.

Wheezing is an unreliable sign to gauge the severity of an attack. Many patients with minor attacks wheeze loudly, whereas others with severe attacks do not wheeze. The patient with severe asthma attacks may have no audible wheezing because of the marked reduction in airflow. For wheezing to occur, the patient must be able to move enough air to produce the sound. Wheezing usually occurs first on exhalation. As asthma progresses, the patient may wheeze during inspiration and expiration. The term *wheezing* may also be used to describe sounds arising from the nose and upper airways.

**SAFETY ALERT Silent Chest**
- If the patient has been wheezing and then there is an absence of a wheeze (i.e., silent chest) and the patient is obviously struggling, this is a life-threatening situation that may require mechanical ventilation.

Diminished or absent breath sounds may indicate a significant decrease in air movement resulting from exhaustion and an inability to generate enough muscle force to ventilate. Severely diminished breath sounds, often referred to as the "silent chest," are an ominous sign, indicating severe obstruction and impending respiratory failure.

A sputum specimen for culture and sensitivity may be obtained to rule out bacterial infection, especially if the patient has purulent sputum, a history of upper respiratory tract infection, a fever, or an elevated white blood cell (WBC) count. However, the vast majority of asthma exacerbations are viral, and sputum cultures are rarely done on an outpatient basis.

## TABLE 28-7 Classification of Acute Asthma Exacerbations

| Degree of Severity | Manifestations | Initial PEF (or $FEV_1$) | Clinical Course |
|---|---|---|---|
| **Mild** | Dyspnea occurs with activity and patient may feel that he or she "can't get enough air." | PEF ≥70% of predicted or personal best | • Usually treated at home<br>• Prompt relief with inhaled SABA such as albuterol (delivered via a nebulizer or MDI with a spacer)<br>• Patients instructed to take 2 to 4 puffs albuterol every 20 min three times to gain rapid control of symptoms<br>• Occasionally short course of oral corticosteroids is needed. |
| **Moderate** | Dyspnea interferes with or limits usual activities. | PEF 40%-69% of predicted or personal best | • Usually requires office or ED visit<br>• Relief is provided with frequent inhaled SABA.<br>• Oral systemic corticosteroids. (Symptoms may persist for several days even after corticosteroids are started.) |
| **Severe** | Dyspnea at rest. Speaks in words, not sentences, because of difficulty of breathing. Feeling of suffocation. | PEF <40% of predicted or personal best | • Usually requires ED visit and likely hospitalization<br>• Partial relief from frequent inhaled SABA<br>• Oral systemic corticosteroids. Some symptoms last for >3 days after treatment is begun.<br>• Adjunctive therapy: ipratropium, IV magnesium |
| **Life-threatening*** | Too dyspneic to speak. May be drowsy or confused. Perspiring | PEF <25% predicted or personal best | • Requires ED visit/hospitalization. Possible ICU<br>• Minimal or no relief from frequent inhaled SABA<br>• IV corticosteroids<br>• Adjunctive therapy: ipratropium, IV magnesium |

Source: Adapted from National Asthma Education and Prevention Program, National Heart, Lung, and Blood Institute: *Expert Panel Report 3: guidelines for the diagnosis and management of asthma*, NIH pub no 08-4051, Bethesda, Md, 2007, National Institutes of Health. Retrieved from *www.nhlbi.nih.gov/guidelines*.
*ED*, Emergency department, *$FEV_1$*, forced expiratory volume; *PEF*, peak expiratory flow.
*May be considered a subset of severe exacerbations

A hand-held, point-of-care device measuring fractional exhaled nitric oxide (FENO) can be used to measure airway inflammation related to asthma. Nitric oxide levels are increased in the breath of people with asthma associated with eosinophilic-induced airway inflammation. FENO may be a used to predict loss of asthma control and exacerbations, to assess a patient's adherence to therapy or to determine if he or she needs more inhaled or oral antiinflammatory medication.[7]

In severe and life-threatening asthma, adjunctive medications such as IV magnesium sulfate may be administered to patients with a very low $FEV_1$ or peak flow (less than 40% of predicted or personal best) or those who fail to respond to initial treatment. IV magnesium has a bronchodilator effect.

Occasionally, asthma exacerbations are life-threatening, and respiratory arrest is pending or actually occurring. The patient requires intubation and mechanical ventilation if there is no response to treatment. The patient is provided with 100% $O_2$, hourly or continuously nebulized SABA, IV corticosteroids, and possibly other adjunctive therapies as noted previously.

Antibiotics are not recommended for asthma treatment unless there are signs of pneumonia, fever, and purulent sputum, suggesting bacterial infections. Chest physiotherapy is generally not recommended for asthma because it is too stressful for the breathless patient.

Epinephrine is not routinely indicated for treatment in asthma exacerbations. However, a subcutaneous or IM injection of epinephrine may be indicated for acute treatment of anaphylaxis. If epinephrine is administered, patients need their BP and electrocardiogram (ECG) monitored closely.

Bronchial thermoplasty is a novel approach that may be used in severe asthma along with conventional therapy. A catheter is introduced via fiberoptic bronchoscopy and directly applies heat and reduces the muscle mass in the bronchial wall. This benefits the patient by reversing the accumulation of excessive tissue that is part of the remodeling process that causes narrowing of the airway size and adds to bronchoconstriction.[8]

## Drug Therapy

A stepwise approach to drug therapy is based initially on the asthma severity and then on the level of control. Persistent asthma requires daily long-term therapy in addition to appropriate medications to manage acute symptoms. Medications are divided into two general classifications: (1) *quick-relief* or *rescue medications* to treat symptoms and exacerbations, such as SABAs and (2) *long-term control medications* to achieve and maintain control of persistent asthma, such as ICSs (Table 28-6). Some of the controllers are used in combination with long-acting bronchodilators (LABA) to gain better asthma control (Table 28-8).

### Antiinflammatory Drugs

***Corticosteroids.*** Chronic inflammation is a primary component of asthma. Corticosteroids are antiinflammatory medications that reduce bronchial hyperresponsiveness, block the late-phase response, and inhibit migration of inflammatory cells. Corticosteroids are more effective in improving asthma control than any other long-term drug. ICSs are first-line therapy for patients with persistent asthma requiring step 2 through 6 therapies (Fig. 28-4). Usually, ICSs must be administered for 1 to 2 weeks before maximum therapeutic effects can be seen. Some ICSs (e.g., fluticasone, budesonide [Pulmicort Flexhaler]) begin to have a therapeutic effect in 24 hours. ICSs must be administered on a fixed schedule.

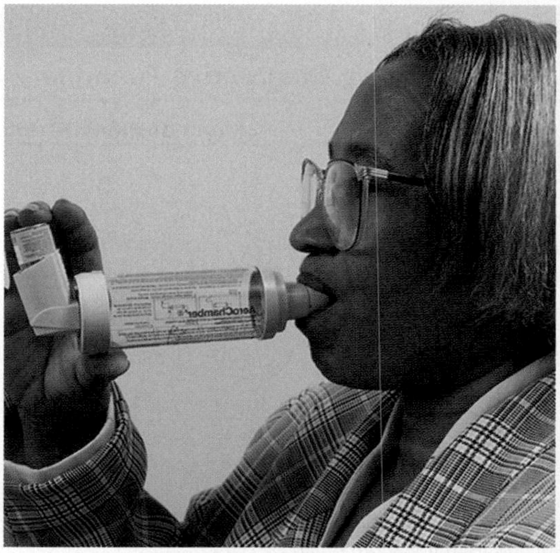

**FIG. 28-5** Example of an AeroChamber spacer used with a metered-dose inhaler. (From Potter PA, Perry AG, Stockert P, et al: *Basic nursing: essentials for practice,* ed 7, St. Louis, 2011, Mosby.)

When ICSs are administered, asthma can usually be controlled without significant systemic side effects, since little systemic drug absorption occurs from these drugs. However, ICSs at the highest dosage levels have been associated with side effects (e.g., easy bruising, decreased bone mineral density).[4] Oropharyngeal candidiasis, hoarseness, and dry cough are local side effects caused by inhalation of corticosteroids. These problems can be reduced or prevented by using a spacer (Fig. 28-5) with the MDI and by gargling with water or mouthwash after each use. Using a spacer or holding device for inhalation of corticosteroids can be helpful in getting more medication into the lungs. However, drugs that are activated in the lungs (not the pharynx) (e.g., ciclesonide [Alvesco]) appear to minimize these side effects without the need for a spacer or mouth rinsing.[4]

To gain prompt control, orally administered corticosteroids are used for acute exacerbations of asthma. Maintenance doses of oral corticosteroids may be necessary to control asthma in patients with severe chronic asthma when long-term therapy is required. These patients should be under the care of a specialized pulmonary HCP. (Side effects of long-term corticosteroid therapy are discussed in Chapter 49.)

Women, especially postmenopausal women, who have asthma and who use corticosteroids should take adequate amounts of calcium and vitamin D and participate in regular weight-bearing exercise. (Osteoporosis is discussed in Chapter 63.)

***Leukotriene Modifiers.*** Leukotriene modifiers include leukotriene receptor blockers (antagonists) (zafirlukast [Accolate], montelukast [Singulair]) and leukotriene synthesis inhibitors (zileuton [Zyflo CR]). These drugs interfere with the synthesis or block the action of leukotrienes. Leukotrienes are inflammatory mediators produced from arachidonic acid metabolism (see Fig. 11-2). Leukotrienes are potent bronchoconstrictors, and some also cause airway edema and inflammation, thus contributing to the symptoms of asthma. Because these drugs block the release of some substances from mast cells and eosinophils, they have both bronchodilator and antiinflammatory effects.

These drugs are not indicated for use in the reversal of bronchospasm in acute asthma attacks. They are used for

## TABLE 28-8 Drug Therapy

### *Asthma and Chronic Obstructive Pulmonary Disease (COPD)*

| Drug | Route of Administration | Comments† |
|---|---|---|
| **Corticosteroids** | | |
| hydrocortisone (Solu-Cortef) | IV | Alternate-day therapy minimizes side effects. Oral dose should be taken in morning with food or milk. When given in high dosages, observe for epigastric distress. Long-term corticosteroid therapy requires supplementation with vitamin D and calcium to prevent osteoporosis. Discontinue gradually over time to prevent adrenal insufficiency. If symptoms recur during tapering, notify HCP. |
| methylprednisolone (Medrol, Solu-Medrol) | Oral, IV | |
| prednisone | Oral | |
| fluticasone (Flovent HFA, Flovent Diskus, Arnuity Ellipta) | MDI, DPI | Not recommended for acute asthma attack. Rinse mouth with water or mouthwash after use to prevent oral fungal infections. Use of spacer device with MDI may decrease incidence of oral candidiasis. With ICSs, may not see effects until after at least 2 wk of regular treatment |
| beclomethasone (Qvar) | MDI | Same as fluticasone except less oral candidiasis because of very small particle size, which is deposited deeper in the airways |
| budesonide (Pulmicort Flexhaler) | DPI | Same as above |
| mometasone (Asmanex Twisthaler) | DPI | Same as above |
| ciclesonide (Alvesco) | MDI | Oral candidiasis and other localized oropharyngeal effects (e.g., hoarseness). Fewer side effects than other ICSs because of small particle size with minimal activation in oropharynx |
| **Phosphodiesterase Inhibitor Type 4 (PDE-4)** | | |
| roflumilast (Daliresp) | Oral | Only used in severe COPD to reduce exacerbation frequency. Not to be used for acute bronchospasm. GI symptoms occur within 6 mo of initiating medication. Patients to report any psychiatric symptoms (e.g., anxiety, depression, suicidal thoughts). Not to be used with theophylline |
| **Anticholinergics** | | |
| ***Short Acting (SAMA)**** | | |
| ipratropium (Atrovent HFA) | Nebulizer, MDI | Approved for COPD. May provide additive benefit to SABA in moderate to severe asthma exacerbations (used in emergency department with no benefit beyond that). Use in asthma as alternative for patients with intolerable side effects with SABA. Temporary blurred vision if sprayed in eyes. Use cautiously in patients with narrow-angle glaucoma or prostatic enlargement. |
| ***Long Acting (LAMA)**** | | |
| tiotropium (Spiriva HandiHaler) | DPI | Only approved for COPD. Blurred vision if powder comes in contact with eyes. Must discontinue use of ipratropium while on tiotropium. Patients with COPD must use SABA or short-acting anticholinergics for quick-relief medication. Maximum effect 1 wk after initiation of drug. Dosed once daily |
| aclidinium bromide (Tudorza, Pressair) | DPI | Only approved for COPD. Do not administer with other anticholinergics. Not for acute relief of bronchospasm. Dosed twice daily |
| umeclidinium (Incruse Ellipta) | DPI | Only approved for COPD. Used once daily as maintenance treatment of airflow obstruction |
| **Monoclonal Antibodies** | | |
| ***Anti-IgE*** | | |
| omalizumab (Xolair) | Subcutaneous | Only for moderate to severe, persistent, allergic asthma with symptoms not adequately controlled by ICSs. Not for acute bronchospasm. Administer only under direct medical supervision biweekly or monthly, depending on IgE levels and weight, and observe patient for a minimum of 2 hr after administration because anaphylaxis has been reported with use. |
| ***Anti-Interleukin 5*** | | |
| mepolizumab (Nucala) | Subcutaneous | Only used for maintenance in patients with severe asthma attacks despite receiving current asthma medications. Administered once every 4 wk by health care professional |
| reslizumab (Cinqair) | IV only | |
| **Leukotriene Modifiers** | | |
| ***Leukotriene Receptor Blocker*** | | |
| zafirlukast (Accolate) | Oral tablets | Take at least 1 hr before or 2 hr after meals. Affects metabolism of erythromycin and theophylline. Not used to treat acute asthma episodes |
| montelukast (Singulair) | Oral tablets, chewable tablets, oral granules | Not used to treat acute asthma episodes |
| ***Leukotriene Inhibitor*** | | |
| zileuton (Zyflo, Zyflo CR) | Oral tablets | Monitor liver enzymes. May interfere with metabolism of warfarin (Coumadin) and theophylline. Not used to treat acute asthma episodes |

*Anticholinergics are muscarinic antagonists. Thus the abbreviations short-acting muscarinic antagonist (SAMA) and long-acting muscarinic antagonist (LAMA).

## TABLE 28-8 Drug Therapy

### Asthma and Chronic Obstructive Pulmonary Disease (COPD)—cont'd

| Drug | Route of Administration | Comments† |
|---|---|---|
| **$\beta_2$-Adrenergic Agonists** | | |
| ***Inhaled: Short Acting (SABA)*** | | |
| albuterol (Proventil HFA, Ventolin HFA, ProAir HFA, AccuNeb, VoSpire ER [oral only]) | Nebulizer, MDI, oral tablets, including extended release<br>NOTE: Oral tablets not for acute use, only long acting | Use with caution in patients with cardiac disorders because β-agonists may cause ↑ BP and heart rate, CNS stimulation/excitation, and ↑ risk of dysrhythmias. Has rapid onset of action (1-3 min). Duration of action is 4-8 hr. Ventolin HFA is the only albuterol MDI with a counter. |
| levalbuterol (Xopenex, Xopenex HFA) | Nebulizer, MDI | Too frequent use can result in loss of effectiveness. Efficacy no better than other SABA |
| ***Inhaled: Long Acting (LABA)*** | *In asthma:* Never use as monotherapy. Use in combination with ICSs.<br>*In COPD:* Can be used as monotherapy. Not used for rapid relief of dyspnea | |
| salmeterol (Serevent Diskus) | DPI | Not to exceed 2 puffs q12hr. Not used for acute exacerbations. Has a counter |
| formoterol (Foradil Aerolizer, Perforomist) | DPI, nebulizer (Perforomist) | Can affect blood glucose levels. Use with caution in patients with diabetes. |
| arformoterol (Brovana) | Nebulizer | See formoterol. For chronic COPD use |
| indacaterol (Arcapta Neohaler) | DPI | Only once-daily LABA. For chronic COPD use. Not intended to treat asthma |
| olodaterol (Striverdi Respimat) | MDI | 2 puffs daily. Less expensive than other LABAs |
| **Methylxanthines** | | |
| *IV agent:* aminophylline (second-line therapy)<br>*Oral:* theophylline | Oral tablets, IV, elixir, sustained-release tablets | Wide variety of response to drug metabolism exists. Half-life is ↓ by smoking and ↑ by heart failure and liver disease. Cimetidine, ciprofloxacin, erythromycin, and other drugs may rapidly ↑ theophylline levels. Taking drug with food or antacids may help GI effects. Use usually limited to situations when other long-term bronchodilation not available or not affordable |
| **Combination Agents** | | **Also see each component of medications for SE.** |
| ***SAMA/SABA*** | | |
| ipratropium/albuterol (Combivent Respimat, DuoNeb) | Nebulizer (DuoNeb), inhalation spray (Combivent Respimat) | Patients must be careful not to overuse. Respimat is an inhaler, but propellant free, unlike an MDI. Respimat is independent of inspiratory flow. Has dose indicator |
| ***ICS/LABA*** | | |
| fluticasone/salmeterol (Advair Diskus or HFA) | DPI, MDI | See salmeterol and fluticasone. Has a counter. Comes in three different strengths |
| budesonide/formoterol (Symbicort) | MDI | See budesonide and formoterol. Has a counter |
| mometasone furoate/formoterol fumarate (Dulera) | MDI | Not for relief of acute bronchospasm |
| fluticasone/vilanterol (Breo Ellipta) | DPI | Dose once daily. |
| ***LAMA/LABA*** | | |
| umeclidinium/vilanterol (Anoro Ellipta) | DPI | Anticholinergic/LABA for COPD. Not for relief of acute bronchospasm |

*DPI,* Dry powder inhaler; *HFA,* hydrofluoroalkane (propellant); *ICSs,* inhaled corticosteroids; *MDI,* metered-dose inhaler.
†For patient instructions in English and Spanish for the devices, see *www.chestnet.org/accp/patient-guides/patient-instructions-inhaled-devices-english-and-spanish.*

prophylactic and maintenance therapy. One advantage of leukotriene modifiers is that they are administered orally.

***Anti-IgE.*** Omalizumab (Xolair) is a monoclonal antibody to IgE that decreases circulating free IgE levels. Omalizumab prevents IgE from attaching to mast cells, thus preventing the release of chemical mediators. This drug is indicated for patients with moderate to severe persistent, allergic asthma, or those requiring step 5 or 6 care with persistent asthma that cannot be controlled with ICSs. Omalizumab is administered subcutaneously every 2 to 4 weeks. The drug has a risk of anaphylaxis, and patients must receive the medication in an HCP's office, where this potential emergency problem can be handled.

***Anti-Interleukin 5.*** Mepolizumab (Nucala) and reslizumab (Cinqair) are monoclonal antibodies to interleukin-5 (IL-5). IL-5 is a major cytokine involved in the inflammatory response in asthma by promoting eosinophil activity. By inhibiting IL-5, these drugs inhibit the production and survival of eosinophils. They are used for patients who have a history of severe asthma attacks despite using current asthma medication.

**Bronchodilators.** Three classes of bronchodilator drugs currently used in asthma therapy are $\beta_2$-adrenergic agonists (also referred to as $\beta_2$-agonists), methylxanthines and derivatives, and anticholinergics (Table 28-8).

***$\beta_2$-Adrenergic Agonist Drugs.*** These drugs may be short-acting $\beta_2$-adrenergic agonists (SABAs) or long-acting $\beta_2$-adrenergic agonists (LABAs). Because inhaled SABAs are the most effective drugs for relieving acute bronchospasm (as seen in acute exacerbations of asthma), they are known as *rescue medications.* These drugs have an onset of action within minutes and are effective for 4 to 8 hours. These drugs act by stimulating β-adrenergic receptors in the bronchioles, thus producing bronchodilation. They also increase mucociliary clearance.

**DRUG ALERT $\beta_2$-Adrenergic Agonists**
- Use with caution in patients with cardiac disorders, since both SABAs and LABAs may cause elevated BP and heart rate, central nervous system stimulation or excitation, and increased risk of dysrhythmias.
- Any MDI is only effective if taken properly. Review MDI technique during each visit as a standard component of care (Fig. 28-6).

$\beta_2$-Adrenergic agonists are also useful in preventing bronchospasm precipitated by exercise and other stimuli because they prevent the release of inflammatory mediators from mast

Using an inhaler seems simple, but most patients do not use it the right way. When you use your inhaler the wrong way, less medicine gets to your lungs. (Your physician may give you other types of inhalers.)

For the next 2 weeks, read these steps aloud as you do them or ask someone to read them to you. Ask your physician or nurse to check how well you are using your inhaler.

Use your inhaler in one of the three ways pictured below (**A** or **B** is best, but **C** can be used if you have trouble with **A** or **B**).

**Steps for Using Your Inhaler**

Getting ready
1. Take off the cap and shake the inhaler.
2. Breathe out all the way.
3. Hold your inhaler the way your doctor said (**A, B,** or **C** below).

Breathe in slowly
4. As you start breathing in **slowly** through your mouth, press down on the inhaler **one** time. (If you use a holding chamber, first press down on the inhaler. Within 5 seconds, begin to breathe in slowly.)
5. Keep breathing in **slowly,** as deeply as you can.

Hold your breath
6. Hold your breath as you count to 10 slowly, if you can.
7. For inhaled quick-relief medicine ($\beta_2$-agonists), wait about 1 minute between puffs. There is no need to wait between puffs for other medicines.

**A.** Hold inhaler 1 to 2 inches in front of your mouth (about the width of two fingers).

**B.** Use a spacer/holding chamber. These come in many shapes and can be useful to any patient.

**C.** Put the inhaler in your mouth.

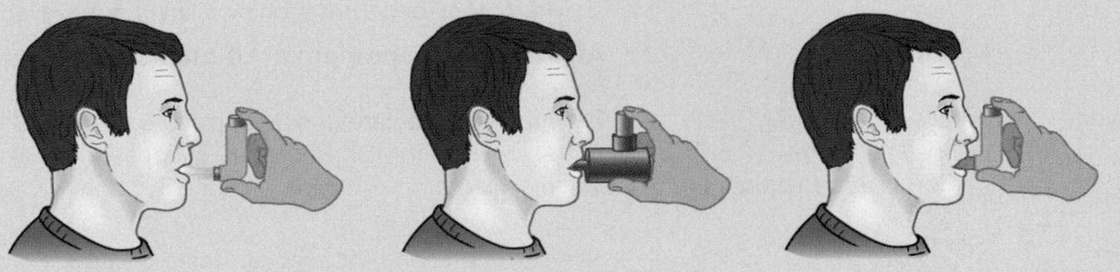

**Clean Your Inhaler as Needed**

Look at the hole where the medicine sprays out from your inhaler. If you see "powder" in or around the hole, clean the inhaler. Remove the metal canister from the L-shaped plastic mouthpiece. Rinse only the mouthpiece and cap in warm water. Let them dry overnight. In the morning, put the canister back inside. Put the cap on.

**Know When to Replace Your Inhaler**

**For medicines you take each day (an example):** Say your new canister has 200 puffs (number of puffs is listed on canister) and you are told to take 8 puffs per day.

25 days
8 puffs per day) 200 puffs in canister

So this canister will last 25 days. If you started using this inhaler on May 1, replace it on or before May 25.
You can write the date on your canister.

For **quick-relief medicine take as needed** and count each puff.

Do not put your canister in water to see if it is empty as water may enter MDI and impair inhaler.

**FIG. 28-6** How to use your metered-dose inhaler correctly.

cells. They do not inhibit the late-phase response of asthma or have antiinflammatory effects. If used frequently, inhaled $\beta_2$-adrenergic agonists may produce tremors, anxiety, tachycardia, palpitations, and nausea.

Too frequent use of $\beta_2$-adrenergic agonists indicates poor asthma control, may mask asthma severity, and may lead to reduced drug effectiveness. The use of SABAs should be limited to less than two times weekly. In other words, regularly scheduled, daily, or chronic use of inhaled SABA is not recommended for long-term control of asthma. SABA inhalers should last for months. Use of long-term bronchodilators with inhaled corticosteroids or other medications can achieve this goal if prescribed and used properly. In summary, SABAs are not used for long-term control, and they should not be used alone for persistent asthma.

LABAs, including salmeterol (Serevent Diskus) and formoterol (Foradil), are effective for 12 hours. LABAs are added to a daily dose of ICSs for long-term control of moderate to severe persistent asthma (i.e., step 3 or higher for long-term control; see Fig. 28-4) and prevention of symptoms, particularly at night. When LABAs are added to a patient's daily regimen of corticosteroids, they decrease the need for SABAs and allow patients to achieve better asthma control with a lower dosage of ICSs.

LABAs should never be used as monotherapy for asthma and should only be used if the patient is on ICS. Tell patients that these drugs should not be used to treat acute symptoms or to obtain quick relief from bronchospasm. Teach the patient that these drugs are used only once every 12 hours.

**DRUG ALERT Long-Acting $\beta_2$-Adrenergic Agonists (LABAs)**
- Should not be the first medicine used to treat asthma
- Should never be used as the only medication to treat asthma but should be added to the treatment plan only if other controller medicines do not control asthma
- Should not be used to treat wheezing that is getting worse
- Always use an SABA to treat sudden wheezing.

Combination therapy using an ICS and LABA is available in several inhalers (e.g., fluticasone/salmeterol [Advair] and budesonide/formoterol [Symbicort]). The combinations are more convenient, improve adherence, and ensure that patients receive the LABA together with an ICS.

***Methylxanthines.*** Sustained-release methylxanthine (theophylline) preparations are not a first-line controller medication. They are used only as an alternative therapy for step 2 care in mild persistent asthma. Methylxanthine is a bronchodilator with mild antiinflammatory effects, but the exact mechanism of action is unknown.

**DRUG ALERT Theophylline**

- Instruct patient to report signs of toxicity: nausea, vomiting, seizures, insomnia.
- Avoid caffeine to prevent intensifying adverse effects.

The main problems with theophylline are the relatively high incidence of interaction with other drugs and the side effects, which include nausea, headache, insomnia, gastrointestinal distress, tachycardia, dysrhythmias, and seizures. Because theophylline has a narrow margin of safety, monitor serum blood levels regularly to determine if the drug is within therapeutic range.

***Anticholinergic Drugs.*** Anticholinergic drugs are another group of bronchodilators that are different from SABA. β-agonists affect the bronchioles (small airways), whereas anticholinergics affect the muscles around the bronchi (large airways). When the lungs are irritated, these bands of muscle can tighten, causing bronchoconstriction via the parasympathetic nervous system. Anticholinergics work by preventing these muscles from tightening. Thus these drugs promote bronchodilation.

Anticholinergic drugs are less effective than equivalent doses of SABAs in asthma. However, they are more effective in COPD patients. Therefore short-acting anticholinergic drugs are not used in the routine management of asthma, except for the management of severe acute asthma exacerbations.

**Inhalation Devices for Drug Delivery.** The multiple devices for asthma drug administration can be confusing. The majority of asthma drugs are administered only or preferably by inhalation because systemic side effects are reduced and the onset of action is faster. Inhalation devices include metered-dose inhalers (MDIs), dry powder inhalers (DPIs), and nebulizers.

***Inhalers.*** MDIs are small, hand-held, pressurized devices that deliver a measured dose of drug with each activation. Dosing is usually accomplished with one or two puffs. Depending on the specific MDI, a spacer or holding chamber (e.g., AeroChamber or InspirEase [Fig. 28-5]) is used to reduce the amount of drug delivered to the oropharynx and improve the amount of drug delivered to the lungs. In addition, spacers assist people who have hand-breath coordination problems.

All MDIs are mandated by international law to have an ozone-friendly propellant, which is a hydrofluoroalkane (HFA). This propellant is nontoxic, evaporates almost instantly once it forces medicine out of the MDI canister, and is not harmful to the patient. The number of times an MDI must be primed and the frequency of priming vary widely, so read the package insert with the patient.

The MDI should be cleaned by removing the dust cap and rinsing the holder (not the medication chamber) in warm water at least two times per week (Fig. 28-6). The patient who needs to use several MDIs is often unclear about the order in which to take the medications. Historically it had been recommended that SABAs should be used first to open up the airway and improve the delivery of subsequent medications. However, this technique is not evidence based. It is a potential source of confusion to patients because the SABAs are usually used on an as-needed (PRN) basis.

One of the major problems with metered-dose drugs is the potential for overuse (more than two canisters per month) rather than seeking needed medical care (Table 28-9). As a patient develops additional asthmatic symptoms, he or she may use the $\beta_2$-adrenergic agonist MDI repeatedly. $\beta_2$-Adrenergic agonists help by relieving bronchospasm. They do not treat the inflammatory response. Therefore teach the patient the correct therapeutic use of these drugs. The patient also needs to know the correct way to determine whether the MDI is empty (Fig. 28-6).

DPIs are simpler to use than MDIs (Fig. 28-7 and Table 28-10). The DPI contains dry, powdered medication and is breath activated. No propellant is used. Instead, an aerosol is created when the patient inhales through a reservoir containing a dose of powder. The convenient-to-carry diskus has several advantages over MDIs: (1) less manual dexterity is needed, (2) there is no need to coordinate device puffs with inhalation, and (3) no spacer is required. Disadvantages are that some commonly prescribed drugs are not yet available in DPIs, and the medication may clump if exposed to humidity. Since the medicine is delivered only by the patient's inspiratory effort, patients with a low $FEV_1$ (less than 1 L) may not be able to inspire the medication adequately.

Differences between MDIs and DPIs are presented in Table 28-11. Aerosolized medication delivery systems, when used with comparable drug doses, provide equivalent efficacy. Therefore patients should use the device best suited to their needs.

***Nebulizers.*** Nebulizers are small machines used to convert drug solutions into mists. The mist can be inhaled through a face mask or mouthpiece held between the teeth. Nebulizers are

**INFORMATICS IN PRACTICE**

***Home Monitoring of Asthma***

- To reduce the rate of readmission to hospital, the patient with asthma may be discharged with a home monitoring system. These systems provide an easy and inexpensive approach to remotely monitoring patients' lung functions.
- Asthma home monitoring usually consists of peak flow rate, pulse oximetry, vital signs, and lung sounds. This information is sent to the HCP so that problems are quickly detected.
- As part of your discharge planning, assist the patient with receiving a system and reviewing its proper use.

**TABLE 28-9 Problems Using a Metered-Dose Inhaler (MDI)**

- Failing to coordinate activation with inspiration
- Activating MDI in the mouth while breathing through nose
- Inspiring too rapidly
- Not holding the breath for 10 sec (or as close to 10 sec as possible)
- Holding MDI upside down or sideways
- Inhaling more than 1 puff with each inspiration
- Not shaking MDI before use (if indicated)
- Not waiting a sufficient amount of time between each puff
- Not opening mouth wide enough (if using open mouth technique), causing medication to bounce off teeth, tongue, or palate
- Not having adequate strength to activate MDI
- Being unable to understand and follow directions

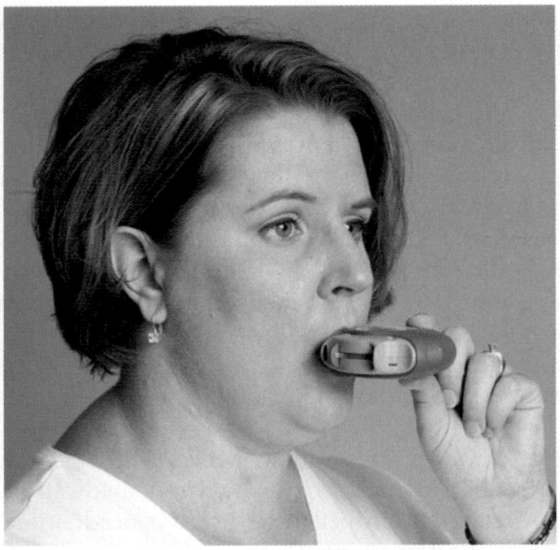

**FIG. 28-7** Example of a dry powder inhaler (DPI). (From Potter PA, Perry AG, Stockert P, et al: *Basic nursing: essentials for practice*, ed 7, St. Louis, 2011, Mosby.)

### TABLE 28-10 Patient Teaching
#### *How to Use a Dry Powder Inhaler (DPI)*

*Include the following instructions when teaching a patient to use a DPI.*

1. Remove mouthpiece cap or open the device according to manufacturer's instructions. Check for dust or dirt. If there is an external counter, note the number of doses remaining.
2. Load the medicine into the inhaler or engage the lever to allow the medicine to become available. Some DPIs should be held upright while loading. Others should be held sideways or in a horizontal position.
3. Do not shake your medicine.
4. Tilt your head back slightly and breathe out, getting as much air out of your lungs as you can. Do not breathe into your inhaler because this could affect the dose.
5. Close your lips tightly around the mouthpiece of the inhaler.
6. Breathe in deeply and quickly. This will ensure that the medicine moves down deeply into your lungs. You may not taste or sense the medicine going into your lungs.
7. Hold your breath for 10 seconds or as long as you can to disperse the medicine into your lungs.
8. If there is an external counter, note the number of doses remaining. It should be one less than the number in step 1 above.
9. Do not keep your DPI in a humid place such as a shower room because the medicine may clump.

usually used for individuals who have severe asthma or difficulty with the MDI inhalation since they do not provide better delivery of medication than a spacer with an inhaler.

Nebulizers are usually powered by a compressed air or $O_2$ generator. At home, the patient may have an air-powered compressor. In the hospital, wall $O_2$ or compressed air is used to power the nebulizer.

Aerosolized medication orders must include the medication, dose, diluent, and whether it is to be nebulized with $O_2$ or compressed air. The advantage of nebulization therapy is that it is easy to use. Medications that are routinely nebulized include albuterol and ipratropium.

The patient is placed in an upright position that allows for most efficient breathing to ensure adequate penetration and deposition of the aerosolized medication. The patient must breathe slowly and deeply through the mouth and hold

### TABLE 28-11 Comparison of Metered-Dose and Dry Powder Inhalers

| | Metered-Dose Inhaler (MDI)* | Dry Powder Inhaler (DPI) |
|---|---|---|
| Shake before use | May be needed for some (e.g., albuterol), but not for others (Read package insert) | No |
| Inspiration | Slow | Rapid |
| Spacer | May be used with inhaled corticosteroids or for more effective delivery (Read package insert) | None permitted |
| Counting device | Many have an external device, but some do not | Most preloaded forms include counter |
| Inhalations/dose | Often 2/dose | Often 1/dose |
| Cleaning | Use water for plastic case | Avoid moisture |

For additional information, see National Jewish Hospital: *Instructions for Inhaler and Spacer Use Videos for various devices.* Available at *www.nationaljewish.org/healthinfo/medications/lung-diseases/devices/instructional-videos.*
*MDIs use hydrofluoroalkane (HFA) as a propellant.

inspirations for 2 or 3 seconds. Deep diaphragmatic breathing helps ensure deposition of the medication. Instruct the patient to breathe normally in between these large forced breaths to prevent alveolar hypoventilation and dizziness. After the treatment instruct the patient to cough effectively.

A disadvantage of nebulizer equipment use is the potential for bacterial growth. Review cleaning procedures for home respiratory equipment with the patient. A frequently used, effective home-cleaning method is to wash the nebulizer daily in soap and water, rinse it with water, and soak it for 20 to 30 minutes in a 1:1 white vinegar–water solution, followed by a water rinse and air drying.

**Patient Teaching Related to Drug Therapy.** When teaching patients about their medications, include the name, purpose, dosage, method of administration, and schedule. Take into consideration the patient's activities of daily living (ADLs) that require energy expenditure and thus $O_2$ (e.g., bathing). Teach about side effects, appropriate action if side effects occur, how to properly use and clean devices, how to prime and the frequency, and consequences of not taking medications as prescribed. One of the major factors determining success in asthma management is the correct administration of drugs.

Several factors can affect the correct use of inhalation devices. These include advanced age, alterations in physical dexterity (e.g., arthritis in hands, coordination), psychologic state (e.g., cognition), affordability, convenience, and administration time and preference.[7]

Poor adherence with asthma therapy is a major challenge in the long-term management of chronic asthma. Lack of adherence often occurs in chronic asthma because the patient is symptom free and does not use the long-term therapy (e.g., ICS) regularly because no immediate benefit is felt. The patient does not realize that ICSs are needed to treat the ongoing inflammatory process.

Explain the importance and purpose of taking the long-term therapy regularly, emphasizing that maximum improvement may take longer than 1 week. Tell the patient that, without regular use, the swelling in the airways may progress and the asthma will likely worsen over time. Become familiar with the vast array of compassionate-use programs offered by pharmaceutical companies to help lower-income patients obtain medications (e.g., *www.needymeds.com*).

Make sure that patients understand exactly how to use their inhaler device, and give them printed instructions. At every clinic visit or hospitalization, reassess the patient's inhaler technique. If package inserts are available, you can review them before teaching the patient. Drug company websites have numerous excellent teaching videos available.

**Nonprescription Combination Drugs.** Several nonprescription combination drugs are available OTC. They are usually combinations of a bronchodilator (ephedrine) and an expectorant (guaifenesin). Inhalers containing epinephrine may be available.[9] These agents are advertised as medications to relieve bronchospasm. Often patients seek OTC drugs because they are less expensive than prescription medication. Many people consider these drugs safe because they can be obtained without a prescription. In general, they should be avoided due to their potential side effects.

Drugs containing ephedrine and epinephrine are dangerous because they stimulate the central nervous and cardiovascular systems, causing nervousness, heart palpitations and dysrhythmias, tremors, insomnia, and increases in BP. Many respiratory products containing ephedrine are located behind the counter at pharmacies or require a prescription. This limited access is to prevent the diversion of ephedrine to the production of methamphetamine. Also many of the OTC products have been reformulated with phenylephrine, instead of ephedrine, which works well topically but has modest effects in the oral form.

An important teaching responsibility is to warn patients about the dangers associated with nonprescription combination drugs. These drugs are especially dangerous to a patient with underlying cardiac problems because elevated BP and tachycardia often occur. Caution the patient who persists in taking these medications to read and follow the directions on the label.

## NURSING MANAGEMENT: ASTHMA

### Nursing Assessment

If a patient is not in acute distress, take a detailed health history, including information about precipitating factors and what has helped alleviate asthma attacks in the past. When completing the health history, ask about specific herbs or supplements that a patient may be using.

Subjective and objective data that should be obtained from a patient with asthma are presented in Table 28-12. You may also assess the patient's asthma control using one of the validated self-administered questionnaires (e.g., ACT).

### Nursing Diagnoses

Nursing diagnoses for the patient with asthma may include, but are not limited to, the following:

- Ineffective airway clearance *related to* bronchospasm, excessive mucus production, tenacious secretions, and fatigue
- Anxiety *related to* difficulty breathing, perceived or actual loss of control, and fear of suffocation
- Deficient knowledge *related to* lack of information and education about asthma and its treatment

Additional information on nursing diagnoses is presented in eNursing Care Plan 28-1 on the website for this chapter.

**TABLE 28-12 Nursing Assessment**

***Asthma***

**Subjective Data**

***Important Health Information***

*Past health history:* Allergic rhinitis, sinusitis, or skin allergies. Previous asthma attack and hospitalization or intubation. Symptoms worsened by triggers in the environment. Gastroesophageal reflux disease (GERD). Occupational exposure to chemical irritants (e.g., paints, dust)

*Medications:* Adherence to medication, inhaler technique. Use of antibiotics. Pattern and amount of short-acting $\beta_2$-adrenergic agonist used per week. Medications that may precipitate an attack in susceptible asthmatics such as aspirin, nonsteroidal antiinflammatory drugs, $\beta$-adrenergic blockers

***Functional Health Patterns***

*Health perception–health management:* Family history of allergies or asthma. Recent upper respiratory tract or sinus infection

*Activity-exercise:* Fatigue, decreased or absent exercise tolerance. Dyspnea, cough (especially at night), productive cough with yellow or green sputum or sticky sputum. Chest tightness, feelings of suffocation, air hunger, talking in short sentences or words or phrases, sitting upright to breathe

*Sleep-rest:* Awakened from sleep because of cough or breathing difficulties, insomnia

*Coping–stress tolerance:* Emotional distress, stress in work environment or home

**Objective Data**

***General***

Restlessness or exhaustion, confusion, upright or forward-leaning body position

***Integumentary***

Diaphoresis, cyanosis (circumoral, nail bed), eczema

***Respiratory***

Nasal discharge, nasal polyps, mucosal swelling. Crackles, diminished or absent breath sounds, and wheezes on auscultation. Hyperresonance on percussion. Sputum (thick, white, tenacious), ↑ work of breathing with use of accessory muscles. Intercostal and supraclavicular retractions. Tachypnea with hyperventilation. Prolonged expiration

***Cardiovascular***

Tachycardia, pulsus paradoxus, jugular venous distention, hypertension or hypotension, premature ventricular contractions

***Possible Diagnostic Findings***

Abnormal ABGs during attacks, ↓ $O_2$ saturation, serum and sputum eosinophilia, ↑ serum IgE, positive skin tests for allergens, chest x-ray demonstrating hyperinflation with attacks, abnormal pulmonary function tests showing ↓ flow rates; FVC, $FEV_1$, PEFR, and $FEV_1$/FVC ratio that improve between attacks and with bronchodilators

*ABGs,* Arterial blood gases; *$FEV_1$,* forced expiratory volume in 1 sec; *FVC,* forced vital capacity; *IgE,* immunoglobulin E; *PEFR,* peak expiratory flow rate.

### Planning

The overall goals are that the patient with asthma will have asthma control as evidenced by (1) minimal symptoms during the day and night, (2) acceptable activity levels (including exercise and other physical activity), (3) maintenance of greater than 80% of personal best PEFR, (4) few or no adverse effects of therapy, (5) no acute exacerbations of asthma, and

(6) adequate knowledge to participate in and carry out the plan of care.

## Nursing Implementation

**Health Promotion.** Your role in preventing asthma attacks or decreasing their severity focuses primarily on teaching the patient and caregiver. Teach the patient to identify and avoid known personal triggers for asthma (e.g., cigarette smoke, pet dander) and irritants (e.g., cold air, aspirin, foods, cats, indoor air pollution) (Table 28-1). Washing bedclothes in hot water or cooler water with detergent and bleach has some effect on allergen levels. Avoidance of furred animals is suggested, but pet allergens are nearly impossible to avoid. Pet allergens can be found in many public areas for months even after removal of the animal. Many people are allergic to cockroach remains and the dried droppings, so measures to avoid or control cockroaches are partly effective in removing allergens.

If cold air cannot be avoided, dressing properly with scarves or using a mask helps reduce the risk of an asthma attack. Aspirin and NSAIDs should be avoided if they are known to precipitate an attack. Many OTC drugs contain aspirin. Therefore teach the patient to read the labels carefully. Nonselective β-blockers (e.g., propranolol [Inderal]) are contraindicated because they inhibit bronchodilation. Selective β-blockers (e.g., atenolol [Tenormin]) should be used with caution. Desensitization (immunotherapy) may be partially effective in decreasing the patient's sensitivity to known allergens (see Chapter 13).

Prompt diagnosis and treatment of upper respiratory tract infections and sinusitis may prevent an asthma exacerbation. If occupational irritants are involved as etiologic factors of asthma, the patient may need to consider changing jobs. Individuals who are obese often find that weight loss improves control of asthma. Encourage the patient to maintain a fluid intake of 2 to 3 L/day, good nutrition, and adequate rest. If exercise is planned or if the patient has asthma only with exercise, the HCP can suggest a medication regimen for pretreatment or long-term control of symptoms to prevent bronchospasm.

**Acute Care.** A goal in asthma care is to maximize the patient's ability to safely manage acute asthma using an asthma action plan developed in conjunction with the HCP (Fig. 28-8). Action plans are particularly important for individuals with moderate to severe persistent asthma or acute exacerbations. The action plan dictates what symptoms or peak flow reading necessitates a change in asthma care to gain control.

The patient can take 2 to 4 puffs of an SABA every 20 minutes three times as a rescue plan. Depending on the response (e.g., alleviation of symptoms or improved peak flow), continued SABA use and/or oral corticosteroids may be a part of the home management plan at this point. If symptoms persist or if the patient's peak flow is less than 50% of the personal best, the HCP or emergency medical services (EMS) must be immediately contacted.

When the patient is in the health care facility with an acute exacerbation, it is important to monitor the patient's respiratory and cardiovascular systems. This includes (1) auscultating lung sounds; (2) taking the heart and respiratory rates and BP; and (3) monitoring pulse oximetry, peak expiratory flow rates, and ABGs.

Louder wheezing may actually occur in airways that are responding to the therapy as airflow increases. As improvement continues and airflow increases, breath sounds increase and wheezing decreases. Remember that, despite the disappearance of most of the bronchospasms, the edema and cellular infiltration of the airway mucosa and the viscous mucous plugs may take several days to improve. Thus intensive therapy must be continued even after clinical improvement.

**TABLE 28-13 Patient Teaching**

***Pursed-Lip Breathing (PLB)***

*Teach the patient how to do PLB using the following guidelines.*

1. Use PLB before, during, and after any activity causing you to be short of breath.
2. Inhale slowly and deeply through the nose.
3. Exhale slowly through pursed lips, almost as if whistling.
4. Relax your facial muscles without puffing your cheeks—like whistling—while you are exhaling.
5. Make breathing out (exhalation) three times as long as breathing in (inhalation).
6. The following activities can help you get the "feel" of PLB:
   - Blow through a straw in a glass of water with the intent of forming small bubbles.
   - Blow a lit candle enough to bend the flame without blowing it out.
   - Steadily blow a table-tennis ball across a table.
   - Blow a tissue held in the hand until it gently flaps.
7. Practice 8-10 repetitions of PLB three or four times a day.

An important nursing goal during an acute attack is to decrease the patient's anxiety and sense of panic. A calm, quiet, reassuring attitude may help the patient relax. Position the patient comfortably (usually sitting) to maximize chest expansion. Stay with the patient and be available to provide additional comfort. A technique called "talking down" can help the patient remain calm. In talking down, you gain eye contact with the patient. In a firm, calm voice coach the patient to use pursed-lip breathing, which keeps the airways open by maintaining positive pressure (Table 28-13), and abdominal breathing, which slows the respiratory rate and encourages deeper breaths (see Table 6-6). You or the caregiver should stay with the patient until the respiratory rate (with the assistance of the medications) has slowed.

When the acute attack subsides, provide rest and a quiet, calm environment for the patient. When the patient has recovered from exhaustion, try to obtain a health history and do a physical assessment. If the caregiver and other family members are present, they may be able to provide information about the patient's health history (Table 28-12). This information is important in planning an individualized nursing care plan.

**Ambulatory Care.** Control of symptoms can also be achieved by teaching the patient about medications. However, the drug regimen itself can be confusing and complex. Teach patients the importance of monitoring their response to medication. It is easy to undermedicate or overmedicate unless careful monitoring is ongoing. Some patients may benefit from keeping a diary to record medication use, wheezing or coughing, peak flow, side effects of drugs, and activity level. This information will help the HCP adjust the medication if needed.

Good nutrition is important. Physical exercise (e.g., swimming, walking, stationary cycling) within the patient's limit of tolerance is also beneficial and may require pretreatment with an SABA (as noted previously). Sleep that is uninterrupted by asthma symptoms is an important goal. If patients with asthma wake up because of asthma symptoms, their asthma is not under good control and their therapeutic plan should be reevaluated.

Together with the patient and caregiver, develop a written asthma action plan (Fig. 28-8). Base these plans on the patient's asthma symptoms and PEFR. To follow the management plan,

## Asthma Action Plan

For: ______________________ Doctor: ______________________ Date: __________

Doctor's Phone Number ______________________ Hospital/Emergency Department Phone Number ______________________

**GREEN ZONE**

### Doing Well

- No cough, wheeze, chest tightness, or shortness of breath during the day or night
- Can do usual activities

**And, if a peak flow meter is used,**

**Peak flow:** more than __________ (80 percent or more of my best peak flow)

My best peak flow is: __________

**Take these long-term control medicines each day (include an antiinflammatory).**

| Medicine | How much to take | When to take it |
|---|---|---|
| | | |
| | | |
| | | |
| | | |
| | | |

| Before exercise | ❒ __________ | ❒ 2 or ❒ 4 puffs __________ | 5 minutes before exercise |
|---|---|---|---|

**YELLOW ZONE**

### Asthma Is Getting Worse

- Cough, wheeze, chest tightness, or shortness of breath, or
- Waking at night due to asthma, or
- Can do some, but not all, usual activities

**-Or-**

**Peak flow:** ________ to ________ (50 to 79 percent of my best peak flow)

**First** — **Add: quick-relief medicine—and keep taking your GREEN ZONE medicine.**

__________________ (short-acting beta$_2$-agonist) ❒ 2 or ❒ 4 puffs, every 20 minutes for up to 1 hour
❒ Nebulizer, once

**Second** — **If your symptoms (and peak flow, if used) return to GREEN ZONE after 1 hour of above treatment:**

❒ Continue monitoring to be sure you stay in the green zone.

**-Or-**

**If your symptoms (and peak flow, if used) do not return to GREEN ZONE after 1 hour of above treatment:**

❒ Take: __________________ (short-acting beta$_2$-agonist) ❒ 2 or ❒ 4 puffs or ❒ Nebulizer

❒ Add: __________________ (oral steroid) mg per day For ________ (3–10) days

❒ Call the doctor ❒ before/ ❒ within ____ hours after taking the oral steroid.

**RED ZONE**

### Medical Alert!

- Very short of breath, or
- Quick-relief medicines have not helped, or
- Cannot do usual activities, or
- Symptoms are same or get worse after 24 hours in Yellow Zone

**-Or-**

**Peak flow:** less than __________ (50 percent of my best peak flow)

### Take this medicine:

❒ __________________ (short-acting beta$_2$-agonist) ❒ 4 or ❒ 6 puffs or ❒ Nebulizer

❒ __________________ (oral steroid) mg

**Then call your doctor NOW.** Go to the hospital or call an ambulance if:

- You are still in the red zone after 15 minutes AND
- You have not reached your doctor.

### DANGER SIGNS

- **Trouble walking and talking due to shortness of breath**
- **Lips or fingernails are blue**

- **Take ❒ 4 or ❒ 6 puffs of your quick-relief medicine AND**
- **Go to the hospital or call for an ambulance __________ (phone) NOW!**

**FIG. 28-8** Asthma action plan. (Source: National Heart, Lung, and Blood Institute.)

the patient must measure his or her peak flow at least daily. Some patients may want to just monitor symptoms for self-management. Patients with asthma frequently do not perceive changes in their breathing. Therefore peak flow monitoring, when done correctly, can be a reliable, objective measurement of asthma control (Table 28-14).

If a patient's PEFR is within the green zone (usually 80% to 100% of the individual's personal best), the patient should remain on her or his usual medications. If the PEFR is within the yellow zone (usually 50% to 80% of personal best), it indicates caution. Something is triggering the patient's asthma (e.g., viral infection).

The patient should have a written asthma action plan that prescribes a step increase in medications during the acute phase of an infection (usually viral). The dose is stepped down once the viral infection symptoms subside. Based on the asthma

## TABLE 28-14 Patient Teaching

### *How to Use Your Peak Flow Meter*

*Include the following instructions when teaching the patient to use a peak flow meter.*

**Why Use a Peak Flow Meter?**

- Peak flow meters are used to check your asthma the way that BP cuffs are used to check BP. A peak flow meter is a device that measures how well air moves out of your lungs.
- During an asthma episode, the airways of the lungs usually begin to narrow slowly. The peak flow meter may tell you if there is narrowing in the airways hours, sometimes even days, before you have any asthma symptoms.
- By taking your medicines early (before symptoms), you may be able to stop the episode quickly and avoid a severe asthma episode.
- The peak flow meter also can be used to help you and your HCP:
  - Learn what makes your asthma worse.
  - Decide if your treatment plan is working well.
  - Decide when to add or stop medicine.
  - Decide when to seek emergency care.

**How to Use Your Peak Flow Meter**

Do the following five steps with your peak flow meter:

1. Move the indicator to the bottom of the numbered scale.
2. Stand up.
3. Take a deep breath, filling your lungs completely.
4. Place the mouthpiece in your mouth and close your lips around it. Do not put your tongue inside the hole.
5. Blow out as hard and fast as you can in a single blow.
   - Write down the number you get. But if you cough or make a mistake, do not write down the number. Do it over again.
   - Repeat steps 1 through 5 two more times, and write down the best of the three blows in your asthma diary.

**Find Your Personal Best Peak Flow Number**

- Your personal best peak flow number is the highest peak flow number you can achieve over a 2-week period when your asthma is under good control. Good control is when you feel good and do not have any asthma symptoms.
- Each patient's asthma is different, and your best peak expiratory flow (PEF) may be higher or lower than the peak flow of someone of your height, weight, and gender. This means that it is important for you to find your own personal best peak flow number, which is the basis for your treatment plan.
- To find your personal best peak flow number, take peak flow readings:
  - At least twice a day for 2-3 wk, between 12 noon and 2 PM when your peak flow is the highest
  - 15-20 min after taking inhaled short-acting $\beta_2$-agonist (SABA) for quick relief
  - As instructed by your HCP

**The Peak Flow Zone System**

Once you know your personal best peak flow number, your HCP will put the peak flow numbers into zones that are set up like a traffic light. This will help you know what to do when your peak flow number changes. For example:

Green Zone (more than __L/min [80% of your personal best number]) signals good control. No asthma symptoms are present. Take your medicines as usual.

Yellow Zone (between __ and __L/min [50% to <80% of your personal best number]) signals caution. If you remain in the yellow zone after several measures of peak flow, take an inhaled SABA. If you continue to register peak flow readings in the yellow zone, your asthma may not be under good control. Ask your HCP if you need to change or increase your daily medicines.

Red Zone (<__L/min [<50% of your personal best number]) signals a medical alert. Take an inhaled SABA (quick-relief medicine) right away. Call your HCP or the emergency department and ask what to do, or go directly to the emergency department.

**Use the Diary to Keep Track of Your Peak Flow**

- Record your personal best peak flow number and peak flow zones in your asthma diary.
- Measure your peak flow when you wake up, *before* taking medicine. Write down your peak flow number in the diary every day, or as instructed by your HCP.

**Actions to Take When Peak Flow Numbers Change**

- PEF goes between __ and __L/min (50% to <80% of personal best, yellow zone).

***ACTION:*** Take an inhaled SABA (quick-relief medicine) as prescribed by your HCP.

- PEF increases ≥20% when measured before and after taking an inhaled SABA (quick-relief medicine).

***ACTION:*** Talk to your HCP about adding more medicine to control your asthma better (e.g., an antiinflammatory medication).

Source: Adapted from National Asthma Education and Prevention Program, National Heart, Lung, and Blood Institute: *Expert Panel Report 3: guidelines for the diagnosis and management of asthma*, NIH pub no 08-4051, Bethesda, Md, 2007, National Institutes of Health. Retrieved from *www.nhlbi.nih.gov/guidelines*.

management plan, the patient can use different strategies, such as using the SABA more frequently.

If the PEFR is in the red zone (50% or less of personal best), it indicates a serious problem. A rescue plan should be a part of the asthma action plan. Teach the patient and caregiver to take definitive action. Emphasize to the patient the need to monitor PEFR daily or several times a day to have an objective measure that can be correlated with symptoms. Although it may happen, it is unusual for a patient's PEFR to drop from the green zone to the red zone quickly. Usually the patient has time to make changes in medications, avoid triggers, and notify the HCP.

It is important to involve the patient's caregiver or family. They should know where the patient's inhalers, oral medications, and emergency phone numbers are located. Instruct the caregiver or family on how to decrease the patient's anxiety if an asthma attack occurs. When the patient is stabilized or controlled, the caregiver can gently remind the patient about doing daily PEFR by asking questions such as, "What zone are you in? How's your peak flow today?" A patient and caregiver teaching guide for the patient with asthma is presented in Table 28-15.

**CHECK YOUR PRACTICE**

A 32-yr-old man is admitted to the emergency department for an acute exacerbation of asthma. It is his third admission in the past 2 months. He had been watching his 6-yr-old son play soccer when his attack started. He says to you, "I am just not a good father. My son is going to think I am just a 'sicky.' I cannot participate in his sports. I cannot even watch them without something happening."

- How would you respond to this man?

An increased number of older adults are diagnosed with asthma. This is a special concern because they have more complicated health issues than younger patients with asthma. Issues that face older adults are costly medications, nonadherence to medical regimen, and difficulty accessing the health care system.

**TABLE 28-15 Patient & Caregiver Teaching**
***Asthma***

*Include the following information in a teaching plan for the patient with asthma and the caregiver. It will help to improve the patient's quality of life and promote lifestyle changes that support successful living with asthma.*

**What is Asthma?**
- Basic anatomy and physiology of lung
- Pathophysiology of asthma
- Relationship of pathophysiology to signs and symptoms
- Measurement and correlation of spirometry and peak expiratory flow rate

**What Is Good Asthma Control?**
- Personal ideas of good control
- Use Asthma Control Test available at *www.asthmacontroltest.com*

**Hindrances to Asthma Treatment and Control**
- Discuss with patient and caregiver about possible hindrances (e.g., denial, poor perception of asthma severity by patient)

**Environmental and Trigger Control**
- Identifications of possible triggers and possible preventive measures (use trigger diary)
- Avoidance of allergens and other triggers
- Need to maintain good hydration

**Medications**
- Types (include mechanism of action)
- $\beta_2$-Agonists
- Corticosteroids
- Methylxanthines
- Anti-IgE
- Leukotriene modifiers
- Combination drugs
- Use of preventive and maintenance (e.g., antiinflammatory) agents
- Write out medication list and schedule
- Asthma Action Plan (Fig. 28-8)

**Correct Use of Inhalers, Spacer, and Nebulizer**
- Demonstration–return demonstration with placebo devices (Figs. 28-5 to 28-7 and Tables 28-9 to 28-11)

**Breathing Techniques**
- Pursed-lip breathing (Table 28-13)

**Correct Use of Peak Flow Meter**
See Table 28-14.

**Asthma Action Plan** (Fig. 28-8)
- Peak flow zones
- Individualize plan
- Patient completes asthma action plan and discusses it with HCP.
- Early recognition of infection
- Building a partnership with your HCP
- Questions patients may have about asthma, but patient cannot reach the HCP

For additional information, see the American Lung Association at *http://www.lung.org/lung-disease/asthma.*

Keep these factors in mind when implementing a management plan for older adults.

A variety of factors may contribute to why African Americans and Hispanics (especially those from Puerto Rico) have higher rates of poorly controlled asthma and deaths compared with whites. Some factors may be disparities in socioeconomic status and access to proper health care, cultural beliefs about the management of asthma, and underutilization of the long-term controller medications because of high costs.[10] Seek to explore and eliminate any barriers to health care. Also seek out culturally appropriate resources and educational material in languages other than English to improve asthma control for these individuals.

Relaxation therapies (e.g., yoga, meditation, relaxation techniques, breathing techniques) may help a patient relax respiratory muscles and decrease the respiratory rate. (Chapter 6 discusses relaxation breathing and other relaxation strategies.) A healthy emotional outlook is also important in preventing asthma attacks. Some communities have asthma support groups.

### ◆ Evaluation

The expected outcomes are that the patient with asthma will
- Maintain clear airway with removal of excessive secretions
- Have normal (for the individual) breath sounds and respiratory rate
- Report decreased anxiety with increased control of respirations
- Describe the disease process and treatment regimen
- Demonstrate correct administration of inhaled drugs
- Express confidence in ability for long-term management of asthma

Additional information on expected outcomes for the patient with asthma is presented in eNursing Care Plan 28-1 available on the website for this chapter.

## CHRONIC OBSTRUCTIVE PULMONARY DISEASE

**Chronic obstructive pulmonary disease (COPD)** is a preventable and treatable disease characterized by persistent airflow limitation that is usually progressive. COPD is associated with an enhanced chronic inflammatory response in the airways and lungs, primarily caused by cigarette smoking and other noxious particles and gases. COPD exacerbations and other coexisting illnesses or co-morbidities contribute to the overall severity of the disease.[11]

Previous definitions of COPD have included such terms as *chronic bronchitis* and *emphysema,* but neither term is part of the current definition of COPD. **Chronic bronchitis**, the presence of cough and sputum production for at least 3 months in each of 2 consecutive years, is an independent disease that may precede or follow the development of airflow limitation. **Emphysema** is the destruction of the alveoli and is a pathologic term that explains only one of several structural abnormalities in COPD patients.

An estimated 12.7 million adults in the United States over age 18 have COPD.[2] An additional 24 million people have evidence of impaired lung function. The number of people with COPD is greatly underestimated because the disease is usually not diagnosed until it is moderately advanced. COPD is the third leading cause of death in the United States, resulting in more than 133,000 deaths in Americans each year.[12]

**GENDER DIFFERENCES**

***Chronic Obstructive Pulmonary Disease (COPD)***

**Men**

- COPD is more common in men than in women, but the incidence is not increasing in men.
- Fewer men die from COPD than women.

**Women**

- The number of women with COPD is increasing.
- Increase is probably due to increased number of women smoking cigarettes and increased susceptibility (e.g., smaller lungs and airways, lower elastic recoil).
- Women with COPD have lower quality of life, more exacerbations, increased dyspnea, and better response to $O_2$ therapy compared with men.

## Etiology

Many factors can influence the development and progression of COPD. The following discussion addresses these numerous factors.

**Cigarette Smoking.** The major risk factor for developing COPD is cigarette smoking.[12,13] COPD affects about 15% of smokers.[14] An intriguing question is why some smokers develop COPD and others do not. COPD should be considered in any person who is over the age of 40 with a smoking history of 10 or more pack-years.

Cigarette smoke has several direct effects on the respiratory tract (Table 28-16). The irritating effect of the smoke causes hyperplasia of cells, including goblet cells, thereby increasing the production of mucus. Hyperplasia reduces airway diameter and increases the difficulty in clearing secretions. Smoking reduces the ciliary activity and may cause actual loss of cilia. Smoking also produces abnormal dilation of the distal air space with destruction of alveolar walls. Many cells develop large, atypical nuclei, which are considered a precancerous condition.

**TABLE 28-16 Effects of Tobacco Smoke on Respiratory System**

| Area of Defect | Acute Effects | Long-Term Effects |
|---|---|---|
| Respiratory mucosa | | |
| • Nasopharyngeal | ↓ Sense of smell | Cancer |
| • Tongue | ↓ Sense of taste | Cancer |
| • Vocal cords | Hoarseness | Chronic cough, cancer |
| • Bronchus and bronchioles | Bronchospasm, cough | Chronic bronchitis, asthma, cancer |
| Cilia | Paralysis, sputum accumulation, cough | Chronic bronchitis, cancer |
| Mucous glands | ↑ Secretions, ↑ cough | Hyperplasia and hypertrophy of glands, chronic bronchitis |
| Alveolar macrophages | ↓ Function | ↑ Incidence of infection |
| Elastin and collagen fibers | ↑ Destruction by proteases<br>↓ Function of antiproteases ($\alpha_1$-antitrypsin)<br>↓ Synthesis and repair of elastin | Emphysema |

Smoking causes chronic, enhanced inflammation of various parts of the lung with structural changes and repair (called *remodeling*). The reasons for the inflammatory response are not clearly understood but may be genetically determined, since patients who have never smoked can develop COPD.

Cigarette smoking causes oxidative stress, as well as an imbalance between proteases that break down connective tissue in the lung and antiproteases that protect the lungs. These changes resulting from cigarette smoking increase with more severe disease and persist even after smoking cessation. (See Chapter 10 for more details about cigarette smoking.)

*Passive smoking* is the exposure of nonsmokers to cigarette smoke, also known as *environmental tobacco smoke* (ETS) or secondhand smoke. In adults, involuntary smoke exposure is associated with decreased pulmonary function, increased respiratory symptoms, and severe lower respiratory tract infections (e.g., pneumonia). ETS is also associated with increased risk for lung cancer and nasal sinus cancer.

**Occupational Chemicals and Dusts.** If a person has intense or prolonged exposure to various dusts, vapors, irritants, or fumes in the workplace, symptoms of lung impairment consistent with COPD can develop. If a person has occupational exposure and smokes, the risk of COPD increases.[11]

**Air Pollution.** High levels of urban air pollution are harmful to people with existing lung disease. However, the effect of outdoor air pollution as a risk factor for the development of COPD is unclear. Another risk factor for COPD development is coal and other biomass fuels that are used for indoor heating and cooking. Many people who have never smoked are at significant risk for developing COPD because of cooking with these fuels in poorly ventilated areas.[11]

**Infection.** Infections are a risk factor for developing COPD. Severe recurring respiratory tract infections in childhood have been associated with reduced lung function and increased respiratory symptoms in adulthood. It is unclear whether the development of COPD can be related to recurrent infections in adults. People who smoke and also have human immunodeficiency virus (HIV) infection have an accelerated development of COPD. Tuberculosis is also a risk factor for COPD development.

**Genetics.** The fact that a relatively small percentage of smokers get COPD strongly suggests that genetic factors influence which smokers get the disease. Because of the genetic-environmental interaction, two people may have the same smoking history, but only one develops COPD. To date, one genetic factor has been clearly identified (see next section).

**$\alpha_1$-Antitrypsin (AAT) Deficiency.** **$\alpha_1$-Antitrypsin (AAT) deficiency** is an autosomal recessive disorder that may affect the lungs or liver. AAT deficiency is a genetic risk factor for COPD. Approximately 3% of all people diagnosed with COPD may have undetected AAT deficiency. AAT is a serum protein produced by the liver and normally found in the lungs. The main function of AAT, an $\alpha_1$-protease inhibitor, is to protect normal lung tissue from attack by proteases during inflammation related to cigarette smoking and infections. Severe AAT deficiency leads to premature bullous emphysema in the lungs found on x-ray. Smoking greatly exacerbates the disease process in these patients.

### Genetic Link

AAT deficiency is an autosomal recessive disorder (see Figs. 12-4 and 12-5 and the Genetics in Clinical Practice box on p. 184).

The severity of AAT deficiency depends on which forms of the gene are inherited. The most common abnormal genes are the S and Z alleles. The normal genotype is MM. The most common genotype associated with AAT disease is ZZ (also referred to as *PI-ZZ*). Other variations include MZ (slightly increased risk of poor lung function) and SZ (higher risk of lung and liver problems in smokers). Some individuals with MZ and SZ genotypes may never seek health care because they have minimal manifestations of the disorder.[15]

## GENETICS IN CLINICAL PRACTICE

### *$\alpha_1$-Antitrypsin (AAT) Deficiency*

**Genetic Basis**

- Autosomal recessive disorder
- Mutations in *SERPINA1* gene (located on chromosome 14) cause AAT deficiency.
- Gene provides instructions for the liver to make the protein AAT, which protects the lungs and liver from powerful proteolytic enzymes.
- Without enough functional AAT, proteolytic enzymes destroy alveoli and cause lung disease.

**Incidence**

- Occurs in 1 in 1700 to 3500 live births in the United States
- People of northern European descent most affected

**Genetic Testing**

- DNA testing is available.
- Screening of siblings is useful.
- Serum assay is available to measure the amount of AAT.

**Clinical Implications**

- AAT deficiency can cause lung and liver disease.
- Onset of disease is between ages 20 and 40 yr.
- Treatment includes AAT replacement (Prolastin).
- Disease predisposes to early-onset emphysema.

Although 100,000 people in the United States are suspected of having the ZZ phenotype, fewer than 10% have been detected. Clues to AAT deficiencies are the onset of symptoms often occurring by age 40, minimal to no tobacco use, and family history of COPD and/or liver disease. Chronic liver disease as an infant or adult with increased liver enzyme levels may also be seen. Individuals with this type of COPD are primarily of northern European origin.[15]

A simple blood test can determine low levels of AAT. Those with borderline or low levels can then be genetically tested.

IV-administered AAT (e.g., Prolastin-C) augmentation therapy is used for people with AAT deficiency. The infusions are usually administered weekly. Its effectiveness in slowing the progression of the disease and the results of this treatment continue to be evaluated.

**Aging.** Although aging is often considered a risk factor for COPD, the evidence is unclear. Does the aging process lead to COPD, or is COPD a result of the cumulative exposures that occur over a long life? Normal aging results in loss of elastic recoil, stiffening of the chest wall, gas exchange alteration, and decrease in exercise tolerance. As people age, the lungs gradually lose their elastic recoil. Thoracic cage changes result from osteoporosis and calcification of the costal cartilages. The thoracic cage becomes stiff and rigid, and the ribs are less mobile. The shape of the rib cage gradually changes because of the increased residual volume (RV), causing it to expand and become rounded. Decreased chest compliance and elastic recoil of the lungs caused by aging affect the mechanical aspects of ventilation and increase the work of breathing.

As one ages, the number of functional alveoli decreases as peripheral airways lose supporting tissues. The surface area for gas exchange decreases, and the $PaO_2$ decreases. Changes in the elasticity of the lungs reduce the ventilatory reserve. These changes are similar to those seen in the patient with COPD.

**Asthma.** Patients with COPD may have asthma. Asthma may be a risk factor for the development of COPD. There is a considerable pathologic and functional overlap between these disorders, particularly among older adults, who may have components of both diseases. Recently this disorder has been called *asthma-COPD overlap syndrome.*

**Gender.** In the past, COPD prevalence and mortality were greater in men than women. Now the prevalence is almost equal, reflecting the changing patterns of cigarette smoking. Women may be more susceptible to the adverse effects of smoking.[16]

### Pathophysiology

COPD is characterized by chronic inflammation of the airways, lung parenchyma (respiratory bronchioles and alveoli), and pulmonary blood vessels (Fig. 28-9). The pathogenesis of COPD is complex and involves many mechanisms. The defining feature of COPD is not fully reversible airflow limitation during forced exhalation. This is caused by loss of elastic recoil and airflow obstruction caused by mucus hypersecretion, mucosal edema, and bronchospasm.

In COPD, various processes occur, such as airflow limitation, air trapping, gas exchange abnormalities, and mucus hypersecretion. In severe disease, pulmonary hypertension and systemic manifestations occur (Fig. 28-9). COPD has an uneven distribution of pathologic changes, with severely destroyed lung areas existing together with areas of relatively normal lung.

The inflammatory process starts with inhalation of noxious particles and gases (e.g., cigarette smoke) but is magnified in the person with COPD. The abnormal inflammatory process causes tissue destruction and disrupts the normal defense mechanisms and repair process of the lung. The mechanisms for the enhanced inflammatory response are not clearly understood but may be genetically determined.

The predominant inflammatory cells in COPD are neutrophils, macrophages, and lymphocytes. This pattern of inflammatory cells is different from that in asthma. (In asthma, the inflammatory cells are eosinophils, mast cells, neutrophils, lymphocytes, and macrophages.) These inflammatory cells attract other inflammatory mediators (e.g., leukotrienes) and proinflammatory cytokines (e.g., tumor necrosis factor). The end result of the inflammatory process is structural changes in the lungs.

The inflammatory process may also be magnified by oxidants, which are produced by cigarette smoke and other inhaled particles and released from the inflammatory cells. The oxidants adversely affect the lungs as they inactivate antiproteases (which prevent the natural destruction of the lungs), stimulate mucus secretion, and increase fluid in the lungs.

After the inhalation of oxidants in tobacco or air pollution, the activity of proteases (which break down the connective tissue of the lungs) increases and the antiproteases (which protect against the breakdown) are inhibited. Therefore the natural balance of protease/antiprotease is tipped in favor

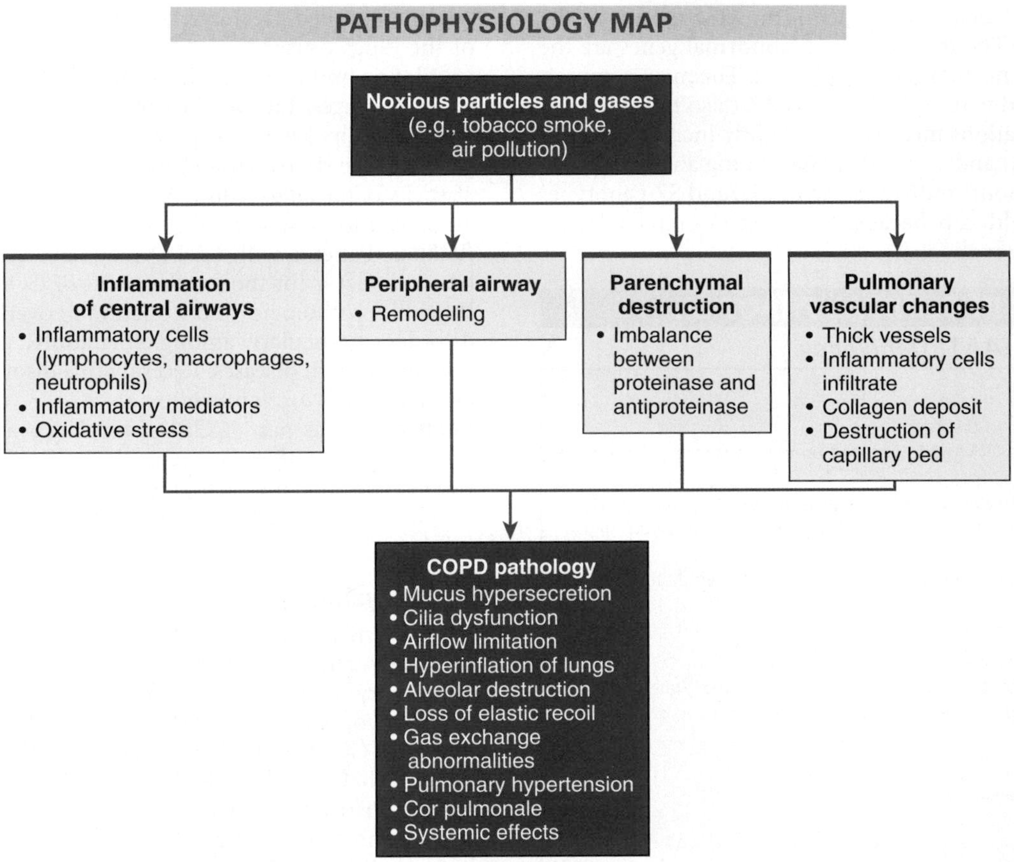


**FIG. 28-9** Pathophysiology of chronic obstructive pulmonary disease *(COPD)*.

of destruction of the alveoli and loss of the lungs' elastic recoil.

Inability to expire air is a main characteristic of COPD. The primary site of the airflow limitation is in the smaller airways. As the peripheral airways become obstructed, air is progressively trapped during expiration. The volume of residual air becomes greatly increased in severe disease as alveolar attachments (similar to rubber bands) to small airways are destroyed. The residual air, combined with the loss of elastic recoil, makes passive expiration of air difficult. As air is trapped in the lungs, the chest hyperexpands and becomes barrel shaped because the respiratory muscles are not able to function effectively. The functional residual capacity is increased. The patient is now trying to breathe in when the lungs are in an "overinflated" state. Thus the patient appears dyspneic and exercise capacity is limited.

Gas exchange abnormalities result in hypoxemia and hypercapnia (increased $CO_2$) as the disease worsens. As the air trapping increases, walls of alveoli are destroyed (Fig. 28-10), and bullae (large air spaces in the parenchyma) and blebs (air spaces adjacent to pleurae) can form.

Bullae and blebs are not effective in gas exchange because they do not contain the capillary bed that normally surrounds each alveolus. Therefore a significant ventilation-perfusion (V/Q) mismatch and hypoxemia result. Peripheral airway obstruction also results in V/Q imbalance and, combined with the respiratory muscle impairment, can lead to $CO_2$ retention, particularly in severe disease.

Excess mucus production, resulting in a chronic productive cough, is a feature of individuals with predominant chronic bronchitis. However, not all COPD patients have sputum production. When present, excess mucus production is multifactorial, including (1) an increased number of mucus-secreting goblet cells, (2) enlarged submucosal glands, (3) dysfunction of cilia, and (4) stimulation from inflammatory mediators.

Pulmonary vascular changes resulting in mild to moderate pulmonary hypertension may occur late in the course of COPD. The small pulmonary arteries vasoconstrict due to hypoxia. As the disease advances, the structure of the pulmonary arteries changes, resulting in thickening of the vascular smooth muscle. Because of the loss of alveolar walls and the capillaries surrounding them, pressure in the pulmonary circulation increases.

Typically, the patient does not have difficulty with hypoxemia at rest until late in the disease. However, hypoxemia may develop during exercise, and the patient may benefit from supplemental $O_2$. Pulmonary hypertension may progress and lead to hypertrophy of the right ventricle of the heart (**cor pulmonale**). The right ventricle dilates and may eventually lead to right-sided heart failure.

In addition to lung disease, COPD is a systemic disease. Chronic inflammation is an underlying etiology for these systemic effects. Cardiovascular diseases commonly exist in COPD (smoking is a primary risk factor for both of them). Other common systemic diseases include cachexia (skeletal muscle wasting), osteoporosis, diabetes, and metabolic syndrome, which cannot be readily related to smoking.

## Clinical Manifestations

Clinical manifestations of COPD typically develop slowly. A clinical diagnosis of COPD should be considered in any patient

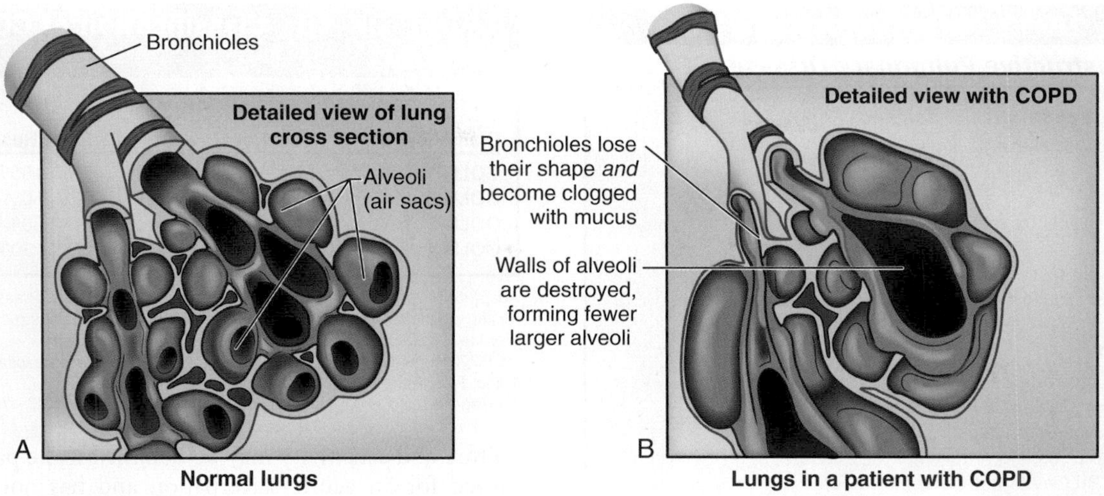


**FIG. 28-10** **A,** Normal lungs showing bronchioles and alveoli. **B,** Changes in the bronchioles and alveoli in the lungs of a patient with chronic obstructive pulmonary disease *(COPD).*

who has chronic cough or sputum production, dyspnea, and a history of exposure to risk factors for the disease (e.g., tobacco smoke, occupational dusts, and chemicals).

A chronic intermittent cough, which is often the first symptom to develop, may be present every day as the disease progresses. The cough is often dismissed by patients as they expect it with smoking or environmental exposures. The cough may be unproductive of mucus. However, significant airflow limitation may exist without sputum or cough. Typically dyspnea is progressive, usually occurs with exertion, and is present every day.

Patients may complain of not being able to take a deep breath, heaviness in the chest, gasping, increased effort to breathe, and air hunger. Patients usually ignore the symptoms and rationalize that "I'm getting older" and "I'm out of shape." They change behaviors to avoid dyspnea, such as taking the elevator instead of the stairs. Gradually the dyspnea interferes with daily activities, such as carrying grocery bags. They cannot walk as fast as their partners or peers. However, as symptoms worsen and interfere with daily activity or they have their first COPD exacerbation, patients usually seek medical care.

In late stages of COPD, dyspnea may be present at rest. As more alveoli become overdistended, increasing amounts of air are trapped. This causes the diaphragm to flatten, and the patient must breathe from partially inflated lungs. Effective abdominal breathing is decreased because of the flattened diaphragm from the overinflated lungs. The person becomes more of a chest breather, relying on the intercostal and accessory muscles. However, chest breathing is not efficient.

Wheezing and chest tightness may be present but may vary by time of the day or from day to day, especially in patients with more severe disease. Wheezes may arise from the laryngeal area, or wheezes may not be present on auscultation. Chest tightness, which often follows activity, may feel similar to muscular contraction.

The person with advanced COPD frequently experiences fatigue, weight loss, and anorexia. Even with adequate caloric intake, the patient still loses weight. Fatigue is a highly prevalent symptom that affects the patient's activities of daily living.[17] Paroxysms of coughing may be so severe that the patient faints or fractures a rib.

During physical examination a prolonged expiratory respiratory phase, wheezes, or decreased breath sounds are noted in all lung fields. The patient may need to breathe louder than normal for auscultated breath sounds to be heard. The anteroposterior diameter of the chest is increased ("barrel chest") from the chronic air trapping. The patient may sit upright with arms supported on a fixed surface such as an overbed table *(tripod position)*. The patient may naturally purse lips on expiration (pursed-lip breathing) and use accessory muscles, such as those in the neck, to aid with inspiration. Edema in the ankles may be the only clue to right-sided heart involvement (cor pulmonale).

Over time, hypoxemia ($PaO_2$ less than 60 mm Hg or $O_2$ saturation less than 88%) may develop with hypercapnia ($PaCO_2$ over 45 mm Hg). The bluish-red color of the skin results from polycythemia and cyanosis. Polycythemia develops as a result of increased production of red blood cells as the body attempts to compensate for chronic hypoxemia. Hemoglobin concentrations may reach 20 g/dL (200 g/L) or more. However, the person may also have lowered hemoglobin and hematocrit because of chronic anemia.

It is sometimes difficult to distinguish COPD from asthma, especially if the individual has a history of cigarette smoking. However, some clinical features are different (Table 28-3).

## Complications

Complications that can occur in patients with COPD include cor pulmonale, acute exacerbations, and acute respiratory failure. These complications and their causes and treatment are discussed in the section on Interprofessional Care on p. 563.

## Diagnostic Studies

A history and physical examination are extremely important in a diagnostic workup. Spirometry is required to confirm the diagnosis in individuals suspected of having COPD. Spirometry confirms the presence of airflow obstruction and determines the severity of COPD.

In spirometry, the patient is given a short-acting bronchodilator, and postbronchodilator values are compared with a normal reference value. A diagnosis of COPD is made when the $FEV_1/FVC$ ratio is less than 70%. The value of $FEV_1$ provides

## TABLE 28-17 Interprofessional Care

### *Chronic Obstructive Pulmonary Disease (COPD)*

**Diagnostic Assessment**

- History and physical examination
- Spirometry
- Chest x-ray
- Serum $\alpha_1$-antitrypsin levels
- ABGs
- Six-minute walk test
- COPD Assessment Test (CAT)* or Clinical COPD Questionnaire (CCQ)†

**Management**

- Cessation of cigarette smoking
- Drug therapies (Tables 28-8 and 28-19)
- Airway clearance techniques
- Breathing exercises and retraining
- Hydration of 3 L/day (if not contraindicated)
- Immunizations
  - Influenza yearly
  - Pneumococcal vaccine (see Table 27-5 for guidelines)
- Long-term $O_2$ (if indicated)
- Progressive plan of exercise, especially walking and upper body strengthening
- Pulmonary rehabilitation program
- Nutritional supplementation if low BMI
- Treatment of complications
  - Cor pulmonale
  - Acute exacerbations
  - Acute respiratory failure
- Surgical therapy
  - Lung volume reduction
  - Bullectomy
  - Lung transplantation

*ABGs,* Arterial blood gases; *BMI,* body mass index.
*See *www.catestonline.org.*
†See *www.ccq.nl.*

a guideline for the degree of severity of COPD. $FEV_1$ can be expressed as a percentage compared with a normal reference value (percent predicted). The lower the $FEV_1$, the more obstructed are the airways.

In addition to spirometry, other diagnostic studies may be performed (Table 28-17). Chest x-rays are not diagnostic but may show a flat diaphragm because of the hyperinflated lungs. Patients often have exercise-induced hypoxemia, and a 6-minute walk test may be done by a physical or respiratory therapist, with pulse oximetry readings taken when the patient is walking and at rest. If values of $O_2$ saturation are 88% or lower when at rest and the patient is breathing room air, he or she qualifies for supplemental $O_2$.

Validated questionnaires such as the COPD Assessment Test (CAT) *(www.catestonline.org)* and Clinical COPD Questionnaire (CCQ) *(www.ccq.nl)* are recommended for a comprehensive assessment of symptoms.

ABGs are usually assessed in the severe stages ($FEV_1$ less than 50%) and monitored in patients hospitalized with acute exacerbations. In the later stages of COPD, typical findings are low $PaO_2$, elevated $PaCO_2$, decreased or low-normal pH, and increased $HCO_3^-$ levels (Table 28-3). In early stages, there may be a normal or only slightly decreased $PaO_2$ and a normal $PaCO_2$. An ECG may be normal or show signs of right ventricular failure.

An echocardiogram or multigated acquisition (MUGA) (cardiac blood pool) scan (see Table 31-6) can be used to evaluate right- and left-sided ventricular function. Sputum for

## TABLE 28-18 Classification of COPD Severity*

*The following classification is based on postbronchodilator $FEV_1$.*

| Classification | Level of Severity | $FEV_1$ Results |
|---|---|---|
| **GOLD 1** | Mild | $FEV_1$ ≥80% predicted |
| **GOLD 2** | Moderate | $FEV_1$ 50%-80% predicted |
| **GOLD 3** | Severe | $FEV_1$ 30%-50% predicted |
| **GOLD 4** | Very severe | $FEV_1$ <30% predicted |

Adapted from Global Initiative for Chronic Obstructive Lung Disease: Global strategy for the diagnosis, management, and prevention of chronic obstructive pulmonary disease (updated 2015). Retrieved from *www.goldcopd.org.*
*COPD,* Chronic obstructive pulmonary disease; *$FEV_1$,* forced expiratory volume in 1 sec; *FVC,* forced vital capacity.
*A diagnosis of COPD is made when a patient has a $FEV_1$/FVC <70%.

culture and sensitivity may be obtained if the patient is hospitalized for an acute exacerbation and has not responded to antibiotic therapy.

### Classification of COPD

COPD can be classified as mild, moderate, severe, and very severe (Table 28-18). An $FEV_1$/FVC ratio of less than 70% establishes the diagnosis of COPD, and the severity of obstruction (as indicated by $FEV_1$) determines the stage of COPD. The management of COPD is based on the patient's symptoms, classification, and exacerbation history.

### Interprofessional Care: Stable COPD

Most patients with COPD are treated as outpatients. They are hospitalized for complications such as acute exacerbations and acute respiratory failure.

Evaluate the patient's exposure to environmental or occupational irritants, and determine ways to control or avoid them. For example, teach the patient to avoid aerosol hair sprays and smoke-filled rooms. The patient with COPD is extremely susceptible to pulmonary infections. The patient with COPD should receive an influenza immunization yearly. The pneumococcal vaccine is recommended for all smokers ages 19 or older and all patients with COPD. (The guidelines for pneumococcal vaccine are presented in Table 27-5.)

**Smoking Cessation.** Cessation of cigarette smoking in any person with COPD at any level of severity is the most important intervention that can affect the natural history of COPD. After a person discontinues smoking, the accelerated decline in pulmonary function found with smoking slows to almost nonsmoking levels. Thus the sooner the smoker stops, the less pulmonary function is lost and the sooner the symptoms decrease, especially cough and sputum production. (Smoking cessation techniques are discussed in Chapter 10 and in Tables 10-4 to 10-6.)

**Drug Therapy.** Medications for COPD can reduce symptoms, increase exercise capacity, improve overall health, and reduce the number and severity of exacerbations. Bronchodilator drug therapy relaxes smooth muscles in the airway and improves the ventilation of the lungs, thus reducing the degree of breathlessness. Patients with COPD do not respond as dramatically to bronchodilator therapy as those with asthma. However, bronchodilator therapy reduces dyspnea and increases $FEV_1$. The inhaled route of medication is preferred and given on a PRN or regular basis.

Patients commonly do not properly administer inhaled medications. Therefore it is important for you to demonstrate

**TABLE 28-19 Drug Therapy**

***Medication Guidelines for Stable COPD***

*The treatment guidelines are based on the $FEV_1$ results.*

| $FEV_1$ Results | Treatment Guidelines* |
|---|---|
| **$FEV_1$ 60%-80% predicted (with respiratory symptoms)** | Treatment with inhaled bronchodilators may be used. |
| **$FEV_1$ <60% predicted (with respiratory symptoms)** | Treat with inhaled bronchodilators: anticholinergics or long-acting $\beta_2$–agonist<br>OR<br>Monotherapy with long-acting inhaled anticholinergics or long-acting $\beta_2$-agonist<br>OR<br>Combination therapy with long-acting inhaled anticholinergics, long-acting $\beta_2$-agonist, or inhaled corticosteroids |

Source: Qaseem A, Wilt T, Weinberger S, et al: Diagnosis and management of stable chronic obstructive pulmonary disease: a clinical practice guideline update from the American College of Physicians, American College of Chest Physicians, American Thoracic Society, and European Respiratory Society, *Ann Intern Med* 155:179, 2011.
*$FEV_1$,* Forced expiratory volume in 1 sec.
*NOTE: Occasional use of short-acting inhaled bronchodilator for acute symptoms is not addressed in these recommendations.

and talk with patients about inhaler use. Give the patient clear, readable instructions.

Medications are given in a stepwise fashion according to the level of airflow obstruction determined from spirometry ($FEV_1$) and symptoms. Medications are stepped up but usually not stepped down, as in asthma, because in COPD continual symptoms are probably present (Table 28-19).

Bronchodilator medications commonly used are $\beta_2$-adrenergic agonists; anticholinergic agents; and, to a much lesser extent, methylxanthines (Table 28-8). The choice of a bronchodilator depends on the patient's response. These medications are given on a PRN or scheduled basis. When the patient has mild COPD or fewer symptoms, a short-acting bronchodilator is used. Albuterol or ipratropium may be used as single agents, but combining bronchodilators improves their effect and decreases the risk of adverse effects. Albuterol and ipratropium can be nebulized together (DuoNeb) or delivered by inhalation spray (Combivent Respimat).

In the moderate stage of COPD ($FEV_1$ less than 60%), a long-acting bronchodilator may be used (Tables 28-8 and 28-19). A short-acting bronchodilator may still be used PRN as a "rescue" for dyspnea. Salmeterol and formoterol are widely used LABAs, and they can be used in COPD as monotherapy (unlike drug therapy for asthma).

In COPD patients with $FEV_1$ of less than 60%, regular treatment with ICS is often prescribed and used in addition to LABA. Examples of combinations of ICSs with LABAs are fluticasone/salmeterol (Advair) and budesonide/formoterol (Symbicort).

Inhaled long-acting anticholinergics, LABAs, and ICSs all reduce COPD exacerbations. However, in COPD, unlike asthma, ICSs are not used as monotherapy because of the concerns about side effects. Some patients are on triple therapy with Advair and tiotropium. Oral corticosteroids should not be used for long-term therapy in COPD but are effective for short-term use to treat exacerbations.

The use of long-acting theophylline in the treatment of COPD is controversial because it interacts with many drugs. A low dose of theophylline with an ICS may benefit a few patients with COPD who do not respond to other inhaled medications.

Roflumilast (Daliresp) is an oral medication used to decrease the frequency of exacerbations in patients with severe COPD and the presence of chronic bronchitis. This drug is a phosphodiesterase inhibitor, which is an antiinflammatory drug that suppresses the release of cytokines and other inflammatory mediators and inhibits the production of reactive $O_2$ radicals.

New drug delivery devices are becoming available at a rapid pace. One example is Respimat, which is an easy-to-use, handheld device that provides a high deposition of drug to the lungs and low mouth and throat deposition. Respimat simplifies coordination between activation of the medication and inhalation without propellant, and it is independent of inspiratory flow. It also has a dose indicator. Combivent Respimat (ipratropium and albuterol) inhalation aerosol is available.

### Interprofessional Care: COPD Complications

**Cor Pulmonale.** *Cor pulmonale* results from pulmonary hypertension, which is caused by diseases affecting the lungs or pulmonary blood vessels (Fig. 28-11). Cor pulmonale is a late manifestation of COPD, yet not all patients with COPD develop cor pulmonale. Once the patient develops cor pulmonale, the prognosis worsens.

In COPD, pulmonary hypertension is caused primarily by constriction of the pulmonary vessels in response to alveolar hypoxia. Chronic hypoxia also stimulates erythropoiesis, which causes polycythemia. This results in increased viscosity of the blood. These patients have increased pulmonary vascular resistance and thus develop pulmonary hypertension.

Normally the right ventricle and pulmonary circulatory system are low-pressure systems compared with the left ventricle and systemic circulation. When pulmonary hypertension develops, the pressures on the right side of the heart must increase to push blood into the lungs. Eventually, right-sided heart failure develops.

Dyspnea is the most common symptom of chronic cor pulmonale. Lung sounds are normal, or crackles may be heard in the bases of the lungs bilaterally. Heart sound changes occur but are usually masked by the underlying lung disease. Other manifestations of right-sided heart failure may develop, including distended neck veins (jugular venous distention), hepatomegaly with right upper quadrant tenderness, peripheral edema, and weight gain.

Typically the patient has large pulmonary vessels on chest x-ray and increased pressure on a right-sided heart cardiac catheterization. Echocardiogram may reflect right-sided heart enlargement. B-type natriuretic peptide (BNP) levels, which are used to diagnose heart failure, may be elevated in cor pulmonale secondary to the stretching of the right ventricle. Normally BNP levels are used to distinguish cardiac from respiratory causes of dyspnea, but in cor pulmonale the cause of the heart failure is the lung disease.

Treatment of cor pulmonale is initially targeted at managing the COPD, including bronchodilator and continuous low-flow, long-term $O_2$ therapy (for more than 15 hr/day), which improves survival.[18] Diuretics are generally administered, similar to their use with chronic heart failure. (Cor pulmonale is also discussed in Chapter 27.)

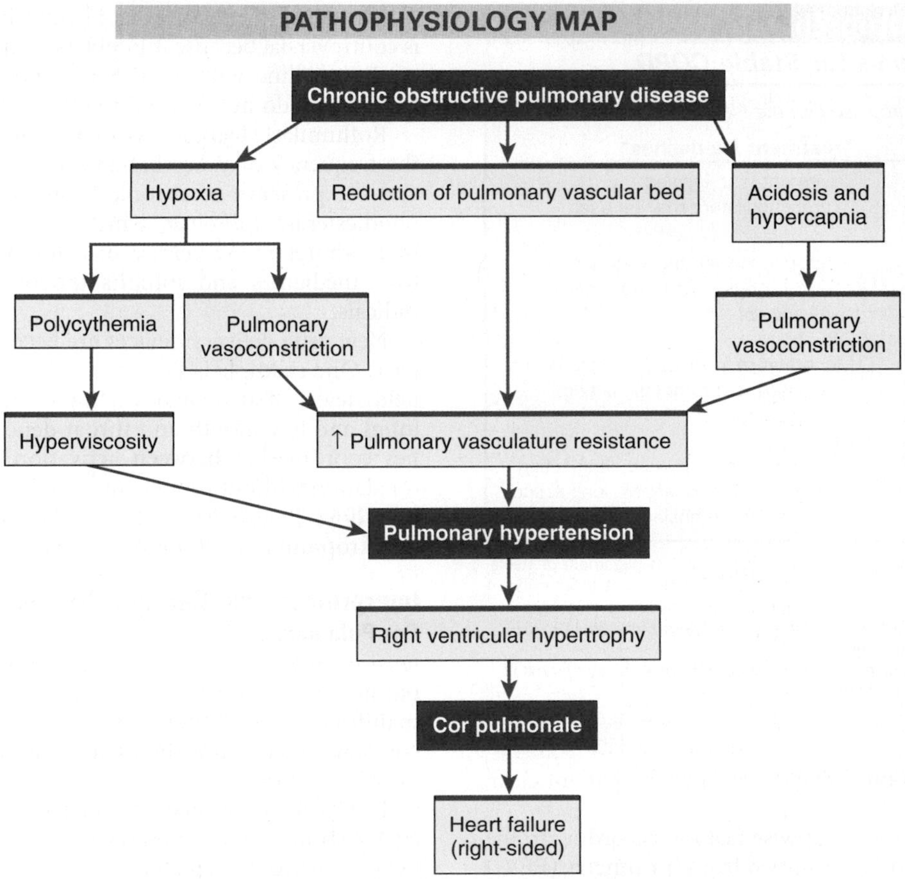


**FIG. 28-11** Mechanisms involved in the pathophysiology of pulmonary hypertension and cor pulmonale secondary to chronic obstructive pulmonary disease.

**Acute Exacerbations.** An exacerbation of COPD is an acute event characterized by a worsening of the patient's respiratory symptoms. Exacerbations are signaled by an acute change in the patient's usual dyspnea, cough, and/or sputum (i.e., something different from the usual daily patterns). The primary causes of exacerbations are bacterial or viral infections.[11] Exacerbations of COPD are typical and increase in frequency (average one or two a year) as the disease progresses.

Assess patients for the classic manifestations of exacerbation: increased dyspnea, increased sputum volume, or increased sputum purulence. They may also have nonspecific complaints of malaise, insomnia, fatigue, depression, confusion, decreased exercise tolerance, increased wheezing, or fever without other causes.

As the severity of COPD increases, exacerbations of COPD are associated with poorer outcomes. Exacerbations may be treated at home or in the hospital, depending on the severity. The severity is determined by the patient's medical history before the exacerbation, the presence of other diseases, current symptoms, ABGs, and other laboratory tests. Typically in the later stages of COPD the patient has a low-normal pH, high-normal or above-normal $PaCO_2$, and high-normal bicarbonate ($HCO_3^-$). This indicates compensated respiratory acidosis as the patient has chronically retained $CO_2$ and the kidneys have conserved $HCO_3^-$ to increase the pH to within the normal range (Table 28-3).

Carefully assess the patient's ABGs for any movement toward respiratory acidosis and further hypoxemia, indicating respiratory failure. Also assess the patient's medical history for the stage of COPD as noted by the level of $FEV_1$. Assess for new symptoms or worsening of usual symptoms. Determine the number of previous exacerbations per year and if treatment occurred in the home or hospital. The presence of other co-morbid conditions complicates the exacerbation. In addition, the current treatment affects its management. Be alert for signs of severity such as use of accessory muscles, central cyanosis, edema in the lower extremities, unstable BP, right-sided heart failure, and altered alertness. These manifestations affect whether the patient is treated as an inpatient or outpatient.

Short-acting bronchodilators, oral systemic corticosteroids, and antibiotics are the typical therapies for exacerbations. SABAs with or without short-acting anticholinergics are preferred for those who are breathless. Drug administration via MDI or nebulizer works equally well, although sicker patients often prefer the nebulizer. Antibiotics are used for the treatment of exacerbations caused by bacterial infections.[19]

Therapies used to treat exacerbations of COPD in the hospital are similar to home management, except supplemental $O_2$ therapy titrated by ABG measurement may be used. Attempts are made to use noninvasive mechanical methods (e.g., continuous positive airway pressure [CPAP] or bi-level positive airway pressure [BiPap] to support ventilation rather than invasive ventilatory support [e.g., intubation and mechanical ventilation]).

Teach the patient and caregiver early recognition of the three cardinal manifestations of exacerbations (increased dyspnea, increased sputum volume, or increased sputum purulence) to promote early treatment. This may prevent hospitalization and possible respiratory failure.

**Acute Respiratory Failure.** Patients with severe COPD who have exacerbations are at risk for acute respiratory failure. Frequently, COPD patients wait too long to contact their HCP when they first develop symptoms suggestive of an exacerbation. Discontinuing bronchodilator or corticosteroid medication may also precipitate respiratory failure.[20] (Respiratory failure is discussed in Chapter 67.)

## Interprofessional Care: Other COPD Treatments

**Oxygen Therapy.** $O_2$ therapy is frequently used in the treatment of COPD and other problems associated with hypoxemia. $O_2$ is a colorless, odorless, tasteless gas that constitutes 21% of the atmosphere. Administering supplemental $O_2$ increases the partial pressure of $O_2$ ($PO_2$) in inspired air. Used clinically, it is considered a prescribed medication and the only one that has been proven to improve survival of COPD patients.

$O_2$ is usually administered to treat hypoxemia caused by a variety of problems such as COPD, shock, pulmonary emboli, and many others. Goals for $O_2$ therapy are to keep the $SaO_2$ greater than 90% during rest, sleep, and exertion or the $PaO_2$ greater than 60 mm Hg.

***Methods of Administration.*** There are various methods of $O_2$ administration (Table 28-20 and Fig. 28-12). The method selected depends on factors such as the fraction of inspired $O_2$ ($FIO_2$) required by the patient and delivered by the device, the patient's mobility, humidification required, patient cooperation, comfort, cost, and financial resources.

$O_2$ delivery systems are classified as low- or high-flow systems. Most methods of $O_2$ administration are low-flow devices that deliver $O_2$ in concentrations that vary with the person's respiratory pattern. In contrast, the Venturi mask is a high-flow device that delivers fixed concentrations of $O_2$ (e.g., 24%, 28%) independent of the patient's respiratory pattern. Mechanical ventilators are another example of a high-flow $O_2$ delivery system. Because room air is mixed with $O_2$ in low-flow systems, the percentage of $O_2$ delivered to the patient is not as precise as with high-flow systems.

***Humidification and Nebulization.*** $O_2$ obtained from cylinders or wall systems is dry. Dry $O_2$ has an irritating effect on mucous membranes and dries secretions. Therefore it is important that a high liter flow of $O_2$, delivering more than 35% to 50% $O_2$, be humidified, either by humidification or nebulization. A common device used for humidification when the patient has a cannula or a mask is a small plastic jar filled with distilled water called a *bubble-through humidifier.* It is attached to the $O_2$ source by means of a flowmeter.

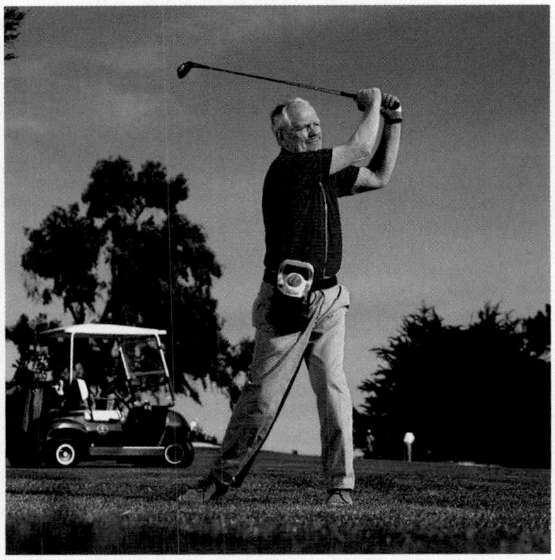

**FIG. 28-12** Golfer uses Helios liquid portable $O_2$ system. (Courtesy Nellcor Puritan Bennett, Inc, Pleasanton, Calif.)

***Complications***

**Combustion.** $O_2$ supports combustion and increases the rate of burning, so it is important to prohibit smoking or have open flames in the area in which $O_2$ is being used. A "No Smoking" sign should be prominently displayed on the patient's door. Also caution the patient against smoking cigarettes with an $O_2$ cannula in place as it can cause significant burns.

**$CO_2$ narcosis.** The chemoreceptors in the respiratory center that control the drive to breathe respond to $CO_2$ and $O_2$. Normally, $CO_2$ accumulation is a major stimulant of the respiratory center. Over time some COPD patients with hypercapnia develop a tolerance for high $CO_2$ levels (the respiratory center loses its sensitivity to the elevated $CO_2$ levels). Theoretically, for these individuals a major "drive" to breathe is hypoxemia. Thus there has been concern regarding the dangers of administering $O_2$ to COPD patients and reducing their drive to breathe. However, the "hypoxic drive" is complex and involves other factors, including ventilation and perfusion. In addition, not all patients with COPD retain $CO_2$.

Pulse oximetry and/or ABGs are used as a guide to determine what $FIO_2$ level is sufficient and can be tolerated. Safe administration of $O_2$ can be achieved by gradually increasing the concentration of $O_2$ with close monitoring of both $PaO_2$ and $PaCO_2$. Venturi masks may be used to have tighter regulation of the maximal $FIO_2$ that is administered. With nasal cannulas, the $O_2$ flow rate is generally increased by 1 L per minute at a time. The goal is a pulse $O_2$ saturation ($SpO_2$) of at least 90% or a $PaO_2$ of at least 60 mmHg. Always remember to assess the patient's mental status and vital signs before starting $O_2$ therapy and frequently thereafter.

**$O_2$ toxicity.** Pulmonary $O_2$ toxicity may result from prolonged exposure to a high level of $O_2$ ($PaO_2$). High concentrations of $O_2$ can result in a severe inflammatory response because of $O_2$ radicals and damage to alveolar-capillary membranes resulting in severe pulmonary edema, shunting of blood, and hypoxemia. Although rare, these individuals can develop acute respiratory distress syndrome (ARDS) (see Chapter 67).

Prevention of $O_2$ toxicity is important for the patient who is receiving $O_2$. The amount of $O_2$ administered should be just enough to maintain the $PaO_2$ within a normal or acceptable range for the patient. Monitor ABGs frequently to evaluate the effectiveness of therapy and guide the tapering of supplemental $O_2$. A safe limit of $O_2$ concentrations has not yet been established. All levels above 60% and $O_2$ used for longer than 24 hours should be considered potentially toxic. Levels of 40% and below used for short periods may be regarded as relatively nontoxic and probably will not result in significant $O_2$ toxicity.

**Infection.** Infection can be a major hazard of $O_2$ administration. Heated nebulizers present the highest risk. The constant use of humidity supports bacterial growth, with the most common organism being *Pseudomonas aeruginosa.* Disposable equipment that operates as a closed system, such as the Ballard closed suctioning system, should be used. Each hospital has a policy on the required frequency of equipment changes based on the type of equipment used.

## TABLE 28-20 Methods of Oxygen Administration

| Description | Nursing Interventions | |
|---|---|---|
| **Low-Flow Delivery Devices** | | |
| ***Nasal Cannula*** | | |
| • Most commonly used device<br>• $O_2$ delivered via plastic nasal prongs<br>• Safe and simple method that allows some freedom of movement. Patient can eat, talk, or cough while wearing device.<br>• Useful for a patient requiring low $O_2$ concentrations<br>• $O_2$ concentrations of 24% (at 1 L/min) to 44% (at 6 L/min) can be obtained. | • Stabilize nasal cannula when caring for a restless patient.<br>• Amount of $O_2$ inhaled depends on room air and patient's breathing pattern.<br>• Most patients with COPD can tolerate 2 L/min via cannula.<br>• Assess patient's nares and ears for skin breakdown. May need to pad cannula where it sits on ears<br>• If flow rates are >5 L/min, nasal membranes may dry and may cause pain in frontal sinuses. | 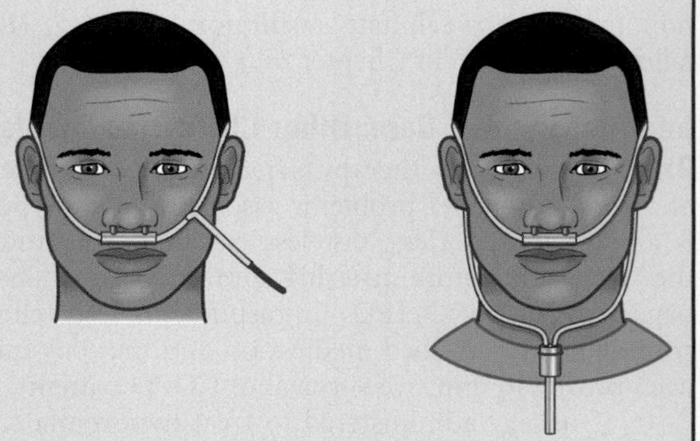 |
| ***Simple Face Mask*** | | |
| • Covers patient's nose and mouth<br>• Used only for short periods, especially when transporting patients<br>• Longer use is typically not tolerated because of tight seal and heat generated around nose and mouth from mask.<br>• $O_2$ concentrations of 35%-50% can be achieved with flow rates of 6-12 L/min.<br>• Mask provides adequate humidification of inspired air. | • Wash and dry under mask q2hr.<br>• Mask must fit snugly.<br>• Nasal cannula may be provided while patient is eating.<br>• Watch for pressure necrosis at top of ears from elastic straps if patient wears for a longer time. (Gauze or other padding may alleviate this problem.) | 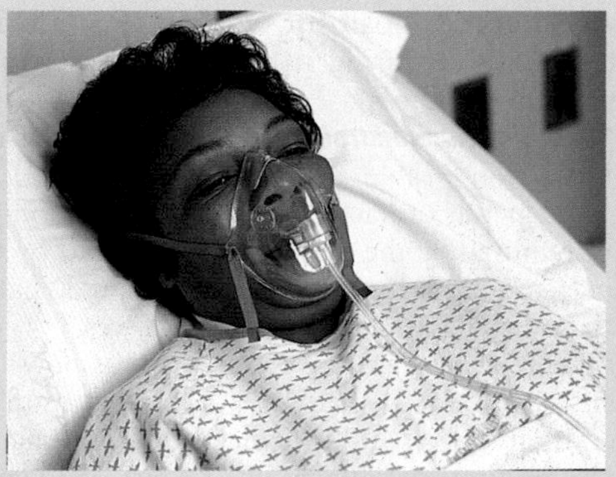 |
| ***Partial and Non-Rebreather Masks*** | | |
| • Useful for short-term (24 hr) therapy for patients needing higher $O_2$ concentrations (60%-90% at 10-15 L/min)<br>• $O_2$ flows into reservoir bag and mask during inhalation.<br>• This bag allows patient to rebreathe about first third of exhaled air (rich in $O_2$) in conjunction with flowing $O_2$.<br>• Vents remain open on partial mask only. Some facilities prefer this over non-rebreather as a safety issue. | • $O_2$ flow rate must be sufficient to keep bag from collapsing during inspiration to avoid $CO_2$ buildup.<br>• If deflation occurs, increase liter flow to keep bag inflated.<br>• Mask should fit snugly.<br>• With non-rebreather masks, make sure valves are open during expiration and closed during inhalation to prevent drastic decrease in $FIO_2$.<br>• Monitor patient closely, since more advanced interventions may be required such as CPAP, BiPAP, or intubation with mechanical ventilation. | 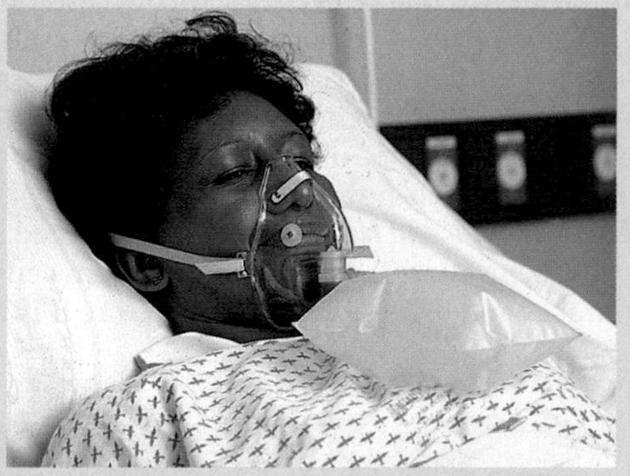 |
| ***Oxygen-Conserving Cannula*** | | |
| • Generally indicated for long-term $O_2$ therapy at home vs. during hospitalization (e.g., pulmonary fibrosis, pulmonary hypertension)<br>• May be "moustache" (Oxymizer) or "pendant" type<br>• Cannula has a built-in reservoir that ↑ $O_2$ concentration and allows patient to use lower flow, usually 30%-50%, which increases comfort, lowers cost, and can be increased with activities.<br>• Can deliver $O_2$ up to 8L/min. | • May cause necrosis over tops of ears. Can be padded<br>• Cannula cannot be cleaned. Manufacturer recommends changing cannula every week.<br>• It is more expensive than standard cannulas and requires evaluation with ABGs and oximetry to determine correct flow for patient.<br>• Cannula is highly visible. | 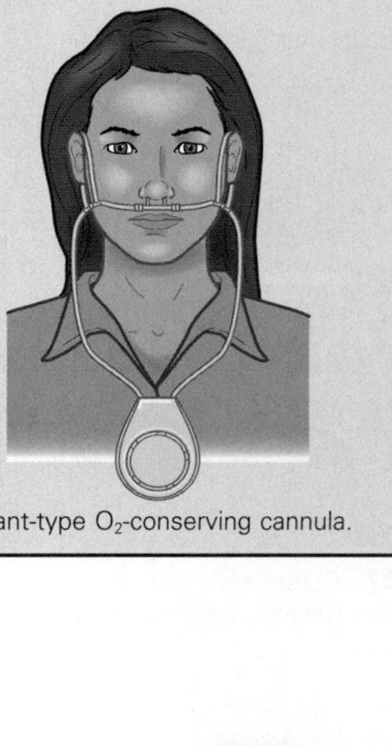<br>Pendant-type $O_2$-conserving cannula. |

*ABGs,* Arterial blood gases; *BiPAP,* biphasic positive airway pressure; *CPAP,* continuous positive airway pressure;

## TABLE 28-20 Methods of Oxygen Administration—cont'd

| Description | Nursing Interventions |
|---|---|
| **High-Flow Delivery Devices** | |
| ***Tracheostomy Collar*** | |
| • Collar attaches to neck with elastic strap and can deliver high humidity and $O_2$ via tracheostomy.<br>• $O_2$ concentration is lost into atmosphere because collar does not fit tightly.<br>• Venturi device can be attached to flowmeter and thus can deliver exact amounts of $O_2$ via collar. | • Secretions collect inside collar and around tracheostomy. Remove collar and clean at least q4hr to prevent aspiration of fluid and infection.<br>• Because condensation occurs in tubing, periodically drain distally to tracheostomy. |
| ***Tracheostomy T Bar*** | |
| • Almost identical to tracheostomy collar, but it has a vent and a T connector that allow an inline catheter (e.g., Ballard catheter) to be connected for suctioning.<br>• Tight fit allows better $O_2$ and humidity delivery than tracheostomy collar. | • Empty as necessary.<br>• Because T bars disconnect easily, monitor closely.<br>• T bar may pull on a patient's tracheostomy tube, causing irritation and potential tissue damage. Monitor this closely.<br>• See tracheostomy collar above. |
| ***Venturi Mask*** | |
| • Mask can deliver precise, high-flow rates of $O_2$.<br>• Lightweight plastic, cone-shaped device is fitted to face.<br>• Masks are available for delivery of 24%, 28%, 31%, 35%, 40%, and 50% $O_2$.<br>• Method is especially helpful for administering low, constant $O_2$ concentrations to patients with COPD.<br>• Adaptors can be applied to increase humidification. | • Entrainment device on mask must be changed to deliver higher concentrations of $O_2$.<br>• Air entrainment ports must not be occluded.<br>• Mask is uncomfortable. Remove when patient eats.<br>• Patient can talk but voice may be muffled.<br>• See other applicable nursing interventions under simple face mask above. |
| ***High-Flow Nasal Cannula*** | |
| • Blends $O_2$ with compressed air to generate $FIO_2$ up to 1.0 at flow rate of up to 60 L/min and PEEP 7.4 cm $H_2O$<br>• Active heated humidifier capable of providing 100% body humidity<br>• Soft and flexible nasal prongs. More comfortable than mask | • Nasal cannula must be smaller than 50% of nares to allow flow during exhalation and flush out end-expiratory $CO_2$.<br>• Patients can eat and drink with device in place.<br>• PEEP drops about 2 cm $H_2O$ when patient's mouth is open. |

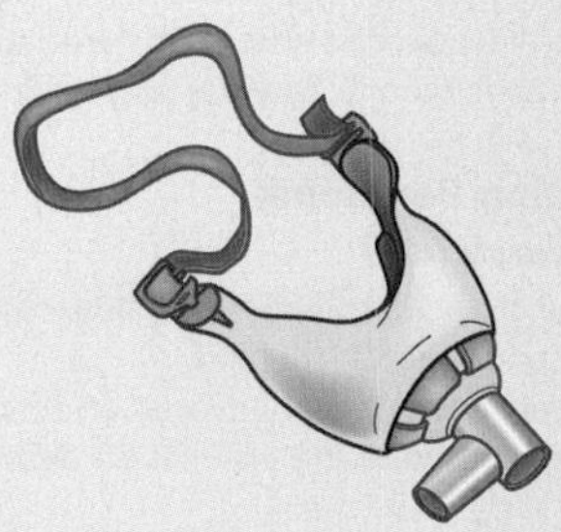

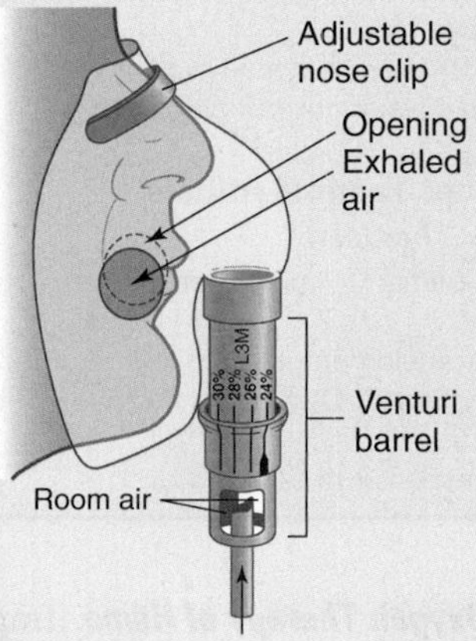


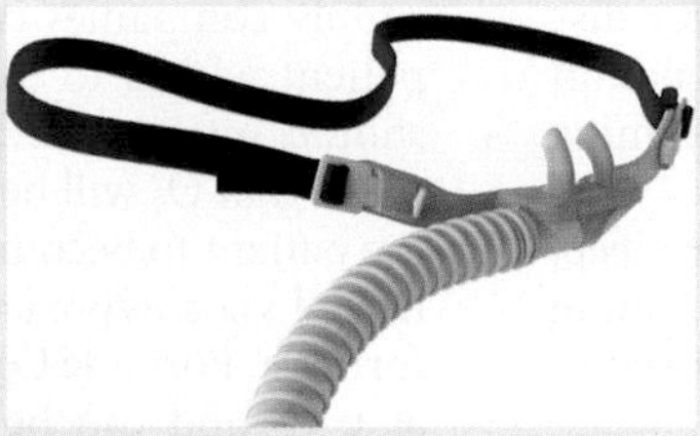

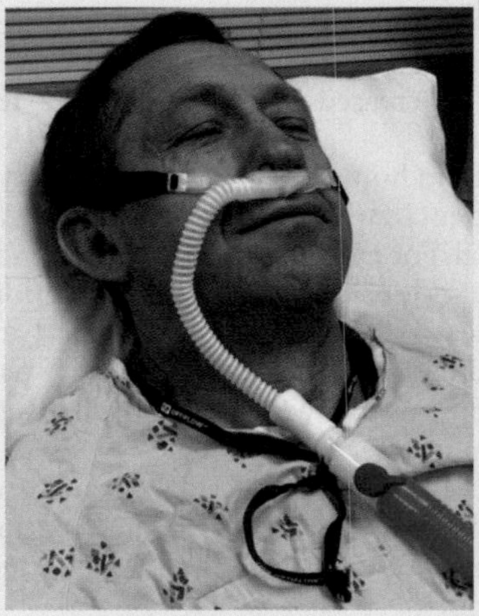

$FIO_2$, Fraction of inspired $O_2$.

## TEAMWORK & COLLABORATION
### *Oxygen Administration*

All members of the health care team should be alert to possible problems with gas exchange in patients who are receiving oxygenation. Patients who are hypoxemic should be cared for by the registered nurse (RN) until they consistently have $O_2$ saturations ≥90%.

**Role of Nursing Personnel**

***Registered Nurse (RN)***

- Assess need for adjustments in $O_2$ flow rate.
- Evaluate response to $O_2$ therapy.
- Monitor patient for signs of adverse effects of $O_2$ therapy.
- In many cases, choose the optimal $O_2$ delivery device (e.g., a nasal cannula or simple face mask).
- Teach patient and caregivers about home $O_2$ use.

***Licensed Practical/Vocational Nurse (LPN/LVN)***

- For stable patients, adjust $O_2$ flow rate depending on desired $O_2$ saturation level.

***Unlicensed Assistive Personnel (UAP)***

- Use pulse oximetry to measure $O_2$ saturation.
- Report $O_2$ saturation level to RN.
- Assist patient with adjustment of $O_2$ delivery devices (e.g., nasal cannula, face mask).
- Report to RN any change in patient level of consciousness or complaints of shortness of breath.

**Role of Other Team Members**

***Respiratory Therapist***

- Assist in optimal $O_2$ delivery device (e.g., nasal cannula or simple face mask).
- Make sure equipment is clean and replaced as needed.
- Check accuracy of $O_2$ delivery and assess need for adjustments in $O_2$ flow rate.
- Evaluate response to $O_2$ therapy.

***Chronic Oxygen Therapy at Home.*** Improved survival occurs in patients with COPD who receive long-term $O_2$ therapy (LTOT) (more than 15 hr/day) to treat hypoxemia. The benefits of LTOT include improved mental status, sleep, and exercise tolerance; decreased hematocrit; and reduced pulmonary hypertension.[11]

Short-term home $O_2$ therapy (7 to 30 days) may be indicated for the patient in whom hypoxemia persists after discharge from the hospital. For example, a patient with underlying COPD who develops a serious respiratory tract infection may need continued $O_2$ therapy to treat hypoxemia for 4 to 6 weeks after discharge from the hospital. Measure the patient's oxygenation status by $SpO_2$ 2 to 4 weeks after an acute episode to determine if the $O_2$ is still needed.

Patients may only receive $O_2$ during exercise and/or sleep. Evaluate the need for $O_2$ during these periods with a 6-minute walk test or overnight oximetry. (Pulse oximetry is discussed in Chapter 25.)

Periodic reevaluations are necessary for the patient who is using chronic supplemental $O_2$. Generally, the patient should be reevaluated every 30 to 90 days during the first year of therapy and annually after that, as long as the patient remains stable.

Nasal cannulas, either regular or the $O_2$-conserving type (Table 28-20), are usually used to deliver $O_2$ from a central source in the home. The source may be a liquid $O_2$ storage system, compressed $O_2$ in tanks, or an $O_2$ concentrator or extractor, depending on the patient's home environment, insurance coverage, activity level, and proximity to an $O_2$ supply company (Table 28-21). To increase mobility in the home, the patient can use extension tubing (up to 50 ft) without adversely affecting the $O_2$ flow delivery. Small, portable systems, such as liquid $O_2$, may be provided for the patient who remains active outside the home (Fig. 28-12).

**TABLE 28-21 Home Oxygen Delivery Systems**

- Liquid $O_2$
- Compressed $O_2$ cylinders
- Concentrator or extractor
- Portable $O_2$ concentrator
- $O_2$ conserving or pulsed devices

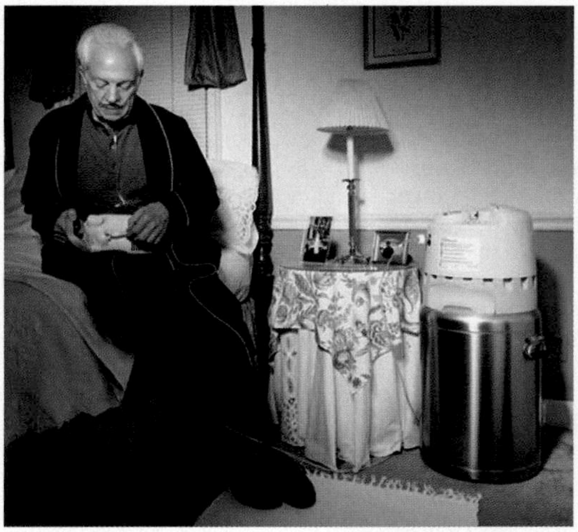

**FIG. 28-13** A portable liquid $O_2$ unit can be refilled from a liquid $O_2$ reservoir unit. (Courtesy Nellcor Puritan Bennett, Inc, Pleasanton, Calif.)

Home $O_2$ systems are usually rented from a company that sends a respiratory therapist to the patient's home (Fig. 28-13). The therapist teaches the patient and caregiver how to use the $O_2$ system, how to care for it, and how to recognize when the supply is running low and must be reordered. A patient and caregiver teaching guide for the use of $O_2$ at home is presented in Table 28-22.

Encourage the patient who uses home $O_2$ to remain active and travel normally. If travel is by automobile, arrangements can be made for $O_2$ to be available at the destination point. $O_2$ supply companies can often assist in these arrangements. If a patient wishes to travel by bus, train, or airplane, the patient should inform the appropriate people when reservations are made that $O_2$ will be needed for travel. If there is a potential for the patient to become hypoxic, $O_2$ needs for flying can be determined via a hypoxia inhalation test or through a mathematical formula. Portable $O_2$ concentrators are a ready source of renewable $O_2$ and can be available by recharging at home or with a DC (e.g., auto) power supply. These systems are widely approved by airlines for in-flight use. The patient should contact the airline to determine the particular accommodations and policies for in-flight $O_2$.

**Breathing Retraining.** The patient with COPD has dyspnea with an increased respiratory rate. In addition, the accessory muscles of breathing in the neck and upper part of the chest are used excessively to promote chest wall movement. These

**TABLE 28-22 Patient & Caregiver Teaching**

***Home Oxygen Use***

*The company that provides the prescribed $O_2$ therapy equipment will instruct the patient on equipment care. The following are some general instructions that you may include when teaching the patient and caregiver about the use of home $O_2$.*

**Decreasing Risk for Infection**

- Brush teeth or use mouthwash several times a day.
- Wash nasal cannula (prongs) with a liquid soap and thoroughly rinse once or twice a week.
- Replace cannula every 2-4 wk.
- If you have a cold, replace the cannula after your symptoms pass.
- Always remove secretions that are coughed out.
- If you use an $O_2$ concentrator, every day unplug the unit and wipe down the cabinet with a damp cloth and dry it.
- Ask the company providing the equipment how often to change the filter.

**Safety Issues**

- Post "No Smoking" warning signs outside the home.
- $O_2$ will not "blow up," but it will increase the rate of burning, since it is a fuel for the fire.
- Do not allow smoking in the home, and do not smoke yourself while wearing $O_2$. Nasal cannulas and masks can catch fire and cause serious burns to face and airways.
- Do not use flammable liquids such as paint thinners, cleaning fluids, gasoline, kerosene, oil-based paints, or aerosol sprays while using $O_2$.
- Do not use blankets or fabrics that carry a static charge, such as wool or synthetics.
- Inform the staff at your electric company if you are using a concentrator. In case of a power failure, they will know the medical urgency of restoring your power.

Adapted from *www.YourLungHealth.org.*

muscles are not designed for long-term use, and as a result, the patient experiences increased fatigue.

The main types of breathing retraining exercises are (1) pursed-lip breathing and (2) diaphragmatic breathing. The purpose of **pursed-lip breathing (PLB)** is to prolong exhalation and thereby prevent bronchiolar collapse and air trapping. PLB is simple and easy to teach and learn, and it gives the patient more control over breathing, especially during exercise and periods of dyspnea (Table 28-13). Patients should be taught to use "just enough" positive pressure with the pursed lips because excessive resistance may increase the work of breathing.

*Diaphragmatic (abdominal) breathing* focuses on using the diaphragm instead of the accessory muscles of the chest to (1) achieve maximum inhalation and (2) slow the respiratory rate. However, the use of diaphragmatic breathing in patients with COPD may increase the work of breathing and dyspnea. Patients with moderate to severe COPD with marked hyperinflation may be poor candidates for diaphragmatic breathing.[21]

PLB slows the respiratory rate and is easier to learn than diaphragmatic breathing. In the setting of extreme acute dyspnea, it is most important to focus on helping the patient slow the respiratory rate by using the principles of PLB. Other techniques that decrease breathing frequency, such as yoga, may also be used to reduce dyspnea.

**Airway Clearance Techniques.** Many patients with COPD or other conditions (e.g., cystic fibrosis, bronchiectasis) who retain secretions require help to adequately clear their airways. Airway clearance techniques (ACTs) loosen mucus and secretions so they can be cleared by coughing. A variety of techniques can be used to achieve airway clearance.

**TABLE 28-23 Patient & Caregiver Teaching**

***Effective Huff Coughing***

*When teaching effective huff coughing:*

1. Help the patient assume a sitting position with head slightly flexed, shoulders relaxed, knees flexed, forearms supported by pillow, and, if possible, feet on the floor.

*Then you should instruct the patient to:*

2. Inhale slowly through the mouth while breathing deeply from the diaphragm.
3. Hold the breath for 2-3 seconds.
4. Forcefully exhale quickly as if one is fogging up a mirror with one's breath (thus creating a "huff"). (This moves the secretions to larger airways.)
5. Repeat the "huff" one or two more times while refraining from a "regular" cough.
6. Cough when mucus is felt in the breathing tubes.
7. Rest for five to ten regular breaths.
8. Repeat the huffs (three to five cycles) until you feel you have cleared mucus or you become tired.

ACTs are especially beneficial in patients who have a COPD exacerbation. Respiratory therapists, physical therapists, and nurses are involved in performing these techniques. ACTs are often used with other treatments. Typically the patient receives bronchodilator therapy via an inhaled device (e.g., nebulization) before ACT. Then the ACT is used, followed by effective coughing (e.g., huff coughing). ACTs include effective coughing, chest physiotherapy, airway clearance devices, and high-frequency chest ventilation.

***Effective Coughing.*** Many patients with COPD have developed ineffective coughing patterns that do not adequately clear their airways of sputum. They also fear developing spastic coughing, resulting in increased dyspnea. Although other techniques (e.g., chest physiotherapy) are used to loosen secretions and mucus, the patient must cough effectively to bring the secretions to the central airways to expectorate them.

*Huff coughing* is an effective forced expiratory technique that you can easily teach the patient. Before starting, ensure that the patient is breathing deeply from the diaphragm. Place the patient's hands on the lower lateral chest wall and then ask the patient to breathe deeply through the nose. You should feel the patient's hands move outward, which represents a breath from the diaphragm. Guidelines for effective huff coughing are presented in Table 28-23.

***Chest Physiotherapy.*** **Chest physiotherapy (CPT)** is primarily used for patients with excessive bronchial secretions who have difficulty clearing them (e.g., cystic fibrosis, bronchiectasis). CPT consists of postural drainage, percussion, and vibration. CPT should be performed by an individual who has been properly trained.

*Percussion* and *vibration* are manual or mechanical techniques used to augment postural drainage. These techniques are used after the patient has assumed a postural drainage position to assist in loosening the mobilized secretions. Percussion, vibration, and postural drainage assist in bringing secretions into larger, more central airways. Effective coughing (huff coughing) is then necessary to help raise these secretions.

Complications associated with improperly performed CPT include fractured ribs, bruising, hypoxemia, and discomfort.

CPT may be stressful for some patients, and some may develop hypoxemia and bronchospasms.

**Postural drainage.** Postural drainage is the use of positioning techniques that drain secretions from specific segments of the lungs and bronchi into the trachea. The postural drainage positions used depend on the areas of lung that are involved. This is determined by patient assessment (including the patient's preference), chest x-rays, and chest auscultation. For example, some patients with left lower lobe involvement require postural drainage of only the affected region, whereas a person with cystic fibrosis may require postural drainage of all segments.

The purpose of various positions in postural drainage is to drain each segment toward the larger airways. A side-lying position can be used for the patient who cannot tolerate a head-down position. Aerosolized bronchodilators and hydration therapy are usually administered before postural drainage. The chosen postural drainage position is maintained for about 5 minutes during percussion and vibration. A common order is two to four times a day. In acute situations, postural drainage may be performed as frequently as every 4 hours. Schedule the procedure to be completed at least 1 hour before meals or 3 hours after meals.

Beds are available that can rotate and percuss in various postural drainage positions, and these are quite effective. Some positions for postural drainage (e.g., Trendelenburg) should not be performed on the patient with chest trauma, hemoptysis, heart disease, pulmonary embolus, or head injury, and in other situations in which the patient's condition is not stable.

**Percussion.** *Percussion* is performed in the appropriate postural drainage position with the hands in a cuplike position, with the fingers and thumbs closed (Fig. 28-14). The cupped hand should create an air pocket between the patient's chest and the hand. Both hands are cupped and used in an alternating rhythmic fashion. If it is performed correctly, a hollow sound should be heard. The air-cushion impact facilitates the movement of thick mucus. Place a thin towel over the area to be percussed, or the patient may choose to wear a T-shirt or hospital gown.

**Vibration.** *Vibration* is accomplished by tensing the hand and arm muscles repeatedly and pressing mildly with the flat of the hand on the affected area while the patient slowly exhales a deep breath. The vibrations facilitate movement of secretions to larger airways. Commercial mechanical vibrators are available for hospital and home use.

***Airway Clearance Devices.*** Various *airway clearance devices* are available to mobilize secretions, are easier to tolerate than CPT, and take less time than conventional CPT sessions. These devices include the Flutter, Acapella, and TheraPEP Therapy System. These devices use the principle of positive expiratory pressure (PEP) and may provide greater benefit to patients with COPD than other ACTs.

The Flutter mucus clearance device is a hand-held device that is shaped like a small, fat pipe. It provides PEP treatment for patients with mucus-producing conditions. The Flutter has a mouthpiece, a high-density stainless steel ball, and a cone that holds the ball. When the patient exhales through the Flutter, the steel ball moves, which causes oscillations (vibrations) in the airways and loosens mucus to allow improved expectoration. The patient must be upright, and the angle at which the Flutter is held is critical.

The Acapella is another small hand-held device (Fig. 28-15) that combines the benefits of both PEP therapy and airway vibrations to mobilize pulmonary secretions. It can be used in virtually any setting, since patients are free to sit, stand, or recline.

TheraPEP Therapy System can also provide sustained PEP and can simultaneously deliver aerosols so that the patient can inhale and exhale through it. TheraPEP has a mouthpiece attached to tubing connected to a small cylindric resistor and a pressure indicator. The pressure indicator provides visual feedback about the pressure that the patient needs to hold in an exhalation to receive the PEP. (A description and photo of this system are available at *www.smiths-medical.com/catalog/bronchial-hygiene/therapep/therapep-system.html.*)

***High-Frequency Chest Wall Oscillation.*** High-frequency chest wall oscillation uses an inflatable vest (e.g., the Vest Airway system or the SmartVest) with hoses connected to a high-frequency pulse generator. (A description and photo are available at *www.thevest.com/products.*) The pulse generator delivers air to the vest, which vibrates the chest. The high-frequency airwaves dislodge mucus from the airways, mobilize the mucus, and move it toward larger airways. The vest can be used without the aid of another person. The units weigh 23 to 30 lb and are quiet. They come in a suitcase and are portable.

**Nutritional Therapy for COPD.** Many COPD patients in the advanced stages are underweight with loss of muscle mass and cachexia. Weight loss is a predictor of a poor prognosis and increased frequency of COPD exacerbations. Malnutrition in COPD patients is multifactorial, including increased inflammatory mediators, increased metabolic rate due to the ventilatory effort, and lack of appetite. Other factors that contribute to malnutrition in COPD include altered taste caused by chronic mouth breathing, excessive sputum, fatigue, anxiety, depression, increased energy needs, numerous infections, and side effects of polypharmacy.

To decrease dyspnea and conserve energy, the patient should rest for at least 30 minutes before eating and use a bronchodilator before meals. Teach the patient to avoid exercise and treatments for at least 1 hour before and after eating. If a patient has $O_2$ therapy prescribed, use of supplemental $O_2$ by nasal cannula while eating may be beneficial. Assess the patient's dentition because broken or missing teeth or loose dentures make eating more difficult. Activity such as walking or getting out of bed during the day can stimulate the appetite and promote weight

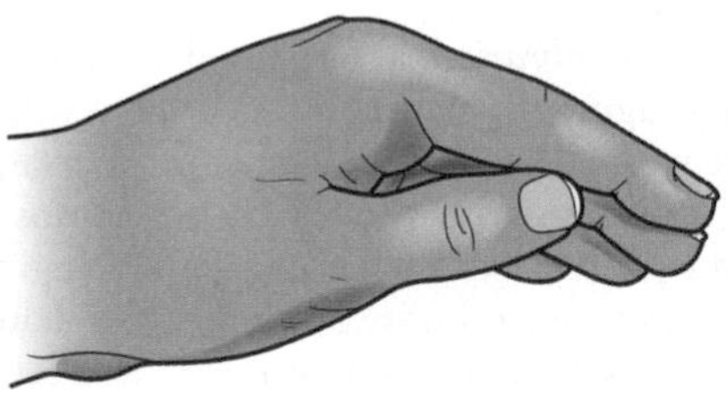

FIG. 28-14 Cupped-hand position for percussion. The hand should be cupped as though scooping up water.

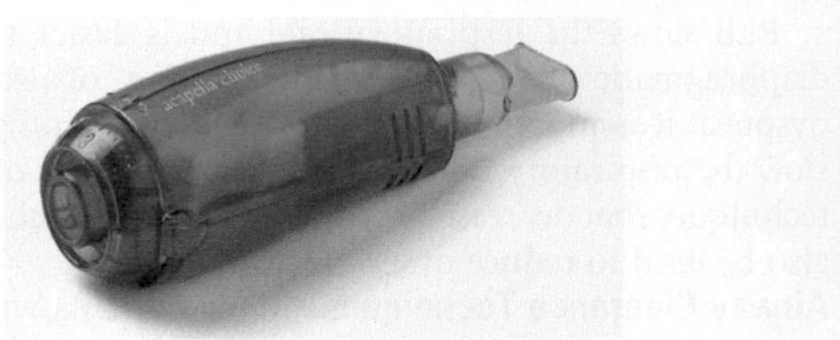

FIG. 28-15 Acapella airway clearance device. (Courtesy Smiths Medical North America.)

## TABLE 28-24 Nutritional Therapy

### Maximizing Food Intake in COPD

*Sometimes it is difficult for patients with COPD to consume adequate amounts of nutrients. Teach the patients to make mealtimes easier and more nutritious by increasing calories and protein without increasing the amount of food eaten.*

- Eat high-calorie foods first.
- Limit liquids at mealtimes.
- Rest before meals.
- Try more frequent meals and snacks.
- Increase calories by adding margarine, butter, mayonnaise, sauces, gravies, and peanut butter to foods.
- Keep favorite foods and snacks on hand.
- Try cold foods, which can make you feel less full than hot foods.
- Keep ready-prepared meals available for times when you have increased shortness of breath.
- Eat larger meals when you are not as tired.
- Avoid foods that you know cause gas (e.g., cabbage, beans, cauliflower).
- Add skim milk powder (2 Tbsp) to regular milk (8 oz) to add protein and calories.
- Use milk or half-and-half instead of water when making soups, cereals, instant puddings, cocoa, or canned soups.
- Add grated cheese to sauces, vegetables, soups, and casseroles.
- Choose dessert recipes that contain egg (e.g., sponge cake, angel food cake, egg custard, bread pudding, rice pudding).

Source: Grodner M, Roth S, Walkingshaw B: *Nutritional foundations and clinical applications: a nursing approach*, ed 5, St Louis, 2011, Mosby.

gain. Sensations of bloating and early satiety when eating can be attributed to swallowing air while eating, side effects of medication (especially corticosteroids and theophylline), and the abnormal position of the diaphragm relative to the stomach in association with hyperinflation of the lungs.

Getting the patient to eat adequate amounts of nutritionally sound foods may be difficult even though well-balanced meals are available. Give the patient or meal preparer printed information that can make mealtime easier and more nutritious (Table 28-24).

Underweight patients with COPD need extra protein and calories. They may need 25 to 45 kcal/kg body weight and more than 1.5 g of protein/kg body weight to maintain their weight. The patient with excessive malnutrition may need up to 2.5 g of protein/kg of body weight to restore muscle mass.

A diet high in calories and protein, moderate in carbohydrate, and moderate to high in fat is recommended and can be divided into five or six small meals a day.[22] High-protein, high-calorie nutritional supplements can be offered between meals (Table 28-24). The dietitian is the best resource to determine what combination of nutrients and what supplements are best for the patient. (Nutritional supplements are discussed in Chapter 39.)

**Surgical Therapy for COPD.** Four different surgical procedures are being used to treat severe COPD. One type of surgery is *lung volume reduction surgery* (LVRS). The goal of this surgery is to reduce the size of the lungs by removing the most diseased lung tissue so that the remaining healthy lung tissue can perform better. Reducing the size of the hyperinflated lungs results in decreased airway obstruction and increased room for the remaining normal alveoli (very small air sacs at the end of each bronchiole) to expand and function. The procedure reduces lung volume and improves lung and chest wall mechanics. LVRS can also allow the diaphragm (the strong wall of muscle that separates the chest cavity from the abdominal cavity; by moving downward, it creates suction in the chest to draw in air and expand the lungs) to return to its normal shape, allowing the patient to breathe more efficiently.

The second type of surgical procedure is *bronchoscopic lung volume reduction surgery* that works by placing one-way valves in the airways leading to the diseased parts of the lung. The valves let air out, but not in. This collapses a certain segment of the lung and produces a result similar to LVRS.[23]

The third surgical procedure is *bullectomy*. In this procedure, one or more very large bullae (large air sacs that form from destroyed alveoli) are removed. These air spaces can become so large that they interfere with breathing.

A fourth surgical procedure is *lung transplantation*, which benefits carefully selected patients with advanced COPD. Although single-lung transplant is the most commonly used technique because of a shortage of donors, bilateral transplantation can be performed. (Lung transplantation is discussed in Chapter 27.)

## Gerontologic Considerations: COPD

Older adults have physiologic changes, including reduced lean body mass and decreased respiratory muscle strength that may increase the burden of disease from COPD, including more dyspnea and lower exercise tolerance. This causes a poorer ADL status and a higher incidence of acute exacerbations, which require hospitalization.[24] Smoking cessation is a key intervention but can be difficult to achieve.

COPD is frequently complicated by the presence of co-morbidities such as cardiovascular disease, serious infections, osteoporosis, psychologic problems (depression, anxiety), impaired cognition, and lung cancer.[25] The presence of co-morbidities can make it difficult for patients to cope with the stress of an exacerbation. Thus assessment of co-morbidities can assist in ensuring comprehensive and safe management, especially during an exacerbation.

Older patients may have difficulty in handling the increased secretions during an acute COPD exacerbation. The use of additional medications to manage the acute exacerbation can complicate disease management and increase the likelihood of adverse events. Assess for potential drug-drug interactions, especially in patients being treated for co-morbidities.

Some medications used to treat common disorders in older adults, such as hypertension, can worsen COPD symptoms. Nonspecific β-blockers should be avoided since they can also block the $\beta_2$ receptors in the airway and cause bronchoconstriction. Angiotensin-converting enzyme (ACE) inhibitors may cause a dry cough or worsen a present cough.

Older adults may not be adherent to drug therapies due to cognitive impairment and complexity of the polypharmacy prescribed. Arthritis in the hands can hinder the person from using proper technique for MDIs. It is important to review MDI technique during clinic visits and have DPI or spacers prescribed (if possible) because they are easier to use. An attempt to simplify the medication regimen with written large font action plans can be an important intervention in patients with poor memory and visual impairment. Long-term use of ICSs has the potential of causing local and systemic side effects, including cataracts, glaucoma, and osteoporosis. Monitoring of ocular pressures, bone densitometry, and using the lowest possible ICS dose should be recommended.[26]

Older patients with COPD generally have impaired QOL.[27] An important role for you is to focus on things that will improve these patients' quality of life. Psychologic and emotional support becomes imperative to help them achieve successful outcomes. In the later stages of COPD, get palliative and hospice care involved to help manage symptoms and improve the quality of the remainder of their lives.[28]

## NURSING MANAGEMENT: CHRONIC OBSTRUCTIVE PULMONARY DISEASE

### Nursing Assessment

Subjective and objective data that should be obtained from a person with COPD are presented in Table 28-25.

### Nursing Diagnoses

The nursing diagnoses for the patient with COPD may include, but are not limited to, the following:

- Ineffective breathing pattern *related to* alveolar hypoventilation, anxiety, chest wall alterations, and hyperventilation
- Ineffective airway clearance *related to* expiratory airflow obstruction, ineffective cough, decreased airway humidity, and tenacious secretions
- Impaired gas exchange *related to* alveolar hypoventilation

Additional information on nursing diagnoses is presented in eNursing Care Plan 28-2 available on the website for this chapter.

### Planning

The overall goals are that the patient with COPD will have (1) prevention of disease progression, (2) ability to perform ADLs and improved exercise tolerance, (3) relief from symptoms, (4) no complications related to COPD, (5) knowledge and ability to implement a long-term treatment regimen, and (6) overall improved quality of life.

### Nursing Implementation

**Health Promotion.** The incidence of COPD would decrease dramatically if people would not begin smoking or would stop smoking. (Techniques to help patients stop smoking are discussed in Chapter 10 and Tables 10-4 to 10-6.) Avoiding or controlling exposure to occupational and environmental pollutants and irritants is another preventive measure to maintain healthy lungs. (These factors are discussed in the section on nursing management of lung cancer in Chapter 27.)

Counseling the patient in smoking cessation is vital, because it is the only way to slow the progression of COPD. As health care professionals, nurses who smoke should reevaluate their own smoking behavior and its relationship to their health. Nurses and other HCPs who smoke should be aware that the odor of smoke is obvious on their clothes, and it can be offensive or tempting to patients.

Early diagnosis and treatment of respiratory tract infections and exacerbations of COPD help prevent progression of the disease. People with COPD should avoid others who are sick, practice good hand-washing techniques, take medications as prescribed, exercise regularly, and maintain a healthy weight. Influenza and pneumococcal pneumonia vaccines are recommended for patients with COPD.

**TABLE 28-25 Nursing Assessment**

***Chronic Obstructive Pulmonary Disease***

| Subjective Data | Objective Data |
|---|---|
| ***Important Health Information*** | ***General*** |
| *Past health history:* Long-term exposure to chemical pollutants, respiratory irritants, occupational fumes, dust; recurrent respiratory tract infections; previous hospitalizations | Debilitation, restlessness, assumption of upright position |
| *Medications:* Use of $O_2$ and duration of $O_2$ use, bronchodilators, corticosteroids, antibiotics, anticholinergics, OTC drugs, herbs, medications purchased outside United States | ***Integumentary*** Cyanosis (bronchitis), pallor or ruddy color, poor skin turgor, thin skin, digital clubbing, easy bruising; peripheral edema (cor pulmonale) |
| ***Functional Health Patterns*** | ***Respiratory*** |
| *Health perception–health management:* Smoking (pack-years, including passive smoking, willingness to stop smoking, and previous attempts); family history of respiratory disease (especially $\alpha_1$-antitrypsin deficiency) | Rapid, shallow breathing; inability to speak; prolonged expiratory phase; pursed-lip breathing; wheezing; crackles, diminished or bronchial breath sounds; ↓ chest excursion and diaphragm movement; use of accessory muscles; hyperresonant or dull chest sounds on percussion |
| *Nutritional-metabolic:* Anorexia, weight loss or gain | ***Cardiovascular*** Tachycardia, dysrhythmias, jugular venous distention, distant heart tones, right-sided $S_3$ (cor pulmonale), edema (especially in feet) |
| *Activity-exercise:* Increasing dyspnea and/or increase in sputum volume or purulence (to detect exacerbation); fatigue, ability to perform ADLs; swelling of feet; progressive dyspnea, especially on exertion; ability to walk up one flight of stairs without stopping; wheezing; recurrent cough; sputum production (especially in the morning); orthopnea | ***Gastrointestinal*** Ascites, hepatomegaly (cor pulmonale) |
| *Elimination:* Constipation, gas, bloating | ***Musculoskeletal*** Muscle atrophy, ↑ anteroposterior diameter (barrel chest) |
| *Sleep-rest:* Insomnia; sitting up position for sleeping, paroxysmal nocturnal dyspnea | ***Possible Diagnostic Findings*** |
| *Cognitive-perceptual:* Headache, chest or abdominal soreness | Abnormal ABGs (compensated respiratory acidosis, ↓ $PaO_2$ or $SaO_2$, ↑ $PaCO_2$), polycythemia, pulmonary function tests showing expiratory airflow obstruction (e.g., low $FEV_1$, low $FEV_1$/FVC, large RV), chest x-ray showing flattened diaphragm and hyperinflation or infiltrates |
| *Coping–stress tolerance:* Anxiety, depression | |

*ABGs,* Arterial blood gases; *$FEV_1$,* forced expiratory volume in 1 sec; *FVC,* forced vital capacity; *RV,* residual volume.

Families with a history of COPD, as well as AAT deficiency, should be aware of the genetic nature of the disease. These individuals should consult a pulmonologist about regular spirometry screening, even though they do not have symptoms. Genetic counseling is appropriate for the patient with AAT deficiency who is planning to have children.

◆ **Acute Care.** The patient with COPD requires acute care for complications such as acute exacerbations of COPD, pneumonia, cor pulmonale, and acute respiratory failure. (The nursing care for these conditions is discussed in Chapters 27 and 67.) Once the crisis in these situations has been resolved, assess the degree and severity of the underlying respiratory problem. The information obtained will help in planning the nursing care.

◆ **Ambulatory Care.** By far the most important aspect in the long-term care of the patient with COPD is teaching. (A patient and caregiver teaching guide is presented in Table 28-26.)

◆ ***Pulmonary Rehabilitation.*** Pulmonary rehabilitation (PR) can be done in an inpatient or outpatient setting or in the home. Components of PR vary but usually include exercise training, smoking cessation, nutrition counseling, and education. A mandatory component of any PR program is exercise that focuses on the muscles used in ambulation, but upper limb exercises may be included also. Smoking cessation is critical to the patient's success. In PR an interprofessional team works together to individualize the treatment plan for COPD patients. Physical therapists or nurses who have experience in pulmonary care are often responsible for the management of pulmonary rehabilitation centers. A large part of your role is to teach patients self-management of their disease.

PR should not be viewed as a "last ditch" effort for patients with severe COPD since it is indicated for any degree of airway obstruction or GOLD classification. PR works best if the patient starts it when COPD is in a moderate stage. However, even people who have advanced COPD can benefit from PR. PR relieves dyspnea and fatigue, improves emotional function, and enhances the sense of control that individuals have over their COPD.[29,30]

PR may be inaccessible to some because of cost, disability, transportation, or geographic location. One alternative program to PR uses the Internet or gaming technology to deliver daily motivational messages and provide cardiopulmonary benefits.[31] However, these types of programs must be approved by the HCP to ensure safety.

## INFORMATICS IN PRACTICE

### Texting for Chronic Obstructive Pulmonary Disease (COPD) Patients

- Sometimes patients with COPD or those requiring $O_2$ therapy experience difficulty speaking because of shortness of breath.
- Encourage your patient to use typed messages displayed on a monitor to communicate.
- Texting and instant messaging family and friends are good alternatives to having phone conversations.

◆ ***Activity Considerations.*** Exercise training leads to energy conservation, which is an important component in COPD rehabilitation. The patient with severe COPD typically uses upper thoracic and neck muscles to breathe rather than the diaphragm. Thus the patient has difficulty performing upper-extremity activities, particularly those that require raising the arm above the head. Exercise training of the upper extremities may improve muscle function and help to reduce dyspnea.

## TABLE 28-26 Patient & Caregiver Teaching

### Chronic Obstructive Pulmonary Disease

*Include the following information in the teaching plan to assist the patient with COPD and the caregiver to improve quality of life through teaching and promotion of lifestyle practices that support successful living with chronic obstructive pulmonary disease (COPD).*

**What is COPD?**
- Basic anatomy and physiology of lung
- Basic pathophysiology of COPD
- Signs and symptoms of COPD, exacerbation, cold, flu, pneumonia
- Tests to assess breathing

**Breathing and Airway Clearance Exercises**
- Pursed-lip breathing (Table 28-13)
- Airway clearance technique: huff cough (Table 28-23)

**Energy Conservation Techniques**
- Daily activities (e.g., waking up, bathing, grooming, shopping, traveling)
- Consult with physical therapist and occupational therapist

**Medications**

Types (include mechanism of action and types of devices)
- Methylxanthines
- $\beta_2$-Adrenergic agonists
- Corticosteroids
- Anticholinergics
- Antibiotics
- Other medications

Establishing medication schedule

**Correct Use of Inhalers, Spacer, and Nebulizer**
- Demonstration–return demonstration with placebo devices (Figs. 28-5 to 28-7 and Tables 28-9 to 28-11)

**Home Oxygen**
- Explanation of rationale for use
- Guide for home $O_2$ use and equipment

**Psychosocial/Emotional Issues**

Open discussion (sharing with patient, caregiver, and family)
- Concerns about interpersonal relationships (e.g., intimacy)
- Problems with emotions (e.g., depression, anxiety, panic)
- Dependency

Treatment decisions
- Support and rehabilitation groups

End-of-life issues

**COPD Management Plan**

Nurse and patient develop and write up COPD management plan that meets individual needs.
- Focus on self-management
- Need to report changes
- Cause of flare-ups or exacerbation
- Recognition of signs and symptoms of respiratory infection, heart failure
- Reduce risk factors, especially smoking cessation
- Exercise program of walking and arm strengthening
- Yearly follow-up

**Healthy Nutrition** (Table 28-24)
- Strategies to lose weight (if overweight)
- Strategies to gain weight (if underweight)
- Consultation with dietitian

For additional information, see American Lung Association at *www.lung.org/lung-disease/copd.*

Frequently the patient has already adapted alternative energy-saving practices for ADLs. Alternative methods of hair care, shaving, showering, and reaching may have to be explored. An occupational therapist may help with ideas in these areas. Assuming a tripod posture (elbows supported on a table, chest in fixed position) and placing a mirror on the table while using an electric razor or hair dryer conserve much more energy than when the patient stands in front of a mirror to shave or blow-dry hair.

If the patient uses home $O_2$ therapy, $O_2$ should be used during activities of hygiene because these are energy consuming. Encourage the patient to make a schedule and plan daily and weekly activities to leave plenty of time for rest periods. The patient should also try to sit as much as possible when performing activities. Another energy-saving tip is to exhale when pushing, pulling, or exerting effort during an activity and inhale during rest.

Regular physical exercise is important for patients with COPD. To ensure long-term adherence, the exercise must be individualized and easy to perform. Walking or other endurance exercises (e.g., cycling) combined with strength training are the best interventions to strengthen muscles and improve the patient's endurance. Teach the patient coordinated walking with slow, pursed-lip breathing (Table 28-13). Many patients with moderate or severe COPD are anxious and fearful of walking or performing exercise. These patients and their caregivers require support while they build the confidence they need to walk or perform daily exercises.

Developing a patient's exercise endurance is very important. If it takes longer than 5 minutes to return to baseline, the patient most likely has overdone it and should proceed at a slower pace during the next exercise period. The patient may benefit from keeping a diary or log of the exercise program. Stationary cycling can also be used either alone or with walking. Cycles and treadmills are particularly good when weather prevents walking outside.

Fatigue, sleep disturbances, and dyspnea are common complaints of patients with COPD. Of these symptoms, dyspnea appears to be the one that affects the patient's ability to carry out daily activities. Therefore you and other members of the interprofessional team should focus your interventions on improving dyspnea, which would then improve the patient's functional performance.

Patients frequently ask whether moving to a warmer or drier climate will help. In general, such a move is not significantly beneficial. Discourage moves to places with an elevation of 4000 ft or more because of the lower partial pressure of $O_2$ found in the air at higher elevations. A disadvantage of moving may be that a person leaves a job, friends, and familiar environment, which could be psychologically stressful. Any advantage gained from a different climate may be outweighed by the psychologic effects of the move.

◆ ***Psychosocial Considerations.*** Healthy coping is a challenge for the COPD patient and family. People with COPD frequently have to deal with many lifestyle changes that may involve decreased ability to care for themselves, decreased energy for social activities, and loss or change in a job.

When a patient with COPD is first diagnosed or has complications that require hospitalization, expect a variety of emotional responses. Emotions frequently encountered include guilt, loneliness from social isolation, denial, and frustration from increased dependence. Guilt may result from the knowledge that the disease was caused primarily by cigarette smoking.

## EVIDENCE-BASED PRACTICE

### *Applying the Evidence*

**Physical Activity and COPD**

You are working as a nurse in the pulmonary clinic with R.P., a 65-yr-old man who has been recently discharged from the hospital after being newly diagnosed with COPD. He tells you he has been mostly inactive for the past few months because his breathing seems to worsen with activity.

***Making Clinical Decisions***

***Best Available Evidence.*** Patients with COPD who participate in regular moderate physical activity (e.g., brisk walking) have fewer severe flare-ups and are less likely to be readmitted to the hospital.

***Clinician Expertise.*** Physical inactivity is common in patients with COPD. You know that persistent inactivity may place a patient at greater risk for hospital readmissions.

***Patient Preference and Values.*** R.P. tells you that he misses taking walks every day with his wife and is wondering if he would be able to resume this activity at a slow pace.

***Implications for Practice***

1. What important factors will you discuss with R.P. about physical activity and COPD?
2. How would you assess R.P.'s willingness and motivation to engage in physical activity?
3. How would you involve the interprofessional team members to assist R.P. in regular physical activity?

***Reference for Evidence***

Nguyen H, Chu L, Liu I, et al: Associations between physical activity and 30-day readmission risk in chronic obstructive pulmonary disease, *Ann Amer Thorac Soc* 11:695, 2014.

Patients with COPD experience many losses as the disease progresses. Because many patients with COPD experience depression and anxiety, assess for both. Ask patients if they "feel down or blue" most of the time. Do they appear anxious about being able to control their breathlessness or know what to do if they have an exacerbation? Are they exhibiting concern over more difficulty in self-care activities such as bathing? How is the family coping with the patient's disease?

It is important to convey a sense of understanding and caring to the patient. The patient with COPD may benefit from stress management techniques (e.g., massage, muscle relaxation [see Chapter 6]). In addition, teach patients about the treatment and disease, which can give them a sense of control of their disease and complex treatment regimens. It is important to include the patient's caregiver in the teaching so that he or she can help the patient cope physically and emotionally. Support groups at local American Lung Association chapters (such as the Better Breathers Club), hospitals, and clinics can also be helpful.

A consultation with a therapist may be needed for proper screening and diagnosis of depression or other mental health problems. Cognitive and behavioral therapy along with COPD teaching may improve the quality of life. Medications may be used to treat both depression and anxiety. Buspirone (BuSpar), which is used to treat anxiety, has few if any respiratory depression effects. Benzodiazepines should be avoided because they may depress the respiratory drive and may be habit forming. When the patient becomes anxious because of dyspnea, the use of pursed-lip breathing (Table 28-13) and short-acting bronchodilators may be appropriate.

***Sexuality and Sexual Activity.*** Modifying but not abstaining from sexual activity can also contribute to healthy psychologic well-being. Most patients with COPD are older. Assess and reflect on your own attitudes and feelings about sexuality, sexual functioning, and aging before exploring sexual issues with the older COPD patient. First assess the patient's concerns related to sexuality and functioning. Ask open-ended questions to determine if the patient wants to discuss any of these concerns. You could ask, "How has your breathing problem affected how you see yourself as a woman or man?" Another question could be, "How does your shortness of breath affect your desire for intimacy with your partner?" These types of questions give the person an opening to discuss concerns. Much of the sexual performance issues experienced by the patient with COPD are changes related to aging, and if you are aware of these changes, you can teach the patient the "normalcy" of the changes.

Dyspnea, the predominant symptom in COPD, should not be a major problem with success in sexual functioning, except for those patients in severe stages. If the patient can walk up two flights of stairs or walk briskly, he or she likely has sufficient energy for sexual activity. Erectile dysfunction can occur with COPD as with many chronic diseases. Using an inhaled bronchodilator before sexual activity can help ventilation. The patient with COPD may also find these suggestions helpful: (1) plan sexual activity during the part of the day when breathing is best, which is usually late morning or early afternoon (plus older men often achieve an erection more easily in the morning); (2) use slow pursed-lip breathing; (3) refrain from sexual activity after eating or drinking alcohol; (4) choose less stressful positions during intercourse (missionary position for men is the worst); (5) use $O_2$ if prescribed; and (6) understand that cigarettes can increase male impotence. Often the patient has coexisting cardiac disease and should obtain advice from a or an HCP related to appropriate levels of activity. These aspects of sexual activity require open communication between partners regarding their needs and expectations and the changes that may be necessary as the result of a chronic disease (e.g., changes in body image, role reversal).[32]

***Sleep.*** Adequate sleep is extremely important to maintain quality of life and productivity. Patients with COPD have an increased prevalence of sleep disorders. The hyperinflation of the lungs and reduction in ventilation can result in severe drops in $O_2$ saturation (down to 60% or less) during sleep. This leads to a strain on the heart. In addition, hypercapnia may develop with more frequent awakening. The net result is sleeping poorly and awakening unrefreshed and fatigued.

Current tobacco use, depression, and anxiety are all common in COPD and lead to more trouble sleeping. $\beta_2$-Agonists may cause restlessness and insomnia. Many patients with COPD have postnasal drip or nasal congestion that may cause coughing and wheezing at night. Nasal saline sprays or rinses before sleep and in the morning may help. If the patient is prescribed $O_2$ therapy, using it at night will decrease insomnia. If the patient is a restless sleeper, snores, stops breathing while asleep, and has a tendency to fall asleep during the day, the patient may need to be tested for sleep apnea (see Chapter 7).

***End-of-Life Considerations.*** The trajectory of COPD is a gradual decline in health characterized by increasing exacerbations that are associated with an increased risk of death. Palliative, end-of-life, and hospice care are important components of care for the patient with advanced COPD.[33]

Patients need to know that symptoms can be managed, but COPD cannot be cured. End-of-life issues and advance directives are important topics for discussion in the terminal stages of COPD. However, this may be difficult for the patient and family to consider because of the uncertainty of the disease. (Palliative care and end-of-life care are discussed in Chapter 9.)

## ETHICAL/LEGAL DILEMMAS

### *Advance Directives*

**Situation**

L.H., a 79-yr-old man with COPD, is in respiratory failure when he is admitted to the hospital. He is placed on a ventilator and responds occasionally by opening his eyes. His advance directives (ADs) were drawn up 5 years ago, and copies were given to his wife and HCP at that time. The patient's wife brings the documents to the intensive care unit and tells you that the hospital must stop treating her husband and allow him to die as he requested. However, the patient's oldest son is threatening the hospital with a lawsuit if the staff does not provide full care to his father.

**Ethical/Legal Points for Consideration**

- A Living Will, one form of AD, permits individuals to state their own preferences and refusals should the individual become terminally ill or be in a situation in which there is no hope of recovery, and the person is not able to speak for himself or herself.*
- The Durable Power Attorney for Health Care, another form of AD, permits individuals to identify a proxy to make health care decisions in the event the individual is incapacitated.
- The National POLST Paradigm is an approach to end-of-life planning that emphasizes patients' wishes about the care they receive. The POLST Paradigm is an approach to end-of-life planning emphasizing the medical orders and includes coverage, regardless of location (e.g., hospital, home, assisted living).[1]
- AD laws vary from state to state concerning the need for witnesses and who the proxy is.
- You have an obligation to check your state requirements.[2]
- Some families are deeply divided about decisions for their loved ones, and conflicts often arise when money and property are involved. This conflict situation requires the nurse to call for a consult from the ethics committee in the organization.
- HCPs are obligated to follow the patient's ADs when a patient is no longer able to speak for himself or herself.
- In your scope of nursing practice, you need to (1) be informed about the decision-making laws and regulations in your state, (2) make AD documents available to patients, (3) teach patients and their families about ADs, (4) determine if all involved health care providers are aware of the existence of ADs, (5) assist the patient and family in communicating with the health care providers when a "no code" order is requested, and (6) assist the conflicted family in obtaining appropriate counseling whenever necessary.

**Discussion Questions**

1. What should you do next with the information provided by L.H.'s wife?
2. How should you address the needs of each member of this family in L.H.'s plan of care?
3. What resources can you use to facilitate decision making in this situation?

**References**

1. Physician Orders for Life Sustaining Treatment (POLST) Program. *www.polst.org.*
2. *www.caringinfo.org/i4a/pages/index.cfm?pageid=3289.*

*Advance directives are listed in Table 9-6.

### ◆ Evaluation

The expected outcomes are that the patient with COPD will

- Return to pre-exacerbation baseline respiratory function
- Demonstrate an effective rate, rhythm, and depth of respirations
- Experience clear breath sounds
- Maintain clear airway by effectively coughing
- Have $PaCO_2$ and $PaO_2$ values that return to normal for patient

Additional information on expected outcomes for the patient with COPD is presented in eNursing Care Plan 28-2 available on the website for this chapter.

## CYSTIC FIBROSIS

Cystic fibrosis (CF) is an autosomal recessive, multisystem disease characterized by altered transport of sodium and chloride ions in and out of epithelial cells. This defect primarily affects the lungs, gastrointestinal tract (pancreas and biliary tract), and reproductive tract.

CF was first described in 1938 when autopsies of young children revealed multiple cysts in the pancreas, so the disease was called "cystic fibrosis of the pancreas."[34] Once advances in care allowed children to live into later childhood, the lung disease became the more significant problem.

Approximately 30,000 children and adults in the United States have CF. About 10 million (about 1 in every 31) Americans are carriers of the CF gene but do not have the disease. Of the CF patients in the Cystic Fibrosis Patient Registry, over 49% are 18 years of age or older.

The first signs and symptoms typically occur in children, but some patients are not diagnosed until they are adults; some live to over 80 years old. The severity and progression of the disease vary. With early diagnosis and improvements in therapy, the prognosis of patients with CF has significantly improved. The median predicted survival was 16 years in 1970 but has increased to more than 41 years.[35]

### Etiology and Pathophysiology

**Genetic Link.** CF is an autosomal recessive disorder (see Figs. 12-4 and 12-5 and the Genetics in Clinical Practice box on this page). The CF gene is located on chromosome 7 and produces a protein called *CF transmembrane conductance regulator (CFTR)*. The CFTR protein localizes to the epithelial surface of the airways, gastrointestinal tract, and ducts of the liver, pancreas, and sweat glands. CFTR regulates sodium and chloride movement in and out of epithelial cells. Mutations in the *CFTR* gene alter this protein in such a way that the channels are blocked. As a result, cells that line the passageways of the lungs, pancreas, intestines, and other organs produce secretions that are low in sodium chloride content (thus low in water content), making mucus abnormally thick and sticky (Fig. 28-16). This mucus plugs up the ducts in these organs, thus causing scarring in the organs, ultimately resulting in organ failure. The high concentrations of sodium and chloride in the sweat of the patient with CF result from decreased chloride reabsorption in the sweat duct.

In the respiratory system, both the upper and lower respiratory tracts can be affected. Upper respiratory tract manifestations may include chronic sinusitis and nasal polyposis. The hallmark of respiratory involvement in CF is its effect on the airways. The disease progresses from being a disease of the

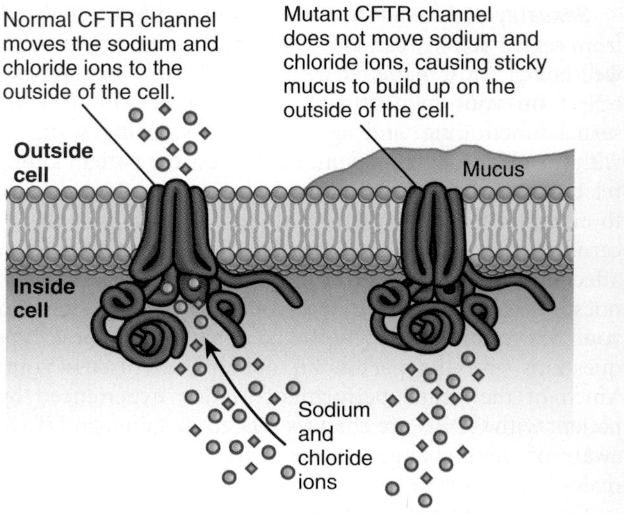


**FIG. 28-16** People with cystic fibrosis inherit a defective gene on chromosome 7 called *cystic fibrosis transmembrane conductance regulator (CFTR)*. The protein produced by this gene normally helps sodium and chloride move in and out of cells. If the protein does not work correctly, then the movement of sodium and chloride is blocked and an abnormally thick sticky mucus is produced on the outside of the cell.

### GENETICS IN CLINICAL PRACTICE

#### *Cystic Fibrosis (CF)*

**Genetic Basis**

- Autosomal recessive disorder
- Caused by mutations in CF transmembrane regulator *(CFTR)* gene on chromosome 7
- Many different mutations of *CFTR* gene have been identified.
- *CFTR* gene provides instructions for making protein that controls the channel that transports sodium and chloride.
- Mutations in the *CFTR* gene disrupt the function of the channels, preventing them from regulating the flow of sodium, chloride, and water across cell membranes.

**Incidence**

- In the United States 1 in 3000 white births
- Less common in other ethnic populations (1 in 17,000 African Americans and 1 in 31,000 Asian Americans)
- One in 20 to 25 whites are carriers of the gene.
- If both parents carry the affected gene, there is a 25% chance each offspring will have the disease (see Figs. 12-4 and 12-5).

**Genetic Testing**

- Blood-based DNA testing is available for disease and carrier states.
- All 50 states have passed legislation requiring that all newborns be screened for CF.
- Testing is usually done in children if CF is suspected or if parents are possible carriers.
- In parents who are known carriers, amniocentesis or chorionic villus sampling in pregnant women may be useful for prenatal testing.

**Clinical Implications**

- CF is the most common autosomal recessive disease in whites.
- CF has a wide range of clinical expression of disease.
- CF requires long-term medical management.
- Advances in medical care have improved life expectancy.
- Most people who have a child with CF are not aware of a family history of disease.
- CF screening should be offered to all individuals of reproductive age regardless of family history.

small airways *(chronic bronchiolitis)* to involvement of the larger airways and finally causes destruction of lung tissue. The mucus becomes dehydrated and tenacious due to the defect in the chloride secretion and excess sodium absorption. Cilia motility is decreased, thus allowing mucus to adhere to the airways. The bronchioles become obstructed with thick mucus, leading to scarring of the airways (bronchiectasis), air trapping, and hyperinflation of the lungs.

CF is characterized by chronic airway infection that cannot be eradicated. Organisms commonly cultured from the sputum of a patient with CF are *Staphylococcus aureus, Haemophilus influenzae,* and *Pseudomonas aeruginosa,* and less commonly but more seriously, *Burkholderia cepacia. Pseudomonas* is by far the most common organism in adults. Antibiotic resistance develops after multiple exposure to antibiotics. Pulmonary inflammation is associated with the chronic infection and can cause a decrease in respiratory function, thus further narrowing the lumen of the airways. Inflammatory mediators (e.g., interleukins, oxidants, proteases released by neutrophils) are increased and contribute to the progression of lung disease.

Lung disorders that initially occur are chronic bronchiolitis and bronchitis. However, after months or years, changes in the bronchial walls lead to bronchiectasis (Fig. 28-17). Over a long period, pulmonary vascular remodeling occurs because of local hypoxia and arteriolar vasoconstriction. Pulmonary hypertension, enlarged pulmonary arteries, and cor pulmonale occur in the later phases of the disease. Blebs and large cysts in the lung are also severe manifestations of lung destruction, and pneumothorax may develop. Other pulmonary complications include hemoptysis, which is caused by proliferation of capillaries in response to chronic infection. During exacerbations, erosion of these capillaries occurs. Hemoptysis may range from scant streaking to major bleeding, which can sometimes be fatal.

Pancreatic insufficiency is caused primarily by mucous plugging of the pancreatic exocrine ducts, which results in atrophy of the gland and progressive fibrotic cyst formation. The pancreas's exocrine function may be completely lost. Because of the exocrine dysfunction, pancreatic enzymes such as lipase, amylase, and proteases (trypsin, chemotrypsin) are not made in sufficient amounts to allow for absorption of nutrients. Malabsorption of fat, protein, and fat-soluble vitamins (A, D, E, and K) occurs. Fat malabsorption results in steatorrhea, and protein malabsorption results in failure to grow and gain weight.

CF-related diabetes mellitus (CFRD) is thought to be caused by underdevelopment of pancreatic islet cells (in utero) as well as destruction of islet cells over the individual's lifetime. CFRD is a unique type of diabetes with characteristics of both type 1 and type 2 diabetes. The pancreas in people with CF produces insulin but too late to fully respond to carbohydrate intake.

Other common disorders that develop in CF include osteopenia and osteoporosis. These disorders are related to malnutrition, malabsorption of vitamin D, insufficient testosterone levels, and chronically elevated inflammatory cytokines.

Individuals with CF often have other gastrointestinal problems, including GERD, which is often related to excessive coughing. The liver and gallbladder can be damaged by mucus deposits in the ducts. The liver enzymes may become chronically elevated, with cirrhosis developing over time. Gallstones, pancreatitis, and portal hypertension can also occur. Distal intestinal obstruction syndrome (DIOS) results from intermittent obstruction commonly occurring in the terminal ileum at the point of the ileocecal junction. It is caused by thickened, dehydrated stool and mucus. The patient may appear to have a small bowel obstruction. DIOS develops because of chronic malabsorption related to exocrine dysfunction, under- or overdosing of pancreatic replacement enzyme supplementation, dehydration, swallowing of mucus, and use of opioids.

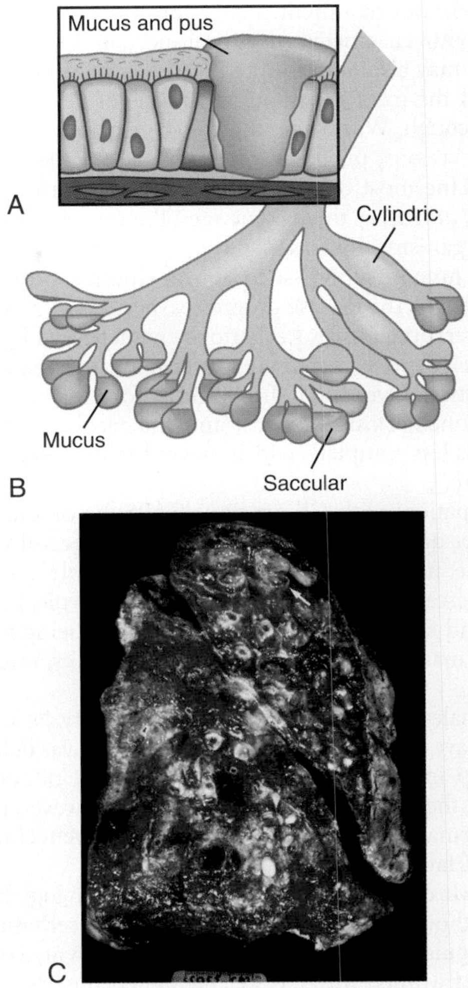


**FIG. 28-17** Pathologic changes in bronchiectasis. **A,** Longitudinal section of bronchial wall where chronic infection has caused damage. **B,** Collection of purulent material in dilated bronchioles, leading to persistent infection. **C,** Bronchiectasis in a patient with cystic fibrosis who underwent lung transplantation. Cut surfaces of lung show markedly distended peripheral bronchi filled with mucopurulent secretions. (***C,*** From Kumar V, Abbas AK, Aster JC, et al: *Robbins and Cotran pathologic basis of disease,* ed 8, Philadelphia, 2010, Saunders.)

## Clinical Manifestations

The clinical manifestations of CF vary depending on the severity of the disease. Carriers are not affected by the mutation. The disease severity may vary greatly, both within families and among different families.

The median age at diagnosis of CF is 5 months of age; 72% are diagnosed in the first year of life.[35] Currently every state has mandatory newborn screening for CF, which has allowed for early intervention. An initial finding of meconium ileus in the newborn infant prompts the diagnosis in 20% of people with CF. Other signs that suggest a CF diagnosis are acute or persistent respiratory symptoms (wheezing, coughing, frequent pneumonia), failure to thrive or malnutrition, steatorrhea (large, oily, frequent bowel movements), and family history. Without treatment, a large, protuberant abdomen may develop with an emaciated appearance of the extremities. A diagnosis may also be prompted by findings of bronchiectasis.

One of the most common symptoms of CF in the adult is frequent cough. With time, the cough becomes persistent and produces viscous, purulent, often yellow or greenish sputum. Although the most common bacteria in the airways in childhood is *S. aureus*, as the patient ages, the prevalence of *Pseudomonas* organisms increases. Other respiratory problems are recurring lung infections such as bronchiolitis, bronchitis, and pneumonia. As the disease progresses, periods of clinical stability are interrupted by exacerbations characterized by increased cough, weight loss, increased sputum, and decreased pulmonary function. Over time, the exacerbations become more frequent, bronchiectasis worsens, and the recovery of lost lung function is less complete, which may ultimately lead to respiratory failure.

If the patient with CF develops DIOS, he or she may have right lower quadrant pain (the area of the ileocecal valve), loss of appetite, nausea, emesis, and often a palpable mass. Insufficient pancreatic enzyme release causes the typical pattern of protein and fat malabsorption with a person being thin with a low body mass index (BMI) and frequent, bulky, foul-smelling stools.

Both males and females have delayed puberty. Nearly all men with CF have reproductive issues because their vas deferens fails to develop in utero, so there is no transport of sperm from storage in the testes to the penile urethra. However, they make sperm normally, and with assisted reproductive technology are capable of fathering a child.

Some women with CF have difficulty conceiving; the cervical mucus is thought to be thickened. During exacerbations, menstrual irregularities and secondary amenorrhea are common. A majority of women with CF are able to become pregnant. Most pregnancies result in viable infants.

## Complications

Complications in CF include CFRD, bone disease, sinus disease, and liver disease. Pneumothorax, a relatively uncommon but serious complication, is caused by the formation of bullae and blebs. A small amount of blood in sputum is common in the CF patient because of chronic lung infection. Massive hemoptysis, which is relatively uncommon, can be life-threatening. With advanced lung disease, digital clubbing occurs. Respiratory failure and cor pulmonale caused by pulmonary hypertension are late complications of CF.

## Diagnostic Studies

The diagnostic criteria for CF include a combination of clinical presentation, family history, laboratory testing, and genetic testing. The sweat glands of CF patients secrete normal volumes of sweat, but sodium chloride cannot be absorbed from sweat as it moves through the sweat duct. Therefore four times the normal amount of sodium and chloride is excreted in sweat. This abnormality usually does not directly affect the person's general health, but it is the main diagnostic test for CF.

The sweat chloride test is considered the gold standard for the diagnosis of CF and is performed with the pilocarpine iontophoresis method. Pilocarpine is placed on the skin and carried by a small electric current to stimulate sweat production. This part of the process takes about 5 minutes, and the patient feels a slight tingling or warmth. The sweat is collected on filter paper or gauze and then analyzed for sweat chloride concentrations. The test takes approximately 1 hour. Sweat chloride values above 60 mmol/L are considered positive for the diagnosis of CF. A second sweat chloride test is obtained at the same time (one test in each arm) to confirm the diagnosis.

A genetic test is often used if the results from a sweat chloride test are unclear. A blood sample or cells taken inside the cheek (buccal smear) are sent to a laboratory that specializes in genetic testing. Most laboratories test for only the most common mutations of the CF gene. Because more than 1700 mutations cause CF, screening for all mutations is difficult and is performed in a specialty laboratory.

## Interprofessional Care

An interprofessional team should be involved in the care of a patient with CF. The Cystic Fibrosis Foundation provides funding for and accredits more than 100 CF care centers nationwide. The high quality of specialized care available throughout the care center network has led to the improved length and quality of life for people with CF. These care centers offer the best care, treatments, and support for those with CF (see *www.cff.org/LivingWithCF/CareCenterNetwork/CFFoundation-accreditedCareCenters*). The teams at these care centers include a nurse, physician, respiratory therapist, physical therapist, dietitian, social worker, and often a nurse practitioner.

Management of pulmonary problems in CF aims at relieving airway obstruction and controlling infection. Drainage of thick bronchial mucus is assisted by aerosol and nebulization treatments of medications used to dilate the airways, liquefy mucus, and facilitate clearance. The abnormal viscosity of CF secretions is increased by concentrated deoxyribonucleic acid (DNA) from neutrophils involved in chronic infection. Agents that degrade the DNA in CF sputum (e.g., dornase alfa [Pulmozyme]) increase airflow and reduce the number of acute pulmonary exacerbations. Inhaled hypertonic saline (7%) is effective in clearing mucus and also decreases the frequency of exacerbations. Hypertonic saline is safe, but some patients require concomitant bronchodilators to avoid bronchospasm. Bronchodilators (e.g., $\beta_2$-adrenergic agonists) may be used to control bronchospasm, but the long-term benefit is not proven.

Airway clearance techniques are critical, since the normal ciliary motion in CF airways is impaired. CPT (including postural drainage with percussion and vibration) and high-frequency chest wall oscillation loosen mucus. Clearance is achieved by the specialized expiratory techniques aimed at using airflow to remove the loosened secretions. Examples of clearance techniques and devices are PEP devices (e.g., Flutter device, Acapella [Fig. 28-15]), breathing exercises (autogenic drainage [*http://hospitals.unm.edu/cf/autogenic_drainage.shtml*]), pursed-lip breathing (Table 28-13), and huff coughing (Table 28-23). Individuals with CF may prefer a certain technique or device that works well for them in a daily routine. No clear evidence exists that any of the airway clearance techniques are superior to the others. (Airway clearance techniques are discussed on p. 569.)

Most patients with CF die of complications from lung infection. Standard treatment of infections includes antibiotics for exacerbations and may include chronic suppressive therapy in conjunction with airway clearance. The use of antibiotics should be carefully guided by sputum culture results. Early intervention with antibiotics is useful, and long courses of antibiotics are the usual treatment. Prolonged high-dose therapy may be necessary because many drugs are abnormally metabolized and rapidly excreted in the patient with CF.

Most patients have *Pseudomonas* infection, which can be difficult to treat because over time the organism develops resistance to antibiotics. The organism also has the ability to form a biofilm that must be penetrated to kill it. One commonly used antibiotic to treat patients who are chronically infected with *Pseudomonas* is aerosolized tobramycin (TOBI) given every other month, twice a day. Tobramycin inhalation powder is also available for treatment of *Pseudomonas*.[36]

Oral agents commonly used for mild exacerbations (i.e., increased cough and sputum) are oral antibiotics such as a semisynthetic penicillin or trimethoprim/sulfamethoxazole (to treat *S. aureus*) or oral quinolones, especially ciprofloxacin (Cipro) (to treat *P. aeruginosa*). The quinolones are used judiciously because of the rapid development of resistant strains. Azithromycin, used chronically (longer than 6 months), decreases the frequency of pulmonary exacerbations in CF, especially in those infected with *Pseudomonas*. It is thought that it acts as an antiinflammatory.

If home support and resources are adequate, the CF patient and caregiver may choose to continue IV antibiotic therapy at home after hospital discharge.[37] The usual treatment is two antibiotics with different mechanisms of action (e.g., cephalosporin and an aminoglycoside). The patient with cor pulmonale or hypoxemia may require home $O_2$ therapy. ($O_2$ therapy is discussed on p. 565.) Patients with a large pneumothorax require chest tube drainage, perhaps repeatedly. Sclerosing of the pleural space or partial pleural stripping and pleural abrasion performed surgically may be indicated for recurrent episodes of pneumothorax. With massive hemoptysis, bronchial artery embolization is performed. CF has become a leading indication for lung transplantation. (Lung transplants are discussed in Chapter 27.)

The management of pancreatic insufficiency includes pancreatic enzyme replacement of lipase, protease, and amylase (e.g., pancrelipase [Pancreaze, Creon, Ultresa, Viokace, Zenpep, Pertzye]) administered before each meal and snack. Adequate intake of fat, calories, protein, and vitamins is important. Fat-soluble vitamins (A, D, E, and K) must be supplemented, since they are malabsorbed. Use of caloric supplements improves nutritional status. Added dietary salt is indicated whenever sweating is excessive, such as during hot weather, when fever is present, or from intense physical activity. Hyperglycemia may require insulin treatment.

If the patient develops DIOS with complete bowel obstruction, gastric decompression may be needed. This complication is most often managed medically. If DIOS does not resolve with medical treatment, surgery may be needed to prevent the development of ischemic bowel. Partial and uncomplicated episodes of DIOS are treated with ingestion of a balanced polyethylene glycol (PEG) electrolyte solution (MiraLax, GoLYTELY) used to hydrate bowel contents. In addition, water-soluble contrast enemas may be used. Careful monitoring of bowel habits and patterns is essential for CF patients.

Ivacaftor (Kalydeco) is used to treat patients who have mutations in the *CFTR* gene.[38] Ivacaftor, rather than treating the effects of the basic chloride ion channel defect (e.g., pancreatic insufficiency), targets the function of the gene itself, assisting this mutation to open the chloride channel. This drug proves that it is possible to alter the function of a mutation.

Ivacaftor is not effective in patients with CF who have two copies (homozygous) of the *F508* mutation in the *CFTR* gene, which is the most common mutation that results in CF. If a patient's genotype is unknown, a CF mutation test should be performed to detect the presence of a CFTR mutation. Ivacaftor/lumicaftor (Orkambi) is a combination drug used to treat patients who have *F508* mutations.

Aerobic exercise is effective in clearing the airways. Important needs to consider when planning an aerobic exercise program for the patient with CF are (1) meeting increased nutritional demands of exercise, (2) observing for dehydration, and (3) drinking large amounts of fluid and replacing salt losses.

There is a higher incidence of depression among individuals with CF than their unaffected peers. CF imposes a significant burden on the individual and family. Issues related to fertility, decreased life expectancy, costs of health care, burden of self-care, and career choices may lead to depression.

## NURSING MANAGEMENT: CYSTIC FIBROSIS

### Nursing Assessment

Subjective and objective data that should be obtained from the patient with CF are presented in Table 28-27.

### Nursing Diagnoses

Nursing diagnoses for the patient with CF may include, but are not limited to, the following:

- Ineffective airway clearance *related to* abundant, thick bronchial mucus, weakness, and fatigue
- Ineffective breathing pattern *related to* bronchoconstriction, anxiety, and airway obstruction
- Impaired gas exchange *related to* recurring lung infections
- Imbalanced nutrition: less than body requirements *related to* dietary intolerances, intestinal gas, and altered pancreatic enzyme production
- Ineffective coping *related to* multiple life stressors such as decreased life expectancy, cost of treatment, and limitation on career choices

### Planning

The overall goals are that the patient with CF will have (1) adequate airway clearance, (2) reduced risk factors associated with respiratory infections, (3) adequate nutritional support to maintain appropriate BMI, (4) ability to perform ADLs, (5) recognition and treatment of complications related to CF, and (6) active participation in planning and implementing a therapeutic regimen.

### Nursing Implementation

Assist young adults in gaining independence by helping them assume responsibility for their care and vocational or school goals. An important issue to discuss is sexuality. Delayed or irregular menstruation is not uncommon. There may be delayed development of secondary sex characteristics, such as breasts in girls. The person with CF may use the illness to avoid certain events or relationships. Other crises and life transitions that must be dealt with in the young adult include building confidence and self-respect on the basis of achievements, persevering with employment goals, developing motivation to achieve, learning to cope with the treatment program, and adjusting to the need for dependence if health fails. Disclosing the CF diagnosis to friends, potential spouses, or employers may pose emotional and financial challenges.

The issue of marrying and having children is difficult. Genetic counseling is an appropriate suggestion for the couple considering having children. Another concern is the uncertainty surrounding the shortened life span of the parent with CF. In

**TABLE 28-27 Nursing Assessment**

***Cystic Fibrosis***

**Subjective Data**

***Important Health Information***

*Past health history:* Recurrent respiratory and sinus infections, persistent cough with excessive sputum production

*Medications:* Use of and compliance with bronchodilators, antibiotics, herbs

***Functional Health Patterns***

*Health perception–health maintenance:* Family history of cystic fibrosis, diagnosis of cystic fibrosis in childhood, genetic testing in offspring

*Nutritional-metabolic:* Dietary intolerances, voracious appetite, weight loss, heartburn

*Elimination:* Intestinal gas. Large, frequent bowel movements, constipation

*Activity-exercise:* Fatigue, ↓ exercise tolerance, amount and type of exercise. Dyspnea, cough, excessive mucus or sputum production, coughing up blood, airway clearance techniques

*Cognitive-perceptual:* Abdominal pain

*Sexuality-reproductive:* Delayed menarche, menstrual irregularities, problems conceiving or fathering a child

*Coping–stress tolerance:* Anxiety, depression, problems adapting to diagnosis

**Objective Data**

***General***

Restlessness; failure to thrive

***Integumentary***

Cyanosis (circumoral, nail bed), digital clubbing; salty skin

***Eyes***

Scleral icterus

***Respiratory***

Sinus congestion, postnasal drip, persistent runny nose. Diminished breath sounds, adventitious breath sounds (crackles, wheezes). Sputum (thick, light or dark, tenacious), hemoptysis, ↑ work of breathing, use of accessory muscles of respiration, barrel chest

***Cardiovascular***

Tachycardia

***Gastrointestinal***

Protuberant abdomen; abdominal distention; foul, fatty stools

***Possible Diagnostic Findings***

Abnormal ABGs and pulmonary function tests; abnormal sweat chloride test, chest x-ray, fecal fat analysis

*ABGs,* Arterial blood gases.

addition, the parent's ability to care for the child must be taken into consideration.

Acute care for the patient with CF includes relief of bronchoconstriction, airway obstruction, and airflow limitation. Interventions include aggressive CPT, antibiotics, and $O_2$ therapy in severe disease. Good nutrition is important. Advances in long-term vascular access (e.g., implanted ports) and inhaled antibiotics have made administration of medication much easier. This has also eased the transition for treatment at home.

The family and person with CF have a great financial and emotional burden. The cost of drugs, special equipment, and health care is often a financial hardship. The burden of living with a chronic disease at a young age can be emotionally overwhelming. Community resources are often available to help the family. In addition, the Cystic Fibrosis Foundation can be of assistance. As the person continues toward and into adulthood, you and other skilled health professionals should be available to help the patient and the family cope with complications resulting from the disease.

## BRONCHIECTASIS

### Etiology and Pathophysiology

**Bronchiectasis** is characterized by permanent, abnormal dilation of medium-sized bronchi that is a result of inflammatory changes that destroy elastic and muscular structures supporting the bronchial wall. Infection is the primary reason for the continuing cycle of inflammation, airway damage, and remodeling. Bronchiectasis can follow a single episode of severe pneumonia, with a wide variety of infectious agents initiating the condition. Airways can become colonized with microorganisms (e.g., *Pseudomonas*), which causes the bronchial walls to weaken and pockets of infection begin to form (Fig. 28-17).

When the walls of the bronchial system are injured, the mucociliary mechanism is damaged, allowing bacteria and mucus to accumulate within the pockets. Stasis of thickened mucus occurs due to impaired clearance of mucus by the cilia. This results in a reduced ability to clear mucus from the lungs and decreased expiratory airflow. Thus bronchiectasis is classified as an obstructive lung disease. Large connections (anastomoses) develop between the blood vessels in the lungs, and hemoptysis is often the result.

A variety of pathophysiologic processes can result in bronchiectasis. CF is the main cause of bronchiectasis in children. In adults, the main cause is bacterial infections of the lungs that are either not treated or receive delayed treatment. Other causes of bronchiectasis are obstruction of an airway with mucus plugs or generalized impairment of pulmonary defenses. A number of systemic diseases such as inflammatory bowel disease, rheumatoid arthritis, or immune disorders (e.g., acquired immunodeficiency syndrome [AIDS]) may be associated with bronchiectasis.

### Clinical Manifestations

The hallmark of bronchiectasis is persistent cough with consistent production of thick, tenacious, purulent sputum. However, some patients with severe disease and upper lobe involvement may have no sputum production and little cough. Recurrent infections injure blood vessels, and hemoptysis occurs. In severe cases it may be life-threatening. The other manifestations of bronchiectasis are pleuritic chest pain, dyspnea, wheezing, clubbing of digits, weight loss, and anemia. On auscultation of the lungs, a variety of adventitious sounds can be heard (e.g., crackles, wheezes).

### Diagnostic Studies

An individual with a chronic productive cough with copious purulent sputum (which may be blood streaked) should be suspected of having bronchiectasis. Chest x-rays may show some nonspecific abnormalities. A high-resolution CT scan of the chest is the preferred method for diagnosing bronchiectasis.

Sputum may provide additional information regarding the severity of impairment and the presence of active infection.

Patients frequently have *H. influenzae, S. aureus,* or *P. aeruginosa,* with the latter leading to more frequent exacerbations and rapid decline in lung function. Spirometry usually shows an obstructive pattern, including a decrease in $FEV_1$ and $FEV_1/FVC$.

### Interprofessional Care

Bronchiectasis is difficult to treat. Therapy is aimed at treating acute flare-ups and preventing a decline in lung function. Antibiotics are the mainstay of treatment and are often given empirically, but attempts are made to culture the sputum. Long-term suppressive therapy with antibiotics is reserved for those patients who have symptoms that recur a few days after stopping antibiotics. Antibiotics may be given orally, IV, or inhaled.

Concurrent bronchodilator therapy with LABAs, SABAs, or anticholinergics is given to prevent bronchospasm and stimulate mucociliary clearance. Hyperosmolar agents (e.g., hypertonic saline) may be given via a nebulizer to liquefy secretions. In addition, oral and inhaled corticosteroids may be used.

Maintaining good hydration is important to liquefy secretions. CPT and other airway clearance techniques are important to facilitate expectoration of sputum. Teach the patient to reduce exposure to excessive air pollutants and irritants, avoid cigarette smoking, and obtain pneumococcal and influenza vaccinations.

Surgical resection of parts of the lungs, which was common in the past, has largely been replaced by more effective supportive and antibiotic therapy. For selected patients who are disabled in spite of maximal therapy, lung transplantation is an option. Massive hemoptysis may require surgical resection or embolization of the bronchial artery.

## NURSING MANAGEMENT: BRONCHIECTASIS

Early detection and treatment of lower respiratory tract infections help prevent complications such as bronchiectasis. Any obstructing lesion or foreign body should be removed promptly.

An important nursing goal is to promote drainage and removal of mucus. Various airway clearance techniques can be effectively used to facilitate secretion removal. CPT with postural drainage is widely used.

Administration of the prescribed medications is important. The patient needs to understand the importance of taking the prescribed regimen of drugs to obtain maximum effectiveness. Rest is important to prevent overexertion.

If hemoptysis occurs, patients should be given explicit instructions on when they should contact the HCP. Some patients may periodically expectorate a "spot" of blood that is usual for them. In the acute care setting, if the patient has hemoptysis, contact the HCP immediately, elevate the head of the bed, and place the patient in a side-lying position with the suspected bleeding side down.

Good nutrition is important and may be difficult to maintain because the patient is often anorexic. Oral hygiene to cleanse the mouth and remove dried sputum crusts may improve the patient's appetite. Offer foods that are appealing, since they may increase the patient's desire to eat.

Adequate hydration to help liquefy secretions and thus make it easier to remove them is extremely important. Unless there are contraindications, instruct the patient to drink at least 3 L of fluid daily. To accomplish this, advise the patient to increase fluid consumption by increasing intake by one glass per day until the goal is reached. Generally, the patient should be counseled to use low-sodium fluids to avoid systemic fluid retention.

Direct hydration of the respiratory system may also prove beneficial in the expectoration of secretions. Often nebulized hypertonic saline may be ordered for a more aggressive effect. At home, a steamy shower can prove effective. Expensive equipment that requires frequent cleaning is usually unnecessary. Teach the patient and caregiver to recognize significant clinical manifestations to report to the HCP. These manifestations include increased sputum production, bloody sputum, increasing dyspnea, fever, chills, and chest pain.

## BECOMING A NURSE LEADER

### *Coaching in Nursing*

#### Situation

You are a new graduate nurse on a busy pulmonary medical unit. You learn from Mr. Boyd, your patient, that he is to be discharged this morning. You are upset because discharge planning would go so much better if Dr. Gooding, his pulmonary physician, would include the nurses when he makes rounds on patients. Your nurse manager coaches you about how you could approach Dr. Gooding about including the nurses in patient rounds. She helps you refocus this scenario as a patient safety issue and develop a plan to discuss it with the physician. You find an opportunity to talk with Dr. Gooding, and he agrees that it would help communication all around if nurses could round with him. You are pleased and you tell your nurse manager of your success.

#### Points for Consideration

- Often when the word *coaching* is mentioned in the workplace, it has negative connotations related to dealing with a problem. Coaching is not about disciplinary action.
- Coaching is a leadership style in which managers provide individualized feedback and assistance to improve an employee's performance and development. It is a technique that can be used by nurse managers to get the best from their staff and thus the best results for the whole organization.[1]
- Coaches can help new nurses identify areas for improvement and work with them to set personal and career goals.
- Coaches ideally focus on professional development, teamwork, leadership, and preparation for increased responsibility. They encourage growth and risk taking.[2]
- Coaches need to be nurturing, have a firm commitment to finding special talents in young nurses, and encourage the growth of every nurse.[3]

#### Discussion Questions

1. What have you learned from the coaching that you have received from your nurse manager? From your teachers?
2. How can you help others learn from your success related to dealing with Dr. Gooding?

#### References

1. Routson J: Coaching—an essential skill for nursing leaders. Retrieved from *www.healthecareers.com/article/coaching-an-essential-skill-for-nursing-leaders/158373.*
2. Hancock B: Developing new nurse leaders, *AJN* 114:59, 2014.
3. Hess V: Coaching communication: tips for nurse managers. Retrieved from *www.americannursetoday.com/coaching-communication-tips-for-nurse-managers.*

## CASE STUDY

### Chronic Obstructive Pulmonary Disease

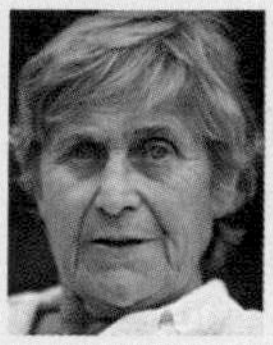

(©iStockphoto/ Thinkstock)

**Patient Profile**

H.M. is a 68-year-old white, married, female, retired traffic police officer. She has been in the hospital for 3 days with an acute COPD exacerbation and will be discharged tomorrow.

**Subjective Data**

- Before admission had 7 days of exceptional shortness of breath and increased volume of sputum, which turned greenish
- Had increased Ventolin HFA use at home to five or six times a day for dyspnea
- Had jitters and racing heart
- Had three or four bouts of exacerbations of COPD in the past year that she treated at home
- Thirty pack-year history of smoking; smokes half a pack per day now to "clear out lungs" in the morning
- Eats a regular diet but "gets full fast"
- Cannot climb one flight of stairs without stopping; walks down the flat driveway 10 yards without difficulty
- Awakens two or three times per night coughing and short of breath

**Objective Data**

***Physical Examination***

- Weight 129 lb, height 5 ft 8 in, BMI 20 kg/m$^2$
- BP 136/76 mm Hg, pulse 86, respiratory rate 28
- Increased anteroposterior diameter of chest (barrel shaped)
- Slight use of accessory (neck) muscles with breathing
- Distant breath sounds with occasional wheezes
- No peripheral edema

***Diagnostic Studies***

- Last spirometry: decreased $FEV_1$ (48%) and $FEV_1/FVC$ (62%)
- ABGs on admission: pH 7.34, $PaCO_2$ 49 mm Hg, $HCO_3^-$ 27 mEq/L, $PaO_2$ 70 mm Hg
- WBC: 14,000/μL on admission
- Chest x-ray: hyperinflation, flat diaphragm, no sign of pneumonia
- Sputum: negative for *Pseudomonas*

**Interprofessional Care**

- GOLD 3 (severe) COPD with acute exacerbation
- $O_2$ 2 L via nasal catheter while in hospital
- Prednisone 40 mg daily PO for 5 days
- Levofloxacin 750 mg PO
- Ipratropium HFA MDI 2 puffs four times a day
- At discharge: Advair Diskus 250/50 one inhalation q12hr

**Discussion Questions**

1. What classic manifestations indicate the patient had a COPD exacerbation?
2. What are some likely causes of her COPD?
3. What symptoms indicate the overuse of inhalers, and which drug would cause the symptoms described?
4. ***Patient-Centered Care:*** What is the only way H.M. can halt the progression of her lung disease?
5. Why would H.M. "feel full fast" when eating? What could you do to minimize this issue?
6. Interpret the ABGs. What pattern do you see?
7. ***Priority Decision:*** What are nursing priorities for discharge planning and teaching?
8. ***Priority Decision:*** Based on the assessment data presented, what are the priority nursing diagnoses? Are there any collaborative problems?
9. ***Evidence-Based Practice:*** H.M.'s son has been trying to convince his mother to quit smoking for many years without success. He asks you to tell his mother the results of her spirometry to convince her it is time to quit. Will this approach work?

Answers available at *http://evolve.elsevier.com/Lewis/medsurg.*

## BRIDGE TO NCLEX EXAMINATION

The number of the question corresponds to the same-numbered outcome at the beginning of the chapter.

1. A patient is concerned that he may have asthma. Of the symptoms that he relates to the nurse, which ones suggest asthma or risk factors for asthma *(select all that apply)*?
   **a.** Allergic rhinitis
   **b.** Prolonged inhalation
   **c.** History of skin allergies
   **d.** Cough, especially at night
   **e.** Gastric reflux or heartburn
2. In evaluating an asthmatic patient's knowledge of self-care, the nurse recognizes that additional instruction is needed when the patient says,
   **a.** "I use my corticosteroid inhaler when I feel short of breath."
   **b.** "I get a flu shot every year and see my HCP if I have an upper respiratory tract infection."
   **c.** "I use my inhaler before I visit my aunt who has a cat, but I only visit for a few minutes because of my allergies."
   **d.** "I walk 30 minutes every day but sometimes I have to use my bronchodilator inhaler before walking to prevent me from getting short of breath."
3. A plan of care for the patient with COPD could include *(select all that apply)*
   **a.** exercise such as walking.
   **b.** high flow rate of $O_2$ administration.
   **c.** low-dose chronic oral corticosteroid therapy.
   **d.** use of peak flow meter to monitor the progression of COPD.
   **e.** breathing exercises such as pursed-lip breathing that focus on exhalation.
4. The effects of cigarette smoking on the respiratory system include
   **a.** hypertrophy of capillaries causing hemoptysis.
   **b.** hyperplasia of goblet cells and increased production of mucus.
   **c.** increased proliferation of cilia and decreased clearance of mucus.
   **d.** proliferation of alveolar macrophages to decrease the risk for infection.
5. The major advantage of a Venturi mask is that it can
   **a.** deliver up to 80% $O_2$.
   **b.** provide continuous 100% humidity.
   **c.** deliver a precise concentration of $O_2$.
   **d.** be used while a patient eats and sleeps.

6. Which guideline would be a part of teaching patients how to use a metered-dose inhaler (MDI)?
   - **a.** After activating the MDI, breathe in as quickly as you can.
   - **b.** Estimate the amount of remaining medicine in the MDI by floating the canister in water.
   - **c.** Disassemble the plastic canister from the inhaler and rinse both pieces under running water every week.
   - **d.** To determine how long the canister will last, divide the total number of puffs in the canister by the puffs needed per day.
7. Which treatments in CF would the nurse expect to implement in the management plan of patients with CF *(select all that apply)*?
   - **a.** Sperm banking
   - **b.** IV corticosteroids on a chronic basis
   - **c.** Airway clearance techniques (e.g., Acapella)
   - **d.** GoLYTELY given PRN for severe constipation
   - **e.** Inhaled tobramycin to combat *Pseudomonas* infection
8. A patient who has bronchiectasis asks the nurse, "What conditions would warrant a call to the clinic?"
   - **a.** Blood clots in the sputum
   - **b.** Sticky sputum on a hot day
   - **c.** Increased shortness of breath after eating a large meal
   - **d.** Production of large amounts of sputum on a daily basis

1. a, c, d, e; 2. a; 3. a, e; 4. b; 5. c; 6. d; 7. a, c, d, e; 8. a

For rationales to these answers and even more NCLEX review questions, visit *http://evolve.elsevier.com/Lewis/medsurg.*

## EVOLVE WEBSITE

http://evolve.elsevier.com/Lewis/medsurg

**Review Questions (Online Only)**

**Key Points**

**Answer Keys for Questions**

- Rationales for Bridge to NCLEX Examination Questions
- Answer Guidelines for Case Study on p. 582
- Answer Guidelines for Managing Care of Multiple Patients Case Study (Section 5) on p. 585

**Student Case Studies**

- Patient With Asthma
- Patient With Chronic Obstructive Pulmonary Disease (COPD)
- Patient With Cystic Fibrosis

**Nursing Care Plans**

- eNursing Care Plan 28-1: Patient With Asthma
- eNursing Care Plan 28-2: Patient With Chronic Obstructive Pulmonary Disease

**Conceptual Care Map Creator**

- Conceptual Care Map for Case Study on p. 582

**Audio Glossary**

**Content Updates**

## REFERENCES


1. American Lung Association: Trends in asthma morbidity and mortality, Epidemiology and Statistics Unit, Research and Health Education Division. Retrieved from *www.lungusa.org.*
2. American Lung Association: Trends in COPD (chronic bronchitis and emphysema): morbidity and mortality, Epidemiology and Statistics Unit, Research and Health Education Division. Retrieved from *www.lungusa.org.*
*3. National Heart, Lung, and Blood Institute and National Asthma Education and Prevention Program: Expert Panel Report 3: guidelines for the diagnosis and management of asthma, NIH pub no 08-4051, Bethesda, Md, 2007, National Institutes of Health. Retrieved from *www.nhlbi.nih.gov/guidelines.*
*4. Global Initiative for Asthma: Global strategy for asthma management and prevention, 2015. Retrieved from *www.ginasthma.org.*
5. Baur X, Sigsgaard T, Aasen TB, et al: Guidelines for management of work-related asthma, *Eur Respir J* 39:529, 2012.
6. Sandur V, Murugesh M, Banait V, et al: Prevalence of gastroesophageal reflux in patients with difficult to control asthma and effect of proton pump inhibitor therapy on asthma symptoms, reflux symptoms, pulmonary function and requirement for asthma medications, *J Postgrad Med* 60(3):282, 2014.
7. Lareau SC, Hodder R: Teaching inhaler use in chronic obstructive pulmonary disease patients, *J Am Acad Nurs Pract* 24:113, 2012.
8. Kane B, Fowler SJ, Niven R: Refractory asthma—beyond step 5, the role of new and emerging adjuvant therapies, *Chron Respir Dis* 12(1):69, 2015.
9. US Food and Drug Administration: Epinephrine CFC metered-dose inhalers: questions and answers. Retrieved from *www.fda.gov/Drugs/DrugSafety.informationbydrugclass/ucm080427.htm.*
10. Rosser FJ, Forno E, Cooper PJ, et al: Asthma in Hispanics: An 8-year update, *Am J Respir Crit Care Med* 189(11):1316, 2014.
*11. Global Initiative for Chronic Obstructive Lung Disease: Global strategy for the diagnosis, management, and prevention of chronic obstructive pulmonary disease (updated 2015). Retrieved from *www.goldcopd.org.*
12. National Heart, Lung, and Blood Institute: COPD: are you at risk? Retrieved from *www.nhlbi.nih.gov/health/public/lung/copd/campaign-materials/html/copd-atrisk.htm.*
13. National Institute on Drug Abuse: Info facts: cigarettes and other tobacco products. Retrieved from *www.drugabuse.gov/publications/infofacts/cigarettes-other-tobacco-products.*
14. Health 24: How many smokers develop COPD? Retrieved from *www.health24.com/medical/Condition_centres/777-792-805-1535,28674.asp.*
15. Alpha-1 Foundation: Healthcare providers: what is alpha-1? Retrieved from *www.alphaone.org.*
16. Rycroft CE, Heyes A, Lanza L, et al: Epidemiology of chronic obstructive pulmonary disease: a literature review, *Int J Chron Obstruct Pulmon Dis* 7:457, 2012.
17. Evans RA, Morgan MD: The systemic nature of chronic lung disease, *Clin Chest Med* 35(2): 283, 2014.
18. McDonald CF. Oxygen therapy for COPD, *J Thorac Dis* 6(11):1632, 2014.
19. Miravitlles M, Anzueto A: Antibiotics for acute and chronic respiratory infection in patients with chronic obstructive pulmonary disease, *Am J Respir Crit Care Med* 188(9):1052, 2013.
20. Farland MZ, Peters CJ, Williams JD, et al: β-Blocker use and incidence of chronic obstructive pulmonary disease exacerbations, *Ann Pharmacother* 47(5):651, 2013.
*21. Borge CR, Hagen KB, Mengshoel AM, et al: Effects of controlled breathing exercises and respiratory muscle training in people with chronic obstructive pulmonary disease: results from evaluating the quality of evidence in systematic reviews, *BMC Pulm Med* 14:184, 2014.
22. Seo SH: Medical nutrition therapy based on nutrition intervention for a patient with chronic obstructive pulmonary disease, *Clin Nutr Res* 3(2):150, 2014.
23. Taneja A: Bronchoscopic interventions in the management of chronic obstructive pulmonary disease, *Curr Opin Pulm Med* 19(2):145, 2013.
24. Kobayashi S, Yanai M, Hanagmana M, et al: The burden of chronic obstructive pulmonary disease in the elderly population, *Resp Investig* 52(5):296, 2014.
25. Areias V, Carreira S, Anciaes M, et al: Co-morbidities in patients with Gold stage 4 chronic obstructive lung disease, *Rev Port Pneumol* 20(1):5, 2014.

26. Battaglia S, Cardillo I, Lavorini F, et al: Safety considerations of inhaled corticosteroids in the elderly, *Drugs Aging* 31(11):787, 2014.
27. Rinaudo M, Ferrer M, Terraneo S, et al: Impact of chronic obstructive pulmonary disease in the outcome of intensive care unit-acquired pneumonia with and without previous intubation, *Chest* 147(6):1530, 2015.
28. Batzlaff CM, Karpman C, Afessa B, et al: Predicting 1-year mortality rate for patients admitted with an acute exacerbation of chronic obstructive pulmonary disease to an intensive care unit: an opportunity for palliative care, *Mayo Clin Proc* 85(9):638, 2014.
*29. McCarthy B, Casey D, Devane D: Pulmonary rehabilitation for chronic obstructive pulmonary disease, *Cochrane Database Syst Rev* 2:CD003793, 2015.
30. Who needs pulmonary rehabilitation? Retrieved from *www.nhlbi.nih.gov/health/health-topics/topics/pulreh/whoneeds.*
31. LeGear T, LeGear M, Preradovic D, et al: Does a Nintendo Wii exercise program provide similar exercise demands as a traditional pulmonary rehabilitation program in adults with COPD? *Clin Respir J* 10(3):303, 2016.
32. Theander K, Hasselgren M, Luhr K: Symptoms and impact of symptoms on function and health in patients with chronic obstructive pulmonary disease and chronic heart failure in primary health care, *Int J Chron Obstruct Pulmon Dis* 9:785, 2014.
33. Schroedl C, Yount S, Szmuilowicz E, et al: Outpatient palliative care for chronic obstructive pulmonary disease: a case series, *J Palliat Med* 17(11):1256, 2014.
34. Andersen D: Cystic fibrosis of the pancreas and its relation to celiac disease, *Am J Dis Child* 56:344, 1938. (Classic)
35. Cystic Fibrosis Foundation Patient Registry: *2013 annual data report*, Bethesda, Md, 2014, Cystic Fibrosis Foundation. Retrieved from *www.cff.org.*
36. Somayaji R, Parkins MD: Tobramycin inhalation powder: an efficient and efficacious therapy for the treatment of *Pseudomonas aeruginosa* infection in cystic fibrosis, *Ther Deliv* 6(2):12, 2015.
*37. Langton Hewer SC, Smyth AR: Antibiotic strategies for eradicating *Pseudomonas aeruginosa* in people with cystic fibrosis, *Cochrane Database Syst Rev* 10:11, 2014.
*38. Whiting P, Al M, Burgers L, et al: Ivacaftor for the treatment of patients with cystic fibrosis and the G551D mutation: a systematic review and cost-effectiveness analysis, *Health Technol Assess* 18(18):1, 2014.

*Evidence-based guidelines for clinical practice.

## CASE STUDY

### *Managing Care of Multiple Patients*

You are assigned to care for the following four patients on a medical-surgical unit. You are sharing one unlicensed assistive personnel (UAP) with another RN.

**Patients**

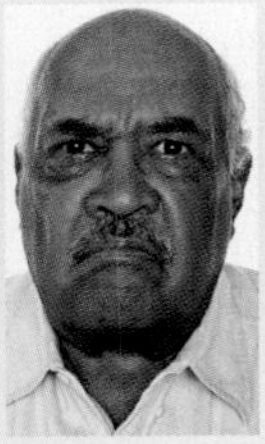
(©Fuse/Thinkstock)

F.T. is a 70-yr-old man with a history of COPD who was admitted yesterday with bilateral lower lobe pneumonia. He is receiving $O_2$ at 2 L/min via nasal cannula and IV antibiotics. His last pulse oximetry reading was 92%.

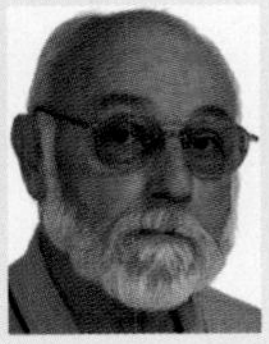
(©iStockphoto/Thinkstock)

M.R. is a 60-yr-old man who is 3 days postoperative following a total laryngectomy with tracheostomy for treatment of laryngeal cancer. He is receiving intermittent tube feeding via a percutaneous endoscopic gastrostomy (PEG) tube and last received pain medication 4 hours ago.

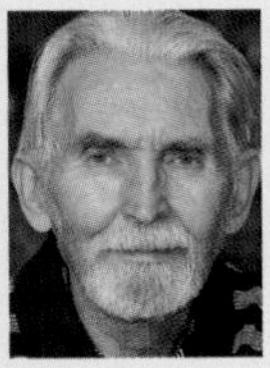
(©iStockphoto/Thinkstock)

J.H. is a 52-yr-old man admitted with right lower lobe pneumonia. A bronchoscopy with biopsy revealed small cell lung carcinoma. He is intermittently confused and anxious with rapid, shallow respirations. He and his family are currently considering his treatment options.

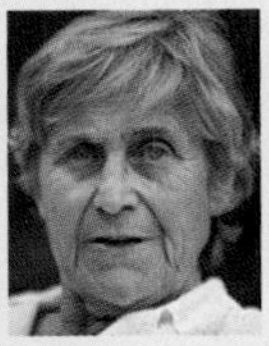
(©iStockphoto/Thinkstock)

H.M. is a 68-yr-old white woman admitted 3 days ago with a COPD exacerbation. She has not been able to ambulate much because of her shortness of breath. She is on oral prednisone and ipratropium. She is anticipating discharge later today. She is to start Advair Diskus and chronic $O_2$ therapy at home after discharge.

**Discussion Questions**

1. ***Priority Decision:*** After receiving report, which patient should you see first? Provide a rationale for your decision.
2. ***Teamwork and Collaboration:*** Which morning tasks can you delegate to the UAP *(select all that apply)*?
   a. Take a pulse oximetry reading on F.T.
   b. Assess M.R.'s pain level and show him how to administer his tube feeding.
   c. Assist H.M. with AM care and gather belongings in anticipation of discharge.
   d. Teach F.T. how to use the incentive spirometer and titrate $O_2$ to obtain pulse oximetry >95%.
   e. Provide coffee and emotional support for J.H.'s family as they await a family meeting with the physician.
3. ***Priority Decision and Teamwork and Collaboration:*** While you are assessing J.H., the UAP tells you that H.M. is complaining of chest pain and worsening shortness of breath. M.R. is also requesting pain medication. What should you do *first*?
   a. Ask the UAP to get H.M.'s vital signs while you give M.R. pain medication.
   b. Ask the UAP to increase H.M.'s $O_2$ to 4 L/min while you assess M.R.'s pain.
   c. Ask the UAP to obtain a stat 12-lead ECG on H.M. while you perform a focused assessment.
   d. Ask the UAP to have another RN give M.R. his pain medication while you go directly to H.M.'s room.

**Case Study Progression**

After assessing H.M., you notify her HCP. A stat 12-lead ECG is obtained and a blood sample is drawn to check cardiac enzymes. H.M.'s chest pain is not relieved by sublingual nitroglycerin. You then administer 4 mg IV morphine. H.M. states that her pain is "a little better" but continues to complain of dyspnea. The 12-lead ECG and cardiac enzyme results are all within normal limits.

4. Because of H.M.'s reduced mobility, you recognize that she is at risk for ____________ and anticipate the HCP will order which tests to determine the cause of her current symptoms?
   a. BNP and echocardiogram
   b. D-dimer and spiral CT scan
   c. CBC and abdominal flat-plate x-ray
   d. Serum electrolytes and renal ultrasound
5. While the charge nurse accompanies H.M. to radiology, you turn your attention back to your remaining three patients. Prior to administering M.R.'s 8 AM tube feeding, you aspirate 300 mL of gastric contents from his PEG tube. Which action should you take *next*?
   a. Discard the aspirated contents and administer the tube feeding as ordered.
   b. Replace the aspirated contents and administer half of ordered tube feeding volume.
   c. Discard the aspirated contents and withhold the next two scheduled tube feedings.
   d. Replace the aspirated contents and notify the HCP prior to administering any further tube feedings.
6. When preparing F.T.'s AM medications, you note that he is scheduled to receive the following antibiotics at 8 AM: levofloxacin (Levaquin) 750 mg in 150 mL normal saline over 90 minutes (give once q24hr) and cefazolin (Kefzol) 1 g in 100 mL normal saline over 30 minutes (give q8hr). He has only one IV site. Which action is *most* appropriate?
   a. Obtain a second peripheral IV site.
   b. Call the HCP to change the administration times.
   c. Check with pharmacy to see if they can be mixed together in the same IV bag.
   d. Administer the cefazolin first because it takes the least amount of time to infuse.
7. ***Management Decision:*** J.H.'s son calls you on the telephone to inquire about his father's current condition and long-term prognosis. Which initial response would be *most* appropriate?
   a. Ask the person calling what the code word is to identify himself or herself as family.
   b. Tell the caller that you are not allowed to discuss any information over the telephone.
   c. Empathize with the son's need to know his father's prognosis while acknowledging that no one really knows.
   d. Ask J.H.'s son what the physician has explained to him in order to clarify his current understanding of the situation.

Answers available at *http://evolve.elsevier.com/Lewis/medsurg*.

# SECTION 6

# Problems of Oxygenation: Transport

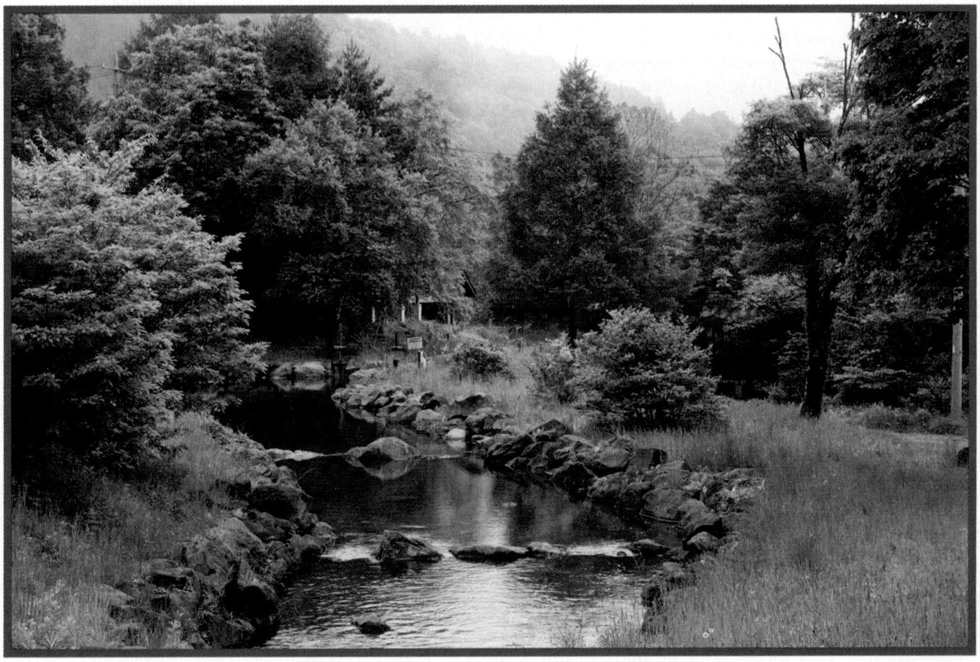



*What makes a river so restful to people is that it doesn't have any doubt—it is sure to get where it is going, and it doesn't want to go anywhere else.*

***Hal Boyle***

29

# Assessment of Hematologic System

Sandra Irene Rome

*There's a lot of blood, sweat, and guts between dreams and success.*

*Paul Bryant*

http://evolve.elsevier.com/Lewis/medsurg/

## LEARNING OUTCOMES

1. Describe the structures and functions of the hematologic system.
2. Differentiate among the different types of blood cells and their functions.
3. Explain the process of hemostasis.
4. Link the age-related changes in the hematologic system to differences in findings of hematologic studies.
5. Obtain significant subjective and objective assessment data related to the hematologic system from a patient.
6. Perform a physical assessment of the hematologic system using the appropriate techniques.
7. Differentiate normal from common abnormal findings of a physical assessment of the hematologic system.
8. Describe the purpose, significance of results, and nursing responsibilities related to diagnostic studies of the hematologic system.

## KEY TERMS



*Hematology* is the study of blood and blood-forming tissues. This includes the bone marrow, blood, spleen, and lymph system. A basic knowledge of hematology is useful in clinical settings to evaluate the patient's ability to transport $O_2$ and $CO_2$, maintain intravascular volume, coagulate blood, and combat infections. Assessment of the hematologic system is based on the patient's health history, physical examination, and results of diagnostic studies.

## STRUCTURES AND FUNCTIONS OF HEMATOLOGIC SYSTEM

### Bone Marrow

Blood cell production (**hematopoiesis**) occurs within the bone marrow. *Bone marrow* is the soft material that fills the central core of bones. Although there are two types of bone marrow (yellow [adipose] and red [hematopoietic]), the red marrow actively produces blood cells. In the adult, the red marrow is found primarily in the flat and irregular bones, such as the ends of long bones, pelvic bones, vertebrae, sacrum, sternum, ribs, flat cranial bones, and scapulae.

All three types of blood cells (red blood cells [RBCs], white blood cells [WBCs], and platelets) develop from a common hematopoietic stem cell within the bone marrow. The hematopoietic *stem cell* is best described as an immature blood cell that is able to self-renew and differentiate into hematopoietic progenitor cells. As the cells mature and differentiate, several different types of blood cells are formed (Fig. 29-1). The marrow responds to increased demands for various types of blood cells by increasing production via a negative feedback system. The bone marrow is stimulated by various factors or cytokines (e.g., erythropoietin, granulocyte colony-stimulating factor [G-CSF], stem cell factor, thrombopoietin) that cause differentiation of the stem cells into one of the committed hematopoietic cells (e.g., RBC). For example, when tissue hypoxia occurs, erythropoietin is secreted by the kidney and liver. It circulates to the bone marrow and causes differentiation of proerythroblasts in the bone marrow.[1]

### Blood

Blood is a type of connective tissue that performs three major functions: transportation, regulation, and protection (Table 29-1). Blood has two major components: plasma and blood cells. In an adult weighing between 150 and 180 lb, the volume of blood is usually between 4.7 and 5.5 L (5 to 6 quarts).

**Plasma.** Approximately 55% of blood is plasma[1] (Fig. 29-2). Plasma is composed primarily of water, but it also contains proteins, electrolytes, gases, nutrients (e.g., glucose, amino acids, lipids), and waste. The term *serum* refers to plasma minus its clotting factors. Plasma proteins include albumin, globulin, and clotting factors (mostly fibrinogen). Most plasma proteins

Reviewed by Judy Carlyle, RN, MNSc, Faculty/Clinical Liaison, Arkansas Rural Nursing Education Consortium (ARNEC), Nashville, Arkansas; and Allison J. Terry, RN, PhD, Associate Professor of Nursing, Assistant Dean of Clinical Practice, School of Nursing, Auburn University Montgomery, Montgomery, Alabama.

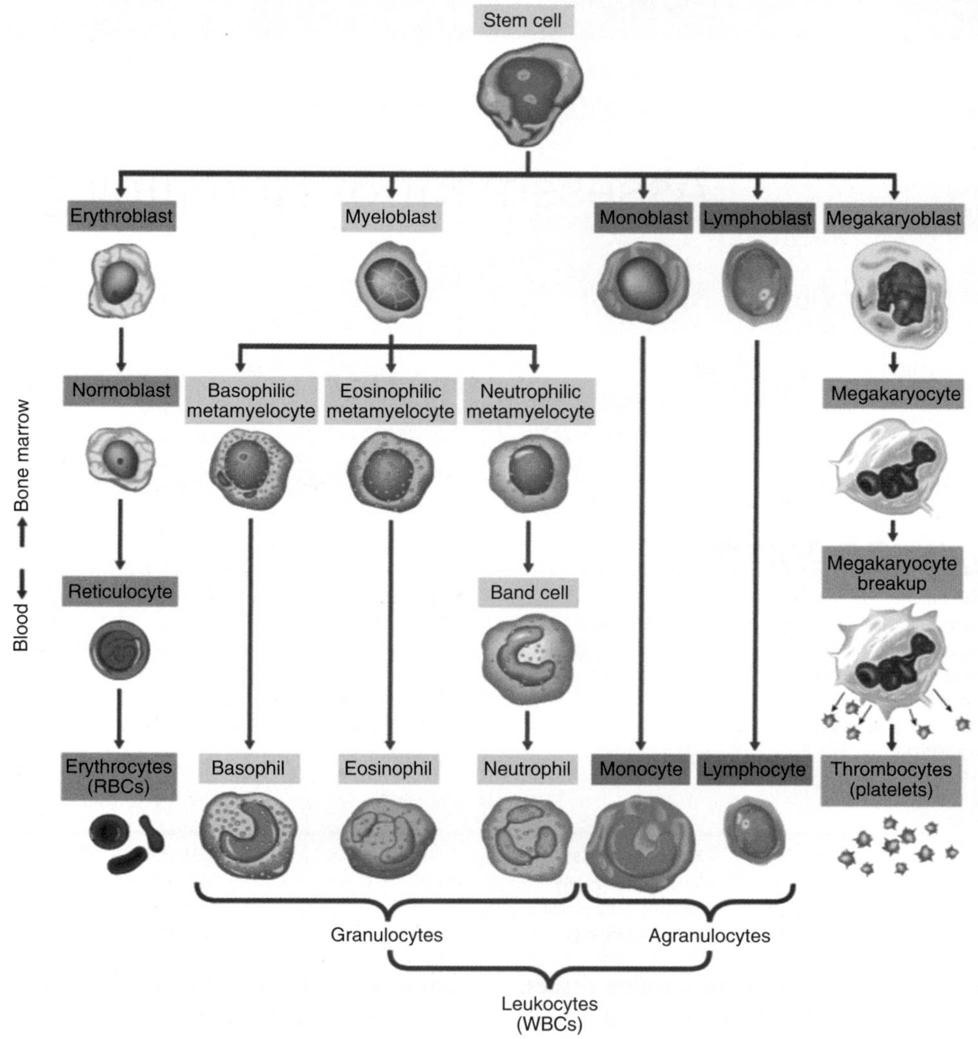


**FIG. 29-1** Development of blood cells. *RBCs,* Red blood cells; *WBCs,* white blood cells.

are produced by the liver, except for antibodies (immunoglobulins), which are produced by plasma cells. Albumin is a protein that helps maintain oncotic pressure in the blood.[1]

**Blood Cells.** About 45% of the blood (Fig. 29-2) is composed of formed elements, or blood cells. The three types of blood cells are *erythrocytes* (RBCs), *leukocytes* (WBCs), and *thrombocytes* (platelets). The primary function of erythrocytes is $O_2$ transportation, whereas the leukocytes are involved in protecting the body from infection. Platelets promote blood coagulation.

***Erythrocytes.*** The primary functions of RBCs include transport of gases (both $O_2$ and $CO_2$) and assistance in maintaining acid-base balance. RBCs are flexible cells with a unique biconcave shape. Flexibility enables the cell to alter its shape so that it can easily pass through tiny capillaries. The cell membrane is thin to facilitate diffusion of gases.

Erythrocytes are primarily composed of a large molecule called *hemoglobin*. Hemoglobin, a complex protein-iron compound composed of heme (an iron compound) and globin (a simple protein), binds with $O_2$ and $CO_2$. As RBCs circulate through the capillaries surrounding alveoli within the lung, $O_2$ attaches to iron on the hemoglobin. The $O_2$-bound hemoglobin is referred to as *oxyhemoglobin* and is responsible for giving arterial blood its bright red appearance. As RBCs flow to body tissues, $O_2$ detaches from the hemoglobin and diffuses from the capillary into tissue cells. $CO_2$ diffuses from tissue cells into the capillary, attaches to the globin portion of hemoglobin, and is transported to the lungs for removal. Hemoglobin also acts as a buffer and plays a role in maintaining acid-base balance. This buffering function is described further in Chapter 16.

**TABLE 29-1 Functions of Blood**

| Function | Examples |
|---|---|
| **Transportation** | • $O_2$ from lungs to cells<br>• Nutrients from GI tract to cells<br>• Hormones from endocrine glands to tissues and cells<br>• Metabolic waste products (e.g., $CO_2$, $NH_3$, urea) from cells to lungs, liver, and kidneys |
| **Regulation** | • Fluid and electrolyte balance<br>• Acid-base balance<br>• Body temperature<br>• Maintaining intravascular oncotic pressure |
| **Protection** | • Maintaining homeostasis of blood coagulation<br>• Combating invasion of pathogens and other foreign substances |

**Erythropoiesis** (the process of RBC production) is regulated by cellular $O_2$ requirements and general metabolic activity.

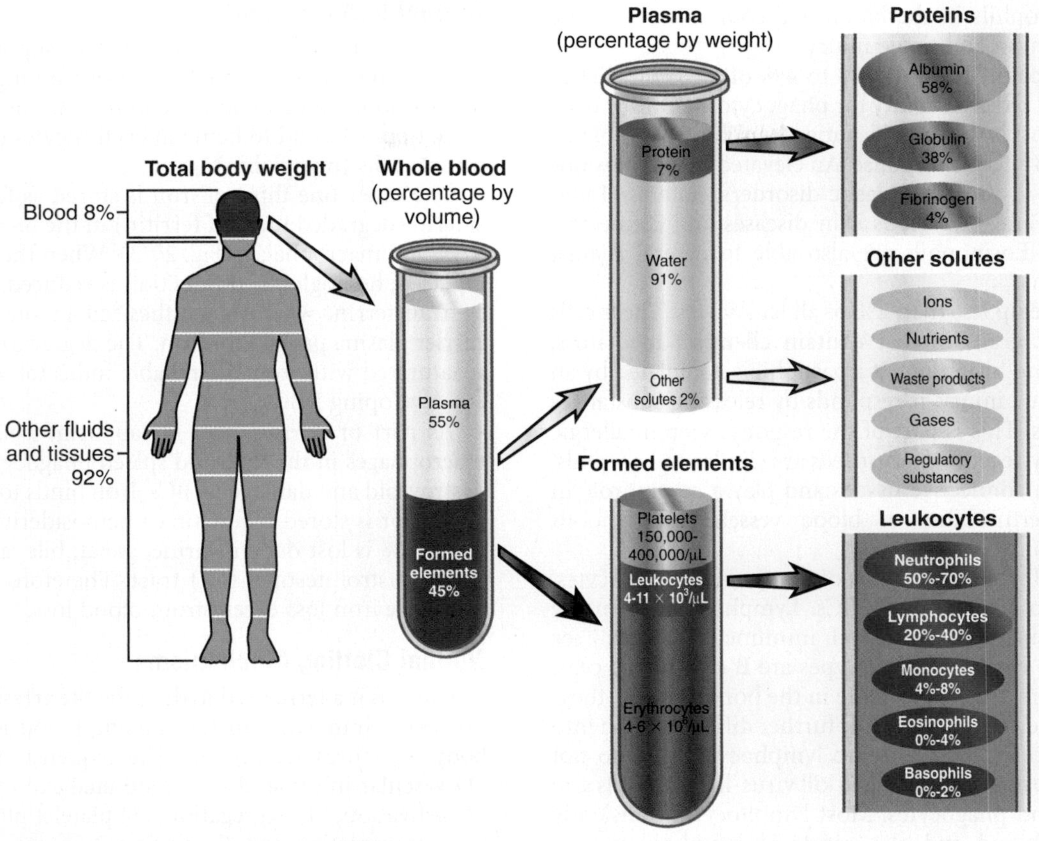


**FIG. 29-2** Approximate values for the components of blood in the adult. Normally, 45% of the blood is composed of blood cells and 55% is composed of plasma.

Erythropoiesis is stimulated by hypoxia and controlled by *erythropoietin,* a glycoprotein growth factor synthesized and released primarily by the kidney. Erythropoietin stimulates the bone marrow to increase erythrocyte production. Approximately 2.5 million erythrocytes are produced per second. The normal life span of an erythrocyte is about 120 days. Erythropoiesis is also influenced by the availability of nutrients. Many essential nutrients are necessary for erythropoiesis, including protein, iron, folate (folic acid), cobalamin (vitamin $B_{12}$), riboflavin (vitamin $B_2$), pyridoxine (vitamin $B_6$), pantothenic acid, niacin, ascorbic acid (vitamin C), and vitamin E. Erythrocyte production is also affected by endocrine hormones, such as thyroxine, corticosteroids, and testosterone. For example, hypothyroidism is often associated with anemia.[1]

Several distinct cell types evolve during erythrocyte maturation (Fig. 29-1). The **reticulocyte** is an immature erythrocyte. Reticulocytes can develop into mature RBCs within 48 hours of release into the circulation. Therefore assessing the number of reticulocytes is a useful means of evaluating the rate and adequacy of erythrocyte production.

**Hemolysis** (destruction of RBCs) by monocytes and macrophages removes abnormal, defective, damaged, and old RBCs from circulation. Hemolysis normally occurs in the bone marrow, liver, and spleen. Because one of the components of RBCs is bilirubin, hemolysis of these cells results in increased bilirubin to be processed by the body. When hemolysis occurs via normal mechanisms, the liver is able to conjugate and excrete all bilirubin that is released (Fig. 30-2).

***Leukocytes.*** *Leukocytes* (WBCs) appear white when separated from blood. Like the RBCs, leukocytes originate from stem cells within the bone marrow (Fig. 29-1) but may eventually reside in the thymus or secondary lymphoid tissues, such as the spleen, lymph nodes, and Peyer patches. There are different types of leukocytes, each with a different function. Leukocytes containing granules within the cytoplasm are called *granulocytes* (also known as *polymorphonuclear leukocytes*). Granulocytes include three types: neutrophils, basophils, and eosinophils.

Leukocytes that do not have granules within the cytoplasm are called *agranulocytes* and include lymphocytes and monocytes. Lymphocytes and monocytes are also referred to as *mononuclear cells* because they have only one discrete nucleus. Leukocytes have a widely variable life span. Granulocytes may only live for hours, yet some T lymphocytes may live for years.

***Granulocytes.*** The primary function of the granulocytes is *phagocytosis,* a process by which WBCs engulf any unwanted organism and then digest and kill it. They can migrate through vessel walls and to the sites where they are needed. The *neutrophil* is the most common type of granulocyte, accounting for 50% to 70% of all WBCs. Neutrophils are the primary phagocytic cells involved in acute inflammatory responses. Once they engulf the pathogen, they die in 1 to 2 days. Neutrophil production and maturation are stimulated by hematopoietic growth factors (e.g., G-CSF, granulocyte-macrophage colony-stimulating factor [GM-CSF]) (see Table 13-3).

A mature neutrophil is called a *segmented neutrophil,* or "seg" or "polysegmented neutrophil," because the nucleus is segmented into two to five lobes connected by strands. An immature neutrophil is called a *band* (for the band appearance of the nucleus). Although band cells are sometimes found in the peripheral circulation of normal people and are capable of phagocytosis, the mature neutrophil is much more effective. An increase in neutrophils in the blood is a common diagnostic indicator of infection and tissue injury.

*Eosinophils* account for only 0% to 4% of all WBCs. They have a similar but reduced ability for phagocytosis. One of their primary functions is to engulf antigen-antibody complexes formed during an allergic response. An elevated level of eosinophils is also seen in some neoplastic disorders, such as Hodgkin's lymphoma, and in various skin diseases and connective tissue disorders.[2] Eosinophils are also able to defend against parasitic infections.

*Basophils* make up less than 2% of all leukocytes. These cells have cytoplasmic granules that contain chemical mediators, such as heparin and histamine. If a basophil is stimulated by an antigen or by tissue injury, it responds by releasing substances from the granules. This is part of the response seen in allergic and inflammatory reactions. *Mast cells* are similar to basophils, but they reside in connective tissues and play a central role in inflammation, permeability of blood vessels, and smooth muscle contraction.

***Lymphocytes.*** Lymphocytes, one of the agranular leukocytes, constitute 20% to 40% of the WBCs. Lymphocytes form the basis of the cellular and humoral immune responses (see Chapter 13). Two lymphocyte subtypes are B cells and T cells. Although T cell precursors originate in the bone marrow, these cells migrate to the thymus gland for further differentiation into T cells. *Natural killer (NK) cells* are lymphocytes that do not require prior exposure to antigens to kill virus-infected cells and activate T cells and phagocytes. Most lymphocytes transiently circulate in the blood and also reside in lymphoid tissues. (Details of lymphocyte function are presented in Chapter 13.)

***Monocytes.*** Monocytes, the other type of agranular leukocytes, account for approximately 4% to 8% of the total WBCs. Monocytes are potent phagocytic cells that ingest small or large masses of matter, such as bacteria, dead cells, tissue debris, and old or defective RBCs. These cells are only present in the blood for a short time before they migrate into the tissues and become macrophages (see Chapter 13). In addition to macrophages that have differentiated from monocytes, tissues also contain resident macrophages. These resident macrophages are given special names (e.g., Kupffer cells in the liver, osteoclasts in the bone, alveolar macrophages in the lung). These macrophages protect the body from pathogens at these entry points and are more phagocytic than monocytes. Macrophages also interact with lymphocytes to facilitate the humoral and cellular immune responses (see Chapter 13).

***Thrombocytes.*** The primary function of thrombocytes, or *platelets*, is to initiate the clotting process by producing an initial platelet plug at a site of injury. Platelets must be available in sufficient numbers and must be structurally and metabolically sound for blood clotting to occur. At the site of any capillary damage, platelet activation is initiated. Increasing numbers of platelets accumulate to form an initial platelet plug that is stabilized with clotting factors. Platelets are also important in the process of clot shrinkage and retraction.

Platelets also originate from stem cells within the bone marrow (Fig. 29-1). The stem cell undergoes differentiation by transforming into a *megakaryocyte*, which fragments into platelets. About one third of the platelets in the body reside in the spleen.

Platelet production is partly regulated by *thrombopoietin*, a growth factor that acts on bone marrow to stimulate platelet production. It is produced in the liver, kidneys, smooth muscle, and bone marrow. Typically, platelets have a life span of only 8 to 10 days.

## Normal Iron Metabolism

Iron is obtained from food and dietary supplements. Approximately 1 mg of every 10 to 20 mg of iron ingested is absorbed in the duodenum and upper jejunum. About two thirds of total body iron is bound to heme in erythrocytes (hemoglobin) and muscle cells (myoglobin).

The other one third of iron is stored as ferritin and hemosiderin (degraded form of ferritin) in the bone marrow, spleen, liver, and macrophages (Fig. 29-3). When the stored iron is not replaced, hemoglobin production is reduced.

Transferrin, which is synthesized in the liver, serves as a carrier plasma protein for iron. The degree to which transferrin is saturated with iron is a reliable indicator of the iron supply for developing RBCs.

As part of normal iron metabolism, iron is recycled after macrophages in the liver and spleen phagocytize, or ingest and destroy, old and damaged RBCs. Iron binds to transferrin in the plasma or is stored as ferritin or hemosiderin (Fig. 29-3). Only about 3% is lost daily in urine, sweat, bile, and epithelial cells in the gastrointestinal (GI) tract. Therefore there is normally very little iron loss except from blood loss.

## Normal Clotting Mechanisms

*Hemostasis* is a term used to describe the arrest of bleeding. This process is important in minimizing blood loss when various body structures are injured. The sequence of events includes (1) vascular injury and subendothelial exposure, (2) adhesion, (3) activation, (4) aggregation, (5) platelet plug formation, and (6) clot retraction and dissolution.

**Vascular Injury and Subendothelial Exposure.** When a blood vessel is injured, an immediate local vasoconstrictive response occurs. Vasoconstriction reduces the leakage of blood from the vessel not only by restricting the vessel size but also by pressing the endothelial surfaces together. The latter reaction enhances vessel wall stickiness and maintains closure of the vessel even after vasoconstriction subsides. Vascular spasm may last for 20

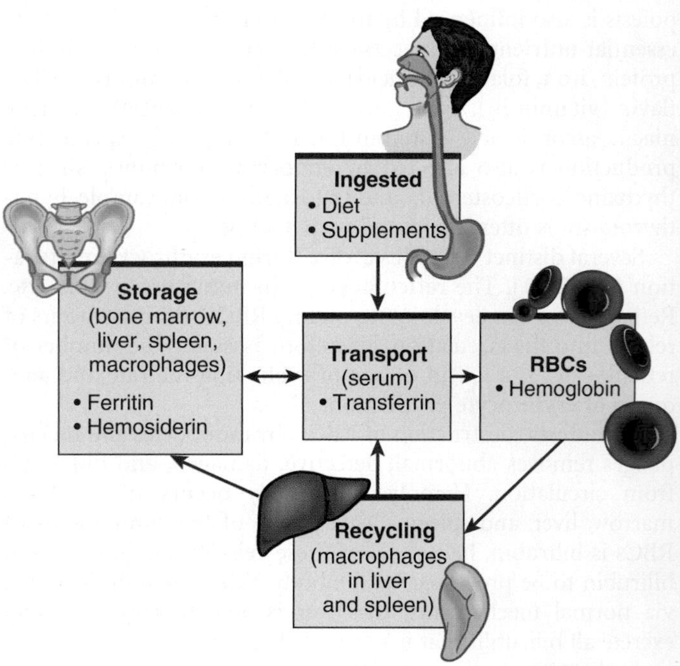


**FIG. 29-3** Normal iron metabolism. Iron is ingested in the diet or from supplements. Macrophages break down ingested red blood cells *(RBCs)*. Iron is returned to blood bound to transferrin or stored as ferritin or hemosiderin.

to 30 minutes, allowing time for the platelet response and plasma clotting factors to be activated. The platelet response and plasma clotting factors are triggered by endothelial injury and the release of substances such as thromboxane $A_2$ ($TXA_2$).

**Platelet Adhesion.** The loss of endothelial cells exposes adhesive glycoproteins such as collagen and von Willebrand factor (vWF), to which the platelets adhere. The stickiness is termed *adhesiveness,* and the formation of clumps is termed *aggregation* or *agglutination.*

**Platelet Activation.** The interaction above causes the platelets to undergo an activation process. This leads to changes in platelet shape. The platelets then have the ability to bind adhesive proteins, including fibrinogen and von Willebrand factor. Release of various platelet granules (including adenosine phosphate [ADP]) also recruits and activates other platelets, clotting factors, and growth factors. As Fig. 29-4 shows, platelet lipoproteins stimulate necessary conversions in the clotting process.

**Platelet Aggregation.** Platelet aggregation is stimulated by $TXA_2$ and ADP, which induce fibrinogen receptors on the platelet. The formation of a visible fibrin clot on the platelet plug is the conclusion of a complex series of reactions involving different clotting (coagulation) factors. The plasma clotting factors are labeled with both names and Roman numerals (Table 29-2).

Plasma proteins circulate in inactive forms until stimulated to initiate clotting through one of two pathways, intrinsic or extrinsic (Fig. 29-4). The *intrinsic pathway* is activated by collagen exposure from endothelial injury when the blood vessel is damaged. The *extrinsic pathway* is initiated when tissue factor or tissue thromboplastin is released extravascularly from injured tissues.

Regardless of whether clotting is initiated by substances internal or external to the blood vessel, coagulation ultimately follows the same final common pathway of the clotting cascade. Thrombin, in the common pathway, is the most powerful enzyme in the coagulation process (Fig. 29-4). It converts fibrinogen to fibrin, which is an essential component of a blood clot.

**Platelet Plug Formation.** The final blood clot is a meshwork of protein strands that stabilizes the platelet plug and traps other cells, such as erythrocytes, phagocytes, and microorganisms.

**Clot Retraction and Dissolution.** Just as some blood elements foster coagulation *(procoagulants),* others interfere with clotting *(anticoagulants).* This counter mechanism to blood clotting keeps blood in its fluid state.

Anticoagulation may be achieved by antithrombin activity, vessel and platelet activity, and fibrinolysis. As the name implies, antithrombins keep blood in a fluid state by antagonizing thrombin, a powerful coagulant. Endogenous heparin, antithrombin III, protein C, and protein S are examples of anticoagulants.

The second means of maintaining blood in its fluid form is **fibrinolysis,** a process resulting in the dissolution of the fibrin

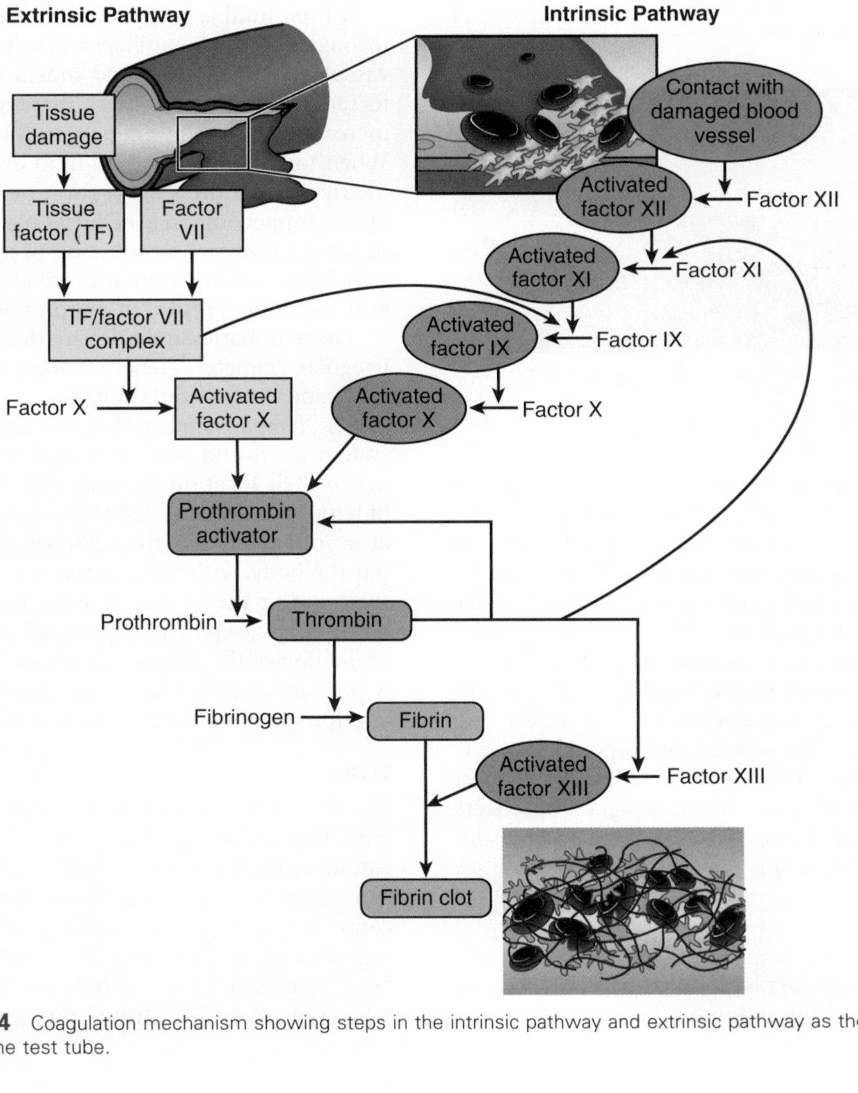


**FIG. 29-4** Coagulation mechanism showing steps in the intrinsic pathway and extrinsic pathway as they would occur in the test tube.

TABLE 29-2 **Coagulation Factors**

| Coagulation Factor | Action |
|---|---|
| **I** Fibrinogen | Source of fibrin to form a clot. Made in liver |
| **II** Prothrombin | Converted to thrombin, which then activates fibrinogen into fibrin as well as factors V, VII, VIII, XI, XIII, protein C, platelets |
| **III** Tissue factor, tissue thromboplastin | Released from damaged endothelial cells and activates the extrinsic pathway by reacting with factor VII |
| **IV** Calcium | Required cofactor at several points in the coagulation cascade |
| **V** Labile factor | Binds with factor X to activate prothrombin |
| **VI** | Not in use (now obsolete) |
| **VII** Stable factor, proconvertin | Forms a complex with factor III and activates factors IX and X |
| **VIII** Antihemophilic factor | Works with factor IX and calcium to activate factor X |
| **IX** Christmas factor | Together with factor VIII, activates factor X |
| **X** Stuart-Prower factor | Activates conversion of factor II (prothrombin) to thrombin |
| **XI** Plasma thromboplastin antecedent | Activates factor IX when calcium is present |
| **XII** Hageman factor | Activates factor XI, which starts the intrinsic pathway |
| **XIII** Fibrin-stabilizing factor | Cross-links fibrin strands and stabilizes fibrin clot |

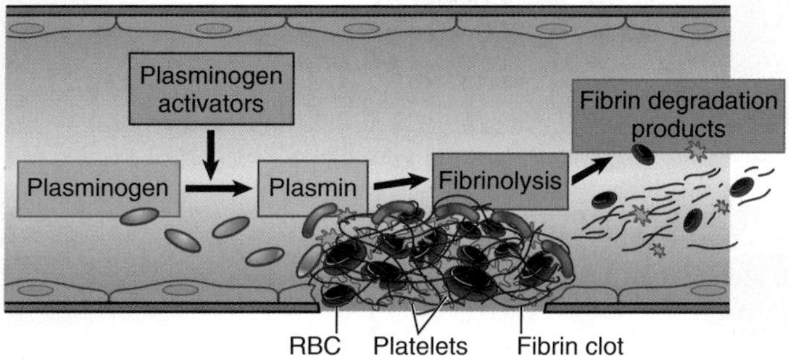


**FIG. 29-5** Fibrinolytic system.

clot. The fibrinolytic system is initiated when plasminogen is activated to plasmin (Fig. 29-5). Thrombin is one of the substances that can activate the conversion of plasminogen to plasmin, thereby promoting fibrinolysis. The plasmin attacks either fibrin or fibrinogen by splitting the molecules into smaller elements known as *fibrin split products* (FSPs) or *fibrin degradation products* (FDPs). (More information about FSPs can be found in Table 29-7 later in this chapter and in the discussion of disseminated intravascular coagulation in Chapter 30.)

If fibrinolysis is excessive, the patient is predisposed to bleeding. In such a situation, bleeding results from the destruction of fibrin in platelet plugs or from the anticoagulation effects of increased FSPs. Increased FSPs lead to impaired platelet aggregation, reduced prothrombin, and an inability to stabilize fibrin.

## Spleen

The spleen is the largest secondary lymphoid organ. It is located in the upper left quadrant of the abdomen. The spleen has four major functions: hematopoietic, filtration, immunologic, and storage. *Hematopoietic function* is manifested by the spleen's ability to produce RBCs during fetal development. The *filtration function* is demonstrated by the spleen's ability to remove old and defective RBCs from the circulation by the mononuclear phagocyte system. Filtration also involves the reuse of iron. The spleen is able to catabolize hemoglobin released by hemolysis and return the iron component of the hemoglobin to the bone marrow for reuse. The spleen also plays an important role in filtering circulating bacteria, especially encapsulated organisms such as gram-positive cocci. The *immunologic function* is demonstrated by the spleen's rich supply of lymphocytes, monocytes, and stored immunoglobulins. The *storage function* is reflected in its role as a storage site for RBCs and platelets. More than 300 mL of blood can be stored. About one third of platelets are stored in the spleen. A person who has had a splenectomy has higher circulating levels of platelets than a person who still has a spleen.

## Lymph System

The lymph system, consisting of lymph fluid, lymphatic capillaries, ducts, and lymph nodes, carries fluid from the interstitial spaces to the blood. It is by means of the lymph that proteins and fat from the gastrointestinal (GI) tract and certain hormones are able to return to the circulatory system. The lymph system also returns excess interstitial fluid to the blood, which is important in preventing edema.

Lymph fluid is pale yellow interstitial fluid that has diffused through lymphatic capillary walls. It circulates through a special vasculature, much as blood moves through blood vessels. The formation of lymph fluid increases when interstitial fluid increases, thereby forcing more fluid into the lymph system. When too much interstitial fluid develops or when something interferes with the reabsorption of lymph, *lymphedema* develops. Lymphedema may occur as a complication of mastectomy or lumpectomy with dissection of axillary nodes. In this situation, lymphedema is often caused by the obstruction of lymph flow from the removal of lymph nodes.

The lymphatic capillaries are thin-walled vessels that have an irregular diameter. They are somewhat larger than blood capillaries and do not contain valves.

The *lymph nodes,* which are also a part of the lymphatic system, are round, oval, or bean shaped and vary in size according to their location. Structurally, the nodes are small clumps of lymphatic tissue and are found in groups along lymph vessels at various sites. More than 200 lymph nodes are found throughout the body, with the greatest number being in the abdomen surrounding the GI tract. Lymph nodes are situated both superficially and deep. The superficial nodes can be palpated, but evaluation of the deep nodes requires radiologic examination.[3,4] A primary function of lymph nodes is filtration of pathogens and foreign particles that are carried by lymph to the nodes.

## Liver

The liver functions as a filter. It also produces all the procoagulants that are essential to hemostasis and blood coagulation. Additionally, it stores iron that is in excess of tissue needs, which can occur with frequent blood transfusions or diseases that cause iron overload. *Hepcidin*, produced by the liver, is a key regulator of iron balance. The synthesis of hepcidin is stimulated by iron overload or inflammation. Hepcidin inhibits the release of stored iron from enterocytes (in the intestines) and macrophages. Thus when iron is deficient, hepatocytes produce less hepcidin. This results in the release of stored iron and an increase in dietary absorption. Other functions of the liver are described in Chapters 38 and 43.

### Gerontologic Considerations: Effects of Aging on Hematologic System

Physiologic aging is a gradual process that involves cell loss and organ atrophy. Aging leads to a decrease in bone marrow mass and cellularity and an increase in bone marrow fat. However, peripheral blood cell concentrations in healthy older adults are similar to those of younger adults. Although the older adult is still capable of maintaining adequate blood cell levels, the reserve capacity leaves the older adult more vulnerable to possible problems with clotting, transporting $O_2$, and fighting infection, especially during periods of increased demand. This results in a diminished ability of an older adult to compensate for an acute or chronic illness.

Hemoglobin levels begin to decrease in both men and women after middle age, with the low-normal levels seen in most older people. Total serum iron, total iron-binding capacity, and intestinal iron absorption are all decreased in older adults. Iron deficiency is usually responsible for the low hemoglobin levels. Healthy older patients are not able to produce reticulocytes in response to hemorrhage or hypoxemia as well as younger adults.

The RBC plasma membranes are more fragile in the older person. This may account for a slight increase in mean corpuscular volume (MCV) and a slight decrease in mean corpuscular hemoglobin concentration (MCHC) of RBCs in some older individuals. It is essential to assess for signs of disease processes such as GI bleeding before concluding that decreased hemoglobin levels are caused solely by aging. Thus iron deficiency anemia is a diagnosis that should be made after other causes have been ruled out.

The total WBC count and differential are generally not affected by aging. However, decreases in lymphocyte function occurs. During an infection, the older adult may have only a minimal elevation in the total WBC count. These laboratory findings suggest a diminished bone marrow reserve of granulocytes in older adults and reflect the possible impaired stimulation of hematopoiesis. The number of platelets is unaffected by the aging process, but functionally they may have increased adhesiveness. Changes in vascular integrity related to aging can manifest as easy bruising.

The effects of aging on hematologic studies are presented in Table 29-3. Immune changes related to aging are presented in Chapter 13.

**TABLE 29-3 Gerontologic Assessment Differences**

***Effects of Aging on Hematologic Studies***

| Study | Changes |
|---|---|
| **CBC Studies** | |
| Hgb | Normal; possibly slight decrease |
| MCV | May be slightly increased |
| MCHC | May be slightly decreased |
| WBC count | Diminished response to infection |
| Platelets | Unchanged but possible increase in adhesiveness |
| **Clotting Studies** | |
| Partial thromboplastin time | Decreased |
| Fibrinogen | May be elevated |
| Factors V, VII, IX | May be elevated |
| ESR | Increased significantly |
| D-dimers | Increased |
| **Iron Studies** | |
| Serum iron | Decreased |
| Total iron-binding capacity | Decreased |
| Ferritin | Increased |
| Erythropoietin | May be decreased |

*ESR,* Erythrocyte sedimentation rate; *MCHC,* mean corpuscular hemoglobin concentration; *MCV,* mean corpuscular volume.

**CASE STUDY**

***Patient Introduction***

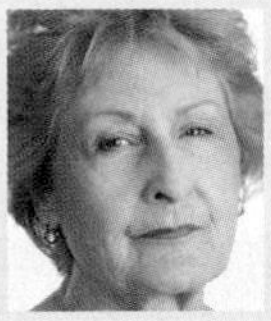

(©Lisa F. Young/iStock)

A.J. is a 63-year-old white woman who is brought to the emergency department by her husband. He came home from work and found his wife at home, weak and lying in bed after she returned from work. She says she has been slowly getting more and more "cold and tired" but "that is what happens when you continue to work at this age." Her husband states that she has become more and more tired over the last couple of weeks and has been having difficulty working all day and even gets short of breath when doing simple errands. She also recently had a "bad cold and sinus infection" that only improved after two courses of antibiotics. A.J. also states, "I've noticed I've had a lot of bruising lately."

**Discussion Questions**

1. What are the possible causes of A.J.'s weakness, pallor, and shortness of breath?
2. Is her condition stable or an emergency?

You will learn more about A.J. and her condition as you read through this assessment chapter. (See p. 596 for more information on A.J.)

Answers available at *http://evolve.elsevier.com/Lewis/medsurg.*

## ASSESSMENT OF HEMATOLOGIC SYSTEM

Much of the evaluation of the hematologic system is based on a thorough health history. You need to be knowledgeable about what to include in the health history so that you can phrase questions to elicit the most information.[5]

### Subjective Data

#### Important Health Information

***Past Health History.*** Determine if the patient has had prior hematologic problems. Ask about previous problems with anemia, bleeding disorders, and blood diseases such as leukemia. Document other related medical conditions such as malabsorption or liver (e.g., hepatitis, cirrhosis), kidney, or spleen disorders. Patients may have received a kidney transplant, may have lost a spleen to traumatic injury, or may have a history of IV drug or alcohol use that affects their risk for hematologic disorders. A history of recent or recurrent infections or problems with blood clotting is also important to note.

***Medications.*** A complete medication history of prescription and over-the-counter drugs is an important component of a hematologic assessment. Inquire about the use of vitamins, herbal products, or dietary supplements because many patients may not consider them to be drugs. Many drugs may interfere with normal hematologic function.[6,7] Herbs can interfere with clotting (see Complementary & Alternative Therapies box in

Chapter 37 on p. 820). Chemotherapy drugs used to treat cancer (see Chapter 15) and antiretroviral agents used to treat human immunodeficiency virus (HIV) infection (see Chapter 14) may cause bone marrow depression. A patient previously treated with chemotherapy agents, particularly alkylating agents, has a higher risk of developing a secondary malignancy of leukemia or lymphoma. A patient on long-term anticoagulant therapy such as warfarin (Coumadin) could be at risk for bleeding problems.

***Surgery or Other Treatments.*** Ask the patient about specific past surgical procedures, including splenectomy, tumor removal, prosthetic heart valve placement, surgical excision of the duodenum (where iron absorption occurs), partial or total gastrectomy (which removes parietal cells, thus reducing intrinsic factor needed for the absorption of cobalamin [vitamin $B_{12}$]), gastric bypass (where the duodenum may be bypassed and parietal cell surface area decreased), and ileal resection (where cobalamin absorption takes place). Also assess how wound healing progressed postoperatively and if and when any bleeding problems occurred in relation to the surgery. Discuss wound healing and bleeding as responses to past injuries (including minor trauma) and dental extractions. Also determine the number of previous blood transfusions and possible complications during administration, since the risk of transfusion reactions and iron overload increases with the number of blood transfusions.

**Functional Health Patterns.** Key questions to ask a patient with a hematologic problem are presented in Table 29-4.

***Health Perception–Health Management Pattern.*** Ask the patient to describe the usual and present state of health. Gather complete demographic data, including age, gender, race, and ethnic background. Ask if there is any family history of hematologic problems.

> **GENETIC RISK ALERT**
>
> - Hematologic problems that have a strong genetic link include sickle cell anemia, hemophilia, thalassemia, and hemochromatosis.
> - People with a family history of these hematologic problems have a much greater risk of developing them.
> - Other hematologic problems, such as leukemia, pernicious anemia, and clotting disorders, may have a genetic predisposition.

When taking a family health history, explore the following health problems: jaundice, anemia, malignancies, RBC disorders such as sickle cell disease, bleeding disorders such as hemophilia, and clotting disorders.

Assess risk factors such as alcohol and cigarette use that may disrupt the hematologic system. Alcohol is a caustic agent to the GI mucosa and can cause damage that results in GI bleeding, esophageal varices, and decreased absorption of cobalamin and other nutrients.

Chronic alcohol users frequently have vitamin deficiencies. Alcohol also exerts a damaging effect on platelet function and the liver, where clotting factors are produced. Consequently, bleeding problems can develop and should be anticipated in cases of known chronic alcohol use. Illicit drug use is also important to document, since many of these drugs may affect hematopoiesis.

Cigarette smoking increases low-density lipoprotein (LDL) cholesterol and levels of $CO_2$, leading to hypoxia and altering the anticoagulant properties of the endothelium. Smoking increases platelet reactivity, plasma fibrinogen, hematocrit, and blood viscosity.

***Nutritional-Metabolic Pattern.*** Obtain the patient's weight and determine if the patient has experienced anorexia, nausea, vomiting, or oral discomfort. A dietary history may provide clues about the cause of anemia. Iron, cobalamin, and folic acid are necessary for the development of RBCs. Iron and folic acid deficiencies are associated with inadequate intake of foods such as liver, meat, eggs, whole-grain and enriched breads and cereals, potatoes, leafy green vegetables, dried fruits, legumes, and citrus fruits. Folic acid deficiencies may be offset by a diet including foods that are also high in iron.[8]

*Hematemesis* (bright red, brown, or black vomitus) is a manifestation of an underlying problem and should always be investigated. Peptic ulcer disease is a common cause of hematemesis.

Explore any changes in the skin's texture, color, or temperature. Ask about bleeding of gum tissue or bleeding from anywhere on the body. Also ask about any lumps or swelling in the neck, armpits, or groin. Specifically, ask what the lumps feel like (i.e., hard or soft, tender or nontender) and if they are mobile or fixed. Primary lymph tumors are usually not painful. A nontender, consistently swollen lymph node may be a sign of a malignancy, such as Hodgkin's or non-Hodgkin's lymphoma. Lymph nodes that are enlarged and tender are usually associated with an acute infection.[3] Explore any reports of fever. Determine if the patient currently has a fever, recurring fevers, chills, or night sweats.

Ask patients if they have a history of cardiac or pulmonary diseases. Cardiovascular disorders such as valvular disease or hypertension may predispose patients to hemolysis. Many of the medications used to treat cardiovascular disease can also cause abnormalities in hematopoietic cell production or coagulation. Pulmonary disorders that lead to hypoxemia may cause chronic stimulation of erythropoietin and result in *polycythemia* (excessive RBCs).

***Elimination Pattern.*** Ask if blood has been noted in the urine or stool or if black, tarry stools have occurred. Ask the patient if he or she has had a recent stool tested for occult blood or colonoscopy. Document any decrease in urine output or diarrhea.

***Activity-Exercise Pattern.*** Because fatigue is a prominent symptom in many hematologic disorders, ask about feelings of tiredness. Also determine any weakness or complaints of heavy extremities. Document symptoms of apathy, malaise, dyspnea, or palpitations. Note any change in the patient's ability to perform regular exercise and/or activities of daily living (ADLs), especially as they relate to patient safety and a history of falling.

***Sleep-Rest Pattern.*** Determine whether the patient feels rested after a night's sleep. Fatigue secondary to a hematologic problem often does not resolve after sleep.

***Cognitive-Perceptual Pattern.*** *Arthralgia* (joint pain) may be caused by a hematologic problem and should be assessed. Pain in the joint may indicate an autoimmune disorder, such as rheumatoid arthritis, or may be caused by gout secondary to increased uric acid production as a result of a hematologic malignancy or hemolytic anemia. Aching bones may result from pressure of expanding bone marrow with diseases such as leukemia. *Hemarthrosis* (blood in a joint) occurs in the patient with bleeding disorders and can be painful.

Paresthesias, numbness, and tingling may be related to a hematologic disorder and should be noted. Also assess any changes in vision, hearing, taste, or mental status.

***Self-Perception–Self-Concept Pattern.*** Determine the effect of the health problem on the patient's perception of self and personal abilities. Also assess the effect of certain problems,

## TABLE 29-4 Health History

### Hematologic System

**Health Perception–Health Management**
- Do you have any difficulty performing daily activities because of a lack of energy?*
- Do you smoke cigarettes or drink alcohol?*
- Do you take any prescribed or over-the-counter medications?*
- Are you taking any herbs?* Home remedies?*
- Have you in the past or are you currently consuming illegal drugs? What agents? What route? How frequently? When did you last use?
- Have you ever received a blood transfusion?*
- Is there any family history of anemia, cancer, bleeding, or clotting problems?*
- Have you had any surgeries?*

**Nutritional-Metabolic**
- Do you have any difficulties with eating, chewing, or swallowing?*
- Have you had any mouth sores, sore tongue, swollen or sore gums, excessive oral bleeding?*
- What kind of diet do you follow? If a vegetarian, do you eat eggs, milk products, fish?
- How has your appetite been?
- Have you had any changes in your weight in the past year?*
- Do you take any vitamins, nutritional supplements, or iron?*
- Is nausea and vomiting a problem for you?*
- Have you ever experienced any unusual bleeding or bruising?*
- Have there been recent changes in the condition or color of your skin?*
- Have you experienced night sweats or cold intolerance?*
- Have you noticed any swelling in your armpits, neck, or groin?*

**Elimination**
- Have you had black or tarry stools?* Have you had light, clay-colored stools?*
- Have you noticed any blood or dark "tea color" in your urine?*
- Has your urine had a foul odor or cloudiness?
- Have you had any decrease in urine output?*
- Do you ever have diarrhea or change in bowel patterns?*

**Activity-Exercise**
- Do you have any shortness of breath at rest? With activity?*
- Do you have any limitations in joint motion?* Have any of your joints been swollen?*
- Do you have a problem with unsteady gait? Have you fallen recently?*
- Do you exercise regularly? What type and how frequently?*
- After activity, do you ever notice bleeding or bruising?*

**Sleep-Rest**
- Have you experienced excessive fatigue recently?*
- Are you more fatigued than usual?*
- Do you feel rested on awakening? If no, explain.

**Cognitive-Perceptual**
- Have you experienced any numbness or tingling?*
- Have you had any problems with your vision, hearing, or taste?*
- Have you noticed any changes in your mental function?*
- Do you have any pain, such as bone, joint, or abdominal pain, or abdominal fullness?*
- Do you have pain when moving your joints?*
- Have your muscles been sore or achy recently?*

**Self-Perception–Self-Concept**
- Does your health problem make you feel differently about yourself?*
- Do you have any physical changes that cause you distress?*

**Role-Relationship**
- Does your occupation bring you into contact with hazardous substances?*
- Has your present illness caused a change in your roles and relationships?*

**Sexuality-Reproductive**
- Has your hematologic problem caused any sexual or intimacy problems that concern you?*
- *Women:* When was your last menses? Do you consider your cycle normal? How long does your bleeding usually last? Have you had any increase in cramping or clotting?* Have there been any changes in the amount of flow?*
- *Men:* Do you experience impotence?*
- Have you had unprotected sex in the past 6 months?* Was your partner someone new or a person with whom you have had a long-term sexual relationship?

**Coping–Stress Tolerance**
- Do you have a support system to assist you when needed?
- What coping strategies do you use during exacerbation of symptoms?
- Do you experience any specific symptoms when you feel stressed?*

**Value-Belief**
- Do you have any personal or religious objection to receiving blood or blood products?*
- Do you have any conflicts between your planned therapy and your value-belief system?*

*If yes, describe.

such as bruising, petechiae, and lymph node swelling, on the patient's personal appearance.

***Role-Relationship Pattern.*** Question the patient about any past or present occupational or household exposures to radiation or chemicals. If such exposure has occurred, determine the type, amount, and duration of the exposure.

A person who has been exposed to radiation, as a treatment modality or by accident, has a higher incidence of certain hematologic problems. The same is true of a person who has been exposed to certain chemicals (e.g., benzene, lead, naphthalene, phenylbutazone). These chemicals are commonly used by potters, dry cleaners, and individuals involved with occupations that use adhesives. Ask the patient about a history in the military. Many Vietnam War veterans were exposed to a dioxin-containing defoliant (Agent Orange), which has been linked with leukemia and lymphoma. Also assess the effect of the present illness on the patient's usual roles and responsibilities.

***Sexuality-Reproductive Pattern.*** Obtain a careful menstrual history from women, including the age at which menarche and menopause began, duration and amount of bleeding, incidence of clotting and cramping, and any associated problems. Ask men if they have any problems related to impotence, since this is common in men with hematologic problems. Also question the patient about sexual behavior because HIV infection is potentially a concern, particularly among high-risk groups.

***Coping–Stress Tolerance Pattern.*** The patient with a hematologic problem often needs assistance with ADLs. Ask the patient if adequate support is available to meet daily needs. Determine the patient's usual methods of handling stress. In the patient with platelet disorders or hemophilia, the potential for hemorrhage can be so frightening that usual life patterns may be drastically curtailed, affecting the person's quality of life. Explore the patient's understanding of the problem and provide teaching.

***Value-Belief Pattern.*** Some hematologic problems are treated with blood transfusions or a bone marrow transplant. Determine if these types of treatments conflict with the patient's value-belief system, including the patient's cultural and religious beliefs related to blood and blood transfusions. If conflicts are identified, notify the HCP.

## CASE STUDY

### *Subjective Data*

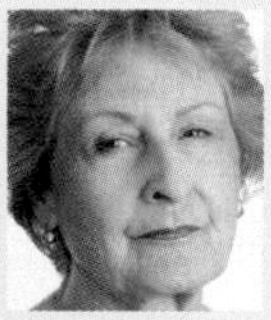

(©Lisa F. Young/iStock)

A focused subjective assessment of A.J. revealed the following information:

***PMH:*** History of mild osteoarthritis. No surgical history. Prefers to take care of self with "natural therapy" and has not seen an HCP for 5 years, except for the recent sinus infection.

***Medications:*** Metamucil 1 Tbsp PO daily; vitamins C, E, and D with calcium.

***Health Perception–Health Management:*** A.J. denies family or personal history of anemia, cancer, or bleeding disorders. She believes she comes from a family with great genes for longevity because they "eat organic foods." She admits to drinking one glass of red wine with her evening meal "because it's good for your heart." She is a nonsmoker and just can't understand her gradual increase in shortness of breath with exertion. She states she really can't do anything anymore without having to stop and catch her breath. She says, "It's tough getting old."

***Nutritional-Metabolic:*** A.J. and her husband eat a lot of pasta "because it is cheap." She uses a lot of garlic for flavoring and the "health benefit of it." Although not a vegetarian, she states that she eats little meat.

***Elimination:*** Denies black or tarry stool. Occasional constipation. No problems with urination. Urine without odor.

***Activity-Exercise:*** As noted above, A.J. is having difficulty performing ADLs without having to stop and catch her breath. Denies dyspnea at rest. States joints are stiff on arising in morning and after sitting but able to get around OK and work at her secretarial job. States her walking is steady but weak. No history of falling.

***Sleep-Rest:*** Typically sleeps 8-9 hr/night with no difficulty falling asleep. However, she still feels tired and needs to nap during her lunch break and during her days off.

***Cognitive-Perceptual:*** Denies any numbness or tingling. Admits to being a little hard-of-hearing but can still see "pretty good."

***Value-Belief:*** Prefers natural therapies over traditional medication.

**Discussion Questions**

1. What type of assessment would be most appropriate for A.J.: comprehensive, focused, or emergency? On what basis did you make that decision? What would be your priority?
2. What assessment questions would you ask A.J.?
3. How will you individualize the physical assessment based on the information from A.J. and her husband?
4. What subjective assessment findings are of most concern to you?
5. Based on these subjective assessment findings, what type of physical assessment should be performed?

You will learn more about the physical examination of the hematologic system in the next section. (See p. 599 for more information on A.J.)

Answers available at *http://evolve.elsevier.com/Lewis/medsurg.*

### Objective Data

**Physical Examination.** A complete physical examination is necessary to accurately examine all systems that affect or are affected by the hematologic system (see Chapter 3). Be aware that disorders of the hematologic system can manifest in various ways. Thus a patient's presenting symptoms may not immediately point to a hematologic problem (Table 29-5). For example, paresthesias of the lower extremities may not immediately appear to reflect a hematologic problem, but when combined with other clinical findings or risk factors, they may indicate cobalamin deficiency and resulting pernicious anemia. Although a full examination should be performed on patients suspected of a hematologic disorder, certain aspects of the physical examination are specifically relevant. These include skin, lymph nodes, spleen, and liver. Examination of the skin is discussed in Chapter 22; spleen and liver examination is found in Chapter 38.

***Lymph Node Assessment.*** Lymph nodes are distributed throughout the body. Superficial lymph nodes can be evaluated by light palpation (Fig. 29-6). Deep lymph nodes cannot be palpated and are best evaluated by radiologic examination. Assess lymph nodes symmetrically and take note of location, size (in centimeters), degree of fixation (e.g., movable, fixed), tenderness, and texture. To assess superficial lymph nodes, lightly palpate the nodes using the pads of the fingers. Then gently roll the skin over the area and concentrate on feeling for possible lymph node enlargement.

Ordinarily, lymph nodes are not palpable in adults. If a node is palpable, it should be small (0.5 to 1 cm), mobile, firm, and nontender to be considered a normal finding. A node that is tender, hard, fixed, or enlarged (regardless if it is tender or not) is an abnormal finding and warrants further investigation. Tender nodes are usually a result of inflammation, whereas hard or fixed nodes suggest malignancy.[3]

Develop a sequence when examining the lymph nodes. A convenient sequence is to start at the head and neck. First,

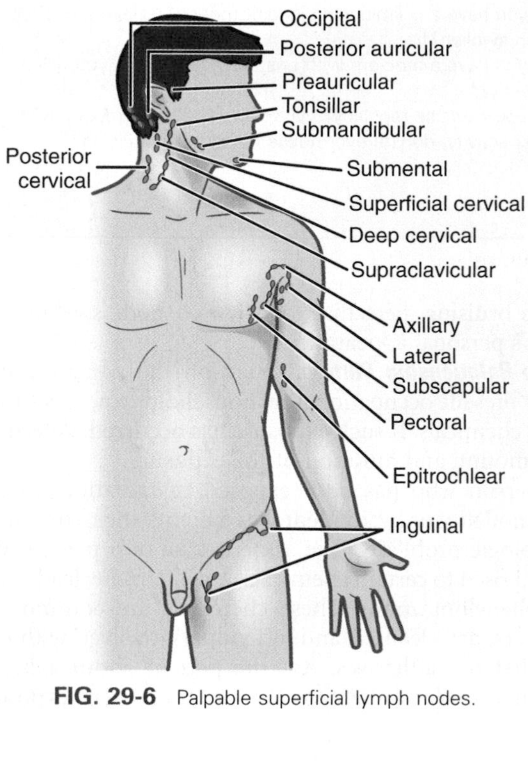


**FIG. 29-6** Palpable superficial lymph nodes.

## TABLE 29-5 Assessment Abnormalities

### *Hematologic System*

| Finding | Description | Possible Etiology and Significance |
|---|---|---|
| **Skin** | | |
| **Pallor of skin or nail beds** | Paleness. Decreased or absence of skin coloration. | Low Hgb level (anemia). |
| **Flushing** | Transient, episodic redness of skin (usually around face and neck). | Increase in Hgb (polycythemia), congestion of capillaries. Flushing of palms of hands or soles of feet possible indication of anemia. |
| **Jaundice** | Yellow appearance of skin and mucous membranes. | Accumulation of bile pigment caused by rapid or excessive hemolysis or liver damage. |
| **Cyanosis** | Bluish discoloration of skin and mucous membranes | Reduced Hgb, excessive concentration of deoxyhemoglobin in blood. |
| **Excoriation** | Scratch or abrasion of skin. | Scratching from intense pruritus. |
| **Pruritus** | Unpleasant cutaneous sensation that provokes the desire to rub or scratch skin. | Hodgkin's lymphoma, cutaneous lymphomas, infiltrative leukemias, increased bilirubin. |
| **Leg ulcers** | Prominent on the malleoli on the ankles. | Sickle cell disease. |
| **Angioma** | Benign tumor consisting of blood or lymph vessels. | Most are congenital. Some may disappear spontaneously. |
| **Telangiectasia** | Small angioma with tendency to bleed. Focal red lesions, coarse or fine red lines. | Dilation of small vessels. |
| **Spider nevus** | Form of telangiectasia characterized by a round red central portion and branching radiations resembling profile of a spider. Usually develop on face, neck, or chest. | Elevated estrogen levels as in pregnancy or liver disease. |
| **Purpura** | Any of a small group of conditions characterized by ecchymosis or other small hemorrhages in skin and mucous membranes. | Decreased platelets or clotting factors resulting in hemorrhage into skin. Vascular abnormalities. Break in blood vessel walls resulting from trauma. |
| **Petechiae** | Pinpoint, nonraised, perfectly round area >2 mm. Purple, dark red, or brown. | Same as above |
| **Ecchymosis (bruise)** | Small hemorrhagic spot, larger than petechiae. Nonelevated. Round or irregular. | Same as above. |
| **Hematoma** | A localized collection of blood, usually clotted. | Same as above. |
| **Chloroma** | A tumor arising from myeloid tissue and containing a pale green pigment. | Acute myelogenous leukemia that has infiltrated the skin. |
| **Plasmacytoma** | Tumor arising from abnormal plasma cells. | Multiple myeloma that has infiltrated tissue. |
| **Eyes** | | |
| **Jaundiced sclera** | Yellow appearance of sclera. | Accumulation of bile pigment resulting from rapid or excessive hemolysis or liver disease or infiltration. |
| **Conjunctival pallor** | Paleness. Decreased or absence of coloration in the conjunctiva. | Low Hgb level (anemia). |
| **Blurred vision, diplopia, visual field cuts** | Decreased visual acuity or areas of blindness (field cuts). | Anemia, extreme leukocytosis, polycythemia may cause visual abnormalities. Thrombocytopenia may cause intraocular hemorrhage with visual abnormalities. Excessive clotting may cause thromboses in circulation to the brain that cause visual field cuts. |
| **Nose** | | |
| **Epistaxis** | Spontaneous bleeding from nares. | May occur with low platelet counts, especially if patient bends down for a long time, tries to lift a heavy item, or performs an intense Valsalva maneuver. |
| **Mouth** | | |
| **Gingival and mucous membrane changes** | Pallor. | Low Hgb level (anemia). |
| | Gingival and mucosal ulceration, swelling, or bleeding. | Neutropenia. Inability of impaired leukocytes to combat oral infections. Thrombocytopenia. Gingival hyperplasia may be present with some types of leukemia. |
| **Smooth tongue** | Tongue surface smooth and shiny. Mucosa thin and red from decreased papillae. | Pernicious anemia, iron-deficiency anemia. |
| **Musculoskeletal System** | | |
| **Bone pain** | Pain in pelvis, ribs, spine, sternum. | Multiple myeloma related to enlarged tumors that stretch periosteum. Bone invasion by leukemia cells. Bone demineralization resulting from various malignancies. Sickle cell disease. |
| **Joint swelling** | Fluid-filled spaces surrounding joints. | Occurs with hemophilia and sickle cell anemia as bleeding occurs into joint (hemarthrosis), causing inflammation. |
| **Arthralgia** | Joint pain. | Sickle cell disease from hemarthrosis. |
| **Lymph Nodes** | | |
| **Lymphadenopathy** | Lymph nodes enlarged (>1 cm). May be tender to touch. | Infection; foreign infiltrations. Systemic disease such as leukemia, lymphoma, Hodgkin's lymphoma, and metastatic cancer. |

*Continued*

**TABLE 29-5 Assessment Abnormalities**
***Hematologic System—cont'd***

| Finding | Description | Possible Etiology and Significance |
|---|---|---|
| **Heart and Chest** | | |
| **Tachycardia** | Heart rate >100 beats/min. | Compensatory mechanism in anemia to increase cardiac output. |
| **Palpitations** | Feeling the heartbeat, flutter, or pound in chest. | Anemia, fluid volume overload, hypotension with impending syncope, hypertension, dysrhythmias. |
| **Altered blood pressure** | *Orthostasis:* heart rate >20 beats/min increase or blood pressure >20 mm Hg decrease from baseline when moving from a lying position to either sitting or standing. | Orthostasis is a common manifestation in anemia, especially if also accompanied by low blood volume. |
| | *Hypotension:* <90 mm Hg systolic or >40 mm Hg drop from baseline. | Hypotension may indicate an infectious process, blood loss, or compromised cardiovascular compensatory mechanisms. |
| | *Hypertension:* >140/90 mm Hg. | Hypertension may occur initially as a compensatory mechanism for anemia. |
| **Sternal tenderness** | Abnormal sensitivity to touch or pressure on sternum. | Leukemia resulting from increased bone marrow cellularity, causing increase in pressure and bone erosion. Multiple myeloma as a result of stretching of periosteum |
| **Low $O_2$ saturation** | $O_2$-carrying capacity as reflected by $O_2$ saturation by pulse oximetry. | $O_2$ saturation may be decreased in cases of severe anemia. |
| **Abdomen** | | |
| **Hepatomegaly** | Palpable liver. | Leukemia, cirrhosis, or fibrosis secondary to iron overload from sickle cell disease or thalassemia. |
| **Splenomegaly** | Palpable spleen. | Anemia, thrombocytopenia, leukemia, lymphomas, leukopenia, mononucleosis, malaria, cirrhosis, trauma, portal hypertension. |
| **Distended abdomen** | A larger than normal abdominal profile. May be soft or firm, tender or nontender, and accompanied by other symptoms such as nausea, vomiting, or rebound tenderness. | Lymphoma may manifest as abdominal adenopathy, mass(es), or bowel obstruction. |
| **Nervous System** | | |
| **Paresthesias of feet and hands, ataxia** | Numbness sensation and extreme sensitivity experienced in central and peripheral nerves. Impaired muscle movement. | Cobalamin (vitamin $B_{12}$) deficiency or folate deficiency. |
| **Weakness** | Lacking physical strength or energy. | Low Hgb level (anemia). |
| **Headache, nuchal rigidity** | Pain in the cranium, potentially involving one area or extending from frontal area to back of neck. | Generalized headache is a common manifestation of mild to moderate anemia. Severe headache with or without visual disturbances may signal intracranial hemorrhage due to thrombocytopenia. |

palpate the preauricular, posterior auricular, occipital, tonsillar, submandibular, submental, superficial cervical, posterior cervical chain, deep cervical chain, and supraclavicular nodes. Next, palpate the axillary lymph nodes and pectoral, subscapular, and lateral groups of nodes. Then examine the epitrochlear nodes, located in the antecubital fossa between the biceps and triceps muscles. Last, palpate the inguinal lymph nodes, found in the groin.

***Palpation of Liver or Spleen.*** Both the liver and spleen are normally not detectable by palpating the abdomen. When they are enlarged, they may be detectable by percussion or palpation. Measure the degree of enlargement of the liver by the number of fingerbreadths it extends below the rib border. The spleen may be more difficult to detect because of its deep location in the left abdomen. Specific techniques for palpating the liver and spleen are described in Chapter 38.

***Skin Assessment.*** In hematologic disorders, assessment of the skin may be a valuable source of information about the hematologic system. Examine the skin over the entire body in a systematic manner (e.g., starting with the face and oral cavity and moving downward over the body). In patients with RBC disorders the skin may be pale or pasty, or it may have a cyanotic tinge in severe anemia. Erythrocytosis often produces small vessel occlusions causing a purple, mottled appearance of the face, nose, fingers, or toes. *Clubbing of the fingers* (discussed in Chapter 25) can be seen with chronic anemia such as in patients with sickle cell disease.

Leukocyte disorders may cause infectious skin lesions or malignant nodular lesions. These may occur anywhere and have a variable distribution pattern. During the physical assessment of the skin, look carefully for **petechiae** (small purplish red pinpoint lesions), **ecchymoses** (bruising), and *spider nevus* (a form of *telangiectasia*) (Table 29-5), because these findings can indicate bleeding disorders. The location of petechiae can indicate an accumulation of blood in the skin or mucous membranes. Small vessels leak under pressure, and the platelet numbers are insufficient to stop the bleeding. Petechiae are more likely to occur where clothing constricts the circulation. In general, skin and mucosal bleeding indicates a platelet disorder, whereas spontaneous bleeding into joints or muscles indicates a coagulation factor problem.

A *focused assessment* is used to evaluate the status of previously identified hematologic problems and to monitor for signs of new problems (see Table 3-6). A focused assessment of the hematologic system is presented in the box on p. 599.

## CASE STUDY

### *Objective Data: Physical Examination*

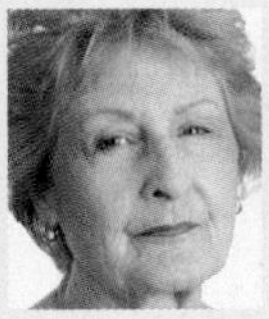

(©Lisa F. Young/iStock)

Physical examination findings of A.J. are as follows: BP 100/70 (lying), 88/60 (standing); apical pulse 110 (lying), 124 (standing), but regular in rhythm. Respiratory rate 26, temperature 96.8° F (36° C), $O_2$ saturation 90% on room air. No jugular venous distention. Weight: 106 lb (48 kg). Height: 5 ft 1 in. Skin pale and two ecchymoses on her arms and one on her left lower leg. A few scattered petechiae on both ankles. No jaundice noted. Conjunctivae pale. Tongue smooth and shiny. Lungs clear but diminished breath sounds in the bases bilaterally. No visible bleeding. No enlarged lymph nodes, spleen, or liver noted. General weakness with dyspnea on exertion. No numbness or tingling or peripheral edema.

**Discussion Questions**

1. What should be included in the physical assessment? For what would you be looking?
2. Which physical assessment findings are of most concern to you?
3. Based on the results of the subjective and physical assessment findings, what diagnostic studies do you think may be ordered for A.J.?

You will learn more about diagnostic studies in relation to the hematologic system in the next section. (See p. 605 for more information on A.J.)

Answers available at *http://evolve.elsevier.com/Lewis/medsurg.*

## FOCUSED ASSESSMENT

### *Hematologic System*

Use this checklist to make sure the key assessment steps have been done.

**Subjective**

*Ask the patient about any of the following and note responses.*

| | | |
|---|---|---|
| Unusual bleeding or bruising | Y | N |
| Black, tarry stool | Y | N |
| Blood in vomitus | Y | N |
| Swelling in neck, armpits, or groin | Y | N |
| Dark-colored urine | Y | N |
| Fatigue | Y | N |
| Heart palpitations | Y | N |

**Objective: Diagnostic**

*Check the following laboratory results for critical values.*

| | |
|---|---|
| CBC | ✓ |
| WBC count with differential | ✓ |
| Clotting: PT, INR, aPTT, platelets | ✓ |
| Hgb, Hct | ✓ |

**Objective: Physical Examination**

***Inspect***

| | |
|---|---|
| Skin for lesions or color changes | ✓ |

***Auscultate***

| | |
|---|---|
| BP for alteration or orthostasis | ✓ |

***Palpate***

| | |
|---|---|
| Pulse for tachycardia | ✓ |
| Liver and spleen for enlargement | ✓ |
| Lymph nodes for lymphadenopathy | ✓ |

*aPTT*, Activated partial thromboplastin time; *INR*, international normalized ratio; *PT*, prothrombin time.

## DIAGNOSTIC STUDIES OF HEMATOLOGIC SYSTEM

The most direct means of evaluating the hematologic system is through laboratory analysis (Tables 29-6, 29-7, 29-9) and other diagnostic studies (Table 29-10).

### Laboratory Studies

**Complete Blood Count.** The complete blood count (CBC) involves several laboratory tests (Table 29-6). In addition to the CBC, a *peripheral smear* may be ordered. The smear is used to look at the *morphology* (shape and appearance) of the blood cells and may assist with the diagnosis. For example, a large number of immature *blast* WBCs may indicate acute leukemia.

Although the status of each cell type is important, the entire system may be disrupted by diseases or by treatment of diseases. When the entire CBC is suppressed, a condition termed **pancytopenia** (marked decrease in the number of RBCs, WBCs, and platelets) exists.

***Red Blood Cells.*** Normal values of some RBC tests are reported separately for men and women because normal values are based on body mass, and men usually have a larger body mass than women.

The *hemoglobin (Hgb) value* is reduced in cases of anemia, hemorrhage, and hemodilution, such as that occurring when the fluid volume is excessive. Increases in hemoglobin are found in polycythemia or in states of hemoconcentration, which can develop from volume depletion (dehydration).

The *hematocrit (Hct) value* is determined by spinning blood in a centrifuge, which causes RBCs and plasma to separate. The RBCs, being the heavier elements, settle to the bottom (Fig. 29-2). The hematocrit value represents the percentage of RBCs compared with the total blood volume. Reductions and elevations of the hematocrit value are seen in the same conditions that raise and lower the hemoglobin value. The hematocrit value generally is three times the hemoglobin value.

The total RBC count is reported as RBC × $10^6$/μL. However, the total RBC count is not always reliable in determining the adequacy of RBC function. Consequently, other data, such as hemoglobin, hematocrit, and RBC indices, must also be evaluated. The RBC count is altered by the same conditions that raise and lower the hemoglobin and hematocrit values.

*RBC indices* are special indicators that reflect RBC volume, color, and hemoglobin saturation (Table 29-6). These parameters may provide insight into the cause of anemia. (The significance of these parameters is discussed further in Chapter 30.)

***White Blood Cells.*** The WBC count provides two different sets of information. The first is a total count of WBCs in 1 μL of peripheral blood. Elevations in WBC count over 11,000/μL are associated with infection, inflammation, tissue injury or death, and malignancies (e.g., leukemia, lymphoma). Although the degree of WBC elevation does not necessarily predict the severity of illness, it can provide clues to the etiology. Certain types of leukemias are more likely to produce extremely high WBC counts (e.g., greater than 25,000/μL). A WBC count less than 4000/μL (**leukopenia**) is associated with bone marrow depression, severe or chronic illness, and some types of leukemia.

The second aspect of the WBC count, the *differential count,* measures the percentage of each type of leukocyte. The WBC differential provides valuable clues in determining the cause of illness. When infections are severe, more granulocytes are released from the bone marrow as a compensatory mechanism. To meet the increased demand, many young, immature polymorphonuclear neutrophils *(bands)* are released into circulation. More

## TABLE 29-6 Diagnostic Studies

### *Complete Blood Count Studies*

| Study | Description and Purpose | Reference Intervals |
|---|---|---|
| **Hemoglobin (Hgb)** | Measurement of gas-carrying capacity of RBC | *Female:* 11.7-15.5 g/dL (117-155 g/L)<br>*Male:* 13.2-17.3 g/dL (132-173 g/L) |
| **Hematocrit (Hct)** | Measure of packed cell volume of RBCs expressed as a percentage of the total blood volume | *Female:* 35%-47% (0.35-0.47)<br>*Male:* 39%-50% (0.39-0.50) |
| **Total RBC count** | Number of circulating RBCs | *Female:* 3.8-5.1 × $10^6$/µL (3.8-5.1 × $10^{12}$/L)<br>*Male:* 4.3-5.7 × $10^6$/µL (4.3-5.7 × $10^{12}$/L) |
| **Red cell indices** | | |
| | Determination of relative size of RBCs. Low MCV reflection of microcytosis, high MCV reflection of macrocytosis | 80-100 fL |
| | Measurement of average weight of Hgb/RBCs. Low MCH indication of microcytosis or hypochromia, high MCH indication of macrocytosis | 27-34 pg |
| | Evaluation of RBC saturation with Hgb. Low MCHC indication of hypochromia, high MCHC evident in spherocytosis | 32%-37% (0.32-0.37) |
| **RBC morphology** | Examination of shape and size of RBCs | No variation in RBC morphology |
| **WBC count** | Measurement of total number of WBCs | 4000-11,000/µL (4-11 × $10^9$/L) |
| **WBC differential** | Determination of whether each kind of WBC is present in proper proportion<br>Absolute value of each type of WBC can be determined by multiplying the percentage of cell type by total WBC count and dividing by 100. | *Neutrophils:* 50%-70% (0.50-0.70)<br>*Eosinophils:* 0%-4% (0-0.04)<br>*Basophils:* 0%-2% (0-0.02)<br>*Lymphocytes:* 20%-40% (0.20-0.40)<br>*Monocytes:* 4%-8% (0.04-0.08) |
| **Platelet count** | Number of platelets available to maintain platelet clotting functions (not measurement of quality of platelet function) | 150,000-400,000/µL (150-400 × $10^9$/L) |

*MCH,* Mean corpuscular hemoglobin; *MCHC,* mean corpuscular hemoglobin concentration; *MCV,* mean corpuscular volume.

mature neutrophils are called *polymorphonuclear segmented neutrophils (segs)*. Together bands and segs make up the *absolute neutrophil count* (ANC). The usual laboratory procedure is to report the WBCs in order of maturity, with the less mature forms on the left side of the written report. Consequently, the existence of many immature cells is termed a *"shift to the left."*

The WBC differential is of considerable significance because it is possible for the total WBC count to remain essentially normal despite a marked change in one type of leukocyte. For example, a patient may have a normal WBC count of 8800/µL, but the differential count may show that the proportion of lymphocytes is reduced to 10%. This is an abnormal finding that warrants further investigation.

When the bone marrow does not produce enough neutrophils, neutropenia occurs. **Neutropenia** is a condition in which the ANC is less than 1000 cells/µL; severe neutropenia is associated with an ANC of less than 500 cells/µL. The ANC is determined by multiplying the total WBC count by the percentage of neutrophils. Neutropenia results from a number of disease processes, such as leukemia, or from bone marrow depression (see Chapter 30), and is associated with a high risk of infection and death from sepsis.

***Platelet Count.*** The platelet count is the number of platelets per microliter of blood. Normal platelet counts are between 150,000 and 400,000/µL. Counts below 100,000/µL signify a condition termed **thrombocytopenia**. Bleeding may occur with thrombocytopenia. Spontaneous hemorrhage is possible once platelet counts fall below 10,000/µL.[2] A more extensive description of clotting studies is presented in Table 29-7.

**Thrombocytosis** is defined as excessive platelets, a disorder that occurs with inflammation and some malignant disorders (see Chapter 30). The most likely complication related to thrombocytosis is excessive clotting.

**Blood Typing and Rh Factor.** Blood group antigens (A and B) are found only on RBC membranes and form the basis for the ABO blood typing system. The presence or absence of one or both of the two inherited antigens is the basis for the four blood groups: A, B, AB, and O. Blood group A has A antigens, group B has B antigens, group AB has both antigens, and group O has neither A nor B antigens. Each person has antibodies in the serum termed *anti-A* and *anti-B* that react with A or B antigens. These antibodies are found when the corresponding antigen is absent from the RBC surface. For example, B antibodies are found in the serum of people with blood group A (Table 29-8).

Blood reactions based on ABO incompatibilities result from intravascular hemolysis of the RBCs. RBCs *agglutinate* (or clump) when a serum antibody is present to react with the antigens on the RBC membrane. For example, agglutination would occur in the blood of a person with type A blood when he or she receives blood transfused from a person with B antigens (i.e., type B or AB). The anti-B antibodies in the type A blood would react with the B antigens, thus initiating the process that results in RBC hemolysis. (Blood component compatibilities for transfusions are presented in Table 30-32.)

The *Rh system* is based on a third antigen, D, which is also on the RBC membrane. Rh-positive people have the D antigen, whereas Rh-negative people do not. Rh-positive blood is indicated with a "+" after the ABO group (e.g., AB+). A Coombs test is used to evaluate the person's Rh status (Table 29-9).

As a result of transfusion therapy or during childbirth, an Rh-negative person may be exposed to Rh-positive blood. After exposure during childbirth, the mother forms an antibody, anti-D, which acts against Rh antigens. (Rh-positive people normally have no anti-D.) In subsequent pregnancies the mother's anti-D antibodies can cross the placenta and attack the RBCs of a fetus who is Rh-positive, thus causing hemolysis of the RBCs. A pregnant Rh-negative woman should receive Rho(D) immune globulin (RhoGAM) injections to prevent anti-D antibodies from forming.

## TABLE 29-7 Diagnostic Studies

### Clotting Studies

| Study | Description and Purpose | Reference Intervals |
|---|---|---|
| **Activated clotting time (ACT)** | Evaluation of intrinsic coagulation status. More accurate than aPTT. Used during dialysis, coronary artery bypass procedure, arteriograms | 70-120 sec |
| **Activated partial thromboplastin time (aPTT)** | Assessment of intrinsic coagulation by measuring factors I, II, V, VIII, IX, X, XI, XII. Longer in patients using heparin | 25-35 sec |
| **Antithrombin** | Naturally occurring protein synthesized by liver that inhibits coagulation through inactivation of thrombin and other factors. Depleted in DIC and hypercoagulable disorders | 21-30 mg/dL (210-300 mg/L) or 80%-120% of standard |
| **Capillary fragility test (tourniquet test, Rumpel-Leede test)** | Reflection of capillary integrity when positive or negative pressure is applied to various areas of the body. Positive test indication of thrombocytopenia, toxic vascular reactions | No petechiae or negative |
| **D-dimer** | Assay to measure a fragment of fibrin that is formed as a result of fibrin degradation and clot lysis. Used as an adjunctive measure in diagnosis of hypercoagulable conditions (e.g., DIC, pulmonary embolism) | <250 ng/mL (<250 mcg/L) |
| **Fibrin split products (FSPs) or fibrin degradation products (FDPs)** | Reflection of degree of fibrinolysis and predisposition to bleed (if present). Screening test for DIC. Elevated levels associated with DIC, advanced malignancy, severe inflammation | <10 mcg/mL (<10 mg/L) |
| **Fibrinogen (Factor I)** | Reflection of level of fibrinogen. Increase in fibrinogen possible indication of enhancement of fibrin formation, making patient hypercoagulable. Decrease in fibrinogen indicates that patient possibly predisposed to bleeding. | 200-400 mg/dL (2-4 g/L) |
| **International normalized ratio (INR)** | Standardized system of reporting PT based on a reference calibration model and calculated by comparing patient's PT with a control value | 2-3* |
| **Plasminogen** | Assessment of adequacy of plasminogen in patients who have multiple thromboembolic episodes | 2.4-4.4 units/mL |
| **Platelet count** | Number of circulating platelets | 150,000-400,000/μL |
| **Prothrombin time (PT)** | Assessment of extrinsic coagulation by measurement of factors I, II, V, VII, X | 11-16 sec |
| **Thrombin time** | Reflection of adequacy of thrombin. Prolonged thrombin time indicates that coagulation is inadequate secondary to decreased thrombin activity. | 17-23 sec |

*DIC,* Disseminated intravascular coagulation.
*Desired therapeutic level with warfarin (Coumadin).

## TABLE 29-8 ABO and Rh Blood Groups

| | ANTIGENS PRESENT ON RBC | | ANTIBODIES POSSIBLY PRESENT IN PLASMA | | |
|---|---|---|---|---|---|
| **Blood Type** | **A or B** | **Rh (D)** | **A or B** | **Rh (D)** | **Percent of General Population** |
| O* | — | — | A, B | Rh† | 35 |
| O+ | — | Rh | A, B | — | 7 |
| A | A | — | B | Rh† | 35 |
| A+ | A | Rh | B | — | 7 |
| B | B | — | A | Rh† | 8 |
| B+ | B | Rh | A | — | 2 |
| AB‡ | A, B | — | — | Rh† | 4 |
| AB+ | A, B | Rh | — | — | 2 |

*Blood type O is considered universal donor.
†Rh (D) antibodies may develop if Rh– person has been exposed to Rh+ blood.
‡Blood type AB is considered universal recipient.

**Iron Metabolism.** The laboratory tests used to evaluate iron metabolism include serum iron, total iron-binding capacity (TIBC), serum ferritin, and transferrin saturation. Additional tests for nutritional deficiencies leading to defective RBC production may also be done (Table 29-9).

Serum iron is a measurement of the amount of protein-bound iron circulating in the serum. TIBC provides a measurement of all proteins that act to bind or transport iron between the tissues and bone marrow. Although this indirect measurement is a general reflection of the amount of transferrin present in the circulation, it overestimates transferrin levels by 16% to 20% because it also measures other proteins that can bind iron. These alternative proteins bind iron only when transferrin is more than half saturated. Also, TIBC varies inversely with tissue iron stores; it is higher when iron stores are low and lower when iron stores are high.

*Transferrin saturation* is a better indicator of the availability of iron for erythropoiesis than serum iron because, unlike serum iron, the iron bound to transferrin is readily available for the body to use. Transferrin saturation is calculated by dividing serum iron by TIBC and multiplying by 100. For example, a patient with a serum iron level of 100 mcg/dL and a TIBC of 300 mcg/dL would have a transferrin saturation of about 33%.

**TABLE 29-9 Diagnostic Studies**

***Miscellaneous Blood Studies***

| Study | Description and Purpose | Normal Values |
|---|---|---|
| **Bilirubin** | Measurement of degree of RBC hemolysis or liver's inability to excrete normal quantities of bilirubin. Increase in indirect bilirubin with hemolytic problems. Increase in direct bilirubin with obstructive problems (e.g., gallstones, liver tumor, etc.) | *Total:* 0.2-1.2 mg/dL (3.0-21.0 μmol/L)<br>*Direct:* 0.1-0.3 mg/dL (1.7-5.1 μmol/L)<br>*Indirect:* 0.1-1.0 mg/dL (1.7-17.0 μmol/L) |
| **Blood smear (peripheral blood smear)** | Reviews color, size, shape, quantity of cells in peripheral blood. Can provide significant amount of information regarding disorders affecting RBCs, WBCs, or platelets | Normal quantity of each cell type, normal size, shape and color of RBCs, normal WBC differential count |
| **Coombs test** | Differentiation among types of hemolytic anemias. Detection of immune antibodies and Rh factor | Negative |
| • Direct | Detection of antibodies that are attached to RBCs | Negative |
| • Indirect | Detection of circulating antibodies against red cells in serum | Negative |
| **Cobalamin (vitamin $B_{12}$)** | Level of cobalamin available for production of new RBCs | 200-835 pg/mL (148-616 pmol/L) |
| **Erythrocyte sedimentation rate (ESR)** | Measurement of sedimentation or settling of RBCs in 1 hr. Inflammatory process causes an alteration in plasma proteins, resulting in aggregation of RBCs and making them heavier. The faster the sedimentation rate, the higher the ESR | <30 mm/hr (some gender variation) |
| **Erythropoietin** | Measurement of degree of hormonal stimulation to bone marrow to stimulate the release of RBCs | 5-35 mU/mL (5-30 U/L) |
| **Ferritin** | Major iron storage protein. Is normally present in blood in concentrations directly related to iron storage | 10-250 ng/mL (10-250 mcg/L) |
| **Folic acid (folate)** | Amount of folic acid (folate) available for RBC production | 3-16 ng/mL (7-36 nmol/L) |
| **Hemoglobin (Hgb) electrophoresis** | Proteins involved in development of Hgb molecule have a definitive pattern of separation on electrophoresis. This pattern is altered with abnormal Hgb synthesis (e.g., thalassemia) or sickle cell anemia (where Hgb S is increased). | *Normal Hb A1:* >95%<br>*Hb A2:* 1.5%-3.7%<br>*Hb F:* <2%<br>*Hb S:* 0<br>*Hb C:* 0 |
| **Homocysteine** | Amino acid formed from methionine. Rapidly metabolized through pathways that require cobalamin (vitamin $B_{12}$) and folic acid. Increased in cobalamin and folic acid deficiency | *Male:* 5.2-12.9 μmol/L<br>*Female:* 3.7-10.4 μmol/L |
| **Iron** | | |
| • Serum iron | Reflection of amount of iron combined with proteins in serum. Accurate indication of status of iron storage and use | 50-175 mcg/dL (9-31.3 μmol/L) |
| • Total iron-binding capacity (TIBC) | Measurement of all proteins available for binding iron. Transferrin represents the largest quantity of iron-binding proteins. Therefore TIBC is an indirect measure of transferrin, an evaluation of amount of extra iron that can be carried. | 250-425 mcg/dL (45-76 μmol/L) |
| **Lactic dehydrogenase (LDH)** | Intracellular enzyme that is present in almost all body tissues. Levels rise in response to cell damage. Increased levels confirm diagnosis of injury or disease. May be used as a nonspecific marker of hematologic malignancy growth and response to treatment | 140-280 U/L (0.83-2.5 μkat/L) |
| **Methylmalonic acid (MMA)** | Indirect test for cobalamin (Vitamin $B_{12}$). MMA metabolism requires cobalamin. Decreased levels with cobalamin deficiency. Helps differentiate cobalamin deficiency from folic acid deficiency | <0.2 μmol/L (<2.4 mcg/dL) |
| **Microglobulin (Beta$_2$ microglobulin)** | Protein that is found on the surface of all cells. It is increased in patients with malignancies such as lymphoma, leukemia, or multiple myeloma and may be used as a tumor marker. | Blood: 0.7-1.8 mcg/mL<br>Urine: ≤300 mcg/L<br>Spinal fluid: ≤2.4 mg/L |
| **Reticulocyte count** | Measurement of immature RBCs, a reflection of bone marrow activity in producing RBCs | 0.5%-1.5% of RBC count (0.005-0.015 of RBC count) |
| **Serum protein electrophoresis (SPEP)** | Separates proteins in blood on basis of electric charge. Helps detect hyperglobulinemic states, such as in multiple myeloma or some lymphomas | Normal banding pattern of albumin and globulins. Increase in any protein *(protein spike)* is abnormal. |
| **Transferrin** | Largest of proteins that bind to iron. Increased in most people with iron-deficiency anemia | 190-380 mg/dL (1.9-3.8 g/L) |
| **Transferrin saturation (%)** | Decreased in iron-deficiency anemia and increased in hemolytic and megaloblastic anemia | 15%-50% |

Under normal conditions, the serum ferritin concentration correlates closely with body iron stores. In normal patients, 1 ng/mL of ferritin corresponds to 8 to 10 mg of stored iron.

## Biopsies

Biopsy procedures specific to hematologic assessment are bone marrow examination and lymph node biopsy. In general, these procedures are done because a peripheral blood smear is nonspecific and usually a diagnosis cannot be established from a peripheral blood smear. Furthermore, a biopsy provides additional information about a hematologic problem that is needed for diagnosis and treatment planning.

**Bone Marrow Examination.** Bone marrow examination is important in the evaluation of many hematologic disorders.

## TABLE 29-10 Diagnostic Studies

### Hematologic System

| Study | Description and Purpose | Nursing Responsibility |
|---|---|---|
| **Blood Studies** | See Tables 29-6, 29-7, and 29-9. | |
| **Urine Studies** | | |
| **Bence Jones protein** | An electrophoretic measurement is used to detect Bence Jones protein, which is found in most cases of multiple myeloma. Negative finding is considered normal. | *During:* Acquire random urine specimen early in the morning. If a 24-hr urine collection is ordered, discard first specimen and collect all urine voided during the 24 hr, keeping on ice or refrigerated. Remind patient not to put toilet paper in urine collection container. |
| **Radioisotope Studies** | | |
| **Bone scan** | Same procedure as for spleen scan except used for evaluating structure of bones | *During:* Patient needs to lie still during imaging. Patient may be asked to drink 4-6 glasses of water and then void before imaging (to see pelvic bones). |
| **SPECT scan (single-photon emission computed tomography)** | Radioactive isotope is injected IV. Images from radioactive emissions are used to evaluate the structures such as spleen, liver, and bone and possible tumors. Patient is not a source of radioactivity. | No specific nursing responsibilities. |
| **Radiologic Studies** | | |
| **Skeletal x-ray** | X-rays done as a bone survey to detect lytic lesions associated with multiple myeloma. Bone scans do not identify lesions in this condition because there is no uptake of radioactive isotopes due to lack of blood supply. | No specific nursing responsibilities. |
| **Liver, spleen, or abdominal ultrasound** | Noninvasive probe is lubricated and slid across the abdomen to detect density and borders of the abdominal organs. Can detect irregular borders, masses, vascular structure, fluid collections, and biliary tree | *During:* Patients must be comfortable lying flat and having probe compress abdomen. |
| **Positron emission tomography (PET)** | Nuclear tracer substance is injected and is taken up by metabolically active cells. Follow-up scan shows different-colored tissues based on metabolic rate. "Hot spots" reflect increased glucose consumption indicating presence of tumor.<br>Valuable diagnostic tool to detect active malignancy because it highlights areas with increased metabolism. CT scanning may also be done in conjunction or images fused. | *Before:* IV access is required for injection of the tracer substance. Patients should be NPO, except for water and medications, for at least 4 hr before the test. IV solutions containing glucose should be held or changed to normal saline. Patients who are glucose intolerant or diabetic may need adjustments in their medications. Bowel preparation may also be needed, depending on area being studied. |
| **Computed tomography (CT) scan** | Noninvasive radiologic examination using computer-assisted x-ray evaluates the lymph nodes. Contrast medium often is used in abdominal studies of liver or spleen. Spiral (helical) CT scans are used to evaluate lymph nodes. | *Before:* Investigate iodine sensitivity if contrast medium used. IV and/or oral contrast may be given prior to procedure, depending on the area being studied. Patient may need to be NPO 4 hr prior to study.<br>*After:* Encourage patient to drink fluids to avoid renal problems with contrast, if ordered. |
| **Magnetic resonance imaging (MRI)** | Noninvasive procedure produces sensitive images of soft tissue without using contrast media. No ionizing radiation is required. Technique is used to evaluate central nervous system, neck and back, bones and joints, heart, breasts. Provides a better contrast between normal tissue and pathologic tissue than CT. | *Before:* Instruct patient to remove all metal objects and ask about any history of surgical insertion of staples, plates, or other metal appliances. Inform patient of need to lie still in small chamber. |
| **Biopsies/Procedures** | | |
| **Bone marrow** (Fig. 29-7) | Technique involves removal of bone marrow through a locally anesthetized site to evaluate status of blood-forming tissue. Used to diagnose and monitor multiple myeloma, myelodysplastic syndromes, leukemia, and some lymphomas and to stage some solid tumors (e.g., breast cancer). | *Before*: Explain procedure to patient. Obtain signed consent form. Ensure that a *time-out** is done before procedure. Analgesic administration may be done to enhance patient comfort and cooperation.<br>*After:* Apply pressure dressing after procedure. Assess biopsy site for bleeding and apply pressure as needed. |
| **Lumbar puncture (LP)** | Purpose is to obtain cerebrospinal fluid for testing for malignancy or infection. It may also be used to administer chemotherapy to central nervous system. | *During:* Assist in positioning patient and provide support.<br>*After:* Observe site for bleeding and signs of infection. Spinal headaches may occur but are not minimized by patient lying flat afterwards. |
| **Lymph node biopsy** | Purpose is to obtain lymph tissue for histologic examination to determine diagnosis and therapy. | *Before:* Explain procedure to patient. Obtain signed consent form.<br>*After:* Observe site for bleeding and monitor vital signs, especially if platelet count is low. Sterile dressing should be changed as ordered, and wound should be inspected for healing and infection. |
| • Open | Performed in operating room or procedure area using either local or general anesthesia. An incision is made, and the lymph node and surrounding tissue are dissected (excised) whenever possible. | |
| • Closed (needle) or fine needle | Performed by a physician at bedside or in an outpatient area. An extremely small needle is used to reduce risk of tracking malignant cells through normal subcutaneous tissue. | |
| **Molecular, Cytogenetic, and Gene Analysis Studies** | | |
| **Fluorescence in situ hybridization (FISH)**<br>**Comparative genomic hybridization (CGH)**<br>**Spectral karyotyping (SKY)** | Tests are performed on malignant cells, either peripheral blood (e.g., leukemia) or biopsy specimen (bone marrow, lymph node), or cerebrospinal fluid. Used to assess genetic or chromosomal abnormalities of cancer cells. May be useful in confirming diagnosis and determining treatment modalities and prognosis | *Before:* Explain purpose of testing to patient. |

*Time-out is done just before the procedure starts to verify patient identification, surgical procedure, and surgical site.

The examination of the marrow may involve aspiration only or aspiration with biopsy. The benefits gained from bone marrow examination are (1) a full evaluation of hematopoiesis and (2) the ability to obtain specimens for cytopathologic and chromosomal abnormalities. The preferred site for both aspiration and biopsy of bone marrow is the posterior iliac crest. Bone marrow aspiration and biopsy are performed by a physician or specially credentialed nurse. Local anesthesia and sedation may be used to minimize anxiety and pain that the patient may experience.

For bone marrow aspiration, the skin over the puncture site is cleansed with a bactericidal agent. The skin, subcutaneous tissue, and periosteum are infiltrated with a local anesthetic agent. The patient may be uncomfortable when the periosteum is penetrated. Once the area is anesthetized, a bone marrow needle is inserted through the cortex of the bone. The stylet of the needle is then removed, the hub is attached to a 10-mL syringe, and 0.2 to 0.5 mL of the fluid marrow is aspirated (Fig. 29-7). The patient experiences pain with aspiration. Although it lasts only a few seconds, the pain may be quite uncomfortable. After the marrow aspiration, the needle is removed. Pressure is applied over the aspiration site to ensure hemostasis.

Although complications of bone marrow aspiration are minimal, there is a possibility of damaging underlying structures. Other complications include hemorrhage (especially if the patient is thrombocytopenic) and infection (especially if the patient is leukopenic).

The needle aspiration or biopsy site is covered with a sterile pressure dressing. Monitor the patient's vital signs until stable, and assess the site for excess drainage or bleeding. If bleeding is present, advise the patient to lie on the side for 30 to 60 minutes to maintain pressure on the site. If the bed is too soft, have the patient lie on a rolled towel to provide additional pressure.

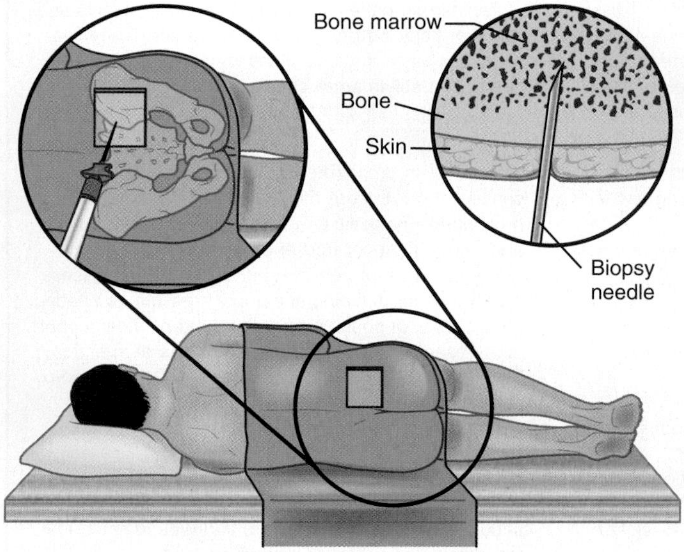


**FIG. 29-7** Bone marrow aspiration from the posterior iliac crest.

Analgesics for postprocedure pain may be administered. Soreness over the puncture site for 3 to 4 days after the procedure is normal.

**Lymph Node Biopsy.** Lymph node biopsy involves obtaining lymph tissue for histologic examination to determine the diagnosis and help plan therapy. This may be accomplished by either an open biopsy or a closed (needle) biopsy.

If the results from a needle biopsy are negative, it may only indicate that the cancer cells were not part of the tissue in the biopsy specimen. However, a positive finding is sufficient evidence for confirming a diagnosis. This technique is rarely used to confirm an initial diagnosis because larger specimens are usually required to perform cytopathologic tests, but it may be used to validate disease recurrence or a new site of disease.

## Molecular Cytogenetics and Gene Analysis

Testing for specific genetic or chromosomal variations in hematologic conditions is often helpful in diagnosis and staging. These results also help determine the treatment options and prognosis. If a large number of abnormal cells are circulating in the blood, such as in acute leukemia, these tests may be done by obtaining peripheral blood. However, testing is usually done on samples from bone marrow, lymph node biopsies, and sometimes cerebrospinal fluid. For example, fluorescence in situ hybridization (FISH) can identify specific areas by attaching a probe to a targeted region of deoxyribonucleic acid (DNA). It may be used to illuminate an abnormal extra chromosome 8, which is common in certain leukemias. Spectral karyotyping (SKY) allows each set of chromosomes to be painted different colors. It can be used to identify the translocation of chromosome 22 to 9 in the Philadelphia chromosome of chronic myelogenous leukemia. More information on genetics is in Chapter 12.

## CASE STUDY

### *Objective Data: Diagnostic Studies*

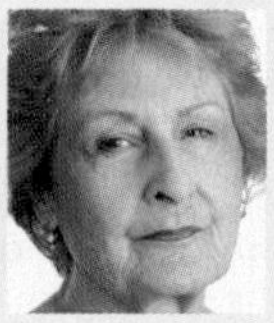

(©Lisa F. Young/iStock)

The HCP orders the following initial diagnostic studies for A.J.:

- CBC, basic metabolic panel (electrolytes, BUN, creatinine), PT/PTT
- Arterial blood gases
- Chest x-ray

A.J.'s CBC reveals a Hgb of 5.9 g/dL, Hct of 18.2%, WBC of 2600/μL (2.6 × $10^9$/L), platelet count of 72,000/μL, PT = 18 sec, aPTT = 37. The arterial blood gases are normal as well as the chest x-ray. The HCP orders more blood work, including a WBC differential, RBC indices, and admits her to the hospital for further evaluation.

**Discussion Questions**

1. Are these the diagnostic studies that you expected to be ordered?
2. Which diagnostic study results are abnormal?
3. Which diagnostic study results are of most concern to you? What additional studies may be ordered on admission?

This case study is continued in Chapter 30 on p. 652.

Answers available at *http://evolve.elsevier.com/Lewis/medsurg.*

## BRIDGE TO NCLEX EXAMINATION

The number of the question corresponds to the same-numbered outcome at the beginning of the chapter.

1. An individual who lives at a high altitude may normally have an increased Hgb and RBC count because
   - **a.** high altitudes cause vascular fluid loss, leading to hemoconcentration.
   - **b.** hypoxia caused by decreased atmospheric $O_2$ stimulates erythropoiesis.
   - **c.** the function of the spleen in removing old RBCs is impaired at high altitudes.
   - **d.** impaired production of leukocytes and platelets leads to proportionally higher red cell counts.
2. Malignant disorders that arise from granulocytic cells in the bone marrow will have the primary effect of causing
   - **a.** risk for hemorrhage.
   - **b.** altered oxygenation.
   - **c.** decreased production of antibodies.
   - **d.** decreased phagocytosis of bacteria.
3. An anticoagulant such as warfarin (Coumadin) that interferes with prothrombin production will alter the clotting mechanism during
   - **a.** platelet aggregation.
   - **b.** activation of thrombin.
   - **c.** the release of tissue thromboplastin.
   - **d.** stimulation of factor activation complex.
4. When reviewing laboratory results of an older patient with an infection, the nurse would expect to find
   - **a.** minimal leukocytosis.
   - **b.** decreased platelet count.
   - **c.** increased hemoglobin and hematocrit levels.
   - **d.** decreased erythrocyte sedimentation rate (ESR).
5. Significant information obtained from the patient's health history that relates to the hematologic system includes
   - **a.** jaundice.
   - **b.** bladder surgery.
   - **c.** early menopause.
   - **d.** multiple pregnancies.
6. While assessing the lymph nodes, the nurse should
   - **a.** apply gentle, firm pressure to deep lymph nodes.
   - **b.** palpate the deep cervical and supraclavicular nodes last.
   - **c.** lightly palpate superficial lymph nodes with the pads of the fingers.
   - **d.** use the tips of the second, third, and fourth fingers to apply deep palpation.
7. If a lymph node is palpated, what is a normal finding?
   - **a.** Hard, fixed nodes
   - **b.** Firm, mobile nodes
   - **c.** Enlarged, tender nodes
   - **d.** Hard, nontender nodes
8. Nursing care for a patient immediately after a bone marrow biopsy and aspiration includes *(select all that apply)*
   - **a.** administering analgesics as necessary.
   - **b.** preparing to administer a blood transfusion.
   - **c.** instructing on need to lie still with a sterile pressure dressing intact.
   - **d.** monitoring vital signs and assessing the site for excess drainage or bleeding.
   - **e.** instructing on the need for preprocedure and postprocedure antibiotic medications.
9. You are taking care of a male patient who has the following laboratory values from his CBC: WBC 6.5 × $10^3$/μL, Hgb 13.4 g/dL, Hct 40%, platelets 50 × $10^3$/μL. What are you *most* concerned about?
   - **a.** Your patient is neutropenic.
   - **b.** Your patient has an infection.
   - **c.** Your patient is at risk for bleeding.
   - **d.** Your patient is at fall risk due to his anemia.

1. b, 2. d, 3. b, 4. a, 5. a, 6. c, 7. b, 8. a, c, d, 9. c

For rationales to these answers and even more NCLEX review questions, visit *http://evolve.elsevier.com/Lewis/medsurg.*

## EVOLVE WEBSITE

http://evolve.elsevier.com/Lewis/medsurg

**Review Questions (Online Only)**

**Key Points**

**Answer Keys for Questions**

- Rationales for Bridge to NCLEX Examination Questions
- Answer Guidelines for Case Studies on pp. 593, 596, 599, and 604

**Conceptual Care Map Creator**

**Audio Glossary**

**Content Updates**

## REFERENCES


1. McCance KL, Huether SE: *Pathophysiology: the biologic basis for disease in adults and children*, ed 6, St Louis, 2014, Mosby.
2. Hoffman R, Benz EJ, Silberstein LE, et al: *Hematology: basic principles and practice*, ed 6, Philadelphia, 2013, Elsevier.
3. Ball JW, Dains JE, Flynn JA, et al: *Seidel's physical examination handbook*, ed 8, St Louis, 2014, Mosby.
4. Pagana KD, Pagana TJ: *Mosby's manual of diagnostic and laboratory tests*, ed 5, St Louis, 2014, Mosby.
5. Rosenzweig MQ, Gardner D, Griffith B: The history and physical in cancer care: a primer for the oncology advanced practitioner, *J Adv Pract Onc* 5:262, 2014.
6. Rodgers GP, Young NS: *The Bethesda handbook of clinical hematology*, ed 3, Philadelphia, 2013, Lippincott Williams & Wilkins.
7. Micromedex 2.0. Truven Health Analytics, Inc. Retrieved from *www.microedexsolutions.com.*
8. American Dietetic Association: Food and Nutrition Topics. Retrieved from *www.eatright.org.*

# 30

# Hematologic Problems

*Sandra Irene Rome*

*We must let go of the life we have planned, so as to accept the one that is waiting for us.*

***Joseph Campbell***

http://evolve.elsevier.com/Lewis/medsurg/

## LEARNING OUTCOMES

1. Describe the general clinical manifestations and complications of anemia.
2. Differentiate the etiologies, clinical manifestations, diagnostic findings, and nursing and interprofessional management of iron-deficiency, megaloblastic, and aplastic anemias and anemia of chronic disease.
3. Explain the nursing management of anemia secondary to blood loss.
4. Describe the pathophysiology, clinical manifestations, and nursing and interprofessional management of anemia caused by increased erythrocyte destruction, including sickle cell disease and acquired hemolytic anemias.
5. Describe the pathophysiology and nursing and interprofessional management of polycythemia.
6. Explain the pathophysiology, clinical manifestations, and nursing and interprofessional management of various types of thrombocytopenia.
7. Describe the types, clinical manifestations, diagnostic findings, and nursing and interprofessional management of hemophilia and von Willebrand disease.
8. Explain the pathophysiology, diagnostic findings, and nursing and interprofessional management of disseminated intravascular coagulation.
9. Describe the etiology, clinical manifestations, and nursing and interprofessional management of neutropenia.
10. Describe the pathophysiology, clinical manifestations, and nursing and interprofessional management of myelodysplastic syndrome.
11. Compare and contrast the major types of leukemia regarding distinguishing clinical and laboratory findings.
12. Explain the nursing and interprofessional management of acute and chronic leukemias.
13. Compare Hodgkin's lymphoma and non-Hodgkin's lymphomas in terms of clinical manifestations, staging, and nursing and interprofessional management.
14. Describe the pathophysiology, clinical manifestations, and nursing and interprofessional management of multiple myeloma.
15. Describe the spleen disorders and related interprofessional care.
16. Describe the nursing management of the patient receiving transfusions of blood and blood components.

## KEY TERMS

**anemia**, p. 606
**aplastic anemia**, p. 614
**disseminated intravascular coagulation (DIC)**, p. 629
**hemochromatosis**, p. 619
**hemolytic anemia**, p. 615
**hemophilia**, p. 626
**Hodgkin's lymphoma**, p. 640
**iron-deficiency anemia**, p. 609
**leukemia**, p. 635
**lymphomas**, p. 640
**megaloblastic anemias**, p. 612
**multiple myeloma**, p. 645
**myelodysplastic syndrome (MDS)**, p. 634
**neutropenia**, p. 632
**non-Hodgkin's lymphomas (NHLs)**, p. 642
**pernicious anemia**, p. 612
**polycythemia**, p. 620
**sickle cell disease (SCD)**, p. 616
**thalassemia**, p. 611
**thrombocytopenia**, p. 622

## ANEMIA

### Definition and Classification

**Anemia** is a deficiency in the number of erythrocytes (red blood cells [RBCs]), the quantity or quality of hemoglobin, and/or volume of packed RBCs (hematocrit). It is a prevalent condition with many diverse causes, such as blood loss, impaired production of erythrocytes, or increased destruction of erythrocytes (Fig. 30-1). Because RBCs transport $O_2$, erythrocyte disorders can lead to tissue hypoxia. This hypoxia accounts for many of the signs and symptoms of anemia. Anemia is not a specific disease. It is a manifestation of a pathologic process.

Anemia is diagnosed based on a complete blood count (CBC), reticulocyte count, and peripheral blood smear. Once anemia is identified, further investigation is done to determine its specific cause.[1]

Anemia can result from primary hematologic problems or can develop as a secondary consequence of diseases or disorders of other body systems. The various types of anemia can be classified according to either *morphology* (cellular characteristic) or *etiology* (cause). Morphologic classification is based on RBC size and color (Table 30-1). Etiologic classification is related to the clinical conditions causing the anemia[2] (Table 30-2). Although the morphologic system is the most accurate means of classifying anemias, it is easier to discuss patient care by focusing on the etiology of the anemia.

Reviewed by Judy Carlyle, RN, MNSc, Faculty/Clinical Liaison, Arkansas Rural Nursing Education Consortium (ARNEC), Nashville, Arkansas; and Allison J. Terry, RN, PhD, Associate Professor of Nursing, Assistant Dean of Clinical Practice, School of Nursing, Auburn University Montgomery, Montgomery, Alabama.

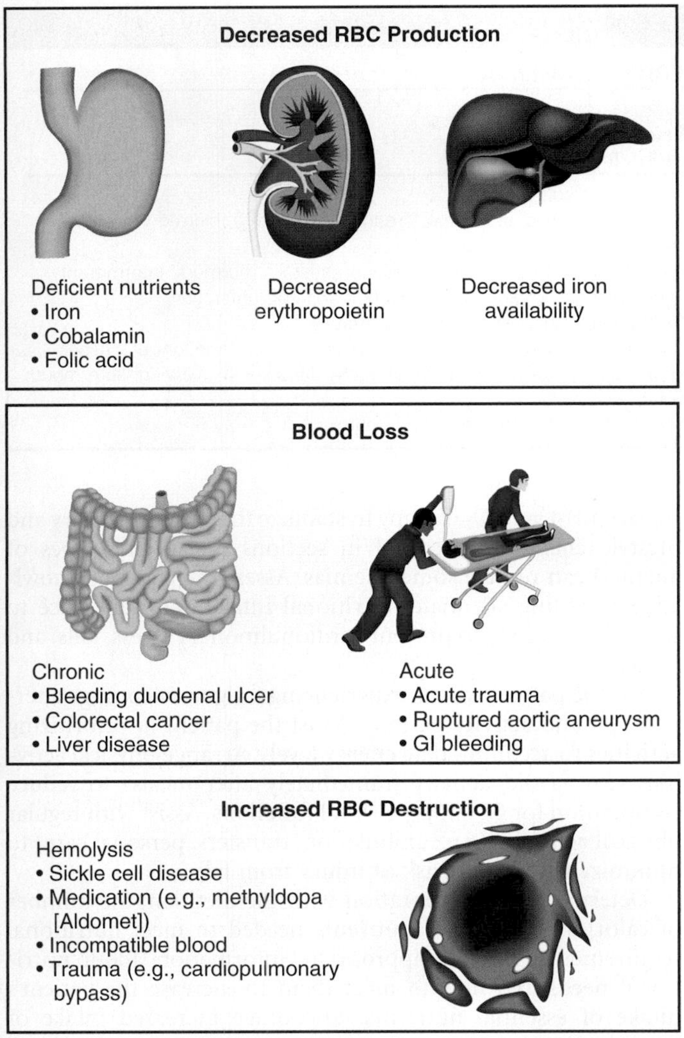


**FIG. 30-1** Causes of anemia.

## CULTURAL & ETHNIC HEALTH DISPARITIES

### *Hematologic Problems*

- Sickle cell disease has a high incidence among African Americans.
- Thalassemia has a high incidence among African Americans and people of Mediterranean origin.
- Tay-Sachs disease has the highest incidence in families of Eastern European Jewish origin, especially the Ashkenazi Jews.
- Pernicious anemia has a high incidence among Scandinavians and African Americans.

## Clinical Manifestations

The clinical manifestations of anemia are caused by the body's response to tissue hypoxia. Specific manifestations vary depending on the rate at which the anemia has evolved, its severity, and any coexisting disease. Hemoglobin (Hgb) levels are often used to determine the severity of anemia.

Mild states of anemia (Hgb 10 to 12 g/dL [100 to 120 g/L]) may exist without causing symptoms. If symptoms develop, it is because the patient has an underlying disease or is experiencing a compensatory response to heavy exercise. Symptoms include palpitations, dyspnea, and mild fatigue.

In moderate anemia (Hgb 6 to 10 g/dL [60 to 100 g/L]) the above cardiopulmonary symptoms are increased. The patient may experience them while resting, as well as with activity.

**TABLE 30-1 Morphologic Classification of Anemia**

| Morphology | Etiology |
|---|---|
| **Normocytic, normochromic** (normal size and color) MCV 80-100 fL, MCH 27-34 pg | Acute blood loss, hemolysis, chronic kidney disease, chronic disease, cancers, sideroblastic anemia, endocrine disorders, starvation, aplastic anemia, sickle cell anemia, pregnancy |
| **Microcytic, hypochromic** (small size, pale color) MCV <80 fL, MCH <27 pg | Iron-deficiency anemia, vitamin $B_6$ deficiency, copper deficiency, thalassemia, lead poisoning |
| **Macrocytic (megaloblastic), normochromic** (large size, normal color) MCV >100 fL, MCH >34 pg | Cobalamin (vitamin $B_{12}$) deficiency, folic acid deficiency, liver disease (including effects of alcohol abuse) |

*MCH,* Mean corpuscular hemoglobin; *MCV,* mean corpuscular volume.

**TABLE 30-2 Etiologic Classification of Anemia**

**Decreased RBC Production**

***Decreased Hemoglobin Synthesis***
- Iron deficiency
- Thalassemias (decreased globin synthesis)
- Sideroblastic anemia (decreased porphyrin)

***Defective DNA Synthesis***
- Cobalamin (vitamin $B_{12}$) deficiency
- Folic acid deficiency

***Decreased Number of RBC Precursors***
- Aplastic anemia and inherited disorders (e.g., Fanconi syndrome)
- Anemia of myeloproliferative diseases (e.g., leukemia) and myelodysplasia
- Chronic diseases or disorders
- Medications and chemicals (e.g., chemotherapy, lead)
- Radiation

**Blood Loss**

***Acute***
- Trauma
- Blood vessel rupture
- Splenic sequestration crisis

***Chronic***
- Gastritis
- Menstrual flow
- Hemorrhoids

**Increased RBC Destruction (Hemolytic Anemias)**

***Hereditary (Intrinsic)***
- Abnormal hemoglobin (sickle cell disease)
- Enzyme deficiency (G6PD)
- Membrane abnormalities (paroxysmal nocturnal hemoglobinuria, hereditary spherocytosis)

***Acquired (Extrinsic)***
- Physical destruction
  - Prosthetic heart valves
  - Extracorporeal circulation
  - Disseminated intravascular coagulopathy (DIC)
  - Thrombotic thrombocytopenic purpura (TTP)
- Antibodies against RBCs
- Infectious agents (e.g., malaria) and toxins

*G6PD,* Glucose-6-phosphate dehydrogenase.

In severe anemia (Hgb less than 6 g/dL [60 g/L]) the patient has many clinical manifestations involving multiple body systems (Table 30-3).

**Integumentary Manifestations.** Integumentary manifestations include pallor, jaundice, and pruritus. Pallor results from reduced amounts of hemoglobin and reduced blood flow to the skin. Jaundice occurs when hemolysis of RBCs results in an increased concentration of serum bilirubin. Pruritus occurs because of increased serum and skin bile salt concentrations. In addition to the skin, the sclera of the eyes and mucous

**TABLE 30-3 Manifestations of Anemia**

| | SEVERITY OF ANEMIA | | |
|---|---|---|---|
| **Body System** | **Mild (Hgb 10-12 g/dL [100-120 g/L])** | **Moderate (Hgb 6-10 g/dL [60-100 g/L])** | **Severe (Hgb <6 g/dL [<60 g/L])** |
| **Integument** | None | None | Pallor, jaundice,* pruritus* |
| **Eyes** | None | None | Icteric conjunctiva and sclera,* retinal hemorrhage, blurred vision |
| **Mouth** | None | None | Glossitis, smooth tongue |
| **Cardiovascular** | Palpitations | Increased palpitations, "bounding pulse" | Tachycardia, increased pulse pressure, systolic murmurs, intermittent claudication, angina, heart failure, myocardial infarction |
| **Pulmonary** | Exertional dyspnea | Dyspnea | Tachypnea, orthopnea, dyspnea at rest |
| **Neurologic** | None | "Roaring in the ears" | Headache, vertigo, irritability, depression, impaired thought processes |
| **Gastrointestinal** | None | None | Anorexia, hepatomegaly, splenomegaly, difficulty swallowing, sore mouth |
| **Musculoskeletal** | None | None | Bone pain |
| **General** | None or mild fatigue | Fatigue | Sensitivity to cold, weight loss, lethargy |

*Caused by hemolysis.

membranes should be evaluated for jaundice because they reflect the integumentary changes more accurately, especially in a dark-skinned individual.

**Cardiopulmonary Manifestations.** Cardiopulmonary manifestations of severe anemia result from additional attempts by the heart and lungs to provide adequate amounts of $O_2$ to the tissues. Cardiac output is maintained by increasing the heart rate and stroke volume. The low viscosity of the blood contributes to the development of systolic murmurs and bruits. In extreme cases or when concomitant heart disease is present, angina pectoris and myocardial infarction (MI) may occur if myocardial $O_2$ needs cannot be met. Heart failure (HF), cardiomegaly, pulmonary and systemic congestion, ascites, and peripheral edema may develop if the heart is overworked for an extended period.

## NURSING AND INTERPROFESSIONAL MANAGEMENT: ANEMIA

This section discusses general management of anemia. Specific care related to various types of anemia is discussed later in this chapter.

### Nursing Assessment

Subjective and objective data that should be obtained from a patient with anemia are presented in Table 30-4.

### Nursing Diagnoses

Nursing diagnoses for the patient with anemia include, but are not limited to, the following:

- Fatigue *related to* inadequate oxygenation of the blood
- Imbalanced nutrition: less than body requirements *related to* inadequate nutritional intake and anorexia
- Ineffective health management *related to* lack of knowledge about appropriate nutrition and medication regimen

Additional information on nursing diagnoses are presented in eNursing Care Plan 30-1.

### Planning

The overall goals are that the patient with anemia will (1) assume normal activities of daily living, (2) maintain adequate nutrition, and (3) develop no complications related to anemia.

### Nursing Implementation

Correcting the cause of the anemia is ultimately the goal of therapy. Acute interventions may include blood transfusions, drug therapy (e.g., erythropoietin, vitamin supplements), RBC replacement, and $O_2$ therapy to stabilize the patient. Dietary and lifestyle changes (described in sections on specific types of anemia) can reverse some anemias. Assess the patient's knowledge regarding adequate nutritional intake and adherence to safety precautions to prevent cardiopulmonary stress, falls, and injury.

For the patient who is experiencing fatigue, encourage alternate rest and activity periods. Assist the patient in prioritizing activities to accommodate energy levels. Arrange physical activities (e.g., avoid activity immediately after meals) to reduce competition for $O_2$ supply to vital functions. Assist with regular physical activities (e.g., ambulation, transfers, personal care) to minimize fatigue and risk of injury from falls.

Determine, in collaboration with the dietitian, the number of calories and type of nutrients needed to meet nutritional requirements. Provide appropriate information about nutritional needs and how to meet them to increase the patient's intake of essential nutrients. Encourage increased intake of foods high in iron.

The numerous causes of anemia necessitate different nursing interventions specific to the patient's needs. General nursing interventions for patients with anemia are presented in eNursing Care Plan 30-1 (available on the website for this chapter).

### Gerontologic Considerations: Anemia

Modest changes in RBC mass occur in older adults. Healthy older men have a modest decline in hemoglobin of about 1 g/dL between ages 70 and 88 years, in part because of the decreased production of testosterone. Only a minimal decrease in hemoglobin (about 0.2 g/dL) occurs between these ages in healthy women.[1]

Anemia is not a normal finding in older adults. However, the prevalence increases starting from the seventh decade of life. For the majority, anemia is related to an underlying cause such as iron deficiency, bleeding, chronic disease/inflammation, renal insufficiency, or a hematologic cancer. For many patients with anemia, there is no identifiable cause.[3]

Clinical manifestations of anemia in older adults may include pallor, confusion, ataxia, fatigue, and worsening cardiovascular and respiratory problems. Unfortunately, anemia may go unrecognized in older adults because these manifestations may be mistaken for normal aging changes or overlooked because of another health problem. By recognizing signs of anemia, you can play a pivotal role in health assessment and related interventions for older adults.

## TABLE 30-4 Nursing Assessment
### Anemia

| Subjective Data | Objective Data |
|---|---|
| **Important Health Information**<br>*Past health history:* Recent blood loss or trauma; chronic liver, endocrine, or renal disease (including dialysis); GI disease (malabsorption syndrome, ulcers, gastritis, or hemorrhoids); inflammatory disorders (especially Crohn's disease); smoking, exposure to radiation or chemical toxins (arsenic, lead, benzenes, copper); infectious diseases (HIV) or recent travel with possible exposure to infection; angina, myocardial infarction; history of falling<br>*Medications:* Use of vitamin and iron supplements; aspirin, anticoagulants, oral contraceptives, phenobarbital, penicillins, nonsteroidal antiinflammatory drugs, omeprazole, phenacetin, phenytoin (Dilantin), sulfonamides, herbal products<br>*Surgery or other treatments:* Recent surgery, small bowel resection, gastrectomy, prosthetic heart valves, chemotherapy, radiation therapy<br>*Dietary history:* General dietary patterns, consumption of alcohol<br><br>**Functional Health Patterns**<br>*Health perception–health management:* Family history of anemia; malaise<br>*Nutritional-metabolic:* Nausea, vomiting, anorexia, weight loss; dysphagia, dyspepsia, heartburn; night sweats, cold intolerance<br>*Elimination:* Hematuria, decreased urine output; diarrhea, constipation, flatulence, tarry stools, bloody stools<br>*Activity-exercise:* Fatigue, muscle weakness and decreased strength; dyspnea, orthopnea, cough, hemoptysis; palpitations; shortness of breath with activity<br>*Cognitive-perceptual:* Headache; abdominal, chest, and bone pain; painful tongue; paresthesias of feet and hands; pruritus; disturbances in vision, taste, or hearing; vertigo; hypersensitivity to cold; dizziness<br>*Sexuality-reproductive:* Menorrhagia, metrorrhagia; recent or current pregnancy; male impotence | **General**<br>Lethargy, apathy, general lymphadenopathy, fever<br><br>**Integumentary**<br>Pale skin and mucous membranes; blue, pale white, or icteric sclera; cheilitis (inflammation of the lips); poor skin turgor; brittle, spoon-shaped fingernails; jaundice; petechiae; ecchymoses; nose or gingival bleeding; poor healing; dry, brittle, thinning hair<br><br>**Respiratory**<br>Tachypnea<br><br>**Cardiovascular**<br>Tachycardia, systolic murmur, dysrhythmias; postural hypotension, widened pulse pressure, bruits (especially carotid); intermittent claudication, ankle edema<br><br>**Gastrointestinal**<br>Hepatosplenomegaly; glossitis; beefy, red tongue; stomatitis; abdominal distention; anorexia<br><br>**Neurologic**<br>Headache, roaring in the ears, confusion, impaired judgment, irritability, ataxia, unsteady gait, paralysis, loss of vibration sense<br><br>**Possible Diagnostic Findings**<br>↓ RBCs, ↓ Hgb; ↓ Hct; ↑ or ↓ reticulocytes, ↑ or ↓ MCV; possible ↓ serum iron, ferritin, folate, or cobalamin (vitamin $B_{12}$); heme (guaiac)–positive stools; ↓ serum erythropoietin level; ↑ or ↓ LDH, bilirubin, transferrin (Table 30-6) |

*LDH,* Lactate dehydrogenase; *MCV,* mean corpuscular volume.

## ANEMIA CAUSED BY DECREASED ERYTHROCYTE PRODUCTION

Normally RBC production (termed *erythropoiesis*) is in equilibrium with RBC destruction and loss. This balance ensures that an adequate number of erythrocytes is available at all times. The normal life span of an RBC is 120 days. Three alterations in erythropoiesis may occur that decrease RBC production: (1) decreased hemoglobin synthesis may lead to iron-deficiency anemia, thalassemia, and sideroblastic anemia; (2) defective deoxyribonucleic acid (DNA) synthesis in RBCs (e.g., cobalamin deficiency, folic acid deficiency) may lead to megaloblastic anemias; and (3) diminished availability of erythrocyte precursors may result in aplastic anemia and anemia of chronic disease (Table 30-2).

## IRON-DEFICIENCY ANEMIA

**Iron-deficiency anemia** is the most common nutritional disorder in the world. Those most susceptible to iron-deficiency anemia are the very young, those on poor diets, and women in their reproductive years.[4] Normally 1 mg of iron is lost daily in urine, bile, sweat, sloughing of epithelial cells from the skin and intestinal mucosa, and minor bleeding.[5]

### Etiology

Iron-deficiency anemia may develop as a result of inadequate dietary intake, malabsorption, blood loss, or hemolysis. (Normal iron metabolism is discussed in Chapter 29 on pp. 590-592.) Normal dietary iron intake is usually sufficient to meet the needs of men and older women, but it may be inadequate for individuals with higher iron needs (e.g., menstruating or pregnant women). Table 30-5 lists nutrients needed for erythropoiesis.[6,7]

Malabsorption of iron may occur after certain types of gastrointestinal (GI) surgery and in malabsorption syndromes. Surgical procedures may involve removal or bypass of the duodenum. As iron absorption occurs in the duodenum, malabsorption syndromes may involve disease of the duodenum in which the absorption surface is altered or destroyed.

Blood loss is a major cause of iron deficiency in adults. Two milliliters of whole blood contain 1 mg of iron. The major sources of chronic blood loss are from the GI and genitourinary (GU) systems. GI bleeding is often not apparent and therefore may exist for a considerable time before the problem is identified. Loss of 50 to 75 mL of blood from the upper GI tract is required for stools to appear black *(melena)*. The black color results from the iron in the RBCs.

Common causes of GI blood loss are peptic ulcer, gastritis, esophagitis, diverticula, hemorrhoids, and neoplasia. GU blood loss occurs primarily from menstrual bleeding. The average monthly menstrual blood loss is about 45 mL and causes the loss of about 22 mg of iron. Postmenopausal bleeding can contribute to anemia in a susceptible older woman. In addition to anemia of chronic kidney disease, dialysis treatment may cause iron-deficiency anemia because of the blood lost in the dialysis equipment and frequent blood sampling.

## TABLE 30-5 Nutritional Therapy

### Nutrients for Erythropoiesis

| Role in Erythropoiesis | Food Sources |
|---|---|
| **Cobalamin (Vitamin $B_{12}$)** | |
| RBC maturation | Red meats, especially liver, eggs, enriched grain products, milk and dairy foods, fish |
| **Copper** | |
| Mobilization of iron from tissues to plasma* | Shellfish, whole grains, beans, nuts, potatoes, organ meats |
| **Folic Acid** | |
| RBC maturation | Green leafy vegetables, liver, meat, fish, legumes, whole grains, orange juice, peanuts, avocado |
| **Iron** | |
| Hemoglobin synthesis | Liver and muscle meats, dried fruits, legumes, dark green leafy vegetables, whole-grain and enriched bread and cereals, beans |
| **Niacin** | |
| RBC maturation | Peanut butter, beans, meats, avocado; enriched and fortified grains |
| **Pantothenic Acid (Vitamin $B_5$)** | |
| Heme synthesis | Meats, vegetables, cereal grains, legumes, eggs, milk |
| **Pyridoxine (Vitamin $B_6$)** | |
| Heme synthesis | Meats, fortified cereals, whole grains, legumes, potatoes, cornmeal, bananas, nuts |
| **Riboflavin (Vitamin $B_2$)** | |
| Oxidative reactions | Milk and dairy foods, enriched bread and other grain products, salmon, chicken, eggs, green leafy vegetables |
| **Vitamin E** | |
| Heme synthesis. Protection against oxidative damage to RBCs | Vegetable oils, meat, eggs, wheat germ, whole-grain products, seeds, nuts, peanut butter |
| **Amino Acids** | |
| Heme and plasma membrane synthesis | Eggs, meat, milk and milk products (cheese, ice cream), poultry, fish, legumes, nuts, tofu |
| **Ascorbic Acid (Vitamin C)** | |
| Conversion of folic acid to its active forms, aids in iron absorption | Citrus fruits, green leafy vegetables, strawberries, potatoes, kiwi fruit |

*Supplementation rarely needed and large amounts of copper are poisonous.

### Clinical Manifestations

In the early course of iron-deficiency anemia, the patient may not have any symptoms. As the disease becomes chronic, any of the general manifestations of anemia may develop (Table 30-3). In addition, specific clinical manifestations may occur related to iron-deficiency anemia. Pallor is the most common finding, and *glossitis* (inflammation of the tongue) is the second most common. Another finding is *cheilitis* (inflammation of the lips). In addition, the patient may report headache, paresthesias, and a burning sensation of the tongue, all of which are caused by lack of iron in the tissues.

### Diagnostic Studies

Laboratory abnormalities characteristic of iron-deficiency anemia are presented in Table 30-6. Other diagnostic studies (e.g., stool occult blood test) are done to determine the cause of the iron deficiency. Endoscopy and colonoscopy may be used to detect GI bleeding. A bone marrow biopsy may be done if other tests are inconclusive.

### Interprofessional Care

The main goal is to treat the underlying disease that is causing reduced intake (e.g., malnutrition, alcoholism) or absorption of iron. In addition, efforts are directed toward replacing iron (Table 30-7). Teach the patient which foods are good sources of iron (Table 30-5). If nutrition is already adequate, increasing iron intake by dietary means may not be practical. Consequently, oral or occasionally parenteral iron supplements are used. If the iron deficiency is from acute blood loss, the patient may require a transfusion of packed RBCs.

**Drug Therapy.** Oral iron should be used whenever possible because it is inexpensive and convenient. Many iron preparations are available. When administering iron, consider the following five factors:

1. Iron is absorbed best from the duodenum and proximal jejunum. Therefore enteric-coated or sustained-release capsules, which release iron farther down in the GI tract, are counterproductive and expensive.
2. The daily dose should provide 150 to 200 mg of elemental iron. This can be ingested in three or four daily doses, with each tablet or capsule of the iron preparation containing between 50 and 100 mg of iron (e.g., a 300-mg tablet of ferrous sulfate contains 60 mg of elemental iron).
3. Iron is best absorbed as ferrous sulfate ($Fe^{2+}$) in an acidic environment. For this reason and to avoid binding the iron with food, iron should be taken about an hour before meals,

## TABLE 30-6 Laboratory Results in Anemia

| Etiology of Anemia | Hgb/Hct | MCV | Reticulocytes | Serum Iron | TIBC | Transferrin | Ferritin | Bilirubin | Serum $B_{12}$ | Folate |
|---|---|---|---|---|---|---|---|---|---|---|
| **Iron deficiency** | ↓ | ↓ | N or slight ↓ or ↑ | ↓ | ↑ | N or ↓ | ↓ | N or ↓ | N | N |
| **Thalassemia major** | ↓ | N or ↓ | ↑ | ↑ | ↓ | ↓ | N or ↑ | ↑ | N | ↓ |
| **Cobalamin deficiency** | ↓ | ↑ | N or ↓ | N or ↑ | N | Slight ↑ | ↑ | N or slight ↑ | ↓ | N |
| **Folic acid deficiency** | ↓ | ↑ | N or ↓ | N or ↑ | N | Slight ↑ | ↑ | N or slight ↑ | N | ↓ |
| **Aplastic anemia** | ↓ | N or slight ↑ | ↓ | N or ↑ | N or ↑ | N | N | N | N | N |
| **Chronic disease** | ↓ | N or ↓ | N or ↓ | N or ↓ | ↓ | N or ↓ | N or ↑ | N | N | N |
| **Acute blood loss** | ↓ | N or ↓ | N or ↑ | N | N | N | N | N | N | N |
| **Chronic blood loss** | ↓ | ↓ | N or ↑ | ↓ | ↓ | N | N | N or ↓ | N | N |
| **Sickle cell anemia** | ↓ | N | ↓ | N or ↑ | N or ↓ | N | N | ↑ | N | ↓ |
| **Hemolytic anemia** | ↓ | N or ↑ | ↑ | N or ↑ | N or ↓ | N | N or ↑ | ↑ | N | N |

*MCV,* Mean corpuscular volume; *N,* normal; *TIBC,* total iron-binding capacity.

**TABLE 30-7 Interprofessional Care**
***Iron-Deficiency Anemia***

| Diagnostic Assessment | Management |
|---|---|
| • History and physical examination<br>• Hct and Hgb levels<br>• RBC count, including morphology<br>• Reticulocyte count<br>• Serum iron<br>• Serum ferritin<br>• Serum transferrin<br>• Total iron-binding capacity (TIBC)<br>• Stool examination for occult blood | • Identification and treatment of underlying cause<br>• Drug therapy<br>  • Oral: Ferrous sulfate or ferrous gluconate<br>  • IM or IV: Iron dextran, sodium ferrous gluconate, iron sucrose<br>• Nutritional therapy (Table 30-5)<br>• Transfusion of packed RBCs |

when the duodenal mucosa is most acidic. Taking iron with vitamin C (ascorbic acid) or orange juice, which contains ascorbic acid, enhances iron absorption. Gastric side effects, however, may necessitate ingesting iron with meals.

4. Undiluted liquid iron may stain the patient's teeth. Therefore it should be diluted and ingested through a straw.
5. GI side effects of iron administration may occur, including heartburn, constipation, and diarrhea. If side effects develop, the dose and type of iron supplement may be adjusted. For example, many individuals who need supplemental iron cannot tolerate ferrous sulfate because of the effects of the sulfate base. However, ferrous gluconate may be an acceptable substitute. Tell patients that the use of iron preparations will cause their stools to become black because the GI tract excretes excess iron. Constipation is common, and the patient should be started on stool softeners and laxatives, if needed, when started on iron.

**DRUG ALERT Iron**
- Some preparations of IV iron have a risk of an allergic reaction, and the patient should be monitored accordingly.
- Oral iron should be taken about 1 hr before meals.
- Vitamin C (ascorbic acid) enhances iron absorption.

In some situations it may be necessary to administer iron parenterally. Parenteral use of iron is indicated for malabsorption, intolerance of oral iron, a need for iron beyond oral limits, or poor patient adherence in taking the oral preparations of iron. Parenteral iron can be given IM or IV. An iron-dextran complex (INFeD) contains 50 mg/mL of elemental iron available in 2-mL single-dose vials. Sodium ferrous gluconate and iron sucrose are alternatives and may carry less risk of life-threatening anaphylaxis.[8]

Because IM iron solutions may stain the skin, separate needles should be used for withdrawing the solution and for injecting the medication. Use a Z-track injection technique.

## NURSING MANAGEMENT: IRON-DEFICIENCY ANEMIA

Certain groups of individuals are at an increased risk for the development of iron-deficiency anemia. These include premenopausal and pregnant women, persons from low socioeconomic backgrounds, older adults, and individuals experiencing blood loss. Diet teaching, with an emphasis on foods high in iron and ways to maximize absorption, is important for these groups.

Discuss with the patient the need for diagnostic studies to identify the cause. Reassess the hemoglobin and RBC counts to evaluate the response to therapy. Emphasize adherence with dietary and drug therapy. To replenish the body's iron stores, the patient needs to take iron therapy for 2 to 3 months after the hemoglobin level returns to normal. Patients who require lifelong iron supplementation should be monitored for potential liver problems related to the iron storage. (Nursing measures for anemia are presented in eNursing Care Plan 30-1.)

## THALASSEMIA

### Etiology

**Thalassemia** is a group of diseases involving inadequate production of normal hemoglobin, and therefore decreased erythrocyte production. Thalassemia is due to an absent or reduced globulin protein. $\alpha$-Globin chains are absent or reduced in $\alpha$-thalassemia, and $\beta$-globin chains are absent or reduced in $\beta$-thalassemia. Hemolysis also occurs in thalassemia, but insufficient production of normal hemoglobin is the predominant problem. Thalassemia is commonly found in members of ethnic groups whose origins are near the Mediterranean Sea and equatorial or near-equatorial regions of Asia, the Middle East, and Africa.

**Genetic Link.** Thalassemia has an autosomal recessive genetic basis (see Fig. 12-4 and Table 12-2). An individual with thalassemia may have a heterozygous or homozygous form of the disease. A person who is heterozygous has one thalassemic gene and one normal gene and has *thalassemia minor* (or thalassemic trait), which is a mild form of the disease. A homozygous person has two thalassemic genes, causing a severe condition known as *thalassemia major.*[9]

### Clinical Manifestations

The patient with thalassemia minor is frequently asymptomatic. The patient has mild to moderate anemia with *microcytosis* (small cells) and *hypochromia* (pale cells).

Thalassemia major is a life-threatening disease in which growth, both physical and mental, is often retarded. The person who has thalassemia major is pale and displays other general symptoms of anemia (Table 30-3). The symptoms develop in childhood by 2 years of age and can cause growth and developmental deficits. Jaundice from the hemolysis of RBCs is prominent. In addition, the person has pronounced splenomegaly, since the spleen continuously tries to remove the damaged red cells. Hepatomegaly and cardiomyopathy may occur from iron deposition.

As the bone marrow responds to the reduced $O_2$-carrying capacity of the blood, RBC production is stimulated and the marrow becomes packed with immature erythroid precursors that die. This stimulates further erythropoiesis, leading to chronic bone marrow hyperplasia and expansion of the marrow space. This may cause thickening of the cranium and maxillary cavity. Thrombocytosis after spleen dysfunction and/or removal may occur.

Patients with thalassemia may have hepatitis C because of having received blood transfusions before donated blood was screened for hepatitis C virus (screening started in 1992). Hepatitis C may result in cirrhosis and hepatocellular carcinoma.

Cardiac complications from iron overload, pulmonary disease, and hypertension also contribute to early death. Endocrinopathies (hypogonadotrophic hypogonadism) and thrombosis may also be complications of the disease.

### Interprofessional Care

The laboratory abnormalities of thalassemia major are summarized in Table 30-6. No specific drug or diet therapies are effective in treating thalassemia. Thalassemia minor requires no treatment because the body adapts to the reduction of normal hemoglobin.

Thalassemia major is managed with blood transfusions or exchange transfusions in conjunction with chelating agents that bind to iron: oral deferasirox (Exjade) or deferiprone (Ferriprox) or IV or subcutaneous deferoxamine (Desferal). These agents reduce the iron overloading (hemochromatosis) that occurs with chronic transfusion therapy.[10] Folic acid is given if there is evidence of hemolysis. Transfusions are administered to keep the hemoglobin level at approximately 10 g/dL (100 g/L) to maintain the patient's own erythropoiesis without causing the spleen to enlarge. Zinc supplementation may be needed since zinc is reduced with chelation therapy. Ascorbic acid supplementation may be needed during chelation therapy, since it increases urine excretion of iron. Other than during chelation therapy, ascorbic acid should not be taken because it increases the absorption of dietary iron. Iron supplements should not be given.

Because RBCs are sequestered in the enlarged spleen, thalassemia major may be treated by splenectomy. Hepatic, cardiac, and pulmonary organ function should be monitored and treated as appropriate.

Although hematopoietic stem cell transplantation (HSCT) remains the only cure for patients with thalassemia, the risk of this procedure may outweigh its benefits. With proper iron chelation therapy, patients are living longer.

## MEGALOBLASTIC ANEMIAS

**Megaloblastic anemias** are a group of disorders caused by impaired DNA synthesis and characterized by the presence of large RBCs. When DNA synthesis is impaired, defective RBC maturation results. The RBCs are large *(macrocytic)* and abnormal and are referred to as *megaloblasts.* Macrocytic RBCs are easily destroyed because they have fragile cell membranes. Although the overwhelming majority of megaloblastic anemias result from cobalamin and folic acid deficiencies, this type of RBC deformity can also occur from suppression of DNA synthesis by drugs, inborn errors of cobalamin and folic acid metabolism, and *erythroleukemia* (malignant blood disorder characterized by a proliferation of erythropoietic cells in bone marrow) (Table 30-8).

**TABLE 30-8 Classification of Megaloblastic Anemia**

**Cobalamin (Vitamin $B_{12}$) Deficiency**
- Dietary deficiency
- Deficiency of gastric intrinsic factor
  - Pernicious anemia
  - Gastrectomy
  - Gastric bypass
  - Celiac disease
  - *Helicobacter pylori*
- Intestinal malabsorption
- Increased requirement (pregnancy)
- Chronic alcoholism

**Folic Acid Deficiency**
- Dietary deficiency (e.g., leafy green vegetables, citrus fruits)
- Malabsorption syndromes
  - Celiac disease
  - Crohn's disease
  - Small bowel resection
- Drugs interfering with absorption or use of folic acid
  - Methotrexate
  - Antiseizure drugs (e.g., phenobarbital, phenytoin [Dilantin])
- Increased requirement (pregnancy)
- Chronic alcoholism
- Chronic hemodialysis (folic acid lost during dialysis)

**Drug-Induced Suppression of DNA Synthesis**
- Folate antagonists
- Metabolic inhibitors
- Alkylating agents

**Inborn Errors**
- Defective folate metabolism
- Defective transport of cobalamin

**Erythroleukemia**

### Megaloblastic Anemia: Cobalamin (Vitamin $B_{12}$) Deficiency

Normally, a protein termed *intrinsic factor* (IF) is secreted by the parietal cells of the gastric mucosa. IF is required for cobalamin (extrinsic factor) absorption. (Cobalamin is normally absorbed in the distal ileum.) Therefore if IF is not secreted, cobalamin will not be absorbed.

### Etiology

**Pernicious Anemia.** The most common cause of cobalamin deficiency is **pernicious anemia**, which is caused by an absence of IF. In pernicious anemia the gastric mucosa is not secreting IF because of either gastric mucosal atrophy or autoimmune destruction of parietal cells. In the autoimmune process antibodies are directed against the gastric parietal cells and/or IF itself. Because parietal cells also secrete hydrochloric (HCl) acid, in pernicious anemia there is a decrease in HCl in the stomach. An acid environment in the stomach is required for the secretion of IF.

Pernicious anemia is a disease of insidious onset that begins in middle age or later (usually after age 40), with 60 years being the most common age at diagnosis. Pernicious anemia occurs frequently in persons of Northern European ancestry (particularly Scandinavians) and African Americans. In African Americans the disease tends to begin early, occurs with higher frequency in women, and is often severe.

**Other Causes of Cobalamin Deficiency.** Cobalamin deficiency can also occur in patients who have had GI surgery (e.g., gastrectomy, gastric bypass); patients who have had a small bowel resection involving the ileum; and patients with Crohn's disease, ileitis, celiac disease, diverticula of the small intestine, or chronic atrophic gastritis (Table 30-8). In these cases, cobalamin deficiency results from the loss of IF-secreting gastric mucosal cells or impaired absorption of cobalamin in the distal ileum. Cobalamin deficiency is also found in excessive alcohol or hot tea ingestion, smoking, long-term users of $H_2$-histamine receptor blockers and proton pump inhibitors, and those who are strict vegetarians.[11]

### Clinical Manifestations

General manifestations of anemia related to cobalamin deficiency develop because of tissue hypoxia (Table 30-3). GI manifestations include a sore, red, beefy, and shiny tongue; anorexia, nausea, and vomiting; and abdominal pain. Typical neuromuscular manifestations include weakness, paresthesias of the feet and hands, reduced vibratory and position senses, ataxia, muscle weakness, and impaired thought processes ranging from confusion to dementia. Because cobalamin deficiency–related anemia has an insidious onset, it may take several months for these manifestations to develop.

### Diagnostic Studies

Laboratory data reflective of cobalamin deficiency anemia are presented in Table 30-6. The RBCs appear large (macrocytic) and have abnormal shapes. This structure contributes to erythrocyte destruction because the cell membrane is fragile. Serum cobalamin levels are reduced.

Serum folate levels are also obtained. If they are normal and cobalamin levels are low, it suggests that megaloblastic anemia is due to a cobalamin deficiency. A serum test for anti-IF antibodies may be done that is specific for pernicious anemia. Because the potential for gastric cancer is increased in patients with pernicious anemia, an upper GI endoscopy and biopsy of the gastric mucosa may also be done.

Testing of serum methylmalonic acid (MMA) (elevated mainly in cobalamin deficiency) and serum homocysteine (elevated in both cobalamin and folic acid deficiencies) helps determine the cause of this type of anemia.

### Interprofessional Care

Regardless of how much is ingested, the patient is not able to absorb cobalamin if IF is lacking or if absorption in the ileum is impaired. For this reason, increasing dietary cobalamin does not correct this anemia. However, instruct the patient on adequate dietary intake to maintain good nutrition (Table 30-5).

Parenteral vitamin $B_{12}$ (cyanocobalamin or hydroxocobalamin) or intranasal cyanocobalamin (Nascobal, CaloMist) is the treatment of choice. Without cobalamin administration, these individuals will die in 1 to 3 years. A typical treatment schedule consists of 1000 mcg/day of cobalamin IM for 2 weeks and then weekly until the hemoglobin is normal, and then monthly for life. High-dose oral cobalamin and sublingual cobalamin are also available for those in whom GI absorption is intact. As long as supplemental cobalamin is used, the anemia can be reversed. However, if the person has had long-standing neuromuscular complications that may not be reversible, physical therapy may be warranted.

### Megaloblastic Anemia: Folic Acid Deficiency

*Folic acid (folate) deficiency* also causes megaloblastic anemia. Folic acid is required for DNA synthesis leading to RBC formation and maturation. Common causes of folic acid deficiency are listed in Table 30-8.

The clinical manifestations of folic acid deficiency are similar to those of cobalamin deficiency. The disease develops insidiously, and the patient's symptoms may be attributed to other coexisting problems (e.g., cirrhosis, esophageal varices). GI disturbances include dyspepsia and a smooth, beefy red tongue. The absence of neurologic problems is an important diagnostic finding and differentiates folic acid deficiency from cobalamin deficiency.

The diagnostic findings for folic acid deficiency are presented in Table 30-6. In addition, the serum folate level is low (normal is 3 to 16 ng/mL [7 to 36 nmol/L]) and the serum cobalamin level is normal.

Folic acid deficiency is treated by replacement therapy. The usual dosage is 1 mg/day by mouth. In malabsorption states or with chronic alcoholism, up to 5 mg/day may be required. The duration of treatment depends on the reason for the deficiency. Encourage the patient to eat foods containing large amounts of folic acid (Table 30-5).

## ❖ NURSING MANAGEMENT: MEGALOBLASTIC ANEMIA

Because of the familial predisposition for pernicious anemia, the most common type of cobalamin deficiency, patients who have a positive family history of pernicious anemia should be evaluated for symptoms. Although the disease cannot be prevented, early detection and treatment can lead to reversal of symptoms. Also consider signs and symptoms of other possible megaloblastic anemias and bring them to the attention of the HCP. Ongoing care focuses on ensuring good patient adherence with treatment. Carefully assess for neurologic difficulties that were not fully corrected by replacement therapy. Because the potential for gastric cancer may be increased in patients with atrophic gastritis-related pernicious anemia, the patient should have frequent and careful appropriate screenings.

The nursing measures presented in eNursing Care Plan 30-1 for the patient with anemia are appropriate for the patient with cobalamin or folic acid deficiency anemia. In addition to these measures, ensure that injuries are not sustained because of the diminished sensitivity to heat and pain resulting from the neurologic impairment. Protect the patient from falling, burns, and trauma. If heat therapy is required, evaluate the patient's skin at frequent intervals to detect redness.

## ANEMIA OF CHRONIC DISEASE

Anemia of chronic disease (also called *anemia of inflammation*) can be caused by chronic inflammation, autoimmune and infectious disorders (human immunodeficiency virus [HIV], hepatitis, malaria), HF, or malignant diseases. Bleeding episodes can also contribute to anemia of chronic disease.

Anemia of chronic disease is associated with an underproduction of RBCs and mild shortening of RBC survival. The RBCs are usually normocytic, normochromic, and hypoproliferative. The anemia is usually mild, but it can become more severe if the underlying disorder is not treated.

This type of anemia, which usually develops after 1 to 2 months of disease activity, has an immune basis. The cytokines released in these conditions, particularly interleukin 6 (IL-6), cause an increased uptake and retention of iron within macrophages (see Fig. 29-3). This leads to a diversion of iron from circulation into storage sites with subsequent limited iron available for erythropoiesis. There is also reduced RBC life span, suppressed production of erythropoietin, and an ineffective bone marrow response to erythropoietin.

For any chronic disease, additional factors may contribute to the anemia. For example, with renal disease, the primary factor causing anemia is decreased erythropoietin, a hormone made in the kidneys that stimulates erythropoiesis. With impaired renal function, erythropoietin production is decreased (see Chapter 46).

Anemia of chronic disease must first be recognized and differentiated from anemia of other etiologies. Findings of elevated serum ferritin and increased iron stores distinguish it from iron-deficiency anemia. Normal folate and cobalamin blood levels distinguish it from megaloblastic anemias secondary to folate and cobalamin deficiencies.

The best treatment of anemia of chronic disease is correction of the underlying disorder. If the anemia is severe, blood transfusions may be indicated, but they are not recommended for long-term treatment. Erythropoietin therapy is used for anemia related to renal disease (see Chapter 46) and may be used for anemia related to cancer and its therapies (see Chapter 15 and Table 15-15). However, erythropoietin therapy must be used conservatively because of the increased risk of thromboembolism and death in some patients.

## APLASTIC ANEMIA

**Aplastic anemia** is a disease in which the patient has peripheral blood *pancytopenia* (decrease of all blood cell types—RBCs, white blood cells [WBCs], and platelets) and hypocellular bone marrow. The spectrum of the anemia can range from a chronic condition managed with erythropoietin or blood transfusions to a critical condition with hemorrhage and sepsis. The incidence of aplastic anemia is rare with an annual rate of 2 to 5 new cases per million per year.[2]

### Etiology

Aplastic anemias, which are usually acquired, are idiopathic and thought to have an autoimmune basis[12] (Table 30-9).

### Clinical Manifestations

Aplastic anemia can manifest abruptly (over days) or insidiously over weeks to months and can vary from mild to severe. Clinically the patient may have symptoms caused by suppression of any or all bone marrow elements. General manifestations of anemia such as fatigue and dyspnea, as well as cardiovascular and cerebral responses, may be seen (Table 30-3). The patient with neutropenia (low neutrophil count) is susceptible to infection and is at risk for septic shock and death. Even a low-grade fever (above 100.4° F [38° C]) should be considered a medical emergency. Thrombocytopenia is manifested by a predisposition to bleeding (e.g., petechiae, ecchymosis, epistaxis).

### Diagnostic Studies

The diagnosis is confirmed by laboratory studies. Because all marrow elements are affected, hemoglobin, WBC, and platelet values are often decreased in aplastic anemia. Other RBC indices are generally normal (Table 30-6). The condition is therefore classified as a normocytic, normochromic anemia. The reticulocyte count is low.

Aplastic anemia can be further evaluated by assessing various iron studies. The serum iron and total iron-binding capacity (TIBC) may be elevated as initial signs of erythropoiesis suppression. Bone marrow biopsy, aspiration, and pathologic examination may be done for any anemic state. However, the findings are especially important in aplastic anemia because the marrow is hypocellular with increased yellow marrow (fat content).

**TABLE 30-9 Causes of Acquired Aplastic Anemia**

- Idiopathic or autoimmune
- Chemical agents and toxins (e.g., benzene, insecticides, arsenic, alcohol)
- Drugs (e.g., alkylating agents, antiseizure drugs, antimetabolites, antimicrobials, gold, nonsteroidal antiinflammatory drugs, antithyroid medications, allopurinol)
- Radiation
- Viral and bacterial infections

### ❖ NURSING AND INTERPROFESSIONAL MANAGEMENT: APLASTIC ANEMIA

Management of aplastic anemia is based on identifying and removing the causative agent (when possible) and providing supportive care until the pancytopenia reverses. Nursing interventions appropriate for the patient with pancytopenia from aplastic anemia are presented in eNursing Care Plan 30-1 for anemia and eNursing Care Plan 30-2 for thrombocytopenia and eNursing Care Plan 30-3 for neutropenia (available on the website for this chapter). Nursing actions are directed at preventing complications from infection and hemorrhage.

The prognosis of severe untreated aplastic anemia is poor. However, advances in medical management, including HSCT and immunosuppressive therapy with antithymocyte globulin (ATG) and cyclosporine or high-dose cyclophosphamide, have improved outcomes significantly. ATG is a horse serum that contains polyclonal antibodies against human T cells. It can cause anaphylaxis and serum sickness. The rationale for this therapy is that idiopathic aplastic anemia is considered an autoimmune disorder resulting from activated cytotoxic T cells that target and destroy the patient's own hematopoietic stem cells. (ATG and cyclosporine are discussed in Chapter 13 and Table 13-16.) Alemtuzumab (Campath) (a monoclonal antibody) and eltrombopag (Promacta) (an oral thrombopoietin receptor agonist) are also options for select patients who do not respond to other therapies.[13]

The treatment of choice for adults younger than 55 years of age who do not respond to the immunosuppressive therapy and who have a human leukocyte antigen (HLA)–matched donor is an HSCT. The best results occur in younger patients who have not had previous blood transfusions. Prior transfusions increase the risk of graft rejection. (HSCT is discussed in Chapter 15.)

For older adults without an HLA-matched donor, the treatment of choice is immunosuppression with ATG or cyclosporine or high-dose cyclophosphamide. High-dose corticosteroids may also be used. However, this therapy may be only partially beneficial. Patients who need ongoing supportive blood transfusion should be on an iron-binding agent to prevent iron overload.

## ANEMIA CAUSED BY BLOOD LOSS

Anemia resulting from blood loss may be caused by either acute or chronic problems.

## ACUTE BLOOD LOSS

*Acute blood loss* occurs as a result of sudden hemorrhage. Causes of acute blood loss include trauma, complications of surgery, and conditions or diseases that disrupt vascular integrity. There are two clinical concerns in such situations. First, a sudden reduction in the total blood volume can lead to hypovolemic shock. Second, if the acute loss is more gradual, the body maintains its blood volume by slowly increasing the plasma volume. Although the circulating fluid volume is preserved, the number of RBCs available to carry $O_2$ is significantly diminished.

### Clinical Manifestations

The clinical manifestations of anemia from acute blood loss are caused by the body's attempts to maintain an adequate blood volume and meet $O_2$ requirements. Table 30-10 summarizes the clinical manifestations of patients with varying degrees of blood volume loss. It is essential to understand that the clinical signs and symptoms the patient is experiencing are more important than the laboratory values. For example, an adult with a bleeding peptic ulcer who had a 750-mL hematemesis (15% of a normal total blood volume) within the past 30 minutes may have postural hypotension but have normal values for hemoglobin and hematocrit. Over the next 36 to 48 hours, most of the blood volume deficit will be replaced by the movement of fluid from the extravascular into the intravascular space. Only then will the hemoglobin and hematocrit reflect the blood loss.

Assess the patient's expression of pain. Internal hemorrhage may cause pain because of tissue distention, organ displacement, and nerve compression. Pain may be localized or referred. In the case of retroperitoneal bleeding, the patient may not experience abdominal pain. Instead the patient may have numbness and pain in a lower extremity secondary to compression of the lateral cutaneous nerve, which is located in the region of the first to third lumbar vertebrae. The major complication of acute blood loss is shock (see Chapter 66).

### Diagnostic Studies

When blood volume loss is sudden, plasma volume has not yet had a chance to increase, the loss of RBCs is not reflected in laboratory data, and values may seem normal or high for 2 to 3 days. However, once the plasma volume is replaced, the RBC mass is less concentrated. At this time, RBC, hemoglobin, and hematocrit levels are low and reflect the actual blood loss.

### Interprofessional Care

Interprofessional care is initially concerned with (1) replacing blood volume to prevent shock and (2) identifying the source of the hemorrhage and stopping the blood loss. IV fluids used in emergencies include dextran, hetastarch, albumin, and crystalloid electrolyte solutions such as lactated Ringer's solution. The amount of infusion varies with the solution used. (Management of shock is discussed in Chapter 66.)

Once volume replacement is established, attention can be directed to correcting the RBC loss. The body needs 2 to 5 days to manufacture more RBCs in response to increased erythropoietin. Consequently, blood transfusions (packed RBCs) may be needed if the blood loss is significant. In addition, if the bleeding is related to a platelet or clotting disorder, replacement of that deficiency is addressed. If a large volume of blood is lost, platelets, plasma, and possibly cryoprecipitate will also be infused, because large volumes of RBCs would dilute the patient's own coagulation system.

The patient may also need supplemental iron because the availability of iron affects the marrow production of erythrocytes. When anemia exists after acute blood loss, dietary sources of iron will probably not be adequate to maintain iron stores. Therefore oral or parenteral iron preparations are administered.

**TABLE 30-10 Manifestations of Acute Blood Loss**

| VOLUME LOST* % | VOLUME LOST* mL | Manifestations |
|---|---|---|
| 10 | 500 | None or rare vasovagal syncope |
| 20 | 1000 | No detectable signs or symptoms at rest. Tachycardia with exercise and slight postural hypotension |
| 30 | 1500 | Normal supine blood pressure and pulse at rest. Postural hypotension and tachycardia with exercise |
| 40 | 2000 | Blood pressure, central venous pressure, and cardiac output below normal at rest; air hunger; rapid, thready pulse and cold, clammy skin |
| 50 | 2500 | Shock, lactic acidosis, and potential death |

*Based on an adult with a total blood volume of 5 L.

## NURSING MANAGEMENT: ACUTE BLOOD LOSS

In the case of trauma, it may be impossible to prevent the loss of blood. For the postoperative patient, carefully monitor the blood loss from various drainage tubes and dressings and implement appropriate actions. The nursing care for the patient with anemia resulting from acute blood loss most likely includes administration of blood products (described at the end of this chapter on pp. 647-652).

The anemia should begin to correct itself once the source of hemorrhage is identified, blood loss is controlled, and fluid and blood volumes are replaced. There should be no need for long-term treatment of this type of anemia.

## CHRONIC BLOOD LOSS

The sources of chronic blood loss are similar to those of iron-deficiency anemia (e.g., bleeding ulcer, hemorrhoids, menstrual and postmenopausal blood loss). The effects of chronic blood loss are usually related to the depletion of iron stores and considered as iron-deficiency anemia. Management of chronic blood loss anemia involves identifying the source and stopping the bleeding. Supplemental iron may be required.

## ANEMIA CAUSED BY INCREASED ERYTHROCYTE DESTRUCTION

The third major cause of anemia is termed **hemolytic anemia**, a condition caused by the destruction or hemolysis of RBCs at a rate that exceeds production. Hemolysis can occur because of problems intrinsic or extrinsic to the RBCs. *Intrinsic hemolytic anemias*, which are usually hereditary, result from defects in the RBCs themselves (Table 30-2).

More common are the *acquired hemolytic anemias*. In this type of anemia the RBCs are normal, but damage is caused by external factors (Table 30-2). The spleen is the primary site of the destruction of RBCs that are old, defective, or moderately damaged. Fig. 30-2 indicates the sequence of events involved in extravascular hemolysis.

The patient with hemolytic anemia has the general manifestations of anemia and specific manifestations related to this type of anemia (Table 30-3). Jaundice is likely because the increased

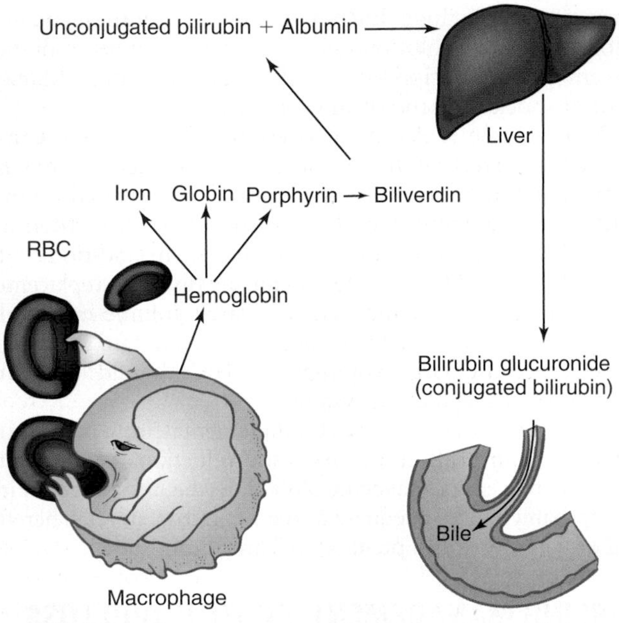


**FIG. 30-2** Sequence of events in extravascular hemolysis.

destruction of RBCs causes an elevation in bilirubin levels. The spleen and liver may enlarge because of their hyperactivity, which is related to macrophage phagocytosis of the defective erythrocytes.

In all causes of hemolysis, a major focus of treatment is to maintain renal function. When RBCs are hemolyzed, the hemoglobin molecule is released and filtered by the kidneys. The accumulation of hemoglobin molecules can obstruct the renal tubules and lead to acute tubular necrosis (see Chapter 46).

## SICKLE CELL DISEASE

Sickle cell disease (SCD) is a group of inherited, autosomal recessive disorders characterized by an abnormal form of hemoglobin in the RBC. (Autosomal recessive genetic disorders are discussed in Chapter 12.) Because this is a genetic disorder, SCD is usually identified during routine neonatal screening. It is an incurable disease that is often fatal by middle age because of renal failure, infection, pulmonary failure, and/or stroke.[9]

### Etiology and Pathophysiology

**Genetic Link.** In SCD the abnormal hemoglobin, *hemoglobin S* (Hgb S), results from the substitution of valine for glutamic acid on the β-globin chain of hemoglobin (see Fig. 12-3). Hgb S causes the erythrocyte to stiffen and elongate, taking on a sickle shape in response to low $O_2$ levels (Fig. 30-3).

Types of SCD disorders include sickle cell anemia, sickle cell–thalassemia, sickle cell Hgb C disease, and sickle cell trait. *Sickle cell anemia*, the most severe of the SCD syndromes, occurs when a person is homozygous for hemoglobin S (Hgb SS); the person has inherited Hgb S from both parents. *Sickle cell–thalassemia* and *sickle cell Hgb C* occur when a person inherits Hgb S from one parent and another type of abnormal hemoglobin (such as thalassemia or hemoglobin C) from the other parent. Both of these forms of SCD are less common and less severe than sickle cell anemia. *Sickle cell trait* occurs when a person is heterozygous for hemoglobin S (Hgb AS); the person has inherited hemoglobin S from one parent and normal hemoglobin (Hgb A) from the other parent. Sickle cell trait is typically a mild to asymptomatic condition.

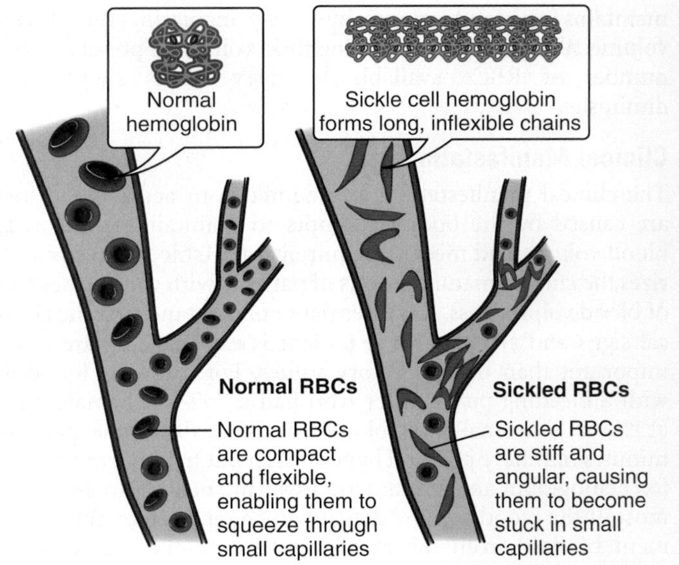


**FIG. 30-3** In sickle cell, the hemoglobin forms long inflexible chains and alters the shape of the red blood cells (RBCs). The sickled RBCs can become stuck in the capillaries and occlude the blood flow.

### GENETICS IN CLINICAL PRACTICE

#### *Sickle Cell Disease*

**Genetic Basis**
- Autosomal recessive disorder.
- Mutation in β-globin *(HBB)* gene located on chromosome 11.
- Various versions of β-globin result from different mutations in the *HBB* gene.
- Hgb S variant involves substitution of valine for glutamic acid in the β-globin gene in sickle cell anemia.

**Incidence**
- Most common inherited blood disorder in the United States.
- Affects 8 of every 100,000 people.
- Affects 1 in 350 to 500 African Americans.
- Affects 1 in 1000 to 1400 Hispanic Americans.
- Also affects people of Mediterranean, Caribbean, Arabian, and East Indian descent.

**Genetic Testing**
- DNA testing is available.
- Electrophoresis of hemoglobin and sickling screening test are more commonly used.

**Clinical Implications**
- Requires ongoing continuity of care and extensive patient teaching.
- Sickle cell trait is the carrier state for sickle cell disease and represents a mild type of sickle cell disease; 1 in 10 to 12 African Americans and 1 in 25 Hispanics have sickle cell trait.
- If both parents have the trait, there is a 1 in 4 chance that their baby will have sickle cell disease.
- Management of sickle cell disease should focus on the prevention of sickle cell crisis (e.g., prevention of dehydration and infection).
- Genetic counseling is recommended for individuals with a family history of sickle cell disease. Individuals should understand the risks of transmitting the genetic mutation.

**Sickling Episodes.** The major pathophysiologic event of SCD is the sickling of RBCs (Fig. 30-3). Sickling episodes are most commonly triggered by low $O_2$ tension in the blood. Hypoxia or deoxygenation of the RBCs can be caused by viral or bacterial infection, high altitude, emotional or physical stress, surgery, and blood loss. Infection is the most common precipitating factor. Other events that can trigger or sustain a sickling episode include dehydration, increased hydrogen ion concentration (acidosis), increased plasma osmolality, decreased plasma volume, and low body temperature. A sickling episode can also occur without an obvious cause.

Sickled RBCs become rigid and take on an elongated, crescent shape (Fig. 30-3). Sickled cells cannot easily pass through capillaries or other small vessels and can cause vascular occlusion, leading to acute or chronic tissue injury. The resulting hemostasis promotes a self-perpetuating cycle of local hypoxia, deoxygenation of more erythrocytes, and more sickling. Circulating sickled cells are hemolyzed by the spleen, leading to anemia. Initially the sickling of cells is reversible with reoxygenation, but it eventually becomes irreversible because of cell membrane damage from recurrent sickling. Thus vaso-occlusive phenomena and hemolysis are the clinical hallmarks of SCD.

*Sickle cell crisis* is a severe, painful, acute exacerbation of RBC sickling, causing a vaso-occlusive crisis. As blood flow is impaired by sickled cells, vasospasm occurs, further restricting blood flow. Severe capillary hypoxia causes changes in membrane permeability, leading to plasma loss, hemoconcentration, thrombi, and further circulatory stagnation. Tissue ischemia, infarction, and necrosis eventually occur from lack of $O_2$. Shock is a possibly life-threatening consequence of sickle cell crisis because of severe $O_2$ depletion of the tissues and a reduction of the circulating fluid volume. Sickle cell crisis can begin suddenly and persist for days to weeks.

The frequency, extent, and severity of sickling episodes are highly variable and unpredictable but largely depend on the percentage of Hgb S present. Individuals with sickle cell anemia have the most severe form because the erythrocytes contain a high percentage of Hgb S.

### Clinical Manifestations

The effects of SCD vary greatly from person to person, the severity of which may be due to genetic polymorphisms. Many people with sickle cell anemia are in reasonably good health the majority of the time. However, they may have chronic health problems and pain because of organ tissue hypoxia and damage (e.g., involving the kidneys or liver).

The typical patient is anemic but asymptomatic except during sickling episodes. Because most individuals with sickle cell anemia have dark skin, pallor is more readily detected by examining the mucous membranes. The skin may have a grayish cast. Because of the hemolysis, jaundice is common and patients are prone to gallstones (cholelithiasis).

The primary symptom associated with sickling is pain. The pain severity can range from trivial to excruciating. During sickle cell crisis the pain is severe because of ischemia of tissue. The episodes can affect any area of the body or several sites simultaneously, with the back, chest, extremities, and abdomen being most commonly affected. Pain episodes are often accompanied by clinical manifestations such as fever, swelling, tenderness, tachypnea, hypertension, nausea, and vomiting.

### Complications

With repeated episodes of sickling, there is gradual involvement of all body systems, especially the spleen, lungs, kidneys, and brain. Organs that have a need for large amounts of $O_2$ are most often affected and form the basis for many of the complications of SCD (Fig. 30-4). Infection is a major cause of morbidity and mortality in patients with SCD. One reason for this is the failure of the spleen to phagocytize foreign substances as it becomes infarcted and dysfunctional (usually by 2 to 4 years of age) from the sickled RBCs. The spleen becomes small because of repeated scarring, a phenomenon termed *autosplenectomy.*

Pneumonia is the most common infection and often is of pneumococcal origin. Infections can be so severe that they cause an aplastic and hemolytic crisis and gallstones. *Aplastic crisis* can be so severe that it causes a temporary shutdown of RBC production in the bone marrow.

*Acute chest syndrome* is a term used to describe acute pulmonary complications that include pneumonia, tissue infarction, and fat embolism. It is characterized by fever, chest pain, cough, pulmonary infiltrates, and dyspnea. Pulmonary infarctions may cause pulmonary hypertension, MI, HF, and ultimately cor pulmonale. The heart may become ischemic and enlarged, leading to HF. Retinal vessel obstruction may result in hemorrhage, scarring, retinal detachment, and blindness. The kidneys may be injured from the increased blood viscosity and the lack of $O_2$, and renal failure may occur. Pulmonary embolism or stroke can result from thrombosis and infarction of cerebral blood vessels. Bone changes may include osteoporosis and osteosclerosis after infarction. Chronic leg ulcers can result from the hypoxia and are especially prevalent around the ankles. *Priapism* (persistent penile erection) may occur if penile veins become occluded.

### Diagnostic Studies

A peripheral blood smear may reveal sickled cells and abnormal reticulocytes. The presence of Hgb S can be diagnosed by the sickling test, which uses RBCs (in vitro) and exposes them to a deoxygenation agent.

As a result of the accelerated RBC breakdown, the patient has characteristic clinical findings of hemolysis (jaundice, elevated serum bilirubin levels) and abnormal laboratory test results (Table 30-6). Hemoglobin electrophoresis may be done to determine the amount of hemoglobin S. Skeletal x-rays demonstrate bone and joint deformities and flattening. MRI may be used to diagnose a stroke caused by blocked cerebral vessels from sickled cells. Doppler studies may be used to assess for deep vein thromboses. Other tests may be indicated, such as a chest x-ray, to diagnose infection or organ malfunction.

## ❖ NURSING AND INTERPROFESSIONAL MANAGEMENT: SICKLE CELL DISEASE

Interprofessional care for a patient with SCD is directed toward (1) prevention of sequelae from the disease; (2) alleviating the manifestations from the complications of the disease; (3) minimizing end-organ damage; and (4) promptly treating serious sequelae, such as acute chest syndrome, that can lead to immediate death.[14] Teach patients with SCD to avoid high altitudes, maintain adequate fluid intake, and treat infections promptly. Screening for retinopathy should begin at age 10. Immunizations such as pneumococcal, *Haemophilus influenzae,* influenza, and hepatitis should be administered. Sickle cell crises may require hospitalization. $O_2$ may be administered to treat hypoxia and control sickling. Because respiratory failure is a most common cause of death, vigilantly assess for any changes in respiratory status. Rest may be instituted to reduce metabolic

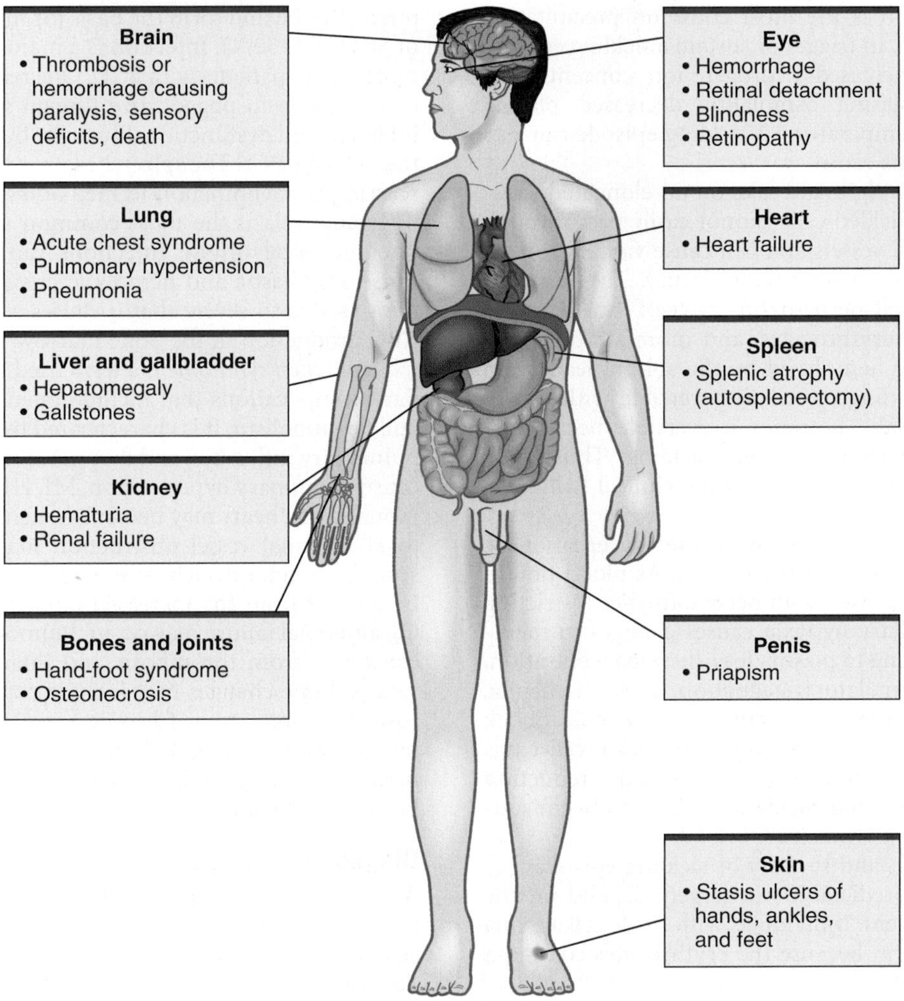


**FIG. 30-4** Clinical manifestations and complications of sickle cell disease. (Modified from McCance KL, Huether SE: *Pathophysiology: the biologic basis for disease in adults and children*, ed 7, St Louis, 2014, Mosby.)

requirements, and deep vein thrombosis prophylaxis (using anticoagulants) should be prescribed. Fluids and electrolytes are administered to reduce blood viscosity and maintain renal function. Priapism is managed with pain medication, fluids, and nifedipine (Procardia). If it does not resolve within a few hours, a urologist can be called to inject the corpus cavernosum with a dilute solution of epinephrine to preserve penile function.

Transfusion therapy is indicated when an aplastic crisis occurs. Aggressive total RBC exchange transfusion programs may be implemented for patients who have frequent crises or serious complications, such as acute chest syndrome. These patients, like those with thalassemia major, may require iron chelation therapy to reduce transfusion-produced iron overload.

Undertreatment of sickle cell pain is a major problem. Lack of understanding can lead HCPs to underestimate how much pain these patients suffer. Patients, because of their prior opioid treatment, may be tolerant, and thus large doses may be needed to reduce the pain to a tolerable level. During an acute crisis, optimal pain control usually includes large doses of continuous (rather than as-needed [PRN]) opioid analgesics along with breakthrough analgesia, often in the form of patient-controlled analgesia (PCA). (PCA is discussed in Chapter 8.) Morphine and hydromorphone are the drugs of choice.

Because patients may be experiencing different types and sites of pain, as well as acute and chronic pain, a holistic approach should be used that addresses the pain and its impact on the patient's psychologic, social, and spiritual well-being[15] (see Chapter 8). In addition to opioids, adjunctive measures, such as nonsteroidal antiinflammatory agents, antineuropathic pain medications (e.g., tricyclic antidepressants, antiseizure medications), local anesthetics, or nerve blocks may be used. Occupational and physical therapy can optimize functioning. Referral to social and chaplain services can assist in addressing social, emotional, and spiritual needs.

Although pain is the most common symptom of patients with SCD, infection is a frequent complication and must be treated. Infections, such as chronic leg ulcers, may be treated with rest, antibiotics, warm saline soaks, mechanical or enzyme debridement, and grafting if necessary. Patients with acute chest syndrome are treated with broad-spectrum antibiotics, $O_2$ therapy, fluid therapy, and possibly exchange transfusion. Blood transfusions have little if any role in the treatment between crises, since patients develop antibodies to RBCs and iron overload. However, because chronic hemolysis results in increased use of folic acid stores, routine oral folic acid should be taken.

Although many antisickling agents have been tried, hydroxyurea (Hydrea) is the only one that has been shown to be clinically beneficial. This drug increases the production of hemoglobin F (fetal hemoglobin) and alters the adhesion of sickled RBCs to the endothelium. The increase in Hgb F is accompanied by a reduction in hemolysis, an increase in hemoglobin concentration, and a decrease in sickled cells and painful crises.[14]

HSCT is the only available treatment that can cure some patients with SCD. The selection of appropriate recipients, scarcity of appropriate donors, risk, and cost-effectiveness limit the use of HSCT for SCD. (HSCT is discussed in Chapter 15.)

## CHECK YOUR PRACTICE

A 21-year-old African American graduate student was just admitted to the ED following a ski trip to Colorado. She is in excruciating pain in her chest and abdomen. She is also short of breath and her $O_2$ saturation is 86%. Your examination reveals that her heart rate is 110 bpm and respiratory rate 28/minute. She has crackles in the lungs. She has a history of six previous ED admissions for sickle cell crises.

- What are your priorities for her nursing care?

Patient teaching and support are important in the long-term care of the patient with SCD. The patient and caregiver must understand the basis of the disease and the reasons for supportive care and ongoing pertinent screening tailored to SCD manifestations, such as eye examinations. Teach the patient ways to avoid crises, including taking steps to avoid dehydration and hypoxia, such as avoiding high altitudes and seeking medical attention quickly to counteract problems such as upper respiratory tract infections. Teaching about pain control is also needed because the pain during a crisis may be severe and often requires considerable analgesia. Minor pain episodes that are not associated with infection or other symptoms warranting medical attention can sometimes be managed at home.

## ETHICAL/LEGAL DILEMMAS

### *Pain Management*

**Situation**

N.C., a 21-year-old African American man, is admitted to the emergency department (ED) in sickle cell crisis with complaints of excruciating pain. He is known to several of the nurses and HCPs in the ED. One of the nurses remarks to you that it must be time for his "fix" of pain drugs.

**Ethical/Legal Points for Consideration**

- The standard of care for pain requires that (1) a pain assessment is done based on the patient's self-report, (2) the best possible relief of pain is provided under the circumstances, and (3) competent and compassionate care is provided to all patients.
- The pain assessment also includes reviewing the patient's medical record to determine if there are health care issues or conditions (e.g., frequent ED visits to request pain medication) that may affect the patient's response to pain and pain management.
- As a nurse, you have a duty to notify the HCP of those issues or conditions. You also need to document behaviors exhibited by the patient related to pain management. Make sure that the documentation is objective (factual observations) rather than labeling (the patient was in withdrawal).
- When pain relief is inadequate, as a nurse, you are responsible for notifying the HCP. Efforts to notify must continue and be appropriately documented until the managing HCP has assessed the patient and made a plan of care based on that assessment.

**Discussion Questions**

1. How can you educate your colleagues regarding pain assessment and management?
2. What important factors would need to be included in your assessment and management of N.C.?

## ACQUIRED HEMOLYTIC ANEMIA

*Acquired hemolytic anemia* results from hemolysis of RBCs from extrinsic factors. These factors include (1) physical destruction, (2) antibody reactions, and (3) infectious agents and toxins (Table 30-2).

*Physical destruction* of RBCs results from the exertion of extreme force on the cells. Traumatic events causing disruption of the RBC membrane include hemodialysis, extracorporeal circulation used in cardiopulmonary bypass, and prosthetic heart valves. In addition, the force needed to push blood through abnormal vessels, such as those that have been burned, irradiated, or affected by vascular disease (e.g., diabetes mellitus), may also physically damage RBCs.

RBCs can also be fragmented and destroyed as they try to pass through abnormal arterial or venous microcirculation. The RBCs are sheared as they try to pass by excessive platelet aggregation and/or fibrin polymer formation, such as is seen in thrombotic thrombocytopenic purpura (TTP) and disseminated intravascular coagulation (DIC) (discussed later in this chapter).

*Antibodies* may destroy RBCs by the mechanisms involved in antigen-antibody reactions. In blood transfusion reactions, the recipient's antibodies attack and hemolyze donor cells. Autoimmune antibody reactions occur when individuals develop antibodies against their own RBCs. This can be an idiopathic (no prior hemolytic history) or secondary to other autoimmune diseases (e.g., systemic lupus erythematosus), leukemia, lymphoma, or medications (penicillin, ibuprofen, metformin, chlorpromazine, procainamide).

*Infectious agents* cause hemolysis in three ways: (1) by invading the RBC and destroying its contents (e.g., parasites such as in malaria), (2) by releasing hemolytic substances (e.g., *Clostridium perfringens*), and (3) by generating an antigen-antibody reaction (e.g., *Mycoplasma pneumoniae*). Various agents may be toxic to RBCs and cause hemolysis. These hemolytic toxins involve chemicals such as oxidative drugs, arsenic, lead, copper, and bee stings or spider bites.

Laboratory findings in hemolytic anemia are presented in Table 30-6. Treatment and management of acquired hemolytic anemias involve general supportive care until the causative agent can be eliminated or at least made less injurious to the RBCs. Because a hemolytic crisis is a potential consequence, be ready to institute appropriate emergency therapy. This includes aggressive hydration and electrolyte replacement to reduce the risk of kidney injury caused by hemoglobin (from RBC lysis) clogging the kidney tubules and subsequent shock. Additional supportive care may include administering corticosteroids and blood products or removing the spleen.

For chronic hemolytic anemia, folate may have to be replaced. To suppress the RBC destruction, immunosuppressive agents may be used, such as rituximab (Rituxan) (monoclonal antibody to B-cell CD20) and eculizumab (Soliris) (monoclonal antibody to complement protein C5).

# OTHER RED BLOOD CELL DISORDERS

## HEMOCHROMATOSIS

**Hemochromatosis** is an iron overload disorder. Although it is caused primarily by a genetic defect, hemochromatosis may occur secondary to diseases such as sideroblastic anemia. It may also be caused by liver disease and chronic blood transfusions that are used to treat thalassemia and SCD.

**Genetic Link.** The genetic disorder *(hereditary hemochromatosis)* is an autosomal recessive disorder characterized by increased intestinal iron absorption and, as a result, increased tissue iron deposition. (Autosomal recessive disorders are discussed in Chapter 12 and Table 12-2.)

## GENETICS IN CLINICAL PRACTICE

### *Hemochromatosis*

**Genetic Basis**

- Autosomal recessive disorder
- Caused by mutations in the *HAMP, HFE, HFE2, SLC40A1*, and *TFR2* genes
- These genes play an important role in regulating the absorption, transport, and storage of iron.
- Mutations in these genes impair the control of iron absorption during digestion and alter the distribution of iron to other parts of the body. As a result, iron accumulates in tissues and organs.

**Incidence**

- Most common genetic disease in people of European ancestry
- One in 8 are carriers of the single HH gene mutation.
- Affects 1 in 200 to 500 in the United States
- Very low prevalence in other ethnic populations

**Genetic Testing**

- DNA testing is available and recommended for all first-degree relatives of people with the disease.
- American Hemochromatosis Society recommends genetic testing regardless of family history.
- Useful diagnostic tests include serum iron concentration, total iron-binding capacity, and transferrin saturation.

**Clinical Implications**

- Most of the 33 million Americans who have the gene mutation do not know it.
- Clinical expression is variable depending on dietary iron, blood loss, and other modifying factors.
- Early treatment can prevent serious complications.
- If untreated, progressive iron deposits can lead to multiple organ failure.

The normal range for total body iron is 2 to 6 g. Individuals with hemochromatosis accumulate iron at a rate of 0.5 to 1.0 g/yr and may exceed total iron concentrations of 50 g. Symptoms of hemochromatosis usually develop between 40 and 60 years of age.

Early symptoms are nonspecific and include fatigue, arthralgia, impotence, abdominal pain, and weight loss. Later, the excess iron accumulates in the liver and causes liver enlargement and eventually cirrhosis. Excess iron is deposited in the liver, pancreas, heart, joints, and endocrine glands, resulting in diabetes mellitus, skin pigment changes (bronzing), cardiac changes (e.g., cardiomyopathy), arthritis, and testicular atrophy. Physical examination reveals an enlarged liver and spleen and pigmentation changes in the skin.

Laboratory values demonstrate an elevated serum iron, TIBC, and serum ferritin. Testing for known genetic mutations confirms the diagnosis. Liver biopsy can quantify the amount of iron and establish the degree of organ damage.

The goal of treatment is to remove excess iron from the body and minimize any symptoms the patient may have. Iron removal is achieved by removing 500 mL of blood each week for 2 to 3 years until the iron stores in the body are depleted. Then blood is removed less frequently to maintain iron levels within normal limits.

Iron chelating agents may be used. Deferoxamine, which chelates and removes accumulated iron via the kidneys, can be administered IV or subcutaneously. Deferasirox and deferiprone are oral agents that chelate iron. Chelating agents form a complex with iron and promote its excretion from the body.[8]

Management of organ involvement (e.g., diabetes mellitus, HF) is the same as conventional treatment for these problems. Iron accumulation can also be reduced by dietary modifications such as avoidance of vitamin C and iron supplements, uncooked seafood, and iron-rich foods. The most common causes of death are cirrhosis, liver failure, hepatocellular cancer, and cardiac failure. With early diagnosis and treatment, life expectancy is normal. However, many cases go undetected and untreated.

## POLYCYTHEMIA

**Polycythemia** is the production and presence of increased numbers of RBCs. The increase in RBCs can be so great that blood circulation is impaired as a result of the increased blood viscosity *(hyperviscosity)* and volume *(hypervolemia)*.

### Etiology and Pathophysiology

The two types of polycythemia are primary polycythemia, or polycythemia vera, and secondary polycythemia (Fig. 30-5). Their etiologies and pathogenesis differ, although their complications and clinical manifestations are similar.

**Primary Polycythemia.** *Polycythemia vera* is a chronic myeloproliferative disorder. Therefore not only RBCs are involved but also WBCs and platelets, leading to increased production of each of these blood cells. The disease develops insidiously and follows a chronic, vacillating course. The median age at diagnosis is 60 years old, with a slight male predominance. In polycythemia vera there is enhanced blood viscosity and blood volume and congestion of organs and tissues with blood. Splenomegaly (which occurs in 90% of patients) and hepatomegaly are common. These patients have hypercoagulopathies that predispose them to clotting.

**Genetic Link.** Polycythemia vera is associated with mutations in the *Janus kinase-2 (JAK2)* gene. The *JAK2* gene provides instructions for making a protein that promotes proliferation of cells, especially blood cells from hematopoietic stem cells. Polycythemia vera begins with one or more DNA mutations of a single hematopoietic stem cell. Most cases of polycythemia vera are not inherited. This condition is associated with genetic changes that are somatic, which means they are acquired during a person's lifetime and are present only in certain cells.

**Secondary Polycythemia.** *Secondary polycythemia* can be either hypoxia driven or hypoxia independent. In hypoxia-driven secondary polycythemia, hypoxia stimulates erythropoietin (EPO) production in the kidney, which in turn stimulates RBC production. The need for $O_2$ may result from high altitude, pulmonary disease, cardiovascular disease, alveolar hypoventilation, defective $O_2$ transport, or tissue hypoxia.

EPO levels may return to normal once the hemoglobin is stabilized at a higher level. In this situation, secondary polycythemia is a physiologic response in which the body tries to compensate for a problem, rather than a pathologic response. (Hypoxia-driven secondary polycythemia is discussed

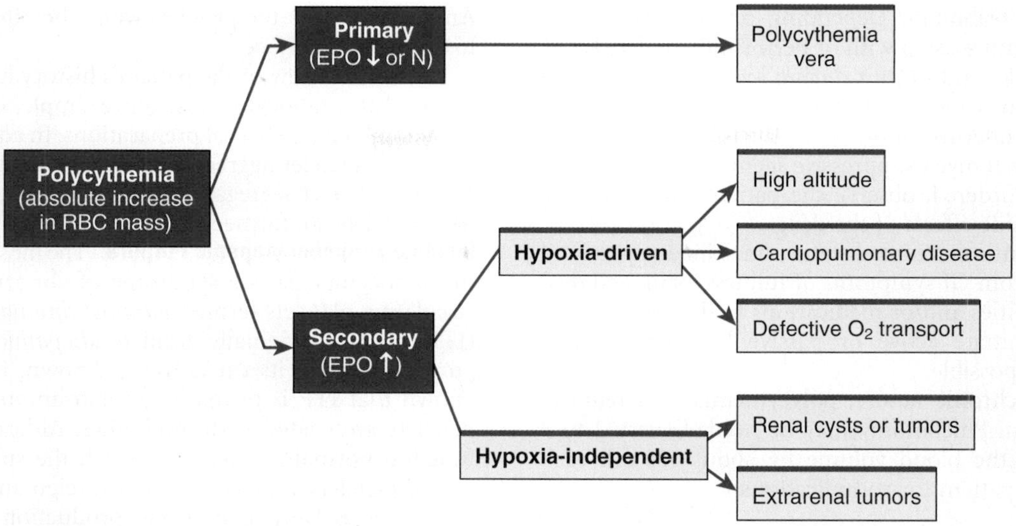


**FIG. 30-5** Differentiating between primary and secondary polycythemia. *EPO,* Erythropoietin; *N,* normal.

in the section on chronic obstructive pulmonary disease in Chapter 28.)

In hypoxia-independent secondary polycythemia, EPO is produced by a malignant or benign tumor tissue. Serum EPO levels often remain elevated in these situations. Splenomegaly does not accompany secondary polycythemia.

## Clinical Manifestations and Complications

Circulatory manifestations of polycythemia vera occur because of the hypertension caused by hypervolemia and hyperviscosity. They are often the first manifestations and include subjective complaints of headache, vertigo, dizziness, tinnitus, and visual disturbances. Generalized pruritus (often exacerbated by a hot bath) may be a striking symptom and is related to histamine release from an increased number of basophils. Paresthesias and *erythromelalgia* (painful burning and redness of the hands and feet) may also be present. In addition, the patient may experience angina, HF, intermittent claudication, and thrombophlebitis, which may be complicated by embolization. These manifestations are caused by blood vessel distention, impaired blood flow, circulatory stasis, thrombosis, and tissue hypoxia caused by the hypervolemia and hyperviscosity. The most common serious acute complication is stroke secondary to thrombosis.

Hemorrhagic phenomena caused by either vessel rupture from overdistention or inadequate platelet function may result in petechiae, ecchymoses, epistaxis, or GI bleeding. Hemorrhage can be acute and catastrophic. Hepatomegaly and splenomegaly from organ engorgement may contribute to patient complaints of satiety and fullness. The patient may also experience pain from peptic ulcer caused either by increased gastric secretions or by liver and spleen engorgement. *Plethora* (ruddy complexion) may also be present. Hyperuricemia is caused by the increase in RBC destruction that accompanies excessive RBC production. Uric acid is one of the products of cell destruction. As RBC destruction increases, uric acid production also increases, thus leading to hyperuricemia and possible gout.

Although the incidence is low, myelofibrosis and leukemia develop in some patients with polycythemia vera. These disorders may be caused by the chemotherapeutic drugs used to treat the disease, or they may be secondary to a disorder in the stem cells that progresses to erythroleukemia. The major cause of morbidity and mortality from polycythemia vera is related to thrombosis (e.g., stroke).

## Diagnostic Studies

The following laboratory manifestations are seen in a patient with polycythemia vera: (1) elevated hemoglobin and RBC count with microcytosis; (2) low to normal EPO level (secondary polycythemia has a high level); (3) elevated WBC count with basophilia; (4) elevated platelet count (thrombocytosis) and platelet dysfunction; (5) elevated leukocyte alkaline phosphatase, uric acid, and cobalamin levels; and (6) elevated histamine levels. Bone marrow examination in polycythemia vera shows hypercellularity of RBCs, WBCs, and platelets.

## Interprofessional Care

Treatment is directed toward reducing blood volume and viscosity and bone marrow activity. Phlebotomy is the mainstay of treatment. The aim of phlebotomy is to reduce the hematocrit and keep it less than 45% in men and 42% in women. Generally, at the time of diagnosis 300 to 500 mL of blood may be removed every other day until the hematocrit is reduced to normal levels. An individual managed with repeated phlebotomies eventually becomes deficient in iron, although this effect is rarely symptomatic. Avoid iron supplementation. Hydration therapy is used to reduce the blood's viscosity. Myelosuppressive agents such as hydroxyurea (Hydrea), busulfan (Myleran), and chlorambucil (Leukeran) are used.

Ruxolitinib (Jakafi), which inhibits the expression of the *JAK2* mutation, is used for patients who have not responded to hydroxyurea.[16] Low-dose aspirin is used to prevent clotting. α-Interferon (α-IFN) is of particular use in women of childbearing age or those with intractable pruritus. Anagrelide (Agrylin) may be used to reduce the platelet count and inhibit platelet aggregation. Allopurinol (Zyloprim) may reduce the number of acute gouty attacks.[17] (Gout may occur because of increased uric acid levels from the destruction of cells.)

# ❖ NURSING MANAGEMENT: POLYCYTHEMIA VERA

Primary polycythemia (polycythemia vera) is not preventable. When acute exacerbations of polycythemia vera develop, you have several responsibilities. Depending on the institution's policies, you may either assist with or perform the phlebotomy. Evaluate fluid intake and output during hydration therapy to avoid fluid overload (which further complicates the circulatory congestion) and underhydration (which can make the blood even more viscous). If myelosuppressive agents are used, administer the drugs as ordered, observe the patient, and teach the patient about the side effects of the drugs.

Assess the patient's nutritional status, since inadequate food intake can result from GI symptoms of fullness, pain, and dyspepsia. Begin activities and/or medications to decrease thrombus formation. Initiate active or passive leg exercises and ambulation when possible.

Because of its chronic nature, polycythemia vera requires ongoing evaluation. Phlebotomy may be needed every 2 to 3 months, reducing the blood volume by about 500 mL each time. Evaluate the patient for complications.

## PROBLEMS OF HEMOSTASIS

Hemostasis involves the vascular endothelium, platelets, and coagulation factors, which normally function together to stop hemorrhage and repair vascular injury. (These mechanisms are described in Chapter 29.) Disruption in any of these components may result in bleeding or thrombotic disorders.

Three major disorders of hemostasis discussed in this section are (1) thrombocytopenia (low platelet count), (2) hemophilia and von Willebrand disease (inherited disorders of specific clotting factors), and (3) disseminated intravascular coagulation (DIC).

## THROMBOCYTOPENIA

### Etiology and Pathophysiology

**Thrombocytopenia** is a reduction of platelets below 150,000/μL ($150 \times 10^9$/L). Acute, severe, or prolonged decreases from this normal range can result in abnormal hemostasis that manifests as prolonged bleeding from minor trauma or spontaneous bleeding without injury.

Platelet disorders can be inherited (e.g., Wiskott-Aldrich syndrome), but the majority are acquired (Table 30-11). A common cause of acquired disorders is the ingestion of certain drugs, often in high doses.[18,19] Although some agents are directly myelosuppressive (e.g., chemotherapy, ganciclovir [Cytovene]), the usual mechanism of thrombocytopenia caused by drugs is accelerated platelet destruction caused by antibodies. Antibodies attack the platelets when the offending agent binds to the platelet surface.

**TABLE 30-11 Causes of Acquired Thrombocytopenia**

- Immune thrombocytopenic purpura (ITP)
- Thrombotic thrombocytopenic purpura (TTP)
- Heparin-induced thrombocytopenia (HIT)
- Disseminated intravascular coagulation (DIC)
- Drugs
  - Chemotherapy drugs
  - Aspirin
- Quinine
- Infections
  - Viral infection (hepatitis C virus, HIV, cytomegalovirus)
  - Bacterial infection
- Hematologic malignancy (leukemia, lymphoma, myeloma)

A careful review of the patient's history helps to identify the cause of thrombocytopenia. For example, quinine is in tonic water and in many herbal preparations. In addition, some drugs can affect platelet aggregation. Aspirin doses as low as 81 mg can alter platelet aggregation. Normal function is restored when new platelets are formed.

**Immune Thrombocytopenic Purpura.** The most common acquired thrombocytopenia is a syndrome of abnormal destruction of circulating platelets termed *immune thrombocytopenic purpura* (ITP). It was originally termed *idiopathic thrombocytopenic purpura* because its cause was unknown. However, it is now known that ITP is primarily an autoimmune disease. In ITP, platelets are coated with antibodies. Although these platelets function normally, when they reach the spleen the antibody-coated platelets are recognized as foreign and are destroyed by macrophages. Decreased platelet production contributes to ITP. Sometimes infection, such as *Helicobacter pylori* or viral infection, contributes to this disorder.[18]

Platelets normally survive 8 to 10 days. However, in ITP survival of platelets is shortened. Generally, the clinical syndrome manifests as an acute condition in children and a chronic condition in adults.

**Thrombotic Thrombocytopenic Purpura.** *Thrombotic thrombocytopenic purpura* (TTP) is an uncommon syndrome characterized by hemolytic anemia, thrombocytopenia, neurologic abnormalities, fever (in the absence of infection), and renal abnormalities; not all features are present in all patients. Because it is almost always associated with hemolytic-uremic syndrome (HUS), it is often referred to as *TTP-HUS*. The disease is associated with enhanced aggregation of platelets, which form microthrombi that deposit in arterioles and capillaries.

In most cases the syndrome is caused by the deficiency of a plasma enzyme (ADAMTS13) that usually breaks down the von Willebrand clotting factor (vWF) into normal size. (vWF is the most important protein-mediating platelet adhesion to damaged endothelial cells.) Without the enzyme, unusually large amounts of vWF attach to activated platelets, thereby promoting platelet aggregation.

TTP is seen primarily in previously healthy adults, with a slight female predominance. The syndrome may be idiopathic (thought to be due to an autoimmune disorder against ADAMTS13), but it may be due to certain drug toxicities (e.g., chemotherapy, cyclosporine, quinine, oral contraceptives, valacyclovir [Valtrex], clopidogrel [Plavix]), pregnancy or preeclampsia, infection, or a known autoimmune disorder such as systemic lupus erythematosus or scleroderma.[20] TTP is a medical emergency because bleeding and clotting occur simultaneously.

**Heparin-Induced Thrombocytopenia.** One of the risks associated with the broad and increasing use of heparin is the development of the life-threatening condition called *heparin-induced thrombocytopenia* (HIT), also called *heparin-induced thrombocytopenia and thrombosis syndrome* (HITTS). Typically, patients develop thrombocytopenia 5 to 10 days after the onset of heparin therapy. HIT should be suspected if the platelet count falls by more than 50% or falls to below 150,000/μL. As many as 3% of patients on heparin therapy develop HIT.[21]

Although the major clinical problem of HIT is venous thrombosis, arterial thrombosis can also develop. Deep vein thromboses and pulmonary emboli most commonly result as a complication of the thromboses. Additional complications may include arterial vascular infarcts, resulting in skin necrosis, stroke, and end-organ damage (e.g., kidneys). Symptoms of bleeding are unusual because the platelet count rarely drops below 20,000/μL.

In HIT, platelet destruction and vascular endothelial injury are the two major responses to an immune-mediated response to heparin. Platelet factor 4 (PF4) (protein made and released by platelets) binds to heparin. This PF4-heparin complex then binds to the platelet surface, leading to further platelet activation and release of more PF4, thus creating a positive feedback loop. Antibodies are created against the PF4-heparin-platelet complex, and they are removed prematurely from circulation, leading to thrombocytopenia and platelet-fibrin thrombi. Platelet aggregation also induces heparin to be neutralized.

## Clinical Manifestations

Many patients with thrombocytopenia are asymptomatic. The most common symptom is bleeding, usually mucosal or cutaneous. Mucosal bleeding may manifest as epistaxis and gingival bleeding, and large bullous hemorrhages may appear on the buccal mucosa because of the lack of vessel protection by the submucosal tissue.

Bleeding into the skin is manifested as petechiae, purpura, or superficial ecchymoses (Fig. 30-6). *Petechiae* are small, flat, pinpoint, red or reddish brown microhemorrhages. When the platelet count is low, RBCs may leak out of the blood vessels and into the skin to cause petechiae. When petechiae are numerous, the resulting reddish skin bruise is called *purpura.* Larger purplish lesions caused by hemorrhage are termed *ecchymoses.* Ecchymoses may be flat or raised; pain and tenderness sometimes are present.

Prolonged bleeding after routine procedures such as venipuncture or IM injection may indicate thrombocytopenia. Because the bleeding may be internal, be aware of manifestations that reflect this type of blood loss, including weakness, fainting, dizziness, tachycardia, abdominal pain, and hypotension.

The major complication of thrombocytopenia is hemorrhage. The hemorrhage may be insidious or acute, and internal or external. It may occur in any area of the body, including the joints, retina, and brain. Cerebral hemorrhage may be fatal. Insidious hemorrhage may first be detected by discovering the anemia that accompanies blood loss.

Because thrombocytopenia can be accompanied by vascular thromboses, signs and symptoms of vascular ischemic problems can manifest (see Chapter 37). For example, subtle confusion, headache, or even serious manifestations such as seizures and coma due to TTP-related thrombosis may be seen. Because signs and symptoms may be subtle, astute and thorough assessment of the patient is essential.

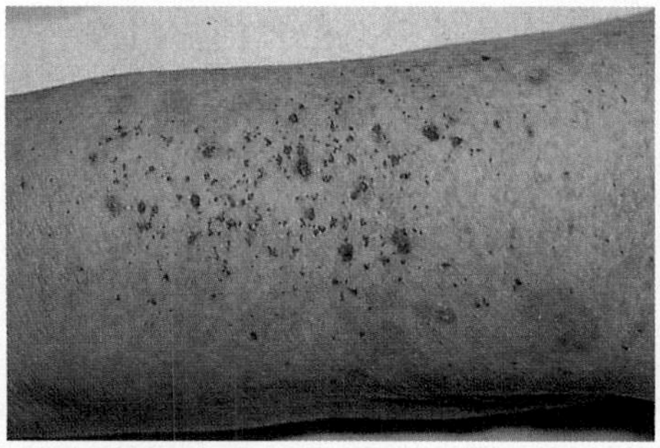

**FIG. 30-6** Acute immune thrombocytopenic purpura commonly manifests with purpuric lesions of this kind, although they may often be widespread by the time medical attention is sought. (From Forbes CD, Jackson WF: *Colour atlas and text of clinical medicine,* ed 3, London, 2003, Mosby.)

## Diagnostic Studies

The platelet count is decreased in thrombocytopenia. Any reduction below 150,000/μL (150 × $10^9$/L) may be termed *thrombocytopenia.* However, prolonged bleeding from trauma or injury does not usually occur until platelet counts are less than 50,000/μL (50 × $10^9$/L). When the count drops below 20,000/μL (20 × $10^9$/L), spontaneous, life-threatening hemorrhages (e.g., intracranial bleeding) can occur. Platelet transfusions are generally not recommended until the count is below 10,000/μL (10 × $10^9$/L), unless the patient is actively bleeding.

The patient's medical history and clinical examination, along with comparisons of laboratory parameters, help to determine the etiology of the thrombocytopenia. Table 30-12 compares the types of thrombocytopenia.[18]

Laboratory tests that assess secondary hemostasis or coagulation, such as the prothrombin time (PT) and aPTT, can be normal even in severe thrombocytopenia. If they are elevated, this may point toward DIC. Bone marrow examination is done to rule out production problems as the cause of thrombocytopenia (e.g., leukemia, aplastic anemia, other myeloproliferative disorders).

Specific assays, such as ITP antigen-specific assay, platelet activation/function assay, or PF4-heparin complex for HIT, can be done to assist with the diagnosis. In TTP, testing for deficiency of ADAMTS13 is not always diagnostic, so an increase of lactate dehydrogenase (LDH) may help establish the diagnosis. When thrombocytopenia occurs with anemia characterized by altered RBC morphology, including *spherocytes* (small, globular, completely hemoglobinated erythrocytes), fragmented cells (schistocytes), and pronounced reticulocytosis, a diagnosis of TTP should be suspected. These findings are partially a result

**TABLE 30-12 Laboratory Results in Thrombocytopenia and DIC**

| Laboratory Test | ITP | TTP | HIT | DIC |
|---|---|---|---|---|
| **Platelets** | ↓↓↓ | ↓↓↓ | ↓↓ | ↓↓↓ |
| **Hemolysis** | | | | |
| Hgb | N | ↓↓ | N | N or ↓ |
| LDH | N | ↑↑↑ | N | ↑ |
| Reticulocytes | N | ↑ | N | N or ↑ |
| Haptoglobin | N | ↓ | N | ↓ |
| Indirect bilirubin | N | ↑ | N | N or ↑ |
| Schistocytes | N | ↑↑↑ | N or ↑ | N or ↑ |
| **Coagulopathy** | | | | |
| PT | N | N | N | ↑ |
| aPTT | N | N | N | ↑ |
| D-dimer | N | N or ↑ | ↑ | ↑↑ |
| Other tests | ITP antigen-specific assay, platelet activation/function assay, *Helicobacter pylori,* bone marrow biopsy | ADAMTS13 | Platelet activation/function assay, PF4-heparin complex | |

*aPTT,* Activated partial thromboplastin time; *LDH,* lactate dehydrogenase; *N,* normal; *PF4,* platelet factor 4; *PT,* prothrombin time.

of intravascular fibrin deposition causing a "slicing" of RBCs. In TTP, thrombocytopenia may be severe, but coagulation studies are normal.

Bone marrow analysis is performed if other test results are inconclusive. When destruction of circulating platelets is the cause, bone marrow analysis shows *megakaryocytes* (precursors of platelets) to be normal or increased, even though circulating platelets are reduced. The absence or decreased number of megakaryocytes on bone marrow biopsy is consistent with thrombocytopenia caused by decreased bone marrow production (e.g., aplastic anemia).

## Interprofessional Care

Interprofessional care of thrombocytopenia differs based on the etiology. Removal or treatment of the underlying cause or disorder is sometimes sufficient. The patient with thrombocytopenia should avoid aspirin and other medications that affect platelet function or production. The following sections discuss management strategies for the different causes of thrombocytopenia (Table 30-13).

**Immune Thrombocytopenic Purpura.** Multiple therapies are used to manage the patient with ITP. If the patient is asymptomatic, therapy may not be used unless the patient's platelet count is below 10,000/μL. Corticosteroids (e.g., prednisone, methylprednisolone) are used initially to treat ITP because of their ability to suppress the phagocytic response of splenic macrophages. This alters the spleen's recognition of platelets and increases the life span of the platelets. In addition, corticosteroids depress antibody formation and reduce capillary leakage.

High doses of IV immunoglobulin (IVIG) and a component of IVIG, anti-$Rh_o$(D) (anti-D, WinRho), may be used in the patient who is unresponsive to corticosteroids or splenectomy, or for whom splenectomy is not an option. It is believed that one way these agents work is by competing with the antiplatelet antibodies for macrophage receptors in the spleen. Rituximab (Rituxan) may be used for its ability to lyse activated B cells, thereby reducing the immune recognition of platelets.

Splenectomy may be indicated if the patient does not respond to the above treatments. Splenectomy can usually be done laparoscopically, and 60% to 70% of patients benefit from splenectomy, resulting in a complete or partial remission.[18] The effectiveness of splenectomy is based on four factors. First, the spleen contains an abundance of the macrophages that sequester and destroy platelets. Second, structural features of the spleen enhance the interaction between antibody-coated platelets and macrophages. Third, some antibody synthesis occurs in the spleen; thus antiplatelet antibodies decrease after splenectomy. Fourth, the spleen normally sequesters approximately one third of the platelets, so its removal increases the number of platelets in circulation.

Romiplostim (Nplate) and eltrombopag (Promacta) are used for patients with chronic ITP who have had an insufficient response to the other treatments or who have a contraindication to splenectomy. These drugs are thrombopoietin receptor agonists, thus increasing platelet production. Danazol, an androgen, may be used along with corticosteroids in some patients. Although the mechanism is not totally understood, danazol reduces the ability of the body to remove antibody-coated platelets from the blood. Immunosuppressive therapy may be used in refractory cases[18] (Table 30-14).

Platelet transfusions may be used to increase platelet counts in cases of life-threatening hemorrhage. Platelets should not be administered prophylactically because of the possibility of antibody formation. The usual indication for administering platelets is for a platelet count less than 10,000/μL or if there is anticipated bleeding before a procedure. Epsilon-aminocaproic acid (EACA, Amicar), an antifibrinolytic agent, may be used for severe bleeding.

**Thrombotic Thrombocytopenic Purpura.** TTP may be treated in a variety of ways. The first step is to treat the underlying disorder (e.g., infection) or remove the causative agent, if identified. If untreated, TTP usually results in irreversible renal failure and death. Plasma exchange (plasmapheresis) (see Chapter 13) is used to aggressively reverse platelet consumption by supplying the appropriate vWF and enzyme (ADAMTS13) and removing the large vWF molecules that bind with platelets. Treatment should be continued daily until the patient's platelet counts normalize and hemolysis has ceased. Corticosteroids may be added to this treatment.

Rituximab is used for patients refractory to plasma exchange; it decreases the level of inhibitory ADAMTS13 IgG antibodies. Other immunosuppressants such as cyclosporine or cyclophosphamide may also be used. Splenectomy may be considered in patients who are refractory to plasma exchange or immunosuppression. The administration of platelets is generally

### TABLE 30-13 Nursing Assessment
### *Thrombocytopenia*

**Subjective Data**

***Important Health Information***

*Past health history:* Recent hemorrhage, excessive bleeding, or viral illness; HIV infection; cancer (especially leukemia or lymphoma); aplastic anemia; systemic lupus erythematosus; cirrhosis; exposure to radiation or toxic chemicals; disseminated intravascular coagulation

*Medications:* Many medications including chemotherapy agents, valproic acid (Depakote), furosemide (Lasix), gold, nonsteroidal antiinflammatory drugs, penicillin

***Functional Health Patterns***

*Health perception–health management:* Family history of bleeding problems; malaise

*Nutritional-metabolic:* Bleeding gingiva; coffee-ground or bloody vomitus; easy bruising

*Elimination:* Hematuria, dark or bloody stools

*Activity-exercise:* Fatigue, weakness, fainting; epistaxis, hemoptysis; dyspnea

*Cognitive-perceptual:* Pain and tenderness in bleeding areas (e.g., abdomen, head, extremities); headache

*Sexuality-reproductive:* Menorrhagia, metrorrhagia

**Objective Data**

***General***

Fever, lethargy

***Integumentary***

Petechiae, ecchymoses, purpura

***Gastrointestinal***

Splenomegaly, abdominal distention; guaiac-positive stools

***Possible Diagnostic Findings***

Platelet count <150,000/μL (150 × $10^9$/L), prolonged bleeding time, ↓ hemoglobin and hematocrit; normal or ↑ megakaryocytes in bone marrow examination

**TABLE 30-14 Interprofessional Care**

***Thrombocytopenia***

**Diagnostic Assessment**
- History and physical examination
- Bone marrow aspiration and biopsy
- CBC, including platelet count
- Specific laboratory studies (Table 30-12)

**Management**

***Immune Thrombocytopenic Purpura***
- Corticosteroids
- IV immunoglobulin (IVIG)
- Anti-$Rh_o$(D)
- Rituximab (Rituxan)
- Splenectomy
- Romiplostim (Nplate)
- Eltrombopag (Promacta)
- Danazol
- Immunosuppressives (e.g., cyclosporine, cyclophosphamide, azathioprine [Imuran], mycophenolate mofetil [CellCept])
- Platelet transfusions

***Thrombotic Thrombocytopenic Purpura***
- Identification and treatment of cause
- Plasmapheresis (plasma exchange)
- Corticosteroids
- Rituximab (Rituxan)
- Immunosuppressives (e.g., cyclophosphamide)
- Chemotherapy (vincristine, vinblastine)
- Splenectomy

***Heparin-Induced Thrombocytopenia***
- Direct thrombin inhibitor (lepirudin [Refludan], argatroban [Acova])
- Indirect thrombin inhibitor (fondaparinux [Arixtra])
- Warfarin (Coumadin)
- Plasmapheresis (plasma exchange)
- Thrombolytic agents

***Decreased Platelet Production***
- Identification and treatment or removal of cause
- Corticosteroids
- Platelet transfusions

contraindicated because this may lead to new vWF-platelet complexes and increased clotting.

**Heparin-Induced Thrombocytopenia.** Heparin must be discontinued when HIT is first recognized. Heparin flushes for vascular catheters should also be stopped.

To maintain anticoagulation, the patient should be started on a direct thrombin inhibitor, such as lepirudin (Refludan) or argatroban (Acova). Fondaparinux (Arixtra), a factor Xa inhibitor (indirect thrombin inhibitor), may be used. Warfarin should be started only when the platelet count has reached 150,000/μL. If the clotting is severe, the most commonly used treatment modalities are plasmapheresis to clear the platelet-aggregating IgG from the blood, protamine sulfate to interrupt the circulating heparin, thrombolytic agents to treat the thromboembolic events, and surgery to remove clots. Platelet transfusions are not effective because they may enhance thromboembolic events.[21]

Patients who have had HIT should never be given heparin or low-molecular-weight heparin (LMWH). This should be clearly marked in the patient's medical record.

**Thrombocytopenia From Decreased Platelet Production.** The management of acquired thrombocytopenia is based on identifying the cause and treating the disease or removing the causative agent. If the precipitating factor is unknown, the patient may receive corticosteroids. Platelet transfusions are given if life-threatening hemorrhage develops.

Often acquired thrombocytopenia is caused by another underlying condition (e.g., aplastic anemia, leukemia) or therapy used to treat another problem. For example, in acute leukemia all blood cell types may be depressed. Additionally, the patient may receive chemotherapeutic drugs that cause bone marrow suppression. If the patient can be adequately supported throughout the course of chemotherapy-induced thrombocytopenia, the thrombocytopenia will also resolve.

## NURSING MANAGEMENT: THROMBOCYTOPENIA

### Nursing Assessment

Subjective and objective data that should be obtained from a patient with thrombocytopenia are presented in Table 30-13.

### Nursing Diagnoses

Nursing diagnoses for the patient with thrombocytopenia may include, but are not limited to, the following.
- Impaired oral mucous membrane *related to* low platelet counts and/or effects of pathologic conditions and treatment
- Risk for bleeding *related to* decreased platelets
- Deficient knowledge *related to* lack of information regarding the disease process and treatment

### Planning

The overall goals are that the patient with thrombocytopenia will (1) have no gross or occult bleeding, (2) maintain vascular integrity, and (3) manage home care to prevent any complications related to an increased risk for bleeding.

### Nursing Implementation

**Health Promotion.** Discourage excessive use of over-the-counter (OTC) medications known to be possible causes of acquired thrombocytopenia. Many medications contain aspirin as an ingredient. Aspirin reduces platelet adhesiveness, thus contributing to bleeding.

Encourage persons to have a complete medical evaluation if manifestations of bleeding tendencies (e.g., prolonged epistaxis, petechiae) develop. Observe for early signs of thrombocytopenia in the patient receiving cancer chemotherapy drugs.

**Acute Care.** The goal during acute episodes of thrombocytopenia is to prevent or control hemorrhage (see eNursing Care Plan 30-2 on the website for this chapter). In the patient with thrombocytopenia, bleeding is usually from superficial sites. Deep bleeding (into muscles, joints, and abdomen) usually occurs only when clotting factors are diminished. Emphasize that a seemingly minor nosebleed or new petechiae may indicate potential hemorrhage and the HCP should be notified.

Bleeding from the posterior nasopharynx may be difficult to detect because the blood may be swallowed. If a subcutaneous injection is unavoidable, the use of a small-gauge needle and application of direct pressure for at least 5 to 10 minutes after injection is indicated, or application of an ice pack may be helpful. Avoid IM injections. Help the patient understand the importance of adherence to self-care measures that reduce the risk of bleeding (Table 30-15).

Note that many of these disorders may be accompanied by vascular clotting, and appropriate assessment and management should be taken (see Chapter 37). As bleeding occurs, RBC and coagulation factors are consumed along with platelets, so it is important to monitor all blood cell and coagulation studies.

In a woman with thrombocytopenia, menstrual blood loss may exceed the usual amount and duration. Counting sanitary napkins used during menses is another important intervention to detect excess blood loss. Blood loss of 50 mL will completely soak a sanitary napkin. Suppression of menses with hormonal agents may be indicated during predictable periods of thrombocytopenia (e.g., during chemotherapy and HSCT) to reduce blood loss from menses.

Closely monitor the platelet count, coagulation studies, hemoglobin, and hematocrit. Together these provide important information regarding potential or actual bleeding.

The proper administration of platelet transfusions is an important nursing responsibility. This is discussed under Blood Component Therapy later in this chapter.

◆ **Ambulatory Care.** Monitor the patient with ITP who is receiving treatment for the response to therapy. Teach the person with acquired thrombocytopenia to avoid causative agents when possible (Table 30-11). If the causative agents cannot be avoided (e.g., chemotherapy), teach the patient to avoid injury or trauma during these periods and to be aware of the clinical signs and symptoms of bleeding caused by thrombocytopenia (Table 30-15).

**TABLE 30-15 Patient & Caregiver Teaching**

***Thrombocytopenia***

Include the following instructions when teaching a patient or caregiver the precautions to take when the platelet count is low.

1. Notify your HCP of any manifestations of bleeding. These include the following:
   - Black, tarry, or bloody bowel movements
   - Black or bloody vomit, sputum, or urine
   - Bruising or small red or purple spots on the skin
   - Bleeding from the mouth or anywhere in the body
   - Headache or changes in how well you can see
   - Difficulty talking, sudden weakness of an arm or leg, confusion
2. Ask your HCP regarding restrictions in your normal activities, such as vigorous exercise or lifting weights. Generally, walking can be done safely and should be done with sturdy shoes or slippers. If you are weak and at risk for falling, get help or supervision when getting out of bed or chair.
3. Do not blow your nose forcefully; gently pat it with a tissue if needed. For a nosebleed, keep your head up and apply firm pressure to the nostrils and bridge of your nose. If bleeding continues, place an ice bag over the bridge of your nose and the nape of your neck. If you are unable to stop a nosebleed after 10 min, call your HCP.
4. Do not bend down with your head lower than your waist.
5. Prevent constipation by drinking plenty of fluids. Do not strain when having a bowel movement. Your HCP may prescribe a stool softener. Do not use a suppository, an enema, or a rectal thermometer without the permission of your HCP.
6. Shave only with an electric razor. Do not use blades.
7. Do not tweeze your eyebrows or other body hair.
8. Do not puncture your skin, such as getting tattoos or body piercing.
9. Avoid using any medication that can prolong bleeding, such as aspirin. Other medications and herbs can have similar effects. If you are unsure about any medication, ask your HCP or pharmacist about it in relation to your thrombocytopenia.
10. Use a soft-bristle toothbrush to prevent injuring the gums. Flossing is usually safe if it is done gently using the thin tape floss. Do not use alcohol-based mouthwashes, since they can dry your gums and increase bleeding.
11. Women who are menstruating should keep track of the number of pads that are used per day. When you start using more pads per day than usual or bleed more days, notify your HCP. Do not use tampons; only use sanitary pads.
12. Ask your HCP before you have any invasive procedures done, such as a dental cleaning, manicure, or pedicure.

Patients with either ITP or acquired thrombocytopenia should have planned periodic medical evaluations to assess their status. These regular evaluations can be used to assess and treat situations in which exacerbations and bleeding are likely to occur. The impact of either an acute or a chronic condition on the patient's quality of life should also be addressed appropriately.

### ◆ Evaluation

The expected outcomes are that the patient with thrombocytopenia will

- Have no evidence of bleeding or bruising
- Verbalize required knowledge and skills to manage disease process at home

## HEMOPHILIA AND VON WILLEBRAND DISEASE

**Hemophilia** is an X-linked recessive genetic disorder caused by a defective or deficient coagulation factor. The two major types of hemophilia, which can occur in mild to severe forms, are *hemophilia A* (classic hemophilia, factor VIII deficiency) and *hemophilia B* (Christmas disease, factor IX deficiency). *von Willebrand disease* is a related disorder involving a deficiency of the von Willebrand coagulation protein. Factor VIII is synthesized in the liver and circulates as a complex with von Willebrand factor (vWF).

Hemophilia A is the most common form of hemophilia, accounting for about 80% to 85% of all hemophilia cases. Although rare, there are cases of *acquired hemophilia A*, which is due to the development of antibodies against the body's own factor VIII. von Willebrand disease is considered the most common congenital bleeding disorder.[22]

**Genetic Link.** The inheritance patterns of hemophilia and von Willebrand disease are compared in Table 30-16. (X-linked genetic disorders are discussed in Chapter 12 and Table 12-2.)

### Clinical Manifestations and Complications

All clinical manifestations relate to bleeding, and any bleeding episode in persons with hemophilia may lead to a life-threatening hemorrhage. Clinical manifestations and complications related to hemophilia include (1) slow, persistent, prolonged bleeding from minor trauma and small cuts; (2) delayed bleeding after minor injuries (the delay may be several hours or days); (3) uncontrollable hemorrhage after dental extractions or irritation of the gingiva with a hard-bristle toothbrush; (4) epistaxis,

**TABLE 30-16 Types of Hemophilia**

| Type | Inheritance Pattern |
|---|---|
| **Hemophilia A** | |
| Factor VIII | Recessive sex-linked (transmitted by female carriers, displayed almost exclusively in men) |
| **Hemophilia B** | |
| Factor IX | Recessive sex-linked (transmitted by female carriers, displayed almost exclusively in men) |
| **von Willebrand Disease** | |
| vWF, variable factor VIII deficiencies and platelet dysfunction | Autosomal dominant, seen in both genders<br>Recessive (in severe forms of the disease) |

*vWF*, von Willebrand factor.

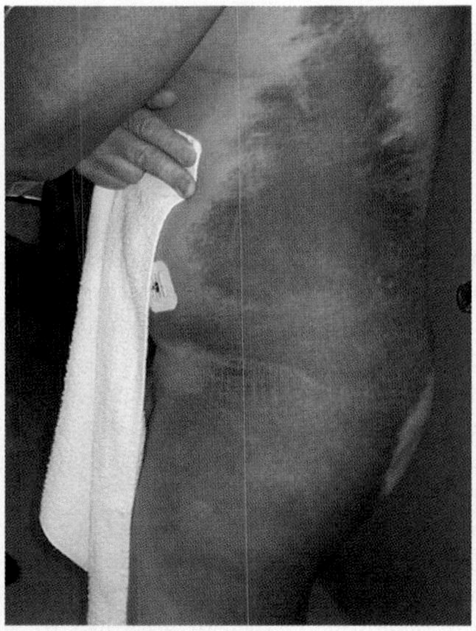

**FIG. 30-7** Severe ecchymoses in a person with hemophilia after a fall. (Courtesy Peter Bonner.)

## GENETICS IN CLINICAL PRACTICE

### *Hemophilia A and B*

**Genetic Basis**
- X-linked recessive disorder
- *Hemophilia A:* Caused by mutations in the *F8* gene that provides instructions for making coagulation factor VIII
- *Hemophilia B:* Caused by mutations in the *F9* gene that provides instructions for making coagulation factor IX
- Mutations in the *F8* or *F9* gene lead to the production of an abnormal version or reduced amounts of these coagulation factors.

**Incidence**
- *Hemophilia A:* 1 in 5000 to 10,000 male births
- *Hemophilia B:* 1 in 30,000 to 50,000 male births

**Genetic Testing**
- DNA testing is available.

**Clinical Implications**
- Female carriers transmit the genetic defect to 50% of their sons, and 50% of their daughters are carriers.
- Males with hemophilia do not transmit the genetic defect to their sons, but all of their daughters are carriers.
- Female hemophilia can occur if a male with hemophilia mates with a female carrier. However, this is a rare situation.
- Clinical manifestations of hemophilia A and B are similar.
- Replacement therapy is available for factors VIII and IX (Table 30-19).

especially after a blow to the face; (5) GI bleeding from ulcers and gastritis; (6) hematuria and potential renal failure from GU trauma and splenic rupture resulting from falls or abdominal trauma; (7) ecchymoses and subcutaneous hematomas (Fig. 30-7) and possible compartment syndrome; (8) neurologic signs, such as pain, anesthesia, and paralysis, which may develop from nerve compression caused by hematoma formation; and (9) hemarthrosis (bleeding into the joints) (Fig. 30-8), which may lead to joint injury and deformity severe enough to cause crippling (most commonly in knees, elbows, shoulders, hips, and ankles).[23]

In children these manifestations may lead to the diagnosis. In adults these developments may be the first sign of a newly

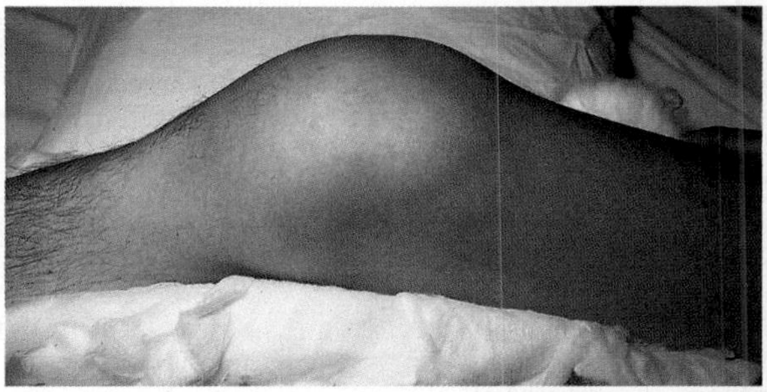

**FIG. 30-8** Acute hemarthrosis of the knee is a common complication of hemophilia. (From Forbes CD, Jackson WF: *Colour atlas and text of clinical medicine,* ed 3, London, 2003, Mosby.)

**TABLE 30-17 Laboratory Results in Hemophilia**

| Test | Results |
|---|---|
| **Prothrombin time** | Normal. No involvement of extrinsic system |
| **Thrombin time** | Normal. No impairment of thrombin-fibrinogen reaction |
| **Platelet count** | Normal. Adequate platelet production |
| **Partial thromboplastin time** | Prolonged because of deficiency in intrinsic clotting system factor |
| **Bleeding time** | Prolonged in von Willebrand disease because of structurally defective platelets. Normal in hemophilia A and B because platelets not affected |
| **Factor assays** | Reductions of factor VIII in hemophilia A, factor IX in hemophilia B, vWF in von Willebrand disease |

*vWF,* von Willebrand factor.

diagnosed mild form of the disease that escaped detection through a childhood free of major injuries, dental procedures, or surgeries.

### Diagnostic Studies

Laboratory studies are used to determine the type of hemophilia present. Any factor deficiency within the intrinsic system (factor VIII, IX, XI, or XII or vWF) will yield the laboratory results presented in Table 30-17.

### Interprofessional Care

The goals of interprofessional care are to prevent and treat bleeding. Care for persons with hemophilia or von Willebrand disease requires (1) preventive care, (2) the use of replacement therapy during acute bleeding episodes and as prophylaxis, and (3) the treatment of the complications of the disease and its therapy. Today most patients can expect almost normal life spans free of bloodborne illnesses because of improved preparation of replacement products, improved screening of blood donor populations, and use of recombinant replacement factors.[23]

Replacement of deficient clotting factors is the primary means of supporting a patient with hemophilia. In addition to treating acute crises, replacement therapy may be given before surgery and dental care as a prophylactic measure.[24] Examples of replacement therapy[25] are listed in Table 30-18. Fresh frozen plasma, once commonly used for replacement therapy, is rarely used today.

**TABLE 30-18 Drug Therapy**

***Replacement Factors for Hemophilia****

| Factor VIII | Factor IX | Von Willebrand | For Patients Who Have Inhibitors |
|---|---|---|---|
| Advate | Alphanine SD | Vonvendi | NovoSeven (factor VIIa) |
| Alphanate | Alprolix | | Autoplex T |
| Eloctate | Bebulin VH | | FEIBA (factor VIII inhibitor bypassing activity) |
| Helixate FS | BeneFIX | | |
| Hemofil M | Mononine | | |
| Humate-P | Profilnine SD | | |
| Koāte-DVI | ProplexT | | |
| Kogenate FS | | | |
| Monoclate P | | | |
| Obizur† | | | |
| Recombinate | | | |
| Xyntha | | | |

*List is not all inclusive.
†For acquired hemophilia A.

For mild hemophilia A and certain subtypes of von Willebrand disease, desmopressin acetate (also known as *DDAVP*), a synthetic analog of vasopressin, may be used to stimulate an increase in factor VIII and vWF. This drug acts on platelets and endothelial cells to cause the release of vWF, which subsequently binds with factor VIII, thus increasing its concentration. It can be administered IV, subcutaneously, or by intranasal spray. Beneficial effects (e.g., decreased bleeding time) of DDAVP, when administered IV, are seen within 30 minutes and can last for more than 12 hours. Because the effect of DDAVP is relatively short lived, the patient must be closely monitored and repeated doses may be necessary. It is an appropriate therapy for minor bleeding episodes and dental procedures. The intranasal form may be indicated for home therapy for some patients with mild to moderate forms of the disease.

Antifibrinolytic therapy (tranexamic acid [Cyklokapron] and epsilon-aminocaproic acid) inhibits fibrinolysis by inhibiting plasminogen activation in the fibrin clot, thereby enhancing clot stability. These agents are used to stabilize clots in areas of increased fibrinolysis, such as the oral cavity, and in patients with difficult episodes of epistaxis and menorrhagia. Topical thrombin and fibrin sealants may also be used for mucosal bleeding.

Complications of the treatment of hemophilia include development of inhibitors to factors VIII or IX, transfusion-transmitted infectious disorders (hepatitis, HIV), allergic reactions, and thrombotic complications with the use of factor IX because it contains activated coagulation factors. Patients with vWF may also develop antibodies against vWF concentrates, the infusion of which could cause life-threatening anaphylaxis. Thus replacement factors for these patients should not contain vWF.

The most common difficulties with acute management are starting factor replacement therapy too late and stopping it too soon. Generally, minor bleeding episodes should be treated for at least 72 hours. Surgery and traumatic injuries may require more prolonged therapy. Chronically, development of inhibitors to the factor products has occurred and requires individualized expert patient management. Designated treatment centers in the United States and many other countries provide interprofessional care of hemophilia and related disorders. Gene therapy has been used on an experimental basis to treat hemophilia.[23]

## NURSING MANAGEMENT: HEMOPHILIA

### Nursing Implementation

**Health Promotion.** Because of the hereditary nature of hemophilia, referral of affected persons for genetic counseling before reproduction is an important measure. This is especially important because many persons with hemophilia live into adulthood. Reproductive concerns and long-term effects are issues that you should include in the patient's care plan.

**Acute Care.** Interventions are related primarily to controlling bleeding and include the following:

1. Stop the topical bleeding as quickly as possible by applying direct pressure or ice, packing the area with Gelfoam or fibrin foam, and applying topical hemostatic agents such as thrombin.
2. Administer the specific coagulation factor to raise the patient's level of the deficient coagulation factor. Monitor the patient for signs and symptoms, such as hypersensitivity.
3. When joint bleeding occurs, in addition to administering replacement factors, it is important to totally rest the involved joint to prevent crippling deformities from hemarthrosis. Pack the joint in ice. Give analgesics (e.g., acetaminophen, codeine) to reduce severe pain. Aspirin and aspirin-containing compounds should never be used. As soon as bleeding ceases, encourage mobilization of the affected area through range-of-motion exercises and physical therapy. Weight bearing is avoided until all swelling has resolved and muscle strength has returned.
4. Manage any life-threatening complications that may develop as a result of hemorrhage or side effects from coagulation factors. Examples include nursing interventions to prevent or treat airway obstruction from hemorrhage into the neck and pharynx, recognition of compartment syndrome in an extremity, and early assessment and treatment of intracranial bleeding.

**Ambulatory Care.** Home management is a primary consideration for the patient with hemophilia because the disease follows a progressive, chronic course. The quality and length of life may be significantly affected by the patient's knowledge of the illness and how to live with it. The patient and caregiver can be referred to a local chapter of the Hemophilia Federation of America to encourage associations with other individuals who are dealing with the problems of hemophilia. Provide ongoing assessment of the patient's adaptation to the illness. Psychosocial support and assistance should be readily available as needed.

Most of the long-term care measures are related to patient teaching. Teach the patient to recognize disease-related problems and to learn which problems can be resolved at home and which require hospitalization. Immediate medical attention is required for severe pain or swelling of a muscle or joint that restricts movement or inhibits sleep and for a head injury, swelling in the neck or mouth, abdominal pain, hematuria, melena, and skin wounds in need of suturing.

Teach the patient to perform daily oral hygiene without causing trauma. Understanding how to prevent injuries is another consideration. Advise the patient to participate only in noncontact sports (e.g., golf) and to wear gloves when doing household chores to prevent cuts or abrasions from knives, hammers, and other tools. The patient should wear a Medic Alert tag to ensure that HCPs know about the hemophilia in case of an accident. Many patients or their caregivers can be taught to self-administer the factor replacement therapies at home.

### ◆ Evaluation

The overall expected outcomes are similar to those for the patient with thrombocytopenia (see p. 626).

## DISSEMINATED INTRAVASCULAR COAGULATION

**Disseminated intravascular coagulation** (DIC) is a serious bleeding and thrombotic disorder that results from abnormally initiated and accelerated clotting. Subsequent decreases in clotting factors and platelets ensue, which may lead to uncontrollable hemorrhage. The term *disseminated intravascular coagulation* can be misleading, because it suggests that blood is clotting. However, this condition is characterized by the profuse bleeding that results from the depletion of platelets and clotting factors. DIC is always caused by an underlying disease or condition. The underlying problem must be treated for the DIC to resolve.

### Etiology and Pathophysiology

DIC is not a disease. It is an abnormal response of the normal clotting cascade stimulated by a disease process or disorder.[26,27] The diseases and disorders known to predispose a patient to DIC are listed in Table 30-19. DIC can occur as an acute, catastrophic condition or it may exist at a subacute or chronic level. Each condition may have one or multiple triggering mechanisms to start the clotting cascade. For example, tumors and traumatized or necrotic tissue release tissue factors into circulation. Endotoxin from gram-negative bacteria activates several steps in the coagulation cascade.

Tissue factor is released at the site of tissue injury and by some malignancies, such as leukemia, and enhances normal coagulation mechanisms. Abundant intravascular thrombin, the most powerful coagulant, is produced (Fig. 30-9). It catalyzes the conversion of fibrinogen to fibrin and enhances platelet aggregation. There is widespread fibrin and platelet deposition in capillaries and arterioles, resulting in thrombosis. This process can lead to multiorgan failure.

In addition, clotting inhibitory mechanisms, such as antithrombin III (AT III) and protein C, are depressed. Excessive clotting activates the fibrinolytic system, which in turn breaks down the newly formed clot, creating fibrin split products (FSPs). These products have anticoagulant properties and inhibit normal blood clotting. Ultimately, as FSPs accumulate and clotting factors are depleted, the blood loses its ability to clot. Therefore a stable clot cannot be formed at injury sites, which predisposes the patient to hemorrhage.

Chronic and subacute DIC is most commonly seen in patients with long-standing illnesses such as malignant disorders or autoimmune diseases. Occasionally these patients have

**TABLE 30-19 Risk Factors for DIC**

| | |
|---|---|
| **Acute DIC**<br>Shock<br>• Hemorrhagic<br>• Cardiogenic<br>• Anaphylactic<br>Septicemia (bacterial, viral, fungal, parasitic)<br>Hemolytic processes<br>• Transfusion of mismatched blood<br>• Acute hemolysis from infection or immunologic disorders<br>Obstetric conditions<br>• Abruptio placentae<br>• Amniotic fluid embolism<br>• Septic abortion<br>• HELLP syndrome<br>Malignancies<br>• Acute leukemia<br>• Metastatic solid tumors<br>Tissue damage<br>• Extensive burns and trauma<br>• Heatstroke<br>• Severe head injury | • Transplant rejections<br>• Postoperative damage, especially after extracorporeal membrane oxygenation<br>• Fat and pulmonary emboli<br>• Snakebites<br>• Glomerulonephritis<br>• Acute anoxia (e.g., after cardiac arrest)<br>• Prosthetic devices<br>• Fulminant hepatitis<br>**Subacute DIC**<br>Malignancy<br>• Myeloproliferative/lymphoproliferative malignancies<br>• Metastatic cancer<br>Obstetric<br>• Retained dead fetus<br>**Chronic DIC**<br>Liver disease<br>Systemic lupus erythematosus<br>Malignancy |

*DIC,* Disseminated intravascular coagulation; *HELLP syndrome,* a life-threatening liver disorder thought to be a type of severe preeclampsia, it is characterized by **H**emolysis (destruction of red blood cells), **E**levated **L**iver enzymes (which indicate liver damage), and **L**ow **P**latelet count.

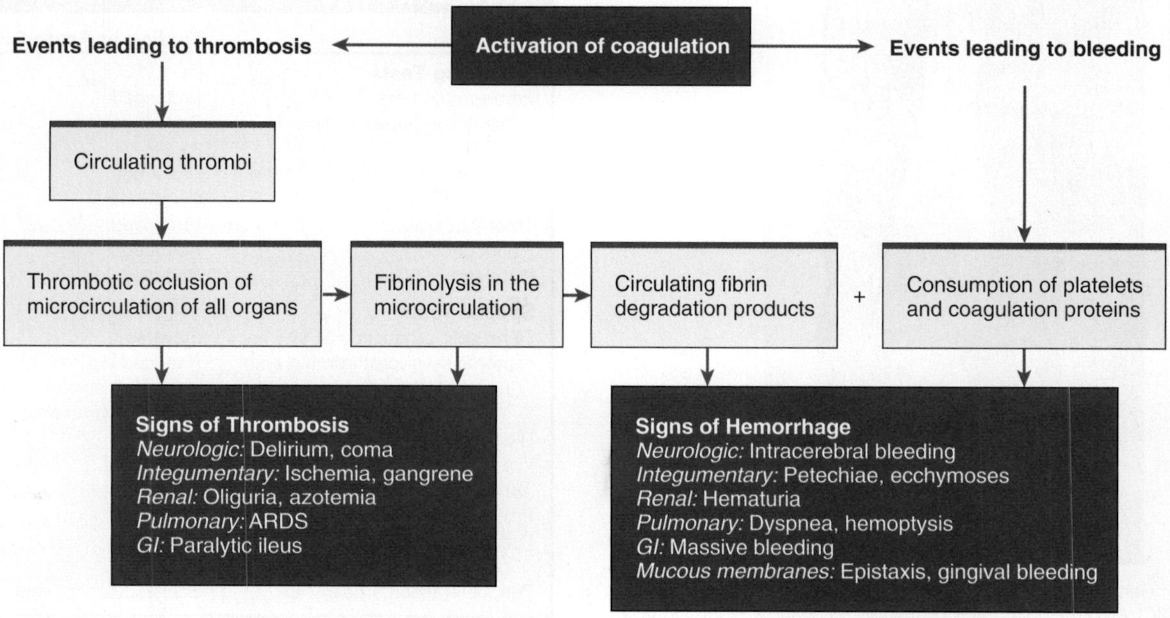


**FIG. 30-9** Sequence of events that occur during disseminated intravascular coagulation (DIC).

subclinical disease manifested only by laboratory abnormalities. However, the clinical spectrum ranges from easy bruising to hemorrhage, and from hypercoagulability to thrombosis.

## Clinical Manifestations

DIC has both bleeding and thrombotic manifestations. Multiple factors cause bleeding manifestations of DIC (Fig. 30-9) and result from consumption and depletion of platelets and coagulation factors, as well as clot lysis and formation of FSPs that have anticoagulant properties. Bleeding in a person with no previous history or obvious cause should be questioned because it may be one of the first manifestations of acute DIC.

*Bleeding manifestations* include (1) integumentary manifestations such as pallor, petechiae, purpura (Fig. 30-10), oozing blood, venipuncture site bleeding, hematomas, and occult hemorrhage; (2) respiratory manifestations such as tachypnea, hemoptysis, and orthopnea; (3) cardiovascular manifestations such as tachycardia and hypotension; (4) GI manifestations such as upper and lower GI bleeding, abdominal distention, and bloody stools; (5) urinary manifestations such as hematuria; (6) neurologic manifestations such as vision changes, dizziness, headache, changes in mental status, and irritability; and (7) musculoskeletal complaints such as bone and joint pain.

*Thrombotic manifestations* are a result of fibrin or platelet deposition in the microvasculature (Fig. 30-9). They include (1) integumentary manifestations, such as cyanosis, ischemic tissue necrosis (e.g., gangrene), and hemorrhagic necrosis; (2) respiratory manifestations, such as tachypnea, dyspnea, pulmonary emboli, and acute respiratory distress syndrome (ARDS); (3) cardiovascular manifestations, such as electrocardiogram (ECG) changes and venous distention; (4) GI manifestations, such as abdominal pain and paralytic ileus; and (5) kidney damage and oliguria, leading to failure.

## Diagnostic Studies

Tests to diagnose acute DIC are listed in Table 30-20. As more clots are made in the body, more breakdown products from fibrinogen and fibrin are also formed. These are termed *fibrin split products* (FSPs), and they interfere with blood coagulation by (1) coating the platelets and interfering with platelet function; (2) interfering with thrombin and thus disrupting coagulation; and (3) attaching to fibrinogen, which interferes with the polymerization process necessary to form a stable clot. D-dimer, a polymer resulting from the breakdown of fibrin (and not fibrinogen), is a specific marker for the degree of fibrinolysis. In general, tests that measure raw materials needed for coagulation (e.g., platelets, fibrinogen) are reduced, and values that measure clotting times are prolonged. Fragmented erythrocytes (schistocytes), indicative of partial occlusion of small vessels by fibrin thrombi, may be found on blood smears.

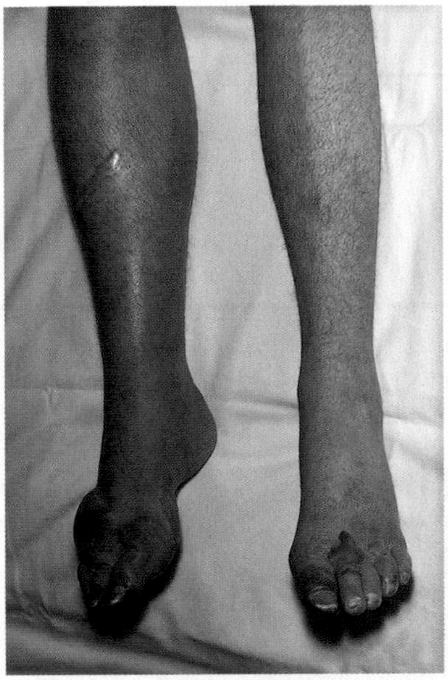

**FIG. 30-10** Gangrene resulting from severe disseminated intravascular coagulation (DIC). (From Howard MR, Hamilton PJ: *Haematology: an illustrated colour atlas,* ed 4, London, 2013, Churchill Livingston.)

## Interprofessional Care

It is important to diagnose DIC quickly, stabilize the patient (e.g., oxygenation, volume replacement), treat the underlying causative disease or problem, and control the ongoing thrombosis and bleeding. Depending on its severity, a variety of different methods are used to manage DIC (Fig. 30-11). First, if chronic DIC is diagnosed in a patient who is not bleeding, no therapy for DIC is necessary. Treatment of the underlying disease may be sufficient to reverse the DIC (e.g., chemotherapy when DIC is caused by malignancy). Second, when the patient with DIC is bleeding, therapy is directed toward providing support with necessary blood products while treating the primary disorder.

The blood products are administered cautiously based on specific component deficiencies to patients who have serious bleeding, are at high risk for bleeding (e.g., surgery), or require invasive procedures. Blood product support with platelets, cryoprecipitate, and fresh frozen plasma (FFP) is usually reserved for a patient with life-threatening hemorrhage. Therapy stabilizes a patient, prevents exsanguination or massive thrombosis, and permits institution of definitive therapy to treat the underlying cause. Cryoprecipitate replaces factor VIII and fibrinogen and is given if the fibrinogen level is below 80 to 100 mg/dL.[22] Fresh frozen plasma is given only to patients with

**TABLE 30-20 Laboratory Results in Acute DIC**

| Test | Finding in Acute DIC |
|---|---|
| **Screening Tests** | |
| Prothrombin time (PT) | Prolonged |
| Partial thromboplastin time (PTT) | Prolonged |
| Activated partial thromboplastin time (aPTT) | Prolonged |
| Thrombin time | Prolonged |
| Fibrinogen | Reduced |
| Platelets | Reduced |
| **Special Tests** | |
| Fibrin split products (FSPs) | Elevated |
| Factor assays (prothrombin and factors V, VIII, X, XIII) | Reduced but may give misleading results, since V and VIII rise with inflammation |
| D-dimers (cross-linked fibrin fragments) | Elevated |
| Antithrombin III (AT III) | Reduced |
| Proteins C and S | Reduced |
| Plasminogen, tissue plasminogen activator | Reduced |
| Peripheral blood smear | Schistocytes present |

*DIC,* Disseminated intravascular coagulation.

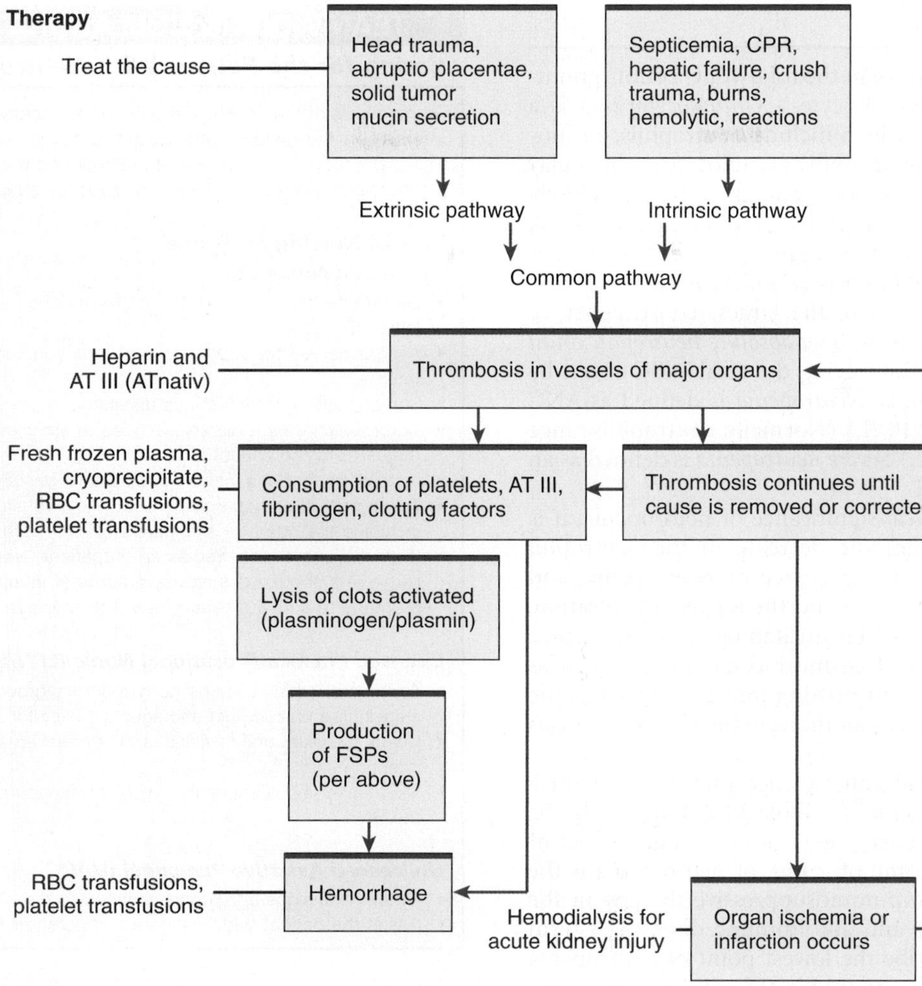


**FIG. 30-11** Sites of action for therapies in disseminated intravascular coagulation (DIC). *AT III,* Antithrombin III; *FSPs,* fibrin split products.

significant bleeding and a prolonged PT and aPTT. It replaces all clotting factors except platelets and provides a source of antithrombin.

A patient with manifestations of thrombosis is often treated by anticoagulation with heparin or low-molecular-weight heparin. Heparin is used in the treatment of DIC only when the benefit (reduce clotting) outweighs the risk (further bleeding). Antithrombin III (ATnativ) may be useful in fulminant DIC, although it increases the risk of bleeding. Chronic DIC does not respond to oral anticoagulants, but it can be controlled with long-term use of heparin.

## ❖ NURSING MANAGEMENT: DISSEMINATED INTRAVASCULAR COAGULATION

### ◆ Nursing Diagnoses

Nursing diagnoses for the patient with DIC may include, but are not limited to, the following:

- Ineffective peripheral tissue perfusion *related to* bleeding and sluggish or diminished blood flow secondary to thrombosis
- Acute pain *related to* bleeding into tissues and diagnostic procedures
- Decreased cardiac output *related to* fluid volume deficit
- Anxiety *related to* fear of the unknown, disease process, diagnostic procedures, and therapy

### ◆ Nursing Implementation

Be alert to the possible development of DIC and especially to the precipitating factors listed in Table 30-19. Remember that because DIC is secondary to an underlying disease, the causative problem must be managed while providing supportive care for the manifestations of DIC.

Appropriate nursing interventions are essential to the survival of a patient with acute DIC. Astute ongoing assessment, active attention to manifestations of DIC, and prompt administration of prescribed therapies are crucial. Table 30-14 and eNursing Care Plan 30-2 (available on the website for this chapter) provide assessments and interventions appropriate for the patient with DIC.

Early detection of bleeding and clotting, both occult and overt, must be a primary goal. Assess for signs of external bleeding (e.g., petechiae, oozing at IV or injection sites), signs of internal bleeding (e.g., increased heart rate, changes in mental status, increasing abdominal girth, pain), and any indications that microthrombi may be causing clinically significant organ damage (e.g., decreased renal output). Minimize tissue damage and protect the patient from additional sources of bleeding.

An additional nursing responsibility is to administer blood products and medications correctly. (Blood product transfusion is discussed later in this chapter on pp. 647-652.)

## NEUTROPENIA

*Leukopenia* refers to a decrease in the total WBC count (granulocytes, monocytes, and lymphocytes). *Granulocytopenia* is a deficiency of granulocytes, which include neutrophils, eosinophils, and basophils. The neutrophilic granulocytes, which play a major role in phagocytizing pathogenic microbes, are closely monitored in clinical practice as an indicator of a patient's risk for infection. A reduction in neutrophils is termed **neutropenia**. (Some clinicians use the terms *granulocytopenia* and *neutropenia* interchangeably because the largest constituency of granulocytes is the neutrophils.) The *absolute neutrophil count* (ANC) is determined by multiplying the total WBC count by the percentage of neutrophils. *Neutropenia* is defined as ANC less than 1000 cells/μL ($1 \times 10^9$/L). (Normally, neutrophils range from 2200 to 7700 cells/μL.) *Severe neutropenia* is defined as an ANC less than 500 cells/μL.

In considering the clinical significance of neutropenia, it is important to know whether the decrease in the neutrophil count was gradual or rapid, the degree of neutropenia, and the duration. The faster the drop and the longer the duration, the greater the likelihood of life-threatening infection, sepsis, and death. Other factors and co-morbid conditions, such as being older than 60, having an existing infection, being in the hospital, and having diabetes, can increase the risk of a serious infection.

Neutropenia is a clinical consequence that occurs with a variety of conditions or disease[28,29] (Table 30-21). It can also be an expected effect, a side effect, or an unintentional effect of certain drugs. The most common cause of neutropenia is the use of chemotherapy and immunosuppressive therapy in the treatment of malignancies and autoimmune diseases. A term that is often used to describe the lowest point of neutropenia (and other blood cells) in a patient treated with chemotherapy is *nadir.*

### Clinical Manifestations

The patient with neutropenia is predisposed to infection with opportunistic pathogens and nonpathogenic organisms from the normal body flora. When the WBC count is depressed or immature WBCs are present, normal phagocytic mechanisms are impaired. Also the classic manifestations of inflammation—redness, heat, and swelling—may not occur. WBCs are the major component of pus. Therefore in the patient with neutropenia, pus formation (e.g., as a visible skin lesion or as pulmonary infiltrates on a chest x-ray) is also absent.

**! SAFETY ALERT Neutropenia**

- A low-grade fever in neutropenic patients is of great significance because it may indicate infection and lead to septic shock and death unless treated promptly.
- Neutropenic fever (≥100.4° F [38° C] and a neutrophil count <500/μL) is a medical emergency.
- Blood cultures should be drawn STAT and antibiotics started within 1 hr.

When fever occurs in a neutropenic patient, it is assumed to be caused by infection and requires immediate attention. The immunocompromised, neutropenic patient has little or no ability to fight infection. Thus minor infections can lead rapidly to sepsis. The mucous membranes of the throat and mouth, skin, perineal area, and pulmonary system are common entry points for pathogenic organisms in susceptible hosts.

Clinical manifestations related to infection at these sites include complaints of sore throat and dysphagia, ulcerative lesions of the pharyngeal and buccal mucosa, diarrhea, rectal tenderness, vaginal itching or discharge, shortness of breath, and nonproductive cough. Any minor complaint of pain or any other symptom by the patient may be significant and should be reported to the HCP immediately. These seemingly minor complaints can progress to fever, chills, sepsis, septic shock, and death if not recognized and treated early.

Systemic infections caused by bacterial, fungal, and viral organisms are common in patients with neutropenia. The patient's own flora (normally nonpathogenic) contributes significantly to life-threatening infections such as pneumonia. Organisms known to be common sources of infection include gram-positive coagulase-negative staphylococci and *Staphylococcus aureus* and gram-negative organisms such as *Escherichia coli* and *Pseudomonas aeruginosa*.[30] Fungi involved include *Candida* (usually *C. albicans*) and *Aspergillus* organisms. Viral infections caused by reactivation of herpes simplex and zoster are common after prolonged periods of neutropenia, such as in HSCT patients.

**TEAMWORK & COLLABORATION**

***Caring for the Patient With Neutropenia***

All members of the health care team have important roles in preventing infection in the patient with neutropenia. Careful hand washing is an important preventive measure and should be done before, during, and after patient care by everyone caring for the patient.

**Role of Nursing Personnel**

***Registered Nurse (RN)***

- Determine the type of isolation precautions that need to be initiated, if any.
- Assess patient for subtle signs of infection such as confusion or fatigue.
- Screen visitors for infectious diseases.
- Communicate with dietary services to eliminate undercooked meats from the patient's diet.
- Instruct patient and visitors about hand washing.
- Teach patient and caregivers about how to avoid infection, including the need for skin care and oral hygiene.
- If the patient is managed as an outpatient, teach the patient and caregivers about signs and symptoms of infection and to report promptly to a health care facility if they occur.

***Licensed Practical/Vocational Nurse (LPN/LVN)***

- Administer antibiotics and hematopoietic growth factors (consider state nurse practice act and agency policy for IV medications).
- Check the skin, oral mucosa, and perineal area for signs of infection.
- Monitor for signs and symptoms of infection and report them to the RN.

***Unlicensed Assistive Personnel (UAP)***

- Obtain vital signs and report changes to the RN.
- Assist the patient with oral care and personal hygiene.

### Diagnostic Studies

The primary diagnostic tests for assessing neutropenia are the peripheral WBC count and bone marrow aspiration and biopsy (Table 30-22). A total WBC count of less than 4000/μL ($4 \times 10^9$/L) reflects leukopenia. However, only a differential count can confirm the presence of neutropenia (neutrophil count less than 1000/μL [$1 \times 10^9$/L]). If the differential WBC count reflects an absolute neutropenia of 500 to 1000/μL ($0.5$ to $1.0 \times 10^9$/L),

## TABLE 30-21 Causes of Neutropenia

**Drugs***
- Antitumor antibiotics (daunorubicin [Cerubidine], doxorubicin [Adriamycin])
- Alkylating agents (nitrogen mustard, busulfan [Myleran])
- Antimetabolites (methotrexate, 6-mercaptopurine [6-MP], cytarabine)
- Antiinflammatory drugs (phenylbutazone)
- Cardiovascular drugs (captopril [Capoten], procainamide [Pronestyl])
- Diuretics (furosemide [Lasix])
- Miscellaneous (gold, penicillamine)
- Antimicrobial agents (ganciclovir, penicillin G, trimethoprim/sulfamethoxazole [Bactrim])

**Hematologic Disorders**
- Idiopathic neutropenia
- Congenital (cyclic neutropenia)
- Aplastic anemia
- Fanconi syndrome
- Leukemia
- Myelodysplastic syndrome

**Autoimmune Disorders**
- Systemic lupus erythematosus
- Felty syndrome
- Rheumatoid arthritis

**Infections**
- Viral (e.g., hepatitis, influenza, HIV, measles)
- Fulminant bacterial infection (e.g., typhoid fever, miliary tuberculosis)
- Parasitic
- Rickettsial

**Others**
- Severe sepsis
- Bone marrow infiltration (e.g., carcinoma, tuberculosis, lymphoma)
- Hypersplenism (e.g., portal hypertension, storage diseases [e.g., Gaucher disease])
- Nutritional deficiencies (cobalamin, folic acid)
- Transfusion reaction
- Hemodialysis

*Not all inclusive.

the patient is at moderate risk for a bacterial infection. An absolute neutropenia of less than 500/μL ($0.5 \times 10^9$/L) places the patient at severe risk. Note that patients with acute leukemia who present with a high WBC may in fact have neutropenia, because the majority of the WBCs are ineffective leukemia blasts cells.

A peripheral blood smear is used to assess for immature forms of WBCs (e.g., bands). The hematocrit level, reticulocyte count, and platelet count are done to evaluate bone marrow function. Also review the patient's recent past and current drug history. If the cause of neutropenia is unknown, bone marrow aspirations and biopsies are done to examine cellularity and cell morphology. Additional studies may be done as indicated to assess spleen and liver function.

## NURSING AND INTERPROFESSIONAL MANAGEMENT: NEUTROPENIA

The factors involved in the nursing and interprofessional care of neutropenia include (1) determining the cause of the neutropenia, (2) instituting antibiotic therapy promptly, (3) identifying the offending organisms if an infection has developed, (4) administering hematopoietic growth factors prophylactically after chemotherapy, and (5) implementing protective practices (e.g., strict hand washing, skin and oral hygiene)[30-32] (Table 30-22).

## TABLE 30-22 Interprofessional Care

### *Neutropenia*

**Diagnostic Assessment**
- History and physical examination
- Risk assessment for severity and duration of neutropenia
- WBC count with differential count
- WBC morphology
- Hct and Hgb
- Reticulocyte and platelet count
- Bone marrow aspiration or biopsy
- Cultures of nose, throat, sputum, urine, stool, obvious lesions, blood (as indicated)
- Chest x-ray or other diagnostic tests

**Management**
- Identification and removal of cause of neutropenia (if possible)
- Identification of site of infection (if present) and causative organism
- Antimicrobial therapy (prophylactically or empiric)*
- Blood cultures drawn STAT, immediately before antibiotics
- Prophylactic hematopoietic growth factors (G-CSF, GM-CSF, pegfilgrastim [Neulasta]) after myelosuppressive chemotherapy
- Strict hand washing
- Patient hygiene (daily skin and frequent oral care; chlorhexidine bathing should be done in the inpatient setting if the patient has a central venous catheter)
- Single-patient room, positive-pressure or high-efficiency particulate air (HEPA) filtration, depending on risk
- Community isolation and home precautions (if outpatient)
  - Nutritional therapy (dietary instruction) on foods to avoid and safe food handling
  - Safe activity and ambulation to maintain physical and pulmonary function

*G-CSF,* Granulocyte colony-stimulating factor; *GM-CSF,* granulocyte-macrophage colony-stimulating factor.
*Prompt initiation of empiric broad-spectrum antibiotic therapy at any sign of infection, even a low-grade fever (100.4°F [38°C]), is essential.

Occasionally the cause of the neutropenia can be easily treated (e.g., nutritional deficiencies). However, neutropenia can also be a side effect that must be tolerated as a necessary step in therapy (e.g., chemotherapy, radiation therapy). In some situations the neutropenia resolves when the primary disease or disorder is treated.

Monitor the neutropenic patient for signs and symptoms of infection (e.g., any fever 100.4°F [38°C] or greater) and early septic shock. Early identification of a potentially infective organism depends on acquiring cultures from various sites. Serial blood cultures (at least two) or one from a peripheral site and one from a venous access device should be done promptly and antibiotics started immediately (within 1 hour).

Administration of broad-spectrum antibiotics is usually by the IV route because of the rapidly lethal effects of infection. However, some oral antibiotics are highly effective and routinely used for prophylaxis against infection in some neutropenic patients. The use of a third- or fourth-generation cephalosporin with broad microorganism coverage (e.g., cefepime [Maxipime], ceftazidime [Ceptaz]), a carbapenem (e.g., imipenem/cilastatin [Primaxin]), will be initiated and augmented depending on the patient's response and/or results of the diagnostic tests.[30,33]

Regardless of the combination, initiate therapy promptly and observe the patient for side effects of antimicrobial agents. Additionally, ongoing febrile episodes or a change in the patient's assessment requires a call to the HCP for assessment, additional cultures, diagnostic tests, or additional antimicrobial therapies. The longer the neutropenia, the greater the risk of a fungal infection. Antifungal therapy is initiated whenever a culture is positive, or in patients who do not become afebrile with broad-spectrum antibiotic coverage.

Cultures of sputum, throat, lesions, wounds, urine, and feces may also be ordered in the surveillance of the patient. Depending on the clinical situation, it may also be necessary to do CT scans, bronchoscopy with bronchial brushings, or lung biopsy to diagnose the cause of pneumonic infiltrates. Invasive diagnostic studies are often contraindicated because of the concern of introducing infection and the fact that these patients are also often thrombocytopenic. Despite these many tests, the causative organism is identified in only approximately one half of neutropenic patients. Thus the priority is to obtain the blood cultures and administer the antibiotic STAT.

Granulocyte colony-stimulating factor (G-CSF) (filgrastim [Neupogen], pegfilgrastim [Neulasta]), and granulocyte-macrophage colony-stimulating factor (GM-CSF) (sargramostim [Leukine, Prokine]) (see Table 15-15) can be used to prevent neutropenia or to reduce its severity and duration.[34] Once neutropenia has occurred, these agents are generally not as effective. G-CSF stimulates the production and function of neutrophils. GM-CSF stimulates the production and function of neutrophils and monocytes. These agents can be given IV or subcutaneously. Keratinocyte growth factor (palifermin [Kepivance]) may also be used to reduce the duration and severity of mucositis that may contribute to infection. (G-CSF, GM-CSF, and palifermin are discussed in Chapter 15.)

Keep the following care principles in mind: (1) the patient's normal flora is the most common source of microbial colonization and infection; (2) transmission of organisms from humans most commonly occurs by direct contact with the hands; (3) air, food, water, and equipment provide additional opportunities for infection transmission; and (4) HCPs with transmissible illnesses and other patients with infections can also be sources of infection transmission under certain conditions.

Hand washing is the single most important preventive measure to minimize the risk of infection in the neutropenic patient. Strict hand washing by staff and visitors using an antiseptic hand wash, before and after contact, is the major method to prevent transmission of harmful pathogens.

Separate immunocompromised patients from those who are infected or have conditions that increase the probability of transmitting infections (e.g., poor hygiene caused by lack of understanding or cognitive dysfunction). Often patients can be managed on an outpatient basis if the patient and caregiver can astutely monitor for fever and other signs of infection and then report promptly to a nearby health care facility (Table 30-23). If the patient is hospitalized, a private room should be used. High-efficiency particulate air (HEPA) filtration is an air-handling method with a high-flow filtering system that can reduce or eliminate the number of aerosolized pathogens in the environment used for hematopoietic stem cell transplant patients. Care routines in a HEPA environment are essentially the same as care in any other private room. Additional neutropenic precaution guidelines may also be employed, such as prophylactic antibiotics and antifungals. The patient and caregiver should be instructed on a diet that restricts potentially hazardous foods, such as raw and undercooked meats and eggs and soft cheeses with molds. The nursing measures presented in eNursing Care Plan 30-3 (available on the website for this chapter) are important in the treatment of the patient with neutropenia.

Quality-of-life issues for the patient with neutropenia should not be overlooked. Fatigue, malaise, a decrease in functioning, and social isolation require coaching on safe activity.

**TABLE 30-23 Patient & Caregiver Teaching**

***Neutropenia***

*Include the following instructions when teaching a patient or caregiver the precautions to take when the neutrophil count is low.*

1. WASH YOUR HANDS frequently and make sure those around you wash their hands frequently, particularly if they help with your care. An antibacterial hand gel may also be used.
2. Notify your nurse or HCP if you have any of the following:
   - Fever ≥100.4° F (38° C)*
   - Chills or feeling hot
   - Redness, swelling, discharge, or new pain on or in your body
   - Changes in urination or bowel movements
   - Cough, sore throat, mouth sores, or blisters
3. If you are at home, take your temperature as directed and follow instructions on what to do if you have a fever.
4. Avoid crowds and people with colds, flu, or infections. If you are in a public area, wear a mask and use hand sanitizing gel frequently.
5. Avoid uncooked meats, seafood, or eggs and unwashed fruits and vegetables. Ask your HCP about specific dietary guidelines for you.
6. Bathe or shower daily. A moisturizer may be used to prevent skin from drying and cracking.
7. Maintain some daily activity as instructed by your health care team. This may include walking and moderate exercise while avoiding crowds.
8. Brush your teeth with a soft toothbrush four times daily. You may floss once daily if it does not cause excessive pain or bleeding. Avoid alcohol-based mouthwashes.
9. Do not perform gardening or clean up after pets. Feeding and petting your dog or cat are fine as long as you wash your hands well after handling.

*Need to verify cut-off temperature with HCP.

## MYELODYSPLASTIC SYNDROME

**Myelodysplastic syndrome (MDS)** is a group of related hematologic disorders characterized by peripheral blood cytopenias (from ineffective blood cell production) and changes in the cellularity of the bone marrow with dysplastic changes. In MDS, *hematopoiesis* is disorderly and ineffective. It is estimated that the incidence is 4.5 per 100,000 people per year in the United States. Although it can occur in all age groups, the highest prevalence is in people over 80 years of age, at which point the rate increases to 51.5 per 100,000.[35]

### Etiology and Pathophysiology

The etiology of MDS is unknown. People who have received radiation therapy, had chemotherapy with alkylating agents (e.g., chlorambucil, cyclophosphamide, melphalan), or have been exposed to industrial solvents (e.g., benzene) have a higher risk of developing MDS than people who have not had these exposures. Rarely, genetic disorders are responsible for the disease. Nevertheless, in 85% of MDS patients, no specific cause can be identified.[36]

## INFORMATICS IN PRACTICE

### *Use of Internet to Access Information on Unfamiliar Diseases*

- If you are assigned to take care of a patient with a disease or disorder that you are not familiar with, such as thalassemia, access the Internet and perform a quick search.
- Within minutes, you can learn the pathophysiology of thalassemia, treatment options, possible complications that you will need to monitor, and recommended medical and nursing interventions.
- Using this readily available information will help you deliver high-quality, evidence-based care.

MDS is referred to as a *clonal disorder,* because some bone marrow stem cells continue to function normally, whereas others (a specific clone) do not. The abnormal clone of the stem cells is usually found in the bone marrow but eventually may be found in the circulation.

Occasionally one type of MDS transforms into another. Depending on the subtype, MDS may progress to acute myelogenous leukemia (AML).[36] In contrast to AML, in which the leukemic cells show little normal maturation, the clonal cells in MDS always display some degree of maturity. Disease progression is slower than in AML, and sometimes treatment is not required.

### Clinical Manifestations

Manifestations result from neoplastic transformation of the pluripotent hematopoietic stem cells in the bone marrow. MDS commonly manifests as infection and bleeding caused by inadequate numbers of ineffectively functioning circulating granulocytes or platelets. MDS is often discovered in the older adult during testing for the symptoms of anemia, thrombocytopenia, or neutropenia. It may also be diagnosed incidentally from a routine CBC. During the advanced stage of MDS, life-threatening anemia, thrombocytopenia, and neutropenia occur.

### Diagnostic Studies

Bone marrow biopsy with aspirate analysis is essential for both the diagnosis and classification of the specific type of myelodysplasia. In MDS the patient has peripheral cytopenia and changes in the bone marrow (hypocellular or hypercellular). Laboratory data and bone marrow studies help rule out other causes of the dysplasia, such as nonmalignant disorders, cobalamin and folate deficiencies, and infections.

## NURSING AND INTERPROFESSIONAL MANAGEMENT: MYELODYSPLASTIC SYNDROME

Supportive treatment of MDS is based on the premise that the aggressiveness of treatment should match the aggressiveness of the disease. This is based on the amount and type of dysplasia in the bone marrow as well as genetic mutations.[35] Supportive treatment consists of hematologic monitoring (serial bone marrow and peripheral blood examinations); antibiotic therapy; or transfusions with blood products, along with iron chelators to prevent iron overload.

Low-risk patients can often be treated with erythropoietin and G-CSF. Only about one third of high-risk patients are treated with intensive chemotherapy and/or HSCT. Azacitidine (Vidaza) and decitabine (Dacogen) are drugs that help restore normal growth control and differentiation of hematopoietic cells and reduce the frequency of transformation of MDS to acute leukemia. Side effects include myelosuppression, nausea, vomiting, constipation or diarrhea, renal dysfunction, and injection site erythema.

Lenalidomide (Revlimid) or thalidomide may also be used. Other treatments for MDS include cytarabine (Cytosar, Ara-C) with or without antitumor antibiotics (anthracyclines), antithymocyte globulin, and cyclosporine. Nonmyeloablative (does not suppress bone marrow) chemotherapy and allogeneic HSCT have been used in patients with high-risk features to treat bone marrow dysfunction of MDS and restore it with normal hematopoiesis.

Nursing care of a patient with MDS is similar to that of a patient with manifestations of anemia, thrombocytopenia, and neutropenia. (See eNursing Care Plan 30-1 for the patient with anemia, eNursing Care Plan 30-2 for the patient with thrombocytopenia, and eNursing Care Plan 30-3 for the patient with neutropenia. The eNursing Care Plans are available on the website for this chapter.)

## LEUKEMIA

**Leukemia** is the general term used to describe a group of malignant disorders affecting the blood and blood-forming tissues of the bone marrow, lymph system, and spleen. Leukemia occurs in all age groups. It results in an accumulation of dysfunctional cells because of a loss of regulation in cell division. It follows a progressive course that is eventually fatal if untreated. An estimated 52,380 new cases are diagnosed each year. Although often thought of as a disease of children, leukemia affects approximately 9 times more adults than children.[37]

### Etiology and Pathophysiology

Regardless of the specific type, leukemia has no single cause. It is now known that all cancers, including leukemia, begin as a mutation in the DNA of certain cells. Most leukemias result from a combination of factors, including genetic and environmental influences. Abnormal genes *(oncogenes)* are capable of causing many types of cancers, including leukemias (see Chapter 15). Chemical agents (e.g., benzene), chemotherapeutic agents (e.g., alkylating agents), viruses, radiation, and immunologic deficiencies have all been associated with the development of leukemia. The incidence of leukemia is increased in radiologists, persons who have lived near nuclear bomb test sites or nuclear reactor accidents (e.g., Chernobyl), and persons previously treated with radiation therapy or chemotherapy.

Although ribonucleic acid (RNA) retroviruses cause a number of leukemias in animals, a viral cause for a human leukemia has been established only for some patients with adult T-cell leukemia. This form of leukemia is endemic in southwestern Japan and parts of the Caribbean and is caused by the human T-cell leukemia virus type 1 (HTLV-1).[37]

### Classification

Leukemia can be classified based on acute versus chronic disease and on the type of WBC involved. The terms *acute* and *chronic* refer to cell maturity and nature of disease onset. Acute leukemia is characterized by the clonal proliferation of immature hematopoietic cells. The leukemia develops after malignant transformation of a single type of immature hematopoietic cell, followed by cellular replication and expansion of that malignant clone. Chronic leukemias involve more mature forms of the WBC, and the disease onset is more gradual.

Leukemia can also be classified by identifying the type of leukocyte involved, whether it is of myelogenous or lymphocytic origin. By combining the acute and chronic categories with the cell type involved, one can identify four major types of leukemia: acute lymphocytic leukemia (ALL), acute myelogenous leukemia (AML), chronic myelogenous (granulocytic) leukemia (CML), and chronic lymphocytic leukemia (CLL).[38-41] Other defining features of these leukemic subtypes are presented in Table 30-24.

**Acute Myelogenous Leukemia.** AML represents only one fourth of all leukemias, but it makes up approximately 80% of the acute leukemias in adults.[37] Its onset is often abrupt and dramatic. A patient may have serious infections and abnormal bleeding from the onset of the disease.

AML is characterized by uncontrolled proliferation of myeloblasts, the precursors of granulocytes. There is hyperplasia of the bone marrow. The clinical manifestations are usually related to replacement of normal hematopoietic cells in the marrow by leukemic myeloblasts and, to a lesser extent, to infiltration of other organs and tissue (Table 30-24).

**Acute Lymphocytic Leukemia.** ALL is the most common type of leukemia in children and accounts for about 20% of acute leukemia cases in adults.[37] In ALL, immature small lymphocytes proliferate in the bone marrow; most are of B-cell origin. The majority of patients have fever at the time of diagnosis. Signs and symptoms may appear abruptly with bleeding or fever, or they may be insidious with progressive weakness, fatigue, bone and/or joint pain, and bleeding tendencies.

Central nervous system (CNS) manifestations are especially common in ALL and represent a serious problem. Leukemic meningitis caused by arachnoid infiltration occurs in many patients with ALL.

**Chronic Myelogenous Leukemia.** CML is caused by excessive development of mature neoplastic granulocytes in the bone marrow. The excess neoplastic granulocytes move into the peripheral blood in massive numbers and ultimately infiltrate the liver and spleen.

The natural history of CML is a chronic stable phase, followed by the development of a more acute, aggressive phase referred to as the *blastic phase*. The chronic phase of CML can last for several years and can usually be well controlled with treatment. Even with treatment, the chronic phase of the disease eventually progresses to the accelerated phase, ending in a blastic phase. Once CML transforms to an acute or blastic phase, it must be treated more aggressively, similar to an acute leukemia.

**Genetic Link.** The *Philadelphia chromosome* originates from the translocation between the *BCR* gene on chromosome 22 and the *ABL* gene on chromosome 9. The protein that is encoded by the newly created *BCR-ABL* gene on the Philadelphia chromosome interferes with normal cell cycle events, such as the regulation of cell proliferation.

The Philadelphia chromosome, which is present in 90% to 95% of patients with CML, is a diagnostic hallmark of CML. In addition, its presence is an important indicator of residual disease or relapse after treatment. However, the presence of the Philadelphia chromosome is not specific to diagnose CML, since it is also found in ALL and occasionally in AML.

**Chronic Lymphocytic Leukemia.** CLL is the most common leukemia in adults.[37] CLL is characterized by the production and

**TABLE 30-24 Types of Leukemia**

| Age of Onset | Clinical Manifestations | Diagnostic Findings |
|---|---|---|
| **Acute Myelogenous Leukemia (AML)** | | |
| Accounts for 15%-20% of acute leukemia in children and 80% in adults. Increase in incidence with advancing age after 60 yr | Fatigue and weakness, headache, mouth sores, anemia, bleeding, fever, infection, sternal tenderness, gingival hyperplasia, mild hepatosplenomegaly (one third of patients) | Low RBC count, Hgb, Hct, platelet count. Low to high WBC count with myeloblasts. High LDH. Hypercellular bone marrow with myeloblasts |
| **Acute Lymphocytic Leukemia (ALL)** | | |
| Peak prevalence occurs between ages 2 and 5 and after age 50. | Fever, pallor, bleeding, anorexia, fatigue, and weakness. Bone, joint, and abdominal pain. Generalized lymphadenopathy, infections, weight loss, hepatosplenomegaly, headache, mouth sores, neurologic manifestations: CNS involvement, increased intracranial pressure (nausea, vomiting, lethargy, cranial nerve dysfunction) secondary to meningeal infiltration | Low RBC count, Hgb, Hct, platelet count. Low, normal, or high WBC count. High LDH. Transverse lines of rarefaction at ends of metaphysis of long bones on x-ray. Hypercellular bone marrow with lymphoblasts. Lymphoblasts also possible in cerebrospinal fluid. Presence of Philadelphia chromosome (20%-25% of patients) |
| **Chronic Myelogenous Leukemia (CML)** | | |
| Increase in incidence with advancing age with median age at diagnosis of 65. Rare in children | No symptoms early in disease. Fatigue and weakness, fever, sternal tenderness, weight loss, joint pain, bone pain, massive splenomegaly, increase in sweating | Low RBC count, Hgb, Hct. High platelet count early, lower count later. ↑ banded neutrophils and myeloblasts and often basophils, normal number of lymphocytes, and normal or low number of monocytes. Nucleated red cells are common. Low leukocyte alkaline phosphatase. Presence of Philadelphia chromosome in 90% of patients |
| **Chronic Lymphocytic Leukemia (CLL)** | | |
| Increase in incidence with advancing age after 65 yr, with predominance in men | Frequently no symptoms. Detection of disease often during examination for unrelated condition, chronic fatigue, anorexia, splenomegaly and lymphadenopathy, hepatomegaly. May progress to fever, night sweats, weight loss, fatigue, and frequent infections | Mild anemia and thrombocytopenia with disease progression. Total WBC count >100,000/μL. Increase in peripheral lymphocytes and lymphocytes in bone marrow. May have autoimmune hemolytic anemia, idiopathic thrombocytopenic purpura, and hypogammaglobulinemia |

*LDH*, Lactate dehydrogenase.

accumulation of functionally inactive but long-lived, small, mature-appearing lymphocytes. B cells are usually involved. The lymphocytes infiltrate the bone marrow, spleen, and liver. Lymph node enlargement (lymphadenopathy) is present throughout the body.

Complications are rare in early stage CLL but may develop as the disease advances. Pressure on nerves from enlarged lymph nodes causes pain and even paralysis. Mediastinal node enlargement leads to pulmonary symptoms. Because CLL is usually a disease of older adults, treatment decisions must be made by considering the progression of the disease and the side effects of treatment. Many individuals in the early stages of CLL require no treatment. Others may be followed closely and receive treatment only when the disease progresses. Approximately one third require immediate intervention at the time of diagnosis.

**Other Leukemias.** Occasionally the subtype of leukemia cannot be identified. The malignant leukemic cells may have lymphoid, myeloid, or mixed characteristics. Frequently these patients do not respond to treatment and have a poor prognosis. Other rare types include hairy cell and biphenotypic (both abnormal myeloid and lymphoid clones) leukemias.

**Overlap Between Leukemia and Lymphoma.** Overlap exists between leukemia and non-Hodgkin's lymphoma (NHL) because both involve proliferation of lymphocytes or their precursors. A leukemia-like picture with peripheral lymphocytosis and bone marrow involvement may be present in about 20% of adults with some types of NHL. Although differentiation can be difficult, generally patients with more extensive nodal involvement (especially mediastinal), fewer circulating abnormal cells, and fewer blast forms in the marrow are considered to have lymphoma. A prominent leukemic phase is less common in aggressive lymphomas, except Burkitt's and lymphoblastic lymphomas.[42]

## Clinical Manifestations

Although the clinical manifestations of leukemia are varied (Table 30-24), they relate to problems caused by bone marrow failure and the formation of leukemic infiltrates (Fig. 30-12). Bone marrow failure results from (1) bone marrow overcrowding by abnormal cells and (2) inadequate production of normal marrow elements. The patient is predisposed to anemia, thrombocytopenia, and decreased number and function of WBCs.

As leukemia progresses, fewer normal blood cells are produced. The abnormal WBCs continue to accumulate because they do not go through the normal cell life cycle to death *(apoptosis)*. The leukemic cells may infiltrate the patient's organs, leading to problems such as splenomegaly, hepatomegaly, lymphadenopathy, bone pain, meningeal irritation, and oral lesions. Solid masses resulting from collections of leukemic cells called *chloromas* can also occur. A high leukemic white count in the peripheral blood (more than 100,000 cells/μL) can cause the blood to thicken and potentially block circulatory pathways. This is called *leukostasis* and can be life threatening.

## Diagnostic Studies

Peripheral blood evaluation and bone marrow examination are the primary methods of diagnosing and classifying the types of leukemia. Morphologic, histochemical, immunologic, and cytogenetic methods are all used to identify leukemic cell types and stage of development. Identifying the type of leukemia is important because the various types have different prognoses and

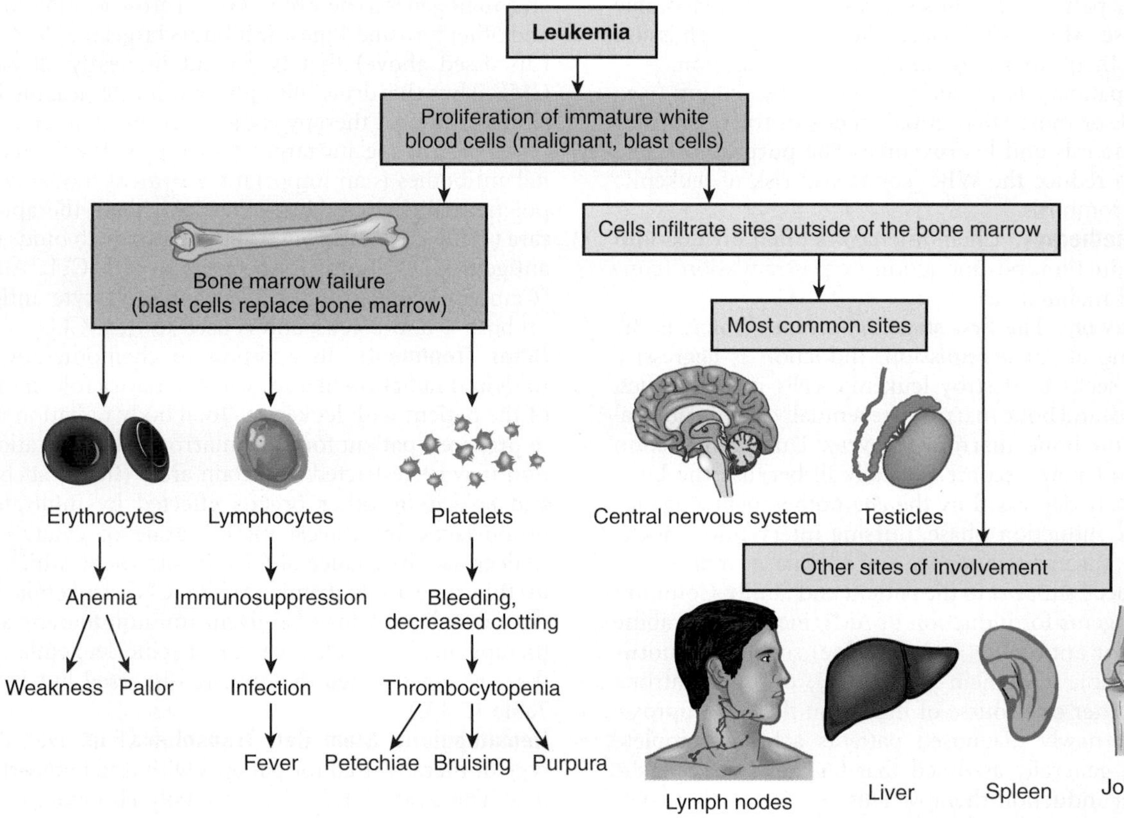


**FIG. 30-12** Pathophysiology of leukemia. (Modified from McKinney ES, James SR, Murray SS, Nelson K: *Maternal-child nursing,* Philadelphia, 2000, Saunders.)

chemotherapeutic regimens. Other studies such as lumbar puncture and CT scan can detect leukemic cells outside of the blood and bone marrow.

The malignant cells in most patients with leukemia have specific cytogenetic abnormalities that are associated with distinct subsets of the disease. These cytogenetic abnormalities have diagnostic, prognostic, and therapeutic importance. For example, in CML, the finding of the Philadelphia chromosome is an important diagnostic indicator.

## Interprofessional Care

Once a diagnosis of leukemia has been made, care is focused on the initial goal of attaining remission. Age and cytogenetic analysis often help form the basis of important treatment decisions. Because chemotherapy is the mainstay of the treatment, you need to understand the principles of cancer chemotherapy. (See the section on chemotherapy in Chapter 15.)

In some cases, such as nonsymptomatic patients with CLL, watchful waiting with active supportive care may be appropriate. Although a patient may not be cured, attaining remission or disease control is a realistic option for the majority of patients. In some cases, cure is a realistic goal. In *complete remission* there is no evidence of overt disease on physical examination, and the bone marrow and peripheral blood appear normal. A lesser state of control is known as partial remission. *Minimal residual disease* is defined as tumor cells that cannot be detected by morphologic examination but can be identified by molecular testing. *Partial remission* is characterized by a lack of symptoms and a normal peripheral blood smear but still evidence of disease in the bone marrow. *Molecular remission* indicates that all molecular studies are negative for residual leukemia. The patient's prognosis is directly related to the ability to maintain a remission. The patient's prognosis becomes more unfavorable with each relapse. After each relapse, the succeeding remission may be more difficult to achieve and shorter in duration.

Sometimes patients have such a high WBC count (e.g., 100,000 cells/μL or more) that initial emergent treatment may include leukapheresis and hydroxyurea. The purpose of these treatments is to reduce the WBC count and risk of leukemia cell–induced thrombosis.

**Stages of Chemotherapy.** Chemotherapy is often divided into three stages: induction, postinduction or postremission (consolidation), and maintenance.

***Induction Therapy.*** The first stage, *induction therapy,* is the attempt to bring about a remission. Induction is aggressive treatment that seeks to destroy leukemic cells in the tissues, peripheral blood, and bone marrow to eventually restore normal hematopoiesis on bone marrow recovery. During induction therapy, a patient may become critically ill because the bone marrow is severely depressed by the chemotherapeutic agents. Throughout the induction phase, nursing interventions focus on neutropenia, thrombocytopenia, and anemia, as well as providing psychosocial support to the patient and family. Common chemotherapy agents for induction of AML include cytarabine and an antitumor antibiotic (anthracycline) such as daunorubicin (Cerubidine), idarubicin (Idamycin), or mitoxantrone (Novantrone). After one course of induction therapy, approximately 70% of newly diagnosed patients achieve complete remission. It is generally assumed that leukemic cells persist undetected after induction therapy. This could lead to relapse within a few months if no further therapy is administered.[38]

***Postinduction or Postremission Therapy.*** Terms used to describe postinduction or postremission chemotherapy include *intensification* and *consolidation. Intensification therapy,* or high-dose therapy, may be given immediately after induction therapy for several months. Other drugs that target the cell in a different way than those administered during induction may also be added.

*Consolidation therapy* is started after a remission is achieved. It may consist of one or two additional courses of the same drugs given during induction or involve high-dose therapy (intensive consolidation). The purpose of consolidation therapy is to eliminate remaining leukemic cells that may not be clinically or pathologically evident.

***Maintenance Therapy.*** *Maintenance therapy* is treatment with lower doses of the same drugs used in induction or other drugs given every 3 to 4 weeks for a prolonged period. Like consolidation or intensification, the goal is to keep the body free of leukemic cells. Each type of leukemia requires different maintenance therapy. In AML, maintenance therapy is rarely effective and therefore rarely administered.

**Drug Therapy Regimens.** The therapeutic agents used to treat leukemia vary. Table 30-25 gives examples of treatment regimens used in various types of leukemia.[16,42-45]

Combination therapy is the mainstay of treatment for leukemia. The three purposes for using multiple drugs are to (1) decrease drug resistance, (2) minimize the drug toxicity to the patient by using multiple drugs with varying toxicities, and (3) interrupt cell growth at multiple points in the cell cycle.

Some therapeutic drugs are aimed at small molecules that promote the growth and differentiation of leukemic cells. For example, arsenic trioxide (Trisenox), which is used to treat acute promyelocytic leukemia (a type of AML), causes DNA fragmentation and cell death. In addition, it inhibits cell proliferation and angiogenesis (new blood vessel growth). Imatinib (Gleevec) and other tyrosine-kinase inhibitors target the *BCR-ABL* protein (discussed above) that is present in nearly all patients with CML. Thus this drug kills only cancer cells, leaving healthy cells alone. (Targeted therapy is discussed in Chapter 15.)

The use of specific targeted therapy in the form of monoclonal antibodies is an important treatment modality in hematopoietic malignancies, but cures with these therapies alone are rare (Table 15-13 and Fig. 15-16). Rituximab binds to the B-cell antigen (CD20) and has been used with CLL. Alemtuzumab (Campath) binds to CD52, a panlymphocyte antigen present on both T and B cells, and is used to treat CLL.

**Other Treatments.** In addition to chemotherapy, corticosteroids and radiation therapy can also have a role in the treatment of the patient with leukemia. Total body radiation may be used to prepare a patient for bone marrow transplantation, or radiation may be restricted to certain areas (fields) such as the liver and spleen or other organs affected by infiltrates. In ALL, prophylactic intrathecal methotrexate or cytarabine is given to decrease the chance of CNS involvement, which is common in this type of leukemia. When CNS leukemia does occur, cranial radiation may be given. Immunotherapy and targeted therapy may be indicated for specific leukemias. (Immunotherapy and targeted therapy are discussed in Chapter 15 and Table 15-13.)

**Hematopoietic Stem Cell Transplantation.** HSCT is another type of therapy used for patients with different forms of leukemia. The goal of HSCT is to totally eliminate leukemic cells from the body using combinations of chemotherapy with or without total body irradiation. This treatment also eradicates the patient's hematopoietic stem cells, which are then replaced with those of an HLA-matched sibling or volunteer donor *(allogeneic)* or an identical twin *(syngeneic)*, or with the patient's own *(autologous)* stem cells that were removed (harvested) before the intensive therapy. (HSCT is discussed in Chapter 15.)

The primary complications for patients with allogeneic HSCT are graft-versus-host disease (GVHD), relapse of leukemia (especially ALL), and infection (especially interstitial pneumonia). GVHD is discussed in Chapter 13. Because HSCT has serious associated risks, the patient must weigh the significant risks of treatment-related death or treatment failure (relapse) with the hope of cure.

**TABLE 30-25 Drug Therapy**
***Leukemia****

| Drug Therapy | Other Therapy |
|---|---|
| **Acute Myelogenous Leukemia** | |
| cytarabine (Cytosar),† daunorubicin (Cerubidine),† idarubicin, mitoxantrone, arsenic trioxide (Trisenox),† tretinoin,† clofarabine (Clolar), decitabine (Dacogen), fludarabine, azacitidine (Vidaza)<br>Combination chemotherapy of cytarabine and antitumor antibiotic (most common) | Autologous or allogeneic hematopoietic stem cell transplant (HSCT) (see Chapter 15) |
| **Acute Lymphocytic Leukemia** | |
| daunorubicin, doxorubicin, vincristine, prednisone, dexamethasone, L-asparaginase (Elspar), ponatinib (Iclusig), pegaspargase (Oncaspar), dasatinib (Sprycel), cyclophosphamide, methotrexate, 6-mercaptopurine, cytarabine, nelarabine (Arranon), imatinib (Gleevec), clofarabine (Clolar), blinatumomab (Blincyto), rituximab (Rituxan)<br>Combination chemotherapy of several agents is common over a prolonged time | Cranial radiation therapy, intrathecal methotrexate or cytarabine, allogeneic HSCT (see Chapter 15) |
| **Chronic Myelogenous Leukemia** | |
| bosutinib (Bosulif), imatinib (Gleevec), dasatinib (Sprycel), nilotinib (Tasigna), omacetaxine (Synribo), ponatinib (Iclusig), hydroxyurea (Hydrea)<br>Combination chemotherapy including any of the following: cytarabine, daunorubicin, methotrexate, prednisone, vincristine, L-asparaginase, 6-mercaptopurine, busulfan (Myleran) | Radiation, HSCT, α-interferon, leukapheresis |
| **Chronic Lymphocytic Leukemia** | |
| chlorambucil (Leukeran), cyclophosphamide, prednisone, vincristine, fludarabine, rituximab (Rituxan), alemtuzumab (Campath), pentostatin (Nipent), bendamustine (Treanda), oxaliplatin (Eloxatin), methotrexate, ofatumumab (Arzerra), idelalisib (Zydelig), obinutuzumab (Gazyva), ibrutinib (Imbruvica), lenalidomide (Revlimid), venetoclax (Venclexta) | Radiation, splenectomy, colony-stimulating factors, allogeneic HSCT |

*The classification and mechanisms of action of these drugs are presented in Table 15-7.
†Used for acute promyelocytic leukemia.

## NURSING MANAGEMENT: LEUKEMIA

### Nursing Assessment

Subjective and objective data that should be obtained from a patient with leukemia are presented in Table 30-26.

**TABLE 30-26 Nursing Assessment**
***Leukemia***

**Subjective Data**

***Important Health Information***

*Past health history:* Exposure to chemical toxins (e.g., benzene, arsenic), radiation, or viruses (Epstein-Barr, HTLV-1); chromosome abnormalities (Down syndrome, Klinefelter syndrome, Fanconi syndrome), immunologic deficiencies; organ transplantation; frequent infections; bleeding tendencies

*Medications:* Chemotherapy

*Surgery or other treatments:* Radiation exposure; prior radiation and chemotherapy for cancer

***Functional Health Patterns***

*Health perception–health management:* Family history of leukemia; malaise

*Nutritional-metabolic:* Mouth sores, weight loss; chills, night sweats; nausea, vomiting, anorexia, dysphagia, early satiety; easy bruising

*Elimination:* Hematuria, decreased urine output; diarrhea, dark or bloody stools

*Activity-exercise:* Fatigue with progressive weakness; dyspnea, epistaxis, cough

*Cognitive-perceptual:* Headache; muscle cramps; sore throat; generalized sternal tenderness, bone, joint, abdominal pain; paresthesias, numbness, tingling, visual disturbances

*Sexuality-reproductive:* Prolonged menses, menorrhagia, metrorrhagia, impotence

**Objective Data**

***General***

Fever, generalized lymphadenopathy, lethargy

***Integumentary***

Pallor or jaundice; petechiae, ecchymoses, purpura, reddish brown to purple cutaneous infiltrates, macules, and papules

***Cardiovascular***

Tachycardia, systolic murmurs

***Gastrointestinal***

Gingival bleeding and hyperplasia; oral ulcerations, herpes and *Candida* infections; perirectal irritation and infection; hepatomegaly, splenomegaly

***Neurologic***

Seizures, disorientation, confusion, decreased coordination, cranial nerve palsies, papilledema

***Musculoskeletal***

Muscle wasting, bone pain, joint pain

***Possible Diagnostic Findings***

Low, normal, or high WBC count with shift to the left (↑ blast cells) and neutropenia; anemia, ↓ hematocrit and hemoglobin, thrombocytopenia, Philadelphia chromosome; hypercellular bone marrow aspirate or biopsy with myeloblasts, lymphoblasts, and markedly ↓ normal cells

*HTLV-1,* Human T-cell leukemia virus, type 1.

## Nursing Diagnoses

Nursing diagnoses for the patient with leukemia include those for anemia (see p. 608), thrombocytopenia (see p. 625), and neutropenia (see eNursing Care Plan 30-3, available on the website).

## Planning

The overall goals are that the patient with leukemia will (1) understand and adhere to the treatment plan; (2) experience minimal side effects and complications associated with both the disease and its treatment; and (3) establish realistic hope and goals, feeling supported during periods of treatment, relapse, or remission.

## Nursing Implementation

**Acute Care.** The nursing role during acute phases of leukemia is extremely challenging because the patient has many physical and psychosocial needs. As with other forms of cancer, the diagnosis of leukemia can evoke great fear and be equated with death. It may be viewed as a hopeless, horrible disease with many painful and undesirable consequences. The treatment and prognosis of each patient with leukemia are driven by many factors, such as age and type of leukemia. Therefore you must understand the patient's type of leukemia, prognosis, treatment plan, and goals. By doing this, you can help the patient realize that, although the future may be uncertain, one can have a meaningful quality of life while in remission or with disease control, and that, in some cases, there is reasonable hope for cure.

The family also needs help adjusting to the stress of this abrupt onset of serious illness and the losses imposed by the sick role (e.g., dependence, withdrawal, changes in role responsibilities, alterations in body image). The diagnosis of leukemia often brings with it the need to make difficult decisions at a time of profound stress for the patient and family.

Patients may have co-morbid conditions that affect treatment decisions. Important nursing interventions include (1) maximizing the patient's physical functioning, (2) teaching patients that acute side effects of treatment are usually temporary, and (3) encouraging patients to discuss their quality-of-life issues. You are an important advocate in helping the patient and family understand the complexities of treatment decisions and manage the side effects and toxicities. A patient may require a long hospitalization or may need to temporarily relocate to an appropriate treatment center. This situation can lead a patient to feel deserted and isolated at a time when support is most needed. You have contact with a patient many hours a day and can help reverse feelings of abandonment and loneliness by balancing the demanding technical needs with a humanistic, caring approach. The needs of the patient with leukemia are best met by an interprofessional team (e.g., psychiatric and oncology clinical nurse specialists, case managers, dietitians, chaplains, and social workers).

From a physical care perspective, you are challenged to make astute assessments and plan care to help the patient manage the severe side effects of chemotherapy. The life-threatening results of bone marrow suppression (neutropenia, thrombocytopenia, and anemia) require aggressive nursing interventions. These patients may be at risk for oncologic emergencies such as tumor lysis syndrome, DIC, and leukostasis. Additional complications of chemotherapy may affect the patient's GI tract, nutritional status, skin and mucosa, cardiopulmonary status, liver, kidneys, and neurologic system. (Nursing interventions related to chemotherapy are discussed in Chapter 15.)

Review all drugs being administered, including the mechanism of action, purpose, routes of administration, usual doses, potential side effects, safe handling considerations, and toxic effects. Assess laboratory data reflecting the effects of the drugs and sequelae of the disease. Unlike treatments for solid tumors, chemotherapy is administered to patients with leukemia even if they have severe myelosuppression, since the underlying disorder is causing the problem and will not resolve unless treated. Patient survival and comfort during aggressive chemotherapy are significantly affected by the quality of nursing care.

**Ambulatory Care.** Ongoing care for the patient with leukemia is necessary to monitor for signs and symptoms of disease control or relapse. For a patient requiring long-term or maintenance chemotherapy, the fatigue of long-term chronic disease management can become discouraging. Therefore teach the patient and caregiver the importance of continued diligence in disease management and the need for follow-up care. Also teach them about the drugs, self-care measures, and when to seek medical attention.

The goals of rehabilitation for long-term survivors of leukemia are to manage the physical, psychologic, social, and spiritual consequences and delayed effects from the disease and its treatment. (Delayed effects are discussed in Chapter 15.) Assistance may be needed to reestablish the various relationships that are a part of the patient's life. Involving the patient in survivor networks and support groups or services may help the patient adapt to living after a life-threatening illness. Exploring resources in the community (e.g., American Cancer Society, Leukemia & Lymphoma Society) may reduce the financial burden and the feelings of dependence. Also provide the resources for spiritual support.

Vigilant follow-up care helps to ensure that the cancer survivor's unique needs are recognized and treated. Often these needs may require a referral or consultation. For example, physical therapy personnel may be asked to develop an exercise program to prevent posttreatment deficits caused by drug-induced peripheral neuropathy. Most patients should receive a pneumococcal vaccine and an annual influenza vaccine.[30] These needs can also include other concerns such as vocational retraining and reproductive concerns for a patient of childbearing age.

## Evaluation

The expected outcomes are that the patient with leukemia will

- Cope effectively with the diagnosis, treatment regimen, and prognosis
- Experience no complications related to the disease or its treatment
- Feel comfortable and supported throughout treatment

# LYMPHOMAS

**Lymphomas** are malignant neoplasms originating in the bone marrow and lymphatic structures resulting in the proliferation of lymphocytes. Lymphomas make up 4% of all cancers in the United States.[37] Two major types of lymphoma are Hodgkin's lymphoma and non-Hodgkin's lymphoma (NHL). A comparison of these two types of lymphoma is presented in Table 30-27.

# HODGKIN'S LYMPHOMA

**Hodgkin's lymphoma**, also called *Hodgkin's disease*, makes up about 11% of all lymphomas. It is a malignant condition

**TABLE 30-27 Comparison of Hodgkin's and Non-Hodgkin's Lymphoma**

| | Hodgkin's Lymphoma | Non-Hodgkin's Lymphoma |
|---|---|---|
| **Cellular origin** | B lymphocytes | B lymphocytes (88%)<br>T or natural killer lymphocytes (12%) |
| **Extent of disease** | Localized to regional, but may be more widespread | Disseminated |
| **B symptoms*** | Common | Uncommon |
| **Extranodal involvement** | Rare | Common |

*B symptoms include fever (>100.4° F [38° C]), drenching night sweats, and weight loss (>10% from baseline within 6 mo).

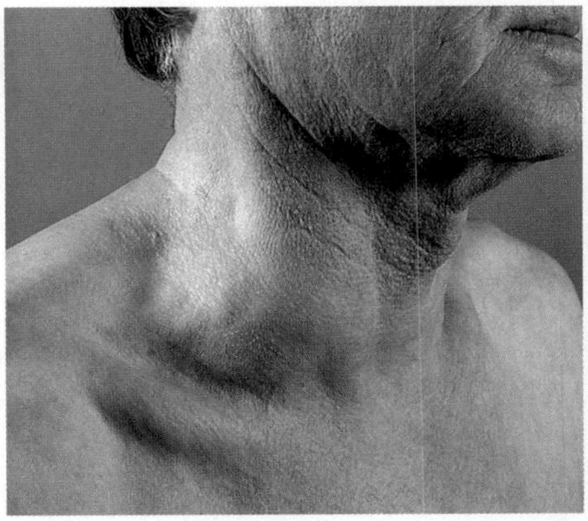

**FIG. 30-13** Enlarged cervical lymph node in the neck of a man with Hodgkin lymphoma. (From Howard MR, Hamilton PJ: *Haematology: an illustrated colour atlas,* ed 4, London, 2013, Churchill Livingston.)

characterized by proliferation of abnormal giant, multinucleated cells, called *Reed-Sternberg cells,* which are located in lymph nodes. The disease has a bimodal age-specific incidence, occurring most frequently in persons from 15 to 30 years of age and above 55 years of age.[46] In adults, it is twice as prevalent in men as in women. Each year, approximately 9190 new cases of Hodgkin's lymphoma are diagnosed and approximately 1100 deaths occur. However, long-term survival exceeds 80% for all stages.[47]

## Etiology and Pathophysiology

Although the cause of Hodgkin's lymphoma remains unknown, several key factors are thought to play a role in its development. The main interacting factors include infection with Epstein-Barr virus (EBV), genetic predisposition, and exposure to occupational toxins. The incidence of Hodgkin's lymphoma is increased in patients who have HIV infection.

Normally, the lymph nodes are composed of connective tissues that surround a fine mesh of reticular fibers and cells. In Hodgkin's lymphoma the normal structure of lymph nodes is destroyed by hyperplasia of monocytes and macrophages. The main diagnostic feature of Hodgkin's lymphoma is the presence of Reed-Sternberg cells in lymph node biopsy specimens. The disease is believed to arise in a single location (it originates in cervical lymph nodes in 80% of patients) and then spreads along adjacent lymphatics. However, in recurrent disease, it may be more diffuse and not necessarily contiguous. It eventually infiltrates other organs, especially lungs, spleen, and liver. When the disease begins above the diaphragm, it remains confined to lymph nodes for a variable time. Disease originating below the diaphragm frequently spreads to extralymphoid sites such as the liver.

## Clinical Manifestations

The onset of symptoms in Hodgkin's lymphoma is usually insidious. The initial development is most often enlargement of cervical, axillary, or inguinal lymph nodes (Fig. 30-13); a mediastinal node mass is the second most common location. This lymphadenopathy affects discrete nodes that remain movable and nontender. The enlarged nodes are not painful unless they exert pressure on adjacent nerves.

The patient may notice weight loss, fatigue, weakness, fever, chills, tachycardia, or night sweats. A group of initial findings including fever (in excess of 100.4° F [38° C]), drenching night sweats, and weight loss (exceeding 10% in 6 months) are termed *B symptoms* and correlate with a worse prognosis. After the ingestion of even small amounts of alcohol, individuals with Hodgkin's lymphoma may complain of a rapid onset of pain at the site of disease. The cause for the alcohol-induced pain is unknown. Generalized pruritus without skin lesions may develop. Cough, dyspnea, stridor, and dysphagia may all reflect mediastinal node involvement.

In more advanced disease, there may be hepatomegaly and splenomegaly. Anemia results from increased destruction and decreased production of erythrocytes. Other physical signs vary depending on where the disease is located. For example, intrathoracic involvement may lead to superior vena cava syndrome, enlarged retroperitoneal nodes may cause palpable abdominal masses or interfere with renal function, jaundice may occur from liver involvement, spinal cord compression leading to paraplegia may occur with extradural involvement, and bone pain occurs as a result of bone involvement.

## Diagnostic and Staging Studies

Peripheral blood analysis, excisional lymph node biopsy, bone marrow examination, and radiologic studies are important means of evaluating Hodgkin's lymphoma. Abnormalities in the CBC, such as a microcytic hypochromic anemia, are variable and not diagnostic. Leukopenia and thrombocytopenia may develop, but they are usually a consequence of treatment, advanced disease, or superimposed hypersplenism. Other blood studies may show elevated erythrocyte sedimentation rate, elevated leukocyte alkaline phosphatase from liver and bone involvement, hypercalcemia from bone involvement, and hypoalbuminemia from liver involvement.

Radiologic evaluation can help define all sites and determine the clinical stage of the disease. Positron emission tomography (PET) with CT scan is used to stage and then assess the response to therapy and to differentiate residual tumor from fibrotic masses after treatment. These scans may show increased uptake (by PET) and masses (by CT) such as mediastinal lymphadenopathy; renal displacement caused by retroperitoneal node enlargement; abdominal lymph node enlargement; and liver, spleen, bone, and brain infiltration.

# NURSING AND INTERPROFESSIONAL MANAGEMENT: HODGKIN'S LYMPHOMA

Using all of the information from the various diagnostic studies, one can determine a clinical stage of disease (Fig. 30-14). The

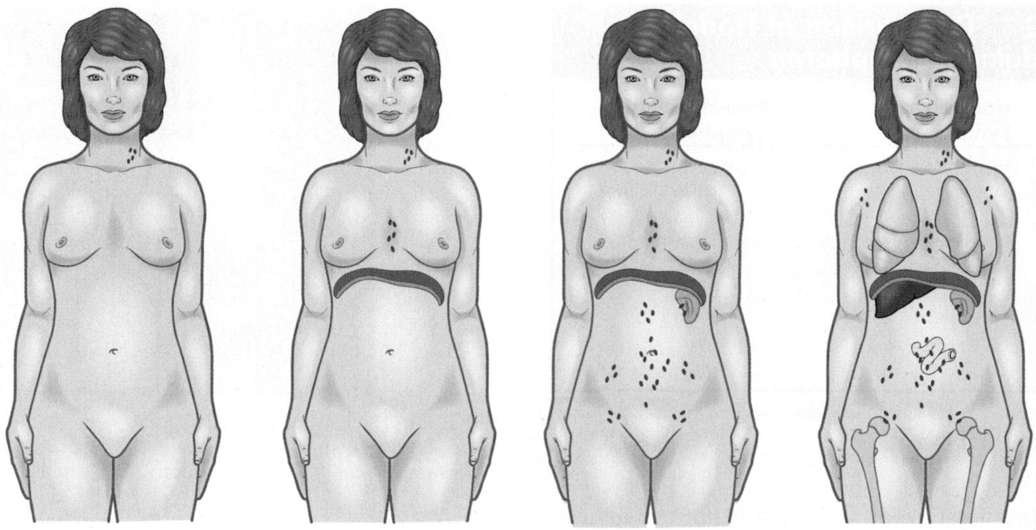


**FIG. 30-14** Staging system for Hodgkin's lymphoma and non-Hodgkin's lymphoma. *Stage I,* involvement of single lymph node (e.g., cervical node). *Stage II,* involvement of two or more lymph nodes on one side of diaphragm. *Stage III,* lymph node involvement above and below the diaphragm. *Stage IV,* involvement outside of diaphragm (e.g., liver, bone marrow). The stage is followed by the letter *A* (absence) or *B* (presence) to indicate significant systemic symptoms (e.g., fever, night sweats, weight loss).

final staging is based on the clinical stage (extent of the disease), presence of B symptom, and other unfavorable prognostic features. Treatment depends on the nature and extent of the disease. The nomenclature used in staging involves an A or B classification, depending on whether symptoms are present when the disease is found, and a Roman numeral (I to IV) that reflects the location and extent of the disease.[46,47]

Once the stage of Hodgkin's lymphoma is established, management focuses on selecting a treatment plan. The standard for chemotherapy is the ABVD regimen: doxorubicin (**A**driamycin), **b**leomycin, **v**inblastine, and **d**acarbazine. Patients with favorable early stage disease receive two to four cycles of chemotherapy. Patients with early stage disease but unfavorable prognostic features (e.g., B symptoms) or intermediate-stage disease are treated with four to six cycles of chemotherapy. Advanced-stage Hodgkin's lymphoma is treated more aggressively using six to eight cycles of chemotherapy. A common regimen is BEACOPP (**b**leomycin, **e**toposide, doxorubicin (**A**driamycin), **c**yclophosphamide, vincristine (**O**ncovin), **pro**carbazine, and **p**rednisone).[46,47] The role of radiation as a supplement to chemotherapy varies depending on sites of disease and the presence of resistant disease after chemotherapy. Response to therapy is determined by PET and CT scans and other diagnostic tests (e.g., bone marrow biopsy).

A variety of chemotherapy regimens and newer agents, such as brentuximab vedotin (Adcetris), are used to treat patients who have relapsed or refractory disease. Ideally, once remission is obtained, a hope for curative option may be intensive chemotherapy with the use of autologous or allogeneic HSCT.[46] HSCT has allowed patients to receive higher, potentially curative doses of chemotherapy while reducing life-threatening leukopenia (see Chapter 15). Combination chemotherapy works well because, as in leukemia, the drugs used have an additive antitumor effect without increasing side effects. As with leukemia, therapy must be aggressive. Therefore potentially life-threatening problems are encountered in an attempt to achieve a remission.

Maintenance chemotherapy does not contribute to increased survival once a complete remission is achieved. Occasionally, single drugs may be administered palliatively to patients who cannot tolerate intensive combination therapy. A serious consequence of the treatment for Hodgkin's lymphoma is the later development of secondary malignancies (see Chapter 15), as well as potential long-term toxicities from the treatment, such as endocrine, cardiac, and pulmonary dysfunction.[47] Secondary cancers occur 10 years after treatment for Hodgkin's lymphoma. The most common secondary malignancies are lung and breast cancer. Patients should have close follow-up and screening for early detection of these problems.[46]

The nursing care for Hodgkin's lymphoma is largely based on managing problems related to the disease (e.g., pain caused by a tumor, superior vena cava syndrome), pancytopenia, and other side effects of therapy. Because the survival of patients with Hodgkin's lymphoma depends on their response to treatment, supporting the patient through the consequences of treatment is extremely important.

Psychosocial considerations are as important as they are with leukemia. However, the prognosis for Hodgkin's lymphoma is better than that for many forms of cancer. The physical, psychologic, social, and spiritual consequences of the patient's disease must be addressed. Fertility issues may be of particular concern because this disease is frequently seen in adolescents and young adults. Help to ensure that these issues have been addressed soon after diagnosis. Evaluation of patients for long-term effects of therapy is important because delayed consequences of disease and treatment may not be apparent for many years. (Secondary malignancies and delayed effects are discussed in Chapter 15.)

## NON-HODGKIN'S LYMPHOMA

**Non-Hodgkin's lymphomas (NHLs)** are a heterogeneous group of malignant neoplasms of primarily B-, T-, or natural killer (NK) cell origin affecting all ages. B-cell lymphomas

## EVIDENCE-BASED PRACTICE

### *Applying the Evidence*

**Exercise and Hematologic Cancer**

You are a nurse caring for G.R., a 59-year-old male patient with non-Hodgkin's lymphoma who is receiving chemotherapy. Due to a decrease in red blood cells and platelets, he was advised to rest and avoid the high level of physical exercise he once enjoyed. He misses his active lifestyle and now admits to you that he is "somewhat depressed."

***Making Clinical Decisions***

***Best Available Evidence.*** Aerobic exercise, especially walking and stretching, to maintain mobility may improve physical functioning, fatigue, and depression in patients with hematologic cancers.

***Clinician Expertise.*** You know recommendations to decrease intensive physical exercise may result in a diminished quality of life for many patients, especially for individuals who are used to being physically active.

***Patient Preferences and Values.*** G.R. is considering joining a neighborhood bicycling club so that he can "feel better."

***Implications for Nursing Practice***

1. Why is intensive or extreme exercise contraindicated in someone who is getting chemotherapy or acutely ill?
2. What precautions would you discuss with G.R. before he increases his exercise level?
3. How would you involve G.R. in monitoring his fatigue?
4. As G.R. seeks ways to improve his quality of life, how would you support him?

***Reference for Evidence***

Bergenthal N, Will A, Streckmann F, et al: Aerobic physical exercise for adult patients with haematological malignancies, *Cochrane Database Syst Rev* 11:CD009075, 2014.

constitute about 88% of all NHLs. They are categorized by the level of differentiation, cell of origin, and rate of cellular proliferation.[42,48] A variety of clinical presentations and courses are recognized, from indolent (slowly developing) to rapidly progressive disease. NHL is the most commonly occurring hematologic cancer and is responsible for 3% of cancer-related deaths. Each year approximately 70,800 new cases of NHL are diagnosed and approximately 18,990 deaths occur.[37]

### Etiology and Pathophysiology

As with Hodgkin's lymphoma, the cause of NHL is usually unknown. NHLs may result from chromosomal translocations, infections, environmental factors, and immunodeficiency states. Chromosomal translocations have an important role in the pathogenesis of many NHLs. Some viruses and bacteria are implicated in the pathogenesis of NHL, including HTLV-1, EBV, human herpesvirus 8, hepatitis B and C, *Helicobacter pylori*, *Chlamydophila psittaci*, *Campylobacter jejuni*, and *Borrelia burgdorferi*. Environmental factors linked to the development of NHL include chemicals (e.g., pesticides, herbicides, solvents, organic chemicals, wood preservatives). NHL is also more common in individuals who have inherited immunodeficiency syndromes and who have used immunosuppressive medications (e.g., to prevent rejection after an organ transplant or to treat autoimmune disorders) or received chemotherapy or radiation therapy.

NHL does not have a hallmark feature that parallels the Reed-Sternberg cell of Hodgkin's lymphoma. However, all NHLs involve lymphocytes arrested in various stages of

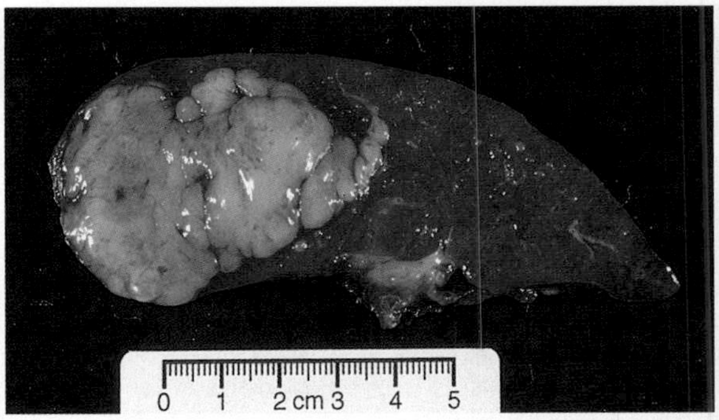


**FIG. 30-15** Non-Hodgkin's lymphoma involving the spleen. The presence of an isolated mass is typical. (From Cotran RS, Kumar V, Abbas AK: *Robbins pathologic basis of disease,* ed 6, Philadelphia, 1999, Saunders.)

development and may mimic a leukemia. For example, small lymphocytic lymphoma (SLL) and chronic lymphocytic leukemia (CLL) result from malignant proliferation of small B lymphocytes, with CLL having the majority of disease within the bone marrow (versus the lymph nodes).[42] (The overlap among leukemia and NHLs is discussed on p. 637.)

Diffuse large B-cell lymphoma, the most common aggressive lymphoma, is a neoplasm that originates in the lymph nodes, usually in the neck or abdomen. Burkitt's lymphoma is the most highly aggressive disease and is thought to originate from B-cell blasts in the lymph nodes.

### Clinical Manifestations

NHLs can originate outside the lymph nodes, the method of spread can be unpredictable, and the majority of patients have widely disseminated disease at the time of diagnosis (Fig. 30-15). The primary clinical manifestation is painless lymph node enlargement. The lymphadenopathy can wax and wane in indolent disease. Because the disease is usually disseminated when it is diagnosed, other symptoms are present depending on where the disease has spread (e.g., hepatomegaly with liver involvement, neurologic symptoms with CNS disease). NHL can also manifest in nonspecific ways, such as an airway obstruction, hyperuricemia and renal failure from tumor lysis syndrome, pericardial tamponade, and GI complaints.

Patients with high-grade lymphomas may have lymphadenopathy and constitutional symptoms (B symptoms) such as fever, night sweats, and weight loss. The peripheral blood is usually normal, but some lymphomas manifest in a "leukemic" phase.

### Diagnostic and Staging Studies

Diagnostic studies used for NHL resemble those used for Hodgkin's lymphoma. However, because NHL is more often in extranodal sites, more diagnostic studies may be done, such as an MRI or lumbar puncture to rule out CNS disease, a bone marrow biopsy to determine bone marrow infiltration, or a barium enema, upper endoscopy, to visualize suspected GI involvement. Clinical staging, as described for Hodgkin's lymphoma, is used to help guide therapy (Fig. 30-14), but establishment of the precise histologic subtype is extremely important. Lymph node excisional biopsy establishes the cell type and pattern. NHL is classified based on morphologic, genetic, immunophenotypic (cell surface antigens, CD20, CD52), and clinical features.

The World Health Organization has categorized more than 60 unique types of NHL.[42] A simplified modification of the classification system is presented in Table 30-28.

**TABLE 30-28 Classification of Non-Hodgkin's Lymphoma***

| B-Cell Lymphomas | T-Cell and NK-Cell Lymphomas |
|---|---|
| • Diffuse large B-cell lymphoma (DBLCL)<br>• Follicular lymphoma<br>• Marginal zone B-cell lymphoma (MALT)<br>• Small lymphocytic lymphoma/chronic lymphocytic leukemia<br>• Mantle cell lymphoma<br>• Burkitt's lymphoma<br>• Plasmablastic lymphoma<br>• AIDS-related B-cell lymphomas | • Lymphoblastic lymphoma<br>• T-cell lymphoma<br>• Mycosis fungoides and Sézary syndrome<br>• Anaplastic large T-cell lymphoma<br>• Natural killer cell lymphomas<br><br>**Posttransplant Lymphoproliferative Disorders (PTLD)** |

*MALT,* Mucosa-associated lymphoid tissue.
*This is only a partial list.

Treatment is guided by the cell type, cytogenetic studies, and clinical behavior: *indolent* (low grade), aggressive (high grade), or *highly aggressive* (very high grade). Additional factors, known as the International Prognostic Index (IPI), may be considered for each subtype to help select the appropriate treatment for these patients. Factors considered may include the clinical stage, number of extranodal sites, serum LDH, WBC count, hemoglobin, and patient's age and performance status.[48] Immunologic, cytogenetic, and molecular studies are also useful for making therapeutic decisions and assessing prognosis. Other studies might include blood tests for tumor lysis (see Chapter 15); screening for hepatitis, HIV, and *H. pylori*; skin biopsies; bone marrow biopsies; and lumbar punctures. The prognosis for NHL is based on the histopathology.

## NURSING AND INTERPROFESSIONAL MANAGEMENT: NON-HODGKIN'S LYMPHOMA

Treatment for NHL involves chemotherapy and sometimes radiation therapy[42,48] (Table 30-29). Ironically, more aggressive lymphomas (diffuse large B cell) are more responsive to treatment and more likely to be cured. In contrast, indolent lymphomas (e.g., follicular lymphomas have a naturally long course but are difficult to effectively treat).[48]

Patients with low-grade (indolent) lymphoma may live 10 years or more without treatment. However, some initial therapies can be well tolerated and have been shown to reduce the time to progression of the disease. Lymphomas that have an infectious basis, such as *H. pylori* gastric lymphomas, may be treated with antibiotic or antiviral therapy. HSCT may have some benefit in certain subtypes of aggressive or refractory lymphomas.

Rituximab, a monoclonal antibody against the CD20 antigen on the surface of normal and malignant B cells, is used to treat NHL. Once bound to the cells, rituximab causes lysis and cell death. Numerous chemotherapy combinations have been used to try to overcome the resistant nature of this disease (Table 30-29). Complete remissions are uncommon, but the majority of patients respond with improvement in symptoms.

**DRUG ALERT Rituximab (Rituxan)**
- Monitor patient for signs of severe hypersensitivity infusion reactions, especially with first infusion.
- Manifestations may include hypotension, bronchospasm, dysrhythmias, angioedema, and cardiogenic shock.
- Screen for history of hepatitis because the drug may reactivate hepatitis.

**TABLE 30-29 Treatment of Non-Hodgkin's Lymphoma*†**

| Recommended Therapies | Common Chemotherapy Combinations |
|---|---|
| **Indolent** (Low Grade) (e.g., Follicular Lymphoma, Marginal Zone B-Cell Lymphoma [MALT]) | |
| • Observation until disease progression for asymptomatic patients with low-volume tumors and normal blood counts<br>• External beam irradiation for local, limited disease<br>• Single-agent rituximab (Rituxan)<br>• Single-agent chemotherapy (chlorambucil, cyclophosphamide, bendamustine) or idelalisib)<br>• Rituximab with another agent (bendamustine, cyclophosphamide, fludarabine, cladribine, lenalidomide, chlorambucil)<br>• Combination chemotherapy (R-CHOP or other)<br>• Radioimmunotherapy<br>• Hematopoietic stem cell transplant (HSCT) | **R-CHOP:** **r**ituximab, **c**yclophosphamide, doxorubicin **h**ydrochloride, vincristine (**O**ncovin), **p**rednisone<br>**FCMR:** **f**ludarabine, **c**yclophosphamide **m**itoxantrone, **r**ituximab<br>**R-CVP:** **r**ituximab, **c**yclophosphamide, **v**incristine, **p**rednisone<br>**RFND:** **r**ituximab, **f**ludarabine, mitoxantrone (**N**ovantrone), **d**examethasone ± rituximab<br>**FC:** **f**ludarabine, **c**yclophosphamide |
| **Aggressive** (Intermediate or High Grade) (e.g., Mantle Cell, Diffuse Large B-Cell, Peripheral T-Cell, Natural Killer Cell Lymphomas) | |
| • Combination chemotherapy with localized radiation if needed<br>• Aggressive combination chemotherapy for 3-8 cycles with rituximab with local radiation if needed<br>• Intrathecal chemotherapy if needed<br>• Single agent or other combination treatment, depending on subtype and response (e.g., bendamustine, bortezomib, cladribine, ibrutinib, lenalidomide, belinostat, gemcitabine, alemtuzumab, oxaliplatin, belinostat, romidepsin)<br>• HSCT | **R-CHOP** (see above)<br>**ICE** (or "RICE" with rituximab): **i**fosfamide, **c**yclophosphamide, **e**toposide<br>**R-EPOCH:** **r**ituximab, **e**toposide, **p**rednisone, vincristine (**O**ncovin), **c**yclophosphamide, doxorubicin **h**ydrochloride<br>**ESHAP ± R:** **e**toposide, methylprednisolone (**S**olu-Medrol), **h**igh-dose cytarabine (**A**ra-C), cisplatin (**P**latinol), with or without **r**ituximab<br>**Hyper-CVAD ± R:** hyperfractionated **c**yclophosphamide, **v**incristine, doxorubicin (**A**driamycin), **d**examethasone alternating with high-dose methotrexate and cytarabine with or without rituximab<br>**DHAP ± R:** **d**examethasone, **h**igh-dose cytarabine (**A**ra-C), cisplatin (**P**latinol), with our without **r**ituximab<br>**SMILE:** **s**teroids, **m**ethotrexate, **i**fosfamide, **L**-asparaginase, **e**toposide<br>High-dose cytarabine and high-dose methotrexate with leucovorin rescue |
| **Highly Aggressive** (e.g., Burkitt's Lymphoma, AIDS-Related B-Cell Lymphomas) | |
| • Aggressive combination chemotherapy for 3-8 cycles<br>• HSCT | **Hyper-CVAD ± R** ( see above)<br>**CODOX-M:** **c**yclophosphamide, vincristine (**O**ncovin), **dox**orubicin, high-dose **m**ethotrexate, with or without rituximab (includes intrathecal methotrexate) |

MALT, Mucosa-associated lymphoid tissue.
*Not all inclusive.
†The acronym for some drug regimens use the trade name of chemotherapy agents. In some cases the trade name has been discontinued, and the drug currently used is the generic version.

Other therapies for some types of NHL include the monoclonal antibody ibritumomab tiuxetan (Zevalin). This antibody linked to a radioactive isotope (yttrium-90) (see Table 15-13). The monoclonal antibody targets the CD20 antigen, which is on the surface of mature B cells and B-cell tumors. This targeting allows for the delivery of radiation directly to the malignant cells. Side effects of this type of treatment include pancytopenia. Use radiation precautions in caring for these patients. Teach patients about safety issues and how to minimize the risk of radiation exposure to staff and others.

In general T-cell lymphomas are more difficult to treat and are often treated aggressively up front often followed by an HSCT. Cutaneous T-cell lymphomas may be treated with topical corticosteroids or topical chemotherapy for limited-stage disease. For more diffuse disease, treatment may include phototherapy, α-interferon, bexarotene (Targretin), vorinostat (Zolinza), or others.[42]

The nursing care for NHL is similar to that for Hodgkin's lymphoma. It is largely based on managing problems related to the disease (e.g., pain caused by the tumor, spinal cord compression, tumor lysis syndrome), pancytopenia, and other side effects of therapy. However, because NHL can be more extensive and involve specific organs (e.g., CNS, spleen, liver, GI tract, bone marrow), it is important to understand the subtype and extent of the disease. For example, a patient with known involvement of the colon may complain of acute abdominal pain. The patient most likely would have abdominal guarding and an enlarged and tympanic abdomen. This could indicate a bowel perforation and be considered a medical emergency. A patient with a Burkitt's NHL beginning chemotherapy would be at high risk for tumor lysis syndrome and would require frequent laboratory studies and monitoring, as well as strict documentation of intake and output. (Cancer-related therapies and side effects are discussed in Chapter 15.)

The patient undergoing external beam radiation therapy has special nursing needs. The skin in the radiation field requires attention. Concepts related to safety issues regarding radiation therapy are important to include in the plan of care (see Chapter 15).

Psychosocial considerations are important. Help the patient and family understand the disease, treatment, and expected and potential side effects. Some aggressive treatments require close follow-up and even inpatient admission. Fertility issues may be of concern in young patients. As in Hodgkin's lymphoma, evaluation of patients with NHL for long-term effects of therapy is important because the delayed consequences of disease and treatment may not become apparent for many years. (Secondary malignancies and delayed effects are discussed in Chapter 15.)

## MULTIPLE MYELOMA

**Multiple myeloma**, or *plasma cell myeloma,* is a condition in which neoplastic plasma cells infiltrate the bone marrow and destroy bone. Multiple myeloma accounts for about 1% of all malignancies and for about 15% of all hematologic malignancies.[37] The disease is twice as common in men as in women and usually develops after 40 years of age, with an average age of 69 years. Multiple myeloma occurs in African Americans more commonly than in whites. Although it was previously not considered curable, the 5-year survival rate is close to 45% because of the variety of treatments that can be provided throughout the course of the disease.[49]

### Etiology and Pathophysiology

The cause of multiple myeloma is unknown. It is possible that exposure to radiation, organic chemicals (such as benzene), metals, herbicides, and insecticides may play a role. Obesity and genetic factors and viral infection may also influence the risk of developing multiple myeloma.

The disease process involves excessive production of plasma cells. Plasma cells are activated B cells, which produce immunoglobulins (antibodies) that normally protect the body. However, in multiple myeloma instead of a variety of plasma cells producing antibodies to fight different infections, myeloma tumors produce monoclonal antibodies. *Monoclonal* means they are all of one kind, making them ineffective and even harmful. Not only do they not fight infections, but they also infiltrate the bone marrow. These monoclonal proteins (called *M proteins*) are made up of two light chains and two heavy chains. *Bence-Jones proteins* are the light chain part of these monoclonal antibodies. They show up in the urine in many patients with multiple myeloma.

Furthermore, plasma cell production of excessive and abnormal amounts of cytokines (interleukins [ILs]; IL-4, IL-5, and IL-6) also plays an important role in the pathologic process of bone destruction. As myeloma protein increases, normal plasma cells are reduced, which further compromises the body's normal immune response. Proliferation of malignant plasma cells and the overproduction of immunoglobulin and proteins result in the end-organ effects of myeloma on the bone marrow, bone, and kidneys and possibly the spleen, lymph nodes, liver, and even heart muscle.

### Clinical Manifestations

Multiple myeloma develops slowly and insidiously. The patient often does not manifest symptoms until the disease is advanced, at which time skeletal pain is the major manifestation. Pain in the pelvis, spine, and ribs is particularly common and is triggered by movement. Diffuse osteoporosis develops as the myeloma protein destroys bone. Osteolytic lesions are seen in the skull, vertebrae, and ribs. Vertebral destruction can lead to collapse of vertebrae with ensuing compression of the spinal cord. Loss of bone integrity can lead to the development of pathologic fractures.

Bony degeneration also causes calcium to be lost from bones, eventually causing hypercalcemia. Hypercalcemia may cause renal, GI, or neurologic manifestations such as polyuria, anorexia, confusion, and ultimately seizures, coma, and cardiac problems. A serum *hyperviscosity syndrome* leading to cerebral, pulmonary, renal, and other organ dysfunction can occur in some patients. Even without hyperviscosity, high protein levels caused by the myeloma protein can result in renal tubular obstruction, interstitial nephritis, and renal failure. The patient may also display manifestations of anemia, thrombocytopenia, neutropenia, and immune dysfunction, all of which are related to the replacement of normal bone marrow with plasma cells. Neurologic abnormalities may be caused by regional myeloma cell growth compressing the spinal cord or cranial nerves, or by perineuronal or perivascular deposition.[50]

### Diagnostic Studies

Evaluating multiple myeloma involves laboratory, radiologic, and bone marrow examination. M protein is found in the blood and urine. Possible findings include pancytopenia, hypercalcemia, Bence Jones protein in the urine, and an elevated serum creatinine.

Skeletal bone surveys, MRI, and/or PET and CT scans show distinct lytic areas of bone erosions; generalized thinning of the bones; or fractures, especially in the vertebrae, ribs, pelvis, and bones of the thigh and upper arms. Bone marrow analysis shows significantly increased numbers of plasma cells in the bone marrow. The simplest measure of staging and prognosis in multiple myeloma is based on blood levels of two markers: $\beta_2$-microglobulin and albumin. In general, higher levels of $\beta_2$-microglobulin and lower levels of albumin are associated with a poorer prognosis.

### Interprofessional Care

Interprofessional care involves managing both the disease and its symptoms. The current treatment options include corticosteroids, chemotherapy, immunotherapy, and targeted therapy, and HSCT.[51] Multiple myeloma is seldom cured, but treatment can relieve symptoms, produce remission, and prolong life. Ambulation and adequate hydration are used to treat hypercalcemia, dehydration, and potential renal damage. Weight bearing helps the bones resorb some calcium, and fluids dilute calcium and prevent protein precipitates from causing renal tubular obstruction. Control of pain and prevention of pathologic fractures are other goals of management. Analgesics, orthopedic supports, and localized radiation help reduce the skeletal pain.

Kyphoplasty is sometimes used to control spine vertebral disease. *Kyphoplasty* is a minimally invasive procedure (usually done in an interventional radiology area) that injects cement to stabilize the vertebral compression.

Bisphosphonates, such as pamidronate (Aredia) and zoledronic acid (Zometa), inhibit bone breakdown and are used for the treatment of skeletal pain and hypercalcemia. They inhibit bone resorption without inhibiting bone formation and mineralization. They are given monthly by IV infusion.

**DRUG ALERT Zoledronic Acid (Zometa)**

- Patient should be adequately rehydrated before administering drug.
- Renal toxicity may occur if IV infusion of drug is administered in less than 15 min.

Chemotherapy with corticosteroids is usually the first treatment recommended for multiple myeloma. It is used to reduce the number of plasma cells. Initial treatment depends on whether the patient is a future bone marrow transplant candidate and anticipated tolerance of therapy. The treatment usually includes a corticosteroid (dexamethasone or prednisone) plus one or two chemotherapy agents, such as melphalan (Alkeran), vincristine (Oncovin), cyclophosphamide (Cytoxan), doxorubicin, and bendamustine (Treanda). High-dose chemotherapy followed by HSCT has evolved as the standard of care in eligible patients.[51]

Immunotherapy and targeted therapy are also used to treat multiple myeloma. Immunomodulator drugs (described in Chapter 15) include thalidomide (Thalidomide), lenalidomide (Revlimid), and pomalidomide (Pomalyst). Proteosome inhibitors include bortezomib (Velcade), carfilzomib (Kyprolis), and ixazomib (Ninlaro). Panobinostat (Farydak) is a drug that can affect which genes are active inside of cells. Daratumumab (Darzalex) is a monoclonal antibody against CD38, which is expressed on the surface of myeloma cells.

Drugs may also be used to treat complications of multiple myeloma. For example, allopurinol may be given to reduce hyperuricemia, and IV furosemide (Lasix) promotes renal excretion of calcium. In some patients, the levels of plasma proteins are so high that it causes a hyperviscosity syndrome leading to neurologic changes, renal insufficiency, and other problems related to lack of blood flow. In this instance plasmapheresis is used.

## BECOMING A NURSE LEADER

### *Importance of Being a Leader*

**Situation**

You are a senior nursing student who is doing a clinical rotation on a busy hematology unit. You are working with Gayla, who is an experienced RN. Gayla is a hardworking, dedicated, experienced nurse whom you greatly admire. You hear her discussing that she has just been appointed to the State Board of Nursing. Why, you wonder, is she getting involved in something like that when she is so busy at work and in her personal life?

**Points for Consideration**

- Leadership is needed from nurses at all levels and across all health care settings.
- The Institute of Medicine's Future of Nursing report recommends that opportunities be provided for nurses to assume leadership positions and serve as full partners in health care improvement.[1]
- Nurses must step up to be leaders to be full partners with HCPs and other health care professionals to assist in health care improvements.
- The Future of Nursing report states that nurses will need a leadership style that works in full partnership with others respectfully and collaboratively. This leadership style helps to improve patient outcomes, reduces errors, and results in less staff turnover.

**Discussion Questions**

1. What may be Gayla's motivation for getting involved with the State Board of Nursing?
2. What benefit will Gayla gain from her experience with the State Board of Nursing? How will her colleagues in her work setting benefit from her experience?
3. What leadership skills do you have? How can these leadership skills be used to promote improvements in health care?

**Reference**

1. Institute of Medicine. The future of nursing: leading change, advancing health. Retrieved from *http://thefutureofnursing.org/sites/default/files/Summary%20%281-14%29.pdf*

## NURSING MANAGEMENT: MULTIPLE MYELOMA

A major focus of care relates to the bone involvement and sequelae from bone breakdown. Maintaining adequate hydration is a primary nursing consideration to minimize problems from hypercalcemia. IV fluids may be administered to attain a urine output of 1.5 to 2 L/day if the patient does not already have renal compromise. Although tumor lysis is rare, once chemotherapy is initiated, allopurinol may be given to prevent any renal damage from uric acid accumulation (from cell breakdown). Because of the myeloma proteins, the patient is at additional risk of renal dysfunction and electrolyte and fluid imbalances.

Because of the potential for pathologic fractures, use caution when moving and ambulating the patient. A slight twist or strain in the wrong area (e.g., a weak area in the patient's bones) may be sufficient to cause a fracture. In addition, the development of peripheral neuropathy is common with several therapies for multiple myeloma and can contribute to discomfort, the inability to perform basic activities of daily living, and the risk of injury from falling. Pain medications and therapies can also lead to severe constipation.

Pain management requires innovative and knowledgeable nursing interventions. Analgesics, such as nonsteroidal antiinflammatory drugs, acetaminophen, or an acetaminophen/opioid combination, may be more effective than opioids alone in diminishing bone pain. Braces, especially for the spine, may also help control pain. As in any pain management situation, assess the patient and implement necessary measures to alleviate the pain. (Pain management is discussed in Chapter 8.) Patients may also be at risk for deep vein thrombosis related to chemotherapy and immobility and should have appropriate preventive measures employed.[50]

Assessment and prompt treatment of infection are important in the care of patients with multiple myeloma. These recurrent infections may be due to a decrease in the production of normal immunoglobulins, the ineffectiveness of the overproduced and abnormal immunoglobulins, corticosteroids, and/or neutropenia as a result of the bone marrow infiltration or side effects of treatment.

The patient's psychosocial needs require sensitive, skilled management. Help the patient and significant others adapt to changes fostered by chronic illness and adjust to the losses related to the disease process, while helping to maximize functioning and quality of life. The patient with multiple myeloma may experience remissions and exacerbations. Patients may be on dialysis because of myeloma-induced renal failure. Consequently acute care is needed at various times during the course of the illness.

The final, acute phase is unresponsive to treatment and usually short in duration. The way in which patients and families confront death may be affected by the manner in which they have learned to accept and live with the chronic disease.

## DISORDERS OF THE SPLEEN

The spleen can be affected by many illnesses, most of which can cause some degree of *splenomegaly* (enlarged spleen)[52] (Table 30-30). However, an enlarged spleen may be present in certain individuals without any evidence of disease. The term *hypersplenism* refers to the occurrence of splenomegaly and peripheral cytopenias (anemia, leukopenia, and thrombocytopenia).[26] The degree of splenic enlargement varies with the disease. For example, massive splenic enlargement occurs with infectious mononucleosis, chronic myelogenous leukemia, and thalassemia major. Mild splenic enlargement occurs with HF and systemic lupus erythematosus. The normal spleen contains 350 mL of blood, and about one third of the platelet mass is sequestered in the spleen.

When the spleen enlarges, its normal filtering and sequestering capacity increases. Consequently, there is often a reduction in the number of circulating blood cells as they engorge the spleen. In addition, there are unusual findings in the peripheral smear, such as pitted or pocked erythrocytes or Howell-Jolly bodies. These findings assist in diagnosing a malfunctioning spleen. A slight to moderate enlargement of the spleen is usually asymptomatic and found during routine examination of the abdomen. Even massive splenomegaly can be well tolerated, but the patient may complain of abdominal discomfort and early satiety. In addition to physical examination, other techniques to assess the size of the spleen include radionuclide colloid liver-spleen scan, CT or PET scan, MRI, and ultrasound scan.

Occasionally a splenectomy is done either via laparoscopy or open laparotomy as part of the evaluation or treatment of splenomegaly. Another major indication for splenectomy is splenic rupture. The spleen may rupture from trauma; inadvertent tearing during other surgical procedures; and diseases such as mononucleosis, malaria, and lymphoid neoplasms. After a splenectomy, there can be a dramatic increase in peripheral RBC, WBC, and platelet counts.

Nursing responsibilities for the patient with spleen disorders vary depending on the problem. Splenomegaly may be painful and may require analgesic administration; care in moving, turning, and positioning; and evaluation of lung expansion because spleen enlargement may impair diaphragmatic excursion. If anemia, thrombocytopenia, or leukopenia develops from splenic enlargement, institute nursing measures to support the patient and prevent life-threatening complications. If splenectomy is performed, observe the patient for hemorrhage and shock.

After splenectomy, immunologic deficiencies may develop, such as low IgG levels. Postsplenectomy patients have a lifelong risk for infection, especially from encapsulated organisms such as *Pneumococcus* species. This risk is reduced by immunization with pneumococcal vaccine.[52]

**TABLE 30-30 Causes of Splenomegaly**

**Infections and Inflammations**
- Bacterial infections: endocarditis, salmonella
- Mycobacterial infections: tuberculosis
- Spirochetes: syphilis, Lyme disease
- Viral infections: hepatitis, human immunodeficiency virus, cytomegalovirus, mononucleosis
- Parasitic infections: malaria, trypanosomiasis, schistosomiasis, leishmaniasis, toxoplasmosis
- Rickettsial infections: Rocky Mountain spotted fever, typhoid fever
- Fungal infections: histoplasmosis
- Autoimmune diseases: systemic lupus erythematosus, rheumatoid arthritis

**Infiltrative Diseases and Tumors or Cysts**
- Acute and chronic leukemia
- Lymphomas
- Polycythemia vera
- Multiple myeloma, amyloidosis
- Other primary or secondary neoplasms and cysts
- Sarcoidosis
- Gaucher disease

**Congestion**
- Cirrhosis of the liver
- Heart failure (portal hypertension)
- Portal or splenic vein thrombosis
- Sickle cell disease
- Thalassemia
- Acquired hemolytic anemia
- Immune thrombocytopenia

## BLOOD COMPONENT THERAPY

Blood component therapy is frequently used to manage hematologic diseases. Many therapeutic and surgical procedures depend on blood product support. However, blood component therapy only temporarily supports the patient until the underlying problem is resolved. Because transfusions are not free from hazards, they should be used only if necessary.

Avoid developing a complacent attitude about this common but potentially dangerous therapy. Make sure that the HCP has

**TABLE 30-31 Blood Products***

| Description | Special Considerations | Indications for Use |
|---|---|---|
| **Packed RBCs** | | |
| Packed RBCs are prepared from whole blood by sedimentation or centrifugation. One unit contains 250-350 mL. They can be stored up to 35 days depending on processing. | Use of RBCs for treatment allows remaining components of blood (e.g., platelets, albumin, plasma) to be used for other purposes. There is less danger of fluid overload. Packed RBCs are preferred RBC source because they are more component specific.<br>Leukocyte depletion (leukoreduction) by filtration, washing, or freezing is frequently used. Decreases hemolytic febrile or mild allergic reactions in patients who receive frequent transfusions | Severe or symptomatic anemia, acute blood loss. One unit of RBCs can be expected to increase Hgb by 1 g/dL or Hct by 3% in a typical adult. One unit of RBCs can replace a blood loss of 500 mL. |
| **Frozen RBCs** | | |
| Frozen RBCs are prepared from RBCs using glycerol for protection and frozen. They can be stored for 10 yr. | Must be used within 24 hr of thawing. Successive washings with saline solution remove majority of WBCs and plasma proteins. | Autotransfusion. Stockpiling or rare donors for patients with alloantibodies |
| **Platelets** | | |
| Platelets are prepared from fresh whole blood. One donor unit contains $3 \times 10^{11}$ platelets (from whole blood). Platelets may also be pooled from multiple donors. (One apheresed unit is roughly equivalent to 4-6 random donor-pooled platelets). An apheresed single donation is usually 200-400 mL in volume. | Multiple units of platelets can be obtained from one donor by plateletpheresis. They can be kept at room temperature for 1-5 days depending on type of collection and storage bag used. Bag should be agitated periodically. For patients who receive frequent transfusions and become refractory, may give leukocyte reduced, HLA, or type specific to prevent alloimmunization to HLA antigens | Bleeding caused by thrombocytopenia. May be contraindicated in thrombotic thrombocytopenic purpura and heparin-induced thrombocytopenia except in life-threatening hemorrhage<br>Expected increase is 5,000/μL/U. Failure to have an increase may be due to fever, sepsis, splenomegaly, or DIC or development of antibodies *(refractory)*. |
| **Fresh Frozen Plasma** | | |
| Liquid portion of whole blood is separated from cells and frozen. One unit contains approximately 250 mL. Plasma is rich in clotting factors but contains no platelets. May be stored for ≥1 yr, depending on storage. Must be used within 24 hr after thawing | Use of plasma in treating hypovolemic shock is being replaced by pure preparations such as albumin and plasma expanders. | Bleeding caused by deficiency in clotting factors (e.g., DIC, hemorrhage, massive transfusion, liver disease, vitamin K deficiency, excess warfarin) |
| **Albumin** | | |
| Albumin is prepared from plasma. It can be stored for 5 yr. It is available in 5% or 25% solution. | Albumin 25 g/dL is osmotically equal to 500 mL of plasma. Hyperosmolar solution acts by moving water from extravascular to intravascular space. It is heat treated and does not transmit viruses. | Hypovolemic shock, hypoalbuminemia |
| **Cryoprecipitates and Commercial Concentrates** | | |
| Cryoprecipitate is prepared from fresh frozen plasma, with 10-20 mL/bag. It can be stored for 1 yr. Once thawed, must be used within 5 days | Table 30-18 | Replacement of clotting factors, especially factor VIII, von Willebrand factor, and fibrinogen |

DIC, Disseminated intravascular coagulation; *HLA,* human leukocyte antigen.
*Component therapy has replaced the use of whole blood, which is infrequently used. Granulocyte transfusions are not included here because they are rarely used.

discussed the risks, benefits, and alternatives with the patient and that this is documented in the patient's medical record.

Traditionally, the term *blood transfusion* meant the administration of whole blood. Blood transfusion now has a broader meaning because of the ability to administer specific components of blood such as platelets, packed red blood cells (PRBCs), or plasma. Usually a specific component is ordered, although whole blood may be rarely used with massive hemorrhage or for an exchange transfusion[53,54] (Table 30-31).

## Administration Procedure

Blood components may be administered with a 22-gauge IV needle, cannula, or catheter.[55] However, larger sizes (e.g., 18- or 16-gauge) may be preferred if rapid transfusions are given or if the infusion is sluggish. Smaller needles can be used for platelets, albumin, and clotting factor replacement. Whatever type of venous access is used, verify its patency before requesting the blood component from the blood bank. Most blood product administration tubing is of a "Y type" with a microaggregate filter (filters out particulate), with one arm of the Y for the isotonic saline solution and the other arm of the Y for the blood product. Infusion pumps may be used if approved for blood administration and according to institution policy.

**! SAFETY ALERT Blood Transfusions**

- Do not use dextrose solutions or lactated Ringer's solution for administering blood because they will cause RBC hemolysis.
- Do not give any additives (including medications) via the same tubing as the blood unless the tubing is first cleared with saline solution.

After obtaining the blood or blood components from the blood bank, make a positive identification of the donor blood and recipient. Improper product-to-patient identification is the most common cause of hemolytic transfusion reactions, thus placing a great responsibility on nurses to carry out the

## ETHICAL/LEGAL DILEMMAS

### *Religious Beliefs*

**Situation**

W.D., an 81-year-old woman with dementia, is transferred from a nursing home to a hospital because of gastrointestinal bleeding from an unknown cause. Some of her family members tell you that she is a Jehovah's Witness and must not receive blood products. If she does not have exploratory surgery and transfusions, the surgeon believes that she will die.

**Ethical/Legal Points for Consideration**

- Competent adults have the right to make health care decisions, including the right to refuse treatment, based on their religious beliefs.
- If the patient is determined to be incompetent and a guardian has been appointed, the guardian has the legal right to make the consent or refusal.
- If the HCP believes that the treatment is essential to preserve life and health and there is no legal decision maker, a request is made for a legal determination of whether the patient is incapable of consent or refusal. If the judge agrees, the patient is made a ward of the court for this issue. Usually the HCP is directed to make a decision based on the patient's best interests.
- Courts tend to defer to any past information coming directly from patients about their own personal desires, even if that information is not in valid advance directives.[1]

**Discussion Questions**

1. What resources do you have available to consult about religious practices?
2. How could you make a determination if the family were acting in W.D.'s best interest or their own?
3. What nonblood alternatives are available for Jehovah's Witnesses?

identification procedure appropriately. Follow the policy and procedures at your place of employment. Many institutions have implemented a dual-checking system with two licensed individuals checking the patient identification with the labeled blood component. The blood bank is responsible for typing and crossmatching the donor's blood with the recipient's blood. The result of the compatibility testing should be noted on the product bag or tag, if pertinent. Table 30-32 outlines blood component compatibilities for transfusions.[53,56]

ABO compatibility is not a prerequisite for platelet transfusions. However, after multiple platelet transfusions, a patient may develop anti-HLA antibodies to the transfused platelets. With the use of lymphocyte typing to match HLA types of the donor and recipient, multiple platelet transfusions can be given with fewer complications to those who develop antibodies to platelets. The patient may be premedicated with an antihistamine (e.g., diphenhydramine [Benadryl]) and hydrocortisone to decrease the possibility of reacting to platelet transfusions if he or she has a history of reactions.[54,57]

Take the patient's vital signs before beginning the transfusion so that you have a baseline measure. If the patient has abnormal vital signs (e.g., high fever), call the HCP to clarify when the blood component may be administered. Administer the blood as soon as it is brought to the patient. Do not refrigerate it on the nursing unit. If the blood is not used within 30 minutes, return it to the blood bank. During the first 15 minutes or 50 mL of blood infusion, remain with the patient. If there are any untoward reactions, they are most likely to occur at this time. The rate of infusion during this period should be no more than 2 mL/minute. Do not infuse PRBCs quickly except in an emergency. Rapid infusion of cold blood may cause the patient to become chilled. If rapid replacement of large amounts of blood is necessary, a blood-warming device may be used. Other blood components, such as fresh frozen plasma and platelets, may be infused over 15 to 30 minutes. Refer to your institution's policy and procedure.

After the first 15 minutes, vital signs are usually retaken, and the rate of infusion is determined by the patient's clinical condition and the product being infused. Observe the patient

## TEAMWORK & COLLABORATION

### *Blood Transfusions*

**Role of Nursing Personnel**

***Registered Nurse (RN)***

- Ensure that an IV line is being used with a large-bore needle, catheter, or cannula, preferably 19 gauge or larger.
- Double-check patient identification and blood product identification data with another licensed nurse (consider state nurse practice act and agency policy).
- Adjust infusion rate of transfusion according to patient needs.
- Evaluate patient for signs of transfusion reactions.
- Evaluate for therapeutic effect of blood product (improvement in complete blood count, increased blood pressure, improved patient color, decreased bleeding).
- Monitor for signs of circulatory overload (e.g., shortness of breath) if the transfusion must be given rapidly.

***Licensed Practical/Vocational Nurse (LPN/LVN)***

- Assist with checking patient identification and blood product identification data with the RN (consider state nurse practice act and agency policy).
- Monitor blood transfusion rate (consider state nurse practice act and agency policy).

***Unlicensed Assistive Personnel (UAP)***

- Obtain blood products from the blood bank as directed by the RN.
- Take vital signs before the transfusion and after the first 15 min.

**Role of Other Team Members**

***Blood Bank Personnel***

- Responsible for typing and crossmatching the donor's blood with the recipient's blood.
- Result of the compatibility testing should be noted on the product bag or tag.
- When handing off the blood or blood component to nursing personnel, ensure that a positive identification is made with product and patient's information.

**TABLE 30-32 Blood Component Compatibilities for Transfusions**

| | DONOR PRODUCT | | | |
|---|---|---|---|---|
| **Recipient's Type** | **Packed Red Blood Cells** | **Plasma** | **Platelets** | **Cryoprecipitate** |
| O+ | O+ , O– | All groups | O, B, A, AB | Any group is safe to transfuse |
| O– | O– | | | |
| A+ | A+, A–, O+, O– | A, AB | A, AB, B, O | |
| A– | A–, O– | | | |
| B+ | B+, B–, O+, O– | B, AB | B, AB, A, O | |
| B– | B–, O+ | | | |
| AB+ | All groups | Only AB | Any group | |
| AB– | AB–, B–, A–, O– | | | |

periodically throughout the transfusion (e.g., every 30 minutes) and up to 1 hour after the transfusion. Most patients not in danger of fluid overload can tolerate the infusion of 1 unit of PRBCs over 2 hours. The transfusion should not take more than 4 hours to administer because of the increased risk of bacterial growth in the product once it is out of refrigeration. Never store blood components in unmonitored refrigerators in nursing units.

## Blood Transfusion Reactions

A *blood transfusion reaction* is an adverse reaction to blood transfusion therapy that can range in severity from mild symptoms to a life-threatening condition. Because complications of transfusion therapy may be significant, judicious evaluation of the patient is required. Blood transfusion reactions can be classified as acute or delayed[53,57,58] (Tables 30-33 and 30-34).

If a transfusion reaction occurs, take the following steps: (1) stop the transfusion; (2) maintain a patent IV line with saline solution; (3) notify the blood bank and the HCP

### CHECK YOUR PRACTICE

Your 82-yr-old male patient with severe iron deficiency anemia is receiving his second unit of packed RBCs. He received his first transfusions without any problems. He is now complaining of chills and feeling like his heart is racing.

- What should you do?

### TABLE 30-33 Acute Transfusion Reactions

| Cause | Manifestations | Management | Prevention |
|---|---|---|---|
| **Acute Hemolytic Reaction** | | | |
| Infusion of ABO-incompatible whole blood, RBCs, or components containing ≥10 mL of RBCs<br>Antibodies in the recipient's plasma attach to antigens on transfused RBCs, causing RBC destruction. | Reactions usually develop in first 15 min. Fever with or without chills; low back, abdominal, chest or flank pain; flushing, tachycardia, dyspnea, tachypnea, hypotension, vascular collapse, hemoglobinuria, acute jaundice, dark urine, bleeding, acute kidney injury, shock, cardiac arrest, DIC, death | • Treat shock and DIC if present.<br>• Draw blood samples for serologic testing slowly to avoid hemolysis from the procedure. Send urine specimen to the laboratory.<br>• Maintain BP with IV colloid solutions. Give diuretics as prescribed to maintain urine flow.<br>• Insert indwelling urinary catheter or measure voided amounts to monitor hourly urine output. Dialysis may be required if renal failure occurs.<br>• Do not transfuse additional RBC-containing components until blood bank has provided newly crossmatched units. | Meticulously verify and document patient identification from sample collection to component infusion (e.g., visually compare label on sample collection and blood component with patient identification). |
| **Febrile, Nonhemolytic Reaction (Most Common)** | | | |
| Sensitization to donor WBCs (most common), platelets, or plasma proteins | Sudden chills, rigors, and fever (rise in temperature of >1°C), headache, flushing, anxiety, vomiting, muscle pain | • Give antipyretics as prescribed (acetaminophen). Avoid aspirin in thrombocytopenic patients.<br>• Do not restart transfusion unless HCP orders. | Consider leukocyte-reduced blood products (filtered, washed, or frozen) for patients with a history of two or more such reactions.<br>Give acetaminophen or diphenhydramine (Benadryl) 30 min before transfusion. |
| **Mild Allergic Reaction** | | | |
| Sensitivity to foreign plasma proteins<br>More common in people with history of allergies | Flushing, itching, pruritus, urticaria (hives) | • Give antihistamine, corticosteroid, epinephrine, as ordered.<br>• If symptoms are mild and transient, transfusion may be restarted slowly with HCP's order.<br>• Do not restart transfusion if fever or pulmonary symptoms develop. | Treat prophylactically with antihistamines or steroids.<br>Consider washed RBCs and platelets. |
| **Anaphylactic and Severe Allergic Reaction** | | | |
| Sensitivity to donor plasma proteins<br>Infusion of IgA proteins to IgA-deficient recipient who has developed IgA antibody | Anxiety, urticaria, dyspnea, wheezing, progressing to cyanosis, bronchospasm, hypotension, shock, and possible cardiac arrest | • Initiate CPR, if indicated. Administer $O_2$.<br>• Have epinephrine ready for injection.<br>• Antihistamines, corticosteroids, $\beta_2$-agonists may also be prescribed.<br>• Do not restart transfusion. | Transfuse extensively washed RBC products from which all plasma has been removed.<br>Use blood from IgA-deficient donor.<br>Use autologous components. |
| **Circulatory Overload Reaction** | | | |
| Fluid administered faster than the circulation can accommodate<br>People with cardiac or renal disease at risk | Cough, dyspnea, pulmonary congestion, adventitious breath sounds, headache, hypertension, tachycardia, distended neck veins | • Place patient upright with feet in dependent position.<br>• Obtain chest x-ray STAT if ordered.<br>• Administer prescribed diuretics, $O_2$, morphine.<br>• Phlebotomy may be indicated. | Adjust transfusion volume and flow rate based on patient size and clinical status.<br>Have blood bank divide future units into smaller aliquots for better spacing of fluid infused. |
| **Sepsis** | | | |
| Transfusion of bacterially infected blood components | Rapid onset of chills, high fever, vomiting, diarrhea, marked hypotension, or shock | • Obtain culture of patient's blood.<br>• Treat septicemia as directed—antibiotics, IV fluids, vasopressors. | Collect, process, store, and transfuse blood products according to blood banking standards and complete the transfusion within 4 hr of starting time. |

**TABLE 30-33 Acute Transfusion Reactions—cont'd**

| Cause | Manifestations | Management | Prevention |
|---|---|---|---|
| **Transfusion-Related Acute Lung Injury (TRALI) Reaction** | | | |
| Reaction between transfused antileukocyte antibodies and recipient's leukocytes, causing pulmonary inflammation and capillary leak | Fever, chills, hypotension, tachypnea, frothy sputum, dyspnea, hypoxemia, respiratory failure. Noncardiogenic pulmonary edema<br>Leading cause of transfusion-related deaths. Arises within 1-6 hours of transfusion | • Draw blood for arterial blood gases and HLA or antileukocyte antibodies. Obtain chest x-ray STAT.<br>• Provide $O_2$ and administer corticosteroids (diuretics of no value) as ordered.<br>• Initiate CPR if needed and provide ventilatory and BP support if needed. | Provide leukocyte-reduced products. Identify donors who are implicated in TRALI reactions and do not allow them to donate. |
| **Massive Blood Transfusion Reaction** | | | |
| Can occur with replacement of 10 or more RBC units within 24 hr<br>RBC transfusions do not contain clotting factors, albumin, and platelets. | Hypothermia and cardiac dysrhythmias (from rapid infusion of large quantities of cold blood)<br>Citrate toxicity and hypocalcemia (from the use of citrate as a storage solution)<br>Hypocalcemia (citrate binds calcium) manifested as muscle tremors and ECG changes<br>Hyperkalemia (from potassium leaking from stored RBCs). Manifested as muscle weakness, diarrhea, paresthesias, paralysis of the cardiac or respiratory muscles, and cardiac arrest | • When patients receive massive transfusions of blood products, monitor clotting status and electrolyte levels. | Use blood-warming equipment.<br>Infusion of 10% calcium gluconate (10 mL with every 1 L of citrated blood). Because of dilution effect on coagulation due to massive RBC transfusion, platelets and plasma will also be administered. |

*DIC,* Disseminated intravascular coagulation; *HLA,* human leukocyte antigen; *IgA,* immunoglobulin A.

**TABLE 30-34 Delayed Transfusion Reactions**

| Manifestations | Prevention and Management | Manifestations | Prevention and Management |
|---|---|---|---|
| **Delayed Hemolytic**<br>Fever, mild jaundice, decreased hemoglobin. Occurs as early as 3 days or as late as several months posttransfusion as the result of destruction of transfused RBCs by alloantibodies not detected during crossmatch | Generally, no acute treatment is required. Hemolysis may be severe enough to warrant further transfusions. | **Iron Overload**<br>Excess iron is deposited in heart, liver, pancreas, and joints, causing dysfunction. Heart failure, dysrhythmias, impaired thyroid and gonadal function, diabetes, arthritis, cirrhosis. Occurs in patients receiving >100 units for chronic anemia (e.g., sickle cell anemia, β-thalassemia) over time | Treat symptomatically. Deferoxamine (Desferal), which chelates and removes accumulated iron via the kidneys, administered IV or subcutaneously. Deferasirox (Exjade) and deferiprone (Ferriprox) are oral agents that chelate iron and should be started before more than 50 units of red cells are transfused. |
| **Hepatitis B***<br>Elevated liver enzymes (AST and ALT), anorexia, malaise, nausea and vomiting, fever, dark urine, jaundice<br>Usually resolves spontaneously within 4-6 wk. Chronic carrier state can develop and result in permanent damage to the liver. | Hepatitis B virus can be detected in donated blood by the presence of hepatitis B surface antigen (HBsAg).<br>Treat symptomatically. | **Other**<br>Cytomegalovirus (CMV), HIV, human herpesvirus type 6 (HSV-6), Epstein-Barr virus (EBV), human T cell leukemia virus, HTLV-1, and malaria<br>Most recent threats have been agents that primarily affect animals, but have been transmitted to the blood supply through the food supply, or vectors such as mosquitoes or ticks. These include *Plasmodium* species (malaria), dengue fever virus, West Nile virus, *Trypanosoma cruzi* (Chagas' disease), *Babesia* species (babesiosis), human herpesvirus 8 (KS virus), and variant Creutzfeldt-Jakob disease ("mad cow disease"). | Treatment based on the cause<br>Ways of detecting some of these agents are now available and required, such as the nucleic acid test for West Nile virus, HIV, and *T. cruzi.* Donor screening has been the only available method to reduce the risk of donor-contaminated blood for others. |
| **Hepatitis C***<br>Similar to hepatitis B, but symptoms are usually less severe. Chronic liver disease and cirrhosis may develop. | Before testing of anti-HCV in donated blood, accounted for 90%-95% of all posttransfusion hepatitis. Treat symptomatically. | | |

*ALT,* Alanine aminotransferase; *AST,* aspartate aminotransferase; *HCV,* hepatitis C virus; *HTLV-1,* human T-cell leukemia virus, type 1; *KS,* Kaposi sarcoma.
*New cases of transfusion-related hepatitis B and C are not common.

immediately; (4) recheck identifying tags and numbers; (5) monitor vital signs and urine output; (6) treat symptoms per HCP order; (7) save the blood bag and tubing and send them to the blood bank for examination; (8) collect required blood and urine specimens at intervals based on the hospital policy to evaluate for hemolysis; and (9) document on transfusion reaction form and patient chart. The blood bank and laboratory are responsible for identifying the type of reaction.

A transfusion reaction is a *serious reportable event* (SRE) and a *sentinel event.* (These events are discussed in Chapter 1.)

**Acute Transfusion Reactions.** The most common cause of hemolytic reactions is transfusion of ABO-incompatible blood (Table 30-33). This is an example of a type II cytotoxic hypersensitivity reaction (see Chapter 13). Severe hemolytic reactions are rare. Mislabeling specimens and administering blood to the wrong individual cause most acute hemolytic reactions. This again points to the importance of using proper patient identifiers when drawing blood samples and when administering medications and blood products.

**Delayed Transfusion Reactions.** Delayed transfusion reactions include delayed hemolytic reactions (discussed previously), infections, and iron overload (Table 30-34).

## Autotransfusion

*Autotransfusion,* or autologous transfusion, involves removing whole blood from a person and transfusing that blood back into the same person. The problems of incompatibility, allergic reactions, and transmission of disease can be avoided. Methods of autotransfusion include the following:

- *Autologous donation* or *elective phlebotomy* (predeposit transfusion). A person donates blood before a planned surgical procedure. The blood can be frozen and stored for up to 10 years. Usually the blood is stored without being frozen and is given to the person within a few weeks of donation. This technique is especially beneficial to the patient with a rare blood type or for any patient who may be expected to require limited blood product support during a major surgical procedure (e.g., elective orthopedic surgery).
- *Autotransfusion.* A newer method for replacing blood volume involves safely and aseptically collecting, filtering, and returning the patient's own blood lost during a major surgical procedure or from a traumatic injury. This system was originally developed in response to patients' concerns about the safety of blood from blood products. However, today it provides an important way to safely replace volume and stabilize bleeding patients. Collection devices are most often used during surgeries. Some systems allow blood to be automatically and continuously reinfused. Others require collecting the blood for a time (usually no longer than 4 hours) and then reinfusing it.

Drainage after the first 24 hours or drainage that is suspected to contain pathogens should not be reinfused. Anticoagulants may or may not be added before reinfusion. Development of clots after blood is filtered through the collection system can sometimes prevent reinfusion of the blood. Sometimes blood that has been collected has become depleted of its normal coagulation factors. Therefore monitoring coagulation studies in the patient receiving an autotransfusion is important.

## CASE STUDY

### *Leukemia*

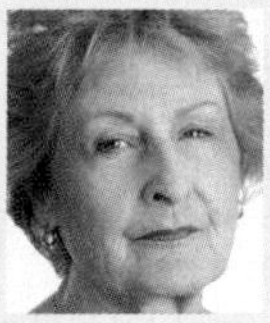

(©Lisa F. Young/iStock)

**Patient Profile**

A.J. is a 63-year-old white woman who is brought to the emergency department by her husband (see Chapter 29 case study on p. 593). She has become progressively weaker and was admitted for further evaluation.

**Subjective Data**

- Complains of progressive weakness over the last couple of weeks
- Has had a recent sinus infection that resolved after two courses of antibiotics
- Complains of shortness of breath
- Has noticed a lot of bruising lately

**Objective Data**

***Physical Examination***

- Has scattered petechiae on both ankles and two ecchymoses on her arms and one on her left lower leg
- Her skin is very pale
- BP 100/70 (lying), temperature 96.8° F (36° C), respiratory rate 26/min, pulse 110/min

***Laboratory Results***

- Hct 18.2%
- Hgb 5.9 g/dL, WBC count 2600/μL (2.6 × $10^9$/L)
- Platelet count 72,000/μL (72 × $10^9$/L)
- Peripheral blood smear indicates that 80% of the WBCs are blasts
- PT 18 sec, aPTT 37 sec
- LDH 560 units/L

***Bone Marrow Biopsy***

- Multiple myeloblasts (>50%)

**Interprofessional Care**

- Consultation with a hematologist-oncologist
- Two units of packed red blood cells
- *Diagnosis:* Acute myelogenous leukemia

**Discussion Questions**

1. What components of the laboratory test results and bone marrow biopsy suggest acute leukemia?
2. How is acute myelogenous leukemia treated?
3. What is A.J.'s prognosis?
4. What are the life-threatening problems that can occur as a result of this disease and treatment? How can you anticipate and assess for these problems?
5. ***Priority Decision:*** What are the priority nursing interventions for A.J.?
6. ***Patient-Centered Care:*** What are the priorities for patient teaching with a newly diagnosed adult with leukemia?
7. ***Priority Decision:*** Based on the assessment data presented, what are the priority nursing diagnoses? Are there any collaborative problems?
8. ***Teamwork and Collaboration:*** What nursing interventions can the registered nurse (RN) delegate to unlicensed assistive personnel (UAP) while A.J. is getting her blood transfusions?
9. ***Evidence-Based Practice:*** A.J. becomes fatigued after starting chemotherapy. She wants to know if she can still work and do household chores even if she is so fatigued. What is your best advice for her?

Answers available at *http://evolve.elsevier.com/Lewis/medsurg.*

## BRIDGE TO NCLEX EXAMINATION

The number of the question corresponds to the same-numbered outcome at the beginning of the chapter.

1. In a severely anemic patient, the nurse would expect to find
   a. dyspnea and tachycardia.
   b. cyanosis and pulmonary edema.
   c. cardiomegaly and pulmonary fibrosis.
   d. ventricular dysrhythmias and wheezing.
2. When obtaining assessment data from a patient with a microcytic, hypochromic anemia, the nurse would question the patient about
   a. folic acid intake.
   b. dietary intake of iron.
   c. a history of gastric surgery.
   d. a history of sickle cell anemia.
3. Nursing interventions for a patient with severe anemia related to peptic ulcer disease include *(select all that apply)*
   a. instructions for high-iron diet.
   b. taking vital signs every 8 hours.
   c. monitoring stools for occult blood.
   d. teaching self-injection of erythropoietin.
   e. administration of cobalamin (vitamin $B_{12}$) injections.
4. The nursing management of a patient in sickle cell crisis includes *(select all that apply)*
   a. monitoring CBC.
   b. optimal pain management and $O_2$ therapy.
   c. blood transfusions if required and iron chelation.
   d. rest as needed and deep vein thrombosis prophylaxis.
   e. administration of IV iron and diet high in iron content.
5. A complication of the hyperviscosity of polycythemia is
   a. thrombosis.
   b. cardiomyopathy.
   c. pulmonary edema.
   d. disseminated intravascular coagulation (DIC).
6. When caring for a patient with thrombocytopenia, the nurse instructs the patient to
   a. dab his or her nose instead of blowing.
   b. be careful when shaving with a safety razor.
   c. continue with physical activities to stimulate thrombopoiesis.
   d. avoid aspirin because it may mask the fever that occurs with thrombocytopenia.
7. The nurse would anticipate that a patient with von Willebrand disease undergoing surgery would be treated with administration of vWF and
   a. thrombin.
   b. factor VI.
   c. factor VII.
   d. factor VIII.
8. DIC is a disorder in which
   a. the coagulation pathway is genetically altered, leading to thrombus formation in all major blood vessels.
   b. an underlying disease depletes hemolytic factors in the blood, leading to diffuse thrombotic episodes and infarcts.
   c. a disease process stimulates coagulation processes with resultant thrombosis, as well as depletion of clotting factors, leading to diffuse clotting and hemorrhage.
   d. an inherited predisposition causes a deficiency of clotting factors that leads to overstimulation of coagulation processes in the vasculature.
9. Priority nursing actions when caring for a hospitalized patient with a new-onset temperature of 102.2° F (39° C) and severe neutropenia include *(select all that apply)*
   a. administering the prescribed antibiotic STAT.
   b. drawing peripheral and central line blood cultures.
   c. ongoing monitoring of the patient's vital signs for septic shock.
   d. taking a full set of vital signs and notifying the physician immediately.
   e. administering transfusions of WBCs treated to decrease immunogenicity.
10. Because myelodysplastic syndrome arises from the pluripotent hematopoietic stem cell in the bone marrow, laboratory results the nurse would expect to find include a(n)
    a. excess of T cells.
    b. excess of platelets.
    c. deficiency of granulocytes.
    d. deficiency of all cellular blood components.
11. The most common type of leukemia in older adults is
    a. acute myelocytic leukemia.
    b. acute lymphocytic leukemia.
    c. chronic myelocytic leukemia.
    d. chronic lymphocytic leukemia.
12. Multiple drugs are often used in combinations to treat leukemia and lymphoma because
    a. there are fewer toxic and side effects.
    b. the chance that one drug will be effective is increased.
    c. the drugs are more effective without causing side effects.
    d. the drugs work by different mechanisms to maximize killing of malignant cells.
13. The nurse is aware that a major difference between Hodgkin's lymphoma and non-Hodgkin's lymphoma is that
    a. Hodgkin's lymphoma occurs only in young adults.
    b. Hodgkin's lymphoma is considered potentially curable.
    c. non-Hodgkin's lymphoma can manifest in multiple organs.
    d. non-Hodgkin's lymphoma is treated only with radiation therapy.
14. A patient with multiple myeloma becomes confused and lethargic. The nurse would expect that these clinical manifestations may be explained by diagnostic results that indicate
    a. hyperkalemia.
    b. hyperuricemia.
    c. hypercalcemia.
    d. CNS myeloma.
15. When reviewing the patient's hematologic laboratory values after a splenectomy, the nurse would expect to find
    a. leukopenia.
    b. RBC abnormalities.
    c. decreased hemoglobin.
    d. increased platelet count.
16. Complications of transfusions that can be decreased by the use of leukocyte depletion or reduction of RBC transfusion are
    a. chills and hemolysis.
    b. leukostasis and neutrophilia.
    c. fluid overload and pulmonary edema.
    d. transmission of cytomegalovirus and fever.

1. a, 2. b, 3. a, c, 4. a, b, c, d, 5. a, 6. a, 7. d, 8. c, 9. a, b, c, d, 10. d,
11. d, 12. d, 13. c, 14. c, 15. d, 16. d

For rationales to these answers and even more NCLEX review questions, visit *http://evolve.elsevier.com/Lewis/medsurg.*

## EVOLVE WEBSITE

http://evolve.elsevier.com/Lewis/medsurg

**Review Questions (Online Only)**

**Key Points**

**Answer Keys for Review Questions**

- Rationales for Bridge to NCLEX Examination Questions
- Answer Guidelines for Case Study on p. 652
- Answer Guidelines for Managing Care of Multiple Patients Case Study (Section 6) on p. 656

**Student Case Studies**

- Patient With Chronic Myelogenous Leukemia Including End-of-life Care
- Patient With Sickle Cell Anemia

**Nursing Care Plans**

- eNursing Care Plan 30-1: Patient With Anemia
- eNursing Care Plan 30-2: Patient With Thrombocytopenia
- eNursing Care Plan 30-3: Patient With Neutropenia

**Conceptual Care Map Creator**

- Conceptual Care Map for Case Study on p. 652

**Audio Glossary**

**Content Updates**

## REFERENCES

1. Marks PW: Approach to anemia in the adult and child. In Hoffman R, Benz EJ, Silberstein LE, et al, editors: *Hematology: basic principles and practice*, ed 6, Philadelphia, 2013, Saunders.
2. Rote NS, McCance KL: Alterations of erythrocyte function. In McCance KL, Huether SE, editors: *Pathophysiology: the biologic basis for disease in adults and children*, ed 7, St Louis, 2014, Mosby.
3. Artz AS, Ershler WB: Hematology in aging. In Hoffman R, Benz EJ, Silberstein LE, et al, editors: *Hematology: basic principles and practice*, ed 6, Philadelphia, 2013, Saunders.
4. World Health Organization. Retrieved from *www.who.int*.
5. Rote NS, McCane KL: Structure and function of the hematologic system. In McCance KL, Huether SE, editors: *Pathophysiology: the biologic basis for disease in adults and children*, ed 7, St Louis, 2014, Mosby.
6. American Dietetic Association. Retrieved from *www.eatright.org*.
7. WebMD. Retrieved from *www.webmd.com*.
8. Micromedex 2.0. Truven Analytics, Inc. Retrieved from *www.micromedexsolutions.com*.
9. Kline NE: Alterations of hematologic function in children. In McCance KL, Huether SE, editors: *Pathophysiology: the biologic basis for disease in adults and children*, ed 7, St Louis, 2014, Mosby.
10. Carson SM, Martin MB: Effective iron chelation practice for patients with β-thalassemia major, *Clin J Oncol Nurs* 18:102, 2014.
11. Townsley DM, Rodgers GP: Deficiencies of vitamin $B_{12}$ and folate. In Rodgers GP, Young NS: *The Bethesda handbook of clinical hematology*, ed 3, Philadelphia, 2013, Lippincott.
12. Scheinberg P, Young NS, Liu JM: Bone marrow failure syndromes: aplastic anemia, acquired and constitutional; paroxysmal nocturnal hemoglobinuria; pure red blood cell aplasia; and agranulocytosis. In Rodgers GP, Young NS: *The Bethesda handbook of clinical hematology*, ed 3, Philadelphia, 2013, Lippincott.
13. Willis L, Rexwinkle A, Bryan J, et al: Recent developments in drug therapy for aplastic anemia, *Ann Pharmacother* 48:1469, 2014.
*14. Yawn BP, Buchanan GR, Afenyi-Annan AN, et al: Management of sickle cell disease: Summary of the 2014 evidence-based report by expert panel members, *J Am Med Assoc* 312:1033, 2014.
15. Taylor LV, Stotts NA, Humphreys J, et al: A biopsychosocial-spiritual model of chronic pain in adults with sickle cell disease, *Pain Manag Nurs* 14:287, 2013.
16. Food and Drug Administration. Retrieved from *www.FDA.gov*.
17. Parikh AR, Olnes MJ: The myeloproliferative neoplasms: polycythemia vera, essential thrombocythemia, and primary myelofibrosis. In Rodgers GP, Young NS: *The Bethesda handbook of clinical hematology*, ed 3, Philadelphia, 2013, Lippincott.
18. Fogarty PF, Dunbar CE: Thrombocytopenia. In Rodgers GP, Young NS: *The Bethesda handbook of clinical hematology*, ed 3, Philadelphia, 2013, Lippincott.
19. Diz-Kucukkaya R, Lopez JA: Acquired disorders of platelet function. In Hoffman R, Benz EJ, Silberstein LE, et al, editors: *Hematology: basic principles and practice*, ed 6, Philadelphia, 2013, Saunders.
20. McCrae KR, Sadler JE, Cines DB: Thrombotic thrombocytopenic purpura and the hemolytic uremic syndrome. In Hoffman R, Benz EJ, Silberstein LE, et al, editors: *Hematology: basic principles and practice*, ed 6, Philadelphia, 2013, Saunders.
21. Warkentin TE: Heparin-induced thrombocytopenia. In Hoffman R, Benz EJ, Silberstein LE, et al, editors: *Hematology: basic principles and practice*, ed 6, Philadelphia, 2013, Saunders.
22. Fogarty PF: Disorders of hemostasis II. In Rodgers GP, Young NS: *The Bethesda handbook of clinical hematology*, ed 3, Philadelphia, 2013, Lippincott.
23. Carcao M, Moorehead P, Lillicrap D: Hemophilia A and B. In Hoffman R, Benz EJ, Silberstein LE, et al, editors: *Hematology: basic principles and practice*, ed 6, Philadelphia, 2013, Saunders.
*24. Oldenburg J, Brackmann H: Prophylaxis in adult patients with severe haemophilia A, *Thromb Res* 134:S33, 2014.
25. Kempton CL, Meeks SL: Toward optimal therapy for inhibitors in hemophilia, *Blood* 124:3365, 2014.
26. Schwartz A, Rote NS: Alterations of leukocyte, lymphoid, and hemostatic function. In McCance KL, Huether SE. editors: *Pathophysiology: the biologic basis for disease in adults and children*, ed 7, St Louis, 2014, Mosby.
27. Levi M: Disseminated intravascular coagulation. In Hoffman R, Benz EJ, Silberstein LE, et al, editors: *Hematology: basic principles and practice*, ed 6, Philadelphia, 2013, Saunders.
28. Noel P, Jaben EA: Consultative hematology. In Rodgers GP, Young NS: *The Bethesda handbook of clinical hematology*, ed 3, Philadelphia, 2013, Lippincott.
29. Maciejewski JP, Tiu RV: Acquired disorders of red cell, white cell, and platelet production. In Hoffman R, Benz EJ, Silberstein LE, et al, editors: *Hematology: basic principles and practice*, ed 6, Philadelphia, 2013, Saunders.
*30. Baden LR, Bensinger W, Angarone M, et al: Prevention and treatment of cancer-related infections, NCCN Clinical Practice Guidelines, version 2, 2014. Retrieved from *www.nccn.org*.
*31. Boubekri A: Reducing central line-associated bloodstream infections in the blood and marrow transplantation population: a review of the literature, *Clin J Oncol Nurs* 17:297, 2013.
*32. Foster M: Re-evaluating the neutropenic diet: time to change, *Clin J Oncol Nurs* 18:239, 2014.
*33. Freifeld AG, Bow EJ, Sepkowitz KA: Clinical practice guideline for the use of antimicrobial agents in neutropenic patients with cancer: 2010 Update by the Infectious Diseases Society of America, *Clin Infect Dis* 52:e56, 2011. (Classic)
*34. Crawford J, Becker PS, Armitage J, et al: Myeloid growth factors, NCCN Clinical Practice Guidelines, version 2, 2014. Retrieved from *www.nccn.org*.
*35. Greenberg PL, Stone RM, Bejar R: Myelodysplastic Syndromes, NCCN Clinical Practice Guidelines, version 1, 2015. Retrieved from *www.nccn.org*.
36. Klotz J, Parikh AR, Battiwalla M: The myelodysplastic syndromes. In Rodgers GP, Young NS: *The Bethesda handbook of clinical hematology*, ed 3, Philadelphia, 2013, Lippincott.
37. American Cancer Society. *Cancer Facts and Figures 2014*. Atlanta: American Cancer Society, 2014. Retrieved from *www.cancer.org*.
38. Yin F, Malkovska V: Acute myeloid leukemia. In Rodgers GP, Young NS: *The Bethesda handbook of clinical hematology*, ed 3, Philadelphia, 2013, Lippincott.
39. Shah NN, Wayne AS: Acute lymphoblastic leukemia. In Rodgers GP, Young NS: *The Bethesda handbook of clinical hematology*, ed 3, Philadelphia, 2013, Lippincott.
40. Yong AS, Barrett AJ: Chronic myelogenous leukemia. In Rodgers GP, Young NS: *The Bethesda handbook of clinical hematology*, ed 3, Philadelphia, 2013, Lippincott.

41. Farooqui MZ, Wiestner A, Aue G: Chronic lymphocytic leukemia. In Rodgers GP, Young NS: *The Bethesda handbook of clinical hematology*, ed 3, Philadelphia, 2013, Lippincott.
*42. Zelenetz AD, Gordon LI, Wierda WG, et al: Non-Hodgkin's lymphomas, NCCN Clinical Practice Guidelines, version 5, 2014. Retrieved from *www.nccn.org*.
*43. O'Donnell MR, Tallman MS, Abboud CH, et al: Acute myeloid leukemia, NCCN Clinical Practice Guidelines, version 2, 2014. Retrieved from *www.nccn.org*.
*44. Alvarnas JC, Brown PA, Aoun P, et al: Acute lymphoblastic leukemia, NCCN Clinical Practice Guidelines, version 1, 2014. Retrieved from *www.nccn.org*.
*45. O'Brien S, Radich JP, Abboud CN, et al: Chronic myelogenous leukemia, NCCN Clinical Practice Guidelines, version 1, 2015. Retrieved from *www.nccn.org*.
*46. Hoppe RT, Advani RH, Ai WZ, et al: Hodgkin lymphoma, NCCN Clinical Practice Guidelines, version 2, 2014. Retrieved from *www.nccn.org*.
47. Kanate AS, Craig M, Abraham J, et al: Hodgkin lymphoma. In Rodgers GP, Young NS: *The Bethesda handbook of clinical hematology*, ed 3, Philadelphia, 2013, Lippincott.
48. Little RF, Wilson WH: Non-Hodgkin lymphomas. In Rodgers GP, Young NS: *The Bethesda handbook of clinical hematology*, ed 3, Philadelphia, 2013, Lippincott.
49. Surveillance, Epidemiology, and End Results Program (SEER): SEER Stat Fact Sheets: Myeloma. Retrieved from *www.seer.cancer.gov*.
50. Manasanch EE, Tageja N, Landgren CO: Multiple myeloma. In Rodgers GP, Young NS: *The Bethesda handbook of clinical hematology*, ed 3, Philadelphia, 2013, Lippincott.
*51. Anderson KC, Bensinger W, Alsina M, et al: Multiple myeloma, NCCN Clinical Practice Guidelines, version 2, 2015. Retrieved from *www.nccn.org*.
52. Connell NT, Shurin SB, Schiffman FJ: The spleen and its disorders. In Hoffman R, Benz EJ, Silberstein LE, et al, editors: *Hematology: basic principles and practice*, ed 6, Philadelphia, 2013, Saunders.
53. Desmond R, Klein HG: Blood transfusion. In Rodgers GP, Young NS: *The Bethesda handbook of clinical hematology*, ed 3, Philadelphia, 2013, Lippincott.
54. Maynard K: Administration of blood components. In Fung MK, Grossman BJ, Hillyer CD, et al, editors: *Technical manual: standards for blood banks and transfusion services*, ed 18, Bethesda, 2014, AABB.
*55. Stupnyckyj C, Smolarek S, Reeves C, et al: Changing blood transfusion policy and practice, *Am J Nurs* 114:50, 2014.
56. Pagana KD, Pagana TJ: *Mosby's manual of diagnostic and laboratory tests*, ed 5, St Louis, 2014, Mosby.
57. Mazzei CA, Popovsky MA, Kopko PM: Noninfectious complications of blood transfusion. In Fung MK, Grossman BJ, Hillyer CD, et al, editors: *Technical manual: standards for blood banks and transfusion services*, ed 18, Bethesda, 2014, AABB.
58. Galel SA: Infectious disease screening. In Fung MK, Grossman BJ, Hillyer CD, et al, editors: *Technical manual: standards for blood banks and transfusion services*, ed 18, Bethesda, 2014, AABB.

*Evidence-based information for clinical practice.

## CASE STUDY

### *Managing Care of Multiple Patients*

You are working on the oncology unit and have been assigned to care for the following four patients. You have one UAP who is assigned to help you, and there are two other RNs on your clinical unit.

#### Patients

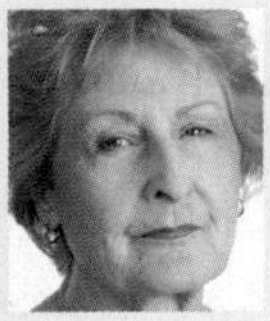

(©Lisa F. Young/iStock)

A.J. is a 63-yr-old white woman who is admitted with severe anemia (Hgb 5.9 g/dL and Hct 18.2%). Her WBC count is 2600/µL and platelet count is 72,000/µL. She prefers to take care of herself with "natural therapy" and has not seen an HCP for 5 years. A.J. is having difficulty performing ADLs without having to stop and catch her breath. She received 2 units of RBCs. After a further workup, she is diagnosed with acute myelocytic leukemia (AML). She remains hospitalized as she starts chemotherapy.

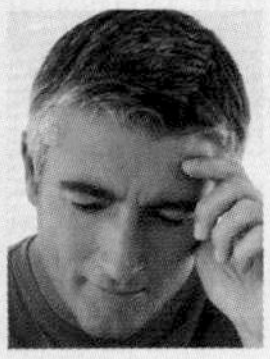

(©g-stockstudio/iStock/Thinkstock)

J.J. is a 52-yr-old white man newly diagnosed with acute lymphocytic leukemia (ALL). His most recent vital signs are BP 100/70, temperature 102.2°F (39°C), respiratory rate 26/min, pulse 110. Laboratory results reveal Hgb 6.9 g/dL, Hct 20%, WBC count 120,000/µL ($120 \times 10^9$/L), and platelet count 25,000/µL ($25 \times 10^9$/L). He is admitted for blood transfusions and induction therapy.

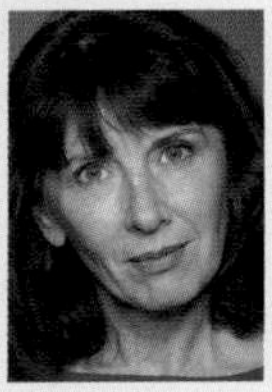

(©Studio Grand Ouest/iStock/Thinkstock)

P.H. is a 45-yr-old woman who is currently receiving chemotherapy for treatment of ovarian cancer. She is admitted with fever and chills. Her WBC count is 2200/µL ($2.2 \times 10^9$/L) with an absolute neutrophil count (ANC) of 400/µL ($0.4 \times 10^9$/L). She is admitted for IV antibiotic therapy and is in isolation. Her most recent vital signs are BP 118/60, temperature 99.2°F (37.3°C), respiratory rate 20/min, pulse 98.

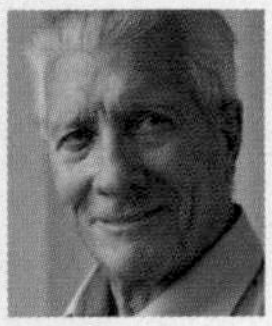

(©Ridofranz/iStock)

G.L. is a 67-yr-old man who came to the ED yesterday evening with complaints of abdominal pain. A CT scan of the abdomen revealed several masses in his lymphatic system. The HCP suspects non-Hodgkin's lymphoma and admits him for a diagnostic workup. He currently rates his pain as a 3 on a scale of 0 to 10.

#### Discussion Questions

1. ***Priority Decision:*** After receiving report, which patient should you see first? Provide a rationale for your decision.
2. ***Teamwork and Collaboration:*** Which task could you delegate to the UAP *(select all that apply)*?
   a. Assist A.J. to a chair after completing her AM care.
   b. Obtain the first unit of blood for J.J. from the blood bank.
   c. Explain the importance of isolation to P.H. and her family.
   d. Ask A.J. why she has not been willing to get any medical care for 5 years.
   e. Ask G.L. about the presence of additional clinical manifestations of non-Hodgkin's lymphoma.
3. ***Priority and Delegation Decision:*** When you enter J.J.'s room, you find him somewhat confused and lethargic. His family states he had just had a severe coughing episode. What initial action would be the *most* appropriate?
   a. Perform a focused neurologic examination.
   b. Call respiratory therapy to give him a breathing treatment.
   c. Ask his family members if they have a copy of his living will.
   d. Have the UAP stay with J.J. while you page the HCP stat.

#### Case Study Progression

J.J.'s HCP orders a repeat CBC and an emergency CT scan of the head. Your supervisor makes arrangements for another RN to accompany J.J. to the CT scan while you prepare to administer the first unit of RBCs.

4. The HCP orders ferrous sulfate 325 mg TID for A.J. You teach A.J. to take her iron *(select all that apply)*
   a. at breakfast time in the morning.
   b. with orange juice to increase absorption.
   c. 1 hour before meals to facilitate absorption.
   d. 2 hours after eating to minimize side effects.
   e. whenever she feels tired or is short of breath with activity.
5. When teaching P.H.'s family about neutropenic precautions, you emphasize that the *most* important intervention to prevent infection is
   a. hand washing.
   b. wearing a mask.
   c. keeping P.H. in a private room.
   d. limiting the number of visitors in her room.
6. G.L. asks you to explain the diagnostic testing he can expect to undergo related to the suspected lymphoma. Which tests will you explain to him *(select all that apply)*?
   a. PET scan
   b. Bone marrow biopsy
   c. Peripheral blood smear
   d. Excisional lymph node biopsy
   e. Lymphangiography of internal lymph nodes
7. ***Management Decision:*** An RN from the float pool arrives to accompany J.J. to CT scan at the same time the UAP arrives with his first unit of RBCs. Which intervention would be *most* appropriate?
   a. Put the unit of RBCs in the refrigerator to start when J.J. returns to the floor.
   b. Ask the RN to verify the correct unit of RBCs with you and start the infusion.
   c. Give the RN an SBAR report on J.J. and ask her to start the blood on the way to her CT scan.
   d. Ask the RN if she would prefer to give the blood or hold it for J.J.'s return to the unit.

Answers available at *http://evolve.elsevier.com/Lewis/medsurg.*

# SECTION 7

# Problems of Oxygenation: Perfusion

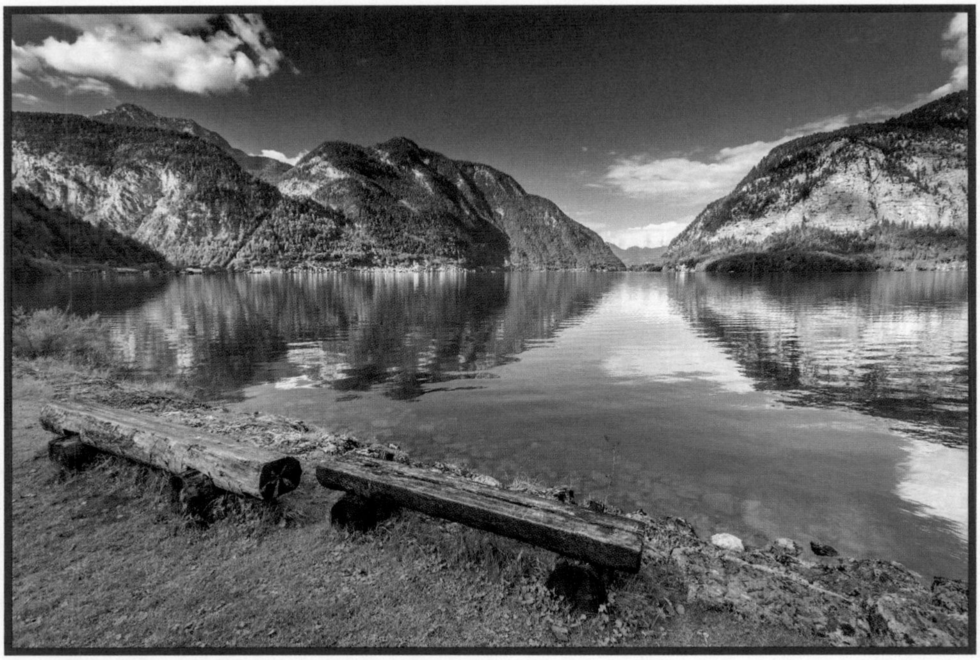

©Shaiith/iStock/Thinkstock

*Sit by a river. Find peace and meaning in the rhythm of the lifeblood of the Earth.*

***Anonymous***

# 31

# Assessment of Cardiovascular System

*Angela DiSabatino Herman, Linda Bucher*

*The only way to do great work is to love what you do.*

***Steve Jobs***

http://evolve.elsevier.com/Lewis/medsurg/

## LEARNING OUTCOMES

1. Differentiate the anatomic location and function of the following structures of the heart: pericardial layers, atria, ventricles, and valves.
2. Relate the coronary circulation to the areas of heart muscle supplied by the major coronary arteries.
3. Differentiate the structure and function of arteries, veins, capillaries, and endothelium.
4. Describe the mechanisms involved in the regulation of blood pressure.
5. Relate the various waveforms on a normal electrocardiogram to the associated cardiac events.
6. Obtain significant subjective and objective assessment data related to the cardiovascular system from a patient and/or caregiver.
7. Perform a physical assessment of the cardiovascular system using the appropriate techniques.
8. Differentiate normal from abnormal findings of a physical assessment of the cardiovascular system.
9. Link the age-related changes of the cardiovascular system to the differences in assessment findings.
10. Describe the purpose, significance of results, and nursing responsibilities related to diagnostic studies of the cardiovascular system.

## KEY TERMS

action potential, p. 659
afterload, p. 661
arterial blood pressure, p. 662
cardiac index (CI), p. 660
cardiac output (CO), p. 660
cardiac reserve, p. 661
coronary angiography, p. 678
diastole, p. 659
diastolic blood pressure (DBP), p. 662
ejection fraction (EF), p. 671
heaves, p. 667
Korotkoff sounds, p. 662
mean arterial pressure (MAP), p. 662
murmur, p. 662
point of maximal impulse (PMI), p. 667
preload, p. 660
pulse pressure, p. 662
systole, p. 660
systolic blood pressure (SBP), p. 662

## STRUCTURES AND FUNCTIONS OF CARDIOVASCULAR SYSTEM

### Heart

**Structure.** The heart is a four-chambered hollow muscular organ normally about the size of a fist. It lies within the thorax in the mediastinal space that separates the right and left pleural cavities. The heart is composed of three layers: a thin inner lining, the *endocardium;* a layer of muscle, the *myocardium;* and an outer layer, the *epicardium.* The heart is covered by a fibroserous sac called the *pericardium.* This sac consists of two layers: the inner *(visceral)* layer of the pericardium (part of the epicardium) and the outer *(parietal)* layer. A small amount of pericardial fluid (approximately 10 to 15 mL) lubricates the space between the pericardial layers *(pericardial space)* and prevents friction between the surfaces as the heart contracts.[1]

The heart is divided vertically by the septum. The interatrial septum creates a right and left atrium, and the interventricular septum creates a right and left ventricle. The thickness of the wall of each chamber is different. The atrial myocardium is thinner than that of the ventricles, and the left ventricular wall is two or three times thicker than the right ventricular wall.[1] The thickness of the left ventricle is necessary to produce the force needed to pump the blood into the systemic circulation.

**Blood Flow Through Heart.** The blood flow through the heart is illustrated in Fig. 31-1.

***Heart Valves.*** The four valves of the heart keep blood flowing in a forward direction. The cusps of the mitral and tricuspid valves are attached to thin strands of fibrous tissue termed *chordae tendineae* (Fig. 31-2). Chordae are anchored in the papillary muscles of the ventricles. This support system prevents the eversion of the leaflets into the atria during ventricular contraction. The pulmonic and aortic valves (also known as *semilunar valves*) prevent blood from regurgitating into the ventricles at the end of each ventricular contraction.

**Blood Supply to Myocardium.** The myocardium has its own blood supply, the *coronary circulation* (Fig. 31-3). Blood flow

Reviewed by Janie Corbitt, RN, MLS, Retired Instructor of Nursing, Milledgeville, Georgia; Cynthia Hambach, RN, MSN, CCRN, Assistant Clinical Professor, Drexel University, Philadelphia, Pennsylvania; and Jennifer Saylor, RN, PhD, ACNS-BC, Assistant Professor, University of Delaware, Newark, Delaware.

into the two major coronary arteries occurs primarily during **diastole** (relaxation of the myocardium). The left coronary artery arises from the aorta and divides into two main branches: the left anterior descending artery and left circumflex artery. These arteries supply the left atrium, left ventricle, interventricular septum, and a portion of the right ventricle. The right coronary artery also arises from the aorta, and its branches supply the right atrium, right ventricle, and a portion of the posterior wall of the left ventricle. In 90% of people the atrioventricular (AV) node and the bundle of His receive blood supply from the right coronary artery. For this reason, blockage of this artery often causes serious defects in cardiac conduction.

The divisions of coronary veins parallel the coronary arteries. Most of the blood from the coronary system drains into the coronary sinus (a large channel), which empties into the right atrium near the entrance of the inferior vena cava.

**Conduction System.** The conduction system consists of specialized tissue responsible for creating and transporting the electrical impulse, or **action potential.** This impulse starts depolarization of the heart cells and subsequently heart contraction (Fig. 31-4, *A*). The electrical impulse normally begins in the sinoatrial (SA) node (pacemaker of the heart). Each impulse coming from the SA node travels through interatrial pathways to depolarize the atria, resulting in a contraction.

The electrical impulse travels from the atria to the AV node through internodal pathways. The signal then moves through

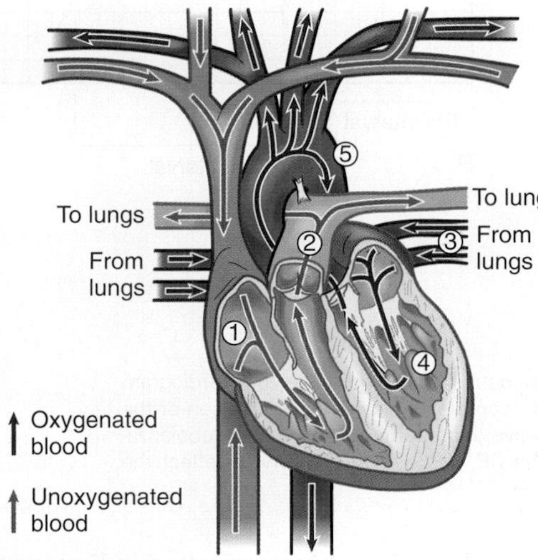


**FIG. 31-1** Schematic representation of blood flow through the heart. *Arrows* indicate direction of flow. *1,* The right atrium receives venous blood from the inferior and superior venae cavae and the coronary sinus. The blood then passes through the tricuspid valve into the right ventricle. *2,* With each contraction, the right ventricle pumps blood through the pulmonic valve into the pulmonary artery and to the lungs. *3,* Oxygenated blood flows from the lungs to the left atrium by way of the pulmonary veins. *4,* It then passes through the mitral valve and into the left ventricle. *5,* As the heart contracts, blood is ejected through the aortic valve into the aorta and thus enters the systemic circulation.

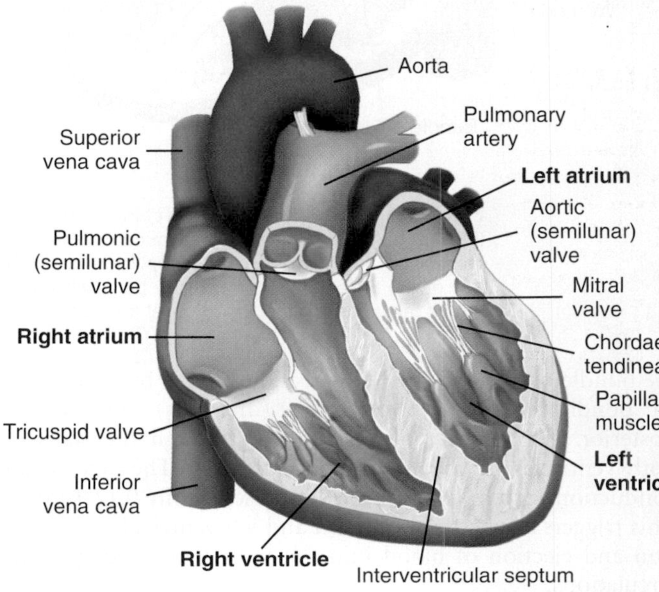


**FIG. 31-2** Anatomic structures of the heart and heart valves.

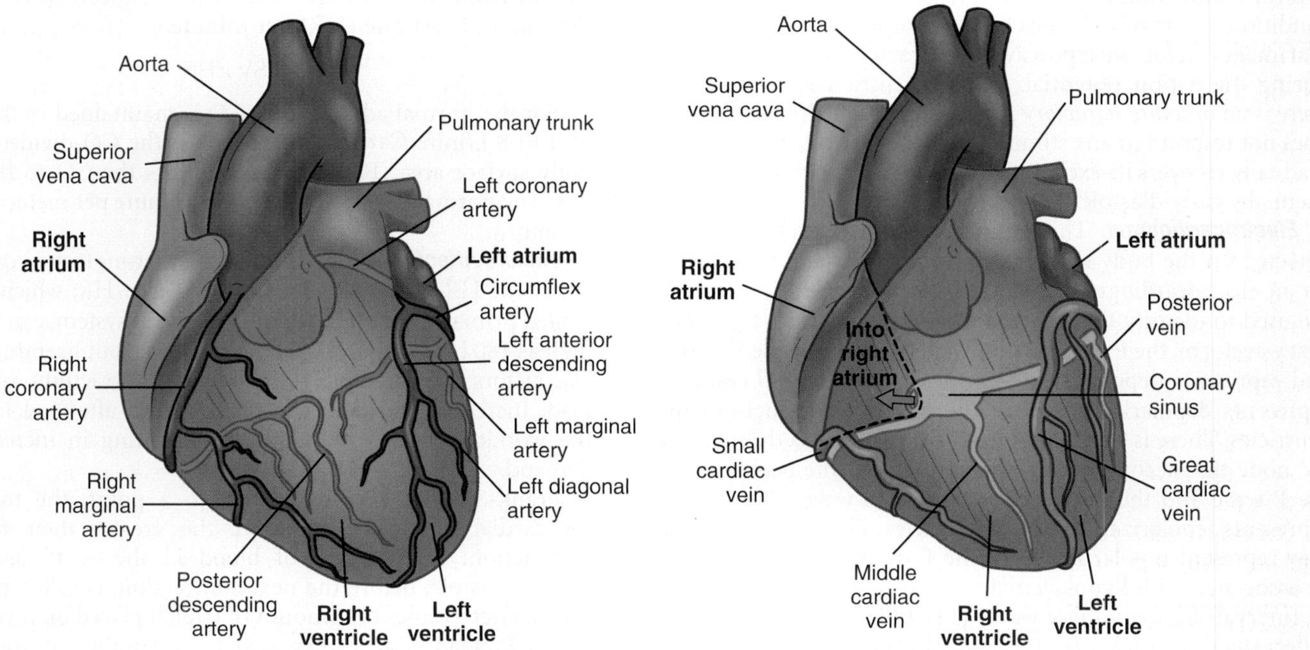


**FIG. 31-3** Coronary arteries and veins.

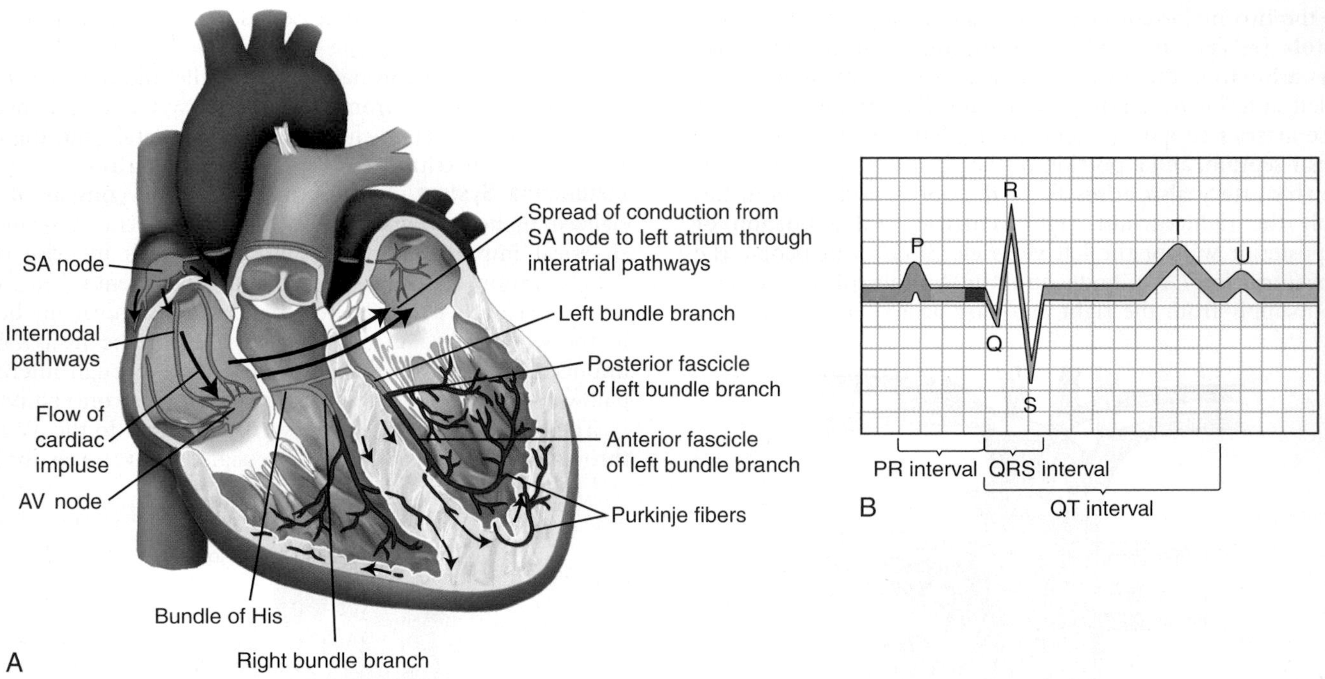


**FIG. 31-4** **A,** Conduction system of the heart. *AV,* Atrioventricular; *SA,* sinoatrial. **B,** The normal electrocardiogram (ECG) pattern. The P wave represents depolarization of the atria. The QRS complex indicates depolarization of the ventricles. The T wave represents repolarization of the ventricles. The U wave, if present, may represent repolarization of the Purkinje fibers, or it may be associated with hypokalemia. The PR, QRS, and QT intervals reflect the time it takes for the impulse to travel from one area of the heart to another.

the bundle of His and the left and right bundle branches. The left bundle branch has two fascicles (divisions): anterior and posterior. The action potential moves through the walls of both ventricles by means of *Purkinje fibers.* The ventricular conduction system delivers the impulse within 0.12 second. This triggers a synchronized right and left ventricular contraction and ejection of blood into the pulmonary and systemic circulations.

Last, repolarization occurs when the contractile fiber cells and the conduction pathway cells regain their resting polarized condition. Heart muscle cells have a compensatory mechanism that makes them unresponsive or refractory to restimulation during the action potential. During ventricular contraction, there is an *absolute refractory period* during which heart muscle does not respond to any stimuli. After this period, heart muscle gradually recovers its excitability, and a *relative refractory period* occurs by early diastole.

***Electrocardiogram.*** The electrical activity of the heart can be detected on the body surface using electrodes and is recorded on an electrocardiogram (ECG). The letters *P, QRS, T,* and *U* are used to identify the separate waveforms (Fig. 31-4, *B*). The first waveform, the P wave, begins with the firing of the SA node and represents depolarization of the atria. The QRS complex represents depolarization from the AV node throughout the ventricles. There is a delay of impulse transmission through the AV node that accounts for the time between the beginning of the P wave and the beginning of the QRS wave. The T wave represents repolarization of the ventricles. The U wave, if seen, may represent repolarization of the Purkinje fibers, or it may be associated with hypokalemia.[2]

Intervals between these waves (PR, QRS, and QT intervals) reflect the time it takes for the signal to travel from one area of the heart to another. These time intervals are measured, and changes from these time references often indicate pathologic conditions. (See Chapter 35 for a complete discussion of ECG monitoring.)

**Mechanical System.** *Depolarization* triggers mechanical activity. **Systole**, contraction of the heart muscle, results in ejection of blood from the ventricles. Relaxation of the heart muscle, *diastole*, allows for filling of the ventricles. **Cardiac output (CO)**, the amount of blood pumped by each ventricle in 1 minute, is calculated by multiplying the amount of blood ejected from the ventricle with each heartbeat: *stroke volume* (SV) times heart rate (HR) per minute:

$$CO = SV \times HR$$

For the normal adult at rest, CO is maintained in the range of 4 to 8 L/min. **Cardiac index (CI)** is the CO divided by the body surface area (BSA). The CI adjusts the CO to the body size. The normal CI is 2.8 to 4.2 L per minute per meter squared ($L/min/m^2$).

***Factors Affecting Cardiac Output.*** Numerous factors can affect either the HR or SV, and thus the CO. The HR, which is controlled primarily by the autonomic nervous system, can reach as high as 180 beats/min for short periods without harmful effects. The factors affecting the SV are preload, contractility, and afterload. Increasing preload, contractility, and afterload increases the workload of the heart muscle, resulting in increased $O_2$ demand.

Frank-Starling law states that, to a point, the more the myocardial fibers are stretched, the greater their force of contraction. The volume of blood in the ventricles at the end of diastole, before the next contraction, is called **preload.** Preload determines the amount of stretch placed on myocardial fibers. Preload can be increased by a number of conditions such as hypertension, aortic valve disease, and hypervolemia.[3]

Contractility can be increased by epinephrine and norepinephrine released by the sympathetic nervous system. Increasing contractility raises the SV by increasing ventricular emptying.

**Afterload** is the peripheral resistance against which the left ventricle must pump. Afterload is affected by the size of the ventricle, wall tension, and arterial blood pressure (BP). If the arterial BP is elevated, the ventricles meet increased resistance to ejection of blood, increasing the work demand. Eventually this results in *ventricular hypertrophy,* an enlargement of the heart muscle without an increase in CO or the size of chambers (Fig. 35-1, *B*).

**Cardiac Reserve.** The cardiovascular system must respond to numerous situations in health and illness (e.g., exercise, stress, hypovolemia). The ability to respond to these demands by altering CO is termed **cardiac reserve.**

## Vascular System

**Blood Vessels.** The three major types of blood vessels in the vascular system are the arteries, veins, and capillaries. Arteries, except for the pulmonary artery, carry oxygenated blood away from the heart. Veins, except for the pulmonary veins, carry deoxygenated blood toward the heart. Small branches of arteries and veins are arterioles and venules, respectively. Blood circulates from the left side of the heart into arteries, arterioles, capillaries, venules, and veins, and then back to the right side of the heart.

***Arteries and Arterioles.*** The arterial system differs from the venous system by the amount and type of tissue that make up arterial walls (Fig. 31-5). The large arteries have thick walls composed mainly of elastic tissue. This elastic property cushions the impact of the pressure created by ventricular contraction and provides recoil that propels blood forward into the circulation. Large arteries also contain some smooth muscle. Examples of large arteries are the aorta and pulmonary artery.

Arterioles have relatively little elastic tissue and more smooth muscle. Arterioles serve as the major control of arterial BP and distribution of blood flow. They respond readily to local conditions such as low $O_2$ and increasing levels of $CO_2$ by dilating or constricting.

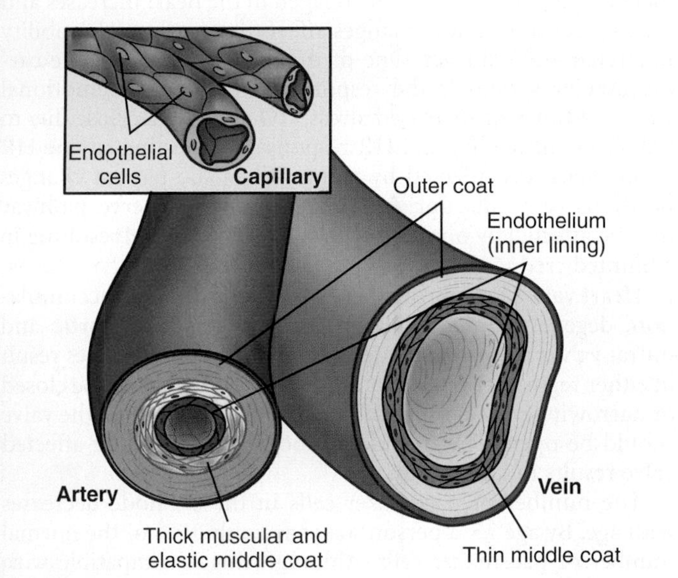


**FIG. 31-5** Comparative thickness of layers of the artery, vein, and capillary.

The innermost lining of the arteries is the endothelium. The endothelium maintains hemostasis, promotes blood flow, and, under normal conditions, inhibits blood coagulation. When the endothelial surface is disrupted (e.g., rupture of an atherosclerotic plaque), the coagulation cascade is initiated and results in the formation of a fibrin clot.

***Capillaries.*** The thin capillary wall, made up of endothelial cells, has no elastic or muscle tissue (Fig. 31-5). The exchange of cellular nutrients and metabolic end products takes place through these thin-walled vessels. Capillaries connect the arterioles and venules.

***Veins and Venules.*** Veins are large-diameter, thin-walled vessels that return blood to the right atrium (Fig. 31-5). The venous system is a low-pressure, high-volume system. The larger veins contain semilunar valves at intervals to maintain the blood flow toward the heart and to prevent backward flow. The amount of blood in the venous system is affected by a number of factors, including arterial flow, compression of veins by skeletal muscles, alterations in thoracic and abdominal pressures, and right atrial pressure.

The largest veins are the *superior vena cava,* which returns blood to the heart from the head, neck, and arms, and the *inferior vena cava,* which returns blood to the heart from the lower part of the body. These large-diameter vessels are affected by the pressure in the right side of the heart. Elevated right atrial pressure can cause distended neck veins or liver engorgement as a result of resistance to blood flow.

Venules are relatively small vessels made up of a small amount of muscle and connective tissue. Venules collect blood from the capillary beds and channel it to the larger veins.

## Regulation of Cardiovascular System

**Autonomic Nervous System.** The autonomic nervous system consists of the sympathetic nervous system and parasympathetic nervous system (see Chapter 55).

***Effect on Heart.*** Stimulation of the sympathetic nervous system increases the HR, speed of impulse conduction through the AV node, and force of atrial and ventricular contractions. This effect is mediated by specific sites in the heart called *beta ($\beta$)-adrenergic receptors,* which are receptors for norepinephrine and epinephrine.

In contrast, stimulation of the parasympathetic system (mediated by the vagus nerve) slows the HR by decreasing the impulses from the SA node and thus conduction through the AV node.

***Effect on Blood Vessels.*** The source of neural control of blood vessels is the sympathetic nervous system. The alpha$_1$ ($\alpha_1$)-adrenergic receptors are located in vascular smooth muscles. Stimulation of $\alpha_1$-adrenergic receptors results in vasoconstriction. Decreased stimulation to $\alpha_1$-adrenergic receptors causes vasodilation. (Sympathetic nervous system receptors that influence BP are presented in Table 32-1.)

The parasympathetic nerves have selective distribution in the blood vessels. For example, blood vessels in skeletal muscle do not receive parasympathetic input.

**Baroreceptors.** *Baroreceptors* in the aortic arch and carotid sinus (at the origin of the internal carotid artery) are sensitive to stretch or pressure within the arterial system. Stimulation of these receptors (e.g., volume overload) sends information to the vasomotor center in the brainstem. This results in temporary inhibition of the sympathetic nervous system and enhancement of the parasympathetic influence, causing a decreased HR and peripheral vasodilation. Decreased arterial pressure causes the opposite effect.

**Chemoreceptors.** *Chemoreceptors* are located in the aortic and carotid bodies and the medulla. They are capable of causing changes in respiratory rate and BP in response to increased arterial $CO_2$ pressure (hypercapnia) and, to a lesser degree, decreased plasma pH (acidosis) and arterial $O_2$ pressure (hypoxia). When the chemoreceptors in the medulla are triggered, they stimulate the vasomotor center to increase BP.[3]

### Blood Pressure

The **arterial blood pressure** is a measure of the pressure exerted by blood against the walls of the arterial system. The **systolic blood pressure (SBP)** is the peak pressure exerted against the arteries when the heart contracts. The **diastolic blood pressure (DBP)** is the residual pressure in the arterial system during ventricular relaxation (or filling).

The two main factors influencing BP are CO and *systemic vascular resistance* (SVR):

$$BP = CO \times SVR$$

SVR is the force opposing the movement of blood. This force is created primarily in small arteries and arterioles. Normal blood pressure is SBP <120 mm Hg and DBP <80 mm Hg[4] (see Chapter 32).

**Measurement of Arterial Blood Pressure.** BP can be measured by invasive and noninvasive techniques. The invasive technique consists of catheter insertion into an artery. The catheter is attached to a transducer, and the pressure is measured directly (see Chapter 65).

Noninvasive, indirect measurement of BP can be done with a sphygmomanometer and stethoscope. The sphygmomanometer consists of an inflatable cuff and a pressure gauge. The BP is measured by auscultating for sounds of turbulent blood flow through a compressed artery (termed **Korotkoff sounds**). The brachial artery is the recommended site for taking a BP.

After placing the appropriate size cuff on the upper arm, inflate the cuff to a pressure 20 to 30 mm Hg above the SBP. This causes blood flow in the artery to cease. If the SBP is not known, estimate the pressure by palpating the brachial pulse and inflating the cuff until the pulse ceases. The pressure noted at this time is the estimated SBP. Inflate the BP cuff 20 to 30 mm Hg above this number.

As the pressure in the cuff is lowered, auscultate the artery for Korotkoff sounds. There are five phases of Korotkoff sounds. The first phase is a tapping sound caused by the spurt of blood into the constricted artery as the pressure in the cuff is gradually deflated. This sound is noted as the SBP. The fifth phase occurs when the sound disappears, which is noted as the DBP.[5]

BP is recorded as the ratio of SBP to DBP (e.g., 120/80 mm Hg). Sometimes, an *auscultatory gap* occurs, which is a loss of sound between the SBP and DBP. Proper BP technique (e.g., using the correct cuff size, positioning arm at heart level) is essential for accurate readings (see Table 32-11).

Another noninvasive way to measure BP indirectly is an automated device that uses oscillometric measurements to assess BP. Though this method does not involve auscultation, the same attention to proper technique is essential for accuracy. SBP (and pulse) can be assessed using a Doppler ultrasonic flowmeter. The hand-held transducer is positioned over the artery (identified by audible, pulsatile sounds). The cuff is applied above the artery, inflated until the sounds disappear, and then another 20 to 30 mm Hg beyond that point. The cuff is then slowly deflated until sounds return. This point is the SBP.

**Pulse Pressure and Mean Arterial Pressure.** **Pulse pressure** is the difference between the SBP and DBP. It is normally about one third of the SBP. If the BP is 120/80 mm Hg, the pulse pressure is 40 mm Hg. An increased pulse pressure due to an increased SBP may occur during exercise or in individuals with atherosclerosis of the larger arteries. A decreased pulse pressure may be found in heart failure or hypovolemia.

Another measurement related to BP is **mean arterial pressure (MAP)**. The MAP refers to the average pressure within the arterial system that is felt by organs in the body. It is not the average of the DBP and SBP, because the length of diastole exceeds that of systole at normal HRs. MAP is calculated as follows:

$$MAP = (SBP + 2\,DBP) \div 3$$

A person with a BP of 120/60 mm Hg has an estimated MAP of 80 mm Hg. In patients with invasive BP monitoring, this value is automatically calculated and takes the patient's HR into consideration (see Chapter 65).

A MAP greater than 60 mm Hg is needed to adequately perfuse and sustain the vital organs of an average person under most conditions. When the MAP falls below this number for a period of time, vital organs are underperfused and will become ischemic.

### Gerontologic Considerations: Effects of Aging on the Cardiovascular System

One of the greatest risk factors for cardiovascular disease (CVD) is age. CVD remains the leading cause of death in adults older than age 65. The most common cardiovascular problem is coronary artery disease (CAD) due to atherosclerosis. It is difficult to separate normal aging changes from the pathophysiologic changes of atherosclerosis. Many of the physiologic changes in the cardiovascular system of older adults are a result of the combined effects of the aging process, disease, environmental factors, and lifetime health behaviors rather than just age alone.[6]

Age-related changes in the cardiovascular system and differences in assessment findings are found in Table 31-1. With increased age, the amount of collagen in the heart increases and elastin decreases. These changes affect the heart muscle's ability to stretch and contract. One of the major changes in the cardiovascular system is the response to physical or emotional stress. In times of increased stress, CO and SV decrease due to reduced contractility and HR response. The resting supine HR is not markedly affected by aging. When the patient changes positions (e.g., sits upright), the sympathetic nerve pathway may be affected by fibrous tissue and fatty deposits, resulting in a blunted (reduced) HR response.[6]

Heart valves become thicker and stiffer from lipid accumulation, degeneration of collagen, and fibrosis. The aortic and mitral valves are most frequently affected. These changes result in either regurgitation of blood when the valve should be closed or narrowing of the orifice of the valve *(stenosis)* when the valve should be open. The turbulent blood flow across the affected valve results in a **murmur**.

The number of pacemaker cells in the SA node decreases with age. By age 75, a person may have only 10% of the normal number of pacemaker cells. Although this is compatible with adequate SA node function, it may account for the frequency of some sinus dysrhythmias in older adults. Similar decreases

## TABLE 31-1 Gerontologic Assessment Differences

### *Cardiovascular System*

| Changes | Differences in Assessment Findings |
|---|---|
| **Chest Wall** | |
| Kyphosis | Altered chest landmarks for palpation, percussion, and auscultation. Distant heart sounds. |
| **Heart** | |
| Myocardial hypertrophy, ↑ collagen and scarring, ↓ elastin | ↓ Cardiac reserve, heart failure. |
| Downward displacement | Difficulty in isolating apical pulse. |
| ↓ CO, HR, SV in response to exercise or stress | ↓ Response to exercise and stress. Slowed recovery from activity. |
| Cellular aging and fibrosis of conduction system | ↓ Amplitude of QRS complex and slight lengthening of PR, QRS, and QT intervals. Irregular cardiac rhythms, ↓ maximal HR, ↓ HR variability. |
| Valvular rigidity from calcification, sclerosis, or fibrosis, impeding complete closure of valves | Systolic murmur (aortic or mitral) possible without an indication of cardiovascular disease. |
| **Blood Vessels** | |
| Arterial stiffening caused by loss of elastin in arterial walls, thickening of intima of arteries, and progressive fibrosis of media | ↑ In SBP and possible ↑ or ↓ in DBP. Possible widened pulse pressure. Pedal pulses diminished. ↑ In intermittent claudication. |
| Venous tortuosity increased | Inflamed, painful, or cordlike varicosities. Dependent edema. |

also occur in the number of conduction cells in the internodal tracts, bundle of His, and bundle branches. These changes contribute to the development of atrial dysrhythmias and heart blocks. About 50% of older adults have an abnormal resting ECG that shows increases in the PR, QRS, and/or QT intervals.[7]

The autonomic nervous system control of the cardiovascular system changes with aging. The number and function of β-adrenergic receptors in the heart decrease with age. So the older adult not only has a decreased response to physical and emotional stress but also is less sensitive to β-adrenergic agonist drugs. The lower maximum HR during exercise results in only a twofold increase in CO compared with the three or four times increase seen in younger adults.

Arterial and venous blood vessels thicken and become less elastic with age. Arteries increase their sensitivity to vasopressin (antidiuretic hormone). With aging both of these changes contribute to a progressive increase in SBP and a decrease or no change in DBP. Thus an increase in the pulse pressure is found. Valves in the large veins in the lower extremities have a reduced ability to return the blood to the heart, often resulting in dependent edema.

Orthostatic hypotension, which is estimated to be present in more than 30% of patients over age 70 with systolic hypertension, may be related to drugs and/or decreased baroreceptor function. *Postprandial hypotension* (decrease in BP of at least 20 mm Hg that occurs within 75 minutes after eating) may also occur in about a third of otherwise healthy older adults. Both orthostatic and postprandial hypotension may be related to falls in older adults. Despite the changes associated with aging, the heart is able to function adequately under most circumstances.

## CASE STUDY

### *Patient Introduction*

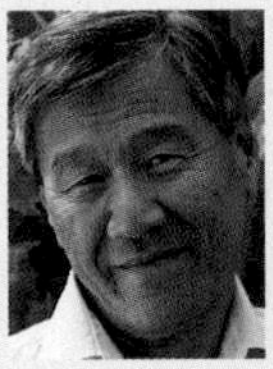

(©Jupiterimages/ Banana-Stock/ Thinkstock)

L.P., a 63-year-old Asian American male, is brought to the emergency department by ambulance at 6 AM with complaints of chest tightness, shortness of breath (SOB), and palpitations. The paramedics have started an IV and $O_2$ at 2 L/min via nasal cannula. They also administered four chewable baby ASA and a nitroglycerin tablet, and they obtained a 12-lead ECG. L.P. is pain free on arrival but still complains of palpitations.

**Discussion Questions**

1. What are the possible causes of L.P.'s chest tightness, SOB, and palpitations?
2. What would be your major priorities when assessing L.P.?
3. Is L.P.'s condition stable or unstable?

You will learn more about L.P. and his condition as you read through this assessment chapter.

(See p. 666 for more information on L.P.)

Answers available at *http://evolve.elsevier.com/Lewis/medsurg.*

## ASSESSMENT OF CARDIOVASCULAR SYSTEM

### Subjective Data

A careful health history and physical examination will help you distinguish symptoms that reflect a cardiovascular problem from problems of other body systems. Explore and record all cues that alert you to the possibility of underlying CVD.

#### Important Health Information

***History of Present Illness.*** Ask the patient what problem has brought him or her to the health care facility or provider. Fully explore all symptoms the patient is experiencing (Table 31-1).

***Past Health History.*** Many illnesses affect the cardiovascular system directly or indirectly. Ask the patient about a history of chest pain, shortness of breath, fatigue, alcohol and tobacco use, anemia, rheumatic fever, streptococcal throat infections, congenital heart disease, stroke, palpitations, dizziness with position changes, syncope, hypertension, thrombophlebitis, intermittent claudication, edema, and varicosities.

***Medications.*** Assess the patient's current and past use of medications. This includes over-the-counter (OTC) drugs, herbal supplements, and prescription drugs. For example, aspirin prolongs the blood clotting time and is found in many drugs used to treat cold symptoms. List all of the patient's drugs. Include dose, time last taken, and the patient's understanding of the drug's purpose and side effects. Many noncardiac drugs can adversely affect the cardiovascular system and should be assessed (Table 31-2).

***Surgery or Other Treatments.*** Ask the patient about specific treatments, past surgeries, or hospital admissions related to cardiovascular problems. Explore any admissions or procedures performed for cardiovascular symptoms. Note whether an ECG or a chest x-ray has been done for baseline data.

**Functional Health Patterns.** The strong correlation between components of a patient's lifestyle and cardiovascular health supports the need to review each functional health pattern. Key questions to ask a person with a cardiovascular problem are listed in Table 31-3.

**TABLE 31-2 Cardiovascular Effects of Noncardiac Drugs***

| Drug Classification | Examples | Cardiovascular Effects |
|---|---|---|
| Anticancer agents | daunorubicin (Cerubidine) doxorubicin | Dysrhythmias, cardiomyopathy |
| Antipsychotics | chlorpromazine haloperido | Dysrhythmias, orthostatic hypotension |
| Corticosteroids | cortisone prednisone | Hypotension, edema, potassium depletion |
| Hormone therapy, oral contraceptives | estrogen + progestin (Prempro) | Myocardial infarction, thromboembolism, stroke, hypertension |
| Nonsteroidal antiinflammatory drugs (NSAIDs) | ibuprofen celecoxib (Celebrex) diclofenac (Voltaren) | Myocardial infarction, stroke, hypertension, heart failure |
| Psychostimulants | cocaine amphetamines | Tachycardia, angina, myocardial infarction, hypertension, dysrhythmias |
| Tricyclic antidepressants | amitriptyline doxepin (Sinequan) | Dysrhythmias, orthostatic hypotension |

*List is not all-inclusive.

***Health Perception–Health Management Pattern.*** Ask the patient about the presence of major cardiovascular risk factors. These include abnormal serum lipids, hypertension, sedentary lifestyle, diabetes, obesity, and tobacco use. If a patient uses tobacco, estimate the number of pack-years of tobacco use (number of packs smoked per day multiplied by the number of years the patient has smoked). Record the patient's attitude about tobacco use and attempts and methods used to stop. Record any alcohol use. Include information about the type of alcohol, amount, frequency, and any changes in the reaction to it. Also note any use of habit-forming drugs, including recreational drugs.

Question the patient about any drug allergies, including food and environmental allergies. Determine whether the patient has ever experienced a drug reaction or an allergic or anaphylactic reaction. Ask specifically about any allergic reaction to contrast media.

**GENETIC RISK ALERT**

**Coronary Artery Disease**

- Specific genetic links, especially related to lipoprotein genes, have been identified for some families with CAD.
- The clustering of CAD in families is strong if there is early age of onset affecting several relatives.

**Cardiomyopathy**

- Hypertrophic cardiomyopathy can be caused by autosomal dominant mutations.
- Dilated cardiomyopathy can be caused by autosomal and X-linked dominant mutations.

**Hypertension**

- Hypertension results from a complex interplay between genetic and environmental factors.
- Lifestyle choices (e.g., smoking, lack of exercise) may trigger genetic tendencies to hypertension.

Confirmed illnesses of blood relatives can highlight any genetic or familial tendencies toward CAD, hypertension, bleeding, diabetes, atherosclerosis, and stroke. Note any family members who had heart disease at an early age (<50 years of age for men; <55 years of age for women). In addition, disorders affecting the vascular system, such as intermittent claudication and varicosities, may be familial. Last, assess any family health history of noncardiac problems such as lung, kidney, or liver disease and obesity, because they can affect the cardiovascular system.

***Nutritional-Metabolic Pattern.*** Being underweight or overweight may indicate potential cardiovascular problems. It is important to assess the patient's weight history (e.g., over the past year) in relation to height. Determine the amount of salt and saturated fats in the patient's typical diet. In addition to actual food habits, which may be influenced by culture, explore the patient's attitudes and plans relative to diet and weight management.

***Elimination Pattern.*** The patient on diuretics may report increased voiding and/or nocturia. Ask about any history of incontinence or constipation, including any use of drugs (prescribed and OTC) for constipation. Teach patients with heart problems to avoid straining during a bowel movement *(Valsalva maneuver)*. Ask patients if they have any swelling of the lower extremities and if it resolves when their feet are elevated or after an overnight sleep.

***Activity-Exercise Pattern.*** The benefit of exercise for cardiovascular health is clear, with aerobic exercise being most beneficial. Record the types of exercise done and the duration, intensity, and frequency of each. Ask about and note the occurrence of any symptoms during exercise (e.g., chest pain, shortness of breath, claudication) that may indicate a cardiovascular problem.

***Sleep-Rest Pattern.*** Cardiovascular problems often disrupt sleep. *Paroxysmal nocturnal dyspnea* (attacks of shortness of breath, especially at night that awaken the patient) and *Cheyne-Stokes respiration* (periods of very shallow breaths to alternating periods of apnea and deep, rapid breathing) are associated with heart failure. Many patients with heart failure need to sleep with several pillows or upright in a chair. Note the number of pillows needed to sleep or the need to sleep upright *(orthopnea)* and whether this has changed recently.

Sleep apnea has been associated with an increased risk of life-threatening dysrhythmias, especially in patients with heart failure. Nocturia, a common finding with cardiovascular patients, also interrupts normal sleep patterns. Fully explore both conditions.

***Cognitive-Perceptual Pattern.*** It is important to ask both the patient and caregiver about cognitive-perceptual problems. Cardiovascular problems such as dysrhythmias, hypertension, and stroke may cause problems with syncope, language, and memory. Report any pain associated with the cardiovascular system (e.g., chest pain, claudication).

***Self-Perception–Self-Concept Pattern.*** If a cardiovascular event is acute, the patient's self-perception may be affected. Invasive diagnostic procedures often lead to body image concerns for the patient. When CVD is chronic, the patient may not be able to identify the cause but can often describe the inability to "keep up" previous levels of activity. This may also affect the patient's quality of life, so ask about the effects of the illness on the patient.

***Role-Relationship Pattern.*** The patient's gender, race, and age are all related to cardiovascular health. In addition, the patient's marital status, role in the household, employment status,

## TABLE 31-3 Health History

***Cardiovascular System***

**Health Perception–Health Management**
- Do you practice any preventive measures to decrease risk factors for heart disease?*
- Have you noticed an increase in heart symptoms such as chest pain or dyspnea?*
- Does your heart problem cause you to be less able to care for yourself?*
- Do you foresee any potential self-care problems because of your heart problem?*
- Have you ever used tobacco? If yes, in what form, how much, and for how long? Have you tried to quit? If yes, what methods have you tried? Are you interested in more information about quitting?
- How often and how much alcohol do you drink?

**Nutritional-Metabolic**
- Describe your usual daily diet, including salt, fat, and liquid intake.
- What is your present weight? What was your weight 1 year ago? If different, explain.
- Does eating cause fatigue or shortness of breath?*

**Elimination**
- Do your feet or ankles ever swell?* If yes, how far up your legs? Does it go away after sleeping all night?
- Have you ever taken drugs to help you get rid of excess fluid or to relieve constipation?*
- Are you having any problems related to urination?*
- Do you ever strain to have a bowel movement?

**Activity-Exercise**
- Are your daily activities or exercise limited because of your heart problem?*
- When were you last able to comfortably perform your usual activities or exercise?
- Do you experience any discomfort or symptoms as a result of exercise or any activity?*
- Can you comfortably walk and talk at the same time?
- How often do you attend activities outside your home?
- What was your most strenuous activity in the last few weeks compared with 6 months ago?

**Sleep-Rest**
- How many pillows do you sleep on at night? Has this changed recently?*
- Do you ever wake up suddenly and feel as if you cannot catch your breath?*
- Do you have a history of sleep apnea?*
- Do you ever sleep in a chair at night? Is yes, how often?
- How many times a night do you awaken to urinate?

**Cognitive-Perceptual**
- Do you ever experience dizziness or fainting?*
- Do you ever find it difficult to express yourself or to remember things?*
- Do you experience any pain (e.g., chest pain, leg pain with activity) as a result of your heart problem?*

**Self-Perception–Self-Concept**
- Have your perceptions of yourself changed since you were diagnosed with heart disease?*
- How has your heart disease affected the quality of your life?

**Role-Relationship**
- Has this illness affected any of the roles that you play in your daily life?*
- How have your significant others been affected by your heart disease?

**Sexuality-Reproductive**
- Has your heart disease caused a change in your sexual activity?*
- Do you experience any heart-related symptoms during sexual activity?*
- Do any of your drugs affect your ability to participate in sexual activities?*
- Females: Are you currently taking oral contraceptives, hormonal therapy, or drug therapy for breast cancer?

**Coping–Stress Tolerance**
- Describe your normal coping mechanisms during times of stress or anxiety.
- To whom or where would you turn during a time of stress? Are these people or services helping you now?*
- Do you practice any stress reduction techniques?*
- Do you have a history of depression?*
- Do you feel capable of handling your present health situation?
- Do you experience any heart symptoms (e.g., chest pain, palpitations) during times of stress or anger?*

**Values-Beliefs**
- What influence have your values or beliefs had during your illness?
- Do you feel any conflicts between your values or beliefs and the plan of care?*
- Describe any cultural or religious beliefs that may influence the management of your heart problem.

*If yes, describe.

number of children and their ages, living environment, and caregivers help you to identify strengths and support systems in the patient's life. Assess the patient's level of satisfaction or dissatisfaction with life roles, since this may alert you to possible areas of stress or conflict.

***Sexuality-Reproductive Pattern.*** Ask the patient about the effect of the cardiovascular problem on sexual activity. Because some patients often fear sudden death during sexual intercourse, it may lead to changes in their sexual behavior. Fatigue, chest pain, or shortness of breath may also limit sexual activity. Erectile dysfunction (ED) may be a symptom of peripheral vascular disease and/or a side effect of some drugs used to treat CVD (e.g., β-blockers, diuretics). Ask about the use of drugs for ED (e.g., sildenafil [Viagra]). These drugs are contraindicated if the patient is also taking a nitrate because the combination can cause significant hypotension.[8] Decide if counseling may be helpful.

Ask female patients if they use oral contraceptives, hormone therapy (HT) for symptoms of menopause, or drug therapy for breast cancer. Women who smoke tobacco and use oral contraceptives are at increased risk for blood clots (e.g., venous thromboembolism). Similarly, there is an increased risk for CVD with the use of HT and selective estrogen-receptor modulators (e.g., tamoxifen [Novaldex]).[9]

***Coping–Stress Tolerance Pattern.*** Ask the patient to identify areas that cause stress and the usual methods of coping with stress. Potentially stressful areas include health concerns, marital relationships, family and friends, occupation, and finances.

Work-related stress, depression, and inadequate social support are risk factors for CVD and heart events. Ask the patient about each of these factors. Information about support systems such as family, extended family and friends, counselors, or religious groups can provide vital insight when planning care.

***Values-Belief Pattern.*** Individual values and beliefs, which are greatly affected by culture, may play a major role in the real or potential conflict that a patient faces when dealing with CVD. Some patients may attribute their illness to punishment from God; others may think that a "higher power" can help them. Information about a patient's values and beliefs will help you intervene during periods of crisis.

## CASE STUDY

### *Subjective Data*

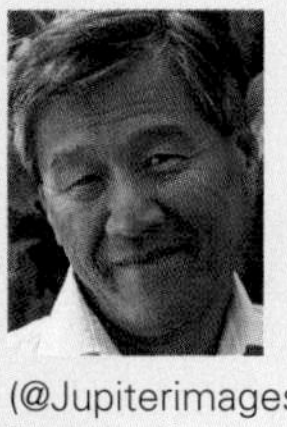

(@Jupiterimages/ Banana-Stock/ Thinkstock)

A focused subjective assessment of L.P. revealed the following information:

- ***PMH:*** History of hypertension, mitral valve prolapse with mild regurgitation, heart failure, and type 2 diabetes.
- ***Medications:*** Lisinopril (Prinivil) 10 mg/day PO, metoprolol (Lopressor) 50 mg PO BID, ASA 81 mg/day PO, furosemide (Lasix) 40 mg/day PO, and glipizide (Glucotrol) 5 mg/day PO.
- ***Health Perception–Health Management:*** L.P. denies any previous history of chest pain or CAD. He was feeling fine until this morning when he awoke and experienced SOB, chest tightness, and palpitations while walking to the bathroom. He became frightened that he was having a heart attack, so his wife called 911. Denies smoking or alcohol intake. SOB and chest tightness are now gone, but he continues to feel palpitations.
- ***Elimination:*** Denies any edema. States takes Lasix in the morning and typically "passes urine until lunchtime." Denies nocturia.

**Discussion Questions**

1. What type of assessment would be most appropriate for L.P.: emergency, focused, or comprehensive? On what basis did you make that decision?
2. What assessment questions will you ask him?
3. How will you individualize the assessment based on his age, ethnic/cultural background, and condition?
4. Is this an appropriate time to teach him about the proper use of nitroglycerin tablets? Why or why not?

You will learn more about the physical examination of the cardiovascular system in the next section.

(See p. 669 for more information on L.P.)

Answers available at *http://evolve.elsevier.com/Lewis/medsurg.*

## Objective Data

### Physical Examination

***Vital Signs.*** After you observe the patient's general appearance, obtain vital signs. Measure BP bilaterally. These readings can vary from 5 to 15 mm Hg. Use the arm with the highest BP for subsequent measurements. Take orthostatic (postural) BPs and HRs while the patient is supine, sitting with legs dangling, and standing. SBP should not decrease more than 20 mm Hg from the supine to the standing position. HR should not increase more than 20 beats/minute from the supine to the standing position.

***Peripheral Vascular System***

**Inspection.** Inspect the skin for color, hair distribution, and venous pattern. Check the extremities for conditions such as edema, dependent rubor, clubbing of the nail beds, varicosities, and lesions such as stasis ulcers. Edema in the legs can be caused by gravity, varicosities, or right-sided heart failure.

Inspect the large veins in the neck (internal and external jugular) while the patient is gradually moved from a supine position to an upright (30 to 45 degrees) position. Distention and prominent pulsations of these neck veins, referred to as *jugular venous distention,* can be caused by right-sided heart failure.

**Palpation.** Palpate the upper and lower extremities for temperature, moisture, pulses, and edema bilaterally to assess for symmetry. Look for edema by depressing the skin over the tibia or medial malleolus for 5 seconds. Normally, there is no depression after releasing pressure. If pitting edema is present, grade it from 1+ (mild pitting, slight brief indentation) to 4+ (very deep pitting, indentation that lasts a long time).[5]

Palpate the pulses in the neck and extremities for information on arterial blood flow. Assess the rhythm (e.g., regular, irregular) and force. It is important to palpate each carotid pulse separately to avoid vagal stimulation and possible dysrhythmias. Compare the characteristics of the arteries on the right and left extremities simultaneously to determine symmetry.

When palpating the arteries identified in Fig. 31-6, rate the force of the pulse using the following scale:

0 = Absent
1+ = Weak
2+ = Normal
3+ = Increased, full, bounding

The rigidity (hardness) of the vessel should also be noted. The normal pulse feels like a tap, whereas a vessel wall that is narrowed or bulging vibrates. The term for a palpable vibration is *thrill.*

*Capillary refill* is used to assess arterial flow to the extremities. Position the patient's hands near the level of the heart and

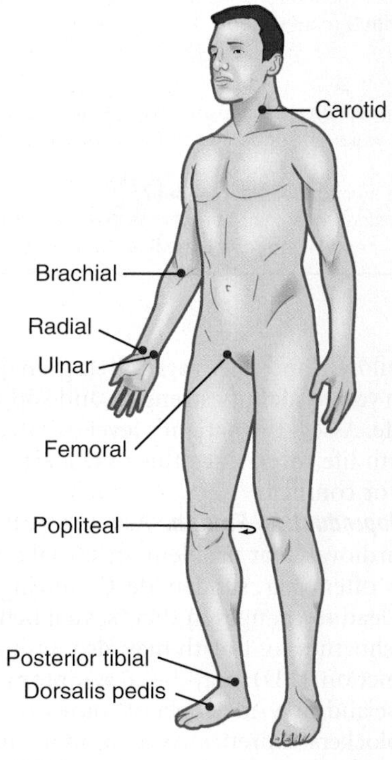


**FIG. 31-6** Common sites for palpating arteries.

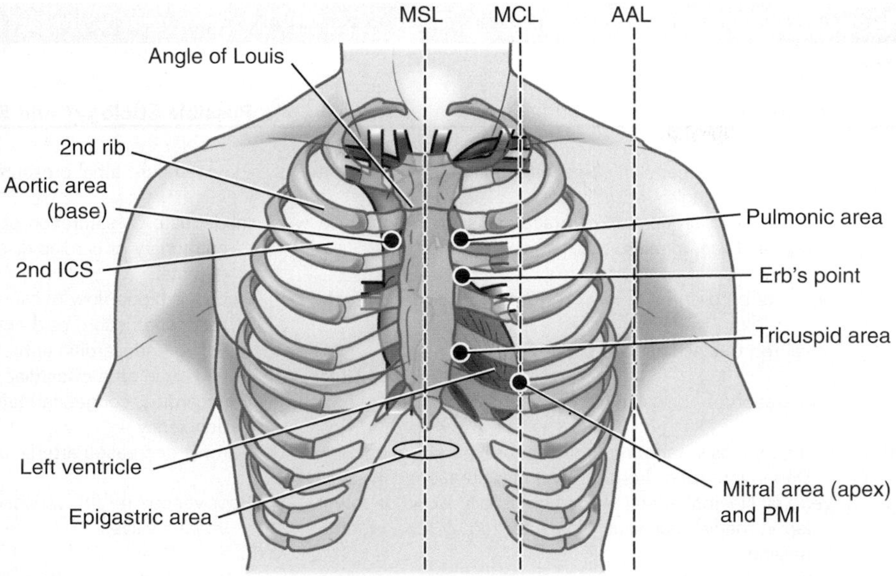


**FIG. 31-7** Orientation of the heart within the thorax and cardiac auscultatory areas. *Red lines* indicate the midsternal line *(MSL)*, midclavicular line *(MCL)*, and anterior axillary line *(AAL)*. *ICS*, Intercostal space; *PMI*, point of maximal impulse.

squeeze a nail bed to produce blanching. Observe for the return of color. This should occur in less than 2 seconds with normal tissue perfusion and CO.

**Auscultation.** An artery that is narrowed or has a bulging wall may create turbulent blood flow. This abnormal flow can cause a buzzing or humming termed a *bruit.* This is heard with the bell of the stethoscope placed over the vessel. Auscultation of major arteries such as the carotid arteries, abdominal aorta, and femoral arteries should be part of the initial cardiovascular assessment. Abnormalities of the cardiovascular system are described in Table 31-4.

***Thorax***

**Inspection and Palpation.** An overall inspection and palpation of the thorax are the first steps in the examination. Next, inspect and palpate the areas where the heart valves project their sounds by identifying the intercostal spaces (ICSs). The raised notch, the *angle of Louis,* is where the manubrium and body of the sternum are joined. It is located at the level of the second rib. It is palpable in the midline of the sternum. It is used to count ICSs and locate specific auscultatory areas (Fig. 31-7).

Locate the following auscultatory areas: aortic area in the second ICS to the right of the sternum, pulmonic area in the second ICS to the left of the sternum, tricuspid area in the fifth left ICS close to the sternum, and mitral area in the left midclavicular line at the fifth ICS. A fifth auscultatory area is *Erb's point,* located at the third left ICS near the sternum. Normally, no pulsations are felt in these areas unless the patient has a thin chest wall.

A heart valve disorder may be suspected if abnormal pulsations or thrills are felt. Next, inspect and palpate the epigastric area, which lies on either side of the midline just below the xiphoid process. In a thin person, you may see the pulsation of the abdominal aorta. Normally, you can palpate it here. Next, inspect the precordium, which is located over the heart, for heaves. **Heaves** are sustained lifts of the chest wall in the precordial area that can be seen or palpated. They may be caused by left ventricular hypertrophy. Normally no pulsations are seen or felt here.

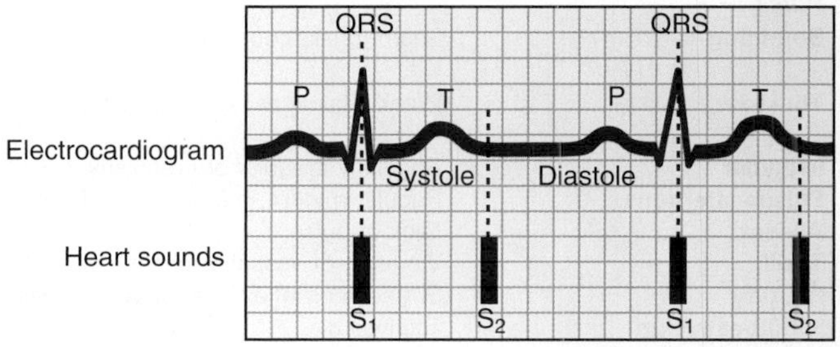


**FIG. 31-8** Relationship of electrocardiogram, cardiac cycle, and heart sounds.

When the patient is supine, palpate the mitral valve area for the **point of maximal impulse (PMI)** (also called the *apical pulse*). This reflects the pulsation of the apex of the heart. The PMI lies medial to the midclavicular line in the fourth or fifth ICS. If you can palpate the PMI, record its position in relation to the midclavicular line and ICSs. When the PMI is below the fifth ICS and left of the midclavicular line, the heart may be enlarged.

**Auscultation.** Normal heart sounds are made by the movement of blood through the heart valves. These sounds can be heard through a stethoscope placed on the chest wall. The first heart sound ($S_1$) is associated with closure of the tricuspid and mitral valves. It has a soft lubb sound. The second heart sound ($S_2$) is associated with closure of the aortic and pulmonic valves. It has a sharp dupp sound. $S_1$ signals the beginning of systole. $S_2$ signals the beginning of diastole (Fig. 31-8). Listen to the auscultatory areas in sequence (Fig. 31-7).

$S_1$ and $S_2$ are heard best with the diaphragm of the stethoscope because they are high pitched. Extra heart sounds ($S_3$ or $S_4$), if present, are heard best with the bell of the stethoscope because they are low pitched. Have the patient lean forward while sitting to enhance the sounds from the second ICSs (aortic and pulmonic areas). Place the patient in a left side-lying position to enhance the sounds at the mitral area.

When auscultating the apical area, simultaneously palpate the radial pulse. Determine whether the rhythm is regular or

## TABLE 31-4 Assessment Abnormalities

### *Cardiovascular System*

| Finding* | Description | Possible Etiology* and Significance |
|---|---|---|
| **Inspection** | | |
| **Jugular venous distention** | Distended neck (jugular) veins with patient sitting at 30- to 45-degree angle | Elevated right atrial pressure, right-sided heart failure |
| **Central cyanosis** | Bluish or purplish tinge in central areas such as tongue, conjunctivae, inner surface of lips | Inadequate $O_2$ saturation of arterial blood because of pulmonary or cardiac disorders (e.g., congenital defects) |
| **Peripheral cyanosis** | Bluish or purplish tinge in extremities or in nose and ears | Reduced blood flow because of heart failure, vasoconstriction, cold environment |
| **Splinter hemorrhages** | Small red to black streaks under fingernails | Infective endocarditis (infection of endocardium, usually in area of cardiac valves) |
| **Clubbing of nail beds** | Obliteration of normal angle between base of nail and skin | Endocarditis, congenital defects, prolonged $O_2$ deficiency |
| **Color changes in extremities with postural change** | Pallor, cyanosis, mottling of skin after limb elevation. Dependent rubor (reddish blue discoloration). Glossy skin | Chronic decreased arterial perfusion |
| **Ulcers** | *Venous:* Necrotic crater-like lesion usually found on lower leg at medial malleolus. Characterized by slow wound healing | Poor venous return, varicose veins, incompetent venous valves. |
| | *Arterial:* Pale ischemic base, well-defined edges usually found on toes, heels, lateral malleoli | Arteriosclerosis, diabetes |
| **Varicose veins** | Visible dilated, discolored, tortuous vessels in lower extremities | Incompetent valves in vein |
| **Palpation** | | |
| ***Pulse*** | | |
| **Bounding** | Sharp, brisk, pounding pulse | Hyperkinetic states (e.g., anxiety, fever), anemia, hyperthyroidism |
| **Thready** | Weak, slowly rising pulse easily obliterated by pressure | Blood loss, decreased cardiac output, aortic valve disease, peripheral arterial disease |
| **Irregular** | Regularly irregular or irregularly irregular. Skipped beats | Cardiac dysrhythmias |
| **Pulsus alternans** | Regular rhythm, but strength of pulse varies with each beat | Heart failure, cardiac tamponade |
| **Absent** | Lack of pulse | Atherosclerosis, trauma, embolus |
| **Thrill** | Vibration of vessel or chest wall | Aneurysm, aortic regurgitation, arteriovenous fistula |
| **Rigidity** | Stiffness or inflexibility of vessel wall | Atherosclerosis |
| **>100 beats/min** | Tachycardia | Exercise, anxiety, shock, need for increased cardiac output, hyperthyroidism |
| **<60 beats/min** | Bradycardia | Rest or sleeping, SA or AV node damage, athletic conditioning, side effect of drugs (e.g., β-blockers), hypothyroidism |
| **Displaced point of maximal impulse (apical pulse)** | Point of maximal impulse is palpated (or auscultated) below the fifth ICS and to the left of the MCL | Cardiac enlargement as a result of coronary artery disease, heart failure, cardiomyopathy |
| ***Extremities*** | | |
| **Unusually warm extremities** | Hands and feet warmer than normal | Possible thyrotoxicosis |
| **Cold extremities** | Hands and/or feet cold to touch. External covering necessary for comfort | Intermittent claudication, peripheral arterial disease, low cardiac output, severe anemia |
| **Pitting edema of lower extremities or sacral area** | Visible finger indentation after application of firm pressure, weight gain, tightening of clothing (including shoes), marks or indentations from constricting garments | Interruption of venous return to heart, right-sided heart failure |
| **Abnormal capillary refill** | Blanching of nail bed for ≥2 sec after release of pressure | Possible reduced arterial capillary perfusion, anemia |
| **Asymmetry in limb circumference** | Measurable swelling of involved limb | Venous thromboembolism, varicose veins, lymphedema |
| **Auscultation** | | |
| **Pulse deficit** | Apical heart rate exceeding peripheral pulse rate | Cardiac dysrhythmias, most often atrial fibrillation/flutter or premature ventricular contractions |
| **Arterial bruit** | Turbulent flow sound in peripheral artery | Arterial obstruction or aneurysm |
| **Third heart sound ($S_3$)** | Extra heart sound, low pitched, heard in early diastole. Similar to sound of a gallop | Left ventricular failure. Volume overload. Mitral, aortic, or tricuspid regurgitation. Hypertension (possible) |
| **Fourth heart sound ($S_4$)** | Extra heart sound, low pitched, heard in late diastole. Similar to sound of a gallop | Forceful atrial contraction from resistance to ventricular filling (e.g., in left ventricular hypertrophy, aortic stenosis, hypertension, coronary artery disease) |
| **Heart murmurs** | Turbulent sounds occurring between normal heart sounds. Characterized by loudness, pitch, shape, quality, duration, timing | Heart valve disorder, abnormal blood flow patterns |
| **Pericardial friction rub** | High-pitched, scratchy sound heard during $S_1$ and/or $S_2$ at the apex. Heard best with patient sitting and leaning forward, and while holding breath at the end of expiration | Pericarditis |

*Limited to common abnormal assessment findings and etiologic factors. (Further discussion of conditions listed may be found in Chapters 32 to 37, 65, and 66.)

irregular while listening and feeling. If the apical and radial pulses are not equivalent, count the apical pulse while a second person simultaneously counts the radial pulse for 1 full minute. The difference between the two numbers is called a *pulse deficit* and can indicate dysrhythmias.

Normally no sound is heard between $S_1$ and $S_2$. Sounds heard during these periods may represent abnormalities and should be described. An exception to this is a normal splitting of $S_2$, which is best heard at the pulmonic area during inspiration. Splitting of this heart sound can be abnormal if it is heard during expiration or if it is constant (fixed) during the respiratory cycle.

The $S_3$ heart sound is a low-intensity vibration of the ventricular walls usually associated with decreased compliance of the ventricles during filling. An $S_3$ heart sound may be normal (physiologic) in young adults. It is pathologic in patients with left-sided heart failure or mitral valve regurgitation. $S_3$ is heard closely after $S_2$ and is known as a *ventricular gallop.* The $S_4$ heart sound is a low-frequency vibration caused by atrial contraction. It precedes $S_1$ of the next cycle, and is known as an *atrial gallop.* An $S_4$ heart sound may be normal in older adults with no evidence of heart disease. It is pathologic in patients with CAD, cardiomyopathy, left ventricular hypertrophy, or aortic stenosis.

Murmurs, if heard, are graded on a six-point Roman numeral scale of loudness and recorded as a ratio. I/VI indicates a murmur that is barely audible with the stethoscope, heard only in a quiet room and then not easily. VI/VI indicates a murmur that can be heard with the stethoscope lifted just off the chest wall.

*Pericardial friction rubs* are sounds caused by friction that occurs when inflamed surfaces of the pericardium (pericarditis) move against each other. They are high-pitched, scratchy sounds that may be intermittent and may last several hours to days. Friction rubs are heard best at the apex, with patients upright and leaning forward, and while holding their breath following expiration.[5]

Record any abnormal sounds. This includes the timing (during systole or diastole), location (the anatomic site on the chest where it is heard the loudest), position (heard best when the patient is supine, sitting and leaning forward, or in the left side-lying position), and any other abnormal findings (irregular apical pulse or palpable chest wall heaves) associated with the sound.

Abnormal assessment findings are described in Table 31-4. A method of recording data from the cardiovascular assessment is presented in Table 31-5.

A *focused assessment* is used to evaluate the status of previously identified cardiovascular problems and to monitor for signs of new problems (see Table 3-7). A focused assessment of the cardiovascular system is presented in the box in right column.

## DIAGNOSTIC STUDIES OF CARDIOVASCULAR SYSTEM

Numerous diagnostic tests are available to assess the cardiovascular system. Table 31-6 identifies the most common studies. Select studies are described in more detail below.

### Blood Studies

Many blood studies provide information about the cardiovascular system. For example, some reflect the $O_2$-carrying capacity (red blood cell count and hemoglobin) and coagulation properties (clotting times) of the blood. (See Chapter 29 and Tables 29-6, 29-7, and 26-9 for hematology studies.)

**Cardiac Biomarkers.** When cells are injured, they release their contents, including enzymes and other proteins, into the circulation. These *biomarkers* are useful in the diagnosis of acute coronary syndrome (ACS).

## CASE STUDY

### *Objective Data: Physical Examination*

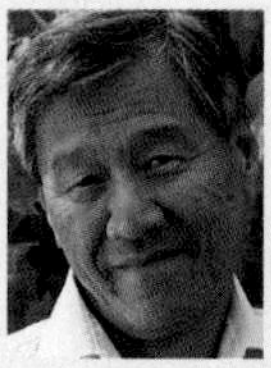

(©Jupiterimages/ Banana-Stock/ Thinkstock)

Physical examination findings of L.P. are as follows:

- BP 100/54, apical-radial pulse 154, pulse irregular, respiratory rate 20, temperature 98.2° F (36.8° C), $O_2$ saturation 94% on room air
- Awake, alert, and oriented ×3
- Lungs clear on auscultation; systolic murmur present
- Heart monitor shows atrial fibrillation with a rapid ventricular response
- +1 pedal pulses bilaterally
- No peripheral edema, jugular venous distention, or heaves noted

**Discussion Questions**

1. What should be included in the physical assessment?
2. Which physical assessment findings are of most concern to you?
3. Based on the results of the subjective and physical assessment findings, what diagnostic studies do you think will be ordered for L.P.?

You will learn more about diagnostic studies related to the cardiovascular system in the next section.

(See p. 679 for more information on L.P.)

Answers available at *http://evolve.elsevier.com/Lewis/medsurg.*

## FOCUSED ASSESSMENT

### *Cardiovascular System*

*Use this checklist to make certain the key assessment steps have been done.*

**Subjective**

Ask the patient about any of the following and note responses.

| | | |
|---|---|---|
| Chest pain, discomfort | Y | N |
| Palpitations | Y | N |
| Shortness of breath (especially when lying down or at rest) | Y | N |
| Edema in legs or any part of body | Y | N |
| Leg pain during exercise | Y | N |
| Excess urination at night | Y | N |

**Objective: Diagnostic**

Check the following for critical values or changes.

| | |
|---|---|
| Cardiac biomarkers | ✓ |
| Hematocrit, hemoglobin, platelets | ✓ |
| Glucose, electrolytes, BUN, creatinine | ✓ |
| Electrocardiogram | ✓ |
| Chest x-ray | ✓ |

**Objective: Physical Examination**

***Inspect and Palpate***

| | |
|---|---|
| Anterior chest wall for pulsations and heaves | ✓ |
| Pulses for symmetry, quality, and rhythm | ✓ |

***Auscultate***

| | |
|---|---|
| Bilateral blood pressures | ✓ |
| Heart for rate, rhythm, and sounds | ✓ |

**TABLE 31-5 Normal Physical Assessment of Cardiovascular System**

| | |
|---|---|
| **Inspection** | Skin warm, normal color. PMI not visible. No JVD with patient at 45-degree angle. |
| **Palpation** | Capillary refill <2 sec. PMI palpable in fourth ICS at left MCL. No thrills or heaves. Slight palpable pulsations of abdominal aorta in epigastric area. Carotid and extremity pulses 2+ and equal bilaterally. No pedal edema. |
| **Auscultation** | $S_1$ and $S_2$ heard. Apical-radial pulse rate equal, 72, and regular. No murmurs or extra heart sounds. |

*ICS*, Intercostal space; *JVD*, jugular venous distention; *MCL*, midclavicular line; *PMI*, point of maximal impulse.

Cardiac-specific troponin is a heart muscle protein released into circulation after injury or infarction. Two subtypes, cardiac-specific troponin T (cTnT) and cardiac-specific troponin I (cTnI), are specific to heart muscle. Normally the level in the blood is very low, so a rise in level is diagnostic of myocardial infarction (MI) or injury. cTnT and cTnI are detectable within hours (on average 4 to 6 hours) of MI or injury, peak at 10 to 24 hours, and can be detected for up to 10 to 14 days (see Fig. 33-10). Troponin is the biomarker of choice in the diagnosis of ACS. High-sensitivity troponin (hs-cTnT, hs-cTnI) assays may provide even earlier detection of a heart event.[10]

Creatine kinase (CK) enzymes are found in a variety of organs and tissues and occur as three isoenzymes. These isoenzymes are specific to skeletal muscle (CK-MM), brain and nervous tissue (CK-BB), and the heart (CK-MB). CK-MB rise is specific for MI or injury. Levels begin to increase 3 to 6 hours after symptom onset, peak in 12 to 24 hours, and return to baseline within 12 to 48 hours after MI.[11] The peak level and return to normal can be delayed in a patient with a large MI. Levels drop more rapidly in patients who are quickly and successfully treated for an MI. (Fig. 33-10 depicts the changes in cardiac markers related to an MI.)

Copeptin, a substitute marker for arginine vasopressin (AVP), is an additional diagnostic test that can be used for patients presenting with signs of ACS. In patients with an acute MI, it can be detected immediately. A combination of troponin and copeptin provide increased sensitivity for diagnosing an acute MI.[12]

Myoglobin is a low-molecular-weight heme protein found in heart and skeletal muscle. Myoglobin elevation is a sensitive indicator of very early myocardial injury but lacks specificity for MI. Its usefulness in diagnosing MI is limited.[11]

Correct interpretation of diagnostic tests requires consideration of the time from onset of symptoms and the time of the expected presence and elevation of the biomarkers. Additional data (patient symptoms, history, and ECG changes) complete the diagnostic picture for the patient with suspected ACS.

**C-Reactive Protein.** C-reactive protein (CRP) is a protein produced by the liver during periods of acute inflammation. CRP can be measured using a high-sensitivity test (hs-CRP). An increased level of CRP has been linked with the presence of atherosclerosis and the first occurrence of a heart event. In addition, the level of CRP may predict the risk for future heart events in patients with MI. However, studies on the usefulness of assessing CRP have produced conflicting results, and measuring CRP routinely in patients with and without CVD is not done.[13]

**Homocysteine.** Homocysteine (Hcy) is an amino acid that is produced during protein catabolism. Elevated Hcy levels can be either hereditary or acquired from dietary deficiencies of vitamin $B_6$, vitamin $B_{12}$, or folate. Elevated levels of Hcy have been linked to a higher risk of CVD, peripheral vascular disease, and stroke. It is recommended that Hcy testing be done in patients with a familial predisposition for early CVD or a history of CVD in the absence of other common risk factors.[14]

**Cardiac Natriuretic Peptide Markers.** There are three natriuretic peptides: (1) atrial natriuretic peptide (ANP) from the atrium, (2) b-type natriuretic peptide (BNP) from the ventricles, and (3) c-type natriuretic peptide from endothelial and renal epithelial cells. BNP is the marker of choice for distinguishing a cardiac or respiratory cause of dyspnea. N-terminal pro-brain natriuretic peptide (NT-pro-BNP) is also secreted in the ventricles and is more sensitive but less specific than BNP as a diagnostic marker of heart failure.[11] When DBP increases (e.g., heart failure), BNP and NT-pro-BNP are released and increase natriuresis (excretion of sodium in the urine). (ANP and BNP are also discussed in Chapter 32 on p. 683 and in Chapter 34 on p. 740.)

**Serum Lipids.** Serum lipids consist of triglycerides, cholesterol, and phospholipids. They circulate in the blood bound to protein. Thus they are often referred to as *lipoproteins.*

Triglycerides are the main storage form of lipids and make up about 95% of fatty tissue. Cholesterol, a structural component of cell membranes and plasma lipoproteins, is a precursor of corticosteroids, sex hormones, and bile salts. In addition to being absorbed from food in the gastrointestinal tract, cholesterol can also be synthesized in the liver. Phospholipids contain glycerol, fatty acids, phosphates, and a nitrogenous compound. Although formed in most cells, phospholipids usually enter the circulation as lipoproteins synthesized by the liver. Apoproteins are water-soluble proteins that combine with most lipids to form lipoproteins.

Different classes of lipoproteins contain varying amounts of the naturally occurring lipids. These include the following:

1. *Chylomicrons:* primarily exogenous triglycerides from dietary fat
2. *Low-density lipoproteins (LDLs):* mostly cholesterol with moderate amounts of phospholipids
3. *High-density lipoproteins (HDLs):* about 50% protein and 50% phospholipids and cholesterol
4. *Very-low-density lipoproteins (VLDLs):* primarily endogenous triglycerides with moderate amounts of phospholipids and cholesterol

A lipid panel usually measures cholesterol, triglyceride, LDL, and HDL. Elevations in triglycerides and LDL are strongly associated with CAD. An increased HDL level is associated with a decreased risk of CAD. High levels of HDLs serve a protective role by mobilizing cholesterol from tissues.

Although an association exists between elevated serum cholesterol levels and CAD, a measure of total cholesterol alone is not sufficient for an assessment of CAD. A risk assessment is calculated by comparing the total cholesterol to HDL ratio over time. An increase in the ratio indicates increased risk. This provides more information than either value alone.

Plasma levels of apolipoprotein A-I (apo A-I) (the major HDL protein) and the ratio of apo A-I to apolipoprotein B (apo B) (the major LDL protein) are stronger predictors of CAD than the HDL cholesterol level alone. Measurements of these lipoproteins can be useful in identifying patients at risk for CAD.[11]

Lipoprotein (a), or Lp(a), has been studied for its role as a risk factor for CAD. Increased levels of Lp(a), especially with increased levels of lactate dehydrogenase (LDH), have been linked with the progression of atherosclerosis, especially in women.

**Lipoprotein-Associated Phospholipase $A_2$.** Lipoprotein-associated phospholipase $A_2$ (Lp-$PLA_2$) is an inflammatory enzyme expressed in atherosclerotic plaques. Elevated levels of Lp-$PLA_2$ are related to an increased risk of CAD, especially in African American women.[15]

## Chest X-Ray

A radiographic picture of the chest can show heart shape and size, and anatomic changes in individual chambers (Fig. 31-9). The chest x-ray records any displacement or enlargement of the heart, extra fluid around the heart (pericardial effusion), and pulmonary congestion.

## Electrocardiogram

The basic P, QRS, and T waveforms (Fig. 31-4, *B*) are used to assess heart activity. Deviations from the normal sinus rhythm can indicate problems in heart function. There are many types of ECG monitoring, including a resting 12-lead ECG, ambulatory ECG monitoring, and exercise or stress testing (Table 31-6). Continuous ambulatory ECG (Holter monitoring) provides diagnostic information over a period of time. (See Chapter 35 for a complete discussion of ECG monitoring.)

**Event Monitor or Loop Recorder.** An event monitor or loop recorder is used to record less frequent ECG events. An event monitor is a portable unit that uses electrodes to store ECG data once triggered by the patient. A disadvantage of this type of monitoring is that, if symptoms occur for only a brief time, they may be over before the patient puts on the device and triggers it to record. Likewise, if patients are extremely symptomatic (e.g., syncopal), they may not be physically able to trigger the ECG recording. These devices can be used for routine pacemaker checks over the phone to the HCP.[16]

An implantable loop recorder is used for patients who may have serious yet infrequent dysrhythmias. This small recorder is implanted though a small incision into the chest wall. It is activated to record either by the patient using a remote device or automatically if the HR exceeds or goes below a set rate. External loop recorders are worn for a month and require electrodes continuously placed on the skin. This device only records when activated by the patient when symptoms occur.

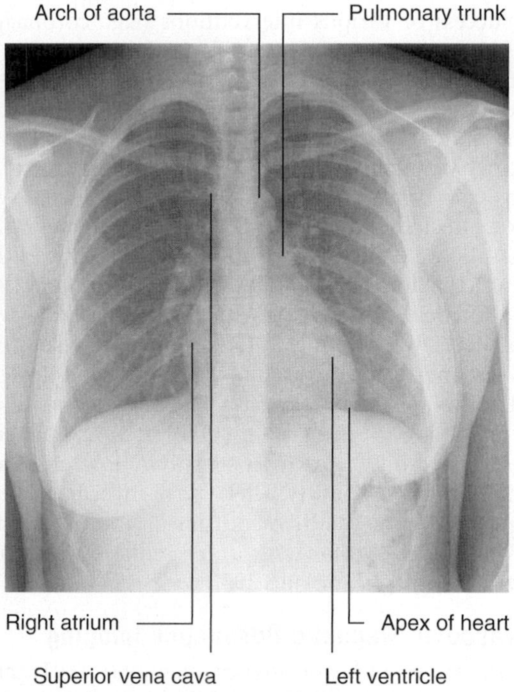


**FIG. 31-9** Chest x-ray: standard posterior-anterior view. (From Drake RL, Vogl AW, Mitchell AWM: *Gray's anatomy for students,* ed 2, Philadelphia, 2010, Churchill Livingstone.)

## Exercise or Stress Testing

Heart symptoms frequently occur only with activity because of the demand on the coronary arteries to provide more $O_2$. Exercise testing is used to evaluate the heart's response to physical stress. This helps to assess CVD and set limits for exercise programs. Exercise testing is used for persons who are able to walk unassisted or use a bicycle. It is also helpful for those with normal ECGs that limit diagnostic interpretation (e.g., pacemakers) (Table 31-6).

## Echocardiogram

The echocardiogram uses ultrasound (US) waves to record the movement of the structures of the heart. In the normal heart, US waves directed at the heart are reflected back in typical patterns. *Contrast echocardiography* involves the addition of an IV contrast agent (e.g., agitated saline) to assist in defining the images, especially in technically difficult patients (e.g., obese).

The echocardiogram provides information about abnormalities of (1) valvular structures and motion, (2) heart chamber size and contents, (3) ventricular and septal motion and thickness, (4) pericardial sac, and (5) ascending aorta. The **ejection fraction (EF)**, or the percentage of end-diastolic blood volume that is ejected during systole, can also be measured. The EF provides information about the function of the left ventricle during systole.

Two commonly used types of echocardiograms are the *motion-mode (M-mode) echocardiogram* and the *two-dimensional (2-D) echocardiogram.* In the M-mode, a single US beam is directed toward the heart, recording the motion of the intracardiac structures and detecting wall thickness and chamber size. The 2-D echocardiogram sweeps the US beam through an arc, producing a cross-sectional view. This shows correct spatial relationships among the structures.

Doppler technology allows for sound evaluation of the flow or motion of the scanned object (heart valves, ventricular walls, blood flow). *Color-flow imaging (duplex)* is the combination of 2-D echocardiography and Doppler technology (Fig. 31-10). It uses color changes to demonstrate the speed and direction of blood flow. Pathologic conditions, such as valvular leaks and congenital defects, can be diagnosed more effectively.

*Real-time three-dimensional (3-D) ultrasound* is a technology that uses multiple 2-D echo images with computer technology to provide a reconstruction of the heart. This technique produces information about the structures of the heart and how these structures change during the cardiac cycle.

*Stress echocardiography,* a combination of treadmill test or pharmacologic test and US images, evaluates wall motion abnormalities. With the use of a digital computer to compare images before and after exercise, wall motion and function are revealed. This test combines the information from a stress test with the information from an echocardiogram. For those individuals unable to exercise, IV drugs are used. These include dobutamine [Dobutrex], which produces pharmacologic stress on the heart and dipyridamole (Persantine), which promotes vasodilation of healthy arteries. Unhealthy arteries do not respond as well, which is seen on the echocardiogram.

*Transesophageal echocardiography (TEE)* provides more precise echocardiography of the heart than surface 2-D

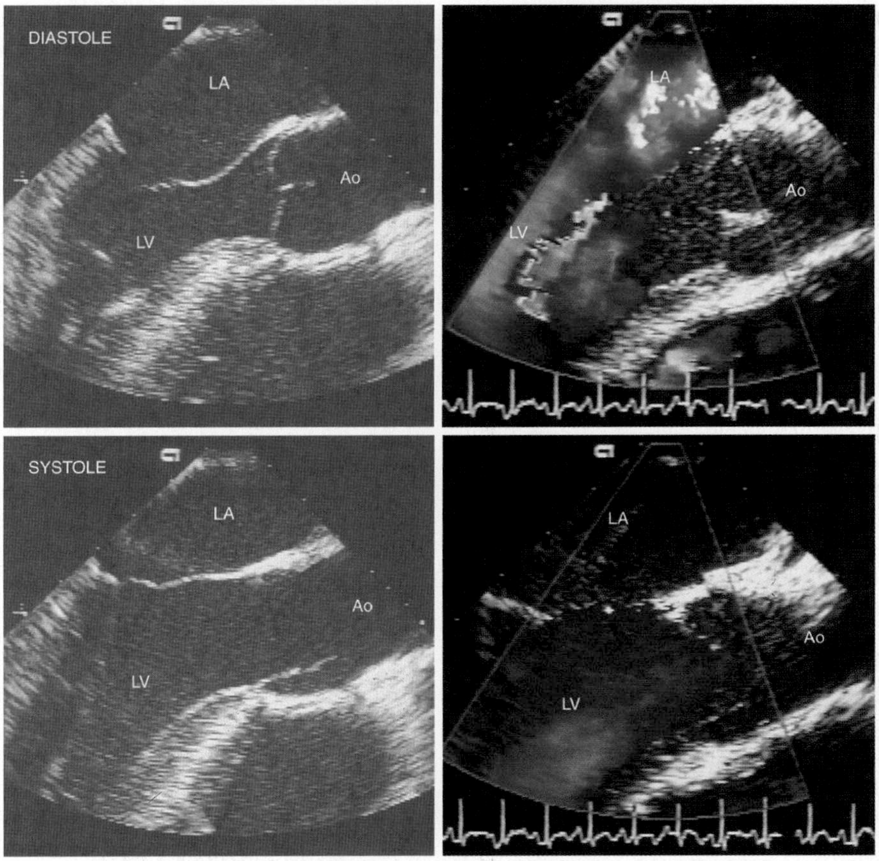


**FIG. 31-10** Long-axis images of the aortic and mitral valve with the depth adjusted to optimize evaluation of valve anatomy and motion. The 2-D images *(left)* in diastole *(top)* and systole *(bottom)* show normal aortic and mitral opening and closure. The color flow images *(right)* show normal left ventricular inflow with no aortic regurgitation in diastole *(top)* and normal antegrade flow in the left ventricular outflow tract and no mitral regurgitation in systole *(bottom)*. (From Otto C: *Textbook of clinical echocardiography,* ed 3, St Louis, 2004, Saunders.)

echocardiography by removing interference from the chest wall and lungs. The TEE uses a flexible endoscope with an US transducer in the tip for imaging of the heart and great vessels. The scope is passed into the esophagus to the level of the heart, and M-mode, 2-D, Doppler, and color-flow imaging can be obtained.

TEE is used frequently in an outpatient setting for evaluation of mitral valve disease and for identification of endocarditis vegetation, thrombus before cardioversion, or the source of heart emboli. In addition, TEE is used in the operating room to assess intraoperative heart function and in the emergency department to detect suspected aortic dissection.

The risks of TEE are low. However, complications may include perforation or tearing of the esophagus, hemorrhage, dysrhythmias, vasovagal reactions, and transient hypoxemia. TEE is contraindicated if the patient has a history of esophageal disorders, dysphagia, or radiation therapy to the chest wall. Patients require sedation during a TEE.

## Nuclear Cardiology

One of the most common nuclear imaging tests is the multigated acquisition (MUGA) or cardiac blood pool scan. This test provides information on wall motion during systole and diastole, heart valves, and EF (Table 31-6).

Perfusion imaging is also used with exercise testing to determine whether the coronary blood flow changes with increased activity. Stress perfusion imaging may show an abnormality even when a resting image is normal. This procedure is used to diagnose CAD, make a prognosis in existing CAD, differentiate viable heart muscle from scar tissue, and determine the potential for success of various interventions (e.g., coronary artery bypass surgery, percutaneous coronary intervention)[17] (see Chapter 33).

Exercise stress perfusion imaging is always preferred but, if a patient cannot exercise, IV regadenoson (Lexiscan), dipyridamole, or adenosine (Adenocard) can be given to dilate the coronary arteries and simulate the effect of exercise. After the drug takes effect, the isotope is injected and the imaging is done.

Single-photon emission computed tomography (SPECT) uses technetium, thallium, or sestamibi as an imaging agent (isotope). Both obese patients and women with large breasts can have attenuation artifacts, which can lead to false-positive results. Patients with severe multi-vessel coronary disease or blockages in their left main coronary artery may have false-negative results.

Positron emission tomography (PET) stress testing is increasingly being used due to its high sensitivity for revealing myocardial ischemia and viability. This type of myocardial perfusion imaging is commonly performed using $^{82}$rubidium. This agent allows for quicker studies with lower radiation exposure and provides better diagnostic quality.[18]

## Cardiovascular Magnetic Resonance Imaging

Cardiovascular magnetic resonance imaging (CMRI) can detect and find areas of MI in a 3-D view. It is sensitive enough to find

*Text continued on p. 678*

## TABLE 31-6 Diagnostic Studies

### *Cardiovascular System*

| Study | Description and Purpose | Nursing Responsibility |
|---|---|---|
| **Blood Studies*** | | |
| **Troponin (cardiac)** | Contractile proteins that are released after an MI. Both troponin T and troponin I are highly specific to cardiac tissue.<br>*Reference intervals:*<br>*Troponin I (cTnI)*<br>Negative: <0.5 ng/mL (<0.5 mcg/L)<br>Indeterminate or suspicious for injury to myocardium: 0.5-2.3 ng/mL (0.5-2.3 mcg/L)<br>Positive for myocardial injury: >2.3 ng/mL (>2.3 mcg/L)<br>*Troponin T (cTnT)*<br><0.1 ng/mL (<0.1 mcg/L) | *Before:* Explain purpose of serial sampling (e.g., q6hr × 3) in conjunction with CK-MB and serial ECGs.<br>*During:* Rapid point-of-care (bedside) assays are available. |
| **CK-MB** | Cardiospecific isoenzyme that is released from cells when myocardial tissue is injured. Concentrations >4%-6% of total creatine kinase (CK) are highly indicative of MI. Serum levels increase within 4-6 hr after MI. | *Before:* Explain purpose of serial sampling that is often done in conjunction with troponin and ECGs. |
| **Copeptin** | Substitute for arginine vasopressin (AVP) that directly reflects AVP concentration. Can be used as a cardiac biomarker for detecting acute MI. Higher in men than women, increased after exercise and stress, and influenced by fasting and water load.<br>*Reference interval:*<br><10 pmol/L | *Before:* Explain to patient that blood is drawn and sent to laboratory. |
| **Myoglobin** | Serum concentrations rise 30-60 min after MI and raidly cleared from circulation. Limited use in the diagnosis of cardiac injury/ infarction.<br>*Reference interval:*<br>*Male:* 15.2-91.2 mcg/L<br>*Female:* 11.1-57.5 mcg/L | *Before:* Explain to patient that blood is drawn and sent to laboratory. |
| **C-reactive protein (CRP)** | Marker of inflammation. May have value in predicting risk of cardiac disease and cardiac events. High-sensitivity (hs) CRP assay used.<br>*Lowest risk:* <1 mg/L<br>*Moderate risk:* 1-3 mg/L<br>*High risk:* >3 mg/L | *Before:* Explain to patient that blood is drawn and sent to laboratory. |
| **Homocysteine** | Amino acid produced during protein catabolism that has been identified as a risk factor for cardiovascular disease. Homocysteine may cause damage to the endothelium or have a role in formation of thrombi.<br>*Reference interval:*<br>*Male:* 5.2-12.9 μmol/L<br>*Female:* 3.7-10.4 μmol/L | *Before:* Explain to patient that blood is drawn and sent to laboratory. |
| **b-Type natriuretic peptide (BNP)** | Peptide that causes natriuresis. Elevation helps to distinguish cardiac vs. respiratory cause of dyspnea. Infusion of nesiritide (Natrecor) elevates levels temporarily.<br>*Reference interval:*<br>*BNP* (diagnostic for heart failure) >100 pg/mL (28.8 pmol/L) | *Before:* Explain to patient that blood is drawn and sent to laboratory. |
| **NT-Pro-BNP** | Aids in assessing the severity of heart failure in symptomatic and asymptomatic patients. In patients with renal insufficiency, concentrations may increase and may not correlate with New York Heart Association functional classification of heart failure.<br>*Reference interval:*<br>*≤74 yr:* 124 pg/mL<br>*>75 yr:* 449 pg/mL | *Before:* Explain to patient that blood is drawn and sent to laboratory. |
| **Serum Lipids** | | |
| **Cholesterol** | A blood lipid. Elevated cholesterol is considered a risk factor for cardiovascular heart disease.<br>*Reference interval:*<br><200 mg/dL (<5.18 mmol/L) (varies with age and gender) | *Before:* Explain to patient that blood is drawn and sent to laboratory.<br>*During:* Can be obtained in a nonfasting state. |
| **Triglycerides** | Mixtures of fatty acids. Elevations are associated with cardiovascular disease and diabetes.<br>*Reference interval:*<br><150 mg/dL (<1.7 mmol/L) (varies with age) | *Before:* Explain to patient that blood is drawn and sent to laboratory. Alcohol should be withheld for 24 hr before testing.<br>*During:* Can be obtained in a nonfasting state. Some protocols continue to recommend obtaining results in a fasting state. |

*Reference ranges for the laboratory tests vary by institution because of differences in equipment and reagents used.

*Continued*

## TABLE 31-6 Diagnostic Studies

***Cardiovascular System—cont'd***

| Study | Description and Purpose | Nursing Responsibility |
|---|---|---|
| **Serum Lipids—cont'd** | | |
| **Lipoproteins (HDL, LDL)** | Electrophoresis is done to separate lipoproteins into HDL and LDL. There are marked day-to-day fluctuations in serum lipid levels. More than one determination is needed for accurate diagnosis and treatment.<br>*Reference intervals* (vary with age):<br>HDL<br>*Recommended*<br>*Male:* >40 mg/dL (>1.04 mmol/L)<br>*Female:* >50 mg/dL (>1.3 mmol/L)<br>*Low risk for CAD:* ≥60 mg/dL (>1.55 mmol/L)<br>*High risk for CAD:* <40 mg/dL (<1.04 mmol/L)<br>LDL<br>*Recommended:* <100 mg/dL (<2.6 mmol/L)<br>*Near optimal:* 100-129 mg/dL (2.6-3.34 mmol/L)<br>*Moderate risk for CAD:* 130-159 mg/dL (3.37-4.12 mmol/L)<br>*High risk for CAD:* >160 mg/dL (>4.14 mmol/L) | *Before:* Explain to patient that blood is drawn and sent to laboratory.<br>*During:* Can be obtained in a nonfasting state. Some protocols continue to recommend obtaining results in a fasting state.<br>*After:* Risk for heart disease is assessed by dividing the total cholesterol level by the HDL level and obtaining a ratio.<br>*Low risk:* Ratio <3<br>*Average risk:* Ratio 3-5<br>*Increased risk:* Ratio >5 |
| **Lipoprotein (a) (Lp[a])** | Increased levels are associated with an increased risk of CAD and stroke.<br>*Reference interval:*<br><30 mg/dL (<0.3 g/L) | *Before:* Explain to patient that blood is drawn and sent to laboratory.<br>*During:* Can be obtained in a nonfasting state. |
| **Lipoprotein-associated phospholipase $A_2$ (Lp-$PLA_2$)** | Elevated levels of Lp-$PLA_2$ are associated with vascular inflammation and increased risk for CAD. Serum levels of Lp-$PLA_2$ are measured by the PLAC test.<br>*Reference intervals:*<br>*Low risk:* ≤151 ng/mL<br>*Moderate risk:* 152-194 ng/mL<br>*High risk:* ≥195 ng/mL | *Before:* Explain to patient that blood is drawn and sent to laboratory.<br>*During:* Can be obtained in a nonfasting state. |
| **Chest X-Ray** | Patient is placed in two upright positions to examine lung fields and heart size. The two common positions are posteroanterior (PA) (Fig. 31-9) and lateral. Normal heart size and contour for the individual's age, sex, and size are noted. | *Before:* Ask about frequency of recent x-rays and possibility of pregnancy. Provide lead shielding to areas not being viewed. Remove any jewelry or metal objects that may obstruct the view of heart and lungs. |
| **12-Lead ECG** | Electrodes are placed on the chest and extremities, allowing the ECG machine to record cardiac electrical activity from 12 different views. A resting 12-lead ECG can identify conduction problems, dysrhythmias, position of heart, cardiac hypertrophy, pericarditis, myocardial ischemia or infarction, pacemaker activity, and effectiveness of drug therapy at one point in time. | *Before:* Prepare skin and apply electrodes and leads. Place patient supine (or with head of bed elevated, if short of breath). Tell patient that no discomfort is involved and to lie still to decrease motion artifact. |
| **Signal-averaged ECG (SAECG)** | A high-resolution ECG that can identify electrical activity called late potentials, indicating a patient is at risk for developing ventricular dysrhythmias (e.g., ventricular tachycardia). | Same as for 12-lead ECG. |
| **Ambulatory ECG Monitoring** | | |
| **Holter monitoring** | Recording of ECG rhythm for 24-48 hr and then correlating rhythm changes with symptoms and activities recorded in diary. Normal patient activity is encouraged to simulate conditions that produce symptoms. Electrodes are placed on chest, and a recorder is used to store information until it is recalled, printed, and analyzed for any rhythm disturbance. | *Before:* Prepare skin and apply electrodes and leads. Explain importance of keeping an accurate diary of activities and symptoms. Tell patient that bathing and showering are prohibited during monitoring. Skin irritation may develop from electrodes. |
| **Event monitor or loop recorder** | Records rhythm disturbances that are not frequent enough to be recorded in one 24-hr period. It allows more freedom than a regular Holter monitor. Some units have electrodes that are attached to chest and have a loop of memory that captures the onset and end of an event. Other types are placed directly on patient's wrist, chest, or fingers and have no loop of memory but record the patient's ECG in real time. Recordings may be transmitted over the phone to a receiving unit. | *Before:* Instruct in the use of equipment for recording and transmitting (if appropriate) of events. Teach patient about skin preparation for lead placement or steady skin contact for units not requiring electrodes. This will ensure the best transmission of quality ECG tracings for analysis. Tell patient to start recording as soon as symptoms begin or as soon thereafter as possible. |

**TABLE 31-6 Diagnostic Studies**

***Cardiovascular System—cont'd***

| Study | Description and Purpose | Nursing Responsibility |
|---|---|---|
| **Exercise or Stress Testing** | Various protocols are used to evaluate the effect of exercise tolerance on cardiovascular function. A common protocol uses 3-min stages at set speeds and elevation of treadmill belt. The patient can exercise to either predicted peak HR (calculated by subtracting the person's age from 220) or to peak exercise tolerance, at which time the test is ended. The test is also ended for chest discomfort, significant changes in vital signs from baseline, or significant ECG changes (e.g., ischemia, dysrhythmias). Vital signs and ECG are monitored. The ECG is monitored after exercise for rhythm disturbances or, if ECG changes occurred with exercise, for return to baseline.<br>Continual monitoring of vital signs and ECG for ischemic changes is important in the diagnosis of CAD. An exercise bike may be used if the patient is unable to walk on the treadmill. | *Before:* Tell patient to wear comfortable clothes and shoes that can be used for walking or running. Tell patient about procedure and importance of reporting any symptoms that occur.<br>β-Blockers may be held 24 hr before the test because they blunt the HR and limit the patient's ability to achieve maximal HR. Caffeine-containing food and fluids are held for 24 hr. Patients must refrain from smoking and strenuous exercise for 3 hr before test.<br>*During:* Monitor vital signs and obtain 12-lead ECG before exercise, during each stage of exercise, and after exercise until all vital signs and ECG changes have returned to normal or baseline. Monitor patient's response throughout procedure for any signs of distress (e.g., angina, shortness of breath). |
| **6-Minute Walk Test** | Distance patient is able to walk on a flat surface in 6 min. Used to measure response to treatments and determine functional capacity for activities of daily living. Useful in people who are unable to perform treadmill or exercise bike testing. May be a better measure of fitness for older adults than exercise testing. | *Before:* Tell patient to wear comfortable shoes. Inform patient to carry or pull $O_2$ if used routinely.<br>*During:* Encourage patient to walk as quickly as possible. |
| **Echocardiogram**<br>• Contrast<br>• M-mode<br>• Two-dimensional<br>• Color-flow imaging (duplex)<br>• Real-time three-dimensional | Transducer that emits and receives ultrasound waves is placed in four positions on the chest above the heart. Transducer records sound waves that are bounced off the heart. Also records direction and flow of blood through the heart and transforms it to audio and graphic data that measure valve abnormalities, congenital heart defects, wall motion, EF, and heart function. IV contrast agent may be used to enhance images (Fig. 31-10). | *Before:* Place patient in a left side-lying position. Tell patient about procedure and sensations (pressure and mechanical movement from head of transducer). No contraindications to procedure exist. |
| **Stress echocardiogram** | Combination of exercise test and echocardiogram. Resting images of the heart are taken with ultrasound, and then the patient exercises. Postexercise images are taken within 1 min of stopping exercise. Differences in left ventricular wall motion and thickening before and after exercise are evaluated. | *Before:* Prepare patient for treadmill or exercise bicycle. Tell patient of importance of timely return to examination table for imaging after exercise. |
| **Pharmacologic echocardiogram** | Used as a substitute for the exercise stress test in individuals unable to exercise. IV adenosine, dobutamine, or dipyridamole is given over several minutes or regadenoson (Lexiscan) is given as a single bolus over 10 sec while echocardiogram is performed to detect wall motion abnormalities. | *Before:* Explain procedure to patient. Obtain IV access for injection of drugs.<br>*During:* Give drugs per protocol. Monitor vital signs before, during, and after test until baseline achieved. Monitor patient for signs and symptoms of distress during procedure. Observe patient for any side effects (e.g., shortness of breath, dizziness, nausea). Aminophylline may be given to prevent or reverse side effects of dipyridamole. Contraindications include any known allergies to the drugs. |
| **Transesophageal echocardiogram (TEE)** | A probe with an ultrasound transducer at the tip is swallowed while the physician controls angle and depth. As it passes down the esophagus, it sends back clear images of heart size, wall motion, valve abnormalities, endocarditis vegetation, and possible source of thrombi without interference from lungs or chest ribs. A contrast medium may be injected IV for evaluating direction of blood flow if an atrial or ventricular septal defect is suspected. Doppler ultrasound and color-flow imaging can also be used concurrently. | *Before:* Tell patient to fast for at least 6 hr before test. Remove dentures.<br>*During:* IV sedation is given and throat locally anesthetized. A bite block is placed in the mouth. Monitor vital signs and $O_2$ saturation levels and perform suctioning as needed during procedure. Assist patient to relax.<br>*After:* Patient may not eat or drink until gag reflex returns. Sore throat is temporary. A designated driver is needed if test is done in the outpatient department. |
| **Nuclear Cardiology** | Study involves IV injection of radioactive isotopes ($^{99m}$technetium-sestamibi [Cardiolite]). Radioactive uptake is counted over the heart by scintillation camera. It supplies information about heart contractility, myocardial perfusion, and acute injury. | *Before:* Explain procedure to patient. Women must remove bras to decrease breast attenuation. Obtain IV access for injection of isotopes. Explain that radioactive isotope used is a small, diagnostic amount and will lose most of its radioactivity in a few hours. Tell patient that he or she will be lying still on back with arms extended overhead for 20 min.<br>*During:* Repeat scans are done within a few minutes to hours after the injection. |

*Continued*

TABLE 31-6 **Diagnostic Studies**

***Cardiovascular System—cont'd***

| Study | Description and Purpose | Nursing Responsibility |
|---|---|---|
| **Nuclear Cardiology—cont'd** | | |
| **Multigated acquisition (MUGA) (cardiac blood pool) scan** | Small amount of the patient's blood is removed, mixed with a radioactive isotope (e.g., $^{99m}$technetium-sestamibi), and reinjected IV. With the ECG used for timing, images are obtained during the cardiac cycle. Indicated for patients with MI, heart failure, or valve disease. Can be used to evaluate the effect of various cardiac or cardiotoxic drugs on the heart. | *Before:* Explain procedure to patient. Obtain IV access for removal of blood sample and reinjection of isotope. Start ECG monitoring. Tell patient that procedure involves little risk. |
| **Single-photon emission computed tomography (SPECT)** | Used to determine size or risk of infarction and to determine infarction size. Small amounts of a radioactive isotope (e.g., $^{99m}$technetium-tetrofosmin [Myoview], thallium-201) are injected IV and recordings are made of the radioactivity emitted over a specific area of the body. Circulation of the isotope can be used to detect coronary artery blood flow, intracardiac shunts, motion of ventricles, EF, and size of the heart chambers. | *Before:* Explain procedure to patient. Obtain IV access for injection of isotope. Start ECG monitoring. Tell patient that procedure involves little risk. |
| **Exercise (stress) nuclear imaging** | Nuclear imaging images are taken at rest and after exercise. Injection is given at maximum HR (usually 85% of age-predicted maximum) on bicycle or treadmill. Patient is then required to continue exercise for 1 min to circulate the radioactive isotope. Scanning is done 15-60 min after exercise. A resting scan is performed 60-90 min after initial infusion or 24 hr later. | *Before:* Explain procedure to patient. Tell patient to eat only a light meal between scans. Certain drugs may need to be held for 1-2 days before the scan. Patients should not have caffeine 12 hr prior. Obtain IV access.<br>*During:* If targeted maximum HR is not achieved with exercise, test may be changed to pharmacologic imaging. |
| **Pharmacologic nuclear imaging** | Regadenoson, dipyridamole, or adenosine is used to produce vasodilation when patients are unable to tolerate exercise. Vasodilation increases blood flow to well-perfused coronary arteries. Scanning procedure is same.<br>Aminophylline may be given to prevent or reverse side effects of dipyridamole (e.g., shortness of breath, dizziness, nausea). Dobutamine is used if vasodilators are contraindicated. | *Before:* Explain procedure to patient. Tell patient to hold all caffeine products and theophylline (for regadenoson or dipyridamole testing) for 12 hr before procedure. Calcium channel blockers and β-blockers should be held 24 hr before the test. Obtain IV access.<br>*During:* Observe patient for any side effects (e.g., shortness of breath, dizziness, nausea). |
| **Positron emission tomography (PET)** | Highly sensitive in distinguishing viable and nonviable heart tissue. Uses two radionuclides. Nitrogen-13-ammonia is injected IV first and scanned to evaluate myocardial perfusion. A second radioactive isotope, fluoro-18-deoxyglucose, is then injected and scanned to show myocardial metabolic function. In the normal heart, both scans match, but in an ischemic or damaged heart, they differ. The patient may or may not be stressed. A baseline resting scan is usually obtained for comparison. | *Before:* Explain that patient will be scanned by a machine and will need to stay still for a time. If exercise is included as part of testing, patient needs to fast and refrain from tobacco and caffeine for 24 hr before test. Obtain IV access.<br>*During:* Patient's glucose level must be between 60-140 mg/dL (3.3-7.8 μmol/L) for accurate glucose metabolic activity. |
| **Cardiovascular Magnetic Resonance Imaging (CMRI)** | Noninvasive imaging technique obtains information about heart tissue, EF, aneurysms, cardiac output, and patency of proximal coronary arteries. It does not involve ionizing radiation and is an extremely safe procedure. Provides images in multiple planes with uniformly good resolution. | *Before:* Explain procedure to patient. Tell patient that the small diameter of the cylinder, along with loud noise of the procedure, may cause anxiety or panic. Antianxiety drugs and distraction strategies (e.g., music) may be provided. Patient must lie still during test. Contraindicated for persons with implanted metallic devices or other metal fragments unless noted to be MRI safe. Discuss any implants before scan. |
| **Magnetic resonance angiography (MRA)** | Used for imaging vascular occlusive disease and abdominal aortic aneurysms. Same as MRI but with use of gadolinium as IV contrast medium. | *Before:* Contraindications include any known allergies to contrast medium and persons with implanted metallic devices or other metal fragments unless noted to be MRA safe. Discuss any implants before scan. Obtain IV access. |
| **Cardiac Computed Tomography (CT)** | Cardiac CT is heart-specific CT imaging technology with or without IV contrast medium used to visualize heart anatomy, coronary circulation, and blood vessels. | *Before:* Explain procedure to patient. |
| **Coronary CT angiography (CTA)** | Use of CT with injected IV contrast medium to obtain images of blood vessels and diagnose CAD. | *Before:* Explain procedure to patient. Obtain IV access. Metal objects should be removed before examination. The patient may need to fast for several hours before the procedure. A β-blocker may be given before the test to control HR.<br>*During:* Patients must have a regular heart rhythm for accurate testing. |

## TABLE 31-6 Diagnostic Studies

### *Cardiovascular System—cont'd*

| Study | Description and Purpose | Nursing Responsibility |
|---|---|---|
| **Calcium-scoring CT scan**<br>• Electron beam computed tomography (EBCT) | EBCT, also known as *ultrafast CT,* uses a scanning electron beam to quantify calcification in coronary arteries and heart valves (Fig. 31-11). Primarily used for risk assessment in asymptomatic patients and to assess for heart disease in patients with atypical symptoms potentially related to cardiac causes. | *Before:* Explain procedure to patient. Tell patient that procedure is quick and involves little or no risk. |
| **Cardiac Catheterization** | Involves insertion of catheter into heart to obtain information about $O_2$ levels and pressure readings within heart chambers. Contrast medium is injected to assist in seeing structures and motion of heart. Procedure is done by insertion of catheter into a vein (for right side of heart) and/or an artery (for left side of heart). | *Before:* Check for sensitivity to contrast media. Withhold food and fluids for 6-12 hr before procedure. Explain the procedure to the patient including use of local anesthesia at insertion site, placement of catheter, flushed feeling when dye is injected, and possible fluttering sensation of heart as catheter is passed. Note that patient may be asked to cough or take a deep breath when dye is injected and that patient is monitored by ECG throughout procedure. Give sedative and other drugs, as ordered.<br>*After:* Frequently assess circulation to extremity used for catheter insertion. Check peripheral pulses, color, and sensation of extremity per agency protocol. Observe insertion site for hematoma and bleeding. Place compression device over arterial site to achieve hemostasis, if indicated. Monitor vital signs and ECG. Assess for hypotension or hypertension, dysrhythmias, and signs of pulmonary emboli (e.g., respiratory difficulty). |
| **Coronary angiography** | During a cardiac catheterization, contrast medium is injected directly into coronary arteries. Used to evaluate patency of coronary arteries and collateral circulation. | Same as for cardiac catheterization. |
| **Intravascular ultrasound (IVUS)** | During cardiac catheterization a small ultrasound probe is introduced into coronary arteries. Used to assess size and consistency of plaque, arterial walls, and effectiveness of intracoronary artery treatment. | Same as for cardiac catheterization. |
| **Fractional flow reserve (FFR)** | During cardiac catheterization a specialized wire is inserted into coronary arteries to measure pressure and flow. Information is used to determine need for angioplasty or stenting on nonsignificant blockages. | Same as for cardiac catheterization. |
| **Electrophysiology Study (EPS)** | Invasive study used to record intracardiac electrical activity using catheters (with multiple electrodes) inserted via the femoral or jugular veins into right side of heart. Catheter electrodes record the electrical activity in different heart structures. In addition, dysrhythmias can be induced and terminated. | *Before:* Antidysrhythmic drugs may be stopped several days before study. Keep patient NPO 6-8 hr before test. Give premedication to promote relaxation if ordered. Obtain IV access. IV sedation often used during procedure.<br>*After:* Assess vital signs frequently and monitor ECG continuously after the procedure per agency protocol. |
| **Peripheral Arteriography and Venography** | Peripheral vessel blood flow is assessed by injecting contrast media into appropriate arteries or veins (arteriography and venography). Serial x-ray studies done to detect and visualize any atherosclerotic plaques, occlusion, aneurysms, venous abnormalities, or traumatic injury. See Table 37-9 for additional peripheral vascular diagnostic studies. | *Before:* Check for allergy to contrast media. Give mild sedative, if ordered.<br>*During:* Observe patient for allergic reactions to contrast media.<br>*After:* Check extremity with puncture site for pulsation, warmth, color, and motion. Inspect insertion site for bleeding or swelling. |
| **Hemodynamic Monitoring** | Invasive and minimally invasive bedside hemodynamic monitoring is done using intraarterial, pulmonary artery, and central vein catheters to monitor arterial BP, stroke volume variation, pulmonary artery pressure, pulmonary artery wedge pressure, cardiac output, and central venous pressure. Used to evaluate cardiovascular status and response to treatment. | Patients requiring hemodynamic monitoring are critically ill and are monitored in intensive care units. See Chapter 65 for complete information on hemodynamic monitoring. |

even small MIs that are not apparent with SPECT. CMRI aids in the final diagnosis of MI and the assessment of EF. It also plays a role in prediction of recovery from MI and in the diagnosis of congenital heart and aortic disorders and CAD.[19] One major advantage of CMRI is that it does not require any radiation to the patient.

Patients with coronary stents can undergo CMRI 6 weeks after stent placement.[20] In patients with older-model pacemakers and ICDs, CMRI is discouraged because the magnets can change the function of the devices. However, when there is a strong clinical need and the benefits outweigh the risks, CMRI should only be performed in these patients at centers experienced in this procedure.[19] Many newer models of pacemakers and ICDs are approved for use with MRI.

### Cardiac Computed Tomography

Cardiac computed tomography (CT) is a heart-imaging test that uses CT technology with or without IV contrast (dye) to see the heart anatomy, coronary circulation, and great blood vessels (e.g., aorta, pulmonary veins, artery). This technology is often called *multidetector CT (MDCT) scanning*. Types of CT scans used to diagnose heart disease include coronary CT angiography (CTA) and calcium-scoring CT scan (Table 31-6).

Coronary CTA is a noninvasive test. It can be done faster than a cardiac catheterization with less risk and discomfort to the patient.[21] Patients must have a normal sinus rhythm for this test. Although the use of coronary CTA is increasing, cardiac catheterization (discussed in the next section) remains the gold standard to diagnose CAD. Further, when a cardiac catheterization is done, procedures (e.g., angioplasty, stent placement) can be done if coronary blockages are found. Last, the radiation exposure during a cardiac catheterization is less than the exposure during a CTA.

The calcium-scoring CT scan is used to find calcium deposits in plaque in the coronary arteries. The most common method used is the electron beam CT (EBCT) (Fig. 31-11). It can detect early coronary calcification before symptoms develop and confirm CAD in patients with suspected CAD. The amount of coronary calcium is a predictor of future cardiac events. The calcium score can be used in the risk analysis of patients without known CVD.[22]

### Cardiac Catheterization

Cardiac catheterization is a common procedure. It provides information about CAD, coronary spasm, congenital and valvular heart disease, and ventricular function. Cardiac catheterization is also used to measure intracardiac pressures and $O_2$ levels, as well as CO and EF. With injection of contrast media and fluoroscopy, the coronary arteries can be seen, chambers of the heart can be outlined, and wall motion can be observed.

Cardiac catheterization is done by inserting a radiopaque catheter into the right and/or left side of the heart. For the right side of the heart, a catheter is inserted through an arm vein (basilic or cephalic) or a leg vein (femoral). Pressures are recorded as the catheter is moved into the vena cava, right atrium, right ventricle, and pulmonary artery. The catheter is then moved until it is wedged or lodged in position. This blocks the blood flow and pressure from the right side of the heart and looks ahead through the pulmonary capillary bed to the pressure in the left side of the heart *(pulmonary artery wedge pressure)*. This pressure is used to assess the function of the left side of the heart.

Left-sided heart catheterization is done by inserting a catheter into a radial, femoral, or brachial artery. The catheter is passed in a retrograde manner up to the aorta, across the aortic valve, and into the left ventricle.

**Coronary angiography** is done with a left-sided heart catheterization. The catheter is positioned at the origin of the coronary arteries (Fig. 31-3), and contrast medium is injected into the arteries. Patients often feel a temporary flushed sensation with dye injection. The images identify the location and severity of any coronary blockages (see Figs. 31-12 and 33-6). Complications of cardiac catheterization include bleeding or hematoma at the puncture site; allergic reactions to the contrast media; looping or kinking of the catheter; infection; thrombus formation; aortic dissection; dysrhythmias; MI; stroke; and puncture of the ventricles, septum, or lung tissue.

**Intravascular Ultrasound.** Intravascular ultrasound (IVUS), also known as intracoronary ultrasound (ICUS), is an invasive procedure performed in the catheterization laboratory with coronary angiography. The 2-D or 3-D US images provide a cross-sectional view of the arterial walls of the coronary arteries. In this procedure a miniature transducer attached to a small catheter is moved to the artery to be studied. Once it is

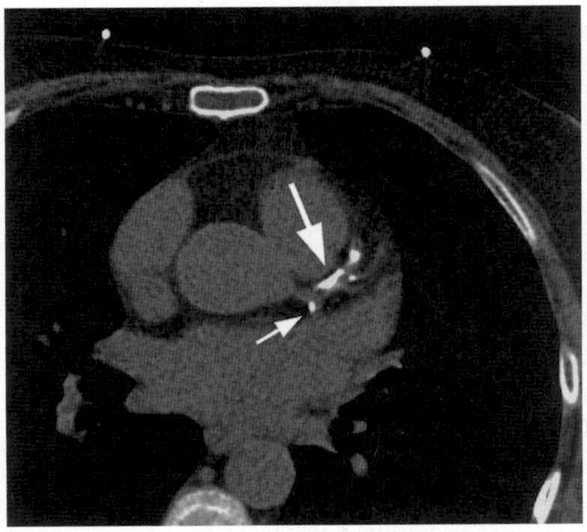

**FIG. 31-11** Examples of coronary calcification of the left anterior descending coronary artery *(large arrow)* and left circumflex artery *(small arrow)* as seen on electron beam computed tomography. (From Libby P, Bonow R, Zipes D, et al: *Braunwald's heart disease: a textbook of cardiovascular medicine,* ed 8, St Louis, 2008, Saunders.)

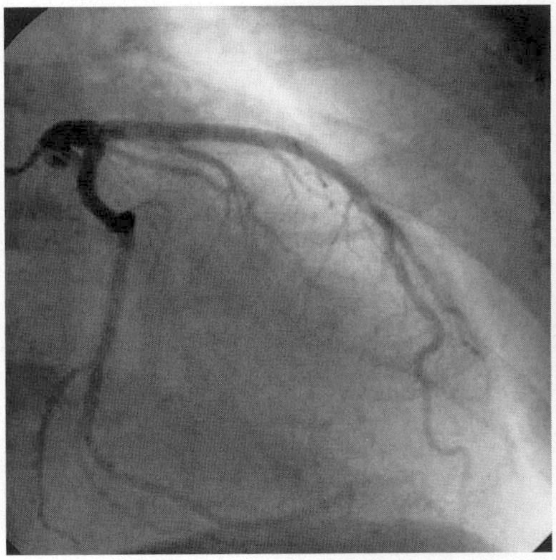

**FIG. 31-12** Angiogram showing a normal left coronary and circumflex artery. (From Drake RL, Vogl AW, Mitchell AWM: *Gray's anatomy for students,* ed 2, Philadelphia, 2010, Churchill Livingstone.)

in the artery, US images are obtained. The health of the arterial layers is assessed, including the composition, location, and thickness of any plaque. IVUS can evaluate vessel response to treatments such as stent placement and atherectomy, as well as any complications that may have occurred during the procedure (see Chapter 33). Patients often have IVUS in addition to angiography or a coronary intervention. Thus nursing care is similar to that following cardiac catheterization (Table 31-6).

**Fractional Flow Reserve.** Fractional flow reserve (FFR) is a procedure that is done during a cardiac catheterization. It involves using a special wire that can measure pressure and flow in the coronary artery. FFR helps to determine the need to perform angioplasty or stenting on nonsignificant blockages.

## Electrophysiology Study

The electrophysiology study (EPS) records and manipulates the heart's electrical activity using electrodes placed inside the heart chambers. It provides information on SA node, AV node, and ventricular conduction. It is particularly helpful in determining the source and treatment of dysrhythmias. Patients with symptomatic tachydysrhythmias are at risk for sudden cardiac death. Information from an EPS helps to make an accurate diagnosis and guides treatment decisions.

In EPS, catheters are inserted in a manner similar to that used in a right-sided heart catheterization. These catheters are placed at specific anatomic sites within the heart to record electrical activity. Nursing care for patients after EPS is similar to the care of patients after cardiac catheterization (Table 31-6).

## CASE STUDY

### *Objective Data: Diagnostic Studies*

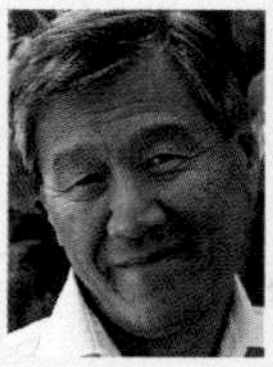

(©Jupiterimages/ Banana-Stock/ Thinkstock)

The HCP orders the following initial diagnostic studies for L.P.:

- 12-lead ECG
- CBC, basic metabolic panel (glucose, electrolytes, BUN, creatinine)
- PTT, PT, INR
- Pro-BNP
- Troponin, CK-MB
- TSH, free $T_4$
- Chest x-ray

L.P.'s initial troponin and CK-MB levels are within normal limits. The ECG demonstrates atrial fibrillation with a rapid ventricular response. Chest x-ray, CBC, and coagulation studies are all within normal limits. The potassium level is 3.1 mEq/L and pro-BNP is elevated (1204 pg/mL). The HCP orders 250 mL NSS IV bolus; a po dose of potassium, a loading dose of IV diltiazem (Cardizem) followed by a continuous infusion, and weight-based heparin to be started in the emergency department. L.P. will be admitted to the progressive care unit and will have a consult with a cardiologist.

**Discussion Questions**

1. Are these the diagnostic studies that you expected to be ordered?
2. Which diagnostic study results are abnormal?
3. Which diagnostic study results are of most concern to you?

Answers available at *http://evolve.elsevier.com/Lewis/medsurg.*

## BRIDGE TO NCLEX EXAMINATION

The number of the question corresponds to the same-numbered outcome at the beginning of the chapter.

1. A patient with a tricuspid valve disorder will have impaired blood flow between the
   **a.** vena cava and right atrium.
   **b.** left atrium and left ventricle.
   **c.** right atrium and right ventricle.
   **d.** right ventricle and pulmonary artery.
2. A patient has a severe blockage in his right coronary artery. Which heart structures are *most* likely to be affected by this blockage *(select all that apply)*?
   **a.** AV node
   **b.** Left ventricle
   **c.** Coronary sinus
   **d.** Right ventricle
   **e.** Pulmonic valve
3. The portion of the vascular system responsible for hemostasis is the
   **a.** thin capillary vessels.
   **b.** endothelial layer of the arteries.
   **c.** elastic middle layer of the veins.
   **d.** smooth muscle of the arterial wall.
4. When a person's blood pressure rises, the homeostatic mechanism to compensate for an elevation involves stimulation of
   **a.** baroreceptors that inhibit the sympathetic nervous system, causing vasodilation.
   **b.** chemoreceptors that inhibit the sympathetic nervous system, causing vasodilation.
   **c.** baroreceptors that inhibit the parasympathetic nervous system, causing vasodilation.
   **d.** chemoreceptors that stimulate the sympathetic nervous system, causing an increased heart rate.
5. A P wave on an ECG represents an impulse arising at the
   **a.** SA node and repolarizing the atria.
   **b.** SA node and depolarizing the atria.
   **c.** AV node and depolarizing the atria.
   **d.** AV node and spreading to the bundle of His.
6. When collecting subjective data related to the cardiovascular system, which information should be obtained from the patient *(select all that apply)*?
   **a.** Annual income
   **b.** Smoking history
   **c.** Religious preference
   **d.** Number of pillows used to sleep
   **e.** Blood for basic laboratory studies
7. The auscultatory area in the left midclavicular line at the level of the fifth ICS is the best location to hear sounds from which heart valve?
   **a.** Aortic
   **b.** Mitral
   **c.** Tricuspid
   **d.** Pulmonic
8. When assessing a patient, you note a pulse deficit of 23 beats. This finding may be caused by
   **a.** dysrhythmias.
   **b.** heart murmurs.
   **c.** gallop rhythms.
   **d.** pericardial friction rubs.
9. When assessing the cardiovascular system of a 79-year-old patient, you may expect to find
   **a.** a narrowed pulse pressure.
   **b.** diminished carotid artery pulses.
   **c.** difficulty in isolating the apical pulse.
   **d.** an increased heart rate in response to stress.

10. Which nursing responsibilities are priorities when caring for a patient returning from a cardiac catheterization *(select all that apply)*?
    a. Monitoring vital signs and ECG
    b. Checking the catheter insertion site and distal pulses
    c. Assisting the patient to ambulate to the bathroom to void
    d. Informing the patient that he will be sleepy from the general anesthesia
    e. Instructing the patient about the risks of the radioactive isotope injection

1. c, 2. a, b, d, 3. b, 4. a, 5. b, 6. b, c, d, 7. b, 8. a, 9. c, 10. a, b

For rationales to these answers and even more NCLEX review questions, visit *http://evolve.elsevier.com/Lewis/medsurg.*

## EVOLVE WEBSITE

http://evolve.elsevier.com/Lewis/medsurg

**Review Questions (Online Only)**

**Key Points**

**Answer Keys for Questions**

- Rationales for Bridge to NCLEX Examination Questions
- Answer Guidelines for Case Studies on pp. 663, 666, 669, and 679

**Conceptual Care Map Creator**

**Audio Glossary**

**Supporting Media**

- Animations
  - Auscultation of Heart Valves
  - Blood Flow: Circulatory System
  - Cardiac Cycle During Systole and Diastole
  - Pulse Variations
- Audio
  - Diastolic Murmur
  - Fourth Heart Sound ($S_4$)
  - Murmurs: Blowing, Harsh or Rough, and Rumble
  - Murmurs: High, Medium, and Low
  - $S_1$ at Various Locations
  - $S_2$ at Various Locations
  - Single $S_1$
  - Single $S_2$
  - Systolic Murmur
  - Third Heart Sound ($S_3$)

**Content Updates**

## REFERENCES

1. Patton KT, Thibodeau GA: *Anatomy and physiology*, ed 8, St Louis, 2013, Mosby.
2. Wesley K: *Huszar's basic dysrhythmias and acute coronary syndromes*, ed 4, St Louis, 2011, Mosby Jems.
3. McCance K, Huether S: *Pathophysiology: biologic basis for disease in adults and children*, ed 7, St Louis, 2014, Elsevier.
4. American Heart Association: Understanding blood pressure readings, 2014. Retrieved from *www.heart.org/HEARTORG/Conditions/HighBloodPressure/AboutHighBloodPressure/Understanding-Blood-Pressure-Readings_UCM_301764_Article.jsp*.
5. Ball JW, Dains JE, Flynn JA, et al: *Seidel's physical examination*, ed 8, St Louis, 2015, Elsevier.
6. North BJ, Sinclair DA: The intersection between aging and cardiovascular disease, *Circ Res* 110:1097, 2012.
7. National Institute on Aging: Aging heart and arteries: a scientific quest, 2014. Retrieved from *www.nia.nih.gov/health/publication/aging-hearts-and-arteries/preface*.
8. Skidmore-Roth L: *Mosby's 2015 nursing drug reference*, ed 28, St Louis, 2015, Elsevier.

*9. Mosca L, Benjamin EJ, Berry K, et al: Effectiveness-based guidelines for cardiovascular disease prevention in women: 2011 update, *Circulation* 123:1243, 2011.

10. Sherwood MW, Newby LK: High-sensitivity troponin assay: evidence, indications, and reasonable use, *J Am Heart Assoc* 3:1, 2014.
11. Pagana KD, Pagana TJ: *Mosby's manual of diagnostic and laboratory tests*, ed 5, St Louis, 2014, Elsevier.

*12. Lipenski LJ, Escarcego RO, D'Ascenzo F, et al: A systematic review and collaborative meta-analysis to determine the incremental value of copeptin for rapid rule-out of acute myocardial infarction, *Am J Cardiol* 113:1581, 2014.

13. Makrygiannis SS, Ampartzidou OS, Zairis MN, et al: Prognostic usefulness of serial C-reactive protein measurements in ST-elevation acute myocardial infarction, *Am J Cardiol* 111:26, 2013.
14. American Heart Association: Homocysteine, folic acid and cardiovascular disease. Retrieved from *www.heart.org/HEARTORG/GettingHealthy/NutritionCenter/Homocysteine-Folic-Acid-and-Cardiovascular-Disease_UCM_305997_Article.jsp*.
15. Ridker PM, Lüscher TF: Anti-inflammatory therapies for cardiovascular disease, *Eur Heart J* 35:1782, 2014.
16. American Heart Association: Cardiac event recorder, 2014. Retrieved from *http://www.heart.org/HEARTORG/Conditions/Arrhythmia/PreventionTreatmentofArrhythmia/Cardiac-Event-Recorder_UCM_447317_Article.jsp*.
17. Zaret BL, Beller GA: *Clinical nuclear cardiology*, ed 4, St Louis, 2010, Mosby.
18. Li Y, Zhang W, Wu H, et al: Advanced tracers in PET imaging of cardiovascular disease, *BioMed Res Intern* 2014:1, 2014.

*19. Hundley WG, Bluemke DA, Finn JP, et al: ACCF/ACR/AHA/NASCI/SCMR 2010 expert consensus document on cardiovascular magnetic resonance: a report of the American College of Cardiology Foundation Task Force on Expert Consensus Documents, *Circulation* 121:2462, 2010.

20. Ramos LM: Cardiac diagnostic testing: what bedside nurses need to know, *Crit Care Nurse* 34:16, 2014.

*21. Mark DB, Berman DS, Budoff MJ, et al: ACCF/ACR/AHA/NASCI/SAIP/SCAI/SCCT 2010 expert consensus document on coronary computed tomographic angiography: a report of the American College of Cardiology Foundation Task Force on Expert Consensus Documents, *Circulation* 121:2509, 2010.

*22. Mieres JH, Gulati M, Merz NB, et al: Role of noninvasive testing in the clinical evaluation of women with suspected ischemic heart disease: a consensus statement from the American Heart Association, *Circulation* 130:350, 2014.

*Evidence-based information for clinical practice.

32

# Hypertension

*Melissa L. Hutchinson*

*One way to get high blood pressure is to go mountain climbing over molehills.*

*Earl Wilson*

http://evolve.elsevier.com/Lewis/medsurg/

## LEARNING OUTCOMES

1. Relate the pathophysiologic mechanisms associated with primary hypertension to the clinical manifestations and complications.
2. Select appropriate strategies for the prevention of primary hypertension.
3. Describe the interprofessional care for primary hypertension, including drug therapy and lifestyle modifications.
4. Explain the interprofessional care of the older adult with primary hypertension.
5. Prioritize the nursing management of the patient with primary hypertension.
6. Describe the nursing and interprofessional care of a patient with a hypertensive crisis.

## KEY TERMS

**blood pressure (BP), p. 681**
**hypertension, p. 684**
**hypertensive crisis, p. 698**
**isolated systolic hypertension (ISH), p. 684**
**orthostatic hypotension, p. 695**
**prehypertension, p. 684**
**primary hypertension, p. 684**
**secondary hypertension, p. 684**
**systemic vascular resistance (SVR), p. 681**

Hypertension, or high blood pressure (BP), is one of the most important modifiable risk factors that can lead to the development of cardiovascular disease (CVD). As BP increases, so does the risk of myocardial infarction (MI), heart failure, stroke, and renal disease. This chapter discusses the nursing and interprofessional care of patients at risk for or who have hypertension.

Hypertension affects one in three adults in the United States. Heart disease, often directly related to hypertension, accounts for 23.7% of all deaths each year in the United States.[1,2] *Healthy People 2020* lists the number of adults with hypertension whose BP is under control as one of the 26 high-priority, leading health indicators for the coming decade.[3] The National Health and Nutrition Examination Survey (NHANES) tracks prevention, treatment, and control of hypertension. Data from NHANES showed that 83% of people 20 years of age and older with hypertension were aware that they had high BP. Of these people, 76% were being treated. Of those aware of their hypertension, 48% did not currently have their BP well controlled.[4,5]

The American College of Cardiology Foundation and the American Heart Association (AHA) provide performance measures for hypertension management that address not only treatment but also control of BP to target goals. Target goals have been updated with new information from the evidence-based Guideline for the Management of High Blood Pressure in Adults report from the Eighth Joint National Committee (JNC 8) and the Systolic Blood Pressure Intervention Trial (SPRINT). Target goals take into consideration both age and co-morbidities when recommending treatment options.[6,7]

National guidelines are designed to apply to all racial and ethnic groups. However, certain groups have a higher incidence of risk factors[6-8] (see boxes on Cultural & Ethnic Health Disparities and Gender Differences on p. 682).

## NORMAL REGULATION OF BLOOD PRESSURE

**Blood pressure (BP)** is the force exerted by the blood against the walls of the blood vessel. It must be adequate to maintain tissue perfusion during activity and rest. The maintenance of normal BP and tissue perfusion requires the integration of both systemic factors and local peripheral vascular effects. BP is primarily a function of cardiac output (CO) and systemic vascular resistance (SVR) (Fig. 32-1).

CO is the total blood flow through the systemic or pulmonary circulation per minute. It is described as the stroke volume (SV) or the amount of blood pumped out of the left ventricle per beat (approximately 70 mL) multiplied by the heart rate (HR).

**Systemic vascular resistance (SVR)** is the force opposing the movement of blood within the blood vessels. The radius of the small arteries and arterioles is the principal factor determining SVR. As arteries narrow, resistance to blood flow increases. As arteries dilate, resistance to blood flow decreases. A small change in the radius of the arterioles creates a major change in the SVR.

Reviewed by Elisabeth G. Bradley, MS, APN, ACNS-BC, AGPCNP-BC, Clinical Leader, Cardiovascular Prevention Program, Christiana Care Health System, Newark, Delaware; Janie Corbitt, RN, MLS, Retired Instructor of Nursing, Milledgeville, Georgia; and Susan J. Eisel, RN, MSEd, Associate Professor of Nursing, Mercy College of Ohio, Toledo, Ohio.

## CULTURAL & ETHNIC HEALTH DISPARITIES

### Hypertension

**African Americans**

- Have the highest prevalence of hypertension in the world
- Develop hypertension at a younger age than whites
- Have a higher incidence of hypertension among women than among men
- Demonstrate more nocturnal non-dipping BP than whites
- Hypertension is more aggressive and results in more severe end-organ damage.
- Have a higher death rate resulting from hypertension than whites
- Produce less renin and do not respond well to renin-inhibiting drugs
- Calcium channel blockers and diuretics provide better BP control, especially with monotherapy.
- Have a higher risk of angioedema with angiotensin-converting enzyme inhibitors than whites

**Mexican Americans**

- Are less likely to receive treatment for hypertension than whites and African Americans
- Have lower rates of BP control than whites and African Americans
- Have lower levels of awareness of hypertension and its treatment than whites and African Americans

## GENDER DIFFERENCES

### Hypertension

**Men**

- Before early middle age, hypertension is more common in men than in women.

**Women**

- Hypertension is two to three times more common in women who take oral contraceptives than in women who do not.
- A history of preeclampsia may be an early sign of risk for cardiovascular disease.
- After age 64, hypertension is more common in women than in men. Part of the rise in BP in women is attributed to menopause-related factors such as estrogen withdrawal, overproduction of pituitary hormones, and weight gain.
- It is more difficult to control hypertension in older women (ages 70-79) than in women ages 50-69, despite having similar rates of treatment.

If SVR is increased and CO remains constant or increases, arterial BP will increase.

The mechanisms that regulate BP can affect either CO or SVR, or both. Regulation of BP is a complex process involving both short-term (seconds to hours) and long-term (days to weeks) mechanisms. Short-term mechanisms, including the sympathetic nervous system (SNS) and vascular endothelium, are active within a few seconds. Long-term mechanisms include renal and hormonal processes that regulate arteriolar resistance and blood volume. In a healthy person these regulatory mechanisms function in response to the body's demands.

### Sympathetic Nervous System

The nervous system, which reacts within seconds after a drop in BP, increases BP primarily by activating the SNS. Increased SNS activity increases HR and cardiac contractility, produces widespread vasoconstriction in the peripheral arterioles, and promotes the release of renin from the kidneys. The net effect of SNS activation is to increase BP by increasing both CO and SVR.

Specialized nerve cells called *baroreceptors (pressoreceptors)* are located in the carotid arteries and arch of the aorta. These cells sense changes in BP and transmit this information to the vasomotor centers in the brainstem. The brainstem sends this information through complex networks of neurons that excite or inhibit efferent nerves. SNS efferent nerves innervate cardiac and vascular smooth muscle cells. Under normal conditions, a low level of continuous SNS activity maintains vascular tone. BP may be reduced by withdrawal of SNS activity or by stimulation of the parasympathetic nervous system (PNS). The PNS decreases the HR (via the vagus nerve) and thereby decreases CO.

The neurotransmitter norepinephrine (NE) is released from SNS nerve endings. NE activates receptors located in the sinoatrial node, myocardium, and vascular smooth muscle. The response to NE depends on the type of receptors present. SNS receptors are classified as $\alpha_1$, $\alpha_2$, $\beta_1$, and $\beta_2$ (Table 32-1). The smooth muscle of the blood vessels has $\alpha$-adrenergic and $\beta_2$-adrenergic receptors. $\alpha$-Adrenergic receptors located in the peripheral vasculature cause vasoconstriction when stimulated by NE. $\beta_1$-Adrenergic receptors in the heart respond to NE and epinephrine with increased HR (chronotropic), increased force of contraction (inotropic), and increased speed of conduction (dromotropic). $\beta_2$-Adrenergic receptors are activated primarily

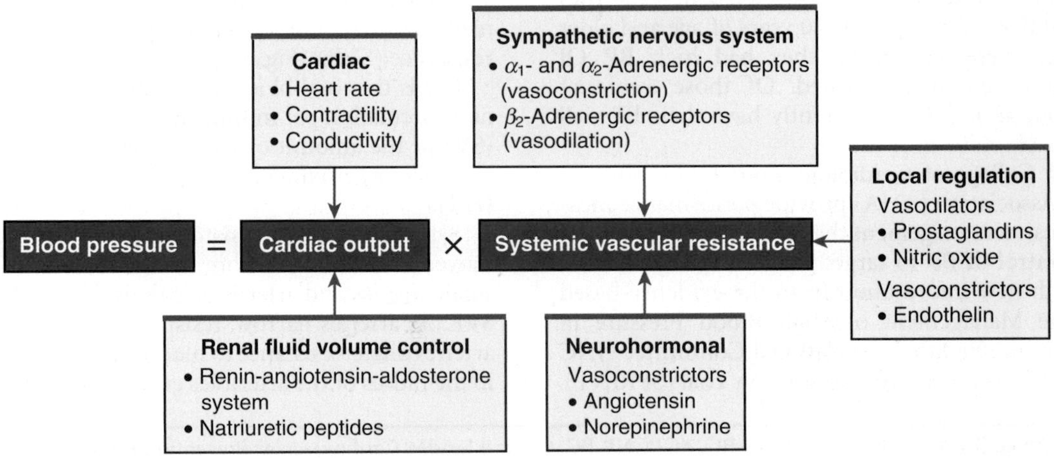


**FIG. 32-1** Factors influencing blood pressure (BP). Hypertension develops when one or more of the BP-regulating mechanisms are defective.

**TABLE 32-1 Sympathetic Nervous System Receptors Affecting BP**

| Receptor | Location | Response When Activated |
|---|---|---|
| $\alpha_1$ | Vascular smooth muscle | Vasoconstriction |
| | Heart | Increased contractility (positive inotropic effect) |
| $\alpha_2$ | Presynaptic nerve terminals | Inhibition of norepinephrine release |
| | Vascular smooth muscle | Vasoconstriction |
| $\beta_1$ | Heart | Increased contractility (positive inotropic effect) |
| | | Increased heart rate (positive chronotropic effect) |
| | | Increased conduction (positive dromotropic effect) |
| | Juxtaglomerular cells of the kidney | Increased renin secretion |
| $\beta_2$ | Smooth muscle of blood vessels in heart (e.g., coronary arteries), lungs (e.g., bronchi), and skeletal muscle | Vasodilation |
| **Dopamine receptors** | Primarily renal blood vessels | Vasodilation |

by epinephrine released from the adrenal medulla and cause vasodilation (Fig. 32-1).

The sympathetic vasomotor center interacts with many areas of the brain to maintain normal BP under various conditions. It is activated during times of pain, stress, and exercise. The SNS response causes an appropriate increase in CO and BP to adjust to the body's increased $O_2$ demands. During postural change from lying to standing, there is a transient decrease in BP. The vasomotor center is stimulated, and the SNS response causes peripheral vasoconstriction and increased venous return to the heart. If this response did not occur, blood flow to the brain would be inadequate, resulting in dizziness or syncope.

**Baroreceptors.** *Baroreceptors* have an important role in the maintenance of BP stability during normal activities. They are sensitive to stretching and, when stimulated by an increase in BP, send inhibitory impulses to the sympathetic vasomotor center. Inhibition of the SNS results in decreased HR, decreased force of contraction, and vasodilation in peripheral arterioles.

When a fall in BP is sensed by the baroreceptors, the SNS is activated. The result is constriction of the peripheral arterioles, increased HR, and increased contractility of the heart. In long-standing hypertension, the baroreceptors become adjusted to elevated BP levels and recognize this level as their new "normal."

## Vascular Endothelium

The vascular endothelium is a single-cell layer that lines the blood vessels. For years the endothelium was thought to be inert, serving only as a passive lining for the vessels. Now information shows that the endothelium is very active and responsible for a number of different critical functions. These include platelet adhesion, coagulation regulation, immune function, and regulation of fluid control within the vessel and extravascular space. The endothelium can also cause adhesion and aggregation of neutrophils and stimulate smooth muscle growth.

One of the most important findings was the discovery that the endothelium was essential to the regulation and maintenance of the vasodilating and vasoconstricting substances.[9] Endothelium-derived vasoactive substances include *nitric oxide* (NO) and *prostacyclin*, which are both vasodilators. Another product of the endothelium is *endothelin* (ET), which is a potent vasoconstrictor (Fig. 32-1). A disruption or dysfunction of arterial tone (either through excessive constriction or dilation) is an early warning signal of CVD.

## Renal System

The kidneys contribute to BP regulation by controlling sodium excretion and extracellular fluid (ECF) volume (see Chapter 44). Sodium retention results in water retention, which causes an increase in ECF volume. This increases the venous return to the heart and stroke volume. Together these increase CO and BP.

The renin-angiotensin-aldosterone system (RAAS) also plays an important role in BP regulation (Fig. 32-1). The juxtaglomerular apparatus in the kidney secretes renin in response to SNS stimulation, decreased blood flow through the kidneys, or decreased serum sodium concentration. Renin is an enzyme that converts angiotensinogen to angiotensin I. Angiotensin I is then converted to angiotensin II (A-II) by angiotensin-converting enzyme (ACE). A-II increases BP by two different mechanisms (see Fig. 44-4). First, A-II is a potent vasoconstrictor and increases SVR. This results in an immediate increase in BP. Second, over a period of hours or days, A-II increases BP indirectly by stimulating the adrenal cortex to secrete aldosterone (discussed below).

A-II also acts at a local level within the heart and blood vessels. These effects include vasoconstriction and tissue growth that result in remodeling of the vessel walls, which can be due to or caused by endothelial dysfunction. These changes are linked to the development of primary hypertension and also the long-term effects of hypertension (e.g., atherosclerosis, renal disease, cardiac hypertrophy).

Prostaglandins ($PGE_2$ and $PGI_2$) secreted by the renal medulla have a vasodilator effect on the systemic circulation. This results in decreased SVR and lowering of BP. (Prostaglandins are discussed in Chapter 11.) The natriuretic peptides (atrial natriuretic peptide [ANP] and b-type natriuretic peptide [BNP]) are secreted by heart cells. They antagonize the effects of antidiuretic hormone (ADH) and aldosterone. This results in *natriuresis* (excretion of sodium in urine) and diuresis, resulting in reduced blood volume and BP.

## Endocrine System

Stimulation of the SNS results in release of epinephrine along with a small fraction of NE by the adrenal medulla. Epinephrine increases the CO by increasing the HR and myocardial contractility. Epinephrine activates $\beta_2$-adrenergic receptors in peripheral arterioles of skeletal muscle, causing vasodilation. In peripheral arterioles with only $\alpha_1$-adrenergic receptors (skin and kidneys), epinephrine causes vasoconstriction.

A-II stimulates the adrenal cortex to release aldosterone. (Release of aldosterone is also regulated by other factors [see Chapters 47 and 49].) Aldosterone stimulates the kidneys to retain sodium and water. This increases blood volume and CO (see Fig. 44-4).

An increased blood sodium and osmolarity level stimulates the release of ADH from the posterior pituitary gland. ADH increases the ECF volume by promoting the reabsorption of water in the distal and collecting tubules of the kidneys. The resulting increase in blood volume causes an increase in CO and BP.

## HYPERTENSION

### Classification of Hypertension

**Hypertension** is defined as a persistent systolic BP (SBP) of 140 mm Hg or more, diastolic BP (DBP) of 90 mm Hg or more, or current use of antihypertensive medication.[9] **Prehypertension** is defined as SBP of 120 to 139 mm Hg or DBP of 80 to 89 mm Hg.

**Isolated systolic hypertension (ISH)** is defined as an average SBP of 140 mm Hg or more, coupled with an average DBP of less than 90 mm Hg.[10] SBP increases with aging. DBP rises until approximately age 55 and then declines. Control of ISH decreases the incidence of stroke, heart failure, and death.

BP classification is based on the confirmation of office BP readings with ambulatory BP monitoring.[11] Table 32-2 presents the BP classification for people 18 years of age and older.

### Etiology

Hypertension can result from either primary or secondary causes.

**Primary Hypertension.** **Primary *(essential* or *idiopathic)* hypertension** is elevated BP without an identified cause, and it accounts for 90% to 95% of all cases of hypertension. Although the exact cause of primary hypertension is unknown, there are several contributing factors. These include changes in endothelial function related to either vasoconstricting or vasodilating agents, increased SNS activity, overproduction of sodium-retaining hormones, increased sodium intake, greater-than-ideal body weight, diabetes, tobacco use, and excessive alcohol intake.

**Secondary Hypertension.** **Secondary hypertension** is elevated BP with a specific cause that often can be identified and corrected (Table 32-3). This type of hypertension accounts for 5% to 10% of hypertension in adults. Secondary hypertension should be suspected in people who suddenly develop high BP, especially if it is severe. Clinical findings that suggest secondary hypertension relate to the underlying cause. For example, an abdominal bruit heard over the renal arteries may indicate renal disease. Treatment of secondary hypertension is aimed at removing or treating the underlying cause. Secondary hypertension is a contributing factor to hypertensive crisis (discussed later in this chapter).

**TABLE 32-2 Classification of Hypertension**

| Category | SBP (mm Hg) | | DBP (mm Hg) |
|---|---|---|---|
| **Normal** | <120 | and | <80 |
| **Prehypertension** | 120-139 | or | 80-89 |
| **Hypertension, stage 1** | 140-159 | or | 90-99 |
| **Hypertension, stage 2** | ≥160 | or | ≥100 |

From the National Heart, Lung, and Blood Institute: Seventh report of the Joint National Committee on Detection, Evaluation, and Treatment of High Blood Pressure (JNC-7), NIH Publication No. 04-5230, Bethesda, Md, 2004, The Institute. Retrieved from *www.nhlbi.nih.gov/guidelines/hypertension/jnc7full.pdf.*
*DBP,* Diastolic blood pressure; *SBP,* systolic blood pressure.

**TABLE 32-3 Causes of Secondary Hypertension***

- Cirrhosis
- Coarctation or congenital narrowing of the aorta
- Drug-related: estrogen replacement therapy, oral contraceptives, corticosteroids, nonsteroidal antiinflammatory drugs (e.g., cyclooxygenase-2 inhibitors), sympathetic stimulants (e.g., cocaine, monoamine oxidase)
- Endocrine disorders (e.g., pheochromocytoma, Cushing syndrome, thyroid disease)
- Neurologic disorders (e.g., brain tumors, quadriplegia, traumatic brain injury)
- Pregnancy-induced hypertension
- Renal disease (e.g., renal artery stenosis, glomerulonephritis)
- Sleep apnea

*List is not all-inclusive.

### Pathophysiology of Primary Hypertension

BP rises with any increase in CO or SVR. Increased CO is sometimes found in the person with prehypertension. Later in the course of hypertension, the SVR rises and CO returns to normal. The hemodynamic hallmark of hypertension is persistently increased SVR. This persistent elevation in SVR may occur in various ways. Table 32-4 presents factors that relate to the development of primary hypertension or contribute to its consequences. Abnormalities of any of the mechanisms involved in the maintenance of normal BP can result in hypertension (Fig. 32-1).

### Genetic Link

Different sets of genes may regulate BP at different times throughout the life span.[2] Genetic variations are associated with the development of hypertension. For example, genetic abnormalities have been associated with a rare form of hypertension characterized by excess levels of potassium. Several genetic variants of substances on the endothelium affect BP and the development of hypertension by influencing the body's sensitivity to salt.[12] When endothelial surface proteins are activated, proinflammatory properties are stimulated. This impairs the endothelial cells' ability to activate vasodilatory effects, which leads to hypertension.

More research is needed to understand the connection among genetics, endothelial function, and hypertension. In practice, children and siblings of persons with hypertension should be screened and strongly advised to adopt healthy lifestyles to reduce their risk of hypertension.[12]

**Water and Sodium Retention.** Excessive sodium intake is linked to the development of hypertension. Although most people consume a high-sodium diet, only one in three will develop hypertension. When sodium is restricted in many people with hypertension, their BP falls. This suggests that some degree of sodium sensitivity may exist for high sodium intake to trigger the development of hypertension. A high sodium intake may activate a number of systemic mechanisms. Figure 32-2 shows the relationship among salt intake, BP, and changes in structure of the heart.

In clinical practice, there is not an easy or simple test to identify individuals whose BP will rise with even a small increase in salt intake *(salt sensitive)* versus those who can ingest large amounts of sodium without much change in BP *(salt resistant)*. Ongoing research may help to understand the most effective treatment options for people based on genetic predisposition. What is known is that the effect of sodium on BP has a strong genetic component. Additionally, the effect of sodium is greater in African Americans and in middle-aged and older adults.[13,14]

**Altered Renin-Angiotensin-Aldosterone Mechanism.** High plasma renin activity (PRA) increases the conversion of angiotensinogen to angiotensin I (see Fig. 44-4). This alteration in the RAAS may contribute to the development of hypertension. Any rise in BP inhibits the release of renin from the renal juxtaglomerular cells. Based on this feedback loop, low levels of PRA would be expected in patients with primary hypertension. However, only about 30% have low PRA, 50% have normal levels, and 20% have high PRA. These normal or high PRA levels may be related to excess renin secretion from ischemic nephrons.

**Stress and Increased Sympathetic Nervous System Activity.** It has long been recognized that BP is influenced by factors such as anger, fear, and pain. Physiologic responses to stress, which are normally protective, may persist to a pathologic degree, resulting in a prolonged increase in SNS activity. Increased SNS stimulation produces increased vasoconstriction, increased HR, and increased renin release. Increased renin activates the RAAS, leading to elevated BP. People exposed to high levels of repeated psychologic stress develop hypertension to a greater extent than those who experience less stress.

**Insulin Resistance and Hyperinsulinemia.** Defects in glucose, insulin, and lipoprotein metabolism are common in primary hypertension. These defects are not present in secondary hypertension and do not improve when primary hypertension is treated. Insulin resistance is a risk factor in the development of hypertension and CVD. High insulin levels stimulate SNS activity and impair nitrous oxide–mediated vasodilation. Additional pressor effects of insulin include vascular hypertrophy and increased renal sodium reabsorption.

**Endothelial Dysfunction.** Endothelial dysfunction is recognized as a marker for CVD, including primary hypertension.[12] Hypertension can present as a prolonged vasoconstriction response or as a reduced vasodilator response. Prolonged vasoconstriction may be caused by high levels of ET. Vasodilation effects can be altered by oxygen free radicals, which impair the bioavailability of NO. This leads to cellular dysfunction and an imbalance of the vasodilation and vasoconstriction mechanisms in the endothelium.

**TABLE 32-4 Risk Factors for Primary Hypertension**

| Risk Factor | Description |
|---|---|
| **Age** | • SBP rises progressively with increasing age, although DBP may decrease with age.<br>• After age 50, SBP >140 mm Hg is a more important cardiovascular risk factor than DBP. |
| **Alcohol** | • Excessive alcohol intake is strongly associated with hypertension.<br>• Moderate intake of alcohol has cardioprotective properties; males with hypertension should limit their daily intake of alcohol to 2 drinks per day, and 1 drink per day for females with hypertension. |
| **Tobacco use** | • Smoking tobacco greatly ↑ risk of cardiovascular disease.<br>• People with hypertension who smoke tobacco are at even greater risk for cardiovascular disease. |
| **Diabetes mellitus** | • Hypertension is more common in patients with diabetes.<br>• When hypertension and diabetes coexist, complications (e.g., target organ disease) are more severe. |
| **Elevated serum lipids** | • ↑ Levels of cholesterol and triglycerides are primary risk factors in atherosclerosis.<br>• Hyperlipidemia is more common in people with hypertension. |
| **Excess dietary sodium** | • High sodium intake can<br>  • Contribute to hypertension in salt-sensitive patients.<br>  • Decrease the effectiveness of certain antihypertensive medications. |
| **Gender** | • Hypertension is more prevalent in men in young adulthood and early middle age.<br>• After age 64, hypertension is more prevalent in women. (See Gender Differences box on p. 682.) |
| **Family history** | • History of a close blood relative (e.g., parents, sibling) with hypertension is associated with an ↑ risk for developing hypertension. |
| **Obesity** | • Weight gain is associated with increased frequency of hypertension.<br>• Risk increases with central abdominal obesity. |
| **Ethnicity** | • Incidence of hypertension is 2 times higher in African Americans than in whites. (See Cultural & Ethnic Health Disparities box on p. 682.) |
| **Sedentary lifestyle** | • Regular physical activity can help control weight and reduce cardiovascular risk.<br>• Physical activity may ↓ BP. |
| **Socioeconomic status** | • Hypertension is more prevalent in lower socioeconomic groups and among the less educated. |
| **Stress** | • People exposed to repeated stress may develop hypertension more frequently than others.<br>• People who develop hypertension may respond differently to stress than those who do not develop hypertension. |

*DBP*, Diastolic blood pressure; *SBP*, systolic blood pressure.

## Clinical Manifestations

Hypertension is often called the "silent killer" because it is frequently asymptomatic until it becomes severe and target organ disease occurs. A patient with severe hypertension may experience a variety of symptoms secondary to the effects on blood vessels in the various organs and tissues or to the increased workload of the heart. These secondary symptoms include fatigue, dizziness, palpitations, angina, and dyspnea.

In the past, symptoms of hypertension were thought to include headache and nosebleeds. Unless BP is very high, these symptoms are no more frequent in people with hypertension than in the general population. However, patients with hypertensive crisis (discussed later in the chapter) may experience severe headaches, dyspnea, anxiety, and nosebleeds.[15]

## Complications

The most common complications of hypertension are *target organ diseases* occurring in the heart (hypertensive heart disease), brain (cerebrovascular disease), peripheral vessels (peripheral vascular disease), kidneys (nephrosclerosis), and eyes (retinal damage) (Table 32-5).

### Hypertensive Heart Disease

***Coronary Artery Disease.*** Hypertension is a major risk factor for coronary artery disease (CAD). The mechanisms by which hypertension contributes to the development of atherosclerosis are not fully known. The "response-to-injury" theory of atherogenesis suggests that hypertension disrupts the coronary artery endothelium (see Fig. 33-1). This results in a stiff arterial wall with a narrowed lumen, and accounts for a high rate of CAD, angina, and MI.

***Left Ventricular Hypertrophy.*** Sustained high BP increases the cardiac workload and produces left ventricular hypertrophy (LVH) (Fig. 32-3). Initially, LVH is a compensatory mechanism that strengthens cardiac contraction and increases CO. However, increased contractility increases myocardial work and $O_2$

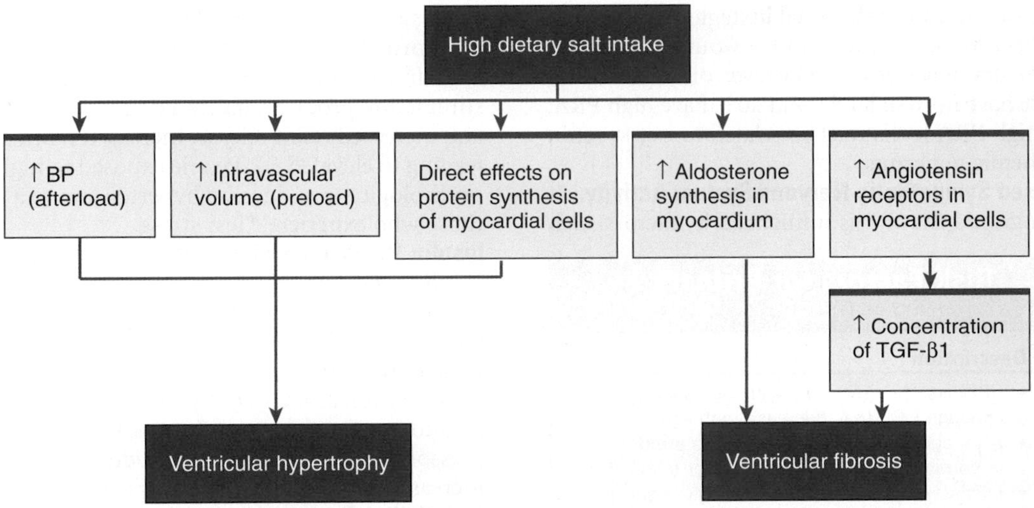


**FIG. 32-2** Proposed link among salt intake, blood pressure, and changes in the heart. High dietary salt intake exerts hypertrophic effects on the left (and potentially also on right) ventricle. Ventricular fibrosis can also result from the high salt intake through mechanisms mediated by the renin-angiotensin-aldosterone system (RAAS). Transforming growth factor-β1 (TGF-β1) is a multifunctional cytokine with fibrogenic properties. Overproduction of TGF-β1 (in part mediated by angiotensin II) results in fibrosis and ventricular dysfunction. (Modified from Frisoli TM, Schmieder RE, Grodzicki T, et al: Salt and hypertension: Is salt dietary reduction worth the effort? *Am J Med* 125:433, 2012.)

**TABLE 32-5 Manifestations of Target Organ Disease**

| Organ | Manifestations |
|---|---|
| **Cardiac** | • Clinical, electrocardiographic, or radiologic evidence of coronary artery disease (e.g., previous MI, coronary revascularization)<br>• Left ventricular hypertrophy by ECG or echocardiography<br>• Left ventricular dysfunction or heart failure |
| **Cerebrovascular** | • Transient ischemic attack<br>• Stroke |
| **Peripheral vascular** | • One or more major pulses in the extremities (except for dorsalis pedis) faint or absent<br>• Intermittent claudication<br>• Abdominal or carotid bruits or thrills<br>• Aneurysm |
| **Renal** | • Serum creatinine ≥1.5 mg/dL (130 μmol/L)<br>• Proteinuria (≥1+)<br>• Microalbuminuria |
| **Retinopathy** | • Generalized or focal narrowing of retinal arterioles<br>• Arteriovenous nicking<br>• Hemorrhages or exudates with or without papilledema |

Source: National Heart, Lung, and Blood Institute: Seventh report of the Joint National Committee on Detection, Evaluation, and Treatment of High Blood Pressure (JNC-7), NIH Publication No. 04-5230, Bethesda, Md, 2004, The Institute. Retrieved from *www.nhlbi.nih.gov/guidelines/hypertension/jnc7full.pdf*.

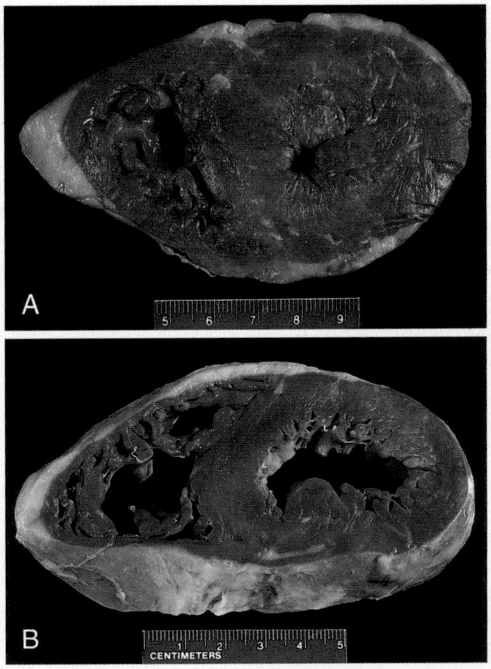


**FIG. 32-3** **A,** Massively enlarged heart caused by hypertrophy of the muscle in the left ventricle. **B,** Compare with the thickness of the normal left ventricle. The patient suffered from severe hypertension. (From Kumar V, Cotran RS, Robbins SL: *Robbins basic pathology,* ed 8, Philadelphia, 2007, Saunders.)

demand. Progressive LVH, especially in the presence of CAD, is associated with the development of heart failure.

***Heart Failure.*** Heart failure occurs when the heart's compensatory mechanisms are overwhelmed and the heart can no longer pump enough blood to meet the body's demands (see Chapter 34). Contractility is depressed, and stroke volume and CO are decreased. The patient may complain of shortness of breath on exertion, paroxysmal nocturnal dyspnea, and fatigue.

**Cerebrovascular Disease.** Atherosclerosis is the most common cause of cerebrovascular disease. Hypertension is a major risk factor for cerebral atherosclerosis and stroke. Even in mildly hypertensive people, the risk of stroke is four times higher than in normotensive people. Adequate control of BP diminishes the risk of stroke.

Atherosclerotic plaques are commonly found at the bifurcation of the common carotid artery and in the internal and external carotid arteries. Portions of the atherosclerotic plaque or the blood clot that forms with disruption of the plaque may break off and travel to cerebral vessels, producing a thromboembolism. The patient may experience transient ischemic attacks or a stroke. (These conditions are discussed in Chapter 57.)

Hypertensive encephalopathy may occur after a marked rise in BP if the cerebral blood flow is not decreased by autoregulation. *Autoregulation* is a physiologic process that maintains constant cerebral blood flow despite fluctuations in BP. Normally, as pressure in the cerebral blood vessels rises, the vessels constrict to maintain constant flow. When BP exceeds the body's ability to autoregulate, the cerebral vessels suddenly dilate, capillary permeability increases, and cerebral edema develops. This produces a rise in intracranial pressure. If left untreated, patients can die quickly from brain damage. (Chapter 56 discusses cerebral blood flow and autoregulation.)

**Peripheral Vascular Disease.** Hypertension speeds up the process of atherosclerosis in the peripheral blood vessels. This leads to the development of peripheral vascular disease, aortic aneurysm, and aortic dissection (see Chapter 37). *Intermittent claudication* (ischemic leg pain precipitated by activity and relieved with rest) is a classic symptom of peripheral vascular disease.

**Nephrosclerosis.** Hypertension is one of the leading causes of chronic kidney disease, especially among African Americans. Some degree of renal disease is usually present in the hypertensive patient, even those with minimally elevated BP. Renal disease results from ischemia caused by the narrowing of the renal blood vessels. This leads to atrophy of the tubules, destruction of the glomeruli, and eventual death of nephrons. Initially intact nephrons can compensate, but these changes may eventually lead to renal failure. Laboratory indications of renal disease are albuminuria, proteinuria, microscopic hematuria, and elevated serum creatinine and blood urea nitrogen (BUN) levels. An early manifestation of renal disease is usually nocturia (see Chapter 46).

**Retinal Damage.** The appearance of the retina provides important information about the severity and duration of hypertension. The blood vessels of the retina can be directly visualized with an ophthalmoscope. Damage to the retinal vessels provides an indication of related vessel damage in the heart, brain, and kidneys. Manifestations of severe retinal damage include blurring of vision, retinal hemorrhage, and loss of vision.

## Diagnostic Studies

Measurement of BP is essential in assessing and monitoring hypertension. Chapter 31 (p. 662) and the Nursing Management section later in this chapter discuss BP measurement.

Some controversy exists over the diagnostic workup in the initial assessment of a person with hypertension. Most hypertension is classified as primary hypertension and testing for secondary causes is not routinely done. Basic laboratory studies are performed to (1) identify or rule out causes of secondary hypertension, (2) evaluate target organ disease, (3) determine overall cardiovascular risk, or (4) establish baseline levels before initiating therapy.

Table 32-6 lists basic diagnostic studies performed in a person with hypertension. Routine urinalysis, BUN, and serum creatinine levels are used to screen for renal involvement and provide baseline information about kidney function. Creatinine clearance reflects the glomerular filtration rate. Decreases in creatinine clearance indicate renal insufficiency. (Chapter 44 discusses serum creatinine and creatinine clearance.)

Measurement of serum electrolytes, especially potassium, is important to detect hyperaldosteronism, a cause of secondary hypertension. Blood glucose levels assist in the diagnosis of diabetes. A lipid profile provides information about additional risk factors related to atherosclerosis and CVD. Uric acid levels establish a baseline, since the levels often rise with diuretic therapy. An electrocardiogram (ECG) provides baseline information about heart status. It can identify the presence of LVH, cardiac ischemia, or previous MI. If LVH is suspected, echocardiography is often performed. If the patient's age, history, physical examination, or severity of hypertension points to a secondary cause, further diagnostic testing is indicated.

**TABLE 32-6 Interprofessional Care**

***Hypertension***

**Diagnostic Assessment**

- History and physical examination, including an ophthalmic examination
- Routine urinalysis
- Basic metabolic panel (serum glucose, sodium, potassium, chloride, carbon dioxide, BUN, and creatinine)
- Complete blood count
- Serum lipid profile (total lipids, triglycerides, HDL and LDL cholesterol, total-to-HDL cholesterol ratio)
- Serum uric acid, calcium, and magnesium
- 12-lead electrocardiogram (ECG)

*Optional:*

- 24-hr urinary creatinine clearance
- Echocardiography
- Liver function studies
- Serum thyroid-stimulating hormone (TSH)

**Management**

- Periodic monitoring of BP
  - Home BP monitoring
  - Ambulatory BP monitoring
  - Every 3-6 months by a HCP once goal BP is achieved and stabilized
- Nutritional therapy
  - Restrict salt and sodium
  - Restrict cholesterol and saturated fats
  - Maintain adequate intake of potassium, calcium, and magnesium
  - Weight management
- Regular, moderate physical activity
- Tobacco cessation (see Tables 10-4 through 10-6)
- Moderation of alcohol intake
- Stress management techniques (see Chapter 6)
- Antihypertensive drugs (Tables 32-7 and 32-8)
- Patient and caregiver teaching

*HDL*, High-density lipoprotein; *LDL*, low-density lipoprotein.

**Ambulatory Blood Pressure Monitoring.** Some patients have elevated BP readings in a clinical setting and normal readings when BP is measured elsewhere. This phenomenon is referred to as *"white coat"* hypertension. Ambulatory BP monitoring (ABPM) is the best method for diagnosing hypertension.[11] It is a noninvasive, fully automated system that measures BP at preset intervals over a 12-24-hour period. The equipment includes a BP cuff and a microprocessing unit that fits into a pouch worn on a shoulder strap or belt. Tell patients to hold their arm still by their side when the device is taking a reading. Also ask them to maintain a diary of activities that may affect BP. Other potential applications for ABPM include suspected antihypertensive drug resistance, hypotensive symptoms with antihypertensive drugs, episodic hypertension, or SNS dysfunction.

BP demonstrates diurnal variability expressed as sleep-wakefulness difference. For day-active people, BP is highest in the early morning, decreases during the day, and is lowest at night. BP at night (during sleep) usually drops by 10% or more from daytime (awake) BP.[10] The presence of diurnal variability is confirmed with ABPM.

Some patients with hypertension do not show a normal nocturnal dip in BP and are referred to as "nondippers." Patients at highest risk of CVD are "reverse dippers." These patients demonstrate an increase in nighttime systolic BP. Current research is focused on the use of drugs to optimize cardioprotective effects and convert non-dippers and reverse dippers to dippers.

## EVIDENCE-BASED PRACTICE

### Applying the Evidence

**Lifestyle Changes and Uncontrolled Hypertension**

You are caring for F.H., a 43-year-old female patient with a history of poorly controlled hypertension and chronic kidney disease (CKD). She is taking three antihypertensive drugs and tells you she no longer can tolerate the side effects of the drugs (e.g., fatigue, peripheral edema, dry mouth, frequent voiding). She wants to stop taking the drugs and control her hypertension by weight loss, exercise, and reducing her salt intake.

***Making Clinical Decisions***

***Best Available Evidence.*** Antihypertensive drugs reduce the risk of cerebrovascular events, heart failure, and overall mortality in patients with concurrent risk for cardiovascular disease (e.g., diabetes, kidney disease). Most patients with hypertension will need to take two or more drugs on a long-term basis to achieve their goal BP in addition to lifestyle changes.

***Clinician Expertise.*** You know lifestyle changes can help reduce and control BP in many patients. However, patients with poorly controlled hypertension and target organ disease require drugs to control BP and prevent further complications.

***Patient Preferences and Values.*** F.H. wants to stop her antihypertensive drugs because of unacceptable side effects.

***Implications for Nursing Practice***

1. What important factors would you discuss with F.H. related to hypertension treatment and preventing further target organ disease?
2. Would you support F.H. in her desire to stop taking hypertensive drugs? Why or why not?
3. How can you help F.H. with her intentions to make lifestyle changes?

***References for Evidence***

Eckel RH, Jakicic JM, Ard JD, et al: 2013 AHA/ACC guideline on lifestyle management to reduce cardiovascular risk: a report of the American College of Cardiology/American Heart Association Task Force on Practice Guidelines, *J Am Coll Cardiol* 63:2960, 2014.

James PA, Oparil S, Carter BL, et al: 2014 Evidence-based guideline for the management of high blood pressure in adults: report from the panel members appointed to the Eighth Joint National Committee (JNC 8), *JAMA* 311:507, 2014.

## Interprofessional Care

Table 32-6 summarizes the interprofessional care for a patient with hypertension. Goals include achieving and maintaining goal BP and reducing cardiovascular risk and target organ disease. Lifestyle modifications are indicated for all patients with prehypertension and hypertension.

**Lifestyle Modifications.** Lifestyle modifications are directed toward reducing the patient's BP and overall cardiovascular risk. Modifications include (1) weight reduction, (2) Dietary Approaches to Stop Hypertension (DASH) eating plan, (3) dietary sodium reduction, (4) moderation of alcohol intake, (5) regular physical activity, (6) avoidance of tobacco use (smoking and chewing), and (7) management of psychosocial risk factors.

***Weight Reduction.*** Overweight persons have an increased incidence of hypertension and increased risk for CVD. Weight reduction has a significant effect on lowering BP in many people, and the effect is seen with even moderate weight loss. A weight loss of 22 lb (10 kg) may decrease SBP by approximately 5 to 20 mm Hg.[10] When a person decreases caloric intake, sodium and fat intake are usually also reduced. Although reducing the fat content of the diet has not been shown to produce sustained benefits in BP control, it may slow the progress of atherosclerosis and reduce overall CVD risk (see Chapter 33). Weight reduction through a combination of calorie restriction and moderate physical activity is recommended for overweight patients with hypertension (see Chapter 40).

***DASH Eating Plan.*** The DASH eating plan emphasizes fruits, vegetables, fat-free or low-fat milk and milk products, whole grains, fish, poultry, beans, seeds, and nuts. Compared with the typical American diet, the plan contains less red meat, salt, sweets, added sugars, and sugar-containing beverages. The DASH eating plan significantly lowers BP, and these decreases compare with those achieved with BP-lowering medication. Additional benefits also include lowering of low-density lipoprotein (LDL) cholesterol.[13]

***Dietary Sodium Reduction.*** Healthy adults should restrict sodium intake to less than or equal to 2300 mg/day. African Americans; people middle aged and older; and those with hypertension, diabetes, or chronic kidney disease should restrict sodium to less than or equal to 1500 mg/day.[13] This involves avoiding foods known to be high in sodium (e.g., canned soups, frozen dinners) and not adding salt in the preparation of foods or at meals (see Table 34-8).

Most adults exceed the recommended limits for sodium. Average sodium intake is approximately 4200 mg/day in men and 3300 mg/day in women.[13] The patient and caregiver, especially the person who prepares the meals, need to learn about sodium-restricted diets. Instruction should include reading labels of over-the-counter drugs, packaged foods, and health products (e.g., toothpaste containing baking soda) to identify hidden sources of sodium (see Fig. 34-6). Review the patient's normal diet to identify foods high in sodium.

Sodium restriction may be enough to control BP in some patients. If drug therapy is needed, a lower dosage may be effective if the patient also restricts sodium intake. Further, moderate sodium restriction lessens the risk of hypokalemia associated with diuretic therapy. However, the response differs between patients who are salt sensitive or salt resistant.

The significance of other dietary elements for the control of hypertension is not certain. Increased levels of dietary potassium, calcium, vitamin D, and omega-3 fatty acids are associated with lower BP in the general population and in those with hypertension. People with hypertension should maintain adequate potassium, calcium, and vitamin D intake from food sources. Calcium supplements are not recommended to lower BP. Omega-3 fatty acids found in certain fish oils can contribute to a reduction in BP and triglycerides (see Complementary & Alternative Therapies box).

***Moderation of Alcohol Intake.*** Excessive alcohol intake is strongly associated with hypertension. Drinking three or more alcoholic drinks daily is also a risk factor for CVD and stroke. Men should limit their intake of alcohol to no more than two

## COMPLEMENTARY & ALTERNATIVE THERAPIES

### *Fish Oil and Omega-3 Fatty Acids*

Dietary sources of omega-3 fatty acids include fish oil and certain plant and nut oils. Fish oil contains both docosahexaenoic acid (DHA) and eicosapentaenoic acid (EPA). Some nuts and vegetable oils contain α-linolenic acid (ALA).

**Scientific Evidence**

- Reduce blood triglyceride levels
- May cause a small reduction in BP
- Although studies have not shown significant benefits of fish oil and omega-3 fatty acid supplementation to hypertension management, no studies have shown harm or adverse effects.
- May reduce the risk of heart attack, stroke, and death among people with cardiovascular disease. There is concern that omega-3 fatty acids in fish oil may be related to increases in prostate cancer.

**Nursing Implications**

- For healthy adults with no history of heart disease, the American Heart Association recommends eating fish at least two times per week. Fatty fish such as anchovies, bluefish, carp, catfish, halibut, lake trout, mackerel, pompano, salmon, striped sea bass, albacore tuna, and whitefish are recommended.
- Fish oil is generally safe in recommended dosages. Higher doses may result in increased risk of bleeding.
- There is no evidence to support the safety of fish oil consumption in persons with shellfish allergies.

Sources: *www.naturalstandard.com* and *http://nccam.nih.gov/health/providers/digest/omega3.*

drinks per day and women and lighter-weight men to no more than one drink per day. One drink is defined as 12 oz of regular beer, 5 oz of wine (12% alcohol), or 1.5 oz of 80-proof distilled spirits. Excessive alcohol intake that results in cirrhosis is the most frequent cause of secondary hypertension.

***Physical Activity.*** A physically active lifestyle is essential to promote and maintain good health. The AHA and American College of Sports Medicine recommend that adults perform moderate-intensity aerobic physical activity for at least 30 minutes most days (i.e., more than 5 days per week) with a goal of at least 150 minutes per week. Exercise goals can be accomplished by performing shorter periods of exercise that last at least 10 minutes. Additionally, combinations of moderate and vigorous activity are acceptable (e.g., walking briskly for 30 minutes on 2 days of the week and jogging for 20 minutes on 2 other days).[16]

Differences in physical activity guidelines exist for adults age 18 to 65 years, adults over 65 years, and adults age 50 to 64 years with functional limitations. The differences relate to the definition of moderate and vigorous aerobic activity. For adults ages 18 to 65, walking briskly at a pace that noticeably increases the pulse defines moderate-intensity aerobic activity. Jogging at a pace that substantially increases the pulse and causes rapid breathing is an example of vigorous activity for this age group. For all other adults, individual fitness levels guide aerobic intensity.[16]

All adults should perform muscle-strengthening activities using the major muscles of the body at least twice a week. This helps to maintain or increase muscle strength and endurance. Additionally, flexibility and balance exercises are recommended at least twice a week for older adults, especially for those at risk for falls.[17] Moderate-intensity activities can lower BP, promote relaxation, and decrease or control body weight. Regular activity of this type can reduce SBP by approximately 4 to 9 mm Hg.[10]

Generally, physical activity is more likely to become a habit if it is safe and enjoyable, fits easily into one's daily schedule, and is inexpensive. Many shopping malls open early in the morning and provide a warm, safe, flat area for walking. Some health clubs offer special "off-peak" rates to encourage physical activity among older adults. Some health insurance carriers offer health club discounts as a benefit to encourage member fitness. Cardiac rehabilitation programs offer supervised exercise and education about cardiovascular risk factor reduction.

Help people with hypertension to increase their physical activity by explaining the need for physical activity, describing the different types of physical activities, and assisting in starting an exercise plan. Advise sedentary people to increase activity levels gradually. Individuals with CVD or other serious health problems need a thorough examination and possibly a stress test before beginning an exercise program.

***Avoidance of Tobacco Products.*** Nicotine contained in tobacco causes vasoconstriction and increases BP, especially in people with hypertension. Smoking tobacco is also a major risk factor for CVD. The cardiovascular benefits of stopping tobacco use are seen within 1 year in all age-groups. Strongly encourage everyone, especially patients with hypertension, to avoid tobacco use. Advise those who continue to use tobacco products to monitor their BP during use. (Chapter 10 discusses tobacco use and smoking cessation.)

***Management of Psychosocial Risk Factors.*** Psychosocial risk factors can contribute to the risk of developing CVD, and to a poorer prognosis and clinical course in patients with CVD. These risk factors include low socioeconomic status, social isolation and lack of support, stress at work and in family life, and negative emotions such as depression and hostility. Frequently, these risk factors are clustered together. For example, rates of depression tend to be higher in individuals with job stress.

Psychosocial risk factors have direct effects on the cardiovascular system by activating the SNS and stress hormones. This can cause a wide variety of pathophysiologic responses, including hypertension and tachycardia, inflammation, endothelial dysfunction, increased platelet aggregation, insulin resistance, and central obesity.[18]

Psychosocial risk factors can contribute to CVD indirectly as well, simply by their impact on lifestyle behaviors and choices. Screening for psychosocial risk factors is important. Make appropriate referrals (e.g., counseling), when indicated. Suggest behavioral interventions such as relaxation training, stress management courses, support groups, and exercise training for individuals who are not in acute psychologic distress.[18]

**Drug Therapy.** The following are recommendations for antihypertensive drug therapy from the JNC 8.[6]

- In patients 60 years or over, start drug treatment for BP greater than or equal to 150 mm Hg systolic or greater than or equal to 90 mm Hg diastolic and treat to goal BP less than those thresholds.
- In patients less than 60 years, treatment initiation and goals should be 140/90 mm Hg, the same threshold used in patients 18 years or older with either chronic kidney disease (CKD) or diabetes.

Findings from the SPRINT indicate that treatment of systolic BP to less than 120 mm Hg (rather than 140 mm Hg) reduced the rates of major cardiovascular events by almost one-third and the risk of death by almost one-fourth.[7] These data may result in changes to the JNC 8 guidelines.

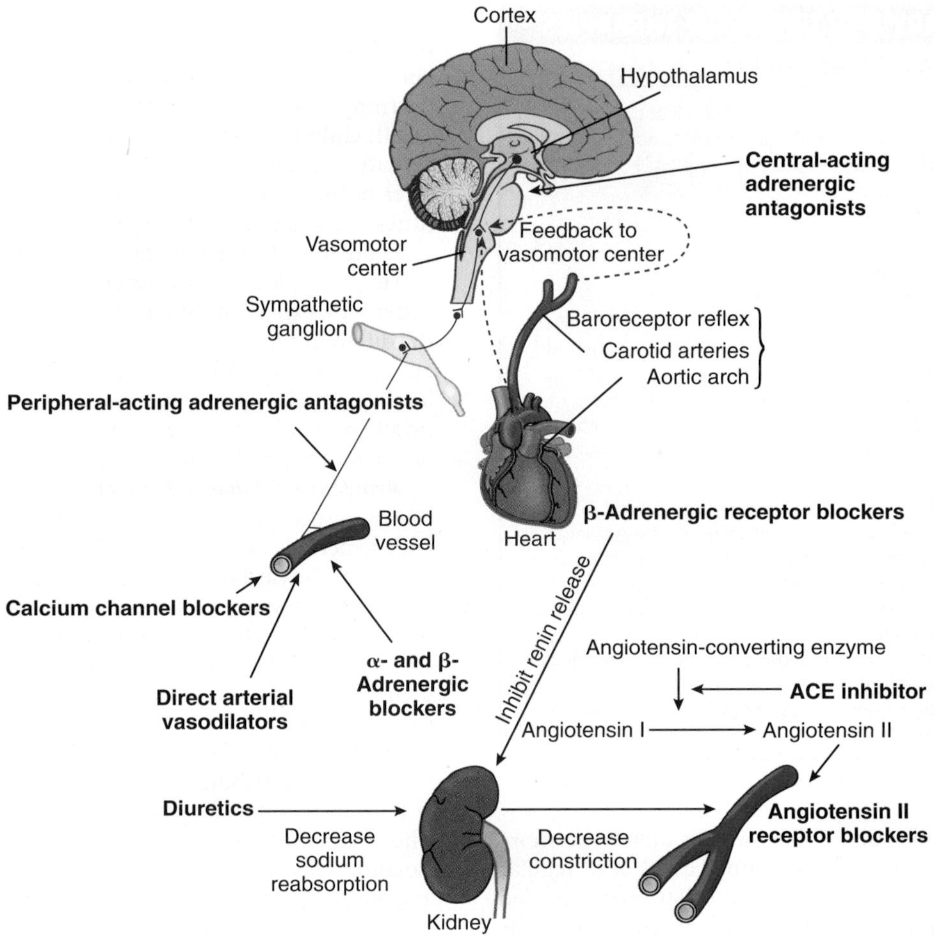


**FIG. 32-4** Site and method of action of various antihypertensive drugs *(bold type). ACE,* Angiotensin-converting enzyme. (From US Department of Health and Human Services: *Seventh report of the Joint National Committee on Prevention, Detection, Evaluation, and Treatment of High Blood Pressure [JNC 7],* Washington, DC, 2003, National Institutes of Health.)

The drugs currently available for treating hypertension have two main actions: (1) decrease the volume of circulating blood and (2) reduce SVR[19,20] (Table 32-7). Fig. 32-4 presents the various sites and methods of action of antihypertensive drugs. The drugs used in the treatment of hypertension include the following:

- *Diuretics* promote sodium and water excretion, reduce plasma volume, and reduce the vascular response to catecholamines.
- *Adrenergic-inhibiting agents* act by diminishing the SNS effects that increase BP. Adrenergic inhibitors include drugs that act centrally on the vasomotor center and peripherally to inhibit norepinephrine release or to block the adrenergic receptors on blood vessels.
- *Direct vasodilators* decrease the BP by relaxing vascular smooth muscle and reducing SVR.
- *Calcium channel blockers* increase sodium excretion and cause arteriolar vasodilation by preventing the movement of extracellular calcium into cells.
- *Angiotensin-converting enzyme (ACE) inhibitors* prevent the conversion of angiotensin I to angiotensin II and reduce angiotensin II (A-II)–mediated vasoconstriction and sodium and water retention.
- *A-II receptor blockers (ARBs)* prevent angiotensin II from binding to its receptors in the walls of the blood vessels.

Most patients who are hypertensive require two or more antihypertensive drugs to achieve their goal BP. The addition of a second drug from a different class is started when use of a single drug in adequate doses fails to achieve the goal BP. These can be separate prescriptions or combination therapy (Table 32-8). If a drug is not tolerated or is contraindicated, then a drug from another class is used.

Once antihypertensive therapy is started, patients should return for follow-up and adjustment of drugs at monthly intervals until the goal BP is reached. More frequent visits are necessary for patients with stage 2 hypertension or with co-morbidities. After BP is at goal and stable, follow-up visits can usually be at 3- to 6-month intervals. Co-morbidities (e.g., heart failure), associated diseases (e.g., diabetes), and the need for ongoing monitoring (e.g., laboratory testing) influence the frequency of visits.

***Patient and Caregiver Teaching Related to Drug Therapy.*** Side effects of antihypertensive drugs are common and may be so severe or undesirable that the patient does not adhere to the therapy[19,20] (Table 32-7). Patient and caregiver teaching related to drug therapy helps them to identify and minimize side effects. This may help the patient adhere to therapy. Side effects may be an initial response to a drug and may decrease over time. Telling the patient about side effects that may decrease with time may help the person to continue taking the drug. The

## TABLE 32-7 Drug Therapy

### *Hypertension*

| Drug | Mechanism of Action | Nursing Considerations |
|---|---|---|
| **Diuretics** | | |
| ***Thiazide and Related Diuretics*** | | |
| chlorothiazide (Diuril)<br>chlorthalidone<br>hydrochlorothiazide<br>indapamide<br>metolazone (Zaroxolyn) | Inhibit NaCl reabsorption in the distal convoluted tubule. Increase excretion of $Na^+$ and $Cl^-$. Initial decrease in ECF. Sustained decrease in SVR. Lower BP moderately in 2-4 wk. | Monitor for orthostatic hypotension, hypokalemia, and alkalosis. Thiazides may potentiate cardiotoxicity of digoxin by producing hypokalemia. Dietary sodium restriction reduces the risk of hypokalemia. NSAIDs can decrease diuretic and antihypertensive effect of thiazide diuretics and potentially cause renal impairment. Advise patient to supplement with potassium-rich foods. |
| ***Loop Diuretics*** | | |
| bumetanide (Bumex)<br>furosemide (Lasix)<br>torsemide (Demadex) | Inhibit NaCl reabsorption in the ascending limb of the loop of Henle. Increase excretion of $Na^+$ and $Cl^-$. More potent diuretic effect than thiazides, but shorter duration of action. Less effective for hypertension. | Monitor for orthostatic hypotension and electrolyte abnormalities. Loop diuretics remain effective despite renal insufficiency. Diuretic effect of drug increases at higher doses. |
| ***Potassium-Sparing Diuretics*** | | |
| amiloride (Midamor)<br>triamterene (Dyrenium) | Reduce $K^+$ and $Na^+$ exchange in the distal and collecting tubules. Reduce excretion of $K^+$, $H^+$, $Ca^{++}$, and $Mg^{++}$. | Monitor for orthostatic hypotension and hyperkalemia. Contraindicated in patients with renal failure. Use with caution in patients on ACE inhibitors or angiotensin II blockers. Avoid potassium supplements. |
| ***Aldosterone Receptor Blockers*** | | |
| spironolactone (Aldactone)<br>eplerenone (Inspra) | Inhibit the $Na^+$-retaining and $K^+$-excreting effects of aldosterone in the distal and collecting tubules. | Monitor for orthostatic hypotension and hyperkalemia. Do not combine with potassium-sparing diuretics or potassium supplements. Use with caution in patients on ACE inhibitors or angiotensin II blockers. These drugs are also classified as potassium-sparing diuretics. |
| **Adrenergic Inhibitors** | | |
| ***Central-Acting $\alpha$-Adrenergic Agonist*** | | |
| clonidine (Catapres)<br>clonidine patch (Catapres-TTS) | Reduce sympathetic outflow from CNS. Reduce peripheral sympathetic tone, produces vasodilation, decreases SVR and BP. | Sudden discontinuation may cause withdrawal syndrome, including rebound hypertension, tachycardia, headache, tremors, apprehension, sweating. Chewing gum or hard candy may relieve dry mouth. Alcohol and sedatives increase sedation. Transdermal patch may be related to fewer side effects and better adherence. |
| guanabenz<br>guanfacine (Tenex) | Same as clonidine. | Same as clonidine, but not available in transdermal formulation. |
| methyldopa | Same as clonidine. | Instruct patient about daytime sedation and avoidance of hazardous activities. Taking a single daily dose at bedtime minimizes sedative effect. |
| ***Peripheral-Acting $\alpha$-Adrenergic Agonist*** | | |
| reserpine | Depletes central and peripheral stores of norepinephrine. Results in peripheral vasodilation (decreases SVR and BP). | Must be given twice daily. Contraindicated in patients with history of depression. Monitor mood and mental status regularly. Advise patient to avoid barbiturates, alcohol, opioids. |
| ***$\alpha_1$-Adrenergic Blockers*** | | |
| doxazosin (Cardura)<br>prazosin (Minipress)<br>terazosin | Block $\alpha_1$-adrenergic effects, producing peripheral vasodilation (decreases SVR and BP). Beneficial effects on lipid profile. | Reduced resistance to the outflow of urine in benign prostatic hyperplasia. Taking drug at bedtime reduces risks associated with orthostatic hypotension. |
| phentolamine (Regitine) | Blocks $\alpha_1$-adrenergic receptors, resulting in peripheral vasodilation (decreases SVR and BP). | Used in short-term management of pheochromocytoma. Also used locally to prevent necrosis of skin and subcutaneous tissue after extravasation of adrenergic drug. No oral formulation. |
| ***$\beta$-Adrenergic Blockers*** | | |
| ***Cardioselective Blockers*** | | |
| acebutolol (Sectral)<br>atenolol (Tenormin)<br>betaxolol<br>bisoprolol (Zebeta)<br>esmolol (Brevibloc)<br>metoprolol (Lopressor)<br>nebivolol (Bystolic) | Cardioselective agents block $\beta_1$-adrenergic receptors (Table 32-1). Reduce BP by blocking $\beta$-adrenergic effects. Decrease CO and reduce sympathetic vasoconstrictor tone. Decrease renin secretion by kidneys. | Monitor pulse and BP regularly. Use with caution in patients with diabetes because drug may depress the tachycardia associated with hypoglycemia and may adversely affect glucose metabolism.<br>Drug of choice for patients with a history of an MI or heart failure. Less effective BP reduction in African American patients. Esmolol is for IV use only. Cardioselective agents lose cardioselectivity at higher doses. |

*Continued*

TABLE 32-7 **Drug Therapy**

***Hypertension—cont'd***

| Drug | Mechanism of Action | Nursing Considerations |
|---|---|---|
| **Adrenergic Inhibitors—cont'd** | | |
| ***β-Adrenergic Blockers—cont'd*** | | |
| ***Non-cardioselective Blockers*** | | |
| nadolol (Corgard)<br>pindolol<br>propranolol (Inderal) | Nonselective agents block $\beta_1$- and $\beta_2$-adrenergic receptors (Table 32-1). Reduce BP by blocking $\beta_1$- and $\beta_2$-adrenergic effects. | Same as cardioselective, except nonselective agents may cause bronchospasm, especially in patients with a history of asthma. |
| ***Mixed α- and β-Blockers*** | | |
| carvedilol (Coreg)<br>labetalol | $\alpha_1$-, $\beta_1$-, and $\beta_2$-adrenergic blocking properties producing peripheral vasodilation and decreased heart rate (Table 32-1). Reduce CO, SVR, and BP. | Same as β-blockers. IV form available for hypertensive crisis in hospitalized patients. Patients must be kept supine during IV administration. Assess patient tolerance of upright position (severe orthostatic hypotension) before allowing upright activities (e.g., commode). |
| **Direct Vasodilators** | | |
| fenoldopam (Corlopam) | Activates dopamine receptors, resulting in systemic and renal vasodilation. | IV use only for hypertensive crisis in hospitalized patients. Use cautiously in patients with glaucoma. Patient should remain flat for 1 hr after administration. |
| hydralazine | Reduces SVR and BP by direct arterial vasodilation. | IV use for hypertensive crisis in hospitalized patients. Twice-daily oral dosage. Not used as monotherapy because of side effects. Contraindicated in patients with coronary artery disease. |
| minoxidil | Reduces SVR and BP by direct arterial vasodilation. | Reserved for treatment of severe hypertension associated with renal failure and resistant to other therapy. Once- or twice-daily dosage. |
| nitroglycerin | Relaxes arterial and venous smooth muscle, reducing preload and SVR. At low dose, venous dilation predominates; at higher dose, arterial dilation is present. | IV use for hypertensive crisis in hospitalized patients with myocardial ischemia. Given by continuous IV infusion with pump or control device. |
| sodium nitroprusside | Direct arterial vasodilation reduces SVR and BP. | IV use for hypertensive crisis in hospitalized patients. Given by continuous IV infusion with pump or control device. Arterial monitoring of BP recommended. Wrap IV solutions with an opaque material to protect from light. Stable for 24 hr. Metabolized to cyanide, then thiocyanate. Monitor thiocyanate levels with prolonged use (>3 days) or doses ≥4 mcg/kg/min. |
| **Angiotensin Inhibitors** | | |
| ***Angiotensin-Converting Enzyme Inhibitors*** | | |
| benazepril (Lotensin)<br>captopril<br>enalapril (Vasotec)<br>fosinopril<br>lisinopril (Zestril)<br>moexipril (Univasc)<br>perindopril (Aceon)<br>quinapril (Accupril)<br>ramipril (Altace)<br>trandolapril (Mavik) | Inhibit ACE, reduce conversion of angiotensin I to angiotensin II (A-II). Inhibit A-II–mediated vasoconstriction. | Aspirin and NSAIDs may reduce drug effectiveness. Addition of diuretic enhances drug effect. Should not be used with potassium-sparing diuretics. Can cause increase in serum creatinine. Inhibit breakdown of bradykinin, which may cause a dry, hacking cough that can occur at any point during treatment, even years later. Captopril may be given orally for hypertensive crisis. |
| ***Angiotensin II Receptor Blockers*** | | |
| azilsartan (Edarbi)<br>candesartan (Atacand)<br>eprosartan (Teveten)<br>irbesartan (Avapro)<br>losartan (Cozaar)<br>olmesartan (Benicar)<br>telmisartan (Micardis)<br>valsartan (Diovan) | Prevent action of A-II and produce vasodilation and increased $Na^+$ and water excretion. | Full effect on BP may not be seen for 3-6 wk. Do not affect bradykinin levels, therefore acceptable alternative to ACE inhibitors in people who develop dry cough. In patients with kidney disease, ACE inhibitors and ARBs should not be used together due to adverse renal effects. |
| **Renin Inhibitors** | | |
| aliskiren (Tekturna) | Directly inhibits renin, thus reducing conversion of angiotensinogen to angiotensin I. | May cause angioedema of the face, extremities, lips, tongue, glottis, and/or larynx.<br>Not to be used in pregnancy. |

TABLE 32-7 **Drug Therapy**
***Hypertension—cont'd***

| Drug | Mechanism of Action | Nursing Considerations |
|---|---|---|
| **Calcium Channel Blockers** | | |
| ***Non-Dihydropyridines*** | | |
| diltiazem extended release (Cardizem LA)<br>verapamil intermediate release (Calan)<br>verapamil long-acting (Covera-HS)<br>verapamil timed-release (Verelan PM) | Inhibit movement of $Ca^{++}$ across cell membrane, resulting in vasodilation<br>Cardioselective resulting in decrease in heart rate and slowing of AV conduction. | Use with caution in patients with heart failure. Serum concentrations and toxicity of certain calcium channel blockers may be increased by grapefruit juice; avoid concurrent use. Used for supraventricular tachydysrhythmias. Avoid in patients with second- or third-degree AV block or left ventricular systolic dysfunction. |
| ***Dihydropyridines*** | | |
| amlodipine (Norvasc)<br>clevidipine (Cleviprex)<br>felodipine<br>isradipine<br>nicardipine sustained release<br>nifedipine long acting (Procardia XL)<br>nisoldipine (Sular) | Cause vascular smooth muscle relaxation resulting in decreased SVR and arterial BP. | More potent peripheral vasodilators.<br>Clevidipine is for IV use only.<br>Use of sublingual short-acting nifedipine in hypertensive emergencies is unsafe and not effective. Serious adverse events (e.g., stroke, acute MI) have been reported.<br>IV nicardipine available for hypertensive crisis in hospitalized patients. Change peripheral IV infusion sites every 12 hr. |

*ACE,* Angiotensin-converting enzyme; *AV,* atrioventricular; *CO,* cardiac output; *DBP,* diastolic blood pressure; *ECF,* extracellular fluid; *HDL,* high-density lipoprotein; *LDL,* low-density lipoprotein; *SBP,* systolic blood pressure; *SVR,* systemic vascular resistance.

number or severity of side effects may relate to the dose. It may be necessary to change the drug or decrease the dose. Advise the patient to report all side effects to the HCP.

A common side effect of several of the antihypertensive drugs is orthostatic hypotension. This condition results from an alteration of the autonomic nervous system's mechanisms for regulating BP, which are needed for position changes. Consequently, the patient may feel dizzy and faint when assuming an upright position after sitting or lying down. Table 32-12 (later in this chapter) presents specific measures to control or decrease orthostatic hypotension.

Sexual problems may occur with many of the antihypertensive drugs. This can be a major reason that patients do not adhere to the treatment plan. Problems can range from reduced libido to erectile dysfunction. Rather than discussing a sexual problem with an HCP, the patient may decide just to stop taking the drug. Approach the patient on this sensitive subject and encourage discussion of any sexual problem that may be experienced. The sexual problems may be easier for the patient to discuss once you explain that the drug may be the source of the problem.

Changing to another antihypertensive drug can decrease or remove these side effects. Encourage the patient to discuss sexual issues with the HCP. If the patient is reluctant to do so, offer to alert the HCP to the side effects that the patient is experiencing. There are many drug options for treating hypertension and a plan that is acceptable to the patient should be the goal.[20]

Some unpleasant side effects of drugs result from their therapeutic effect, but these can be decreased. For example, diuretics cause dry mouth and frequent voiding. Sugarless gum or hard candy may help ease the dry mouth. Taking diuretics earlier in the day may limit frequent voiding during the night and preserve sleep.

***Resistant Hypertension.*** Carefully explore all reasons why a patient may not be at goal BP (Table 32-9). *Resistant hypertension* is the failure to reach goal BP in patients who are taking full doses of an appropriate three-drug therapy regimen that includes a diuretic. Overactive renal nerves can be one cause of resistant hypertension. Percutaneous catheter-based radiofrequency ablation of the renal nerves (known as *renal denervation*) lowers BP and sympathetic nerve activity in patients with resistant hypertension.[21]

## ❖ NURSING MANAGEMENT: PRIMARY HYPERTENSION

### ◆ Nursing Assessment

Table 32-10 presents subjective and objective data to obtain from a patient with hypertension.

### ◆ Nursing Diagnoses

Nursing diagnoses and collaborative problems for the patient with hypertension include, but are not limited to, the following.

- Ineffective health management *related to* lack of knowledge of pathology, complications, and management of hypertension
- Anxiety *related to* complexity of management regimen
- Sexual dysfunction *related to* side effects of antihypertensive medication
- Risk for decreased cardiac tissue perfusion
- Risk for ineffective cerebral tissue perfusion
- Risk for ineffective renal perfusion
- Potential complication: stroke, MI

### ◆ Planning

The overall goals for the patient with hypertension are that the patient will (1) achieve and maintain the goal BP; (2) follow the therapeutic plan, including appointments with the HCP; (3) experience minimal side effects of therapy; and (4) manage and cope with this condition.

### ◆ Nursing Implementation

◆ **Health Promotion.** Primary prevention of hypertension is a cost-effective approach. Current recommendations for primary

**TABLE 32-8 Drug Therapy**

***Combination Therapy for Hypertension****

| Combinations | Trade Names |
|---|---|
| **Angiotensin-Converting Enzyme Inhibitors and Diuretics** | |
| benazepril/hydrochlorothiazide | Lotensin HCT |
| enalapril/hydrochlorothiazide | Vaseretic |
| lisinopril/hydrochlorothiazide | Zestoretic |
| **Angiotensin II Receptor Blockers and Diuretics** | |
| candesartan/hydrochlorothiazide | Atacand HCT |
| losartan/hydrochlorothiazide | Hyzaar |
| olmesartan medoxomil/ hydrochlorothiazide | Benicar HCT |
| valsartan/hydrochlorothiazide | Diovan HCT |
| **β-Blockers and Diuretics** | |
| metoprolol/hydrochlorothiazide | Lopressor HCT |
| nadolol/bendroflumethiazide | Corzide |
| **Angiotensin-Converting Enzyme Inhibitors and Calcium Channel Blockers** | |
| amlodipine/benazepril | Lotrel |
| **Angiotensin II Receptor Blockers and Calcium Channel Blockers** | |
| telmisartan/amlodipine | Twynsta |
| valsartan/amlodipine | Exforge |
| olmesartan/amlodipine | Azor |
| **Diuretics and Diuretics** | |
| spironolactone/hydrochlorothiazide | Aldactazide |
| triamterene/hydrochlorothiazide | Dyazide, Maxzide |
| **Angiotensin II Receptor Blocker, Calcium Channel Blocker, and Diuretic** | |
| olmesartan medoxomil/amlodipine/ hydrochlorothiazide | Tribenzor |
| amlodipine/hydrochlorothiazide/valsartan | Exforge HCT |

*List is not all inclusive and only contains examples of the various categories.

prevention include lifestyle modifications that prevent or delay the rise in BP in at-risk people. Following the DASH diet and reducing sodium can lower BP. This diet is recommended for primary prevention in the general population. Dietary changes by the food industry (e.g., reducing the amount of salt in processed foods) may also be effective.

The National Heart, Lung, and Blood Institute provides web-based educational materials for HCPs, patients, and the public to raise awareness about the dangers of high BP. (See Your Guide to Lowering High Blood Pressure at *www.nhlbi.nih.gov/health/resources/heart/hbp-guide-to-lower*.)

◆ ***Individual Patient Evaluation.*** Hypertension is usually identified through routine screening for insurance, preemployment, and military physical examinations. You are in an ideal position to assess for the presence of hypertension, identify the risk factors for hypertension and CAD, and teach patients about these conditions. In addition to BP measurement, a health assessment should include such factors as age, gender, and race; diet history (including salt and alcohol intake); weight patterns; tobacco use; and family history of CVD, stroke, renal disease, and diabetes. Note all drugs taken, both prescribed and over-the-counter. Last, ask the patient about a previous history of high BP and the results of treatment (if any) (Table 32-10).

◆ ***Blood Pressure Measurement.*** BP can be measured using the oscillatory or auscultatory method.[22] First, take the BP in both arms to note any differences. Atherosclerosis in the subclavian artery can cause a falsely low reading on the side where the narrowing occurs. Use the arm with the highest BP and take at least two readings, a minimum of 1 minute apart (Table 32-11). Waiting for at least 1 minute between readings allows the blood to drain from the arm and prevents inaccurate readings. Record the average pressure as the value for that visit.

Proper size and correct placement of the BP cuff are critical for accurate measurement. Place the cuff snugly around the patient's bare upper arm with the midline of the bladder of the cuff (usually marked on the cuff by the manufacturer) placed in line with the brachial artery. Place the patient's arm at the level of the heart during BP measurement. For BP measurements taken in the sitting position, raise and support the arm at the level of the heart. For measurements taken in a supine position, raise and support (e.g., with a small pillow) the arm at heart level. If the arm is resting on the bed, it will be below heart level.

**EVIDENCE-BASED PRACTICE**

***Translating Research Into Practice***

**Can Home-Based Blood Pressure Monitoring Improve Hypertension Screening?**

***Clinical Question***

In adults screened for hypertension (P), what is the effect of home-based blood pressure (BP) monitoring (I) on the validation of office-based BP results (O)?

***Synthesis of Best Available Evidence***

- Systematic review of randomized controlled trials (RCTs), diagnostic accuracy and cohort BP studies.
- More than 60 studies examining high BP screening among adults (n >150,000). Review summarized BP measurement methods including office-based and home-based (ambulatory) monitoring, diagnostic and predictive accuracy of BP methods on cardiovascular outcomes, and rescreening intervals.
- Home-based BP monitoring with multiple measurements over time in a nonmedical setting may reduce measurement error and the misdiagnosis and overtreatment of isolated clinic hypertension.
- Home-based BP monitoring predicted long-term cardiovascular outcomes independent of office monitoring.
- Rescreening intervals of up to 6 years found persons at higher risk for hypertension were older age, African Americans, and those with high-normal BP and/or above-normal body mass index.

***Conclusions***

- Unless immediate treatment is needed, hypertension detected by office-based measurements should be confirmed by home-based BP monitoring.
- Persons with identified risk factors should be screened more often for hypertension.

***Implications for Nursing Practice***

1. Why is it important for HCPs to be aware of the importance of home-based BP monitoring as an adjunct to office-based monitoring?
2. What information will you share with patients who are worried about a newly elevated BP detected in the office?
3. How will you determine if patients are accurately monitoring their BP at home?

***Reference for Evidence***

Piper MA, Evans CV, Burda BU, et al: Diagnostic and predictive accuracy of blood pressure screening methods with consideration of rescreening intervals: a systematic review for the U.S. Preventive Services Task Force, *Ann Intern Med* 162:192, 2015.

*P*, Patient population of interest; *I*, intervention or area of interest; *C*, comparison of interest or comparison group; *O*, outcomes of interest; *T*, timing (see p. 15).

**TABLE 32-9 Causes of Resistant Hypertension**

- **Improper BP measurement**
- **Volume overload**
  - Excess salt intake
  - Volume retention from kidney disease
  - Inadequate diuretic therapy
- **Drug-induced or other causes**
  - Nonadherence (e.g., due to drug side effects, finances)
  - Illegal drugs (e.g., cocaine, amphetamines)
  - Inadequate drug dosages
  - Inappropriate combinations of drug therapy
  - Nonsteroidal antiinflammatory drugs
  - Sympathomimetics (e.g., decongestants, diet pills)
  - Oral contraceptives
  - Corticosteroids
  - Cyclosporine and tacrolimus (Prograf)
  - Erythropoietin
  - Licorice
  - Some chewing tobacco
  - Selected over-the-counter dietary or herbal supplements and drugs (e.g., ma huang, bitter orange)
- **Associated conditions**
  - Increasing obesity
  - Excess alcohol intake
- **Identifiable causes of secondary hypertension**

Source: National Heart, Lung, and Blood Institute: Seventh Report of the Joint National Committee on Detection, Evaluation, and Treatment of High Blood Pressure (JNC-7), NIH Publication No. 04-5230, Bethesda, Md, 2004, The Institute. Retrieved from *www.nhlbi.nih.gov/guidelines/hypertension/jnc7full.pdf.*

If neither upper arm can be used to measure the BP (e.g., presence of IV lines, fistula), or if a maximum size BP cuff does not fit the upper arm, use the forearm. In this case, position the proper size cuff midway between the elbow and the wrist. Auscultate Korotkoff sounds over the radial artery or use a Doppler device to note SBP. Use of an oscillometric device on the forearm is acceptable. Forearm and upper arm BPs are not interchangeable.[22]

**SAFETY ALERT Blood Pressure Measurement**

- If using the forearm for BP measurement, always document the site.
- BP cuffs that are too small or too large will result in readings that are falsely high or low, respectively.
- If bilateral BP measurements are not equal, document this finding and use the arm with the highest BP for all future measurements.

Assess for orthostatic (or postural) changes in BP and HR in older adults, in people taking antihypertensive drugs, and in patients who report symptoms consistent with reduced BP on standing (e.g., light-headedness, dizziness, syncope). Measure serial BP and HR with the patient in the supine, sitting, and standing positions. First, measure BP and HR with the patient in the supine position after at least 2 to 3 minutes of rest. Reposition the patient in the sitting position with legs dangling and measure BP and HR again within 1 to 2 minutes. Last, reposition the patient to the standing position and measure the BP and HR within 1 to 2 minutes. Usually the SBP decreases slightly (less than 10 mm Hg) on standing, whereas the DBP and pulse increase slightly. **Orthostatic hypotension** occurs when a patient moves from a supine to standing position, and there is a decrease of 20 mm Hg or more in SBP, a decrease of 10 mm Hg or more in DBP, and/or an increase in the HR of 20 beats/minute. Common causes of orthostatic hypotension include dehydration and inadequate vasoconstrictor mechanisms related to disease or drugs.

**TABLE 32-10 Nursing Assessment**

***Hypertension***

**Subjective Data**

***Important Health Information***

*Past health history:* Known duration and past workup of high BP; cardiovascular, cerebrovascular, renal, or thyroid disease; diabetes mellitus; pituitary disorders; obesity; dyslipidemia; menopause or hormone replacement status

*Medications:* Use of any prescription or over-the-counter, illicit, or herbal drugs or products; previous use of antihypertensive drug therapy

***Functional Health Patterns***

*Health perception–health management:* Family history of hypertension or cardiovascular disease; tobacco use, alcohol use; sedentary lifestyle; health literacy; readiness for change

*Nutritional-metabolic:* Usual salt and fat intake; weight gain or loss

*Elimination:* Nocturia

*Activity-exercise:* Fatigue; dyspnea on exertion, palpitations, exertional chest pain; intermittent claudication, muscle cramps; usual pattern and type of exercise

*Cognitive-perceptual:* Dizziness; blurred vision; paresthesias

*Sexual-reproductive:* Erectile dysfunction, decreased libido

*Coping–stress tolerance:* Stressful life events

**Objective Data**

***Cardiovascular***

SBP consistently >140 mm Hg or DBP >90 mm Hg for patients <60 yr old or >150 mm Hg or DBP >90 mm Hg for patients >60 years old. Orthostatic changes in BP and HR; bilateral BPs significantly different; abnormal heart sounds; laterally displaced apical pulse; diminished or absent peripheral pulses; carotid, renal, or femoral bruits; peripheral edema

***Gastrointestinal***

Obesity (BMI ≥30 kg/m$^2$); abnormal waist-hip ratio

***Neurologic***

Mental status changes

***Possible Diagnostic Findings***

Abnormal serum electrolytes (especially potassium); ↑ BUN, creatinine, glucose, cholesterol, and triglyceride levels; proteinuria, albuminuria, microscopic hematuria; evidence of ischemic heart disease and left ventricular hypertrophy on ECG; evidence of structural heart disease and left ventricular hypertrophy on echocardiogram; evidence of arteriovenous nicking, retinal hemorrhages, and papilledema on funduscopic examination

*BMI,* Body mass index; *DBP,* diastolic blood pressure; *HR,* heart rate; *SBP,* systolic blood pressure.

**DRUG ALERT Doxazosin (Cardura)**

- Use caution when giving the first dose. It is recommended to give the first dose at bedtime to reduce the first dose BP drop.
- Syncope occasionally occurs 30 to 90 min after the first dose, a too-rapid increase in dose, or addition of another antihypertensive agent to therapy.
- Drug interactions (severe low BP) can occur with patients taking phosphodiesterase inhibitors such as sildenafil (Viagra).

In acute care settings, BP measurement is usually done to evaluate vital signs, volume status, and effects of drugs, rather than to diagnose hypertension. Trends in BP are more important

**TABLE 32-11 Blood Pressure Measurement**

The patient should not have smoked, exercised, or ingested caffeine within 30 min before measurement.

1. Seat patient with legs uncrossed, feet on the floor, and back supported. Bare patient's arm and support it at heart level.
2. Begin measurement after patient has rested quietly for 5 min. Ask patient to relax as much as possible and not to talk during the measurement.
3. Measure and record BP in both arms initially.
4. Select the appropriate cuff size, following instructions for fit and placement according to manufacturer's recommendations.
5. Take the BP with a recently calibrated aneroid or mercury sphygmomanometer, or electronic oscillometric device. Accuracy of oscillometric devices may be limited if patients are hypertensive, hypotensive, or have heart dysrhythmias (e.g., atrial fibrillation).
6. For auscultatory measurement, estimate SBP by palpating the radial pulse and inflating the cuff until the pulse disappears. Inflate the cuff 20-30 mm Hg above this level.
7. Deflate the cuff at a rate of 2-3 mm Hg/sec.
8. Record the SBP and DBP. Note the SBP when the first of two or more Korotkoff sounds is heard and the DBP when sound disappears.
9. Average two or more readings (taken at intervals of at least 1 min). Obtain additional readings if the first two readings differ by more than 5 mm Hg.
10. Provide the patient (verbally and in writing) with the BP reading, BP goal, and recommendations for follow-up.
11. Clean BP cuffs between patients according to agency policy.

Sources: National Heart, Lung, and Blood Institute: Seventh report of the Joint National Committee on Detection, Evaluation, and Treatment of High Blood Pressure (JNC-7), NIH Publication No. 04-5230, Bethesda, Md, 2004, The Institute. Retrieved from *www.nhlbi.nih.gov/guidelines/hypertension/jnc7full.pdf* and Martin B: AACN practice alert: non-invasive blood pressure monitoring, 2010. Retrieved from *www.aacn.org/wd/practice/docs/practicealerts/non-invasive-bp-monitoring.pdf?menu=aboutus*

*DBP*, Diastolic blood pressure; *SBP*, systolic blood pressure.

than a single value. Inform the HCP of any patient with a persistent elevated BP. These patients should be evaluated for hypertension before discharge, if appropriate, or after discharge.[10]

◆ ***Screening Programs.*** Screening programs in the community are widely used to identify persons who have a high BP. At the time of the BP measurement, give each person a written, numeric value of the reading. Explain why further evaluation is needed.

Focus efforts on the following: (1) controlling BP in persons already identified as having hypertension; (2) identifying and controlling BP in at-risk groups such as African Americans, obese people, and blood relatives of people with hypertension; (3) screening those with limited access to health care; and (4) connecting persons with an HCP and/or health insurance (e.g., Marketplace at *www.healthcare.gov*) if needed.

◆ ***Cardiovascular Risk Factor Modification.*** Teaching regarding CVD risk factors is appropriate for all persons and during targeted screening programs. Modifiable CVD risk factors include hypertension, obesity, diabetes, tobacco use, and physical inactivity. Discuss lifestyle modifications based on identified risk factors. (Table 33-2 discusses health-promoting behaviors for risk factor reduction.)

◆ **Ambulatory Care.** Your primary roles in long-term management of hypertension are to assist the patient to reach the goal BP and adhere to the treatment plan. Your actions include evaluating therapeutic effectiveness, detecting and reporting any adverse treatment effects, assessing and enhancing adherence, and patient and caregiver teaching (Table 32-12).

◆ ***Home BP Monitoring.*** Most patients with known or suspected hypertension should monitor their BP at home. Home BP monitoring reduces the white coat effect of measurement by an HCP. The readings are often lower than those taken in the office setting and are a better predictor of CVD risk.

Patient teaching is critical to ensure accuracy. Tell patients to buy an oscillometric BP monitor that uses a cuff for the upper arm or wrist. The patient should bring the BP monitor to the office to verify proper cuff size, accuracy of the device, and the patient's technique.

## TEAMWORK & COLLABORATION

### *Caring for the Patient With Hypertension*

You will work with many members of the health care team to care for a patient with hypertension. You will need to collaborate with the team members to deliver, delegate, and coordinate care based on the patient's status.

**Role of Nursing Personnel**

***Registered Nurse (RN)***

- Develop and conduct hypertension screening programs.
- Assess patients for hypertension risk factors and develop risk modification plans.
- Teach patients about lifestyle management and drug use.
- Evaluate the effectiveness of lifestyle management and drugs in decreasing BP to acceptable levels.
- Teach about home BP monitoring, including the correct use of automatic BP monitors. Check that the device selected by the patient meets the Association for the Advancement of Medical Instrumentation standards (*www.dableducational.org/sphygmomanometers/devices_1_clinical.html#ClinTable*).
- Make appropriate referrals to other HCPs, such as dietitians or stress management programs.
- Monitor for complications of hypertension such as coronary artery disease, heart failure, cerebrovascular disease, peripheral vascular disease, and renal disease.
- Assess the patient with hypertensive crisis for evidence of target organ disease (e.g., encephalopathy, renal insufficiency, cardiac decompensation).
- Manage the patient with hypertensive urgency or emergency, including administration of drugs and evaluation for resolution of the crisis.

***Licensed Practical/Vocational Nurse (LPN/LVN)***

- Give antihypertensive drugs to stable patients.
- Monitor for adverse effects of antihypertensive drugs.
- Reinforce teaching about drugs and lifestyle management.

***Unlicensed Assistive Personnel (UAP)***

- Obtain accurate BP readings in outpatient and inpatient settings.
- Report high or low BP readings immediately to RN.
- Check for postural changes in BP as directed.

**Role of Other Team Members**

***Dietitian***

- Obtain a diet history from the patient.
- Teach the components of the DASH diet.
- Provide instructions for dietary changes as needed.

***Physical Therapist***

- Assess patient's current level of fitness.
- Develop an exercise plan with the patient.

## TABLE 32-12 Patient & Caregiver Teaching

### *Hypertension*

*When teaching the patient and/or caregiver about hypertension, include the following information.*

**General Instructions**

1. Provide the patient's BP reading and explain what it means (e.g., high, low, goal, borderline). Encourage patient to monitor BP at home and instruct the patient to call the HCP if BP exceeds high or low limits set by HCP.
2. Hypertension is usually asymptomatic and symptoms (e.g., nosebleeds) do not reliably indicate BP levels.
3. Hypertension means high BP and does not relate to a "hyper" personality.
4. Long-term therapy and follow-up care are necessary to treat hypertension. Therapy involves lifestyle changes (e.g., weight management, sodium reduction, smoking cessation, regular physical activity) and, in most cases, drugs.
5. Therapy will not cure, but should control, hypertension.
6. Controlled hypertension usually results in an excellent prognosis and a normal lifestyle.
7. Explain the potential dangers of uncontrolled hypertension (e.g., stroke, heart attack).

**Instructions Related to Medications**

1. Be specific about the names, actions, dosages, and side effects of prescribed drugs.
2. Help the patient plan regular and convenient times for taking drugs and measuring BP.
3. Do not stop drugs abruptly because withdrawal may cause a severe hypertensive reaction.
4. Do not double up on dose when a dose is missed.
5. If BP increases or decreases, do not adjust the drug dose without consulting the HCP.
6. Do not take any drugs belonging to someone else.
7. Supplement diet with foods high in potassium (e.g., citrus fruits, green leafy vegetables) if taking potassium-wasting diuretics.
8. Avoid hot baths, excessive amounts of alcohol, and strenuous exercise within 3 hours of taking drugs that promote vasodilation.
9. Many drugs cause orthostatic hypotension. Reduce the effects of orthostatic hypotension by rising slowly from bed, sitting on the side of the bed for a few minutes, standing slowly, and beginning to move if no symptoms develop (e.g., dizziness, light-headedness). Do not stand still for prolonged periods, do leg exercises to increase venous return, or sleep with the head of the bed raised. Do lie or sit down when dizziness occurs.
10. Some drugs cause sexual problems (e.g., erectile dysfunction, decreased libido). Consult with the HCP about changing drugs or dosages if sexual problems develop.
11. Some side effects of drug(s) may decrease with time (e.g., fatigue, diarrhea).
12. Be careful about taking potentially high-risk over-the-counter drugs, such as high-sodium antacids, NSAIDs, appetite suppressants, and cold and sinus medications. Read warning labels and consult with a pharmacist.

Teach the patient to obtain a BP according to the steps in Table 32-11. Tell the patient to measure BP in the nondominant arm, or arm with the higher BP if there is a known difference between arms. Tell the patient to measure BP first thing in the morning (if possible, before taking medications) and at night before going to bed. Have the patient record all BP measurements and bring the record to office visits.

For clinical decision making (e.g., changes in dosage, start of new drug), tell patients to take BP readings as described for 1 week. Stable, normotensive patients should measure morning and evening BP for at least 1 week every 3 months. Devices that have memory or printouts of the readings are recommended to ensure accurate reporting.[10]

## CHECK YOUR PRACTICE

You are making a home visit for a 78-year-old woman who is recovering from a hip replacement after she fractured her femur. She currently takes a combination of lisinopril/hydrochlorothiazide. The patient's daughter (her caregiver) tells you that her BP that morning was 150/88 and then she took it two more times and it was the same. They are both worried and anxious that something is wrong because they heard that BP over 120/80 is very bad.

- What should you do? What teaching would you provide?

## INFORMATICS IN PRACTICE

### *Monitoring Blood Pressure*

- Smartphones and computer applications can be used to help patients manage their care, including BP self-monitoring, drug history, and appointment tracking. Patients can enter a variety of variables including: SBP and DBP, HR, time of day, arm or wrist used, and position (e.g., lying, sitting).
- Remote BP monitoring using telehealth technology can also be used for patients who have limited access to health care services.
- Reports can be generated to evaluate how well the patient's BP has been controlled.

*DBP,* Diastolic BP; *HR,* heart rate; *SBP,* systolic BP.

Home BP readings may help achieve patient adherence by reinforcing the need to remain on therapy. However, some patients become overly concerned with the BP readings. Discourage too frequent checking of their BP. Generally, home BP monitoring should reassure the patient that the treatment is effective. It is also important for patients to know what their goal or target BP is.

◆ ***Patient Adherence.*** A major problem in the long-term management of the patient with hypertension is poor adherence with the treatment plan. The reasons for nonadherence are complex and can include inadequate patient teaching, low health literacy, unpleasant side effects of drugs, return of BP to normal range while on drugs, high cost of drugs, and lack of insurance.

It is important to determine the reasons why a patient is not adhering to treatment. Also assess the patient's diet, activity level, and lifestyle as additional indicators of adherence. Develop a plan with the patient and caregiver to improve adherence. The plan should be compatible with the patient's habits, cultural beliefs, and lifestyle. Active patient participation increases the chance of adherence to the plan. Measures include involving the patient in selecting drugs that are affordable and involving caregivers to help increase patient adherence.

Substituting combination drugs for multiple drugs once the BP is stable may also facilitate adherence. Combination drugs reduce the number of pills that the patient has to take each day and may reduce costs. (Combination drugs are presented in Table 32-8.)

It is important to help the patient and caregiver understand that hypertension is a chronic illness that cannot be cured. Emphasize that it can be controlled with drug therapy, diet changes, physical activity, periodic follow-up, and other relevant lifestyle modifications.

### ◆ Evaluation

The overall expected outcomes are that the patient with hypertension will:

- Achieve and maintain goal BP as defined for the individual
- Understand, accept, and implement the treatment plan
- Report minimal side effects of drug therapy

### Gerontologic Considerations: Hypertension

The prevalence of hypertension increases with age. The lifetime risk of developing hypertension is approximately 90% for middle-aged (ages 55 to 65) and older (over 65) normotensive men and women.[19] ISH is the most common form of hypertension in people over 50 years of age. Additionally, older adults are more likely to have white coat hypertension.[10]

The pathophysiology of hypertension in the older adult involves the following age-related physical changes: (1) loss of elasticity in large arteries from atherosclerosis, (2) increased collagen content and stiffness of the myocardium, (3) increased peripheral vascular resistance, (4) decreased adrenergic receptor sensitivity, (5) blunting of baroreceptor reflexes, (6) decreased renal function, and (7) decreased renin response to sodium and water depletion.

In the older adult who is taking antihypertensive drugs, absorption of some drugs may be altered as a result of decreased blood flow to the gut. Metabolism and excretion of drugs may also be prolonged.

Careful technique is important in assessing BP in older adults. Some older people have a wide gap between the first Korotkoff sound and subsequent beats. This is called the *auscultatory gap.* Failure to inflate the cuff high enough may result in underestimating SBP (Table 32-11).

Current recommendations for target BP goals in people older than 60 years of age are controversial and range from less than 120/80 mm Hg[7] to less than 150/90 mm Hg.[6] The preferred three first-line antihypertensive drugs are a thiazide diuretic, a calcium channel blocker, and an ACE inhibitor or ARB. A diuretic should always be the first or second drug ordered for most patients.[14]

Orthostatic hypotension often occurs in older adults because of varying degrees of impaired baroreceptor reflexes, especially in those with ISH. Orthostatic hypotension in this age group is often associated with volume depletion or chronic disease states, such as decreased renal and hepatic function or electrolyte imbalance.

Additionally, older adults experience postprandial drops in BP. The greatest decrease occurs approximately 1 hour after eating. BP returns to preprandial levels 3 to 4 hours after eating. To reduce the likelihood of orthostatic hypotension, antihypertensive drugs should be started at low doses and increased slowly. Measure BP and HR in the supine, sitting, and standing positions at every visit.

After CVD, arthritis is the second most prevalent disease in older adults. The most frequently taken drugs by older adults are nonsteroidal antiinflammatory drugs (NSAIDs), both prescription and over-the-counter. Nonselective NSAIDs (e.g., ibuprofen [Advil]) and selective NSAIDs (e.g., celecoxib [Celebrex]) cause loss of BP control and heart failure. Additionally, there is the potential for adverse renal effects and/or hyperkalemia when NSAIDs are used with ACE inhibitors, ARBs, or aldosterone antagonists.[20]

## HYPERTENSIVE CRISIS

**Hypertensive crisis** is a term used to indicate either a hypertensive urgency or emergency. Hypertensive crisis occurs at systolic BP greater than 180 mm Hg and/or diastolic BP greater than 110 mm Hg. BPs can often be greater than 220/140 mm Hg. The difference between a hypertensive urgency and emergency is the absence or presence of target organ damage.

*Hypertensive urgency* develops over hours to days and does not have clinical evidence of target organ disease. It may not require hospitalization to correct.

*Hypertensive emergencies* have target organ disease and most often require hospitalization for prompt, controlled reduction of BP. If prompt treatment is not obtained, a hypertensive emergency can produce severe problems. These include encephalopathy, intracranial or subarachnoid hemorrhage, heart failure, MI, renal failure, dissecting aortic aneurysm, and retinopathy.[23]

The rate of increase of BP is more important than the absolute value in determining the need for emergency treatment. Patients with chronic hypertension can tolerate much higher BPs than normotensive people. Prompt recognition and management of a hypertensive crisis are essential to decrease the threat to organ function and life.

Hypertensive crisis occurs more often in patients with a history of hypertension who have not adhered to their drug regimens or who have been undermedicated. Rapidly increasing BP can cause shearing of the endothelial surface due to turbulent blood flow within the vessels. This can lead to further vascular damage and the release of additional vasoconstricting substances. A vicious cycle of BP elevation follows, leading to life-threatening damage to target organs.

Hypertensive crisis related to cocaine or crack use is a frequent problem. Other drugs, such as amphetamines, phencyclidine (PCP), and lysergic acid diethylamide (LSD), can also cause hypertensive crisis that may be complicated by drug-induced seizures, stroke, MI, or encephalopathy. Table 32-13 lists causes of hypertensive crisis.

### Clinical Manifestations

A hypertensive emergency is often manifested as *hypertensive encephalopathy*, a syndrome in which a sudden rise in BP is associated with severe headache, nausea, vomiting, seizures, confusion, and coma. The manifestations of encephalopathy are the result of increased cerebral capillary permeability. This leads to cerebral edema and a disruption in cerebral function. On retinal examination, exudates, hemorrhages, and/or papilledema are found (Fig. 32-5).

Renal insufficiency ranging from minor injury to complete renal failure can occur. Rapid cardiac decompensation ranging

**TABLE 32-13 Causes of Hypertensive Crisis**

- Exacerbation of chronic hypertension
- Renovascular hypertension
- Preeclampsia, eclampsia
- Pheochromocytoma
- Drugs (cocaine, amphetamines)
- Monoamine oxidase inhibitors taken with tyramine-containing foods
- Rebound hypertension (from abrupt withdrawal of some antihypertensive drugs such as clonidine [Catapres] or β-blockers)
- Head injury
- Acute aortic dissection

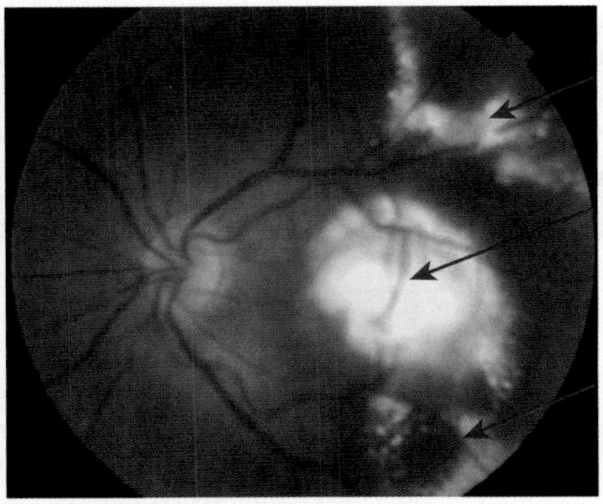

FIG. 32-5 Massive retinal exudates (indicated by *arrows*) from hypertensive retinopathy. To see what a normal retina looks like on ophthalmoscopic examination, see Fig. 20-5 on p. 359. (From Kliegman RM, Behrman RE, Jenson HB, Stanton B: *Nelson textbook of pediatrics,* ed 18, Philadelphia, 2011, Saunders.)

from unstable angina to MI and pulmonary edema is also possible. Patients can have chest pain and dyspnea. Aortic dissection can develop and will cause sudden, excruciating chest and back pain and possibly reduced or absent pulses in the extremities.

Patient assessment is extremely important. Monitor for signs of neurologic deficits, retinal damage, heart failure, pulmonary edema, and renal failure. The neurologic changes are often similar to those related to a stroke. However, a hypertensive crisis does not show focal or lateralizing signs often seen with a stroke. (In a stroke, focal impairments affect a specific region of the body [e.g., weakness in the left arm, right leg]. Lateralizing signs are restricted to one side of the body [e.g., weakness of an arm or leg].)

## NURSING AND INTERPROFESSIONAL MANAGEMENT: HYPERTENSIVE CRISIS

Hypertensive emergencies require hospitalization, IV administration of antihypertensive drugs, and intensive care monitoring.

BP level alone is a poor marker of the seriousness of the patient's condition. It is not the major factor in deciding the treatment for a hypertensive crisis. The link between elevated BP and signs of new or progressive target organ disease determines the seriousness of the situation.

When treating hypertensive emergencies, the mean arterial pressure (MAP) is often used instead of BP readings to guide and evaluate drug therapy. MAP is calculated as follows:

$$MAP = (SBP + 2\,DBP) \div 3$$

The initial goal is to decrease MAP by no more than 20% to 25%, or to decrease MAP to 110 to 115 mm Hg. If the patient is clinically stable, drugs can be titrated to gradually lower BP over the next 24 hours. Lowering the BP too quickly or too much may decrease cerebral, coronary, or renal perfusion. This could cause a stroke, MI, or renal failure.

Special circumstances include patients with aortic dissection. These patients should have their SBP lowered to less than 100 to 120 mm Hg as soon as possible (if tolerated). Another exception is patients with acute ischemic stroke, in whom BP is lowered to allow the use of thrombolytic agents. Last, an elevated BP in the immediate poststroke period may be a compensatory response to improve cerebral perfusion to ischemic brain tissue. There is no clear evidence supporting the use of antihypertensive drugs in these patients[10] (see Chapter 57).

### CHECK YOUR PRACTICE

A 68-yr-old male patient is admitted to the emergency department with a BP 210/118 and complaining of a severe headache and vomiting. You know that his BP is dangerously high and must be lowered.

- Calculate his MAP.
- What treatments would you expect to be ordered for this patient?

IV drugs used for hypertensive emergencies include vasodilators (e.g., sodium nitroprusside, fenoldopam [Corlopam], nicardipine [Cardene]), adrenergic inhibitors (e.g., phentolamine [Regitine], labetalol, esmolol [Brevibloc]), and the calcium channel blocker clevidipine (Cleviprex)[24] (Table 32-7). Sodium nitroprusside is the most effective IV drug to treat hypertensive emergencies. Oral agents may be given along with IV drugs to help make an earlier transition to long-term therapy.

**DRUG ALERT Labetalol**

- Instruct patient not to discontinue drug abruptly.
- Abrupt cessation may precipitate angina or heart failure.

Antihypertensive drugs given IV have a rapid (within seconds to minutes) onset of action. Assess the patient's BP and HR every 2 to 3 minutes during the initial administration of these drugs. Use an arterial line (see Chapter 65) or an automated, noninvasive BP machine to monitor the BP. Titrate the drug according to MAP or BP as ordered. Monitor the ECG for dysrhythmias and signs of ischemia or MI. Use extreme caution in treating the patient with CAD or cerebrovascular disease. Measure urine output hourly to assess renal perfusion. Patients receiving IV antihypertensive drugs may be restricted to bed. Getting up (e.g., to use the commode) may cause severe cerebral ischemia and fainting.

Ongoing assessment is essential to evaluate the effectiveness of these drugs and the patient's response to therapy. Frequent neurologic checks, including level of consciousness, pupillary size and reaction, and movement of extremities, help detect any changes in the patient's condition. Monitor cardiac, pulmonary, and renal systems for decompensation caused by the severe elevation in BP (e.g., angina, pulmonary edema, renal failure).

Hypertensive urgencies usually do not require IV drugs but can be managed with oral agents. The patient with hypertensive urgency may not need hospitalization but will require follow-up. The oral drugs most frequently used for hypertensive urgencies are captopril, labetalol, clonidine (Catapres), and amlodipine (Norvasc)[24] (Table 32-7). The disadvantage of oral drugs is the inability to regulate the dosage moment to moment, as can be done with IV drugs. If a patient with hypertensive urgency is not hospitalized, outpatient follow-up care should be arranged within 24 hours.

Once the hypertensive crisis is resolved, it is important to determine the cause. The patient will need appropriate management and teaching to avoid future crises.

**DRUG ALERT Clonidine (Catapres)**

- Instruct patient to change positions slowly to limit orthostatic hypotension.
- Hazardous activities should be avoided since the drug may cause drowsiness.
- Drug should not be stopped abruptly as this may cause rebound hypertension.

Not every patient with an elevated BP and no target organ disease will require emergent drug therapy or hospitalization. Allowing the patient to sit for 20 or 30 minutes in a quiet environment may significantly reduce BP. Oral drugs may be started or adjusted. Additional nursing interventions include encouraging the patient to verbalize any concerns or fears, answering questions regarding hypertension, and eliminating any adverse stimuli (e.g., excess noise) in the patient's environment.

## CASE STUDY

### *Primary Hypertension*

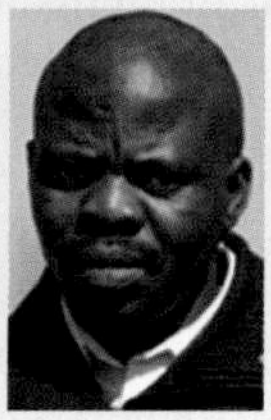

(©iStockphoto/ Thinkstock)

#### Patient Profile

R.L. is a 45-year-old African American man with no previous history of hypertension. At a screening clinic 2 months ago, his BP was found to be 150/95 mm Hg. His HCP has followed him for the past month. During this time he has been taking hydrochlorothiazide 12.5 mg/day. He is here today for a follow-up visit.

#### Subjective Data

- Father died of stroke at age 60
- Mother is alive but has hypertension and a history of MI
- States that he feels fine and is not a "hyper" person
- Smokes one pack of cigarettes daily for the past 28 yr
- Drinks 1-2 six-packs of beer on most Friday and Saturday nights
- Has heard that BP drugs "make you impotent"

#### Objective Data

***Physical Examination***

- Mild retinopathy (retinal arteriolar narrowing on ophthalmoscopic examination)
- BP: 166/108 mm Hg (average of two readings, 2 min apart)
- Sustained apical impulse palpable in the fourth intercostal space just lateral to the midclavicular line

***Diagnostic Studies***

- ECG: mild left ventricular hypertrophy
- Urinalysis: protein 30 mg/dL (0.3 g/L)
- Serum creatinine level: 1.6 mg/dL (141 mmol/L)

#### Interprofessional Care

- Low-sodium, DASH diet
- Hydrochlorothiazide 25 mg/day PO (dose increase)
- Nicardipine (Cardene) sustained release 30 mg PO bid (second drug added)

#### Discussion Questions

1. What risk factors for hypertension does R.L. have?
2. What evidence of target organ disease is present?
3. ***Patient-Centered Care:*** What misconceptions about hypertension should be corrected?
4. ***Priority Decision:*** Based on the assessment data, what are the priority nursing diagnoses and interventions? What are the collaborative problems?
5. ***Evidence-Based Practice:*** R.L. wants to know the most effective nonpharmacologic strategies to lower his BP. What would you tell him?
6. ***Patient-Centered Care:*** What lifestyle preferences should be addressed in R.L's plan of care?
7. ***Teamwork and Collaboration:*** What referrals may be indicated for this patient?
8. ***Safety:*** What safety precautions should be considered when changing antihypertensive drugs for R.L.?
9. ***Quality Improvement:*** What outcomes would indicate that interprofessional care was successful?

Answers available at *http://evolve.elsevier.com/Lewis/medsurg.*

## BRIDGE TO NCLEX EXAMINATION

The number of the question corresponds to the same-numbered outcome at the beginning of the chapter.

1. Which BP-regulating mechanism(s) can result in the development of hypertension if defective *(select all that apply)*?
   **a.** Release of norepinephrine
   **b.** Secretion of prostaglandins
   **c.** Stimulation of the sympathetic nervous system
   **d.** Stimulation of the parasympathetic nervous system
   **e.** Activation of the renin-angiotensin-aldosterone system
2. While obtaining subjective assessment data from a patient with hypertension, the nurse recognizes that a modifiable risk factor for the development of hypertension is
   **a.** a low-calcium diet.
   **b.** excessive alcohol intake.
   **c.** a family history of hypertension.
   **d.** consumption of a high-protein diet.
3. In teaching a patient with hypertension about controlling the illness, the nurse recognizes that
   **a.** all patients with elevated BP require medication.
   **b.** obese persons must achieve a normal weight to lower BP.
   **c.** it is not necessary to limit salt in the diet if taking a diuretic.
   **d.** lifestyle modifications are indicated for all persons with elevated BP.
4. A *priority* consideration in the management of the older adult with hypertension is to
   **a.** prevent primary hypertension from converting to secondary hypertension.
   **b.** recognize that the older adult is less likely to adhere to the drug therapy regimen than a younger adult.
   **c.** ensure that the patient receives larger initial doses of antihypertensive drugs because of impaired absorption.
   **d.** use careful technique in assessing the BP of the patient because of the possible presence of an auscultatory gap.
5. A patient with newly discovered high BP has an average reading of 158/98 mm Hg after 3 months of exercise and diet modifications. Which management strategy will be a *priority* for this patient?
   **a.** Medication will be required because the BP is still not at goal.
   **b.** BP monitoring should continue for another 3 months to confirm a diagnosis of hypertension.
   **c.** Lifestyle changes are less important, since they were not effective, and medications will be started.
   **d.** More vigorous changes in the patient's lifestyle are needed for a longer time before starting medications.

6. A patient is admitted to the hospital in hypertensive emergency (BP 244/142 mm Hg). Sodium nitroprusside is started to treat the elevated BP. Which management strategy(ies) would be *most* appropriate for this patient *(select all that apply)*?
   **a.** Measuring hourly urine output
   **b.** Decreasing the MAP by 50% within the first hour
   **c.** Continuous BP monitoring with an arterial line
   **d.** Maintaining bed rest and providing tranquilizers to lower the BP
   **e.** Assessing the patient for signs and symptoms of heart failure and changes in mental status

1. a, c, e, 2. b, 3. d, 4. d, 5. a, 6. a, c, e

For rationales to these answers and even more NCLEX review questions, visit *http://evolve.elsevier.com/Lewis/medsurg.*

## EVOLVE WEBSITE

http://evolve.elsevier.com/Lewis/medsurg
**Review Questions (Online Only)**
**Key Points**
**Answer Keys for Questions**
- Rationales for Bridge to NCLEX Examination Questions
- Answer Guidelines for Case Study on p. 700

**Student Case Study**
- Patient With Hypertension and Stroke

**Conceptual Care Map Creator**
**Audio Glossary**
**Content Updates**

## REFERENCES


1. Centers for Disease Control and Prevention: High blood pressure facts. Retrieved from *www.cdc.gov/bloodpressure/facts.htm.*
2. Go AS, Mozaffarian D, Roger VL, et al: Heart disease and stroke statistics—2014 update: a report from the American Heart Association, *Circulation* 129:e28, 2013.
3. US Department of Health and Human Services: Healthy People 2020. Retrieved from *www.healthypeople.gov.*
4. Nwankwo R, Yoon SS, Burt V, et al: *Hypertension among adults in the United States*, 2011–2012, NCHS Data Brief, 133, Hyattsville, Md: National Center for Health Statistics.
5. Johnson N, Hayes L, Hoo E, et al: CDC National Health Report: leading causes of morbidity and mortality and associated behavioral risk and protective factors—United States, 2005-2013, *MMWR Surveillance Summary*, 2014.
*6. James PA, Oparil S, Carter BL, et al: 2014 Evidence-based guideline for the management of high blood pressure in adults: report from the panel members appointed to the Eighth Joint National Committee (JNC 8), *JAMA* 311:507, 2014.
*7. National Heart, Lung, and Blood Institute. Landmark NIH study shows intensive blood pressure management may save lives. Retrieved from *www.nhlbi.nih.gov/news/press-releases/2015/landmark-nih-study-shows-intensive-blood-pressure-management-may-save-lives.*
*8. Mosca L, Benjamin EJ, Berra K, et al: Effectiveness-based guidelines for the prevention of cardiovascular disease in women—2011 update, *Circulation* 123:1243, 2011.
9. Flammer AJ, Anderson T, Celermajer DS, et al: The assessment of endothelial function: from research into clinical practice, *Circulation* 126:6, 2012.
*10. National Heart, Lung, and Blood Institute: *Seventh report of the Joint National Committee on Detection, Evaluation, and Treatment of High Blood Pressure (JNC-7), NIH Publication No. 04-5230*, Bethesda, Md, 2004, The Institute. Retrieved from *www.nhlbi.nih.gov/health-pro/guidelines/current/hypertension-jnc-7/complete-report.*
*11. Piper MA, Evans CV, Burda BU, et al: Diagnostic and predictive accuracy of blood pressure screening methods with consideration of rescreening intervals: a systematic review for the U.S. Preventive Services Task Force, *Ann Intern Med* 162:192, 2015.
12. Liu F, He J, Gu D, et al: Associations of endothelial system genes with blood pressure changes and hypertension incidence: the GenSalt study, *Am J Hypertens* 27:1370, 2014.
13. National Heart, Lung, and Blood Institute: *Your guide to lowering your blood pressure with DASH, NIH Pub No 06-5834*, Bethesda, Md, 2006. Retrieved from *http://catalog.nhlbi.nih.gov/catalog/product/In-Brief-Your-Guide-to-Lowering-Your-Blood-Pressure-With-DASH/06-5834.*
*14. Weber MA, Schiffrin EL, White WB, et al: Clinical practice guidelines for the management of hypertension in the community: a statement by the American Society of Hypertension and the International Society of Hypertension, *J Hypertens* 32:1, 2014.
15. American Heart Association: What are the symptoms of high blood pressure? Retrieved from *www.heart.org/HEARTORG/Conditions/HighBloodPressure/SymptomsDiagnosisMonitoringofHighBloodPressure/What-are-the-Symptoms-of-High-Blood-Pressure_UCM_301871_Article.jsp.*
*16. Haskell WL, Lee I-M, Pate RR, et al: Physical activity and public health: updated recommendations for adults from the American College of Sports Medicine and the American Heart Association, *Circulation* 116:1081, 2007.
*17. Nelson ME, Rejeski WJ, Blair SN, et al: Physical activity and public health in older adults: recommendation from the American College of Sports Medicine and the American Heart Association, *Circulation* 116:1094, 2007. (Classic)
18. Rozanski A, Blumenthal JA, Davidson KW, et al: The epidemiology, pathophysiology, and management of psychosocial risk factors in cardiac practice, *J Am Coll Cardiol* 45:637, 2005. (Classic)
*19. Aronow WS, Fleg JL, Pepine CJ, et al: ACCF/AHA 2011 expert consensus document on hypertension in the elderly, *J Am Coll Cardiol* 57:2037, 2011.
20. Lehne RA: *Pharmacology for nursing care*, ed 8, St Louis, 2013, Saunders.
*21. Krum H, Schlaich M, Sobotka P, et al: Percutaneous renal denervation in patients with treatment-resistant hypertension: final 3-year report of the Simplicity HTN-1 study, *Lancet* 383:9917, 2014.
*22. Martin B: AACN practice alert: non-invasive blood pressure monitoring, 2010. Retrieved from *www.aacn.org/wd/practice/docs/practicealerts/non-invasive-bp-monitoring.pdf?menu=aboutus.*
23. Rafey MA: Hypertension, Cleveland Clinic Center for Continuing Education. Retrieved from *www.clevelandclinicmeded.com/medicalpubs/diseasemanagement/nephrology/arterial-hypertension.*
24. Smithburger PL, Kane-Gill SL, Nestor BL, et al: Recent advances in the treatment of hypertensive emergencies, *Crit Care Nurse* 30:24, 2010.

*Evidence-based information for clinical practice.

# 33

# Coronary Artery Disease and Acute Coronary Syndrome

*Rose Shaffer and Linda Bucher*

*The best and most beautiful things in the world*
*cannot be seen or even touched—they must be felt with the heart.*

***Helen Keller***

http://evolve.elsevier.com/Lewis/medsurg/

## LEARNING OUTCOMES

1. Relate the etiology and pathophysiology of coronary artery disease (CAD) and acute coronary syndrome (ACS) to the clinical manifestations of each disorder.
2. Describe the nursing role in the promotion of therapeutic lifestyle changes in patients at risk for CAD.
3. Differentiate the precipitating factors, clinical manifestations, interprofessional care, and nursing management of the patient with CAD and chronic stable angina.
4. Explain the clinical manifestations, diagnostic studies, complications, and interprofessional care of the patient with ACS.
5. Evaluate commonly used drug therapy in treating patients with CAD and ACS.
6. Prioritize key components to include in the rehabilitation of patients recovering from ACS and coronary revascularization procedures.
7. Differentiate the precipitating factors, clinical presentation, and interprofessional care of patients who are at risk for or have experienced sudden cardiac death.

## KEY TERMS

acute coronary syndrome (ACS), p. 718
angina, p. 712
atherosclerosis, p. 702
chronic stable angina, p. 712
collateral circulation, p. 703
coronary artery disease (CAD), p. 702
coronary revascularization, p. 717
metabolic equivalent (MET), p. 731
myocardial infarction (MI), p. 719
percutaneous coronary intervention (PCI), p. 717
Prinzmetal's angina, p. 713
silent ischemia, p. 713
stent, p. 717
sudden cardiac death (SCD), p. 733
unstable angina (UA), p. 719

Cardiovascular disease (CVD) is the major cause of death in the United States. Coronary artery disease (CAD) is the most common type of CVD and accounts for approximately 1.1 million of these deaths.[1] Patients with CAD can be asymptomatic or develop chronic stable angina (or chest pain). CAD may also evolve to more serious conditions of unstable angina (UA) and myocardial infarction (MI), which are called acute coronary syndrome (ACS). This chapter discusses the care of patients with CAD and ACS.

## CORONARY ARTERY DISEASE

**Coronary artery disease (CAD)** is a type of blood vessel disorder that is included in the general category of atherosclerosis. The term **atherosclerosis** comes from two Greek words: *athere,* meaning "fatty mush," and *skleros,* meaning "hard." This combination means that atherosclerosis begins as soft deposits of fat that harden with age. Consequently, atherosclerosis is commonly referred to as "hardening of the arteries." Although this disease can occur in any artery in the body, the *atheromas* (fatty deposits) prefer the coronary arteries. The terms *arteriosclerotic heart disease, cardiovascular heart disease, ischemic heart disease, coronary heart disease,* and *CAD* all describe this disease process.

### Etiology and Pathophysiology

Atherosclerosis is the major cause of CAD. It is characterized by lipid deposits within the intima of the artery. Endothelial injury and inflammation play a central role in the development of atherosclerosis.

The endothelium (inner lining of the vessel wall) is normally nonreactive to platelets and leukocytes, as well as coagulation, fibrinolytic, and complement factors. However, the endothelial lining can be injured as a result of tobacco use, hyperlipidemia, hypertension, toxins, diabetes, hyperhomocysteinemia, and infection causing a local inflammatory response[2] (Fig. 33-1, *A*).

C-reactive protein (CRP), a protein produced by the liver, is a nonspecific marker of inflammation. It is increased in many patients with CAD[3] (see Table 31-6). CRP levels rise when there

Reviewed by Marylee Bressie, RN, DNP, CCRN, CCNS, CEN, Core Faculty/Nurse Planner, Department of Nursing, School of Public Service Leadership, Capella University, Minneapolis, Minnesota; Christina D. Keller, RN, MSN-Ed, Instructor, Clinical Simulation Center, Radford University, Radford, Virginia; and Bonnie Tong, MSN, ACNP-BC, Nurse Practitioner, Mount Sinai Hospital, New York, New York.

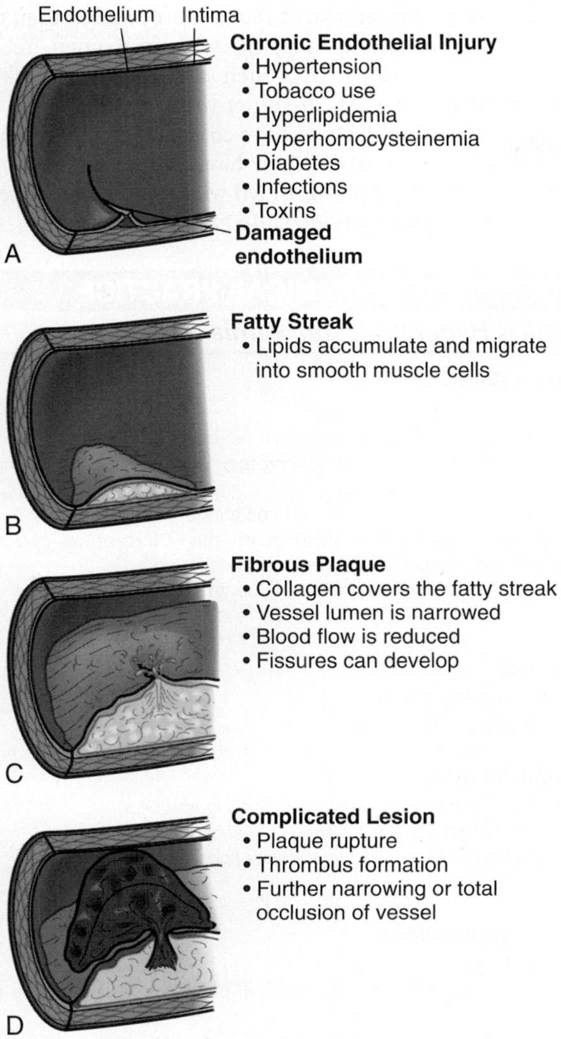


**FIG. 33-1** Pathogenesis of atherosclerosis. **A,** Damaged endothelium. **B,** Fatty streak and lipid core formation. **C,** Fibrous plaque. Raised plaques are visible: some are yellow; others are white. **D,** Complicated lesion: thrombus is red; collagen is blue. Plaque is complicated by red thrombus deposition.

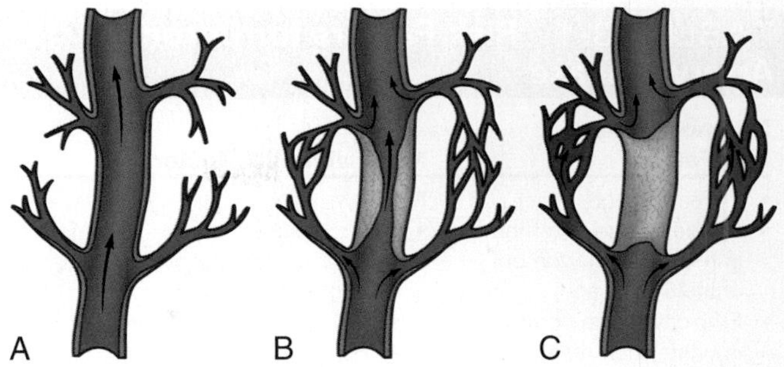


**FIG. 33-2** Vessel occlusion with collateral circulation. **A,** Open, functioning coronary artery. **B,** Partial coronary artery closure with collateral circulation being established. **C,** Total coronary artery occlusion with collateral circulation bypassing the occlusion to supply blood to the myocardium.

is systemic inflammation. Chronic elevations of CRP are linked with unstable plaques and the oxidation of low-density lipoprotein (LDL) cholesterol.

**Developmental Stages.** CAD is a progressive disease that develops over many years. When it becomes symptomatic, the disease process is usually well advanced. The stages of development in atherosclerosis are (1) fatty streak, (2) fibrous plaque, and (3) complicated lesion.

***Fatty Streak.*** *Fatty streaks,* the earliest lesions of atherosclerosis, are characterized by lipid-filled smooth muscle cells. As streaks of fat develop within the smooth muscle cells, a yellow tinge appears. Fatty streaks can be seen in the coronary arteries by age 20 and involve an increasing amount of surface area as one ages. Treatment that lowers LDL cholesterol may reverse this process (Fig. 33-1, *B*).

***Fibrous Plaque.*** The *fibrous plaque* stage is the beginning of progressive changes in the endothelium of the arterial wall. These changes can appear in the coronary arteries by age 30 and increase with age.

Normally the endothelium repairs itself immediately. This does not occur in the person with CAD. LDLs and growth factors from platelets stimulate smooth muscle proliferation and thickening of the arterial wall. Once endothelial injury has taken place, lipoproteins (carrier proteins within the bloodstream) transport cholesterol and other lipids into the arterial intima. Collagen covers the fatty streak and forms a fibrous plaque with a grayish or whitish appearance. These plaques can form on one portion of the artery or in a circular fashion involving the entire lumen. The borders can be smooth or irregular with rough, jagged edges. The result is a narrowing of the vessel lumen and a reduction in blood flow to the distal tissues (Fig. 33-1, *C*).

***Complicated Lesion.*** The final stage in the development of the atherosclerotic lesion is the most dangerous. As the fibrous plaque grows, continued inflammation can result in plaque instability, ulceration, and rupture. Once the integrity of the artery's inner wall is compromised, platelets accumulate in large numbers, leading to a thrombus. The thrombus may adhere to the wall of the artery, leading to further narrowing or total occlusion of the artery. Activation of the exposed platelets causes expression of glycoprotein IIb/IIIa receptors that bind fibrinogen. This, in turn, leads to further platelet aggregation and adhesion, further enlarging the thrombus. At this stage the plaque is referred to as a *complicated lesion* (Fig. 33-1, *D*).

**Collateral Circulation.** Normally some arterial anastomoses or connections, called **collateral circulation**, exist within the coronary circulation. Two factors contribute to the growth and extent of collateral circulation: (1) inherited predisposition to develop new blood vessels *(angiogenesis)* and (2) presence of chronic ischemia. When plaque blocks the normal flow of blood through a coronary artery and the resulting *ischemia* is chronic, increased collateral circulation develops (Fig. 33-2). When blockages in coronary arteries occur slowly over a long period, there is a greater chance of collateral circulation developing, and the heart muscle may still receive an adequate amount of blood and $O_2$.

However, with rapid-onset CAD (e.g., familial hypercholesterolemia) or coronary spasm, time is inadequate for collateral development. Consequently, a reduced blood flow results in a more severe ischemia or infarction.

## Risk Factors for Coronary Artery Disease

Risk factors are characteristics or conditions that are linked with a high incidence of a disease. Many risk factors have been associated with CAD. They are grouped as nonmodifiable and modifiable (Table 33-1). *Nonmodifiable risk factors* are age, gender, ethnicity, family history, and genetics. *Modifiable risk factors* include elevated serum lipids, elevated BP, tobacco use,

TABLE 33-1 **Risk Factors for Coronary Artery Disease**

| Nonmodifiable Risk Factors | Modifiable Risk Factors |
|---|---|
| • Increasing age<br>• Gender (more common in men than in women until 75 yr of age)<br>• Ethnicity (more common in white men than in African Americans)<br>• Genetic predisposition and family history of heart disease | **Major**<br>• Serum lipids:<br>  • Total cholesterol >200 mg/dL<br>  • Triglycerides ≥150 mg/dL*<br>  • LDL cholesterol >160 mg/dL<br>  • HDL cholesterol <40 mg/dL in men or <50 mg/dL in women*<br>• BP ≥140/90 mm Hg*<br>• Diabetes<br>• Tobacco use<br>• Physical inactivity<br>• Obesity: Waist circumference ≥102 cm (≥40 in) in men and ≥88 cm (≥35 in) in women*<br>**Contributing**<br>• Fasting blood glucose ≥100 mg/dL*<br>• Psychosocial risk factors (e.g., depression, hostility, anger, stress)<br>• Elevated homocysteine levels |

*Three or more of these risk factors meet the criteria for metabolic syndrome (discussed in Chapter 40).

physical inactivity, obesity, diabetes, metabolic syndrome, psychologic states, and elevated homocysteine level.

### Nonmodifiable Risk Factors

***Age, Gender, and Ethnicity.*** The incidence of CAD is highest among middle-aged men. After age 75, the incidence of serious heart events in men and women equalizes, although CAD causes more deaths in women than men.[1] Additionally, CAD is present in African American women at rates higher than those of their white counterparts.[4] (See Cultural & Ethnic Health Disparities box for additional differences in CAD among ethnic groups.)

## CULTURAL & ETHNIC HEALTH DISPARITIES

### *Coronary Artery Disease*

**Whites**
- White men have the highest incidence of coronary artery disease (CAD).

**African Americans**
- African Americans have an early age of onset of CAD.
- Deaths from cardiovascular diseases (e.g., CAD, stroke) are higher for African Americans than for the overall population in the United States.
- African American women have a higher incidence and death rate related to CAD than white women.

**Native Americans**
- Native Americans die from heart disease earlier than expected. Mortality rates for those under 65 yr old are twice as high as those of other Americans.
- Major modifiable cardiovascular risk factors for Native Americans are tobacco use, hypertension, obesity, and diabetes.

**Hispanics**
- Hispanics have slightly lower rates of CAD than either non-Hispanic whites or African Americans.
- Hispanics have lower death rates from CAD than non-Hispanic whites.

Heart disease kills almost 10 times more women than breast cancer and is the leading cause of death in women. Yet most women do not consider CAD their greatest health risk.[4] On average, women with CAD are older than men who have CAD, and women are more likely to have co-morbidities (e.g., hypertension, diabetes). Most women have atypical symptoms of angina rather than symptoms of MI when they experience their first heart event[5] (see Gender Differences box).

## GENETICS IN CLINICAL PRACTICE

### *Familial Hypercholesterolemia*

**Genetic Basis**
- Autosomal dominant disorder
- Mutation in low-density lipoprotein receptor *(LDLR)* gene
- Gene codes for low-density lipoprotein (LDL) receptor that binds to LDLs.
- LDLs are the primary carriers of cholesterol in the blood. By removing LDLs from the bloodstream, the LDL receptors play a critical role in regulating cholesterol levels.
- Exists in both heterozygous (most common) and homozygous forms

**Incidence**
- Heterozygotes: 1 in 500
- Homozygotes: rare

**Genetic Testing**
- Disorder is characterized by elevated serum LDLs.
- Serum lipid profile can be used to measure total cholesterol, triglycerides, LDLs, and high-density lipoproteins (HDLs).
- DNA testing is available.

**Clinical Implications**
- Common genetic disease
- High cholesterol levels are a result of defective function of the LDL receptors.
- Elevated plasma levels of LDLs throughout life
- Develop severe atherosclerosis in early to middle years
- Develop xanthomas
- Treatment strategies include low-fat diet, exercise, and lipid-lowering drugs (e.g., PCSK9 inhibitors).*
- Homozygous familial hypercholesterolemia is much more severe than the heterozygous form. Cholesterol levels may exceed 600 mg/dL in these patients.

*See Table 33-5.

### Genetic Link

Genetic predisposition is an important factor in the occurrence of CAD. Family history is a risk factor for CAD and MI. Often, patients with angina or MI can name a parent or sibling who died of CAD.

The genetic basis of CAD/MI is complex and poorly understood. It is estimated that the genetic contribution to CAD/MI is as high as 40% to 60%. This proportion relates mainly to genes that control known risk factors (e.g., lipid metabolism).[6] (See Genetics in Clinical Practice box.)

### Major Modifiable Risk Factors

***Elevated Serum Lipids.*** An elevated serum lipid level is one of the four most firmly established risk factors for CAD.[7] The risk of CAD is associated with a serum cholesterol level greater than 200 mg/dL (5.2 mmol/L) or a fasting triglyceride level greater than 150 mg/dL (3.7 mmol/L). (See Table 31-6 for normal serum lipid values.)

## GENDER DIFFERENCES

### Coronary Artery Disease and Acute Coronary Syndrome

| Men | Women |
|---|---|
| **Coronary Artery Disease** | |
| • First heart event for men is more often MI than angina.<br>• Men report more typical signs and symptoms of angina and MI.<br>• Men receive more evidence-based therapies (e.g., aspirin, statins, diagnostic catheterization, PCI) when acutely ill from CAD (e.g., MI) than women.<br>• Mortality rates from CAD have decreased more rapidly for men than women. | • Women experience the onset of heart disease approximately 10 yr later than men.<br>• CAD is the leading cause of death for women, regardless of race or ethnicity.<br>• More women with MI (compared to men with MI) die of sudden cardiac death before reaching the hospital.<br>• Before menopause, women have higher HDL cholesterol levels and lower LDL cholesterol levels than men. After menopause LDL levels increase. |
| **Acute Coronary Syndrome** | |
| • After age 75, the incidence of MI in men and women equalizes.<br>• Men present more frequently than women with an acute MI as the first manifestation of CAD.<br>• Men develop greater collateral circulation than women.<br>• Men have larger-diameter coronary arteries than women. Vessel diameter is inversely related to risk of restenosis after interventions.<br>• Standard screening for risk of sudden cardiac death (e.g., EP studies) is more predictive in men. | • Women are older than men when seen with first MI and often have more co-morbidities.<br>• Women seek medical care later in the CAD process and often are more ill on presentation than men.<br>• First heart event for women is more often unstable angina than MI.<br>• Once a woman reaches menopause, her risk for an MI quadruples.<br>• Fewer women than men manifest the "classic" signs and symptoms of UA or MI.<br>• Fatigue is often the first symptom of ACS in women.<br>• Women experience more "silent" MIs compared with men.<br>• Among those who have an MI, women are more likely to suffer a fatal heart event within 1 yr than men.<br>• Women report more disability after a heart event than men.<br>• Women who have coronary artery bypass graft surgery have a higher mortality rate and more complications after surgery than men. |

*ACS,* Acute coronary syndrome; *CAD,* coronary artery disease; *EP,* electrophysiology; *HDL,* high-density lipoprotein; *LDL,* low-density lipoprotein; *PCI,* percutaneous coronary intervention, *UA,* unstable angina.

For lipids to be used and transported by the body, they must become soluble in blood by combining with proteins. Lipids combine with proteins to form lipoproteins. Lipoproteins are vehicles for fat mobilization and transport and vary in composition. Three major lipoproteins are high-density lipoproteins (HDLs), LDLs, and very-low-density lipoproteins (VLDLs).

HDLs contain more protein by weight and fewer lipids than any other lipoprotein. HDLs carry lipids away from arteries and to the liver for metabolism. This process of HDL transport prevents lipid accumulation within the arterial walls. Therefore high serum HDL levels are desirable and lower the risk of CAD.

There are several types of HDLs. They differ by their density and apolipoprotein composition. Apolipoproteins are found on lipoproteins and activate enzyme or receptor sites that promote the removal of fat from plasma. Several types of apolipoproteins exist (e.g., apo A-I, apo B-100, apo C-I). Women have more apo A-I than men, and premenopausal women have HDL levels approximately three times greater than men. This is thought to be related to the protective effects of natural estrogen. After menopause, women's HDL levels decrease and quickly near those of men. In general, HDL levels are higher in women, decrease with age, and are low in individuals with CAD. Physical activity and moderate alcohol intake increase HDL levels.

LDLs contain more cholesterol than any of the lipoproteins and have an attraction for arterial walls. VLDLs contain both cholesterol and triglycerides and may deposit cholesterol directly on the walls of arteries. Elevated LDL levels correlate closely with an increased incidence of atherosclerosis and CAD. Therefore low serum LDL levels are desirable.[7]

Certain diseases (e.g., type 2 diabetes, chronic kidney disease), drugs (e.g., corticosteroids, hormone therapy), and genetic disorders have been associated with elevated triglyceride levels. Lifestyle factors that can contribute to elevated triglycerides include high alcohol intake, high intake of refined carbohydrates and simple sugars, and physical inactivity. When a high triglyceride level is combined with a high LDL level, a smaller, denser LDL particle is formed, which favors deposition on arterial walls. People with insulin resistance often have this pattern.

Guidelines for treating elevated LDL cholesterol are based on a person's 10-year and lifetime risk for having heart disease or stroke. The following data generate a risk score: (1) age, (2) gender, (3) race, (4) use of tobacco, (5) diabetes, (6) systolic BP, (7) diastolic BP, (8) use of BP drugs, (9) total cholesterol level, and (10) HDL cholesterol level.[8] A 10-year risk calculator is available at *http://www.cvriskcalculator.com/* as well as for smartphones (e.g., ASCVD Risk Estimator app).

In general, individuals with no or only one risk factor are considered at low risk for the development of CAD, and their LDL goal is less than 160 mg/dL (4.14 mmol/L). Those at very high risk for developing CAD have multiple risk factors. They have an LDL goal of less than 70 mg/dL (1.8 mmol/L).[7]

***Hypertension.*** The second major risk factor in CAD is hypertension, which is defined as a BP greater than 140/90 mm Hg. For people older than 60 years, a goal BP of less than 150/90 mm Hg has been recommended to prevent stroke, CVD, and heart failure.[9] Newer findings recommend a goal of less than 120/80 mm Hg.[10] Hypertension increases the risk of death from CAD 10-fold in all people. In postmenopausal women, hypertension is associated with a higher incidence of CAD than in men and premenopausal women.

BP is classified as (1) normal (BP less than 120/80 mm Hg), (2) *prehypertension* (BP of 120 to 139/80 to 89 mm Hg), (3) stage 1 hypertension (140 to 159/90 to 99 mm Hg), and (4) stage 2 hypertension (BP greater than or equal to 160/100 mm Hg).[11] The cause of hypertension in 90% of those affected is unknown, but it is usually controllable with drugs and/or diet. Therapeutic lifestyle changes should begin in people with prehypertension. Those with stage 1 or 2 hypertension often require more than one drug to reach therapeutic goals (see Table 32-7). Teach all people with elevated systolic or diastolic BP the importance of achieving and maintaining target BP goals.

The stress of an elevated BP increases the rate of atherosclerosis. This relates to the shearing stress that causes endothelial injury. Atherosclerosis, in turn, causes narrowed, thickened arterial walls and decreases the distensibility and elasticity of vessels. More force is required to pump blood through diseased arteries. This increased force is reflected in a higher BP. This added workload results in left ventricular (LV) hypertrophy and decreased stroke volume with each contraction. Salt intake positively correlates with elevated BP, adding volume and increasing systemic vascular resistance (SVR) to the heart's workload. (See Chapter 32 for a complete discussion of hypertension.)

***Tobacco Use.*** A third major risk factor in CAD is tobacco use. The risk of developing CAD is two to six times higher in those who smoke tobacco or use smokeless tobacco than in those who do not. Further, tobacco smoking decreases estrogen levels, placing premenopausal women at greater risk for CAD. Risk is proportional to the number of cigarettes smoked.

Nicotine in tobacco smoke causes catecholamine (i.e., epinephrine, norepinephrine) release. These neurohormones cause an increased heart rate (HR), peripheral vasoconstriction, and increased BP. These changes increase the heart's workload. Tobacco smoke is also related to an increase in LDL level, a decrease in HDL level, and release of toxic $O_2$ radicals. All of these add to vessel inflammation and thrombosis.

Carbon monoxide, found in tobacco smoke, affects the $O_2$-carrying capacity of hemoglobin by reducing the sites available for $O_2$ transport. Thus the effects of an increased cardiac workload and the $O_2$-depleting effect of carbon monoxide significantly decrease the $O_2$ available to the heart muscle. There is also some indication that carbon monoxide is a chemical irritant and causes injury to the endothelium.

The benefits of smoking cessation are dramatic and almost immediate. CAD mortality rates drop to those of nonsmokers within 12 months. However, nicotine is highly addictive, and often intensive intervention is needed to assist people to quit. Individual and group counseling, nicotine replacement therapy, smoking cessation drugs (e.g., bupropion [Zyban], varenicline [Chantix]), and hypnosis are examples of smoking cessation strategies. (See Chapter 10, Tables 10-4 through 10-6 for information on smoking cessation.)

Chronic exposure to environmental tobacco (secondhand) smoke also increases the risk of CAD.[7] People who live in the same house as the person who smokes should encourage that person to quit. This reinforces the person's effort and decreases the risk of ongoing exposure to environmental smoke. Pipe and cigar smokers, who often do not inhale, have an increased risk of CAD similar to those exposed to secondhand smoke.

***Physical Inactivity.*** Physical inactivity is the fourth major modifiable risk factor. Physical inactivity implies a lack of adequate physical exercise on a regular basis. An example of health-promoting regular physical activity is brisk walking (3 to 4 miles per hour) for at least 30 minutes five or more times a week.[12]

The mechanism by which physical inactivity predisposes a person to CAD is still unclear. Physically active people have increased HDL levels. Exercise improves thrombolytic activity, thus reducing the risk of clot formation. Exercise may also encourage the development of collateral circulation in the heart.

Exercise training for those who are physically inactive reduces the risk of CAD through more efficient lipid metabolism, increased HDL production, and more efficient $O_2$ extraction by the muscles, thereby decreasing the heart's workload. For individuals with CAD, regular physical activity reduces symptoms, improves functional capacity, and improves other risk factors such as insulin resistance and glucose intolerance.

***Obesity.*** The death rate from CAD is higher in obese individuals. Obesity is defined as a body mass index (BMI) of greater than 30 kg/m$^2$ and a waist circumference more than 40 inches for men and more than 35 inches for women. BMI is a measure of body fat based on height and weight. It can be calculated online *(http://www.nhlbi.nih.gov/health/educational/lose_wt/BMI/bmicalc.htm)*.

The increased risk for CAD is proportional to the degree of obesity. Obese individuals may produce increased levels of LDLs and triglycerides, which are strongly related to atherosclerosis. Obesity is often linked with hypertension and insulin resistance. People who tend to store fat in the abdomen (an "apple" figure) rather than in the hips and buttocks (a "pear" figure) have a higher incidence of CAD (see Table 40-2).

**Contributing Modifiable Risk Factors**

***Diabetes Mellitus.*** The incidence of CAD is two to four times greater among people who have diabetes, even those with well-controlled blood glucose levels, than the general population. The patient with diabetes manifests CAD not only more often but also at an earlier age. There is no age difference between male or female patients with diabetes in the onset of symptoms of CAD. Diabetes virtually eliminates the lower incidence of CAD in premenopausal women.

Undiagnosed diabetes is frequently discovered at the time a person has an MI. The person with diabetes has an increased tendency toward endothelial dysfunction. This may account for the development of fatty streaks in these patients. Patients with diabetes also have changes in lipid metabolism and tend to have high cholesterol and triglyceride levels. Management of diabetes should include lifestyle changes and drug therapy to achieve a glycosylated hemoglobin (A1C or Hb A1C) level of less than 7%.[7]

***Metabolic Syndrome.*** *Metabolic syndrome* refers to a cluster of risk factors for CAD whose underlying pathophysiology may be related to insulin resistance. These risk factors include central obesity, hypertension, abnormal serum lipids, and an elevated fasting blood glucose (see Table 40-11). These interrelated risk factors appear to promote the development of CAD. (Chapter 40 discusses metabolic syndrome.)

***Psychologic States.*** Certain behaviors and lifestyles may contribute to the development of CAD. One type of behavior, referred to as type A, includes perfectionism and a hardworking, driven personality. The type A person often suppresses anger and hostility, has a sense of time urgency, is impatient, and creates stress and tension. This person may be more prone to MIs than a type B person, who is more easygoing, takes upsets in stride, knows personal limitations, takes time to relax, and is not an overachiever. However, the relationship between behaviors and the risk for CAD/MI remains controversial and complex.

Psychologic risk factors thought to increase the risk of CAD include depression, acute and chronic stress (e.g., poverty, serving as a caregiver), anxiety, hostility and anger, and lack of social support.[13,14] In particular, depression is a risk factor for both the development and worsening of CAD. Depressed patients have elevated levels of circulating catecholamines. This may contribute to endothelial injury and inflammation and platelet activation. Higher levels of depression are also associated with an increased number of adverse heart events.[13]

Stressful states can contribute to the development of CAD.[14] Sympathetic nervous system (SNS) stimulation and its effect on the heart are the physiologic mechanisms by which stress predisposes a person to the development of CAD. SNS stimulation causes an increased release of catecholamines (i.e., epinephrine, norepinephrine). This stimulation increases HR and the force of myocardial contraction. Both results increase myocardial $O_2$ demand. Also, stress-induced mechanisms can cause elevated lipid and glucose levels and changes in blood coagulation, which can lead to increased atherosclerosis.

***Homocysteine.*** High blood levels of homocysteine have been linked to an increased risk for CAD and other CVDs.[15] Homocysteine is produced by the breakdown of the essential amino acid methionine, which is found in dietary protein. High homocysteine levels may contribute to atherosclerosis by (1) damaging the inner lining of blood vessels, (2) promoting plaque buildup, and (3) altering the clotting mechanism to make clots more likely to occur.

Research to determine if a decline in homocysteine can reduce the risk of CVD is ongoing. B-complex vitamins ($B_6$, $B_{12}$, folic acid) have been shown to lower blood levels of homocysteine. Generally, a screening test for homocysteine is limited to those suspected of having elevated levels. These include older patients with pernicious anemia or people who develop CAD at an early age.

***Substance Abuse.*** The use of illegal drugs, such as cocaine and methamphetamine, can produce coronary spasm resulting in myocardial ischemia and chest pain. Most patients seen in the emergency department (ED) with drug-induced chest pain are initially indistinguishable from those with CAD. Although MI can occur, these patients often have sinus tachycardia, high BP, angina, and anxiety.[16]

The U.S. Food and Drug Administration (FDA) prohibits the sale of dietary supplements containing ephedrine alkaloids. These compounds should be avoided because they can cause high BP, MI, and stroke.

## NURSING AND INTERPROFESSIONAL MANAGEMENT: CORONARY ARTERY DISEASE

### Health Promotion

The appropriate management of risk factors in CAD may prevent, modify, or slow the progression of the disease. In the United States, there has been a gradual decline in CVD-related deaths over the past 35 years. This relates to people's efforts to become generally healthier, as well as advances in the treatment of CAD. Prevention and early treatment of heart disease must involve a multifaceted approach and must be ongoing throughout the life span.

**Identification of High-Risk Individuals.** Clinical signs of CAD are not apparent in the early stages of the disease. Therefore regardless of the health care setting, it is critical to identify people at risk for CAD. Risk screening involves obtaining a thorough health history. Ask the patient about a family history of heart disease in parents and siblings. Note the presence of any cardiovascular symptoms. Assess environmental factors, such as eating habits, type of diet, and level of exercise, to elicit lifestyle patterns. Include a psychosocial history to determine tobacco use, alcohol intake, recent stressful events (e.g., loss of a spouse), and any negative psychologic states (e.g., anxiety, depression, anger). The place and type of employment provide important information on the kind of activity performed, exposure to pollutants or toxins, and the degree of stress associated with work.

Identify the patient's attitudes and beliefs about health and illness. This information can give you insight to how disease and lifestyle changes may affect the patient. It also can reveal possible misconceptions about heart disease. Knowing the

## EVIDENCE-BASED PRACTICE

### *Translating Research Into Practice*

**Do Cardiac Rehabilitation Programs Improve Outcomes?**

***Clinical Question***

In patients with coronary artery disease (P), do cardiac rehabilitation programs (I) versus usual care (C) reduce readmissions, improve quality of life, and affect mortality rates (O)?

***Synthesis of Best Available Evidence***

- Six Cochrane reviews of randomized controlled trials (RCTs)
- 148 RCTs ($n$ = 93,093) of patients with MI who underwent heart surgery or had chronic heart failure (HF). Cardiac rehabilitation programs may include exercise, healthy lifestyle education, and/or psychologic interventions such as stress reduction counseling. Programs were conducted in supervised centers or home-based. Outcomes included hospital readmission, health-related quality of life, and mortality. Program uptake (attendance or enrollment) and adherence were also determined.
- Participants in exercise-based programs compared to individuals receiving usual care had reduced hospital admissions, improved quality of life, and no increase in short-term mortality.
- Although programs with only education or psychologic interventions had minimal impact on readmissions or mortality, quality of life may be improved.
- Positive changes to program uptake were noted with structured nurse-led contacts, appointments made soon after discharge, and motivational letters.
- Adherence improved with self-monitoring and tailored counseling.
- Home-based and center-based programs were equally effective on outcomes measured with financial costs of the two programs similar.

***Conclusions***

- Patients with HF or after MI or PCI may safely engage in cardiac rehabilitation programs with no increased mortality.
- Cardiac rehabilitation programs may reduce hospital admissions and improve quality of life.

***Implications for Nursing Practice***

1. What strategies may be useful in motivating patients to stay engaged in a program?
2. Why is it important to reinforce the benefits of adhering to a recommended exercise program, and what actions would you take to positively affect adherence?
3. What would you suggest to patients who are not able to travel to a supervised center–based program?

***Reference for Evidence***

Anderson L, Taylor RS: Cardiac rehabilitation for people with heart disease: an overview of Cochrane systematic reviews, *Cochrane Database Syst Rev* 12:CD011273, 2014.

*P*, Patient population of interest; *I*, intervention or area of interest; *C*, comparison of interest or comparison group; *O*, outcomes of interest; *T*, timing (see p. 15).

patient's educational background and health literacy can help to identify teaching needs. If the patient has prescribed drugs, it is important to know the names and dosages and if the patient adheres to the drug regimen.

◆ **Management of High-Risk Individuals.** Recommend preventive measures for all individuals at risk for CAD. Risk factors such as age, gender, ethnicity, and genetics cannot be modified. However, the person with any of these risk factors can still reduce the risk of CAD by controlling the additive effects of modifiable risk factors. For example, a young man with a family history of heart disease can decrease the risk of CAD by maintaining an ideal body weight, getting adequate physical exercise, reducing intake of saturated fats, and avoiding tobacco and illicit drug use.

Encourage people who have modifiable risk factors to make lifestyle changes to reduce their risk of CAD. You can play a major role in teaching health-promoting behaviors (Table 33-2). For highly motivated individuals, knowing how to reduce this risk may be the information they need to get started.

For individuals who are less motivated to take charge of their health, the idea of reducing risk factors may be so remote that they are unable to perceive a threat of CAD. Few people desire to make lifestyle changes, especially in the absence of symptoms. First help these patients to clarify their personal values. Then, discuss risk factors and have them identify their individual risks. This can help patients set realistic goals and choose which risk factor(s) to change first. Some individuals are reluctant to change until they begin to have symptoms or actually suffer an MI. Others, having suffered an MI, may find the idea of changing lifelong habits still unacceptable. Help them identify their choices and respect their final decision.

### ◆ Physical Activity

A physical activity program should be designed to improve physical fitness by following the FITT formula: Frequency (how often), Intensity (how hard), Type (isotonic), and Time (how long). Everyone should aim for at least 30 minutes of moderate physical activity on most days of the week. In addition, adding weight training to an exercise program two days a week can help treat metabolic syndrome and improve muscle strength. Examples of moderate physical activity include brisk walking, hiking, biking, and swimming. Regular physical activity helps with weight reduction, reduces systolic BP, and, in some men more than women, increases HDL cholesterol. The AHA has developed a program to encourage people, especially women, to increase their daily physical activity (My Heart, My Life at *www.startwalkingnow.org*).

### ◆ Nutritional Therapy

*Therapeutic lifestyle changes* are recommended for all people to reduce the risk of CAD by lowering LDL cholesterol. These recommendations emphasize a decrease in saturated fat and cholesterol and an increase in complex carbohydrates (e.g., whole grains, fruit, vegetables) and fiber (Tables 33-3 and 33-4). Fat intake should be about 25% to 35% of total calories, with most coming from mono- and polyunsaturated fats. Red meat, egg yolks, and whole milk products are major sources of saturated fat and cholesterol and should be reduced or

**TABLE 33-2 Patient & Caregiver Teaching**

***Reducing Risk Factors for Coronary Artery Disease***

*Include the following instructions when teaching risk reduction for coronary artery disease.*

| Risk Factor | Health-Promoting Behaviors |
|---|---|
| **Hypertension** | • Monitor home-based BP and obtain regular checkups.<br>• Take prescribed drugs for BP control.<br>• Reduce salt intake.<br>• Stop tobacco use. Avoid exposure to environmental tobacco (secondhand) smoke.<br>• Control or reduce weight.<br>• Perform physical activity daily. |
| **Elevated serum lipids** | • Reduce total fat intake.<br>• Reduce animal (saturated) fat intake.<br>• Take prescribed drugs for lipid reduction.<br>• Adjust total caloric intake to achieve and maintain ideal body weight.<br>• Engage in daily physical activity.<br>• Increase amount of complex carbohydrates, fiber, and vegetable proteins in diet. |
| **Tobacco use*** | • Begin a tobacco cessation program.<br>• Change daily routines associated with tobacco use to reduce desire to smoke.<br>• Substitute other activities for smoking.<br>• Ask caregivers to support efforts to stop smoking.<br>• Avoid exposure to environmental tobacco smoke. |
| **Physical inactivity** | • Develop and maintain at least 30 min of moderate physical activity daily (minimum 5 days a week).<br>• Increase activities to a fitness level. |
| **Psychologic state** | • Increase awareness of behaviors that are harmful to health.<br>• Alter patterns that add to stress (e.g., get up 30 min earlier so that breakfast is not eaten on way to work).<br>• Set realistic goals for self.<br>• Reassess priorities in light of identified risk factors.<br>• Learn effective stress management strategies (see Chapter 6).<br>• Seek professional help if feeling depressed, angry, anxious, etc.<br>• Plan time for adequate rest and sleep (see Chapter 7). |
| **Obesity†** | • Change eating patterns and habits.<br>• Reduce caloric intake to achieve body mass index of 18.5–24.9 kg/m$^2$.<br>• Increase physical activity to increase caloric expenditure.<br>• Avoid fad and crash diets, which are not effective over time.<br>• Avoid large, heavy meals. Consider smaller, more frequent meals. |
| **Diabetes‡** | • Follow the recommended diet.<br>• Control or reduce weight.<br>• Take prescribed drugs for diabetes.<br>• Monitor blood glucose levels regularly. |

*Smoking cessation is discussed in Chapter 10 and Tables 10-4 through 10-6.
†See Chapter 40 for additional health-promoting behaviors.
‡See Chapter 48 for additional health-promoting behaviors.

**TABLE 33-3 Nutritional Therapy**

***Therapeutic Lifestyle Changes Diet***

| Dietary Recommendations | Recommended Daily Intake |
|---|---|
| Combined total fat calories from:<br>• *Saturated fats:* found in fats that are usually solid at room temperature (e.g., bacon, lard, butter, egg yolks) and should be limited)<br>• *Trans fats:* found mainly in foods made with hydrogenated vegetable oils, such as many hard margarines and shortenings<br>• *Monounsaturated fats:* found in greatest amounts in foods from plants including olive, canola, sunflower, and peanut oils<br>• *Polyunsaturated fats:* found in greatest amounts in many kinds of nuts and in foods from plants including safflower, sunflower, corn, soybean, cottonseed oils | 25%-35% of total daily calories (including <7% from saturated fat) |
| Cholesterol | <200 mg |
| Plant stanols or sterols (e.g., margarines, nuts, seeds, legumes, vegetable oils)* | 2 g |
| Dietary fiber* | 10-25 g of soluble fiber |
| Total calories | Only enough calories to reach or maintain a healthy weight |

**Physical Activity**

In addition to diet, teach the patient to get at least 30 minutes of a moderate intensity physical activity, such as brisk walking, on most, and preferably all, days of the week.

Source: U.S. Department of Health and Human Services: Your Guide to Lowering Your Cholesterol with TLC. Retrieved from *www.nhlbi.nih.gov/health/public/heart/chol/chol_tlc.pdf*.
*Diet options for additional lowering of low-density lipoprotein (LDL).

eliminated from diets. If the serum triglyceride level is elevated, alcohol and simple sugars should be reduced or eliminated.

Omega-3 fatty acids reduce the risks associated with CAD when eaten regularly. For individuals without CAD, the AHA recommends eating fatty fish twice a week. Fatty fish such as salmon and tuna contain two types of omega-3 fatty acids: eicosapentaenoic acid (EPA) and docosahexaenoic acid (DHA). Patients with CAD are encouraged to take EPA and DHA supplements with their diet. The AHA also recommends eating tofu and other forms of soybean, canola, walnut, and flaxseed because these products contain alpha-linolenic acid, which becomes omega-3 fatty acid in the body.

Lifestyle changes such as a low-saturated-fat, high-fiber diet; avoidance of tobacco; and increase in physical activity can promote the reversal of CAD and reduce heart events.

## ◆ Lipid-Lowering Drug Therapy

An estimated 31.9 million American adults have cholesterol levels greater than or equal to 240 mg/dL (6.2 mmol/L).[1] Guidelines for treatment of high cholesterol focus on LDL cholesterol. A complete lipid profile is recommended every 5 years beginning at age 20. Guidelines recommend the following groups of people receive statin therapy: (1) patients with known CVD, (2) patients with primary elevations of LDL cholesterol levels greater than or equal to 190 mg/dL (e.g., familial hypercholesterolemia), (3) patients between 40 and 75 years old with diabetes and LDL cholesterol levels between 70 and 189 mg/dL, and (4) patients between 40 and 75 years old with LDL

**TABLE 33-4 Nutritional Therapy**

***Tips to Make Diet and Lifestyle Changes***

**General Tips**

1. Know your calorie needs to achieve and maintain a healthy weight.
2. Know the calorie content of the foods and beverages you eat.
3. Track your weight, physical activity, and calorie intake.
4. Prepare and eat smaller, more frequent meals.
5. Track your activities and, whenever possible, decrease sedentary activities (e.g., watching television, computer time).
6. Incorporate physical movement into daily activities (e.g., take stairs and extra steps whenever possible).
7. Do not smoke or use tobacco products.
8. If you drink alcohol, do so in moderation (i.e., no more than one drink for women or two drinks for men a day).

**Tips Related to Food Choices and Preparation**

1. Use the Nutrition Facts panel on food labels and ingredients list when choosing foods to buy.
2. Use fresh vegetables and fruits in place of canned vegetables and fruits.
3. Replace high-calorie foods with fresh fruits and vegetables.
4. Increase fiber intake by eating beans (legumes), whole-grain products, fruits, and vegetables.
5. Use liquid vegetable oils in place of solid fats.
6. Limit beverages and foods high in added sugars (e.g., sucrose, glucose, fructose, maltose, dextrose, corn syrups, concentrated fruit juice, honey).
7. Choose foods made with whole grains (e.g., whole wheat, oats, rye, barley, brown rice, wild rice, buckwheat).
8. Avoid pastries and high-calorie bakery products (e.g., muffins, doughnuts).
9. Select milk and dairy products that are either fat free or low fat.
10. Reduce salt intake by
    - Comparing the sodium content of similar products (e.g., different brands of tomato sauce) and choosing products with less sodium.
    - Choosing versions of processed foods that are reduced in salt, including cereals, canned products, and baked goods.
    - Limiting condiments (e.g., soy sauce, ketchup).
11. Use lean cuts of meat and remove skin from poultry before cooking or eating.
12. Avoid processed meats that are high in saturated fat and sodium (e.g., deli meats).
13. Grill, bake, or broil fish, meat, and poultry.
14. Incorporate plant-based meat substitutes into recipes (e.g., soy, tofu, quinoa).
15. Consume whole vegetables and fruits in place of juices.

Adapted from Gidding SS, Lichtenstein AH, Faith MS, et al: Implementing American Heart Association pediatric and adult nutrition guidelines, *Circulation* 119:1161, 2009.

cholesterol levels between 70 and 189 mg/dL and a 10-year risk for CVD of at least 7.5%.[8]

Treatment also includes weight loss (if overweight), decreased dietary fat and cholesterol intake, and increased physical activity. Serum lipid levels should be reassessed after 6 weeks of therapy. If they remain elevated, changes in drug therapy (Table 33-5) and additional dietary options (see the Complementary & Alternative Therapies box on the following page) should be considered.

### ◆ Drugs That Restrict Lipoprotein Production

◆ ***HMG-CoA Reductase Inhibitors (Statins).*** The statin drugs are the most widely used lipid-lowering drugs. These drugs inhibit the synthesis of cholesterol in the liver. An unexplained result of the inhibition of cholesterol synthesis is an increase in hepatic LDL receptors. Consequently, the liver is able to remove more

### COMPLEMENTARY & ALTERNATIVE THERAPIES
**Lipid-Lowering Agents**

| Agent | Evidence for Use |
|---|---|
| **Garlic** | Inconsistent scientific evidence for reductions in total cholesterol and low-density lipoproteins (LDLs) over short periods |
| **Flaxseed** | Some evidence for reducing risk of heart disease, diabetes, and stroke |
| **Niacin** | Evidence for increased high-density lipoproteins. Less dramatic reduction of LDLs |
| **Omega-3 fatty acids** | Strong scientific evidence for reduction of triglyceride levels |
| **Psyllium** | Strong scientific evidence for modest reduction in total cholesterol and LDLs |
| **Plant sterols** | Strong scientific evidence for reduction of total cholesterol |
| **Red yeast rice** | Strong scientific evidence for reduction of total cholesterol, LDLs, and triglycerides |
| **Soy** | Strong scientific evidence for moderate reduction in total cholesterol and LDLs |

Source: *www.naturalstandard.com.*

LDLs from the blood. In addition, statins produce a small increase in HDLs and lower CRP levels. Serious adverse effects of these drugs are rare and include liver damage and myopathy that can progress to rhabdomyolysis (breakdown of skeletal muscle). Liver enzymes (e.g., aspartate aminotransferase, alanine aminotransferase) are initially monitored and rechecked with any increase in dosage. Creatine kinase isoenzymes (e.g., CK-MM) should be assessed if symptoms of myopathy (e.g., muscle aches, weakness) occur.

**DRUG ALERT Simvastatin (Zocor)**
- Increased risk for rhabdomyolysis when also used with gemfibrozil (Lopid) or niacin (Niaspan)
- Signs of rhabdomyolysis: ↑ creatine kinase levels, muscle pain

◆ ***Niacin.*** Niacin, a water-soluble B vitamin, is highly effective in lowering LDL and triglyceride levels by interfering with their synthesis. Niacin also increases HDL levels better than many other lipid-lowering drugs. Unfortunately, side effects of this drug are common and may include severe flushing, pruritus, gastrointestinal (GI) symptoms, and orthostatic hypotension.

**DRUG ALERT Niacin (Niaspan)**
- Instruct patient that flushing (especially of face and neck) may occur within 20 minutes after taking drug and may last for 30 to 60 minutes.
- Patient can premedicate with aspirin 30 minutes before taking to reduce flushing.
- Use of extended-release niacin may decrease side effects.

◆ ***Fibric Acid Derivatives.*** The *fibric acid derivatives* (Table 33-5) work by aiding the removal of VLDLs and increasing the production of apolipoproteins A-I and A-II. They are the most effective drugs for lowering triglycerides and increasing HDL levels. They have no effect on LDLs. Although most patients tolerate the drugs well, complaints may include GI irritability. These drugs should be used with caution when combined with statin medications.

**DRUG ALERT Gemfibrozil (Lopid)**
- May increase the risk of bleeding in patients taking warfarin (Coumadin)
- May increase the effects of antihyperglycemic drugs (e.g., repaglinide [Prandin])

### ◆ Drugs That Increase Lipoprotein Removal

◆ ***Bile Acid Sequestrants.*** The major route of elimination of cholesterol is by conversion to bile acids in the liver. Bile-acid sequestrants increase conversion of cholesterol to bile acids and decrease hepatic cholesterol (Table 33-5). The primary effect is a decrease in total cholesterol and LDL levels.

These drugs have been associated with complaints related to taste and a variety of upper and lower GI symptoms. These include belching, heartburn, nausea, abdominal pain, and constipation. The bile-acid sequestrants interfere with absorption of many other drugs (e.g., warfarin, thiazides, thyroid hormones, β-adrenergic blockers [β-blockers]). Separating the time of administration of these drugs from that of other drugs decreases this adverse effect.[17]

◆ ***Proprotein Convertase Subtilisin/Kexin 9 (PCSK9) Inhibitors.*** PCSK9 inhibitors are a new class of cholesterol-lowering drugs (Table 33-5). PCSK9 reduces the number of receptors on the liver that remove LDL cholesterol from the blood. By blocking PCSK9's ability to work, more receptors are available and can get rid of LDL, thus decreasing circulating LDL levels. Evolocumab (Repatha) and alirocumab (Praluent) are two PCSK9 inhibitors. These drugs are used in addition to diet and maximum statin therapy in adults with familial hypercholesterolemia or clinical evidence of atherosclerotic heart disease who need increased lowering of LDL.[18]

◆ **Drugs That Decrease Cholesterol Absorption.** Ezetimibe (Zetia) selectively inhibits the absorption of dietary and biliary cholesterol across the intestinal wall (Table 33-5). It serves as an adjunct to dietary changes, especially in patients with primary hypercholesterolemia. When it is combined with a statin (e.g., ezetimibe and simvastatin [Vytorin]), even greater reductions in LDLs are found.

Drug therapy for hyperlipidemia often continues for a lifetime. New combination drug therapy (e.g., atorvastatin/ezetimibe [Liptruzet]) is available and may be considered. Concurrent diet modification is essential to reduce the need for drug therapy. The patient must fully understand the rationale and goals of treatment, as well as the safety and side effects of lipid-lowering drugs.

### ◆ Antiplatelet Therapy

Aspirin is recommended for most people at risk for CVD. Low-dose aspirin (81 mg) is recommended for adults 50 to 59 years old who have a calculated 10-year CVD risk of 10% or more, are not at increased risk for bleeding (e.g., history of GI bleeding), have a life expectancy of at least 10 years, and are willing to take low-dose aspirin for at least 10 years. For adults 60 to 69 years old who have a calculated 10-year CVD risk of 10% or more, the decision to take low-dose aspirin is an individual one. Adults who have no contraindications (e.g., history of stroke), have a life expectancy of at least 10 years, and are willing to take low-dose aspirin daily for at least 10 years are more likely to benefit. Currently there is insufficient evidence to recommend low-dose aspirin for those younger than 50 or older than 70.[19]

### Gerontologic Considerations: Coronary Artery Disease

The incidence of heart disease is greatly increased in older adults and is the leading cause of death in older individuals.[1] In the older adult, CAD is often a result of the complex interaction of nonmodifiable risk factors (e.g., age) and lifelong modifiable risk behaviors (e.g., inactivity, tobacco use). Strategies to reduce CAD risk and to treat CAD are effective in this age group.

**TABLE 33-5 Drug Therapy**

***Hyperlipidemia***

| Drug | Mechanism of Action | Side Effects | Nursing Considerations |
|---|---|---|---|
| **Restrict Lipoprotein Production** | | | |
| ***HMG-CoA Reductase Inhibitors (Statins)*** | | | |
| atorvastatin (Lipitor)<br>fluvastatin (Lescol)<br>lovastatin<br>pravastatin (Pravachol)<br>simvastatin (Zocor)<br>rosuvastatin (Crestor) | Block synthesis of cholesterol and increase LDL receptors in liver<br>↓ LDL<br>↓ Triglycerides<br>↑ HDL | Rash, GI disturbances, elevated liver enzymes, myopathy, rhabdomyolysis | Well tolerated with few side effects. Monitor liver enzymes and creatine kinase (if muscle weakness or pain occurs). |
| ***Niacin*** | | | |
| niacin (Niaspan) | Inhibits synthesis and secretion of VLDL and LDL<br>↓ LDL<br>↓ Triglycerides<br>↑ HDL | Flushing and pruritus in upper torso and face, GI disturbances (e.g., nausea and vomiting, dyspepsia, diarrhea), orthostatic hypotension, elevated homocysteine levels | Most side effects subside with time. Decreased liver function may occur with high doses.<br>Taking aspirin or NSAID 30 min before drug may prevent flushing. Take drug with food.<br>Treat elevated homocysteine levels with folic acid. |
| ***Fibric Acid Derivatives*** | | | |
| fenofibrate (Tricor)<br>gemfibrozil (Lopid) | Decrease hepatic synthesis and secretion of VLDL. Reduce triglycerides by ↓ VLDL<br>↓ LDL<br>↓ Triglycerides<br>↑ HDL | Rashes, mild GI disturbances (e.g., nausea, diarrhea), elevated liver enzymes | May ↑ effects of warfarin (Coumadin) and some antihyperglycemic drugs.<br>When used in combination with statins, may increase adverse effects of statins, especially myopathy. |
| ***Omega-3 Fatty Acid*** | | | |
| icosapent ethyl (Vascepa) | Inhibits synthesis and/or secretion of triglycerides | Arthralgia | Used for patients with severe hypertriglyceridemia (levels ≥500 mg/dL) |
| **Increase Lipoprotein Removal** | | | |
| ***Bile-Acid Sequestrants*** | | | |
| cholestyramine (Prevalite)<br>colesevelam (WelChol)<br>colestipol (Colestid) | Bind with bile acids in intestine, forming insoluble complex and excreted in feces<br>Binding results in removal of LDL and cholesterol<br>↓ LDL | Unpleasant quality to taste, GI disturbances (e.g., indigestion, constipation, bloating) | Effective and safe for long-term use. Side effects diminish with time.<br>Interfere with absorption of many drugs (e.g., digoxin, thiazide diuretics, warfarin, some antibiotics [e.g., penicillins]) |
| ***Proprotein Convertase Subtilisin/Kexin 9 (PCSK9) Inhibitors*** | | | |
| evolocumab (Repatha)<br>alirocumab (Praluent) | Inactivate PCSK9 protein<br>↓ LDL | Injection-site reactions, muscle pain, limb pain, and fatigue | Used with diet and maximum statin therapy to treat familial hypercholesterolemia and for those who need LDL lowering and are statin intolerant<br>Drugs are given by injection every 2-4 wk. |
| **Decrease Cholesterol Absorption** | | | |
| ***Cholesterol Absorption Inhibitor*** | | | |
| ezetimibe (Zetia) | Inhibits the intestinal absorption of cholesterol<br>↓ LDL<br>↑ HDL | Infrequent, but may include headache and mild GI distress | When used with a statin, LDL is further reduced.<br>Should not be used by patients with liver impairment |

Aggressive treatment of hypertension and hyperlipidemia stabilizes plaques in the coronary arteries of older adults, and cessation of tobacco use helps to decrease the risk for CAD at any age. Similarly, encourage the older patient to consider a planned program of physical activity. Activity performance, endurance, and ability to tolerate stress are improved in the older adult with physical training. Positive psychologic benefits from physical activity can include increased self-esteem and emotional well-being and improved body image. For the older adult who is obese, making modest dietary changes and slowly increasing physical activity (e.g., walking) results in more positive benefits than aiming for a significant weight loss.

When planning a physical activity program for the older adult, recommend the following: (1) longer warm-up periods, (2) longer periods of low-level activity, or (3) longer rest periods between sessions. Heat intolerance in the older adult results from a decreased ability to sweat efficiently. Teach the patient to avoid physical activity in extremes of temperature and to maintain a moderate pace. The older adult should exercise a minimum of 30 minutes on most days of the week as able.

Encouraging the older patient to adopt a healthy lifestyle may increase the quality of life and reduce the risk of CAD and fatal heart events. Older adults face many of the same challenges as younger individuals when it comes to making lifestyle changes. Older adults are more likely to consider change at two points in time: (1) when hospitalized and (2) when symptoms (e.g., chest pain) are the result of CAD and not normal aging (see Table 31-1). First, assess the older adult for readiness to change and health literacy. Then help the patient select the lifestyle changes most likely to produce the greatest reduction in risk for CAD.

## CHRONIC STABLE ANGINA

CAD is a chronic and progressive disease. Patients may be asymptomatic for many years or may develop chronic stable chest pain. When the demand for myocardial $O_2$ exceeds the ability of the coronary arteries to supply the heart with $O_2$, *myocardial ischemia* occurs. **Angina**, or chest pain, is the clinical manifestation of myocardial ischemia. It is caused by either an increased demand for $O_2$ or a decreased supply of $O_2$ (Table 33-6). The most common reason for angina to develop is narrowing of one or more coronary arteries by atherosclerosis. This leads to insufficient blood flow to the heart muscle. For ischemia secondary to atherosclerotic plaque to occur, the artery is usually blocked (stenosed) 70% or more (50% or more for the left main coronary artery).[5,20]

**Chronic stable angina** refers to chest pain that occurs intermittently over a long period of time with a similar pattern of onset, duration, and intensity of symptoms. It is often provoked by physical exertion, stress, or emotional upset. When asked, some patients may deny feeling pain but describe a pressure, heaviness, or discomfort in the chest (Table 33-7). This discomfort is often described as a squeezing, heavy, tight, or suffocating sensation. It may be associated with other symptoms such as dyspnea or fatigue. Chronic angina pain usually does not change with position or breathing and is rarely described as sharp or stabbing.

Although most angina pain occurs substernally, it may radiate to other locations, including the jaw, neck, shoulders, and/or arms. Many people with angina complain of indigestion or a burning sensation in the epigastric region. The sensation may also be felt between the shoulder blades (Fig. 33-3). Often people who complain of pain between the shoulder blades or indigestion type pain dismiss it as not being heart related. Some patients, especially women and older adults, report atypical symptoms of angina including dyspnea, nausea, and/or fatigue.[4] This is referred to as *angina equivalent.*

The pain of chronic stable angina usually lasts for only a few minutes and commonly subsides when the precipitating factor is resolved (e.g., resting, calming down, using sublingual nitroglycerin (SL NTG) (Nitrostat) (Table 33-8). Pain at rest is unusual and often a symptom of UA. A 12-lead electrocardiogram (ECG) often shows ST segment depression and/or T wave

**TABLE 33-6 Factors Influencing Myocardial $O_2$ Needs***

| Decreased $O_2$ Supply | Increased $O_2$ Demand or Consumption |
|---|---|
| **Cardiac** | |
| • Coronary artery atherosclerosis | • Aortic stenosis |
| • Coronary artery spasm | • Cardiomyopathy |
| • Coronary artery thrombosis | • Dysrhythmias |
| • Dysrhythmias | • Left ventricular hypertrophy |
| • Heart failure | • Tachycardia |
| • Valve disorders | |
| **Noncardiac** | |
| • Anemia | • Anxiety |
| • Asthma | • Hypertension |
| • Chronic obstructive pulmonary disease | • Hyperthermia |
| • Hypovolemia | • Hyperthyroidism |
| • Hypoxemia | • Physical exertion |
| • Pneumonia | • Substance (stimulant) abuse (e.g., cocaine, amphetamines) |
| • Substance (stimulant) abuse (e.g., cocaine, amphetamines) | |

*Lists are not all-inclusive.

**TABLE 33-7 PQRST Assessment of Angina**

*Use the following memory aid to obtain information from the patient who has chest pain.*

| | Factor | Questions to Ask Patient |
|---|---|---|
| P | Precipitating events | What events or activities precipitated the pain or discomfort (e.g., argument, exercise, resting)? |
| Q | Quality of pain | What does the pain or discomfort feel like (e.g., pressure, dull, aching, tight, squeezing, heaviness)? |
| R | Region (location) and radiation of pain | Can you point to where the pain or discomfort is located? Does the pain or discomfort radiate to other areas (e.g., back, neck, arms, jaw, shoulder, elbow)? |
| S | Severity of pain | On a scale of 0 to 10, with 0 indicating no pain and 10 being the most severe pain you could imagine, what number would you give the pain or discomfort? |
| T | Timing | When did the pain or discomfort begin? Has it changed since this time? Have you had pain/discomfort like this before? |

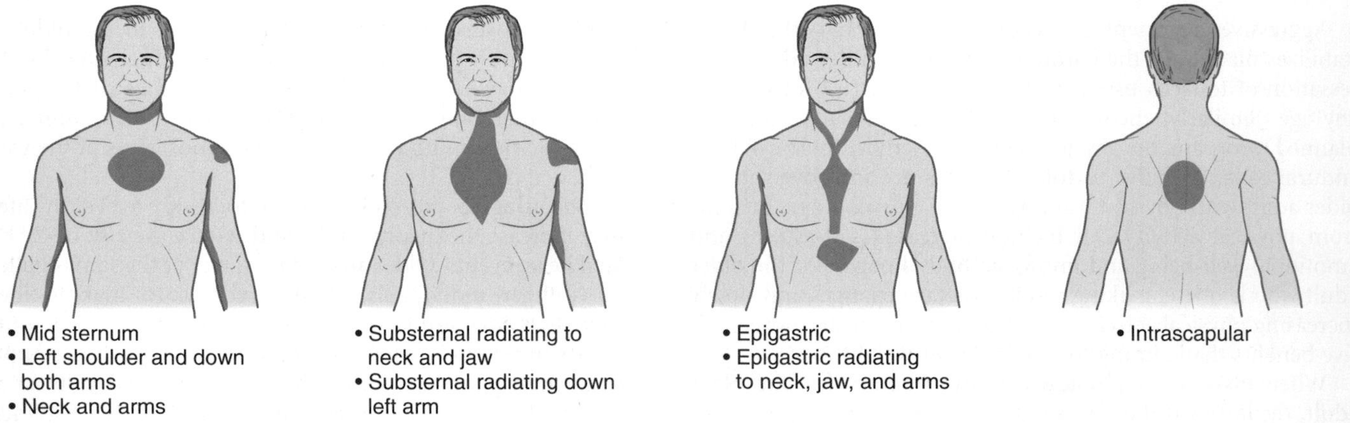


**FIG. 33-3** Common locations and patterns of pain during angina or myocardial infarction.

**TABLE 33-8 Precipitating Factors of Angina**

**Physical Exertion**
- Increases HR, reducing the time the heart spends in diastole (the time of greatest coronary blood flow), resulting in an increase in myocardial $O_2$ demand.
- Isometric exercise of the arms (e.g., raking, lifting heavy objects, snow shoveling) can cause exertional angina.

**Temperature Extremes**
- Increase the workload of the heart.
- Blood vessels constrict in response to a cold stimulus.
- Blood vessels dilate and blood pools in the skin in response to a hot stimulus.

**Strong Emotions**
- Stimulate the sympathetic nervous system, activating the stress response.
- Increase the workload of the heart.

**Consumption of Heavy Meal (e.g., holiday meals)**
- Can increase the workload of the heart.
- During the digestive process, blood is diverted to the GI system, reducing blood flow in the coronary arteries.

**Tobacco Use and Environmental Tobacco Smoke**
- Diminish available $O_2$ by increasing the level of carbon monoxide.
- Nicotine stimulates catecholamine release, causing vasoconstriction and an increased HR.

**Sexual Activity**
- Increases the cardiac workload and sympathetic stimulation.
- In a person with CAD, the extra cardiac workload may precipitate angina.

**Stimulants (e.g., cocaine, amphetamines)**
- Increase HR and BP and subsequently increases myocardial $O_2$ demand.
- Stimulate vasoconstriction and subsequently decreases myocardial $O_2$ supply.
- May precipitate dysrhythmias

**Circadian Rhythm Patterns**
- Manifestations of CAD tend to occur in the early morning after awakening.

inversion indicating ischemia (see Chapter 35). The ECG returns to baseline when the pain is relieved.

Chronic stable angina is controlled with drugs on an outpatient basis. Because chronic stable angina is often predictable, drugs are timed to provide peak effects during the time of day when angina is likely to occur. For example, if angina occurs when rising, the patient can take medication as soon as awakening and wait 30 minutes to 1 hour before engaging in activity. (A comparison of the major types of angina is presented in Table 33-9.)

**Silent ischemia** refers to ischemia that occurs in the absence of any subjective symptoms. Patients with diabetes have an increased prevalence of silent ischemia. This is most likely due to diabetic neuropathy affecting the nerves that innervate the cardiovascular system. When patients are monitored (e.g., Holter monitor) and silent ischemia occurs, ECG changes are revealed. Ischemia with pain or without pain has the same prognosis.

**TABLE 33-9 Comparison of Major Types of Angina**

| Type | Etiology | Characteristics |
|---|---|---|
| **Chronic stable angina** | Myocardial ischemia (usually secondary to CAD) caused by an $O_2$ supply/demand mismatch | • Episodic pain lasting a few minutes<br>• Provoked by exertion or stress<br>• Relieved by rest or nitroglycerin |
| **Prinzmetal's angina** | Coronary vasospasm | • Occurs primarily at rest<br>• Triggered by smoking and increased levels of some substances (e.g., histamine, epinephrine, cocaine)<br>• May occur in presence or absence of CAD |
| **Microvascular angina** | Myocardial ischemia secondary to microvascular disease affecting the small, distal branches of coronary arteries | • More common in women<br>• Triggered by activities of daily living (e.g., shopping, work) vs. physical exercise (exertion)<br>• Treatment may include nitroglycerin |
| **Unstable angina** | Rupture of unstable plaque, exposing thrombogenic surface | • New-onset angina<br>• Chronic stable angina that increases in frequency, duration, or severity<br>• Occurs at rest or with minimal exertion<br>• Lasts more than 10 min |

## Prinzmetal's Angina

**Prinzmetal's angina** *(variant angina)* is a rare form of angina that often occurs at rest and not with increased physical demand. It is sometimes seen in patients with a history of migraine headaches, Raynaud's phenomenon, and heavy smoking. It is usually due to spasm of a major coronary artery. The spasm may occur in the presence or absence of CAD. Strong contraction (spasm) of smooth muscle in the coronary artery results from increased intracellular calcium.[21]

Factors contributing to coronary artery spasm include increased myocardial $O_2$ demand and increased levels of certain substances (e.g., tobacco smoke, alcohol, cocaine). When spasm occurs, the patient experiences angina and transient ST segment elevation (see Chapter 35). The pain may occur during rapid-eye-movement (REM) sleep when myocardial $O_2$ consumption increases or when exposed to cold temperatures. The pain may be relieved by moderate exercise, with SL NTG, or it may disappear spontaneously. Cyclic, short bursts of pain at a usual time each day may also occur with this type of angina. Calcium channel blockers and/or nitrates are used to control the pain, as well as stopping any offending substances.

## Microvascular Angina

In *microvascular angina,* chest pain occurs in the absence of significant CAD or coronary spasm of a major coronary artery. In these patients, chest pain is related to myocardial ischemia associated with atherosclerosis or spasm of the small distal branch vessels of the coronary microcirculation. This is known as *coronary microvascular disease* (MVD). It is also referred to as *Syndrome X*.[4] It is more common in postmenopausal women. Often the angina in these patients is prolonged and brought on by physical exertion. These patients usually have positive stress test results and have an inconsistent response to nitrates. Prevention and treatment of coronary MVD follow the same recommendations as for CAD.[22]

## INTERPROFESSIONAL CARE: CHRONIC STABLE ANGINA

The treatment of chronic stable angina aims to decrease $O_2$ demand and/or increase $O_2$ supply. The reduction of risk factors is a priority and should include those strategies discussed for patients with CAD (see pp. 707-712). In addition to antiplatelet and lipid-lowering drug therapy, the most common therapeutic interventions for the management of chronic stable angina are the use of nitrates, angiotensin-converting enzyme (ACE) inhibitors, β-blockers, and calcium channel blockers to optimize myocardial perfusion (Table 33-10 and Fig. 33-4).

### Drug Therapy

Drug therapy for chronic stable angina aims to reduce symptoms and the risk of MI and death. Aspirin (previously discussed) is given in the absence of contraindications (Table 33-11).

**Short-Acting Nitrates.** Short-acting nitrates are first-line therapy for the treatment of angina. Nitrates produce their principal effects by the following mechanisms:

*Dilating peripheral blood vessels:* This results in decreased SVR, venous pooling, and decreased venous blood return to the

**TABLE 33-10 Treatment of Chronic Stable Angina**

*Strategies for the patient with chronic stable angina should address all the treatment elements and related patient teaching in the following mnemonic:**

| Element | Treatment |
|---|---|
| A | Antiplatelet/anticoagulant therapy<br>Antianginal therapy<br>ACE inhibitor/angiotensin receptor blocker |
| B | β-blocker<br>BP control |
| C | Cigarette smoking cessation<br>Cholesterol (lipid) management<br>Calcium channel blockers<br>Cardiac rehabilitation |
| D | Diet (weight management)<br>Diabetes management<br>Depression screening |
| E | Education<br>Exercise |
| F | Flu vaccination |

*Modified from Smith SC, Benjamin EJ, Bonow RO, et al: AHA/ACCF secondary prevention and risk reduction therapy for patients with coronary and other atherosclerotic vascular disease: 2011 update, *J Am Coll Cardiol* 58:2432, 2011.

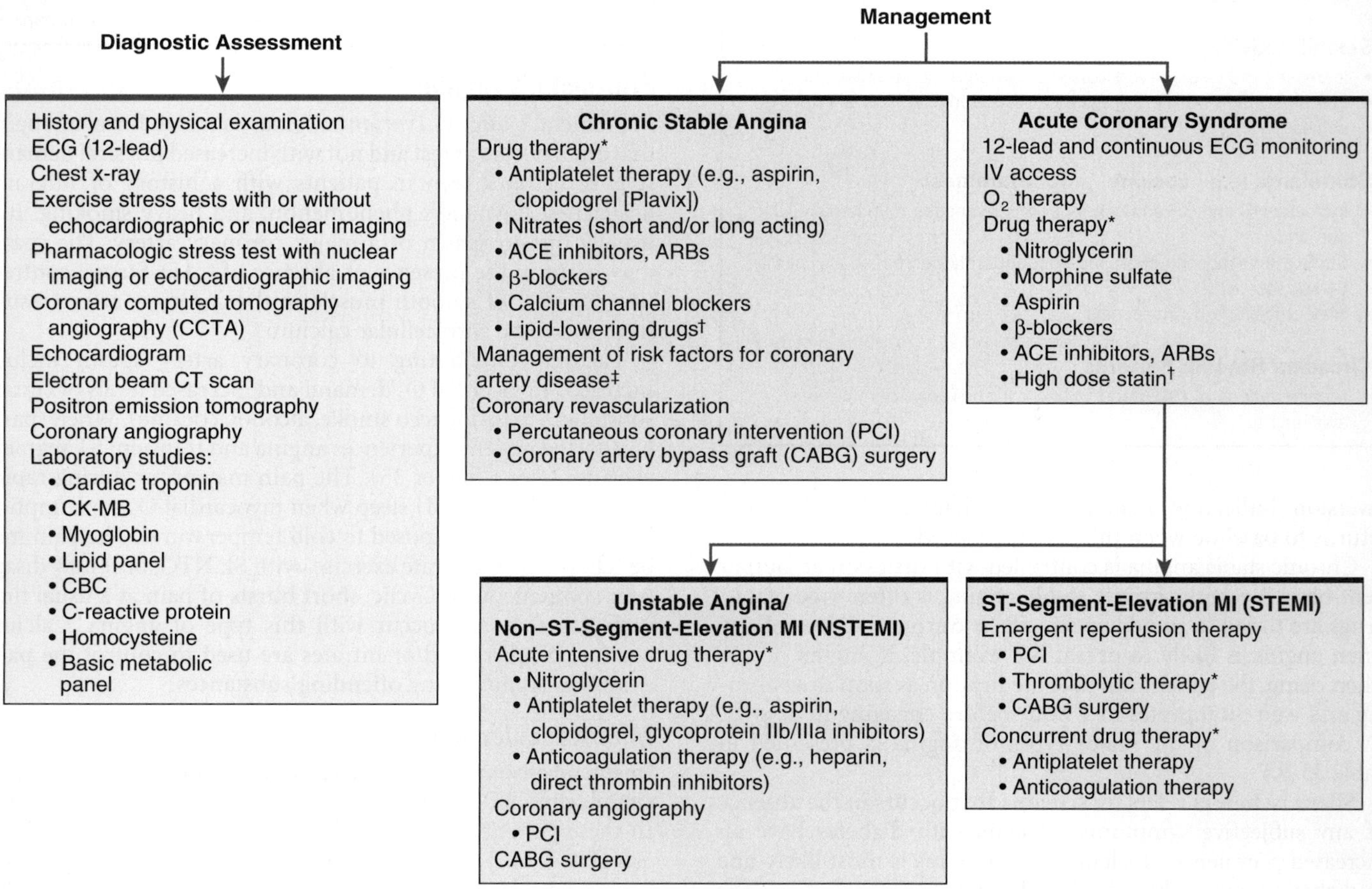


**FIG. 33-4** Interprofessional care: chronic stable angina and acute coronary syndrome. *ACE,* Angiotensin-converting enzyme; *ARBs,* angiotensin II receptor blockers; *CK,* creatine kinase.
*Table 33-11.
†Table 33-5.
‡Tables 33-2, 33-3, and 33-4.

## TABLE 33-11 Drug Therapy

### *Chronic Stable Angina and Acute Coronary Syndrome*

| Drug | Mechanism of Action and Comments |
|---|---|
| **Antiplatelet Agents** | |
| aspirin | • Inhibits cyclooxygenase, which in turn produces thromboxane $A_2$, a potent platelet activator<br>• Should be administered as soon as ACS is suspected, unless truly allergic<br>• Initial dose 162-325 mg, then 81-325 mg daily |
| cangrelor (Kengreal) | • Inhibits platelet aggregation<br>• Given IV<br>• Approved for use in patients having PCI |
| clopidogrel (Plavix) | • Inhibits platelet aggregation<br>• Alternative for patients who cannot take aspirin<br>• Used to treat ACS with medical therapy alone or used in combination with aspirin after PCI for chronic stable angina or ACS |
| prasugrel (Effient) | • Inhibits platelet aggregation<br>• Used as an alternative to clopidogrel in combination with aspirin for patient with ACS who have PCI<br>• Not indicated to treat ACS with medical therapy alone |
| ticagrelor (Brilinta) | • Inhibits platelet aggregation<br>• Alternative for patient who cannot take aspirin<br>• Used to treat ACS with medical therapy alone or used in combination with aspirin after PCI for ACS<br>• If used in combination with aspirin, effectiveness may be decreased by aspirin dosages >100 mg/day (according to a boxed warning) |
| vorapaxar (Zontivity) | • Inhibits platelet aggregation<br>• Increases risk of bleeding, including life-threatening and fatal bleeding (according to a boxed warning)<br>• Must not be used in people who have had a stroke, transient ischemic attack (TIA), or bleeding in the head, because the risk of bleeding in the head is too great |
| ***Glycoprotein IIb/IIIa Inhibitors*** | |
| abciximab (ReoPro)<br>eptifibatide (Integrilin)<br>tirofiban (Aggrastat) | • Prevent the binding of fibrinogen to platelets, thereby blocking platelet aggregation<br>• May be used in combination with aspirin for patients with ACS |
| **Anticoagulant Agents** | |
| ***Unfractionated Heparin**** | |
| heparin | • Prevents conversion of fibrinogen to fibrin and prothrombin to thrombin |
| ***Low-Molecular-Weight Heparin**** | |
| dalteparin (Fragmin)<br>enoxaparin (Lovenox) | • Bind to antithrombin III, enhancing its effect<br>• Heparin–antithrombin III complex inactivates activated factor X and thrombin.<br>• Prevent conversion of fibrinogen to fibrin |
| ***Vitamin K Antagonist**** | |
| warfarin (Coumadin) | • Interferes with hepatic synthesis of vitamin K–dependent clotting factors<br>• Used for patients with atrial fibrillation or those who are risk for thromboembolism (large anterior wall infarctions or ventricular aneurysms)<br>• Closely monitor for bleeding when taking with antiplatelet drugs. |
| ***Direct Thrombin Inhibitors*** | |
| bivalirudin (Angiomax)<br>argatroban | • Direct inhibition of the clotting factor thrombin |
| **Nitrates** | |
| Sublingual nitroglycerin (Nitrostat)<br>Translingual spray nitroglycerin (Nitrolingual)<br>nitroglycerin ointment (Nitro-Bid)<br>Transdermal nitroglycerin (Transderm-Nitro)<br>isosorbide dinitrate (Isordil)<br>Isosorbide mononitrate<br>IV nitroglycerin | • Promote peripheral vasodilation, decreasing preload and afterload<br>• Promote coronary artery vasodilation<br>• May prevent or control coronary vasospasm |
| **Angiotensin-Converting Enzyme (ACE) Inhibitors†** | |
| captopril<br>enalapril (Vasotec)<br>lisinopril (Zestril) | • Prevent conversion of angiotensin I to angiotensin II, resulting in vasodilation<br>• May prevent or limit ventricular remodeling<br>• Decrease endothelial dysfunction<br>• Useful with heart failure, decreased LV function, tachycardia, MI, hypertension, diabetes, and chronic kidney disease |
| **Angiotensin II Receptor Blockers†** | |
| losartan (Cozaar)<br>valsartan (Diovan) | • Inhibit binding of angiotensin II to angiotensin I receptors, resulting in vasodilation<br>• Used for patients intolerant of ACE inhibitors |
| **β-Adrenergic Blockers†** | |
| atenolol (Tenormin)<br>carvedilol (Coreg)<br>metoprolol (Lopressor)<br>nadolol (Corgard) | • Inhibit sympathetic nervous stimulation of the heart<br>• Reduce heart rate, contractility, and BP<br>• Reduce ischemia<br>• Decrease afterload |
| **Calcium Channel Blockers†** | |
| amlodipine (Norvasc)<br>diltiazem (Cardizem)<br>felodipine<br>nicardipine (Cardene)<br>verapamil (Calan)<br>nifedipine (Procardia) | • Prevent calcium entry into vascular smooth muscle cells and myocytes (cardiac cells)<br>• May prevent or control coronary vasospasm<br>• Promote coronary and peripheral vasodilation<br>• Reduce heart rate, contractility, and BP |

*See Table 37-10.
†See Table 32-7.

*Continued*

TABLE 33-11 **Drug Therapy**

***Chronic Stable Angina and Acute Coronary Syndrome—cont'd***

| Drug | Mechanism of Action and Comments | Drug | Mechanism of Action and Comments |
|---|---|---|---|
| **Opioid**<br>morphine | • Functions as an analgesic and sedative<br>• Acts as a vasodilator to reduce preload and myocardial $O_2$ consumption | **Thrombolytic Agents**<br>reteplase (Retavase)<br>alteplase (Activase)<br>tenecteplase (TNKase) | • Break up fibrin meshwork in clots<br>• Used only in ST-segment–elevation MI when access to a hospital with PCI capability is not available |
| | | **Lipid-Lowering Agents**<br>Drugs listed in Table 33-5 | • Have been shown to reduce morbidity and mortality from CAD |

*PCI,* Percutaneous coronary intervention.

heart (preload). Therefore myocardial $O_2$ demand is decreased because of the reduced cardiac workload.

*Dilating coronary arteries and collateral vessels:* This may increase blood flow to the ischemic areas of the heart. However, when the coronary arteries are severely atherosclerotic, coronary dilation is difficult to achieve.

***Sublingual Nitroglycerin.*** SL NTG or translingual spray (Nitrolingual) usually relieves pain in about 5 minutes and lasts approximately 30 to 40 minutes. The recommended dose of NTG is one tablet taken sublingually (SL) or one metered spray on the tongue for symptoms of angina. If symptoms are unchanged or worse after 5 minutes, tell the patient or caregiver to repeat NTG every 5 minutes for a maximum of three doses and contact emergency response system (ERS) if symptoms have not resolved completely.

Instruct the patient in the proper use of NTG. It should be easily accessible to the patient at all times. The patient should store the tablets away from light and heat sources, including body heat, to protect them from degradation. Tablets are packaged in light-resistant bottles with metal caps. Once opened, the tablets lose potency, and should be replaced every 6 months.

Tell the patient to sit down and place a NTG tablet under the tongue and allow it to dissolve. If using the spray, the patient should direct it on the tongue, not inhale it. SL NTG should cause a tingling sensation when taken; otherwise it may be outdated. Warn the patient that a headache, dizziness, or flushing may occur. Caution the patient to change positions slowly after NTG use because orthostatic hypotension may occur.

Patients can use NTG prophylactically before starting an activity that is known to cause angina. In these cases the patient can take a tablet or spray 5 to 10 minutes before beginning the activity. Tell the patient to report to the HCP any changes in the usual pattern of pain, especially increasing frequency, nighttime angina, or angina at rest.

**Long-Acting Nitrates.** Nitrates, such as isosorbide dinitrate (Isordil) and isosorbide mononitrate, are longer acting than SL or translingual NTG. They are used to reduce the frequency of anginal attacks. The main side effect of all nitrates is headache from the dilation of cerebral blood vessels. Tell patients to take acetaminophen (Tylenol) to relieve the headache. Over time, the headaches may decrease, but the antianginal effects are still present.

Orthostatic hypotension is a complication of all nitrates. Monitor BP after the first dose, since the venous dilation that occurs may cause a drop in BP, especially in volume-depleted patients. Finally, tolerance to long-acting NTG can develop. To limit this, patients are often scheduled a 10- to 14-hour nitrate-free period every day. Remind patients that taking a long-acting NTG preparation should not keep them from using translingual or SL NTG if angina develops.

***Nitroglycerin Ointment.*** Nitropaste is a 2% NTG topical ointment dosed by the inch. It is placed on the upper body or arm, over a flat muscular area that is free of hair and scars. Once absorbed, it produces anginal prophylaxis for 3 to 6 hours. It is especially useful for nighttime and UA. The ointment should be wiped off to allow for a 10- to 14-hour nitrate-free interval in order to prevent nitrate tolerance.

***Transdermal Controlled-Release Nitrates.*** Currently two systems are available for transdermal NTG drug delivery: silicone gel and polymer matrix. These systems allow timed release of NTG over a 24-hour period. These preparations should also be removed in the evening to allow for a 10- to 14-hour nitrate-free interval.

**DRUG ALERT Nitrates**

- NTG tablets must be kept in a dark, airtight container to maintain potency.
- SL NTG must be placed under the tongue.
- Translingual NTG should be sprayed on the tongue, not under the tongue.
- Tell patient not to combine with drugs used for erectile dysfunction (e.g., sildenafil [Viagra]) as severe hypotension can occur.
- Monitor for orthostatic hypotension because it may occur after administration.
- Headaches are common after taking any NTG preparation.
- Use gloves to apply and remove NTG ointment or transdermal patches to avoid contact with drug.
- Never discharge a cardioverter-defibrillator over NTG ointment or transdermal patch.
- When using long-acting nitrates, provide a 10- to 14-hour nitrate-free period.

**Angiotensin-Converting Enzyme (ACE) Inhibitors and Angiotensin Receptor Blockers (ARBs).** Patients with chronic stable angina who have an ejection fraction (EF) of 40% or less, diabetes, hypertension, or chronic kidney disease should take an ACE inhibitor (e.g., lisinopril [Zestril]) indefinitely, unless contraindicated. Patients with chronic stable angina and a normal EF, diabetes, and one other CAD risk factor should also take an ACE inhibitor to decrease the risk of MI, stroke, and death.

These drugs result in vasodilation and reduced blood volume. Most important, they can prevent or reverse ventricular remodeling in patients who have had an MI (see pp. 725-726). For patients who are intolerant of ACE inhibitors (e.g., cough, angioedema), ARBs (e.g., losartan [Cozaar]) are used. (ACE inhibitors and ARBs are discussed later in the chapter and in Chapter 32 and Table 32-7).

**β-Adrenergic Blockers.** β-Blockers are ordered for relief of angina symptoms in patients with chronic stable angina. Patients who have LV dysfunction, elevated BP, or have had an MI should start and continue β-blockers indefinitely, unless contraindicated. These drugs decrease myocardial contractility, HR, SVR, and BP, all of which reduce the myocardial $O_2$ demand. β-Blockers that have been shown to reduce the risk of death in patients with LV dysfunction, heart failure (HF), or MI are carvedilol (Coreg), metoprolol (Lopressor, Toprol XL), and bisoprolol (Zebeta).[5]

β-Blockers have many side effects and can be poorly tolerated. Side effects may include bradycardia, hypotension, wheezing from bronchospasm, and GI complaints. Many patients also complain of weight gain, depression, fatigue, and sexual dysfunction. Absolute contraindications to using β-blockers include severe bradycardia and acute HF. Patients with asthma should avoid β-blockers. They are used cautiously in patients with diabetes, since they mask signs of hypoglycemia. β-Blockers should not be stopped abruptly without medical supervision, as this may result in an increase in the number and intensity of angina attacks.

**Calcium Channel Blockers.** If β-blockers are contraindicated, are poorly tolerated, or do not control anginal symptoms, calcium channel blockers are used. The primary effects of calcium channel blockers are (1) systemic vasodilation with decreased SVR, (2) decreased myocardial contractility, (3) coronary vasodilation, and (4) decreased HR.

There are two groups of calcium channel blockers. The dihydropyridines (e.g., amlodipine [Norvasc]), which have more vasodilatory effects, and the nondihydropyridines (e.g., verapamil [Calan], diltiazem [Cardizem]), which have more rate and contractility effects.

Calcium channel blockers enhance the action of digoxin by increasing serum digoxin levels (see Chapter 34). Therefore serum digoxin levels should be closely monitored after starting calcium channel blockers. Teach the patient the signs and symptoms of digoxin toxicity. Verapamil can cause severe constipation, especially in older adults.[5]

**Lipid-Lowering Drugs.** Although patients with chronic stable angina are encouraged to follow a diet low in saturated fat and cholesterol, a moderate or high dose of a lipid-lowering drug should be ordered, unless contraindicated.

**Sodium Current Inhibitor.** Ranolazine (Ranexa), a sodium current inhibitor, is used to treat chronic angina in patients who have not had an adequate response with other antianginals. It is not a first-line drug for chronic stable angina. Because ranolazine prolongs the QT interval, patients with a long QT interval or who are taking QT-prolonging drugs (e.g., fluoxetine [Prozac]) should not use it (see Chapter 35). Common side effects of ranolazine include dizziness, nausea, constipation, and headache.

## Diagnostic Studies

When CAD is suspected in a patient or when a patient with chronic stable angina has a change in the anginal pattern, a variety of studies are completed (Fig. 33-4). After a detailed health history and physical examination, a chest x-ray is done to look for cardiac enlargement, aortic calcifications, and pulmonary congestion. A 12-lead ECG is done and compared with a previous ECG whenever possible to look for any changes. Laboratory tests (e.g., lipid profile, C-reactive protein) are done to identify specific risk factors for CAD. An echocardiogram may be done to look for resting LV wall motion abnormalities, which may suggest evidence of CAD. An exercise stress test with or without echocardiography or nuclear imaging may be ordered. For patients with physical limitations in walking, a pharmacologic (adenosine [Adenocard] or dipyridamole [Persantine]) stress test with nuclear imaging, or a pharmacologic (dobutamine [Dobutrex]) stress echocardiogram may be ordered. Coronary blockages less than 70% are not usually detected with stress testing.[5] (See Chapter 31 and Table 31-6 for a discussion of these studies, including nursing considerations.)

The electron beam computed tomography (EBCT) scan locates and measures coronary calcification (see Fig. 31-11). However, additional testing (e.g., stress testing or heart catheterization) is needed to further assess the impact of the lesion on coronary blood flow. Further studies are needed to determine the accuracy of the EBCT scan to diagnose high-grade blockages because many atherosclerotic plaques are not calcified.

Coronary computed tomography angiography (CCTA) may be considered. Using IV contrast and radiation, CCTA can detect calcified and noncalcified plaques in the artery, as well as other heart conditions. Limitations of using CCTA include patients with rapid HRs (greater than 90 beats per minute), extensive coronary artery calcifications, obesity, and a history of prior coronary artery stent. Patients allergic to IV contrast dye must be premedicated with corticosteroids. Patients with chronic kidney disease need hydration pre- and postprocedure. A baseline serum creatinine level should be obtained as the IV contrast dye can cause or worsen renal dysfunction.

**Cardiac Catheterization.** For patients with increasing angina symptoms, a cardiac catheterization is ordered. Cardiac catheterization and coronary angiography use radiation and IV contrast dye to provide images of the coronary circulation and identify the location and severity of any blockage. A patient who is allergic to IV contrast dye must be premedicated with corticosteroids. Patients with chronic kidney disease need hydration pre- and postprocedure. A baseline serum creatinine level is obtained because the IV contrast dye can cause or worsen renal dysfunction. Monitor renal function closely after the procedure. This procedure should only be done if the patient is a candidate for percutaneous or surgical coronary revascularization.

If a coronary blockage is amenable to treatment, **coronary revascularization** with an elective **percutaneous coronary intervention (PCI)** may be recommended. PCI may be done at the same time as the catheterization or at a later date. During PCI, a catheter with a deflated balloon tip is inserted into the appropriate coronary artery. The deflated balloon is positioned in the blockage and inflated. This compresses the plaque against the artery wall, resulting in vessel dilation and a larger vessel diameter. This procedure is called *balloon angioplasty.*

Intracoronary stents are usually placed along with balloon angioplasty. A **stent** is an expandable mesh-like structure designed to keep the vessel open after balloon angioplasty. It provides support to the arterial wall (Figs. 33-5 and 33-6). Because stents are thrombogenic, many different types of drugs are used to prevent platelet aggregation within the stent. Drugs commonly used during PCI are unfractionated heparin (UH) or low-molecular-weight heparin (LMWH), a direct thrombin inhibitor (e.g., bivalirudin [Angiomax]), and/or a glycoprotein IIb/IIIa inhibitor (e.g., eptifibatide [Integrilin]) (Table 33-11).

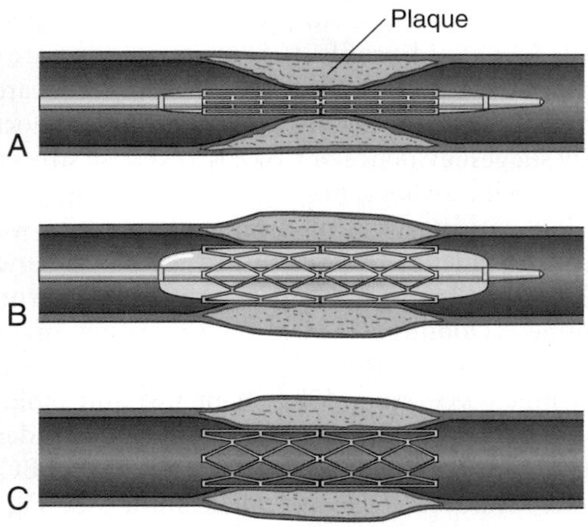


**FIG. 33-5** Placement of a coronary artery stent. **A,** The stent is positioned at the site of the lesion. **B,** The balloon is inflated, expanding the stent. The balloon is then deflated and removed. **C,** The implanted stent is left in place.

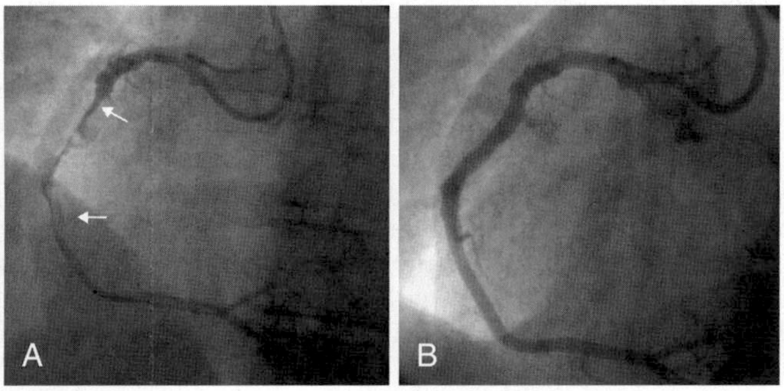


**FIG. 33-6** **A,** A thrombotic occlusion of the right coronary artery is noted *(arrows).* **B,** Right coronary artery is opened and blood flow restored following angioplasty and placement of a 4-mm stent. (From Zipes DB, Libby P, Bonow RO, Braunwald E: *Braunwald's heart disease: a textbook of cardiovascular medicine,* ed 7, St Louis, 2005, Saunders.)

After PCI, the patient is treated with dual antiplatelet drugs (e.g., aspirin [indefinitely] and clopidogrel) up to 12 months or longer, until the intimal lining grows over the stent and provides a smooth vascular surface.

There are two types of stents: bare metal stents (BMS) and drug-eluting stents (DES). DESs are coated with a drug (e.g., paclitaxel, everolimus) to reduce the risk of overgrowth of the intimal lining *(neointimal hyperplasia)* within the stent. This is the primary cause of in-stent restenosis (ISR). Following DES placement, dual antiplatelet drugs are taken to prevent thrombus formation within the stent (stent thrombosis) for a minimum of 12 months or longer. The duration of dual antiplatelet drugs for patients with BMS is a minimum of 1 month but ideally 1 full year after PCI.[20] Some DES are gradually absorbed by the body in approximately 3 years.

Potential complications from cardiac catheterization with PCI include abrupt closure from coronary artery dissection, vascular injury at the artery access site (e.g., femoral, radial), acute MI, stent embolization, coronary spasm, dye allergy, renal compromise, bleeding (e.g., retroperitoneal), infection, stroke, and emergent coronary artery bypass graft (CABG) surgery. The possibility of dysrhythmias during and after the procedure is always present.

PCI may not be a feasible option for all patients (e.g., patients with three-vessel CAD [three different coronary arteries] and/or significant left main coronary artery disease). Coronary revascularization with CABG surgery may be recommended and is discussed later in the chapter.

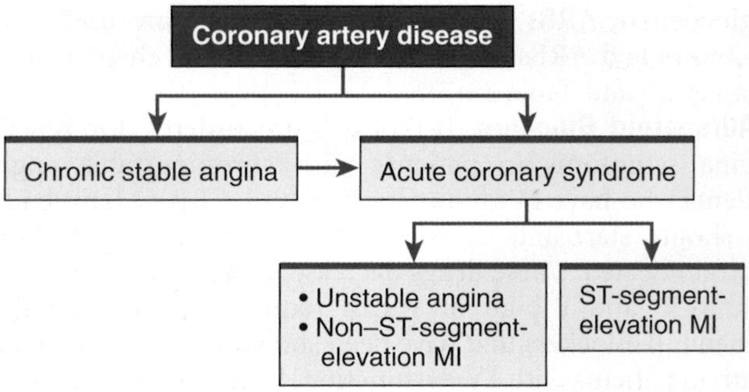


**FIG. 33-7** Relationships among coronary artery disease, chronic stable angina, and acute coronary syndrome.

### Alternative Therapies for Refractory Chronic Stable Angina

For patients with refractory stable angina, *enhanced external counterpulsation* (EECP) may be used. EECP consists of placing inflatable BP cuffs around the legs. The cuffs sequentially inflate during diastole and deflate during systole from the calves to the thighs. This action is thought to increase venous return and augment diastolic BP in order to increase coronary perfusion, improve LV diastolic filling, and help with collateral circulation. Patients get treatments 5 days a week for a total of 35 treatments. EECP is contraindicated in patients with decompensated HF, severe peripheral arterial disease, and severe aortic insufficiency.

Spinal cord stimulation may also help relieve symptoms in patients who are refractory to drugs or revascularization. The stimulation lead is placed in the epidural space between T1 and T2 and is connected to an implanted subcutaneous pulse generator. The mechanism by which angina is reduced is not well understood.

## ACUTE CORONARY SYNDROME

When ischemia is prolonged and not immediately reversible, **acute coronary syndrome (ACS)** develops. ACS includes the spectrum of UA, *non–ST-segment-elevation myocardial infarction* (NSTEMI), and *ST-segment-elevation myocardial infarction* (STEMI) (Fig. 33-7). When patients first present with chest pain, ST-elevations on the 12-lead ECG are most likely indicative of a STEMI. The ECG should always be compared to a previous ECG whenever possible. For patients with chest pain who do not show ST segement elevation or ST-T wave changes on the ECG, it is difficult to distinguish between UA and NSTEMI until serum cardiac biomarkers are measured.[23]

On the cellular level, the heart muscle becomes hypoxic within the first 10 seconds of a total coronary occlusion. Heart cells are deprived of $O_2$ and glucose needed for aerobic metabolism and contractility. Anaerobic metabolism begins and lactic acid accumulates. In ischemic conditions, heart cells are viable for approximately 20 minutes. Irreversible heart damage starts after 20 minutes if there is no collateral circulation[21] (Fig. 33-2). With restoration of blood flow (reperfusion), aerobic metabolism resumes, contractility is restored, and cellular repair begins.

ACS is caused by the decline of a once-stable atherosclerotic plaque. The previously stable plaque ruptures, releasing substances into the vessel. This causes platelet aggregation and thrombus formation. The vessel may be partially blocked by a thrombus (manifesting as UA or NSTEMI) or totally blocked by a thrombus (manifesting as STEMI). What causes the plaque to suddenly become unstable is not well understood, but systemic inflammation (described earlier) is thought to play a role. Patients with suspected ACS need immediate hospitalization.

## UNSTABLE ANGINA

**Unstable angina (UA)** is chest pain that is new in onset, occurs at rest, or occurs with increasing frequency, duration, or with less effort than the patient's chronic stable angina pattern. The pain usually lasts 10 minutes or more. Prompt treatment is needed for patients with suspected UA.

The patient with chronic stable angina may develop UA, or UA may be the first clinical sign of CAD. Unlike chronic stable angina, UA is unpredictable. The patient with previously diagnosed chronic stable angina describes a significant change in the pattern of angina. It occurs with increasing frequency and is easily provoked by minimal or no exertion, during sleep, or even at rest. The patient without previously diagnosed angina describes anginal pain that has progressed rapidly in the past few hours, days, or weeks, often ending in pain at rest.

Women seek medical attention for symptoms of UA more often than men. Despite efforts to increase awareness, women's symptoms continue to be underrecognized as heart related. These symptoms include fatigue, shortness of breath, indigestion, and anxiety. Fatigue is the most prominent symptom.[4] However, all these symptoms can relate to many different diseases and syndromes. Thus women often present with UA before CAD is diagnosed. (See Gender Differences box on p. 705 earlier in this chapter.)

## MYOCARDIAL INFARCTION: ST-ELEVATION AND NON–ST-ELEVATION

A **myocardial infarction (MI)** occurs because of abrupt stoppage of blood flow through a coronary artery from a thrombus caused by platelet aggregation. This causes irreversible myocardial cell death (necrosis) in the heart muscle beyond the blockage (Figs. 33-8 and 33-9). Most MIs occur in the setting of preexisting CAD.[21]

A STEMI caused by an occlusive thrombus creates ST-elevation in the ECG leads facing the area of infarction (see Figs. 35-28 and 35-30). A STEMI is an emergency situation. In order to limit the infarct size, the artery must be opened within 90 minutes of presentation. This can be done either by PCI or thrombolytic (fibrinolytic) therapy. PCI is the first-line treatment if a hospital is capable of performing PCI.

NSTEMI, caused by a nonocclusive thrombus, does not cause ST segment elevation on the 12-lead ECG. Patients may or may not develop ST-T wave changes in the leads affected by the infarction. NSTEMI patients do not go to the catheterization laboratory emergently but usually undergo the procedure within 12 to 72 hours if there are no contraindications. Thrombolytic therapy is not indicated for NSTEMI patients.

With either a NSTEMI or STEMI, an echocardiogram may show *hypokinesis* (worsening myocardial contractility) or *akinesis* (absent myocardial contractility) in the necrotic area(s). The degree of LV dysfunction depends on the area of the heart involved and size of the infarction.

The acute MI process evolves over time. The earliest tissue to become ischemic is the subendocardium (the innermost layer of tissue in the heart muscle). If ischemia persists, it takes approximately 4 to 6 hours for the entire thickness of the heart muscle to become necrosed. If the thrombus is not completely blocking the artery, the time to complete necrosis may be as long as 12 hours.

The majority of MIs affect the LV and are usually described based on the location of damage (e.g., anterior, inferior, lateral, septal, or posterior wall infarction). The location of the MI and ECG changes correlate with the involved coronary artery (see Table 35-14). For example, in most people, the right coronary artery provides blood to the inferior and posterior LV walls. Blockage of the right coronary artery results in an inferior wall and/or posterior wall MI. Anterior wall infarctions result from blockages in the left anterior descending artery. Blockages in the left circumflex artery usually cause lateral LV wall MIs. Damage can occur in more than one location, especially if more than one coronary artery is involved (e.g., anterolateral MI). Right ventricular MIs are much less common and treated differently than LV MIs.

Not everyone develops collateral circulation, but if present, the degree of collateral circulation influences the severity of the MI (Fig. 33-2). A person with a long history of CAD may develop good collateral circulation to provide the area surrounding the infarction site with a blood supply. This is one

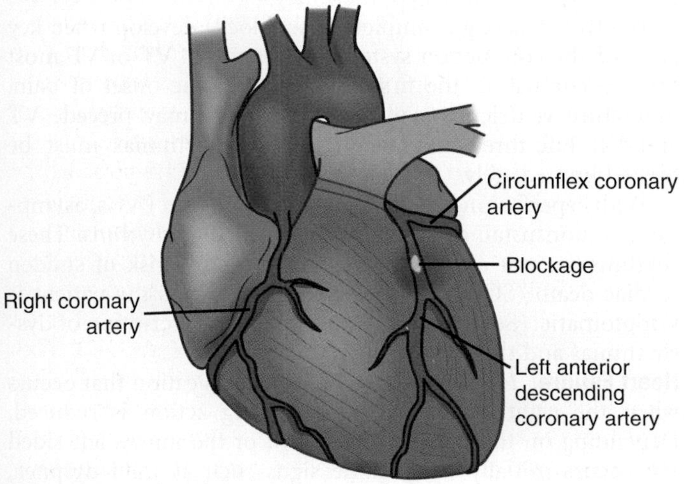


**FIG. 33-8** Occlusion of the left anterior descending coronary artery, resulting in a myocardial infarction.

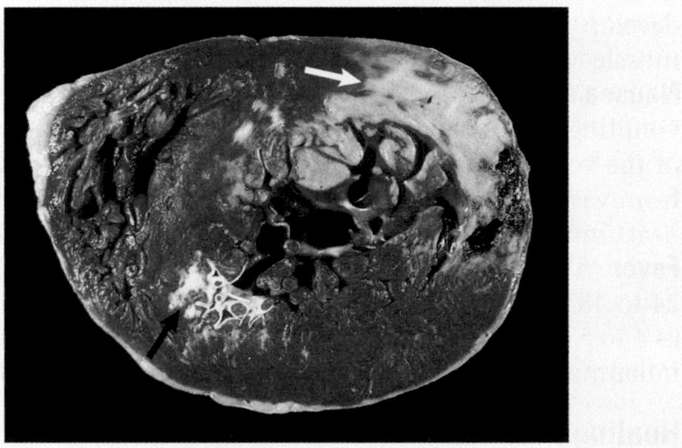

**FIG. 33-9** Acute myocardial infarction in the posterolateral wall of the left ventricle. This is demonstrated by the absence of staining in the areas of necrosis *(white arrow)*. Note the scarring from a previous anterior wall myocardial infarction *(black arrow)*. (From Kumar V, Abbas AK, Aster JC, Fausto N: *Robbins and Cotran pathologic basis of disease,* ed 8, Philadelphia, 2010, Saunders.)

reason why a younger person may have a more serious first MI than an older person with the same degree of blockage.

### Clinical Manifestations of Myocardial Infarction

**Pain.** Severe chest pain not relieved by rest, position change, or nitrate administration is the hallmark of an MI. Persistent and unlike any other pain, it is usually described as heavy, pressure, tight, burning, constricted, or crushing feeling. Common locations are substernal or epigastric areas. The pain may radiate to the neck, lower jaw, and arms or to the back (Fig. 33-3). When epigastric pain is present, the patient may relate it to indigestion and take antacids without relief. It may occur while the patient is active or at rest, asleep, or awake. However, it often occurs in the early morning hours. It usually lasts for 20 minutes or longer and is more severe than usual anginal pain.

Not everyone who has an MI has classic symptoms. Some patients may not experience pain but may have "discomfort," weakness, nausea, indigestion, or shortness of breath. Although women and men have more similarities than differences in their acute MI symptoms, some women may experience atypical discomfort, shortness of breath, or fatigue. Patients with diabetes may experience silent (asymptomatic) MIs because of cardiac neuropathy or may manifest atypical symptoms (e.g., dyspnea). An older patient may experience a change in mental status (e.g., confusion), shortness of breath, pulmonary edema, dizziness, or a dysrhythmia.

**Sympathetic Nervous System Stimulation.** During the initial phase of MI, the ischemic heart cells release catecholamines (norepinephrine and epinephrine) that are normally found in these cells. This results in release of glycogen, diaphoresis, increased HR and BP, and vasoconstriction of peripheral blood vessels. On physical examination, the patient's skin may be ashen, clammy, and cool to touch.

**Cardiovascular Manifestations.** In response to the release of catecholamines, BP and HR may be elevated initially. Later, the BP may drop because of decreased cardiac output (CO). If severe enough, this may result in decreased renal perfusion and urine output. Crackles, if present, may persist for several hours to several days, suggesting LV dysfunction. Jugular venous distention, hepatic engorgement, and peripheral edema may indicate right ventricular dysfunction.

Examination may reveal abnormal heart sounds that may seem distant. Other abnormal sounds suggesting LV dysfunction are $S_3$ and $S_4$. In addition, a loud holosystolic murmur may develop. This may indicate a ventricular septal defect, papillary muscle rupture, or valve dysfunction.

**Nausea and Vomiting.** The patient may experience nausea and vomiting. These symptoms can result from reflex stimulation of the vomiting center by the severe pain. They can also result from vasovagal reflexes initiated from the area of the infarcted heart muscle.

**Fever.** The temperature may increase to 100.4° F (38° C) within 24 to 48 hours. The temperature elevation may last for as long as 4 to 5 days. This increase in temperature is due to a systemic inflammatory process caused by the death of heart cells.

### Healing Process

The body's response to cell death is the inflammatory process (see Chapter 11). Within 24 hours, leukocytes infiltrate the area. The dead heart cells release enzymes that are important diagnostic indicators of MI (see serum cardiac biomarkers later in this chapter). The proteolytic enzymes of the neutrophils and macrophages begin to remove necrotic tissue by the fourth day. During this time the necrotic muscle wall is thin. Once infarction takes place, catecholamine-mediated lipolysis and glycogenolysis occur. These processes allow the increased plasma glucose and free fatty acids to be used by the $O_2$-depleted myocardium for anaerobic metabolism. For this reason, serum glucose levels are frequently elevated after MI.

The necrotic zone of an STEMI is identified by ECG changes (e.g., lowering of the ST segments, T wave inversion plus a pathologic Q wave) within a day or two. At this point, the neutrophils and monocytes have cleared the necrotic debris from the injured area, and the collagen matrix that will eventually form scar tissue is laid down.

At 10 to 14 days after MI, the new scar tissue is still weak. The heart muscle is vulnerable to increased stress during this time because of the unstable state of the healing heart. At the same time the patient's activity level may be increasing, so special caution and assessment are necessary. By 6 weeks after MI, scar tissue has replaced necrotic tissue and the injured area is considered healed. Often the scarred area is less compliant than the surrounding area. This condition may be manifested by abnormal wall motion on an echocardiogram or nuclear imaging, LV dysfunction, altered conduction patterns, or HF.

These changes in the infarcted heart muscle also cause changes in the unaffected areas. In an attempt to compensate for the damaged muscle, the normal myocardium hypertrophies and dilates. This process is called *ventricular remodeling.* Remodeling of normal myocardium can lead to the development of late HF, especially in the person with atherosclerosis of other coronary arteries and/or an anterior MI. ACE inhibitors are given to limit ventricular remodeling.

### Complications of Myocardial Infarction

**Dysrhythmias.** Any condition that affects the heart cells' sensitivity to nerve impulses (e.g., ischemia, electrolyte imbalances, SNS stimulation) can cause dysrhythmias that adversely affect the damaged heart muscle. Dysrhythmias are the most common complication after an MI. They occur in 80% to 90% of patients. Ventricular tachycardia (VT) and ventricular fibrillation (VF) are the most common cause of death in patients in the prehospital period. If a patient survives a cardiac arrest, start therapeutic hypothermia (also known as targeted temperature management) as soon as possible.[20] (See Chapter 68 for a discussion of therapeutic hypothermia.)

Bradycardias (e.g., complete heart block) develop when key areas of the conduction system are destroyed. VT or VF most often occur within the first 4 hours after the onset of pain. Premature ventricular contractions (PVCs) may precede VT and VF. Life-threatening ventricular dysrhythmias must be treated immediately.

With reperfusion, it is not uncommon to see PVCs, asymptomatic nonsustained VT, and idioventricular rhythms. These rhythms are not associated with an increased risk of sudden cardiac death (SCD) and are not treated unless the patient is symptomatic. (See Chapter 35 for a detailed description of dysrhythmias and their management.)

**Heart Failure.** *Heart failure* (HF) is a complication that occurs when the right or left heart's pumping action is reduced. Depending on the severity and extent of the injury, left-sided HF occurs initially with subtle signs such as mild dyspnea, restlessness, agitation, or slight tachycardia. Other signs indicating the onset of left-sided HF include pulmonary congestion on chest x-ray, $S_3$ or $S_4$ heart sounds on auscultation of the heart, crackles on auscultation of the lungs, paroxysmal nocturnal dyspnea (PND), and orthopnea. Signs of right-sided HF include jugular venous distention, hepatic congestion, or lower extremity edema. (The treatment of acute decompensated HF is discussed in Chapter 34.)

**Cardiogenic Shock.** *Cardiogenic shock* occurs when $O_2$ and nutrients supplied to the tissues are inadequate because of severe LV failure, papillary muscle rupture, ventricular septal rupture, LV free wall rupture, or right ventricular infarction. This occurs less often with the early and rapid treatment of STEMI with PCI or thrombolytic therapy. When cardiogenic shock does occur, it is associated with a high death rate. Cardiogenic shock requires aggressive management. This includes control of dysrhythmias, intraaortic balloon pump (IABP) therapy, and support of contractility with vasoactive drugs. Goals of therapy are to maximize $O_2$ delivery, reduce $O_2$ demand, and prevent complications (e.g., acute kidney injury). (Cardiogenic shock is discussed in Chapter 66.)

**Papillary Muscle Dysfunction or Rupture.** *Papillary muscle dysfunction* may occur if the infarcted area includes or is near the papillary muscle that attaches to the mitral valve (see Fig. 31-2). Suspect papillary muscle dysfunction if you hear a new murmur at the cardiac apex. An echocardiogram confirms the diagnosis.

Papillary muscle rupture is a rare and life-threatening complication. It causes immediate and massive mitral valve regurgitation with no time for the heart to compensate. This is not the case with mitral regurgitation, which has a gradual onset. Dyspnea, pulmonary edema, and decreased CO result from the backup of blood in the left atrium. This condition aggravates an already damaged LV by reducing CO even further. The patient undergoes rapid clinical decline. Treatment includes afterload reduction with nitroprusside (Nipride) and/or IABP therapy and immediate cardiac surgery with mitral valve repair or replacement. (See Chapter 36 for discussion of valve disorders.)

**Left Ventricular Aneurysm.** *Left ventricular aneurysm* results when the infarcted heart wall is thin and bulges out during contraction. This can develop within a few days, weeks, or months. It is more common with anterior MIs. The patient with a ventricular aneurysm may experience HF, dysrhythmias, and angina. Besides ventricular rupture, which is usually fatal, ventricular aneurysms can hide thrombi that can lead to an embolic stroke. Anticoagulation therapy is recommended for these patients if not contraindicated.

**Ventricular Septal Wall Rupture and Left Ventricular Free Wall Rupture.** A new loud systolic murmur heard in patients with acute MI may signal ventricular septal wall rupture. Depending on the size of the defect and degree of right and LV dysfunction, HF and cardiogenic shock may occur. The patient must receive emergency repair, either surgically or percutaneously. The defect can quickly expand and lead to hemodynamic compromise.

LV free wall rupture is an emergent clinical situation. Rapid hemodynamic compromise and death ensues if not treated immediately. Although this is a rare complication, death rates are high. Free wall rupture is seen more frequently in patients suffering their first MI, patients with anterior MIs, older adults, and women.[20]

**Pericarditis.** *Acute pericarditis,* an inflammation of the visceral and/or parietal pericardium, may occur 2 or 3 days after an acute MI. Pericarditis is characterized by mild to severe chest pain that increases with inspiration, coughing, and movement of the upper body. Sitting in a forward position often relieves the pain. The pain is usually different from pain associated with an MI.

Assess the patient with suspected pericarditis for the presence of a friction rub over the pericardium. The sound is best heard with the diaphragm of the stethoscope at the mid to lower left sternal border. It may be persistent or intermittent. Fever may also be present. The patient may have hypotension and/or a narrow pulse pressure if it is complicated by a pericardial effusion or cardiac tamponade.

Diagnosis of pericarditis can be made with serial 12-lead ECGs. Typical ECG changes include diffuse ST segment elevations. This reflects the inflammation of the pericardium. Treatment includes pain relief with high doses of aspirin (e.g., 650 mg every 4 to 6 hours). (Pericarditis is discussed in Chapter 36.)

**Dressler Syndrome.** *Dressler syndrome* is pericarditis and fever that develop 1 to 8 weeks after MI. Although the cause is unclear, it may be an autoimmune reaction to the necrotic heart muscle. The patient experiences chest pain, fever, malaise, a pericardial friction rub, and arthralgia. A pericardial effusion may be present. Laboratory findings include an elevated white blood cell count and sedimentation rate. High-dose aspirin is the treatment of choice. Nonsteroidal antiinflammatory drugs (NSAIDs) and corticosteroids are avoided in the first 4 weeks following MI because they can interfere with myocardial scar formation.

## DIAGNOSTIC STUDIES: ACUTE CORONARY SYNDROME

In addition to the patient's history of pain, risk factors, and health history, the primary diagnostic studies used to determine whether a person has UA or an MI include an ECG and serum cardiac biomarkers (Fig. 33-4).

### Electrocardiogram Findings

The ECG is one of the primary tools to diagnose UA or an MI (STEMI or NSTEMI). Whenever possible, it should be compared to a previous ECG. Changes in the QRS complex, ST segment, and T wave caused by ischemia and infarction can develop slowly or quickly with UA and MI.

The ECG must be read carefully, since changes can be absent or subtle at first. For this reason, serial 12-lead ECGs are done. For diagnostic and treatment purposes, it is important to distinguish between STEMI and NSTEMI/UA. STEMI patients usually have a complete coronary occlusion. ST elevation is first seen on the 12-lead ECG. Within a few hours to days, T wave inversion and pathologic Q waves develop. Patients with NSTEMI or UA usually have transient thrombosis or incomplete coronary occlusion. These patients often develop ST depression or T wave inversion on the initial ECG. They usually do not develop pathologic Q waves. Because MI is a dynamic process that evolves over time, serial ECGs are done to show the evolution of ischemia, injury, infarction, and resolution of the infarction. (See Chapter 35 for discussion of ECG changes associated with ischemia and MI and Fig. 35-29.)

### Serum Cardiac Biomarkers

*Serum cardiac biomarkers* are proteins released into the blood from necrotic heart muscle after an MI (see Table 31-6). These

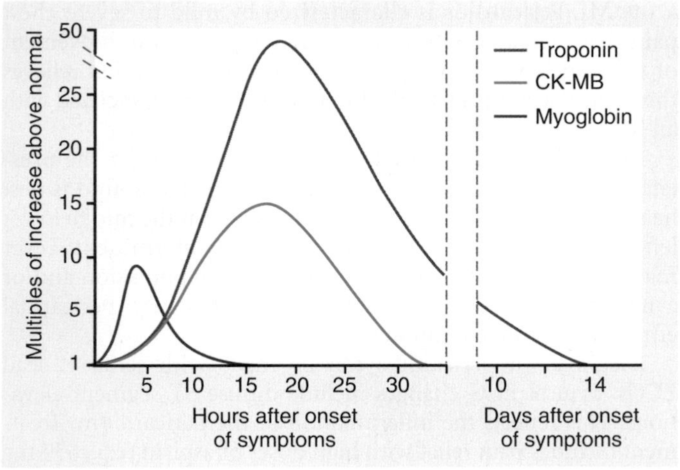


**FIG. 33-10** Serum cardiac biomarkers found in the blood after myocardial infarction.

biomarkers are important in the diagnosis of MI. The onset, peak, and duration of levels of these biomarkers are shown in Fig. 33-10.

*Cardiac-specific troponin* has two subtypes: cardiac-specific troponin T (cTnT) and cardiac-specific troponin I (cTnI). These biomarkers are highly specific indicators of MI and have greater sensitivity and specificity for myocardial injury than creatine kinase MB (CK-MB). Serum levels of cTnI and cTnT increase 4 to 6 hours after the onset of MI, peak at 10 to 24 hours, and return to baseline over 10 to 14 days. Serial cardiac biomarkers are drawn over 24 hours (e.g., every 6 hours × 3). The presence of biomarkers helps to differentiate between a diagnosis of UA (negative biomarkers) and NSTEMI (positive biomarkers).

CK levels begin to rise about 6 hours after an MI, peak at about 18 hours, and return to normal within 24 to 36 hours. The CK enzymes are fractionated into bands. The CK-MB band is specific to heart muscle cells and helps to quantify myocardial damage.

Myoglobin is released into the circulation within 2 hours after an MI and peaks in 3 to 15 hours. Although it is one of the first serum cardiac biomarkers to appear after an MI, it lacks cardiac specificity. Its role in diagnosing MI is limited.

### Coronary Angiography

The patient with a STEMI must undergo coronary angiography within 90 minutes of presentation or receive thrombolytic therapy within 30 minutes in agencies without PCI capability. This will open the totally occluded artery and limit the infarction size. The patient with UA or NSTEMI may or may not undergo coronary angiography to evaluate the extent of the disease. Guidelines suggest that it is reasonable to do coronary angiography on stable but high-risk patients with UA or NSTEMI within 12 to 72 hours after presentation. If appropriate, a PCI is performed at this time. Some patients may be treated only with conservative medical management.[23]

### Other Measures

When the ECG and serum cardiac biomarkers do not confirm MI, other measures for diagnosing CAD are considered (see Table 31-6). To assess for ischemia or infarction, pharmacologic stress testing may be done when a patient has an abnormal but nondiagnostic ECG and negative biomarkers. (See Chapter 31 for additional information on cardiac assessment.)

## INTERPROFESSIONAL CARE: ACUTE CORONARY SYNDROME

It is extremely important to quickly diagnose and treat a patient with ACS to preserve heart muscle. Initial management of the patient with chest pain most often occurs in the ED. Table 33-12 presents the emergency care of the patient with chest pain. Obtain a 12-lead ECG and start continuous ECG monitoring. Position the patient in an upright position unless contraindicated, and start $O_2$ by nasal cannula to keep $O_2$ saturation above 93%. Obtain IV access for drug administration. Give SL NTG and 162 to 325 mg of aspirin (chewable) if not given before arrival at the ED. A high-dose statin (atorvastatin [Lipitor]) is started if not already taking prior to the hospitalization. Morphine sulfate is given for pain unrelieved by NTG.

The patient is usually transferred to a critical care unit where ongoing care including continuous ECG monitoring is available. Dysrhythmias are treated according to agency protocols. Some patients are started on glycoprotein IIb/IIIa inhibitors (e.g., eptifibatide) either before catheterization or at the time of PCI. Fig. 33-4 on p. 714 presents the interprofessional care of ACS.

Monitor vital signs (including pulse oximetry) frequently (e.g., every hour) during the first few hours after admission and closely thereafter, according to agency protocol. Maintain bed rest and limit activity for 12 to 24 hours, with a gradual increase in activity unless contraindicated.

For patients with UA and NSTEMI, aspirin and heparin (UH or LMWH) are recommended. Dual antiplatelet therapy (e.g., aspirin and clopidogrel) (Table 33-11) and heparin are recommended for NSTEMI patients. Cardiac catheterization with possible PCI is considered for both UA and NSTEMI patients once the patient is stabilized and angina is controlled or if angina returns or increases in severity.

For patients with STEMI, reperfusion therapy is started (Figs. 33-6 and 33-7). *Reperfusion therapy* includes emergent PCI (preferred) or thrombolytic therapy for STEMI. The goal in the treatment of STEMI is to save as much heart muscle as possible. Dual antiplatelet therapy and heparin are also used.

### Emergent PCI

Emergent PCI is the first line of treatment for patients with confirmed STEMI (i.e., ST-elevation on the ECG and/or positive cardiac biomarkers). The goal is to open the blocked artery within 90 minutes of arrival to a facility that has an interventional cardiac catheterization laboratory. In this case the patient undergoes a cardiac catheterization to locate and assess the severity of the blockage(s), determine the presence of collateral circulation, and evaluate LV function. During the procedure, a bare metal stent (BMS) or drug-eluting stent (DES) is inserted into the blocked coronary artery. Additional arteries may also be stented at this time if appropriate.[20] Patients with severe LV dysfunction may require the addition of IABP therapy and/or inotropes (e.g., dobutamine). A small percentage of patients may require emergent CABG surgery.

The advantages of PCI (compared to thrombolytic therapy) include the following: (1) it provides an alternative to surgical

**TABLE 33-12 Emergency Management**

***Chest Pain***

| Etiology | Assessment Findings | Interventions |
|---|---|---|
| **Cardiovascular**<br>• Myocardial ischemia<br>• Myocardial infarction<br>• Dysrhythmia<br>• Pericarditis<br>• Aortic aneurysm<br>• Aortic valve disease<br>**Respiratory**<br>• Costochondritis<br>• Pleurisy<br>• Pneumonia<br>• Pneumothorax, hemothorax<br>• Pulmonary edema<br>• Pulmonary embolus<br>**Chest Trauma**<br>• Rib/sternal fracture<br>• Flail chest<br>• Cardiac tamponade<br>• Hemothorax<br>• Pulmonary contusion<br>• Great vessel injury<br>**Gastrointestinal**<br>• Esophagitis<br>• GERD<br>• Hiatal hernia<br>• Peptic ulcer<br>• Cholecystitis<br>**Others**<br>• Stress<br>• Strenuous exercise<br>• Drugs (e.g., cocaine)<br>• Acute anxiety | • Pain in chest, neck, jaw, arm, or shoulder<br>• Cold, clammy skin<br>• Diaphoresis<br>• Nausea and vomiting<br>• Epigastric pain<br>• Indigestion, heartburn<br>• Dyspnea, tachypnea<br>• Weakness<br>• Anxiety<br>• Feeling of impending doom<br>• Tachycardia, bradycardia<br>• Irregular HR, murmurs<br>• Palpitations<br>• Dysrhythmias<br>• Decreased or increased BP<br>• Narrowed pulse pressure<br>• Unequal BP readings in upper extremities<br>• Syncope, loss of consciousness<br>• Decreased $O_2$ saturation<br>• Decreased or absent breath sounds<br>• Pericardial friction rub | **Initial**<br>• If unresponsive, assess circulation, airway, and breathing.<br>• If responsive, monitor airway, breathing, and circulation.<br>• Position patient upright unless contraindicated and give $O_2$ by nasal cannula or non-rebreather mask.<br>• Obtain baseline vital signs, including $O_2$ saturation.<br>• Auscultate heart and breath sounds.<br>• Obtain 12-lead ECG.<br>• Insert two IV catheters.<br>• Assess pain using PQRST mnemonic (Table 33-7).<br>• Medicate for pain as ordered (e.g., nitroglycerin, morphine).<br>• Start continuous ECG monitoring and identify underlying rhythm.<br>• Obtain baseline blood work (e.g., cardiac biomarkers, CBC, basic metabolic panel, coagulation studies).<br>• Obtain portable chest x-ray.<br>• Assess for contraindications for antiplatelet, anticoagulant, or thrombolytic therapy, or PCI as appropriate.<br>• Give aspirin for heart-related chest pain unless contraindicated.<br>• Give a high-dose statin.<br>• Give antidysrhythmic drugs for life-threatening dysrhythmias.<br>**Ongoing Monitoring**<br>• Monitor ABCs, vital signs, level of consciousness, heart and breath sounds, heart rhythm, and $O_2$ saturation.<br>• Assess and record response to drugs (e.g., decrease in chest pain) and remedicate or titrate drugs (e.g., nitroglycerin) as needed.<br>• Provide reassurance and emotional support to patient and caregiver.<br>• Explain all interventions and procedures to patient and caregiver in simple terms.<br>• Anticipate need for intubation if respiratory distress is evident.<br>• Prepare for CPR and defibrillation if cardiac arrest is evident.<br>• Anticipate need for transcutaneous pacing for symptomatic bradycardia or heart block. |

*GERD,* Gastroesophageal reflux disease; *PCI,* percutaneous coronary intervention.

intervention; (2) it is performed with local anesthesia; (3) the patient is ambulatory shortly after the procedure; (4) the length of hospital stay is approximately 3 to 4 days after MI compared with the 4 to 6 days with CABG surgery, thus reducing hospital costs; and (5) the patient can return to work several weeks sooner after PCI, compared with a 6- to 8-week convalescence after CABG.

Advances in PCI techniques have significantly reduced the need for emergent CABG. More PCIs are performed in the U.S. than CABGs.[1] Complications of PCI that may lead to emergent CABG include dissection of the coronary artery, abrupt artery closure, coronary artery rupture, acute stent thrombosis, and failure to cross the blockage with a balloon or stent. There is a risk that the infarction could be extended should a part of the plaque dislodge and block the vessel distal to the catheter. Coronary spasm from the mechanical irritation of the catheter or balloon can occur, as well as renal dysfunction or an allergic reaction from the contrast dye used in the procedure. Other complications of PCI include vascular access-site bleeding or other vascular complications, stroke, and infection.

In-stent restenosis (ISR) is a potential problem whenever stents are placed in a coronary artery. ISR usually occurs within a few months to a year after stent placement. Nursing care of the patient following PCI is similar to that after cardiac catheterization (see Table 31-6).

### Thrombolytic Therapy

Thrombolytic (fibrinolytic) therapy is indicated only for patients with a STEMI. Advantages include the availability and rapid administration in agencies that do not have an interventional cardiac catheterization laboratory or when one is too far away to transfer the patient safely. Treatment of STEMI with thrombolytic therapy aims to limit the infarction size by dissolving the thrombus in the coronary artery and reperfusing the heart muscle. The goal is to give the thrombolytic within 30 minutes of the patient's arrival to the ED. Patients who are taken to non–PCI-capable hospitals can be moved to a PCI capable hospital if the first medical contact to balloon inflation (PCI) time can be done within 120 minutes.[20]

**Indications and Contraindications.** All thrombolytics are given IV (Table 33-11). The cost, efficacy, and ease of administration guide the choice of a thrombolytic agent. Although these drugs have different pharmacokinetics, they all open the blocked artery by lysis of the thrombus. Because all thrombolytics lyse the pathologic clot, they may also lyse other clots (e.g., a post-operative site). Therefore patient selection is important because minor or major bleeding can be a complication of therapy.

Inclusion criteria for thrombolytic therapy are (1) chest pain less than 12 hours with 12-lead ECG findings consistent with acute STEMI and (2) no absolute contraindications (Table 33-13). Patients with chest pain lasting 12 to 24 hours with ECG

**TABLE 33-13 Contraindications for Thrombolytic Therapy**

**Absolute Contraindications**
- Any prior history of intracranial hemorrhage
- Known structural or vascular abnormality (e.g., arteriovenous malformation)
- Known intracranial neoplasm (primary or metastatic)
- Recent (within past 3 mo) ischemic stroke
- Significant closed-head or facial trauma within past 3 mo
- Intracranial or intraspinal surgery within 2 mo
- Severe uncontrolled hypertension
- Active internal bleeding or bleeding diathesis (excluding menstruation)
- Suspected aortic dissection
- For streptokinase, prior treatment within the past 6 months

**Relative Contraindications**
- Active peptic ulcer disease
- Current use of oral anticoagulants
- Pregnancy
- Prior ischemic stroke (>3 mo ago)
- Dementia
- Known intracranial pathology not covered in absolute contraindications
- Noncompressible vascular punctures
- Recent (within 2-4 wk) internal bleeding
- Major surgery (<3 wk)
- History of chronic, severe, poorly controlled hypertension
- Significant hypertension on presentation (SBP >180 mm/Hg or DBP >110 mm/Hg)
- Traumatic or prolonged (>10 min) cardiopulmonary resuscitation

Source: O'Gara PT, Kushner FG, Ascheim DD, et al: 2013 ACCF/AHA guideline for the management of ST-elevation myocardial infarction: a report of the American College of Cardiology Foundation/American Heart Association Task Force on Practice Guidelines, *Circulation* 127:e362, 2013.

changes supporting STEMI may be considered for thrombolytic therapy.[20]

**Procedure.** Each hospital has a protocol for giving thrombolytic therapy, but several factors are common. Draw blood to obtain baseline laboratory values and start two or three lines for IV therapy. All other invasive procedures are done before the thrombolytic agent is given to reduce the possibility of bleeding.

Depending on the drug selected, therapy is given in one IV bolus or over time (30 to 90 minutes). Note the time at which therapy begins, and monitor the patient during and after giving the thrombolytic. Assess heart rhythm, vital signs, and pulse oximetry. Assess the heart and lungs frequently to evaluate the patient's response to therapy. Regularly assess for changes in neurologic status, since this may indicate cerebral bleeding.

When reperfusion occurs (i.e., the coronary artery that was blocked is opened and blood flow is restored to the heart muscle), several clinical signs may be seen. The most reliable sign is the return of the ST segment to baseline on the ECG. Other signs include a resolution of chest pain and an early, rapid rise of the serum cardiac biomarkers within 3 hours of therapy, peaking within 12 hours. These levels increase as the necrotic heart cells release proteins into the circulation after perfusion is restored to the area. The presence of *reperfusion dysrhythmias* (e.g., accelerated idioventricular rhythm) is a less reliable sign of reperfusion. These dysrhythmias are generally self-limiting and do not require aggressive treatment. (See Chapter 35 for management of dysrhythmias.)

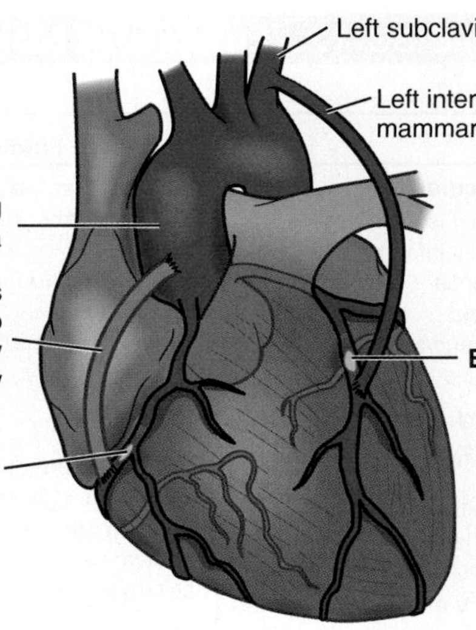


**FIG. 33-11** Distal end of the left internal mammary artery is grafted below the area of blockage in the left anterior descending artery. Proximal end of the saphenous vein is grafted to the aorta, and the distal end is grafted below the area of blockage in the right coronary artery.

A major concern with thrombolytic therapy is reocclusion of the artery. The site of the thrombus is unstable, and formation of another clot or spasm of the artery may occur. Therefore IV heparin therapy is started. If another clot develops, the patient will have similar complaints of chest pain and ECG changes will return. Patients receiving thrombolytic therapy should be moved to a facility with PCI capabilities as soon as possible so PCI can be performed if thrombolytic therapy fails.

The major complication with thrombolytic therapy is bleeding. Ongoing nursing assessment is essential. Minor bleeding (e.g., surface bleeding from IV sites or gingival bleeding) is expected and controlled by applying a pressure dressing or ice packs.

**SAFETY ALERT Thrombolytic Therapy**
- Minor or major bleeding can occur with thrombolytic drugs.
- Place two or three IV lines before thrombolytic therapy is started.
- If signs and symptoms of major bleeding occur (e.g., drop in BP, increase in HR, sudden change in the patient's mental status, blood in the urine or stool), stop the drug and notify the HCP.

## Coronary Surgical Revascularization

Coronary revascularization with CABG surgery is recommended for patients who (1) fail medical management, (2) have left main coronary artery or three-vessel disease, (3) are not candidates for PCI (e.g., blockages are long or difficult to access), or (4) have failed PCI and continue to have chest pain. CABG may also be the option for patients with diabetes, LV dysfunction, or chronic kidney disease.[24] CABG surgery and PCI are considered palliative treatment for CAD and not a cure.

**Traditional Coronary Artery Bypass Graft Surgery.** CABG surgery consists of the placement of arterial or venous grafts to provide blood between the aorta or other major arteries and the heart muscle distal to the blocked coronary artery (or arteries). The procedure may involve one or more grafts using the internal mammary (thoracic) artery (IMA or ITA), saphenous vein, radial artery, gastroepiploic artery, and/or inferior epigastric artery (Fig. 33-11).

CABG surgery requires a sternotomy (opening of the chest cavity) and *cardiopulmonary bypass* (CPB). During CPB, blood is diverted from the patient's heart to a machine. Here it is oxygenated and returned (via a pump) to the patient. This allows the surgeon to operate on a quiet, nonbeating, bloodless heart while perfusion to vital organs is maintained. CPB is associated with postoperative neurologic dysfunction, renal dysfunction and systemic inflammatory response syndrome (SIRS).[24]

The IMA is the most common artery used for bypass graft. It is left attached to its origin (the subclavian artery) but then dissected from the chest wall. Next, it is *anastomosed* (connected with sutures) to the coronary artery distal to the blockage.

Saphenous veins are also used for bypass grafts. The surgeon endoscopically removes the saphenous vein from one or both legs. A section is sutured into the ascending aorta near the native coronary artery opening and then sutured to the coronary artery distal to the blockage. Saphenous vein grafts are more prone to develop diffuse intimal hyperplasia. This contributes to future stenosis and graft occlusion. The use of antiplatelet and statin therapy after surgery improves vein graft patency.

The radial artery, another potential graft, is a thick muscular artery that is prone to spasm. Perioperative calcium channel blockers and long-acting nitrates can control the spasms. Patency rates are not as good as the IMA but better than saphenous veins. Serious extremity complications (e.g., hand ischemia, wound infection) are rare after removal of the radial artery. Paresthesia and impaired sensation are common side effects after radial artery harvest.[25]

Other potential grafts include the gastroepiploic or inferior epigastric artery. Like the radial artery, these also are prone to spasms.

Women have higher periprocedural mortality and morbidity rates than men. This has been attributed to the late treatment of CAD in women because women first present with CAD at an older age and have more co-morbidities at the time of surgery. Other possible factors include smaller-diameter coronary vessels, smaller body surface area, and the fact that women are less likely to be referred for catheterization and PCI.[24]

**Minimally Invasive Direct Coronary Artery Bypass.** *Minimally invasive direct coronary artery bypass* (MIDCAB) offers patients with disease of the left anterior descending or right coronary artery an approach to surgical treatment that does not involve a sternotomy and CPB. The technique requires several small incisions between the ribs or a mini-thoracotomy. A thoracoscope or robotic assistance is used to dissect the IMA from the chest. A mechanical stabilizer immobilizes the operative site. The IMA is then sutured to the left anterior descending or right coronary artery. Some patients undergo hybrid procedures in which they have a MIDCAB for the left anterior descending artery and undergo a PCI of a second or third artery at a later time.

**Off-Pump Coronary Artery Bypass.** The *off-pump coronary artery bypass* (OPCAB) procedure uses a median sternotomy to access all coronary vessels. OPCAB is performed on a beating heart (no CPB) using mechanical stabilizers. OPCAB is associated with less blood loss, less renal dysfunction, less postoperative atrial fibrillation, and fewer neurologic complications. It is estimated that less than 20% of CABG procedures are OPCAB procedures. OPCAB is primarily used for patients with multiple co-morbidities who should avoid CPB.[25]

**Robotic or Totally Endoscopic Coronary Artery Bypass (TECAB).** This technique uses a robot in performing CABG surgery. This procedure is done without the use of CPB or with the use of CPB using femoral access. TECAB is used for limited bypass grafting. The benefits include increased precision, smaller incisions, decreased blood loss, less pain, and shorter recovery time.[25]

**Transmyocardial Laser Revascularization.** *Transmyocardial laser revascularization* is an indirect revascularization procedure. It is used for patients with advanced CAD who are not candidates for traditional CABG surgery and who have persistent angina despite maximum medical therapy. The procedure involves the use of a high-energy laser to create channels in the heart muscle to allow blood flow to ischemic areas. The procedure can be done using a left thoracotomy approach or in combination with CABG surgery. It is as an adjunctive therapy when bypass grafts cannot be placed.

## Drug Therapy

When a patient presents with suspected ACS, dual antiplatelet therapy (e.g., chewable aspirin, clopidogrel), IV NTG, atorvastatin, and systemic anticoagulation with either subcutaneous LMWH or IV UH are drug treatments of choice. Glycoprotein IIb/IIIa inhibitors may also be used if PCI is anticipated. Oral β-blockers are given within the first 24 hours if there are no contraindications (e.g., HF, heart block, hypotension). ACE inhibitors are added for select patients following MI if there are no contraindications. Calcium channel blockers are added if the patient cannot tolerate β-blockers. These drugs must be used cautiously after MI because of their effect on contractility.[26] Nitrates may be used if the patient has persistent chest pain.

Table 33-11 and Fig. 33-4 present drug therapy for patients with ACS. These drugs are discussed on pp. 714-717. Drugs that are specifically used to treat ACS are discussed in this section.

**IV Nitroglycerin.** IV NTG is used in the initial treatment of the patient with ACS. The goal of therapy is to reduce anginal pain and improve coronary blood flow. IV NTG decreases preload and afterload while increasing the myocardial $O_2$ supply. The onset of action is immediate. Titrate NTG to control and stop chest pain. Because hypotension is a common side effect, closely monitor BP during this time. Patients who do become hypotensive are often volume depleted and can benefit from an IV fluid bolus.

**Morphine.** Morphine sulfate is the drug of choice for chest pain that is unrelieved by NTG. As a vasodilator, it decreases cardiac workload by lowering myocardial $O_2$ consumption, reducing contractility, and decreasing BP and HR. In addition, morphine can help reduce anxiety and fear. In rare situations, morphine can depress respirations. Monitor patients for signs of bradypnea or hypotension, which are conditions to avoid in myocardial ischemia and infarction.

**β-Adrenergic Blockers.** β-Blockers decrease myocardial $O_2$ demand by reducing HR, BP, and contractility. The use of these drugs in patients who are not at risk for complications of MI (e.g., cardiogenic shock, bradycardia, hypotension) reduces the risk of reinfarction and the development of HF. β-blockers are continued indefinitely. (See Table 33-11, Chapter 32 and Table 32-7 for a discussion of β-blockers.)

**Angiotensin-Converting Enzyme Inhibitors and Angiotensin Receptor Blockers.** ACE inhibitors should be started within the first 24 hours if the BP is stable and there are no contraindications. They are continued indefinitely in patients recovering from STEMI or NSTEMI, with heart failure, or an EF of 40% or less. The use of ACE inhibitors can help prevent ventricular remodeling and prevent or slow the progression of HF. For patients who cannot tolerate ACE inhibitors (e.g., angioedema, cough), ARBs should be considered. (See Tables 33-11 and 32-7.)

**Antidysrhythmic Drugs.** Dysrhythmias are the most common complications after an MI. In general, they are self-limiting and not treated aggressively unless they are life threatening (e.g., sustained ventricular tachycardia). (Chapter 35 discusses the drugs used in the treatment of dysrhythmias.)

**Lipid-Lowering Drugs.** A lipid panel is obtained on all patients with ACS. All patients with ACS or diagnosed with CAD should receive lipid-lowering drugs indefinitely, unless contraindicated (Table 33-5).

**Stool Softeners.** After an MI, the patient may be predisposed to constipation because of bed rest and use of opioid drugs. Stool softeners (e.g., docusate sodium [Colace]) are given to aid bowel movements. This prevents straining and the resultant vagal stimulation from the *Valsalva maneuver*. Vagal stimulation produces bradycardia and can provoke dysrhythmias.

### Nutritional Therapy

Initially, patients may be NPO (nothing by mouth) except for water until stable (e.g., pain free, nausea resolved). Advance the diet as tolerated to a low-salt, low-saturated-fat, and low-cholesterol diet (Tables 33-3 and 33-4).

## NURSING MANAGEMENT: CHRONIC STABLE ANGINA AND ACUTE CORONARY SYNDROME

### Nursing Assessment

Table 33-14 presents the subjective and objective data to obtain from a patient with ACS.

**TABLE 33-14 Nursing Assessment**
***Acute Coronary Syndrome***

**Subjective Data**

***Important Health Information***

*Past health history:* Previous history of CAD, chest pain/angina, MI, valve disease (e.g., aortic stenosis), heart failure, or cardiomyopathy. Hypertension, diabetes, anemia, lung disease, hyperlipidemia

*Medications:* Use of antiplatelets or anticoagulants, nitrates, angiotensin-converting enzyme inhibitors, β-blockers, calcium channel blockers, antihypertensive drugs, lipid-lowering drugs, over-the-counter drugs (e.g., vitamin and herbal supplements)

*History of present illness:* Description of events related to current illness (Table 33-8), including any self-treatments and response

***Functional Health Patterns***

*Health perception–health management:* Family history of heart disease. Sedentary lifestyle, tobacco use, exposure to environmental smoke

*Nutritional-metabolic:* Indigestion, heartburn, nausea, belching, vomiting

*Elimination:* Urinary urgency or frequency, straining at stool

*Activity-exercise:* Palpitations, dyspnea, dizziness, weakness

*Cognitive-perceptual:* Substernal chest pain or pressure (squeezing, constricting, aching, sharp, tingling), possible radiation to jaw, neck, shoulders, back, or arms (Table 33-7)

*Coping–stress tolerance:* Stressful lifestyle, depression; anger, anxiety. Feeling of impending doom

**Objective Data**

***General***

Anxious, fearful, restless, distressed

***Integumentary***

Cool, clammy, pale skin

***Cardiovascular***

Tachycardia or bradycardia, pulsus alternans (alternating weak and strong heartbeats), pulse deficit, dysrhythmias (especially ventricular), $S_3$, $S_4$, ↑ or ↓ BP, murmur

***Possible Diagnostic Findings***

Positive serum cardiac biomarkers, ↑ serum lipids; ↑ WBC count. Positive exercise or pharmacologic stress test and thallium scans. Pathologic Q wave, ST segment elevation, and/or T wave abnormalities on ECG. Cardiac enlargement, calcifications, or pulmonary congestion on chest x-ray. Abnormal wall motion with stress echocardiogram. Positive coronary angiography.

### Nursing Diagnoses

Nursing diagnoses for the patient with ACS may include, but are not limited to, the following:

- Decreased cardiac output *related to* altered contractility and altered heart rate and rhythm
- Acute pain *related to* an imbalance between myocardial $O_2$ supply and demand
- Anxiety *related to* perceived or actual threat of death, pain, and/or possible lifestyle changes
- Activity intolerance *related to* general weakness secondary to decreased cardiac output and poor lung and tissue perfusion
- Ineffective health management *related to* lack of knowledge of disease process, risk factor reduction, rehabilitation, home activities, and medications

More information on nursing diagnoses of patients with ACS is presented in eNursing Care Plan 33-1 available on the website for this chapter.

### Planning

The overall goals for a patient with ACS include (1) relief of pain, (2) preservation of heart muscle, (3) immediate and appropriate treatment, (4) effective coping with illness-associated anxiety, (5) participation in a rehabilitation plan, and (6) reduction of risk factors. In addition, the Joint Commission has identified a core measure related to the timing of thrombolytics in the management of patients with an acute MI to reflect standards of evidence-based care (available at *www.jointcommission.org/acute_myocardial_infarction/default.aspx*).

### Nursing Implementation: Chronic Stable Angina

**Health Promotion.** Behaviors to reduce the risk for CAD are presented in Table 33-2 and discussed on pp. 707-712.

**Acute Care.** If your patient experiences angina, perform the following measures: (1) position patient upright unless contraindicated and apply supplemental $O_2$, (2) assess vital signs, (3) obtain a 12-lead ECG, (4) provide prompt pain relief first with NTG followed by an opioid analgesic if needed, and (5) assess heart and breath sounds. The patient will most likely be anxious and may have pale, cool, clammy skin. The BP and HR may be elevated. Auscultation of the heart may reveal an atrial ($S_4$) or a ventricular ($S_3$) gallop. A new murmur heard during an anginal attack may indicate ischemia of a papillary muscle of the mitral valve. The murmur is likely to be transient and disappear when symptoms stop.

Ask the patient to describe the pain and to rate it on a scale of 0 to 10 before and after treatment to evaluate the effectiveness of the interventions (Table 33-7). It is important to use the same words that patients use to describe their symptoms (e.g., tightness, pressure). Assess for other signs of pain, such as restlessness; ECG changes; elevated HR, respiratory rate, or BP; clutching of the bed linens; or other nonverbal cues. Support and reassure the patient. Use a calm approach to help reduce the patient's anxiety during an anginal attack.

**CHECK YOUR PRACTICE**

A visitor finds you in the hallway and tells you that her father is having chest pain. The patient is not assigned to you.

- How would you proceed?

◆ **Ambulatory Care.** Reassure the patient with a history of angina that a long, active life is possible. Prevention of angina is preferable to its treatment. This is why teaching is important. Give the patient information about CAD, angina, precipitating factors for angina, risk factor reduction, and drugs.

Patient teaching can be done in a variety of ways. One-on-one contact between you and the patient is often the most effective approach. Time spent providing daily care (e.g., giving drugs) offers many teachable moments. Teaching aids such as DVDs, heart models, and printed information are important parts of patient and caregiver teaching (see Chapter 4).

Help the patient to identify factors that precipitate angina (Table 33-8). Tell the patient how to avoid or control these factors. For example, teach the patient to avoid exposure to extremes of weather and eating large, heavy meals. If a heavy meal is eaten, tell the patient to rest for 1 to 2 hours after the meal because blood is shifted to the GI tract to aid digestion and absorption.

Help the patient to identify personal risk factors for CAD. Then discuss the various ways modifiable risk factors can be reduced (Table 33-2). Teach the patient and caregiver about diets that are low in salt and saturated fats (Tables 33-3 and 33-4). Maintaining ideal body weight is important in controlling angina because excess weight increases the heart's workload.

It is important that the patient has a regular, individualized program of physical activity that conditions rather than stresses the heart. For example, tell patients that walking briskly on a flat surface at least 30 minutes a day, most days of the week is recommended.

It is important to teach the patient and caregiver the proper use of NTG (see pp. 714 and 716). NTG may be used prophylactically before an emotionally stressful situation, sexual intercourse, or physical exertion (e.g., climbing a long flight of stairs).

If needed, arrange for counseling to assess the psychologic adjustment of the patient and caregiver to the diagnosis of CAD and the resulting angina. Many patients feel a threat to their identity and self-esteem and may be unable to fill their usual roles in society. These emotions are normal and real.

## ◆ Nursing Implementation: Acute Coronary Syndrome

◆ **Acute Care.** Priorities for nursing interventions in the initial phase of ACS include (1) pain assessment and relief, (2) physiologic monitoring, (3) promotion of rest and comfort, (4) alleviation of stress and anxiety, and (5) understanding of the patient's emotional and behavioral reactions. Patients with increased anxiety levels have a greater risk for adverse outcomes such as recurrent ischemic events and dysrhythmias. Proper management of these priorities decreases the $O_2$ needs of a compromised heart muscle and reduces the risk of complications. In addition, start measures to avoid the hazards of immobility while encouraging periods of rest.

◆ ***Pain.*** Provide NTG, morphine, and supplemental $O_2$ as needed to eliminate or reduce chest pain. Ongoing evaluation and documentation of the effectiveness of the interventions are important. Once pain is relieved, you may have to deal with denial in a patient who interprets the absence of pain as an absence of heart disease.

◆ ***Monitoring.*** Maintain continuous ECG monitoring while the patient is in the ED and ICU and after transfer to a step-down or general unit. Dysrhythmias must be identified quickly and treated. During the initial period after MI, ventricular fibrillation is the most common lethal dysrhythmia. In many patients, premature ventricular contractions or ventricular tachycardia precedes this dysrhythmia. Monitor the patient for reinfarction or ischemia by monitoring the ST segment for shifts above or below the baseline of the ECG. Silent ischemia can occur without subjective symptoms (e.g., chest pain). It is noted by ST segment changes only. Notify the HCP if you see ST segment changes without any clinical symptoms. (See Chapter 35 for a complete discussion of ECG monitoring.)

Perform a physical assessment to detect changes from the patient's baseline findings. Assess heart and breath sounds and any signs of early HF (e.g., dyspnea, tachycardia, pulmonary congestion, distended neck veins). In addition to routine vital signs, monitor intake and output at least once a shift.

Assessment of the patient's oxygenation status is important, especially if the patient is receiving $O_2$. If a nasal cannula is used to deliver $O_2$, check the nares for irritation or dryness, which can cause considerable discomfort.

◆ ***Rest and Comfort.*** It is important to promote rest and comfort with any degree of heart damage. Bed rest may be ordered for the first few days after an MI that involves a large portion of the LV. A patient with an uncomplicated MI (e.g., angina resolved, no signs of complications) may rest in a chair within 8 to 12 hours after the event. The use of a commode or bedpan is based on patient preference.

When sleeping or resting, the body requires less work from the heart than it does when active. It is important to plan nursing and other interventions to ensure adequate rest periods free from interruption. Comfort measures that can promote rest include a quiet environment, use of relaxation techniques (e.g., music therapy, guided imagery), and assurance that staff are nearby and responsive to the patient's needs.

It is important that the patient understand the reasons why activity is limited but not completely restricted. Gradually increase the patient's heart workload through more demanding physical tasks. It is important that the patient achieve a discharge activity level adequate for home care. Table 33-15 outlines the phases of cardiac rehabilitation.

◆ ***Anxiety.*** To some degree anxiety is present in all patients with ACS. Your role is to identify the source of anxiety and assist the patient in reducing it. If the patient is afraid of being alone, allow a caregiver to sit by quietly or check in with the patient frequently. If a source of anxiety is fear of the unknown, explore these concerns with the patient. For anxiety caused by lack of information, provide teaching based on the patient's stated need and level of understanding. Answer the patient's questions with clear, simple explanations.

**TABLE 33-15 Phases of Rehabilitation After Acute Coronary Syndrome**

**Phase I: Hospital**
- Occurs while the patient is still hospitalized
- Activity level depends on severity of angina or MI.
- Patient may first sit up in bed or chair, perform range-of-motion exercises and self-care (e.g., washing, shaving), and progress to walking in hallway and limited stair climbing.
- Attention focuses on management of chest pain, anxiety, dysrhythmias, and complications.

**Phase II: Early Recovery**
- Begins after the patient is discharged
- Usually lasts from 2-12 wk and is held in an outpatient facility
- Activity level is gradually increased under the supervision of the cardiac rehabilitation team and with ECG monitoring.
- Team may suggest that physical activity (e.g., walking) be started at home.
- Information regarding risk factor reduction is provided at this time.

**Phase III: Late Recovery**
- Long-term maintenance program
- Individual physical activity programs are designed and implemented at home, a local gym, or the rehabilitation center.
- Patient and caregiver possibly restructure lifestyles and roles.
- Therapeutic lifestyle changes should become lifelong habits.
- Medical supervision is still recommended.

**CHECK YOUR PRACTICE**

You are walking in the hallway with a 64-yr-old woman who had an MI 3 days ago. She is scheduled to be discharged tomorrow. She is visibly anxious and irritable, wringing her hands, and talking very fast. She tells you, "My heart is pounding." You do not know if she is anxious or about to have another MI.
- What should you do?

It is important to start teaching at the patient's level rather than to present a prepackaged program. For example, patients generally are not ready to learn about the pathology of CAD. The earliest questions usually relate to how the disease affects perceived control and independence. Examples include the following.
- When will I leave the intensive care unit?
- When can I be out of bed?
- When will I be discharged?
- When can I return to work?
- How many changes will I have to make in my life?
- Will this happen again?

Tell the patient that more complete teaching will begin once the patient is feeling stronger. Often the patient may not be able to ask the most serious concern of ACS patients: Am I going to die? Even if a patient denies this concern, it is helpful for you to start a conversation by remarking that fear of dying is a common concern among most patients who have experienced ACS. This gives the patient "permission" to talk about an uncomfortable and fearful topic.

◆ ***Emotional and Behavioral Reactions.*** Patients' emotional and behavioral reactions vary, but often follow a predictable response pattern (Table 33-16). Your role is to understand what the patient is currently experiencing and to support the use of constructive coping styles.

**TABLE 33-16 Psychosocial Responses to Acute Coronary Syndrome**

**Denial**
- May have history of ignoring signs and symptoms related to heart disease
- Minimizes severity of health condition
- Ignores activity restrictions
- Avoids discussing illness or its significance

**Depression**
- Mourns loss of health, altered body function, and changes in lifestyle
- Realizes seriousness of situation
- Begins to worry about future implications of health problem
- Shows manifestations of withdrawal, crying, apathy
- May be more evident after discharge

**Anger and Hostility**
- Is commonly expressed as, "Why did this happen to me?"
- May be directed at family, staff, or medical regimen

**Anxiety and Fear**
- Fears long-term disability and death
- Overtly displays apprehension, restlessness, insomnia, tachycardia
- Less overtly displays increased verbalization, projection of feelings to others, hypochondriasis
- Fears activity
- Fears recurrent chest pain, heart attacks, and sudden death

**Dependency**
- Is totally reliant on staff
- Is unwilling to perform tasks or activities unless approved by HCP
- Wants to be monitored by ECG at all times
- Is hesitant to leave the intensive care or telemetry unit or hospital

**Realistic Acceptance**
- Focuses on optimum rehabilitation
- Plans changes compatible with altered cardiac function
- Actively engages in lifestyle changes to address modifiable risk factors

Assess the support structure of the patient and caregiver. Determine how you can help maximize the support system. Often the patient is separated from the most significant support system at the time of hospitalization. Your role can include talking with the caregiver(s), informing them of the patient's progress, allowing the patient and caregivers to interact as necessary, and supporting the caregivers who will provide the necessary support to the patient. Open visitation is helpful in decreasing anxiety and increasing support for the patient with ACS.[27] It is important for you to help the patient identify additional support systems (e.g., spiritual care, Mended Hearts) that can assist after discharge.

◆ **Coronary Revascularization.** Patients with ACS may undergo coronary revascularization with PCI or CABG surgery. The major nursing responsibilities for patient care after PCI involve monitoring for signs of recurrent angina; frequent assessment of vital signs, including HR and rhythm; evaluation of the catheter insertion site for signs of bleeding; neurovascular assessment of the involved extremity; and maintenance of bed rest per agency policy.

For patients having CABG surgery, care is provided in the ICU for the first 24 to 36 hours. Ongoing and intensive monitoring of the patient's hemodynamic status is critical. The

## TEAMWORK & COLLABORATION

### *Cardiac Catheterization and Percutaneous Coronary Intervention (PCI)*

Before and after cardiac catheterization and PCI, patients require frequent interventions by RNs. The RN is responsible for assessing the patient, developing and implementing an individualized plan of care, evaluating the patient, and providing discharge teaching. Much of the care can be delegated to LPN/LVNs and UAP. Respiratory therapy may also have a role in the patient's care depending on the patient's past medical history.

**Role of Nursing Personnel**

***Registered Nurse (RN)***

*Preprocedure*

- Assess for allergies, especially to contrast dye. Perform baseline assessment, including vital signs, pulse oximetry, heart and breath sounds, neurovascular assessment of extremities (e.g., distal pulses, skin temperature, skin color, sensation).
- Assess baseline laboratory values (e.g., cardiac biomarkers, creatinine).
- Teach patient and caregiver about procedure and postprocedure care.

*Postprocedure*

- Perform assessment and compare to baseline: vital signs, pulse oximetry, heart and breath sounds, neurovascular assessment of extremity used for procedure, assessment of catheter insertion site for hematoma, bleeding, and bruit.
- Monitor ECG for dysrhythmias or other changes (e.g., ST segment elevation).
- Monitor patient for chest pain and other sources of pain or discomfort.
- Monitor IV infusions of anticoagulants, antiplatelets.
- Teach patient and caregiver about discharge drugs (e.g., aspirin, clopidogrel, antianginal drugs).
- Teach patient and caregiver about discharge care including signs and symptoms to report to HCP (e.g., site complications, return of chest pain).

***Licensed Practical/Vocational Nurse (LPN/LVN)***

- Give drugs before and after the procedure (consider state nurse practice act and agency policy).
- Assess neurovascular status of involved extremity every 15 min for the first hour, then according to agency policy (consider state nurse practice act and agency policy).
- Check for bleeding at catheter insertion site every 15 min for the first hour, then according to agency policy.
- Report changes in neurovascular status of involved extremity or any bleeding to the RN.

***Unlicensed Assistive Personnel (UAP)***

- Take vital signs and report increases or decreases in HR or BP to RN.
- Report decreases in pulse oximetry to the RN.
- Report patient complaints of chest pain, shortness of breath, and/or any other discomfort or distress to RN.
- Assist with oral hygiene and hydration, meals, and toileting.
- Record oral intake and urine output as ordered.
- Perform related skills as ordered (e.g., capillary blood glucose).

**Role of Other Team Members**

***Respiratory Therapist***

- Provide respiratory therapies (e.g., nebulizer treatments) as ordered and per agency policy.

patient will have numerous invasive lines for monitoring heart status and other vital organs (see Chapter 65). These include (1) a pulmonary artery catheter for hemodynamic monitoring (e.g., CO), (2) an arterial line for continuous BP monitoring, (3) pleural and mediastinal chest tubes for chest drainage, (4) continuous ECG monitoring, (5) an endotracheal tube connected to mechanical ventilation, (6) epicardial pacing wires for emergency pacing of the heart, (7) a urinary catheter to monitor urine output, and (8) a nasogastric tube for gastric decompression. Most patients are extubated within 6 hours and transferred to a step-down unit within 24 hours for continued monitoring of heart status.

Many of the postoperative complications that develop after CABG surgery relate to the use of cardiopulmonary bypass (CPB). Major consequences of CPB are systemic inflammation. This includes complications of bleeding and anemia from damage to red blood cells and platelets, fluid and electrolyte imbalances, hypothermia as blood is cooled as it passes through the CPB machine, and infections. Focus your care on assessing the patient for bleeding (e.g., chest tube drainage, incision sites), hemodynamic monitoring, checking fluid status, replacing blood and electrolytes as needed, and restoring temperature (e.g., warming blankets).

Postoperative dysrhythmias, especially atrial dysrhythmias (e.g., atrial fibrillation [AF]), are common in the first 3 days after CABG surgery.[24] β-Blockers should be restarted as soon as possible after surgery (unless contraindicated) to reduce the incidence of AF. Discharge is often delayed in these patients in order to begin anticoagulation therapy. (See Chapter 35 for information on treatment of AF.)

Nursing care for the patient with a CABG involves caring for the surgical sites (e.g., leg, chest, arm). Care of the leg incision is minimal since endoscopy is used to harvest the vein. Chest incisions are usually closed with Dermabond and do not require dressings. Management of the chest wound, which involves a sternotomy, is similar to that of other chest surgeries (see Chapter 27).

Care of the radial artery harvest site includes monitoring sensory and motor function of the hand. The patient with radial artery harvest should take a calcium channel blocker for approximately 3 months to reduce the incidence of arterial spasm at the arm or anastomosis site.

After CABG other interventions include strategies to manage pain and prevent venous thromboembolism (e.g., early ambulation, sequential compression device) and respiratory complications (e.g., use of incentive spirometer, splinting during coughing and deep-breathing exercises). (See Chapter 19 for care of the postoperative patient.)

Postoperatively, patients may experience some cognitive dysfunction. This includes impairment of memory, concentration, language comprehension, and social integration. Patients may cry or become teary. *Postoperative cognitive dysfunction* (POCD) can manifest days to weeks to months after surgery and may become a chronic disorder.[28] (POCD is discussed in Chapter 19.)

In the older patient, elective CABG is generally well tolerated. However, the incidence of postoperative complications (e.g., dysrhythmias, stroke, POCD, infection) is high. Although the benefits of treatment may outweigh risks in this group, complications are higher than in younger individuals.

Postoperative nursing care of the patient with a MIDCAB, OPCAB, or TECAB procedure is similar to that for CABG surgery patients. The recovery time is somewhat shorter with these procedures, and patients often resume routine activities sooner than patients who have CABG surgery. However, pain control is important regardless of the procedure. Patients have higher levels of pain with a thoracotomy incision than a sternotomy incision.

◆ **Ambulatory Care.** *Cardiac rehabilitation* is the restoration of a person to an optimal state of function in six areas: physiologic, psychologic, mental, spiritual, economic, and vocational. Many patients recover from ACS physically but do not attain psychologic well-being. All patients (e.g., those with ACS, chronic stable angina, heart surgery) need to be referred to a cardiac rehabilitation program. In considering rehabilitation, the patient must recognize that CAD is a chronic disease. It is not curable. Therefore basic changes in lifestyle must be made to promote recovery and future health. These changes often are needed when a person is middle aged or older. The patient must realize that recovery takes time. Tell patients that resuming physical activity after ACS or heart surgery is slow and gradual. However, with appropriate and adequate supportive care, recovery is more likely to occur.

◆ ***Patient Teaching.*** Patient teaching must occur at every stage of the patient's hospitalization and recovery (e.g., ED, telemetry unit, home care). The purpose of teaching is to give the patients and caregivers the tools they need to make informed decisions about their health. For teaching to be meaningful, the patient must be aware of the need to learn. Careful assessment of the patient's health literacy and learning needs helps you set goals that are realistic (see Chapter 4).

The timing of the teaching is important. When patients and caregivers are in crisis (either physiologic or psychologic), they may not be ready to learn new information. Answer the patient's questions in simple, brief terms. The answers often require repetition. When the shock accompanying a crisis subsides, the patient and caregiver are better able to focus on new and more detailed information.

## EVIDENCE-BASED PRACTICE

### *Translating Research Into Practice*

**Do Behavioral Interventions Reduce Cardiovascular Risk Factors?**

***Clinical Question***

In adults with cardiovascular risk factors (P), what is the effect of behavioral intervention (I) versus control group (C) on cardiovascular health outcomes (O) at 12 to 24 months (T)?

***Synthesis of Best Available Evidence***

- Systematic review of randomized controlled trials (RCTs) or controlled clinical trials
- 74 trials of adults (*n* >33,000) with at least one cardiovascular risk factor, including hypertension, dyslipidemia, impaired fasting glucose or glucose tolerance, metabolic syndrome, and cigarette smoking. Intervention was intensive behavioral counseling on diet or physical activity delivered alone or part of a multicomponent program with follow-up of at least 6 months. Control group was usual care, minimal intervention or attention. Physiologic outcomes included BP, weight, cholesterol and glucose levels, and diabetes incidence. Depression and quality of life were also measured.
- After 1 to 2 years, weight, systolic and diastolic BP, cholesterol and fasting glucose levels had decreased with lowered incidence of diabetes in the intervention group.
- Improvements in diet and physical activity were consistent with positive physiologic changes in the intervention group.
- Inconclusive if depression and quality of life significantly improved in the intervention group

***Conclusions***

- Intensive behavioral counseling for up to 2 years resulted in positive decreases in cardiovascular risk factors.

***Implications for Nursing Practice***

1. What would you advise an overweight patient with hypertension who asks if a lifestyle counseling program may be helpful to her?
2. What information would you offer a patient who after 3 weeks of counseling is discouraged that the test results did not show significant improvements in total cholesterol or fasting glucose levels?

***Reference for Evidence***

Lin JS, O'Connor E, Evans CV, et al: Behavioral counseling to promote a healthy lifestyle in individuals with cardiovascular risk factors: A systematic review for the U.S. Preventive Services Task Force, *Ann Intern Med* 161:568, 2014.

*P*, Patient population of interest; *I*, intervention or area of interest; *C*, comparison of interest or comparison group; *O*, outcomes of interest; *T*, timing (see p. 15).

## BECOMING A NURSE LEADER

### *Bullying in the Workplace*

**Situation**

Laura is a nursing student who is doing her cardiac rotation. Although sensitive about her inexperience, Laura was unprepared to deal with the negative attitude and disrespect of her preceptor. Laura's preceptor referred to her as "Hey, student!" and "Little newbie!" throughout her 3-day clinical rotation while continually rolling her eyes and acting perturbed when Laura asked her questions about the care of patients. Laura was very upset and felt bullied and put-down by her preceptor.

**Points for Consideration**

- Bullying is the use of force, threat, or coercion to abuse, intimidate, or aggressively dominate others. The behavior, which is often repeated and habitual, is used to gain control and power.
- This type of behavior may involve hidden or open acts of verbal and nonverbal aggression, such as verbal abuse, criticism, sarcasm, demeaning statements, false accusations, and gossiping.
- *Horizontal* or *lateral violence* refers to acts between peers or colleagues.
- *Bullying* is often described as acts perpetrated by one in a higher level of authority *(vertical violence).*
- Such demeaning behavior makes the work place stressful and unpleasant. These types of behavior also result in enough psychologic distress for nurses to cause them to leave the profession.
- Bullying ultimately places patient safety at risk.
- New standards address disruptive and inappropriate behaviors in health care workplaces.[1]

**Discussion Questions**

1. What would you do if you were Laura and were treated this way by your preceptor?
2. What damaging effects can bullying have on you? On your patients?
3. What strategies can you use to prevent and/or deal with bullying behavior?

**Reference**

1. American Nurses Association Position Statement on Incivility, Bullying, and Workplace Violence. Retrieved from *www.nursingworld.org/MainMenuCategories/Policy-Advocacy/Positions-and-Resolutions/ANAPositionStatements/Position-Statements-Alphabetically/Incivility-Bullying-and-Workplace-Violence.html.*

## TABLE 33-17 Patient & Caregiver Teaching

### *Acute Coronary Syndrome*

*Include the following information in the teaching plan for the patient with acute coronary syndrome and the caregiver.*

- Signs and symptoms of angina and MI and what to do should they occur (e.g., take nitroglycerin)*
- When and how to seek help (e.g., contact ERS)
- Anatomy and physiology of the heart and coronary arteries
- Cause and effect of CAD
- Definition of terms (e.g., CAD, angina, MI, sudden cardiac death, heart failure)
- Identification of and plan to decrease risk factors* (Tables 33-2, 33-3, and 33-4)
- Reasons for tests and treatments (e.g., ECG monitoring, lab work, angiography), activity limitations and rest, diet, and drugs*
- Appropriate expectations about recovery (anticipatory guidance)
- Resumption of work, physical activity, sexual activity
- Measures to promote recovery and health (e.g., cardiac rehabilitation)
- Importance of the gradual, progressive resumption of activity*

*Identified by patients as most important to learn before discharge.

Limit your use of medical terms. For example, you are caring for a patient with unstable angina and he asks you why he has chest tightness when he climbs stairs. Begin by explaining that the heart is a muscle that works as a pump. Like all muscles, it needs $O_2$ to work (or pump) properly. When blood vessels supplying the heart muscle with $O_2$ are blocked by plaque, less $O_2$ is available to the muscle. As a result, the pump cannot work well. Tell the patient that the chest tightness (angina) is the heart's message that it is having trouble doing its work. Use a model of the heart to support what you are explaining to the patient. Provide an angina log for the patient to use that is available from the AHA.[29]

Anticipatory guidance involves preparing the patient and caregiver for what to expect in the course of recovery and rehabilitation. By learning what to expect during treatment and recovery, the patient gains a sense of control over his or her life.

The idea of perceived control is operationalized as the process by which the patient makes decisions by cutting back. Cutting back is one way of reducing the psychologic and physiologic losses after ACS (or any other life-changing event). For example, a middle-aged man who smokes two packs of cigarettes a day, is 20 pounds overweight, and gets no physical exercise has a seemingly overwhelming task. He may decide that he can live with a weight reduction plan and will get more exercise (although perhaps not daily) but that it is not possible for him to quit smoking. He believes that because he is changing two of his three risk factors, he will be healthier. Ideally, the tobacco risk factor should be a priority for this patient. If the information regarding risks and effects of tobacco use is not accepted, you must respect the patient's choices.

In addition to teaching the patient and caregiver what they wish to know, several types of information are essential in achieving optimal health. Table 33-17 presents a teaching guide for the patient with ACS and the caregiver.

◆ ***Physical Activity.*** Physical activity, an integral part of rehabilitation, is necessary for optimal physiologic functioning and psychologic well-being. It has a direct, positive effect on maximal $O_2$ uptake, increasing CO, decreasing blood lipids, decreasing BP, increasing blood flow through the coronary arteries, increasing muscle mass and flexibility, improving the psychologic state, and assisting in weight loss and control. A regular schedule of physical activity, even after many years of sedentary living, is beneficial.[12]

## TABLE 33-18 Energy Expenditure in Metabolic Equivalents

**Low-Energy Activities (<3 METs or <3 cal/min)**

***Activities in Hospital***
- Resting supine
- Eating
- Washing hands, face

***Activities Outside Hospital***
- Sweeping floor
- Painting, seated
- Driving a car
- Sewing by machine

**Moderate-Energy Activities (3-6 METs or 3-5 cal/min)**

***Activities in Hospital***
- Sitting on bedside commode
- Showering
- Using bedpan
- Walking at 3-4 mph

***Activities Outside Hospital***
- Ironing, standing
- Cycling at 5.5 mph on level ground
- Golfing
- General gardening
- Painting, standing
- Ascending a flight of stairs

**High-Energy Activities (6-8 METs or 6-8 cal/min)**
- Walking 5 mph
- Performing carpentry
- Mowing lawn using walking mower

**Very-High-Energy Activities (>9 METs or >9 cal/min)**
- Cross-country skiing
- Running at >6 mph
- Cycling at >13 mph
- Shoveling heavy snow

One method of identifying levels of physical activity is by using **metabolic equivalent (MET)** units: 1 MET is the amount of $O_2$ needed by the body at rest—3.5 mL of $O_2$ per kilogram per minute, or 1.4 cal/kg of body weight per minute. The MET determines the energy costs of various exercises (Table 33-18).

In the hospital, the activity level is gradually increased so that by the time of discharge the patient can tolerate moderate-energy activities of 3 to 6 METs. Many patients with UA that has resolved or an uncomplicated MI are in the hospital for approximately 3 or 4 days. By day 2, the patient can walk in the hallway and begin stair climbing (e.g., three or four steps). Many HCPs order low-level exercise stress tests before discharge to assess readiness for discharge, optimal HR for an exercise program, and potential for ischemia or reinfarction. If tests are positive (i.e., ischemia at a low level of energy expenditure), the patient is evaluated for cardiac catheterization before discharge. If the test is negative, a catheterization may still be done before discharge or several weeks after discharge. Because of the short hospital stay, it is critical to give the patient specific guidelines for physical activity so that overexertion will not occur. Tell the patient to always "listen to what your body is saying"—the most important aspect of recovery.

Teach patients to check their HR. The patient should know the limits within which to exercise. Tell the patient the maximum HR that should be present at any point. If the HR exceeds this level or does not return to the resting HR within a few minutes, tell the patient to stop and rest. Also tell the patient to stop exercising and rest if chest pain or shortness of breath occurs.

In a normal, healthy person the minimum goal for improving cardiopulmonary fitness is 60% of the age-predicted maximum HR (calculate by subtracting the person's age from 220). The ideal training target HR is 80% of maximum HR. The patient who has been physically inactive and is just starting an exercise program should do so under supervision whenever possible.

**TABLE 33-19 Patient & Caregiver Teaching**

***FITT Activity Guidelines After Acute Coronary Syndrome***

*Include the following information in the teaching plan for the patient with acute coronary syndrome and the caregiver:*

**Warm-Up/Cool-Down**

Perform mild stretching for 3-5 min before the physical activity and 5 min after the activity. Activity should not be started or stopped abruptly.

**Frequency**

Perform physical activity on most days of the week.

**Intensity**

Activity intensity is determined by the patient's HR. If an exercise stress test has not been performed, the HR of the patient recovering from an MI should not exceed 20 beats/min over the resting HR.

**Type of Physical Activity**

Select physical activity that is regular, rhythmic, and repetitive, using large muscles to build up endurance (e.g., walking, cycling, swimming, rowing).

**Time**

Physical activity sessions should be at least 30 min long. Begin slowly at personal tolerance (perhaps only 5-10 min) and build up to 30 min.

The more important factor is the patient's response to physical activity in terms of symptoms rather than absolute HR, especially since many patients are taking β-blockers and may not be able to reach a target HR. This point cannot be overstressed. Basic physical activity guidelines for patients after ACS follow the FITT formula (Table 33-19).

The basic categories of physical activity are isometric (static) and isotonic (dynamic). Most daily activities are a mixture of the two. *Isometric activities* involve the development of tension during muscular contraction but produce little or no change in muscle length or joint movement. Lifting, carrying, and pushing heavy objects are isometric activities. These activities are associated with the Valsalva maneuver and may cause a vasovagal response. Because the HR and BP change rapidly during isometric work, isometric exercises should be limited.

*Isotonic activities* involve changes in muscle length and joint movement with rhythmic contractions at relatively low muscular tension. Walking, jogging, swimming, bicycling, and jumping rope are examples of activities that are mostly isotonic. Isotonic exercise can put a safe, steady load on the heart and lungs and improve the circulation in many organs.

Discuss participation in an outpatient cardiac rehabilitation program with all patients (Table 33-15). These programs are helpful, but not all patients choose or are able to participate in them (e.g., location and travel limitations). Home-based cardiac rehabilitation programs can provide an alternative. Physical activity guidelines are developed for the patient, and staff maintains ongoing contact with the patient (e.g., telehealth, exercise logs, Internet). Maintaining contact with the patient is one key to the success of these programs.

Older women (65 years or older) who experience MI may frequently have poor adherence to a regular physical activity program. Often these women describe continued fatigue post-MI that is poorly understood. Another factor that has been linked to poor adherence to a physical activity program after MI is depression. Depression is common among patients with CAD, especially in women.[30] Routinely screen for depression in all patients with CAD and recommend treatment as appropriate.

◆ **Resumption of Sexual Activity.** It is important to include sexual counseling for heart patients and their partners. This often-neglected area of discussion may be difficult for both the patient and HCP to approach. However, the patient's concern about resumption of sexual activity after hospitalization for ACS often produces more stress than the physiologic act itself. Most patients change their sexual behavior not because of physical problems, but because they are concerned about sexual inadequacy, death during intercourse, and impotence. A concerned and knowledgeable HCP could clarify any misconceptions with specific counseling.

Before providing guidelines on resumption of sexual activity, it is important to know the patient's physiologic status, physiologic effects of sexual activity, and psychologic effects of having an MI. Sexual activity for most middle-aged men and women with their usual partners is considered a moderate-energy activity equivalent to climbing two flights of stairs.[31]

You may be uncertain of how and when to begin counseling about resumption of sex. It is helpful to consider sex as a physical activity and to discuss or explore feelings in this area when other physical activities are discussed. One helpful approach is, "Many people who have had a heart attack wonder when they will be able to resume sexual activity. Has this been of concern to you?" You may also state, "Sexual activity, like other forms of activity, should be gradually resumed after MI. If your ability to perform sexually is concerning you, the energy you use is no more than walking briskly." Facilitate discussion by providing the patient with reading material on resumption of sexual activity. Say something like, "If resuming sexual activity has been of concern to you, this information should be helpful." This type of nonthreatening statement brings up the topic, allows the patient to explore personal feelings, and gives the patient an opportunity to raise questions with you or another HCP. Common guidelines are presented in Table 33-20.

Tell the patient that the inability to perform sexually after MI is common and that sexual dysfunction usually disappears after several attempts. Reinforce the idea that patience and understanding usually solve the problem. However, many male patients may be interested in using drugs to correct erectile dysfunction. Warn the patient that these drugs are not to be used with nitrates because severe hypotension and even death have been reported. Tell patients to discuss the use of these drugs with their HCP.

It is common for a patient who experiences chest pain on physical exertion to have some angina during sexual stimulation or intercourse. The patient may be told to take NTG prophylactically. Tell the patient to delay sex after a heavy meal or excessive intake of alcohol, when extremely tired or stressed, or with unfamiliar partners. Patients should also avoid anal intercourse because of the likelihood of eliciting a vasovagal response.

Tell the patient that resumption of sex depends on the patient and his or her partner's emotional readiness and on the HCP's assessment of the extent of recovery. It is generally safe to resume sexual activity 7 to 10 days after an uncomplicated

**TABLE 33-20 Patient & Partner Teaching**

***Sexual Activity After Acute Coronary Syndrome***

*Include the following information in the teaching plan for the patient and his/her partner after an acute coronary syndrome:*

- Sexual activity should be resumed at a level that relates to sexual activity before experiencing ACS.
- Physical training may improve the physiologic response to intercourse. Encourage daily physical activity during recovery.
- Consumption of food and alcohol should be reduced before intercourse is anticipated (e.g., waiting 3-4 hr after ingesting a large meal before engaging in sexual activity).
- Familiar surroundings and a familiar partner reduce anxiety.
- Masturbation may be a useful sexual outlet and may reassure the patient that sexual activity is still possible.
- Hot or cold showers should be avoided just before and after intercourse.
- Foreplay is desirable because it allows a gradual increase in heart rate before orgasm.
- Positions during intercourse are a matter of individual choice.
- Orogenital sex places no undue strain on the heart.
- A relaxed atmosphere free of fatigue and stress is optimal.
- Prophylactic use of nitrates to decrease chest pain during sexual activity may be suggested.
- Use of erectile agents (e.g., sildenafil) is contraindicated if taking nitrates in any form.
- Anal intercourse should be avoided because of the possibility of inducing a vasovagal response.

MI. However, some HCPs believe that the patient should decide when he or she is ready to resume sex. Others believe patients must be asymptomatic when performing moderate-energy activities before resuming sexual activity.[31]

### Evaluation

The expected outcomes are that the patient with ACS will

- Maintain stable signs of adequate cardiac output
- Report relief of pain
- Report decreased anxiety and increased sense of self-control
- Achieve a realistic program of activity that balances physical activity with energy-conserving activities
- Describe the disease process, measures to reduce risk factors, and rehabilitation activities necessary to manage the therapeutic regimen

Additional information on expected outcomes for the patient with ACS is presented in eNursing Care Plan 33-1 available on the website for this chapter.

## SUDDEN CARDIAC DEATH

**Sudden cardiac death (SCD)** is unexpected death resulting from a variety of cardiac causes. Almost 400,000 people experience SCD yearly.[1]

### Etiology and Pathophysiology

In SCD a sudden disruption in heart function produces an abrupt loss of CO and cerebral blood flow. The affected person may or may not have a known history of heart disease. SCD is often the first sign of illness for 25% of those who die of heart disease.[32]

Acute ventricular dysrhythmias (e.g., ventricular tachycardia, ventricular fibrillation) cause the majority of cases of SCD. Structural heart disease accounts for 10% of the cases of SCD. Patients in this group include those with LV hypertrophy, myocarditis, and hypertrophic cardiomyopathy. Hypertrophic cardiomyopathy is a risk factor for SCD, especially in young, athletic people.

Some cases of SCD (especially in people less than age 45) occur in the absence of structural heart disease. These involve disturbances in the conduction system (e.g., prolonged QT syndrome, Wolff-Parkinson-White syndrome).

It is difficult to know who is at high risk for SCD. However, LV dysfunction (EF less than 30%) and ventricular dysrhythmias following MI have been found to be the strongest predictors.[32] Other risk factors include history of syncope, LV outflow tract obstruction (e.g., aortic stenosis), male gender (especially African American men), and family history of ventricular dysrhythmias.

### Clinical Manifestations and Complications

Individuals who experience SCD because of CAD fall into two groups: (1) those who did not have an acute MI and (2) those who did have an acute MI. The first group accounts for the majority of cases of SCD.[32] These people usually have no warning signs or symptoms. Patients who survive SCD are at risk for another SCD event because of the continued electrical instability of the heart that caused the first event to occur.

The second, smaller group of patients includes those who have had an MI and have suffered SCD. Such patients usually have prodromal symptoms, such as chest pain, palpitations, and dyspnea. Death often occurs within 1 hour of the onset of acute symptoms.

## NURSING AND INTERPROFESSIONAL MANAGEMENT: SUDDEN CARDIAC DEATH

People who survive an episode of SCD require a diagnostic workup to determine whether they have had an MI. Serial analysis of cardiac biomarkers and ECGs are done, and the patient is treated accordingly. (See section on interprofessional care of ACS.) In addition, because most individuals with SCD have CAD, cardiac catheterization is done to determine the possible location and extent of coronary artery occlusion. PCI or CABG surgery may be indicated.

Most SCD patients have a lethal ventricular dysrhythmia that is associated with a high incidence of recurrence. It is useful to know when those individuals are most likely to have a recurrence and what drug therapy is the most effective treatment. Assessment of dysrhythmias in these patients includes 24-hour Holter monitoring or other type of event recorder, exercise stress testing, signal-averaged ECG, and electrophysiology study (EPS).

EPS is performed under fluoroscopy. Pacing electrodes are placed in various intracardiac areas, and stimuli are selectively used in an attempt to produce dysrhythmias. The patient's response to various antidysrhythmic drugs is determined and monitored in a controlled environment. (See Chapters 31 and 35 for a discussion of EPS.)

The most common approach to preventing a recurrence of SCD is the use of an implantable cardioverter-defibrillator (ICD). It has been shown that an ICD improves survival compared with drug therapy alone.[32] (See Chapter 35 for a discussion of ICDs.) Drug therapy with amiodarone (Cordarone) may be used with an ICD to decrease episodes of ventricular dysrhythmias.

Some patients at risk for SCD may consider using a LifeVest as a bridge to ICD or heart transplantation[33] (see Chapter 35). A LifeVest is a personal external defibrillator that has two main parts: a garment and monitor. The garment is worn under clothing and has electrodes that continuously record the patient's ECG. The monitor is worn around the waist or from a shoulder strap. If the patient has ventricular tachycardia or ventricular fibrillation, the device sounds an alarm to confirm that the patient is unresponsive. If the patient is conscious, the patient can press two buttons to stop the shock. If the patient does not respond, the device warns bystanders that a shock is about to be delivered. If the dysrhythmia continues and the patient still does not respond, a treatment shock is delivered through the electrodes.[33]

Teaching people about the symptoms of impending cardiac arrest and the actions to take can save lives. Rapid cardiopulmonary resuscitation (CPR) (see Appendix A) and defibrillation with an automatic external defibrillator (AED), combined with early advanced cardiac life support, have improved long-term survival rates for a witnessed arrest.

When caring for these patients, be alert to the patient's psychosocial adaptation to this sudden "brush with death." Many of these patients develop a "time bomb" mentality. They fear the recurrence of cardiac arrest and may become anxious, angry, and depressed. Their caregivers are likely to experience the same feelings. Patients and caregivers may also need to deal with additional issues such as possible driving restrictions, role reversal, and change in occupation. The grief response varies among patients and caregivers. Be attuned to the specific needs of the patient and caregiver. Teach them accordingly while providing appropriate emotional support.

## CASE STUDY

### *Myocardial Infarction*

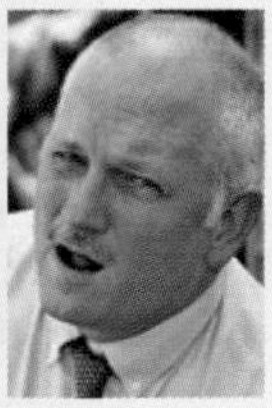

(©iStockphoto/ Thinkstock)

#### Patient Profile

D.M., a 51-year-old, white, successful executive, is rushed to the hospital by ambulance after experiencing crushing, substernal chest pain that radiates down his left arm. He also complains of dizziness and nausea.

#### Subjective Data

- Has a history of chronic stable angina and hypertension
- States he is "borderline diabetic"
- Overweight but recently lost 10 pounds
- Rarely exercises
- Has three teenage children who are causing "problems"
- Recently experienced loss of best friend and business partner, who died from cancer

#### Objective Data

##### *Physical Examination*

- Diaphoretic, short of breath, nauseous
- BP 165/100 mm Hg, pulse rate 120/min, respiratory rate 26/min

##### *Diagnostic Studies*

- 12-lead ECG shows sinus tachycardia with occasional premature ventricular contractions and ST elevation in leads II, III, aVF, $V_5$, $V_6$ consistent with an inferolateral wall MI
- Cardiac-specific troponin I level elevated
- Total cholesterol 350 mg/dL (9.1 mmol/L)
- Hb A1C 9.0%

#### Interprofessional Care

Emergency Department: Notify the cardiac catheterization laboratory of patient with STEMI:

- $O_2$ 2 L/min via nasal cannula, titrate to keep $O_2$ saturation above 93%
- Continuous ECG monitoring
- 2 IV access sites
- Aspirin 325 mg (chewable)
- Atorvastatin (Lipitor) 80 mg PO
- Eptifibatide (Integrilin) IV
- Weight-based heparin IV
- Nitroglycerin IV, titrate to relieve chest pain; hold for systolic BP below 100 mm Hg
- Morphine 2 mg IV q5-15 min PRN for chest pain unrelieved by nitroglycerin
- Vital signs (including pulse oximetry) every 10 minutes
- Prepare patient for transfer to cardiac catheterization laboratory for possible PCI

#### Discussion Questions

1. Which coronary artery(ies) is (are) most likely occluded in D.M.'s coronary circulation?
2. Explain the pathogenesis of CAD. What risk factors contribute to its development? What risk factors were present in D.M.'s life?
3. What is angina? How does chronic stable angina differ from angina associated with acute coronary syndrome?
4. Explain the pathophysiologic basis for the clinical manifestations that D.M. exhibited.
5. Explain the significance of the results of the laboratory tests and the 12-lead ECG findings.
6. Provide a rationale for each treatment measure ordered for D.M.
7. ***Priority Decision:*** Based on the assessment data presented, what are the priority nursing diagnoses? Identify any collaborative problems.
8. ***Priority Decision:*** What are the priority nursing interventions for D.M. before PCI? Immediately after his PCI?
9. ***Teamwork and Collaboration:*** Identify activities that can be delegated to unlicensed assistive personnel (UAP).
10. ***Evidence-Based Practice:*** Two days after an uncomplicated PCI and the placement of two stents, D.M. wants to know what the most effective strategies are to prevent another MI. Based on his clinical situation, what would you tell him?
11. ***Quality Improvement:*** What outcomes would indicate that the interdisciplinary care was successful?

Answers and a corresponding conceptual care map available at *http://evolve.elsevier.com/Lewis/medsurg.*

## BRIDGE TO NCLEX EXAMINATION

The number of the question corresponds to the same-numbered outcome at the beginning of the chapter.

1. In teaching a patient about coronary artery disease, the nurse explains that the changes that occur in this disorder include *(select all that apply)*
   - **a.** diffuse involvement of plaque formation in coronary veins.
   - **b.** abnormal levels of cholesterol, especially low-density lipoproteins.
   - **c.** accumulation of lipid and fibrous tissue within the coronary arteries.
   - **d.** development of angina due to a decreased blood supply to the heart muscle.
   - **e.** chronic vasoconstriction of coronary arteries leading to permanent vasospasm.
2. After teaching about ways to decrease risk factors for CAD, the nurse recognizes that additional instruction is needed when the patient says
   - **a.** "I would like to add weight lifting to my exercise program."
   - **b.** "I can only keep my blood pressure normal with medication."
   - **c.** "I can change my diet to decrease my intake of saturated fats."
   - **d.** "I will change my lifestyle to reduce activities that increase my stress."
3. A hospitalized patient with a history of chronic stable angina tells the nurse that she is having chest pain. The nurse bases his actions on the knowledge that ischemia
   - **a.** will always progress to myocardial infarction.
   - **b.** will be relieved by rest, nitroglycerin, or both.
   - **c.** indicates that irreversible myocardial damage is occurring.
   - **d.** is frequently associated with vomiting and extreme fatigue.
4. The nurse is caring for a patient who is 2 days post MI. The patient reports that she is experiencing chest pain. She states, "It hurts when I take a deep breath." Which action would be a *priority*?
   - **a.** Notify the physician STAT and obtain a 12-lead ECG.
   - **b.** Obtain vital signs and auscultate for a pericardial friction rub.
   - **c.** Apply high-flow $O_2$ by face mask and auscultate breath sounds.
   - **d.** Medicate the patient with PRN analgesic and reevaluate in 30 minutes.
5. A patient is admitted to the ICU with a diagnosis of unstable angina. Which drugs(s) would the nurse expect the patient to receive *(select all that apply)*?
   - **a.** ACE inhibitor
   - **b.** Antiplatelet therapy
   - **c.** Thrombolytic therapy
   - **d.** Prophylactic antibiotics
   - **e.** Intravenous nitroglycerin
6. A patient is recovering from an uncomplicated MI. Which rehabilitation guideline is a *priority* to include in the teaching plan?
   - **a.** Refrain from sexual activity for a minimum of 3 weeks.
   - **b.** Plan a diet program that aims for a 1- to 2-pound weight loss per week.
   - **c.** Begin an exercise program that aims for at least five 30-minute sessions per week.
   - **d.** Consider the use of erectile agents and prophylactic NTG before engaging in sexual activity.
7. The most common finding in individuals at risk for sudden cardiac death is
   - **a.** aortic valve disease.
   - **b.** mitral valve disease.
   - **c.** left ventricular dysfunction.
   - **d.** atherosclerotic heart disease.

1. b, c, d, 2. a, 3. b, 4. b, 5. a, b, e, 6. c, 7. c

For rationales to these answers and even more NCLEX review questions, visit *http://evolve.elsevier.com/Lewis/medsurg*.

### EVOLVE WEBSITE

*http://evolve.elsevier.com/Lewis/medsurg*

**Review Questions (Online Only)**

**Key Points**

**Answer Keys for Questions**

- Rationales for Bridge to NCLEX Examination Questions
- Answer Guidelines for Case Study on p. 734

**Student Case Study**

- Patient With Coronary Artery Disease and Acute Coronary Syndrome

**Nursing Care Plan**

- eNursing Care Plan 33-1: Patient With Acute Coronary Syndrome

**Conceptual Care Map Creator**

- Conceptual Care Map for Case Study on p. 734

**Audio Glossary**

**Content Updates**

## REFERENCES

1. Go AS, Mozaffarian D, Roger VL, et al: Heart disease and stroke statistics: 2014 update: a report from the American Heart Association, *Circulation* 129:e28, 2014.
2. McCance KL, Huether SE: *Pathophysiology*, ed 7, St Louis, 2014, Mosby.
3. Strang F, Schunkert H: C-reactive protein and coronary heart disease: all said—is not it? *Mediators Inflamm* 2014:757123, 2014. doi: 10.1155/2014/757123.

*4. McSweeney JC, Rosenfeld AG, Abel WM, et al: Preventing and experiencing ischemic heart disease as a woman: state of the science a scientific statement from the American Heart Association, *Circulation* 133:00, 2016. DOI: 10.1161/CIR.0000000000000381.

*5. Fihn SD, Blankenship JC, Alexander KP, et al: 2014 CC/AHA/AATS/PCNA/SCAI/STS focused update of the guideline for the diagnosis and management of patients with stable ischemic heart disease: a report of the American College of Cardiology Foundation/American Heart Association Task Force on Practice Guidelines and the American College of Physicians, American Association for Thoracic Surgery, Preventive Cardiovascular Nurses Association, Society for Cardiovascular Angiography and Interventions, and Society of Thoracic Surgeons, *Circulation* 130:1749,2014.

6. Sasidhar MV, Reddy S, Naik A, et al: Genetics of coronary artery disease—a clinician's perspective, *Indian Heart J* 66(6):663, 2014.

*7. Eckel RH, Jakicic JM, Ard JD, et al: 2013 AHA/ACC guideline on lifestyle management to reduce cardiovascular risk - a report of the American College of Cardiology/American Heart Association Task Force on Practice Guidelines, *Circulation* 129(suppl 2):S76, 2014.

*8. Goff DC, Lloyd-Jones DM, Bennett G, et al: 2013 ACC/AHA guideline on the assessment of cardiovascular risk: a report of the American College of Cardiology/American Heart Association Task Force on Practice Guidelines, *Circulation* 12(suppl 2):S49, 2014.

*9. James PA, Oparil S, Carter BL, et al: 2014 evidence-based guideline for the management of high blood pressure in adults: report from the panel

members appointed to the eighth Joint National Committee (JNC 8), *JAMA* 311:507, 2014.
*10. National Heart, Lung, and Blood Institute. Landmark NIH study shows intensive blood pressure management may save lives. Retrieved from *http://www.nhlbi.nih.gov/news/press-releases/2015/landmark-nih-study-shows-intensive-blood-pressure-management-may-save-lives.*
*11. National Institutes of Health: *Seventh report of the Joint National Committee on Prevention, Detection, Evaluation, and Treatment of High Blood Pressure (JNC 7), pub no 03-5233*, Bethesda, Md, 2003, US Department of Health and Human Services.
*12. Jhamnani S, Patel D, Heimlich L, et al: Meta-analysis of the effects of lifestyle modifications on coronary and carotid atherosclerotic burden, *Am J Cardiol* 115(2):268, 2015.
*13. Burg MM, Edmondson D, Shimbo D, et al: The "perfect storm" and acute coronary syndrome onset: do psychosocial factors play a role? *Prog Cardiovasc Dis* 55(6):601, 2013.
*14. Cohen BE, Edmondson D, Kronish IM: State of the art review: depression, stress, anxiety, and cardiovascular disease, *Am J Hypertens* 28(11):1295, 2015.
15. American Heart Association: Homocysteine, folic acid, and cardiovascular disease. Retrieved from *http://www.heart.org/HEARTORG/GettingHealthy/NutritionCenter/Homocysteine-Folic-Acid-and-Cardiovascular-Disease_UCM_305997_Article.jsp.*
16. National Institute on Drug Abuse: Drug facts: cocaine. Retrieved from *http://www.drugabuse.gov/publications/drugfacts/cocaine.*
17. Lehne RA: *Pharmacology for nursing care*, ed 8, St Louis, 2013, Saunders.
18. Pietrangelo A: PCSK9 inhibitors: what you need to know. Retrieved from *http://www.healthline.com/health/pcsk9-inhibitors-what-you-need-to-know#Overview1*
*19. Bibbins-Domingo K, Grossman DC, Curry SJ, et al: Aspirin use for the primary prevention of cardiovascular disease and colorectal cancer: U.S. preventive services task force recommendation statement, *Ann Intern Med* doi:10.7326/M16-0577 Retrieved from *http://annals.org/article.aspx?articleid=2513179*, 2016.
*20. Levine GN, O'Gara PT, Bates ER, et al: 2015 ACC/AHA/SCAI focused update on primary percutaneous coronary intervention for patients with ST-elevation myocardial infarction: an update of the 2011 ACCF/AHA/SCAI guideline for percutaneous coronary intervention and the 2013 ACCF/AHA guideline for the management of ST-elevation myocardial infarction, *Circulation* 133:1135, 2016.
21. Mann DL, Zipes DP, Libby P, et al: *Braunwald heart disease: a textbook of cardiovascular medicine*, ed 10, St Louis, 2015, Saunders.
22. Fiore DP, Beltrame JF: Chest pain in patients with 'normal angiography': could it be cardiac? *Int J Evid-Based Health* 11:56, 2013.
*23. Amsterdam EA, Wenger NK, Brindis RG, et al: 2014 AHA/ACC guideline for the management of patients with non-ST-elevation acute coronary syndromes: executive summary, *JACC* 64:2645, 2014.
*24. Hillis LD, Smith PK, Anderson JL, et al: 2011 ACCF/AHA guideline for coronary artery bypass graft surgery: a report of the American College of Cardiology Foundation/American Heart Association Task Force on Practice Guidelines, *Circulation* 124:e652, 2011.
25. Bojar RM: *Manual of perioperative care in adult cardiac surgery*, ed 5, Hoboken, NJ, 2011, Wiley-Blackwell.
*26. Jneid H, Anderson JL, Wright RS, et al: 2012 ACCF/AHA focused update of the guidelines for the management of patients with unstable angina/non-ST-elevation myocardial infarction (updating the 2007 guideline and replacing the 2011 focused update), *J Am Coll Cardiol* 126:875, 2012.
*27. American Association of Critical-Care Nurses: Family presence: visitation in the adult ICU (2011). Retrieved from *www.aacn.org/WD/practice/docs/practicealerts/family-visitation-adult-icu-practicealert.pdf.*
28. Rovai D, Giannessi D, Andreassi MG, et al: Mind injuries after cardiac surgery, *J Cardiovasc Med (Hagerstown)*. 16(12):844, 2015.
29. American Heart Association: Angina log. Retrieved from *https://www.heart.org/idc/groups/heart-public/@wcm/@hcm/documents/downloadable/ucm_307470.pdf.*
30. European Society of Cardiology: Women more likely to develop anxiety and depression after heart attack (2014). Retrieved from *www.escardio.org/about/press/press-releases/pr-14/Pages/women-develop-anxiety-post-infarction.aspx.*
*31. Levine GN, Steinke EE, Bakaeen FG, et al: Sexual activity and cardiovascular disease: a scientific statement from the American Heart Association, *Circulation* 125:1058, 2012.
32. Mitrani RD, Myerburg RJ: Ten advances defining sudden cardiac death, *Trends Cardiovasc Med* 26(1):23, 2016.
33. Cleveland Clinic: LifeVest. Retrieved from *http://my.clevelandclinic.org/services/heart/services/lifevest.*

*Evidence-based information for clinical practice.

34

# Heart Failure

Carolyn Moffa

*Wherever you go, go with all your heart.*
**Confucius**

http://evolve.elsevier.com/Lewis/medsurg/

## LEARNING OUTCOMES

1. Compare the pathophysiology of systolic and diastolic heart failure (HF).
2. Relate the compensatory mechanisms involved in HF to the development of acute decompensated heart failure (ADHF) and chronic HF.
3. Select appropriate nursing and interprofessional care to manage the patient with ADHF.
4. Select appropriate nursing and interprofessional care to manage the patient with chronic HF.
5. Describe the indications for heart transplantation and the nursing care of heart transplant recipients.

## KEY TERMS

diastolic failure, p. 738
heart failure (HF), p. 737
heart transplantation, p. 753
paroxysmal nocturnal dyspnea (PND), p. 742
pulmonary edema, p. 741
systolic failure, p. 738

## HEART FAILURE

**Heart failure (HF)** is a complex clinical syndrome that results in the inability of the heart to provide sufficient blood to meet the $O_2$ needs of tissues and organs. It is a major health problem in the United States. This chapter discusses the nursing and interprofessional care of patients experiencing this syndrome.

A defect in either ventricular filling (diastolic dysfunction) or ventricular ejection (systolic dysfunction) are the key manifestations of HF. The amount of blood pumped by the left ventricle with each heart beat is called the *ejection fraction* (EF). The American Academy of Cardiology Foundation (ACCF) has adopted the terms *heart failure with reduced EF* (HFrEF) and *heart failure with preserved EF* (HFpEF) to describe systolic and diastolic HF.[1]

HF is associated with numerous cardiovascular diseases (CVDs), particularly long-standing hypertension, coronary artery disease (CAD), and myocardial infarction (MI). Unlike other CVDs, HF is increasing in incidence and prevalence. This is in part due to better survival after cardiac events and the aging population. HF is primarily a disease of older adults. The incidence is similar in men and women.[2]

The American Heart Association (AHA) estimates that more than 650,000 new cases of HF are diagnosed each year.[2] It is the most common reason for hospital admission in adults over the age of 65. This places a significant economic burden on the health care system.[1] The complex, progressive nature of HF often results in poor outcomes, the most costly being hospital readmissions. Approximately 25% of patients discharged with a primary diagnosis of HF are readmitted within 30 days. The total cost of HF care in the United States exceeds $40 billion annually, with over half of these costs spent on hospitalizations.[2]

### Etiology

Hypertension and CAD are the primary risk factors for HF. Hypertension is a modifiable risk factor that should be aggressively treated and managed. Long-term treatment of hypertension reduces the incidence of HF by 50%.[1] Other co-morbidities, such as diabetes, metabolic syndrome, advanced age, tobacco use, and vascular disease, also contribute to the development of HF. (Metabolic syndrome is discussed in Chapter 40.)

HF may be caused by any interference with the normal mechanisms regulating cardiac output (CO). CO depends on (1) preload, (2) afterload, (3) myocardial contractility, and (4) heart rate (HR). (Preload and afterload are discussed in Chapter 31.) Any changes in these factors can lead to decreased ventricular function and HF.

The major causes of HF may be divided into two subgroups: (1) primary causes (Table 34-1) and (2) precipitating causes

Reviewed by Vera Barton-Caro, RN, PhD, FNP-BC, CHFN, Assistant Professor of Nursing, Wheeling Jesuit University, Wheeling, West Virginia; Carla V. Hannon, MS, APRN, CCRN, CCNS, Clinical Nurse Specialist, Medical Intensive Care Unit, Yale–New Haven Hospital, New Haven, Connecticut; Patricia Lea, RN, DNP, CCRN, Assistant Professor, University of Texas Medical Branch School of Nursing, Galveston, Texas; and Rebecca Personett, RN, PhD, NEA-BC, Professor of Nursing, North Central Texas College, Gainesville, Texas and Brookhaven College, Dallas, Texas.

### TABLE 34-1 Primary Causes of Heart Failure

- Hypertension, including hypertensive crisis
- Coronary artery disease, including myocardial infarction
- Rheumatic heart disease
- Congenital heart defects (e.g., ventricular septal defect)
- Pulmonary hypertension
- Cardiomyopathy (e.g., viral, postpartum, substance abuse)
- Hyperthyroidism
- Valvular disorders (e.g., mitral stenosis)
- Myocarditis

### CULTURAL & ETHNIC HEALTH DISPARITIES
#### *Heart Failure*

- African Americans have a higher incidence of HF, develop HF at an earlier age, and experience higher mortality rates related to HF than whites.
- African Americans may experience more ACE inhibitor–related angioedema than whites.
- Isosorbide dinitrate/hydralazine (BiDil) is used for the treatment of HF in African Americans. This combination drug is approved for use only in this ethnic group.
- Asians have an extremely high risk (15%-50%) for ACE inhibitor–related cough.

*ACE,* Angiotensin-converting enzyme; *HF,* heart failure.

### TABLE 34-2 Precipitating Causes of Heart Failure*

| Cause | Mechanism |
|---|---|
| **Anemia** | ↓ $O_2$-carrying capacity of the blood stimulating ↑ in CO to meet tissue demands, leading to increase in cardiac workload and increase in size of LV |
| **Infection** | ↑ $O_2$ demand of tissues, stimulating ↑ CO |
| **Thyrotoxicosis** | Changes the tissue metabolic rate, ↑ HR and workload of the heart |
| **Hypothyroidism** | Indirectly predisposes to ↑ atherosclerosis. Severe hypothyroidism decreases myocardial contractility. |
| **Dysrhythmias** | May ↓ CO and ↑ workload and $O_2$ requirements of myocardial tissue |
| **Bacterial endocarditis** | *Infection:* ↑ metabolic demands and $O_2$ requirements<br>*Valvular dysfunction:* causes stenosis or regurgitation |
| **Obstructive sleep apnea** | Frequent nighttime apnea results in ↑ afterload, intermittent hypoxia, and ↑ sympathetic nervous system activity. |
| **Pulmonary embolism** | ↑ Pulmonary pressure resulting from obstruction leads to pulmonary hypertension, ↓ CO. |
| **Paget's disease** | ↑ Workload of the heart by ↑ vascular bed in the skeletal muscle |
| **Nutritional deficiencies** | May ↓ cardiac function by ↑ myocardial muscle mass and myocardial contractility |
| **Hypervolemia** | ↑ Preload causing volume overload on the RV |

*CO,* Cardiac output; *LV,* left ventricle; *RV,* right ventricle.
*List is not all inclusive.

(Table 34-2). Precipitating causes often increase the workload of the heart, resulting in an acute condition and decreased heart function.

## Genetic Link

Specific genes and gene mutations have been linked to the development of hypertension, CAD, and cardiomyopathy (weakening of the heart muscle) (see Chapters 32, 33, and 36). These CVDs are known risk factors for HF. Cardiomyopathy, a common cause of HF, may be attributed to as many as 40 different defective genes. The body's largest protein is a muscle protein called *titin,* which is found in cardiac sarcomeres (part of the heart muscle that contracts). Mutations in the titin gene are the most common known genetic cause of dilated cardiomyopathy.[3] More research into the effects of these gene mutations, as well as other genetic mutations, is needed.

## Pathophysiology

**Left-Sided Heart Failure.** The most common form of HF is left-sided HF. Left-sided HF results either from the inability of the left ventricle (LV) to (1) empty adequately during systole or (2) fill adequately during diastole. Left-sided HF can be further classified as systolic, diastolic, or mixed systolic and diastolic failure.

***Systolic Failure or Heart Failure with Reduced EF.*** Systolic failure, also known as HFrEF, results from an inability of the heart to pump blood effectively. The hallmark of systolic failure is a decrease in the EF. Normal EF is 55% to 60%. Patients with HFrEF generally have an EF less than 45%. It can be as low as 5% to 10%. HFrEF is caused by impaired contractile function (e.g., MI), increased afterload (e.g., hypertension), cardiomyopathy, and mechanical abnormalities (e.g., valvular heart disease).

The LV in systolic failure loses its ability to generate enough pressure to eject blood forward through the aorta. Over time, the LV becomes dilated and hypertrophied. The weakened heart muscle cannot generate adequate stroke volume, which affects CO. Because the LV cannot effectively push blood forward, end diastolic volumes and pressures in the LV increase. When the LV fails, blood backs up into the left atrium. This causes fluid accumulation in the lungs. The increased pulmonary hydrostatic pressure causes fluid leakage from the pulmonary capillary bed into the interstitium and then the alveoli. This results in pulmonary congestion and edema (Fig. 34-1, *A* through *D*).

***Diastolic Failure or Heart Failure With Preserved EF.*** Diastolic failure, or HFpEF, is the inability of the ventricles to relax and fill during diastole. Approximately 50% of patients with HF have HFpEF. Hypertension is the most important cause of diastolic failure.[1] Other risk factors include older age, female gender, diabetes, and obesity (see Gender Differences box). In diastolic failure, the LV is generally stiff and noncompliant. Diastolic failure is characterized by high filling pressures because of stiff ventricles. Decreased filling of the ventricles results in decreased stroke volume and CO. The end result of diastolic failure is the same as systolic failure (e.g., pulmonary congestion). HFpEF is diagnosed by the following criteria: (1) signs and symptoms of HF, (2) normal EF, and (3) evidence of LV diastolic dysfunction by echocardiography or cardiac catheterization. Therapies for HFpEF are targeted at reducing underlying risk factors and treating co-morbidities.

***Mixed Systolic and Diastolic Failure.*** Mixed systolic and diastolic failure is seen in disease states such as *dilated cardiomyopathy* (DCM). DCM is a condition in which poor systolic function is further compromised by a dilated LV that is unable

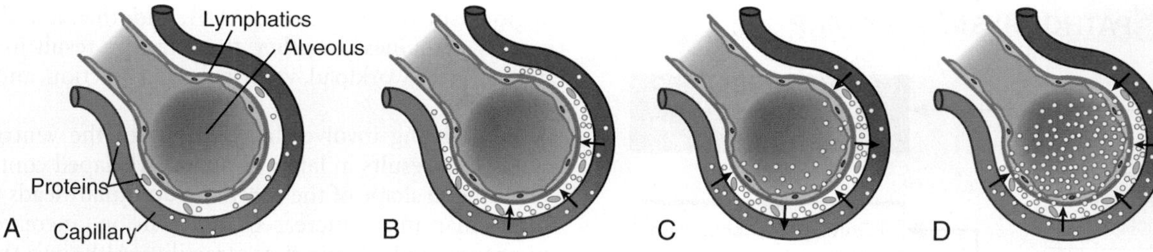


**FIG. 34-1** As pulmonary edema progresses, it inhibits $O_2$ and $CO_2$ exchange at the alveolar-capillary interface. **A,** Normal relationship. **B,** Increased pulmonary capillary hydrostatic pressure causes fluid to move from the vascular space into the pulmonary interstitial space. **C,** Lymphatic flow increases in an attempt to pull fluid back into the vascular or lymphatic space. **D,** Failure of lymphatic flow and worsening of left-sided heart failure result in further movement of fluid into the interstitial space and into the alveoli. (Modified from Urden LD, Stacy KM, Lough ME: *Critical care nursing: diagnosis and management,* ed 6, St Louis, 2010, Mosby.)

## GENDER DIFFERENCES

### *Heart Failure*

| Men | Women |
|---|---|
| • Men experience systolic failure more frequently than women.<br>• Men with asymptomatic systolic failure experience greater mortality benefit from ACE inhibitor therapy than women. | • Women experience diastolic failure more frequently than men.<br>• Women have a higher risk of ACE inhibitor–related cough than men.<br>• Women experience more digitalis-related death than men.<br>• Women with diabetes are more predisposed to HF than men. |

*ACE,* Angiotensin-converting enzyme; *HF,* heart failure.

to relax (see Chapter 36). These patients often have extremely low EFs (less than 35%), high pulmonary pressures, and *biventricular failure* (both ventricles are dilated and have poor filling and emptying capacity).

The patient with ventricular failure of any type may have low BP, low CO, and poor renal perfusion. Poor exercise tolerance and heart dysrhythmias are also common. The patient may arrive at this point acutely from an MI or chronically from worsening cardiomyopathy or hypertension. In both acute and chronic causes of HF, the body's response to low CO is to mobilize its compensatory mechanisms to maintain CO and BP.

**Right-Sided Heart Failure.** Right-sided HF occurs when the right ventricle (RV) fails to pump effectively. When the RV fails, fluid backs up into the venous system. This causes movement of fluid into the tissues and organs (e.g., peripheral edema, abdominal ascites, hepatomegaly, jugular venous distention).

The most common cause of right-sided HF is left-sided HF (Fig. 34-2). As the LV fails, fluid backs up into the pulmonary system, causing increased pressures in the lungs. The RV has to work harder to push blood to the pulmonary system. Over time, this increased workload weakens the RV and gradually it fails. Other causes of right-sided HF (independent of the function of the LV) include RV infarction, pulmonary embolism, and *cor pulmonale* (RV dilation and hypertrophy caused by pulmonary disease) (see Chapter 27).

**Compensatory Mechanisms.** HF can have an abrupt onset as with acute MI, or it can be a subtle process resulting from slow, progressive changes. The overloaded heart uses compensatory mechanisms to try to maintain adequate CO. The main compensatory mechanisms include (1) neurohormonal responses: renin-angiotensin-aldosterone system (RAAS) and the sympathetic nervous system (SNS), (2) ventricular dilation, and (3) ventricular hypertrophy.

#### *Neurohormonal Response*

**Renin-angiotensin-aldosterone system.** The RAAS is a regulatory system that works to maintain normal homeostasis. The activation of the RAAS results in BP control and fluid and electrolyte balance. In response to stress, the role of the RAAS is to promote retention of fluid and sodium and cause vasoconstriction to raise BP. However, recurrent activation of the RAAS in HF is what is responsible for the signs and symptoms that develop.

As CO falls, blood flow to the kidneys decreases. This is sensed by the juxtaglomerular apparatus in the kidneys as decreased volume. In response, the kidneys release renin, which converts angiotensinogen to angiotensin I (see Chapter 44 and Fig. 44-4). Angiotensin I is next converted to angiotensin II by a converting enzyme made in the lungs. Angiotensin II causes (1) activation of the SNS to increase BP and HR; (2) release of aldosterone from the adrenal cortex, which results in sodium and water retention; (3) increased peripheral vasoconstriction, which increases BP; and (4) stimulation of the pituitary gland, which releases antidiuretic hormone (ADH), which results in water reabsorption. The outcome of the cascade results in further water and sodium retention in an already overloaded state and increased workload of the failing heart.

Other factors also contribute to the development of HF. The production of *endothelin,* a potent vasoconstrictor produced by the vascular endothelial cells, is stimulated by ADH, angiotensin II, and catecholamines. This results in further arterial vasoconstriction and an increase in cardiac contractility and hypertrophy.

Locally, proinflammatory cytokines are released by heart cells in response to various forms of heart injury (e.g., MI). Two cytokines, tumor necrosis factor (TNF) and interleukin-1 (IL-1), further depress heart function by causing hypertrophy, contractile dysfunction, and cell death. Over time, a systemic inflammatory response also occurs.

**Sympathetic nervous system.** In response to an inadequate stroke volume and CO, the SNS is activated, resulting in the release of catecholamines (epinephrine and norepinephrine). The circulating catecholamines enhance peripheral vasoconstriction and cause an increase in the HR *(chronotropy)* and

**PATHOPHYSIOLOGY MAP**

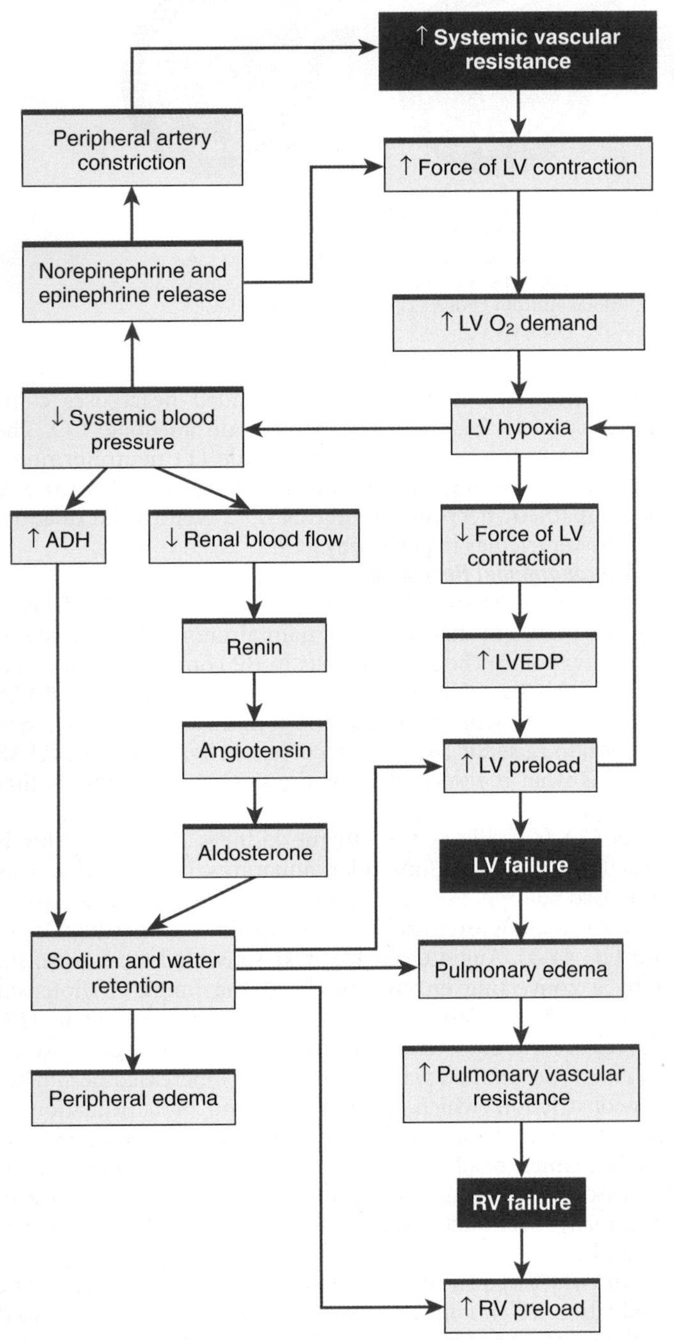


**FIG. 34-2** Pathophysiology of heart failure. Elevated systemic vascular resistance results in left-sided heart failure that leads to right-sided heart failure. Systemic vascular resistance and preload are exacerbated by the renin-angiotensin-aldosterone system. *ADH,* Antidiuretic hormone; *LA,* left atrium; *LV,* left ventricle; *LVEDP,* left ventricular end-diastolic pressure; *RV,* right ventricle. (Modified from Huether SE, McCance KL: *Understanding pathophysiology,* ed 3, St Louis, 2004, Mosby.)

myocardial contractility *(inotropy)*. Initially, the compensatory mechanisms are beneficial with a result of increased CO. However, over time these factors become harmful and counterproductive, as they increase the workload, preload (volume), and $O_2$ requirement in an already failing heart.

In HF, continuous activation of the neurohormonal responses (RAAS and SNS) leads to elevated levels of norepinephrine, angiotensin II, aldosterone, ADH, endothelin, and proinflammatory cytokines. Together, these factors result in an increase in the heart's workload, ventricular dysfunction, and *ventricular remodeling.*

Remodeling involves hypertrophy of the ventricular myocytes. This results in large, abnormally shaped contractile cells. This altered shape of the ventricles eventually leads to increased ventricular mass, increased wall tension, increased $O_2$ consumption, and impaired contractility. Although the ventricles become larger, they become less effective pumps. Ventricular remodeling is a risk factor for life-threatening dysrhythmias and sudden cardiac death (SCD). Drug therapies to prevent or reverse remodeling and decrease mortality are recommended. These include ACE inhibitors, β-adrenergic blockers (β-blockers), and aldosterone antagonists.

***Dilation.*** *Dilation* is an enlargement of the chambers of the heart (Fig. 34-3, *A*). It occurs when pressure in the heart chambers (usually the LV) is elevated over time. The heart muscle fibers stretch in response to the volume of blood in the heart at the end of diastole. The degree of stretch is directly related to the force of the contraction (systole) (this is the *Frank-Starling law*). This increased contraction initially leads to increased CO and maintenance of BP and perfusion. Dilation starts as an adaptive mechanism to cope with increasing blood volume. Eventually this mechanism becomes inadequate, because the elastic elements of the muscle fibers are overstretched and can no longer contract effectively, thereby decreasing the CO.

***Hypertrophy.*** *Hypertrophy* is an increase in the muscle mass and heart wall thickness in response to overwork and strain (Fig. 34-3, *B*). It occurs slowly because it takes time for this increased muscle tissue to develop. Initially, the increased contractile power of the muscle fibers leads to an increase in CO and maintenance of tissue perfusion. Over time, hypertrophic heart muscle has poor contractility, requires more $O_2$ to perform work, has poor coronary artery circulation (tissue becomes ischemic more easily), and is prone to dysrhythmias.

**Counterregulatory Mechanisms.** The body's attempts to maintain balance are demonstrated by several counterregulatory processes. Natriuretic peptides (atrial natriuretic peptide [ANP] and brain [b-type] natriuretic peptide [BNP]) are hormones produced by the heart muscle. ANP is released from the atria, and BNP is released from the ventricles in response to increased blood volume in the heart.[4]

The natriuretic peptides have renal, cardiovascular, and hormonal effects. Renal effects include (1) increased glomerular filtration rate and diuresis and (2) excretion of sodium (natriuresis). Cardiovascular effects include vasodilation and decreased BP. Hormonal effects include (1) inhibition of aldosterone and renin secretion and (2) interference with ADH release. The combined effects of ANP and BNP help to counter the adverse effects of the SNS and RAAS in patients with HF.[4]

Nitric oxide (NO) and prostaglandin are counterregulatory substances released from the vascular endothelium in response to the compensatory mechanisms activated in HF. Like the natriuretic peptides, NO and prostaglandin work to relax the arterial smooth muscle, resulting in vasodilation and decreased afterload.

Compensated HF occurs when compensatory mechanisms succeed in maintaining an adequate CO that is needed for tissue perfusion. Decompensated HF occurs when these mechanisms can no longer maintain adequate CO and inadequate tissue perfusion results.

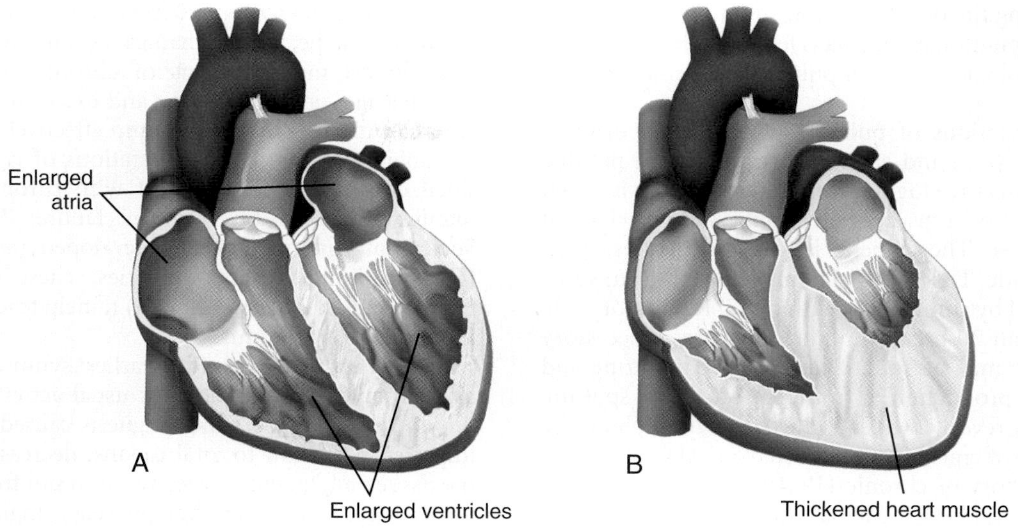


**FIG. 34-3** **A,** Dilated heart chambers. **B,** Hypertrophied heart chambers.

## Classification of Heart Failure

The New York Heart Association (NYHA) developed functional guidelines for classifying people with heart disease based on tolerance to physical activity. Because this system only reflected exercise capacity, the American College of Cardiology Foundation/AHA (ACCF/AHA) developed a staging system that identified disease progression and treatment strategies.[1] This system allows for identification of people at risk for developing HF but who do not currently have heart disease. The ACCF/AHA system encourages clinicians to actively address the patient's risk factors and treat any existing conditions to prevent further disease progression. This may help reduce the growing number of HF patients.

Patients may move between levels in the NYHA classification system based on worsening or improving symptoms. However, the ACCF/AHA staging system is progressive. Patients can only advance to a higher (worse) stage as the disease progresses (Table 34-3).

## Clinical Manifestations: Acute Decompensated Heart Failure

*Acute decompensated HF* (ADHF) is defined as the sudden onset of signs and symptoms of HF, requiring urgent medical care. The universal finding in ADHF is pulmonary and systemic congestion due to elevated left-sided and right-sided filling pressures. In ADHF, an increase in pulmonary venous pressure is caused by failure of the LV. This results in engorgement of the pulmonary vascular system (Fig. 34-1, *A* and *B*). As a result, the lungs become less compliant, and there is increased resistance in the small airways. To help compensate, the lymphatic system increases its flow to help maintain a constant volume of the pulmonary extravascular fluid. This early stage is clinically associated with a mild increase in the respiratory rate and a decrease in partial pressure of $O_2$ in arterial blood ($PaO_2$).

If pulmonary venous pressure continues to increase, the increase in intravascular pressure causes more fluid to move into the interstitial space than the lymphatics can remove. *Interstitial edema* occurs at this point (Fig. 34-1, *C*). Tachypnea develops, and the patient becomes symptomatic (e.g., short of breath). If the pulmonary venous pressure increases further, the alveoli lining cells are disrupted, and a fluid containing red blood cells (RBCs) moves into the alveoli *(alveolar edema)*. As the disruption becomes worse from further increases in the pulmonary venous pressure, the alveoli and airways are flooded with fluid. This is accompanied by a worsening of the arterial blood gas values (i.e., lower $PaO_2$ and possible increased partial pressure of $CO_2$ in arterial blood [$PaCO_2$] and progressive respiratory acidosis).

ADHF can manifest as **pulmonary edema**. This is an acute, life-threatening situation, in which the lung alveoli become

**TABLE 34-3 Comparison of ACCF/AHA Stages of Heart Failure and NYHA Functional Classifications**

| ACCF/AHA Stages of Heart Failure (HF) | NYHA Functional Classifications |
|---|---|
| **A** At high risk for HF, but without structural heart disease or symptoms of HF | None |
| **B** Structural heart disease, but without signs or symptoms of HF | **I** No limitation of physical activity. Ordinary physical activity does not cause symptoms of HF. |
| **C** Structural heart disease with prior or current symptoms of HF | **I** No limitation of physical activity. Ordinary physical activity does not cause symptoms of HF. |
| | **II** Slight limitation of physical activity. Comfortable at rest, but ordinary physical activity results in symptoms of HF. |
| | **III** Marked limitation of physical activity. Comfortable at rest, but less than ordinary activity causes symptoms of HF. |
| | **IV** Unable to carry on any physical activity without symptoms of HF, or symptoms of HF at rest |
| **D** Refractory HF requiring specialized interventions | **IV** Unable to carry on any physical activity without symptoms of HF, or symptoms of HF at rest |

Reprinted with permission. *Circulation* 128:e240-e327, 2013. ©2013 American Heart Association, Inc.
*ACCF,* American College of Cardiology Foundation; *AHA,* American Heart Association; *HF,* heart failure; *NYHA,* New York Heart Association.

filled with serosanguineous fluid (Fig. 34-1, *D*). The most common cause of pulmonary edema is left-sided HF secondary to CAD. (Other etiologic factors for pulmonary edema are listed in Table 27-25.)

Clinical manifestations of pulmonary edema are distinct. The patient has dyspnea and *orthopnea* (unable to lie flat due to shortness of breath). Jugular venous distention is often present and is the most sensitive and specific sign for elevated LV filling pressures. The patient is usually anxious, pale, and possibly cyanotic. The skin is clammy and cold from vasoconstriction caused by stimulation of the SNS. Respiratory rate is often greater than 30 breaths/minute, and use of accessory muscles to breathe may be seen. There may be wheezing and coughing with the production of frothy, blood-tinged sputum. Breath sounds may reveal crackles and wheezes throughout the lungs. The absence of crackles does not rule out ADHF as many patients with a history of chronic HF develop increased lymphatic drainage of the alveolar edema. The patient's HR is rapid, and an abnormal $S_3$ or $S_4$ heart sound may be auscultated (see Table 31-4). BP may be elevated or decreased depending on the severity of the HF.

**CHECK YOUR PRACTICE**

You are assigned to a patient with ADHF who has been admitted to the Heart Failure Unit. Your assessment reveals that the patient has bilateral crackles in the mid-lower lung fields and dyspnea on exertion (e.g., moving from the bed to the commode). The patient's skin is warm and pulses are present in all extremities. Your preceptor asks you to categorize your patient based on the classification system in Table 34-4.

- In what category would you put your patient?

Patients with ADHF can be categorized into one of four groups based on hemodynamic and clinical status: dry-warm, dry-cold, wet-warm, and wet-cold[1] (Table 34-4). The most common presentation in patients with ADHF is the wet and warm patient. A patient is "wet" due to volume overload (e.g., congestion, dyspnea) but "warm" due to adequate perfusion (warm skin, positive pulses).

## Clinical Manifestations: Chronic Heart Failure

Chronic HF is characterized as a progressive worsening of ventricular function and chronic neurohormonal activation that results in ventricular remodeling. This process involves changes in the size, shape, and mechanical performance of the ventricle. The clinical manifestations of chronic HF depend on the patient's age, underlying type and extent of heart disease, and which ventricle is failing to pump effectively.

Table 34-5 lists the manifestations of right-sided and left-sided chronic HF. The patient with chronic HF usually has manifestations of biventricular failure. The Heart Failure Society of America (HFSA) developed the acronym *FACES* (*F*atigue, limitation of *A*ctivities, chest *C*ongestion/cough, *E*dema, and *S*hortness of breath) to help teach patients to identify early HF symptoms.[5]

**Fatigue.** Fatigue is one of the earliest symptoms of chronic HF. The patient notes fatigue after usual activities and eventually limits these activities. The fatigue is caused by decreased CO, impaired perfusion to vital organs, decreased oxygenation of the tissues, and anemia. Anemia can result from poor nutrition, renal disease, or drug therapy (e.g., angiotensin-converting enzyme [ACE] inhibitors).

**Dyspnea.** Dyspnea is a common manifestation of chronic HF. It is caused by increased pulmonary pressures secondary to interstitial and alveolar edema. Dyspnea can occur with mild exertion or at rest. Orthopnea often accompanies dyspnea. Careful questioning of patients often reveals adaptive behaviors such as sleeping with two or more pillows or in a chair to aid breathing.

**Paroxysmal nocturnal dyspnea (PND)** occurs when the patient is asleep. The patient awakens in a panic and has feelings of suffocation and a strong desire to sit or stand to aid breathing. PND is caused by the reabsorption of fluid from dependent body areas when the patient is flat. A cough is often associated

**TABLE 34-4 Clinical Profile in Acute Decompensated Heart Failure**

| | | CONGESTION (WET) | |
|---|---|---|---|
| | | **No** | **Yes** |
| **LOW PERFUSION (COLD)** | **No** | **Dry-Warm**<br>• PAWP normal<br>• CO normal<br>• Signs and symptoms: none | **Wet-Warm**<br>• PAWP ↑<br>• CO normal<br>• Possible signs and symptoms: dyspnea, edema, orthopnea |
| | **Yes** | **Dry-Cold**<br>• PAWP ↓ or normal<br>• CO ↓<br>• Possible signs and symptoms: edema, hypotension, cool extremities | **Wet-Cold**<br>• PAWP ↑<br>• CO ↓<br>• Possible signs and symptoms: altered mental status, decreased $O_2$ saturation, reduced urine output, shock |

*CO,* Cardiac output; *PAWP,* pulmonary artery wedge pressure.

**TABLE 34-5 Manifestations of Heart Failure**

| Right-Sided Heart Failure | Left-Sided Heart Failure |
|---|---|
| **Signs** | |
| • RV heaves<br>• Murmurs<br>• Jugular venous distention<br>• Edema (e.g., pedal, scrotum, sacrum)<br>• Weight gain<br>• ↑ HR<br>• Ascites<br>• Anasarca (massive generalized body edema)<br>• Hepatomegaly (liver enlargement) | • LV heaves<br>• Pulsus alternans (alternating pulses: strong, weak)<br>• ↑ HR<br>• PMI displaced inferiorly and left of the midclavicular line (LV hypertrophy)<br>• ↓ $PaO_2$, slight ↑ $PaCO_2$ (poor $O_2$ exchange)<br>• Crackles (pulmonary edema)<br>• $S_3$ and $S_4$ heart sounds<br>• Pleural effusion<br>• Changes in mental status<br>• Restlessness, confusion |
| **Symptoms** | |
| • Fatigue<br>• Anxiety, depression<br>• Dependent, bilateral edema<br>• Right upper quadrant pain<br>• Anorexia and GI bloating<br>• Nausea | • Weakness, fatigue<br>• Anxiety, depression<br>• Dyspnea<br>• Shallow respirations up to 32-40/min<br>• Paroxysmal nocturnal dyspnea<br>• Orthopnea<br>• Dry, hacking cough<br>• Nocturia<br>• Frothy, pink-tinged sputum (advanced pulmonary edema) |

*LV,* Left ventricle; *$PaCO_2$,* partial pressure of $CO_2$ in arterial blood; *$PaO_2$,* partial pressure of $O_2$ in arterial blood; *PMI,* point of maximal impulse; *RV,* right ventricle.

with HF and may be the first clinical symptom. It begins as a dry, nonproductive cough and may be misdiagnosed as asthma or other lung disease. The cough is not relieved by position change or over-the-counter cough medicine.

**Tachycardia.** Tachycardia is an early clinical sign of HF. One of the body's first responses to compensate for a failing heart is to increase the HR via activation of the SNS. This works to increase CO. Initially this response is favorable, but over time, persistent tachycardia is harmful and may exacerbate HF. Adequate HR control in patients with chronic HF has been associated with better clinical outcomes, including decreased hospitalizations and mortality.[6]

**Edema.** Edema is a common sign of HF. It may occur in dependent body areas (peripheral edema), liver (hepatomegaly), abdominal cavity (ascites), and lungs (pulmonary edema and pleural effusion). If the patient is in bed, sacral and scrotal edema may develop. Pressing the edematous skin with the finger may leave a depression *(pitting edema)*. The development of dependent edema or a sudden weight gain of more than 3 lb (1.4 kg) in 2 days is often a sign of ADHF. It is important to note that not all lower-extremity edema is a result of HF. Hypoproteinemia, immobility, venous insufficiency, and certain drugs can cause peripheral edema.

**Nocturia.** Nocturia is the tendency to urinate excessively during the night. Chronic HF is frequently associated with poor renal perfusion and function. Patients develop increased peripheral and systemic edema. At night when lying flat, extravascular fluid is reabsorbed from the interstitial spaces back into the circulatory system. This results in increased perfusion to the kidneys. The increased renal blood flow results in diuresis. The patient may complain of having to urinate frequently throughout the night.

**Skin Changes.** Because tissue capillary $O_2$ extraction is increased in a person with chronic HF, the skin may appear dusky. Often the lower extremities are shiny and swollen, with diminished or absent hair growth. Chronic swelling may result in pigment changes. This causes the skin to appear brown or brawny in areas covering the ankles and lower legs.

**Behavioral Changes.** Cerebral circulation may be reduced with chronic HF secondary to decreased CO. The patient or caregiver may report unusual behavior, including restlessness, confusion, and decreased attention span or memory. This may also be secondary to poor gas exchange and worsening HF. It is often seen in the late stages of HF. Coexisting psychologic disorders, especially depression and anxiety, contribute a twofold risk of mortality and higher readmission rates and health care costs in patients with HF. Approximately 1 in 5 patients with HF have clinical depression.[7] In addition, patients with psychologic disorders have poorer adherence to treatment plans. Assess patients with HF for depression and anxiety and, if needed, initiate appropriate consults.

**Chest Pain.** HF can precipitate chest pain (angina) because of decreased coronary artery perfusion from decreased CO and increased myocardial work. Chest pain may accompany either ADHF or chronic HF.

**Weight Changes.** Many factors contribute to weight changes. First, a progressive weight gain may occur because of fluid retention. Renal failure may also contribute to fluid retention. Abdominal fullness from ascites and hepatomegaly frequently causes anorexia and nausea. As HF advances, the patient may have cardiac *cachexia* with muscle wasting and fat loss. This can be masked by the patient's edematous condition and may not be seen until after the edema subsides.

## Complications of Heart Failure

**Pleural Effusion.** *Pleural effusion* is a common complication in HF. There are two pleural layers or membranes: the visceral pleura lines the lungs, while the parietal pleura lines the chest cavity. Normally there is a small amount of fluid between the two layers for lubrication and to aid breathing. A pleural effusion occurs when excess fluid builds up in the pleural cavity of the lungs secondary to increasing pressure in the pleural capillaries. Fluid then moves from these capillaries into the pleural space. Pleural effusions may result in symptoms of dyspnea, cough, and chest pain. (Pleural effusion is discussed in Chapter 27.)

**Dysrhythmias.** Chronic HF causes enlargement of the chambers of the heart. This enlargement can cause changes in the normal electrical pathways. Patients with HF are at high risk for atrial dysrhythmias. The prevalence of atrial fibrillation in patients with HF increases as the severity of HF increases. Atrial fibrillation occurs when numerous sites in the atria fire spontaneously and rapidly, and the organized atrial depolarization (contraction) no longer occurs. Loss of "atrial kick" during systole may contribute to decreased CO and worsening HF symptoms.

Atrial fibrillation also promotes thrombus formation within the atria. Thrombi can break loose and form emboli. This places patients with atrial fibrillation at risk for stroke. Treatment with anticoagulation should be considered if there are no significant contraindications. Treatment with drugs to achieve HR control is a primary goal. Restoring normal sinus rhythm with cardioversion, ablation, and antidysrhythmic drugs may be considered.

Patients with HF are also at risk for ventricular dysrhythmias (e.g., ventricular tachycardia [VT], ventricular fibrillation [VF]). Sudden cardiac death (SCD) is a major cause of death in the HF population. Patients with decreased LV function are at the greatest risk for SCD. Guidelines recommend implantation of a prophylactic implantable cardioverter-defibrillator (ICD) for patients with an EF less than 35%, who are NYHA Class II or III.[8] (SCD is discussed in Chapter 33, and dysrhythmias are discussed in Chapter 35.)

**Left Ventricular Thrombus.** With ADHF or chronic HF, the enlarged LV and decreased CO combine to increase the risk of thrombus formation in the LV. Once a thrombus has formed, it may also decrease LV contractility, decrease CO, and worsen the patient's perfusion. The development of emboli from the thrombus also places the patient at risk for stroke.

**Hepatomegaly.** HF can lead to severe hepatomegaly, especially with RV failure. The liver becomes congested with venous blood. The hepatic congestion leads to impaired liver function. Eventually liver cells die, fibrosis occurs, and cirrhosis can develop (see Chapter 43).

**Renal Failure.** The decreased CO that accompanies chronic HF results in decreased perfusion to the kidneys and can lead to renal insufficiency or failure (see Chapter 46).

## Diagnostic Studies

Diagnosing HF is often difficult. Patient signs and symptoms are not highly specific and may mimic those associated with many other medical conditions (e.g., anemia, lung disease). Diagnostic tests for ADHF and chronic HF are presented in Table 34-6. A primary goal in diagnosis is to find the underlying cause of HF.

An echocardiogram is a common diagnostic tool used in patients with HF. It provides information on the EF. This helps

**TABLE 34-6 Interprofessional Care**

***Heart Failure***

| Both ADHF and Chronic HF | ADHF | Chronic HF |
|---|---|---|
| **Diagnostic Assessment** | | |
| • History and physical examination<br>• Determination of underlying cause<br>• Serum chemistries, cardiac biomarkers, BNP or NT-proBNP level (see Table 31-6), liver function tests, thyroid function tests, CBC, lipid profile, kidney function tests, urinalysis<br>• Chest x-ray<br>• 12-lead ECG<br>• 2-dimensional echocardiogram (see Table 31-6)<br>• Nuclear imaging studies (see Table 31-6)<br>• Cardiac catheterization (see Table 31-6) | • Measurement of LV function<br>• Hemodynamic monitoring<br>• Endomyocardial biopsy in select patients | • Cardiopulmonary exercise stress test<br>• 6-minute walk test<br>• Sleep studies in select patients |
| **Management** | | |
| • Treatment of underlying cause<br>• Circulatory assist devices (e.g., ventricular assist device)<br>• Daily weights<br>• Sodium- and possibly fluid-restricted diet | • High Fowler's position<br>• $O_2$ by mask or nasal cannula<br>• Noninvasive positive pressure ventilation<br>• Circulatory assist device: intraaortic balloon pump<br>• Endotracheal intubation and mechanical ventilation<br>• Vital signs, urine output at least q1hr until stable<br>• Continuous ECG and pulse oximetry monitoring<br>• Hemodynamic monitoring (e.g., intraarterial BP, PAWP, CO)<br>• Drug therapy (Table 34-7)<br>• Possible cardioversion (e.g., atrial fibrillation)<br>• Ultrafiltration | • $O_2$ therapy by nasal cannula if indicated<br>• Drug therapy (Table 34-7)<br>• Cardiac resynchronization therapy with biventricular pacing and internal cardioverter-defibrillator<br>• LVAD<br>• Heart transplantation<br>• Rest-activity periods<br>• Dietitian consult<br>• Physical/occupational therapy consult<br>• Cardiac rehabilitation<br>• Home health nursing care (e.g., telehealth monitoring)<br>• Palliative and end-of-life care |

*ADHF,* Acute decompensated heart failure; *BNP,* b-type natriuretic peptide; *CO,* cardiac output; *HF,* heart failure; *LVAD,* left ventricular assist device; *NT-proBNP,* N-terminal prohormone of BNP; *PAWP,* pulmonary artery wedge pressure.

to differentiate between HFpEF and HFrEF. An echocardiogram also provides information on the structure and function of the heart valves. Heart chamber enlargement or stiffness can also be assessed. Other useful tests include electrocardiogram (ECG), chest x-ray, 6-minute walk test, multi-gated acquisition (MUGA) scan, cardiopulmonary exercise stress test, and heart catheterization. Studies for obstructive sleep apnea may be done in select patients. An endomyocardial biopsy (EMB) may be done as part of a heart catheterization in select acutely ill patients who develop unexplained, new-onset HF that is unresponsive to usual care.[9]

Laboratory studies also aid in the diagnosis of HF. In general, BNP levels correlate positively with the degree of LV failure. Many agencies routinely measure the N-terminal prohormone of BNP (NT-proBNP). This is a more precise test to aid in the diagnosis of HF. Levels are temporarily higher in patients receiving nesiritide (Natrecor) and may be high in patients with chronic, stable HF. Increases in BNP or NT-proBNP levels can be caused by conditions other than HF. These include pulmonary embolism, renal failure, and acute coronary syndrome.

## Interprofessional Care: Acute Decompensated Heart Failure

Patients with ADHF need continuous monitoring and assessment. If unstable, these patients are managed in an intensive care unit (ICU). In the ICU, monitor heart rhythm and $O_2$ saturation continuously. Assess vital signs and urine output at least every hour. The patient may have hemodynamic monitoring, including arterial BP and pulmonary artery pressures. If a pulmonary artery catheter is placed, evaluate CO and pulmonary artery wedge pressure (PAWP). Therapy is titrated to maximize CO and reduce PAWP. A normal PAWP is generally between 8 and 12 mm Hg. Patients with ADHF may have a PAWP as high as 30 mm Hg. (Hemodynamic monitoring is discussed in Chapter 65.)

Provide supplemental $O_2$ to help increase the percentage of $O_2$ in inspired air. ($O_2$ therapy is discussed in Chapter 28.) In severe pulmonary edema, the patient may need noninvasive positive pressure ventilation (e.g., bilevel positive airway pressure [BiPAP]) or intubation and mechanical ventilation. BiPAP is also effective in decreasing preload. (Ventilatory support is discussed in Chapter 65.)

More stable patients with ADHF may require hospitalization but do not need to be in an ICU. They are often admitted to a telemetry or stepdown unit for treatment. Assess these patients every 4 hours (e.g., vital signs, pulse oximetry) for adequate oxygenation. Record intake and output and daily weights to evaluate fluid status.

If the patient has dyspnea, place in a high Fowler's position with the feet horizontal in the bed or dangling at the bedside. This position helps decrease venous return because of the pooling of blood in the extremities. This position also increases the thoracic capacity, allowing for improved breathing.

*Ultrafiltration* (UF), or *aquapheresis,* is an option for the patient with volume overload.[1] It is a process to remove excess salt and water from the patient's blood. UF can rapidly remove intravascular fluid volume while maintaining hemodynamic stability. The ideal patients for UF are those with major pulmonary or systemic volume overload who have shown resistance to diuretics and are hemodynamically stable. UF also may be an appropriate adjunctive therapy for patients with HF and coexisting renal failure. (UF is discussed in Chapter 46.)

In the ICU, circulatory assist devices are used to manage patients with worsening HF. The intraaortic balloon pump (IABP) is a device that increases coronary blood flow to the heart muscle and decreases the heart's workload through a process called *counterpulsation*. The IABP is useful in hemodynamically unstable patients because it decreases pulmonary artery pressures and systemic vascular resistance (SVR), leading to improved CO.

Ventricular assist devices (VADs) can be used to maintain the pumping action of a heart that cannot effectively pump. A VAD is a mechanical pump that is surgically implanted. (IABPs and VADs are discussed in Chapter 65.) Once the patient is more stable, determination of the cause of ADHF is important. Diagnosis of systolic or diastolic HF will then direct further treatment protocols.

**Drug Therapy.** Drug therapy is essential in treating ADHF (Table 34-7).

***Diuretics.*** Diuretics are the mainstay of treatment in patients with volume overload. They decrease sodium reabsorption at various sites within the nephrons, thereby enhancing sodium and water loss. Decreasing intravascular volume with the use of diuretics reduces venous return (preload) and subsequently the volume returning to the LV. This allows the LV to pump more efficiently. CO is increased, pulmonary vascular pressures are decreased, and gas exchange is improved. Loop diuretics (e.g., furosemide [Lasix]) can be given by IV push and act rapidly in the kidneys.

***Vasodilators.*** IV nitroglycerin is a vasodilator that reduces circulating blood volume. It also improves coronary artery blood flow by dilating the coronary arteries. Therefore nitroglycerin reduces preload, slightly reduces afterload (in high doses), and increases myocardial $O_2$ supply. When titrating IV nitroglycerin, monitor BP frequently (every 5 to 10 minutes) to avoid hypotension.

Sodium nitroprusside (Nitropress) is a potent IV vasodilator that reduces both preload and afterload, thus improving myocardial contraction, increasing CO, and reducing pulmonary congestion. Complications of IV sodium nitroprusside include hypotension and thiocyanate toxicity, which can develop after 48 hours of use. Sodium nitroprusside is given in an ICU, since symptomatic hypotension is the main adverse effect.

**DRUG ALERT Sodium Nitroprusside (Nitropress)**

- Arterial BP monitoring is recommended during drug infusion.
- Record baseline BP and continuously monitor during administration.
- Too rapid rate of IV infusion can reduce BP too quickly and cause hypotension.
- Headache, dizziness, nausea, agitation, and restlessness can occur.
- Monitor thiocyanate (drug by-product) levels if infusion is greater than 3 mcg/kg/min, as toxicity can occur.

Nesiritide, given IV, is a recombinant form of BNP. It causes both arterial and venous dilation. The main hemodynamic effects of nesiritide include a (1) reduction in PAWP and (2) decrease in systemic BP. Although classified as a vasodilator, nesiritide is also a neurohormonal blocking agent. It can be used for short-term treatment of ADHF. Nesiritide does not need titration after the initial IV bolus. It can be given in the emergency department (ED) and non-ICU setting. Because the

**TABLE 34-7 Drug Therapy**

***Heart Failure***

| Drug | Mechanism of Action |
|---|---|
| **Diuretics** (see Table 32-7)<br>***Loop Diuretics***<br>furosemide (Lasix)<br>bumetanide (Bumex)<br>***Thiazide Diuretics****<br>• hydrochlorothiazide<br>• metolazone (Zaroxolyn)<br>***Potassium-Sparing Diuretics***<br>• spironolactone (Aldactone)<br>• eplerenone (Inspra) | • Decrease fluid volume<br>• Decrease preload<br>• Decrease pulmonary venous pressure<br>• Relieve symptoms of heart failure (e.g., edema) |
| **Renin-Angiotensin-Aldosterone System Inhibitors** (see Table 32-7)<br>***ACE Inhibitors***<br>• captopril<br>• benazepril (Lotensin)<br>• enalapril (Vasotec)<br>***Angiotensin II Receptor Blockers***<br>• losartan (Cozaar)<br>• valsartan (Diovan)<br>• valsartan/sacubitril (Entresto) | • Dilate venules and arterioles<br>• Improve renal blood flow<br>• Decrease fluid volume<br>• Relieve symptoms of heart failure<br>• Promote reverse remodeling<br>• Decrease morbidity and mortality |
| **Vasodilators**<br>• hydralazine*<br>• isosorbide dinitrate/hydralazine (BiDil)*<br>• nitrates (e.g., nitroglycerin [Nitro-Bid], isosorbide dinitrate [Isordil])<br>• nesiritide (Natrecor)†<br>• nitroprusside (Nitropress)† | • Reduce cardiac afterload, leading to increased CO<br>• Dilate the arterioles of the kidneys, leading to increased renal perfusion and fluid loss<br>• Decrease BP<br>• Decrease preload<br>• Relieve symptoms of heart failure (e.g., dyspnea) |
| **β-Adrenergic Blockers*** (see Table 32-7)<br>• metoprolol (Toprol XL)<br>• bisoprolol (Zebeta)<br>• carvedilol (Coreg) | • Promote reverse remodeling<br>• Decrease afterload<br>• Inhibit SNS<br>• Decrease morbidity and mortality |
| **Positive Inotropes**<br>***β-Adrenergic Agonists***†<br>• dopamine<br>• dobutamine<br>***Phosphodiesterase Inhibitor***†<br>• milrinone<br>***Digitalis Glycoside****<br>• digoxin | • Increase contractility (positive inotropic effect)<br>• Increase CO<br>• Increase heart rate (positive chronotropic effect)<br>• Produce mild vasodilation<br>• Increase stroke volume and CO<br>• Promote vasodilation |
| **Cardiac Sinus Node Inhibitor***<br>• ivabradine (Corlanor) | • Decreases heart rate |
| **Morphine**† | • Decreases anxiety<br>• Decreases preload and afterload |
| **Antidysrhythmic Drugs** (see Table 35-9) | • Prevent or treat dysrhythmias |
| **Anticoagulants** | • Prevent thromboembolism<br>• Recommended for patients with an ejection fraction <20% and/or atrial fibrillation |

*ACE,* Angiotensin-converting enzyme; *ADHF,* acute decompensated heart failure; *CO,* cardiac output; *SNS,* sympathetic nervous system.
*Used for chronic HF only.
†Used for ADHF only.

main adverse effect of nesiritide is symptomatic hypotension, monitor BP closely.

***Morphine.*** Morphine sulfate reduces preload and afterload. It is frequently used in the treatment of HF and acute coronary syndrome (see Chapter 33). It dilates both pulmonary and systemic blood vessels. Results include a decrease in pulmonary pressures and myocardial $O_2$ needs and an improvement in gas exchange. When morphine is used, the patient often experiences relief from dyspnea and, consequently, the anxiety often associated with dyspnea.

Use morphine cautiously in patients with ADHF. Morphine is related to more adverse events, including a greater need for mechanical ventilation, more ICU admissions, prolonged hospitalization, and higher mortality rates in these patients.[10]

***Positive Inotropes.*** Inotropic therapy increases myocardial contractility. Drugs include β-agonists (e.g., dopamine, dobutamine, norepinephrine [Levophed]), the phosphodiesterase inhibitor milrinone, and digitalis. The β-agonists are only used as a short-term treatment of ADHF. In addition to increasing myocardial contractility and SVR, dopamine dilates the renal blood vessels and enhances urine output. Unlike dopamine, dobutamine is a selective β-agonist and works mainly on the $\beta_1$-receptors in the heart. Dobutamine does not increase SVR and is preferred for short-term treatment of ADHF.[11]

**DRUG ALERT Dopamine**
- Monitor IV site for signs of extravasation.
- Tissue necrosis with sloughing can occur with drug extravasation.
- High dosages may produce ventricular dysrhythmias.

Milrinone is a phosphodiesterase inhibitor that has been called an inodilator. It increases myocardial contractility (inotropic effect) and promotes peripheral vasodilation. Inhibition of phosphodiesterase increases cyclic adenosine monophosphate (cAMP). This enhances calcium entry into the cell and improves myocardial contractility. Milrinone increases CO and reduces BP (decrease afterload). Like dopamine and dobutamine, this drug is available only for IV use. Adverse effects include dysrhythmias, thrombocytopenia, and hepatotoxicity.

Digitalis is a positive inotrope that improves LV function. Digitalis increases contractility but also increases myocardial $O_2$ consumption. Because digitalis requires a loading dose and time to work, it is not recommended for the initial treatment of ADHF.[11]

Currently, inotropic therapy is only recommended for use in the short-term management of patients with ADHF who have not responded to conventional drug therapy (e.g., diuretics, vasodilators, morphine).[1]

**SAFETY ALERT Infusion Pumps**
- To control the rate and assist with titration, use an infusion pump whenever you are giving IV vasodilators and inotropes.
- Ideally, pumps that contain drug libraries can help to avoid rates and dosages that are out of the safe range for the drug being given.

### Interprofessional Care: Chronic Heart Failure

With the addition of new drugs and devices, the management of HF has dramatically changed in the past few years. Because of the large number of patients and the high cost of care related to hospital readmissions, strategies to improve outcomes have been developed. One example is the use of guideline-directed medical therapy as defined by the AACF/AHA.[1] Another example is specialized HF inpatient units with transitional programs to the outpatient setting to help manage these patients. These units are staffed with multidisciplinary HF teams, including nurses who are educated in the care of these patients (Table 34-6).

The main goals in the treatment of chronic HF are to treat the underlying cause and contributing factors, maximize CO, reduce symptoms, improve ventricular function, improve quality of life, preserve target organ function, and reduce mortality and morbidity. The management of hypertension is discussed in Chapter 32, CAD in Chapter 33, dysrhythmias in Chapter 35, and valvular disorders in Chapter 36.

In a person with HF, $O_2$ saturation of the blood can be reduced because the blood is not adequately oxygenated in the lungs. The use of supplemental $O_2$ improves saturation and assists in meeting tissue $O_2$ needs. This helps to relieve dyspnea and fatigue. Optimally pulse oximetry is used to monitor the need for and effectiveness of $O_2$ therapy.

Physical and emotional rest allows the patient to conserve energy and decreases the need for additional $O_2$. The degree of rest recommended depends on the severity of HF. A patient with severe HF may be on bed rest with limited activity. A patient with mild to moderate HF can be ambulatory with restriction of strenuous activity. Tell the patient to participate in prescribed activities with adequate recovery periods. A structured exercise program, such as cardiac rehabilitation (CR), should be considered for all patients with chronic HF. CR has been associated with decreased hospitalizations and reduced mortality. Patients enrolled in CR programs have also reported improved quality of life and less depression.[1,12]

The CardioMems system is a new device to help monitor patients' pulmonary pressures. It is implanted in a patient's distal pulmonary artery during a right heart catheterization. The permanent device is approved for patients with NYHA Class III HF symptoms. It allows for close monitoring of changes in pulmonary pressures. Data are sent wirelessly from the patient's home to a secure website. The data are reviewed by the HCP. Early interventions such as drug adjustments can be started. This may help prevent worsening of HF symptoms and possibly hospitalizations.[13]

Nonpharmacologic therapies are an integral part of the care of HF patients. Patients with an EF less than 35% are at an increased risk of SCD from VT or VF. An ICD is recommended for SCD prophylaxis. In HF, neurohormonal effects and cardiac remodeling can result in dyssynchrony of the LV and RV. This contributes to poor CO. In these patients, biventricular pacing, known as *cardiac resynchronization therapy (CRT)*, is recommended.[1] In CRT an extra pacing lead is placed through the coronary sinus to a coronary vein of the LV. This lead coordinates right and left ventricular contractions (Fig. 34-4). The ability to have normal electrical conduction (synchrony) between the RV and the LV increases left ventricular function and CO. At times, patients may need both CRT and an ICD. (Pacemakers and defibrillators are discussed in Chapter 35.)

**CHECK YOUR PRACTICE**

Your patient is scheduled for a biventricular pacemaker for her worsening HF. She currently has a demand pacemaker and asks you why she needs this new one.
- How would you respond to her question?

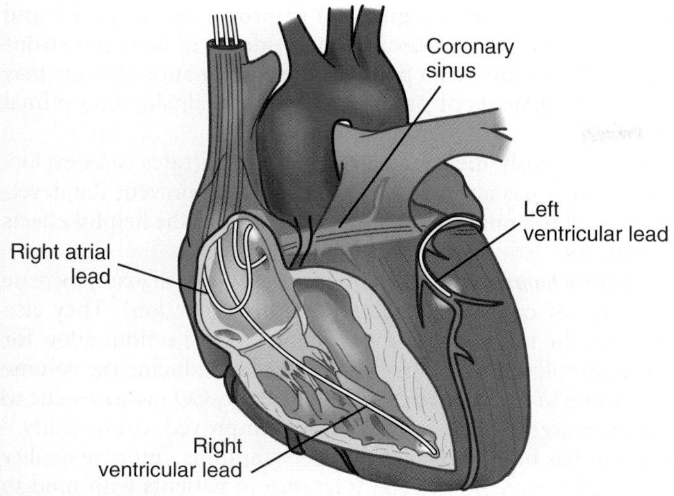


**FIG. 34-4** Placement of pacing leads in cardiac resynchronization therapy.

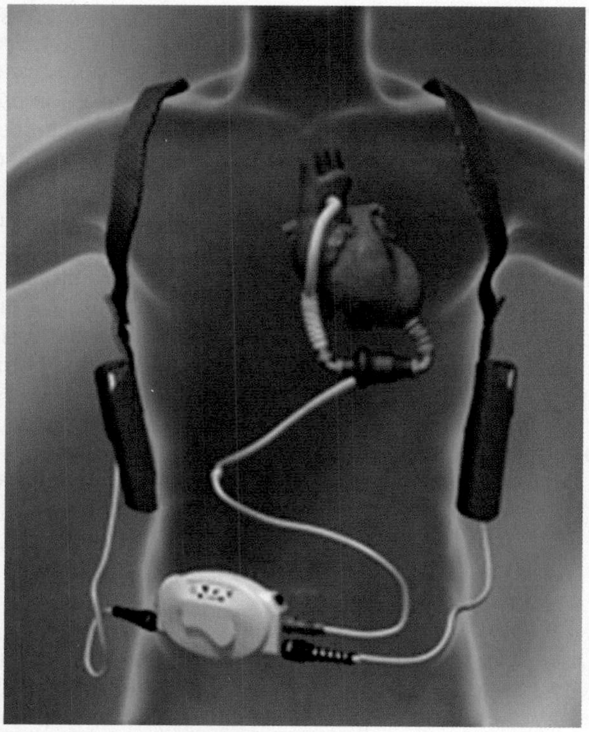

**FIG. 34-5** Left ventricular assist device. (Reprinted with the permission of Thoratec Corporation.)

Several mechanical options are available to sustain HF patients with deteriorating conditions, especially those awaiting heart transplantation. These include the IABP and VADs. However, the limitations of bed rest and the risk of infection and vascular complications preclude long-term use of the IABP. VADs provide highly effective long-term support and have become standard care in many heart transplant centers. The heart pump is operated via a driveline that exits the abdominal wall and is attached to a system controller with patient specific settings. VADs operate on AC current or batteries (Fig. 34-5). They may be used as a bridge to transplant (BTT), or as destination therapy (DT) in patients who do not meet criteria for heart transplant. (IABPs and VADs are discussed in Chapter 65.)

**Drug Therapy.** Drug therapy for chronic HF is presented in Table 34-7.

***Diuretics.*** Diuretics are used to reduce edema, pulmonary venous pressure, and preload (see Table 32-7). If excess extracellular fluid is removed, blood volume returning to the heart can be reduced and cardiac function improved.

Diuretics act on the kidney by promoting excretion of sodium and water. Many varieties of diuretics are available. Loop diuretics (e.g., bumetanide [Bumex]) are potent diuretics. These drugs act on the ascending loop of Henle to promote sodium, chloride, and water excretion. Problems in using loop diuretics include reduction in serum potassium levels, ototoxicity, and possible allergic reaction in patients sensitive to sulfa-type drugs.

Thiazide diuretics inhibit sodium reabsorption in the distal tubule, thus promoting excretion of sodium and water. They can be added to loop diuretics to obtain results if patients become resistant to loop diuretics. Thiazide diuretics also can cause severe reductions in potassium levels.

Diuretics are effective in relieving the congestive symptoms of HF. However, their use does activate the SNS and RAAS, which can exacerbate the HF syndrome. In chronic HF, the lowest effective dose of diuretic should be used.

***Renin-Angiotensin-Aldosterone System Inhibitors***

**Angiotensin-converting enzyme inhibitors.** ACE inhibitors are the primary drug of choice for blocking the RAAS system in HF patients with systolic failure.[1] Examples of ACE inhibitors are listed in Table 34-7. Other examples of ACE inhibitors are discussed in Chapter 32 and listed in Table 32-7.

The conversion of angiotensin I to the potent vasoconstrictor angiotensin II requires ACE. ACE inhibitors block this enzyme, resulting in reduced levels of angiotensin II. The end result of the neurohormonal blockade is decreased plasma aldosterone levels, decreased SNS activity, vasodilation, and sodium and water excretion. ACE inhibitors also decrease the development of ventricular remodeling by inhibiting ventricular hypertrophy.

**DRUG ALERT Captopril**

- Excessive hypotension and hyperkalemia may occur.
- Monitor patient for first-dose hypotension (first-dose syncope).
- Skipping doses or discontinuing the drug can result in rebound hypertension.
- Angioedema, a rare adverse effect, can develop suddenly and can be life-threatening.

Major side effects of ACE inhibitors include symptomatic hypotension, intractable cough, hyperkalemia, *angioedema* (allergic reaction involving edema of the face and airways), and renal insufficiency (when ACE inhibitors are used in high doses). Aging and renal insufficiency slow the metabolism of ACE inhibitors and may lead to increased serum drug levels. Carefully monitor patients taking ACE inhibitors for potential adverse effects. For example, a cough may be attributed to ACE inhibitors when, in fact, it is also a common symptom of an exacerbation of HF. It is critical that the exact cause of cough and other side effects be confirmed before stopping ACE inhibitor therapy.

**Angiotensin II receptor blockers.** For patients who are unable to tolerate ACE inhibitors, angiotensin II receptor blockers (ARBs) (see Table 32-7) are recommended.[14] These agents prevent the vasoconstrictor and aldosterone-secreting effects of angiotensin II by binding to the angiotensin II receptor sites.

**Combination therapy.** Combination therapy with valsartan/sacubitril (Entresto), an ARB/neprilysin inhibitor, is recommended for HF patients with reduced EF. Inhibition of neprilysin increases several endogenous vasoactive peptides, including natriuretic peptides, bradykinin, and adrenomedullin (vasodilator peptide hormone). The combination of these two drugs is used as an alternative to an ACE inhibitor (or single agent ARB) therapy in these patients.[15]

**Aldosterone antagonists.** Spironolactone (Aldactone) and eplerenone (Inspra) are aldosterone antagonists. They block the harmful neurohormonal effects of aldosterone on the heart blood vessels. Aldosterone antagonists may prolong survival in patients with HFrEF.[16] They are also potassium-sparing diuretics that promote sodium and water excretion while retaining potassium. These effects occur because these agents bind to receptors at the aldosterone-dependent sodium-potassium exchange site in the distal renal tubule.

**DRUG ALERT Spironolactone (Aldactone)**
- Monitor potassium levels during treatment.
- Use with caution in patients taking digoxin, since hyperkalemia may reduce the effects of digoxin.
- Instruct patient to avoid foods high in potassium (e.g., bananas, oranges, dried apricots).
- Assess male patients for gynecomastia, a common side effect of long-term use of spironolactone.

***β-Adrenergic Blockers.*** β-Blockers directly block the negative effects of the SNS (e.g., increased HR) on the failing heart. Three β-blockers have been shown to decrease mortality in patients with HFrEF: metoprolol succinate (Toprol XL), bisoprolol (Zebeta), and carvedilol (Coreg). These β-blockers may also increase EF. The improvement in EF is dose-related, and therefore the highest tolerated dose should be given.[1,14] However, because β-blockers can reduce myocardial contractility, care must be taken to start at a low dose. Dosage is increased every 2 weeks as tolerated by the patient. Major adverse effects include edema, worsening of HF, hypotension, fatigue, and bradycardia.

**DRUG ALERT Carvedilol (Coreg)**
- Overdosage can produce profound bradycardia, hypotension, bronchospasm, and cardiogenic shock.
- Obtain standing BP 1 hr after dosing to assess tolerance.
- Abrupt withdrawal may result in sweating, palpitations, and headaches.

#### *Vasodilators*

**Nitrates.** Nitrates cause vasodilation by acting directly on the smooth muscle of the vessel wall. Nitrates can be used in combination with hydralazine for chronic HF management in patients who cannot tolerate ACE inhibitors or ARBs. Nitrates are of particular benefit in the management of myocardial ischemia related to HF because they promote vasodilation of the coronary arteries.

Long-term use of nitrates may result in tolerance to the drug, making it less effective. Nitrates are contraindicated in patients who take phosphodiesterase inhibitors (PDE5 inhibitors) (e.g., sildenafil [Viagra], tadalafil [Cialis]). These drugs are used to treat pulmonary artery hypertension and erectile dysfunction. The combined use of nitrates and PDE5 inhibitors may result in symptomatic hypotension.

**Combination therapy.** Combination therapy with hydralazine and isosorbide dinitrate (Bidil) may be helpful in African American patients with HF who are getting optimal therapy with ACE inhibitors and β-blockers. The same benefit is not found in white patients. The combination of the two drugs is also associated with a significant improvement in LV EF and exercise tolerance.[1,17] Although the evidence of benefit is stronger in African American patients, the combination therapy may be used in patients of other races who are already on optimal therapy.

As previously mentioned, tolerance to nitrates can develop. Hydralazine has antioxidant properties that prevent the development of tolerance to nitrates and preserves the helpful effects of nitrates.[17]

***Positive Inotropes.*** Digitalis preparations (e.g., digoxin) increase the force of cardiac contraction (inotropic action). They also decrease the HR (chronotropic action). These actions allow for more complete emptying of the ventricles, reducing the volume remaining in the ventricles during diastole. CO increases due to the increased stroke volume from improved contractility.[11] Digoxin has been shown to reduce symptoms, improve quality of life, and increase exercise tolerance in patients with mild to moderate HF. It has not been shown to decrease mortality in patients with HF.[1]

Patients taking a digitalis preparation are at risk for digitalis toxicity. Hypokalemia, secondary to the use of potassium-depleting diuretics (e.g., thiazides, loop diuretics), is one of the most common causes of digitalis toxicity. Low serum potassium enhances the action of digitalis, causing a therapeutic dose to reach toxic levels. Similarly, hyperkalemia inhibits the action of digitalis, resulting in a subtherapeutic dose. Both hypokalemia and hyperkalemia can also cause dysrhythmias. Monitor serum potassium levels of all patients taking digitalis preparations and potassium-depleting and potassium-sparing diuretics. Other electrolyte imbalances, such as hypercalcemia and hypomagnesemia, can also trigger digitalis toxicity. (Manifestations of electrolyte imbalances are discussed in Chapter 16.)

**DRUG ALERT Digoxin**
- Monitor for signs of hypokalemia and hyperkalemia, since these can increase or decrease the effects of digoxin, respectively.
- Monitor for early signs of toxicity: anorexia, nausea and vomiting, fatigue, headache, depression, visual changes.
- Monitor for late signs of toxicity, such as dysrhythmias (e.g., bradycardia, atrioventricular block).

Diseases of the kidney and liver increase the risk of digitalis toxicity, because most preparations are metabolized and eliminated by these organs. An older adult is especially prone to digitalis toxicity. This is because digitalis accumulation occurs sooner with decreased liver and kidney function and slowed body metabolism.

The usual treatment of toxicity consists of withholding the drug until the symptoms subside. In the case of life-threatening toxicity, IV digoxin immune Fab (ovine) (DigiFab) is an antidote. The treatment of life-threatening dysrhythmias is started as needed (see Chapter 35).

***Cardiac Sinus Node Inhibitor.*** Ivabradine (Corlanor) is a new category of oral drug that inhibits the sinus node and reduces HR. It is used for patients who have symptoms of chronic HF. They must be in sinus rhythm with a resting HR of at least 70 beats per minute and taking β-blockers at the highest dose tolerated. Ivabradine also reduces the risk of hospitalization for worsening HF.[18]

The most common side effects of ivabradine include symptomatic bradycardia, high BP, atrial fibrillation, and vision disturbance (i.e., flashes of light). Tell patients to call their HCP if they experience symptoms of an irregular HR, feel that their heart is pounding or racing, or have chest pressure or worsened dyspnea. Low HR is a common side effect of ivabradine and can be serious. Patients should tell their HCP if they experience dizziness, weakness, or fatigue.[18]

## COMPLEMENTARY & ALTERNATIVE THERAPIES

### *Hawthorn*

**Scientific Evidence***
- Strong evidence for its use in mild to moderate HF
- May have a diuretic effect
- May inhibit angiotensin-converting enzyme
- May reduce incidence of sudden cardiac death in patients with ejection fractions >25%

**Nursing Implications**
- Potentially beneficial treatment for patients who cannot or will not take prescription drugs
- May add to the effects of established therapies (e.g., cardiac glycosides, antihypertensives, lipid-lowering drugs)

*Source: *www.naturalstandard.com.*

## Nutritional Therapy

Poor adherence to a low-sodium diet and failure to take prescribed drugs as directed are the two most common reasons for readmissions of HF patients to the hospital. Therefore it is critical that you accurately assess a patient's diet and teach both the patient and caregiver about the importance of diet.

Diet teaching and weight management are essential to the patient's control of chronic HF. You or a dietitian should obtain a detailed diet history. Determine not only what foods the patient eats but also when, where, and how often the patient dines out. In addition, assess the cultural value of food. Use this information to assist the patient in making appropriate dietary choices when developing a diet plan. The National Heart, Lung, and Blood Institute provides helpful dietary guidelines for heart-healthy food preparation for people of various cultures (e.g., Hispanics, Asian Americans). These are available online at *www.nhlbi.nih.gov/health/educational/lose_wt/menuplanner.html.* Diet and weight management recommendations must be individualized and culturally sensitive if the necessary changes are to be made.

The edema associated with chronic HF is often treated by dietary restriction of sodium. Teach the patient what foods are low and high in sodium and ways to enhance food flavors without the use of salt (e.g., substituting lemon juice, various spices). The degree of sodium restriction depends on the severity of the HF and the effectiveness of diuretic therapy. The Dietary Approaches to Stop Hypertension (DASH) diet is effective as a first-line therapy for many individuals with hypertension. (The DASH diet is discussed in Chapter 32.) This diet is now also widely used for the patient with HF, with or without hypertension.

The average American adult's daily intake of sodium ranges from 7 to 15 g. A commonly ordered diet for a patient with HF is a 2-g sodium diet (Table 34-8). All foods high in sodium (more than 400 mg/serving) should be avoided. On this diet, processed meats, cheese, bread, cereals, canned soups, and canned vegetables must be limited. Teach the patient and caregiver how to read labels to look for sodium content (Fig. 34-6).

## TABLE 34-8 Nutritional Therapy

### *Low-Sodium Diets*

**General Principles**

Do not add salt or seasonings containing sodium when preparing foods.*
Do not use salt at the table.*
Avoid high-sodium foods (e.g., canned soups, processed meats, cheese, frozen meals).
Limit milk products to 2 cups daily.

**Sample Menu Plans for 2400-mg Sodium Diet**

| *Breakfast* | *Sodium (mg)* |
|---|---|
| ⅔ cup bran cereal | 161 |
| (⅔ cup Shredded Wheat cereal)† | 3 |
| 1 slice whole-wheat bread | 149 |
| 1 medium banana | 1 |
| 6 oz fruit yogurt, fat free | 85 |
| 1 cup fat-free milk | 126 |
| 2 Tbsp jelly | 5 |
| Coffee, 8 oz | 5 |
| ***Lunch*** | |
| Chicken breast sandwich | |
| 2 slices (3 oz) chicken breast, skinless | 65 |
| 2 slices whole wheat bread | 299 |
| 1 slice (¾ oz) American cheese | 328 |
| (1 slice [¾ oz] Swiss cheese, natural)† | 54 |
| Large-leaf romaine lettuce | 1 |
| 2 slices tomato | 90 |
| 1 Tbsp mayonnaise, low fat | 90 |
| 1 medium peach | 7 |
| ***Dinner*** | |
| ¾ cup vegetarian spaghetti sauce | 459 |
| (6 oz no-salt-added tomato paste)† | 260 |
| 1 cup spaghetti | 1 |
| 3 Tbsp parmesan cheese | 349 |
| Spinach salad | |
| 1 cup fresh spinach leaves | 24 |
| ¼ cup fresh carrots (grated) | 10 |
| ¼ cup fresh mushrooms (sliced) | 1 |
| 2 Tbsp vinaigrette dressing | 0 |
| ½ cup canned pears, juice pack | 4 |
| ½ cup corn, cooked from frozen | 4 |
| ***Snack*** | |
| ⅓ cup almonds | 4 |
| ¼ cup dried apricots | 3 |
| 6 oz fruit yogurt, fat free | 85 |

*1 tsp of salt equals 2.3 g of sodium.
†Substitutes to reduce to 1500-mg sodium diet.

The patient and caregiver should also be aware of the high sodium content of most restaurant foods.

Fluid restrictions are not commonly ordered for the patient with mild to moderate HF. However, in moderate to severe HF and renal insufficiency, fluids are limited to less than 2 L/day.[14] Helping patients deal with thirst as a side effect of the drugs is important. Suggest ice chips, gum, hard candy, or ice pops.

To monitor fluid status, tell patients to weigh themselves at the same time each day. Ideally this should be before breakfast, using the same scale, and wearing the same type of clothing. This helps ensure valid comparisons from day to day and helps identify early signs of fluid retention. For patients with visual limitations, suggest scales with larger numbers or an audible response. Tell patients to call the HCP if they see a weight gain of 3 lb (1.4 kg) over 2 days or a 3- to 5-lb (2.3-kg) gain over a week.[14]

Chicken Noodle Soup

**Nutrition Facts**

Serving Size 1/2 cup (120 mL) condensed soup
Servings Per Container about 2.5

| Amount Per Serving | |
|---|---|
| **Calories** 60 | Calories from Fat 15 |
| | **% Daily Value*** |
| **Total Fat** 1.5 g | 2% |
| Saturated Fat 0.5 g | 3% |
| *Trans* Fat 0 g | |
| **Cholesterol** 15 mg | |
| **Sodium** 890 mg | 37% |
| **Total Carbohydrate** 8 g | 3% |
| Dietary Fiber 1 g | 4% |
| Sugars 1 g | |
| **Protein** 3 g | |

| | | | |
|---|---|---|---|
| **Vitamin A** | 4% | **Calcium** | 0% |
| **Vitamin C** | 0% | **Iron** | 2% |

*Percent Daily Values are based on a 2,000 calorie diet Your Daily Values may be higher or lower depending on your calorie needs.

| | Calories | 2000 | 2500 |
|---|---|---|---|
| Total Fat | Less than | 65 g | 80 g |
| Sat Fat | Less than | 20 g | 25 g |
| Cholesterol | Less than | 300 g | 300 g |
| Sodium | Less than | 2400 mg | 2400 mg |
| Total Carbohydrate | | 300 g | 375 g |
| Dietary Fiber | | 25 g | 30 g |

**FIG. 34-6** Typical nutrition label. Note that a single serving (½ cup) provides more than one third of the daily recommended intake of sodium.

## ❖ NURSING MANAGEMENT: HEART FAILURE

### ◆ Nursing Assessment

Subjective and objective data that you should obtain from a patient with HF are presented in Table 34-9. Carefully review the patient's current prescription and over-the-counter drugs. Assess for use of any nonsteroidal antiinflammatory drugs (NSAIDs), since they can contribute to sodium retention and an exacerbation of HF. In addition, review the patient's dietary habits to identify issues related to an exacerbation of HF.

Explore the patient's chronic health problems as they may act as exacerbating factors, affecting the plan of care and the timing and selection of therapies. For example, a patient with sleep apnea may not regularly use his or her continuous positive airway pressure device at night. This can worsen pulmonary or systemic hypertension and lead to an exacerbation of HF.

### ◆ Nursing Diagnoses

Nursing diagnoses for the patient with HF include, but are not limited to, the following:

- Impaired gas exchange *related to* increased preload and alveolar-capillary membrane changes
- Decreased cardiac output *related to* altered contractility, altered preload, and/or altered stroke volume
- Excess fluid volume *related to* increased venous pressure and decreased renal perfusion secondary to heart failure
- Activity intolerance *related to* imbalance between $O_2$ supply and demand secondary to cardiac insufficiency and pulmonary congestion

Additional information on nursing diagnoses for the patient with HF is presented in eNursing Care Plan 34-1 on the website for this chapter.

**TABLE 34-9 Nursing Assessment**

***Heart Failure***

**Subjective Data**

***Important Health Information***

*Past health history:* CAD (including recent MI), hypertension, cardiomyopathy, valvular or congenital heart disease, diabetes mellitus, hyperlipidemia, renal disease, thyroid or lung disease, rapid or irregular heart rate

*Medications:* Use of and adherence with any heart drugs. Use of diuretics, estrogens, corticosteroids, nonsteroidal antiinflammatory drugs, over-the-counter drugs, herbal supplements

***Functional Health Patterns***

*Health perception–health management:* Fatigue, depression, anxiety

*Nutritional-metabolic:* Usual sodium intake. Nausea, vomiting, anorexia, stomach bloating. Weight gain, ankle swelling

*Elimination:* Nocturia, decreased daytime urine output, constipation

*Activity-exercise:* Dyspnea, orthopnea, cough (e.g., dry, productive). Palpitations, dizziness, fainting

*Sleep-rest:* Number of pillows used for sleeping. Paroxysmal nocturnal dyspnea, insomnia, sleep apnea

*Cognitive-perceptual:* Chest pain or heaviness. RUQ pain, abdominal discomfort. Behavioral changes, visual changes

**Objective Data**

***Integumentary***

Cool, diaphoretic skin. Cyanosis or pallor. Peripheral edema (right-sided heart failure)

***Respiratory***

Tachypnea, crackles, wheezes. Frothy, blood-tinged sputum

***Cardiovascular***

Tachycardia, $S_3$, $S_4$, murmurs. Pulsus alternans. PMI displaced inferiorly and posteriorly, lifts and heaves, jugular venous distention

***Gastrointestinal***

Abdominal distention, hepatosplenomegaly, ascites

***Neurologic***

Restlessness, confusion, decreased attention or memory

***Possible Diagnostic Findings***

Altered serum electrolytes (especially $Na^+$ and $K^+$), ↑ BUN, creatinine, or liver function tests. ↑ NT-proBNP or BNP. Chest x-ray demonstrating cardiomegaly, pulmonary congestion, and interstitial pulmonary edema. Echocardiogram showing increased chamber size, decreased wall motion, decreased EF or normal EF with evidence of diastolic failure. Atrial and ventricular enlargement on ECG. ↓ $O_2$ saturation

*BNP,* b-Type natriuretic peptide; *BUN,* blood urea nitrogen; *EF,* ejection fraction; *NT-proBNP,* N-terminal prohormone of BNP; *PMI,* point of maximal impulse; *RUQ,* right upper quadrant.

### ◆ Planning

The overall goals for the patient with HF include (1) a decrease in symptoms (e.g., shortness of breath, fatigue), (2) a decrease in peripheral edema, (3) an increase in exercise tolerance, (4) adherence with the treatment regimen, and (5) no complications related to HF.

### ◆ Nursing Implementation

◆ **Health Promotion.** Communication and joint decision making among the patient, caregiver, and interprofessional team are integral to selection and delivery of high-quality, patient-centered care. Currently, the emphasis is on aggressively identifying and treating risk factors for HF to prevent or slow the progression of the disease.[19] For example, teach a patient with hypertension or hyperlipidemia ways to manage BP or cholesterol with drugs, diet, and exercise. Encourage patients to obtain the flu and pneumococcal vaccinations. Patients with valvular disease should be evaluated for valve replacement procedures if they are contributing to HF and symptoms. Coronary revascularization procedures should be considered in patients with CAD. The use of antidysrhythmic drugs or pacing therapy is indicated for patients with serious dysrhythmias or conduction disturbances.

◆ **Acute Care.** Many persons with HF experience one or more episodes of ADHF. When they do, they are usually admitted through the ED, first stabilized, and then cared for in an ICU, an intermediate care unit, or a specialized HF unit with continuous ECG monitoring capability.

Successful HF care depends on several important principles: (1) HF is a progressive disease, and treatment plans are established along with quality-of-life goals; (2) symptom management is controlled by the patient with self-management tools (e.g., daily weights, drug regimens, diet and exercise plans); (3) salt and, at times, water must be restricted; (4) energy must be conserved; and (5) support systems are essential to the success of the entire treatment plan.

Reduction of anxiety is an important nursing function, since anxiety may increase the SNS response and further increase myocardial workload. Reducing anxiety may be aided by a variety of nursing interventions (e.g., imagery) and the use of sedatives (e.g., benzodiazepines).

In the past, the Joint Commission had identified core measures in the management of patients with HF to reflect standards of evidence-based care.[20] Currently, the AHA has developed a program, Get With the Guidelines—Heart Failure, to improve adherence to standards of evidence-based care of patients hospitalized with HF.[21] These approaches work to ensure high-quality care for patients with HF.

◆ **Ambulatory Care.** HF is a chronic illness. When a patient is diagnosed with HF, care should focus on slowing the progression of the disease. Your important nursing responsibilities include (1) teaching the patient about the physiologic changes that have occurred, (2) helping the patient adapt to both physiologic and psychologic changes, and (3) including the patient and caregiver in the overall care plan. Review the signs and symptoms of HF exacerbations with the patient and caregiver. Give them a clear action plan to follow should symptoms occur.[14] Early detection of worsening HF may help prevent an acute episode requiring hospitalization. A patient and caregiver guide for the patient with HF is presented in Table 34-10 below.

## TABLE 34-10 Patient & Caregiver Teaching

### *Heart Failure*

*Include the following instructions when teaching the patient and caregiver about the management of heart failure.*

**Dietary Therapy**
- Consult the diet plan and list of permitted and restricted foods.
- Examine labels to determine sodium content. Also examine the labels of over-the-counter drugs such as laxatives, cough medicines, and antacids for sodium content.
- Avoid using salt when preparing foods or adding salt to foods.
- Weigh yourself at the same time each day, preferably in the morning, using the same scale and wearing similar clothes.
- Eat small, frequent meals.

**Activity Program**
- Increase walking and other activities gradually, provided they do not cause fatigue or dyspnea.
- Consider a cardiac rehabilitation program.
- Avoid extremes of heat and cold.

**Ongoing Monitoring**
- Know the signs and symptoms of worsening heart failure (Think *FACES*: *F*atigue, limitation of *A*ctivities, chest *C*ongestion/cough, *E*dema, and *S*hortness of breath).
- Recall the symptoms experienced when illness began. Reappearance of previous symptoms may indicate a recurrence.
- Report immediately any of the following to the HCP:
  - Weight gain of 3 lb (1.4 kg) in 2 days, or 3-5 lb (2.3 kg) in a wk
  - Difficulty breathing, especially with activity or when lying flat
  - Waking up breathless at night
  - Frequent dry, hacking cough, especially when lying down
  - Fatigue, weakness
  - Swelling of ankles, feet, or abdomen. Swelling of face or difficulty breathing (if taking ACE inhibitors)
  - Nausea with abdominal swelling, pain, and tenderness
  - Dizziness or fainting
- Follow up with HCP on regular basis.
- Consider joining a local support group with your family members and/or caregiver(s).

**Health Promotion**
- Obtain annual flu vaccination.
- Obtain pneumococcal vaccine (see Table 27-5 for guidelines on pneumococcal vaccination).
- Develop plan to reduce risk factors (e.g., BP control, tobacco cessation, weight reduction).

**Rest**
- Plan a regular daily rest and activity program.
- After exertion, such as exercise and ADLs, plan a rest period.
- Consider shorter working hours or schedule rest period during working hours
- Avoid emotional upsets. Share any concerns, fears, feelings of depression, etc. with HCP.

**Drug Therapy**
- Take each drug as ordered.
- Develop a system (e.g., daily chart, weekly pillbox) to ensure drugs have been taken.
- Count pulse rate each day before taking drugs (if appropriate). Know the limits that your HCP wants for your pulse rate.
- Take BP at determined intervals (if appropriate). Know your target BP limits.
- Know signs and symptoms of orthostatic hypotension and how to prevent them (see Table 32-12).
- If taking anticoagulants, know signs and symptoms of internal bleeding (bleeding gums, increased bruises, blood in stool or urine) and what to do.
- Know your INR and target range if taking warfarin (Coumadin) and how often to have blood checked.

*ACE*, Angiotensin-converting enzyme; *INR*, international normalized ratio.

Patients with HF are at risk for anxiety and depression.[7] Emphasize to the patient that it is possible to live a productive life with this chronic illness. Patients with HF usually need to take drugs for the rest of their lives. This often becomes difficult because a patient may be asymptomatic when HF is under control. You must stress that the disease is chronic, and that drugs must be continued to keep the HF under control.

Teach the patient the expected actions of the ordered drugs and the signs of drug toxicity. Also teach the patient and caregiver how to take a pulse rate. The pulse should always be taken for 1 full minute. A pulse less than 50 beats/minute may be a contraindication to taking a β-blocker or a digitalis preparation unless directed by the HCP. However, in the absence of symptoms (e.g., heart block, ventricular ectopy, syncope), a pulse less than 50 beats/minute may be acceptable. Include clear information about when a drug, especially β-blockers and digitalis, should be held and an HCP called.

Teach the patient the symptoms of hypokalemia and hyperkalemia if diuretics that deplete or spare potassium are ordered. Weakness, fatigue, constipation, and muscle cramping may occur, but often there are no physical signs of hypo- or hyperkalemia. Frequently the patient who takes thiazide or loop diuretics is given supplemental potassium. It may also be appropriate to teach patients home BP monitoring, especially those with hypertension.

The physical therapist, occupational therapist, or you can instruct the patient in energy-conserving and energy-efficient behaviors after an evaluation of daily activities has been done. For example, once you understand the patient's daily routine, make suggestions to simplify work or modify an activity.

Exercise training (e.g., cardiac rehabilitation) improves symptoms of chronic HF but is often underprescribed. Exercise for patients with HF has been found to be safe and to improve the overall sense of well-being. It has also been related to a decrease in mortality.[1,12]

Frequently the patient needs a prescription for rest after an activity. Many hard-driving persons need the "permission" to not feel "lazy." Sometimes the patient may need to stop an activity that he or she enjoys. In such cases, help the patient explore alternative activities that cause less physical stress. Changes may be needed if some situations produce an increased cardiac workload (e.g., frequent climbing of stairs). Help a patient identify areas where changes can be made and outside assistance obtained if needed.

Managing HF patients out of the hospital is a priority. Effective home health care can prevent or limit future hospitalizations by providing ongoing assessments (e.g., monitoring vital signs and weight, evaluating response to therapies).[21] Many agencies offer specialized programs designed to manage HF patients at home. For example, these programs may include the use of telehealth monitoring technology (e.g., electronic scale, BP cuff, pulse oximeter) to collect physiologic data (Fig. 34-7). The technology may also audibly ask the patient questions such as, "Are you short of breath today?" Results are transmitted via the telephone or computer to the HCP. After the data are reviewed, the patient may be called to further assess the situation or schedule a visit.

Home health nurses frequently work with protocols set up with the patient's HCP. The protocols enable you and the patient to identify problems, such as an increase in weight or dyspnea, as evidence of worsening HF. To prevent hospitalization, interventions can be started such as changing drugs or dosages and restricting fluids. Home health nursing care of HF patients is vital in reducing the number of hospitalizations, increasing functional capacity, and improving the quality of life.

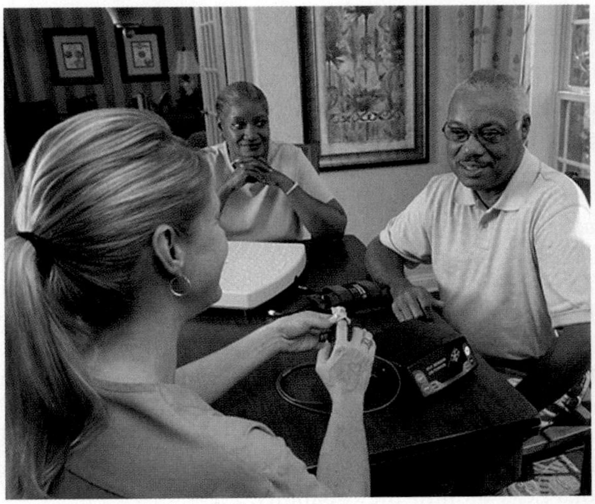

**FIG. 34-7** Home-based telehealth monitoring unit. (Used with permission from Honeywell HomMed.)

## EVIDENCE-BASED PRACTICE

### *Applying the Evidence*

**Home Care and Heart Failure**

B.H. is a 68-yr-old Hispanic female with chronic heart failure (HF) who is being discharged home tomorrow. You have made arrangements for the interprofessional home health care team to resume visits. B.H. tells you that since her hospitalization she does not feel the home visits have been helpful and that she is now considering home care from "family" only. She also tells you her heart is not getting better. B.H.'s daughter is her caregiver and she wants to continue the home care visits.

***Making Clinical Decisions***

***Best Available Evidence.*** In patients with HF, transitional home health care programs result in decreased readmissions and mortality compared to the usual care.

***Clinician Expertise.*** You know it is important for patients to receive home visits to avoid preventable adverse outcomes after hospitalization (e.g., readmission). You also understand that HF is a progressive illness and is often not predictable.

***Patient Preferences and Values.*** B.H. believes that continuation of home health care visits will not be beneficial.

***Implications for Nursing Practice***

1. What will you discuss with B.H. related to the purpose of the home visits?
2. Why is it important for you to determine B.H.'s understanding of HF?
3. How will you involve B.H.'s daughter if B.H. remains undecided about home health care visits?
4. How will you engage B.H. in her own care before she is discharged home?

***Reference for Evidence***

Feltner C, Jones CD, Cené CW, et al: Transitional care interventions to prevent readmissions for people with heart failure. AHRQ comparative effectiveness reviews, Rockville, Md, 2014, Agency for Healthcare Research and Quality (US).

◆ **Palliative and End-of-Life Care.** HCPs are often reluctant to refer patients with advanced HF for palliative or end-of-life care.

The unpredictable trajectory of HF during the last few months of life makes assessing the prognosis of the disease difficult.[22] In addition, patients and caregivers may have a poor understanding of the disease and may fail to recognize HF as a terminal illness.[23]

The ACCF/AHA provides guidelines for patients with end-stage HF (stage D).[1] HCPs in collaboration with the patient and caregiver can select either advanced treatment interventions (e.g., heart transplant, VAD), or palliative care for symptom management and hospice care. The guidelines recommend (1) ongoing patient and caregiver teaching regarding prognosis and survival, (2) patient and caregiver teaching about options for composing advance directives (e.g., deactivation of ICD), and (3) continuity of medical care (e.g., continuous infusion of inotropes for symptom control).[1]

Patients are eligible for hospice when an HCP certifies that they are likely to have a life expectancy of 6 months or less. Unfortunately, many eligible patients are not referred to hospice. There are a number of reasons for this. These include a lack of understanding of the role of hospice, lack of an identifiable terminal phase for HF, and concerns about meeting hospice referral criteria. African American and Hispanic patients with HF use hospice less than whites.[24]

The seriousness of the prognosis and the actual knowledge of the expected short life span are misunderstood by many HF patients and caregivers. Many HCPs and HF patients overestimate the life expectancy. When caring for these patients, attempt to identify those who may be eligible for hospice and initiate a discussion among the patient, caregiver, and HCP.

Because patients with end-stage HF have multiple symptoms, your care should involve ongoing assessment and evaluation of interventions for effectiveness. Strategies involve patient and caregiver support, drug therapies, and nondrug therapies. Drugs are continued unless they are not tolerated. The goals of providing comfort and relieving suffering remain priorities in the care of patients with end-stage HF. (Palliative and end-of-life care are discussed in Chapter 9.)

### Evaluation

The expected outcomes are that the patient with HF will

- Maintain adequate $O_2/CO_2$ exchange at the alveolar-capillary membrane to meet $O_2$ needs of the body
- Maintain adequate blood pumped by the heart to meet metabolic demands of the body
- Experience reduction or absence of edema and stable baseline weight
- Achieve a realistic program of activity that balances physical activity with energy-conserving activities

Additional information on expected outcomes for the patient with HF is presented in eNursing Care Plan 34-1 on the website for this chapter.

## HEART TRANSPLANTATION

**Heart transplantation** is the transfer of a healthy donor heart to a patient with a diseased heart. This surgery is used to treat a variety of terminal or end-stage heart conditions (Table 34-11). Retransplantation (i.e., a second or third heart transplant) is also done. In the United States, approximately 3000 patients are listed for heart transplants. However, on average only 2000 hearts become available. The 1-year transplant survival rate is 85% to 90%, whereas the 3-year survival rate is approximately 75%.[25]

**TABLE 34-11 Indications and Contraindications for Heart Transplantation***

**Indications**
- End-stage HF refractory to medical care
- Severe, decompensated, inoperable, valvular heart disease
- Recurrent life-threatening dysrhythmias not responsive to maximal interventions, including defibrillators
- Any other heart abnormalities that severely limit normal function and/or have a mortality risk of more than 50% at 2 yr

**Absolute Contraindications**
- Chronologic age over 70 yr or physiologic age over 65 yr
- Life-threatening illness (e.g., malignancy) that will limit survival to <5 yr despite therapy
- Advanced cerebral or peripheral vascular disease not amenable to correction
- Active infection, including HIV infection
- Severe pulmonary disease that will likely result in the patient being ventilator dependent after transplant

**Relative Contraindications**
- Severe obesity
- Psychologic impairment
- Active substance abuse (e.g., alcohol, drugs, tobacco)
- Uncontrolled diabetes with vascular and neurologic complications
- Irreversible liver or kidney dysfunction not explained by HF
- Evidence of noncompliance with accepted medical practices
- Lack of social support network that can make long-term commitment for patient's welfare
- Unrealistic expectations by the patient or caregiver regarding transplant, its risks, and its benefits

*These are representative examples from various heart transplant centers.

### Criteria for Selection

A careful selection process ensures that hearts are distributed fairly and to those who will benefit most from the donor heart. The United Network for Organ Sharing (UNOS) is in charge of a system that gives organs fairly to people. (UNOS is discussed in Chapter 13.)

Indications and contraindications for heart transplantation are identified in Table 34-11. Once a person meets the criteria for heart transplantation, a complete physical examination and diagnostic workup are done. In addition, the patient and caregiver undergo a comprehensive psychologic evaluation. This includes assessing coping skills, support systems, and commitment to follow the rigorous regimen that is essential to a successful transplantation. The complexity of the transplant process may be overwhelming to a patient with inadequate support systems and a poor understanding of the lifestyle changes needed after transplant.

Donor and recipient matching is based on body and heart size and an immunologic evaluation. The immunologic assessment includes ABO blood type, antibody screen, panel of reactive antibody (PRA) level, and human leukocyte antigen typing (explained in Chapter 13).

Once a person is accepted as a transplant candidate (this may happen quickly during an acute illness or after a longer period), he or she is placed on a transplant list. Patients may wait at home and receive ongoing medical care if their condition is stable. If not, they may require hospitalization for more intensive therapy. Unfortunately, the overall waiting period for a new heart is long. Many patients die while waiting for a transplant.

### Bridge to Transplantation

Several devices are available as a bridge to transplantation (BTT), but only two have received FDA approval for heart recovery after a life-threatening cardiac event. The AB5000 Circulatory Support System and the BVS 5000 Biventricular Support System provide temporary support for one or both sides of the heart in situations in which the heart has failed but has the potential to recover (e.g., reversible HF, myocarditis, acute MI). Patients with these devices are critically ill and require close observation in an ICU.

The Thoratec HeartMate II and the HeartWare LVAD are permanent pumps that support the heart. After the initial surgery and recovery period, patients do not require ongoing hospitalization. The HeartMate II is approved as a BTT or destination therapy (DT) for those patients who do not meet criteria for a heart transplant. The HeartWare device is currently only approved as a BTT.

### Surgical Procedure

The surgical procedure actually involves two surgeries. First, the donor heart is retrieved. The donor is someone who has suffered irreversible brain injury *(brain death).* A surgical team goes to the hospital of the donor to remove donated organs once brain death has been determined. The retrieved organs are transported on ice until they can be implanted. For the heart, this is optimally less than 4 hours. Often the donor heart is flown to the recipient's hospital.

Next, the donor heart is implanted into the recipient. Two different approaches are used in this surgery. In the biatrial approach, the recipient's damaged heart is removed at the midatrial level and the donor heart connected at the left atrium, pulmonary artery, aorta, and right atrium. In the bicaval approach, the right atrium of the recipient's heart (with the sinoatrial node and atrial conduction intact) is preserved, and then the donor heart is connected. Cardiopulmonary bypass is needed during the surgical procedure to maintain oxygenation and perfusion to vital organs.

### Posttransplantation

After the transplant a variety of complications can occur, including a risk for SCD. Acute rejection is an immediate posttransplant complication, and immunosuppressive therapy is the key in posttransplant management. In the first year after transplantation, the major causes of death are acute rejection and infection. Later, malignancy (especially lymphoma) and cardiac vasculopathy (accelerated CAD) are major causes of death.[26]

Most immunosuppressive regimens include corticosteroids, calcineurin inhibitors (tacrolimus [Prograf]), and antiproliferative drugs (mycophenolate mofetil [CellCept]). (The mechanisms of action and side effects of these and other immunosuppressants are discussed in Chapter 13 and Table 13-16.) Because of the use of immunosuppressive therapy, infection is a primary complication after transplant surgery. On a long-term basis, immunosuppressive therapy increases the risk for cancer.[26]

To detect rejection, an EMB is obtained on a weekly basis for the first month, monthly for the following six months, and yearly thereafter. In this procedure, a catheter is inserted into the jugular vein and moved into the RV. The catheter uses a bioptome, a device with two small cups that can be closed, to remove small samples of heart muscle.[26]

Nursing management throughout the posttransplant period focuses on promoting patient adaptation to the transplant process, monitoring heart function, managing lifestyle changes, and providing ongoing teaching of the patient and caregiver.

## ETHICAL/LEGAL DILEMMAS

### *Competence*

**Situation**

M.T., a 60-yr-old man, has been awaiting heart transplantation for 6 months. He has been a patient in intensive care for 1 month, since he has required a ventricular assist device for his failing heart. He recently suffered a stroke, which is a complication of the device. It left him paralyzed on his right side. He is only able to answer yes/no questions by shaking his head. He has required mechanical ventilation since his stroke. For the past 2 weeks, he has needed hemodialysis because of renal failure. Recently, when you suction him, he turns his head away from you and bites down on the endotracheal tube. Although he does not have an advance directive, his wife and daughter tell you that, on numerous occasions before these events, he expressed that he would not want to live if he lost his independence. His wife and daughter request to have the mechanical ventilator withdrawn.

**Ethical/Legal Points for Consideration**

- Decisional capacity for informed consent related to treatment decisions involves four elements: (1) information provided about possible treatment options must be understandable to patients, (2) patients must have the capacity to deliberate about the treatment choices and their consequences, (3) patients' treatment decisions must be freely chosen and made without coercion, and (4) patients must be able to communicate their decisions.
- Legal competence, as determined by the courts, has a fairly low threshold. The ability to respond to questions by signaling a yes or no may be enough to demonstrate understanding of the questions, ability to discriminate between choices, and ability to communicate choices, providing that the answers make sense and are appropriate. You need to know how legal competence is defined in your state.
- Next of kin are the legal decision makers in the absence of advance directives if he is unable to make decisions for himself. However, decisional capacity should be tested without assuming it is absent.
- Some courts have accepted past assertions of preferences, past behavior, and assertions of their parties as evidence to support end-of-life preferences in the absence of advance directives.
- You must be knowledgeable of your agency's policies and about the local jurisdiction's laws and regulations regarding informed consent and end-of-life decision making.

**Discussion Questions**

1. What would you do next given M.T.'s behavior and the information you obtained from his wife?
2. What are your feelings and concerns about participating in the care of a patient for whom withdrawal of treatment will result in death?

## CASE STUDY

### *Heart Failure*

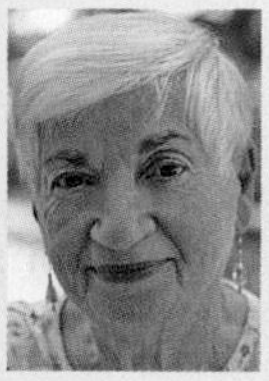

(©iStockphoto/ Thinkstock)

**Patient Profile**

J.E. is a 70-yr-old Hispanic woman who was admitted to the intermediate care unit with complaints of increasing shortness of breath, fatigue, and weight gain.

**Subjective Data**

- History of hypertension for 20 yr
- History of MI at 58 yr of age
- Has experienced increasing shortness of breath, fatigue, and an unexplained 11-lb weight gain during the past 2 wk
- Had a respiratory tract infection 2 wk ago; has persistent cough and edema in legs
- Cannot climb a flight of stairs without getting short of breath
- Sleeps with head elevated on three pillows
- Lives alone, does not always remember to take medication

**Objective Data**

***Physical Examination***

- Moderate respiratory distress, use of accessory muscles, respiratory rate 36 breaths/minute
- Systolic heart murmur
- Bilateral crackles in all lung fields
- Cyanotic lips and extremities
- Skin cool and diaphoretic

***Diagnostic Studies***

- Chest x-ray results: cardiomegaly with right and left ventricular hypertrophy; fluid in lower lung fields
- Echocardiogram results: EF 20%

**Interprofessional Care**

- Furosemide (Lasix) 40 mg IV bid
- Potassium 40 mEq PO bid
- Enalapril (Vasotec) 5 mg/day PO
- Nesiritide (Natrecor) 2 mcg/kg IV bolus followed by a continuous infusion of 0.01 mcg/kg/min
- Continuous ECG monitoring
- Diet: 2-g sodium diet
- Titrate $O_2$ to keep $O_2$ saturation >93%
- Monitor intake and output, and daily weights
- Serum electrolytes; cardiac biomarkers q8hr × 3

**Discussion Questions**

1. Explain the pathophysiology of J.E.'s heart disease and symptoms.
2. What clinical manifestations of ADHF did J.E. exhibit?
3. What is the significance of the findings of the diagnostic studies?
4. How would a serum NT-proBNP be beneficial in the diagnosis of ADHF?
5. Provide the rationale for each of the HCP's orders prescribed for J.E.
6. ***Priority Decision:*** Based on the assessment data presented, what are the priority nursing diagnoses? Identify any collaborative problems.
7. ***Priority Decision:*** What are your priority nursing interventions for J.E.?
8. ***Teamwork and Collaboration:*** Which interventions could be delegated to unlicensed assistive personnel (UAP) or other members of the interprofessional team?
9. ***Patient-Centered Care:*** What priority patient teaching measures should be instituted to prevent recurrence of ADHF and prepare J.E. for discharge?
10. ***Evidence-Based Practice:*** J.E. asks you why it is so important to "watch her salt." She tells you that food tastes better with salt. How would you respond to her?

Answers and a corresponding concept map available at *http://evolve.elsevier.com/Lewis/medsurg.*

## BRIDGE TO NCLEX EXAMINATION

The number of the question corresponds to the same-numbered outcome at the beginning of the chapter.

1. The nurse recognizes that *primary* manifestations of systolic failure include
   - **a.** ↓ EF and ↑ PAWP.
   - **b.** ↓ PAWP and ↑ EF.
   - **c.** ↓ pulmonary hypertension associated with normal EF.
   - **d.** ↓ afterload and ↓ left ventricular end-diastolic pressure.
2. A compensatory mechanism involved in HF that leads to inappropriate fluid retention and additional workload of the heart is
   - **a.** ventricular dilation.
   - **b.** ventricular hypertrophy.
   - **c.** neurohormonal response.
   - **d.** sympathetic nervous system activation.
3. You are caring for a patient with ADHF who is receiving IV dobutamine (Dobutrex). You know that this drug is ordered because it *(select all that apply)*
   - **a.** increases SVR.
   - **b.** produces diuresis.
   - **c.** improves contractility.
   - **d.** dilates renal blood vessels.
   - **e.** works on the $\beta_1$-receptors in the heart.
4. A patient with chronic HF and atrial fibrillation is treated with a digitalis glycoside and a loop diuretic. To prevent possible complications of this combination of drugs, what does the nurse need to do *(select all that apply)*?
   - **a.** Monitor serum potassium levels.
   - **b.** Teach the patient how to take a pulse rate.
   - **c.** Keep an accurate measure of intake and output.
   - **d.** Teach the patient about dietary restriction of potassium.
   - **e.** Withhold digitalis and notify health care provider if pulse is irregular.
5. Patients with a heart transplantation are at risk for which complications in the first year after transplantation *(select all that apply)*?
   - **a.** Cancer
   - **b.** Infection
   - **c.** Rejection
   - **d.** Vasculopathy
   - **e.** Sudden cardiac death

1. a, 2. c, 3. c, e, 4. a, b, 5. b, c, e

For rationales to these answers and even more NCLEX review questions, visit *http://evolve.elsevier.com/Lewis/medsurg.*

## EVOLVE WEBSITE

http://evolve.elsevier.com/Lewis/medsurg

**Review Questions (Online Only)**

**Key Points**

**Answer Keys for Questions**

- Rationales for Bridge to NCLEX Examination Questions
- Answer Guidelines for Case Study on p. 755

**Student Case Study**

- Patient With Heart Failure

**Nursing Care Plan**

- eNursing Care Plan 34-1: Patient With Heart Failure

**Conceptual Care Map Creator**

- Conceptual Care Map for Case Study on p. 755

**Audio Glossary**

**Content Updates**

## REFERENCES


*1. Yancy CW, Jessup M, Bozkurt B, et al: 2013 ACCF/AHA guideline for the management of heart failure: executive summary: a report of the American College of Cardiology Foundation/American Heart Association Task Force on practice guidelines, *Circulation* 128:1810, 2013.

2. Go AS, Mozaffarian D, Roger VL, et al: Heart disease and stroke statistics—2014 update: a report from the American Heart Association, *Circulation* 129:e28, 2013.

3. LeWinter M, Granzier H: Titin is a major human disease gene, *Circulation* 127:938, 2013.

*4. Silver MA, Maisel A, Yancy CW, et al: BNP Consensus Panel 2004: a clinical approach for the diagnostic, prognostic, screening, treatment monitoring, and therapeutic roles of natriuretic peptides in cardiovascular diseases, *Congest Heart Fail* 10(5 Suppl 3):1, 2004. (Classic)

5. Heart Failure Society of America: Who is the patient with heart failure? Think FACES, 2002. Retrieved from *www.hfsa.org/hfsa-wp/content/uploads/2014/10/faces_card.pdf.* (Classic)

6. Nawarskas JJ, Bowman BN, Anderson JR: Ivabradine: a unique and intriguing medication for treating cardiovascular disease, *Cardiol Rev* 23(4):201, 2015.

7. Newhouse A, Jiang W: Heart failure and depression, *Heart Fail Clin* 10(2):295, 2014.

*8. Tracy CM, Epstein AE, Darbar D, et al: 2012 ACCF/AHA/HRS Focused update incorporated into the ACCF/AHA/HRS 2008 Guidelines for Device-Based Therapy of Cardiac Rhythm Abnormalities: a report of the American College of Cardiology Foundation/American Heart Association Task Force on Practice Guidelines and the Heart Rhythm Society, *J Am Coll Cardiol* 61(3):e6, 2013.

*9. Thiene G, Bruneval P, Veinot J, Leone O: Diagnostic use of the endomyocardial biopsy: a consensus statement, *Virchows Arch* 463(1):1, 2013.

10. Coons JC, McGraw M, Murali S: Pharmacotherapy for acute heart failure syndromes, *Am J Health Syst Pharm* 68(1):21, 2011.

11. Key JL, Hayes ER, McCuistion LE: *Pharmacology: a patient centered nursing process approach,* ed 8, St Louis, 2015, Elsevier.

12. Ades PA, Keteyian SJ, Balady GJ, et al: Cardiac rehabilitation exercise and self-care for chronic heart failure, *JCHF* 1(6):540, 2013.

*13. Abraham WT, Adamson PB, Bourge RC, et al: Wireless pulmonary artery haemodynamic monitoring in chronic heart failure: a randomised controlled trial, *Lancet* 377:658, 2011.

*14. Lindenfeld J, Albert NM, Boehmer JP, et al: Executive summary: HFSA 2010 comprehensive heart failure practice guidelines, *J Card Fail* 16:475, 2010.

15. O'Riordan M: FDA approves valsartan/sacubitril (Entresto) combination for heart failure. Retrieved from *www.medscape.com/viewarticle/847619.*

*16. Lee D, Wilson K, Akehurst R, et al: Eplerenone in Mild Patients Hospitalization and Survival Study in Heart Failure (EMPHASIS-HF) Study: cost-effectiveness of eplerenone in patients with systolic heart failure and mild symptoms, *Heart* 100(21):1681, 2014.

*17. Ferdinand KC, Elkayam U, Mancini D, et al: Use of isosorbide dinitrate and hydralazine in African-Americans with heart failure 9 years after the African-American Heart Failure Trial, *Am J Cardiol* 114(1):151, 2014.

18. U.S. Food and Drug Administration: FDA approves Corlanor. Retrieved from *www.drugs.com/history/corlanor.html.*

*19. Schocken DD, Benjamin EJ, Fonarow G, et al: Prevention of heart failure: a scientific statement from the American Heart Association councils on epidemiology and prevention, clinical cardiology, cardiovascular nursing, and high blood pressure research, *Circulation* 117:2544, 2008.

20. The Joint Commission: Advanced certification in heart failure: standardized performance measures. Retrieved from *www.jointcommission.org/adv_certification_heart_failure_standardized_performance_measures.*

21. American Heart Association: Get with the guidelines—heart failure: fact sheet. Retrieved from *www.heart.org/idc/groups/heart-public/@wcm/@private/@hcm/@gwtg/documents/downloadable/ucm_310967.pdf.*

*22. Huynh B, Rovner A, Rich M: Identification of older patients with heart failure who may be candidates for hospice care: development of a simple four-item risk score, *J Am Geriatr Soc* 56:1111, 2008. (Classic)

*23. Allen LA, Stevenson l, Grady KL, et al: Decision making in advanced heart failure: a scientific statement from the American Heart Association, *Circulation* 125:1928, 2012.

24. Givens JL, Tjia J, Zhou C, et al: Racial and ethnic differences in hospice use among patients with heart failure, *Arch Intern Med* 170:427, 2010.

25. Stehlik J, Edwards LB, Kucheryavaya AY, et al: The registry of the International Society of Heart and Lung Transplantation: Twenty eighth Adult Heart Transplant Report—2011, *J Heart Lung Transplant* 30(10):1078, 2011.

*26. Taylor D, Meiser B, Webber S, et al: The International Society of Heart and Lung Transplantation Guidelines for the Care of Heart Transplant Recipients: task force 2: immunosuppression and rejection, *J Heart Lung Transplant* 29(8):926, 2010.


*Evidence-based information for clinical practice.

35

# Dysrhythmias

*Linda Bucher*

*The greatest test of courage on earth is to bear defeat without losing heart.*

***Robert Green Ingersoll***

http://evolve.elsevier.com/Lewis/medsurg/

## LEARNING OUTCOMES

1. Examine the nursing care of patients needing continuous electrocardiographic (ECG) monitoring.
2. Distinguish the clinical characteristics and ECG patterns of normal sinus rhythm, common dysrhythmias, and acute coronary syndrome (ACS).
3. Compare the nursing and interprofessional management of patients with common dysrhythmias and ECG changes associated with ACS.
4. Differentiate between defibrillation and cardioversion, including indications for use and physiologic effects.
5. Describe the nursing and interprofessional management of patients with pacemakers and implantable cardioverter-defibrillators.
6. Select appropriate interventions for patients undergoing electrophysiologic testing and radiofrequency catheter ablation therapy.

## KEY TERMS

asystole, p. 765
atrial fibrillation, p. 766
atrial flutter, p. 765
automatic external defibrillator (AED), p. 771
cardiac pacemaker, p. 773
complete heart block, p. 768
dysrhythmias, p. 757
premature atrial contraction (PAC), p. 764
premature ventricular contraction (PVC), p. 768
telemetry monitoring, p. 760
ventricular fibrillation (VF), p. 770
ventricular tachycardia (VT), p. 769

This chapter describes basic principles of electrocardiographic monitoring and recognition and treatment of common dysrhythmias. In addition, it presents ECG changes that are associated with acute coronary syndrome (ACS).

## RHYTHM IDENTIFICATION AND TREATMENT

Your ability to recognize normal and abnormal heart rhythms, called **dysrhythmias**, is an essential nursing skill.[1] Prompt assessment of dysrhythmias and the patient's response to the rhythm is critical.

### Conduction System

Four properties of heart cells allow the conduction system to start an electrical impulse, send it through the heart tissue, and stimulate muscle contraction (Table 35-1). The heart's conduction system consists of specialized neuromuscular tissue located throughout the heart (see Fig. 31-4, *A*). A normal impulse starts in the sinoatrial (SA) node in the upper right atrium near the entrance of the vena cava. It spreads over the atrial myocardium via interatrial and internodal pathways, causing atrial contraction. The impulse then travels to the atrioventricular (AV) node, through the bundle of His, and down the left and right bundle branches. It ends in the Purkinje fibers, which transmit the impulse to the ventricles.

### Nervous Control of the Heart

The autonomic nervous system plays an important role in the rate of impulse formation, speed of conduction, and strength of cardiac contraction. The components of the autonomic nervous system that affect the heart are the vagus nerve fibers of the parasympathetic nervous system and nerve fibers of the sympathetic nervous system.

Stimulation of the vagus nerve causes a decreased rate of firing of the SA node and slowed impulse conduction of the AV node. Stimulation of the sympathetic nerves increases SA node firing, AV node impulse conduction, and cardiac contractility.[2]

### Electrocardiographic Monitoring

The *electrocardiogram* (ECG) is a graphic tracing of the electrical impulses produced in the heart. The waveforms on the ECG represent electrical activity produced by the movement of ions across the membranes of heart cells, representing depolarization and repolarization (see Fig. 31-4, *B*).

The membrane of a heart cell is semipermeable. This allows it to maintain a high concentration of potassium and a low

Reviewed by Linda R. Lewis, MSN, RN-BC, Faculty Specialist, Nursing, University of Scranton, Scranton, Pennsylvania; and Tamekia L. Thomas, MSN, APN, PCCN, ACNS-BC, Critical Care Education Coordinator, Christiana Care Health System, Newark, Delaware.

**TABLE 35-1 Properties of Heart Cells**

| Property | Definition |
|---|---|
| Automaticity | Ability to initiate an impulse spontaneously and continuously |
| Excitability | Ability to be electrically stimulated |
| Conductivity | Ability to transmit an impulse along a membrane in an orderly manner |
| Contractility | Ability to respond mechanically to an impulse |

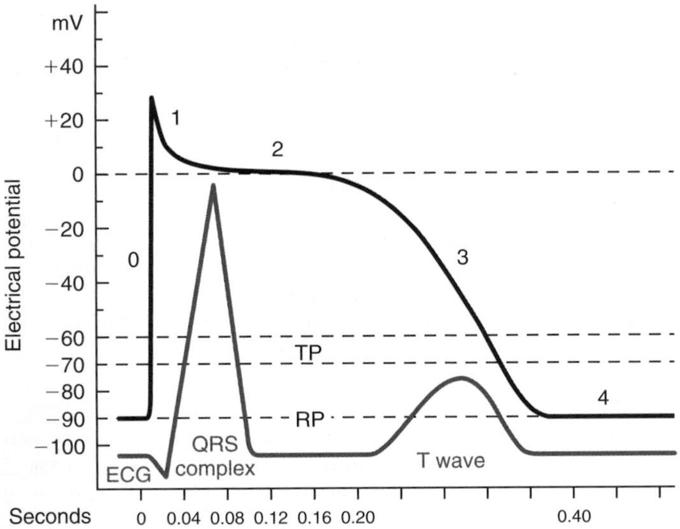


**FIG. 35-1** Phases of the cardiac action potential. The electrical potential, measured in millivolts (mV), is indicated along the vertical axis of the graph. Time, measured in seconds (sec), is indicated along the horizontal axis. The action potential has five phases, labeled *0* through *4*. Each phase represents a particular electrical event or combination of electrical events. Phase 0 is the upstroke of rapid depolarization and corresponds with ventricular contraction. Phases 1, 2, and 3 represent repolarization. Phase 4 is known as complete repolarization (or the polarized state) and corresponds to diastole. *RP,* Resting membrane potential; *TP,* threshold membrane potential.

concentration of sodium inside the cell. Outside the cell a high concentration of sodium and a low concentration of potassium exist. The inside of the cell, when at rest, or in the polarized state, is negative compared with the outside. When a cell or groups of cells are stimulated, the cell membrane changes its permeability. This allows sodium to move rapidly into the cell, making the inside of the cell positive compared with the outside *(depolarization)*. A slower movement of ions across the membrane restores the cell to the polarized state, called *repolarization*. Fig. 35-1 describes the phases of the cardiac action potential.[2]

The ECG has 12 recording leads. Six of the leads measure electrical forces in the frontal plane. These are bipolar (positive and negative) leads I, II, and III and unipolar (positive) leads aVR, aVL, and aVF (Fig. 35-2, *A* and *B*). The remaining six unipolar leads ($V_1$ through $V_6$) measure the electrical forces in the horizontal plane (precordial leads) (Fig. 35-2, *C*). The 12-lead ECG may show changes suggesting structural changes, conduction disturbances, damage (e.g., ischemia, infarction), electrolyte imbalance, or drug toxicity. Obtaining 12-lead ECG views of the heart is also helpful in the assessment of dysrhythmias. Fig. 35-3 is an example of a normal 12-lead ECG.

One or more ECG leads can be used to continuously monitor a patient. The most common leads selected are leads II and $V_1$ (Fig. 35-4). A modified chest lead ($MCL_1$) is used when only three leads are available for monitoring. $MCL_1$ is similar to $V_1$. Accurate interpretation of an ECG depends on the correct placement of the leads on the patient. The monitoring leads selected are determined by the patient's clinical status.[3,4]

The monitor continuously displays the heart rhythm. ECG paper attached to the monitor records the ECG (i.e., rhythm strip). This provides a record of the patient's rhythm. It also allows for measurement of complexes and intervals, and for assessment of dysrhythmias.

To correctly interpret an ECG, measure time and voltage on the ECG paper. ECG paper consists of large (heavy lines) and small (light lines) squares (Fig. 35-5). Each large square consists of 25 smaller squares (five horizontal and five vertical). Horizontally, each small square (1 mm) represents 0.04 second. This means that one large square equals 0.20 second and that 300 large squares equal 1 minute. Vertically, each small square

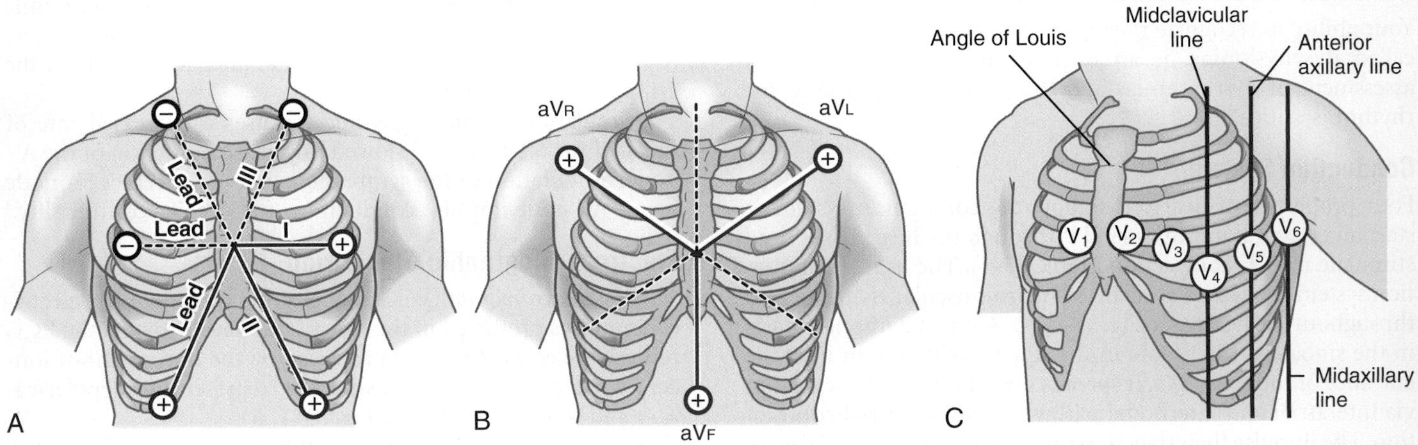


**FIG. 35-2 A,** Limb leads I, II, and III. These bipolar leads are located on the extremities. Illustrated are the angles from which these leads view the heart. **B,** Limb leads aVR, aVL, and aVF. These unipolar leads use the center of the heart as their negative electrode. **C,** Placement for the unipolar chest leads: *$V_1$,* fourth intercostal space at the right sternal border; *$V_2$,* fourth intercostal space at the left sternal border; *$V_3$,* halfway between $V_2$ and $V_4$; *$V_4$,* fifth intercostal space at the left midclavicular line; *$V_5$,* fifth intercostal space at the left anterior axillary line; *$V_6$,* fifth intercostal space at the left midaxillary line.

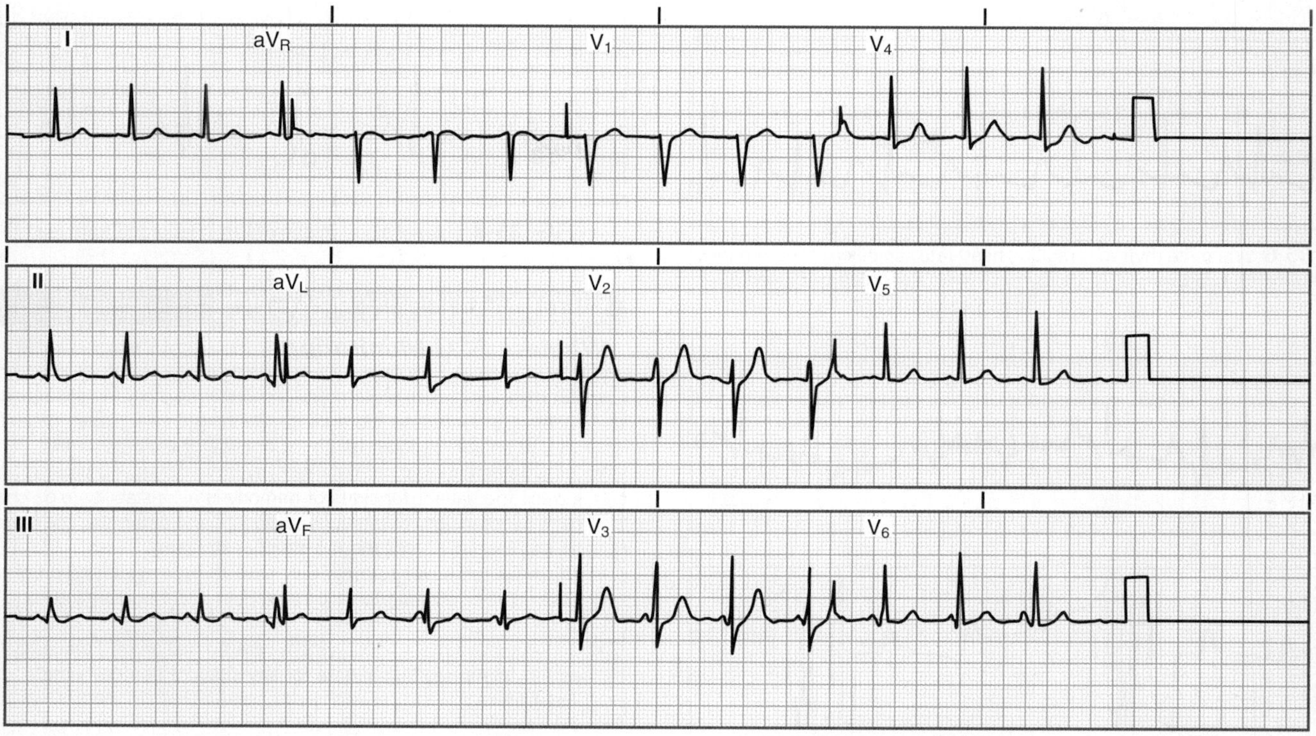


**FIG. 35-3** Twelve-lead electrocardiogram showing a normal sinus rhythm.

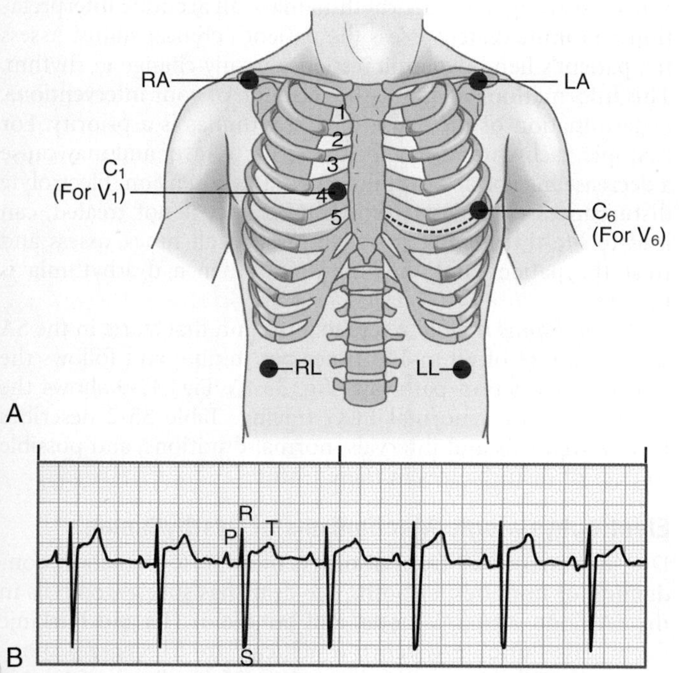


**FIG. 35-4 A,** Lead placement for $V_1$ or $V_6$ using a five-lead system. **B,** Typical ECG tracing in lead $V_1$. *C,* Chest; *LA,* left arm; *LL,* left leg; *RA,* right arm; *RL,* right leg.

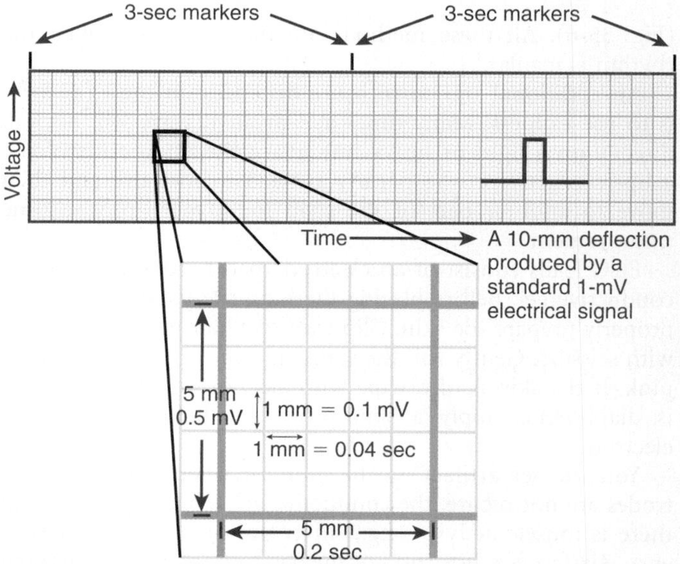


**FIG. 35-5** Time and voltage on the electrocardiogram; 6-sec strip. (Modified from Wesley K: *Basic dysrhythmias and acute coronary syndromes,* ed 4, St Louis, 2011, Mosby JEMS.)

(1 mm) represents 0.1 millivolt (mV). This means that one large square equals 0.5 mV. Use these squares to calculate the heart rate (HR) and measure time intervals for the different ECG complexes.

You can use a variety of methods to calculate the HR from an ECG. The most accurate way is to count the number of QRS complexes in 1 minute. However, because this method is time consuming, a simpler process is used. Note that every 3 seconds a marker appears on the ECG paper (Fig. 35-5). Count the number of R-R intervals in 6 seconds and multiply that number by 10. (An R wave is the first upward [or positive] wave of the QRS complex.) This is the estimated number of beats per minute (Fig. 35-6).

Another method is to count the number of small squares between one R-R interval. Divide this number into 1500 to get the HR. Last, you can count the number of large squares between one R-R interval and divide this number into 300 to get the HR

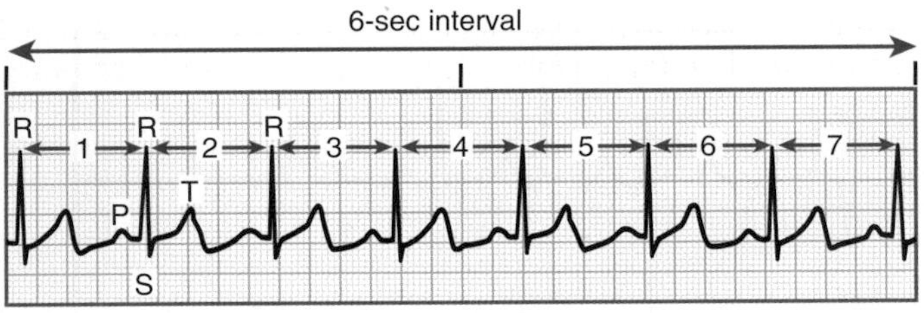


**FIG. 35-6** When the rhythm is regular, heart rate can be easily determined. The estimated heart rate is 70 beats/min. NOTE: Recorded from lead II.

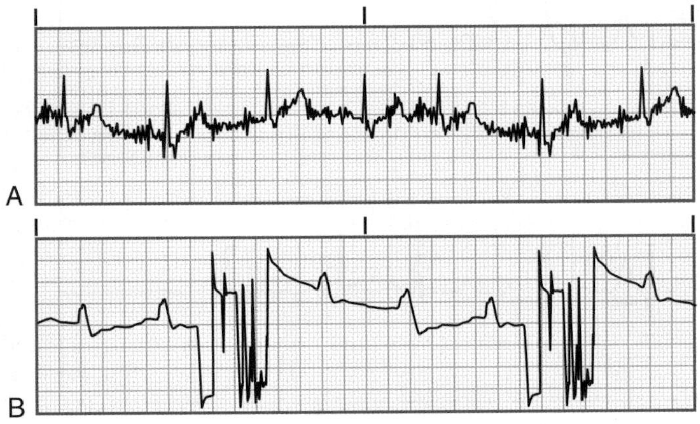


**FIG. 35-7** Artifact. **A,** Muscle tremor. **B,** Loose electrodes.

(Fig. 35-6). All these methods are most accurate when the rhythm is regular.[1]

An additional way to measure distances on the ECG strip is to use calipers. Many times a P or an R wave will not fall directly on a light or heavy line. Place the fine points of the calipers exactly on the parts you need to measure and then move to another part of the strip for a more precise time measurement.

ECG leads consist of an electrode pad fixed with electrical conductive gel. Before placing these on the patient, you must properly prepare the skin. Clip excessive hair on the chest wall with scissors. Gently rub the skin with dry gauze until slightly pink. If the skin is oily, wipe with alcohol first. If the patient is diaphoretic, apply a skin protectant before placing the electrode.

You will see artifact on the monitor when leads and electrodes are not secure, the conductive gel is becoming dry, and there is muscle activity (e.g., shivering) or electrical interference. *Artifact* is a distortion of the baseline and waveforms seen on the ECG (Fig. 35-7). Accurate interpretation of heart rhythm is difficult when artifact is present. If artifact occurs, check the connections in the equipment. Replace the electrodes if the conductive gel has dried out.

**Telemetry Monitoring.** Telemetry monitoring is the observation of a patient's HR and rhythm at a site distant from the patient. The use of this technology can help rapidly identify dysrhythmias, ischemia, or infarction. Two types of systems are used for telemetry monitoring. The first type, a centralized monitoring system, requires you or a telemetry technician to continuously observe a group of patients' ECGs at a central location. The second system of telemetry monitoring does not require constant surveillance. These systems have the capability of detecting and storing data. Advanced alarm systems provide different levels of detection of dysrhythmias, ischemia, or infarction.

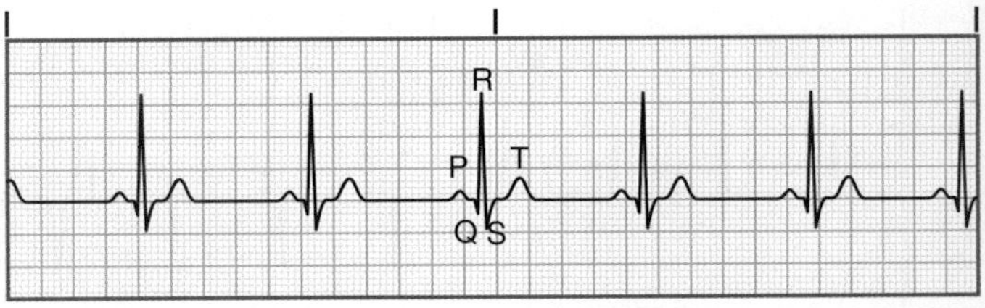


**FIG. 35-8** Normal sinus rhythm. NOTE: Recorded from lead II.

## INFORMATICS IN PRACTICE

### *Wireless ECG Monitoring*

- Wireless electrocardiogram (ECG) monitoring systems continuously monitor and interpret the findings, sending an alert when patient rhythm and/or measurements fall outside of set parameters.
- Early detection of abnormal heart rhythms allows you time to assess the patient for signs of hemodynamic instability (e.g., chest pain, hypotension, palpitations, dyspnea) and determine the need to intervene (e.g., call the rapid response team).
- These systems can automatically save the pre-event portion of the ECG while continuing to record the post-event portion and send all of the information to the HCP.
- Computerized monitoring systems are not fail-proof. Frequently assess all monitored patients for any signs of hemodynamic instability.

## Assessment of Heart Rhythm

When assessing the heart rhythm, make an accurate interpretation and immediately assess the patient's clinical status. Assess the patient's hemodynamic response to any change in rhythm. This information will guide the selection of your interventions. Determination of the cause of dysrhythmias is a priority. For example, tachycardias may be the result of fever and may cause a decrease in cardiac output (CO) and hypotension. Electrolyte disturbances can cause dysrhythmias and, if not treated, can lead to life-threatening dysrhythmias. At all times, assess and treat the patient, not the "monitor" when a dysrhythmia is noted.

*Normal sinus rhythm* refers to a rhythm that starts in the SA node at a rate of 60 to 100 times per minute and follows the normal conduction pathway (Fig. 35-8). Fig. 35-9 shows the components of a normal ECG tracing. Table 35-2 describes ECG waveforms and intervals, normal durations, and possible sources of disturbances in these features.

## Electrophysiologic Mechanisms of Dysrhythmias

Dysrhythmias result from disorders of impulse formation, conduction of impulses, or both. The heart has specialized cells in the SA node, atria, AV node, and bundle of His and Purkinje fibers (His-Purkinje system), which can fire (discharge) spontaneously. This is termed *automaticity.* Normally, the SA node is the pacemaker of the heart. It spontaneously fires 60 to 100 times per minute (Table 35-3). A secondary pacemaker from another site may fire in two ways. If the SA node fires more slowly than a secondary pacemaker, the electrical signals from the secondary pacemaker may "escape." The secondary pacemaker will then fire automatically at its intrinsic rate. These secondary pacemakers may start from the AV node at a rate of 40 to 60 times per minute or the His-Purkinje system at a rate of 20 to 40 times per minute.

Another way that secondary pacemakers can start is when they fire more rapidly than the normal pacemaker of the SA node. *Triggered beats* (early or late) may come from an *ectopic focus* or *accessory pathway* (area outside the normal conduction pathway) in the atria, AV node, or ventricles. This results in a dysrhythmia, which replaces the normal sinus rhythm.

The impulse started by the SA node or an ectopic focus must be conducted to the entire heart. The property of myocardial tissue that allows it to be depolarized by a stimulus is called *excitability.* This is an important part of the transmission of the impulse from one cell to another. The level of excitability is determined by the length of time after depolarization that the tissues can be restimulated. The recovery period after stimulation is the *refractory phase* or period. The *absolute refractory phase* or period occurs when excitability is zero and the heart cannot be stimulated. The *relative refractory period* occurs slightly later in the cycle, and excitability is more likely. In states of *full excitability,* the heart is completely recovered. Fig. 35-10 shows the relationship between the refractory period and ECG.

If conduction is depressed and some areas of the heart are blocked (e.g., by infarction), the unblocked areas are activated earlier than the blocked areas. When the block is unidirectional, this uneven conduction may allow the initial impulse to reenter areas that were previously not excitable but have recovered. The reentering impulse may be able to depolarize the atria and ventricles, causing a premature beat. If the reentrant excitation continues, tachycardia occurs.

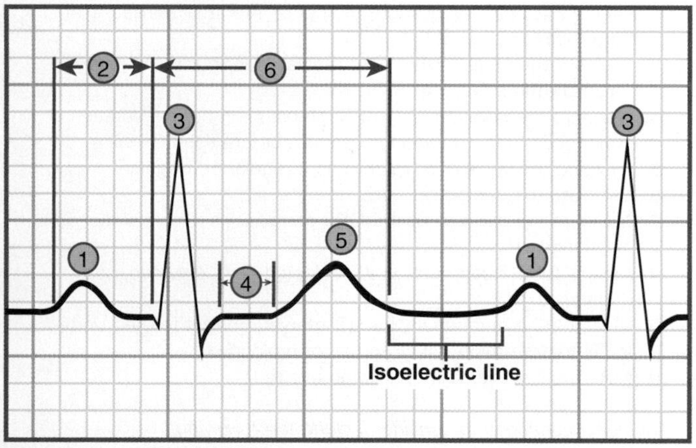


**FIG. 35-9** The ECG tracing as seen in normal sinus rhythm. *1,* P wave; *2,* PR interval; *3,* QRS complex: Q wave, R wave, S wave; *4,* ST segment; *5,* T wave; *6,* QT interval. Isoelectric (flat) line or baseline represents the absence of electrical activity in the heart cells. (Table 35-2 for timing of intervals.)

## Evaluation of Dysrhythmias

Dysrhythmias occur as the result of various abnormalities and disease states. The cause of a dysrhythmia influences the patient's treatment. Table 35-4 presents common causes of

**TABLE 35-2 ECG Waveforms and Intervals***

| Description | Normal Duration (sec) | Source of Possible Variation |
|---|---|---|
| **P Wave** | | |
| Represents time for the passage of the electrical impulse through the atrium causing atrial depolarization (contraction). Should be upright | 0.06-0.12 | Disturbance in conduction within atria |
| **PR Interval** | | |
| Measured from beginning of P wave to beginning of QRS complex. Represents time taken for impulse to spread through the atria, AV node and bundle of His, bundle branches, and Purkinje fibers, to a point immediately before ventricular contraction | 0.12-0.20 | Disturbance in conduction usually in AV node, bundle of His, or bundle branches but can be in atria as well |
| **QRS Complex** | | |
| ***Q wave:*** First negative (downward) deflection after the P wave, short and narrow, not present in several leads | <0.03 | MI may result in development of a pathologic Q wave that is wide (≥0.03 sec) and deep (≥25% of the height of the R wave) |
| ***R wave:*** First positive (upward) deflection in the QRS complex | Not usually measured | |
| ***S wave:*** First negative (downward) deflection after the R wave | Not usually measured | |
| **QRS Interval** | | |
| Measured from beginning to end of QRS complex. Represents time taken for depolarization (contraction) of both ventricles (systole) | <0.12 | Disturbance in conduction in bundle branches or in ventricles |
| **ST Segment** | | |
| Measured from the S wave of the QRS complex to the beginning of the T wave. Represents the time between ventricular depolarization and repolarization (diastole). Should be isoelectric (flat) | 0.12 | Disturbances (e.g., elevation, depression) usually caused by ischemia, injury, or infarction |
| **T Wave** | | |
| Represents time for ventricular repolarization. Should be upright | 0.16 | Disturbances (e.g., tall, peaked; inverted) usually caused by electrolyte imbalances, ischemia, or infarction |
| **QT Interval†** | | |
| Measured from beginning of QRS complex to end of T wave. Represents time taken for entire electrical depolarization and repolarization of the ventricles. Normal adult women have slightly longer QT intervals than men. | 0.34-0.43 | Disturbances usually affecting repolarization more than depolarization and caused by drugs, electrolyte imbalances, and changes in heart rate |

*AV,* Atrioventricular.
*Heart rate influences the duration of these intervals, especially the PR and QT intervals (e.g., QT interval shortens in duration as heart rate increases).
†A corrected QT interval (QTc) is calculated to account for the influence of heart rate.

**TABLE 35-3 Intrinsic Rates of the Conduction System**

| Part of Conduction System | Rate |
|---|---|
| **SA node and atria** | 60-100 times/min |
| **AV node and bundle of His** | 40-60 times/min |
| **Bundle branches and Purkinje fibers** | 20-40 times/min |

*AV,* Atrioventricular; *SA,* sinoatrial.

**TABLE 35-4 Common Causes of Dysrhythmias***

**Heart Conditions**
- Accessory pathways
- Cardiomyopathy
- Conduction defects
- Heart failure
- Myocardial ischemia, infarction
- Valve disease

**Other Conditions**
- Acid-base imbalances
- Alcohol
- Caffeine, tobacco
- Connective tissue disorders
- Drug effects (e.g., antidysrhythmia drugs, stimulants, β-blockers) or toxicity
- Electric shock
- Electrolyte imbalances (e.g., hyperkalemia, hypocalcemia)
- Emotional crisis
- Herbal supplements (e.g., areca nut, wahoo root bark, yerba maté)
- Hypoxia
- Metabolic conditions (e.g., thyroid dysfunction)
- Drowning
- Sepsis, shock
- Toxins

*List is not all-inclusive.

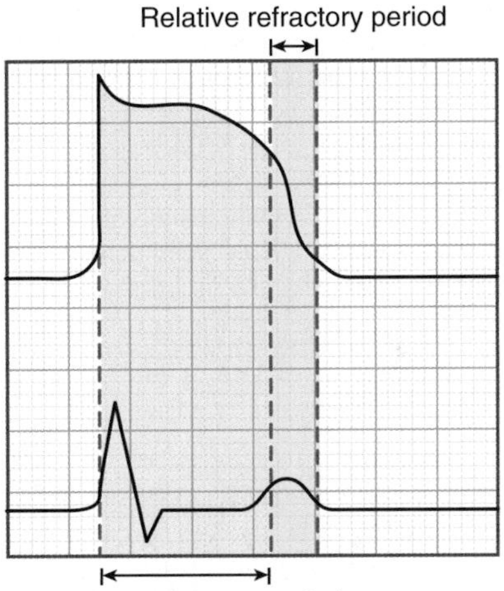


**FIG. 35-10** Absolute and relative refractory periods correlated with the heart muscle's action potential and with an ECG tracing. (Modified from Urden LD, Stacy KM, Lough ME: *Critical care nursing: diagnosis and management,* ed 6, St Louis, 2010, Mosby.)

dysrhythmias. Table 35-5 presents a systematic approach to assessing a heart rhythm.

Dysrhythmias occurring in nonmonitored settings present management challenges. If the patient becomes symptomatic (e.g., chest pain, syncope), determination of the rhythm by heart monitoring is a high priority. Activate the emergency

**TABLE 35-5 Approach to Assessing Heart Rhythm**

*When assessing a heart rhythm, use a consistent and systematic approach. One such approach includes the following:*
1. Look for the P wave. Is it upright or inverted? Is there one for every QRS complex or more than one? Are atrial fibrillatory or flutter waves present?
2. Evaluate the atrial rhythm. Is it regular or irregular?
3. Calculate the atrial rate.
4. Measure the duration of the PR interval. Is it normal duration or prolonged? Is the duration consistent before each QRS?
5. Evaluate the ventricular rhythm. Is it regular or irregular?
6. Calculate the ventricular rate.
7. Measure the duration of the QRS complex. Is it normal duration or prolonged?
8. Assess the ST segment. Is it isoelectric (flat), elevated, or depressed?
9. Measure the duration of the QT interval. Correct for heart rate (cQT) to determine if it is normal or prolonged.*
10. Note the T wave. Is it upright or inverted?

*Additional questions to consider include the following:*
1. What is the dominant or underlying rhythm and/or dysrhythmia?
2. What is the clinical significance of your findings?
3. What is the treatment for the particular rhythm?

*A website for calculating the cQT interval for heart rate can be found at *www.mdcalc.com/corrected-qt-interval-qtc.*

response system (ERS). Table 35-6 outlines the emergency care of the patient with a dysrhythmia.

In addition to continuous ECG monitoring during hospitalization, several other tests can assess dysrhythmias and the effectiveness of antidysrhythmia drug therapy. An electrophysiologic study, Holter monitoring, event monitoring (or loop recorder), exercise treadmill testing, and signal-averaged ECG can be performed on an inpatient or outpatient basis (see Table 31-6 for nursing care related to these tests).

An *electrophysiologic study* (EPS) can identify the causes of heart blocks, tachydysrhythmias (dysrhythmias with rates greater than 100 beats/minute), bradydysrhythmias (dysrhythmias with rates less than 60 beats/minute), and syncope. An EPS study can also locate accessory pathways and determine the effectiveness of antidysrhythmia drugs.

The Holter monitor continuously records the ECG while the patient is ambulatory and performing daily activities. The patient keeps a diary and records activities and any symptoms. Events in the diary are correlated with any dysrhythmias seen on the ECG. Use of event monitors has improved the evaluation of dysrhythmias in outpatients. Event monitors are recorders that the patient activates only when he or she experiences symptoms. New technology using smart phone apps can obtain and save ECG recordings and even detect some dysrhythmias (e.g., AliveECG at *https://itunes.apple.com/us/app/aliveecg/id579769143?mt=8*).

Exercise treadmill testing evaluates the patient's heart rhythm during exercise. If exercise-induced dysrhythmias or ECG changes occur, they are reviewed. If needed, drug therapy can be started and evaluated.

The signal-averaged ECG identifies *late potentials,* strongly suggesting that the patient may be at risk for developing serious ventricular dysrhythmias. (See Chapter 31 for a discussion of diagnostic procedures for assessment of the cardiovascular system and related nursing care.)

## TABLE 35-6 Emergency Management

### *Dysrhythmias*

| Etiology | Assessment Findings | Interventions |
|---|---|---|
| Table 35-4 | • Irregular rate and rhythm; tachycardia, bradycardia<br>• Decreased or increased BP<br>• Decreased $O_2$ saturation<br>• Chest, neck, shoulder, back, jaw, or arm pain<br>• Dizziness, syncope<br>• Dyspnea<br>• Extreme restlessness, anxiety<br>• Decreased level of consciousness, confusion<br>• Feeling of impending doom<br>• Numbness, tingling of arms<br>• Weakness and fatigue<br>• Cold, clammy skin<br>• Diminished peripheral pulses<br>• Diaphoresis<br>• Pallor<br>• Palpitations<br>• Nausea and vomiting | **Initial**<br>• If unresponsive, assess circulation, airway, and breathing (CAB).<br>• If responsive, monitor airway, breathing, and circulation (ABC).<br>• Apply $O_2$ via nasal cannula or non-rebreather mask.<br>• Obtain baseline vital signs, including $O_2$ saturation.<br>• Obtain 12-lead ECG.<br>• Begin continuous ECG monitoring.<br>• Identify underlying rate and rhythm.<br>• Identify dysrhythmia.<br>• Establish IV access.<br>• Obtain baseline laboratory studies (e.g., CBC, electrolytes).<br>**Ongoing Monitoring**<br>• Monitor ABCs, vital signs, level of consciousness, $O_2$ saturation, and heart rhythm.<br>• Anticipate need for antidysrhythmia drugs and analgesics.<br>• Anticipate need for intubation if respiratory distress is evident.<br>• Anticipate need to begin advanced cardiovascular life support (e.g., CPR, defibrillation, transcutaneous pacing). |

## Types of Dysrhythmias

Figs. 35-11 to 35-19 provide examples of the ECG tracings of common dysrhythmias. Table 35-7 presents the descriptive characteristics.

**Sinus Bradycardia.** In *sinus bradycardia* the conduction pathway is the same as that in sinus rhythm, but the SA node fires at a rate less than 60 beats/minute (Fig. 35-11, *A*). *Symptomatic bradycardia* refers to an HR that is less than 60 beats/minute and is inadequate for the patient's condition. This causes the patient to experience symptoms (e.g., fatigue, dizziness, chest pain, syncope).

***Clinical Associations.*** Sinus bradycardia may be a normal sinus rhythm in aerobically trained athletes and in some people during sleep. It also occurs in response to carotid sinus massage, Valsalva maneuver, hypothermia, increased intraocular pressure, vagal stimulation, and certain drugs (e.g., β-blockers, calcium channel blockers). Common disease states associated with sinus bradycardia are hypothyroidism, increased intracranial pressure, and inferior myocardial infarction (MI).

***ECG Characteristics.*** In sinus bradycardia, the HR is less than 60 beats/minute and rhythm is regular. The P wave precedes each QRS complex and has a normal shape and duration. The PR interval is normal and the QRS complex has a normal shape and duration.

***Clinical Significance.*** The clinical significance of sinus bradycardia depends on how the patient tolerates it. Manifestations of symptomatic bradycardia include pale, cool skin; hypotension; weakness; angina; dizziness or syncope; confusion or disorientation; and shortness of breath.

***Treatment.*** For the patient with symptoms, treatment consists of giving IV atropine (anticholinergic drug). If atropine is ineffective, transcutaneous pacing or a dopamine or epinephrine (Adrenalin) infusion is considered. Permanent pacemaker therapy may be needed. If bradycardia is due to drugs, these may have to be held, discontinued, or reduced.

**Sinus Tachycardia.** The conduction pathway is the same in *sinus tachycardia* as that in normal sinus rhythm. The discharge rate from the sinus node increases because of vagal inhibition or sympathetic stimulation. The sinus rate is 101 to 200 beats/minute (Fig. 35-11, *B*).

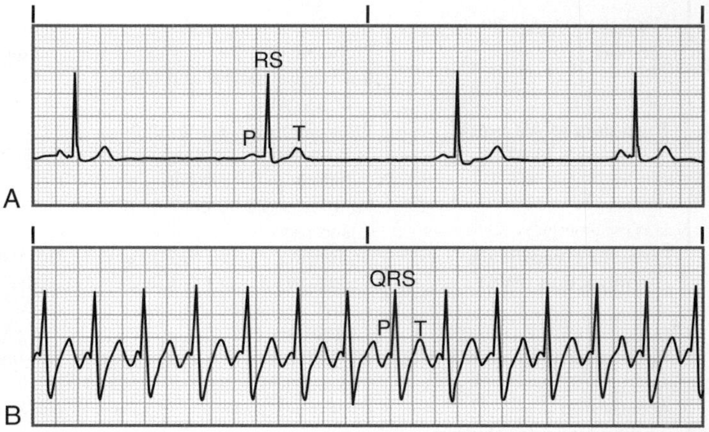


**FIG. 35-11** **A,** Sinus bradycardia. **B,** Sinus tachycardia.

***Clinical Associations.*** Sinus tachycardia is associated with physiologic and psychologic stressors such as exercise, fever, pain, hypotension, hypovolemia, anemia, hypoxia, hypoglycemia, myocardial ischemia, heart failure (HF), hyperthyroidism, anxiety, and fear. It can also be an effect of drugs such as epinephrine, norepinephrine (Levophed), atropine, caffeine, theophylline, or hydralazine. In addition, many over-the-counter cold remedies have active ingredients (e.g., pseudoephedrine [Sudafed]) that can cause tachycardia.

***ECG Characteristics.*** In sinus tachycardia, the HR is 101 to 200 beats/minute and rhythm is regular. The P wave is normal, precedes each QRS complex, and has a normal shape and duration. The PR interval is normal and the QRS complex has a normal shape and duration.

***Clinical Significance.*** The clinical significance of sinus tachycardia depends on the patient's tolerance of the increased HR. The patient may have dizziness, dyspnea, and hypotension because of decreased CO. Increased myocardial $O_2$ consumption is associated with an increased HR. Angina or an increase

**TABLE 35-7 Characteristics of Common Dysrhythmias**

| Pattern | Rate and Rhythm | P Wave | PR Interval | QRS Complex |
|---|---|---|---|---|
| **Normal sinus rhythm (NSR)** | 60-100 beats/min and regular | Normal | Normal | Normal |
| **Sinus bradycardia** | <60 beats/min and regular | Normal | Normal | Normal |
| **Sinus tachycardia** | 101-200 beats/min and regular | Normal | Normal | Normal |
| **Premature atrial contraction (PAC)** | Usually 60-100 beats/min and irregular | Abnormal shape | Normal | Normal (usually) |
| **Paroxysmal supraventricular tachycardia (PSVT)** | 150-220 beats/min and regular | Abnormal shape, may be hidden in the preceding T wave | Normal or shortened | Normal (usually) |
| **Atrial flutter** | *Atrial:* 200-350 beats/min and regular<br>*Ventricular:* > or <100 beats/min and may be regular or irregular | Flutter (F) waves (sawtoothed pattern); more flutter waves than QRS complexes; may occur in a 2:1, 3:1, 4:1, etc., pattern | Not measurable | Normal (usually) |
| **Atrial fibrillation** | *Atrial:* 350-600 beats/min and irregular<br>*Ventricular:* > or <100 beats/min and irregular | Fibrillatory (f) waves | Not measurable | Normal (usually) |
| **Junctional dysrhythmias** | 40-180 beats/min and regular | Inverted, may be hidden in QRS complex | Shortened, if present | Normal (usually) |
| **First-degree AV block** | Normal and regular | Normal | >0.20 sec | Normal |
| **Second-degree AV block** | | | | |
| • **Type I** (Mobitz I, Wenckebach heart block) | *Atrial:* Normal and regular<br>*Ventricular:* Slower and irregular | Normal | Progressive lengthening | Normal QRS width, with pattern of one nonconducted (blocked) QRS complex |
| • **Type II** (Mobitz II heart block) | *Atrial:* Usually normal and regular<br>*Ventricular:* Slower and regular or irregular | More P waves than QRS complexes (e.g., 2:1, 3:1) | Normal or prolonged but consistent for every QRS | Widened QRS, preceded by ≥2 P waves, with nonconducted (blocked) QRS complex |
| **Third-degree AV block** (complete heart block) | *Atrial:* Regular but may appear irregular due to P waves hidden in QRS complexes<br>*Ventricular:* 20-60 beats/min and regular | Normal, but no connection with QRS complex | Inconsistent | Normal or widened, no relationship with P waves |
| **Premature ventricular contraction (PVC)** | Underlying rhythm can be any rate, regular or irregular rhythm, PVCs occur at variable rates | Not usually visible, hidden in the PVC | Not measurable | Wide and distorted |
| **Ventricular tachycardia (VT)** | 150-250 beats/min and regular or irregular | Not usually visible | Not measurable | Wide and distorted |
| **Accelerated idioventricular rhythm** | 40-100 beats/min and regular | Not usually visible | Not measurable | Wide and distorted |
| **Ventricular fibrillation (VF)** | Not measurable and irregular | Absent | Not measurable | Not measurable |

*AV,* Atrioventricular.

in infarction size may accompany sinus tachycardia in patients with coronary artery disease (CAD) or an acute MI.

***Treatment.*** The underlying cause of tachycardia guides the treatment. For example, if the patient is experiencing tachycardia from pain, effective pain management is important to treat the tachycardia. In clinically stable patients, vagal maneuvers can be attempted. In addition, IV β-blockers (e.g., metoprolol [Lopressor]), adenosine (Adenocard), or calcium channel blockers (e.g., diltiazem [Cardizem]) can be given to reduce HR and decrease myocardial $O_2$ consumption. In clinically unstable patients, synchronized cardioversion is used. (Cardioversion is discussed on p. 772.)

**Premature Atrial Contraction.** A premature atrial contraction (PAC) is a contraction starting from an ectopic focus in the atrium (i.e., a location other than the SA node) and coming sooner than the next expected sinus beat. The ectopic signal starts in the left or right atrium and travels across the atria by an abnormal pathway. This creates a distorted P wave (Fig. 35-12). At the AV node, it may be stopped (nonconducted PAC), delayed (lengthened PR interval), or conducted normally. If the signal moves through the AV node, in most cases it is conducted normally through the ventricles.

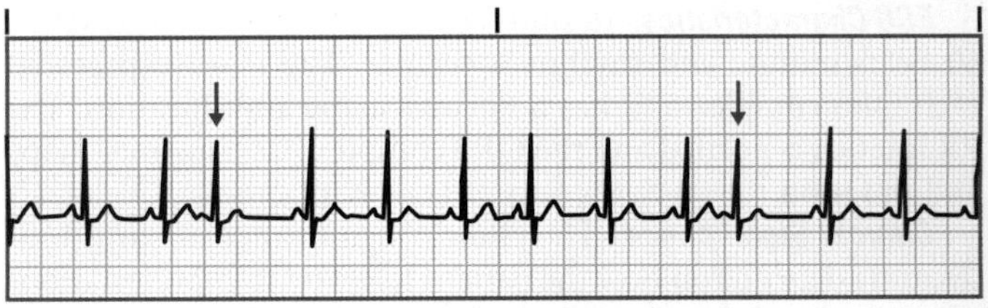

**FIG. 35-12** Premature atrial contractions *(arrows)*.

***Clinical Associations.*** In a normal heart, a PAC can result from emotional stress or physical fatigue or from the use of caffeine, tobacco, or alcohol. A PAC can also result from hypoxia; electrolyte imbalances; and disease states such as hyperthyroidism, chronic obstructive pulmonary disease (COPD), and heart disease, including CAD and valvular disease.

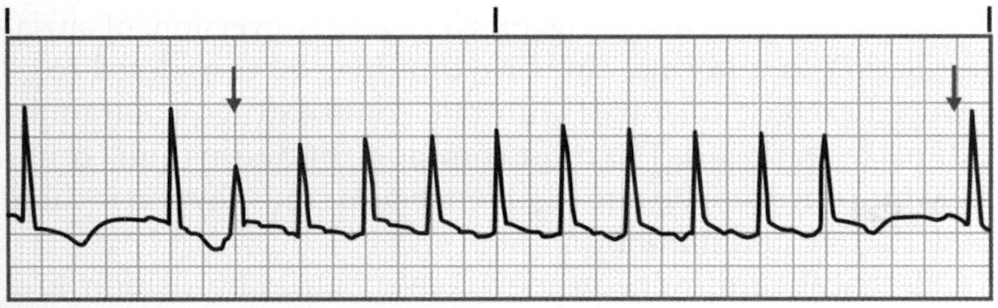

**FIG. 35-13** Paroxysmal supraventricular tachycardia (PSVT). *Arrows* indicate beginning and ending of PSVT.

***ECG Characteristics.*** HR varies with the underlying rate and frequency of the PAC. The rhythm is irregular. The P wave has a different shape from that of a P wave originating in the SA node, or it may be hidden in the preceding T wave. The PR interval may be shorter or longer than the PR interval coming from the SA node, but it is within normal limits. The QRS complex is usually normal. If the QRS interval is 0.12 second or more, abnormal conduction through the ventricles occurs.

***Clinical Significance.*** In persons with healthy hearts, isolated PACs are not significant. Patients may report palpitations or a sense that their hearts "skipped a beat." In persons with heart disease, frequent PACs may indicate enhanced automaticity of the atria or a reentry mechanism. Such PACs may warn of or start more serious dysrhythmias (e.g., supraventricular tachycardia).

***Treatment.*** Treatment depends on the patient's symptoms. Withdrawal of sources of stimulation such as caffeine or sympathomimetic drugs may be needed. β-Blockers may be used to decrease PACs.

**Paroxysmal Supraventricular Tachycardia.** *Paroxysmal supraventricular tachycardia* (PSVT) is a dysrhythmia starting in an ectopic focus anywhere above the bifurcation of the bundle of His (Fig. 35-13). Identification of the ectopic focus is often difficult even with a 12-lead ECG, since it requires recording the dysrhythmia as it starts.

PSVT occurs because of a reentrant phenomenon (reexcitation of the atria when there is a one-way block). Usually a PAC triggers a run of repeated premature beats. *Paroxysmal* refers to an abrupt onset and ending. Termination is sometimes followed by a brief period of **asystole** (absence of all cardiac electrical activity). Some degree of AV block may be present. PSVT can occur in the presence of Wolff-Parkinson-White (WPW) syndrome or "preexcitation." In this syndrome, there is extra conduction or accessory pathways.

***Clinical Associations.*** In the normal heart, PSVT is associated with overexertion, emotional stress, deep inspiration, and stimulants such as caffeine and tobacco. PSVT is also associated with rheumatic heart disease, digitalis toxicity, CAD, and cor pulmonale.

***ECG Characteristics.*** In PSVT, the HR is 150 to 220 beats/minute and rhythm is regular or slightly irregular. The P wave is often hidden in the preceding T wave. If seen, it may have an abnormal shape. The PR interval may be shortened or normal and the QRS complex is usually normal.

***Clinical Significance.*** The clinical significance of PSVT depends on the associated symptoms. A prolonged episode and HR greater than 180 beats/minute will cause decreased CO because of reduced stroke volume. Manifestations include hypotension, palpitations, dyspnea, and angina.

***Treatment.*** Treatment for PSVT includes vagal stimulation and drug therapy. Common vagal maneuvers include Valsalva, carotid massage, and coughing. IV adenosine is the drug of

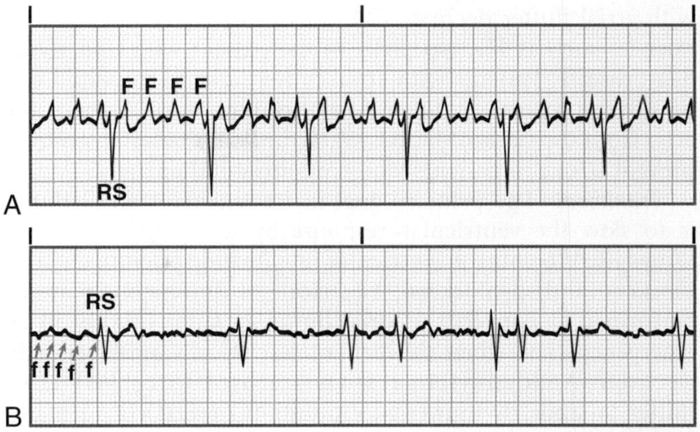


**FIG. 35-14** **A,** Atrial flutter with a 4 : 1 conduction (four flutter *[F]* waves to each QRS complex). **B,** Atrial fibrillation with a controlled ventricular response. Note the chaotic fibrillatory *(f)* waves *(arrows)* between the RS complexes. NOTE: Recorded from lead $V_1$.

choice to convert PSVT to a normal sinus rhythm. This drug has a short half-life (10 seconds) and is well tolerated.[5] IV β-blockers and calcium channel blockers (diltiazem and verapamil [Calan]) can also be used. If vagal stimulation and drug therapy are ineffective and the patient becomes hemodynamically unstable, synchronized cardioversion is used.[6] (Cardioversion is discussed on p. 772.)

**DRUG ALERT Adenosine (Adenocard)**

- Injection site should be as close to the heart as possible (e.g., antecubital area).
- Give IV dose rapidly (over 1 to 2 sec) and follow with a rapid 20 mL normal saline flush.
- Monitor patient's ECG continuously. Brief period of asystole is common.
- Observe patient for flushing, dizziness, chest pain, or palpitations.

Ongoing treatment of recurring PSVT and PSVT in patients with WPW syndrome includes radiofrequency catheter ablation of the accessory pathway.[6] (Catheter ablation therapy is discussed on p. 775.)

**Atrial Flutter.** **Atrial flutter** is an atrial tachydysrhythmia identified by recurring, regular, sawtooth-shaped flutter waves that originate from a single ectopic focus in the right atrium or, less commonly, the left atrium (Fig. 35-14, *A*).

***Clinical Associations.*** Atrial flutter rarely occurs in a healthy heart. It is associated with CAD, hypertension, mitral valve disorders, pulmonary embolus, chronic lung disease, cor pulmonale, cardiomyopathy, hyperthyroidism, and the use of drugs such as digoxin, quinidine, and epinephrine.

***ECG Characteristics.*** Atrial rate is 200 to 350 beats/minute. The ventricular rate varies based on the conduction ratio. In 2 : 1 conduction, the ventricular rate is typically found to be approximately 150 beats/minute. Atrial rhythm is regular and ventricular rhythm is usually regular. The atrial flutter waves represent atrial depolarization followed by repolarization. The PR interval is variable and not measurable. The QRS complex is usually normal. Because the AV node can delay signals from the atria, there is usually some AV block in a fixed ratio of flutter waves to QRS complexes.

***Clinical Significance.*** The high ventricular rates (greater than 100 beats/minute) and loss of the atrial "kick" (atrial contraction reflected by a sinus P wave) that are associated with atrial flutter decrease CO. This can cause serious consequences such as HF, especially in the patient with underlying heart disease. Patients with atrial flutter have an increased risk of stroke because of the risk of thrombus formation in the atria from the stasis of blood. Warfarin (Coumadin) is given to prevent stroke in patients who have atrial flutter.[6]

***Treatment.*** The primary goal in treatment of atrial flutter is to slow the ventricular response by increasing AV block. Drugs used to control ventricular rate include calcium channel blockers and β-blockers. Electrical cardioversion may be performed to convert the atrial flutter to sinus rhythm in an emergency (i.e., when the patient is clinically unstable) and electively. Antidysrhythmia drugs are used to convert atrial flutter to sinus rhythm (e.g., ibutilide [Corvert]) or to maintain sinus rhythm (e.g., amiodarone, flecainide, dronedarone [Multaq]).[5]

Radiofrequency catheter ablation is the treatment of choice for atrial flutter.[7] The procedure is done in an EPS laboratory and involves placing a catheter in the right atrium. With the use of a low-voltage, high-frequency form of electrical energy, the ectopic foci are ablated (or destroyed), dysrhythmia is ended, and normal sinus rhythm is restored. (Catheter ablation is discussed on p. 775.)

**Atrial Fibrillation.** Atrial fibrillation is characterized by a total disorganization of atrial electrical activity because of multiple ectopic foci, resulting in loss of effective atrial contraction (Fig. 35-14, *B*). The dysrhythmia may be paroxysmal (i.e., beginning and ending spontaneously) or persistent (lasting more than 7 days).[1] Atrial fibrillation is the most common, clinically significant dysrhythmia with respect to morbidity and mortality rates and economic impact. Its prevalence increases with age.[8]

***Clinical Associations.*** Atrial fibrillation usually occurs in a patient with underlying heart disease, such as CAD, valvular heart disease, cardiomyopathy, hypertensive heart disease, HF, and pericarditis. It often develops acutely with thyrotoxicosis, alcohol intoxication, caffeine use, electrolyte disturbances, stress, and heart surgery.

***ECG Characteristics.*** During atrial fibrillation, the atrial rate may be as high as 350 to 600 beats/minute. P waves are replaced by chaotic, fibrillatory waves. Ventricular rate varies and the rhythm is usually irregular. When the ventricular rate is between 60 and 100 beats/minute, it is atrial fibrillation with a *controlled ventricular response.* Atrial fibrillation with a ventricular rate greater than 100 beats/minute is atrial fibrillation with a *rapid (or uncontrolled) ventricular response.* The PR interval is not measurable, and the QRS complex usually has a normal shape and duration. At times, atrial flutter and atrial fibrillation may coexist.[1]

***Clinical Significance.*** Atrial fibrillation results in a decrease in CO because of ineffective atrial contractions (loss of atrial kick) and/or a rapid ventricular response. Thrombi (clots) form in the atria because of blood stasis. An embolized clot may develop and move to the brain, causing a stroke. Atrial fibrillation accounts for as many as 17% of all strokes.[9]

***Treatment.*** The goals of treatment of atrial fibrillation include a decrease in ventricular response (to less than 100 beats/minute), prevention of stroke, and conversion to sinus rhythm, if possible. Ventricular rate control is a priority for patients with atrial fibrillation. Drugs used for rate control include calcium channel blockers (e.g., diltiazem), β-blockers (e.g., metoprolol), dronedarone, and digoxin (Lanoxin).

For some patients, drug or electrical conversion of atrial fibrillation to a normal sinus rhythm may be considered (e.g., reduced exercise tolerance with rate control drugs, contraindications to warfarin). The most common antidysrhythmia drugs used for conversion to and maintenance of sinus rhythm include amiodarone and ibutilide.[8]

Electrical cardioversion may convert atrial fibrillation to a normal sinus rhythm. If a patient is in atrial fibrillation for longer than 48 hours, anticoagulation therapy with warfarin is needed for 3 to 4 weeks before the cardioversion and for several weeks after successful cardioversion.[5] Anticoagulation therapy is necessary because the procedure can cause the clots to dislodge, placing the patient at risk for stroke. A transesophageal echocardiogram may be performed to rule out clots in the atria. If no clots are present, anticoagulation therapy may not be needed before the cardioversion.

If drugs or cardioversion does not convert atrial fibrillation to normal sinus rhythm, long-term anticoagulation therapy is needed (Table 35-8). Warfarin is the drug of choice, and patients are monitored for therapeutic levels (e.g., international normalized ratio [INR]). Alternatives to warfarin are available for anticoagulation therapy in patients with nonvalvular atrial fibrillation. Examples include dabigatran (Pradaxa), apixaban (Eliquis), and rivaroxaban (Xarelto). These drugs do not require routine laboratory testing.[8] (See Chapter 37 for discussion of anticoagulation therapy.)

For patients with drug-refractory atrial fibrillation or who do not respond to electrical conversion and remain symptomatic, radiofrequency catheter ablation (similar to procedure for atrial flutter), AV nodal ablation, and the Maze procedure are further options. AV nodal ablation involves the destruction of the AV node and insertion of a permanent ventricular pacemaker.[8]

The Maze procedure is a surgical intervention that stops atrial fibrillation by interrupting the ectopic foci that are

**TABLE 35-8 Drug Therapy**

***Antithrombotic Therapy for Atrial Fibrillation****

| Risk Category | Recommended Therapy |
|---|---|
| Mechanical heart valve | Warfarin (target INR 2.5-3.5) |
| $CHA_2DS_2$-VASc† score of 0 | No therapy recommended |
| $CHA_2DS_2$-VASc score of 1 | No therapy recommended or an oral anticoagulant or aspirin (e.g., 81-325 mg/day) may be considered |
| $CHA_2DS_2$-VASc score of ≥2 | Warfarin<br>Dabigatran (Pradaxa)‡<br>Apixaban (Eliquis)‡<br>Rivaroxaban (Xarelto)‡ |
| $CHA_2DS_2$-VASc score of ≥2 and end-stage kidney disease or on hemodialysis | Warfarin |

Source: January CT, Wann LS, Albert JS, et al: 2014 AHA/ACC/HRS guideline for the management of patients with atrial fibrillation: executive summary: a report of the American College of Cardiology/American Heart Association Task Force on Practice Guidelines and the Heart Rhythm Society, *J Am Coll Cardiol* 64(21):e1, 2014.
*$CHA_2DS_2$-VASc,* Congestive heart failure; hypertension; age ≥75 [doubled]; diabetes; prior stroke, transient ischemic attack, thromboembolism [doubled]; vascular disease; age 65-74; sex, *INR,* international normalized ratio.
*For atrial flutter, antithrombotic therapy is recommended as for atrial fibrillation.
†The $CHA_2DS_2$-VASc score for nonvalvular atrial fibrillation stroke risk can be calculated at *www.mdcalc.com/cha2ds2-vasc-score-for-atrial-fibrillation-stroke-risk/*
‡Renal function should be assessed prior to starting direct thrombin inhibitor (e.g., dabigatran) or factor Xa inhibitor (e.g., apixaban, rivaroxaban) and regularly thereafter.

responsible for the dysrhythmia. Incisions are made in both atria, and *cryoablation* (cold therapy) is used to stop the formation and conduction of these signals and restore normal sinus rhythm.

**Left atrial appendage occlusion.** The left atrial appendage (LAA) is a pouch that extends off the left atrium. The LAA is known to trigger atrial fibrillation and is a common source of blood clots in patients with atrial fibrillation. LAA occlusion is a treatment strategy to prevent blood clot formation in patients who have atrial fibrillation. By removing or occluding the LAA, the incidence of strokes can be decreased.

A special stapler can be used to remove the LAA or sutures can be used to manually occlude the LAA. In addition, LAA occlusion devices (e.g., AtriClip, Watchman) are available. These devices are positioned around the LAA and then closed, similar to a clamp that is used to shut off the blood supply. This prevents blood from flowing into and out of the LAA. LAA occlusion can be used as an alternative for patients who cannot use oral anticoagulants such as warfarin.[10]

### CHECK YOUR PRACTICE

You are assigned to a 72-yr-old female patient who was admitted with chest pain. She has continuous EGG monitoring. You notice that her ECG tracing is difficult to interpret. Your preceptor tells you that there is a lot of artifact.

- How would you proceed to improve her tracing?

**Junctional Dysrhythmias.** *Junctional dysrhythmias* refer to dysrhythmias that start in the area of the AV node to the bundle of His known as the AV junction. They result because the SA node fails to fire or the signal is blocked. When this occurs, the AV node becomes the pacemaker of the heart. The impulse from the AV node usually moves in a retrograde (backward) fashion. This produces an abnormal P wave that occurs just before or after the QRS complex or that is hidden in the QRS complex. The impulse usually moves normally through the ventricles. Junctional premature beats may occur, and they are treated in a manner similar to that for PACs. Other junctional dysrhythmias include junctional escape rhythm (Fig. 35-15), accelerated junctional rhythm, and junctional tachycardia. These dysrhythmias are treated according to the patient's tolerance of the rhythm and the patient's clinical condition.

***Clinical Associations.*** Junctional dysrhythmias are often associated with CAD, HF, cardiomyopathy, electrolyte imbalances, inferior MI, and rheumatic heart disease. Certain drugs (e.g., digoxin, nicotine, amphetamines, caffeine) can also cause junctional dysrhythmias.

***ECG Characteristics.*** In junctional escape rhythm, the HR is 40 to 60 beats/minute. It is 61 to 100 beats/minute in accelerated junctional rhythm and 101 to 180 beats/minute in junctional tachycardia. Rhythm is regular. The P wave is abnormal in shape and inverted, or it may be hidden in the QRS complex (Fig. 35-15). The PR interval is less than 0.12 second when the P wave precedes the QRS complex. The QRS complex is usually normal.

***Clinical Significance.*** Junctional escape rhythms serve as a safety mechanism when the SA node has not been effective. Escape rhythms such as this should not be suppressed. Accelerated junctional rhythm is due to sympathetic stimulation to improve CO. Junctional tachycardia indicates a more serious problem. This rhythm may reduce CO, causing the patient to become hemodynamically unstable (e.g., hypotensive).

***Treatment.*** Treatment varies according to the type of junctional dysrhythmia. If a patient has symptoms with a junctional escape rhythm, atropine can be used. In accelerated junctional rhythm and junctional tachycardia caused by drug toxicity, the drug is stopped. In the absence of digitalis toxicity, β-blockers, calcium channel blockers, and amiodarone are used for rate control. Cardioversion should not be used.

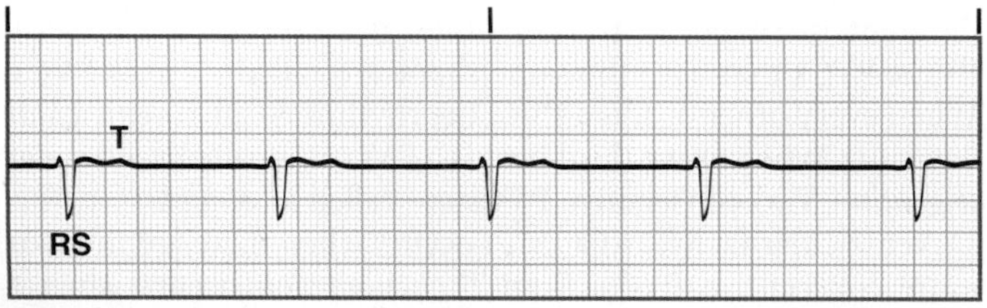


**FIG. 35-15** Junctional escape rhythm. P wave is hidden in the RS complex. NOTE: Recorded from lead $V_1$.

**First-Degree AV Block.** *First-degree AV block* is a type of AV block in which every impulse is conducted to the ventricles but the time of AV conduction is prolonged (Fig. 35-16, *A*). After the impulse moves through the AV node, the ventricles usually respond normally.

***Clinical Associations.*** First-degree AV block is associated with MI, CAD, rheumatic fever, hyperthyroidism, electrolyte

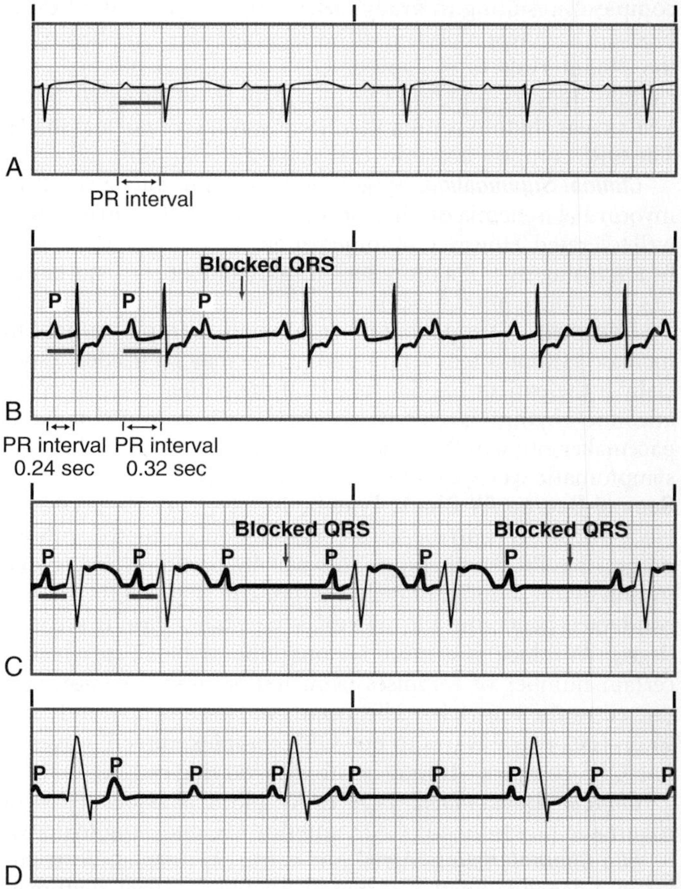


**FIG. 35-16** Heart block. **A,** First-degree atrioventricular (AV) block with a PR interval of 0.40 sec. **B,** Second-degree AV block, type I, with progressive lengthening of the PR interval until a QRS complex is blocked. **C,** Second-degree AV block, type II, with constant PR intervals and variable blocked QRS complexes. **D,** Third-degree AV block. Note that there is no relationship between P waves and QRS complexes.

imbalances (e.g., hypokalemia), vagal stimulation, and drugs such as digoxin, β-blockers, calcium channel blockers, and flecainide.

***ECG Characteristics.*** In first-degree AV block, the HR is normal and rhythm is regular. The P wave is normal, the PR interval is prolonged (greater than 0.20 second), and the QRS complex usually has a normal shape and duration.

***Clinical Significance.*** First-degree AV block is usually not serious but can be a sign of higher degrees of AV block. Patients with first-degree AV block are asymptomatic.

***Treatment.*** There is no treatment for first-degree AV block. Changes to potentially causative situations may be considered. Monitor patients for any new changes in heart rhythm (e.g., more serious AV block).

**Second-Degree AV Block, Type I.** *Type I second-degree AV block (Mobitz I* or *Wenckebach heart block)* includes a gradual lengthening of the PR interval. It occurs because of a prolonged AV conduction time until an atrial impulse is nonconducted and a QRS complex is blocked (missing) (Fig. 35-16, *B*). Type I AV block most commonly occurs in the AV node, but it can also occur in the His-Purkinje system.

***Clinical Associations.*** Type I AV block may result from drugs such as digoxin or β-blockers. It may also be associated with CAD and other diseases that can slow AV conduction.

***ECG Characteristics.*** Atrial rate is regular, but ventricular rate may be slower because of nonconducted or blocked QRS complexes resulting in bradycardia. Once a ventricular beat is blocked, the cycle repeats itself with progressive lengthening of the PR intervals until another QRS complex is blocked. The rhythm appears on the ECG in a pattern of grouped beats. Ventricular rhythm is irregular. The P wave has a normal shape. The QRS complex has a normal shape and duration.

***Clinical Significance.*** Type I AV block is usually a result of myocardial ischemia or inferior MI. It is generally transient and well tolerated. However, in some patients (e.g., acute MI) it may be a warning sign of a more serious AV conduction disturbance (e.g., complete heart block).

***Treatment.*** If the patient is symptomatic, atropine is used to increase HR, or a temporary pacemaker may be needed, especially if the patient has had an MI. If the patient is asymptomatic, the rhythm is closely observed with a transcutaneous pacemaker on standby. Bradycardia is more likely to become symptomatic when hypotension, HF, or shock is present.

**Second-Degree AV Block, Type II.** In *type II second-degree AV block (Mobitz II heart block),* a P wave is nonconducted without progressive PR lengthening. This usually occurs when a block in one of the bundle branches is present (Fig. 35-16, *C*). On conducted beats, the PR interval is constant. Type II second-degree AV block is a more serious type of block in which a certain number of impulses from the SA node are not conducted to the ventricles. This occurs in ratios of 2 : 1, 3 : 1, and so on (i.e., two P waves to one QRS complex, three P waves to one QRS complex). It may occur with varying ratios.

***Clinical Associations.*** Type II AV block is associated with rheumatic heart disease, CAD, anterior MI, and drug toxicity.

***ECG Characteristics.*** Atrial rate is usually normal. Ventricular rate depends on the degree of AV block. Atrial rhythm is regular, but ventricular rhythm may be irregular. The P wave has a normal shape. The PR interval may be normal or prolonged in duration and remains constant on conducted beats. The QRS complex is usually greater than 0.12 second because of bundle branch block.

***Clinical Significance.*** Type II AV block often progresses to third-degree AV block and is associated with a poor prognosis. The reduced HR frequently results in decreased CO with subsequent hypotension and myocardial ischemia. Type II AV block is an indication for therapy with a permanent pacemaker.

***Treatment.*** Transcutaneous pacing or the insertion of a temporary pacemaker may be necessary before the insertion of a permanent pacemaker if the patient becomes symptomatic (e.g., hypotension, angina).[11] (Temporary pacemakers are discussed on pp. 774 to 775.) Atropine is not an effective drug for this dysrhythmia.

**Third-Degree AV Block.** Third-degree AV block, or complete heart block, constitutes one form of AV dissociation in which no impulses from the atria are conducted to the ventricles (Fig. 35-16, *D*). The atria are stimulated and contract independently of the ventricles. The ventricular rhythm is an escape rhythm, and the ectopic pacemaker may be above or below the bifurcation of the bundle of His.

***Clinical Associations.*** Third-degree AV block is associated with severe heart disease, including CAD, MI, myocarditis, cardiomyopathy, and some systemic diseases such as amyloidosis and progressive systemic sclerosis (scleroderma). Some drugs can also cause third-degree AV block, such as digoxin, β-blockers, and calcium channel blockers.

***ECG Characteristics.*** The atrial rate is usually a sinus rate of 60 to 100 beats/minute. The ventricular rate depends on the site of the block. If it is in the AV node, the rate is 40 to 60 beats/minute, and if it is in the His-Purkinje system, it is 20 to 40 beats/minute. Atrial and ventricular rhythms are regular but unrelated to each other. The P wave has a normal shape. The PR interval is variable, and there is no relationship between the P wave and the QRS complex. The QRS complex is normal if an escape rhythm is initiated at the bundle of His or above. It is widened if an escape rhythm is initiated below the bundle of His.

***Clinical Significance.*** Third-degree AV block usually results in reduced CO with subsequent ischemia, HF, and shock. Syncope from third-degree AV block may result from severe bradycardia or even periods of asystole.

***Treatment.*** For symptomatic patients, a transcutaneous pacemaker is used until a temporary transvenous pacemaker can be inserted.[7] (Types of temporary pacemakers are discussed on pp. 774-775.) The use of drugs such as dopamine and epinephrine is a temporary measure to increase HR and support BP until temporary pacing is started.[11] Patients need a permanent pacemaker as soon as possible. Atropine is not an effective drug for this dysrhythmia.

**Premature Ventricular Contractions.** A premature ventricular contraction (PVC) is a contraction coming from an ectopic focus in the ventricles. It is the premature (early) occurrence of a QRS complex. A PVC is wide and distorted in shape compared with a QRS complex coming down the normal conduction pathway (Fig. 35-17). PVCs that arise from different foci appear different in shape from each other and are called *multifocal* PVCs. PVCs that have the same shape are called *unifocal* PVCs. When every other beat is a PVC, the rhythm is called *ventricular bigeminy.* When every third beat is a PVC, it is called *ventricular trigeminy.* Two consecutive PVCs are called a *couplet.*

Ventricular tachycardia (VT) occurs when there are three or more consecutive PVCs. *R-on-T phenomenon* occurs when a PVC falls on the T wave of a preceding beat. This is especially dangerous because the PVC is firing during the relative

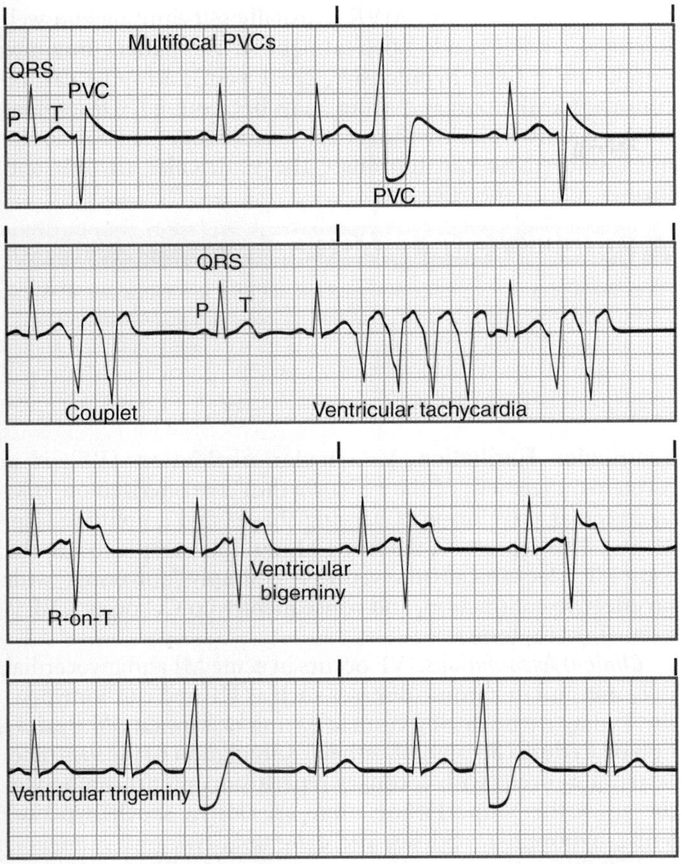


**FIG. 35-17** Various types of premature ventricular contractions (PVCs).

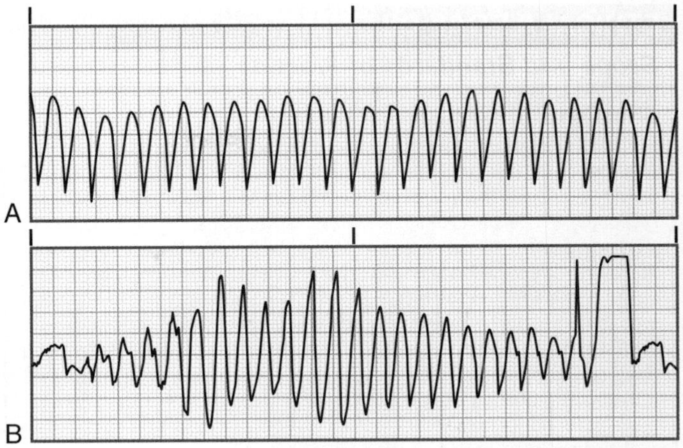


**FIG. 35-18** Ventricular tachycardia. **A,** Monomorphic. **B,** Torsades de pointes (polymorphic).

refractory phase of ventricular repolarization. Excitability of the heart cells increases during this time, and the risk for the PVC to start VT or ventricular fibrillation (VF) is great.

***Clinical Associations.*** PVCs are associated with stimulants such as caffeine, alcohol, nicotine, aminophylline, epinephrine, isoproterenol, and digoxin. They are also associated with electrolyte imbalances, hypoxia, fever, exercise, and emotional stress. Disease states associated with PVCs include MI, mitral valve prolapse, HF, cardiomyopathy, and CAD.

***ECG Characteristics.*** HR varies according to intrinsic rate and number of PVCs. Rhythm is irregular because of premature beats. The P wave is rarely visible and is usually lost in the QRS complex of the PVC. Retrograde conduction may occur and the P wave may be seen after the ectopic beat. The PR interval is not measurable. The QRS complex is wide and distorted in shape, lasting more than 0.12 second. The T wave is generally large and opposite in direction to the major direction of the QRS complex.

***Clinical Significance.*** PVCs are usually not harmful in a patient with a normal heart. In heart disease, PVCs may reduce the CO and lead to angina and HF depending on the frequency. Because PVCs in CAD or acute MI indicate ventricular irritability, assess the patient's physiologic response to PVCs. Obtain the patient's apical-radial pulse rate, since PVCs often do not generate a sufficient ventricular contraction to result in a peripheral pulse. This can lead to a pulse deficit.

***Treatment.*** Treatment relates to the cause of the PVCs (e.g., $O_2$ therapy for hypoxia, electrolyte replacement). Assessment of the patient's hemodynamic status is important to determine if treatment with drug therapy is needed. Drug therapy includes β-blockers, procainamide, or amiodarone.

**Ventricular Tachycardia.** A run of three or more PVCs defines **ventricular tachycardia (VT)**. It occurs when an ectopic focus or foci fire repeatedly and the ventricle takes control as the pacemaker. Different forms of VT exist, depending on QRS configuration. *Monomorphic* VT (Fig. 35-18, *A*) has QRS complexes that are the same in shape, size, and direction. *Polymorphic* VT occurs when the QRS complexes gradually change back and forth from one shape, size, and direction to another over a series of beats. *Torsades de pointes* (French for "twisting of the points") is polymorphic VT associated with a prolonged QT interval of the underlying rhythm (Fig. 35-18, *B*).

VT may be sustained (longer than 30 seconds) or nonsustained (less than 30 seconds). The development of VT is an ominous sign. It is a life-threatening dysrhythmia because of decreased CO and the possibility of development of VF, which is lethal.

***Clinical Associations.*** VT is associated with MI, CAD, significant electrolyte imbalances, cardiomyopathy, long QT syndrome, drug toxicity, and central nervous system disorders. This dysrhythmia can be seen in patients who have no evidence of heart disease.

***ECG Characteristics.*** Ventricular rate is 150 to 250 beats/minute. Rhythm may be regular or irregular. AV dissociation may be present, with P waves occurring independently of the QRS complex. The atria may be depolarized by the ventricles in a retrograde fashion. The P wave is usually buried in the QRS complex, and the PR interval is not measurable. The QRS complex is distorted in appearance and wide (greater than 0.12 second in duration). The T wave is in the opposite direction of the QRS complex (Fig. 35-18).

***Clinical Significance.*** VT can be stable (patient has a pulse) or unstable (patient is pulseless). Sustained VT causes a severe decrease in CO because of decreased ventricular diastolic filling times and loss of atrial contraction. This results in hypotension, pulmonary edema, decreased cerebral blood flow, and cardiopulmonary arrest. The dysrhythmia must be treated quickly, even if it occurs only briefly and stops abruptly. Episodes may recur if prophylactic treatment is not started. VF may also develop.

**Treatment.** Precipitating causes (e.g., electrolyte imbalances, ischemia) must be identified and treated. If the VT is monomorphic and the patient is clinically stable (i.e., pulse is present)

## ETHICAL/LEGAL DILEMMAS

### *Scope and Standards of Practice*

**Situation**

A young woman is admitted to the intensive care unit (ICU) from the emergency department after experiencing several episodes of nonsustained ventricular tachycardia (VT) attributed to a history of viral cardiomyopathy. While she is being stabilized in the ICU, she codes (pulseless VT) and intubation is indicated. A nurse anesthetist attempts to intubate her three times unsuccessfully. There is an unforeseen delay in the arrival of the anesthesiologist. P.F., an ICU nurse and former paramedic who is certified in advanced trauma life support (ATLS) and advanced cardiovascular life support (ACLS), attempts to intubate the patient and does so successfully. The next day the nursing supervisor questions P.F. about intubating the patient, since this is not within the scope of practice for an ICU nurse.

**Ethical/Legal Points for Consideration**

- The RN *Scope of Practice,* including rules and regulations that guide practice, are defined by individual state Boards of Nursing and can vary from state to state.
- Individual agencies also have policies and procedures that describe the scope of practice for nurses. These can be more restrictive than those of the state.
- *Scope and Standards of Practice* are also defined by professional nursing organizations (e.g., American Nurses Association, American Association of Critical-Care Nurses). These are authoritative statements that serve to define expected competent practice in various registered nurse (RN) roles (e.g., Scope and Standards for Nursing Administration).
- P.F. has had training, education, and certification beyond the usual nursing role.
- A life-threatening situation provides for extenuating circumstances.
- Negligence may have been a factor if P.F., who is a nurse with training and experience, had not acted.

**Discussion Questions**

1. What would you have done in this situation?
2. How would you respond to the nursing supervisor?
3. What are the legal ramifications for P.F. in this situation?
4. What are the ethical issues in this situation?

and has preserved left ventricular function, IV procainamide, sotalol, or amiodarone is used. These drugs can also be used if the VT is polymorphic with a normal baseline QT interval.

Polymorphic VT with a prolonged baseline QT interval is treated with IV magnesium, isoproterenol, phenytoin (Dilantin), or antitachycardia pacing (discussed later in this chapter). Drugs that prolong the QT interval (e.g., dofetilide [Tikosyn]) should be discontinued. Cardioversion is used if drug therapy is ineffective.

VT without a pulse is a life-threatening situation. It is treated in the same manner as VF. Cardiopulmonary resuscitation (CPR) and rapid defibrillation are the first lines of treatment, followed by the administration of vasopressors (e.g., epinephrine) and antidysrhythmics (e.g., amiodarone) if defibrillation is unsuccessful.[11]

An *accelerated idioventricular rhythm* (AIVR) can develop when the intrinsic pacemaker rate (SA node or AV node) becomes less than that of a ventricular ectopic pacemaker. The rate is between 40 and 100 beats/minute. It is most commonly associated with acute MI and reperfusion of the myocardium after thrombolytic therapy or percutaneous coronary interventions (e.g., angioplasty). It can be seen with digitalis toxicity. In the setting of acute MI, AIVR is usually self-limiting and well tolerated, and it needs no treatment. If the patient becomes symptomatic (e.g., hypotensive, chest pain), atropine can be considered. Temporary pacing may be required. Drugs that suppress ventricular rhythms (e.g., amiodarone) should not be used, since these can terminate the ventricular rhythm and further reduce the HR.

## CHECK YOUR PRACTICE

You are assigned to a 69-yr-old male patient on a telemetry unit who is recovering from colon surgery. He has a history of two MIs and he has three stents in place. You hear his ECG monitor alarm and see what looks like ventricular tachycardia on the screen.

- What should you do?

**Ventricular Fibrillation.** Ventricular fibrillation (VF) is a severe derangement of the heart rhythm characterized on ECG by irregular waveforms of varying shapes and amplitude (Fig. 35-19). This represents the firing of multiple ectopic foci in the ventricle. Mechanically the ventricle is simply "quivering," with no effective contraction, and consequently no CO occurs. VF is a lethal dysrhythmia.

***Clinical Associations.*** VF occurs in acute MI and myocardial ischemia and in chronic diseases such as HF and cardiomyopathy. It may occur during cardiac pacing or cardiac catheterization procedures because of catheter stimulation of the ventricle. It may also occur with coronary reperfusion after thrombolytic therapy. Other clinical associations are electric shock, hyperkalemia, hypoxemia, acidosis, and drug toxicity.

***ECG Characteristics.*** HR is not measurable. Rhythm is irregular and chaotic. The P wave is not visible, and the PR interval and the QRS interval are not measurable.

***Clinical Significance.*** VF results in an unresponsive, pulseless, and apneic state. If it is not rapidly treated, the patient will not recover.

***Treatment.*** Treatment consists of immediate initiation of CPR and advanced cardiovascular life support (ACLS) with the use of defibrillation and definitive drug therapy (e.g., epinephrine, vasopressin). There should be no delay in starting chest compressions and using a defibrillator once available.

**Asystole.** Asystole represents the total absence of ventricular electrical activity. Occasionally, P waves are seen. No ventricular contraction occurs because depolarization does not occur. Patients are unresponsive, pulseless, and apneic. Asystole is a lethal dysrhythmia that requires immediate treatment. VF may masquerade as asystole. Always assess the rhythm in more than one lead. The prognosis of a patient with asystole is extremely poor.

***Clinical Associations.*** Asystole is usually a result of advanced heart disease, a severe cardiac conduction system disturbance, or end-stage HF.

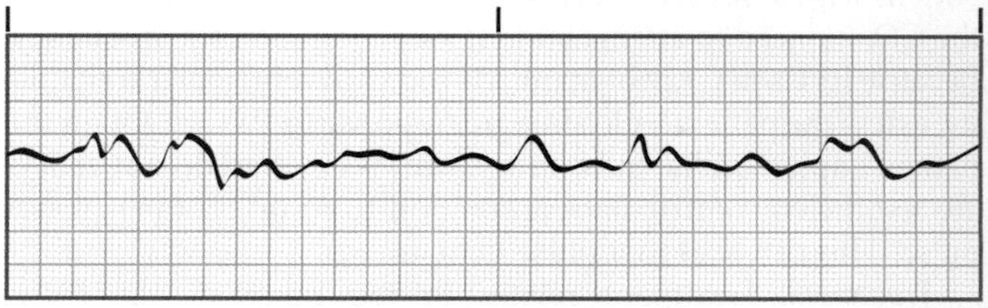

**FIG. 35-19** Ventricular fibrillation.

***Clinical Significance.*** Generally the patient with asystole has end-stage heart disease or has a prolonged arrest and cannot be resuscitated.

***Treatment.*** Treatment consists of CPR with initiation of ACLS measures. These include definitive drug therapy with epinephrine and/or vasopressin, and intubation.

**Pulseless Electrical Activity.** *Pulseless electrical activity* (PEA) is a situation in which organized electrical activity is seen on the ECG, but there is no mechanical heart activity and the patient has no pulse. It is the most common dysrhythmia seen after defibrillation. Prognosis is poor unless the underlying cause is quickly identified and treated. The most common causes of PEA include hypovolemia, hypoxia, metabolic acidosis, hyperkalemia, hypokalemia, hypoglycemia, hypothermia, toxins (e.g., drug overdose), cardiac tamponade, thrombosis (e.g., MI, pulmonary embolus), tension pneumothorax, and trauma. Treatment begins with CPR followed by drug therapy (e.g., epinephrine) and intubation. Correcting the underlying cause is critical to prognosis.

**Sudden Cardiac Death.** The term *sudden cardiac death* (SCD) refers to death from a cardiac cause. Most SCDs result from ventricular dysrhythmias, specifically VT or VF. (SCD is discussed in Chapter 33.)

**Prodysrhythmia.** Antidysrhythmia drugs can cause life-threatening dysrhythmias similar to those for which they are given. This concept is termed *prodysrhythmia.* The patient who has severe left ventricular dysfunction is the most susceptible to prodysrhythmias. Digoxin and class IA, IC, and III antidysrhythmia drugs can cause a prodysrhythmic response.[5] The first several days of drug therapy are the vulnerable period for developing prodysrhythmias. For this reason, many oral antidysrhythmia drug regimens are started in a monitored hospital setting.

## Antidysrhythmia Drugs

Table 35-9 categorizes antidysrhythmia drugs by their primary effects on the heart cells and the ECG.

**TABLE 35-9 Drug Therapy**

***Antidysrhythmia Drugs***

| Drug | Actions* | Effects on ECG |
|---|---|---|
| **Class I: Sodium Channel Blockers** | Decrease impulse conduction in the atria, ventricles, and His-Purkinje system | |
| ***Class IA***<br>disopyramide (Norpace)<br>procainamide<br>quinidine | Delay repolarization | Widened QRS and prolonged QT interval |
| ***Class IB***<br>mexiletine<br>phenytoin (Dilantin) | Accelerate repolarization | Little or no effect on ECG |
| ***Class IC***<br>flecainide<br>propafenone (Rythmol) | Decrease impulse conduction | Pronounced prodysrhythmic actions, widened QRS, prolonged QT interval |
| **Class II: β-Adrenergic Blockers**<br>esmolol (Brevibloc)<br>metoprolol (Lopressor)<br>propranolol (Inderal) | Decrease automaticity of the SA node, slow impulse conduction in AV node, reduce atrial and ventricular contractility | Bradycardia, prolonged PR interval, AV block |
| **Class III: Potassium Channel Blockers**<br>amiodarone (Cordarone)<br>dofetilide (Tikosyn)<br>ibutilide (Corvert)<br>sotalol† (Betapace) | Delay repolarization, resulting in prolonged duration of action potential and refractory period | Prolonged PR and QT intervals, widened QRS, bradycardia |
| **Class IV: Calcium Channel Blockers**<br>diltiazem (Cardizem)<br>verapamil (Calan) | Decrease automaticity of SA node, delay AV node conduction; reduce myocardial contractility | Bradycardia, prolonged PR interval, AV block |
| **Other Antidysrhythmia Drugs** | | |
| adenosine (Adenocard)<br>digoxin (Lanoxin) | Decrease conduction through AV node, reduce automaticity of SA node | Prolonged PR interval, AV block |
| dronedarone (Multaq)‡ | Suppresses atrial dysrhythmias though mechanism is unknown | Prolonged QT interval |
| magnesium | Decreases impulse conduction through AV node | AV block |

*AV,* Atrioventricular; *SA,* sinoatrial.

*Antidysrhythmia drugs have a direct effect on the various phases of the action potential (Fig. 35-1).
†Sotalol has both class II and class III properties.
‡Dronedarone has class I through IV properties.

## Defibrillation

*Defibrillation* is the treatment of choice to end VF and pulseless VT. It is most effective when the myocardial cells are not anoxic or acidotic. Rapid defibrillation (within 2 minutes) is critical to a successful patient outcome. Defibrillation involves the passage of an electric shock through the heart to depolarize the myocardial cells. The goal is that the following repolarization of heart cells will allow the SA node to resume the role of pacemaker.

Defibrillators deliver energy using a monophasic or biphasic waveform. Monophasic defibrillators deliver energy in one direction, and biphasic defibrillators deliver energy in two directions (Fig. 35-20). Biphasic defibrillators deliver shocks at lower energies and with fewer postshock ECG dysrhythmias than monophasic defibrillators.

The output of a defibrillator is measured in *joules,* or watts per second. The recommended energy for initial shocks in defibrillation depends on the type of defibrillator. Biphasic defibrillators deliver the first and any successive shocks using 120 to 200 joules. Recommendations for monophasic defibrillators include an initial shock at 360 joules. After the first shock, start CPR immediately beginning with chest compressions. (CPR is discussed in Appendix A of this book.)

Rapid defibrillation can be performed using a manual or automatic device (Fig. 35-21). Manual defibrillators require you to interpret heart rhythms, determine the need for a shock, and deliver a shock. An **automatic external defibrillator (AED)** can detect heart rhythms and advise the user to deliver a shock using hands-free defibrillator pads. Proficiency in the use of the

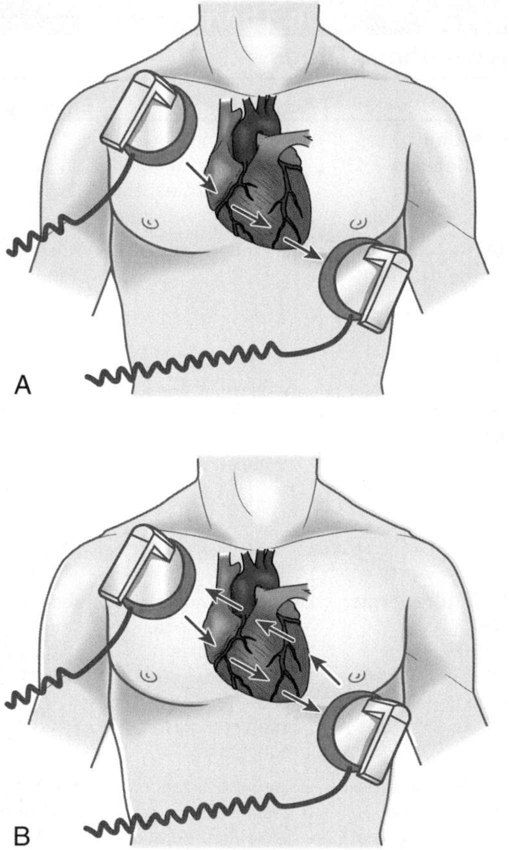


**FIG. 35-20** Paddle placement and current flow in monophasic defibrillation **(A)** and biphasic defibrillation **(B)**.

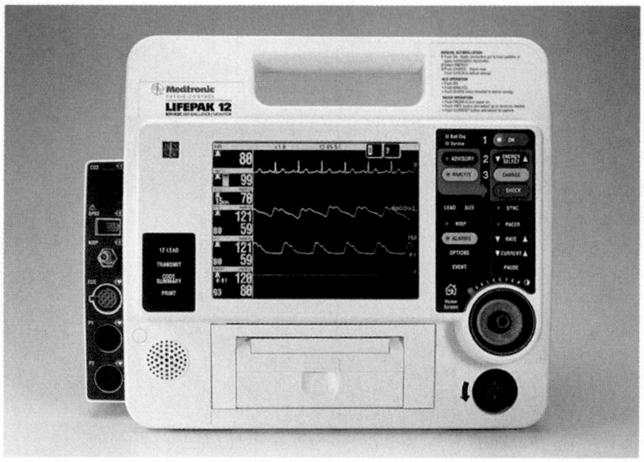


**FIG. 35-21** LifePak contains a monitor, defibrillator, and transcutaneous pacemaker. (Courtesy Medtronic Physio-Control, Redmond, Wash.)

AED is part of the basic life support course for health care professionals. You must be familiar with the operation of the type of defibrillator used in your clinical setting.

The following general steps are taken for defibrillation: (1) CPR should be in progress until the defibrillator is available; (2) turn the defibrillator on, and select the proper energy level; (3) check to see that the synchronizer switch is turned off (discussed later); (4) apply conductive materials (e.g., defibrillator gel pads) to the chest, one to the right of the sternum just below the clavicle, and the other to the left of the apex; (5) charge the defibrillator using the button on the defibrillator or the paddles; (6) position the paddles firmly on the chest wall over the conductive material (Fig. 35-20); (7) call and look to see that everyone is "all clear" to ensure that staff are not touching the patient or the bed at the time of discharge; and (8) deliver the charge by depressing buttons on both paddles simultaneously.

Hands-free, multifunction defibrillator pads are available and are placed on the chest as described earlier. Connect the cables from the pads to the defibrillator. Charge and discharge the defibrillator using buttons on the defibrillator. It is still essential to ensure that all staff are clear before discharging the defibrillator.

**Synchronized Cardioversion.** *Synchronized cardioversion* is the therapy of choice for the patient with ventricular tachydysrhythmias (e.g., VT with a pulse) or supraventricular tachydysrhythmias (e.g., atrial flutter with a rapid ventricular response). A synchronized circuit in the defibrillator delivers a shock that is programmed to occur on the R wave of the QRS complex of the ECG. The synchronizer switch must be turned on when cardioversion is planned.

The procedure for synchronized cardioversion is the same as for defibrillation with the following exceptions. If synchronized cardioversion is done on a nonemergency basis (i.e., the patient is awake and hemodynamically stable), the patient is sedated (e.g., IV midazolam) before the procedure. Strict attention to maintaining the patient's airway is critical. If a patient with supraventricular tachycardia or VT with a pulse becomes hemodynamically unstable, synchronized cardioversion should be performed as quickly as possible. Start the initial energy for synchronized cardioversion at 50 to 100 joules (biphasic defibrillator) and 100 joules (monophasic defibrillator), and increase if needed. If the patient becomes pulseless or the rhythm changes to VF, turn the synchronizer switch off and perform defibrillation.

**! SAFETY ALERT Defibrillation and Cardioversion**

- Check that the synchronizer switch is OFF when defibrillation is planned.
- Turn the synchronizer switch ON when cardioversion is planned.
- Never apply the defibrillator pads over a pacemaker or implantable cardioverter-defibrillator.
- Be certain that personnel are "all clear" before discharging the device.

**Implantable Cardioverter-Defibrillator.** The *implantable cardioverter-defibrillator* (ICD) is an important technology for patients who (1) have survived SCD, (2) have spontaneous sustained VT, (3) have syncope with inducible VT or VF during EPS, or (4) are at high risk for future life-threatening dysrhythmias (e.g., have cardiomyopathy). The use of ICDs has significantly decreased mortality rates in these patients.[12]

The ICD consists of a lead system placed via a subclavian vein to the endocardium. A battery-powered pulse generator is implanted subcutaneously, usually over the pectoral muscle on the patient's nondominant side. The pulse generator is similar in size to a pacemaker. Most systems are single-lead systems (Fig. 35-22). The ICD sensing system monitors the HR and rhythm and identifies VT or VF. After the sensing system detects a lethal dysrhythmia, the device delivers a 25-joule or less shock to the patient's heart. If the first shock is unsuccessful, the device recycles and can continue to deliver shocks.

In addition to defibrillation capabilities, ICDs are equipped with *antitachycardia* and *antibradycardia pacing* capabilities.

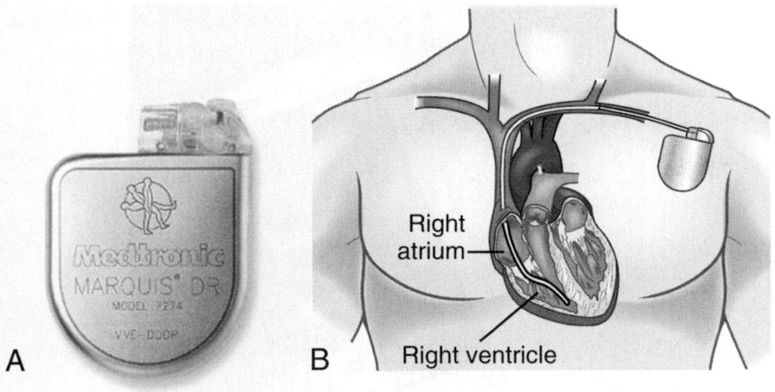


**FIG. 35-22** **A,** The implantable cardioverter-defibrillator (ICD) pulse generator from Medtronic, Inc. (Courtesy Medtronic, Inc., Minneapolis, Minn.) **B,** The ICD is placed in a subcutaneous pocket over the pectoral muscle. A single-lead system is placed transvenously from the pulse generator to the endocardium. The single lead detects dysrhythmias and delivers an electric shock to the heart muscle.

These devices use algorithms that detect dysrhythmias and determine the appropriate response. They can initiate *overdrive pacing* of supraventricular tachycardia and VT, sparing the patient painful defibrillator shocks. They also provide backup pacing for bradydysrhythmias that may occur after defibrillation. Preprocedure and postprocedure nursing care of the patient undergoing ICD placement is similar to the care of a patient undergoing permanent pacemaker implantation (see p. 775).

Recent research has focused on a totally subcutaneous ICD (S-ICD). The S-ICD pulse generator is placed under the skin on the left side of the chest and the electrode is placed under the skin above the sternum. The system delivers a shock when VT or VF is detected. Since the S-ICD does not have any electrodes implanted in the heart, it has no pacing capability.[13]

Teaching the patient who is receiving an ICD and the caregiver is extremely important. Patients experience a variety of emotions, including fear of body image change, fear of recurrent dysrhythmias, expectation of pain with ICD discharge (described as a feeling of a blow to the chest), and anxiety about going home. Encourage patients and caregivers to participate in local or online ICD support groups[14] *(www.facebook.com/ICD.pacemaker)*. Table 35-10 presents a teaching guide for the patient with an ICD and the caregiver.

## Pacemakers

The artificial **cardiac pacemaker** is an electronic device used to pace the heart when the normal conduction pathway is damaged. The basic pacing circuit consists of a power source (battery-powered pulse generator) with programmable circuitry, one or more pacing leads, and the myocardium. The electrical signal (stimulus) travels from the pulse generator, through the leads, to the wall of the myocardium. The heart muscle is "captured" and stimulated to contract (Fig. 35-23). Recently a leadless pacemaker that is fully implanted in the right ventricle has been approved by the FDA.

Current pacemakers are small, sophisticated, and physiologically precise. They pace the atrium and/or one or both of the ventricles. Most pacemakers are *demand pacemakers.* This means that they sense the heart's electrical activity and fire only when the HR drops below a preset rate. Demand pacemakers have two distinct features: (1) a sensing device that inhibits the pacemaker when the HR is adequate and (2) a pacing device that triggers the pacemaker when no QRS complexes occur within a preset time.[1]

In addition to antibradycardia pacing, devices now include antitachycardia and overdrive pacing. *Antitachycardia pacing* involves the delivery of a stimulus to the ventricle to end tachydysrhythmias (e.g., VT). Overdrive pacing involves pacing the atrium at rates of 200 to 500 impulses per minute in an attempt to terminate atrial tachycardias (e.g., atrial flutter with a rapid ventricular response). You can refer to textbooks on pacemaker therapy for more detailed information.[15]

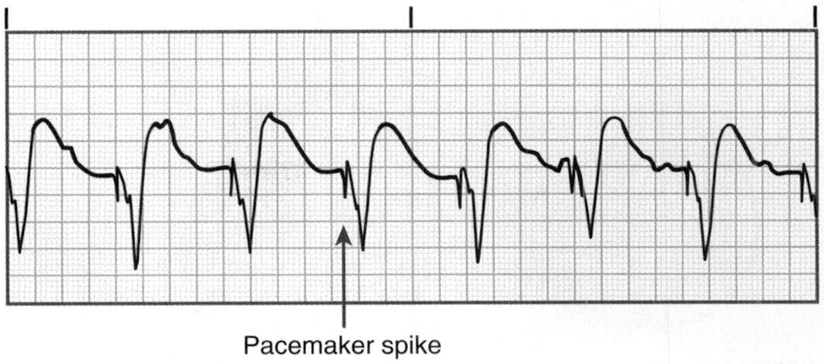


**FIG. 35-23** Ventricular capture (depolarization) secondary to signal *(pacemaker spike)* from pacemaker lead in the right ventricle.

### TABLE 35-10 Patient & Caregiver Teaching
### *Implantable Cardioverter-Defibrillator (ICD)*

*Include the following information in the teaching plan for a patient receiving an ICD and the patient's caregiver.*

1. Follow up with an HCP for routine checks of the function of the ICD. This is often done by interrogating the device using a telephone.
2. Report any signs of infection at incision site (e.g., redness, swelling, drainage) or fever to your HCP immediately.
3. Keep incision dry for 4 days after insertion or as instructed.
4. Avoid lifting arm on ICD side above shoulder until approved.
5. Discuss resuming sexual activity with your HCP. It is usually safe to resume sexual activity once your incision is healed.
6. Avoid driving until cleared by your HCP. This decision is usually based on the ongoing presence of dysrhythmias, the frequency of ICD firings, your overall health, and state laws regarding drivers with ICDs.
7. Avoid direct blows to ICD site.
8. Avoid large magnets and strong electromagnetic fields because these may interfere with the device.
9. You should not have magnetic resonance imaging (MRI) unless the ICD is approved as MRI safe or there is a protocol in place for patient safety during the procedure.
10. Travel is not restricted. Inform security (e.g., airport, train station, public buildings) of presence of ICD because it may set off the metal detector. If hand-held screening wand is used, it should not be placed directly over the ICD. Manufacturer information may vary regarding the effect of metal detectors on the function of the ICD.
11. Avoid standing near antitheft devices in doorways of stores and public buildings. You should walk through them at a normal pace.
12. If your ICD fires, call your HCP immediately.
13. If your ICD fires and you feel sick, contact the emergency response system (ERS).
14. If your ICD fires more than once, contact ERS.
15. You should obtain and wear a Medic Alert ID device at all times.
16. Always carry the ICD identification card and a current list of your drugs.
17. Consider joining an ICD support group (e.g., *www.facebook.com/ICD.pacemaker*).
18. Caregivers should learn cardiopulmonary resuscitation (CPR).

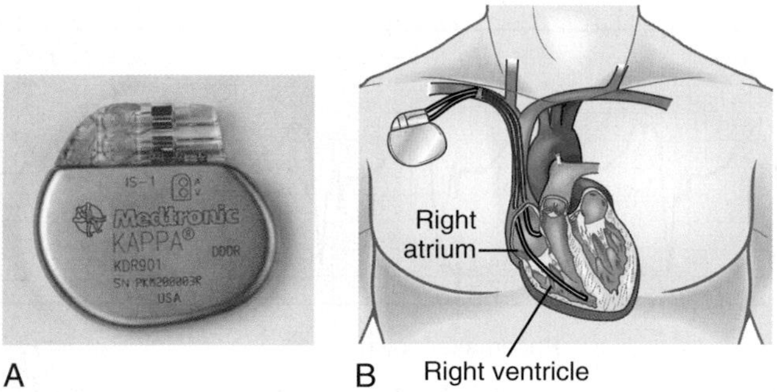


**FIG. 35-24** **A,** A dual-chamber rate-responsive pacemaker from Medtronic, Inc., is designed to treat patients with chronic heart problems in which the heart beats too slowly to adequately support the body's circulation needs. (Courtesy Medtronic, Inc., Minneapolis, Minn.) **B,** Pacing leads in both the atrium and the ventricle enable a dual-chamber pacemaker to sense and pace in both heart chambers.

**TABLE 35-11 Indications for Permanent Pacemakers**

- Acquired AV block
- Second-degree AV block
- Third-degree AV block
- Atrial fibrillation with a slow ventricular response
- Bundle branch block
- Cardiomyopathy
  - Dilated
  - Hypertrophic
- Heart failure
- SA node dysfunction
- Tachydysrhythmias (e.g., ventricular tachycardia)

*AV,* Atrioventricular; *SA,* sinoatrial.

**Permanent Pacemaker.** A *permanent pacemaker* is implanted totally within the body (Fig. 35-24). The power source is placed subcutaneously, usually over the pectoral muscle on the patient's nondominant side. The pacing leads are placed transvenously to the right atrium and/or one or both ventricles and attached to the power source. Common reasons for insertion of a permanent pacemaker are found in Table 35-11.

New technology and research are focused on miniaturized, leadless permanent pacemakers. Most candidates for the new device are patients who need single-chamber pacing for atrial fibrillation with AV block. The device is placed in the right ventricle. The lack of a transvenous lead and subcutaneous pulse generator is a major shift in cardiac pacing.[16]

**Cardiac Resynchronization Therapy.** *Cardiac resynchronization therapy* (CRT) is a pacing technique that resynchronizes the heart cycle by pacing both ventricles *(biventricular pacing).* This promotes improvement in ventricular function (Fig. 34-4). Most HF patients have intraventricular conduction delays causing abnormal ventricular contraction. This causes dyssynchrony between the right and left ventricles and results in reduced systolic function, pump inefficiency, and worsened HF. For patients with severe left ventricular dysfunction, CRT is combined with an ICD for maximum therapy.[17] (HF is discussed in Chapter 34.)

**Temporary Pacemaker.** A *temporary pacemaker* is one that has the power source outside the body (Fig. 35-25). There are three types of temporary pacemakers: transvenous, epicardial, and transcutaneous. Table 35-12 lists common reasons for temporary pacing.

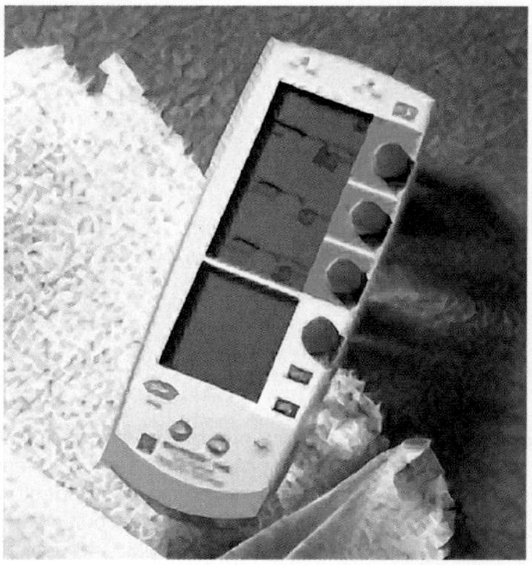

**FIG. 35-25** Temporary external, dual-chamber demand pacemaker. (Courtesy Medtronic, Inc., Minneapolis, Minn.)

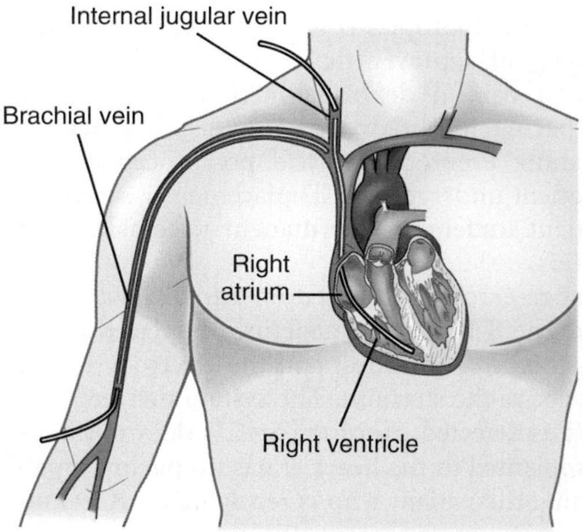


**FIG. 35-26** Temporary transvenous pacemaker catheter insertion. A single lead is positioned in the right ventricle through the brachial, subclavian, jugular, or femoral vein.

**TABLE 35-12 Indications for Temporary Pacemakers***

- Maintenance of adequate HR and rhythm during special circumstances such as surgery and postoperative recovery, during cardiac catheterization or coronary angioplasty, during drug therapy that may cause bradycardia, and before implantation of a permanent pacemaker
- As prophylaxis after open heart surgery
- Acute anterior MI with second- or third-degree AV block or bundle branch block
- Acute inferior MI with symptomatic bradycardia and AV block
- Electrophysiologic studies to evaluate patient with bradydysrhythmias and tachydysrhythmias

*List is not all-inclusive.
*AV,* Atrioventricular; *HR,* heart rate; *MI,* myocardial infarction.

A *transvenous pacemaker* consists of a lead or leads that are threaded transvenously to the right atrium and/or right ventricle and attached to the external power source (Fig. 35-26). Most temporary transvenous pacemakers are inserted in emergency departments and critical care units in emergency situations. They provide a bridge to insertion of a permanent

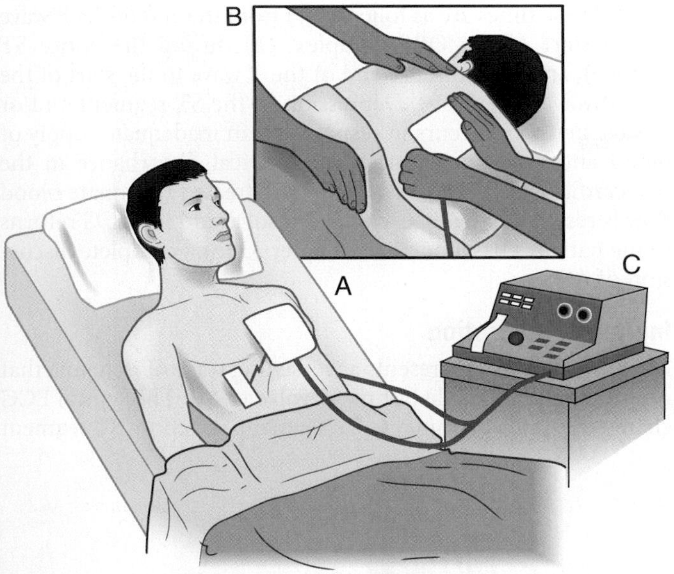


**FIG. 35-27** Transcutaneous pacemaker. Pacing electrodes are placed on the patient's anterior *(A)* and posterior *(B)* chest walls and attached to an external pacing unit *(C)*.

pacemaker or until the underlying cause of the dysrhythmia is resolved.

*Epicardial pacing* involves attaching an atrial and ventricular pacing lead to the epicardium during heart surgery. The leads are passed through the chest wall and attached to the external power source. Epicardial pacing leads are placed prophylactically in case any bradydysrhythmias or tachydysrhythmias occur in the early postoperative period.[7]

A *transcutaneous pacemaker* (TCP) is used to provide adequate HR and rhythm to the patient in an emergency situation. Placement of the TCP is a noninvasive, temporary procedure used until a transvenous pacemaker is inserted or until more definitive therapy is available.[7]

The TCP consists of a power source and a rate- and voltage-control device that attaches to two large, multifunction electrode pads. Position one pad on the anterior part of the chest, usually on the $V_4$ lead position, and the other pad on the back between the spine and left scapula at the level of the heart (Fig. 35-27). When programming the TCP, always use the lowest current that results in a ventricular contraction (capture) to minimize patient discomfort.

Before starting TCP therapy, it is important to tell the patient what to expect. Explain that the muscle contractions created by the pacemaker when the current passes through the chest wall are uncomfortable. Reassure the patient that the TCP is temporary and that it will be replaced by a transvenous pacemaker as soon as possible. Whenever possible, provide analgesia and/or sedation while the TCP is in use.

**Monitoring of Patients With Pacemakers.** Patients with temporary or permanent pacemakers are ECG monitored to evaluate the status of the pacemaker. Pacemaker malfunction primarily involves a failure to sense or a failure to capture. *Failure to sense* occurs when the pacemaker fails to recognize spontaneous atrial or ventricular activity, and it fires inappropriately. This can result in the pacemaker firing during the excitable period of the cardiac cycle, resulting in VT. Failure to sense is caused by fibrosis around the tip of the pacing lead, battery failure, sensing set too high, or dislodgment of the electrode.

*Failure to capture* occurs when the electrical charge to the myocardium is insufficient to produce atrial or ventricular contraction. This can result in serious bradycardia or asystole. Failure to capture is caused by pacer lead damage, battery failure, dislodgment of the electrode, electrical charge set too low, or fibrosis at the electrode tip.

Complications of invasive temporary (i.e., transvenous) or permanent pacemaker insertion include infection and hematoma formation at the insertion site, pneumothorax, failure to sense or capture, perforation of the atrial or ventricular septum by the pacing lead, and appearance of "end-of-life" battery power on testing the pacemaker. Several measures can prevent or assess for complications. These include prophylactic IV antibiotic therapy before and after insertion, postinsertion chest x-ray to check lead placement and to rule out a pneumothorax, careful observation of insertion site, and continuous ECG monitoring of the patient's rhythm.

After the pacemaker has been inserted, the patient can be out of bed once stable. Have the patient limit arm and shoulder activity on the operative side to prevent dislodging the newly implanted pacing leads. Observe the insertion site for signs of bleeding, and check that the incision is intact. Note any temperature elevation or pain at the insertion site and treat as ordered. Most patients are discharged the next day if stable.

Provide teaching in addition to observing for complications after pacemaker insertion. The patient with a newly implanted pacemaker and the caregiver may have questions about activity restrictions and fears concerning body image after the procedure. The goals of pacemaker therapy include enhancing physiologic functioning and quality of life. Emphasize this to the patient and caregiver, and provide specific advice on activity restrictions. Table 35-13 outlines patient and caregiver teaching for the patient with a pacemaker.

After discharge, patients need to check pacemaker function on a regular basis. This can include outpatient visits to a pacemaker clinic or home monitoring using telephone transmitter devices. Another method to evaluate pacemaker performance is noninvasive program stimulation. This procedure is done on an outpatient basis in the EPS laboratory.

### Radiofrequency Catheter Ablation Therapy

*Radiofrequency catheter ablation therapy* uses electrical energy to "burn" or ablate areas of the conduction system as definitive treatment of tachydysrhythmias. Ablation therapy is done after EPS has identified the source of the dysrhythmia. An electrode-tipped ablation catheter ablates accessory pathways or ectopic sites in the atria, AV node, and ventricles. Catheter ablation is considered the nonpharmacologic treatment of choice for atrial dysrhythmias resulting in rapid ventricular rates and AV nodal reentrant tachycardia refractory to drug therapy.[8]

The ablation procedure is an effective treatment with a low complication rate. Care of the patient after ablation therapy is similar to that of a patient undergoing cardiac catheterization (see Chapter 31 and Table 31-6).

## ECG CHANGES ASSOCIATED WITH ACUTE CORONARY SYNDROME

The 12-lead ECG is a major diagnostic tool used to evaluate patients with ACS. ECG changes that occur with ACS direct many treatment decisions. The ECG changes are in response to ischemia, injury, or infarction (necrosis) of heart cells. The leads facing the area of involvement demonstrate the definitive ECG changes (Fig. 35-28). The leads facing opposite the area involved in ACS often demonstrate reciprocal (opposite) ECG changes. In addition, the pattern of ECG changes among the 12 leads provides information on the coronary artery involved in ACS (Table 35-14).

### Ischemia

Typical ECG changes that are seen in myocardial ischemia include ST segment depression and/or T wave inversion (Fig. 35-29, *A*). ST segment depression is significant if it is at least 1 mm (one small box) below the isoelectric line in at least two contiguous (neighboring) leads (Fig. 35-5). The isoelectric line is flat and represents those normal times in the cardiac cycle when the ECG is not recording any electrical activity in the heart. These times are as follows: (1) from the end of the P wave to the start of the QRS complex, (2) during the entire ST segment, and (3) from the end of the T wave to the start of the next P wave (Fig. 35-9). Depression in the ST segment and/or T wave inversion occurs in response to an inadequate supply of blood and $O_2$, which causes an electrical disturbance in the myocardial cells.[6,7] Once the patient is treated (adequate blood flow is restored), the ECG changes resolve and the ECG returns to the patient's baseline. (See Chapter 33 for a complete discussion of ACS.)

### Injury and Infarction

Myocardial injury represents a worsening stage of ischemia that is potentially reversible but may evolve to MI. The typical ECG change seen during injury is ST segment elevation. ST segment

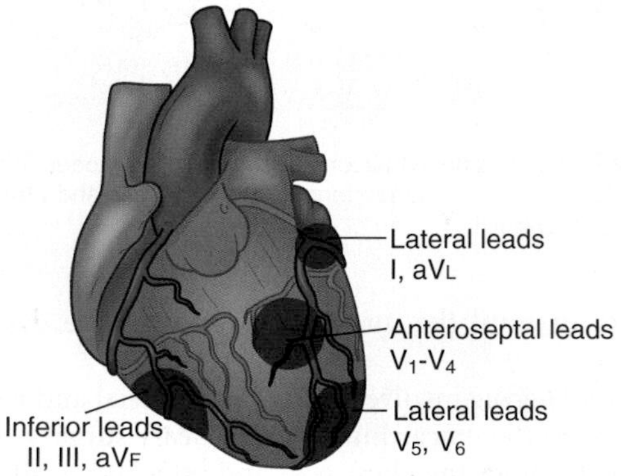


**FIG. 35-28** Definitive ECG changes occur in leads that face the area of ischemia, injury, or infarction. Reciprocal changes may occur in leads facing opposite the area of ischemia, injury, or infarction.

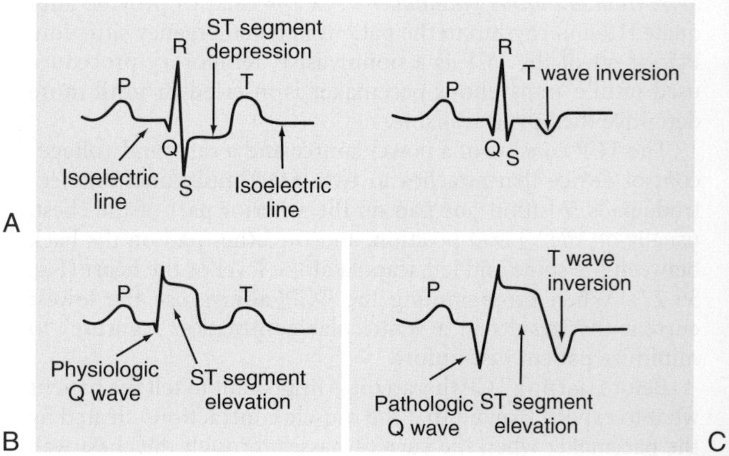


**FIG. 35-29** ST segment, T wave, and Q wave changes associated with myocardial ischemia **(A)**, injury **(B)**, and infarction **(C)**. (From Bucher L, Melander S: *Critical care nursing,* Philadelphia, 1999, Saunders.)

## TABLE 35-13 Patient & Caregiver Teaching

### *Pacemaker*

*Include the following information in the teaching plan for a patient with a pacemaker and the patient's caregiver.*

1. Maintain follow-up care with your HCP to begin regular pacemaker function checks. This is often done by interrogating the device using a telephone.
2. Report any signs of infection at incision site (e.g., redness, swelling, drainage) or fever to your HCP immediately.
3. Keep incision dry for 4 days after implantation, or as ordered.
4. Avoid lifting arm on pacemaker side above shoulder until approved by your cardiologist.
5. Avoid direct blows to pacemaker site.
6. Avoid close proximity to high-output electric generators, since these can interfere with the function of the pacemaker.
7. You should not have magnetic resonance imaging (MRI) unless the pacemaker is approved as MRI safe or there is a protocol in place for patient safety during the procedure.
8. Microwave ovens are safe to use and do not interfere with pacemaker function.
9. Avoid standing near antitheft devices in doorways of department stores and public libraries. You should walk through them at a normal pace.
10. Travel is not restricted. Inform security (e.g., airport, train station, public buildings) of presence of pacemaker because it may set off the metal detector. If hand-held screening wand is used, it should not be placed directly over the pacemaker. Manufacturer information may vary regarding the effect of metal detectors on the function of the pacemaker.
11. Monitor pulse and inform HCP if heart rate drops below predetermined rate.
12. Carry pacemaker information card and a current list of your drugs at all times.
13. Obtain and wear a Medic Alert ID device at all times.
14. Consider joining a pacemaker support group (e.g., *www.facebook.com/ICD.pacemaker*).

## TABLE 35-14 ECG Evidence in Acute Coronary Syndrome

| Left Ventricle Involvement | ECG EVIDENCE: Leads Facing Area | ECG EVIDENCE: Leads Opposite Area (Reciprocal Changes) | Associated Coronary Artery |
|---|---|---|---|
| Septal wall | $V_1$, $V_2$ | II, III, aVF | Left anterior descending |
| Anterior wall | $V_2$-$V_4$ | II, III, aVF | Left anterior descending |
| Lateral wall, low | $V_5$, $V_6$ | II, III, aVF | Left anterior descending or circumflex |
| Lateral wall, high | I, aVL | II, III, aVF | Circumflex |
| Inferior wall | II, III, aVF | I, aVL, $V_5$, $V_6$ | Right coronary artery, posterior descending coronary artery |

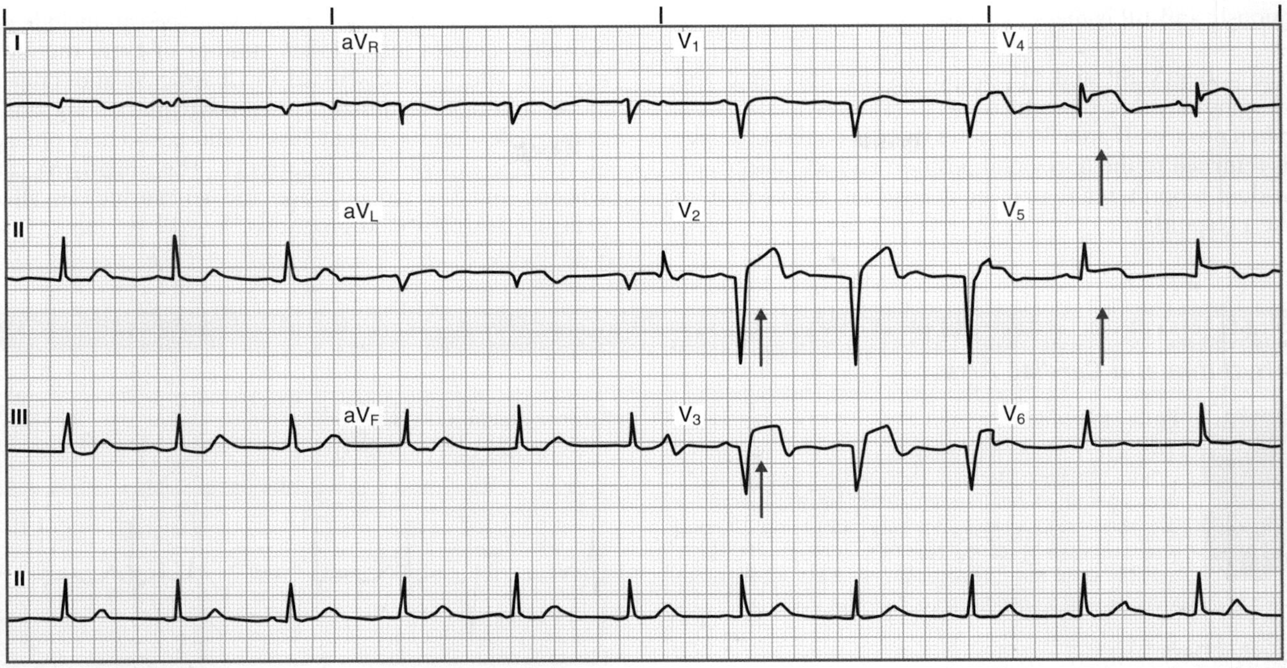


**FIG. 35-30** ECG findings with anteroseptal lateral wall myocardial infarction. Normally, leads I, aVL, and $V_1$ to $V_3$ have a positive R wave. Note the pathologic Q waves in these leads and the ST segment elevation in leads $V_2$ to $V_5$ *(arrows)*.

elevation is significant if it is 1 mm or more above the isoelectric line in at least two contiguous leads (Fig. 35-29, *B*). If treatment is fast and effective, it is possible to restore $O_2$ to the heart muscle and avoid or limit infarction. The absence of serum cardiac biomarkers confirms this.

In addition to ST segment elevation, a pathologic Q wave may be seen on the ECG in patients with MI (Fig. 35-29, *C*). A physiologic Q wave is the first negative deflection (wave) following the P wave. It is normally very short and narrow (Fig. 35-9 and Table 35-2). A pathologic Q wave that develops during MI is wide (greater than 0.03 second in duration) and deep (greater than or equal to 25% of the height of the R wave).[1,7] This is referred to as a *Q wave MI.* The pathologic Q wave may remain on the ECG indefinitely.

T wave inversion related to MI occurs within hours following the event and may persist for months. The ECG changes seen in injury and MI reflect electrical disturbances in the heart cells caused by a prolonged lack of blood and $O_2$ leading to necrosis (Fig. 35-30).

### Patient Monitoring

Monitoring guidelines for patients who are suspected of having ACS include continuous, multilead ECG and ST segment monitoring.[3] The leads selected for monitoring should minimally include the leads that reflect the area of ischemia, injury, or infarction.

## SYNCOPE

*Syncope,* a brief lapse in consciousness accompanied by a loss in postural tone (fainting), is a common diagnosis of patients coming to the emergency department. The causes of syncope can be cardiovascular or noncardiovascular. The most common cause of syncope is cardioneurogenic syncope, or "vasovagal" syncope (e.g., carotid sinus sensitivity). Other cardiovascular causes relate to dysrhythmias (e.g., tachycardias, bradycardias), prosthetic valve malfunction, pulmonary emboli, and HF. Noncardiovascular causes vary and include stress, hypoglycemia, dehydration, stroke, and seizure.[17]

A diagnostic workup for a patient with syncope from a suspected heart cause begins with ruling out structural and ischemic heart disease. This is done with echocardiography and stress testing. In the older patient, who is more likely to have structural and ischemic heart disease, EPS is used to diagnose atrial and ventricular tachydysrhythmias and conduction disturbances causing bradydysrhythmias, all of which can cause syncope. These problems can be treated with antidysrhythmia drug therapy, pacemakers, ICDs, and/or catheter ablation therapy.

In patients without structural heart disease or in whom EPS testing is not diagnostic, the *head-up tilt-test* may be performed. Normally, an upright position results in gravity displacing 300 to 800 mL of blood to the lower extremities. Specialized nerve fibers called mechanoreceptors are located throughout the vascular system. These respond to the increased blood volume by starting a reflex increase in sympathetic stimulation and decrease in parasympathetic output. The end results are a slight increase in HR and diastolic BP, and a slight decrease in systolic BP.[18]

In cardioneurogenic syncope, the increase in venous pooling that occurs in the upright position reduces venous return to the heart. This results in a sudden, compensatory increase in ventricular contraction. This is mistaken by the brain as a hypertensive state, and consequently sympathetic stimulation is withdrawn. This produces a paradoxical vasodilation and bradycardia (vasovagal response). The end results are bradycardia, hypotension, cerebral hypoperfusion, and syncope.

In the head-up tilt-test the patient is placed on a table supported by a belt across the torso and feet. Baseline ECG, BP, and HR are obtained in the horizontal position. Next, the table is tilted 60 to 80 degrees and the patient is kept in this upright position for 20 to 60 minutes. ECG and HR are recorded continuously and BP is measured every 3 minutes throughout the test.

If the patient's BP and HR responses are abnormal and clinical symptoms are reproduced (e.g., faintness), the test is considered positive. If after 30 minutes there is no response, the table is returned to the horizontal position and an IV infusion of low-dose isoproterenol may be started in an attempt to provoke a response.

Additional diagnostic tests for syncope can include various recording devices (e.g., Holter monitor or event monitor/loop recorder, which are discussed in Chapter 31 and Table 31-6), blood volume determination, hemodynamic testing, and autonomic reflex testing. About 30% of those who have one episode of syncope experience a recurrence. The underlying cause of syncope and the patient's age and co-morbidities affect the patient's treatment and prognosis.[18]

## CASE STUDY

### *Dysrhythmia and Cardiac Arrest*

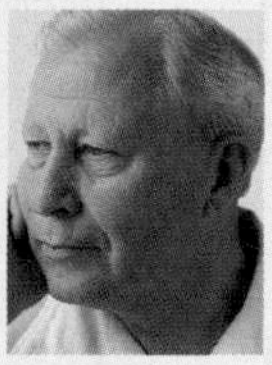

(©iStockphoto/ Thinkstock)

**Patient Profile**

J.M., a 68-yr-old white, retired postal worker, was admitted to the telemetry unit with a diagnosis of acute decompensated heart failure (HF). He experienced a cardiac arrest (pulseless ventricular tachycardia [VT]) and was successfully defibrillated after one shock. He is transferred to the cardiac care unit. J.M. is awake but lethargic and responds appropriately to questions.

**Subjective Data**

- History of hypertension, coronary artery disease, two MIs, and chronic HF
- Reports shortness of breath at rest and even in an upright position

**Objective Data**

***Physical Examination***

- Appears weak, anxious
- BP 102/60 mm Hg, pulse 70/min, respirations 26/min
- Lungs: bilateral coarse crackles in the bases
- Heart: $S_3$ gallop at apex

***Diagnostic Studies***

- Echocardiogram: severe left ventricular dysfunction with ejection fraction of 24%
- Serum potassium: 2.9 mEq/L (2.9 mmol/L)
- Serum cardiac biomarkers: negative
- Serum b-type natriuretic peptide (BNP): 1852 pg/mL

**Interprofessional Care**

- Continuous ECG monitoring

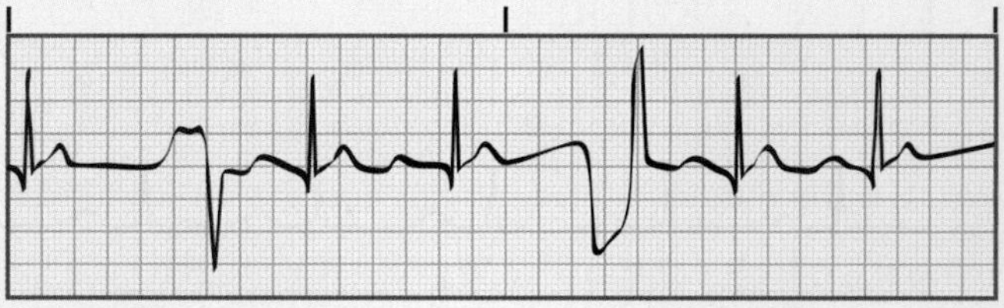

- Amiodarone infusion
- Cardiac rehabilitation consult
- Dietary consult

**Discussion Questions**

1. Why is J.M. at risk for sudden cardiac death?
2. Explain the rationale for using amiodarone after cardiac arrest.
3. What methods are used to assess the effectiveness of the antidysrhythmia therapy?
4. Interpret the rhythm strip.
5. Explain the significance of the diagnostic studies and other interprofessional care orders.
6. Why would J.M. be a candidate for CRT and an ICD?
7. ***Priority Decision:*** Based on the assessment data provided, what are the priority nursing diagnoses?
8. ***Priority Decision:*** Based on these nursing diagnoses, what are the priority nursing interventions for J.M.?
9. ***Teamwork and Collaboration:*** Which tasks could be delegated to unlicensed assistive personnel (UAP)?
10. ***Evidence-Based Practice:*** Once J.M. is stable, he is scheduled for the insertion of a CRT/ICD. On your rounds, he asks you why he needs two devices.

Answers available at *http://evolve.elsevier.com/Lewis/medsurg.*

## BRIDGE TO NCLEX EXAMINATION

The number of the question corresponds to the same-numbered outcome at the beginning of the chapter.

**1.** A patient admitted with ACS has continuous ECG monitoring. An examination of the rhythm strip reveals the following characteristics: atrial rate 74 beats/min and regular; ventricular rate 62 beats/min and irregular; P wave normal shape; PR interval lengthens progressively until a P wave is not conducted; QRS normal shape. The *priority* nursing intervention would be to
   **a.** perform synchronized cardioversion.
   **b.** administer epinephrine 1 mg IV push.
   **c.** observe for symptoms of hypotension or angina.
   **d.** apply transcutaneous pacemaker pads on the patient.

**2.** The nurse is monitoring the ECG of a patient admitted with ACS. Which ECG characteristics would be *most* suggestive of myocardial ischemia?
   **a.** Sinus rhythm with a pathologic Q wave
   **b.** Sinus rhythm with an elevated ST segment
   **c.** Sinus rhythm with a depressed ST segment
   **d.** Sinus rhythm with premature atrial contractions

**3.** The ECG monitor of a patient in the cardiac care unit after an MI indicates ventricular bigeminy with a rate of 50 beats/min. The nurse would anticipate
   **a.** performing defibrillation.
   **b.** treating with IV amiodarone.
   **c.** inserting a temporary transvenous pacemaker.
   **d.** assessing the patient's response to the dysrhythmia.

**4.** The nurse prepares a patient for synchronized cardioversion knowing that cardioversion differs from defibrillation in that
  **a.** defibrillation requires a lower dose of electrical energy.
  **b.** cardioversion is indicated to treat atrial bradydysrhythmias.
  **c.** defibrillation is synchronized to deliver a shock during the QRS complex.
  **d.** patients should be sedated if cardioversion is done on a nonemergency basis.

**5.** Which patient teaching points should the nurse include when providing discharge instructions to a patient with a new permanent pacemaker and the caregiver *(select all that apply)*?
  **a.** Avoid or limit air travel.
  **b.** Take and record a daily pulse rate.
  **c.** Obtain and wear a Medic Alert ID device at all times.
  **d.** Avoid lifting arm on the side of the pacemaker above shoulder.
  **e.** Avoid microwave ovens because they interfere with pacemaker function.

**6.** Important teaching for the patient scheduled for a radiofrequency catheter ablation procedure includes explaining that
  **a.** ventricular bradycardia may be induced and treated during the procedure.
  **b.** a catheter will be placed in both femoral arteries to allow double-catheter use.
  **c.** the procedure will destroy areas of the conduction system that are causing rapid heart rhythms.
  **d.** a general anesthetic will be given to prevent the awareness of any "sudden cardiac death" experiences.

1. c, 2. c, 3. d, 4. d, 5. b, c, d, 6. c

For rationales to these answers and even more NCLEX review questions, visit *http://evolve.elsevier.com/Lewis/medsurg.*

## EVOLVE WEBSITE

http://evolve.elsevier.com/Lewis/medsurg

**Review Questions (Online Only)**

**Key Points**

**Answer Keys for Questions**

- Rationales for Bridge to NCLEX Examination Questions
- Answer Guidelines for Case Study on p. 778

**Case Study**

- Patient With Atrial Fibrillation

**Conceptual Care Map Creator**

**Audio Glossary**

**Content Updates**

## REFERENCES


1. Wesley K: *Huszar's basic dysrhythmias and acute coronary syndrome,* ed 4, St Louis, 2011, Mosby Jems.
2. Patton KT, Thibodeau GA: *Anatomy and physiology,* ed 8, St Louis, 2013, Mosby.
*3. American Association of Critical-Care Nurses: AACN practice alert: ST segment monitoring. Retrieved from *www.aacn.org/wd/practice/docs/practicealerts/st-segment-monitoring.pdf?menu=aboutus.*
*4. American Association of Critical-Care Nurses: AACN practice alert: dysrhythmia monitoring. Retrieved from *www.aacn.org/wd/practice/docs/practicealerts/dysrhythmia-monitoring.pdf?menu=aboutus.*
5. Lehne RA: *Pharmacology for nursing care,* ed 8, St Louis, 2013, Saunders.
*6. Page RL, Joglar JA, Caldwell MA, et al: 2015 ACC/AHA/HRS Guideline for the management of adult patients with supraventricular tachycardia: executive summary, *Circulation* 133:e471, 2016.
7. Alspach JG: *Core curriculum for critical care nursing,* ed 6, St Louis, 2011, Saunders.
*8. January CT, Wann LS, Albert JS, et al: 2014 AHA/ACC/HRS guideline for the management of patients with atrial fibrillation: executive summary: a report of the American College of Cardiology/American Heart Association Task Force on Practice Guidelines and the Heart Rhythm Society, *J Am Coll Cardiol* 64(21):e1, 2014.
9. Go AS, Mozaffarian D, Roger VL, et al: Heart disease and stroke statistics—2013 update: a report from the American Heart Association, *Circulation* 127:e6, 2013.
10. FDA U.S. Food and Drug Administration: WATCHMAN LAA Closure Technology—P130013. Retrieved from *www.fda.gov/MedicalDevices/ProductsandMedicalProcedures/DeviceApprovalsandClearances/Recently-ApprovedDevices/ucm440621.htm.*
11. Sinz E, Navarro K, Soderberg ES, editors: *Advanced cardiovascular life support: provider manual,* Dallas, 2011, American Heart Association.
*12. Tracy CM, Epstein AE, Darbar D, et al: 2012 ACCF/AHA/HRS focused update of the 2008 guidelines for device-based therapy of cardiac rhythm abnormalities: a report of the American College of Cardiology Foundation/American Heart Association Task Force on Practice Guidelines, *Circulation* 126:1784, 2012.
*13. Burke MC, Gold MR, Knight BP: Safety and efficacy of the totally subcutaneous implantable defibrillator: 2-year results from a pooled analysis of the IDE study and EFFORTLESS registry, *J Am Coll Cardiol* 65(16):1605, 2015.
*14. Dunbar SB, Dougherty CM, Sears SF, et al: Educational and psychological interventions to improve outcomes for recipients of implantable cardioverter defibrillators and their families: a scientific statement from the American Heart Association, *Circulation* 126:2146, 2012.
15. Burri H, Deharo J-C, Israel C: *The EHRA book of pacemaker, ICD, and CRT troubleshooting: case-based learning with multiple-choice questions,* Oxford, United Kingdom, 2015, Oxford University Press.
*16. Knops RE, Tjong FV, Neuzil P, et al: Chronic performance of a leadless cardiac pacemaker: 1-year follow-up of the LEADLESS trial, *J Am Coll Cardiol* 65(15):1497, 2015.
17. McAlister FA, Ezekowitz J, Dryden DM, et al: Cardiac resynchronization therapy and implantable cardiac defibrillators in left ventricular systolic dysfunction, AHRQ Pub No 07-E009. Retrieved from *http://archive.ahrq.gov/downloads/pub/evidence/pdf/defib/defib.pdf.* (Classic)
18. Cleveland Clinic: Syncope. Retrieved from *http://my.clevelandclinic.org/services/heart/disorders/syncope.*

*Evidence-based information for clinical practice.

# 36

# Inflammatory and Structural Heart Disorders

*Nancy Kupper, De Ann F. Mitchell*

*A kind heart is a fountain of gladness, making everything in its vicinity freshen into smiles.*

***Washington Irving***

http://evolve.elsevier.com/Lewis/medsurg/

## LEARNING OUTCOMES

1. Differentiate the etiology, pathophysiology, and clinical manifestations of infective endocarditis and pericarditis.
2. Describe the interprofessional care and nursing management of the patient with infective endocarditis and pericarditis.
3. Describe the etiology, pathophysiology, and clinical manifestations of myocarditis.
4. Describe the interprofessional care and nursing management of the patient with myocarditis.
5. Differentiate the etiology, pathophysiology, and clinical manifestations of rheumatic fever and rheumatic heart disease.
6. Describe the interprofessional care and nursing management of the patient with rheumatic fever and rheumatic heart disease.
7. Relate the pathophysiology to the clinical manifestations and diagnostic studies for the various types of valvular heart disease.
8. Describe the interprofessional care and nursing management of the patient with valvular heart disease.
9. Relate the pathophysiology to the clinical manifestations and diagnostic studies for the different types of cardiomyopathy.
10. Compare the nursing and interprofessional management of patients with different types of cardiomyopathy.

## KEY TERMS

aortic regurgitation (AR), p. 792
aortic stenosis (AS), p. 792
cardiac tamponade, p. 785
cardiomyopathy (CMP), p. 796
chronic constrictive pericarditis, p. 787
dilated cardiomyopathy, p. 796
hypertrophic cardiomyopathy, p. 798
infective endocarditis (IE), p. 780
mitral valve prolapse (MVP), p. 791
myocarditis, p. 787
pericardiocentesis, p. 786
pericarditis, p. 784
regurgitation, p. 791
rheumatic fever (RF), p. 788
rheumatic heart disease, p. 788
stenosis, p. 791

This chapter describes the pathophysiology and management of patients experiencing select inflammatory and structural heart disorders. In addition, the interprofessional care and nursing management of these patients is presented.

## INFLAMMATORY DISORDERS OF HEART

## INFECTIVE ENDOCARDITIS

**Infective endocarditis (IE)** is an infection of the endocardial layer of the heart. The *endocardium* is the innermost layer of the heart (Fig. 36-1) and heart valves. Therefore IE affects the valves. Treatment of IE with antibiotic therapy has improved the prognosis of this disease. Although relatively uncommon, an estimated 10,000 to 15,000 new cases of IE are diagnosed in the United States each year.[1]

### Classification

IE was traditionally classified as subacute or acute. The *subacute form* affects those with preexisting valve disease and has a clinical course that may extend over months. In contrast, the *acute form* affects those with healthy valves and manifests as a rapidly progressive illness. Today IE is more often classified based on the cause (e.g., IV drug abuse IE [IVDA IE], fungal endocarditis) or site of involvement (e.g., prosthetic valve endocarditis [PVE]).

### Etiology and Pathophysiology

The most common causative organisms of IE, *Staphylococcus aureus* and *Streptococcus viridans,* are bacterial. Other possible pathogens include fungi and viruses.[2] IE occurs when blood flow within the heart allows the causative organism to infect previously damaged valves or other endothelial surfaces. IE can occur in persons with a variety of underlying cardiac and noncardiac conditions (Table 36-1).

*Vegetations,* the primary lesions of IE, consist of fibrin, leukocytes, platelets, and microbes that stick to the valve surface or endocardium (Fig. 36-2). The loss of parts of these fragile vegetations into the circulation results in *emboli.* Many persons with IE will develop systemic embolization. This occurs when left-sided heart vegetation moves to various organs (e.g., brain, kidneys, spleen) and to the extremities, causing limb infarction.

Reviewed by Vickie Lee Doscher, MSN, FNP-C, APRN, Family Nurse Practitioner, Chesapeake Regional Medical Center, Chesapeake, Virginia; Tracy H. Knoll, RN, MSN, Nursing Instructor, Chamberlain College of Nursing, St. Louis, Missouri; and Rebecca Personett, RN, PhD, NEA-BC, Professor of Nursing, North Central Texas College, Gainesville, Texas and Brookhaven College, Dallas, Texas.

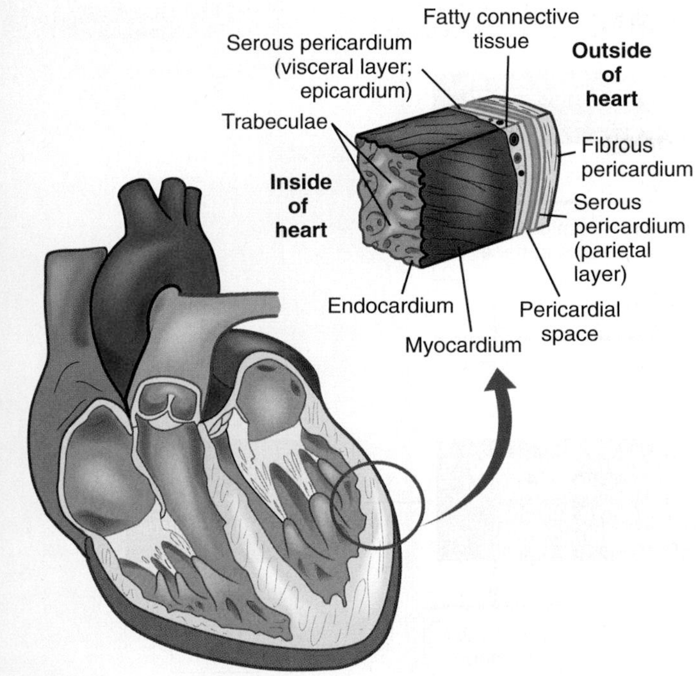


**FIG. 36-1** Layers of the heart muscle and pericardium. The section of the heart wall shows the fibrous pericardium, the parietal and visceral layers of the serous pericardium (with the pericardial sac between them), the myocardium, and the endocardium. (Modified from Patton KT, Thibodeau GA: *The human body in health and disease,* ed 5, St Louis, 2010, Mosby.)

| TABLE 36-1 **Risk Factors for Endocarditis*** |
|---|
| **Cardiac Conditions** |
| • Prior endocarditis |
| • Prosthetic heart valve(s) |
| • Acquired valve disease (e.g., mitral valve prolapse with regurgitation, calcified aortic stenosis) |
| • Heart lesions (e.g., ventricular septal defect, asymmetric septal hypertrophy) |
| • Rheumatic heart disease (e.g., mitral valve regurgitation) |
| • Congenital heart disease |
| • Pacemaker |
| • Marfan's syndrome |
| • Cardiomyopathy |
| **Noncardiac Conditions** |
| • Hospital-acquired bacteremia |
| • IV drug abuse |
| **Procedure-Associated Risks** |
| • Intravascular devices (e.g., central venous catheter) |
| • Procedures listed in Table 36-2 |

*List is not all-inclusive.

Right-sided heart lesions move to the lungs, resulting in pulmonary emboli.

The infection may spread locally and damage the valves or their supporting structures. This causes dysrhythmias, valve dysfunction, and eventual invasion of the myocardium, leading to heart failure (HF), sepsis, and heart block (Fig. 36-3).

At one time rheumatic heart disease was the most common cause of IE. Now it accounts for less than 20% of cases. The main contributing factors to IE include (1) aging (more than 50% of older people have calcified aortic stenosis [AS]), (2) IVDA, (3) use of prosthetic valves, (4) use of intravascular devices

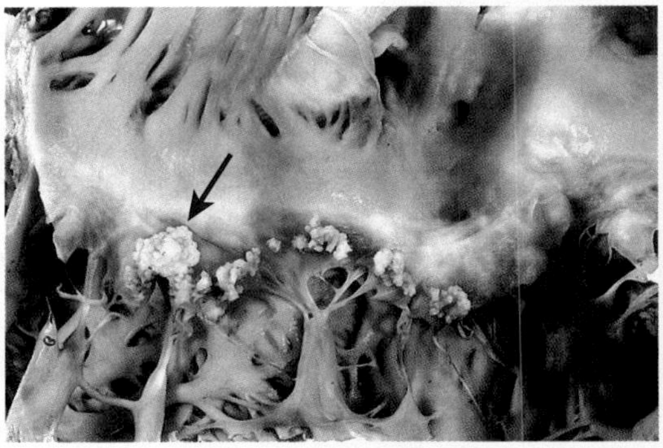

**FIG. 36-2** Bacterial endocarditis of the mitral valve. The valve is covered with large, irregular vegetations *(arrow).* (From Damjanov I, Linder J: *Pathology: a color atlas,* St Louis, 2000, Mosby.)

resulting in health care–associated infections (e.g., methicillin-resistant *S. aureus* [MRSA]), and (5) renal dialysis.[1]

## Clinical Manifestations

The clinical manifestations of IE are nonspecific and can involve multiple organ systems. Symptoms include fever, chills, weakness, malaise, fatigue, and anorexia. Arthralgias, myalgias, back pain, abdominal discomfort, weight loss, headache, and clubbing of fingers may occur in subacute forms of IE. Fever may be absent in older adults or those who are immunocompromised.

Vascular signs of IE include *splinter hemorrhages* (black longitudinal streaks) that may occur in the nail beds. Petechiae may result from fragmentation and microembolization of vegetative lesions. They can occur on the conjunctivae, lips, buccal mucosa, and palate and over the ankles, feet, and antecubital and popliteal areas. *Osler's nodes* (painful, tender, red or purple, pea-size lesions) may be found on the fingertips or toes. *Janeway's lesions* (flat, painless, small, red spots) may be seen on the fingertips, palms, soles of feet, and toes. Eye examination may reveal hemorrhagic retinal lesions called *Roth's spots.*

The onset of a new or worsening systolic murmur is noted in most patients with IE. The aortic and mitral valves are most often affected. Murmurs are usually absent in tricuspid endocarditis because right-sided heart sounds are too low to be heard. HF occurs in up to 80% of patients with aortic valve endocarditis and approximately 50% of patients with mitral valve endocarditis.[3]

Clinical signs secondary to embolization may be present in various body organs. Embolization to the spleen may cause sharp, left upper quadrant pain and splenomegaly, local tenderness, and abdominal rigidity. Embolization to the kidneys may cause flank pain, hematuria, and renal failure. Emboli may lodge in small peripheral blood vessels of the arms and legs and may cause ischemia and gangrene. Embolization to the brain may cause neurologic damage, resulting in hemiplegia, ataxia, aphasia, visual changes, and change in mental status. Pulmonary emboli may occur in right-sided endocarditis and cause dyspnea, chest pain, hemoptysis, and respiratory arrest.

## Diagnostic Studies

The patient's health history is important in assessing IE. Ask patients if they have had any recent (within the past 3 to 6 months) dental, urologic, surgical, or gynecologic procedures, including normal or abnormal obstetric delivery. Note any previous history of IVDA, heart disease, recent heart

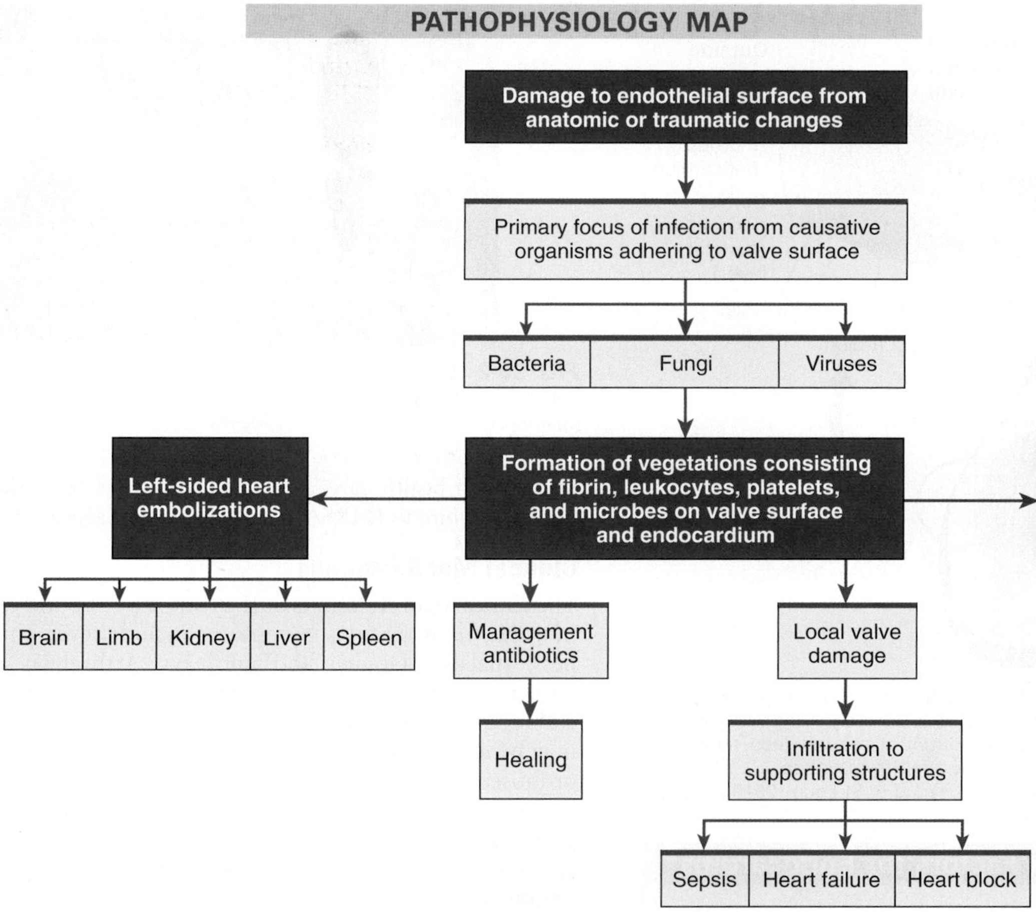


**FIG. 36-3** Pathogenesis of infective endocarditis.

catheterization, heart surgery, intravascular device placement, renal dialysis, or infections (e.g., skin, respiratory, urinary tract).

Three blood cultures drawn over a period of 1 hour from three different sites will be positive in most patients.[3] Culture-negative endocarditis is often associated with antibiotic usage within the previous 2 weeks, or results from a pathogen not easily detected by standard culture tests. Cultures that are negative should be kept for 3 weeks if the clinical diagnosis remains IE because of the possibility of slow-growing organisms. A mild leukocytosis occurs in acute IE (uncommon in subacute). The erythrocyte sedimentation rate (ESR) and C-reactive protein (CRP) levels may also be elevated.

Major criteria to diagnose IE include at least two of the following: two positive blood cultures 12 hours apart, nonvalvular regurgitation, or intracardiac mass or vegetation noted on echocardiography.[3] Echocardiography (e.g., transesophageal echocardiogram, two- or three-dimensional [2-D or 3-D] transthoracic echocardiogram) is critical in the diagnostic workup of a patient suspected of having IE and should be done in a timely manner.[3]

A chest x-ray is done to detect *cardiomegaly* (an enlarged heart). An electrocardiogram (ECG) may show first- or second-degree atrioventricular (AV) block. Heart block occurs because the heart valves lie close to conductive tissue, especially the AV node. Heart catheterization may be used to assess valve function and the coronary arteries when surgery is being considered.[4]

## Interprofessional Care

**Prophylactic Treatment.** The situations and conditions requiring antibiotic prophylaxis are presented in Table 36-2.

**Drug Therapy.** Accurate identification of the causative organism is the key to successful treatment of IE. Long-term treatment is necessary to kill dormant bacteria within the valvular vegetations. Complete removal of the organism generally takes weeks, and relapses are common.[3]

Patients are hospitalized and IV antibiotic therapy, based on blood cultures, is started. The effectiveness of therapy is assessed with subsequent blood cultures. Cultures that remain positive indicate inadequate or inappropriate selection of antibiotic, aortic root or myocardial abscess, or the wrong diagnosis (e.g., an infection elsewhere).

Fungal endocarditis and PVE respond poorly to antibiotic therapy alone. Early valve replacement followed by prolonged (6 weeks or more) antibiotics is needed in these situations. Valve replacement (discussed later in this chapter) has become an important adjunct procedure in the management of IE.[3]

Fever may persist for several days after treatment has been started. It can be treated with aspirin, acetaminophen (Tylenol), fluids, and rest. Complete bed rest is usually not needed unless the temperature remains elevated, or there are signs of HF. Endocarditis with HF responds poorly to drug therapy and valve replacement and is often life threatening.

**! SAFETY ALERT Communicating Test Results**

- The results of a blood culture on a patient diagnosed with IE indicate that the causative organism is not susceptible to the ordered antibiotic.
- Immediately share this information with the HCP.
- A National Patient Safety Goal stresses the importance of communicating critical test results to the right HCP in a timely manner.

**TABLE 36-2 Antibiotic Prophylaxis to Prevent Endocarditis**

**Target Groups for Prophylactic Antibiotics**

*People with the following heart conditions should receive prophylactic antibiotics when they have the conditions or procedures listed below.*

- Prosthetic heart valve or prosthetic material used to repair heart valve
- Previous history of infectious endocarditis
- Congenital heart disease (CHD)*
  - Unrepaired cyanotic CHD (including palliative shunts and conduits)
  - Repaired congenital heart defect with prosthetic material or device for 6 mo after the procedure
  - Repaired CHD with residual defects at the site or adjacent to the site of prosthetic patch or prosthetic device
- Heart transplantation recipients who develop heart valve disease

**Conditions or Procedures Requiring Antibiotic Prophylaxis***

*When the target groups have the following conditions or procedures, they need prophylactic antibiotics.*

- Oral
  - Dental manipulation involving the gums or roots of the teeth
  - Dental manipulation involving puncture of the oral mucosa
- Respiratory
  - Respiratory tract incisions (e.g., biopsy)
  - Tonsillectomy and adenoidectomy
- Surgery
  - Procedures that involve infected skin, skin structures, or musculoskeletal tissue

Sources: Habib G, Hoen B, Tornos P, et al: Guidelines on the prevention, diagnosis and treatment of infective endocarditis (new version 2009): the Task Force on the Prevention, Diagnosis, and Treatment of Infective Endocarditis of the European Society of Cardiology, *Eur Heart J* 30:2369, 2009. Nishimura RA, Otto CM, Bonow RO, et al: 2014 AHA/ACC Guidelines for the management of patients with valvular heart disease: executive summary: a report of the American College of Cardiology/American Heart Association Task Force on Practice Guidelines, *Circulation* 129:2440, 2014.
*Except for the conditions listed above, prophylaxis is no longer recommended for any form of CHD or for patients undergoing gastrointestinal or genitourinary tract procedures.

## NURSING MANAGEMENT: INFECTIVE ENDOCARDITIS

### Nursing Assessment

Subjective and objective data that you should obtain from a patient with IE are found in Table 36-3. Assess vital signs together with heart sounds to detect a murmur, a change in a preexisting murmur, and extra sounds (e.g., $S_3$).

*Arthralgia* is common in IE. It may involve multiple joints and be accompanied by myalgias. Assess the patient for joint tenderness, decreased range of motion (ROM), and muscle tenderness. Examine the patient for petechiae, splinter hemorrhages, and Osler's nodes. Complete a general systems assessment to determine any hemodynamic or embolic complications.

### Nursing Diagnoses

Nursing diagnoses for the patient with IE may include, but are not limited to, the following:

- Decreased cardiac output *related to* altered heart rhythm, valvular insufficiency, and fluid overload
- Activity intolerance *related to* generalized weakness, arthralgia, and alteration in $O_2$ transport secondary to valvular dysfunction

Additional information on nursing diagnoses is presented in eNursing Care Plan 36-1 available on the website for this chapter.

**TABLE 36-3 Nursing Assessment**

***Infective Endocarditis***

**Subjective Data**

***Important Health Information***

*Past health history:* Valvular, congenital, or syphilitic heart disease, including valve repair or replacement. Previous endocarditis, childbirth, staphylococcal or streptococcal infections, hospital-acquired bacteremia

*Medications:* Immunosuppressive therapy

*Surgery or other treatments:* Recent obstetric or gynecologic procedures. Invasive procedures, including catheterization, cystoscopy. Recent dental or surgical procedures, GI procedures (e.g., endoscopy)

***Functional Health Patterns***

*Health perception–health management:* IV drug abuse, alcohol abuse. Malaise

*Nutritional-metabolic:* Weight gain or loss, anorexia. Chills, diaphoresis

*Elimination:* Bloody urine

*Activity-exercise:* Exercise intolerance, generalized weakness, fatigue. Cough, dyspnea on exertion, orthopnea, palpitations

*Sleep-rest:* Night sweats

*Cognitive-perceptual:* Chest, back, or abdominal pain. Headache, joint tenderness, muscle tenderness

**Objective Data**

***General***

Fever

***Integumentary***

Osler's nodes on extremities, splinter hemorrhages under nail beds, Janeway's lesions on fingertips, palms, soles of feet, and toes. Petechiae of skin, mucous membranes, or conjunctivae. Purpura, peripheral edema, finger clubbing

***Respiratory***

Tachypnea, crackles

***Cardiovascular***

Dysrhythmia, tachycardia, new murmurs, $S_3$, $S_4$. Retinal hemorrhages

***Possible Diagnostic Findings***

Leukocytosis, anemia, ↑ ESR, ↑ CRP and cardiac biomarkers. Positive blood cultures, hematuria. Echocardiogram showing chamber enlargement, valvular dysfunction, and vegetations. Chest x-ray showing cardiomegaly and pulmonary infiltrates. ECG demonstrating ischemia and conduction defects. Signs of systemic embolization or pulmonary embolism

*CRP*, C-reactive protein; *ESR*, erythrocyte sedimentation rate.

### Planning

The overall goals for the patient with IE include (1) normal or baseline heart function, (2) performance of activities of daily living (ADLs) without fatigue, and (3) knowledge of the therapeutic regimen to prevent recurrence of endocarditis.

### Nursing Implementation

**Health Promotion.** The incidence of IE can be decreased by identifying individuals who are at risk for the disease (Tables 36-1 and 36-2). Assessment of the patient's history and an understanding of the disease are crucial for planning and implementing appropriate health promotion strategies.

Teaching the patient at high risk for IE helps to reduce the incidence and recurrence of the disease. Teaching is important for the patient's understanding of and adherence to the treatment regimen. Tell the patient to avoid people with infections, especially upper respiratory tract infections, and to report cold, flu, and cough symptoms. Stress the importance of avoiding excessive fatigue, and the need to plan rest periods before and after activity. Good oral hygiene, including daily care and regular dental visits, is critical.[3]

Tell the patient to inform HCPs performing certain invasive procedures of the history of IE. Be certain the patient understands the importance of prophylactic antibiotic therapy before certain invasive procedures. Refer the patient with a history of IVDA for drug rehabilitation.

◆ **Ambulatory Care.** A patient with IE has many problems that require nursing management (see eNursing Care Plan 36-1 on the website for this chapter). IE generally requires treatment with antibiotics for 4 to 6 weeks. After initial treatment in the hospital, the patient may continue treatment at home if hemodynamically stable and adherent. Assess the home setting for adequate support. Patients who receive outpatient IV antibiotics require vigilant home nursing care.

Assessment findings are often nonspecific (Table 36-3) but can help with the treatment plan. Fever, chronic or intermittent, is a common early sign. Tell the patient and caregiver about the importance of monitoring body temperature. Persistent temperature elevations may mean that the antibiotic is ineffective. Patients with IE are at risk for life-threatening complications, such as stroke, pulmonary edema, and HF. Teach patients and caregivers to recognize signs and symptoms of these complications (e.g., change in mental status, dyspnea, chest pain, unexplained weight gain).

The patient with IE needs adequate periods of physical and emotional rest. Bed rest may be necessary when the patient has fever or complications (e.g., heart damage). Otherwise the patient may walk and perform moderate activity. To prevent problems related to decreased mobility, teach the patient to wear elastic compression stockings, perform ROM exercises, and deep breathe and cough every 2 hours. The patient may experience anxiety and fear associated with the illness. You must recognize this and begin strategies to help the patient cope with the illness.

Monitor laboratory data to determine the effectiveness of the antibiotic therapy. Ongoing monitoring of the patient's blood cultures is necessary to ensure destruction of the infecting organism. Assess IV lines for patency and signs of complications (e.g., phlebitis). Give antibiotics as ordered, and monitor the patient for any adverse drug reactions.

Management also focuses on teaching the patient and caregiver the nature of the disease and on reducing the risk of reinfection. Explain to the patient the relationship of follow-up care, good nutrition and dental care, and early treatment of common infections (e.g., colds) to stay healthy. Teach the patient about symptoms that may indicate another infection (e.g., fever, fatigue, chills). Tell the patient to notify the HCP if any of these symptoms occur. Finally, tell the patient about the importance of prophylactic antibiotic therapy before certain invasive procedures (Table 36-2).

### ◆ Evaluation

The expected outcomes are that the patient with IE will

- Maintain adequate tissue and organ perfusion
- Maintain normal body temperature
- Report an increase in physical and emotional comfort

Additional information on expected outcomes for the patient with IE is presented in eNursing Care Plan 36-1 on the website for this chapter.

## ACUTE PERICARDITIS

**Pericarditis** is a condition caused by inflammation of the pericardial sac (pericardium).The pericardium is composed of the inner serous membrane (visceral pericardium) and the outer fibrous (parietal) layer (Fig. 36-1). The pericardial space is the cavity between these two layers. Normally it contains 10 to 15 mL of serous fluid. The pericardium serves an anchoring function, provides lubrication to decrease friction between heart contractions, and helps to prevent excessive dilation of the heart during diastole. It may be congenitally absent or surgically removed.

### Etiology and Pathophysiology

Common causes of acute pericarditis are listed in Table 36-4. Most often the cause of acute pericarditis is *idiopathic* (unknown), with a variety of suspected viral causes. The coxsackievirus B is the most commonly identified virus.[5]

Pericarditis in the patient with an MI may be described as two distinct syndromes. The first is *acute pericarditis,* which may occur within the first 48 to 72 hours after an MI. The second is *Dressler syndrome* (late pericarditis), which occurs 4 to 6 weeks after an MI (see Chapter 33). An inflammatory response is the characteristic pathologic finding in acute pericarditis. There is an influx of neutrophils, increased pericardial vascularity, and eventually fibrin deposition on the epicardium (Fig. 36-4).

**TABLE 36-4 Common Causes of Pericarditis**

**Infectious**

- Viral: Coxsackie A and B virus, echovirus, adenovirus, mumps, hepatitis, Epstein-Barr, varicella zoster, human immunodeficiency virus
- Bacterial: Pneumococci, staphylococci, streptococci, *Neisseria gonorrhoeae, Legionella pneumophila, Mycobacterium tuberculosis,* septicemia from gram-negative organisms
- Fungal: *Histoplasma, Candida* species
- Others: Toxoplasmosis, Lyme disease

**Noninfectious**

- Renal failure
- Acute myocardial infarction
- Neoplasms: Lung cancer, breast cancer, leukemia, Hodgkin's lymphoma, non-Hodgkin's lymphoma
- Trauma: Thoracic surgery, pacemaker insertion, cardiac diagnostic procedures
- Radiation
- Dissecting aortic aneurysm
- Myxedema

**Hypersensitive or Autoimmune**

- Dressler syndrome
- Postpericardiotomy syndrome
- Rheumatic fever
- Drug reactions (e.g., procainamide, hydralazine)
- Rheumatologic diseases: Rheumatoid arthritis, systemic lupus erythematosus, systemic sclerosis (scleroderma), ankylosing spondylitis

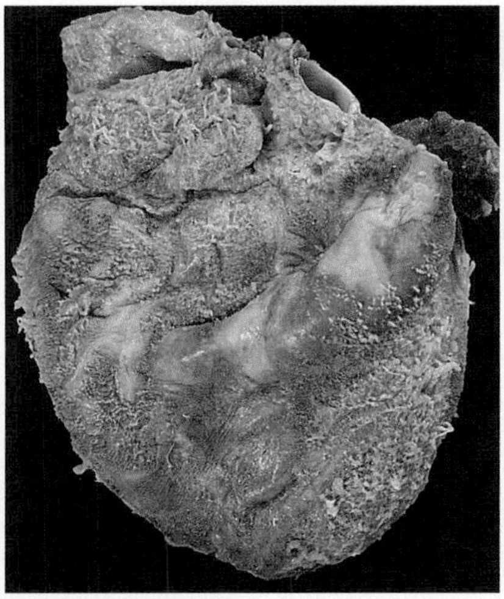

**FIG. 36-4** Acute pericarditis. Note shaggy coat of fibers covering surface of heart. (From Damjanov I, Linder J: *Pathology: a color atlas,* St Louis, 2000, Mosby.)

## Clinical Manifestations

In acute pericarditis, clinical symptoms include progressive, frequently severe, sharp chest pain. The pain is generally worse with deep inspiration and when lying flat. It is relieved by sitting up and leaning forward. The pain may radiate to the neck, arms, or left shoulder, making it difficult to differentiate from angina. One distinction is that the pain from pericarditis can be referred to the trapezius muscle (shoulder, upper back). The dyspnea that accompanies acute pericarditis is related to the patient's need to breathe in rapid, shallow breaths to avoid chest pain. Dyspnea may be aggravated by fever and anxiety.

The hallmark finding in acute pericarditis is the *pericardial friction rub.* The rub is a scratching, grating, high-pitched sound believed to result from friction between the roughened pericardial and epicardial surfaces. It is best heard with the stethoscope placed at the lower left sternal border of the chest with the patient leaning forward. Since it is difficult to tell a pericardial friction rub from a pleural friction rub, ask the patient to hold his or her breath. If you still hear the rub, then it is cardiac. Pericardial friction rubs may require frequent attempts to identify because they are often intermittent and short lived.

## Complications

Two major complications that may result from acute pericarditis are pericardial effusion and cardiac tamponade. *Pericardial effusion* is a build-up of fluid in the pericardium. It can occur rapidly (e.g., chest trauma) or slowly (e.g., tuberculosis pericarditis). Large effusions may compress nearby structures. Pulmonary tissue compression can cause cough, dyspnea, and tachypnea. Phrenic nerve compression can cause hiccups, and compression of the laryngeal nerve may result in hoarseness. Heart sounds are generally distant and muffled, although BP is usually maintained.

**Cardiac tamponade** develops as the pericardial effusion increases in volume. This results in compression of the heart. The speed of fluid accumulation affects the severity of clinical manifestations. Cardiac tamponade can occur acutely (e.g., rupture of heart, trauma) or subacutely (e.g., secondary to renal failure, malignancy).

The patient with cardiac tamponade may report chest pain and is often confused, anxious, and restless. As the compression of the heart increases, there is decreased cardiac output (CO), muffled heart sounds, and narrowed pulse pressure. The patient develops tachypnea and tachycardia. Neck veins are usually markedly distended because of increased jugular venous pressure.

*Pulsus paradoxus,* which may be present, is a decrease in systolic BP during inspiration that is exaggerated in cardiac tamponade (Table 36-5). In a patient with a slow onset of a cardiac tamponade, dyspnea may be the only clinical manifestation.

**TABLE 36-5 Measurement of Pulsus Paradoxus**

1. Position the patient in a semirecumbent position.
2. Instruct patient to breathe normally.*
3. Using a manually operated BP cuff, determine systolic BP.
4. Inflate BP cuff at least 20 mm Hg above systolic BP.
5. Deflate cuff slowly until you hear sounds throughout the respiratory cycle (inspiration and expiration), and note the pressure.
6. Determine the difference between the measurements taken in steps 4 and 5. This will equal the amount of paradox:

| | |
|---|---|
| Sounds heard on expiration at | 110 mm Hg |
| Sounds heard throughout cycle at | –82 mm Hg |
| Amount of paradox | 28 mm Hg |

The difference is normally <10 mm Hg. If the difference is >10 mm Hg, cardiac tamponade may be present.

*Ask the patient to breathe slowly and deeply to reveal this finding when pulsus paradoxus is not severe.

## Diagnostic Studies

The ECG is useful in the diagnosis of acute pericarditis, with changes noted in approximately 90% of cases. The most sensitive ECG changes include diffuse (widespread) ST segment elevations. This reflects the abnormal repolarization that develops secondary to the pericardial inflammation. You need to differentiate these changes from the ST changes seen in MI. (See Chapter 35 for more information on ECG monitoring.)

Echocardiographic findings are most useful in determining the presence of a pericardial effusion or cardiac tamponade. Methods such as Doppler imaging and color M-mode assess diastolic function and diagnose constrictive pericarditis (discussed later in the chapter). A CT scan and MRI provide for visualization of the pericardium and pericardial space. Chest x-ray findings are generally normal, but cardiomegaly may be seen in a patient who has a large pericardial effusion (Fig. 36-5).

Common laboratory findings include leukocytosis and elevation of CRP and ESR. Troponin levels may be elevated in patients with ST segment elevation and acute pericarditis, which could indicate concurrent heart damage. HIV and antinuclear antibody testing may be done. The fluid obtained during pericardiocentesis or the tissue from a pericardial biopsy may be studied to determine the cause of the pericarditis.

## Interprofessional Care

Management of acute pericarditis is aimed at identifying and treating the underlying problem and symptoms (Table 36-6). Antibiotics treat bacterial pericarditis, and nonsteroidal antiinflammatory drugs (NSAIDs) (e.g., salicylates [aspirin], ibuprofen) control the pain and inflammation. Corticosteroids are generally reserved for patients with pericarditis secondary to systemic lupus erythematosus, patients already taking corticosteroids for rheumatologic or other autoimmune conditions, or patients who do not respond to NSAIDs. They are used

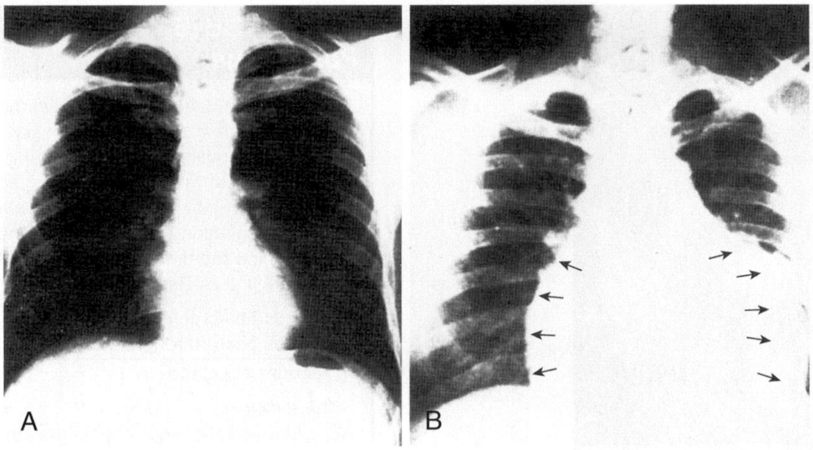


**FIG. 36-5** **A,** X-ray of a normal chest. **B,** Pericardial effusion is present, and the cardiac silhouette is enlarged with a globular shape *(arrows)*. (From Guzzetta CE, Dossey BM: *Cardiovascular nursing: holistic practice,* St Louis, 1992, Mosby.)

**TABLE 36-6 Interprofessional Care**

***Acute Pericarditis***

| Diagnostic Assessment | Management |
|---|---|
| • History and physical examination (assess for pericardial friction rub, pulsus paradoxus)<br>• Laboratory: CRP, ESR, white blood cell count<br>• Electrocardiogram<br>• Chest x-ray<br>• Echocardiogram<br>• CT scan<br>• MRI<br>• Pericardiocentesis, pericardial window<br>• Pericardial biopsy | • Treatment of underlying disease<br>• Bed rest<br>• Drug therapy<br>  • Nonsteroidal antiinflammatory drugs<br>  • Corticosteroids<br>• Pericardiocentesis (for tamponade)<br>• Pericardial window (for tamponade or ongoing pericardial effusion) |

*CRP,* C-reactive protein; *ESR,* erythrocyte sedimentation rate.

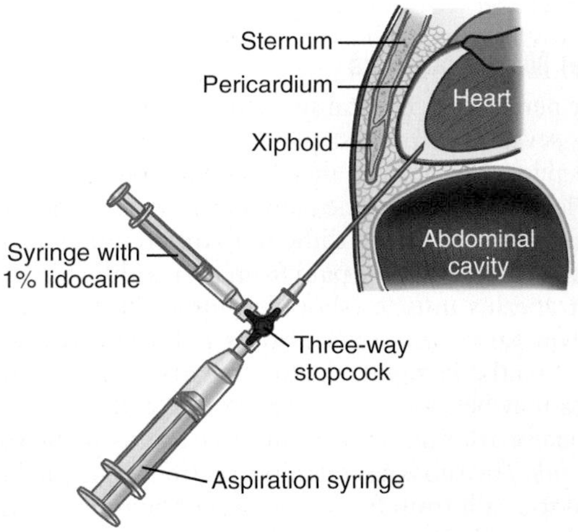


**FIG. 36-6** Pericardiocentesis performed under sterile conditions in conjunction with electrocardiogram (ECG) and hemodynamic measurements.

cautiously because of their numerous side effects (see Chapter 49). Colchicine, an antiinflammatory drug used for gout, can be used for patients who have recurrent pericarditis.[5]

**Pericardiocentesis** is usually done for pericardial effusion with acute cardiac tamponade, purulent pericarditis, and suspected neoplasm. Hemodynamic support for the patient being prepared for the pericardiocentesis may include giving volume expanders and inotropic agents (e.g., dopamine) and discontinuing any anticoagulants. The procedure is done rapidly and safely using a percutaneous approach that is guided by echocardiography (Fig. 36-6). A needle is inserted into the pericardial space to remove fluid for analysis and to relieve heart pressure. Complications from pericardiocentesis include dysrhythmias, further cardiac tamponade, pneumomediastinum, pneumothorax, myocardial laceration, and coronary artery laceration.

A *pericardial window* can be used for diagnosis or for drainage of excess fluid. This involves cutting a "window" or portion of the pericardium. This allows the fluid to drain continuously into the peritoneum or chest.

## ❖ NURSING MANAGEMENT: ACUTE PERICARDITIS

The management of the patient's pain and anxiety during acute pericarditis is your primary nursing consideration. Assess the pain to distinguish angina (myocardial ischemia) (see Table 33-7) from the pain of pericarditis. Pericarditis pain is usually located in the precordium or left trapezius region and has a sharp, pleuritic quality that increases with inspiration. Pain is often relieved when the patient sits up or leans forward and is worse when lying flat.

An ECG can help to distinguish the cause of pain. In acute pericarditis, there are diffuse ST segment changes. In myocardial ischemia, there are usually localized ST segment changes. In addition, in acute pericarditis serial ECGs do not show evolving changes such as those with MI.

Pain relief measures include keeping the patient on bed rest with the head of the bed raised to 45 degrees and providing an overbed table for support. Antiinflammatory drugs can help control the pain. However, because of the risk of gastrointestinal (GI) bleeding, give these drugs with food or milk and tell the patient to avoid alcohol. Other drugs, such as a proton pump inhibitor (e.g., pantoprazole [Protonix]), may be given to reduce stomach acid.

Anxiety-reducing measures for the patient with acute pericarditis include providing simple, complete explanations of all procedures and possible causes of the pain. These explanations are particularly important for the patient whose diagnosis of acute pericarditis is being established and for the patient who has previously experienced angina or an MI.

The patient with acute pericarditis is at risk for cardiac tamponade and decreased CO. Monitor for manifestations of tamponade and prepare for possible pericardiocentesis.

**CHECK YOUR PRACTICE**

You are assigned to a 58-yr-old male patient who had an MI 3 days ago. He has now developed pericarditis. When you are making your rounds, you assess that the patient is slightly confused, has a rapid heart rate, and has prominent neck veins.

- What should you do next?

## CHRONIC CONSTRICTIVE PERICARDITIS

### Etiology and Pathophysiology

**Chronic constrictive pericarditis** results from scarring of the pericardium with consequent loss of elasticity of the pericardial sac. It usually begins with an initial episode of acute pericarditis. It is characterized by fibrin deposition with a clinically undetected pericardial effusion. Reabsorption of the effusion slowly follows, with progression toward the chronic stage. This involves fibrous scarring, thickening of the pericardium from calcium deposition, and eventual destruction of the pericardial space. The fibrotic, thickened, and adherent pericardium encases the heart. This impairs the ability of the atria and ventricles to stretch adequately.

### Clinical Manifestations and Diagnostic Studies

Manifestations of chronic constrictive pericarditis occur over time and mimic those of HF and cor pulmonale. Decreased CO accounts for many of the clinical manifestations. These include dyspnea on exertion, peripheral edema, ascites, fatigue, anorexia, and weight loss. The most prominent finding on physical examination is jugular venous distention (JVD). Unlike with cardiac tamponade, the presence of pulsus paradoxus (greater than 10 mm Hg) is not common.

ECG changes are often nonspecific in chronic constrictive pericarditis. The heart on the chest x-ray may be normal or enlarged depending on the degree of pericardial thickening and the presence of a pericardial effusion. 2-D echocardiography findings may reveal a thickened pericardium but without a large pericardial effusion. CT and MRI provide measurement of pericardial thickness and assessment of diastolic filling patterns.

## NURSING AND INTERPROFESSIONAL MANAGEMENT: CHRONIC CONSTRICTIVE PERICARDITIS

Unless the patient is free of symptoms or the condition is inoperable, the treatment of choice for chronic constrictive pericarditis is a *pericardiectomy.* This involves complete resection of the pericardium through a median sternotomy with the use of cardiopulmonary bypass (see Chapter 33). Some patients show immediate improvement after, but others may take weeks. The prognosis improves when surgery is done before the patient becomes clinically unstable.

## MYOCARDITIS

### Etiology and Pathophysiology

**Myocarditis** is a focal or diffuse inflammation of the myocardium. Possible causes include viruses, bacteria, fungi, radiation therapy, and pharmacologic and chemical factors. Coxsackie A and B viruses are the most common causative agents. Autoimmune disorders (e.g., polymyositis) have been linked with the development of myocarditis. It may also be idiopathic. Myocarditis is one of the most common causes of dilated cardiomyopathy[6] (discussed later in this chapter).

When the myocardium becomes infected, the causative agent invades the myocytes and causes cellular damage and necrosis. The immune response is activated, and cytokines and $O_2$ free radicals are released. As the infection progresses, an autoimmune response is activated. This causes further destruction of myocytes. Myocarditis results in heart dysfunction.

### Clinical Manifestations

The clinical features of myocarditis are variable, ranging from a benign course without any overt symptoms to severe heart involvement or sudden cardiac death (SCD). Fever, fatigue, malaise, myalgias, pharyngitis, dyspnea, lymphadenopathy, and nausea and vomiting are early manifestations of the viral illness.

Early cardiac signs appear 7 to 10 days after viral infection. These include pleuritic chest pain with a pericardial friction rub and effusion because pericarditis often accompanies myocarditis. Late cardiac signs relate to the development of HF and may include an $S_3$ heart sound, crackles, JVD, syncope, peripheral edema, and angina.

### Diagnostic Studies and Interprofessional Care

The ECG changes for a patient with myocarditis are often nonspecific but may reflect associated pericardial involvement (e.g., diffuse ST segment changes). Dysrhythmias and conduction disturbances may be present. Laboratory findings are often inconclusive. They may include mild to moderate leukocytosis and atypical lymphocytes, increased ESR and CRP levels, elevated levels of cardiac biomarkers such as troponin, and elevated viral titers. The virus is generally present in tissue and pericardial fluid samples only during the initial 8 to 10 days of illness.

Histologic confirmation of myocarditis is through an *endomyocardial biopsy.* A biopsy done during the first 6 weeks of acute illness is most diagnostic. This is the period in which lymphocytic infiltration and myocyte damage are present. Nuclear scans, echocardiography, and MRI are used to assess heart function.

Treatment for myocarditis consists of managing associated heart symptoms. Angiotensin-converting enzyme (ACE) inhibitors and β-adrenergic blockers (β-blockers) are used if the heart is enlarged or to treat HF (see Chapter 34). Diuretics reduce fluid volume and decrease preload. If hypotension is not present, IV drugs such as nitroprusside (Nitropress) and milrinone reduce afterload and improve CO by decreasing systemic vascular resistance. Digoxin (Lanoxin) improves heart contractility and reduces heart rate. However, it is used cautiously in patients with myocarditis because of the heart's increased sensitivity to the adverse effects of this drug (e.g., dysrhythmias) and the potential toxicity. Anticoagulation therapy reduces the risk of clot formation from blood stasis in patients with a low ejection fraction (EF).

**DRUG ALERT Digoxin (Lanoxin)**

- Use cautiously in patients with myocarditis.
- Myocarditis predisposes to drug-related dysrhythmias and toxicity.

Some types of myocarditis have an autoimmune basis and are treated with immunosuppressive agents. These drugs reduce heart inflammation and prevent irreversible heart damage. However, the use of these drugs for the treatment of myocarditis remains controversial since they may also lead to recurrence.[6]

General supportive measures for management of myocarditis include $O_2$ therapy, bed rest, and restricted activity. In cases of severe HF, intraaortic balloon pump therapy and ventricular assist devices may be required (see Chapters 34 and 65).

## ❖ NURSING MANAGEMENT: MYOCARDITIS

Decreased CO is an ongoing problem in the care of the patient with myocarditis. Focus your interventions on managing the signs and symptoms of HF. Select nursing measures to decrease cardiac workload. These include placing the patient in a semi-Fowler's position, spacing activity and rest periods, and providing a quiet environment. Carefully monitor drugs that increase the heart's contractility and decrease preload, afterload, or both. Evaluate the effectiveness of your interventions on an ongoing basis.

The patient may be anxious about the diagnosis of myocarditis and recovery. Assess the level of anxiety, take measures to decrease anxiety, and keep the patient and caregiver informed about the therapeutic plan.

The patient who receives immunosuppressive therapy is at increased risk for infection. Monitor for complications and provide the patient with proper infection control procedures.

Although most patients with myocarditis recover spontaneously, some may develop dilated cardiomyopathy (discussed later in this chapter). If severe HF occurs, the patient may require heart transplantation.

## RHEUMATIC FEVER AND RHEUMATIC HEART DISEASE

**Rheumatic fever (RF)** is an acute inflammatory disease of the heart potentially involving all layers (endocardium, myocardium, and pericardium). **Rheumatic heart disease** is a chronic condition resulting from RF that is characterized by scarring and deformity of the heart valves.

### Etiology and Pathophysiology

RF is a complication that occurs as a delayed result (usually after 2 to 3 weeks) of a group A streptococcal pharyngitis. Manifestations of RF appear to be related to an abnormal immunologic response to group A streptococcal cell membrane antigens.[7] RF affects the heart, skin, joints, and central nervous system (CNS). Rheumatic heart disease, caused by RF, primarily affects young adults.

RF has declined in developed countries because of the effective use of antibiotics to treat streptococcal infections. However, it remains an important public health problem in developing countries.[7]

**Cardiac Lesions and Valve Deformities.** About 40% of RF episodes are marked by pancarditis, meaning that all layers of the heart (endocardium, myocardium, and pericardium) are involved (Fig. 36-1). This gives rise to the term *rheumatic pancarditis.*

Rheumatic endocarditis is found mainly in the valves, with swelling and erosion of the valve leaflets. Vegetation forms from deposits of fibrin and blood cells in areas of erosion. The lesions initially create thickening of the valve leaflets, fusion of commissures and chordae tendineae, and fibrosis of the papillary muscle. Valve leaflets may become calcified, resulting in stenosis. The less mobile valve leaflets may not close properly, resulting in regurgitation. The mitral and aortic valves are most commonly affected.

Nodules, called *Aschoff's bodies,* are formed by a reaction to inflammation with swelling and destruction of collagen fibers. As the Aschoff's bodies age, they become more fibrous, and scar tissue forms in the myocardium. Rheumatic pericarditis develops and affects both layers of the pericardium. The layers become thick and covered with a fibrinous exudate. A serosanguineous pericardial effusion may develop. When healing occurs, fibrosis and adhesions develop that partially or completely destroy the pericardial sac. These pathophysiologic changes in the heart can begin during an initial attack of RF. Recurrent infections cause further structural damage.

**Extracardiac Lesions.** The lesions of RF are systemic and involve the skin, joints, and CNS. Painless subcutaneous nodules, arthralgias or arthritis, and chorea may develop.

### Clinical Manifestations

A cluster of signs and symptoms, including laboratory findings, leads to the diagnosis of acute RF. Established criteria provide a basis for diagnosis.[8] The presence of two major criteria or one major and two minor criteria plus evidence of a preceding group A streptococcal infection indicate a high probability of acute RF (Table 36-7).

**Major Criteria.** *Carditis* is the most important manifestation of RF and results in three signs: (1) heart murmur or murmurs of mitral or aortic regurgitation, or mitral stenosis; (2) heart enlargement and HF secondary to myocarditis; and (3) pericarditis resulting in muffled heart sounds, chest pain, pericardial friction rub, or signs of effusion.

*Monoarthritis* or *polyarthritis* is the most common finding in RF. The inflammatory process affects the synovial

**TABLE 36-7 Revised Jones Criteria for Diagnosing Rheumatic Fever***

**Major Criteria**
- Carditis: clinical and/or subclinical†
- Arthritis
  - Monoarthritis or polyarthritis
  - Polyarthralgia
- Sydenham's chorea
- Erythema marginatum
- Subcutaneous nodules

**Minor Criteria**
- Monoarthralgia
- Fever
- Laboratory findings: ↑ ESR and/or ↑ CRP
- ECG findings: Prolonged PR interval after accounting for age variability (unless carditis is a major criterion)

**Evidence of Group A Streptococcal Infection**
- Laboratory findings
- ↑ Antistreptolysin-O titer, positive throat culture, or positive rapid antigen test for group A streptococci

Modified from Gewitz MH, Baltimore RS, Tani LY, et al: Revision of the Jones criteria for the diagnosis of acute rheumatic fever in the era of Doppler echocardiography: a scientific statement from the American Heart Association, *Circulation* 131:1806, 2015.
*CRP,* C-reactive protein; *ESR,* erythrocyte sedimentation rate.
*Criteria apply to initial episodes of rheumatic fever in moderate or high risk populations as defined by an all age prevalence of rheumatic heart disease of ≥1 per 1000 population per year.
†Subclinical carditis is defined by echocardiographic valvulitis.

membranes of the joints. This causes swelling, heat, redness, tenderness, and limitation of motion. The larger joints, particularly the knees, ankles, elbows, and wrists, are most frequently affected.

*Sydenham's chorea* is the major CNS manifestation of RF. It is often a delayed sign occurring several months after the initial infection. It is characterized by involuntary movements, especially of the face and limbs; muscle weakness; and disturbances of speech and gait.

*Erythema marginatum* lesions are a less common feature of RF. The bright pink, nonpruritic, maplike macular lesions occur mainly on the trunk and proximal extremities and may be exacerbated by heat (e.g., warm bath).

*Subcutaneous nodules,* usually associated with severe carditis, are firm, small, hard, painless swellings located over extensor surfaces of joints, particularly the knees, wrists, and elbows.

**Minor Criteria.** Minor clinical manifestations (Table 36-7) are frequently present and are helpful in diagnosing the disease. The minor criteria are used as supplemental information to confirm the presence of RF when only one major criterion is present.

**Evidence of Infection.** In addition to the major and minor criteria, there must also be evidence of a preceding group A streptococcal infection. Table 36-7 lists the various laboratory tests used to confirm evidence of infection.

### Complications

A complication that can result from RF is *chronic rheumatic carditis.* It results from changes in valvular structure that may occur months to years after an episode of RF. Rheumatic endocarditis can result in fibrous tissue growth in valve leaflets and chordae tendineae with scarring and contractures. The mitral valve is most frequently involved. The aortic and tricuspid valves may also be affected.

### Diagnostic Studies and Interprofessional Care

No single diagnostic test exists for RF. An echocardiogram may show valvular insufficiency and pericardial fluid or thickening.[9] A chest x-ray may show an enlarged heart if HF is present. The most consistent ECG change is delayed AV conduction as evidenced by a prolonged PR interval.

Treatment consists of drug therapy and supportive measures (Table 36-8). Antibiotic therapy does not change the course of the acute disease or the development of carditis. It does eliminate residual group A streptococci remaining in the tonsils and pharynx and prevents the spread of organisms to close contacts. Salicylates, NSAIDs, and corticosteroids are the anti-inflammatory agents most widely used in the management of RF. All are effective in controlling the fever and joint manifestations. Salicylates or NSAIDs are used when arthritis is the main manifestation, and corticosteroids are used if severe carditis is present.

**TABLE 36-8 Interprofessional Care**

***Rheumatic Fever***

| Diagnostic Assessment | Management |
|---|---|
| • History and physical examination<br>• Laboratory studies (Table 36-7)<br>  • Chest x-ray<br>  • Echocardiogram<br>  • Electrocardiogram | • Bed rest or limited activity<br>• Drug therapy<br>  • Antibiotics<br>  • Nonsteroidal antiinflammatory drugs<br>  • Salicylates<br>  • Corticosteroids |

## NURSING MANAGEMENT: RHEUMATIC FEVER AND RHEUMATIC HEART DISEASE

### Nursing Assessment

Table 36-9 presents the subjective and objective data that you should obtain from a patient with RF and rheumatic heart disease.

Inspect the patient's skin for subcutaneous nodules and erythema marginatum. This involves palpating for subcutaneous nodules over all bony surfaces and along extensor tendons of the hands and feet. The nodules range in size from 1 to 4 cm and are hard, painless, and freely movable. Erythema marginatum can occur on the trunk and inner aspects of the upper arm and thigh. The erythematous maculae do not itch and are flat. Assess for these bright pink maculae in good light because the rash is difficult to observe, especially in dark-skinned patients.

**TABLE 36-9 Nursing Assessment**

***Rheumatic Fever and Rheumatic Heart Disease***

**Subjective Data**

***Important Health Information***

*Past health history:* Recent streptococcal infection, previous history of rheumatic fever or rheumatic heart disease

***Functional Health Patterns***

*Health perception–health management:* Family history of rheumatic fever. Malaise

*Nutritional-metabolic:* Anorexia, weight loss

*Activity-exercise:* Palpitations, generalized weakness, fatigue, ataxia

*Cognitive-perceptual:* Chest pain, widespread joint pain and tenderness (especially large joints)

**Objective Data**

***General***

Fever

***Integumentary***

Subcutaneous nodules and erythema marginatum

***Cardiovascular***

Tachycardia, pericardial friction rub, muffled heart sounds, murmurs, peripheral edema

***Neurologic***

Chorea (involuntary, purposeless, rapid motions; facial grimaces)

***Musculoskeletal***

Signs of monoarthritis or polyarthritis, including swelling, heat, redness, limitation of motion (especially of knees, ankles, elbows, shoulders, wrists)

***Possible Diagnostic Findings***

Cardiomegaly on chest x-ray. Prolonged PR interval on ECG. Valve abnormalities, chamber dilation, and pericardial effusion on echocardiogram. ↑ antistreptolysin-O titer, positive throat culture, positive rapid antigen test for group A streptococci, ↑ ESR, ↑ CRP, leukocytosis

*CRP,* C-reactive protein; *ESR,* erythrocyte sedimentation rate.

### Nursing Diagnoses

Nursing diagnoses for the patient with RF and rheumatic heart disease may include, but are not limited to, the following:

- Decreased CO *related to* valve dysfunction or HF
- Activity intolerance *related to* arthralgia or arthritis secondary to joint pain, pain from pericarditis, and HF
- Ineffective health management *related to* lack of knowledge concerning possible disease sequelae and the need for long-term prophylactic antibiotic therapy

### Planning

The goals for a patient with RF and rheumatic heart disease include (1) normal or baseline heart function, (2) resumption of daily activities without joint pain, and (3) verbalization of the ability to manage the disease sequelae.

### Nursing Implementation

**Health Promotion.** RF is a preventable heart disease. It involves early detection and immediate treatment of group A streptococcal pharyngitis. Adequate treatment of streptococcal pharyngitis prevents initial attacks of RF. Treatment with oral penicillin V (Penicillin VK) or amoxicillin (Moxatag) for 10 days is recommended. If the patient is allergic to penicillin, a narrow-spectrum cephalosporin (e.g., cephalexin [Keflex]), clindamycin (Cleocin), azithromycin (Zithromax) is used.[10] Therapy requires strict adherence to the full course of treatment. Your role is to teach people in the community to seek medical attention for symptoms of streptococcal pharyngitis and to emphasize the need for prompt and adequate treatment.

**Acute Care.** The primary goals of managing a patient with RF are to (1) control and remove the infecting organism; (2) prevent heart complications; and (3) relieve joint pain, fever, and other symptoms. Give antibiotics as ordered to treat the streptococcal infection. Teach the patient that completing the full course of antibiotics is vital to successful treatment. Give salicylates, NSAIDs, and corticosteroids as ordered and monitor fluid intake as appropriate.

Promoting optimal rest is essential to reduce cardiac workload and the body's metabolic needs. A priority nursing goal is relief of joint pain. Position painful joints for comfort and proper alignment. Apply heat and give drugs as ordered for joint pain.

After the acute symptoms have subsided, the patient without carditis can walk. If the patient has carditis with HF, bed rest restrictions may apply (see Chapter 34 for care of a patient with HF). Stress the importance of nonstrenuous activities once recovery has begun.

> **CHECK YOUR PRACTICE**
>
> Your 28-year-old male patient is recovering from carditis secondary to RF. You are preparing him for discharge from the hospital. When you walk into his room, you notice that he is pacing the floor and seems quite upset. You ask him to sit down so you can talk. He tells you, "I'm a cardiac cripple. I'll never be able to play ball with my sons or go skiing again. I might as well just go to bed and stay there."
>
> - What are the key elements that you should include in your teaching plan?

**Ambulatory Care.** The aim of secondary prevention is to stop the recurrence of RF. Teach the patient with a history of RF about the disease process, possible sequelae, and the need for ongoing antibiotic prophylaxis.

Prior history of RF makes the patient more susceptible to a second attack after a streptococcal infection. The best prevention is treatment with prophylactic antibiotics. Patients with RF without carditis require prophylaxis until age 20 and for a minimum of 5 years. Patients with rheumatic carditis and residual heart disease (e.g., persistent valve disease) need longer-term and even lifelong prophylaxis.[10]

Teach the patient about good nutrition, hygienic practices, and adequate rest. Caution the patient about the possible development of heart valve disease. Tell the patient to seek medical attention if symptoms such as excessive fatigue, dizziness, palpitations, unexplained weight gain, or exertional dyspnea develop.[11]

### Evaluation

The expected outcomes are that the patient with RF and rheumatic heart disease will

- Be able to perform ADLs with minimal fatigue and pain
- Adhere to treatment regimen
- Express confidence in managing disease
- Use measures to prevent complications

## VALVULAR HEART DISEASE

The heart contains two AV valves (mitral and tricuspid) and two semilunar valves (aortic and pulmonic), which control blood flow through the heart (see Fig. 31-1). Valvular heart disease is defined according to the valve or valves affected and the type of dysfunction: stenosis or regurgitation (Fig. 36-7).

The pressure on either side of an open valve is normally equal. However, in a stenotic valve, the valve opening is smaller. The forward flow of blood is impaired. This creates a difference

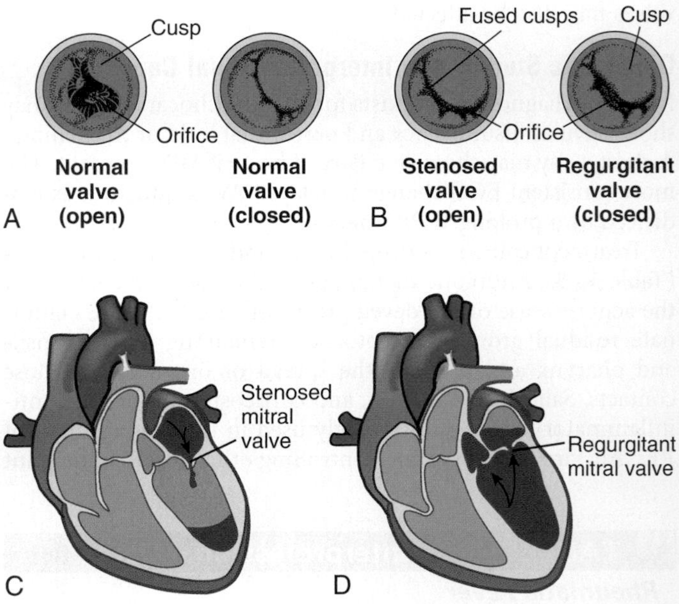


**FIG. 36-7** Valvular stenosis and regurgitation. **A,** Normal position of the valve leaflets, or cusps, when the valve is open and closed. **B,** Open position of a stenosed valve *(left)* and closed position of regurgitant valve *(right)*. **C,** Hemodynamic effect of mitral stenosis. The stenosed valve is unable to open sufficiently during left atrial systole, inhibiting left ventricular filling. **D,** Hemodynamic effect of mitral regurgitation. The mitral valve does not close completely during left ventricular systole, permitting blood to reenter the left atrium. At the same time, blood is moving forward through the aortic valve. (From McCance KL, Huether SE: *Pathophysiology: the biologic basis for disease in adults and children*, ed 6, St Louis, 2010, Mosby.)

in pressure on the two sides of the open valve. The amount of **stenosis** (constriction or narrowing) is seen in the pressure differences (i.e., the higher the difference, the greater the stenosis). When **regurgitation** occurs (referred to as *incompetence* or *insufficiency*), there is incomplete closure of the valve. This results in the backward flow of blood.

Congenital heart conditions are the most common cause of valve disorders in children and adolescents. Valvular heart disease remains prevalent because of an increased number of older adults who have some form of heart disease. AS and mitral regurgitation (MR) are common valve disorders in older adults. Other causes of valve disease in adults include disorders related to acquired immunodeficiency syndrome and the use of some antiparkinsonian drugs.[12]

## MITRAL VALVE STENOSIS

### Etiology and Pathophysiology

Most cases of adult mitral valve stenosis result from rheumatic heart disease. Rheumatic mitral stenosis is widespread in developing countries. Less common causes are congenital mitral stenosis, rheumatoid arthritis, and systemic lupus erythematosus. Rheumatic endocarditis causes scarring of the valve leaflets and the chordae tendineae. Contractures and adhesions develop between the commissures (the junctional areas). The stenotic mitral valve takes on a "fish mouth" shape because of the thickening and shortening of the mitral valve structures.

These deformities block the blood flow and create a pressure difference between the left atrium and left ventricle during diastole. As a result, left atrial pressure and volume increase, causing higher pulmonary vasculature pressure. The overloaded left atrium places the patient at risk for atrial fibrillation. In chronic mitral stenosis, pressure overload occurs in the left atrium, pulmonary bed, and right ventricle.

### Clinical Manifestations

The primary symptom of mitral stenosis is exertional dyspnea caused by reduced lung compliance (Table 36-10). Heart sounds include a loud first heart sound and a low-pitched, diastolic murmur (best heard at the apex with the stethoscope). Less often, patients may have hoarseness (from atrial enlargement pressing on the laryngeal nerve), hemoptysis (from pulmonary hypertension), and chest pain (from decreased CO and coronary perfusion). Emboli can form in the left atrium secondary to atrial fibrillation and cause a stroke.[12] Fatigue and palpitations from atrial fibrillation may also occur.

## MITRAL VALVE REGURGITATION

### Etiology and Pathophysiology

Mitral valve function depends on intact mitral leaflets, mitral annulus, chordae tendineae, papillary muscles, left atrium, and left ventricle. A defect in any of these structures can result in regurgitation. Most cases of mitral regurgitation (MR) are caused by MI, chronic rheumatic heart disease, mitral valve prolapse, ischemic papillary muscle dysfunction, and IE. MI with left ventricular failure increases the risk for rupture of the chordae tendineae and acute MR.

MR allows blood to flow backward from the left ventricle to the left atrium because of incomplete valve closure during systole. Both the left ventricle and left atrium must work harder to preserve an adequate CO. In acute MR the sudden increase in pressure and volume transmits to the pulmonary bed. This results in pulmonary edema and, if not treated, cardiogenic shock. In chronic MR the additional volume results in left atrial enlargement, left ventricular dilation and hypertrophy, and, finally, a decrease in CO.

**TABLE 36-10 Manifestations of Valvular Heart Disease**

| Type | Manifestations |
|---|---|
| **Mitral valve stenosis** | Dyspnea on exertion, hemoptysis, fatigue. Atrial fibrillation on ECG. Palpitations. Loud, accentuated $S_1$. Low-pitched, diastolic murmur |
| **Mitral valve regurgitation** | *Acute:* Generally poorly tolerated. New systolic murmur with pulmonary edema and cardiogenic shock develop rapidly.<br>*Chronic:* Weakness, fatigue, exertional dyspnea, palpitations, $S_3$ gallop, holosystolic murmur |
| **Mitral valve prolapse** | Palpitations, dyspnea, chest pain, activity intolerance, syncope, holosystolic murmur |
| **Aortic valve stenosis** | Angina, syncope, dyspnea on exertion, heart failure, normal or soft $S_1$, diminished or absent $S_2$, systolic murmur, prominent $S_4$ |
| **Aortic valve regurgitation** | *Acute:* Abrupt onset of profound dyspnea, chest pain, left ventricular failure and cardiogenic shock<br>*Chronic:* Fatigue, exertional dyspnea, orthopnea, PND. Water-hammer pulse, heaving precordial impulse, diminished or absent $S_1$, $S_3$, or $S_4$. Soft high-pitched diastolic murmur, Austin Flint murmur |
| **Tricuspid and pulmonic stenosis** | *Tricuspid:* Peripheral edema, ascites, hepatomegaly. Diastolic low-pitched murmur with increased intensity during inspiration<br>*Pulmonic:* Fatigue, loud midsystolic murmur |

*PND,* Paroxysmal nocturnal dyspnea.

### Clinical Manifestations

The clinical course of MR is determined by the nature of its onset (Table 36-10). Patients with acute MR have thready, peripheral pulses and cool, clammy extremities. A low CO may mask a new systolic murmur. Rapid assessment (e.g., heart catheterization) and intervention (e.g., valve repair or replacement) are critical.

Patients with chronic MR may remain asymptomatic for many years. Early symptoms of left ventricular failure may include weakness, fatigue, palpitations, and dyspnea. These gradually progress to orthopnea, paroxysmal nocturnal dyspnea, and peripheral edema. Increased left ventricular volume leads to an audible third heart sound ($S_3$), even with normal left ventricular function. The murmur is a loud holosystolic murmur at the apex radiating to the left axilla. Patients with asymptomatic MR must be monitored carefully. Surgery (valve repair or replacement) should be considered before significant left ventricular failure or pulmonary hypertension develops.[12]

## MITRAL VALVE PROLAPSE

### Etiology and Pathophysiology

**Mitral valve prolapse (MVP)** is an abnormality of the mitral valve leaflets and the papillary muscles or chordae that allows the leaflets to prolapse, or buckle, back into the left atrium during systole (Fig. 36-8). It is the most common form of valvular heart disease in the United States. It affects both genders equally.[13]

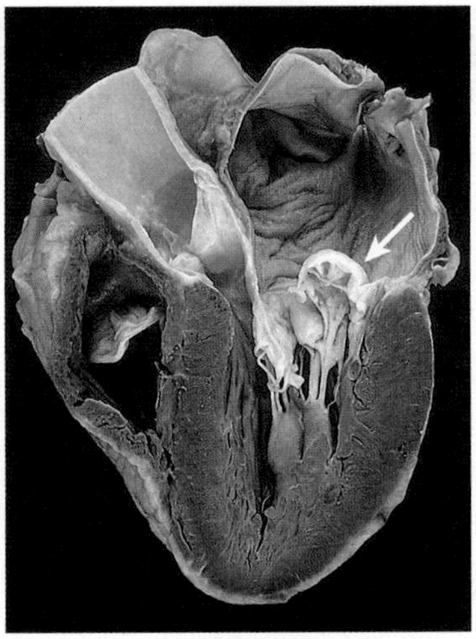

**FIG. 36-8** Mitral valve prolapse. In this valvular abnormality, the mitral leaflets have prolapsed back into the left atrium. They also demonstrate hooding *(arrow)*. The left ventricle is on the right. (From Kumar V, Abbas AK, Aster JC, et al: *Robbins and Cotran pathologic basis of disease,* ed 8, Philadelphia, 2010, Saunders.)

The use of the term *prolapse* can be misleading because it is used even when the valve is working normally. MVP is usually benign, but serious complications can occur, including MR, IE, SCD, HF, and cerebral ischemia.

### Genetic Link

Although the etiology of MVP is unknown, some patients have an increased familial incidence. The genetic inheritance is frequently autosomal dominant (see Chapter 12). MVP in this group results from a connective tissue defect affecting only the valve, or as part of Marfan's syndrome or other hereditary conditions that affect the structure of collagen in the body.

### Clinical Manifestations

MVP covers a broad range of severity. Most patients are asymptomatic and remain so for their entire lives. About 10% of those with MVP become symptomatic. A characteristic of MVP is a murmur from regurgitation that is louder during systole. MVP does not alter $S_1$ or $S_2$ heart sounds. Severe MR is an uncommon but serious complication of MVP.

M-mode and 2-D echocardiography are used to confirm MVP. Dysrhythmias such as premature ventricular contractions, paroxysmal supraventricular tachycardia, and ventricular tachycardia may cause palpitations, light-headedness, and syncope. IE may occur in patients with MR associated with MVP.

Patients may or may not have chest pain. The cause of the chest pain is not known. It may be the result of abnormal tension on the papillary muscles. If chest pain occurs, episodes tend to occur in clusters, especially during periods of emotional stress. Dyspnea, palpitations, and syncope may occasionally accompany the chest pain and do not respond to antianginal treatment (e.g., nitrates). β-Blockers may be given to control palpitations and chest pain. Encourage the patient to stay hydrated, exercise regularly, and avoid caffeine.

The majority of patients with MVP generally have a benign, manageable course. For those who develop symptomatic MR, no accepted medical therapy appears to delay the need for valve surgery.[13] A teaching plan for patients with MVP is presented in Table 36-11.

**TABLE 36-11 Patient & Caregiver Teaching**

***Mitral Valve Prolapse***

*Include the following information in the teaching plan for a patient with mitral valve prolapse (MVP) and the patient's caregiver.*

- Take drugs as prescribed (e.g., β-blockers to control palpitations, chest pain).
- Adopt healthy eating habits.
- Avoid caffeine because it is a stimulant and may exacerbate symptoms.
- If you use diet pills or other over-the-counter drugs, check for common ingredients that are stimulants (e.g., caffeine, ephedrine), since these can exacerbate symptoms.
- Begin (or maintain) an exercise program to achieve optimal health.
- Contact the HCP or emergency response system (ERS) if symptoms develop or worsen (e.g., palpitations, fatigue, shortness of breath, anxiety).

## AORTIC VALVE STENOSIS

### Etiology and Pathophysiology

Congenital **aortic stenosis (AS)** is generally found in childhood, adolescence, or young adulthood. In older adults, AS is a result of RF or degeneration that may have an etiology similar to that of coronary artery disease. It affects 3% of people over 65 years of age.[14] In rheumatic valve disease, fusion of the commissures and secondary calcification cause the valve leaflets to stiffen and retract, resulting in stenosis. AS due to rheumatic heart disease accompanies mitral valve disease. Isolated AS is usually nonrheumatic in origin. The incidence of rheumatic aortic valve disease has been decreasing, but degenerative stenosis is increasing as the population ages.

AS causes obstruction of blood flow from the left ventricle to the aorta during systole. The effect is left ventricular hypertrophy and increased myocardial $O_2$ consumption because of the increased myocardial mass. As the disease progresses and compensatory mechanisms fail, reduced CO leads to decreased tissue perfusion, pulmonary hypertension, and HF. Left untreated, severe AS has approximately a 50% mortality rate at 1 year.[14]

### Clinical Manifestations

Manifestations of AS (Table 36-10) develop when the valve orifice becomes about one third its normal size. These manifestations include the classic triad of angina, syncope, and exertional dyspnea, reflecting left ventricular failure.[14]

The prognosis is poor for patients who exhibit manifestations and those whose valve obstruction is not fixed. Nitroglycerin is used cautiously to treat angina, since the drug can significantly reduce BP and worsen chest pain. Auscultation of AS often reveals a normal or soft $S_1$, a diminished or absent $S_2$, a systolic murmur, and a prominent $S_4$.

**DRUG ALERT Nitroglycerin**

- Use cautiously in patients with AS, since significant hypotension may occur.
- When the drug is used, chest pain can worsen due to a decrease in preload and drop in BP.

## AORTIC VALVE REGURGITATION

### Etiology and Pathophysiology

**Aortic regurgitation (AR)** may be the result of primary disease of the aortic valve leaflets, the aortic root, or both. Trauma, IE, or aortic dissection can cause acute AR, which constitutes a life-threatening emergency. Chronic AR is generally the result of rheumatic heart disease, a congenital bicuspid aortic valve, syphilis, or chronic rheumatic conditions, such as ankylosing spondylitis or reactive arthritis.

AR causes retrograde (backward) blood flow from the ascending aorta into the left ventricle during diastole. This results in volume overload. The left ventricle initially compensates for chronic AR by dilation and hypertrophy. Myocardial contractility eventually declines, and blood volume in the left atrium and pulmonary bed increases. This leads to pulmonary hypertension and right ventricular failure.

### Clinical Manifestations

Patients with acute AR have sudden signs of cardiovascular collapse (Table 36-10). The left ventricle is exposed to aortic pressure during diastole. The patient develops severe dyspnea, chest pain, and hypotension indicating left ventricular failure and cardiogenic shock, a life-threatening emergency.

Patients with chronic, severe AR develop a *water-hammer pulse* (strong, quick beat that collapses immediately). Heart sounds may include a soft or absent $S_1$, $S_3$, or $S_4$ and a soft, high-pitched diastolic murmur.

The patient with chronic AR generally remains asymptomatic for years. Exertional dyspnea, orthopnea, and paroxysmal nocturnal dyspnea develop only after considerable heart dysfunction has occurred (Table 36-10). Angina occurs less frequently than in AS.

## TRICUSPID AND PULMONIC VALVE DISEASE

### Etiology and Pathophysiology

Diseases of the tricuspid and pulmonic valves are uncommon, with stenosis occurring more frequently than regurgitation. *Tricuspid stenosis* occurs almost exclusively in patients who have RF or who abuse IV drugs. Tricuspid stenosis results in right atrial enlargement and elevated systemic venous pressures. *Pulmonic stenosis* is almost always congenital and results in right ventricular hypertension and hypertrophy (Table 36-10).

## DIAGNOSTIC STUDIES: VALVULAR HEART DISEASE

Diagnosis of valvular heart disease includes information from the patient's history and physical examination and a variety of tests (Table 36-12). A CT scan of the chest with contrast is the gold standard for evaluating aortic disorders. An echocardiogram reveals valve structure, function, and heart chamber size. Transesophageal echocardiography and Doppler color-flow imaging help diagnose and monitor valvular heart disease progression. Real-time 3-D echocardiography can help assess mitral valve and congenital heart disease.

Chest x-ray reveals the heart size, altered pulmonary circulation, and valve calcification. An ECG identifies heart rate, rhythm, and any ischemia or ventricular hypertrophy. Heart catheterization detects pressure changes in the heart chambers, records pressure differences across the valves, and measures the size of valve openings.

## INTERPROFESSIONAL CARE: VALVULAR HEART DISEASE

### Conservative Therapy

An important aspect of conservative management of valvular heart disease is prevention of recurrent RF and IE (Table 36-12). Treatment depends on the valve involved and disease severity. It focuses on preventing exacerbations of HF, acute pulmonary edema, thromboembolism, and recurrent endocarditis. HF is treated with vasodilators, positive inotropes, β-blockers, diuretics, and a low-sodium diet (see Chapter 34).

Anticoagulant therapy prevents and treats systemic or pulmonary emboli. It is used prophylactically in patients with atrial fibrillation. Atrial dysrhythmias are common and treated with calcium channel blockers, β-blockers, antidysrhythmic drugs, or electrical cardioversion (see Chapter 35).

**Percutaneous Transluminal Balloon Valvuloplasty.** An alternative treatment for some patients with valvular heart disease is *percutaneous transluminal balloon valvuloplasty* (PTBV). During PTBV, the fused commissures are split open. Balloon valvuloplasty is used for mitral, tricuspid, and pulmonic stenosis, and less often for AS.

The procedure is done in the heart catheterization laboratory. It involves threading a balloon-tipped catheter from the femoral artery or vein to the stenotic valve. The balloon is inflated in an attempt to separate the valve leaflets. A single- or double-balloon technique may be used for the PTBV procedure. Currently, the use of a single Inoue balloon with hourglass shape allows sequential inflation (Fig. 36-9). This technique is the most popular because it is easy and has good results with few complications (e.g., left ventricular perforation). The PTBV procedure is generally indicated for older adults and for those who are poor surgery candidates. The long-term results of PTBV are similar to those of surgical commissurotomy.

Similar to PTBV, the Sapien Transcatheter Heart Valve (THV) is used for select patients with AS. The THV is inserted

**TABLE 36-12 Interprofessional Care**

***Valvular Heart Disease***

**Diagnostic Assessment**
- History and physical examination
- Chest x-ray
- CBC
- Electrocardiogram
- Echocardiography (Doppler and transesophageal)
- Heart catheterization

**Management**

***Conservative Therapy***
- Prophylactic antibiotic therapy (Table 36-2)
  - Rheumatic fever
  - Infective endocarditis
- Sodium restriction
- Drug therapy to treat or control HF
- Vasodilators* (e.g., nitrates, ACE inhibitors)
  - Positive inotropes (e.g., digoxin)
  - Diuretics
  - β-Blockers
- Anticoagulation therapy (see Table 37-10)
- Antidysrhythmic drugs
- Percutaneous transluminal balloon valvuloplasty
- Percutaneous valve replacement

***Surgical Therapy***
- Valve repair
  - Commissurotomy (valvulotomy)
  - Valvuloplasty
  - Annuloplasty
- Valve replacement

*ACE*, Angiotensin-converting enzyme; *HF*, heart failure.
*Use cautiously in patients with aortic stenosis.

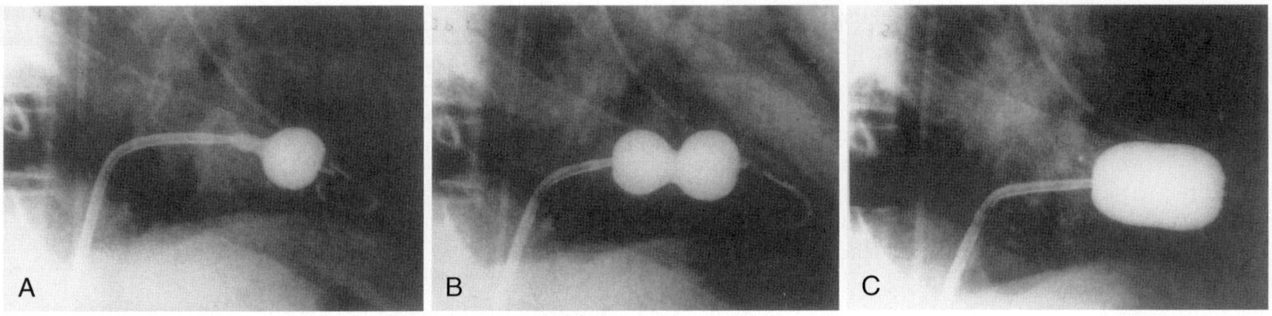


**FIG. 36-9** Mitral valvuloplasty performed by the Inoue technique. The catheter is placed in the mitral valve and the distal part of the Inoue balloon inflated **(A)**. The balloon is then pulled back in the mitral valve and inflated for 10 to 15 sec under fluoroscopic control **(B)** until the waist of the balloon is no longer visible **(C)** and the balloon falls back into the left atrium. (From Crawford MH, DiMarco JP, Paulus WJ: *Cardiology,* ed 3, Edinburgh, 2010, Mosby Ltd.)

through the femoral artery and moved to the heart. It is released and expanded with a balloon in the location of the aortic valve. This procedure is limited to patients who are eligible for surgery but who are at high risk for surgical complications (e.g., patients with multiple co-morbidities).

### Surgical Therapy

The decision for surgical intervention depends on the patient's clinical state using the New York Heart Association classification system for functional disability (see Table 34-3). The type of surgery can be valve repair or valve replacement. The procedure that is used depends on the (1) valves involved, (2) pathology and severity of the disease, and (3) patient's clinical condition. All types of valve surgery are palliative, not curative, and patients require lifelong health care.

**Valve Repair.** Valve repair is usually the surgical procedure of choice. It has a lower operative mortality rate than valve replacement and is often used in mitral or tricuspid valvular heart disease.[14] Although valve repair avoids the risks of replacement, it may not restore total valve function.

Mitral *commissurotomy (valvulotomy)* is the procedure of choice for patients with pure mitral stenosis. The less precise closed method of commissurotomy has generally been replaced by the open method. In the *closed procedure* the surgeon inserts a transventricular dilator through the apex of the left ventricle into the opening of the mitral valve. The direct vision procedure, or *open procedure,* requires the use of cardiopulmonary bypass. The surgeon removes thrombi from the atrium and makes a commissure incision. Next, the fused chordae are separated by splitting the papillary muscle and debriding the calcified valve.

Open surgical *valvuloplasty* involves repair of the valve by suturing the torn leaflets, chordae tendineae, or papillary muscles. It is primarily used to treat mitral or tricuspid regurgitation.

*Minimally invasive valvuloplasty* surgery involves a ministernotomy or parasternal approach. It may include robotic and thoracoscopic surgical systems. Results compare with those of the open procedure. In addition, shorter lengths of stay, fewer blood transfusions, less pain, and lower risk of sternal infection and postoperative atrial fibrillation have been reported.[15]

For patients with mitral or tricuspid regurgitation, further valve repair or reconstruction using annuloplasty is an option. *Annuloplasty* involves reconstruction of the annulus, with or without the aid of prosthetic rings.

**Valve Replacement.** Valve replacement may be required for mitral, aortic, tricuspid, and occasionally pulmonic valve disease.

## ETHICAL/LEGAL DILEMMAS

### *Do Not Resuscitate*

**Situation**

J.L., a 68-yr-old man, is admitted for a second mitral valve surgery and coronary artery bypass graft surgery. He did not adhere to the treatment plan after his original surgery 7 years ago. You are worried about his future adherence with drugs, diet, and exercise. His kidneys are failing and he is on dialysis, making him a high-risk surgical patient. The patient and his caregiver want all possible treatment and refuse to discuss advance directives (ADs) or do not resuscitate (DNR) orders.

**Ethical/Legal Points for Consideration**

- Based on their expertise, HCPs have the right to refuse to provide treatment that offers no benefit to the patient.
- ADs do not include a DNR order. If the patient is unable to speak for himself or herself, a DNR order can be started only by the HCP after conversation with the health care proxy and/or nearest kin. The decision usually depends on evidence of the patient's preferences (substituted judgment standard) or what is in the best interest of the patient.
- If there is an AD refusing resuscitation, the HCP is required to act accordingly but is not compelled to enact a DNR without clear direction from the patient or proxy.
- Patient adherence with past treatment plans is not a factor that must be considered in DNR decisions. Many circumstances related to nonadherence are outside the patient's control, such as finances, transportation, availability of assistance, and declining physical and medical capabilities.
- If the involved parties disagree about the patient's treatment plan, a referral can be made to an ethics committee, they can seek treatment from another HCP, or they may seek legal intervention by way of a court order.

**Discussion Questions**

1. How can a lack of understanding or limited financial resources contribute to nonadherence with the plan of care?
2. What type of information should be provided to a patient and caregiver in discussions about ADs and DNR orders? Who should provide this information?
3. Who can initiate a referral to an ethics committee?

A wide variety of prosthetic valves are currently available. Desirable valves are nonthrombogenic and durable, and create minimal stenosis. Prosthetic valves are categorized as mechanical or biologic (tissue) valves (Fig. 36-10).

*Mechanical valves* are manufactured from artificial materials and consist of combinations of metal alloys, pyrolytic carbon, and Dacron. *Biologic valves* are constructed from bovine, porcine, and human (cadaver) heart tissue and usually contain

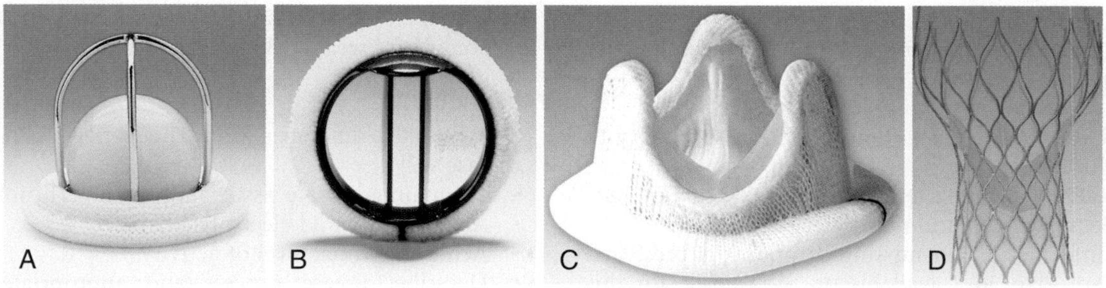


**FIG. 36-10** Types of prosthetic heart valves. **A,** Starr-Edwards caged ball valve. **B,** St. Jude bi-leaflet valve. **C,** Carpentier-Edwards porcine valve. **D,** CoreValve transcatheter aortic valve (CV26 Hero), Medtronic 2015. (A through C, From Bonow RO, Mann DL, Zipes DP, et al: *Braunwald's heart disease: a textbook of cardiovascular medicine,* ed 9, Philadelphia, 2012, Saunders.)

## INFORMATICS IN PRACTICE

### *Heart Surgery DVD/TV*

- Many patients prefer to watch DVDs or the patient education channel of the hospital's TV system instead of reading educational pamphlets. For a patient facing heart surgery, these formats can be effective tools to teach the patient and caregiver what to expect before and after the procedure.
- Remember that the DVD or TV is not the teacher.
- Beforehand discuss what the DVD or TV will cover.
- Encourage the patient and caregiver to write down questions or note what they do not understand.
- After the patient and caregiver view the material, answer any questions they have. Reinforce important information.

some man-made materials. A "decellularizing" process removes the cadaver cells from the valve. This lowers the risk of immune response and tissue rejection. Biologic valves are asymmetric in shape and produce a more natural pattern of blood flow compared with mechanical valves. Asymmetric mechanical valve prototypes are being tested.

Mechanical prosthetic valves are more durable and last longer than biologic valves. However, they have an increased risk of thromboembolism and require long-term anticoagulation therapy.[13] The main risk of mechanical valves is bleeding from the use of anticoagulants. Biologic valves do not require anticoagulation therapy because of their low thrombogenicity. However, they are less durable and tend to cause early calcification, tissue degeneration, and stiffening of the leaflets. Either type of prosthetic valve can leak and cause endocarditis.

Minimally invasive aortic valve replacement uses a transcatheter or transapical approach and is the surgical choice for patients at high risk for traditional surgery.[16] The CoreValve transcatheter aortic valve is made of tissue obtained from the heart of a pig[17] (Fig. 36-10, *D*). Prolonged waiting time for aortic valve replacement is associated with greater mortality, and surgery should be done on a semi-urgent basis.[18]

Long-term anticoagulation is needed for those patients with biologic valves who have atrial fibrillation. Some patients with biologic valves or annuloplasty with prosthetic rings may need anticoagulation the first few months after surgery until the suture lines are covered by endothelial cells (endothelialized).

The choice of valves depends on many factors. For example, if a patient cannot take an anticoagulant (e.g., women of childbearing age), a biologic valve is considered. A mechanical valve may be best for a younger patient because it is more durable. For patients over age 65, durability is less important than the risks of bleeding from anticoagulants, so most receive a biologic valve.

## TABLE 36-13 Nursing Assessment

### *Valvular Heart Disease*

**Subjective Data**

***Important Health Information***

- *Past health history:* Rheumatic fever, infective endocarditis; congenital defects, heart attack, chest trauma, cardiomyopathy; syphilis, Marfan's syndrome, streptococcal infections

***Functional Health Patterns***

*Health perception–health management:* IV drug abuse, fatigue
*Activity-exercise:* Palpitations, generalized weakness, activity intolerance, dizziness, fainting, dyspnea on exertion, cough, hemoptysis, orthopnea
*Sleep-rest:* Paroxysmal nocturnal dyspnea
*Cognitive-perceptual:* Angina or atypical chest pain

**Objective Data**

***General***

Fever

***Integumentary***

Diaphoresis, flushing, cyanosis, clubbing, peripheral edema

***Respiratory***

Crackles, wheezes, hoarseness

***Cardiovascular***

Abnormal heart sounds, including murmurs, $S_3$, and $S_4$. Dysrhythmias, including atrial fibrillation, premature ventricular contractions. Tachycardia. ↑ or ↓ in pulse pressure, hypotension, water-hammer or thready peripheral pulses

***Gastrointestinal***

Ascites, hepatomegaly, unexplained weight gain

***Possible Diagnostic Findings***

Cardiomegaly on chest x-ray. ECG abnormalities specific to involved valve. Echocardiogram (valve disorders and chamber dilation), heart catheterization (abnormal valves, chamber pressures, cardiac output, and blood flow depending on involved valve)

## NURSING MANAGEMENT: VALVULAR DISORDERS

### Nursing Assessment

Table 36-13 presents the subjective and objective data to obtain from a patient with valve disease.

### Nursing Diagnoses

Nursing diagnoses for the patient with valvular heart disease may include, but are not limited to, the following:

- Decreased CO *related to* valvular incompetence
- Excess fluid volume *related to* fluid retention secondary to valvular-induced HF
- Activity intolerance *related to* insufficient oxygenation secondary to decreased CO and pulmonary congestion

Additional information on nursing diagnoses is presented in eNursing Care Plan 36-2 available on the website for this chapter.

### Planning

The overall goals for the patient with valve disease include (1) normal heart function, (2) improved activity tolerance, and (3) an understanding of the disease process and health maintenance measures.

### Nursing Implementation

**Health Promotion.** Diagnosing and treating streptococcal infections and providing prophylactic antibiotics for patients with a history of RF are critical to prevent acquired rheumatic valve disease. The patient at risk for endocarditis and any patient with certain heart conditions must also receive prophylactic antibiotics (Table 36-2).

The patient must adhere to ordered therapies. The person with a history of RF, endocarditis, and congenital heart disease should know the symptoms of valvular heart disease so that early medical treatment may begin.

**Acute Care and Ambulatory Care.** A patient with progressive valvular heart disease may need outpatient care or hospitalization for management of HF, endocarditis, embolic disease, or dysrhythmias. HF is the most common reason for ongoing medical care.

Your role is to implement therapeutic interventions and evaluate their effects. Design activities considering the patient's limitations. An appropriate exercise plan can increase cardiac tolerance, but activities that cause fatigue and dyspnea should be limited. Discourage tobacco use. Tell the patient to avoid strenuous physical exercise because damaged valves may not handle the increased CO demand. Develop your patient's care plan to emphasize conserving energy, setting priorities, and taking planned rest periods. Consider a referral to a vocational counselor if the patient has a physically or emotionally demanding job.

Perform ongoing cardiac assessments to monitor the effectiveness of drugs. Teach the actions and side effects of drugs to increase adherence. The patient must understand the importance of prophylactic antibiotic therapy to prevent IE (Table 36-2). If the valve disease was caused by RF, ongoing prophylaxis to prevent recurrence is necessary.

When valvular heart disease can no longer be managed medically, surgery is necessary (see Chapter 33 for the care of a patient having heart surgery). The patient on anticoagulation therapy (e.g., warfarin [Coumadin]) after surgery for valve replacement must have the international normalized ratio (INR) checked regularly to determine proper dosage and adequacy of therapy. INR values of 2.5 to 3.5 are therapeutic for patients with mechanical valves.

A teaching guide related to anticoagulation therapy is found in Table 37-14. The patient must know that valve surgery is not a cure and that regular follow-up with an HCP is needed. Also, teach the patient when to seek medical care. Any signs of infection, HF, or bleeding and any planned invasive or dental work require the patient to notify the HCP. Last, encourage patients to obtain and wear a Medic Alert device.

### Evaluation

The expected outcomes are that a patient with valvular heart disease will

- Maintain adequate tissue and organ perfusion
- Achieve fluid and electrolyte balance
- Achieve optimal level of activity
- Describe disease process and appropriate measures to prevent complications

Additional information on expected outcomes is presented in eNursing Care Plan 36-2 available on the website for this chapter.

# CARDIOMYOPATHY

**Cardiomyopathy (CMP)** is a group of diseases that directly affect myocardial structure or function. A diagnosis of CMP is based on the patient's clinical manifestations and noninvasive and invasive diagnostic procedures.

CMP can be classified as primary or secondary. *Primary CMP* refers to those conditions in which the etiology of the disease is idiopathic. The heart muscle in this case is the only part of the heart involved, and other heart structures are unaffected. In *secondary CMP* the cause of the myocardial disease is known and is secondary to another disease process. Common causes of secondary CMP are listed in Table 36-14.

Three major types of CMP are dilated, hypertrophic, and restrictive. Each type has its own pathogenesis, clinical presentation, and treatment protocols (Tables 36-15 and 36-16). CMP can lead to cardiomegaly and HF. It is the primary reason that heart transplants are done.

*Takotsubo cardiomyopathy (TCM)* is a transient heart syndrome that mimics acute coronary syndrome. Patients often have chest pain, ST segment elevation on ECG, and elevated cardiac biomarkers consistent with an MI. However, when the patient undergoes heart catheterization, there is no significant coronary artery disease. TCM is an acute, stress-related syndrome that is more common in postmenopausal women. Normal heart function returns in days or weeks after supportive therapy.[19]

## DILATED CARDIOMYOPATHY

### Etiology and Pathophysiology

**Dilated cardiomyopathy** is the most common type of CMP, with a prevalence of 5 to 8 cases per 100,000 people in the

**TABLE 36-14 Causes of Cardiomyopathy**

| Dilated | Hypertrophic |
|---|---|
| • Cardiotoxic agents: alcohol, cocaine, doxorubicin | • Aortic stenosis |
| • Coronary artery disease | • Genetic (autosomal dominant) |
| • Genetic (autosomal dominant) | • Hypertension |
| • Hypertension | **Restrictive** |
| • Metabolic disorders | • Amyloidosis |
| • Muscular dystrophy | • Endomyocardial fibrosis |
| • Myocarditis | • Neoplastic tumor |
| • Pregnancy | • Post-radiation therapy |
| • Valve disease | • Sarcoidosis |
| | • Ventricular thrombus |

**TABLE 36-15 Types of Cardiomyopathy**

| Dilated | Hypertrophic | Restrictive |
|---|---|---|
| **Major Manifestations** | | |
| Fatigue, weakness, palpitations, dyspnea | Exertional dyspnea, fatigue, angina, syncope, palpitations | Dyspnea, fatigue |
| **Cardiomegaly** | | |
| Moderate to severe | Mild to moderate | Mild |
| **Contractility** | | |
| Decreased | Increased or decreased | Normal or decreased |
| **Valvular Incompetence** | | |
| Atrioventricular (AV) valves, especially mitral | Mitral valve | AV valves |
| **Dysrhythmias** | | |
| Sinus tachycardia, atrial and ventricular dysrhythmias | Atrial and ventricular dysrhythmias | Atrial and ventricular dysrhythmias |
| **Cardiac Output** | | |
| Decreased | Normal or decreased | Normal or decreased |
| **Outflow Tract Obstruction** | | |
| None | Increased | None |

**TABLE 36-16 Interprofessional Care**

***Cardiomyopathy***

**Diagnostic Assessment**

- History and physical examination
- Electrocardiogram
- b-Type natriuretic peptide (BNP)
- Chest x-ray
- Echocardiogram
- Nuclear imaging studies
- Heart catheterization
- Endomyocardial biopsy

**Management**

- Drug therapy
  - Nitrates (except in hypertrophic CMP)
  - β-Blockers
  - Antidysrhythmics
  - ACE inhibitors
  - Diuretics
  - Digitalis (except in hypertrophic CMP unless used to treat atrial fibrillation)
  - Anticoagulants (if indicated)
- Ventricular assist device
- Cardiac resynchronization therapy
- Implantable cardioverter-defibrillator
- Surgical repair
- Heart transplantation
- Cardiac rehabilitation
- Palliative and hospice care

*ACE*, Angiotensin-converting enzyme; *CMP*, cardiomyopathy.

United States. It causes HF in 25% to 40% of cases, occurs more frequently in middle-aged African Americans and men, and has a genetic link in 30% of cases. Dilated CMP often follows an infectious myocarditis. Some evidence links dilated CMP with an autoimmune process.[20] Alcoholic dilated CMP is under-recognized and has a unique presentation, treatment, and

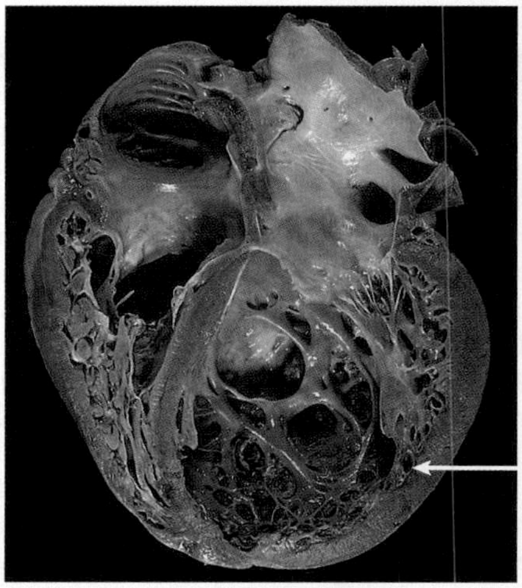

**FIG. 36-11** Dilated cardiomyopathy. The dilated left ventricular wall has thinned *(arrow)*, and the chamber size and volume are increased. (From Kumar V, Abbas AK, Aster JC, et al: *Robbins and Cotran pathologic basis of disease*, ed 8, Philadelphia, 2010, Saunders.)

outcomes.[21] Other common causes of dilated CMP are listed in Table 36-14.

Dilated CMP is characterized by a diffuse inflammation and rapid degeneration of heart fibers. This results in ventricular dilation, impaired systolic function, atrial enlargement, and stasis of blood in the left ventricle. SCD from ventricular dysrhythmias is a leading cause of death in idiopathic dilated CMP.[22] *Cardiomegaly* results from ventricular dilation (Fig. 36-11). This causes contractile dysfunction in spite of an enlarged chamber size. In contrast to HF, the walls of the ventricles do not hypertrophy.

## Clinical Manifestations

The signs and symptoms of dilated CMP may develop acutely after an infection or slowly over time. Most people eventually develop HF. Symptoms can include decreased exercise capacity, fatigue, dyspnea at rest, paroxysmal nocturnal dyspnea, and orthopnea. As the disease progresses, the patient may experience dry cough, palpitations, abdominal bloating, nausea, vomiting, and anorexia. Signs can include an abnormal $S_3$ and/or $S_4$, dysrhythmias, heart murmurs, pulmonary crackles, edema, weak peripheral pulses, pallor, hepatomegaly, and JVD. Decreased blood flow through an enlarged heart promotes stasis and blood clot formation and may lead to systemic embolization.

## Diagnostic Studies

The diagnosis of dilated CMP is based on the patient's history and exclusion of other causes of HF. Doppler echocardiography is the basis for the diagnosis of dilated CMP in the majority of patients. The chest x-ray may show cardiomegaly with signs of pulmonary venous hypertension and pleural effusion. The ECG may reveal tachycardia, bradycardia, and dysrhythmias with conduction disturbances. Laboratory studies may show elevated serum levels of b-type natriuretic peptide (BNP) in the presence of HF.

Heart catheterization confirms or rules out coronary artery disease, and multiple gated acquisition (MUGA) nuclear scan determines EF. EF less than 20% is associated with a 50% mortality rate within 1 year. Endomyocardial biopsy is done at the time of the right-sided heart catheterization to identify any infectious organisms in heart tissue.

## ❖ NURSING AND INTERPROFESSIONAL MANAGEMENT: DILATED CARDIOMYOPATHY

Interventions focus on controlling HF by enhancing heart contractility and decreasing preload and afterload. This is similar to the management of chronic HF. Treatment guidelines are based on the specific stage of disease progression (see Table 34-3). Treatment of patients with Class IV (stage D) HF is more palliative than curative.

Several different types of drugs are available to manage HF (see Table 34-7). Nitrates (e.g., nitroglycerin [Nitrol]) and diuretics (e.g., furosemide [Lasix]) decrease preload, and ACE inhibitors (e.g., captopril [Capoten]) reduce afterload. β-Blockers (e.g., metoprolol [Lopressor]) and aldosterone antagonists (e.g., spironolactone [Aldactone]) control the neurohormonal stimulation that occurs in HF. Dysrhythmias are treated with antidysrhythmics (e.g., amiodarone) as indicated (see Chapter 35). Anticoagulation therapy reduces the risk of systemic embolization from clots. These may form in the heart chambers secondary to atrial fibrillation.

Drug and nutritional therapy and cardiac rehabilitation may help (1) alleviate symptoms of HF and (2) improve CO and quality of life. A patient with secondary dilated CMP must be treated for the underlying disease process. For example, the patient with alcohol-related dilated CMP must abstain from all alcohol. (See Chapter 10 for a discussion on addictive behaviors and Chapter 34 for a discussion on HF.)

Unfortunately, dilated CMP does not respond well to therapy, and patients experience multiple episodes of HF. Patients are often hospitalized for infusions of dobutamine (Dobutrex) or milrinone followed by aggressive diuresis. Sometimes these treatments are done in an outpatient setting or in the home under nursing supervision. After treatment, many patients experience an improvement in symptoms that lasts several weeks. The use of statins (e.g., atorvastatin [Lipitor]) in ischemic and idiopathic dilated CMP increases survival, improves heart function, and reduces inflammatory markers[23] (see Table 33-5).

Patients also may benefit from nondrug therapies. A ventricular assist device (VAD) allows the heart to rest and recover from acute HF. It may also serve as a bridge to heart transplantation. Additionally, cardiac resynchronization therapy and an implantable cardioverter-defibrillator are used in appropriate patients (see Chapter 34).

The patient with terminal or end-stage CMP may consider heart transplantation. The use of a permanent, implantable VAD, known as *destination therapy,* is an option for patients with advanced disease who are not candidates for heart transplantation (see Chapter 34). Currently, approximately 50% of heart transplantations that are performed are for treatment of CMP. Heart transplant recipients have a good prognosis. However, donor hearts are difficult to obtain, and many patients with dilated CMP die before receiving a heart.

Patients with dilated CMP are very ill and have a grave prognosis. Your expert nursing care is critical. Observe for signs and symptoms of worsening HF, dysrhythmias, embolus formation, and drug effectiveness. The goals of therapy are to keep the patient at an optimal level of functioning and out of the hospital. Always include caregivers when planning a patient's care. Encourage caregivers to learn cardiopulmonary resuscitation (CPR). Teach them when and how to access emergency care.

Home health and hospice nursing can provide the patient and caregiver with palliative care. This includes strategies to maximize and maintain functional status or end-of-life care to prepare for a peaceful death.

## HYPERTROPHIC CARDIOMYOPATHY

### Etiology and Pathophysiology

**Hypertrophic cardiomyopathy** is asymmetric left ventricular hypertrophy without ventricular dilation.[24] In one form of the disease the septum between the two ventricles becomes enlarged and blocks the blood flow from the left ventricle. It is termed *hypertrophic obstructive cardiomyopathy* (HOCMP) or *asymmetric septal hypertrophy* (ASH).

Although hypertrophic CMP can be idiopathic, about half of all cases have a genetic basis characterized by inappropriate myocardial hypertrophy. Early identification is important (Table 36-14). Hypertrophic CMP occurs less commonly than dilated CMP. It is more common in men than in women. It is usually diagnosed in young adults and, most often, in active, athletic individuals. Hypertrophic CMP is the most common cause of SCD in otherwise healthy young people. It accounts for 3% of deaths in young competitive athletes.[25]

The four main characteristics of hypertrophic CMP are (1) massive ventricular hypertrophy; (2) rapid, forceful contraction of the left ventricle; (3) impaired relaxation (diastole); and (4) obstruction to aortic outflow (not present in all patients). Ventricular hypertrophy is associated with a thickened intraventricular septum and ventricular wall (Fig. 36-12). The end result is impaired ventricular filling as the ventricle becomes noncompliant and unable to relax. The primary defect of hypertrophic CMP is diastolic dysfunction from left ventricular stiffness. Decreased ventricular filling and obstruction to outflow can result in decreased CO, especially during exertion.

### Clinical Manifestations

Patients with hypertrophic CMP may be asymptomatic or may have exertional dyspnea, fatigue, angina, and syncope. The most common symptom is dyspnea, which is caused by an elevated left ventricular diastolic pressure. Fatigue occurs because of the resultant decrease in CO and in exercise-induced flow obstruction. Angina can occur and is most often caused by the increased left ventricular mass or compression of the small coronary arteries by the hypertrophic ventricular myocardium. The

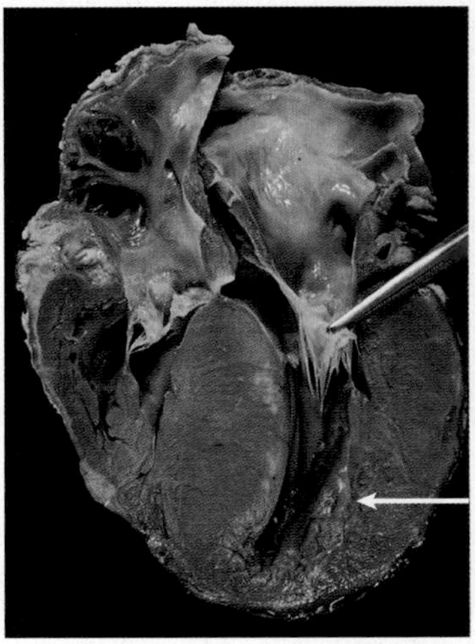

**FIG. 36-12** Hypertrophic cardiomyopathy. There is marked left ventricular hypertrophy *(arrow),* and the chamber size and volume are decreased. (From Kumar V, Abbas AK, Aster JC, et al: *Robbins and Cotran pathologic basis of disease,* ed 8, Philadelphia, 2010, Saunders.)

patient may also have syncope, especially during exertion. Syncope is most often caused by an increase in obstruction to aortic outflow during increased activity. This results in decreased CO and cerebrovascular circulation. Syncope can also be caused by dysrhythmias. Common dysrhythmias include supraventricular tachycardia, atrial fibrillation, ventricular tachycardia, and ventricular fibrillation. Any of these dysrhythmias may lead to syncope or SCD (see Chapters 33 and 35).

### Diagnostic Studies

Clinical findings on examination may be unremarkable. However, on palpation of the chest the apical impulse can be exaggerated and displaced to the left. Auscultation may reveal an $S_4$ and a systolic murmur between the apex and sternal border at the fourth intercostal space. ECG findings usually indicate ventricular hypertrophy, ST-T wave abnormalities, prominent Q waves in the inferior or precordial leads, and ventricular and atrial dysrhythmias (see Chapter 35).

The echocardiogram is the primary diagnostic tool used to confirm hypertrophic CMP. The echocardiogram may also demonstrate wall motion abnormalities and diastolic dysfunction. Heart catheterization and nuclear stress testing may also be helpful in diagnosing and guiding the treatment of hypertrophic CMP.

## ❖ NURSING AND INTERPROFESSIONAL MANAGEMENT: HYPERTROPHIC CARDIOMYOPATHY

Goals of care are to improve ventricular filling by reducing ventricular contractility and relieving left ventricular outflow obstruction. These can be done with the use of β-blockers (e.g., metoprolol) or calcium channel blockers (e.g., verapamil [Calan]). Digitalis is considered if needed to treat atrial fibrillation. Amiodarone or sotalol (Betapace) are effective antidysrhythmic drugs. However, their use does not prevent SCD. For patients at risk for SCD, a cardioverter-defibrillator is needed (see Chapter 35).

AV pacing is helpful for patients with hypertrophic CMP and outflow obstruction. When the ventricles are paced from the apex of the right ventricle, septal depolarization occurs first. This allows the septum to move away from the left ventricular wall and reduces the degree of obstruction of the outflow tract.

Some patients may be candidates for surgical treatment of their hypertrophied septum. The indications for surgery include severe symptoms unresponsive to therapy with marked obstruction to aortic outflow. The surgery is termed a *ventriculomyotomy and myectomy.* It involves cutting into the thickened septal muscle and removing some of the ventricular muscle. Most patients have an improvement in symptoms and exercise tolerance after surgery.

An alternative nonsurgical procedure to reduce symptoms and the left ventricular outflow obstruction is alcohol-induced, *percutaneous transluminal septal myocardial ablation* (PTSMA). This procedure consists of injecting alcohol into the first septal artery branching off the left anterior descending artery. This causes ischemia and septal wall infarction. Ablation of the septal wall decreases the obstruction to flow, and the patient's symptoms decrease. The procedure improves HF symptoms and exercise capacity 3 months after ablation.[26] Potential complications of PTSMA include conduction disturbances (e.g., heart block) and MI.

Nursing interventions for hypertrophic CMP focus on relieving symptoms, observing for and preventing complications, and providing emotional support. Focus your teaching on helping patients avoid strenuous activity and dehydration. Any activity that causes an increase in systemic vascular resistance (thus increasing the obstruction to forward flow) is dangerous and should be avoided. Rest and elevation of the feet to improve venous return to the heart can manage chest pain in these patients. Vasodilators such as nitroglycerin may worsen the chest pain by decreasing venous return and further increasing obstruction of blood flow from the heart.

## RESTRICTIVE CARDIOMYOPATHY

### Etiology and Pathophysiology

*Restrictive cardiomyopathy* is the least common type of CMP. It is a disease of the myocardium that impairs diastolic filling and stretch. Systolic function remains unchanged. Although the specific etiology of restrictive CMP is unknown, a number of pathologic processes may be involved in its development. Myocardial fibrosis, hypertrophy, and infiltration produce stiffness of the ventricular wall with loss of ventricular compliance. Secondary causes of restrictive CMP include amyloidosis, endocardial fibrosis, sarcoidosis, fibrosis of different etiology, and radiation to the thorax. With restrictive CMP, the ventricles are resistant to filling and therefore demand high diastolic filling pressures to maintain CO.

### Clinical Manifestations and Diagnostic Studies

Classic manifestations of restrictive CMP are fatigue, exercise intolerance, and dyspnea. These occur because the heart cannot increase CO by increasing the heart rate without further compromising ventricular filling. Additional symptoms may include angina, orthopnea, syncope, and palpitations. The patient may have signs of HF, including dyspnea, peripheral edema, weight gain, ascites, hepatomegaly, and JVD.

The chest x-ray may be normal, or it may show cardiomegaly from right and left atrial enlargement. Pleural effusions and pulmonary congestion may be seen in the patient with progression to HF. The ECG may reveal a mild tachycardia at rest. The most common dysrhythmias are supraventricular (atrial fibrillation) or AV block. Echocardiography may reveal a left ventricle that is normal size with a thickened wall, slightly dilated right ventricle, and dilated atria. Endomyocardial biopsy, CT scan, and nuclear imaging may help in the diagnosis.

## ❖ NURSING AND INTERPROFESSIONAL MANAGEMENT: RESTRICTIVE CARDIOMYOPATHY

Currently, there is no specific treatment for restrictive CMP. Interventions are aimed at improving diastolic filling and the underlying disease process. Treatment includes conventional therapy for HF and dysrhythmias. Heart transplant may also be a consideration. Nursing care is similar to the care of a patient with HF. As in the treatment of patients with hypertrophic CMP, teach the patient to avoid situations that impair ventricular filling and increase systemic vascular resistance, such as strenuous activity and dehydration.

Nursing care of a patient with CMP includes individualized teaching based on the patient's clinical manifestations. All patients with CMP are at risk for IE from any procedure that may cause bacteremia. Instruct the patient on the need for prophylactic antibiotics (Table 36-2). A guide for patient and caregiver teaching is presented in Table 36-17.

## TABLE 36-17 Patient & Caregiver Teaching

### *Cardiomyopathy*

*Include the following information in the teaching plan for a patient with cardiomyopathy and the patient's caregiver.*

1. Take all drugs as prescribed and regularly follow up with HCP.
2. Follow a low-sodium diet (if ordered) and read all product labels (food and over-the-counter drugs) for sodium content.
3. Drink 6 to 8 glasses of water a day unless fluids are restricted.
4. Achieve and maintain a reasonable weight and avoid large meals.
5. Avoid alcohol, caffeine, diet pills, and over-the-counter cold medicines that may contain stimulants.
6. Balance activity and rest periods.
7. Avoid heavy lifting or vigorous isometric exercises, and check with HCP for exercise guidelines.
8. Use stress management techniques: relaxation breathing, guided imagery.
9. Report any signs of heart failure to HCP, including weight gain, edema, shortness of breath, and increased fatigue.
10. Encourage caregivers to learn CPR because of the potential for cardiac arrest (see Appendix A).
11. Access emergency response system (ERS) according to the HCP's instructions.

*CPR,* Cardiopulmonary resuscitation.

## CASE STUDY

### *Valvular Heart Disease*

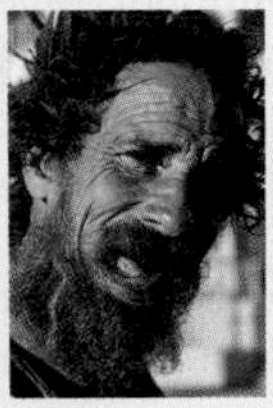

(©JennaDub/ iStock/ Thinkstock)

**Patient Profile**

R.B., a 50-yr-old white man, is admitted to the hospital for acute decompensated heart failure due to valvular heart disease.

**Subjective Data**

- Reports past history of IV drug abuse
- Reports current regular alcohol intake approximately 1 pint of whiskey per day
- Complains of chest pain with minimal exertion
- Recently unemployed
- States, "I'm short of breath all the time. I can't sleep when I lay down."
- States, "I'm always tired."
- States, "The drugs are too expensive. I can't afford them."
- Smokes a pack of cigarettes a day for past 35 years

**Objective Data**

***Physical Examination***

- Third heart sound ($S_3$)
- Loud holosystolic murmur of mitral regurgitation
- Edentulous (secondary to periodontal disease)
- Vital signs: temperature 99.0° F (37.2° C); apical-radial pulse equal at 110 beats per min, irregular; respirations 24; BP 104/58

***Diagnostic Studies***

- ECG shows atrial fibrillation with a rapid ventricular response
- Chest x-ray reveals pulmonary congestion and cardiomegaly
- Transesophageal echocardiography shows left atrial and ventricular hypertrophy and mitral and aortic regurgitation. Ejection fraction 30%

**Discussion Questions**

1. Identify the cause and course of R.B.'s disease based on his history and current examination.
2. Differentiate between mitral and aortic regurgitation.
3. What medical treatments or surgical procedures will R.B. probably require as his condition worsens?
4. ***Priority Decision:*** On the basis of the assessment data provided, what are the priority nursing diagnoses?
5. ***Priority Decision:*** Identify the priority nursing interventions for R.B.
6. ***Safety:*** What safety precautions should be initiated for R.B.?
7. ***Teamwork and Collaboration:*** Identify the tasks that you could delegate to unlicensed assistive personnel (UAP).
8. ***Evidence-Based Practice:*** R.B. asks you why he needs to be on "blood thinners" after his valves are replaced.

Answers are available at *http://evolve.elsevier.com/Lewis/medsurg.*

## BRIDGE TO NCLEX EXAMINATION

The number of the question corresponds to the same-numbered outcome at the beginning of the chapter.

1. Assessment of an IV cocaine user with infective endocarditis should focus on which signs and symptoms *(select all that apply)*?
   a. Retinal hemorrhages
   b. Splinter hemorrhages
   c. Presence of Osler's nodes
   d. Painless nodules over bony prominences
   e. Painless erythematous macules on the palms and soles
2. The nurse is caring for a patient with chronic constrictive pericarditis. Which assessment finding reflects a *more* serious complication of this condition?
   a. Fatigue
   b. Peripheral edema
   c. Jugular venous distention
   d. Thickened pericardium on echocardiography
3. A patient is admitted with myocarditis. While performing the initial assessment, the nurse may find which clinical signs and symptoms *(select all that apply)*?
   a. Angina
   b. Pleuritic chest pain
   c. Splinter hemorrhages
   d. Pericardial friction rub
   e. Presence of Osler's nodes
4. *Priority* nursing management for a patient with myocarditis includes interventions related to
   a. meticulous skin care.
   b. antibiotic prophylaxis.
   c. tight glycemic control.
   d. oxygenation and ventilation.
5. When teaching a patient about the long-term consequences of rheumatic fever, the nurse should discuss the possibility of
   a. valvular heart disease.
   b. pulmonary hypertension.
   c. superior vena cava syndrome.
   d. hypertrophy of the right ventricle.

6. Which is a *priority* nursing intervention for a patient during the acute phase of rheumatic fever?
   a. Administration of antibiotics as ordered
   b. Management of pain with opioid analgesics
   c. Encouragement of fluid intake for hydration
   d. Performance of frequent active range-of-motion exercises
7. Which clinical finding would *most* likely indicate decreased cardiac output in a patient with aortic valve regurgitation?
   a. Reduction in peripheral edema and weight
   b. Carotid venous distention and new-onset atrial fibrillation
   c. Significant pulsus paradoxus and diminished peripheral pulses
   d. Shortness of breath on minimal exertion and a diastolic murmur
8. A patient is diagnosed with mitral stenosis and new-onset atrial fibrillation. Which interventions could the nurse delegate to unlicensed assistive personnel (UAP) *(select all that apply)*?
   a. Obtain and record daily weight.
   b. Determine apical-radial pulse rate.
   c. Observe for overt signs of bleeding.
   d. Obtain and record vital signs, including pulse oximetry.
   e. Teach the patient how to purchase a Medic Alert device.
9. Which diagnostic study *best* differentiates the various types of cardiomyopathy?
   a. Echocardiography
   b. Arterial blood gases
   c. Heart catheterization
   d. Endomyocardial biopsy
10. The nurse is caring for a patient newly admitted with heart failure secondary to dilated cardiomyopathy. Which intervention would be a *priority*?
   a. Encourage caregivers to learn CPR.
   b. Consider a consultation with hospice for palliative care.
   c. Monitor the patient's response to prescribed medications.
   d. Arrange for the patient to enter a cardiac rehabilitation program.

1. a, b, c, e, 2. c, 3. a, b, d, 4. d, 5. a, 6. a, 7. d, 8. a, c, d, 9. a, 10. c

For rationales to these answers and even more NCLEX review questions, visit *http://evolve.elsevier.com/Lewis/medsurg*.

## EVOLVE WEBSITE

http://evolve.elsevier.com/Lewis/medsurg

**Review Questions (Online Only)**

**Key Points**

**Answer Keys for Questions**

- Rationales for Bridge to NCLEX Examination Questions
- Answer Guidelines for Case Study on p. 800

**Student Case Study**

- Patient With Rheumatic Fever and Heart Disease

**Nursing Care Plans**

- eNursing Care Plan 36-1: Patient With Infective Endocarditis
- eNursing Care Plan 36-2: Patient With Valvular Heart Disease

**Conceptual Care Map Creator**

**Audio Glossary**

**Supporting Media**

- Audio
  - Pericardial Friction Rub

**Content Updates**

## REFERENCES


1. Keynan Y, Singal R, Kumar K, et al: Infective endocarditis in the intensive care unit, *Crit Care Clin* 29(4):923, 2013.
2. Josephson L: Infective endocarditis: a review for nurses, *Dimens Crit Care Nurs* 33(6):327, 2014.
*3. Baddour LM, Wilson WR, Bayer AS, et al: Infective endocarditis in adults: diagnosis, antimicrobial therapy, and management of complications. A scientific statement for healthcare professionals from the American Heart Association, *Circulation* 132:e215, 2015.
4. Gupta A, Gupta A, Kaul U, et al: Infective endocarditis in an Indian setup: are we entering the 'modern' era? *Indian J Crit Care Med* 17(3):140, 2013.
5. Eun J, Smith A: Safety and efficacy of colchicine therapy in the prevention of recurrent pericarditis, *Am J Health-Syst Pharm* 71(15):1277, 2014.
6. Kindermann I, Barth C, Mahfoud F, et al: Update on myocarditis, *J Am Coll Cardiol* 59(9):779, 2012.
7. Kumar RK, Tandon R: Rheumatic fever & rheumatic heart disease: the last 50 years, *Indian J Med Res* 137(4):643, 2013.
*8. Gewitz MH, Baltimore RS, Tani LY, et al: Revision of the Jones criteria for the diagnosis of acute rheumatic fever in the era of Doppler echocardiography: a scientific statement from the American Heart Association, *Circulation* 131:1806, 2015.
9. Texas Heart Institute Heart Information Center: Rheumatic fever. Retrieved from *www.texasheart.org/HIC/Topics/Cond/rheufev.cfm*.
10. Woods CJ, Levy CS: Medscape: Streptococcus Group B infections treatment & management. Retrieved from *http://emedicine.medscape.com/article/229091-treatment*.
*11. Nishimura RA, Otto CM, Bonow RO, et al: 2014 AHA/ACC Guideline for the management of patients with valvular heart disease: executive summary: a report of the American College of Cardiology/American Heart Association Task Force on Practice Guidelines, *Circulation* 129:2440, 2014.
*12. Meziani F, Debbal S, Atbi A: Analysis of the pathological severity degree of aortic stenosis (AS) and mitral stenosis (MS) using the discrete wavelet transform (DTW), *J Med Eng Tech* 37(1):61, 2013.
13. Mitral Valve Repair Center at the Mount Sinai Hospital: Mitral repair, 2015. Retrieved from *www.mitralvalverepair.org/content/view/64*.
14. Teehan S, McKee G, Dempsey O: Management of severe aortic stenosis, *WIN* 22(10):61, 2014/2015.
15. Mitral Valve Repair Center at the Mount Sinai Hospital: Minimally invasive heart surgery center, 2015. Retrieved from *www.mitralvalverepair.org/content/view/16*
16. Zhang P, Melander S: Transcatheter aortic valve replacement for severe aortic stenosis, *Crit Care Nurs Q* 37(4):346, 2014.
17. Medtronic: An advanced TAVR Design. CoreValve® Transcatheter Aortic Valve Implantation (TAVI) platform. Retrieved from *www.corevalve.com/intl/product/index.htm*.
18. Malaisrie SC, McDonald E, Kruse J, et al: Mortality while waiting for aortic valve replacement, *Ann Thorac Surg* 98(5):1564, 2014.
19. Padilla H, Paltoo B, Edsall R, et al: Recognizing and treating Takotsubo cardiomyopathy, *Nursing* 44(8):50, 2014.
20. Frustaci A, Petrosillo N, Farancone M, et al: Biopsy-proven autoimmune myocarditis in HIV-associated dilated cardiomyopathy, *BMC Infect Dis* 14:729, 2014.
21. Nicholson C: Chronic heart failure: pathophysiology, diagnosis and treatment, *Nurs Older People* 26(7):29, 2014.
*22. Al-Zaiti SS, Fallavollita JA, Cantry JM, et al: Electrocardiographic predictors of sudden and non-sudden cardiac death in patients with ischemic cardiomyopathy, *Heart Lung* 43:527, 2014.
23. American Heart Association: Prevention and treatment of cardiomyopathy. Retrieved from *www.heart.org/HEARTORG/Conditions/More/Cardiomyopathy/Prevention-and-Treatment-of-Cardiomyopathy_UCM_444176_Article.jsp*.
24. Hensley N, Deitrich J, Nyhan D, et al: Hypertrophic cardiomyopathy: a review, *Anesth Analg* 120(3):554, 2015.
25. Caselli S, Maron MS, Pandian NG, et al: Differentiating left ventricular hypertrophy in athletes from that in patients with hypertrophic cardiomyopathy, *Am J Cardiol* 114(9):1383, 2013.
*26. Chen YZ, Qiao SB, Hu FH, et al: Biventricular reverse remodeling after successful alcohol septal ablation for obstructive hypertrophic cardiomyopathy, *Am J Cardiol* 115(4):493, 2015.

*Evidence-based information for clinical practice.

# 37

# Vascular Disorders

*Deidre D. Wipke-Tevis, Kathleen A. Rich*

*Hardening of the heart ages people more quickly than hardening of the arteries.*

**Unknown**

http://evolve.elsevier.com/Lewis/medsurg/

## LEARNING OUTCOMES

1. Relate the major risk factors to the etiology and pathophysiology of peripheral artery disease (PAD).
2. Describe the clinical manifestations, interprofessional care, and nursing management of the patient with PAD of the lower extremities.
3. Plan appropriate nursing and interprofessional management for the patient with acute arterial ischemic disorders of the lower extremities.
4. Differentiate the pathophysiology, clinical manifestations, and nursing and interprofessional management of the patient with thromboangiitis obliterans (Buerger's disease) and Raynaud's phenomenon.
5. Differentiate the pathophysiology, clinical manifestations, interprofessional care, and nursing management of patients with different types of aortic aneurysms.
6. Select appropriate nursing interventions for a patient undergoing an aortic aneurysm repair.
7. Describe the pathophysiology, clinical manifestations, interprofessional care, and nursing management of the patient with aortic dissection.
8. Evaluate the risk factors predisposing patients to the development of superficial vein thrombosis and venous thromboembolism (VTE).
9. Differentiate between the clinical characteristics of superficial vein thrombosis and VTE.
10. Compare and contrast the interprofessional care and nursing management of patients with superficial vein thrombosis and VTE.
11. Prioritize the key aspects of nursing management of the patient receiving anticoagulant therapy.
12. Relate the pathophysiology and clinical manifestations to the interprofessional care, drug therapy, and interventional/surgical therapies of patients with varicose veins, chronic venous insufficiency, and venous leg ulcers.

## KEY TERMS

acute arterial ischemia, p. 808
aneurysm, p. 810
aortic dissection, p. 814
chronic venous insufficiency (CVI), p. 826
critical limb ischemia, p. 804
deep vein thrombosis (DVT), p. 816
intermittent claudication, p. 803
peripheral artery disease (PAD), p. 802
post-thrombotic syndrome (PTS), p. 818
Raynaud's phenomenon, p. 809
superficial vein thrombosis, p. 816
thromboangiitis obliterans (Buerger's disease), p. 809
varicose veins, p. 825
venous thromboembolism (VTE), p. 816
venous thrombosis, p. 816
Virchow's triad, p. 816

Problems of the vascular system include disorders of the arteries, veins, and lymphatic vessels. Arterial disorders are classified as atherosclerotic, aneurysmal, and nonatherosclerotic vascular diseases. Atherosclerotic vascular disease is divided into coronary, cerebral, peripheral, mesenteric, and renal artery disease.[1] This chapter discusses peripheral artery disease, aortic aneurysm and dissection, and venous diseases.

## PERIPHERAL ARTERY DISEASE

**Peripheral artery disease (PAD)** involves thickening of artery walls. This results in a progressive narrowing of the arteries of the upper and lower extremities. PAD prevalence increases with age. It typically becomes symptomatic in the sixth to eighth decades of life. In people with diabetes mellitus, PAD occurs earlier. In the United States, PAD prevalence is higher in those of lower socioeconomic status, women, and African Americans.[2]

PAD is strongly related to other types of cardiovascular disease (CVD) and their risk factors. Patients with PAD have a significantly higher risk of mortality (in general), CVD mortality, major coronary events, and stroke.[3] PAD is a marker of advanced systemic atherosclerosis. Patients with PAD are more likely to have coronary artery disease (CAD) and/or cerebral artery disease.

Unfortunately, low levels of public awareness of PAD and its risk factors exist in the United States. In general, PAD remains underdiagnosed and undertreated.

### Etiology and Pathophysiology

The leading cause of PAD is *atherosclerosis,* a gradual thickening of the *intima* (the innermost layer of the arterial wall) and *media*

Reviewed by Rebecca Personett, RN, PhD, NEA-BC, Professor of Nursing, North Central Texas College, Gainesville, Texas and Brookhaven College, Dallas, Texas; Tara McMillan-Queen, RN, MSN, ANP, GNP, Faculty II, Mercy School of Nursing, Charlotte, North Carolina; and Janet M. Riggs, RN, MSN, DrNP, Clinical Research Coordinator, University of Pennsylvania, Philadelphia, Pennsylvania.

(middle layer of the arterial wall). This results from the deposit of cholesterol and lipids within the vessel walls and leads to progressive narrowing of the artery (see Fig. 33-1). Although the exact cause of atherosclerosis is unknown, inflammation and endothelial injury play a major role (see Chapter 33).

Risk factors for PAD are similar, but not identical, to coronary artery disease. Important risk factors for PAD are tobacco use (most important), chronic kidney disease, diabetes, hypertension, and hypercholesterolemia.[2] The additive presence of risk factors dramatically increases the risk of PAD, especially in women and African Americans.[2] Other risk factors include elevated C-reactive protein, family history, hypertriglyceridemia, increasing age, hyperhomocysteinemia, hyperuricemia, obesity, sedentary lifestyle, and stress.[4]

Atherosclerosis more commonly affects certain segments of the arterial tree. These include the coronary (see Chapter 33), carotid (see Chapter 57), and lower extremity arteries. Clinical symptoms occur when vessels are 60% to 75% blocked.

## PERIPHERAL ARTERY DISEASE OF THE LOWER EXTREMITIES

Lower extremity PAD may affect the iliac, femoral, popliteal, tibial, or peroneal arteries, or any combination of these arteries (Fig. 37-1). The femoral popliteal area is the most common site in nondiabetic patients. Patients with diabetes tend to develop PAD in the arteries below the knee. In advanced PAD, multiple levels of occlusions are found.

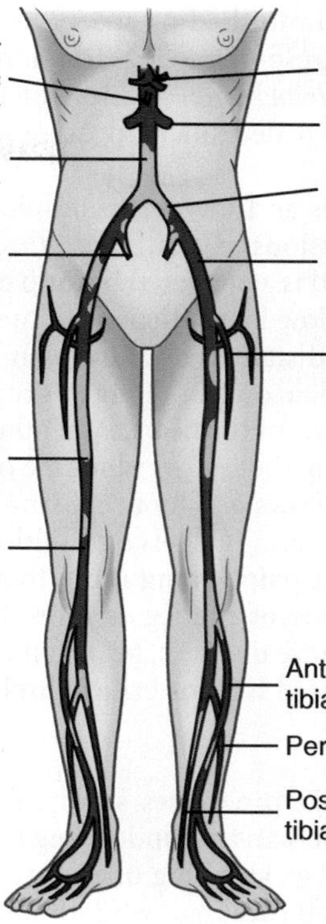


**FIG. 37-1** Common anatomic locations of atherosclerotic lesions (shown in *yellow*) of the abdominal aorta and lower extremities.

### GENDER DIFFERENCES
***Vascular Disorders***

**Men**

- Thromboangiitis obliterans (Buerger's disease) occurs predominantly in men <40 yr of age.
- Abdominal aortic aneurysms (AAAs) are more common in men than women.
- Men with AAAs are more likely to undergo endovascular aneurysm repair or open aneurysm repair than women.
- Sexual dysfunction in male patients is common after aortic surgery.
- Aortic dissection affects men more often than women.

**Women**

- Peripheral artery disease (PAD) prevalence is higher in women.
- Women with low lifetime recreational activity are at greater risk for PAD than similar men.
- Older women experience the classic signs of intermittent claudication less often than men.
- Women with PAD experience faster functional decline and greater mobility loss than men with PAD.
- Raynaud's phenomenon occurs primarily in women between 15 and 40 yr of age.
- Risk for venous thromboembolism (VTE) is greater in women over age 35 who use tobacco and oral contraceptives or oral hormone therapy, are pregnant or postpartum, or have a family history of VTE.
- Primary varicose veins are more common and more symptomatic in women than men.
- Risk for varicose veins is greater in multiparous women.
- Women with AAAs are at higher risk for rupture.
- In-hospital mortality is higher in women undergoing revascularization than men, regardless of disease severity or procedure performed.
- Women develop surgical site infections more often than men.
- Women, particularly African American and Hispanic women, experience more graft thrombosis and amputation after lower extremity bypass surgery than men.

### Clinical Manifestations

Generally, the severity of the clinical manifestations depends on the site and extent of the blockage and the amount of collateral circulation. The classic symptom of lower extremity PAD is **intermittent claudication**. This ischemic muscle pain is caused by exercise, resolves within 10 minutes or less with rest, and is reproducible. The ischemic pain is a result of the buildup of lactic acid from anaerobic metabolism. Once the patient stops exercising, the lactic acid is cleared and the pain subsides. PAD of the iliac arteries produces claudication in the buttocks and thighs. Calf claudication indicates femoral or popliteal artery involvement.

As many as one third of patients with PAD report classic claudication symptoms. The remaining either have no symptoms or present with atypical leg symptoms (e.g., burning, heaviness, pressure, soreness, tightness, weakness) in atypical locations (e.g., ankle, foot, hamstring, hip, knee, shin). Older women experience classic claudication less often than men.[5] If PAD involves the internal iliac arteries, erectile dysfunction may result.

*Paresthesia,* or numbness or tingling, in the toes or feet may result from nerve tissue ischemia. True peripheral neuropathy occurs more often in patients with diabetes (see Chapter 48) and in those with long-standing ischemia. Neuropathy produces severe shooting or burning pain in the extremity. It does not follow particular nerve roots and may be present near ulcerated areas. Gradual, reduced blood flow to neurons produces loss of both pressure and deep pain sensations. Thus patients may not notice lower extremity injuries.

The limb's physical appearance provides important information about blood flow. The skin becomes thin, shiny, and taut, and hair loss occurs on the lower legs. Pedal, popliteal, or femoral pulses are diminished or absent. Pallor (blanching of the foot) develops in response to leg elevation *(elevation pallor)*. Conversely, *reactive hyperemia* (redness of the foot) develops when the limb is in a dependent position *(dependent rubor)* (Table 37-1).

As PAD progresses and involves multiple arterial segments, continuous pain develops at rest. *Rest pain* most often occurs in the foot or toes and is aggravated by limb elevation. Rest pain occurs when blood flow is insufficient to meet basic metabolic requirements of the distal tissues. Rest pain occurs more often at night because cardiac output tends to drop during sleep and the limbs are at the level of the heart. Patients often try to achieve pain relief by dangling the leg over the side of the bed or sleeping in a chair. This allows gravity to maximize blood flow.

Critical limb ischemia (CLI) is a condition characterized by chronic ischemic rest pain lasting more than 2 weeks, arterial leg ulcers, or gangrene of the leg as a result of PAD. Patients with PAD who also have diabetes, heart failure, and a history of a stroke are at increased risk for critical limb ischemia.[6]

## Complications

Lower extremity PAD progresses slowly. Prolonged ischemia leads to atrophy of the skin and underlying muscles. Even minor trauma to the feet (e.g., stubbing one's toe, blister from shoes) can result in delayed healing, wound infection, and tissue necrosis, especially in the patient with diabetes. Arterial (ischemic) ulcers most often occur over bony prominences on the toes, feet, and lower legs (Table 37-1). Nonhealing arterial ulcers and gangrene are the most serious complications. If PAD is present for an extended period, collateral circulation may prevent gangrene of the extremity.

Amputation may be needed if adequate blood flow is not restored or if severe infection occurs. Uncontrolled pain and severe, spreading infection are indicators that an amputation is needed in people who are not candidates for revascularization.

## Diagnostic Studies

Various tests can assess blood flow and the vascular system (Table 37-2). Doppler ultrasound with duplex imaging maps blood flow throughout the entire region of an artery. When palpation of a peripheral pulse is difficult because of severe PAD, the Doppler ultrasound can determine the degree of blood flow. A palpable pulse and a Doppler pulse are not equivalent, and the terms are not interchangeable.

*Segmental blood pressures* (BPs) are obtained (using Doppler ultrasound and a sphygmomanometer) at the thigh, below the knee, and at ankle level while the patient is supine. A drop in

### TABLE 37-1 Comparison of Peripheral Artery and Venous Disease

| Characteristic | Peripheral Artery Disease | Venous Disease |
|---|---|---|
| **Peripheral pulses** | Decreased or absent | Present, may be difficult to palpate with edema |
| **Capillary refill** | >3 sec | <3 sec |
| **Ankle-brachial index** | ≤0.90 | >0.90 |
| **Edema** | Absent unless leg constantly in dependent position | Lower leg edema |
| **Hair** | Loss of hair on legs, feet, toes | Hair may be present or absent |
| **Ulcer** | | |
| • Location | Tips of toes, foot, or lateral malleolus | Near medial malleolus |
| • Margin | Rounded, smooth, looks "punched out" | Irregularly shaped |
| • Drainage | Minimal | Moderate to large amount |
| • Tissue | Black eschar or pale pink granulation | Yellow slough or dark red, "ruddy" granulation |
| **Pain** | Intermittent claudication or rest pain in foot<br>Ulcer may or may not be painful | Dull ache or heaviness in calf or thigh<br>Ulcer often painful |
| **Nails** | Thickened; brittle | Normal or thickened |
| **Skin color** | Dependent rubor, elevation pallor | Bronze-brown pigmentation<br>Varicose veins may be visible |
| **Skin texture** | Thin, shiny, taut | Skin thick, hardened, and indurated |
| **Skin temperature** | Cool, temperature gradient down the leg | Warm, no temperature gradient |
| **Dermatitis** | Rarely occurs | Frequently occurs |
| **Pruritus** | Rarely occurs | Frequently occurs |

### TABLE 37-2 Interprofessional Care
#### *Peripheral Artery Disease*

**Diagnostic Assessment**
- Health history and physical examination, including palpation of peripheral pulses
- Doppler ultrasound studies
- Segmental blood pressures
- Ankle-brachial index (Table 37-3)
- Duplex imaging
- Angiography
- Magnetic resonance angiography

**Management**
- Cardiovascular disease risk factor modification
  - Tobacco cessation
  - Regular physical exercise
  - Achieve or maintain ideal body weight
  - Follow Dietary Approaches to Stop Hypertension (DASH) diet
  - Tight glucose control in diabetics including A1C monitoring
  - Tight BP control
  - Treatment of hyperlipidemia and hypertriglyceridemia (see Table 33-5)
  - Antiplatelet agent (aspirin or clopidogrel [Plavix])
  - Angiotensin-converting enzyme inhibitors (see Table 32-7)
- Treatment of claudication symptoms
  - Structured walking or exercise program
  - Cilostazol (Pletal) or pentoxifylline
- Nutritional therapy
- Physical/occupational therapy
- Proper foot care (see Table 48-21)

***Surgical Therapy***
- Percutaneous transluminal balloon angioplasty with or without stent
- Percutaneous transluminal atherectomy
- Percutaneous transluminal cryoplasty
- Peripheral artery bypass surgery
- Patch graft angioplasty, often in conjunction with bypass surgery
- Endarterectomy (for localized stenosis but rarely done as a stand-alone procedure)
- Thrombolytic therapy or mechanical clot extraction therapy (for acute ischemia only)
- Sympathectomy (for pain management only)
- Amputation

**TABLE 37-3 Interpreting Ankle-Brachial Index Results**

| Ankle-Brachial Index (ABI) | Clinical Significance |
|---|---|
| >1.30 | Noncompressible arteries |
| 1.00-1.30 | Normal ABI |
| 0.91-0.99 | Borderline ABI |
| ≤0.90 | Abnormal ABI |
| **Classification of PAD Severity** | |
| 0.90-0.71 | Mild PAD |
| 0.70-0.41 | Moderate PAD |
| ≤0.40 | Severe PAD |

*PAD,* Peripheral artery disease.

segmental BP of greater than 30 mm Hg suggests PAD. Angiography and magnetic resonance angiography delineate the location and extent of PAD (see Table 31-6).

The *ankle-brachial index* (ABI) is a PAD screening tool. It is performed using a hand-held Doppler. The ABI is calculated by dividing the ankle systolic BPs by the higher of the left and right brachial systolic BPs. PAD guidelines recommend uniform reporting of ABI results[6] (Table 37-3). In older patients and those with diabetes, the arteries often are calcified and noncompressible. This results in a falsely elevated ABI.

## Interprofessional Care

Table 37-2 summarizes the interprofessional care for a patient with PAD.

**Risk Factor Modification.** The first treatment goal in treating PAD is to reduce CVD risk factors in all patients with PAD regardless of the severity of symptoms. Risk factors must be modified with both drug therapy and lifestyle changes (see Tables 33-1 to 33-4).

Tobacco cessation is essential to reduce the risk of CVD events, PAD progression, and death. This is a complex and difficult process with a high incidence of relapse. Comprehensive tobacco cessation strategies are recommended (see Tables 10-4 to 10-6).

Diabetes is a major risk factor for PAD and increases the risk of amputation in these patients. It is recommended that patients with diabetes maintain a glycosylated hemoglobin (A1C) below 7.0% and, optimally, as near as possible to 6.0%.[7] (Chapter 48 discusses diabetes mellitus.)

Aggressive lipid management is essential for all patients with PAD. Both dietary interventions and drug therapy are needed. Statins (e.g., simvastatin [Zocor]) and a fibric acid derivative (gemfibrozil [Lopid]) may be used (see Table 33-5).

Hypertension is a well-known risk factor for PAD progression, as well as other CVD events (e.g., stroke, myocardial infarction [MI], heart failure). Current guidelines for the management of hypertension in people with PAD include BP less than 140/90 mm Hg.[6] In PAD patients with diabetes or renal insufficiency, BP less than 130/80 mm Hg is recommended.

Angiotensin-converting enzyme (ACE) inhibitors (e.g., ramipril [Altace]) are used for symptomatic patients with PAD. Lifestyle changes are encouraged and include reducing dietary sodium and following the Dietary Approaches to Stop Hypertension (DASH) diet. (Chapter 32 discusses hypertension.)

**Drug Therapy.** Antiplatelet agents are critical for reducing the risks of CVD events and death in PAD patients. Oral antiplatelet therapy should include 75 to 325 mg/day of aspirin. Aspirin-intolerant patients may take 75 mg of clopidogrel (Plavix) daily.

Combination antiplatelet therapy with aspirin and clopidogrel is not typically recommended. However, it may be used in select high-risk PAD patients. Anticoagulants (e.g., warfarin [Coumadin]) are not recommended for prevention of CVD events in PAD patients.

**DRUG ALERT Clopidogrel (Plavix) and Omeprazole (Prilosec)**

- Antiplatelet effect of clopidogrel is reduced by about half when given with omeprazole.
- This increases the risk of MI and stroke.

Two drugs are available to treat intermittent claudication: cilostazol (Pletal) and pentoxifylline. Cilostazol, a phosphodiesterase inhibitor, inhibits platelet aggregation and increases vasodilation. Pentoxifylline, a xanthine derivative, improves the deformability of RBCs and WBCs and decreases fibrinogen concentration, platelet adhesiveness, and blood viscosity.

**DRUG ALERT Cilostazol (Pletal)**

- Contraindicated in patients with heart failure of any severity.

**Exercise Therapy.** A supervised exercise program is recommended as an initial treatment for all patients with intermittent claudication. Exercise should be performed for 30 to 45 minutes/day, at least 3 times/week, for a minimum of 3 months. Although walking is the most commonly prescribed exercise for PAD patients, alternative modes of exercise (e.g., cycling) also improve walking ability and quality of life in patients with PAD.[8]

Encouragement of participation in exercise is particularly important for women with PAD, since women experience faster functional decline and greater mobility loss than men with PAD. Overall, patients with PAD who have higher levels of daily physical activity also have better survival rates.[6]

**Nutritional Therapy.** Teach patients with PAD to maintain a body mass index (BMI) less than 25 kg/m$^2$ and a waist circumference less than 40 inches for men and less than 35 inches for women. Even modest, sustained weight loss of 3% to 5% yields important reductions in triglycerides, glucose, A1C, and the risk of developing type 2 diabetes. Greater weight loss produces greater benefits.[9] Recommend a diet reduced in calories and salt for obese or overweight individuals with PAD.[10]

**Complementary and Alternative Therapies.** Patients taking antiplatelet agents, nonsteroidal antiinflammatory drugs (NSAIDs) (e.g., ibuprofen), and anticoagulants (e.g., warfarin) should consult with their HCP before taking any dietary or herbal supplements because of potential interactions and bleeding risks[11] (see the Complementary & Alternative Therapies box on p. 820).

**Care of the Leg With Critical Limb Ischemia.** Optimal therapy for the patient with critical limb ischemia is revascularization via bypass surgery using an *autogenous* (native) vein. If this is not feasible, percutaneous transluminal angioplasty (PTA) is recommended.[6] Patients with CLI who are not candidates for surgery or PTA may be treated with IV prostanoids (e.g., iloprost [Ventavis]). These drugs may decrease rest pain and improve ulcer healing. Patients with CLI should continue optimal drug therapy (e.g., statin, antiplatelet, ACE inhibitor, β-blocker) to reduce the risk of a CVD event.

Conservative management of critical limb ischemia includes protecting the extremity from trauma, decreasing ischemic pain, preventing and controlling infection, and improving perfusion. Carefully inspect, cleanse, and lubricate feet to prevent cracking of the skin and infection. Avoid lubrication between the toes and soaking the patient's feet to prevent skin *maceration* (or breakdown). If ulceration is present, keep the affected foot clean and dry. Cover any ulcers with a dry, sterile dressing to maintain cleanliness. Deep ulcers can be treated with a variety of wound care products, but healing is unlikely without increased blood flow. Systemic antibiotics are used in patients with CLI, skin ulcerations, and limb infection.[6]

Encourage the patient to select soft, roomy, and protective footwear and avoid extremes of heat and cold. Keep the patient's heels free of pressure. You can do this by placing a pillow under the calves so that the heels are off the mattress. Commercially available devices can also provide heel protection. Giving opioid analgesics and placing the bed in the reverse Trendelenburg position may control pain and increase perfusion to the lower extremities.

Spinal cord stimulation may be helpful in managing pain and preventing amputation in patients with CLI. Other promising strategies include growth factors and gene and stem cell therapy to stimulate blood vessel growth *(angiogenesis)*. Unfortunately, almost half of the patients with CLI will die within 5 years.[12]

**Interventional Radiology Catheter-Based Procedures.** Interventional radiology catheter-based procedures are alternatives to open surgical approaches for treatment of lower extremity PAD. These procedures take place in a catheterization laboratory rather than in an operating room. Determining which intervention to use depends on blockage location and lesion type and severity.

All these procedures are similar to angiography in that they involve the insertion of a specialized catheter into the femoral artery. The *percutaneous transluminal angioplasty* (PTA) procedure uses a catheter that contains a balloon at the tip. The end of the catheter is moved to the narrowed (stenotic) area of the artery. The balloon is then inflated, compressing the atherosclerotic intimal lining.[13]

*Stents,* expandable metallic devices, are placed within the artery immediately after the balloon angioplasty is done. The stent acts as a scaffold to keep the artery open. Both angioplasty balloons and peripheral stents may be coated with a drug-eluting agent (e.g., paclitaxel) to reduce restenosis. These drugs work by limiting the growth of new tissue in the treated stenotic area and improve long-term patency rates.[14]

*Atherectomy* is the removal of the obstructing plaque. A directional atherectomy device uses a high-speed cutting disk that cuts long strips of the atheroma. Laser atherectomy uses ultraviolet energy to break up the atheroma. Other types of atherectomy catheters have a diamond-coated tip that rotates at a high speed (similar to a dentist drill). These crush the calcium within the atheroma into particles smaller than a blood cell.[15]

*Cryoplasty* combines two procedures: PTA and cold therapy. A specialized balloon is filled with liquid nitrous oxide, which changes from liquid to gas as it enters the balloon. Expansion of the gas results in cooling to 14° F (−10° C). The cold temperature limits restenosis by reducing smooth muscle cell activity.[16]

Pre- and postprocedure nursing care is the same as for a diagnostic angiography (see Table 31-6). Antiplatelet agents are needed postprocedure to reduce the risk of restenosis. Long-term, low-dose aspirin therapy or clopidogrel is recommended.

**Surgical Therapy.** Various surgical approaches can be used to improve blood flow beyond a blocked artery. When possible, peripheral artery bypass surgery should be done with an autogenous vein to bypass (carry blood around) the lesion (Fig. 37-2).

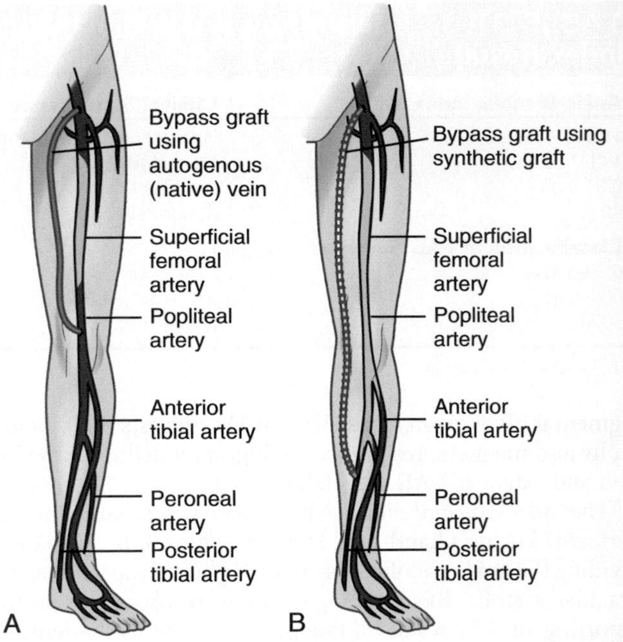


**FIG. 37-2** **A,** Femoral-popliteal bypass graft around an occluded superficial femoral artery. **B,** Femoral–posterior tibial bypass graft around occluded superficial femoral, popliteal, and proximal tibial arteries.

Synthetic grafts typically are used for long bypasses such as an axillary-femoral bypass. When a person's own vein is not available, human umbilical vein or a composite sequential bypass graft (native vein plus synthetic graft) is an alternative.[6] PTA with stenting may also be used in combination with bypass surgery.

Other surgical options include *endarterectomy* (opening the artery and removing the obstructing plaque) and *patch graft angioplasty* (opening the artery, removing plaque, and sewing a patch to the opening to widen the lumen). In-hospital mortality is higher in women undergoing revascularization than men, regardless of disease severity or procedure performed.[17]

Amputation may be required if tissue necrosis is extensive, gangrene or osteomyelitis develops, or all major arteries in the limb are blocked, precluding the possibility of successful surgery. Every effort is made to preserve as much of the limb as possible to improve the potential for rehabilitation. (Amputation is discussed in Chapter 62.)

## ❖ NURSING MANAGEMENT: LOWER EXTREMITY PERIPHERAL ARTERY DISEASE

### ◆ Nursing Assessment

Table 37-4 presents subjective and objective data that you should obtain from a patient with PAD.

### ◆ Nursing Diagnoses

Nursing diagnoses for the patient with PAD may include, but are not limited to, the following:

- Ineffective peripheral tissue perfusion *related to* deficient knowledge of contributing factors
- Activity intolerance *related to* imbalance between $O_2$ supply and demand
- Chronic pain *related to* ischemia, inflammation, and swelling
- Ineffective health management *related to* lack of knowledge of disease and self-care measures

**TABLE 37-4 Nursing Assessment**

***Peripheral Artery Disease***

**Subjective Data**

***Important Health Information***

*Past health history:* Tobacco use, diabetes mellitus, hypertension, hyperlipidemia, hypertriglyceridemia, hyperuricemia, impaired renal function, obesity. ↑ high-sensitivity C-reactive protein, homocysteine, or lipoprotein (a) [Lp(a)] levels. Positive family history, sedentary lifestyle, stress

***Functional Health Patterns***

*Health perception–health management:* Family history of cardiovascular disease. Tobacco use, including exposure to environmental smoke

*Nutritional-metabolic:* High sodium, saturated fat, and cholesterol intake. Elevated A1C

*Activity-exercise:* Exercise intolerance

*Cognitive-perceptual:* Buttock, thigh, or calf pain that is precipitated by exercise and that subsides with rest (intermittent claudication) or progresses to pain at rest. Burning pain in feet and toes at rest. Numbness, tingling, sensation of cold in legs or feet. Progressive loss of sensation and deep pain in extremities

*Sexuality-reproductive:* Erectile dysfunction

**Objective Data**

***Integumentary***

Loss of hair on legs and feet. Thick toenails. Pallor with elevation. Dependent rubor. Thin, cool, shiny skin with muscle atrophy. Skin breakdown and arterial ulcers, especially over bony areas. Gangrene

***Cardiovascular***

Decreased or absent peripheral pulses. Feet cool to touch. Capillary refill >3 sec. Bruits may be present at pulse sites.

***Neurologic***

Mobility or sensation impairment

***Possible Diagnostic Findings***

Arterial stenosis evident with duplex imaging, ↓ Doppler pressures, ↓ ankle-brachial index, angiography indicative of peripheral atherosclerosis

Additional information on nursing diagnoses for the patient with PAD of the lower extremities is presented in eNursing Care Plan 37-1 on the website for this chapter.

## ◆ Planning

The overall goals for the patient who has lower extremity PAD include (1) adequate tissue perfusion; (2) relief of pain; (3) increased exercise tolerance; (4) intact, healthy skin on the extremities; and (5) increased knowledge of disease and treatment plan.

## ◆ Nursing Implementation

◆ **Health Promotion.** Assess the patient for CVD risk factors and provide instructions on how to control them (see Tables 33-1 to 33-2). Also teach diet modification to reduce the intake of cholesterol, saturated fat, and refined sugars (see Tables 33-3 to 33-4); proper care of the feet; and avoidance of injury to the extremities. Encourage patients with positive family histories of cardiac, diabetic, or vascular disease to obtain regular follow-up care.

◆ **Acute Care.** After surgical or radiologic intervention, the patient is moved to a recovery area for observation. Check the operative extremity every 15 minutes initially and then hourly for color, temperature, capillary refill, presence of peripheral pulses, and sensation and movement. Loss of palpable pulses or a change in the Doppler sound over a pulse requires immediate notification of the HCP and prompt intervention. Postoperative ABI measurements are not recommended as they place the patient at risk for graft thrombosis. Compare all assessment findings with the patient's baseline and with findings in the opposite limb.

Many PAD patients have a history of chronic ischemic rest pain and may have developed a tolerance to opioids. Thus aggressive pain management may be needed postoperatively.

After the patient leaves the recovery area, continue to monitor perfusion to the extremities. Assess for potential complications such as bleeding, hematoma, thrombosis, embolization, and compartment syndrome. A dramatic increase in pain, loss of previously palpable pulses, extremity pallor or cyanosis, numbness or tingling, or a cold extremity suggests blockage of the graft or stent. Report these findings to the HCP immediately.

Avoid placing the patient in a knee-flexed position except for exercise. Turn the patient and position frequently with pillows to support the incision. On postoperative day 1, assist the patient out of bed several times daily. Discourage prolonged sitting with leg dependency, since it may cause pain and edema, increase the risk of venous thrombosis, and place stress on the suture lines. If edema develops, position the patient supine and elevate the leg above heart level.

**CHECK YOUR PRACTICE**

You are caring for a 74-yr-old male patient who is recovering from left femoral-popliteal bypass graft surgery. When responding to the patient's call bell, the patient reports severe pain in the operative leg. On assessment, you note that the dorsalis pedis and posterior tibial pulses are no longer palpable and the foot is cold to touch.

- What are your next actions?

Graduated compression stockings may be used to help control leg edema. Walking even short distances is desirable. The use of a walker may be helpful, especially in frail, older patients.

Surgical site infection (SSI) occurs in about 5% of cases. Women develop SSIs more often than men.[18] Careful postoperative assessment and wound care are important. SSIs are associated with early graft loss, longer hospitalizations, reoperation, and sepsis. If no complications occur, discharge can be anticipated 3 to 5 days after surgery.

◆ **Ambulatory Care.** Assess for CVD risk factors and be alert for opportunities to teach health promotion strategies to patients and their caregivers (see Chapters 4 and 33). Continued tobacco use dramatically decreases the long-term patency rates of grafts and stents and increases the risk of an MI or stroke. Long-term antiplatelet therapy with aspirin or clopidogrel is recommended for patients after surgery. Patients having distal peripheral bypass surgery (i.e., below the knee) using synthetic graft materials are given dual antiplatelet therapy (clopidogrel plus aspirin) for 1 year, followed by lifelong single antiplatelet therapy.[19]

Encourage supervised exercise training after a successful revascularization. Explain that exercise decreases CVD risk

**TABLE 37-5 Patient & Caregiver Teaching**
***Peripheral Artery Bypass Surgery***

*Include the following information in the teaching plan for a patient undergoing peripheral artery bypass surgery and the patient's caregiver.*

1. Reduce risk factors by stopping the use of all tobacco products, controlling blood glucose levels (if diabetic) and blood pressure, lowering cholesterol and triglyceride levels, achieving or maintaining ideal body weight, and exercising regularly.
2. Provide teaching about the basic mechanism of action and side effects of drugs such as antiplatelets, antihypertensives, lipid-lowering therapy, and pain medication.
3. Eat healthy—it is essential to recovery. Drink plenty of fluids, eat a well-balanced diet (e.g., foods high in protein, vitamins C and A, and zinc; high-fiber foods; fresh fruits and vegetables), eat fewer high-fat foods, and reduce salt intake.
4. Participate in a supervised exercise program or take a daily walk. In the beginning, take several short walks a day and rest between activities. Gradually increase your walking to 30 to 40 min/day, 3 to 5 days/wk.
5. Care for feet and legs. Inspect feet and wash them daily. Wear clean cotton or wool socks and well-fitting shoes. File toenails straight across. Avoid sitting with legs crossed, extreme hot and cold temperatures, and prolonged standing.
6. Follow routine postoperative wound care that includes keeping incision clean and dry; do not disturb Steri-Strips (if present).
7. Monitor for signs and symptoms of impaired healing or infection of the leg incision, and notify HCP if any of the following occur:
   - Prolonged drainage or pus from the incision
   - Increased redness, warmth, pain, or hardness along incision
   - Separation of wound edges
   - Temperature >100° F (37.8° C)
8. Keep all follow-up appointments with HCP.
9. Notify HCP immediately of increased leg or foot pain or a change in the color or temperature of leg or foot.

factors, including hypertension, hyperlipidemia, obesity, and glucose levels. Teach foot care to all patients with PAD. Meticulous foot care is especially important in the patient with diabetes and PAD (see Table 48-21). Diabetic neuropathy increases the patient's risk for injury and results in delay in seeking treatment. Tell patients to inspect their legs and feet daily for mottling, changes in skin color or texture, and reduction in hair growth. Show patients how to check skin temperature and capillary refill and to palpate pulses. Stress that they must report any changes in these findings or the development of ulceration or inflammation to their HCP.

Thick or overgrown toenails and calluses are potentially serious and require regular attention by an HCP (e.g., podiatrist). Patients who have poor eyesight, back problems, obesity, or arthritis may need help with foot care. Encourage patients to wear clean, all-cotton or all-wool socks and comfortable shoes with rounded (not pointed) toes and soft insoles. Tell patients to lace shoes loosely and to break in new shoes gradually (Table 37-5).

### ◆ Evaluation

The expected outcomes are that a patient with PAD of the lower extremities will have:

- Adequate peripheral tissue perfusion
- Increased activity tolerance
- Effective pain management
- Knowledge of disease and treatment plan

Additional information on the expected outcomes for the patient with PAD of the lower extremities is presented in eNursing Care Plan 37-1 (available on the website for this chapter).

## ACUTE ARTERIAL ISCHEMIC DISORDERS

### Etiology and Pathophysiology

**Acute arterial ischemia** is a sudden interruption in the arterial blood supply to a tissue, an organ, or an extremity that, if left untreated, can result in tissue death. It is caused by embolism, thrombosis of a preexisting atherosclerotic artery, or trauma. *Embolization* of a thrombus from the heart is the most frequent cause of acute arterial occlusion. Heart conditions in which thrombi can develop include infective endocarditis, mitral valve disease, atrial fibrillation, cardiomyopathies, and prosthetic heart valves. Noncardiac sources of emboli include aneurysms, ulcerated atherosclerotic plaque, recent endovascular procedures, and venous thrombi.

The thrombi become dislodged and may travel anywhere in the systemic circulation if they originate in the left side of the heart. Most emboli block an artery of the lower extremity in areas where vessels branch (e.g., iliofemoral, popliteal, tibial) or there is atherosclerotic narrowing. Sudden local thrombosis may occur at the site of an atherosclerotic plaque. Hypovolemia (e.g., shock), hyperviscosity (e.g., polycythemia), and hypercoagulability (e.g., chemotherapy) predispose an individual to thrombotic arterial occlusion.

*Traumatic injury* to the extremity itself may cause partial or total blockage. Acute arterial occlusion may also develop as a result of arterial dissection in the carotid artery or aorta or as a result of a procedure-related arterial injury (e.g., after angiography).

### Clinical Manifestations

Clinical manifestations of acute arterial ischemia include the *six Ps: pain, pallor, pulselessness, paresthesia, paralysis,* and *poikilothermia* (adaptation of the limb to the environmental temperature, most often cool). Without immediate intervention, ischemia may progress to tissue necrosis and gangrene within a few hours. If you detect these signs, immediately notify the HCP.

Paralysis is a late sign of acute arterial ischemia and signals the death of nerves supplying the extremity. Foot drop occurs as a result of nerve damage. Because nerve tissue is extremely sensitive to hypoxia, limb paralysis or ischemic neuropathy may persist even after revascularization.

### Interprofessional Care

Early diagnosis and treatment are essential to keep the affected limb viable during acute arterial ischemia. Anticoagulant therapy with IV unfractionated heparin (UH) is started to prevent thrombus growth and inhibit further embolization. In patients undergoing embolectomy, UH should be followed by long-term anticoagulation with warfarin (see discussion of other anticoagulant options later in this chapter).

To restore blood flow, the thrombus is removed as soon as possible. Options consist of surgical thrombectomy (recommended procedure), percutaneous catheter-directed thrombolytic therapy, percutaneous mechanical thrombectomy with or without thrombolytic therapy, or surgical bypass. A mechanical catheter that is used with a thrombolytic is known as a *pharmacomechanical device.*[20]

Percutaneous catheter-directed thrombolytic therapy using tissue plasminogen activator (tPA [alteplase]) or urokinase

(Kinlytic) is recommended for acute arterial ischemia of duration less than 14 days.[6] A catheter is inserted into the femoral artery and moved to the site of the clot, and the thrombolytic drug is continuously infused. Thrombolytic agents work by directly dissolving the clot over a period of 24 to 48 hours. (Chapter 33 discusses thrombolytic therapy.)

The mechanical thrombectomy device is designed to extract or fragment the thrombus. Surgical revascularization may be used in a patient with trauma (e.g., laceration of the artery) or with significant arterial blockage. Amputation is reserved for patients with ischemic rest pain and tissue loss in whom limb salvage is not possible. If the patient remains at risk for further embolization from a persistent source (e.g., chronic atrial fibrillation), long-term anticoagulation is recommended to prevent further acute arterial ischemic episodes[21] (see Table 37-10 on p. 820).

## THROMBOANGIITIS OBLITERANS

**Thromboangiitis obliterans (Buerger's disease)** is a nonatherosclerotic, segmental, recurrent inflammatory disorder of the small and medium arteries and veins of the upper and lower extremities. Rarely, systemic manifestations of the disease may involve cerebral, coronary, mesenteric, pulmonary, and/or renal arteries. The disease occurs mostly in young men (younger than 45 years of age) with a long history of tobacco and/or marijuana use and chronic periodontal infection but without other CVD risk factors (e.g., hypertension, hyperlipidemia, diabetes).[22]

In the acute phase of Buerger's disease, an inflammatory thrombus forms and blocks the vessel. Over time, the thrombus becomes more organized and the inflammation in the vessel wall subsides.[22]

During the chronic phase, thrombosis and fibrosis occur in the vessel, causing tissue ischemia. The symptoms of Buerger's disease often are confused with PAD and other autoimmune diseases (e.g., scleroderma). Patients may have intermittent claudication of the feet, hands, or arms. As the disease progresses, rest pain and ischemic ulcerations develop. Other signs and symptoms may include color and temperature changes of the limbs, paresthesia, superficial vein thrombosis, and cold sensitivity.

There are no laboratory or diagnostic tests specific to Buerger's disease. Diagnosis is made based on age of onset; history; clinical symptoms; involvement of distal vessels; presence of ischemic ulcerations; and exclusion of autoimmune disease, diabetes, thrombophilia (inherited tendency to clot), and other sources of emboli, such as atherosclerosis and aneurysm.[22]

The primary treatment for Buerger's disease is the complete cessation of tobacco and marijuana use in any form. Use of nicotine replacement products is contraindicated. Patients must choose between their tobacco or marijuana and their affected limb, but not both.

Conservative management includes avoiding limb exposure to cold temperatures, a supervised walking program, antibiotics to treat any infected ulcers, and analgesics to manage the ischemic pain. Teach patients to avoid trauma to the extremities.

A variety of drugs have been tried to treat Buerger's disease (e.g., calcium channel blockers, cilostazol, sildenafil [Viagra]). Although these drugs do not stop disease progression, they can be used to decrease pain.

One promising drug used to manage pain has been IV iloprost (Ventavis), a prostaglandin analog that promotes vasodilation. This drug improves rest pain, promotes healing of ischemic ulcers, and decreases the need for amputation.[22]

Surgical options include *sympathectomy* (transection of a nerve, ganglion, and/or plexus of the sympathetic nervous system), implantation of a spinal cord stimulator, and bypass surgery. Sympathectomy and implantation of a spinal cord stimulator can improve distal blood flow, reduce pain, and decrease the rate of amputation but neither alters the inflammatory process. Bypass surgery typically is not an option because of the involvement of smaller, distal vessels but may be used in selected patients with severe ischemia.

Painful ulcerations may require finger or toe amputations. Amputation below the knee may be needed in severe cases. The rate of amputation in patients who continue tobacco or marijuana use after diagnosis is much higher than in those who stop.[22]

## RAYNAUD'S PHENOMENON

**Raynaud's phenomenon** is an episodic vasospastic disorder of small cutaneous arteries, most often involving the fingers and toes. It occurs primarily in young women (typically between 15 and 40 years of age), and it is more common in women than men. The pathogenesis of Raynaud's phenomenon is due to abnormalities in the vascular, intravascular, and neuronal mechanisms that cause an imbalance between vasodilation and vasoconstriction.[23]

Raynaud's phenomenon may occur in isolation *(primary Raynaud's phenomenon)* or in association with an underlying disease (e.g., rheumatoid arthritis, scleroderma, systemic lupus erythematosus) *(secondary Raynaud's phenomenon)*. Other contributing factors include occupation-related conditions, such as the use of vibrating machinery or work in cold environments, exposure to heavy metals (e.g., lead), and hyperhomocysteinemia.

Diagnosis is based on persistent symptoms for at least 2 years. Patients with Raynaud's phenomenon should have routine follow-up to monitor for development of connective tissue or autoimmune diseases.

Raynaud's phenomenon is characterized by vasospasm-induced color changes of fingers, toes, ears, and nose (white, blue, and red). Decreased perfusion results in pallor (white). The digits then appear cyanotic (bluish purple) (Fig. 37-3). These changes are followed by rubor (red), caused by the hyperemic response that occurs when blood flow is restored. The patient usually describes coldness and numbness in the vasoconstrictive phase. This is followed by throbbing, aching pain,

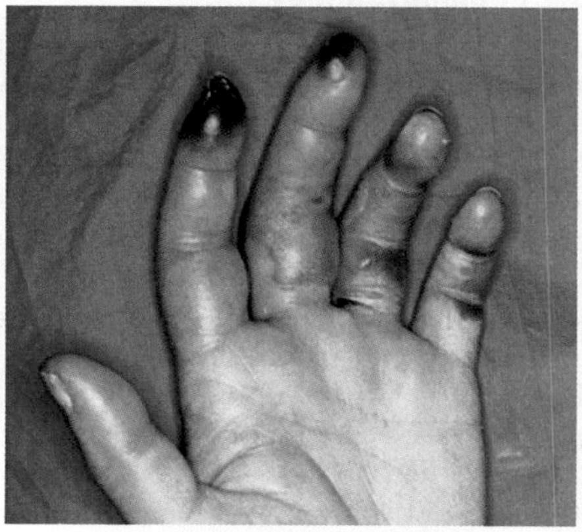

**FIG. 37-3** Raynaud's phenomenon. (From Kamal A, Brockelhurst JC: *Colour atlas of geriatric medicine*, ed 2, 1991, Mosby-Year Book-Europe.)

tingling, and swelling in the hyperemic phase. An episode usually lasts only minutes but in severe cases may persist for several hours. Exposure to cold, emotional upsets, tobacco use, and caffeine often bring on symptoms.

After frequent, prolonged attacks the skin may become thickened and the nails brittle. Occasionally, complications include *punctate* (small hole) lesions of the fingertips and superficial gangrenous ulcers in advanced stages.

The primary focus of nursing management of Raynaud's phenomenon is patient teaching. Focus your instructions on preventing recurrent episodes. Tell patients to wear loose, warm clothing as protection from the cold, including gloves when handling cold objects. At all times, patients should avoid temperature extremes. Immersing hands in warm water often decreases the vasospasm. The patient should stop using all tobacco products and avoid caffeine and other drugs that have vasoconstrictive effects (e.g., cocaine, amphetamines, ergotamine, pseudoephedrine). Finally, provide patients with stress management strategies as appropriate.

When conservative management is ineffective, drug therapy is considered. Sustained-release calcium channel blockers (e.g., nifedipine [Procardia]) are the first-line drug therapy. Calcium channel blockers relax smooth muscles of the arterioles by blocking the influx of calcium into the cells. This reduces the frequency and severity of vasospastic attacks. If calcium channel blockers are not sufficient treatment, other vasodilators (e.g., transdermal glyceryl trinitrate [Nitro-Dur]) may be used.[24]

Prompt intervention is needed for patients with digital ulceration and/or critical ischemia. Treatment options include prostacyclin infusion therapy (e.g., iloprost), antibiotics, analgesics, and possibly an endothelin receptor antagonist (e.g., bosentan [Tracleer]) and surgical debridement of necrotic tissue. Statins may also lessen the severity of Raynaud's phenomenon.[24] Sympathectomy is considered only in advanced cases.

## AORTIC ANEURYSMS

The aorta is the largest artery and supplies $O_2$, nutrients, and blood to all vital organs. One of the most common problems affecting the aorta is an **aneurysm**, which is a permanent, localized outpouching or dilation of the vessel wall. Aneurysms occur in men more often than in women and in whites more often than African Americans. The incidence increases with age.[25] Aneurysms may occur in more than one location. Peripheral artery aneurysms can also develop but are not common.

### Etiology and Pathophysiology

Aortic aneurysms may involve the aortic arch and thoracic and/or abdominal aorta. Three fourths of aortic aneurysms occur in the abdominal aorta (Fig. 37-4) and one fourth in the thoracic aorta. Most abdominal aortic aneurysms (AAAs) occur below the renal arteries. Growth rates are higher in patients who smoke tobacco.[25] The larger the aneurysm, the greater the risk of rupture.

A variety of disorders are associated with aortic aneurysms. The primary causes are classified as degenerative, congenital, mechanical (e.g., penetrating or blunt trauma), inflammatory (e.g., aortitis [Takayasu's arteritis]), or infectious (e.g., aortitis [*Chlamydia pneumoniae,* human immunodeficiency virus]).

Risk factors for aortic aneurysms include age, male gender, hypertension, CAD, family history, tobacco use, high cholesterol,

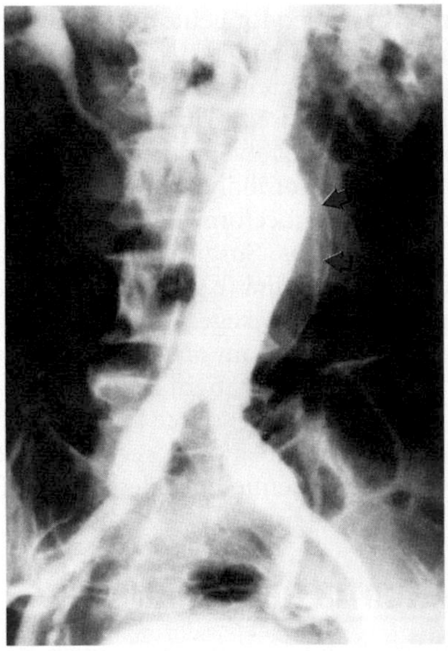

**FIG. 37-4** Angiography demonstrating fusiform abdominal aortic aneurysm. Note calcification of the aortic wall *(arrows)* and extension of the aneurysm into the common iliac arteries. (Courtesy Jo Menzoian, Boston, Mass.)

lower extremity PAD, carotid artery disease, previous stroke, and excess weight or obesity. Tobacco use is the most important modifiable risk factor.[25]

### Genetic Link

The development of both aortic aneurysm and aortic dissection has a strong genetic component. The familial tendency is related to a number of congenital anomalies. Examples include bicuspid aortic valve, coarctation of the aorta, Turner syndrome, autosomal dominant polycystic kidney disease, specific collagen defects (e.g., Ehlers-Danlos syndrome), and premature breakdown of vascular elastic tissue (e.g., Marfan's syndrome).[26]

### Classification

Aneurysms are classified as true or false aneurysms (Fig. 37-5, *A* to *C*). A *true aneurysm* is one in which the wall of the artery forms the aneurysm, with at least one vessel layer still intact. True aneurysms are further subdivided into fusiform and saccular types. A *fusiform aneurysm* is circumferential and relatively uniform in shape. A *saccular aneurysm* is pouchlike with a narrow neck connecting the bulge to one side of the arterial wall.

A *false aneurysm,* or *pseudoaneurysm,* is not an aneurysm but a disruption of all arterial wall layers with bleeding that is contained by surrounding anatomic structures. False aneurysms may result from trauma, infection, peripheral artery bypass graft surgery (at the site of the graft-to-artery anastomosis), or arterial leakage after removal of cannulae (e.g., femoral artery catheters, intraaortic balloon pump devices).

### Clinical Manifestations

Thoracic aortic aneurysms (TAAs) are often asymptomatic. When present, symptoms include deep, diffuse chest pain that may extend to the interscapular area. Ascending aorta and aortic arch aneurysms can cause (1) angina from decreased blood flow to the coronary arteries; (2) transient ischemic attacks from decreased blood flow to the carotid arteries; and (3) coughing, shortness of breath, hoarseness, and/or dysphagia

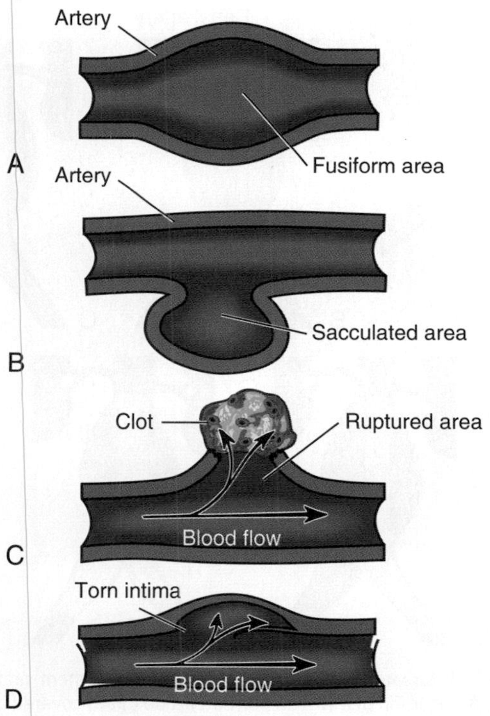


**FIG. 37-5** **A,** True fusiform abdominal aortic aneurysm. **B,** True saccular aortic aneurysm. **C,** False aneurysm, or pseudoaneurysm. **D,** Aortic dissection.

(difficulty swallowing) from pressure on the laryngeal nerve. If the aneurysm presses on the superior vena cava, decreased venous return can result in jugular venous distention (distended neck veins) and edema of the face and arms.

AAAs are often asymptomatic and frequently found during routine physical examinations or evaluations for an unrelated problem (e.g., abdominal x-ray, CT scan). A pulsatile mass in the periumbilical area slightly to the left of the midline may be present. Bruits may be auscultated over the aneurysm. Physical findings may be more difficult to detect in obese individuals.

AAA symptoms may mimic pain associated with abdominal or back disorders. Compression of nearby anatomic structures and nerves may cause symptoms such as back pain, epigastric discomfort, altered bowel elimination, and intermittent claudication. Occasionally, aneurysms spontaneously embolize plaque, causing *"blue toe syndrome"* (patchy mottling of the feet and toes in the presence of palpable pedal pulses).

## Complications

Rupture of an aneurysm is the most serious complication. It is more likely to occur in people who smoke tobacco.[3,25] If rupture occurs into the retroperitoneal space, bleeding may be controlled by surrounding anatomic structures, preventing exsanguination and death. In this case the patient often has severe back pain and may or may not have back or flank ecchymosis *(Grey Turner's sign)*.

If rupture occurs into the thoracic or abdominal cavity, patients can die from massive hemorrhage. The patient who reaches the hospital will be in hypovolemic shock with tachycardia, hypotension, pale clammy skin, decreased urine output, altered level of consciousness, and abdominal tenderness. (Shock is discussed in Chapter 66.) In this situation, simultaneous resuscitation and immediate surgical repair are necessary. For patients admitted to the hospital with a ruptured AAA, in-hospital mortality is high at 53%.[3,26]

## Diagnostic Studies

Chest x-rays are done to reveal abnormal widening of the thoracic aorta. An abdominal x-ray may show calcification within the aortic wall. An electrocardiogram (ECG) may rule out MI, since thoracic aneurysm or dissection symptoms can mimic angina. Echocardiography assesses the function of the aortic valve. Ultrasound is useful for aneurysm screening and to monitor aneurysm size. A CT scan is the most accurate test to determine the length and cross-sectional diameter and the presence of thrombus in the aneurysm. MRI may also be used to diagnose and assess the location and severity of aneurysms. Angiography provides helpful information by using contrast imaging to map the entire aortic system. (Chapter 31 and Table 31-6 discuss angiography.)

## Interprofessional Care

The primary goal of interprofessional care is to prevent the rupture of an aneurysm. Early detection and prompt treatment are essential. Conservative medical therapy of small, asymptomatic AAAs (4.0 to 5.4 cm) is the best practice.[6] This consists of risk factor modification (ceasing tobacco use, decreasing BP, optimizing lipid profile, gradually increasing physical activity) and monitoring of aneurysm size using ultrasound or CT every 6 to 12 months. Growth rates may be lowered with β-blockers (e.g., propranolol [Inderal]), ACE inhibitors (e.g., captopril [Capoten]), and angiotensin II receptor blockers (e.g., losartan [Cozaar]), statins (e.g., simvastatin [Zocor]), and antibiotics (e.g., doxycycline [Acticlate]).[26] Monitoring by ultrasound every 2 to 3 years is recommended for patients with AAAs smaller than 4.0 cm in diameter.[6]

Surgical repair is recommended in patients with asymptomatic aneurysms 5.5 cm in diameter or larger. Surgical intervention may occur sooner if the patient has a genetic disorder (e.g., Marfan's, Ehlers-Danlos syndrome), the aneurysm expands rapidly, it becomes symptomatic, or the risk of rupture is high.[6] A careful review of body systems is necessary to identify any co-morbidities, especially of the lungs, heart, or kidneys, because they affect the patient's surgical risk. Correction of existing carotid or coronary artery blockages may be needed before the aneurysm is repaired.

**Surgical Therapy.** For elective surgery, the patient needs to be well hydrated, and any electrolyte, coagulation, and hematocrit abnormalities are corrected preoperatively. If the aneurysm has ruptured, emergent surgical intervention is required.

The open aneurysm repair (OAR) involves a large abdominal incision through which the surgeon (1) cuts into the diseased aortic segment, (2) removes any thrombus or plaque, (3) sutures a synthetic graft to the aorta proximal and distal to the aneurysm, and (4) sutures the native aortic wall around the graft to act as a protective cover (Fig. 37-6). If the iliac arteries are also aneurysmal, a bifurcated graft replaces the entire diseased segment. With saccular aneurysms, it may be possible to excise only the bulbous lesion, repairing the artery by primary closure (suturing the artery together) or by application of an autogenous or synthetic patch graft.

All OARs require aortic cross-clamping proximal and distal to the aneurysm. Most resections are done in 30 to 45 minutes, after which the clamps are removed and blood flow is restored. If the cross clamp must be applied above the renal arteries,

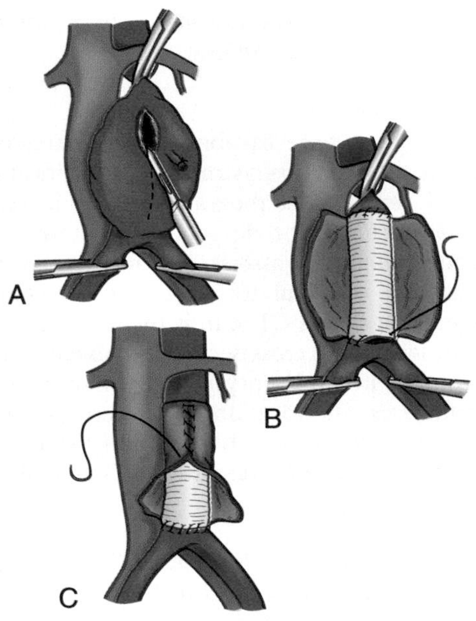


**FIG. 37-6** Surgical repair of an abdominal aortic aneurysm. **A,** Incising the aneurysmal sac. **B,** Insertion of synthetic graft. **C,** Suturing native aortic wall over synthetic graft.

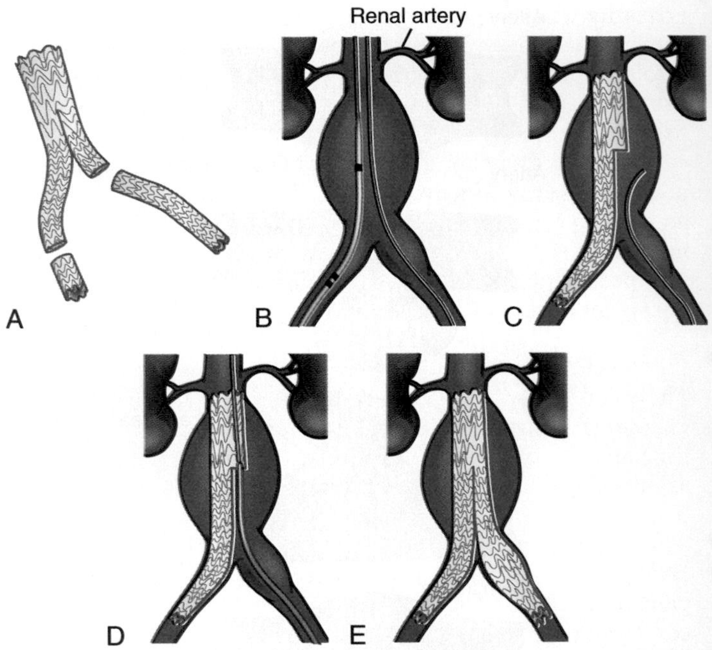


**FIG. 37-7** Bifurcated (two-branched) endovascular stent grafting of an aneurysm. **A,** Insertion of a woven polyester tube (graft) covered by a tubular metal web (stent). **B,** The stent graft is inserted through a large blood vessel (e.g., femoral artery) using a delivery catheter. The catheter is positioned below the renal arteries in the area of the aneurysm. **C,** The stent graft is slowly released (deployed) into the blood vessel. When the stent comes in contact with the blood vessel, it expands to a preset size. **D,** A second stent graft can be inserted in the contralateral (opposite) vessel if necessary. **E,** Fully deployed bifurcated stent graft.

adequate renal blood flow after clamp removal should be determined before closure of the abdominal incision. The risk of postoperative renal complications such as acute kidney injury increases in patients who have OAR of AAAs above the level of the renal arteries.

***Endovascular Graft Procedure.*** Minimally invasive endovascular aneurysm repair (EVAR) is an alternative to OAR for select patients. Eligibility criteria include iliofemoral vessels that allow for safe graft insertion and vessels of sufficient length and width to support the graft.[26]

EVAR involves the placement of a sutureless aortic graft into the abdominal aorta inside the aneurysm via the femoral artery. The grafts are made of various materials, such as a Dacron cylinder consisting of several sections, and are supported with multiple rings of flexible wire (Fig. 37-7).

The main section of the graft is bifurcated and delivered through a femoral artery catheter. The second part of the graft is inserted through the opposite femoral artery. When all graft components are in place, they are released (deployed) against the vessel wall by balloon inflation. The blood then flows through the endovascular graft, thus preventing further expansion of the aneurysm.

Postprocedure angiography is done to check for any leaks and to confirm patency of all stent-graft components. The aneurysmal wall will shrink over time because the blood is being diverted through the endograft.

***Complications.*** EVAR is less invasive than OAR. EVAR also has fewer complications, such as paraplegia and death. In addition, hospital stays are shorter with EVAR.[27] Women have a higher rate of complications after EVAR compared to men. However, there are no gender differences in mortality rates.[28]

The most common complication of AAA repair is *endoleak,* the seepage of blood back into the old aneurysm. This may be the result of an inadequate seal at either graft end, a tear through the graft fabric, or leakage between overlapping graft segments. Repair may require coil embolization (insertion of beads) for hemostasis.

Other potential complications include aneurysm growth above or below the graft, aneurysm rupture, aortic dissection, bleeding, renal artery occlusion caused by stent migration, graft thrombosis, incisional site hematoma, and incisional infection. Patients undergoing EVAR require periodic imaging for the rest of their lives to monitor for an endoleak, document stability of the aneurysm sac, and determine the need for surgical intervention.

A potentially lethal complication in an emergency repair of a ruptured AAA is the development of *intraabdominal hypertension* (IAH) with associated *abdominal compartment syndrome* (ACS). Persistent IAH reduces blood flow to the viscera. ACS refers to the impaired organ perfusion caused by IAH and resulting multisystem organ failure.[29] IAH is confirmed by measuring the patient's intraabdominal pressure indirectly through a catheter and transducer system, typically by using an indwelling urinary catheter.

Treatment goals include control of situations that lead to IAH. Interventions include open (surgical) decompression, percutaneous drainage, and percutaneous drainage combined with tPA infusion. Conservative measures such as intubation, ventilation, patient positioning, gastric decompression, cautious fluid resuscitation, pain management, and temporary hemofiltration are also used.

## NURSING MANAGEMENT: AORTIC ANEURYSMS

### Nursing Assessment

Begin by performing a thorough history and physical assessment. Because atherosclerosis is a systemic disease, look for signs of coexisting cardiac, pulmonary, cerebral, and lower extremity vascular problems. Monitor the patient for signs of aneurysm rupture, such as diaphoresis; pallor; weakness; tachycardia; hypotension; abdominal, back, groin, or periumbilical pain; changes in level of consciousness; or a pulsating abdominal mass.

Establishing baseline data is critical for comparison with later postoperative assessments. Pay special attention to the character and quality of the patient's peripheral pulses, and renal and neurologic status. Before surgery, mark pedal pulse sites (dorsalis pedis and posterior tibial) with a single-use marker and document any skin lesions on the lower extremities.

## ◆ Planning

The overall goals for a patient undergoing aortic surgery include (1) normal tissue perfusion; (2) intact motor and sensory function; and (3) no complications related to surgical repair, such as thrombosis, infection, or rupture.

## ◆ Nursing Implementation

◆ **Health Promotion.** To promote overall health, encourage the patient to reduce CVD risk factors (see Table 33-2), including controlling BP, ceasing tobacco use (see Chapter 10), increasing physical activity, and maintaining normal body weight and serum lipid levels. These measures also help ensure continued graft patency after surgical repair.

◆ **Acute Care.** During the preoperative period, provide emotional support and teaching to the patient and caregiver. Preoperative teaching includes a brief explanation of the disease process, the planned surgical procedure(s), preoperative routines, what to expect immediately after surgery (e.g., recovery room, tubes and drains), and usual postoperative timelines. Specific preoperative routines vary by agency and surgeon. In general, aortic surgery patients have a bowel preparation (e.g., laxatives, enemas) and skin cleansing with an antimicrobial agent the day before surgery, have nothing by mouth (NPO) after midnight the day of surgery, and receive IV antibiotics immediately before the incision is made. If appropriate, a preoperative visit to the intensive care unit (ICU) may be helpful to the patient and caregiver. Patients with a history of CVD should receive a β-blocker (e.g., metoprolol [Lopressor]) preoperatively.

Postoperatively, aortic surgery patients typically go to an ICU for 24 to 48 hours for close monitoring. When the patient arrives in the ICU, various devices are in place. These include an endotracheal tube for mechanical ventilation, an arterial line, a central venous pressure (CVP) or pulmonary artery (PA) catheter, peripheral IV lines, an indwelling urinary catheter, and a nasogastric (NG) tube. The patient needs continuous ECG and pulse oximetry monitoring. If the thorax is opened during surgery, chest tubes will be in place. Pain medication is given via epidural catheter or patient-controlled analgesia (PCA).

In addition to the usual goals of care for a postoperative patient (e.g., maintaining adequate respiratory function, fluid and electrolyte balance, and pain control [see Chapter 19]), check for graft patency and renal perfusion. Also watch for and intervene to limit or treat cardiac ischemia, dysrhythmias, infections, VTE, and neurologic complications. eNursing Care Plan 37-2 for the patient with an aneurysm repair or other aortic surgery is available on the website for this chapter.

◆ ***Graft Patency.*** An adequate BP is important to maintain graft patency. Prolonged low BP may result in graft thrombosis. Give IV fluids and blood components as ordered to maintain adequate blood flow. Monitor CVP or PA pressures and urine output hourly in the immediate postoperative period to assess the patient's hydration and perfusion status.

Avoid severe hypertension, since it may cause undue stress on the arterial anastomoses, resulting in leakage of blood or rupture at the suture lines. Drug therapy with IV diuretics (e.g., furosemide [Lasix]) or IV antihypertensive agents (e.g., labetalol [Normodyne], metoprolol, hydralazine [Apresoline], sodium nitroprusside [Nipride]) may be indicated.

◆ ***Cardiovascular Status.*** Myocardial ischemia or infarction may occur in the perioperative period because of decreased myocardial $O_2$ supply or increased myocardial $O_2$ demands. Cardiac dysrhythmias may occur because of electrolyte imbalances, hypoxemia, hypothermia, or myocardial ischemia. Nursing interventions include continuous ECG monitoring; frequent electrolyte and arterial blood gas determinations; administration of $O_2$, IV antidysrhythmic and antihypertensive drugs, and electrolytes as needed; adequate pain control; and resumption of cardiac drugs.

◆ ***Infection.*** A prosthetic vascular graft infection is a relatively rare but potentially life-threatening complication. Nursing interventions to prevent infection include giving a broad-spectrum antibiotic as prescribed. Assess temperature regularly, and promptly report elevations. Monitor laboratory data for an elevated white blood cell (WBC) count, which may be the first indication of an infection. Ensure adequate nutrition and assess the surgical incision for signs of infection (e.g., redness, swelling, drainage). Keep surgical incisions clean and dry and perform wound care as ordered.

Use strict aseptic technique in the care of all peripheral, arterial, and CVP or PA catheter insertion sites, since these are ports of entry for bacteria. Meticulous perineal care for the patient with an indwelling urinary catheter and early catheter removal are essential to minimize the risk of urinary tract infection.

◆ ***Gastrointestinal Status.*** After OAR, postoperative ileus may develop as a result of anesthesia and the handling of the bowel during surgery. The intestines may become swollen and bruised, and peristalsis ceases for variable intervals. A retroperitoneal surgical approach can be used to decrease the risk of bowel complications.

An NG tube may be placed during surgery and connected to low, intermittent suction to decompress the stomach, prevent aspiration of stomach contents, and decrease pressure on suture lines. Record the amount and character of the NG output. While the patient is NPO, provide oral care frequently. Ice chips or lozenges can help soothe a dry or irritated throat. Assess for bowel sounds every 4 hours. The passing of flatus signals returning bowel function and should be noted. Encourage early ambulation, since this can help the return of bowel function. A postoperative ileus rarely lasts beyond the fourth postoperative day.

If the blood supply to the bowel is disrupted during surgery, temporary ischemia or infarction (death) of intestinal tissue may result. Clinical manifestations of this rare but serious complication include absent bowel sounds, fever, abdominal distention and pain, diarrhea, and bloody stools. If bowel infarction occurs, immediate reoperation is necessary to restore blood flow, with likely resection of the infarcted bowel.

◆ ***Neurologic Status.*** Neurologic complications can occur after aortic surgery. When the ascending aorta and aortic arch are involved, assess the patient's level of consciousness, pupil size and response to light, facial symmetry, tongue position, speech, upper extremity movement, and quality of hand grasps (see

Chapter 55). When the descending aorta is involved, perform a neurovascular assessment of the lower extremities. Record all assessments and report changes from baseline to the HCP immediately.

◆ ***Peripheral Perfusion Status.*** The location of the aneurysm determines what type of peripheral perfusion assessment is done. Check and record all peripheral pulses hourly for several hours and then routinely (based on agency policy). When the ascending aorta and aortic arch are involved, assess the carotid, radial, and temporal artery pulses. For surgery of the descending aorta, assess the femoral, popliteal, posterior tibial, and dorsalis pedis pulses (see Fig. 31-6). You may need a Doppler to assess peripheral pulses. Check skin temperature and color, capillary refill time, and sensation and movement of the extremities (see Chapter 31).

Occasionally, lower extremity pulses may be absent for a short time after surgery because of vasospasm and hypothermia. A decreased or absent pulse together with a cool, pale, mottled, or painful extremity may indicate embolization or graft occlusion. Report these findings to the HCP immediately. Graft occlusion requires reoperation if identified early. Thrombolytic therapy may also be considered. In some patients, pulses may have been absent before surgery because of coexistent PAD. It is essential to compare your findings with the preoperative status to determine the cause of a decreased or absent pulse and the proper treatment.

◆ ***Renal Perfusion Status.*** The patient will have an indwelling urinary catheter after surgery. In the immediate postoperative period, record hourly urine output. Further evaluate renal function by monitoring daily blood urea nitrogen (BUN) and serum creatinine levels. CVP and PA pressures also provide important information about hydration status. Maintain accurate fluid intake and output and record daily weights until the patient resumes a regular diet.

Decreased renal perfusion can occur from embolization of the aortic thrombus or plaque to one or both of the renal arteries. This causes ischemia of one or both kidneys. Hypotension, dehydration, prolonged aortic clamping during surgery, or blood loss can also lead to decreased renal perfusion. Irreversible renal failure may occur after surgery, particularly in high-risk people (e.g., patients with diabetes). (Acute kidney injury is discussed in Chapter 46.)

◆ **Ambulatory Care.** Instruct the patient and caregiver to gradually increase activities once home. Fatigue, poor appetite, and irregular bowel habits are common. Teach the patient to avoid heavy lifting for 6 weeks after surgery. Any redness, swelling, increased pain, drainage from incisions, or fever greater than 100° F (37.8° C) should be reported to an HCP.

Teach the patient and caregiver to look for changes in color or warmth of the extremities. Patients and caregivers can learn to palpate peripheral pulses to assess changes in their quality.

Sexual dysfunction in male patients is common after aortic surgery. Preoperatively, document baseline sexual function and recommend counseling as appropriate. A referral to a urologist may be useful if erectile dysfunction occurs.

### ◆ Evaluation

Expected outcomes are that the patient who undergoes aortic surgery will have:

- Patent arterial graft with adequate distal perfusion
- Adequate urine output
- No signs of infection

## AORTIC DISSECTION

**Aortic dissection,** often misnamed *"dissecting aneurysm,"* is not a type of aneurysm. Rather, dissection results from the creation of a false lumen between the intima (inner lining) and the media (middle layer) of arterial wall (Figs. 37-5, *D* and 37-8). Aortic dissection is classified based on the location of the dissection and duration of onset. *Type A dissection* affects the ascending aorta and arch. *Type B dissection* begins in the descending aorta. Dissections are also classified as acute (first 14 days), subacute (14 to 90 days), or chronic (greater than 90 days) based on symptom onset.[26] Approximately two thirds of dissections involve the ascending aorta and are acute in onset.[30] Chronic dissections are almost always Type B.

### Etiology and Pathophysiology

Nontraumatic aortic dissection is caused by degenerated elastic fibers in the arterial wall. Chronic hypertension hastens this process. In aortic dissection a tear develops in the inner layer of the aorta. Blood surges through this tear into the middle layer of the aorta, causing the inner and middle layers to separate (dissect). If the blood-filled channel ruptures through the outside aortic wall, aortic dissection is often fatal.

As the heart contracts, each pulsation increases the pressure on the damaged area, which further increases the dissection. Extension of the dissection may cut off blood supply to critical areas such as the brain, kidneys, spinal cord, and extremities. The false lumen may remain patent, become thrombosed (clotted), rejoin the true lumen by way of a distal tear, or rupture.

Aortic dissection affects men 2 to 5 times more often than women and occurs most frequently in the sixth and seventh decades of life.[30] Predisposing factors include age, aortic diseases (e.g., aortitis, coarctation, arch hypoplasia), atherosclerosis, blunt or iatrogenic trauma, tobacco use, cocaine or methamphetamine use, congenital heart disease (e.g., bicuspid aortic valve), connective tissue disorders (e.g., Marfan's or Ehlers-Danlos syndrome), family history, history of heart surgery, male gender, pregnancy, and poorly controlled hypertension.[26] Nearly half of all acute aortic dissections in patients younger than 40 years of age occur in patients with Marfan's syndrome.[30]

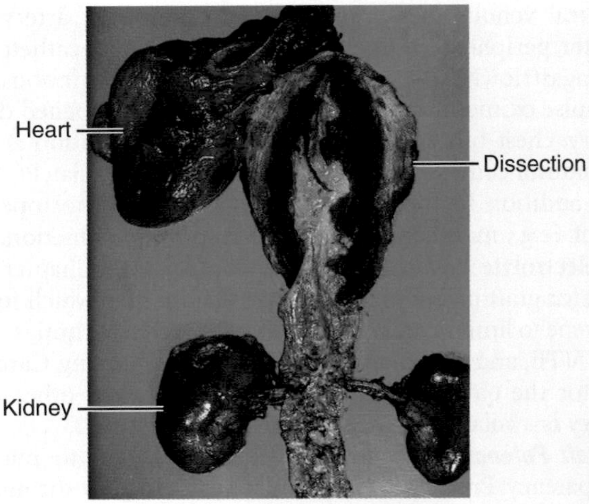


**FIG. 37-8** Aortic dissection of the thoracic aorta. (From Damjanov I, Linder J, editors: *Anderson's pathology,* ed 10, St Louis, 1996, Mosby.)

## Clinical Manifestations

About 80% of patients with an acute Type A aortic dissection report an abrupt onset of excruciating anterior chest pain. Patients with acute Type B aortic dissection are more likely to report pain located in their back, abdomen, or legs. Pain location may overlap between Type A and B dissections. The pain is frequently described as "sharp" and "worst ever," or as "tearing," "ripping," or "stabbing."

Dissection pain can be differentiated from MI pain, which is more gradual in onset and has increasing intensity. As the dissection progresses, pain may migrate and follow the path of the dissection. Older patients are less likely to have abrupt onset of chest or back pain and more likely to have hypotension and vague symptoms. Some patients have a painless aortic dissection, emphasizing the importance of the physical examination.

If the aortic arch is involved, the patient may exhibit neurologic deficits. These include altered level of consciousness, weakened or absent carotid and temporal pulses, and dizziness or syncope. Type A aortic dissection usually produces some degree of disruption in blood flow in the coronary arteries and aortic valve insufficiency. The patient may develop angina; MI; and a new, high-pitched heart murmur. In severe cases, these complications can result in left heart failure (e.g., dyspnea, orthopnea, pulmonary edema), cardiogenic shock, and death.[26] When either subclavian artery is involved, radial, ulnar, and brachial pulse quality and BP readings may be different between the left and right arms. As the dissection progresses down the aorta, the abdominal organs and lower extremities demonstrate evidence of decreased tissue perfusion.

## Complications

A severe and life-threatening complication of an acute ascending aortic dissection is *cardiac tamponade.* This occurs when blood from the dissection leaks into the pericardial sac. Clinical manifestations of tamponade include hypotension, narrowed pulse pressure, jugular venous distention, muffled heart sounds, and pulsus paradoxus (see Chapter 36).

The aorta may rupture because it is weakened by the dissection. Hemorrhage may occur into the mediastinal, pleural, or abdominal cavities. Aortic rupture typically results in exsanguination and death. Dissection can lead to occlusion of the blood supply to vital organs. Spinal cord ischemia leads to weakness and decreased sensation and rarely to complete lower extremity paralysis. Renal ischemia can lead to renal failure. Abdominal (mesenteric) ischemia can occur and cause abdominal pain, decreased bowel sounds, altered bowel function, and bowel necrosis.

## Diagnostic Studies

Diagnostic studies to detect aortic dissection are similar to those for suspected aneurysms (Table 37-6). An ECG can help rule out cardiac ischemia. A chest x-ray may show a widening of the mediastinum and pleural effusion. Three-dimensional (3-D) CT scanning, MRI, and transesophageal echocardiography (TEE) are equally reliable for the diagnosis of acute aortic dissection. A CT scan or MRI can provide more detailed information on the severity of the dissection and related complications (e.g., pericardial effusions, carotid dissection). TEE is preferred in very unstable patients or those with contraindications to CT or MRI (e.g., those with metal implants, allergies to contrast material).[26]

**TABLE 37-6 Interprofessional Care**

***Aortic Dissection***

| Diagnostic Assessment | Management |
| --- | --- |
| • Health history and physical examination<br>• ECG<br>• Chest x-ray<br>• CT scan<br>• Transesophageal echocardiogram<br>• MRI | • Bed rest<br>• Pain relief with opioids<br>• Blood transfusion (if needed)<br><br>***Drug Therapy*** *(see Table 32-7)*<br>• IV β-blockers<br>• IV calcium channel blockers<br>• Angiotensin-converting enzyme inhibitors<br><br>***Surgical Therapy***<br>• Endovascular aortic dissection repair<br>• Open surgical repair |

## Interprofessional Care

Patients with acute aortic dissection are managed in the ICU. The initial goals of therapy for acute aortic dissection without complications are heart rate (HR) and BP control and pain management. HR and BP control reduces aortic wall stress by decreasing systolic BP and myocardial contractility (Table 37-6). An IV β-blocker (e.g., esmolol [Brevibloc]) is titrated to a target HR of 60 beats/minute or less or to a systolic BP between 100 and 110 mm Hg.

A calcium channel blocker (e.g., diltiazem [Cardizem]) can be used to lower HR if a β-blocker is contraindicated. Reducing the HR, BP, and myocardial contractility limits extension of the dissection. Morphine is the preferred analgesic. It decreases sympathetic nervous system stimulation and relieves pain. Supportive treatment for an acute aortic dissection serves as a bridge to surgery.

**Conservative Therapy.** The patient with an acute or chronic Type B aortic dissection without complications can be treated conservatively. Conservative treatment includes pain relief, HR and BP control, and CVD risk factor modification along with close surveillance imaging with CT or MRI.

**Endovascular Dissection Repair.** Endovascular repair of acute Type B aortic dissections with complications (e.g., hemodynamic instability) and chronic Type B aortic dissection with complications (e.g., peripheral ischemia) is a treatment option. Thoracic endovascular aortic repair (TEVAR) is similar to EVAR. However, a temporary lumbar drain may be inserted for cerebrospinal fluid removal to reduce spinal cord edema and help prevent paralysis.[31] If a lumbar drain is used, strict aseptic techniques are essential to avoid introducing infection.

**Surgical Therapy.** An acute Type A aortic dissection is a surgical emergency. Mortality rate is 50% within 48 hours of symptom onset. Otherwise, surgery is indicated when conservative therapy is ineffective or when complications (e.g., heart failure) occur. Open surgical repair is recommended for patients with a chronic dissection who have a connective tissue disorder and a descending thoracic aortic diameter greater than 5.5 cm.[26]

The aorta is fragile after dissection. Thus surgery is delayed for as long as possible to allow time for edema to decrease and to permit clotting of the blood in the false lumen. Surgery involves resection of the aortic segment containing the intimal tear and replacement with a synthetic graft. Even with prompt surgical intervention, the in-hospital mortality and neurologic complications are high.[26] Causes of death include aortic rupture, mesenteric ischemia, MI, sepsis, stroke, and multiorgan failure.

## ❖ NURSING MANAGEMENT: AORTIC DISSECTION

Preoperatively, nursing management includes keeping the patient in bed in a semi-Fowler's position and maintaining a quiet environment. These measures help to keep the HR and systolic BP at the lowest possible level that maintains vital organ perfusion (typically HR less than 60 beats/minute; systolic BP between 110 and 120 mm Hg). Give opioids and sedatives as ordered. To prevent extension of the dissection, manage pain and anxiety because they can cause elevations in the HR and systolic BP.

Titrating IV antihypertensive agents requires careful supervision, including continuous ECG and arterial BP monitoring (see Chapters 32 and 65). Monitor vital signs frequently, sometimes as often as every 2 to 3 minutes, until target HR and BP are reached. Look for any changes in peripheral pulses and signs of increasing pain, restlessness, and anxiety. If the arteries branching off the aortic arch are involved, monitor the patient's level of consciousness, cranial nerve functions, and limb movement, sensation, and strength.[31] Postoperative care is similar to that after OAR (see earlier section on nursing management of aortic aneurysms on p. 813).

In preparation for discharge, focus on patient and caregiver teaching. All patients with a history of aortic dissection, regardless of location or treatment approach, require long-term health care to control HR and BP. Patients must understand that they need to take antihypertensive drugs daily for the rest of their lives. β-Blockers are used to control HR and BP and decrease myocardial contractility. It is important that patients understand the drug regimen and potential side effects (e.g., dizziness, depression, fatigue, erectile dysfunction). Tell the patient to discuss any side effects with the HCP before stopping the drug.

Follow-up with regularly scheduled MRIs or CTs is essential. The most common cause of death in long-term survivors is aortic rupture from redissection or aneurysm formation. Tell patients that if the pain or other symptoms return, they should activate emergency response system (ERS) for immediate care.

# ACUTE AND CHRONIC VENOUS DISORDERS

## PHLEBITIS

Generally, every hospitalized patient has an IV catheter inserted for giving fluids and/or drugs. *Phlebitis* is an acute inflammation of the walls of small cannulated veins of the hand or arm. Clinical manifestations include pain, tenderness, warmth, erythema, swelling, and a palpable cord. Phlebitis risk factors are mechanical irritation from the catheter, infusion of irritating drugs, and catheter location. Severe phlebitis is more likely to occur in the antecubital area, and IV catheter insertion in this area should be avoided when possible.[32]

Phlebitis is rarely infectious and usually resolves quickly after catheter removal. If edema is present, elevate the extremity to promote reabsorption of fluid into the vasculature. Apply warm, moist heat and give oral NSAIDs (e.g., diclofenac [Voltaren]) or topical NSAIDs (e.g., diclofenac gel [Solaraze]) to relieve pain and inflammation. In rare cases, surgical intervention may be needed.[32]

## VENOUS THROMBOSIS

**Venous thrombosis** involves the formation of a *thrombus* (blood clot) in association with inflammation of the vein. It is the most common disorder of the veins and is classified as either superficial vein thrombosis or deep vein thrombosis. **Superficial vein thrombosis** is the formation of a thrombus in a superficial vein, usually the greater or lesser saphenous vein. **Deep vein thrombosis (DVT)** involves a thrombus in a deep vein, most commonly the iliac and/or femoral veins. **Venous thromboembolism (VTE)** is the preferred terminology and represents the spectrum of pathology from DVT to pulmonary embolism (PE) (Table 37-7). (Chapter 27 discusses PE.)

Superficial vein thrombosis has been considered a benign disorder. However, superficial vein thrombosis is serious. Nearly 25% of patients with superficial vein thrombosis may also have a DVT or PE at the time of diagnosis. Further, between 5% and 10% of these patients are at risk for developing recurrent VTE with the greatest risk being in the first 3 months after having the superficial vein thrombosis.[33]

### Etiology

Three important factors (called **Virchow's triad**) in the etiology of venous thrombosis are (1) venous stasis, (2) damage of the endothelium (inner lining of the vein), and (3) hypercoagulability of the blood (Fig. 37-9). The patient at risk for the development of VTE usually has predisposing conditions to these three disorders (Table 37-8).

**TABLE 37-7 Comparison of Superficial Vein Thrombosis and Venous Thromboembolism**

| | Superficial Vein Thrombosis | Venous Thromboembolism (VTE) |
|---|---|---|
| **Usual location** | Typically, superficial leg veins (e.g., varicosities). Occasionally superficial arm veins. | Deep veins of arms (e.g., axillary, subclavian), legs (e.g., femoral), pelvis (e.g., iliac), vena cava, and pulmonary system. |
| **Clinical findings** | Tenderness, itchiness, redness, warmth, pain, inflammation, and induration along the course of superficial vein. Vein appears as a palpable cord. Edema rarely occurs. | Tenderness to pressure over involved vein, induration of overlying muscle, venous distention. Edema. May have mild to moderate pain, deep reddish color to area caused by venous congestion. NOTE: Some patients may have no obvious physical changes in the affected extremity. |
| **Sequelae** | If untreated, clot may extend to deeper veins and VTE may occur. | Embolization to lungs (pulmonary embolism) may occur and may result in death.* Pulmonary hypertension and post-thrombotic syndrome with or without venous leg ulceration may develop. |

*See Chapter 27 for clinical findings related to pulmonary embolism.

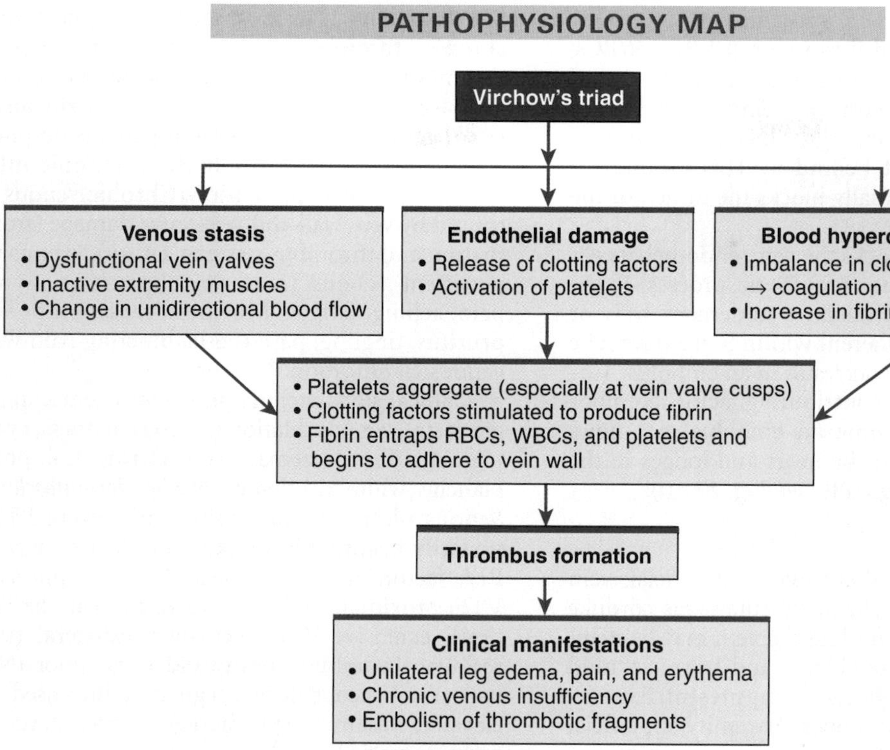


**FIG. 37-9** Pathophysiology of venous thromboembolism.

## TABLE 37-8 Risk Factors for Venous Thromboembolism

**Venous Stasis**

- Advanced age
- Atrial fibrillation
- Bed rest
- Chronic heart failure
- Fractured leg or hip
- Long trips without adequate exercise
- Obesity
- Orthopedic surgery (especially hip or lower extremity)
- Pregnancy and postpartum period
- Prolonged immobility
- Spinal cord injury or limb paralysis
- Stroke
- Varicose veins

**Endothelial Damage**

- Abdominal and pelvic surgery (e.g., gynecologic or urologic surgery)
- Caustic or hypertonic IV drugs
- Fractures of the pelvis, hip, or leg
- History of previous venous thromboembolism
- Indwelling, peripherally inserted central vein catheter
- IV drug abuse
- Trauma

**Hypercoagulability of Blood**

- Antiphospholipid antibody syndrome
- Antithrombin III deficiency
- Dehydration or malnutrition
- Elevated (clotting) factor VIII or lipoprotein (a)
- Erythropoiesis-stimulating drugs (e.g., epoetin alfa [Procrit])
- High altitudes
- Hormone therapy
- Hyperhomocysteinemia
- Cancer (especially breast, brain, hepatic, pancreatic, and gastrointestinal)
- Nephrotic syndrome
- Oral contraceptives, especially in women >35 yr who use tobacco
- Polycythemia vera
- Pregnancy and postpartum period
- Protein C deficiency
- Protein S deficiency
- Sepsis
- Severe anemias
- Tobacco use

**Venous Stasis.** Normal venous blood flow depends on the action of muscles in the extremities and the functional adequacy of venous valves, which allow flow in one direction. *Venous stasis* occurs when the valves are dysfunctional or the muscles of the extremities are inactive. Venous stasis occurs more frequently in people who are obese or pregnant, have chronic heart failure or atrial fibrillation, have been traveling on long trips without regular exercise, have a prolonged surgical procedure, or are immobile for long periods (e.g., spinal cord injury, fractured hip, limb paralysis).[34]

**Endothelial Damage.** Damage to the endothelium of the vein may be caused by direct (e.g., surgery, intravascular catheterization, trauma, burns, prior VTE) or indirect (chemotherapy, diabetes, sepsis) injury to the vessel. Damaged endothelium stimulates platelet activation and starts the coagulation cascade. This predisposes the patient to thrombus development.

**Hypercoagulability of Blood.** Hypercoagulability of blood occurs in many disorders. These include severe anemias; polycythemia; malignancies (e.g., cancers of the breast, brain, pancreas, and gastrointestinal tract); nephrotic syndrome; hyperhomocysteinemia; protein C, protein S, and antithrombin deficiency.[34] A patient with sepsis is predisposed to hypercoagulability because of endotoxins that are released. Some drugs (e.g., corticosteroids, estrogens) predispose a patient to thrombus formation.

Women of childbearing age who take estrogen-based oral contraceptives or postmenopausal women on oral hormone therapy are at increased risk for VTE. Women who use oral contraceptives and tobacco double their risk. Smoking causes hypercoagulability by increasing plasma fibrinogen and homocysteine levels and activating the intrinsic coagulation pathway. Women who use tobacco and oral contraceptives, are over 35 years old, and have a family history of VTE are at an extremely high risk for VTE.[34]

### Pathophysiology

Localized platelet aggregation and fibrin entrap RBCs, WBCs, and more platelets to form a thrombus. A frequent site of thrombus formation is the valve cusps of veins, where venous stasis occurs. As the thrombus enlarges, increased numbers of blood cells and fibrin collect behind it. This produces a larger clot with a "tail" that eventually blocks the lumen of the vein.

If a thrombus only partially blocks the vein, endothelial cells cover the thrombus and stop the thrombotic process. If the thrombus does not become detached, it undergoes lysis or becomes firmly organized and adherent within 5 to 7 days. The organized thrombus may detach and result in an embolus. Turbulence of blood flow is a major contributing factor to embolization. The thrombus can become an embolus that flows through the venous circulation to the heart and lodges in the pulmonary circulation, becoming a PE (see Fig. 27-10).

### Superficial Vein Thrombosis

**Clinical Manifestations.** The patient with superficial vein thrombosis may have a palpable, firm, subcutaneous cordlike vein (Table 37-7). The area surrounding the vein may be itchy, tender or painful to the touch, reddened, and warm. A mild temperature elevation and leukocytosis may be present. Extremity edema may or may not occur. Lower extremity superficial vein thrombosis often involves one or more varicose veins.

Risk factors for superficial vein thrombosis include increased age, pregnancy, obesity, malignancy, recent fracture(s), and thrombophilia; estrogen therapy; recent sclerotherapy (e.g., treatment for varicose veins); recent surgery or long-distance travel; and a history of chronic venous insufficiency (CVI), superficial vein thrombosis, or VTE.[33] It also can occur in people with endothelial alterations (e.g., Buerger's disease), or it may be unprovoked.

**Interprofessional Care.** Duplex ultrasound is used to confirm the diagnosis (clot 5 cm or larger) and to rule out clot extension to a deep vein.[34] For patients with a lower leg superficial vein thrombosis, subcutaneous fondaparinux (Arixtra) reduces symptomatic VTE, and superficial vein thrombosis extension and recurrence without causing major bleeding problems.[35]

If the superficial vein thrombosis affects a very short vein segment (less than 5 cm) and is not near the saphenofemoral junction, anticoagulants may not be necessary and oral NSAIDs can ease symptoms. Additional interventions to relieve symptoms include telling the patient to wear graduated compression stockings or bandages, elevate the affected limb above level of heart, apply topical NSAIDS, and perform mild exercise such as walking.

### Venous Thromboembolism

**Clinical Manifestations.** The patient with lower extremity VTE may or may not have unilateral leg edema, pain, tenderness with palpation, dilated superficial veins, a sense of fullness in the thigh or the calf, paresthesias, warm skin, erythema, or a systemic temperature greater than 100.4° F (38° C) (Table 37-7). If the inferior vena cava is involved, both legs may be edematous and cyanotic. About 5% to 10% of VTEs involve the upper extremity veins and may extend into the internal jugular vein or superior vena cava. If the superior vena cava is involved, similar symptoms may occur in the arms, neck, back, and face. Diagnosis of an initial VTE is based on clinical assessment combined with D-dimer testing and/or duplex ultrasound.

**Complications.** The most serious complications of VTE are PE, chronic thromboembolic pulmonary hypertension, post-thrombotic syndrome, and phlegmasia cerulea dolens. (See Chapter 27 for discussion of PE.) **Post-thrombotic syndrome (PTS)** occurs in 20% to 50% of patients despite adequate anticoagulant therapy. It results from chronic inflammation and chronic venous hypertension. Chronic venous hypertension is caused by vein wall and vein valve damage (from acute inflammation and thrombus reorganization), venous valve reflux, and persistent venous (outflow) obstruction. Symptoms include pain, aching, fatigue, heaviness, sensation of swelling, cramps, pruritus, tingling, paresthesia, bursting pain with exercise, and venous claudication.[36]

Clinical signs include persistent edema, spider veins (telangiectasia), venous dilation (ectasia), redness, cyanosis, increased pigmentation, eczema, pain during compression, atrophie blanche (white scar tissue), and *lipodermatosclerosis* (Fig. 37-10). Venous ulceration can occur with severe PTS. Signs of PTS typically begin within a few months to a few years of a VTE. Risk factors include persistent leg symptoms 1 month after VTE, proximal VTE location (e.g., near the iliofemoral junction), extensive VTE, recurrent ipsilateral (same side) VTE, residual thrombus, obesity, older age, poor INR control, daily use of tobacco before pregnancy, increased D-dimer levels, elevated inflammatory markers, varicose veins, and possibly asymptomatic VTE.[36]

*Phlegmasia cerulea dolens* (swollen, blue, painful leg), a rare complication, may develop in a patient in the advanced stages of cancer. It results from severe lower extremity VTE(s) that involve(s) the major leg veins, causing near-total occlusion of venous outflow. Patients typically experience sudden, massive swelling; deep pain; and intense cyanosis of the extremity. If untreated, the venous obstruction causes arterial occlusion and gangrene and requires amputation.

**Diagnostic Studies.** Table 37-9 presents the various diagnostic studies used to determine the site or location and extent of a VTE.

#### Interprofessional Care

***Prevention and Prophylaxis.*** VTE prophylaxis is a core measure of high-quality health care in high-risk hospitalized patients developed by the Joint Commission and the National Quality

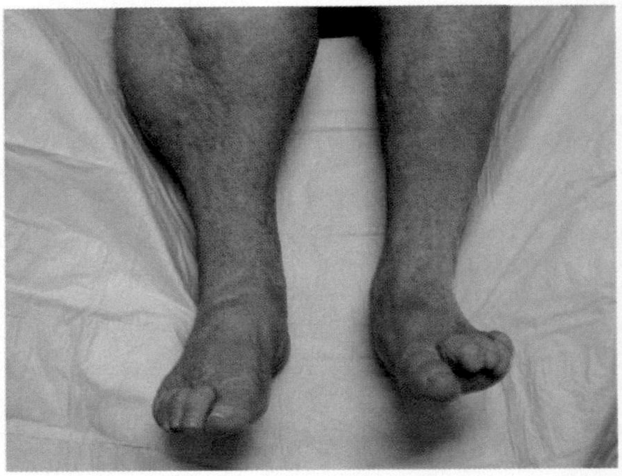

**FIG. 37-10** Lipodermatosclerosis. Skin on lower leg becomes scarred, and the leg becomes tapered like an "inverted bottle." Hallmark signs of lipodermatosclerosis are leathery skin, brown discoloration, hyperpigmentation and hypopigmentation, and circumferential or near circumferential scarring and shrinking of the extremity. (From Etufugh CN, Phillips TJ: Venous ulcers, *Clin Dermatol* 25[1]:125, 2007.)

**TABLE 37-9 Diagnostic Studies**

***Venous Thromboembolism****

| Study | Description and Abnormal Findings |
|---|---|
| **Blood Laboratory Studies** | |
| **ACT, aPTT, INR, bleeding time, Hgb, Hct, platelet count** | Alterations if patient has underlying blood dyscrasia (e.g., increased Hgb and Hct in patient with polycythemia). |
| **D-dimer** | Fragment of fibrin formed as result of fibrin degradation and clot lysis. Elevated results suggest venous thromboembolism (VTE). *Normal results:* <250 ng/mL (<250 mcg/L) |
| **Fibrin monomer complex** | Forms when concentration of thrombin exceeds that of antithrombin. Presence is evidence of thrombus formation and suggests VTE. *Normal results:* <6.1 mg/L |
| **Noninvasive Venous Studies** | |
| **Venous compression ultrasound** | Evaluation of deep femoral, popliteal, and posterior tibial veins. *Normal finding:* Veins collapse with application of external pressure. *Abnormal finding:* Veins fail to collapse with application of external pressure. Failure to collapse suggests a thrombus. |
| **Duplex ultrasound** | Combination of compression ultrasound with spectral and color flow Doppler. Veins examined for compressibility and intraluminal filling defects to help determine location and extent of thrombus (most widely used test to diagnose VTE). |
| **Invasive Venous Studies** | |
| **Computed tomography venography (CTV)** | Uses spiral CT to evaluate veins in the pelvis, thighs, and calves after injection of contrast material. May be performed simultaneously with CT angiography of pulmonary vessels for patients being evaluated for VTE. |
| **Magnetic resonance venography** | Uses MRI with specialized software to evaluate blood flow through veins. Can be done with or without contrast. Highly accurate for pelvic and proximal veins. Less accurate for calf veins. Can distinguish acute and chronic thrombus. |
| **Contrast venography (phlebogram)** | X-ray determination of location and extent of clot using contrast media to outline filling defects. Identifies the presence of collateral circulation. Once the gold standard, but currently rarely performed. |

*ACT,* Activated clotting time; *aPTT,* activated partial thromboplastin time; *INR,* international normalized ratio.
*See Table 27-26 for diagnostic studies for pulmonary embolism.

Forum. There are six VTE measures. These can be found at *www.jointcommission.org/venous_thromboembolism/default.aspx.* In addition, it is recommended that hospitals have a thromboprophylaxis policy that addresses VTE prevention on admission of all adult patients. As many as 80% of medically ill patients at risk for VTE do not receive appropriate thromboprophylaxis.[37]

In patients at risk for VTE, a variety of interventions are used. These are based on such factors as bleeding and thrombosis risk, past medical history, current drugs, medical diagnoses, scheduled procedures, and patient preferences.

Early and aggressive mobilization based on the patient's condition is the easiest and most cost-effective method to decrease VTE risk. Patients on bed rest should change position at least every 2 hours. Unless contraindicated, teach patients to flex and extend their feet, knees, and hips at least every 2 to 4 hours while awake. Patients who can get out of bed need to be in a chair for meals and walk at least four to six times per day as able. Tell the patient and caregiver about the importance of these measures. Early and frequent ambulation is sufficient prophylaxis for very low VTE–risk patients undergoing minor surgical procedures.[38] Anticoagulation and mechanical prophylaxis are not recommended for acutely ill medical patients at low risk for VTE.

*Graduated compression stockings* (e.g., thromboembolic deterrent [TED] hose) are a part of VTE prevention in hospitalized patients. When fitted correctly (both size and length) and worn properly and consistently from admission until discharge or full mobility, these stockings decrease VTE risk in surgical patients.[39] Proper use means the toe hole is under the toes, the heel patch is over the heel, the thigh gusset is on the inner thigh (thigh length only), and there are no wrinkles. The stockings are not to be rolled down, cut, or otherwise altered.

Knee-length stockings seem to be as effective as thigh-length stockings in the prevention of VTE in surgical patients. However, additional research is needed.[40] If the stockings are not fitted and worn correctly, venous return is impeded. This may promote the development of arterial ischemia, edema, skin breakdown, and VTE. VTE prevention is enhanced if graduated compression stockings are used along with anticoagulation.

*Intermittent pneumatic compression devices* (IPCs) use inflatable sleeves or boots to compress the calf and thigh and/or foot and ankle to improve venous return. The sleeves apply external pressure by means of an electric pump. IPCs may or may not be used with graduated compression stockings. Like graduated compression stockings, ensure correct fit by accurately measuring the extremities. IPCs will not be effective if they are not applied correctly, if the fit is incorrect, or if the patient does not wear the device continuously. Exceptions include during bathing, skin assessment, and ambulation. IPCs are not worn when a patient has an active VTE because of the risk of PE.[41]

***Drug Therapy.*** Anticoagulants are used routinely for VTE prevention and treatment. The regimen depends on the patient's VTE risk. The goal of anticoagulant therapy for VTE prophylaxis is to prevent clot formation. The goals for treatment of a confirmed VTE are to prevent new clot development, spread of the clot, and embolization.[42]

Three major classes of anticoagulants are available: (1) vitamin K antagonists (VKA), (2) thrombin inhibitors (both indirect and direct), and (3) factor Xa inhibitors[43] (Table 37-10). Anticoagulant therapy does not dissolve the clot. Clot lysis begins naturally through the body's intrinsic fibrinolytic system (see Chapter 29).

**Vitamin K antagonists.** The oral anticoagulant for long-term or extended anticoagulation is warfarin, a VKA. Warfarin

## TABLE 37-10 Drug Therapy
### *Anticoagulant Therapy*

| Drug | Route of Administration | Comments |
|---|---|---|
| **Vitamin K Antagonists (VKA)** | | |
| warfarin (Coumadin) | PO | INR is used for monitoring therapeutic levels. Administer at the same time each day. Variations of certain genes (e.g., *CYP2CP, VKORC1*) may influence response to drug. *Antidote:* Vitamin K. For major VKA-related bleeding, treatment with four-factor prothrombin complex concentrate and IV vitamin K is recommended over fresh frozen plasma. |
| **Thrombin Inhibitors: Indirect** | | |
| ***Unfractionated Heparin (UH)*** heparin sodium | Continuous IV Intermittent IV Subcutaneous | Therapeutic effects measured at regular intervals by the aPTT or ACT. Monitor CBC counts at regular intervals and titrate according to parameters. If administering subcutaneously, inject deep into subcutaneous tissue (preferably into the abdominal fatty tissue or above the iliac crest), inserting the entire length of the needle. Hold skinfold during injection but release before removing needle. Do not aspirate. Do not inject IM. Do not rub site after injection. Rotate sites. *Antidote:* Protamine neutralizes the effect of UH. |
| ***Low-Molecular-Weight Heparin (LMWH)*** enoxaparin (Lovenox) dalteparin (Fragmin) | Subcutaneous | Routine coagulation tests typically not required. Monitor CBC count at regular intervals. Do not expel air bubble before administering subcutaneously. Follow remaining administration guidelines as described above for UH. Reduced dosage needed in patients with renal impairment. Use extreme caution in patients with a history of HIT. *Antidote:* Protamine neutralizes the effects of LMWH. |
| **Thrombin Inhibitors: Direct** | | |
| ***Hirudin Derivatives*** | | |
| bivalirudin (Angiomax) desirudin (Iprivask) | IV Subcutaneous | Therapeutic effect measured by ACT or aPTT. Used in patients with HIT when anticoagulation is still required. *Antidote:* None. |
| ***Synthetic Thrombin Inhibitors*** | | |
| argatroban dabigatran (Pradaxa) | IV PO | Therapeutic effect measured by aPTT. Used in patients at risk for or with HIT. Used for VTE prevention in joint replacement surgery. VTE treatment option and for stroke prevention in nonvalvular atrial fibrillation. *Antidote:* idarucizumab (Praxbind) neutralizes the effect of dabigatran only. |
| ***Factor Xa Inhibitors*** | | |
| fondaparinux (Arixtra) rivaroxaban (Xarelto) apixaban (Eliquis) edoxaban (Savaysa) | Subcutaneous PO PO PO | Routine coagulation tests not required. Monitor complete blood count and creatinine at regular intervals. Do not expel air bubble before administering. Follow remaining administration guidelines as described for UH. All are approved for VTE prophylaxis and treatment. For surgical patients, initial dose should be given no earlier than 6 hr postoperatively. Use with caution in older patients. Assess creatinine level before giving fondaparinux. May cause thrombocytopenia. If uncontrollable bleeding occurs, treatment with recombinant factor VIIa may be effective. *Antidote:* Andexanet alfa is currently under FDA priority review. Andexanet alfa has been shown to reverse the effects of Factor Xa inhibitors. |

*ACT,* Activated clotting time; *aPTT,* activated partial thromboplastin time; *HIT,* heparin-induced thrombocytopenia; *INR,* international normalized ratio; *VTE,* venous thromboembolism.

inhibits activation of the vitamin K–dependent coagulation factors II, VII, IX, and X, as well as the anticoagulant proteins C and S. (Fig. 29-4 displays the clotting pathways, and clotting factors are listed in Table 29-2.) Warfarin begins to take effect in 48 to 72 hours. It then takes several more days to achieve a maximum effect. Thus an overlap of a parenteral anticoagulant (e.g., UH or LMWH) and warfarin typically is required for 5 days. The level of anticoagulation is monitored daily using the international normalized ratio (INR). The INR is a standardized system of reporting prothrombin time (PT) (Table 37-11). The antidote for warfarin-related bleeding is vitamin K or Kcentra (Prothrombin Complex Concentrate [Human]).

Take a careful history before starting warfarin. Do not give antiplatelets or NSAIDs with warfarin, since these drugs increase bleeding risk.[43] Many other drugs, vitamins, minerals, and dietary and herbal supplements also interact with warfarin (see the Complementary & Alternative Therapies box on this page). A diet that frequently varies in vitamin K intake (e.g., green leafy vegetables) can make it hard to achieve and maintain a target INR level.

## COMPLEMENTARY & ALTERNATIVE THERAPIES
### *Herbal and Dietary Supplements That May Affect Clotting*

**Scientific Evidence**

The following herbs and dietary supplements may affect blood clotting: bilberry, black cohosh, chamomile, chondroitin sulfate, DHEA, feverfew, garlic, ginger, ginkgo biloba, ginseng, goldenseal, grapeseed extract, green tea, horse chestnut seed extract, melatonin, niacin, omega-3 fatty acids, psyllium, red yeast rice extract, saw palmetto, soy, turmeric.

**Nursing Implications**

- Inform patients that taking these herbs or dietary supplements may increase their risk of bleeding.
- Caution patients with bleeding disorders about the use of these herbs and dietary supplements. Advise them that they should consult with their HCP before using these substances.

*DHEA,* Dehydroepiandrosterone.

**TABLE 37-11 Blood Coagulation Tests**

| Test and Drugs Monitored | Normal Value | Therapeutic Value |
|---|---|---|
| **International normalized ratio (INR)** | 0.75-1.25 | 2-3 |
| • Vitamin K antagonists (e.g., warfarin [Coumadin]) | | |
| **Activated partial thromboplastin time (aPTT)** | 25-35 sec | 46-70 sec |
| • Unfractionated heparin (e.g., heparin [Hep-Lock]) | | |
| • Hirudin derivatives (e.g., bivalirudin [Angiomax]) | | |
| • Synthetic thrombin inhibitors (e.g., argatroban [Acova], dabigatran [Pradaxa]) | | |
| **Activated clotting time (ACT)** | 70-120 sec* | >300 sec |
| • Unfractionated heparin | | |
| • Hirudin derivatives | | |
| • Synthetic thrombin inhibitors | | |
| **Anti–factor Xa** | | |
| • Low-molecular-weight heparin (e.g., enoxaparin [Lovenox]) | 0 U/mL | 0.6-1.0 U/mL |
| • Factor Xa inhibitors (e.g., fondaparinux [Arixtra], rivaroxaban [Xarelto]) | 0 U/mL | 0.2-1.5 U/mL |

*Varies based on type of system and test reagent or activator used.

Genetic variants in the genes *VKORC1* and cytochrome P450 2C9 *(CYP2C9)* may influence how some people respond to warfarin (see Table 12-5). Although genetic testing is available, pharmacogenetic-based dosing is not recommended in clinical practice at this time.[44]

**Thrombin inhibitors.** *Indirect thrombin inhibitors* are divided into two major classes: UH and LMWHs. UH (e.g., heparin) affects both the intrinsic and common pathways of blood coagulation by way of the plasma antithrombin. Antithrombin inhibits thrombin-mediated conversion of fibrinogen to fibrin by affecting factors II (prothrombin), IX, X, XI, and XII (see Fig. 29-4).

Heparin can be given subcutaneously for VTE prophylaxis or by continuous IV infusion for VTE treatment. When given IV, heparin requires frequent monitoring of clotting status as measured by activated partial thromboplastin time (aPTT) (Table 37-11). Protamine sulfate reverses the effect of heparin.

One serious side effect of heparin is *heparin-induced thrombocytopenia* (HIT). HIT is an immune reaction to heparin. It causes a severe, sudden reduction in the platelet count along with a paradoxical increase in venous or arterial thrombosis. HIT is diagnosed by measuring the presence of heparin antibodies in the blood. Treatment requires immediately stopping heparin therapy and, if further anticoagulation is required, using a non-heparin anticoagulant (e.g., fondaparinux).[45] Another side effect of long-term heparin therapy is osteoporosis.

LMWHs (e.g., enoxaparin [Lovenox]) are derived from UH. They have more bioavailability, more predictable dose response, longer half-life, and fewer bleeding complications than UH. LMWHs are less likely to cause HIT and osteoporosis. LMWHs typically do not require ongoing anticoagulant monitoring and dose adjustment and their antiinflammatory properties may help prevent PTS and venous ulcer development.[36] Protamine neutralizes the effect of LMWH.

*Direct thrombin inhibitors* are classified as hirudin derivatives or synthetic thrombin inhibitors. Hirudin is made using recombinant deoxyribonucleic acid (DNA) technology. It binds specifically with thrombin and directly inhibits its function without causing plasma protein and platelet interactions. Hirudin derivatives (e.g., bivalirudin [Angiomax]) are given by continuous IV infusion. Bivalirudin is approved for patients with or at risk for HIT having a percutaneous coronary intervention. Anticoagulant activity is monitored using aPTT or activated clotting time (ACT) (Table 37-11). If bleeding occurs, there is no antidote for hirudin derivatives.

Argatroban, a synthetic direct thrombin inhibitor, inhibits thrombin. Like bivalirudin, it is used as an alternative to heparin for the prevention and treatment of HIT and for patients with or at risk for HIT needing percutaneous coronary interventions. Dabigatran (Pradaxa), an oral direct thrombin inhibitor, is used for VTE prevention after elective joint replacement, for stroke prevention in nonvalvular atrial fibrillation, and as a treatment option in VTE. The effect of argatroban is not reversible. Anticoagulant effect is monitored for both drugs using aPTT or ACT. Idarucizumab (Praxbind) neutralizes the effect of dabigatran. There are no similar drugs for any other synthetic direct thrombin inhibitor.

**Factor Xa inhibitors.** *Factor Xa inhibitors* inhibit factor Xa directly or indirectly, producing rapid anticoagulation. These include fondaparinux (Arixtra), rivaroxaban (Xarelto), apixaban (Eliquis), and edoxaban (Savaysa). All are used for both VTE treatment and prophylaxis. Fondaparinux is given subcutaneously. Rivaroxaban, apixaban, and edoxaban are oral drugs. Although coagulation monitoring or dose adjustment is not needed, the drug's anticoagulant activity can be measured using anti-Xa assays (Table 37-11). If uncontrollable bleeding occurs, recombinant factor VIIa may be useful. Fondaparinux is contraindicated in patients with severe renal disease.

**Anticoagulant therapy for VTE prophylaxis.** For VTE prophylaxis in the hospitalized medical patient at risk for thrombosis who is not bleeding, low-dose UH, LMWH, or fondaparinux is used. If the patient is at low VTE risk, drug prophylaxis is not needed. Patients with moderate VTE risk (e.g., general, gynecologic, urologic surgery) should receive either UH or LMWH. Patients with high VTE risk (e.g., trauma) should receive UH or LMWH until discharge. Patients having abdominal or pelvic surgery for cancer or major orthopedic surgery (e.g., total knee or hip replacement) should be prescribed VTE prophylaxis.[44]

**Anticoagulant therapy for VTE treatment.** Patients with confirmed VTE should receive initial treatment with either LMWH, UH, or an oral Factor Xa drug. Oral VKA therapy may be considered. A therapeutic INR is maintained between 2.0 and 3.0 if VKA therapy is used. Subtherapeutic INR, especially in the first few months of therapy, is linked with PTS development.[36] Active treatment of VTE should continue for at least 3 months and may continue longer in some patients.[46]

Patients with multiple co-morbidities, complex medical issues, or a very large VTE usually are hospitalized for treatment. Parenteral administration of UH is the typical initial treatment. Depending on the clinical presentation and home situation, patients may be safely and effectively managed as outpatients.

**Thrombolytic therapy for VTE treatment.** Another treatment option for patients with a thrombus is catheter-directed administration of a thrombolytic drug (e.g., urokinase, tPA). It dissolves the clot(s), reduces the acute symptoms, improves deep venous flow, reduces valvular reflux, and may help to decrease the incidence of PTS. Catheter-directed thrombolysis is recommended for select patients who are at a low bleeding risk and present with an acute, extensive, symptomatic, proximal VTE. Systemic anticoagulation is recommended before, during, and after catheter-directed thrombolysis. (Chapter 33 discusses thrombolytic therapy.)

**CHECK YOUR PRACTICE**

Your 55-yr-old female patient is admitted with an extensive VTE in her right leg. She is receiving weight-based IV heparin per agency protocol: 18 U/kg/hr. You receive the following critical laboratory result: aPTT 122 seconds.

- Describe your next actions.

***Surgical and Interventional Radiology Therapies.*** Although most VTE patients are managed medically, a small number of patients with extensive, acute, proximal VTE who are not candidates for catheter-directed thrombolysis and/or interventional radiology therapies (due to bleeding risk) may undergo surgery.[36] Surgical options include open venous thrombectomy and inferior vena cava interruption. *Venous thrombectomy* involves the removal of a thrombus through an incision in the vein. Anticoagulant therapy is recommended after venous thrombectomy.

*Vena cava interruption* devices (e.g., Greenfield, Vena Tech, TrapEase filters) can be placed percutaneously through the right femoral or right internal jugular veins. The filter device is opened, and the spokes penetrate the vessel walls (Fig. 37-11). The filters act as a "sieve-type" device, permitting filtration of clots without interruption of blood flow. Complications after the insertion are rare but include air embolism, improper placement, migration of the filter, and perforation of the vena cava with retroperitoneal bleeding. Over time, clots can clog the filter and completely block the vena cava, requiring filter removal and replacement. A filter device is recommended with acute PE or proximal VTE of the leg in patients with active bleeding or if anticoagulant therapy is contraindicated or ineffective. Patients with a filter device alone are at increased risk of developing a VTE. If the active bleeding or anticoagulation contraindication resolves, a course of anticoagulant therapy is suggested.[47]

Percutaneous endovascular interventional radiology procedures can be used along with catheter-directed thrombolytic therapy, especially for severely symptomatic patients with iliocaval or iliofemoral obstruction.[36] The interventional radiology procedures are similar to those used in the treatment of lower-extremity PAD. The difference is accessing an occluded vein instead of an artery. They include mechanical thrombectomy, pharmacomechanical devices, and post-thrombus extraction, angioplasty, and/or stenting.[47] Anticoagulation therapy is recommended after an iliofemoral interventional radiology procedure. Postprocedure nursing care focuses on (1) maintenance of catheter systems (if continuous infusions); (2) monitoring for bleeding, embolization, and impaired perfusion; and (3) VTE prevention teaching.[48]

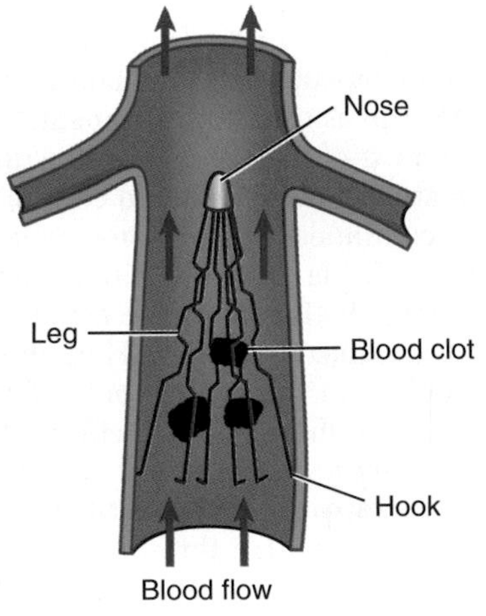


**FIG. 37-11** Inferior vena caval interruption technique using Greenfield stainless steel filter to prevent pulmonary embolism. As blood travels up the vena cava, clots are trapped in the filter.

## NURSING MANAGEMENT: VENOUS THROMBOEMBOLISM

### Nursing Assessment

Table 37-12 presents the subjective and objective data to obtain from a patient with VTE.

**TABLE 37-12 Nursing Assessment**
***Venous Thromboembolism***

**Subjective Data**

***Important Health Information*** *(Table 37-8)*

*Past health history:* Trauma to vein, intravascular catheter (e.g., peripherally inserted central catheter), varicose veins, pregnancy or recent childbirth, bacteremia, obesity, prolonged bed rest, irregular heartbeat (e.g., atrial fibrillation), COPD, HF, cancer, coagulation disorders and hypercoagulable states, systemic lupus erythematosus, MI, spinal cord injury, stroke, prolonged travel, recent bone fracture, dehydration

*Medications:* Use of estrogens (including oral contraceptives, hormone therapy), tamoxifen, raloxifene (Evista), corticosteroids, excessive amounts of vitamin E, erythropoiesis-stimulating drugs

*Surgery or other treatments:* Any recent surgery, especially orthopedic, gynecologic, gastric, or urologic. Previous surgery involving veins. Central venous catheter

***Functional Health Patterns***

*Health perception–health management:* IV drug abuse, tobacco use, obesity

*Activity-exercise:* Inactivity

*Cognitive-perceptual:* Pain in area on palpation or ambulation

**Objective Data**

***General***

Fever, anxiety, pain

***Integumentary***

Increased size of extremity when compared with other side. Taut, shiny, warm skin, erythematous, tender to palpation. No physical changes in the affected extremity in some patients

***Cardiovascular***

Distention and warmth of superficial veins in affected area. Edema and cyanosis of extremities, neck, back, and face (if superior vena cava involvement)

***Possible Diagnostic Findings***

Leukocytosis, abnormal coagulation, anemia or ↑ hematocrit and RBC count, ↑ D-dimer level, positive venous compression on duplex ultrasound study; positive CTV, magnetic resonance venogram, or contrast venogram study

*COPD,* Chronic obstructive pulmonary disease; *CTV,* computed tomography venogram; *HF,* heart failure; *MI,* myocardial infarction.

## Nursing Diagnoses

Nursing diagnoses and collaborative problems for the patient with VTE include, but are not limited to, the following:

- Acute pain *related to* venous congestion, impaired venous return, and inflammation
- Ineffective health management *related to* lack of knowledge about disorder and its treatment
- Risk for impaired skin integrity *related to* altered peripheral tissue perfusion
- Potential complication: bleeding *related to* anticoagulant therapy
- Potential complication: PE *related to* embolization of thrombus, dehydration, and immobility

## Planning

The overall goals for the patient with VTE include (1) pain relief, (2) decreased edema, (3) increased knowledge of disorder and treatment plan, (4) no skin ulceration, (5) no bleeding complications, and (6) no evidence of PE.

## Nursing Implementation

**Acute Care.** Focus your nursing care for the patient with VTE on prevention of emboli formation and reduction of inflammation. Review with the patient any drugs, vitamins, minerals, and dietary and herbal supplements being taken that may interfere with anticoagulant therapy (see the Complementary & Alternative Therapies box on p. 820). Depending on the anticoagulant ordered, monitor INR, aPTT, ACT, anti–factor Xa levels, complete blood count (CBC), creatinine, factor X levels, hemoglobin, hematocrit, platelet levels, and/or liver enzymes.[49] Monitor platelet counts for patients getting UH or LMWH to assess for HIT. Titrate doses of UH, warfarin, and direct thrombin inhibitors based on results of blood studies and agency protocols. Direct thrombin inhibitors may need adjustment for patients with renal or liver disease. Always check the results of appropriate tests before starting, giving, or changing anticoagulant therapy.

Monitor for and reduce the risk of bleeding that may occur with anticoagulant therapy (Table 37-13). Be aware that the risk of bleeding is greater in people receiving LMWH or UH with an active gastroduodenal ulcer, prior bleeding history, low platelet count, hepatic or renal failure, rheumatic disease, cancer, or age greater than 85 years.[50] Patients receiving warfarin with an INR of 5.0 or more are also at increased risk for bleeding. In the event of anticoagulation above target goals, give reversal agents (e.g., protamine, vitamin K) or make dosage adjustments as ordered. In the event of major VKA-related bleeding, rapid treatment with four-factor prothrombin complex concentrate and IV vitamin K is recommended over fresh frozen plasma.

**DRUG ALERT Anticoagulant Therapy**

- Avoid IM injections.
- Observe closely for any signs of bleeding: hypotension, tachycardia, hematuria, melena, hematemesis, petechiae, ecchymosis, oozing or visible bleeding from trauma site or surgical incision.
- Tell patients to report any signs of bleeding: black or bloody stools, bleeding gums, bloody urine or sputum, coffee-ground or bloody vomit, excessive bruising, nosebleeds, excessive menstrual bleeding.
- Assess for mental status changes, especially in the older patient, since this may indicate cerebral bleeding.
- Tell patients to avoid taking aspirin, NSAIDs, fish oil supplements, garlic supplements, ginkgo biloba, and certain antibiotics (e.g., sulfamethoxazole and trimethoprim [Bactrim]).

### TABLE 37-13 Nursing Interventions for Patients Taking Anticoagulants

**Assessment**

- Monitor vital signs as indicated.
- Examine urine and stool for overt and occult signs of blood.
- Inspect skin frequently, especially under any splinting devices.
- Evaluate platelet count for signs of heparin-induced thrombocytopenia.
- Evaluate appropriate laboratory coagulation tests for target therapeutic levels.
- Evaluate lower extremity for ecchymosis or hematoma development if intermittent pneumatic compression device used.
- Perform assessments frequently to observe for signs and symptoms of bleeding (e.g., hypotension, tachycardia) or clotting.
- Notify the HCP of any abnormalities in assessments, vital signs, or laboratory values.

**Injections**

- Avoid IM injections.
- Minimize venipunctures.
- Use small-gauge needles for venipunctures unless therapy requires a larger gauge.
- Apply manual pressure for at least 10 min (or longer if needed) on venipuncture sites.

**Patient Care**

- Avoid restrictive clothing.
- Apply moisturizing lotion to skin.
- Use electric razors, not straight razors.
- Perform physical care in a gentle manner.
- Tell patient not to forcefully blow nose.
- Avoid removing or disrupting established clots.
- Humidify $O_2$ source if supplemental $O_2$ is ordered.
- Use soft toothbrushes or foam swabs for oral care.
- Reposition the patient carefully at regular intervals.
- Limit tape application. Use paper tape as appropriate.
- Give stool softeners to avoid hard stools and straining.
- Lubricate tubes (e.g., suction catheter) adequately before insertion.
- Avoid restraints if possible. Use only soft, padded restraints if needed.
- Use support pads, mattresses, bed cradles, and therapeutic beds as indicated.
- Apply graduated compression stockings or intermittent pneumatic compression devices (if ordered) and with attention to proper size, application, and use.
- Perform risk for fall and skin breakdown assessments per agency policy and implement safety and preventive measures as needed.

Early ambulation when compared with bed rest does not increase the short-term risk of a PE in patients with VTE. In addition, early ambulation after acute VTE results in a more rapid decrease in edema and limb pain, fewer PTS symptoms, and better quality of life. Teach the patient and caregiver the importance of physical activity and assist the patient to ambulate several times a day. For patients with acute VTE with severe edema and limb pain, bed rest with limb elevation may initially be prescribed.

**Ambulatory Care.** Focus discharge teaching on modification of VTE risk factors, importance of monitoring laboratory values, dietary and drug instructions, and guidelines for follow-up. If appropriate, tell the patient to stop smoking and avoid all nicotine products. Instruct the patient to avoid constrictive clothing. If appropriate, tell women with a history of VTE to stop oral contraceptives or HT. Teach patients to limit standing or sitting in a motionless, leg-dependent position.

## TEAMWORK & COLLABORATION

### *Caring for the Patient With Venous Thromboembolism (VTE)*

*All members of the interprofessional team have important roles in VTE prevention and management of a patient with VTE..*

**Role of Nursing Personnel**

***Registered Nurse (RN)***

- Assess patients for VTE risk and monitor for VTE in at-risk patients.
- Teach patients who are at risk for VTE about preventive measures such as increasing mobility, using graduated compression stockings and intermittent pneumatic compression devices, and taking anticoagulant drugs.
- Assess for the use of dietary supplements or herbs that may affect the coagulation status before the start of anticoagulant therapy.
- Evaluate the effect of anticoagulant drugs by monitoring appropriate laboratory results and side effects of therapy.
- Assess for complications of VTE, including pulmonary embolism (PE) and chronic venous insufficiency.
- Teach the patient and caregiver the clinical manifestations of PE and the need to contact the ERS if these occur.
- Provide discharge teaching about use of graduated compression stockings, anticoagulant drugs, diet, laboratory testing, and administration of subcutaneous anticoagulants (if needed).
- Teach safety precautions to prevent falls or other injuries that might result in bleeding.
- Provide instructions about the use of pressure to stop bleeding and that the ERS should be contacted for persistent bleeding.
- Teach the patient about lifestyle measures to prevent VTE, including leg exercises, ambulation, and avoidance of nicotine and oral contraceptives.

***Licensed Practical/Vocational Nurse (LPN/LVN)***

- Give prescribed oral, subcutaneous, and IV anticoagulants (consider state nurse practice act and agency policies regarding administration of high-alert medications and IV medications).
- Measure patients for graduated compression stockings and/or intermittent pneumatic compression devices.

***Unlicensed Assistive Personnel (UAP)***

- Reposition patients who are on bed rest at least every 2 hr.
- Remind patients about the need to flex and extend the legs and feet at least every 2 hr while in bed.
- Help ambulatory patients to walk at least 4 to 6 times daily.
- Help patients with putting on graduated compression stockings.
- Apply intermittent pneumatic compression devices.

**Role of Other Team Members**

***Physical Therapist***

- Assess patient's mobility status.
- Develop exercise/muscle strengthening program as needed.

***Dietitian***

- Assess patient's diet and nutritional status.
- Provide diet teaching as needed.

When traveling long distances, tell patients to frequently exercise the calf muscles, take short walks, and drink nonalcoholic, noncaffeinated beverages. For those at high risk for VTE who are planning a long trip, recommend properly fitted, knee-high graduated compression stockings during travel to decrease edema and VTE risk. Aspirin or anticoagulant use is not suggested for long-distance travelers. Teach the patient and caregiver about signs and symptoms of PE such as sudden onset of dyspnea, tachypnea, and pleuritic chest pain. (Chapter 27 discusses PE.) They should contact ERS if these symptoms occur.

Teach the patient and caregiver about drug dosage, actions, and side effects; the need for routine blood tests; and what symptoms need immediate medical attention (Table 37-14). Devices are available for home monitoring of INR. Teach patients taking LMWH or fondaparinux and their caregivers how to give the drug subcutaneously. Active or young patients need to avoid contact sports and high-risk (for trauma) activities (e.g., skiing). Teach older patients about safety precautions to prevent falls (e.g., avoid use of throw rugs). Tell the patient and caregiver to apply pressure for 10 to 15 minutes if bleeding occurs (e.g., nosebleed).

A well-balanced diet is important. Teach patients taking warfarin to follow a consistent diet of foods containing vitamin K and to avoid any supplements containing vitamin K (e.g., vitamins, green tea). Tell the patient to avoid excessive amounts of vitamin E and alcohol. Encourage proper hydration to prevent additional hypercoagulability of the blood, which may occur with dehydration.

The overweight patient needs to limit carbohydrates and total caloric intake and increase physical activity to achieve and maintain desired weight. Exercise does not harm and may benefit patients with VTE and PTS.[36] Help the patient develop

## TABLE 37-14 Patient & Caregiver Teaching

### *Anticoagulant Therapy*

*Include the following information in the teaching plan for a patient receiving anticoagulant therapy and the patient's caregiver.*

1. Give reasons for and action of anticoagulant drug and how long therapy will last.
2. Take drug at the same time each day (preferably in afternoon or evening).
3. Depending on drug prescribed, obtain blood tests to assess therapeutic effect of the drug and whether change in dosage is needed.
4. Contact ERS immediately for any of the following adverse side effects of drug therapy:
   - Blood in urine or stool; or black, tarry stools
   - Vomiting blood, coffee-ground emesis
   - Unusual bleeding from gums, skin, or nose, or heavy menstrual bleeding
   - Severe headaches or stomach pain
   - Chest pain, shortness of breath, palpitations (heart racing)
   - Weakness, dizziness, mental status changes
   - Cold, blue, or painful feet
5. Avoid any trauma or injury that may cause bleeding (e.g., vigorous brushing of teeth, contact sports, rollerblading, use of straight razor).
6. Avoid all aspirin-containing drugs and nonsteroidal antiinflammatory drugs.
7. Limit alcohol intake to small to moderate amounts (12 oz beer, 4 oz wine, 1 oz hard liquor/day).
8. Wear a Medic Alert device indicating what anticoagulant drug is being taken.
9. If taking warfarin (Coumadin), avoid frequent or dramatic changes in eating foods high in vitamin K (e.g., broccoli, spinach, kale, greens). Do not take supplemental vitamin K.
10. Consult with HCP before beginning or discontinuing any drug, vitamin, mineral, or dietary or herbal supplement (see Complementary & Alternative Therapies box on p. 820).
11. Inform all HCPs, including dentist, of anticoagulant therapy.
12. Correct dosing is essential. Provide supervision if patient experiences confusion or cognitive impairment.

an exercise program with an emphasis on leg strength training and aerobic activity. An exercise program also improves the patient's quality of life.

Graduated compression stockings reduce symptomatic swelling in patients with a diagnosis of proximal VTE.[36] Alternatively, IPCs may be used for patients with significant edema and moderate to severe PTS. The long-term use of graduated compression stockings may not prevent PTS development.

### Evaluation

The expected outcomes are that the patient with VTE will have:

- Minimal to no pain
- Intact skin
- Increased knowledge of disorder and treatment plan
- No signs of hemorrhage or occult bleeding

## VARICOSE VEINS

**Varicose veins**, or *varicosities,* are dilated (3 mm or larger in diameter), tortuous superficial veins commonly found in the saphenous vein system. Varicosities may be small and harmless or large and bulging. *Primary varicose veins* (idiopathic) are due to a weakness of the vein walls and are more common in women. *Secondary varicose veins* result from direct injury, a previous VTE, or excessive vein distension. Secondary varicose veins may also occur in the esophagus (esophageal varices), vulva, spermatic cords (varicoceles), and anorectal area (hemorrhoids), and as abnormal arteriovenous (AV) connections.

*Congenital varicose veins* result from chromosomal defects which cause abnormal development of the venous system.[51] *Reticular veins* are smaller varicose veins that appear flat, less tortuous, and blue-green in color. *Telangiectasias* (often referred to as spider veins), are small visible vessels (generally less than 1 mm in diameter) that appear bluish black, purple, or red.

### Etiology and Pathophysiology

The etiology of varicose veins is multifactorial. Superficial veins in the lower extremities become dilated and tortuous in response to backward (retrograde) blood flow and increased venous pressure. Risk factors include family history of chronic venous disease, weakness of the vein structure, female gender, Hispanic ethnicity, tobacco use, increasing age, obesity, multiparity, history of VTE, venous obstruction resulting from extrinsic pressure by tumors, thrombophilia, phlebitis, previous leg injury, and occupations that require prolonged standing or sitting.[52]

In primary varicose veins, weak vein walls allow the vein valve ring to enlarge, so the leaflets no longer fit together properly (incompetent). Incompetent vein valves allow backward blood flow, particularly when the patient is standing. This results in increased venous pressure and further venous distention. High pressure in the superficial veins can also be caused by vein valve dysfunction in the deep veins or perforator veins (veins that perforate the deep fascia of muscles to connect the superficial veins to the deep veins).

### Clinical Manifestations and Complications

Discomfort from varicose veins varies among people and tends to be worse after episodes of superficial vein thrombosis. Self-reported symptoms typically are worse in women.[52] The most common varicose vein symptoms include a heavy, achy feeling or pain after prolonged standing or sitting, which is relieved by walking or limb elevation. Some patients feel pressure or complain of an itchy, burning, tingling, throbbing, or cramplike leg sensation. Swelling, restless or tired legs, fatigue, and nocturnal leg cramps also may occur.

Superficial venous thrombosis is the most frequent complication of varicose veins. It may occur spontaneously or after trauma, surgical procedures, or pregnancy. Rare complications include rupture of the varicose veins resulting in external bleeding and skin ulcerations.

### Diagnostic Studies and Interprofessional Care

Superficial varicose veins can often be diagnosed by careful physical examination. Duplex ultrasound imaging is the gold standard to evaluate venous anatomy, valvular competence, and venous obstruction.[52] Conservative treatment involves rest with limb elevation; graduated compression stockings; leg strengthening exercise, such as walking; and weight loss, if indicated.

### Drug Therapy

Venoactive drugs, derived from plant extracts, are powerful antioxidants that work by stimulating release of chemicals within the vein walls to strengthen the circulation and reduce inflammation and edema. Several natural and synthetic venoactive agents have been used to treat varicose veins and advanced chronic venous disease. These include coumarins ($\alpha$-benzopyrenes), defibrotide, flavonoids (e.g., diosmin, hesperidin, micronized purified flavonoid fraction [Daflon]), rutosides (e.g., horse chestnut seed extract *[Aesculus hippocastanum]*), and other plant extracts such as butcher's broom *[Ruscus aculeatus]*), Gotu kola, pine bark, and red vine leaf.[36,52]

Therapeutic benefits of venoactive drugs include pain relief, edema reduction, and decreased leg cramping and restless legs. These drugs have been widely used in Europe. They are not approved by the Federal Drug Administration (FDA) in the United States. However, many are available over-the-counter as dietary or herbal supplements.

**DRUG ALERT Horse Chestnut Seed Extract *(Aesculus hippocastanum)***

- May interact with lithium and antidiabetes, antiplatelet, and anticoagulant drugs.
- Should not be taken by individuals with liver or kidney disease or with a latex allergy.

### Interventional and Surgical Therapies

*Sclerotherapy* involves the direct IV injection of a liquid or foam sclerosing substance (e.g., hypertonic saline, polidocanol, glycerin) that chemically ablates (destroys) the treated veins. Sclerotherapy can be used on telangiectasias, perforator veins, reticular veins, varicose veins 5 mm in diameter or smaller, and venous malformations (Fig. 37-12). This procedure is performed in an office setting and causes minimal discomfort.

The most common complications of sclerotherapy are residual pigmentation and matting (new telangiectasias develop in the area).[53] Less common complications include headaches, migraines, skin necrosis, sensory nerve injury, visual disturbances, and distal VTE. After injection, a graduated compression stocking or compression bandage is recommended. Patients should not travel long distances during the first week after sclerotherapy to minimize the risk of a VTE.[53]

Other noninvasive options include transcutaneous laser therapy for telangiectasias and high-intensity pulsed-light

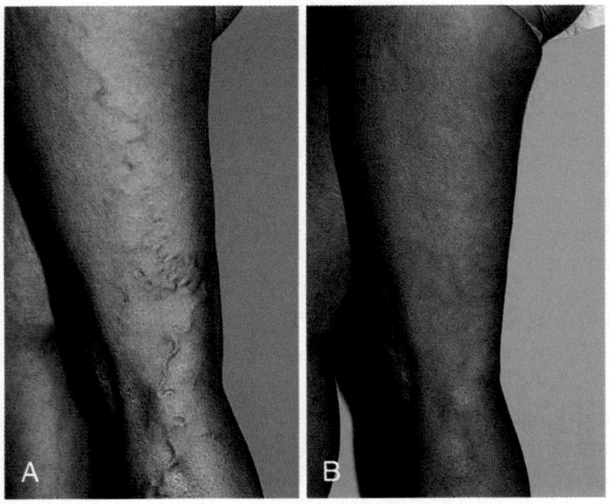


**FIG. 37-12** **A,** Lateral aspect of varicose veins before treatment. **B,** Lateral aspect of varicose veins 2 years after initial treatment with sclerotherapy. (From Goldman MP, Guex JJ, Weiss RA: *Sclerotherapy: treatment of varicose and telangiectatic leg veins,* ed 5, Philadelphia, 2011, Mosby.)

therapy for reticular veins. Transcutaneous laser or light therapy is used for patients in whom sclerotherapy is contraindicated or has been ineffective.[52] Vascular lasers work by heating the hemoglobin in the vessels, resulting in vessel sclerosis. Potential complications of these therapies include pain, blistering, hyperpigmentation, and superficial erosions.

A minimally invasive treatment option for saphenous vein reflux is endovenous ablation using thermal energy from radiofrequency or laser therapy. A catheter is inserted into the vein to heat the vein wall, which then causes the vein to collapse. Potential complications include bruising, skin burns, hyperpigmentation, infection, paresthesia, superficial or deep vein thrombosis, and pulmonary embolism. Graduated compression stockings or bandages are recommended postprocedure. Endovenous thermal ablation may be done in combination with surgical ligation or phlebectomy.

Surgical intervention is indicated for recurrent superficial venous thrombosis or when symptoms cannot be controlled with medical or interventional therapy. The traditional surgical intervention involves ligation of the entire vein (usually the greater saphenous vein) and removal of its incompetent branches. An alternative but time-consuming technique is *ambulatory phlebectomy*. This involves pulling the varicosity through a "stab" incision followed by excision of the vein. *Transilluminated powered phlebectomy* involves the use of a tissue resector to destroy clusters of varicosities and removes the pieces via aspiration. Potential complications include bleeding, bruising, and infection. In up to 30% of patients, a new vein forms to replace the one removed.

## ❖ NURSING MANAGEMENT: VARICOSE VEINS

Prevention is a key factor related to varicose veins. Tell the patient to avoid sitting or standing for long periods, maintain ideal body weight, take precautions against injury to the extremities, avoid wearing constrictive clothing, and walk daily.

After vein ligation surgery, encourage the patient to deep breathe, which promotes venous return. Check the extremities regularly for color, movement, sensation, temperature, edema, and quality of pedal pulses. Some bruising and discoloration are normal. Elevate the legs 15 degrees to limit edema. Apply graduated compression stockings or bandages. Remove them every 8 hours for short periods and then reapply.

Long-term management of varicose veins is directed toward improving circulation and appearance, relieving discomfort, and avoiding complications and ulceration. Varicose veins can recur in other veins after surgery. Teach the patient the proper use and care of custom-fitted graduated compression stockings. The patient should apply stockings in bed before rising in the morning.

Emphasize the importance of periodic positioning of the legs above the heart. The overweight patient may need assistance with weight loss. The patient with a job that requires long periods of standing or sitting needs to frequently flex and extend her or his hips, legs, and ankles and change positions. Remind patients to consult with their HCP before taking any dietary or herbal supplements to avoid drug interactions.

## CHRONIC VENOUS INSUFFICIENCY AND VENOUS LEG ULCERS

Chronic venous insufficiency (CVI), a common problem in older adults, describes long-standing functional abnormalities of the venous system that result in advanced venous signs and symptoms, such as edema, skin changes, and/or venous leg ulcers.[51] CVI can lead to *venous leg ulcers* (formerly called *venous stasis ulcers* or *varicose ulcers*). Although CVI and venous leg ulcers are not life-threatening diseases, they are painful, slow to heal, debilitating, and costly conditions that adversely affect patients' quality of life.

### Etiology and Pathophysiology

Both long-standing primary varicose veins and PTS can progress to CVI. As a result of *ambulatory venous hypertension,* serous fluid and RBCs leak from the capillaries and venules into the tissue. This produces edema and chronic inflammatory changes. Enzymes in the tissue eventually break down RBCs, causing the release of *hemosiderin,* which causes a brownish skin discoloration. Over time, the skin and subcutaneous tissue around the ankle are replaced by fibrous tissue, resulting in thick, hardened, contracted skin. Although the causes of CVI are known, the exact pathophysiology of venous leg ulcers is unknown.

### Clinical Manifestations and Complications

In individuals with CVI, the skin of the lower leg is leathery, with a characteristic brownish or "brawny" appearance from the hemosiderin deposition. Edema usually has been persistent for a prolonged period. Eczema is often present, and itching is a common complaint (Table 37-1).

Venous ulcers classically are located above the medial malleolus (Fig. 37-13). The ulcer is often quite painful, particularly when edema or infection is present. Pain may be worse when the leg is in a dependent position. If the venous ulcer is untreated, the wound becomes wider and deeper, increasing the likelihood of infection. Severe complications can include osteomyelitis and malignant changes.[54] On rare occasions, severe, long-standing CVI may result in the need for amputation.[52]

### Interprofessional Care

Compression is essential for venous ulcer healing and prevention of venous ulcer recurrence.[36,55] A variety of options are available for compression therapy. These include custom-fitted

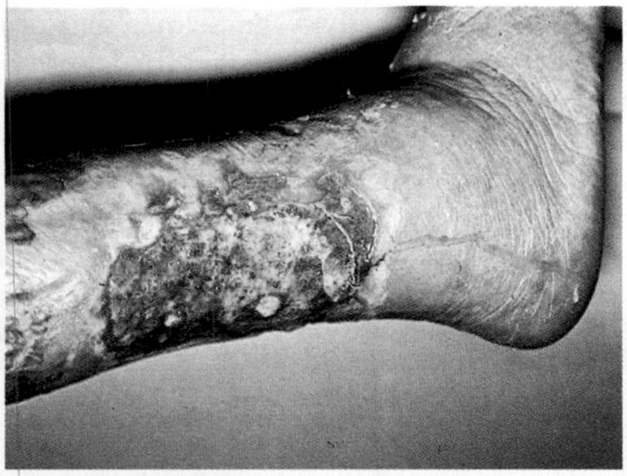

**FIG. 37-13** Venous leg ulcer. (From Kamal A, Brockelhurst JC: *Colour atlas of geriatric medicine,* ed 2, 1991, Mosby-Year Book-Europe.)

graduated compression stockings, elastic tubular support bandages, a Velcro wrap (CircAid), IPCs, a paste bandage (Unna boot) with an elastic wrap, and multilayer (three or four) bandage systems (e.g., Profore).[52] There are benefits to each type of compression therapy. Evaluate patients individually when choosing a compression method. Before starting compression therapy, assess the arterial status to make sure that PAD is not also present. An ABI of 0.4 or less suggests severe PAD, and the patient should not have any type of compression therapy.[55]

Moist environment dressings are the basis of wound care.[50] A variety of these dressings are available, including transparent film dressings, hydrocolloids, hydrogels, foams, alginates, gauze, dextranomer, flax, and combination dressings. Dressing decisions should be based on wound characteristics, cost, best evidence, and clinician judgment. (Chapter 11 and Table 11-9 discuss dressings.)

Evaluate the nutritional status of a patient with a venous ulcer. A balanced diet with adequate protein, calories, and nutrients is essential. Foods high in protein (e.g., meat, beans, cheese, tofu), vitamin A (green leafy vegetables), vitamin C (citrus fruits, tomatoes, cantaloupe), and zinc (meat, seafood) are most important for healing. For patients with diabetes, maintaining normal blood glucose levels assists the healing process.

Venous leg ulcers are colonized by bacteria, but routine use of antibiotics is not indicated.[52] Clinical signs of infection include change in quantity, color, or odor of the drainage; pus; erythema of the wound edges; change in sensation around the wound; warmth around the wound; increased local pain, edema, or both; dark-colored granulation tissue; induration around the wound; delayed healing; and cellulitis. If signs of infection occur, obtain a wound culture. Antibiotic therapy should be guided by wound culture results. The usual treatment for infection is wound debridement, wound excision, and systemic antibiotics. Topical antibiotics are not recommended.

If the ulcer does not heal with conservative therapy, drug therapy should be considered. Pentoxifylline or micronized purified flavonoid fraction (Daflon) is recommended with compression therapy to improve healing.[36] Pentoxifylline minimizes WBC activation and adhesion to capillary endothelium and decreases oxidative stress. Micronized purified flavonoid fraction acts on WBCs to decrease inflammation and edema.[51]

Other treatments are recommended for large venous leg ulcers that do not respond to standard therapy after 4 to 6 weeks. These include coverage with a skin replacement or substitute such as split-thickness skin grafts, cultured keratinocyte grafts, artificial bioengineered skin, or porcine small intestinal submucosal tissue construct.[55] (Chapter 24 discusses skin grafting.) Although grafts may aid with healing, they do not replace the need for lifelong compression therapy. Neovalve reconstruction also may be considered in patients with long-standing, nonhealing ulcers.[36]

## TEAMWORK & COLLABORATION

### *Caring for the Patient With Chronic Venous Insufficiency*

Many patients with chronic venous insufficiency and venous ulcers are cared for in an outpatient setting. The registered nurse (RN) does an initial assessment of the wound, develops and implements the plan of care, and periodically evaluates the patient and venous ulcer. Much of the routine wound care is done by licensed practical/vocational nurses (LPN/LVNs) and unlicensed assistive personnel (UAP).

**Role of Nursing Personnel**

***Registered Nurse (RN)***

- Assess patients with chronic venous insufficiency for increases in edema, eczema, and venous leg ulcers.
- Assess patient's diet and nutritional status and make referrals as necessary.
- Assess for the use of venoactive dietary supplements or herbs that may adversely affect co-morbid conditions and/or prescription drugs.
- Choose appropriate options for compression therapy and wound care.
- Evaluate for the effectiveness of therapies and need for alternative approaches.
- Teach patient and caregiver about the clinical manifestations, complications, and treatment of venous insufficiency.

***Licensed Practical/Vocational Nurse (LPN/LVN)***

- Give prescribed analgesics, antibiotics, or other drugs.
- Apply compression therapy.
- Provide wound care for venous leg ulcers (consider state nurse practice act and agency policy).

***Unlicensed Assistive Personnel (UAP)***

- Assist patients in elevating legs to reduce edema and pain.
- Apply graduated compression stockings.
- Provide wound care for venous leg ulcers (consider state nurse practice act and agency policy).

**Role of Other Team Members**

***Dietitian***

- Assess patient's diet and nutritional status.
- Provide diet education as needed.

## ❖ NURSING MANAGEMENT: CHRONIC VENOUS INSUFFICIENCY AND VENOUS LEG ULCERS

Long-term management of venous leg ulcers should focus on teaching the patient self-care measures. Demonstrate the correct application of graduated compression stockings and have the patient "show back" the skill. Prescription graduated compression stockings should be worn daily to prevent venous leg ulcer recurrence. Stress the importance of regular replacement every 4 to 6 months. Tell the patient and caregiver to avoid trauma to the limbs, and teach them proper foot and leg care to avoid additional skin trauma.

Patients with CVI have dry, flaky, itchy skin because of eczema. Daily moisturizing decreases itching and prevents cracking of the skin. Contact dermatitis may also result from contact with sensitizing products such as topical antimicrobial agents (e.g., gentamicin); additives in bandages or dressings (e.g., adhesives); ointments containing lanolin, alcohols, or benzocaine; and over-the-counter creams or lotions with fragrance or preservatives.[54] Assess the wound for signs of infection with each dressing change.

Be certain to discuss activity guidelines and proper limb positioning. Tell patients with CVI with or without a venous ulcer to avoid standing or sitting for long periods. Standing or sitting with the legs in a dependent position decreases blood flow to the lower extremities. Also tell patients to frequently elevate their legs above the level of the heart to reduce edema. Encourage patients to begin a daily walking program once an ulcer heals.

## CASE STUDY

### Peripheral Artery Disease

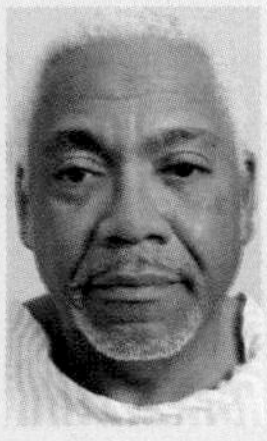

(©IPGGutenberg-UKLtd/iStock/Thinkstock)

**Patient Profile**

S.J., a 73-yr-old African American man, is admitted to the hospital with rest pain in both legs and a nonhealing ulcer of the big toe on the right foot.

**Subjective Data**

- History of a myocardial infarction, stroke, hypertension, heart failure, and type 1 diabetes mellitus
- Underwent a left femoral-popliteal bypass 5 yr ago
- Has a 45-pack-yr history of tobacco use
- Has been using insulin for 30 yr
- Complains of sudden, intense increase in right foot pain for past 2 hr
- Has slept in recliner with right leg in dependent position for several months

***Current Medications***

- Furosemide (Lasix) 40 mg/day PO
- Isosorbide dinitrate/hydralazine hydrochloride (BiDil) 1 tablet q8hr
- Aspart (NovoLog) insulin with meals
- Glargine insulin 50 U/day subcutaneously
- Diltiazem sustained release (Cardizem LA) 240 mg/day PO
- Aspirin 325 mg/day PO
- Fish oil daily (self-prescribed)

**Objective Data**

***Physical Examination***

- BP 148/92 mm Hg, irregular apical HR 90/min, respiratory rate 22/min, temperature 97.9°F (36.6°C)
- Alert and oriented but anxious, no apparent physical or mental deficits from previous stroke
- Has a diminished right femoral pulse, popliteal pulse by Doppler only, posterior tibial pulse by Doppler only, and dorsalis pedis pulse absent (not palpable or present by Doppler). Left leg pulses are weakly palpable
- Right leg ABI: 0.20. Left leg ABI: 0.68
- Has a 2-cm necrotic ulcer on tip of right big toe
- Has thickened toenails. Shiny, thin skin on legs. Hair absent on both lower legs
- Right foot is very cool, pale, and mottled in color with decreased sensation
- No peripheral edema present
- Bedside glucose measurement 298 mg/dL (last meal 4 hr before admission)

**Discussion Questions**

1. Assess S.J.'s risk factors for peripheral artery disease (PAD).
2. Differentiate S.J.'s signs and symptoms of chronic PAD and acute arterial ischemia.
3. Identify the possible cause(s) for the sudden, intense increase in right foot pain.
4. How would you interpret S.J.'s ABI findings?
5. What additional diagnostic tests can be performed to assess the extent of his PAD?
6. Given the physical examination data, what initial drug(s) would you expect the HCP to prescribe?
7. What treatment modalities are possible for S.J.?
8. ***Priority Decision:*** What are the priority nursing responsibilities in caring for S.J.?
9. ***Teamwork and Collaboration:*** Identify activities that can be delegated to unlicensed assistive personnel.
10. ***Priority Decision:*** Based on the assessment data presented, what are the priority nursing diagnoses? Are there any collaborative problems?
11. ***Evidence-Based Practice:*** When teaching S.J., what evidence-based advice would you give him regarding the use of dietary supplements such as fish oil?
12. ***Safety:*** To ensure S.J.'s safety, what nursing interventions are necessary to initiate?

Answers available at *http://evolve.elsevier.com/Lewis/medsurg.*

## BRIDGE TO NCLEX EXAMINATION

The number of the question corresponds to the same-numbered outcome at the beginning of the chapter.

1. A 50-year-old woman weighs 95 kg and has a history of tobacco use, high blood pressure, high sodium intake, and sedentary lifestyle. When developing an individualized care plan for her, the nurse determines that the *most important* risk factors for peripheral artery disease (PAD) that must be modified are
   **a.** weight and diet.
   **b.** activity level and salt intake.
   **c.** tobacco use and high blood pressure.
   **d.** sedentary lifestyle and exercise training.
2. Rest pain is a manifestation of PAD that occurs due to a chronic
   **a.** vasospasm of small cutaneous arteries in the feet.
   **b.** increase in retrograde venous blood flow in the legs.
   **c.** decrease in arterial blood flow to the nerves of the feet.
   **d.** constriction in arterial blood flow to the leg muscles during exercise.
3. A patient with infective endocarditis develops sudden left leg pain with pallor, paresthesia, and a loss of peripheral pulses. The nurse's *initial* action should be to
   **a.** elevate the leg to promote venous return.
   **b.** start anticoagulant therapy with IV heparin.
   **c.** notify the HCP of the change in peripheral perfusion.
   **d.** place the bed in reverse Trendelenburg to promote perfusion.
4. Which clinical manifestations are seen in patients with either Buerger's disease or Raynaud's phenomenon *(select all that apply)*?
   **a.** Intermittent fevers
   **b.** Sensitivity to cold temperatures
   **c.** Gangrenous ulcers on fingertips
   **d.** Color changes of fingers and toes
   **e.** Episodes of superficial vein thrombosis

5. A patient is admitted to the hospital with a diagnosis of abdominal aortic aneurysm. Which signs and symptoms would suggest that his aneurysm has ruptured?
   a. Rapid onset of shortness of breath and hemoptysis
   b. Sudden, severe low back pain and bruising along his flank
   c. Gradually increasing substernal chest pain and diaphoresis
   d. Sudden, patchy blue mottling on feet and toes and rest pain
6. What are the *priority* nursing interventions after an abdominal aortic aneurysm repair?
   a. Assessment of cranial nerves and mental status
   b. Administration of IV heparin and monitoring of PT
   c. Administration of IV fluids and monitoring of kidney function
   d. Elevation of the legs and application of graduated compression stockings
7. The *first* priority of interprofessional care of a patient with a suspected acute aortic dissection is to
   a. reduce anxiety.
   b. monitor for chest pain.
   c. control blood pressure.
   d. increase myocardial contractility.
8. The patient at *highest* risk for venous thromboembolism (VTE) is
   a. a 62-year-old man with spider veins who is having arthroscopic knee surgery.
   b. a 32-year-old woman who smokes, takes oral contraceptives, and is planning a trip to Europe.
   c. a 26-year-old woman who is 3 days postpartum and received maintenance IV fluids for 12 hours during her labor.
   d. an active 72-year-old man at home recovering from transurethral resection of the prostate for benign prostatic hyperplasia.
9. Which are clinical findings in a person with an acute lower extremity VTE *(select all that apply)*?
   a. Pallor and coolness of foot and calf
   b. Mild to moderate calf pain and tenderness
   c. Grossly diminished or absent pedal pulses
   d. Unilateral edema and induration of the thigh
   e. Palpable cord along a superficial varicose vein
10. The recommended treatment for an initial VTE in an otherwise healthy person with no significant co-morbidities would include
   a. IV argatroban (Acova) as an inpatient.
   b. IV unfractionated heparin as an inpatient.
   c. subcutaneous unfractionated heparin as an outpatient.
   d. subcutaneous low-molecular-weight heparin as an outpatient.
11. A *key* aspect of teaching for the patient on anticoagulant therapy includes which instructions?
   a. Monitor for and report any signs of bleeding.
   b. Do not take acetaminophen (Tylenol) for a headache.
   c. Decrease your dietary intake of foods containing vitamin K.
   d. Arrange to have blood drawn twice a week to check drug effects.
12. In planning care and patient teaching for the patient with venous leg ulcers, the nurse recognizes that the *most* important intervention in healing and control of this condition is
   a. discussing activity guidelines.
   b. using moist environment dressings.
   c. taking horse chestnut seed extract daily.
   d. applying graduated compression stockings.

1. c, 2. c, 3. c, 4. b, c, d, 5. b, 6. c, 7. c, 8. b, 9. b, d, 10. d, 11. a, 12. d

For rationales to these answers and even more NCLEX review questions, visit *http://evolve.elsevier.com/Lewis/medsurg.*

## EVOLVE WEBSITE

http://evolve.elsevier.com/Lewis/medsurg

**Review Questions (Online Only)**
**Key Points**
**Answer Keys for Questions**
- Rationales for Bridge to NCLEX Examination Questions
- Answer Guidelines for Case Study on p. 828
- Answer Guidelines for Managing Care of Multiple Patients Case Study (Section 7) on p. 831

**Student Case Studies**
- Patient With Abdominal Aortic Aneurysm
- Patient With Chronic Peripheral Artery Disease

**Nursing Care Plans**
- eNursing Care Plan 37-1: Patient With Peripheral Artery Disease of the Lower Extremities
- eNursing Care Plan 37-2: Patient After Surgical Repair of the Aorta

**Conceptual Care Map Creator**
**Audio Glossary**
**Content Updates**

## REFERENCES


*1. Creager MA, Belkin B, Bluth EI, et al: 2012 ACCF/AHA/ACR/SCAI/SIR/STS/SVM/SVN/SVS key data elements and definitions for peripheral atherosclerotic vascular disease: a report of the American College of Cardiology Foundation/American Heart Association Task Force on Clinical Data Standards, *Circulation* 125:395, 2012. (Classic)
2. Eraso LH, Fukaya E, Mohler ER, et al: Peripheral arterial disease, prevalence, and cumulative risk factor profile analysis, *Eur Prevent Cardiol* 21:704, 2014.
3. Mozaffarian D, Benjamin EJ, Go AS, et al: Heart disease and stroke statistics—2015 update: a report from the American Heart Association, *Circulation* 131:29, 2015.
4. Rein P, Saely CH, Silbernagel G, et al: Systemic inflammation is higher in peripheral artery disease than in stable coronary artery disease, *Atherosclerosis* 239:299, 2015.
5. Schorr EN, Peden-McAlpine C, Treat-Jacobson D, et al: Characterization of the peripheral artery disease symptom experience, *Geriatric Nurs* 36(4):293, 2015.
*6. Anderson JL, Halperin JL, Albert NM, et al: Management of patients with peripheral artery disease (compilation of 2005 and 2011 ACCF/AHA guideline recommendations): a report of the American College of Cardiology Foundation/American Heart Association Task Force on Practice Guidelines, *J Am Coll Cardiol* 61:1555, 2013.
*7. American Diabetes Association: Standards of medical care in diabetes, *Diabetes Care* 38(Suppl):S1, 2015.
*8. Lauret GJ, Fakhry F, Fokkenrood HJP, et al: Modes of exercise training for intermittent claudication, *Cochrane Database Syst Rev* (7):CD009638, 2014.
*9. Jensen MD, Ryan DH, Apovian CM, et al: 2013 AHA/ACC/TOS guideline for the management of overweight and obesity in adults: a report of the American College of Cardiology/American Heart Association Task Force on Practice Guidelines and The Obesity Society, *J Am Coll Cardiol* 1:2985, 2014.
10. Nosova EV, Conte MS, Grenon SM: Advancing beyond the "heart-healthy diet" for peripheral artery disease, *J Vasc Surg* 61:265, 2015.
11. Kirk J, Dunker KS: Dietary counseling: the ingredient for successfully addressing the use of herbal supplements and probiotics in chronic kidney disease, *Adv Chronic Kidney Dis* 21:377, 2014.
*12. Rollins KE, Jackson D, Coughlin PA: Meta-analysis of contemporary short- and long-term mortality rates in patients diagnosed with critical limb ischaemia, *Br J Surg* 100:1002, 2013.

*13. Chowdhury MM, McLain AD, Twine CP: Angioplasty versus bare metal stenting for superficial femoral artery lesions, *Cochrane Database Syst Rev* (6):CD006767, 2014.
*14. Dake MD, Ansel GM, Jaff MR, et al: Sustained safety and effectiveness of paclitaxel-eluting stents for femoropopliteal lesions: 2-year follow-up from the Zilver PTX randomized and single-arm clinical studies, *J Am Coll Cardiol* 61:2417, 2013.
*15. Ambler GK, Radwan R, Hayes PD, et al: Atherectomy for peripheral arterial disease, *Cochrane Database Syst Rev* (3):CD006680, 2014.
*16. McCaslin JE, Andras A, Stansby G: Cryoplasty for peripheral arterial disease, *Cochrane Database Syst Rev* (8):CD005507, 2013.
17. Lo RC, Bensley RP, Dahlberg SE, et al: Presentation, treatment, and outcome differences between men and women undergoing revascularization or amputation for lower extremity peripheral arterial disease, *J Vasc Surg* 59:409, 2014.
18. Kalish JA, Farber A, Homa K, et al: Factors associated with surgical site infection after lower extremity bypass in the Society for Vascular Surgery (SVS) Vascular Quality Initiative (VQI), *J Vasc Surg* 60:1248, 2014.
*19. Alonso-Coello P, Bellmunt S, McGorrian C, et al: Antithrombotic therapy in peripheral artery disease: antithrombotic therapy and prevention of thrombosis, ed 9: American College of Chest Physicians evidence-based clinical practice guidelines, *Chest* 141:e669S, 2012. (Classic)
20. Byrne R, Taha A, Avgerinos E, et al: Contemporary outcomes of endovascular interventions for acute limb ischemia, *J Vasc Surg* 59:988, 2014.
*21. January C, Wann L, Alpert J, et al: 2014 AHA/ACC/HRS guideline for the management of patients with atrial fibrillation: executive summary, *J Am Coll Cardiol* 64:2246, 2014.
22. Vijayakumar A, Tiwari R, Prabhuswamy VK: Thromboangiitis obliterans (Buerger's disease)—current practices, *Int J Inflam* 2013:156905, 2013.
*23. Nietert PJ, Shaftman SR, Silver RM, et al: Raynaud phenomenon and mortality: 20+ years of follow-up of the Charleston Heart Study cohort, *Clin Epidemiol* 7:161, 2015.
24. Sinnathurai P, Schrieber L: Treatment of Raynaud phenomenon in systemic sclerosis, *Intern Med J* 43:476, 2013.
*25. Jahangir E, Lipworth L, Edwards TL, et al: Smoking, sex, risk factors and abdominal aortic aneurysms: a prospective study of 18782 persons aged above 65 years in the Southern Community Cohort Study, *J Epidemiol Community Health* 69:481, 2015.
*26. Erbel R, Aboyans V, Boileau C, et al: 2014 ESC guidelines on the diagnosis and treatment of aortic diseases, *Euro Heart J* 35:2873, 2014.
*27. Abraha I, Romagnoli C, Montedori A, et al: Thoracic stent graft versus surgery for thoracic aneurysm, *Cochrane Database Syst Rev* (9): CD006796, 2013.
28. Gloviczki P, Huang Y, Oderich GS, et al: Clinical presentation, comorbidities, and age, but not female gender predict survival after endovascular repair of abdominal aortic aneurysm, *J Vasc Surg* 61:853, 2015.
29. Rubenstein C, Bietz G, Davenport D, et al: Abdominal compartment syndrome associated with endovascular and open repair of ruptured abdominal aortic aneurysms, *J Vasc Surg* 61:648, 2015.
30. Conrad MF, Cambria RP: Aortic dissection. In Cronenwett JL, Johnston KW, editors: *Rutherford's vascular surgery*, ed 8, Philadelphia, 2014, Saunders.
31. Chen T, Crozier JA: Endovascular repair of thoracic aortic pathologies: postoperative nursing implications, *J Vasc Nurs* 32:63, 2014.
*32. Dunda SE, Demir E, Muffel OJ, et al: Management, clinical outcomes, and complications of acute cannula-related peripheral vein phlebitis of the upper extremity: a retrospective study, *Phlebology* 30:381, 2015.
*33. Cannegieter SC, Horváth-Puhó E, Schmidt M, et al: Risk of venous and arterial thrombotic events in patients diagnosed with superficial vein thrombosis: a nationwide cohort study, *Blood* 125:229, 2015.
34. Ver Hage A: Acute venous thromboembolism in critically ill patients, *Nursing Crit Care* 10:22, 2015.
*35. Di Nisio M, Wichers IM, Middledorp S: Treatment for superficial thrombophlebitis of the leg, *Cochrane Database Syst Rev* (4):CD004982, 2013.
*36. Kahn SR, Comerota AJ, Cushman M, et al: The postthrombotic syndrome: evidence-based prevention, diagnosis, and treatment strategies: a scientific statement from the American Heart Association, *Circulation* 130:1636, 2014.
37. Pendergraft T, Liu X, Edelsberg J, et al: Prophylaxis against venous thromboembolism in hospitalized medically ill patients, *Circ Cardiovasc Qual Outcomes* 6:75, 2013.
*38. Gould MK, Garcia DA, Wren SM, et al: Prevention of VTE in nonorthopedic surgical patients: antithrombotic therapy and prevention of thrombosis, ed 9: American College of Chest Physicians evidence-based clinical practice guidelines, *Chest* 141:e227S, 2012. (Classic)
*39. Sachdeva A, Dalton M, Amaragiri SV, et al: Graduated compression stockings for prevention of deep vein thrombosis, *Cochrane Database Syst Rev* (12):CD001484, 2014.
*40. Sajid MS, Desai M, Morris RW, et al: Knee length versus thigh length graduated compression stockings for prevention of deep vein thrombosis in postoperative surgical patients, *Cochrane Database Syst Rev* (5):CD007162, 2012. (Classic)
*41. Zhao JM, He ML, Xiao ZM, et al: Different types of intermittent pneumatic compression devices for preventing venous thromboembolism in patients after total hip replacement, *Cochrane Database Syst Rev* (12):CD009543, 2014.
*42. Garcia DA, Baglin TP, Weitz JI, et al: Parenteral anticoagulants: antithrombotic therapy and prevention of thrombosis, ed 9: American College of Chest Physicians evidence-based clinical practice guidelines, *Chest* 141:e24S, 2012. (Classic)
*43. Ageno W, Gallus AS, Wittkowsky A, et al: Oral anticoagulant therapy: antithrombotic therapy and prevention of thrombosis, ed 9: American College of Chest Physicians evidence-based clinical practice guidelines, *Chest* 141:e44S, 2012. (Classic)
*44. Guyatt GH, Akl EA, Crowther M, et al: Executive summary: antithrombotic therapy and prevention of thrombosis, ed 9: American College of Chest Physicians evidence-based clinical practice guidelines, *Chest* 141:7S, 2012. (Classic)
*45. Linkins LA, Dans AL, Moores LK, et al: Treatment and prevention of heparin-induced thrombocytopenia: antithrombotic therapy and prevention of thrombosis, ed 9: American College of Chest Physicians evidence-based clinical practice guidelines, *Chest* 141:e495S, 2012. (Classic)
46. Kearon C, Aki E: Duration of anticoagulation therapy for deep vein thrombosis and pulmonary embolism, *Blood* 123:1794, 2014.
47. Jenkins JS, Michael P: Deep venous thrombosis: an interventionalist's approach, *Ochsner J* 14:633, 2014.
48. Rich K: Iliofemoral deep vein thrombosis: percutaneous endovascular treatment options, *J Vasc Nurs* 23:47, 2015.
*49. Holbrook A, Schulman S, Witt DM, et al: Evidence-based management of anticoagulant therapy: antithrombotic therapy and prevention of thrombosis, ed 9: American College of Chest Physicians evidence-based clinical practice guidelines, *Chest* 141:e152S, 2012. (Classic)
50. Shoeb M, Fang M: Assessing bleeding risk in patients taking anticoagulants, *J Thromb Thrombolysis* 35:312, 2013.
51. Raffetto JD, Eberhardt RT: Chronic venous disorders. In Cronenwett JL, Johnston KW, editors: *Rutherford's vascular surgery*, ed 8, Philadelphia, 2014, Saunders.
*52. Wittens C, Davies AH, Baekgaard R, et al: Management of chronic venous disease: clinical practice guidelines of the European Society for Vascular Surgery (ESVS) 2015 European chronic venous disease guidelines, *Eur J Vasc Endovasc Surg* 49:678, 2015.
*53. Rabe E, Breu FX, Cavezzi A, et al: European guidelines for sclerotherapy in chronic venous disorders, *Phlebology* 29:338, 2014.
54. Vasudevan B: Venous leg ulcers: pathophysiology and classification, *Indian Dermatol Online J* 5:366, 2014.
*55. O'Donnell TF, Passman TA, Marston WA, et al: Management of venous leg ulcers: clinical practice guidelines of the Society for Vascular Surgery and the American Venous Forum, *J Vasc Surg* 60:3S, 2014.

*Evidence-based information for clinical practice.

## CASE STUDY

### *Managing Care of Multiple Patients*

You are working on the cardiovascular stepdown unit and have been assigned to care for the following six patients. You have one LPN and a UAP assigned to help you.

#### Patients

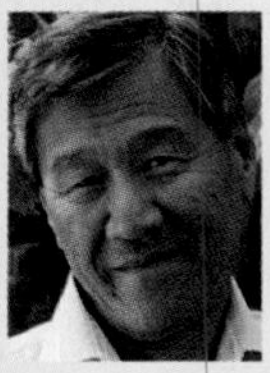

(©Jupiterimages/Banana-Stock/Thinkstock)

L.P. is a 63-yr-old man who was brought to the ED with complaints of chest pain, shortness of breath, palpitations, and dizziness. L.P.'s CK-MB and troponin levels are within normal limits. His ECG showed atrial fibrillation with a rapid ventricular response. He has been on IV diltiazem and IV heparin for 24 hr. Although his heart rate has decreased to 102 bpm, the atrial fibrillation persists.

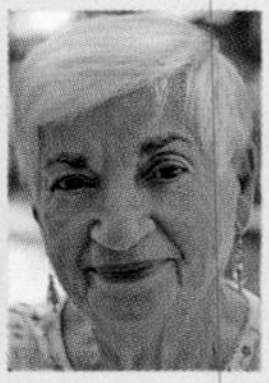

(©iStockphoto/Thinkstock)

J.E. is a 70-yr-old woman admitted with complaints of increasing shortness of breath, fatigue, and weight gain. She has a systolic murmur and bilateral crackles. Her ejection fraction is 20%. She is currently receiving IV furosemide, oral potassium and enalapril (Vasotec), and a continuous infusion of nesiritide (Natrecor). She is receiving $O_2$ at 6 L via nasal cannula to keep her $O_2$ saturation >93%. Normal initial set of cardiac enzymes.

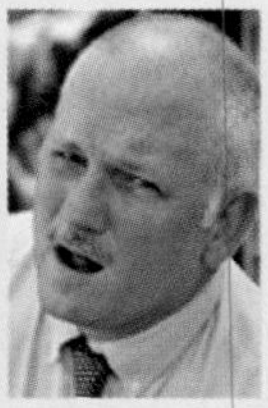

(©iStockphoto/Thinkstock)

D.M. is a 51-yr-old man who was rushed to the hospital by ambulance after experiencing crushing substernal chest pain that radiated down his left arm. His ECG demonstrated marked ST segment elevation in the inferior leads. Cardiac catheterization showed a 90% blockage of his left anterior descending (LAD) artery. Coronary angioplasty was performed and a stent inserted. He is now 2 days post-PTCA, has had no recurrence of his chest pain, and is to be discharged today.

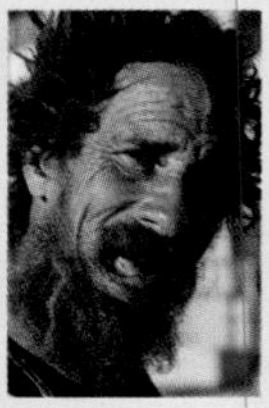

(©JennaDub/iStock/Thinkstock)

R.B. is a 50-yr-old man admitted for heart failure due to valvular heart disease. He has a history of IV drug and alcohol abuse. He complains of chest pain with minimal exertion. He has atrial fibrillation with a rapid ventricular response. His rhythm converted to normal sinus rhythm after receiving IV amiodarone. Transesophageal echocardiography shows left atrial and ventricular hypertrophy and mitral and aortic regurgitation.

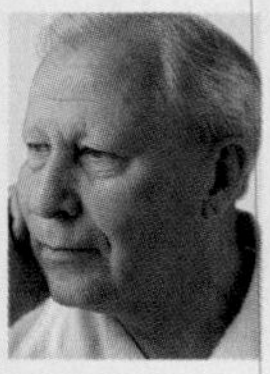

(©iStockphoto/Thinkstock)

J.M. is a 68-yr-old man admitted 3 days ago with a diagnosis of acute decompensated HF. He had a cardiac arrest (pulseless VT) and was successfully defibrillated after one shock. He underwent electrophysiology studies and implantation of an implantable cardiodefibrillator (ICD). He now is being treated for his heart failure.

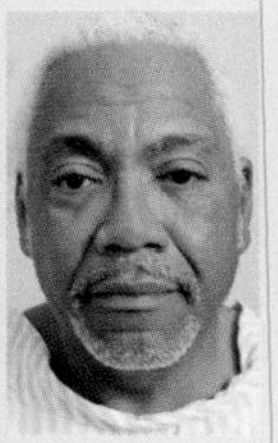

(©IPGGutenberg-UKLtd/iStock/Thinkstock)

S.J. is a 73-yr-old man admitted with rest pain in both legs and a nonhealing ulcer of the big toe on the right foot. He has history of an MI, stroke, hypertension, heart failure, and type 1 diabetes mellitus. He underwent a left femoral-popliteal bypass 5 years ago. His right foot is cool, pale, and mottled in color with decreased sensation. He has a diminished right femoral pulse, right popliteal and posterior tibial pulses only obtained by Doppler, and his right dorsalis pedis pulse is absent (not palpable or present by Doppler). His left leg pulses are weak but palpable. His right leg ABI: 0.20; left leg ABI: 0.68.

#### Discussion Questions

1. ***Priority Decision:*** After receiving report, which patient should you see first? Second? Provide a rationale for your decision.
2. ***Teamwork and Collaboration:*** Which tasks could you delegate to the LPN *(select all that apply)*?
   a. Monitor L.P.'s heparin infusion.
   b. Report changes in pain or sensation of S.J.'s legs.
   c. Teach D.M. about activity restriction post-PTCA.
   d. Administer prescribed medications to R.B. and J.M.
   e. Hook up J.M. to 12-lead ECG and monitor for any dysrhythmias.
3. ***Priority Decision and Teamwork and Collaboration:*** As you are assessing L.P., the LPN informs you that S.J. is diaphoretic and complaining of chest pain. Which initial action would be *most* appropriate?
   a. Ask the LPN to notify S.J.'s HCP.
   b. Have the LPN administer prescribed nitroglycerin to S.J.
   c. Leave L.P.'s room to perform a focused assessment on S.J.
   d. Finish assessing L.P. while the UAP obtains a 12-lead ECG on S.J.

#### Case Study Progression

S.J. rates his chest pain as a 9/10. His blood pressure is 110/70, heart rate 110, respiratory rate 26, and $O_2$ saturation 93% on room air. You obtain a 12-lead ECG and administer 0.4 mg SL nitroglycerin with minimal pain relief after 5 minutes. The 12-lead ECG demonstrates new ST elevation in leads II, III, and aVF.

4. Which interventions would you expect the HCP to order for S.J. *(select all that apply)*?
   a. IV nitroglycerin
   b. IV morphine sulfate
   c. Emergent cardiac catheterization
   d. Furosemide 40 mg IV push stat
   e. Increase $O_2$ flow rate to 12 L/minute
5. Which statement would you include in patient teaching regarding ICDs with J.M. and his family?
   a. Avoid air travel.
   b. Avoid driving for 6 weeks.
   c. Avoid any sexual activity in case the ICD discharges.
   d. Avoid standing near antitheft devices in doorways of stores and public buildings.
6. Knowing the mechanism of action for nesiritide, you prioritize monitoring of J.E.'s
   a. blood pressure.
   b. respiratory rate.
   c. b-natriuretic peptide (BNP) level.
   d. troponin and CK-MB laboratory values.
7. ***Management Decision:*** You ask the UAP to take D.M.'s vital signs before and after having him walk 300 feet. When reviewing the patient's chart, you note documentation of the patient's walk but not his vital signs. What is your *best* initial action?
   a. Report the incident to the charge nurse for follow-up.
   b. Talk to the UAP to discuss why the vital signs were not documented.
   c. Walk D.M. yourself again and take his vital signs pre- and post-activity.
   d. Ask the LPN to ambulate D.M. and obtain his vital signs before and after.

Answers and rationales available at *http://evolve.elsevier.com/Lewis/medsurg*.

# SECTION 8

# Problems of Ingestion, Digestion, Absorption, and Elimination

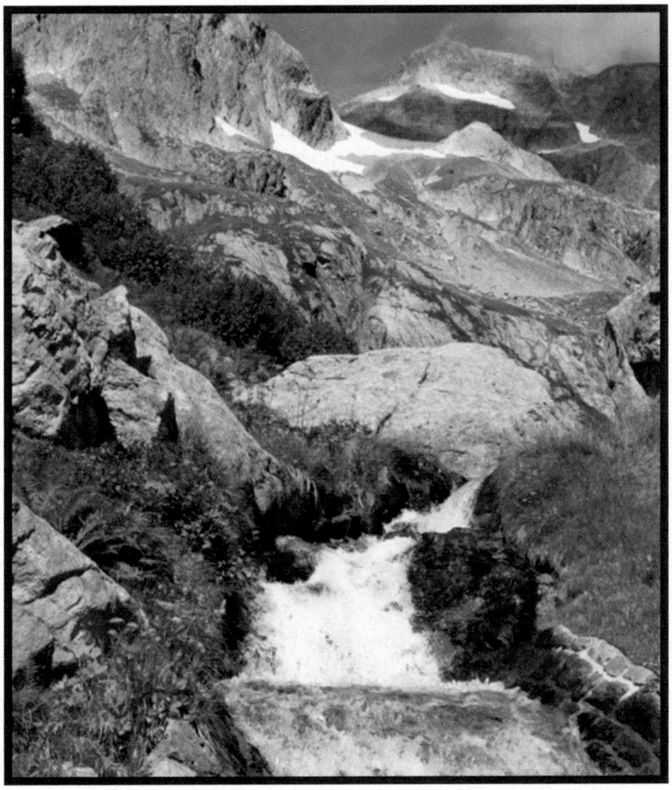

Peter Bonner

*Let the mountains talk, let the river run. Once more, and forever.*

***David Brower***

38

# Assessment of Gastrointestinal System

*Paula Cox-North*

*Nothing compares to the stomach ache you get from laughing with your best friends.*

***Unknown author***

http://evolve.elsevier.com/Lewis/medsurg/

## LEARNING OUTCOMES

1. Describe the structures and functions of the organs of the gastrointestinal tract.
2. Describe the structures and functions of the liver, gallbladder, biliary tract, and pancreas.
3. Differentiate the processes of ingestion, digestion, absorption, and elimination.
4. Explain the processes of biliary metabolism, bile production, and bile excretion.
5. Link the age-related changes of the gastrointestinal system to the differences in assessment findings.
6. Obtain significant subjective and objective assessment data related to the gastrointestinal system from a patient.
7. Perform a physical assessment of the gastrointestinal system using appropriate techniques.
8. Differentiate normal from abnormal findings of a physical assessment of the gastrointestinal system.
9. Describe the purpose, significance of results, and nursing responsibilities related to diagnostic studies of the gastrointestinal system.

## KEY TERMS

**absorption, p. 835**
**bilirubin, p. 837**
**borborygmi, Table 38-10, p. 847**
**cheilosis, Table 38-10, p. 846**
**deglutition, p. 834**
**digestion, p. 835**
**endoscopy, p. 851**
**hematemesis, Table 38-10, p. 846**
**Kupffer cells, p. 837**
**melena, Table 38-10, p. 847**
**pyorrhea, Table 38-10, p. 846**
**pyrosis, Table 38-10, p. 846**
**steatorrhea, Table 38-10, p. 847**
**tenesmus, Table 38-10, p. 847**
**Valsalva maneuver, p. 836**

The gastrointestinal (GI) system, also called the *digestive system,* consists of the GI tract and its associated organs and glands. Included in the GI tract are the mouth, esophagus, stomach, small intestine, large intestine, rectum, and anus. The associated organs are the liver, pancreas, and gallbladder (Fig. 38-1).

## STRUCTURES AND FUNCTIONS OF GASTROINTESTINAL SYSTEM

The GI tract extends approximately 30 ft (9 m) from the mouth to the anus. The GI tract is essentially a tube composed of four layers. From the inside to the outside, these layers are (1) mucosa lining; (2) submucosa connective tissue, which contains glands, blood vessels, and lymph nodes; (3) muscle; and (4) serosa (Fig. 38-1). The muscular coat has two layers: circular (inner) layer and longitudinal (outer) layer.

Parasympathetic and sympathetic branches of the autonomic nervous system (ANS) innervate the GI tract. The parasympathetic (cholinergic) system is mainly excitatory. The sympathetic (adrenergic) system is mainly inhibitory. For example, parasympathetic stimulation increases peristalsis and sympathetic stimulation decreases it. Both sympathetic and parasympathetic afferent fibers relay sensory information.

The GI tract has its own nervous system: the enteric nervous system (ENS) or intrinsic nervous system. The ENS system regulates motility and secretion along the entire GI tract. The ENS is composed of two networks: (1) Meissner plexus in the submucosa and (2) Auerbach (myenteric) plexus between the muscle layers. The submucosal plexus controls secretion and is involved in many sensory functions. The myenteric plexus is the major nerve supply to the GI tract and controls GI movements. Although the ENS receives innervation from the ANS, it operates independently of the brain and spinal cord.

Circulation in the GI system is unique in that venous blood draining the GI tract organs empties into the portal vein, which then perfuses the liver. This allows the liver to clean the blood of bacteria and toxins from the GI tract. The celiac artery, superior mesenteric artery (SMA), and the inferior mesenteric artery (IMA) supply arterial blood to the GI tract. The stomach and duodenum receive their blood supply from the celiac axis. The distal small intestine to mid large intestine receives its blood supply from branches of the hepatic and SMA. The distal large

Reviewed by Barbara Brunow, RN, MSN, MEd, CNS, CNE, Assistant Director, Firelands Regional Medical Center, School of Nursing, Sandusky, Ohio; and Christina D. Keller, RN, MSN-Ed, Instructor, Radford University, Radford, Virginia.

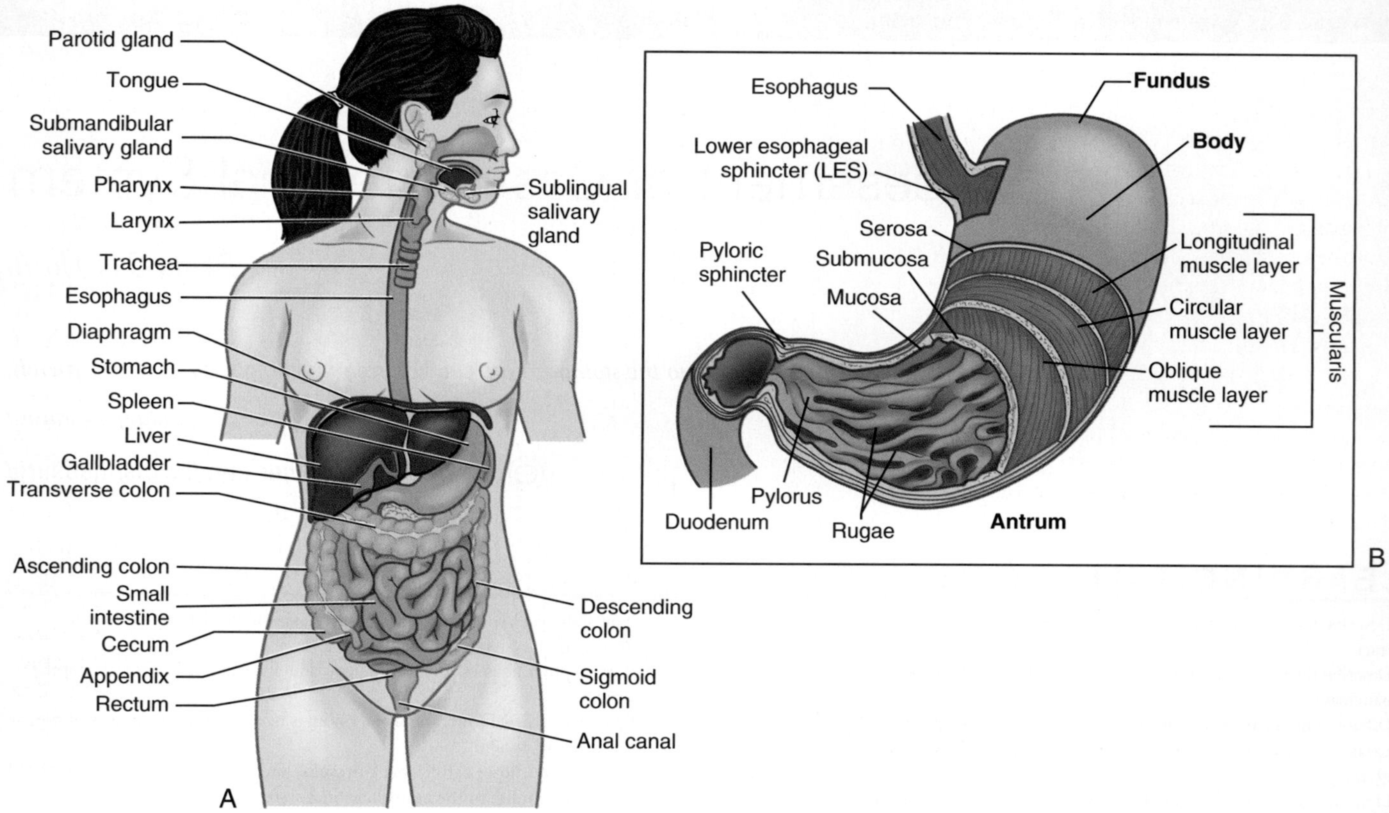


**FIG. 38-1** **A,** Location of organs of the gastrointestinal system. **B,** Parts of the stomach.

intestine through the anus receives its blood supply from the IMA. The GI tract and accessory organs receive approximately 25% to 30% of the cardiac output at rest and 35% or more after eating. Because such a large percentage of the cardiac output perfuses these organs, the GI tract is a major source from which to divert blood flow during exercise, stress, or injury.

The peritoneum almost completely covers the abdominal organs. The two layers of the peritoneum are the *parietal layer,* which lines the abdominal cavity wall, and the *visceral layer,* which covers the abdominal organs. The peritoneal cavity is the potential space between the parietal and visceral layers. The two folds of the peritoneum are the mesentery and omentum. The mesentery attaches the small intestine and part of the large intestine to the posterior abdominal wall and contains blood and lymph vessels. The omentum hangs like an apron from the stomach to the intestines and contains fat and lymph nodes.

The main function of the GI system is to supply nutrients to body cells. This is accomplished through the processes of (1) *ingestion* (taking in food), (2) *digestion* (breaking down food), and (3) *absorption* (transferring food products into circulation). *Elimination* is the process of excreting the waste products of digestion.

## Ingestion

*Ingestion* is the intake of food. *Appetite,* the desire to ingest food, influences how much food a person eats. An appetite center is located in the hypothalamus. A number of factors, including hypoglycemia, an empty stomach, and a decrease in body temperature, stimulate appetite. The hormone *ghrelin* released from the stomach mucosa plays a role in appetite stimulation. Another hormone, *leptin,* is involved in appetite suppression. (See Chapter 40 for a discussion of ghrelin and leptin.) The sight, smell, and taste of food frequently stimulate appetite. Stomach distention, illness (especially accompanied by fever), hyperglycemia, nausea and vomiting, and certain drugs (e.g., amphetamines) inhibit appetite.

**Deglutition**, or swallowing, is the mechanical component of ingestion. The organs involved in the deglutition of food are the mouth, pharynx, and esophagus.

**Mouth.** The mouth consists of the lips and oral (buccal) cavity. The lips surround the opening of the mouth and function in speech. The hard and soft palates form the roof of the oral cavity. The oral cavity contains the teeth, used in *mastication* (chewing), and the tongue. The tongue is a solid muscle mass and assists in chewing and moving food to the back of the throat for swallowing. The taste receptors (taste buds) are on the sides and tip of the tongue. The tongue is also important in speech.

Within the oral cavity are three pairs of salivary glands: parotid, submaxillary, and sublingual glands. These glands produce saliva, which consists of water, protein, mucin, inorganic salts, and salivary amylase.

**Pharynx.** The pharynx is a muscular tube lined with mucous membrane. It has three divisions: nasopharynx, oropharynx, and laryngeal pharynx. The mucous membrane is continuous with the nasal cavity, mouth, auditory tubes, and larynx. During ingestion, the oropharynx provides a route for food from the mouth to the esophagus. Food or liquid stimulates receptors in the oropharynx, initiating the swallowing reflex. During swallowing, the epiglottis closes over the opening to the larynx and prevents food from entering the respiratory tract. The tonsils and adenoids, composed of lymphoid tissue, assist the body in preventing infection.

**Esophagus.** The esophagus is a hollow, muscular tube that receives food from the pharynx and moves it to the stomach. It is 7 to 10 in (18 to 25 cm) long and 0.8 in (2 cm) in diameter. The esophagus is located in the thoracic cavity. It is structurally composed of four layers: inner mucosa, submucosa, muscularis propria, and outermost adventitia. The upper third of the esophagus is composed of striated skeletal muscle. The distal two thirds are composed of smooth muscle.

Between swallows, the esophagus remains collapsed and the *upper esophageal sphincter* (UES) closed. With swallowing, the UES relaxes and a peristaltic wave moves the bolus into the esophagus. The muscular layers contract *(peristalsis)* and propel the food to the stomach. The *lower esophageal sphincter* (LES) at the distal end of the esophagus controls the opening of the esophagus into the stomach. It remains contracted except during swallowing, belching, or vomiting. The LES is an important barrier that normally prevents reflux of acidic gastric contents into the esophagus.

## Digestion and Absorption

**Stomach.** The stomach's functions are to store food, mix food with gastric secretions, and empty contents in small boluses into the small intestine. The stomach absorbs only small amounts of water, alcohol, electrolytes, and certain drugs.

The stomach is usually J shaped and lies obliquely in the epigastric, umbilical, and left hypochondriac regions of the abdomen (Fig. 38-5 later in the chapter). It always contains gastric fluid and mucus. The three main parts of the stomach are the fundus (cardia), body, and antrum (Fig. 38-1). The pylorus is a small portion of the antrum proximal to the pyloric sphincter. The LES and pyloric sphincter guard the entrance to and exit from the stomach.

The stomach wall has four layers. The serous (outer) layer of the stomach is continuous with the peritoneum. The muscular layer consists of the longitudinal (outer) layer, circular (middle) layer, and oblique (inner) layer. The mucosal layer forms folds called *rugae* that contain many small glands. In the fundus the glands contain (1) chief cells, which secrete pepsinogen and (2) parietal cells, which secrete hydrochloric (HCl) acid, water, and intrinsic factor. The secretion of HCl acid makes gastric juice acidic. This acidic pH aids in the protection against ingested organisms. Intrinsic factor promotes cobalamin (vitamin $B_{12}$) absorption in the small intestine.

**Small Intestine.** The two primary functions of the small intestine are digestion and **absorption**, the uptake of nutrients from the gut lumen to the bloodstream. The small intestine is a coiled tube approximately 23 ft (7 m) in length and 1 to 1.1 in (2.5 to 2.8 cm) in diameter. It extends from the pylorus to the ileocecal valve. The small intestine is composed of the duodenum, jejunum, and ileum. The ileocecal valve prevents reflux of large intestine contents into the small intestine.

The mucosa of the small intestine is thick, vascular, and glandular. The functional units of the small intestine are *villi,* which are minute, fingerlike projections in the mucous membrane. Villi contain epithelial cells that produce the intestinal digestive enzymes. The epithelial cells on the villi also have *microvilli.* The circular folds in the mucous and submucous layers, along with the villi and microvilli, increase the surface area for digestion and absorption.

The digestive enzymes on the brush border of the microvilli chemically break down nutrients for absorption. Between the bases of the villi lie the crypts of Lieberkühn, which contain the multipotent stem cells that are the precursors for the other epithelial cell types. Brunner's glands in the submucosa of the duodenum secrete an alkaline fluid containing bicarbonate that neutralizes acidic fluids and protects the mucosa. Intestinal goblet cells secrete mucus that also protects the mucosa.

**Physiology of Digestion.** **Digestion** is the physical and chemical breakdown of food into absorbable substances. The timely movement of food through the GI tract and the secretion of specific enzymes facilitate digestion. These enzymes break down foodstuffs to particles of appropriate size for absorption (Table 38-1).

The process of digestion begins in the mouth, where food is chewed, mechanically broken down, and mixed with saliva. Saliva facilitates swallowing by lubricating food. Saliva contains amylase, which breaks down starches to maltose. Chewing and the sight, smell, thought, and taste of food stimulate the release of saliva. A person produces about 1 L of saliva each day. After swallowing, food moves through the esophagus to the stomach. No digestion or absorption occurs in the esophagus.

Both GI secretion and motility are under neural and hormonal control. Food entering the stomach and small intestine triggers the release of hormones into the bloodstream (Tables 38-2 and 38-3). These hormones play important roles in the control of HCl acid secretion, production and release of digestive enzymes, and motility.

**TABLE 38-1 Gastrointestinal Secretions**

| Daily Amount (mL) | Secretions, Enzymes | Action |
|---|---|---|
| **Salivary Glands** | | |
| 1000-1500 | Salivary amylase | Initiation of starch digestion |
| **Stomach** | | |
| 2500 | Pepsinogen | Protein digestion |
| | HCl acid | Activation of pepsinogen to pepsin |
| | Lipase | Fat digestion |
| | Intrinsic factor | Essential for cobalamin absorption in ileum |
| **Small Intestine** | | |
| 3000 | Enterokinase | Activation of trypsinogen to trypsin |
| | Amylase | Carbohydrate digestion |
| | Peptidases | Protein digestion |
| | Aminopeptidases | Protein digestion |
| | Maltase | Maltose to two glucose molecules |
| | Sucrase | Sucrose to glucose and fructose |
| | Lactase | Lactose to glucose and galactose |
| | Lipase | Fat digestion |
| **Pancreas** | | |
| 700 | Trypsinogen | Protein digestion |
| | Chymotrypsin | Protein digestion |
| | Amylase | Starch to disaccharides |
| | Lipase | Fat digestion |
| **Liver and Gallbladder** | | |
| 1000 | Bile | Emulsification of fats and aid in absorption of fatty acids and fat-soluble vitamins (A, D, E, K) |

In the stomach, muscle action mixes the food with gastric secretions to form *chyme*, which is now ready for absorption. Protein digestion begins with the release of pepsinogen from chief cells. The stomach's acidic environment results in the conversion of pepsinogen to its active form, pepsin. Pepsin begins the breakdown of proteins. There is minimal digestion of starches and fats. The stomach also serves as a reservoir for food, releasing it slowly into the small intestine. The length of time that food remains in the stomach depends on the composition of the food. The average meal remains in the stomach for 3 to 4 hours.

In the small intestine, the physical presence and chemical nature of chyme stimulates motility and secretion. Secretions involved in digestion include enzymes from the pancreas, bile from the liver, and enzymes from the small intestine (Table 38-1). Carbohydrates are broken down to monosaccharides, fats to glycerol and fatty acids, and proteins to amino acids. Enzymes on the brush border of the microvilli complete the digestion process. These enzymes break down disaccharides to monosaccharides and peptides to amino acids for absorption.

The absorption of most of the end products of digestion occurs in the small intestine. The movement of the villi enables these end products to come in contact with the absorbing membrane. Monosaccharides, fatty acids, amino acids, water, electrolytes, vitamins, and minerals are absorbed.

## Elimination

**Large Intestine.** The large intestine is a hollow, muscular tube approximately 5 to 6 ft (1.5 to 1.8 m) long and 2 in (5 cm) in diameter. The four parts of the large intestine are shown in Fig. 38-2.

The most important function of the large intestine is the absorption of water and electrolytes. The large intestine also forms feces and serves as a reservoir for the fecal mass until defecation occurs. Feces are composed of water (75%), bacteria, unabsorbed minerals, undigested foodstuffs, bile pigments, and desquamated (shed) epithelial cells. The large intestine secretes mucus, which acts as a lubricant and protects the mucosa.

Microorganisms in the colon contribute to digestion by (1) producing vitamin K and some B vitamins and (2) breaking down proteins that are not digested or absorbed in the small intestine into amino acids. Bacteria deaminate the amino acids, resulting in ammonia. Ammonia is carried to the liver, where it is converted to urea, which is excreted by the kidneys. Bacteria produce gas that escapes the colon through the anus, a phenomenon called *flatulence* or *flatus*. If an infection or antibiotics alter the normal microbiome, an overgrowth of pathogenic bacteria can occur and cause disease.

The movements of the large intestine are usually slow. However, propulsive (mass movements) peristalsis also occurs. Food entering the stomach and duodenum triggers gastrocolic and duodenocolic reflexes, resulting in peristalsis in the colon. These reflexes are more active after the first daily meal and frequently result in bowel evacuation.

*Defecation* is a reflex action involving voluntary and involuntary control. Feces in the rectum stimulate sensory nerve endings that produce the desire to defecate. The reflex center for defecation is in the parasympathetic nerve fibers in the sacral portion of the spinal cord. These fibers produce contraction of the rectum and relaxation of the internal anal sphincter. When a person feels the desire to defecate, he or she can voluntarily relax the external anal sphincter. An acceptable environment for defecation is usually necessary, or the urge to defecate will be ignored. If defecation is suppressed over long periods, problems can occur, such as constipation or fecal impaction.

The **Valsalva maneuver**, often referred to as "bearing down," can facilitate defecation. During this maneuver, the person inspires deeply and holds the breath, closing the airway, while contracting abdominal muscles and bearing down. This increases both intraabdominal and intrathoracic pressures and reduces venous return to the heart. The heart rate temporarily decreases along with a decrease in cardiac output. This results in a transient drop in BP. When the patient relaxes, thoracic pressure falls, resulting in a sudden flow of blood into the heart, increased heart rate, and an immediate rise in BP. The Valsalva maneuver may be contraindicated in the patient with a head injury, eye surgery, cardiac problems,

**TABLE 38-2 Phases of Gastric Secretion**

| Stimulus to Secretion | Secretion |
|---|---|
| **Cephalic** (nervous) | |
| Sight, smell, taste of food (before food enters stomach). Initiated in the CNS and mediated by the vagus nerve. | HCl acid, pepsinogen, mucus |
| **Gastric** (hormonal and nervous) | |
| Food in antrum of stomach, vagal stimulation. | Release of gastrin from antrum into circulation to stimulate gastric secretions and motility |
| **Intestinal** (hormonal) | |
| Presence of chyme in small intestine. | Acidic chyme (pH <2): Release of secretin, gastric inhibitory polypeptide, cholecystokinin into circulation to decrease HCl acid secretion<br>Chyme (pH >3): Release of gastrin from duodenum to increase acid secretion |

**TABLE 38-3 Hormones Controlling GI Secretion and Motility**

| Hormone | Source | Activating Stimuli | Function |
|---|---|---|---|
| **Gastrin** | Gastric and duodenal mucosa | Stomach distention, partially digested proteins in pylorus | Stimulates gastric acid secretion and motility. Maintains lower esophageal sphincter tone. |
| **Secretin** | Duodenal mucosa | Acid entering small intestine | Inhibits gastric motility and acid secretion. Stimulates pancreatic bicarbonate secretion. |
| **Cholecystokinin** | Duodenal mucosa | Fatty acids and amino acids in small intestine | Contracts gallbladder and relaxes sphincter of Oddi. Allows increased flow of bile into duodenum. Release of pancreatic digestive enzymes. |
| **Gastric inhibitory peptide** | Duodenal mucosa | Fatty acids and lipids in small intestine | Inhibits gastric acid secretion and motility. |

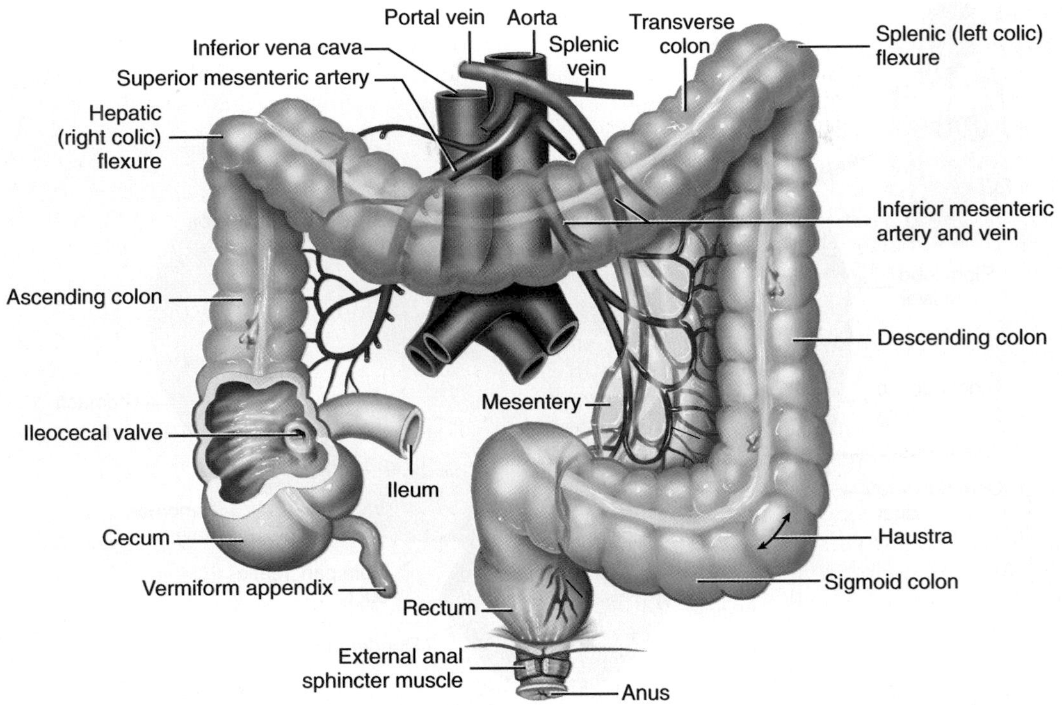


**FIG. 38-2** Anatomic locations of the large intestine. (From Patton KT, Thibodeau GA: *Anatomy and physiology,* ed 8, St Louis, 2013, Mosby.)

hemorrhoids, abdominal surgery, or liver cirrhosis with portal hypertension.

## Liver, Biliary Tract, and Pancreas

**Liver.** The liver is the largest internal organ in the body, weighing approximately 3 lb (1.36 kg). It lies in the right epigastric region (Fig. 38-5 later in the chapter). Most of the liver is enclosed in peritoneum. It has a fibrous capsule that divides it into right and left lobes (Fig. 38-3).

The functional units of the liver are lobules. A lobule consists of rows of hepatic cells *(hepatocytes)* arranged in cords that radiate out from a central vein. Capillaries called *sinusoids* are located between the rows of hepatocytes. Sinusoids are lined with Kupffer cells, which carry out phagocytic activity, removing bacteria and toxins from the blood. The hepatic cells secrete bile into tiny canals called *canaliculi.* These merge with other canals to form larger, interlobular bile ducts, which unite into the two main left and right hepatic ducts.

The liver has a rich blood supply. The portal circulatory system brings blood to the liver from the stomach, intestines, spleen, and pancreas. About one fourth of the blood supply comes from the hepatic artery, a branch of the celiac artery. Three fourths comes from the portal vein. The portal vein carries absorbed products of digestion directly to the liver. Once in the liver, the portal vein branches and comes in contact with each lobule.

The liver performs numerous functions and is essential for life. It has metabolic, secretory, vascular, and storage functions (Table 38-4). The hepatic cells constantly make bile. Bile consists of water, cholesterol, bile salts, electrolytes, fatty acids, and bilirubin. It provides the alkaline medium needed for the action of pancreatic lipase. Bile salts are needed for fat emulsification and digestion.

***Bilirubin Metabolism.*** Bilirubin, a pigment derived from the breakdown of hemoglobin, is constantly produced (Fig. 38-4). When released into the bloodstream, it binds to albumin. This

**TABLE 38-4 Functions of Liver**

| Function | Description |
|---|---|
| **Metabolic Functions** | |
| Carbohydrate metabolism | Performs glycogenesis (conversion of glucose to glycogen), glycogenolysis (process of breaking down glycogen to glucose), gluconeogenesis (formation of glucose from amino acids and fatty acids). |
| Protein metabolism | Synthesis of nonessential amino acids, synthesis of plasma proteins (except gamma globulin), synthesis of clotting factors, urea formation ($NH_4$) from ammonia ($NH_3$). $NH_3$ formed from deamination of amino acids by action of bacteria in colon. |
| Fat metabolism | Synthesis of lipoproteins, breakdown of triglycerides into fatty acids and glycerol, formation of ketone bodies, synthesis of fatty acids from amino acids and glucose, synthesis and breakdown of cholesterol. |
| Detoxification | Inactivation of drugs and harmful substances and excretion of their breakdown products. |
| Blood clotting | Synthesis of prothrombin (factor I), fibrinogen (factor II) and factors V, VII, IX, and X. |
| **Secretory Functions** | |
| Bile production | Formation of bile, containing bile salts, bile pigments (mainly bilirubin), and cholesterol. |
| Bilirubin | Conjugation and secretion of bilirubin. |
| **Vascular Functions** | |
| Blood filtration | Breakdown of old RBCs, WBCs, bacteria, and other particles. Breakdown of hemoglobin from old RBCs to bilirubin and biliverdin. |
| Blood reservoir | Serves as temporary storage for blood within general circulation. |
| **Storage Functions** | |
| Storage | Stores glucose in form of glycogen; vitamins, including fat-soluble (A, D, E, K) and water-soluble ($B_1$, $B_2$, cobalamin, folic acid); fatty acids; minerals (iron, copper); and amino acids in form of albumin and beta-globulins. |

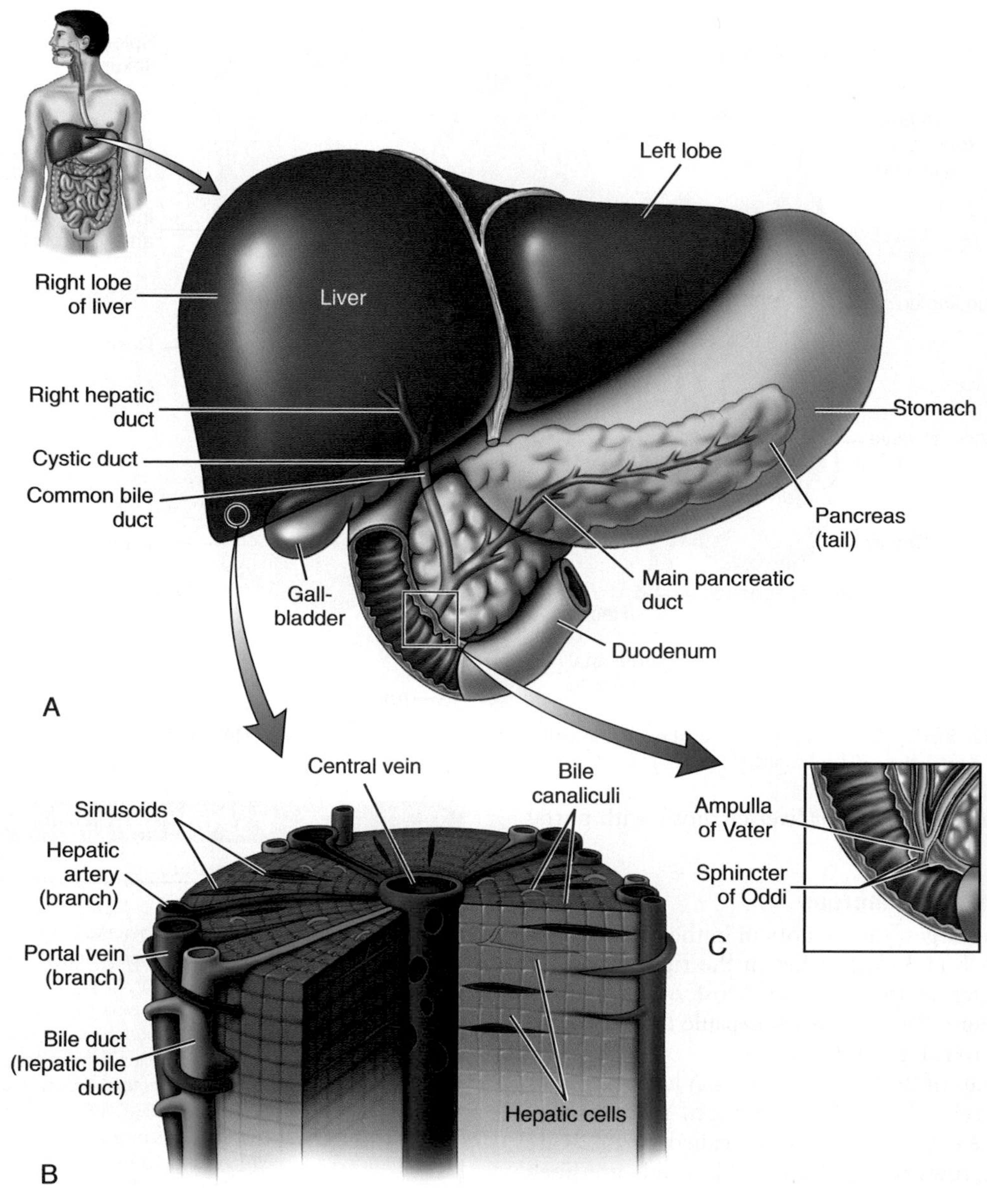


**FIG. 38-3** **A,** Gross structure of the liver, gallbladder, pancreas, and duct system. **B,** Liver lobule. **C,** Entrance of the common bile duct into the duodenum.

form of bilirubin is referred to as *unconjugated.* It is insoluble in water and transported to the liver. In the liver, unconjugated bilirubin is conjugated with glucuronic acid and is excreted in bile into the intestine. *Conjugated* bilirubin is soluble in water. In the intestines, bacterial action reduces bilirubin to stercobilinogen and urobilinogen. Stercobilinogen accounts for the brown color of stool. A small amount of urobilinogen is reabsorbed into the blood, where it is returned to the liver through the portal circulation. There, it is excreted again in the bile or entered into circulation and excreted by the kidneys.

**Biliary Tract.** The biliary tract consists of the gallbladder and ducts that connect the liver, gallbladder, and duodenum. The gallbladder is a pear-shaped sac located below the liver. The gallbladder's function is to concentrate and store bile. It holds approximately 45 mL of bile. The presence of fat in the upper duodenum triggers the release of cholecystokinin, which causes the gallbladder to contract and release bile.

The hepatic ducts receive bile from the canaliculi in the liver lobules. The left and right hepatic ducts merge with the cystic duct from the gallbladder to form the common bile duct. Bile moves down the common bile duct to enter the duodenum at the ampulla of Vater (Fig. 38-3). The pancreatic duct also enters the duodenum at this point.

**Pancreas.** The pancreas is a long, slender gland lying behind the stomach and in front of the first and second lumbar vertebrae. It consists of a head, body, and tail. The peritoneum covers the anterior surface of the pancreas. The pancreas contains lobes and lobules. The pancreatic duct extends along the gland and enters the duodenum through the common bile duct at the ampulla of Vater (Fig. 38-3).

The pancreas has both exocrine and endocrine functions. The exocrine function contributes to digestion through the production and release of enzymes (Table 38-1). The endocrine function occurs in the islets of Langerhans, whose β cells secrete

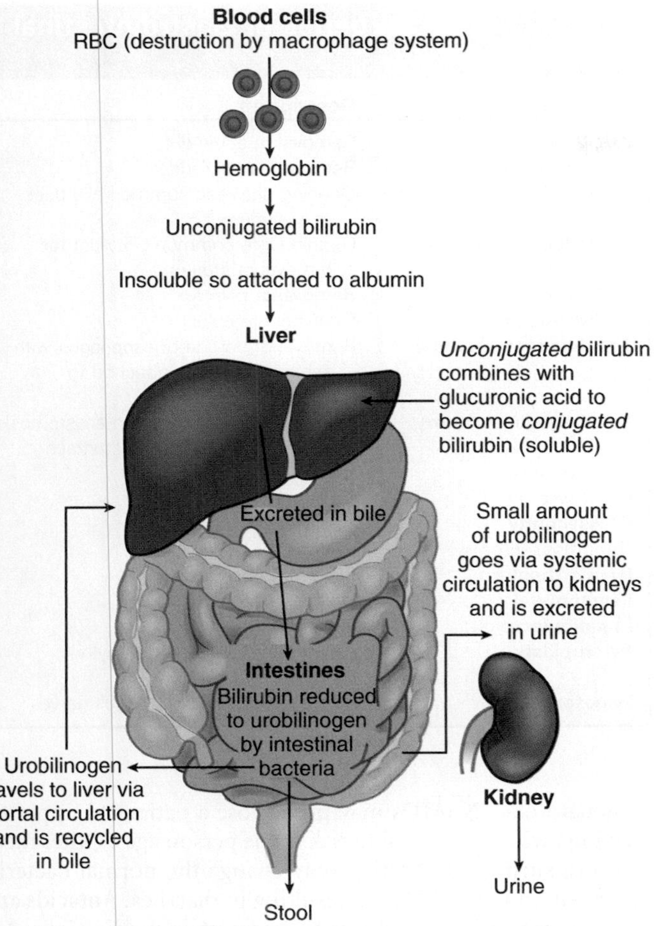


**FIG. 38-4** Bilirubin metabolism and conjugation.

insulin and amylin; α cells secrete glucagon; δ cells secrete somatostatin; and F cells secrete pancreatic polypeptide.

### Gerontologic Considerations: Effects of Aging on Gastrointestinal System

The process of aging changes the functional ability of the GI system. Diet, alcohol intake, and obesity affect organs of the GI system, making it a challenge to separate the sole effects of aging from lifestyle. Many factors can lead to a decrease in appetite and make eating less pleasurable. Caries and periodontal disease can lead to loss of teeth. Taste buds decline in number and the sense of smell lessens, leading to decreased ability to taste. With less saliva, a very dry mouth *(xerostomia)* is common.

Age-related changes in the esophagus include delayed emptying, resulting from smooth muscle weakness, reduced UES opening, and an incompetent LES.[1] Although motility of the GI system decreases with age, secretion and absorption are affected to a lesser extent. The older patient often has a decrease in HCl acid secretion *(hypochlorhydria)* and a reduction in the secretion of intrinsic factor.

The prevalence of constipation in adults over age 60 is about 34%.[2] Factors that may increase the risk for constipation include slower peristalsis, anorectal dysfunction, inactivity, decreased dietary fiber, inadequate fluid intake, constipating medications, and laxative abuse. Neurologic, cognitive, and metabolic disorders may also play a role.[3] (See Chapter 42 for a detailed discussion of constipation.)

The liver size decreases after 50 years of age, but results of liver function tests remain within normal ranges. Age-related enzyme changes in the liver decrease the liver's ability to metabolize drugs and hormones.

The size of the pancreas is unaffected by aging, but it does undergo structural changes, such as fibrosis, fatty acid deposits, and atrophy. Gallbladder diseases increase with age.[4]

Older adults, especially those over 85, are at risk for decreased food intake. The economic inability to purchase food supplies affects nutritional intake, especially in the older adult. Economic constraints may reduce the number of fresh fruits and vegetables consumed and thus the amount of fiber. Immobility limits the ability to obtain and prepare meals. Age-related changes in the GI system and differences in assessment findings are presented in Table 38-5.

## ASSESSMENT OF GASTROINTESTINAL SYSTEM

### Subjective Data

#### Important Health Information

***Past Health History.*** Obtain information from the patient about the history or existence of the problems related to GI functioning and fully explore any symptoms. Inquire about any abdominal pain, nausea, vomiting, diarrhea, constipation, abdominal distention, jaundice, heartburn, dyspepsia, changes in appetite, hematemesis, indigestion, excessive gas, bloating, melena, trouble swallowing, or rectal bleeding. Document related conditions such as food intolerance or allergies, lactose intolerance, and anemia. Ask the patient about a history or existence of diseases such as reflux, gastritis, hepatitis, colitis, gallstones, hemorrhoids, peptic ulcer, cancer, diverticuli, or hernias.

Question the patient about weight history. Explore in detail any unexplained or unplanned weight loss or gain within the past 6 to 12 months. Document a history of chronic dieting and repeated weight loss and gain.

***Medications.*** Assess the patient's past and current use of medications. Ask about the reason for taking the medication, its name, the dose and frequency, length of time taken, its effect, and any

**CASE STUDY**

***Patient Introduction***

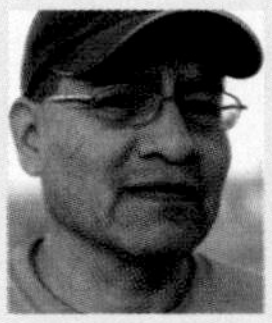

(©iStockphoto/ Thinkstock)

**Patient Profile**

L.C. is a 58-yr-old Native American man from a Pueblo tribe in northern New Mexico. L.C.'s wife and family drove 50 miles to take him to the Indian Health Service hospital. He comes into the emergency department (ED) doubled over with abdominal pain. He is grimacing and holding his abdomen with both arms. You are working as the triage nurse that morning.

**Discussion Questions**

1. What are the possible causes for L.C.'s acute abdominal pain?
2. Is his condition stable or is it an emergency?
3. What type of assessment should you do: comprehensive, focused, or emergency?
4. What assessment questions will you ask him?
5. How will you individualize the assessment based on his ethnic/cultural background?

You will learn more about L.C. and his condition as you read through this assessment chapter.

(See p. 843 for more information on L.C.)

Answers available at *http://evolve.elsevier.com/Lewis/medsurg.*

## TABLE 38-5 Gerontologic Assessment Differences

### *Gastrointestinal System*

| Expected Aging Changes | Differences in Assessment Findings |
|---|---|
| **Mouth** | |
| Gingival retraction | Loss of teeth, dental implants, dentures, difficulty chewing |
| Decreased taste buds, decreased sense of smell | Diminished sense of taste (especially salty and sweet) |
| Decreased volume of saliva | Dry oral mucosa |
| Atrophy of gingival tissue | Poor-fitting dentures |
| **Esophagus** | |
| Lower esophageal sphincter pressure decreased, motility decreased | Epigastric distress, dysphagia, potential for hiatal hernia and aspiration |
| **Abdominal Wall** | |
| Thinner and less taut | More visible peristalsis, easier palpation of organs |
| Decreased number and sensitivity of sensory receptors | Less sensitivity to surface pain |
| **Stomach** | |
| Atrophy of gastric mucosa, decreased blood flow | Food intolerances, signs of anemia as result of cobalamin malabsorption, slower gastric emptying |
| **Small Intestines** | |
| Slightly decreased motility and secretion of most digestive enzymes | Complaints of indigestion, slowed intestinal transit, delayed absorption of fat-soluble vitamins |
| **Liver** | |
| Decreased size and lowered position | Easier palpation because of lower border extending past costal margin |
| Decreased protein synthesis, ability to regenerate decreased | Decreased drug and hormone metabolism |
| **Large Intestine, Anus, Rectum** | |
| Decreased anal sphincter tone and nerve supply to rectal area | Fecal incontinence |
| Decreased muscular tone, decreased motility | Flatulence, abdominal distention, relaxed perineal musculature |
| Increased transit time, decreased sensation to defecation | Constipation, fecal impaction |
| **Pancreas** | |
| Pancreatic ducts distended, lipase production decreased, pancreatic reserve impaired | Impaired fat absorption, decreased glucose tolerance |

## TABLE 38-6 Surgeries of Gastrointestinal System

| Procedure | Description |
|---|---|
| **Appendectomy** | Removal of appendix |
| **Cholecystectomy** | Removal of gallbladder |
| **Choledochojejunostomy** | Opening between common bile duct and jejunum |
| **Choledocholithotomy** | Opening into common bile duct for removal of stones |
| **Colectomy** | Removal of colon |
| **Colostomy** | Opening into colon |
| **Esophagoenterostomy** | Removal of portion of esophagus with segment of colon attached to remaining portion |
| **Esophagogastrostomy** | Removal of esophagus and anastomosis of remaining portion to stomach |
| **Gastrectomy** | Removal of stomach |
| **Gastrostomy** | Opening into stomach |
| **Glossectomy** | Removal of tongue |
| **Hemiglossectomy** | Removal of half of tongue |
| **Herniorrhaphy** | Repair of a hernia |
| **Ileostomy** | Opening into ileum |
| **Mandibulectomy** | Removal of mandible |
| **Pyloroplasty** | Enlargement and repair of pyloric sphincter area |
| **Vagotomy** | Resection of branch of vagus nerve |

side effects. Include information about over-the-counter (OTC) medications, prescription drugs, herbal products, vitamins, probiotics, and nutritional supplements. This is a critical aspect of history taking. Many medications not only affect the GI system, but they are also affected by abnormalities of the GI system.

Many chemicals and drugs are potentially hepatotoxic (see *livertox.nih.gov*) and result in significant harm unless monitored closely. For example, chronic high doses of acetaminophen and nonsteroidal antiinflammatory drugs (NSAIDs) may be hepatotoxic. NSAIDs may predispose a patient to upper GI bleeding, with an increasing risk as the person ages. Other medications, such as antibiotics, may change the normal bacterial composition in the GI tract, resulting in diarrhea. Antacids and laxatives may affect the absorption of certain medications. Ask the patient about laxative or antacid use, including the kind and frequency.

***Surgery or Other Treatments.*** Obtain information about hospitalizations for any problems related to the GI system. Document data related to any abdominal or rectal surgery, including the year, reason for surgery, postoperative course, and possible blood transfusions. Terms related to surgery of the GI system are listed in Table 38-6.

**Functional Health Patterns.** Key questions to ask a patient with a GI problem are presented in Table 38-7.

***Health Perception–Health Management Pattern.*** Ask about the patient's health practices related to the GI system, such as maintenance of normal body weight, proper dental care, adequate nutrition, and effective elimination habits.

Query the patient about recent foreign travel with possible exposure to hepatitis or parasitic infestation. Ask about risk behaviors for hepatitis exposure. Document whether the patient has received hepatitis A and B vaccination.

Assess the patient for habits that directly affect GI functioning. The intake of alcohol in large quantities or for long periods has detrimental effects on the stomach mucosa. Chronic alcohol exposure causes fatty infiltration of the liver and can cause damage, leading to cirrhosis and hepatocellular carcinoma. Obtain a history of cigarette smoking. Nicotine is irritating to the GI tract mucosa. Cigarette smoking is related to GI cancers (especially mouth and esophageal cancers), esophagitis, and ulcers. Smoking delays the healing of ulcers.

Family history is an important component of this health pattern. About one third of cases of colorectal cancer occur in patients with a family history. Because of the relationship

## TABLE 38-7 Health History

### *Gastrointestinal System*

**Health Perception–Health Management**
- Describe any measures used to treat GI symptoms such as diarrhea or constipation.
- Do you smoke?* Do you drink alcohol?*
- Are you exposed to any chemicals on a regular basis?* Have you been exposed in the past?*
- Have you recently traveled outside the United States?*

**Nutritional-Metabolic**
- Describe your usual daily food and fluid intake.
- Do you take any supplemental vitamins or minerals?*
- Have you experienced any changes in appetite or food tolerance?*
- Has there been a weight change in the past 6-12 mo?*
- Are you allergic to any foods?*

**Elimination**
- Describe the frequency and time of day you have bowel movements. What is the consistency of the bowel movement?
- Do you use laxatives or enemas?* If so, how often?
- Have there been any recent changes in your bowel pattern?*
- Do you have any pain with bowel movements or pain relieved by bowel movements?
- Describe any skin problems caused by GI problems.
- Do you need any assistive equipment, such as ostomy equipment, raised toilet seat, commode?

**Activity-Exercise**
- Do you have limitations in mobility that make it difficult for you to obtain and prepare food?*

**Sleep-Rest**
- Do you experience any difficulty sleeping because of a GI problem?*
- Are you awakened by symptoms such as gas, abdominal pain, diarrhea, or heartburn?*

**Cognitive-Perceptual**
- Have you experienced any change in taste or smell that has affected your appetite?*
- Do you have any heat or cold sensitivity that affects eating?*
- Does pain interfere with food preparation, appetite, or chewing?*
- Do pain medications cause constipation, diarrhea, or appetite suppression?*

**Self-Perception–Self-Concept**
- Describe any changes in your weight that have affected how you feel about yourself.
- Have you had any changes in normal elimination that have affected how you feel about yourself?*
- Have any symptoms of GI disease caused physical changes that are a problem for you?*

**Role-Relationship**
- Describe the impact of any GI problem on your usual roles and relationships.
- Have any changes in elimination affected your relationships?*
- Do you live alone? Describe how your family or others assist you with your GI problems.

**Sexuality-Reproductive**
- Describe the effect of your GI problem on your sexual activity.

**Coping–Stress Tolerance**
- Do you experience GI symptoms in response to stressful or emotional situations?
- Describe how you deal with any GI symptoms that result.

**Value-Belief**
- Describe any culturally specific health beliefs regarding food and food preparation that may influence the treatment of your GI problem.

*If yes, describe.

## GENETIC RISK ALERT

### *Colorectal Cancer*

- Colorectal cancer may run in families if first-degree relatives (parents, siblings) or many other family members (grandparents, aunts, uncles) have had colorectal cancer. This is especially true when family members are diagnosed with colorectal cancer before age 50.
- Genetic conditions associated with an increased risk of colorectal cancer include:
  - Hereditary nonpolyposis colorectal cancer (HNPCC), which is caused by mutations in several different genes.
  - Familial adenomatous polyposis (FAP), which is characterized by multiple polyps that are noncancerous at first but eventually develop into cancer if not treated. Most cases of FAP are due to mutations of the adenomatous polyposis coli *(APC)* gene.

## GENETIC RISK ALERT

### *Inflammatory Bowel Disease (IBD)*

- People with IBD have a genetic predisposition or susceptibility to the disease.
- First-degree relatives have a 5- to 20-fold increased risk of developing IBD.

between colorectal and breast cancer, inquire about a history of either type of cancer in the family.

***Nutritional-Metabolic Pattern.*** A thorough nutritional assessment is essential. Take a diet history and inquire about both content and amount or portion size. Food preferences and preparation may vary by culture. Open-ended questions allow the patient to express beliefs and feelings about the diet. For example, you can say, "Please tell me about your food and beverage intake over the past 24 hours." A 24-hour dietary recall can be used to analyze the adequacy of the diet. Assist the patient in recalling the preceding day's food intake, including early morning and nighttime intake, snacks, liquids, and vitamin supplements. You can then evaluate the diet in relation to recommended servings for dietary intake using a guide such as MyPlate *(www.choosemyplate.gov)*. A 1-week recall may provide additional information on usual dietary patterns. Compare weekday and weekend dietary intake patterns in relation to both the quality and quantity of food.

Ask the patient about the use of sugar and salt substitutes, use of caffeine, and amount of fluid and fiber intake. Note any changes in appetite, food tolerance, and weight. Anorexia and weight loss may indicate cancer or inflammation. Decreased food intake can also be the consequence of economic problems or depression.

Ask about food allergies and dietary intolerances, including lactose and gluten. Have the patient describe the allergic response and any GI symptoms.

***Elimination Pattern.*** Elicit a detailed account of the patient's bowel elimination pattern. Note the frequency, time of day, and usual stool consistency. Ask about the presence of pain with bowel movements or if bowel movements relieve pain. Document the use of laxatives and enemas, including type, frequency, and results. Investigate any recent change in bowel patterns.

Document the amount and type of fluid and fiber intake because these influence the frequency and consistency of stools. Inadequate fiber intake can be associated with constipation. Investigate the possible association between a skin problem and a GI problem. Food allergies can cause skin lesions, pruritus, and edema. Diarrhea can result in redness, irritation, and pain in the perianal area. External drainage systems, such as an ileostomy or ileal conduit, may cause local skin irritation.

***Activity-Exercise Pattern.*** Activity and exercise affect GI motility. Immobility is a risk factor for constipation. Assess ambulatory status to determine if the patient is capable of securing and preparing food. If the patient is unable to do these tasks, determine if a family member or an outside agency is meeting this need.

Note any limitation in the ability to feed oneself. Assess for access to a toilet. Identify the use of and access to supplies such as a commode or ostomy supplies.

***Sleep-Rest Pattern.*** GI symptoms can interfere with the quality of sleep. Nausea, vomiting, diarrhea, indigestion, and bloating can produce sleep problems. Ask the patient if GI symptoms affect sleep or rest. For example, a patient with gastroesophageal reflux disease (GERD) may wake with burning, epigastric pain.

A patient may have a bedtime ritual that involves a particular food or beverage. Herbal teas may be sleep inducing. Document individual routines and comply with these whenever possible to avoid sleeplessness. Hunger can prevent sleep and a light, easily digested snack may be helpful.

***Cognitive-Perceptual Pattern.*** Sensory alterations can result in problems related to the acquisition, preparation, and ingestion of food. Changes in taste or smell can affect appetite and eating pleasure. Vertigo can make shopping and standing at a stove difficult and dangerous. Heat or cold sensitivity can make certain foods painful to eat. Problems in expressive communication limit the patient's ability to state personal dietary preferences. If a patient has a GI disorder, ask questions to determine his or her understanding of the illness and its treatment.

Both acute and chronic pain influence dietary intake. Behaviors associated with pain include avoiding activity, fatigue, and disrupted eating patterns. For patients receiving opioid medications, assess for constipation, nausea, sedation, and appetite suppression.

***Self-Perception–Self-Concept Pattern.*** Many GI and nutritional problems affect the patient's self-perception. Overweight and underweight persons may have problems related to self-esteem and body image. Repeated attempts to achieve a personally acceptable weight can be discouraging and depressing for some people. The way a person recounts a weight history can alert you to potential problems in this area.

The need for external devices to manage elimination, such as a colostomy or an ileostomy, may be challenging for some patients. The patient's willingness to engage in self-care and to discuss this situation provides you with valuable information related to body image and self-esteem.

The altered physical changes often associated with advanced liver disease can be disturbing for the patient. Jaundice and ascites cause significant changes in external appearance. Assess the patient's attitude about these changes.

***Role-Relationship Pattern.*** Problems related to the GI system such as cirrhosis, hepatitis, ostomies, obesity, and carcinoma may alter the patient's ability to maintain usual roles and relationships. A chronic illness may necessitate leaving a job or reducing work hours. Changes in body image and self-esteem can affect relationships.

***Sexuality-Reproductive Pattern.*** Changes related to sexuality and reproductive status can result from problems of the GI system. For example, obesity, jaundice, anorexia, and ascites could decrease the acceptance of a potential sexual partner. An ostomy could affect the patient's confidence related to sexual activity. Your sensitive questioning can identify potential problems.

Anorexia can affect the reproductive status of a female patient. Obesity leads to reduced fertility and increased miscarriage rates in women.

***Coping–Stress Tolerance Pattern.*** Determine what is stressful for the patient and what coping mechanisms the patient uses. Factors outside the GI tract can influence its functioning. Both psychologic and emotional factors, such as stress and anxiety, influence GI functioning in many people. Stress can manifest as anorexia, nausea, epigastric and abdominal pain, or diarrhea. It can also aggravate some diseases of the GI system, such as peptic ulcer disease, irritable bowel syndrome, and IBD. However, never attribute GI symptoms solely to psychologic factors.

***Value-Belief Pattern.*** Assess the patient's spiritual and cultural beliefs regarding food and food preparation. Whenever possible, respect these preferences. Determine if any value or belief could interfere with planned interventions. For example, if the patient with anemia is a vegetarian, you will need to consider how to increase dietary intake of iron-rich foods other than meat. Thoughtful assessment and consideration of the patient's beliefs and values usually increase adherence and satisfaction.

## Objective Data

### Physical Examination

#### *Mouth*

**Inspection.** Inspect the mouth for symmetry, color, and size. Observe for abnormalities such as pallor or cyanosis, cracking, ulcers, or fissures. The dorsum (top) of the tongue should have a thin white coating. The undersurface should be smooth. Observe for any lesions. Using a tongue blade, inspect the buccal mucosa and note the color, any areas of pigmentation, and any lesions. Dark-skinned individuals normally have patchy areas of pigmentation. In assessing the teeth and gums, look for caries; loose teeth; abnormal shape and position of teeth; and swelling, bleeding, discoloration, or gingival inflammation. Note any distinctive breath odor.

Inspect the pharynx by tilting the patient's head back and depressing the tongue with a tongue blade. Observe the tonsils, uvula, soft palate, and anterior and posterior pillars. Instruct the patient to say "ah." The uvula and soft palate should rise and remain in the midline.

**Palpation.** Palpate any suspicious areas in the mouth. Note ulcers, nodules, indurations, and areas of tenderness. The mouth of the older adult requires careful assessment. Give particular attention to dentures (e.g., fit, condition), ability to swallow, the tongue, and lesions. Ask the patient with dentures to remove them during an oral examination to allow for good visualization and palpation of the area.

***Abdomen.*** Two systems are used to anatomically describe the surface of the abdomen. One system divides the abdomen into four quadrants by a perpendicular line from the sternum to the pubic bone and a horizontal line across the abdomen at the umbilicus (Fig. 38-5, *A*, and Table 38-8). The other system divides the abdomen into nine regions (Fig. 38-5, *B*). Only the epigastric, umbilical, and suprapubic or hypogastric regions are commonly assessed.

For the abdominal examination, good lighting should shine across the abdomen. The patient should be in the supine position and as relaxed as possible. To help relax the abdominal muscles, have the patient slightly flex the knees and raise the head of the bed slightly. The patient should have an empty bladder. Use warm hands when doing the abdominal examination to avoid eliciting muscle guarding. Ask the patient to breathe slowly through the mouth.

The standard approach for examining the abdomen is appropriate for an older adult. The abdomen may be thinner and more lax unless the patient is obese.

**Inspection.** Assess the abdomen for skin changes (color, texture, scars, striae, dilated veins, rashes, lesions), umbilicus (location and contour), symmetry, contour (flat, rounded [convex], concave, protuberant, distended), observable hernias or masses, and movement (pulsations and peristalsis). A normal aortic pulsation may be seen in the epigastric area. Look across the abdomen tangentially (across the abdomen in a line) for peristalsis. Peristalsis is not normally visible in an adult but may be visible in a thin person.

**Auscultation.** When you examine the abdomen, auscultate before percussion and palpation because these latter procedures may alter the bowel sounds. Use the diaphragm of the stethoscope to auscultate bowel sounds because they are relatively high pitched. Use the bell of the stethoscope to detect lower-pitched sounds. Warm the stethoscope in your hands before auscultating to help prevent abdominal muscle contraction. Listen in the epigastrium and in all four quadrants. Start in the right lower quadrant because bowel sounds are normally present there. Listen for bowel sounds for at least 2 minutes. Do not count bowel sounds. Determine if they are normal, hypoactive, or hyperactive.

The frequency and intensity of bowel sounds vary depending on the phase of digestion. Normal sounds are relatively high pitched and gurgling. Stomach growling or loud gurgles

## CASE STUDY

### *Subjective Data*

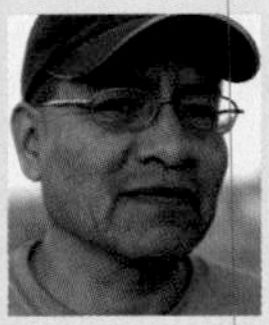

(©iStockphoto/ Thinkstock)

A focused subjective assessment of L.C. revealed the following information:

- ***PMH:*** Negative history for medical or surgical problems.
- ***Medications:*** None.
- ***Health Perception–Health Management:*** L.C. states he has not been feeling well for the past several weeks. He feels weak and is easily fatigued. Denies exposure to chemicals. No recent travel outside of the United States. Smokes approximately 1 pack of cigarettes/day for 20 yr. Drinks beer on a daily basis, typically 3 or 4 bottles per day.
- ***Nutritional-Metabolic:*** L.C. is 5 ft, 9 in tall and weighs 140 lb (BMI: 20.7 kg/m$^2$). States has been losing weight over the past several months and does not have an appetite. No food allergies.
- ***Elimination:*** States has had alternating episodes of constipation and diarrhea. He noticed some bright red blood in stools. Has not had a bowel movement for 4 days.
- ***Cognitive-Perceptual:*** Rates pain as a 9 on a scale of 0 to 10. States pain comes and goes in waves. Prefers to lie still with knees flexed and drawn into his abdomen.

**Discussion Questions**

1. Which subjective assessment findings are of most concern to you?
2. Based on these subjective assessment findings, what should be included in the physical assessment? What would you be looking for?
3. What would be your priority assessment?

You will learn more about physical examination of the gastrointestinal system in the next section.

(See p. 845 for more information on L.C.)

Answers available at *http://evolve.elsevier.com/Lewis/medsurg.*

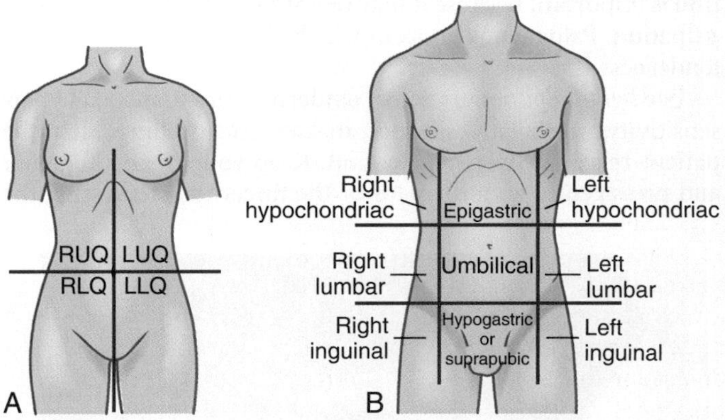


**FIG. 38-5** **A,** Abdominal quadrants. **B,** Abdominal regions. *LLQ,* Left lower quadrant; *LUQ,* left upper quadrant; *RLQ,* right lower quadrant; *RUQ,* right upper quadrant.

### TABLE 38-8 Structures Located in Abdominal Regions

| Right Upper Quadrant | Left Upper Quadrant | Right Lower Quadrant | Left Lower Quadrant |
|---|---|---|---|
| • Liver and gallbladder | • Left lobe of liver | • Lower pole of right kidney | • Lower pole of left kidney |
| • Pylorus | • Spleen | • Cecum and appendix | • Sigmoid flexure |
| • Duodenum | • Stomach | • Portion of ascending colon | • Portion of descending colon |
| • Head of pancreas | • Body of pancreas | • Bladder (if distended) | • Bladder (if distended) |
| • Right adrenal gland | • Left adrenal gland | • Right ovary and salpinx | • Left ovary and salpinx |
| • Portion of right kidney | • Portion of left kidney | • Uterus (if enlarged) | • Uterus (if enlarged) |
| • Hepatic flexure of colon | • Splenic flexure of colon | • Right spermatic cord | • Left spermatic cord |
| • Portion of ascending and transverse colon | • Portion of transverse and descending colon | • Right ureter | • Left ureter |

*(borborygmi)* indicate hyperperistalsis. The bowel sounds are more high pitched (rushes and tinkling) when the intestines are under tension, as in intestinal obstruction. Listen for decreased or absent bowel sounds. A perfectly "silent abdomen" is uncommon.[5] If you are patient and listen for several minutes, you will frequently find the bowel sounds are not absent but are hypoactive. If you do not hear bowel sounds, note the amount of time you listened in each quadrant without hearing bowel sounds.

Listen for vascular sounds. A *bruit,* best heard with the bell of the stethoscope, is a swishing or buzzing sound and indicates turbulent blood flow. Normally you should not hear aortic bruits.

**Percussion.** The purpose of percussing the abdomen is to estimate the size of the liver and determine the presence of fluid, distention, and masses. Sound waves vary according to the density of underlying tissues. Air produces a higher-pitched, hollow sound termed *tympany.* Fluid or masses produce a short, high-pitched sound with little resonance termed *dullness.* Lightly percuss all four quadrants of the abdomen and assess the distribution of tympany and dullness (Fig. 38-6). Tympany is the predominant percussion sound of the abdomen.

To percuss the liver, start below the umbilicus in the right midclavicular line and percuss lightly upward until you hear dullness, thus determining the lower border of the liver. Next, start at the nipple line in the right midclavicular line and percuss downward between ribs to the area of dullness indicating the upper border of the liver. Measure the height or vertical space between the two borders to determine the size of the liver. The normal range of liver height in the right midclavicular line is 2.4 to 5 in (6 to 12.7 cm).

**Palpation.** Use palpation to assess the abdominal organs and detect any tenderness, distension, masses, or fluid. Palpation is important because it may reveal a tumor. Begin with light palpation. Palpate any areas in which the patient complains of tenderness last.

Use *light palpation* to detect tenderness or cutaneous hypersensitivity, muscular resistance, masses, and swelling. Help the patient relax for deeper palpation. Keep your fingers together and press gently with the pads of the fingertips, depressing the abdominal wall about 0.4 in (1 cm). Use smooth movements and palpate all quadrants (Fig. 38-7, *A*).

Use *deep palpation* to delineate abdominal organs and masses (Fig. 38-7, *B*). Use the palmar surfaces of your fingers to press more deeply. Again, palpate all quadrants and note the location, size, and shape of masses, as well as the presence of tenderness. During these maneuvers, observe the patient's facial expression because it will provide nonverbal cues of discomfort or pain.

An alternative method for deep abdominal palpation is the two-hand method. Place one hand on top of the other and apply pressure to the bottom hand with the fingers of the top hand. With the fingers of the bottom hand, feel for organs and masses. Practice both methods of palpation to determine which one is most effective.

Check a problem area on the abdomen for rebound tenderness by pressing in slowly and firmly over the painful site. Withdraw the palpating fingers quickly. Pain on withdrawal of the fingers indicates peritoneal inflammation. Because assessing for rebound tenderness may produce pain and severe muscle spasm, it should be done at the end of the examination and only by an experienced practitioner.

To palpate the liver, place your left hand behind the patient to support the right eleventh and twelfth ribs (Fig. 38-8). The patient may relax on your hand. Press the left hand forward and place the right hand on the patient's right abdomen lateral to the rectus muscle. The fingertips should be below the lower border of liver dullness and pointed toward the right costal margin. Gently press in and up. The patient should take a deep breath with the abdomen so that the liver drops and is in a better position for palpation. Try to feel the liver edge as it comes down to the fingertips. During inspiration, the liver edge should feel firm, sharp, and smooth. Describe the surface and contour and any tenderness. If the patient has chronic obstructive pulmonary disease, large lungs, or a low diaphragm, the liver may be palpated 0.4 to 0.8 in (1 to 2 cm) below the right costal margin.

To palpate the spleen, move to the patient's left side. Place your right hand under the patient, and support and press the patient's left lower rib cage forward. Place your left hand below the left costal margin, and press it in toward the spleen. Ask the patient to breathe deeply. The fingertips can feel the tip or edge of an enlarged spleen. The spleen is normally not palpable. If it is palpable, do not continue because manual compression of an enlarged spleen may cause it to rupture.

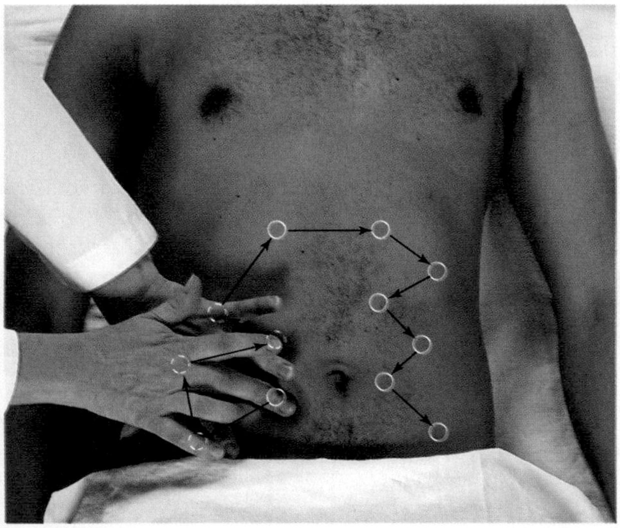

**FIG. 38-6** Technique for percussion of the abdomen. Moving clockwise, percuss lightly in all four quadrants. (From Jarvis C: *Physical examination and health assessment,* ed 6, St Louis, 2012, Saunders.)

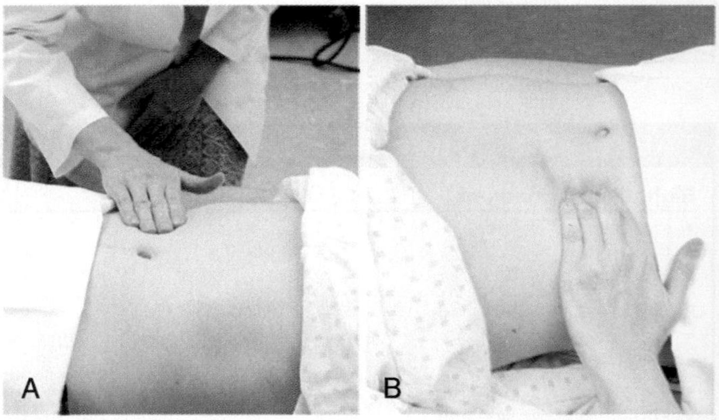


**FIG. 38-7** **A,** Technique for light palpation of the abdomen. **B,** Technique for deep palpation.

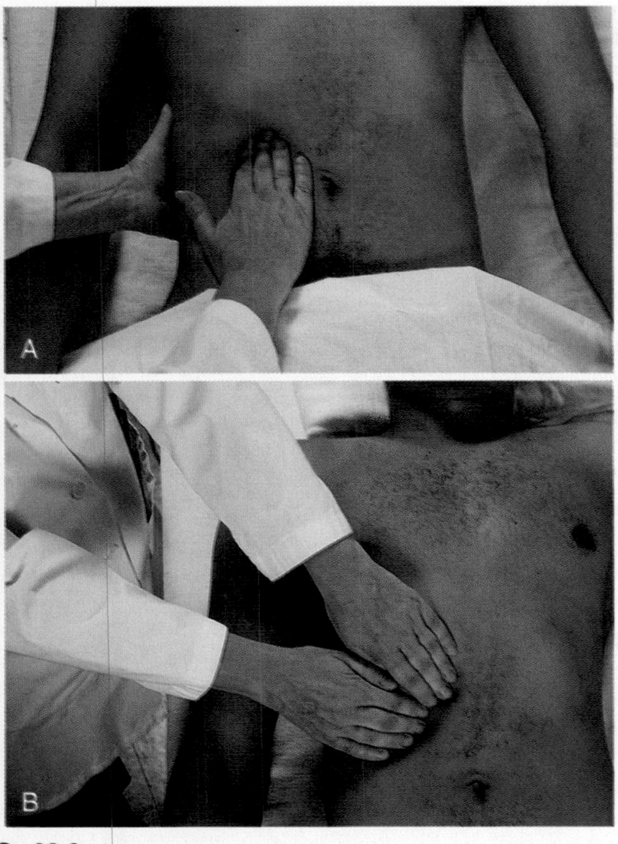


**FIG. 38-8** **A,** Technique for liver palpation. **B,** Alternative technique to palpate liver with fingers hooked over the costal region. (From Jarvis C: *Physical examination and health assessment*, ed 6, St Louis, 2012, Saunders.)

***Rectum and Anus.*** Inspect perianal and anal areas for color, texture, masses, rashes, scars, erythema, fissures, and external hemorrhoids. Palpate any masses or unusual areas with a gloved hand.

For the digital examination of the rectum, place a gloved, lubricated index finger against the anus while having the patient gently bear down (Valsalva maneuver). Then, as the sphincter relaxes, insert the finger. Point the finger toward the umbilicus. Try to get the patient to relax. Insert the finger into the rectum as far as possible, and palpate all surfaces. Assess any nodules, tenderness, or irregularities. Use the gloved finger to remove a stool sample and check it for occult blood. However, a single guaiac-based fecal occult blood test has limited sensitivity in detecting colorectal cancer.

Findings of a normal physical assessment of the GI system are given in Table 38-9. Table 38-10 outlines assessment abnormalities. Gerontologic differences in the GI system and differences in assessment findings are described in Table 38-5. A *focused assessment* is used to evaluate the status of previously identified GI problems and to monitor for signs of new problems. A focused assessment of the GI system is presented on p. 846.

## DIAGNOSTIC STUDIES OF GASTROINTESTINAL SYSTEM

Table 38-11 presents common diagnostic studies of the GI system. Selected diagnostic studies are described in more detail below.

### CASE STUDY

#### *Objective Data: Physical Examination*

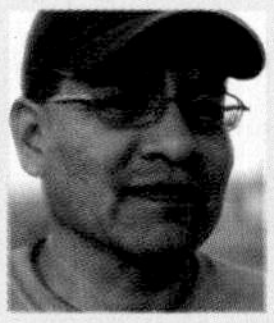

(©iStockphoto/ Thinkstock)

A focused assessment of L.C. reveals the following: BP 120/74, heart rate 110, respiratory rate 24, temp 100.4° F (38° C). Abdomen firm and slightly distended. High-pitched bowel sounds in upper quadrants. No bowel sounds auscultated in left lower quadrant. Mild abdominal palpation elicits pain.

**Discussion Questions**

1. Which physical assessment findings are of most concern to you?
2. Based upon the subjective and objective assessment data presented so far, what would be three priority nursing diagnoses?
3. What diagnostic studies do you think may be ordered for L.C.?

You will learn more about diagnostic studies related to the gastrointestinal system in the next section.

(See p. 852 for more information on L.C.)

Answers available at *http://evolve.elsevier.com/Lewis/medsurg.*

For most diagnostic studies, make sure a signed consent form for the procedure has been completed and is in the medical record. The HCP doing the procedure is responsible for explaining the procedure and obtaining written consent. You play an important role in teaching patients about the procedures. When preparing the patient, it is important to ask about any known allergies to drugs, iodine, shellfish, or contrast media.

Many GI system diagnostic procedures require (1) measures to cleanse the GI tract and (2) ingestion or injection of a contrast medium or a radiopaque tracer. Often the patient has a series of GI diagnostic tests done. Monitor the patient closely to ensure adequate hydration and nutrition during the testing period.

Some diagnostic studies are especially difficult and uncomfortable for the older adult. Adjustments may be needed during the preparation to avoid dehydration or worsening renal function. Make sure to consider any physical limitations when positioning the older patient during testing. Close monitoring is needed to avoid problems such as dehydration from prolonged fluid restriction and diarrhea from bowel-cleansing procedures.

### Radiologic Studies

**Upper Gastrointestinal Series.** An upper GI series with small bowel follow-through provides visualization of the oropharyngeal area, esophagus, stomach, and small intestine. The procedure consists of the patient swallowing contrast medium (a thick barium solution or gastrograffin) and then assuming different positions on the x-ray table. The movement of the contrast medium is observed with fluoroscopy and a series of x-rays are taken. An upper GI series is useful in identifying esophageal strictures, polyps, tumors, hiatal hernias, foreign bodies, and ulcers.

**Lower Gastrointestinal Series.** The purpose of a lower GI series, or a barium enema, is to observe (using fluoroscopy) the colon filling with contrast medium and to observe (by x-ray) the filled colon. It consists of administering an enema of contrast medium to the patient. This procedure identifies polyps, tumors, and other lesions in the colon. Adding air contrast after

*Text continued on p. 851*

## TABLE 38-9 Normal Physical Assessment of Gastrointestinal System

**Mouth**

- Moist and pink lips
- Pink and moist buccal mucosa and gingivae without plaques or lesions
- Teeth in good repair
- Protrusion of tongue in midline without deviation or fasciculations
- Pink uvula (in midline), soft palate, tonsils, and posterior pharynx
- Swallows smoothly without coughing or gagging

**Abdomen**

- Flat without masses or scars. No bruises
- Bowel sounds in all quadrants
- No abdominal tenderness; nonpalpable liver and spleen
- Liver 10 cm in right midclavicular line
- Generalized tympany

**Anus**

- Absence of lesions, fissures, and hemorrhoids
- Good sphincter tone
- Rectal walls smooth and soft
- No masses
- Stool soft, brown, and heme negative

## FOCUSED ASSESSMENT

### *Gastrointestinal System*

*Use this checklist to make sure the key assessment steps have been done.*

**Subjective**

*Ask the patient about any of the following and note responses.*

| | | |
|---|---|---|
| Loss of appetite | Y | N |
| Abdominal pain | Y | N |
| Changes in stools (e.g., color, blood, consistency, frequency, pain) | Y | N |
| Nausea, vomiting | Y | N |
| Painful swallowing | Y | N |

**Objective: Diagnostic**

*Check the following results for critical values.*

| | |
|---|---|
| Endoscopy: colonoscopy, sigmoidoscopy, esophagogastroduodenoscopy | ✓ |
| CT scan | ✓ |
| Radiologic series: upper GI, lower GI | ✓ |
| Stool for occult blood or ova and parasites | ✓ |
| Liver function tests | ✓ |

**Objective: Physical Examination**

***Inspect***

| | |
|---|---|
| Skin for color, lesions, scars, petechiae, etc. | ✓ |
| Abdominal contour for symmetry and distention | ✓ |
| Perianal area for intact skin, hemorrhoids | ✓ |

***Auscultate****

| | |
|---|---|
| Bowel sounds | ✓ |

***Palpate***

| | |
|---|---|
| Abdominal quadrants using light touch | ✓ |
| Abdominal quadrants using a deep technique | ✓ |

*NOTE: Do auscultation before palpation.

## TABLE 38-10 Assessment Abnormalities

### *Gastrointestinal System*

| Finding | Description | Possible Etiology and Significance |
|---|---|---|
| **Mouth** | | |
| **Ulcer, plaque on lips or in mouth** | Sore or lesion | Carcinoma, viral infections |
| **Cheilosis** | Softening, fissuring, and cracking of lips at angles of mouth | Riboflavin deficiency |
| **Cheilitis** | Inflammation of lips (usually lower) with fissuring, scaling, crusting | Often unknown |
| **Geographic tongue** | Scattered red, smooth (loss of papillae) areas on dorsum of tongue | Unknown |
| **Smooth tongue** | Red, slick appearance | Cobalamin deficiency |
| **Leukoplakia** | Thickened white patches | Premalignant lesion |
| **Pyorrhea** | Recessed gingivae, purulent pockets | Periodontitis |
| **Herpes simplex** | Benign vesicular lesion | Herpesvirus |
| **Candidiasis** | White, curdlike lesions surrounded by erythematous mucosa | *Candida albicans* |
| **Glossitis** | Reddened, ulcerated, swollen tongue | Exposure to streptococci, irritation, injury, vitamin B deficiencies, anemia |
| **Acute marginal gingivitis** | Friable, edematous, painful, bleeding gingivae | Irritation from ill-fitting dentures or orthodontic appliances, calcium deposits on teeth, food impaction |
| **Esophagus and Stomach** | | |
| **Dysphagia** | Difficulty swallowing, sensation of food sticking in esophagus | Esophageal problems, cancer of esophagus |
| **Hematemesis** | Vomiting of blood | Esophageal varices, bleeding peptic ulcer |
| **Pyrosis** | Heartburn, burning in epigastric or substernal area | Hiatal hernia, esophagitis, incompetent lower esophageal sphincter |
| **Dyspepsia** | Burning or indigestion | Peptic ulcer disease, gallbladder disease |
| **Odynophagia** | Painful swallowing | Cancer of esophagus, esophagitis |
| **Eructation** | Belching | Gallbladder disease |
| **Nausea and vomiting** | Feeling of impending vomiting, expulsion of gastric contents through mouth | GI infections, common manifestation of many GI diseases; stress, fear, and pathologic conditions |

## TABLE 38-10 Assessment Abnormalities

### *Gastrointestinal System—cont'd*

| Finding | Description | Possible Etiology and Significance |
|---|---|---|
| **Abdomen** | | |
| **Distention** | Excessive gas accumulation, enlarged abdomen, generalized tympany | Obstruction, paralytic ileus |
| **Ascites** | Accumulated fluid within abdominal cavity, eversion of umbilicus (usually) | Peritoneal inflammation, heart failure, metastatic carcinoma, cirrhosis |
| **Bruit** | Humming or swishing sound heard through stethoscope over vessel | Partial arterial obstruction (narrowing of vessel), turbulent flow (aneurysm) |
| **Hyperresonance** | Loud, tinkling rushes | Intestinal obstruction |
| **Borborygmi** | Waves of loud, gurgling sounds | Hyperactive bowel as result of eating |
| **Absent bowel sounds** | No bowel sounds on auscultation | Peritonitis, paralytic ileus, obstruction |
| **Absence of liver dullness** | Tympany on percussion | Air from viscus (e.g., perforated ulcer) |
| **Masses** | Lump on palpation | Tumors, cysts |
| **Rebound tenderness** | Sudden pain when fingers withdrawn quickly | Peritoneal inflammation, appendicitis |
| **Nodular liver** | Enlarged, hard liver with irregular edge or surface | Cirrhosis, carcinoma |
| **Hepatomegaly** | Enlargement of liver, liver edge >1-2 cm below costal margin | Metastatic carcinoma, hepatitis, venous congestion |
| **Splenomegaly** | Enlarged spleen | Chronic leukemia, hemolytic states, portal hypertension, some infections |
| **Hernia** | Bulge or nodule in abdomen, usually appearing on straining | Inguinal (in inguinal canal), femoral (in femoral canal), umbilical (herniation of umbilicus), or incisional (defect in muscles after surgery) |
| **Rectum and Anus** | | |
| **Hemorrhoids** | Thrombosed veins in rectum and anus (internal or external) | Portal hypertension, chronic constipation, prolonged sitting or standing, pregnancy |
| **Mass** | Firm, nodular edge | Tumor, carcinoma |
| **Pilonidal cyst** | Opening of sinus tract, cyst in midline just above coccyx | Probably congenital |
| **Fissure** | Ulceration in anal canal | Straining, irritation |
| **Melena** | Abnormal, black, tarry stool containing digested blood | Cancer, bleeding in upper GI tract from ulcers, varices |
| **Tenesmus** | Painful and ineffective straining at stool. Sense of incomplete evacuation | Inflammatory bowel disease, irritable bowel syndrome, diarrhea secondary to GI infection (e.g., food poisoning) |
| **Steatorrhea** | Fatty, frothy, foul-smelling stool | Chronic pancreatitis, biliary obstruction, malabsorption problems |

## TABLE 38-11 Diagnostic Studies

### *Gastrointestinal System*

| Study | Description and Purpose | Nursing Responsibility |
|---|---|---|
| **Radiology** | | |
| **Upper gastrointestinal (GI) or barium swallow** | Fluoroscopic x-ray study using contrast medium. Used to diagnose structural abnormalities of esophagus, stomach, and duodenum. | *Before:* Explain procedure including the need to drink contrast medium and assume various positions on x-ray table. Keep patient NPO for at least 8 hr. Tell patient to avoid smoking after midnight.<br>*After:* Take measures to prevent contrast medium impaction (fluids, laxatives). Tell patient that stool may be white for up to 72 hr. |
| **Small bowel series** | Contrast medium is ingested and films taken every 30 min until medium reaches terminal ileum. | Same as for upper GI. |
| **Lower GI or barium enema** | Fluoroscopic x-ray examination of colon using contrast medium, which is administered rectally (enema) (Fig. 38-9). Double-contrast or air-contrast barium enema is test of choice. Air is infused after the barium flows through transverse colon. Used to detect the presence of tumors, diverticula, and polyps. | *Before:* Administer laxatives and enemas until colon is clear of stool evening before procedure. Administer clear liquid diet evening before procedure. Keep patient NPO for 8 hr before test. Instruct patient about barium being given by enema. Explain that cramping and urge to defecate may occur during procedure and patient may be placed in various positions on tilt table.<br>*After:* Give fluids, laxatives, or suppositories to assist in expelling barium. Observe stool for passage of contrast medium. Tell patient that stool may be white for up to 72 hr. |

*Continued*

## TABLE 38-11 Diagnostic Studies

*Gastrointestinal System—cont'd*

| Study | Description and Purpose | Nursing Responsibility |
|---|---|---|
| **Radiology—cont'd** | | |
| **Cholangiography** | | |
| • Percutaneous transhepatic (PTC) | Under local anesthesia and monitored anesthesia care, a long needle is passed into liver (under fluoroscopy) and into bile duct. Bile is removed and radiopaque contrast medium directly injected into biliary system. Used to determine filling of hepatic and biliary ducts. | *Before:* Assess patient's medications for possible contraindications, precautions, or complications with use of contrast medium. Keep patient NPO for 8-12 hr before test. Initiate prophylactic IV antibiotics 1 hr prior.<br>*After:* Observe patient for signs of hemorrhage, bile leakage, and infection. Observe safety precautions until sedation wears off. Maintain bed rest for 6 hr. |
| • Surgical cholangiogram | Contrast medium is injected into common bile duct during surgery on biliary structures. | *Before:* Explain that anesthetic will be used. Assess patient's medications for possible contraindications, precautions, or complications with use of contrast medium. |
| • Magnetic resonance cholangiopancreatography (MRCP) | Use of MRI technology to obtain images of biliary and pancreatic ducts. | *Before:* Explain procedure to patient. Assess for contraindications, including pregnancy and presence of metal implants (e.g., pacemaker). |
| **Ultrasound** | Noninvasive procedure using high-frequency ultrasound waves, which are passed into body structures and recorded as they are reflected.<br>Used to show size and configuration of an organ. | |
| • Abdominal ultrasound | A conductive gel is applied to skin and a transducer is placed on the area. Detects abdominal masses (tumors, cysts), gallstones, biliary and liver disease. | *Before:* Instruct patient to be NPO for 8-12 hr. Air or gas can reduce quality of images. Food intake can cause gallbladder contraction, resulting in suboptimal study. |
| • Endoscopic ultrasound (EUS) | Small ultrasound transducer is installed on tip of endoscope. Because EUS transducer gets close to the organ(s) being examined, images obtained are more accurate and detailed than those provided by traditional ultrasound.<br>Detects and stages esophageal, gastric, rectal, biliary, and pancreatic tumors and abnormalities. | Same as esophagogastroduodenoscopy (EGD). |
| • Ultrasound elastography (Fibroscan) | Transient elastography uses an ultrasound transducer to assess level of liver fibrosis. Used to monitor patients with chronic liver disease. | *Before:* Explain the need to lie in dorsal decubitus position with right arm in extreme abduction. |
| **Nuclear imaging scans (scintigraphy)** | Tracer doses of a radioactive isotope are injected IV and a scanning device picks up radioactive emission, which is recorded on paper. Shows size, shape, and position of organ. Functional disorders and structural defects may be identified. | *Before:* Tell patient that the substance used contains only traces of radioactivity and poses little to no danger. Schedule no more than one radionuclide test a day. Explain to patient need to lie flat during scanning. |
| • Gastric emptying studies | Radionuclide study (scintigraphy) is used to assess ability of stomach to empty solids. Patient eats cooked egg containing Tc-99m and toast with water. Images are obtained at 0, 1, 2, and 4 hr later. Study is used in patients with gastric emptying disorders caused by ulcers, ulcer surgery, diabetes, gastric malignancies, or functional disorders. | Same as above. |
| • Hepatobiliary scintigraphy (HIDA) | Patient is given IV injection of Tc-99m and positioned under camera to record distribution of tracer dose in liver, biliary tree, gallbladder, and proximal small intestine. Used to identify obstructions of bile ducts (gallstones, tumors), diseases of gallbladder, and bile leaks. | Same as above. |
| • Scintigraphy of GI bleeding | Tc-99m–labeled sulfur colloid or Tc-99m labeling of the patient's own RBCs to determine the site of active GI blood loss. Sulfur colloid or patient's RBCs are injected, and images of abdomen are obtained at intermittent intervals. | Same as above. |
| **Gastric emptying breath test (GEBT)** | Noninvasive test that measures $CO_2$ in a patient's breath. Used to diagnose delayed gastric emptying (gastroparesis). Baseline breath test done and then patient eats a special test meal that includes a scrambled egg–mix and *Spirulina platensis,* a type of protein that has been enriched with carbon-13, which can be measured in breath samples.<br>Both carbon-12 and a very small amount of carbon-13 are normally found in exhaled $CO_2$. By adding carbon-13 to the test meal, the GEBT can determine how fast the stomach empties the meal by measuring the ratio of carbon-13 to carbon-12 collected in breath samples at multiple time points after the meal is consumed compared to baseline. | *Before:* Instruct patient to be NPO after midnight and that the test takes 4 hr.<br>*During:* Can be done in any clinical setting since it does not require the special training or special precautions related to radiation (as does scintigraphy). |

**TABLE 38-11 Diagnostic Studies**
***Gastrointestinal System—cont'd***

| Study | Description and Purpose | Nursing Responsibility |
|---|---|---|
| **Computed tomography (CT) scan** | Noninvasive radiologic examination allows for exposures at different depths. Using oral and IV contrast medium accentuates density differences. Detects biliary tract, liver, and pancreatic disorders. | *Before:* Explain procedure. Determine sensitivity to iodine or shellfish if contrast material used. |
| **Magnetic resonance imaging (MRI)** | Noninvasive procedure using radiofrequency waves and a magnetic field. IV contrast medium (gadolinium) may be used. Used to detect hepatobiliary disease, hepatic lesions, and sources of GI bleeding and stage colorectal cancer. | *Before:* Explain procedure to patient. Assess for contraindications, including pregnancy and presence of metal implants (e.g., pacemaker). |
| **Virtual colonoscopy** | Combines CT scanning or MRI with computer virtual reality software. Air is introduced via a tube placed in rectum to enlarge colon to enhance visualization. Images obtained while patient is on back and abdomen. Computer combines images to form 2-D and 3-D pictures that are viewed on monitor. Detects intestine and colon diseases, including polyps, cancer, diverticulosis, and lower GI bleeding. | *Before:* Bowel preparation similar to colonoscopy (see Colonoscopy). |
| **Defecography** | Uses fluoroscopy or MRI to assess the shape and position of the rectum during defecation. Using a lubricated small plastic tip, fill rectum and anus with barium. Oral barium allows small bowel to be visualized. The person then sits on a toilet-like seat attached to the x-ray table, and is asked to push and empty the rectum. Images are taken while person is sitting at rest, straining, squeezing, and during defecation. Detects pelvic floor abnormalities. | *Before:* Keep patient NPO for 2 hr. Two enemas are given 2 hr before, 15 minutes apart. Oral barium is given 1 hr before. |
| **Endoscopy** | | |
| **Esophagogastroduodenoscopy (EGD)** | Directly visualizes mucosal lining of esophagus, stomach, and duodenum with flexible endoscope. Test may use video imaging to visualize stomach motility. Detects inflammation, ulcerations, tumors, varices, or Mallory-Weiss tears. Biopsies may be taken. Varices can be treated with band ligation or sclerotherapy. | *Before:* Keep patient NPO for 8 hr. Make sure signed consent is on chart. Give preoperative medication if ordered. Explain to patient that local anesthesia may be sprayed on throat before insertion of scope and that patient will be sedated during procedure.<br>*After:* Keep patient NPO until gag reflex returns. Gently tickle back of throat to determine reflex. Use warm saline gargles for relief of sore throat. Check temperature q15-30min for 1-2 hr (sudden temperature spike is sign of perforation). |
| **Colonoscopy** | Directly visualizes entire colon up to ileocecal valve with flexible fiberoptic scope. Patient's position is changed frequently during procedure to assist with advancement of scope to cecum. Used to diagnose or detect inflammatory bowel disease, polyps, tumors, and diverticulosis and dilate strictures. Procedure allows for biopsy and removal of polyps without laparotomy. | *Before:* Bowel preparation prior varies depending on HCP. For example, patient follows either a low-residue or full liquid diet the day before until bowel cleansing begins. Bowel cleansing follows a split-dose regimen. The evening before the procedure the patient drinks 2 L of oral polyethylene glycol (PEG) lavage solution. The second 2 L dose begins 4-6 hr before procedure. Explain to patient that a flexible scope will be inserted while patient in side-lying position and sedation will be given.<br>*After:* Patient may experience abdominal cramps caused by stimulation of peristalsis because the bowel is constantly inflated with air during procedure. Observe for rectal bleeding and manifestations of perforation (e.g., malaise, abdominal distention, tenesmus). Check vital signs. |
| **Video capsule endoscopy (VCE)** | Patient swallows a vitamin-sized capsule with camera, which provides endoscopic visualization of GI tract (Fig. 38-11). Camera takes >50,000 images during 8-hr examination, relaying images to monitoring device that patient wears on belt. Afterwards, images are downloaded to a workstation.<br>Used to visualize small intestine and diagnose diseases such as Crohn's disease, small bowel tumors, small bowel injury due to NSAIDs, celiac disease, and malabsorption syndrome and to identify sources of possible GI bleeding in areas not accessible by upper endoscopy or colonoscopy. | *Before:* Instruct patient to fast overnight. May have bowel preparation similar to colonoscopy. Video capsule is swallowed, and clear liquids resumed after 2 hr and food and medications after 4 hr.<br>*During:* 8 hr after swallowing the capsule, the patient returns to have the monitoring device removed. A patency capsule may be used first in patients assessed to be high risk for capsule retention due to strictures.<br>*After:* Peristalsis causes passage of the disposable capsule with a bowel movement. |

*Continued*

TABLE 38-11 **Diagnostic Studies**

***Gastrointestinal System—cont'd***

| Study | Description and Purpose | Nursing Responsibility |
|---|---|---|
| **Endoscopy—cont'd** | | |
| **Sigmoidoscopy** | Directly visualizes rectum and sigmoid colon with lighted flexible endoscope. Sometimes a special table is used to tilt patient into knee-chest position.<br>Used to detect tumors, polyps, inflammatory and infectious diseases, fissures, hemorrhoids. | *Before:* Bowel preparation similar to colonoscopy (see Colonoscopy). Explain to patient knee-chest position (unless patient is older or very ill), need to take deep breaths during insertion of scope, and possible urge to defecate as scope is passed. Encourage patient to relax and let abdomen go limp.<br>*After:* Observe for rectal bleeding after polypectomy or biopsy. |
| **Endoscopic retrograde cholangiopancreatography (ERCP)** | Fiberoptic endoscope (using fluoroscopy) is orally inserted into descending duodenum. Then common bile and pancreatic ducts are cannulated. Contrast medium is injected into ducts and allows for direct visualization of structures. Can be used to retrieve a gallstone from distal common bile duct, dilate strictures, biopsy, and diagnose pseudocysts. | *Before:* Explain procedure. Keep patient NPO 8 hr before. Ensure consent form signed. Administer sedation immediately before and during procedure. Administer antibiotics if ordered.<br>*After:* Check vital signs. Check for signs of perforation or infection. Be aware that pancreatitis is most common complication. Check for return of gag reflex. |
| **Laparoscopy (peritoneoscopy)** | Visualize peritoneal cavity and contents with laparoscope. Double-puncture peritoneoscopy permits better visualization of abdominal cavity, especially liver. Done in operating room. Can obtain biopsy specimen. | *Before:* Make sure signed consent is on chart. Keep patient NPO 8 hr. Administer preoperative sedative medication. Ensure bladder and bowels are emptied.<br>*After:* Observe for possible complications of bleeding and bowel perforation after the procedure. |
| **Blood Studies** | | |
| **Amylase** | Enzyme secreted by pancreas. Important in diagnosing acute pancreatitis. Level of amylase peaks in 24 hr and then drops to normal in 48-72 hr.<br>Depending on method, *reference interval* is 30-122 U/L (0.51-2.07 μkat/L). | *Before:* Explain procedure to patient. |
| **Lipase** | Enzyme secreted by pancreas. Important in diagnosing pancreatitis. Level stays elevated longer than serum amylase in acute pancreatitis.<br>*Reference interval:* 31-186 U/L (0.5-3.2 μkat/L). | *Before:* Explain procedure to patient. |
| **Gastrin** | Hormone secreted by cells of the antrum of the stomach, the duodenum, and the pancreatic islets of Langerhans.<br>*Reference interval:* 25-100 pg/mL when fasting. | *Before:* Explain procedure to patient. |
| **Liver Biopsy** | Percutaneous procedure uses needle inserted between 6th and 7th or 8th and 9th intercostal spaces on the right side to obtain specimen of hepatic tissue. Often done with ultrasound or CT guidance | *Before:* Check patient's coagulation status (prothrombin time, clotting or bleeding time). Ensure patient's blood is typed and crossmatched. Take baseline vital signs. Explain need to hold breath after expiration when needle is inserted. Ensure informed consent has been signed.<br>*After:* Check vital signs to detect internal bleeding q15min × 2, q30min × 4, q1hr × 4. Keep patient lying on right side for minimum of 2 hr to splint puncture site. Keep patient in bed in flat position for 12-14 hr. Assess patient for complications such as bile peritonitis, shock, pneumothorax. |
| **Fecal Tests** | | |
| **Fecal analysis** | Form, consistency, and color are noted. Specimen examined for mucus, blood, pus, parasites, and fat content. May test for occult blood (guaiac test, Hemoccult, Hemoccult II, Hemoccult-SENSA, Hematest) and DNA testing (PreGen-Plus, Cologuard) to detect colorectal cancer | *Before*: Keep diet free of red meat for 24-48 hr before occult blood test.<br>*During:* Observe patient's stools. Collect stool specimens. Check stools for blood. |
| **Stool culture** | Tests for the presence of bacteria, including *Clostridium difficile* | *During:* Collect stool specimen. |

the barium provides better visualization (Fig. 38-9). Because it requires the patient to retain the barium, an older or immobile patient may not tolerate it very well.

**Virtual Colonoscopy.** *Virtual colonoscopy* combines CT scanning or MRI with computer software to produce images of the colon and rectum. The test is less invasive than a conventional colonoscopy and the patient does not need sedation. It does require radiation and prior cleansing of the colon.

Compared to conventional colonoscopy, virtual colonoscopy provides a better view inside the colon that is narrow from inflammation or a growth.[6] There are a few disadvantages of virtual colonoscopy. If a polyp is found, it will have to be biopsied or removed by conventional colonoscopy. Virtual colonoscopy may be less sensitive in obtaining information on the details and color of the mucosa and in detecting small (less than 10 mm) or flat polyps.

## Endoscopy

**Endoscopy** refers to the direct visualization of a body structure through an endoscope. An endoscope is a fiberoptic instrument with a light and camera attached, allowing the ability to take video and still pictures (Fig. 38-10). Some endoscopes contain a channel through which to pass instruments, such as biopsy forceps and cytology brushes.

GI structures that can be examined by endoscopy include the esophagus, stomach, duodenum, and colon. An *endoscopic retrograde cholangiopancreatography* (ERCP) is used to visualize the pancreatic, hepatic, and common bile ducts. Endoscopy is often combined with diagnostic procedures, including biopsy and cytologic studies and invasive and therapeutic procedures. Examples include polypectomy, sclerosis or banding of varices, laser treatment, cauterization of bleeding sites, papillotomy, common bile duct stone removal, and balloon dilation.

The major complication of GI endoscopy is perforation through the structure being scoped. Many endoscopic procedures require short-acting IV sedation. All endoscopic procedures require informed, written consent. Specific endoscopy procedures are discussed in Table 38-11.

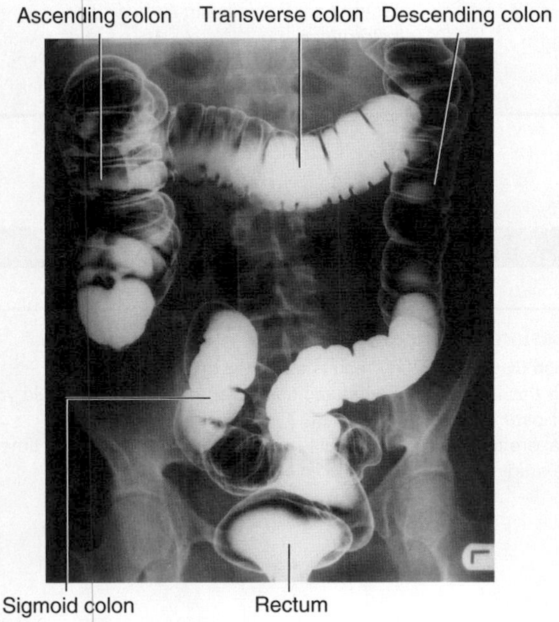


**FIG. 38-9** Barium enema x-ray showing the large intestine. (From Drake RL, Vogl W, Mitchell AWM: *Gray's anatomy for students,* ed 3, Edinburgh, 2014, Churchill Livingstone.)

*Capsule endoscopy* is a noninvasive approach to visualize the GI tract (Fig. 38-11). Colon capsule endoscopy may be useful in monitoring inflammation in patients with inflammatory bowel disease. Its sensitivity in detecting small lesions, colonic polyps, and colorectal cancer is under investigation.[7]

## Liver Biopsy

The purpose of a liver biopsy is to obtain hepatic tissue to use in establishing a diagnosis of cancer or assessing and staging fibrosis. It may also be useful for following the progress of liver disease, such as chronic hepatitis.

The two types of liver biopsy are open and closed. The *open method* involves making an incision and removing a wedge of tissue. It is done in the operating room with the patient under general anesthesia, often concurrently with another surgical procedure. The *closed,* or *needle, biopsy* is a percutaneous procedure. The site is infiltrated with a local anesthetic and a needle

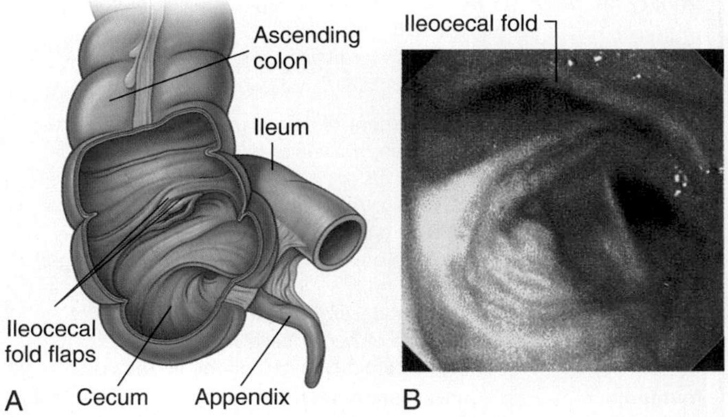


**FIG. 38-10** **A,** Illustration showing the ileocecal junction and the ileocecal fold. **B,** Endoscopic image of the ileocecal fold. (From Drake RL, Vogl W, Mitchell AWM: *Gray's anatomy for students,* ed 3, Edinburgh, 2015, Churchill Livingstone.)

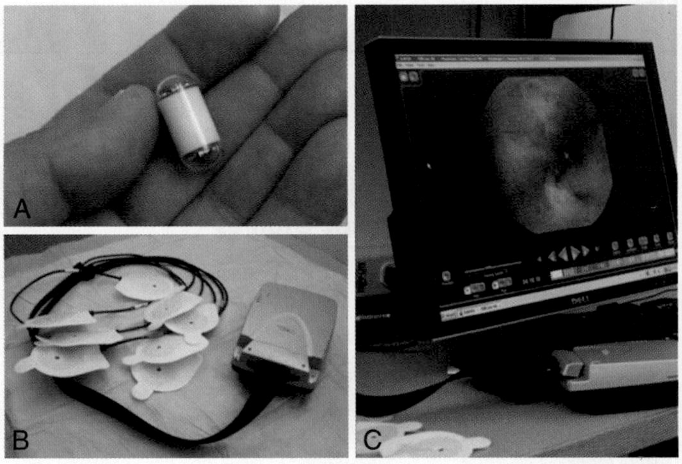


**FIG. 38-11** Capsule endoscopy. **A,** The pill-sized video capsule has its own camera and light source. **B,** As it travels through the GI tract, it sends messages through sensing electrodes placed on the chest and abdomen to a data recorder worn on a waist belt. **C,** After the test, the images are viewed on a computer. (From Dye CE, Gaffney RR, Dykes TM, et al: Endoscopic and radiographic evaluation of the small bowel in 2012, *Am J Med* 125:1228e1, 2012.)

inserted between the sixth and seventh or eighth and ninth intercostal spaces on the right side. The patient lies supine with the right arm over the head. Instruct the patient to expire fully and not breathe when the needle is inserted.

### Liver Function Studies

Liver function tests (LFTs) are laboratory (blood) studies that reflect hepatic disease. Table 38-12 describes the most common LFTs.

**TABLE 38-12 Diagnostic Studies**

***Liver Function Tests***

| Test | Description and Purpose |
|---|---|
| **Bile Formation and Excretion** | |
| **Serum bilirubin** | Measurement of liver's ability to conjugate and excrete bilirubin, allowing differentiation between unconjugated (indirect) and conjugated (direct) bilirubin in plasma |
| • Total | Measurement of direct and indirect total bilirubin<br>*Reference interval:* 0.2-1.2 mg/dL (3-21 µmol/L) |
| • Direct | Measurement of conjugated bilirubin. Elevated in obstructive jaundice<br>*Reference interval:* 0.1-0.3 mg/dL (1.7-5.1 µmol/L) |
| • Indirect | Measurement of unconjugated bilirubin. Elevated in hepatocellular and hemolytic conditions<br>*Reference interval:* 0.1-1.0 mg/dL (1.7-17 µmol/L) |
| **Urinary bilirubin** | Measurement of urinary excretion of conjugated bilirubin<br>*Reference interval:* 0 or negative |
| **Protein Metabolism** | |
| **Protein (serum)** | Measurement of serum proteins made by liver<br>• Albumin, *reference interval:* 3.5-5.0 g/dL (35-50 g/L)<br>• Globulin, *reference interval:* 2.0-3.5 g/dL (20-35 g/L)<br>• Total protein, *reference interval:* 6.4-8.3 g/dL (64-83 g/L)<br>• A/G ratio, *reference interval:* 1.5:1-2.5:1 |
| **α-Fetoprotein** | Indication of hepatocellular cancer<br>*Reference interval:* <10 ng/mL (<10 mcg/L) |
| **Ammonia** | Conversion of ammonia to urea normally occurs in liver. Increase can result in hepatic encephalopathy secondary to liver cirrhosis.<br>*Reference interval:* 15-45 mcg N/dL (11-32 µmol N/L) |
| **Hemostatic Function** | |
| **Prothrombin time (PT)** | Determination of prothrombin activity<br>*Reference interval:* 11-16 sec |
| **International normalized ratio (INR)** | Standardized system of reporting PT based on a reference calibration model and calculated by comparing the patient's PT with a control value<br>*Reference interval:* In general, 2-3 is the desired therapeutic level with warfarin (Coumadin), depending on laboratory. |
| **Vitamin K** | Essential cofactor for many clotting factors<br>*Reference interval:* 0.1-2.2 ng/mL (0.22-4.88 nmol/L) |
| **Serum Enzymes** | |
| **Alkaline phosphatase (ALP)** | Originates from bone and liver. Serum levels rise when excretion is impaired because of obstruction in biliary tract.<br>*Reference interval:* 38-126 U/L (0.65-2.14 µkat/L), depending on method and age |
| **Aspartate aminotransferase (AST)** | Elevated in liver damage and inflammation<br>*Reference interval:* 10-30 U/L (0.17-0.51 µkat/L) |
| **Alanine aminotransferase (ALT)** | Elevated in liver damage and inflammation<br>*Reference interval:* 10-40 U/L (0.17-0.68 µkat/L) |
| **γ-Glutamyl transpeptidase (GGT)** | Present in biliary tract (not in skeletal or cardiac muscle). Increase in hepatitis and alcoholic liver disease. More sensitive for liver dysfunction than ALP<br>*Reference interval:* 0-30 U/L (0-0.5 µkat/L) |
| **Lipid Metabolism** | |
| **Cholesterol (serum)** | Synthesis and excretion by liver. Increase in biliary obstruction. Decrease in cirrhosis and malnutrition<br>*Reference interval:* <200 mg/dL (<5.2 mmol/L), varying with age |

*A/G,* Albumin/globulin.

**CASE STUDY**

***Objective Data: Diagnostic Studies***

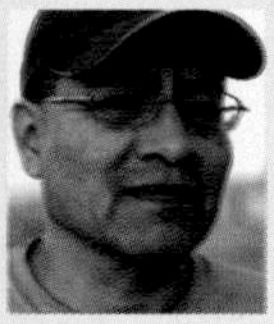

(©iStockphoto/Thinkstock)

The ED physician performs a rectal examination and finds a palpable mass. The following diagnostic tests are ordered:

- CBC
- Electrolytes
- Liver function tests
- Urinalysis
- CT scan of the abdomen
- Colonoscopy

The CBC reveals an Hgb of 6.8 g/dL and Hct of 20%. The WBC count is normal. The electrolytes, liver function tests, and urinalysis are within normal limits. The CT scan reveals pockets of gas and fluid in the ascending colon and two medium-sized tumors in the transverse colon.

**Discussion Questions**

1. Which diagnostic study results are of most concern to you?
2. With this information, what additional diagnostic studies would you anticipate being ordered for L.C.?
3. What are the interprofessional team's priorities for L.C. at this time?

Case study continued in Chapter 42 on p. 971.

Answers available at *http://evolve.elsevier.com/Lewis/medsurg.*

## BRIDGE TO NCLEX EXAMINATION

The number of the question corresponds to the same-numbered outcome at the beginning of the chapter.

1. A patient is admitted to the hospital with a diagnosis of diarrhea with dehydration. The nurse recognizes that increased peristalsis resulting in diarrhea can be related to
   **a.** sympathetic inhibition.
   **b.** mixing and propulsion.
   **c.** sympathetic stimulation.
   **d.** parasympathetic stimulation.
2. A patient has an elevated blood level of indirect (unconjugated) bilirubin. One cause of this finding is that
   **a.** the gallbladder is unable to contract to release stored bile.
   **b.** bilirubin is not being conjugated and excreted into the bile by the liver.
   **c.** the Kupffer cells in the liver are unable to remove bilirubin from the blood.
   **d.** there is an obstruction in the biliary tract preventing flow of bile into the small intestine.
3. As gastric contents move into the small intestine, the bowel is normally protected from the acidity of gastric contents by the
   **a.** inhibition of secretin release.
   **b.** release of bicarbonate by the pancreas.
   **c.** release of pancreatic digestive enzymes.
   **d.** release of gastrin by the duodenal mucosa.
4. A patient is jaundiced and her stools are clay colored (gray). This is *most* likely related to
   **a.** decreased bile flow into the intestine.
   **b.** increased production of urobilinogen.
   **c.** increased bile and bilirubin in the blood.
   **d.** increased production of cholecystokinin.
5. An 80-year-old man states that, although he adds a lot of salt to his food, it still does not have much taste. The nurse's response is based on the knowledge that the older adult
   **a.** should not experience changes in taste.
   **b.** has a loss of taste buds, especially for sweet and salt.
   **c.** has some loss of taste but no difficulty chewing food.
   **d.** loses the sense of taste because the ability to smell is decreased.
6. When the nurse is assessing the health perception–health maintenance pattern as related to GI function, an appropriate question to ask is
   **a.** "What is your usual bowel elimination pattern?"
   **b.** "What percentage of your income is spent on food?"
   **c.** "Have you traveled to a foreign country in the last year?"
   **d.** "Do you have diarrhea when you are under a lot of stress?"
7. During an examination of the abdomen the nurse should
   **a.** position the patient in the supine position with the bed flat and knees straight.
   **b.** listen for bowel sounds in the epigastrium and all four quadrants for 2 minutes.
   **c.** describe bowel sounds as absent if no sound is heard in a quadrant after 2 minutes.
   **d.** use the following order of techniques: inspection, palpation, percussion, auscultation.
8. Normal physical assessment findings of the GI system are *(select all that apply)*
   **a.** nonpalpable liver and spleen.
   **b.** borborygmi in upper right quadrant.
   **c.** tympany on percussion of the abdomen.
   **d.** liver edge 2 to 4 cm below the costal margin.
   **e.** finding of a firm, nodular edge on the rectal examination.
9. In preparing a patient for a colonoscopy, the nurse explains that
   **a.** a signed permit is not necessary.
   **b.** sedation will be used during the procedure.
   **c.** one cleansing enema is necessary for preparation.
   **d.** light meals should be eaten for 3 days before the procedure.

1. d, 2. b, 3. b, 4. a, 5. b, 6. c, 7. b, 8. a, c, 9. b

For rationales to these answers and even more NCLEX review questions, visit *http://evolve.elsevier.com/Lewis/medsurg.*

## EVOLVE WEBSITE

http://evolve.elsevier.com/Lewis/medsurg

**Review Questions (Online Only)**
**Key Points**
**Answer Keys for Questions**
- Rationales for Bridge to NCLEX Examination Questions
- Answer Guidelines for Case Studies on pp. 839, 843, 845, and 852

**Conceptual Care Map Creator**
**Audio Glossary**
**Supporting Media**
- Animation
  - Rectal Examination

**Content Updates**

## REFERENCES

1. Omari T, Kritas S, Fraser R, et al: Swallowing dysfunction in healthy older people using pharyngeal pressure-flow analysis, *Neurogastroenterol Motil* 26:59, 2014.
*2. Bharucha A, Pemberton J, Locke G: American Gastroenterological Association technical review on constipation, *J Gastro* 144:218, 2013.
3. Bailes B, Reeve K: Constipation in older adults, *Nurs Pract* 38:21, 2013.
4. McArthur T, Planz V, Fineberg N, et al: The common duct dilates after cholecystectomy and with advancing age: reality or myth? *J Ultrasound Med* 32:8, 2013.
5. Jarvis C: *Physical examination and health assessment*, ed 6, St Louis, 2012, Saunders.
6. National Digestive Diseases Information Clearinghouse: virtual colonoscopy. Retrieved from *www.niddk.nih.gov/health-information/health-topics/diagnostic-tests/virtual-colonoscopy/Pages/diagnostic-test.aspx.*
7. Tal A, Vermehren J, Albert J: Colon capsule endoscopy: current status and future directions, *World J Gastroenterol* 20:44, 2014.

*Evidence-based information for clinical practice.

# Nutritional Problems

*Rose Ann DiMaria-Ghalili*

*Let thy food be thy medicine and thy medicine be thy food.*

***Hippocrates***

http://evolve.elsevier.com/Lewis/medsurg/

## LEARNING OUTCOMES

1. Relate the essential components of a well-balanced diet to their impact on health outcomes.
2. Describe the common etiologic factors, clinical manifestations, and management of malnutrition.
3. Describe the components of a nutritional assessment.
4. Explain the indications, complications, and nursing management principles related to the use of enteral nutrition.
5. Explain the indications, complications, and nursing management related to the use of parenteral nutrition.
6. Compare the etiologic factors, clinical manifestations, and nursing management of eating disorders.

## KEY TERMS

**anorexia nervosa, p. 871**
**bulimia nervosa, p. 872**
**enteral nutrition (EN), p. 865**
**malabsorption syndrome, p. 857**
**malnutrition, p. 856**
**parenteral nutrition (PN), p. 869**
**refeeding syndrome, p. 870**
**tube feeding, p. 865**

This chapter focuses on problems related to nutrition. A review of normal nutrition provides a basis for evaluating nutritional status. Malnutrition and types of supplemental nutrition, including enteral and parenteral nutrition, are discussed.

## NUTRITIONAL PROBLEMS

*Nutrition* is the sum of processes by which one takes in and uses nutrients.[1] Nutritional status can be viewed on a continuum from undernutrition to normal nutrition to overnutrition. Any alteration in the process of nutrient intake or use can cause nutritional problems. Nutritional problems occur in all ages, cultures, ethnic groups, socioeconomic classes, and across all educational levels.

Many factors influence nutritional status. A person establishes attitudes towards food and eating habits early. Dietary intake frequently reflects cultural or religious preferences. The financial status of a person or family influences the type and amount of nutritionally sound food that can be purchased.[2]

## NORMAL NUTRITION

Nutrition is important for energy, growth, and maintaining and repairing body tissues. Optimal nutrition (in the absence of any underlying disease process) results from eating a balanced diet. The major components of the basic food groups are macronutrients (carbohydrates, fats, proteins), micronutrients (vitamins, minerals, electrolytes), and water. Optimal nutrition and daily physical activity are essential for a healthy lifestyle.

Body type, age, gender, medications, physical activity, and the presence or absence of disease influence a person's daily caloric requirements. Adjustments in caloric intake are necessary depending on changes in health status and daily activity level. There are several ways to estimate caloric need. The Mifflin–St. Jeor equation calculates daily adult energy (calorie) requirements based on resting metabolic rate[3] (Table 39-1). A simpler way to estimate daily calories needed is by kilocalories per kilogram (kcal/kg). An average adult should consume 20 to 25 cal/kg body weight to lose weight, 25 to 30 cal/kg to maintain body weight, and 30 to 35 cal/kg to gain weight.[4] Energy needs may be greater during illness.

Carbohydrates, the body's primary source of energy, yield approximately 4 cal/g. They are classified as either simple or complex, depending on the number of sugars they contain. Simple carbohydrates come in two forms: monosaccharides (e.g., glucose, fructose), which are found in fruits and honey, and disaccharides (e.g., sucrose, maltose, lactose), which are found in foods such as table sugar, malted cereal, and milk,

Reviewed by Karen Gilbert, RN, MSN, CNSC, CRNP, Nutrition Support Clinical Nurse Specialist, Thomas Jefferson University Hospital, Riverton, New Jersey; and Allison J. Terry, RN, PhD, Associate Professor of Nursing, Assistant Dean of Clinical Practice, School of Nursing, Auburn University Montgomery, Montgomery, Alabama.

**TABLE 39-1 Estimating Daily Energy (Calorie) Requirements**

**Mifflin–St. Jeor Equation**

For each gender, use the formula below to calculate energy expenditure:

*Men:* 10 × weight (kg) + 6.25 × height (cm) − 5 × age (yr) + 5

*Women:* 10 × weight (kg) + 6.25 × height (cm) − 5 × age (yr) − 161

To determine total daily calorie needs, the energy expenditure has to be multiplied by the appropriate activity factor, as follows:

1.200 = sedentary (little or no exercise)
1.375 = lightly active (light exercise/sports 1-3 days/wk)
1.550 = moderately active (moderate exercise/sports 3-5 days/wk)
1.725 = very active (hard exercise/sports 6-7 days a wk)
1.900 = extra active (very hard exercise/sports and physical job)

***Example***

*Man:* Weight 180 lb (82 kg), height 5 ft 10 in (178 cm), age 50, very active

Energy expenditure = 10 (82) + 6.25 (178) − 5 (50) + 5 × 1.725 = 2911

*Woman:* Weight 150 lb (68 kg), height 5 ft 6 in (168 cm), age 60, lightly active

Energy expenditure = 10 (68) + 6.25 (168) − 5 (60) −161 × 1.375 = 1745

respectively. Complex carbohydrates or polysaccharides include starches, such as cereal grains, potatoes, and legumes.

Carbohydrates are the chief protein-sparing ingredient in a nutritionally sound diet. The Dietary Reference Intake (DRI) recommendations are that 45% to 65% of total calories should come from carbohydrates.[4] A person should take approximately 14 g of dietary fiber per 1000 calories eaten per day from fruits, vegetables, and whole grains. This equates to roughly 28 to 30 g for a typical 2000-calorie diet. Individuals should choose food and beverages with little added sugar or caloric sweeteners.

*Fats* are a major source of energy for the body. One gram of fat yields 9 calories. Fats are stored in adipose tissue and the abdominal cavity. They act as carriers of essential fatty acids and fat-soluble vitamins. Fats provide a feeling of satiety after eating. Fat intake should be no more than 20% to 35% of total calories.[4]

Fats can be divided into (1) potentially harmful (saturated fat and *trans* fat) and (2) healthier dietary fat (monounsaturated and polyunsaturated fat). One type of polyunsaturated fat, omega-3 fatty acids, may be especially beneficial to your heart. Omega-3 fatty acids (found in some types of fatty fish) appear to decrease the risk of coronary artery disease.

Diets high in excess calories, usually in the form of fats, contribute to the development of obesity. Individuals should consume less than 10% of calories from saturated fatty acids (approximately 20 g of saturated fat per day in a 2000-calorie diet and choose foods with no *trans*-fatty acids.

*Proteins* are an essential component of a well-balanced diet. They are required for tissue growth, repair, and maintenance; body regulatory functions; and energy production. Ideally, 10% to 35% of daily caloric needs should come from protein.[4] The recommended daily protein intake is 0.8 to 1 g/kg of body weight. One gram of protein yields 4 calories. Amino acids are the fundamental units of protein structure. The 22 amino acids are classified as essential and nonessential. The body can synthesize nonessential amino acids if an adequate supply of protein is available. The body cannot synthesize the 9 essential amino acids. Their availability depends totally on dietary sources. We obtain them from both animal and plant sources. *Complete proteins* contain all the essential amino acids. Proteins that lack one or more of the essential amino acids are *incomplete proteins.* Table 39-2 lists foods high in protein.

**TABLE 39-2 Nutritional Therapy**

***Foods High in Protein***

| Complete Proteins | Incomplete Proteins |
|---|---|
| • Milk and milk products (e.g., cheese)<br>• Eggs<br>• Fish<br>• Meats<br>• Poultry | • Grains (e.g., corn)<br>• Legumes (e.g., navy beans, soybeans, peas)<br>• Nuts (e.g., peanuts)<br>• Seeds (e.g., sesame seeds, sunflower seeds) |

*Vitamins* are organic compounds required in small amounts for normal metabolism. Vitamins function primarily in enzyme reactions that facilitate amino acid, fat, and carbohydrate metabolism. A diet consisting of foods from the five basic food groups is essential for obtaining the recommended dietary allowances of essential vitamins. Vitamins are divided into two categories: *water-soluble* vitamins (vitamin C and the B-complex vitamins) and *fat-soluble* vitamins (vitamins A, D, E, and K). Since the body stores excess fat-soluble vitamins, consuming too much can result in toxicity. Upper limits have been established for vitamins A, D, and E.

**HEALTHY PEOPLE**

***Health Impact of a Well-Balanced Diet***

- Reduces incidence of anemia
- Maintains normal body weight and prevents obesity
- Maintains good bone health and reduces risk of osteoporosis
- Lowers the risk of developing elevated cholesterol and type 2 diabetes mellitus
- Decreases the risk of heart disease, hypertension, and certain types of cancers

*Mineral salts* (e.g., magnesium, iron, calcium) make up approximately 4% of the total body weight. Minerals are necessary for the body to build and repair tissues, regulate body fluids, and assist in various functions. Minerals required in amounts greater than 100 mg/day are called *major minerals.* Minerals present in minute amounts are *trace elements.* Table 39-3 lists the major minerals and trace elements. Some minerals are stored and can be toxic if taken in excess amounts. The amount of minerals needed daily varies greatly, from a few micrograms of trace minerals to 1 g or more of the major minerals, such as calcium, phosphorus, and sodium. A well-balanced diet usually meets the daily requirements of minerals. However, deficiency and excess states can occur.

## VEGETARIAN DIET

The common element among all vegetarians is the exclusion of red meat from the diet. There are many types of vegetarians and no strict definition of the word "vegetarian." Many vegetarians are *vegans,* who are pure or total vegetarians and eat only plants, and *lacto-ovo-vegetarians,* who eat plants, dairy products, and eggs.

**TABLE 39-3 Major Minerals and Trace Elements**

| Major Minerals | Trace Elements |
|---|---|
| • Calcium | • Chromium |
| • Chloride | • Copper |
| • Magnesium | • Fluoride |
| • Phosphorus | • Iodine |
| • Potassium | • Iron |
| • Sodium | • Manganese |
| • Sulfur | • Molybdenum |
| | • Selenium |
| | • Zinc |

**TABLE 39-4 Nutritional Therapy**

***Foods High in Iron***

*These foods provide 25%-39% of the Dietary Reference Intake (DRI) of iron.*

| Food | Selected Serving Size |
|---|---|
| **Breads, Cereals, and Grain Products** | |
| Farina, regular or quick cooked (enriched) | ⅔ cup |
| Oatmeal, instant, fortified, prepared (enriched) | ⅔ cup |
| Ready-to-eat cereals, fortified (enriched) | 1 oz |
| **Meat, Poultry, Fish, and Alternatives** | |
| Beef liver, braised | 3 oz |
| Pork liver, braised | 3 oz |
| Chicken or turkey liver, braised | ½ cup diced |
| Clams: steamed, boiled, or canned (drained) | 3 oz |
| Oysters: baked, broiled, steamed, or canned (undrained) | 3 oz |
| Soybeans, cooked | ½ cup |

Without a well-planned diet, vegetarians can have vitamin or protein deficiencies. Plant protein, although a lesser quality than animal protein, fulfills most of the protein requirements. Combinations of vegetable protein foods (e.g., cornmeal, kidney beans) can increase the nutritional value. Milk made from soybeans or almonds is an excellent protein source and should be calcium fortified. Other deficiencies that may be present in a vegan diet include calcium, zinc, and vitamins A and D.

The primary deficiency for a strict vegan is lack of cobalamin (vitamin $B_{12}$). Cobalamin is only obtained from animal protein, special supplements, or foods fortified with the vitamin. Vegans not using cobalamin supplements are susceptible to the development of megaloblastic anemia and the neurologic signs of cobalamin deficiency.

Strict vegetarians and lacto-ovo-vegetarians are at risk for iron deficiency. Table 39-4 lists examples of foods high in iron.

### Culturally Competent Care: Nutrition

People have unique cultural heritages that may affect eating customs and nutritional status. Each culture has its own beliefs and behaviors related to food and the role that food plays in the etiology and treatment of disease. In addition, culture and religion can influence what food is considered edible, how it is prepared, when it is eaten, and how and who prepares it. For example, some religions, such as Judaism and Islam, have specific laws regarding food. Assess the extent to which Jewish or Muslim patients adhere to Kosher or Halal dietary practices to ensure that appropriate meals are served. The websites for Kosher Quest *(www.kosherquest.org)* and the Islamic Food and Nutrition Council of America *(www.ifanca.org)* provide detailed information.

Assess the patient's diet history and implement necessary dietary changes. Avoid *cultural stereotyping* by not making assumptions or generalizations about diet based on a person's cultural background. Dietary habits differ considerably within and among ethnic groups. Acculturation (extent to which immigrants adopt attributes of a new culture) can also affect dietary practices.[5]

It is important to know whether the patient eats "traditional foods" associated with the culture. Assess the impact of eating traditional foods on health. For example, many traditional foods eaten by some African Americans tend to be high in fat, cholesterol, and sodium. Traditional foods eaten by some Asian Americans may be high in fiber and low in fat and cholesterol. The diet may be low in calcium because of limited dairy product intake.

Considering cultural beliefs is important when planning and monitoring acceptance of dietary changes. Culture can also influence perception of body weight and size. Ask the patient or family about how culture affects dietary choices and weight maintenance. For example, in some cultures obesity does not carry the stigma that it does in Western cultures. This may make teaching regarding weight reduction more challenging. A Jewish patient who eats only Kosher food may be comforted in knowing that an enteral nutrition formula is Kosher. Another example of culturally sensitive planning is adjusting meal plans for the Muslim patient observing Ramadan (the Islamic month of *fasting,* in which Muslims refrain from eating and drinking during daylight hours).

## MALNUTRITION

**Malnutrition** is a deficit, excess, or imbalance of essential nutrients. It may occur with or without inflammation. Malnutrition affects body composition and functional status.[6] Other terms used to describe malnutrition include *undernutrition* and *overnutrition.*

*Undernutrition* describes a state of poor nourishment because of inadequate diet or diseases that interfere with normal appetite and assimilation of ingested food. *Overnutrition* refers to the ingestion of more food than is required for body needs, as in obesity.

Malnutrition is a problem in both developing and developed countries across the care continuum (community, hospital, long-term care). Prevalence rates for malnutrition in the hospital setting range from 30% to 50%.[7] The prevalence of malnutrition in older adults based on the Mini Nutritional Assessment (MNA) ranges from approximately 6% (community-dwelling older adults) to 50% (rehabilitation settings).[8]

### Etiology of Malnutrition

Several terms describe the types and causes of adult malnutrition. Older terms still used in some settings include *primary* or *secondary protein-calorie malnutrition* (PCM), *marasmus,* and *kwashiorkor.* Marasmus and kwashiorkor describe forms of malnutrition seen in children in developing countries. These terms should not be used to describe malnutrition in adults.

The following etiology-based terms are the preferred ones to use in clinical practice settings, since they indicate the interaction and importance of inflammation on nutritional status.[6]

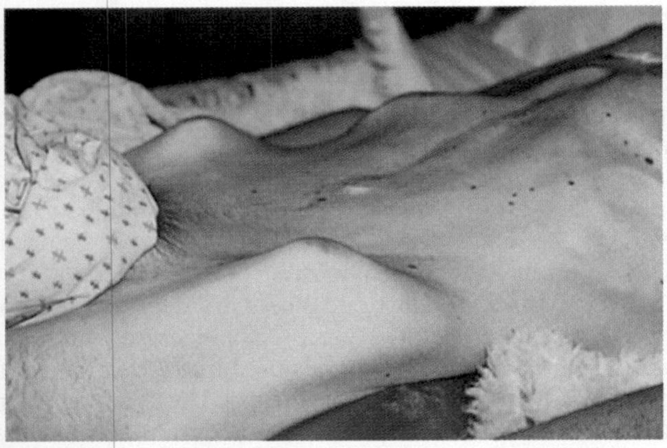

**FIG. 39-1** Patient with malnutrition. (From Morgan SL, Weinsier RL: *Fundamentals of clinical nutrition,* ed 2, St Louis, 1998, Mosby.)

**TABLE 39-5 Conditions That Increase the Risk for Malnutrition**

- Dementia
- Depression
- Chronic alcoholism
- Excessive dieting to lose weight
- Swallowing disorders (e.g., head and neck cancer)
- Decreased mobility that limits access to food or its preparation
- Nutrient losses from malabsorption, dialysis, diarrhea, or wounds
- Drugs with antinutrient or catabolic properties such as corticosteroids and oral antibiotics
- Extreme need for nutrients because of hypermetabolism or stresses such as infection, burns, trauma, or fever
- No oral intake and/or receiving standard IV solutions (5% dextrose) for 10 days (adults) or for 5 days (older adults)

- *Starvation-related malnutrition,* or primary PCM, occurs when nutritional needs are not met (Fig. 39-1). In primary PCM, there is chronic starvation without inflammation (e.g., anorexia nervosa).
- *Chronic disease–related malnutrition,* or secondary PCM, is associated with conditions that have sustained mild to moderate inflammation. This occurs when dietary intake does not meet tissue needs, although it would under normal conditions. Examples of conditions associated with this type of malnutrition include organ failure, cancer, rheumatoid arthritis, obesity, and metabolic syndrome.
- *Acute disease– or injury-related malnutrition* is associated with acute disease or injury states with marked inflammatory response (e.g., major infection, burns, trauma, surgery).

## Contributing Factors to Malnutrition

Many factors contribute to the development of malnutrition, including socioeconomic factors, physical illnesses, incomplete diets, and drug-nutrient interactions. Table 39-5 lists conditions that increase the risk for malnutrition.

**Socioeconomic Factors.** Persons or families with limited financial resources may have *food insecurity* (inadequate access).[2] Food insecurity is a major public health problem. It affects the overall quality of food that is available in both quantity and nutritional value. Those with food insecurity usually choose less expensive "filling" foods, which are more energy dense (high fat) and lack nutritional value. This type of diet increases the risk of nutrient deficiencies.

To help obtain food, people may use "safety net programs." These include food assistance programs; housing and energy subsidies; and in-kind contributions from relatives, friends, food pantries, or charitable organizations. Consult with social workers to help patients gain access to government and local programs such as Meals on Wheels that deliver nutritious meals to homebound people.

The "heat or eat" phenomenon is problematic, as those with limited economic resources struggle to pay household utility bills or put food on the table. Older adults on a fixed income have an added burden of deciding on whether to pay for medications or food. You and the dietitian can assist patients in making food choices that meet nutritional requirements while staying within their limited resources.

**Physical Illnesses.** Malnutrition is a common consequence of illness, surgery, injury, or hospitalization. The hospitalized patient, especially the older adult, is at risk of becoming malnourished. Prolonged illness, major surgery, sepsis, draining wounds, burns, hemorrhage, fractures, and immobilization can all contribute to malnutrition. Undernutrition can aggravate a pathologic condition. An existing deficiency state is likely to become more severe during illness.

Anorexia, nausea, vomiting, diarrhea, abdominal distention, and abdominal cramping may accompany GI disease. Any combination of these symptoms interferes with normal food consumption and metabolism. In addition, a patient may restrict intake to a few foods or fluids that may not be nutritionally sound out of fear of aggravating an existing GI problem.

**Malabsorption syndrome** is the impaired absorption of nutrients from the GI tract. Decreases in digestive enzymes or in bowel surface area can quickly lead to a deficiency state. Many drugs have undesirable GI side effects and alter normal digestive and absorptive processes. For example, antibiotics change the normal flora of the intestines, decreasing the body's ability to synthesize biotin.

Fever accompanies many illnesses, injuries, and infections, with a concomitant increase in the body's basal metabolic rate (BMR) and nitrogen loss. Each degree of temperature increase on the Fahrenheit scale raises the BMR by about 7%. Without an increase in caloric intake, the body uses protein stores to supply calories, and protein depletion develops. After the body temperature returns to normal, the rate of protein breakdown and resynthesis may be increased for several weeks.

Consider the nutritional requirements of a patient who is not overtly ill but is undergoing diagnostic studies. This patient may be nutritionally fit on entering the hospital but can become malnourished because of the dietary restrictions imposed by multiple diagnostic studies.

**Incomplete Diets.** Vitamin deficiencies are rare in most developed countries. When vitamin imbalances do occur, they usually involve several vitamins, rather than a single one. This may happen with persons with a pattern of alcohol and drug abuse, those who are chronically ill, and those who follow poor dietary practices. Persons who had surgery on the GI tract may be at risk for vitamin deficiencies. For example, resection of the terminal ileum poses a risk for deficiencies of fat-soluble vitamins. After a gastrectomy, patients require cobalamin supplementation because intrinsic factor (normally made in the stomach) is not available to bind with cobalamin so that this vitamin can be absorbed in the ileum. Followers of fad diets or poorly planned vegetarian diets are also at risk.

**TABLE 39-6 Recommended Daily Vitamin Intake and Manifestations of Deficiencies**

| Vitamin | Dietary Reference Intake | Manifestations of Deficiencies |
|---|---|---|
| A (retinol) | *Men:* 900 mcg/retinol equivalents* *Women:* 700 mcg/ retinol equivalents | Dry, scaly skin. Increased susceptibility to infection, night blindness, anorexia, eye irritation, keratinization of respiratory and GI mucosa, bladder stones, anemia, retarded growth |
| D | *Adults ages 19-70:* 600 IU *Adults age >70:* 800 IU | Muscular weakness, excessive sweating, diarrhea and other GI disturbances, bone pain, active or healed rickets, osteomalacia |
| E | *Adults:* 15 mg | Neurologic deficits |
| K | *Men:* 120 mcg *Women:* 90 mcg | Defective blood coagulation |
| $B_1$ (thiamine) | *Men:* 1.2 mg *Women:* 1.1 mg | Anorexia, fatigue, nervous irritability, constipation, paresthesias, insomnia |
| $B_6$ (pyridoxine) | *Men ages 19-50:* 1.3-1.7 mg *Men age >51:* 1.7 mg *Women ages 19-50:* 1.3-1.5 mg *Women age >51:* 1.5 mg | Seizures, dermatitis, anemia, neuropathy with motor weakness, anorexia |
| $B_{12}$ (cobalamin) | *Adults:* 2.4 mcg | Megaloblastic anemia, anorexia, glossitis, sore mouth and tongue, pallor, neurologic problems such as depression and dizziness, weight loss, nausea, constipation |
| C | *Men:* 90 mg *Women:* 75 mg | Bleeding gums, loose teeth, easy bruising, poor wound healing, scurvy, dry, itchy skin |
| Folate (folic acid) | *Adults:* 400 mcg | Impaired cell division and protein synthesis, megaloblastic anemia, anorexia, fatigue, sore tongue, diarrhea, forgetfulness |

*1 retinol equivalent = 10 international units vitamin A activity from β-carotene or 3.33 international units vitamin A activity from retinol.

Clinical manifestations of vitamin imbalances range from skin conditions to neurologic signs. The recommended dietary allowances for essential vitamins and manifestations of imbalances are presented in Table 39-6.

**Drug-Nutrient Interactions.** A *drug-nutrient interaction* occurs when a drug affects the use of nutrients in the body. Many drug and food or beverage interactions may occur. Potential adverse interactions include incompatibilities, altered drug effectiveness, and impaired nutritional status. For example, many drugs produce side effects such as changes in taste, appetite, and nausea. Grapefruit juice can increase the absorption of some drugs, enhancing their effect. Drug-nutrient interactions can also occur with the use of herbs and dietary supplements. Monitor and prevent these potential interactions for patients in the hospital and at home.

## Pathophysiology of Starvation

Knowing the pathophysiology of the starvation process will help you understand the physiologic changes that occur in malnutrition. Initially, the body selectively uses carbohydrates (glycogen) rather than fat and protein to meet metabolic needs. These carbohydrate stores, found in the liver and muscles, are minimal. They may be totally depleted within 18 hours. During the early phase of starvation, protein is used only in its normal participation in cellular metabolism.

However, once carbohydrate stores are depleted, the body converts skeletal protein to glucose for energy. Alanine and glutamine are the first amino acids used in *gluconeogenesis,* the process by which the liver forms glucose. The resulting plasma glucose allows metabolic processes to continue. When these amino acids are used as energy sources, the person may be in negative nitrogen balance (nitrogen excretion exceeds nitrogen intake).

Within 5 to 9 days, the body mobilizes fat to supply much of the needed energy. In prolonged starvation, fat provides up to 97% of calories, conserving protein. Depletion of fat stores depends on the amount available. Fat stores are generally used up in 4 to 6 weeks. Once fat stores are gone, the body uses visceral and body proteins, including those in internal organs and plasma. They rapidly decrease because they are the only remaining body source of energy available.

If a malnourished patient has surgery, experiences physical trauma, or has an infection, the stress response is superimposed on the starvation response. The body uses protein stores for energy to meet the increased metabolic energy expenditure.

As protein depletion continues, liver function becomes impaired, and protein synthesis decreases. The decrease in protein synthesis lowers plasma oncotic pressure. A major function of plasma proteins, primarily albumin, is to maintain the osmotic pressure of blood. When the oncotic pressure decreases, body fluids shift from the vascular space into the interstitial compartment. Eventually albumin leaks into the interstitial space along with the fluid. Edema becomes clinically observable. Often edema in the patient's face and legs masks the underlying muscle wasting.

As the total blood volume decreases, the skin appears dry and wrinkled. As fluids shift to the interstitial space, ions also move. Sodium (a predominant extracellular ion) increases in amount within the cell. Potassium (a predominant intracellular ion) and magnesium shift to the extracellular space. The sodium-potassium exchange pump has high-energy needs, using 20% to 50% of all calories ingested. When the diet is extremely deficient in calories and essential proteins, the pump will fail. This leaves sodium inside the cell (along with water), and the cell expands.

The liver is the body organ that loses the most mass during protein deprivation. Fat gradually infiltrates the liver due to decreased synthesis of lipoproteins. If dietary protein and other necessary nutrients are not given, death will rapidly ensue.

**Impact of Inflammation.** Inflammation affects nutrient metabolism and is an important component of nutritional status. During the starvation process, there is a decreased BMR, sparing of skeletal muscle, and decreased protein breakdown. However, in inflammatory states, there are alterations in the expression of proinflammatory (e.g., interleukin-6) and antiinflammatory cytokines (e.g., interleukin-10). These cytokine changes result in increased protein and skeletal muscle breakdown, increased BMR, increased glucose turnover, decreased negative acute

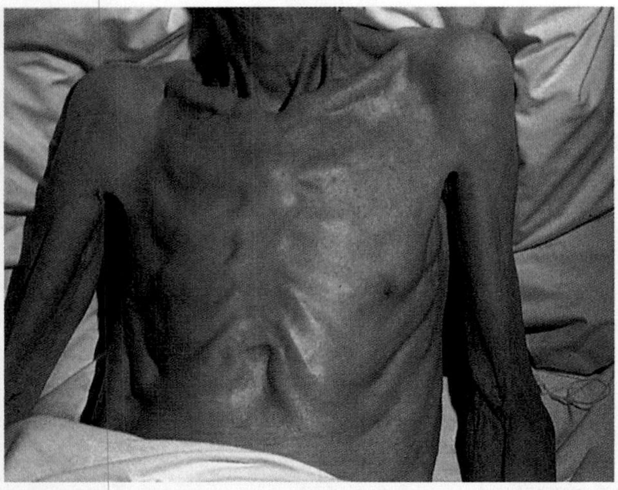

**FIG. 39-2** Severe malnutrition that results in wasting and extensive loss of adipose tissue. (From Kamal A, Brockelhurst JC: *Color atlas of geriatric medicine,* ed 2, St Louis, 1991, Mosby.)

phase protein (albumin, prealbumin) production, and increased positive acute phase protein (e.g., C-reactive protein [CRP]) production.[6,7,9]

## Clinical Manifestations

The clinical manifestations of malnutrition range from mild to emaciation and death (Fig. 39-2). The most obvious signs on physical examination are apparent in the skin (dry and scaly skin, brittle nails, rashes, hair loss), mouth (crusting and ulceration, changes in tongue), muscles (decreased mass and weakness), and CNS (mental changes such as confusion, irritability). The speed at which malnutrition develops depends on the quantity and quality of the protein intake, caloric value, illness, and the person's age.

The manifestations of malnutrition result from numerous interactions at the cellular level. As protein intake declines, the muscles (which are the largest store of protein in the body) become wasted and flabby. This leads to weakness and fatigability. Decreased protein is available for tissue repair, causing delayed wound healing. The person is more susceptible to infections. Both humoral and cell-mediated immunity are deficient. Leukocytes decrease in the peripheral blood. Impaired phagocytosis occurs because of the lack of energy needed to drive the process. Many malnourished persons are anemic, generally because of nutritional deficiencies in iron and folic acid (necessary building blocks for red blood cells [RBC]).

## Diagnostic Studies

**History and Physical Examination.** The diagnosis of malnutrition is best determined by body composition, including a thorough history of weight loss, nutrient intake, and measures of functional status. A dietary history of foods eaten over the past week reveals a great deal about the patient's diet habits and knowledge of good nutrition. In addition to height, weight, and vital signs, assess and document the patient's physical state and each body system. Table 39-7 summarizes the assessment and findings of the patient with malnutrition.

**Laboratory Studies.** Serum albumin has a half-life of approximately 20 to 22 days. In the absence of marked fluid loss (e.g., from hemorrhage or burns), the serum albumin value lags behind actual protein changes by more than 2 weeks. This makes albumin a poor indicator of acute changes in nutritional status. Prealbumin, a protein synthesized by the liver, has a half-life of 2 days. It is a better indicator of recent or current nutritional status. However, the extent to which visceral proteins, including albumin and prealbumin, are true markers of malnutrition is questionable.

Albumin and prealbumin are *negative acute phase proteins.* This means that during an inflammatory response, the liver decreases synthesis of these proteins. So low or below normal levels of these negative acute phase proteins may indicate an inflammatory state rather than accurately depicting nutritional status. One way to determine if low albumin and prealbumin levels are due to malnutrition is to measure CRP, a *positive acute phase protein.* CRP is typically elevated during inflammation. A high CRP and low albumin or prealbumin suggests that inflammation is driving the change in albumin and prealbumin levels.[9]

Serum electrolyte levels reflect changes taking place between the intracellular and extracellular spaces. The serum potassium level is often elevated. The RBC count and hemoglobin level indicate the presence and degree of anemia. The total lymphocyte count decreases with malnutrition. Calculate it by multiplying the percent of lymphocytes times the total white blood cell (WBC) count. Liver enzyme levels may be elevated during malnutrition. Serum levels of both fat-soluble and water-soluble vitamins are usually decreased. Low serum levels of fat-soluble vitamins correlate with the clinical signs of *steatorrhea* (fatty stools).

**Anthropometric Measurements.** Anthropometric measurements are gross measures of fat and muscle contents. They consist of measures of skinfold thickness at various sites (indicators of subcutaneous fat stores) and midarm muscle circumference (indicator of protein stores). The sites most reflective of body fat are those over the biceps and triceps, below the scapula, above the iliac crest, and over the upper thigh. The measures obtained are compared with standards for healthy persons of the same age and gender.

Anthropometric measurements are most beneficial when done serially and by persons trained in anthropometry. They evaluate the long-term effects of malnutrition or responses to nutritional interventions. Both skinfold thickness and midarm circumference decrease in malnutrition. Shifts in hydration status influence these measurements. The exact relationship of the midarm circumference measure to morbidity and mortality remains to be established.

Waist circumference and hip-to-waist ratio are commonly used to reflect nutritional status. These measures are discussed in Chapter 40.

**Functional Measurements.** Functional assessment focuses on performance of activities of daily living (ADL) tools.[10] The most frequently used tools are the Katz Index and Lawton Scale.[11] Measuring muscle strength can assess physical functional status, an important outcome of nutrition status. Handgrip strength is measured with a hand dynamometer. Timed gait and chair stands are markers of lower extremity strength.[10]

## ❖ NURSING AND INTERPROFESSIONAL MANAGEMENT: MALNUTRITION

### ◆ Nursing Assessment

As a nurse, you are responsible for nutritional screening across care settings. Nutritional screening identifies those who are

## TABLE 39-7 Nursing Assessment
### *Malnutrition*

**Subjective Data**

***Important Health Information***

*Past health history:* Severe burns, major trauma, hemorrhage, draining wounds, bone fractures with prolonged immobility, chronic renal or liver disease, cancer, malabsorption syndromes, GI obstruction, infectious diseases, acute (e.g., trauma, sepsis) or chronic inflammatory condition (e.g., rheumatoid arthritis)

*Medications:* Corticosteroids, chemotherapy, diet pills, dietary supplements, herbs

*Surgery or other treatments:* Recent surgery, radiation

***Functional Health Patterns***

*Health perception–health management:* Alcohol or drug abuse. Malaise, apathy

*Nutritional-metabolic:* Increase or decrease in weight, weight problems. Increase or decrease in appetite, typical dietary intake, food preferences and aversions, food allergies or intolerance. Ill-fitting or absent dentures. Dry mouth, difficulty in chewing or swallowing, bloating, or gas. ↑ sensitivity to cold, delayed wound healing

*Elimination:* Constipation, diarrhea, nocturia, decreased urine output

*Activity-exercise:* Increase or decrease in activity patterns. Weakness, fatigue, decreased endurance

*Cognitive-perceptual:* Pain in mouth. Paresthesias, loss of position and vibratory sense

*Role-relationship:* Change in family (e.g., loss of a spouse), financial resources

*Sexual-reproductive:* Amenorrhea, impotence, decreased libido

**Objective Data**

***General***

Listless, cachectic, underweight for height

***Eyes***

Pale or red conjunctivae, gray keratinized epithelium on conjunctiva (Bitot's spots). Dryness and dull appearance of conjunctivae and cornea, soft cornea. Blood vessel growth in cornea. Redness and fissuring of eyelid corners

***Integumentary***

Dry, brittle, sparse hair with color changes and lack of luster, alopecia. Dry, scaly lips. Fever blisters, angular crusts and lesions at corners of mouth (cheilosis). Brittle, ridged nails. Decreased tone and elasticity of skin. Cool, rough, dry, scaly skin with brown-gray pigment changes. Reddened, scaly dermatitis, scrotal dermatitis. Slight cyanosis, peripheral edema

***Respiratory***

Decreased respiratory rate, ↓ vital capacity, crackles, weak cough

***Cardiovascular***

Increased or decreased heart rate, ↓ BP, dysrhythmias

***Gastrointestinal***

Swollen, smooth, raw, beefy red tongue (glossitis), hypertrophic or atrophic papillae. Dental cavities, absent or loose teeth, discolored tooth enamel. Spongy, pale, receded gums with a tendency to bleed easily, periodontal disease. Ulcerations, white patches or plaques. Redness, swelling of oral mucosa. Distended, tympanic abdomen. Ascites, hepatomegaly, decreased bowel sounds, steatorrhea

***Neurologic***

Decreased or loss of reflexes, tremor; irritability, confusion, syncope, peripheral neuropathy

***Musculoskeletal***

Decreased muscle mass with poor tone, "wasted" appearance, bowlegs, knock-knees, beaded ribs, chest deformity, prominent bony structures

***Possible Diagnostic Findings***

↓ Hemoglobin and hematocrit, ↓ MCV (mean corpuscular volume), MCH (mean corpuscular hemoglobin), or MCHC (mean corpuscular hemoglobin concentration). Altered serum electrolyte levels, especially hyperkalemia. ↓ BUN and creatinine, ↓ serum albumin, transferrin, and prealbumin. ↑ CRP, ↓ lymphocytes, ↑ liver enzymes, ↓ serum vitamin levels

malnourished or at risk for malnutrition. The Joint Commission requires nutritional screening for all patients within 24 hours of admission, with a detailed nutrition assessment if a patient is at risk. Following a standard approach to nutritional screening, using valid and reliable tools, will accurately identify those at risk. Many nutritional screening and assessment tools are available. Hospital-specific screening tools review common admission assessment data, including history of weight loss, intake before admission, use of nutritional support, chewing or swallowing issues, and skin breakdown.[12]

The Mini Nutritional Assessment (MNA) assesses nutrition status in older adults. In long-term care, the Minimum Data Set (MDS) form is used to obtain nutrition information.[13] In home care settings, the Outcome and Assessment Information Set (OASIS) is used to collect information on diet, oral intake, dental health, swallowing difficulties, and any need for meal assistance.[13]

If screening identifies a person at nutritional risk, perform a full nutritional assessment. A nutritional assessment is a comprehensive approach that includes medical, nutritional, and medication histories; physical examination; anthropometric measurements; and laboratory data (Table 39-8). Nutritional assessment provides the basis for nutritional intervention.

Across all care settings, be aware of the patient's nutritional status. Obtaining an accurate measure of body weight and height and recording this information are critical components of this assessment. When assessing weight, obtain a detailed weight history, noting weight loss. Ask whether the weight loss was intentional or unintentional and the period over which it took place. A loss of more than 5% of usual body weight over 6 months (whether intentional or unintentional) is a critical indicator for further assessment, especially in the older adult.[13] If an involuntary weight loss exceeds 10% of the usual weight, determine the reason. Unintentional weight loss is important to consider in the obese person. Latent malnutrition may be present despite excess body weight. Determine the patient's current weight in relation to ideal body weight.

When possible, measure the patient's actual height rather than using the patient's self-report. Alternatives to standing height (stature) measurements include arm demi-span and knee-height measurements. The *arm demi-span* is the distance from a point on the midline at the suprasternal notch to the

**TABLE 39-8 Components of Nutritional Assessment**

| | |
|---|---|
| **Anthropometric Measurements**<br>• Height and weight<br>• Body mass index (BMI)<br>• Rate of weight change<br>• Amount of weight loss | **Diet History**<br>• Chewing and swallowing ability<br>• Changes in appetite or taste<br>• Food and nutrient intake<br>• Availability of food |
| **Physical Examination**<br>• Physical appearance<br>• Muscle mass and strength<br>• Dental and oral health | **Laboratory Data**<br>• Glucose<br>• Electrolytes<br>• Lipid profile<br>• Blood urea nitrogen (BUN)<br>• Albumin, prealbumin, CRP |
| **Health History**<br>• Personal and family history<br>• Acute or chronic illnesses<br>• Current medications, herbs, supplements<br>• Cognitive status, depression | **Functional Status**<br>• Ability to perform basic and instrumental activities of daily living<br>• Handgrip strength<br>• Performance tests (e.g., timed walk tests) |

web between the middle and ring fingers with the arm horizontally outstretched. For persons confined to bed, using a Luft ruler is an alternative to standing height.

*Body mass index* (BMI) is a measure of weight for height (see Fig. 40-2). A BMI of less than 18.5 kg/m$^2$ is considered underweight, normal weight is a BMI between 18.5 and 24.9 kg/m$^2$, and overweight is a BMI between 25 and 29.9 kg/m$^2$. A BMI of 30 kg/m$^2$ or greater is obese. BMIs outside the normal weight range are associated with increased morbidity and mortality.

Obtain a complete diet history from the patient or caregiver. Often the patient's nutritional state is not the reason for seeking medical care. However, it may be a contributing factor to the disease and have an impact on management and recovery.

## ◆ Nursing Diagnoses

Nursing diagnoses for the patient with malnutrition include, but are not limited to, the following:

- Imbalanced nutrition: less than body requirements *related to* decreased access, ingestion, digestion, or absorption of food or *related to* anorexia, dysphagia, or increased metabolic needs
- Feeding self-care deficit *related to* decreased strength and endurance, fatigue, and apathy
- Deficient fluid volume *related to* factors affecting access to or absorption of fluids
- Risk for impaired skin integrity *related to* poor nutritional state
- Noncompliance *related to* alteration in perception, lack of motivation, or incompatibility of regimen with lifestyle or resources

## ◆ Planning

The overall goals are that the patient with malnutrition will (1) achieve an appropriate weight, (2) consume a specified number of calories per day on an individualized diet; and (3) have no adverse consequences related to malnutrition or nutritional therapies.

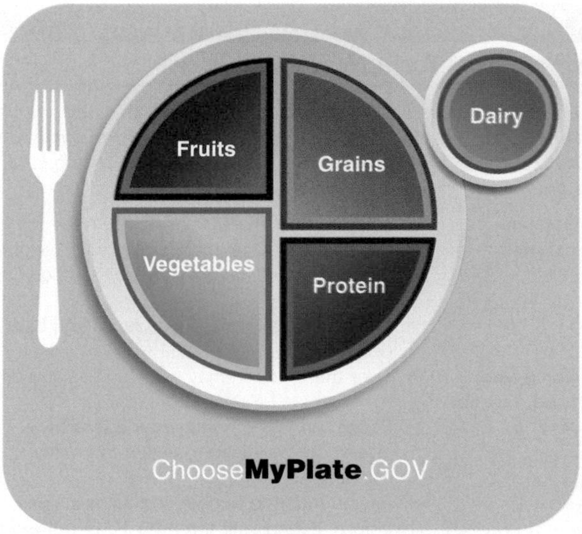


**FIG. 39-3** MyPlate is the primary food group symbol that serves as a reminder to make healthy food choices and to build a healthy plate at mealtimes. It is a visual cue that identifies the five basic food groups from which to select healthy foods. The plate is divided into four slightly different-sized quadrants, with fruits and vegetables taking up half the space and grains and protein making up the other half. The vegetables and grains portions are the largest of the four. Next to the plate is a blue circle for dairy, which could be a glass of milk or a food such as cheese or yogurt. For more information, see *www.choosemyplate.gov*. (US Department of Agriculture, Center for Nutrition Policy and Promotion: Guidance on Use of USDA's MyPlate and Statements about Amounts of Food Groups Contributed by Foods on Food Product Labels, Washington, DC.)

## ◆ Nursing Implementation

**◆ Health Promotion.** It is part of your role to teach and reinforce healthy eating habits. Use MyPlate, Dietary Guidelines for Americans 2015, and Nutrition Facts food labels to promote healthy nutrition. The MyPlate approach provides a visual guide for sensible meal planning. It helps Americans eat healthfully and make good food choices. MyPlate focuses on the proportions of five food groups (grains, protein, fruits, vegetables, and dairy) that you should eat at each meal (Fig. 39-3, Table 39-9). At the health professionals' link at *www.choosemyplate.gov*, you can download daily food plans, sample menus, and tips for how to be physically active. These materials are valuable to use in patient teaching. MyPlate materials for older adults are available at *www.nutrition.tufts.edu/research/myplate-older-adults*.

There are many resources to help people eat a nutritious diet and maintain a healthy weight. Electronic and print sources are available for determining nutritional information in commonly consumed foods. Many food products have Nutrition Facts labels (Fig. 39-4). Consumer and health professional education materials on Nutrition Facts labels are available on the U.S. Food and Drug Administration (FDA) website *(www.fda.gov/Food/IngredientsPackagingLabeling/LabelingNutrition)*.

Interactive web-based programs and mobile device applications are available to track physical activity, calories, nutrients, and foods eaten. Mobile device applications assist with making healthy eating choices easier. Some use built-in barcode scanners to scan foods quickly and give individual food items' nutrition facts. Users can compare items for their nutrition benefit and cost. Other applications give information on portion sizes and adjustments needed to reduce calories, sodium, or fat in the diet based on the user's height, weight, and activity level.

## TABLE 39-9 Nutritional Therapy

### *MyPlate Tips for a Healthy Lifestyle*

*Making food choices for a healthy lifestyle can be as simple as using these 10 tips. Use the ideas in this list to (1) balance your calories, (2) choose foods to eat more often, and (3) cut back on foods to eat less often.*

| | |
|---|---|
| 1. **Balance calories** | • Find out how many calories you need for a day as a first step in managing your weight. Go to *www.choosemyplate.gov* to find your calorie level.<br>• Being physically active also helps you balance calories. |
| 2. **Enjoy your food, but eat less** | • Take the time to enjoy your food as you eat it.<br>• Eating too fast or when your attention is elsewhere may lead to eating too many calories.<br>• Pay attention to hunger and fullness cues before, during, and after meals. Use them to recognize when to eat and when you have had enough. |
| 3. **Avoid oversized portions** | • Use a smaller plate, bowl, and glass.<br>• Portion out foods before you eat.<br>• When eating out, choose a smaller size option, share a dish, or take home part of your meal. |
| 4. **Foods to eat more often** | • Eat more vegetables, fruits, whole grains, and fat-free or 1% milk and dairy products.<br>• These foods have the nutrients you need for health, including potassium, calcium, vitamin D, and fiber.<br>• Make them the basis for meals and snacks. |
| 5. **Make half your plate fruits and vegetables** | • Choose red, orange, and dark-green vegetables such as tomatoes, sweet potatoes, and broccoli, along with other vegetables, for your meals.<br>• Add fruit to meals as part of main or side dishes or as dessert. |
| 6. **Switch to fat-free or low-fat (1%) milk** | • They have the same amount of calcium and other essential nutrients as whole milk.<br>• They have fewer calories and less saturated fat. |
| 7. **Make half your grains whole grains** | • To eat more whole grains, substitute a whole-grain product for a refined product.<br>• For example, eat whole-wheat bread instead of white bread, or brown rice instead of white rice. |
| 8. **Foods to eat less often** | • Cut back on foods high in solid fats, added sugars, and salt.<br>• They include cakes, cookies, ice cream, candies, sweetened drinks, pizza, and fatty meats like ribs, sausages, bacon, and hot dogs.<br>• Use these foods as occasional treats, not everyday foods. |
| 9. **Compare sodium in foods** | • Use the Nutrition Facts label (Fig. 39-4) to choose lower sodium versions of foods such as soup, bread, and frozen meals.<br>• Select foods labeled "low sodium," "reduced sodium," or "no salt added." |
| 10. **Drink water instead of sugary drinks** | • Cut calories by drinking water or unsweetened beverages.<br>• Soda, energy drinks, and sports drinks are a major source of added sugar and calories in American diets. |

Source: US Department of Agriculture Center for Nutrition Policy and Promotion: Nutrition education series, DG Tips Sheet No 1, June 2011. Retrieved from *www.choosemyplate.gov* and *www.health.gov/dietaryguidelines*.

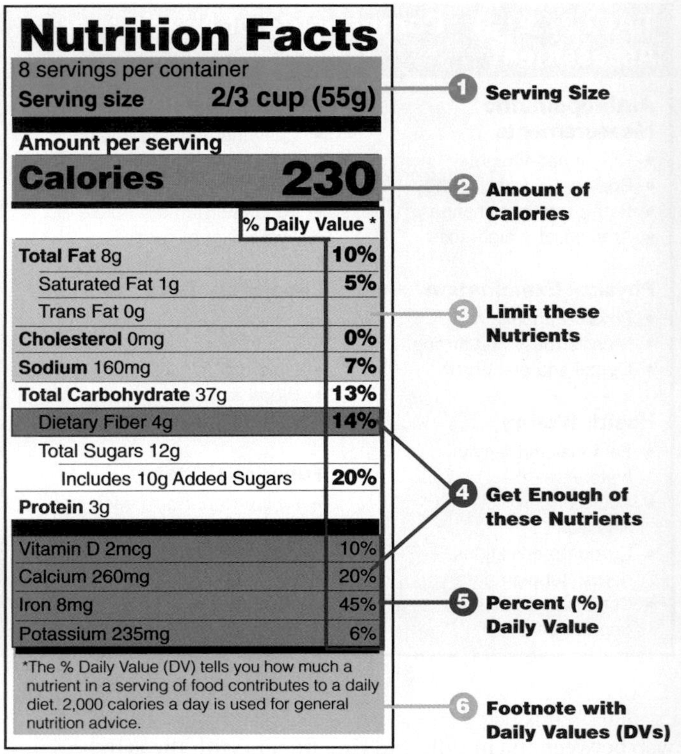


For educational purposes only. This label does not meet the labeling requirements described in 21 CFR 101.9.

**FIG. 39-4** Sample of a Nutrition Facts label. (US Department of Health and Human Services, Nutrition Facts Label, Silver Spring, Md.)

◆ **Acute Care.** Collaborate with the HCP and dietitian to identify malnutrition and implement appropriate interventions to meet the patient's nutritional needs. Assess the patient's nutritional state during your assessment of the patient's other physical problems. Identify risk factors for malnutrition and why they exist. With increased stress, such as surgery, severe trauma, and sepsis, the patient needs more calories and protein. Wound healing requires increased protein synthesis. The patient undergoing major surgery who is malnourished or is at risk for malnutrition needs several weeks of increased protein and calorie intake preoperatively to promote healing postoperatively.

Teach the patient and caregiver the importance of good nutrition and the rationale for recording the daily weight, intake, and output. Measure weight and height on admission, and routinely assess and document the person's weight. Daily weights give an ongoing record of body weight gain or loss. Rapid gains and losses are usually the result of shifts in fluid balance. In conjunction with accurate recording of food and fluid intake, the body weight provides a clearer picture of the patient's fluid and nutritional state.

If the patient is able to take food by mouth, obtain a daily calorie count and diet diary to give an accurate record of food intake. You and the dietitian can assist the patient and family in selecting high-calorie and high-protein foods (unless medically contraindicated). Table 39-10 gives examples of high-calorie, high-protein foods. Offering foods preferred by the patient enhances intake. Encourage the family to bring the patient's favorite foods from home.

Make sure the environment is conducive to eating. Provide a quiet environment. Offer oral hygiene and provide hand

**TABLE 39-10 Nutritional Therapy**

***High-Calorie, High-Protein Diet***

*Suggestions for high-calorie, high-protein foods include the following.*

**Breads and Cereals**
- Hot cereals (oatmeal, cream of wheat) prepared with milk, added fat (butter or margarine), and sugar
- Potatoes prepared with added fat (butter and whole milk)
- Granola and other cereals with dried fruit
- Croissants, buttermilk biscuits, muffins, banana bread, zucchini bread

**Vegetables**
- Vegetables prepared with added fat (margarine, butter)
- Fried vegetables

**Fruits**
- Canned fruit in heavy syrup
- Dried fruit

**Meat**
- Fried meats
- Meats covered in cream sauces or gravy
- Casseroles

**Milk and Milk Products**
- Milkshakes
- Whole milk and milk products (yogurt, ice cream, cheese)
- Whipping cream or heavy cream
- Whole milk with added nutritional supplements

hygiene. Assist the patient to a comfortable position and place the bedside table at the appropriate height. Clear the bedside table of clutter. Place urinals, bedpans, and emesis basins out of sight. If needed, open cartons and packages. Protect mealtime from unnecessary interruptions by performing non-urgent care before or after mealtime.

The undernourished patient usually needs to have between-meal supplements. These may consist of items prepared in the dietary department or commercially prepared products. Eating these items provides extra calories, proteins, fluids, and nutrients. If the patient is unable to consume enough nutrition with a high-calorie, high-protein diet, consider adding oral liquid nutritional supplements.

Some patients may benefit from appetite stimulants such as megestrol acetate (Megace) or dronabinol (Marinol) to improve nutritional intake. If the patient is still unable to take in enough calories, enteral feedings may be considered (Fig. 39-5). Contraindications for enteral nutrition include GI obstruction, prolonged ileus, severe diarrhea or vomiting, and enterocutaneous fistula. If enteral feedings are not feasible, consider initiating parenteral nutrition (PN).

**Ambulatory Care.** Many patients are discharged on a therapeutic diet. Discharge preparation for both the patient and caregiver is essential. Teach them about the cause of the undernourished state and ways to avoid the problem in the future. They need to be aware that undernourishment, whatever the cause, can recur and that adhering to a diet high in protein and calories for a few weeks cannot fully restore a normal nutritional state. It may take many months to reach this goal.

Assess their ability to comply with the dietary instructions in light of past eating habits, religious and ethnic preferences, age, income, other resources, and state of health. Emphasize the need for continual follow-up care to accomplish and maintain rehabilitation. In the discharge planning, ensure proper follow-up such as visits by the home health nurse and outpatient dietitian referrals.

Determine the need for nutritious meals and snacks after discharge from the hospital. Access to a dietitian may be limited and you may be the primary source of nutritional information. In your assessment, consider the availability and acceptability of community resources that provide meals such as Meals on Wheels, senior congregate feeding sites, and the Supplemental Nutrition Assistance Program (SNAP, formerly known as Food Stamps). Help the patient identify reliable Internet sources that provide evidence-based food and nutrition recommendations.

Keeping a diet diary for 3 days at a time is one way to analyze and reinforce healthful eating patterns. These records are also helpful to the interprofessional care team in the follow-up care. Encourage self-assessment of progress by having the patient weigh himself or herself once or twice a week and keep a weight record.

## Evaluation

The expected outcomes are that the patient who is malnourished will

- Achieve and maintain optimal body weight
- Consume a well-balanced diet
- Experience no adverse outcomes related to malnutrition
- Maintain optimal physical functioning

## Gerontologic Considerations: Malnutrition

Nutrition affects quality of life, functional status, and health in older adults. They are particularly vulnerable to malnutrition across care settings. You play an important role in assessing the physiologic, functional, environmental, dietary, psychologic, and social factors related to nutritional risk in older adults.[10] Older hospitalized adults with malnutrition are more likely to have poor wound healing, pressure ulcers, infections, decreased muscle strength, postoperative complications, and increased morbidity and mortality risks. They are less able to regain body weight after periods of undernutrition due to illness or surgery.

Older adults may report little or no appetite, problems with eating or swallowing, inadequate servings of nutrients, and fewer than two meals per day. Limited incomes may cause them to restrict the number of meals or the dietary quality of meals eaten. Social isolation is a problem in older adults. Those who live alone may lose their desire to cook and report decreased appetite. Functional limitations may affect the ability to feed oneself, purchase food, or cook and prepare meals.[10] Some may lack transportation to buy food.

Chronic illnesses associated with aging can also affect nutritional status. For example, depression and dysphagia (secondary to stroke) can affect intake. Poor oral health from cavities, gum disease (gingivitis), and missing teeth, as well as *xerostomia* (dry mouth), can impair the older adult's ability to lubricate, masticate, and swallow food. Medications can cause dry mouth, alter the taste of food, or decrease appetite.

Physiologic changes associated with aging include a decrease in lean body mass and redistribution of fat around internal organs, which can decrease caloric requirements. Sarcopenia (loss of lean body mass with aging) affects muscle strength and function.[14] Older adults on bed rest or prolonged inactivity lose more lean body mass than younger adults.[15] Changes in odor and taste perception (from medications, nutrient deficiencies, or taste-bud atrophy) can alter nutritional status.

Daily requirements for healthy older adults for maintaining weight include 30 cal/kg of body weight and 0.8 to 1 g/kg of protein per day, with no more than 30% of calories from fat. Requirements may differ depending on the degree of malnutrition and physiologic stress. To prevent loss of muscle mass and

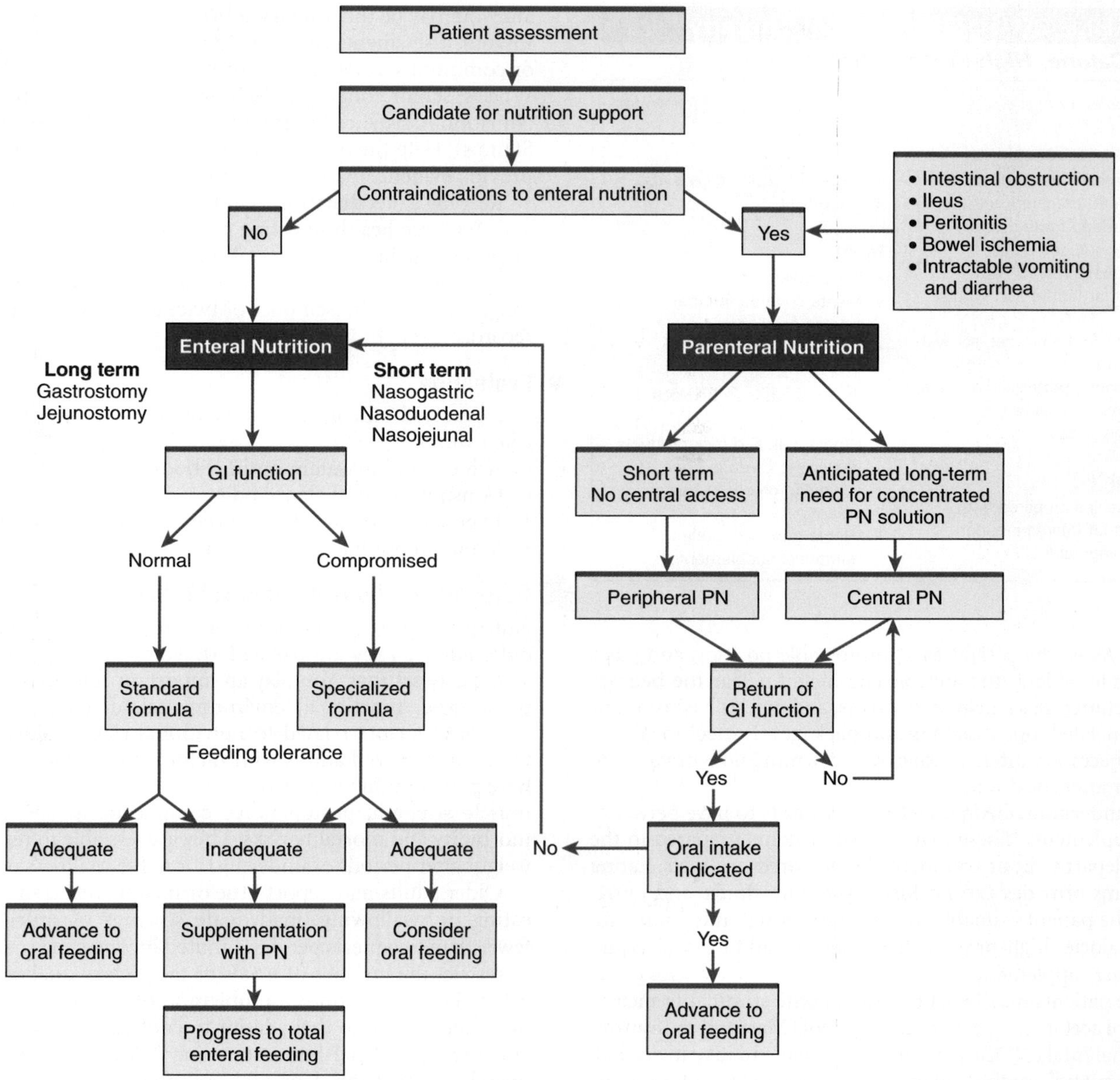


**FIG. 39-5** Nutritional support algorithm. (Adapted from Ukleja A, Freeman KL, Gilbert K, and the ASPEN Board of Directors: Standards for nutrition support: adult hospitalized patients, *Nutr Clin Pract* 25:403, 2010.)

maintain function, older adults should consume a moderate amount of high-quality protein at each meal.[14] Daily vitamin D requirements are higher for older adults (Table 39-6).

Focus your initial care strategies on improving oral intake and providing a stimulating environment for meals. Special strategies, such as use of adaptive devices (e.g., such as large-handled eating utensils often are helpful in increasing the patient's dietary intake).

Oral liquid supplements have a role in improving the nutritional status of older adults. Do not use supplements as meal substitutes, rather use them as snacks between meals. In long-term care, using these beverages instead of water for oral medication administration increases caloric intake. Some older adults may require nutritional support therapies until their strength and general health improve. Before starting any nutritional support therapy (e.g., enteral or parenteral nutrition) for an older patient unable to give consent, review his or her advance directives regarding the use of artificial nutrition and hydration.

Malnourished or nutritionally at-risk older adults are vulnerable when discharged from the hospital to the home. Older adults may not be able to shop for or prepare foods during the initial recovery period.[10] Consult with the social worker and dietitian to ensure the older adult has access to food on discharge. Home-delivered meals or senior congregate feeding programs are an appropriate referral. Many community nutritional programs are available to the older person to make mealtime a pleasant, social event. Improving the social setting of a meal frequently improves dietary intake. SNAP is another alternative that allows low-income households, regardless of age, to buy more food of a greater variety.

Older adults with dementia or a stroke present unique nursing challenges with regard to eating and feeding. (Dementia is discussed in Chapter 59; strokes are discussed in Chapter 57.)

## SPECIALIZED NUTRITIONAL SUPPORT

If patients are unable to maintain or achieve adequate nutritional status, nutritional support may be necessary. For a decision-making plan related to nutritional support, see Fig. 39-5.

Some institutions have nutritional support teams composed of a physician, nurse, dietitian, and pharmacist. The team's function is to oversee the nutritional support of select inpatients and outpatients. The nutritional support nurse on that team is a key resource for issues regarding patients' nutrition and nutritional access.

### Oral Feeding

Oral supplements are used as an adjunct to meals and fluid intake in the patient whose nutritional intake is deficient. They provide advanced nutrition and calories and are relatively inexpensive. These include milkshakes, puddings, or commercially available products (e.g., Carnation Instant Breakfast, Ensure, Boost).

### Enteral Nutrition

**Enteral nutrition (EN)**, also known as **tube feeding**, is nutrition (e.g., a nutritionally balanced liquefied food or formula) delivered into the GI tract distal to the oral cavity via a tube, catheter, or stoma. EN is used with the patient who has a functioning GI tract but is unable to take any or enough oral nourishment, or when it is unsafe to do so.

Indications for EN include persons with anorexia, orofacial fractures, head and neck cancer, neurologic or psychiatric conditions that prevent oral intake, extensive burns, or critical illness (especially if mechanical ventilation is required), and those receiving chemotherapy or radiation therapy. EN is easily administered, safer, more physiologically efficient, and less expensive than parenteral nutrition (PN).

There is a wide variety of enteral formulas. Their concentration, flavor, osmolality, and amounts of protein, sodium, and fat vary. There are special formulas for patients with diabetes and liver, kidney, or lung disease. Most are lactose free. Concentrations range from 1 to 2 cal/mL. Most standard formulas provide between 1 and 1.5 cal/mL. The more calorically dense the formula, the less water it contains. The number and size of particles in the formula determines its osmolality. The more hydrolyzed or broken down the nutrients, the greater the osmolality.

A formula with a high sodium content is contraindicated in the patient with cardiovascular problems, such as heart failure. Those with short bowel syndrome or ileocecal resection should not receive one with a high fat content because of impaired fat absorption. Patients receiving feedings with a protein content greater than 16% require supplemental fluids through the feeding tube or by mouth (if permitted) to avoid dehydration.

Common delivery options are continuous infusion or cyclic feedings by infusion pump, intermittent infusion by gravity, and intermittent bolus by syringe. Critically ill patients often receive EN by continuous infusion. Intermittent feeding may be preferred as the patient improves or is receiving EN at home.[16]

Nasally and orally placed tubes (orogastric, nasogastric [NG], nasoduodenal, or nasojejunal) are appropriate for short-term feeding (less than 4 weeks). Nasoduodenal and nasojejunal tubes are transpyloric tubes. They are used when pathophysiologic conditions such as risk of aspiration warrant feeding the patient below the pyloric sphincter. If feedings are necessary for an extended time, tubes are placed in the stomach or small bowel by surgical, endoscopic, or fluoroscopic procedures. Fig. 39-6 shows the locations of commonly used enteral feeding tubes.

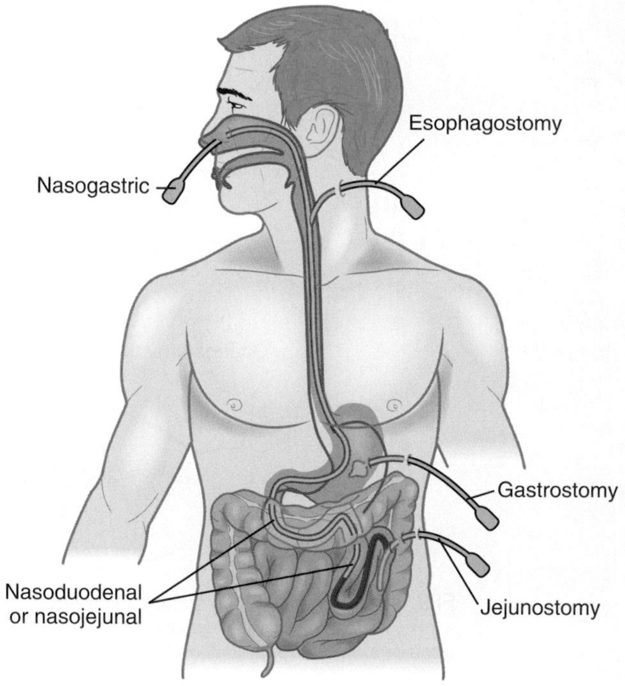


**FIG. 39-6** Common enteral feeding tube placement locations.

**Orogastric, Nasogastric, and Nasointestinal Tubes.** Polyurethane or silicone feeding tubes are long, small in diameter, soft, and flexible. This design decreases the risk of mucosal damage from prolonged placement. These tubes are radiopaque, making their position readily identified by x-ray. Placement into the small intestine decreases the chance of regurgitating gastric contents into the esophagus and subsequent aspiration.[16] However, the patient can still aspirate gastric secretions if the stomach is not emptying properly. A stylet is used for tube placement in a comatose patient because the ability to swallow is not essential during insertion. A complication that can result from using a stylet is increased risk for perforation.

Although smaller feeding tubes have many advantages over wider-lumen tubes, such as the standard decompression NG tube, there are some disadvantages. Because of the small diameter, these tubes clog easily when feedings are thick. They are more difficult to use for checking residual volumes. They are particularly prone to obstruction if you do not thoroughly crush and dissolve oral drugs before administration. Failure to flush the tubing before and after both drug administration and residual volume determination can result in tube clogging. Vomiting or coughing can dislodge the tubes. They can become knotted or kinked. Problems with a tube may necessitate removal and insertion of a new tube, which adds to cost and patient discomfort.

**Gastrostomy and Jejunostomy Tubes.** A gastrostomy tube may be used when a patient requires EN for an extended time (Fig. 39-6). Gastrostomy tubes can be placed surgically, radiologically, or endoscopically. The patient must have an intact, unobstructed GI tract. The esophageal lumen must be wide enough to pass the endoscope for percutaneous endoscopic gastrostomy (PEG) tube placement (Fig. 39-7). PEG tube and radiologically placed gastrostomy tube procedures have fewer risks than

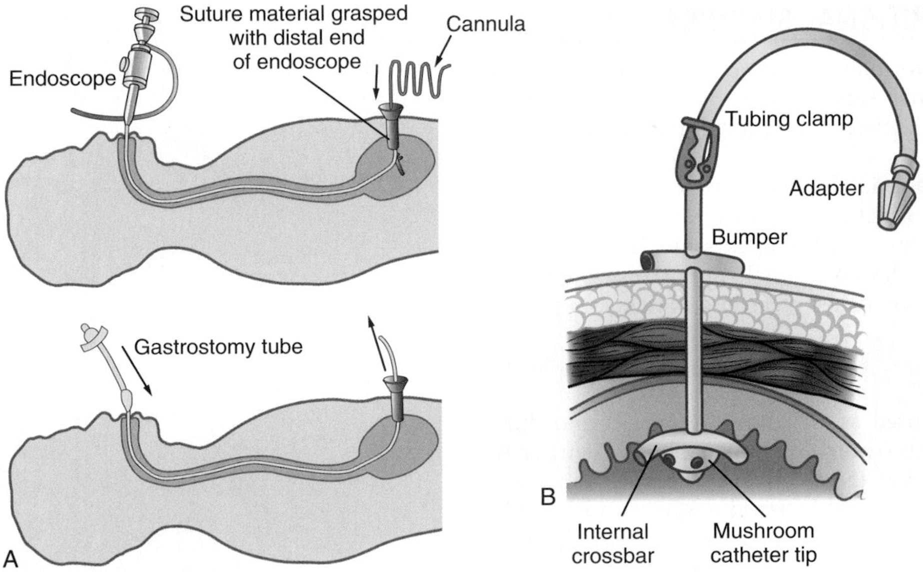


**FIG. 39-7** Percutaneous endoscopic gastrostomy. **A,** Gastrostomy tube placement via percutaneous endoscopy. With use of endoscopy, a gastrostomy tube is inserted through the esophagus into the stomach and then pulled through a stab wound made in the abdominal wall. **B,** A retention disk and bumper secure the tube.

surgical placement. The procedure requires IV sedation and local anesthesia. IV antibiotics are given before the procedure.

For the patient with chronic reflux, feeding through a jejunostomy (J-tube) may be necessary to reduce the risk of aspiration. Jejunostomy tubes are placed either endoscopically or with open or laparoscopic surgery. Combination gastrojejunostomy (G-J) tubes allow for simultaneous gastric decompression and small bowel feeding. When a patient has a G-J tube, it is important to know which port is the gastric and which is the jejunal.

Enteral feedings can start within 24 to 48 hours after a surgically placed gastrostomy or jejunostomy tube without waiting for flatus or a bowel movement. Most PEG tube feeding can start within 2 hours of insertion, although the institution's policies may vary.[17] The feeding tube is either premarked or marked at the skin insertion site.

**Tube Feedings and Safety.** You have a critical role in ensuring that tube feedings are administered safely. Aspiration and dislodged tubes are two important safety concerns. Nursing management of tube feedings is addressed in Table 39-11.

Accidental tube removal can result in delayed feedings and potential discomfort with tube replacement. The management of common problems in patients receiving tube feedings is presented in Table 39-12. A nursing care plan for the patient receiving enteral nutrition (eNCP 39-1) is available on the website for this chapter.

Specific care and teaching related to feeding tubes and enteral nutrition are summarized in the following section. Remember that is important to teach the patient and caregiver how to care for the feeding tube and properly administer enteral nutrition.

***Patient Position.*** Proper patient positioning decreases the risk of aspiration. To prevent aspiration, elevate the head of bed to a minimum of 30 degrees, but preferably 45 degrees. If the patient does not tolerate a backrest elevation, use a reverse Trendelenburg position to elevate the head of the bed, unless contraindicated. If you need to lower the head of the bed for a procedure, return the patient to an elevated position as soon as possible. Follow the institution's policy for suspending feeding while the patient is supine. If intermittent delivery is used, the head should remain elevated for 30 to 60 minutes after feeding.

**TABLE 39-11 Nursing Management of Tube Feedings**

1. Check tube placement before feeding and before each drug administration.
2. Assess for bowel sounds before feeding.
3. Use liquid medications rather than pills.
   - Dilute viscous liquid medications.
   - Do not add medications to enteral feeding formula.
4. If using tablets, crush drugs to a fine powder and dissolve in water to avoid clogging feeding tubes.
5. Follow measures to decrease aspiration risk:
   - Keep head of bed elevated to 30- to 45-degree angle.
   - Check for residual volumes per facility policy.
6. Assess regularly for complications (e.g., aspiration, diarrhea, abdominal distention, hyperglycemia, constipation, and fecal impaction).

***Aspiration Risk.*** Evaluate all enterally fed patients for risk of aspiration. Before starting tube feedings, ensure the tube is in the proper position. Maintain head-of-bed elevation as described above. Checking gastric residual volumes is important when giving feedings into the stomach. An increased residual volume increases the risk for aspiration of the formula into the lungs.[16]

Check gastric residual volumes every 4 hours during the first 48 hours for gastrically fed patients. After attaining the enteral feeding rate goal, decrease gastric residual monitoring to every 6 to 8 hours in non–critically ill patients or continue every 4 hours in critically ill patients. Promotility drugs such as erythromycin or metoclopramide improve gastric emptying and may reduce aspiration risk. Feeding tubes may need to be advanced below the ligament of Treitz (jejunostomy) if gastric residual volumes consistently measure more than 500 mL. Do not obtain residual volumes for EN delivered through a jejunostomy tube.

### TABLE 39-12 Management of Tube Feeding Problems

| Problems and Causes | Management |
|---|---|
| **Vomiting** | |
| Improper placement of tube | • Replace tube in proper position.<br>• Check tube position before beginning feeding and every 4 hr if continuous feedings. |
| Delayed gastric emptying, increased residual volume | • If gastric residual volume is ≥250 mL after second gastric residual check, consider a promotility drug.<br>• If gastric residual volume is >500 mL, hold feeding and reassess patient tolerance.<br>• Advance tube below the ligament of Treitz if gastric residual volume consistently remains >500 mL. |
| **Dehydration** | |
| Excessive diarrhea, vomiting | • Decrease rate or change formula.<br>• Check drugs that patient is receiving, especially antibiotics.<br>• Avoid bacterial contamination of formula and equipment. |
| Poor fluid intake | • Increase intake and check amount and number of feedings.<br>• Increase amount of fluid intake if appropriate. |
| High-protein formula | • Change formula to one with less protein. |
| Hyperosmotic diuresis | • Check blood glucose levels frequently.<br>• Change formula to one with less glucose. |
| **Diarrhea** | |
| Feeding too fast | • Dilute or decrease rate of feeding.<br>• Change to continuous drip feedings.<br>• Discontinue excess water boluses. |
| Infection | • Obtain stool culture for fecal leukocyte determination, *C. difficile,* and/or toxin assay. |
| Medications | • Check for drugs that may cause diarrhea (e.g., sorbitol in liquid medications, antibiotics). |
| Low-fiber formula | • Change to formula with more fiber. |
| Tube moving distally | • Properly secure tube before beginning feeding.<br>• Check placement before each feeding or at least every 24 hr if continuous feedings. |
| Contaminated formula | • Refrigerate unused formula and record date opened.<br>• Discard outdated formula.<br>• Discard formula left standing for longer than manufacturer's guidelines.<br>  • 8 hr for ready-to-feed formulas (cans)<br>  • 4 hr for reconstituted formula<br>  • 24-48 hr for closed-system enteral formulas<br>• Use closed system to prevent contamination. |
| **Constipation** | |
| Formula components | • Change formula to one with more fiber content.<br>• Give as-needed laxative. |
| Poor fluid intake | • Increase fluid intake if not contraindicated.<br>• Give total fluid intake of 30 mL/kg body weight. |
| Drugs | • Check for drugs that may be constipating. |
| Impaction | • Perform rectal examinations and manually remove feces if present. |
| Inactivity | • Encourage ambulation unless contraindicated.<br>• Collaborate with physical therapy to promote activity. |

## TEAMWORK & COLLABORATION

### *Nasogastric and Gastric Tubes and Enteral Feedings*

**Role of Nursing Personnel**

***Registered Nurse (RN)***

- Insert nasogastric (NG) tube for unstable patient.
- Irrigate NG or gastrostomy tube for unstable patient.
- Insert nasointestinal tube.
- Give bolus or continuous enteral feeding for unstable patient.
- Give medications through the NG or gastrostomy tube to unstable patient.
- Evaluate nutritional status of patient receiving enteral feedings.
- Monitor for complications related to tubes and enteral feedings.
- Develop plan for gastrostomy or jejunostomy tube care.
- Teach patient and caregiver about home enteral feeding and gastrostomy or jejunostomy tube care.
- Evaluate for therapeutic effect of NG tube connected to suction (e.g., decreased nausea or distention).

***Licensed Practical/Vocational Nurse (LPN/LVN)***

- Insert NG tube for stable patient.
- Irrigate NG and gastrostomy tubes.
- Give bolus or continuous enteral feeding for stable patient.
- Remove NG tube.
- Give medications through NG or gastrostomy tube to stable patient.
- Provide skin care around gastrostomy or jejunostomy tubes.

***Unlicensed Assistive Personnel (UAP)***

- Provide oral care to patient with NG, gastrostomy, or jejunostomy tube.
- Weigh patient who is receiving enteral feeding.
- Position and maintain patient receiving enteral feeding with the head of bed elevated.
- Notify RN or LPN about patient symptoms (e.g., nausea, diarrhea) that may indicate problems with enteral feedings.
- Alert RN or LPN about enteral feeding infusion pump alarms.
- Empty drainage devices and measure output.

**Role of Other Team Members**

***Dietitian***

- Evaluate nutritional status of patient receiving enteral feedings.
- Select appropriate enteral feeding formula.
- Monitor for and manage complications related to enteral feedings.
- Teach patient and caregiver about home enteral feedings.

***Tube Position.*** Obtain x-ray confirmation of newly inserted nasal or orogastric tubes (small bore or large bore) to confirm proper position in the GI tract before administering feedings or medications. Smaller feeding tubes can pass directly into the bronchus on insertion without any obvious respiratory manifestations. Do not rely on the auscultation method to differentiate between gastric and respiratory or gastric and small bowel placement. Placing a tube under electromagnetic guidance is associated with reduced tube misplacement.[18] Capnography, a direct monitor of breath-to-breath $CO_2$ level, can determine tube placement in the respiratory tract. However, it still requires x-ray confirmation to verify location before feeding.[16]

Maintain proper placement of the tube after starting feedings. A small bowel tube may dislocate upward into the stomach or the tube's tip can dislocate upward into the esophagus. To determine if a feeding tube is still in the proper position, mark the exit site of the feeding tube at the time of the initial x-ray and check the tube external length at regular intervals.

Observe for negative pressure when attempting to withdraw fluid from the feeding tube.[17] You are more likely to feel negative pressure during attempts to aspirate fluid from a small bowel than from a gastric tube. Observe for unexpected changes in residual volume. An increase in gastric residual volume may indicate displacement of a small intestine tube into the stomach.[17] If you see a significant increase in the external length, use other bedside tests to help determine whether the tube has become dislocated. These measures include assessing aspirate color and pH. Because each of these measures has limitations, confirm placement with more than one test. Consider applying a nasal bridle in patients who attempt to pull out a tube or for whom taping the nose is difficult.

***Site Care.*** Skin care around gastrostomy and jejunostomy tube sites is important because the action of digestive juices irritates the skin. Daily assess the skin around the feeding tube for signs of redness and maceration. Monitor bumper tension and routinely check for pressure injury.

## BECOMING A NURSE LEADER

### Practicing Safe Delegation

**Situation**

It is the beginning of a hectic shift on a medical-surgical unit. You are a new RN and have a full patient care assignment. You observe Janet, a fellow RN, whispering something to Tony, the unlicensed assistive personnel (UAP). Immediately thereafter, you see Tony going into Mr. Jade's room with his enteral feeding and a medication cup. You carefully watch from the hallway as you see Tony inserting the medication and enteral feeding into Mr. Jade's NG tube. Although you realize that all of you are very busy, Tony is not qualified to administer medications or enteral feedings.

**Points for Consideration**

- The RN may delegate components of care but certain nursing functions cannot be delegated or assigned to UAP.[1]
- The RN uses critical thinking and professional judgment when following the Five Rights of Delegation (see Table 1-7) to be sure that the delegation or assignment is:
  - The right task
  - Under the right circumstances
  - To the right person
  - With the right directions and communication
  - Under the right supervision and evaluation
- RNs decide what patient care interventions are necessary and how, when, and by whom these interventions need to be provided.
- Effective delegation is based on one's state nurse practice act and an understanding of the concepts of responsibility, authority, and accountability.
- Each person involved in the delegation process is accountable for his or her own actions or inaction and is potentially liable if competent and safe care is not provided.[2]

**Discussion Questions**

1. Why is it inappropriate to delegate the administrations of medication or enteral feedings via an NG tube to Tony?
2. Who could be liable in this situation? Why?
3. What action should you take after you witnessed what Tony did?

**References**

1. American Nurses Association (ANA) and the National Council of State Boards of Nursing (NCSBN). Retrieved from *www.ncsbn.org/Delegation_joint_statement_NCSBN-ANA.pdf.*
2. Anderson L: General guidelines to effective delegation in nursing. Retrieved from *www.nursetogether.com/guidelines-to-effective-nursing-delegation.*

To keep the skin clean and dry, initially rinse it with sterile water and dry it. Apply a dressing until the site is healed. After that, wash with mild soap and water. A protective ointment (zinc oxide, petroleum gauze) or a skin barrier (Karaya, Stomahesive) may be used on the skin around the tube. If the skin is irritated, consider using other types of drain or tube pouches. A wound, ostomy, and continence nurse (WOCN) can provide assistance if issues arise.

***Tube Patency.*** All enteral feedings require routine flushing. Flush feedings tubes in adults with 30 mL of warm tap water every 4 hours during continuous feedings or before and after each intermittent feeding. Use sterile water in immunocompromised and critically ill patients. Always flush tubes between each medication and after all medications are given. Try to only use liquid medications and do not mix medications.[17] Flush clogged tubes with warm water, using a back-and-forth motion.

***Misconnection.*** An *enteral feeding misconnection* is an inadvertent connection between an enteral feeding system and a nonenteral system such as an IV line, a peritoneal dialysis catheter, or a tracheostomy tube cuff. With an enteral feeding misconnection, nutritional formula intended for the GI tract is given IV or into the respiratory tract. Severe patient injury and death can result from tubing misconnection. Table 39-13 provides tips to decrease the risk of enteral feeding misconnections.

### Gerontologic Considerations: Enteral Nutrition

EN feeding strategies are used in the older patient to improve nutritional status. Because of physiologic changes associated with aging, the older adult is more vulnerable to complications associated with nutritional interventions, especially fluid and

**TABLE 39-13 Decreasing Enteral Feeding Misconnections**

*The following are tips to help you decrease your risk of making an enteral tube feeding misconnection.*

1. Teach visitors, LPN/LVNs, and UAP to notify nurse if an enteral feeding line becomes disconnected and not to reconnect any line.
2. Do not modify or adapt IV or feeding devices, because you may compromise the safety features incorporated into their design.
3. Do not use an IV pump or IV tubing to deliver an enteral feeding.
4. When making a reconnection or connecting any new device or infusion, trace lines back to their origins and ensure connections are secure.
5. When patient arrives on a new unit or setting or during shift handoff, recheck connections and trace all tubes.
6. Route tubes and catheters that have different purposes in unique and standardized directions (e.g., route IV lines toward the patient's head and enteral lines toward the feet).
7. Package together all parts needed for enteral feeding and reduce the availability of additional adapters and connectors. This will minimize the availability of dissimilar tubes or catheters that could be improperly connected.
8. Label or color-code feeding tubes and connectors. Teach staff about the labeling or color-coding process in the institution's enteral feeding system.
9. When there are several access points and/or several bags hanging, place proximal and distal labels on all tubings.
10. Check the patient's vital signs after making any connection.
11. Identify and confirm a solution's label, since a three-in-one parenteral nutrition solution can appear similar to an enteral nutrition formulation bag. Label the bags with large, bold statements such as "WARNING! For Enteral Use Only—NOT for IV Use."
12. Make all connections under proper lighting conditions.

**TABLE 39-14 Common Indications for Parenteral Nutrition**

| | |
|---|---|
| • Chronic severe diarrhea and vomiting | • Severe anorexia nervosa |
| • Complicated surgery or trauma | • Severe malabsorption |
| • GI obstruction | • Short bowel syndrome |
| • Intractable diarrhea | • GI tract anomalies and fistulae |

electrolyte imbalances. Complications such as diarrhea can leave the patient dehydrated. Decreased thirst perception or impaired cognitive function decreases the patient's ability to seek additional fluids.

With aging, there is an increased risk of glucose intolerance. As a result, the older patient may be more susceptible to hyperglycemia in response to the high carbohydrate load of some EN formulas. The older adult with compromised cardiovascular function (e.g., heart failure) will have a decreased ability to handle large volumes of formula. If this happens, the patient may need a more concentrated formula (2.0 cal/mL). The older adult has an increased risk for aspiration caused by gastroesophageal reflux disease (GERD), delayed gastric emptying, hiatal hernia, or diminished gag reflex. Physical mobility, fine motor movement, and visual system changes associated with aging may contribute to difficulties in managing EN in the home setting.

## Parenteral Nutrition

**Parenteral nutrition (PN)** is the administration of nutrients directly into the bloodstream. PN is used when the GI tract cannot be used for the ingestion, digestion, and absorption of essential nutrients. Table 39-14 lists common indications for the use of PN. PN is a relatively safe method of providing complete nutritional support.

**Composition.** PN is customized to meet the needs of each patient. The composition is reformulated as the patient's condition changes. This requires you to collaborate with the interprofessional team in delivering PN to the patient.

Commercially prepared PN base solutions are available. These base solutions contain dextrose and protein in the form of amino acids. The pharmacy adds prescribed electrolytes (e.g., sodium, potassium, chloride, calcium, magnesium, and phosphate), vitamins, and trace elements (e.g., zinc, copper, chromium, and manganese) to meet the patient's needs. A three-in-one or total nutrient admixture containing an IV fat emulsion, dextrose, and amino acids is widely used. Premixed PN solutions are relatively new and require manipulation of the dextrose and amino acid chambers prior to use. Standard electrolytes are available in some premixed solutions; multivitamins are added prior to use.[19]

**Calories.** Calories in PN are supplied primarily by carbohydrates in the form of dextrose and by fat in the form of fat emulsion. The administration of 100 to 150 g of dextrose daily (1 g provides approximately 3.4 calories, as opposed to oral carbohydrates, which provide 4 calories) has a protein-sparing effect. Providing adequate nonprotein calories in the form of glucose and fat allows the use of amino acids for wound healing and not for energy. However, overfeeding can lead to metabolic complications. To minimize these problems, the recommended energy intake is 25 to 35 cal/kg/day in a nonobese patient.

Fat-emulsion solutions of 10%, 20%, and 30% are available. Fat emulsions provide approximately 1 cal/mL (10% solution) or 2 cal/mL (20% solution). Fat emulsions primarily contain soybean or safflower triglycerides with egg phospholipids added as an emulsifier. They provide a large number of calories in a relatively small amount of fluid. This is beneficial when the patient is at risk for fluid overload.

IV fat emulsions should provide up to 20% to 30% of total calories of PN. Most stable patients receive 1 g/kg/day. The maximum daily lipid dose is 2.5 g/kg/day. Critically ill patients may not tolerate this dose and may receive less than 1 g/kg/day. Serum triglyceride levels are done at the beginning of PN and then closely monitored. Give IV fat emulsions administered separately over 8 to 10 hours. The infusion rate should not exceed 0.11 g/kg/hr.[19]

Nausea, vomiting, and elevated temperature may occur, especially when lipids are infused quickly. Fat emulsions are contraindicated in the patient with a disturbance in fat metabolism such as hyperlipidemia. They are used cautiously in the patient at risk for fat embolism (e.g., fractured femur) and the patient with an allergy to eggs or soybeans.

**Protein.** The normal healthy person of average body size needs approximately 45 to 65 g of protein daily. Protein is provided at the rate of 1 to 1.5 g/kg/day depending on the patient's needs. In a nutritionally depleted patient who is under the stress of illness or surgery, protein requirements can exceed 150 g/day (1.5 to 2 g/kg/day) to ensure a positive nitrogen balance. Burn patients, who are often on PN, EN, and oral food, may need upward of 2 g/kg protein. Protein needs may be lower than 1 g/kg and restricted in those with end-stage renal disease who are not on dialysis.

**Electrolytes.** The exact amount of electrolytes needed depends on the patient's health problem and on serum electrolyte levels. Assess individual requirements daily at the beginning of therapy and then several times a week as the treatment progresses. The following are ranges for average daily electrolyte requirements for adult patients without renal or liver impairment:[19]

- Sodium: 1 to 2 mEq/kg
- Potassium: 1 to 2 mEq/kg
- Chloride: as needed to maintain acid-base balance
- Magnesium: 8 to 20 mEq
- Calcium: 10 to 15 mEq
- Phosphate: 20 to 40 mmol

**Trace Elements and Vitamins.** Zinc, copper, chromium, manganese, selenium, molybdenum, and iodine supplements may be added according to the patient's condition and needs. Monitor levels of these elements. The HCP may order additional amounts added to the PN. The daily addition of a multivitamin preparation to the PN generally meets the vitamin requirements.

**Methods of Administration.** PN is administered as central PN or peripheral parenteral nutrition (PPN). Central PN and PPN differ in nutrient content and tonicity, which is measured in milliosmoles (mOsm; the concentration of particles in a fluid).

***Central Parenteral Nutrition.*** *Central PN* is indicated when long-term support is necessary or when the patient has high protein and caloric requirements. Central PN is administered through a central venous catheter or a peripherally inserted central catheter (PICC) whose tip lies in the superior vena cava (see Chapter 16). Central PN solutions are hypertonic, measuring at least 1600 mOsm/L. The high glucose content ranges from 20% to 50%. Central PN must be infused in a large central vein so that rapid dilution can occur. The use of a peripheral vein for hypertonic, central PN solutions would cause irritation and thrombophlebitis.

***Peripheral Parenteral Nutrition.*** PPN is administered through a peripherally inserted catheter or vascular access device into a large vein. PPN is used when (1) nutritional support is needed for only a short time, (2) protein and caloric requirements are not high, (3) the risk of a central catheter is too great, or (4) PN is used to supplement inadequate oral intake.

Compared with central PN, PPN contains fewer nutrients. Although this makes PPN less hypertonic, it still has an osmolality of up to 800 mOsm/L. This increases the risk of phlebitis. Another potential complication is fluid overload. PPN requires large volumes of fluid, which many patients cannot tolerate.

## NURSING MANAGEMENT: PARENTERAL NUTRITION

Nursing management of patients receiving PN is presented in Table 39-15 and eNursing Care Plan 39-2 (available on the website for this chapter).

### Complications

Complications associated with PN are related either to the catheter or to the PN infusion itself (Table 39-16).

**Refeeding syndrome** is characterized by fluid retention a nd electrolyte imbalances (hypophosphatemia, hypokalemia,

**TABLE 39-15 Management of Parenteral Nutrition Infusions**

**Preparation of Parenteral Nutrition (PN) Solutions**
- All PN solutions must be prepared by a pharmacist or a trained technician using strict aseptic techniques under a laminar flow hood.
- Add nothing to PN solutions after they are prepared in the pharmacy. Danger of drug incompatibilities and contamination is high.
- Limit number of personnel involved in preparing and administering PN to reduce risk of infection.
- PN solutions are ordered daily to adjust to the patient's current needs.
- PN solution label indicates the nutrient content, all additives, time mixed, and date and time of expiration. In general, solutions are good for 24 hr and must be refrigerated until 30 min before use.

**Maintaining PN Infusions**
- Follow proper aseptic techniques to reduce infection risk.
- Use a 0.22-micron Millipore filter with parenteral solutions not containing fat emulsion and a 1.2-micron filter with solutions containing fat emulsion.
- Change filters and IV tubing q24 hr if giving PN with lipids and q72 hr for PN with amino acids and dextrose.
- Label tubing and filter with date and time they are put into use.
- If a multilumen catheter is present, use a dedicated line for PN.
- Control the infusion rate. Give PN using an infusion pump.
- Set an alarm to alert for tubing obstruction.
- Periodically check the volume infused because pump malfunctions can alter the rate.

**Catheter Site Care**
- Change dressings covering catheter site according to the institution's protocol.
- Carefully observe the catheter site for signs of inflammation and infection. Phlebitis can readily occur in the vein because of the hypertonic infusion, and the area can become infected.
- After the catheter is removed, change dressing daily and assess for wound healing.
- If an infection is suspected during a dressing change, send a culture specimen of the site and drainage and notify the HCP immediately.

**Ensuring Patient Safety**
- Before starting PN, check label and ingredients in solution to make sure they match what the HCP ordered.
- Examine the solution for leaks, color changes, particulate matter, clarity, and fat emulsions cracking (separating into layers). If present, promptly return it to the pharmacy for replacement.
- Discontinue a PN solution and replace it with a new solution if bag is not empty at the end of 24 hr. At room temperature, the solution (especially when containing fat emulsion) is a good medium for microorganism growth.
- If fat emulsions are infused separately from the PN solution, the preferred delivery method is a continuous low volume, such as 20% lipids delivered over 12 hr.
- Monitor for adverse reactions, including allergic manifestations, dyspnea, cyanosis, fever, flushing, phlebitis, chest and back pain, and pain at IV site.

**Hypoglycemia**
- If a PN formula bag should empty before the next solution is available, a 10% or 20% dextrose solution (based on the amount of dextrose in the central PN solution) or 5% dextrose solution (based on the amount of dextrose in the peripheral PN solution) can be given to prevent hypoglycemia.

**Hyperglycemia**
- Check glucose blood levels at bedside q4-6hr with glucose-testing meter.
- Maintain a glucose range of 110-150 mg/dL. Give sliding scale doses of insulin to keep the glucose level in normal range.
- Insulin can be added to the PN admixture, but the dosage will not be able to be changed for 24 hr.

**Catheter-Related Infections**
- Catheter-related infection and septicemia can occur. Local manifestations: erythema, tenderness, and exudate at the catheter insertion site. Systemic manifestations: fever, chills, nausea, vomiting, and malaise
- If no other causes can be identified, a catheter-related infection is suspected. Blood cultures are drawn. A chest x-ray is taken to detect changes in pulmonary status.
- Immunosuppressed patients are at high-risk for infection. Note subtle signs in patients receiving chemotherapy, corticosteroids, or antibiotics, which can mask signs of infection.
- To reduce the risk of infection, catheters with antibiotic or antiseptic surfaces may be used. Follow institutional central line infection prevention measures (see Chapter 16).
- Antibiotics may be prescribed. A new central line may or may not be placed depending on the patient's condition.

**Transitioning to Oral Nutrition**
- Encourage oral nourishment and maintain a careful record of intake. A general rule is that 60% of caloric needs should be met orally before discontinuation of PN.
- Begin with clear liquids and advance as tolerated to a soft diet.
- Limit full liquids because of an increased risk of lactose deficiency resulting in nausea, diarrhea, and bloating.

**Assessing Effectiveness**
- Monitor initial vital signs q4-8hr in the patient receiving PN.
- Weigh patient daily as a measure of the patient's hydration status.
- Maintain an accurate intake and output record.
- Determine the cause of any weight changes (e.g., fluid gained from edema, actual increase or decrease in tissue weight).
- Assess blood levels of glucose, electrolytes, and urea nitrogen.
- Complete blood count and hepatic enzyme studies are followed a minimum of three times per week until stable and then weekly as the patient's condition warrants.

**TABLE 39-16 Complications of Parenteral Nutrition**

| Metabolic Problems | Catheter-Related Problems |
|---|---|
| • Refeeding syndrome<br>• Hyperglycemia, hypoglycemia<br>• Altered renal function<br>• Essential fatty acid deficiency<br>• Liver dysfunction<br>• Hyperlipidemia | • Air embolus<br>• Pneumothorax, hemothorax, and hydrothorax<br>• Hemorrhage<br>• Dislodgment<br>• Thrombosis of vein<br>• Phlebitis<br>• Catheter-related sepsis<br>• Occlusion |

hypomagnesemia). Hypophosphatemia is the hallmark of refeeding syndrome and is associated with serious outcomes, including cardiac dysrhythmias, respiratory arrest, and neurologic disturbances (e.g., paresthesias). Conditions that predispose patients to refeeding syndrome include long-standing malnutrition states, such as chronic alcoholism, vomiting and diarrhea, chemotherapy, and major surgery. Refeeding syndrome can occur any time a malnourished patient starts aggressive nutritional support.

### Home Nutritional Support

Home PN or EN is an accepted mode of nutritional therapy for the person who does not require hospitalization but needs continued nutritional support. Some patients successfully receive home therapy for many months, even years. It is important for you to teach the patient and caregiver about catheter or tube care, proper technique in mixing and handling of the solutions and tubing, and side effects and complications.

Home nutritional therapies are expensive. Specific criteria must be met for expenses to be reimbursed. The discharge planning team must be involved early to help plan for such issues. Home nutritional support may be a burden for the patient and caregivers and affect quality of life. Tell the family about support groups such as the Oley Foundation *(www.oley.org)* that provide peer support and advocacy.

## EATING DISORDERS

*Eating disorders* are psychiatric conditions associated with physiologic alterations and risk for death. The manifestations of eating disorders vary across gender, age, socioeconomic status, and race and ethnicity.[20] Patients with eating disorders may be hospitalized for fluid and electrolyte alterations; cardiac dysrhythmias; and nutritional, endocrine, and metabolic disorders.[20]

Menstrual problems may be reported in women of childbearing age. A number of nutritional problems associated with these disorders require you to implement a nutritional plan of care.

The three most common types of eating disorders are anorexia nervosa, bulimia nervosa, and binge-eating disorder. *Binge-eating disorder* is less severe than bulimia nervosa and anorexia nervosa. Those with binge-eating disorder do not have a distorted body image and are often overweight or obese.

Eating disorders also occur in some who are health conscious. For example, men with *bigorexia* or muscle dysmorphia (an extreme concern with becoming more muscular) may use steroids or other drugs to increase muscle mass. They may also use supplements and protein shakes to increase their body weight and mass.

The *female athlete triad* is a syndrome in which eating disorders, amenorrhea, and osteoporosis are present.[21] The triad is seen in females participating in sports that emphasize leanness and low body weight.

### Anorexia Nervosa

**Anorexia nervosa** is characterized by self-starvation, an intense fear of being fat, and disrupted self-image.[20] Anorexia nervosa clinically manifests as extreme thinness, unwillingness to maintain a healthy weight, intense fear of gaining weight, distorted body image, *lanugo* (soft, downy hair covering the body except the palms and soles), refusal to eat, continuous dieting, hair loss, sensitivity to cold, compulsive exercise, dry and yellowish skin, constipation, and absent or irregular menstruation in women of childbearing age.[20] Signs of malnutrition are noted during the physical examination.

Diagnostic studies often show osteopenia or osteoporosis, iron-deficiency anemia, an elevated blood urea nitrogen level from marked intravascular volume depletion, and abnormal renal function. A lack of dietary potassium and potassium loss in the urine lead to potassium deficiency. Manifestations of potassium deficiency include muscle weakness, cardiac dysrhythmias, and renal failure. Leukopenia, hypoglycemia, hyponatremia, hypomagnesemia, and hypophosphatemia may be present.

Interprofessional treatment must involve a combination of nutritional support and psychiatric care. Nutritional care

**EVIDENCE-BASED PRACTICE**

***Translating Research Into Practice***

**What Is the Effect of Internet-Based Interventions on Eating Disorders?**

***Clinical Question***

In persons with eating disorders (P), are Internet-based interventions (I) effective in the treatment of eating-disorder behaviors (O)?

***Synthesis of Best Available Evidence***

- Systematic review of randomized controlled trials (RCTs) and nonrandomized controlled studies
- 8 studies of persons (*n* = 609) diagnosed with bulimia nervosa, binge eating, or more than one eating disorder. Participants were mainly females (97%) with average age of 24 to 45 years old. In most studies, cognitive behavioral therapy (CBT) with a guided self-help component was the basis of the intervention. Planned contact between coach and participant averaged once per week. Outcomes were symptoms of eating disorder–behaviors (e.g., binge eating and purging), anxiety, depression, and quality of life.
- Significant reductions were noted in binge eating and purging. Improvements in depressive symptoms, anxiety, and quality of life were also reported.

***Conclusions***

- Internet-based interventions using CBT have positive effects on reducing bulimia nervosa and binge eating.

***Implications for Nursing Practice***

- Why is it important for health care providers to facilitate alternative methods of treatment delivery other than face-to-face?
- How would you help a patient with an eating disorder who resides in a rural area who regularly misses clinic appointments because of transportation problems?

***Reference for Evidence***

Dolemeyer R, Tietjen A, Kersting A, et al: Internet-based interventions for eating disorders in adults: a systematic review, *BMC Psychiatry* 13:207, 2013.

*P*, Patient population of interest; *I*, intervention or area of interest; *C*, comparison of interest or comparison group; *O*, outcomes of interest; *T*, timing (see p. 15).

focuses on reaching and maintaining a healthy weight, normal eating patterns, and perception of hunger and satiety. Hospitalization may be necessary if the patient has medical complications that cannot be managed in an outpatient therapy program. Nutritional repletion must be closely supervised to ensure consistent and ongoing weight gains. Refeeding syndrome is a rare but serious complication of refeeding programs. The use of EN or PN may be necessary.

Improved nutrition, however, is not a cure for anorexia nervosa. The underlying psychiatric problem must be addressed by identifying disturbed patterns of personal and family interactions, followed by personal and family counseling.

### Bulimia Nervosa

**Bulimia nervosa** is a disorder characterized by episodes of binge eating, inappropriate behaviors to avoid weight gain (vomiting, laxative abuse, over exercise), and a persistent concern with body image.[20] Those with bulimia nervosa may have normal weight for height or their weight may fluctuate with bingeing and purging. They may abuse laxatives, diuretics, exercise, or diet drugs. They may have signs of frequent vomiting, such as macerated knuckles, swollen salivary glands, broken blood vessels in the eyes, and dental problems. The person with bulimia nervosa goes to great lengths to conceal abnormal eating habits. Abnormal laboratory parameters, including hypokalemia, metabolic alkalosis, and elevated serum amylase, may occur with frequent vomiting.[20]

The cause of bulimia remains unclear. It is thought to be similar to that of anorexia nervosa. Substance abuse, anxiety, affective disorders, and personality disturbances have been reported among persons with bulimia. Over time, problems associated with bulimia become increasingly hard to deal with effectively. A treatment combination of psychologic counseling (i.e., cognitive behavioral therapy) and nutritional counseling is essential.

Fluoxetine (Prozac) is the only FDA-approved antidepressant for treating bulimia nervosa. It may not be appropriate in all patients with bulimia. Education and emotional support for the patient and family are vital. Support groups such as the National Association of Anorexia Nervosa and Associated Disorders (ANAD) (*www.anad.org*) are helpful to those affected by these disorders.

## CASE STUDY

### *Undernutrition*

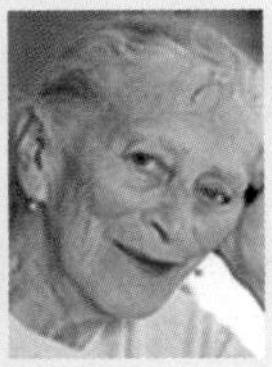

(©iStockphoto/ Thinkstock)

#### Patient Profile

M.S. is a 70-yr-old white woman who is 5 ft 4 in tall and weighs 100 lb. She was recently admitted to the inpatient medical unit.

#### Subjective Data

- Reports 30-lb weight loss in past 2 mo
- Recently had a thrombotic stroke with hemiparesis and dysphagia
- Has a history of rheumatoid arthritis
- Has had nothing by mouth for the past 24 hr and just started enteral nutrition via PEG tube
- Lives with her daughter, who is at her bedside

#### Objective Data

***Physical Examination***

- Has left-sided weakness
- BP is 150/90 mm Hg
- A PEG tube was recently placed

***Laboratory Results***

- Serum albumin 2.9 g/dL
- Prealbumin 11.0 mg/dL
- C-reactive protein 0.9 mg/L

#### Discussion Questions

1. What are M.S.'s risk factors for malnutrition?
2. What is her BMI?
3. What are contributing factors to her developing dysphagia and malnutrition?
4. What should you include in a successful weight gain program for M.S.?
5. For which possible complications of enteral nutrition could M.S. be at risk?
6. ***Priority Decision:*** What is the priority of the nursing care for M.S.?
7. ***Priority Decision:*** Based on the assessment data presented, write one or more appropriate nursing diagnoses. Are there any collaborative problems?
8. ***Teamwork and Collaboration:*** How would you use unlicensed assistive personnel (UAP) to care for M.S.?
9. ***Evidence-Based Practice:*** M.S.'s daughter tells you that her mother's abdomen appears bloated and she wonders if she should massage it.
10. ***Teamwork and Collaboration:*** What is the interprofessional team's top priority at this time for M.S.?
11. ***Safety:*** To ensure M.S.'s safety, what nursing interventions are necessary considering M.S.'s recent weight loss?

Answers available at *http://evolve.elsevier.com/Lewis/medsurg.*

## BRIDGE TO NCLEX EXAMINATION

The number of the question corresponds to the same-numbered outcome at the beginning of the chapter.

1. The percentage of daily calories for a healthy person consists of
   **a.** 50% carbohydrates, 25% protein, 25% fat, and <10% of fat from saturated fatty acids.
   **b.** 65% carbohydrates, 25% protein, 25% fat, and >10% of fat from saturated fatty acids.
   **c.** 50% carbohydrates, 40% protein, 10% fat, and <10% of fat from saturated fatty acids.
   **d.** 40% carbohydrates, 30% protein, 30% fat, and >10% of fat from saturated fatty acids.
2. Place in order the substrates the body uses for energy during starvation, beginning with 1 for the first component and ending with 4 for the last component.
   ___ **a.** skeletal protein.
   ___ **b.** glycogen.
   ___ **c.** visceral protein.
   ___ **d.** fat stores.

3. A complete nutritional assessment including anthropometric measurements is *most* important for the patient who
   a. has a BMI of 25.5 kg/m$^2$.
   b. complains of frequent nocturia.
   c. reports a 5-year history of constipation.
   d. reports an unintentional weight loss of 10 lb in 2 months.
4. Which method is *best* to use when confirming initial placement of a blindly inserted small-bore NG feeding tube?
   a. x-ray.
   b. air insufflation.
   c. observing patient for coughing.
   d. pH measurement of gastric aspirate.
5. A patient is receiving peripheral parenteral nutrition. The parenteral nutrition solution is completed before the new solution arrives on the unit. The nurse gives
   a. 20% intralipids.
   b. 5% dextrose solution.
   c. 0.45% normal saline solution.
   d. 5% lactated Ringer's solution.
6. A patient with anorexia nervosa shows signs of malnutrition. During initial refeeding, the nurse carefully assesses the patient for
   a. hyperkalemia.
   b. hypoglycemia.
   c. hypercalcemia.
   d. hypophosphatemia.

1. a, 2. b, a, d, c, 3. d, 4. a, 5. b, 6. d

For rationales to these answers and even more NCLEX review questions, visit *http://evolve.elsevier.com/Lewis/medsurg.*

## EVOLVE WEBSITE

http://evolve.elsevier.com/Lewis/medsurg
**Review Questions (Online Only)**
**Key Points**
**Answer Keys for Questions**
- Rationales for Bridge to NCLEX Examination Questions
- Answer Guidelines for Case Study on p. 872

**Nursing Care Plans**
- eNursing Care Plan 39-1: Patient Receiving Enteral Nutrition
- eNursing Care Plan 39-2: Patient Receiving Parenteral Nutrition

**Conceptual Care Map Creator**
**Audio Glossary**
**Content Updates**

## REFERENCES


1. American Society for Parenteral and Enteral Nutrition (A.S.P.E.N.) Board of Directors and Clinical Practice Committee: Definition of terms, style, and conventions used in A.S.P.E.N. Retrieved from *www.nutritioncare.org/uploadedFiles/Home/Guidelines_and_Clinical_Practice/DefinitionsStyleConventions.pdf.*
2. United States Department of Agriculture: Scientific report of the 2015 Dietary Guidelines Advisory Committee. Retrieved from *www.health.gov/dietaryguidelines/2015-scientific-report.*
3. Mifflin MD, St. Jeor ST, Hill LA, et al: A new predictive equation for resting energy expenditure in healthy individuals, *Am J Clin Nutr* 51:242, 1990. (Classic)
4. U.S. Department of Health and Human Services and U.S. Department of Agriculture: *2015-2020 Dietary Guidelines for Americans,* ed 8. Retrieved from *www.health.gov/dietaryguidelines/2015-scientific-report.*
5. Colby SE: Multicultural food perspectives: Strategies for health care providers, *Am J Lifestyle Med* 7:13, 2013.
6. White JV, Guenter P, Jensen G, et al: Consensus statement of the Academy of Nutrition and Dietetics/American Society for Parenteral and Enteral Nutrition: Characteristics recommended for the identification and documentation of adult malnutrition, *J Acad Nutr Diet* 112:730, 2012. (Classic)
7. Jensen GL: Malnutrition and inflammation—"Burning Down the House" inflammation as an adaptive physiologic response versus self-destruction, *J Parenter Enteral Nut* 39:56, 2015.
8. Kaiser MJ, Bauer JM, Ramsch C, et al: Frequency of malnutrition in older adults: A multinational perspective using the Mini Nutritional Assessment, *J Am Geriatr Soc* 58:1734, 2010. (Classic)
9. Jensen GL, Hsiao PY, Wheeler D: Adult nutrition assessment tutorial, *J Parenter Enteral Nutr* 36:267, 2012. (Classic)
10. DiMaria-Ghalili RA: Integrating nutrition in the comprehensive geriatric assessment, *Nutr Clin Pract* 29:420, 2014.
11. Russell MK: Functional assessment of nutrition status, *Nutr Clin Pract* 30:211, 2015.
*12. Guenter P, DiMaria-Ghalli RA: Survey of nurses' nutrition screening and assessment practices in hospitalized patients, *MedSurg Matters* 22:10, 2013.
13. Bales C, Locher J, Slatzman E: *Handbook of clinical nutrition and aging,* New York, 2015, Springer Publishing.
14. Litchford MD: Counteracting the trajectory of frailty and sarcopenia in older adults, *Nutr Clin Pract* 29:428, 2014.
*15. Deutz NE, Pereira SL, Hays NP, et al: Effect of β-hydroxy-β-methylbutyrate (HMB) on lean body mass during 10 days of bed rest in older adults, *Clin Nutr* 32:704, 2013.
16. Enteral Nutrition Practice Recommendations Task Force: Enteral nutrition practice recommendations, *J Parenter Enteral Nutr* 33:122, 2009. (Classic)
17. Boullata J, Carney LN, Guenter P: *A.S.P.E.N. enteral nutrition handbook,* Silver Springs, Md, 2010, ASPEN. (Classic)
18. Taylor S, Allen K, McWilliam H, et al: Confirming nasogastric tube position with electromagnetic tracking versus pH or x-ray and tube radio-opacity, *Br J Nurs* 23:352, 2014.
19. Ayers P, Guenter P, Holcombe B, et al: *A.S.P.E.N. parenteral nutrition handbook,* ed 2, Silver Spring, Md, 2014, ASPEN.
20. Dickstein LP, Franco KN, Rome ES, et al: Recognizing, managing medical consequences of eating disorders in primary care, *Cleve Clin J Med* 81:255, 2014.
21. De Souza MJ, Nattiv A, Joy E, et al: 2014 Female Athlete Triad Coalition consensus statement on treatment and return to play of the female athlete triad, *Br J Sports Med* 48:289, 2014.


*Evidence-based information for clinical practice.

# Obesity

*Sharon L. Lewis*

*Our greatest weakness lies in giving up. The most certain way to succeed is always to try just one more time.*

*Thomas A. Edison*

http://evolve.elsevier.com/Lewis/medsurg/

## LEARNING OUTCOMES

1. Discuss the epidemiology and etiology of obesity.
2. Compare the classification systems for determining a person's body size.
3. Explain the health risks associated with obesity.
4. Discuss nutritional therapy and exercise plans for the obese patient.
5. Differentiate among the bariatric surgical procedures used to treat obesity.
6. Describe the nursing and interprofessional management related to conservative and surgical therapies for obesity.
7. Describe the etiology, clinical manifestations, and nursing and interprofessional management of metabolic syndrome.

## KEY TERMS

bariatric surgery, p. 885
body mass index (BMI), p. 874
extreme obesity, p. 874
lipectomy, p. 890
metabolic syndrome, p. 890
obese, p. 874
obesity, p. 874
overweight, p. 874
waist-to-hip ratio (WHR), p. 875

## OBESITY

**Obesity** is an excessively high amount of body fat or adipose tissue (Fig. 40-1). Obesity is a major health problem because it increases the risk of many other diseases such as diabetes and cancer.[1] Whether obesity should be labeled as a disease has been controversial. In 2008 the Obesity Society announced their support for calling obesity a disease. In 2013 the American Medical Association designated obesity as a disease.[2]

Attitudes about obesity can create biases and discrimination against people who are obese. Obesity must be viewed and treated as a chronic disease similar to other chronic diseases, such as diabetes and hypertension.

### Classifications of Body Weight and Obesity

An important part of your patient assessment is to determine and classify a patient's body weight. A number of assessment methods are available, including body mass index (BMI), waist circumference, waist-to-hip ratio (WHR), and body shape. The most widely used and endorsed measures are BMI and waist circumference. These measures are cost-effective, reliable, and easily used in all practice settings.

**Body Mass Index.** The most common measure of obesity is the **body mass index (BMI)**. BMI is calculated by dividing a person's weight (in kilograms) by the square of the height in meters (Fig. 40-2). Individuals with a BMI less than 18.5 kg/m$^2$ are considered underweight, whereas those with a BMI between 18.5 and 24.9 kg/m$^2$ reflect a normal body weight. A BMI of 25 to 29.9 kg/m$^2$ is classified as being **overweight,** and those with values at 30 kg/m$^2$ or above are considered **obese**. The term **extreme obesity** *(morbid* or *severe obesity)* is used for those with a BMI greater than 40 kg/m$^2$.

Table 40-1 shows the classification of overweight and obesity by BMI. The BMI, which provides an overall assessment of fat mass, must be considered in relation to the patient's age, gender, and body build. For example, a body builder may have a BMI associated with obesity, but because of a high muscle mass, the BMI would not be an accurate assessment. In contrast, in individuals who have lost body mass (e.g., older adults), the BMI would underestimate the degree of obesity. For this reason, other measures must be combined with the BMI for an accurate evaluation of a person's weight.

**Waist Circumference.** *Waist circumference* is another way to assess and classify a person's weight (Table 40-1). The average waist size has increased by more than 1 inch (from 37.6 inches to 38.8 inches) in the past decade. Health risks increase if the waist circumference is greater than 40 inches in men and greater than 35 inches in women.[3] People who have visceral

Reviewed by Geraldine M. Budd, RN, PhD, FNP-BC, FAANP, Assistant Dean and Professor, Widener University School of Nursing, Harrisburg, Pennsylvania; Lorraine Nowakowski-Grier, MSN, APRN, BC, CDE, Diabetes Nurse Practitioner, Christiana Care Health Services, Nursing Development & Education, Newark, Delaware; Sarah Byram Poppe, MSN, ANP-BC, Nurse Practitioner, Gastroenterology Associates, Olympia, Washington; and Daryle Wane, PhD, ARNP, FNP-BC, RN to BSN Coordinator, Professor of Nursing, Department of Health Occupations, Pasco-Hernando Community College, New Port Richey, Florida.

**TABLE 40-1 Classification of Overweight and Obesity**

| | BMI (kg/m²) | Obesity Class | DISEASE RISK* RELATIVE TO NORMAL WEIGHT AND WAIST CIRCUMFERENCE: Men ≤40 in (102 cm) Women ≤35 in (89 cm) | Men >40 in (102 cm) Women >35 in (89 cm) |
|---|---|---|---|---|
| **Underweight** | <18.5 | — | — | — |
| **Normal†** | 18.5-24.9 | — | — | — |
| **Overweight** | 25.0-29.9 | — | Increased | High |
| **Obesity** | 30.0-34.9 | Class I | High | Very high |
| | 35.0-39.9 | Class II | Very high | Very high |
| **Extreme obesity** | ≥40.0 | Class III | Extremely high | Extremely high |

Source: National Heart, Lung, and Blood Institute: Classification of overweight and obesity by BMI, waist circumference, and associated disease risks. Retrieved from *www.nhlbi.nih.gov/health/public/heart/obesity/lose_wt/bmi_dis.htm.*
*BMI*, Body mass index.
*Disease risk for type 2 diabetes, hypertension, and cardiovascular disease.
†Increased waist circumference can also be a marker for increased risk in persons of normal weight.

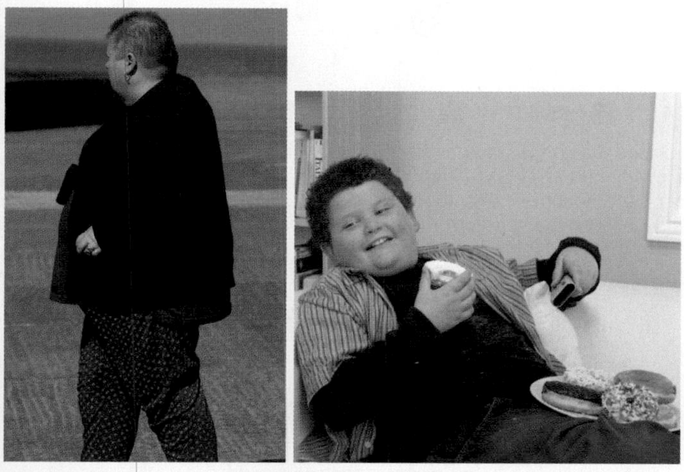

A B

**FIG. 40-1** The obesity epidemic has taken its toll on both adults **(A)** and children **(B)** in the United States. (Source: *A*, Marilyn Barbone/Hemera/Thinkstock; *B*, IPGGutenbergUKLtd/iStock/Thinkstock.)

fat with truncal obesity are at an increased risk for cardiovascular disease and metabolic syndrome (discussed later in this chapter).

**Waist-to-Hip Ratio.** The waist-to-hip ratio (WHR) is another method used to assess obesity. This ratio is a method of describing the distribution of both subcutaneous and visceral adipose tissue. The ratio is calculated by using the waist measurement divided by the hip measurement. A WHR less than 0.8 is optimal. A WHR greater than 0.8 indicates more truncal fat, which puts the individual at a greater risk for health complications.

**Body Shape.** *Body shape* is another method of identifying those who are at a higher risk for health problems (Table 40-2). Individuals with fat located primarily in the abdominal area, an *apple-shaped body,* have *android obesity.* Those with fat distribution in the upper legs, a *pear-shaped body,* have *gynoid obesity.* Genetics has an important role in determining a person's body shape and weight.[4]

## Epidemiology of Obesity

The magnitude of the obesity problem is a public health crisis. After decades of rising obesity rates among adults, the rate of increase is beginning to slow, but rates remain far too high. Currently, about 34% of adults in the United States are obese. Women have a slightly higher incidence of obesity than men.[1]

$$\text{BMI (kg/m}^2\text{)} = \frac{\text{Weight (pounds)} \times 703}{\text{Height (inches)}^2}$$

**Weight in Pounds**

| Height in Feet and Inches | 120 | 130 | 140 | 150 | 160 | 170 | 180 | 190 | 200 | 210 | 220 | 230 | 240 | 250 |
|---|---|---|---|---|---|---|---|---|---|---|---|---|---|---|
| 4'6 | 29 | 31 | 34 | 36 | 39 | 41 | 43 | 46 | 48 | 51 | 53 | 56 | 58 | 60 |
| 4'8 | 27 | 29 | 31 | 34 | 36 | 38 | 40 | 43 | 45 | 47 | 49 | 52 | 54 | 56 |
| 4'10 | 25 | 27 | 29 | 31 | 34 | 36 | 38 | 40 | 42 | 44 | 46 | 48 | 50 | 52 |
| 5'0 | 23 | 25 | 27 | 29 | 31 | 33 | 35 | 37 | 39 | 41 | 43 | 45 | 47 | 49 |
| 5'2 | 22 | 24 | 26 | 27 | 29 | 31 | 33 | 35 | 37 | 38 | 40 | 42 | 44 | 46 |
| 5'4 | 21 | 22 | 24 | 26 | 28 | 29 | 31 | 33 | 34 | 36 | 38 | 40 | 41 | 43 |
| 5'6 | 19 | 21 | 23 | 24 | 26 | 27 | 29 | 31 | 32 | 34 | 36 | 37 | 39 | 40 |
| 5'8 | 18 | 20 | 21 | 23 | 24 | 26 | 27 | 29 | 30 | 32 | 34 | 35 | 37 | 38 |
| 5'10 | 17 | 19 | 20 | 22 | 23 | 24 | 26 | 27 | 29 | 30 | 32 | 33 | 35 | 36 |
| 6'0 | 16 | 18 | 19 | 20 | 22 | 23 | 24 | 26 | 27 | 28 | 30 | 31 | 33 | 34 |
| 6'2 | 15 | 17 | 18 | 19 | 21 | 22 | 23 | 24 | 26 | 27 | 28 | 30 | 31 | 32 |
| 6'4 | 15 | 16 | 17 | 18 | 20 | 21 | 22 | 23 | 24 | 26 | 27 | 28 | 29 | 30 |
| 6'6 | 14 | 15 | 16 | 17 | 19 | 20 | 21 | 22 | 23 | 24 | 25 | 27 | 28 | 29 |
| 6'8 | 13 | 14 | 15 | 17 | 18 | 19 | 20 | 21 | 22 | 23 | 24 | 25 | 26 | 28 |

Underweight · Normal weight · Overweight · Obese · Extreme obesity

**FIG. 40-2** Body mass index (BMI) chart. Healthy weight: BMI 18 to 24.9 kg/m²; overweight: BMI 25 to 29.9 kg/m²; obesity: BMI 30 kg/m². BMI = weight (kg)/height (m²).

Significant geographic, racial and ethnic, and income disparities exist. Obesity rates are highest in the South (Fig. 40-3) and among African Americans, Hispanics, and lower-income, less-educated Americans[1] (Fig. 40-4).

Obesity in adulthood is often a problem that begins in childhood or adolescence. One in ten children becomes obese as early as age 2 to 5.[1] Reversing the childhood obesity crisis is key to addressing the overall obesity epidemic.

## Etiology and Pathophysiology

Obesity is an increase in body weight beyond the body's physical requirements. This results in an abnormal increase and

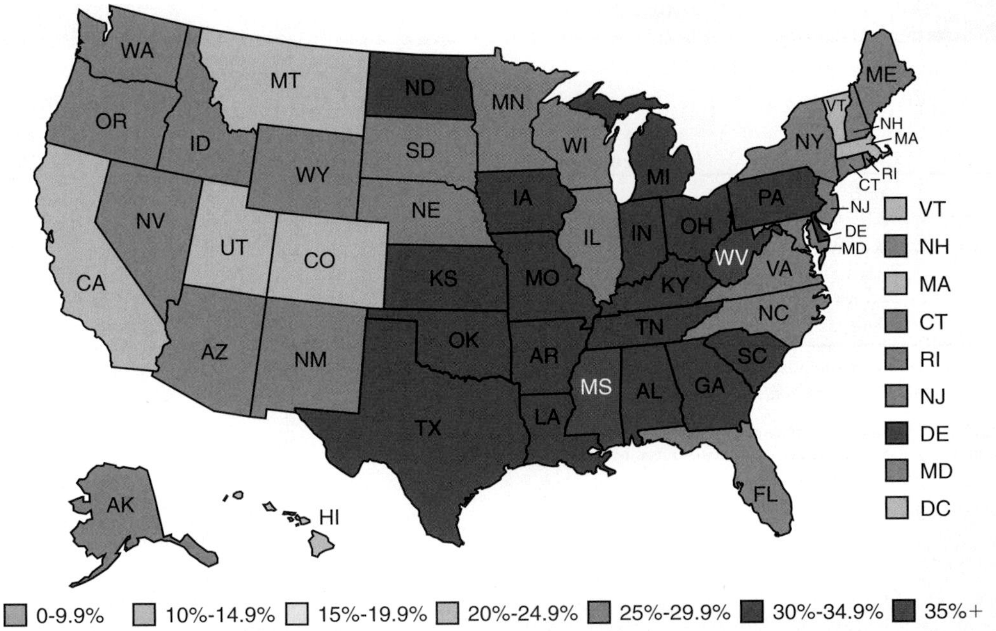


**FIG. 40-3** Percent of obese adults (BMI >30 kg/m²) in the United States. Mississippi and West Virginia have the highest rates of obesity at 35.1%, whereas Colorado has the lowest rate at 21.3%. Twenty states have rates at or above 30%, 43 states have rates of at least 25%, and every state is above 20%. (Source: Trust for America's Health, Robert Wood Johnson Foundation. The state of obesity. 2014. Retrieved from *http://stateofobesity.org.*)

## TABLE 40-2 Relationship Between Body Shape and Health Risks

| Body Shape | Characteristics | Health Risks |
|---|---|---|
| **Gynoid (pear)** 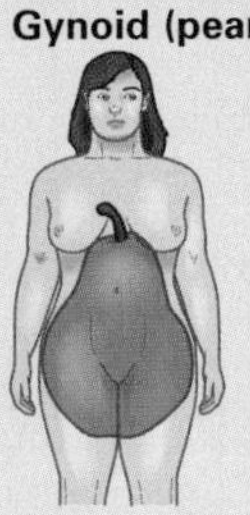 | • Fat mainly located in the upper legs<br>• Has a better prognosis but difficult to treat | • Osteoporosis<br>• Varicose veins<br>• Cellulite<br>• Subcutaneous fat traps and stores dietary fat<br>• Trapped fatty acids stored as triglycerides |
| **Android (apple)** 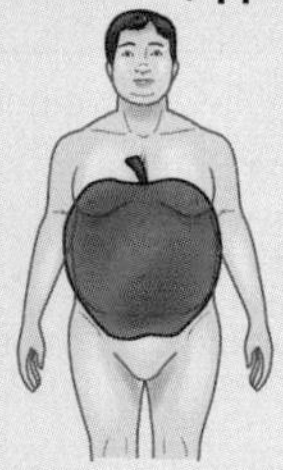 | • Fat primarily located in abdominal area<br>• Fat also distributed over upper body (neck, arms, shoulders)<br>• Greater risk for obesity-related complications | • Heart disease<br>• Diabetes mellitus<br>• Breast cancer<br>• Endometrial cancer<br>• Visceral fat more active, causing ↓ insulin sensitivity<br>• ↑ Triglycerides<br>• ↓ HDL cholesterol<br>• ↑ BP<br>• ↑ Free fatty acid release into blood |

*HDL,* High-density lipoprotein.

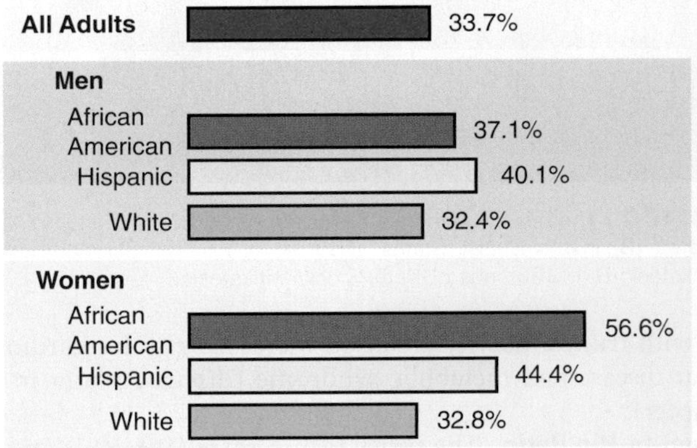


**FIG. 40-4** Obesity affects some groups disproportionately. Among U.S. adults, African American and Hispanic populations have substantially higher rates of obesity than do white populations. This is true among both men and women. (Source: Trust for America's Health, Robert Wood Johnson Foundation. The state of obesity. 2014. Retrieved from *http://stateofobesity.org.*)

accumulation of fat cells. However, the processes leading to and sustaining the obese state are complex and still undergoing investigation.

In obesity, there is an increase in the number of adipocytes *(hyperplasia)* and an increase in their size *(hypertrophy)*. Adipocyte *hypertrophy* is a process by which adipocytes can increase their volume several thousand–fold to accommodate large increases in lipid storage. In addition, preadipocytes are triggered to become adipocytes once storage of existing fat cells is exceeded. This process occurs primarily in the visceral (intraabdominal) and subcutaneous tissues. The process of *hyperplasia* (increase in numbers) of adipocytes is greatest from infancy through adolescence.

The majority of obese persons have *primary obesity,* which is excess calorie intake over energy expenditure for the body's metabolic demands. Others have *secondary obesity,* which can result from various congenital anomalies, chromosomal anomalies, metabolic problems, central nervous system lesions and disorders, or drugs (e.g., corticosteroids, antipsychotics).

The cause of obesity involves significant genetic and biologic factors that are highly influenced by environmental and psychosocial factors. Each of these factors can and should be considered individually, but in reality they are interrelated.

## Genetic Link

Studies of twins suggest the existence of genetic factors in obesity.[5] However, genetic factors do not totally account for the etiology of obesity. Estimates of obesity as an inherited problem are more than 50%.[6]

A number of genes have been identified as being linked to obesity. Genes actually may influence how calories are stored and energy released. "Energy-thrifty" genes, once protective against long periods when food was not available, are now maladaptive in societies in which food availability is no longer a primary issue. Genes may be responsible for why two individuals living in the same environment can vary considerably in body size.

A strong link exists between a gene known as *FTO* (fat mass and obesity-associated gene) and BMI. Variants of this gene may explain why some people become overweight, whereas others do not. People with two copies of a certain allele at the *FTO* gene weigh 7 to 8 lb more and have a greater risk of obesity than those who do not have the risk allele.[7] More research is needed to better understand the role of genes in obesity.

**Physiologic Regulatory Mechanisms in Obesity.** Research has focused on the physiologic regulatory processes that control eating behavior, energy metabolism, and body fat metabolism. Knowing how appetite is triggered and energy is expended provides important information for understanding obesity and specific targets for the development of drugs.

The hypothalamus, gut, and adipose tissue synthesize hormones and peptides that stimulate or inhibit the appetite (Fig. 40-5). The hypothalamus is a major site for regulating appetite. Neuropeptide Y, produced in the hypothalamus, is a powerful appetite stimulant. When it is imbalanced, it leads to overeating and obesity. Hormones and peptides produced in the gut and adipocyte cells affect the hypothalamus and have a critical role in appetite and energy balance (Table 40-3).

Leptin, secreted from adipocytes when they fill with fat, acts in the hypothalamus to suppress appetite and increase fat metabolism. A genetic deficiency of leptin causes extreme obesity. In obesity the level of leptin is actually increased, which has raised the question of whether obese people are insensitive to leptin. Possible causes of obesity include failure to produce enough leptin receptors or production of receptors that are faulty.

**TABLE 40-3 Hormones and Peptides in Obesity**

| Where Produced | Normal Function | Alteration in Obesity |
|---|---|---|
| **Anorexins (Suppress Appetite)** | | |
| ***Leptin*** | | |
| Adipocytes | Suppresses appetite and hunger<br>Regulates eating behavior | Obesity is associated with high levels. Leptin resistance develops; thus obese people may lose the effect of appetite suppression. |
| ***Insulin*** | | |
| Pancreas | Decreases appetite | Increased insulin secretion which stimulates ↑ liver synthesis of triglycerides and ↓ HDL production |
| ***Peptide YY*** | | |
| Colon | Inhibits appetite by slowing GI motility and gastric emptying | Circulating levels are decreased. ↓ Release after eating |
| ***Cholecystokinin*** | | |
| Small intestine | Inhibits gastric emptying<br>Sends satiety signals to hypothalamus | Unknown role |
| ***Glucagon-Like Peptide-1 (GLP-1)*** | | |
| Small intestine | Stimulates insulin secretion from pancreas<br>Increases satiety (mediated by GLP-1 receptors in brain) | Unknown role |
| **Orexins (Stimulate Appetite)** | | |
| ***Neuropeptide Y*** | | |
| Hypothalamus | Stimulates appetite | Imbalance causes increased appetite |
| ***Ghrelin*** | | |
| Stomach (primarily) | Stimulates appetite<br>↑ After food deprivation<br>↓ In response to food in the stomach | Normal postprandial decline does not occur, which can lead to increased appetite and overeating |

*HDL,* High-density lipoprotein.

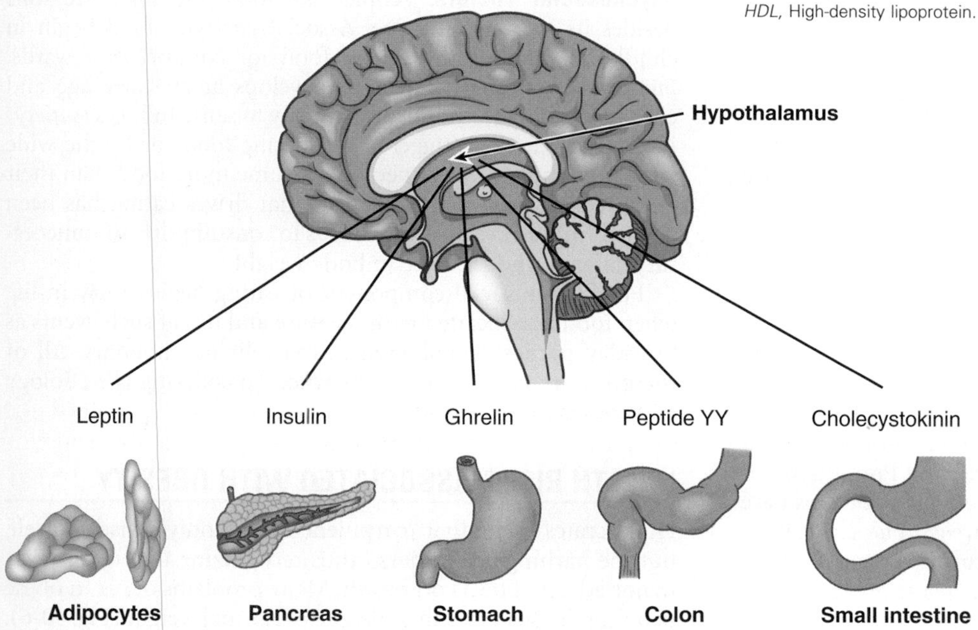


**FIG. 40-5** Some of the common hormones and peptides that interact with the hypothalamus to control and influence eating patterns, metabolic activities, and digestion. Obesity disrupts this balance (Table 40-3).

## CULTURAL & ETHNIC HEALTH DISPARITIES

### *Obesity*

- African Americans and Hispanics have a higher prevalence of obesity than whites.
- Among women, African Americans have the highest prevalence of being overweight or obese, and 15% have extreme obesity.
- Among men, Hispanics have the highest prevalence of being overweight or obese.
- African American and Hispanic women with low incomes have the greatest likelihood of being overweight when compared with other socioeconomic groups.
- Native Americans have a higher prevalence of being overweight than the general population.
- Among Native Americans ages 45 to 74, more than 30% of women are overweight and more than 40% are obese.
- Asian Americans have the lowest prevalence of being overweight and obese compared with the general population.

## HEALTHY PEOPLE

### *Health Impact of Maintaining a Healthy Weight*

- Reduces the risk of developing type 2 diabetes mellitus
- Increases chance of longevity and better quality of life
- Lowers the risk of hypertension and elevated cholesterol
- Reduces the risk of heart disease, stroke, and gallbladder disease
- Reduces the likelihood of breathing problems, including sleep apnea and asthma
- Decreases the risk of developing osteoarthritis, low back pain, and certain types of cancers

Ghrelin, a gut hormone, regulates appetite through inhibition of leptin. In a fasting state, ghrelin is increased. Ghrelin acts in the hypothalamus by working on the reward system that triggers overeating. Ghrelin is thought to play a part in compulsive eating. In gastric bypass surgery, ghrelin is decreased significantly, which helps suppress appetite.[8]

The two major consequences of obesity are due to the sheer increase in fat mass and production of adipokines produced by fat cells. Adipocytes produce at least 100 different proteins. These proteins, secreted as enzymes, adipokines, growth factors, and hormones, contribute to the development of insulin resistance and atherosclerosis.

An increased release of cytokines from fat cells may disrupt immune factors, thus predisposing the person to certain cancers. Because visceral fat accumulation is associated with more alterations of these adipokines, people with abdominal obesity have more complications of obesity.[8]

**Environmental Factors.** Environmental factors play an important role in obesity. In today's culture, people have greater access to food (particularly prepackaged and fast foods) and soft drinks, which have poor nutritional quality. In addition, eating outside of the home interferes with the ability to control the quality and quantity of food.

Portion size of meals has increased dramatically (Table 40-4). Underestimating portion sizes and therefore caloric intake is common. The Centers for Disease Control and Prevention has developed visual programs that demonstrate how portions have increased over time *(www.cdc.gov/healthyweight/index.html)*.

Lack of physical exercise is another factor that contributes to weight gain and obesity. With increases in the use of technology, labor-saving devices, and cars, Americans are expending less

**TABLE 40-4 Portion Sizes: 30 Years Ago vs. Today**

| | 30 Yr Ago | Today |
|---|---|---|
| **Turkey sandwich** | 320 cal | 820 cal |
| | 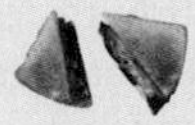 | 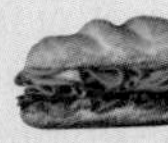 |
| **Bagel** | 3-in diameter, 140 cal | 6-in diameter, 350 cal |
| | 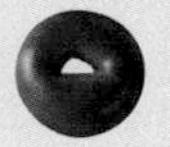 | 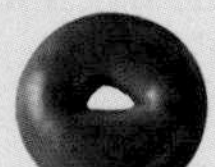 |
| **Cheeseburger** | 333 cal | 590 cal |
| | 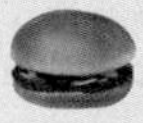 | 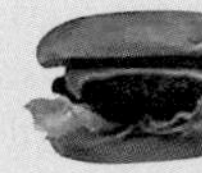 |
| **Soda** | 6½ oz, 85 cal | 20 oz, 250 cal |
| | 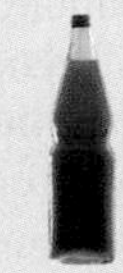 | 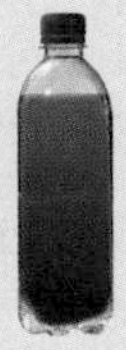 |

energy in their everyday lives. Elimination of physical education programs in schools, along with increased time spent playing video games and watching TV, has contributed to the increase in sedentary habits.

Socioeconomic status is a known risk factor for obesity in a variety of ways.[1] People with low incomes may attempt to stretch their food dollars by purchasing less expensive foods that often have poor nutritional quality with a greater caloric content. For example, people with low incomes are more likely to purchase pasta, bread, and canned fruit packed with sugar rather than chicken and fresh fruits and vegetables. Low-income residents may also live in environments that do not accommodate outdoor activities (e.g., safe playgrounds, walking tracks, tennis, swimming pools).

**Psychosocial Factors.** People use food for many reasons besides its nutritional value. Associations with food begin in childhood, such as the use of food for comfort or rewards. Furthermore, when overeating develops at an early age and continues into adulthood, one's ability to sense fullness *(satiety)* is altered. Whether triggered by specific foods or by the wide variety of choices, some people consume more food than their bodies need. The lack of hunger that drives eating has been termed "mindless eating" and leads to consumption of unnecessary calories and increase in body weight.

Finally, the social component of eating begins early in life when food is associated with pleasure and fun at such events as birthday parties, Thanksgiving, and religious holidays. All of these factors must be included when considering the etiology and treatment of obesity.

## HEALTH RISKS ASSOCIATED WITH OBESITY

Hippocrates wrote that "corpulence is not only a disease itself, but the harbinger of others," thus recognizing that obesity has major adverse effects on health. Many problems occur in obese people at higher rates than people of normal weight (Fig. 40-6).

Mortality rates rise as obesity increases, especially when obesity is associated with visceral fat.[9] In addition to these problems, obese patients have a reduced quality of life. Fortunately, most of these conditions can improve if an individual loses weight.

## Cardiovascular Problems

Obesity is a significant risk factor for cardiovascular disease in both men and women. Android obesity is the best predictor of these risks and is linked with increased low-density lipoproteins (LDLs), high triglycerides, and decreased high-density lipoproteins (HDLs).[10] Obesity is also associated with hypertension, which can occur because of increased circulating blood volume, abnormal vasoconstriction, increased inflammation (damaging blood vessels), and increased risk of sleep apnea (raises BP). Altered lipid metabolism and hypertension can increase the long-term risk of heart disease and stroke. Excess body fat can also lead to chronic inflammation throughout the body, especially in blood vessels, thus increasing the risk of heart disease.

## Diabetes Mellitus

Obesity is a major risk factor for the development of type 2 diabetes.[11] Hyperinsulinemia and insulin resistance, common features of type 2 diabetes, are also found in obesity. The term *diabesity* reflects the combined effects of diabetes and obesity.

Excess weight decreases the effectiveness of insulin. When insulin does not work effectively, too much glucose stays in the bloodstream. Thus more insulin is made to compensate. Pancreatic β cells (cells that make insulin) may get overworked and become worn out. Over time, the pancreas is no longer able to keep blood glucose in normal range. Adiponectin, a peptide that increases insulin sensitivity, is decreased in obese people.

Obesity complicates the management of type 2 diabetes by increasing insulin resistance and glucose intolerance. These factors make drug treatment for diabetes less effective.

## Gastrointestinal and Liver Problems

Gastroesophageal reflux disease (GERD) and gallstones are more prevalent in obese people. Gallstones occur due to supersaturation of the bile with cholesterol. Nonalcoholic steatohepatitis (NASH) is a condition in which lipids are deposited in the liver, resulting in a fatty liver. NASH is associated with elevated hepatic glucose production. NASH can eventually progress to cirrhosis and can be fatal. Weight loss can improve NASH.

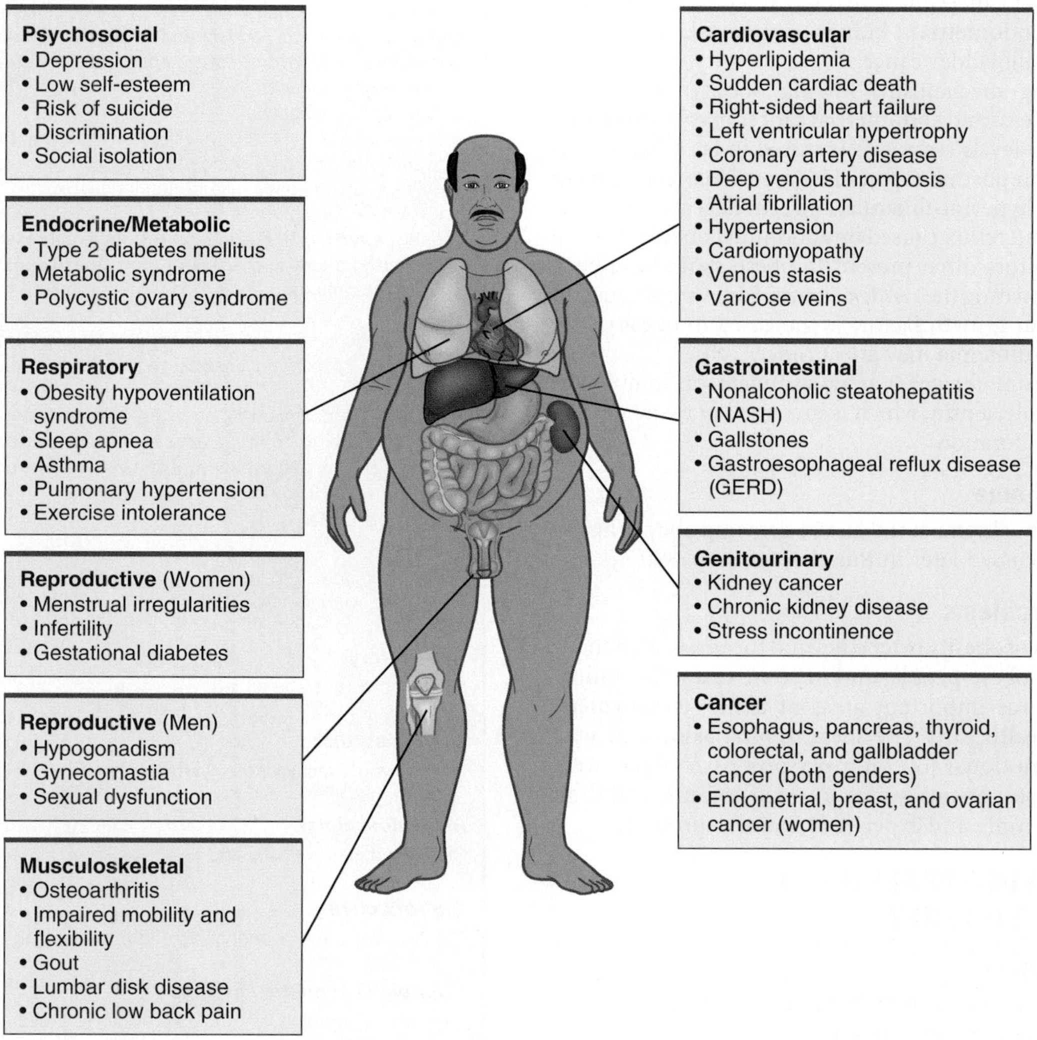


**FIG. 40-6** Health risks associated with obesity.

### Respiratory and Sleep Problems

The increased fat mass associated with obesity may lead to sleep apnea and obesity hypoventilation syndrome. The increased distribution of fat around the diaphragm causes a reduced chest wall compliance, increased work of breathing, and decreased total lung capacity. Sleep apnea results from increased fat around the neck, leading to snoring and hypoventilation while sleeping. Weight loss can improve lung function.

Poor sleep and sleep deprivation may increase appetite. Sleep deprivation has been associated with obesity. Building up a sleep debt over a matter of days can impair metabolism and disrupt hormone levels. The level of leptin falls in people who are sleep deprived, thus promoting appetite.

### Musculoskeletal Problems

Obesity is associated with an increased incidence of osteoarthritis because of the stress put on weight-bearing joints, especially the knees and hips. Increased body fat also triggers inflammatory mediators and contributes to deterioration of cartilage. Hyperuricemia and gout are often found in people who are obese and in those who have metabolic syndrome (discussed later in this chapter).

### Cancer

Obesity is one of the most important preventable causes of cancer. The types of cancer most strongly linked to excess body fat are breast, endometrial, kidney, colorectal, pancreatic, esophageal, and gallbladder cancer.[12]

The underlying mechanisms linking obesity and cancer remain unclear. Breast and endometrial cancer may be due to the increased estrogen levels (estrogen is stored in fat cells) associated with obesity in postmenopausal women. Colorectal cancer has been linked to hyperinsulinemia, and esophageal cancer may be secondary to acid reflux caused by abdominal obesity. Several hormones and factors often present in obese states have been identified as potentiating the risk for cancer. For example, insulin (a powerful cellular growth factor) is increased in obesity. The resulting hyperinsulinemia may affect cancer cells.

Adipokines (from fat cells) may stimulate or inhibit cell growth. For example, leptin, which is increased in obese people, promotes cell proliferation.

### Metabolic Syndrome

Metabolic syndrome is one of the fastest-growing obesity health concerns. It is discussed later in this chapter on p. 890.

### Psychosocial Problems

The consequences of obesity extend beyond the physical changes. Stigmatization of obese people, and in some cases discrimination, occurs in three important areas of living: employment, education, and health care. The social stigma associated with obesity has an emotional toll on a person's psychologic well-being. Many obese persons suffer low self-esteem, withdraw from social interaction, and experience major depression.[13]

## NURSING AND INTERPROFESSIONAL MANAGEMENT: OBESITY

### Nursing Assessment

The first step in the treatment of obesity is to determine whether any physical conditions are present that may be causing or contributing to obesity. This requires a thorough history and physical examination.

Table 40-5 lists information that can assist you in understanding an obese patient and provides a basis for intervention. When assessing an individual who is overweight or obese, be sensitive and nonjudgmental in asking specific and leading questions about weight, diet, and exercise (Table 40-6). In doing so, you can often obtain information that the patient may have withheld out of embarrassment or shyness. Patients need to understand the rationale for questions asked about weight or dietary habits, and you must be ready to respond to their concerns.

**TABLE 40-5 Nursing Assessment**
***Obese Patient***

**Subjective Data**

***Important Health Information***

*Past health history:* Time of obesity onset; diseases related to metabolism and obesity, such as hypertension, cardiovascular problems, stroke, cancer, chronic joint pain, respiratory problems, diabetes mellitus, cholelithiasis, metabolic syndrome

*Medications:* Thyroid preparations, diet pills, herbal products

*Surgery or other treatments:* Prior weight-reduction procedures (bariatric surgery)

***Functional Health Patterns***

*Health perception–health management:* Family history of obesity; perception of problem; methods of weight loss attempted

*Nutritional-metabolic:* Amount and frequency of eating; overeating in response to boredom, stress, specific times, or activities; history of weight gain and loss

*Elimination:* Constipation

*Activity-exercise:* Typical physical activity; drowsiness, somnolence; dyspnea on exertion, orthopnea, paroxysmal nocturnal dyspnea

*Sleep-rest:* Sleep apnea, use of continuous positive airway pressure (CPAP)

*Cognitive-perceptual:* Feelings of rejection, depression, isolation, guilt, or shame; meaning or value of food; adherence to prescribed reducing diets, degree of long-term commitment to a weight loss program

*Role-relationship:* Change in financial status or family relationships; personal, social, and financial resources to support a reducing diet

*Sexuality-reproductive:* Menstrual irregularity, heavy menstrual flow in women, birth control practices, infertility; effect of obesity on sexual activity and attractiveness to significant other

**Objective Data**

***General***

Body mass index ≥30 kg/m$^2$; waist circumference: woman >35 in (89 cm), man >40 in (102 cm)

***Respiratory***

Increased work of breathing; wheezing; rapid, shallow breathing

***Cardiovascular***

Hypertension, tachycardia, dysrhythmias

***Musculoskeletal***

Decreased joint mobility and flexibility; knee, hip, and low back pain

***Reproductive***

Gynecomastia and hypogonadism in men

***Possible Diagnostic Findings***

Elevated serum glucose, cholesterol, triglycerides; chest x-ray demonstrating enlarged heart; electrocardiogram showing dysrhythmia; abnormal liver function tests

**TABLE 40-6 Assessing Patients With Obesity**

*When assessing patients with obesity and before selecting a weight loss strategy, ask the following questions.*

- What is your history with weight gain and weight loss?
- Are other family members overweight?
- How has your health been affected by your body weight?
- What do you think contributes to your weight?
- What does food mean to you? How do you use food (e.g., to relieve stress, provide comfort)?
- What is your motivation for losing weight?
- What have you already tried to lose weight? Was it successful? If not, why not?
- Would you like to manage your weight differently? If so, how?
- What sort of barriers do you think impede your weight loss efforts?
- Are there any major stresses that will make it difficult to focus on weight control?
- How much time can you devote to exercise on a daily or weekly basis?
- What type of support do you have from family and/or friends for losing weight?

**CHECK YOUR PRACTICE**

You are working in the hypertension clinic, and the attending physician has asked you to do an assessment on a 54-yr-old man for possible referral to a weight loss program. He is 5′9″ and weighs 242 pounds. His BP has been difficult to control with drugs and diet. While trying to do an assessment (using the questions in Table 40-6), he interrupts you and asks you if he can leave. He angrily tells you, "I do not want to give up my favorite foods, quit drinking, or exercise. Do you understand that?"

- How would you respond to him?

Assess a patient's willingness to change and potential for change. If people are not ready for change, offer them the opportunity to return for further discussion when they are ready to discuss their weight again and make lifestyle changes.

When obtaining the history, explore genetic and endocrine factors such as hypothyroidism, hypothalamic tumors, Cushing syndrome, hypogonadism in men, and polycystic ovary syndrome in women. Laboratory tests of liver function and thyroid function, a fasting glucose level, and a lipid panel (triglyceride level, LDL and HDL cholesterol levels) assist in evaluating the cause and effects of obesity. When no organic cause (e.g., hypothyroidism) is associated with obesity, the disorder should be considered a chronic, complex disease.

As part of the initial nursing history and physical examination, examine each body system with particular attention to the organ system in which the patient has expressed a problem or concern. Measurements used with the obese person may include height (without shoes), weight (obtain in a private location and in a gown if possible), waist circumference, and BMI. Have the right equipment to take these measurements. Provide special chairs, examination tables, and scales that can accommodate an obese person.

Also assess for any co-morbid diseases associated with obesity (e.g., hypertension, sleep apnea). These obesity-related complications require special treatment.

## Planning

The overall goals are that the obese patient will (1) modify eating patterns, (2) participate in a regular physical activity program, (3) achieve and maintain weight loss to a specified level, and (4) minimize or prevent health problems related to obesity.

## Nursing Implementation

Obesity is one of the most challenging health problems. For the majority of patients who are obese, successful weight management will be a difficult, lifelong project. Obesity treatment begins with patients understanding their weight history and deciding on a plan that is best for them.

Together with other members of the interprofessional care team, you have a major role in planning for and managing the care of an obese patient. First, examine your own personal beliefs and any potential biases related to obesity. If you associate obesity with a lack of willpower and overindulgence, your attitude may be conveyed to patients. They may experience shame in a setting that claims to be a caring one.

You are in a pivotal position to help overweight and obese individuals. Interventions include (1) helping obese patients explore and deal with their negative experiences and (2) teaching other health professionals about stigma and biases experienced by obese patients.

Although health care for obese people has greater demands, HCPs often fail to address these needs. In addition, obese people underutilize health care opportunities available to them. HCPs are often reluctant to counsel patients about obesity for a variety of reasons, including (1) time constraints during appointments make it difficult, (2) weight management may be viewed as professionally unrewarding, (3) reimbursement for weight management services is difficult to obtain, and (4) many HCPs do not feel knowledgeable about giving weight loss advice.

Despite the known benefits of weight loss, it is a difficult process for most individuals. Achieving an "ideal" BMI is not necessary and may not be a realistic goal. Modest weight loss of even 3% to 5% of starting weight can have clinical benefits, and greater weight losses produce greater benefits.[14] In general, the average weight loss program (except for bariatric surgery) results in a 10% reduction of body weight. This average reduction should not be considered a failure, since it is associated with significant health benefits.[15]

Exploring an individual's motivation for weight loss is essential for overall success. Using principles from motivational interviewing (discussed in Chapter 4 on p. 47), you can help patients understand their desire to lose weight and gain confidence in achieving weight loss.

Focusing on the reasons for wanting to lose weight may help patients develop strategies for a weight loss program. Any supervised plan of care must be directed at two different processes: (1) successful weight loss, which requires a short-term energy deficit, and (2) successful weight control, which requires long-term behavior changes.

A multicomponent approach for weight loss must be used that includes nutritional therapy, exercise, behavior modification, and for some, drugs or surgical intervention (Table 40-7). Focusing on more than one aspect provides for more effective weight loss and weight control efforts. While teaching patients, stress healthy eating habits and adequate physical activity as lifestyle patterns to develop and maintain.

**Nutritional Therapy.** There are no "magic" diets for weight loss. No one diet is superior for weight loss. All diets can work if they achieve a reduced caloric intake relative to expenditure.[14]

Restricting dietary intake so that it is below energy requirements is a cornerstone for any weight loss or maintenance program. A good weight loss plan should contain foods from

## TABLE 40-7 Interprofessional Care

### *Obesity*

| Diagnostic Assessment | Management |
|---|---|
| • History and physical examination<br>• Family history<br>• BMI, waist circumference, waist-to-hip ratio<br>• Assessment of health risks and co-morbidities | • Management of co-morbidities<br>• Lifestyle interventions<br>  • Participation in weight loss program<br>  • Support groups<br>  • Behavior modification<br>• Nutritional therapy<br>• Exercise<br>• Behavior modification<br>• Support groups<br>• Drug therapy (Table 40-9)<br>• Surgical therapy (Table 40-10) |

*BMI,* Body mass index.

## TABLE 40-8 Nutritional Therapy

### *1200-Calorie–Restricted Weight-Reduction Diet**

**General Principles**

1. Eat regularly. Do not skip meals.
2. Measure foods to determine the correct portion size.
3. Avoid concentrated sweets, such as sugar, candy, honey, pies, cakes, cookies, and regular sodas.
4. Reduce fat intake by baking, broiling, or steaming foods.
5. Maintain a regular exercise program for successful weight loss.

| Meal | Exchanges | Menu Plan |
|---|---|---|
| **Breakfast** | 1 meat | 1 hard-boiled egg |
| | 2 bread | 1 slice toast |
| | | ¾ cup dry cereal (unsweetened) |
| | 1 fruit | ½ small banana |
| | 1 fat | 1 tsp margarine |
| | 1 dairy† | 1 cup low-fat milk |
| | Beverage | Coffee |
| **Lunch** | 2 meat | Cheese enchiladas (made with 2 oz |
| | 2 bread | cheese, two corn tortillas, lettuce, |
| | Vegetable | chili sauce) |
| | 1 fruit | Fresh grapes (12) |
| | Beverage | Diet soda |
| **Dinner** | 2 meat | 2 oz baked chicken |
| | 1 bread | Corn on the cob with 1 tsp margarine |
| | Vegetable | Tossed salad and 1 Tbsp salad dressing |
| | 1 fruit | ¾ cup strawberries |
| | 1 milk | 1 cup low-fat milk |

*For 1000 cal, omit 1 fruit exchange and change low-fat milk to skim milk. For 1500 cal, add 1 meat exchange, 1 fruit exchange, and 2 fat exchanges; change low-fat milk to whole milk. For 1800 cal, add 2 bread exchanges, 3 meat exchanges, 3 fat exchanges, and 1 fruit exchange; change low-fat milk to whole milk.
†One extra fat exchange allowed for each cup of 2% low-fat milk; 2 extra fat exchanges allowed for each cup of skim milk.

the basic food groups (MyPlate is presented in Fig. 39-1 and Table 39-1). (Table 40-8 presents an example of a 1200-calorie diet.)

A supervised diet plan may be prescribed that limits calories to a total of 800 or less per day (very-low-calorie diet), but this is not sustainable on a long-term basis. These diets should be provided only by trained professionals in a medical care setting. Persons on very-low-calorie diets need frequent professional monitoring, because the severe energy restriction places them at risk for multiple health complications.[14]

In general, it is best to recommend a diet that includes adequate amounts of fruits and vegetables, provides enough bulk to prevent constipation, and meets daily vitamin A and vitamin C requirements. Lean meat, fish, and eggs provide sufficient protein and the B-complex vitamins.

It is rare to find an obese person who has not at some time attempted to lose weight. Some people have met with limited and temporary success, and others have met only with failure. Many individuals attempt weight loss by trying one of the many fad diets that offer the enticement of quick weight loss with little effort. Often these quick weight-reduction diets (found in the popular media) advocate the elimination of one category of foods (e.g., carbohydrates). Therefore these should be discouraged. Low-carbohydrate diets do produce a rapid weight loss but reduce the opportunity to get adequate amounts of fiber, vitamins, and minerals. These restrictive diets are difficult to maintain on a long-term basis. The more restrictive the regimen, the greater the demand for intense discipline in the face of an intense desire to eat foods not allowed on the diet.

It is best to recommend a dietary approach in which calorie restriction includes all food groups (e.g., MyPlate). Patients will

## EVIDENCE-BASED PRACTICE

### *Translating Research Into Practice*

**What Types of Diet Programs Result in Weight Loss?**

***Clinical Question***

For adults who are overweight or obese (P), what is the effect of low-fat and low-carbohydrate diet programs (I) versus control group (C) on weight loss at 6 and 12 months (T)?

***Synthesis of Best Available Evidence***

- Meta-analysis of randomized controlled trials (RCTs)
- 48 RCTs ($n$ = 7286) of overweight or obese adults (BMI ≥25 kg/m$^2$). Interventions were popular branded diet programs (e.g., Atkins low-carbohydrate diet, Ornish low-fat diet) with and without exercise and/or behavioral support such as counseling. Control groups included wait-listed controls, no specific diet, or competing dietary programs. Outcomes were weight loss measurements at 6 and 12 months.
- At 6-month follow-up, all diet programs resulted in some weight loss with low-carbohydrate and low-fat diets having the greatest weight loss.
- At 12-month follow-up, weight loss for all diets was about 1 to 2 kg less than after 6-month follow-up. Low-carbohydrate and low-fat diets had strongest effect on weight loss.
- Exercise and behavioral support were related to increased weight loss.

***Conclusions***

- Low-carbohydrate and low-fat diets are associated with significant weight loss.
- Differences in weight loss among types of low-carbohydrate and low-fat diets were small.

***Implications for Nursing Practice***

- What factors are important to discuss with a patient who asks what diet will help the most in losing weight?
- How will you assist the patient on a diet incorporate exercise into his or her lifestyle?
- What strategies will you use to help patients maintain weight loss after 6 months?

***Reference for Evidence***

Johnston BC, Kanters S, Bandayrel K, et al: Comparison of weight loss among named diet programs in overweight and obese adults: a meta-analysis, *JAMA* 312: 923, 2014.

*P,* Patient population of interest; *I,* intervention or area of interest; *C,* comparison of interest or comparison group; *O,* outcomes of interest; *T,* timing (see p. 15).

find it easier to incorporate such a change into their lifestyle and not become as bored with their food options. However, the ability to adhere to a diet and degree of weight loss strongly depends on the patient's motivation.

The degree of success of any diet depends in part on the amount of weight to be lost. A moderately obese person will obviously attain his or her goal more easily than a person with extreme obesity. Because men have a higher percentage of lean body mass, they are often able to lose weight more quickly than women. Women have a higher percentage of body fat, which is metabolically less active than muscle tissue. Postmenopausal women are particularly prone to weight gain, especially increased abdominal fat.

The obese patient must recognize the advantages of weight loss and weight control. You can assist by helping the patient track eating patterns with a diet diary. Through a frank discussion of eating patterns, the patient often realizes that eating is "mindless" and the result of bad habits picked up over time. These eating behaviors must be changed, or any weight loss will only be temporary.

Setting a realistic and healthy goal, such as losing 1 to 2 lb/wk, should be mutually agreed on at the beginning of a weight loss program. Trying to lose too much too fast usually results in a sense of frustration and failure for the patient. You can help patients understand that losing large amounts of weight in a short period causes skin and underlying tissue to lose elasticity and tone. Slower weight loss offers better cosmetic results.

Inevitably, the patient reaches plateau periods during which no weight is lost. These plateaus may last from several days to several weeks. Remind the patient that plateaus are normal occurrences during weight reduction. A weekly check of body weight is a good method of monitoring progress. Daily weighing is not recommended because of the frequent fluctuations resulting from retained water (including urine) and elimination of feces. Instruct the patient to record the weight at the same time of the day, wearing the same type of clothing.

There is no clear consensus on the number of meals to be eaten when a person is on a diet. Some nutritionists advocate several small meals per day because the body's metabolic rate is temporarily increased immediately after eating. However, when eating several small meals a day, patients may consume more calories unless they carefully adhere to portion sizes and total daily calorie allotment.

When a person first starts a weight loss program, food portion sizes must be carefully determined to stay within the dietary guidelines. Portion sizes over the past 30 years have increased considerably (Table 40-4). Food portions can be weighed using a scale, or everyday objects can be used as a visual cue to determine portion sizes. The size of a woman's fist or a baseball is equivalent to a serving of vegetables or fruit. A serving of meat is about the size of a person's palm or a deck of cards. A serving of cheese is about the size of a thumb or six dice. A portion size quiz is available at *www.nhlbi.nih.gov/health/educational/wecan/eat-right/distortion.htm*.

Another aspect of the American diet that must be considered is which foods contribute the most calories—animal sources, fruits, grains, or vegetables. Two thirds or more of an individual's diet should be plant-source foods, and the other one third or less should be from animal protein. Being aware of personal consumption habits and striving for the two-thirds to one-third ratio is a simple goal that can be achieved without weighing and measuring foods at every meal. Once this ratio has been adopted into the patient's meal planning, portions can gradually be reduced as activity levels are gradually increased to achieve healthy weight loss. The recommended portion size of animal protein is 3 oz. The standard size for chopped vegetables is ½ cup, according to MyPlate guidelines (Table 39-1).

A list of healthy or low-calorie foods serves as a good reference and permits an occasional meal to be eaten at a restaurant. Furthermore, the patient who carefully follows the prescribed diet may not need to take vitamin supplements.

Encourage the appropriate fluid intake in the form of water. Alcoholic and sugary beverages should be limited or avoided, since they increase caloric intake and are low in nutritional value.

◆ **Exercise.** Exercise is an essential part of a weight loss program. Patients should exercise daily, preferably 30 minutes to an hour. There is no evidence that increased activity promotes an increase in appetite or leads to dietary excess. In fact, exercise frequently has the opposite effect. The addition of exercise produces more weight loss than does dieting alone and has a favorable effect on body fat distribution. With regular exercise, WHR is reduced. Finally, exercise is especially important in maintaining weight loss.

When large muscles are involved in the exercise program, a primary benefit is cardiovascular conditioning. Exercise is of benefit to overweight and obese persons even if it does not make them lean. Many psychologic benefits can be derived from an increased physical activity program. Exercise decreases tension and stress, promotes better-quality sleep and rest, increases stamina and energy, improves self-concept and self-confidence, improves attitudes, and increases optimism about the future.[16]

Explore with patients possible ways to incorporate exercise in daily routines. It may be as simple as parking farther from their place of employment or taking the stairs versus an elevator. Encourage individuals to wear a pedometer to track their activity with a goal of 10,000 steps a day. However, success may be walking one third of the recommended steps with incremental increases over time. Although joining a health club can be one way of getting exercise, it is not necessary. Patients can walk, swim, and cycle, all of which have long-term benefits. Stress to patients that engaging in weekend exercise only or in spurts of strenuous activity is not advantageous and can actually be dangerous.

◆ **Behavior Modification.** The assumption behind behavior modification is twofold: (1) obesity is a learned disorder caused by overeating and (2) often the critical difference between an obese person and a person of normal weight is the cues that regulate eating behavior. Therefore most behavior-modification programs deemphasize the diet and focus on how and when to eat. Ideally, behavior intervention should begin with counseling sessions with a trained interventionist.[14]

Teach people to restrict their eating to designated meals and to increase the amount of physical activity in their lives. Persons who participate in a behavioral therapy program are more successful in maintaining their losses over an extended time than those who do not participate in such training.

Various behavioral techniques for patients engaged in a weight loss program include (1) self-monitoring, (2) stimulus control, and (3) rewards. *Self-monitoring* may involve keeping a record of the type and time food was consumed and how the person was feeling when eating. *Stimulus control* is aimed at separating events that trigger eating from the act of eating. *Rewards* may be used as incentives for weight loss. Short- and long-term goals are useful benchmarks for earning rewards. It is important that the reward for a specified weight loss not be associated with food, such as dinner out or a favorite treat. Reward items do not have to have a monetary component. For example, time for a hot bath or an hour of pleasure reading would be an enjoyable reward for many people.

Praise your patient's successes, even small ones, at every opportunity. Changing existing behaviors is difficult.

◆ **Support Groups.** People who are on a weight management plan are often encouraged to join a group in which others are also trying to modify their eating habits. Many self-help groups are available that offer support and information on dieting tips. For example, Take Off Pounds Sensibly (TOPS) *(www.tops.org)* is the oldest nonprofit organization of this type. Behavior modification is an integral part of the program, along with nutrition education. Weight Watchers International, Inc. *(www.weightwatchers.com)*, Jenny Craig *(www.jennycraig.com)*, and Nutrisystems *(www.nutrisystem.com)* are probably the most successful commercial weight-loss programs.[17] Weight Watchers offers a food plan that is nutritionally balanced and practical to follow. Group leaders, all of whom have successfully lost weight with Weight Watchers, teach members various behavior-modification techniques.

Commercial weight-reduction centers have proliferated across the nation. Many of these programs are staffed by nurses and dietitians. These weight-reduction centers are cost prohibitive for those with limited financial resources. Many of these programs also offer special prepackaged foods and supplements that must be purchased as part of the weight-reduction plan. Only these prescribed foods and drinks are to be consumed until an agreed-on amount of weight is lost. The patient is encouraged to buy the same type of foods for the maintenance phase of the program, lasting from 6 months to 1 year. Behavior-modification training is incorporated in these programs as well. Individuals must learn how to adjust their diet once they are no longer using the commercial products. This can be challenging for many, and the weight lost may be regained once the restricted food program is completed.[18]

In recent years, a number of employers have begun weight loss programs at the workplace. The rationale for such programs is that better health repays the cost of the programs through improved work performance, decreased absenteeism, less hospitalization, and lower insurance costs. Such programs have been well accepted by both employees and employers.

## ◆ Drug Therapy

Drugs should never be used alone. Rather, they should be part of a comprehensive weight loss program that includes reduced-calorie diet, exercise, and behavior modification.[19-21] Drugs should be reserved for adults with a BMI of 30 kg/m$^2$ or greater (obese), or adults with a BMI of 27 kg/m$^2$ or greater (overweight) who have at least one weight-related condition, such as hypertension, type 2 diabetes, or dyslipidemia. The drugs currently approved by the U.S. Food and Drug Administration (FDA) for obesity are presented in Table 40-9.

◆ **Appetite-Suppressing Drugs.** The sympathomimetic amines suppress appetite by increasing the availability of norepinephrine in the brain, thus stimulating the central nervous system. The sympathomimetics fall into two groups: amphetamines and nonamphetamines. The amphetamines have a much higher abuse potential than the nonamphetamines. Amphetamines are not recommended, nor are they approved by the FDA for either short- or long-term weight loss.

**TABLE 40-9 Drug Therapy**
***Obesity***

| Drug | Mechanism of Action | Nursing Considerations |
|---|---|---|
| orlistat (Xenical, Allī [low-dose form available over the counter]) | • Blocks fat breakdown and absorption in intestine<br>• Inhibits the action of intestinal lipases, resulting in undigested fat excreted in feces | • Associated with leakage of stool, flatulence, diarrhea, and abdominal bloating, especially if a high-fat diet is consumed<br>• Severe liver injury may occur.<br>• Fat-soluble vitamin levels may have to be supplemented. |
| lorcaserin (Belviq) | • Selective serotonin (5-HT) agonist<br>• Suppresses appetite and creates a sense of satiety | • Common side effects are headache, dizziness, fatigue, nausea, dry mouth, and constipation. |
| bupropion/ naltrexone (Contrave) | *bupropion:* antidepressant<br>*naltrexone:* opioid antagonist | • Common side effects are nausea, constipation, headache, vomiting, dizziness, insomnia, dry mouth, and diarrhea.<br>• Suicidal thoughts and behaviors and neuropsychiatric reactions can occur.<br>• Can increase BP and heart rate and should not be used in patients with uncontrolled hypertension<br>• Can cause seizures and must not be used in patients who have seizure disorder |
| phentermine/ topiramate (Qsymia) | *phentermine:* sympathomimetic anorectic<br>*topiramate:* antiseizure drug that induces satiety | • Common side effects are paresthesias, dizziness, insomnia, constipation, dry mouth.<br>• Must not be used in patients with glaucoma or hyperthyroidism<br>• Can increase heart rate, and should not be used in patients with uncontrolled hypertension or heart disease |
| liraglutide (Saxenda) | • Glucagon-like peptide 1 (GLP-1) agonist<br>• Induces satiety | • Used to treat type 2 diabetes<br>• Must be injected<br>• Side effects include thyroid tumors and pancreatitis. |

Nonamphetamines are not usually recommended for weight loss because of the potential for abuse. If used, these drugs should only be used short term (for 3 months or less).

Nonamphetamines include phentermine (Adipex-P, Fastin, Ionamin), diethylpropion (Tenuate), phendimetrazine (Bontril), and benzphetamine (Didrex). Adverse effects of these drugs include palpitations, tachycardia, overstimulation, restlessness, dizziness, insomnia, weakness, and fatigue.

◆ **Nursing Interventions Related to Drug Therapy.** Drugs will not cure obesity, and individuals must understand that without substantial changes in food intake and increased physical activity, they will gain weight when drug therapy is stopped.

As with any drug treatment, there are side effects (Table 40-9). Careful evaluation for other medical conditions can help determine which drugs, if any, would be advisable for a given patient. Many insurance companies do not cover the cost of weight loss drugs.

Your role related to drug therapy is to teach the patient about proper administration, side effects, and how the drugs fit into the overall weight loss plan. The modification of dosage without consultation with the HCP can have detrimental effects. Emphasize that diet and exercise regimens are the cornerstones of permanent weight loss. Finally, discourage the purchase of over-the-counter diet aids except for Allī.

## BARIATRIC SURGICAL THERAPY

**Bariatric surgery**, surgery on the stomach and/or intestines to help a person with extreme obesity lose weight, has become a viable option for treating obesity. Surgery is currently the only treatment that has been found to have a successful and lasting impact for sustained weight loss for individuals with extreme obesity.[14]

Criteria guidelines for bariatric surgery include having a BMI of 40 $kg/m^2$ or more or a BMI of 35 $kg/m^2$ or more with other significant co-morbidities (e.g., hypertension, type 2 diabetes mellitus, heart failure, sleep apnea).

The majority of people who undergo bariatric surgery successfully improve their overall quality of life. In addition to losing weight, patients often experience resolution of co-morbidities such as diabetes. Although overall mortality is very low, a number of complications can arise from surgery. Therefore the option to have surgery must be carefully considered.[22]

Many insurance carriers do not cover the cost of bariatric surgery. If they do consider reimbursing for the surgery, most of them require documentation of a medically supervised weight loss program for approximately 6 months.

Before being considered candidates for surgery, patients must be screened for psychologic, physical, and behavioral conditions that have been associated with poor surgical outcomes. These include untreated depression, binge eating disorders, and drug and alcohol abuse that may interfere with a commitment to lifelong behavioral changes. Other contraindications to surgery include illnesses that are known to reduce life expectancy and are not likely to be improved with weight reduction. These conditions include advanced cancer; end-stage kidney, liver, and cardiopulmonary disease; severe coagulopathy; or inability to comply with nutritional recommendations.

Bariatric surgeries fall into one of three broad categories: restrictive, malabsorptive, or a combination of malabsorptive and restrictive (Table 40-10 and Fig. 40-7). In *restrictive procedures* the stomach is reduced in size (less food eaten), and in *malabsorptive procedures* the small intestine is shortened or bypassed (less food absorbed). The majority of procedures are performed laparoscopically, thus decreasing postoperative recuperation as compared to an open procedure. With laparoscopy, patients have fewer wound infections, shorter hospital stays, and a faster recovery period.

### Restrictive Surgeries

Restrictive bariatric surgery reduces either the size of the stomach, which causes the patient to feel full more quickly, or the amount allowed to enter the stomach. In these surgeries, digestion is not altered, so the risk of anemia or cobalamin deficiency is low. The most common restrictive surgeries include adjustable gastric banding and sleeve gastrectomy.

**Adjustable Gastric Banding.** Laparoscopic *adjustable gastric banding* (AGB), the most common restrictive procedure done, involves limiting the stomach size with an inflatable band placed around the fundus of the stomach (Fig. 40-7, *A*). This restrictive procedure can be done using a Lap-Band or Realize Band system. The band is connected to a subcutaneous port and can be inflated or deflated (by fluid injection in the HCP's office) to change the stoma size to meet the patient's needs as weight is lost. The restrictive effect of the band creates a sense of fullness as the upper portion of the stomach now accommodates less than the average stomach. The band then causes a delay in stomach emptying, providing patients with further satiety.

The procedure can be either modified or reversed at a later date if necessary. AGB is the preferred option for patients who are surgical risks, because it is a less invasive approach.

**Sleeve Gastrectomy (Gastric Sleeve).** In the sleeve gastrectomy (gastric sleeve), about 75% of the stomach is removed, leaving a sleeve-shaped stomach (Fig. 40-7, *B*). Although the stomach is drastically reduced in size, its function is preserved. The removal of the majority of the stomach also results in the elimination of hormones produced in the stomach that stimulate hunger, such as ghrelin.

Research is ongoing on a procedure called *endoscopic sleeve gastroplasty*. It involves using an endoscope rather than making a surgical incision. When the endoscope reaches the stomach, the surgeon places sutures in the stomach, making it smaller and changing its shape.

**Gastric Plication.** Gastric plication is a minimally invasive weight-loss surgery that reduces the size of the stomach. It is done by folding the stomach wall inward, and then sutures are placed to secure the folded stomach wall. This reduces the stomach volume by as much as 70%.

**Intragastric Balloons.** Intragastric balloons involve a weight-loss system (Orbera, ReShape) that uses a gastric balloon that occupies space in the stomach. The balloon is placed into the stomach through the mouth, using a minimally invasive endoscopic procedure, while the patient is under mild sedation. Once in place, the balloon is filled with saline so that it expands. The balloon can be filled with different amounts of saline (from 400 to 700 mL). When it is time to remove the balloon, it is first deflated and then removed using another endoscopic procedure.

The intragastric balloon does not change or alter the stomach's natural anatomy. It is designed to help patients feel more full, curb the appetite, and reduce food intake. Patients are advised to follow a diet and exercise plan to assist with their weight loss efforts.

The balloons are less invasive than having gastric bypass surgery. This device should not be used in patients who have had previous gastrointestinal or bariatric surgery or who have been diagnosed with inflammatory bowel disease, large hiatal hernia, symptoms of delayed gastric emptying, or active *Helicobacter pylori* infection.

Once the device is placed in the stomach, patients may experience vomiting, nausea, abdominal pain, and feelings of indigestion. Other potential risks are gastric ulcers and balloon deflation.

### Combination of Restrictive and Malabsorptive Surgery

**Roux-en-Y Gastric Bypass.** The Roux-en-Y gastric bypass (RYGB) procedure is a combination of restrictive and

TABLE 40-10 **Surgical Therapy for Obesity***

| Description | Advantages | Disadvantages |
|---|---|---|
| **Restrictive Surgery** | | |
| ***Adjustable Gastric Banding (AGB) (Lap-Band, Realize Band)*** | | |
| • Inflatable band encircles stomach<br>• Creation of gastric pouch with about 30 mL (1 oz) capacity<br>• Later stretches to 60-90 mL (2-3 oz)<br>• Upper gastric pouch connected by very narrow channel to lower section of stomach | • Food digestion occurs through normal process<br>• Band can be adjusted to ↑ or ↓ restriction<br>• Surgery can be reversed<br>• Absence of dumping syndrome<br>• Lack of malabsorption<br>• Low complication rate | • Some nausea and vomiting initially (eating too much too quickly)<br>• Problems with adjustment device<br>• Band may slip or erode into stomach wall<br>• Gastric perforation<br>• Weight loss may be more limited than with other types of surgery |
| ***Sleeve Gastrectomy (Gastric Sleeve)*** | | |
| • About 75% of stomach removed<br>• Creation of sleeve-shaped stomach with 60-150 mL (2-5 oz) capacity | • Function of stomach preserved<br>• No bypass of intestine<br>• Avoids complications of obstruction, anemia, vitamin deficiencies | • Weight loss may be more limited than with other types of surgery<br>• Leakage related to stapling<br>• Irreversible |
| ***Gastric Plication*** | | |
| • Adapted version of sleeve gastrectomy (gastric sleeve)<br>• Sleeve created by suturing rather than removing stomach | • Minimal surgery compared to sleeve gastrectomy<br>• No rerouting of intestines<br>• Natural nutrient absorption capabilities maintained | • Requires hospital stay of 24-48 hr<br>• Nausea common after procedure<br>• Risks include stomach leakage from sutured areas, blockage of stomach from swelling or fold too tight |
| ***Intragastric Balloon*** | | |
| • Involves placing a deflated balloon into stomach using an endoscope<br>• Balloon then filled with saline and occupies space in stomach | • Does not require invasive surgery<br>• Done as outpatient procedure | • Can only be left in place for 6 months<br>• Once device in stomach, patients may experience nausea, vomiting, abdominal pain, indigestion, and gastric ulcers |
| **Malabsorptive Surgery** | | |
| ***Biliopancreatic Diversion (BPD) With or Without Duodenal Switch*** | | |
| • 70% of the stomach removed horizontally<br>• Anastomosis between stomach and intestine<br>• Decreases the amount of small intestine available for nutrient absorption<br>• Duodenal switch cuts the stomach vertically and is shaped like a tube | • Able to eat larger meals than with gastric bypass or banding procedures<br>• Less food intolerance<br>• Rapid weight loss<br>• Greater long-term weight loss | • Abdominal bloating, diarrhea, and foul-smelling gas (steatorrhea)<br>• Three or four loose bowel movements a day<br>• Malabsorption of fat-soluble vitamins<br>• Iron deficiency<br>• Protein-calorie malnutrition<br>• Dumping syndrome<br>• Most complicated of weight loss surgeries |
| **Combination of Restrictive and Malabsorptive Surgery** | | |
| ***Roux-en-Y Gastric Bypass (RYGB)*** | | |
| • Surgery on stomach to create a pouch (restrictive)<br>• Small gastric pouch connected to jejunum<br>• Remaining stomach and first segment of small intestine are bypassed (malabsorptive) | • Better weight loss results than with restrictive procedures<br>• Lower incidence of malnutrition and diarrhea<br>• Rapid improvement of weight-related co-morbidities<br>• Good long-term results | • Leak at site of anastomosis<br>• Anemia: iron deficiency, cobalamin deficiency, folic acid deficiency<br>• Calcium deficiency<br>• Dumping syndrome<br>• Irreversible |
| **Implanted Gastric Stimulation Device** | | |
| ***Maestro Rechargeable System*** *(Fig. 40-8)* | | |
| • Device implanted into abdomen<br>• Works like pacemaker to deliver electrical impulses to vagus nerve, which tells brain when stomach is full. | • Least invasive of weight loss surgeries<br>• Procedure done on outpatient basis | • Device must be charged 1-2 times/week<br>• If battery completely drained, device needs to be reprogrammed<br>• Side effects include nausea, vomiting, heartburn, belching, swallowing problems |

*Fig. 40-7.

malabsorptive surgery. This surgical procedure is the most common bariatric procedure performed in the United States. It is considered the gold standard among bariatric procedures.[14]

This procedure involves creating a small gastric pouch and attaching it directly to the small intestine using a Y-shaped limb of the small bowel (Fig. 40-7, *D*). After the procedure, food bypasses 90% of the stomach, the duodenum, and a small segment of jejunum.

Overall, it has low complication rates, has excellent patient tolerance, and sustains long-term weight loss. Outcomes include improved glucose control with improvement or reversal of diabetes, normalization of BP, decreased total cholesterol and triglycerides, decreased GERD, and decreased sleep apnea.

A complication of the RYGB is *dumping syndrome,* in which gastric contents empty too rapidly into the small intestine, overwhelming its ability to digest nutrients. Symptoms can include vomiting, nausea, weakness, sweating, faintness, and, on occasion, diarrhea. Patients are discouraged from eating sugary foods after surgery to avoid dumping syndrome. Because sections of the small intestine are bypassed, poor absorption of iron can cause iron-deficiency anemia. Patients need to take a multivitamin with iron and calcium supplements. Chronic anemia caused

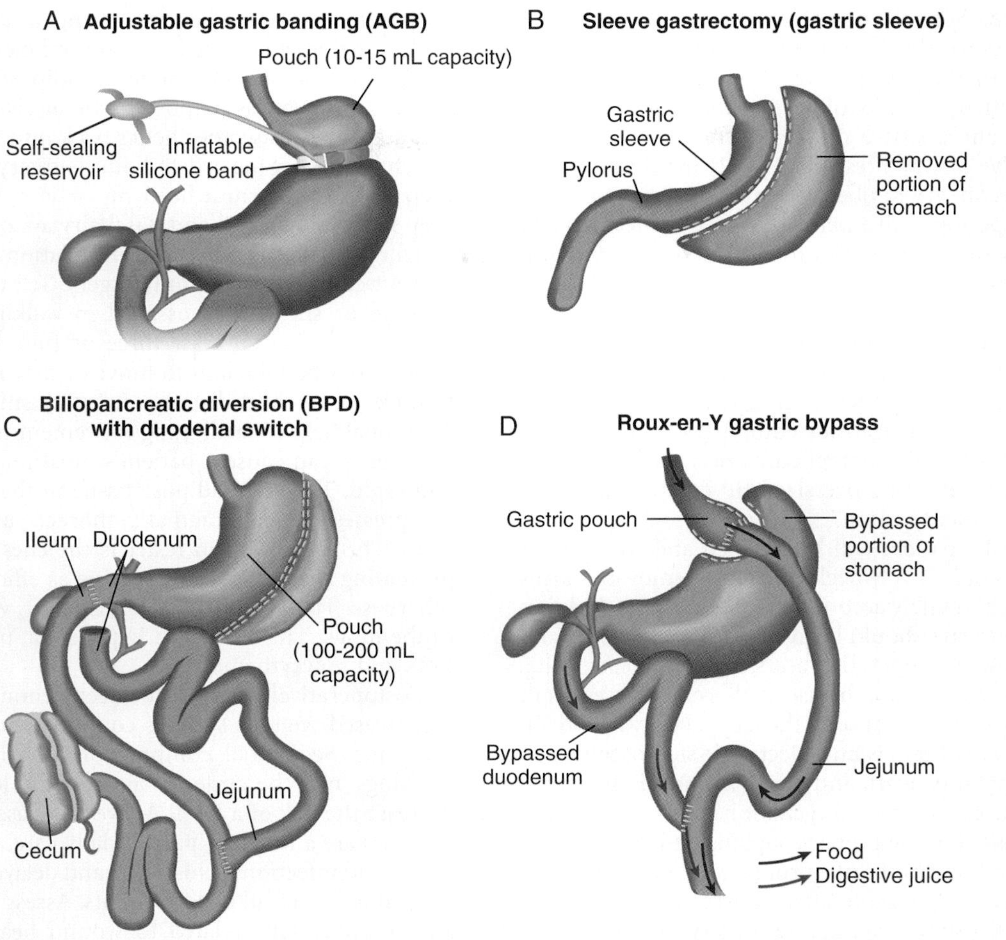


**FIG. 40-7** Bariatric surgical procedures. **A,** Adjustable gastric banding (AGB) uses a band to create a gastric pouch. **B,** Sleeve gastrectomy involves creating a sleeve-shaped stomach by removing about 75% of the stomach. **C,** Biliopancreatic diversion (BPD) with duodenal switch procedure creates an anastomosis between the stomach and intestine. **D,** Roux-en-Y gastric bypass procedure involves constructing a gastric pouch whose outlet is a Y-shaped limb of small intestine.

by cobalamin deficiency may also occur. This problem can usually be managed with parenteral or intranasal cobalamin.

### Implantable Gastric Stimulation

An implantable gastric stimulation device (e.g., Maestro Rechargeable System) consists of a pacemaker-like electrical pulse generator, wire leads, and electrodes that are implanted in the abdomen (Fig. 40-8). The Maestro System works by sending intermittent electrical pulses to the vagus nerve, which is involved in regulating stomach emptying and signaling to the brain that the stomach feels empty or full. External controllers allow the patient to charge the device and allow HCPs to adjust the device's settings in order to provide optimal therapy.

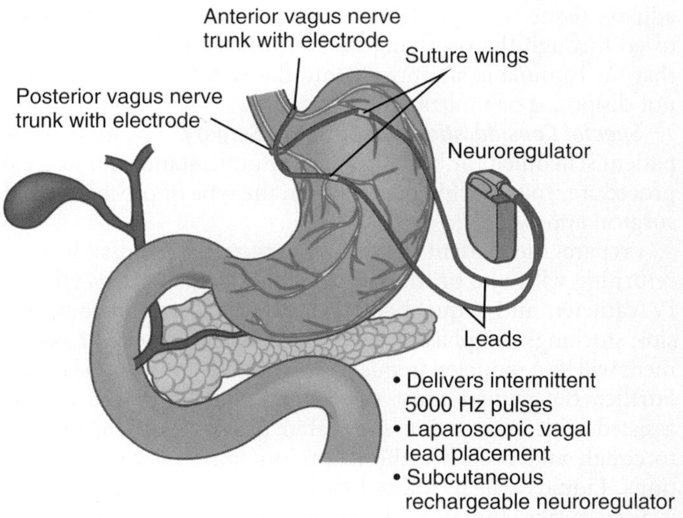


**FIG. 40-8** The Maestro Rechargeable System is an electrical stimulator that is surgically implanted into the abdomen. It works by sending intermittent electrical pulses to the vagus nerve, which is involved in regulating stomach emptying and signaling to the brain that the stomach feels empty or full.

## NURSING MANAGEMENT: PERIOPERATIVE CARE OF THE OBESE PATIENT

### Nursing Implementation

This section discusses general nursing considerations for the care of the obese patient who is having surgery. Special nursing considerations are described for the patient who is having bariatric surgery. (Care of the surgical patient is discussed in Chapters 17 to 19.)

**Preoperative Care.** Special considerations are necessary for the obese patient, especially the individual with extreme obesity, who is admitted to the hospital for surgery. Before surgery, interview the patient to identify past and current health information and any assistive devices currently in use (e.g., continuous positive airway pressure [CPAP] for sleep apnea). Co-morbidities secondary to obesity increase the risk for complications in the perioperative period. It may be necessary to coordinate care with the patient's cardiologist, pulmonologist, gynecologist, gastroenterologist, or other specialists.

Have a plan in place before the patients arrive so that they receive optimal care and do not feel like they are a burden to the nursing staff. Nursing units must have available appropriate size hospital gowns, beds that accommodate an increased body size, and necessary patient transfer equipment.[23] To correctly measure BP in obese people, a larger cuff size is needed to avoid artifactual errors. Ensure that oversized BP cuffs are available and placed in the patient's room.

Consider how the patient will be weighed and transported throughout the hospital. A wheelchair with removable arms that is large enough to safely accommodate the patient and pass easily through doorways should be available.

Preoperative and postoperative assessment of heart, lung, and bowel sounds may require the use of alternative assessment techniques. For example, because of the large chest wall, breath and heart sounds are often distant. Electronic stethoscopes can be used to amplify lung, heart, and bowel sounds. Pulse oximetry may also be used to assess oxygenation status.

Instruct the patient in the proper coughing and deep breathing techniques and methods of turning and positioning to prevent pulmonary complications after surgery. If possible, demonstrate the use of a spirometer before surgery. Use of the spirometer helps prevent and treat postoperative lung congestion. Practicing these strategies preoperatively can help the patient perform them correctly postoperatively. Furthermore, if the patient uses CPAP at home for sleep apnea, make arrangements for the use of a machine while the patient is hospitalized.

Obtaining venous access may be complicated by excess adipose tissue. A longer IV catheter is helpful (longer than 1 in) to go through the overlying tissue to the vein. It is important that the cannula is far enough into the vein to ensure that it is not dislodged or infiltrated.

***Special Considerations for Bariatric Surgery.*** Ensure that the patient scheduled for bariatric surgery understands the surgical procedure. Your teaching depends on the type of procedure and surgical approach.[24]

Prepare the patient before surgery for the possibility of returning with one or more of the following: urinary catheter, IV catheter, and sequential compression device or compression stockings. Emphasize that vital signs and a general assessment will be conducted frequently to monitor for complications. Further, the patient must understand that he or she will be assisted with ambulation soon after surgery and encouraged to cough and deep breathe to prevent pulmonary complications. Liquids will be started early, but only after the patient is fully awake and there is no evidence of any anastomosis leaks.

**Postoperative Care.** The initial postoperative care focuses on careful assessment and immediate intervention for cardiopulmonary complications, thrombus formation, anastomosis leaks, and electrolyte imbalances. The transfer from surgery may require many trained staff members. During the transfer, the patient's airway should remain stabilized and attention given to managing the patient's pain. Maintain the patient's head at a 35- to 40-degree angle to reduce abdominal pressure and increase lung expansion.

The body stores anesthetics in adipose tissue, thus placing patients with excess adipose tissue at risk for re-sedation. As adipose cells release anesthetics back into the bloodstream, the patient may become sedated after surgery. If this happens, be prepared to perform a head-tilt or jaw-thrust maneuver and keep the patient's oral and nasal airways open.

Diligence in turning and ambulation postoperatively will prevent complications from surgery. Tell the patient that typically he or she will be assisted in walking the evening after surgery and then at least three or four times each day. The patient may be reluctant to move or may not have the stamina to walk even a short distance. In either situation, you will need additional help in facilitating movement in an obese patient.

Obesity can cause a patient's breathing to become shallow and rapid. The extra adipose tissue in the chest and abdomen compresses the diaphragmatic, thoracic, and abdominal structures. This compression restricts the chest's ability to expand, preventing the lungs from working as efficiently as they would otherwise. The patient retains more $CO_2$ with less $O_2$ delivered to the lungs. This results in hypoxemia, pulmonary hypertension, and polycythemia.

Postoperatively the risk for deep venous thrombosis (DVT) is increased. Venous stasis is common due to the pressure on the veins. Sequential compression stockings or compression stockings may be ordered along with low-dose heparin to decrease the risk of a DVT. Active and passive range-of-motion exercises are a frequent part of daily care.

Wound infection, dehiscence, and delayed healing are potential problems for all obese patients. Assess the patient's skin for any complications related to wound healing. Keep skinfolds clean and dry to prevent dermatitis and secondary bacterial or fungal infections.

***Special Considerations for Bariatric Surgery.*** Patients experience considerable abdominal pain after bariatric surgery. Give pain medications as necessary during the immediate postoperative period (first 24 hours). Be aware that pain could be from an anastomosis leak rather than typical surgical pain.

Abdominal wounds require frequent observation for the amount and type of drainage, condition of the incision, and signs of infection. Protect the incision against undue straining that accompanies turning and coughing. Monitor vital signs to assist in identifying problems such as infection.

During the immediate postoperative period water and sugar-free clear liquids are given (30 mL every 2 hours while awake). Before discharge, instruct patients on a measured amount of a high-protein liquid diet. The patient is taught to eat slowly, stop eating when feeling full, and not consume liquids with solid food. Vomiting is a common complication during this time. A dietitian is usually part of the bariatric team and assists the patient with the transition to the new diet.

**Ambulatory and Home Care**

***Special Considerations for Bariatric Surgery.*** The patient who has undergone major surgical treatment for obesity has not been successful in the past in following or maintaining a prescribed diet. Now the patient is forced to reduce oral intake because of the anatomic changes from the surgical procedure. The patient's adherence to a reduced intake is necessary because of the concern for abdominal distention, cramping abdominal pain, and perhaps diarrhea.

Weight loss is considerable during the first 6 to 12 months. During this time the patient must learn to adjust intake sufficiently to maintain a stable weight. Although behavior modification is not necessarily an intended outcome with these surgical procedures, it becomes an unexpected secondary gain. For example, a person who has had bariatric surgery cannot overeat or binge eat without consequences.

The diet generally prescribed should be high in protein and low in carbohydrates, fat, and roughage and consist of six small feedings daily. Fluids should not be ingested with the meal, and in some cases, fluids should be restricted to less than 1000 mL/day. Fluids and foods high in carbohydrate tend to promote diarrhea and symptoms of the dumping syndrome. Generally, calorically dense foods (foods high in fat) should be avoided to permit more nutritionally sound food to be consumed.[25]

The patient must clearly understand the proper diet. Late complications can be anticipated after bariatric surgery, including anemia, vitamin deficiencies, diarrhea, and psychologic problems. Failure to lose weight or loss of too much weight may be caused by the surgical formation of too large a stomach pouch or of an outlet that is much too small, respectively. Peptic ulcer formation, dumping syndrome, and small bowel obstruction may be seen late in the recovery and rehabilitation stage.

Emphasize the importance of long-term follow-up care, in part because of potential complications late in the recovery period. Encourage patients to adhere strictly to the prescribed diet and to inform the HCP of any changes in their physical or emotional condition. Some patients have been known to overeat when they return home and gain rather than lose weight.

## INFORMATICS IN PRACTICE

### *Use of Cell Phone for Weight Loss*

- Cell phone apps (e.g., My Fitness Pal) are available to help track calories, weight, exercise, and eating patterns.
- Apps are popular for accountability, reflection, and motivation.
- Tracking systems may provide immediate access to nutritional information for better dietary decision making.
- Some apps (e.g., Foodmeter) can be used to scan the barcode of foods in the grocery store and give nutritional information.
- Calorie tracker apps can be used to monitor daily calorie intake and keep a record of weight loss progress.
- With text messaging, a phone "buddy" can be used to provide support when a person's will power is lacking.
- Share progress with friends and family. Some weight loss apps for cell phones sync with social media accounts so that a person can share milestones by adding them to Twitter and Facebook.

## CHECK YOUR PRACTICE

You are working in the bariatric surgery outpatient clinic. When you walk into the clinic room where a 36-yr-old woman is waiting for her follow-up visit, you find her distraught and crying. You ask her what is wrong. She responds, "I am a total failure. I have been fat all my life and I had to have this horrible surgery to help me. Why couldn't I do it on my own?"

- What is an effective way for you to handle this situation?

Several potential psychologic problems may arise after surgery. Some patients express guilty feelings that weight loss was achieved by surgical interventions rather than by the "sheer willpower" of reduced dietary intake and exercise. Be ready to provide support and assist the patient in moving away from such negative feelings.

By 6 to 8 months after surgery, considerable weight loss has usually occurred, and patients are able to see how much their appearance has changed. Discussion of this possible outcome with the patient before surgery and again during the rehabilitation phase facilitates the patient's adjustment to a new body image. Do not hesitate to encourage counseling for unresolved psychologic issues.

Massive weight loss often leaves the patient with large quantities of flabby skin that can result in problems related to altered body image (Fig. 40-9). Cosmetic surgery may alleviate this situation.

Often one result of bariatric surgery is the return of fertility in women. Pregnancy complications can result from anemia and nutritional deficiencies. Furthermore, depending on the type of surgery, intestinal obstructions and hernias are commonly experienced in pregnancy. Women must carefully consider the risk of pregnancy after bariatric surgery. In general, encourage women to postpone pregnancy for 12 to 18 months after bariatric surgery.

## EVIDENCE-BASED PRACTICE

### *Applying the Evidence*

**Obesity Interventions in Faith-Based Organizations**

J.W. is a 39-year-old African American woman who is 5 ft 6 in tall and weighs 196 lb. You work in the outpatient clinic that she visits for health care. Your clinic is referring patients who would benefit from losing weight to weight loss programs. She tells you she has been trying to lose weight by "watching what she eats" and that she is "not sure what else she can do." In further conversations with her, you learn she is an active member of her neighborhood church.

***Making Clinical Decisions***

***Best Available Evidence.*** Faith-based organizations are places where effective programs have helped obese individuals improve weight-related behaviors and lose weight.

***Clinician Expertise.*** You know it is important for J.W. to engage in a weight loss program that will assist her in adopting healthy behaviors. You also know churches can play a major role in providing health promotion programs in African American communities.

***Patient Preferences and Values.*** J.W. indicates she is interested in learning about a weight loss program at her church.

***Implications for Nursing Practice***

1. Why is it important to discuss with J.W. her motivation for attending the program at her church?
2. How will you help J.W. to set realistic short- and long-term goals related to weight loss? How may these goals differ?
3. At each clinic visit, how will you support J.W.'s efforts to lose weight?

***Reference for Evidence***

Lancaster K, Carter-Edwards L, Grilo S, et al: Obesity interventions in African American faith-based organizations: a systematic review, *Obes Rev* 15:159, 2014.

## ◆ Evaluation

The expected outcomes are that the obese patient will

- Experience long-term weight loss
- Have improvement in obesity-related co-morbidities
- Integrate healthy practices into daily routines
- Monitor for adverse side effects of surgical therapy
- Have an improved self-image

## Gerontologic Considerations: Obesity in Older Adults

The prevalence of obesity is increasing in all age groups, including older people. The number of obese older persons has markedly risen because of increases in both the total number of older persons and the percentage of the older adults who are obese. Obesity is more common in older women than in older men.

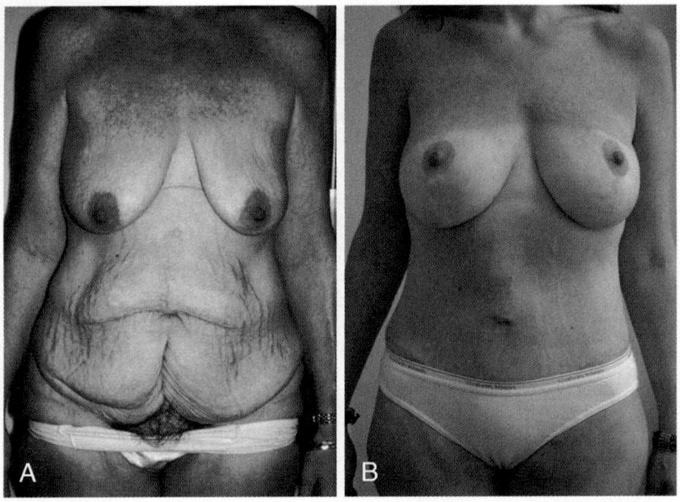


**FIG. 40-9** **A,** Preoperative view of a 37-year-old woman with massive weight loss who had gastric bypass surgery. **B,** Postoperative view 2½ years after abdominoplasty. She also underwent breast surgery, thighlift, backlift with excision of excess skin of the lower back and upper buttocks, and upper arm surgery. (From Shermak MA: Contouring the epigastrium, *Aesthet Surg J* 25:506, 2005.)

A decrease in energy expenditure is an important contributor to a gradual increase in body fat with age.

Obesity in older adults can exacerbate age-related declines in physical function and lead to frailty and disability. Obesity is associated with decreased survival. Individuals who are obese live 6 to 7 years less than people of normal weight.

Many of the changes associated with aging are exacerbated by obesity. Excess body weight places more demands on arthritic joints. The mechanical strain on weight-bearing joints can lead to premature immobility. Excess weight also affects other body systems. Older adults may find that excess intraabdominal weight causes problems with urinary incontinence. In addition, excess weight may contribute to hypoventilation and sleep apnea.

Obesity affects the quality of life for older adults. Weight loss can improve physical functioning and obesity-related health complications. The same therapeutic approaches for obesity as were discussed earlier also apply to the older adult.

## COSMETIC SURGICAL THERAPY

### Lipectomy

**Lipectomy** (adipectomy) is performed to remove unsightly flabby folds of adipose tissue (Fig. 40-9). There is no evidence that a regeneration of adipose tissue occurs at the surgical sites. However, emphasize to the patient that surgical removal does not prevent obesity from recurring, especially if lifetime eating habits remain the same. Although body image and self-esteem may be enhanced by such procedures, these operations are not without complications. The dangerous effects of anesthesia and the potential for poor wound healing in the obese patient cannot be overemphasized.

### Liposuction

Another cosmetic surgical procedure is liposuction, or suction-assisted lipectomy. It is used for cosmetic purposes and not for weight reduction. This surgical intervention helps improve facial appearance or body contours. A good candidate for this type of surgery is a person who has achieved weight reduction but who has excess fat under the chin, along the jaw line, in the nasolabial folds, over the abdomen, or around the waist and upper thighs. A long, hollow, stainless steel cannula is inserted through a small incision over the fatty tissue to be suctioned. This surgical procedure is not usually recommended for the older person because the skin is less elastic and will not accommodate the new underlying shape.

**TABLE 40-11 Criteria for Metabolic Syndrome***

| Measure | Criteria |
|---|---|
| **Waist circumference** | ≥40 in (102 cm) in men<br>≥35 in (89 cm) in women |
| **Triglycerides** | >150 mg/dL (1.7 mmol/L)<br>OR<br>Drug treatment for elevated triglycerides |
| **High-density lipoprotein (HDL) cholesterol** | <40 mg/dL (0.9 mmol/L) in men<br><50 mg/dL (1.1 mmol/L) in women<br>OR<br>Drug treatment for elevated cholesterol |
| **BP** | ≥130 mm Hg systolic BP<br>OR<br>≥85 mm Hg diastolic BP<br>OR<br>Drug treatment for hypertension |
| **Fasting blood glucose** | ≥110 mg/dL<br>OR<br>Drug treatment for elevated glucose |

Source: National Heart, Lung, and Blood Institute: How is metabolic syndrome diagnosed? Retrieved from *www.nhlbi.nih.gov/health/dci/Diseases/ms/ms_diagnosis.html.*
*Any three of the five measures are needed for a diagnosis of metabolic syndrome.

## METABOLIC SYNDROME

**Metabolic syndrome** is a group of metabolic risk factors that increase an individual's chance of developing cardiovascular disease, stroke, and diabetes mellitus. About one in three adults have metabolic syndrome. The syndrome is more prevalent in those 60 years of age and older.[26]

Metabolic syndrome is characterized by a cluster of health problems, including obesity, hypertension, abnormal lipid levels, and high blood glucose. Metabolic syndrome is diagnosed if an individual has three or more of the conditions listed in Table 40-11.

Currently health professionals are debating whether metabolic syndrome should be viewed as a distinct condition. Since there is not one standard treatment for the syndrome itself, interventions are focused on each risk factor.

### Etiology and Pathophysiology

The main underlying risk factor for metabolic syndrome is insulin resistance related to excessive visceral fat (Fig. 40-10). Insulin resistance is the body's cells diminished ability to respond to the action of insulin. The pancreas compensates by secreting more insulin, resulting in hyperinsulinemia.

Other characteristics of metabolic syndrome include hypertension, increased risk for clotting, and abnormalities in cholesterol levels. The net effect of these conditions is an increased prevalence of coronary artery disease.

### Clinical Manifestations and Diagnostic Studies

The signs of metabolic syndrome are impaired fasting blood glucose, hypertension, abnormal cholesterol levels, and obesity.

PATHOPHYSIOLOGY MAP

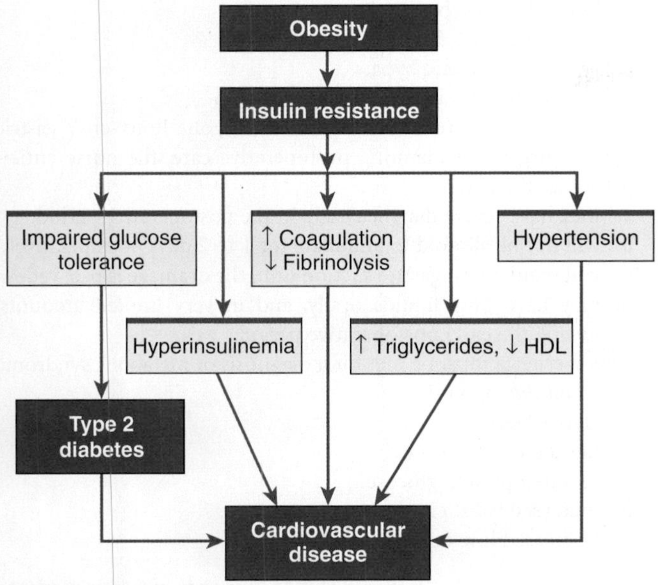


**FIG. 40-10** Relationship among insulin resistance, obesity, diabetes mellitus, and cardiovascular disease. *HDL,* High-density lipoprotein.

Medical problems develop over time if the condition remains unaddressed. Patients with this syndrome are at a higher risk of heart disease, stroke, diabetes, renal disease, and polycystic ovary syndrome. Patients who have metabolic syndrome and smoke are at an even higher risk.

## NURSING AND INTERPROFESSIONAL MANAGEMENT: METABOLIC SYNDROME

Lifestyle modifications are the first-line interventions to reduce the risk factors for metabolic syndrome. Management or reversal of metabolic syndrome can be achieved by reducing the major risk factors of cardiovascular disease: reducing LDL cholesterol, stopping smoking, lowering BP, and reducing glucose levels. For long-term risk reduction, weight should be decreased, physical activity increased, and healthy dietary habits established.

There is no specific management of metabolic syndrome. You can assist patients by providing information on healthy diets, exercise, and positive lifestyle changes. The diet, which should be low in saturated fats, should promote weight loss. Weight reduction and maintenance of a lower weight should be the first priority in those with abdominal obesity and metabolic syndrome.

Because sedentary lifestyles contribute to metabolic syndrome, increasing regular physical activity will lower a patient's risk factors. In addition to assisting in weight reduction, regular exercise has been found to decrease the triglyceride level and increase the HDL cholesterol level in patients with metabolic syndrome.[26]

Patients unable to lower risk factors with lifestyle therapies alone or those at high risk for a coronary event or diabetes may be considered for drug therapy. Although there is no specific medication for metabolic syndrome, cholesterol-lowering and antihypertensive drugs can be used. Metformin (Glucophage) has also been used to prevent diabetes by lowering glucose levels and enhancing the cells' sensitivity to insulin.

## CASE STUDY

### *Obesity*

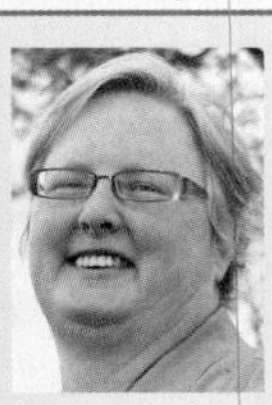

(©Thinkstock)

**Patient Profile**

S.R. is a 48-yr-old white woman who comes to the clinic with complaints of hip pain.

**Subjective Data**

- States that it is "getting hard to get around"
- Reports gradual weight gain of 40 lb over past 40 yr
- Lives in a rural community with no sidewalks
- Spends most of her free time watching television
- Reports health problems related to type 2 diabetes mellitus, shortness of breath, hypertension, and osteoarthritis
- Had knee replacement surgery at age 46 for osteoarthritis
- Has tried orlistat (Xenical) but hated the side effects

**Objective Data**

***Physical Examination***

- 5 ft 6 in tall; weighs 230 lb; BMI 37 kg/m², waist circumference of 40 in
- Has obese, nontender, soft round, abdomen
- BP 160/100 mm Hg

***Laboratory Results***

- Fasting blood glucose 250 mg/dL (13.9 mmol/L)
- Total cholesterol 205 mg/dL (5.3 mmol/L)
- Triglyceride 298 mg/dL (3.36 mmol/L)
- HDL cholesterol 31 mg/dL (0.8 mmol/L)
- LDL cholesterol 114 mg/dL

**Interprofessional Care**

- Referral to a community weight loss program
- Consultation with bariatric surgeon

**Discussion Questions**

1. What are S.R.'s risk factors for obesity?
2. Of the possible complications of obesity, which ones does S.R. have? Why did she develop them?
3. ***Patient-Centered Care:*** How would you assist S.R. in designing a successful weight loss and weight management program?
4. ***Teamwork and Collaboration:*** How could a comprehensive community weight loss program be beneficial to S.R.?
5. What are S.R.'s risk factors for metabolic syndrome?
6. Is S.R. a candidate for bariatric surgery? Why or why not?
7. ***Evidence-Based Practice:*** S.R. tells you that she is not sure surgery will work for her. She asks you, "What is the best surgery for me?"

Answers available at *http://evolve.elsevier.com/Lewis/medsurg.*

## BRIDGE TO NCLEX EXAMINATION

The number of the question corresponds to the same-numbered outcome at the beginning of the chapter.

1. Which statement *best* describes the etiology of obesity?
   - **a.** Obesity primarily results from a genetic predisposition.
   - **b.** Psychosocial factors can override the effects of genetics in the etiology of obesity.
   - **c.** Obesity is the result of complex interactions between genetic and environmental factors.
   - **d.** Genetic factors are more important than environmental factors in the etiology of obesity.
2. The obesity classification that is *most* often associated with cardiovascular health problems is
   - **a.** primary obesity.
   - **b.** secondary obesity.
   - **c.** gynoid fat distribution.
   - **d.** android fat distribution.
3. Health risks associated with obesity include *(select all that apply)*
   - **a.** colorectal cancer.
   - **b.** rheumatoid arthritis.
   - **c.** polycystic ovary syndrome.
   - **d.** nonalcoholic steatohepatitis.
   - **e.** systemic lupus erythematosus.
4. The *best* nutritional therapy plan for a person who is obese is
   - **a.** the Zone diet.
   - **b.** the Atkins diet.
   - **c.** Sugar Busters.
   - **d.** foods from the basic food groups.
5. This bariatric surgical procedure involves creating a gastric pouch that is reversible and no malabsorption occurs. What surgical procedure is this?
   - **a.** Vertical gastric banding
   - **b.** Biliopancreatic diversion
   - **c.** Roux-en-Y gastric bypass
   - **d.** Adjustable gastric banding
6. A patient with extreme obesity has undergone Roux-en-Y gastric bypass surgery. In planning postoperative care, the nurse anticipates that the patient
   - **a.** may have severe diarrhea early in the postoperative period.
   - **b.** will not be allowed to ambulate for 1 to 2 days postoperatively.
   - **c.** will require nasogastric suction until the drainage is pale yellow.
   - **d.** may have only liquids orally, and in very limited amounts, during the early postoperative period.
7. Which criteria must be met for a diagnosis of metabolic syndrome *(select all that apply)*?
   - **a.** Hypertension
   - **b.** Elevated triglycerides
   - **c.** Elevated plasma glucose
   - **d.** Increased waist circumference
   - **e.** Decreased low-density lipoproteins

1. c, 2. d, 3. a, c, d, 4. d, 5. d, 6. d, 7. a, b, c, d

For rationales to these answers and even more NCLEX review questions, visit *http://evolve.elsever.com/Lewis/medsurg.*

## EVOLVE WEBSITE

http://evolve.elsevier.com/Lewis/medsurg

**Review Questions (Online Only)**

**Key Points**

**Answer Keys for Questions**

- Rationales for Bridge to NCLEX Examination Questions
- Answer Guidelines for Case Study on p. 891

**Student Case Study**

- Patient With Obesity and Osteoarthritis

**Conceptual Care Map Creator**

**Audio Glossary**

**Content Updates**

## REFERENCES


1. Trust for America's Health, Robert Wood Johnson Foundation. The state of obesity. 2014. Retrieved from *http://stateofobesity.org.*
2. Breymaier SOB: AMA adopts new policies on second day of voting at annual meeting. 2013. Retrieved from *www.ama-assn.org/ama/pub/news/news/2013/2013-06-18-new-ama-policies-annual-meeting.page.*
*3. Ford ES, Maynard LM, Li C: Trends in mean waist circumference and abdominal obesity among US adults, 1999-2012, *JAMA* 312(11):1151, 2014.
4. Modern Genetics: Genetics of body shape: apple or pear? Retrieved from *http://sirens-space.blogspot.com/2012/03/genetics-of-body-shape-apple-or-pear.html.*
*5. Naukkarinen J, Rissanen A, Kaprio J, et al: Causes and consequences of obesity: the contribution of recent twin studies, *Int J Obes (Lond)* 36(8):1017, 2012.
6. Malis C, Rasmussen EL, Foulsen P, et al: Total and regional fat distribution is strongly influenced by genetic factors in young and elderly twins, *Obesity Res* 13:2139, 2005. (Classic)
7. Tung YC, Yeo GS, O'Rahilly S, et al: Obesity and FTO: changing focus at a complex locus, *Cell Metab* 20(5):710, 2014.
8. Troke RC, Tan TM, Bloom SR: The future role of gut hormones in the treatment of obesity, *Ther Adv Chronic Dis* 5(1):4, 2014.
*9. Flegal KM, Kit BK, Orpana H, et al: Association of all-cause mortality with overweight and obesity using standard body mass index categories: a systematic review and meta-analysis, *JAMA* 309(1):71, 2013.
10. Lavie CJ, McAuley PA, Church TS, et al: Obesity and cardiovascular diseases: implications regarding fitness, fatness, and severity in the obesity paradox, *J Am Coll Cardiol* 63(14):1345, 2014.
11. Gregg EW, Zhuo X, Cheng YJ, et al: Trends in lifetime risk and years of life lost due to diabetes in the USA, 1985-2011: a modelling study, *Lancet Diabetes Endocrinol* 2(11):867, 2014.
12. Gallagher EJ, LeRoith D: Obesity and diabetes: the increased risk of cancer and cancer-related mortality, *Physiol Rev* 95(3):727, 2015.
13. Budd GM, Peterson JA: The obesity epidemic, Part 1: Understanding the origins, *AJN* 114:40, 2014.
*14. Jensen MD, Ryan DH, Donato KA, et al: Guidelines (2013) for managing overweight and obesity in adults, *Obesity* 22(S2):S1, 2014.
15. The National Weight Control Registry. NWCR facts. Retrieved from *www.nwcr.ws/Research/default.htm.*
16. Budd GM, Peterson JA: The obesity epidemic, Part 2: Nursing assessment and intervention, *AJN* 115:38, 2015.
17. Gudzune KA, Doshi RS, Mehta AK, et al. Efficacy of commercial weight-loss programs: an updated systematic review, *Ann Intern Med* 162(7):501, 2015.
18. Wee CC: The role of commercial weight-loss programs, *Ann Intern Med* 162(7):522, 2015.
19. Schumacher D: Pharmacological management of the obese patient, *Am J Lifestyle Med* 9(2):137, 2015.
*20. Apovian CM, Aronne LJ, Bessesen DH, et al: Pharmacological management of obesity: an Endocrine Society Clinical Practice Guideline, *J Clin Endocrinol Metab* 100(2):342, 2015.
21. Pucci A, Finer N: New medications for treatment of obesity: metabolic and cardiovascular effects, *Can J Cardiol* 31(2):142, 2015.
22. Dunham M: Caring for patients undergoing bariatric surgery, *Nursing* 43:45, 2013.
23. Gardner LA: Caring for Class III obese patients, *AJN* 113:66, 2013.
24. Idzik S, Troeleman N, Mielke A: Be prepared for bariatric patients in the OR, *OR Nurse J* 7:13, 2013.
25. Dietary Guidelines After Bariatric Surgery. Retrieved from *www.ucsfhealth.org/education/dietary_guidelines_after_gastric_bypass.*
26. National Heart, Lung, and Blood Institute. What is metabolic syndrome? Retrieved from *www.nhlbi.nih.gov/health/health-topics/topics/ms.*

*Evidence-based information for clinical practice.

# Upper Gastrointestinal Problems

*Paula P. Cox-North*

*As with stomachs, we should pity minds that do not eat.*

**Victor Hugo**

http://evolve.elsevier.com/Lewis/medsurg/

## LEARNING OUTCOMES

1. Describe the etiology, complications, interprofessional care, and nursing management of nausea and vomiting.
2. Describe the etiology, clinical manifestations, and treatment of common oral inflammations and infections.
3. Describe the etiology, clinical manifestations, complications, interprofessional care, and nursing management of oral cancer.
4. Explain the types, pathophysiology, clinical manifestations, complications, and interprofessional care (including surgical therapy and nursing management) of gastroesophageal reflux disease (GERD) and hiatal hernia.
5. Describe the pathophysiology, clinical manifestations, complications, and interprofessional care of esophageal cancer, diverticula, achalasia, and esophageal strictures.
6. Differentiate between acute and chronic gastritis, including the etiology, pathophysiology, interprofessional care, and nursing management.
7. Compare and contrast gastric and duodenal ulcers, including the etiology, pathophysiology, clinical manifestations, complications, interprofessional care, and nursing management.
8. Describe the clinical manifestations, interprofessional care, and nursing management of stomach cancer.
9. Explain the common etiologies, clinical manifestations, interprofessional care, and nursing management of upper gastrointestinal bleeding.
10. Identify common types of foodborne illnesses and nursing responsibilities related to food poisoning.

## KEY TERMS



## NAUSEA AND VOMITING

Nausea and vomiting are the most common manifestations of gastrointestinal (GI) disease. Although nausea and vomiting can occur independently, they are closely related and usually treated as one problem. **Nausea** is a feeling of discomfort in the epigastrium with a conscious desire to vomit. **Vomiting** is the forceful ejection of partially digested food and secretions *(emesis)* from the upper GI tract.

### Etiology and Pathophysiology

Nausea and vomiting occur in a wide variety of GI disorders and in many conditions unrelated to GI disease. These include pregnancy; infection; central nervous system (CNS) disorders (e.g., meningitis, tumor); cardiovascular problems (e.g., myocardial infarction, heart failure); metabolic disorders (e.g., diabetes mellitus, Addison's disease, renal failure); postoperatively after general anesthesia; side effects of drugs (e.g., chemotherapy, opioids); psychologic factors (e.g., stress, fear); and conditions in which the GI tract becomes overly irritated, excited, or distended. Women are more likely to have nausea and vomiting associated with anesthesia and motion sickness.[1]

A vomiting center in the medulla coordinates the multiple components involved in vomiting. This center receives input from various stimuli. Neural impulses reach the vomiting center via afferent pathways through branches of the autonomic nervous system. Receptors for these afferent fibers are located in the GI tract, kidneys, heart, and uterus. When stimulated, these receptors relay information to the vomiting center, which then initiates the vomiting reflex (Fig. 41-1).

Vomiting is a complex act. It requires the coordinated activity of several structures: closure of the glottis, deep inspiration with contraction of the diaphragm in the inspiratory position, closure of the pylorus, relaxation of the stomach and lower esophageal sphincter (LES), and contraction of the abdominal muscles with increasing intraabdominal pressure. These

Reviewed by Susan C. Landis, RN, MN, Senior Lecturer, University of Washington School of Nursing, Seattle, Washington; Heidi E. Monroe, MSN, RN-BC, CPAN, CAPA, Assistant Professor of Nursing, Bellin College and Bellin Hospital, Green Bay, Wisconsin; Sarah Byram Poppe, MSN, ANP-BC, Nurse Practitioner, Gastroenterology Associates, Olympia, Washington; and Andrea H. Thurler, RN, DNP, FNP-BC, Nurse Practitioner, Massachusetts General Hospital, Harvard University, Massachusetts General Institute of Health Professions, Boston, Massachusetts.

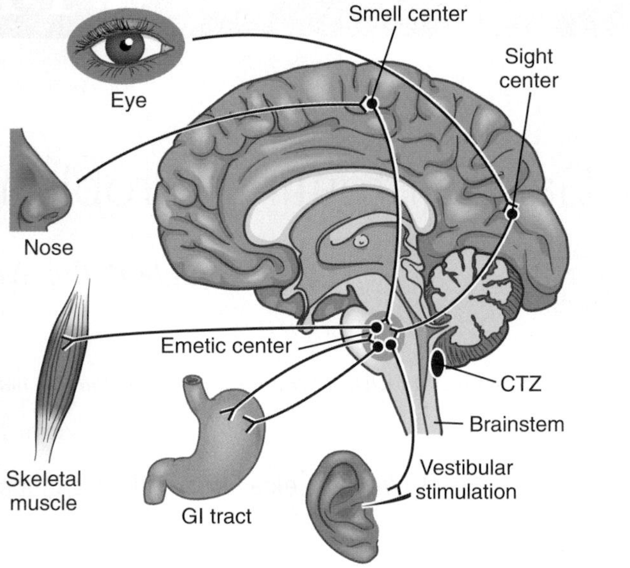


**FIG. 41-1** Stimuli involved in the act of vomiting. *CTZ,* Chemoreceptor trigger zone. (Modified from McKenry L, Tessier E, Hogan M: *Mosby's pharmacology in nursing,* ed 22, St Louis, 2006, Mosby.)

simultaneous activities force the stomach contents up through the esophagus, into the pharynx, and out the mouth.

The *chemoreceptor trigger zone* (CTZ) located in the brainstem responds to chemical stimuli from drugs, toxins, and labyrinthine stimulation (e.g., motion sickness). Once stimulated, the CTZ transmits impulses directly to the vomiting center. This action activates the autonomic nervous system, resulting in both parasympathetic and sympathetic stimulation. Sympathetic activation produces tachycardia, tachypnea, and diaphoresis. Parasympathetic stimulation causes relaxation of the LES, an increase in gastric motility, and a pronounced increase in salivation.

## Clinical Manifestations

Nausea is a subjective complaint. *Anorexia* (lack of appetite) usually accompanies nausea. When nausea and vomiting occur over a long period, dehydration can develop rapidly. Water and essential electrolytes (e.g., potassium, sodium, chloride, hydrogen) are lost. As vomiting persists, the patient may have severe electrolyte imbalances, extracellular fluid volume loss, decreased plasma volume, and eventually circulatory failure.

Metabolic alkalosis can result from loss of gastric hydrochloric (HCl) acid. When contents of the small intestine are vomited, metabolic acidosis can occur. However, metabolic acidosis is less common than metabolic alkalosis. Weight loss resulting from fluid loss can occur in a short time with severe vomiting.

## Interprofessional Care

The goals of interprofessional care are to determine and treat the underlying cause of the nausea and vomiting and provide symptomatic relief. Assess the patient for precipitating factors, and describe the contents of the emesis.

It is important to differentiate among vomiting, regurgitation, and projectile vomiting. *Regurgitation* is an effortless process in which partially digested food slowly comes up from the stomach. Retching or vomiting rarely occurs before it. *Projectile vomiting* is a forceful expulsion of stomach contents without nausea. It is characteristic of CNS (brain and spinal cord) tumors.

Emesis containing partially digested food several hours after a meal indicates gastric outlet obstruction or delayed gastric emptying. The presence of fecal odor and bile after prolonged vomiting suggests intestinal obstruction below the level of the pylorus. Bile in the emesis suggests obstruction below the ampulla of Vater.

The color of the emesis aids in identifying the presence and source of any bleeding. Bright red blood indicates active bleeding. This could be due to a **Mallory-Weiss tear** (disruption of the mucosal lining near the esophagogastric junction), esophageal varices, gastric or duodenal ulcer, or cancer. Vomitus with a "coffee-ground" appearance is related to gastric bleeding. The blood changes to dark brown because of its interaction with HCl acid.

The timing of nausea and vomiting can help determine its cause. Early morning vomiting is common in pregnancy. Emotional stressors with no evident pathologic disorder may elicit vomiting during or immediately after eating. Those with *cyclic vomiting syndrome* have recurring episodes of nausea, vomiting, and fatigue that last from a few hours up to 10 days.

**Drug Therapy.** The use of drugs to treat nausea and vomiting depends on the cause of the problem (Table 41-1). Many antiemetic drugs act in the CNS via the CTZ to block the neurochemicals that trigger nausea and vomiting. Because the cause cannot always be readily determined, use drugs with caution. Using antiemetics before determining the cause can mask the underlying disease process and delay diagnosis and treatment.

**DRUG ALERT Promethazine Injection**
- Do not administer into an artery or under the skin because of the risk of severe tissue injury, including gangrene.
- When given IV, it can leach out of the vein and cause serious damage to surrounding tissue.
- Deep muscle injection is the preferred route of injection administration.

**DRUG ALERT Metoclopramide (Reglan)**
- Chronic use or high doses carry the risk of tardive dyskinesia.
- Tardive dyskinesia is a neurologic condition characterized by involuntary and repetitive movements of the body (e.g., extremity movements, lip smacking).
- Tardive dyskinesia may persist after discontinuing the drug.

Serotonin (5-$HT_3$) receptor antagonists are effective in reducing chemotherapy-induced vomiting caused by delayed gastric emptying and nausea and vomiting related to migraine headache, anesthesia, and anxiety.[2] They are effective in preventing and treating postoperative nausea and vomiting. Dexamethasone is given in combination with other antiemetics to manage acute and delayed chemotherapy-induced vomiting. Aprepitant (Emend) and rolapitant (Varubi), neurokinin-1 receptor antagonists ($NK_1RA$), are used to prevent chemotherapy-induced and postoperative nausea and vomiting.

Dronabinol (Marinol) is an orally active cannabinoid. It is used alone or in combination with other antiemetics for preventing chemotherapy-induced vomiting. Because of the potential for abuse as well as drowsiness and sedation, it is used only when other therapies are not effective.

**Nutritional Therapy.** The patient with severe vomiting requires IV fluid therapy with electrolyte and glucose replacement until able to tolerate oral intake. Some patients may need a nasogastric (NG) tube and suction to decompress the stomach. Start oral nutrition beginning with clear liquids once symptoms

## TABLE 41-1 Drug Therapy

### *Nausea and Vomiting*

| Drug | Mechanism of Action | Side Effects |
|---|---|---|
| **Serotonin (5-$HT_3$) Antagonists** | | |
| dolasetron (Anzemet)<br>granisetron<br>ondansetron (Zofran)<br>palonosetron (Aloxi) | Block action of serotonin (causes nausea and vomiting) | Constipation, diarrhea, headache, fatigue, malaise, elevated liver function tests |
| **Phenothiazines** | | |
| chlorpromazine<br>perphenazine<br>prochlorperazine<br>trifluoperazine<br>promethazine | Act in the CNS level of the chemoreceptor trigger zone (CTZ)<br>Block dopamine receptors that trigger nausea and vomiting | Dry mouth, hypotension, sedative effects, rashes, constipation |
| **Antihistamines** | | |
| meclizine (Antivert)<br>dimenhydrinate (Dramamine)<br>hydroxyzine (Vistaril)<br>diphenhydramine | Block histamine receptors that trigger nausea and vomiting | Dry mouth, hypotension, sedative effects, rashes, constipation |
| **Prokinetic Agents** | | |
| metoclopramide (Reglan) | Inhibit action of dopamine<br>↑ Gastric motility and emptying | CNS side effects ranging from anxiety to hallucinations<br>Extrapyramidal side effects, including tremor and dyskinesias (similar to Parkinson's disease) |
| **Anticholinergic (Antimuscarinic)** | | |
| scopolamine transdermal<br>trimethobenzamide (Tigan) | Block cholinergic pathways to vomiting center | Xerostomia, somnolence |
| **Butyrophenone** | | |
| droperidol | Block neurochemicals that trigger nausea and vomiting | Dry mouth, hypotension, sedative effects, rashes, constipation |
| **Neurokinin-1 Receptor Antagonist** | | |
| aprepitant (Emend)<br>netupitant and palonosetron (Akynzeo)<br>rolapitant (Varubi) | Block interaction of Substance P at NK-1 receptor preventing nausea and vomiting | Headache, hiccups, fatigue, constipation, diarrhea, anorexia |
| **Corticosteroids** | | |
| dexamethasone | Not well understood how it prevents nausea and vomiting | Hyperglycemia, insomnia, euphoria |
| **Cannabinoids** | | |
| dronabinol (Marinol)<br>nabilone (Cesamet) | Inhibit vomiting control mechanism in the medulla oblongata | Xerostomia, amnesia, ataxia, confusion, coordination problems, dizziness, and somnolence |

have subsided. Water is the initial fluid of choice for oral rehydration. Have the patient sip small amounts of fluid (5 to 15 mL) every 15 to 20 minutes. Other options include carbonated beverages with the carbonation removed at room temperature and warm tea. Extremely hot or cold liquids are often difficult to tolerate. Broth and sports drinks (e.g., Gatorade) are high in sodium, so give them with caution. Dry toast or crackers may be helpful.

As the patient's condition improves, provide a diet high in carbohydrates and low in fat. Items such as a baked potato, plain gelatin, rice, and cereal are ideal. Many patients do not tolerate coffee, spicy foods, highly acidic foods, and those with strong odors. Tell the patient to eat food slowly and in small amounts to prevent overdistending the stomach. Liquids taken between meals rather than with meals also reduce overdistention. Consult a dietitian about nutritious foods that are well tolerated by the patient.

**Nondrug Therapy.** For some patients, acupressure or acupuncture at specific points is effective in reducing postoperative nausea and vomiting.[3] Some patients use herbs such as ginger and peppermint oil. Relaxation breathing exercises, changes in body position, or exercise may help some patients.

### COMPLEMENTARY & ALTERNATIVE THERAPIES

#### *Ginger*

**Scientific Evidence**

- May be effective for nausea and vomiting of pregnancy when used at recommended doses for short periods
- If taken 1 hr before surgery, may reduce nausea and vomiting for up to 24 hr

**Nursing Implications**

- Few adverse effects reported with short-term use
- May inhibit platelet aggregation and increase risk of bleeding
- Possibly lowers blood glucose levels

Source: Based on a systematic review of scientific literature. Retrieved from *www.nlm.nih.gov/medlineplus/druginfo/natural/961.html.*

## NURSING MANAGEMENT: NAUSEA AND VOMITING

### Nursing Assessment

Each patient with a history of prolonged and persistent nausea or vomiting requires a thorough nursing assessment before you

**TABLE 41-2 Nursing Assessment**

***Nausea and Vomiting***

**Subjective Data**

***Important Health Information***

*Past health history:* GI disorders, chronic indigestion, food allergies, pregnancy, infection, CNS disorders, recent travel, eating disorders, metabolic disorders, cancer, cardiovascular disease, renal disease

*Medications:* Antiemetics, digitalis, opioids, ferrous sulfate, aspirin, aminophylline, alcohol, antibiotics, chemotherapy. General anesthesia.

*Surgery or other treatments:* Recent surgery

***Functional Health Patterns***

*Nutritional-metabolic:* Amount, frequency, character, and color of vomitus. Dry heaves. Anorexia, weight loss

*Activity-exercise:* Weakness, fatigue

*Cognitive-perceptual:* Abdominal tenderness or pain

*Coping–stress tolerance:* Stress, fear

**Objective Data**

***General***

Lethargy, sunken eyeballs

***Integumentary***

Pallor, dry mucous membranes, poor skin turgor

***Gastrointestinal***

Amount, frequency, character (e.g., projectile), content (undigested food, blood, bile, feces), and color of vomitus (red, "coffee ground," green-yellow)

***Urinary***

Decreased output, concentrated urine

***Possible Diagnostic Findings***

Altered serum electrolytes (especially hypokalemia), metabolic alkalosis, abnormal upper GI findings on endoscopy or abdominal x-rays

develop a specific plan of care. Although many conditions are associated with nausea and vomiting, you should have a basic understanding of the common conditions and be able to identify the patient who is at high risk. Knowing the physiologic mechanisms involved in nausea and vomiting is important in the assessment process. Table 41-2 presents subjective and objective data to obtain from a patient with nausea and vomiting.

## ◆ Nursing Diagnoses

Nursing diagnoses for the patient with nausea and vomiting may include, but are not limited to, the following:

- Nausea *related to* multiple etiologies
- Deficient fluid volume *related to* prolonged vomiting
- Imbalanced nutrition: less than body requirements *related to* nausea and vomiting

Additional information on nursing diagnoses is presented in eNursing Care Plan 41-1 (available on the website for this chapter).

## ◆ Planning

The overall goals are that the patient with nausea and vomiting will (1) experience minimal or no nausea and vomiting, (2) have normal electrolyte levels and hydration status, and (3) return to a normal pattern of fluid balance and nutrient intake.

## ◆ Nursing Implementation

◆ **Acute Care.** Most people with nausea and vomiting remain at home. When nausea and vomiting persist, hospitalization may be necessary for diagnosis of the underlying problem. Until a diagnosis is confirmed, the patient is on nothing-by-mouth (NPO) status and given IV fluids. The patient with persistent vomiting, a possible bowel obstruction, or paralytic ileus may need an NG connected to suction. Secure the NG tube to prevent its movement in the nose and back of the throat, because this can stimulate nausea and vomiting.

With prolonged vomiting, there is a chance of dehydration and acid-base and electrolyte imbalances. Record intake and output, monitor vital signs, and assess for signs of dehydration. Provide physical and emotional support. Maintain a quiet, odor-free environment. Observe for changes in the patient's physical comfort and mentation. The risk of pulmonary aspiration is a concern when vomiting occurs in older or unconscious patients or in patients with conditions that impair the gag reflex. To prevent aspiration, put the patient who cannot adequately manage self-care in a semi-Fowler's or side-lying position.

**CHECK YOUR PRACTICE**

You are caring for a newly admitted 76-yr-old man who reports vomiting for the past 3 days. He says, "I cannot keep anything down, not even water."

- What assessment findings do you need to monitor in this man?
- What findings would indicate that he is experiencing dehydration?
- What are your priority nursing interventions for him?

◆ **Ambulatory Care.** Teach the patient and caregiver (1) how to manage the unpleasant sensation of nausea, (2) methods to prevent nausea and vomiting, and (3) strategies to maintain fluid and nutritional intake. Tell them to keep the immediate environment quiet, free of noxious odors, and well ventilated. Avoiding sudden changes of position and unnecessary activity are helpful. Encourage the use of relaxation techniques, frequent rest periods, effective pain management strategies, and diversional tactics. Cleansing the face and hands with a cool washcloth and providing mouth care between episodes increase the person's comfort level. When symptoms occur, stop all foods and drugs until the acute phase is over.

If you suspect a medication is the cause, notify the HCP immediately. The HCP can change the drug dose or prescribe a new drug. Advise the patient that stopping the drug without consulting the HCP may have detrimental effects on the person's health. The patient should take an antiemetic drug only if prescribed by the HCP. Taking over-the-counter (OTC) drugs to relieve symptoms may make the problem worse.

When food is the precipitating cause of nausea and vomiting, help the patient identify the specific food. Determine when it was eaten, prior history with the food, and whether anyone else who ate the food is sick. A patient may be reluctant to resume fluid intake because of fear of symptoms recurring. Suggest that he or she begin with clear liquids or cola beverages, sports drinks (e.g., Gatorade), tea or broth, dry crackers or toast, and plain gelatin. Bland foods, such as cereal, rice, baked potato, and cooked chicken, are generally tolerated in small amounts.

### Evaluation

The expected outcomes are that the patient with nausea and vomiting will

- Be comfortable with minimal or no nausea and vomiting
- Have electrolyte levels within normal range
- Be able to maintain adequate intake of fluids and nutrients

### Gerontologic Considerations: Nausea and Vomiting

The older adult experiencing nausea and vomiting requires careful assessment and monitoring, particularly during periods of fluid loss and subsequent rehydration therapy. Older patients are more likely to have cardiac or renal insufficiency that places them at greater risk for life-threatening fluid and electrolyte imbalances. Excessive fluid and electrolytes replacement may result in adverse consequences for a person with heart failure or renal disease. The older adult with a decreased level of consciousness is at high risk for aspirating vomitus. Close monitoring of the patient's physical status and level of consciousness during episodes of vomiting is important.

Older adults are particularly susceptible to the CNS side effects of antiemetic drugs. These drugs may produce confusion and increase their risk for falls. Dosages should be reduced and efficacy closely evaluated. Use safety precautions for these patients (e.g., removing rugs that may cause slipping).

## ORAL INFLAMMATION AND INFECTIONS

Oral inflammation and infections may be due to specific mouth diseases or secondary to systemic disorders such as leukemia or vitamin deficiency. Common inflammations and infections of the oral cavity are presented in Table 41-3. The patient who is immunosuppressed (e.g., receiving chemotherapy for cancer) or using corticosteroid inhalant treatment for asthma is at risk for oral infections (e.g., candidiasis). Oral infections may predispose the patient to infections in other body organs. For example, the oral cavity is a potential reservoir for respiratory pathogens. Oral pathogens have been associated with diabetes and heart disease.[4]

Managing these conditions focuses on identifying the cause, eliminating infection, providing comfort measures, and maintaining nutritional intake. Oral inflammation and infections can severely impair oral ingestion. Regular and good oral and dental hygiene reduces oral infections and inflammation.

**TABLE 41-3 Infections and Inflammation of the Mouth**

| Infection or Inflammation | Etiology | Manifestations | Treatment |
|---|---|---|---|
| **Gingivitis** | • Neglected oral hygiene, malocclusion, missing or irregular teeth, faulty dentistry<br>• Eating of soft rather than fibrous foods | • Inflamed gingivae and interdental papillae<br>• Bleeding during tooth brushing<br>• Development of pus, formation of abscess with loosening of teeth (periodontitis) | • Prevention through health teaching, dental care, gingival massage, professional cleaning of teeth<br>• Eat fibrous foods<br>• Conscientious brushing habits with flossing |
| **Vincent's infection** (acute necrotizing ulcerative gingivitis, trench mouth) | • Fusiform bacteria, Vincent spirochetes<br>• Predisposing factors of stress, excessive fatigue, poor oral hygiene<br>• Nutritional deficiencies (B and C vitamins) | • Painful, bleeding gingivae<br>• Eroding necrotic lesions of interdental papillae<br>• Ulcerations that bleed<br>• Increased saliva with metallic taste, fetid mouth odor<br>• Anorexia, fever, general malaise | • Rest (physical and mental)<br>• Avoidance of smoking and alcohol<br>• Soft, nutritious diet<br>• Correct oral hygiene habits<br>• Topical applications of antibiotics<br>• Mouth irrigations with chlorhexidine (Hibiclens) and saline solutions |
| **Oral candidiasis** (moniliasis or thrush) | • *Candida albicans* (a yeastlike fungus)<br>• Debilitation<br>• Prolonged high-dose antibiotic or corticosteroid therapy | • Pearly, bluish white "milk-curd" membranous lesions on mucosa of mouth and larynx<br>• Sore mouth, yeasty halitosis | • Miconazole buccal tablets (Oravig)<br>• Nystatin or amphotericin B as oral suspension or buccal tablets<br>• Good oral hygiene |
| **Herpes simplex** (cold sore, fever blister) (see Table 23-6) | • Herpes simplex virus (type 1 or 2)<br>• Predisposing factors of upper respiratory tract infections, excessive exposure to sunlight, food allergies, emotional tension, onset of menstruation | • Lip lesions, mouth lesions, vesicle formation (single or clustered)<br>• Shallow, painful ulcers | • Spirits of camphor, corticosteroid cream, mild antiseptic mouthwash, viscous lidocaine<br>• Removal or control of predisposing factors<br>• Antiviral agents (e.g., acyclovir [Zovirax], famciclovir [Famvir], valacyclovir [Valtrex]) |
| **Aphthous stomatitis** (canker sore) | • Recurrent and chronic form of infection<br>• Secondary to systemic disease, trauma, stress, or unknown causes | • Ulcers of mouth and lips, causing extreme pain<br>• Ulcers surrounded by erythematous base | • Corticosteroids (topical or systemic)<br>• Tetracycline oral suspension |
| **Parotitis** (inflammation of parotid gland, surgical mumps) | • *Staphylococcus* species usually<br>• *Streptococcus* species occasionally<br>• Debilitation and dehydration with poor oral hygiene<br>• Extended NPO status | • Pain in area of gland and ear<br>• Absence of salivation<br>• Purulent exudate from gland, erythema, ulcers | • Antibiotics, mouthwashes, warm compresses<br>• Preventive measures such as chewing gum, sucking on hard candy (lemon drops)<br>• Adequate fluid intake |
| **Stomatitis** (inflammation of mouth) | • Trauma, pathogens, irritants (tobacco, alcohol)<br>• Renal, liver, and hematologic diseases<br>• Side effect of chemotherapy and radiation | • Excessive salivation<br>• Halitosis<br>• Sore mouth | • Removal or treatment of cause<br>• Oral hygiene with soothing solutions, topical medications<br>• Soft, bland diet |

## ORAL CANCER

There are two types of oral cancer: *oral cavity cancer,* which starts in the mouth, and *oropharyngeal cancer,* which develops in the part of the throat just behind the mouth (the oropharynx). *Head and neck squamous cell carcinoma* (HNSCC) is a broad term used for cancers of the oral cavity, pharynx, and larynx, which account for 90% of malignant oral tumors. Annually 42,440 Americans are diagnosed with oral cancer. An estimated 8,390 people die from the disease.[5]

Oral cancer is more prevalent in African American men, and their survival rate is lower than that of white men. Oral cancer is more common after age 35. The average age at diagnosis is 65 years. It is two times more common in men than in women. The 5-year survival rate is 83% for localized cancer and 61% for all stages of cancer of the oral cavity and pharynx combined.[5]

Most oral cancer lesions occur on the lower lip. Other common sites are the lateral border and undersurface of the tongue, labial commissure, and buccal mucosa. Lip cancer has the most favorable prognosis of any of the oral tumors. The visibility of lip lesions usually leads to an earlier diagnosis.

### Etiology and Pathophysiology

Although the definitive cause of oral cancer is unknown, it has a number of predisposing factors (Table 41-4). Of those with oral cancer, 75% to 90% report either using tobacco or a history of frequent alcohol consumption. More than 30% of patients with cancer of the lip have outdoor occupations, indicating that prolonged exposure to sunlight is a risk factor. Irritation from the pipe stem resting on the lip is a factor in pipe smokers. Human papillomavirus (HPV) contributes to 25% of oral cancer cases.[5] HPV-associated oropharyngeal cancer is associated with multiple sexual partners, especially multiple oral sex partners.[6]

### CULTURAL & ETHNIC HEALTH DISPARITIES

***Oral, Pharyngeal, and Esophageal Problems***

**Nausea and Vomiting**

- Asian Americans, Middle Easterners, and African Americans are more likely to experience nausea and vomiting than whites.

**Cancers of Oral Cavity and Pharynx**

- Incidence and mortality rates are higher in African American men than in whites.
- Death rates from oral cancer are decreasing in whites but increasing in nonwhites.

**Esophageal Cancer**

- Highest incidence is in non-Hispanic white men.
- Higher incidence occurs in Alaska Natives than in whites.

**Stomach Cancer**

- Asian Americans and Pacific Islanders, Hispanics, and African Americans have higher rates of stomach cancer than non-Hispanic whites.
- Asian Americans show significantly higher survival rates than other ethnic groups.

### Clinical Manifestations

The common manifestations of oral cancer are shown in Table 41-4. Patients may report nonspecific symptoms such as chronic sore throat, sore mouth, and voice changes. *Leukoplakia,* called "smoker's patch," is a white patch on the mouth mucosa or tongue. It is a precancerous lesion, although less than 15% actually transform into cancer cells. The patch becomes *keratinized* (hard and leathery) and is sometimes described as hyperkeratosis. Leukoplakia is the result of chronic irritation, especially from smoking. *Erythroplasia* (erythroplakia), which is a red velvety patch on the mouth or tongue, is another precancerous lesion. More than 50% of cases of erythroplakia progress to squamous cell carcinoma. About 30% of patients with oral cancer have an asymptomatic neck mass.

Cancer of the lip usually appears as an indurated, painless ulcer on the lip. The first sign of cancer of the tongue is an ulcer or area of thickening. Soreness or pain of the tongue may occur, especially when eating hot or highly seasoned foods. Lesions are most likely to develop in the proximal half of the tongue. Some patients have limited tongue movement. Later symptoms of cancer of the tongue include increased salivation, slurred speech, **dysphagia** (difficulty swallowing), toothache, and earache.

### Diagnostic Studies

Diagnostic tests are done to identify oral dysplasias, which are precursors to oral cancer (Table 41-5). Oral exfoliative cytologic

**TABLE 41-5 Interprofessional Care**

***Oral Cancer***

| Diagnostic Assessment | Management |
|---|---|
| • History and physical examination<br>• Biopsy<br>• Oral exfoliative cytology<br>• Toluidine blue test<br>• CT, MRI, PET | • Surgical therapy<br>  • Surgical excision of the tumor<br>  • Radical neck dissection<br>• Radiation (internal or external) therapy<br>• Combined surgical and radiation therapy<br>• Chemotherapy |

**TABLE 41-4 Types and Characteristics of Oral Cancer**

| Location | Predisposing Factors | Clinical Manifestations | Treatment |
|---|---|---|---|
| **Lip** | Constant overexposure to sun, ruddy and fair complexion, recurrent herpetic lesions, irritation from pipe stem, syphilis, immunosuppression | Indurated, painless ulcer | Surgical excision, radiation |
| **Tongue** | Tobacco, alcohol, chronic irritation, syphilis | Ulcer or area of thickening, soreness or pain<br>Increased salivation, slurred speech, dysphagia, toothache, earache (later signs) | Surgery (hemiglossectomy or glossectomy), radiation |
| **Oral cavity** | Poor oral hygiene, tobacco usage (pipe and cigar smoking, snuff, chewing tobacco), chronic alcohol intake, chronic irritation (jagged tooth, ill-fitting prosthesis, chemical or mechanical irritants), human papillomavirus (HPV) | Leukoplakia, erythroplakia, ulcerations, sore spot, rough area, pain, dysphagia, a lump or thickening in the cheek<br>A sore throat or a feeling that something is stuck<br>Difficulty chewing and speaking (later signs) | Surgery (mandibulectomy, radical neck dissection, resection of buccal mucosa), internal and external radiation |

study involves scraping the suspicious lesion and spreading the scraping on a slide for microscopic examination. The toluidine blue test is a screening test for oral cancer. When toluidine blue is applied topically to stain an area, cancer cells preferentially take up the dye. A negative cytologic smear or negative toluidine blue test does not necessarily rule out a malignant condition. Once cancer is diagnosed, CT scan, MRI, and positron emission tomography (PET) are used for staging of the cancer.[7]

### Interprofessional Care

Management of the patient with oral cancer usually consists of surgery, radiation, chemotherapy, or a combination of these. The curative treatments are usually surgery and radiation.

**Surgical Therapy.** Surgery remains the most effective treatment, especially for early-stage disease. The procedure done depends on the location and extent of the tumor. Some patients with small tumors in the mouth and throat are candidates for minimally invasive robotic-assisted surgery. However, many of the operations are radical procedures involving extensive resections. Some examples are partial *mandibulectomy* (removal of the mandible), *hemiglossectomy* (removal of half of the tongue), *glossectomy* (removal of the tongue), resections of the buccal mucosa and floor of the mouth, and radical neck dissection.

Radical neck dissection includes wide excision of the primary lesion with removal of the regional lymph nodes, the deep cervical lymph nodes, and their lymphatic channels. The following structures are removed or transected depending on the extent of the primary lesion: sternocleidomastoid muscle and other closely associated muscles, internal jugular vein, mandible, submaxillary gland, part of the thyroid and parathyroid glands, and spinal accessory nerve. The patient usually has a tracheostomy. Drainage tubes are inserted into the surgical area and connected to suction to remove fluid and blood. (Head and neck surgery is described in more detail in Chapter 26.)

**Nonsurgical Therapy.** Radiation therapy may be used alone to treat small cancers or when lesions cannot be removed. Patients usually do not have radiation before surgery because it is difficult to remove radiated tissue. The tissue becomes fibrotic and heals slower.[8] Most patients begin radiation about 6 weeks after surgery.

Chemotherapy can shrink lesions before surgery, decrease metastasis, sensitize cancer cells to radiation, or treat distant metastases. Chemotherapy drugs include 5-fluorouracil (5-FU), methotrexate, cisplatin, carboplatin, paclitaxel, docetaxel, ifosfamide (Ifex), and bleomycin. A commonly used combination is cisplatin and 5-FU. This combination is more effective than either drug alone. (Chemotherapy is discussed in Chapter 15.)

Palliative treatment is the best management when the prognosis is poor, the cancer is inoperable, or the patient decides against surgery. Palliation aims to treat the symptoms and make the patient more comfortable. If it becomes difficult for the patient to swallow, placing a gastrostomy tube will allow for adequate nutritional intake. Give analgesic medications freely. Frequent suctioning of the oral cavity is necessary when swallowing becomes difficult. (Other palliative and end-of-life nursing measures are discussed in Chapter 9.)

**Nutritional Therapy.** Many patients are malnourished before surgery. They may require placement of a percutaneous endoscopic gastrostomy (PEG) and enteral nutrition before radiation treatment or surgery. After radical neck surgery, the patient may be unable to ingest nutrients orally because of mucositis, swelling, location of sutures, or difficulty swallowing. Parenteral fluids are given for the first 24 to 48 hours. After that time, enteral nutrition is given via NG, gastrostomy, or jejunostomy. (See Chapter 39 for information on PEG and parenteral and enteral feedings.) Cervical esophagostomy and pharyngostomy are options for some patients.

Observe for feeding tolerance and adjust the amount, time, and formula if nausea, vomiting, diarrhea, or distention occurs. Give small amounts of water when the patient can swallow. Observe for choking. Suctioning may be necessary to prevent aspiration.

## NURSING MANAGEMENT: ORAL CANCER

### Nursing Assessment

Subjective and objective data to obtain from a patient with oral cancer are presented in Table 41-6.

### Nursing Diagnoses

Nursing diagnoses for the patient with oral cancer may include, but are not limited to, the following:

- Imbalanced nutrition: less than body requirements *related to* oral pain, difficulty chewing and swallowing, surgical resection, and radiation treatment
- Chronic pain *related to* the tumor, surgery, or radiation
- Anxiety *related to* diagnosis of cancer, uncertain future, potential for disfiguring surgery, and prognosis

### Planning

The overall goals are that the patient with cancer of the oral cavity will (1) have a patent airway, (2) be able to communicate, (3) have adequate nutritional intake to promote wound healing, and (4) have relief of pain and discomfort.

**TABLE 41-6 Nursing Assessment**

***Oral Cancer***

**Subjective Data**

***Important Health Information***

*Past health history:* Recurrent oral herpetic lesions, human papillomavirus (HPV) infection or vaccination, syphilis, exposure to sunlight

*Medications:* Immunosuppressants

*Surgery or other treatments:* Removal of prior tumors or lesions

***Functional Health Patterns***

*Health perception–health management:* Use of alcohol and tobacco, pipe smoking. Poor oral hygiene

*Nutritional-metabolic:* Reductions in oral intake, weight loss, difficulty chewing food, increased salivation, intolerance to certain foods or temperatures of food

*Cognitive-perceptual:* Mouth or tongue soreness or pain, toothache, earache, neck stiffness, dysphagia, difficulty speaking

**Objective Data**

***Integumentary***

Indurated, painless ulcer on lip. Painless neck mass

***Gastrointestinal***

Areas of thickening or roughness, ulcers, leukoplakia, or erythroplakia on the tongue or oral mucosa. Limited movement of the tongue. Increased salivation, drooling. Slurred speech. Foul breath odor

***Possible Diagnostic Findings***

Positive exfoliative smear cytology (microscopic examination of cells removed by scraping), positive biopsy

### HEALTHY PEOPLE

**Health Impact of Good Oral Hygiene**

- Improves quality of life
- Lowers risk of teeth loss
- Reduces pain and disability
- Decreases cost of care needed from dental professionals
- Assists in early detection of oral and craniofacial cancers
- Decreases risk of developing periodontal disease, gingivitis, and dental caries

### ◆ Nursing Implementation

You have a significant role in early detection and treatment of oral cancer. Identify patients at risk (Table 41-4) and provide information about predisposing factors. Inform the patient who smokes about smoking cessation programs available in the community. Warn adolescents and teenagers about the danger of using snuff or chewing tobacco. (Smoking cessation is discussed in Chapter 10 and Tables 10-3 to 10-6.)

Because early detection of oral cancer is important, teach the patient to report unexplained pain or soreness of the mouth, unusual bleeding, dysphagia, sore throat, voice changes, or swelling or lump in the neck. Refer any person with an ulcerative lesion that does not heal within 2 to 3 weeks to the HCP.

Preoperative care for the patient who will have a radical neck dissection must consider the patient's physical and psychosocial needs. Physical preparation is the same as that for any major surgery, with special emphasis on oral hygiene. Explanations and emotional support should include information on postoperative communication and feeding. Explain the surgical procedure, and ensure that the patient understands the information. (See Chapter 26 and eNursing Care Plan 26-2 for more information about the nursing management of a patient undergoing a radical neck dissection).

### ◆ Evaluation

The expected outcomes are that the patient with oral cancer will

- Have no respiratory complications
- Be able to communicate
- Maintain an adequate nutritional intake to promote wound healing
- Experience minimal pain and discomfort with eating, drinking, and talking

# ESOPHAGEAL DISORDERS

## GASTROESOPHAGEAL REFLUX DISEASE

**Gastroesophageal reflux disease (GERD)** is a chronic symptom of mucosal damage caused by reflux of stomach acid into the lower esophagus. GERD is not a disease but a syndrome. GERD is the most common upper GI problem. Approximately 10% to 20% of the U.S. population experience GERD symptoms (heartburn or regurgitation) at least once a week.[9]

### Etiology and Pathophysiology

GERD has no one single cause (Fig. 41-2). GERD results when the reflux of acidic gastric contents into the esophagus overwhelms the esophageal defenses. Gastric HCl acid and pepsin secretions in refluxate cause esophageal irritation and inflammation *(esophagitis)*. If the refluxate contains intestinal

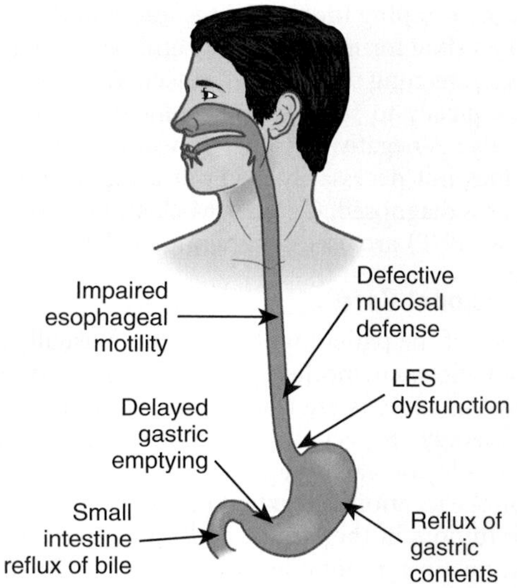


**FIG. 41-2** Factors involved in the pathogenesis of gastroesophageal reflux disease (GERD). *LES,* Lower esophageal sphincter.

**TABLE 41-7 Factors Affecting Lower Esophageal Sphincter Pressure**

| | |
|---|---|
| **Increase Pressure**<br>• bethanechol (Urecholine)<br>• metoclopramide (Reglan)<br><br>**Decrease Pressure**<br>• Alcohol<br>• Chocolate (theobromine)<br>• Fatty foods<br>• Nicotine<br>• Peppermint, spearmint | • Tea, coffee (caffeine)<br>• Drugs<br>  • Anticholinergics<br>  • β-Adrenergic blockers<br>  • Calcium channel blockers<br>  • Diazepam (Valium)<br>  • Morphine sulfate<br>  • Nitrates<br>  • Progesterone<br>  • Theophylline |

proteolytic enzymes (e.g., trypsin) and bile, this further irritates the esophageal mucosa. The degree of inflammation depends on the amount and composition of the gastric reflux and on the esophagus's mucosal defense mechanisms.

One of the primary etiologic factors in GERD is an incompetent LES. Under normal conditions, the LES acts as an antireflux barrier. An incompetent LES lets gastric contents move from the stomach to the esophagus when the patient is supine or has an increase in intraabdominal pressure.

Decreased LES pressure can be due to certain foods and drugs (Table 41-7). Obesity is a risk factor for GERD.[10] In an obese person the intraabdominal pressure is increased, which can exacerbate GERD. Cigarette and cigar smoking can contribute to GERD. Hiatal hernia, discussed in the next section, commonly causes GERD.

### Clinical Manifestations

The symptoms of GERD vary from person to person. The persistence of mild symptoms (i.e., more than twice a week) or moderate to severe symptoms once a week is considered GERD.

Heartburn *(pyrosis)* is the most common manifestation. Heartburn is a burning, tight sensation felt intermittently beneath the lower sternum and spreading upward to the throat or jaw. It may occur after ingesting food or drugs that decrease the LES pressure or directly irritate the esophageal mucosa. An HCP should evaluate heartburn that occurs more than twice a week, is severe, is associated with dysphagia, or occurs at night and wakes a person from sleep. Older adults who complain of recent onset of heartburn should receive medical evaluation.

Patients may complain of dyspepsia or regurgitation. *Dyspepsia* is pain or discomfort centered in the upper abdomen (mainly in or around the midline as opposed to the right or left hypochondrium). Regurgitation is often described as hot, bitter, or sour liquid coming into the throat or mouth.

A person with GERD may report respiratory symptoms, including wheezing, coughing, and dyspnea. Nocturnal discomfort and coughing can awaken the person, resulting in disturbed sleep patterns. Otolaryngologic symptoms include hoarseness, sore throat, a *globus sensation* (sense of a lump in the throat), hypersalivation, and choking.

GERD-related chest pain can mimic angina. It is described as burning; squeezing; or radiating to the back, neck, jaw, or arms. Complaints of chest pain are more common in older adults with GERD. Unlike angina, GERD-related chest pain is relieved with antacids.

## Complications

Complications of GERD are due to the direct local effects of gastric acid on the esophageal mucosa. **Esophagitis** (inflammation of the esophagus) is a common complication of GERD. Esophagitis with esophageal ulcerations is shown in Fig. 41-3. Repeated esophagitis may lead to scar tissue formation, stricture, and dysphagia.

Another complication of chronic GERD is **Barrett's esophagus** (esophageal metaplasia). *Metaplasia* is the reversible change from one type of cell to another type because of an abnormal stimulus. In Barrett's esophagus, the flat epithelial cells in the distal esophagus change into columnar epithelial cells. These cell changes are primarily due to GERD. However, some people with no history of GERD develop Barrett's esophagus.

Barrett's esophagus is a precancerous lesion that increases the patient's risk for esophageal adenocarcinoma. About 5% to 20% of people with chronic GERD have Barrett's esophagus.[11] Compared with whites, African Americans and Asians are at lower risk for Barrett's esophagus. Because of the risk for esophageal cancer, a surveillance endoscopy every 2 to 3 years or radiofrequency ablation is recommended.[11]

Respiratory complications of GERD include cough, bronchospasm, laryngospasm, and cricopharyngeal spasm. These complications are due to gastric secretions irritating the upper airway. Asthma, chronic bronchitis, and pneumonia may develop from aspiration into the respiratory system. Dental erosion, especially in the posterior teeth, may result from acid reflux into the mouth.[12]

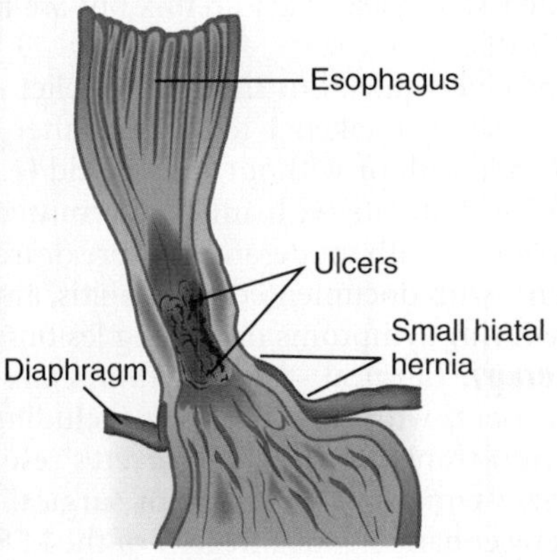


**FIG. 41-3** Esophagitis with esophageal ulcerations.

## Diagnostic Studies

GERD is usually diagnosed based on symptoms and the patient's response to behavioral and drug therapies. Diagnostic tests are done when usual therapy is ineffective or when complications are suspected. Diagnostic studies done to determine the cause of the GERD are shown in Table 41-8.

Endoscopy is useful in assessing the LES competence and the degree of inflammation (if present), potential scarring, and strictures. Biopsy and cytologic specimens can be used to distinguish stomach or esophageal cancer from Barrett's esophagus. In addition, the degree of dysplasia (low grade versus high grade) is determined. Manometric studies measure pressure in the esophagus and LES and esophageal motility function. Ambulatory esophageal pH monitoring may be done for patients with refractory symptoms and no evidence of mucosal inflammation. Radionuclide tests can detect reflux of gastric contents and the rate of esophageal clearance.

## Interprofessional Care

Most patients with GERD can successfully manage the condition through lifestyle modifications and drug therapy. These approaches require patient teaching and adherence to therapies. When these therapies are ineffective, surgery is an option (Table 41-8).

**Lifestyle Modifications.** Teach the patient with GERD to avoid factors that trigger symptoms. Give particular attention to food and drugs that may affect the LES, acid secretion, or gastric emptying. Recommend weight reduction if the patient is overweight. A patient and caregiver teaching guide is provided in Table 41-9.

Encourage patients who smoke to stop. If needed, refer the patient to community resources for assistance in stopping smoking. (See Chapter 10 for more information related to smoking cessation.) If stress seems to cause symptoms, discuss measures to cope with stress. (See Chapter 6 for stress management techniques.)

### TABLE 41-8 Interprofessional Care

***Gastroesophageal Reflux Disease (GERD) and Hiatal Hernia***

**Diagnostic Assessment**
- History and physical examination
- Upper GI endoscopy with biopsy and cytologic analysis
- Esophagram (barium swallow)
- Motility (manometry) studies
- pH monitoring (laboratory or 24 hr ambulatory)
- Radionuclide studies

**Management**

***Conservative***
- Elevate head of bed on 4- to 6-in blocks
- Avoid reflux-inducing foods (fatty foods, chocolate, peppermint)
- Avoid alcohol
- Reduce or avoid acidic pH beverages (colas, red wine, orange juice)

*Drug Therapy (Table 41-10)*
- Proton pump inhibitors
- $H_2$-receptor blockers
- Prokinetic drug therapy
- Cholinergic drugs
- Antacids

***Surgical Therapy***
- Nissen fundoplication
- Toupet fundoplication

***Endoscopic Therapy***
- Intraluminal valvuloplasty
- Radiofrequency therapy

## TABLE 41-9 Patient & Caregiver Teaching
### *Gastroesophageal Reflux Disease (GERD)*

*Include the following instructions when teaching the patient and caregiver about management of GERD.*

1. Explain the reason for a low-fat diet.
2. Encourage the patient to eat small, frequent meals to prevent gastric distention.
3. Explain the reason for avoiding alcohol, smoking (causes an almost immediate, marked decrease in lower esophageal sphincter pressure), and beverages that contain caffeine.
4. Advise the patient to not lie down for 2-3 hr after eating, wear tight clothing around the waist, or bend over (especially after eating).
5. Have the patient avoid eating within 3 hr of bedtime.
6. Encourage the patient to sleep with head of bed elevated on 4- to 6-in blocks (gravity fosters esophageal emptying).
7. Provide information about drugs, including reason for their use and common side effects.
8. Discuss strategies for weight reduction if appropriate.
9. Encourage patient and caregiver to share concerns about lifestyle changes and living with a chronic problem.

**Nutritional Therapy.** Diet does not cause GERD, but food can aggravate symptoms. No specific diet is necessary. Some patients may need to avoid foods that decrease LES pressure, such as chocolate, peppermint, fatty foods, coffee, and tea (Table 41-7), which predispose them to reflux. Certain foods (e.g., tomato-based products, orange juice, cola, red wine) may irritate the esophagus. Tell the patient to avoid late evening meals, nocturnal snacking, and milk, especially at bedtime, since it increases gastric acid secretion. Small, frequent meals and drinking fluids between meals help prevent overdistention of the stomach. Increased saliva production by chewing gum and oral lozenges may help with mild symptoms.

**Drug Therapy.** Drug therapy for GERD focuses on decreasing the volume and acidity of reflux, improving LES function, increasing esophageal clearance, and protecting the esophageal mucosa[13] (Table 41-10). Proton pump inhibitors (PPIs) and histamine ($H_2$)-receptor blockers are the most common and effective treatments for symptomatic GERD. The goal of HCl acid suppression treatment is to reduce the acidity of the gastric refluxate. Patients who are symptomatic with GERD but do not have evidence of esophagitis *(nonerosive GERD)* achieve symptom relief with PPIs and $H_2$-receptor blockers.

PPIs are more effective in healing esophagitis than $H_2$-receptor blockers. PPIs are also beneficial in decreasing the incidence of esophageal strictures, a complication of chronic GERD. PPIs are available in prescription or OTC preparations. Therapy should start with once a day dosing, before the first meal of the day. Long-term use of PPIs has been associated with decreased bone density, chronic hypochlorhydria, and increased risk of pneumonia.[14]

**DRUG ALERT Proton Pump Inhibitors (PPIs)**
- Long-term use or high doses may increase the risk of fractures of hip, wrist, and spine.
- Patients should take the lowest dose for the shortest duration needed to treat their condition.
- Use is associated with an increased risk of new and recurrent *Clostridium difficile* infection in hospitalized patients.[15]

$H_2$-receptor blockers reduce symptoms and promote esophageal healing in 50% of patients. These drugs are available in OTC and prescription formulations. Some formulations include an $H_2$-receptor blocker plus antacid combination. For example,

## EVIDENCE-BASED PRACTICE
### *Translating Research Into Practice*

**Do Proton Pump Inhibitors Increase Gastric Cancer Risk?**
In adults with acid-related gastric problems (P), what is the effect of taking proton pump inhibitors (I) for at least 6 months (T) versus endoscopy or no treatment (C) and the risk of developing gastric cancer (O)?

***Synthesis of Best Available Evidence***
- Systematic review of randomized controlled trials (RCTs)
- Seven RCTs of patients ($n$ = 1789) taking proton pump inhibitors (PPIs) for at least 6 months and without gastric cancer at start of trial. Intervention was taking PPIs for an acid-related gastric disorder. Comparison groups received no treatment or surgery/endoscopic treatment only. Outcome was to examine development and progression of gastric precancerous lesions.
- PPIs are commonly prescribed worldwide and are the most effective drugs to reduce gastric acid secretion.
- PPIs did not increase risk of atrophy or metaplasia of gastric mucosa.
- Higher incidence of developing focal cell hyperplasia (thickening of stomach lining) with PPIs
- No participants had dysplastic or neoplastic gastric mucosa changes.

***Conclusions***
- Taking PPIs for $\geq$6 months does not appear to promote development of precancerous gastric lesions.

***Implications for Nursing Practice***
1. How would you counsel a patient who is concerned about the long-term effects of taking a PPI?
2. What information would you provide to a patient who due to reported adverse effects with PPIs is self-treating frequent heartburn with OTC medications that are not effective?

***Reference for Evidence***
Song H, Zhu J, Lu D: Long-term proton pump inhibitor (PPI) use and the development of gastric pre-malignant lesions, *Cochrane Database Syst Rev* 12: CD010623, 2014.

*P*, Patient population of interest; *I*, intervention or area of interest; *C*, comparison of interest or comparison group; *O*, outcomes of interest; *T*, timing (see p. 15).

Pepcid Complete includes famotidine, calcium carbonate, and magnesium hydroxide.

Cholinergic drugs (e.g., bethanechol [Urecholine]) increase LES pressure, improve esophageal emptying in the supine position, and increase gastric emptying. However, cholinergic drugs increase HCl acid secretion. Prokinetic (motility-enhancing) drugs (metoclopramide [Reglan]) promote gastric emptying and reduce the risk of gastric acid reflux but are not a primary therapy for GERD.

Antacids produce quick but short-lived relief of heartburn. They are most effective taken 1 to 3 hours after meals and at bedtime. Antacids with or without alginic acid (e.g., Gaviscon) may be useful in patients with mild, intermittent heartburn. However, in patients with moderate to severe or frequent symptoms or patients with documented esophagitis, antacids are not effective in relieving symptoms or healing lesions.

**Surgical Therapy.** Surgical therapy (*antireflux* surgery) is reserved for patients with complications, including esophagitis, medication intolerance, stricture, Barrett's esophagus, and persistent severe symptoms. The goal of surgical therapy is to reduce reflux by enhancing the integrity of the LES. Most surgical procedures are done laparoscopically. The fundus of the

TABLE 41-10 **Drug Therapy**

***Gastroesophageal Reflux Disease (GERD) and Peptic Ulcer Disease (PUD)***

| Drug | Mechanism of Action | Side Effects |
|---|---|---|
| **Proton Pump Inhibitors (PPIs)** | | |
| dexlansoprazole (Dexilant)<br>esomeprazole (Nexium)<br>lansoprazole (Prevacid)<br>omeprazole (Prilosec)<br>pantoprazole (Protonix)<br>rabeprazole (Aciphex)<br>omeprazole and sodium bicarbonate (Zegerid) | ↓ HCl acid secretion by inhibiting the proton pump ($H^+$-$K^+$-ATPase) responsible for the secretion of $H^+$<br>↓ Irritation of the esophageal and gastric mucosa | Headache, abdominal pain, nausea, diarrhea, vomiting, flatulence |
| **Histamine ($H_2$)-Receptor Blockers** | | |
| cimetidine<br>famotidine (Pepcid)<br>nizatidine (Axid)<br>ranitidine (Zantac) | Block the action of histamine on the $H_2$ receptors to ↓ HCl acid secretion<br>↓ Conversion of pepsinogen to pepsin<br>↓ Irritation of the esophageal and gastric mucosa | Headache, abdominal pain, constipation, diarrhea |
| **Prokinetic Agents** | | |
| metoclopramide (Reglan) | Block effect of dopamine<br>↑ Gastric motility and emptying<br>Reduce reflux | CNS side effects ranging from anxiety to hallucinations<br>Extrapyramidal side effects (tremor and dyskinesias similar to Parkinson's disease) |
| **Antiulcer, Protectants** | | |
| sucralfate (Carafate) | Act to form a protective layer and serve as a barrier against acid, bile salts, and enzymes in the stomach | Constipation |
| **Cholinergic** | | |
| bethanechol (Urecholine) | ↑ Lower esophageal sphincter pressure, improve esophageal emptying, increase gastric emptying | Lightheadedness, syncope, flushing, diarrhea, stomach cramps, dizziness |
| **Antacids, Acid Neutralizers** | | |
| ***Single Substance***<br>aluminum hydroxide<br>calcium carbonate (Tums, Titralac)<br>magnesium oxide (MagOx)<br>sodium bicarbonate (Alka-Seltzer)<br>sodium citrate (Bicitra)<br>***Aluminum and Magnesium***<br>Gelusil, Maalox, Mylanta<br>aluminum/magnesium trisilicate (Gaviscon) | Neutralize HCl acid<br>Taken 1-3 hr after meals and at bedtime | *Aluminum hydroxide:* Constipation, phosphorus depletion with chronic use<br>*Calcium carbonate:* Constipation or diarrhea, hypercalcemia, milk-alkali syndrome, renal calculi<br>*Magnesium preparations:* Diarrhea, hypermagnesemia<br>*Sodium preparations:* Milk-alkali syndrome if used with large amounts of calcium. Use with caution in patients on sodium restrictions |
| **Prostaglandin (Synthetic)** | | |
| misoprostol (Cytotec) | Protect lining of stomach<br>*Cytoprotective:* Increase production of gastric mucus and mucosal secretion of bicarbonate<br>*Antisecretory:* ↓ HCl acid secretion | Abdominal pain, diarrhea, GI bleeding, uterine rupture if pregnant |

stomach is wrapped around the lower portion of the esophagus to reinforce and repair the defective barrier. Nissen and Toupet fundoplications are common laparoscopic antireflux surgeries (Fig. 41-4).

A LINX Reflux Management System is an option for patients who have symptoms despite maximum medical management. A LINX system is a ring of small, flexible magnets enclosed in titanium beads and connected by titanium wires. Once implanted laparoscopically into the LES, the ring provides strength to a weakened LES. Under resting (nonswallowing) conditions, the magnetic attraction between the beads helps keep a weak LES closed to prevent reflux. When the person swallows, the force of pressure associated with the movement of fluids or foods overwhelms the magnetic forces and the fluid or food passes to the stomach. Adverse events with the system include difficulty swallowing, vomiting, nausea, chest pain, and

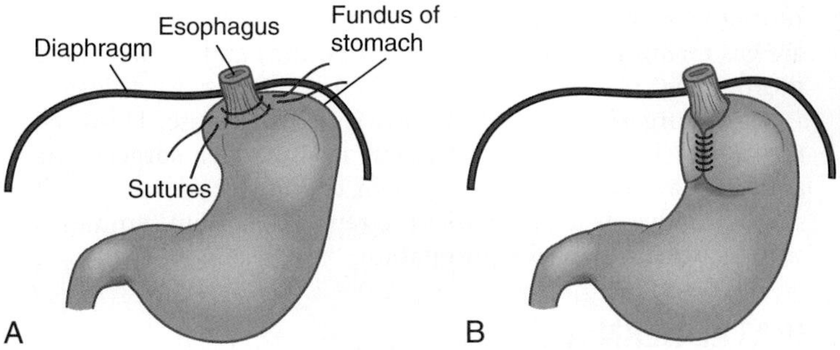


**FIG. 41-4** Nissen fundoplication for repair of hiatal hernia. **A,** Fundus of stomach is wrapped around distal esophagus. **B,** The fundus is then sutured to itself. (Modified from Doughty DB, Jackson DB: *Mosby's clinical nursing series: gastrointestinal disorders,* St Louis, 1993, Mosby.)

pain when swallowing food. Tell patients who have a LINX system not to have an MRI as it could cause serious harm.

**Endoscopic Therapy.** Alternatives to surgical therapy include endoscopic mucosal resection (EMR), photodynamic therapy, cryotherapy, and radiofrequency ablation (image-guided technique that kills cells through heating). For patients with high-grade dysplasia, EMR can be used as a diagnostic test to obtain biopsy samples. The results of the biopsy can determine whether cancer is present.

## NURSING MANAGEMENT: GASTROESOPHAGEAL REFLUX DISEASE

Nursing care for the patient with acute symptoms of GERD consists of encouraging the patient to follow the necessary regimen. The head of the bed is elevated to approximately 30 degrees. This can be done using pillows or with 4- to 6-in blocks under the bed. The patient should not be supine for 2 to 3 hours after a meal. Teach the patient to avoid food and activities that cause reflux (e.g., late night eating). Have patients contact the HCP if symptoms persist.

The patient on a PPI needs to take the medication before the first meal of the day. Teach the patient about possible medication side effects. Tell the patient on a prescription $H_2$-receptor agent to take the medication as prescribed and not to stop without checking with the HCP.

Postoperative care focuses on preventing respiratory complications, maintaining fluid and electrolyte balance, and preventing infection. Laparoscopic fundoplication is often an outpatient procedure. However, patients at risk for complications, including those with prior upper abdominal surgeries or co-morbidities (e.g., cardiac disease, obesity), may be hospitalized after the procedure. A small percentage of patients experience complications, including gastric or esophageal injury, splenic injury, pneumothorax, perforation, bleeding, infection, and pneumonia.

Since most procedures are done laparoscopically, the risk of respiratory complications is reduced. If an open high abdominal incision is used, respiratory complications can occur. Respiratory assessment includes respiratory rate and rhythm, pulse rate and rhythm, and signs of pneumothorax (e.g., dyspnea, chest pain, cyanosis). Have the patient cough and deep breathe to expand the lungs. Patients may require medications to prevent nausea and vomiting and to control pain. Measure and record the intake and output. When peristalsis returns, only give fluids initially. Solids are added gradually with the goal of resuming a normal diet. Teach the patient to avoid foods that are gas forming (prevents gastric distention) and to chew food thoroughly.

After surgery, reflux symptoms should decrease. However, recurrence is possible. In the first month after surgery, the patient may report mild dysphagia caused by edema, but it should resolve. Teach the patient to report persistent symptoms such as heartburn and regurgitation.

## HIATAL HERNIA

**Hiatal hernia** is herniation of a portion of the stomach into the esophagus through an opening, or hiatus, in the diaphragm. It is also referred to as *diaphragmatic hernia* and *esophageal hernia*. Hiatal hernias are the most common abnormality found on x-ray examination of the upper GI tract. They are common in older adults and occur more often in women.

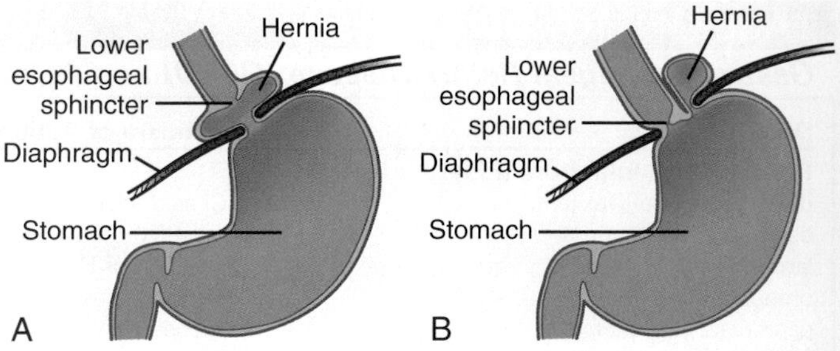


**FIG. 41-5** **A,** Sliding hiatal hernia. **B,** Rolling or paraesophageal hernia.

There are two types of hiatal hernias (Fig. 41-5):

1. *Sliding:* The junction of the stomach and esophagus is above the diaphragm, and a part of the stomach slides through the hiatal opening in the diaphragm. This occurs when the patient is supine. The hernia usually goes back into the abdominal cavity when the patient is standing upright. This is the most common type of hiatal hernia.
2. *Paraesophageal* or *rolling:* The fundus and greater curvature of the stomach roll up through the diaphragm, forming a pocket alongside the esophagus. The esophagogastric junction remains in the normal position. Acute paraesophageal hernia is a medical emergency.

### Etiology and Pathophysiology

Many factors contribute to the development of a hiatal hernia. Structural changes (weakening of the muscles in the diaphragm around the esophagogastric opening) occur with aging. Factors that increase intraabdominal pressure may predispose patients to developing a hiatal hernia. These include obesity, pregnancy, ascites, tumors, intense physical exertion, and heavy lifting on a continual basis.

### Clinical Manifestations and Complications

Some people with hiatal hernia are asymptomatic. When present, manifestations of hiatal hernia are similar to those described for GERD on pp. 900-901.

Complications that may occur with hiatal hernia include GERD, esophagitis, hemorrhage from erosion, stenosis (narrowing of the esophagus), ulcerations of the herniated portion of the stomach, strangulation of the hernia, and regurgitation with tracheal aspiration.

### Diagnostic Studies

An esophagram (barium swallow) may show the protrusion of gastric mucosa through the esophageal hiatus. Endoscopic visualization of the lower esophagus provides information on the degree of mucosal inflammation or other abnormalities. Other tests done are the same as those for GERD (Table 41-8).

## NURSING AND INTERPROFESSIONAL MANAGEMENT: HIATAL HERNIA

Conservative therapy of hiatal hernia is similar to that described for GERD (pp. 901-904). Teach the patient to reduce intraabdominal pressure by eliminating constricting garments and avoiding lifting and straining.

Surgical approaches to hiatal hernias can include reduction of the herniated stomach into the abdomen, *herniotomy* (excision of the hernia sac), *herniorrhaphy* (closure of the hiatal defect), an antireflux procedure, and *gastropexy* (attachment of the stomach subdiaphragmatically to prevent reherniation). The goals are to reduce the hernia, provide an acceptable LES pressure, and prevent movement of the gastroesophageal junction.

Surgery to repair hiatal hernia is often done laparoscopically by either Nissen or Toupet techniques (Fig. 41-4). The approach used (thoracic or abdominal) depends on the patient.

### Gerontologic Considerations: GERD and Hiatal Hernia

The incidence of hiatal hernia and GERD increases with age. Hiatal hernia is associated with weakening of the diaphragm, obesity, kyphosis, or other factors (e.g., wearing girdles) that increase intraabdominal pressure. Older patients may take medications known to decrease LES pressure (e.g., nitrates, calcium channel blockers, antidepressants). Other agents such as nonsteroidal antiinflammatory drugs (NSAIDs) and potassium can irritate the esophageal mucosa *(medication-induced esophagitis)*.

Some older adults with hiatal hernia and GERD are asymptomatic or have less severe symptoms. The first indication may be a serious problem such as esophageal bleeding secondary to esophagitis or respiratory complications (e.g., aspiration pneumonia) related to aspiration of gastric contents.

The clinical course and management of GERD and hiatal hernia in the older adult are similar to those for the younger adult. Changes in lifestyle, including eliminating dietary factors (such as caffeine-containing beverages and chocolate) and elevating the head of the bed on blocks may be challenging for the older adult.

Laparoscopic procedures reduce the risk associated with surgical repair. An older patient with cardiovascular and pulmonary problems may not be a good candidate for surgical intervention.

## ESOPHAGEAL CANCER

**Esophageal cancer** is not common. However, the rates are increasing. In the United States, approximately 16,980 new cases are diagnosed and 15,590 deaths occur from esophageal cancer each year.[5] The 5-year survival rate is 37% for localized cancer and 18% for regional cancer.

Most esophageal cancers are adenocarcinomas. The others are squamous cell tumors. Adenocarcinomas arise from the glands lining the esophagus and resemble cancers of the stomach and small intestine. The incidence of esophageal cancer increases with age. Those between 70 and 84 are at greatest risk. There is a higher incidence in non-Hispanic white men and Alaska Natives compared with other ethnic groups. The incidence is higher in men than in women.

### Etiology and Pathophysiology

The cause of esophageal cancer is unknown. Several important risk factors include Barrett's esophagus, smoking, excessive alcohol intake, and obesity. For example, current smoking or a history of smoking is associated with a twofold higher risk of esophageal cancer. Those with injury to the esophageal mucosa (e.g., from occupational exposure to asbestos and cement dust) are at greater risk. *Achalasia,* a condition marked by delayed emptying of the lower esophagus, is associated with squamous cell cancer.

Most esophageal tumors are located in the middle and lower portions of the esophagus. The tumor usually appears as an ulcerated lesion. It may penetrate the muscular layer and extend outside the wall of the esophagus. The majority of patients have advanced disease at the time of diagnosis. The cancer spreads via the lymph system, with the liver and lung being common sites of metastasis.

### Clinical Manifestations and Complications

By the time the patient experiences symptoms, the tumor is often advanced. Progressive dysphagia is the most common symptom. It may be described as a substernal feeling that food is not passing. Initially the dysphagia occurs only with meat, then with soft foods, and eventually with liquids.

Pain develops late. It occurs in the substernal, epigastric, or back areas and usually increases with swallowing. The pain may radiate to the neck, jaw, ears, and shoulders. If the tumor is in the upper third of the esophagus, symptoms such as sore throat, choking, and hoarseness may occur. Most patients lose weight. When esophageal stenosis (narrowing) is severe, regurgitation of blood-flecked esophageal contents is common.

Hemorrhage occurs if the cancer erodes through the esophagus and into the aorta. Esophageal perforation with fistula formation into the lung or trachea sometimes develops. The tumor may enlarge enough to cause esophageal obstruction, particularly in the later stages.

### Diagnostic Studies

Endoscopic biopsy is necessary to make a definitive diagnosis of esophageal cancer. Endoscopic ultrasonography (EUS) is an important tool used to stage esophageal cancer. Esophagram (barium swallow) may show narrowing of the esophagus at the tumor site (Table 41-11).

### Interprofessional Care

The treatment of esophageal cancer depends on the tumor's location and whether invasion or metastasis is present. Esophageal cancer usually has a poor prognosis because it is often not diagnosed until the disease is advanced. The best results are obtained with a multimodal approach, including surgery, endoscopic ablation, chemotherapy, and radiation therapy. Depending on the location and cancer spread, only chemotherapy and radiation may be used. Palliative therapy consists of restoring swallowing function and maintaining nutrition and hydration.

**Surgical Therapy.** The types of surgical procedures done are (1) removal of part or all of the esophagus *(esophagectomy)* with use of a Dacron graft to replace the resected part, (2) resection of a portion of the esophagus and anastomosis of the remaining

**TABLE 41-11 Interprofessional Care**

***Esophageal Cancer***

| Diagnostic Assessment | Management |
|---|---|
| • History and physical examination<br>• Endoscopy of esophagus with biopsy<br>• Endoscopic ultrasonography<br>• Esophagram (barium swallow)<br>• Bronchoscopy<br>• CT, MRI | • Surgical therapy<br>  • Esophagectomy<br>  • Esophagogastrostomy<br>  • Esophagoenterostomy<br>• Endoscopic therapy<br>  • Photodynamic therapy<br>  • Endoscopic mucosal resection<br>  • Radiofrequency ablation<br>  • Laser therapy<br>  • Dilation<br>  • Stent or prosthesis placement<br>• Radiation therapy<br>• Chemotherapy |

portion to the stomach *(esophagogastrostomy)*, and (3) resection of a portion of the esophagus and anastomosis of a segment of colon to the remaining portion *(esophagoenterostomy)*. The surgical approaches may be open (thoracic, abdominal incision) or laparoscopic.

Minimally invasive esophagectomy (e.g., laparoscopic vagal nerve–sparing surgery) is being done more frequently. It has the advantage of using smaller incisions, decreasing intensive care unit (ICU) and hospital stays, and producing fewer pulmonary complications.

**Endoscopic Therapy.** Endoscopic therapy includes photodynamic therapy, endoscopic mucosal resection (EMR), and radiofrequency ablation. In photodynamic therapy, the patient receives an IV injection of porfimer sodium (Photofrin), which is a photosensitizer. Although most tissues absorb porfimer, cancer tissue absorbs it to a greater degree. The HCP directs light towards the cancerous area using a fiber passed through an endoscope. The light reacts with porfimer, starting a reaction that destroys the cancer cells. Warn patients to avoid direct sunlight for up to 4 weeks after the procedure.

Endoscopic mucosal resection (EMR) is an option for some small, very early stage cancers. It involves the removal of malignant tissue using an endoscope. Radiofrequency ablation is used to kill cancer cells using electric current.

Dilation, stent placement, or both can relieve obstruction. Dilation increases the lumen of the esophagus. It often relieves dysphagia and allows for improved nutrition. There are various types of dilators. Placement of stents or expandable stents may help when dilation is no longer effective.[16] Stents allow food and liquid to pass through the stenotic area of the esophagus. Self-expandable metal stents are available with features to prevent stent migration and tumor ingrowth. Stents may be placed before surgery to improve the patient's nutritional status.

Endoscopic laser therapy may be used in combination with dilation. Laser therapy can be repeated if obstruction recurs as the tumor grows. Sometimes these procedures are combined with radiation therapy.

**Radiation Therapy.** Depending on the type and stage of esophageal cancer, chemotherapy with or without radiation therapy may be given. Concurrent radiation and chemotherapy are given for palliation of symptoms, especially dysphagia, and to increase survival. Some patients receive radiation therapy before surgery.

**Chemotherapy.** Many different chemotherapy drugs can be used to treat esophageal cancer. Common combination regimens are carboplatin and paclitaxel, cisplatin and 5-fluorouracil (5-FU), ECF (epirubicin [Ellence], cisplatin, and 5-FU), DCF (docetaxel, cisplatin, and 5-FU), cisplatin with capecitabine (Xeloda), and oxaliplatin with either 5-FU or capecitabine. Other chemotherapy drugs that have been used include bleomycin, mitomycin, methotrexate, vinorelbine (Navelbine), topotecan, and irinotecan (Camptosar). (Chemotherapy is discussed in Chapter 15.)

**Targeted Therapy.** Some esophageal cancers have too much HER-2 protein on their cell surfaces, which helps cancer cells to grow. Trastuzumab (Herceptin) is a drug that targets the HER-2 protein and kills the cancer cells.

Ramucirumab (Cyramza), an angiogenesis inhibitor, binds to the receptor for *vascular endothelial growth factor* (VEGF), a compound that stimulates blood vessel growth. Thus ramucirumab prevents VEGF from binding to the receptor and signaling the body to make more blood vessels. This can help slow or stop the growth and spread of cancer. Ramucirumab is used to treat advanced cancers that start at the gastroesophageal (GE) junction. (Targeted therapies are discussed in Chapter 15.)

**Nutritional Therapy.** After esophageal surgery parenteral fluids are given. A jejunostomy, gastrostomy, or esophagostomy feeding tube may be placed to feed the patient depending on the type of surgery (e.g., esophagogastrectomy) performed. A swallowing study is often done before allowing the patient to have oral fluids. When starting fluids, give water (30 to 60 mL) hourly and gradually progress to small, frequent, bland meals. Place the patient in an upright position to prevent regurgitation. With tube feeding, observe the patient for signs of intolerance to the feeding or leakage of the feeding into the mediastinum. Symptoms that indicate leakage are pain, increased temperature, and dyspnea. (Enteral nutrition is discussed in Chapter 39.)

## NURSING MANAGEMENT: ESOPHAGEAL CANCER

### Nursing Assessment

Ask the patient about a history of GERD, hiatal hernia, achalasia, Barrett's esophagus, and tobacco and alcohol use. Assess the patient for progressive dysphagia and *odynophagia* (burning, squeezing pain while swallowing). Ask about the type of substances (e.g., meats, soft foods, liquids) that cause dysphagia. Assess the patient for pain (substernal, epigastric, or back areas), choking, heartburn, hoarseness, cough, anorexia, weight loss, and regurgitation.

### Nursing Diagnoses

Nursing diagnoses for the patient with esophageal cancer include, but are not limited to, the following:

- Chronic pain *related to* the compression of tumor on surrounding tissues, esophageal stenosis
- Imbalanced nutrition: less than body requirements *related to* dysphagia, odynophagia, weakness, chemotherapy, and radiation therapy
- Risk for aspiration *related to* difficulty swallowing, choking, and regurgitation
- Anxiety and grieving *related to* diagnosis of cancer, uncertain future, and prognosis

### Planning

The overall goals are that the patient with esophageal cancer will (1) have relief of symptoms, including pain and dysphagia; (2) achieve optimal nutritional intake; and (3) experience a quality of life appropriate to stage of disease and prognosis.

### Nursing Implementation

**Health Promotion.** Counsel the patient with GERD, Barrett's esophagus, or hiatal hernia about the importance of regular follow-up evaluation. Health counseling should focus on elimination of smoking and excessive alcohol intake, as well as other risk factors for GERD (Table 41-7). Maintaining good oral hygiene and dietary habits (e.g., intake of fresh fruits and vegetables) is important. Encourage patients to seek medical attention for any esophageal problems, especially dysphagia.

**Acute Care**

***Preoperative Care.*** The patient and caregiver usually react with shock, disbelief, and depression when they are told about a diagnosis of esophageal cancer. Provide emotional and physical support, provide information, clarify test results, and maintain a positive attitude with respect to the patient's immediate recovery and long-term survival.

In addition to general preoperative teaching and preparation, pay particular attention to the patient's nutritional needs. Many patients are poorly nourished because of the inability to ingest adequate amounts of food and fluids. A high-calorie, high-protein diet is recommended. Some patients require a liquid form of this diet. Others may need IV fluid replacement or parenteral nutrition. Teach the patient and caregiver how to keep an intake and output record and assess for signs of fluid and electrolyte imbalance. Some treatment protocols require preoperative radiation and chemotherapy.

Meticulous oral care is essential. Cleanse the mouth thoroughly, including the tongue, gingivae, and teeth or dentures. It may be necessary to use swabs or a gauze pad and to scrub the mouth, including the tongue. Milk of magnesia with mineral oil helps remove crust formation.

Teaching should include information about chest tubes (if an open thoracic approach is used), IV lines, NG tubes, pain management, gastrostomy or jejunostomy feeding, turning, coughing, and deep breathing. (General preoperative care is discussed in Chapter 17.)

***Postoperative Care.*** The patient usually has an NG tube in place and may have bloody drainage for 8 to 12 hours. The drainage gradually changes to greenish yellow. Assessing the drainage, maintaining the tube, and providing oral and nasal care are nursing responsibilities. Do not reposition the NG tube or reinsert it without consulting the surgeon.

Because of the location of the surgery and the patient's general condition, emphasize preventing respiratory complications. Have the patient turn, cough, and deep breathe, and use an incentive spirometer every 2 hours.

Cardiac dysrhythmias may result from the proximity of the pericardium to the surgical site. Other complications that can occur after esophagectomy include esophageal anastomotic leaks, fistula formation, interstitial pulmonary edema, and acute respiratory distress related to the disruption of the mediastinal lymph nodes.

Position the patient in a semi-Fowler's or Fowler's position to prevent reflux and aspiration of gastric secretions. When the patient can drink fluids or eat, maintain the upright position for at least 2 hours after eating to assist with gastric emptying.

**Ambulatory Care.** Many patients require long-term follow-up care after surgery for esophageal cancer. The patient may undergo chemotherapy and radiation treatment after surgery. Encourage and assist the patient in maintaining adequate nutrition. A permanent feeding gastrostomy may be required. The patient usually has fears and anxieties about a diagnosis of cancer. Know what the HCP has told the patient about the prognosis and provide appropriate counseling.

Referral to a palliative care or home health nurse may be needed. (See Chapter 15 for the care of the cancer patient and Chapter 9 for a discussion of palliative and end-of-life care.)

### Evaluation

The expected outcomes are that the patient with esophageal cancer will

- Maintain a patent airway
- Have relief of pain
- Be able to swallow comfortably and consume adequate nutritional intake
- Experience a quality of life appropriate to stage of disease and prognosis

## OTHER ESOPHAGEAL DISORDERS

### Eosinophilic Esophagitis

*Eosinophilic esophagitis* (EoE) is characterized by swelling of the esophagus from an infiltration of *eosinophils.* People with EoE frequently have a personal or family history of other allergic diseases. The most common food triggers are milk, egg, wheat, rye, and beef. Environmental allergens, such as pollens, molds, cat, dog, and dust mite allergens, may be involved in the development of EoE.

Clinical manifestations include severe heartburn, difficulty swallowing, food impaction in the esophagus, nausea, vomiting, and weight loss. The diagnosis is based on symptoms and biopsy findings of eosinophils infiltrating esophageal tissue obtained from endoscopy.

Allergy skin testing helps to determine the person's allergens. A trial of avoidance of the foods to which the person has positive allergy tests is the initial form of treatment. Other common treatments include the use of PPIs (Table 41-10) and corticosteroids. Corticosteroids are frequently used to treat EoE when avoiding allergic triggers does not relieve symptoms.

Corticosteroids may be used orally (prednisone) or as a topical therapy with inhaled corticosteroids (e.g., fluticasone [Flovent]). The patient takes a puff of fluticasone, and rather than inhaling it, swallows the medication. This directly delivers the drug to the esophagus. The most common side effect is a yeast infection of the throat (esophageal candidiasis).

### Esophageal Diverticula

**Esophageal diverticula** are saclike outpouchings of one or more layers of the esophagus. They occur in three main areas: (1) above the upper esophageal sphincter *(Zenker's diverticulum)*, which is the most common location; (2) near the esophageal midpoint (traction diverticulum); and (3) above the LES (epiphrenic diverticulum) (Fig. 41-6). Pharyngeal pouches (Zenker's diverticula) occur commonly in people over 60 years.

Typical symptoms include dysphagia, regurgitation, chronic cough, aspiration, and weight loss. Food becomes trapped in the outpouches. This causes tasting sour food and smelling a foul odor. Complications include malnutrition, aspiration, and perforation. Endoscopy or barium studies can easily establish a diagnosis.

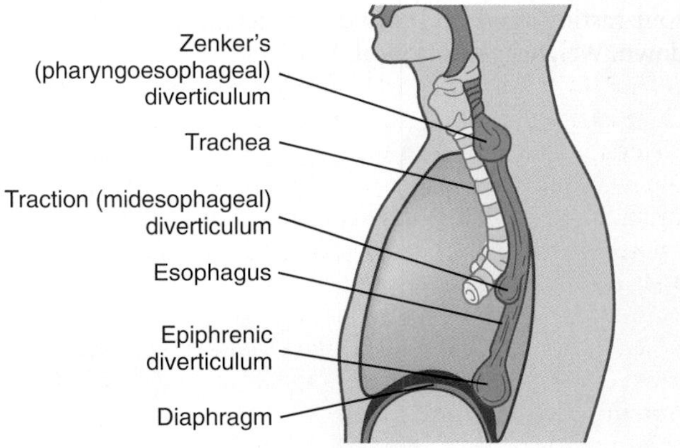


**FIG. 41-6** Possible sites for esophageal diverticula. These hollow outpouchings may occur just above the upper esophageal sphincter (Zenker's, the most common type of pulsion diverticulum), near the midpoint of the esophagus (traction), and just above the lower esophageal sphincter (epiphrenic). (Modified from Price SA, Wilson LM: *Pathophysiology: clinical concepts of disease processes,* ed 6, St Louis, 2003, Mosby.)

There is no specific treatment for esophageal diverticula. Some patients find that they can empty the pocket of food that collects by applying pressure at a point on the neck. The diet may have to be limited to foods that pass more readily (e.g., blenderized foods). Surgical treatment may be necessary if nutrition is disrupted. Treatment by endoscopic stapling diverticulotomy or diverticulostomy is associated with decreased complications compared with the open approaches. The most serious surgical complication is esophageal perforation.

### Esophageal Strictures

The most common cause of *esophageal strictures* (or narrowing) is chronic GERD. The ingestion of strong acids or alkalis, external beam radiation, and surgical anastomosis can also create strictures. Trauma such as throat lacerations and gunshot wounds can lead to strictures because of scar formation. Strictures can result in dysphagia, regurgitation, and ultimately weight loss.

Strictures can be dilated using mechanical *bougies* (dilating instruments) or balloons. Dilation may be done with or without endoscopy, or with fluoroscopy. Surgical excision with anastomosis is sometimes necessary. The patient may have a temporary or permanent gastrostomy.

### Achalasia

In **achalasia**, peristalsis of the lower two thirds (smooth muscle) of the esophagus is absent. Achalasia is a rare, chronic disorder. The exact cause is unknown. With achalasia, the pressure in the LES increases along with incomplete relaxation. Esophageal obstruction at or near the diaphragm occurs. Food and fluid accumulate in the lower esophagus. The result is dilation of the esophagus proximal to (above) the tapering affected segment of the lower esophagus (Fig. 41-7). There is a selective loss of inhibitory neurons, resulting in unopposed contraction of the LES.

The onset of achalasia is usually insidious. Dysphagia is the most common symptom and occurs with both liquids and solids. Patients may report a globus sensation and/or substernal chest pain (similar to angina pain) during or immediately after a meal. About a third of the patients experience nocturnal regurgitation. *Halitosis* (foul-smelling breath) and the inability to eructate (belch) are other symptoms. Patients with achalasia may report symptoms of GERD and regurgitation of sour-tasting food and liquids, especially when they are lying down. Weight loss is typical.

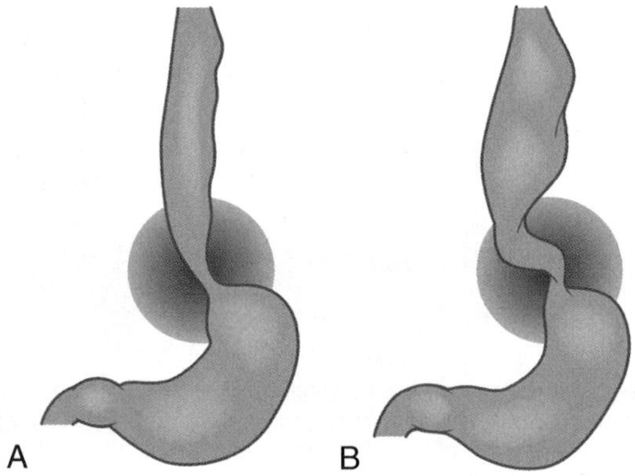


**FIG. 41-7** Esophageal achalasia. **A,** Early stage, showing tapering of lower esophagus. **B,** Advanced stage, showing dilated, tortuous esophagus.

Diagnosis is made with esophagram (barium swallow), manometric evaluation (high-resolution manometry), and/or endoscopic evaluation. Treatment focuses on symptom management. The goals of treatment are to relieve dysphagia and regurgitation, improve esophageal emptying by disrupting the LES, and prevent the development of megaesophagus (enlargement of the lower esophagus).

Endoscopic pneumatic dilation involves dilating the LES muscle using balloons of progressively larger diameter (3.0, 3.5, and 4.0 cm) (Fig. 41-8). It is an outpatient procedure. If this is ineffective, the next option is a Heller myotomy, done laparoscopically. In this procedure, the surgeon cuts through the muscles of the LES, allowing food to pass. Because GERD with esophagitis and stricture is a common complication, the patient often has antireflux surgery at the same time. The patient typically returns to usual activities 1 to 2 weeks afterwards.

Medical therapy is less effective than invasive procedures. The injection of botulinum toxin endoscopically into the LES gives short-term relief of symptoms and improves esophageal emptying. It works by promoting relaxation of the smooth muscle. This treatment is used for older patients for whom surgery and pneumatic dilation may not be appropriate due to other chronic illnesses.

Smooth muscle relaxants, such as nitrates (isosorbide dinitrate [Isordil]) and calcium channel blockers (e.g., nifedipine [Procardia]), taken sublingually 30 to 45 minutes before meals may improve dysphagia. Side effects (e.g., headache), drug tolerance, and short duration of action limit their use. Symptomatic treatment consists of eating a semisoft diet, eating slowly and drinking fluid with meals, and sleeping with the head elevated.

### Esophageal Varices

*Esophageal varices* are dilated, tortuous veins occurring in the lower portion of the esophagus because of portal hypertension. Esophageal varices are a common complication of liver cirrhosis. They are discussed in Chapter 43.

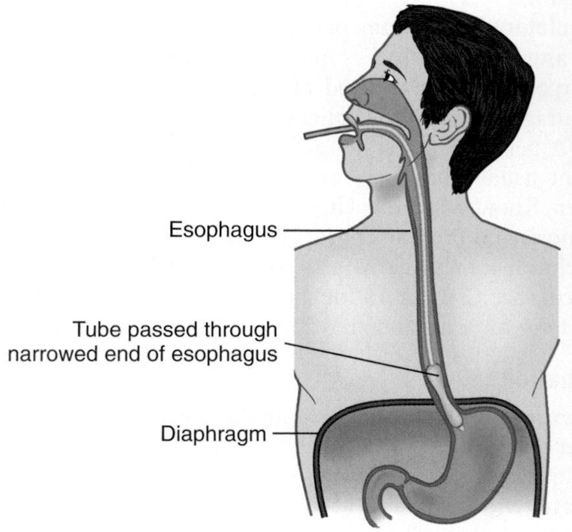


**FIG. 41-8** Pneumatic dilation attempts to treat achalasia by maintaining an adequate lumen and decreasing lower esophageal sphincter (LES) tone. (Modified from Price SA, Wilson LM: *Pathophysiology: clinical concepts of disease processes,* ed 6, St Louis, 2003, Mosby.)

# DISORDERS OF THE STOMACH AND UPPER SMALL INTESTINE

## GASTRITIS

Gastritis, an inflammation of the gastric mucosa, is one of the most common problems affecting the stomach. Gastritis may be acute or chronic and diffuse or localized.

### Etiology and Pathophysiology

Gastritis occurs as the result of a breakdown in the normal gastric mucosal barrier. This mucosal barrier normally protects the stomach tissue from the corrosive action of HCl acid and pepsin. When the barrier is broken, HCl acid and pepsin can diffuse back into the mucosa. This back diffusion results in tissue edema, disruption of capillary walls with loss of plasma into the gastric lumen, and possible hemorrhage.

**Risk Factors.** Risk factors and causes of gastritis are listed in Table 41-12. Some of the risk factors are discussed in this section.

***Drug-Related Gastritis.*** Drugs contribute to the development of acute and chronic gastritis. NSAIDs, including aspirin, and corticosteroids inhibit the synthesis of prostaglandins that are protective to the gastric mucosa. This makes the mucosa more susceptible to injury. NSAID-related gastritis is associated with many drugs, including piroxicam (Feldene), naproxen (Naprosyn), indomethacin, diclofenac (Voltaren), and ibuprofen.[17]

Risk factors for NSAID-induced gastritis include being female; being over age 60; having a history of ulcer disease; taking anticoagulants, other NSAIDs (including low-dose aspirin), or other ulcerogenic drugs (including corticosteroids); and having a chronic debilitating disorder such as cardiovascular disease. Some drugs such as digitalis (digoxin) and alendronate (Fosamax) have direct irritating effects on the gastric mucosa.

***Diet.*** Dietary indiscretions can result in acute gastritis. After an alcoholic drinking binge, acute damage to the gastric mucosa can range from localized injury of superficial epithelial cells to destruction of the mucosa with mucosal congestion, edema, and hemorrhage. Prolonged damage induced by repeated alcohol abuse results in chronic gastritis. Eating large quantities of spicy, irritating foods can cause acute gastritis.

**Helicobacter pylori.** An important cause of chronic gastritis is *Helicobacter pylori* infection. *H. pylori* infection causes acute gastritis in most infected persons. In some patients, chronic gastritis develops. Prolonged inflammation leads to functional changes in the stomach and in some cases, stomach cancer. *H. pylori* is discussed later in this chapter on p. 911.

***Other Risk Factors.*** Although not as common as *H. pylori,* other bacterial, viral, and fungal infections are associated with chronic gastritis. Gastritis can occur from reflux of bile salts from the duodenum into the stomach because of anatomic changes following surgical procedures (e.g., gastroduodenostomy, gastrojejunostomy). Prolonged vomiting may cause reflux of bile salts. Intense emotional responses and CNS lesions may produce inflammation of the mucosal lining from hypersecretion of HCl acid.

**Autoimmune Gastritis.** Autoimmune metaplastic atrophic gastritis (also called *autoimmune atrophic gastritis*) is an inherited condition in which there is an immune response directed against parietal cells. It most commonly affects women of northern European descent. Patients often have other autoimmune disorders. The loss of parietal cells leads to low chloride levels, inadequate production of intrinsic factor, cobalamin (vitamin $B_{12}$) malabsorption, and pernicious anemia. It is associated with an increased risk of stomach cancer.

**TABLE 41-12 Causes of Gastritis**

| | |
|---|---|
| **Drugs**<br>• Aspirin<br>• Bisphosphonates<br>• Corticosteroids<br>• Iron supplements<br>• Nonsteroidal antiinflammatory drugs (NSAIDs) | **Environmental Factors**<br>• Radiation<br>• Smoking |
| **Diet**<br>• Alcohol<br>• Large quantities of spicy, irritating foods | **Diseases/Disorders**<br>• Burns<br>• Large hiatal hernia<br>• Physiologic stress<br>• Crohn's disease<br>• Reflux of bile and pancreatic secretions<br>• Renal failure<br>• Sepsis<br>• Shock |
| **Microorganisms**<br>• *Helicobacter pylori*<br>• Mycobacterium species<br>• Salmonella organisms<br>• Staphylococcus organisms<br>• Cytomegalovirus<br>• Syphilis | **Other Factors**<br>• Endoscopy procedures<br>• Nasogastric tube<br>• Psychologic stress |

### Clinical Manifestations

The symptoms of *acute gastritis* include anorexia, nausea and vomiting, epigastric tenderness, and a feeling of fullness. Hemorrhage is commonly associated with alcohol abuse and at times is the only symptom. Acute gastritis is self-limiting, lasting from a few hours to a few days. Complete healing of the mucosa is expected.

The manifestations of *chronic gastritis* are similar to those of acute gastritis. Some patients are asymptomatic. However, when parietal cells are lost because of atrophy, the source of intrinsic factor is also lost. *Intrinsic factor* is essential for the absorption of cobalamin in the terminal ileum. Once the body's cobalamin stores in the liver are depleted, a state of cobalamin deficiency exists. Because it is essential for the growth and maturation of red blood cells (RBCs), the lack of cobalamin results in pernicious anemia and neurologic complications. (Cobalamin deficiency anemia is discussed in Chapter 30.)

### Diagnostic Studies

Acute gastritis is usually diagnosed based on the patient's symptoms and a history of drug or alcohol use. Occasionally, an endoscopic examination with biopsy is necessary to provide a definitive diagnosis. Breath, urine, serum, stool, and gastric tissue biopsy tests are available to assess for *H. pylori* infection. A complete blood count (CBC) may show anemia from blood loss or lack of intrinsic factor. Stools are tested for occult blood. Serum tests for antibodies to parietal cells and intrinsic factor may be done. A tissue biopsy can rule out gastric cancer.

## ❖ NURSING AND INTERPROFESSIONAL MANAGEMENT: GASTRITIS

### ◆ Acute Gastritis

Eliminating the cause and preventing or avoiding it in the future are generally all that is needed to treat acute gastritis. The

**TABLE 41-13 Drug Therapy**
***Helicobacter pylori Infection***

| Treatment | Duration | Eradication Rate |
|---|---|---|
| **Triple-drug therapy**<br>proton pump inhibitor (PPI)<br>amoxicillin<br>clarithromycin (Biaxin) | 7-14 days | 70%-85% |
| **Quadruple therapy**<br>PPI<br>bismuth<br>tetracycline<br>metronidazole (Flagyl) | 10-14 days | 85% |

plan of care is supportive and similar to that described for nausea and vomiting. If vomiting accompanies acute gastritis, rest, NPO status, and IV fluids may be prescribed. Antiemetics are given (Table 41-1). Monitor for dehydration. It can occur rapidly in acute gastritis with vomiting.

In severe cases of acute gastritis, an NG tube may be used to (1) monitor for bleeding, (2) lavage the precipitating agent from the stomach, or (3) keep the stomach empty and free of noxious stimuli. Clear liquids are resumed when symptoms have subsided. Reintroduce solids gradually.

If the patient is at risk for hemorrhage, frequently check vital signs and test the vomitus for blood. All of the management strategies discussed in the section on upper GI bleeding apply to the patient with severe gastritis (see pp. 923-925).

Drug therapy focuses on reducing irritation of the gastric mucosa and providing symptomatic relief. $H_2$-receptor blockers (e.g., ranitidine, cimetidine) or PPIs (e.g., omeprazole, lansoprazole) reduce gastric HCl acid secretion (Table 41-10). Teach the patient about the therapeutic effects of PPIs and $H_2$-receptor blockers.

### ◆ Chronic Gastritis

The treatment of chronic gastritis focuses on evaluating and eliminating the specific cause (e.g., cessation of alcohol intake, abstinence from drugs, *H. pylori* eradication). Antibiotic combinations are used to eradicate *H. pylori* (Table 41-13). The patient with pernicious anemia needs lifelong cobalamin therapy (see Chapter 30).

The patient undergoing treatment for chronic gastritis may have to adapt to lifestyle changes and strictly adhere to a drug regimen. Some patients find a nonirritating diet consisting of six small feedings a day helpful. Smoking is contraindicated in all forms of gastritis. An interprofessional team approach in which the HCP, nurse, dietitian, and pharmacist provide consistent information and support will increase the patient's success in making these changes.

## PEPTIC ULCER DISEASE

**Peptic ulcer disease (PUD)** is a condition characterized by erosion of the GI mucosa from the digestive action of HCl acid and pepsin. Any portion of the GI tract that is in contact with gastric secretions is susceptible to ulcer development. This includes the lower esophagus, stomach, duodenum, and margin of a gastrojejunal anastomosis after surgical procedures. About 25 million people in the United States are affected by PUD in their lifetime.[18]

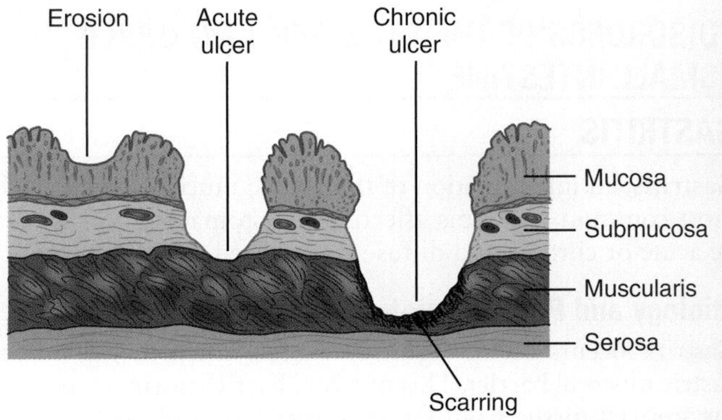


**FIG. 41-9** Peptic ulcers, including an erosion, an acute ulcer, and a chronic ulcer. Both the acute ulcer and the chronic ulcer may penetrate the entire wall of the stomach. (Modified from Price SA, Wilson LM: *Pathophysiology: clinical concepts of disease processes,* ed 6, St Louis, 2003, Mosby.)

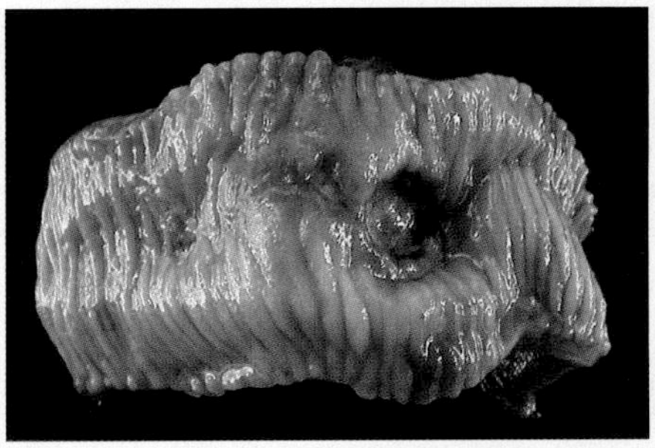

**FIG. 41-10** Peptic ulcer of the duodenum. (From Kumar V, Abbas AK, Aster JC, Fausto N: *Robbins and Cotran pathologic basis of disease,* ed 8, Philadelphia, 2010, Saunders.)

### Types

Peptic ulcers are classified as acute or chronic, depending on the degree and duration of mucosal involvement, and gastric or duodenal, according to the location. The *acute ulcer* (Fig. 41-9) is associated with superficial erosion and minimal inflammation. It is of short duration and resolves quickly when the cause is identified and removed. A chronic ulcer (Fig. 41-10) is one of long duration, eroding through the muscular wall with the formation of fibrous tissue. It is present continuously for many months or intermittently throughout the person's lifetime. Chronic ulcers are more common than acute erosions.

Although gastric and duodenal ulcers are both considered PUD, they are different in their incidence and presentation (Table 41-14). Generally, the treatment of all types of ulcers is similar.

### Etiology and Pathophysiology

Peptic ulcers develop only in an acid environment. However, an excess of HCl acid may not be necessary for ulcer development. Pepsinogen, the precursor of pepsin, changes to pepsin in the presence of HCl acid and a pH of 2 to 3. When food or antacids neutralize the stomach acid level or drugs block acid secretion, the pH increases to 3.5 or more. At a pH of 3.5 or more, pepsin has little or no proteolytic activity.

The pathophysiology of ulcer development is outlined in Fig. 41-11. The back diffusion of HCl acid into the gastric mucosa results in cellular destruction and inflammation. Histamine is released from the damaged mucosa, resulting in vasodilation and increased capillary permeability and further secretion of acid and pepsin. Fig. 41-12 depicts the interrelationship between

**TABLE 41-14 Comparison of Gastric and Duodenal Ulcers**

| Gastric Ulcers | Duodenal Ulcers |
|---|---|
| **Lesion** | |
| Superficial, smooth margins. Round, oval, or cone shaped | Penetrating (associated with deformity of duodenal bulb from healing of recurrent ulcers) |
| **Location of Lesion** | |
| Predominantly antrum, also in body and fundus of stomach | First 1-2 cm of duodenum |
| **Gastric Secretion** | |
| Normal to decreased | Increased |
| **Incidence** | |
| Greater in women | Greater in men, but increasing in women (especially postmenopausal) |
| Peak age 50-60 yr | Peak age 35-45 yr |
| Increased cancer risk | No increase in cancer risk |
| *H. pylori* infection in 80% | *H. pylori* infection in 90% |
| ↑ With incompetent pyloric sphincter and bile reflux | Associated with other diseases (e.g., chronic obstructive pulmonary disease, pancreatic disease, hyperparathyroidism, Zollinger-Ellison syndrome, chronic renal failure) |
| **Clinical Manifestations** | |
| Burning or gaseous pressure in epigastrium | Burning, cramping, pressure-like pain across midepigastrium and upper abdomen. Back pain with posterior ulcers |
| Pain 1-2 hr after meals. If penetrating ulcer, aggravation of discomfort with food | Pain 2-5 hr after meals and midmorning, midafternoon, middle of night. Periodic and episodic. Pain relief with antacids and food |
| **Recurrence Rate** | |
| High | High |

the mucosal blood flow and disruption of the gastric mucosal barrier. As described in the section on gastritis, a number of factors damage the mucosal barrier.

***Helicobacter pylori.*** *H. pylori* is associated with PUD. About 70% of people in developing countries and 40% in the U.S. and industrialized countries are infected with *H. pylori*.[18] Infection likely occurs during childhood with transmission from family members to the child, possibly through a fecal-oral or oral-oral route. In the United States, those more likely to be infected are people born before 1940 and those of low socioeconomic status.

In the stomach, the bacteria can survive a long time by colonizing the gastric epithelial cells within the mucosal layer. The bacteria produce urease, which metabolizes urea-producing ammonium chloride and other damaging chemicals. Urease activates the immune response with both antibody production and the release of inflammatory cytokines. This leads to increased gastric secretion and produces tissue damage, leading to PUD.

Although most people with *H. pylori* never develop ulcers, it appears that those infected with *CagA*-positive strains are more likely to have PUD. Other factors influencing risk for PUD include genetics, smoking, NSAID use, and diet. It is thought that the higher risk of PUD among persons of lower socioeconomic status is due to their having a higher prevalence of *H. pylori* infection.

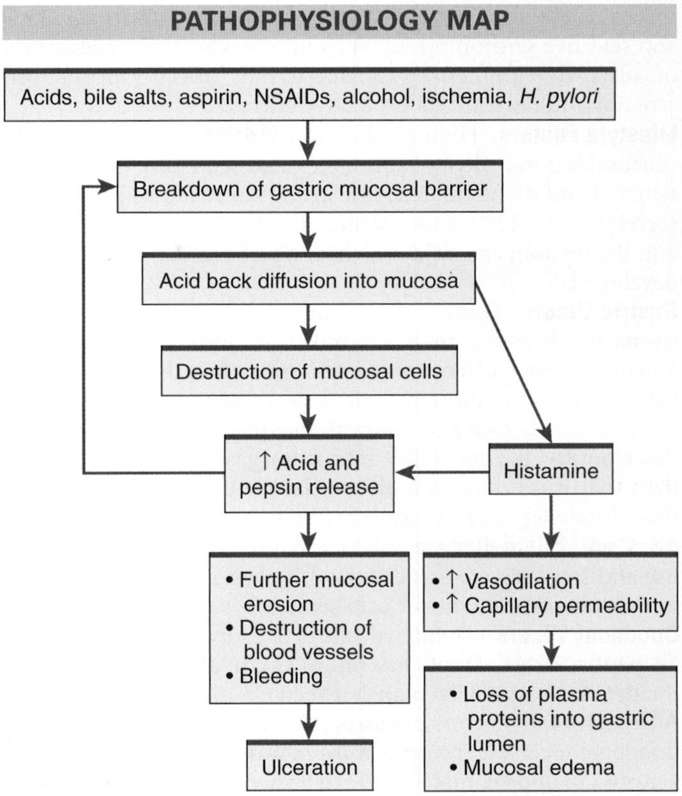


**FIG. 41-11** Disruption of gastric mucosa and pathophysiologic consequences of back diffusion of acids.

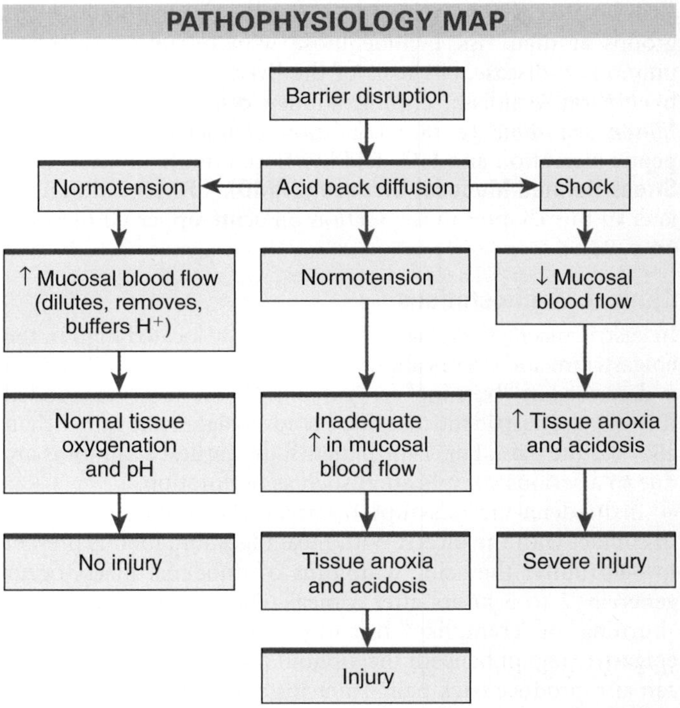


**FIG. 41-12** Relationship between mucosal blood flow and disruption of the gastric mucosal barrier.

**Medication-Induced Injury.** Ulcerogenic drugs, such as aspirin and NSAIDs, inhibit prostaglandin synthesis, increase gastric acid secretion, and reduce the integrity of the mucosal barrier. The use of NSAIDs is responsible for the majority of non–*H. pylori* peptic ulcers. NSAIDs in the presence of *H. pylori* increase the risk of PUD.[17] Patients on corticosteroids, anticoagulants, and selective serotonin reuptake inhibitors are at increased risk of ulcer development.[19] Corticosteroids affect mucosal cell renewal and decrease its protective effects.

**Lifestyle Factors.** High alcohol intake is associated with acute mucosal lesions. Alcohol stimulates acid secretion. Coffee (caffeinated and decaffeinated) is a strong stimulant of gastric acid secretion. Smoking and psychologic distress, including stress and depression, can delay the healing of ulcers once they have developed.

**Gastric Ulcers.** Gastric ulcers can occur in any portion of the stomach. However, they are most commonly found in the antrum. Gastric ulcers are less common than duodenal ulcers. Gastric ulcers are more prevalent in women and those over 50 years of age. Because of the peak incidence of gastric ulcers in older adults, the mortality rate from gastric ulcers is greater than that from duodenal ulcers. Gastric ulcers are more likely than duodenal ulcers to result in obstruction. *H. pylori,* medications, and bile reflux are risk factors for gastric ulcers. Alcohol use and smoking are associated with ulcer formation. They are both known stimulants of acid secretion.

**Duodenal Ulcers.** Duodenal ulcers account for about 80% of all peptic ulcers. Duodenal ulcers occur at any age, but the incidence is especially high between 35 and 45 years of age. Although many factors are associated with the development of duodenal ulcers, *H. pylori* is most common. *H. pylori* infection is found in approximately 90% to 95% of patients with duodenal ulcers.

The development of duodenal ulcers is often associated with a high HCl acid secretion. Alcohol ingestion and smoking are also associated with duodenal ulcer formation. Several patient groups at high risk include those with chronic obstructive pulmonary disease, cirrhosis of the liver, chronic pancreatitis, hyperparathyroidism, chronic kidney disease, and *Zollinger-Ellison syndrome* (a rare condition characterized by severe peptic ulceration and HCl acid hypersecretion).

**Stress-Related Mucosal Disease (SRMD).** SRMD is described later in this chapter in the section on acute upper GI bleeding on p. 922.

## Clinical Manifestations

In gastric ulcers, the discomfort is generally located high in the epigastrium and occurs about 1 to 2 hours after meals. The pain is described as "burning" or "gaseous." If the ulcer has eroded through the gastric mucosa, food tends to aggravate rather than alleviate the pain. For some patients, the earliest symptoms are due to a serious complication such as perforation.

In duodenal ulcers, symptoms occur when gastric acid comes in contact with the ulcers. With meal ingestion, food is present to help buffer the acid. Symptoms of duodenal ulcers occur generally 2 to 5 hours after a meal. The pain is described as "burning" or "cramplike." It is most often located in the mid-epigastric region beneath the xiphoid process. Duodenal ulcers can also produce back pain. Antacids alone or in combination with an $H_2$-receptor blocker, as well as food, neutralize the acid to provide relief. A characteristic of duodenal ulcer is its tendency to occur continuously for a few weeks or months and then disappear for a time, only to recur some months later.

Some patients experience bloating, nausea, vomiting, and early feelings of fullness. Not all patients with ulcers experience pain or discomfort. *Silent* peptic ulcers are more likely to occur in older adults and those taking NSAIDs. The presence or absence of symptoms is not directly related to the size of the ulcer or the degree of healing.

## Complications

The three major complications of chronic PUD are hemorrhage, perforation, and gastric outlet obstruction. All these complications are considered emergency situations and may require surgical intervention.

**Hemorrhage.** Hemorrhage is the most common complication of PUD. Duodenal ulcers account for a greater percentage of upper GI bleeding episodes than gastric ulcers.

**Perforation.** Perforation is considered the most lethal complication of PUD. Perforation is commonly seen in large penetrating duodenal ulcers (Fig. 41-13). Even though duodenal ulcers are more prevalent and perforate more often, mortality rates associated with perforation of gastric ulcers are higher. The patient with gastric ulcers is older and often has concurrent medical problems, which accounts for the higher mortality rate.

With perforation, the ulcer penetrates the serosal surface with spillage of either gastric or duodenal contents into the peritoneal cavity. Larger perforations require immediate surgical closure. Small perforations may spontaneously seal themselves and symptoms cease. Spontaneous sealing occurs because of fibrin production in response to the perforation. This can lead to fibrinous fusion of the duodenum or gastric curvature to adjacent tissue (mainly the liver) and strictures that can obstruct the flow of intestinal contents and the passage of stool.

The clinical manifestations of perforation are sudden and dramatic in onset. During the initial phase (0 to 2 hours after perforation), the patient has sudden, severe upper abdominal pain that quickly spreads throughout the abdomen. The pain radiates to the back and shoulders. Food or antacids do not relieve the pain. The abdomen appears rigid and boardlike as the abdominal muscles attempt to protect from further injury. The patient's respirations become shallow and rapid. The heart rate is elevated (tachycardia), and the pulse is weak. Bowel sounds are usually absent. Nausea and vomiting may occur.

The contents entering the peritoneal cavity from the stomach or duodenum may contain air, saliva, food particles, HCl acid, pepsin, bacteria, bile, and pancreatic fluid and enzymes. If the condition is untreated, bacterial peritonitis may occur within 6 to 12 hours. The intensity of peritonitis is proportional to the amount and duration of the spillage through the perforation. It is difficult to determine from the symptoms alone whether a

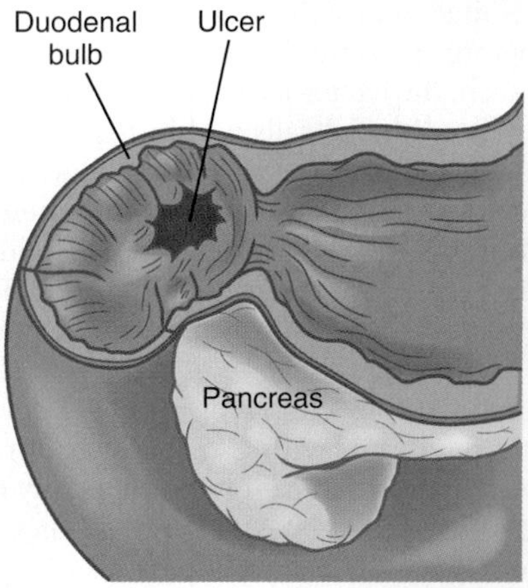


**FIG. 41-13** Duodenal ulcer of the posterior wall penetrating into the head of the pancreas, resulting in walled-off perforation.

gastric or duodenal ulcer has perforated, because the manifestations of peritonitis are the same (see Chapter 42).

**Gastric Outlet Obstruction.** Both acute and chronic PUD can result in gastric outlet obstruction. Obstruction in the distal stomach and duodenum is the result of edema, inflammation, or pylorospasm and fibrous scar tissue formation. With obstruction the patient reports discomfort or pain that is worse toward the end of the day as the stomach fills and dilates. Belching or self-induced vomiting may provide some relief. Vomiting is common and often projectile. The vomitus may contain food particles that were ingested hours or days before. Constipation occurs because of dehydration and decreased diet intake secondary to anorexia. Over time dilation of the stomach and visible swelling in the upper abdomen may occur.

## Diagnostic Studies

The diagnostic tests used to determine the presence and location of an ulcer are similar to those used for acute upper GI bleeding. Endoscopy is the most accurate diagnostic procedure. Endoscopy allows for direct viewing of the gastric and duodenal mucosa (Fig. 41-14). During endoscopy, tissue specimens are obtained to determine if *H. pylori* is present and rule out stomach cancer. Endoscopy can also be used to determine the degree of ulcer healing after treatment.

Several noninvasive and invasive tests are available to confirm *H. pylori* infection. The gold standard for diagnosing *H. pylori* infection is a biopsy of the antral mucosa with testing for urease (rapid urease testing). Noninvasive tests include serology, stool, and breath testing. The urea breath test can identify active infection. Urea is a by-product of the metabolism of *H. pylori* bacteria. Stool antigen tests are not as accurate as the urea breath test. Serum or whole blood antibody tests, particularly immunoglobulin G (IgG), do not distinguish between past and current infection.

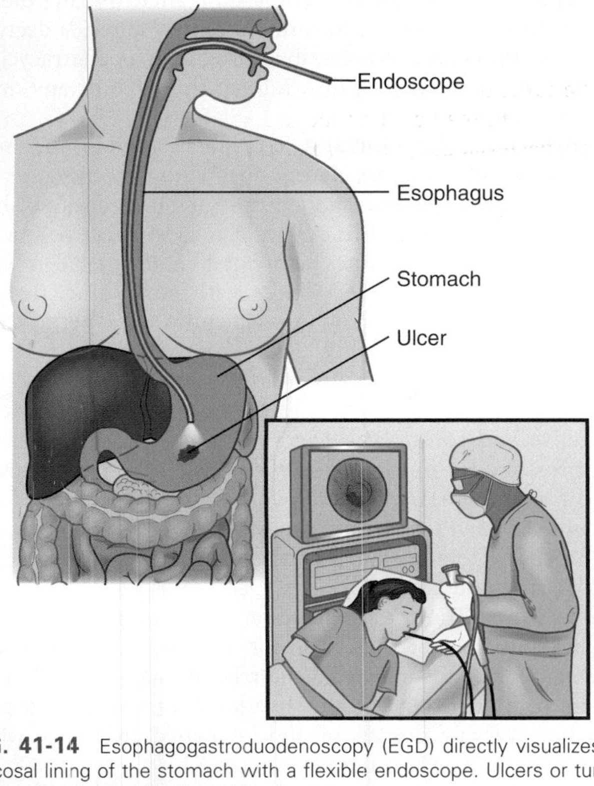


**FIG. 41-14** Esophagogastroduodenoscopy (EGD) directly visualizes the mucosal lining of the stomach with a flexible endoscope. Ulcers or tumors can be directly visualized and biopsies taken.

A barium contrast study may be used to diagnose gastric outlet obstruction or for ulcer detection in those who cannot undergo endoscopy. Elevated fasting serum gastrin levels may indicate the presence of a possible gastrinoma (Zollinger-Ellison syndrome). A secretin stimulation test can discern patients with gastrinomas from those with other causes of hypergastrinemia.

Laboratory tests, including a CBC, liver enzyme studies, serum amylase, and stool examination, should be done. A CBC may indicate anemia secondary to ulcer bleeding. Liver enzyme studies help detect any liver problems (e.g., cirrhosis) that may complicate ulcer treatment. Stools are tested for blood. A serum amylase evaluates pancreatic function when posterior duodenal ulcer penetration of the pancreas is suspected.

## Interprofessional Care: Conservative Therapy

A treatment regimen begins after diagnostic studies confirm the presence of PUD (Table 41-15). The regimen consists of adequate rest, drug therapy, smoking cessation, dietary modifications (if needed), and long-term follow-up care. The aim of treatment is to decrease gastric acidity and enhance mucosal defense mechanisms.

Patients are generally treated in ambulatory care clinics. Pain disappears after 3 to 6 days, but ulcer healing is much slower. Complete healing may take 3 to 9 weeks, depending on ulcer size, treatment regimen, and patient adherence. Endoscopic examination is the most accurate method to monitor ulcer healing. The usual follow-up endoscopic evaluation is done 3 to 6 months after diagnosis and treatment.

Aspirin and nonselective NSAIDs are discontinued for 4 to 6 weeks. When aspirin must be continued, co-administration with a PPI, $H_2$-receptor blocker, or misoprostol (Cytotec) may be prescribed. Patients receiving low-dose aspirin for cardiovascular and stroke risk who have a history of ulcer disease or complications may need to receive long-term treatment with a PPI.[20] Enteric-coated aspirin decreases localized irritation but has not been proved to reduce the overall risk for GI bleeding.

Smoking has an irritating effect on the mucosa and delays mucosal healing. The patient should either stop or severely reduce smoking. (See Chapter 10 for ways to enhance patient smoking cessation.) Adequate rest, both physical and emotional, is important for ulcer healing and may require some modifications in the patient's daily routine. Avoiding or restricting alcohol intake will enhance healing.

**Drug Therapy.** Drugs are a vital part of therapy (Table 41-10). Drug therapy focuses on reducing gastric acid secretion and, if needed, eliminating *H. pylori* infection. Patients with *H. pylori* infection need treatment with antibiotics and a PPI. After the ulcer has healed, many patients can stop $H_2$-receptor blocker and PPI therapy. Some may need to continue low-dose maintenance therapy.

Because ulcers frequently recur, interrupting or discontinuing therapy can have harmful results. Strict adherence to the prescribed drug regimen is important. Encourage the patient to adhere to therapy and continue with follow-up care as prescribed. Teach the patient and caregiver about each drug prescribed, why it is ordered, and the expected benefits. Review what to do if pain and discomfort recur or there is blood in vomitus or stools.

***Antibiotic Therapy.*** Eradicating *H. pylori* is the most important part of treating PUD in patients positive for *H. pylori*. Antibiotic therapy is prescribed concurrently with a PPI for 7

**TABLE 41-15 Interprofessional Care**

***Peptic Ulcer Disease***

**Diagnostic Assessment**

- History and physical examination
- Upper GI endoscopy with biopsy
- Endoscopic ultrasound
- *Helicobacter pylori* testing of breath, urine, blood, tissue
- Complete blood cell count
- Liver enzymes
- Serum amylase
- Stool testing for blood

**Management**

***Conservative Therapy***

- Adequate rest
- Smoking and alcohol cessation
- Stress management (see Chapter 6)

*Drug Therapy (Tables 41-10 and 41-13)*

- Antibiotics for *H. pylori*
- Proton pump inhibitors
- $H_2$-receptor blockers
- Cytoprotective drugs
- Antacids

***Acute Exacerbation Without Complications***

- NPO
- NG suction
- Adequate rest
- IV fluid replacement

*Drug Therapy*

- Proton pump inhibitors
- $H_2$-receptor blockers
- Antacids
- Sedatives

***Acute Exacerbation With Complications (Hemorrhage, Perforation, Obstruction)***

- NPO
- NG suction
- IV proton pump inhibitor
- Bed rest
- IV fluid replacement (lactated Ringer's solution)
- Blood transfusions
- Stomach lavage (possible)

***Surgical Therapy***

- *Perforation:* Simple closure with omentum graft
- Gastric outlet obstruction: Pyloroplasty and vagotomy
- Ulcer removal or reduction
  - Billroth I and II
  - Vagotomy and pyloroplasty

to 14 days (Table 41-13). If the patient has a penicillin allergy, metronidazole is used instead of amoxicillin in the triple-drug regimen. Bismuth can be given alone or as part of a combination capsule (Pylera) containing bismuth, tetracycline, and metronidazole. Because of the existence of antibiotic-resistant organisms, a growing number of patients do not have *H. pylori* eradicated with a single round of therapy.

***Proton Pump Inhibitors.*** PPIs are more effective than $H_2$-receptor blockers in reducing gastric acid secretion and promoting ulcer healing. PPIs are used in combination with antibiotics to treat ulcers caused by *H. pylori*. Several PPIs are available as both prescription and OTC preparations.

***Histamine ($H_2$)-Receptor Blockers.*** $H_2$-receptor blockers promote ulcer healing. The onset of action of $H_2$-receptor blockers is 1 hour. Depending on the specific drug, therapeutic effects last up to 12 hours. Several $H_2$ receptor blockers are available as both prescription and OTC preparations. Famotidine, ranitidine, and cimetidine can be given orally or IV. Nizatidine is only available orally.

***Antacids.*** Antacids are sometimes used as adjunct therapy for PUD. They increase gastric pH by neutralizing the HCl acid. As a result, they reduce the acid content of chyme reaching the duodenum. In addition, some antacids (e.g., aluminum hydroxide) can bind to bile salts, thus decreasing the damaging effects of bile on the gastric mucosa.

Common antacids consist of magnesium hydroxide or aluminum hydroxide as single preparations or in various combinations (Table 41-10). The neutralizing effects of antacids taken on an empty stomach last only 20 to 30 minutes. When antacids are taken after meals, the effects may last as long as 3 to 4 hours. After an acute phase of bleeding, antacids may be given hourly, either orally or through the NG tube. If an NG tube is in place, the stomach contents should be aspirated and tested periodically for pH level. If pH is less than 5, intermittent suction may be used, or the frequency or dosage of the antacid or antisecretory agent increased.

The type and dosage of antacid given depend on side effects and potential drug interactions. Antacids high in sodium (e.g., sodium citrate [Bicitra]) are used cautiously in older adults and patients with liver cirrhosis, hypertension, heart failure, and renal disease. Patients with renal failure should not take magnesium preparations because of the risk of magnesium toxicity. An antacid combination of aluminum and magnesium seems to decrease the side effects of both.

Antacids can interact unfavorably with many drugs. They can enhance the absorption of drugs such as dicumarol and amphetamines. Calcium and magnesium antacids can potentiate the effects of digitalis. In some instances, antacids decrease the absorption rates of prescribed drugs, such as tetracycline. Before antacid therapy begins, inform the HCP of any drugs that a patient is taking.

***Cytoprotective Drug Therapy.*** Sucralfate is used for the short-term treatment of ulcers. It provides cytoprotection for the esophagus, stomach, and duodenum. Sucralfate does not have acid-neutralizing capabilities. Since it is most effective at a low pH, give it at least 60 minutes before or after an antacid. Adverse side effects are minimal. It binds with cimetidine, digoxin, warfarin (Coumadin), phenytoin (Dilantin), and tetracycline, reducing their bioavailability.

Misoprostol is a synthetic prostaglandin analog prescribed to prevent gastric ulcers caused by NSAIDs and aspirin. It has protective and some antisecretory effects on gastric mucosa. Misoprostol does not interfere with the therapeutic effects of aspirin and NSAIDs. People who require chronic NSAID therapy, such as those with osteoarthritis, may benefit from its use. Since it is teratogenic, it is used with caution in women of childbearing potential.

***Other Drugs.*** Tricyclic antidepressants (e.g., imipramine [Tofranil], doxepin) may be prescribed for some patients. Antidepressants may contribute to overall pain relief through their effects on afferent pain fiber transmission. In addition, tricyclic antidepressants have varying degrees of anticholinergic properties, which result in reduced acid secretion.

Anticholinergic drugs are occasionally used for PUD treatment. Anticholinergics are associated with a number of side effects, such as dry mouth, warm skin, flushing, thirst, tachycardia, dilated pupils, blurred vision, and urine retention.

**Nutritional Therapy.** There is no specific recommended dietary modification for PUD. Patients should eat and drink foods and fluids that do not cause any distressing symptoms. Foods that commonly cause gastric irritation include pepper, carbonated beverages, broth (meat extract), and hot, spicy foods. Caffeine-containing beverages and foods can increase symptoms in some patients. Teach the patient to avoid alcohol use because it can delay healing.

**Therapy Related to Complications of Peptic Ulcer Disease**

***Acute Exacerbation.*** Patients with an acute exacerbation frequently experience bleeding, increased pain and discomfort, and nausea and vomiting. Management is similar to that described for upper GI bleeding later in this chapter (see pp. 923-925).

***Perforation.*** The immediate focus of managing a patient with a perforation is to stop the spillage of gastric or duodenal contents into the peritoneal cavity and restore blood volume. An NG tube can provide continuous aspiration and gastric decompression to stop spillage through the perforation. For duodenal aspiration, the tube is placed as near to the perforation site as possible to facilitate decompression.

Circulating blood volume is replaced with lactated Ringer's and albumin solutions. These solutions substitute for the fluids lost from the vascular and interstitial space as peritonitis develops. Blood replacement in the form of packed RBCs may be necessary. A central venous pressure line and an indwelling urinary catheter may be inserted and monitored hourly. The patient with a history of cardiac disease requires electrocardiographic (ECG) monitoring or placement of a pulmonary artery catheter for accurate assessment of left ventricular function. Broad-spectrum antibiotic therapy is started immediately to treat bacterial peritonitis.

Either open or laparoscopic procedures are used for perforation repair depending on the location of the ulcer and surgeon preference. The procedure involving the least risk to the patient is simple oversewing of the perforation and reinforcement of the area with a graft of omentum. Excess gastric contents are suctioned from the peritoneal cavity during the surgical procedure.

***Gastric Outlet Obstruction.*** The aim of therapy for obstruction is to decompress the stomach, correct any existing fluid and electrolyte imbalances, and improve the patient's general state of health. An NG tube is used as described previously. With continuous decompression for several days, the ulcer can begin healing, and the inflammation and edema will subside. Pain relief results from the decompression.

IV fluids and electrolytes are replaced according to the degree of dehydration, vomiting, and electrolyte imbalance indicated by laboratory studies. A PPI or $H_2$-receptor blocker is used if the obstruction is due to an active ulcer as determined by endoscopy. Pyloric obstruction may be treated endoscopically by balloon dilations. Surgical intervention may be needed to remove scar tissue.

## NURSING MANAGEMENT: PEPTIC ULCER DISEASE

### Nursing Assessment

Subjective and objective data to obtain from a patient with PUD are presented in Table 41-16.

### Nursing Diagnoses

Nursing diagnoses related to PUD may include, but are not limited to, the following:

**TABLE 41-16 Nursing Assessment**

***Peptic Ulcer Disease***

**Subjective Data**

***Important Health Information***

*Past health history:* Chronic kidney disease, pancreatic disease, chronic obstructive pulmonary disease, serious illness or trauma, hyperparathyroidism, cirrhosis of the liver, Zollinger-Ellison syndrome

*Medications:* Aspirin, corticosteroids, nonsteroidal antiinflammatory drugs

*Surgery or other treatments:* Complicated or prolonged surgery

***Functional Health Patterns***

*Health perception–health management:* Chronic alcohol abuse, smoking, caffeine use. Family history of peptic ulcer disease

*Nutritional-metabolic:* Weight loss, anorexia, nausea and vomiting, hematemesis, dyspepsia, heartburn, belching

*Elimination:* Black, tarry stools

*Cognitive-perceptual*

- *Duodenal ulcers:* Burning, midepigastric or back pain occurring 2-5 hr after meals and relieved by food; nocturnal pain common
- *Gastric ulcers:* High epigastric pain occurring 1-2 hr after meals. Pain may be precipitated or aggravated by food.

*Coping–stress tolerance:* Acute or chronic stress

**Objective Data**

***General***

Anxiety, irritability

***Gastrointestinal***

Epigastric tenderness

***Possible Diagnostic Findings***

Anemia. Guaiac-positive stools. Positive blood, urine, breath, or stool tests for *Helicobacter pylori*. Abnormal upper gastrointestinal endoscopic and barium studies

- Acute pain *related to* increased gastric secretions
- Ineffective health management *related to* lack of knowledge of long-term management of PUD
- Nausea *related to* acute exacerbation of disease process

Additional information on nursing diagnoses for the patient with PUD is presented in eNursing Care Plan 41-2 available on the website for this chapter.

### Planning

The overall goals are that the patient with PUD will (1) adhere to the prescribed therapeutic regimen, (2) experience a reduction in or absence of discomfort, (3) exhibit no signs of GI complications, (4) have complete healing of the peptic ulcer, and (5) make appropriate lifestyle changes to prevent recurrence.

### Nursing Implementation

**Health Promotion.** You play an important role in identifying patients at risk for PUD. Early detection and effective treatment of ulcers are important aspects of reducing morbidity risks associated with PUD. Patients who are taking ulcerogenic drugs (e.g., aspirin, NSAIDs) are at risk for PUD. Encourage patients to take these drugs with food. Teach patients to report symptoms related to gastric irritation, including epigastric pain, to their HCP.

**Acute Care.** During an acute exacerbation, the patient often complains of increased pain, nausea, and vomiting. Some may have evidence of bleeding. Initially many patients attempt to cope with the symptoms at home before seeking medical assistance.

During the acute phase, the patient may be NPO for a few days, have an NG tube inserted and connected to intermittent suction, and have IV fluid replacement. Explain to the patient and caregiver the reasons for these therapies so they understand that the advantages far outweigh any temporary discomfort. Regular mouth care alleviates the dry mouth. Cleaning and lubricating the nares facilitate breathing and decrease soreness. Analysis of gastric contents may include pH testing and analysis for blood, bile, or other substances. When the stomach is empty of gastric secretions, pain diminishes and ulcer healing begins.

The volume of fluid lost, the patient's signs and symptoms, and laboratory test results (hemoglobin, hematocrit, and electrolytes) determine the type and amount of IV fluids administered. Take vital signs initially and then at least hourly to detect and treat shock. Give IV fluids as ordered and record intake and output.

Physical and emotional rest is helpful to ulcer healing. The patient's environment should be quiet and restful. Give pain medications as ordered. A mild sedative or tranquilizer has beneficial effects when the patient is anxious and apprehensive. Use good judgment before sedating a person who is becoming increasingly restless because the drug could mask the signs of shock secondary to upper GI bleeding.

◆ ***Hemorrhage.*** Changes in vital signs and an increase in the amount and redness of aspirate often signal massive upper GI bleeding. With bleeding, the patient's pain often decreases because the blood helps neutralize the acidic gastric contents. It is important to maintain the patency of the NG tube so that blood clots do not obstruct the tube. If the tube becomes blocked, the patient can develop abdominal distention. Use interventions similar to those described for upper GI bleeding on pp. 923-925.

◆ ***Perforation.*** With perforation, the patient complains of sudden, severe upper abdominal pain that quickly becomes generalized throughout the abdomen. Other manifestations include a rigid, boardlike abdomen; severe back and shoulder pain; shallow respirations; and a weak, rapid heart rate. Bowel sounds that may have been previously normal or hyperactive may diminish and become absent. When the patient with an ulcer demonstrates these changes, suspect perforation and notify the HCP immediately.

Take vital signs promptly and record them every 15 to 30 minutes. Temporarily stop all oral or NG drugs and feedings. If perforation exists, anything taken orally can add to the spillage into the peritoneal cavity and increase discomfort. If you are giving IV fluid, maintain the rate or increase it per institutional protocol to replace the depleted plasma volume. Giving pain medications provides comfort.

Those with confirmed perforation start on antibiotic therapy. If the perforation fails to seal spontaneously, surgical closure is necessary. Since surgery is done as soon as possible, there may not be time to adequately prepare the patient and family.

◆ ***Gastric Outlet Obstruction.*** Gastric outlet obstruction can happen at any time. It is most likely to occur in the patient whose ulcer is located close to the pylorus. The onset of symptoms is usually gradual. Constant NG aspiration of stomach contents can help relieve symptoms. This allows edema and inflammation to subside and permits normal flow of gastric contents through the pylorus.

Regularly irrigate the NG tube with a normal saline solution per institutional policy to assist proper functioning. It may be helpful to reposition the patient from side to side so that the tube tip is not constantly lying against the mucosal surface. It is important to maintain accurate intake and output records, especially of the gastric aspirate.

To check for ongoing obstruction, clamp the NG tube intermittently and measure the gastric residual volume. The frequency and amount of time the tube remains clamped are related to the amount of aspirate obtained and the patient's comfort level. A method commonly followed is to clamp the tube overnight (approximately 8 to 12 hours) and measure the gastric residual volume in the morning. When the aspirate falls below 200 mL, it is within a normal range and the patient can begin oral intake of clear liquids. Oral fluids begin at 30 mL/hr and then gradually increase in amount. As the amount of gastric residual decreases, solid foods are added and the tube removed.

If the patient has resumed oral feedings and you note symptoms of obstruction, promptly inform the HCP. Generally, all that is necessary to treat the problem is to resume gastric aspiration so that the edema and inflammation resulting from the acute episode resolve. IV fluids with electrolyte replacement keep the patient hydrated during this period. If conservative treatment is not successful, surgery is done after the acute phase has passed.

◆ **Ambulatory Care.** Patients with PUD have specific needs to prevent recurrence and complications. Teaching should cover aspects of the disease process, drugs, possible changes in lifestyle (alcohol intake, smoking), and regular follow-up care. Table 41-17 provides a patient and caregiver teaching guide for PUD.

Knowing the etiology and pathophysiology of PUD may motivate the patient to become involved in care and improve adherence to therapy. Work with the dietitian to elicit a dietary history and plan ways to incorporate any needed dietary modifications into the patient's home and work setting.

Teach the patient about prescribed drugs, including their actions, side effects, and dangers if omitted for any reason.

**TABLE 41-17 Patient & Caregiver Teaching**

***Peptic Ulcer Disease (PUD)***

*Include the following instructions when teaching the patient and caregiver about management of PUD.*

1. Follow dietary modifications, including avoiding foods that may cause epigastric distress such as acidic foods.
2. Avoid cigarettes. In addition to promoting ulcer development, smoking delays ulcer healing.
3. Reduce or eliminate alcohol intake.
4. Avoid OTC drugs unless approved by the HCP. Many preparations contain ingredients, such as aspirin, that should not be taken unless approved by the HCP. Check with the HCP about the use of nonsteroidal antiinflammatory drugs.
5. Do not interchange brands of antacids, $H_2$-receptor blockers, and proton pump inhibitors that can be purchased OTC without checking with the HCP. This can lead to harmful side effects.
6. Take all medications as prescribed. This includes both antisecretory and antibiotic drugs. Failing to take medications as prescribed can result in relapse.
7. It is important to report any of the following:
   - Increased nausea or vomiting
   - Increased epigastric pain
   - Bloody emesis or tarry stools
8. Stress can be related to signs and symptoms of PUD. Learn and use stress management strategies (see Chapter 6).
9. Share concerns about lifestyle changes and living with a chronic illness.

Make sure the patient knows not to take OTC drugs (e.g., aspirin, NSAIDs) unless approved by the HCP.[20] Because you can buy several $H_2$-receptor blockers and PPIs without a prescription, tell the patient that substituting prescription with OTC preparations without checking with the HCP can lead to harmful side effects.

Try to obtain information about the patient's psychosocial status. Knowledge of lifestyle, occupation, and coping behaviors can be helpful in planning care. The patient may be reluctant to talk about personal subjects, the stress experienced at home or on the job, the usual methods of coping, or dependence on drugs or alcohol.

The patient may not be honest about habitual use of alcohol or cigarettes. Provide information about the negative effects of alcohol and cigarettes on PUD and ulcer healing. Changes, such as smoking cessation and alcohol abstinence, are difficult for many people. The patient may do better in reducing, rather than totally eliminating, use of these substances. However, the goal should always be total cessation.

PUD is often a chronic, recurring disorder. Inform patients with chronic PUD about potential complications, the clinical manifestations indicating their presence, and what to do until they see the HCP. Emphasize the need for long-term follow-up care. Encourage the patient to seek immediate intervention if symptoms return. The patient may be frustrated, especially if the patient followed prescribed therapy and it failed to prevent a recurrence.

Some patients do not adhere to the plan of care and experience repeated exacerbations. Patients quickly learn that they often experience no discomfort when they omit prescribed drugs, smoke, or drink alcohol. Consequently, they make no or little alterations in their lifestyle. After an acute exacerbation, the patient is likely to be more amenable to following the plan of care and open to suggestions for changes in lifestyle.

## Evaluation

Expected outcomes are that the patient with PUD will

- Have pain controlled without the use of analgesics
- Verbalize an understanding of the treatment regimen
- Commit to self-care and management of the disease
- Have no complications (hemorrhage, perforation)

Additional information on expected outcomes for the patient with PUD is presented in eNursing Care Plan 41-2 (available on the website for this chapter).

## Interprofessional Care: Surgical Therapy for Peptic Ulcer Disease

With the use of drug therapy and endoscopic therapy to treat PUD, surgery is used less frequently. Surgery is done on patients with complications that are unresponsive to medical management or concerns about stomach cancer.

Surgical procedures include partial gastrectomy, vagotomy, and pyloroplasty. Partial gastrectomy with removal of the distal two thirds of the stomach and anastomosis of the gastric stump to the duodenum is called a *gastroduodenostomy* or *Billroth I* operation (Fig. 41-15, *A*). If the gastric stump is anastomosed to the jejunum, the surgery is a *gastrojejunostomy* or *Billroth II* operation (Fig. 41-15, *B*).

*Vagotomy* is the severing of the vagus nerve, either totally *(truncal)* or selectively *(highly selective vagotomy)*. These procedures decrease gastric acid secretion. *Pyloroplasty* consists of surgical enlargement of the pyloric sphincter to facilitate the easy passage of contents from the stomach. It is commonly done after vagotomy or to enlarge an opening that is constricted from scar tissue.

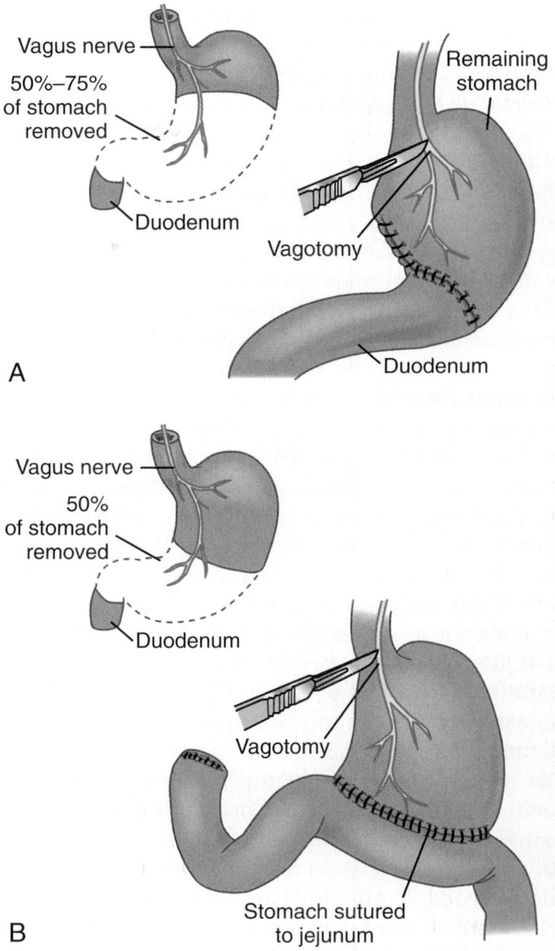


**FIG. 41-15** **A,** Billroth I procedure (subtotal gastric resection with gastroduodenostomy anastomosis). **B,** Billroth II procedure (subtotal gastric resection with gastrojejunostomy anastomosis).

**Postoperative Complications.** As with all surgeries, acute postoperative bleeding at the surgical site can occur. Monitoring of patients is similar to that described under acute upper GI bleeding. The most common long-term postoperative complications from PUD surgery are (1) dumping syndrome, (2) postprandial hypoglycemia, and (3) bile reflux gastritis.

***Dumping Syndrome.*** *Dumping syndrome* is the direct result of surgical removal of a large portion of the stomach and pyloric sphincter. Approximately 20% of patients experience dumping syndrome after PUD surgery.

Normally, gastric chyme enters the small intestine in small amounts. After surgery, the stomach no longer has control over the amount of gastric chyme entering the small intestine. Therefore a large bolus of hypertonic fluid enters the intestine and causes fluid to be drawn into the bowel lumen. This creates a decrease in plasma volume, distention of the bowel lumen, and rapid intestinal transit.

Symptoms begin within 15 to 30 minutes after eating. The patient usually describes feelings of generalized weakness, sweating, palpitations, and dizziness. These symptoms are due to the sudden decrease in plasma volume. The patient complains of abdominal cramps, *borborygmi* (audible abdominal sounds produced by hyperactive intestinal peristalsis), and the urge to defecate. These manifestations usually last less than 1 hour after eating. A short rest period after each meal reduces the chance of dumping syndrome.

***Postprandial Hypoglycemia.*** *Postprandial hypoglycemia* is considered a variant of dumping syndrome. It is the result of uncontrolled gastric emptying of a bolus of fluid high in carbohydrate into the small intestine. The bolus of concentrated carbohydrate results in hyperglycemia and the release of excess amounts of insulin into the circulation. This results in reflex hypoglycemia. Symptoms are similar to those of any hypoglycemic reaction and include sweating, weakness, mental confusion, palpitations, tachycardia, and anxiety. Symptoms generally occur 2 hours after eating.

***Bile Reflux Gastritis.*** Gastric surgery that involves either reconstruction or removal of the pylorus can result in reflux of bile into the stomach. Prolonged contact with bile causes damage to the gastric mucosa, chronic gastritis, and recurrence of PUD.

The main symptom is continuous epigastric distress that increases after meals. Vomiting relieves the distress, but only temporarily. Although only a small number of patients experience bile reflux gastritis, caution the patient to notify the HCP of any continuous epigastric distress after meals. Cholestyramine (Questran), given before or with meals, has been used successfully to treat this problem. Cholestyramine binds with the bile salts that are the source of gastric irritation.

**Nutritional Therapy.** Understanding the surgery performed and the patient's resulting anatomy are important. Nutrition interventions help minimize the occurrence of expected complications and maximize nutrient intake (Table 41-18). Start nutrition teaching as soon as the immediate postoperative period has passed. The dietitian usually provides dietary instructions. You must reinforce them. Reassure the patient that unpleasant symptoms are usually of short duration. Following dietary measures will decrease symptoms within a few months and is essential to long-term adherence.

Because gastric resection decreases the stomach's reservoir, patients must reduce their meal size accordingly. Teach the patient to limit drinking fluids with meals. Initially, dry foods with a low carbohydrate content and moderate protein and fat content are better tolerated. To avoid hypoglycemic episodes, teach the patient to limit the amount of sugar consumed with each meal and eat small, frequent meals with moderate amounts of protein and fat. The immediate ingestion of sugared fluids or candy relieves hypoglycemic symptoms.

**TABLE 41-18 Nutritional Therapy**

***Postgastrectomy Dumping Syndrome***

**Purposes**

- To slow the rapid passage of food into the intestine
- To control symptoms of dumping syndrome (dizziness, sense of fullness, diarrhea, tachycardia), which sometimes occurs after a partial or total gastrectomy

**Diet Principles**

- Divide meals into six small feedings to avoid overloading the stomach and intestine at mealtimes.
- Do not take fluids with meals but at least 30-45 min before or after meals. This helps prevent distention or a feeling of fullness.
- Avoid concentrated sweets (e.g., honey, sugar, jelly, jam, candies, sweet pastries, sweetened fruit) because they sometimes cause dizziness, diarrhea, and a sense of fullness.
- Increase protein and fats to promote rebuilding of body tissues and to meet energy needs. Meat, cheese, and eggs are specific foods to increase in the diet.
- Amount of time these restrictions should be followed varies. The HCP decides the proper amount of time to remain on this prescribed diet according to the patient's clinical condition and progress.

## NURSING MANAGEMENT: SURGICAL THERAPY FOR PEPTIC ULCER DISEASE

### Preoperative Care

Surgery can involve either laparoscopic or open surgery techniques. The surgeon will provide the necessary information about the procedure and expected outcomes so that the patient can make an informed decision. Help the patient and caregiver by clarifying and interpreting their questions. Teach them what to expect after surgery, including comfort measures, pain relief, coughing and breathing exercises, use of an NG tube, and IV fluid administration (see Chapter 17).

### Postoperative Care

Care of the patient after major abdominal surgery is similar to the postoperative care after abdominal laparotomy (see Chapter 42). An NG tube is used to decompress the remaining portion of the stomach. This decreases pressure on the suture line and allows edema and inflammation resulting from surgical trauma to resolve.

Observe the gastric aspirate for color, amount, and odor. The aspirate is usually bright red at first, with a gradual darkening within the first 24 hours after surgery. Normally the color changes to yellow-green within 36 to 48 hours. If the tube becomes clogged, the HCP may order periodic gentle irrigations with normal saline solution. It is essential that the NG suction is working and that the tube remains patent so that accumulated gastric secretions do not put a strain on the anastomosis. This can lead to distention of the remaining portion of the stomach and result in (1) rupture of the sutures, (2) leakage of gastric contents into the peritoneal cavity, (3) hemorrhage, and (4) possible abscess formation. If the tube must be replaced or repositioned, call the HCP to perform this task because of the danger of perforating the gastric mucosa or disrupting the suture line.

Observe the patient for signs of decreased peristalsis, including abdominal distention and lower abdominal discomfort, which may indicate intestinal obstruction. Monitor and record accurate intake and output every 4 hours.

Keep the patient comfortable and free of pain by giving analgesics and frequently changing position. In an open surgical approach, the incision is relatively high in the epigastrium and may interfere with deep breathing and coughing. Splinting the area with a pillow while encouraging the patient to deep breathe helps prevent pulmonary complications. Splinting also protects the abdominal suture line from rupturing during coughing. Observe the dressing for signs of bleeding or odor and drainage indicative of an infection. Encourage early ambulation.

While the NG tube is connected to suction, maintain IV therapy. Administer potassium and vitamin supplements as ordered until oral feedings are resumed. Before the NG tube is removed, the patient begins clear liquids to determine the tolerance level. The stomach may be aspirated within 1 or 2 hours to assess the amount remaining and its color and consistency. When fluids are well tolerated, the NG tube is removed. Fluids are increased in frequency, with a slow progression to regular foods. The patient begins a regimen of six small meals a day.

Pernicious anemia is a long-term complication of total gastrectomy and may occur after partial gastrectomy. Pernicious anemia is due to the loss of intrinsic factor, which is produced by the parietal cells. The patient will require cobalamin replacement therapy (see Chapter 30). PUD is a chronic problem, and ulcers can recur, especially at the site of the anastomosis.

### Gerontologic Considerations: Peptic Ulcer Disease

The morbidity and mortality rates associated with PUD in older adults are higher than for younger adults because of concurrent health problems and a decreased ability to withstand hypovolemia. Monitor older adults who use NSAIDs for osteoarthritis for signs and symptoms of PUD. In older patients, pain may not be the first symptom associated with an ulcer. For some patients the first manifestation is frank gastric bleeding or a decrease in hematocrit.

The treatment and management of PUD in older adults are similar to those in younger adults. An emphasis is placed on preventing gastritis and PUD. This includes teaching the patient to take NSAIDs and other gastric-irritating drugs with food, milk, or antacids. Teach the patient to avoid irritating substances, adhere to the PPI or $H_2$-receptor blocker therapy as prescribed, and report abdominal pain or discomfort to the HCP.

## STOMACH CANCER

**Stomach (gastric) cancer** is an adenocarcinoma of the stomach wall (Fig. 41-16). It accounts for more than 24,590 new cancer cases and 10,720 deaths annually.[5] The rate of stomach (particularly distal) cancer has been steadily declining in the United States. However, cancer in the proximal gastric and gastroesophageal junction is increasing.

Asian Americans, Pacific Islanders, Hispanics, and African Americans have higher rates of stomach cancer than non-Hispanic whites. In the U.S., the incidence is higher in men than in women by a 2 : 1 ratio. Stomach cancer mostly affects older people. The average age of people when they are diagnosed is 69.

At the time of diagnosis, only 10% to 20% of patients have disease confined to the stomach. More than 50% have advanced metastatic disease. The 5-year survival rate is 71% in persons with early stage disease (confined to the stomach). The overall 5-year survival rate of all people with stomach cancer is about 29%.[5]

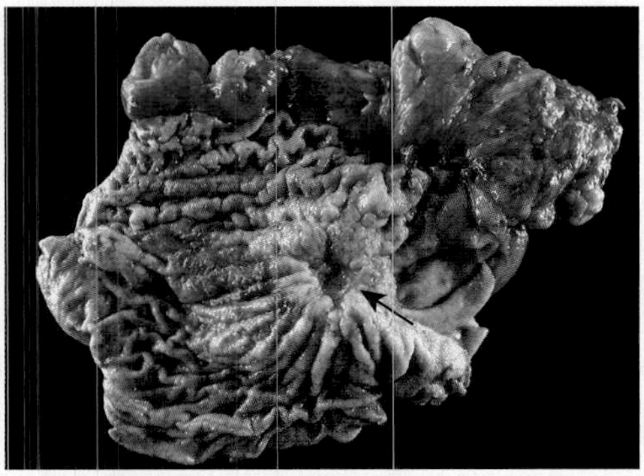

**FIG. 41-16** Stomach cancer. Gross photograph showing an ill-defined, excavated central ulcer surrounded by irregular, heaped-up borders. (From Kumar V, Abbas AK, Aster JC, Fausto N: *Robbins and Cotran pathologic basis of disease,* ed 8, Philadelphia, 2010, Saunders.)

### Etiology and Pathophysiology

While many factors are implicated in the development of stomach cancer, no single causative agent has been identified. Stomach cancer probably begins with a nonspecific mucosal injury because of infection *(H. pylori),* autoimmune-related inflammation, or repeated exposure to irritants such as bile, antiinflammatory agents, and tobacco use.

Stomach cancer has been associated with diets containing smoked foods, salted fish and meat, and pickled vegetables. Whole grains and fresh fruits and vegetables are associated with reduced rates of stomach cancer. Infection with *H. pylori,* especially at an early age, is a risk factor for stomach cancer. It is possible that *H. pylori* and resulting cell changes can induce a sequence of transitions from dysplasia to cancer. People with lymphoma of the stomach (mucosa-associated lymphoid tissue [MALT]) are at higher risk of stomach cancer.

Other predisposing factors include atrophic gastritis, pernicious anemia, adenomatous polyps, hyperplastic polyps, and achlorhydria. Smoking and obesity both increase the risk of stomach cancer. Although first-degree relatives of patients with stomach cancer are at increased risk, only 8% to 10% of stomach cancers have an inherited component.[21]

Stomach cancer spreads by direct extension and typically infiltrates rapidly to the surrounding tissue and liver. Seeding of tumor cells into the peritoneal cavity occurs late in the course of the disease.

### Clinical Manifestations

Stomach cancers often spread to adjacent organs before any distressing symptoms occur. Clinical manifestations include unexplained weight loss, indigestion, abdominal discomfort or pain, and signs and symptoms of anemia. The patient may report *early satiety,* or a sense of being full sooner than usual. Anemia is common. It is caused by chronic blood loss as the lesion erodes through the mucosa or from pernicious anemia (caused by loss of intrinsic factor). The person appears pale and weak and complains of fatigue, weakness, dizziness, and, in extreme cases, shortness of breath. The stool may be positive for occult blood. Supraclavicular lymph nodes that are hard and enlarged suggest metastasis via the thoracic duct. The presence of ascites is a poor prognostic sign.

### Diagnostic Studies

The diagnostic studies for stomach cancer are presented in Table 41-19. Upper GI endoscopy is the best diagnostic tool. The stomach can be distended with air during the procedure, stretching the mucosal folds. Tissue biopsy and subsequent histologic examination are important in diagnosing stomach cancer.

Endoscopic ultrasound, CT, and PET scanning can be used to stage the disease. Barium studies do not always detect small lesions of the cardia and fundus. Laparoscopy is done to determine peritoneal spread.

Blood studies detect anemia and determine its severity. Elevations in liver enzymes and serum amylase levels may indicate liver and pancreatic involvement. Stool examination provides evidence of occult or gross bleeding. The presence of tumor markers can help diagnose cancer.

### Interprofessional Care

The treatment of choice for stomach cancer is surgical removal of the tumor. Preoperative management focuses on correcting nutritional deficits and treating anemia. Transfusions of packed

**TABLE 41-19 Interprofessional Care**

***Stomach Cancer***

| Diagnostic Assessment | Management |
|---|---|
| • History and physical examination<br>• Endoscopy and biopsy<br>• CT and PET scans<br>• Upper GI barium study<br>• Exfoliative cytologic study<br>• Endoscopic ultrasonography<br>• Complete blood count<br>• Urinalysis<br>• Stool examination<br>• Liver enzymes<br>• Serum amylase<br>• Tumor markers<br>• Carcinoembryonic antigen (CEA)<br>• Carbohydrate antigen (CA)–19-9, CA-125, CA 72-4<br>• α-Fetoprotein | • Surgical therapy<br>  • Subtotal gastrectomy (Billroth I or II procedure)<br>  • Total gastrectomy with esophagojejunostomy<br>• Radiation therapy<br>• Chemotherapy<br>• Targeted therapy |

RBCs correct the anemia. If gastric outlet obstruction occurs, gastric decompression may be necessary before surgery.

**Surgical Therapy.** The surgical interventions used in the treatment of stomach cancer are the same procedures used for PUD. The location and extent of the lesion, the patient's physical condition, and the surgeon's preference determine the specific surgery used (e.g., open versus laparoscopic).

The surgical aim is to remove as much of the stomach as necessary to remove the tumor and a margin of normal tissue. Lesions located in the antrum or pyloric region are generally treated by either a Billroth I or II procedure (Fig. 41-15). When the lesion is located in the fundus, a total gastrectomy with esophagojejunostomy is performed (Fig. 41-17). When metastasis has occurred to adjacent organs, such as the spleen, ovaries, or bowel, the surgical procedure is extended as necessary. If the tumor extends into the transverse colon, partial colon resection is required.

**Chemotherapy and Radiation Therapy.** A number of chemotherapy drugs can be used to treat stomach cancer. These include 5-FU (fluorouracil) (often given with leucovorin [folinic acid]), capecitabine (Xeloda), carboplatin, cisplatin, docetaxel (Taxotere), epirubicin (Ellence), irinotecan (Camptosar), oxaliplatin (Eloxatin), and paclitaxel. Combination therapies are commonly used as the drugs affect different phases of the cell cycle. Examples of combination therapy include ECF (epirubicin, cisplatin, and 5-FU) and DCF (docetaxel, cisplatin, and 5-FU). Intraperitoneal administration of chemotherapy agents may also be used to treat metastatic disease. (Chemotherapy is discussed in Chapter 15.)

Radiation therapy may be used together with chemotherapy to reduce the recurrence or as a palliative measure to decrease tumor mass and provide temporary relief of obstruction.

**Targeted Therapy.** Trastuzumab (Herceptin) and ramucirumab (Cyramza) are targeted therapies used to treat stomach cancer. About 20% of patients with stomach cancer have too much HER-2 (growth-promoting protein) on the surface of the cancer cells. Trastuzumab (Herceptin) targets the HER-2 protein and kills the cancer cells.[22] Ramucirumab (Cyramza) binds to the receptor for VEGF and prevents VEGF from binding to the receptor, thus preventing the growth and spread of cancer. These drugs are also used for esophageal cancer as discussed on p. 906. (Targeted therapies are discussed in Chapter 15.)

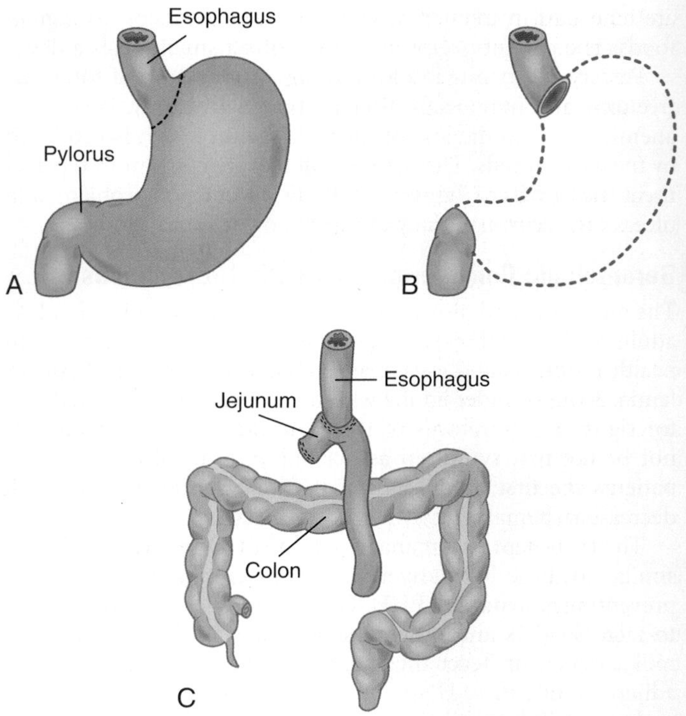


**FIG. 41-17** Total gastrectomy for stomach cancer. **A,** Normal anatomic structure of the stomach. **B,** Removal of the stomach (total gastrectomy). **C,** Anastomosis of the esophagus with the jejunum (esophagojejunostomy).

## NURSING MANAGEMENT: STOMACH CANCER

### Nursing Assessment

The assessment of a person with possible stomach cancer is similar to that for PUD (Table 41-16). Important data to obtain from the patient and caregiver include a nutritional assessment, a psychosocial history, the patient's perceptions of the health problem and need for care, and a physical examination.

The nutritional assessment obtains information about appetite and changes in eating patterns over the previous 6 months. Determine the patient's normal weight and any recent changes in it. Unexplained weight loss is common. Evaluate the patient's nutritional status. Cachexia may be evident if oral intake has been reduced for an extended period. A malnourished patient does not respond well to chemotherapy or radiation therapy and is a poor surgical risk. The patient may report a history of vague abdominal symptoms, including dyspepsia and intestinal gas discomfort or pain. If the patient reports pain, explore where and when it occurs and how it is relieved.

Determine the patient's personal perception of the health problem and method of coping with hospitalization, diagnostic tests, and procedures. The possibility of a diagnosis of cancer and a treatment regimen that may include surgery, chemotherapy, or radiation treatment is stressful. Support the patient, caregiver, and family. If surgery is planned, assess the patient's expectations regarding surgery (cure or palliation) and how the patient has responded to previous surgical procedures.

### Nursing Diagnoses

Nursing diagnoses for the patient with stomach cancer include, but are not limited to, the following:

- Imbalanced nutrition: less than body requirements *related to* inability to ingest, digest, or absorb nutrients

- Acute pain *related to* underlying disease process and side effects of surgery, chemotherapy, or radiation therapy
- Anxiety and grieving *related to* diagnosis of cancer, uncertain future, and prognosis

### Planning

The overall goals are that the patient with stomach cancer will (1) experience minimal discomfort, (2) achieve optimal nutritional status, and (3) maintain a degree of spiritual and psychologic well-being appropriate to the disease stage.

### Nursing Implementation

**Health Promotion.** Your role in the early detection of stomach cancer focuses on identifying the patient at risk because of specific disorders such as *H. pylori* infection, pernicious anemia, and achlorhydria. Be aware of symptoms associated with stomach cancer and the significant findings on physical examination. Symptoms often occur late and mimic other conditions, such as PUD. Poor appetite, weight loss, fatigue, and persistent stomach distress are symptoms of stomach cancer. Encourage patients with a positive family history of stomach cancer to undergo diagnostic evaluation if anemia, PUD, or vague epigastric distress are present. It is important that you recognize the possibility of stomach cancer in a patient who is treated for PUD and fails to have relief with prescribed therapy.

**Acute Care**

***Preoperative Care.*** When diagnostic tests confirm cancer, the patient and family generally react with shock, disbelief, and depression. Provide emotional and physical support, provide information, clarify test results, and maintain a positive attitude with respect to the patient's immediate recovery and long-term survival.

Because of changes in appetite and early satiety, the patient's current nutritional status may be poor. Surgery may be delayed until the patient is more physically able to withstand it. A positive nutritional state enhances wound healing and the ability to deal with infection and other possible postoperative complications. The patient may better tolerate several small meals a day than three regular meals. It may be challenging to persuade the patient to eat when he or she has no appetite and is depressed. Getting the patient's caregiver to assist with meals and encourage intake may be beneficial. The diet may be supplemented by a variety of commercial liquid supplements and vitamins. If the patient is unable to ingest oral feedings, the HCP may prescribe enteral (tube feeding) or parenteral nutrition (see Chapter 39).

If needed, packed RBCs and fluid volume restoration may be given during the preoperative period. Closely observe for transfusion reactions. Monitor hemoglobin and hematocrit levels.

The preoperative teaching plan before stomach cancer surgery is similar to that for PUD (see the section on surgical therapy for PUD on pp. 918).

***Postoperative Care.*** Postoperative care is similar to that following a procedure for PUD (see the section on surgical therapy for PUD earlier in this chapter). If the patient had a Billroth I or II procedure, the postoperative care is similar to that of the patient having this procedure for PUD. When the surgical intervention involves a total gastrectomy, the plan of care is somewhat different. A total gastrectomy requires resection of the lower esophagus, removal of the entire stomach, and anastomosis of the esophagus to the jejunum. If the chest cavity is entered, postoperative drainage is accomplished by the insertion of chest tubes. (Chest surgery and drainage tubes are discussed in Chapter 27.)

After total gastrectomy, the NG tube does not drain a large quantity of secretions because removal of the stomach has eliminated the reservoir capacity. The NG tube is removed when intestinal peristalsis has resumed. Small amounts of clear fluid are then started. Closely observe the patient for signs of fluid leakage at the anastomosis site as evidenced by an elevation in the temperature and increasing dyspnea. When the patient tolerates fluids without distress, fluid intake is increased and some solid foods added.

After a total gastrectomy, the patient experiences symptoms of dumping syndrome. Weight loss often occurs. Postoperative wound healing may be impaired because of poor nutritional intake. This necessitates IV or oral replacement of vitamins C, D, and K; the B-complex vitamins; and cobalamin. These vitamins (with the exception of cobalamin) must be replaced because they are normally absorbed in the duodenum.

Radiation therapy or chemotherapy is used as an adjuvant to surgery or for palliation. Your role is to provide detailed instructions, reassure the patient, and ensure completion of the designated number of treatments. Start by assessing the patient's knowledge of these therapies. Teach the patient about skin care, need for nutrition and fluid intake during therapy, and appropriate use of antiemetic drugs. (Specific care of the patient receiving chemotherapy and radiation therapy is discussed in Chapter 15.)

**Ambulatory Care.** Most dietary measures useful after PUD surgery are applicable after stomach cancer surgery. Make plans for pain relief, including comfort measures and the judicious use of analgesics. Teach wound care (if needed) to the primary caregiver in the home setting. Dressings, special equipment, or special services may be required. Provide the patient with a list of community agencies (e.g., American Cancer Society) that are available for assistance before the patient goes home.

When chemotherapy or radiation treatment is continuing after discharge, a referral to home health care may be beneficial. The home health nurse can assist with recovery, determine the degree of patient adherence, and provide consultation to the patient and caregiver. Encourage the patient to adhere to the prescribed therapies, keep appointments for chemotherapy administration or radiation treatments, and keep the HCP informed of changes in physical condition. (Long-term management of the cancer patient is discussed in Chapter 15.)

### Evaluation

Expected outcomes are that the patient with stomach cancer will

- Experience no or minimal discomfort, pain, or nausea
- Achieve optimal nutritional status
- Maintain a degree of psychologic well-being appropriate to the disease stage

## UPPER GASTROINTESTINAL BLEEDING

In the United States approximately 300,000 hospital admissions occur each year for upper GI bleeding. Approximately 60% of these are adults over age 65. Despite advances in drug management of predisposing conditions and identification of risk factors, the mortality rate for upper GI bleeding has remained at approximately 6% to 13% for the past 45 years.[23]

### Etiology and Pathophysiology

Although the most serious loss of blood from the upper GI tract is characterized by a sudden onset, insidious occult bleeding can be a major problem. The severity of bleeding depends on whether the origin is venous, capillary, or arterial. Types of upper GI bleeding are presented in Table 41-20. Bleeding from an arterial source is profuse, and the blood is bright red, indicating it has not been in contact with gastric HCl acid secretion. In contrast, "coffee-ground" vomitus indicates that the blood has been in the stomach for some time. *Melena* (black, tarry stools) indicates slow bleeding from an upper GI source. The longer the passage of blood through the intestines, the darker the stool color because of the breakdown of hemoglobin and release of iron.

Discovering the cause of the bleeding is not always easy. A variety of areas in the GI tract may be involved. Table 41-21 lists the common causes of upper GI bleeding.

**Stomach and Duodenal Origin.** Bleeding peptic ulcers account for 40% of the cases of upper GI bleeding. Drugs are a major cause of upper GI bleeding. Aspirin, NSAIDs, and corticosteroids can cause irritation and disruption of the gastroduodenal mucosa. About 25% of people on chronic NSAIDs (e.g., ibuprofen) develop ulcer disease; of these, 2% to 4% will bleed. Even low-dose aspirin is associated with a risk for GI bleeding. Many OTC preparations contain aspirin. A careful history of all commonly used drugs is necessary whenever upper GI bleeding is suspected.

**Stress-related mucosal disease (SRMD)**, also called *physiologic stress ulcers,* is a continuum of conditions ranging from stress-related injury (superficial mucosal damage) to stress ulcers (focal deep mucosal damage). SRMD is most commonly seen in critically ill patients who have had severe burns, trauma, or major surgery. Patients with coagulopathy and those who experience respiratory failure resulting in mechanical ventilation for more than 48 hours are at highest risk for SRMD.[24]

**Esophageal Origin.** Bleeding from the esophagus is most likely due to chronic esophagitis, Mallory-Weiss tear, or esophageal varices. Chronic esophagitis can be caused by GERD, smoking, alcohol use, and the ingestion of drugs irritating to the mucosa. Esophageal varices most often occur from cirrhosis of the liver. (Esophageal varices are discussed in Chapter 43.)

**TABLE 41-20 Types of Upper Gastrointestinal Bleeding**

| Type | Manifestations |
|---|---|
| **Obvious bleeding** | |
| • Hematemesis | Bloody vomitus appearing as fresh, bright red blood or "coffee-ground" appearance (dark, grainy digested blood). |
| • Melena | Black, tarry stools (often foul smelling) caused by digestion of blood in the GI tract. Black appearance is from the presence of iron. |
| **Occult bleeding** | Small amounts of blood in gastric secretions, vomitus, or stools not apparent by appearance. Detectable by guaiac test |

**TABLE 41-21 Causes of Upper Gastrointestinal Bleeding**

**Stomach and Duodenum**
- Stomach cancer
- Erosive gastritis
- Peptic ulcer disease
- Polyps
- Stress-related mucosal disease
- Drug-induced
  - Corticosteroids
  - Nonsteroidal antiinflammatory drugs (NSAIDs)
  - Salicylates

**Esophagus**
- Esophageal varices
- Esophagitis
- Mallory-Weiss tear

**Systemic Diseases**
- Blood dyscrasias (e.g., leukemia, aplastic anemia)
- Renal failure

### Diagnostic Studies

Endoscopy is the primary tool for diagnosing the source (e.g., esophageal or gastric varices, gastritis) of upper GI bleeding. Angiography is used when endoscopy cannot be done or when bleeding persists after endoscopic therapy. Angiography is a procedure requiring preparation and setup time and may not be appropriate for a high-risk, unstable patient. In this procedure, a catheter is inserted into the femoral artery and advanced to the left gastric or superior mesenteric artery until the site of bleeding is found.

Laboratory studies include CBC, blood urea nitrogen (BUN), serum electrolytes, prothrombin time, partial thromboplastin time, liver enzymes, arterial blood gases (ABGs), and a type and crossmatch for possible blood transfusions. All vomitus and stools are tested for gross and occult blood.

Monitor the patient's laboratory studies to estimate the effectiveness of therapy. The hemoglobin and hematocrit values are not of immediate help in estimating the degree of blood loss, but they provide a baseline for guiding further treatment. The initial hematocrit may be normal and may not reflect the loss until 4 to 6 hours after fluid replacement, since initially the loss of plasma and RBCs is equal.

Assess the patient's BUN level. During a significant hemorrhage, GI tract bacteria break down proteins, resulting in elevated BUN levels. An elevated BUN level may also indicate renal hypoperfusion or renal disease.

### Interprofessional Care

A massive upper GI hemorrhage is a loss of more than 1500 mL of blood or 25% of intravascular blood volume. Although 80% to 85% of patients with massive hemorrhage spontaneously stop bleeding, the cause must be identified and treatment started immediately.

**Emergency Assessment and Management.** A complete history of events leading to the bleeding episode is deferred until emergency care has been started. To facilitate early intervention, focus your physical examination on identifying signs and symptoms of shock, such as tachycardia, weak pulse, hypotension, cool extremities, prolonged capillary refill, and apprehension. (Shock is discussed in Chapter 66.)

Urine output is one of the best measures of vital organ perfusion. An indwelling urinary catheter is inserted so that hourly output can be accurately assessed. Hemodynamic monitoring provides an accurate and quick assessment of blood flow and pressure in the cardiovascular system (see Chapter 65). A central venous pressure line may be used for fluid volume status assessment. If the patient has a history of valvular heart disease, coronary artery disease, or heart failure, a pulmonary artery catheter may be necessary. Administer supplemental $O_2$ to increase blood $O_2$ saturation.

The patient is at risk for perforation and peritonitis. Do a thorough abdominal examination. Note the presence of a tense, rigid, boardlike abdomen and the presence or absence of bowel sounds.

The type and amount of fluids infused are based on physical and laboratory findings. Generally, an isotonic crystalloid solution (e.g., lactated Ringer's solution) is started. Whole blood, packed RBCs, and fresh frozen plasma may be used for volume replacement in massive hemorrhage. When upper GI bleeding is less profuse, infusion of isotonic saline solution followed by packed RBCs restores the hematocrit more quickly and does not create complications related to fluid volume overload. (The use of blood transfusions and volume expanders is discussed in Chapter 30.)

**Endoscopic Therapy.** The first-line management of upper GI bleeding is endoscopy. Endoscopy performed within the first 24 hours of bleeding is important for diagnosis, determining the need for surgical intervention, and providing treatment.

The goal of endoscopic hemostasis is to coagulate or thrombose the bleeding vessel. Several techniques are used including (1) thermal (heat) probe, (2) multipolar and bipolar electrocoagulation probe, (3) argon plasma coagulation (APC), (4) neodymium:yttrium-aluminum-garnet (Nd:YAG) laser, and (5) mechanical therapy with endoscopic clips or bands. Multipolar electrocoagulation and thermal probe are the two most commonly used procedures. The heat probe coagulates tissue by directly applying a heating element to the bleeding site. The APC is a noncontact coagulation that delivers monopolar current to tissue. Endoscopic clips and bands directly compress the bleeding vessel. For variceal bleeding, other strategies include variceal ligation, injection sclerotherapy, and balloon tamponade (see Chapter 43).

**Surgical Therapy.** Surgical intervention is indicated when bleeding continues regardless of the therapy provided and when the site of the bleeding has been identified. Surgical therapy may be necessary when the patient continues to bleed after rapid transfusion of up to 2000 mL of whole blood or remains in shock after 24 hours. The site of the hemorrhage determines the choice of surgery. Mortality rates increase considerably in older patients.

**Drug Therapy.** During the acute phase of upper GI bleeding, drugs are used to decrease bleeding, decrease HCl acid secretion, and neutralize the HCl acid that is present. Empiric PPI therapy with high-dose IV bolus and subsequent infusion to decrease acid secretion is often started before endoscopy (Table 41-10). Efforts are made to reduce acid secretion because the acidic environment can alter platelet function and interfere with clot stabilization. This may decrease the amount of bleeding and need for endoscopic therapy.

Injection therapy with epinephrine (1:10,000 dilution) during endoscopy is effective for acute hemostasis. Epinephrine produces tissue edema and, ultimately, pressure on the source of bleeding (Table 41-22). Octreotide (Sandostatin) or vasopressin may be given when upper GI bleeding is from esophageal or gastric varices (Chapter 43).

## NURSING MANAGEMENT: UPPER GASTROINTESTINAL BLEEDING

### Nursing Assessment

A thorough and accurate nursing assessment is an essential first step as you begin care of the patient admitted with upper GI bleeding. The patient may not be able to provide specific information about the cause of the bleeding until immediate physical needs are met. Perform an immediate nursing assessment while you are getting the patient ready for initial treatment. The assessment includes the patient's level of consciousness, vital signs, skin color, and capillary refill. Check the abdomen for distention, guarding, and peristalsis. Immediate determination of vital signs indicates whether the patient is in shock from blood loss and provides a baseline BP and pulse for monitoring the progress of treatment. Signs and symptoms of shock include low BP; rapid, weak pulse; increased thirst; cold, clammy skin; and restlessness. Monitor the patient's vital signs every 15 to 30 minutes. Inform the HCP of any significant changes.

Once the immediate interventions have begun, the patient or caregiver should answer the following questions: Is there a history of previous bleeding episodes? Has the patient received blood transfusions in the past? Were there any transfusion reactions? Are there any other illnesses (e.g., liver disease, cirrhosis)

**TABLE 41-22 Nursing Assessment**

***Upper Gastrointestinal Bleeding***

**Subjective Data**

***Important Health Information***

*Past health history:* Precipitating events before bleeding episode, previous bleeding episodes and treatment, peptic ulcer disease, esophageal varices, esophagitis, acute and chronic gastritis, stress-related mucosal disease

*Medications:* Aspirin, nonsteroidal antiinflammatory drugs, corticosteroids, anticoagulants

***Functional Health Patterns***

*Health perception–health management:* Family history of bleeding, smoking, alcohol use

*Nutritional-metabolic:* Nausea, vomiting, weight loss, thirst

*Elimination:* Diarrhea. Black, tarry stools. Decreased urine output. Sweating

*Activity-exercise:* Weakness, dizziness, fainting

*Cognitive-perceptual:* Epigastric pain, abdominal cramps

*Coping–stress tolerance:* Acute or chronic stress

**Objective Data**

***General***

Fever

***Integumentary***

Clammy, cool, pale skin. Pale mucous membranes, nail beds, and conjunctivae. Spider angiomas, jaundice, peripheral edema

***Respiratory***

Rapid, shallow respirations

***Cardiovascular***

Tachycardia, weak pulse, orthostatic hypotension, slow capillary refill

***Gastrointestinal***

Red or "coffee-ground" vomitus. Tense, rigid abdomen, ascites. Hypoactive or hyperactive bowel sounds. Black, tarry stools

***Urinary***

Decreased urine output, concentrated urine

***Neurologic***

Agitation, restlessness. Decreasing level of consciousness

***Possible Diagnostic Findings***

↓ Hematocrit and hemoglobin, hematuria. Guaiac-positive stools, emesis, or gastric aspirate. ↓ Levels of clotting factors, ↑ liver enzymes, abnormal endoscopy results or medications that may contribute to bleeding or interfere with treatment? Does the patient have a religious preference that prohibits the use of blood or blood products?

Subjective and objective data to obtain from the patient or caregiver are presented in Table 41-22.

## Nursing Diagnoses

Nursing diagnoses for the patient with upper GI bleeding include, but are not limited to, the following:

- Risk for decreased cardiac output *related to* loss of blood
- Deficient fluid volume *related to* acute loss of blood and gastric secretions
- Ineffective peripheral tissue perfusion *related to* loss of circulatory volume
- Anxiety *related to* upper GI bleeding, hospitalization, uncertain outcome, source of bleeding

## Planning

The overall goals are that the patient with upper GI bleeding will (1) have no further GI bleeding, (2) have the cause of the bleeding identified and treated, (3) experience a return to a normal hemodynamic state, and (4) experience minimal or no symptoms of pain or anxiety.

## Nursing Implementation

**Health Promotion.** Although not all cases of upper GI bleeding can be prevented, you have an important role in identifying patients at high risk. Always consider the patient with a history of chronic gastritis, cirrhosis, or PUD at high risk. The patient who has had a previous upper GI bleeding episode is more likely to have another bleed. Patients on daily low-dose aspirin to reduce cardiovascular disease risk are at risk for upper GI bleeding, especially those over 60 years old with a history of PUD.

Teach the at-risk patient to avoid known gastric irritants such as alcohol and smoking and to take only prescribed medications. OTC drugs can be harmful because they may contain ingredients (e.g., aspirin) that increase the risk of bleeding. Review how to test vomitus or stools for occult blood. Teach them to report positive results promptly to the HCP. Stress the importance of treating an upper respiratory tract infection promptly. Severe coughing or sneezing can increase pressure on the already fragile varices and may result in massive hemorrhage (see Chapter 43).

The patient who requires regular doses of drugs that produce gastroduodenal toxicity (peptic ulcer formation, bleeding), such as aspirin, corticosteroids, or NSAIDs, needs to be taught about the potential for GI bleeding. Taking these drugs with meals or snacks lessens their direct irritation. Patients receiving low-dose aspirin who have a history of ulcer disease or complications may need to receive long-term treatment with a PPI, $H_2$-receptor blocker, or misoprostol (Cytotec).[20]

Patients with blood dyscrasias (e.g., aplastic anemia), liver dysfunction, or those who are taking chemotherapy drugs are at risk due to a decrease in clotting factors and platelets. Teach patients about their disease process, drugs, and increased risk of GI bleeding.

**Acute Care.** Emergency management of acute GI bleeding is presented in Table 41-23. Place IV lines, preferably two, with a 16- or 18-gauge needle for fluid and blood replacement. Administer fluid or blood replacement as ordered. An accurate intake and output record is essential so that the patient's hydration status can be assessed. Measure the urine output hourly. If the patient has a central venous pressure line or pulmonary artery catheter in place, record these readings every 1 to 2 hours. Use ECG monitoring to evaluate cardiac function. Close monitoring of vital signs, especially in the patient with cardiovascular disease, is important because dysrhythmias may occur.

Observe the older adult or the patient with a history of cardiovascular problems closely for signs of fluid overload. However, volume overload and pulmonary edema are concerns in all patients who are receiving large amounts of IV fluids within a short time. Auscultate breath sounds and closely observe the respiratory effort. Keep the head of the bed elevated to provide comfort and prevent aspiration.

When an NG tube is present, pay special attention to keeping it in proper position and observe the aspirate for blood. Although gastric lavage (room temperature, cool, or iced) is used in some institutions, its effectiveness as a treatment for upper GI bleeding is questionable. When lavage is used, approximately 50 to 100 mL of fluid is instilled at a time into the stomach. The lavage fluid may be aspirated from the stomach or drained by gravity. When aspiration is the method used, it is important not to aspirate if you feel resistance. The tip of the NG tube may be up against the gastric mucosal lining. When resistance is a factor, use the gravity method.

Approach the patient in a calm manner to help decrease the level of anxiety. Use caution when administering sedatives for

**TABLE 41-23 Emergency Management**
***Acute Gastrointestinal Bleeding***

| Assessment Findings | Interventions |
|---|---|
| **Abdominal and GI Findings**<br>• Hematemesis<br>• Melena<br>• Nausea<br>• Abdominal pain<br>• Abdominal rigidity<br>**Hypovolemic Shock**<br>• ↓ BP<br>• ↓ Pulse pressure<br>• Tachycardia<br>• Cool, clammy skin<br>• ↓ Level of consciousness<br>• ↓ Urine output (<0.5 mL/kg/hr)<br>• Slow capillary refill | **Initial**<br>• If unresponsive, assess circulation, airway, and breathing.<br>• If responsive, monitor airway, breathing, and circulation.<br>• Establish IV access with large-bore catheter and start fluid replacement therapy. Insert additional large-bore catheter if shock present.<br>• Give $O_2$ via nasal cannula or non-rebreather mask.<br>• Initiate ECG monitoring.<br>• Obtain blood for CBC, clotting studies, and type and crossmatch as appropriate.<br>• Insert NG tube as needed.<br>• Insert indwelling urinary catheter.<br>• Give IV proton pump inhibitor (PPI) therapy to decrease acid secretion.<br>**Ongoing Monitoring**<br>• Monitor vital signs, level of consciousness, $O_2$ saturation, ECG, bowel sounds, and intake/output.<br>• Assess amount and character of emesis.<br>• Keep patient NPO.<br>• Provide reassurance and emotional support to patient and caregiver. |

**CHECK YOUR PRACTICE**

You are admitting a 71-yr-old man to the clinical unit from the emergency department. He has a diagnosis of upper GI bleeding. He complains of heartburn and pain (6 on a scale of 10) in the upper epigastric region and has just had a 250 mL coffee-ground emesis.

- What assessment data do you need to obtain?
- What are the priority nursing interventions for this man?

restlessness because it is one of the warning signs of shock and may be masked by the drugs.

Assess the stools for blood (hematochezia, black-tarry, bright red). Black, tarry stools are not usually associated with a brisk hemorrhage but are indicative of prolonged bleeding. Determine if menses or bleeding are possible sources of blood in the stools. When vomitus contains blood but the stool contains no gross or occult blood, the hemorrhage is considered to be of short duration.

When beginning oral nourishment, observe the patient for symptoms of nausea and vomiting and a recurrence of bleeding. Feedings initially consist of clear fluids. They are given hourly until tolerance is determined. Gradually introduce foods if the patient exhibits no signs of discomfort.

When hemorrhage is the result of chronic alcohol abuse, closely observe the patient for delirium tremens as alcohol withdrawal takes place. Symptoms indicating the onset of delirium tremens are agitation, uncontrolled shaking, sweating, and vivid hallucinations. (Alcohol withdrawal is discussed in Chapter 10.)

**Ambulatory Care.** Teach the patient and caregiver how to avoid future bleeding episodes. Ulcer disease, drug or alcohol use, and liver and respiratory diseases can all result in upper GI bleeding. Help the patient and caregiver to be aware of the consequences of not adhering to drug therapy.

Emphasize not to take any drugs (especially aspirin, NSAIDs) other than those prescribed by the HCP. Support the patient in smoking and alcohol cessation because they are sources of irritation and interfere with tissue repair. Long-term follow-up care may be necessary because of possible recurrence. Teach the patient and caregiver what to do if an acute hemorrhage occurs in the future.

### Evaluation

The expected outcomes are that the patient with upper GI bleeding will

- Have no upper GI bleeding
- Maintain normal fluid volume
- Experience a return to a normal hemodynamic state
- Understand potential etiologic factors and make appropriate lifestyle modifications

## FOODBORNE ILLNESS

*Foodborne illness* (food poisoning) is a nonspecific term that describes acute GI symptoms such as nausea, vomiting, diarrhea, and cramping abdominal pain caused by the intake of contaminated food or liquids.[25] There are 31 known foodborne pathogens. Each year one out of six Americans, approximately 48 million, experiences a foodborne illness. Of these, 128,000 are hospitalized and approximately 3000 die.[26]

Bacteria account for most foodborne illnesses. The most common source is raw foods that become contaminated during growing, harvesting, processing, storing, shipping, or final preparation. When food is uncooked and left out for more than 2 hours at room temperature, bacteria can multiply quickly. One example is prepackaged cookie dough. The most common bacterial food poisonings are presented in Table 41-24.

Focus interventions on preventing infection. Teaching includes correct food preparation and cleanliness, adequate cooking, and refrigeration (Table 41-25). For the hospitalized patient, emphasize correcting fluid and electrolyte imbalances from diarrhea and vomiting. With botulism, additional assessment and care relative to neurologic symptoms are indicated (see Chapter 60).

### *Escherichia coli* O157:H7 Poisoning

*Escherichia coli* O157:H7 causes hemorrhagic colitis and kidney failure. In the very young and older adults, *E. coli* O157:H7 can be life threatening. *E. coli* O157:H7 is found primarily in undercooked meats, particularly poultry and hamburger.[26] *E. coli* outbreaks have been observed with contaminated leafy vegetables, fruits, and nuts. Infection can occur after drinking raw milk, unpasteurized juice, or contaminated fruit juices and after swimming in or drinking sewage-contaminated water.

**TABLE 41-24 Bacterial Food Poisoning**

| Type and Cause | Sources | Manifestations | Treatment and Prevention |
|---|---|---|---|
| **Staphylococcal**<br>Toxin from *Staphylococcus aureus* | Meat, bakery products, cream fillings, salad dressings, milk. Skin and respiratory tract of food handlers | *Onset:* 30 min to 7 hr<br>Vomiting, nausea, abdominal cramping, diarrhea | *Treat:* Symptomatic, fluid and electrolyte replacement, antiemetics<br>*Prevent:* Immediate refrigeration of foods, monitoring of food handlers |
| **Clostridial**<br>*Clostridium perfringens* | Meat or poultry dishes cooked at lower temperature (stew, pot pie), rewarmed meat dishes, gravies, improperly canned vegetables | *Onset:* 8-24 hr<br>Diarrhea, nausea, abdominal cramps, vomiting (rare), midepigastric pain | *Treat:* Symptomatic, fluid replacement<br>*Prevent:* Correct preparation of meat dishes. Serving food immediately after cooking or rapid cooling of food |
| **Salmonella**<br>*Salmonella typhimurium* (grows in gut) | Improperly cooked poultry, pork, beef, lamb, and eggs | *Onset:* 8 hr to several days<br>Nausea and vomiting, diarrhea, abdominal cramps, fever and chills | *Treat:* Symptomatic, fluid and electrolyte replacement<br>*Prevent:* Correct preparation of food |
| **Botulism**<br>Toxin from *Clostridium botulinum;* ingested toxin absorbed from gut and blocks acetylcholine at neuromuscular junction | Improperly canned or preserved food, home-preserved vegetables (most common), preserved fruits and fish, canned commercial products | *Onset:* 12-36 hr<br>*GI:* Nausea, vomiting, abdominal pain, constipation, distention<br>*Central nervous system:* Headache, dizziness, muscular incoordination, weakness, inability to talk or swallow, diplopia, breathing difficulties, paralysis, delirium, coma | *Treat:* Maintenance of ventilation, polyvalent antitoxin, guanidine hydrochloric acid (enhances acetylcholine release)<br>*Prevent:* Correct processing of canned foods, boiling of suspected canned foods for 15 min before serving |
| ***Escherichia coli***<br>*E. coli* O157:H7 | Contaminated beef, pork, milk, cheese, fish, cookie dough | *Onset:* 8 hr to 1 wk (varies by strain)<br>Bloody stools, hemolytic uremic syndrome, abdominal cramping, profuse diarrhea | *Treat:* Symptomatic, fluid and electrolyte replacement<br>*Prevent:* Correct preparation of food |

### TABLE 41-25 Patient & Caregiver Teaching

**Prevention of Food Poisoning**

*Include the following instructions when teaching the patient and caregiver how to prevent food poisoning.*

1. Cook all ground beef and hamburger thoroughly.
   - Use a digital instant-read meat thermometer to ensure thorough cooking (ground beef can turn brown before disease-causing bacteria are killed).
   - Cook ground beef until a thermometer inserted into several parts of the patty, including the thickest part, reads at least 160° F.
   - People who cook ground beef without using a thermometer can decrease their risk of illness by not eating ground beef patties that are still pink in the middle.
2. If you are served an undercooked hamburger or other ground beef product in a restaurant, send it back for further cooking. Also ask for a new bun and a clean plate.
3. Avoid spreading harmful bacteria. Keep raw meat separate from ready-to-eat foods. Wash hands, counters, and utensils with hot soapy water after they touch raw meat. Never place cooked hamburgers or ground beef on the unwashed plate that held raw patties. Wash meat thermometers in between tests of patties that require further cooking.
4. Drink only pasteurized milk, juice, or cider. Commercial juice with an extended shelf-life that is sold at room temperature (e.g., juice in cardboard boxes, vacuum-sealed juice in glass containers) has been pasteurized. Juice concentrates are heated sufficiently to kill pathogens.
5. Wash fruits and vegetables thoroughly, especially those that will not be cooked.
6. Do not eat raw food products that are supposed to be cooked. Follow package directions for cooking at proper temperatures.
7. People who are immunocompromised should avoid eating alfalfa sprouts until the safety of the sprouts can be ensured.

Person-to-person contact in families, nursing homes, and child-care centers is an important mode of transmission.

Most strains of *E. coli* are harmless and live in the intestines of healthy humans and animals. *E. coli* O157:H7 produces a powerful toxin and can cause severe illness. The manifestations of *E. coli* O157:H7 include diarrhea (often bloody) and abdominal cramping pain for 2 to 8 days (average 3 to 4 days) after swallowing the organism. The diarrhea is variable, ranging from mild to bloody. It may start out as watery but may progress to bloody. Systemic complications, including hemolytic uremia and thrombocytopenic purpura, and even death can occur.

Infection with *E. coli* O157:H7 is diagnosed by detecting the bacteria in the stool. All people who suddenly have diarrhea with blood should have a stool culture for *E. coli* O157:H7.

Treatment involves supportive care to maintain blood volume. Antibiotic therapy remains controversial. Most people recover without antibiotics or other specific treatment. There is no evidence that antibiotics improve the course of disease. It is thought that treatment with some antibiotics may precipitate kidney complications. Patients should avoid antidiarrheal agents, such as loperamide (Imodium). Other therapies may include dialysis and plasmapheresis.

In a small percentage of infections, particularly in young children and older adults, hemolytic uremic syndrome (HUS) occurs. With HUS, the RBCs are destroyed and the kidneys fail. It is a life-threatening condition usually treated in an ICU. Blood transfusions and kidney dialysis are often required. Approximately 3% to 5% of patients with HUS die. About one third of people with HUS have abnormal kidney function for years after. A few require long-term dialysis. Additional long-term complications of HUS include hypertension, seizures, blindness, and paralysis.

## CASE STUDY

**Peptic Ulcer Disease**

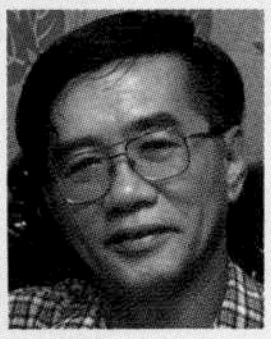

(©iStockphoto/Thinkstock)

### Patient Profile

F.H., a 40-yr-old male immigrant from Vietnam, has a 1-yr history of epigastric distress. Increasingly, it is not relieved by over-the-counter omeprazole (Prilosec). He is scheduled for an upper endoscopy this morning.

### Subjective Data

- Reports increasing substernal pain, especially 2 to 3 hr after eating
- Currently avoids alcohol and is taking an over-the-counter PPI
- Smoking history of 1 pack of cigarettes per day for 20 yr
- Complains of increasing fatigue with exercise
- Reports occasional black bowel movement
- Takes Chinese medicine for frequent back pain

### Objective Data

***Physical Examination***

- Height 5 ft, 5 in tall and weight 140 lb

***Diagnostic Studies***

- Endoscopy reveals a duodenal ulcer
- Hgb 10.2 g/dL; Hct 30%
- Histology of biopsied tissue reveals *Helicobacter pylori* infection

### Interprofessional Care

- omeprazole 20 mg bid × 10 days
- clarithromycin 500 mg bid × 10 days
- amoxicillin 1 gram bid × 10 days

### Discussion Questions

1. Explain the pathophysiology of peptic ulcer disease.
2. What are the risk factors for duodenal ulcers? Which of these did F.H. have?
3. What is the pathophysiology of *H. pylori*?
4. ***Priority Decision:*** Based on the assessment data provided, what are the priority nursing diagnoses? Are there any collaborative problems?
5. ***Patient-Centered Care:*** How will you consider F.H.'s cultural preferences in planning care?
6. ***Priority Decision:*** What are the priority nursing interventions for F.H.?
7. ***Teamwork and Collaboration:*** For the interventions that you identified in question 6, which of the following personnel could be responsible for implementing them: registered nurse (RN), licensed practical nurse (LPN), unlicensed assistive personnel (UAP)?
8. What lifestyle interventions would you recommend for F.H.?
9. ***Evidence-Based Decision:*** F.H. asks you if the treatment will work and this will be the end of his problems. How will you respond?
10. ***Teamwork and Collaboration:*** What referrals may be indicated?

Answers available at *http://evolve.elsevier.com/Lewis/medsurg.*

## BRIDGE TO NCLEX EXAMINATION

The number of the question corresponds to the same-numbered outcome at the beginning of the chapter.

1. M.J. calls the clinic and tells the nurse that her 85-year-old mother has been nauseated all day and has vomited twice. Before the nurse hangs up and calls the HCP, she should tell M.J. to
   - **a.** administer antiemetic drugs and observe skin turgor.
   - **b.** give her mother sips of water and elevate the head of her bed to prevent aspiration.
   - **c.** offer her mother a high-protein liquid supplement to drink to maintain her nutritional needs.
   - **d.** offer her mother large quantities of Gatorade to decrease the risk of sodium depletion.
2. The nurse explains to the patient with Vincent's infection that treatment will include
   - **a.** tetanus vaccinations.
   - **b.** viscous lidocaine rinses.
   - **c.** amphotericin B suspension.
   - **d.** topical application of antibiotics.
3. The nurse teaching young adults about behaviors that put them at risk for oral cancer includes
   - **a.** discouraging use of chewing gum.
   - **b.** avoiding use of perfumed lip gloss.
   - **c.** avoiding use of smokeless tobacco.
   - **d.** discouraging drinking of carbonated beverages.
4. Which instructions would the nurse include in a teaching plan for a patient with mild gastroesophageal reflux disease (GERD)?
   - **a.** "The best time to take an as-needed antacid is 1 to 3 hours after meals."
   - **b.** "A glass of warm milk at bedtime will decrease your discomfort at night."
   - **c.** "Do not chew gum; the excess saliva will cause you to secrete more acid."
   - **d.** "Limit your intake of foods high in protein because they take longer to digest."
5. A patient who has undergone an esophagectomy for esophageal cancer develops increasing pain, fever, and dyspnea when a full liquid diet is started postoperatively. The nurse recognizes that these symptoms are *most* indicative of
   - **a.** an intolerance to the feedings.
   - **b.** extension of the tumor into the aorta.
   - **c.** leakage of fluids into the mediastinum.
   - **d.** esophageal perforation with fistula formation into the lung.
6. The pernicious anemia that may accompany gastritis is due to
   - **a.** chronic autoimmune destruction of cobalamin stores in the body.
   - **b.** progressive gastric atrophy from chronic breakage in the mucosal barrier and blood loss.
   - **c.** a lack of intrinsic factor normally produced by acid-secreting cells of the gastric mucosa.
   - **d.** hyperchlorhydria from an increase in acid-secreting parietal cells and degradation of RBCs.
7. The nurse is teaching the patient and family that peptic ulcers are
   - **a.** caused by a stressful lifestyle and other acid-producing factors such as *H. pylori*.
   - **b.** inherited within families and reinforced by bacterial spread of *Staphylococcus aureus* in childhood.
   - **c.** promoted by factors that tend to cause oversecretion of acid, such as excess dietary fats, smoking, and *H. pylori*.
   - **d.** promoted by a combination of factors that may result in erosion of the gastric mucosa, including certain drugs and alcohol.
8. An optimal teaching plan for an outpatient with stomach cancer receiving radiation therapy should include information about
   - **a.** cancer support groups, alopecia, and stomatitis.
   - **b.** nutrition supplements, ostomy care, and support groups.
   - **c.** prosthetic devices, wound and skin care, and grief counseling.
   - **d.** wound and skin care, nutrition, drugs, and community resources.
9. The teaching plan for the patient being discharged after an acute episode of upper GI bleeding includes information concerning the importance of *(select all that apply)*
   - **a.** limiting alcohol intake to one serving per day.
   - **b.** only taking aspirin with milk or bread products.
   - **c.** avoiding taking aspirin and drugs containing aspirin.
   - **d.** only taking drugs prescribed by the health care provider.
   - **e.** taking all drugs 1 hour before mealtime to prevent further bleeding.
10. Several patients are seen at an urgent care center with symptoms of nausea, vomiting, and diarrhea that began 2 hours ago while attending a large family reunion potluck dinner. You question the patients specifically about foods they ingested containing
    - **a.** beef.
    - **b.** meat and milk.
    - **c.** poultry and eggs.
    - **d.** home-preserved vegetables.

1. b, 2. d, 3. c, 4. a, 5. c, 6. c, 7. d, 8. d, 9. c, d, 10. b

For rationales to these answers and even more NCLEX review questions, visit *http://evolve.elsevier.com/Lewis/medsurg.*

## EVOLVE WEBSITE

http://evolve.elsevier.com/Lewis/medsurg

**Review Questions (Online Only)**

**Key Points**

**Answer Keys for Questions**

- Rationales for Bridge to NCLEX Examination Questions
- Answer Guidelines for Case Study on p. 926

**Student Case Studies**

- Patient With Oral Cancer
- Patient With Peptic Ulcer Disease

**Nursing Care Plans**

- eNursing Care Plan 41-1: Patient With Nausea and Vomiting
- eNursing Care Plan 41-2: Patient With Peptic Ulcer Disease

**Conceptual Care Map Creator**

**Audio Glossary**

**Content Updates**

## REFERENCES


*1. Gang TJ, Diemunsch P, Habib AS, et al: Consensus guidelines for the management of postoperative nausea and vomiting, *Anesthes Analg* 118:85, 2014.

2. National Comprehensive Cancer Network (NCCN): NCCN Clinical practice guidelines in oncology. Retrieved from *www.nccn.org/professionals/physician_gls/f_guidelines.asp.*

*3. Song HJ, Seo HJ, Lee H, et al: Effect of self-acupressure for symptom management: a systematic review, *Complement Ther Med* 23:68, 2015.

*4. Linden GJ, Lyons A, Scannapieco FA: Periodontal systemic associations: review of the evidence, *J Periodontol* 84:S8, 2013.

5. National Cancer Institute: SEER stat fact sheets. Retrieved from *http://seer.cancer.gov/statfacts/html.*

6. Chai RC, Lambie D, Verma M, et al: Current trends in the etiology and diagnosis of HPV-related head and neck cancers, *Cancer Med* 4:596, 2015.

7. Fedele S: Diagnostic aids in the screening of oral cancer, *Head Neck Oncol* 1:5, 2009. (Classic)

*8. Omura K: Current status of oral cancer treatment strategies, *Int J Clin Oncol* 19:423, 2014.

9. Badillo R, Francis D: Diagnosis and treatment of gastroesophageal reflux disease, *World J Gastrointest Pharmacol Ther* 5:105, 2014.

10. Chang P, Friedenberg F: Obesity and GERD, *Gastroenterol Clin North Am* 43:795, 2014.

*11. Spechler SJ, Sharma P, Souza RF, et al: American Gastroenterological Association medical position statement on the management of Barrett's esophagus, *Gastroenterol* 140:1084, 2011. (Classic)

*12. Kosalram K, Whittle T, Byth K, et al: An investigation of risk factors associated with tooth surface loss: A pilot study, *J Oral Rehabil* 41:675, 2014.

*13. Katz PO, Gersen LB, Vela MF: American College of Gastroenterology: Diagnosis and management of gastroesophageal reflux disease, *Am J Gastroenterol* 108:308, 2013.

*14. Leontiadis GI, Moayyedi P: Proton pump inhibitors and risk of bone fractures, *Curr Treat Options Gastroenterol* 12:414, 2014.

*15. Deshpande A, Pasupuleti V, Thota P, et al: Risk factors for recurrent *Clostridium difficile* infection: A systematic review and meta-analysis, *Infect Control Hosp Epidemiol* 36:452, 2015.

*16. Dai Y, Li C, Xie Y, et al: Interventions for dysphagia in esophageal cancer, *Cochrane Database Syst Rev* (10):CD005048, 2014.

17. Goldstein JL, Cryer B: Gastrointestinal injury associated with NSAID use: a case study and review of risk factors and preventative strategies, *Drug Healthcare Patient Saf* 7:31, 2015.

18. Centers for Disease Control and Prevention: *Helicobacter pylori* and peptic ulcer disease: the key to cure. Retrieved from *www.cdc.gov/ulcer/keytocure.htm.*

*19. Jiang HY, Chen HZ, Hu XJ, et al: Use of selective serotonin reuptake inhibitors and risk of upper gastrointestinal bleeding: a systematic review and meta-analysis, *Clin Gastroenterol Hepatol* 13:42, 2015.

20. Yasuda H, Matsuo Y, Sato Y: Treatment and prevention of gastrointestinal bleeding in patients receiving antiplatelet therapy, *World J Crit Care Med* 4:40, 2015.

21. Oliveira C, Pinheiro H, Figueiredo J, et al: Familial gastric cancer: Genetic susceptibility, pathology, and implications for management, *Lancet Oncol* 16:e60, 2015.

22. Lordick F, Lorenzen S, Yamada Y: Optimal chemotherapy for advanced gastric cancer: is there a global consensus? *Gastric Cancer* 17:213, 2014.

*23. Lu Y, Loffroy R, Lau JY: Multidisciplinary management strategies for acute non-variceal upper gastrointestinal bleeding, *Br J Surg* 10:e34, 2014.

24. Bardou M, Quenot JP, Barkun A: Stress-related mucosal disease in the critically ill patient, *Nat Rev Gastroenterol Hepatol* 12:98, 2015.

25. National Digestive Diseases Information Clearinghouse: Bacteria and foodborne illness. Retrieved from *www.niddk.nih.gov/health-information/health-topics/digestive-diseases/foodborne-illnesses/Pages/facts.aspx.*

26. Centers for Disease Control and Prevention: *Escherichia coli* O157:H7. Retrieved from *www.cdc.gov/Features/EcoliInfection.*

*Evidence-based information for clinical practice.

# Lower Gastrointestinal Problems

*Diana L. Gallagher, Mariann M. Harding*

*In this life we cannot do great things. We can only do small things with great love.*

***Mother Teresa***

http://evolve.elsevier.com/Lewis/medsurg/

## LEARNING OUTCOMES

1. Explain the common etiologies, interprofessional care, and nursing management of diarrhea, fecal incontinence, and constipation.
2. Describe common causes of acute abdominal pain and nursing management of the patient after an exploratory laparotomy.
3. Describe the interprofessional care and nursing management of acute appendicitis, peritonitis, and gastroenteritis.
4. Compare and contrast the inflammatory bowel diseases of ulcerative colitis and Crohn's disease, including pathophysiology, clinical manifestations, complications, interprofessional care, and nursing management.
5. Differentiate among mechanical and nonmechanical bowel obstructions, including causes, interprofessional care, and nursing management.
6. Describe the clinical manifestations and interprofessional care of colorectal cancer.
7. Explain the anatomic and physiologic changes and nursing management of the patient with a fistula and a fecal diversion.
8. Differentiate between diverticulosis and diverticulitis, including clinical manifestations, interprofessional care, and nursing management.
9. Compare and contrast the types of hernias, including etiology and surgical and nursing management.
10. Describe the types of malabsorption syndromes and interprofessional care of celiac disease, lactase deficiency, and short bowel syndrome.
11. Describe the types, clinical manifestations, interprofessional care, and nursing management of anorectal conditions.

## KEY TERMS

anal fistula, p. 970
appendicitis, p. 942
celiac disease, p. 966
constipation, p. 934
Crohn's disease, p. 944
diarrhea, p. 929
diverticulitis, p. 963
fecal incontinence, p. 933
fistula, p. 962
gastroenteritis, p. 944
hemorrhoids, p. 968
hernia, p. 964
inflammatory bowel disease (IBD), p. 944
intestinal obstruction, p. 950
irritable bowel syndrome (IBS), p. 940
lactase deficiency, p. 967
ostomy, p. 958
paralytic ileus, p. 950
peritonitis, p. 943
short bowel syndrome (SBS), p. 967
steatorrhea, p. 965
stoma, p. 958
ulcerative colitis, p. 944

The wide variety of intestinal problems presented in this chapter include the disorders of diarrhea, constipation, and fecal incontinence; inflammatory and infectious bowel disorders; bowel trauma; bowel obstructions; colorectal cancer; abdominal and bowel surgery (including ostomy formation); and malabsorption disorders.

## DIARRHEA

**Diarrhea** is the passage of at least three loose or liquid stools per day. It may be acute, lasting 14 days or less, or persistent, lasting greater than 14 days. Chronic diarrhea lasts 30 days or longer.[1]

### Etiology and Pathophysiology

The primary cause of acute diarrhea is ingesting infectious organisms (Table 42-1). Viruses cause most cases of infectious diarrhea in the United States. While some viral infections can be deadly, most are mild and last less than 24 hours. Therefore most patients rarely seek treatment.

Bacterial infection with *Escherichia coli* O157:H7, a type of enterohemorrhagic *E. coli*, is the most common cause of bloody diarrhea in the United States. It is transmitted by undercooked beef or chicken contaminated with the bacteria or in fruits and vegetables exposed to contaminated manure. Other pathologic *E. coli* strains are endemic in developing countries and commonly cause traveler's diarrhea. *Giardia lamblia* is the most

Reviewed by Janica Barnett, JD, AGPCNP-BC, Adult Gerontology Nurse Practitioner, Mt. Sinai Hospital, New York, New York; Janet L. Hannah, RN, CGRN, Staff Nurse, Inova Loudoun ASC, Leesburg, Virginia; Susan C. Landis, RN, MN, Senior Lecturer, University of Washington School of Nursing, Seattle, Washington; Sarah Byram Poppe, MSN, ANP-BC, Nurse Practitioner, Gastroenterology Associates, Olympia, Washington; Andrea H. Thurler, RN, DNP, FNP-BC, Nurse Practitioner, Massachusetts General Hospital, Harvard University, Massachusetts General Institute of Health Professions, Boston, Massachusetts; and Daryle Wane, PhD, ARNP, FNP-BC, RN to BSN Coordinator, Professor of Nursing, Department of Health Occupations, Pasco-Hernando State College, New Port Richey, Florida.

## TABLE 42-1 Causes and Manifestations of Acute Infectious Diarrhea

| Type of Organism | Manifestations | Source of Infection/Susceptibility |
|---|---|---|
| **Viral** | | |
| Rotavirus | • Fever, vomiting, and profuse watery diarrhea<br>• Lasts 3 to 8 days | • Highly contagious<br>• Transmitted mainly by fecal-oral route |
| Norovirus (also called *Norwalk-like virus*) | • Nausea, vomiting, diarrhea, stomach cramping<br>• Rapid onset. Lasts 1-2 days | • Very contagious<br>• Virus is present in stool and emesis |
| **Bacterial** | | |
| Enterotoxigenic *Escherichia coli* | • Watery or bloody diarrhea, abdominal cramps<br>• Nausea, vomiting, and fever may be present<br>• Mean duration >60 hr | • Most common cause of traveler's diarrhea<br>• Transmitted in water or food contaminated with infected feces |
| Enterohemorrhagic *E. coli* (e.g., *E. coli* O157:H7) | • Severe abdominal cramping, bloody diarrhea, and vomiting<br>• Low-grade fever<br>• Usually lasts 5-7 days | • Can cause serious illness, especially in older adults<br>• May progress to life-threatening renal failure<br>• Transmitted in water or food contaminated with infected feces |
| *Shigella* | • Diarrhea (sometimes bloody), fever, and stomach cramps<br>• Usually lasts 5-7 days<br>• Postinfection arthritis may occur | • Transmitted via fecal-oral route or in food or water contaminated with infected feces<br>• Can contaminate recreational water |
| *Salmonella* | • Diarrhea, fever, and abdominal cramps<br>• Lasts 4-7 days | • Reservoir is poultry, reptiles, and other animals (especially turtles, lizards, snakes, chicks, and young birds)<br>• Can be transmitted by handling animals<br>• Found in undercooked poultry, meat, and foods prepared with raw eggs |
| *Staphylococcus* | • Nausea, vomiting, abdominal cramps, and diarrhea<br>• Usually mild<br>• May cause illness in as little as 30 min<br>• Lasts 1-3 days | • 25%-50% of people are carriers in mucous membranes, skin, or hair<br>• Transmitted in food contaminated by food workers who are carriers or through contaminated milk and cheese |
| *Campylobacter jejuni* | • Diarrhea, abdominal cramps, and fever. Sometimes nausea and vomiting<br>• Lasts about 7 days | • Undercooked poultry and unpasteurized milk<br>• Most frequent in summer months |
| *Clostridium perfringens* | • Diarrhea, abdominal cramps, nausea, and vomiting<br>• Occurs 6-24 hr after eating contaminated food and lasts approximately 24 hr | • Associated with meats, gravies, and stews. Commonly associated with dried or pre-cooked foods<br>• Can cause serious illness in anyone, especially older adults |
| *Clostridium difficile* | • Watery diarrhea, fever, anorexia, nausea, abdominal pain | • Prolonged use of antibiotics followed by exposure to feces-contaminated surfaces<br>• Spores on hands and environmental surfaces are extremely difficult to kill |
| **Parasitic** | | |
| *Giardia lamblia* | • Abdominal cramps, nausea, diarrhea<br>• May interfere with nutrient absorption | • Highly contagious<br>• Transmitted via fecal-oral route<br>• Found in fresh lakes and rivers. Has been transmitted in swimming pools, water parks, and hot tubs |
| *Entamoeba histolytica* | • Diarrhea, abdominal cramping<br>• Only 10%-20% are ill, and symptoms are usually mild | • Fecally contaminated food, water, or hands<br>• Most common in developing countries<br>• In the United States, high-risk groups include travelers, recent immigrants, and homosexual men |
| *Cryptosporidium* | • Watery diarrhea<br>• Lasts about 2 wk<br>• May have abdominal cramps, nausea, vomiting, fever, dehydration, weight loss<br>• May be fatal in those who are immunocompromised (e.g., AIDS) | • Lives in human intestines and is transmitted in stool of infected human or animal<br>• Outer shell allows it to live for long periods outside of body and makes it resistant to chlorine<br>• Common cause of waterborne disease (swimming pools, lakes, drinking water, food contaminated with feces) |

common intestinal parasite that causes diarrhea in the United States.

Infectious organisms attack the intestines in different ways. Some organisms (e.g., *Rotavirus A*, *Norovirus*, *G. lamblia*) alter secretion and/or absorption of the enterocytes of the small intestine without causing inflammation. Other organisms (e.g., *Clostridium difficile*) impair absorption by destroying cells, cause inflammation in the colon, and produce toxins that cause damage.

*Secretory diarrhea* is a common result of bacterial or viral infections. It occurs when ingested pathogens survive in the GI tract long enough to absorb into the enterocytes. The resulting chain reaction changes cell permeability and results in the oversecretion of water and sodium and chloride ions into the bowel.

Organisms enter the body in contaminated food (e.g., *Salmonella* in undercooked eggs and chicken) or contaminated drinking water (*G. lamblia* in contaminated lakes or pools). Travelers often get diarrhea, especially if they travel to countries with poorer sanitation than their own. Infection can spread from one person to another via the fecal-oral route. For example, adult day care workers can transmit infection from one resident to another if they do not wash their hands thoroughly after changing soiled diapers and linens.

A person's age, gastric acidity, intestinal microflora, and immune status influence susceptibility to pathogenic organisms. Older adults are most likely to suffer life-threatening diarrhea. Since stomach acid kills ingested pathogens, taking medications designed to decrease stomach acid (e.g., proton pump inhibitors and histamine [$H_2$]-receptor blockers) increases the likelihood that pathogens will survive.[2]

The healthy human colon contains short-chain fatty acids and bacteria such as *E. coli.* These organisms aid in fermentation and provide a microbial barrier against pathogenic bacteria. Antibiotics kill off the normal flora, making the person more susceptible to pathogenic organisms. For example, patients receiving broad-spectrum antibiotics (e.g., clindamycin [Cleocin], cephalosporins, fluoroquinolones) are susceptible to pathogenic strains of *C. difficile. C. difficile* infection (CDI) causes the most serious antibiotic-associated diarrhea and is the most common cause of hospital-related GI illness in the United States.[2] Probiotics such as *Saccharomyces boulardii* and *Lactobacillus* may be helpful in preventing antibiotic-induced diarrhea in some patients.

People who are immunocompromised because of disease (e.g., human immunodeficiency virus [HIV]) or immunosuppressive medications are susceptible to gastrointestinal (GI) tract infection. Immunocompromised patients receiving jejunal enteral nutrition are especially prone to CDI and other foodborne infections. Jejunostomy and nasointestinal feedings, which bypass the stomach's acid environment, do not contain the poorly digestible fiber that is necessary for the survival of normal colonic bacteria.

Diarrhea is not always due to infection. Drugs and specific food intolerances can cause diarrhea. Large amounts of undigested carbohydrate in the bowel, lactose intolerance, and certain laxatives (e.g., lactulose, sodium phosphate, magnesium citrate) produce osmotic diarrhea. *Osmotic diarrhea* results from rapid GI transit that prevents absorption of fluid and electrolytes. Bile salts and undigested fats lead to excessive fluid secretion into the GI tract. Diarrhea from celiac disease and short bowel syndrome results from malabsorption in the small intestine.

## Clinical Manifestations

Infections that attack the upper GI tract (e.g., *Norovirus, G. lamblia*) usually produce large-volume, watery stools, cramping, and periumbilical pain (Table 42-1). Patients have either a low-grade or no fever and often experience nausea and vomiting before the diarrhea begins. Infections of the colon and distal small bowel (e.g., *Shigella, Salmonella, C. difficile*) produce fever and frequent bloody diarrhea with a small volume.

Leukocytes, blood, and mucus may be present in the stool, depending on the causative agent. Severe diarrhea produces life-threatening dehydration, electrolyte disturbances (e.g., hypokalemia), and acid-base imbalances (metabolic acidosis). CDI can progress to fulminant colitis and intestinal perforation.

## Diagnostic Studies

Since most cases of diarrhea resolve quickly, stool cultures are done only in patients who are very ill, have a high fever, or have had diarrhea longer than 3 days. Stools are examined for blood, mucus, white blood cells (WBCs), and parasites. Cultures reliably identify infectious organisms. Multiple-pathogen tests can concurrently detect common viral, parasitic, and bacterial organisms from a single stool sample. Toxins produced by *C. difficile* can usually be detected in a stool sample.

Testing for ova and parasites is reserved for people who have had diarrhea more than 2 weeks. The WBC count may be elevated. People with long-standing diarrhea can develop anemia from iron and folate deficiencies. Increased hematocrit, blood urea nitrogen (BUN), and creatinine levels are signs of fluid deficit.

In patients with chronic diarrhea, measuring stool electrolytes, pH, and osmolality helps determine whether the diarrhea is from decreased fluid absorption or increased fluid secretion. Measuring stool fat and undigested muscle fibers may indicate fat and protein malabsorption conditions, including pancreatic insufficiency. Some patients with secretory diarrhea have elevated serum levels of GI hormones such as vasoactive intestinal polypeptide and gastrin.

## Interprofessional Care

Treatment of diarrhea depends on the cause. Acute infectious diarrhea is usually self-limiting. The major concerns are preventing transmission, replacing fluid and electrolytes, and protecting the skin. Patients usually tolerate oral fluids. Solutions containing glucose and electrolytes (e.g., Pedialyte) may be sufficient to replace losses from mild diarrhea. If losses are severe, parenteral administration of fluids, electrolytes, vitamins, and nutrition is necessary. Teach the patient to avoid foods and drugs that cause diarrhea. Insoluble fiber (psyllium) may be helpful in thickening the stool.

Antidiarrheal agents are sometimes used short term. They coat and protect mucous membranes, absorb irritating substances, inhibit intestinal transit, decrease intestinal secretions, or decrease central nervous system stimulation of the GI tract (Table 42-2). Antidiarrheal agents are contraindicated in treating some infectious diarrheas because they potentially prolong exposure to the organism. They are used cautiously in

**TABLE 42-2 Drug Therapy**

***Antidiarrheal Drugs***

| Drug | Mechanism of Action |
|---|---|
| bismuth subsalicylate (Pepto-Bismol) | Decreases secretions and has weak antibacterial activity. Used to prevent traveler's diarrhea |
| calcium polycarbophil (Mitrolan) | Bulk-forming agent that absorbs excessive fluid from diarrhea to form a gel. Used when intestinal mucosa cannot absorb fluid |
| loperamide (Imodium, Pepto Diarrhea Control) | Inhibits peristalsis, delays transit, increases absorption of fluid from stools |
| diphenoxylate with atropine (Lomotil) | Opioid and anticholinergic. Decreases peristalsis and intestinal motility |
| paregoric (camphorated tincture of opium) | Opioid. Decreases peristalsis and intestinal motility |
| Donnagel-PG (combination of kaolin, pectin, and paregoric) | Decreases peristalsis and intestinal motility |
| octreotide acetate (Sandostatin) | Suppresses serotonin secretion, stimulates fluid absorption from GI tract, decreases intestinal motility |

inflammatory bowel disease (IBD) because of the danger of causing *toxic megacolon* (colonic dilation greater than 5 cm).

Antibiotics are rarely used to treat acute diarrhea. They are used for certain infections or when the infected person is severely ill or immunosuppressed. For example, a nonabsorbable antibiotic, rifaximin (Xifaxan), is used to treat traveler's diarrhea caused by *E. coli.*[1]

***Clostridium difficile* Infection.** CDI is a particularly hazardous health care–associated infection (HAI). The risk for contracting CDI is highest in patients receiving antimicrobial, chemotherapy, or immunosuppressive agents. Additional risk factors include an ICU stay, a prolonged hospital stay, having surgery, and receiving drugs that suppress gastric acid.[2] *C. difficile* spores can survive for up to 70 days on objects, including commodes, telephones, thermometers, bedside tables, and floors. Health care workers who do not adhere to strict infection control precautions can transmit *C. difficile* from patient to patient. Meticulous hand washing with soap and water and frequently changing gloves are extremely important in limiting the spread of *C. difficile.*

CDI is treated with either metronidazole (Flagyl) or vancomycin (Vancocin).[2] Metronidazole is the first line of treatment of mild to moderate CDI. Vancomycin is used for severe CDI or in patients who do not respond to metronidazole therapy within 5 to 7 days. Vancomycin is given orally or by enema. All nonessential antibiotics, stool softeners, laxatives, and antidiarrheal agents should be stopped. Patients who are at risk for relapse from certain strains of *C. difficile* or have recurrent CDI may receive the antibiotic fidaxomicin (Dificid).

Recurrent CDI occurs in about 20% of patients. The risk increases with the use of additional antibiotics and subsequent CDI recurrences.[2] *Fecal microbiota transplantation* (FMT) is emerging as the most effective treatment for recurrent CDI.[3] FMT reestablishes healthy intestinal flora by infusing fecal bacteria obtained from healthy donor stool into the patient's colon. To perform an FMT, feces obtained from the donor is pureed into a liquid, slurry consistency using saline, water, or pasteurized cow's milk. The donor stool is then placed in the GI tract via an enema, nasoenteral tube, or during colonoscopy. The major concern with FMT is the potential for transmitting infectious agents in the donor stool. Using feces from donors who have intimate physical contact with the recipient and careful screening minimize this risk. Most patients have diarrhea immediately after the procedure.

## NURSING MANAGEMENT: ACUTE INFECTIOUS DIARRHEA

### Nursing Assessment

Begin the nursing assessment with a thorough history and physical examination (Table 42-3). Ask the patient to describe his or her stool pattern and associated symptoms. Focus on the duration, frequency, character, and consistency of stool, and the relationship to other symptoms such as pain and vomiting. Inquire about medical conditions that may cause diarrhea and whether the person is taking medications such as antibiotics and laxatives that are known to cause diarrhea, decrease stomach acidity, or cause immunosuppression. Determine whether the patient has traveled to a foreign country, been at a day care facility recently, and if other family members are ill. Ask about food preparation practices, food intolerances (e.g., milk), and changes in diet and appetite.

**TABLE 42-3 Nursing Assessment**

***Diarrhea***

**Subjective Data**

***Important Health Information***

*Past health history:* Recent travel, hospitalization, infections, stress. Diverticulitis or malabsorption, metabolic disorders, inflammatory bowel disease, irritable bowel syndrome

*Medications:* Laxatives or enemas, magnesium-containing antacids, sorbitol-containing suspensions or elixirs, antibiotics, methyldopa, digitalis, colchicine; OTC antidiarrheal medications

*Surgery or other treatments:* Stomach or bowel surgery, radiation

***Functional Health Patterns***

*Health perception–health management:* Chronic laxative abuse, malaise

*Nutritional-metabolic:* Ingestion of fatty and spicy foods, food intolerances. Anorexia, nausea, vomiting, weight loss. Thirst

*Elimination:* Increased stool frequency, volume, and looseness. Change in color and character of stools. Steatorrhea, abdominal bloating. Decreased urine output

*Cognitive-perceptual:* Abdominal tenderness, abdominal pain and cramping, tenesmus

**Objective Data**

***General***

Lethargy, sunken eyeballs, fever, malnutrition

***Integumentary***

Pallor, dry mucous membranes, poor skin turgor, perianal irritation

***Gastrointestinal***

Frequent soft to liquid stools that may alternate with constipation, altered stool color. Abdominal distention, hyperactive bowel sounds. Pus, blood, mucus, or fat in stools. Fecal impaction

***Urinary***

Decreased output, concentrated urine

***Possible Diagnostic Findings***

Abnormal serum electrolyte levels. Anemia, leukocytosis, eosinophilia, hypoalbuminemia. Positive stool cultures. Ova, parasites, leukocytes, blood, or fat in stool. Abnormal sigmoidoscopy or colonoscopy findings. Abnormal lower GI series

Assess for fever and signs of dehydration (dry skin, low-grade fever, orthostatic changes in pulse and BP, decreased and concentrated urine). Assess the abdomen for distention, pain, and guarding. Inspect the perineal skin for signs of redness and breakdown from the diarrhea.

### Nursing Diagnoses

Nursing diagnoses for the patient with acute infectious diarrhea may include, but are not limited to, the following:

- Diarrhea *related to* acute infectious process
- Deficient fluid volume *related to* excessive fluid loss and decreased fluid intake

For additional information on nursing diagnoses for diarrhea, see eNursing Care Plan 42-1 on the website for this chapter.

### Planning

The overall goals are that the patient with diarrhea will have (1) no transmission of the microorganism causing the infectious diarrhea; (2) cessation of diarrhea and resumption of normal bowel patterns; (3) normal fluid, electrolyte, and acid-base balance; (4) normal nutritional status; and (5) no perianal/perineal skin breakdown.

### Nursing Implementation

Consider all cases of acute diarrhea as infectious until the cause is known. Strict infection control precautions are necessary to prevent the illness from spreading to others. Wash your hands before and after contact with each patient and when handling body fluids of any kind. Flush vomitus and stool in the toilet. Teach the patient and caregiver to wash contaminated clothing immediately with soap and water. Teach them the principles of hygiene, infection control precautions, and the potential dangers of an illness that is infectious to themselves and others. Discuss proper food handling, cooking, and storage with the patient and caregiver (see Tables 41-24 and 41-25).

Viruses and *C. difficile* spores are extremely difficult to kill. Alcohol-based hand cleaners and ammonia-based disinfectants are ineffective, and even vigorous cleaning with soap and water does not kill everything. Immediately put patients with CDI in isolation, and ensure that visitors and health care providers wear gloves and gowns. Give infected patients their own disposable stethoscopes and thermometers. Consider all objects in the room contaminated. Ensure surfaces and equipment are disinfected with a 10% bleach solution or a disinfectant labeled as *C. difficile* sporicidal.[2]

## FECAL INCONTINENCE

### Etiology and Pathophysiology

**Fecal incontinence** is the involuntary passage of stool. It occurs when the normal structures that maintain continence are damaged or disrupted. Defecation is a voluntary action when the neuromuscular system is intact (see Chapter 38). Problems with motor function (contraction of sphincters and rectal floor muscles) and/or sensory function (ability to perceive the presence of stool or to experience the urge to defecate) can result in fecal incontinence. Contributing factors include weakness or disruption of the internal or external anal sphincter, damage to the pudendal nerve or other nerves that innervate the anorectum, damage to the anal tissue, and trauma to the puborectalis muscle (Table 42-4).

For women, obstetric trauma is the most common cause of sphincter disruption. Childbirth, aging, and menopause contribute to the development of fecal incontinence. With diarrhea, the likelihood is increased that stool will be accidentally discharged. Chronic constipation can lead to *fecal impaction,* a collection of hardened feces in the rectum or sigmoid colon that a person cannot expel. Incontinence occurs as liquid stool seeps around the hardened feces. Fecal impaction is a common problem in older adults with limited mobility. Constipated individuals tend to strain during defecation. Straining contributes to incontinence because it weakens the pelvic floor muscles.

Anorectal surgery can damage the sphincters and pudendal nerves. Radiation for prostate cancer decreases rectal compliance. Neurologic conditions, including stroke, spinal cord injury, and multiple sclerosis, interfere with defecation. Even people with normally functioning defecation experience incontinence if immobility prevents timely access to a toilet.

### Diagnostic Studies and Interprofessional Care

The diagnosis and effective management of fecal incontinence require a thorough health history and physical examination.

**TABLE 42-4 Causes of Fecal Incontinence**

| Traumatic | Neurologic |
|---|---|
| • Anorectal surgery for hemorrhoids, fistula, and fissures<br>• Childbirth injury (episiotomy is a risk factor)<br>• Perineal trauma or pelvic fracture | • Brain tumor<br>• Cauda equina nerve injury<br>• Congenital abnormalities (e.g., spina bifida, myelomeningocele)<br>• Dementia<br>• Diabetes mellitus (secondary to neuropathy)<br>• Multiple sclerosis<br>• Rectal surgery<br>• Spinal cord injuries<br>• Stroke |
| **Inflammatory**<br>• Infection<br>• Inflammatory bowel disease<br>• Radiation | |
| **Pelvic Floor Dysfunction**<br>• Medications<br>• Rectal prolapse | **Other**<br>• Chronic constipation<br>• Denervation of pelvic muscles from chronic excessive straining<br>• Fecal impaction<br>• Loss of rectal elasticity<br>• Rapid transit of large diarrheal stools |
| **Functional**<br>• Physical or mobility impairments affecting toileting ability (e.g., frail older person who cannot get to the bathroom in time) | |

Ask the patient about the number of incontinent episodes per week, stool consistency and volume, and the degree that incontinence interferes with work and social activities. A rectal examination can reveal reduced anal canal muscle tone and contraction strength of the external sphincter, as well as detect internal prolapse, rectocele, hemorrhoids, fecal impaction, and masses. If the impaction is higher in the colon, an abdominal x-ray or a CT scan may be helpful. Other tests include anorectal manometry, anorectal ultrasonography, and defecography. Sigmoidoscopy or colonoscopy can identify inflammation, tumors, fissures, and other pathologic conditions.

Treatment of incontinence depends on the underlying cause. Fecal incontinence from fecal impaction usually resolves after manual removal of the hard feces and cleansing enemas. To prevent recurrence, maintaining normal stool consistency and a bowel management program are important. This includes regular defecation, a high-fiber diet, and increased intake of caffeine free fluids. Patients with dehydration will need fluid replacement therapy.

Dietary fiber supplements or bulk-forming laxatives such as psyllium (Metamucil, Konsyl) increase stool bulk, firm consistency, and promote the sensation of rectal filling. Patients may need to reduce or eliminate foods that cause diarrhea and rectal irritation. Common food triggers include coffee, dried fruit, onions, mushrooms, green vegetables, fruit with peels, spicy foods, and foods with monosodium glutamate. Antidiarrheal agents (e.g., loperamide [Imodium]) are useful in slowing intestinal transit.

Kegel exercises (see Table 45-18) can strengthen and coordinate the pelvic floor muscles to improve continence. Biofeedback therapy can improve awareness of rectal sensation, coordinate internal and external anal sphincters, and increase the strength of external sphincter contraction. Biofeedback training requires intact sensory and motor nerves and motivation to learn. It is a safe, painless, and effective treatment.[4]

Mild electrical stimulation of the sacral nerves targets communication problems between the brain and nerves that control the pelvic floor muscles and sphincters. Electrical stimulation can improve quality of life, and some patients may achieve complete continence.[4]

For patients who do not respond to conservative treatment, treatment with dextranomer/hyaluronic acid gel (Solesta) may be used. In this treatment, the gel is injected into the deep submucosa of the patient's anal canal. It works by building up tissue in the anal area, narrowing the anal canal and allowing muscles to more adequately close. No anesthesia is required. Postinjection pain and bleeding may occur.

Surgery (e.g., sphincter repair procedures) is an option when other conservative treatments fail, the patient has a full-thickness prolapse, or the anal sphincter needs repair. A colostomy is sometimes necessary.

## NURSING MANAGEMENT: FECAL INCONTINENCE

### Nursing Assessment

Fecal incontinence is embarrassing, uncomfortable, and irritating to the skin. Its unpredictable nature makes it difficult to maintain school and work activities and hampers social or intimate contact. Be sensitive to the patient's feelings when discussing incontinence. Ask about daily activities (mealtimes and work), diet, and family and social activities.

If the underlying cause cannot be corrected, help the patient reestablish a predictable pattern of defecation. Ask about bowel patterns before the incontinence developed; current bowel habits; stool consistency and frequency; and symptoms, including pain during defecation and a feeling of incomplete evacuation *(tenesmus)*. Assess whether the patient has a sensation of urgency to evacuate the bowel or sensation of passing flatus and leaking stool. Check the perineal area for irritation or breakdown. The Bristol Stool Scale is helpful to assess stool consistency *(www.poopreport.com/Poll/bristol_scale.html)*.

Patients who have fecal incontinence are at risk for *incontinence-associated dermatitis* (IAD).[5] IAD results from chemical irritants in the feces causing skin damage. It is characterized by location, redness, skin loss, and rash. The location of IAD is usually the perianal or perineal area, buttocks, or upper thighs. Fungal infection is common and frequently seen as a dark red center surrounded by satellite lesions. Your assessment is important in differentiating IAD from pressure ulcer development.

### Nursing Implementation

Regardless of the cause of fecal incontinence, bowel training is an effective strategy for many patients. Bowel elimination occurs at regular intervals in most people. Knowing the patient's usual bowel pattern can assist you in planning a bowel program that will achieve optimal stool consistency and predictable bowel elimination patterns. For the hospitalized patient, placement on a bedpan, assistance to a bedside commode, or walks to the bathroom at a regular time daily help to establish regular defecation. A good time to schedule elimination is within 30 minutes after breakfast.

If these techniques are ineffective in reestablishing bowel regularity, administer bisacodyl (Dulcolax), a glycerin suppository, or a small phosphate enema 15 to 30 minutes before the usual evacuation time. These preparations stimulate the anorectal reflex. Since stimulation will not occur unless the suppository or enema touches the rectal wall, first check for stool in the rectum and digitally remove it before inserting the laxative. Once a regular pattern is established, discontinue these drugs. Digital stimulation is another method for stimulating the anorectal reflex and is commonly included in bowel programs for people with neurogenic bowels (e.g., from spinal cord injury). Irrigating the rectum and colon (usually with tap water) at regular intervals is another way to achieve continence in patients with neurogenic bowel.

Maintaining perineal skin integrity is of utmost importance, especially in the bedridden patient. Feces can contaminate wounds, damage skin, cause bladder infections, and spread infections such as *C. difficile*. Containment of the feces is essential. One option to contain stool is a fecal management system (e.g., Flexi-Seal, DignaCare, Actiflo, Instaflo). A fecal management system funnels liquid stool from the rectum into a containment system. Common features include a retention cuff that sits above the anal sphincter and soft tubing that extends from this cuff to a secure hub that allows a person to change the containment canister when it is full. A system can remain in place for weeks. Fecal management systems may decrease the risk of CDI, skin damage from exposure to stool, IAD, and pressure ulcer development.[6] Avoid the use of rectal tubes or urinary catheters. They can reduce the responsiveness of the rectal sphincter and potentially irritate or ulcerate the rectal mucosa.

Perform frequent skin assessments when absorbent products are used. Incontinence briefs may help minimize risk of developing IAD, but only if changed promptly after each episode of incontinence. Use absorbent products in combination with a defined skin care program. This includes prompt cleansing, moisturizing, and skin protection. Soap is not an ideal product since it can be drying. Cleanse the perineal skin gently with tap water or a pH-balanced cleanser to remove feces. Apply a moisture barrier and, if needed, a skin barrier cream for more protection. For patients unable to care for themselves at home, you should teach caregivers how to maintain skin integrity.

Fecal incontinence is an overwhelming burden for most patients. Be sensitive to their fears. Teach strategies to help patients reduce incontinent episodes and better cope with them when they do occur. Help patients identify food triggers that may worsen symptoms. Encourage them to avoid those foods and exercise after meals. Tell them to try to use bathrooms when they are available. Patients may be more confident when they use discreet, disposable briefs or pads. Have them wear dark-colored clothing that they can quickly remove for toileting. Ready access to a spare set of clothing and cleansing cloths is important.

## CONSTIPATION

**Constipation** is a syndrome defined by difficult or infrequent stools; hard, dry stools that are difficult to pass; or a feeling of incomplete evacuation.[7] Because people vary, it is important to compare the current symptoms with the patient's normal pattern of elimination.

### Etiology and Pathophysiology

Common causes of constipation include taking in insufficient dietary fiber or fluids, decreasing physical activity, and ignoring the defecation urge (Table 42-5). Many drugs, especially opioids, cause constipation. Constipation occurs with diseases that slow GI transit and hamper neurologic function such as diabetes mellitus, Parkinson's disease, and multiple sclerosis. Emotions, including anxiety, depression, and stress, affect the GI tract and can contribute to constipation.

Some people believe that they are constipated if they do not have a daily bowel movement. This can result in chronic laxative

## TABLE 42-5 Causes of Constipation

**Colonic Disorders**
- Diverticular disease
- Inflammation-induced strictures
- Intussusception
- Irritable bowel syndrome
- Luminal or extraluminal obstructing lesions
- Rectocele
- Volvulus

**Drug-Induced Causes**
- Antacids (calcium and aluminum)
- Anticholinergics
- Antidepressants
- Antihypertensives
- Antipsychotics
- Barium sulfate
- Bismuth
- Calcium supplements
- Iron supplements
- Laxative abuse
- Opioids

**Systemic Disorders**

***Metabolic/Endocrine***
- Celiac disease
- Diabetes mellitus
- Hypercalcemia/hyperparathyroidism
- Hypokalemia
- Hypothyroidism
- Pheochromocytoma
- Pregnancy

***Collagen Vascular Disease***
- Amyloidosis
- Systemic sclerosis (scleroderma)

***Neurologic Disorders***
- Autonomic neuropathy (resulting from diabetes mellitus)
- Hirschsprung's megacolon
- Multiple sclerosis
- Neurofibromatosis
- Parkinson's disease
- Spinal cord lesions or injury
- Stroke

use and subsequent *cathartic colon syndrome,* a condition in which the colon becomes dilated and atonic (lacking muscle tone). Ultimately, the person cannot defecate without a laxative.

Ignoring the urge to defecate for a prolonged period can cause the muscles and mucosa of the rectum to become insensitive to the presence of feces. In addition, the prolonged retention of feces results in drying of stool due to water absorption. The harder and drier the feces, the more difficult it is to expel.

### Clinical Manifestations

The clinical presentation of constipation may vary from a mild discomfort to a more severe event mimicking an "acute abdomen." Stools are absent or hard, dry, and difficult to pass. Abdominal distention, bloating, increased flatulence, and increased rectal pressure may be present.

Hemorrhoids are the most common complication of chronic constipation. They result from venous engorgement caused by repeated *Valsalva maneuvers* (straining) and venous compression from hard, impacted stool. Valsalva maneuver may have serious outcomes for patients with heart failure, cerebral edema, hypertension, and coronary artery disease. During straining, the patient inspires deeply and holds the breath while contracting abdominal muscles and bearing down. This increases both intraabdominal and intrathoracic pressures and reduces venous return to the heart. The heart rate temporarily decreases along with a decrease in cardiac output. This results in a transient drop in arterial pressure. When the patient relaxes, thoracic pressure falls, resulting in a sudden flow of blood into the heart, increased heart rate, and an immediate rise in arterial pressure. These changes may be fatal for the patient who cannot compensate for the sudden increased blood flow returning to the heart.

In the presence of *obstipation* (severe constipation with no passage of gas or stool) or fecal impaction secondary to constipation, colonic perforation may occur. Perforation, which is life threatening, causes abdominal pain, nausea, vomiting, fever,

## EVIDENCE-BASED PRACTICE

### *Applying the Evidence*

**Probiotics and Constipation**

L.R. is an 82-yr-old female patient with decreased mobility after a recent hip fracture. During a check-up visit at the orthopedic clinic, L.R. mentions she is experiencing discomfort due to constipation. She tells you she is following her discharge instructions and is drinking "lots of water all day and trying to increase fiber in her diet."

***Making Clinical Decisions***

***Best Available Evidence.*** In adults with constipation, there is an association between the use of probiotics, especially products containing *Bifidobacterium lactis,* and significant improvements in gut transit time, stool frequency, and stool consistency. Quality of life diminishes with increased severity in constipation symptoms.

***Clinician Expertise.*** You recently read about the potential benefit of probiotics in relieving constipation. You also understand that diet can play a major role in treating and preventing constipation.

***Patient Preferences and Values.*** L.R. asks if you know of anything else she can do as she does not want to take any more of those "constipation" drugs.

***Implications for Nursing Practice***

1. What information would you share with L.R. related to probiotics and constipation?
2. What additional data would you obtain from L.R. related to her diet, mobility, and fluid intake?
3. Why is it important for you to know about alternative therapies? What is your role in supporting patients who desire alternatives to drug therapy?

***Reference for Evidence***

Dimidi E, Christodoulides S, Fragkos K, et al: The effect of probiotics on functional constipation in adults: a systematic review and meta-analysis of randomized controlled trials, *Am J Clin Nutr* 100:1075, 2014.

and an elevated WBC count. Rectal mucosal ulcers and fissures may occur from stool stasis or straining. Diverticulosis is another potential complication of chronic constipation. These complications are most common in older patients.

### Diagnostic Studies and Interprofessional Care

Perform a thorough history and physical examination to identify the underlying cause of constipation. Ask the patient about usual defecation patterns and habits, diet, exercise, laxative use, and past history such as obstetric injuries that could contribute to difficulties with defecation. Diagnostic testing may include abdominal x-rays, barium enema, colonoscopy, sigmoidoscopy, rectal balloon expulsion test, anorectal manometry, defecography with barium or fluoroscopy, and colonic transit tests.

Increasing dietary fiber, maintaining adequate fluid intake, and exercise can prevent many cases of constipation. Laxatives (Table 42-6) and enemas are an option in treating acute constipation. They are used cautiously because overuse leads to chronic constipation. The choice of laxative or enema depends on the severity of the constipation and the patient's health. Daily bulk-forming laxatives (psyllium) can prevent constipation because they work like dietary fiber and do not cause dependence. Bisacodyl tablets and suppositories, milk of magnesia, and lactulose act more rapidly but are more likely to cause dependence. Enemas are fast acting and beneficial for immediate treatment of constipation but must be used cautiously. Soapsuds enemas produce inflammation of colon mucosa, tap water enemas can potentially lead to water intoxication, and

## TABLE 42-6 Drug Therapy
### *Constipation*

| Mechanism of Action | Example | Comments |
|---|---|---|
| **Bulk Forming** | | |
| Absorbs water. Increases bulk, thereby stimulating peristalsis<br>*Action:* Usually within 24 hr | methylcellulose (Citrucel)<br>psyllium (Metamucil, Perdiem, Konsyl, Hydrocil, Fiberall) | Contraindicated in patients with abdominal pain, nausea, and vomiting and in patients suspected of having appendicitis, biliary tract obstruction, or acute hepatitis. Must be taken with fluids (≥8 oz). Best choice for initial treatment of constipation |
| **Stool Softeners and Lubricants** | | |
| Lubricate intestinal tract and soften feces, making hard stools easier to pass. Do not affect peristalsis<br>*Action:* Softeners in 72 hr, lubricants in 8 hr | *Softeners:* docusate (Colace, Surfak, Peri-Colace)<br>*Lubricants:* mineral oil (Fleet's Oil Retention Enema, Kondremul Plain) | Can block absorption of fat-soluble vitamins such as vitamin K, which may increase risk of bleeding in patients on anticoagulants |
| **Saline and Osmotic Solutions** | | |
| Cause retention of fluid in intestinal lumen caused by osmotic effect<br>*Action:* Within 15 min-3 hr | Magnesium salts (magnesium citrate, Milk of Magnesia)<br>Sodium phosphates (Fleet Enema, Phospho-soda)<br>lactulose (Constulose)<br>polyethylene glycol (MiraLAX, GoLYTELY, CoLyte) | Magnesium-containing products may cause hypermagnesemia in patients with renal insufficiency |
| **Stimulants** | | |
| Increase peristalsis by irritating colon wall and stimulating enteric nerves<br>*Action:* Usually within 12 hr | cascara sagrada, senna (Senokot)<br>phenolphthalein: sennosides (Ex-Lax), bisacodyl (Correctol, Feen-a-Mint, Dulcolax), docusate/phenolphthalein (Doxidan) | Cause melanosis coli (brown or black pigmentation of colon). Are most widely abused laxatives. Should not be used in patients with impaction or obstipation |
| **Selective Chloride Channel Activator** | | |
| Increases intestinal fluid secretion and motility<br>*Action:* Usually within 24 hr | lubiprostone (Amitiza) | Used in the treatment of idiopathic constipation and irritable bowel syndrome with constipation (women only). Contraindicated in patients with history of mechanical GI obstruction |
| **Intestinal Secretagogue** | | |
| Increases fluid secretion and accelerates intestinal transit<br>*Action:* Usually within 24 hr | linaclotide (Linzess) | Used in the treatment of idiopathic constipation and irritable bowel syndrome with constipation |

sodium phosphate (e.g., Fleet) enemas may cause electrolyte imbalances in patients with cardiac and renal problems.

Intestinal secretagogues, lubiprostone (Amitiza) and linaclotide (Linzess), increase intestinal chloride and water secretion, accelerating transit and easing evacuation. They are useful in treating chronic idiopathic constipation.[7]

Newer medications include methylnaltrexone (Relistor) and naloxegol (Movantik), peripherally acting opioid receptor antagonists that decrease constipation caused by opioid use. These drugs do not block the analgesic effects of opioids.

Other therapies target specific patient needs. Biofeedback therapy may benefit patients who have constipation because of *anismus* (uncoordinated contraction of the anal sphincter during straining).

A patient with severe constipation related to bowel motility or mechanical disorders may require more intense treatment. Diagnostic studies include anorectal manometry, GI tract transit studies, and sigmoidoscopic rectal biopsies. A patient with unrelenting constipation may need a colostomy, ileostomy, or continent fecal diversion. (These procedures are discussed later in this chapter.)

**Nutritional Therapy.** Diet is an important factor in preventing and treating constipation. Many patients experience improved symptoms when they increase their dietary fiber intake. Dietary fiber is found in fruits, vegetables, and grains (Table 42-7). Wheat bran and prunes are especially effective for preventing and treating constipation. Whole wheat and bran are high in insoluble fiber.

Dietary fiber adds to the stool bulk directly by attracting water. Therefore adequate fluid intake (2 L/day) is essential. Large, bulky stools move through the colon much more quickly than small stools. However, the recommended fluid intake may be contraindicated in a patient with cardiac disease or renal failure. Tell the patient that increasing fiber intake may initially increase gas production because of fermentation in the colon, but this effect decreases over several days.

## NURSING MANAGEMENT: CONSTIPATION

### Nursing Assessment

Table 42-8 outlines the subjective and objective data you should obtain from a patient with constipation.

### Nursing Implementation

Tailor the nursing management of constipation to your assessment of the patient's symptoms. Teach the patient about the importance of diet, fluids, and activity in the prevention and treatment of constipation (Table 42-9). Emphasize the importance of a high-fiber diet, adequate fluid intake, and regular exercise. Teach the patient to establish a regular time to defecate and not to suppress the urge to defecate. Discourage the use of laxatives and enemas to achieve fecal elimination.

Defecation is easiest when the person is sitting on a commode with the knees higher than the hips. The sitting position allows gravity to aid defecation, and flexing the hips straightens the angle between the anal canal and rectum so that stool flows out

## TABLE 42-7 Nutritional Therapy

### High-Fiber Foods

*High-fiber foods are recommended for patients with diverticulosis, irritable bowel syndrome, constipation, hemorrhoids, atherosclerosis, hyperlipidemia, and diabetes mellitus.*

| | Fiber/ Serving (g) | Serving Size | Calories/ Serving |
|---|---|---|---|
| **Vegetables** | | | |
| Asparagus | 3.5 | ½ cup | 18 |
| Beans | | | |
| • Navy | 8.4 | ½ cup | 80 |
| • Kidney | 9.7 | ½ cup | 94 |
| • Lima | 8.3 | ½ cup | 63 |
| • Pinto | 8.9 | ½ cup | 78 |
| • String | 2.1 | ½ cup | 18 |
| Broccoli | 3.5 | ½ cup | 18 |
| Carrots, raw | 1.8 | ½ cup | 15 |
| Corn | 2.6 | ½ medium ear | 72 |
| Peas, canned | 6.7 | ½ cup | 63 |
| Potatoes | | | |
| • Baked | 1.9 | ½ medium | 72 |
| • Sweet | 2.1 | ½ medium | 79 |
| Squash, acorn | 7.0 | 1 cup | 82 |
| Tomato, raw | 1.5 | 1 small | 18 |
| **Fruits** | | | |
| Apple | 2.0 | ½ large | 42 |
| Blackberries | 6.7 | ¾ cup | 40 |
| Orange | 1.6 | 1 small | 35 |
| Peach | 2.3 | 1 medium | 38 |
| Pear | 2.0 | ½ medium | 44 |
| Raspberries | 9.2 | 1 cup | 42 |
| Strawberries | 3.1 | 1 cup | 45 |
| **Grain Products** | | | |
| Bread, whole wheat | 1.3 | 1 slice | 59 |
| Cereal | | | |
| • All Bran (100%) | 8.4 | ⅓ cup | 70 |
| • Corn Flakes | 2.6 | ¾ cup | 70 |
| • Shredded Wheat | 2.8 | 1 biscuit | 70 |
| Popcorn | 3.0 | 3 cups | 62 |

## TABLE 42-8 Nursing Assessment

### Constipation

**Subjective Data**

***Important Health Information***

*Past health history:* Colorectal disease, neurologic dysfunction, bowel obstruction, environmental changes, cancer, irritable bowel syndrome, diabetes mellitus

*Medications:* Aluminum and calcium antacids, anticholinergics, antidepressants, antihistamines, antipsychotics, diuretics, opioids, iron, laxatives, enemas

***Functional Health Patterns***

*Health perception–health management:* Chronic laxative or enema abuse. Rigid beliefs regarding bowel function. Malaise

*Nutritional-metabolic:* Changes in diet or mealtime. Inadequate fiber and fluid intake. Anorexia, nausea

*Elimination:* Change in usual elimination patterns. Hard, difficult-to-pass stool, decrease in frequency and amount of stools. Flatus, abdominal distention. Tenesmus, rectal pressure. Fecal incontinence (if impacted)

*Activity-exercise:* Change in daily activity routines. Immobility, sedentary lifestyle

*Cognitive-perceptual:* Dizziness, headache, anorectal pain. Abdominal pain on defecation

*Coping–stress tolerance:* Acute or chronic stress

**Objective Data**

***General***

Lethargy

***Integumentary***

Anorectal fissures, hemorrhoids, abscesses

***Gastrointestinal***

Abdominal distention. Hypoactive or absent bowel sounds. Palpable abdominal mass. Fecal impaction. Small, hard, dry stool. Stool with blood

***Possible Diagnostic Findings***

Guaiac-positive stools. Abdominal x-ray demonstrating stool in lower colon

## TABLE 42-9 Patient & Caregiver Teaching

### Constipation

*Include the following instructions when teaching the patient and caregiver about management of constipation.*

**1. Eat Dietary Fiber**

Eat 20 to 30 g of fiber per day. Gradually increase the amount of fiber eaten over 1 to 2 wk. Fiber softens hard stool and adds bulk to stool, promoting evacuation.

- Foods high in fiber: raw vegetables and fruits, beans, breakfast cereals (All Bran, oatmeal)
- Fiber supplements: Metamucil, Citrucel, FiberCon

Eat prunes or drink prune juice daily. Prunes stimulate defecation.

**2. Drink Fluids**

Fluid softens hard stools. Drink 2 L per day. Drink water or fruit juices. Avoid caffeinated coffee, tea, and cola. Caffeine stimulates fluid loss through urination.

**3. Exercise Regularly**

Walk, swim, or bike at least three times per wk. Contract and relax abdominal muscles when standing or by doing sit-ups to strengthen muscles and prevent straining. Exercise stimulates bowel motility and moves stool through the colon.

**4. Establish a Regular Time to Defecate**

First thing in the morning or after the first meal of the day is a good time because people often have the urge to defecate at this time.

**5. Do Not Delay Defecation**

Respond to the urge to have a bowel movement as soon as possible. Delaying defecation results in hard stools and a decreased "urge" to defecate. Water is absorbed from stool by the intestine over time. The colon becomes less sensitive to the presence of stool in the rectum.

**6. Record Your Bowel Elimination Pattern**

Develop a habit of recording when you have a bowel movement on your calendar. Regular monitoring of bowel movement will assist in early identification of a problem.

**7. Avoid Laxatives and Enemas**

Do not overuse laxatives and enemas because they cause dependence. People who overuse them are unable to have a bowel movement without them.

more easily. Place a footstool in front of the toilet to promote flexion of the thighs. It is challenging to defecate while sitting on a bedpan. For a patient in bed, elevate the head of the bed as high as the patient can tolerate.

The sights, odors, and sounds of defecation embarrass most people. Provide as much privacy as possible and use an odor eliminator. Encourage patients to maintain abdominal muscle tone. Prompt patients to contract abdominal muscles several times a day. Sit-ups and straight-leg raises can help improve abdominal muscle tone.

For the patient whose perceived constipation is related to rigid beliefs regarding bowel function, initiate a discussion about these concerns. Give appropriate information on normal bowel function and discuss the adverse consequences of excessive use of laxatives and enemas.

## ACUTE ABDOMINAL PAIN

### Etiology and Pathophysiology

Acute abdominal pain is pain of recent onset. It may signal a life-threatening problem and therefore requires immediate attention. Causes include damage to organs in the abdomen and pelvis, which leads to inflammation, infection, obstruction, bleeding, and perforation (Fig. 42-1). Perforation of the GI tract results in irritation of the *peritoneum* (serous membrane lining the abdominal cavity) and peritonitis. Hypovolemic shock occurs from bleeding or obstruction and peritonitis causing large amounts of fluid to move from the vascular space into the abdomen.

### Clinical Manifestations

Pain is the most common symptom of an acute abdominal problem. The patient may have nausea, vomiting, diarrhea, constipation, flatulence, fatigue, fever, rebound tenderness, and bloating.

### Diagnostic Studies and Interprofessional Care

Diagnosis begins with a complete history and physical examination. Description of the pain (frequency, timing, duration, location), accompanying symptoms, and sequence of symptoms (e.g., pain before or after vomiting) provide vital clues about the origin of the problem. Note the patient's position. The fetal posture is common with peritoneal irritation (e.g., appendicitis), a supine posture with outstretched legs with visceral pain, and restlessness with a seated posture with bowel obstructions or obstructions from kidney stones and gallstones.

Physical examination includes examination of the abdomen, rectum, and pelvis. A complete blood count (CBC), urinalysis, abdominal x-ray, and electrocardiogram are done, along with an ultrasound or CT scan. Women of childbearing age may need a pregnancy test to rule out an ectopic pregnancy.

Emergency management of the patient with acute abdominal pain is presented in Table 42-10. The goal of management is to identify and treat the cause, and monitor and treat complications, especially shock. Careful use of pain medications (e.g., morphine) provides pain relief without interfering with diagnostic accuracy when patients have nontraumatic acute abdominal pain.

In patients with acute abdominal pain, an immediate surgical consult is needed. The surgeon may perform a diagnostic

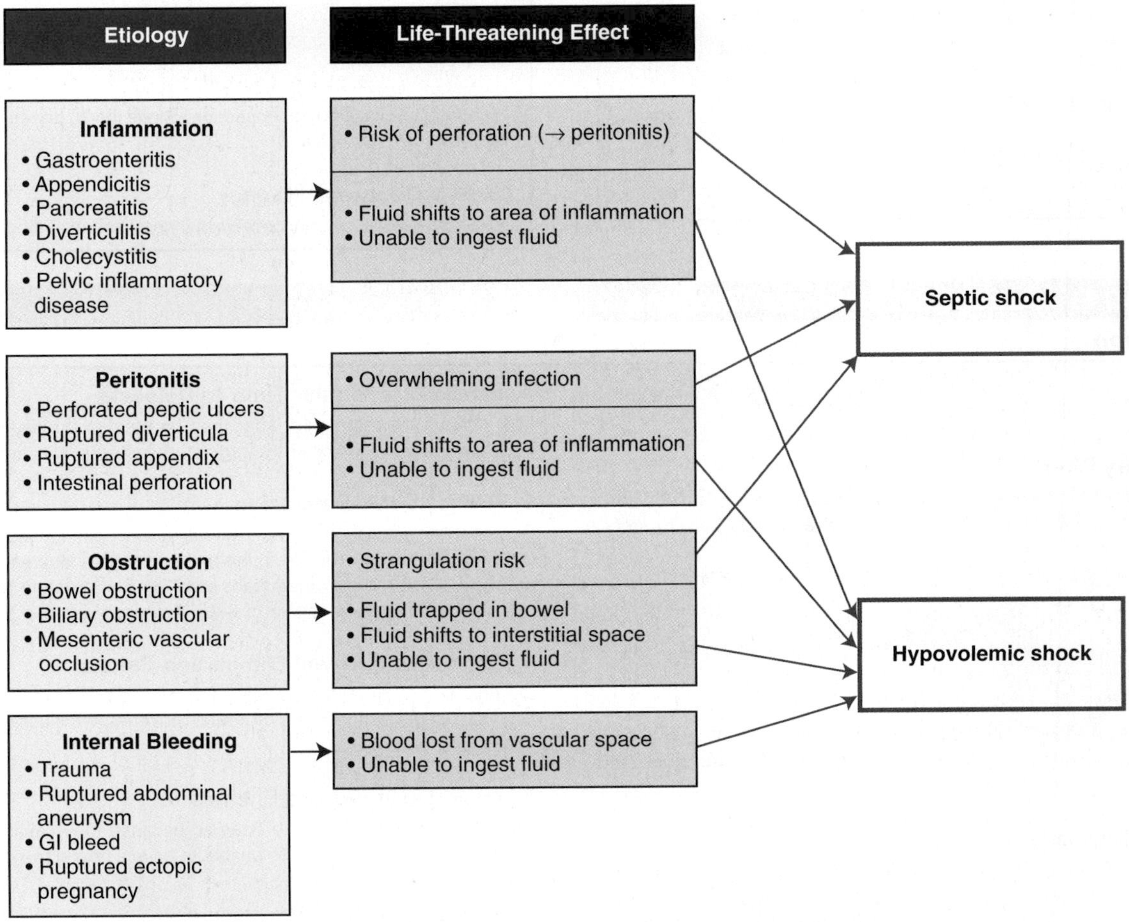


**FIG. 42-1** Etiology of acute abdominal pain and pathophysiologic sequelae.

**TABLE 42-10 Emergency Management**

***Acute Abdominal Pain***

| Etiology | Assessment Findings | Interventions |
|---|---|---|
| **Inflammation**<br>• Appendicitis<br>• Cholecystitis<br>• Crohn's disease<br>• Gastritis<br>• Pancreatitis<br>• Pyelonephritis<br>• Ulcerative colitis<br>**Vascular Problems**<br>• Ruptured aortic aneurysm<br>• Mesenteric vascular occlusion<br>**Gynecologic Problems**<br>• Pelvic inflammatory disease<br>• Ruptured ectopic pregnancy<br>• Ruptured ovarian cyst<br>**Infectious Disease**<br>• *Escherichia coli* O157:H7<br>• *Giardia*<br>• *Salmonella*<br>**Other**<br>• Obstruction or perforation of abdominal organ<br>• Gastrointestinal bleeding or ischemia<br>• Trauma | **Abdominal and GI Findings**<br>• Diffuse, localized, dull, burning, or sharp abdominal pain or tenderness<br>• Rebound tenderness<br>• Abdominal distention<br>• Abdominal rigidity<br>• Nausea and vomiting<br>• Diarrhea<br>• Hematemesis<br>• Melena<br>**Hypovolemic Shock**<br>• ↓ BP<br>• ↓ Pulse pressure<br>• Tachycardia<br>• Cool, clammy skin<br>• ↓ Level of consciousness<br>• ↓ Urine output (<0.5 mL/kg/hr) | **Initial**<br>• Ensure patent airway.<br>• Administer $O_2$ via nasal cannula or non-rebreather mask.<br>• Establish IV access with large-bore catheter and infuse warm normal saline or lactated Ringer's solution. Insert additional large-bore catheter if shock present.<br>• Obtain blood for CBC and electrolyte levels.<br>• Anticipate order for amylase level, pregnancy tests, clotting studies, and type and crossmatch as appropriate.<br>• Insert indwelling urinary catheter.<br>• Obtain urinalysis.<br>• Insert NG tube as needed.<br>**Ongoing Monitoring**<br>• Monitor vital signs, level of consciousness, $O_2$ saturation, and intake/output.<br>• Assess quality and amount of pain.<br>• Assess amount and character of emesis.<br>• Anticipate surgical intervention.<br>• Keep patient NPO. |

laparoscopy to inspect the surface of abdominal organs, obtain biopsy specimens, perform laparoscopic ultrasounds, and remove organs. A laparotomy is used when laparoscopic techniques are inadequate. If the cause of the acute abdomen can be surgically removed (e.g., inflamed appendix) or surgically repaired (e.g., ruptured abdominal aneurysm), surgery is considered definitive therapy.

## NURSING MANAGEMENT: ACUTE ABDOMINAL PAIN

### Nursing Assessment

For the patient complaining of acute abdominal pain, take vital signs immediately and again at frequent intervals. Increased pulse and decreasing BP indicate impending shock. An elevated temperature suggests an inflammatory or infectious process. Intake and output measurement provides essential information about the adequacy of vascular volume. Altered mental status indicates poor cerebral perfusion. Skin color, skin temperature, and peripheral pulse strength provide information about perfusion.

Inspect the abdomen for distention, masses, abnormal pulsation, symmetry, hernias, rashes, scars, and pigmentation changes. Apply light pressure when inspecting the abdomen to help determine the level of a patient's pain. Auscultate bowel sounds. Diminished or absent bowel sounds in a quadrant may indicate a bowel obstruction, acute peritonitis, or paralytic ileus. Perform palpation gently. Determine pain from peritoneal irritation by asking the person to cough, gently palpating the abdomen, or shaking the bed.

Ask the patient about the onset, location, intensity, duration, frequency, and character of pain. Note whether the pain has spread or moved to new sites (quadrants) and what makes the pain worse or better. Is the pain associated with other symptoms, such as nausea, vomiting, changes in bowel and bladder habits, or vaginal discharge in women? Assessment of vomiting includes the amount, color, consistency, and odor of the emesis. Ask about usual and changes in bowel patterns and habits.

### Nursing Diagnoses

Nursing diagnoses for the patient with acute abdominal pain include, but are not limited to, the following:

- Acute pain *related to* inflammation of the peritoneum and abdominal distention
- Risk for deficient fluid volume *related to* collection of fluid in peritoneal cavity secondary to inflammation or infection
- Anxiety *related to* pain and uncertainty of cause or outcome of condition

### Planning

The overall goals are that the patient with acute abdominal pain will have (1) relief of abdominal pain, (2) resolution of inflammation, (3) freedom from complications (especially hypovolemic shock), and (4) normal nutritional status.

### Nursing Implementation

General care for the patient with acute abdominal pain involves management of fluid and electrolyte imbalances, pain, and anxiety. Assess the quality and intensity of pain at regular intervals, and provide medication and other comfort measures. Maintain a calm environment and provide information to help decrease anxiety. A nasogastric (NG) tube with low suction may decrease vomiting and relieve discomfort from gastric distention. Conduct ongoing assessments of vital signs, intake and output, and level of consciousness, which are key indicators of hypovolemic shock.

### Acute Care

***Preoperative Care.*** Preoperative care includes the emergency care of the patient described in Table 42-10 and general care of the preoperative patient (see Chapter 17).

◆ ***Postoperative Care.*** Postoperative care depends on the type of surgical procedure performed. See eNursing Care Plan 19-1, a general plan for the postoperative patient, on the website for Chapter 19.

Postoperatively some patients will have an NG tube with low suction to empty the stomach and prevent gastric dilation. If the upper GI tract was entered, drainage from the NG tube may be dark brown to dark red for the first 12 hours. Later it should be light yellowish brown, or it may have a greenish tinge because of bile. If a dark red color continues or you observe bright red blood, notify the surgeon because of the possibility of hemorrhage. "Coffee-ground" granules in the drainage indicate blood that has been changed by acidic gastric secretions.

Nausea and vomiting are common after a laparotomy and result from the surgery, decreased peristalsis, or pain medications. Antiemetics such as ondansetron (Zofran), promethazine (Phenergan), and prochlorperazine (Compazine) may be ordered. Monitor fluid and electrolyte status along with BP, heart rate, and respirations. (See Chapter 41 for further discussion of managing nausea and vomiting.)

Swallowed air and reduced peristalsis from decreased mobility, manipulation of the abdominal organs during surgery, and anesthesia can result in abdominal distention and gas pains. Early ambulation helps restore peristalsis, expel flatus, and reduce gas pain. Gradually, as intestinal activity increases, distention and gas pain disappear.

◆ **Ambulatory Care.** Preparation for discharge begins soon after surgery. Teach the patient and caregiver about any modifications in activity, care of the incision, diet, and drug therapy. Initially the patient starts on clear liquids after surgery and then, if tolerated, progresses to a regular diet.

Early ambulation speeds recovery, but normal activities are resumed gradually, with planned rest periods. Patients generally have restrictions not to lift anything heavier than a few pounds. The patient and caregiver should be aware of possible complications after surgery. Teach them to notify the surgeon immediately if fever greater than 101° F (38.6° C), vomiting, pain, weight loss, incisional drainage, or changes in bowel function occur.

### ◆ Evaluation

The expected outcomes are that the patient with acute abdominal pain will have

- Resolution of the cause of the acute abdominal pain
- Relief of abdominal pain and discomfort
- Freedom from complications, especially hypovolemic shock and septicemia
- Normal fluid, electrolyte, and nutritional status

## CHRONIC ABDOMINAL PAIN

*Chronic abdominal pain* may originate from abdominal structures or be referred from a site with the same or a similar nerve supply. The pain is often described as dull, aching, or diffuse. Common causes of chronic abdominal pain include irritable bowel syndrome (IBS), peptic ulcer disease, chronic pancreatitis, hepatitis, pelvic inflammatory disease, adhesions, and vascular insufficiency.

Diagnosing the cause of chronic abdominal pain begins with a thorough history and description of specific pain characteristics, including severity, location, frequency, duration, and onset. The assessment includes factors that increase or decrease the pain, such as eating, defecation, and activities.

Endoscopy, CT scan, MRI, laparoscopy, and barium studies may be done. Treatment for chronic abdominal pain depends on the underlying cause.

## IRRITABLE BOWEL SYNDROME

**Irritable bowel syndrome (IBS)** is a disorder characterized by chronic abdominal pain or discomfort and alteration of bowel patterns. Diarrhea or constipation may predominate, or they may alternate. As a functional GI disorder, IBS has no known organic cause.

The manifestations of IBS are intermittent and may occur for years. Patients often report a history of GI infections and food intolerances. However, the role of food allergies in IBS is unclear. Other dietary factors that may contribute to symptoms include fermentable oligo-, di-, and monosaccharides and polyols (FODMAPs). Examples include fructans (found in wheat, rye, onions, garlic, and legumes), galactans, lactose (found in milk and yogurt), fructose (found in honey, apples, pears, and high-fructose corn syrup), sorbitol, and xylitol. Psychologic stressors (e.g., depression, anxiety, sexual abuse, posttraumatic stress disorder) are associated with development and exacerbation of IBS.

IBS is diagnosed solely on symptoms. The Rome III criteria for diagnosing IBS require the presence of abdominal pain and/or discomfort at least 3 months that is associated with two or more of the following: improvement with defecation, change in stool frequency at onset, or change in the stool appearance at onset.[8] Depending on the stool patterns, IBS is categorized as IBS with constipation, IBS with diarrhea, IBS mixed, and IBS unsubtyped. Other common symptoms include abdominal distention, nausea, flatulence, bloating, urgency, mucus in the stool, and sensation of incomplete evacuation. Non-GI symptoms may include fatigue, headache, and sleep disturbances.

### GENDER DIFFERENCES
#### *Irritable Bowel Syndrome (IBS)*

| Men | Women |
|---|---|
| • More likely to have IBS with diarrhea<br>• Less likely to admit to symptoms or seek help for them<br>• Experience more interpersonal difficulties | • Affects women 2 to 2.5 times more often than men<br>• More likely to have IBS with constipation<br>• Report more extraintestinal co-morbidities (e.g., migraine headache, insomnia, fibromyalgia) |

The key to accurate diagnosis is a thorough history and physical examination. Ask patients to describe symptoms, past health history (including psychosocial factors such as stress and anxiety), family history, and drug and diet history. Determine if and how IBS symptoms interfere with school, work, or recreational activities. Diagnostic tests are selectively used to rule out other disorders such as colorectal cancer, IBD, endometriosis, and malabsorption disorders (lactose intolerance, celiac disease).

No single therapy is effective for all patients with IBS. Treatment may include dealing with psychologic factors, dietary changes, and drugs to regulate stool output and reduce discomfort. Patients may benefit from keeping a diary of symptoms, diet, and episodes of stress to help identify any factors that trigger the IBS symptoms. Cognitive behavior therapy and stress management techniques may help a patient cope. Participating in regular exercise reduces bloating and constipation as well as reduces symptoms of anxiety and depression. Acupuncture and hypnosis can also be used.

Review with the patient foods that are high in FODMAPs and teach them to follow a low FODMAP diet.[9] Advise the patient whose primary symptoms are abdominal distention and flatulence to avoid common gas-producing foods such as broccoli and cabbage. If dairy products tend to cause symptoms, yogurt may be the best option because of the lactobacillus bacteria it contains. Some patients benefit from certain probiotic combinations. For those with constipation, encourage an intake of enough dietary fiber to produce soft, painless bowel movements.

Drug therapy is individualized. Antispasmodic medications (hyoscyamine, dicyclomine [Bentyl]) decrease GI motility and smooth muscle spasms, reducing pain and diarrhea. An option for women with severe pain and diarrhea is alosetron (Lotronex). Because of serious side effects (e.g., severe constipation, ischemic colitis), it is available only in a restricted access program for those who have not responded to other IBS therapies.

**DRUG ALERT Alosetron (Lotronex)**

- Patients taking this drug may experience severe constipation and ischemic colitis (reduced blood flow to intestines).
- Teach the patient to discontinue the drug and contact the HCP if constipation, rectal bleeding, bloody diarrhea, or abdominal pain occurs.

Loperamide (Imodium), a synthetic opioid that slows intestinal transit, is another option for those with diarrhea. Eluxadoline (Viberzi) is used to treat the symptoms of diarrhea and abdominal pain.

Women with IBS with constipation may benefit from lubiprostone (Amitiza). Men or women with constipation symptoms can take linaclotide (Linzess). It is contraindicated in patients with a history of mechanical obstruction or prior bowel surgery. Low doses of tricyclic antidepressants and selective serotonin reuptake inhibitors (SSRIs) may reduce symptoms.[8]

## ABDOMINAL TRAUMA

### Etiology and Pathophysiology

Injuries to the abdominal area usually are a result of blunt trauma or penetrating injuries. Common injuries of the abdomen include lacerated liver, ruptured spleen, mesenteric artery tears, diaphragm rupture, urinary bladder rupture, great vessel tears, renal or pancreas injury, and stomach or intestine rupture.

*Blunt trauma* commonly occurs with motor vehicle accidents, direct blows, and falls and may not be obvious because it does not leave an open wound. Both compression injuries (e.g., direct blow to the abdomen) and shearing injuries (e.g., rapid deceleration in a motor vehicle crash allowing some tissue to move forward while other tissues stay stationary) occur with blunt trauma. *Penetrating injuries* occur when a gunshot or stabbing produces an obvious, open wound into the abdomen.

When solid organs (liver, spleen) are injured, bleeding can be profuse, resulting in hypovolemic shock. When contents from hollow organs (e.g., bladder, stomach, intestines) spill into the peritoneal cavity, the patient is at risk for peritonitis. In addition, abdominal compartment syndrome can develop.

*Abdominal compartment syndrome*, or abdominal hypertension, is excessively high pressure in the abdomen. Anything that increases the volume in the abdominal cavity (e.g., edematous organs, bleeding) increases abdominal pressure. High abdominal pressure restricts ventilation, potentially leading to respiratory failure. The high pressure decreases cardiac output, venous return, and arterial perfusion of organs. Decreased perfusion to the kidneys can lead to renal failure.

### Clinical Manifestations

Careful assessment provides important clues to the type and severity of injury. Intraabdominal injuries are often associated with rib fractures, fractured pelvis, spinal injury, and thoracic injury. If the patient was in an automobile accident, a contusion or abrasion across the lower abdomen may indicate internal organ trauma due to seat belt use. Seat belts can produce blunt trauma to abdominal organs by pressing the intestine and pancreas into the spinal column.

Classic manifestations of abdominal trauma are (1) guarding and splinting of the abdominal wall (indicating peritonitis); (2) a hard, distended abdomen (indicating intraabdominal bleeding); (3) decreased or absent bowel sounds; (4) abrasions or bruising over the abdomen; (5) abdominal pain; (6) hematemesis or hematuria; and (7) signs of hypovolemic shock (Table 42-11). Ecchymosis around the umbilicus *(Cullen's sign)* or flanks *(Grey Turner's sign)* may indicate retroperitoneal hemorrhage. Loss of bowel sounds occurs with peritonitis. If the diaphragm ruptures, you can hear bowel sounds (if present) in the chest. Auscultation of bruits is indicative of arterial damage.

### Diagnostic Studies

Laboratory tests include a baseline CBC and urinalysis. Even when bleeding, the patient will have normal hemoglobin and hematocrit because fluids are lost at the same rate as the red blood cells. Deficiencies are evident after fluid resuscitation begins. Blood in the urine may be a sign of kidney or bladder damage. Additional laboratory work includes arterial blood gases, prothrombin time, electrolytes, BUN and creatinine, and type and crossmatch (in anticipation of possible blood transfusions). An abdominal CT scan and focused abdominal ultrasound are the most common diagnostic methods, but the patient must be stable before going for CT.

Diagnostic peritoneal lavage can be used to detect blood, bile, intestinal contents, and urine in the peritoneal cavity. It is generally used only for unstable patients to identify blood in the peritoneum.

## ❖ NURSING AND INTERPROFESSIONAL MANAGEMENT: ABDOMINAL TRAUMA

Emergency management of abdominal trauma is presented in Table 42-11. IV access is established, and volume expanders or blood given if the patient is hypotensive. An NG tube with low suction will decompress the stomach and prevent aspiration. Frequent ongoing assessment is necessary to monitor fluid status, detect deterioration in condition, and determine the necessity for surgery. Do not remove an impaled object until skilled care is available. Removal may cause further injury and bleeding. The decision about whether to do surgery depends on clinical findings, diagnostic test results, and the patient's response to conservative management.

## TABLE 42-11 Emergency Management

### *Abdominal Trauma*

| Etiology | Assessment Findings | Interventions |
|---|---|---|
| **Blunt**<br>• Falls<br>• Motor vehicle collisions<br>• Pedestrian event<br>• Assault with blunt object<br>• Crush injuries<br>• Explosions<br>**Penetrating**<br>• Knife<br>• Gunshot wounds<br>• Impalement<br>• Other missiles | **Hypovolemic Shock**<br>• ↓ Level of consciousness<br>• Tachypnea<br>• Tachycardia<br>• ↓ BP<br>• ↓ Pulse pressure<br>**Surface Findings**<br>• Abrasions or ecchymoses on abdominal wall, flank, or peritoneum<br>• Open wounds: lacerations, eviscerations, puncture wounds, gunshot wounds<br>• Impaled object<br>**Abdominal and GI Findings**<br>• Nausea and vomiting<br>• Hematemesis<br>• Absent or decreased bowel sounds<br>• Hematuria<br>• Abdominal distention<br>• Abdominal rigidity<br>• Abdominal pain with palpation<br>• Rebound tenderness | **Initial**<br>• If unresponsive, assess circulation, airway, and breathing.<br>• If responsive, monitor airway, breathing, and circulation.<br>• Administer appropriate $O_2$ therapy.<br>• Control external bleeding with direct pressure or sterile pressure dressing.<br>• Establish IV access with two large-bore catheters and infuse normal saline or lactated Ringer's solution.<br>• Obtain blood for type and crossmatch and CBC.<br>• Remove clothing.<br>• Stabilize impaled objects with bulky dressing—*do not remove.*<br>• Cover protruding organs or tissue with sterile saline dressing.<br>• Insert indwelling urinary catheter if there is no blood at the meatus, pelvic fracture, or boggy prostate.<br>• Obtain urine for urinalysis.<br>• Insert NG tube if no evidence of facial trauma.<br>• Anticipate diagnostic peritoneal lavage.<br>**Ongoing Monitoring**<br>• Monitor vital signs, level of consciousness, $O_2$ saturation, and urine output.<br>• Maintain patient warmth using blankets, warm IV fluids, or warm humidified $O_2$. |

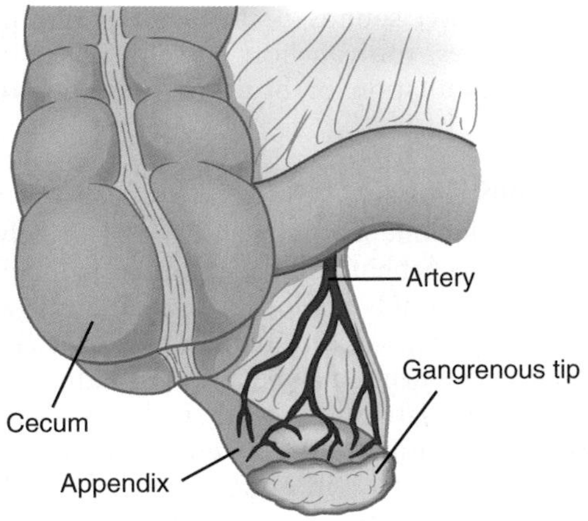


**FIG. 42-2** In appendicitis the blood supply of the appendix is impaired by inflammation and bacterial infection, which may result in gangrene.

# INFLAMMATORY DISORDERS

## APPENDICITIS

**Appendicitis** is inflammation of the appendix, a narrow blind tube that extends from the inferior part of the cecum (Fig. 42-2). It is the most common reason for emergency abdominal surgery.

### Etiology and Pathophysiology

About 7% of people will develop appendicitis sometime during their lifetime.[10] It is most common in individuals 10 to 30 years of age. A common cause of appendicitis is obstruction of the lumen by a fecalith (accumulated feces). Obstruction results in distention; venous engorgement; and the accumulation of mucus and bacteria, which can lead to gangrene, perforation, and peritonitis.

### Clinical Manifestations

Diagnosis can be difficult because many patients do not have classic symptoms. Appendicitis typically begins with dull periumbilical pain, followed by anorexia, nausea, and vomiting. The pain is persistent and continuous, eventually shifting to the right lower quadrant and localizing at *McBurney's point* (halfway between the umbilicus and right iliac crest). A low-grade fever may develop. Further assessment reveals localized tenderness, rigidity, rebound tenderness, and muscle guarding. Coughing, sneezing, and deep inhalation worsen pain. The patient usually prefers to lie still, often with the right leg flexed. The older adult may report less severe pain, slight fever, and discomfort in the right iliac fossa.

### Diagnostic Studies and Interprofessional Care

Patient examination includes a complete history, physical examination, and a differential WBC count. Most patients have a mildly to moderately elevated WBC count. A urinalysis is done to rule out genitourinary conditions that mimic appendicitis. CT scan is the preferred diagnostic procedure. However, ultrasound and MRI are also used.

If there is a delay in diagnosis and treatment, the appendix can rupture and the resulting peritonitis can be fatal. The treatment of appendicitis is an immediate *appendectomy* (surgical removal of appendix). If the inflammation is localized, surgery should be done as soon as the diagnosis is made. Antibiotics and fluid resuscitation are started before surgery.

If the appendix has ruptured and there is evidence of peritonitis or an abscess, giving parenteral fluids and antibiotic therapy for 6 to 8 hours before the appendectomy helps prevent dehydration and sepsis.

## NURSING MANAGEMENT: APPENDICITIS

Managing the patient presenting with manifestations of appendicitis focuses on preventing fluid volume deficit, relieving pain, and preventing complications. To ensure the stomach is empty in case surgery is needed, keep the patient on nothing-by-mouth (NPO) status until the HCP evaluates the patient. Monitor vital signs and perform ongoing assessment to detect any deterioration in condition. Administer IV fluids, analgesics, and antiemetics as ordered. Provide comfort measures.

Postoperative care for the patient who had an appendectomy is similar to the patient after a laparotomy. Patients are usually discharged within 24 hours following an uncomplicated laparoscopic appendectomy. Ambulation begins a few hours after surgery and the diet advanced as tolerated. Most patients resume normal activities 2 to 3 weeks after surgery.

**CHECK YOUR PRACTICE**

A 28-yr-old female patient comes to the emergency department with acute abdominal pain.

- What manifestations would make you suspect appendicitis is the cause of the patient's abdominal pain rather than other causes of abdominal pain?

## PERITONITIS

### Etiology and Pathophysiology

**Peritonitis** results from a localized or generalized inflammatory process of the peritoneum. Causes of peritonitis are listed in Table 42-12. Primary peritonitis occurs when blood-borne organisms enter the peritoneal cavity. For example, the ascites that occurs with cirrhosis of the liver provides an excellent liquid environment for bacteria to flourish. Organisms can enter the peritoneum during peritoneal dialysis. (Peritoneal dialysis is described in Chapter 46.)

Secondary peritonitis is much more common. It occurs when abdominal organs perforate or rupture and release their contents (bile, enzymes, and bacteria) into the peritoneal cavity. Common causes include a ruptured appendix, perforated gastric or duodenal ulcer, severely inflamed gallbladder, and trauma from gunshot or knife wounds.

Intestinal contents and bacteria irritate the normally sterile peritoneum and produce an initial chemical peritonitis. Bacterial peritonitis develops a few hours later. The resulting inflammatory response leads to massive fluid shifts (peritoneal edema) and adhesions as the body attempts to wall off the infection.

### Clinical Manifestations

Abdominal pain is the most common symptom of peritonitis. A universal sign is tenderness over the involved area. Rebound tenderness, muscular rigidity, and spasm are other signs of peritoneal irritation. Patients may lie still and take only shallow breaths because movement worsens the pain. Abdominal distention, fever, tachycardia, tachypnea, nausea, vomiting, and altered bowel habits may be present. These manifestations vary, depending on the severity and acuteness of the underlying condition. Complications of peritonitis include hypovolemic shock, sepsis, intraabdominal abscess formation, paralytic ileus, and acute respiratory distress syndrome. Peritonitis can be fatal if treatment is delayed.

**TABLE 42-12 Causes of Peritonitis**

| Primary | Secondary |
|---|---|
| • Blood-borne organisms<br>• Genital tract organisms<br>• Cirrhosis with ascites | • Appendicitis with rupture<br>• Blunt or penetrating trauma to abdominal organs<br>• Diverticulitis with rupture<br>• Ischemic bowel disorders<br>• Pancreatitis<br>• Perforated intestine<br>• Perforated peptic ulcer<br>• Peritoneal dialysis<br>• Postoperative (breakage of anastomosis) |

### Diagnostic Studies and Interprofessional Care

A CBC is done to determine elevations in WBC count and hemoconcentration from fluid shifts (Table 42-13). Peritoneal aspiration may be performed and the fluid analyzed for blood, bile, pus, bacteria, fungus, and amylase content. An abdominal x-ray may show dilated loops of bowel consistent with paralytic ileus, free air if perforation has occurred, or air and fluid levels if an obstruction is present. Ultrasound and CT scans may be useful in identifying ascites and abscesses. Peritoneoscopy may be helpful in the patient without ascites. It allows for direct examination of the peritoneum and the ability to obtain biopsy specimens for diagnosis.

Patients with milder cases of peritonitis or those who are poor surgical risks receive conservative care. Treatment consists of antibiotics, NG suction, analgesics, and IV fluid administration. Surgery is indicated to locate the cause of the inflammation, drain purulent fluid, and repair any damage (e.g., perforated organs).

## NURSING MANAGEMENT: PERITONITIS

### Nursing Assessment

Assessment of the patient's pain, including the location, is important and may help to determine the cause of peritonitis.

**TABLE 42-13 Interprofessional Care**

***Peritonitis***

**Diagnostic Assessment**

- History and physical examination
- CBC, including WBC differential
- Serum electrolytes
- Abdominal x-ray
- Abdominal paracentesis and culture of fluid
- CT scan or ultrasound
- Peritoneoscopy

**Management**

***Preoperative or Nonoperative***

- NPO status
- IV fluid replacement
- NG to low-intermittent suction
- $O_2$ PRN
- Parenteral nutrition as needed

*Drug Therapy*

- Antibiotic therapy
- Analgesics (e.g., morphine)
- Antiemetics as needed

***Postoperative***

- NPO status
- NG to low-intermittent suction
- Semi-Fowler's position
- IV fluids with electrolyte replacement
- Parenteral nutrition as needed
- Blood transfusions as needed

*Drug Therapy*

- Antibiotic therapy
- Sedatives and opioids
- Antiemetics as needed

Assess the patient for the presence and quality of bowel sounds, increasing abdominal distention, abdominal guarding, nausea, fever, and manifestations of hypovolemic shock.

### ◆ Nursing Diagnoses

Nursing diagnoses for the patient with peritonitis include, but are not limited to, the following:

- Acute pain *related to* inflammation of the peritoneum and abdominal distention
- Risk for deficient fluid volume *related to* fluid shifts into the peritoneal cavity secondary to trauma, infection, or ischemia
- Anxiety *related to* uncertainty of cause or outcome of the condition and pain

### ◆ Planning

The overall goals are that the patient with peritonitis will have (1) resolution of inflammation, (2) relief of abdominal pain, (3) freedom from complications (especially sepsis and hypovolemic shock), and (4) normal nutritional status.

### ◆ Nursing Implementation

The patient with peritonitis is extremely ill and needs skilled supportive care. Establish IV access so that you can administer replacement fluids lost to the peritoneal cavity and have access for antibiotic therapy. Monitor the patient for pain and response to analgesics. You may position the patient with knees flexed to increase comfort. Sedatives may be given to relieve anxiety.

Accurate monitoring of fluid intake and output and electrolyte status is necessary to determine replacement therapy. Frequently monitor vital signs. Administer antiemetics to decrease nausea and vomiting and prevent further fluid and electrolyte losses. Place the patient on NPO status. The patient may need an NG tube to decrease gastric distention and further leakage of bowel contents into the peritoneum. Administer low-flow oxygen therapy as needed.

If the patient had an open surgical procedure, drains are inserted to remove purulent drainage and excess fluid. Postoperative care is similar to that of the patient who had a laparotomy.

## GASTROENTERITIS

Gastroenteritis is an inflammation of the mucosa of the stomach and small intestine. Features of *acute gastroenteritis* are sudden diarrhea accompanied by nausea, vomiting, fever, and abdominal cramping. Viruses are the most common cause of gastroenteritis (Table 42-1).

*Norovirus* is a leading cause of foodborne outbreaks of acute gastroenteritis. Laboratory testing to identify norovirus is useful when a number of people have simultaneously contracted gastroenteritis and there is a clear avenue for virus transmission, such as a shared location or food.

Most cases of gastroenteritis are self-limiting. Encourage oral fluids containing glucose and electrolytes (e.g., Pedialyte) to prevent and treat dehydration. Older adults and chronically ill patients may be unable to consume enough fluids to compensate for fluid loss. If dehydration occurs, IV fluid replacement may be necessary. Nursing management of the patient with gastroenteritis is the same as for the patient with acute diarrhea (see pp. 932-933).

## INFLAMMATORY BOWEL DISEASE

Inflammatory bowel disease (IBD) is a chronic inflammation of the GI tract characterized by periods of remission interspersed with periods of exacerbation. The exact cause is unknown, and there is no cure. IBD is classified as either Crohn's disease or ulcerative colitis based on clinical manifestations (Table 42-14). As the name suggests, ulcerative colitis is usually limited to the colon. Crohn's disease can involve any segment of the GI tract from the mouth to the anus.

Both ulcerative colitis and Crohn's disease commonly occur during the teenage years and early adulthood, and both have a second peak in the sixth decade. IBD occurs more commonly in people of white and Ashkenazic Jewish origin than in other racial and ethnic groups. Many people with IBD have a family member with the disorder.

### Etiology and Pathophysiology

IBD is an autoimmune disease involving an immune reaction to a person's own intestinal tract. Some agent or a combination of agents triggers an overactive, inappropriate, sustained immune response. The resulting inflammation causes widespread tissue destruction.

IBD is caused by a combination of factors, including environmental factors, genetic predisposition, and alterations in immune function. Environmental factors such as diet, exposure to air pollution, stress, and smoking increase susceptibility by influencing the environment of the GI microbial flora and the immune system. IBD is more prevalent in industrialized countries. Dietary factors unique to these countries contribute to the development of IBD. High dietary intake of total fats, polyunsaturated fatty acid (PUFA), omega-6 fatty acids, and meat is associated with an increased risk of IBD. High fiber and fruit intake is associated with a decreased risk of Crohn's disease, whereas a high vegetable intake is associated with a decreased risk of ulcerative colitis.[11] Oral contraceptives and nonsteroidal antiinflammatory drugs (NSAIDs) exacerbate Crohn's disease.

### Genetic Link

IBD occurs more frequently in family members of people with IBD, especially monozygotic twins. Numerous genome-wide association studies have confirmed a genetic predisposition. Certain genetic mutations are associated with Crohn's disease, others are associated with ulcerative colitis, and many are associated with both. IBD is more likely to occur in those with other genetic syndromes, including cystic fibrosis. An increased prevalence occurs in the presence of other inflammatory disorders with genetic susceptibility, such as psoriasis and multiple sclerosis.[12]

The recent identification of the first gene associated with Crohn's disease, the *NOD2* gene, was a major breakthrough. *NOD2* gene changes are associated with a form of Crohn's disease that affects the ileum in persons of northern European descent. Changes in the *NOD2* gene trigger an abnormal immune response that allows bacteria to grow unchecked and invade intestinal cells, causing chronic inflammation and digestive problems.[13]

The discovery of numerous gene variations suggests that IBD is a group of diseases that produce similar types of mucosal destruction. A genetically susceptible person who is not exposed to a triggering agent will not become ill, and a person who is not genetically susceptible will not develop IBD even if exposed to a triggering agent. The pathway from genetic mutation to

**TABLE 42-14 Comparison of Ulcerative Colitis and Crohn's Disease**

| Characteristic | Ulcerative Colitis | Crohn's Disease |
|---|---|---|
| **Clinical** | | |
| Usual age at onset | Teens to mid-30s. After 60 | Teens to mid-30s. After 60 |
| Diarrhea | Common | Common |
| Abdominal pain | Common, severe constant | Common, cramping |
| Fever (intermittent) | During acute attacks | Common |
| Weight loss | Rare | Common, may be severe |
| Rectal bleeding | Common | Sometimes |
| Tenesmus | Common | Rare |
| Malabsorption and nutritional deficiencies | Minimal incidence | Common |
| **Pathologic** | | |
| Location | Usually starts in rectum and spreads in a continuous pattern up the colon | Occurs anywhere along GI tract. Most frequent site is distal ileum. |
| Small bowel involvement | Minimal | Common |
| Distribution | Continuous areas of inflammation | Healthy tissue interspersed with areas of inflammation (skip lesions) |
| Depth of involvement | Mucosa | Entire thickness of bowel wall (transmural) |
| Cobblestoning of mucosa | Rare | Common |
| Pseudopolyps | Common | Rare |
| **Complications** | | |
| Perianal abscess and fistulas | Rare | Common |
| Strictures | Occasional | Common |
| *C. difficile* infection | Increased incidence and severity | Increased incidence and severity |
| Perforation | Common (because of toxic megacolon) | Common (because inflammation involves entire bowel wall) |
| Toxic megacolon | More common | Rare |
| Carcinoma | Increased incidence of colorectal cancer after 10 yr of disease | Increased incidence of small intestinal cancer<br>Increased incidence of colorectal cancer but not as much as with ulcerative colitis |

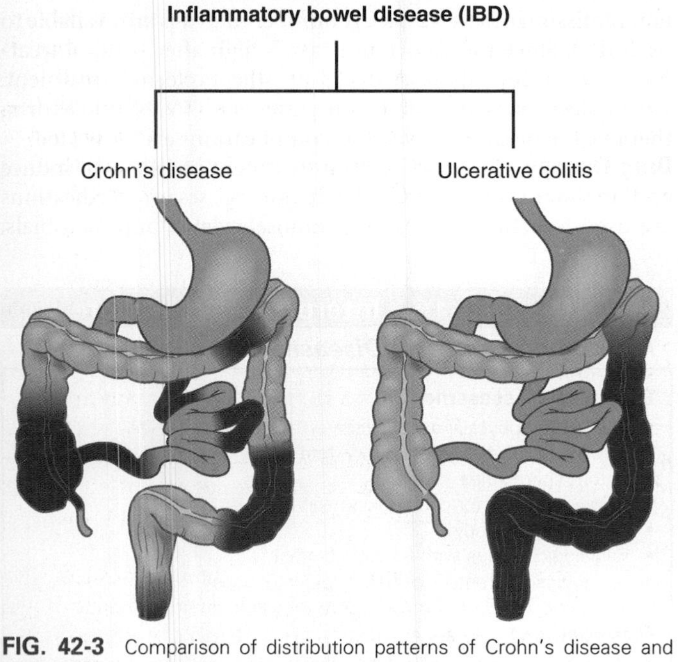


**FIG. 42-3** Comparison of distribution patterns of Crohn's disease and ulcerative colitis.

abnormal immune responses varies depending on which gene or genes are affected. This genetic variation may explain differences in patient responses to various drug therapies for IBD.

**Pattern of Inflammation in Ulcerative Colitis vs. Crohn's Disease.** The pattern of inflammation differs between Crohn's disease and ulcerative colitis (Fig. 42-3). Crohn's disease can occur anywhere in the GI tract from the mouth to the anus but most commonly involves the distal ileum and proximal colon. Segments of normal bowel can occur between diseased portions, so-called "skip" lesions (Table 42-14). The inflammation in Crohn's disease involves all layers of the bowel wall. Typically, ulcerations are deep and longitudinal and penetrate between islands of inflamed edematous mucosa, causing the classic cobblestone appearance. Strictures at the areas of inflammation can cause bowel obstruction. Since the inflammation goes through the entire wall, microscopic leaks can allow bowel contents to enter the peritoneal cavity and form abscesses or produce peritonitis. In active Crohn's disease, fistulas are common.

Ulcerative colitis usually starts in the rectum and moves in a continual fashion toward the cecum. Although mild inflammation may occur in the terminal ileum, ulcerative colitis is a disease of the colon and rectum. The inflammation and ulcerations occur in the mucosal layer, the innermost layer of the bowel wall. Fistulas and abscesses are rare since inflammation does not extend through all bowel wall layers. Because water and electrolytes are not absorbed through inflamed mucosa, diarrhea with large fluid and electrolyte losses is common. Breakdown of cells results in protein loss through the stool. Areas of inflamed mucosa form *pseudopolyps,* tongue-like projections into the bowel lumen.

## Clinical Manifestations

Both forms of IBD are chronic disorders with mild to severe acute exacerbations that occur at unpredictable intervals over many years. Although the manifestations of Crohn's disease and ulcerative colitis are similar (diarrhea, weight loss, abdominal pain, fever, and fatigue), there are differences (Table 42-14).

In Crohn's disease, diarrhea and cramping abdominal pain are common symptoms. If the small intestine is involved, weight loss occurs from inflammation of the small intestine causing malabsorption. Rectal bleeding sometimes occurs with Crohn's disease, although not as often as with ulcerative colitis.

In ulcerative colitis, the primary manifestations are bloody diarrhea and abdominal pain. Pain may vary from the mild lower abdominal cramping associated with diarrhea to severe, constant pain associated with acute perforations. With *mild disease,* diarrhea may consist of no more than four semi-formed stools daily that contain small amounts of blood. The patient may have no other manifestations. In *moderate disease,* the patient has increased stool output (up to 10 stools/day), increased bleeding, and systemic symptoms (fever, malaise, mild anemia, anorexia). In *severe disease,* diarrhea is bloody, contains mucus, and occurs 10 to 20 times a day. In addition, fever, rapid weight loss greater than 10% of total body weight, anemia, tachycardia, and dehydration are present.

## Complications

Patients with IBD experience both local (confined to the GI tract) and systemic (extraintestinal) complications (Table 42-15). GI tract complications include hemorrhage, strictures, perforation (with possible peritonitis), abscesses, fistulas, CDI, and colonic dilation (toxic megacolon). Patients with toxic megacolon are at risk of perforation and may need an emergency colectomy. Toxic megacolon is more common with ulcerative colitis. Perineal abscess and fistulas occur in up to a third of patients with Crohn's disease. CDI increases in frequency and severity in patients with IBD.[14]

Hemorrhage may lead to anemia. Blood transfusions and iron supplements are used to treat the anemia. Nutritional problems are especially common in Crohn's disease when the terminal ileum is involved. Bile salts and cobalamin are exclusively absorbed in the terminal ileum. Thus disease in the terminal ileum can result in fat malabsorption and anemia.

Patients with a history of IBD have an increased risk for colorectal cancer. Those with Crohn's disease are at increased risk for small intestinal cancer. Cancer screening at regular intervals is important in persons with IBD.

Some people with IBD suffer from systemic complications, including joint, eye, mouth, kidney, bone, vascular, and skin problems (Table 42-15). Circulating factors such as cytokines trigger inflammation in these areas. Routine liver function tests are important because primary sclerosing cholangitis, a complication of IBD, can lead to liver failure.

## Diagnostic Studies

The diagnosis of IBD includes ruling out other diseases with similar symptoms and then determining whether the patient has Crohn's disease or ulcerative colitis. The symptoms of early Crohn's disease are similar to those of IBS. Diagnostic studies provide information about disease severity and complications. A CBC typically shows iron-deficiency anemia from blood loss. An elevated WBC count may be an indication of toxic megacolon or perforation. Decreased serum sodium, potassium, chloride, bicarbonate, and magnesium levels occur due to fluid and electrolyte losses from diarrhea and vomiting. Hypoalbuminemia is present with severe disease because of poor nutrition or protein loss. Elevated erythrocyte sedimentation rate, C-reactive protein, and WBCs reflect inflammation. The stool is examined for blood, pus, and mucus. Stool cultures can determine if infection is present.

Imaging studies such as double-contrast barium enema, small bowel series (small bowel follow through), transabdominal ultrasound, CT, and MRI are useful for diagnosing IBD. Colonoscopy allows for examination of the entire large intestine lumen and sometimes the most distal ileum. The extent of inflammation, ulcerations, pseudopolyps, and strictures is determined, and biopsy specimens taken for a definitive diagnosis. Since a colonoscope can enter only the distal ileum, capsule endoscopy (see Chapter 38) may be used to diagnose Crohn's disease in the small intestine.

### TABLE 42-15 Extraintestinal Complications of IBD

| | |
|---|---|
| **Joints** | **Eye** |
| • Peripheral arthritis (colitic) | • Conjunctivitis |
| • Ankylosing spondylitis | • Uveitis |
| • Sacroiliitis | • Episcleritis |
| • Finger clubbing | |
| **Skin** | **Other** |
| • Erythema nodosum | • Gallstones |
| • Pyoderma gangrenosum | • Kidney stones |
| | • Liver disease: primary sclerosing cholangitis |
| **Mouth** | • Osteoporosis |
| • Aphthous ulcers | • Thromboembolism |

## Interprofessional Care

The goals of treatment of IBD are to (1) rest the bowel, (2) control the inflammation, (3) combat infection, (4) correct malnutrition, (5) alleviate stress, (6) provide symptomatic relief, and (7) improve quality of life. Since the cause is unknown, treatment relies on drugs to treat the inflammation and maintain remission (Table 42-16). A number of drugs are available to treat IBD. Since the recurrence rate is high after surgical treatment of Crohn's disease, drugs are the preferred treatment. Hospitalization is indicated if the patient fails to respond to drug therapy, the disease is severe, or complications are suspected.

**Drug Therapy.** The goal of drug treatment in IBD is to induce and maintain remission. Five major classes of medications are used to achieve this goal: aminosalicylates, antimicrobials,

### TABLE 42-16 Interprofessional Care
#### *Inflammatory Bowel Disease*

**Diagnostic Assessment**
- History and physical examination
- CBC, erythrocyte sedimentation rate
- Serum chemistries
- Testing of stool for occult blood and infection
- Capsule endoscopy
- Radiologic studies with barium contrast
- Sigmoidoscopy and/or colonoscopy with biopsy

**Management**
- High-calorie, high-vitamin, high-protein, low-residue, lactose-free (if lactase deficiency) diet
- Elemental diet or parenteral nutrition
- Drug therapy (Table 42-17)
  - Aminosalicylates
  - Antimicrobials
  - Corticosteroids
  - Immunosuppressants
  - Biologic and targeted therapy (immunomodulators)
- Physical and emotional rest
- Referral for counseling or support group
- Surgical therapy (Table 42-18)

**TABLE 42-17 Drug Therapy**
***Inflammatory Bowel Disease***

| Class | Action | Examples |
|---|---|---|
| **5-Aminosalicylates (5-ASA)** | Decrease inflammation by suppressing proinflammatory cytokines and other inflammatory mediators | *Systemic:* sulfasalazine (Azulfidine), mesalamine (Asacol, Pentasa), olsalazine (Dipentum), balsalazide (Colazal)<br>*Topical:* 5-ASA enema (Rowasa), mesalamine suppositories (Canasa) |
| **Antimicrobials** | Prevent or treat secondary infection | metronidazole (Flagyl), ciprofloxacin (Cipro), clarithromycin (Biaxin) |
| **Corticosteroids** | Decrease inflammation | *Systemic:* corticosteroids (prednisone, budesonide [Uceris]) (oral); hydrocortisone or methylprednisolone (IV for severe IBD)<br>*Topical:* hydrocortisone suppository or foam (Cortifoam) or enema (Cortenema) |
| **Immunosuppressants** | Suppress immune response | azathioprine (Imuran), 6-mercaptopurine (6-MP), methotrexate, cyclosporine |
| **Biologic and targeted therapy (immunomodulators)** | Inhibit the cytokine tumor necrosis factor (TNF) | infliximab (Remicade), adalimumab (Humira), certolizumab pegol (Cimzia), golimumab (Simponi) |
| | Prevent migration of leukocytes from bloodstream to inflamed tissue | natalizumab (Tysabri), vedolizumab (Entyvio) |

corticosteroids, immunosuppressants, and biologic and targeted therapy (Table 42-17). Drug selection depends on the location and severity of inflammation. Patients are treated with either a "step-up" or a "step-down" approach. With the step-up approach, the patient begins with less toxic therapies (e.g., aminosalicylates and antimicrobials) and is started on more toxic medications (e.g., biologic and targeted therapy) when initial therapies do not work. The step-down approach uses biologic and targeted therapy first.

Medications containing 5-aminosalicylic acid (5-ASA) remain a mainstay in achieving and maintaining remission and preventing flare-ups of IBD. They include sulfasalazine (Azulfidine) and the new generation of sulfa-free drugs (olsalazine [Dipentum], mesalamine [Pentasa]). Aminosalicylates are more effective for ulcerative colitis. However, they are first-line therapies for mild to moderate Crohn's disease, especially when the colon is involved.

The exact mechanism of action of 5-ASA is unknown, but topical application to the intestinal mucosa suppresses proinflammatory cytokines and other inflammatory mediators. The benefits of these drugs usually depend on the dose: the larger the dose, the more likely patients will improve during the acute phase and remain in remission. However, many people cannot tolerate the side effects of sulfasalazine. Headaches, nausea, and fatigue occur at the higher doses. In men, long-term sulfasalazine treatment may cause abnormal sperm production, leading to infertility. These effects are reversible if sulfasalazine is discontinued.

**DRUG ALERT Sulfasalazine (Azulfidine)**
- May cause yellowish orange discoloration of skin and urine
- Avoid exposure to sunlight and ultraviolet light until photosensitivity is determined.

The sulfa-free drugs are as effective as sulfasalazine and better tolerated when administered orally. Topical 5-ASA preparations include rectal suppositories and enemas. Topical treatment offers the advantage of delivering the 5-ASA directly to the affected tissue and minimizing systemic effects. The combination of oral and rectal therapy is better than oral or rectal therapy alone.

Corticosteroids are used to achieve remission in IBD. They are given for the shortest possible time because of side effects associated with long-term use. Patients with disease in the left colon, sigmoid, and rectum benefit from suppositories, enemas, and foams because they deliver the corticosteroid directly to the inflamed tissue with minimal systemic effects. Oral prednisone is given to patients with mild to moderate disease who did not respond to either 5-ASA or topical corticosteroids. Those with severe inflammation may require a short course of IV corticosteroids. Corticosteroids must be tapered to very low levels when surgery is planned to prevent postoperative complications (e.g., infection, delayed wound healing, fistula formation).

Immunosuppressants (6-mercaptopurine, azathioprine [Imuran]) are given to maintain remission after corticosteroid induction therapy. These drugs require regular CBC monitoring because they can suppress the bone marrow and lead to inflammation of the pancreas or liver. They have a delayed onset of action and are therefore not useful for acute flare-ups.

Methotrexate is most useful in patients with Crohn's disease who cannot stop corticosteroid use without a flare-up or in whom other medications have been ineffective. Many patients have flu-like symptoms with use, and some develop bone marrow depression and liver dysfunction. Correct dosing is critical to minimize the risk of toxicity. Careful monitoring of the CBC and liver enzymes is essential. Advise women of childbearing age to avoid pregnancy because use causes birth defects and fetal death.

Currently there are six biologic and targeted medications.[15] Four are antitumor necrosis factor (TNF) agents: infliximab (Remicade), adalimumab (Humira), certolizumab pegol (Cimzia) and golimumab (Simponi). Infliximab is a monoclonal antibody to TNF (proinflammatory cytokine). This drug is given IV to induce and maintain remission in patients with Crohn's disease and in patients with draining fistulas who do not respond to conventional drug therapy. The other TNF agents are given subcutaneously and have effects similar to those of infliximab.

The anti-TNF agents have similar side effects. The most common adverse effects are upper respiratory and urinary tract infections, headaches, nausea, joint pain, and abdominal pain. More serious effects include reactivation of hepatitis and tuberculosis (TB); opportunistic infections; and malignancies, especially lymphoma. Patients need to know the risks before starting therapy. They are tested for TB and hepatitis before treatment begins and cannot receive live virus immunizations. Teaching includes how to prevent infection and recognize early signs and symptoms (e.g., fever, cough, malaise, dyspnea).

Two biologic and targeted medications are integrin receptor antagonists: natalizumab (Tysabri) and vedolizumab (Entyvio). They inhibit leukocyte adhesion by blocking $\alpha_4$-integrin, an adhesion molecule. The use of integrin receptor antagonists is limited to those who have not had an adequate response with other therapies (corticosteroids, immunosuppressants, or TNF agents). Both are given by IV infusion. Their use is associated

**TABLE 42-18 Indications for Surgical Therapy for IBD**

- Drainage of abdominal abscess
- Failure to respond to conservative therapy
- Fistulas
- Inability to decrease corticosteroids
- Intestinal obstruction
- Massive hemorrhage
- Perforation
- Severe anorectal disease
- Suspicion of carcinoma

with increased risk of infection, hepatotoxicity, and hypersensitivity reactions. Because of the risk of progressive multifocal leukoencephalopathy, natalizumab is available only through a restricted program.

The biologic and targeted agents do not work for everyone. They are costly and may produce allergic reactions. They are immunogenic, meaning that patients receiving them frequently produce antibodies against them. Immunogenicity leads to acute infusion reactions and delayed hypersensitivity-type reactions. The drugs are most effective when given at regular intervals. Infusion reactions are more likely if a drug is stopped and then restarted.

### Surgical Therapy

***Ulcerative Colitis.*** Indications for surgery for ulcerative colitis are presented in Table 42-18. Since ulcerative colitis affects only the colon, a total proctocolectomy is curative. Surgical procedures used to treat ulcerative colitis include (1) total proctocolectomy with ileal pouch/anal anastomosis and (2) total proctocolectomy with permanent ileostomy. These procedures can be performed laparoscopically.

**Total proctocolectomy with ileal pouch/anal anastomosis (IPAA).** The most commonly used surgical procedure for ulcerative colitis is a total proctocolectomy with ileal pouch/anal anastomosis (IPAA). In this procedure, a diverting ileostomy is performed, and an ileal pouch is created and anastomosed directly to the anus (Fig. 42-4). It requires two surgical procedures performed approximately 8 to 12 weeks apart. The first procedure includes colectomy, rectal mucosectomy, ileal pouch (reservoir) construction, ileoanal anastomosis, and temporary ileostomy. The second surgery involves closure of the ileostomy to direct stool toward the new pouch. Initially, patients may have 4 to 6 stools or more daily, but adaptation over the next 3 to 6 months will result in a decreased number of bowel movements. The patient is able to control defecation at the anal sphincter. The major complication of this procedure is acute or chronic pouchitis. A permanent ileostomy may be done if pouchitis does not resolve.

**Total proctocolectomy with permanent ileostomy.** A proctocolectomy with a permanent ileostomy is a one-stage surgery involving the removal of the colon, rectum, and anus with closure of the anal opening. The end of the terminal ileum is brought out through the abdominal wall to form a stoma (ostomy). The stoma is usually placed in the right lower quadrant below the belt line. With a permanent ileostomy, continence is not possible.

***Crohn's Disease.*** Surgery for Crohn's disease is usually performed for complications such as strictures, obstructions, bleeding, and fistula (Table 42-18). Most patients with Crohn's disease eventually require surgery. The most common surgery involves resection of the diseased segments with reanastomosis of the remaining intestine. Unfortunately, the disease often recurs at the anastomosis site. Repeated removal of sections of small intestine can lead to short bowel syndrome. *Short bowel syndrome (SBS)* occurs when either surgery or disease leaves too little small intestine surface area to maintain normal nutrition and hydration. Lifetime fluid boluses and parenteral nutrition may be needed. For more detail, see the discussion on short bowel syndrome later in this chapter on p. 967.

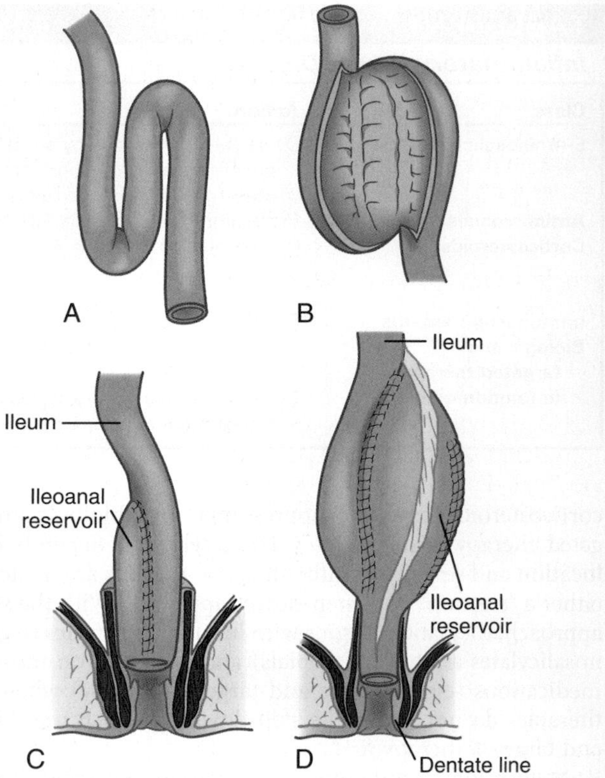


**FIG. 42-4** Ileoanal pouch (reservoir). **A,** Formation of a pouch. **B,** Posterior suture lines completed. **C,** J-shaped configuration for ileoanal pouch (J-pouch). **D,** S-shaped configuration for ileoanal pouch (S-pouch).

The other common surgery for Crohn's disease is a strictureplasty, which opens up narrowed areas obstructing the bowel. Since the intestine remains intact, it reduces the risk of developing short-bowel syndrome and its associated complications. Recurrences at the site of the strictureplasty are uncommon.

***Postoperative Care.*** Postoperative care after surgical procedures for IBD is similar to that described in the general nursing care plan for the postoperative patient (see eNursing Care Plan 19-1 on the website for Chapter 19). If an ileostomy is formed, monitor stoma viability, the mucocutaneous juncture (the area where the mucous membrane of the bowel interfaces with the skin), and peristomal skin integrity. Your patient should return from surgery with a clear ileostomy pouch in place. Replace pouches if feces leak onto the skin. (See the later discussion on ileostomy care on pp. 961-962.)

Immediately after surgery, ileostomy output initially may be as high as 1500 to 1800 mL/24 hr. Observe the patient for signs of fluid and electrolyte imbalance, hemorrhage, abdominal abscess, small bowel obstruction, dehydration, and other related complications. If an NG tube is used, remove it when bowel function returns. Over a period of days to weeks, the proximal small bowel adapts and increases fluid absorption. Then, feces will thicken to a paste-like consistency and the volume decrease. Patients, especially those with Crohn's disease, are at risk for developing a bowel obstruction during the first 30 days postoperatively.

Transient incontinence of mucus is a result of intraoperative manipulation of the anal canal. Initial drainage through the ileoanal anastomosis will be liquid. Have the patient start Kegel exercises about 4 weeks after surgery to strengthen the pelvic floor and sphincter muscles (see Table 45-18). Perianal skin care is important to protect the epidermis from mucous drainage and maceration. Instruct the patient to gently clean the skin with a mild cleanser, rinse well, and dry thoroughly. A moisture barrier ointment and a perineal pad may be used.

**Nutritional Therapy.** An individualized diet is an important component in the treatment of IBD. It is essential that people with IBD eat a balanced, healthy diet with sufficient calories, protein, and nutrients. Consult a dietitian regarding dietary recommendations. The goals of diet management are to (1) provide adequate nutrition without exacerbating symptoms, (2) correct and prevent malnutrition, (3) replace fluid and electrolyte losses, and (4) prevent weight loss.

Nutritional deficiencies are due to decreased oral intake, blood loss, and, depending on the location of the inflammation, malabsorption of nutrients. Patients may reduce food intake in an effort to reduce diarrhea. Inflammatory mediators reduce appetite. Bloody diarrhea leads to iron-deficiency anemia, which may require treatment with supplemental iron (ferrous sulfate or ferrous gluconate). Parenteral or IV iron may be needed for patients who cannot tolerate oral iron or if anemia is severe.

Disease of the terminal ileum reduces absorption of cobalamin and bile acids. Reduced cobalamin contributes to anemia, and bile salts are important for fat absorption and contribute to osmotic diarrhea. Those who develop anemia should receive cobalamin injections. Cholestyramine, an ion-exchange resin that binds unabsorbed bile salts, helps control diarrhea. Zinc deficiency can result from severe or chronic diarrhea, and supplementation may be necessary.

Medications can contribute to nutritional problems. Patients receiving sulfasalazine should receive folate (folic acid) daily. Those receiving corticosteroids are prone to osteoporosis and need calcium supplements. Potassium supplements may be necessary with corticosteroids. Vitamin D deficiency requiring supplementation is common. This may be due to malabsorption due to inflammation, surgical resection of intestine, reduced sunlight exposure, and decreased dietary intake.[16]

During an acute exacerbation, patients with IBD may not be able to tolerate a regular diet. Liquid enteral feedings are preferred over parenteral nutrition because atrophy of the gut and bacterial overgrowth occur when the GI tract is not used. (Enteral and parenteral nutrition are discussed in Chapter 39.) Enteral nutrition is high in calories and nutrients, lactose free, and easily absorbed. Enteral feedings help achieve remission and improve nutritional status. Restarting regular foods gradually will help identify food intolerances or sensitivities.

There are no universal food triggers for IBD, but some may find that certain foods cause diarrhea. A food diary helps to identify problem foods to avoid. Because many patients with IBD are lactose intolerant, avoiding milk and milk products improves symptoms. Lactose-intolerant patients can use yogurt as a substitute. High-fat foods, cold foods, and high-fiber foods (cereal with bran, nuts, raw fruits with peels) may trigger diarrhea.

## NURSING MANAGEMENT: INFLAMMATORY BOWEL DISEASE

### Nursing Assessment

Table 42-19 outlines the subjective and objective data you should obtain from a patient with IBD.

**TABLE 42-19 Nursing Assessment**
***Inflammatory Bowel Disease***

**Subjective Data**

***Important Health Information***

*Past health history:* Infection, autoimmune disorders
*Medications:* Antidiarrheal medications

***Functional Health Patterns***

*Health perception–health management:* Family history of ulcerative colitis or Crohn's disease. Fatigue, malaise
*Nutritional-metabolic:* Nausea, vomiting; anorexia. Weight loss
*Elimination:* Diarrhea. Blood, mucus, or pus in stools
*Cognitive-perceptual:* Lower abdominal pain (worse before defecation), cramping, tenesmus

**Objective Data**

***General***

Intermittent fever, emaciated appearance, fatigue

***Integumentary***

Pale skin with poor turgor, dry mucous membranes. Skin lesions, anorectal irritation, skin tags, cutaneous fistulas

***Gastrointestinal***

Abdominal distention, hyperactive bowel sounds, abdominal cramps

***Cardiovascular***

Tachycardia, hypotension

***Possible Diagnostic Findings***

Anemia, leukocytosis. Electrolyte imbalance, hypoalbuminemia, vitamin and trace metal deficiencies. Guaiac-positive stool. Abnormal sigmoidoscopic, colonoscopic, and/or barium enema findings

### Nursing Diagnoses

Nursing diagnoses for the patient with IBD include, but are not limited to, the following:

- Diarrhea *related to* bowel inflammation and intestinal hyperactivity
- Imbalanced nutrition: less than body requirements *related to* decreased absorption and increased nutrient loss through diarrhea
- Ineffective coping *related to* chronic disease, lifestyle changes, inadequate confidence in ability to cope

For additional information on nursing diagnoses on IBD, see eNursing Care Plan 42-2 on the website for this chapter.

### Planning

The overall goals are that the patient with IBD will (1) have fewer and less severe acute exacerbations, (2) maintain normal fluid and electrolyte balance, (3) be free from pain or discomfort, (4) adhere to medical regimens, (5) maintain nutritional balance, and (6) have an improved quality of life.

### Nursing Implementation

During the acute phase, focus your attention on hemodynamic stability, pain control, fluid and electrolyte balance, and nutritional support. Maintain accurate intake and output records, and monitor the number and appearance of stools. Assess for the presence of blood in stools and emesis. Administer IV fluids, electrolytes, analgesics, and antiinflammatory medications as ordered. Monitor serum electrolytes, CBC, and vital signs, being alert for any changes related to diarrhea and dehydration. If the patient experiences orthostatic hypotension, teach the patient to change position slowly and use safety precautions.

Until diarrhea is controlled, help the patient stay clean, dry, and free of odor. Place a deodorizer in the room. Meticulous perianal skin care using plain water (no harsh soap) together with a moisturizing skin barrier cream prevents skin breakdown. Dibucaine (Nupercainal), witch hazel, sitz baths, and other soothing compresses or ointments may reduce irritation and discomfort of the anus.

Calculate the adequacy of the daily calorie intake. Obtain a daily weight. Assess the abdomen, including bowel sounds, as needed. Consult with a dietitian regarding diet modifications and the need for nutritional supplements.

IBD is a chronic illness. Assist the patient in accepting the chronicity of IBD and learning strategies to cope with its recurrent, unpredictable nature. Teaching includes (1) the importance of rest and diet management, (2) perianal care, (3) drug action and side effects, (4) symptoms of recurrence of disease, (5) when to seek medical care, and (6) ways to reduce stress. Excellent teaching resources, written in easily comprehensible language are available from the Crohn's and Colitis Foundation of America *(www.ccfa.org)*.

It is important to establish rapport and encourage the patient to talk about self-care strategies. Ask patients what you can do to facilitate their self-care. An explanation of all procedures and treatments helps to build trust, decrease apprehension, and increase self-control. Once you have established a therapeutic relationship, talk with smokers who have Crohn's disease about quitting since smoking is associated with more severe disease.[17]

The patient and caregiver may need your help setting realistic short- and long-term goals. Patients may suffer severe fatigue, which limits their energy for physical activity. Rest is important. Patients may lose sleep because of frequent episodes of diarrhea and abdominal pain. Nutritional deficiencies and anemia leave the patient feeling weak and listless. Teach them to schedule activities around rest periods.

Many patients experience intermittent exacerbations and remissions of symptoms. Given the chronicity and uncertainty related to the frequency and severity of flares, the patient may experience frustration, depression, and anxiety. Psychotherapy and behavioral therapies may help patients deal with their feelings about the disease and help to manage their symptoms. Because of the relationship between emotions and the GI tract, teach the patient strategies for managing stress (see Chapter 6). Suggest that your patient seek support through a local or online support group from the Crohn's and Colitis Foundation of America.

### ◆ Evaluation

The expected outcomes are that the patient with IBD will

- Experience a decrease in the number of diarrhea stools
- Maintain body weight within a normal range
- Be free from pain and discomfort
- Demonstrate the use of effective coping strategies

For additional information on expected outcomes for IBD, see eNursing Care Plan 42-2 on the website for this chapter.

### Gerontologic Considerations: Inflammatory Bowel Disease

A second peak in occurrence of IBD is in the sixth decade. The etiology, natural history, and clinical course of IBD are similar to those observed in younger patients. However, in the older patient, proctitis and left-sided ulcerative colitis are more common. Diagnosis is sometimes difficult in older adults, since IBD can be confused with CDI and the colitis associated with diverticulosis or NSAID ingestion.

For the healthy older adult, the interprofessional care of IBD is similar to that of the younger patient. For the frail older patient with IBD, the usual treatments may increase the risk of adverse events, hospitalization, or mortality.[18] Older adults are more prone to adverse events from corticosteroids. Immunosuppressants and biologic therapy have a higher risk of infection and malignancy in older patients. Those with diminished renal and cardiovascular function are more vulnerable to the consequences of volume depletion from diarrhea. Those with physical limitations may have difficulty handling fecal urgency and multiple trips to the bathroom without assistance.

In addition to Crohn's disease and ulcerative colitis, older adults are vulnerable to inflammation of the colon (colitis) from drug use and systemic vascular disease. Drugs such as NSAIDs, digitalis, sumatriptan (Imitrex), vasopressin, estrogen, and allopurinol (Zyloprim) have been associated with the development of colitis in the older patient. Colitis may also be secondary to ischemic bowel disease related to atherosclerosis and heart failure.

## INTESTINAL OBSTRUCTION

**Intestinal obstruction** occurs when intestinal contents cannot pass through the GI tract. The obstruction may occur in the small intestine or colon and can be partial or complete, simple or strangulated. Partial obstructions do not completely occlude the intestinal lumen, allowing for some fluid and gas to pass through. They usually resolve with conservative treatment. A complete obstruction totally occludes the lumen and usually requires surgery. A simple obstruction has an intact blood supply; a strangulated one does not.

### Types of Intestinal Obstruction

The causes of intestinal obstruction are classified as mechanical or nonmechanical.

**Mechanical.** In *mechanical obstruction,* there is a physical obstruction of the intestinal lumen. Most intestinal obstructions occur in the small intestine.[19] Surgical adhesions are the most common cause of small bowel obstructions and can occur within days of surgery or several years later (Fig. 42-5). Other causes of small bowel obstruction are hernia, strictures from Crohn's disease, and intussusception after bariatric abdominal surgery. The most common cause of colon obstruction is colorectal cancer (malignant obstruction) followed by diverticular disease and sigmoid volvulus. A *volvulus* is an intestinal obstruction that occurs by the bowel twisting on itself.

**Nonmechanical.** A *nonmechanical obstruction* occurs with reduced or absent peristalsis due to altered neuromuscular transmission of the parasympathetic innervation to the bowel.[19] It may result from a neuromuscular or vascular disorder. **Paralytic ileus** (lack of intestinal peristalsis and bowel sounds) is the most common form of nonmechanical obstruction. It occurs to some degree after any abdominal surgery. It can be difficult to know whether postoperative obstruction is due to paralytic ileus or adhesions. One clue is that bowel sounds usually return before postoperative adhesions develop. Other causes of paralytic ileus include peritonitis, inflammatory responses (e.g., acute pancreatitis, acute appendicitis), electrolyte abnormalities

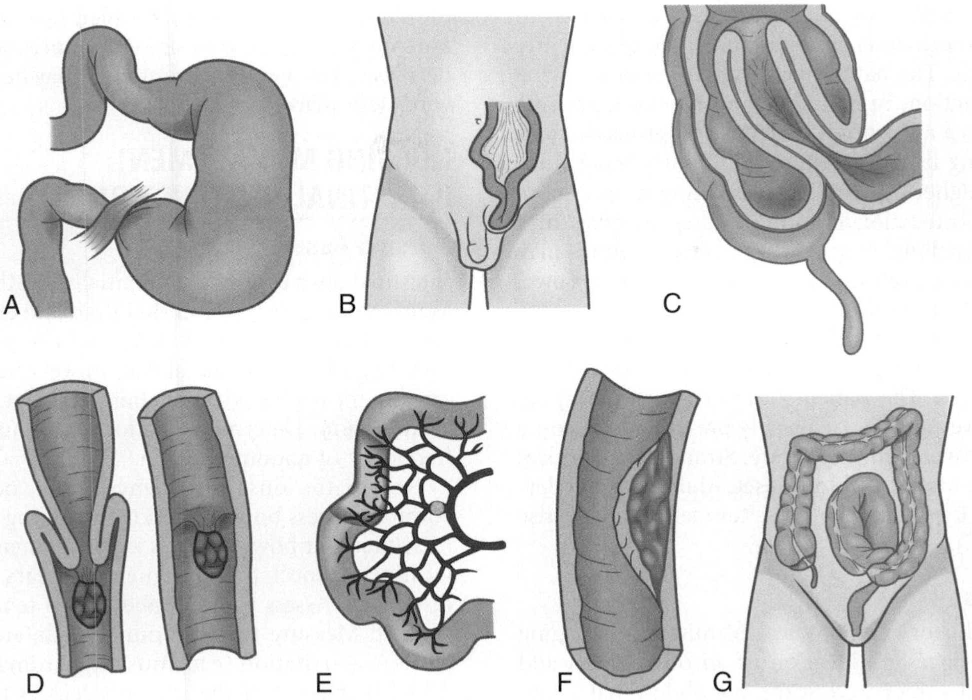


**FIG. 42-5** Bowel obstructions. **A,** Adhesions. **B,** Strangulated inguinal hernia. **C,** Ileocecal intussusception. **D,** Intussusception from polyps. **E,** Mesenteric occlusion. **F,** Neoplasm. **G,** Volvulus of the sigmoid colon.

(especially hypokalemia), and thoracic or lumbar spinal fractures.

*Pseudo-obstruction* is a mechanical obstruction of the intestine without any cause found on radiologic imaging. There are several conditions that are associated with a pseudo-obstruction. These include myocardial infarction, renal failure, Parkinson's disease, trauma, recent major orthopedic surgery, opiate use, and metabolic disturbances (e.g., hypokalemia).[19]

Vascular obstructions are rare and are the result of an interference with the blood supply to a portion of the intestines. The most common causes are emboli and atherosclerosis of the mesenteric arteries. Emboli may originate from thrombi in patients who have chronic atrial fibrillation, diseased heart valves, and prosthetic valves. Venous thrombosis may occur in conditions of low blood flow, such as heart failure and shock.

## Etiology and Pathophysiology

About 6 to 8 L of fluid enter the small intestine daily. Most of the fluid is absorbed before it reaches the colon. Approximately 75% of intestinal gas is swallowed air. When an obstruction occurs, fluid, gas, and intestinal contents accumulate proximal to the obstruction. Distention reduces fluid absorption and initially stimulates intestinal secretions. Distal to the obstruction, the bowel empties and then collapses. As distention increases in the proximal bowel, intraluminal bowel pressure rises. The increased pressure leads to an increase in capillary permeability and extravasation of fluids and electrolytes into the peritoneal cavity. Eventually the intestinal muscle becomes fatigued, and peristalsis stops. Retention of fluids in the intestine and peritoneal cavity leads to a severe reduction in circulating blood volume. This leads to hypotension and hypovolemic shock.

If blood flow is inadequate, bowel tissue becomes ischemic, then necrotic, and the bowel may perforate. In the most dangerous situation the bowel becomes so distended that the blood flow stops, causing edema, cyanosis, and gangrene of a bowel segment. This is called *intestinal strangulation* or *intestinal infarction.* If not quickly corrected, the bowel will become necrotic and rupture, leading to infection, septic shock, and death.

**TABLE 42-20 Manifestations of Small and Large Intestinal Obstructions**

| Manifestation | SMALL INTESTINE Proximal | SMALL INTESTINE Distal | Large Intestine |
|---|---|---|---|
| Onset | Rapid | Rapid | Gradual |
| Vomiting | Frequent and copious | Less frequent | Late or absent |
| Pain | Colicky, cramping, occurs at frequent intervals | Colicky, occurs more intermittently | Persistent, cramping |
| Bowel movement | Feces for a short time | Gradual constipation | Absolute constipation |
| Abdominal distention | Minimal | Increased | Increased |

The location of the obstruction determines the extent of fluid, electrolyte, and acid-base imbalances. If the obstruction is high (e.g., upper duodenum), metabolic alkalosis may result from the loss of gastric hydrochloric (HCl) acid through vomiting or NG intubation and suction. When the obstruction is located in the small intestine, dehydration occurs rapidly. Dehydration and electrolyte imbalances do not occur early in large bowel obstruction. If the obstruction is below the proximal colon, solid fecal material accumulates until symptoms of discomfort appear.

## Clinical Manifestations

The four hallmark clinical manifestations of an obstruction are abdominal pain, vomiting, distention, and constipation. The order and degree these appear vary by the location and type of the obstruction (Table 42-20). Colicky abdominal pain is usually the first manifestation of an obstruction. In small bowel obstruction, the pain is often of sudden onset. It occurs at 4- to 5-minute intervals for proximal obstructions and less frequently for distal obstructions. The nature of the vomiting gives a clue to the level of obstruction. In a proximal obstruction, patients rapidly develop nausea and vomiting. It may be projective and contain bile. Vomiting usually provides temporary relief from abdominal pain in higher obstructions. Vomiting from a more distal small bowel obstruction is more gradual in onset and more fecal and foul smelling. Auscultation of bowel sounds may reveal high-pitched sounds above the area of obstruction. Bowel sounds are usually absent with paralytic ileus.

Signs of colonic obstruction include abdominal distention, either absolute constipation or a marked change in bowel function, and lack of flatus. The patient has persistent, cramping abdominal pain. Bowel sounds are usually present and become progressively hypoactive. Vomiting is rare. Strangulation causes severe, constant pain that is rapid in onset. Abdominal tenderness and rigidity occur and the patient's temperature may rise above 100° F (37.8° C).

### Diagnostic Studies

Perform a thorough history and physical examination. Imaging can identify the presence and location of an obstruction and guide decisions about surgery. CT scans and abdominal x-rays are ordered. Sigmoidoscopy or colonoscopy may provide direct visualization of an obstruction in the colon.

Blood tests include a CBC and blood chemistries. An elevated WBC count may indicate strangulation or perforation. Elevated hematocrit values may reflect hemoconcentration. Decreased hemoglobin and hematocrit values may indicate bleeding from a neoplasm or strangulation with necrosis. Serum electrolytes, BUN, and creatinine are monitored frequently to assess the degree of dehydration. Metabolic alkalosis can develop from vomiting.

### Interprofessional Care

Treatment of a bowel obstruction depends on the cause. If a strangulated obstruction or perforation is present, the patient will require emergency surgery to relieve the obstruction and survive. In some, especially those due to surgical adhesions, an obstruction may resolve without surgery.

The initial medical treatment includes placing the patient on NPO status, inserting an NG tube for decompression, providing IV fluid therapy with either normal saline or lactated Ringer's solution (since fluid losses from the GI tract are isotonic), adding potassium to IV fluids after verifying renal function, and administering analgesics for pain control. Some patients require parenteral nutrition to allow bowel rest and improve nutritional status before surgery.

Surgery may involve simply resecting the obstructed segment of bowel and anastomosing the remaining healthy bowel back together. Partial or total colectomy, colostomy, or ileostomy may be required when extensive obstruction or necrosis is present. Occasionally, an obstruction can be removed nonsurgically. Colonoscopy offers a means to remove polyps, dilate strictures, and remove and destroy tumors with a laser.

The treatment goal for a patient with a malignant bowel obstruction is to regain patency and resolve the obstruction. Stents can be placed via endoscopic or fluoroscopic procedures. They are used for palliative purposes or as "a bridge to surgery," allowing a patient to avoid emergency surgery. This gives the interprofessional care team time to correct fluid volume problems and treat other problems, thus improving surgical outcomes. Corticosteroids with antiemetic properties that decrease edema and inflammation may be used in combination with stent placement.

## NURSING MANAGEMENT: INTESTINAL OBSTRUCTION

### Nursing Assessment

Intestinal obstruction is a potentially life-threatening condition. Major concerns are preventing fluid and electrolyte deficiencies and early recognition of deterioration in the patient's condition (e.g., hypovolemic shock, bowel strangulation). Nursing assessment begins with a detailed patient history and physical examination. Determine the location, duration, intensity, and frequency of abdominal pain.

Record the onset, frequency, color, odor, and amount of vomitus. Assess bowel function, including the passage of flatus. Auscultate for bowel sounds and document their character and location. Inspect the abdomen for scars, visible masses, and distention. Assess whether abdominal tenderness or rigidity is present. Measure the abdominal girth, and check for signs of peritoneal irritation (e.g., muscle guarding, rebound pain, pain if bed is shaken). If the surgeon decides to wait and see if the obstruction resolves on its own, assess the patient regularly and notify the surgeon of changes in vital signs, changes in bowel sounds, decreased urine output, increased abdominal distention, and pain.

Maintain a strict intake and output record, including emesis and tube drainage. A urinary catheter allows for hourly monitoring of urine output. Immediately report if the urine output is less than 0.5 mL/kg of body weight per hour, because this indicates inadequate vascular volume and the potential for acute kidney injury. Rising serum creatinine and BUN levels are additional indicators of acute kidney injury.

### Nursing Diagnoses

Nursing diagnoses for the patient with intestinal obstructions include, but are not limited to, the following:

- Acute pain *related to* abdominal distention and increased peristalsis
- Deficient fluid volume *related to* a decrease in intestinal fluid absorption, third space fluid shifts into the bowel lumen and peritoneal cavity, NG suction, and vomiting

### Planning

The overall goals are that the patient with an intestinal obstruction will have (1) relief of the obstruction and return to normal bowel function, (2) minimal to no discomfort, and (3) normal fluid and electrolyte and acid-base status.

### Nursing Implementation

Monitor the patient closely for signs of dehydration and electrolyte imbalances. Administer IV fluids as ordered. Watch for signs and symptoms of fluid overload, since some patients, especially older adults, may not tolerate rapid fluid replacement. Monitor serum electrolyte levels closely. A patient with a high intestinal obstruction is more likely to have metabolic alkalosis. A patient with a low obstruction is at greater risk for metabolic acidosis. The patient is often restless and constantly changes position to relieve the pain. Provide comfort measures and promote a restful environment. Nursing care of the patient after surgery for an intestinal obstruction is similar to care of the patient after a laparotomy (see p. 940).

With an NG tube in place, oral care is extremely important. Vomiting leaves an unpleasant taste in the patient's mouth, and fecal odor may be present. The patient breathes through the mouth, drying the mouth and lips. Encourage and help the patient to brush the teeth frequently. Mouthwash and water for rinsing the mouth and water-soluble lubricant for the lips should be readily available to the patient. Check the nose for signs of irritation from the NG tube. Clean and dry this area daily, apply water-soluble lubricant, and retape the tube. Check the NG tube every 4 hours for patency.

## POLYPS OF LARGE INTESTINE

Colonic polyps arise from the mucosal surface of the colon and project into the lumen. They may be *sessile* (flat, broad based, and attached directly to the intestinal wall) or *pedunculated* (attached to the intestinal wall by a thin stalk). Polyps tend to be sessile when small and become pedunculated as they enlarge (Fig. 42-6). They may be found anywhere in the large intestine. As patients age, polyps are increasingly present in the proximal colon. Rectal bleeding and occult blood in the stool are the most common signs, but most patients with polyps are asymptomatic.

### Types of Polyps

The most common types of polyps are hyperplastic and adenomatous. *Hyperplastic polyps* are non-neoplastic growths. They rarely grow larger than 5 mm and never cause clinical symptoms. Other benign (nonneoplastic) polyps include inflammatory polyps, lipomas, and juvenile polyps.

*Adenomatous polyps* are neoplastic and closely linked to colorectal adenocarcinoma. There are three types of adenomatous polyps: tubular, tubulovillous, and villous. Large or villous adenomatous polyps are more likely to have cancers develop in them. Removing adenomatous polyps decreases the occurrence of colorectal cancer.

### Genetic Link

*Familial adenomatous polyposis* (FAP) is the most common polyposis syndrome (see the Genetics in Clinical Practice box).

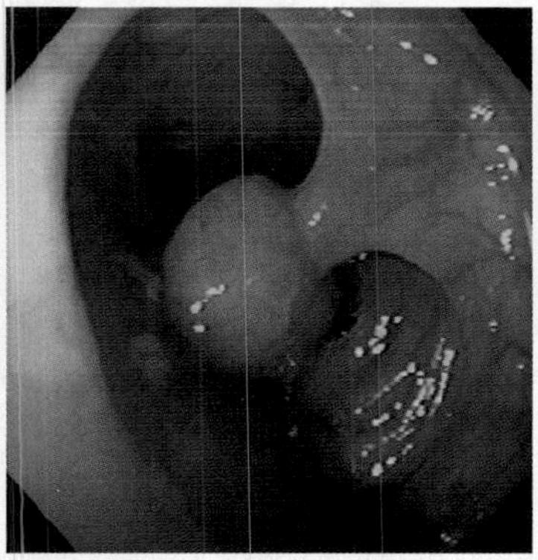

**FIG. 42-6** Endoscopic image of pedunculated polyp in descending colon. (Courtesy David Bjorkman, MD, University of Utah School of Medicine, Department of Gastroenterology. In McCance KL, Huether SE: *Pathophysiology: the biologic basis for disease in adults and children,* ed 6, St Louis, 2010, Mosby.)

**GENETICS IN CLINICAL PRACTICE**

***Familial Adenomatous Polyposis (FAP)***

**Genetic Basis**

- Classic form of disease
  - Autosomal dominant disorder
  - Mutations in adenomatous polyposis coli *(APC)* gene
  - Normally this is a tumor suppressor gene involved in DNA repair.
  - Normally this gene produces a special substance (a protein) that keeps polyps from developing in the colon.
- Autosomal recessive FAP
  - Autosomal recessive disorder
  - Mutations in the *mutY* homolog *(MUTYH)* gene
  - Normally this gene is involved in DNA repair.

**Incidence**

- Affects 1 in 7000 to 22,000 people
- Equally affects men and women

**Genetic Testing**

- DNA testing is available.

**Clinical Implications**

- FAP accounts for about 1% of all colorectal cancers.
- Persons with classic FAP have hundreds to thousands of colorectal polyps.
- Polyps are not present at birth but appear during adolescence and early adulthood.
- Autosomal recessive FAP is characterized by fewer polyps, typically <100.
- If untreated, almost all persons with classic FAP will develop colorectal cancer before age 40.
- With classic FAP, there are other benign and malignant tumors sometimes present, especially in the small intestine, stomach, liver, thyroid, and other tissues.
- Many deaths related to FAP can be prevented with early and aggressive monitoring and treatment, including frequent colonoscopies and total colectomy.
- Individuals with a family history of FAP can benefit from genetic counseling.

FAP is a genetic disorder characterized by hundreds or sometimes thousands of polyps in the colon that eventually become cancerous, usually by age 40. Since it is autosomal dominant, 50% of the offspring of a patient with FAP carry the FAP gene. Anyone with a family history of FAP should undergo genetic testing during childhood. If the FAP gene is present, colorectal screening begins at puberty, and annual colonoscopy begins at age 16. Since cancer is inevitable, the colon and rectum are removed, usually by age 25, and proctocolectomy with an IPAA or an ileostomy is performed (see p. 948). Patients with FAP are at risk for cancers of the thyroid, small intestine, liver, and brain, so lifetime cancer surveillance is essential.

### Diagnostic Studies and Interprofessional Care

Colonoscopy, sigmoidoscopy, barium enema, and virtual colonoscopy (CT or MRI colonography) are used to discover polyps. Colonoscopy is preferred because it allows evaluation of the total colon. All polyps are considered abnormal and should be removed. Polyps can be removed immediately *(polypectomy)* with colonoscopy or sigmoidoscopy. They cannot be removed during barium enema and virtual colonoscopy. After polypectomy, observe the patient for rectal bleeding, fever, severe abdominal pain, and abdominal distention, which may indicate hemorrhage or perforation.

## COLORECTAL CANCER

Of cancers that affect both men and women, colorectal cancer (CRC) is the second leading cause of cancer-related deaths and is the third most common cancer in men and women. Annually about 136,800 people in the United States are diagnosed with CRC and 50,300 people die from CRC.[20]

CRC is more common in men than in women. Mortality rates are highest among African American men and women. The risk of CRC increases with age, with about 90% of new CRC cases detected in people older than 50. However, while the incidence of CRC in people over 50 years is decreasing due to increased screening efforts to detect precancerous lesions, the number of cases in people aged 20 to 49 years is rising and expected to continue to do so.

### CULTURAL & ETHNIC HEALTH DISPARITIES

#### *Colorectal Cancer*

- African Americans are more likely to develop colorectal cancer (CRC) when compared with other ethnic groups.
- Incidence of CRC is declining in the United States except among Native American men.
- African Americans are more likely to die of CRC than any other ethnic group.
- Cancer may occur at an earlier age in African Americans and Hispanics.
- Those least likely to undergo screening include Hispanics, Native Indians, and Alaska natives.

### Etiology and Pathophysiology

Unlike some other cancers, no single risk factor accounts for most cases of CRC (Table 42-21). The risk is highest in those with first-degree relatives with CRC and people with IBD. About one third of cases of CRC occur in patients with a family history of CRC. Hereditary forms of CRC, including FAP and hereditary nonpolyposis colorectal cancer (HNPCC) syndrome (Lynch syndrome), account for 5% to 10% of those cases.

About 30% to 50% of people with CRC have an abnormal *KRAS* gene.[21] The *KRAS* gene, which is primarily involved in regulating cell division, belongs to a class of genes known as *oncogenes*. When mutated, oncogenes have the potential to cause normal cells to become cancerous.

Physical exercise and a diet with large amounts of fruits, vegetables, and grains may decrease the risk of CRC. Long-term use of NSAIDs (e.g., aspirin) is associated with reduced CRC risk.

Adenocarcinoma is the most common type of CRC. Approximately 85% of CRCs arise from adenomatous polyps. As the tumor grows, the cancer invades and penetrates the muscularis mucosae (Fig. 42-7). Eventually tumor cells gain access to the regional lymph nodes and vascular system and spread to distant sites. Since venous blood leaving the colon and rectum flows through the portal vein and the inferior rectal vein, the liver is a common site of metastasis. The cancer spreads from the liver to other sites, including the lungs, bones, and brain. CRC can also spread directly into adjacent structures.

**TABLE 42-21 Risk Factors for Colorectal Cancer**

- Family history of colorectal cancer (first-degree relative)
- Personal history of inflammatory bowel disease
- Personal history of colorectal cancer
- Family or personal history of familial adenomatous polyposis (FAP)
- Family or personal history of hereditary nonpolyposis colorectal cancer (HNPCC) syndrome
- Obesity (body mass index ≥30 kg/m²)
- Red meat (≥7 servings/wk)
- Cigarette smoking
- Alcohol (≥4 drinks/wk)
- Personal history of diabetes mellitus

### GENETICS IN CLINICAL PRACTICE

#### *Hereditary Nonpolyposis Colorectal Cancer (HNPCC) or Lynch Syndrome*

**Genetic Basis**
- Autosomal dominant disorder
- Mutations in *MSH2, MLH1, MSH6,* or *PMS2* genes
- These genes are involved in repair of mistakes when DNA is replicated.

**Incidence**
- Affects 1 in 500 to 2000 people

**Genetic Testing**
- DNA testing is available.

**Clinical Implications**
- Accounts for 3% of all CRC
- Depending on the genetic mutation present, the risk of developing CRC ranges from 50% to 80%.
- Occasionally, people with HNPCC have colon polyps, which occur at an earlier age than do colon polyps in the general population and are more prone to become malignant.
- Cancers of the uterus, ovaries, stomach, urinary tract, small bowel, and bile ducts occur more often in affected persons.
- People with HNPCC need to be have a colonoscopy every year.
- Women with HNPCC should undergo screening for ovarian and endometrial cancer by having a yearly pelvic examination, ultrasound, and endometrial biopsy.

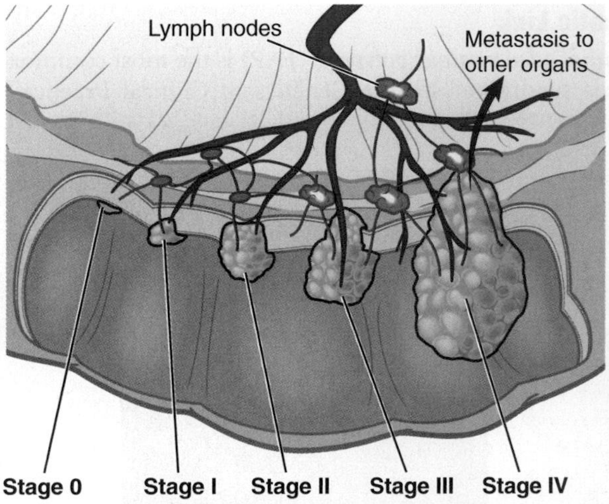


**FIG. 42-7** The five stages of colorectal cancer. Stage 0 cancer has not grown beyond the mucosal layer. Stage I cancer has grown beyond the mucosa into the submucosa, but no lymph nodes are involved. Stage II cancer has grown beyond the submucosa into the muscle but there is no lymph node involvement or metastasis. Stage III cancer is any tumor with lymph node involvement but no metastasis. Stage IV cancer is any tumor with lymph node involvement and metastasis.

### Clinical Manifestations

CRC has an insidious onset, and symptoms do not appear until the disease is advanced. Common clinical manifestations include iron-deficiency anemia, rectal bleeding, abdominal pain, change in bowel habits, and intestinal obstruction or perforation.

Physical findings may include the following:

- *Early disease:* Nonspecific findings (fatigue, weight loss) or none at all
- *More advanced disease:* Abdominal tenderness, palpable abdominal mass, hepatomegaly, ascites

Bleeding can occur with both right- and left-sided CRC. Bleeding on the right side, which is more common than the left side, is often unrecognized and an early manifestation is often anemia. Hematochezia (fresh blood in the stool) is more often caused by left-sided CRC than right-sided CRC.

Right-sided lesions are more likely to cause diarrhea, while left-sided tumors are usually detected later and could present with bowel obstruction (Fig. 42-8). Complications of CRC include obstruction, bleeding, perforation, peritonitis, and fistula formation.

### Diagnostic Studies

Obtain a thorough history with close attention to family history (Table 42-22). Since symptoms of CRC do not become evident until the disease is advanced, there is an increased emphasis on screening. Beginning at age 50 and continuing until age 75, men and women at average risk for developing CRC should have screening tests to detect both polyps and cancer based on one of these testing schedules:

- Flexible sigmoidoscopy (every 5 years)
- Colonoscopy (every 10 years)
- Double-contrast barium enema (every 5 years)
- CT colonography (virtual colonoscopy) (every 5 years)
- Tests that primarily find cancer include the following:
  - High sensitivity fecal occult blood test (FOBT) (every year), or
  - Fecal immunochemical test (FIT) (every year)

Colonoscopy is the gold standard for CRC screening, because the entire colon is examined (only 50% of CRCs are detected by sigmoidoscopy), biopsies can be obtained, and polyps can be immediately removed and sent to the laboratory for examination. People at average risk of CRC should have a colonoscopy every 10 years beginning at age 50.

Persons at risk (Table 42-21) should begin screening earlier and have screening done more often. African Americans should have their first colonoscopy at age 45. Those who have a first-degree relative who developed CRC before age 60 or have two first-degree relatives with CRC should have a colonoscopy every 5 years beginning at age 40 or 10 years earlier than when the youngest relative developed cancer. Those who have one first-degree relative who had CRC after age 60 should have a colonoscopy every 10 years beginning at age 40.[22]

Less favorable, but acceptable, screening methods include stool testing for fecal blood. The FOBT and FIT look for blood in the stool. Stool tests must be done frequently, since tumor bleeding occurs at intervals and may easily be missed if a single test is done. In addition to testing for blood in human stool, new tests (PreGen-Plus, Cologuard) can detect DNA mutations that may indicate the presence of CRC.

Once tissue biopsies confirm the diagnosis of CRC, additional laboratory studies include a CBC to check for anemia and liver function tests. A CT scan or MRI of the abdomen may be helpful in detecting liver metastases, retroperitoneal and pelvic disease, and depth of penetration of tumor into the bowel wall. However, liver function tests may be normal even when metastasis has occurred.

Carcinoembryonic antigen (CEA) is a complex glycoprotein sometimes produced by CRC cells. It may be used to monitor for disease recurrence after surgery or chemotherapy but is not a good screening tool because of the large number of false positives. CEA levels may also be increased in non-colon carcinomas (e.g., gastric, pancreatic, lung carcinoma, breast, and thyroid carcinoma) as well as some non-neoplastic conditions, such as IBD, pancreatitis, cirrhosis, and COPD.

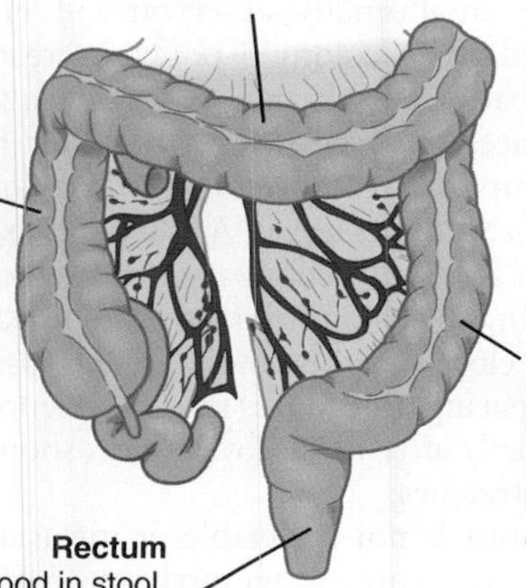


**FIG. 42-8** Signs and symptoms of colorectal cancer by location of primary cancer. (Modified from McCance KL, Huether SE: *Pathophysiology: the biologic basis for disease in adults and children,* ed 6, St Louis, 2010, Mosby.)

**TABLE 42-22 Interprofessional Care**

***Colorectal Cancer***

| Diagnostic Assessment | Management |
|---|---|
| • History and physical examination<br>• Digital rectal examination<br>• Testing of stool for occult blood<br>• CBC<br>• Liver function tests<br>• Barium enema<br>• Sigmoidoscopy and/or colonoscopy with biopsy<br>• Abdominal CT scan, ultrasound, or MRI<br>• Carcinoembryonic antigen (CEA) test | • Surgery<br>  • Right hemicolectomy<br>  • Left hemicolectomy<br>  • Abdominal-perineal resection<br>  • Laparoscopic colectomy<br>• Chemotherapy<br>• Targeted therapy<br>• Radiation therapy |

### Interprofessional Care

The prognosis and treatment of CRC correlate with pathologic staging of the disease. The most commonly used staging system is the tumor, node, metastasis (TNM) staging (Table 42-23). As with other cancers, prognosis worsens with greater size and depth of tumor, lymph node involvement, and metastasis (Table 42-24).

**Surgical Therapy.** Goals of surgical therapy include (1) complete resection of the tumor, (2) a thorough exploration of the abdomen to determine if the cancer has spread, (3) removing all lymph nodes that drain the area where the cancer is located,

**TABLE 42-23 TNM Classification of Colorectal Cancer**

| T | Primary Tumor |
|---|---|
| $T_x$ | Primary tumor cannot be assessed because of incomplete information. |
| $T_{is}$ | Carcinoma in situ. Cancer is in earliest stage and has not grown beyond mucosa layer. |
| $T_1$ | Tumor has grown beyond mucosa into the submucosa. |
| $T_2$ | Tumor has grown through submucosa into muscularis propria. |
| $T_3$ | Tumor has grown through the muscularis propria into the subserosa but not to neighboring organs or tissues. |
| $T_4$ | Tumor has spread completely through the colon or rectal wall and into nearby tissues or organs. |
| **N** | **Lymph Node Involvement** |
| $N_x$ | Lymph nodes cannot be assessed. |
| $N_0$ | No regional lymph node involvement is found. |
| $N_1$ | Cancer is found in one to three nearby lymph nodes. |
| $N_2$ | Cancer is found in four or more nearby lymph nodes. |
| **M** | **Metastasis** |
| $M_x$ | Presence of distant metastasis cannot be assessed. |
| $M_0$ | No distant metastasis is seen. |
| $M_1$ | Distant metastasis is present. |

**TABLE 42-24 Classification System Used to Stage Colorectal Cancer**

| Stage* | TNM† | Duke's | 5-Yr Survival Rate |
|---|---|---|---|
| 0 | $T_{is}$ $N_0$ $M_0$ | | >96% |
| I | $T_1$ $N_0$ $M_0$ | A | >90% |
| | $T_2$ $N_0$ $M_0$ | $B_1$ | 85% |
| II | $T_3$ $N_0$ $M_0$ | $B_2$ | 70%-80% |
| III | Any T, $N_1$ $M_0$ | C | 64% |
| IV | Any T, any N, $M_1$ | D | 8% |

*Staging system is shown in Fig. 42-7.
†See Table 42-23.

(4) restoring bowel continuity so that normal bowel function will return, and (5) preventing surgical complications.

Some polyps can be removed during colonoscopy, whereas others require surgery. Polypectomy during colonoscopy can be used to resect CRC in situ and is considered successful when the resected margin of the polyp is free of cancer, the cancer is well differentiated, and there is no apparent lymphatic or blood vessel involvement.

The decision for surgical treatment of CRC depends on the staging and location of the cancer and ability to restore normal bowel function and continence. Surgical removal of stage I cancer includes removal of the tumor and at least 5 cm of intestine on either side of the tumor, plus removal of nearby lymph nodes. The remaining cancer-free ends are sewn back together (anastomosis). Laparoscopic surgery is sometimes used for stage I tumors, especially those in the left colon. Low-risk stage II tumors are treated with wide resection and reanastomosis, and chemotherapy is used in addition to surgery for high-risk stage II tumors. Stage III tumors are treated with surgery and chemotherapy. Radiation and chemotherapy may be done before surgery to reduce tumor size. Once the cancer has spread to distant sites (stage IV), any surgery is usually palliative, with chemotherapy and radiation used to control the spread and provide pain relief. Select patients with limited lung or liver metastases can achieve a cure after primary and metastatic tumor resection and chemotherapy.[23] A patient who has a perforation, peritonitis, or is hemodynamically unstable may need a temporary colostomy or ileostomy.

In rectal cancer, the location and size of the tumor determines the course of treatment. Local excision may be an option. If the tumor is in the distal rectum (1 to 2 cm from the anorectal junction) and the sphincters cannot be preserved, the patient will undergo an *abdominal-perineal resection (APR)*. An APR involves removing the entire rectum with the tumor, and the patient will have a permanent colostomy. The perineal wound may be closed around a drain or left open with packing to allow healing by granulation. Complications that can occur include delayed wound healing, hemorrhage, persistent perineal sinus tracts, infections, and urinary tract and sexual dysfunction.

If the tumor is in the mid or proximal rectum, it may be possible to preserve the sphincters. In this situation, a low anterior resection (LAR) can be done. A LAR involves removing the rectum and anastomosing the colon to the anal canal. A temporary ileostomy or colostomy may be done to divert stool and allow time for the anastomosis to heal, usually about 8 to 12 weeks. Then the ostomy can be "taken down," and the ends of the colon surgically reconnected. An LAR is increasingly common because of advancements in laparoscopy and stapling techniques. End-to-end anastomosis stapling involves less tissue (less than 5 cm from anus) and is more secure with less leakage.

Another option if the anal sphincters remain is for the surgeon to create an alternative reservoir with either a colonic J-pouch or coloplasty. A colonic J-pouch is created by folding the distal colon back on itself and suturing it to form a pouch. The pouch replaces the rectum as a reservoir for stool. The patient has a temporary ostomy to allow the J-pouch sutures time to heal before stool enters it. A coloplasty is made by slitting the side of a section of colon a short distance proximal to the anus, stretching the colon transversely to make it wider, and then suturing it closed in the new widened position. Patients with sphincter-sparing procedures may experience urgency and frequency, especially after meals. Symptoms should improve as the new pouch stretches.

When the tumor is not resectable or metastasis is present, palliative surgery can control hemorrhage or relieve a malignant bowel obstruction.

**Chemotherapy and Targeted Therapy.** Chemotherapy can be used to shrink the tumor before surgery, as an adjuvant therapy after colon resection, and as palliative treatment for nonresectable cancer. Adjuvant chemotherapy is recommended for patients with stage III tumors and high-risk stage II tumors. Current chemotherapy protocols include varying doses of 5-fluorouracil (5-FU) and folinic acid (leucovorin) alone or in combination with oxaliplatin (Eloxatin) or irinotecan (Camptosar). The preferred protocol includes oxaliplatin. It is omitted if patients have too many side effects. Oral fluoropyrimidines (e.g., capecitabine [Xeloda]) in combination with oxaliplatin are an alternative to 5-FU/folinic acid therapy.[24]

Several targeted therapies have a role in treating metastatic CRC. Angiogenesis inhibitors, which inhibit the blood supply to tumors, include aflibercept (Zaltrap), bevacizumab (Avastin), and ramucirumab (Cyramza). Bevacizumab is often added to a combination chemotherapy regimen (e.g., 5-FU and irinotecan or 5-FU, leucovorin, oxaliplatin) to treat metastatic CRC. Regorafenib (Stivarga) is a multikinase inhibitor that blocks several enzymes that promote cancer growth. Cetuximab (Erbitux) and panitumumab (Vectibix) block the epidermal growth factor receptor.

Lonsurf, which is a combination of trifluridine and tipiracil, is used in patients with metastatic CRC who are no longer responding to other therapies. Trifluridine impairs DNA function and angiogenesis. Tipiracil prevents the rapid metabolism of trifluridine, thus increasing its bioavailability.

**Radiation Therapy.** Some patients may receive radiation therapy as an adjuvant to surgery and chemotherapy or as a palliative measure for those with metastatic cancer. As a palliative measure, the primary objective is to reduce tumor size and provide symptomatic relief. Radiation therapy is described in Chapter 15.

## NURSING MANAGEMENT: COLORECTAL CANCER

### Nursing Assessment

Table 42-25 outlines the subjective and objective data you should obtain from a patient with CRC.

### Nursing Diagnoses

Nursing diagnoses for the patient with CRC include, but are not limited to, the following:

- Diarrhea or constipation *related to* altered bowel elimination patterns
- Fear and anxiety *related to* diagnosis of CRC, surgical or therapeutic interventions, and possible terminal illness
- Ineffective coping *related to* diagnosis of cancer and side effects of treatment

**TABLE 42-25 Nursing Assessment**

***Colorectal Cancer***

**Subjective Data**

***Important Health Information***

*Past health history:* Previous breast or ovarian cancer, familial polyposis, villous adenoma, adenomatous polyps, inflammatory bowel disease

*Medications:* Use of any medications affecting bowel function (e.g., laxatives, antidiarrheal drugs)

***Functional Health Patterns***

*Health perception–health management:* Family history of colorectal, breast, or ovarian cancer; weakness, fatigue

*Nutritional-metabolic:* High-calorie, high-fat, low-fiber diet. Anorexia, nausea and vomiting, weight loss

*Elimination:* Change in bowel habits, alternating diarrhea and constipation, defecation urgency. Rectal bleeding, mucoid stools. Black, tarry stools. Increased flatus, decrease in stool caliber. Feelings of incomplete evacuation

*Cognitive-perceptual:* Abdominal and low back pain, tenesmus

**Objective Data**

***General***

Pallor, cachexia, lymphadenopathy (later signs)

***Gastrointestinal***

Palpable abdominal mass, distention, ascites, and hepatomegaly (liver metastasis)

***Possible Diagnostic Findings***

Anemia. Guaiac-positive stools, palpable mass on digital rectal examination. Positive sigmoidoscopy, colonoscopy, barium enema, or CT scan. Positive biopsy

### Planning

The overall goals are that the patient with CRC will have (1) normal bowel elimination patterns, (2) quality of life appropriate to the disease progression, (3) relief of pain, and (4) feelings of comfort and well-being.

### Nursing Implementation

**Health Promotion.** Encourage all persons over 50 to have regular CRC screening. Help identify those at high risk who need screening at an earlier age. Discuss with patients how participating in early cancer screening helps decrease mortality rates. Realize that barriers exist, including lack of accurate information and fear of diagnosis.

Endoscopic and radiographic procedures can only reveal polyps when the bowel has been adequately prepared to eliminate stool. Provide teaching about bowel cleansing for outpatient diagnostic procedures, and administer cleansing preparations to inpatients. The patient should follow either a low-residue or a full liquid diet the day before the procedure until bowel cleansing begins. Bowel cleansing should follow a split-dose regimen. The evening before the procedure, the patient should drink 2 L of oral polyethylene glycol (PEG) lavage solution. The second 2 L dose should begin 4 to 6 hours before the procedure. A split-dose regimen started early morning the day of a procedure provides better cleansing for patients scheduled in the afternoon. Because many people find the PEG lavage solution difficult to drink and experience nausea and bloating, manufacturers have modified the PEG solutions to improve taste and palatability. Magnesium citrate solution or bisacodyl tablets or suppositories are sometimes given before the PEG lavage to remove the bulk of stool so that only 2 L of solution are needed.[25] Encourage the patient to drink all of the solution. Stools will be clear or clear yellow liquid when the colon is clean.

**Acute Care.** Depending on your practice setting and surgeon preference, you may see patients undergoing a preoperative bowel cleansing routine prior to elective bowel surgeries. In the past, many patients underwent a cleansing routine with polyethylene glycol solutions (e.g., MiraLAX, GoLYTELY), enemas, and/or laxatives to reduce bacterial counts. There is very little evidence that supports this practice. There is no difference in surgical outcome between those who underwent a preoperative cleansing routine and those who did not.[25]

Nursing care for the patient after a colon resection is similar to care of the patient after a laparotomy (see p. 940). If enough healthy bowel remained that the surgeon could reconnect the bowel ends, normal bowel function is maintained and routine postoperative care is appropriate. Patients with more extensive surgery (e.g., APR) may have an open wound and drains (e.g., Jackson-Pratt, Hemovac) and a permanent ostomy. Postoperative care includes sterile dressing changes, care of drains, and patient and caregiver teaching about the ostomy.

A patient who has open and packed wounds requires meticulous care. Reinforce dressings and change them frequently during the first several hours postoperatively when drainage is likely to be profuse. Carefully assess all drainage for amount, color, and consistency. The drainage is usually serosanguineous. Examine the wound regularly and record bleeding, excessive drainage, and unusual odor. Use aseptic technique with dressing changes. Some patients experience phantom rectal pain or still feel as if they need to have a bowel movement. This is normal and often subsides over time. Be astute in distinguishing phantom sensations from perineal abscess pain. Consult with a wound, ostomy, and continence nurse (WOCN) if available. Ostomy care is discussed in depth in the next section on pp. 960-962.

If the patient's wound is closed or partially closed, assess the incision for suture integrity and signs and symptoms of wound inflammation and infection. Examine the drainage for amount, color, and characteristics. Observe the skin around the drain for signs of inflammation, and keep the area around the drain clean and dry. Monitor for edema, erythema, and drainage around the suture line, as well as fever and an elevated WBC count.

Sexual dysfunction is a possible complication after APR. The likelihood of sexual dysfunction depends on the surgical technique used. The surgeon should discuss the possibility with the patient. Members of the interprofessional care team should be available to address the patient's questions and concerns. Erection, ejaculation, and orgasm involve different nerve pathways, and a dysfunction of one does not mean complete sexual dysfunction. The WOCN is an important source of information concerning sexual dysfunction resulting from an APR.

◆ **Ambulatory Care.** Psychologic support for the patient and caregiver dealing with the diagnosis of cancer is important. Discuss the patient's feelings about his or her prognosis and future screening. Patients need much emotional support because recurrent cancer is painful, debilitating, and demoralizing. The special needs of the cancer patient are discussed in Chapter 15. You may need to address issues surrounding palliative care, end-of-life issues, and hospice (see Chapter 9).

Patients with CRC need to know how to manage changes that are the result of the cancer and cancer treatment. Those who had sphincter-sparing surgery may experience diarrhea and incontinence of feces and gas. They may need antidiarrheal drugs or bulking agents to control the diarrhea, but overuse can result in constipation. A consult with a dietitian or WOCN may help patients and caregivers understand how to manage food and fluid options. Ostomy rehabilitation, including teaching and ongoing support, should be available for all ostomy patients. Patients with skin changes from incontinence and/or radiation therapy will need assistance in managing these conditions.

### ◆ Evaluation

The expected outcomes for the patient with CRC are that the patient will have

- Minimal alterations in bowel elimination patterns
- Optimal nutritional intake
- Quality of life appropriate to disease progression
- Feelings of comfort and well-being

## OSTOMY SURGERY

### Types

An **ostomy** is a surgically created opening on the abdomen that allows the discharge of body waste. The outermost portion that is visible is a **stoma**. The stoma is the result of the large or small bowel being brought to the outside of the abdomen and sutured in place. When a stoma is created as a fecal diversion, feces will drain through the stoma instead of the anus.

An ostomy is necessary when the normal elimination route is no longer possible. For example, if a person has Stage III CRC, the surgeon will remove the diseased portion of the colon along with a certain margin of healthy tissue. If the tumor involves the rectum and is large enough to necessitate the removal of the anal sphincters, the anus will be sutured shut and a permanent ostomy created. Patients at high risk for CRC, such as those with FAP, and patients with ulcerative colitis may have a total colectomy and an ileostomy.

Ostomies are named according to their location and type (Fig. 42-9). An ostomy in the ileum is called an *ileostomy*. An ostomy in the colon is called a *colostomy*. The ostomy is further characterized by its anatomic site (e.g., ascending, transverse, or sigmoid colostomy). The more distal the ostomy, the more the functioning bowel remains and the more likely that the intestinal contents will resemble the feces that would have been eliminated from an intact colon and rectum. Ileostomy output will be a liquid to thin paste since it did not enter the colon. Patients have no control over ileostomy drainage; it is involuntary. An ileostomy drains frequently, and the patient must wear an ostomy appliance (pouch) to collect the drainage (effluent). In contrast, output from a sigmoid colostomy resembles normal formed stool. Some patients are able to regulate emptying time with colostomy irrigation and may not need to wear a pouch. See Table 42-26 for a comparison of colostomies and ileostomies.

Ostomies may be temporary or permanent. For example, the person with a draining fistula may need a temporary ostomy to prevent stool from reaching the diseased area. Patients who have trauma to the intestines (e.g., gunshot wound, stabbing) may need a temporary ostomy. Cancer involving the rectum requires a permanent ostomy if all bowel distal to the ostomy is removed.

Permanent ostomies may be continent or traditional. *Continent ileostomies* (e.g., Koch pouch, Barnett Continent Ileal Reservoir) use 40 to 45 cm of the terminal ileum to fashion an internal pouch, nipple valve, and abdominal stoma. The internal pouch can hold approximately 500 mL or more of material. Continent ostomies are an option for patients who have had a prior APR with ileostomy for ulcerative colitis or FAP. They are not normally done for Crohn's disease because of the risk of disease reoccurrence and the loss of a significant length of small bowel. Appropriate patients must be motivated and compliant. Patients must drain the pouch manually by inserting a catheter through the nipple valve. Initially, this is needed every 1 to 2 hours. As the pouch enlarges, the frequency decreases to four times daily and as needed. They must keep the stool consistency relatively fluid by following a low-residue diet.

The major types of traditional ostomies include end, double-barreled, and loop ostomy.

**End Stoma.** An end stoma is constructed by dividing the bowel and bringing out the proximal end as a single stoma, making a colostomy or ileostomy. The distal portion of the GI tract is either surgically removed or the distal segment is oversewn and left in the abdominal cavity with its mesentery intact. If the distal bowel is removed, the stoma is permanent. When the distal bowel is oversewn and not removed, the procedure is called a *Hartmann's pouch* (Fig. 42-10). With a Hartmann's pouch, the potential exists for the bowel to be reanastomosed and the stoma closed (referred to as a *takedown*).

**Loop Stoma.** A loop stoma is constructed by bringing a loop of bowel to the abdominal surface and then opening the anterior wall of the bowel to provide fecal diversion. This results in one stoma with a proximal opening for feces and a distal opening for mucus drainage from the distal colon. An intact posterior wall separates the two openings. A plastic rod holds the loop of bowel in place for 7 to 10 days after surgery to prevent it from slipping back into the abdominal cavity (Fig. 42-11). A loop stoma is usually temporary.

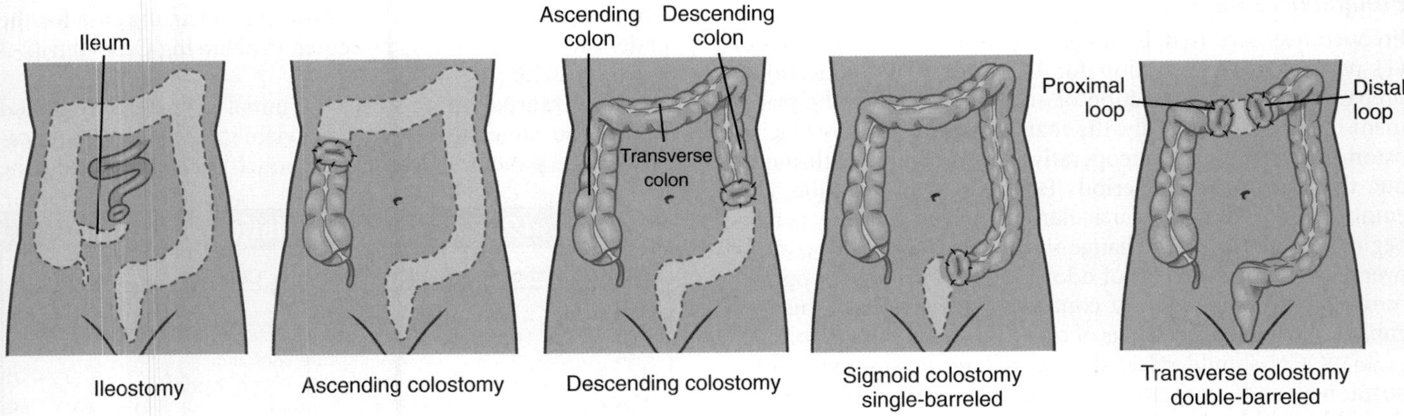


**FIG. 42-9** Types of ostomies.

**TABLE 42-26 Comparison of Ileostomy and Colostomy**

| | | COLOSTOMY | | |
|---|---|---|---|---|
| **Characteristic** | **Ileostomy** | **Ascending** | **Transverse** | **Sigmoid** |
| **Stool consistency** | Liquid to semiliquid | Semiliquid | Semiliquid to semiformed | Formed |
| **Fluid requirement** | Increased | Increased | Possibly increased | No change |
| **Bowel regulation** | No | No | No | Yes (if there is a history of a regular bowel pattern) |
| **Pouch and skin barriers** | Yes | Yes | Yes | Dependent on regulation |
| **Irrigation** | No | No | No | Possibly every 24-48 hr (if patient meets criteria) |
| **Indications for surgery** | Ulcerative colitis, Crohn's disease, diseased or injured colon, familial polyposis, trauma, cancer | Perforating diverticulum in lower colon, trauma, rectovaginal fistula, inoperable tumors of colon, rectum, or pelvis | Same as for ascending | Cancer of the rectum or rectosigmoid area, perforating diverticulum, trauma |

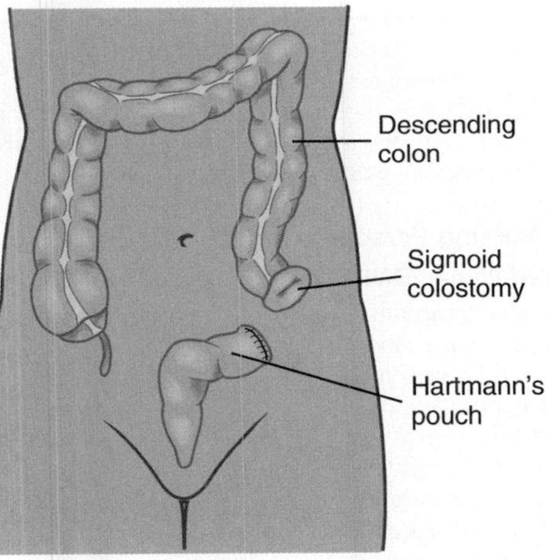


**FIG. 42-10** Sigmoid colostomy. Distal bowel is oversewn and left in place to create Hartmann's pouch.

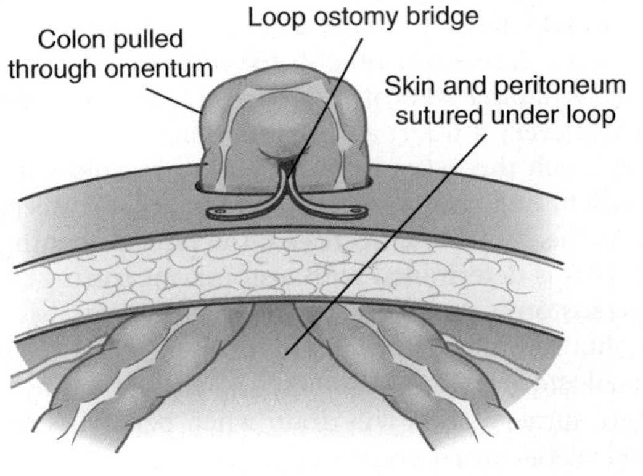


**FIG. 42-11** Loop colostomy.

**Double-Barreled Stoma.** To create a double-barreled stoma, the surgeon divides the bowel and both the proximal and distal ends are brought through the abdominal wall as two separate stomas (Fig. 42-9). The proximal one is the functioning stoma. The distal, nonfunctioning stoma is referred to as the *mucus fistula.* The double-barreled stoma is usually temporary.

## NURSING MANAGEMENT: OSTOMY SURGERY

Two major aspects of nursing care for the patient with an ostomy are (1) emotional support as the patient copes with a radical change in body image and (2) patient and caregiver teaching about ostomy care. Accurate information, emotional support, and mastering basic skills will help patients learn to live a full life with an ostomy and accept the changes in body appearance and function. Without accurate information, fear and misconceptions can be overwhelming. People with ostomies lose control over flatus and feces and worry about odor and leakage. They question the patency of ostomy pouches and wonder how the ostomy will change their lives. With time and proper support, people learn to manage the stoma and resume work, social, and sexual activities. Adjusting to any major change in health status and personal appearance is highly individualized. People with new ostomies need time and support to adjust to the changes but should be reassured they can adjust and resume their previous lifestyle.

## ◆ Preoperative Care

Preoperative care that is unique to ostomy surgery includes (1) psychologic preparation for the ostomy, (2) educational preparation, and (3) selection of an optimal site for the placement of the stoma. Ideally, the management of patients facing ostomy surgery begins preoperatively and continues throughout the postoperative period. Psychologic preparation and emotional support are particularly important as the person begins to cope with the change in body image, loss of control over elimination, and fear of odors. Provide the patient opportunities for verbalization of concerns and questions. This will enhance the patient's feelings of control and thus ability to cope.

A WOCN should select the site where the ostomy will be positioned and mark the abdomen preoperatively. The site should be within the rectus muscle, on a flat surface, and in a place that the patient is able to see. Stomas placed outside the rectus muscle may increase the chance of developing a hernia. A flat site makes it much easier to create a good seal and avoid leakage from the bag. Being able to see the stoma makes caring for it easier. Whenever possible, it should be discreetly hidden under clothing and appropriate for normal activities.

It is normal for the patient and caregiver to have questions concerning the procedures. If available, a WOCN should visit with the patient and caregiver to determine the patient's ability to perform self-care, identify support systems, and determine any modifications that could facilitate learning during rehabilitation. The patient and caregiver should understand the extent of surgery, the type of stoma planned, and basic stoma care.

## ◆ Postoperative Care

Postoperative nursing care includes assessment of the stoma and provision of an appropriate pouching system that protects the skin and contains drainage and odor. The stoma should be rosy pink to red. A dusky blue stoma indicates ischemia, and a brown-black stoma indicates necrosis. Assess and document stoma color every 4 hours and ensure that there is no excessive bleeding. Teach the patient that the stoma is mildly to moderately swollen. Edema will resolve over the first 6 weeks (Table 42-27). As the stoma size decreases, the pouch opening will be smaller. This is determined with a stoma-measuring card.

The colostomy starts functioning when peristalsis returns. Record the volume, color, and consistency of the drainage. When a colostomy is performed on a colon that was not cleaned out before surgery, stool will drain when peristalsis returns. If the bowel was cleansed preoperatively, it will not begin producing stool until a few days after the patient is eating again. Excessive amounts of gas are common during the first 2 weeks. Because this can be distressing to patients, assure them this is temporary.

## ◆ Colostomy Care

An appropriate pouching system is vital to protect the skin and provide dependable stool collection. Most pouching systems have an adhesive skin barrier and a pouch to collect the feces. Most skin barriers are made of pectin-based or karaya mediums with hydrocolloid properties. Adhesion occurs in two phases. First, the wafer's backing has adhesive material that forms an immediate bond with the skin. Second, the hydrocolloids interface with the moisture on the skin to form a tighter seal. If the abdominal stoma site has bends or creases, it is difficult to get a good seal and the skin barrier will pull away faster. Since excessive weight of collected stool pulls the wafer away from the skin, empty ostomy bags when one-third full. (Nursing care for the patient with an ostomy is presented in eNursing Care Plan 42-3 on the website.)

Use a transparent pouch in the initial postoperative period so that you can easily assess stoma viability and pouch application by the patient. Each time the pouch is changed, assess the

### TABLE 42-27 Characteristics of Stoma

| Characteristic | Description or Cause |
|---|---|
| **Color*** | |
| Rose to brick-red | Viable stoma mucosa. |
| Pale | May indicate anemia. |
| Blanching, dark red to purple | Indicates inadequate blood supply to the stoma or bowel. |
| **Edema†** | |
| Mild to moderate edema | Normal in initial postoperative period. Trauma to the stoma. |
| Moderate to severe edema | Obstruction of the stoma, allergic reaction to food, gastroenteritis. |
| **Bleeding** | |
| Small amount | Oozing from stoma mucosa when touched is normal because of its high vascularity. |
| Moderate to large amount | Could indicate lower gastrointestinal bleeding, coagulation factor deficiency, stomal varices secondary to portal hypertension. |

*Report sustained color changes to surgeon.
†Closely observe and report to the surgeon and adjust the stoma opening size in the pouch.

### TEAMWORK & COLLABORATION

### *Ostomy Care*

Although licensed practical/vocational nurses (LPN/LVNs) and unlicensed assistive personnel (UAP) provide much of the ostomy care for patients with established ostomies, patients with new ostomies have complex needs and require frequent assessment, planning, intervention, and evaluation by a registered nurse (RN).

#### Role of Nursing Personnel

***Registered Nurse (RN)****

- Assess and document stoma appearance.
- For patient with a new ostomy, assess patient's psychologic preparation for ostomy care.
- Choose appropriate ostomy pouching system (skin barrier and bag or pouch) for patient.
- Place ostomy pouching system for a new ostomy.
- Develop plan of care for skin care around the ostomy.
- Teach ostomy care and skin care to patient and caregiver.
- Irrigate new colostomy.
- Teach colostomy irrigation to patient and caregiver.
- Teach patient and caregivers about appropriate dietary choices.

***Licensed Practical/Vocational Nurse (LPN/LVN)***

- Monitor the volume, color, and odor of the ostomy drainage.
- Monitor the skin around the ostomy for breakdown.
- Provide skin care around the ostomy.
- Irrigate colostomy in stable patient.

***Unlicensed Assistive Personnel (UAP)***

- Empty ostomy bag and measure liquid contents.
- Place the ostomy pouching system for an established ostomy.
- Assist stable patient with colostomy irrigation.

*In agencies where a wound, ostomy, and continence nurse (WOCN) is available, many of these roles will be assumed by that person.

skin for irritation. If the peristomal skin is irritated and raw, additional products may have to be applied. Do not allow feces to remain on the skin or irritation will quickly develop. If a pouch has failed, it must be changed immediately.

A colostomy in the ascending and transverse colon has semiliquid stools. Have the patient use a drainable pouch. A drainable pouch may last up to 4 to 7 days.

A colostomy in the sigmoid or descending colon has semiformed or formed stools. The patient can use a drainable pouch or choose a disposable, closed end pouch changed every day. Another option is irrigation. Patients who irrigate may not need a regular pouch as they may be able to regulate when the colon empties. Optional charcoal filters can deodorize and automatically release flatus. They are available for both drainable and nondrainable pouches.

With shorter hospital stays, patient teaching should focus on the critical aspects that patients need to master. Teaching must include (1) basic skills about managing the ostomy (e.g., emptying and changing the pouch), (2) food and fluid requirements, and (3) how to get help for problems. Additional teaching should include expanded information on these topics plus skin care, managing gas and odor, care of the stoma, potential complications, resuming activities of daily living, and sources for support and assistance.[26] Teach the patient when to seek health care. Home care and outpatient follow-up may be helpful, especially if there is access to a WOCN. Provide written information about the particular ostomy, instructions for pouch changes, basic supplies needed, where to purchase supplies (including retailers' names and phone numbers), any follow-up appointments, and contact information for the surgeon and WOCN. Patient and caregiver teaching is presented in Table 42-28.

Teach the patient about the importance of fluids and a healthy diet. A well-balanced diet and adequate fluid intake are important. The effect of food on stoma output is individual. Most patients with colostomies can eat anything they want. However, some choose to avoid certain foods because of possible increased gas, odor, or stoma output[27] (Table 42-29). Teach patients to chew their food very well to reduce the chance of blockage.

The patient can resume activities of daily living within 6 to 8 weeks but should avoid heavy lifting. The patient's physical condition determines when he or she can resume sports. Swimming with an ostomy pouch intact is not a problem. The patient can bathe and shower with or without the pouching system in place because water does not harm the stoma.

◆ **Colostomy Irrigations.** Colostomy irrigations may be used to stimulate emptying of the colon. Regularity is possible only when the stoma is in the distal colon. If the colon is irrigated and emptied on a regular basis, the bowel can be trained, and little or no spillage should occur between irrigations. The patient may need to wear only a pad or small pouch over the stoma. Irrigation requires manual dexterity and adequate vision. People who irrigate regularly should still have ostomy bags readily available in case they develop diarrhea from foods or illness.

## ◆ Ileostomy Care

Nursing care for a patient with an ileostomy is similar to that for a patient with a colostomy. Because the stool from an ileostomy is caustic to the skin, a secure pouching system is important. This is easier with stoma protrusion of at least 1 to 1.5 cm. When the stoma is flat, recessed, or in a crease, seepage occurs and results in altered skin integrity. The patient must wear a pouch at all times since regularity is not possible with an ileostomy. An open-ended, drainable pouch is needed so that drainage can be easily emptied. A drainable pouch usually lasts for 4 to 7 days before having to be changed. If leakage occurs, the pouch must be promptly removed, the skin cleansed, and a new pouch applied. The skin barrier should completely protect the skin from any exposure to stool. Caulking strips or "paste" around the stoma may help ensure a secure seal.

Observe the patient with an ileostomy for signs and symptoms of fluid and electrolyte imbalance, particularly potassium, sodium, and fluid deficits. In the first 24 to 48 hours after surgery, the amount of drainage from the stoma may be negligible. Patients with new ileostomies lose the absorptive

### TABLE 42-28 Patient & Caregiver Teaching

***Ostomy Self-Care***

*Include the following instructions when teaching the patient and/or caregiver about self-care of an ostomy.*

1. Explain what an ostomy is and how it functions.
2. Describe the underlying condition that resulted in the need for an ostomy.
3. Demonstrate and allow the patient and caregiver to practice the following activities:
   - Remove the old skin barrier, cleanse the skin, and correctly apply new skin barriers.
   - Apply, empty, clean, and remove the pouch.
   - Empty the pouch before it is one-third full to prevent leakage.
4. Irrigate the colostomy to regulate bowel elimination (optional).
5. Explain how to contact the wound, ostomy, and continence nurse with questions.
6. Describe how to obtain additional ostomy supplies.
7. Explain dietary and fluid management.
   - Identify a well-balanced diet and dietary supplements to prevent nutritional deficiencies.
   - Identify foods to avoid to reduce diarrhea or gas.
   - Promote fluid intake of least 3000 mL/day to prevent dehydration (unless contraindicated).
   - Increase fluid intake during hot weather, excessive perspiration, and diarrhea to replace losses and prevent dehydration.
   - Describe symptoms of fluid and electrolyte imbalance.
   - Explain how to contact the dietitian with questions.
   - Explain how to recognize problems (fluid and electrolyte deficits, fever, diarrhea, skin irritation, stomal problems) and how to contact the appropriate health care provider.
8. Describe community resources to assist with emotional and psychologic adjustment to the ostomy.
9. Explain the importance of follow-up care.
10. Describe the ostomy's potential effects on sexual activity, social life, work, and recreation and strategies to manage these changes.

### TABLE 42-29 Nutritional Therapy

***Effects of Food on Stoma Output***

| Odor Producing | Gas Forming | Diarrhea Causing |
|---|---|---|
| Eggs | Beans | Alcohol |
| Garlic | Cabbage family | Beer |
| Onions | Onions | Cabbage family |
| Fish | Beer | Spinach |
| Asparagus | Carbonated beverages | Green beans |
| Cabbage | Cheeses (strong) | Coffee |
| Broccoli | Sprouts | Spicy foods |
| Alcohol | | Fruits (raw) |

functions provided by the colon and the delay provided by the ileocecal valve. As a result, they may experience a period of high-volume output of 1500 to 1800 mL/day when peristalsis returns. Later, as the proximal small bowel adapts, the average amount can be 500 mL/day. If the small bowel was been shortened by surgery, drainage from the ileostomy may be greater. Patients need to increase fluid intake to at least 2 to 3 L/day or more when there are excessive fluid losses from heat and sweating. They may also need to ingest additional sodium. Patients must learn signs and symptoms of fluid and electrolyte imbalance so that they can take appropriate action.

The ileostomy patient is susceptible to obstruction because the lumen is less than 1 inch in diameter. It may narrow further at the point where the bowel passes through the fascia/muscle layer of the abdomen. Foods such as nuts, raisins, popcorn, coconut, mushrooms, olives, stringy vegetables, foods with skins, dried fruits, and meats with casings must be chewed extremely well before swallowing.[27] If the terminal ileum was removed, the patient may need cobalamin treatment.

### ◆ Psychologic Adaptation to an Ostomy

The patient's response to a new ostomy is highly individualized. Some have minimal difficulty and view their ostomy positively. It may be curative if their presenting condition was ulcerative colitis or a step toward remission if the diagnosis was CRC. Other patients may experience a grief reaction from the loss of a body part and an alteration in body image. They may be angry, depressed, or resentful. Anxiety and fear are normal. Concerns about stool leaking, odor, sounds of flatus, pouch reliability, and changes in normal life style are all valid worries.

The patient's emotional state may limit his or her ability to participate in teaching and ostomy care. Emotional support, interventions from skillful WOCNs, and visits from people who have successfully learned to manage their ostomies will help patients learn to cope with and manage the new stoma.

Discuss with the patient the psychologic impact of the stoma and its effect on body image and self-esteem. Assist the patient in identifying ways of coping with depression and anxiety resulting from the illness, surgery, or postoperative problems. Support from the caregiver, family, and friends is vital and reassures the patient that he or she is still cherished and valued despite having the ostomy. Encourage patients to share their concerns and ask questions. Provide information in an easily understood manner and help patients develop confidence and competence in managing the stoma.

New ostomy patients will have questions on a variety of topics ranging from managing gas to intimacy to travel. Provide the names and contact information for support groups. The Wound Ostomy Continence Nurses Society *(www.wocn.org)*, local support groups, and United Ostomy Associations of America *(www.ostomy.org)* provide practical information about living with an ostomy. Online support groups are also available. Ask the patient if he or she would like to meet with a person who has adjusted to an ostomy. Most hospitals have a visitor's program. Visitor's programs give the patient and caregiver an opportunity to talk with a person who has adjusted well to an ostomy and has experienced some of the same feelings and concerns they have.

### ◆ Sexual Function After Ostomy Surgery

Sexual function and sexuality concerns affect both men and women with an ostomy. The patient with a stoma may fear rejection by a partner or that others will not find him or her desirable. Incorporate a discussion of sexuality and sexual function in the plan of care. Help the patient realize that it takes time to adjust to the pouch and to body changes before feeling secure in his or her sexual functioning.

Help the patient understand if specific aspects of surgery and treatment have the potential for sexual dysfunction. Pelvic surgery can disrupt nerve and vascular supplies to the genitalia. Radiation therapy, chemotherapy, and medications can alter sexual function. The patient's overall physical health influences sexual desire. Generalized fatigue caused by illness can decrease desire. Understanding this information can help patients plan the timing of sexual activity.

For men, the main concern may be erection and ejaculation. Erection of the penis depends on intact parasympathetic and nonadrenergic noncholinergic nerves as well as adequate blood supply. Nerve-sparing surgical techniques are used when possible to preserve sexual function. Unfortunately, any pelvic surgery that removes the rectum has the potential of damaging the parasympathetic nerve plexus. Sympathetic nerve damage in the presacral area can disrupt the ability to ejaculate. This can occur with the APR procedure. Sexual dysfunction may be temporary and resolve in 3 to 12 months. Pelvic radiation can reduce blood flow to the pelvis by causing scarring in the small blood vessels.

For women, the main issues may be vaginal lubrication, clitoral congestion, and dyspareunia. Nerve damage can result in vaginal dryness and decreased sensation in the vagina and clitoris, making arousal and achieving orgasm more challenging. Experimenting with positions and using lubrication may help. A woman with an ostomy can still become pregnant.

Teach the patient to empty the pouch before sexual activities. Some may apply a smaller pouch during sexual activity. Women may consider wearing open panties, a short slip, or similar lingerie. Men may consider wearing a wrap or cummerbund around the midsection to secure the pouch. There are many types of pouch covers that patients can make or purchase.

## FISTULAS

A **fistula** is an abnormal tract between two hollow organs or a hollow organ and the skin. Fistulas are named by the track that they take from one body part to another. For example, an enterocutaneous fistula is an opening between the small intestine and skin. An enterovaginal fistula is between the small intestine and vagina, allowing stool and gas to drain through the vagina.

A GI fistula occurs between the lumen of the GI tract and another organ. GI fistulas are a serious complication associated with increased morbidity and mortality, extended hospital stays, and increased costs. Most fistulas occur after surgery, or are associated with IBD, cancer, or adhesions. Fistulas can form in the presence of diverticulitis, pancreatitis, trauma, hypotension, sepsis, and corticosteroid use. Fistulas are classified as simple or complex and by the amount of output. A simple fistula has only one short, direct tract. A complex fistula is associated with an abscess, involves multiple organs, and may open into the base of a wound. High output fistulas drain more than 500 mL/day, moderate output fistulas drain 200 to 500 mL/day, and low output fistulas drain less than 200 mL/day.[28]

Fever and abdominal pain are early indicators of a fistula. Other manifestations vary depending on the type of fistula.

With an enterocutaneous fistula, there may be pus or intestinal contents draining through the skin opening. Patients with a colocutaneous (colon to skin) fistula may have stool or pus draining through the opening. If a colovesical (colon to urinary tract) fistula is present, manifestations include fecaluria (passing stool with urination), recurrent urinary tract infections, dysuria, and hematuria.

## NURSING AND INTERPROFESSIONAL MANAGEMENT: GASTROINTESTINAL FISTULAS

The development of a draining fistula can be disheartening for the patient and caregiver and a time-consuming challenge for HCPs. Managing a fistula requires (1) identifying the fistula tract, (2) maintaining fluid and electrolyte balance, (3) controlling infection, (4) protecting the surrounding skin, (5) managing output, and (6) providing nutritional support.[28] Most fistulas heal spontaneously. Surgery may be necessary to treat the complications.

Appropriate fluid and electrolyte replacement can be challenging, especially when the patient has a high output fistula. Monitor the volume of fistula output as this guides replacement therapies and nutritional support. Assess the character of the drainage, noting the color, consistency, and odor. Monitor laboratory values. Hypokalemia, hypomagnesemia, and hypophosphatemia from the loss of GI fluids are common. Administer IV fluids and electrolyte replacement as ordered. Keep an accurate intake and output record. To reduce intestinal output, many patients require NPO status and receive somatostatin or octreotide to decrease GI secretions. Measure vital signs frequently and be alert for signs of dehydration.

Malnutrition is a significant problem, particularly if the patient is on NPO status or has a small intestinal fistula. Consult a dietitian. High-calorie, high-protein parenteral or enteral nutrition is necessary for providing enough calories and protein to replace losses and support healing. Many patients require trace element (e.g., copper, zinc, magnesium) and vitamin supplements.

**CHECK YOUR PRACTICE**

A 51-yr-old female is 4 days postop following a proctocolectomy for ulcerative colitis. You note a 2.5 cm of erythema in the center of her incision with heavy, foul-smelling tan drainage pooling on her skin. Suspecting she is developing an enterocutaneous fistula, you notify the surgeon and WOCN.

- What will you do to protect her skin?

Maintaining skin integrity and optimizing healing is essential. Consult a WOCN if available. Although low output fistulas may be managed with a simple absorbent dressing, a high-output enterocutaneous fistula often requires advanced techniques, including specialty pouches; barrier creams, powders, and sealants to protect the skin; and negative pressure wound therapy.

## DIVERTICULOSIS AND DIVERTICULITIS

*Diverticula* are saccular dilations or outpouchings of the mucosa that develop in the colon (Fig. 42-12). Diverticulosis is the presence of multiple noninflamed diverticula. **Diverticulitis** is inflammation of one or more diverticula, resulting in perforation into the peritoneum. Clinically, diverticular disease covers a spectrum from asymptomatic, uncomplicated diverticulosis to diverticulitis with complications such as perforation, abscess, fistula, and bleeding. Diverticula are common, especially in older adults, but most people never develop diverticulitis.[29]

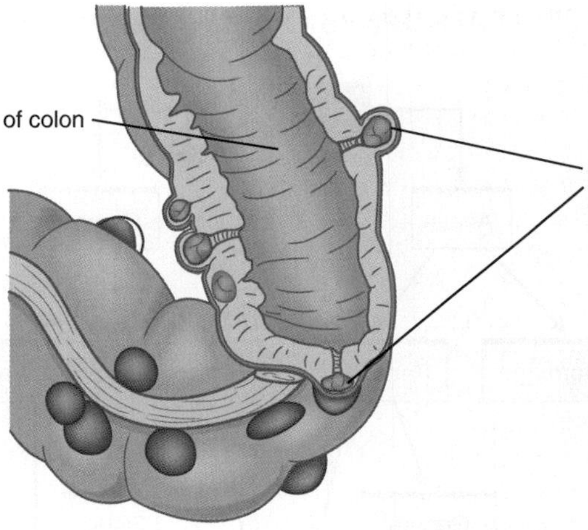


**FIG. 42-12** Diverticula are outpouchings of the colon. When they become inflamed, the condition is diverticulitis. The inflammatory process can spread to the surrounding area in the intestine.

### Etiology and Pathophysiology

Diverticula may occur anywhere in the GI tract but are most common in the left (descending, sigmoid) colon. They seem to occur at weak points in the intestinal wall, such as where the blood vessels pass through the muscle layer. The main factor thought to contribute to the development of diverticulosis is a lack of dietary fiber intake. The disease is more prevalent in Western, industrialized populations, where people tend to consume diets low in fiber and high in refined carbohydrates. Inadequate dietary fiber slows transit time, allowing more water to be absorbed from the stool, making it more difficult to pass through the lumen. Decreased stool size increases intraluminal pressure. This places stress on the weakened areas and promotes diverticula formation. Diverticula are uncommon in vegetarians. Other risk factors for diverticula are obesity, inactivity, smoking, excessive alcohol use, and immunosuppression.

### Clinical Manifestations and Complications

The majority of patients with diverticulosis have no symptoms. Those with symptoms typically have abdominal pain, bloating, flatulence, and changes in bowel habits. In more serious situations, the diverticula bleed or diverticulitis develops. The most common signs and symptoms of diverticulitis are acute pain in the left lower quadrant (location of sigmoid colon), a palpable abdominal mass, nausea, vomiting, and systemic symptoms of infection (fever, increased C-reactive protein, leukocytosis with a shift to the left). Older adults with diverticulitis may be afebrile, with a normal WBC count and little, if any, abdominal tenderness. Diverticulitis can cause erosion of the bowel wall and perforation into the peritoneum (Fig. 42-13). A localized abscess develops when the body is able to wall off the area of perforation. Peritonitis develops if it cannot be contained. Bleeding can be extensive but usually stops spontaneously.

### Diagnostic Studies

Diverticular disease can be asymptomatic and is typically discovered during routine sigmoidoscopy or colonoscopy. Diagnosis of diverticulitis is based on the history and physical

PATHOPHYSIOLOGY MAP

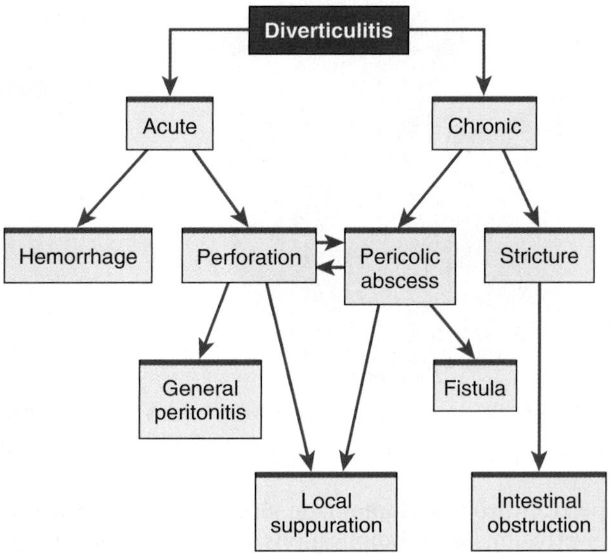


**FIG. 42-13** Complications of diverticulitis.

examination (Table 42-30). The preferred diagnostic test is a CT scan with oral contrast. Abdominal and chest x-ray rule out other causes of acute abdominal pain.

## NURSING AND INTERPROFESSIONAL MANAGEMENT: DIVERTICULOSIS AND DIVERTICULITIS

A high-fiber diet, mainly from fruits and vegetables, with a decreased intake of fat and red meat is the best way to prevent diverticular disease. High levels of physical activity also seem to decrease the risk. Currently there is no evidence to support the theory that diverticulitis can be prevented by avoiding nuts and seeds.

In acute diverticulitis, the goal of treatment is to let the colon rest and the inflammation subside. Some patients can be managed at home with oral antibiotics and a clear liquid diet. Hospitalization is necessary if symptoms are severe, the patient is unable to tolerate oral fluids, there are systemic manifestations of infection (fever, significant leukocytosis), or the patient has co-morbid conditions (e.g., immunosuppression).

If hospitalized, the patient is kept on NPO status and IV fluids and antibiotics are given. Observe for signs of abscess, bleeding, and peritonitis, and monitor the WBC count. Administer analgesics as needed. When the acute attack subsides, give oral fluids first and then progress the diet to semisolids.

Patients with frequently reoccurring diverticulitis or complications, such as an abscess or obstruction, may need surgery. The usual surgical procedure involves resection of the involved colon with a primary anastomosis. If the surgeon is not able to anastomose the colon, then the patient will have a temporary diverting colostomy. After the colon heals, the temporary colostomy can be "taken down" and the ends of the colon reconnected.

Provide the patient with diverticular disease with a full explanation of the condition. Patients who understand the disease process well and adhere to the prescribed regimen are less likely to experience an exacerbation of the disease and complications. Teach them the importance of following a high-fiber diet (Table 42-7) and encourage a fluid intake of at least 2L/day.

Weight reduction is important for the obese person with diverticular disease. A patient with diverticular disease should avoid increased intraabdominal pressure because it may precipitate an attack. Factors that increase intraabdominal pressure are straining at stool, vomiting, bending, heavy lifting, and wearing tight, restrictive clothing.

**TABLE 42-30 Interprofessional Care**

***Diverticulosis and Diverticulitis***

**Diagnostic Assessment**
- History and physical examination
- Testing of stool for occult blood
- CBC
- Urinalysis
- Barium enema
- Sigmoidoscopy and/or colonoscopy with biopsy
- Blood culture
- CT scan with oral contrast
- Abdominal and/or chest x-ray

**Management**

***Conservative Therapy***
- High-fiber diet
- Dietary fiber supplements
- Stool softeners
- Anticholinergics
- Clear liquid diet
- Oral antibiotics
- Mineral oil
- Bulk laxatives
- Weight reduction (if overweight)

***Acute Care: Diverticulitis***
- Antibiotic therapy
- NPO status
- IV fluids
- NG suction
- Surgery
- Possible resection of involved colon
- Possible temporary colostomy

## HERNIAS

A **hernia** is a protrusion of the viscus (internal organ such as the intestine) through an abnormal opening or a weakened area in the wall of the cavity in which it is normally contained. A hernia may occur in any part of the body, but it usually occurs within the abdominal cavity. *Reducible* hernias easily return into the abdominal cavity. Reducing can be done manually or may occur spontaneously when the person lies supine. *Irreducible,* or *incarcerated,* hernias cannot be placed back into the abdominal cavity and have abdominal contents trapped in the opening. Strangulation occurs if the blood supply to the contents trapped in an irreducible hernia becomes compromised. The result is an acute intestinal obstruction. Gangrene and necrosis of the hernia contents are possible.

### Types

The *inguinal hernia* is the most common type of hernia and occurs at the point of weakness in the abdominal wall where the spermatic cord (in men) or the round ligament (in women) emerges (Fig. 42-14, *C*).

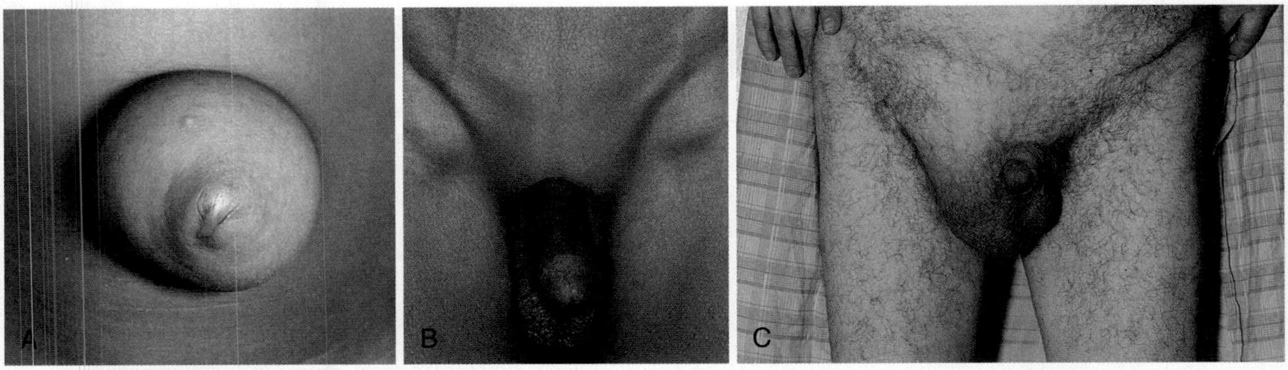


**FIG. 42-14** **A,** Umbilical hernia. **B,** Femoral hernias (note swelling below the inguinal ligaments). **C,** Right inguinal hernia. (*A* and *B*, From Zitelli BJ, McIntire SC, Nowalk AJ: *Zitelli and Davis' atlas of pediatric physical diagnosis*, ed 6, Philadelphia, 2012, Saunders. *C*, From Swartz MH: *Textbook of physical diagnosis: history and examination,* ed 6, Philadelphia, 2010, Saunders.)

**GENDER DIFFERENCES**

***Hernia***

| Men | Women |
|---|---|
| • Inguinal hernias are more common in men.<br>• Men have a 25% lifetime risk of developing a groin hernia.<br>• Men undergo 90% of the 750,000 groin hernia repairs done annually in the United States. | • Femoral hernias are more common in women, particularly older women.<br>• Women have less than a 5% lifetime risk of developing a groin hernia. |

An *umbilical hernia* occurs when the rectus muscle is weak (as with obesity) or the umbilical opening fails to close after birth (Fig. 42-14, *A*). A *femoral hernia* occurs when there is a protrusion through the femoral ring into the femoral canal. It appears as a bulge below the inguinal ligament. Femoral hernias easily strangulate (Fig. 42-14, *B*).

*Ventral* or *incisional hernias* are due to weakness of the abdominal wall at the site of a previous incision. They occur most commonly in patients who are obese, have had multiple surgical procedures in the same area, or have had inadequate wound healing because of poor nutrition or infection. Peristomal hernias are ventral hernias.

### Clinical Manifestations

Pain is the classic symptom of a hernia. It may worsen with activities that increase intraabdominal pressure, such as lifting, coughing, and straining. A hernia may be readily visible, especially when the person tenses the abdominal muscles. If the hernia becomes strangulated, the patient will have severe pain and symptoms of a bowel obstruction such as vomiting, cramping abdominal pain, and distention.

## ❖ NURSING AND INTERPROFESSIONAL MANAGEMENT: HERNIAS

Diagnosis of a hernia is usually based on history and physical examination findings. Ultrasound, CT, and MRI can assist in identifying a hernia and determining the contents. Laparoscopic surgery is the treatment of choice. The surgical repair of a hernia, known as a *herniorrhaphy,* is usually an outpatient procedure. Reinforcing the weakened area with wire, fascia, or mesh is known as a *hernioplasty.* Emergency surgery is required for strangulated hernias or inflamed, irreducible hernias. Surgery for strangulated hernias involves resecting the involved area with possible placement of a temporary colostomy.

After a hernia repair, the patient may have difficulty voiding. Measure intake and output and observe for a distended bladder. Scrotal edema is a painful complication after an inguinal hernia repair. A scrotal support with application of an ice bag and elevating the scrotum may help relieve pain and edema. Encourage deep breathing, but not coughing. Teach patients to splint the incision and keep their mouths open when coughing or sneezing is unavoidable. The patient may be restricted from heavy lifting (>10 lb) for 6 to 8 weeks.

## MALABSORPTION SYNDROME

*Malabsorption* results from impaired absorption of fats, carbohydrates, proteins, minerals, and vitamins. The stomach, small intestine, liver, and pancreas regulate normal digestion and absorption. Digestive enzymes ordinarily break down nutrients so that absorption can take place. Malabsorption may occur if this process is interrupted at any point. Several problems can cause malabsorption (Table 42-31). Lactose intolerance is the most common malabsorption disorder, followed by IBD, celiac disease, tropical sprue, and cystic fibrosis.

The most common signs of malabsorption are weight loss, diarrhea, and **steatorrhea** (bulky, foul-smelling, yellow-gray, greasy stools with putty-like consistency) (Table 42-32). Steatorrhea does not occur with lactose intolerance.

Tests used to determine the cause of malabsorption include qualitative examination of stool for fat (e.g., Sudan III stain), a

**TABLE 42-31 Causes of Malabsorption**

| Biochemical or Enzyme Deficiencies | Bacterial Proliferation |
|---|---|
| • Biliary tract obstruction<br>• Chronic pancreatitis<br>• Cystic fibrosis<br>• Lactase deficiency<br>• Pancreatic insufficiency<br>• Zollinger-Ellison syndrome | • Parasitic infection<br>• Tropical sprue |
| **Disturbed Lymphatic and Vascular Circulation** | **Small Intestinal Mucosal Disruption** |
| • Heart failure<br>• Ischemia<br>• Lymphangiectasia<br>• Lymphoma | • Celiac disease<br>• Crohn's disease<br>• Whipple's disease |
| | **Surface Area Loss** |
| | • Billroth II gastrectomy<br>• Distal ileal resection, disease, or bypass<br>• Short bowel syndrome |

**TABLE 42-32 Manifestations of Malabsorption**

| Manifestations | Pathophysiology |
|---|---|
| **Gastrointestinal** | |
| Weight loss | Malabsorption of fat, carbohydrates, and protein leading to loss of calories. Marked reduction in caloric intake or increased use of calories |
| Diarrhea | Impaired absorption of water, sodium, fatty acids, bile salts, and carbohydrates |
| Flatulence | Bacterial fermentation of unabsorbed carbohydrates |
| Steatorrhea | Undigested and unabsorbed fat |
| Glossitis, cheilosis, stomatitis | Deficiency of iron, riboflavin, cobalamin, folic acid, and other vitamins |
| **Hematologic** | |
| Anemia | Impaired absorption of iron, cobalamin, and folic acid |
| Hemorrhagic tendency | Vitamin C deficiency. Vitamin K deficiency inhibiting production of clotting factors II, VII, IX, and X |
| **Musculoskeletal** | |
| Bone pain | Osteoporosis from impaired calcium absorption. Osteomalacia secondary to hypocalcemia, hypophosphatemia, inadequate vitamin D |
| Tetany | Hypocalcemia, hypomagnesemia |
| Weakness, muscle cramps | Anemia, electrolyte depletion (especially potassium) |
| Muscle wasting | Protein malabsorption |
| **Neurologic** | |
| Altered mental status | Dehydration |
| Paresthesias | Cobalamin deficiency |
| Peripheral neuropathy | Cobalamin deficiency |
| Night blindness | Thiamine deficiency, vitamin A deficiency |
| **Integumentary** | |
| Bruising | Vitamin K deficiency |
| Dermatitis | Fatty acid deficiency, zinc deficiency, niacin and other vitamin deficiencies |
| Brittle nails | Iron deficiency |
| Hair thinning and loss | Protein deficiency |
| **Cardiovascular** | |
| Hypotension | Dehydration |
| Tachycardia | Hypovolemia, anemia |
| Peripheral edema | Protein malabsorption, protein loss in diarrhea |

72-hour stool collection for quantitative measurement of fecal fat, serologic testing for celiac disease, and fecal elastase testing to determine if there is pancreatic insufficiency. Near-infrared reflectance analysis (NIRA) for fecal fat is available at some centers in the United States.

Other diagnostic studies include a CT scan and endoscopy to obtain a small bowel biopsy specimen. A small bowel barium enema can identify abnormal mucosal patterns. Capsule endoscopy is useful in assessing the small intestine for alterations in mucosal integrity and inflammation. Tests for carbohydrate malabsorption include the D-xylose test and the lactose tolerance test. Laboratory studies that are frequently ordered include a CBC, measurement of prothrombin time (to see if vitamin K absorption is adequate), serum vitamin A and carotene levels, serum electrolytes, cholesterol, and calcium. Treatment depends on the cause.

## CELIAC DISEASE

**Celiac disease** is an autoimmune disease characterized by damage to the small intestinal mucosa from ingesting wheat, barley, and rye.[30] It can occur at any age and has a wide variety of symptoms. *Celiac sprue* and *gluten-sensitive enteropathy* are other names for celiac disease.

Celiac disease is not the same disease as *tropical sprue,* a chronic disorder occurring primarily in tropical areas. Tropical sprue causes progressive disruption of jejunal and ileal tissue, resulting in nutritional difficulties. It is treated with folic acid and tetracycline.

Celiac disease is most common in people of European ancestry and affects about 1% of the population of the United States.[30] High-risk groups include first- or second-degree relatives of someone with celiac disease and people with disorders associated with the disease such as migraine and myocarditis. It is slightly more common in women. Symptoms often begin in childhood.

### Etiology and Pathophysiology

Three factors necessary for developing celiac disease are genetic predisposition, gluten ingestion, and an immune-mediated response.

### Genetic Link

About 90% to 95% of patients with celiac disease have human leukocyte antigen (HLA) allele HLA-DQ2. The other 5% to 10% have HLA-DQ8. However, not everyone with these genetic markers develops celiac disease, and some people with celiac disease do not have these HLA alleles.

As with other autoimmune diseases, the tissue destruction that occurs with celiac disease is the result of chronic inflammation. Gluten contains specific peptides called *prolamines.* Partial digestion of gluten releases the prolamine peptides, which are absorbed into the intestinal submucosa. In genetically susceptible individuals, the peptides bind to HLA-DQ2 and/or HLA-DQ8 and activate an inflammatory response. Inflammation damages the microvilli and brush border of the small intestine, ultimately decreasing the amount of surface area available for nutrient absorption. Damage is most severe in the duodenum, probably because it has more exposure to gluten. The inflammation lasts as long as gluten ingestion continues.

### Clinical Manifestations

Classic manifestations of celiac disease include foul-smelling diarrhea, steatorrhea, flatulence, abdominal distention, and malnutrition.[30] Some people have no obvious GI symptoms and may instead have atypical signs and symptoms such as decreased bone density and osteoporosis, dental enamel hypoplasia, iron and folate deficiencies, peripheral neuropathy, and reproductive problems. An intensely pruritic, vesicular skin lesion, called *dermatitis herpetiformis,* is sometimes present and occurs as a rash on the buttocks, scalp, face, elbows, and knees. Celiac disease is also associated with other autoimmune diseases, particularly rheumatoid arthritis, type 1 diabetes mellitus, and thyroid disease.

Protein, fat, and carbohydrate absorption is affected. Weight loss, muscle wasting, and other signs of malnutrition may be present. Abnormal serum folate, iron, and cobalamin levels can occur. Iron-deficiency anemia is common. Patients may exhibit lactose intolerance and need to refrain from lactose-containing products until the disease is under control. Inadequate calcium intake and vitamin D absorption can lead to decreased bone density and osteoporosis.

### Diagnostic Studies and Interprofessional Care

Early diagnosis and treatment can prevent complications. Screening is recommended for close relatives of patients known to have the disease, young patients with decreased bone density, those with anemia once other causes are ruled out, and certain autoimmune diseases.

Celiac disease is confirmed by a combination of findings from the history and physical exam, serology testing, and histologic analysis of small intestine biopsies.[31] Have the patient complete diagnostic testing before starting a gluten-free diet, since the diet will alter the results. Serologic testing for immunoglobulin A (IgA) antitissue transglutaminase and IgA endomysial antibody provides good sensitivity and specificity. Histologic evidence remains the gold standard for confirming the diagnosis. Biopsies show flattened mucosa and noticeable losses of villi. Genotyping involves testing for HLA-DQ2 and/or HLA-DQ8 antigens.

A gluten-free diet (Table 42-33) is the only effective treatment for celiac disease. Most patients need to maintain on a gluten-free diet for the rest of their lives. If the disease is untreated, chronic inflammation and hyperplasia continue. Individuals with celiac disease have an increased risk of non-Hodgkin's lymphoma and GI cancers. Those with refractory disease who do not respond to a gluten-free diet alone may need corticosteroid therapy.

Refer all patients for a dietary consultation. You can work with a dietitian to teach the patient how to eat a nutritionally adequate diet while staying within a budget. Teach the patient to avoid wheat, barley, oats, and rye products. Although pure oats do not contain gluten, wheat, rye, and barley can contaminate oat products during the milling process. Teach the patient to read medication and food labels. Some medications and many food additives, preservatives, and stabilizers contain gluten. The patient needs to know where to purchase gluten-free products. Good sources are health food stores, many grocery stores, and through Internet sites.

Maintaining a gluten-free diet can be difficult, particularly when traveling or eating in restaurants. Many with celiac disease describe feeling embarrassed or like a burden when having to discuss gluten-free menu options with restaurant staff or when dining in other's homes. Mobile phone users will find apps listing gluten-free menu options at popular restaurants helpful. Many restaurants now indicate which food choices are gluten free. The Celiac Sprue Association website *(www.csaceliacs.info)* and the Celiac Disease Foundation *(www.celiac.org)* provide suggestions for maintaining a gluten-free diet and living with celiac disease.

**TABLE 42-33 Nutritional Therapy**

***Celiac Disease***

| Foods to Eat | Foods to Avoid |
|---|---|
| • Butter<br>• Cheese, cottage cheese<br>• Coffee, tea, and cocoa<br>• Corn tortillas<br>• Eggs<br>• Flax, corn, and rice<br>• Fresh fruits<br>• Gluten-free flour breads, crackers, pasta, and cereals<br>• Meat, fish, poultry (not marinated or breaded)<br>• Peanut butter<br>• Potatoes<br>• Soy products<br>• Tapioca<br>• Unflavored milk<br>• Yogurt | • Baked goods, including muffins, cookies, cakes, pies<br>• Barley<br>• Bread, including wheat bread, white bread, "potato" bread<br>• Flour<br>• Gluten stabilizers<br>• Oats<br>• Pasta, pizza, bagels<br>• Rye<br>• Wheat |

## LACTASE DEFICIENCY

**Lactase deficiency** is a condition in which the lactase enzyme is deficient or absent. Lactase is the enzyme that breaks down lactose into two simple sugars: glucose and galactose. Primary lactase insufficiency is most commonly a result of genetic factors. Certain ethnic or racial groups, especially those with Asian or African ancestry, develop low lactase levels in childhood. Less common causes include low lactase levels resulting from premature birth and congenital lactase deficiency, a rare genetic disorder. Lactose malabsorption can occur when conditions leading to bacterial overgrowth promote lactose fermentation in the small bowel or when intestinal mucosal damage interferes with absorption. The latter occurs with IBD and celiac disease.

Symptoms of lactose intolerance include bloating, flatulence, cramping abdominal pain, and diarrhea. Diarrhea results from the excess, undigested lactose in the small intestine attracting water molecules, which prevents them from being properly absorbed. Symptoms generally occur within 30 minutes to several hours after drinking a glass of milk or ingesting a milk product. Lactose intolerance is diagnosed with a lactose tolerance test, a lactose hydrogen breath test, or genetic testing.

Treatment consists of eliminating lactose from the diet by avoiding milk and milk products, and/or replacing lactase with commercially available preparations. A lactose-free diet generally results in prompt resolution of symptoms. Many lactose-intolerant persons are aware of their condition. They likely have been avoiding lactose-containing products and using lactose-free milk products. Lactase enzyme (Lactaid) is available as an over-the-counter product. It breaks down the lactose present in ingested milk. A number of milk products treated with lactase enzyme are readily available.

The diet may gradually advance to a low-lactose diet as tolerated by the patient. Many lactose-intolerant persons may not exhibit symptoms if they have lactose in small amounts. Cheese contains less lactose than milk and ice cream. Live culture yogurt has less lactose because the bacteria help digest the lactose. Teach the patient to read labels to detect any hidden sources of milk products. Some people tolerate lactose better if taken with meals. Teach the patient that adhering to the diet is important. Since avoiding milk and milk products can lead to calcium deficiency, supplements may be necessary to prevent osteoporosis.

## SHORT BOWEL SYNDROME

**Short bowel syndrome (SBS)** is a condition in which the small intestine does not have adequate surface area to absorb enough nutrients. This leaves the person unable to meet energy, fluid, electrolyte, and nutritional needs to stay healthy on a normal diet. Causes of SBS include diseases that damage the intestinal mucosa, surgical removal of too much small intestine (primarily in patients with Crohn's disease), and congenital defects.

SBS is likely to develop in patients with a loss of two-thirds length of the small intestine. The length and area of the remaining small intestine and the presence of the colon affect the patient's outcome. If the terminal ileum and ileocecal valve remain intact, the remaining intestine undergoes adaptive changes that are most pronounced in the ileum. The villi and crypts increase in size, and the absorptive capacity of the remaining intestine increases. When the colon is present, fluid and electrolyte absorption increases. Those with an end jejunostomy often have little to no adaptation. Providing enteral nutrition and a normal diet after surgery stimulates the remaining intestine to adapt and function better.

### Clinical Manifestations

The predominant manifestation of SBS is chronic diarrhea. Other manifestations include abdominal pain, flatulence, and steatorrhea. Signs of malnutrition as well as vitamin and mineral deficiencies include weight loss, cobalamin and zinc deficiency, and hypocalcemia. The patient may develop lactase deficiency and bacterial overgrowth. Oxalate kidney stones may form because of increased colonic absorption of oxalate.

### Interprofessional Care

The treatment goals are that the patient will have fluid and electrolyte balance, normal nutritional status, and control of diarrhea. The main treatment is nutritional support involving parenteral nutrition, enteral nutrition, medications, and a tailored diet. In the immediate period after massive bowel resection, patients receive parenteral nutrition to replace fluid, electrolyte, and nutrient losses and to rest the bowel. Those with severe resections will require parenteral nutrition indefinitely. Enteral nutrition and a normal diet are gradually resumed to stimulate the remaining intestine to function better. Some can eventually discontinue parenteral nutrition.

Refer the patient to a dietitian. The optimal diet is high in protein and complex carbohydrates and low in fat and concentrated sweets. Oral supplements of calcium, zinc, and multivitamins may be required. Soluble fiber is encouraged if the colon is present. The patient should eat at least six small meals per day to increase the time of contact between food and the intestine. Oral intake may be supplemented with elemental nutrient formulas and tube feeding during the night. For patients with severe malabsorption, parenteral nutrition is necessary (see Chapter 39).

Patients often take multiple medications to help control fecal output. Excess fluid secretion is reduced with $H_2$ blockers, proton pump inhibitors, $\alpha$-adrenergic receptor agonists (e.g., clonidine), or octreotide. Opioid antidiarrheal drugs are the most effective in decreasing intestinal motility (Table 42-2). For patients who have limited ileal resections, cholestyramine (Questran) reduces diarrhea resulting from unabsorbed bile acids by increasing their excretion in feces. Bile acids stimulate intestinal fluid secretion and reduce colonic fluid absorption. Antibiotic therapy is used if bacterial overgrowth is contributing to diarrhea.[32]

Three drugs have FDA approval for the treatment of SBS: somatropin (Zorbtive), glutamine, and teduglutide (Gattex). Somatropin enhances intestinal adaption and increases the flow of water, electrolytes, and nutrients into the bowel. Glutamine improves intestinal absorption. Teduglutide helps to increase the surface area of the intestine and improve intestinal absorption of fluids and nutrients.

*Intestinal transplantation* is a procedure performed at a few specialized transplant centers in the United States. It is considered the only long-term treatment option for patients with intestinal failure who have irreversible complications from parenteral nutrition. The leading cause of intestinal failure is SBS. Transplantation may include the intestine alone, liver and intestine, or multivisceral combinations (stomach, duodenum, jejunum, ileum, colon, and/or pancreas).

## GASTROINTESTINAL STROMAL TUMORS

*Gastrointestinal stromal tumors* (GISTs) are a rare form of cancer that originates in cells found in the wall of the GI tract. These cells, known as *interstitial cells of Cajal,* help control the movement of food and liquid through the stomach and intestines. About 55% of GISTs are in the stomach; 35% are in the small intestine; and the rest are in the gallbladder, esophagus, colon, or peritoneum.[33] Most GISTs occur in people between the ages of 50 and 70. While the exact cause of GISTs is unknown, genetic mutations likely play a role. A few GISTs occur in people with familial mutations in either the KIT or platelet-derived growth factor receptor a (PDGFRa) oncogenes or occur in those with neurofibromatosis type 1.[33]

The manifestations of GISTs depend on the part of the GI tract affected. Early manifestations are often subtle, including early satiety, fatigue, bloating, nausea or vomiting, and a change in bowel habits. Because these manifestations are similar to those of many other GI problems, early detection of the cancer is difficult. Later manifestations may include GI bleeding and obstruction caused by growth of the tumor. GISTs are often found during imaging for other problems. Diagnosis is based on histologic examination of biopsied tissue. Endoscopic ultrasound, CT, or MRI are used to determine the extent of disease.

Patients initially undergo surgery to remove the tumor, but the GIST has often metastasized by the time of diagnosis or commonly recurs. GISTs are unresponsive to conventional chemotherapy. However, discovery of genetic mutations led to the development of tyrosine kinase inhibitor drugs (e.g., imatinib mesylate [Gleevec], regorafenib [Stivarga]) that are highly effective against certain GISTs.[33]

# ANORECTAL PROBLEMS

## HEMORRHOIDS

**Hemorrhoids** are dilated hemorrhoidal veins. They may be internal (occurring above the internal sphincter) or external (occurring outside the external sphincter) (Figs. 42-15 and 42-16). In affected persons, hemorrhoids appear periodically, depending on the amount of anorectal pressure.

### Etiology and Pathophysiology

Hemorrhoids develop because of increased anal pressure and weakening of the connective tissue that supports the hemorrhoidal veins. Weakened supporting tissue allows for downward displacement of the hemorrhoidal veins, causing them to dilate. Blood flow through the veins of the hemorrhoidal plexus is impaired. An intravascular clot in the venule results in a thrombosed external hemorrhoid. Many factors increase the risk for hemorrhoids, including pregnancy, prolonged constipation,

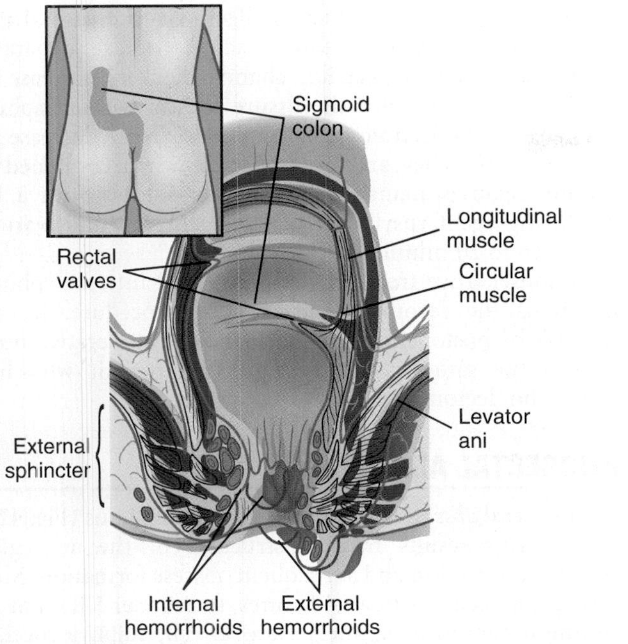


**FIG. 42-15** Anatomic structures of the rectum and anus with external and internal hemorrhoids.

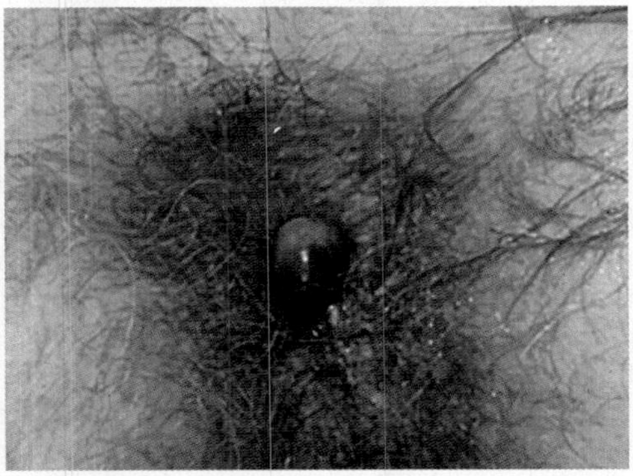

**FIG. 42-16** Thrombosed external hemorrhoids. (From Townsend CM, Beauchamp RD, Evers BM, et al: *Sabiston textbook of surgery: the biological basis of modern surgical practice,* ed 19, Philadelphia, 2012, Saunders.)

straining in an effort to defecate, heavy lifting, prolonged standing and sitting, obesity, and portal hypertension.

## Clinical Manifestations

Hemorrhoids are the most common reason for bleeding with defecation. Other manifestations include anal pruritus, prolapse, and pain. Internal hemorrhoids most often cause painless bright red bleeding with stools, on the toilet paper, or dripping into the toilet water. If internal hemorrhoids become constricted, the patient will report pain. Internal hemorrhoids can prolapse into the anal canal or externally. Symptoms of prolapse include pressure with defecation and a protruding mass.

External hemorrhoids are reddish blue and seldom bleed. There may be itching, burning, and edema. They usually do not cause pain unless thrombosis (blood clots) is present. Thrombosed hemorrhoids are a bluish purple tinge and palpable at the anal orifice. They usually cause pain and inflammation. The clot can erode through the overlying stretched skin, causing bleeding with defecation. Constipation or diarrhea can aggravate these symptoms.

## Diagnostic Studies and Interprofessional Care

Internal hemorrhoids are diagnosed by digital examination, anoscopy, and sigmoidoscopy. External hemorrhoids are easily diagnosed by visual inspection and digital examination.

Therapy is based on the cause and the patient's symptoms. A high-fiber diet and increased fluid intake prevent constipation and reduce straining, which allows engorgement of the veins to subside. The resulting stool bulk may also decrease stool leakage and therefore itching. Ointments such as dibucaine; creams, suppositories, and impregnated pads that contain antiinflammatory agents (e.g., hydrocortisone); or astringents and anesthetics (e.g., witch hazel, benzocaine) may be used to shrink the mucous membranes and relieve discomfort. The use of topical corticosteroids should be limited to 1 week or less to prevent side effects such as contact dermatitis and mucosal atrophy. Stool softeners can keep the stools soft. Sitz baths help relieve pain.

External hemorrhoids are usually managed by conservative therapy unless they become thrombosed. For internal hemorrhoids, nonsurgical approaches (rubber band ligation, infrared coagulation, sclerotherapy, laser treatment) are options.[34] Rubber band ligation is the most widely used technique. The surgeon inserts an anoscope to identify the hemorrhoid and then ligates it with a rubber band. The rubber band around the hemorrhoid constricts circulation, and the tissue becomes necrotic, separates, and sloughs off. There is some local discomfort with this procedure, but no anesthetic is required.

A *hemorrhoidectomy* is the surgical excision of hemorrhoids. Surgery is indicated when there is marked prolapse, excessive pain or bleeding, or large or multiple thrombosed hemorrhoids. Surgical removal is done by cautery, clamp, or excision. After removing the hemorrhoids, the tissue is either sutured and the wound heals by primary intention or the area is left open and healing takes place by secondary intention.

## ❖ NURSING MANAGEMENT: HEMORRHOIDS

Conservative nursing management for the patient with hemorrhoids includes teaching measures to prevent constipation and to avoid prolonged standing or sitting, and proper use of OTC drugs for hemorrhoidal symptoms. Teach the patient to seek medical care for severe symptoms of hemorrhoids (e.g., excessive pain and bleeding, prolapsed hemorrhoids). Sitz baths (15 to 20 minutes, two or three times each day) may help to reduce discomfort and swelling associated with hemorrhoids.

Nursing care after a hemorrhoidectomy focuses on pain control and promoting wound healing. Be aware that although the procedure is minor, the pain is severe and feared by many. There are several analgesic regimens, using a combination of medications. Most patients initially receive an opioid and NSAID in conjunction with topical preparations that provide anesthesia or reduce internal sphincter spasms, such as glyceryl trinitrate (GTN), calcium channel blockers (e.g., nifedipine with lidocaine, diltiazem), or nitroglycerin preparations.

The patient usually dreads the first bowel movement and often resists the urge to defecate. Give pain medication before the bowel movement to reduce discomfort. Stool softeners (e.g., docusate [Colace]) and bulking agents help form a soft, bulky stool that is easier to pass. If the patient does not have a bowel movement within 2 or 3 days, an oil-retention enema is given.

Sitz baths are started 1 or 2 days after surgery and continued for 1 to 2 weeks. A warm sitz bath provides comfort and keeps the anal area clean. A sponge ring in the sitz bath helps relieve pressure on the area. Initially, do not leave the patient alone because of the possibility of weakness or fainting. Instruct the patient that pressure relief cushions are acceptable to ease discomfort when sitting. Tell the patient not to use a pressure relief ring or "doughnut" because they can reduce blood flow to the area.

The patient may have packing in the rectum to absorb drainage, with a T-binder to hold the dressing in place. Packing is usually removed on the first or second postoperative day. Assess for rectal bleeding, especially in patients taking clopidogrel or oral anticoagulants. The patient may be embarrassed when the dressing is changed. Provide as much privacy as possible.

Teach the patient the importance of diet, care of the anal area, symptoms of complications (especially bleeding), and avoidance of constipation and straining. Hemorrhoids may recur. Occasionally, anal strictures develop and dilation is necessary. Regular checkups are important to prevent any further problems.

## ANAL FISSURE

An *anal fissure* is a skin ulcer or a crack in the lining of the anal wall. Many times the initiating factor is the passage of hard stools. Other fissures are related to trauma (anal intercourse, insertion of a foreign body such as endoscope), local infection (syphilis; tuberculosis; gonorrhea; or infection with *Chlamydia,* herpes simplex virus, or HIV), or inflammation (Fig. 42-17). An anal fissure is considered acute when it is of recent onset (less than 6 weeks), and chronic if it has been present for a longer period. Chronic fissures have a characteristic appearance that includes perianal skin tag and fibrotic edges.[35]

Anal tissue ulcerates because of ischemia caused by a combination of high pressure in the internal anal sphincter and poor blood supply to the area. The ischemic tissue may ulcerate spontaneously or when traumatized by factors such as hard stools that would not normally cause tissue breakdown. Ischemia must be corrected for a fissure to heal.

The hallmark of an anal fissure is severe anal pain. It tends to be worse with defecation and with direct pressure on the site (e.g., sitting). Acute fissures tend to bleed slightly, and patients may report red blood on the toilet paper. Constipation results because of fear of pain associated with bowel movements.

Anal fissures are easy to diagnose with a physical examination. Conservative care with fiber supplements, adequate fluid

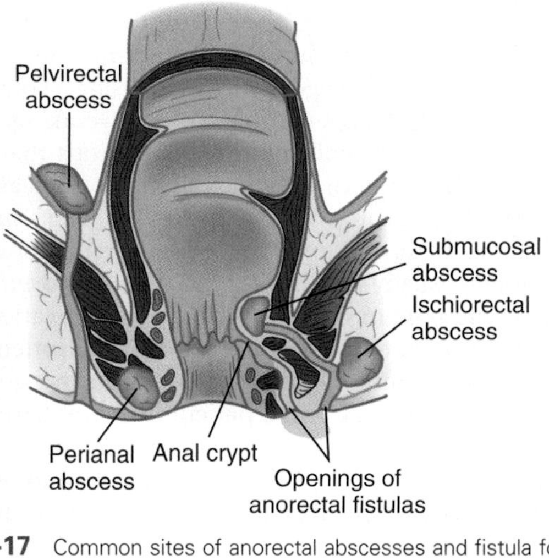


**FIG. 42-17** Common sites of anorectal abscesses and fistula formation.

intake, sitz baths, and topical analgesics is successful in most cases, especially if the fissure is acute. Topical preparations, including nitrates and calcium channel blockers, decrease rectal anal pressure and allow the fissure to heal without sphincter damage. Local injections of botulinum toxin can decrease rectal anal pressure. They are most effective when combined with nitrates. Pain is managed by softening stools with a bulk-producing agent (psyllium) or stool softener, and warm sitz baths (15 to 20 minutes, 3 times per day).[35]

If conservative treatment fails, a lateral internal sphincterotomy is the recommended surgical procedure. It carries the risk of postoperative incontinence. Postoperative nursing care is the same as the care for the patient who had a hemorrhoidectomy.

## ANORECTAL ABSCESS

An *anorectal abscess* is a collection of perianal pus (Fig. 42-17). The abscess results from obstruction of the anal glands, leading to infection and subsequent abscess formation. Abscess formation occurs with anal fissures, trauma, or IBD. The most common causative organisms are *E. coli*, staphylococci, and streptococci. Clinical manifestations include local severe pain and swelling, foul-smelling drainage, tenderness, and elevated temperature. Sepsis can occur as a complication. Anorectal abscesses are diagnosed by rectal examination.

Anorectal abscesses require surgical drainage. Larger abscesses require packing afterwards with impregnated gauze or placement of drains (e.g., Penrose) to promote drainage. The area then heals by granulation. Patients who have diabetes, cellulitis, or are immunocompromised (e.g., chemotherapy) may require antibiotic therapy. Nursing care includes warm, moist heat applications and changing packing daily. The patient is usually more comfortable lying on the abdomen or side. A low-fiber diet is given. The patient may leave the hospital with the wound still open. Teach the patient about wound care and the importance of sitz baths, thorough cleaning after urinating or bowel movements, and follow-up visits with the HCP.

## ANAL FISTULA

An **anal fistula** is an abnormal tunnel leading from the anus or rectum. It may extend to the outside of the skin, vagina, or buttocks and often precedes an abscess. Anal fistulas are a complication of Crohn's disease and may resolve when drug treatment (i.e., with infliximab) achieves remission of the disease. About 50% of anal fistulas are due to anorectal abscess.

Feces may enter the fistula and cause an infection. There may be persistent, bloody, or purulent discharge, or stool leakage from the fistula. The patient may need to wear a pad to avoid staining clothes.

Surgical treatment of an anal fistula depends on the location and nature of the fistula. In a fistulotomy, the surgeon opens the fistula and healthy tissue is allowed to granulate in the wound. Care is the same as that after a hemorrhoidectomy. Options for complex fistulas include ligation of the intersphincteric fistula tract (LIFT), or the use of rectal flaps, setons, plugs, or fibrin glue injections to seal the fistula.

## ANAL CANCER

Anal cancer is uncommon in the general population, but the incidence is increasing. In the United States approximately 7200 people are diagnosed with anal cancer each year.[36] It mainly occurs in older adults, with the average age being in the early 60s. Human papillomavirus (HPV) is associated with about 80% of the cases of anal cancer. Those at high risk for anal cancer include smokers, men who have sex with men, women with cervical or vulvar cancer or precancerous lesions, and people who are immunocompromised (e.g., posttransplantation immunosuppression) or HIV-positive.[37]

The most frequent initial symptom is rectal bleeding. Other symptoms include rectal pain and sensation of a rectal mass. Some patients have no symptoms, which leads to delayed diagnosis and treatment.

It is especially important to screen high-risk individuals using DRE and anal Pap tests. In an anal Pap test, the anal lining is swabbed and the cells examined to identify any cell changes (e.g., dysplasia, neoplasia). High-resolution anoscopy allows for visualization of the mucosa and biopsy. An endoanal *(endorectal) ultrasound* may also be done.

Review with the patient behavior practices used to reduce the risk of sexually transmitted infections. Encourage the use of condoms, avoiding unprotected anal sex, and limiting sexual partners. Two HPV vaccines are available to help prevent cervical, vulvar, vaginal, and anal cancers and associated precancerous lesions. Both Gardasil and Gardasil 9 vaccines protect against HPV types 6, 11, 16, and 18. Gardasil 9 protects against 5 additional HPV types, 31, 33, 45, 52, and 58. After vaccination with HPV vaccine, patients at risk need to continue their recommended screening program.[37]

Treatment of anal cancer depends on the size and depth of the lesions. Topical therapy with bichloroacetic or trichloroacetic acid may be used to remove genital warts and kill the HPV virus. Options for precancerous lesions are surgical removal or treatment with topical imiquimod (Aldara) and 5-FU. Cancer therapy involves surgery or a combination of radiation and chemotherapy. Chemotherapy regimens include combinations of mitomycin, cisplatin, and 5-FU.

## PILONIDAL SINUS

A *pilonidal sinus* is a small tract under the skin between the buttocks in the sacrococcygeal area. It is thought to be of congenital origin. It may have several openings and is lined with epithelium and hair, hence the name *pilonidal* ("a nest of hair"). The skin is moist, and movement of the buttocks causes the short, wiry hair to penetrate the skin. If the irritated skin becomes infected, it forms a pilonidal cyst or abscess. There are no symptoms with a pilonidal sinus unless there is an infection. Then the patient complains of pain and swelling at the base of the spine.

An abscess requires incision and drainage. The wound may be closed, or left open to heal by secondary intention. The wound is packed, and sitz baths are ordered. Nursing care includes warm, moist heat applications when an abscess is present. The patient is usually more comfortable lying on the abdomen or side. Teach the patient to avoid contaminating the dressing when urinating or defecating and to avoid straining whenever possible.

## CASE STUDY

### *Colorectal Cancer*

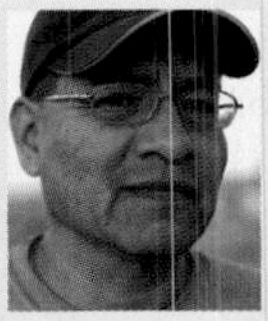

(©iStockphoto/ Thinkstock)

**Patient Profile**

L.C., a 58-yr-old Native American man, is from a Pueblo tribe in northern New Mexico. L.C.'s wife and family drove 50 miles to take him to the Indian Health Service hospital because of his deteriorating health (see the case study in Chapter 38 on p. 839).

**Subjective Data**

See the case study in Chapter 38 on p. 843.

**Objective Data**

***Physical Examination***

See the case study in Chapter 38 on p. 845.

***Laboratory Tests***

- CT scan and colonoscopy show two medium-sized tumors in the transverse colon.

**Interprofessional Care**

***Surgical Procedure***

- Transverse hemicolectomy performed and lymph node biopsies taken.
- Pathology results indicate that the adenocarcinoma tumor has invaded the muscle wall of colon and 2 out of 5 lymph nodes are positive for cancer.

***Postoperative***

- Feels like his life has ended and does not want to leave hospital.
- States that there is "no one" to take care of him at his home and he is far away from the hospital.

**Follow-Up Treatment**

Scheduled for outpatient chemotherapy

**Discussion Questions**

1. What signs and symptoms of colorectal cancer did L.C. manifest (see the case study in Chapter 38 on p. 852)?
2. What stage of CRC does L.C. probably have? What treatment is recommended for this stage of CRC?
3. How could you provide emotional support to L.C. and his family?
4. ***Patient-Centered Care:*** What is a culturally sensitive way for you to support L.C. and his family in making decisions about his continued health care?
5. ***Priority Decision:*** Based on the assessment data, what are the priority nursing diagnoses? Are there any collaborative problems?
6. ***Priority Decision:*** What are the priority nursing interventions for L.C. at this stage of his illness?
7. ***Teamwork and Collaboration:*** What referrals may be indicated at this time?
8. ***Evidence-Based Practice:*** L.C. had not had a previous colonoscopy. He is worried that other members of his family may have colon cancer. What can you tell him about the recommendations for colorectal cancer screening?
9. ***Quality Improvement:*** What outcomes would indicate nursing interventions were successful?

Answers available at *http://evolve.elsevier.com/Lewis/medsurg.*

## BRIDGE TO NCLEX EXAMINATION

The number of the question corresponds to the same-numbered outcome at the beginning of the chapter.

1. The *most* appropriate therapy for a patient with acute diarrhea caused by a viral infection is to
   **a.** increase fluid intake.
   **b.** administer an antibiotic.
   **c.** administer an antimotility drug.
   **d.** quarantine the patient to prevent spread of the virus.
2. A 35-year-old female patient is admitted to the emergency department with acute abdominal pain. Which medical diagnoses should you consider as possible causes of her pain *(select all that apply)*?
   **a.** Gastroenteritis
   **b.** Ectopic pregnancy
   **c.** Gastrointestinal bleeding
   **d.** Irritable bowel syndrome
   **e.** Inflammatory bowel disease
3. Assessment findings suggestive of peritonitis include *(select all that apply)*
   **a.** rebound tenderness.
   **b.** a soft, distended abdomen.
   **c.** dull, intermittent abdominal pain.
   **d.** shallow respirations with bradypnea.
   **e.** observing that the patient is lying still.
4. In planning care for the patient with Crohn's disease, the nurse recognizes that a major difference between ulcerative colitis and Crohn's disease is that Crohn's disease
   **a.** frequently results in toxic megacolon.
   **b.** causes fewer nutritional deficiencies than ulcerative colitis.
   **c.** often recurs after surgery, whereas ulcerative colitis is curable with a colectomy.
   **d.** is manifested by rectal bleeding and anemia more often than is ulcerative colitis.
5. The nurse performs a detailed assessment of the abdomen of a patient with a possible bowel obstruction, knowing that manifestations of an obstruction in the large intestine are *(select all that apply)*
   **a.** persistent abdominal pain.
   **b.** marked abdominal distention.
   **c.** diarrhea that is loose or liquid.
   **d.** colicky, severe, intermittent pain.
   **e.** profuse vomiting that relieves abdominal pain.
6. A patient with stage I colorectal cancer is scheduled for surgery. Patient teaching for this patient would include an explanation that
   **a.** chemotherapy will begin after the patient recovers from the surgery.
   **b.** both chemotherapy and radiation can be used as palliative treatments.
   **c.** follow-up colonoscopies will be needed to ensure that the cancer does not recur.
   **d.** a wound, ostomy, and continence nurse will visit the patient to identify an abdominal site for the ostomy.
7. The nurse determines a patient undergoing ileostomy surgery understands the procedure when the patient states
   **a.** "I should only have to change the pouch every 4 to 7 days."
   **b.** "The drainage in the pouch will look like my normal stools."
   **c.** "I may not need to wear a drainage pouch if I irrigate it daily."
   **d.** "Limiting my fluid intake should decrease the amount of output."
8. In contrast to diverticulitis, the patient with diverticulosis
   **a.** has rectal bleeding.
   **b.** often has no symptoms.
   **c.** has localized cramping pain.
   **d.** frequently develops peritonitis.
9. A nursing intervention that is *most* appropriate to decrease postoperative edema and pain after an inguinal herniorrhaphy is
   **a.** applying a truss to the hernia site.
   **b.** allowing the patient to stand to void.
   **c.** supporting the incision during coughing.
   **d.** applying a scrotal support with an ice bag.
10. The nurse determines that the goals of dietary teaching have been met when the patient with celiac disease selects from the menu
    **a.** scrambled eggs and sausage.
    **b.** buckwheat pancakes with syrup.
    **c.** oatmeal, skim milk, and orange juice.
    **d.** yogurt, strawberries, and rye toast with butter.
11. What should a patient be taught after a hemorrhoidectomy?
    **a.** Take mineral oil before bedtime.
    **b.** Eat a low-fiber diet to rest the colon.
    **c.** Administer oil-retention enema to empty the colon.
    **d.** Use prescribed pain medication before a bowel movement.

1. a, 2. a, b, c, d, 3. a, e, 4. c, 5. a, b, 6. c, 7. a, 8. b, 9. d, 10. a, 11. d

For rationales to these answers and even more NCLEX review questions, visit *http://evolve.elsevier.com/Lewis/medsurg*.

## EVOLVE WEBSITE

http://evolve.elsevier.com/Lewis/medsurg

**Review Questions (Online Only)**

**Key Points**

**Answer Keys for Questions**

- Rationales for Bridge to NCLEX Examination Questions
- Answer Guidelines for Case Study on p. 971

**Student Case Study**

- Patient With Ulcerative Colitis

**Nursing Care Plans**

- eNursing Care Plan 42-1: Patient With Acute Infectious Diarrhea
- eNursing Care Plan 42-2: Patient With Inflammatory Bowel Disease
- eNursing Care Plan 42-3: Patient With a Colostomy/Ileostomy

**Conceptual Care Map Creator**

**Audio Glossary**

**Content Updates**

## REFERENCES

1. Hamilton AC, Moises A: Diarrhea, *Hosp Med Clin* 2:e227, 2013.
*2. Surawicz C, Brandt L, Zuckerbraun B, et al: Guidelines for diagnosis, treatment, and prevention of *Clostridium difficile* infections, *Am J Gastroenterol* 108:478, 2013.
3. Orenstein R, Griesbach CL, DiBaise JK: Moving fecal microbiota transplantation into the mainstream, *Nutr Clin Pract* 28:589, 2013.
*4. Whitehead W, Rao S, Hamilton F, et al: Treatment of fecal incontinence: state of the science summary for the National Institute of Diabetes and Digestive and Kidney Diseases workshop, *Am J Gastroenterol* 110:138, 2015.
*5. Kottner J, Blume-Peytavi U, Lohrmann C, et al: Associations between individual characteristics and incontinence-associated dermatitis, *Int J Nurs Stud* 51:1373, 2014.
6. Whiteley I, Sinclair G: Fecal management systems for disabling incontinence or wounds, *Br J Nurs* 23:881, 2014.

*7. Bharucha A, Pemberton J, Locke G: American Gastroenterological Association technical review on constipation, *Gastroenterol* 144:218, 2013.
8. Peyton L, Greene J: Irritable bowel syndrome: current and emerging treatment options, *P&T* 38:567, 2014.
*9. Anusha T, Eamonn MQ: Diet and irritable bowel syndrome, *Curr Opin Gastroenterol* 31:605, 2015.
10. Teixeira PG, Demetrios D: Appendicitis: changing perspectives, *Adv in Surg* 47:119, 2013.
*11. Hou JK, Lee D, Lewis J: Diet and inflammatory bowel disease: review of patient-targeted recommendations, *Clin Gastroenterol Hepatol* 12:1592, 2014.
12. Ek WE, D'Amato M, Halfvarson J: The history of genetics in inflammatory bowel disease, *Ann Gastroenterol* 27:294, 2014.
13. NOD2. Retrieved from *http://ghr.nlm.nih.gov/gene/NOD2.*
*14. Berg AM, Kelly CP, Farraye FA: Clostridium difficile infection in the inflammatory bowel disease patient, *Inflamm Bowel Dis* 19:194, 2013.
15. Park SC, Jeen YT: Current and emerging biologics for ulcerative colitis, *Gut and Liver* 9:18, 2015.
*16. Pappa H: Vitamin D deficiency and supplementation in patients with IBD, *Gastroenterol Hepatol* 10:127, 2014.
*17. Parkes GC: Smoking in inflammatory bowel disease: impact on disease course and insights into the etiology of its effect, *J Crohns* 8:717, 2014.
*18. Gisbert JP: Systematic review with meta-analysis: inflammatory bowel disease in the elderly, *Aliment Pharmacol Ther* 39:459, 2014.
19. Glancy DG: Intestinal obstruction, *Surgery* 32:204, 2014.
20. Colorectal cancer facts and figures. Retrieved from *www.cancer.org/research/cancerfactsstatistics/colorectal-cancer-facts-figures.*
*21. Brenner H, Matthias K, Christian PP: Effect of screening sigmoidoscopy and colonoscopy on colorectal cancer incidence and mortality, *Lancet* 383:1490, 2014.
22. American Cancer Society recommendations for colorectal cancer early detection. Retrieved from *www.cancer.org/cancer/colonandrectumcancer/moreinformation/colonandrectumcancerearlydetection/colorectal-cancer-early-detection-acs-recommendations.*
23. Brenner H, Kloor M, Pox C: Colorectal cancer, *Lancet* 383:1490, 2014.
24. Colon cancer treatment. Retrieved from *www.cancer.gov/cancertopics/pdq/treatment/colon/HealthProfessional.*
25. Johnson D, Barkun A, Rex D, et al: Optimizing adequacy of bowel cleansing for colonoscopy: recommendations from the US multi-society task force on colorectal cancer, *Gastroenterol* 147:903, 2014.
26. Prinz A, Colwell J, Cross H, et al: Discharge planning for a patient with a new ostomy: best practice for clinicians, *J Wound Ostomy Continence Nurs* 42:79, 2015.
27. Willcutts K, Touger-Decker R: Nutritional management for ostomates, *Top Clin Nutr* 28:373, 2013.
28. Haack C, Galloway JR, Srinivasan S: Enterocutaneous fistulas: a look at causes and management, *Curr Surg Rep* 10:1, 2014.
29. Coyne PE, Kalbassi MR: Diverticular disease, *Surgery* 32:431, 2014.
30. Levy J, Bernstein L, Silber N: Celiac disease: an immune dysregulation syndrome, *Curr Probl Pediatr Adolesc Health Care* 44:324, 2014.
*31. Rubio-Tapia A, Hill ID, Kelly CP, et al: ACG clinical guidelines: diagnosis and management of celiac disease, *Am J Gastroenterol* 108:656, 2013.
32. Kumpf VJ: Pharmacologic management of diarrhea in patients with short bowel syndrome, *J Parenter Enteral Nutr* 38:38S, 2014.
33. Heikki J, Hohenberger P, Corless CL: Gastrointestinal stromal tumor, *Lancet* 382:973, 2013.
34. Rakinic J, Poola VP: Hemorrhoids and fistulas: new solutions to old problems, *Curr Prob Surg* 51:98, 2014.
35. Higuero T: Update on the management of anal fissure, *J Visceral Surg* 152:S37, 2015.
36. American Cancer Society: Anal cancer. Retrieved from *www.cancer.org/cancer/analcancer/detailedguide/anal-cancer-what-is-key-statistics.*
*37. Shridhar R, Shibata D, Chan E, et al: Anal cancer: current standards in care and recent changes in practice, *CA Canc J for Clin* 65:139, 2015.

*Evidence-based information for clinical practice.

# Liver, Pancreas, and Biliary Tract Problems

*Kathy H. Wu*

*Neither should a ship rely on one small anchor, nor should life rest on a single hope.*

***Epictetus***

http://evolve.elsevier.com/Lewis/medsurg/

## LEARNING OUTCOMES

1. Differentiate among the types of viral hepatitis, including etiology, pathophysiology, clinical manifestations, complications, and interprofessional care.
2. Describe the nursing management of the patient with viral hepatitis.
3. Describe the pathophysiology, clinical manifestations, complications, and interprofessional care of the patient with nonalcoholic fatty liver disease.
4. Explain the etiology, pathophysiology, clinical manifestations, complications, interprofessional care, and nursing management of the patient with cirrhosis of the liver.
5. Describe the clinical manifestations and management of liver cancer.
6. Differentiate between acute and chronic pancreatitis related to pathophysiology, clinical manifestations, complications, interprofessional care, and nursing management.
7. Explain the clinical manifestations, interprofessional care, and nursing management of the patient with pancreatic cancer.
8. Describe the pathophysiology, clinical manifestations, complications, and interprofessional care of gallbladder disorders.
9. Describe the nursing management of the patient undergoing surgical treatment of cholecystitis and cholelithiasis.

## KEY TERMS



Nursing management of patients with liver, pancreatic, and gallbladder problems is the focus of this chapter. Viral hepatitis, cirrhosis, acute pancreatitis, cholecystitis, and cholelithiasis are described in detail.

## DISORDERS OF THE LIVER

## HEPATITIS

**Hepatitis** is inflammation of the liver. Hepatitis is most commonly caused by viruses. It can also be caused by substances (e.g., alcohol, medications, chemicals), autoimmune diseases, and metabolic abnormalities.

### Viral Hepatitis

There are several types of viral hepatitis, and each type is designated by a letter (A, B, C, D, E). The different types of viral hepatitis have similar clinical manifestations, but their modes of transmission and disease course vary (Table 43-1). Some types of viral hepatitis infection can lead to chronic liver disease. Other less common viruses can also cause liver disease. These include cytomegalovirus (CMV), Epstein-Barr virus (EBV), herpesvirus, coxsackievirus, and rubella virus.

**Hepatitis A Virus.** Hepatitis A is a self-limiting infection that can cause a mild flu-like illness and jaundice. In more severe cases, it can cause acute liver failure. Hepatitis A virus (HAV) is a ribonucleic acid (RNA) virus that is transmitted primarily through the fecal-oral route. It frequently occurs in small outbreaks caused by fecal contamination of food or drinking water. Poor hygiene, improper handling of food, crowded situations, and poor sanitary conditions are contributing factors.

Transmission occurs between family members, institutionalized individuals, and children in day care centers. Foodborne hepatitis A outbreaks are usually due to food contaminated by

Reviewed by Marian Altman, RN, MS, CNS-BC, ANP, Patient Care Services Safety Manager, Virginia Commonwealth University Health System, Richmond, Virginia; Brian J. Fasolka, RN, MSN, CEN, Assistant Clinical Professor, College of Nursing and Health Professions, Drexel University, Philadelphia, Pennsylvania; Lauren Kemph, RN, DNP, AGPCNP, Nurse Practitioner, Center for Liver Disease and Transplantation at New York Presbyterian, New York, New York; Katherine A. Ladetto, RN, MSN, APRN, ANP-BC, GNP-BC, Nurse Practitioner, North Shore Physicians Group, Peabody, Massachusetts; and Heidi E. Monroe, MSN, RN-BC, CPAN, CAPA, Assistant Professor of Nursing, Bellin College and Bellin Hospital, Green Bay, Wisconsin.

### TABLE 43-1 Characteristics of Hepatitis Viruses

| Incubation Period and Mode of Transmission | Sources of Infection | Infectivity |
|---|---|---|
| **Hepatitis A Virus (HAV)**<br>*Incubation:* 15-50 days (average 28)<br>• Fecal-oral (primarily fecal contamination and oral ingestion) | • Crowded conditions (e.g., day care, nursing home)<br>• Poor personal hygiene<br>• Poor sanitation<br>• Contaminated food, milk, water, shellfish<br>• Persons with subclinical infections, infected food handlers, sexual contact, IV drug users | • Most infectious during 2 wk before onset of symptoms<br>• Infectious until 1-2 wk after the start of symptoms |
| **Hepatitis B Virus (HBV)**<br>*Incubation:* 45-180 days (average 56-96)<br>• Percutaneous (parenteral) or permucosal exposure to blood or blood products<br>• Sexual contact<br>• Perinatal transmission | • Contaminated needles, syringes, and blood products<br>• Sexual activity with infected partners. Asymptomatic carriers<br>• Tattoos or body piercing with contaminated needles<br>• HBV-infected mother (perinatal transmission) | • Before and after symptoms appear<br>• Infectious for 4-6 mo<br>• Carriers continue to be infectious for life |
| **Hepatitis C Virus (HCV)**<br>*Incubation:* 14-180 days (average 56)<br>• Percutaneous (parenteral) or mucosal exposure to blood or blood products<br>• High-risk sexual contact<br>• Perinatal contact | • Blood and blood products<br>• Needles and syringes<br>• Sexual activity with infected partners | • 1-2 wk before symptoms appear<br>• Continues during clinical course<br>• 75%-85% go on to develop chronic hepatitis C and remain infectious |
| **Hepatitis D Virus (HDV)**<br>*Incubation:* 2-26 wk<br>• HBV must precede HDV<br>• Chronic carriers of HBV always at risk | • Same as HBV<br>• Can cause infection only when HBV is present<br>• Routes of transmission same as for HBV | • Blood infectious at all stages of HDV infection |
| **Hepatitis E Virus (HEV)**<br>*Incubation:* 15-64 days (average 26-42 days)<br>• Fecal-oral route<br>• Outbreaks associated with contaminated water supply in developing countries | • Contaminated water, poor sanitation<br>• Found in Asia, Africa, and Mexico<br>• Not common in United States | • Not known<br>• May be similar to HAV |

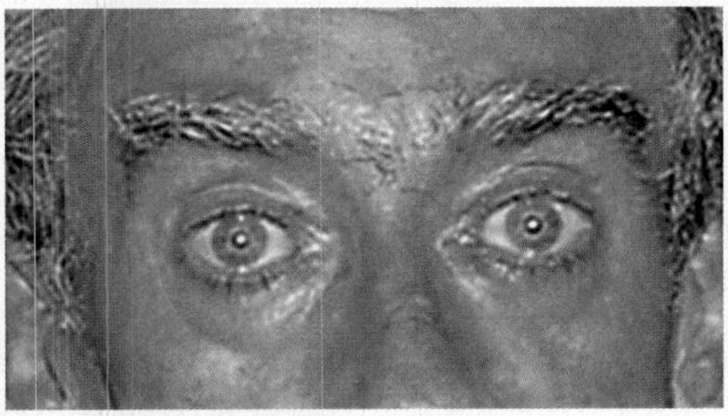

**FIG. 43-1** Jaundiced patient. (From Butcher GP: *Gastroenterology: an illustrated colour text*, London, 2004, Churchill Livingstone.)

an infected food handler. Individuals at increased risk for hepatitis A infection include drug users (both injection and noninjection drugs), men who have sex with men (MSM), and persons traveling to developing countries.

The virus is present in feces during the incubation period. Therefore it can be carried and transmitted by persons who have undetectable, subclinical infections. The greatest risk of transmission occurs before clinical symptoms appear. HAV is found in feces 2 or more weeks before the onset of symptoms and up to 1 week after the onset of jaundice (Fig. 43-1). It is present only briefly in blood.

Anti-HAV (antibody to HAV) immunoglobulin (Ig) M appears in the serum as the stool becomes negative for the virus. Detection of hepatitis A IgM indicates acute hepatitis. Although not commonly tested clinically, hepatitis A IgG indicates past infection. IgG antibody provides lifelong immunity (Fig. 43-2). Hepatitis A vaccination and thorough hand washing are the best measures to prevent outbreaks. In the United States, the

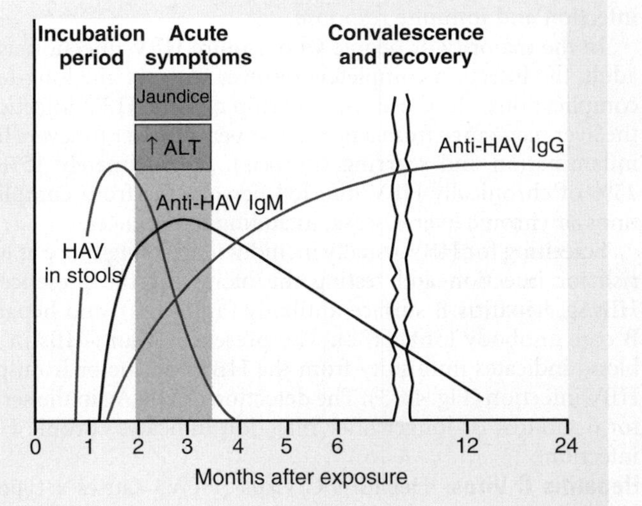


**FIG. 43-2** Course of infection with hepatitis A virus *(HAV). ALT,* Alanine aminotransferase. (From McCance KL, Huether SE: *Pathophysiology: the biologic basis for disease in adults and children,* ed 6, St Louis, 2010, Mosby.)

incidence of hepatitis A viral infection has declined since vaccination was recommended for at-risk persons and children (at the age of 1 year).[1]

**Hepatitis B Virus.** Hepatitis B virus (HBV) is a blood-borne pathogen that can cause either acute or chronic hepatitis. Since the 1990s, the incidence of HBV infection has decreased because of the widespread use of the HBV vaccine.[1]

Asians and Pacific Islanders have a high incidence of HBV hepatitis. Perinatal transmission is the most common mode of transmission in this population and often results in chronic HBV infection.

HBV is a deoxyribonucleic acid (DNA) virus. It can be transmitted several ways: (1) perinatally from mothers infected with HBV to their infants; (2) percutaneously (e.g., IV drug use, accidental needle-stick punctures); or (3) via small cuts on mucosal surfaces and exposure to infectious blood, blood products, or other body fluids (e.g., semen, vaginal secretions, saliva).

Sexual transmission is a common mode of HBV transmission. MSM (especially those practicing unprotected anal intercourse) are at an increased risk for HBV infection. It is generally believed that casual encounters such as hugging, kissing, and sharing utensils do not transmit the disease.

Other at-risk individuals include those who live with chronically HBV-infected persons, patients on hemodialysis, health care personnel, and public safety workers. HBV can live on a dry surface for at least 7 days, and it is 50 to 100 times more infectious than human immunodeficiency virus (HIV).[2]

HBV has been detected in almost every body fluid. Infected semen and saliva contain much lower concentrations of HBV than blood, but the virus can be transmitted via these secretions. If gastrointestinal (GI) bleeding occurs, feces can be contaminated with the virus from the blood. There is no evidence that urine, feces (without GI bleeding), breast milk, tears, and sweat are infectious. Organ and tissue transplantation is another potential source of infection. However, in some patients with acute hepatitis B, there is no readily identifiable risk factor.[1]

HBV is a complex structure with three distinct antigens: surface antigen (HBsAg), core antigen (HBcAg), and e antigen (HBeAg). Each antigen along with its corresponding antibody may appear or disappear in serum depending on the phase of infection and immune response.

In the majority of people who acquire HBV infection as an adult, the infection completely resolves without any long-term complications.[3] In those who develop chronic HBV infections, the liver may range from a normal-appearing liver to severe liver inflammation and scarring (fibrosis). Approximately 15% to 25% of chronically HBV-infected persons die from complications of chronic liver disease, including liver cancer.

Screening for HBV usually includes identifying those at high risk for infection and testing the blood for the presence of HBsAg, hepatitis B surface antibody (anti-HBs), and hepatitis B core antibody (anti-HBc). The presence of anti-HBs in the blood indicates immunity from the HBV vaccine or from past HBV infection (Fig. 43-3). The detection of HBsAg in the serum for 6 months or longer after infection indicates chronic HBV infection.

**Hepatitis C Virus.** Hepatitis C virus (HCV) causes a type of hepatitis that can result in both acute illness as well as chronic infection. Acute hepatitis C, which can be mild in presentation, can be difficult to detect unless a diagnosis is made with laboratory testing. The most common causes of acute hepatitis C outbreaks are among injection drug users and HIV-positive MSM.

HCV is an RNA virus that is primarily transmitted percutaneously. The most common mode of HCV transmission is the sharing of contaminated needles and equipment among injection drug users. High-risk sexual behavior (e.g., unprotected sex, multiple partners), especially among MSM, is associated with increased risk of transmission.

Approximately 10% of all cases of HCV infection in the United States are due to occupational exposure, hemodialysis,

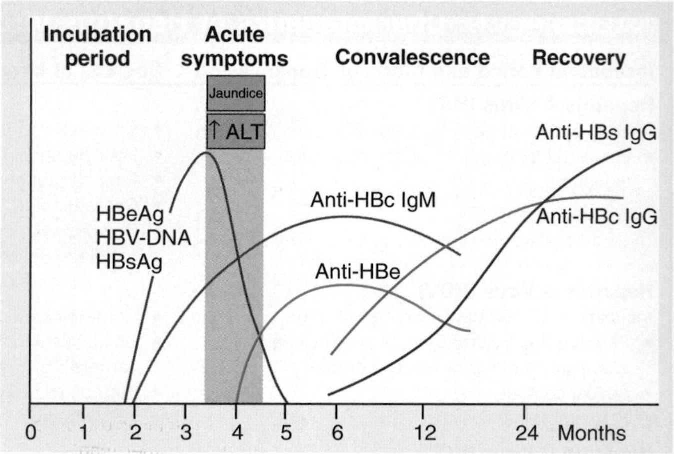


**FIG. 43-3** Course of infection with hepatitis B virus *(HBV). ALT,* Alanine aminotransferase; *anti-HBc,* antibody to hepatitis B core antigen; *anti-HBe,* antibody to HBeAg; *anti-HBs,* antibody to HBsAg; *HBeAg,* hepatitis B e antigen; *HBsAg,* hepatitis B surface antigen. (From McCance KL, Huether SE: *Pathophysiology: the biologic basis for disease in adults and children,* ed 6, St Louis, 2010, Mosby.)

and perinatal transmission.[2] The risk of perinatal HCV transmission is higher in women who are co-infected with both HIV and HCV. Persons who were given blood or blood products before 1992 (when blood product testing for HCV began) are at higher risk for chronic HCV infection and should be routinely tested.[4] Some patients with HCV infection cannot identify a source of infection.

The majority of patients who acquire hepatitis C usually develop chronic infection. However, because signs and symptoms of HCV infection are generally mild, most individuals are unaware of their infection. Hepatitis C is the most common cause of chronic liver disease and liver failure, with 20% to 30% of these patients developing cirrhosis and eventually liver failure and/or liver cancer.[4] Along with chronic HBV, HCV account for 80% of the cases of liver cancer.[5] HCV hepatitis is the most common indication for liver transplantation in the United States.[4]

Because of the 15- to 20-year delay between infection and the clinical manifestations of liver damage, long-term effects of HCV infection pose important health care challenges.

Persons at risk for HCV infection are also at risk for HBV and HIV infections. About 30% to 40% of HIV-infected patients also have HCV. This high rate of co-infection is primarily related to IV drug use. Co-infection with HIV and HCV places the patient at greater risk for progression to cirrhosis.

Screening for HCV infection should be conducted on those at increased risk. This includes individuals who engage in high-risk sexual practices, injection drug users, persons of the "baby boomer" generation born between 1945 and 1965, those who may have had blood or blood products prior to 1992, and/or those who have abnormal liver function tests. A positive antibody test for HCV (anti-HCV) is usually sufficient for a diagnosis.[4]

**Hepatitis D Virus.** Hepatitis D virus (HDV), also called *delta virus,* is uncommon in the United States. HDV is a defective single-stranded RNA virus that cannot survive on its own and requires hepatitis B to replicate. It can be acquired at the same time as HBV, or a person with HBV can be infected with HDV at a later time. HDV is also transmitted percutaneously, similar to HBV. It can cause a spectrum of illness ranging from an asymptomatic chronic carrier state to acute liver failure. There

## EVIDENCE-BASED PRACTICE

### Applying the Evidence

**Screening and Testing for Hepatitis C**

You are caring for S.B., a 32-yr-old man who frequently visits the community clinic when he has health concerns. He arrives today at the clinic saying he feels "tired." He tells you a friend was recently diagnosed with hepatitis C (HCV) and that he wants a shot to prevent getting it. The staff are aware from S.B.'s medical record that he injects drugs and has not previously been tested for HCV.

***Making Clinical Decisions***

***Best Available Evidence.*** Overarching themes of persons who inject drugs and their views on HCV testing and diagnosis include (1) a lack of HCV awareness and missed opportunities by health professionals to provide information contributes to delayed testing, (2) risks of being tested and prioritization of needs other than testing, and (3) unexpected diagnosis that creates anxiety and confusion.

***Clinician Expertise.*** You know a major risk factor for HCV is IV drug use. You also understand that early diagnosis of HCV is important for best outcomes and prevention of transmission.

***Patient Preferences and Values.*** S.B. tells you he is "busy today" and will be back tomorrow for HCV testing.

***Implications for Nursing Practice***

1. What information would you provide to S.B. on HCV symptoms and transmission?
2. Since S.B. is now willing to be tested for HCV, how would you determine barriers to the informed consent process?
3. How would you inform S.B. on the test results?

***Reference for Evidence***

Jones L, Atkinson A, Bates G, et al: Views and experiences of hepatitis C testing and diagnosis among people who inject drugs: systematic review of qualitative research, *Inter J Drug Policy* 25:204, 2014.

is no vaccine for HDV. However, vaccination against HBV reduces the risk of HDV co-infection.

**Hepatitis E Virus.** Hepatitis E virus (HEV) is an RNA virus transmitted by the fecal-oral route. The usual mode of transmission is drinking contaminated water. Hepatitis E infection occurs primarily in developing countries, with epidemics reported in India, Asia, Mexico, and Africa. Only a few cases of HEV have been reported in the United States, primarily in persons who recently traveled to an HEV-endemic area.

## Pathophysiology

**Liver.** In viral hepatitis, hepatocytes become targets of the virus in one of two ways: through direct action of the virus (as in HCV infection) or through a cell-mediated immune response to the virus (as in HBV infection).[5,6]

During acute viral hepatitis, large numbers of infected hepatocytes are destroyed. The destruction of hepatocytes leads to a wide range of liver-related dysfunction. Bile production, coagulation, blood glucose, and protein metabolism can be affected. Detoxification and processing of drugs, hormones, and metabolites (e.g., ammonia from protein catabolism) may also be disrupted.

After resolution of an acute infection, liver cells can regenerate. If no complications occur, the liver can resume its normal appearance and function. In certain cases, the acute hepatitis can become so severe and irreversible that people experience liver failure or even death.

**TABLE 43-2 Manifestations of Hepatitis**

| Acute Hepatitis | Chronic Hepatitis |
|---|---|
| • Anorexia<br>• Dark urine<br>• Decreased sense of taste and smell<br>• Diarrhea or constipation<br>• Fatigue, lethargy, malaise<br>• Flu-like symptoms (e.g., headache)<br>• Hepatomegaly<br>• Jaundice<br>• Clay-colored stools<br>• Low-grade fever<br>• Lymphadenopathy<br>• Myalgias and/or arthralgias<br>• Nausea, vomiting<br>• Pruritus<br>• Right upper quadrant tenderness<br>• Splenomegaly<br>• Weight loss | • ALT, AST elevations (may be normal in some people)<br>• Anemia<br>• Ascites and lower extremity edema<br>• Asterixis ("liver flap")<br>• Bleeding abnormalities (thrombocytopenia, easy bruising, prolonged clotting time)<br>• Fatigue, malaise<br>• Hepatic encephalopathy: confusion, difficulty concentrating, easy agitation<br>• Hepatomegaly<br>• Hyperbilirubinemia<br>• Jaundice<br>• Myalgias and/or arthralgias<br>• Palmar erythema<br>• Spider angiomas |

*ALT,* Alanine aminotransferase; *AST,* aspartate aminotransferase.

Chronic viral hepatitis can be insidious and silent, causing persistent and continual destruction of infected hepatocytes. Over time scar tissue can develop, which leads to fibrosis and compromised liver function. Fibrosis can lead to cirrhosis and liver failure. Cirrhosis is a generally irreversible condition that can increase one's risk for liver dysfunction, portal hypertension, and primary liver cancer. (Cirrhosis is discussed later in this chapter.)

**Systemic Effects.** In the early phases of hepatitis infection, antigen-antibody complexes between the virus and its corresponding antibody form circulating immune complexes. The circulating immune complexes activate the complement system (see Chapter 11). The clinical manifestations of this activation are rash, angioedema, arthritis, fever, and malaise. *Cryoglobulinemia* (abnormal proteins found in the blood), glomerulonephritis, and vasculitis can occur secondary to immune complex activation.

## Clinical Manifestations and Complications

The clinical manifestations of the different viral hepatitis infections can be classified into acute hepatitis and chronic hepatitis (Table 43-2).

**Acute Hepatitis.** Many patients with acute hepatitis have no symptoms and may not even know they have been infected. However, others may have intermittent or ongoing anorexia, lethargy, nausea, vomiting, low-grade fever, skin rashes, diarrhea or constipation, malaise, fatigue, myalgias, arthralgias, other flu-like symptoms, and right upper quadrant tenderness (caused by liver inflammation).

Although the acute phase of viral hepatitis varies depending on the type of hepatitis, it usually lasts from 1 to 6 months. During this time, the patient may have a decreased sense of smell and find food repugnant. Smokers may have distaste for cigarettes. Physical examination often reveals hepatomegaly, lymphadenopathy, abdominal tenderness, and sometimes splenomegaly. The acute phase is the period of maximal infectivity.

A patient in the acute phase of hepatitis may be *icteric* (jaundiced) or anicteric. (Types of jaundice are presented in

**TABLE 43-3 Classification of Jaundice**

| | Hemolytic Jaundice | Hepatocellular Jaundice | Obstructive Jaundice |
|---|---|---|---|
| **Causes** | • Blood transfusion reactions, sickle cell crisis, hemolytic anemia. | • Hepatitis, cirrhosis, hepatocellular carcinoma. | • Hepatitis, cirrhosis, hepatocellular carcinoma.<br>• Common bile duct obstruction from stone(s), biliary strictures, sclerosing cholangitis, and pancreatic cancer. |
| **Description** | • Caused by increased breakdown of RBCs, which produces an increased amount of unconjugated bilirubin in blood.<br>• Liver is unable to handle increased load. | • Results from liver's altered ability to take up bilirubin from blood or to conjugate or excrete it.<br>• In hepatocellular disease, damaged hepatocytes leak bilirubin. | • Results from decreased or obstructed flow of bile through liver or biliary duct system.<br>• Obstruction may occur in intrahepatic or extrahepatic bile ducts.<br>• Intrahepatic obstructions are due to swelling or fibrosis of the liver's canaliculi and bile ducts. |
| **Diagnostic Findings** | | | |
| ***Serum Bilirubin*** | | | |
| Unconjugated (indirect) | ↑ | ↑ | ↑ |
| Conjugated (direct) | Normal | ↑ or ↓ (severe disease) | ↑ |
| Urine Bilirubin | Negative | ↑ | ↑ |
| ***Urobilinogen*** | | | |
| Stool | ↑ | Normal, ↓ | ↓ |
| Urine | ↑ | Normal, ↑ | ↓ |

Table 43-3.) **Jaundice**, a yellowish discoloration of body tissues, results from an alteration in normal bilirubin metabolism or disruption of the flow of bile into the hepatic or biliary duct systems. (Normal bilirubin metabolism is presented in Fig. 38-4.)

The urine may appear darker because of excess bilirubin being excreted by the kidneys. If conjugated bilirubin cannot pass into the intestines from the liver because of obstruction or inflammation of the bile ducts, the stools will be light or clay colored.

*Pruritus* (intense generalized itching) sometimes accompanies jaundice. It occurs as a result of the accumulation of bile salts beneath the skin. The pruritus can be intolerable to the patient.

As jaundice fades, the convalescent phase begins. The convalescent phase can last for weeks to months, with an average of 2 to 4 months. During this period, patients typically experience malaise and easy fatigability. Hepatomegaly remains for several weeks, but splenomegaly (if present) subsides during this period.

Most patients with acute viral hepatitis recover completely. Almost all cases of acute hepatitis A resolve. However, some patients may have a relapse in the first 2 to 3 months after the infection. The disappearance of jaundice does not mean the patient has totally recovered. Some HBV infections and the majority of HCV infections result in chronic hepatitis.

The overall mortality rate for acute hepatitis is less than 1%. The mortality rate is higher in older adults and those with underlying debilitating illnesses (including chronic liver disease).

Complications that can result from acute hepatitis are acute liver failure, chronic hepatitis, cirrhosis of the liver, portal hypertension, and hepatocellular carcinoma.

***Acute Liver Failure.*** Occasionally acute liver failure (fulminant hepatic failure) may occur, which is a serious condition with a poor prognosis. Manifestations include encephalopathy, gastrointestinal bleeding, disseminated intravascular coagulation, fever with leukocytosis, renal manifestations (oliguria, azotemia), ascites, edema, hypotension, respiratory failure, hypoglycemia, bacterial infections, thrombocytopenia, and coagulopathies. Liver transplantation is usually the cure for these patients. (Acute liver failure is discussed in this chapter on p. 996.)

**Chronic Hepatitis.** Manifestations of chronic hepatitis are presented in Table 43-2. Chronic HBV is more likely to develop in infants born to infected mothers and in those who acquire the infection before age 5 than in those who acquire the virus after age 5.[3]

Alterations in the patient's cellular immune response may be important in the development of the chronic HBsAg carrier state and the progression of acute HBV to chronic HBV. For example, persons with chronic kidney disease undergoing dialysis tend to have a depressed cellular immune response, which may explain why they are more at risk for developing chronic infection after acquiring the acute form of HBV.[6]

HCV infection is more likely than HBV to become chronic.[4] As previously mentioned, many patients with chronic HCV infection develop chronic liver disease, cirrhosis, portal hypertension, and liver cancer. Risk factors for progression to cirrhosis include male gender, alcohol consumption, concomitant fatty liver disease, and excess iron deposition in the liver. People with metabolic syndrome (obesity, elevated cholesterol or triglycerides, hypertension, and diabetes mellitus) are also at risk for progression of HCV to cirrhosis.[4] In some patients, co-infection with HIV may also cause complications or require modification of treatment. Manifestations of chronic hepatitis include anemia and coagulation problems (easy bruising and bleeding). The liver is responsible for producing clotting factors, so in persons with liver disease, clotting and bleeding times can be impaired or prolonged.

Skin manifestations may include spider angiomas, palmar erythema, and gynecomastia. Some patients have splenomegaly, hepatomegaly, or cervical lymph node enlargement.

In patients with severe liver damage, *hepatic encephalopathy* is a potentially life-threatening spectrum of neurologic, psychiatric, and motor disturbances. Hepatic encephalopathy results from the liver's inability to remove toxins (especially ammonia) from the blood. (Hepatic encephalopathy is discussed later in this chapter on p. 990.)

*Ascites*, a common manifestation of hepatitis (especially chronic hepatitis), is the accumulation of excess fluid in the peritoneal cavity. Fluid accumulates due to reduced protein levels in the blood, which reduces the plasma oncotic pressure. (Ascites is discussed later in this chapter on p. 988.)

**TABLE 43-4 Diagnostic Studies**
***Viral Hepatitis***

| Virus | Tests | Significance |
|---|---|---|
| A | Anti-HAV immunoglobulin M (IgM)<br>Anti-HAV immunoglobulin G (IgG) | Acute infection<br>Previous infection or immunization. Not routinely done in clinical practice |
| B | HBsAg (hepatitis B surface antigen) | Marker of infectivity<br>Present in acute or chronic infection<br>Positive in chronic carriers |
| | Anti-HBs (hepatitis B surface antibody) | Indicates previous infection with HBV or immunization |
| | HBeAg (hepatitis B e antigen) | Indicates high infectivity<br>Used to determine the clinical management of patients with chronic hepatitis B |
| | Anti-HBe (hepatitis B e antibody) | Indicates previous infection<br>In chronic hepatitis B, indicates a low viral load and low degree of infectivity |
| | Anti-HBc (antibody to hepatitis B core antigen) IgM | Indicates acute infection<br>Does not appear after vaccination |
| | Anti-HBc IgG | Indicates previous infection or ongoing infection with hepatitis B<br>Does not appear after vaccination |
| | HBV DNA quantitation | Indicates active ongoing viral replication<br>Best indicator of viral replication and effectiveness of therapy in patient with chronic hepatitis B |
| | HBV genotyping | Indicates the genotype of HBV |
| C | Anti-HCV (antibody to HCV)<br>HCV RNA quantitation<br>HCV genotyping | Marker for acute or chronic infection with HCV<br>Indicates active ongoing viral replication<br>Indicates the genotype of HCV |
| D | Anti-HDV<br>HDV Ag (hepatitis D antigen) | Present in past or current infection with HDV<br>Present within a few days after infection |
| E* | Anti-HEV IgM and IgG<br>HEV RNA quantitation | Present 1 wk-2 mo after illness onset<br>Indicates active ongoing viral replication |

*A,* Hepatitis A virus (HAV); *B,* hepatitis B virus (HBV); *C,* hepatitis C virus (HCV); *D,* hepatitis D virus (HDV); *E,* hepatitis E virus (HEV).
*Currently, no serologic tests to diagnose HEV infection are commercially available in the United States. However, diagnostic tests are available in research laboratories to detect IgM and IgG anti-HEV and HEV RNA levels.

## Diagnostic Studies

The only definitive way to distinguish among the various types of viral hepatitis is by testing the patient's blood for the specific antigen or antibody. In some types of viral hepatitis, the blood can be tested for the viral load (viral level). Tests for the different types of viral hepatitis are presented in Table 43-4.

In viral hepatitis, many results of liver function tests show significant abnormalities such as those shown in Table 43-5.

Several tests are available to determine the presence of HCV. Initial testing for HCV infection includes HCV antibody testing. If the antibody test is positive, HCV RNA testing is done to assess for chronic infection; a positive result confirms chronic infection. A few patients may have a false-positive HCV antibody result with a negative HCV RNA test. If recent HCV infection is suspected, HCV RNA testing is usually done because it may take several weeks or longer for HCV antibodies to develop.

HCV RNA testing may used for immunocompromised patients (e.g., patient with HIV). Because of altered or delayed antibody response to HCV, these patients may not have detectable antibody levels even though they are infected with HCV.

Viral genotype testing is done in patients undergoing drug therapy for HBV or HCV infection. HBV has at least eight different genotypes (A to H). In some centers, HBV genotyping is performed before starting treatment. HBV genotype may be useful in predicting disease course and treatment outcomes.

HCV has six genotypes and more than 50 subtypes. In the United States, 75% of HCV infections are caused by HCV genotype 1. For patients who test positive for HCV, genotyping is obtained before drug therapy is started.[4] The genotype determines the choice and duration of therapy. It is also one of the strongest predictors of a patient's response to drug therapy.

**TABLE 43-5 Diagnostic Findings in Acute Hepatitis**

| Test | Abnormal Finding | Etiology |
|---|---|---|
| **Aminotransferases** | | |
| • Aspartate aminotransferase (AST) | Increased in acute phase<br>Decreases as jaundice disappears | Liver cell injury |
| • Alanine aminotransferase (ALT) | Increased in acute phase<br>Decreases as jaundice disappears | Liver cell injury |
| **γ-Glutamyl transpeptidase** (GGT) | Increased | Liver cell injury |
| **Alkaline phosphatase** | Moderately increased | Impaired excretory function of liver |
| **Serum proteins** | | |
| • γ-Globulin | Normal or increased | Impaired clearance from liver |
| • Albumin | Normal or decreased | Liver cell injury |
| **Serum bilirubin (total)** | Increased to about 8-15 mg/dL (137-257 μmol/L) | Liver cell injury |
| **Urinary bilirubin** | Increased | Conjugated hyperbilirubinemia |
| **Urinary urobilinogen** | Increased 2-5 days before jaundice | Diminished reabsorption of urobilinogen |
| **Prothrombin time** | Prolonged | Decreased prothrombin production by liver |

A liver biopsy is not indicated in acute hepatitis unless the diagnosis is in doubt. In chronic hepatitis, a liver biopsy may be done for histologic examination of liver cells and characterization of the degree of inflammation, fibrosis, or cirrhosis that may be present. A patient who has a bleeding disorder may not be an appropriate candidate for a percutaneous liver biopsy because of the risk of bleeding. In these patients, a transjugular biopsy may be an alternative. This type of biopsy consists of obtaining liver tissue through a rigid cannula introduced into one of the hepatic veins, typically using jugular venous access.

Techniques for noninvasive assessment of liver fibrosis may eventually replace the need for liver biopsy. Options include the use of ultrasound elastography (FibroScan), which uses an ultrasound transducer to determine the degree of liver fibrosis. FibroSure (FibroTest) is a biomarker that uses the results of serum tests (e.g., liver enzyme levels) to assess the extent of hepatic fibrosis.[7]

## Interprofessional Care

There is no specific treatment for acute viral hepatitis. Most patients can be managed at home. Emphasis is on providing adequate nutrition and measures to rest the body and assist the liver to regenerate and repair (Table 43-6). Rest reduces the metabolic demands on the liver and promotes liver cell regeneration. The degree of rest depends on the severity of symptoms, but usually alternating periods of activity and rest are adequate. Counseling should include the importance of avoiding alcohol and notification of possible contacts for testing and prophylaxis, if indicated.

In patients with chronic viral hepatitis, care may involve hepatologists, infectious disease specialists, pharmacists, dietitians, and mental health or substance abuse specialists. The role and extent of involvement of team members is based on the patient's specific needs.

### TABLE 43-6 Interprofessional Care

#### *Viral Hepatitis*

**Diagnostic Assessment**

- History and physical examination
- Liver function tests
- Alanine aminotransferase (ALT)
- Aspartate aminotransferase (AST)
- Serum bilirubin
- Prothrombin time (PT) and INR
- Alkaline phosphatase
- γ-Glutamyl transpeptidase
- Hepatitis testing
  - *Hepatitis A:* Anti-HAV IgM
  - *Hepatitis B:* HBsAg, anti-HBs, HBeAg, anti-HBe, anti-HBc IgM and IgG, HBV DNA quantitation, HBV genotyping
  - *Hepatitis C:* Anti-HCV, HCV RNA quantitation, HCV genotyping
  - *Hepatitis D:* Anti-HDV, HDV Ag
- FibroScan
- FibroSure (FibroTest)

**Management**

***Acute and Chronic***

- Well-balanced diet
- Vitamin supplements
- Rest (degree of strictness varies)
- Avoidance of alcohol intake and drugs detoxified by liver

***Chronic HBV and HCV***

- Drug therapy (Table 43-7)

*HAV,* Hepatitis A virus; *HB,* hepatitis B; *HBeAg,* hepatitis B e antigen; *HBsAg,* hepatitis B surface antigen; *HBV,* hepatitis B virus; *HCV,* hepatitis C virus; *HDV Ag,* hepatitis D antigen; *HDV,* hepatitis D virus; *INR,* international normalized ratio.

### Drug Therapy

***Acute Hepatitis.*** There are no drug therapies for treating acute HAV infection. Treatment of acute HBV may be indicated only in patients with severe hepatitis and liver failure.

In acute hepatitis C, some patients may choose to be monitored for spontaneous clearance of the infection. For those patients who choose treatment, one of the direct-acting antivirals (DAAs) may be used. (DAAs are discussed later in the section on chronic hepatitis.)

Supportive drug therapy may include antihistamines for generalized itching and antiemetics for nausea. These drugs include promethazine (Phenergan) and ondansetron (Zofran).

### COMPLEMENTARY & ALTERNATIVE THERAPIES

#### *Milk Thistle (Silymarin)*

**Scientific Evidence**

- Previous studies suggested that milk thistle may benefit the liver by protecting and promoting the growth of liver cells and inhibiting inflammation. These studies were small and not well designed.
- A meta-analysis found no real benefit from using milk thistle:
  - Silymarin was no better than placebo for chronic hepatitis C in people who had not responded to standard antiviral treatment.
  - Hepatitis C patients who used silymarin had fewer and milder symptoms of liver disease and somewhat better quality of life but no change in virus activity or liver inflammation.

**Nursing Implications**

- Appears to be well tolerated in recommended doses for up to 6 yr.
- May lower blood glucose.
- May interfere with the liver's cytochrome P450 enzyme system.

Source: National Center for Complementary and Alternative Therapy: Milk thistle. Retrieved from *https://nccih.nih.gov/health/milkthistle/ataglance.htm.*

***Chronic Hepatitis B.*** Drug therapy for chronic HBV is focused on decreasing the hepatitis B viral load and liver enzymes, and in turn slowing the rate of disease progression. Long-term goals are preventing development of cirrhosis, portal hypertension, liver failure, and hepatocellular cancer. Current drug therapies for chronic HBV do not eradicate the virus but suppress viral replication and prevent complications of hepatitis B. First-line therapies now include primarily nucleoside and nucleotide analogs (Table 43-7) and occasionally interferon therapy.[8]

**Nucleoside and nucleotide analogs.** Nucleoside and nucleotide analogs inhibit viral DNA replication. HBV reproduces by making copies of its viral DNA nucleosides and nucleotides. The nucleoside and nucleotide analog drugs mimic normal building blocks for DNA, but are actually faulty viral DNA building blocks. Once they become incorporated into the viral DNA, they halt DNA synthesis.

Nucleoside and nucleotide analogs do not prevent all viral reproduction, but they can substantially lower the amount of virus in the body. These medications include lamivudine (Epivir), adefovir (Hepsera), entecavir (Baraclude), telbivudine (Tyzeka), and tenofovir (Viread). These oral medications are indicated in the treatment of chronic HBV when there is evidence of significant active viral replication and liver inflammation.[8]

Nucleoside and nucleotide analogs also reduce viral load, decrease liver damage, and decrease serum levels of liver

**TABLE 43-7 Drug Therapy**
***Viral Hepatitis B and C***

| Drug Class | Examples | Mechanism of Action | Indication |
|---|---|---|---|
| **Nucleoside and Nucleotide Analogs** | adefovir dipivoxil (Hepsera)<br>entecavir (Baraclude)<br>lamivudine (Epivir HBV)<br>telbivudine (Tyzeka)<br>tenofovir (Viread)<br>ribavirin* (Copegus, Rebetol, Ribasphere) | Inhibits HBV DNA polymerase enzyme by competing with natural substrates. Prevents viral replication | Chronic hepatitis B |
| **Immune Modulator** | pegylated interferon (PegIntron, Pegasys) | Has antiviral, antiproliferative, immune-regulating actions | Chronic hepatitis B and C† |
| **Direct-Acting Antivirals** | | | |
| ***NS3/4A Protease Inhibitors*** | simeprevir (Olysio)<br>grazoprevir‡<br>paritaprevir‡ | Blocks viral protease enzyme. Prevents viral replication in genotype 1 HCV | Chronic hepatitis C |
| ***NS5B Polymerase Inhibitors*** | sofosbuvir (Sovaldi)<br>dasabuvir‡ | Nucleoside and nucleotide inhibitors of HCV polymerase. Prevent replication of RNA HCV | Chronic hepatitis C |
| ***NS5A Inhibitors*** | daclatasvir (Daklinza)<br>ledipasvir‡<br>ombitasvir‡<br>elbasvir‡<br>velpatasvir‡ | Blocks nonstructural protein 5A (NS5A) at early stage in RNA HCV replication | Chronic hepatitis C |
| **Combination Therapy** | sofosbuvir + ledipasvir (Harvoni)<br>ombitasvir + paritaprevir + ritonavir§ + dasabuvir (Viekira Pak)<br>ombitasvir + paritaprevir + ritonavir (Technivie)<br>elbasvir + grazoprevir (Zepatier)<br>sofosbuvir + velpatasvir (Epclusa) | More than one drug combined in single tablet. Drugs may be from the same or different classes. | Chronic hepatitis C |

*Also used for chronic hepatitis C.
†Use of all oral or noninterferon therapies for chronic hepatitis C is preferred.
‡Used only in combination therapy.
§CYP3A inhibitor used to enhance the pharmacokinetics of the other agents.

enzymes. Most patients with HBV require long-term treatment with these medications. Frequently when these drugs are stopped, patients' (except those who have seroconverted) HBV DNA and liver enzyme levels return to pretreatment levels.

Severe exacerbations of hepatitis B can develop after discontinuation of treatment. If these drugs are discontinued for any reason, closely monitor liver function for several months.

**Interferon.** Interferon is a naturally occurring immune protein made by the body during an infection to recognize and respond to pathogens. It has antiviral, antiproliferative, and immune-modulating effects. (Interferon is discussed in Chapter 13 on p. 194.) Pegylated interferon (PegIntron, Pegasys) is given by subcutaneous injection.

The numerous side effects with interferon therapy, including flu-like symptoms (e.g., fever, malaise, fatigue), make adherence to therapy challenging for some patients. Currently the use of interferon is limited due to the availability of better tolerated and more effective oral treatments.

Patients receiving interferon should have blood counts and liver function tests performed every 4 to 6 weeks. Depression is a side effect of interferon. Patients must be screened for depression and other mood disorders before starting interferon treatment and monitored frequently while on therapy.[9]

***Chronic Hepatitis C.*** Treatment of chronic hepatitis C is individualized and based on the genotype of the HCV, severity of liver disease, and presence of other health problems (e.g., HIV). Drug therapy is directed at eradicating the virus and preventing HCV-related complications.[10] Treatment for HCV primarily includes the use of direct-acting antivirals (DAAs) (Table 43-7), which block proteins needed for HCV replication.

With DAAs, patients complete treatment with oral drugs, typically with only 12 weeks of therapy. The majority of individuals who complete treatment with the DAAs are now able to cure their chronic HCV infection.

**DRUG ALERT Ribavirin (Rebetol, Copegus, Ribasphere)**
- May cause severe birth defects. During treatment, pregnancy must be avoided both by women taking the drug and by women whose male partners are taking the drug.
- Monitor hemoglobin and hematocrit as it may cause anemia.

Many patients with HIV also have HCV. Patients who have stable HIV and relatively intact immune systems ($CD4^+$ counts greater than 200/μL) are treated for HCV with the goal of eradicating HCV and reducing the risk of progression to cirrhosis. HCV treatment may reduce $CD4^+$ counts and increase the patient's risk for anemia and leukopenia.

Patients with advanced fibrosis or cirrhosis can undergo drug therapy as long as liver decompensation (e.g., ascites, variceal rupture, jaundice, wasting, encephalopathy) is not present.

**Nutritional Therapy.** No special diet is required in the treatment of viral hepatitis. Emphasis is placed on a well-balanced diet that the patient can tolerate. During acute viral hepatitis, adequate calories are important because the patient usually loses weight. If fat content is poorly tolerated because of decreased bile production, it should be reduced. Vitamin supplements, particularly B-complex vitamins and vitamin K, are frequently used. If anorexia, nausea, and vomiting are severe, IV solutions of glucose or supplemental enteral nutrition therapy may be used. Fluid and electrolyte balance must be maintained.

## NURSING MANAGEMENT: VIRAL HEPATITIS

### Nursing Assessment

Subjective and objective data that should be obtained from a person with hepatitis are presented in Table 43-8.

### Nursing Diagnoses

Nursing diagnoses for the patient with viral hepatitis may include, but are not limited to, the following:

- Imbalanced nutrition: less than body requirements *related to* anorexia and nausea
- Activity intolerance *related to* fatigue and weakness
- Risk for impaired liver function *related to* viral infection

**TABLE 43-8 Nursing Assessment**

***Hepatitis****

**Subjective Data**

***Important Health Information***

*Past health history:* Hemophilia, exposure to infected persons, ingestion of contaminated food or water. Exposure to benzene, carbon tetrachloride, or other hepatotoxic agents. Crowded, unsanitary living conditions. Exposure to contaminated needles. Recent travel, organ transplant recipient, exposure to new drug regimens, hemodialysis, transfusion of blood or blood products before 1992. HIV status (if known)

*Medications:* Use and misuse of acetaminophen, new prescription, over-the-counter, or herbal medications or supplements

***Functional Health Patterns***

*Health perception–health management:* IV drug and chronic alcohol use. Malaise, distaste for cigarettes (in smokers), high-risk sexual behaviors

*Nutritional-metabolic:* Weight loss, anorexia, nausea, vomiting. Feeling of fullness in right upper quadrant

*Elimination:* Dark urine, light-colored stools, constipation or diarrhea, skin rashes, hives

*Activity-exercise:* Fatigue, arthralgias, myalgias

*Cognitive-perceptual:* Right upper quadrant pain and liver tenderness, headache, pruritus

*Role-relationship:* Exposure as health care worker, resident in long-term care institution, incarceration, homelessness

**Objective Data**

***General***

Low-grade fever, lethargy, lymphadenopathy

***Integumentary***

Rash or other skin changes, jaundice, icteric sclera, injection sites

***Gastrointestinal***

Hepatomegaly, splenomegaly

***Possible Diagnostic Findings***

Elevated liver enzyme levels. ↑ serum total bilirubin, hypoalbuminemia, anemia, bilirubin in urine and increased urobilinogen, prolonged prothrombin time, positive tests for hepatitis, including anti-HAV IgM, HBsAg, anti-HBs, HBeAg, anti-HBe, anti-HBc IgM and IgG, HBV DNA quantitation, anti-HCV, HCV RNA quantitation, anti-HDV, HDV Ag. Abnormal liver scan, abnormal results on liver biopsy

*HAV,* Hepatitis A virus; *HBcAg,* hepatitis B core antigen; *HBeAg,* hepatitis B e antigen; *HBsAg,* hepatitis B surface antigen; *HBV,* hepatitis B virus; *HCV,* hepatitis C virus; *HDV Ag,* hepatitis D antigen; *HDV,* hepatitis D virus.

*Hepatitis includes both viral and nonviral causes. History questions should be tailored to the type of hepatitis.

Additional information on nursing diagnoses for the patient with hepatitis is presented in eNursing Care Plan 43-1 available on the website for this chapter.

### Planning

The overall goals are that the patient with viral hepatitis will (1) have relief of discomfort, (2) be able to resume normal activities, and (3) return to normal liver function without complications.

### Nursing Implementation

**Health Promotion.** Viral hepatitis is a public health problem. Your role is important in the prevention and control of this disease. It is helpful to understand the epidemiology of the different types of viral hepatitis before considering appropriate control measures. Preventive and control measures for hepatitis A, B, and C are summarized in Table 43-9.

***Hepatitis A.*** Outbreaks of viral hepatitis are usually due to HAV. Preventive measures include personal and environmental hygiene and health education to promote good sanitation. Hand washing is probably the most important precaution. Teach about careful hand washing after bowel movements and before eating.

Vaccination is the best protection against HAV. All children at 1 year of age should receive the vaccine. Adults at risk should also receive the vaccine. These include people who travel to areas with increased rates of hepatitis A, MSM, injecting and noninjecting drug users, persons with clotting factor disorders (e.g., hemophilia), and persons with chronic liver disease.

HAV vaccine is inactivated HAV. There are currently several forms of HAV vaccine: Havrix, Vaqta, and Avaxim. Primary immunization consists of a single dose administered IM in the deltoid muscle. A booster is recommended 6 to 12 months after the primary dose to ensure adequate antibody titers and long-term protection. The primary immunization provides immunity within 30 days after a single dose in more than 95% of those vaccinated.

Twinrix, a combined HAV and HBV vaccine, is available for people over 18 years of age. Immunization consists of three doses, given on a 0-, 1-, and 6-month schedule, the same schedule as that used for the single HBV vaccine. Twinrix may be given to high-risk individuals, including patients with chronic liver disease, users of illicit IV drugs, patients on hemodialysis, MSM, and people with clotting factor disorders who receive therapeutic blood products. The side effects of the vaccine are mild and usually limited to soreness and redness at the injection site.

Isolation is not required for HAV infection. For a patient with HAV infection, use infection control precautions. A private room is indicated if the patient is incontinent of stool or has poor personal hygiene.

Both hepatitis A vaccine and immune globulin (IG) are used for prevention of HAV infection after exposure to an infected person *(postexposure prophylaxis).* The vaccine is used for pre-exposure prophylaxis, and IG can be used either before or after exposure. IG provides temporary (1 to 2 months) passive immunity and is effective for preventing hepatitis A if given within 2 weeks after exposure. IG is recommended for persons who do not have anti-HAV antibodies and are exposed as a result of close (household, day care center) contact with persons who have HAV or foodborne exposure. Because patients with HAV are most infectious just before the onset of symptoms (the preicteric phase), those exposed through household contact or

**TABLE 43-9 Preventive Measures for Viral Hepatitis***

**Hepatitis A**

***General Measures***

- Hand washing
- Proper personal hygiene
- Environmental sanitation
- Control and screening (signs, symptoms) of food handlers
- Serologic screening for those carrying virus
- Active immunization: HAV vaccine

***Use of Immune Globulin***

- Early administration (1-2 wk after exposure) to those exposed
- Prophylaxis for travelers to areas where hepatitis A is common if not vaccinated with HAV vaccine

***Special Considerations for Health Care Personnel***

- Wash hands after contact with a patient or removal of gloves
- Use infection control precautions

**Hepatitis B and C**

***Percutaneous Transmission***

- Screening of donated blood
- *HBV:* HBsAg
- *HCV:* Anti-HCV
- Use of disposable needles and syringes

***Sexual Transmission***

- Acute exposure: HBIG administration to sexual partner of HBsAg-positive person
- HBV vaccine series administered to uninfected sexual partners
- Condoms used for sexual intercourse

***General Measures***

- Hand washing
- Avoid sharing toothbrushes and razors
- HBIG administration for one-time exposure (needle stick, contact of mucous membranes with infectious material)
- Active immunization: HBV vaccine

***Special Considerations for Health Care Personnel***

- Use infection control precautions
- Reduce contact with blood or blood-containing secretions
- Handle the blood of patients as potentially infective
- Dispose of needles properly
- Use needleless IV access devices when available

*HAV,* Hepatitis A virus; *HBIG,* hepatitis B immune globulin; *HBsAg,* hepatitis B surface antigen; *HBV,* hepatitis B virus; *HCV,* hepatitis C virus.
*A suggested guideline for general practice to prevent you from contracting viral hepatitis from diagnosed and undiagnosed patients and carriers is for you to wear disposable gloves, goggles, and gowns (sometimes) when fecal or blood contamination is likely in handling (1) soiled bedpans, urinals, and catheters and (2) when the patient's bed linens are soiled by body excreta or secretions.

foodborne outbreaks should receive IG. Although IG may not prevent infection in all persons, it may modify the illness to a subclinical infection. When hepatitis A occurs in a food handler, IG should be administered to all other food handlers at the establishment. Patrons may also need to be given IG.

Persons who are exposed to HAV who have received a dose of HAV vaccine more than 1 month previously or who have a history of laboratory-confirmed HAV infection do not require IG.

◆ ***Hepatitis B.*** The best way to reduce HBV infection is to identify those at risk, screen them for HBV, and vaccinate those who have not been infected. Teach individuals at high risk of contracting HBV to reduce risks by maintaining good hygienic practices, including hand washing, and using gloves when expecting contact with blood. Patients should not share razors, toothbrushes, and other personal items. Teach patients to use a condom for sexual intercourse. In addition, the partner should be vaccinated.

The HBV vaccine is the best means of prevention. The HBV vaccines (Recombivax HB, Engerix-B) contain HBsAg, which promotes the synthesis of specific antibodies directed against HBV. The vaccine is given in a series of three IM injections in the deltoid muscle. The second dose is administered within 1 month of the first one, and the third one within 6 months of the first. The vaccine is more than 95% effective. Only minor adverse reactions have been reported with vaccination, including transient fever and soreness at the injection site. The vaccine is not contraindicated in pregnancy.

The first dose of hepatitis B vaccine should be given at birth, with the vaccine series completed by age 6 to 18 months. Older children and adolescents who did not previously receive the hepatitis B vaccine should also be vaccinated.[8] It is also important to vaccinate adults who are in the at-risk groups and are not immune. Household members of the patient with HBV should be tested and vaccinated if they are HBsAg and antibody negative. Hepatitis vaccination is recommended for patients with chronic kidney disease before they start dialysis. Dialysis patients should routinely have their antibody titer levels checked to determine the need for revaccination.

For postexposure prophylaxis, the HBV vaccine and hepatitis B immune globulin (HBIG) are used. HBIG contains antibodies to HBV and confers temporary passive immunity. HBIG is prepared from plasma of donors with a high titer of anti-HBs. HBIG is recommended for postexposure prophylaxis in cases of needle stick, mucous membrane contact, or sexual exposure and for infants born to mothers who are positive for HBsAg. Ideally HBIG should be given within 24 hours of exposure. The vaccine series should also be started.

The Centers for Disease Control and Prevention (CDC) recommends following standard precautions for the patient with HBV (see Table 14-9). This includes using disposable needles and syringes and disposing of them in puncture-resistant units without recapping, bending, or breaking.

◆ ***Hepatitis C.*** No vaccine is currently available for hepatitis C. Therefore it is important to identify individuals at high risk for contracting HCV and teach them how to reduce their risks. Primary measures to prevent HCV transmission include (1) screening of blood, organ, and tissue donors; (2) using infection control precautions; and (3) modifying high-risk behavior.

In the United States there are many people who have undiagnosed hepatitis C. Because of this, the Centers for Disease Control and Prevention (CDC) recommends universal screening for all persons born between 1945 and 1965.[11] The CDC does not recommend IG or antiviral agents (e.g., interferon) for postexposure prophylaxis for HCV infection (e.g., needle-stick exposure from an infected patient). After an acute exposure (e.g., needle stick), the person should have anti-HCV testing done. For the person exposed to HCV, baseline anti-HCV and ALT levels should be measured, with follow-up testing at 4 to 6 months. Testing for HCV RNA may be performed at 4 to 6 weeks.[11]

◆ **Acute Care.** In patients with hepatitis, assess for the presence and degree of jaundice. In light-skinned persons, jaundice is usually observed first in the sclera of the eyes and later in the skin. In dark-skinned persons, jaundice is observed in the hard palate of the mouth and inner canthus of the eyes. The urine may have a dark brown or brownish red color because of bilirubin excretion from the kidneys. Comfort measures to relieve pruritus (if present), headache, and arthralgias are helpful.

**CHECK YOUR PRACTICE**

You are caring for a 32-yr-old man who has acute hepatitis A. He has been having severe nausea and vomiting. He is admitted to the hospital for IV hydration and monitoring. The patient says, "I'm so weak and I feel like I'm going to vomit all the time. Isn't there something you can do to help me?"
- How would handle this situation?
- What information and teaching will you provide him?

Ensuring that the patient receives adequate nutrition is not always easy. The anorexia and distaste for food may cause nutritional problems. Assess the patient's tolerance of specific foods and eating pattern. Small, frequent meals may be preferable to three large ones and may also help prevent nausea. Often a patient with hepatitis finds that anorexia is not as severe in the morning, so it is easier to eat a good breakfast than a large dinner. Measures to stimulate the appetite, such as mouth care, antiemetics, and attractively served meals in pleasant surroundings, should be included in your nursing care plan. Drinking carbonated beverages and avoiding very hot or very cold foods may help alleviate anorexia. Adequate fluid intake (2500 to 3000 mL/day) is also important.

Rest is a critical factor in promoting hepatocyte regeneration. Assess the patient's response to the rest and activity plan, and modify it accordingly. Liver function tests and symptoms are used as a guide to activity level.

Psychologic and emotional rest is as essential as physical rest. Limited activity may produce anxiety and extreme restlessness in some patients. Diversion activities, such as reading and hobbies, may help a patient cope with the plan of care and ensure adequate rest.

**Ambulatory Care.** Most patients with viral hepatitis are cared for at home. Assess the patient's knowledge of nutrition and provide the necessary dietary teaching. Caution the patient about overexertion and the need to follow the HCP's advice about when to return to work. For patients who suffer from fatigue, tell them to plan activities after periods of rest when energy levels are highest. Teach the patient and caregiver how to prevent transmission to other family members. Also teach what symptoms should be reported to the HCP.

Assess the patient for any manifestations of complications. These include bleeding tendencies with increasing prothrombin time values, manifestations of encephalopathy, sudden increase in weight and abdominal girth (may indicate fluid retention and/or ascites), bloody or tarry stools, vomiting of blood, or elevated liver enzymes.

Instruct the patient to have regular follow-ups for at least 1 year after the diagnosis of hepatitis. Because relapses occur with hepatitis B and C, teach the patient the symptoms of recurrence and the need for follow-up evaluations. All patients with chronic HBV or HCV should avoid alcohol, since it can accelerate disease progression.

It should also be noted that patients who are positive for HBsAg (chronic carrier status) or HCV antibody cannot be blood donors.

### Evaluation

Expected outcomes are that the patient with hepatitis will
- Maintain food and fluid intake adequate to meet nutritional needs
- Avoid alcohol and other hepatotoxic agents
- Demonstrate gradual increase in activity tolerance
- Perform daily activities with scheduled rest periods

Additional information on expected outcomes for the patient with hepatitis is presented in eNursing Care Plan 43-1 available on the website for this chapter.

## DRUG- AND CHEMICAL-INDUCED LIVER DISEASES

Alcohol consumption is the most frequent cause of both acute and chronic liver disease. It can cause injury and subsequent necrosis of liver tissue. Alcohol consumption can cause a spectrum of manifestations, ranging from mild elevation in liver enzymes (aspartate aminotransferase [AST] and alanine aminotransferase [ALT]) to acute alcoholic hepatitis. It may also cause advanced fibrosis and cirrhosis, which usually occurs after decades of excessive alcohol intake. Patients may also have serious liver disease caused by another chronic disease (e.g., chronic HCV infection) in combination with alcoholic liver disease, which can significantly compound the problem.

*Acute alcoholic hepatitis* is a syndrome of hepatomegaly, jaundice, elevation of liver enzyme tests (AST, ALT, alkaline phosphate), low-grade fever, and possibly ascites and prolonged prothrombin time. These manifestations may improve with cessation of alcohol intake.

Even at the end-stage of cirrhosis, abstinence can result in significant reversal in some patients. If liver function does not recover after abstaining from alcohol for 6 months or longer, liver transplantation may be considered.

*Chemical hepatotoxicity* is liver injury caused by exposure to certain compounds (e.g., carbon tetrachloride, gold compounds). Some agents can cause hepatotoxicity, while others may induce cholestasis, necrosis, or liver cancer. Fortunately because of the declining use of these agents, the incidence of chemically induced liver toxicity has diminished since the 1980s.

*Drug-induced liver injury* (DILI) is one of the more common causes of jaundice.[12] Many medications (prescription, over-the-counter [OTC], diet and herbal supplements) can cause an increase in liver enzymes and, in severe cases, jaundice and acute liver failure. The pattern of injury depends on the drug causing the reaction. The most common cause of DILI is acetaminophen. In patients with chemical hepatotoxicity or DILI, the agents that are identified as the cause of liver injury should be stopped or discontinued.

**DRUG ALERT Acetaminophen (Tylenol)**
- Drug is safe if taken at recommended levels. However, its prevalence in a variety of pain relievers, fever reducers, and cough medicines may mean that patients do not realize they are taking several drugs that all contain acetaminophen and overdose may occur.
- Acute liver failure can occur as a result of overdosing, either intentionally or unintentionally.
- The FDA has asked drug manufacturers to limit the strength of acetaminophen in prescription drug products to 325 mg per tablet, capsule, or other dosage unit, making these products safer.
- Combining the drug with alcoholic beverages increases the risk of liver damage.

## AUTOIMMUNE, GENETIC, AND METABOLIC LIVER DISEASES

### Autoimmune Hepatitis

*Autoimmune hepatitis* is a chronic inflammatory disorder of the liver in which the patient's own immune system attacks the liver. The cause of this condition is unknown. Autoimmune hepatitis is characterized by the presence of autoantibodies and high levels of serum immunoglobulins. It frequently occurs together with other autoimmune diseases.

The majority of patients with autoimmune hepatitis are women. Laboratory tests useful in the diagnosis include antinuclear antibody (ANA) and/or anti–smooth muscle antibody testing (ASMA). A liver biopsy is usually done to confirm the diagnosis and guide the treatment decision.[13]

Although autoimmune hepatitis can cause acute liver failure, the spectrum of disease is variable, with most patients developing chronic hepatitis. Untreated autoimmune hepatitis can progress to cirrhosis. Prednisone with or without azathioprine (Imuran) is the recommended treatment for active autoimmune hepatitis. Cyclosporine (Gengraf), tacrolimus (Prograf, FK506), budesonide (Entocort), methotrexate, and mycophenolate mofetil (CellCept) have also been used in patients who do not respond to prednisone and azathioprine.[13]

### Wilson's Disease

*Wilson's disease* is an autosomal recessive disorder involving cellular copper transport. A defect in biliary excretion leads to accumulation of copper in the liver, causing progressive liver injury and cirrhosis. Approximately 1 in 40,000 people have Wilson's disease. It affects both men and women equally. Symptoms appear between ages 5 and 35.[14]

Once cirrhosis occurs, copper leaks into the plasma, leading to multiple complications including neurologic, hematologic, and renal disease. The hallmark of Wilson's disease is corneal Kayser-Fleischer rings. These are brownish red rings that can be seen in the cornea near the limbus on eye examination. Low serum ceruloplasmin levels and measurable copper concentrations from liver biopsy samples are also present. Diagnosis is based on clinical findings, including the corneal rings and neurologic symptoms. First-degree relatives of patients with Wilson's disease should be screened for the disease.

The recommended initial treatment of symptomatic patients or those with active disease is chelating agents such as D-penicillamine (Cuprimine) or trientine (Syprine), which promote the excretion of urinary copper. Zinc acetate (Galzin), which has also been used as therapy, interferes with the absorption of copper. Once the amount of copper in the body has been reduced, treatment focuses on preventing copper from building up again. When liver damage is severe, liver transplantation may be required.

### Hemochromatosis

*Hemochromatosis* is a condition in which excessive amounts of iron accumulate in the body. Although it is primarily caused by a genetic defect *(hereditary hemochromatosis),* it may also be caused by liver disease and chronic blood transfusions that are used to treat thalassemia and sickle cell disease. (Hemochromatosis is discussed in Chapter 30.)

### Primary Biliary Cholangitis

*Primary biliary cholangitis* (PBC), formerly known as primary biliary cirrhosis, is a chronic disease of the small bile ducts of the liver. In PBC, there is a T cell–mediated attack of the small bile duct cells, resulting in loss of bile ducts and ultimately *cholestasis* (blockage of bile flow). Over time, this leads to liver fibrosis and cirrhosis.

Most patients diagnosed with PBC are women between ages 30 and 65.[15] The disease is associated with other autoimmune disorders such as rheumatoid arthritis, Sjögren's syndrome, and scleroderma. Elevated serum alkaline phosphatase levels, antimitochondrial antibodies (AMAs), ANAs, and serum lipid levels are seen in patients with PBC.

The goals of treatment are the suppression of ongoing liver damage, prevention of complications, and symptom management. Drugs for PBC include ursodeoxycholic acid (ursodiol [Actigall]), a bile acid, and obeticholic acid (Ocaliva), which decreases the bile in the liver. Management focuses on preventing or minimizing malabsorption, skin disorders such as pruritus and xanthomas (cholesterol deposits in the skin), hyperlipidemia, vitamin deficiencies, anemia, and fatigue. Cholestyramine is used to treat pruritus. Patients are monitored for progression to cirrhosis. Liver transplantation is a treatment option for end-stage liver disease in patients with PBC.

### Primary Sclerosing Cholangitis

*Primary sclerosing cholangitis* (PSC) is a disease of unknown etiology characterized by chronic inflammation, fibrosis, and strictures (narrowing) of the medium and large bile ducts both inside and outside the liver. The majority of patients with PSC also have ulcerative colitis. Complications of PSC can include cholangitis, cholestasis with jaundice, cholangiocarcinoma (bile duct cancer), and cirrhosis.

Drug therapy is not beneficial. Treatment is directed at reducing the incidence of biliary complications and screening for bile duct and colorectal cancer, which is related to the high incidence of ulcerative colitis. Patients with advanced liver disease may require liver transplantation.

### Nonalcoholic Fatty Liver Disease and Nonalcoholic Steatohepatitis

**Nonalcoholic fatty liver disease (NAFLD)** refers to a wide spectrum of liver diseases ranging from a fatty liver (steatosis) to **nonalcoholic steatohepatitis (NASH)** to cirrhosis. The term *nonalcoholic* is used because NAFLD and NASH occur in individuals who do not consume excessive amounts of alcohol. However, a pathologic analysis of liver cells in NAFLD is similar to that found in alcoholic liver disease.

The common characteristic of NAFLD is the accumulation of fatty infiltration in the hepatocytes. In NASH the fat accumulation is associated with varying degrees of inflammation and fibrosis of the liver. If NASH is left untreated, it can become a serious liver disease that can cause cirrhosis, hepatocellular cancer, and liver failure.

Currently, NAFLD affects about 10% to 20% of the U.S. population. This percentage is increasing because of the growing number of people who are obese. NAFLD should be considered in patients with risk factors such as obesity, diabetes, hyperlipidemia, and hypertension (also known as *metabolic syndrome*). NASH affects 2% to 5% of the U.S. population.[16]

Elevations in liver function tests (ALT, AST) are often the first sign of NAFLD. Ultrasound and CT scans can be used to diagnose NAFLD. Definitive diagnosis is by a liver biopsy.

There is no currently approved treatment for NAFLD. The goal of therapy is directed at reducing risk factors, which includes (1) reducing body weight, hyperlipidemia, and hypertension and (2) managing diabetes.

## CULTURAL & ETHNIC HEALTH DISPARITIES

### Liver, Pancreas, and Gallbladder Disorders

**Hepatitis**

- Hepatitis C has a higher incidence among African Americans and Hispanics than whites.
- Hepatitis B has a higher incidence among Asian Americans and African Americans than non-Hispanic whites.
- Deaths caused by viral hepatitis are more common in African Americans.

**Cirrhosis**

- Death from cirrhosis occurs more frequently among African Americans than in other ethnic groups.

**Liver and Pancreatic Cancer**

- Primary liver cancer has a higher incidence among African Americans, Asian Americans, and Alaska Natives than whites.
- Pancreatic cancer occurs more frequently among African Americans and Asian Americans than whites.

**Gallbladder Disease**

- Whites and Native Americans have a higher incidence of gallbladder disease than African Americans or Asian Americans.

## CIRRHOSIS

Cirrhosis is the end-stage of liver disease. Cirrhosis is characterized by extensive degeneration and destruction of the liver cells. This results in the replacement of liver tissue by fibrosis (scar tissue) and regenerative nodules that occur from the liver's attempt to repair itself (Fig. 43-4). The development of cirrhosis usually happens after decades of chronic liver disease. Cirrhosis (combined with chronic liver diseases) ranks as the eighth leading cause of death in the United States. It is twice as common in men as compared to women.

### Etiology and Pathophysiology

Any chronic liver disease, including disease from excessive alcohol intake and NAFLD, can cause cirrhosis. The most common causes of cirrhosis in the United States are chronic hepatitis C infection and alcohol-induced liver disease. In patients with alcohol-induced liver disease, some controversy exists as to whether the cause is the alcohol or the malnutrition that often coexists with alcoholism. Some cases of nutrition-related cirrhosis have resulted from extreme dieting, malabsorption, and obesity. Environmental factors and genetic predisposition may also lead to the development of cirrhosis, regardless of dietary or alcohol intake.

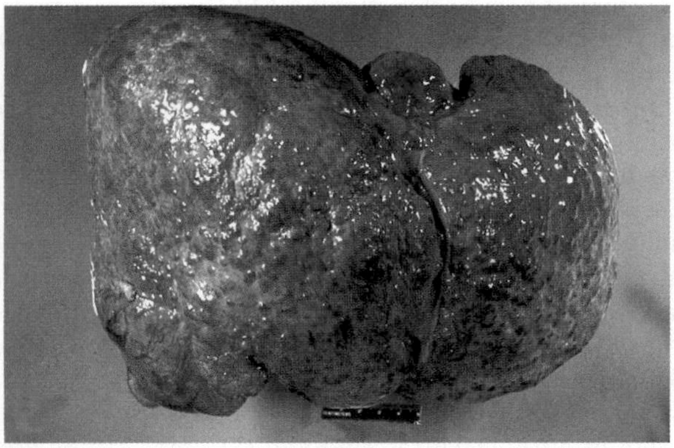

**FIG. 43-4** Cirrhosis that developed secondary to alcoholism. The characteristic diffuse nodularity of the surface is due to the combination of regeneration and scarring of the liver. (From Kumar V, Abbas AK, Aster JC, Fausto N: *Robbins and Cotran pathologic basis of disease*, ed 8, Philadelphia, 2010, Saunders.)

Approximately 20% of patients with chronic hepatitis C and 10% to 20% of those with chronic hepatitis B develop cirrhosis.[17] Chronic inflammation and cell necrosis from viral hepatitis can result in progressive fibrosis and, ultimately, cirrhosis. Chronic hepatitis combined with alcohol ingestion has a synergistic effect in accelerating liver damage.

Biliary causes of cirrhosis include primary biliary cholangitis (PBC) and primary sclerosing cholangitis (PSC). Both are described earlier in this chapter.

*Cardiac cirrhosis* includes a spectrum of hepatic derangements that result from long-standing, severe, right-sided heart failure. It causes hepatic venous congestion, parenchymal damage, necrosis of liver cells, and fibrosis over time. The treatment is aimed at managing the patient's underlying heart failure.

In cirrhosis, the liver cells attempt to regenerate, but the regenerative process is disorganized, resulting in abnormal blood vessel and bile duct architecture. The overgrowth of new and fibrous connective tissue distorts the liver's normal lobular structure, resulting in lobules of irregular size and shape with impeded blood flow. Eventually, irregular and disorganized liver regeneration, poor cellular nutrition, and hypoxia (from inadequate blood flow and scar tissue) result in decreased liver function.

### Clinical Manifestations

**Early Manifestations.** Patients may be unaware of their liver condition because there are relatively few symptoms in early-stage disease. If an individual does have symptoms, it may include fatigue or an enlarged liver. Blood tests may show normal liver function (compensated cirrhosis). The diagnosis of cirrhosis is often made later when a patient manifests symptoms of more advanced liver disease.

**Late Manifestations.** Late manifestations result from liver failure and portal hypertension (Fig. 43-5). Jaundice, peripheral edema, and ascites develop gradually. Other late manifestations include skin lesions, hematologic disorders, endocrine disturbances, and peripheral neuropathies (Fig. 43-6). In the advanced stages, the liver becomes small and nodular. Liver function is dramatically diminished.

***Jaundice.*** Jaundice results from decreased ability to conjugate and excrete bilirubin into the small intestines (Table 43-3). There is an overgrowth of connective tissue in the liver, which compresses the bile ducts and leads to an obstruction. This results in an increase in the bilirubin in the vascular system, and jaundice occurs. (Normal bilirubin metabolism is presented in Fig. 38-4.) The jaundice may be minimal or severe, depending on the degree of liver damage.

***Skin Lesions.*** Various skin manifestations are commonly seen in cirrhosis. Spider angiomas (*telangiectasia* or *spider nevi*) are small, dilated blood vessels with a bright red center point and spiderlike branches. They occur on the nose, cheeks, upper trunk, neck, and shoulders. *Palmar erythema* (a red area that blanches with pressure) is located on the palms of the hands. Both of these lesions are due to an increase in circulating estrogen as a result of the damaged liver's inability to metabolize steroid hormones.

***Hematologic Problems.*** Hematologic problems include thrombocytopenia, leukopenia, anemia, and coagulation disorders.

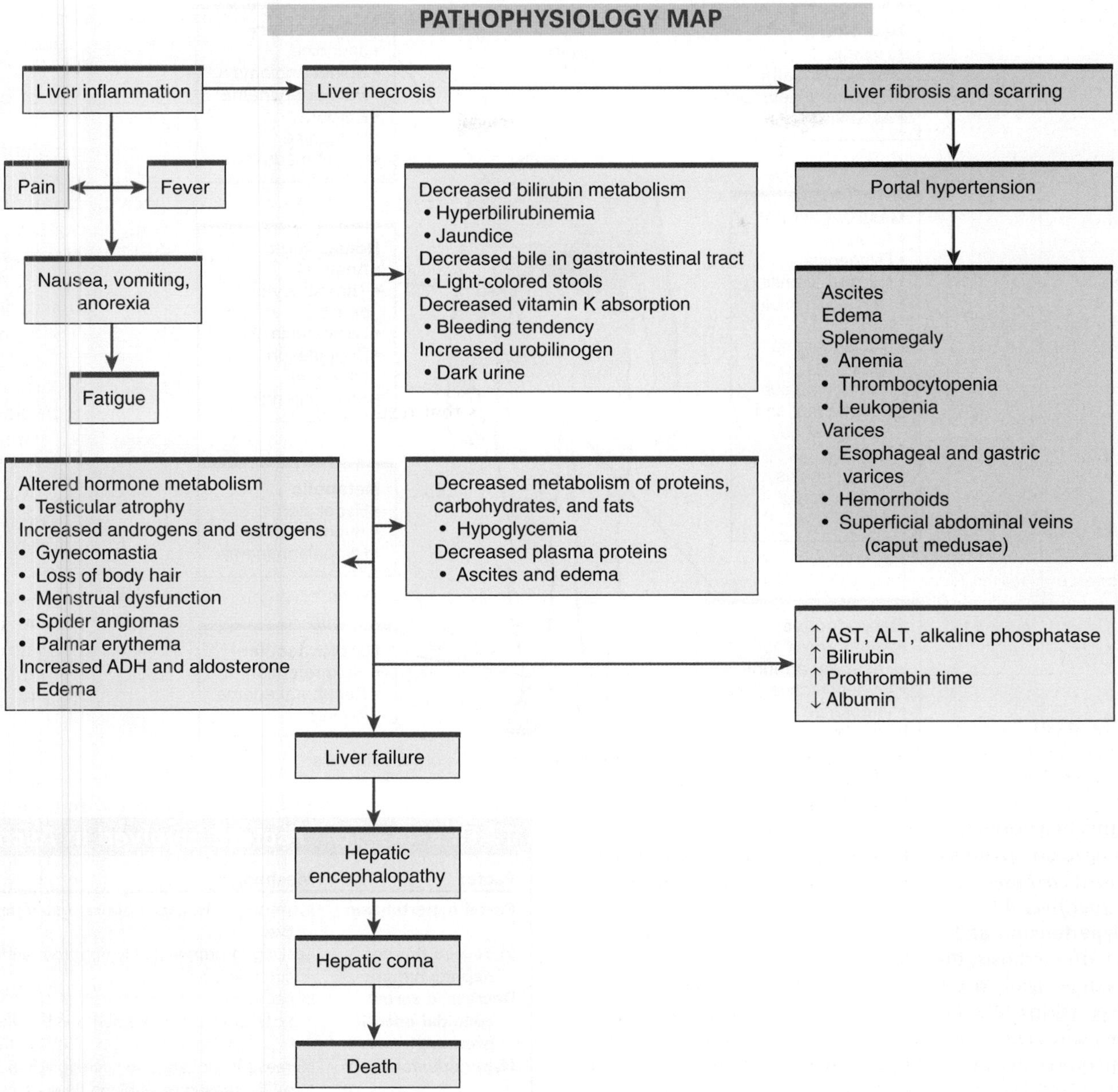


**FIG. 43-5** Continuum of liver dysfunction in cirrhosis and resulting manifestations. *ADH,* Antidiuretic hormone; *ALT,* alanine aminotransferase; *AST,* aspartate aminotransferase. (Adapted from Huether SE, McCance KL: *Understanding pathophysiology,* ed 5, St Louis, 2012, Mosby.)

Thrombocytopenia, leukopenia, and anemia are thought to be caused by the splenomegaly that results from backup of blood from the portal vein into the spleen (portal hypertension). Overactivity of the enlarged spleen results in increased removal of blood cells from circulation. Anemia can result from inadequate red blood cell (RBC) production and survival, poor diet, poor absorption of folic acid, and bleeding from varices.

The coagulation problems result from the liver's inability to produce prothrombin and other factors essential for blood clotting. Manifestations of coagulation problems (bleeding tendencies) include epistaxis, purpura, petechiae, easy bruising, gingival bleeding, and heavy menstrual bleeding.

***Endocrine Problems.*** The liver plays an important role in the metabolism of hormones, such as estrogen and testosterone. In men with cirrhosis, gynecomastia (benign growth of the glandular tissue of the male breast), loss of axillary and pubic hair, testicular atrophy, and impotence with loss of libido may occur because of increased estrogen levels. Younger women with cirrhosis may develop amenorrhea, and older women may have vaginal bleeding. Aldosterone, an important hormone associated with fluid balance, can also be altered. If the liver fails to metabolize aldosterone adequately, it can lead to hyperaldosteronism with subsequent sodium and water retention and potassium loss.

***Peripheral Neuropathy.*** Peripheral neuropathy is a common finding in alcoholic cirrhosis and is probably due to a dietary deficiency of thiamine, folic acid, and cobalamin. The neuropathy usually results in sensory and motor symptoms, but sensory symptoms may predominate.

## Complications

Major complications of cirrhosis are portal hypertension, esophageal and gastric varices, peripheral edema, abdominal ascites, hepatic encephalopathy (mental status changes, including

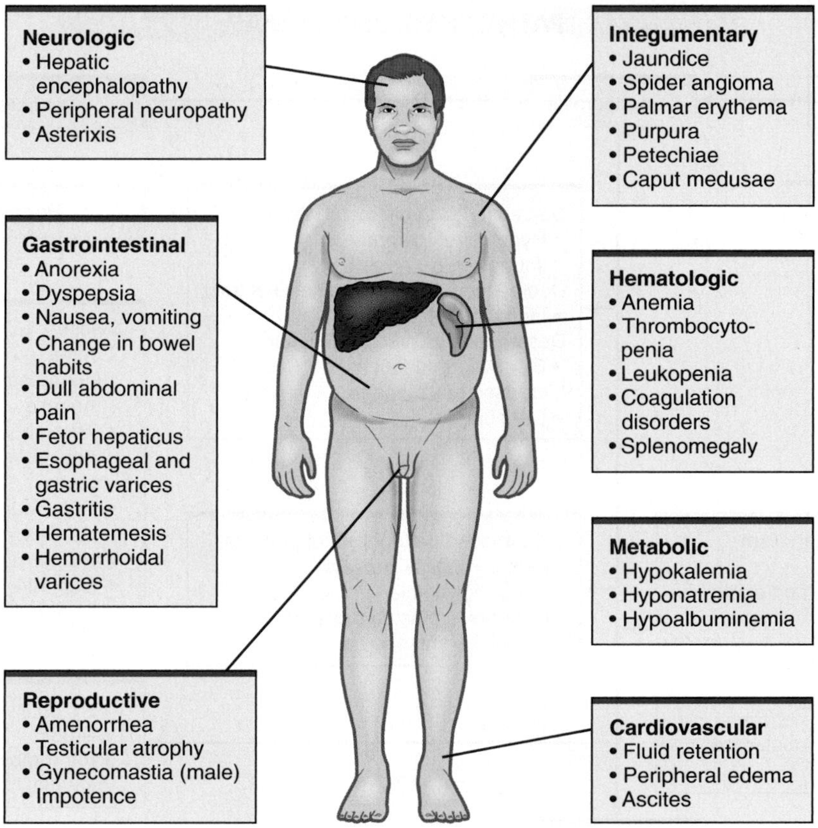


**FIG. 43-6** Systemic clinical manifestations of liver cirrhosis.

coma), and hepatorenal syndrome. Patients who are cirrhotic but who have no obvious complications are considered to have *compensated cirrhosis.* Those who have one or more complications of their liver disease have *decompensated cirrhosis.*

**Portal Hypertension and Esophageal and Gastric Varices.** In patients with cirrhosis, the liver undergoes structural changes. These changes lead to obstruction of blood flow in and out of the liver. Ultimately this results in increased pressure within the liver's circulatory system (portal hypertension). Portal hypertension is characterized by increased venous pressure in the portal circulation, splenomegaly, large collateral veins, ascites, and gastric and esophageal varices.

As a way of reducing pressure, the body develops alternate circulatory pathways, referred to as *collateral circulation.*[18] The collateral channels commonly form in the lower esophagus, anterior abdominal wall, parietal peritoneum, and rectum. Varicosities (distended veins) develop in areas where the collateral and systemic circulations communicate, resulting in esophageal and gastric varices, *caput medusae* (ring of varices around the umbilicus), and hemorrhoids.

Esophageal varices are a complex of tortuous, enlarged veins at the lower end of the esophagus. Gastric varices are located in the upper portion of the stomach. These varices are fragile and do not tolerate high pressure, thus they can bleed easily. Large varices are more likely to bleed. Esophageal varices are responsible for approximately 80% of variceal hemorrhages.[19] The remaining 20% of variceal hemorrhages are due to gastric varices. The patient may present with melena or hematemesis. Ruptured esophageal varices are the most life-threatening complication of cirrhosis and considered a medical emergency.

**TABLE 43-10 Factors Involved in Ascites**

| Factor | Mechanism |
|---|---|
| **Portal hypertension** | Increase in resistance of blood flow through liver. |
| **Increased flow of hepatic lymph** | Leaking of protein-rich lymph from surface of cirrhotic liver. |
| **Decreased serum colloidal oncotic pressure** | Impairment of liver synthesis of albumin. Loss of albumin into peritoneal cavity. |
| **Hyperaldosteronism** | Increase in aldosterone secretion stimulated by decreased renal blood flow. Decreased liver catabolism of circulating aldosterone. |
| **Impaired water excretion** | Increase in antidiuretic hormone (ADH) stimulated by decrease in renal blood flow. |

**Peripheral Edema and Ascites.** Peripheral edema occurs in the lower extremities and presacral area. Peripheral edema can occur before, concurrently with, or after ascites development. Edema results from decreased colloidal oncotic pressure from impaired liver synthesis of albumin and increased portacaval pressure from portal hypertension.

Ascites is the accumulation of serous fluid in the peritoneal or abdominal cavity. It is a common manifestation of cirrhosis. Several mechanisms lead to ascites. One mechanism of ascites occurs with portal hypertension, which causes proteins to shift from the blood vessels into the lymph space (Fig. 43-7). When the lymphatic system is unable to carry off the excess proteins and water, they leak into the peritoneal cavity. The osmotic pressure of the proteins pulls additional fluid into the peritoneal cavity (Table 43-10).

**PATHOPHYSIOLOGY MAP**

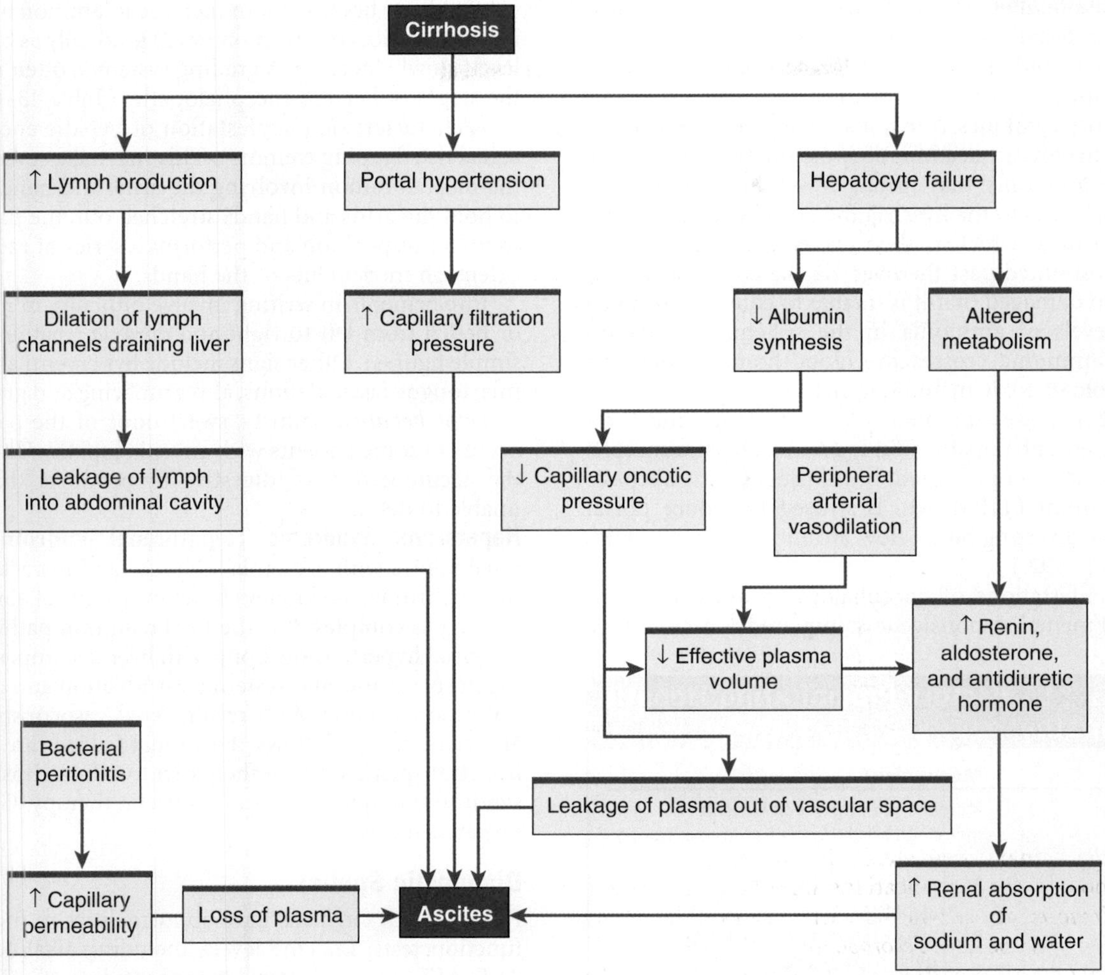


**FIG. 43-7** Mechanisms for development of ascites. (Adapted from Huether SE, McCance KL: *Understanding pathophysiology*, ed 5, St Louis, 2012, Mosby.)

A second mechanism of ascites formation is hypoalbuminemia resulting from the liver's decreased ability to synthesize albumin. The hypoalbuminemia results in decreased colloidal oncotic pressure.

A third mechanism of ascites is hyperaldosteronism, which occurs when the hormone aldosterone is metabolized by damaged hepatocytes. The increased level of aldosterone causes increased sodium reabsorption by the renal tubules. This retention of sodium, combined with an increase in antidiuretic hormone in blood, leads to additional water retention. Because of edema formation, there is decreased intravascular volume and, subsequently, decreased renal blood flow and glomerular filtration.

Ascites is manifested by abdominal distention with weight gain (Fig. 43-8). If the ascites is severe, the increase in abdominal pressure from the fluid accumulation may cause eversion of the umbilicus. Abdominal striae with distended abdominal wall veins may be present. Patients may show signs of dehydration (e.g., dry tongue and skin, sunken eyeballs, muscle weakness) and a decrease in urine output. Hypokalemia is common and is due to an excessive loss of potassium caused by hyperaldosteronism. Low potassium levels can also result from diuretic therapy used to treat the ascites.

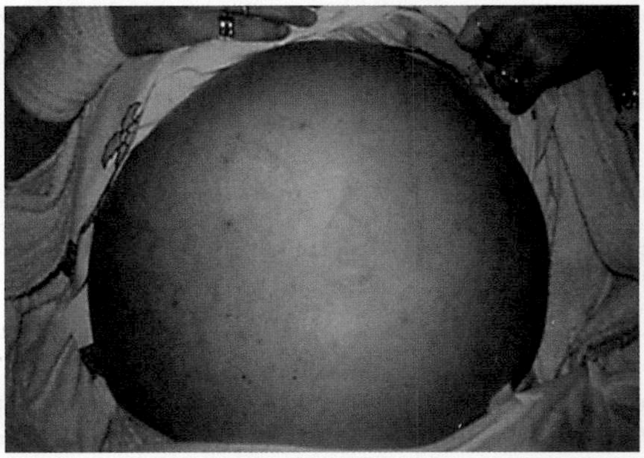

**FIG. 43-8** Gross ascites. (From Butcher GP: *Gastroenterology: an illustrated colour text*, London, 2004, Churchill Livingstone.)

Because of alterations in immune function associated with cirrhosis, patients with ascites are at risk for *spontaneous bacterial peritonitis* (SBP). SBP is a bacterial infection of the ascitic fluid. In SBP, bacteria normally found in the intestines are translocated into the peritoneal space. The bacteria most frequently responsible for the infection are a gram-negative enteric pathogen such as *Escherichia coli*. SBP occurs in approximately

15% to 25% of hospitalized patients with cirrhosis and ascites. It is particularly common after variceal hemorrhage.[20]

**Hepatic Encephalopathy.** Hepatic encephalopathy is a neuropsychiatric manifestation of liver disease. The pathogenesis is multifactorial and includes the neurotoxic effects of ammonia, abnormal neurotransmission, astrocyte swelling, and inflammatory cytokines. A major source of ammonia is the bacterial and enzymatic deamination of amino acids in the intestines. The ammonia that results from this deamination process normally goes to the liver via the portal circulation and is converted to urea, which is then excreted by the kidneys. When blood is shunted past the liver via the collateral vessels or the liver is so damaged that it is unable to convert ammonia to urea, the levels of ammonia in the systemic circulation increase. The ammonia crosses the blood-brain barrier and produces neurologic toxic manifestations.

Factors that increase ammonia in the circulation may precipitate hepatic encephalopathy (Table 43-11). Hepatic encephalopathy can occur after placement of transjugular intrahepatic portosystemic shunt (TIPS), which is used to reduce portal hypertension by diverting blood flow around the liver.[21] (TIPS is discussed on p. 992.)

Clinical manifestations of encephalopathy are changes in neurologic and mental responsiveness; impaired consciousness; and inappropriate behavior, ranging from sleep disturbances to trouble concentrating to deep coma. Changes may occur (1) suddenly because of an increase in ammonia in response to bleeding varices or infection or (2) gradually as blood ammonia levels slowly increase. A grading system is often used to classify the stages of hepatic encephalopathy (Table 43-12).

A characteristic manifestation of hepatic encephalopathy is asterixis (flapping tremors). This may take several forms, with the most common involving the arms and hands. When asked to hold the arms and hands stretched out, the patient is unable to hold this position and performs a series of rapid flexion and extension movements of the hands.

Impairments in writing involve difficulty in moving the pen or pencil from left to right and *apraxia* (inability to construct simple figures). Other signs include hyperventilation, hypothermia, tongue fasciculations, and grimacing and grasping reflexes.

*Fetor hepaticus* (musty, sweet odor of the patient's breath) occurs in some patients with encephalopathy. This odor is from the accumulation of digestive by-products that the liver is unable to degrade.

**Hepatorenal Syndrome.** Hepatorenal syndrome is a type of renal failure with azotemia, oliguria, and intractable ascites. In this syndrome, the kidneys have no structural abnormality. The etiology is complex, but the final common pathway is likely to be portal hypertension along with liver decompensation, resulting in splanchnic and systemic vasodilation and decreased arterial blood volume. As a result, renal vasoconstriction occurs, and renal failure follows. This renal failure can be reversed by liver transplantation. In the patient with cirrhosis, hepatorenal syndrome frequently follows diuretic therapy, GI hemorrhage, or paracentesis.

## Diagnostic Studies

Patients with cirrhosis have abnormalities in most of the liver function tests. Enzyme levels, including alkaline phosphatase, AST, ALT, and γ-glutamyl transpeptidase (GGT), are initially elevated because of their release from inflamed liver cells. However, in end-stage liver disease, AST and ALT levels may be normal due to the death and loss of hepatocytes. Patients with cirrhosis will also have decreased serum total protein and albumin, increased serum bilirubin (Table 43-3) and globulin levels, and prolonged prothrombin time. Alterations in fat metabolism are reflected by decreased cholesterol levels.

Although a liver ultrasound may be able to detect the presence of cirrhosis, it is not a reliable diagnostic test for cirrhosis. Ultrasound elastography (Fibroscan) is a noninvasive test that is used to quantify the degree of liver fibrosis. A liver biopsy, which may be done to identify liver cell changes, is the gold standard for a definitive diagnosis of cirrhosis.

**TABLE 43-11 Factors Precipitating Hepatic Encephalopathy**

| Factor | Mechanism |
|---|---|
| **GI hemorrhage** | Increase in ammonia in GI tract. |
| **Constipation** | Increased production of ammonia from bacterial action on feces. |
| **Hypokalemia** | Potassium is needed by brain to metabolize ammonia. |
| **Hypovolemia** | Increase in blood ammonia because of hepatic hypoxia. Impairment of cerebral, hepatic, and renal function because of decreased blood flow. |
| **Infection** | Increase in metabolic rate and increase in cerebral sensitivity to toxins. |
| **Cerebral depressants** (e.g., opioids) | Decrease in metabolism by liver, causing higher drug levels and cerebral depression. |
| **Metabolic alkalosis** | Facilitation of transport of ammonia across blood-brain barrier. Increase in renal production of ammonia. |
| **Paracentesis** | Loss of sodium and potassium ions. Decrease in blood volume. |
| **Dehydration** | Potentiates ammonia toxicity. |
| **Increased metabolism** | Increase in workload of liver. |
| **Uremia (renal failure)** | Retention of nitrogenous metabolites. |

**TABLE 43-12 Grading Scale for Hepatic Encephalopathy**

| Grade | Level of Consciousness | Intellectual Function | Neurologic Findings |
|---|---|---|---|
| **0** | Normal to minimal change | Subtle to no change in personality, behavior, memory, concentration | Asterixis absent<br>May have abnormal psychometric test |
| **1** | Lack of awareness, sleep disturbance | Short attention span, impaired computational skills, personality change, decrease in short-term memory, mild confusion, depression | Incoordination, asterixis may be absent |
| **2** | Lethargy, drowsiness | Disoriented to time, inappropriate behavior, deficits in executive function | Asterixis, abnormal reflexes |
| **3** | Somnolent, arousable | Disoriented to time, loss of meaningful conversation, marked confusion, incomprehensible speech | Asterixis, abnormal reflexes |
| **4** | Not arousable, comatose | Absent | Decerebrate<br>May be responsive to painful stimuli |

## Interprofessional Care

The goal of treatment is to slow the progression of cirrhosis and to prevent and treat any complications. Interprofessional care measures are listed in Table 43-13. Management of specific problems associated with cirrhosis is described next.

**Ascites.** Management of ascites focuses on sodium restriction, diuretics, and fluid removal. Patients may be encouraged to limit sodium intake to 2 g/day.[22] Patients with severe ascites may need to restrict their sodium intake to 250 to 500 mg/day. Very low sodium intake can result in reduced nutritional intake and subsequent problems associated with malnutrition. The patient is usually not on restricted fluids unless severe ascites develops. When caring for patients with ascites, accurately assess and monitor fluid and electrolyte balance. Albumin infusion may be used to help maintain intravascular volume and adequate urine output by increasing plasma colloid oncotic pressure.

Diuretic therapy is an important part of management. Often a combination of drugs that work at multiple sites of the nephron is more effective than a single agent. Spironolactone (Aldactone) is an effective diuretic, even in patients with severe ascites. Spironolactone is also an antagonist of aldosterone and is potassium sparing. Other potassium-sparing diuretics include amiloride (Midamor) and triamterene (Dyrenium). A high-potency loop diuretic, such as furosemide (Lasix), is frequently used in combination with a potassium-sparing drug.

**TABLE 43-13 Interprofessional Care**

***Cirrhosis of the Liver***

**Diagnostic Assessment**

- History and physical examination
- Liver function tests (ALT, AST, alkaline phosphatase, γ-glutamyl transpeptidase [GGT])
- Liver biopsy (percutaneous needle)
- Upper endoscopy (esophagogastroduodenoscopy)
- CT scan, MRI
- Liver ultrasound (e.g., FibroScan)
- Serum electrolytes
- Prothrombin time
- Total bilirubin
- Serum albumin
- Complete blood count

**Management**

***Conservative Therapy***

- Rest
- B-complex vitamins
- Avoidance of alcohol
- Minimization or avoidance of aspirin, acetaminophen, and NSAIDs

***Ascites***

- Low-sodium diet
- Diuretics
- Paracentesis (if indicated)

***Esophageal and Gastric Varices***

- Endoscopic band ligation or sclerotherapy
- Balloon tamponade
- Transjugular intrahepatic portosystemic shunt (TIPS)

*Drug Therapy*

- Nonselective β-blocker (e.g., propranolol [Inderal])
- octreotide (Sandostatin)
- vasopressin

***Hepatic Encephalopathy***

*Drug Therapy*

- Antibiotics (rifaximin [Xifaxan])
- lactulose

*ALT,* Alanine aminotransferase; *AST,* aspartate aminotransferase.

Tolvaptan (Samsca), a vasopressin-receptor antagonist, is used to correct hyponatremia, which is often seen in patients with cirrhosis. It causes an increase in water excretion, resulting in an increase in serum sodium concentration.

A **paracentesis** is a sterile procedure in which a catheter is used to withdraw fluid from the abdominal cavity. This procedure can be used to diagnose a medical condition or relieve pain, pressure, or difficulty breathing. In the patient with cirrhosis, this procedure is reserved for the person with impaired respiration or abdominal discomfort caused by severe ascites who does not respond to diuretic therapy. It is only a temporary measure of palliation because the fluid tends to reaccumulate rapidly.

TIPS (discussed later in this section) is used to alleviate ascites that does not respond to diuretics. Peritoneovenous shunt is a surgical procedure that provides continuous reinfusion of ascitic fluid into the venous system. Its use has almost been eliminated because of the high rate of complications.

**Esophageal and Gastric Varices.** The main therapeutic goal for esophageal and gastric varices is to prevent bleeding and variceal rupture by reducing portal pressure. The patient who has esophageal and/or gastric varices should avoid ingesting alcohol, aspirin, and nonsteroidal antiinflammatory drugs (NSAIDs).

All patients with cirrhosis should have an upper endoscopy (esophagogastroduodenoscopy [EGD]) to screen for varices. Patients with varices at risk of bleeding are generally started on a nonselective β-blocker (nadolol [Corgard] or propranolol [Inderal]) to reduce the incidence of hemorrhage. β-Blockers decrease high portal pressure, which decreases the risk for rupture.

When variceal bleeding occurs, the first step is to stabilize the patient and manage the airway. IV therapy is initiated and may include administration of blood products. Management that involves a combination of drug therapy and endoscopic therapy is more successful than either approach alone.

Drug therapy for bleeding varices may include the somatostatin analog octreotide (Sandostatin) or vasopressin. The main goal of drug therapy is first to stop the bleeding and identify the source and apply interventions to prevent further bleeding. IV administration of octreotide or vasopressin produces vasoconstriction of the splanchnic arterial bed, decreases portal blood flow, and decreases portal hypertension. Currently, octreotide is more widely used in this setting because of its limited side effect profile when compared with vasopressin.

At the time of endoscopy, band ligation or sclerotherapy of varices may be used to prevent rebleeding. Endoscopic variceal ligation (EVL, or "banding") is performed by placing a small rubber band (elastic O-ring) around the base of the *varix* (enlarged vein). Sclerotherapy involves injection of a sclerosing solution into the swollen veins through an injection needle that is placed through the endoscope.

Balloon tamponade may be used when acute esophageal or gastric variceal hemorrhage cannot be controlled on initial endoscopy. Balloon tamponade controls the hemorrhage by mechanical compression of the varices. Different types of tubes are available. The Sengstaken-Blakemore tube has two balloons, gastric and esophageal, with three lumens: one for the gastric balloon, one for the esophageal balloon, and one for gastric aspiration. Two other types of balloons are the Minnesota tube (a modified Sengstaken-Blakemore tube with an esophageal suction port above the esophageal balloon) and the Linton-Nachlas tube.

**SAFETY ALERT Balloon Tamponade**
- Label each lumen to avoid confusion.
- Secure the tube to prevent movement of the tube that could result in occlusion of the airway.
- Deflate balloons for 5 min every 8-12 hr per institutional policy to prevent tissue necrosis.

Supportive measures during an acute variceal bleed include administration of fresh frozen plasma and packed RBCs, vitamin K, and proton pump inhibitors (e.g., pantoprazole [Protonix]). Lactulose and rifaximin (Xifaxan) may be administered to prevent hepatic encephalopathy from breakdown of blood and the release of ammonia in the intestine. Antibiotics are given to prevent bacterial infection.

Because of the high incidence of recurrent bleeding with each bleeding episode, continued therapy is necessary. Long-term management of patients who have had an episode of bleeding includes nonselective β-blockers, repeated band ligation of the varices, and portosystemic shunts in patients who develop recurrent bleeding.

***Shunting Procedures.*** Nonsurgical and surgical methods of shunting blood away from the varices are available. Shunting procedures tend to be used more after a second major bleeding episode than during an initial bleeding episode. *Transjugular intrahepatic portosystemic shunt (TIPS)* is a nonsurgical procedure in which a tract (shunt) between the systemic and portal venous systems is created to redirect portal blood flow. A catheter is placed in the jugular vein and then threaded through the superior and inferior vena cava to the hepatic vein. The wall of the hepatic vein is punctured, and the catheter is directed to the portal vein. Stents are positioned along the passageway, overlapping in the liver tissue and extending into both veins.

This procedure reduces portal venous pressure and decompresses the varices, thus controlling bleeding. TIPS does not interfere with a future liver transplantation. Limitations of the procedure include the increased risk of hepatic encephalopathy (toxin-containing blood bypasses the liver) and stenosis of the stent. TIPS is contraindicated in patients with severe hepatic encephalopathy, hepatocellular carcinoma, severe hepatorenal syndrome, and portal vein thrombosis.

Various surgical shunting procedures may be used to decrease portal hypertension by diverting some of the portal blood flow while allowing adequate liver perfusion. Currently, the surgical shunts most commonly used are the portacaval shunt and the distal splenorenal shunt (Fig. 43-9).

**Hepatic Encephalopathy.** The goal of management of hepatic encephalopathy is the reduction of ammonia formation. Ammonia formation in the intestines is reduced with lactulose, a drug that traps ammonia in the gut. It can be given orally, as an enema, or through a nasogastric (NG) tube. The laxative effect of the drug expels the ammonia from the colon. Antibiotics such as rifaximin may also be given, particularly in patients who do not respond to lactulose. Constipation should be prevented, and regular and frequent bowel movements are necessary to minimize the ammonia buildup.

Control of hepatic encephalopathy also involves treatment of precipitating causes (Table 43-10). This includes lowering one's dietary protein intake, preventing and controlling GI bleeds, and in the event of a bleed, removing the blood promptly from the GI tract to decrease the protein accumulation in the gut.[23]

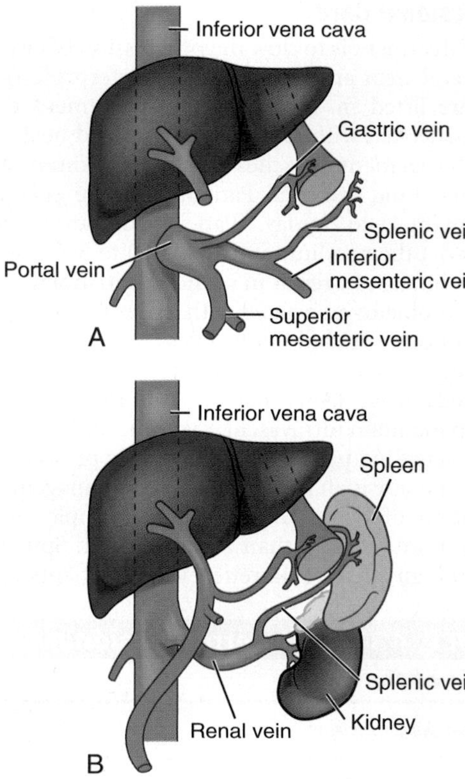


**FIG. 43-9** Portosystemic shunts. **A,** Portacaval shunt. The portal vein is anastomosed to the inferior vena cava, diverting blood from the portal vein to the systemic circulation. **B,** Distal splenorenal shunt. The splenic vein is anastomosed to the renal vein. The portal venous flow remains intact while esophageal varices are selectively decompressed. (The short gastric veins are decompressed.) The spleen conducts blood from the high pressure of the esophageal and gastric varices to the low-pressure renal vein.

**Drug Therapy.** There is no specific drug therapy for cirrhosis. However, a number of drugs are used to treat symptoms and complications of advanced liver disease (Table 43-14).

**Nutritional Therapy.** The diet for the patient who has cirrhosis without complications is high in calories (3000 cal/day) with high carbohydrate content and moderate to low levels of fat. Protein restriction may be appropriate in some patients immediately after a severe flare of symptoms (i.e., episodic hepatic encephalopathy). However, protein restriction is rarely justified in patients with cirrhosis and persistent hepatic encephalopathy. For many patients, malnutrition is a more serious clinical problem than hepatic encephalopathy.[24]

A patient with alcoholic cirrhosis frequently has protein-calorie malnutrition. Oral nutritional supplements containing protein from branched-chain amino acids that are metabolized by the muscles may be recommended. These supplements provide protein that is more easily metabolized by the liver. Parenteral nutrition or enteral nutrition therapy may be required, although rarely used, and only reserved for severe cases of malnutrition.

The patient with ascites and edema is put on a low-sodium diet. The degree of sodium restriction depends on the patient's condition. Instruct the patient and caregiver about the degree of restriction. Table salt is a well-known source of sodium, but sodium is also present in baking soda and baking powder. Foods

**TABLE 43-14 Drug Therapy**
***Cirrhosis***

| Drug | Mechanism of Action |
|---|---|
| octreotide (Sandostatin)<br>vasopressin | Hemostasis and control of bleeding in esophageal and gastric varices, constriction of splanchnic arterial bed |
| propranolol (Inderal)<br>nadolol (Corgard) | Reduction of portal venous pressure and esophageal variceal bleeding |
| lactulose | Acidification of feces in bowel and trapping of ammonia, causing its elimination in feces |
| rifaximin (Xifaxan)<br>neomycin sulfate | Decrease bacterial flora, thus reducing formation of ammonia |
| magnesium sulfate | Magnesium replacement (hypomagnesemia possible with liver dysfunction) |
| Vitamin K | Correction of clotting abnormalities from decreased levels of this vitamin |
| Proton pump inhibitors (e.g., pantoprazole [Protonix]) | Decrease in gastric acidity |
| Diuretics | |
| • spironolactone (Aldactone) | Blocks actions of aldosterone, potassium sparing |
| • furosemide (Lasix) | Acts on distal tubule and loop of Henle to decrease reabsorption of sodium and water |

that are high in sodium content include canned soups and vegetables, many frozen foods, salted snacks (e.g., potato chips), nuts, smoked meats and fish, crackers, breads, olives, pickles, ketchup, and beer. Advise the patient to read labels for sodium content. Provide suggestions to the patient and caregiver about how to make the diet more palatable. Seasonings such as garlic, parsley, onion, lemon juice, and spices may make food more appetizing. Collaborate with a dietitian regarding dietary strategies.

## NURSING MANAGEMENT: CIRRHOSIS

### Nursing Assessment

Subjective and objective data that should be obtained from an individual with cirrhosis are presented in Table 43-15.

### Nursing Diagnoses

Nursing diagnoses for the patient with cirrhosis include, but are not limited to, the following:

- Imbalanced nutrition: less than body requirements *related to* anorexia, nausea, and impaired utilization and storage of nutrients
- Impaired skin integrity *related to* peripheral edema, ascites, and pruritus
- Excess fluid volume *related to* portal hypertension and hyperaldosteronism
- Ineffective health management *related to* ineffective coping and abuse of alcohol

Additional information on nursing diagnoses for the patient with cirrhosis is presented in eNursing Care Plan 43-2 available on the website for this chapter.

### Planning

The overall goals are that the patient with cirrhosis will (1) have relief of discomfort, (2) have minimal to no complications (ascites, esophageal varices, hepatic encephalopathy), and (3) return to as normal a lifestyle as possible.

**TABLE 43-15 Nursing Assessment**
***Cirrhosis***

**Subjective Data**

***Important Health Information***

*Past health history:* Previous viral, toxic, or idiopathic hepatitis. Alcohol intake, metabolic syndrome, chronic biliary obstruction and infection, severe right-sided heart failure

*Medications:* Adverse reaction to any medication. Use of anticoagulants, aspirin, NSAIDs, acetaminophen

***Functional Health Patterns***

*Health perception–health management:* Chronic alcohol abuse. Weakness, fatigue

*Nutritional-metabolic:* Anorexia, weight loss, dyspepsia, nausea and vomiting, gingival bleeding

*Elimination:* Dark urine, decreased urine output, light-colored or black stools, flatulence, change in bowel habits. Dry, yellow skin, bruising

*Cognitive-perceptual:* Dull, right upper quadrant or epigastric pain. Numbness, tingling of extremities. Pruritus

*Sexuality-reproductive:* Impotence, amenorrhea

**Objective Data**

***General***

Fever, cachexia, wasting of extremities

***Integumentary***

Icteric sclera, jaundice, petechiae, ecchymoses, spider angiomas, palmar erythema, alopecia, loss of axillary and pubic hair, peripheral edema

***Respiratory***

Shallow, rapid respirations. Epistaxis

***Gastrointestinal***

Abdominal distention, ascites, distended abdominal wall veins, palpable liver and spleen, foul breath. Hematemesis. Black, tarry stools. Hemorrhoids

***Neurologic***

Altered mentation, asterixis

***Reproductive***

Gynecomastia, testicular atrophy, and impotence (men); loss of libido (men and women); amenorrhea or heavy menstrual bleeding (women)

***Possible Diagnostic Findings***

Anemia, thrombocytopenia; leukopenia. ↓ serum albumin, potassium. Abnormal liver function studies. ↑ INR, ↓ platelets, ↑ ammonia, ↑ bilirubin levels. Abnormal abdominal ultrasound, CT, or MRI

*INR,* International normalized ratio.

### Nursing Implementation

**Health Promotion.** Common risk factors for cirrhosis include alcoholism, malnutrition, viral hepatitis, biliary obstruction, obesity, and right-sided heart failure. Prevention and early treatment of cirrhosis focus on reducing or eliminating these risk factors. Urge patients to abstain from alcohol, and encourage those with a chronic alcohol use history to enroll in Alcoholics Anonymous or other support groups. (The treatment of alcohol dependence is discussed in Chapter 10.)

Adequate nutrition, especially for the person who abuses alcohol and other individuals at risk for cirrhosis, is essential to promote normal liver regeneration. Identify and treat acute hepatitis early so that it does not progress to chronic hepatitis and cirrhosis. Bariatric surgery for morbidly obese individuals reduces the incidence of NAFLD.

◆ **Acute Care.** Nursing care for the patient with cirrhosis focuses on conserving the patient's strength while maintaining muscle strength and tone. When the patient requires complete bed rest, implement measures to prevent pneumonia, thromboembolic problems, and pressure ulcers. Modify the activity and rest schedule according to signs of clinical improvement (e.g., decreasing jaundice, improvement in liver function studies).

Anorexia, nausea and vomiting, pressure from ascites, and poor eating habits all interfere with adequate intake of nutrients. Oral hygiene before meals may improve the patient's taste sensation. Make between-meal snacks available so that the patient can eat them at times when food is best tolerated. Provide food preferences whenever possible. Explain the reason for any dietary restrictions to the patient and caregiver.

Nursing assessment and care should include the patient's physical status. Is jaundice present? Where is it observed—sclera, skin, hard palate? What is the progression of jaundice? If the jaundice is accompanied by pruritus, carry out measures to relieve itching. Cholestyramine or hydroxyzine (Atarax) may be ordered to help relieve the pruritus. Other measures to alleviate pruritus include baking soda or moisturizing bath oils (Alpha Keri), lotions containing calamine, antihistamines, soft or old linens, and control of the temperature (not too hot and not too cold). Keep the patient's nails short and clean. Teach patients to rub with their knuckles rather than scratch with their nails when they cannot resist scratching.

Note the color of urine and stools and assess for improvement or normalization of color. When jaundice is present, the urine is often dark brown and the stool is gray or tan.

Edema and ascites are frequent manifestations of cirrhosis and require nursing assessments and interventions. Accurate calculation and recording of intake and output, daily weights, and measurements of extremities and abdominal girth help in the ongoing assessment of the location and extent of the edema. Mark the abdomen with a permanent marker so that the girth is measured at the same location each time.

Immediately before a paracentesis have the patient void to prevent puncturing of the bladder during the procedure. When the paracentesis is completed, have the patient sit on the side of the bed or place him/her in high Fowler's position. Also monitor for hypovolemia and electrolyte imbalance. Check and monitor BP and heart rate following the procedure. Check the dressing for bleeding and/or leakage of ascitic fluid.

Dyspnea is a frequent problem for the patient with severe ascites and can lead to pleural effusions. A semi-Fowler's or Fowler's position allows for maximal respiratory efficiency. Use pillows to support the arms and chest to increase the patient's comfort and ability to breathe.

Meticulous skin care is essential because the edematous tissues are prone to breakdown. Use an alternating-air pressure mattress or other special mattress. A turning schedule (minimum of every 2 hours) must be adhered to rigidly. Support the abdomen with pillows. If the abdomen is taut, cleanse it gently. The patient will tend to avoid moving because of abdominal discomfort and dyspnea. Range-of-motion exercises are helpful. Implement measures such as coughing and deep breathing to prevent respiratory problems. The lower extremities may be elevated. If scrotal edema is present, a scrotal support provides some comfort.

When the patient is taking diuretics, monitor the serum levels of sodium, potassium, chloride, and bicarbonate. Monitor renal function (blood urea nitrogen [BUN], serum creatinine) routinely and with any change in the diuretic dosage. Observe for signs of fluid and electrolyte imbalance, especially hypokalemia. Hypokalemia may be manifested by cardiac dysrhythmias, hypotension, tachycardia, and generalized muscle weakness. Water excess (hyponatremia) is manifested by muscle cramping, weakness, lethargy, and confusion.

Observe for and provide nursing care for any hematologic problems. These include bleeding tendencies, anemia, and increased susceptibility to infection.

Assess the patient's response to altered body image resulting from jaundice, spider angiomas, palmar erythema, ascites, and gynecomastia. The patient may experience anxiety and embarrassment about these changes. Explain these phenomena and be a supportive listener. Provide nursing care with concern and encouragement to help the patient maintain his or her self-esteem.

## CHECK YOUR PRACTICE

You are caring for a 69-yr-old male patient with advanced cirrhosis who just underwent banding for esophageal varices. The unlicensed assistive personnel (UAP) tells you that the patient's BP is 80/60 mm Hg and he is difficult to arouse.

- What would you do?
- What are your nursing priorities?
- What are you concerned about?

◆ ***Bleeding Varices.*** If the patient has esophageal or gastric varices, observe for any signs of bleeding from the varices, such as hematemesis and melena. If hematemesis occurs, assess the patient for hemorrhage, call the HCP, and be ready to transfer the patient to the endoscopy suite and/or assist with equipment to control the bleeding. The patient's airway must be maintained. Patients with bleeding varices are usually admitted to the ICU.

Balloon tamponade may be used in patients who have bleeding that is unresponsive to band ligation or sclerotherapy. When balloon tamponade is used, explain to the patient and caregiver the use of the tube and how it will be inserted. Check the balloons for patency. It is usually the HCP's responsibility to insert the tube by either the nose or mouth. Then the gastric balloon is inflated with approximately 250 mL of air, and the tube is retracted until resistance (lower esophageal sphincter) is felt. The tube is secured by placement of a piece of sponge or foam rubber at the nostrils (nasal cuff). For continued bleeding, the esophageal balloon is then inflated. A sphygmomanometer is used to measure and maintain the desired pressure at 20 to 40 mm Hg. The position of the balloons is verified by x-ray.

Nursing care includes monitoring for complications of rupture or erosion of the esophagus, regurgitation and aspiration of gastric contents, and occlusion of the airway by the balloon. If the gastric balloon breaks or is deflated, the esophageal balloon will slip upward, obstructing the airway and causing asphyxiation. If this happens, cut the tube or deflate the esophageal balloon. Keep scissors at the bedside. Minimize regurgitation by oral and pharyngeal suctioning and by keeping the patient in a semi-Fowler's position.

The patient is unable to swallow saliva because of the inflated esophageal balloon occluding the esophagus. Encourage the patient to expectorate, and provide an emesis basin and tissues. Frequent oral and nasal care provides relief from the taste of blood and irritation from mouth breathing.

***Hepatic Encephalopathy.*** Nursing care of the patient with hepatic encephalopathy focuses on maintaining a safe environment, sustaining life, and assisting with measures to reduce the formation of ammonia. Patients with hepatic encephalopathy may exhibit confusion and be at risk for falls or other injuries. Assess the patient's (1) level of responsiveness (e.g., reflexes, pupillary reactions, orientation), (2) sensory and motor abnormalities (e.g., hyperreflexia, asterixis, motor coordination), (3) fluid and electrolyte imbalances, (4) acid-base imbalances, and (5) response to treatment measures.

Assess the neurologic status, including an exact description of the patient's behavior at least every 2 hours. Plan your care of the patient based on the severity of the encephalopathy.

Institute measures to prevent falls or injuries. In addition, measures to minimize constipation are important to reduce ammonia production. Give drugs, laxatives, and enemas as ordered. Encourage fluids, if not contraindicated. Any GI bleeding may worsen encephalopathy. Assess the patient taking lactulose for diarrhea and excessive fluid and electrolyte losses.

Control factors known to precipitate encephalopathy as much as possible, including anything that may cause constipation (e.g., dehydration, opioid medications). In patients with altered levels of consciousness or whose airway may become compromised, have safety measures and emergency equipment readily available.

## ETHICAL/LEGAL DILEMMAS

### *Rationing*

**Situation**

T.H., a 43-yr-old female patient with cirrhosis of the liver, is frequently admitted to the hospital. She has been told that her continued alcohol consumption will inevitably lead to her death. Now she has been admitted for GI bleeding and needs blood transfusions. She has a rare blood type that is difficult to match. Should you ask for an ethics consultation?

**Ethical/Legal Points for Consideration**

- *Rationing*, or the controlled distribution of scarce resources, is a difficult ethical problem. The needs of an individual patient or group of patients are weighed against the needs of many patients, who may have a greater chance of recovery, and the availability of the necessary resources.
- Health interests can supersede the interests or rights of an individual. For example, in anticipation of an anthrax attack, the government could confiscate all relevant antibiotics and restrict their use to treat the disease.
- Two individual rights that must be considered with regard to rationing are the (1) constitutional right to privacy and (2) right to consent to or refuse medical procedures and therapy.
- The competent adult is the only person who may consent to or refuse treatment for his or her health care problems.
- If T.H. consents to a blood transfusion, an intervening party may be permitted to refuse that treatment only given substantial intervening circumstances and not as a threat to compel compliant future behavior.
- If involved parties cannot reach an agreement, legal intervention by way of a court order may become necessary.

**Discussion Questions**

1. Do you think patients with diseases that have a behavioral component such as substance abuse, deserve aggressive treatment?
2. Would you request an ethics committee consultation in T.H.'s case?

◆ **Ambulatory Care.** The patient with cirrhosis may be faced with a prolonged course and the possibility of life-threatening problems and complications. The patient and caregiver need to understand the importance of continual health care and medical supervision. Supportive measures include proper diet, rest, avoidance of potentially hepatotoxic OTC drugs such as acetaminophen in high doses, and abstinence from alcohol. Abstinence from alcohol is important and results in improvement in most patients. However, some patients find abstinence extremely difficult and require a lot of emotional support. Explore your own attitude towards the patient whose cirrhosis is secondary to chronic alcohol use. Always provide care without being condescending or judgmental. Treat patients with respect and concern for their well-being (see Chapter 10).

Cirrhosis is a chronic disease and people can live many years with symptoms and complications secondary to cirrhosis. The patient is affected not only physically but also psychologically, socially, and economically. Major lifestyle changes may be required, especially if chronic alcohol use is the primary cause. Provide information regarding community support programs, such as Alcoholics Anonymous, for help with chronic alcohol use.

Teach the patient and caregiver about complications and when to seek medical attention (Table 43-16). Include instructions about adequate rest periods, how to detect early signs of complications, skin care, drug therapy side effects, observation for bleeding, and protection from infection.

Referral to a community or home health nurse may sometimes be necessary to ensure patient adherence to prescribed therapy. Home care for the patient with cirrhosis should focus on helping the patient with activities of daily living while maintaining the highest level of wellness possible.

## ◆ Evaluation

Expected outcomes are that the patient with cirrhosis will

- Maintain food and fluid intake adequate to meet nutritional needs
- Maintain skin integrity with relief of edema and pruritus
- Experience normalization of fluid balance as a result of medical and nursing interventions
- Acknowledge and get treatment for a substance use problem

## TABLE 43-16 Patient & Caregiver Teaching

### *Cirrhosis*

*When teaching the patient and caregiver about management of cirrhosis, do the following.*

1. Explain that cirrhosis is a chronic illness and requires continual health care.
2. Teach the symptoms of complications and when to seek medical attention to enable prompt treatment.
3. Teach the patient to avoid potentially hepatotoxic over-the-counter drugs, because the diseased liver is unable to metabolize them.
4. Encourage abstinence from alcohol because continued use increases the rate of liver disease progression and risk of liver complications.
5. Instruct the patient with esophageal or gastric varices to avoid aspirin and NSAIDs to prevent hemorrhage.
6. Teach the patient with portal hypertension and varices that straining at stool, coughing, sneezing, and retching and vomiting may increase the risk of variceal hemorrhage.

Additional information on expected outcomes for the patient with cirrhosis is presented in eNursing Care Plan 43-2 available on the website for this chapter.

## ACUTE LIVER FAILURE

Acute liver failure, or *fulminant hepatic failure,* is a potentially life-threatening clinical syndrome. It is characterized by a rapid onset of severe liver dysfunction in someone with no prior history of liver disease. It is often accompanied by hepatic encephalopathy.

The most common cause of acute live failure is drugs, usually acetaminophen in combination with alcohol.[25] Other drugs that can cause acute liver failure include isoniazid, halothane, sulfa-containing drugs, and NSAIDs. Drugs can cause hepatocyte damage by disrupting essential intracellular processes or causing an accumulation of toxic metabolic products. Other causes can include viral hepatitis, in particular HBV. Hepatitis A is a less common cause. Although the disease can run its course over 8 weeks, it can last as long as 26 weeks. The survival rate is approximately 60%.[26]

### Clinical Manifestations and Diagnostic Studies

Manifestations of acute liver failure include jaundice, coagulation abnormalities, and encephalopathy. In acute liver failure, changes in cognitive function are the first clinical sign. Patients are susceptible to a wide variety of complications, including cerebral edema, renal failure, hypoglycemia, metabolic acidosis, sepsis, and multiorgan failure.

Serum bilirubin is elevated, and the prothrombin time is prolonged. Liver enzyme levels (AST, ALT) are often markedly elevated. Additional laboratory tests include blood chemistries (especially glucose, since hypoglycemia may be present and require correction), complete blood count (CBC), acetaminophen level, screening for other drugs and toxins, viral hepatitis serology (especially HAV and HBV), serum ceruloplasmin (enzyme synthesized in liver) and $\alpha_1$-antitrypsin levels, iron levels, and autoantibodies (antinuclear and anti–smooth muscle antibodies). Plasma ammonia levels may also be obtained.

CT or MRI is helpful in providing information about the liver size and contour, presence of ascites or tumors, and patency of the blood vessels.

## ❖ NURSING AND INTERPROFESSIONAL MANAGEMENT: ACUTE LIVER FAILURE

Since acute liver failure may progress rapidly, with hour-by-hour changes in consciousness, the patient is usually transferred to the ICU once the diagnosis is made. Planning for transfer to a transplant center should begin in patients with grade 1 or 2 encephalopathy because they may worsen rapidly. Early transfer is important because the risks involved with patient transport may increase or even preclude transfer once stage 3 or 4 encephalopathy develops (Table 43-12).

Renal failure is a frequent complication of liver failure and may be due to dehydration, hepatorenal syndrome, or acute tubular necrosis. The frequency of renal failure may be even greater with acetaminophen overdose or other toxins, with which direct renal toxicity occurs. Although few patients die of renal failure alone, it often increases the mortality risk and may worsen the prognosis. Protect renal function by maintaining adequate fluid balance, avoiding nephrotoxic agents (e.g., aminoglycosides, NSAIDs), and promptly identifying and treating infection.

Liver transplantation is the treatment of choice for and increases survival rates in patients with acute liver failure. Cerebral edema, cerebellar herniation, and brainstem compression are the most common causes of death. Treatment of cerebral edema is described in Chapter 56.

Monitoring and management of hemodynamic and renal function, as well as glucose, electrolytes, and acid-base status, are critical. Conduct frequent neurologic evaluations for signs of elevated intracranial pressure. Position the patient with the head elevated at 30 degrees. Avoid excessive patient stimulation. Maneuvers that cause straining or Valsalva-like movements may increase intracranial pressure (ICP). (ICP monitoring is discussed in Chapter 56.)

Assess the patient regularly for baseline level of consciousness and orientation and report any changes to the HCP. Avoid the use of any sedatives because of their effects on mental status and the effect of their use can be confused with worsening encephalopathy. Only minimal doses of benzodiazepines should be used due to their delayed metabolism by the failing liver. Additional measures include padding bedrails to avoid injury from possible seizures, closely observing the patient to prevent injuries, monitoring intake and output for renal function, and providing good skin and oral care to avoid breakdown and infection.

Alterations in level of consciousness may compromise nutritional intake and vitamin supplementation should be implemented. Factors such as coagulation problems may also influence whether enteral nutrition is initiated. An NG tube may be irritating to the nasal and esophageal mucosa, and cause bleeding.

## LIVER CANCER

*Primary liver cancer* starts in the liver. The most common types of liver cancer are hepatocellular carcinoma [HCC] (75% of cases) and intrahepatic cholangiocarcinoma (bile duct cancer). Annually about 35,660 people in the United States are diagnosed with liver cancer and 24,550 die. Worldwide liver cancer is the fifth most common cancer and second most common cause of cancer death.[27]

Liver cancer is the most common cause of death in patients with cirrhosis. Cirrhosis caused by hepatitis C is the most common cause of HCC in the United States, followed by alcoholic cirrhosis.[27]

Liver cancer incidence rates are higher in men than women. The incidence of HCC is increasing in the United States because of the large number of patients infected with chronic hepatitis C.[27]

In primary liver cancer, lesions may be singular or numerous and nodular or diffusely spread over the entire liver. Some tumors infiltrate other organs such as the gallbladder or move into the peritoneum or the diaphragm. Primary liver cancer commonly metastasizes to the lung.

Metastatic carcinoma of the liver is more common than primary liver cancer (Fig. 43-10). The liver is a common site of metastatic growth because of its high rate of blood flow and extensive capillary network. Cancer cells in other parts of the body are commonly carried to the liver via the portal circulation.

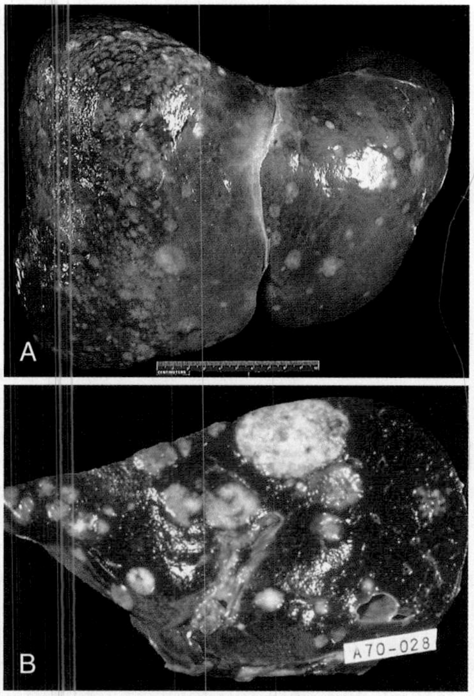

**FIG. 43-10** Multiple hepatic metastases from a primary colon cancer. **A,** Gross specimen showing outside of liver. **B,** Liver section showing metastatic lesions. (*A,* From Kumar V, Abbas AK, Fausto N: *Robbins and Cotran pathologic basis of disease,* ed 7, Philadelphia, 2005, Saunders. *B,* From Kumar V, Abbas AK, Aster JC, Fausto N: *Robbins and Cotran pathologic basis of disease,* ed 8, Philadelphia, 2010, Saunders.)

### Clinical Manifestations and Diagnostic Studies

The clinical manifestations of early liver cancer can be absent or subtle. They are often a result of the underlying cirrhosis rather than from the actual liver tumor(s). The patient may present with hepatomegaly, splenomegaly, fatigue, peripheral edema, ascites, and other complications from portal hypertension. In late stages, patients will commonly have manifestations of fever/chills, jaundice, anorexia, weight loss, palpable mass, and right upper quadrant pain.

Diagnostic and screening for liver cancer are ultrasound, CT, and MRI. Recent advancements in MRI scanning have allowed for accurate diagnosis of liver cancers without the need for a percutaneous biopsy.[28] Occasionally, a biopsy may be performed when the results of diagnostic imaging studies are inconclusive or tissue is needed to guide treatment. Risks of a biopsy include bleeding and potential tumor cell seeding along the needle tract. Therefore a biopsy is generally avoided unless a diagnosis cannot be made by CT or MRI and clinical presentation.

Serum α-fetoprotein (AFP) levels are elevated in approximately 60% of patients with HCC. The level of elevation may not correlate with the clinical features of HCC (e.g., stage or prognosis). (AFP is discussed in Chapter 15.)

## NURSING AND INTERPROFESSIONAL MANAGEMENT: LIVER CANCER

Prevention of liver cancer focuses on identifying and treating chronic hepatitis B and C viral infections. Treatment of chronic alcohol abuse may also lower the risk of liver cancer. Screening for at-risk patients (e.g., those with cirrhosis) usually involves a combination of serum AFP and either CT, MRI, or ultrasound imaging of the liver.

Treatment of liver cancer depends primarily on the stage of cancer: number, size, and location of tumors, involvement of any blood vessels, patient's age and overall health, and extent of underlying liver disease. Surgical liver resection (partial hepatectomy) offers the best chance for a cure. However, only about 15% of people have sufficient healthy liver tissue for this to be an option. The underlying cirrhosis and portal hypertension often compromises liver function and may cause liver failure postoperatively. Furthermore, many patients tend to be diagnosed at an advanced stage of liver cancer, when surgery is not an option. For those patients who have relatively early stage liver cancer and have impaired liver function, liver transplantation offers another option with good prognosis.

Nonsurgical therapies include percutaneous ablation, chemoembolization, radioembolization, and sorafenib (Nexavar) oral therapy.[29] In ablation, a thin needle is inserted into the core of the tumor. Then various substances can be injected (ethanol, acetic acid) and the temperature of the probe (radiofrequency, microwave, cryotherapy) can be altered for ultimate destruction of the tumor. This procedure can be done percutaneously, laparoscopically, or through an open incision. This method is typically limited by the number, size, and location of liver tumors. It is usually offered to patients with early stage liver cancer. Although complications are not common, they can include infection, bleeding, dysrhythmias, and skin burn.

In those patients with multinodular HCC or intermediate stage liver cancer, embolization of the tumors is another intervention. There are two options typically used: transarterial chemoembolization (TACE) or transarterial radioembolization (TARE). TACE and TARE are minimally invasive procedures performed by interventional radiologists. A catheter is placed via the femoral artery or radial artery and advanced to the arterial blood supply of the tumors in the liver. Either a chemotherapy drug (TACE) or radioactive beads (TARE) along with embolizing agents are then injected into the arteries of the tumor(s) region. TACE works by shutting off the blood supply to the tumors and exposing liver tumor cells to the chemotherapy agent. TARE destroys the tumor(s) by slowly releasing radioactive material directly to the site of the tumor. It can take up to 3 months for complete results.

In patients with advanced HCC, sorafenib (Nexavar) is typically the first-line treatment. It is a kinase inhibitor, a type of targeted therapy, that blocks certain proteins (kinases) that play a role in tumor growth and cancer progression (see Table 15-13). This drug has the potential to slow tumor progression and prolong life.

Nursing intervention for the patient with liver cancer focuses on keeping the patient as comfortable as possible. Since these patients manifest the same problems as any patient with advanced liver disease, the nursing interventions discussed for cirrhosis of the liver are used for these patients (see pp. 993-995.) (See Chapter 15 for care of the patient with cancer.)

Although the prognosis for patients with liver cancer is poor, it is improving with early screening and surveillance programs for those with chronic hepatitis and/or cirrhosis. The cancer progresses relatively rapidly, and patients often have complications both from the advancing cancer and declining liver function. Without treatment, death may occur within 6 to 12 months, most commonly as a result of hepatic encephalopathy or massive blood loss from GI bleeding.

## LIVER TRANSPLANTATION

Liver transplantation has become a practical option for many people with end-stage liver disease or localized HCC. Liver disease related to chronic viral hepatitis is the leading indication for liver transplantation. Other indications include congenital biliary abnormalities (biliary atresia), inborn errors of metabolism, sclerosing cholangitis, acute liver failure, and chronic end-stage liver disease. Liver transplants are not recommended for the patient with widespread cancer. Currently about 17,000 people are waiting for liver transplants. However, only 6000 transplants are performed annually.[30]

Liver transplant candidates must go through a rigorous transplant evaluation prior to being listed on the transplant list. This is done to confirm the diagnosis of end-stage liver disease and to assess for other co-morbid conditions (e.g., cardiovascular disease, chronic kidney disease) that may affect the patient's surgical outcome. The evaluation includes physical examination, laboratory tests (CBC, liver function tests), cardiac and pulmonary evaluations, endoscopy, CT scan, and psychologic testing. Potential recipients receive counseling regarding cigarette smoking and alcohol abstinence. Contraindications for liver transplant include severe extrahepatic disease, advanced HCC or other cancer, ongoing drug or chronic alcohol use, and inability to comprehend or comply with the rigorous posttransplant care.

Liver transplantation is performed using both deceased (cadaver) and live donor livers. (See Chapter 13 for a general discussion of organ transplants.) The live donor liver transplant was developed initially for children whose parents wanted to serve as donors. Today, some liver transplant centers are performing live liver transplant procedures for adults. In this procedure, the living person donates a portion of his or her liver to another. However, live liver donation poses potential risks to the donor, including biliary problems, hepatic artery thrombosis, wound infection, postoperative ileus, and pneumothorax.

Because of the limited number of donor livers, when a liver becomes available for transplant it may be divided into two parts (split liver transplant) and implanted into two recipients. The decision to use a split donor liver is based on the donor's size and health. The recipients of the split liver generally are smaller than the donor. The success rate associated with split liver transplantation is somewhat lower than that associated with whole organ transplantation.

Postoperative complications of liver transplant include bleeding, infection, and rejection. However, the liver is subject to a less aggressive immunologic attack than other organs such as the kidneys. (Transplants and immunosuppressive therapy are discussed in Chapter 13.)

Immunosuppressive therapy generally involves a combination of corticosteroids (prednisone), a calcineurin inhibitor (cyclosporine or tacrolimus), and an antiproliferative agent (e.g., azathioprine). (Immunosuppressive therapy is presented in Table 13-16.) Tacrolimus appears to be superior to cyclosporine in liver transplantation. Standard immunosuppressive regimens often change during the course of a liver transplant recipient's life. In addition, corticosteroid withdrawal may be done and is relatively safe to do in liver transplant recipients.

About 80% of patients survive more than 5 years after liver transplant. Long-term survival depends on the cause of liver failure (e.g., localized HCC, chronic hepatitis B or C, biliary disease). Patients who have liver disease secondary to hepatitis B or C often experience reinfection of the transplanted liver. For patients with hepatitis B, treatment after surgery with IV HBIG and one of the nucleoside or nucleotide analogs (used to treat HBV infection) has reduced the rates of reinfection of the transplanted liver.

After a liver transplant, patients with HCV typically have lower survival rates than other patient groups. However, with the new direct-acting antivirals (DAAs) that can cure HCV infection, the need for liver transplant may decrease. For those patients with chronic hepatitis C who still need a transplant, the possibility of reinfection may still exist. Research is ongoing to determine if DAAs should be initiated before or after transplant.

The patient who has had a liver transplant requires highly skilled nursing care, either in an ICU or in some other specialized unit. Postoperative nursing care includes assessing neurologic status; monitoring for signs of hemorrhage; preventing pulmonary complications; monitoring drainage, electrolyte levels, and urine output; and monitoring for manifestations of infection and rejection. Common respiratory problems are pneumonia, atelectasis, and pleural effusions. To prevent these complications, encourage the patient to use measures such as coughing, deep breathing, incentive spirometry, and repositioning. Measure the drainage from the Jackson-Pratt drain, NG tube, and T tube, and note the color and consistency of the drainage at regular intervals.

The first 2 months after surgery are critical for monitoring for infection. Causes of infection can be viral, fungal, or bacterial. Fever may be the only sign of infection. Adherence to the medication regimen can be challenging, especially in the beginning. Emotional support and teaching for the patient and caregiver are essential to the success of the patient with a liver transplant.

### Gerontologic Considerations: Liver Disease in the Older Adult

The incidence of liver disease increases with age. With aging, the liver's size and metabolic breakdown of drugs decrease, and hepatobiliary function is altered. The liver has a decreased capacity to respond to injury. This especially applies to regeneration after injury.[31] Transplanted livers take longer to regenerate in the older adult compared with the younger adult.

Older adults are particularly vulnerable to drug-induced liver injury. This is due to several factors, including the increased use of multiple prescription and OTC drugs, which can lead to drug interactions and potential drug toxicity. Age-related decreases in liver function result in decreased drug metabolism. In addition, with aging the liver is less able to recover from drug-induced injury.

A growing number of older adults have chronic hepatitis C and the resulting cirrhosis. Antibodies to HCV and elevated liver enzymes may be found during a routine health assessment in asymptomatic patients.

Lifetime health behaviors may also influence the development of chronic liver disease in the older adult. Chronic alcohol use and obesity can contribute to cirrhosis, fatty liver inflammation (NASH), and subsequent liver failure and its complications. Because of many older adults' concomitant cardiovascular and pulmonary diseases and possible anticoagulant therapy, variceal bleeding can cause significant morbidity and mortality and needs immediate medical intervention. In the older adult with liver disease, hepatic encephalopathy can sometimes be misdiagnosed as dementia and often overlooked.

PATHOPHYSIOLOGY MAP

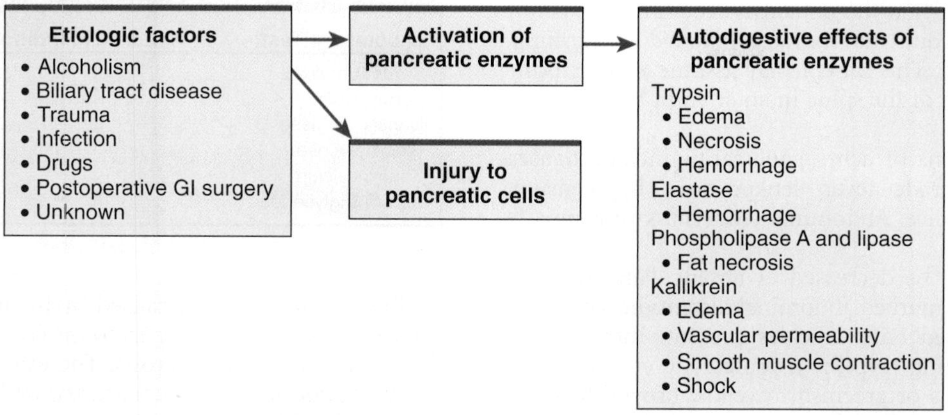


**FIG. 43-11** Pathogenic process of acute pancreatitis.

Because older adults tend to have more co-morbid conditions, transplantation may have more risks for complications. Therefore older adults are not good candidates for liver transplants.

# DISORDERS OF THE PANCREAS

## ACUTE PANCREATITIS

**Acute pancreatitis** is an acute inflammation of the pancreas. Spillage of pancreatic enzymes into surrounding pancreatic tissue causes autodigestion and severe pain. The degree of inflammation varies from mild edema to severe hemorrhagic necrosis. Acute pancreatitis is most common in middle-aged men and women. It affects women and men equally. The rate of pancreatitis in African Americans is three times higher than in whites.

### Etiology and Pathophysiology

Many factors can cause injury to the pancreas. In the United States, the most common cause is gallbladder disease (gallstones), which is more common in women. The second most common cause is chronic alcohol intake, which is more common in men.

Smoking is an independent risk factor for acute pancreatitis. **Biliary sludge**, or microlithiasis, which is a mixture of cholesterol crystals and calcium salts, is found in 20% to 40% of patients with acute pancreatitis.[32] The formation of biliary sludge is seen in patients with bile stasis.

Acute pancreatitis attacks are also associated with hypertriglyceridemia (serum levels over 1000 mg/dL). Other less common causes of acute pancreatitis include trauma (postoperative, postprocedure following an endoscopic retrograde cholangiopancreatography [ERCP]), viral infections (mumps, coxsackievirus B, HIV), penetrating duodenal ulcer, cysts, abscesses, cystic fibrosis, Kaposi sarcoma, certain drugs (corticosteroids, thiazide diuretics, oral contraceptives, sulfonamides, NSAIDs), metabolic disorders (hyperparathyroidism, renal failure), and vascular diseases.[32] In some cases the cause is unknown (idiopathic).

The most common pathogenic mechanism in acute pancreatitis is autodigestion of the pancreas (Fig. 43-11). The etiologic factors injure pancreatic cells or activate the pancreatic enzymes in the pancreas rather than in the intestine. This may be due to reflux of bile acids into the pancreatic ducts through an open or distended sphincter of Oddi. This reflux may be caused by blockage created by gallstones. Obstruction of pancreatic ducts results in pancreatic ischemia.

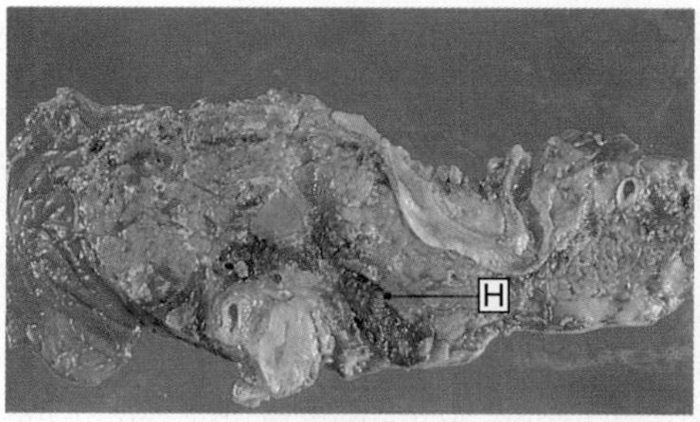


**FIG. 43-12** In acute pancreatitis, the pancreas appears edematous and is commonly hemorrhagic *(H)*. (From Stevens A, Lowe J: *Pathology: illustrated review in colour,* ed 2, London, 2000, Mosby.)

Consuming alcohol is another cause of pancreatitis. The exact mechanism by which chronic alcohol intake predisposes a person to pancreatitis is not known. It is thought that alcohol increases the production of the digestive enzymes in the pancreas. Approximately 5% to 10% of chronic alcohol users develop pancreatitis. This suggests that certain environmental (high-fat diet, smoking) and genetic factors may also be contributing factors.

The pathophysiologic involvement of acute pancreatitis is classified as either *mild pancreatitis* (also known as *edematous* or *interstitial pancreatitis*) or *severe pancreatitis* (also called *necrotizing pancreatitis*) (Fig. 43-12). In severe pancreatitis, approximately half the patients have permanent decreases in pancreatic endocrine and exocrine function. Patients with severe pancreatitis are also at high risk of developing pancreatic necrosis, organ failure, and septic complications, resulting in a 25% mortality rate.[32]

### Clinical Manifestations

Abdominal pain is the predominant manifestation of acute pancreatitis. The pain is due to distention of the pancreas, peritoneal irritation, and obstruction of the biliary tract. The pain is usually located in the left upper quadrant, but it may be mid-epigastric. It commonly radiates to the back because of the retroperitoneal location of the pancreas. The pain has a sudden onset and is described as severe, deep, piercing, and continuous or steady. The pain is aggravated by eating. It frequently has its onset when the patient is recumbent. It is not relieved by vomiting and may be accompanied by flushing, cyanosis, and dyspnea. The patient may assume various positions involving flexion of the spine in an attempt to relieve the severe pain.

Other manifestations of acute pancreatitis include nausea and vomiting, low-grade fever, leukocytosis, hypotension, tachycardia, and jaundice. Abdominal tenderness with muscle guarding is common.

Bowel sounds may be decreased or absent. Paralytic ileus may occur and causes marked abdominal distention. The lungs are frequently involved with crackles present. Intravascular damage from circulating trypsin (a proteolytic enzyme) may cause areas of cyanosis or greenish to yellow-brown discoloration of the abdominal wall. Other areas of ecchymoses are the flanks (*Grey Turner's spots* or *sign,* a bluish flank discoloration) and the periumbilical area (*Cullen's sign,* a bluish periumbilical discoloration). These result from seepage of bloodstained exudate from the pancreas and may occur in severe cases.

Shock may occur because of hemorrhage into the pancreas, toxemia from the activated pancreatic enzymes, or hypovolemia as a result of fluid shift into the retroperitoneal space (massive fluid shifts).

### Complications

The severity of the acute pancreatitis depends on the extent of pancreatic destruction. Acute pancreatitis can be life threatening. Some patients recover completely, others have recurring attacks, and others develop chronic pancreatitis.

Two significant local complications of acute pancreatitis are pseudocyst and abscess. A *pancreatic pseudocyst* is an accumulation of fluid, pancreatic enzymes, tissue debris, and inflammatory exudates surrounded by a wall adjacent to the pancreas. Manifestations of pseudocyst are abdominal pain, palpable epigastric mass, nausea, vomiting, and anorexia. The serum amylase level frequently remains elevated. CT, MRI, and endoscopic ultrasound (EUS) may be used in the detection of a pseudocyst. The cysts usually resolve spontaneously within a few weeks but may perforate, causing peritonitis or rupture into the stomach or the duodenum. Treatment options include surgical drainage, percutaneous catheter placement and drainage, and endoscopic drainage.

When a pseudocyst gets infected, a *pancreatic abscess* results from extensive necrosis in the pancreas. It may rupture or perforate into adjacent organs. Manifestations of an abscess include upper abdominal pain, abdominal mass, high fever, and leukocytosis. Pancreatic abscesses require prompt surgical drainage to prevent sepsis.

The main systemic complications of acute pancreatitis are pulmonary (pleural effusion, atelectasis, pneumonia, and acute respiratory distress syndrome [ARDS]) and cardiovascular (hypotension). The pulmonary complications are likely due to the passage of exudate containing pancreatic enzymes from the peritoneal cavity through transdiaphragmatic lymph channels. Enzyme-induced inflammation of the diaphragm occurs with the result being atelectasis caused by reduced diaphragm movement. Trypsin can activate prothrombin and plasminogen, increasing the patient's risk for intravascular thrombi, pulmonary emboli, and disseminated intravascular coagulation (DIC).

**TABLE 43-17 Diagnostic Findings in Acute Pancreatitis**

| Laboratory Test | Abnormal Finding |
|---|---|
| Serum amylase | ↑ |
| Serum lipase | ↑ |
| Urinary amylase | ↑ |
| Blood glucose | ↑ |
| Serum calcium | ↓ |
| Serum triglycerides | ↑ |

Tetany, which can be caused by hypocalcemia, is a sign of severe disease. It is due in part to the combining of calcium and fatty acids during fat necrosis. The exact mechanisms of how or why hypocalcemia occurs are not well understood.

Patients with severe acute pancreatitis are at risk for abdominal compartment syndrome secondary to intraabdominal hypertension and edema. Abdominal compartment syndrome is discussed in Chapter 42.

### Diagnostic Studies

The primary diagnostic tests for acute pancreatitis are serum amylase and lipase (Table 43-17). The serum amylase level is usually elevated early and remains elevated for 24 to 72 hours. Serum lipase level, which is also elevated in acute pancreatitis, is an important test because other disorders (e.g., mumps, cerebral trauma, renal transplantation) may increase serum amylase levels. Other serum findings include an increase in liver enzymes, triglycerides, glucose, and bilirubin and a decrease in calcium.

Diagnostic evaluation of acute pancreatitis is also directed at determining the cause. An abdominal ultrasound, x-ray, or contrast-enhanced CT scan can be used to identify pancreatic problems. CT scan is the best imaging test for pancreatitis and related complications such as pseudocysts and abscesses. ERCP is used (although ERCP can cause acute pancreatitis), along with EUS, magnetic resonance cholangiopancreatography (MRCP), and angiography. Chest x-rays may show pulmonary changes, including atelectasis and pleural effusions.

### Interprofessional Care

Goals of interprofessional care for acute pancreatitis include (1) relief of pain; (2) prevention or alleviation of shock; (3) reduction of pancreatic secretions; (4) correction of fluid and electrolyte imbalances; (5) prevention or treatment of infections; and (6) removal of the precipitating cause, if possible (Table 43-18).

**Conservative Therapy.** Treatment of acute pancreatitis is primarily focused on supportive care, including aggressive hydration, pain management, management of metabolic complications, and minimization of pancreatic stimulation. Treatment and control of pain are very important. IV morphine may be used. Pain medications may be combined with an antispasmodic agent. However, atropine and other anticholinergic drugs should be avoided when paralytic ileus is present because they can decrease GI mobility, thus further exacerbating the problem. Other medications that relax smooth muscles (spasmolytics), such as nitroglycerin or papaverine, may be used. Supplemental $O_2$ is used to maintain $O_2$ saturation greater than 95%. In patients with severe pancreatitis, serum glucose levels are closely monitored for hyperglycemia.

**TABLE 43-18 Interprofessional Care**
***Acute Pancreatitis***

**Diagnostic Assessment**
- History and physical examination
- Serum amylase and lipase
- Blood glucose
- Serum calcium
- Serum triglycerides
- Flat plate of the abdomen
- Abdominal ultrasound
- Endoscopic ultrasound (EUS)
- Magnetic resonance cholangiopancreatography (MRCP)
- Endoscopic retrograde cholangiopancreatography (ERCP)
- Contrast-enhanced CT of pancreas
- Chest x-ray

**Management**
- NPO with NG tube to suction
- Albumin (if shock present)
- IV calcium gluconate (10%) (if tetany present)
- Lactated Ringer's solution

***Drug Therapy***
- Pain medication (e.g., morphine)
- Proton pump inhibitor (e.g., omeprazole [Prilosec])
- Antibiotics (if necrotizing pancreatitis)

**TABLE 43-19 Drug Therapy**
***Acute and Chronic Pancreatitis***

| Drug | Mechanism of Action |
|---|---|
| **Acute Pancreatitis** | |
| Morphine | Relief of pain |
| Antispasmodics (e.g., dicyclomine [Bentyl]) | ↓ Vagal stimulation, motility, pancreatic outflow (↓ volume and concentration of bicarbonate and enzyme secretion)<br>Contraindicated in paralytic ileus |
| Carbonic anhydrase inhibitor (acetazolamide) | ↓ Volume and bicarbonate concentration of pancreatic secretion |
| Antacids | Neutralization of gastric hydrochloric (HCl) acid secretion<br>↓ Production and secretion of pancreatic enzymes and bicarbonate |
| Proton pump inhibitors (e.g., omeprazole [Prilosec]) | ↓ HCl acid secretion (HCl acid stimulates pancreatic activity) |
| **Chronic Pancreatitis** | |
| Pancreatic enzyme products (pancrelipase [Pancrease, Zenpep, Creon, Viokace]) | Replacement therapy for pancreatic enzymes |
| Insulin | Treatment for diabetes mellitus or hyperglycemia, if needed |

If shock is present, blood volume replacements are used. Plasma or plasma volume expanders such as dextran or albumin may be given. Fluid and electrolyte imbalances are corrected with lactated Ringer's solution or other electrolyte solutions. Central venous pressure readings may be used to assist in determining fluid replacement requirements. Vasoactive drugs such as dopamine (Intropin) may be used to increase systemic vascular resistance in patients with ongoing hypotension.

**CHECK YOUR PRACTICE**

You are a nurse working in the emergency department. Your patient is a 45-yr-old woman who is admitted with acute abdominal pain in her left upper quadrant. She is diagnosed with acute pancreatitis. She tells you, "I've been waiting in this emergency room for 8 hours and I'm starving. Why can't I get something to eat? My pain is so bad; I think it's becoming worse because you won't give me food."
- How would you respond?
- What information and teaching would you provide her?

It is important to reduce or suppress pancreatic enzymes to decrease stimulation of the pancreas and allow it to rest. This is accomplished in several ways. First, the patient is NPO. Second, NG suction may be used to reduce vomiting and gastric distention and to prevent gastric acidic contents from entering the duodenum. In addition, certain drugs may be used to suppress gastric acid secretion (Table 43-19). With resolution of the pancreatitis, the patient resumes oral intake. For the patient with severe acute pancreatitis who does not resume oral intake, enteral nutrition support may be initiated.

The inflamed and necrotic pancreatic tissue is a good medium for bacterial growth. In patients with acute necrotizing pancreatitis, infection is the leading cause of morbidity and mortality. Therefore it is important to prevent infections. Because many of the organisms come from the intestine, enteral feeding reduces the risk of necrotizing pancreatitis. Monitor the patient closely so that antibiotic therapy can be instituted early if necrosis and infection occur. Endoscopic- or CT-guided percutaneous aspiration with Gram stain and culture may be performed.

**Surgical Therapy.** When the acute pancreatitis is related to gallstones, an urgent ERCP plus endoscopic *sphincterotomy* (severing of the muscle layers of the sphincter of Oddi) may be done. This may be followed by laparoscopic cholecystectomy to reduce the potential for recurrence. Surgical intervention may also be indicated when the diagnosis is uncertain and for patients who do not respond to conservative therapy.

Those with severe acute pancreatitis may require drainage of necrotic fluid collections. This is done surgically, under CT guidance, or endoscopically. Percutaneous drainage of a pseudocyst can be performed, and a drainage tube is left in place.

**Drug Therapy.** Several different drugs are used to prevent and treat problems associated with pancreatitis (Table 43-19). Currently there are no drugs that cure pancreatitis.

**Nutritional Therapy.** Initially the patient with acute pancreatitis is on NPO status to reduce pancreatic secretion. Depending on the severity of the pancreatitis, enteral feedings via nasojejunal tube are initiated. Because of infection risk, parenteral nutrition is reserved for patients who cannot tolerate enteral nutrition (see Chapter 39). If IV lipids are ordered, blood triglyceride levels must be monitored. In cases of moderate to severe pancreatitis, the patient may require enteral feeding via a jejunal feeding tube.

When food is allowed, small, frequent feedings are given. The diet is usually high in carbohydrate content because that is the least stimulating to the exocrine portion of the pancreas. Suspect intolerance to oral foods when the patient reports pain, has increasing abdominal girth, or has elevations in serum amylase and lipase levels. Supplemental fat-soluble vitamins may be given.

## NURSING MANAGEMENT: ACUTE PANCREATITIS

### Nursing Assessment

Subjective and objective data that should be obtained from a person with acute pancreatitis are presented in Table 43-20.

**TABLE 43-20 Nursing Assessment**
***Acute Pancreatitis***

**Subjective Data**

***Important Health Information***

*Past health history:* Biliary tract disease, alcohol use, abdominal trauma, duodenal ulcers, infection, metabolic disorders
*Medications:* Thiazides, nonsteroidal antiinflammatory drugs
*Surgery or other treatments:* Surgical procedures on the pancreas, stomach, duodenum, or biliary tract. Endoscopic retrograde cholangiopancreatography (ERCP)

***Functional Health Patterns***

*Health perception–health management:* Chronic alcohol use, fatigue
*Nutritional-metabolic:* Nausea and vomiting, anorexia
*Activity-exercise:* Dyspnea
*Cognitive-perceptual:* Severe midepigastric or left upper quadrant pain that may radiate to the back, aggravated by food and alcohol intake and unrelieved by vomiting

**Objective Data**

***General***

Restlessness, anxiety, low-grade fever

***Integumentary***

Flushing, diaphoresis, discoloration of abdomen and flanks, cyanosis, jaundice. Decreased skin turgor, dry mucous membranes

***Respiratory***

Tachypnea, basilar crackles

***Cardiovascular***

Tachycardia, hypotension

***Gastrointestinal***

Abdominal distention, tenderness, and muscle guarding. Diminished bowel sounds

***Possible Diagnostic Findings***

↑ Serum amylase and lipase, leukocytosis, hyperglycemia, hypocalcemia, abnormal ultrasound and CT scans of pancreas, abnormal ERCP or MRCP

## ◆ Nursing Diagnoses

Nursing diagnoses for the patient with acute pancreatitis may include, but are not limited to, the following:

- Acute pain *related to* distention of pancreas, peritoneal irritation, obstruction of biliary tract, and ineffective pain and comfort measures
- Deficient fluid volume *related to* nausea, vomiting, restricted oral intake, and fluid shift into the retroperitoneal space
- Imbalanced nutrition: less than body requirements *related to* anorexia, dietary restrictions, nausea, loss of nutrients from vomiting, and impaired digestion
- Ineffective health management *related to* lack of knowledge of preventive measures, diet restrictions, alcohol intake restriction, and follow-up care

Additional information on nursing diagnoses for the patient with acute pancreatitis is presented in eNursing Care Plan 43-3 available on the website for this chapter.

## ◆ Planning

The overall goals are that the patient with acute pancreatitis will have (1) relief of pain, (2) normal fluid and electrolyte balance, (3) minimal to no complications, and (4) no recurrent attacks.

## ◆ Nursing Implementation

◆ **Health Promotion.** The major factors involved in health promotion are (1) assessment of the patient for predisposing and etiologic factors and (2) encouragement of early treatment of these factors to prevent acute pancreatitis. Encourage early diagnosis and treatment of biliary tract disease, such as cholelithiasis. Encourage the patient to eliminate alcohol intake, especially if he or she has had any previous episodes of pancreatitis. Recurrent attacks of pancreatitis may become milder or disappear with the discontinuance of alcohol use.

◆ **Acute Care.** During the acute phase, it is important to monitor vital signs. Hemodynamic stability may be compromised by hypotension, fever, and tachypnea. Monitor the response to IV fluids. Also closely monitor fluid and electrolyte balance. Frequent vomiting, along with gastric suction, may result in decreased chloride, sodium, and potassium levels.

Respiratory failure may develop in the patient with severe acute pancreatitis. Assess respiratory function (e.g., lung sounds, $O_2$ saturation levels). If ARDS develops, the patient may require intubation and mechanical ventilation support.

**! SAFETY ALERT Respiratory Distress in Acute Pancreatitis**

- Assess for respiratory distress in the patient with severe acute pancreatitis.
- Listen to lung sounds and monitor $O_2$ saturation on a regular basis.

Because hypocalcemia can also occur, observe for symptoms of tetany, such as jerking, irritability, and muscular twitching. Numbness or tingling around the lips and in the fingers is an early indicator of hypocalcemia. Assess the patient for a positive Chvostek's sign or Trousseau's sign (see Fig. 16-15). Calcium gluconate (as ordered) should be given to treat symptomatic hypocalcemia. Hypomagnesemia may also develop, necessitating the monitoring of serum magnesium levels.

Because abdominal pain is a prominent symptom of pancreatitis, a major focus of your care is the relief of pain. Pain and restlessness can increase the metabolic rate. In addition, acute pain can contribute to hemodynamic instability. Morphine may be used for pain relief. Assess and document the duration of pain relief. Measures such as comfortable positioning, frequent changes in position, and relief of nausea and vomiting assist in reducing the restlessness that usually accompanies the pain. Assuming positions that flex the trunk and draw the knees up to the abdomen may decrease pain. A side-lying position with the head elevated 45 degrees decreases tension on the abdomen and may help ease the pain.

For the patient who is on NPO status or has an NG tube, provide frequent oral and nasal care to relieve the dryness of the mouth and nose. Oral care is essential to prevent parotitis. Also if the patient is taking anticholinergics to decrease GI secretions, the mouth will be especially dry. If the patient is taking antacids to neutralize gastric acid secretion, they should be sipped slowly or inserted in the NG tube.

Observe for fever and other manifestations of infection in the patient with acute pancreatitis. Respiratory tract infections are common, which causes the patient to take shallow, guarded abdominal breaths. Measures to prevent respiratory tract infections include turning, coughing, deep breathing, and assuming a semi-Fowler's position.

Other important assessments are observation for signs of paralytic ileus, renal failure, and mental changes. Determine the blood glucose level to assess damage to the β cells of the islets of Langerhans in the pancreas.

If patients have surgery to drain necrotic fluid or treat a cyst, they may require special wound care for an anastomotic leak or a fistula. To prevent skin irritation, use skin barriers (e.g., Stomahesive, Karaya Paste, or Colly-Seel), pouching, and drains. In addition to protecting the skin, pouching also permits a more accurate determination of fluid and electrolyte losses and increases patient comfort. Sterile pouching systems are available. Consult with a clinical specialist or wound, ostomy, and continence nurse (WOCN).

**Ambulatory Care.** After acute pancreatitis, the patient may require home care follow-up. Because of loss of physical and muscle strength, physical therapy may be needed. Continued care to prevent infection and detect any complications is important. Counseling regarding abstinence from alcohol is important to prevent the patient from experiencing future attacks of acute pancreatitis and development of chronic pancreatitis. Because cigarettes can stimulate the pancreas, smoking should be avoided.

Dietary teaching should include restriction of fats because they stimulate the secretion of cholecystokinin, which then stimulates the pancreas. Carbohydrates are less stimulating to the pancreas and are encouraged. Also instruct the patient to avoid crash dieting and bingeing because they can precipitate attacks.

Teach the patient and caregiver to recognize and report symptoms of infection, diabetes mellitus, or steatorrhea (foul-smelling, fatty stools). These changes indicate possible ongoing destruction of pancreatic tissue and pancreatic insufficiency and may require exogenous enzyme supplementation. Teach the patient and caregiver about the prescribed regimen, including the importance of taking the required medications and following the recommended diet.

### Evaluation

The expected outcomes are that the patient with acute pancreatitis will

- Have adequate pain control
- Maintain adequate fluid balance
- Be knowledgeable about treatment regimen to restore health
- Get help for alcohol dependence and smoking cessation (if appropriate)

Additional information on expected outcomes for the patient with acute pancreatitis is presented in eNursing Care Plan 43-3 available on the website for this chapter.

## CHRONIC PANCREATITIS

**Chronic pancreatitis** is a continuous, prolonged, inflammatory, and fibrosing process of the pancreas. The pancreas is progressively destroyed as it is replaced by fibrotic tissue. Strictures and calcifications may also occur in the pancreas.

### Etiology and Pathophysiology

Chronic pancreatitis can be due to chronic alcohol use; obstruction caused by cholelithiasis (gallstones), tumor, pseudocysts, or trauma; and systemic diseases (e.g., systemic lupus erythematosus), autoimmune pancreatitis, and cystic fibrosis. Some patients may not have an identifiable risk factor (idiopathic pancreatitis). Chronic pancreatitis may follow acute pancreatitis, but it may also occur in the absence of any history of an acute condition.

The most common cause of obstructive pancreatitis is inflammation of the sphincter of Oddi associated with cholelithiasis. Cancer of the ampulla of Vater, duodenum, or pancreas can also cause this type of chronic pancreatitis.

The most common cause of nonobstructive pancreatitis (the most common type of chronic pancreatitis) is chronic alcohol use. There is inflammation and sclerosis, mainly in the head of the pancreas and around the pancreatic duct. In some people who drink alcohol, a genetic factor may predispose them to the direct toxic effect of the alcohol on the pancreas.

### Clinical Manifestations

As with acute pancreatitis, a major manifestation of chronic pancreatitis is abdominal pain. The patient may have episodes of acute pain, but it usually is chronic (recurrent attacks at intervals of months or years). The attacks may become more and more frequent until they are almost constant, or they may diminish as pancreatic fibrosis develops. The pain is located in the same areas as in acute pancreatitis but is usually described as a heavy, gnawing feeling or sometimes as burning and cramp-like. The pain is not relieved with food or antacids.

Other clinical manifestations include symptoms of pancreatic insufficiency, including malabsorption with weight loss, constipation, mild jaundice with dark urine, steatorrhea, and diabetes mellitus. The steatorrhea may become severe, with voluminous, foul-smelling, fatty stools. Some abdominal tenderness may be present.

Chronic pancreatitis is also associated with a variety of complications, including pseudocyst formation, bile duct or duodenal obstruction, pancreatic ascites or pleural effusion, splenic vein thrombosis, pseudoaneurysms, and pancreatic cancer.

### Diagnostic Studies

Confirming the diagnosis of chronic pancreatitis can be challenging. The diagnosis is based on the patient's signs and symptoms, laboratory studies, and imaging. In chronic pancreatitis, the levels of serum amylase and lipase may be elevated slightly or not at all, depending on the degree of pancreatic fibrosis. Serum bilirubin and alkaline phosphatase levels may be increased. There is usually mild leukocytosis and an elevated sedimentation rate.

ERCP is used to visualize the pancreatic and common bile ducts. Imaging studies such as CT, MRI, MRCP, abdominal ultrasound, and EUS are useful in patients with chronic pancreatitis. These procedures show a variety of changes, including calcifications, ductal dilation, pseudocysts, and enlargement of the pancreas.

Stool samples are examined for fecal fat content. Deficiencies of fat-soluble vitamins and cobalamin, glucose intolerance, and possibly diabetes may also be found in those with chronic pancreatitis. A secretin stimulation test may be used to assess the degree of pancreatic dysfunction (see Chapter 38).

### Interprofessional Care

When the patient with chronic pancreatitis experiences an acute attack, the therapy is identical to that for acute pancreatitis. At other times the focus is on prevention of further attacks, relief of pain, and control of pancreatic exocrine and endocrine insufficiency. It sometimes takes frequent doses of analgesics (morphine or fentanyl patch [Duragesic]) to relieve the pain if dietary measures and enzyme replacement are not effective.

Diet, pancreatic enzyme replacement, and control of diabetes are ways to control the pancreatic insufficiency. Small, bland, frequent meals that are low in fat content are recommended to decrease pancreatic stimulation. Smoking is associated with accelerated progression of chronic pancreatitis. Also teach the patient not to consume alcohol and caffeinated beverages.

Pancreatic enzyme products such as pancrelipase (Pancrease, Zenpep, Creon, Viokace) contain amylase, lipase, and trypsin and are used to replace the deficient pancreatic enzymes. They are usually enteric coated to prevent their breakdown or inactivation by gastric acid. Bile salts are sometimes given to facilitate the absorption of the fat-soluble vitamins (A, D, E, and K) and prevent further fat loss. If diabetes develops, it is controlled with insulin (more commonly) or oral hypoglycemic agents. Acid-neutralizing drugs (e.g., antacids) and acid-inhibiting drugs (e.g., $H_2$-receptor blockers, proton pump inhibitors) may be given to decrease hydrochloric (HCl) acid secretion but have little overall effect on patient outcomes. Antidepressants, such as nortriptyline (Aventyl), have been shown to reduce the neuropathic pain associated with chronic pancreatitis.

Treatment of chronic pancreatitis sometimes requires endoscopic therapy or surgery. When biliary disease is present or obstruction or pseudocyst develops, surgery may be indicated. Surgical procedures can divert bile flow or relieve ductal obstruction. A choledochojejunostomy diverts bile around the ampulla of Vater, where there may be spasm or hypertrophy of the sphincter. In this procedure, the common bile duct is anastomosed into the jejunum. Another type of surgical diverting procedure is the Roux-en-Y pancreatojejunostomy, in which the pancreatic duct is opened and an anastomosis is made with the jejunum. Pancreatic drainage procedures can relieve ductal obstruction and are often done with ERCP. Some patients may undergo ERCP with sphincterotomy and/or stent placement at the site of obstruction. These patients require follow-up procedures such as ERCP to either exchange or remove the stent.

## ❖ NURSING MANAGEMENT: CHRONIC PANCREATITIS

Except during an acute episode, nursing management focuses on chronic care and health promotion. Instruct the patient to take measures to prevent further attacks. Dietary control, along with consistency of other treatment measures, such as taking pancreatic enzymes, is essential. The enzymes are usually taken with meals or a snack. Observe the patient's stools for steatorrhea to help determine the effectiveness of the enzymes. Instruct the patient and caregiver to monitor stool quality.

If diabetes has developed, instruct the patient regarding testing of blood glucose levels and drug therapy (see Chapter 48). Ensure that the patient who is taking antisecretory agents or antacids takes them as ordered to control gastric acidity. Antacids should be taken after meals and at bedtime.

The patient must avoid alcohol and may need assistance with this problem. If the patient is dependent on alcohol, referral to other agencies or resources may be necessary (see Chapter 10).

## PANCREATIC CANCER

Annually in the United States an estimated 48,960 people are diagnosed with pancreatic cancer, and 40,560 people die from pancreatic cancer.[33] It is the fourth leading cause of death from cancer in the United States. The risk increases with age, with the peak incidence occurring between 65 and 80 years of age.

Most pancreatic tumors are adenocarcinomas originating from the epithelium of the ductal system. More than half of the tumors occur in the head of the pancreas. As the tumor grows, the common bile duct becomes obstructed, and obstructive jaundice develops. Tumors starting in the body or the tail often remain silent until their growth is advanced. The majority of cancers have metastasized at the time of diagnosis. The signs and symptoms of pancreatic cancer are often similar to those of chronic pancreatitis. The prognosis of a patient with cancer of the pancreas is poor. The majority of patients die within 5 to 12 months of the initial diagnosis, and the 5-year survival rate is less than 5%.[33]

### Etiology and Pathophysiology

The cause of pancreatic cancer remains unknown. Risk factors for pancreatic cancer include chronic pancreatitis, diabetes mellitus, age, cigarette smoking, family history of pancreatic cancer, high-fat diet, and exposure to chemicals such as benzidine. African Americans have a higher incidence of pancreatic cancer than whites. The most firmly established environmental risk factor is cigarette smoking. Smokers are two to three times more likely to develop pancreatic cancer than nonsmokers. The risk is related to both the duration and amount of cigarettes smoked.

### Clinical Manifestations

Common manifestations of pancreatic cancer include abdominal pain (dull, aching), anorexia, rapid and progressive weight loss, nausea, and jaundice. The most common manifestations of cancer of the head of the pancreas are pain, jaundice, and weight loss. Pruritus may accompany obstructive jaundice. In general, pain is common and is related to the location of malignancy. Extreme, unrelenting pain is related to extension of the cancer into the retroperitoneal tissues and nerve plexuses. The pain is frequently located in the upper abdomen or left hypochondrium and often radiates to the back. It is commonly related to eating, and it also occurs at night. Weight loss is due to poor digestion and absorption caused by lack of digestive enzymes from the pancreas.

### Diagnostic Studies

Abdominal ultrasound or endoscopic ultrasound (EUS), spiral CT scan, ERCP, MRI, and MRCP are the most commonly used diagnostic imaging techniques for pancreatic diseases, including cancer. EUS involves imaging the pancreas with the use of an endoscope positioned in the stomach and duodenum. EUS also allows for fine-needle aspiration of the tumor for pathologic examination. CT scan is often the initial study and provides information on metastasis and vascular involvement of the tumor. ERCP allows visualization of the pancreatic duct and biliary system. When ERCP is used, pancreatic secretions and tissue can be collected for analysis of different tumor markers. MRI and MRCP may also be used for diagnosing and staging pancreatic cancer. A positron emission tomography (PET) scan or PET/CT scan may also be obtained to confirm a pancreatic cancer diagnosis and determine the stage at time of diagnosis. It is also used to monitor progress and response to therapy.

Tumor markers are used both for establishing the diagnosis of pancreatic adenocarcinoma and for monitoring the response to treatment. Cancer-associated antigen 19-9 (CA 19-9) is elevated in pancreatic cancer and is the most commonly used tumor marker. However, CA 19-9 can also be elevated in gallbladder cancer or in benign conditions such as acute and chronic pancreatitis, hepatitis, and biliary obstruction.

### Interprofessional Care

Surgery provides the most effective treatment for cancer of the pancreas, but only 15% to 20% of patients have resectable tumors at the time of diagnosis. With the use of neoadjuvant chemotherapy (treatment before surgery), more patients can eventually become surgical candidates. The type of surgery depends on the size and location of the tumor. Pancreatic head tumors require the classic Whipple procedure or pancreaticoduodenectomy (Fig. 43-13), whereas pancreatic body and/or tail tumors require a distal pancreatectomy procedure. In the Whipple surgery, the proximal pancreas (proximal pancreatectomy), along with duodenum (duodenectomy), distal segment of the common bile duct and distal portion of the stomach (partial gastrectomy) are removed together followed by a surgical anastomosis of the pancreatic duct, common bile duct, and stomach to the jejunum. Occasionally, a total pancreatectomy is performed, which would cause diabetes and the patient would be dependent on exogenous insulin and pancreatic enzyme supplementation for life. If the pancreatic tumor cannot be removed surgically, palliative measures such as a cholecystojejunostomy to relieve biliary obstruction and/or endoscopically placed biliary stents can be used.

Radiation therapy alone has little effect on survival but may be effective for pain relief. External radiation is typically used, but implantation of internal radiation seeds into the tumor has also been used. The current role of chemotherapy in pancreatic cancer is limited and can have significant side effect profile. Chemotherapy usually consists of fluorouracil (5-FU) and gemcitabine (Gemzar) either alone or in combination with agents such as capecitabine (Xeloda), paclitaxel (Abraxane), erlotinib (Tarceva), or irinotecan (Onivyde). Erlotinib is a targeted therapy drug (see Table 15-13).

## NURSING MANAGEMENT: PANCREATIC CANCER

Because the patient with pancreatic cancer has many of the same problems as the patient with pancreatitis, nursing care includes many of the same measures (see sections on acute and chronic pancreatitis on pp. 999-1001 and 1003-1004). Provide symptomatic and supportive nursing care. This includes administration of medications and comfort measures to relieve pain. Psychologic support is essential, especially during times of anxiety or depression.

Adequate nutrition is an important part of the nursing care plan. Frequent and supplemental feedings may be necessary. Include measures to stimulate the appetite as much as possible and to manage anorexia, nausea, and vomiting. If the patient is undergoing radiation therapy, observe for adverse reactions such as anorexia, nausea, vomiting, and skin irritation.

The prognosis for a patient with pancreatic cancer is poor. A significant component of the nursing care is helping the patient and caregiver cope with the diagnosis and prognosis. Chapter 9 provides information on palliative and end-of-life care.

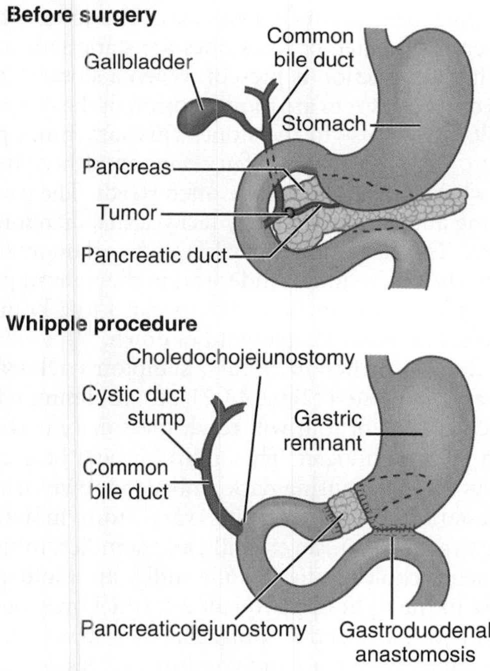


**FIG. 43-13** Whipple procedure or radical pancreaticoduodenectomy. This surgical procedure involves resection of the proximal pancreas, adjoining duodenum, distal portion of the stomach, and distal portion of the common bile duct. An anastomosis of the pancreatic duct, common bile duct, and stomach to the jejunum is done. (From Butcher GP: *Gastroenterology: an illustrated colour text*, London, 2004, Churchill Livingstone.)

# DISORDERS OF THE BILIARY TRACT

## CHOLELITHIASIS AND CHOLECYSTITIS

The most common disorder of the biliary system is **cholelithiasis** (stones in the gallbladder) (Fig. 43-14). The gallstones may get lodged in the neck of the gallbladder or in the cystic duct. **Cholecystitis** (inflammation of the gallbladder wall) is usually associated with cholelithiasis and usually occurs together, but a person can have cholelithiasis without cholecystitis. Cholecystitis may present acutely or chronically.

Gallbladder disease is a common health problem in the United States. It has been estimated that up to 10% of American adults have cholecystitis caused by gallstones. The actual number is not known because many persons with stones are asymptomatic. *Cholecystectomy* (removal of the gallbladder) ranks among the most common surgical procedures performed in the United States.

Cholelithiasis is more common in women, especially multiparous women and women over 40 years of age. Postmenopausal women on estrogen replacement therapy and younger women on oral contraceptives are at an increased risk for gallbladder disease. Oral contraceptives affect cholesterol production and increase the likelihood of gallbladder cholesterol saturation. Other factors that increase the occurrence of gallbladder disease are a sedentary lifestyle, a familial tendency, and obesity. Obesity causes increased secretion of cholesterol in bile. The incidence of gallbladder disease is especially high in the Native American population, particularly in the Navajo and Pima tribes.

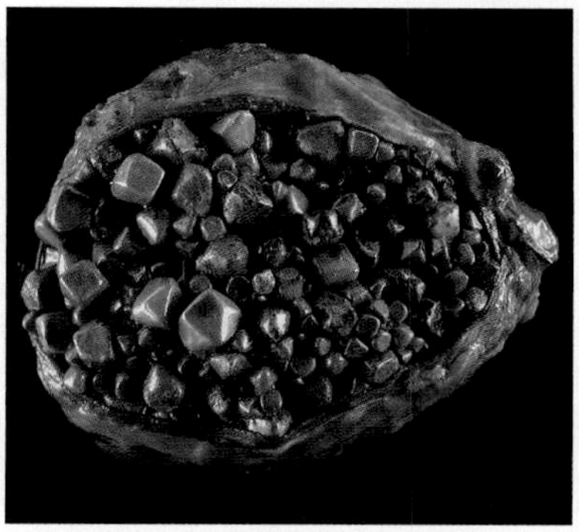

**FIG. 43-14** Cholesterol gallstones in a gallbladder that was removed. (From Kumar V, Abbas AK, Aster JC, Fausto N: *Robbins and Cotran pathologic basis of disease*, ed 8, Philadelphia, 2010, Saunders.)

## GENDER DIFFERENCES

### *Cholelithiasis*

| Men | Women |
|---|---|
| • Incidence of cholelithiasis is lower in men than in women.<br>• Gender differences in incidence decrease after age 50. | • Pregnancy is the greatest risk factor for increased prevalence in women.<br>• Obesity increases the risk, especially for women. |

## Etiology and Pathophysiology

**Cholelithiasis.** The cause of gallstones is unknown. Cholelithiasis develops when the balance that keeps cholesterol, bile salts, and calcium in solution is altered so that these substances precipitate. Conditions that upset this balance include infection and disturbances in the metabolism of cholesterol. In patients with cholelithiasis, the bile secreted by the liver is supersaturated with cholesterol (lithogenic bile). The bile in the gallbladder also becomes supersaturated with cholesterol. When bile is supersaturated with cholesterol, precipitation of cholesterol occurs in the gallbladder.

Other components of bile that precipitate into stones are bile salts, bilirubin, calcium, and protein. Mixed cholesterol stones, which are predominantly cholesterol, are the most common gallstones.

Changes in the composition of bile are significant in the formation of gallstones. Stasis of bile leads to progression of the supersaturation and changes in the chemical composition of the bile (biliary sludge). Immobility, pregnancy, and inflammatory or obstructive lesions of the biliary system decrease bile flow. Hormonal factors during pregnancy may cause delayed emptying of the gallbladder, resulting in stasis of bile.

The stones may remain in the gallbladder or migrate to the cystic duct or the common bile duct. They cause pain as they pass through the ducts, and they may lodge in the ducts and produce an obstruction. Small stones are more likely to move into a duct and cause obstruction. Table 43-21 depicts the changes and manifestations that occur when the stones obstruct the common bile duct. If the blockage occurs in the cystic duct, the bile can continue to flow into the duodenum directly from the liver. However, when the bile in the gallbladder cannot escape, this stasis of bile may lead to cholecystitis.

**Cholecystitis.** Cholecystitis is most commonly associated with obstruction caused by gallstones or biliary sludge. Cholecystitis in the absence of obstruction *(acalculous cholecystitis)* occurs most frequently in older adults and in patients who are critically ill. Acalculous cholecystitis is also associated with prolonged immobility and fasting, prolonged parenteral nutrition, and diabetes mellitus. The main cause of this illness is thought to be bile stasis. Critically ill patients are more predisposed because of increased bile viscosity due to fever and dehydration and because of prolonged absence of oral feeding resulting in a decrease or absence of cholecystokinin-induced gallbladder contraction. Other etiologic factors include adhesions, neoplasms, anesthesia, and opioids.

Once acalculous cholecystitis is established, secondary infection with enteric pathogens, including *Escherichia coli, Enterococcus faecalis, Klebsiella, Pseudomonas,* and *Proteus,* is common. Perforation occurs in severe cases.

Inflammation is the major pathophysiologic condition and may be confined to the mucous lining or involve the entire wall of the gallbladder. During an acute attack of cholecystitis, the gallbladder is edematous and hyperemic, and it may be distended with bile or pus. The cystic duct is also involved and may become occluded. The wall of the gallbladder becomes scarred after an acute attack. Decreased functioning will occur if large amounts of tissue become fibrotic.

**TABLE 43-21 Manifestations of Obstructed Bile Flow**

| Manifestation | Etiology |
|---|---|
| Obstructive jaundice | No bile flow into duodenum, bilirubin accumulates in blood |
| Dark amber to brown urine, which foams when shaken | Increase in water soluble (conjugated) bilirubin elimination in urine |
| No urobilinogen in urine | No bilirubin reaching small intestine to be converted to urobilinogen |
| Clay-colored stools | Same as above |
| Pruritus | Deposition of bile salts in skin tissues |
| Intolerance for fatty foods (nausea, sensation of fullness, anorexia) | No bile in small intestine for fat digestion |
| Bleeding tendencies | Lack of or decreased absorption of vitamin K, resulting in decreased production of prothrombin |
| Steatorrhea | Undigested fatty components of food are eliminated in stool. Occurs because no bile in small intestine, thus preventing emulsion, digestion, and absorption of fat |
| Fever, chills, cholangitis | Bacterial reflux from biliary tract to systemic circulation |

## Clinical Manifestations

Cholelithiasis may produce severe symptoms or none at all. Many patients have "silent cholelithiasis." The severity of symptoms depends on whether the stones are stationary or mobile and whether obstruction is present. When a stone is lodged in the ducts or when stones are moving through the ducts, spasms may result in response to the stone. This sometimes produces severe pain, which is termed *biliary colic,* even though the pain is rarely colicky. The pain is more often steady. The pain can be excruciating and accompanied by tachycardia, diaphoresis, and prostration. The severe pain may last up to an hour, and when it subsides, there is residual tenderness in the right upper quadrant. The attacks of pain frequently occur 3 to 6 hours after a high-fat meal or when the patient lies down.

When total obstruction occurs, symptoms related to bile blockage are manifested (Table 43-21). If the common bile duct is obstructed, no bilirubin will reach the small intestine to be converted to urobilinogen. Thus bilirubin will be excreted by the kidneys instead, causing dark amber to brown urine.

Manifestations of cholecystitis vary from indigestion to moderate to severe pain, fever, chills, and jaundice. Initial symptoms of acute cholecystitis include indigestion and pain and tenderness in the right upper quadrant, which may be referred to the right shoulder and scapula. The pain may be acute and be accompanied by nausea and vomiting, restlessness, and diaphoresis. Manifestations of inflammation include leukocytosis and fever. Physical findings include right upper quadrant or epigastrium tenderness and abdominal rigidity. Manifestations of chronic cholecystitis include a history of fat intolerance, dyspepsia, heartburn, and flatulence.

### Complications

Complications of cholelithiasis and cholecystitis include gangrenous cholecystitis, subphrenic abscess, pancreatitis, *cholangitis* (inflammation of biliary ducts), biliary cirrhosis, fistulas, and rupture of the gallbladder, which can produce bile peritonitis. In older patients and those with diabetes, gangrenous cholecystitis and bile peritonitis are the most common complications of cholecystitis. *Choledocholithiasis* (stone in the common bile duct) may occur, producing symptoms of obstruction.

### Diagnostic Studies

Ultrasound is commonly used to diagnose gallstones (see Table 38-11). It is especially useful for patients with jaundice (because it does not depend on renal function) and for patients who are allergic to contrast medium. ERCP allows for visualization of the gallbladder, cystic duct, common hepatic duct, and common bile duct. Bile taken during ERCP is sent for culture to identify possible infecting organisms.

Percutaneous transhepatic cholangiography is the insertion of a needle directly into the gallbladder duct followed by injection of contrast materials. It is generally done after ultrasound indicates a bile duct blockage.

Laboratory tests may reveal an increased WBC count as a result of inflammation. Both direct and indirect bilirubin levels may also be elevated, as is the urinary bilirubin level if an obstructive process is present (Table 43-3). Serum enzymes, such as alkaline phosphatase, ALT, and AST, may be elevated. Serum amylase is increased if there is pancreatic involvement.

### Interprofessional Care

Once gallstones become symptomatic, definitive surgical intervention with cholecystectomy is usually indicated. However, in some cases, conservative therapy may be considered.

**Conservative Therapy**

***Cholelithiasis.*** The treatment of gallstones depends on the stage of disease. Bile acids (cholesterol solvents) such as ursodeoxycholic acid (ursodiol) and chenodeoxycholic acid (chenodiol) are used to dissolve stones. However, the gallstones may recur. Gallstones are not usually treated with drugs because of the high use and success of laparoscopic cholecystectomy.

ERCP with endoscopic sphincterotomy (papillotomy) may be used for stone removal (Fig. 43-15). ERCP allows for visualization of the biliary system, dilation (balloon sphincteroplasty), and placement of stents and sphincterotomy. Special catheters with wire baskets or inflatable balloon tip may be used for stone removal.[34] When a stent is placed, it is generally removed or changed after a few months.

Extracorporeal shock-wave lithotripsy (ESWL) is an alternative treatment used when stones cannot be removed by endoscopic approaches. In ESWL a lithotriptor uses high-energy shock waves to disintegrate gallstones once they have been located by ultrasound. It usually takes 1 to 2 hours to disintegrate the stones. After they are broken up, the fragments pass through the common bile duct and into the small intestine. Usually ESWL and oral dissolution therapy are used together.

***Cholecystitis.*** During an acute episode of cholecystitis, treatment focuses on pain control, control of possible infection with antibiotics, and maintenance of fluid and electrolyte balance (Table 43-22). Treatment is mainly supportive and focused on symptom management. If nausea and vomiting are severe, NG tube insertion and gastric decompression may be used to prevent further gallbladder stimulation. A cholecystostomy may be used to drain purulent material from the obstructed gallbladder. Opioids are given for pain management. Anticholinergics may be used to decrease GI secretions and counteract smooth muscle spasms.

**Surgical Therapy.** Laparoscopic cholecystectomy is the treatment of choice for symptomatic cholelithiasis. Approximately 90% of cholecystectomies are done laparoscopically. In this procedure, the gallbladder is removed through one to four small

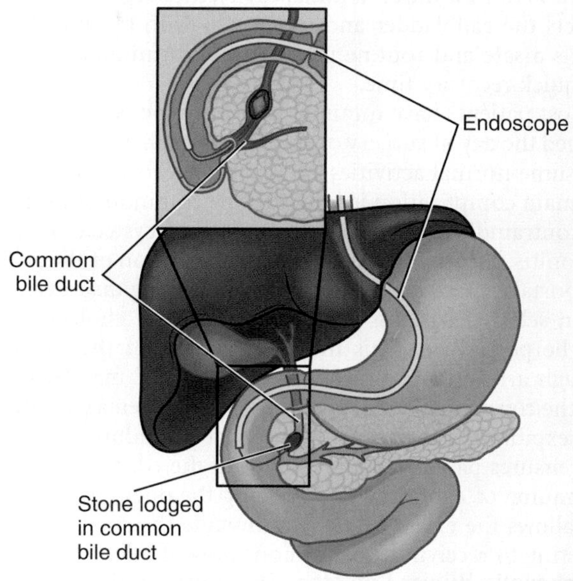


**FIG. 43-15** During endoscopic sphincterotomy, an endoscope is advanced through the mouth and stomach until its tip sits in the duodenum opposite the common bile duct. *Inset,* After widening the duct mouth by incising the sphincter muscle, the physician advances a basket attachment into the duct and snags the stone.

**TABLE 43-22 Interprofessional Care**

***Cholelithiasis and Acute Cholecystitis***

**Diagnostic Assessment**
- History and physical examination
- Ultrasound
- Endoscopic retrograde cholangiopancreatography (ERCP)
- Percutaneous transhepatic cholangiography
- Liver function tests
- White blood cell count
- Serum bilirubin

**Management**

***Conservative Therapy***
- IV fluid
- NPO with NG tube, later progressing to low-fat diet
- Antiemetics
- Analgesics
- Fat-soluble vitamins (A, D, E, and K)
- Anticholinergics (antispasmodics)
- Antibiotics (for secondary infection)
- Transhepatic biliary catheter
- ERCP with sphincterotomy (papillotomy)
- Extracorporeal shock-wave lithotripsy

***Dissolution Therapy***
- ursodeoxycholic acid (ursodiol [Actigall])

***Surgical Therapy***
- Laparoscopic cholecystectomy
- Incisional (open) cholecystectomy

punctures in the abdomen. The surgeon makes a small cut below the umbilicus and inserts a needle into the area. $CO_2$ gas is passed into the abdomen to expand the area, which allows the surgeon to see the organs more clearly and provides more room to work. A laparoscope, which has a camera attached, and grasping forceps are inserted into the abdomen through the punctures. (The incision sites may vary.) Using closed-circuit monitors to view the abdominal cavity, the surgeon retracts and dissects the gallbladder and removes it with grasping forceps. This is a safe and routine procedure with minimal morbidity and quick recovery time.

Most patients have minimal postoperative pain and are discharged the day of surgery or the day after. They are usually able to resume normal activities and return to work within 1 week. The main complication is injury to the common bile duct. The few contraindications to laparoscopic cholecystectomy include peritonitis, cholangitis, gangrene or perforation of the gallbladder, portal hypertension, and serious bleeding disorders.

On selected patients an incisional (open) cholecystectomy may be performed. This involves removal of the gallbladder through a right subcostal incision. A T tube may be inserted into the common bile duct during surgery when a common bile duct exploration is part of the surgical procedure (Fig. 43-16). This ensures patency of the duct until the edema produced by the trauma of exploring and probing the duct has subsided. It also allows the excess bile to drain while the small intestine is adjusting to receiving a continuous flow of bile.

**Transhepatic Biliary Catheter.** The transhepatic biliary catheter can be used preoperatively in biliary obstruction and in hepatic dysfunction secondary to obstructive jaundice. It can also be inserted for palliative care when inoperable liver, pancreatic, or bile duct carcinoma obstructs bile flow. The catheter is used when endoscopic drainage has been unsuccessful. The catheter is inserted percutaneously and allows for decompression of obstructed extrahepatic bile ducts so that bile can flow freely. After placement of the catheter into the obstructed duct internally, the external catheter is connected to a drainage bag. Patients should be encouraged to replace fluids lost in the drainage bag with electrolyte-rich drinks. The skin around the catheter insertion site should be cleansed daily with an antiseptic. Observe for bile leakage at the insertion site and any signs or symptoms of sudden abdominal pain, nausea, fever, or chills that may signal an occluded or malfunctioning drain.

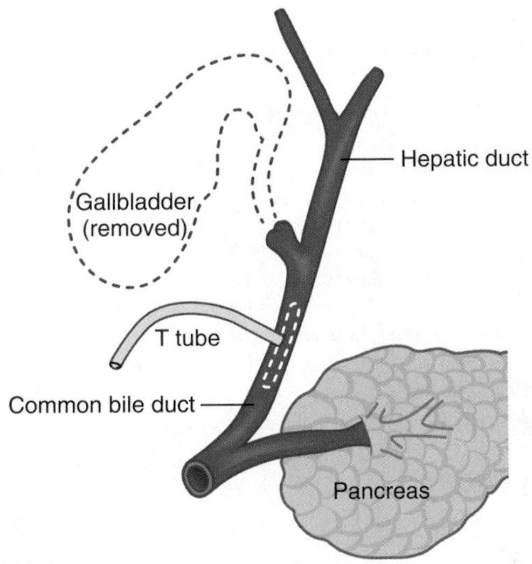


**FIG. 43-16** Placement of T tube. *Dotted lines* indicate parts removed.

**Drug Therapy.** The most common drugs used in the treatment of gallbladder disease are analgesics, anticholinergics (antispasmodics), fat-soluble vitamins, and bile salts. Morphine may be used initially for pain management. Anticholinergics such as atropine and other antispasmodics may be used to relax the smooth muscle and decrease ductal tone.

If the patient has chronic gallbladder disease or any biliary tract obstruction, fat-soluble vitamins (A, D, E, and K) may be given. Bile salts may be administered to facilitate digestion and vitamin absorption.

Cholestyramine may provide relief from pruritus. Cholestyramine is a resin that binds bile salts in the intestine, increasing their excretion in the feces. It is administered in powder form, mixed with milk or juice. Side effects include nausea, vomiting, diarrhea or constipation, and skin reactions. Because cholestyramine may bind with other medications, check drug-to-drug interactions prior to administering.

**Nutritional Therapy.** People have fewer gallbladder problems if they eat smaller, more frequent meals with some fat at each meal to promote gallbladder emptying. If obesity is a problem, a reduced-calorie diet is indicated. The diet should be low in saturated fats (e.g., butter, shortening, lard) and high in fiber and calcium. Rapid weight loss should be avoided because it can promote gallstone formation.

After a laparoscopic cholecystectomy, instruct the patient to have liquids for the rest of the day and eat light meals for a few days. If an incisional cholecystectomy is done, the patient will progress from liquids to a regular diet once bowel sounds have returned. The amount of fat in the postoperative diet depends on the patient's tolerance of fat. A low-fat diet may be helpful if the flow of bile is reduced (usually only in the early postoperative period) or if the patient is overweight. Sometimes the patient is instructed to restrict fats for 4 to 6 weeks. Otherwise, no special dietary instructions are needed other than to eat nutritious meals and avoid excessive fat intake.

## NURSING MANAGEMENT: GALLBLADDER DISEASE

### Nursing Assessment

Subjective and objective data that should be obtained from a person with gallbladder disease are presented in Table 43-23.

### Nursing Diagnoses

Nursing diagnoses for the patient with gallbladder disease treated surgically include, but are not limited to, the following:

- Acute pain *related to* surgical procedure
- Ineffective health management *related to* lack of knowledge of diet and postoperative management

### Planning

The overall goals are that the patient with gallbladder disease will have (1) relief of pain and discomfort, (2) no complications postoperatively, and (3) no recurrent attacks of cholecystitis or cholelithiasis.

### Nursing Implementation

**Health Promotion.** Be aware of predisposing factors for gallbladder disease in general health screening. Teach patients from ethnic groups in which the disease is more common, such as Native Americans, the initial manifestations and to see their HCP if these manifestations occur. Patients with chronic cholecystitis may not have acute symptoms and may not seek help until jaundice and biliary obstruction occur. Earlier detection

**TABLE 43-23 Nursing Assessment**
***Cholecystitis or Cholelithiasis***

**Subjective Data**

***Important Health Information***

*Past health history:* Obesity, multiparity, infection, cancer, extensive fasting, pregnancy
*Medications:* Estrogen or oral contraceptives
*Surgery or other treatments:* Previous abdominal surgery

***Functional Health Patterns***

*Health perception–health management:* Positive family history, sedentary lifestyle
*Nutritional-metabolic:* Weight loss, anorexia, indigestion, fat intolerance, nausea and vomiting, dyspepsia, chills
*Elimination:* Clay-colored stools, steatorrhea, flatulence. Dark urine
*Cognitive-perceptual:* Moderate to severe pain in right upper quadrant that may radiate to the back or scapula. Pruritus

**Objective Data**

***General***

Fever, restlessness

***Integumentary***

Jaundice, icteric sclera, diaphoresis

***Respiratory***

Tachypnea, splinting during respirations

***Cardiovascular***

Tachycardia

***Gastrointestinal***

Palpable gallbladder, abdominal guarding and distention

***Possible Diagnostic Findings***

↑ Serum liver enzymes, alkaline phosphatase, and bilirubin. Absence of urobilinogen in urine, ↑ urinary bilirubin, leukocytosis. Abnormal gallbladder ultrasound

in these patients is important so that they can be managed with a low-fat diet and monitored more closely.

◆ **Acute Care.** Nursing goals for the patient undergoing conservative therapy include treating pain, relieving nausea and vomiting, providing comfort and emotional support, maintaining fluid and electrolyte balance and nutrition, making accurate assessments to ensure effective treatment, and observing for complications.

The patient with acute cholecystitis or cholelithiasis frequently has severe pain. Give the drugs ordered to relieve the pain as required before it becomes more severe. Assess what drugs relieve the pain and how much medication is required. Observe for side effects of the drugs as part of the continued assessment. Nursing comfort measures, such as a clean bed, comfortable positioning, and oral care, are appropriate.

Some patients have more severe nausea and vomiting than others. For these patients, an NG tube and gastric decompression may be ordered. Eliminating intake of food and fluids also prevents further stimulation of the gallbladder. Oral hygiene, care of nares, accurate intake and output measurements, and maintenance of suction should be a part of the nursing care plan for this patient. For patients with less severe nausea and vomiting, antiemetics are usually adequate. When the patient is vomiting, provide comfort measures such as frequent mouth rinses. Remove any vomitus immediately from the patient's view. If pruritus occurs with jaundice, measures to relieve itching are necessary and can include antihistamines or other treatments as previously discussed.

Assess for progression of the symptoms and development of complications. Observe for signs of obstruction of the ducts by stones. These include jaundice; clay-colored stools; dark, foamy urine; steatorrhea; fever; and increased WBC count.

When manifestations of obstruction are present (Table 43-21), bleeding may result from decreased prothrombin production by the liver. Common sites to observe for bleeding are the mucous membranes of the mouth, nose, gingivae, and injection sites. If injections are given, use a small-gauge needle and apply gentle pressure after the injection. Know the patient's prothrombin time and use it as a guide in the assessment process.

Assessment for infections includes monitoring vital signs. A temperature elevation with chills and jaundice may indicate choledocholithiasis.

Your care of the patient after ERCP with papillotomy includes assessment to detect complications such as pancreatitis, perforation, infection, and bleeding. Monitor the patient's vital signs. Abdominal pain, fever, and increasing amylase and lipase may indicate acute pancreatitis. The patient should be on bed rest for several hours and should be NPO until the gag reflex returns. Teach the patient the need for follow-up if the stent is to be removed or changed.

◆ ***Postoperative Care.*** Postoperative nursing care after a laparoscopic cholecystectomy includes monitoring for complications such as bleeding, making the patient comfortable, and preparing the patient for discharge. A common postoperative complaint is referred pain to the shoulder because of the $CO_2$ that is used to inflate the abdominal cavity during surgery. It may not be released or absorbed by the body. The $CO_2$ can irritate the phrenic nerve and diaphragm, causing some difficulty in breathing. Placing the patient in the Sims' position (on left side with right knee flexed) helps move the gas pocket away from the diaphragm. Encourage deep breathing along with movement and ambulation. The pain can usually be relieved by NSAIDs or codeine. The patient is allowed clear liquids and can walk to the bathroom to void. Most patients go home the same day.

Postoperative nursing care for incisional cholecystectomy focuses on adequate ventilation and prevention of respiratory complications. Other nursing care is the same as general postoperative nursing care (see Chapter 19).

If the patient has a T tube (Fig. 43-16), you must maintain bile drainage and monitor T-tube function and drainage. The T tube is usually connected to a closed gravity drainage system. If the Penrose or Jackson-Pratt drain or the T tube is draining large amounts of bile, it is helpful to use a sterile pouching system to protect the skin. Encourage the patient to replace fluids and electrolytes that are lost.

◆ **Ambulatory Care.** When the patient has conservative therapy, nursing management depends on the patient's symptoms and on whether surgical intervention is planned. Dietary teaching is usually necessary. The diet is usually low in fat, and sometimes a weight-reduction diet is also recommended. The patient may need to take fat-soluble vitamin supplements. Instruct the patient on observations that indicate obstruction (e.g., stool and urine changes, jaundice, pruritus). Explain the importance of continued health care follow-up.

The patient who undergoes a laparoscopic cholecystectomy is discharged soon after the surgery, so home care and teaching are important (Table 43-24).

**TABLE 43-24 Patient & Caregiver Teaching**

***Postoperative Laparoscopic Cholecystectomy***

*The patient's postoperative teaching plan should include the following:*

1. Remove the bandages on the puncture sites the day after surgery and you can shower.
2. Notify your surgeon if any of the following signs and symptoms occurs:
   - Redness, swelling, bile-colored drainage or pus from any incision
   - Severe abdominal pain, nausea, vomiting, fever, chills
3. You can gradually resume normal activities.
4. Return to work within 1 wk of surgery.
5. You can resume your usual diet, but a low-fat diet is usually better tolerated for several weeks after surgery.

After an incisional cholecystectomy, instruct the patient to avoid heavy lifting for 4 to 6 weeks. Usual sexual activities, including intercourse, can be resumed as soon as the patient feels ready, unless otherwise instructed by the HCP.

Sometimes the patient is required to remain on a low-fat diet for 4 to 6 weeks. If so, an individualized dietary teaching plan is necessary. A weight-reduction program may be helpful if the patient is overweight. Most patients tolerate a regular diet with no difficulties but should avoid excessive fats.

### ◆ Evaluation

The overall expected outcomes are that the patient with gallbladder disease will

- Appear comfortable and verbalize pain relief
- Verbalize knowledge of activity level and dietary restrictions

## GALLBLADDER CANCER

Primary cancer of the gallbladder is uncommon. The majority of gallbladder carcinomas are adenocarcinomas. Annually an estimated 10,910 new cases of gallbladder cancer occur with an estimated 3700 deaths.[35] A relationship exists between cancer of the gallbladder and chronic cholecystitis and cholelithiasis.

The early symptoms of carcinoma of the gallbladder are insidious and are similar to those of chronic cholecystitis and cholelithiasis, which makes the diagnosis difficult. Later symptoms are usually those of biliary obstruction. Gallbladder cancer is twice as common in women as in men.[35]

Diagnosis and staging of gallbladder cancer are done using EUS, abdominal ultrasound, CT, MRI, and/or MRCP. Unfortunately, gallbladder cancer often is not detected until the disease is advanced. When it is found early, surgery can be curative. Several factors influence successful surgical outcomes, including the depth of cancer invasion, extent of liver involvement, venous or lymphatic invasion, and lymph node metastasis. Extended cholecystectomy with lymph node dissection has improved the outcomes for patients with gallbladder cancer.

When surgery is not an option, endoscopic stenting of the biliary tract can be done to reduce obstructive jaundice. Adjuvant therapies, including radiation therapy and chemotherapy, may be used depending on the disease state. Overall, cancer of the gallbladder has a poor prognosis.

Nursing management involves palliative care with special attention to nutrition, hydration, skin care, and pain relief. Nursing care measures used for patients with cholecystitis and cholelithiasis are frequently applied, as well as nursing care measures for the patient with cancer (see Chapter 15).

## CASE STUDY

***Cirrhosis of the Liver***

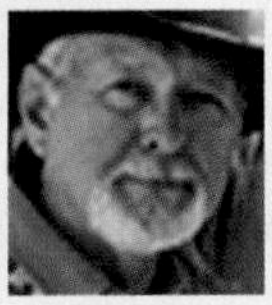

(©sbeagle/ iStock/ Thinkstock)

**Patient Profile**

M.B., a 58-yr-old male rancher who lives in rural Wyoming, is admitted with a diagnosis of cirrhosis of the liver. He has been vomiting for 2 days and noticed blood in the toilet when he vomits. He lives 40 miles from the nearest hospital. He had one of his ranch hands drive him to the hospital.

**Subjective Data**

- Has 2 children who live in New York. He has been estranged from them since his divorce 3 years ago
- Has had cirrhosis for 12 yr
- Acknowledges that he had been drinking heavily for 20 yr but has been sober for the past 2 yr
- Complains of anorexia, nausea, and abdominal discomfort

**Objective Data**

***Physical Examination***

- Has moderate ascites
- Has jaundice of sclera and skin
- Has 4+ pitting edema of the lower extremities
- Liver and spleen are palpable

***Laboratory Values***

- Total bilirubin: 15 mg/dL (257 mmol/L)
- AST: 190 U/L (3.2 μkat/L)
- ALT: 210 U/L (3.5 μkat/L)
- Platelets: 45,000/μL
- ECG is at right:

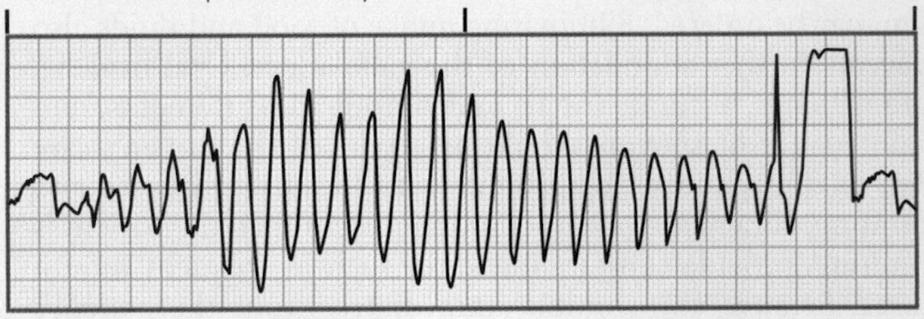

**Discussion Questions**

1. What are possible causes of cirrhosis? What type of cirrhosis does M.B. probably have?
2. Describe the pathophysiologic changes that occur in the liver as cirrhosis develops.
3. List M.B.'s clinical manifestations of liver failure. For each manifestation, explain the pathophysiologic basis.
4. Explain the significance of the results of his laboratory values and ECG findings.
5. If M.B. begins to manifest signs and symptoms of hepatic encephalopathy, what would you monitor? What measures should be instituted to control or decrease the encephalopathy?
6. What are possible causes of his gastrointestinal bleeding?
7. ***Priority Decision:*** Based on the assessment data, what are the priority nursing diagnoses? Are there any collaborative problems?
8. ***Priority Decision:*** What are the priority nursing interventions for a patient at this stage of his illness?
9. ***Evidence-Based Practice:*** M.B. discusses his prognosis with you. He says, "There is no hope. I might as well keep drinking." How would you respond to his statement?
10. ***Safety:*** Given the patient's bleeding history and current laboratory values, identify areas of injury risk and specify actions you will take to ensure patient safety.

Answers and corresponding conceptual care map available at *evolve.elsevier.com/Lewis/medsurg*.

## BRIDGE TO NCLEX EXAMINATION

The number of the question corresponds to the same-numbered outcome at the beginning of the chapter.

1. A patient with hepatitis A is in the acute phase. The nurse plans care for the patient based on the knowledge that
   - **a.** pruritus is a common problem with jaundice in this phase.
   - **b.** the patient is most likely to transmit the disease during this phase.
   - **c.** gastrointestinal symptoms are not as severe in hepatitis A as they are in hepatitis B.
   - **d.** extrahepatic manifestations of glomerulonephritis and polyarteritis are common in this phase.
2. A patient with acute hepatitis B is being discharged in 2 days. The discharge teaching plan should include instructions to
   - **a.** avoid alcohol for the first 3 weeks.
   - **b.** use a condom during sexual intercourse.
   - **c.** have family members get an injection of immunoglobulin.
   - **d.** follow a low-protein, moderate-carbohydrate, moderate-fat diet.
3. A patient has been told that she has elevated liver enzymes caused by nonalcoholic fatty liver disease (NAFLD). The nursing teaching plan should include
   - **a.** having genetic testing done.
   - **b.** recommending a heart-healthy diet.
   - **c.** the necessity to reduce weight rapidly.
   - **d.** avoiding alcohol until liver enzymes return to normal.
4. The patient with advanced cirrhosis asks why his abdomen is so swollen. The nurse's response is based on the knowledge that
   - **a.** a lack of clotting factors promotes the collection of blood in the abdominal cavity.
   - **b.** portal hypertension and hypoalbuminemia cause a fluid shift into the peritoneal space.
   - **c.** decreased peristalsis in the GI tract contributes to gas formation and distention of the bowel.
   - **d.** bile salts in the blood irritate the peritoneal membranes, causing edema and pocketing of fluid.
5. In planning care for a patient with metastatic liver cancer, the nurse should include interventions that
   - **a.** focus primarily on symptomatic and comfort measures.
   - **b.** reassure the patient that chemotherapy offers a good prognosis.
   - **c.** promote the patient's confidence that surgical excision of the tumor will be successful.
   - **d.** provide information necessary for the patient to make decisions regarding liver transplantation.
6. Nursing management of the patient with acute pancreatitis includes *(select all that apply)*
   - **a.** checking for signs of hypocalcemia.
   - **b.** providing a diet low in carbohydrates.
   - **c.** giving insulin based on a sliding scale.
   - **d.** observing stools for signs of steatorrhea.
   - **e.** monitoring for infection, particularly respiratory tract infection.
7. A patient with pancreatic cancer is admitted to the hospital for evaluation of possible treatment options. The patient asks the nurse to explain the Whipple procedure that the surgeon has described. The explanation includes the information that a Whipple procedure involves
   - **a.** creating a bypass around the obstruction caused by the tumor by joining the gallbladder to the jejunum.
   - **b.** resection of the entire pancreas and the distal portion of the stomach, with anastomosis of the common bile duct and the stomach into the duodenum.
   - **c.** removal of part of the pancreas, part of the stomach, the duodenum, and the gallbladder, with joining of the pancreatic duct, the common bile duct, and the stomach into the jejunum.
   - **d.** radical removal of the pancreas, the duodenum, and the spleen, and attachment of the stomach to the jejunum, which requires oral supplementation of pancreatic digestive enzymes and insulin replacement therapy.
8. The nursing management of the patient with cholecystitis associated with cholelithiasis is based on the knowledge that
   - **a.** shock-wave therapy should be tried initially.
   - **b.** once gallstones are removed, they tend not to recur.
   - **c.** the disorder can be successfully treated with oral bile salts that dissolve gallstones.
   - **d.** laparoscopic cholecystectomy is the treatment of choice in most patients who are symptomatic.
9. Teaching in relation to home management after a laparoscopic cholecystectomy should include
   - **a.** keeping the bandages on the puncture sites for 48 hours.
   - **b.** reporting any bile-colored drainage or pus from any incision.
   - **c.** using over-the-counter antiemetics if nausea and vomiting occur.
   - **d.** emptying and measuring the contents of the bile bag from the T tube every day.

1. a, 2. b, 3. b, 4. b, 5. a, 6. a, e, 7. c, 8. d, 9. b

For rationales to these answers and even more NCLEX review questions, visit *evolve.elsevier.com/Lewis/medsurg*.

## EVOLVE WEBSITE

evolve.elsevier.com/Lewis/medsurg

**Review Questions (Online Only)**

**Key Points**

**Answer Keys for Questions**

- Rationales for Bridge to NCLEX Examination Questions
- Answer Guidelines for Case Study on p. 1010
- Answer Guidelines for Managing Care of Multiple Patients Case Study (Section 8) on p. 1013

**Student Case Studies**

- Patient With Acute Pancreatitis and Septic Shock
- Patient With Cholelithiasis/Cholecystitis
- Patient With Cirrhosis
- Patient With Hepatitis

**Nursing Care Plans**

- eNursing Care Plan 43-1: Patient With Acute Viral Hepatitis
- eNursing Care Plan 43-2: Patient With Cirrhosis
- eNursing Care Plan 43-3: Patient With Acute Pancreatitis

**Conceptual Care Map Creator**

- Conceptual Care Map for Case Study on p. 1010

**Audio Glossary**

**Content Updates**

## REFERENCES

1. Centers for Disease Control and Prevention: Viral hepatitis—Hepatitis A Information—United States. Retrieved from *www.cdc.gov/hepatitis/hav/havfaq.htm#general*.

2. Centers for Disease Control and Prevention: Viral hepatitis—Hepatitis B information—United States. Retrieved from *www.cdc.gov/hepatitis/hbv/hbvfaq.htm.*
3. Centers for Disease Control and Prevention: Viral hepatitis—CDC Recommendations for Specific Populations and Settings—United States. Retrieved from *www.cdc.gov/hepatitis/populations/api.htm.*
4. Centers for Disease Control and Prevention: Viral hepatitis—Hepatitis C information—United States. Retrieved from *www.cdc.gov/hepatitis/hcv/hcvfaq.htm#section3.*
5. American Cancer Society: Liver cancer. Retrieved from *www.cancer.org/cancer/livercancer/detailedguide/liver-cancer-risk-factors.*
6. Busch K, Thimme R: Natural history of chronic hepatitis B virus infection, *Med Microbiol Immunol* 204:5, 2015.
7. Castera L: Noninvasive assessment of liver fibrosis, *Dig Dis* 33:498, 2015.
*8. World Health Organization: Guidelines for the prevention, care and treatment for persons with chronic hepatitis B infection. Retrieved from *www.who.int/hiv/pub/hepatitis/hepatitis-b-guidelines/en/.*
9. Lucaciu LA, Dumitrascu DL: Depression and suicide ideation in chronic hepatitis C patients untreated and treated with interferon: prevalence, prevention, and treatment, *Ann Gastro* 28:1, 2015.
*10. American Association for the Study of Liver Diseases: Recommendations for testing, managing, and treating Hepatitis C—United States. Retrieved from *www.hcvguidelines.org/full-report/initial-treatment-hcv-infection.*
11. Centers for Disease Control and Prevention: Testing recommendations for hepatitis C virus infection. Retrieved from *www.cdc.gov/hepatitis/hcv/guidelinesc.htm.*
*12. Chalasani NP, Hayashi PH, Bonkovsky HL, et al: ACG Clinical Guideline: the diagnosis and management of idiosyncratic drug-induced liver injury, *Am J Gastroenterol* 109:950, 2014.
13. Trivedi PJ, Hirschfield GM: Treatment of autoimmune liver disease: current and future therapeutic options, *Ther Adv Chronic Dis* 4:119, 2013.
14. Hahn SH: Population screening for Wilson's disease, *Ann New York Acad Sci* 1:64, 2014.
15. Juran BD, Lazaridis KN: Environmental factors in primary biliary cirrhosis, *Semin Liver Dis* 34: 265, 2014.
16. Schwenger KP, Allard JP: Clinical approaches to non-alcoholic fatty liver disease, *World J Gastroenterol* 20:1712, 2014.
17. Centers for Disease Control and Prevention: Chronic liver disease and cirrhosis. Retrieved from *www.cdc.gov/nchs/fastats/liver-disease.htm.*
18. Iwakiri Y: Pathophysiology of portal hypertension, *Clin Liv Dis* 18:281, 2014.
19. Rajoriya N, Tripathi D: Historical overview and review of current day treatment in the management of acute variceal haemorrhage, *World J Gastroenterol* 20:6481, 2014.
20. Preveden T: Bacterial infections in patients with liver cirrhosis, *Med Pregl* 68:187, 2015.
21. Sharma P, Sharma BC: Management of overt hepatic encephalopathy, *J Clin Exp Hepatol* 5:S82, 2015.
22. Poorad FF: Presentation and complications associated with cirrhosis of the liver, *Curr Med Res Opin* 31:925, 2015.
23. Kodali S, McGuire BM: Diagnosis and management of hepatic encephalopathy in fulminant hepatic failure, *Clin Liver Dis* 19:565, 2015.
24. Toshikuni N, Arisawa T, Tsutsumi M: Nutrition and exercise in the management of liver cirrhosis, *World J Gastroenterol* 20:7286, 2014.
25. Raschi E, De Ponti F: Drug and herb-induced liver injury: progress, current challenges and emerging signals of post-marketing risk, *World J Hepatol* 7:1761, 2015.
26. Bernal W, Wendon J: Acute liver failure, *NEJM* 369:2525, 2013.
27. American Cancer Society: What are the key statistics about liver cancer? Retrieved from *www.cancer.org/cancer/livercancer/detailedguide/liver-cancer-what-is-key-statistics.*
28. You MW, Kim SY, Kim KW, et al: Recent advances in the imaging of hepatocellular carcinoma, *Clin Mol Hepatol* 21:95, 2015.
29. Tejeda-Maldonado J, Garcia-Juarez I, Aguirre-Valadez J, et al: Diagnosis and treatment of hepatocellular carcinoma: an update, *World J Hepatol* 7:362, 2015.
30. American Liver Foundation: More about organ donation. Retrieved from *dwww.liverfoundation.org/patients/organdonor/about.*
31. Kim IH: Aging and liver disease, *Curr Opin Gastroenterol* 31:184, 2015.
32. Talukdar R, Vege SS: Acute pancreatitis, *Curr Opin Gastroenterol* 31:374, 2015.
33. National Cancer Institute: Pancreatic cancer for health professionals. Retrieved from *www.cancer.gov/types/pancreatic/hp.*
34. Guda NM, Freeman ML: *Overview of ERCP complications: prevention and management in ERP and EUS*, New York, 2015, Springer.
*35. Aloia TA, Jarufe N, Javle M, et al: Gallbladder cancer: expert consensus statement, *HPB* 8:681, 2015.

*Evidence-based information for clinical practice.

## CASE STUDY

### *Managing Care of Multiple Patients*

You are working on the medical-surgical unit and have been assigned to care for the following five patients. You have one LPN and one UAP who are assigned to help you.

#### Patients

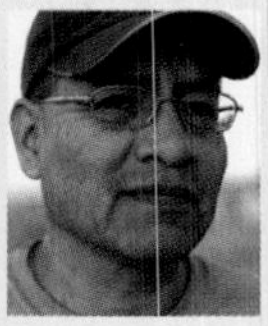

(©iStockphoto/ Thinkstock)

L.C. is a 58-yr-old Native American man admitted from the ED with acute abdominal pain. A CBC showed an Hgb of 6.8 g/dL and Hct of 20%. The WBC count is normal. A CT scan and colonoscopy indicated two medium-size tumors in the transverse colon. A hemicolectomy was performed. The adenocarcinoma had spread to the muscle of the colon wall, and there were two positive lymph nodes.

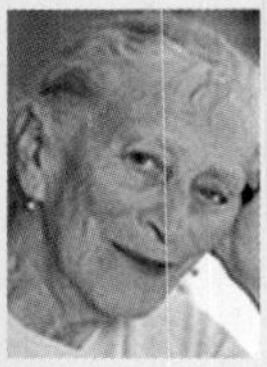

(©iStockphoto/ Thinkstock)

M.S. is a 70-yr-old white woman who was recently admitted to the unit with generalized weakness and malnutrition. She is 5 feet 4 inches tall and weighs 100 lb, with a 30-lb weight loss in past 2 months. Her PMH includes a recent thrombotic stroke with hemiparesis and dysphagia. She has had nothing by mouth for the past 24 hours and just started enteral nutrition via PEG tube.

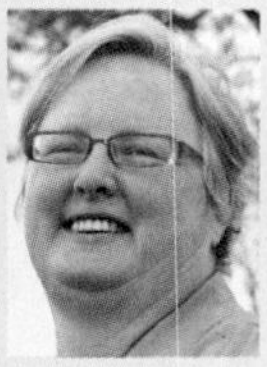

(©Christa Brunt/ iStock/ Thinkstock)

S.R. is a 48-yr-old white woman admitted with hip pain. She has a history of type 2 diabetes mellitus, hypertension, and osteoarthritis. She is 5 feet 4 inches tall and weighs 210 lb. Her most recent BP was 160/110 mm Hg. Her morning laboratory results reveal elevations in fasting blood glucose, total cholesterol, LDL cholesterol, and triglycerides. Her HDL cholesterol is low. Her cardiac enzymes and ECG are all within normal limits. She is scheduled to undergo a cardiac stress test at 10 AM.

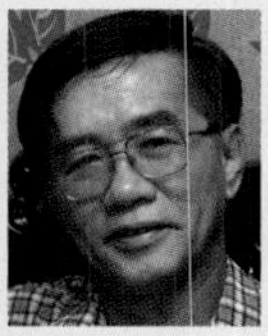

(©iStockphoto/ Thinkstock)

F.H., a 40-yr-old male immigrant from Vietnam, has a 1-yr history of epigastric distress. He underwent an upper endoscopy a few weeks ago, which revealed a duodenal ulcer and *H. pylori.* He was started on omeprazole, clarithromycin, and amoxicillin for 10 days. He came to the ED yesterday with complaints of severe epigastric pain and melena. His Hgb is 10.2 g/dL and Hct is 30%. He was admitted and put on a pantoprazole (Protonix) continuous infusion and is scheduled for a repeat EGD today.

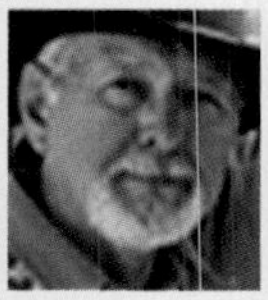

(©sbeagle/ iStock/ Thinkstock)

M.B. is a 58-yr-old man admitted with a diagnosis of upper GI bleeding. He has been vomiting for 2 days and noticed blood in the toilet when he vomits. He has had cirrhosis for 12 yr and admits to drinking heavily for 20 yr but has been sober for the past 2 yr. He currently complains of anorexia, nausea, and abdominal discomfort. He has moderate ascites, jaundice of sclera and skin, 4+ pitting edema of the lower extremities, and palpable liver and spleen. His bilirubin and liver enzymes are all elevated. His platelet and RBC counts are low.

#### Discussion Questions

1. ***Priority Decision:*** After receiving report, which patient should you see first? Provide a rationale for your decision.
2. ***Teamwork and Collaboration:*** Which tasks could you delegate to the LPN *(select all that apply)*?
   a. Assess L.C.'s dressing, pain level, and bowel sounds.
   b. Provide enteral tube feeding for M.S. if gastric residual <500 mL.
   c. Because she speaks Vietnamese, teach F.H.'s wife about his disease.
   d. Call M.B.'s health care provider regarding the morning laboratory results.
   e. Perform bedside glucometer reading and administer oral medications to S.R.
3. ***Priority Decision:*** As you are assessing M.B., the LPN informs you that F.H. just vomited a large amount of bright red blood. What initial action would be *most* appropriate?
   a. Have the LPN administer an antiemetic to F.H.
   b. Ask the LPN to notify F.H.'s health care provider.
   c. Leave M.B.'s room to perform a focused assessment on F.H.
   d. Ask the UAP to obtain a unit of packed RBCs from the blood bank.

#### Case Study Progression

When you enter F.H.'s room, he tells you that his pain actually feels somewhat relieved since he vomited. However, you note that his skin is cool and clammy, his BP is 90/54 mm Hg, and his heart rate is 116 bpm. You notify his HCP.

4. Which interventions would you expect the HCP to order for F.H. *(select all that apply)*?
   a. Stat hemoglobin and hematocrit
   b. Emergent endoscopy and endotherapy
   c. Discontinue the pantoprazole (Protonix) infusion
   d. Start a second IV site and administer 500 mL normal saline bolus
   e. Contact surgeon and notify operating room that patient is unstable and needs surgery
5. ***Priority Decision:*** After administering a bolus feeding of enteral nutrition to M.S., it would be *most* important to
   a. assess for gastric residual.
   b. obtain an abdominal x-ray.
   c. keep head of bed elevated 30 to 45 degrees.
   d. record the total amount of fluid administered.
6. Which intervention to treat ascites would you expect the HCP to order for M.B. *(select all that apply)*?
   a. Paracentesis
   b. 2 g sodium diet
   c. Diuretic therapy
   d. 1800 mL/day fluid restriction
   e. Shunt insertion from peritoneum to heart
7. ***Management Decision:*** As you enter the nurse's station, you overhear derogatory comments made by the UAP to the LPN about S.R.'s weight. Which response would be *most* appropriate?
   a. Report the incident to charge nurse for follow-up.
   b. Talk to the UAP to discuss possible HIPAA violation.
   c. Talk to S.R. to assess impact of UAP's bias on patient's self-image.
   d. Teach staff members to recognize obesity as a disease process.

Answers and rationales available at *http://evolve.elsevier.com/Lewis/medsurg.*

# SECTION 9

# Problems of Urinary Function

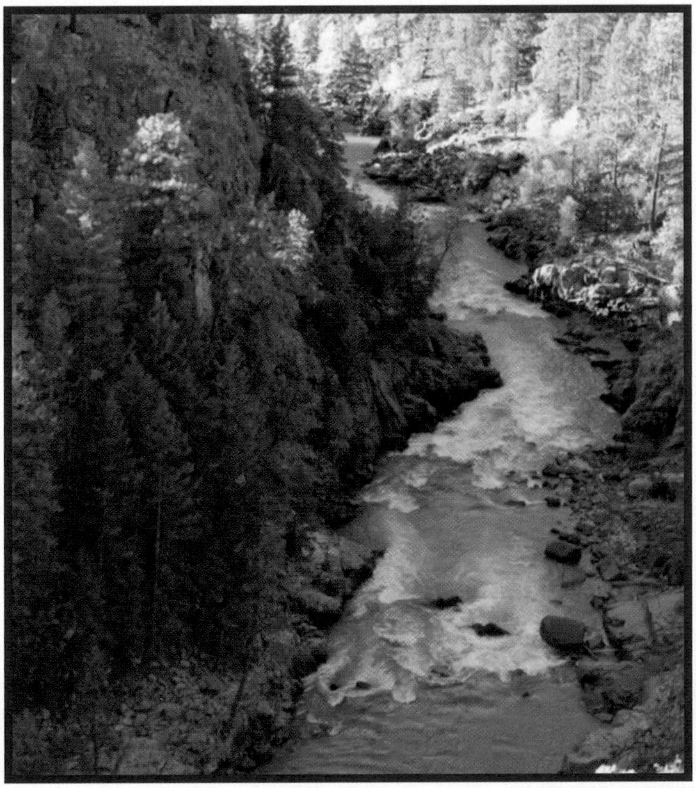

Peter Bonner

*Sometimes ... if you lean over to watch the river slipping slowly away beneath you, you will suddenly know everything there is to be known.*

***Winnie the Pooh***

# Assessment of Urinary System

*Suzanne Teresa Parsell*

*Life is really simple, but we insist on making it complicated.*

*Confucius*

http://evolve.elsevier.com/Lewis/medsurg/

## LEARNING OUTCOMES

1. Differentiate among the anatomic location and functions of the kidneys, ureters, bladder, and urethra.
2. Explain the physiologic events involved in the formation and passage of urine from glomerular filtration to voiding.
3. Obtain significant subjective and objective data related to the urinary system from a patient.
4. Link the age-related changes of the urinary system to the differences in assessment findings.
5. Perform a physical assessment of the urinary system using appropriate techniques.
6. Differentiate normal from abnormal findings of a physical assessment of the urinary system.
7. Describe the purpose, significance of results, and nursing responsibilities related to diagnostic studies of the urinary system.
8. Differentiate normal from abnormal findings of a urinalysis.

## KEY TERMS

costovertebral angle (CVA), p. 1023
creatinine, Table 44-8, p. 1026
cystometrogram, Table 44-8, p. 1029
cystoscopy, Table 44-8, p. 1028
glomerular filtration rate (GFR), p. 1017
glomerulus, p. 1016
nephron, p. 1016
renal biopsy, Table 44-8, p. 1030

Adequate kidney function is essential to the maintenance of a healthy body. If a person has complete kidney failure and treatment is not provided, death is inevitable. This chapter discusses the structures and functions, assessment, and diagnostic studies of the urinary system.

## STRUCTURES AND FUNCTIONS OF URINARY SYSTEM

The *upper urinary system* consists of two kidneys and two ureters. The *lower urinary system* consists of a urinary bladder and urethra (Fig. 44-1). Urine is formed in the kidneys, drains through the ureters to be stored in the bladder, and then passes out of the body through the urethra.

### Kidneys

The kidneys are the principal organs of the urinary system. The primary functions of the kidneys are to (1) regulate the volume and composition of extracellular fluid (ECF) and (2) excrete waste products from the body. The kidneys also function to control BP, produce erythropoietin, activate vitamin D, and regulate acid-base balance.

**Macrostructure.** The paired kidneys are bean-shaped organs located retroperitoneally (behind the peritoneum) on either side of the vertebral column at about the level of the twelfth thoracic (T12) vertebra to the third lumbar (L3) vertebra. Each kidney weighs 4 to 6 oz (113 to 170 g) and is about 5 inches (12.5 cm) long. The right kidney, positioned at the level of the twelfth rib, is lower than the left. An adrenal gland lies on top of each kidney.

Each kidney is surrounded by a considerable amount of fat and connective tissue that cushions, supports, and maintains its position. A thin, smooth layer of fibrous membrane called the *capsule* covers the surface of each kidney. The capsule protects the kidney and serves as a shock absorber when this area is traumatized from a sudden force or strike. The *hilus* on the medial side of the kidney serves as the entry site for the renal artery and nerves and as the exit site for the renal vein and ureter.

The *parenchyma* (actual tissue) of the kidney can be visualized on a longitudinal section of the kidney (Fig. 44-2). The outer layer is the *cortex* and the inner layer is the *medulla.* The medulla consists of a number of pyramids. The apices (tops) of these pyramids are called *papillae,* through which urine passes to enter the calyces. The minor calyces widen and merge to form

Reviewed by Janie Corbitt, RN, MLS, Retired Instructor of Nursing, Milledgeville, Georgia; Deborah Erickson, RN, PhD, Associate Professor and Graduate Coordinator, Department of Nursing, Bradley University, Peoria, Illinois; Shari Gould, RN, MSN, Associate Professor of Nursing, Victoria College, Victoria, Texas; and Marci Langenkamp, RN, MS, Associate Professor of Nursing, Edison Community College, Piqua, Ohio.

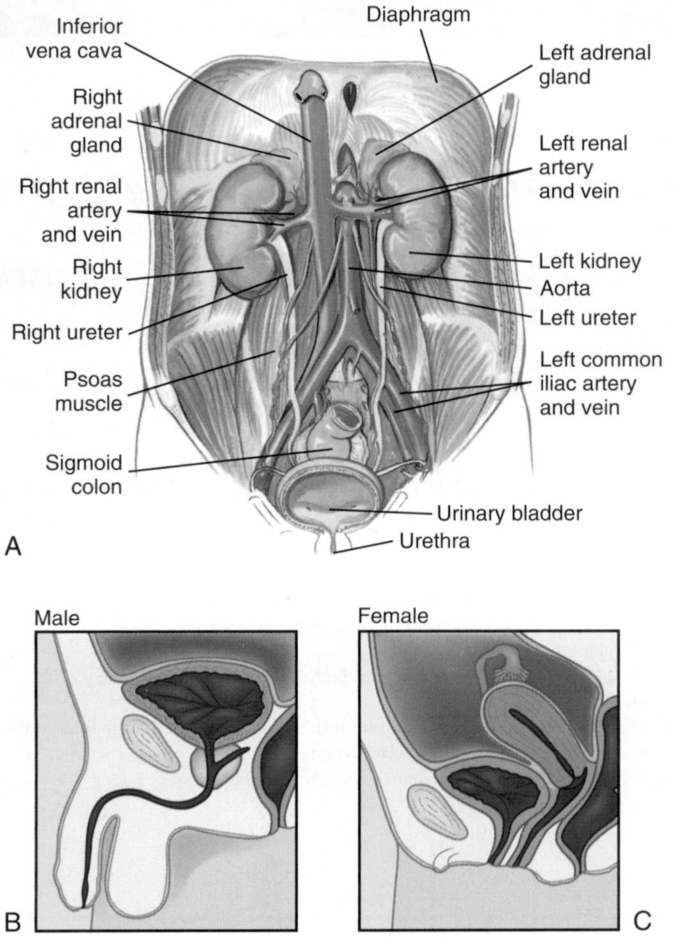


**FIG. 44-1** Organs of the urinary system. **A,** Upper urinary tract in relation to other anatomic structures. **B,** Male urethra in relation to other pelvic structures. **C,** Female urethra.

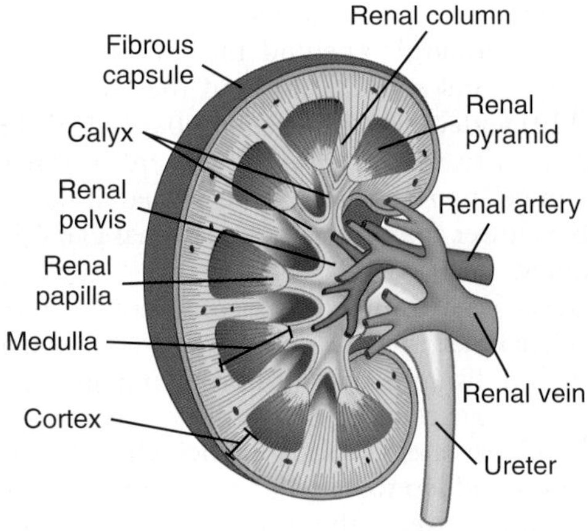


**FIG. 44-2** Longitudinal section of the kidney.

major calyces, which form a funnel-shaped sac called the *renal pelvis.* The minor and major calyces transport urine to the renal pelvis, from which it drains through the ureter to the bladder. The renal pelvis can store a small volume of urine (3 to 5 mL).

**Microstructure.** The **nephron** is the functional unit of the kidney. Each kidney contains approximately 1 million nephrons. Each nephron is composed of the glomerulus, Bowman's capsule, and a tubular system. The tubular system consists of the proximal convoluted tubule, loop of Henle, distal convoluted tubule, and collecting tubules (Fig. 44-3). The glomerulus, Bowman's capsule, proximal tubule, and distal tubule are located in the cortex of the kidney. The loop of Henle and collecting tubules are located in the medulla. Several collecting tubules join to form a single collecting duct. The collecting ducts eventually merge into a pyramid that empties via the papilla into a minor calyx.

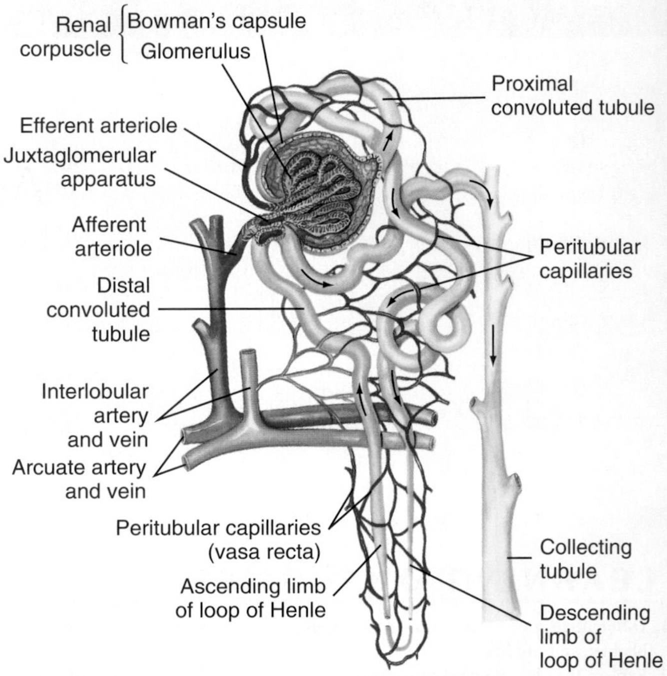


**FIG. 44-3** The nephron is the basic functional unit of the kidney. This illustration of a single nephron unit also shows the surrounding blood vessels. (Modified from Thibodeau GA, Patton KT: *The human body in health and disease,* ed 4, St Louis, 2005, Mosby.)

**Blood Supply.** Blood flow to the kidneys, approximately 1200 mL/min, accounts for 20% to 25% of the cardiac output. Blood reaches the kidneys via the renal artery, which arises from the aorta and enters the kidney through the hilus. The renal artery divides into secondary branches and then into still smaller branches, each of which forms an afferent arteriole. The afferent arteriole divides into a capillary network, the **glomerulus**, which is a collection of up to 50 capillaries (Fig. 44-3). The capillaries of the glomerulus unite in the efferent arteriole. This efferent arteriole splits to form a capillary network, the peritubular capillaries, which surround the tubular system. All peritubular capillaries drain into the venous system; the renal vein empties into the inferior vena cava.

**Physiology of Urine Formation.** Urine formation is the outcome of a complex, multistep process of filtration, reabsorption, secretion, and excretion of water, electrolytes, and metabolic waste products. Although urine formation is the result of this process, the primary functions of the kidneys are to filter the blood and maintain the body's internal homeostasis.

***Glomerular Function.*** Urine formation begins at the glomerulus, where blood is filtered. The glomerulus is a semipermeable membrane that allows filtration (Fig. 44-3). The hydrostatic pressure of the blood within the glomerular capillaries causes a portion of blood to be filtered across the semipermeable membrane into Bowman's capsule, where the filtered portion of the blood (glomerular filtrate) begins to pass down to the tubule. Filtration is more rapid in the glomerulus than in ordinary

**TABLE 44-1 Functions of Nephron Segments**

| Segment | Function |
|---|---|
| **Glomerulus** | Selective filtration. |
| **Proximal tubule** | Reabsorption of 80% of electrolytes and water, glucose, amino acids, $HCO_3^-$. Secretion of $H^+$ and creatinine. |
| **Loop of Henle** | Reabsorption of $Na^+$ and $Cl^-$ in ascending limb and water in descending loop. Concentration of filtrate. |
| **Distal tubule** | Secretion of $K^+$, $H^+$, ammonia. Reabsorption of water (regulated by ADH) and $HCO_3^-$. Regulation of $Ca^{2+}$ and $PO_4^{2-}$ by parathyroid hormone. Regulation of $Na^+$ and $K^+$ by aldosterone. |
| **Collecting duct** | Reabsorption of water (ADH required). |

*ADH,* Antidiuretic hormone.

tissue capillaries because the glomerular membrane is porous. The ultrafiltrate is similar in composition to blood except that it lacks blood cells, platelets, and large plasma proteins. Under normal conditions, the capillary pores are too small to allow the loss of these large blood components. However, in many kidney diseases, capillary permeability is increased, which permits plasma proteins and blood cells to pass into the urine.

The amount of blood filtered each minute by the glomeruli is expressed as the **glomerular filtration rate (GFR)**. The normal GFR is about 125 mL/min. The peritubular capillary network reabsorbs most of the glomerular filtrate before it reaches the end of the collecting duct. Therefore only 1 mL/min (on average) is excreted as urine.

***Tubular Function.*** Since the glomerular membrane is a selective filtration membrane that filters primarily by size, provision is made for the reabsorption of essential materials and excretion of nonessential ones (Table 44-1). The tubules and collecting ducts carry out these functions by means of reabsorption and secretion. *Reabsorption* is the passage of a substance from the lumen of the tubules through the tubule cells and into the capillaries. This process involves both active and passive transport mechanisms. Tubular *secretion* is the passage of a substance from the capillaries through the tubular cells into the lumen of the tubule. Reabsorption and secretion cause numerous changes in the composition of the glomerular filtrate as it moves through the entire length of the tubule.

In the proximal convoluted tubule, about 80% of the electrolytes are reabsorbed. Normally, all the glucose, amino acids, and small proteins are reabsorbed. As reabsorption continues in the loop of Henle, water is conserved, which is important for concentrating the filtrate. The descending loop is permeable to water and moderately permeable to sodium, urea, and other solutes. In the ascending limb, chloride ions ($Cl^-$) are actively reabsorbed, followed by passive reabsorption of sodium ions ($Na^+$). About 25% of the filtered sodium is reabsorbed in the ascending limb.

Two important functions of the distal convoluted tubules are final regulation of water balance and acid-base balance. Antidiuretic hormone (ADH) is required for water reabsorption in the kidney and is important in water balance. ADH makes the distal convoluted tubules and collecting ducts permeable to water. This allows water to be reabsorbed into the peritubular capillaries and eventually returned to the circulation.

Decreases in plasma osmolality are detected in the anterior hypothalamus by osmoreceptors. These osmoreceptors send neural input to *superoptic nuclei cells* in the hypothalamus. These superoptic nuclei cells have neuronal axons that terminate in the posterior pituitary gland and act to inhibit secretion of ADH. In the absence of ADH, the tubules are essentially impermeable to water. Thus any water in the tubules leaves the body as urine.

Aldosterone (released from the adrenal cortex) acts on the distal tubule to cause reabsorption of $Na^+$ and water. In exchange for $Na^+$, potassium ions ($K^+$) are excreted. The secretion of aldosterone is influenced by both circulating blood volume and plasma concentrations of $Na^+$ and $K^+$.

Acid-base regulation involves reabsorbing and conserving most of the bicarbonate ($HCO_3^-$) and secreting excess hydrogen ions ($H^+$). The distal tubule has different ways to maintain the pH of ECF within a range of 7.35 to 7.45 (see Chapter 16).

Myocyte cells in the right atrium secrete a hormone, atrial natriuretic peptide (ANP), in response to atrial distention, which is a result of an increase in plasma volume. ANP acts on the kidneys to increase sodium excretion. At the same time, ANP inhibits renin, ADH, and the action of angiotensin II on the adrenal glands, thereby suppressing aldosterone secretion. These combined effects of ANP result in the production of a large volume of dilute urine. Furthermore, secretion of ANP causes relaxation of the afferent arteriole, thus increasing the GFR.

The renal tubules are also involved in calcium balance. Parathyroid hormone (PTH) is released from the parathyroid gland in response to low serum calcium levels. PTH maintains serum calcium levels by causing increased tubular reabsorption of calcium ions ($Ca^{2+}$) and decreased tubular reabsorption of phosphate ions ($PO_4^{2-}$). In kidney disease, the effects of PTH may have a major effect on bone metabolism.

Vitamin D is a hormone that can be obtained in the diet or synthesized by the action of ultraviolet radiation on cholesterol in the skin. These forms of vitamin D are inactive and require two more steps to become metabolically active. The first step in activation occurs in the liver; the second step occurs in the kidneys. Active vitamin D is essential for the absorption of calcium from the gastrointestinal (GI) tract. The patient with kidney failure (also called *renal failure*) has a deficiency of the active metabolite of vitamin D and manifests problems of altered calcium and phosphate balance (see Chapter 47).

In summary, the basic function of nephrons is to cleanse blood plasma of unnecessary substances. After the glomerulus has filtered the blood, the tubules select the unwanted from the wanted portions of tubular fluid. Essential constituents are returned to the blood, and dispensable substances pass into urine.

**Other Functions of Kidneys.** The kidneys perform vital functions through participation in red blood cell (RBC) production and BP regulation. Erythropoietin is a hormone produced in the kidneys and secreted in response to hypoxia and decreased renal blood flow. Erythropoietin stimulates RBC production in the bone marrow. A deficiency of erythropoietin occurs in kidney failure, leading to anemia.

Renin is important in the regulation of BP. Renin is produced and secreted by the kidney's juxtaglomerular cells (Fig. 44-4). Renin is released into the bloodstream in response to decreased renal perfusion, decreased arterial BP, decreased ECF, decreased serum $Na^+$ concentration, and increased urinary $Na^+$ concentration. The plasma protein angiotensinogen (from the liver) is activated to angiotensin I by renin. Angiotensin I is

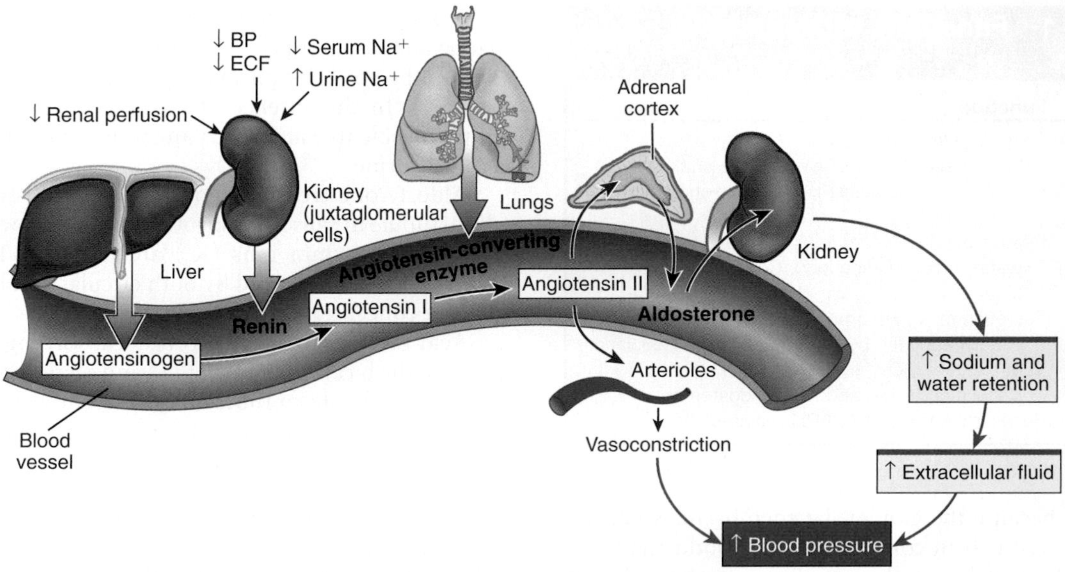


**FIG. 44-4** Renin-angiotensin-aldosterone system. (Modified from Herlihy B, Maebius N: *The human body in health and disease,* ed 4, Philadelphia, 2011, Saunders.)

subsequently converted to angiotensin II by angiotensin-converting enzyme (ACE). ACE is located on the inner surface of all blood vessels, with particularly high levels in the vessels of the lungs. Angiotensin II stimulates the release of aldosterone from the adrenal cortex, which causes $Na^+$ and water retention, leading to increased ECF volume. Angiotensin II also causes increased peripheral vasoconstriction. Release of renin is inhibited by an elevation in BP. Excessive renin production caused by impaired renal perfusion may be a contributing factor in the etiology of hypertension (see Chapter 32).

Most body tissues synthesize prostaglandins (PGs) from the precursor arachidonic acid in response to appropriate stimuli. (See Chapter 11 and Fig. 11-2 for a more detailed discussion of PGs.) In the kidney, PG synthesis (primarily $PGE_2$ and $PGI_2$) occurs primarily in the medulla. These PGs have a vasodilating action, thus increasing renal blood flow, and promoting $Na^+$ excretion. They counteract the vasoconstrictive effect of substances such as angiotensin and norepinephrine. Renal PGs may have a systemic effect in lowering BP by decreasing systemic vascular resistance. The significance of renal PGs is related to the kidneys' role in causing hypertension. In renal failure with a loss of functioning tissue, these renal vasodilator factors are also lost, which may contribute to hypertension (see Chapter 46).

## Ureters

The ureters are tubes that carry urine from the renal pelvis to the bladder (Fig. 44-1). Arranged in a meshlike outer layer, circular and longitudinal smooth muscle fibers contract to promote the peristaltic, one-way flow of urine through the ureters. Distention, neurologic and endocrine influences, and drugs can affect these muscle contractions. Each ureter is approximately 10 to 12 inches (25 to 30.5 cm) long and 0.08 to 0.3 inches (0.2 to 0.8 cm) in diameter.

The narrow area where each ureter joins the renal pelvis is termed the *ureteropelvic junction* (UPJ). Subsequently, the ureters insert into either side of the bladder base at the *ureterovesical junctions* (UVJs). Because the ureteral lumens are narrowest at these junctions, the UPJ and UVJ are often sites of obstruction. The narrow ureteral lumens can be easily obstructed internally (e.g., urinary calculi) or externally (e.g., tumors, adhesions, inflammation). Sympathetic and parasympathetic nerves, along with the vascular supply, surround the mucosal lining of the ureters. Stimulation of these nerves during passage of a stone may cause acute, severe pain, termed *renal colic.*

Because the renal pelvis holds only 3 to 5 mL of urine, kidney damage can result from a backflow of more than that amount of urine. The UVJ relies on the ureter's angle of bladder insertion and muscle fiber attachments with the bladder to prevent the backflow *(reflux)* of urine, which predisposes a person to an ascending infection. The distal ureter enters the bladder laterally at its base, courses along obliquely through the bladder wall for about 1.5 cm, and intermingles with muscle fibers of the bladder base. Circular and longitudinal bladder muscle fibers adjacent to the imbedded ureter help secure it. When bladder pressure rises (e.g., during voiding or coughing), muscle fibers that the ureter shares with the bladder base contract first, promoting ureteral lumen closure. Next, the bladder contracts against its base, ensuring UVJ closure and prevention of urine reflux through the junction.

## Bladder

The urinary bladder is a stretchable (able to fill at relatively low pressures) organ positioned behind the symphysis pubis and anterior to the vagina and rectum (Fig. 44-5). Its primary functions are to serve as a reservoir for urine and to eliminate waste products from the body. Normal adult urine output is approximately 1500 mL/day, which varies with food and fluid intake. The volume of urine produced at night is less than half of that formed during the day because of hormonal influences (e.g., ADH). This diurnal pattern of urination is normal. Typically, an individual will urinate five or six times during the day and occasionally at night.

The *trigone* is the triangular area formed by the two ureteral openings and bladder neck at the base of the bladder. The trigone is attached to the pelvis by many ligaments and does not change its shape during bladder filling or emptying. The bladder muscle *(detrusor)* is composed of layers of intertwined smooth muscle fibers capable of considerable distention during bladder filling and contraction during emptying. It is attached

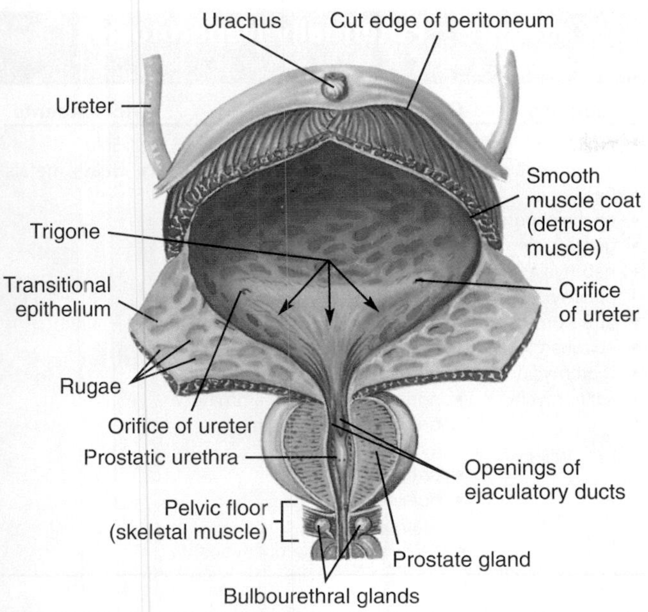


**FIG. 44-5** Urinary bladder of a male. (Modified from Thibodeau GA, Patton KT: *Anatomy and physiology,* ed 6, St Louis, 2007, Mosby.)

to the abdominal wall by an umbilical ligament, the *urachus.* As a result of this attachment, as the bladder fills it rises toward the umbilicus. The dome and the anterior and lateral aspects of the bladder expand and contract.

On average, 200 to 250 mL of urine in the bladder cause moderate distention and the urge to urinate. When the quantity of urine reaches approximately 400 to 600 mL, the person feels uncomfortable. Bladder capacity varies with the individual but generally ranges from 600 to 1000 mL. Evacuation of urine is termed *urination, micturition,* or *voiding.*

The bladder has the same mucosal lining as that of the renal pelvises, ureters, and bladder neck. The bladder is lined by transitional cell epithelium and is referred to as the *urothelium.* Unique to the urinary tract, the urothelium is resistant to absorption of urine. This means that after waste products (produced by the kidneys) have left the kidneys, they cannot be reabsorbed in the urinary system. Microscopically, urothelium is only several cells deep. However, as urine enters the bladder, these calls can stretch to accommodate filling. As the bladder empties, the urothelium resumes its multicellular layer formation.

Transitional cell cancers occurring in one section of the urinary tract can easily metastasize to other urinary tract areas given that the mucosal lining throughout the urinary tract is the same. Malignant cells may move down from upper urinary tract cancers and embed in the bladder, or large bladder tumors can invade the ureter. Cancer recurrence within the bladder is common.

### Urethra

The urethra is a small tube that incorporates the smooth muscle of the bladder neck and extends to the striated muscle of the external meatus. The urethra's primary functions are to (1) control voiding and (2) serve as a conduit for urine from the bladder to the outside of the body during voiding.

The female urethra is 1 to 2 inches (2.5 to 5 cm) long and lies behind the symphysis pubis but anterior to the vagina (Fig. 44-1, *C*). The male urethra, which is about 8 to 10 inches (20 to 25 cm) long, originates at the bladder neck and extends the length of the penis (Fig. 44-1, *B*).

### Urethrovesical Unit

Together, the bladder, urethra, and pelvic floor muscles form what is called the *urethrovesical unit.* Voluntary control of this unit is defined as *continence.* Stimulating and inhibiting impulses are sent from the brain through the thoracolumbar (T11 to L2) and sacral (S2 to S4) areas of the spinal cord to control voiding. Distention of the bladder stimulates stretch receptors within the bladder wall. Impulses are transmitted to the sacral spinal cord and then to the brain, causing a desire to urinate.

If it is not appropriate to void at a given time, inhibitor impulses in the brain are stimulated and transmitted back through the thoracolumbar and sacral nerves innervating the bladder. In a coordinated fashion, the detrusor muscle accommodates to the pressure (does not contract) while the sphincter and pelvic floor muscles tighten (contract) to resist bladder pressure.

If voiding is appropriate, cerebral inhibition is voluntarily suppressed, and impulses are transmitted via the spinal cord for the bladder neck, sphincter, and pelvic floor muscles to relax and for the bladder to contract. The sphincter closes and the detrusor muscle relaxes when the bladder is empty.

Any disease or trauma that affects the function of the brain, spinal cord, or nerves that directly innervate the bladder, bladder neck, external sphincter, or pelvic floor can affect bladder function. These conditions include diabetes mellitus, multiple sclerosis, paraplegia, and tetraplegia (quadriplegia). Drugs affecting nerve transmission also can affect bladder function.

### Gerontologic Considerations: Effects of Aging on Urinary System

Anatomic changes in the aging kidney include a 20% to 30% decrease in size and weight between ages 30 and 90 years. By the seventh decade of life, 30% to 50% of glomeruli have lost their function.[1] Atherosclerosis accelerates the decrease of renal size with age. Despite these changes, older individuals maintain body fluid homeostasis unless they encounter diseases or other physiologic stressors.

Physiologic changes in the aging kidney include decreased renal blood flow, due in part to atherosclerosis, resulting in a decreased GFR. Alterations in hormone levels (including ADH, aldosterone, and ANP) result in decreased urinary concentrating ability and alterations in the excretion of water, sodium, potassium, and acid. Under normal conditions, the aging kidney is able to maintain homeostasis. However, after abrupt changes in blood volume, acid load, or other insults, the kidney may not be able to function effectively because much of its renal reserve has been lost.[2,3]

Physiologic changes also occur in the aging urethra and bladder. The female urethra, bladder, vagina, and pelvic floor undergo a loss of elasticity and muscle support. Consequently, older women are more prone to bladder infections and incontinence.

The prostate surrounds the proximal urethra. As men age, the prostate enlarges and may affect urinary patterns, causing hesitancy, retention, slow stream, and bladder infections.

Constipation, often experienced by older adults, can also affect urination. Partial urethral obstruction may occur because of the rectum's close proximity to the urethra.

### TABLE 44-2 Gerontologic Assessment Differences

***Urinary System***

| Gerontologic Changes | Differences in Assessment Findings |
|---|---|
| **Kidney** | |
| • ↓ Amount of renal tissue | • Less palpable |
| • ↓ Number of nephrons and renal blood vessels. Thickened basement membrane of Bowman's capsule and glomeruli | • ↓ Creatinine clearance, ↑ BUN level, ↑ serum creatinine |
| • ↓ Function of loop of Henle and tubules | • Alterations in drug excretion, nocturia, loss of normal diurnal excretory pattern because of ↓ ability to concentrate urine; less concentrated urine |
| **Ureter, Bladder, and Urethra** | |
| • ↓ Elasticity and muscle tone | • Palpable bladder after urination because of retention |
| • Weakening of urinary sphincter | • Stress incontinence (especially during Valsalva maneuver), dribbling of urine after urination |
| • ↓ Bladder capacity and sensory receptors | • Frequency, urgency, nocturia, overflow incontinence |
| • Estrogen deficiency leading to thin, dry vaginal tissue | • Stress or overactive bladder, dysuria |
| • ↑ Prevalence of unstable bladder contractions | • Overactive bladder |
| • Prostatic enlargement | • Hesitancy, frequency, urgency, nocturia, straining to urinate, retention, dribbling |

Age-related changes in the urinary system and differences in assessment findings are presented in Table 44-2.

## ASSESSMENT OF URINARY SYSTEM

### Subjective Data

#### Important Health Information

***Past Health History.*** Question the patient about the presence or history of diseases that are related to renal or other urologic problems. Some of these diseases are hypertension, diabetes mellitus, gout and other metabolic problems, connective tissue disorders (e.g., systemic lupus erythematosus, systemic sclerosis [scleroderma]), skin or upper respiratory tract infections of streptococcal origin, tuberculosis, viral hepatitis, congenital disorders, neurologic conditions (e.g., stroke, back injury), or trauma. Note specific urinary problems such as cancer, infections, benign prostatic hyperplasia, and calculi.

***Medications.*** An assessment of the patient's current and past use of medications is important. This should include over-the-counter drugs, prescription medications, and herbs. Drugs affect the urinary tract in several ways. Many drugs are known to be nephrotoxic (Table 44-3). Certain drugs may alter the quantity and character of urine output (e.g., diuretics). A number of drugs change the color of urine such as phenazopyridine (Pyridium) (urine turns orange) and nitrofurantoin (Macrodantin) (urine turns dark yellow to brown). Anticoagulants may cause hematuria. Many antidepressants, calcium channel blockers, antihistamines, and drugs used for neurologic and musculoskeletal disorders affect the ability of the bladder or sphincter to contract or relax normally.

### TABLE 44-3 Potentially Nephrotoxic Agents

| Antibiotics | Other Drugs | Other Agents |
|---|---|---|
| • amikacin | • captopril | • Gold |
| • amphotericin B | • cimetidine | • Heavy metals |
| • bacitracin | • cisplatin | |
| • cephalosporins | • cocaine | |
| • gentamicin | • cyclosporine | |
| • neomycin | • ethylene glycol | |
| • polymyxin B | • heroin | |
| • streptomycin | • lithium | |
| • sulfonamides | • methotrexate | |
| • tobramycin | • nitrosoureas (e.g., carmustine) | |
| • vancomycin | • nonsteroidal antiinflammatory drugs (e.g., ibuprofen, indomethacin) | |
| | • phenacetin | |
| | • quinine | |
| | • rifampin | |
| | • salicylates (large quantities) | |

## CASE STUDY

***Patient Introduction***

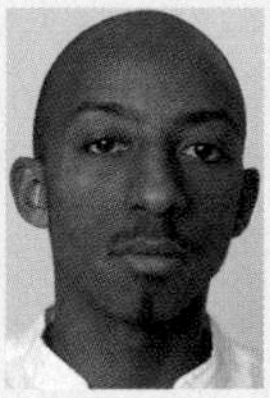

(©iStockphoto/ Thinkstock)

A.K. is a 28-yr-old African American man who comes to the emergency department (ED) in acute distress with complaints of severe abdominal pain. The pain began about 6 hr ago after he finished a 10-mile run as part of his training for a marathon. He says that the pain has steadily increased, he is nauseated, and his urine is a dark, smoky color.

**Discussion Questions**

1. What are the possible causes of A.K.'s abdominal pain, nausea, and urine color?
2. What would be your priority assessment of A.K.?

You will learn more about A.K. and his condition as you read through this assessment chapter.

(See p. 1023 for more information on A.K.)

Answers available at *http://evolve.elsevier.com/Lewis/medsurg.*

***Surgery or Other Treatments.*** Ask the patient about previous hospitalizations related to renal or urologic diseases and all urinary problems during past pregnancies. Inquire about the duration, severity, and patient's perception of any problem and its treatment. Document past surgeries, particularly pelvic surgeries, or urinary tract instrumentation (e.g., catheterization). Ask the patient about any radiation or chemotherapy treatment for cancer.

**Functional Health Patterns.** Key questions to ask a patient with problems related to the renal system are listed in Table 44-4.

***Health Perception–Health Management Pattern.*** Ask about the patient's general health, particularly when a disorder affecting the kidneys is suspected. Abnormal kidney function may be suspected if the patient reports changes in weight or appetite, excess thirst, fluid retention, headache, pruritus, blurred vision, or "feeling tired all the time." Similarly, an older patient may report malaise and nonlocalized abdominal discomfort as the only symptoms of a urinary tract infection (UTI). In older adults with a UTI, family members may report that the patient is disoriented or has increased confusion.

A patient's occupational history is an important consideration, because exposure to certain chemicals can affect the urinary system. Phenol and ethylene glycol are examples of

## TABLE 44-4 Health History

*Urinary System*

**Health Perception–Health Management**
- How is your energy level compared with 1 yr ago?
- Do you notice any visual changes?*
- Have you ever smoked? If yes, how many packs per day?

**Nutritional-Metabolic**
- How is your appetite?
- Has your weight changed over the past yr?*
- Do you take vitamins, herbs, or any other supplements?*
- How much and what kinds of fluids do you drink daily?
- How many dairy products and how much meat do you eat?
- Do you drink coffee? Colas? Tea?
- Do you eat chocolate?
- Do you spice your food heavily?*

**Elimination**
- Are you able to sit through a 2-hr meeting or ride in a car for 2 hr without urinating?
- Do you awaken at night with the desire to urinate? If so, how many times does this occur during an average night?
- Do you ever notice blood in your urine?* If so, at what point in the urination does it occur?
- Do you ever pass urine when you do not intend to? When?
- Do you use special devices or supplies for urine elimination or control?*
- How often do you move your bowels?
- Do you ever experience constipation?
- Do you frequently experience diarrhea? Do you ever have problems controlling your bowels? If so, do you have problems controlling the passage of gas? Watery or liquid stool? Solid stool?

**Activity-Exercise**
- Have you noticed any changes in your ability to perform your usual daily activities?*
- Do certain activities aggravate your urinary problem?*
- Has your urinary problem caused you to alter or stop any activity or exercise?*
- Do you require assistance in moving or getting to the bathroom?*

**Sleep-Rest**
- Do you awaken at night from an urge to urinate?* How does this disturb your sleep?
- Do you awaken at night from pain or other problems and urinate as a matter of routine before returning to sleep?*
- Do you experience daytime sleepiness and fatigue as a result of nighttime urination?*

**Cognitive-Perceptual**
- Do you ever have pain when you urinate?* If so, where is the pain?

**Self-Perception–Self-Concept**
- How does your urinary problem make you feel about yourself?
- Do you perceive your body differently since you have developed a urinary problem?

**Role-Relationship**
- Does your urinary problem interfere with your relationships with family or friends?*
- Has your urinary problem caused a change in your job status or affected your ability to carry out job-related responsibilities?*

**Sexuality-Reproductive**
- Has your urinary problem caused any change in your sexual pleasure or performance?*
- Do hygiene concerns interfere with sexual activities?

**Coping–Stress Tolerance**
- Do you feel able to manage the problems associated with your urinary problem? If not, explain.
- What strategies are you using to cope with your urinary problem?

**Values-Beliefs**
- Has your present illness affected your belief system?*
- Are your treatment decisions related to your urinary problem in conflict with your value system?*

*If yes, describe.

nephrotoxic chemicals. Aromatic amines and some organic chemicals may increase the risk of bladder cancers. Textile workers, painters, hairdressers, and industrial workers have an increased incidence of bladder cancer.[4]

Obtain a smoking history. Cancer occurs more frequently in cigarette smokers than in nonsmokers. Cigarette smoking is a major risk factor for bladder and kidney cancer.

Information about places where a patient has lived is important. Persons living in certain parts of the United States (Great Lakes, Southwest, Southeast) have a higher than normal incidence of urinary calculi, possibly caused by the higher mineral content of the soil and water. A person living in Middle Eastern countries or Africa can acquire certain parasites that can cause cystitis or bladder cancer.

### GENETIC RISK ALERT

- Polycystic kidney disease and congenital urinary tract abnormalities (e.g., Alport syndrome [congenital nephritis]) are genetic disorders.
- A family history of certain renal or urologic problems increases the likelihood of similar problems occurring in the patient.
- For any disease the patient has reported in the health history, ask if other family members also have/had the same or similar diseases.

***Nutritional-Metabolic Pattern.*** The usual quantity and types of fluid a patient drinks are important in relation to urinary tract disease. Dehydration may contribute to UTIs, calculi formation, and kidney failure. Large intake of particular foods, such as dairy products or foods high in proteins, may also lead to calculi formation. Asparagus may cause the urine to smell musty, and red urine caused by beet ingestion may be mistaken for bloody urine. Caffeine, alcohol, carbonated beverages, some artificial sweeteners, or spicy foods often aggravate urinary inflammatory diseases. Green tea and some herbal teas also cause diuresis. An unexplained weight gain may be the result of fluid retention secondary to a renal problem. Anorexia, nausea, and vomiting can dramatically affect fluid status and require careful monitoring. Obtain information related to vitamin and mineral supplements and herbal therapies. The patient may not think of these supplements and therapies when listing over-the-counter drugs.

***Elimination Pattern.*** Questions about urine elimination patterns are the cornerstone of the health history in the patient with a lower urinary tract disorder. This line of inquiry begins with a question of how the patient manages urine elimination. Most patients eliminate urine by spontaneous voiding. Therefore ask about daytime (diurnal) voiding frequency and

**TABLE 44-5 Manifestations of Urinary System Disorders**

| | SPECIFIC MANIFESTATIONS RELATED TO URINARY SYSTEM | | | | |
|---|---|---|---|---|---|
| **General Manifestations** | **Edema** | **Pain** | **Patterns of Urination** | **Urine Output** | **Urine Composition** |
| • Fatigue<br>• Headaches<br>• Blurred vision<br>• Elevated BP<br>• Anorexia<br>• Nausea and vomiting<br>• Chills<br>• Itching<br>• Excessive thirst<br>• Change in body weight<br>• Cognitive changes | • Facial (periorbital)<br>• Ankle<br>• Ascites<br>• Anasarca (generalized edema)<br>• Sacral | • Dysuria<br>• Flank or costovertebral angle<br>• Groin<br>• Suprapubic | • Frequency<br>• Urgency<br>• Hesitancy of stream<br>• Change in stream<br>• Retention<br>• Dysuria<br>• Nocturia<br>• Incontinence<br>• Stress incontinence<br>• Dribbling | • Anuria<br>• Oliguria<br>• Polyuria | • Concentrated<br>• Dilute<br>• Hematuria<br>• Pyuria<br>• Color (red, brown, yellowish green) |

the frequency of nocturia. Pelvic organ prolapse, particularly advanced anterior vaginal prolapse, may cause suprapubic pressure, frequency, urgency, and incontinence secondary to urinary retention. Query patients about additional bothersome lower urinary tract symptoms, including urgency, incontinence, or urinary retention. Table 44-5 lists some of the common manifestations of urinary tract disorders.

Changes in the color and appearance of urine are often significant and should be evaluated. If blood is visible in the urine, determine if it occurs at the beginning of, throughout, or at the end of urination. This is more difficult for the female patient.

Investigate bowel function. Problems with fecal incontinence may signal neurologic causes for bladder problems because of shared nerve pathways. Constipation and fecal impaction can partially obstruct the urethra, causing inadequate bladder emptying, overflow incontinence, and infection.

Determine the patient's method of managing a urinary problem. A patient may already be using a catheter or collection device. Sometimes a patient has to assume a particular position to urinate or perform maneuvers such as pressing on the lower abdomen (Credé's method) or straining (Valsalva maneuver) to empty the bladder.

***Activity-Exercise Pattern.*** Assess the patient's level of activity. A sedentary person is more likely to have stasis of urine than an active individual and thus can be predisposed to infection and calculi. Demineralization of bones in an individual with limited physical activity can cause increased urine calcium precipitation.

An active person may find that increasing activity aggravates the urinary problem. The patient who has had prostate surgery or who has weakened pelvic floor muscles may leak urine when attempting particular activities such as running. Some men develop chronic inflammatory prostatitis or epididymitis after heavy lifting or long-distance driving.

***Sleep-Rest Pattern.*** Nocturia is a common and a particularly bothersome lower urinary tract symptom that often leads to sleep deprivation, daytime sleepiness, and fatigue. It occurs in multiple disorders affecting the lower urinary tract, including urinary incontinence, urinary retention, and interstitial cystitis. Nocturia may also be related to polyuria secondary to kidney disease, poorly controlled diabetes mellitus, alcoholism, excessive fluid intake, liver disease, heart failure, or obstructive sleep apnea.

When assessing nocturia, determine whether the need to urinate causes the person to arise from sleep or whether pain or other symptoms interrupt sleep, and the person urinates as a matter of habit before returning to bed. Up to one episode of nocturia is considered normal in younger adults, and up to two episodes are acceptable in adults ages 65 years or older. If an older adult has more than two voidings during the night, assess the amount and timing of fluid intake. This information will help determine whether further investigation is needed.

***Cognitive-Perceptual Pattern.*** Assess the level of mobility, visual acuity, and dexterity as these are important factors to evaluate in a patient with urologic problems, particularly when urine retention or incontinence is a problem. Determine if the patient is alert, is able to understand instructions, and can recall the instructions when necessary.

If urinary incontinence is present, elicit a thorough history of the problem to help determine the type of incontinence. Ask how the patient has managed the problem in the past. Recognize that incontinence is often distressing and embarrassing. Discuss the problem with the patient with sensitivity in a nonjudgmental manner.

A frequent symptom of renal and urologic problems is pain, including dysuria, groin pain, costovertebral pain, and suprapubic pain. Assess pain and document the location, character, and duration. The absence of pain when other urinary symptoms exist is also significant. Many urinary tract cancers are painless in the early stages.

***Self-Perception–Self-Concept Pattern.*** Problems associated with the urinary system, such as incontinence, urinary diversion procedures, and chronic fatigue (may indicate anemia), can result in loss of self-esteem and a negative body image.

***Role-Relationship Pattern.*** Urinary problems can affect many aspects of a person's life, including the ability to work and relationships with others. These factors have important implications for future treatment and management of the patient's condition.

Urinary system problems may be serious enough to cause problems in job-related and social situations. Chronic dialysis therapy often makes regular employment or management of home and family responsibilities difficult. Concurrent poor health and negative body image can seriously alter existing roles.

***Sexuality-Reproductive Pattern.*** Assess the effect of renal problems on the patient's sexual satisfaction. Problems related to personal hygiene and fatigue can negatively affect sexual relationships. Although urinary incontinence is not directly associated with sexual dysfunction, it often has a devastating effect on self-esteem and social and intimate relationships. Counseling of both the patient and partner may be indicated.

## CASE STUDY—cont'd

### Subjective Data

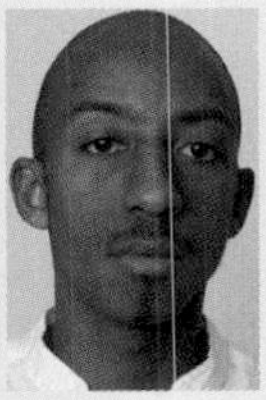

(©iStockphoto/ Thinkstock)

A focused subjective assessment of A.K. revealed the following information:

***PMH:*** History of one isolated incidence of possible gout 6 yr ago. He stopped drinking alcohol with no further occurrence. Appendectomy 12 yr ago.

***Medications:*** None.

***Health Perception–Health Management:*** A.K. states that he is usually healthy. He does not smoke or drink alcohol. He has never experienced this type of pain before. Describes the pain as being sharp and colicky (coming in waves). Rates the pain as 9 on a scale of 0-10.

***Nutritional-Metabolic:*** A.K. is currently on a high-protein diet as he trains for the marathon. He eats a lot of chicken, beef, and seafood. He drinks milk-based protein shakes and water after exercising but admits that he does not think he drinks enough to replace fluid loss from perspiration. He drinks coffee for energy but denies eating chocolate or other sweets. He also avoids sodas.

***Elimination:*** Denies any history of difficulty with urination or constipation or diarrhea. This is the first time he has ever noticed a change of color in his urine.

***Activity-Exercise:*** Prides himself on his ability to exercise and run without difficulty.

***Sleep-Rest:*** Does not awaken at night to urinate.

***Cognitive-Perceptual:*** Denies pain on urination.

***Self-Perception–Self-Concept:*** Believes he is able to monitor self and maintain healthy lifestyle.

***Coping–Stress Tolerance:*** Worried that this pain may interfere with his marathon training.

**Discussion Questions**

1. What type of assessment would be most appropriate for A.K.: comprehensive, focused, or emergency? On what basis did you make that decision?
2. What assessment questions will you ask him?
3. Which subjective assessment findings are of most concern to you?

You will learn more about the physical examination of the urinary system in the next section.

(See p. 1024 for more information on A.K.)

Answers available at *http://evolve.elsevier.com/Lewis/medsurg.*

## Objective Data

### Physical Examination

***Inspection.*** Assess for changes in the following:

- *Skin:* Pallor, yellow-gray cast, excoriations, changes in turgor, bruises, texture (e.g., rough, dry skin) (see Table 22-9 for assessment of dark-skinned individuals)
- *Mouth:* Stomatitis, ammonia breath odor
- *Face and extremities:* Generalized edema, peripheral edema
- *Abdomen:* Abdominal contour for midline mass in lower abdomen (may indicate bladder distention and urinary retention) or unilateral mass (occasionally seen in adults, indicating enlargement of one or both kidneys from large tumor or polycystic kidney)
- *Weight:* Weight gain secondary to edema. Weight loss and muscle wasting in kidney failure
- *General state of health:* Fatigue, lethargy, and diminished alertness

***Palpation.*** The kidneys are posterior organs protected by the abdominal organs, ribs, and heavy back muscles. A landmark useful in locating the kidneys is the **costovertebral angle (CVA)** formed by the rib cage and the vertebral column. The normal-sized left kidney is rarely palpable because the spleen lies directly on top of it. Occasionally the lower pole of the right kidney is palpable.

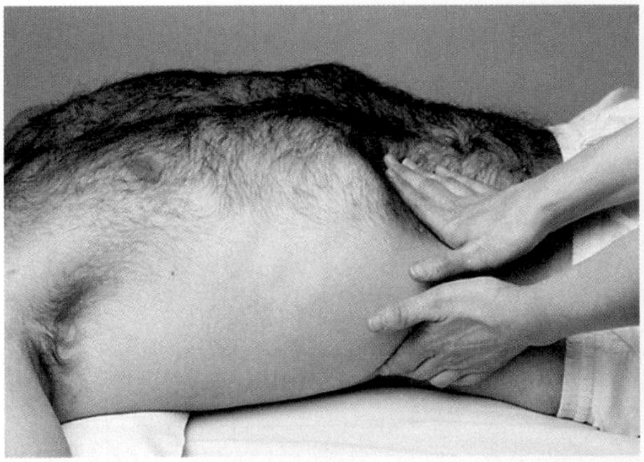

**FIG. 44-6** Palpating the right kidney. (From Brundage DJ: *Renal disorders,* St Louis, 1992, Mosby.)

**TABLE 44-6 Normal Physical Assessment of Urinary System**

- No costovertebral angle tenderness
- Nonpalpable kidney and bladder
- No palpable masses

To palpate the right kidney, place your left (anterior) hand behind and support the patient's right side between the rib cage and the iliac crest (Fig. 44-6). Elevate the right flank with the left hand. Use your right hand to palpate deeply for the right kidney. The lower pole of the right kidney may be felt as a smooth, rounded mass that descends on inspiration. If the kidney is palpable, note its size, contour, and tenderness. Kidney enlargement is suggestive of neoplasm or other serious renal pathologic conditions.

The urinary bladder is normally not palpable unless it is distended with urine. If the bladder is full, it may be felt as a smooth, round, firm organ and is sensitive to palpation.

***Percussion.*** Tenderness in the flank area may be detected by fist percussion *(kidney punch).* This technique is performed by striking the fist of one hand against the dorsal surface of the other hand, which is placed flat along the posterior CVA margin (Fig. 44-7). Normally this type of percussion should not elicit pain. If CVA tenderness and pain are present, it may indicate a kidney infection or polycystic kidney disease.[5]

A bladder is not normally percussible until it contains at least 150 mL of urine. If the bladder is full, dullness is heard above the symphysis pubis. A distended bladder may be percussed as high as the umbilicus.

***Auscultation.*** Use the diaphragm of the stethoscope to auscultate the bowels, since they may also affect the urinary system.

Table 44-6 shows how to record the normal physical assessment findings of the urinary system. Table 44-7 describes assessment abnormalities of the urinary system. Assessment findings may vary in the older adult. Table 44-2 presents the age-related changes in the urinary system and differences in assessment findings. Use a *focused assessment* to evaluate the status of previously identified urinary system problems and to monitor for signs of new problems (see Table 3-7). A focused assessment of the urinary system is presented in the box on p. 1024.

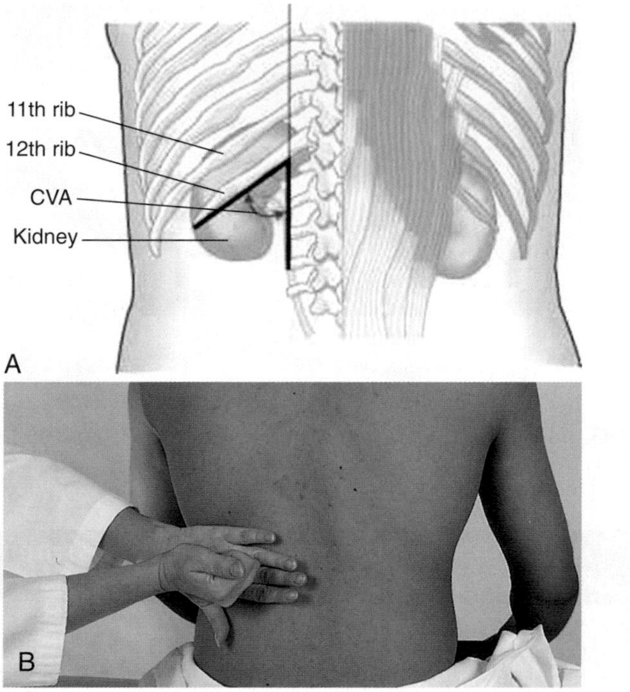


**FIG. 44-7** **A,** Costovertebral angle. **B,** Indirect fist percussion of the costovertebral angle (CVA). To assess the kidney, place one hand over the twelfth rib at the CVA on the back. Thump that hand with the ulnar edge of the other fist. (*A,* From Jarvis C: *Physical examination and health assessment,* ed 7, St Louis, 2016, Saunders. *B,* From Jarvis C: *Physical examination and health assessment,* ed 6, St Louis, 2012, Saunders.)

## FOCUSED ASSESSMENT

### *Urinary System*

*Use this checklist to ensure that the key assessment steps have been done.*

**Subjective**

Ask the patient about any of the following and note responses.

| | | |
|---|---|---|
| Painful urination | Y | N |
| Changes in color of urine (blood, cloudy) | Y | N |
| Change in characteristics of urination (diminished, excessive) | Y | N |
| Problems with frequent nighttime urination (nocturia) | Y | N |

**Objective: Diagnostic**

Check the following laboratory results for critical values.

| | |
|---|---|
| Blood urea nitrogen | ✓ |
| Serum creatinine | ✓ |
| Urinalysis | ✓ |
| Urine culture and sensitivity | ✓ |

**Objective: Physical Examination**

***Inspect***

| | |
|---|---|
| Abdomen | ✓ |
| Urinary meatus for inflammation or discharge | ✓ |

***Palpate***

| | |
|---|---|
| Abdomen for bladder distention, masses, or tenderness | ✓ |

***Percuss***

| | |
|---|---|
| Costovertebral angle for tenderness | ✓ |

## CASE STUDY—cont'd

### *Objective Data: Physical Examination*

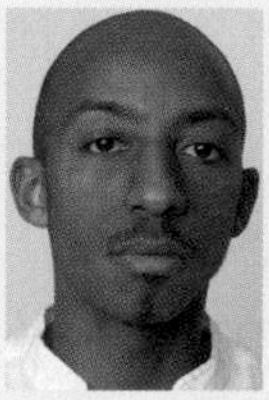

(©iStockphoto/Thinkstock)

A focused assessment of A.K. reveals the following:

A.K. is lying on the ED stretcher with his knees bent and drawn to his abdominal area. He appears restless and keeps moving from back to side in an effort to reduce his discomfort. Vital signs as follows: BP 156/70, apical pulse 108, respiratory rate 24, temperature 37.4° C, $O_2$ saturation 96% on room air. Awake, alert, and oriented × 3. Lungs clear to auscultation. Apical pulse regular. Abdomen nondistended with + bowel sounds in all four quadrants. No rebound tenderness. Positive left costovertebral tenderness. Voiding small amounts of dark, smoky urine.

**Discussion Questions**

1. What should be included in the physical assessment? What would you be looking for?
2. Which physical assessment findings are of most concern to you?
3. Based on the results of the subjective and physical assessment findings, what diagnostic studies do you think may be ordered for A.K.?

You will learn more about diagnostic studies related to the urinary system in the next section.

(See p. 1031 for more information on A.K.)

Answers available at *http://evolve.elsevier.com/Lewis/medsurg.*

## DIAGNOSTIC STUDIES OF URINARY SYSTEM

Numerous diagnostic studies are used to assess problems of the urinary system. Tables 44-8 and 44-9 describe the most common studies, and select studies are described in more detail in the following text.

Many radiologic studies require the use of a bowel preparation the evening before the study to clear the lower GI tract of feces and flatus. Because the kidneys lie in a retroperitoneal location, the contents of the colon may obstruct visualization of the urinary tract. If the bowel preparation fails to adequately evacuate the lower GI tract, the study may be unsuccessful and may have to be rescheduled. Commonly used bowel preparations include enemas, magnesium citrate, and bisacodyl (Dulcolax) tablets or suppositories. In patients with kidney failure, some bowel preparations, such as magnesium citrate and Fleet enema, should not be used because magnesium cannot be excreted by the kidneys (see Chapter 46). Iodine-based contrast media used in some diagnostic studies may cause allergic reactions[6] (Table 44-8).

When a patient has undergone diagnostic studies on consecutive days, it is important to prevent dehydration. The patient is at risk for dehydration related to consecutive days of being NPO, extended time in the radiology department, and bowel preparations. Severe dehydration, especially in debilitated or older patients and patients with diabetes may lead to acute kidney injury. When a patient is scheduled for diagnostic studies, ensure that the patient is properly hydrated and given adequate nourishment between studies. Also check with the HCP regarding insulin dosage for diabetic patients who are placed on NPO status.

### Urine Studies

**Urinalysis.** *Urinalysis* (Tables 44-8 and 44-9) is one of the first studies done to evaluate disorders of the urinary tract. Results

*Text continued on p. 1031*

## TABLE 44-7 Assessment Abnormalities

### Urinary System

| Finding | Description | Possible Etiology and Significance |
|---|---|---|
| **Anuria** | Technically no urination (24-hr urine output <100 mL) | Acute kidney injury, end-stage renal disease, bilateral ureteral obstruction |
| **Burning on urination** | Stinging pain in urethral area | Urethral irritation, urinary tract infection, urethral calculus |
| **Dysuria** | Painful or difficult urination | Sign of urinary tract infection, interstitial cystitis, urethral calculus, and wide variety of pathologic conditions |
| **Enuresis** | Involuntary nocturnal urination | Symptomatic of lower urinary tract disorder |
| **Frequency** | Increased incidence of urination | Acutely inflamed bladder, retention with overflow, excess fluid intake, intake of bladder irritants, urethral calculus |
| **Hematuria** | Blood in the urine | Cancer of genitourinary tract, blood dyscrasias, kidney disease, urinary tract infection, stones in kidney or ureter, medications (anticoagulants) |
| **Hesitancy** | Delay or difficulty in initiating urination | Partial urethral obstruction, benign prostatic hyperplasia |
| **Incontinence** | Inability to voluntarily control discharge of urine | Neurogenic bladder, bladder infection, injury to external sphincter |
| **Nocturia** | Frequency of urination at night | Kidney disease with impaired concentrating ability, bladder obstruction, heart failure, diabetes mellitus, finding after renal transplant, excessive evening and nighttime fluid intake |
| **Oliguria** | Diminished amount of urine in a given time (24-hr urine output of 100-400 mL) | Severe dehydration, shock, transfusion reaction, kidney disease, end-stage renal disease |
| **Pain** | Suprapubic pain (related to bladder), urethral pain (irritation of bladder neck), flank (CVA) pain | Infection, urinary retention, foreign body in urinary tract, urethritis, pyelonephritis, renal colic or stones |
| **Pneumaturia** | Passage of urine containing gas | Fistula connections between bowel and bladder, gas-forming urinary tract infections |
| **Polyuria** | Large volume of urine in a given time | Diabetes mellitus, diabetes insipidus, chronic kidney disease, diuretics, excess fluid intake, obstructive sleep apnea |
| **Retention** | Inability to urinate even though bladder contains excessive amount of urine | Finding after pelvic surgery, childbirth, catheter removal, anesthesia; urethral stricture or obstruction; neurogenic bladder |
| **Stress incontinence** | Involuntary urination with increased pressure (sneezing or coughing) | Weakness of sphincter control, lack of estrogen, urinary retention |

*CVA,* Costovertebral angle.

## TABLE 44-8 Diagnostic Studies

### Urinary System

| Study | Description and Purpose | Nursing Responsibility |
|---|---|---|
| **Urine Studies** | | |
| **Urinalysis** | General examination of urine to establish baseline information or provide data to establish a tentative diagnosis and determine whether further studies are needed (Table 44-9). | *Before:* Wash perineal area before collecting specimen. *During:* Try to obtain first urinated morning specimen. *After:* Ensure specimen is examined within 1 hr of urinating. |
| **Creatinine clearance** | Creatinine is a waste product of protein breakdown (primarily body muscle mass). Clearance of creatinine by kidney approximates the GFR. Creatinine clearance is calculated as follows: $\text{Creatinine clearance} = \frac{\text{Urine creatinine (mg/dL)} \times \text{Urine volume (mL/min)}}{\text{Serum creatinine (mg/dL)}}$ *Reference interval:* 70-135 mL/min/1.73 $m^2$ (corrected for body surface area). | *During:* Collect 24-hr urine specimen. Discard first urination when test is started. Save urine from all subsequent urinations for 24 hr. Instruct patient to urinate at end of 24 hr and add specimen to collection. Ensure that serum creatinine is determined during 24-hr period. |
| **Composite urine collection** | Measures specific components, such as electrolytes, glucose, protein, 17-ketosteroids, catecholamines, creatinine, and minerals. Composite urine specimens are collected over a period ranging from 2 to 24 hr. | *During:* Instruct the patient to urinate and discard this first urine specimen. Note this time as the start of the test. Save all urine from subsequent urinations in a container for designated period. At end of period, ask patient to urinate, and this urine is added to container. Remind patient to save all urine during study period. Specimens may have to be refrigerated or preservatives added to container used for collecting urine. |
| **Urine culture ("clean catch," "midstream")** | Confirms suspected urinary tract infection and identifies causative organisms. *Normally,* bladder is sterile, but urethra contains bacteria and a few WBCs. *Reference interval:* If properly collected, stored, and handled: $<10^3$ organisms/mL usually indicates no infection. $10^3$-$10^5$/mL is usually not diagnostic and test may have to be repeated. $>10^5$/mL indicates infection. | *During:* Use sterile container for collection of urine. Touch only outside of container. *For women:* separate labia with one hand and clean meatus with other hand, using at least three sponges (saturated with cleansing solution) in a front-to-back motion. *For men:* retract foreskin (if present) and cleanse glans with at least three cleansing sponges. (Replace foreskin after cleaning.) After cleaning, instruct patient to start urinating and then continue voiding in sterile container. (The initial voided urine flushes out most contaminants in the urethra and perineal area.) Catheterization may be needed if patient is unable to cooperate with procedure. |

*Continued*

## TABLE 44-8 Diagnostic Studies

### Urinary System—cont'd

| Study | Description and Purpose | Nursing Responsibility |
|---|---|---|
| **Urine Studies—cont'd** | | |
| **Concentration test** | Evaluates renal concentration ability. Measured by specific gravity readings.<br>*Reference interval*: 1.003-1.030. | *Before:* Instruct patient to fast after given time in evening (in usual procedure).<br>*During:* Collect three urine specimens at hourly intervals in morning. |
| **Residual urine** | Determines amount of urine left in bladder after urinating. Finding may be abnormal in problems with bladder innervation, sphincter impairment, BPH, or urethral strictures.<br>*Reference interval:* ≤50 mL urine (increases with age). | *During:* Immediately after patient urinates, catheterize patient or use bladder ultrasound equipment. If a large amount of residual urine is obtained, HCP may want catheter left in bladder. |
| **Protein determination** | | |
| • Dipstick (Albustix, Combistix) | Detects protein (primarily albumin) in urine.<br>*Reference interval:* 0-trace. | *During:* Dip end of stick in urine and read result by comparison with color chart on label as directed. Grading is from 0 to 4+. Interpret with caution. Positive result may not indicate significant proteinuria. Some medications may give false-positive readings. |
| • Quantitative protein test | A 24-hr collection gives a more accurate indication of amount of protein in urine. Persistent proteinuria usually indicates glomerular kidney disease.<br>*Reference interval:* <150 mg/24 hr (mainly albumin). | *During:* Perform 24-hr urine collection as above. |
| **Urine cytologic study** | Identifies abnormal cellular structures that occur with bladder cancer. Also used to follow the progress of bladder cancer after treatment. | *During:* Obtain specimens by voiding, catheterization, or bladder irrigation. Do not use morning's first voided specimen because epithelial cells may change in appearance in urine held in bladder overnight.<br>*After:* Specimen should be fresh or brought to laboratory within the hour. An alcohol-based fixative is then added to preserve the cellular structure. |
| **Blood Studies** | | |
| **Blood urea nitrogen (BUN)** | Used to detect renal problems. Concentration of urea in blood is regulated by rate at which kidney excretes urea. Nonrenal factors may cause an increased BUN (e.g., rapid cell destruction from infections, fever, GI bleeding, trauma, athletic activity and excessive muscle breakdown).<br>*Reference interval:* 6-20 mg/dL (2.1-7.1 mmol/L). | *During:* Explain test and watch for postpuncture bleeding. |
| **Creatinine** | More reliable than BUN as a determinant of renal function. Creatinine is end product of muscle and protein metabolism and is released at a constant rate.<br>*Reference interval:* 0.6-1.3 mg/dL (53-115 μmol/L). | *During:* Explain test and watch for postpuncture bleeding. |
| **BUN/creatinine ratio** | Increased ratio may be due to conditions that decrease blood flow to kidneys (e.g., heart failure, dehydration), GI bleeding, or increased dietary protein. A decreased ratio may occur with liver disease (due to decreased urea formation) and malnutrition.<br>*Reference interval:* 12 : 1 to 20 : 1. | *During:* Explain test and watch for postpuncture bleeding |
| **Uric acid** | Used as screening test for disorders of purine metabolism but can also indicate kidney disease. Values depend on renal function, rate of purine metabolism, and dietary intake of food rich in purines.<br>*Female:* 2.3-6.6 mg/dL (137-393 μmol/L).<br>*Male:* 4.4-7.6 mg/dL (262-452 μmol/L). | *During:* Explain test and watch for postpuncture bleeding. |
| **Sodium** | Main extracellular electrolyte determining blood volume. Values usually stay within normal range until late stages of renal failure.<br>*Reference interval:* 135-145 mEq/L (135-145 mmol/L). | *During:* Explain test and watch for postpuncture bleeding. |
| **Potassium** | Kidneys are responsible for excreting majority of body's potassium. In kidney disease, $K^+$ determinations are critical because $K^+$ is one of the first electrolytes to become abnormal. Elevated $K^+$ levels >6 mEq/L can lead to muscle weakness and cardiac dysrhythmias.<br>*Reference interval:* 3.5-5.0 mEq/L (3.5-5.0 mmol/L). | *During:* Explain test and watch for postpuncture bleeding. |
| **Calcium (total)** | Main mineral in bone and aids in muscle contraction, neurotransmission, and clotting. In kidney disease, decreased reabsorption of $Ca^{2+}$ leads to renal osteodystrophy.<br>*Reference interval:* 8.6-10.2 mg/dL (2.15-2.55 mmol/L). | *During:* Explain test and watch for postpuncture bleeding. |

## TABLE 44-8 Diagnostic Studies

*Urinary System—cont'd*

| Study | Description and Purpose | Nursing Responsibility |
|---|---|---|
| **Phosphorus** | Phosphorus balance is inversely related to $Ca^{2+}$ balance. In kidney disease, phosphorus levels are elevated because the kidney is the primary excretory organ. *Reference interval:* 2.4-4.4 mg/dL (0.78-1.42 mmol/L). | *During:* Explain test and watch for postpuncture bleeding. |
| **Bicarbonate** | Most patients in renal failure have metabolic acidosis and low serum $HCO_3^-$ levels. *Reference interval:* 22-26 mEq/L (22-26 mmol/L). | *During:* Explain test and watch for postpuncture bleeding. |
| **Radiologic Procedures** | | |
| **Kidneys, ureters, bladder (KUB)** | X-ray examination of abdomen and pelvis delineates size, shape, and position of kidneys, ureter, and bladder. Radiopaque stones and foreign bodies can be seen. | *Before:* No special preparation needed. |
| **Computed tomography (CT) scan (CT urogram)** | Provides visualization of kidneys, ureters, and bladder. Can detect tumors, abscesses, suprarenal masses (e.g., adrenal tumors), and obstructions. Can be done with or without contrast media. Contrast is iodine based.* | *Before:* Explain procedure to patient. Ask patient about iodine sensitivity. Corticosteroids (prednisone) may be used to prevent an allergic reaction to contrast. *During:* Instruct the patient to lie still during the procedure while the machine takes precise transaxial images. Sedation may be required if patient is unable to cooperate. |
| **Renal arteriogram (angiogram)** | Visualizes renal blood vessels. Can assist in diagnosing renal artery stenosis (Fig. 44-8), additional or missing renal blood vessels, and renovascular hypertension. Can assist in differentiating between a renal cyst and renal tumor. Also included in workup of a potential renal transplant donor. A catheter is inserted into the femoral artery and passed up the aorta to level of renal arteries (Fig. 44-9). Contrast media is injected to outline renal blood supply.* | *Before:* Cathartic or enema may be used the night before. Before injection of contrast material, assess for iodine sensitivity. Tell patient a transient warm feeling may be felt along the course of blood vessel when contrast media is injected. *After:* Place a pressure dressing over femoral artery injection site. Observe site for bleeding and inflammation. Have patient maintain bed rest with affected leg straight. Take peripheral pulses in the involved leg every 30-60 min to detect occlusion of blood flow (from thrombus or emboli). |
| **Renal ultrasound** | Used to detect renal or perirenal masses (tumors, cysts) and obstructions. Small external ultrasound probe is placed on patient's skin. Conductive gel is applied to skin. Noninvasive procedure involves passing sound waves into body structures and recording images as they are reflected back. Computer interprets tissue density based on sound waves and displays it in picture form. It can be used safely in patients with renal failure. | *Before:* Explain procedure to patient. A bowel preparation is not required. *During:* Because radiation exposure is avoided, a number of images can be obtained and repeat studies can be done over a brief period. Images can be obtained from both prone and supine positions. |
| **Intravenous pyelogram (IVP)** | Visualizes urinary tract after IV injection of contrast media. Size and shape of kidneys, ureters, and bladder can be evaluated. Cysts, tumors, and ureteral obstructions (strictures) cause a distortion in normal appearance of these structures. Patient with decreased renal function should not have IVP because contrast media can be nephrotoxic. (Currently procedure is seldom performed.) | *Before:* Cathartic or enema given night before. Assess patient for iodine sensitivity to avoid anaphylactic reaction. *During:* Procedure involves lying on table and having serial x-rays taken. Advise patient that during injection of contrast material, warmth, flushed face, and a salty taste may be experienced. *After:* Force fluids (if permitted) to flush out contrast media. |

**N*-acetylcysteine, a renal vasodilator and antioxidant, is sometimes administered to reduce the incidence of contrast-induced nephropathy; it can be given by oral or IV route.

*Continued*

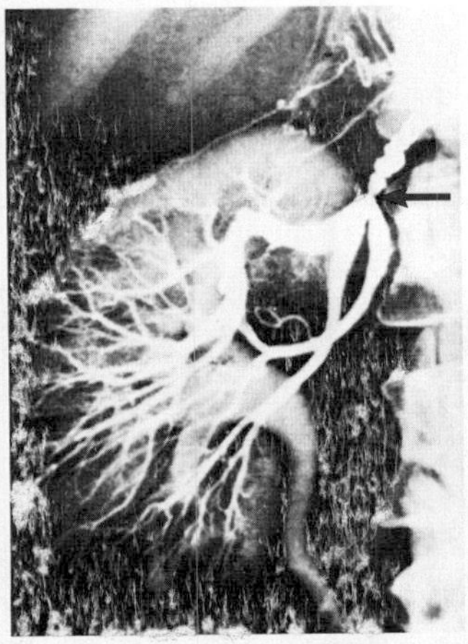

**FIG. 44-8** Renal arteriogram showing stenosis of the right renal artery *(arrow)*. (From Brundage DJ: *Renal disorders,* St Louis, 1992, Mosby.)

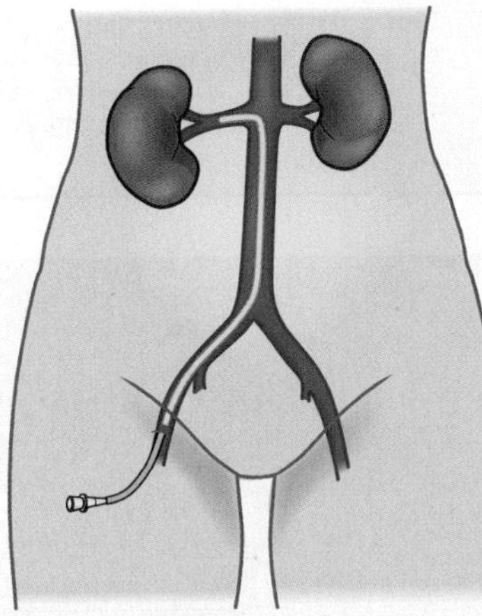

**FIG. 44-9** Catheter insertion for a renal arteriogram.

**TABLE 44-8 Diagnostic Studies**
***Urinary System—cont'd***

| Study | Description and Purpose | Nursing Responsibility |
|---|---|---|
| **Radiologic Procedures—cont'd** | | |
| **Antegrade pyelogram (nephrostogram)** | Evaluates upper urinary tract when patient has allergy to contrast media, decreased renal function, or abnormalities that prevent passage of a ureteral catheter. Contrast media may be injected percutaneously into renal pelvis or via a nephrostomy tube that is already in place when determining tube function or ureteral integrity after trauma or surgery.* | *Before:* Explain procedure and prepare patient as for IVP.<br>*During and after:* Watch for signs of complications (e.g., hematuria, infection, hematoma). |
| **Retrograde pyelogram** | X-ray of urinary tract taken after injection of contrast material into kidneys. It may be done if an IVP does not visualize the urinary tract or if patient is allergic to contrast media or has decreased renal function. A cystoscope is inserted and ureteral catheters are inserted through it into renal pelvis. Contrast media is injected through catheters.* | *Before:* Prepare patient as for IVP. Inform patient that pain may be experienced from distention of pelvis and discomfort from cystoscope. Inform patient that anesthesia may be given for procedure.<br>*After:* Complications are similar to those for cystoscopy (see cystoscopy later in table). |
| **Magnetic resonance imaging (MRI)** | Useful for visualization of kidneys. Not proven useful for detecting urinary calculi or calcified tumors. Computer-generated films rely on radiofrequency waves and alteration in magnetic field. | *Before:* Explain procedure to patient. Have patient remove all metal objects. Patients with a history of claustrophobia may need to be sedated. Contraindications: presence of implanted magnetic clips or prosthesis and pacemakers |
| **Magnetic resonance angiography** | Allows visualization of renal vasculature. Gadolinium-enhanced studies allow visualization of renal artery. | Same as above. Does not require femoral artery puncture |
| **Cystogram** | Visualizes bladder and evaluates vesicoureteral reflux. Evaluates patients with neurogenic bladder and recurrent urinary tract infections. Can also delineate abnormalities of bladder (e.g., diverticula, calculi, tumors). Contrast media is instilled into bladder via cystoscope or catheter. | *Before:* Explain procedure to patient.<br>*During:* If done via cystoscope, follow nursing care related to cystoscopy. |
| **Urethrogram** | Similar to a cystogram. Contrast media is injected retrograde into urethra to identify strictures, diverticula, or other urethral pathologic conditions. When urethral trauma is suspected, a urethrogram is done before catheterization. | *Before:* Explain procedure to patient. |
| **Voiding cystourethrogram (VCUG)** | Voiding study of bladder opening (bladder neck) and urethra. Bladder is filled with contrast media. Fluoroscopic films are taken to visualize bladder and urethra. After urination, another film is taken to assess for residual urine. Can detect abnormalities of lower urinary tract, urethral stenosis, bladder neck obstruction, vesicoureteral reflux, and prostatic enlargement. | *Before:* Explain procedure to patient. |
| **Loopogram** | Detects obstructions, anastomotic leaks, stones, reflux, and other uropathologic features when patient has a urinary pouch or ileal conduit. Because urinary diversions are created with bowel, there is risk of absorption of contrast media. | *Before:* Explain procedure to patient.<br>*During:* Closely monitor patient for reactions to the contrast media. |
| **Endoscopy** | | |
| **Cystoscopy** | Inspects interior of bladder with a tubular lighted scope (cystoscope) (Fig. 44-10). Can be used to insert ureteral catheters, remove calculi, obtain biopsy specimens of bladder lesions, and treat bleeding lesions. Lithotomy position is used. Procedure may be done using local or general anesthesia, depending on patient's needs and condition. Complications include urinary retention, urinary tract hemorrhage, bladder infection, and perforation of bladder. | *Before:* Force fluids or give IV fluids if general anesthesia is to be used. Ensure consent form is signed. Explain procedure to patient. Give preoperative medication.<br>*After:* Explain that burning on urination, pink-tinged urine, and urinary frequency are expected effects. Observe for bright red bleeding, which is not normal. Assist with ambulation because orthostatic hypotension may occur. Offer warm sitz baths, heat, mild analgesics to relieve discomfort. |

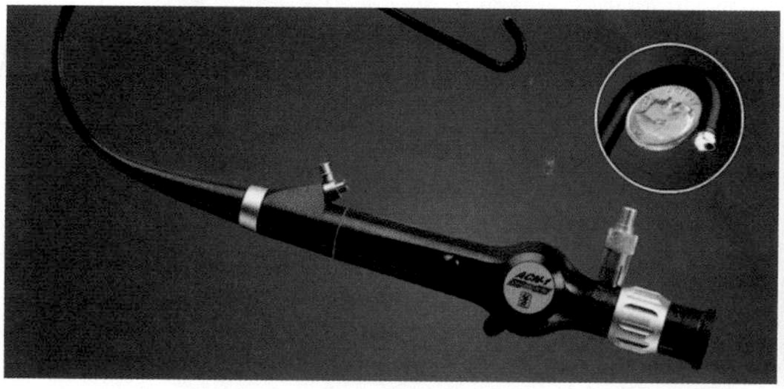
A

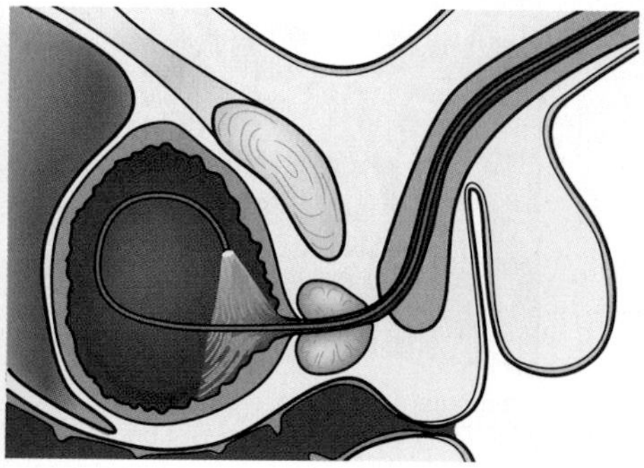
B

**FIG. 44-10** Cystoscopic examination of the bladder in a man. **A,** Flexible cystonephroscope. **B,** Scope inserted into bladder. (*A,* Courtesy Circon Corporation, Santa Barbara, Calif.)

**TABLE 44-8 Diagnostic Studies**

***Urinary System—cont'd***

| Study | Description and Purpose | Nursing Responsibility |
|---|---|---|
| **Urodynamic Studies** | | |
| **Urine flow study (uroflow)** | Measures urine volume in a single voiding expelled in a period of time. Used to (1) assess the degree of outflow obstruction caused by such conditions as BPH or stricture, (2) assess bladder or sphincter dysfunction effects on voiding, and (3) evaluate effects of treatment for lower urinary tract problems. Graphic displays can illustrate straining and intermittent flow patterns or other abnormal voiding disorders.<br>*Normal maximum flow rate:* Men: 20-25 mL/sec; women: 25-30 mL/sec. Volume voided and the patient's age can affect the flow rate. | *Before:* Explain procedure to patient.<br>*During:* Ask the patient to start the test with a comfortably full bladder, urinate into a designated container, and try to empty completely.<br>*After:* Measure residual urine volume immediately after a urinary flow study because this will help identify degree of chronic urinary retention that is often associated with abnormal flow patterns. |
| **Cystometrogram** | Evaluates bladder's capacity to contract and expel urine. Involves insertion of catheter and instillation of water or saline solution into bladder. Measurements of pressure exerted against bladder wall are recorded. If abdominal pressure is measured, a second tube is inserted into rectum or vagina. This tube is attached to a small fluid-filled balloon to allow pressure recording. | *Before:* Explain procedure to patient.<br>*During:* Ask patient about sensations of bladder filling, usually including the first desire (urge) to urinate, a strong desire to urinate, and perception of bladder fullness.<br>*After:* Observe patient for manifestations of urinary tract infection after procedure. |
| **Sphincter electromyography (EMG)** | Recording of electrical activity created when nervous system stimulates muscle tissue. By placing needles, percutaneous wires, or patches near the urethra, pelvic floor muscle activity can be assessed. During the cystometrogram, sphincter EMG is used to identify voluntary pelvic floor muscle contractions and response of these muscles to bladder filling, coughing, and other provocative maneuvers. | *Before:* Explain procedure to patient. |
| **Voiding pressure flow study** | Combines a urinary flow rate, cystometric pressures (intravesical, abdominal, and detrusor pressures), and sphincter EMG for detailed evaluation of micturition. It is completed by assisting the patient to a specialized toilet to urinate while the various pressure tubes and EMG apparatus remain in place. | *Before:* Explain procedure to patient. |
| **Videourodynamics** | Combination of cystometrogram, sphincter EMG, and/or urinary flow study with anatomic imaging of the lower urinary tract, typically via fluoroscopy. Used in selected cases to identify an obstructive lesion and characterize anatomic changes in bladder and lower urinary tract | *Before:* Explain procedure to patient. |
| **Radionuclide cystography (RNC)** | Detects and grades vesicoureteral reflux. Similar to VCUG with a small dose of radioisotope tracer instilled into the bladder via urethral catheter. More sensitive than VCUG, and radiation dose is 1/1000 that of the VCUG. | *Before:* Explain procedure to patient as in VCUG. |
| **Whitaker study** | Measures the pressure differential between renal pelvis and bladder. Ureteral obstruction can be assessed. Percutaneous access is gained to renal pelvis by placing a catheter in renal pelvis. A catheter is also placed in bladder. Fluid is perfused through the percutaneous tube or needle at a rate of 10 mL/min. Pressure data are then collected. Pressure measurements are combined with fluoroscopic imaging to identify the level of obstruction. | *Before:* Explain procedure to patient. |
| **Renal Scan** | Evaluates anatomic structures, perfusion, and function of kidneys. IV radioactive isotopes are injected. Radiation detector probes are placed over kidney and scintillation counter monitors radioactive material in kidney. Radioisotope distribution in kidney is scanned and mapped. Shows location, size, and shape of kidney and assesses blood flow, glomerular filtration, tubular function, and urinary excretion. Abscesses, cysts, and tumors may appear as cold spots because of nonfunctioning tissue. Also monitors function of a transplanted kidney | *Before:* Requires no dietary or activity restriction. Inform patient that no pain or discomfort should be experienced during test. |

*Continued*

## TABLE 44-8 Diagnostic Studies
### Urinary System—cont'd

| Study | Description and Purpose | Nursing Responsibility |
|---|---|---|
| **Renal Biopsy** | Obtains renal tissue for examination to determine type of kidney disease or to follow progress of kidney disease. Technique is usually done as a skin (percutaneous) biopsy through needle insertion into lower lobe of kidney. Can be performed with CT or ultrasound guidance.<br>Absolute contraindications are bleeding disorders, single kidney, and uncontrolled hypertension. Relative contraindications include suspected renal infection, hydronephrosis, and possible vascular lesions. | *Before:* Type and crossmatch patient for blood. Ensure consent form is signed. Assess coagulation status through patient history, medication history, CBC, hematocrit, prothrombin time, and bleeding and clotting time. Patient should not be taking aspirin or warfarin (Coumadin).<br>*After:* Apply pressure dressing and keep patient on affected side for 30-60 min. Bed rest for 24 hr. Vital signs every 5-10 min, first hour. Assess for flank pain, hypotension, decreasing hematocrit, ↑ temperature, chills, urinary frequency, dysuria, and gross or microscopic hematuria. Urine dipstick can be used to test for bleeding in urine. Inspect biopsy site for bleeding. Instruct patient to avoid lifting heavy objects for 5-7 days and to not take anticoagulant drugs until allowed by HCP. |

*BPH,* Benign prostatic hyperplasia, *GFR,* glomerular filtration rate.

## TABLE 44-9 Diagnostic Studies
### Urinalysis

| Test | Normal | Abnormal Finding | Possible Etiology and Significance |
|---|---|---|---|
| **Color** | Amber yellow | Dark, smoky color | Hematuria. |
| | | Yellow-brown to olive green | Excessive bilirubin. |
| | | Orange-red or orange-brown | phenazopyridine (Pyridium). |
| | | Cloudiness of freshly voided urine | Urinary tract infection (UTI). |
| | | Colorless urine | Excessive fluid intake, kidney disease, or diabetes insipidus. |
| **Odor** | Aromatic | Ammonia-like odor | Urine allowed to stand. |
| | | Unpleasant odor | Urinary tract infection. |
| **Protein** | Random protein (dipstick): 0-trace | Persistent proteinuria | Characteristic of acute and chronic kidney disease, especially involving glomeruli. Heart failure. |
| | 24-hr protein (quantitative): <150 mg/day | | In absence of disease: high-protein diet, strenuous exercise, dehydration, fever, emotional stress, contamination by vaginal secretions. |
| **Glucose** | None | Glycosuria | Diabetes mellitus, low renal threshold for glucose reabsorption (if blood glucose level is normal). Pituitary disorders. |
| **Ketones** | None | Present | Altered carbohydrate and fat metabolism in diabetes mellitus and starvation; dehydration, vomiting, severe diarrhea. |
| **Bilirubin** | None | Present | Liver disorders. May appear before jaundice is visible (see Chapter 43). |
| **Specific gravity** | 1.003-1.030 | Low | Dilute urine, excessive diuresis, diabetes insipidus. |
| | Maximum concentrating ability of kidney in morning urine (1.025-1.030) | High | Dehydration, albuminuria, glycosuria. |
| | | Fixed at about 1.010 | Renal inability to concentrate urine; end-stage renal disease. |
| **Osmolality** | 300-1300 mOsm/kg (300-1300 mmol/kg) | <300 mOsm/kg<br>>1300 mOsm/kg | Tubular dysfunction. Kidney lost ability to concentrate or dilute urine (not part of routine urinalysis). |
| **pH** | 4.0-8.0 (average, 6.0) | >8.0 | UTI. Urine allowed to stand at room temperature (bacteria decompose urea to ammonia). |
| | | <4.0 | Respiratory or metabolic acidosis. |
| **RBCs** | 0-4/hpf | >4/hpf | Calculi, cystitis, neoplasm, glomerulonephritis, tuberculosis, kidney biopsy, UTI, trauma. |
| **WBCs** | 0-5/hpf | >5/hpf | UTI or inflammation. |
| **Casts** | None<br>Occasional hyaline | Present | Molds of the renal tubules that may contain protein, WBCs, RBCs, or bacteria. Noncellular casts (hyaline in appearance) occasionally found in normal urine. |
| **Culture for organisms** | No organisms in bladder<br>$<10^4$ organisms/mL result of normal urethral flora | Bacteria counts $>10^5$/mL | Urinary tract infection; most common organisms are *Escherichia coli*, enterococci, *Klebsiella*, *Proteus*, and streptococci. |

*hpf,* High-powered field.

from the urinalysis may indicate possible abnormalities, suggest the need for further studies, or provide evidence of progression in a previously diagnosed disorder.

Although a specimen may be collected at any time of the day for a routine urinalysis, it is best to obtain the first specimen urinated in the morning. This concentrated specimen is more likely to contain abnormal constituents if they are present in the urine. The specimen should be examined within 1 hour of urinating. Otherwise, bacteria multiply rapidly, RBCs hemolyze, *casts* (molds of renal tubules) disintegrate, and the urine becomes alkaline as a result of urea-splitting bacteria. If it is not possible to send the specimen to the laboratory immediately, refrigerate it. However, to obtain the best results, coordinate specimen collection with routine laboratory hours.

**Creatinine Clearance.** A common test used to analyze urinary system disorders is creatinine clearance. **Creatinine** is a waste product produced by muscle breakdown. Urinary excretion of creatinine is a measure of the amount of active muscle tissue in the body, not of body weight. Therefore individuals with larger muscle mass have higher values. Because almost all creatinine in the blood is normally excreted by the kidneys, creatinine clearance is the most accurate indicator of renal function. The result of a creatinine clearance test closely approximates that of the GFR. A blood specimen for serum creatinine determination should be obtained during the period of urine collection.

Creatinine levels remain remarkably constant for each person because they are not significantly affected by protein ingestion, muscular exercise, water intake, or rate of urine production. Normal creatinine clearance values range from 70 to 135 mL/min (Table 44-8). After age 40, the creatinine clearance rate decreases at a rate of about 1 mL/min/yr.

### Urodynamic Studies

*Urodynamic studies* measure urinary tract function. Urodynamic tests study the storage of urine within the bladder and the flow of urine through the urinary tract to the outside of the body.[7] A combination of techniques may be used for a detailed assessment of urinary function (Table 44-8).

## CASE STUDY—cont'd

### *Objective Data: Diagnostic Studies*

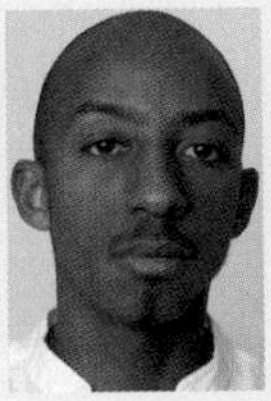

(©iStockphoto/ Thinkstock)

The HCP orders the following initial diagnostic studies for A.K.:

- CBC, basic metabolic panel (electrolytes, BUN, creatinine)
- Urinalysis, culture if indicated
- Renal ultrasound

Although A.K.'s laboratory results are all within normal limits, his renal ultrasound identifies calculi in the left ureter. There is no hydronephrosis at present. The HCP prescribes IV opioids for pain management and admits A.K. to a medical unit for further observation.

**Discussion Questions**

1. Which diagnostic study results are abnormal?
2. Which diagnostic study results are of most concern to you?

Answers available at *http://evolve.elsevier.com/Lewis/medsurg.*

## BRIDGE TO NCLEX EXAMINATION

The number of the question corresponds to the same-numbered outcome at the beginning of the chapter.

1. A renal stone in the pelvis of the kidney will alter the function of the kidney by interfering with the
   - **a.** structural support of the kidney.
   - **b.** regulation of the concentration of urine.
   - **c.** entry and exit of blood vessels at the kidney.
   - **d.** collection and drainage of urine from the kidney.
2. A patient with kidney disease has oliguria and a creatinine clearance of 40 mL/min. These findings most directly reflect abnormal function of
   - **a.** tubular secretion.
   - **b.** glomerular filtration.
   - **c.** capillary permeability.
   - **d.** concentration of filtrate.
3. The nurse identifies a risk for urinary calculi in a patient who relates a past health history that includes
   - **a.** hyperaldosteronism.
   - **b.** serotonin deficiency.
   - **c.** adrenal insufficiency.
   - **d.** hyperparathyroidism.
4. Diminished ability to concentrate urine, associated with aging of the urinary system, is attributed to
   - **a.** a decrease in bladder sensory receptors.
   - **b.** a decrease in the number of functioning nephrons.
   - **c.** decreased function of the loop of Henle and tubules.
   - **d.** thickening of the basement membrane of Bowman's capsule.
5. During physical assessment of the urinary system, the nurse
   - **a.** cannot palpate the left kidney
   - **b.** palpates an empty bladder as a small nodule.
   - **c.** finds a dull percussion sound when 100 mL of urine is present in the bladder.
   - **d.** palpates above the symphysis pubis to determine the level of urine in the bladder.
6. Normal findings expected by the nurse on physical assessment of the urinary system include *(select all that apply)*
   - **a.** nonpalpable left kidney.
   - **b.** auscultation of renal artery bruit.
   - **c.** CVA tenderness elicited by a kidney punch.
   - **d.** no CVA tenderness elicited by a kidney punch.
   - **e.** palpable bladder to the level of the pubic symphysis.
7. A diagnostic study that indicates renal blood flow, glomerular filtration, tubular function, and excretion is a(n)
   - **a.** IVP.
   - **b.** VCUG.
   - **c.** renal scan.
   - **d.** loopogram.
8. On reading the urinalysis results of a dehydrated patient, the nurse would expect to find
   - **a.** a pH of 8.4.
   - **b.** RBCs of 4/hpf.
   - **c.** color: yellow, cloudy.
   - **d.** specific gravity of 1.035.

1. d, 2. b, 3. d, 4. c, 5. a, 6. a, d, 7. c, 8. d

For rationales to these answers and even more NCLEX review questions, visit *http://evolve.elsevier.com/Lewis/medsurg.*

## EVOLVE WEBSITE

http://evolve.elsevier.com/Lewis/medsurg
**Review Questions (Online Only)**
**Key Points**
**Answer Keys for Questions**
- Rationales for Bridge to NCLEX Examination Questions
- Answer Guidelines for Case Study on pp. 1020, 1023, 1024 and 1031

**Conceptual Care Map Creator**
**Audio Glossary**
**Content Updates**

## REFERENCES


1. Baldea AJ: Effect of aging on renal function plus monitoring and support, *Surg Clin North Am* 95(1):71, 2015.
2. Wang X, Bonventre JV, Parrish AR: The aging kidney: increased susceptibility to nephrotoxicity, *Int J Mol Sci* 15(9):15358, 2014.
3. Verma V, Kant R, Sunnoqrot N, et al: Proteinuria in the elderly: evaluation and management, *Int Urol Nephrol* 44(6):1745, 2012.
4. DeSouza K, Chowdhury S, Hughes S: Prompt diagnosis key in bladder cancer, *Practitioner* 258(1767):23, 2014.
5. Jarvis C: *Physical examination and health assessment*, ed 7, St Louis, 2016, Saunders.
6. Prasad V, Gandhi D, Stokum C, et al: Incidence of contrast material-induced nephropathy after neuroendovascular procedures, *Radiology* 273(3):853, 2014.
7. Danforth TL, Ginsberg DA: Neurogenic lower urinary tract dysfunction: how, when, and with which patients do we use urodynamics? *Urol Clin North Am* 41(3):445, 2014.

# 45

# Renal and Urologic Problems

*Suzanne Teresa Parsell*

*Happiness is never stopping to think if you are.*

*Palmer Sondreal*

http://evolve.elsevier.com/Lewis/medsurg/

## LEARNING OUTCOMES

1. Differentiate the pathophysiology, clinical manifestations, interprofessional care, and drug therapy of cystitis, urethritis, and pyelonephritis.
2. Explain the nursing management of urinary tract infections.
3. Describe the immunologic mechanisms involved in glomerulonephritis.
4. Differentiate the clinical manifestations and nursing and interprofessional management of acute poststreptococcal glomerulonephritis, Goodpasture syndrome, and chronic glomerulonephritis.
5. Describe the common causes, clinical manifestations, interprofessional care, and nursing management of nephrotic syndrome.
6. Compare and contrast the etiology, clinical manifestations, interprofessional care, and nursing management of various types of urinary calculi.
7. Differentiate the common causes and management of renal trauma, renal vascular problems, and hereditary kidney diseases.
8. Describe the clinical manifestations and nursing and interprofessional management of kidney cancer and bladder cancer.
9. Describe the common causes and management of urinary incontinence and urinary retention.
10. Differentiate among urethral, ureteral, suprapubic, and nephrostomy catheters with regard to indications for use and nursing responsibilities.
11. Explain the nursing management of the patient undergoing nephrectomy or urinary diversion surgery.

## KEY TERMS

calculus, p. 1045
cystitis, p. 1034
glomerulonephritis, p. 1041
Goodpasture syndrome, p. 1043
hydronephrosis, p. 1044
hydroureter, p. 1044
ileal conduit, p. 1064
interstitial cystitis (IC), p. 1040
lithotripsy, p. 1047
nephrolithiasis, p. 1045
nephrosclerosis, p. 1050
nephrotic syndrome, p. 1043
polycystic kidney disease (PKD), p. 1051
pyelonephritis, p. 1034
renal artery stenosis, p. 1050
stricture, p. 1049
urethritis, p. 1034
urinary incontinence (UI), p. 1055
urinary retention, p. 1059
urosepsis, p. 1034

Renal and urologic disorders encompass a wide spectrum of problems. The diverse causes of these disorders may involve infectious, immunologic, obstructive, metabolic, collagen-vascular, traumatic, congenital, neoplastic, and neurologic mechanisms. This chapter discusses specific disorders of the upper urinary tract (kidneys and ureter) and lower urinary tract (bladder and urethra). Acute kidney injury and chronic kidney disease are discussed in Chapter 46.

## INFECTIOUS AND INFLAMMATORY DISORDERS OF URINARY SYSTEM

### URINARY TRACT INFECTION

*Urinary tract infections (UTIs)* are the most common bacterial infection in women.[1] Inflammation of the urinary tract may be caused by a variety of disorders, but bacterial infection is by far the most common. The bladder and its contents are free from bacteria in the majority of healthy people. Nevertheless, a minority of otherwise healthy individuals have some bacteria colonizing the bladder. This condition is called *asymptomatic bacteriuria* and does not justify screening or treatment except in pregnant women.

*Escherichia coli* (*E. coli*) is the most common pathogen causing a UTI (Table 45-1) and is seen primarily in women.[2] Bacterial counts of $10^5$ colony-forming units per milliliter (CFU/mL) or higher typically indicate a clinically significant UTI. However, counts as low as $10^2$ to $10^3$ CFU/mL in a person with signs and symptoms are indicative of UTI.

Although fungal and parasitic infections may also cause UTIs, this is uncommon. UTIs from these causes are sometimes found in patients who are immunosuppressed, have diabetes mellitus, have kidney problems, or have undergone multiple courses of antibiotic therapy. These types of UTIs may also be

Reviewed by Janie Corbitt, RN, MLS, Retired Instructor of Nursing, Milledgeville, Georgia; Rowena W. Elliott, RN, PhD, CNN, CNE, AGNP-C, FAAN, Associate Professor, University of Southern Mississippi, College of Nursing, Hattiesburg, Mississippi; Deborah Erickson, RN, PhD, Associate Professor and Graduate Coordinator, Department of Nursing, Bradley University, Peoria, Illinois; Shari Gould, RN, MSN, Associate Professor of Nursing, Victoria College, Victoria, Texas; and Marci Langenkamp, RN, MS, Associate Professor of Nursing, Edison Community College, Piqua, Ohio.

found in persons who live in or have traveled to certain developing countries.

## Classification of Urinary Tract Infection

A UTI can be broadly classified as an upper or lower UTI according to its location within the urinary system (Fig. 45-1). Infection of the upper urinary tract (involving the renal parenchyma, pelvis, and ureters) typically causes fever, chills, and flank pain, whereas a UTI confined to the lower urinary tract does not usually have systemic manifestations.

Specific terms are used to further delineate the location of a UTI. For example, **pyelonephritis** implies inflammation (usually caused by infection) of the renal parenchyma and collecting system, **cystitis** indicates inflammation of the bladder, and **urethritis** means inflammation of the urethra. **Urosepsis** is a UTI that has spread systemically and is a life-threatening condition requiring emergency treatment.

Classifying a UTI as complicated or uncomplicated is also useful. *Uncomplicated* UTIs occur in an otherwise normal urinary tract and usually only involve the bladder. *Complicated* UTIs include those infections in which the patient has coexisting obstruction, stones, or catheters; abnormal GU tract; or diabetes or neurologic diseases. They can also occur when a person has developed resistance to antibiotics, is immunocompromised, or has pregnancy-induced changes. The term *complicated UTI* also applies to a recurrent infection. The individual with a complicated infection is at risk for pyelonephritis, urosepsis, and renal damage.

### CULTURAL & ETHNIC HEALTH DISPARITIES

***Urologic Disorders***

- Urinary tract calculi are more common among whites than African Americans.
- Uric acid stones are more common in Jewish men.
- Bladder cancer has a higher incidence among white men than African American men.
- In all ethnic groups, bladder cancer affects men about three times more often than women.
- Urinary incontinence is underreported because culturally it is seen as a social hygiene problem causing patient embarrassment.

### TABLE 45-1 Causes of Urinary Tract Infections

- *Escherichia coli**
- *Enterococcus*
- *Klebsiella*
- *Enterobacter*
- *Proteus*
- *Pseudomonas*
- *Staphylococcus*
- *Serratia*
- *Candida albicans*†

*Causative microorganism for urinary tract infection (UTI) in 80% of cases without urinary tract structural abnormalities or calculi.
†Typically identified as the causative microorganism for UTI associated with the use of broad-spectrum antibiotic therapy or in patients with an indwelling catheter.

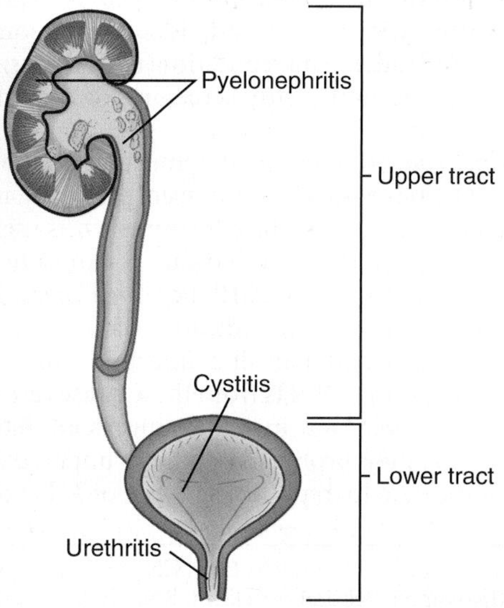


**FIG. 45-1** Sites of infectious processes in the upper and lower urinary tracts.

## Etiology and Pathophysiology

The urinary tract above the urethra is normally sterile. Several mechanical and physiologic defense mechanisms assist in maintaining sterility and preventing UTIs. These defenses include normal voiding with complete emptying of the bladder, ureterovesical junction competence, and ureteral peristaltic activity that propels urine toward the bladder. Antibacterial characteristics of urine are maintained by an acidic pH (less than 6.0), high urea concentration, and abundant glycoproteins that interfere with the growth of bacteria. An alteration in any of these defense mechanisms increases the risk for a UTI (Table 45-2).

The organisms that usually cause UTIs are introduced via the ascending route from the urethra and originate in the perineum. Most infections are caused by gram-negative bacilli normally found in the gastrointestinal (GI) tract. However, gram-positive organisms such as streptococci, enterococci, and *Staphylococcus saprophyticus* can also cause UTIs.

A common factor contributing to ascending infection is urologic instrumentation (e.g., catheterization, cystoscopic examinations). Instrumentation allows bacteria that are normally present at the opening of the urethra to enter into the urethra or bladder. Sexual intercourse promotes "milking" of bacteria from the vagina and perineum and may cause minor urethral trauma that predisposes women to UTIs.

Rarely do UTIs result from a hematogenous route, where blood-borne bacteria secondarily invade the kidneys, ureters, or bladder from elsewhere in the body. There must be prior injury to the urinary tract, such as obstruction of the ureter, damage caused by stones, or renal scars, for a kidney infection to occur from hematogenous transmission.

*Catheter-associated urinary tract infections (CAUTIs)* are the most common health care–associated infection (HAI). The cause of CAUTIs is often *E. coli* and, less frequently, *Pseudomonas* organisms. Most often these infections are underrecognized and undertreated, leading to extended hospital stays, increased health care costs, and patient morbidity and mortality.[3]

## Clinical Manifestations

Clinical manifestations of UTIs range from painful urination in uncomplicated urethritis or cystitis to severe systemic illness associated with abdominal or back pain, fever, sepsis, and decreased kidney function in some cases of pyelonephritis.

*Lower urinary tract symptoms* are experienced in patients who have UTIs of the upper urinary tract, as well as those confined to the lower tract. Symptoms are related to either bladder storage or bladder emptying. These symptoms are presented in Table 45-3.

**TABLE 45-2 Risk Factors for Urinary Tract Infections**

***Factors Increasing Urinary Stasis***

- Intrinsic obstruction (stone, tumor of urinary tract, urethral stricture, BPH)
- Extrinsic obstruction (tumor, fibrosis compressing urinary tract)
- Urinary retention (e.g., neurogenic bladder)
- Renal impairment

**Foreign Bodies**

- Urinary tract calculi
- Catheters (indwelling, external condom catheter, ureteral stent, nephrostomy tube, intermittent catheterization)
- Urinary tract instrumentation (cystoscopy)

**Anatomic Factors**

- Congenital defects leading to obstruction or urinary stasis
- Fistula (abnormal opening) exposing urinary stream to skin, vagina, or fecal stream
- Shorter female urethra and colonization from normal vaginal flora
- Obesity

**Factors Compromising Immune Response**

- Aging
- Human immunodeficiency virus infection
- Diabetes mellitus

**Functional Disorders**

- Constipation
- Voiding dysfunction with detrusor sphincter dyssynergia

**Other Factors**

- Pregnancy
- Menopause
- Multiple sex partners (women)
- Use of spermicidal agents, contraceptive diaphragm (women), bubble baths, feminine sprays
- Poor personal hygiene
- Habitual delay of urination ("nurse's bladder," "teacher's bladder")

These symptoms include dysuria, frequent urination (more than every 2 hours), urgency, and suprapubic discomfort or pressure. The urine may contain grossly visible blood (hematuria) or sediment, giving it a cloudy appearance. Flank pain, chills, and fever indicate an infection involving the upper urinary tract (pyelonephritis). People with significant bacteriuria may have no symptoms or may have nonspecific symptoms such as fatigue or anorexia.

Remember that these symptoms, considered characteristic of a UTI, are often absent in older adults. Older adults tend to experience nonlocalized abdominal discomfort rather than dysuria and suprapubic pain. In addition, they may have cognitive impairment or generalized clinical deterioration. Because older adults are less likely to experience a fever with a UTI, the value of body temperature as an indicator of a UTI is unreliable.[4]

Multiple factors may produce LUTS similar to the symptoms of a UTI. For example, patients with bladder tumors or those receiving intravesical chemotherapy or pelvic radiation usually experience urinary frequency, urgency, and dysuria. Interstitial cystitis/painful bladder syndrome (discussed on pp. 1040-1041) also produces urinary symptoms that are similar to and sometimes confused with a UTI.

**TABLE 45-3 Lower Urinary Tract Symptoms (LUTS)**

| Symptoms | Description |
|---|---|
| **Emptying Symptoms** | |
| **Hesitancy** | • Difficulty starting urine stream<br>• Delay between initiation of urination (because of urethral sphincter relaxation) and beginning of flow of urine<br>• Diminished urinary stream |
| **Intermittency** | • Interruption of urinary stream while voiding |
| **Postvoid dribbling** | • Urine loss after completion of voiding |
| **Urinary retention or incomplete emptying** | • Inability to empty urine from bladder<br>• Caused by atonic bladder or obstruction of urethra<br>• Can be acute or chronic |
| **Dysuria** | • Painful or difficult urination |
| **Storage Symptoms** | |
| **Urinary frequency** | • More than eight times in 24-hr period<br>• Often <200 mL each voiding |
| **Urgency** | • Sudden, strong, or intense desire to void immediately<br>• Commonly accompanied by frequency |
| **Incontinence** | • Involuntary or accidental urine loss or leakage |
| **Nocturia** | • Awakened by urge to void two or more times during sleep<br>• May be diurnal or nocturnal depending on sleep schedule |
| **Nocturnal enuresis** | • Adults: loss of urine during sleep |

## Diagnostic Studies

In a patient suspected of having a UTI, initially obtain a dipstick urinalysis to identify the presence of nitrites (indicating bacteriuria), white blood cells (WBCs), and leukocyte esterase (an enzyme present in WBCs, indicating pyuria). These findings can be confirmed by microscopic urinalysis. After confirmation of bacteriuria and pyuria, a urine culture may be obtained. A urine culture is indicated in complicated or HAI UTIs, persistent bacteriuria, or frequently recurring UTIs (more than two or three episodes per year). Urine may also be cultured when the infection is unresponsive to empiric therapy or the diagnosis is questionable.

A voided midstream technique *(clean-catch urine sample)* is preferred for obtaining a urine culture in most circumstances. For women, teach them to spread the labia and wipe the periurethral area from front to back using a moistened, clean gauze sponge (no antiseptic is used because it could contaminate the specimen and cause false positives). Instruct them to keep the labia spread, start voiding, and collect the specimen 1 to 2 seconds after voiding starts. For men, instruct them to wipe the glans penis around the urethra and collect the specimen 1 to 2 seconds after voiding begins.

Refrigerate urine immediately on collection. The urine should be cultured within 24 hours of refrigeration. A specimen obtained by catheterization provides more accurate results than a clean-catch specimen. When an adequate clean-catch specimen cannot be readily obtained, a catheterization may be necessary.

A urine culture is accompanied by *sensitivity testing* to determine the bacteria's susceptibility to a variety of antibiotic drugs. The results of this test allow the HCP to select an antibiotic known to be capable of destroying the bacteria causing a UTI in a specific patient.

Imaging studies of the urinary tract are indicated in selected cases. An ultrasound or CT scan (CT urogram) may be obtained when obstruction of the urinary system is suspected or UTIs recur.

### Interprofessional Care

Once a UTI has been diagnosed, appropriate antimicrobial therapy is initiated. An antibiotic may be selected based on the HCP's best judgment *(empiric therapy)* or the results of sensitivity testing.

The interprofessional care and drug therapy of UTIs are summarized in Table 45-4. Uncomplicated cystitis can be treated using a short-term course of antibiotics, typically for 3 days. In contrast, complicated UTIs require treatment for a longer period of time, lasting 7 to 14 days or more.[7,8]

Many residents of long-term care facilities, especially women, have chronic asymptomatic bacteriuria. However, usually only symptomatic UTIs are treated.

First-choice drugs to empirically treat uncomplicated or initial UTIs are trimethoprim/sulfamethoxazole (Bactrim), nitrofurantoin (Macrodantin), and fosfomycin (Monurol).[5] Trimethoprim/sulfamethoxazole has the advantages of being relatively inexpensive and taken twice daily. A disadvantage is *E. coli* resistance to trimethoprim/sulfamethoxazole, which is an increasing problem in the United States. Nitrofurantoin is normally given three or four times daily, but a long-acting preparation (Macrobid) is available that is taken twice daily.

Other antibiotics that may be used to treat uncomplicated UTI include ampicillin, amoxicillin, and cephalosporins. The fluoroquinolones are used to treat complicated UTIs. These drugs include ciprofloxacin (Cipro), levofloxacin (Levaquin), ofloxacin, and gatifloxacin. In patients with UTIs secondary to fungi, amphotericin or fluconazole (Diflucan) is the preferred therapy.

**DRUG ALERT Nitrofurantoin (Furadantin, Macrodantin)**
- Avoid sunlight. Use sunscreen and wear protective clothing.
- Notify HCP immediately if fever, chills, cough, chest pain, dyspnea, rash, or numbness or tingling of fingers or toes develops.

A urinary analgesic such as oral phenazopyridine may relieve discomfort caused by severe dysuria. Phenazopyridine is an azo dye excreted in urine, where it exerts a topical analgesic effect on the urinary tract mucosa. Teach patients that this drug causes the urine to turn orange or red.

*Prophylactic* or *suppressive antibiotics* are sometimes given to patients who have repeated UTIs. A low dose of TMP/SMX, nitrofurantoin, or another antibiotic may be taken daily to prevent recurring UTIs, or a single dose may be taken before an event likely to provoke a UTI, such as sexual intercourse. Although suppressive therapy is often effective on a short-term basis, this strategy is limited because of the risk of antibiotic resistance, which ultimately leads to breakthrough infections with increasingly virulent pathogens.

**TABLE 45-4 Interprofessional Care**

***Urinary Tract Infection***

**Diagnostic Assessment**
- History and physical examination
- Urinalysis (obtain midstream, "clean-catch" voided specimen)
- Urine for culture and sensitivity (if indicated)
- Imaging studies of urinary tract (if indicated): CT scan (CT urogram), ultrasound, cystoscopy

**Management**

***Uncomplicated UTI***
- Patient teaching
- Adequate fluid intake (six 8-oz glasses/day)

*Drug Therapy*
- Phenazopyridine
- Antibiotics
  - trimethoprim/sulfamethoxazole (Bactrim)
  - trimethoprim alone (in patients with sulfa allergy)
  - nitrofurantoin (Macrodantin, Macrobid)
  - fosfomycin (Monurol)

***Recurrent UTI***
- Repeat urinalysis
- Urine culture and sensitivity testing
- Adequate fluid intake (six 8-oz glasses/day)
- Repeat patient teaching
- Imaging studies of urinary tract (if indicated): see above

*Drug Therapy*
- Antibiotic: trimethoprim/sulfamethoxazole, nitrofurantoin
- Sensitivity-guided antibiotic therapy: ampicillin, amoxicillin, first-generation cephalosporin, fluoroquinolones
- Consider 3- to 6-mo trial of suppressive or prophylactic antibiotic regimen
- Consider postcoital antibiotic prophylaxis: trimethoprim/sulfamethoxazole, nitrofurantoin, cephalexin

## NURSING MANAGEMENT: URINARY TRACT INFECTION

### Nursing Assessment

Subjective and objective data that should be obtained from a patient with a UTI are presented in Table 45-5.

### Nursing Diagnoses

Nursing diagnoses for the patient with a UTI may include, but are not limited to, the following:
- Impaired urinary elimination *related to* the effects of UTI
- Readiness for enhanced health management

Additional information on nursing diagnoses for the patient with a UTI is presented in eNursing Care Plan 45-1 (available on the website for this chapter).

### Planning

The overall goals are that the patient with a UTI will have (1) relief from bothersome, (2) no upper urinary tract involvement, and (3) no recurrence.

### Nursing Implementation

**Health Promotion.** It is important to recognize individuals who are at risk for a UTI. These people include debilitated persons, older adults, patients who are immunocompromised (e.g., cancer, human immunodeficiency virus [HIV], diabetes mellitus), and patients treated with immunosuppressive drugs or corticosteroids. Health promotion activities, particularly for these individuals, can help decrease the frequency of infections and provide for early detection of infection. Health promotion activities include teaching preventive measures such as (1) emptying the bladder regularly and completely,

**TABLE 45-5 Nursing Assessment**

***Urinary Tract Infection***

**Subjective Data**

***Important Health Information***

*Past health history:* Previous urinary tract infection. Urinary calculi, reflux, strictures, or retention. Neurogenic bladder, pregnancy, benign prostatic hyperplasia, bladder cancer, sexually transmitted infection.

*Medications:* Antibiotics, anticholinergics, antispasmodics

*Surgery or other treatments:* Recent urologic instrumentation (catheterization, cystoscopy)

***Functional Health Patterns***

*Health perception–health management:* Urinary hygiene practices. Lassitude, malaise

*Nutritional-metabolic:* Nausea, vomiting, anorexia. Chills

*Elimination:* Urinary frequency, urgency, hesitancy. Dysuria, nocturia

*Cognitive-perceptual:* Suprapubic or low back pain, costovertebral tenderness, bladder spasms, dysuria, burning on urination

*Sexuality-reproductive:* Multiple sex partners (women), use of spermicidal agents or contraceptive diaphragm (women)

**Objective Data**

***General***

Fever, chills, dysuria

Atypical presentation in older adults: afebrile, absence of dysuria, loss of appetite, altered mental status

***Urinary***

Hematuria. Cloudy, foul-smelling urine. Tender, enlarged kidney

***Possible Diagnostic Findings***

Leukocytosis. UA positive for bacteria, pyuria, RBCs, WBCs, and nitrites. Positive urine culture. Ultrasound, CT scan (CT urogram), VCUG, and cystoscopy indicating urinary tract abnormalities

*VCUG,* Voiding cystourethrogram.

(2) evacuating the bowel regularly, (3) wiping the perineal area from front to back after urination and defecation, and (4) drinking an adequate amount of liquid each day.

To estimate the amount of fluid intake a person should have in 24 hours, take the person's weight in pounds and divide that number in half. The result is the number of ounces of fluid a person should have per day. Thus a 150-pound person would require 75 oz/day. The person will obtain about 20% of this fluid from food, which leaves 60 oz (1775 mL) obtained by drinking, or just over seven 8-oz glasses of fluid.

Daily intake of cranberry juice or cranberry tablets or capsules may reduce the number of UTIs. It is thought that enzymes found in cranberries inhibit attachment of urinary pathogens (especially *E. coli*) to the bladder wall.[6]

Routine and thorough perineal hygiene is important for all hospitalized patients, especially when a bedpan is used, after a bowel movement, or if fecal incontinence is present. Answer call lights quickly and offer the bedpan or urinal to bedridden patients at frequent intervals. These measures can prevent incontinence and decrease the number of incontinent episodes.

◆ ***Prevention of CAUTI.*** All patients undergoing instrumentation of the urinary tract are at risk for developing CAUTI. You have a major role in the prevention of these infections. Avoidance of unnecessary catheterization and early removal of indwelling catheters are the most effective means for reducing CAUTI. Always follow aseptic technique during these procedures. Wash your hands before and after contact with each patient. Wear gloves for care of urinary catheters. The American Nurses Association offers an evidenced-based clinical tool for decreasing CAUTI *(http://nursingworld.org/CAUTI-Tool).* Special measures for the care of urethral catheters are discussed in Table 45-21 later in this chapter on p. 1062.

◆ **Acute Care.** Acute care for a patient with a UTI includes ensuring adequate fluid intake if it is not contraindicated. Maintaining adequate fluid intake may be difficult because of the patient's perception that fluid intake will worsen the discomfort and urinary frequency associated with a UTI. Tell patients that fluids will increase frequency of urination at first but will also dilute the urine, making the bladder less irritable. Fluids will help flush out bacteria before they have a chance to colonize in the bladder. Caffeine, alcohol, citrus juices, chocolate, and highly spiced foods or beverages should be avoided because they are potential bladder irritants.

Application of local heat to the suprapubic area or lower back may relieve the discomfort associated with a UTI. Advise the patient to apply a heating pad (turned to its lowest setting) against the back or suprapubic area. A warm shower or sitting in a tub of warm water filled above the waist can also provide temporary relief.

Instruct the patient about the prescribed drug therapy, including side effects. Emphasize the importance of taking the full course of antibiotics. Often patients stop antibiotic therapy once symptoms disappear. This can lead to inadequate treatment and recurrence of infection or bacterial resistance to antibiotics.

Sometimes a second drug or a reduced dosage of drug is ordered after the initial course to suppress bacterial growth in patients susceptible to recurrent UTI. Instruct the patient to monitor for signs of improvement (e.g., cloudy urine becomes clear) and a decrease in or cessation of symptoms. Teach patients to promptly report any of the following to their HCP: (1) persistence of bothersome LUTS beyond the antibiotic treatment course, (2) onset of flank pain, or (3) fever.

◆ **Ambulatory Care.** Home care for the patient with a UTI should emphasize the importance of adhering to the drug regimen. Your responsibility is to teach the patient and caregiver about the need for ongoing care (Table 45-6). This includes taking

**TABLE 45-6 Patient & Caregiver Teaching**

***Urinary Tract Infection***

*When teaching a patient and caregiver measures to prevent a recurrence of a urinary tract infection (UTI), include the following.*

1. Take all antibiotics as prescribed. Symptoms may improve after 1-2 days of therapy, but organisms may still be present.
2. Practice appropriate hygiene, including the following:
   - Carefully clean the perineal region by separating the labia when cleansing.
   - Wipe from front to back after urinating.
   - Cleanse with warm soapy water after each bowel movement.
3. Empty the bladder before and after sexual intercourse.
4. Urinate regularly, approximately every 3-4 hr during the day.
5. Maintain adequate fluid intake.
6. Avoid vaginal douches and harsh soaps, bubble baths, powders, and sprays in the perineal area.
7. Report to the HCP symptoms or signs of recurrent UTI (e.g., fever, cloudy urine, pain on urination, urgency, frequency).
8. Consider drinking unsweetened cranberry juice (8 oz three times a day) or taking cranberry extract tablets 300-400 mg/day for UTI prevention. (This practice may not be effective with every patient.)

antimicrobial drugs as ordered, maintaining adequate daily fluid intake, voiding regularly (approximately every 3 to 4 hours), urinating before and after intercourse, and temporarily discontinuing the use of a diaphragm.

If treatment is complete and the symptoms are still present, instruct the patient to get follow-up care. Recurrent symptoms because of bacterial persistence or inadequate treatment typically occur within 1 to 2 weeks after completion of therapy. If the patient has followed the treatment regimen, a relapse indicates the need for further evaluation.

### ◆ Evaluation

The expected outcomes are that the patient with a UTI will

- Experience normal urinary elimination patterns
- Report relief of bothersome urinary tract symptoms
- Verbalize knowledge of treatment regimen

Additional information on the expected outcomes for the patient with a UTI is presented in eNursing Care Plan 45-1 (available on the website for this chapter).

## ACUTE PYELONEPHRITIS

### Etiology and Pathophysiology

*Pyelonephritis* is an inflammation of the renal parenchyma (Fig. 45-2) and collecting system (including the renal pelvis). The most common cause is bacterial infection, but fungi, protozoa, or viruses can also infect the kidney.[7]

*Urosepsis* is a systemic infection arising from a urologic source. Its prompt diagnosis and effective treatment are critical because it can lead to septic shock and death unless promptly treated. (Septic shock is discussed in Chapter 65.)

Pyelonephritis usually begins with colonization and infection of the lower urinary tract via the ascending urethral route. Bacteria normally found in the intestinal tract, such as *E. coli* or *Proteus, Klebsiella,* or *Enterobacter* species, frequently cause pyelonephritis. A preexisting factor is often present such as *vesicoureteral reflux* (retrograde [backward] movement of urine from lower to upper urinary tract) or dysfunction of the lower urinary tract (e.g., obstruction from benign prostatic hyperplasia [BPH], stricture, urinary stone). For residents of long-term care facilities, CAUTI is a common cause of pyelonephritis and urosepsis.

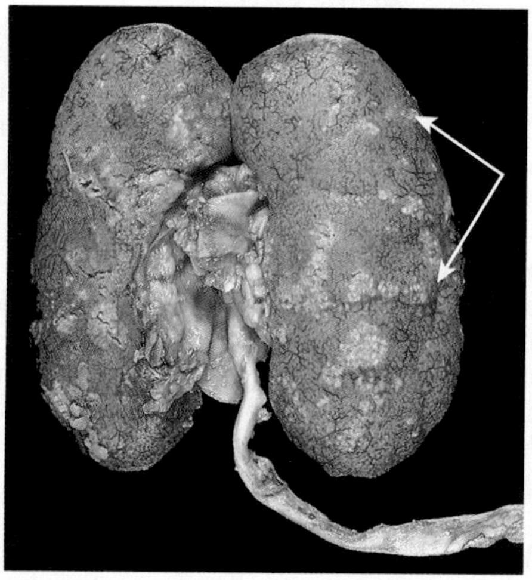

**FIG. 45-2** Acute pyelonephritis. Cortical surface shows grayish white areas of inflammation and abscess formation *(arrows)*. (From Kumar V, Abbas AK, Aster JC, et al: *Robbins and Cotran pathologic basis of disease,* ed 8, Philadelphia, 2010, Saunders.)

Acute pyelonephritis commonly starts in the renal medulla and spreads to the adjacent cortex. One of the most important risk factors for acute pyelonephritis is pregnancy-induced physiologic changes in the urinary system. Recurring episodes of pyelonephritis, especially in the presence of obstructive abnormalities, can lead to *chronic pyelonephritis* (discussed later).

### Clinical Manifestations and Diagnostic Studies

The clinical manifestations of acute pyelonephritis vary from mild fatigue to the sudden onset of chills; fever; vomiting; malaise; flank pain; and the LUTS characteristic of cystitis, including dysuria, urgency, and frequency. *Costovertebral tenderness* to percussion (costovertebral angle [CVA] pain) is typically present on the affected side. Although the clinical manifestations may subside within a few days, even without specific therapy, bacteriuria and pyuria usually persist.

Urinalysis results indicate pyuria, bacteriuria, and varying degrees of hematuria. WBC casts may be found in the urine, indicating involvement of the renal parenchyma. A complete blood count shows leukocytosis and a shift to the left with an increase in bands (immature neutrophils). Urine cultures must be obtained when pyelonephritis is suspected. In patients with more severe illness who are hospitalized, blood cultures are usually done as well.

Ultrasounds of the urinary system may be performed to identify anatomic abnormalities, hydronephrosis, renal abscesses, or an obstructing stone. CT urograms are also used to assess for signs of infection in the kidney and complications of pyelonephritis, such as impaired renal function, scarring, chronic pyelonephritis, or abscesses.

### Interprofessional Care

The diagnostic tests and interprofessional care of acute pyelonephritis are summarized in Table 45-7. Patients with severe infections or complicating factors such as nausea and vomiting with dehydration require hospitalization.

The patient with mild symptoms may be treated as an outpatient with antibiotics for 14 to 21 days (Table 45-7). Parenteral antibiotics are often given initially in the hospital to rapidly establish high serum and urinary drug levels.[7] When initial treatment resolves acute symptoms and the patient is able to tolerate oral fluids and drugs, the person may be discharged on a regimen of oral antibiotics for an additional 14 to 21 days. Symptoms and signs typically improve or resolve within 48 to 72 hours after starting therapy.

Relapses may be treated with a 6-week course of antibiotics. Antibiotic prophylaxis may also be used for recurrent infections. The effectiveness of therapy is evaluated based on the presence or absence of bacterial growth on urine culture.

Urosepsis is characterized by bacteriuria and bacteremia (bacteria in blood). Close observation and vital sign monitoring are essential. Prompt recognition and treatment of septic shock may prevent irreversible damage or death.

## ❖ NURSING MANAGEMENT: ACUTE PYELONEPHRITIS

### ◆ Nursing Assessment

Subjective and objective data that should be obtained from a patient with pyelonephritis are similar to those for the patient with a UTI (Table 45-5).

**TABLE 45-7 Interprofessional Care**

***Acute Pyelonephritis***

**Diagnostic Assessment**

- History and physical examination
- Urinalysis
- Urine for culture and sensitivity
- Imaging studies: ultrasound (initially), CT scan (CT urogram), cystoscopy, VCUG
- CBC count with WBC differential
- Blood culture (if bacteremia is suspected)
- Percussion for flank (costovertebral angle [CVA]) pain

**Management**

***Mild Symptoms***

- Outpatient management or short hospitalization
  - Adequate fluid intake
  - Nonsteroidal antiinflammatory drugs (NSAIDs) or antipyretic drugs
  - Follow-up urine culture and imaging studies

*Drug Therapy*

- Empirically selected broad-spectrum antibiotics: ampicillin, vancomycin combined with an aminoglycoside (e.g., tobramycin, gentamicin)
- Switch to sensitivity-guided therapy: trimethoprim/sulfamethoxazole (Bactrim) when results of urine and blood culture are available
- Fluoroquinolones: ciprofloxacin (Cipro), ofloxacin, gatifloxacin

***Severe Symptoms***

- Hospitalization
- Adequate fluid intake (parenteral initially; switch to oral fluids as nausea, vomiting, and dehydration subside)
- NSAIDs or antipyretic drugs to reverse fever and relieve discomfort
- Follow-up urine culture and imaging studies

*Drug Therapy*

- Parenteral antibiotics
  - Empirically selected broad-spectrum antibiotics: ampicillin, vancomycin combined with an aminoglycoside (e.g., tobramycin, gentamicin)
  - Switch to sensitivity-guided antibiotic therapy when results of urine and blood culture are available
- Oral antibiotics when patient tolerates oral intake

*VCUG,* Voiding cystourethrogram.

### Nursing Diagnoses

Nursing diagnoses for the patient with pyelonephritis include, but are not limited to, those for the patient with a UTI (see p. 1036).

### Planning

The overall goals are that the patient with pyelonephritis will have (1) normal renal function, (2) normal body temperature, (3) no complications, (4) relief of pain, and (5) no recurrence of symptoms.

### Nursing Implementation

Health promotion and maintenance measures are similar to those for cystitis (see pp. 1036-1037). Early treatment for cystitis can prevent ascending infections. Because patients with structural abnormalities of the urinary tract are at high risk for infection, stress the need for regular medical care.

Nursing interventions vary depending on the severity of symptoms. These interventions include teaching the patient about the disease process with emphasis on (1) continuing medications as prescribed, (2) having a follow-up urine culture, and (3) recognizing manifestations of recurrence or relapse (Table 45-6). In addition to antibiotic therapy, encourage the patient to drink at least eight glasses of fluid every day, even after the infection has been treated. Rest will increase patient comfort.

The patient who has frequent relapses or reinfections may be treated with long-term, low-dose antibiotics. Making certain the patient understands the rationale for therapy is important to increase adherence.

### Evaluation

The expected outcomes for the patient with pyelonephritis are the same as for UTI (see p. 1038).

## CHRONIC PYELONEPHRITIS

In *chronic pyelonephritis* the kidneys become small, atrophic, and shrunken and lose function due to fibrosis (scarring). Chronic pyelonephritis is usually the result of recurring infections involving the upper urinary tract. However, it may also occur in the absence of an existing infection, recent infection, or history of UTIs.

Radiologic imaging and a biopsy, rather than clinical features, are used to confirm the diagnosis of chronic pyelonephritis. Imaging studies reveal a small, fibrotic kidney. The collecting system may be small or hydronephrotic. Biopsy results indicate the loss of functioning nephrons, infiltration of the parenchyma with inflammatory cells, and fibrosis.

The level of renal function in chronic pyelonephritis depends on whether one or both kidneys are affected, the extent of scarring, and the presence of coexisting infection. Chronic pyelonephritis often progresses to end-stage renal disease (ESRD) even if the underlying infection is successfully treated. Nursing and interprofessional management of the patient with chronic kidney disease is discussed in Chapter 46.

## URETHRITIS

*Urethritis* is an inflammation of the urethra. Causes of urethritis include a bacterial or viral infection, *Trichomonas* and monilial infection (especially in women), chlamydial infection, and gonorrhea (especially in men).

In men, the causes of urethritis are usually sexually transmitted. Purulent discharge usually indicates a gonococcal urethritis, whereas a clear discharge typically signifies a nongonococcal urethritis. (Sexually transmitted infections are discussed in Chapter 52.) Urethritis also produces bothersome LUTS, including dysuria, urgency, and frequent urination, similar to those seen with cystitis.

In women, urethritis is difficult to diagnose. It often produces bothersome LUTS, but urethral discharge may not be present.

Treatment of urethritis is based on identifying and treating the cause and providing symptomatic relief. Drugs used for bacterial infections include trimethoprim/sulfamethoxazole, doxycycline (Vibramycin), ceftriaxone (Rocephin), and nitrofurantoin. Metronidazole (Flagyl) and clotrimazole (Mycelex) may be used for treating *Trichomonas* infection. Drugs such as nystatin or fluconazole may be used for monilial infections. In chlamydial infections, doxycycline may be used. Women with negative urine cultures and no pyuria usually do not respond to antibiotics.

Warm sitz baths may temporarily relieve bothersome symptoms. Instruct the patient to avoid using vaginal deodorant sprays, properly cleanse the perineal area after bowel movements and urination, and avoid sexual intercourse until symptoms subside. Teach patients with sexually transmitted urethritis to refer their sex partners for evaluation and testing if they had sexual contact in the 60 days preceding the onset of the patient's symptoms or diagnosis.

## URETHRAL DIVERTICULA

*Urethral diverticula* are localized outpouchings of the urethra. Most often they result from enlargement of obstructed periurethral glands. In women, who have a higher incidence than men, the diverticula protrude into the anterior vaginal wall. The rare cases reported in males generally have been associated with lower urinary tract congenital anomalies or surgical trauma.

The periurethral glands are found along the entire length of the urethra, with the majority draining into the distal third of the urethra. Skene's glands are the largest of these glands. Causes of urethral diverticuli include urethral trauma from childbearing, urethral instrumentation, urethral dilation, and infection with gonococcal organisms.

Symptoms of urethral diverticuli include dysuria, postvoid dribbling, frequent urination (more often than every 2 hours), urgency, suprapubic discomfort or pressure, dyspareunia, and a feeling of incomplete bladder emptying. Urinary incontinence is frequently present. However, many women have no symptoms.

The urine may contain gross blood (hematuria) or sediment, which gives it a cloudy appearance. An anterior vaginal wall mass may be felt on physical examination. When palpated, the mass is often quite tender and expresses purulent discharge through the urethra.

Radiographic studies such as voiding cystourethrography (VCUG) can be used to confirm the diagnosis. Additional studies include ultrasound and MRI to determine the size of the diverticulum in relation to the urethral lumen.

Surgical options include transurethral incision of the diverticular neck, marsupialization (creation of a permanent opening) of the diverticular sac into the vagina (often referred to as a *Spence procedure*), and surgical excision. Stress urinary incontinence, infection, bleeding, and urethral-vaginal fistula are potential complications of the surgery.

## INTERSTITIAL CYSTITIS/PAINFUL BLADDER SYNDROME

**Interstitial cystitis (IC)** is a chronic, painful inflammatory disease of the bladder characterized by symptoms of urgency, frequency, and pain in the bladder and/or pelvis. *Painful bladder syndrome* (PBS) is suprapubic pain related to bladder filling. The term *IC/PBS* refers to cases of urinary pain that cannot be attributed to other causes such as infection or urinary calculi. IC/PBS is more common in women than men. It affects about 3.3 million women and 1.6 million men.[8]

The etiology of IC/PBS remains unknown and is likely multifactorial. Possible causes include neurogenic hypersensitivity of the lower urinary tract, alterations in mast cells in the muscle and/or mucosal layers of the bladder, infection with an unusual organism (e.g., slow-growing virus), or production of a toxic substance in the urine.

The bladder wall may be irritated and inflamed and can become scarred. *Glomerulations* (superficial ulcerations with pinpoint bleeding) and Hunner's ulcers may occur on the bladder wall.

### Clinical Manifestations and Diagnostic Studies

The two primary clinical manifestations of IC/PBS are pain and bothersome LUTS (e.g., frequency, urgency). People with severe cases may urinate as often as 60 times in a day including nighttime urination. The pain is usually located in the suprapubic area but may involve the vagina, labia, or entire perineal region, including the rectum and anus. The pain varies from moderate to severe and is exacerbated by bladder filling, postponed urination, physical exertion, pressure against the suprapubic area, certain foods, or emotional distress. The pain is transiently relieved by urination. Bothersome LUTS are similar to a UTI, and the condition is often misdiagnosed as a recurring or chronic UTI or, in men, chronic prostatitis.

The patient experiences periods of remission and exacerbation of the pain and bothersome voiding symptoms. Women often report that pain occurs premenstrually and is aggravated by sexual intercourse or emotional stress. Some patients experience symptoms that disappear altogether after a period of weeks to months, whereas others have persistent symptoms over months to years.

IC/PBS is a diagnosis of exclusion. A careful history and physical examination are necessary to rule out other disorders that produce similar symptoms, such as UTI or endometriosis. Urine cultures do not find any bacteria or other organisms in the urine. Furthermore, people with IC/PBS do not respond to antibiotic therapy. Cystoscopic examination may reveal a small bladder capacity and glomerulations, but these findings are frequently not present in patients with IC/PBS.

### Interprofessional Care

Because the etiology of IC/PBS is unknown, no single treatment consistently reverses or relieves symptoms. Various therapies have been effective, including nutritional and drug therapy. Surgical therapy is rarely indicated.

Elimination of foods and beverages that are likely to irritate the bladder may provide some relief from symptoms. Typical bladder irritants include caffeine; alcohol; citrus products; aged cheeses; nuts; foods containing vinegar, curries, or hot peppers; and foods or beverages likely to lower urinary pH (including fruits such as cranberries). Recipes and menus for a well-balanced diet that is specifically designed to avoid bladder-irritating foods and beverages are available at the website for the Interstitial Cystitis Association *(www.ichelp.org)*.

An over-the-counter (OTC) dietary supplement called *calcium glycerophosphate* (Prelief) alkalinizes the urine and can provide relief from the irritating effects of certain foods. This agent may be particularly helpful when dining away from home, where the patient has less control over food preparation.

Because stress can exacerbate or cause flare-ups of IC/PBS symptoms, stress management techniques such as relaxation breathing and imagery (see Chapter 6) may be helpful. Using lubrication or altering positions may decrease pain associated with sexual intercourse.

Two tricyclic antidepressants, amitriptyline and nortriptyline , are used to reduce the burning pain and urinary frequency. Pentosan (Elmiron) is the only oral agent approved for the treatment of patients with symptoms of IC. It enhances the protective effects of the glycosaminoglycan layer of the bladder and relieves pain associated with IC/PBS by reducing the irritative effects of urine on the bladder wall. These drugs are used to provide relief over time (weeks to months) but do not provide the immediate relief that may be needed for an acute exacerbation of symptoms. A short course of opioid analgesics may be used for immediate relief.

Dimethyl sulfoxide (DMSO) can be directly instilled into the bladder through a small catheter. This drug desensitizes pain receptors in the bladder wall. Heparin and hyaluronic acid also may be instilled into the bladder to relieve IC/PBS symptoms. Like pentosan, they are thought to enhance the protective properties of the glycosaminoglycan layer of the bladder. Instillations are often administered with lidocaine, which rapidly desensitizes the bladder wall, helping the patient tolerate instillation of additional heparin or hyaluronic acid and providing transient relief from pain.

Several surgical procedures can be used to relieve severe, debilitating pain. Fulguration and resection of Hunner's ulcers are possible surgical treatments. Surgical urinary diversion, such as an ileal conduit, is used when other measures fail. Unfortunately, some patients have reported pain within the urinary diversion, possibly indicating that some factor in the urine may contribute to IC/PBS in certain cases.

## NURSING MANAGEMENT: INTERSTITIAL CYSTITIS/PAINFUL BLADDER SYNDROME

Assess the characteristics of the pain associated with IC/PBS. Ask the patient about specific dietary or lifestyle factors that exacerbate or alleviate pain, and assess the intensity of the pain. Instruct the patient to keep a bladder log or voiding diary over a period of at least 3 days to determine voiding frequency and patterns of nocturia. Keeping a pain record at the same time may be useful.

A UTI may occur during the course of IC/PBS management because of diagnostic instrumentation and frequent bladder instillations. A UTI is likely to produce an acute exacerbation of bothersome LUTS and urinary frequency, as well as dysuria (not typically associated with IC/PBS) and odorous urine, possibly with hematuria.

Instruct the patient to maintain good nutrition, particularly in light of the broad dietary restrictions often necessary to control IC-related pain. Advise the patient to take a multivitamin containing no more than the recommended dietary allowance for essential vitamins and to avoid high-potency vitamins, because they may irritate the bladder. Advise the patient to avoid clothing that creates suprapubic pressure, including pants with tight belts or restrictive waistlines. Educational materials about diet, ways to cope with the need for frequent urination, and strategies for coping with the emotional burden of IC/PBS are available from the Interstitial Cystitis Association (*www.ichelp.com*). Reassurance that IC/PBS is a real condition experienced by others and that it can be treated may relieve the anxiety, anger, guilt, and frustration related to experiences of chronic pain and voiding dysfunction in the absence of a clear-cut diagnosis and treatment strategy.

## GENITOURINARY TUBERCULOSIS

*Genitourinary tuberculosis (GUTB)* is usually secondary to TB of the lung. In a small percentage of patients with pulmonary TB, the tubercle bacilli reach the kidneys via the bloodstream. Onset occurs 5 to 8 years after the primary lung infection.[9,10] When the kidney is initially infected with bacilli, the patient is often asymptomatic. Sometimes the patient complains of fatigue and develops a low-grade fever. As the lesions ulcerate, infection descends to the bladder and other genitourinary organs. Then the patient experiences cystitis, frequent urination, burning on voiding, and epididymitis (in men).

Symptoms of a UTI are the first manifestations in the majority of patients with renal TB. However, the urinalysis and urine culture show sterile pyuria (WBCs but no organisms are present). Renal lesions may calcify as they heal. Infrequently, renal colic, lumbar and iliac pain, and hematuria may be present.

Tuberculin skin test results are positive in most patients, but this finding only indicates that the person has had previous inhalation of mycobacteria rather than active disease. A diagnosis of renal TB is based on finding tubercle bacilli in the urine.

Radiographic tests that may be done include CT urogram and voiding cystourethrogram (VCUG). These studies help determine the extent and severity of the disease.

Long-term complications of GUTB depend on the duration of the disease. Scarring of the renal parenchyma, hydronephrosis, and the development of ureteral strictures occur. The earlier treatment is initiated, the less likely renal failure will develop. The patient may require long-term urologic follow-up. Nursing and interprofessional management of the patient with TB is discussed in Chapter 27.

# IMMUNOLOGIC DISORDERS OF KIDNEY

## GLOMERULONEPHRITIS

Immunologic processes involving the urinary tract predominantly affect the renal glomerulus. The disease process results in **glomerulonephritis** (inflammation of the glomeruli), which affects both kidneys equally and is the third leading cause of ESRD in the United States. Although the glomerulus is the primary site of inflammation, tubular, interstitial, and vascular changes also occur.

A variety of conditions can cause glomerulonephritis, ranging from kidney infections to systemic diseases (Table 45-8). Glomerulonephritis can be acute or chronic. With *acute glomerulonephritis,* symptoms come on suddenly and may be temporary or reversible. An example of this is acute poststreptococcal glomerulonephritis (discussed in the next section). *Chronic glomerulonephritis* is slowly progressive glomerulonephritis generally leading to irreversible renal failure (discussed later in this chapter).

### Acute Poststreptococcal Glomerulonephritis

*Acute poststreptococcal glomerulonephritis* (APSGN) is a common type of acute glomerulonephritis. It is most common in children and young adults, but all age groups can be affected. APSGN develops about 1 to 2 weeks after an infection of the tonsils, pharynx, or skin (e.g., streptococcal sore throat, impetigo) by nephrotoxic strains of group A β-hemolytic streptococci.[11] The person produces antibodies to the streptococcal antigen. Although the specific mechanism is not known, tissue injury occurs as the antigen-antibody complexes are deposited in the glomeruli, complement is activated (see Chapter 11), and inflammation results.

The clinical manifestations of APSGN include generalized body edema, hypertension, oliguria, hematuria with a smoky or rusty appearance, and proteinuria. Fluid retention occurs as a

**TABLE 45-8 Causes or Risk Factors for Glomerulonephritis**

| Cause or Risk Factor | Description |
|---|---|
| **Infections** | |
| **Poststreptococcal glomerulonephritis** | • GN may develop 1-2 wk after a streptococcal throat infection or, rarely, a skin infection (impetigo).<br>• Antibodies (Ab) to strep antigen (Ag) develop and the Ag-Ab deposit in the glomeruli, causing inflammation. |
| **Infective endocarditis** | • Bacteria can cause an infection of one or more of the heart valves (see Chapter 36).<br>• People at risk include those with a heart defect, such as a damaged or artificial heart valve.<br>• Bacterial endocarditis is associated with GN, but the exact cause is not known. |
| **Viral infections** | • Viral infections can trigger GN.<br>• Common viruses include human immunodeficiency virus (HIV) and hepatitis B and hepatitis C viruses. |
| **Immune Diseases** | |
| **Systemic lupus erythematosus (SLE)** | • Autoimmune disorder characterized by the involvement of several tissues and organs, particularly joints, skin, and kidneys (see Chapter 64).<br>• GN frequently occurs in SLE and has a poor prognosis. |
| **Scleroderma** | • Disease of unknown etiology characterized by widespread alterations of connective tissue and vascular lesions in many organs (see Chapter 64).<br>• In the kidney, vascular lesions are associated with fibrosis. Severity of renal involvement varies. |
| **Goodpasture syndrome** | • Autoimmune disorder that causes lung and kidney disease.<br>• Causes bleeding into lungs and GN. |
| **IgA nephropathy** | • Results from deposits of immunoglobulin A (IgA) in the glomeruli.<br>• Characterized by recurrent episodes of hematuria. |
| **Vasculitis** | |
| **Polyarteritis** | • Autoimmune disease that affects small and medium blood vessels.<br>• Can affect any organ but common in heart, kidneys, and intestines. |
| **Wegener's granulomatosis** | • Form of vasculitis affecting small and medium blood vessels.<br>• Most commonly affects kidneys, lungs, and upper respiratory tract. |
| **Conditions Causing Scarring of Glomeruli** | |
| **Diabetic nephropathy** | • Primary cause of end-stage renal disease in the United States (see Chapter 46).<br>• Microvascular changes of diffuse glomerulosclerosis involving thickening of the glomerular basement membrane. |
| **Hypertension** | • Nephrosclerosis is a complication of hypertension.<br>• GN can also cause hypertension. |
| **Focal segmental glomerulosclerosis** | • Characterized by scattered scarring of glomeruli.<br>• May result from another disease or occur for unknown reasons. |
| **Other Causes** | |
| **Amyloidosis** | • Caused by infiltration of tissues with amyloid (hyaline substance).<br>• Hyaline bodies consist largely of protein.<br>• Kidney involvement is common, and proteinuria is often the first clinical manifestation. |
| **Illegal drug use** | • People who use these drugs are at increased risk for GN. |

*GN*, Glomerulonephritis.

result of decreased glomerular filtration. Initially edema appears in low-pressure tissues, such as those around the eyes *(periorbital edema)*, but later it progresses to involve the total body as ascites or peripheral edema in the legs. Smoky urine indicates bleeding in the upper urinary tract. The degree of proteinuria varies with the severity of the glomerulonephropathy. Hypertension primarily results from increased extracellular fluid volume. The patient with APSGN may have abdominal or flank pain. In other cases, the patient may be asymptomatic, and the problem is found on routine urinalysis.

More than 95% of patients with APSGN recover completely or improve rapidly with conservative management. Accurate recognition and assessment are critical, since chronic glomerulonephritis can develop if the patient is not treated appropriately.

The diagnosis of APSGN is based on a complete history and physical examination. An immune response to the streptococci is often demonstrated by assessment of antistreptolysin-O (ASO) titers. The finding of decreased complement components (especially C3 and CH50) indicates an immune-mediated response. A renal biopsy may be done to confirm the disease.

Dipstick urinalysis and urine sediment microscopy reveal erythrocytes in significant numbers. Erythrocyte casts are highly suggestive of APSGN. Proteinuria may range from mild to severe. Blood tests include blood urea nitrogen (BUN) and serum creatinine to assess the extent of renal impairment.

## ❖ NURSING AND INTERPROFESSIONAL MANAGEMENT: ACUTE POSTSTREPTOCOCCAL GLOMERULONEPHRITIS

The management of APSGN focuses on symptomatic relief. Rest is recommended until the signs of glomerular inflammation (proteinuria, hematuria) and hypertension subside. Edema is treated by restricting sodium and fluid intake and by administrating diuretics. Severe hypertension is treated with antihypertensive drugs. Dietary protein intake may be restricted if there is evidence of an increase in nitrogenous wastes (e.g., elevated BUN). The dietary protein restriction varies with the degree of proteinuria. Low-protein, low-sodium, fluid-restricted diets are discussed in Chapter 46.

Antibiotics should be given only if the streptococcal infection is still present. Corticosteroids and cytotoxic drugs have not been shown to be of value in the treatment of APSGN.

One of the most important ways to prevent APSGN is to encourage early diagnosis and treatment of sore throats and skin lesions. If streptococci are found in the culture, treatment with appropriate antibiotic therapy (usually penicillin) is essential. Encourage the patient to take the full course of antibiotics to ensure that the bacteria have been eradicated. Good personal hygiene is an important factor in preventing the spread of cutaneous streptococcal infections.

In most cases, recovery from the acute glomerulonephritis is complete. However, if progressive involvement occurs and chronic glomerulonephritis develops, ESRD results.

### Goodpasture Syndrome

Goodpasture syndrome is an autoimmune disease characterized by antibodies that attack the glomerular and alveolar basement membrane. Damage to the kidneys and lungs results when binding of the antibody causes an inflammatory reaction mediated by complement activation (see Chapter 11).

Goodpasture syndrome is a rare disease that is found primarily in young male smokers. The clinical manifestations include flu-like symptoms with pulmonary symptoms such as cough, mild shortness of breath, hemoptysis, crackles, and pulmonary insufficiency. Renal involvement causes hematuria, weakness, pallor, anemia, and renal failure. Pulmonary hemorrhage usually occurs and may precede glomerular abnormalities by weeks or months.

Current management includes corticosteroids, immunosuppressive drugs (e.g., cyclophosphamide, azathioprine [Imuran]), plasmapheresis (see Chapter 13), and dialysis. Plasmapheresis removes the circulating anti–glomerular basement membrane (GBM) antibodies, and immunosuppressive therapy inhibits further antibody production. Renal transplantation can be attempted after the circulating anti-GBM antibody titer decreases. Although the disease may recur in the transplanted kidney, this is not a contraindication to transplantation.

Nursing management appropriate for a critically ill patient who is experiencing acute kidney injury (see Chapter 46) and respiratory distress (see Chapter 67) is instituted. Death is often secondary to hemorrhage in the lungs and respiratory failure.

### Rapidly Progressive Glomerulonephritis

*Rapidly progressive glomerulonephritis* (RPGN) is a type of glomerular disease characterized by rapid, progressive loss of renal function over days to weeks. In contrast, chronic glomerulonephritis develops insidiously and progresses over many years. The manifestations of RPGN are hypertension, edema, proteinuria, hematuria, and red blood cell (RBC) casts.

RPGN can occur in a variety of situations: (1) as a complication of inflammatory or infectious disease (e.g., APSGN), (2) as a complication of a systemic disease (e.g., systemic lupus erythematosus), (3) as an idiopathic disease, or (4) with the use of certain drugs (e.g., penicillamine).

Treatment is directed toward correction of fluid overload, hypertension, uremia, and inflammatory injury to the kidney. Treatment includes corticosteroids, cytotoxic agents, and plasmapheresis. Dialysis therapy and transplantation are used as maintenance therapy for the patient with RPGN. After kidney transplantation, RPGN may recur.

### Chronic Glomerulonephritis

*Chronic glomerulonephritis* is a syndrome that reflects the end stage of glomerular inflammatory disease. Most types of glomerulonephritis and nephrotic syndrome can eventually lead to chronic glomerulonephritis. Some people who develop chronic glomerulonephritis have no history of kidney disease. Frequently the cause of chronic glomerulonephritis is not found. Infrequently, it is an inherited disorder (e.g., Alport syndrome [see p. 1052]).

With chronic glomerulonephritis, symptoms develop slowly over time. Patients are often unaware that progressive kidney impairment is occurring. They do not realize that they have severe kidney impairment until a diagnostic evaluation is done. Chronic glomerulonephritis is often discovered coincidentally with the finding of an abnormality on a urinalysis or elevated BP.

The syndrome is characterized by proteinuria, hematuria, and the slow development of uremia (see Chapter 46) as a result of decreasing renal function. Chronic glomerulonephritis progresses insidiously toward ESRD in 2 to 30 years.

Clinical manifestations of glomerulonephritis include varying degrees of hematuria (ranging from microscopic to gross) and urinary excretion of various formed elements, including RBCs, WBCs, and casts. Proteinuria and elevated BUN and serum creatinine levels are other findings. Sometimes fatigue may be a presenting symptom.

The patient's history provides important information related to glomerulonephritis. Assess exposure to drugs, immunizations, microbial infections, and viral infections such as hepatitis. Also evaluate the patient for more generalized conditions involving immune disorders, such as systemic lupus erythematosus and scleroderma. Commonly the patient has no recollection or history of any renal problems.

Ultrasound and CT scan are generally preferred as diagnostic measures. However, a renal biopsy may be performed to determine the exact cause of the glomerulonephritis.

Treatment is supportive and symptomatic. Management of chronic kidney disease is discussed in Chapter 46.

## NEPHROTIC SYNDROME

Nephrotic syndrome results when the glomerulus is excessively permeable to plasma protein, causing proteinuria that leads to low plasma albumin and tissue edema.

### Etiology and Clinical Manifestations

Some of the common causes of nephrotic syndrome are listed in Table 45-9. About one third of patients with nephrotic syndrome have a systemic disease such as diabetes or systemic lupus erythematosus.[12]

The characteristic manifestations of nephrotic syndrome include peripheral edema, massive proteinuria, hypertension, hyperlipidemia, hypoalbuminemia, and foamy urine. Characteristic laboratory findings include decreased serum albumin, decreased total serum protein, and elevated serum cholesterol. The increased glomerular membrane permeability found in nephrotic syndrome is responsible for the massive excretion of protein in the urine. This results in decreased serum protein and subsequent edema formation. Ascites and *anasarca* (massive generalized edema) develop if there is severe hypoalbuminemia.

The diminished plasma oncotic pressure from the decreased serum proteins stimulates hepatic lipoprotein synthesis, which results in hyperlipidemia. Initially, cholesterol and low-density lipoproteins are elevated. Later the triglyceride level is also increased. Fat bodies (fatty casts), which commonly appear in the urine, cause foamy urine.

Immune responses are altered in nephrotic syndrome. As a result, infection is a primary cause of morbidity and mortality.

**TABLE 45-9 Causes of Nephrotic Syndrome**

| | |
|---|---|
| **Primary Glomerular Disease**<br>• Membranous proliferative glomerulonephritis<br>• Primary nephrotic syndrome<br>• Focal glomerulonephritis<br>• Inherited nephrotic disease | ***Infections***<br>• Bacterial (streptococcal, syphilis)<br>• Viral (hepatitis, human immunodeficiency virus, mononucleosis)<br>• Protozoal (malaria) |
| **Extrarenal Causes**<br>***Multisystem Disease***<br>• Systemic lupus erythematosus<br>• Diabetes mellitus<br>• Amyloidosis | ***Neoplasms***<br>• Hodgkin's lymphoma<br>• Solid tumors of lungs, colon, stomach, breast<br>• Leukemias |
| ***Allergens***<br>• Bee sting<br>• Pollen | ***Drugs***<br>• penicillamine<br>• Nonsteroidal antiinflammatory drugs (NSAIDs)<br>• captopril heroin |

Calcium and skeletal abnormalities may occur, including hypocalcemia, blunted calcium response to parathyroid hormone, hyperparathyroidism, and osteomalacia.

With nephrotic proteinuria, hypercoagulability results from the urinary loss of anticoagulant proteins. Hypercoagulability with thromboembolism is a serious complication of nephrotic syndrome. The renal vein is the most common site for thrombus formation. Pulmonary emboli occur in about 40% of nephrotic patients with thrombosis.

## ❖ NURSING AND INTERPROFESSIONAL MANAGEMENT: NEPHROTIC SYNDROME

Specific treatment of nephrotic syndrome depends on the cause. The goals are to cure or control the primary disease and relieve the symptoms. Corticosteroids and cyclophosphamide may be used for the treatment of nephrotic syndrome. Prednisone has been effective to varying degrees for some causes of nephrotic syndrome (e.g., membranous glomerulonephritis, lupus nephritis). Management of diabetes and treatment of edema are measures used for nephrotic syndrome related to diabetes.

Management of the edema includes the cautious use of angiotensin-converting enzyme inhibitors; nonsteroidal antiinflammatory drugs (NSAIDs); and a low-sodium (2 to 3 g/day), moderate-protein (1 to 2 g/kg/day) diet. If urine protein losses are high (more than 10 g/day), additional protein may be recommended.

Dietary salt restrictions are a key to managing edema. Some individuals may need thiazide or loop diuretics.

The treatment of hyperlipidemia includes lipid-lowering agents, such as colestipol (Colestid) and lovastatin (see Table 33-5). If thrombosis is detected, anticoagulant therapy may be needed.

A major nursing intervention for a patient with nephrotic syndrome focuses on the management of edema. Assess the edema by weighing the patient daily, accurately recording intake and output, and measuring abdominal girth or extremity size. Compare this information on a daily basis to assess the effectiveness of treatment. Clean the edematous skin carefully. Avoid trauma to the skin. Monitor the effectiveness of diuretic therapy.

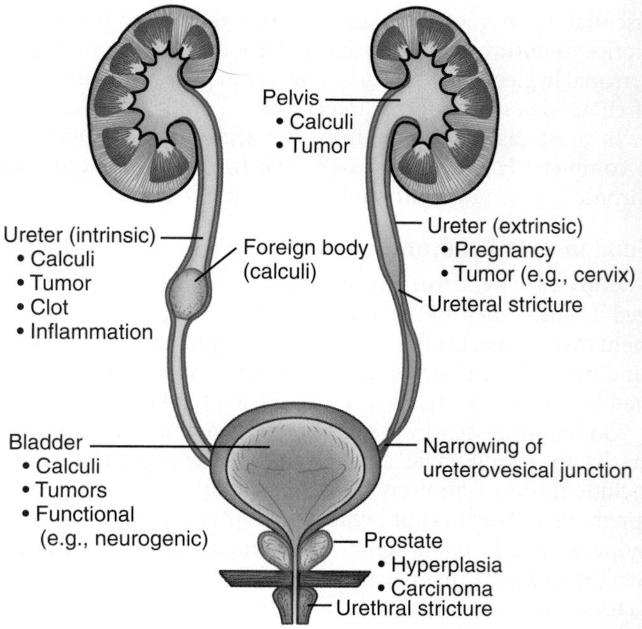


**FIG. 45-3** Sites and causes of upper and lower urinary tract obstruction.

Patients with nephrotic syndrome are usually anorexic and have the potential to become malnourished from the excessive loss of protein in the urine. Serve small, frequent meals in a pleasant setting to encourage better dietary intake.

Because the patient with nephrotic syndrome is susceptible to infection, teach the patient to avoid exposure to persons with known infections. Support for the patient, especially helping them cope with an altered body image, is essential because of the embarrassment and shame often associated with the edematous appearance.

## OBSTRUCTIVE UROPATHIES

*Urinary obstruction* refers to any anatomic or functional condition that blocks or impedes the flow of urine (Fig. 45-3). It may be congenital or acquired. Damaging effects from urinary tract obstruction affect the system above the level of the obstruction. The severity of these effects depends on the location, duration of obstruction, amount of pressure or dilation, and presence of urinary stasis or infection. Infection increases the risk of irreversible damage.[13]

When obstruction occurs at the level of the bladder neck or prostate, significant bladder changes can occur. Detrusor muscle fibers *hypertrophy* (increase in size) to contract harder to push urine out a narrower pathway. Over a long period, the detrusor loses its ability to compensate for this resistance, eventually leading to large residual urine volume in the bladder.

When *bladder outlet obstruction* is present, pressure increases during bladder filling or storage and can be transmitted to the ureter. This pressure leads to *reflux* (backflow of urine), **hydroureter** (ureteral dilation and distention), vesicoureteral reflux (backflow [backward movement] of urine from the lower to upper urinary tract), and **hydronephrosis** (dilation or enlargement of the renal pelvises and calyces) (Fig. 45-4). Chronic pyelonephritis and renal atrophy may develop. If only one kidney is obstructed, the other kidney may try to compensate by hypertrophy.

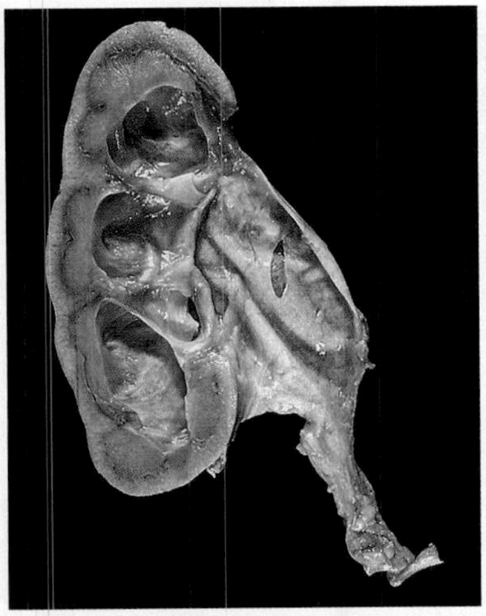

**FIG. 45-4** Hydronephrosis of the kidney. Note the marked dilation of the pelvis and calyces and thinning of the renal parenchyma. (From Kumar V, Abbas AK, Aster JC, et al: *Robbins and Cotran pathologic basis of disease,* ed 8, Philadelphia, 2010, Saunders.)

Partial obstruction may occur in the ureter or at the ureteropelvic junction (UPJ) (where the renal pelvis narrows into the ureter). If the pressure remains low or moderate, the kidney may continue to dilate with no noticeable loss of function. The risk of pyelonephritis is increased because of urinary stasis and reflux. If only one kidney is involved and the other kidney is functioning, the patient may be asymptomatic.

If both kidneys or only one functioning kidney is involved (e.g., if the patient has only one kidney), alterations in renal function (e.g., increased BUN or serum creatinine levels) are found. Progressive obstruction can lead to renal failure. Treatment requires locating and relieving the blockage. This can include insertion of a tube (e.g., urethral or ureteral), surgical correction of the primary problem, or diversion of the urinary stream above the level of blockage.

## URINARY TRACT CALCULI

Each year an estimated 1 million to 2 million people in the United States have **nephrolithiasis** (kidney stone disease). In the United States the incidence of urinary stone disease is highest in the Southeast and Southwest, followed by the Midwest. Except for struvite (magnesium ammonium phosphate) stones associated with UTI, stone disorders are more common in men than in women. The majority of patients are between 20 and 55 years of age.[13]

Stone formation is more frequent in whites than in African Americans. The incidence is also higher in persons with a family history of stone formation. Stones can recur in up to 50% of patients. Stone formation occurs more often in the summer months, thus supporting the role of dehydration in this process.

### GENDER DIFFERENCES

***Urinary Tract Calculi***

| Men | Women |
|---|---|
| • Urinary calculi disorders (except for struvite stones) are more common in men. | • Struvite stones associated with urinary tract infection are more common in women than in men. |

**TABLE 45-10 Risk Factors for Urinary Tract Calculi**

**Metabolic**
- Abnormalities that result in increased urine levels of calcium, oxalate uric acid, or citric acid

**Climate**
- Warm climates that cause increased fluid loss, low urine volume, and increased solute concentration in urine

**Diet**
- Large intake of dietary proteins that increases uric acid excretion
- Excessive amounts of tea or fruit juices that elevate urinary oxalate level
- Large intake of calcium and oxalate
- Low fluid intake that increases urinary concentration

**Genetic Factors**
- Family history of stone formation, cystinuria, gout, or renal acidosis
- Lifestyle
- Sedentary occupation, immobility

### Etiology and Pathophysiology

Many factors are involved in the incidence and type of stone formation, including metabolic, dietary, genetic, climatic, lifestyle, and occupational influences (Table 45-10). Although many theories have been proposed, no single theory can account for stone formation in all cases. Crystals, when in a supersaturated concentration, can precipitate and unite to form a stone. Keeping urine dilute and free flowing reduces the risk of recurrent stone formation in many individuals.

A mucoprotein is formed in the kidneys as a matrix for the stone. Urinary pH, solute load, and inhibitors in the urine affect the formation of stones. The higher the pH (alkaline), the less soluble are calcium and phosphate. The lower the pH (acidic), the less soluble are uric acid and cystine. When a substance is not very soluble in fluid, it is more likely to precipitate out of solution.

Other important factors in the development of stones include obstruction with associated urinary stasis and UTI with urea-splitting bacteria (e.g., *Proteus, Klebsiella, Pseudomonas,* and some species of staphylococci). These bacteria cause the urine to become alkaline and contribute to the formation of struvite stones. Infected stones, entrapped in the kidney (Fig. 45-5), may assume a staghorn configuration as the stone branches to occupy a large portion of the collecting system. These stones can lead to a renal infection, hydronephrosis, and loss of kidney function.

Genetic factors may also contribute to urine stone formation. Cystinuria, an autosomal recessive disorder, is characterized by a markedly increased excretion of cystine.

### Types of Urinary Calculi

The term **calculus** refers to the stone, and *lithiasis* refers to stone formation. The five major categories of stones are (1) calcium phosphate, (2) calcium oxalate, (3) uric acid, (4) cystine, and (5) struvite (magnesium ammonium phosphate) (Table 45-11). Although calcium stones are the most common, stone composition may be mixed. Calculi can be found in various locations in the urinary tract (Figs. 45-3 and 45-5).

**TABLE 45-11 Types of Urinary Tract Calculi**

| Characteristics | Predisposing Factors | Treatment |
|---|---|---|
| **Calcium Oxalate*** | | |
| Small, often possible to get trapped in ureter. More frequent in men than in women. *Incidence:* 35%-40% | Idiopathic hypercalciuria, hyperoxaluria, independent of urinary pH, family history | Increase hydration. Reduce dietary oxalate.† Give thiazide diuretics. Give cellulose phosphate to chelate calcium and prevent GI absorption. Give potassium citrate to maintain alkaline urine. Give cholestyramine to bind oxalate. Give calcium lactate to precipitate oxalate in GI tract. Reduce daily sodium intake. |
| **Calcium Phosphate** | | |
| Mixed stones (typically), with struvite or oxalate stones. *Incidence:* 8%-10% | Alkaline urine, primary hyperparathyroidism | Treat underlying causes and other stones. |
| **Struvite (Magnesium Ammonium Phosphate)** | | |
| Three or four times as common in women as men. Always associated with urinary tract infections. Large staghorn type (usually) (Fig. 45-5). *Incidence:* 10%-15% | Urinary tract infections (usually *Proteus*) | Administer antimicrobial agents, acetohydroxamic acid. Use surgical intervention to remove stone. Take measures to acidify urine. |
| **Uric Acid** | | |
| Predominant in men, high incidence in Jewish men. *Incidence:* 5%-8% | Gout, acidic urine, inherited condition | Reduce urinary concentration of uric acid. Alkalinize urine with potassium citrate. Administer allopurinol. Reduce dietary purines.† |
| **Cystine** | | |
| Genetic autosomal recessive defect. Defective absorption of cystine in GI tract and kidney, excess concentrations causing stone formation. *Incidence:* 1%-2% | Acidic urine | Increase hydration. Give α-penicillamine and tiopronin to prevent cystine crystallization. Give potassium citrate to maintain alkaline urine. |

*Calcium stones can exist as calcium oxalate, calcium phosphate, or a mixture of both. Calcium stones account for the majority of all stones.
†See Table 45-12: Nutritional Therapy: Urinary Tract Calculi.

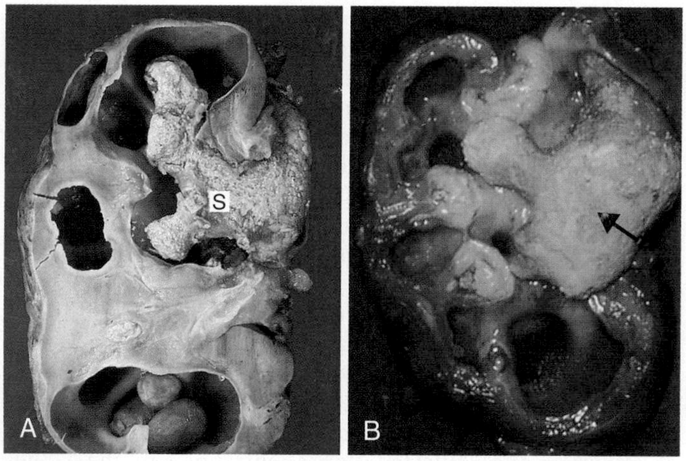


**FIG. 45-5** **A,** Renal staghorn calculus. The renal pelvis is filled with a large calculus that is shaped to its contours, resembling the horns of a stag *(S)*. **B,** Imbedded staghorn calculus *(arrow)* in hydronephrotic, infected, nonfunctioning kidney. (***A,*** From Stevens A, Lowe JS, Scott I: *Core pathology: illustrated review in color,* ed 3, London, 2009, Mosby Ltd. *B,* From Bullock N, Doble A, Turner W, et al: *Urology: an illustrated colour text,* London, 2008, Churchill Livingstone.)

## Clinical Manifestations

The first symptom of a kidney stone is usually severe pain that begins suddenly. Typically, a person feels a sharp pain in the flank area, back, or lower abdomen. People describe the pain as the most excruciating that a person can endure. *Renal colic* is the term used for the sharp, severe pain, which results from the stretching, dilation, and spasm of the ureter in response to the obstructing stone. Nausea and vomiting may occur due to the severe pain.

Urinary stones cause clinical manifestations when they obstruct urinary flow. Common sites of obstruction are at the UPJ and ureterovesical junction (UVJ). The type of pain is determined by the location of the stone. If the stone is nonobstructing, pain may be absent. If the obstruction is in a calyx or at the UPJ, the patient may experience dull costovertebral flank pain or renal colic. Pain resulting from the passage of a calculus down the ureter is intense and colicky.

Patients with renal colic have a hard time being still. They go from walking to sitting to lying down, and then they repeat the process. Some people refer to this as the *kidney stone dance.*

The patient may be in mild shock with cool, moist skin. As a stone nears the UVJ, pain moves around toward the abdomen and down toward the lower quadrant. Men may experience testicular pain, whereas women may complain of labial pain. Both men and women may experience pain in the groin. The patient may also have manifestations of UTI with dysuria, fever, and chills.

## Diagnostic Studies

Noncontrast helical (spiral) CT scan is commonly used in patients with renal colic. It is quick and noninvasive and requires no IV contrast. In some situations, ultrasound is used. A complete urinalysis helps confirm the diagnosis of a urinary stone by assessing for hematuria, crystalluria, and urinary pH.

Retrieval and analysis of the stones are important in the diagnosis of the underlying problem contributing to stone formation. The patient's serum calcium, phosphorus, sodium, potassium, bicarbonate, uric acid, BUN, and creatinine levels are also measured. A careful history should include any previous episodes of stone formation, prescribed and OTC medications, dietary supplements, and family history of urinary calculi. Measurement of urine pH is useful in the diagnosis of struvite stones and renal tubular acidosis (tendency to alkaline or high pH) and uric acid stones (tendency to acidic or low pH). Patients who experience recurrent stone formation should have a 24-hour urinary measurement of calcium, phosphorus, magnesium, sodium, oxalate, citrate, sulfate, potassium, uric acid, and total volume.

### Interprofessional Care

Evaluation and management of a patient with renal calculi consist of two concurrent approaches. The first approach is directed toward management of the acute attack by treating the pain, infection, and/or obstruction. Administer opioids to relieve renal colic pain. Most stones are 4 mm or less in size and will probably pass spontaneously. However, it may take weeks for a stone to pass.

Tamsulosin (Flomax) or terazosin, α-adrenergic blockers that relax the smooth muscle in the ureter, can be used to facilitate stone passage. These drugs are also used to relax the muscle tissue in the prostate in men with BPH.

The second approach is directed toward evaluation of the cause of the stone formation and prevention of further stone development. Obtain information from the patient, including a family history of stone formation; geographic residence; nutritional assessment, including the intake of vitamins A and D; activity pattern (active or sedentary); history of prolonged illness with immobilization or dehydration; and any history of disease or surgery involving the GI or genitourinary tract.

Therapy for active stone formers requires a comprehensive management approach, with the primary emphasis on teaching. Adequate hydration, dietary sodium restrictions, dietary changes, and drugs are used to minimize urinary stone formation (Table 45-11). Depending on the specific problem underlying the stone formation, various drugs are prescribed. These drugs prevent stone formation in various ways, including altering urine pH, preventing excessive urinary excretion of a substance, or correcting a primary disease (e.g., hyperparathyroidism).

Treatment of struvite stones requires control of infection. This may be difficult if the stone remains in place. In addition to antibiotics, acetohydroxamic acid may be used to treat kidney infections that result in the continual formation of struvite stones. Acetohydroxamic acid inhibits the chemical action caused by the persistent bacteria and thus retards struvite stone formation. The stone may have to be removed surgically if the infection cannot be controlled.[14]

Endourology, lithotripsy, or open surgical stone removal may be used in the following situations: (1) stones too large for spontaneous passage (usually greater than 7 mm); (2) stones associated with bacteriuria or symptomatic infection; (3) stones causing impaired renal function; (4) stones causing persistent pain, nausea, or paralytic ileus; (5) inability of patient to be treated medically; and (6) patient with only one kidney.[15]

**Endourologic Procedures.** If the stone is located in the bladder, a cystoscopy is done to remove small stones. For large stones (Fig. 45-6), a *cystolitholapaxy* is done. In this procedure, large stones are broken up with an instrument called a *lithotrite* (stone crusher). The bladder is then irrigated and the crushed stones washed out. A *cystoscopic lithotripsy* uses an ultrasonic lithotrite to pulverize (break up) stones. Complications associated with these cystoscopic procedures include hemorrhage, retained stone fragments, and infection.

Flexible *ureteroscopes,* inserted via a cystoscope, can be used to remove stones from the renal pelvis and upper urinary tract. Ultrasonic, laser, or electrohydraulic lithotripsy may be used in conjunction with the ureteroscope to pulverize the stone.

In *percutaneous nephrolithotomy,* a nephroscope is inserted into the kidney pelvis through a track (using a sheath) in the skin. The track is created in the patient's back. The kidney stones can be fragmented using ultrasound, electrohydraulic, or laser lithotripsy. The stone fragments are removed, and the pelvis is irrigated. A percutaneous nephrostomy tube is usually left in place to make sure that the ureter is not obstructed. Complications include bleeding, injury to adjacent structures, and infection.

**Lithotripsy.** Lithotripsy is a procedure used to eliminate calculi from the urinary tract. Lithotripsy techniques include (1) laser lithotripsy, (2) extracorporeal shock-wave lithotripsy (ESWL), (3) percutaneous ultrasonic lithotripsy, and (4) electrohydraulic lithotripsy. *Laser lithotripsy* is used to fragment ureteral and large bladder stones (bladder stones are described earlier). To access ureteral stones, a ureteroscope is used to get close to the stone. A small fiber is inserted up the endoscope so that the tip (which emits the laser energy) can come in contact with the stone. A holmium laser in direct contact with the stone is commonly used. The intense energy breaks the stone into small pieces, which can be extracted or flushed out. Because of the type of laser energy, no other tissue is affected. This minimally invasive treatment usually requires general anesthesia.

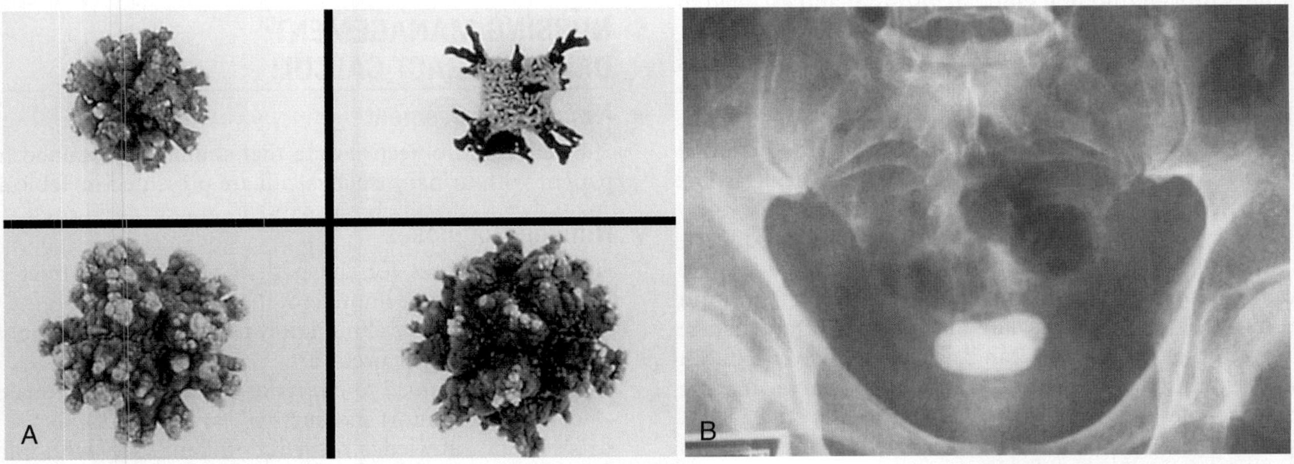


**FIG. 45-6** **A,** Calcium oxalate stones. **B,** Plain abdominal x-ray showing large bladder calculus. (From Bullock N, Doble A, Turner W, et al: *Urology: an illustrated colour text,* London, 2008, Churchill Livingstone.)

## EVIDENCE-BASED PRACTICE

### Applying the Evidence

**Prevention of Recurrent Kidney Stones**

You are caring for K.D., a 51-yr-old male patient, who is being discharged home following successful kidney stone retrieval. This was his first experience with a kidney stone and he states it was "very painful." He asks you if anything can be done to prevent more stones. You note on the medical record that the stone was composed of calcium and that he has a personal history of gout.

***Making Clinical Decisions***

***Best Available Evidence.*** Increased fluid intake (about 3 L/daily) decreases the risk of recurrent calcium stones in patients with a prior stone. Reducing soft-drink consumption may also help. Addition of medication (i.e., thiazide, citrate, allopurinol) for persons with multiple past calcium stones further reduces the risk.

***Clinician Expertise.*** You know risk factors for kidney stone formation include low fluid intake and having conditions such as gout, renal tubular acidosis, obesity, diabetes, and/or primary hyperthyroidism. You understand preventive measures may decrease the likelihood of recurrent kidney stones.

***Patient Preferences and Values.*** K.D. states that he is not a "water drinker," and it may be difficult to increase his fluid intake now that he cannot have sodas. He wants to know if drugs are available instead.

***Implications for Nursing Practice***

1. Why is it important for K.D. to understand the link between increased fluid intake and stone recurrence?
2. How would you help him identify ways to improve his uptake of fluids and why this may be difficult?
3. How would you respond to K.D.'s request for drugs to prevent recurrence?

***Reference for Evidence***

Fink HA, Wilt TJ, Eidman KE, et al: Medical management to prevent recurrent nephrolithiasis in adults: a systematic review for an American College of Physicians Clinical Guideline, *Ann Intern Med* 158:535, 2013.

In *extracorporeal shock-wave lithotripsy (ESWL),* a noninvasive procedure, the patient is anesthetized (spinal or general) to ensure that he or she maintains the same position during the procedure. Fluoroscopy or ultrasound is used to focus the lithotripter on the affected kidney, and a high-voltage spark generator produces high-energy acoustic shock waves that shatter the stone without damaging the surrounding tissues. The stone is broken into fine sand *(steinstrasse)* and excreted in the urine.

In *percutaneous ultrasonic lithotripsy* an ultrasonic probe is placed in the renal pelvis via a percutaneous nephroscope inserted through a small incision in the flank and is then positioned against the stone. The patient is given general or spinal anesthesia for this procedure. The probe produces ultrasonic waves, which break the stone into sandlike particles.

In *electrohydraulic lithotripsy* the probe is positioned directly on a stone, but it breaks the stone into small fragments that are removed by forceps or suction. A continuous saline irrigation flushes out the stone particles, and all of the outflow drainage is strained so that the particles can be analyzed. The calculi can also be removed by basket extraction. Complications are rare but they include hemorrhage, sepsis, and abscess formation. Postoperatively, the patient usually experiences moderate to severe colicky pain. The first few times that the patient urinates, the urine is bright red. As the bleeding subsides, the urine becomes dark red or a smoky color. Antibiotics are usually administered after the procedure to reduce the risk of infection.

Hematuria is common after lithotripsy procedures. A self-retaining ureteral stent is often placed after the procedure to facilitate passage of sand (shattered stone) and prevent sand buildup within the ureter, which may lead to obstruction. The stent is typically removed within 2 weeks following lithotripsy. If a stone is large or positioned in the mid or distal ureter, additional treatment, such as surgery, may be necessary.

**Surgical Therapy.** A small group of patients require open surgical procedures. The primary indications for surgery include pain, infection, and obstruction. The type of open surgery performed depends on the location of the stone. A *nephrolithotomy* is an incision into the kidney to remove a stone. A *pyelolithotomy* is an incision into the renal pelvis for stone removal. If the stone is located within the ureter, a *ureterolithotomy* is performed. A *cystotomy* may be indicated for bladder calculi. For open surgery on the kidney or ureter, a flank incision directly below the diaphragm and across the side is usually preferred. The most common complications after surgical procedures for stone removal are related to hemorrhage.

**Nutritional Therapy.** To manage an obstructing stone, the patient should drink adequate fluids to avoid dehydration. Forcing excessive fluids is not advised, since this has not proved effective in facilitating spontaneous passage (excretion) of stones via the urine. Forcing fluids may also increase the pain or precipitate the development of renal colic.

After an episode of urolithiasis, encourage a high fluid intake (approximately 3 L/day) to produce a urine output of at least 2 L/day. High urine output prevents supersaturation of minerals (i.e., dilutes the concentration of urine) and promotes excretion of minerals within the urine, thus preventing stone formation. Increasing fluid intake is particularly important for patients at risk for dehydration, including those who (1) are active in sports, (2) live in a dry climate, (3) perform physical exercise, (4) have a family history of stone formation, or (5) work outside or in an occupation that requires a great deal of physical activity. Water is the preferred fluid. Limit consumption of colas, coffee, and tea because high intake of these beverages tends to increase the risk of recurring urinary calculi.

A low-sodium diet is recommended, since high-sodium intake increases calcium excretion in the urine. Foods high in calcium, oxalate, and purines are presented in Table 45-12.

## ❖ NURSING MANAGEMENT: URINARY TRACT CALCULI

### ◆ Nursing Assessment

Subjective and objective data that should be obtained from a patient with urinary tract calculi are presented in Table 45-13.

### ◆ Nursing Diagnoses

Nursing diagnoses for the patient with urinary tract calculi include, but are not limited to, the following:

- Impaired urinary elimination *related to* trauma or obstruction of ureters or urethra
- Acute pain *related to* effects of stones and inadequate pain control or comfort measures
- Deficient knowledge *related to* unfamiliarity with information resources and lack of experience with urinary stones

**TABLE 45-12 Nutritional Therapy**

***Urinary Tract Calculi***

*Depending on the type of calculi, modify the diet to decrease foods that are high in the substance that is the cause of the calculi.*

**Purine***

*High:* Sardines, herring, mussels, liver, kidney, goose, venison, meat soups, sweetbreads

*Moderate:* Chicken, salmon, crab, veal, mutton, bacon, pork, beef, ham

**Calcium**

*High:* Milk, cheese, ice cream, yogurt, sauces containing milk; all beans (except green beans), lentils; fish with fine bones (e.g., sardines, kippers, herring, salmon); dried fruits, nuts; Ovaltine, chocolate, cocoa

**Oxalate**

*High:* Dark roughage, spinach, rhubarb, asparagus, cabbage, tomatoes, beets, nuts, celery, parsley, runner beans; chocolate, cocoa, instant coffee, Ovaltine, tea; Worcestershire sauce

*Uric acid is a waste product from purine in food.

Additional information on nursing diagnoses for the patient with urinary tract calculi is presented in eNursing Care Plan 45-2 (on the website for this chapter).

### Planning

The overall goals are that the patient with urinary tract calculi will have (1) relief of pain, (2) no urinary tract obstruction, and (3) knowledge of ways to prevent recurrence of stones.

### Nursing Implementation

Most people who have had urinary stones can lower their risk of recurrence by changing their lifestyle and dietary habits. Adequate fluid intake is important to produce a urine output of approximately 2 L/day. Consult with the HCP about specific recommendations for fluid intake in a given person. The moderately active, ambulatory person should drink about 3 L/day. Fluid intake must be higher in the active person who works outdoors or who regularly engages in athletic activities.

Preventive measures for a person who is on bed rest or is relatively immobile for a prolonged time include maintaining an adequate fluid intake, turning the patient every few hours, and helping the patient sit or stand, if possible, to maximize urinary flow.

Additional preventive measures focus on reducing metabolic or secondary risk factors. For example, dietary restriction of purines may be helpful for the patient at risk for developing uric acid stones. Teach the patient the dosage, scheduling, and potential side effects of drugs used to reduce the risk of stone formation (Table 45-11). Some patients may be taught to self-monitor urinary pH or urine output.

Pain management and patient comfort are primary nursing responsibilities when managing a patient who has an obstructing stone and renal colic (see eNursing Care Plan 45-2). To ensure that any spontaneously passed stones are retrieved, strain all urine voided by the patient using a gauze or a urine strainer. Encourage ambulation to promote movement of the stone from the upper to the lower urinary tract. To ensure safety, tell the patient who is experiencing acute renal colic to ask for assistance when ambulating, particularly if opioid analgesics are being given.

**TABLE 45-13 Nursing Assessment**

***Urinary Tract Calculi***

**Subjective Data**

***Important Health Information***

*Past health history:* Recent or chronic UTI. Immobilization. Previous urinary tract stones, obstruction, or kidney disease with urinary stasis. Gout, benign prostatic hyperplasia (BPH), hyperparathyroidism, chronic diarrhea

*Medications:* Prior use of medication for prevention of stones or treatment of UTI, allopurinol, analgesics, loop diuretics, thiazide diuretics

*Surgery or other treatments:* External urinary diversion, long-term indwelling urinary catheter

***Functional Health Patterns***

*Health perception–health management:* Family history of renal calculi, sedentary lifestyle

*Nutritional-metabolic:* Nausea, vomiting. Dietary intake of purines, excessive calcium ingestion, salt excess, oxalates, phosphates. Low fluid intake. Chills

*Elimination:* Decreased urine output, urinary urgency, frequency, feeling of bladder fullness

*Cognitive-perceptual:* Acute, severe, colicky pain in flank, back, abdomen, groin, or genitalia. Burning on urination, dysuria. Anxiety

**Objective Data**

***General***

Guarding, back pain, fever, dehydration

***Integumentary***

Warm, flushed skin or pallor with cool, moist skin (mild shock)

***Gastrointestinal***

Abdominal distention, absence of bowel sounds

***Urinary***

Oliguria, hematuria, tenderness on palpation of renal areas, passage of stone or stones

***Possible Diagnostic Findings***

↑ BUN and serum creatinine levels. Urinalysis indicating RBCs, WBCs, pyuria, crystals, casts, minerals, bacteria. ↑ Uric acid, calcium, phosphorus, oxalate, or cystine values on 24-hr urine sample. Calculi or anatomic changes on KUB x-ray. Direct visualization of obstruction on cystoureteroscopy

*KUB,* Kidneys, ureters, bladder; *UTI,* urinary tract infection.

### Evaluation

The expected outcomes are that the patient with urinary calculi will

- Maintain free flow of urine with minimal hematuria
- Report satisfactory pain relief
- Verbalize understanding of disease process and measures to prevent recurrence

Additional information on expected outcomes for the patient with urinary calculi is presented in eNursing Care Plan 45-2 (on the website for this chapter).

## STRICTURES

A **stricture** is a narrowing of the lumen of the ureter or urethra.

### Ureteral Strictures

*Ureteral strictures* can affect the entire length of the ureter, from the UPJ to UVJ. These strictures are usually secondary to adhesions or scar formation (following surgery or radiation) or they may be due to extrinsic factors such as large tumors in the peritoneal cavity. Depending on its severity, ureteral obstruction can threaten the function of the kidney.

Clinical manifestations of a ureteral stricture include mild to moderate colic. This pain may be moderate to severe in intensity if the patient consumes a large volume of fluids (such as alcohol) over a brief period. Infection is unusual unless a calculus or foreign object such as a stent or nephrostomy tube is present.

The discomfort and obstruction of a ureteral stricture may be temporarily bypassed by placing a stent using endoscopy or by diverting urinary flow via a nephrostomy tube inserted into the renal pelvis of the affected kidney. Definitive correction requires dilation with a balloon or catheter. If the stricture is severe or recurs after initial balloon or catheter dilation, it is surgically incised using an endoscopic procedure *(endoureterotomy)*. In selected cases an open surgical approach may be required to excise the stenotic area and re-anastomose the ureter to the contralateral ureter *(ureteroureterostomy)* or to the renal pelvis. Alternatively, distal ureteral strictures may be treated by a *ureteroneocystostomy* (reimplantation of the ureter into the bladder wall).

### Urethral Strictures

A *urethral stricture* is the result of fibrosis or inflammation of the urethral lumen. Causes of urethral strictures include trauma, urethritis (particularly after gonococcal infection), surgical intervention or repeated catheterizations (iatrogenic), or a congenital defect of the urethra. Once the process of inflammation and fibrosis begins, the lumen of the urethra narrows and its compliance (ability to close or open in response to bladder filling or micturition) is compromised. Meatal stenosis, a narrowing of the urethral opening, is also common.

Clinical manifestations associated with a urethral stricture include a diminished force of the urinary stream, straining to void, sprayed stream, postvoid dribbling, or a split urine stream. The patient may report feelings of incomplete bladder emptying with urinary frequency and nocturia. Moderate to severe obstruction of the bladder outlet may lead to acute urinary retention. The patient may report a history of urethritis, difficulty with insertion of a urinary catheter, or trauma involving the penis or the perineum. However, many patients are unable to recall any such events, thus leading to a diagnosis of an idiopathic stricture. A history of UTI is common, particularly if the stricture involves the distal urethra. Retrograde urethrography (RUG) and VCUG are used to identify stricture length, location, and caliber.

Initial management of a stricture is focused on dilation. A metal instrument (urethral sound) may be placed, or a series of progressively large stents (filiforms and followers) can be placed into the urethra to expand its lumen in a stepwise fashion. Although this process is initially successful, stenosis frequently recurs. Recurrences may be managed by teaching the patient to repeatedly dilate the urethra by self-catheterization using a soft (coudé-tip, red rubber) catheter every few days. Alternatively, an endoscopic or open surgical procedure *(urethroplasty)* may be a more definitive therapy for an obstructive urethral stricture. Shorter strictures may be treated by resection of the fibrotic area followed by re-anastomosis of the urethra. Longer strictures may require the use of a skin flap as a substitute urethral segment.

## RENAL TRAUMA

Renal trauma can be blunt or penetrating. *Blunt trauma* is the most common cause. Injury to the kidney should be considered in sports injuries, motor vehicle collisions, and falls. Renal trauma is especially likely when the patient injures the abdomen, flank, or back. *Penetrating injuries* may result from violent encounters (e.g., gunshot or stabbing incidents). The majority of incidents occur in men younger than 30 years of age.

Clinical findings include a history of trauma to the area of the kidneys. Gross or microscopic hematuria may be present. Diagnostic studies include urinalysis, ultrasound, CT, or MRI evaluation. Renal arteriography may also be used. Both the injured kidney and the uninvolved kidney should be evaluated. The severity of renal trauma depends on the extent of the injury. Treatments range from bed rest, fluids, and analgesia to exploratory surgery and repair or nephrectomy.

Nursing interventions depend on the type of renal trauma and the extent of any associated injuries. Interventions related to renal trauma include the following: (1) assess the cardiovascular status and monitor for shock, especially in a penetrating injury; (2) ensure adequate fluid intake and monitor intake and output; (3) provide for pain relief and comfort measures; and (4) assess for hematuria and myoglobinuria.

# RENAL VASCULAR PROBLEMS

Vascular problems involving the kidney include (1) nephrosclerosis, (2) renal artery stenosis, and (3) renal vein thrombosis.

## NEPHROSCLEROSIS

**Nephrosclerosis** is sclerosis of the small arteries and arterioles of the kidney. The decreased blood flow results in ischemia and necrosis of parts of the kidney. *Benign nephrosclerosis,* which usually occurs in adults 30 to 50 years of age, is caused by vascular changes resulting from hypertension and from atherosclerosis. Atherosclerotic vascular changes account for most of the loss of renal function associated with aging. The degree of nephrosclerosis is directly related to the severity of hypertension. In the early stages, the patient with benign nephrosclerosis may have normal renal function, with the only detectable abnormality being hypertension.

*Accelerated nephrosclerosis (malignant nephrosclerosis)* is associated with malignant hypertension, which is characterized by a sharp increase in BP with a diastolic pressure greater than 130 mm Hg. The patient is usually a young adult, with a male-to-female predominance of 2:1. Renal insufficiency progresses rapidly.

Treatment for benign nephrosclerosis is the same as that for essential hypertension (see Chapter 32). Malignant nephrosclerosis is treated with aggressive antihypertensive therapy (see Chapter 32). The availability and use of antihypertensive drugs have improved the prognosis for patients with benign and malignant nephrosclerosis. Kidney disease, and subsequent renal failure, is a major complication of hypertension. The prognosis for a patient with untreated or refractive malignant hypertension is poor, with the major cause of death related to renal failure.

## RENAL ARTERY STENOSIS

**Renal artery stenosis** is a partial occlusion of one or both renal arteries and their major branches. It can be due to atherosclerotic narrowing or fibromuscular hyperplasia. Renal artery stenosis, which accounts for 1% to 2% of all cases of hypertension, is a cause of secondary hypertension.

When hypertension develops rather abruptly, renal artery stenosis should be considered as a possible cause, especially in patients under 30 or over 50 years of age and in patients with no family history of hypertension. This contrasts with the age distribution for primary hypertension, which is 30 to 50 years of age.

Diagnostic tests used to assess for renal artery stenosis include a renal ultrasound, CT scan, MRI, and renal arteriogram (the best diagnostic tool).

The goals of therapy are to control BP and restore perfusion to the kidney. Percutaneous transluminal renal angioplasty is the procedure of choice, especially in older patients who are poor surgical risks.

Surgical revascularization of the kidney is indicated when decreased blood flow causes renal ischemia or when renovascular hypertension is present. Revascularization of the kidney may result in the patient becoming normotensive. The surgical procedure usually involves anastomosis between the kidney and another major artery, usually the splenic artery or aorta. In selected cases of unilateral renal involvement, unilateral nephrectomy may be indicated.

## RENAL VEIN THROMBOSIS

*Renal vein thrombosis* may occur unilaterally or bilaterally. Causes include trauma, extrinsic compression (e.g., tumor, aortic aneurysm), renal cell cancer, pregnancy, contraceptive use, and nephrotic syndrome.

The patient has symptoms of flank pain, hematuria, or fever or has nephrotic syndrome. Anticoagulation (e.g., heparin, warfarin [Coumadin]) is important to treat the high incidence of pulmonary emboli. Corticosteroids may be used for the patient with nephrotic syndrome. Surgical thrombectomy may be performed instead of or along with anticoagulation.

# HEREDITARY KIDNEY DISEASES

Hereditary kidney (or renal) diseases involve developmental abnormalities of the renal parenchyma. Most inherited structural abnormalities are cystic. However, cysts may also develop as a result of obstructive uropathies, metabolic problems, or neurologic diseases. Cysts may be evaluated to rule out tumors.

## POLYCYSTIC KIDNEY DISEASE

**Polycystic kidney disease (PKD)** is the most common life-threatening genetic disease in the world, affecting 600,000 people in the United States. PKD accounts for 10% to 15% of chronic kidney disease.[16]

### Genetic Link

PKD has two hereditary forms: manifestations in childhood or adulthood. The childhood form of PKD is a rare autosomal recessive disorder that is often rapidly progressive (see the Genetics in Clinical Practice box). The adult form of PKD is an autosomal dominant disorder (see Figs. 12-4 and 12-5). If one parent has the disease, there is a 50% chance that the disease will pass to the child.

Adult PKD is latent for many years and is usually manifested between 30 and 40 years of age.[17] It involves both kidneys and occurs in both men and women. The cortex and medulla are filled with large, thin-walled cysts that are several millimeters to several centimeters in diameter (Fig. 45-7). The cysts enlarge and destroy surrounding tissue by compression. The cysts are filled

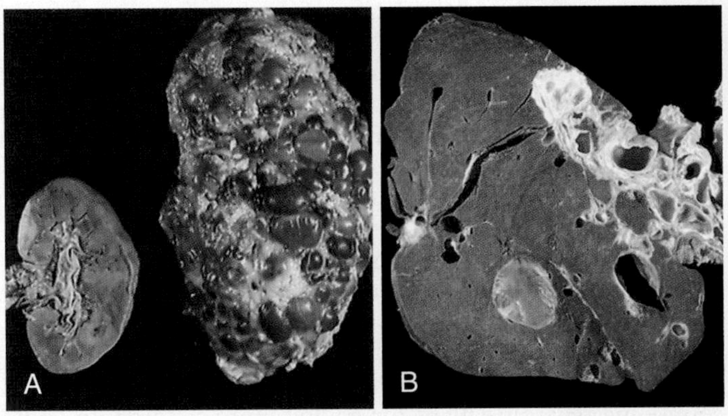


**FIG. 45-7** **A,** Comparison of polycystic kidney with normal kidney. **B,** Cysts in the liver. (*A,* From Brundage DJ: *Renal disorders,* St Louis, 1992, Mosby. *B,* From Kumar V, Abbas AK, Fausto N: *Robbins and Cotran pathologic basis of disease,* ed 7, Philadelphia, 2005, Saunders.)

## GENETICS IN CLINICAL PRACTICE

### *Polycystic Kidney Disease (PKD)*

| | Adult | Child |
|---|---|---|
| **Genetic basis** | Autosomal dominant | Autosomal recessive |
| **Incidence** | 1 in 400-1000 | 1 in 10,000-20,000 |
| **Gene location** | • *PKD1* gene on chromosome 16 and *PKD2* gene on chromosome 4<br>• Genes code for polycystins (proteins that promote normal kidney development and function)<br>• Mutations in genes lead to formation of thousands of cysts that disrupt the normal function of kidneys and other organs | • Polycystic kidney and hepatic disease *(PKHD1)* gene on chromosome 6<br>• Gene codes for fibrocystin<br>• Mutations in gene leads to cyst formation |
| **Genetic testing** | DNA testing available | DNA testing available* |
| **Age of onset** | Ages 30-40 | Infancy or childhood |
| **Clinical implications** | • Multisystem involvement<br>• Systemic hypertension occurs in 60%-80% of patients<br>• Increased risk for cerebral aneurysms<br>• Families at risk should be screened | • Up to 30%-50% of affected newborns die shortly after birth<br>• If infant survives the newborn period, chances of survival are good, but about one third need dialysis or transplantation by age 10 yr |

*Genetic testing is also available on fertilized embryos before implantation. This allows embryos free of the disorder to be placed into the uterus.

with fluid and may contain blood or pus. PKD kidneys examined during autopsy appear as if they are filled with golf balls.

Early in the disease, patients are generally asymptomatic. Symptoms appear when the cysts begin to enlarge. Often the first manifestations of PKD are headaches; hypertension; hematuria (from rupture of cysts); or a feeling of pain or heaviness in the back, side, or abdomen. However, the first manifestation can also be a UTI or urinary calculi.

Chronic pain is one of the most common problems experienced by individuals with PKD. The pain can be constant and severe. Bilateral, enlarged kidneys are often palpable on physical examination. Many people have no symptoms, and the disease is not diagnosed.

PKD can also affect the liver (liver cysts [Fig. 45-7]), heart (abnormal heart valves), blood vessels (aneurysms), and intestines (diverticulosis). The most serious complication is a cerebral aneurysm, which can rupture.

Diagnosis is based on clinical manifestations, family history, ultrasound (best screening measure), or CT scan (provides a more precise scan). The disease usually progresses from loss of kidney function to ESRD by age 60 in 50% of patients.[16]

## ❖ NURSING AND INTERPROFESSIONAL MANAGEMENT: POLYCYSTIC KIDNEY DISEASE

There is no specific treatment for PKD. A major aim of treatment is to prevent or treat infections of the urinary tract. Nephrectomy may be necessary if pain, bleeding, or infection becomes a chronic, serious problem. Dialysis and kidney transplant may be needed to treat ESRD (see Chapter 47).

When the patient begins to experience progressive renal failure, the interventions depend on the remaining renal function. Nursing measures are those used for management of ESRD. They include diet modification, fluid restriction, drugs (e.g., antihypertensives), and assistance for the patient and family in coping with the chronic disease process and financial concerns.

The patient who has adult PKD often has children by the time the disease is diagnosed. The patient needs appropriate counseling regarding plans for having more children. In addition, genetic counseling should be provided for the children.

### CHECK YOUR PRACTICE

You are doing a rotation in the dialysis unit. You have been doing vital sign checks on a 45-yr-old man who receives dialysis three times/week. When you ask him why he is on dialysis, he tells you that he has polycystic kidney disease. After further discussion, he tells you that he only has one son who is now 23 years old, but they are estranged. He does not want to tell him about his medical problems or why he is on dialysis.

- How would you respond to this patient?

## MEDULLARY CYSTIC DISEASE

*Medullary cystic disease* is a hereditary disorder that occurs in two forms. The *autosomal recessive form* is associated with renal failure before age 20. The *autosomal dominant form* is associated with renal failure after age 20.

Most cysts are located in the medulla. The kidneys are asymmetric in shape and are significantly scarred. Defects in the kidneys' concentrating ability result in polyuria. Other clinical manifestations include hypertension, progressive renal failure, severe anemia, and metabolic acidosis. Genetic counseling may be helpful in family planning. Treatment measures are those related to ESRD (see Chapter 46).

## ALPORT SYNDROME

*Alport syndrome,* also known as *chronic hereditary nephritis,* is an inherited disease that primarily affects the glomeruli. The basic defect is a mutation in a gene for collagen that results in altered synthesis of the glomerular basement membrane.[18]

There are three genetic types of Alport syndrome: sex-linked, autosomal recessive type, and autosomal dominant type. In sex-linked (the most common type) the earliest manifestation is hematuria. These patients also have progressive hearing loss and deformities of the lens of the eye. The other types of Alport syndrome cause hematuria but not deafness or lens deformities.

Males are affected earlier and more severely than females. The disease is often diagnosed in the first decade of life. Alport syndrome causes progressive kidney damage, leading to kidney failure. Children with the autosomal recessive type of Alport syndrome develop kidney failure, usually by their teens or young adult years. People with autosomal dominant Alport syndrome usually live well into middle age before kidney failure develops.

Treatment is supportive. Corticosteroids and cytotoxic drugs are not effective. Kidney transplantation is usually very successful in people with Alport syndrome and is considered the best treatment. The disease does not recur after kidney transplantation.

# URINARY TRACT TUMORS

## KIDNEY CANCER

*Kidney cancer* arises from the cortex or pelvis (and calyces). Tumors from these areas may be benign or malignant. However, malignant tumors are more common. In the United States, about 61,560 new cases of kidney cancer are diagnosed each year, and about 14,080 people die from kidney cancer.[19]

Renal cell carcinoma (adenocarcinoma) is the most common type of kidney cancer (Fig. 45-8). This type of tumor occurs

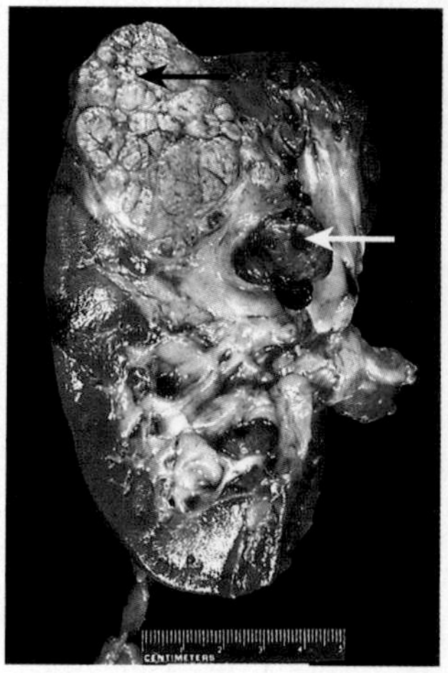

**FIG. 45-8** Cross section of kidney with renal cell carcinoma. The carcinoma *(black arrow)* is on the pole of the kidney. Note that the renal vein is involved and thrombosed *(white arrow).* (From Kumar V, Abbas AK, Fausto N: *Robbins and Cotran pathologic basis of disease,* ed 7, Philadelphia, 2005, Saunders.)

twice as often in men as in women and is typically discovered when the person is 50 to 70 years of age. Cigarette smoking is the most significant risk factor for the development of renal cell carcinoma. An increased incidence has also been found in first-degree relatives of people who have or had renal cell carcinoma. Other risk factors include obesity; hypertension; and exposure to asbestos, cadmium, and gasoline. Risk for kidney cancer is also increased in individuals who have acquired cystic disease of the kidney associated with ESRD (see Chapter 46).

### Clinical Manifestations and Diagnostic Studies

Early stage kidney cancer usually has no symptoms, so many patients go undiagnosed until the disease has significantly progressed. Many kidney cancers are diagnosed as incidental findings on imaging studies used to evaluate symptoms for unrelated conditions.

Kidney tumors can cause symptoms by compressing, stretching, or invading structures near or within the kidney. The most common presenting manifestations are hematuria, flank pain, and a palpable mass in the flank or abdomen. Other clinical manifestations include weight loss, fever, hypertension, and anemia.

About 30% of patients have metastasis at the time of diagnosis. Local extension of kidney cancer into the renal vein and vena cava is common (Fig. 45-8). The most common sites of metastases include lungs, liver, and long bones.

CT scan is commonly used in the diagnosis and can detect small kidney tumors. Ultrasound examinations have improved the ability to differentiate between a solid mass tumor and a cyst. This is significant because the majority of masses detected on imaging are cysts. Angiography, biopsy, and MRI are also used in the diagnosis of renal tumors. Radionuclide isotope scanning is used to detect metastases.

## NURSING AND INTERPROFESSIONAL MANAGEMENT: KIDNEY CANCER

Preventive measures, such as quitting smoking, maintaining a healthy weight, controlling BP, and reducing or avoiding exposure to toxins, can help reduce the incidence of kidney cancer. Patients in high-risk groups should be aware of their increased risk for kidney cancer. Teach them about early manifestations (e.g., hematuria, hypertension). A cure for kidney cancer may be possible when it is detected early and treated.

Interprofessional care of the patient with kidney cancer is presented in Table 45-14. Staging of renal carcinoma provides a basis for determining treatment options. The following is a simple description of staging of kidney cancer:

*Stage I:* The tumor can be up to 7 cm in diameter but is confined to the kidney.

*Stage II:* The tumor is larger than a stage I tumor but is still confined to the kidney.

*Stage III:* The tumor extends beyond the kidney to the surrounding tissue and may also have spread to a nearby lymph node.

*Stage IV:* Cancer spreads outside the kidney to multiple lymph nodes or to distant parts of the body, such as bones, brain, liver, or lung.

The treatment of choice for some renal cancers is a partial nephrectomy (for smaller tumors), simple total nephrectomy, or a radical nephrectomy (for larger tumors). Radical nephrectomy involves removal of the kidney, adrenal gland, surrounding fascia, part of the ureter, and draining lymph nodes. Nephrectomy can be performed by a conventional (open) approach or laparoscopically (see discussion of nephrectomy on p. 1063). Other treatment options include cryoablation (freezing technique) and radiofrequency ablation (destroying tumor by using radiofrequency heat). These procedures can be used when surgery is not an option (e.g., patient has co-morbid conditions) and for small renal tumors.

**TABLE 45-14 Interprofessional Care**

***Renal Cancer***

| Diagnostic Assessment | Management |
|---|---|
| • History and physical examination<br>• Urinalysis<br>• Ultrasound<br>• CT scan (CT urogram)<br>• MRI<br>• Renal biopsy<br>• Renal scan<br>• Angiography | • Surgical therapy<br>  • Partial nephrectomy<br>  • Radical nephrectomy<br>• Ablation<br>• Cryoablation<br>  • Radiofrequency ablation<br>• Radiation therapy<br>• Chemotherapy<br>• Immunotherapy<br>• Targeted therapy |

Kidney cancer is relatively resistant to most chemotherapy drugs and radiation therapy. Chemotherapy is used as a treatment in metastatic disease.[20] These drugs include 5-fluorouracil (5-FU), floxuridine, and gemcitabine (Gemzar). Radiation therapy is used palliatively in inoperable cases and when there is metastasis to bone or lungs.

Immunotherapy, including α-interferon and interleukin-2 (IL-2), is another treatment in metastatic disease. (The use of α-interferon and IL-2 is discussed in Chapter 15.) Another type of drug used as immunotherapy is nivolumab (Opdivo). This drug targets PD-1, a protein on T cells that normally helps keep these cells from attacking other cells in the body. By blocking PD-1, this drug boosts the immune response against cancer cells. This can shrink some tumors or slow their growth.

Targeted therapy is the preferred treatment for metastatic kidney cancer. Kinase inhibitors, one class of targeted therapies, block certain proteins (kinases) that play a role in tumor growth and cancer progression. Kinase inhibitors include sunitinib (Sutent), sorafenib (Nexavar), cabozantinib (Cabometyx), and axitinib (Inlyta). Bevacizumab (Avastin) and pazopanib (Votrient) inhibit the formation of new blood vessel growth to the tumor. Temsirolimus (Torisel) and everolimus (Afinitor) inhibit a specific protein known as the *mechanistic target of rapamycin (mTOR)*. These drugs are presented in Table 15-13, and the mechanisms of action are shown in Fig. 15-16. The diagnosis of cancer is devastating. In kidney cancer the disease can already be metastasized by the time a person is diagnosed. (The nursing care of the patient with cancer is discussed in Chapter 15.)

## BLADDER CANCER

About 74,000 new cases of bladder cancer are diagnosed annually, and about 16,000 deaths related to bladder cancer are reported every year. Cancer of the bladder is most common between ages 60 and 70 years and is four times more common in men than in women.[19]

The most frequent malignant tumor of the urinary tract is transitional cell carcinoma of the bladder. Most bladder tumors are papillomatous growths within the bladder (Fig. 45-9).

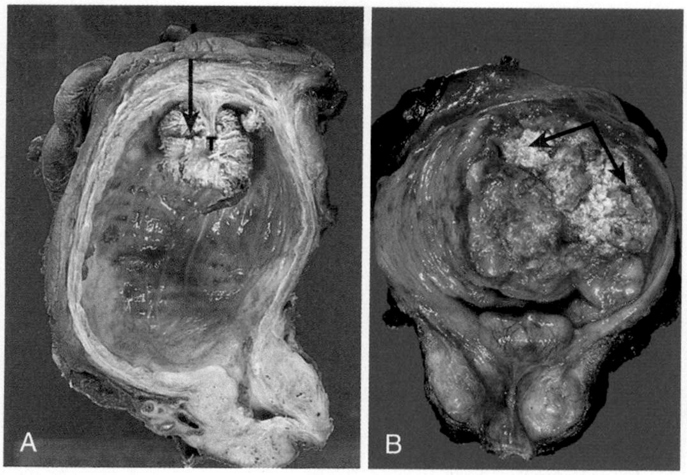


**FIG. 45-9** **A,** Papillary transitional cell carcinoma *(T)* seen arising from the dome of the bladder as a cauliflower-like lesion *(arrow).* **B,** Opened bladder showing bladder cancer at an advanced stage. Yellow areas represent ulcerations and necrosis *(arrows).* (*A,* From Stevens A, Lowe J: *Pathology: illustrated review in colour,* ed 2, London, 2000, Mosby. *B,* From Kumar V, Abbas AK, Fausto N: *Robbins and Cotran pathologic basis of disease,* ed 7, Philadelphia, 2005, Saunders.)

About one half of bladder cancers are related to cigarette smoking. Other risk factors include exposure to dyes used in the rubber and other industries. Also at increased risk for bladder cancer are women treated with radiation for cervical cancer, patients who received cyclophosphamide, and patients who take the diabetes drug pioglitazone (Actos).

Individuals with chronic, recurrent renal calculi (often bladder) and chronic lower UTIs have an increased risk of squamous cell cancer of the bladder. Patients who have indwelling catheters for long periods are also at an increased risk to develop bladder cancer.

### Clinical Manifestations and Diagnostic Studies

Microscopic or gross, painless hematuria (chronic or intermittent) is the most common clinical manifestation of bladder cancer. Bladder irritability with dysuria, frequency, and urgency may also occur.

When cancer is suspected, obtain urine specimens to identify any cancer or atypical cells. Exfoliated cells from the bladder's epithelial surface can be detected in voided specimens. Other urine tests assess for specific factors associated with bladder cancer, such as bladder tumor antigens.

Bladder cancers can be detected using CT, ultrasound, or MRI. The presence of cancer is confirmed by cystoscopy and biopsy. Cystoscopy with biopsy is the most reliable test for detecting bladder tumors.

## NURSING AND INTERPROFESSIONAL MANAGEMENT: BLADDER CANCER

The majority of bladder cancers are diagnosed at an early stage when the cancer is treatable. Before a treatment regimen is started, bladder cancers are graded based on the cell type and staged based on the extent and invasiveness of the cancer. A grading system is used to classify the malignant potential of tumor cells, using a scale from well differentiated (closely resembling the normal tissue) to undifferentiated (poorly differentiated) (see pp. 240-241 in Chapter 15).

The clinical staging of bladder cancer is determined by the depth of invasion of the bladder wall and surrounding tissue.

**TABLE 45-15 Interprofessional Care**

***Bladder Cancer***

| Diagnostic Assessment | Management |
|---|---|
| • History and physical examination<br>• Urinalysis<br>• Urine cytology studies<br>• Cystoscopy with biopsy<br>• Ultrasound<br>• CT scan | • Surgical therapy<br>  • Transurethral resection with fulguration<br>  • Laser photocoagulation<br>  • Open loop resection with fulguration<br>  • Cystectomy (segmental, partial, or radical)<br>• Radiation therapy<br>• Intravesical immunotherapy<br>  • Bacille Calmette-Guérin (BCG)<br>  • α-interferon (Intron A)<br>• Intravesical chemotherapy<br>  • mitomycin<br>  • thiotepa<br>  • valrubicin (Valstar)<br>• Systemic chemotherapy and immunotherapy |

The following is a simple description of staging of bladder cancer:

*Stage I:* Cancer is in the inner lining of the bladder but has not invaded the bladder muscle wall.

*Stage II:* Cancer has invaded the bladder wall but is still confined to bladder.

*Stage III:* Cancer has spread through the bladder wall to surrounding tissue. It may also have spread to the prostate in men or the uterus or vagina in women.

*Stage IV:* Cancer has spread to the lymph nodes and other organs, such as lungs, bones, or liver.

Interprofessional care of bladder cancer includes surgery, radiation, chemotherapy, and intravesical therapy (Table 45-15).

### Surgical Therapy

Surgical therapies include a variety of procedures. *Transurethral resection of the bladder tumor* (TURBT) is used for superficial lesions of the bladder's inner lining. A wire loop inserted through the cystoscope is used to cauterize (with electric current or laser) and kill the cancer cells. This procedure is also used to control bleeding in the patient who is a poor operative risk or who has advanced tumors. The primary disadvantage of this approach is destruction of the tumor so that pathologic evaluation for grading and staging cannot be completed.

A *segmental cystectomy (partial cystectomy)* is used to treat larger tumors or those that involve only one area of the bladder. A portion of the bladder wall containing the tumor is removed along with a margin of normal tissue.

When the tumor is invasive or involves the trigone (the area where the ureters insert into the bladder) and the patient is free from metastasis beyond the pelvic area, a radical cystectomy is the treatment of choice. A *radical cystectomy* involves removal of the bladder, prostate, and seminal vesicles in men and the bladder, uterus, cervix, urethra, and ovaries in women. After a radical cystectomy, a new way must be created for urine to leave the body. This surgical technique is called a *urinary diversion* (discussed on pp. 1064-1065 later in this chapter).

Postoperative instructions for any of these surgical procedures include drinking a large volume of fluid for the first week after the procedure. Teach the patient to monitor the color and consistency of the urine. The urine is pink for the first several days after the procedure, but it should not be bright red or contain blood clots. Approximately 7 to 10 days after tumor resection, the patient may observe dark red or rust-colored flecks in the urine. These may be from the healing tumor resection site.

Administer opioid analgesics for a brief period after the procedure, along with stool softeners. Also help the patient and family cope with fears about cancer, surgery, and sexuality. Emphasize the importance of regular follow-up care. Follow-up cystoscopies are required on a regular basis after surgery for bladder cancer.

### Radiation Therapy, Chemotherapy, and Immunotherapy

Radiation therapy can be used in combination with cystectomy or as the primary therapy when the cancer is inoperable or the patient refuses surgery. Chemotherapy drugs used in treating invasive bladder cancer include cisplatin, vinblastine, doxorubicin, and methotrexate. Atezolizumab (Tecentriq) is a type of immunotherapy that enhances the immune response against the bladder cancer cells.

### Intravesical Therapy

Chemotherapy with local instillation of immunotherapy or chemotherapy can be delivered directly into the bladder by a urethral catheter.[21] *Intravesical therapy* is usually initiated at weekly intervals for 6 to 12 weeks. The drug is instilled directly into the patient's bladder and retained for about 2 hours. The patient's bladder must be empty before instillation. Change the patient's position every 15 minutes during the instillation for maximum contact in all areas of the bladder. Maintenance therapy after the initial induction regimen may be beneficial.

Bacille Calmette-Guérin (BCG), a weakened strain of *Mycobacterium bovis,* is the treatment of choice for carcinoma in situ. BCG stimulates the immune system rather than acting directly on cancer cells in the bladder. When BCG fails, α-interferon in addition to BCG may be used. Other treatments that can be used when BCG fails include mitomycin and valrubicin (chemotherapy antibiotics) and thiotepa (an alkylating agent).[22]

Most patients have irritative voiding symptoms and hemorrhagic cystitis after intravesical therapy. Thiotepa can significantly reduce WBC and platelet counts in some individuals when absorbed into the circulation from the bladder wall. BCG may cause flu-like symptoms, increased urinary frequency, hematuria, or systemic infection. Other side effects of chemotherapy (e.g., nausea, vomiting, hair loss) are not experienced with intravesical chemotherapy.

Encourage patients to increase their daily fluid intake and to quit smoking. Assess the patient for secondary UTI, and stress the need for routine urologic follow-up. The patient may have fears or concerns about sexual activity or bladder function that must be addressed. Because of the high rate of disease recurrence and progression in bladder cancer, follow-up studies are very important.

# BLADDER DYSFUNCTION

## URINARY INCONTINENCE

**Urinary incontinence (UI)** is an involuntary leakage of urine. Although incontinence is more prevalent among older women and older men, it is not a natural consequence of aging. UI has traditionally been viewed as a social or hygienic problem, but it also has a major effect on quality of life and contributes to serious health problems, especially in older adults.

### Etiology and Pathophysiology

UI occurs when bladder pressure exceeds urethral closure pressure. Anything that interferes with bladder or urethral sphincter control can result in UI. Using the acronym *DRIP,* the causes can include *D:* delirium, dehydration, depression; *R:* restricted mobility, rectal impaction; *I:* infection, inflammation, impaction; and *P:* polyuria, polypharmacy. Patients may have more than one type of incontinence (Table 45-16).

**GENDER DIFFERENCES**

***Urinary Incontinence***

| Men | Women |
|---|---|
| • Urinary incontinence is a common manifestation of benign prostatic hyperplasia and prostate cancer in men.<br>• Urinary incontinence in men most often is overflow incontinence caused by urinary retention. | • Prevalence of urinary incontinence is higher in women than men.<br>• Women more frequently experience stress and urge incontinence than men. |

### Diagnostic Studies

The basic evaluation for UI includes a focused history, physical assessment, and bladder log or voiding record whenever possible. Obtain information related to the onset of UI, factors that provoke urinary leakage, and associated conditions. Pay special attention to factors known to produce transient UI, particularly when the onset of urine loss is relatively sudden. Begin the physical examination with an assessment of general health and functional issues associated with urination, including mobility, dexterity, and cognitive function.

A pelvic examination includes careful inspection of the perineal skin for signs of erosion or rashes related to UI and existence of pelvic organ prolapse. Also evaluate local innervation and pelvic floor muscle strength, including a digital examination of the pelvic floor muscle to determine weakness or tension. Whenever possible, ask the patient to keep a bladder log or voiding diary documenting the timing of urinations, episodes of urinary leakage, and frequency of nocturia for a period of 1 to 7 days. This record can be kept by nursing staff if the person is in an inpatient or long-term care facility.

A urinalysis is used to identify possible factors contributing to transient UI (e.g., UTI, diabetes mellitus). Measure postvoid residual (PVR) urine in the patient undergoing evaluation for UI. The PVR volume is obtained by asking the patient to urinate, followed by catheterization or use of a bladder ultrasound within a relatively brief period (preferably 10 to 20 minutes).

Urodynamic testing is indicated in selected cases of UI. Imaging studies of the upper urinary tract (e.g., ultrasound) are obtained when UI is associated with UTIs or evidence of upper urinary tract involvement.

### Interprofessional Care

Many cases of incontinence can be cured or significantly improved. Transient, reversible factors are initially corrected, followed by management of the type of UI (Table 45-16). In general, less invasive treatments are attempted before more invasive methods (e.g., surgery). Nevertheless, the choice of the initial treatment is individualized, based on patient preference, the type and severity of UI, and associated anatomic defects.

Several behavioral therapies may be used to improve UI (Table 45-17). Pelvic floor muscle training (Kegel exercises) is used to manage stress, urge, or mixed UI[23] (Table 45-18). Biofeedback is used to help the patient identify, isolate, contract,

**TABLE 45-16 Types of Urinary Incontinence**

| Description | Causes | Treatment |
|---|---|---|
| **Stress Incontinence*** | | |
| • Sudden increase in intraabdominal pressure causes involuntary passage of urine.<br>• Can occur during coughing, laughing, sneezing, or physical activities such as heavy lifting, exercising.<br>• Leakage usually is in small amounts and may not be daily. | • Most common in women with relaxed pelvic floor musculature (from delivery, use of instrumentation during vaginal delivery, or multiple pregnancies).<br>• Structures of female urethra atrophy when estrogen decreases.<br>• Prostate surgery for BPH or prostate cancer. | • Pelvic floor muscle exercises (e.g., Kegel exercises), weight loss if obese, cessation of smoking, topical estrogen products, external condom catheters or penile clamp in men, surgery<br>• Urethral inserts, patches, or bladder neck support devices (e.g., incontinence pessary) to correct underlying problem |
| **Urge Incontinence*** | | |
| • Often referred to as overactive bladder.<br>• Occurs randomly when involuntary urination is preceded by urinary urgency.<br>• Leakage is periodic but frequent and usually in large amounts.<br>• Nocturnal frequency and incontinence are common. | • Caused by uncontrolled contraction or overactive detrusor muscle.<br>• Bladder escapes central inhibition and contracts reflexively.<br>• Conditions include:<br>  • Nervous system disorders (e.g., stroke, Alzheimer's disease, brain tumor, Parkinson's disease)<br>  • Bladder disorders (e.g., carcinoma in situ, radiation effects, interstitial cystitis)<br>  • Interference with spinal inhibitory pathways (e.g., malignant growth in spinal cord, spondylosis)<br>  • Bladder outlet obstruction or conditions of unknown etiology | • Treatment of underlying cause<br>• Biobehavioral interventions (bladder retraining with urge suppression, decrease in dietary irritants, bowel regularity, pelvic floor muscle exercises)<br>• Anticholinergic drugs (Table 45-19)<br>• Mirabegron (Myrbetriq)<br>• Calcium channel blockers (Table 45-19)<br>• Containment devices (e.g., external condom catheters)<br>• Vaginal estrogen creams<br>• Absorbent products |
| **Overflow Incontinence** | | |
| • Occurs when pressure of urine in overfull bladder overcomes sphincter control.<br>• Leakage of small amounts of urine is frequent throughout day and night.<br>• Urination may also occur frequently in small amounts.<br>• Bladder remains distended and is usually palpable. | • Disorder is caused by bladder or urethral outlet obstruction (bladder neck obstruction, urethral stricture, pelvic organ prolapse) or by underactive detrusor muscle caused by myogenic or neurogenic factors (e.g., herniated disc, diabetic neuropathy).<br>• May also occur after anesthesia and surgery (e.g., hemorrhoidectomy, herniorrhaphy, cystoscopy).<br>• Neurogenic bladder (flaccid type). | • Urinary catheterization to decompress bladder<br>• Implementation of Credé or Valsalva maneuver<br>• 5α-Reductase inhibitors (Table 45-19) to decrease outlet resistance<br>• α-Adrenergic blockers (Table 45-19)<br>• Bethanechol (Urecholine) to enhance bladder contractions<br>• Intravaginal device such as a pessary to support prolapse<br>• Intermittent catheterization<br>• Surgery to correct underlying problem |
| **Reflex Incontinence** | | |
| • Condition occurs when no warning or stress precedes periodic involuntary urination.<br>• Urination is frequent, moderate in volume, and occurs equally during day and night. | • Spinal cord lesion above S2 interferes with central nervous system inhibition.<br>• Disorder results in detrusor hyperreflexia and interferes with pathways coordinating detrusor contraction and sphincter relaxation. | • Treatment of underlying cause<br>• Bladder decompression to prevent ureteral reflux and hydronephrosis<br>• Intermittent self-catheterization<br>• Diazepam (Valium) or baclofen (Lioresal) to relax external sphincter<br>• Prophylactic antibiotics<br>• Surgical sphincterotomy |
| **Incontinence After Trauma or Surgery** | | |
| • In women, vesicovaginal or urethrovaginal fistula may occur.<br>• In men, alteration in continence control involves proximal urethral sphincter (bladder neck and prostatic urethra) and distal urethral sphincter (external striated muscle). | • Fistulas may occur during pregnancy, after delivery of baby, as a result of hysterectomy or invasive cancer of cervix, or after radiation therapy.<br>• Incontinence is a postoperative complication of transurethral, perineal, or retropubic prostatectomy. | • Surgery to correct fistula<br>• Urinary diversion surgery to bypass urethra and bladder<br>• External condom catheter<br>• Penile clamp<br>• Placement of artificial implantable sphincter |
| **Functional Incontinence** | | |
| • Loss of urine resulting from cognitive, functional, or environmental factors. | • Older adults often have problems that affect balance and mobility (e.g., severe arthritis).<br>• Cognitive problems (e.g., dementia). | • Modifications of environment or care plan that facilitates regular, easy access to toilet and promotes patient safety<br>• Includes better lighting, removal of scatter rugs, ambulatory assistance equipment, clothing alterations, timed voiding, different toileting equipment |

*Patients can have a combination of stress and urge incontinence, referred to as mixed incontinence.

**TABLE 45-17 Interventions for Urinary Incontinence**

| Intervention | Description |
|---|---|
| **Lifestyle Modifications** | Self-management strategies to reduce or eliminate risk factors, including the following: • Smoking cessation • Weight reduction • Good bowel regimen • Reduction of bladder irritants (e.g., caffeine, aspartame artificial sweetener, citrus juices) • Fluid modifications for those with urge incontinence |
| **Scheduled Voiding Regimens** | |
| Timed voiding | Toileting on a fixed schedule (typically every 2-3 hr during waking hours). |
| Habit retraining | Scheduled toileting with adjustments of voiding intervals (longer or shorter) based on the individual's voiding pattern. |
| Prompted voiding | Scheduled toileting that requires prompts to void from a caregiver (typically every 3 hr). Used in conjunction with operant conditioning techniques to reward individuals for maintaining continence and appropriate toileting. |
| Bladder retraining and urge-suppression strategies | Scheduled toileting with progressive voiding intervals. Includes teaching of urge-control strategies using relaxation and distraction techniques, self-monitoring, reinforcement techniques, and other strategies such as conscious contraction of pelvic floor muscles. |
| **Pelvic Floor Muscle Rehabilitation** | |
| Pelvic floor muscle (Kegel) exercises or training | Table 45-18. |
| Vaginal weight training | Active retention of vaginal weights (devices designed and shaped to exercise and strengthen pelvic floor muscles) at least twice a day. Typically used in combination with pelvic floor muscle exercises. |
| Biofeedback | See Complementary & Alternative Therapies box on p. 1057. |
| Electrical stimulation | Application of low-voltage electric current to sacral and pudendal afferent fibers through vaginal, anal, or surface electrodes. Used to inhibit bladder overactivity and improve awareness, contractility, and efficiency of pelvic muscle contraction. |
| **Anti-Incontinence Devices** | |
| Intravaginal support devices (pessaries and bladder neck support prostheses) | Devices support bladder neck, relieve minor pelvic organ prolapse, and change pressure transmission to the urethra. |
| Intraurethral occlusive device (urethral plug) | Single-use device that is worn in the urethra to provide mechanical obstruction to prevent urine leakage. Removed for voiding. |
| Intraurethral valve pump | Replaceable urinary prosthesis for use in women who have impaired detrusor contractility (cannot contract muscles necessary to push urine out of the bladder). Draws urine out to empty bladder and blocks urine flow when continence is desired. |
| Incontinence clamps (penile compression devices) | Mechanical fixed compression applied to the penis to prevent any flow or leakage via the urethra. Must be released to void. |
| **Containment Devices** | |
| External collection devices | External catheter (condom) systems (e.g., penile sheaths) direct urine into a drainage bag. Most commonly used by men. |
| Absorbent products | Variety of reusable and disposable pads and undergarment systems. |

## COMPLEMENTARY & ALTERNATIVE THERAPIES

### *Biofeedback*

**Scientific Evidence**

Biofeedback has been shown to be helpful in treating a variety of medical conditions: urinary incontinence, asthma, Raynaud's disease, irritable bowel syndrome, hot flashes, nausea and vomiting associated with chemotherapy, headaches, hypertension, and seizure disorders.

**Nursing Implications**

- Feedback from monitoring equipment can teach patients to control certain involuntary body responses, such as urinary incontinence.
- Although biofeedback is considered safe, patients should consult a qualified professional before using biofeedback.

and relax the pelvic muscles (see the Complementary & Alternative Therapies box on this page).

**Drug Therapy.** Drug therapy varies according to the UI type (Table 45-19). In stress UI, drugs have a limited role in the management. α-Adrenergic agonists can be used to increase bladder sphincter tone and urethral resistance, but they have limited benefit. In urge and reflex UI, drugs play a key management role.

Anticholinergic drugs (muscarinic receptor blockers) block the action of acetylcholine at muscarinic receptors. They relax the bladder muscle and inhibit overactive detrusor contractions (Table 45-19). Side effects of these drugs include dry mouth and eyes, constipation, blurred vision, and sleepiness.

Botox (onabotulinumtoxin A) can be used in the treatment of UI as a result of detrusor overactivity. Botox is injected into the bladder, resulting in relaxation of the bladder, an increase in its storage capacity, and a decrease in UI.

**DRUG ALERT Tolterodine (Detrol)**

- Overdosage can result in severe anticholinergic effects.
- These effects include GI cramping, diaphoresis, blurred vision, and urinary urgency.

**Surgical Therapy.** Surgical techniques also vary depending on the type of UI. Surgical correction of stress UI is aimed at making the urinary structures more receptive to intraabdominal pressure and augmenting the urethral resistance of the internal sphincter. It may involve repositioning the urethra and/or creating a backboard of support to stabilize the urethra and bladder neck and make them more receptive to changes in intraabdominal pressure. Another technique for stress UI

## TABLE 45-18 Patient Teaching

### *Pelvic Floor Muscle (Kegel) Exercises*

*Include the following instructions when teaching the patient to perform Kegel exercises.*

**What Is the Pelvic Floor Muscle?**

- Your pelvic floor muscle provides support for your bladder and rectum and, in women, the vagina and uterus.
- If it weakens or is damaged, it cannot support these organs and their position can change.
- This causes problems with the normal bladder and rectal function.
- If you have a weak pelvic floor muscle, you may want to do special exercises to make the muscle stronger, prevent unwanted urine leakage, and lessen urinary urgency.

**Finding the Pelvic Floor Muscle**

- Without tensing the muscles of your leg, buttocks, or abdomen, imagine that you are trying to control the passing of gas or pinching off a stool.
- Or imagine you are in an elevator full of people and you feel the urge to pass gas. What do you do?
- You tighten or pull in the ring of muscle around your rectum—your pelvic floor muscle.
- You should feel a lifting sensation in the area around the vagina or a pulling in of your rectum.

**How to Do the Exercises**

There are two different kinds of exercises—short squeezes and long squeezes.

1. To do the *short squeezes,* tighten your pelvic floor muscle quickly, squeeze hard for 2 sec, and then relax the muscle. Also, when you have strong urinary urges, try to tighten your pelvic floor muscle quickly and hard several times in a row until the urge passes.
2. To do the *long squeezes,* tighten the muscle for 5-10 sec before you relax.

Do both of these exercises 40-50 times each day.

**When to Do These Exercises**

- You can do these exercises anytime and anywhere.
- You can do these exercises in any position, but sitting or lying down may be the easiest.

**How Long Does It Take Before I Notice a Change?**

After 4-6 wk of doing these exercises, you should start to see less urine leakage and urinary urgency.

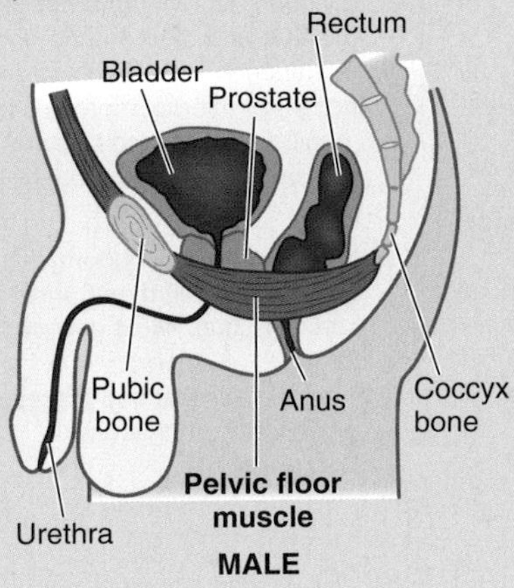


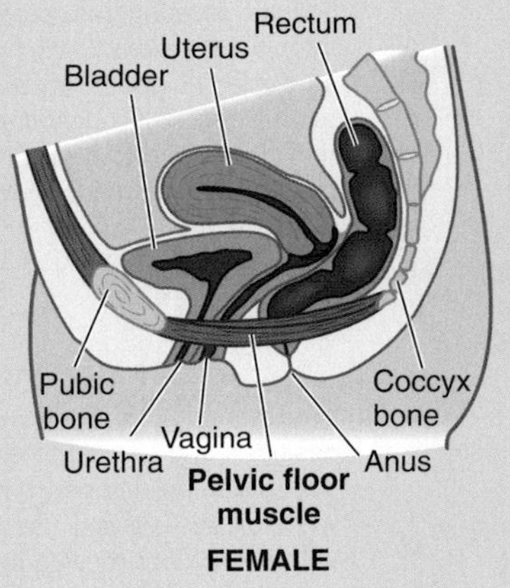


Courtesy Diane Newman.

augments the urethral resistance of the intrinsic sphincter with a sling or periurethral injectable.

Retropubic colposuspension and pubovaginal sling placement appear to be most effective. Typically, both procedures are performed through low transverse incisions. Complications specific to the retropubic suspensions include postoperative voiding dysfunction, urgency, and vaginal prolapse.

Placement of a suburethral sling, using the person's own fascia, cadaveric fascia, or a synthetic material, is also used to correct stress UI in women. Complications include vascular and bowel injury, urinary retention, mesh or sling erosion, infection, urgency, and bladder perforation. Suburethral slings have success rates comparable to those of colposuspensions or slings and are associated with shorter recovery periods. An artificial urethral sphincter can be used in men with intrinsic sphincter deficiency and severe stress UI.

Alternatively, one of several bulking agents can be injected underneath the mucosa of the urethra to correct stress UI in women or men. Bulking agents include glutaraldehyde cross-linked bovine collagen (GAX collagen), small silicone beads (Durasphere), or polytetrafluoroethylene (Teflon). Because of the risk of migration of Teflon particles, GAX collagen or Durasphere injections are most commonly used today. Although treatment with suburethral compounds avoids the risk associated with open surgery, reinjection is typically required after several years.

In artificial sphincter surgery, the bladder sphincter that no longer works is replaced with an artificial one. A silicone inflatable ring is placed around the urethra (internally), and the patient inflates it to stop the flow and deflates it when the need to empty occurs. The patient must be able to work the pump that is placed internally. This procedure is usually used only as a last resort and in a patient who is cognitively aware and able to participate in the use of the artificial sphincter.

## ❖ NURSING MANAGEMENT: URINARY INCONTINENCE

It is important to recognize both the physical and emotional problems associated with UI. Maintain and enhance the patient's dignity, privacy, and feelings of self-worth. This is a two-step approach: (1) containment devices to manage existing urinary leakage and (2) a definitive plan to reduce or resolve the factors leading to UI.

Management options are reviewed in Tables 45-17 and 45-18. They include lifestyle interventions such as teaching the patient about consumption of an adequate volume of fluids

**TABLE 45-19 Drug Therapy**

***Voiding Dysfunction****

| Class and Mechanism of Action | Drug |
|---|---|
| **Anticholinergics (Muscarinic Receptor Blockers)** | |
| Reduce overactive bladder contractions in urge urinary incontinence | oxybutynin (Ditropan XL, Oxytrol Transdermal System) |
| | tolterodine (Detrol, Detrol LA) |
| Relax bladder muscle during filling and improves the storage capacity of bladder | trospium chloride |
| | solifenacin (VESIcare) |
| | darifenacin (Enablex) |
| | flavoxate |
| **α-Adrenergic Blockers** | |
| Reduce urethral sphincter resistance to urinary outflow | doxazosin (Cardura) |
| | terazosin |
| | tamsulosin (Flomax) |
| | alfuzosin (Uroxatral) |
| **5α-Reductase Inhibitors** | |
| Suppress androgen resulting in epithelial atrophy and decrease in prostate size | finasteride (Proscar) |
| | dutasteride (Avodart) |
| **α-Adrenergic Agonists** | |
| Increase urethral resistance | phenylpropanolamine |
| | pseudoephedrine |
| **$\beta_3$-Adrenergic Agonist** | |
| Improves bladder's storage capacity by relaxing bladder muscle during filling | mirabegron (Myrbetriq) |
| **Tricyclic Antidepressants** | |
| Reduce sensory urgency and burning pain of interstitial cystitis | imipramine (Tofranil) |
| | amitriptyline |
| Reduce overactive bladder contractions | |
| **Calcium Channel Blockers** | |
| Reduce smooth muscle contraction strength | nifedipine |
| | diltiazem (Cardizem) |
| May reduce burning pain of interstitial cystitis | verapamil (Calan) |
| **Hormone Therapy** | |
| Local application reduces urethral irritation and increases host defenses against UTI | estrogen cream (Premarin, Estrace) |
| | estrogen vaginal ring (Estring) |
| | estrogen vaginal tablets (Vagifem) |

*The type of drug therapy depends on the type of incontinence.

**CHECK YOUR PRACTICE**

You are doing BP and glucose screening at the community senior center. While you are checking the BP on a 78-year-old woman, she starts to sob quietly. You tell her that her BP is 134/84 and gently place your hand on her arm. You ask her what is wrong. She tells you, "I have to pee all the time. I soak the bed and my husband won't sleep with me anymore. I am washing sheets and my clothes all the time. Our whole house smells like urine."

- How would you respond to her?

and reduction or elimination of bladder irritants (particularly caffeine and alcohol) from the diet. Advise the patient to maintain a regular, flexible schedule of urination (usually every 2 to 3 hours while awake). Advise patients to quit smoking because this habit increases the risk of stress UI. Counsel patients about the relationship among constipation, UI, and urinary retention. Aggressive management of constipation is recommended, beginning with ensuring adequate fluid intake, increasing dietary fiber, lightly exercising, and judiciously using stool softeners. (The management of constipation is discussed in Chapter 42.)

Behavioral treatments include scheduled voiding regimens (timed voiding, habit training, and prompted voiding), bladder retraining, and pelvic floor muscle training. Assess strategies that the patient uses to contain UI and offer alternative devices when indicated. When attempting to manage UI, many women use feminine hygiene pads, and many men and women use household products such as rags, paper towels, or folded toilet tissue. Unfortunately, none of these products is adequately designed to wick urine away from the skin, prevent soiling of clothing, and reduce or eliminate odor.

Instead, provide information on products specifically designed to contain urine. For example, patients with mild to moderate UI often benefit from incontinent pads containing superabsorbent material, designed to absorb many times its weight in water. Patients with higher-volume urine loss or those with both urinary and fecal incontinence may benefit from disposable or reusable incontinence protective underwear, briefs, or pad/pant systems.

In inpatient or long-term care facilities, nursing management of UI includes maximizing toilet access. This assistance may take the form of offering the urinal or bedpan or assisting the patient to the bathroom every 2 to 3 hours or at scheduled times. Ensure that toilets are accessible to patients and provide privacy to allow effective urine elimination.

**TEAMWORK & COLLABORATION**

***Caring for the Incontinent Patient***

All members of the interprofessional care team are responsible for decreasing the risk for incontinence and preventing complications such as skin breakdown in patients who are experiencing incontinence.

**Role of Nursing Personnel**

***Registered Nurse (RN)***

- Assess for risk factors for incontinence or urinary retention.
- Determine type of incontinence that patient is experiencing.
- Develop plan of care to decrease incontinence.
- Teach patient ways to decrease incontinence such as pelvic floor muscle (Kegel) exercises.
- Assist patient in choosing appropriate products to contain urine.

***Licensed Practical/Vocational Nurse (LPN/LVN)***

- Use bladder scanner to estimate the postvoid residual volume (PVR).
- Catheterize patient and measure PVR.
- Administer medications to decrease incontinence or urinary retention.

***Unlicensed Assistive Personnel (UAP)***

- Assist incontinent patient to commode or bedpan at regular intervals.
- Clean patient and provide skin care.
- Notify RN about new-onset incontinence in a previously continent patient.

## URINARY RETENTION

**Urinary retention** is the inability to empty the bladder when a person voids (micturition) or the accumulation of urine in the bladder because of an inability to urinate. In certain cases, it is associated with urinary leakage or postvoid dribbling, called *overflow UI*. *Acute urinary retention* is the total inability to pass urine via micturition. It is a medical emergency. *Chronic urinary retention* is an incomplete bladder emptying despite urination. The postvoid residual (PVR) volumes in patients with chronic urinary retention vary widely. Normal PVR is between 50 and 75 mL. Findings over 100 mL indicate the need to repeat the measurement. An abnormal PVR in the older patient of more than 200 mL obtained on two separate occasions requires further evaluation. Even smaller volumes may justify further evaluation when the patient has recurring UTIs or lower urinary tract symptoms suggestive of UTI.

### Etiology and Pathophysiology

Urinary retention is caused by two different dysfunctions of the urinary system: bladder outlet obstruction and deficient detrusor (bladder muscle) contraction strength. *Bladder outlet obstruction* leads to urinary retention when the blockage is so severe that the bladder can no longer evacuate its contents despite a detrusor contraction. A common cause of obstruction in men is an enlarged prostate.

*Deficient detrusor contraction* strength leads to urinary retention when the muscle is no longer able to contract with enough force or for a sufficient time to completely empty the bladder. Common causes of deficient detrusor contraction strength are neurologic diseases affecting sacral segments 2, 3, and 4; long-standing diabetes mellitus; overdistention; chronic alcoholism; and drugs (e.g., anticholinergic drugs).

### Diagnostic Studies

The diagnostic studies for urinary retention are the same as the ones for UI (see p. 1055).

### Interprofessional Care

Behavioral therapies that were described for UI may also be used in the management of urinary retention. Scheduled toileting and double voiding may be effective in chronic urinary retention with moderate PVR volumes. *Double voiding* is an attempt to maximize bladder evacuation. The patient is asked to urinate, sit on the toilet for 3 to 4 minutes, and urinate again before exiting the bathroom.

For acute or chronic urinary retention, catheterization may be required. Intermittent catheterization allows the patient to remain free of an indwelling catheter with its associated risk of UTI and urethral irritation. In some situations, an indwelling catheter is preferred (e.g., if the patient is unwilling or unable to perform intermittent catheterization). An indwelling catheter is also used when urethral obstruction makes intermittent catheterization uncomfortable or infeasible.

**Drug Therapy.** Several drugs may be administered to promote bladder evacuation. For the patient with obstruction at the level of the bladder neck, an α-adrenergic blocker may be prescribed. These drugs relax the smooth muscle of the bladder neck, the prostatic urethra, and possibly the rhabdosphincter, diminishing urethral resistance. Examples of α-adrenergic blockers are listed in Table 45-19. They are indicated in patients with BPH, bladder neck dyssynergia (muscle incoordination), or detrusor sphincter dyssynergia.

**Surgical Therapy.** Surgical interventions are used to manage urinary retention caused by obstruction. Transurethral or open surgical techniques are used to treat benign or malignant prostatic enlargement, bladder neck contracture, urethral strictures, or dyssynergia of the bladder neck. Pelvic reconstruction using an abdominal or transvaginal approach can correct bladder outlet obstruction in women with severe pelvic organ prolapse.

Unfortunately, surgery has a minimal role in the management of urinary retention caused by deficient detrusor contraction strength. Attempts to create a bladder stimulator (implanted device capable of stimulating micturition) have proved largely unsuccessful because of the difficulty in achieving a coordinated detrusor contraction associated with pelvic muscle and striated sphincter relaxation.

## NURSING MANAGEMENT: URINARY RETENTION

Acute urinary retention is a medical emergency that requires prompt recognition and bladder drainage. Insert a catheter (as ordered) unless otherwise directed. Use a catheter with a retention balloon in anticipation of the need for an indwelling catheter.

Teach the patient with acute urinary retention (and the patient predisposed to these episodes) strategies to minimize risk, including avoiding intake of large volumes of fluid over a brief period. Instead, advise the patient to drink small amounts throughout the day. In addition, instruct the patient (if chilled) to warm up before attempting to urinate and to avoid excessive alcohol intake because it leads to polyuria and a diminished awareness of the need to urinate until the bladder is distended.

Advise the patient who is unable to urinate to drink a cup of coffee or brewed caffeinated tea to create or maximize urinary urgency. Tell patients that sitting in a tub of warm water or taking a warm shower may also help them urinate. If these measures do not lead to successful urination, advise the patient to seek immediate care.

Patients with chronic urinary retention may be managed by behavioral methods, indwelling or intermittent catheterization, surgery, or drugs. Scheduled toileting and double voiding are the primary behavioral interventions used for chronic retention. Scheduled toileting is used to reduce rather than expand bladder capacity. In this case, ask the patient to void every 3 to 4 hours regardless of the desire to urinate. This intervention is particularly useful in the patient with chronic overdistention, diabetes mellitus, or chronic alcoholism characterized by a large bladder capacity and diminished or delayed sensations of bladder filling and urgency.

# CATHETERIZATION

## INDICATIONS FOR AND COMPLICATIONS OF CATHETERIZATION

Indications for short-term urinary catheterization are listed in Table 45-20. Unacceptable reasons for catheterization include (1) routine acquisition of a urine specimen for laboratory analysis and (2) convenience of the nursing staff or the patient's family. The risk of CAUTI is too high to allow catheterization of a patient for the convenience of hospital personnel or family members.

Complications that are seen more frequently with long-term use (more than 30 days) of indwelling catheters include CAUTI, bladder spasms, periurethral abscess, chronic pyelonephritis, urosepsis, urethral trauma or erosion, fistula or stricture formation, and calculi. Catheterization for sterile urine specimens may occasionally be necessary when patients have a history of

**TABLE 45-20 Indications for Urinary Catheterization**

**Indwelling Catheter**
- Relief of urinary retention caused by lower urinary tract obstruction, paralysis, or inability to void
- Bladder decompression preoperatively and operatively for lower abdominal or pelvic surgery
- Facilitation of surgical repair of urethra and surrounding structures
- Splinting of ureters or urethra to facilitate healing after surgery or other trauma in area
- Accurate measurement of urine output in critically ill patient
- Contamination of stage III or IV pressure ulcers with urine that has impeded healing, despite appropriate personal care for the incontinence
- Terminal illness or severe impairment, which makes positioning or clothing changes uncomfortable, or which is associated with intractable pain

**Intermittent (Straight, in and Out) Catheter**
- Relief of urinary retention caused by lower urinary tract obstruction, paralysis, or inability to void
- Study of anatomic structures of urinary system
- Urodynamic testing
- Collection of sterile urine sample in selected situations
- Instillation of medications into bladder
- Measurement of residual urine after urination (postvoid residual [PVR]) if portable ultrasound not available

complicated UTI. A catheter should be the final resort to provide the patient with a dry environment to prevent skin breakdown and protect dressings or skin lesions.

Urinary catheterization is commonly used in the management of the hospitalized patient. However, it is not without serious complications. As previously discussed on p. 1034, CAUTIs are the most common HAI. Scrupulous aseptic technique is mandatory when a urinary catheter is inserted. After insertion, maintenance and protection of the closed drainage system are major nursing responsibilities. Do not routinely irrigate the catheter; this should be done only if ordered.

While the patient has a catheter in place, maintain patency of the catheter, manage fluid intake, provide for the patient's comfort and safety, and prevent infection. Address the psychologic implications of urinary drainage. Patient concerns can include embarrassment related to exposure of the body, an altered body image, and fear that care of the catheter will result in increased dependency.

## CATHETER CONSTRUCTION

Catheter materials include Teflon-coated latex, silicone elastomer, and hydrogel-coated silicone. Catheters coated with silver or antimicrobial agents may prevent UTIs.

Catheters vary in construction materials, tip shape (Fig. 45-10), and size of the lumen. A coudé-tip catheter is commonly used in men. Catheters are sized according to the French scale. Each French unit (F) equals 0.33 mm of diameter. The diameter listed is the internal diameter of the catheter. The size used varies with the patient's size and the purpose of catheterization. In women, urethral catheter sizes 14F to 16F are the most common. In men, sizes 14F to 18F are used. Balloon sizes are either 5 or 30 mL. The primary problem resulting from too large a catheter is tissue erosion secondary to excessive pressure on the meatus or urethra.

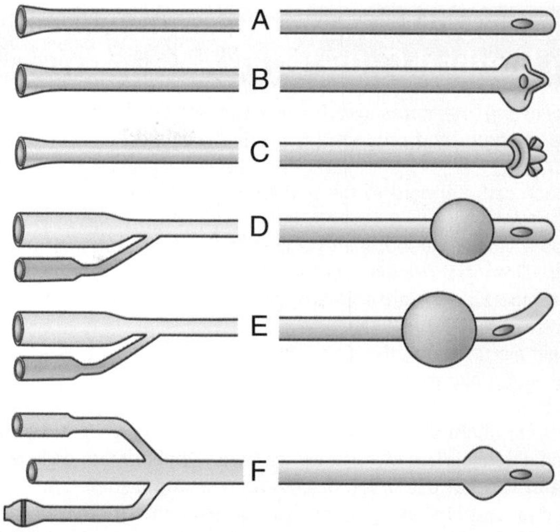


**FIG. 45-10** Types of urinary catheters. **A,** Simple urethral catheter. **B,** Mushroom-tip de Pezzer catheter (can be for suprapubic catheterization). **C,** Wing-tip Malecot catheter (wings hold catheter in place for temporary drainage). **D,** Indwelling urethral catheter with inflated balloon. **E,** Indwelling Tiemann catheter with coudé-tip (slightly curved tip allows for passage past obstruction). **F,** Three-way indwelling catheter (third lumen can be used for irrigation).

## TYPES OF CATHETERS

Four routes are used for urinary tract catheterization: urethral, ureteral, suprapubic, and via a nephrostomy tube.

### Urethral Catheterization

*Urethral catheterization,* the most common route of catheterization, involves the insertion of a catheter through the external meatus into the urethra, past the internal sphincter, and into the bladder. Table 45-21 summarizes important principles in the management of the patient with an indwelling urethral catheter.

**TEAMWORK & COLLABORATION**

***Urinary Catheters***

**Role of Nursing Personnel**

***Registered Nurse (RN)***
- Determine need for catheterization, but HCP must order.
- Choose appropriate type and size of catheter.
- Insert catheter in patient with urethral trauma, pain, or obstruction.
- Develop plan of care to decrease risk for infection in patient with indwelling catheter.

***Licensed Practical/Vocational Nurse (LPN/LVN)***
- Insert intermittent or indwelling catheter for uncomplicated patients.
- Irrigate the catheter if obstruction is suspected in stable patients (e.g., in long-term care).

***Unlicensed Assistive Personnel (UAP)***
- Provide perineal care around the catheter with soap and water.
- Anchor the catheter in place (upper thigh in women and lower abdomen in men).
- Notify RN about changes in skin condition, especially around meatus.

**TABLE 45-21 Management of Patient With Urethral Catheter**

*The following measures can be used to manage the patient with a urethral catheter and prevent a catheter-associated urinary tract infection (CAUTI).*

1. Teach catheter care to the patient, particularly one who is ambulatory.
2. Use a sterile, closed drainage system in short-term catheterization. Do not disconnect the distal urinary catheter and proximal drainage tube except for catheter irrigation (if ordered and indicated).
3. Maintain unobstructed downhill flow of urine. Empty the collecting bag regularly, and keep it below the level of the bladder.
4. Provide perineal care (once or twice a day and when necessary), including cleaning the meatus-catheter junction with soap and water. Do not use lotion or powder near the catheter.
5. Anchor catheter using some type of securement device. Anchor catheter to upper thigh in women and lower abdomen in men to prevent catheter movement and urethral tension.
6. Use sterile technique whenever the collecting system is open. If frequent irrigations are necessary in short-term catheterization to maintain catheter patency, a triple-lumen catheter may be preferable, permitting continuous irrigations within a closed system.
7. If ordered, aspirate small volumes of urine for culture from the catheter sampling port by means of a sterile syringe and needle. First prepare the puncture site with an antiseptic solution.
8. When the patient is catheterized for less than 2 wk, routine catheter change is not necessary. For long-term use of an indwelling catheter, replace the catheter based on patient assessment and not on a routine changing schedule.
9. With long-term use of a catheter, a leg bag may be used. If the collection bag is reused, wash it in soap and water and rinse thoroughly. When it is not reused immediately, fill it with ½ cup of vinegar and drain. The vinegar is effective against *Pseudomonas* and other organisms and eliminates odors.
10. Remove the catheter as early as possible. Intermittent catheterization and external catheters are alternatives that may be associated with fewer cases of bacteriuria and UTI than chronic indwelling urethral catheters.

### Ureteral Catheters

The *ureteral catheter* is placed through the ureters into the renal pelvis. The catheter is inserted either (1) by being threaded up the urethra and bladder to the ureters under cystoscopic observation or (2) by surgical insertion through the abdominal wall into the ureters. The ureteral catheter is used after surgery to splint the ureters and to prevent them from being obstructed by edema. Record the urine volume from the ureteral catheter separately from that of other urinary catheters.

The patient is often kept on bed rest while a ureteral catheter is in place until specific orders indicate that ambulation is permitted. The self-retaining ureteral catheter is often inserted after a lithotripsy procedure or when ureteral obstruction from adjacent tumors or fibrosis threatens renal function. The double-J ureteral catheter is frequently used and allows the patient to ambulate. One end coils up in the kidney pelvis, while the other coils in the bladder.

Check the placement of the ureteral catheter frequently and avoid tension on the catheter. The catheter drains urine from the renal pelvis, which has a capacity of 3 to 5 mL. If the volume of urine in the renal pelvis increases, tissue damage to the pelvis will result from pressure. Do not clamp the ureteral catheter. If the HCP orders irrigation of the ureteral catheter, use strict aseptic technique. If the output is decreased, notify the HCP immediately. Check the drainage often (at least every 1 or 2 hours). It is normal for some urine to drain around the ureteral catheter into the bladder. Accurately record the urine output from the ureteral and urethral catheters. Sometimes a ureteral catheter may be used as a stent and is not expected to drain. It is important to check with the HCP as to the type of catheter and what to expect.

### Suprapubic Catheters

*Suprapubic catheterization* is the simplest and oldest method of urinary diversion. The two methods of insertion of a suprapubic catheter into the bladder are (1) through a small incision in the abdominal wall and (2) by the use of a trocar. A suprapubic catheter is placed while the patient is under general anesthesia for another surgical procedure or at the bedside with a local anesthetic. The catheter may be sutured into place. Tape the catheter to prevent dislodgment. The care of the tube and catheter is similar to that of the urethral catheter. A pectin-base skin barrier (e.g., Stomahesive) is effective in protecting the skin around the insertion site from breakdown.

The suprapubic catheter is used in temporary situations such as bladder, prostate, and urethral surgery. The suprapubic catheter is also used on a long-term basis in selected patients.

A suprapubic catheter is prone to poor drainage because of mechanical obstruction of the catheter tip by the bladder wall, sediment, and clots. To ensure patency of the tube (1) prevent tube kinking by coiling the excess tubing and maintaining gravity drainage, (2) have the patient turn from side to side, and (3) milk the tube. If these measures are not effective, obtain a order from the HCP to irrigate the catheter using sterile technique.

If the patient experiences bladder spasms that are difficult to control, urinary leakage may result. Oxybutynin or other oral antispasmodics or belladonna and opium (B&O) suppositories may be prescribed to decrease bladder spasms.

### Nephrostomy Tubes

The *nephrostomy tube* (catheter) is inserted on a temporary basis to preserve renal function when a ureter is completely obstructed. The tube is inserted through a small flank incision directly into the pelvis of the kidney and attached to connecting tubing for closed drainage. The principle is the same as with the ureteral catheter—that is, the catheter should never be kinked, compressed, or clamped. If the patient complains of excessive pain in the area or if there is excessive drainage around the tube, check the catheter for patency. If irrigation is ordered, use strict aseptic technique. Gently instill no more than 5 mL of sterile saline solution at one time to prevent overdistention of the kidney pelvis and renal damage. Infection and secondary stone formation are complications associated with the insertion of a nephrostomy tube.

### Intermittent Catheterization

An alternative approach to a long-term indwelling catheter is *intermittent catheterization,* often referred to as "straight" catheterization or "in-and-out" catheterization. The main goal of intermittent catheterization is to prevent urinary retention, stasis, and compromised blood supply to the bladder caused by prolonged pressure.[24]

It is being used with increasing frequency in conditions such as neurogenic bladder (e.g., spinal cord injuries, chronic neurologic diseases) or bladder outlet obstruction in men. This type of catheterization is used in the oliguric and anuric phases of acute kidney injury to reduce the possibility of infection from an indwelling catheter. Intermittent catheterization is also used postoperatively after a surgical procedure to treat UI.

The technique consists of inserting a urethral catheter into the bladder every 3 to 5 hours. Some patients perform intermittent catheterization only once or twice a day to measure residual urine and to ensure an empty bladder.

The techniques and protocols for intermittent catheterization vary. Catheters can be sterile (single use) or clean (multiple use). Catheters can be coated (prelubricated) or uncoated. Available data on intermittent catheterization do not provide convincing evidence that any specific technique (sterile or clean), catheter type (coated or uncoated), method (single-use or multiple-use), person (self or other), or strategy is better than any other for all clinical settings.[24]

The design of single-use, self-lubricating, silicone-coated (closed-sterile) systems is useful for patients who have recurrent UTIs or need to catheterize while at work or during travel. Instruct patients to wash and rinse the catheter and their hands with soap and water before and after catheterization. Lubricant is necessary for men and may make catheterization more comfortable for women. The catheter may be inserted by the patient, caregiver, or HCP.

Sterile technique is used for catheterization in the hospital or long-term care facility. For home care, a clean technique that includes good hand washing with soap and water is used. Teach the patient to observe for signs of UTI so that treatment can be started early. If indicated, some patients are placed on a regimen of prophylactic antibiotics. Urethral damage from intermittent catheterization in men is similar to problems seen with indwelling catheterization. Complications include urethritis, urethral sphincter damage (especially if there is a forceful catheterization against a closed sphincter), urethral stricture, and creation of a false passage.

# SURGERY OF THE URINARY TRACT

## RENAL AND URETERAL SURGERY

The most common indications for nephrectomy are a renal tumor, polycystic kidneys that are bleeding or severely infected, massive traumatic injury to the kidney, and the elective removal of a kidney from a donor to be transplanted. Surgery involving the ureters and kidneys is most commonly performed to remove calculi that become obstructive, correct congenital anomalies, and divert urine when necessary.

### Surgical Procedure

Nephrectomy can be performed by a conventional (open) approach or laparoscopically. In the open approach, an incision of about 6 to 10 in is made through several layers of muscle. The incision can be made in the flank or abdominal area.

**Laparoscopic Nephrectomy.** *Laparoscopic nephrectomy* can be performed in selected situations to remove a diseased kidney. Laparoscopic nephrectomy can also be used to obtain a kidney from a living donor to be transplanted into a person with end-stage renal disease (ESRD). A laparoscopic nephrectomy is performed using five puncture sites. One incision is to view the kidney, and another is to dissect it. The laparoscope contains a miniature camera so that the surgeons can watch what they are doing on a video monitor. Once dissected, the kidney is maneuvered into a nylon impermeable sack and then safely removed from the patient. Compared with conventional nephrectomy, the laparoscopic approach is less painful, involves a shorter hospital stay, and has a much faster recovery.

### Preoperative Management

The basic needs of the patient undergoing renal and ureteral surgery are similar to those of any patient who experiences surgery (see Chapters 17 through 19). In addition, it is important preoperatively to ensure adequate fluid intake and a normal electrolyte balance. Tell the patient that, if there is a flank incision, surgery will require a hyperextended, side-lying position. This position frequently causes the patient to experience muscle aches after surgery. If a nephrectomy is planned, it is important that the patient have one working kidney to maintain normal renal function.

### Postoperative Management

Specific postoperative needs of a patient are related to urine output, respiratory status, and abdominal distention.

**Urine Output.** In the immediate postoperative period, measure and record the urine output at least every 1 or 2 hours. Measure drainage from the various catheters and record it separately. Do not clamp or irrigate the catheter or tube without a specific order. The total urine output should be at least 0.5 mL/kg/hr. It is important to assess for urine drainage on the dressing and to estimate this amount. Observe and monitor the color and consistency of urine. Urine with increased amounts of mucus, blood, or sediment may occlude the drainage tubing or catheter.

Weigh the patient daily using the same scale, and have the patient wear similar clothing and dressings each time. A significant change in daily weight can indicate retention of fluids, which places the patient at cardiovascular risk for developing heart failure. Retention of fluids can increase the work required of the remaining kidney to perform its functions.

**Respiratory Status.** A nephrectomy can be performed through a flank incision just below the diaphragm. Postoperatively, it is important to ensure adequate ventilation. The patient is often reluctant to turn, cough, and deep breathe because of the incisional pain. Give adequate pain medication to ensure the patient's comfort and ability to perform coughing and deep-breathing exercises. Frequently, additional respiratory devices such as an incentive spirometer are used every 2 hours while the patient is awake. In addition, early and frequent ambulation helps to maintain adequate respiratory function.

**Abdominal Distention.** Abdominal distention is present to some degree in most patients who have had surgery on their kidneys or ureters. It is most commonly due to paralytic ileus caused by manipulation and compression of the bowel during surgery. Oral intake is restricted until bowel sounds are present (usually 24 to 48 hours after surgery). IV fluids are given until the patient can take oral fluids. Progression to a regular diet follows.

## URINARY DIVERSION

*Urinary diversion* may be performed with or without cystectomy. Urinary diversion procedures are performed to treat cancer of the bladder, neurogenic bladder, congenital anomalies, strictures, trauma to the bladder, and chronic infections

TABLE 45-22 **Urinary Diversion Surgery**

| Description | Advantages | Disadvantages | Special Considerations |
|---|---|---|---|
| **Ileal Conduit** | | | |
| Ureters are implanted into part of ileum or colon that has been resected from intestinal tract. Abdominal stoma is created. | Relatively good urine flow with few physiologic alterations. | External appliance necessary to continually collect urine. | Surgical procedure is complex. Postoperative complications may be increased. Reabsorption of urea by ileum occurs. Meticulous attention is necessary to care for stoma and collecting device. |
| **Cutaneous Ureterostomy** | | | |
| Ureters are excised from bladder and brought through abdominal wall, and stoma is created. Ureteral stomas may be created from both ureters, or ureters may be brought together and one stoma created. | No need for major surgery as required with ileal conduit. | External appliance necessary because of continuous urine drainage. Possibility of stricture or stenosis of small stoma. | Periodic catheterizations may be required to dilate stomas to maintain patency. |
| **Nephrostomy** | | | |
| Catheter is inserted into pelvis of kidney. Procedure may be done to one or both kidneys and may be temporary or permanent. It is most frequently done in advanced disease as palliative procedure. | No need for major surgery. | High risk of renal infection. Predisposition to calculus formation from catheter. | Nephrostomy tube may have to be changed every month. Never clamp the catheter. |

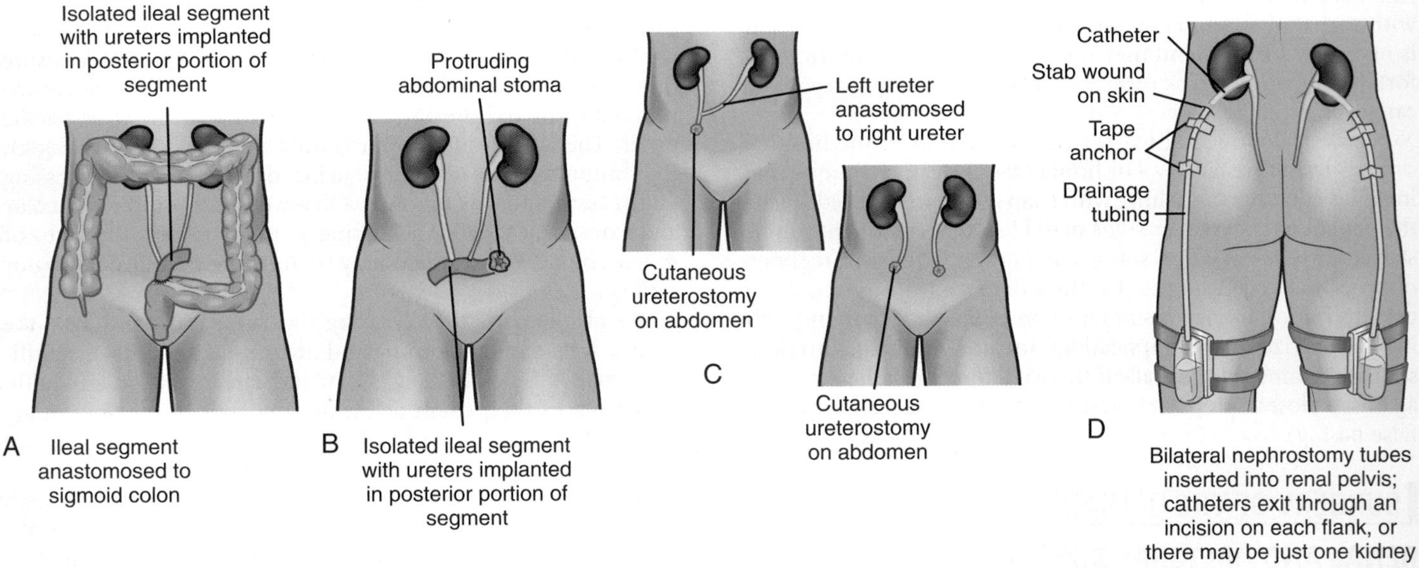


**FIG. 45-11** Methods of urinary diversion. **A,** Ureteroileosigmoidostomy. **B,** Ileal loop (ileal conduit). **C,** Ureterostomy (transcutaneous ureterostomy and bilateral cutaneous ureterostomies). **D,** Nephrostomy.

with deterioration of renal function. Numerous urinary diversion techniques and bladder substitutes are possible, including an incontinent urinary diversion, a continent urinary diversion catheterized by the patient, or an orthotopic bladder so that the patient voids urethrally.[25] Types of surgical procedures for urinary diversion are presented in Table 45-22 and Fig. 45-11.

## Incontinent Urinary Diversion

*Incontinent urinary diversion* is diversion to the skin, requiring an appliance. The simplest form is the cutaneous ureterostomy, but scarring and strictures of the ureter have led to the use of ileal or colonic conduits. The most commonly performed incontinent urinary diversion procedure is the ileal conduit (ileal loop). In this procedure a 6- to 8-in (15- to 20-cm) segment of the ileum is converted into a conduit for urinary drainage. The colon (colon conduit) can be used instead of the ileum. The ureters are anastomosed into one end of the conduit, and the other end of the bowel is brought out through the abdominal wall to form a stoma (Fig. 45-12). Although the

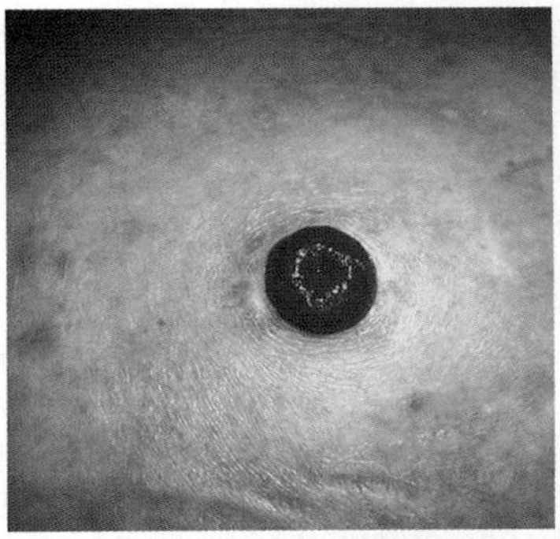

**FIG. 45-12** Urinary stoma. Symmetric, no skin breakdown, protrudes about 1.5 cm. Mucosa is healthy red. This configuration is flat when the patient is upright or supine. (Courtesy Lynda Brubacher, Virginia Mason Hospital, Seattle, Wash.)

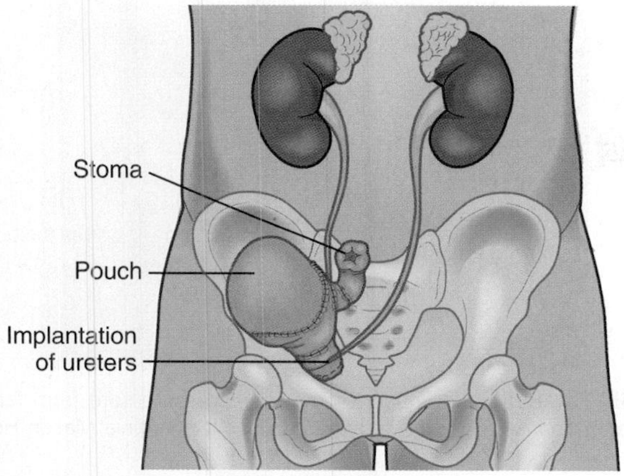


FIG. 45-13 Creation of a Kock pouch with implantation of ureters into one intussuscepted portion of the pouch and creation of a stoma with the other intussuscepted portion.

segment of bowel remains supported by the mesentery, it is completely isolated from the intestinal tract. The bowel is anastomosed and continues to function normally.

Because there is no valve and no voluntary control over the stoma, drops of urine flow from the stoma every few seconds, requiring a permanent external collecting device. The visible stoma and need for external collection devices are disadvantages of this procedure. The lifelong need to care for and deal with the stoma and collection devices may be psychologically difficult. These problems have led to the increasing use of continent diversions and orthotopic bladder substitutes.

### Continent Urinary Diversions

A *continent urinary diversion* is an intraabdominal urinary reservoir that can be catheterized or that has an outlet controlled by the anal sphincter. Continent diversions are internal pouches created similarly to the ileal conduit. Reservoirs are constructed from the ileum, ileocecal segment, or colon. Large segments of bowel are altered to prevent peristaltic action. A continence mechanism is formed between this large, low-pressure reservoir and the stoma by intussuscepting a portion of bowel. In this way, a patient does not leak involuntarily. The patient with a continent reservoir needs to self-catheterize every 4 to 6 hours but does not need to wear external attachments. Patients may wear a small bandage on the stoma to collect any mucous drainage or excess drainage. Examples of continent diversions are the Kock (Fig. 45-13), Mainz, Indiana, and Florida pouches. The main difference among the various diversions is the segment of bowel used. For example, the Indiana pouch uses the right colon as a reservoir and has become a popular form of continent urinary diversion.

### Orthotopic Bladder Reconstruction

*Orthotopic bladder reconstruction,* or orthotopic neobladder, is the construction of a new bladder in the bladder's normal anatomic position, with discharge of urine through the urethra. The reconstruction or neobladder can be derived from various segments of the intestines to create a low-pressure reservoir. An isolated segment of the distal ileum is often preferred. Various procedures include the hemi-Kock pouch, Studer pouch, and W-shaped ileoneobladder. In these procedures the bowel is surgically reshaped to become a neobladder. The ureters and urethra are sutured into the neobladder.

Orthotopic bladder reconstruction has become a more viable option for both men and women if cancer does not involve the bladder neck or urethra. Ideal candidates for this procedure have normal renal and liver function, longer than 1- to 2-year life expectancy, adequate motor skills, and no history of inflammatory bowel disease or colon cancer. Obese patients and those with inflammatory bowel disease are not good candidates for this procedure. The advantage of orthotopic bladder substitution is that it allows for natural micturition. Incontinence is a possible problem with this technique, and intermittent catheterization may be required.

## ❖ NURSING MANAGEMENT: URINARY DIVERSION

### ◆ Preoperative Management

Teaching is important for the patient awaiting cystectomy and urinary diversion surgery. Assess the patient's ability and readiness to learn before initiating a teaching program. If the patient is not ready to learn, modify the teaching plan. The patient's anxiety and fear may be decreased by providing more information. However, the anxiety and fear may also interfere with learning. Involve the patient's caregiver and family in the teaching process.

Discuss the psychosocial aspects of living with a stoma (including clothing, changes in body image and sexuality, exercise, and odor). This may allay some fears. Teach the patient with a continent diversion (e.g., Indiana pouch) to catheterize at least every 6 hours and irrigate the pouch daily. The patient with an orthotopic neobladder may have problems with incontinence. Discuss patient's' concerns about sexual activities and let them know that counseling is available. A wound, ostomy, and continence nurse (WOCN) should be involved in the preoperative phase of the patient's care. A visit from an ostomate can be helpful. Additional interventions are presented in eNursing Care Plan 45-3 for the patient with an ileal conduit (on the website for this chapter).

### ◆ Postoperative Management

Plan the nursing interventions during the postoperative period to prevent surgical complications such as postoperative atelectasis and shock (see Chapter 19). After pelvic surgery, there is an increased incidence of thrombophlebitis, small bowel obstruction, and UTI. With removal of part of the bowel, the incidence of paralytic ileus and small bowel obstruction is increased, the patient is kept on NPO status, and a nasogastric tube may be needed for a few days.

Prevent injury to the stoma and maintain urine output. Advise the patient that mucus in the urine is a normal occurrence. The mucus is secreted by the mucosa of the intestine (which is used to create the ileal conduit) in response to the irritating effect of urine. Encourage a high fluid intake to "flush" the ileal conduit or continent diversion.

When an ileal conduit is created, provide meticulous care for the skin around the stoma. Alkaline encrustations with dermatitis may occur when alkaline urine comes in contact with exposed skin (Fig. 45-14). The urine is kept acidic to prevent alkaline encrustations. Other common peristomal skin problems include yeast infections, product allergies, and shearing-effect excoriations. Changing appliances (pouches) is described in Table 45-23. A properly fitting appliance is essential to prevent skin problems. The appliance should be about 0.1 in (0.2 cm) larger than the stoma. It is normal for the stoma to shrink within the first few weeks after surgery.

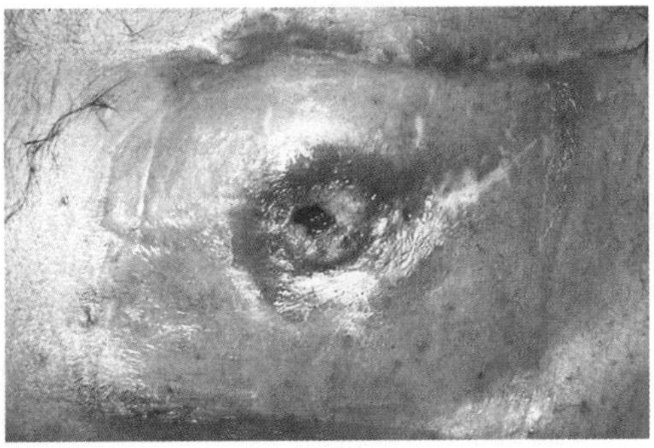

**FIG. 45-14** Ammonia salt encrustation secondary to alkaline urine. (Courtesy Lynda Brubacher, Virginia Mason Hospital, Seattle, Wash.)

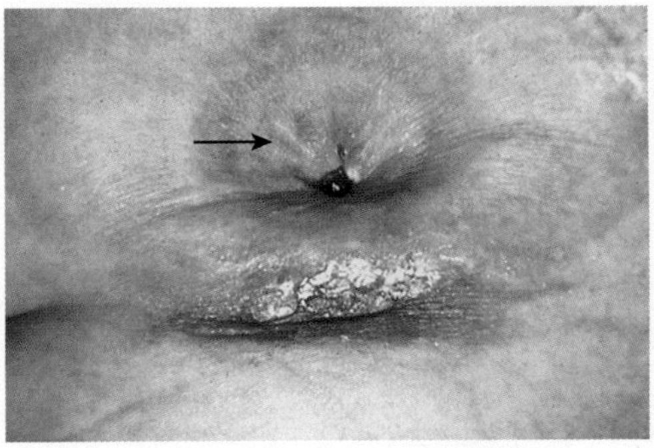

**FIG. 45-15** Retracted urinary stoma with pressure sore from faceplate above stoma *(arrow)*. (Courtesy Lynda Brubacher, Virginia Mason Hospital, Seattle, Wash.)

## TABLE 45-23 Patient & Caregiver Teaching

### *Ileal Conduit Appliances*

*Include the following instructions when teaching a patient or a caregiver how to change an ileal conduit appliance.*

**Temporary Appliance**

1. Cut hole in pouch to fit over stoma (pouch 0.1 in [0.2 cm] larger than stoma).
2. Remove old pouch.
3. Clean area gently and remove old adhesive.
4. Wash area with warm water.
5. Place wick (rolled-up 4 × 4-in pad) over stoma to keep area dry during rest of procedure.
6. Dry skin around stoma.
7. Apply tincture of benzoin or other skin protectant around stoma to area where pouch will be placed.
8. Apply pouch by first smoothing its edges toward side and lower portion of body.
9. Remove wick and complete application of bag.
10. If patient is usually in bed, apply bag so that it lies toward side of body.
11. If patient is ambulatory, apply bag so that it lies vertically.
12. Connect drainage tubing to pouch.
13. Keep drainage pouch on same side of bed as stoma.

**Permanent Appliance***

1. Keep appliance in place for 2-14 days.
2. Change appliance when fluid intake has been restricted for several hours.
3. Sit or stand in front of mirror.
4. Moisten edge of faceplate with adhesive solvent and gently remove.
5. Clean skin with adhesive solvent.
6. Wash skin with warm water (may be done while showering).
7. Dry skin and inspect.
8. Place wick (rolled-up 4 × 4-in pad) over stoma to keep skin free of urine.
9. Apply skin cement to faceplate and skin.
10. Place appliance over stoma.
11. Wash removed appliance with soap and lukewarm water; soak in distilled vinegar; rinse with lukewarm water and air dry.

*Many disposable appliances with self-adhesive backing are used as permanent appliances.

Patients with a neobladder may have postoperative urinary retention and require catheterization. It may take up to 6 months for them to regain bladder control. Patients empty their neobladders by relaxing their outlet sphincter muscles and bearing down with their abdominal muscles. Since there is no longer neurologic feedback between the reservoir and the brain, the patient should not expect a normal desire to void. To avoid bladder overdistention, patients should void at least every 2 to 4 hours, sit during voiding, and practice pelvic floor muscle relaxation to aid voiding. Follow-up x-ray studies include a "pouchogram" 3 to 4 weeks after surgery to assess for healing.

Acceptance of the surgery and of alterations in body image is needed to ensure the patient's best adjustment. Meeting and sharing feelings with similar patients can enhance a patient's adjustment to a urinary diversion. Patient concerns include fear that the stoma will be offensive to others and will interfere with sexual, personal, professional, and recreational activities. Advise the patient that few activities will be restricted as a result of the urinary diversion.

Discharge teaching after an ileal conduit includes instructing the patient about symptoms of obstruction or infection and care of the ostomy. The patient with an ileal conduit is fitted for a permanent appliance 7 to 10 days after surgery. It may have to be refitted at a later time, depending on the degree of stoma healing and shrinkage.

Appliances are made of a variety of products, including natural and synthetic rubbers, plastics, and metals. Most appliances have a faceplate that adheres to the skin, a collecting pouch, and an opening to drain the pouch. The faceplate may be secured to the skin with glues, adhesives, or adherent synthetic wafers. Some appliances do not require adhesives, but their design relies on pressure to keep the pouch in place. If improperly fitted or applied, the faceplate may cause skin problems (Fig. 45-15). Inform the patient and caregiver about where to purchase supplies, emergency telephone numbers, and location of ostomy clubs, and follow-up visits with a WOCN. Follow-up with an HCP is imperative to monitor the patient's recovery, detect any complications, and assess renal function.

## CASE STUDY

### *Painful Bladder and Frequent Urination*

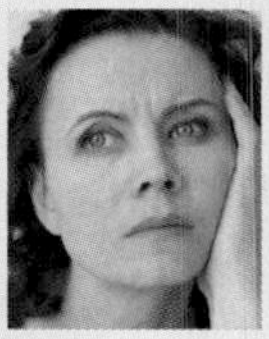

(©marilook/ iStock/ Thinkstock)

**Patient Profile**

L.T., a 38-yr-old white woman, is seen in the nurse practitioner's office for the eighth time in the past year for a history of pelvic pain with urinary frequency during the day, nocturia, and urgency to void. All urine cultures have been negative for bacteria. An evaluation by her gynecologist was negative for possible endometriosis.

**Subjective Data**

- Has a history of suprapubic and vaginal pain and urinary frequency and urgency. Bladder pain increases with bladder filling
- Reports this is her third attack of suprapubic pain and painful urination in 2 months
- Constant pain and discomfort has been physically and emotionally exhausting
- Is worried that she has cancer and no one cares
- Has had four pregnancies with uneventful vaginal deliveries
- Her menstrual cycles are normal. Her husband had a vasectomy, although they rarely have sexual intercourse because she experiences pain with intercourse
- She has a bowel movement every day. Denies constipation and/or diarrhea
- Recalls having many UTIs as a child

**Objective Data**

***Physical Examination***

- Lungs are clear. BP 132/86. Heart rate 86/min. Respiratory rate 18/min. Abdomen soft, tender in suprapubic region.

**Diagnostic Studies**

- Urinalysis: normal
- Urine cytology: ordered to rule out cancer
- Referral to urologist for cystoscopy

**Interprofessional Care**

- Cystoscopy results indicate glomerulations and Hunner's ulcers
- Diagnosis: interstitial cystitis
- Urologist prescribes pentosan (Elmiron)
- Follow-up in 4 weeks

**Discussion Questions**

1. After taking the patient's history, would you consider a UTI as a cause of her symptoms? Why or why not?
2. What additional testing and patient information would help to determine a definitive diagnosis?
3. What is the significance of the cystoscopy findings?
4. What is the rationale for the use of pentosan (Elmiron)?
5. ***Patient-Centered Care:*** How can you help L.T. deal with her diagnosis and treatment regimen?
6. ***Priority Decision:*** What are the priority nursing diagnoses for L.T.?
7. ***Teamwork and Collaboration:*** Why is it important to get a dietitian involved in the care of L.T.?
8. ***Evidence-Based Practice:*** L.T. asks you how she can control her interstitial cystitis. How would you respond?

Answers available at *http://evolve.elsevier.com/Lewis/medsurg.*

## BRIDGE TO NCLEX EXAMINATION

The number of the question corresponds to the same-numbered outcome at the beginning of the chapter.

1. In teaching a patient with pyelonephritis about the disorder, the nurse informs the patient that the organisms that cause pyelonephritis *most* commonly reach the kidneys through
   **a.** the bloodstream.
   **b.** the lymphatic system.
   **c.** a descending infection.
   **d.** an ascending infection.
2. The nurse teaches the female patient who has frequent UTIs that she should
   **a.** take tub baths with bubble bath.
   **b.** urinate before and after sexual intercourse.
   **c.** take prophylactic sulfonamides for the rest of her life.
   **d.** restrict fluid intake to prevent the need for frequent voiding.
3. The immunologic mechanisms involved in acute poststreptococcal glomerulonephritis include
   **a.** tubular blocking by precipitates of bacteria and antibody reactions.
   **b.** deposition of immune complexes and complement along the GBM.
   **c.** thickening of the GBM from autoimmune microangiopathic changes.
   **d.** destruction of glomeruli by proteolytic enzymes contained in the GBM.
4. One of the nurse's *most* important roles in relation to acute poststreptococcal glomerulonephritis is to
   **a.** promote early diagnosis and treatment of sore throats and skin lesions.
   **b.** encourage patients to obtain antibiotic therapy for upper respiratory tract infections.
   **c.** teach patients with APSGN that long-term prophylactic antibiotic therapy is necessary to prevent recurrence.
   **d.** monitor patients for respiratory symptoms that indicate the disease is affecting the alveolar basement membrane.
5. The edema that occurs in nephrotic syndrome is due to
   **a.** increased hydrostatic pressure caused by sodium retention.
   **b.** decreased aldosterone secretion from adrenal insufficiency.
   **c.** increased fluid retention caused by decreased glomerular filtration.
   **d.** decreased colloidal osmotic pressure caused by loss of serum albumin.
6. A patient is admitted to the hospital with severe renal colic. The nurse's *first priority* in management of the patient is to
   **a.** administer opioids as prescribed.
   **b.** obtain supplies for straining all urine.
   **c.** encourage fluid intake of 3 to 4 L/day.
   **d.** keep the patient NPO in preparation for surgery.
7. The nurse recommends genetic counseling for the children of a patient with
   **a.** nephrotic syndrome.
   **b.** chronic pyelonephritis.
   **c.** malignant nephrosclerosis.
   **d.** adult-onset polycystic kidney disease.

8. The nurse identifies a risk factor for kidney and bladder cancer in a patient who relates a history of
   a. aspirin use.
   b. tobacco use.
   c. chronic alcohol abuse.
   d. use of artificial sweeteners.
9. In planning nursing interventions to increase bladder control in the patient with urinary incontinence, the nurse includes
   a. teaching the patient to use Kegel exercises.
   b. clamping and releasing a catheter to increase bladder tone.
   c. teaching the patient biofeedback mechanisms to suppress the urge to void.
   d. counseling the patient concerning choice of incontinence containment device.
10. A patient with a ureterolithotomy returns from surgery with a nephrostomy tube in place. Postoperative nursing care of the patient includes
    a. encouraging the patient to drink fruit juices and milk.
    b. encouraging fluids of at least 2 to 3 L/day after nausea has subsided.
    c. irrigating the nephrostomy tube with 10 mL of normal saline solution as needed.
    d. notifying the physician if nephrostomy tube drainage is more than 30 mL/hr.
11. A patient has had a cystectomy and ileal conduit diversion performed. Four days postoperatively, mucous shreds are seen in the drainage bag. The nurse should
    a. notify the physician.
    b. notify the charge nurse.
    c. irrigate the drainage tube.
    d. document it as a normal observation.

1. d, 2. b, 3. b, 4. a, 5. d, 6. a, 7. d, 8. b, 9. a, 10. b, 11. d

For rationales to these answers and even more NCLEX review questions, visit *http://evolve.elsevier.com/Lewis/medsurg.*

## EVOLVE WEBSITE

http://evolve.elsevier.com/Lewis/medsurg

**Review Questions (Online Only)**

**Key Points**

**Answer Keys for Questions**

- Rationales for Bridge to NCLEX Examination Questions
- Answer Guidelines for Case Study on p. 1067

**Student Case Studies**

- Patient With Bladder Cancer and Urinary Diversion
- Patient With Glomerulonephritis and Acute Kidney Injury

**Nursing Care Plans**

- eNursing Care Plan 45-1: Patient With a Urinary Tract Infection
- eNursing Care Plan 45-2: Patient With Urinary Tract Calculi
- eNursing Care Plan 45-3: Patient With an Ileal Conduit

**Conceptual Care Map Creator**

**Audio Glossary**

**Content Updates**

## REFERENCES

1. National Kidney and Urologic Diseases Information Clearinghouse: Kidney and urologic diseases statistics for the United States. Retrieved from *www.niddk.nih.gov/health-information/health-topics/urologic-disease/urinary-tract-infections-in-adults/Pages/facts.aspx.*
2. Brusch JL, Bavaro MF, Cunha BA, et al: Cystitis in females. Retrieved from *http://emedicine.medscape.com/article/233101-overview.*
3. American Association of Nurses: ANA CAUTI Prevention Tool. Retrieved from *http://nursingworld.org/ANA-CAUTI-Prevention-Tool.*
4. Nazarko L: Recurrent urinary tract infection in older women: an evidence-based approach, *Br J Community Nurs* 18(8):407, 2013.
5. Wang A, Nizran P, Malone MA, et al: Urinary tract infections, *Prim Care* 40(3):687, 2013.
*6. Wang C, Fang C, Chen N, et al: Cranberry-containing products for prevention of urinary tract infections in susceptible populations: a systematic review and meta-analysis of randomized controlled trials, *Arch Intern Med* 172:988, 2012.
7. Neumann I, Moore P: Pyelonephritis (acute) in non-pregnant women, *BMJ Clin Evid* Nov 4, 2014. pii: 0807.
8. National Institute for Diabetes and Digestive and Kidney Diseases: Interstitial cystitis/painful bladder syndrome. Retrieved from *www.niddk.nih.gov/health-information/health-topics/urologic-disease/interstitial-cystitis-painful-bladder-syndrome/Pages/facts.aspx.*
9. Lessnau K, Kim ED, Pais VM: Tuberculosis of the genitourinary system: overview of GUTB. Retrieved from *http://emedicine.medscape.com/article/450651-overview.*
10. Soliman MS: Tuberculosis of the genitourinary system. Retrieved from *http://emedicine.medscape.com/article.*
11. Ralph AP, Carapetis JR: Group A streptococcal diseases and their global burden, *Curr Top Microbiol Immunol* 368:1, 2013.
12. Cohen EP, Batuman V: Nephrotic syndrome clinical presentation. Retrieved from *http://emedicine.medscape.com/article/244631-clinical.*
13. National Institute of Diabetes and Digestive and Kidney Diseases: Kidney stones in adults. Retrieved from *www.niddk.nih.gov/health-information/health-topics/urologic-disease/kidney-stones-in-adults/Pages/facts.aspx.*
14. Flannigan R, Choy WH, Chew B, et al: Renal struvite stones—pathogenesis, microbiology, and management strategies, *Nat Rev Urol* 11(6):333, 2014.
15. Slater RC, Ost M: Percutaneous stone removal: new approaches to access and imaging, *Curr Urol Rep* 16(5):501, 2015.
16. Paul BM, Vanden Heuvel GB: Kidney: polycystic kidney disease, *Wiley Interdiscip Rev Dev Biol* 3(6):465, 2014.
17. Alam A: Risk factors for progression in ADPKD, *Curr Opin Nephrol Hypertens* 24(3): 290, 2015.
18. National Kidney Foundation: Alport syndrome. Retrieved from *www.kidney.org/atoz/content/Alport.*
19. American Cancer Society: Cancer facts and figures 2015. Retrieved from *www.cancer.org/research/cancerfactsstatistics/allcancerfactsfigures/index.*
20. Puente VA, Alonso G, Moreno J, et al: New challenges in kidney cancer management: integration of surgery and novel therapies, *Curr Treat Option Oncol* 16(3):337, 2015.
21. Kim JW, Tomita Y, Trepel J, et al: Emerging immunotherapies for bladder cancer, *Curr Opin Oncol* 27:191, 2015.
*22. Houghton BB, Chalasani V, Hayne D, et al: Intravesical chemotherapy plus bacille Calmette-Guérin in non-muscle invasive bladder cancer: a systematic review with meta-analysis, *BJU Int* 111:977, 2013.
*23. Shin DC, Shin SH, Lee MM, et al: Pelvic floor muscle training for urinary incontinence in female stroke patients: a randomized, controlled and blinded trial, *Clin Rehabil* 30(3):259, 2016.
24. Newman DK, Willson M: Review of intermittent catheterization and current best practices. Retrieved from *www.medscape.com/viewarticle/745908_10.*
25. National Institute for Diabetes and Digestive and Kidney Diseases: Urinary diversion. Retrieved from *www.niddk.nih.gov/health-information/health-topics/urologic-disease/urinary-diversion/Pages/facts.aspx.*

*Evidence-based information for clinical practice.

46

# Acute Kidney Injury and Chronic Kidney Disease

*Hazel A. Dennison*

*The greatest healing therapy is friendship and love.*

**Hubert H. Humphrey**

http://evolve.elsevier.com/Lewis/medsurg/

## LEARNING OUTCOMES

1. Differentiate between acute kidney injury and chronic kidney disease.
2. Identify criteria used in the classification of acute kidney injury using the acronym RIFLE (*R*isk, *I*njury, *F*ailure, *L*oss, *E*nd-stage renal disease).
3. Describe the clinical course of acute kidney injury.
4. Explain the interprofessional care and nursing management of a patient with acute kidney injury.
5. Define chronic kidney disease and delineate its five stages based on the glomerular filtration rate.
6. Identify risk factors that contribute to the development of chronic kidney disease.
7. Summarize the significance of cardiovascular disease in individuals with chronic kidney disease.
8. Explain the conservative interprofessional care for and the related nursing management of the patient with chronic kidney disease.
9. Differentiate among renal replacement therapy options for individuals with end-stage renal disease.
10. Compare and contrast nursing interventions for individuals on peritoneal dialysis and hemodialysis.
11. Discuss the role of nurses in the management of individuals who receive a kidney transplant.

## KEY TERMS

acute kidney injury (AKI), p. 1069
acute tubular necrosis (ATN), p. 1071
anuria, p. 1071
arteriovenous fistula (AVF), p. 1087
arteriovenous grafts (AVGs), p. 1088
automated peritoneal dialysis (APD), p. 1086
azotemia, p. 1069
chronic kidney disease (CKD), p. 1075
CKD mineral and bone disorder (CKD-MBD), p. 1078
continuous ambulatory peritoneal dialysis (CAPD), p. 1086
continuous renal replacement therapy (CRRT), p. 1091
dialysis, p. 1084
end-stage renal disease (ESRD), p. 1076
hemodialysis (HD), p. 1084
oliguria, p. 1071
peritoneal dialysis (PD), p. 1084
uremia, p. 1076

*Kidney failure* (also called *renal failure*) is the partial or complete impairment of kidney function. It results in an inability to excrete metabolic waste products and water, and it contributes to disturbances of all body systems. Kidney failure can be classified as acute or chronic (Table 46-1). Acute kidney injury (AKI) has a rapid onset. Chronic kidney disease (CKD) is linked with the development of cardiovascular (CV) disease.

## ACUTE KIDNEY INJURY

**Acute kidney injury (AKI)** is the term used to encompass the entire scope of the syndrome, ranging from a slight deterioration in kidney function to severe impairment. AKI is characterized by a rapid loss of kidney function. This loss is accompanied by a rise in serum creatinine and/or a reduction in urine output. The severity of dysfunction can range from a small increase in serum creatinine or reduction in urine output to the development of **azotemia** (an accumulation of nitrogenous waste products [urea nitrogen, creatinine] in the blood).

Although AKI is potentially reversible, it has a high mortality rate.[1] AKI usually affects people with other life-threatening conditions[2] (Table 46-2). Most commonly, AKI follows severe, prolonged hypotension or hypovolemia or exposure to a nephrotoxic agent.

AKI can develop over hours or days with progressive elevations of blood urea nitrogen (BUN), creatinine, and potassium with or without a reduction in urine output. Hospitalized patients develop AKI at a high rate (1 in 5) and have a high mortality rate. When AKI develops in patients in intensive care units (ICUs), the mortality rate can be as high as 70% to 80%.[3,4]

Reviewed by Rowena W. Elliott, RN, PhD, CNN, CNE, AGNP-C, FAAN, Associate Professor, University of Southern Mississippi, College of Nursing, Hattiesburg, Mississippi; Shari Gould, RN, MSN, Associate Professor of Nursing, Victoria College, Victoria, Texas; Sharon Haas, RN, MSN, CDN, Instructor, College of Nursing, Cardinal Stritch University, Milwaukee, Wisconsin; and Rebecca Personett, RN, PhD, NEA-BC, Professor of Nursing, North Central Texas College, Gainesville, Texas and Brookhaven College, Dallas, Texas.

### Etiology and Pathophysiology

The causes of AKI, which are multiple and complex, are categorized as prerenal, intrarenal (or intrinsic), and postrenal causes (Table 46-2 and Fig. 46-1).

**Prerenal.** *Prerenal* causes of AKI are factors that reduce systemic circulation, causing a reduction in renal blood flow. The decrease in blood flow leads to decreased glomerular perfusion and filtration of the kidneys.

It is important to distinguish prerenal oliguria from the oliguria of intrarenal AKI. In prerenal oliguria there is no damage to the kidney tissue (parenchyma). The oliguria is caused by a decrease in circulating blood volume (e.g., severe dehydration, heart failure [HF], decreased cardiac output). Prerenal oliguria is readily reversible with appropriate treatment.[5] With a decrease in circulating blood volume, autoregulatory mechanisms that increase angiotensin II, aldosterone, norepinephrine, and antidiuretic hormone attempt to preserve blood flow to essential organs. Prerenal azotemia results in a reduction in the excretion of sodium (less than 20 mEq/L), increased sodium and water retention, and decreased urine output.

**TABLE 46-1 Comparison of Acute Kidney Injury and Chronic Kidney Disease**

| | Acute Kidney Injury | Chronic Kidney Disease |
|---|---|---|
| **Onset** | Sudden | Gradual, often over many years |
| **Most common cause** | Acute tubular necrosis | Diabetic nephropathy |
| **Diagnostic criteria** | Acute reduction in urine output<br>and/or<br>Elevation in serum creatinine | GFR <60 mL/min/1.73 m$^2$ for >3 mo<br>and/or<br>Kidney damage >3 mo |
| **Reversibility** | Potentially | Progressive and irreversible |
| **Primary cause of death** | Infection | Cardiovascular disease |

*GFR,* Glomerular filtration rate.

Prerenal conditions contribute to intrarenal AKI. If decreased perfusion persists for an extended time, the kidneys lose their ability to compensate and damage to kidney parenchyma occurs (intrarenal damage).

**Intrarenal.** *Intrarenal* causes of AKI (Table 46-2) include conditions that cause direct damage to the kidney tissue, resulting in impaired nephron function. The damage from intrarenal causes usually results from prolonged ischemia, nephrotoxins (e.g., aminoglycoside antibiotics, contrast media), hemoglobin released from hemolyzed red blood cells (RBCs), or myoglobin released from necrotic muscle cells.

Nephrotoxins can cause obstruction of intrarenal structures by crystallizing or by causing damage to the epithelial cells of

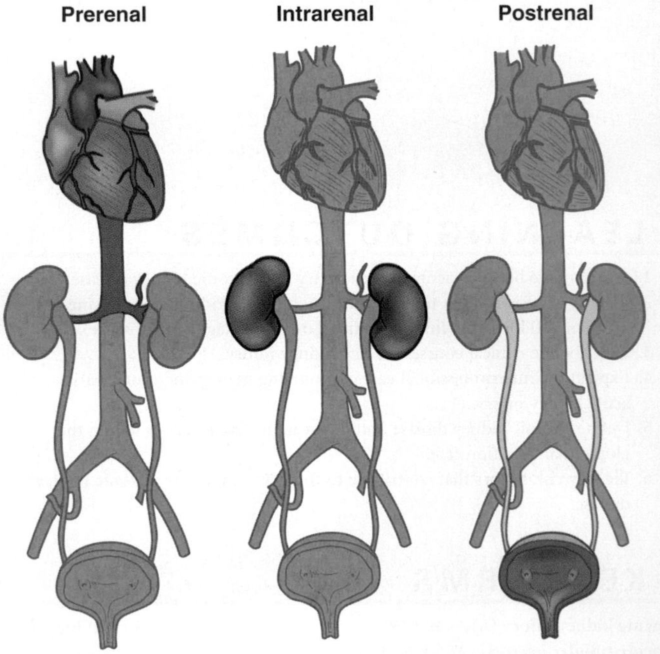


**FIG. 46-1** Prerenal, intrarenal, and postrenal causes of acute kidney injury (AKI).

**TABLE 46-2 Common Causes of Acute Kidney Injury**

| Prerenal | Intrarenal | Postrenal |
|---|---|---|
| **Hypovolemia**<br>• Dehydration<br>• Hemorrhage<br>• GI losses (diarrhea, vomiting)<br>• Excessive diuresis<br>• Hypoalbuminemia<br>• Burns<br>**Decreased Cardiac Output**<br>• Cardiac dysrhythmias<br>• Cardiogenic shock<br>• Heart failure<br>• Myocardial infarction<br>**Decreased Peripheral Vascular Resistance**<br>• Anaphylaxis<br>• Neurologic injury<br>• Septic shock<br>**Decreased Renovascular Blood Flow**<br>• Bilateral renal vein thrombosis<br>• Embolism<br>• Hepatorenal syndrome<br>• Renal artery thrombosis | **Nephrotoxic Injury**<br>• Drugs: aminoglycosides (gentamicin, amikacin), amphotericin B<br>• Contrast media<br>• Hemolytic blood transfusion reaction<br>• Severe crush injury<br>• Chemical exposure: ethylene glycol, lead, arsenic, carbon tetrachloride<br>**Interstitial Nephritis**<br>• Allergies: antibiotics (sulfonamides, rifampin), nonsteroidal antiinflammatory drugs, ACE inhibitors<br>• Infections: bacterial (acute pyelonephritis), viral (CMV), fungal (candidiasis)<br>**Other Causes**<br>• Prolonged prerenal ischemia<br>• Acute glomerulonephritis<br>• Thrombotic disorders<br>• Toxemia of pregnancy<br>• Malignant hypertension<br>• Systemic lupus erythematosus | • Benign prostatic hyperplasia<br>• Bladder cancer<br>• Calculi formation<br>• Neuromuscular disorders<br>• Prostate cancer<br>• Spinal cord disease<br>• Strictures<br>• Trauma (back, pelvis, perineum) |

*ACE,* Angiotensin-converting enzyme; *CMV,* cytomegalovirus.

the tubules. Hemoglobin and myoglobin can block the tubules and cause renal vasoconstriction. Diseases of the kidney such as acute glomerulonephritis and systemic lupus erythematosus may also cause AKI.

**Acute tubular necrosis (ATN)** is the most common intrarenal cause of AKI and is primarily the result of ischemia, nephrotoxins, or sepsis. Ischemic and nephrotoxic ATN is responsible for 90% of intrarenal AKI cases.[6,7] Severe kidney ischemia causes a disruption in the basement membrane and patchy destruction of the tubular epithelium. Nephrotoxic agents cause necrosis of tubular epithelial cells, which slough off and plug the tubules. ATN is potentially reversible if the basement membrane is not destroyed and the tubular epithelium regenerates.

ATN is the most common cause of AKI for hospitalized patients.[7] Risks associated with the development of ATN while in the hospital include major surgery, shock, sepsis, blood transfusion reaction, muscle injury from trauma, prolonged hypotension, and nephrotoxic agents (Table 46-2).

**Postrenal.** *Postrenal* causes of AKI involve mechanical obstruction in the outflow of urine. As the flow of urine is obstructed, urine refluxes into the renal pelvis, impairing kidney function. The most common postrenal causes are benign prostatic hyperplasia, prostate cancer, calculi, trauma, and extrarenal tumors. Bilateral ureteral obstruction leads to *hydronephrosis* (kidney dilation), increase in hydrostatic pressure, and tubular blockage, resulting in a progressive decline in kidney function. If bilateral obstruction is relieved within 48 hours of onset, complete recovery is likely. Prolonged obstruction can lead to tubular atrophy and irreversible kidney fibrosis. Postrenal causes of AKI account for less than 10% of AKI cases.[8]

## Clinical Manifestations

Prerenal and postrenal AKI that has not caused intrarenal damage usually resolves quickly with treatment. When parenchymal damage occurs due to either prerenal or postrenal causes, or when parenchymal damage occurs directly as with intrarenal causes, AKI has a prolonged course. Clinically, AKI may progress through phases: oliguric, diuretic, and recovery. When a patient does not recover from AKI, then CKD may develop.

The RIFLE classification is used to describe the stages of AKI (Table 46-3). *R*isk, the first stage of AKI, is followed by *I*njury, which is the second stage. Then AKI increases in severity to the final, or third, stage, *F*ailure. The two outcome variables are *L*oss and *E*nd-stage renal disease.[9,10]

**Oliguric Phase.** The most common manifestations of AKI are discussed in this section.

***Urinary Changes.*** The most common initial manifestation of AKI is **oliguria**, a reduction in urine output to less than 400 mL/day. Nonoliguria AKI indicates a urine output greater than 400 mL/day. Oliguria usually occurs within 1 to 7 days of the injury to the kidneys. If the cause is ischemia, oliguria often occurs within 24 hours. In contrast, when nephrotoxic drugs are involved, the onset may be delayed for as long as 1 week. The oliguric phase lasts on average about 10 to 14 days but can last months in some cases. The longer the oliguric phase lasts, the poorer the prognosis for complete recovery of kidney function.[1]

About 50% of patients will not be oliguric, making the initial diagnosis more difficult.[7] Changes in urine output generally do not correspond to changes in glomerular filtration rate (GFR). However, changes in urine output are often helpful in differentiating the etiology of AKI. For example, **anuria** (no urine output) is usually seen with urinary tract obstruction, oliguria is commonly seen with prerenal causes, and nonoliguric AKI is seen with acute interstitial nephritis and ATN.[8]

A urinalysis may show casts, RBCs, and white blood cells (WBCs). The casts are formed from mucoprotein impressions of the necrotic renal tubular epithelial cells, which slough

**TABLE 46-3 RIFLE Classification for Staging Acute Kidney Injury**

| Stage | GFR Criteria | Urine Output Criteria | Clinical Example |
|---|---|---|---|
| Risk | Serum creatinine increased × 1.5<br>OR<br>GFR decreased by 25% | Urine output <0.5 mL/kg/hr for 6 hr | • 68-yr-old African American woman with type 2 diabetes, hypertension, CAD, and CKD.<br>• Scheduled to undergo emergency coronary artery bypass graft.<br>• Serum creatinine is 1.8 mg/dL (increased) and she weighs 60 kg.<br>• Calculated GFR is 35 mL/min/1.73 m$^2$.<br>• She has Stage 3b CKD. |
| Injury | Serum creatinine increased × 2<br>OR<br>GFR decreased by 50% | Urine output <0.5 mL/kg/hr for 12 hr | • During surgery, she experiences hypotension for a sustained period.<br>• Acute tubular necrosis is diagnosed.<br>• After surgery: Serum creatinine is 3.6 mg/dL and urine output is reduced to 28 mL/hr |
| Failure | Serum creatinine increased × 3<br>OR<br>GFR decreased by 75%<br>OR<br>Serum creatinine >4 mg/dL with acute rise ≥0.5 mg/dL | Urine output <0.3 mL/kg/hr for 24 hr (oliguria)<br>OR<br>Anuria for 12 hr | • 72 hours after surgery and in ICU develops ventilator-associated pneumonia and sepsis.<br>• Serum creatinine rises to 5.2 mg/dL and urine output drops to 10 mL/hr.<br>• BP remains low despite dopamine therapy. |
| Loss | Persistent acute kidney failure. Complete loss of kidney function >4 wk | — | • Continuous venovenous hemodialysis is started.<br>• After 3 wk of therapy she has a cardiopulmonary arrest and does not survive. |
| End-Stage Renal Disease | Complete loss of kidney function >3 mo | — | — |

*GFR,* Glomerular filtration rate.

into the tubules. Urinary specific gravity (measure of the concentration of solutes in the urine) is normally 1.003 to 1.030. Urine osmolality is used to measure the number of dissolved particles in the urine. Urine osmolality range is 300 to 1300 mOsm/kg. As a measure of urine concentration, it is more accurate than specific gravity.

In kidney failure, a urinalysis may show a specific gravity fixed at around 1.010 and urine osmolality at about 300 mOsm/kg (300 mmol/kg). This is the same specific gravity and osmolality of plasma, thus reflecting tubular damage with a loss of concentrating ability by the kidney. Proteinuria may be present if kidney failure is related to glomerular membrane dysfunction.

***Fluid Volume.*** Hypovolemia (volume depletion) has the potential to exacerbate all forms of AKI. Fluid replacement is often sufficient to treat many forms of AKI, especially prerenal causes. When urine output decreases, fluid retention occurs. The severity of the manifestations depends on the extent of the fluid overload. In the case of reduced urine output (anuria and oliguria), the neck veins may become distended with a bounding pulse. Edema and hypertension may develop. Fluid overload can eventually lead to heart failure, pulmonary edema, and pericardial and pleural effusions.

***Metabolic Acidosis.*** In the normal kidney, excess hydrogen ions are excreted to maintain a physiologic balance of the blood pH. The impaired kidneys cannot excrete hydrogen ions or the acid products of metabolism. Serum bicarbonate production is decreased because of defective reabsorption and regeneration of bicarbonate ions. Serum bicarbonate is depleted through buffering of acidic hydrogen ions and metabolic end products. The patient with severe acidosis may develop Kussmaul respirations (rapid, deep respirations) in an effort to compensate by increasing the exhalation of $CO_2$.

***Sodium Balance.*** Damaged tubules cannot conserve sodium. The urinary excretion of sodium may increase, resulting in normal or below-normal levels of serum sodium. Excessive intake of sodium should be avoided because it can lead to volume expansion, hypertension, and HF. Uncontrolled hyponatremia or water excess can lead to cerebral edema.

***Potassium Excess.*** The kidneys normally excrete 80% to 90% of the body's potassium. In AKI the serum potassium level increases because the kidney's normal ability to excrete potassium is impaired. Hyperkalemia risk is increased if AKI is caused by massive tissue trauma because the damaged cells release additional potassium into the extracellular fluid. Bleeding and blood transfusions may cause cellular destruction, releasing more potassium into the extracellular fluid. Metabolic acidosis worsens hyperkalemia as hydrogen ions enter the cells, and potassium is driven out of the cells into the extracellular fluid.

While patients with hyperkalemia are often asymptomatic, some may complain of weakness with severe hyperkalemia. Because cardiac muscle is intolerant of acute increases in potassium, emergency treatment of hyperkalemia is needed.

Acute or rapid development of hyperkalemia may result in clinical signs that are apparent on electrocardiogram (ECG). These changes include peaked T waves, widening of the QRS complex, and ST segment depression. Progressive changes in the ECG that are related to increasing potassium levels are depicted in Fig. 16-14.

***Hematologic Disorders.*** Several hematologic disorders are found in patients with AKI. Hospital-acquired AKI often occurs in patients who have multiorgan failure. Leukocytosis is often present with AKI. The most common cause of death in AKI is infection. The most common sites of infection are the urinary and respiratory systems.

***Waste Product Accumulation.*** The kidneys are the primary excretory organs for urea (an end product of protein metabolism) and creatinine (an end product of endogenous muscle metabolism). BUN and serum creatinine levels are elevated in kidney disease. An elevated BUN level can also be caused by dehydration; corticosteroids; or catabolism resulting from infections, fever, severe injury, or GI bleeding. The best serum indicator of AKI is creatinine because it is not significantly altered by other factors.

***Neurologic Disorders.*** Neurologic changes can occur as the nitrogenous waste products accumulate in the brain and other nervous tissue. The manifestations can be as mild as fatigue and difficulty concentrating, and escalate to seizures, stupor, and coma.

**Diuretic Phase.** During the diuretic phase of AKI, daily urine output is usually around 1 to 3 L but may reach 5 L or more. The nephrons are still not fully functional even as urine output increases. The high urine volume is caused by osmotic diuresis from the high urea concentration in the glomerular filtrate and the inability of the tubules to concentrate the urine. In this phase, the kidneys have recovered their ability to excrete wastes but not to concentrate the urine. Hypovolemia and hypotension can occur from massive fluid losses.

Patients who develop an oliguric phase will have greater diuresis as kidney function returns. Large losses of fluid and electrolytes require the patient be monitored for hyponatremia, hypokalemia, and dehydration. The diuretic phase may last 1 to 3 weeks. Near the end of this phase, the patient's acid-base, electrolyte, and waste product (BUN, creatinine) values stabilize.

**Recovery Phase.** The recovery phase begins when the GFR increases, allowing the BUN and serum creatinine levels to decrease. Major improvements occur in the first 1 to 2 weeks of this phase, but kidney function may take up to 12 months to stabilize. The outcome of AKI is influenced by the patient's overall health, severity of kidney injury, and number and type of complications. Some individuals do not recover and progress to end-stage renal disease. The older adult is less likely to have a complete recovery of kidney function. Patients who recover may achieve clinically normal kidney function but remain in an early stage of CKD.

## Diagnostic Studies

A thorough history is essential for diagnosing the etiology of AKI. Consider prerenal causes when there is a history of dehydration, hypotension, or blood loss. Suspect intrarenal causes if the patient has been exposed to potentially nephrotoxic drugs or contrast media used in a radiologic study. Postrenal causes are suggested by a history of changes in the urinary stream, stones, benign prostatic hyperplasia, or bladder or prostate cancer.

Although changes in urine output and serum creatinine occur relatively late in the course of AKI, they are known diagnostic indicators. An increase in serum creatinine may not be evident until there is a loss of more than 50% of kidney function. The rate of increase in serum creatinine is also important as a diagnostic indicator in determining the severity of injury.

Urinalysis is an important diagnostic test. Urine sediment containing abundant cells, casts, or proteins suggests intrarenal disorders. The urine osmolality, sodium content, and specific gravity help in differentiating the causes of AKI. Urine sediment may be normal in both prerenal and postrenal AKI. In

**TABLE 46-4 Interprofessional Care**

***Acute Kidney Injury***

**Diagnostic Assessment**

- History and physical examination
- Identification of precipitating cause
- Serum creatinine and BUN levels
- Serum electrolytes
- Urinalysis
- Renal ultrasound
- Renal scan
- CT scan

**Management**

- Treatment of precipitating cause
- Fluid restriction (600 mL plus previous 24-hr fluid loss)
- Nutritional therapy
- Adequate protein intake (0.6-2 g/kg/day) depending on degree of catabolism
- Enteral nutrition
- Parenteral nutrition
- Dietary restrictions (potassium, phosphate, sodium)
- Measures to lower potassium (if elevated) (Table 46-5)
- Calcium supplements or phosphate-binding agents
- Initiation of dialysis (if necessary)
- Continuous renal replacement therapy (if necessary)

intrarenal problems, hematuria, pyuria, and crystals may be seen. To establish a diagnosis of AKI, other testing may be required (Table 46-4). A kidney ultrasound is often the first test done, since it provides imaging without exposure to potentially nephrotoxic contrast agents. It is useful for evaluating for possible kidney disease and obstruction of the urinary collection system. A renal scan can assess abnormalities in kidney blood flow, tubular function, and the collecting system. A CT scan can identify lesions, masses, obstructions, and vascular anomalies. A renal biopsy is considered the best method for confirming intrarenal causes of AKI.

Obtaining an MRI or magnetic resonance angiography (MRA) study with the contrast media gadolinium is not advised in patients with kidney failure. Administration of gadolinium can be potentially fatal.

In patients with normal kidney function, administration of contrast media poses minimal risk. In patients with kidney disease, *contrast-induced nephropathy* (CIN) can occur when contrast media for diagnostic studies causes nephrotoxic injury. In patients with diabetes receiving metformin, the drug should be held for 48 hours prior to and after the use of contrast media to decrease the risk of lactic acidosis. The best way to avoid CIN is to avoid exposure to contrast media by using other diagnostic tests such as ultrasound. If contrast media must be administered to a high-risk patient, the patient needs to have optimal hydration and the lowest possible dose of the contrast agent. Nursing interventions to ensure adequate fluid intake and hydration can decrease the risks associated with contrast media. Other treatment options to prevent CIN remain controversial such as administration of bicarbonate or sodium chloride solutions or prophylactic administration of *N*-acetylcysteine.

## Interprofessional Care

Because AKI is potentially reversible, the primary goals of treatment are to eliminate the cause, manage the signs and symptoms, and prevent complications while the kidneys recover (Table 46-4). The first step is to determine if there is adequate intravascular volume and cardiac output to ensure adequate perfusion of the kidneys. Diuretic therapy may be administered and usually includes loop diuretics (e.g., furosemide [Lasix], bumetanide [Bumex]) or an osmotic diuretic (e.g., mannitol). If AKI is already established, forcing fluids and diuretics will not be effective and may be harmful. Closely monitor fluid intake during the oliguric phase of AKI.

**TABLE 46-5 Therapies for Elevated Potassium Levels**

**Regular Insulin IV**

- Potassium moves into cells when insulin is given.
- IV glucose is given concurrently to prevent hypoglycemia.
- When effects of insulin diminish, potassium shifts back out of cells.

**Sodium Bicarbonate**

- Therapy can correct acidosis and cause a shift of potassium into cells.

**Calcium Gluconate IV**

- Generally used in advanced cardiac toxicity (with evidence of hyperkalemic ECG changes).
- Calcium raises the threshold for excitation, resulting in dysrhythmias.

**Hemodialysis**

- Most effective therapy to remove potassium.
- Works within a short time.

**Sodium Polystyrene Sulfonate (Kayexalate)**

- Cation-exchange resin is administered by mouth or retention enema.
- When resin is in the bowel, potassium is exchanged for sodium.
- Therapy removes 1 mEq of potassium per gram of drug.
- It is mixed in water with sorbitol to produce osmotic diarrhea, allowing for evacuation of potassium-rich stool from body.

**Dietary Restriction**

- Potassium intake is limited to 40 mEq/day.
- Primarily used to prevent recurrent elevation. Not used for acute elevation.

**Patiromer (Veltassa)**

- Oral suspension that binds potassium in GI tract.
- It is used to treat chronic kidney disease.
- It should not be used as an emergency drug for life-threatening hyperkalemia.
- It has a delayed onset of action.

The general rule for calculating the fluid restriction is to add all losses for the previous 24 hours (e.g., urine, diarrhea, emesis, blood) plus 600 mL for insensible losses (e.g., respiration, diaphoresis). For example, if a patient excreted 300 mL of urine on Tuesday with no other losses, the fluid allocation on Wednesday would be 900 mL.

Hyperkalemia is one of the most serious complications in AKI because it can cause life-threatening cardiac dysrhythmias. The various therapies used to treat elevated potassium levels are listed in Table 46-5. Both insulin and sodium bicarbonate serve as temporary measures for treatment of hyperkalemia by promoting a transient shift of potassium into the cells. Potassium will eventually diffuse back into the bloodstream. Calcium gluconate raises the threshold at which dysrhythmias occur, temporarily stabilizing the myocardium. Only sodium polystyrene sulfonate (Kayexalate) and dialysis actually remove potassium from the body. Never give sodium polystyrene sulfonate to a patient with a paralytic ileus as bowel necrosis can occur.

Conservative therapy may be all that is necessary until kidney function improves. If conservative therapy is not effective in treating AKI, then *renal replacement therapy* (RRT) is used. Controversy exists about the timing of RRT in AKI.[11] The most common indications for RRT in AKI are (1) volume overload, resulting in compromised cardiac and/or pulmonary status; (2) elevated serum potassium level; (3) metabolic acidosis (serum bicarbonate level less than 15 mEq/L [15 mmol/L]); (4) BUN level greater than 120 mg/dL (43 mmol/L); (5) significant change in mental status; and (6) pericarditis, pericardial effusion, or cardiac tamponade. Although laboratory values provide rough parameters, the best guideline is the clinical status of the patient.

Of the several RRT therapy options available, there is no consensus regarding the best approach.[10] Even though peritoneal dialysis (PD) is considered a viable option for RRT, it is not frequently used. Intermittent hemodialysis (HD) and continuous renal replacement therapy (CRRT) have both been used effectively.

CRRT is provided continuously over approximately 24 hours through cannulation of a vein or catheter placement. CRRT has much slower blood flow rates compared with intermittent HD. HD is the method of choice when changes are required emergently. It is technically more complicated because specialized staff and equipment and a vascular access are required. It also requires anticoagulation therapy to prevent the patient's blood from clotting when the blood makes contact with the extracorporeal dialysis circuit. Rapid fluid shifts during HD may cause hypotension. (RRT and CRRT are discussed later in this chapter on pp. 1091-1092.)

**Nutritional Therapy.** The goal of nutritional management in AKI is to provide adequate calories to prevent catabolism despite restrictions that prevent electrolyte and fluid disorders and azotemia. Nutritional intake must maintain adequate caloric intake (providing 30 to 35 kcal/kg and 0.8 to 1.0 g of protein per kilogram of desired body weight) to prevent the breakdown of body protein.

Adequate energy should primarily be from carbohydrate and fat sources to prevent ketosis from endogenous fat breakdown and gluconeogenesis from muscle protein breakdown. Essential amino acids may be supplemented. Potassium and sodium are regulated in accordance with plasma levels. Sodium is restricted as needed to prevent edema, hypertension, and HF. Dietary fat intake is increased so that the patient receives at least 30% to 40% of total calories from fat. Fat emulsion IV infusions given as a nutritional supplement provide a good source of nonprotein calories (see Chapter 39). If a patient cannot maintain adequate oral intake, enteral nutrition is the preferred route for nutritional support (see Chapter 39). When the gastrointestinal (GI) tract is not functional, parenteral nutrition is necessary to provide adequate nutrition. The patient treated with parenteral nutrition may need daily HD or CRRT to remove the excess fluid. Concentrated formulas of parenteral nutrition are available to minimize fluid volume.

## NURSING MANAGEMENT: ACUTE KIDNEY INJURY

### Nursing Assessment

Monitor vital signs, weight, and fluid intake and output. Daily monitoring of a patient's urine output has prognostic implications and is crucial for determining therapy and daily fluid volume replacement. Examine the urine for color, specific gravity, glucose, protein, blood, and sediment. Assess the patient's general appearance, including skin color, edema, neck vein distention, and bruises. If a patient is receiving dialysis, observe the access site for inflammation and exudate. Evaluate the patient's mental status and level of consciousness. Examine the oral mucosa for dryness and inflammation. Auscultate the lungs for crackles and wheezes or diminished breath sounds. Monitor the heart for an $S_3$ gallop, murmurs, or a pericardial friction rub. Assess ECG readings for dysrhythmias. Review laboratory values and diagnostic test results. All of the previous data are essential for developing an interprofessional plan of care.[12]

### Nursing Diagnoses

Nursing diagnoses and a potential complication for the patient with AKI include, but are not limited to, the following:

- Risk for infection *related to* invasive lines, uremic toxins, and altered immune responses secondary to kidney injury
- Excess fluid volume *related to* kidney injury and fluid retention
- Fatigue *related to* anemia, metabolic acidosis, and uremic toxins
- Anxiety *related to* disease processes, therapeutic interventions, and uncertainty of prognosis
- Potential complication: dysrhythmias *related to* electrolyte imbalances

### Planning

The overall goals are that the patient with AKI will (1) completely recover without any loss of kidney function, (2) maintain normal fluid and electrolyte balance, (3) have decreased anxiety, and (4) adhere to and understand the need for careful follow-up care.

### Nursing Implementation

**Health Promotion.** Prevention and early recognition of AKI are the most important components of care. Prevention is directed primarily toward identifying and monitoring high-risk populations, controlling exposure to nephrotoxic drugs and industrial chemicals, and preventing prolonged episodes of hypotension and hypovolemia. In the hospital, the factors that increase the risk for developing AKI are preexisting CKD, older age, massive trauma, major surgical procedures, extensive burns, cardiac failure, sepsis, or obstetric complications.

Carefully monitor the patient's weight, intake and output, and fluid and electrolyte balance. Assess and record extrarenal losses of fluid from vomiting, diarrhea, hemorrhage, and increased insensible losses. Prompt replacement of significant fluid losses helps prevent ischemic tubular damage associated with trauma, burns, and extensive surgery. Intake and output records and the patient's weight provide valuable indicators of fluid volume status. Aggressive diuretic therapy for the patient with fluid overload from any cause can lead to a reduction in renal blood flow.

Monitor kidney function in individuals who are taking drugs that are potentially nephrotoxic (see Table 44-3). Nephrotoxic drugs should be used sparingly in the high-risk patient. When these drugs must be used, they should be given in the smallest effective doses for the shortest possible periods. Caution the patient about abuse of over-the-counter analgesics (especially nonsteroidal antiinflammatory drugs [NSAIDs]) as these may worsen kidney function in the patient with mild CKD.

Angiotensin-converting enzyme (ACE) inhibitors can also decrease perfusion pressure and cause hyperkalemia. If other measures such as diet modification, diuretics, and sodium bicarbonate cannot control the hyperkalemia, ACE inhibitors may have to be reduced or eliminated. However, ACE inhibitors are frequently used to prevent proteinuria and progression of kidney disease, especially in patients with diabetes.[13]

◆ **Acute Care.** The patient with AKI is critically ill and may have co-morbid diseases or conditions (e.g., diabetes, CV disease) in addition to kidney injury. Focus on the patient holistically, since he or she will have many physical and emotional needs. Usually the changes caused by AKI arise suddenly. The patient needs assistance in understanding that kidney disease may affect the entire body's functions.

You have an important role in managing fluid and electrolyte balance during the oliguric and diuretic phases. Observe and record accurate intake and output. Take daily weights with the same scale at the same time each day to detect excessive gains or losses of body fluid (1 kg is equivalent to 1000 mL of fluid). Assess for the common signs and symptoms of hypervolemia (in the oliguric phase) or hypovolemia (in the diuretic phase), potassium and sodium disturbances, and other electrolyte imbalances that may occur in AKI (see Chapter 16).

Because infection is the leading cause of death in AKI, meticulous aseptic technique is critical. Protect the patient from other individuals with infectious diseases. Be alert for local manifestations of infection (e.g., swelling, redness, pain) as well as systemic manifestations (e.g., fever, malaise, leukocytosis).

If a patient with renal failure has an infection, it is important to recognize that the temperature may not always be elevated. Patients with kidney failure have a blunted febrile response to an infection (e.g., pneumonia). If antibiotics are used to treat an infection, the type, frequency, and dosage must be carefully considered because the kidneys are the primary route of excretion for many antibiotics. Dosages may be altered depending on the patient's level of kidney function if the drug is primarily eliminated by the kidneys. Nephrotoxic drugs (see Table 44-3) should be used judiciously.

Perform skin care and take measures to prevent pressure ulcers as mobility may be impaired. Mouth care is important to prevent stomatitis, which develops when ammonia (produced by bacterial breakdown of urea) in saliva irritates the mucous membranes.

**INFORMATICS IN PRACTICE**

***Computer Monitoring of Antibiotic Safety***

- Many patients receiving antibiotic therapy are at risk for kidney failure.
- Set the computer to alert you about elevated creatinine levels and, if possible, send you a text message.
- With earlier notification of the HCP, medications can be stopped or doses adjusted and the patient's kidney function preserved.

◆ **Ambulatory Care.** Recovery from AKI is highly variable and depends on whether other body systems fail, the patient's general condition and age, the length of the oliguric phase, and the severity of nephron damage. Protein and potassium intake should be regulated in accordance with kidney function. Regular evaluation of kidney function through appropriate follow-up is necessary. Teach the patient the signs and symptoms of recurrent kidney disease. Emphasize measures to prevent the recurrence of AKI.

The long-term convalescence of 3 to 12 months may cause psychosocial and financial hardships for the patient, caregiver, and family. Make appropriate referrals for counseling. If the kidneys do not recover, the patient will need to transition to life on chronic dialysis or possible future transplantation.

### ◆ Evaluation

The expected outcomes are that the patient with AKI will

- Regain and maintain normal fluid and electrolyte balance
- Adhere to the treatment regimen
- Experience no complications
- Have a complete recovery

### Gerontologic Considerations: Acute Kidney Injury

The glomerular filtration rate declines with age. In older adults, impaired function of other organ systems from CV disease or diabetes mellitus can increase the risk of developing AKI. The aging kidney is less able to compensate for changes in fluid volume, solute load, and cardiac output.

Although the causes of AKI in older adults are similar to younger adults, they are at an increased risk for AKI. Dehydration is a predisposing factor and tends to occur much more frequently in older adults. Dehydration can occur from polypharmacy (diuretics, laxatives, and drugs that suppress appetite or consciousness), acute febrile illnesses, and immobility from being bedridden.

Other common causes of AKI in the older adult include hypotension, diuretic therapy, aminoglycoside therapy, obstructive disorders (e.g., prostatic hyperplasia), surgery, infection, and contrast media. Mortality rates are similar for older and younger patients. Patients over 65 years of age are less likely to recover from AKI. Despite this, a patient's chronologic age is not a barrier to offering renal replacement therapy.[11]

## CHRONIC KIDNEY DISEASE

**Chronic kidney disease (CKD)** involves progressive, irreversible loss of kidney function. More than 26 million American adults have CKD, and a million more are at increased risk. One of every nine Americans has CKD. Over half a million Americans are receiving treatment (dialysis, transplant) for ESRD. Despite all the technologic advances in life-sustaining treatment with dialysis, patients with ESRD have a high mortality rate. As the stage of kidney disease progresses, the mortality rate also increases. Mortality rates are as high as 19% to 24% for individuals with ESRD on dialysis.[14,15]

Although CKD has many different causes, the leading causes are diabetes (about 50%) and hypertension (about 25%). Less common etiologies include glomerulonephritis, cystic diseases, and urologic diseases.[16] (Kidney diseases are discussed in Chapter 45.)

CKD is much more common than AKI (Table 46-1). The increasing prevalence of CKD has been partially attributed to increased risk factors, including an aging population, increased rates of obesity, and increased incidence of diabetes and hypertension.

Because the kidneys are highly adaptive, kidney disease is often not recognized until there has been considerable loss of nephrons. Individuals with CKD are frequently asymptomatic, resulting in CKD being underdiagnosed and untreated. It has

**TABLE 46-6 Stages of Chronic Kidney Disease**

| Description | GFR (mL/min/1.73 m²) | Clinical Action Plan |
|---|---|---|
| **Stage 1** Kidney damage with normal or ↑ GFR | ≥90 | Diagnosis and treatment<br>CVD risk reduction<br>Slow progression |
| **Stage 2** Kidney damage with mild ↓ GFR | 60-89 | Estimation of progression |
| **Stage 3a** Moderate ↓ GFR | 45-59 | Evaluation and treatment of complications |
| **Stage 3b** Moderate ↓ GFR | 30-44 | More aggressive treatment of complications |
| **Stage 4** Severe ↓ GFR | 15-29 | Preparation for renal replacement therapy (dialysis, kidney transplant) |
| **Stage 5** Kidney failure | <15 (or dialysis) | Renal replacement therapy (if uremia present and patient desires treatment) |

Source: Kidney Disease: Improving Global Outcomes (KDIGO) CKD Work Group. KDIGO 2012 Clinical Practice Guideline for the Evaluation and Management of Chronic Kidney Disease, *Kidney Inter Suppl* 3(1):1, 2013.

been estimated that about 70% of people with CKD are unaware that they have the disease.[14]

Kidney Disease Improving Global Outcomes (KDIGO) Clinical Practice Guidelines defines CKD as either the presence of kidney damage or a decreased GFR less than 60 mL/min/1.73 m² for longer than 3 months. The classification of CKD is presented in Table 46-6. The last stage of kidney disease, **end-stage renal disease (ESRD)**, occurs when the GFR is less than 15 mL/min. At this point, renal replacement therapy (dialysis or transplantation) is required to maintain life.

The prognosis and course of CKD are highly variable depending on the etiology, patient's condition and age, and adequacy of health care follow-up. Some individuals live normal, active lives with kidney disease, whereas others may rapidly progress to ESRD (stage 5).

Since 1972, the United States has covered the majority of the costs of providing dialysis through Medicare benefits. Under Title XVIII of the Social Security Act, ESRD was recognized as a disability. Medicare pays for 80% of eligible charges, with the remaining being paid for by state or private insurance or out of pocket.[15]

## Clinical Manifestations

As kidney function deteriorates, all body systems become affected. The clinical manifestations are a result of retained urea, creatinine, phenols, hormones, electrolytes, and water. **Uremia** is a syndrome in which kidney function declines to the point that symptoms may develop in multiple body systems (Fig. 46-2). It often occurs when the GFR is 15 mL/min or less. The manifestations of uremia vary among patients according to the cause of the kidney disease, co-morbid conditions, age, and degree of adherence to the prescribed medical regimen. Many patients are tolerant of the changes caused by declining kidney function because they occur gradually.

**Urinary System.** In the early stages of CKD, patients usually do not report any change in urine output. Since diabetes is the primary cause of CKD, polyuria may be present, but not necessarily as a consequence of kidney disease. As CKD progresses, patients have increasing difficulty with fluid retention and require diuretic therapy. After a period on dialysis, patients may develop anuria.

**Metabolic Disturbances**

***Waste Product Accumulation.*** As the GFR decreases, the BUN and serum creatinine levels increase. The BUN is increased not only by kidney disease but also by protein intake, fever, corticosteroids, and catabolism. For this reason, serum creatinine clearance determinations (calculated GFR) are considered more accurate indicators of kidney function than BUN or creatinine (Table 46-8). Significant elevations in BUN contribute to development of nausea, vomiting, lethargy, fatigue, impaired thought processes, and headaches.

***Altered Carbohydrate Metabolism.*** Defective carbohydrate metabolism is caused by impaired glucose metabolism, resulting from cellular insensitivity to the normal action of insulin. Mild to moderate hyperglycemia and hyperinsulinemia may occur.

**CULTURAL & ETHNIC HEALTH DISPARITIES**

***Chronic Kidney Disease***

- Chronic kidney disease (CKD) has a high incidence in minority populations, especially African Americans and Native Americans.
- Hypertension and diabetes mellitus are also more common in African Americans and Native Americans.

**African Americans**

- The risk of CKD as a complication of hypertension is significantly increased in African Americans.
- African Americans have the highest rate of CKD, nearly four times that of whites.

**Native Americans**

- Native Americans have a rate of CKD twice that of whites.
- The rate of CKD is six times higher among Native Americans with diabetes than among other ethnic groups with diabetes.

**Hispanics**

- The rate of CKD in Hispanics is 1.5 times higher than in non-Hispanic whites.

**CHECK YOUR PRACTICE**

You are working in a community-based dialysis unit. One of your patients is a 56-yr-old woman who has been on HD for 3 weeks. You are reviewing her medications with her and she is surprised that her dose of glargine insulin has been decreased. She tells you, "I have been a diabetic for 30 years, and this is the first time ever that my dose of insulin has been decreased."

- How would you respond?

Insulin and glucose metabolism may improve (but not to normal values) after the initiation of dialysis. Patients with diabetes who develop uremia may require less insulin than before the onset of CKD. Insulin, which depends on the kidneys for excretion, remains in the circulation longer. As a result, individuals who required insulin before starting dialysis may require

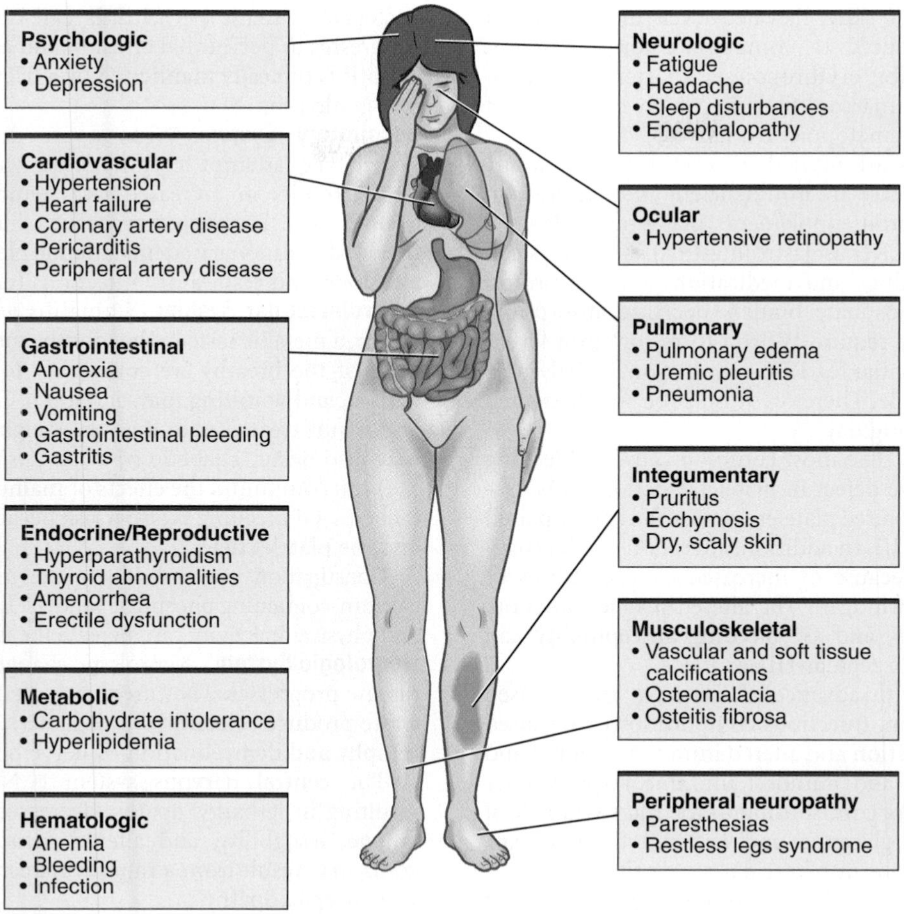


**FIG. 46-2** Possible clinical manifestations of chronic kidney disease.

less insulin therapy when they start dialysis and their kidney disease progresses. Insulin dosing must be individualized and glucose levels monitored carefully.

***Elevated Triglycerides.*** Hyperinsulinemia stimulates hepatic production of triglycerides. Many patients with uremia develop dyslipidemia, with increased very-low-density lipoproteins (VLDLs), increased low-density lipoproteins (LDLs), and decreased high-density lipoproteins (HDLs). The altered lipid metabolism is related to decreased levels of the enzyme lipoprotein lipase, which is important in the breakdown of lipoproteins. Most patients with CKD die from CV disease.[17]

**Electrolyte and Acid-Base Imbalances**

***Potassium.*** Hyperkalemia is a serious electrolyte disorder associated with kidney failure. Fatal dysrhythmias have been reported when the serum potassium level reaches 7 to 8 mEq/L (7 to 8 mmol/L). Hyperkalemia results from the decreased excretion of potassium by the kidneys, the breakdown of cellular protein, bleeding, and metabolic acidosis. Potassium may also come from foods, dietary supplements, drugs, and IV infusions.

***Sodium.*** Sodium may be elevated, normal, or low in kidney disease. Because of impaired sodium excretion, sodium along with water is retained. If large quantities of water are retained, dilutional hyponatremia occurs. Sodium retention can contribute to edema, hypertension, and HF. Sodium intake must be individually determined but is generally restricted to 2 g/day.

***Calcium and Phosphate.*** Calcium and phosphate alterations are discussed in the section on the musculoskeletal system on pp. 1078-1079.

***Magnesium.*** Magnesium is primarily excreted by the kidneys. Hypermagnesemia is generally not a problem unless the patient is ingesting magnesium (e.g., milk of magnesia, magnesium citrate, antacids containing magnesium). Clinical manifestations of hypermagnesemia can include absence of reflexes, decreased mental status, cardiac dysrhythmias, hypotension, and respiratory failure.

***Metabolic Acidosis.*** Metabolic acidosis results from the kidneys' impaired ability to excrete excess acid and from defective reabsorption and regeneration of bicarbonate. The average adult produces 80 to 90 mEq of acid per day. This acid is normally buffered by bicarbonate. In kidney disease, plasma bicarbonate, which is an indirect measure of acidosis, usually falls to a new steady state at around 16 to 20 mEq/L (16 to 20 mmol/L). The decreased plasma bicarbonate reflects its use in buffering metabolic acids. The bicarbonate level generally does not progress below this level because hydrogen ion production is usually balanced by buffering from demineralization of the bone (the phosphate buffering system).

**Hematologic System**

***Anemia.*** A normocytic, normochromic anemia is associated with CKD. Anemia in CKD is due to decreased production of the hormone erythropoietin by the kidneys. Erythropoietin normally stimulates precursor cells in the bone marrow to produce RBCs (erythropoiesis). Other factors contributing to anemia are nutritional deficiencies, decreased RBC life span, increased hemolysis of RBCs, frequent blood samplings, and bleeding from the GI tract. For patients receiving maintenance hemodialysis (HD), blood loss in the dialyzer may also contribute to the anemic state. Elevated levels of parathyroid hormone (PTH) (produced to compensate for low serum calcium levels) can inhibit erythropoiesis, shorten survival of RBCs, and cause bone marrow fibrosis, which can result in decreased numbers of hematopoietic cells.

Sufficient iron stores are needed for erythropoiesis. Many patients with kidney disease are iron deficient and require iron supplementation. Oral iron supplements may not be effective for the individual with CKD as gastrointestinal side effects can cause adherence difficulties and medications such as proton pump inhibitors or phosphate binders decrease absorption. Patients on dialysis may require IV iron to restore iron levels. Folic acid, which is essential for RBC maturation, is dialyzable because it is water soluble. Therefore it must be supplemented in the diet (folic acid 1 mg/day).[18]

***Bleeding Tendencies.*** The most common cause of bleeding in uremia is a qualitative defect in platelet function. This dysfunction is caused by impaired platelet aggregation and impaired release of platelet factor III. In addition, alterations in the coagulation system occur because of increased concentrations of both factor VIII and fibrinogen. The altered platelet function, hemorrhagic tendencies, and GI bleeding susceptibility can usually be corrected with regular HD or PD.

***Infection.*** Patients with advanced CKD have an increased susceptibility to infection. Infectious complications are caused by changes in WBC function and altered immune response and function. Both cellular and humoral immune responses are suppressed. Other factors contributing to the increased risk of infection include hyperglycemia and external trauma (e.g., catheters, needle insertions into vascular access sites).

**Cardiovascular System.** The most common cause of death in patients with CKD is CV disease. Leading causes of death are myocardial infarction, ischemic heart disease, peripheral arterial disease, HF, cardiomyopathy, and stroke.[17] CV disease and CKD are so closely linked that if patients develop cardiac events (e.g., myocardial infarction, HF), kidney function is evaluated. Traditional CV risk factors such as hypertension and elevated lipids are common in CKD patients.

CV disease may also be related to nontraditional CV risk factors such as vascular calcification and arterial stiffness. The calcium deposits in the vascular medial layer are associated with stiffening of the blood vessels. The mechanisms involved are multifactorial. They include (1) vascular smooth muscle cells changing into chondrocytes or osteoblast-like cells, (2) high total body amount of calcium and phosphate resulting from abnormal bone metabolism, (3) impaired renal excretion, and (4) drug therapies to treat the bone disease (e.g., calcium phosphate binders).[19]

Hypertension, which is prevalent in patients with CKD, is both a cause and a consequence of CKD. Hypertension is aggravated by sodium retention and increased extracellular fluid volume.[20] In some individuals, increased renin production contributes to hypertension (see Fig. 44-4). Hypertension and diabetes mellitus are contributing risk factors for vascular complications.[21] Long-standing hypertension, extracellular fluid volume overload, and anemia contribute to development of left ventricular hypertrophy that may eventually lead to cardiomyopathy and HF. Hypertension can cause retinopathy, encephalopathy, and nephropathy. Because of the many effects of hypertension, BP control is one of the most important therapeutic goals in the management of CKD.

Patients with CKD are susceptible to cardiac dysrhythmias that result from hyperkalemia and decreased coronary artery perfusion. Uremic pericarditis can develop and occasionally progresses to pericardial effusion and cardiac tamponade. Pericarditis is typically manifested by a friction rub, chest pain, and low-grade fever.

**Respiratory System.** With severe acidosis, the respiratory system may attempt to compensate with Kussmaul breathing, which results in increased $CO_2$ removal by exhalation (see Chapter 16). Dyspnea may occur as a manifestation of fluid overload, pulmonary edema, uremic pleuritis (pleurisy), pleural effusions, and respiratory infections (e.g., pneumonia).

**Gastrointestinal System.** Stomatitis with exudates and ulcerations, a metallic taste in the mouth, and *uremic fetor* (a urinous odor of the breath) are commonly found in CKD. Anorexia, nausea, and vomiting may develop if CKD progresses to ESRD and is not treated with dialysis. Weight loss and malnutrition may also occur. Diabetic *gastroparesis* (delayed gastric emptying) can compound the effects of malnutrition for patients with diabetes. GI bleeding is also a risk because of mucosal irritation and the platelet defect.

Constipation may be due to the ingestion of iron salts or calcium-containing phosphate binders. Limitations on fluid intake and physical inactivity can increase the risk of constipation.

**Neurologic System.** Neurologic changes are expected as kidney disease progresses. They are the result of increased nitrogenous waste products, electrolyte imbalances, metabolic acidosis, and atrophy and demyelination of nerve fibers.

The central nervous system (CNS) becomes depressed, resulting in lethargy, apathy, decreased ability to concentrate, fatigue, irritability, and altered mental ability. Seizures and coma may result from a rapidly increasing BUN and hypertensive encephalopathy.

*Peripheral neuropathy* is initially manifested by a slowing of nerve conduction to the extremities. Individuals with advanced stage 5 CKD may complain of restless legs syndrome (see Chapter 58), described as "bugs crawling inside the leg." Paresthesias are most often experienced in the feet and legs and may be described by the patient as a burning sensation. Eventually, motor involvement may lead to bilateral footdrop, muscular weakness and atrophy, and loss of deep tendon reflexes. Muscle twitching, jerking, *asterixis* (hand-flapping tremor), and nocturnal leg cramps may occur. In patients with diabetic neuropathy, symptoms can be compounded by uremic neuropathy.[21]

Dialysis should improve general CNS manifestations and may slow or halt the progression of neuropathies. Motor neuropathy may not be reversible. The treatment for neurologic problems is dialysis or transplantation. Altered mental status, a late manifestation of CKD stage 5, rarely occurs unless the patient has chosen not to have renal replacement therapy.

**Musculoskeletal System.** CKD mineral and bone disorder (CKD-MBD) develops as a systemic disorder of mineral and bone metabolism caused by progressive deterioration in kidney function (Fig. 46-3). Activated vitamin D is necessary to optimize absorption of calcium from the GI tract. As kidney function deteriorates, less vitamin D is converted to its active form, resulting in decreased serum levels. Low levels of active vitamin D result in decreased serum calcium levels.[19]

Serum calcium levels are regulated primarily by parathyroid hormone (PTH). When hypocalcemia occurs, the parathyroid gland secretes PTH, which stimulates bone demineralization, releasing calcium from the bones. Phosphate is released as well, leading to elevated serum phosphate levels. Hyperphosphatemia also results from decreased phosphate excretion by the

PATHOPHYSIOLOGY MAP

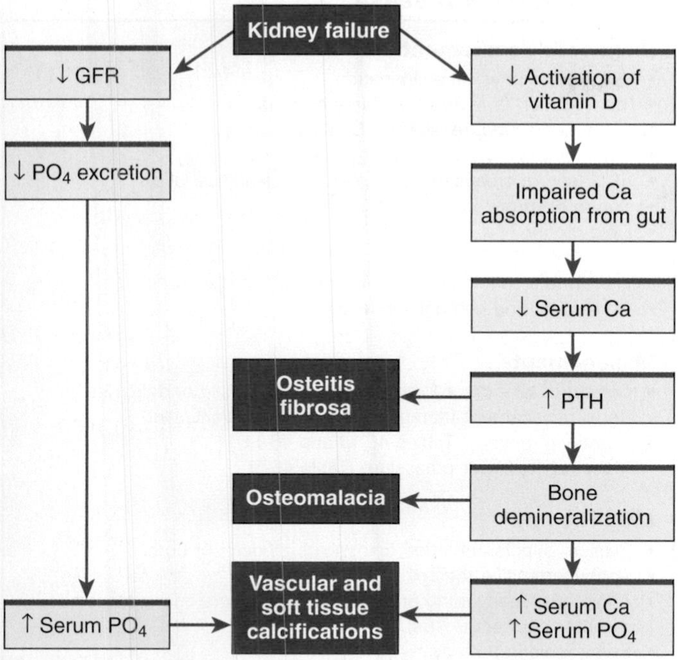


**FIG. 46-3** Mechanisms of chronic kidney disease mineral and bone disorder (CKD-MBD). *GFR,* Glomerular filtration rate; *PTH,* parathyroid hormone.

kidneys. Hyperphosphatemia decreases serum calcium levels and further reduces the kidneys' ability to activate vitamin D.

Low serum calcium, elevated phosphate, and decreased vitamin D contribute to the stimulation of the parathyroid gland and excretion of PTH. PTH acts on the bone to increase remodeling and increase serum calcium levels. The accelerated rate of bone remodeling causes a weakened bone matrix and places the patient at a higher risk for fractures. Normally plasma calcium is found ionized or free (physiologically active form) or bound to protein.

A low ionized calcium level can lead to tetany (see Chapter 16). However, in kidney failure, it is unusual for hypocalcemia to be symptomatic. In the acidotic state associated with kidney failure, more calcium is in the ionized form than is bound to protein.

CKD-MBD is a common complication of CKD and results in skeletal complications, vascular and soft tissue (extraskeletal) complications. Skeletal complications include (1) *osteomalacia* (results from demineralization from slow bone turnover and defective mineralization of newly formed bone) and (2) *osteitis fibrosa* (decalcification of the bone and replacement of bone tissue with fibrous tissue).

Soft tissue complications result from vascular calcifications. Vascular calcifications are a significant contributing factor to CV disease. "Uremic red eye" is caused by the irritation from calcium deposits in the eye. Intracardiac calcifications can disrupt the conduction system and cause cardiac arrest.

**Integumentary System.** A small percentage of patients develop refractory pruritus that can have a devastating impact on their well-being and quality of life. Pruritus has multiple causes, including dry skin, calcium-phosphate deposition in the skin, and sensory neuropathy. Pruritus is more prevalent in patients receiving dialysis than in the earlier stages of CKD. The itching may be so intense that it can lead to bleeding or infection secondary to scratching. Uremic frost is an extremely rare condition in which urea crystallizes on the skin; this is usually seen only when BUN levels are extremely elevated (e.g., over 200 mg/dL).

**Reproductive System.** Both men and women can experience infertility and a decreased libido. Women usually have decreased levels of estrogen, progesterone, and luteinizing hormone, causing anovulation and menstrual changes (usually amenorrhea). Menses and ovulation may return after dialysis is started. Men experience loss of testicular consistency, decreased testosterone levels, and low sperm counts.

Sexual dysfunction may also be caused by anemia, which causes fatigue and decreased libido. In addition, peripheral neuropathy can cause impotence in men and anorgasmy in women. Additional factors that may cause changes in sexual function are psychologic problems (e.g., anxiety, depression), physical stress, and side effects of medications. Sexual function may improve with maintenance dialysis and may become normal with successful transplantation.

Patients who become pregnant while receiving dialysis have been able to carry a fetus to term, but there is significant risk to the mother and infant. Pregnancy in patients with a kidney transplant is more common, but there is still considerable risk to both the mother and fetus.

**Psychologic Changes.** Personality and behavioral changes, emotional lability, withdrawal, and depression are commonly observed in patients with CKD. Fatigue and lethargy contribute to the feeling of illness. The changes in body image caused by edema, integumentary disturbances, and access devices (e.g., fistulas, catheters) may lead to anxiety and depression. Decreased ability to concentrate and slowed mental activity can give the appearance of dullness and disinterest in the environment. The patient must also deal with significant changes in lifestyle, occupation, family responsibilities, and financial status. Long-term survival depends on medications, dietary restrictions, dialysis, and possibly transplantation. The patient also grieves the loss of kidney function and independence.

## Diagnostic Studies

Because persistent proteinuria is usually the first indication of kidney damage, screening for CKD involves a dipstick evaluation of protein in the urine or evaluation for albuminuria, which is not detected with routine urinalysis. The urine of patients with diabetes must be examined for albuminuria if no protein is detected on routine urinalysis. A person with persistent proteinuria (1+ protein on standard dipstick testing two or more times over a 3-month period) should have further assessment of risk factors and a diagnostic workup with blood and urine tests to evaluate for CKD.

A urinalysis can detect RBCs, WBCs, protein, casts, and glucose. An ultrasound of the kidneys is usually done to detect any obstructions and determine the size of the kidneys. Other diagnostic studies (Table 46-7) help establish the diagnosis and cause of CKD. A kidney biopsy may be necessary to provide a definitive diagnosis.

Serum creatinine alone poorly reflects kidney function. GFR is the preferred measure to determine kidney function. Several GFR calculators are available. The two equations used most frequently to estimate GFR are the Cockcroft-Gault formula and Modification of Diet in Renal Disease (MDRD) Study equation (Table 46-8). MDRD is the preferred method.[22]

## Interprofessional Care

The overall goals of CKD therapy are to preserve existing kidney function, reduce the risks of CV disease, prevent

## EVIDENCE-BASED PRACTICE

### *Translating Research Into Practice*

**Do Nonpharmacologic Interventions Improve Sleep in Dialysis Patients?**

***Clinical Question***

Among patients with end-stage renal disease on dialysis (P), what is the effect of cognitive behavioral therapy, physical exercise, and acupressure (I) versus control group (C) on sleep quality (O)?

***Synthesis of Best Available Evidence***

- Systematic review of randomized controlled trials (RCTs) and one prospective cohort study.
- 13 studies of patients ($n = 1518$) with end-stage renal disease dependent on dialysis. Interventions included cognitive behavioral therapy (CBT), physical exercise, and acupressure. Control groups included sleep hygiene and usual care. Outcome was sleep quality.
- Sleep latency and sleep disturbance improved with CBT. Sleep medication use declined with CBT.
- Aerobic exercise during dialysis may improve sleep quality for patients who also have restless leg syndrome.
- Trend was noted for CBT and improved daytime functioning and subjective sleep quality.
- Although acupressure appears promising to help with sleep, there are some concerns regarding the methodological quality of the studies.

***Conclusion***

- Nonpharmacologic interventions such as cognitive behavioral therapy (CBT), physical exercise, and acupressure can improve sleep quality in dialysis patients.

***Implications for Nursing Practice***

1. Why is it important to assess sleep quality in patients on dialysis who report poor quality of life?
2. How would you assist a patient who is on dialysis and experiencing sleep problems at night?
3. When sleep medications are minimally effective, what information would you share with a patient related to nonpharmacologic treatments?

***Reference for Evidence***

Yang B, Xy J, Xue Q, et al: Non-pharmacological interventions for improving sleep quality in patients on dialysis: systematic review and meta-analysis, *Sleep Med Rev* 23:68, 2015.

*P*, Patient population of interest; *I*, intervention or area of interest; *C*, comparison of interest or comparison group; *O*, outcomes of interest; *T*, timing (see p. 15).

complications, and provide for the patient's comfort (Table 46-9). Early recognition, diagnosis, and treatment can prevent the progression of kidney disease. It is important that patients with CKD receive appropriate referral to a nephrologist early in the course of the disease. Every effort is made to detect and treat potentially reversible causes of kidney failure (e.g., HF, dehydration, infections, nephrotoxins, urinary tract obstruction, glomerulonephritis, renal artery stenosis).

Patients with CKD have a high incidence of CV complications. A higher percentage of patients will die from CV disease than live to need dialysis. When a patient is diagnosed as having CKD, therapy is aimed at treating the CV disease in addition to slowing the progression of kidney disease (Table 46-7).

A focus on stages 1 through 4 (Table 46-6) before the need for dialysis (stage 5) includes the control of hypertension, hyperparathyroid disease, CKD-MBD, anemia, and dyslipidemia. The following section focuses primarily on the drug and nutritional aspects of care.

## TABLE 46-7 Interprofessional Care

### *Chronic Kidney Disease*

**Diagnostic Assessment**

- History and physical examination
- Identification of reversible kidney disease
- Renal ultrasound, renal scan, CT scan
- Renal biopsy
- BUN, serum creatinine, and creatinine clearance levels
- Serum electrolytes
- Lipid profile
- Urinalysis
- Protein-to-creatinine ratio in first morning voided specimen
- Hematocrit and hemoglobin levels

**Management**

- Correction of extracellular fluid volume overload or deficit
- Renal replacement therapy (dialysis, kidney transplant)
- Nutritional therapy (Tables 46-10 and 46-11)
- Measures to lower potassium (Table 46-5)

***Drug Therapy***

- Calcium supplementation, phosphate binders, or both
- Antihypertensive therapy
- Angiotensin-converting enzyme (ACE) inhibitors or angiotensin receptor blockers (ARBs)
- Erythropoietin therapy
- Lipid-lowering drugs
- Adjustment of drug dosages to degree of renal function

## TABLE 46-8 Indicators of Kidney Function

*This example shows why serum creatinine alone is a poor indicator of kidney function. Calculation of GFR is considered the best index to estimate kidney function as indicated by the following example.*

| | TYPE OF PATIENT | |
|---|---|---|
| **Estimation of GFR** | **76-Yr-Old African American Woman (Weight 56 kg)** | **28-Yr-Old African American Man (Weight 74 kg)** |
| Serum creatinine | 1.4 mg/dL | 1.4 mg/dL |
| GFR, estimated by the Cockcroft-Gault formula* | 30.2 mL/min | 82.2 mL/min |
| GFR, estimated by MDRD equation† | 47 mL/min/1.73 m² | 64 mL/min/1.73 m² |

*Cr*, Creatinine; *GFR*, glomerular filtration rate; *MDRD*, modification of diet in renal disease.
*Cockcroft-Gault GFR = (140 – Age) × (Weight in kilograms) × (0.85 if female)/(72 × Cr).
†GFR as estimated by MDRD equation calculator can be accessed at *www.mdrd.com*.

### Drug Therapy

***Hyperkalemia.*** Multiple strategies are used to manage hyperkalemia (Table 46-5), including the restriction of high-potassium foods and drugs. Acute hyperkalemia may require treatment with IV glucose and insulin or IV 10% calcium gluconate.

Sodium polystyrene sulfonate, a cation-exchange resin, is commonly used to lower potassium levels in stage 4 CKD and can be administered on an outpatient basis. Sodium polystyrene sulfonate has an osmotic laxative action and ensures evacuation of the potassium from the bowel. Tell the patient to expect some diarrhea. Never give sodium polystyrene sulfonate to a patient with a hypoactive bowel (paralytic ileus) because fluid shifts could lead to bowel necrosis. As sodium polystyrene sulfonate exchanges sodium ions for potassium ions, observe the patient

**TABLE 46-9 Risk Factors for Chronic Kidney Disease**

| Risk Factors | Prevention and Management |
|---|---|
| Diabetes | Achieve optimal glycemic control. |
| Hypertension | Maintain BP in normal range with angiotensin-converting enzyme (ACE) inhibitors or angiotensin receptor blockers (ARBs). |
| Age >60 yr | Prevent insult or injury to kidneys. |
| Cardiovascular disease | Institute aggressive risk factor reduction. |
| Family history of CKD | Teach about increased risk and assist with appropriate screening (BP measurement, urinalysis). |
| Exposure to nephrotoxic drugs | Limit exposure and give sodium bicarbonate as treatment. |
| Ethnic minority (e.g., African American, Native American) | Teach about increased risk and assist with appropriate screening (BP measurement, urinalysis). |

for sodium and water retention. If changes appear in the ECG such as peaked T waves and widened QRS complexes, dialysis may be required to remove excess potassium.

Patiromer (Veltassa) is an oral suspension that binds potassium in the GI tract and is used to treat hyperkalemia in individuals with CKD. It should not be used in emergency situations to treat hyperkalemia because of its delayed onset of action. Because this drug can also bind other oral medications, it needs to be given at least 6 hours before or 6 hours after other oral medications.

***Hypertension.*** For some, the progression of CKD can be delayed by controlling hypertension. (Control and treatment of hypertension are discussed in Chapter 32.) Treatment of hypertension includes (1) weight loss (if indicated), (2) therapeutic lifestyle changes (e.g., exercise, avoidance of alcohol, smoking cessation), (3) diet recommendations (DASH Diet), and (4) administration of antihypertensive drugs. Most patients require two or more drugs to reach target BP.

Prescribed medications depend on whether the patient with CKD has diabetes. The ACE inhibitors and ARBs are used with patients with diabetes and those with nondiabetic proteinuria because they decrease proteinuria and possibly delay the progression of CKD. These medications must be used with caution as they can further decrease the GFR and increase serum potassium levels.

Measure the BP with the patient in the supine, sitting, and standing positions to monitor the effect of antihypertensive drugs. Teach the patient and caregiver how to monitor the BP at home and what readings require immediate intervention.

***CKD-MBD.*** It is difficult to determine what type of bone disease a patient may have by just looking at the serum levels of calcium, phosphorus, PTH, and alkaline phosphatase. The gold standard for diagnosis is a bone biopsy.

Interventions for CKD-MBD include limiting dietary phosphorus, administering phosphate binders, supplementing vitamin D, and controlling hyperparathyroidism.[19] Phosphate intake is not usually restricted until the patient requires RRT. At that time, phosphate is usually limited to about 1 g/day, but dietary control alone is usually inadequate.

Phosphate binders include calcium-based binders: calcium acetate and calcium carbonate. They bind phosphate in the bowel and then are excreted in the stool. The administration of calcium may increase the calcium load and place the patient at increased risk for vascular calcifications. Therefore when calcium levels are increased or there is evidence of existing vascular or soft tissue calcifications, non–calcium-based phosphate binders may be used. These include lanthanum carbonate (Fosrenol), sevelamer carbonate (Renvela), and iron-based, calcium-free phosphate binders such as sucroferric oxyhydroxide (Velphoro) and ferric citrate (Auryxia).

To be most effective, administer phosphate binders with each meal. Constipation is a frequent side effect of phosphate binders, and stool softeners may be needed.

Because bone disease (osteomalacia) is associated with excess aluminum, aluminum preparations should be used with caution in patients with kidney disease. Do not use magnesium-containing antacids (e.g., Maalox, Mylanta) because magnesium depends on the kidneys for excretion.

Hypocalcemia is a problem in the later stages of CKD because of the inability of the GI tract to absorb calcium in the absence of active vitamin D. If hypocalcemia persists even if the serum phosphate levels are normal, then supplemental calcium and vitamin D should be given. Assess vitamin D levels to determine the need for supplementation. If the levels are low (serum values less than 30 ng/mL), vitamin D supplementation is recommended in the form of cholecalciferol.

Treatment of secondary hyperparathyroidism in ESRD patients requires the activated form of vitamin D because the kidneys no longer possess the ability to activate vitamin D. Active vitamin D is available as oral or IV calcitriol (Rocaltrol), IV paricalcitol (Zemplar), or oral or IV doxercalciferol (Hectorol), and can reduce the elevated levels of PTH. Cinacalcet (Sensipar), a calcimimetic agent, is used to control secondary hyperparathyroidism. Calcimimetics mimic calcium and increase the sensitivity of the calcium receptors in the parathyroid glands. As a result, the parathyroid glands detect calcium at lower serum levels and decrease PTH secretion.

If hyperparathyroid disease becomes severe despite medical management, a subtotal or total parathyroidectomy may be performed to decrease the synthesis and secretion of PTH. In most cases, a total parathyroidectomy is performed and parathyroid tissue is transplanted into the forearm. The transplanted cells produce PTH as needed. If production of PTH becomes excessive, some of the cells can be removed from the forearm.

Hypercalcemia may occur with calcium and vitamin D supplementation. If hypercalcemia occurs, vitamin D may be withheld and calcium-based phosphate binders replaced with noncalcium-based phosphate binders.

***Anemia.*** Anemia in CKD is caused by a decreased production of erythropoietin by the kidneys. Exogenous erythropoietin (EPO) is used to treat anemia. It is available as epoetin alfa (Epogen, Procrit), which can be administered IV or subcutaneously, usually two or three times per week. Darbepoetin alfa (Aranesp) is longer acting and can be administered weekly or biweekly.

Hemoglobin and hematocrit levels may take 2 to 3 weeks to increase. Higher hemoglobin levels (more than 12 g/dL) and higher doses of EPO are associated with a higher rate of thromboembolic events and increased risk of death from serious CV events (heart attack, HF, stroke). The recommendation is to use the lowest possible dose of EPO to treat anemia.

Treatment of CKD-related anemia should be individualized with the goal being to reduce the need for blood transfusions.

There is no target hemoglobin or widely accepted EPO dosing strategy. Teach people who are prescribed EPO about the risks and benefits and allow them to make a decision regarding their treatment plan.

EPO can increase BP and is contraindicated in uncontrolled hypertension. The underlying mechanism is related to the hemodynamic changes (e.g., increased whole blood viscosity) that occurs as the anemia is corrected.

EPO therapy may lead to the development of iron deficiency from the increased demand for iron to support erythropoiesis. Iron supplementation is recommended if the plasma ferritin concentrations fall below 100 ng/mL. Most CKD patients receive iron supplementation.

Although iron can be administered by mouth or IV, the enteral route is limited due to GI side effects, which decrease patient adherence. Oral iron should not be taken at the same time as phosphate binders because calcium binds the iron, preventing its absorption. Tell the patient that iron may make the stool dark in color. Most patients receiving HD are prescribed IV iron sucrose injection (Venofer) or sodium ferric gluconate complex in sucrose injection (Ferrlecit). Supplemental folic acid (1 mg/day) is usually given because it is needed for RBC formation and is removed by dialysis.

Blood transfusions should be avoided in treating anemia unless the patient experiences an acute blood loss or has symptomatic anemia (i.e., dyspnea, excess fatigue, tachycardia, palpitations, chest pain). Transfusions increase the development of antibodies, thus making it more difficult to find a compatible donor for kidney transplantation. Multiple blood transfusions may lead to iron overload because each unit of blood contains about 250 mg of iron.

***Dyslipidemia.*** Dyslipidemia, a risk factor for CV disease, is a common problem in CKD. Statins (HMG-CoA reductase inhibitors), such as atorvastatin (Lipitor), are used to lower LDL cholesterol levels (see Table 33-5). Statins should be used in patients with CKD (especially patients with diabetes) not yet on dialysis.

Fibrates (fibric acid derivatives), such as gemfibrozil (Lopid), are used to lower triglyceride levels (see Table 33-5) and can also increase HDLs. Specific drugs used in these classes depend on the individual patient response and HCP recommendation.

***Complications of Drug Therapy.*** Many drugs are partially or totally excreted by the kidneys. CKD causes decreased elimination that leads to an accumulation of drugs and the potential for drug toxicity. Drug doses and frequency of administration are adjusted based on the severity of the kidney disease. Increased sensitivity may result as drug levels increase in the blood and tissues. Drugs of particular concern include digoxin, diabetic agents (metformin, glyburide), antibiotics (e.g., vancomycin, gentamicin), and opioid medications.

### Nutritional Therapy

***Protein Restriction.*** The current diet for the individual with CKD is designed to maintain good nutrition (Table 46-10). Calorie-protein malnutrition is a potential and serious problem that results from altered metabolism, anemia, proteinuria, anorexia, and nausea. Additional factors leading to malnutrition include depression and complex diets that restrict protein, phosphorus, potassium, and sodium. Frequent monitoring of laboratory parameters, especially serum albumin, prealbumin (may be a better indicator of recent or current nutritional status than albumin), and ferritin, and anthropometric measurements are necessary to evaluate nutritional status. All patients with CKD should be referred to a dietitian for nutritional teaching.

For the patient who is undergoing dialysis, protein is not routinely restricted (Table 46-10). For CKD stages 1 through 4, many HCPs encourage a diet with normal protein intake. Teach patients to avoid high-protein diets and supplements because they may overburden the diseased kidneys.[23]

Dietary protein guidelines for PD differ from those for HD because of protein loss through the peritoneal membrane. During PD, protein intake must be high enough to compensate for the losses so that the nitrogen balance is maintained. The recommended protein intake is at least 1.2 g/kg of ideal body weight (IBW) per day. This can be increased depending on the patient's individual needs.

For patients with malnutrition or inadequate caloric or protein intake, commercially prepared products that are high in protein but low in sodium and potassium are available (e.g., Nepro, Amin-Aid). As an alternative, liquid or powder breakfast drinks may be purchased at the grocery store.

***Fluid Restriction.*** Water and any other fluids are not routinely restricted in patients with CKD stages 1 to 5 who are not receiving HD. In an effort to reduce fluid retention, diuretics are often used. Patients on HD have a more restricted fluid intake than patients receiving PD. For those receiving HD, as their urine output diminishes, fluids are restricted. Recommended fluid intake depends on the daily urine output. Generally, 600 mL (from insensible loss) plus an amount equal to the

**TABLE 46-10 Nutritional Therapy**

***Chronic Kidney Disease****

| | Pre-ESRD | Hemodialysis | Peritoneal Dialysis |
|---|---|---|---|
| **Fluid allowance** | As desired or depends on urine output | Urine output plus 600-1000 mL | Unrestricted if weight and BP controlled and residual renal function |
| **Calories** | 30-35 kcal/kg/day | 30-35 kcal/kg/day | 25-35 kcal/kg/day (includes calories from dialysate glucose absorption) |
| **Protein** | Individualized or 0.6-1.0 g/kg/day (low protein) | 1.2 g/kg/day | 1.2-1.3 g/kg/day |
| **Sodium** | Individualized or 1-3 g/day | Individualized or 2-3 g/day | Individualized or 2-4 g/day |
| **Potassium** | Individualized based on laboratory values | Individualized or about 2-4 g/day | Usually not restricted |
| **Phosphorus** | Individualized or 1.0-1.8 g/day | Individualized or about 0.6-1.2 g/day | Individualized or about 0.6-1.2 g/day |
| **Calcium** | About 1000-1500 mg/day | Individualized | Individualized |
| **Iron** | Supplement recommended if receiving erythropoietin | Supplement recommended if receiving erythropoietin | Supplement recommended if receiving erythropoietin |

*Diets must be individualized in accordance with needs.

### TABLE 46-11 Nutritional Therapy

***High-Potassium Foods****

| Fruits | Vegetables | Other Foods |
|---|---|---|
| • Apricot, raw (medium)<br>• Avocado (¼ whole)<br>• Banana (¼ whole)<br>• Cantaloupe<br>• Dried fruits<br>• Grapefruit juice<br>• Honeydew<br>• Orange (medium)<br>• Orange juice<br>• Prunes<br>• Raisins | • Baked beans<br>• Butternut squash<br>• Refried beans<br>• Black beans<br>• Broccoli, cooked<br>• Carrots, raw<br>• Greens, except kale<br>• Mushrooms, canned<br>• Potatoes, white and sweet<br>• Spinach, cooked<br>• Tomatoes or tomato products<br>• Vegetable juices | • Bran or bran products<br>• Chocolate (1.5-2 oz)<br>• Granola<br>• Milk, all types (1 cup)<br>• Nutritional supplements (use only under the direction of physician or dietitian)<br>• Nuts and seeds (1 oz)<br>• Peanut butter (2 Tbsp)<br>• Salt substitutes, Lite Salt<br>• Salt-free broth<br>• Yogurt |

*Contain at least 200 mg/portion. Portion = ½ cup unless otherwise noted.
Source: National Kidney Foundation: Potassium and your CKD diet. *www.kidney.org/atoz/content/potassium.cfm.*

previous day's urine output is allowed for a patient receiving HD.

Foods that are liquid at room temperature (e.g., gelatin, ice) should be counted as fluid intake. The fluid allotment should be spaced throughout the day so that the patient does not become thirsty. Patients are advised to limit fluid intake so that weight gains are no more than 1 to 3 kg between dialyses *(interdialytic weight gain).*

***Sodium and Potassium Restriction.*** Patients with CKD are advised to restrict sodium. Sodium-restricted diets may vary from 2 to 4 g/day. Instruct the patient to avoid high-sodium foods, such as cured meats, pickled foods, canned soups and stews, frankfurters, cold cuts, soy sauce, and salad dressings (see Chapter 34, Table 34-8). Potassium restriction depends on the kidneys' ability to excrete potassium. Salt substitutes should be avoided in potassium-restricted diets because they contain potassium chloride.

Dietary restrictions for potassium range from about 2 to 3 g (39 mg = 1 mEq). Teach patients receiving HD which foods are high in potassium and to avoid them (Table 46-11). Patients using PD do not usually need potassium restrictions and may even be prescribed oral potassium supplementation because of the loss of potassium with dialysis exchanges.

***Phosphate Restriction.*** As kidney function deteriorates, phosphate elimination by the kidneys is diminished and the patient begins to develop hyperphosphatemia. By the time a patient reaches ESRD, phosphate is limited to approximately 1 g/day. Foods that are high in phosphate include meat, dairy products (e.g., milk, ice cream, cheese, yogurt), and foods containing dairy products (e.g., pudding). Many foods that are high in phosphate are also high in protein. Since patients on dialysis are encouraged to eat a diet containing protein, phosphate binders are essential to control the phosphate level.

## NURSING MANAGEMENT: CHRONIC KIDNEY DISEASE

### Nursing Assessment

Obtain a complete history of any existing kidney disease or family history of kidney disease. Some kidney disorders, including Alport syndrome and polycystic kidney disease, have a genetic component. Other disorders that can lead to CKD are diabetes mellitus, hypertension, and systemic lupus erythematosus.

Because many drugs are potentially nephrotoxic, ask the patient about both current and past use of prescription and over-the-counter drugs and herbal preparations. Decongestants and antihistamines that contain pseudoephedrine and phenylephrine cause vasoconstriction and lead to an increase in BP. Magnesium and aluminum from antacids can accumulate in the body because they cannot be excreted. Some antacids contain high levels of salt, contributing to hypertension. In addition, antacids may interfere with the absorption of other medications.

NSAIDs (aspirin, ibuprofen, naproxen) can contribute to the development of AKI and progression of CKD, especially when taken in higher doses than recommended. If taken as prescribed, these analgesics are usually considered safe.

Assess the patient's dietary habits and discuss any problems regarding intake. Measure the patient's height and weight, and evaluate any recent weight changes.

The chronicity of kidney disease and the long-term treatment affect virtually every area of a person's life, including family relationships, social and work activities, self-image, and emotional state. Assess the patient's support systems. The choice of treatment modality may be related to support systems available.

### Nursing Diagnoses

Nursing diagnoses for CKD may include, but are not limited to, the following:

- Excess fluid volume *related to* impaired kidney function
- Risk for electrolyte imbalance *related to* impaired kidney function resulting in hyperkalemia, hypocalcemia, hyperphosphatemia, and altered vitamin D metabolism
- Imbalanced nutrition: less than body requirements *related to* restricted intake of nutrients (especially protein), nausea, vomiting, anorexia, and stomatitis

Additional information on nursing diagnoses for the patient with CKD is presented in eNursing Care Plan 46-1 (available on the website for this chapter).

### Planning

The overall goals are that a patient with CKD will (1) demonstrate knowledge of and ability to comply with the therapeutic regimen, (2) participate in decision making for the plan of care and future treatment modality, (3) demonstrate effective coping strategies, and (4) continue with activities of daily living within physiologic limitations.

### Nursing Implementation

**Health Promotion.** Identify individuals at risk for CKD. At-risk individuals include those diagnosed with diabetes or hypertension and people with a history (or a family history) of kidney disease or repeated urinary tract infections. These individuals should have regular checkups that include a routine urinalysis and calculation of the estimated GFR.

People with diabetes need to have their urine checked for albuminuria if routine urinalysis is negative for protein. Advise patients with diabetes to report any changes in urine appearance (color, odor), frequency, or volume to the HCP. If a patient needs a potentially nephrotoxic drug, it is important to monitor kidney function with serum creatinine and BUN and GFR.

## HEALTHY PEOPLE

### *Prevention and Detection of Chronic Kidney Disease*

- Early detection and treatment are the primary methods for reducing chronic kidney disease.
- Monitor BP to detect elevations so that treatment can be started early.
- Treat hypertension appropriately and aggressively, since it is the second leading cause of chronic kidney disease.
- Ensure proper diagnosis and treatment of diabetes mellitus, since it is the leading cause of chronic kidney disease.

Individuals identified at risk must take measures to prevent or delay the progression of CKD. Most important are measures to reduce the risk or progression of CV disease. These include glycemic control for patients with diabetes (see Chapter 48); BP control (see Chapter 32); and lifestyle modifications, including smoking cessation.

◆ **Acute Care.** Most of the care of the patient with CKD occurs on an outpatient basis. In-hospital care is required for management of complications and for kidney transplantation (if applicable).

◆ **Ambulatory Care.** Encourage patients to participate in their care. Teach the patient and caregiver about the diet, drugs, and follow-up medical care (Table 46-12). The patient needs to understand the drugs and common side effects. Because patients with CKD take many medications, a pillbox organizer or a list of the drugs and the times of administration may be helpful. Instruct the patient to avoid over-the-counter medications such as NSAIDs and aluminum- and magnesium-based laxatives and antacids. Teach the patient to take daily BP readings and identify signs and symptoms of fluid overload, hyperkalemia, and other electrolyte imbalances.

### TABLE 46-12 Patient & Caregiver Teaching

### *Chronic Kidney Disease*

*Include the following information in the teaching plan for the patient and caregiver.*

1. Dietary (protein, sodium, potassium, phosphate) and fluid restrictions.
2. Difficulties in modifying diet and fluid intake.
3. Signs and symptoms of electrolyte imbalance, especially high potassium.
4. Alternative ways of reducing thirst, such as sucking on ice cubes, lemon, or hard candy.
5. Rationales for prescribed drugs and common side effects. *Examples:*
   - Phosphate binders (including calcium supplements used as phosphate barriers) should be taken with meals.
   - Calcium supplements prescribed to treat hypocalcemia should be taken on an empty stomach (but not at the same time as iron supplements).
   - Iron supplements should be taken between meals.
6. The importance of reporting any of the following:
   - Weight gain >4 lb (2 kg)
   - Increasing BP
   - Shortness of breath
   - Edema
   - Increasing fatigue or weakness
   - Confusion or lethargy
7. Need for support and encouragement. Share concerns about lifestyle changes, living with a chronic illness, and decisions about type of dialysis or transplantation.

The dietitian should meet with the patient and caregiver on a regular basis for diet planning. A diet history and consideration of cultural variations facilitate diet planning and adherence. The rate of progression of CKD is dependent on the type of kidney disease and presence of other co-morbid conditions. Specific nursing management of the patient with CKD is presented in eNursing Care Plan 46-1.

The patient can complete an evaluation for a kidney transplant prior to the need to initiate dialysis. Patients may receive a transplant before ever having to start dialysis. Even though transplantation offers the best therapeutic management for many ESRD patients, the critical shortage of donor organs limits this treatment option for many patients.

Most patients require either peritoneal dialysis (PD) or hemodialysis (HD). The majority of patients use HD as a modality. Explain to the patient and caregiver what is involved in PD or HD and home hemodialysis modalities, transplantation, and even the option for palliative care. Offer information about all treatment options so that the patient can be involved in the decision-making process, providing a sense of control over life-altering decisions. Inform the patient that even while on dialysis, transplant remains an option. Let the patient know that if a transplanted organ fails, the patient can return to dialysis.

It is important to respect the patient's choice to not receive treatment. Patients themselves often initiate the conversation about palliative care. Focus the discussion on moving from the curative approach to promotion of comfort care and consideration of hospice care. Listen to the patient and caregiver, allowing them to do most of the talking and pay special attention to their hopes and fears. (Palliative and end-of-life care is discussed in Chapter 9.)

### ◆ Evaluation

The expected outcomes are that the patient with CKD will maintain

- Fluid and electrolyte levels within normal ranges
- An acceptable weight with no more than a 10% weight loss

Additional information on expected outcomes is presented in eNursing Care Plan 46-1 (available on the website).

## DIALYSIS

**Dialysis** is the movement of fluid and molecules across a semipermeable membrane from one compartment to another. Clinically, dialysis is a technique in which substances move from the blood through a semipermeable membrane and into a dialysis solution *(dialysate)*. It is used to correct fluid and electrolyte imbalances and to remove waste products in kidney failure. It can also be used to treat drug overdoses.

The two methods of dialysis available are **peritoneal dialysis (PD)** and **hemodialysis (HD)** (Table 46-13). In PD the peritoneal membrane acts as the semipermeable membrane. In HD an artificial membrane (usually made of cellulose-based or synthetic materials) is used as the semipermeable membrane and is in contact with the patient's blood.

Dialysis is begun when the patient's uremia can no longer be adequately treated with conservative medical management. Generally dialysis is initiated when the GFR is less than 15 mL/min/1.73 $m^2$. This criterion can vary widely in different clinical situations, and the nephrologist determines when to start dialysis based on the patient's clinical status. Certain uremic

**TABLE 46-13 Comparison of Peritoneal Dialysis and Hemodialysis**

| Advantages | Disadvantages |
|---|---|
| **Peritoneal Dialysis (PD)** | |
| • Immediate initiation in almost any hospital<br>• Less complicated than hemodialysis<br>• Portable system with CAPD<br>• Fewer dietary restrictions<br>• Relatively short training time<br>• Usable in patient with vascular access problems<br>• Less cardiovascular stress<br>• Home dialysis possible<br>• Preferable for patient with diabetes | • Bacterial or chemical peritonitis<br>• Protein loss into dialysate<br>• Exit site and tunnel infections<br>• Self-image problems with catheter placement<br>• Hyperglycemia<br>• Surgery for catheter placement<br>• Contraindicated in patient with multiple abdominal surgeries, trauma, unrepaired hernia<br>• Requires completion of education program<br>• Catheter can migrate<br>• Best instituted with willing partner |
| **Hemodialysis (HD)** | |
| • Rapid fluid removal<br>• Rapid removal of urea and creatinine<br>• Effective potassium removal<br>• Less protein loss<br>• Lowering of serum triglycerides<br>• Home dialysis possible<br>• Temporary access can be placed at bedside | • Vascular access problems<br>• Dietary and fluid restrictions<br>• Heparinization may be necessary<br>• Extensive equipment necessary<br>• Hypotension during dialysis<br>• Added blood loss that contributes to anemia<br>• Specially trained personnel necessary<br>• Surgery for permanent access placement<br>• Self-image problems with permanent access |

*CAPD,* Continuous ambulatory peritoneal dialysis.

complications, including encephalopathy, neuropathies, uncontrolled hyperkalemia, pericarditis, and accelerated hypertension, indicate a need for immediate dialysis.

Most patients with ESRD are treated with dialysis because (1) there is a lack of donated organs, (2) some patients are physically or mentally unsuitable for transplantation, or (3) some patients do not want transplants. An increasing number of individuals, including older adults and those with complex medical problems, are receiving maintenance dialysis. A patient's chronologic age is not a factor in determining candidacy for dialysis.

### General Principles of Dialysis

Solutes and water move across the semipermeable membrane from the blood to the dialysate or from the dialysate to the blood in accordance with concentration gradients. The principles of diffusion, osmosis, and ultrafiltration are involved in dialysis (Fig. 46-4). *Diffusion* is the movement of solutes from an area of greater concentration to an area of lesser concentration. In kidney failure, urea, creatinine, uric acid, and electrolytes (potassium, phosphate) move from the blood to the dialysate with the net effect of lowering their concentration in the blood. RBCs, WBCs, and plasma proteins are too large to diffuse through the pores of the membrane. Small-molecular-weight substances can pass from the dialysate into a patient's blood, so the purity of the water used for dialysis is monitored and controlled.

*Osmosis* is the movement of fluid from an area of lesser concentration to an area of greater concentration of solutes.

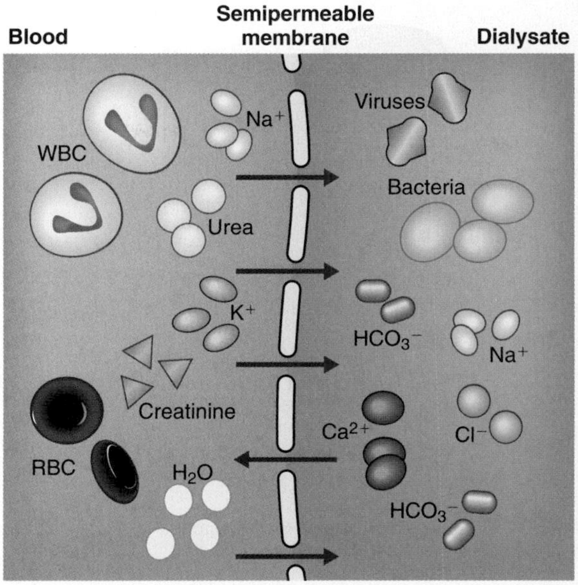


**FIG. 46-4** Osmosis and diffusion across a semipermeable membrane.

Glucose is added to the dialysate and creates an osmotic gradient across the membrane, pulling excess fluid from the blood.

*Ultrafiltration* (water and fluid removal) results when there is an osmotic gradient or pressure gradient across the membrane. In PD, excess fluid is removed by increasing the osmolality of the dialysate (osmotic gradient) with the addition of glucose. In HD, the gradient is created by increasing pressure in the blood compartment (positive pressure) or decreasing pressure in the dialysate compartment (negative pressure). Extracellular fluid moves into the dialysate because of the pressure gradient. The excess fluid is removed by creating a pressure differential between the blood and the dialysate solution with a combination of positive pressure in the blood compartment or negative pressure in the dialysate compartment.

## PERITONEAL DIALYSIS

Although PD was first used in 1923, it did not come into widespread use for chronic treatment until the 1970s with the development of soft, pliable peritoneal solution bags and the introduction of the concept of continuous PD. In the United States, approximately 12% of patients receiving dialysis treatments are on PD.

### Catheter Placement

Peritoneal access is obtained by inserting a catheter through the anterior abdominal wall (Fig. 46-5). The catheter is about 24 inches (60 cm) long and has one or two Dacron cuffs. The cuffs act as anchors and prevent the migration of microorganisms into the peritoneum. Within a few weeks, fibrous tissue grows into the Dacron cuff, holding the catheter in place and preventing bacterial penetration into the peritoneal cavity. The tip of the catheter rests in the peritoneal cavity and has many perforations spaced along the distal end of the tubing, allowing fluid movement through the catheter.

The technique for catheter placement varies. It is usually placed surgically so that the catheter can be directly visualized, minimizing potential complications. Preparation of the patient for catheter insertion includes emptying the bladder and bowel, weighing the patient, and obtaining a signed consent form.

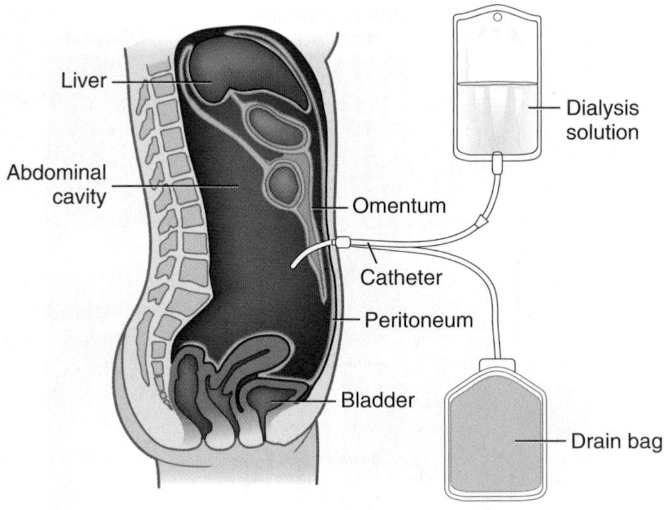


**FIG. 46-5** Peritoneal dialysis showing peritoneal catheter inserted into peritoneal cavity.

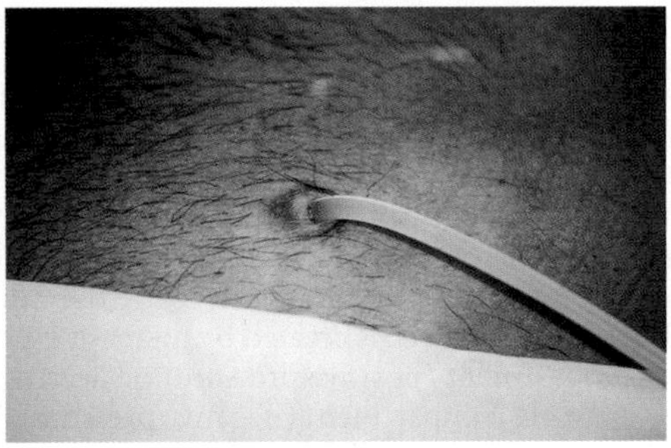

**FIG. 46-6** Peritoneal catheter exit site. (Courtesy Mary Jo Holechek, Baltimore, Md.)

After placement, PD may be initiated immediately with low volume exchanges, or delayed for 2 weeks pending healing and sealing of the exit site. Once the catheter incision site is healed, the patient may shower and then pat the catheter and exit site dry.[24] Daily catheter care varies. Some patients just wash with soap and water and go without a dressing (Fig. 46-6), whereas others require daily dressing changes. Teach all patients to examine their catheter site for signs of infection. Showering is preferred to bathing.

## Dialysis Solutions and Cycles

PD is accomplished by putting dialysis solution into the peritoneal space. The three phases of the PD cycle are inflow (fill), dwell (equilibration), and drain. The three phases are called an *exchange.* For manual PD, a period of about 30 to 50 minutes is required to complete an exchange. During *inflow,* a prescribed amount of solution, usually 2 L, is infused through an established catheter over about 10 minutes. The flow rate may be decreased if the patient has pain. After the solution has been infused, the inflow clamp is closed.

The next part of the cycle is the *dwell* phase, or equilibration, during which diffusion and osmosis occur between the patient's blood and peritoneal cavity. The duration of the dwell time can be brief lasting 20 or 30 minutes or up to 8 or more hours, depending on the method of PD.

*Drain* time takes 15 to 30 minutes and may be facilitated by gently massaging the abdomen or changing position. The cycle starts again with the infusion of another 2 L of solution.

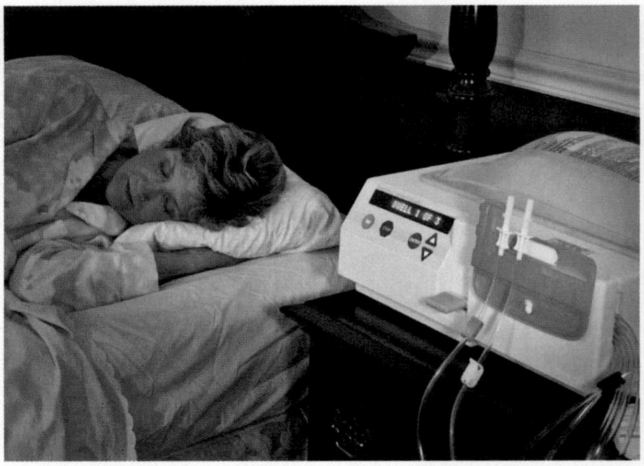

**FIG. 46-7** Automated peritoneal dialysis that can be used while the patient is sleeping.

Dialysis solutions vary, and the choice of the exchange volume is primarily determined by the size of the peritoneal cavity. A larger person may require a 3-L exchange volume without any difficulty, whereas an average-size person typically uses a 2-L exchange. Smaller exchange volumes are used for patients with a smaller body, pulmonary compromise (the added pressure of the large volume may precipitate respiratory difficulty), or inguinal hernias.

*Ultrafiltration* (fluid removal) during PD depends on osmotic forces, with dextrose being the most commonly used osmotic agent in PD solutions. It is relatively safe and inexpensive but is associated with high rates of peritoneal glucose absorption leading to problems with hypertriglyceridemia, hyperglycemia, and long-term peritoneal membrane dysfunction.

Alternatives to dextrose PD solution include icodextrin and amino acid solutions. Icodextrin is a commercially available iso-osmolar preparation and induces ultrafiltration by its oncotic effect. Amino acid PD solutions are also available and used primarily for patients requiring nutritional supplementation.

## Peritoneal Dialysis Systems

**Automated Peritoneal Dialysis.** Automated peritoneal dialysis (APD) is the most popular form of PD because it allows patients to do dialysis while they sleep. An automated device called a *cycler* is used to deliver the dialysate for APD (Fig. 46-7). The size of a cycler is similar to a DVD player. The automated cycler times and controls the fill, dwell, and drain phases. The machine cycles four or more exchanges per night with 1 to 2 hours per exchange. Alarms and monitors are built into the system to make it safe for the patient to sleep while dialyzing. The patient disconnects from the machine in the morning and usually leaves fluid in the abdomen during the day.

It is difficult to achieve the required solute and fluid clearance solely with nighttime APD. One or two daytime manual exchanges may be prescribed to ensure adequate dialysis.

**Continuous Ambulatory Peritoneal Dialysis.** Continuous ambulatory peritoneal dialysis (CAPD) is performed every few hours during the day. The patient may perform an exchange of 2 L of peritoneal dialysate four times daily, with dwell times averaging 4 hours. A common schedule includes exchanges at 7 AM, 12 noon, 5 PM, and 10 PM. In this procedure, the person instills 2 to 3 L of dialysate from a plastic bag into the peritoneal cavity through a disposable administration line.

In CAPD the bag and line can be disconnected after the instillation of the fluid. After the equilibration period, the line is reconnected to the catheter, the dialysate (effluent) is drained from the peritoneal cavity, and a new 2- to 3-L bag of dialysate solution is infused. In PD it is critical to maintain aseptic technique to avoid peritonitis. Several tubing connections and devices are commercially available to help in maintaining an aseptic system.

### Complications of Peritoneal Dialysis

**Exit Site Infection.** Infection of the peritoneal catheter exit site is most commonly caused by *Staphylococcus aureus* or *Staphylococcus epidermidis* (from skin flora). Clinical manifestations of an exit site infection include redness at the site, tenderness, and drainage. Superficial exit site infections caused by these organisms are generally resolved with antibiotic therapy. If not treated immediately, subcutaneous tunnel infections may progress and may cause peritonitis, necessitating catheter removal.

**Peritonitis.** Peritonitis results from contact contamination or an exit site or tunnel infection. Most frequently peritonitis occurs because of improper technique when connections for exchanges are contaminated. Peritonitis is usually caused by *S. aureus* or *S. epidermidis.* Peritonitis infrequently results from bacteria in the intestine crossing into the peritoneal cavity.

The primary clinical manifestations of peritonitis are abdominal pain, rebound tenderness, and cloudy peritoneal effluent with a WBC count greater than 100 cells/μL (more than 50% neutrophils) or demonstration of bacteria in the peritoneal effluent by Gram stain or culture. GI manifestations of peritonitis may include diarrhea, vomiting, abdominal distention, and hyperactive bowel sounds. Fever may or may not be present. To determine if the peritoneal effluent is cloudy, drain the effluent and place the drained bag on reading material such as a newspaper. If you cannot read the print through the effluent, it is cloudy.

Cultures, Gram stain, and a WBC differential of the peritoneal effluent are used to confirm the diagnosis of peritonitis. Antibiotics can be given orally, IV, or intraperitoneally. In most cases, the patient is treated on an outpatient basis.

The formation of adhesions in the peritoneum can result from repeated infections and interferes with the peritoneal membrane's ability to act as a dialyzing surface. Repeated infections may require the removal of the peritoneal catheter and a temporary or permanent change of modality to HD.

**Hernias.** Because of increased intraabdominal pressure secondary to the dialysate volume, hernias can develop in predisposed individuals such as multiparous women and older men. After hernia repair, PD can often be resumed after several days using small dialysate volumes and keeping the patient supine.

**Lower Back Problems.** Increased intraabdominal pressure can cause or aggravate lower back pain. The lumbosacral curvature is increased by intraperitoneal infusion of dialysate. Orthopedic binders and a regular exercise program for strengthening the back muscles have been beneficial for some patients.

**Bleeding.** After peritoneal catheter placement, it is common for the PD effluent drained after the first few exchanges to be pink or slightly bloody secondary to the trauma associated with catheter insertion. Bloody effluent over several days or the new appearance of blood in the effluent can indicate active intraperitoneal bleeding. If this occurs, check the BP and hematocrit. Blood may also be present in the effluent of women who are menstruating or ovulating, and this requires no intervention.

**Pulmonary Complications.** Atelectasis, pneumonia, and bronchitis may occur from repeated upward displacement of the diaphragm, resulting in decreased lung expansion. Longer dwell times increase the likelihood of pulmonary problems. Frequent repositioning and deep-breathing exercises can help. When the patient is lying in bed, elevate the head of the bed to prevent these problems.

**Protein Loss.** The peritoneal membrane is permeable to plasma proteins, amino acids, and polypeptides. These substances are lost in the dialysate fluid. The amount of loss is usually about 0.5 g/L of dialysate drainage, but it can be as high as 10 to 20 g/day. This loss may increase to as much as 40 g/day during episodes of peritonitis as the peritoneal membrane becomes more permeable. Unresolved peritonitis is associated with excessive protein loss that can result in malnutrition and may indicate the need to terminate PD temporarily or sometimes permanently.

### Effectiveness of Chronic Peritoneal Dialysis

Learning the self-management skills required to do PD is usually accomplished in a 3- to 7-day training program. Mortality rates are similar between in-center HD patients and PD patients for the first few years. After about 2 years, mortality rates for patients receiving PD increase, especially for the older person with diabetes and patients with a prior history of CV disease.[24]

The primary advantage of PD is its simplicity and that it is a home-based program, increasing patient participation in their care. There is no need for special water systems, and equipment setup is relatively simple.

## HEMODIALYSIS

### Vascular Access Sites

Obtaining vascular access is one of the most difficult problems associated with HD. To perform HD, a very rapid blood flow is required, and access to a large blood vessel is essential. Enough time is needed for evaluation and consideration of the best arteriovenous access for HD. The types of vascular access include arteriovenous fistulas (AVFs), arteriovenous grafts (AVGs), and temporary vascular access.[25]

**Arteriovenous Fistulas and Grafts.** A subcutaneous **arteriovenous fistula (AVF)** is usually created in the forearm or upper arm with an anastomosis between an artery and a vein (usually cephalic or basilic) (Figs. 46-8, *A,* and 46-9). The fistula allows arterial blood to flow through the vein.

The vein becomes "arterialized," increasing in size and developing thicker walls. The arterial blood flow is essential to provide the rapid blood flow required for HD. As the fistula matures, it is more amenable to repeated venipunctures. Maturation may take 6 weeks to months. AVF should be placed at least 3 months before the need to initiate HD. The fistula is the preferred access for HD.[26]

Normally, a *thrill* (buzzing sensation) can be felt by palpating the fistula, and a *bruit* (rushing sound) can be heard with a stethoscope. The thrill and bruit are created by arterial blood moving at a high velocity through the vein.

AVFs are more difficult to create in patients with a history of severe peripheral vascular disease (e.g., people with diabetes), those with prolonged IV drug use, and obese women. For these individuals, a synthetic graft may be required.

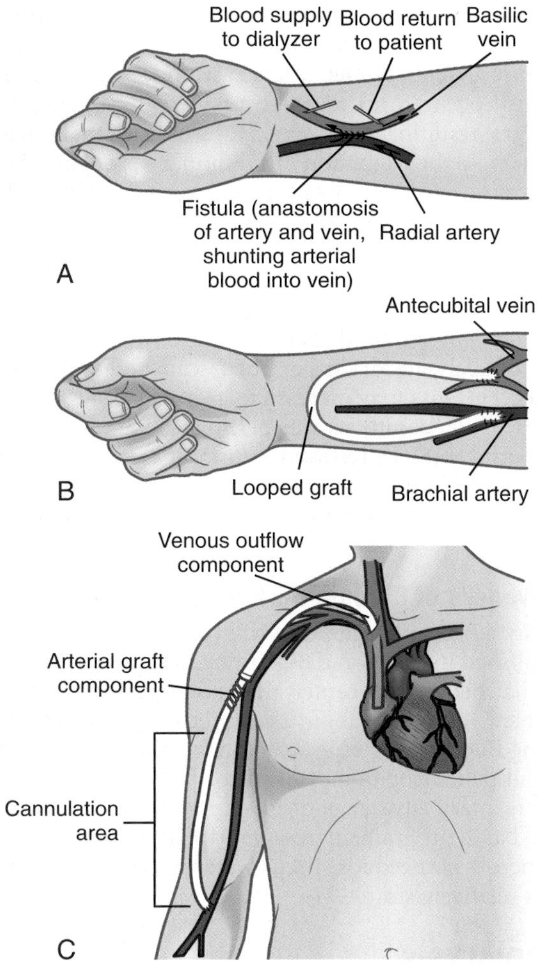


**FIG. 46-8** Vascular access for hemodialysis. **A,** Arteriovenous fistula. **B,** Arteriovenous graft. **C,** HeRO graft.

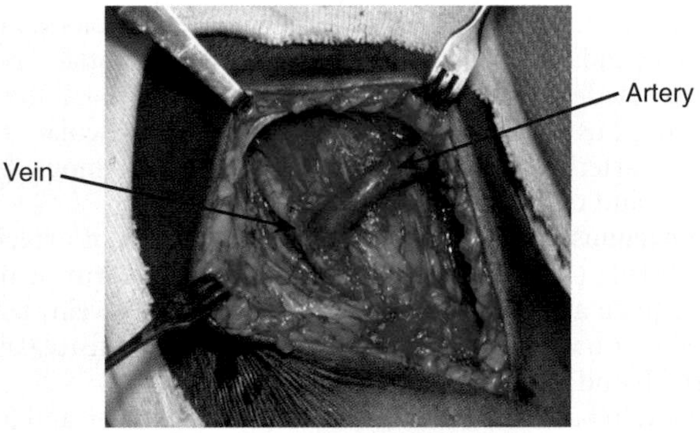


**FIG. 46-9** Arteriovenous fistula created by anastomosing an artery and a vein. (Courtesy Dr. Stephen Van Voorst, MD.)

## CHECK YOUR PRACTICE

You are rotating to the inpatient dialysis unit today. It is your first experience working with HD patients. You are helping a hemodialysis tech "hook-up" a 56-yr-old man to HD. He has been on HD for 5 years secondary to polycystic kidney disease. You take his vital signs, palpate his AV fistula, and then use your stethoscope to auscultate the AV fistula. You are very concerned because you feel a super-strong pulse and hear a very loud "whoosh" sound. The patient turns to you and just smirks, "I bet you have never had a thrill like that."

- You are very flustered and not sure how to respond. What should you say to him?

**Arteriovenous grafts (AVGs)** are made of synthetic materials (polytetrafluoroethylene [PTFE, Teflon]) and form a "bridge" between the arterial and venous blood supplies. Grafts are placed under the skin and are surgically anastomosed between an artery (usually brachial) and a vein (usually antecubital) (Fig. 46-8, *B*). An interval of 2 to 4 weeks is usually necessary to allow the graft to heal but may be used earlier. Because grafts are made of artificial materials, they are more likely than AVFs to become infected, and they also have a tendency to be thrombogenic. When AVG infections occur, they may require surgical removal, since it is difficult to completely resolve the infection from the synthetic material.

A common problem in patients on HD is central venous stenosis (CVS) or occlusion. This is a serious issue and has a greater impact than peripheral venous stenosis because the central veins are the final pathway for blood flow to the heart. As CVS progresses, vascular access for HD is frequently lost.

*HeRO graft* (Hemodialysis Reliable Outflow) is a special bridge access used in patients when other access options are exhausted. It consists of two pieces: a reinforced tube to bypass blockages in veins and a dialysis graft anastomosed to an artery to be accessed for HD (Fig. 46-8, *C*). The *HeRO graft* is placed under the skin, like both a fistula and standard graft. The HeRO Graft bypasses the venous system to provide blood flow directly from a target artery to the heart. HeRO Graft is a graft but differs from a conventional AV graft since it has no venous anastomosis. It may be more difficult to auscultate the bruit or feel the thrill in this type of access because of the absence of a venous anastomosis.

Surgical creation of an arteriovenous access for HD has several risks, including development of distal ischemia *(steal syndrome)* and pain because too much of the arterial blood is being shunted or "stolen" from the distal extremity. Classic manifestations of steal syndrome are pain distal to the access site, numbness or tingling of fingers that may worsen during dialysis, and poor capillary refill. Aneurysms can also develop in the arteriovenous access and can rupture if left untreated.

**SAFETY ALERT Arteriovenous Fistulas and Grafts**

- Never perform BP measurements, insertion of IV lines, and venipuncture in the extremity with the vascular access.
- These special precautions are taken to prevent infection and clotting of the vascular access.
- When a patient is hospitalized, hang signs in patient's room or label the arm with a band that says "No BP, blood draws, or IV in this arm."

**Temporary Vascular Access.** When immediate vascular access is required, catheterization of the internal jugular or femoral vein is performed. A flexible catheter is inserted at the bedside into one of these large veins and provides access to the circulation without surgery (Fig. 46-10). The catheters usually have a double external lumen with an internal septum separating the two internal segments. One lumen is used for blood removal and the other for blood return (Fig. 46-11, *A* and *B*). Temporary catheters have high rates of infection, dislodgment, and malfunction. A patient should not be discharged from the hospital with a temporary catheter in place.

Long-term cuffed HD catheters are often used for temporary vascular access. These catheters provide temporary access while the patient is waiting for fistula placement or as long-term access when other forms of access have failed. This type of catheter exits on the upper chest wall and is tunneled subcutaneously to the internal or external jugular vein (Fig. 46-11, *C*).

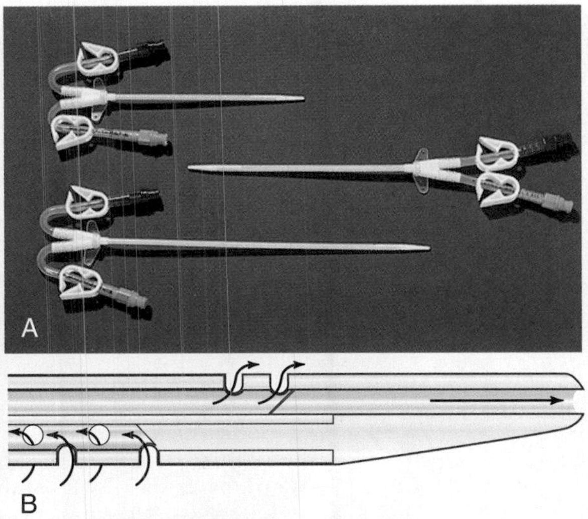


FIG. 46-10 Temporary double-lumen vascular access catheter for acute hemodialysis. **A,** Soft, flexible double-lumen tube is attached to a Y hub. **B,** The distance between the arterial intake lumen and the venous return lumen typically provides recirculation rates of 5% or less. (*A,* Courtesy Quinton Instrument Co., Seattle, Wash.)

The catheter tip rests in the right atrium. It has one or two subcutaneous Dacron cuffs that prevent infection from tracking along the catheter and anchor the catheter, thus eliminating the need for sutures.

## Dialyzers

The HD dialyzer is a plastic cartridge that contains thousands of parallel hollow tubes or fibers. The fibers are semipermeable membranes made of cellulose-based or other synthetic materials. The blood is pumped into the top of the cartridge and is dispersed into all of the fibers. Dialysis fluid *(dialysate)* is pumped into the bottom of the cartridge and bathes the outside of the fibers. Ultrafiltration, diffusion, and osmosis occur across the pores of this semipermeable membrane. When the dialyzed blood reaches the end of the thousands of semipermeable fibers, it converges into a single tube that returns it to the patient. Dialyzers differ in surface area, membrane composition and thickness, clearance of waste products, and removal of fluid.

## Procedure for Hemodialysis

The needles used for HD are large bore, usually 14 to 16 gauge, and are inserted into the fistula or graft to obtain vascular access. One needle is placed to pull blood from the circulation to the HD machine, and the other needle is used to return the dialyzed blood to the patient. The needles are attached via tubing to dialysis lines. If a patient has a catheter, the two blood lines are attached to the two catheter lumens. The needle closer to the fistula (red catheter lumen) is used to pull blood from the patient to the dialyzer using a blood pump. Blood is returned from the dialyzer to the patient through the second needle (blue catheter lumen).

When blood comes in contact with a foreign material (such as the dialyzer), it has a tendency to clot. Heparin is added to the blood to prevent clotting.

In addition to the dialyzer, a dialysate delivery and monitoring system is used (Fig. 46-12). This system pumps the dialysate through the dialyzer, countercurrent to the blood flow. To terminate the treatment, a saline solution is used to return the blood in the extracorporeal circuit back to the patient through the vascular access. The needles are removed from the patient, and firm pressure is applied to the venipuncture sites until the bleeding stops.

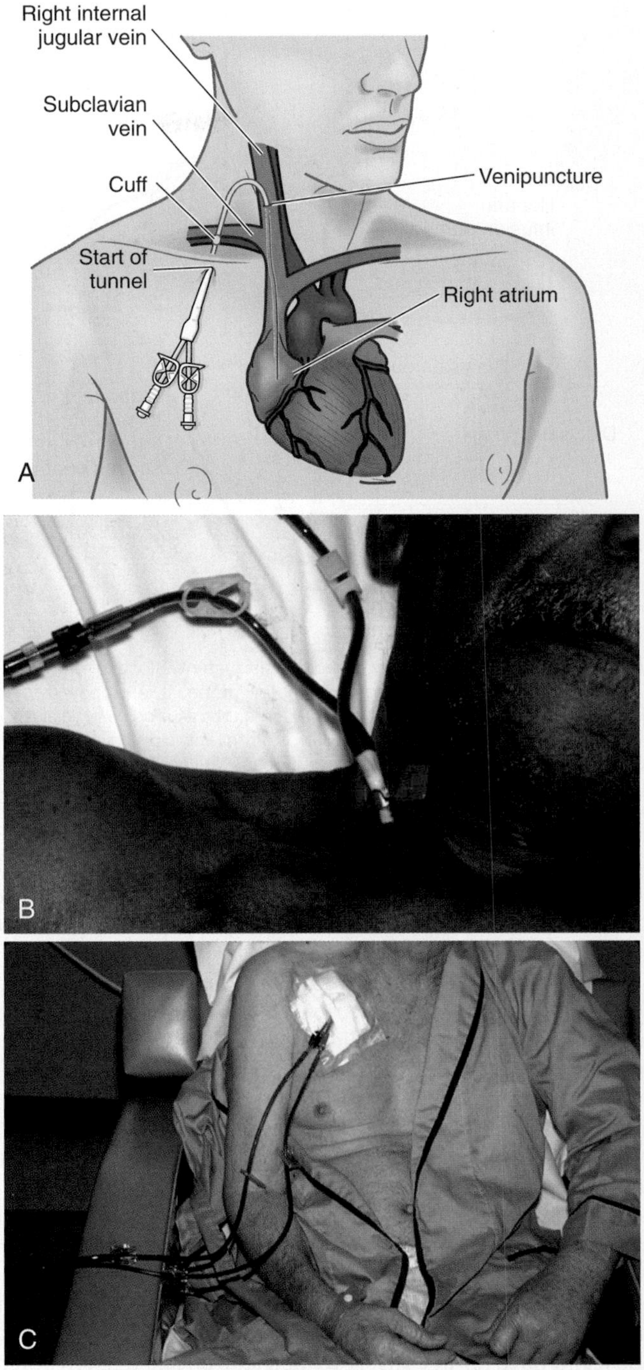


FIG. 46-11 **A,** Right internal jugular placement for a tunneled, cuffed semipermanent catheter. **B,** Temporary hemodialysis catheter in place. **C,** Long-term cuffed hemodialysis catheter. (*B* and *C,* Courtesy Dr. Stephen Van Voorst, MD.)

Before beginning treatment, assess fluid status (weight, BP, peripheral edema, lung and heart sounds), condition of vascular access, and temperature. The difference between the last post-dialysis weight and the present predialysis weight determines the ultrafiltration or the amount of weight (from fluid) to be removed. While the patient is on dialysis, take vital signs at least every 30 to 60 minutes because rapid BP changes may occur.

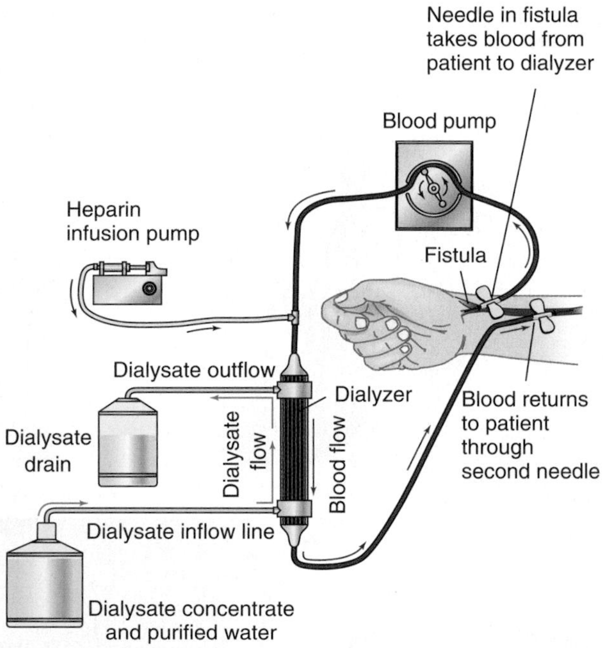


**FIG. 46-12** Components of a hemodialysis system. Blood is removed via a needle inserted in a fistula or via catheter lumen. It is propelled to the dialyzer by a blood pump. Heparin is infused either as a bolus predialysis or through a heparin pump continuously to prevent clotting. Dialysate is pumped in and flows in the opposite direction of the blood. The dialyzed blood is returned to the patient through a second needle or catheter lumen. Old dialysate and ultrafiltrate are drained and discarded.

**Settings and Schedules for Hemodialysis.** The majority of HD patients are treated in a community-based center and dialyze for 3 to 4 hours 3 days per week. Most people sleep, read, talk, or watch television during HD.

Other schedule options for HD are short daily HD and long nocturnal HD. The patient receiving long nocturnal HD has the advantage of sleeping while dialyzing. Each nocturnal treatment lasts 6 to 8 hours, and the patient dialyzes up to six times per week.

In addition to in-center HD, home HD is available (Fig. 46-13). The option for home HD often depends on a patient's family support. One of the main advantages of home HD is that it allows greater freedom in choosing dialysis times. In short daily HD, the patient dialyzes for $2\frac{1}{2}$ to 3 hours per session 5 to 6 days per week. Short daily HD is usually done at home.

Patients who choose daily dialysis or nocturnal dialysis may have fewer uremic symptoms, tend to require fewer medications, and have fewer dialysis-related side effects (e.g., hypotension, cramps). In addition, they have more autonomy. Although daily home HD offers the potential of significant health benefits, only about 2% of HD patients dialyze at home.

## Complications of Hemodialysis

**Hypotension.** Hypotension that occurs during HD primarily results from rapid removal of vascular volume (hypovolemia), decreased cardiac output, and decreased systemic vascular resistance. The drop in BP during dialysis may precipitate lightheadedness, nausea, vomiting, seizures, vision changes, and chest pain from cardiac ischemia. The usual treatment for hypotension includes decreasing the volume of fluid being removed and infusion of 0.9% saline solution.

**Muscle Cramps.** The cause of muscle cramps in HD is poorly understood. Factors associated with the development of muscle

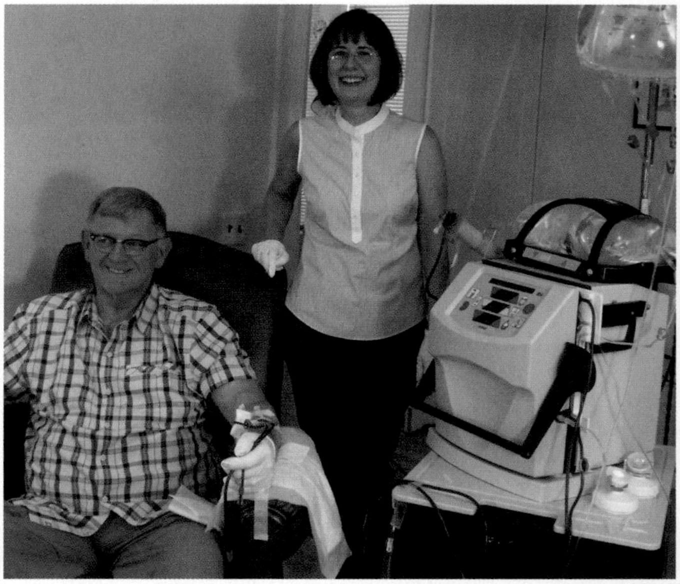

**FIG. 46-13** Home hemodialysis is growing in popularity, and machines are more compact. (From NxStage Medical, Inc, Lawrence, Mass.)

## BECOMING A NURSE LEADER

### *Leadership vs. Management*

**Situation**

Paula and Stacy, two nurses on a large dialysis unit, are discussing their dissatisfaction with their manager. Paula adamantly declares, "I never want to be a manager or a leader. I just want to be a nurse, take care of my patients, and go home at the end of my shift." Stacy responds, "All nurses need to be leaders." Paula fires back, "Not me!"

**Points for Consideration**

- Management and leadership are often lumped together. However, leadership roles are different from management responsibility.
- Both leadership and management are necessary for success in nursing today. You can be a leader without being a manager. Leadership has nothing to do with titles.
- *Leaders* create a vision of the future, communicate that vision effectively, and help team members commit to it. Leadership is an important skill for nurses at all levels.
- *Managers* are responsible for the functioning of their units, focusing on work and tasks. They must ensure there is sufficient staff that can provide safe, quality care. They maintain daily operations, stay within the unit budget, and meet strategic goals. However, the manager must also lead by exemplifying the mission, goals, and values of the organization to his or her staff, which will motivate them to strive for excellence.
- Nurse managers are expected to lead their team so that team members willingly participate, accept guidance, and carry out instruction.
- Education and training are required to be both a successful leader and manager. All too often in nursing, the best clinical nurses are promoted to managers without the benefit of formal training and mentoring.

**Discussion Questions**

1. Identify a situation in which you functioned as a leader.
2. What qualities could you develop personally and professionally to help you become a more effective nurse leader?

**Reference**

Baker J: Leadership from the trenches. Managing and leading in a competitive environment. Retrieved from *www.leadershipfromthetrenches.com/2010/02/doing-the-right-thing*.

cramps include hypotension, hypovolemia, high ultrafiltration rate (large interdialytic weight gain), and low-sodium dialysis solution. Treatment includes reducing the ultrafiltration rate and administering fluids (saline, glucose, mannitol). Hypertonic saline is not recommended since the sodium load can be problematic. Hypertonic glucose administration is preferred.

**Loss of Blood.** Blood loss may result from blood not being completely rinsed from the dialyzer, accidental separation of blood tubing, dialysis membrane rupture, or bleeding after the removal of needles at the end of HD. If a patient has received too much heparin or has clotting problems, postdialysis bleeding can occur. It is essential to rinse back all blood, avoid excess anticoagulation, and hold firm but nonocclusive pressure on access sites until the risk of bleeding has passed.

**Hepatitis.** At one time, hepatitis B had an unusually high prevalence in dialysis patients, but the incidence today is low. Lower transfusion requirements, screening, and recommendations for vaccinations have lowered the incidence. Outbreaks of hepatitis B still occur, since transmission is attributed to breaks in infection control practices. To prevent transmission, all patients and personnel in dialysis units receive hepatitis B vaccine.

Currently, hepatitis C virus (HCV) is responsible for the majority of cases of hepatitis in dialysis patients. (Hepatitis is discussed in more detail in Chapter 43.) Approximately 8% to 10% of patients undergoing dialysis in the United States are positive for anti-HCV, which indicates a previous infection. Infection control precautions are mandated in care of the patient with hepatitis C to protect the patient and staff. (Infection control precautions are discussed in Chapter 14.) Currently no vaccine is available for hepatitis C.

### Effectiveness of Hemodialysis

HD is still an imperfect therapy for management of ESRD. It cannot fully replace the normal functions of the kidneys. It can ease many of the symptoms of CKD and, if started early, can prevent certain complications. It does not alter the accelerated rate of CV disease and the related high mortality rate.

The yearly death rate of patients receiving maintenance dialysis remains high at an estimated 19% to 24%. The majority of deaths are caused by CV disease (stroke or myocardial infarction). Infectious complications are the second leading cause of death.[26]

Individual adaptation to maintenance HD varies considerably. Initially many patients feel positive about the dialysis because it makes them feel better and keeps them alive, but there is often great ambivalence about whether it is worthwhile. Dependence on a machine is a reality. In response to their illness, dialysis patients may be nonadherent or depressed and exhibit suicidal tendencies. The primary nursing goals are to (1) assist the patient to maintain a healthy self-image and (2) return the patient to the highest level of function possible, including returning to work.

## CONTINUOUS RENAL REPLACEMENT THERAPY

Continuous renal replacement therapy (CRRT) is a method for treating AKI. It provides a means by which uremic toxins and fluids are removed while acid-base status and electrolytes are adjusted slowly and continuously in a hemodynamically unstable patient. The principle of CRRT is to dialyze patients in a more physiologic way (over 24 hours), just like the kidneys. CRRT is contraindicated if a patient has life-threatening manifestations of uremia (hyperkalemia, pericarditis) that require rapid treatment. CRRT can be used in conjunction with HD.

Various types of CRRT are available (Table 46-14). CRRT most commonly uses the venovenous approaches of continuous venovenous hemofiltration (CVVH), continuous venovenous hemodialysis (CVVHD), and continuous venovenous hemodiafiltration (CVVHDF).

Vascular access for CRRT is achieved through the use of a double-lumen catheter (as used in HD [Fig. 46-10]) placed in the jugular or femoral vein. A blood pump propels the blood through the circuit. A highly permeable, hollow-fiber hemofilter removes plasma water and nonprotein solutes, which are collectively termed *ultrafiltrate*. The ultrafiltration rate (UFR) may range from 0 to 500 mL/hr. Under the influence of hydrostatic pressure and osmotic pressure, water and nonprotein solutes pass out of the filter into the extracapillary space and drain through the ultrafiltrate port into a collection device (drainage bag) (Fig. 46-14). The remaining fluid continues

**TABLE 46-14 Continuous Renal Replacement Therapies**

| Therapy | Abbreviation | Purpose |
|---|---|---|
| **Continuous venovenous hemofiltration** | CVVH | Removes both fluid and solutes. Replacement fluid required. |
| **Slow continuous ultrafiltration** | SCUF | Simplified version of CVVH. Removes fluid. No fluid replacement required. |
| **Continuous venovenous hemodialysis** | CVVHD | Removes both fluids and solutes. Requires both dialysate and replacement fluid. |
| **Continuous venovenous hemodiafiltration** | CVVHDF | Removes both fluids and solutes. Requires both dialysate and replacement fluid. |

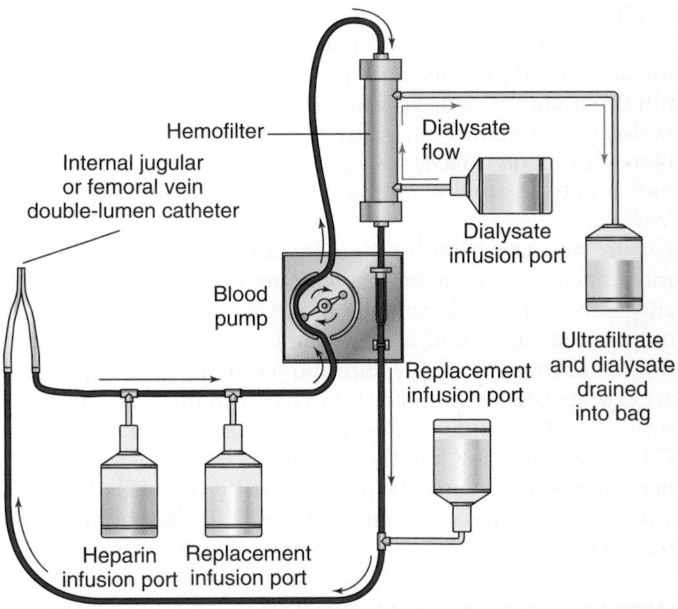


**FIG. 46-14** Basic schematic of continuous venovenous therapies. Blood pump is required to pump blood through the circuit. Replacement ports are used for instilling replacement fluids and can be given prefilter or postfilter. Dialysate port is used for infusing dialysis solution. Regardless of modality, ultrafiltrate is drained via the ultrafiltration drain port.

through the filter and returns to the patient via the return port of the double-lumen catheter.

As ultrafiltrate drains out of the hemofilter, fluid and electrolyte replacements can be infused through a port located before or after the filter as the blood returns to the patient. Replacement fluid is designed to replace volume and solutes such as sodium, chloride, bicarbonate, and glucose. The infusion rate of replacement fluid is determined by the degree of fluid and electrolyte imbalance. Replacement fluid infused into the infusion port before the hemofilter allows for greater clearance of urea and can decrease filter clotting. The use of the infusion port located after the filter dilutes intravascular fluid, decreasing the concentration of unwanted solutes such as BUN, creatinine, and potassium. Anticoagulants are needed to prevent blood clotting and may be infused as a bolus at the initiation of CRRT or through an infusion port before the hemofilter.

The type of CRRT can be customized to the patient's needs. Some types involve the introduction of replacement fluids. CVVHD and CVVHDF use dialysate. Dialysis fluid is attached to the distal end of the hemofilter, and the fluid is pumped countercurrent to the blood flow (Fig. 46-14). As in hemodialysis, diffusion of solutes and ultrafiltration via hydrostatic pressure and osmosis occur. This is an ideal treatment for a patient who needs both fluid and solute control but cannot tolerate the rapid fluid shifts associated with HD.

Several features of CRRT differ from HD:

- It is continuous rather than intermittent. Fluid volume can be removed over days (24 hours to more than 2 weeks) versus hours (3 to 4 hours).
- Solute removal can occur by *convection* (no dialysate required) in addition to osmosis and diffusion.
- It causes less hemodynamic instability (e.g., hypotension).
- It does not require constant monitoring by a specialized HD nurse but does require a trained ICU nurse.
- It does not require complicated HD equipment, but a blood pump is needed for venovenous therapies.

CRRT can be continued as long as 30 to 40 days, but the hemofilter should be changed every 24 to 48 hours because of loss of filtration efficiency or potential for clotting. The ultrafiltrate should be clear yellow. Specimens may be obtained for evaluation of serum chemistries. If the ultrafiltrate becomes bloody or blood tinged, suspect a possible rupture in the filter membrane. Treatment must be terminated to prevent blood loss.

Specific nursing interventions include obtaining weights and monitoring and documenting laboratory values daily to ensure adequate fluid and electrolyte balance. Assess hourly intake and output, vital signs, and hemodynamic status. Although reductions in central venous pressure and pulmonary artery pressure are expected, there should be little change in mean arterial pressure or cardiac output. Assess and maintain the patency of the CRRT system. Care for the patient's vascular access site to prevent infection. Once the patient's AKI is resolved or there is a decision to withdraw treatment, CRRT is discontinued and the needle(s) removed.

## WEARABLE ARTIFICIAL KIDNEY

While many improvements have been made for the care of ESRD patients, none has been able to replace a person's biologic kidneys. The wearable artificial kidney (WAK) has recently been developed and is approved for use to improve the quality of life of an ESRD patient.

The WAK is a miniaturized dialysis machine that can be worn on the body. The carrier resembles a tool belt. The device connects to a patient via a catheter. Like conventional dialysis machines, it is designed to filter the blood of ESRD patients. Unlike current portable or stationary dialysis machines, it can run continuously on batteries and is not plugged into an electrical outlet or attached to a water pipe. The present version weighs about 10 pounds, but future modifications could make it lighter and more streamlined.

## KIDNEY TRANSPLANTATION

Major advances have been made in kidney transplantation since the first live donor kidney transplant was performed in 1954 between identical twins. These advances include organ procurement and preservation, surgical techniques, tissue typing and matching, immunosuppressant therapy, and prevention and treatment of graft rejection. (A general discussion of organ transplantation is in Chapter 13, pp. 207-210).

Even though kidney transplantation is the best treatment option available to patients with ESRD, fewer than 4% ever receive a transplant. This is because of the large disparity between the supply and demand for kidneys. Every year thousands are waiting for kidney transplants (more than 100,000 are currently on the list), yet only about 17,000 transplants take place every year. Most die while waiting. Transplantation from a deceased donor usually requires a prolonged waiting period with differences in waiting time depending on age, gender, and race. Average wait times in the United States for a cadaveric kidney usually range from 2 to 5 years.[27,28]

Kidney transplantation is very successful, with 1-year graft survival rates over 90% for deceased donor transplants and 95% for live donor transplants.[29] An advantage of kidney transplantation when compared with dialysis is that it reverses many of the pathophysiologic changes associated with renal disease. It also eliminates the dependence on dialysis and the accompanying dietary and lifestyle restrictions. Transplantation is also less expensive than dialysis after the first year.

### Recipient Selection

Appropriate recipient selection is important for a successful outcome. Candidacy is determined by a variety of medical and psychosocial factors that vary among transplant centers. Some transplant programs exclude patients who are morbidly obese or who continue to smoke (despite smoking cessation interventions). A careful evaluation is completed in an attempt to identify and minimize potential complications after transplantation. Certain patients, particularly those with CV disease and diabetes mellitus, are considered high risk and must be carefully evaluated and then monitored closely after transplantation.

For a small number of patients who are approaching ESRD, a *preemptive transplant* (before dialysis is required) is possible if they have a living donor. This approach is most advantageous for patients with diabetes, who have a much higher mortality rate on dialysis than nondiabetics.

Contraindications to transplantation include disseminated malignancies, refractory or untreated cardiac disease, chronic respiratory failure, extensive vascular disease, chronic infection, and unresolved psychosocial disorders (e.g., nonadherence to medical regimens, alcoholism, drug addiction). Being HIV-positive or having hepatitis B or C is not a contraindication to transplantation.

Surgical procedures may be required before transplantation based on the results of the recipient evaluation. Coronary artery bypass or coronary angioplasty may be indicated for advanced coronary artery disease. Cholecystectomy may be necessary for patients with a history of gallstones, biliary obstruction, or cholecystitis. On rare occasions, bilateral nephrectomies are necessary for patients with refractory hypertension, recurrent urinary tract infections, or grossly enlarged kidneys from polycystic kidney disease. In general, the recipient's own kidneys do not have to be removed before he or she receives a kidney transplant.

### Histocompatibility Studies

Histocompatibility studies, including human leukocyte antigen (HLA) testing and crossmatching, are discussed in Chapter 13 on pp. 206-207.

### Donor Sources

Kidneys for transplantation may be obtained from compatible blood-type deceased donors, blood relatives, emotionally related (close and distant) living donors (e.g., spouses, distant cousins, etc.), and altruistic living donors who are known (friends) or unknown to the recipient.

Another option is *paired organ donation,* in which one donor/recipient pair who are incompatible or poorly matched with each other find another donor/recipient pair with whom they can exchange kidneys. Thus a spouse (person A) who wants to donate a kidney to his wife (person B) but is incompatible is paired with another donor/recipient pair involving a son with ESRD (person C) and his mother (person D). In this example, person A would donate his kidney to person C, and person D would donate her kidney to person B. Paired organ donation is the practice of matching biologically incompatible donor/recipient pairs to permit transplantation of both candidates with a well-matched organ.

**Live Donors.** Live donors undergo an extensive interprofessional evaluation to ensure that they are in good health and have no history of disease that would place them at risk for developing kidney disease or operative complications. Crossmatches are done at the time of the evaluation and about a week before the transplant to ensure that no antibodies to the donor are present or that the antibody titer is below the allowed level. Advantages of a live donor kidney include (1) better patient and graft survival rates regardless of histocompatibility match, (2) immediate organ availability, (3) immediate function because of minimal *cold time* (kidney out of body and not getting blood supply), and (4) the opportunity to have the recipient in the best possible medical condition because the surgery is elective.

The potential donor sees a nephrologist for a complete history and physical examination and laboratory and diagnostic studies. Laboratory studies include a 24-hour urine study for creatinine clearance and total protein, complete blood count, and chemistry and electrolyte profiles. Hepatitis B and C, HIV, and cytomegalovirus (CMV) testing is done to assess for transmitted diseases. An ECG and chest x-ray are also done. A renal ultrasound and renal arteriogram or three-dimensional CT scan is performed to ensure that the blood vessels supplying each kidney are adequate and that no anomalies exist and to determine selection of the kidney to be used in the transplant.

## ETHICAL/LEGAL DILEMMAS

### *Allocation of Resources*

**Situation**

T.H., a transplant nurse coordinator, is considering her feelings about two patients who are being evaluated for placement on the deceased (cadaveric) kidney transplant waiting list. One patient is a 40-yr-old African American schoolteacher. She is married and has two children. The other patient is a 22-yr-old unemployed white man. He misses three or four dialysis treatments per month and does not take his antihypertensive medications consistently.

**Ethical/Legal Points for Consideration**

- The foundation of this conflict resides in the Constitution, in which the founders made education a free public resource and ignored health care as a right. Health care then became a privilege, a resource to be obtained by persons with the funds to pay for it.
- It took almost 200 yr for health entitlement programs to be developed. Medicare is a federally administrated program. Individuals covered by Medicare are protected by Constitutional laws prohibiting discrimination based on race, gender, religion, and ethnic background.
- Medicaid is a federally sponsored program jointly administered by the various states. The states have the right to set coverage eligibility and limits but may not violate an individual's constitutionally protected rights against discrimination.
- It is highly unlikely that the standard prohibitions against discrimination will change, but it is possible that definitions of unhealthy behavior such as substance abuse, alcoholism, smoking, and obesity may be used to screen out candidates.
- Nurses are concerned about social justice because of their health advocacy role. Today the situation is immensely more complex because of the cost and availability of care.

**Discussion Questions**

1. What does the American Nurses Association (ANA) Code of Ethics say about how you as a nurse should view patients?
2. What are your thoughts about which of the patients should receive the next available kidney transplant?
3. Can you assign value to the lives of various patients? Who is worth more?

A transplant psychologist or social worker determines if the individual is emotionally stable and able to deal with the issues related to organ donation. All donors must be informed about the risks and benefits of donation, the potential short- and long-term complications, and what to expect during the hospitalization and recovery phases. Kidney donation is considered safe without any long-term health consequences. Although the costs of the evaluation and surgery are covered by the recipient's insurance, no compensation is available for lost wages during the posthospitalization recovery period. This period can last 6 weeks or longer.

When there is ABO incompatibility between a donor and recipient, paired donor exchange is a viable alternative. Another option for ABO incompatibility or a positive crossmatch between the donor and recipient is to use plasmapheresis to remove antibodies from the recipient. (Crossmatching is discussed in Chapter 13.) This allows transplant candidates to receive kidneys from live donors with blood types that have traditionally been considered incompatible. After the transplant, the patient undergoes additional plasmapheresis treatments.

**Deceased Donors.** Deceased (cadaver) kidney donors are relatively healthy individuals who have suffered an irreversible brain injury and are declared brain dead. The most common causes of injury are cerebral trauma from motor vehicle accidents or gunshot wounds, intracerebral or subarachnoid hemorrhage, and anoxic brain damage caused by cardiac arrest. The brain-dead donor must have effective CV function and be supported on a ventilator to preserve the organs.

Even if the donor carried a signed donor card, permission from the donor's legal next of kin is still requested after brain death is determined. That is why it is important for you to talk with your family about your wishes before losing the capacity to convey your desires.

In deceased kidney donation, the kidneys are removed and preserved. They can be preserved for up to 72 hours, but most transplant surgeons prefer to transplant kidneys before the cold time (time outside of the body when being transported from the deceased donor to the recipient) reaches 24 hours. Prolonged cold time increases the likelihood that the kidney will not function immediately, and acute tubular necrosis (ATN) may develop.

The United Network for Organ Sharing (UNOS) distributes deceased donor kidneys using an objective computerized point system. The ABO group, HLA typing, age, antibody level, and length of time waiting are entered into the national computer for each candidate. When a donor becomes available, the donor's key information is compared with the data of all patients awaiting transplantation locally and nationwide. Points are given for how close the HLA match is, how long the patient has been waiting, if the antibody level is unusually high, and if the recipient is younger than 19 years old. Extra points are given for high antibody levels because this can severely limit the number of donors with whom the patient will not have a positive crossmatch. The kidney is offered to the recipient with the most points in the local area. If no patients in the local area are suitable, the organ is then offered in the region and then in the nation. When a kidney arrives at the recipient's transplant center, a final crossmatch is done and must be negative for the deceased donor transplantation to proceed. (Crossmatching is discussed in Chapter 13.)

The only exception to the previous plan is if a patient needs an emergency transplant or if a donor and recipient match on all six HLA antigens (zero antigen mismatch). The patient meeting either one of these criteria goes to the top of the list. Emergency transplants are given priority because the patient is facing imminent death if not transplanted. If a zero antigen mismatch patient is identified nationally, since statistically these grafts have better survival rates, one of the donor kidneys must be sent to that recipient's transplant center regardless of location.

## Surgical Procedure

**Live Donor.** Living donation accounts for nearly 27% of all kidney transplants in the United States, and most transplant centers regard them as the preferred donation modality.[27] The donor nephrectomy is performed by a transplant surgeon. The donor's surgery begins 1 to 2 hours before the recipient's surgery. The recipient is surgically prepared for the kidney transplant in a nearby operating room.

*Laparoscopic donor nephrectomy* is the most common technique for removing a kidney in a living donor. (Laparoscopic nephrectomy is discussed in Chapter 45.) After the kidney has been removed, it is flushed with a chilled, sterile electrolyte solution and prepared for immediate transplant into the recipient. The use of a laparoscopic donor nephrectomy procedure is minimally invasive with fewer risks and shorter recovery time than an open procedure. The laparoscopic approach significantly decreases hospital stay, pain, operative blood loss, debilitation, and length of time off work. For these reasons, the number of people willing to donate a kidney has increased significantly.

For an *open (conventional) nephrectomy*, the donor is placed in the lateral decubitus position on the operating table so that the flank is exposed laterally. An incision is made at the level of the eleventh rib. The rib may have to be removed to provide adequate visualization of the kidney.

**Kidney Transplant Recipient.** The transplanted kidney is usually placed extraperitoneally in the iliac fossa. The right iliac fossa is preferred to facilitate anastomoses of the blood vessels and ureter and minimize the occurrence of paralytic ileus. A urinary catheter is placed into the bladder and an antibiotic solution is instilled to distend the bladder and decrease the risk of infection. A crescent-shaped incision is made extending from the iliac crest to the symphysis pubis (Fig. 46-15).

Rapid revascularization is critical to prevent ischemic injury to the kidney. The donor artery is anastomosed to the recipient's internal iliac (hypogastric) or external iliac artery. The donor vein is anastomosed to the recipient's external iliac vein. When the anastomoses are complete, the clamps are released, and blood flow to the kidney is reestablished. The kidney should become firm and pink. Urine may begin to flow from the ureter immediately. The donor ureter in most cases is then tunneled through the bladder submucosa before entering the bladder cavity and being sutured in place. This approach is called

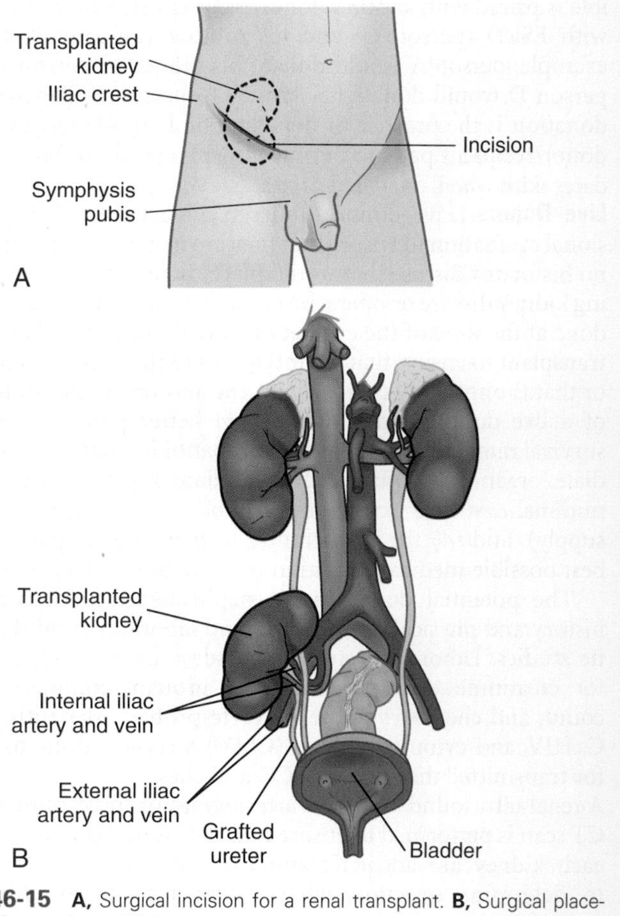


**FIG. 46-15** **A,** Surgical incision for a renal transplant. **B,** Surgical placement of transplanted kidney.

*ureteroneocystostomy.* This allows the bladder wall to compress the ureter as it contracts for micturition, thereby preventing reflux of urine up the ureter into the transplanted kidney. The transplant surgery takes about 3 to 4 hours.

## NURSING MANAGEMENT: KIDNEY TRANSPLANT RECIPIENT

### Preoperative Care

Nursing care of the patient in the preoperative phase includes emotional and physical preparation for surgery. Because the patient and caregiver may have been waiting years for the kidney transplant, a review of the operative procedure and what can be expected in the immediate postoperative recovery period is necessary. Stress that there is a chance the kidney may not function immediately, and dialysis may be required for days to weeks. Review the need for immunosuppressive drugs and measures to prevent infection.

To ensure the patient is in optimal physical condition for surgery, an ECG, chest x-ray, and laboratory studies are ordered. Dialysis may be required before surgery for fluid overload or hyperkalemia. Because dialysis may be required after transplantation, the patency of the vascular access must be maintained. The vascular access extremity should be labeled "dialysis access, no procedures" to prevent use of the affected extremity for BP measurement, blood drawing, or IV infusions. A patient on PD must empty the peritoneal cavity of all dialysate solution before going to surgery and have the PD catheter capped.

### Postoperative Care

**Live Donor.** Postoperative care for the donor is similar to that following open (conventional) or laparoscopic nephrectomy (see Chapter 45). Closely monitor renal function to assess for impairment and monitor the hematocrit to assess for bleeding. Donors usually experience more pain than the recipient. Donors who have had an open surgical approach may experience more pain than when a laparoscopic approach is used.

Donors who had an open approach are usually discharged from the hospital in 4 or 5 days and return to work in 6 to 8 weeks. With a laparoscopic approach, donors are discharged from the hospital in 2 to 4 days and return to work in 4 to 6 weeks. The donor is seen by the surgeon 1 to 2 weeks after discharge.

Nurses caring for the living donor must acknowledge the precious gift that this person has given. The donor has taken physical, emotional, and financial risks to assist the recipient. It is vital that the donor not be forgotten postoperatively. The donor will need support if the donated organ does not work immediately or for some reason fails.

**Kidney Transplant Recipient.** The first priority during the postoperative period is maintenance of fluid and electrolyte balance. Because close monitoring is required, kidney transplant recipients spend the first 12 to 24 hours in the ICU. Large volumes of urine may be produced soon after the blood supply to the transplanted kidney is reestablished. This diuresis is due to the (1) new kidney's ability to filter BUN, which acts as an osmotic diuretic; (2) abundance of fluids administered during the operation; and (3) initial renal tubular dysfunction, which inhibits the kidney from concentrating urine normally. Urine output during this phase may be as high as 1 L/hr and gradually decreases as the BUN and serum creatinine levels return toward normal. Urine output is replaced with fluids milliliter for milliliter hourly for the first 12 to 24 hours.

Central venous pressure readings are essential for monitoring postoperative fluid status. Dehydration must be avoided to prevent subsequent renal hypoperfusion and renal tubular damage. Electrolyte monitoring to assess for the hyponatremia and hypokalemia often associated with rapid diuresis is critical. Treatment with potassium supplements or infusion of 0.9% normal saline may be indicated. IV sodium bicarbonate may also be required if the patient develops metabolic acidosis from a delay in the return of kidney function.

Acute tubular necrosis (ATN) in the transplanted kidney can occur because of prolonged cold times causing ischemic damage and the use of marginal cadaveric donors (those who are medically suboptimal). While the patient is in ATN, dialysis is required to maintain fluid and electrolyte balance. Some patients have high-output ATN with the ability to excrete fluid but not metabolic wastes or electrolytes. Other patients have oliguric or anuric ATN. These patients are at risk for fluid overload in the immediate postoperative period and must be assessed closely for the need for dialysis. The period of ATN can last anywhere from days to weeks, with gradually improving kidney function. Most patients with ATN are discharged from the hospital on dialysis. This is extremely discouraging for the patient, who needs reassurance that renal function usually improves. Dialysis is discontinued when urine output increases and serum creatinine and BUN begin to normalize.

A sudden decrease in urine output in the early postoperative period is a cause for concern. It may be due to dehydration, rejection, a urine leak, or obstruction. A common cause of early obstruction is a blood clot in the urinary catheter. Catheter patency must be maintained, since the catheter remains in the bladder for 3 to 5 days to allow the ureter-bladder anastomosis to heal. If blood clots are suspected, gentle catheter irrigation (if ordered) can reestablish patency.

With a hospital length of stay averaging 4 to 5 days, discharge planning and teaching needs must be identified and addressed early in the hospital course. Patient teaching ensures a smooth transition from the hospital to home and includes how to recognize signs of rejection, infection, and any complications of surgery. Frequent blood tests and clinic visits help detect rejection early.

### Immunosuppressive Therapy

The goal of immunosuppression is to adequately suppress the immune response to prevent rejection of the transplanted kidney while maintaining sufficient immunity to prevent overwhelming infection. Immunosuppressive therapy is discussed in Chapter 13 and in Table 13-16.

### Complications of Transplantation

Complications of PD, HD, and kidney transplantation are compared in Table 46-15.

**Rejection.** Rejection is one of the major problems following kidney transplantation. Rejection can be hyperacute, acute, or chronic. These types of rejection are discussed in Chapter 13 on pp. 208-209. Patients with chronic rejection may be placed on the transplant list to be retransplanted before dialysis is required.

**Infection.** Infection remains a significant cause of morbidity and mortality after transplantation.[29] The transplant recipient is at risk for infection because of suppression of the body's normal defense mechanisms by surgery, immunosuppressive drugs, and the effects of ESRD. Underlying systemic illness such as diabetes mellitus or systemic lupus erythematosus,

**TABLE 46-15 Complications of Dialysis and Transplantation**

| Peritoneal Dialysis (PD) | Hemodialysis (HD) | Transplantation |
|---|---|---|
| • Exit site infection<br>• Peritonitis<br>• Abdominal pain<br>• Catheter outflow<br>• Hernias<br>• Lower back pain<br>• Cardiovascular disease<br>• Pulmonary problems<br>  • Atelectasis<br>  • Pneumonia<br>  • Bronchitis<br>• Protein loss<br>• Carbohydrate abnormalities<br>• Lipid abnormalities<br>• Encapsulating sclerosing peritonitis | • Hypotension<br>• Muscle cramps<br>• Exsanguination<br>• Hepatitis<br>• Infection, including sepsis<br>• Disequilibrium syndrome<br>• Cardiovascular disease | • Rejection of transplant<br>  • Hyperacute<br>  • Acute<br>  • Chronic<br>• Susceptibility to infection<br>• Cardiovascular disease<br>• Malignancies<br>• Recurrence of kidney disease<br>• Corticosteroid-related complications |

malnutrition, and older age can further compound the negative effects on the immune response. The signs and symptoms of infection can be subtle. You must be astute in your observation and assessment of kidney transplant recipients because prompt diagnosis and treatment of infections improve patient outcomes.

The most common infections observed in the first month after transplantation are similar to those acquired by any postoperative patient, such as pneumonia, wound infections, IV line and drain infections, and urinary tract infections. Fungal and viral infections are common because of the patient's immunosuppressed state. Fungal infections include *Candida, Cryptococcus,* and *Aspergillus* organisms and *Pneumocystis jiroveci.* Fungal infections are difficult to treat, require prolonged treatment periods, and often involve the administration of nephrotoxic drugs. Transplant recipients usually receive prophylactic antifungal drugs to prevent these infections, such as clotrimazole, fluconazole (Diflucan), and trimethoprim/sulfamethoxazole (Bactrim).

Viral infections, including CMV, Epstein-Barr virus, herpes simplex virus (HSV), varicella-zoster virus, and polyomavirus (e.g., BK virus), can be primary infections or reactivations of existing disease. Primary infections occur as new infections after transplantation from an exogenous source such as the donated organ or a blood transfusion. Reactivation occurs when a virus exists in a patient and becomes reactivated after transplantation because of immunosuppression.

CMV is one of the most common viral infections. If a recipient has never had CMV and receives an organ from a donor with a history of CMV, antiviral prophylaxis will be administered (e.g., ganciclovir [Cytovene], valganciclovir [Valcyte]). To prevent HSV infections, oral acyclovir (Zovirax) is given for several months after the transplant.

**Cardiovascular Disease.** CV disease is the leading cause of death after renal transplantation.[29] Transplant recipients have an increased incidence of atherosclerotic vascular disease. Hypertension, dyslipidemia, diabetes mellitus, smoking, rejection, infections, and increased homocysteine levels (many of which existed prior to the transplant) can all contribute to CV disease. Immunosuppressants can worsen hypertension and dyslipidemia.

Teach the patient to control risk factors such as elevated cholesterol, triglycerides, and blood glucose and weight gain. Adherence to the prescribed antihypertensive regimen is essential not only to prevent CV events but also to prevent damage to the new kidney. (Hypertension is discussed in Chapter 32.)

**Malignancies.** The overall incidence of malignancies in kidney transplant recipients is greater than in the general population, primarily because of immunosuppressive therapy. Not only do immunosuppressants suppress the immune system to prevent rejection, but they also suppress the ability to fight infection and the production of abnormal cells such as cancer cells.

The most common types of cancer after transplant are (1) skin cancers: basal and squamous cell carcinoma and melanoma and (2) *posttransplant lymphoproliferative disorder (PTLD).* The majority of PTLDs are of B-cell origin, associated with Epstein-Barr virus (EBV), and cause aggressive lymphomas (Hodgkin's and non-Hodgkin's lymphoma). Most cases of PTLD occur within the first year of transplant.

Patients are also at risk for cancers of the colorectum, breast, cervix, liver, stomach, oropharynx, anus, vulva, and penis. Regular screening for cancer is an important part of the transplant recipient's preventive care. Advise the patient to avoid sun exposure by using protective clothing and sunscreens to minimize the incidence of skin cancers.

**Recurrence of Original Kidney Disease.** Recurrence of the original disease that destroyed the native kidneys occurs in some kidney transplant recipients. It is most common with certain types of glomerulonephritis, immunoglobulin A (IgA) nephropathy, diabetic nephropathy, and focal segmental sclerosis. Disease recurrence can result in the loss of a functioning kidney transplant. Patients must be advised before transplantation if they have a disease known to recur.

**Corticosteroid-Related Complications.** Aseptic necrosis of the hips, knees, and other joints can result from chronic corticosteroid therapy and renal osteodystrophy. Other significant problems related to corticosteroids include peptic ulcer disease, glucose intolerance and diabetes, cataracts, dyslipidemia, infections, and malignancies. The use of tacrolimus and other immunosuppressants has allowed corticosteroid doses to be much lower than they were in the past.

Many transplant programs have initiated corticosteroid-free drug regimens because of the problems of long-term corticosteroid use. Other centers withdraw patients from corticosteroids after transplantation. For patients who remain on corticosteroids, vigilant monitoring for side effects and early treatment are essential. (Corticosteroid therapy as immunosuppression is discussed in Chapter 13 on pp. 209-210.)

## Gerontologic Considerations: Chronic Kidney Disease

The incidence of CKD in the United States is increasing most rapidly in older adults. The most common diseases leading to renal disease in older people are hypertension and diabetes.[30]

The care of older patients is particularly challenging, not only because of the normal physiologic changes of aging but also because of the disabilities, chronic diseases, and a number of co-morbid conditions that occur with aging. Physiologic changes include diminished cardiopulmonary function, bone loss, immunodeficiency, altered protein synthesis, impaired cognition, and altered drug metabolism. Malnutrition is common in these patients for a variety of reasons, including lack of mobility, lack of understanding of basic nutritional requirements, social isolation, physical disability, impaired cognitive function, and malabsorption problems.

When conservative therapy for CKD is no longer effective, the older patient needs to consider the best treatment modality based on his or her physical and emotional health, personal preferences, and availability of support. PD allows the patient to be more mobile and to enjoy an increased sense of control over the illness. PD causes less hemodynamic instability than HD but does require self-care or assistance from another person, which may not always be available.

Most individuals 65 years of age or older select treatment with in-center HD because of a lack of assistance in the home and reluctance to manage the technology of home HD or PD. Establishing vascular access for HD may be a concern in an older adult because of atherosclerotic changes. Although transplantation is an option, older adults must be carefully screened to ensure that the benefits of transplantation outweigh the risks.[31] Although a living donor is preferable, this may not be an option for many older patients.

The most common cause of death in older ESRD patients is CV disease (myocardial infarction, stroke), followed by withdrawal from dialysis. If a competent patient decides to withdraw from dialysis, it is essential to support the patient and family. Ethical issues (see the Ethical/Legal Dilemmas box) to consider in this situation include patient competency, benefit versus burden of treatment, and futility of treatment. Withdrawal from treatment is not a failure if the patient is well informed and comfortable with the decision.

Dialysis (especially PD) has been successfully used in older adults. Quality-of-life measures show no justification for excluding the older adult from dialysis programs. Rationing dialysis based on age alone is not a reasonable decision for health care professionals to make.

## ETHICAL/LEGAL DILEMMAS

### *Withdrawing Treatment*

**Situation**

L.R., a 70-yr-old patient with diabetes mellitus and end-stage renal disease, has been on dialysis for 10 yr. He tells you that he wants to discontinue his dialysis. His quality of life has diminished during the past 2 yr since his wife died. He is not a transplant candidate.

**Ethical/Legal Points for Consideration**

- Informed consent includes the legal right to refuse treatment. However, the right to refuse may be more difficult if (1) it is contrary to the wishes of family and friends, (2) the treatment still appears to have some effectiveness, and (3) the treatment has been in place for some time.
- Quality-of-life decisions often outweigh the benefit against the burden of treatment. When a treatment becomes too burdensome, the patient (if competent) may request to withdraw the treatment.
- It must be determined whether some other treatable problem, such as depression, may be clouding the patient's judgment.
- Although there is no ethical or legal difference between withdrawing treatment and withholding treatment, withdrawing treatment feels different because it requires an action.
- Some health care professionals become conflicted when they are asked to withdraw treatment, since they may think they are contributing to the patient's untimely death.
- If a decision is made to withdraw treatment, the interprofessional care team, patient, and family should develop an appropriate follow-up plan that includes palliative care and hospice support.

**Discussion Questions**

1. How should you respond to L.R.'s request?
2. What is the American Nurses Association's position on withdrawing or withholding treatment that no longer benefits the patient or causes suffering?

## CASE STUDY

### *Chronic Kidney Disease*

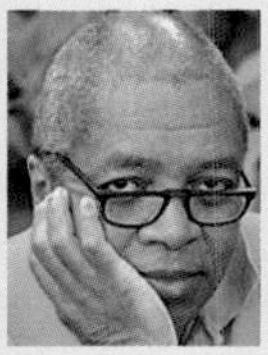

(©iStockphoto/Thinkstock)

**Patient Profile**

M.B. is a 56-yr-old African American college professor. He is seen by his primary care provider for a routine physical examination. He has not been seen by a physician in a little over a year. He complains of generalized malaise, frequent urination, and "increasing thirst." His medical history is significant for borderline hypertension and dyslipidemia. He smokes one pack of cigarettes per day, and his efforts to quit have been unsuccessful.

**Subjective Data**

- Family history: father died of a heart attack at age 62, brother had coronary artery bypass graft (CABG) at age 50, mother died from complications of diabetes
- Becomes "winded" when walking from his car to his office at the university
- Wakes up at night to urinate and has more frequent urination
- Increasing thirst

**Objective Data**

***Laboratory Data***

- Calculated creatinine clearance using the MDRD equation: 42 mL/min/1.73 m$^2$
- Serum creatinine 2.5 mg/dL
- BUN 35 mg/dL
- Serum glucose 264 mg/dL
- Hgb 13 g/dL
- Serum cholesterol 236 mg/dL

**Physical Examination**

- Weight 220 lb, height 5 ft 11 in
- BP 168/104 mm Hg

**Discussion Questions**

1. What do you think caused M.B.'s kidney disease?
2. What stage of chronic kidney disease does he have?
3. ***Teamwork and Collaboration:*** What are the most important treatment measures that the interprofessional team can provide for M.B.?
4. Identify the abnormal diagnostic study results and why each would occur.
5. ***Patient-Centered Care:*** What are the nursing interventions that would help promote M.B.'s self-management of his disease process?
6. ***Priority Decision:*** Based on the assessment data provided, what are the priority nursing diagnoses? Are there any collaborative problems?
7. ***Teamwork and Collaboration:*** How can the interprofessional team work together with M.B. to decide on the best form of renal replacement therapy?
8. ***Evidence-Based Practice:*** M.B. tells you that he has not been taking his BP medications regularly. When he asks you how important they are, what will you tell him?

Answers available at *http://evolve.elsevier.com/Lewis/medsurg.*

## BRIDGE TO NCLEX EXAMINATION

The number of the question corresponds to the same-numbered outcome at the beginning of the chapter.

1. Which descriptions characterize acute kidney injury *(select all that apply)*?
   a. Primary cause of death is infection.
   b. It almost always affects older people.
   c. Disease course is potentially reversible.
   d. Most common cause is diabetic nephropathy.
   e. Cardiovascular disease is most common cause of death.
2. RIFLE defines three stages of AKI based on changes in
   a. blood pressure and urine osmolality.
   b. fractional excretion of urinary sodium.
   c. estimation of GFR with the MDRD equation.
   d. serum creatinine or urine output from baseline.
3. During the oliguric phase of AKI, the nurse monitors the patient for *(select all that apply)*
   a. hypotension.
   b. ECG changes.
   c. hypernatremia.
   d. pulmonary edema.
   e. urine with high specific gravity.
4. If a patient is in the diuretic phase of AKI, the nurse must monitor for which serum electrolyte imbalances?
   a. Hyperkalemia and hyponatremia
   b. Hyperkalemia and hypernatremia
   c. Hypokalemia and hyponatremia
   d. Hypokalemia and hypernatremia
5. A patient is admitted to the hospital with chronic kidney disease. The nurse understands that this condition is characterized by
   a. progressive irreversible destruction of the kidneys.
   b. a rapid decrease in urine output with an elevated BUN.
   c. an increasing creatinine clearance with a decrease in urine output.
   d. prostration, somnolence, and confusion with coma and imminent death.
6. Nurses must teach patients at risk for developing chronic kidney disease. Individuals considered to be at increased risk include *(select all that apply)*
   a. older African Americans.
   b. patients more than 60 years old.
   c. those with a history of pancreatitis.
   d. those with a history of hypertension.
   e. those with a history of type 2 diabetes.
7. Patients with chronic kidney disease experience an increased incidence of cardiovascular disease related to *(select all that apply)*
   a. hypertension.
   b. vascular calcifications.
   c. a genetic predisposition.
   d. hyperinsulinemia causing dyslipidemia.
   e. increased high-density lipoprotein levels.
8. Nutritional support and management are essential across the entire continuum of chronic kidney disease. Which statements would be considered true related to nutritional therapy *(select all that apply)*?
   a. Fluid is not usually restricted for patients receiving peritoneal dialysis.
   b. Sodium and potassium may be restricted in someone with advanced CKD.
   c. Decreased fluid intake and a low-potassium diet are hallmarks of the diet for a patient receiving hemodialysis.
   d. Decreased fluid intake and a low-potassium diet are hallmarks of the diet for a patient receiving peritoneal dialysis.
   e. Decreased fluid intake and a diet with phosphate-rich foods are hallmarks of a diet for a patient receiving hemodialysis.
9. An ESRD patient receiving hemodialysis is considering asking a relative to donate a kidney for transplantation. In assisting the patient to make a decision about treatment, the nurse informs the patient that
   a. successful transplantation usually provides better quality of life than that offered by dialysis.
   b. if rejection of the transplanted kidney occurs, no further treatment for the renal failure is available.
   c. hemodialysis replaces the normal functions of the kidneys, and patients do not have to live with the continual fear of rejection.
   d. the immunosuppressive therapy following transplantation makes the person ineligible to receive other forms of treatment if the kidney fails.
10. To assess the patency of a newly placed arteriovenous graft for dialysis, the nurse should *(select all that apply)*
    a. monitor the BP in the affected arm.
    b. irrigate the graft daily with low-dose heparin.
    c. palpate the area of the graft to feel a normal thrill.
    d. listen with a stethoscope over the graft to detect a bruit.
    e. frequently monitor the pulses and neurovascular status distal to the graft.
11. A major advantage of peritoneal dialysis is
    a. the diet is less restricted and dialysis can be performed at home.
    b. the dialysate is biocompatible and causes no long-term consequences.
    c. high glucose concentrations of the dialysate cause a reduction in appetite, promoting weight loss.
    d. no medications are required because of the enhanced efficiency of the peritoneal membrane in removing toxins.
12. A kidney transplant recipient complains of having fever, chills, and dysuria over the past 2 days. What is the *first* action that the nurse should take?
    a. Assess temperature and initiate workup to rule out infection.
    b. Reassure the patient that this is common after transplantation.
    c. Provide warm cover for the patient and give 1 g acetaminophen orally.
    d. Notify the nephrologist that the patient has developed symptoms of acute rejection.

1. a, c; 2. d; 3. b, d; 4. c; 5. a; 6. a, b, d, e; 7. a, b, d; 8. a, b, c; 9. a;
10. c, d, e; 11. a; 12. a

For rationales to these answers and even more NCLEX review questions, visit *http://evolve.elsevier.com/Lewis/medsurg*.

## EVOLVE WEBSITE

http://evolve.elsevier.com/Lewis/medsurg

**Review Questions (Online Only)**

**Key Points**

**Answer Keys for Questions**

- Rationales for Bridge to NCLEX Examination Questions
- Answer Guidelines for Case Study on p. 1097
- Answer Guidelines for Managing Care of Multiple Patients Case Study (Section 9) on p. 1100

**Student Case Studies**

- Patient With Glomerulonephritis and Acute Kidney Injury
- Patient With Kidney Transplant

**Nursing Care Plan**

- eNursing Care Plan 46-1: Patient With Chronic Kidney Disease

**Conceptual Care Map Creator**

**Audio Glossary**

**Content Updates**

## REFERENCES


1. Workeneh BT, Agraharkar M, Gupta R: Acute kidney injury. 2014. Retrieved from *http://emedicine.medscape.com/article243492*.
2. Fournier M: Stemming the rising tide of acute kidney injury by obtaining a thorough history and conducting a careful assessment, you can help patients avoid this condition, *Am Nurse Today* 8(1):12, 2013.
3. Thakar CV, Christianson A, Almenoff P, et al: Degree of acute kidney injury before dialysis initiation and hospital mortality in critically ill patients, *Int J Nephrol* 2013:827459, 2013.
4. Zeng X, McMahon GM, Brunelli SM, et al: Incidence, outcomes, and comparisons across definitions of AKI in hospitalized individuals, *Clin J Am Soc Nephrol* 9(1):12, 2014.
5. Oh HJ, Shin DH, Lee MJ, et al: Urine output is associated with prognosis in patients with acute kidney injury requiring continuous renal replacement therapy, *J Crit Care* 28(4):379, 2013.
6. Libório AB, Leite TT, Neves FM, et al: AKI complications in critically ill patients: association with mortality rates and RRT, *Clin J Am Soc Nephrol* 10(1):21, 2015.
7. Bagshaw SM, Uchino S, Kellum JA, et al: Association between renal replacement therapy in critically ill patients with severe acute kidney injury and mortality, *J Crit Care* 28(6):1011, 2013.
8. Goldstein SL, Jaber BL, Faubel S, et al: AKI transition of care: a potential opportunity to detect and prevent CKD, *Clin J Am Soc Nephrol* 8(3):476, 2013.
9. Williams LM: Take aim at acute kidney injury with RIFLE criteria, *Nursing* 44:50, 2014.
10. Salgado G, Landa M, Masevicius D, et al: Acute renal failure according to the RIFLE and AKIN criteria: a multicenter study, *Med Intensiva* 38(5):271, 2014.

*11. Schneider AG, Bellomo R, Bagshaw SM, et al: Choice of renal replacement therapy modality and dialysis dependence after acute kidney injury: a systematic review and meta-analysis, *Intens Care Med* 39(6):987, 2013.

*12. Palevsky PM, Liu KD, Brophy PD, et al: KDOQI US commentary on the 2012 KDIGO clinical practice guideline for acute kidney injury, *Am J Kidney Dis* 61(5):649, 2013.

*13. James PA, Oparil S, Carter BL, et al: 2014 evidence-based guideline for the management of high blood pressure in adults: report from the panel members appointed to the Eighth Joint National Committee (JNC 8), *JAMA* 311(5):507, 2014.

*14. Inker LA, Astor BC, Fox CH, et al: KDOQI US commentary on the 2012 KDIGO clinical practice guideline for the evaluation and management of CKD, *Am J Kidney Dis* 63(5):713, 2014.

15. US Department of Health and Human Services: ESRD: general information, Centers for Medicare and Medicaid Services. Retrieved from *www.cms.gov/Medicare/End-Stage-Renal-Disease/ESRDGeneralInformation*.
16. United States Renal Data System: 2014 Annual data report: epidemiology of kidney disease in the United States. Bethesda, Md, 2014. National Institutes of Health, National Institute of Diabetes and Digestive and Kidney Diseases. Retrieved from *www.usrds.org/adr.aspx*.
17. Pilmore H, Dogra G, Roberts M, et al: Cardiovascular disease in patients with chronic kidney disease, *Nephrology* 19(1):3, 2014.
18. Drüeke TB: Anemia treatment in patients with chronic kidney disease, *N Engl J Med* 368:387, 2013.
19. Fang Y, Ginsberg C, Sugatani T, et al: Early chronic kidney disease–mineral bone disorder stimulates vascular calcification, *Kidney Int* 85(1):142, 2014.
20. Taler SJ, Agarwal R, Bakris GL, et al: KDOQI US commentary on the 2012 KDIGO clinical practice guideline for management of blood pressure in CKD, *Am J Kidney Dis* 62(2):201, 2013.
21. Afkarian M, Sachs MC, Kestenbaum B, et al: Kidney disease and increased mortality risk in type 2 diabetes, *J Am Soc Nephrol* 24(2):302, 2013.
22. National Kidney Foundation Kidney Disease Outcomes Quality Initiative (NKF KDOQI). Retrieved from *www.kidney.org/professionals/KDOQI/guidelines_commentaries*. 2015.

*23. Hernández Morante JJ, Sánchez-Villazala A, Cutillas RC, et al: Effectiveness of a nutrition education program for the prevention and treatment of malnutrition in end-stage renal disease, *J Ren Nutr* 24(1):42, 2014.

24. National Kidney and Urologic Diseases Information Clearinghouse: Treatment methods for kidney disease: peritoneal dialysis. Retrieved from *http://kidney.niddk.nih.gov/KUDiseases/pubs/peritoneal/index.aspx*.
25. Drew DA, Lok CE, Cohen JT, et al: Vascular access choice in incident hemodialysis patients: a decision analysis, *J Am Soc Nephrol* 26(1):183, 2015.
26. National Kidney and Urologic Diseases Information Clearinghouse: Treatment methods for kidney disease: hemodialysis. Retrieved from *http://kidney.niddk.nih.gov/KUDiseases/pubs/hemodialysis/index.aspx*.
27. United Network for Organ Sharing: 2012 annual report: the U.S. Scientific registry of transplant recipients and the organ procurement and transplantation network. Bethesda, Md, 2013, US Department of Health and Human Services.
28. Weir MR, Lerma EV: *Kidney transplantation: practical guide to management*, New York, 2014, Springer.
29. Reese PP, Bloom RD, Shults J, et al: Functional status and survival after kidney transplantation, *Transplantation* 97(2):189, 2014.

*30. Bolignano D, Mattace-Raso F, Sijbrands EJ, et al: The aging kidney revisited: a systematic review, *Ageing Res Rev* 14:65, 2014.

31. Haase M, Haase-Fielitz A: *Managing renal injury in the elderly patient*, New York, 2014, Springer.

*Evidence-based information for clinical practice.

## CASE STUDY

### *Managing Care of Multiple Patients*

You are working on the medical-surgical unit and have been assigned to care for the following four patients. You are also assigned to receive a new admission to the clinical unit. You have one UAP on your team to help you.

#### Patients

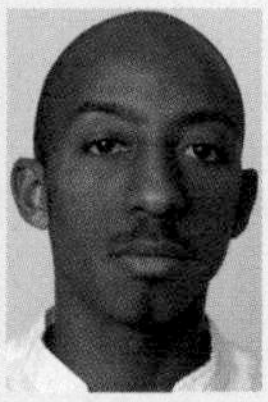

(©iStockphoto/Thinkstock)

A.K., a 28-yr-old African American man, was admitted for observation after a renal ultrasound identified calculi in the left ureter. A.K. came to the ED with complaints of sharp, colicky left flank pain for which the HCP prescribed IV opioids. His last pain medication was given 2 hours ago. His current pain level is 4 on a scale of 1 to 10. He is voiding dark, smoky-colored urine. His vital signs are within normal limits. He has positive costovertebral tenderness.

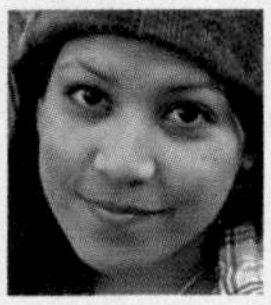

(©iStockphoto/Thinkstock)

S.U., a 29-yr-old Hispanic woman with type 1 diabetes, was admitted with acute pyelonephritis following a recent UTI. She complains of bilateral flank pain and has abdominal tenderness to palpation. Her temperature is 101.5°F (38.6°C). Her urinalysis indicates pyuria and hematuria. Her WBC is elevated at 14,800/μL. Blood culture results are pending. IV antibiotics have been started. Most recent blood glucose is 195 mg/dL.

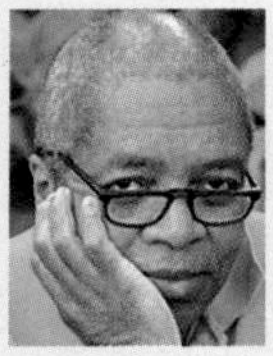

(©iStockphoto/Thinkstock)

M.B., a 56-yr-old African American college professor, was admitted with uncontrolled hypertension. He was recently diagnosed with CKD. He smokes at least one pack of cigarettes per day and is experiencing some nicotine withdrawal symptoms. His BP on admission was 224/102 mm Hg. He is receiving IV metoprolol (Lopressor) 5 mg q4hr prn for SBP >180 mm Hg. His most recent BP 3 hr ago was 174/86 mm Hg. Most recent lab results indicate a BUN of 66 mg/dL and serum creatinine of 3.2 mg/dL.

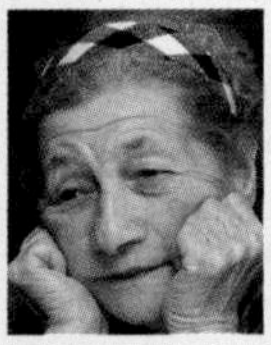

(©iStockphoto/Thinkstock)

D.M., an 82-yr-old woman, was admitted to the ED with severe dehydration, heart failure, and acute kidney injury. Her daughter found her unconscious and lying on the floor. She is confused. Her serum potassium is 5.7 mEq/L. Her urine output for the past 8 hours was 90 mL.

#### Discussion Questions

1. ***Priority Decision:*** After receiving report, which patient should you see first? Second? Provide a rationale for your decision.
2. ***Teamwork and Collaboration:*** Which tasks could you delegate to the UAP *(select all that apply)*?
   a. Obtain vital signs on M.B.
   b. Strain A.K.'s voided urine.
   c. Report D.M.'s potassium level to the HCP.
   d. Measure D.M.'s urine output and report the results to the RN.
   e. Assess S.U. for manifestations of sepsis or diabetic ketoacidosis.
3. ***Priority Decision and Teamwork and Collaboration:*** As you are assessing D.M., the UAP informs you that M.B.'s blood pressure is 190/86. He is asymptomatic. Additionally, the charge nurse informs you that you will be receiving a patient with heart failure from the ED within the next 20 minutes. Which action would be *most* appropriate?
   a. Ask the charge nurse to assign the new admission to someone else.
   b. Have the UAP admit the new patient while you administer M.B.'s IV metoprolol.
   c. Call the ED and have them hold the new admission until after you have assessed all your patients.
   d. Ask the charge nurse to administer M.B.'s IV metoprolol while you complete your assessment of D.M. and then S.U.

#### Case Study Progression

As you complete your assessment of D.M., you notice her apical pulse is irregular. She has 1+ pitting edema in her lower extremities. Her BP is 160/90 mmHg, heart rate 108 bpm, and respiratory rate 28/min. Auscultation of D.M's lungs reveal crackles in the bases and $O_2$ saturation is 92% on room air. You notify her HCP.

4. Which interventions would you expect the HCP to order for D.M. *(select all that apply)*?
   a. Administer IV Kayexalate.
   b. Obtain arterial blood gas levels.
   c. Administer 40 mg of furosemide IV push.
   d. Prepare her for hemodialysis and notify her family.
   e. Obtain a 12-lead ECG and initiate continuous cardiac monitoring.
5. ***Priority Decision:*** Which nursing diagnosis would be of *highest* priority when planning care for A.K.?
   a. Risk for injury
   b. Impaired comfort
   c. Risk for infection
   d. Ineffective health management
6. Which statement would be *most* appropriate when teaching S.U. about her kidney infection?
   a. "The damage to your kidneys will likely require dialysis."
   b. "You will need to be in the hospital for a 2-week course of IV antibiotics."
   c. "It is very important that you maintain adequate hydration to flush your kidneys."
   d. "You will not need further antibiotics once you are discharged from the hospital."
7. ***Management Decision:*** As the UAP prepares the room for the patient being admitted from the ED, you overhear her telling a co-worker that she has to do all your work for you. What is your *best* initial action?
   a. Report the incident to the charge nurse for follow-up.
   b. Ask the UAP to discuss her concerns with you in private.
   c. Tell the UAP how much you appreciate and value her input on your team.
   d. Immediately clarify the situation by telling the UAP all the tasks you are completing.

Answers available at *http://evolve.elsevier.com/Lewis/medsurg.*

SECTION 10

# Problems Related to Regulatory and Reproductive Mechanisms

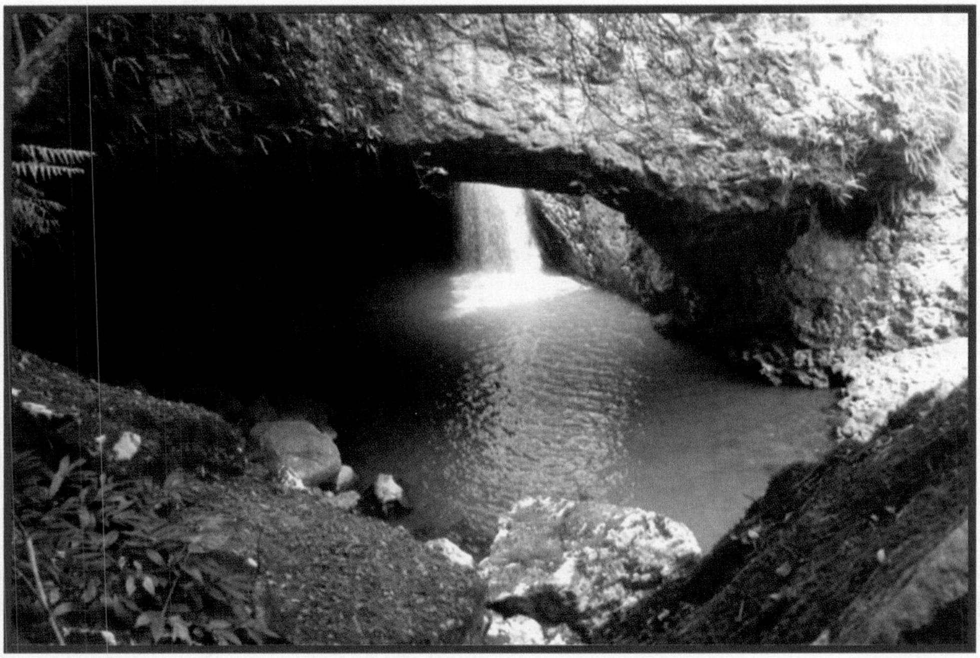

Peter Bonner

*There's a river somewhere that flows through the lives of everyone.*

***Roberta Flack***

47

# Assessment of Endocrine System

*Katherine A. Kelly*

*Success is walking from failure to failure with no loss of enthusiasm.*

***Winston Churchill***

http://evolve.elsevier.com/Lewis/medsurg/

## LEARNING OUTCOMES

1. Describe the common characteristics and functions of hormones.
2. Identify the locations of the endocrine glands.
3. Describe the functions of hormones secreted by the pituitary, thyroid, parathyroid, and adrenal glands and the pancreas.
4. Describe the locations and roles of hormone receptors.
5. Obtain significant subjective and objective assessment data related to the endocrine system from a patient.
6. Perform a physical assessment of the endocrine system using the appropriate techniques.
7. Link age-related changes in the endocrine system to differences in assessment findings.
8. Differentiate normal from common abnormal findings of a physical assessment of the endocrine system.
9. Describe the purpose, significance of results, and nursing responsibilities related to diagnostic studies of the endocrine system.

## KEY TERMS

aldosterone, p. 1108
antidiuretic hormone (ADH), p. 1106
catecholamines, p. 1107
circadian rhythm, p. 1105
corticosteroid, p. 1107
cortisol, p. 1107
glucagon, p. 1108
growth hormone (GH), p. 1105
hormones, p. 1102
insulin, p. 1108
negative feedback, p. 1103
positive feedback, p. 1104
thyroxine ($T_4$), p. 1107
triiodothyronine ($T_3$), p. 1107
tropic hormones, p. 1105

## STRUCTURES AND FUNCTIONS OF ENDOCRINE SYSTEM

### Glands

*Endocrine glands* include the hypothalamus, pituitary, thyroid, parathyroids, adrenals, pancreas, ovaries, testes, and pineal gland (Fig. 47-1). These glands are able to make and release special chemical messengers called *hormones.* The endocrine system has five general functions. It has a role in reproductive and central nervous system development in the fetus, stimulating growth and development during childhood and adolescence, sexual reproduction, maintaining homeostasis, and responding to emergency demands.[1]

### Hormones

**Hormones** are chemical substances produced by endocrine glands that control and regulate the activity of certain target cells or organs. Many are made in one part of the body and control and regulate the activity of certain cells or organs in another part of the body. The thyroid gland makes the hormone thyroxine, which affects many body tissues when released directly into the circulation. Other hormones act locally on cells where they are released and never enter the bloodstream. This local effect is called *paracrine action.* The action of sex steroids on the ovary is an example of paracrine action.

Most hormones have common characteristics, including (1) secretion in small amounts at variable but predictable rates; (2) regulation by feedback systems; and (3) ability to bind to specific target cell receptors. Table 47-1 summarizes the major hormones, the glands or tissues that synthesize the hormones, their target organs or tissues, and their functions.

There is a strong connection between the endocrine system and nervous system. *Catecholamines* (e.g., epinephrine), secreted by the adrenal gland, travel through the bloodstream and affect multiple organ systems. These same substances, when secreted by nerve cells in the brain and peripheral nervous system, act as neurotransmitters, sending important impulses across nerve synapses.[1]

Organs can act as endocrine glands by secreting hormones. For example, the kidneys secrete erythropoietin, a substance

Reviewed by Teresa J. Seright, RN, PhD, CCRN, Associate Teaching Professor, College of Nursing, Montana State University, Bozeman, Montana; and Crystal Sheaves, RN, MSN, APRN, FNP-BC, Senior Lecturer, West Virginia University School of Nursing, Charleston, West Virginia.

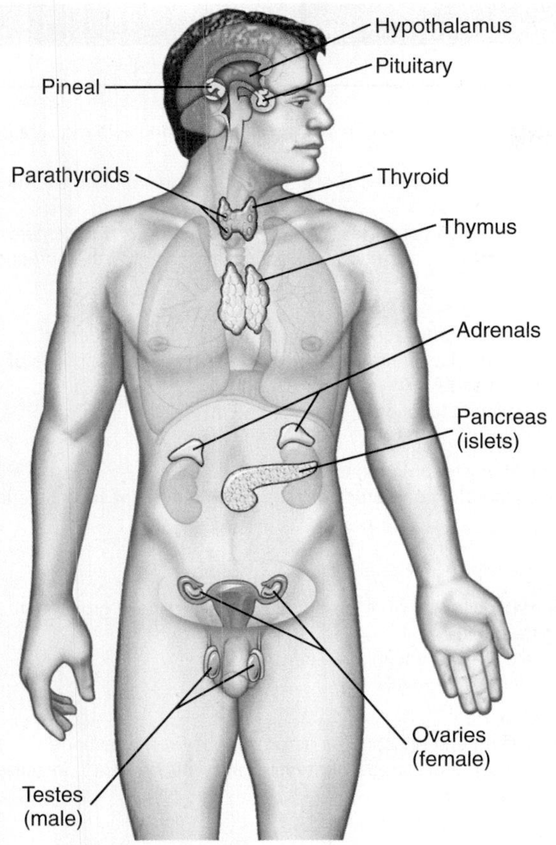


**FIG. 47-1** Location of the major endocrine glands. The parathyroid glands lie on the posterior surface of the thyroid gland. (Modified from Patton KT, Thibodeau GA: *Anatomy and physiology*, ed 8, St Louis, 2013, Mosby.)

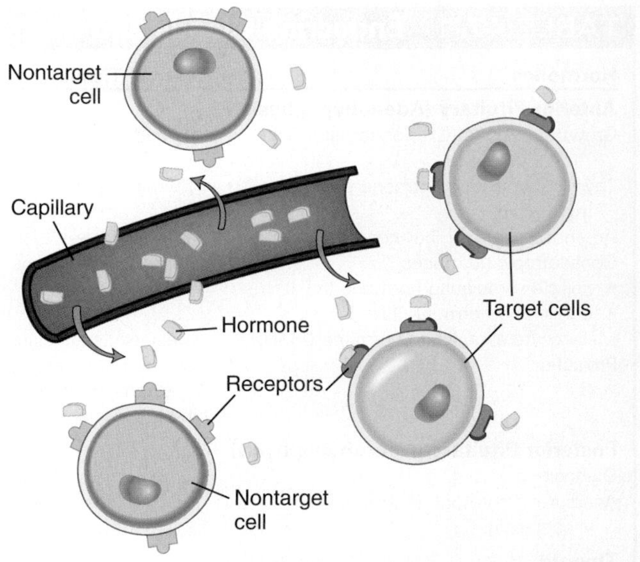


**FIG. 47-2** The target cell concept. Hormones act only on cells that have receptors specific to that hormone, since the shape of the receptor determines which hormone can react with it. This is an example of the lock-and-key model of biochemical reactions.

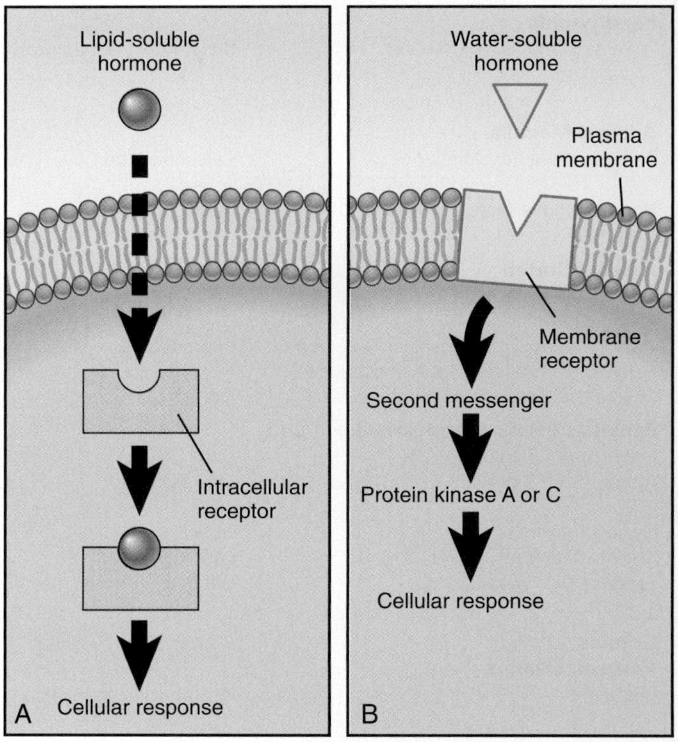


**FIG. 47-3** **A,** Lipid-soluble hormones (e.g., steroid hormones) penetrate the cell membrane and interact with intracellular receptors. **B,** Water-soluble hormones (e.g., protein hormones) bind to receptors located in the cell membrane. The hormone-receptor interaction stimulates various cell responses. (Modified from McCance KL, Huether SE: *Pathophysiology: the biologic basis for disease in adults and children,* ed 6, St Louis, 2010, Mosby.)

that stimulates red blood cell production. The heart secretes atrial natriuretic peptide (ANP). The gastrointestinal (GI) tract secretes numerous peptide hormones (e.g., gastrin), which aid in digestion. These hormones are discussed in their respective assessment chapters.

**Hormone Receptors.** Hormones exert their effects by recognizing their target tissues and attaching to receptor sites in a "lock-and-key" type of mechanism. This means a hormone will act only on cells that have a receptor specific for that hormone (Fig. 47-2).

**Lipid-Soluble and Water-Soluble Hormones.** Hormones are classified by their chemical structure as either lipid soluble or water soluble. The differences in solubility become important in understanding how the hormone interacts with the target cell (Fig. 47-3). Lipid-soluble hormones (steroids, thyroid) are bound to plasma proteins as they travel to target cells. They cross the cell membrane by simple diffusion. Water-soluble hormones (insulin, growth hormone, prolactin) circulate freely in the blood and act directly on target tissues.

**Regulation of Hormonal Secretion.** Endocrine activity is controlled by specific mechanisms that either stimulate or inhibit hormone synthesis and secretion. These include positive and negative feedback, nervous system control, and physiologic rhythms.

***Simple Feedback.*** Negative feedback relies on the blood level of a hormone or other chemical compound regulated by the hormone (e.g., glucose). It is the most common type of endocrine feedback system and results in the gland increasing or decreasing the release of a hormone. Negative feedback is similar to the functioning of a thermostat. Cold air in a room activates the thermostat to release heat. Warm air signals the thermostat to turn off the heater. An example of negative feedback is calcium and parathyroid hormone (PTH) regulation. Low blood levels of calcium stimulate the parathyroid gland to release PTH. PTH acts on the bone, intestine, and kidneys to

**TABLE 47-1 Endocrine Glands and Hormones**

| Hormones | Target Tissue | Functions |
|---|---|---|
| **Anterior Pituitary (Adenohypophysis)** | | |
| Growth hormone (GH), or somatotropin | All body cells | Promotes protein anabolism (growth, tissue repair) and lipid mobilization and catabolism |
| Thyroid-stimulating hormone (TSH), or thyrotropin | Thyroid gland | Stimulates synthesis and release of thyroid hormones, growth and function of thyroid gland |
| Adrenocorticotropic hormone (ACTH) | Adrenal cortex | Fosters growth of adrenal cortex. Stimulates secretion of corticosteroids |
| Gonadotropic hormones<br>• Follicle-stimulating hormone (FSH)<br>• Luteinizing hormone (LH) | Reproductive organs | Stimulate sex hormone secretion, reproductive organ growth, reproductive processes |
| Melanocyte-stimulating hormone (MSH) | Melanocytes in skin | Increases melanin production in melanocytes to make skin darker |
| Prolactin | Ovary and mammary glands in women<br>Testes in men | Stimulates milk production in lactating women. Increases response of follicles to LH and FSH<br>Stimulates testicular function in men |
| **Posterior Pituitary (Neurohypophysis)** | | |
| Oxytocin | Uterus, mammary glands | Stimulates milk secretion, uterine contractility |
| Antidiuretic hormone (ADH), or vasopressin | Renal tubules, vascular smooth muscle | Promotes reabsorption of water from the renal tubules, vasoconstriction |
| **Thyroid** | | |
| Thyroxine ($T_4$) | All body tissues | Precursor to $T_3$ |
| Triiodothyronine ($T_3$) | All body tissues | Regulates metabolic rate of all cells and processes of cell growth and tissue differentiation |
| Calcitonin | Bone tissue | Regulates calcium and phosphorus serum levels<br>Decreases serum $Ca^{2+}$ levels |
| **Parathyroids** | | |
| Parathyroid hormone (PTH), or parathormone | Bone, intestine, kidneys | Regulates calcium and phosphorus serum levels. Promotes bone demineralization and increases intestinal absorption of $Ca^{2+}$. Increases serum $Ca^{2+}$ levels |
| **Adrenal Medulla** | | |
| Epinephrine (adrenaline) | Catecholamine | Increases in response to stress. Enhances and prolongs effects of sympathetic nervous system |
| Norepinephrine (noradrenaline) | Catecholamine | Increases in response to stress. Enhances and prolongs effects of sympathetic nervous system |
| **Adrenal Cortex** | | |
| Corticosteroids (e.g., cortisol, hydrocortisone) | All body tissues | Promote metabolism. Increased in response to stress. Antiinflammatory |
| Androgens (e.g., dehydroepiandrosterone [DGEA], androsterone) and estradiol | Reproductive organs | Promote growth spurt in adolescence, secondary sex characteristics, and libido in both sexes |
| Mineralocorticoids (e.g., aldosterone) | Kidney | Regulate sodium and potassium balance and thus water balance |
| **Pancreas (Islets of Langerhans)** | | |
| Insulin (from β cells) | General | Promotes glucose transport from the blood into the cell |
| Amylin (from β cells) | Liver, stomach | Decreases gastric motility, glucagon secretion, and endogenous glucose release from liver. Increases satiety |
| Glucagon (from α cells) | General | Stimulates glycogenolysis and gluconeogenesis |
| Somatostatin | Pancreas | Inhibits insulin and glucagon secretion |
| Pancreatic polypeptide | General | Influences regulation of pancreatic exocrine function and metabolism of absorbed nutrients |
| **Gonads** | | |
| ***Women: Ovaries*** | | |
| Estrogen | Reproductive system, breasts | Stimulates development of secondary sex characteristics, preparation of uterus for fertilization and fetal development. Stimulates bone growth |
| Progesterone | Reproductive system | Maintains lining of uterus necessary for successful pregnancy |
| ***Men: Testes*** | | |
| Testosterone | Reproductive system | Stimulates development of secondary sex characteristics, spermatogenesis |

increase blood calcium levels. The increased blood calcium level then inhibits further PTH release (Fig. 47-4).

With **positive feedback**, increasing hormone levels cause another gland to release a hormone that then stimulates further release of the first hormone. A means to stop the release of the first hormone (e.g., follicle death) is required or its release will continue. The ovarian hormone estradiol operates by this type of feedback. Increased levels of estradiol produced by the follicle during the menstrual cycle result in the production and release of follicle-stimulating hormone (FSH) by the anterior pituitary. FSH causes further increases in estradiol until the death of the follicle. This results in a drop of FSH serum levels.

***Nervous System Control.*** Nervous system activity directly affects some endocrine glands. Pain, fear, sexual excitement, and other stressors can stimulate the nervous system to modulate hormone secretion. For example, when stress is sensed or

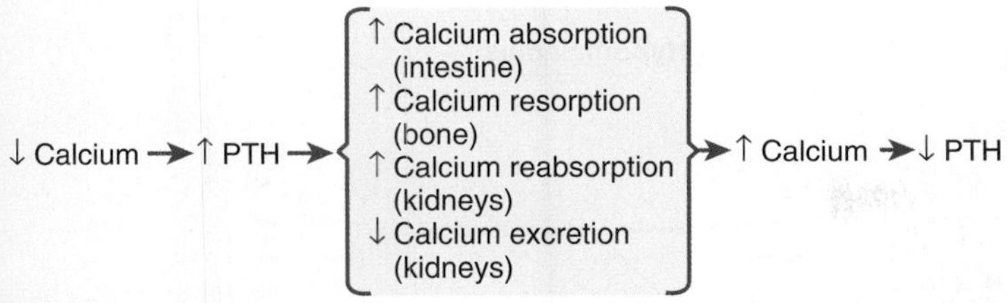


**FIG. 47-4** Feedback mechanism between parathyroid hormone *(PTH)* and calcium.

perceived by the central nervous system (CNS), the sympathetic nervous system (SNS) secretes catecholamines (e.g., epinephrine), which maximize cardiac and lung function and vision to deal with the stress more effectively. Chronic exposure to some stressors can cause persistent elevation in heart rate and BP and changes in the endocrine system. This puts patients at risk for chronic disease such as hypertension and cardiac disease. Stress-related effects are discussed in Chapter 6.

***Rhythms.*** A common physiologic rhythm is the **circadian rhythm**. It is a 24-hour rhythm that can be driven and altered by sleep-wake or dark-light 24-hour (diurnal) cycles. Hormone levels and the responsiveness of target tissues fluctuate predictably during these cycles.[2] Cortisol, produced by the adrenal cortex, rises early in the day, declines toward evening, and rises again toward the end of sleep to peak by morning (Fig. 47-5). Growth hormone (GH), thyroid-stimulating hormone (TSH), and prolactin levels peak during sleep. Reproductive cycles are often longer than 24 hours *(ultradian)*. An example is the menstrual cycle. These rhythms are an important factor when interpreting laboratory results for hormone levels.

## Hypothalamus

Although many refer to the pituitary gland as the "master gland" of the endocrine system, most of its functions rely on its interrelationship with the hypothalamus, which lies adjacent to the pituitary gland. The hypothalamus releases substances that either stimulate or inhibit the formation and release of groups of hormones from the pituitary gland (Table 47-2). Examples of these hormones include corticotropin-releasing hormone and thyrotropin-releasing hormone. Somatostatin inhibits growth hormone release.

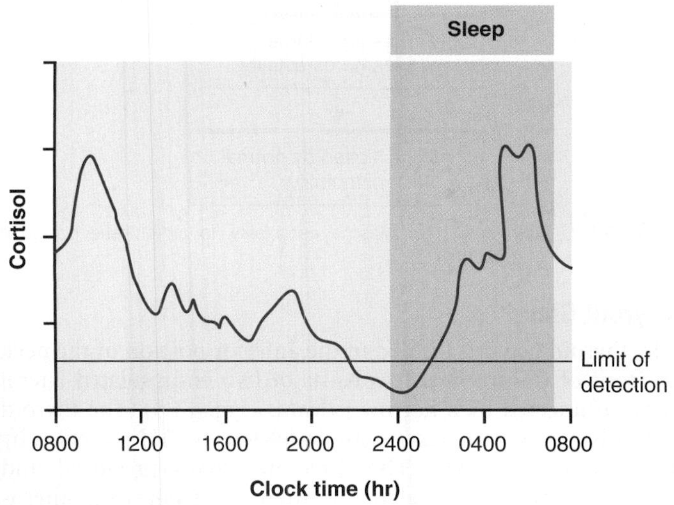


**FIG. 47-5** Circadian rhythm of cortisol secretion.

**TABLE 47-2 Hormones of the Hypothalamus**

*The following hormones from the hypothalamus target the anterior pituitary.*

**Releasing Hormones**

- Corticotropin-releasing hormone (CRH)
- Thyrotropin-releasing hormone (TRH)
- Growth hormone–releasing hormone (GHRH), or somatotropin-releasing hormone
- Gonadotropin-releasing hormone (GnRH)
- Prolactin-releasing factor (PRF)

**Inhibiting Hormones**

- Somatostatin (inhibits growth hormone release)
- Prolactin-inhibiting factor (PIF)

The hypothalamus contains neurons that receive input from the CNS, including the brainstem, limbic system, and cerebral cortex. Neurons from the hypothalamus create a circuit to facilitate coordination of the endocrine system and autonomic nervous system (ANS). The hypothalamus also coordinates the expression of complex behavioral responses, such as anger, fear, and pleasure.

## Pituitary

The pituitary gland *(hypophysis)* is located in the sella turcica under the hypothalamus at the base of the brain above the sphenoid bone (Fig. 47-1). The infundibular *(hypophyseal)* stalk connects the pituitary and hypothalamus. This stalk relays information between the hypothalamus and pituitary, creating a strong neuroendocrine connection. The pituitary consists of two major parts, the anterior lobe *(adenohypophysis)* and posterior lobe *(neurohypophysis)*. A smaller intermediate lobe produces melanocyte-stimulating hormone.

**Anterior Pituitary.** The anterior lobe of the pituitary accounts for 80% of the gland by weight. The hypothalamus regulates the anterior lobe through releasing and inhibiting hormones. These hypothalamic hormones reach the anterior pituitary through a network of capillaries known as the *hypothalamus-hypophyseal portal system*. The releasing and inhibiting hormones in turn affect the secretion of six hormones from the anterior pituitary (Fig. 47-6).

Several hormones secreted by the anterior pituitary are referred to as **tropic hormones**. Tropic hormones control the secretion of hormones by other glands. Thyroid-stimulating hormone (TSH) stimulates the thyroid gland to secrete thyroid hormones. Adrenocorticotropic hormone (ACTH) stimulates the adrenal cortex to secrete corticosteroids. Follicle-stimulating hormone (FSH) stimulates secretion of estrogen and the development of ova in women and sperm in men. Luteinizing hormone (LH) stimulates ovulation in women and secretion of sex hormones in both men and women. In men, LH is sometimes referred to as *interstitial cell–stimulating hormone (ICSH)*.

**Growth hormone (GH)** affects the growth and development of all body tissues. It has numerous biologic actions, including a role in protein, fat, and carbohydrate metabolism. *Prolactin*, or lactogenic hormone, stimulates breast development necessary for lactation after childbirth.

**Posterior Pituitary.** The posterior pituitary is composed of nerve tissue and is essentially an extension of the hypothalamus.

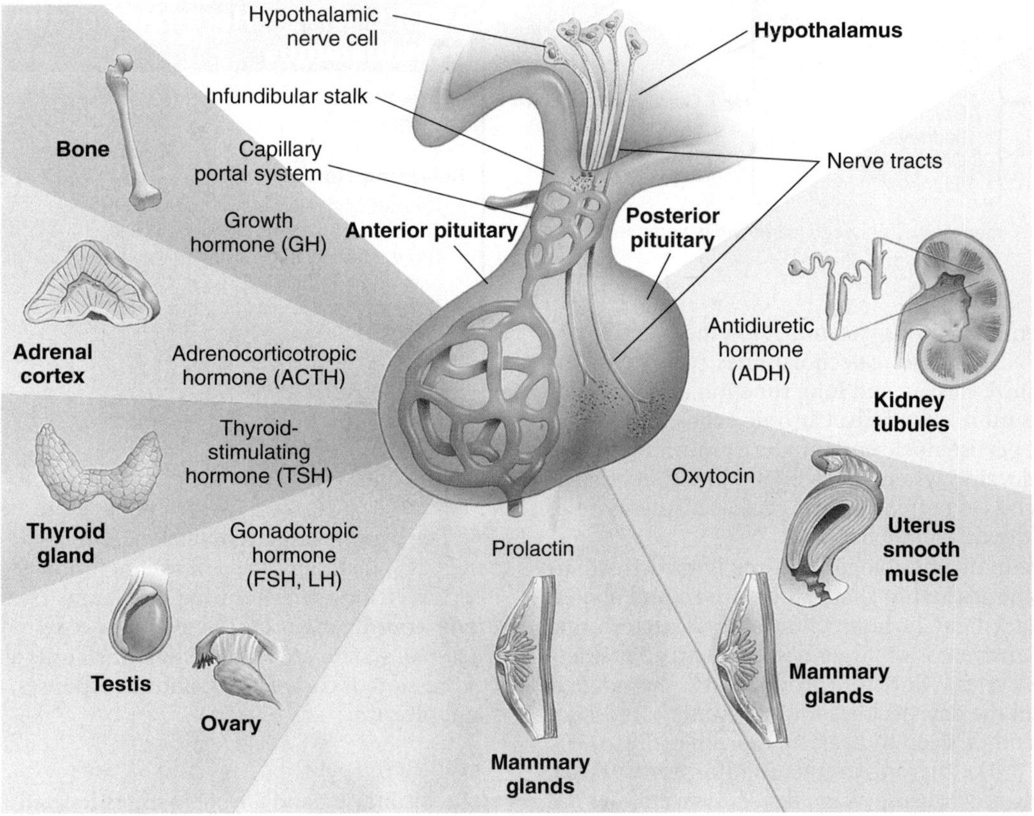


**FIG. 47-6** Relationship between the hypothalamus, pituitary, and target organs. The hypothalamus communicates with the anterior pituitary via a capillary system and with the posterior pituitary via nerve tracts. The anterior and posterior pituitary hormones are shown with their target tissues. *FSH,* Follicle-stimulating hormone; *LH,* luteinizing hormone. (Modified from Patton KT, Thibodeau GA: *Anatomy and physiology,* ed 8, St Louis, 2013, Mosby.)

Communication between the hypothalamus and posterior pituitary occurs through nerve tracts known as the *median eminence.* The hormones secreted by the posterior pituitary, **antidiuretic hormone (ADH)** and oxytocin, are produced in the hypothalamus. These hormones travel down the nerve tracts from the hypothalamus to the posterior pituitary and are stored until the appropriate stimuli trigger their release (Fig. 47-6).

The major physiologic role of ADH (also called *arginine vasopressin*) is to regulate fluid volume. It causes the renal tubules to reabsorb water, making the urine more concentrated. A rise in *plasma osmolality* (a measure of solute concentration of circulating blood) and/or hypovolemia stimulates ADH secretion (Fig. 47-7). Increases in plasma osmolality cause specialized neurons in the hypothalamus, known as *osmoreceptors,* to stimulate ADH release from the posterior pituitary. Volume receptors in large veins, heart atria, and carotid arteries that sense pressure changes (from hypovolemia) also contribute to ADH control. When ADH release is inhibited, renal tubules do not reabsorb water, resulting in a more dilute urine. ADH is also a potent vasoconstrictor.

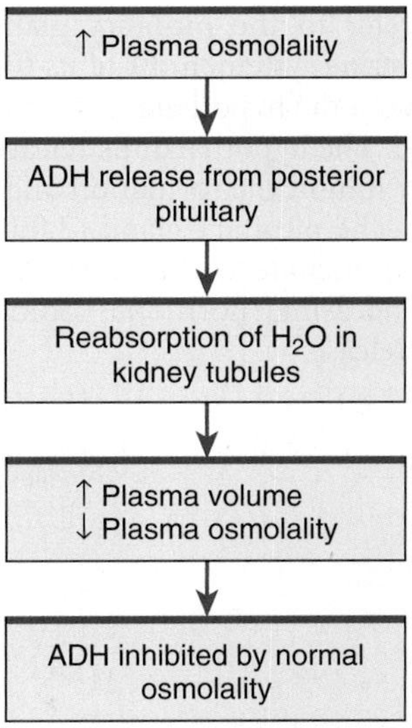


**FIG. 47-7** Relationship of plasma osmolality to antidiuretic hormone *(ADH)* release and action.

## Pineal Gland

The pineal gland is located in the brain. It is composed of photoreceptive cells. Its primary function is the secretion of the hormone *melatonin.* Melatonin secretion increases in response to exposure to the dark and decreases in response to light exposure. The gland helps to regulate circadian rhythms and the reproductive system at the onset of puberty.

## Thyroid Gland

The thyroid gland is located in the anterior portion of the neck in front of the trachea. It consists of two encapsulated lateral lobes connected by a narrow isthmus (Fig. 47-8). The thyroid gland is highly vascular. Its size is related to TSH secretion by the anterior pituitary. The three hormones produced and secreted by the thyroid gland are thyroxine ($T_4$), triiodothyronine ($T_3$), and calcitonin.

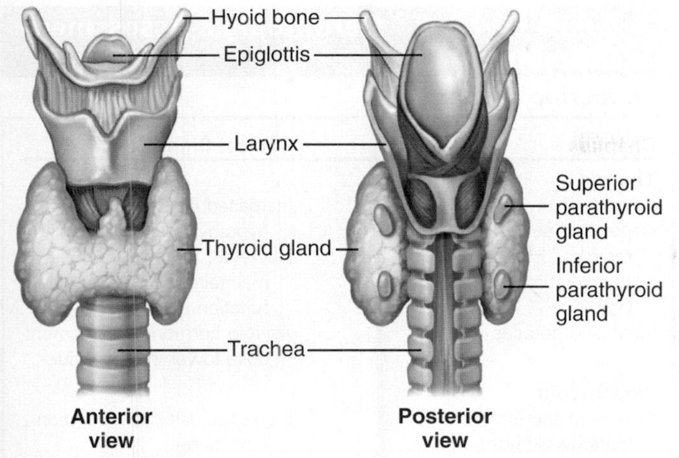


**FIG. 47-8** Thyroid and parathyroid glands. Note the surrounding structures. (From Thibodeau GA, Patton KT: *The human body in health and disease*, ed 4, St Louis, 2005, Mosby.)

**Thyroxine and Triiodothyronine.** Thyroxine ($T_4$) accounts for 90% of thyroid hormone produced by the thyroid gland. However, triiodothyronine ($T_3$) is much more potent and has greater metabolic effects. The thyroid gland directly secretes about 20% of circulating $T_3$. The remainder comes from the conversion of $T_4$ after its release into the bloodstream. Iodine is necessary for the synthesis of both $T_3$ and $T_4$. Both hormones affect metabolic rate, caloric requirements, $O_2$ consumption, carbohydrate and lipid metabolism, growth and development, brain function, and other nervous system activities. More than 99% of thyroid hormones are bound to plasma proteins, especially thyroxine-binding globulin synthesized by the liver. Only the unbound "free" hormones are biologically active.

TSH from the anterior pituitary gland stimulates thyroid hormone production and release. When circulating levels of thyroid hormone are low, the hypothalamus releases thyrotropin-releasing hormone (TRH). TRH causes the anterior pituitary to release TSH. High circulating thyroid hormone levels inhibit the secretion of both TRH from the hypothalamus and TSH from the anterior pituitary gland.

**Calcitonin.** *Calcitonin* is made by C cells (parafollicular cells) of the thyroid gland in response to high circulating calcium levels. Calcitonin lowers serum calcium levels by (1) inhibiting the transfer of calcium from the bone to blood, (2) increasing calcium storage in bone, and (3) increasing renal excretion of calcium and phosphorus. Calcitonin and parathyroid hormone (PTH) regulate calcium balance.

## Parathyroid Glands

Two pairs of parathyroid glands usually lie behind each thyroid lobe (Fig. 47-8). Although there are usually four glands, their number may range from two to six.

**Parathyroid Hormone.** The parathyroid glands secrete parathyroid hormone (PTH), also called *parathormone*. Its major role is to regulate serum calcium levels. PTH increases serum calcium levels by acting on bone, the kidneys, and indirectly on the GI tract. PTH stimulates the transfer of calcium from the bone into the blood. In the kidney, PTH promotes calcium reabsorption (moving calcium from the renal tubules back into the bloodstream) and phosphate excretion. In addition, PTH stimulates the renal conversion of vitamin D to its most active form (1,25-dihydroxyvitamin $D_3$). This form of vitamin D promotes absorption of calcium and phosphorus by the GI tract.

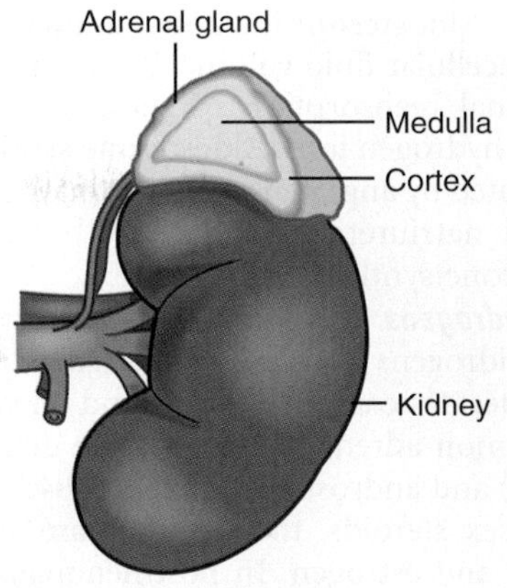


**FIG. 47-9** The adrenal gland is composed of the adrenal cortex and the adrenal medulla.

PTH secretion is regulated by a negative feedback system. When the serum calcium level is low, PTH secretion increases. When the serum calcium level rises, PTH secretion falls. In addition, high levels of active vitamin D inhibit secretion of PTH, and low levels of magnesium stimulate PTH secretion.

## Adrenal Glands

The adrenal glands are small, paired, highly vascular glands located on the upper portion of each kidney. Each gland consists of two parts: medulla and cortex (Fig. 47-9). Each part has distinct functions, and they act independently from one another.

**Adrenal Medulla.** The adrenal medulla is the inner part of the adrenal gland. It consists of sympathetic postganglionic neurons. The medulla secretes the catecholamines *epinephrine* (adrenaline), *norepinephrine* (noradrenaline), and *dopamine*. Catecholamines are considered neurotransmitters when secreted by neurons and hormones when secreted by the adrenal medulla. They are an essential part of the SNS's "fight or flight" response.

**Adrenal Cortex.** The adrenal cortex is the outer part of the adrenal gland. It secretes several steroid hormones, including *glucocorticoids, mineralocorticoids,* and *androgens.* Cholesterol is the precursor for steroid hormone synthesis. Glucocorticoids (e.g., cortisol) are named for their effects on glucose metabolism. They inhibit the inflammatory response and are considered antiinflammatory. Mineralocorticoids (e.g., aldosterone) are essential for maintaining fluid and electrolyte balance. The term corticosteroid refers to hormones synthesized by the adrenal cortex, excluding androgens.

***Cortisol.*** Cortisol, the most abundant and potent glucocorticoid, is necessary to maintain life and protect the body from stress. It is secreted in a diurnal pattern (Fig. 47-5). A negative feedback mechanism controls cortisol secretion. The release of corticotropin-releasing hormone (CRH) from the hypothalamus stimulates the secretion of ACTH by the anterior pituitary.

One major function of cortisol is the regulation of blood glucose concentration by stimulating hepatic glucose formation (*gluconeogenesis*). Cortisol inhibits peripheral glucose use in the fasting state, inhibits protein synthesis, and stimulates the mobilization of glycerol and free fatty acids. It helps maintain vascular integrity and fluid volume through its action on mineralocorticoid receptors. Cortisol decreases the inflammatory response by stabilizing the membranes of cellular lysosomes and preventing increased capillary permeability. Stress, burns, infection, fever, acute anxiety, and hypoglycemia increase cortisol levels.

***Aldosterone.*** Aldosterone is a potent mineralocorticoid that maintains extracellular fluid volume. It acts on the renal tubule to promote renal reabsorption of sodium and excretion of potassium and hydrogen ions. Aldosterone synthesis and secretion are stimulated by angiotensin II, hyponatremia, and hyperkalemia. Atrial natriuretic peptide (ANP) and hypokalemia inhibit aldosterone synthesis and release.

***Adrenal Androgens.*** The adrenal cortex secretes small amounts of androgens that are converted to sex steroids in peripheral tissues: testosterone in men and estrogen in women. The most common adrenal androgens are dehydroepiandrosterone (DHEA) and androstenedione. Because they are precursors to other sex steroids, their actions are similar to those of testosterone and estrogen. In postmenopausal women, the major source of estrogen is from the peripheral conversion of adrenal androgen to estrogen.

### Pancreas

The pancreas is a long, tapered, lobular, soft gland located behind the stomach and anterior to the first and second lumbar vertebrae. The pancreas has both exocrine and endocrine functions. The hormone-secreting portion of the pancreas is the *islets of Langerhans.* The islets account for less than 2% of the gland and consist of four types of hormone-secreting cells: α, β, delta, and F cells. α Cells make and secrete the hormone glucagon. β Cells make and secrete insulin and amylin. Delta cells make and secrete somatostatin. F (or PP) cells secrete pancreatic polypeptide.

**Glucagon.** Glucagon is released from pancreatic α cells and the gut in response to low blood glucose levels, protein ingestion, and exercise. Glucagon increases blood glucose, providing fuel for energy by stimulating glycogenolysis (breakdown of glycogen into glucose), gluconeogenesis (formation of glucose from non-carbohydrate molecules), and ketogenesis.[3] Glucagon and insulin function in a reciprocal manner to maintain normal blood glucose levels.

**Insulin.** Insulin is the principal regulator of metabolism and storage of ingested carbohydrates, fats, and proteins. Insulin facilitates glucose transport into cells, transport of amino acids across muscle membranes, and the synthesis of amino acids into protein in the peripheral tissues. However, the brain, nerves, lens of the eye, hepatocytes, erythrocytes, and cells in the intestinal mucosa and kidney tubules are not dependent on insulin for glucose uptake. After a meal, insulin is responsible for the utilization and storage of nutrients *(anabolism).* An increased blood glucose level is the major stimulus for insulin synthesis and secretion. Low blood glucose levels, glucagon, somatostatin, hypokalemia, and catecholamines usually inhibit insulin secretion.

### Gerontologic Considerations: Effects of Aging on Endocrine System

Normal aging has many effects on the endocrine system (Table 47-3). These include (1) decreased hormone production and secretion, (2) altered hormone metabolism and biologic activity, (3) decreased responsiveness of target tissues to hormones, and (4) alterations in circadian rhythms.

Assessing the effects of aging on the endocrine system may be difficult because the subtle changes of aging may mimic manifestations of endocrine disorders. Endocrine problems may manifest differently in an older adult than in a younger person. Older adults may have multiple co-morbidities and take medications that alter the body's usual response to endocrine function. Symptoms of endocrine dysfunction such as fatigue, constipation, or mental impairment may be attributed to aging, resulting in delayed treatment.

**TABLE 47-3 Gerontologic Assessment Differences**

***Endocrine System***

| Changes | Clinical Significance |
|---|---|
| **Thyroid** | |
| Atrophy of thyroid gland | Increased incidence of hypothyroidism with aging |
| Decreased secretion of triiodothyronine ($T_3$), thyroxine ($T_4$), thyroid-stimulating hormone (TSH) | However, most older adults maintain adequate thyroid function. |
| Increased nodules | Thyroid hormone replacement dose lower in older adults |
| **Parathyroid** | |
| Increased secretion of PTH (parathyroid hormone) | Increased calcium resorption from bone |
| Increased basal level of PTH | Hypercalcemia, hypercalciuria (may reflect defective renal mechanism) |
| **Adrenal Cortex** | |
| Adrenal cortex becomes more fibrotic and slightly smaller | Decreased metabolic clearance rate for glucocorticoids |
| Decreased metabolism of cortisol | |
| Decreased plasma levels of adrenal androgens and aldosterone | |
| **Adrenal Medulla** | |
| Increased secretion and basal level of norepinephrine | Decreased responsiveness to β-adrenergic agonists and receptor blockers |
| Decreased β-adrenergic receptor response to norepinephrine | May partly explain increased incidence of hypertension with aging |
| **Pancreas** | |
| Increase in fibrosis and fatty deposits in pancreas | May partly contribute to increased incidence of diabetes mellitus with advanced aging |
| Increased glucose intolerance with decreased sensitivity to insulin | |
| **Gonads** | |
| *Women:* Decline in estrogen secretion | Experience symptoms associated with menopause<br>Have increased risk for arteriosclerosis and osteoporosis |
| *Men:* Decline in testosterone secretion | Men may or may not experience symptoms |

## ASSESSMENT OF ENDOCRINE SYSTEM

Endocrine dysfunction is generally the result of too much or too little of a specific hormone. The onset of symptoms is often gradual. The subtle or vague symptoms are often attributed to other physiologic or psychologic causes. Consequently, patients with endocrine dysfunction may present with fluid and electrolyte imbalances, altered tissue perfusion, inadequate coping mechanisms, alterations in cardiac rhythm, or changes in skin integrity that can be interpreted as many other conditions. Alternatively, patients may present with acute symptoms that are life threatening and demand immediate intervention.

## CASE STUDY

### *Patient Introduction*

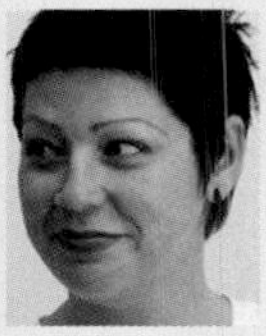

(©iStockphoto/ Thinkstock)

L.M. is a 35-yr-old Hispanic woman who comes to the clinic complaining of "just not feeling well." She is accompanied by H.H., her female partner. L.M. states that she has gained a lot of weight despite trying to watch her diet and just seems to be getting more and more tired. H.H. voices concerns about changes in her partner's energy level.

**Discussion Questions**

1. What are the possible causes of L.M.'s weight gain, fatigue, and irritability?
2. What would be your priority assessment of L.M.?
3. What questions would you ask L.M.?

You will learn more about L.M. and her condition as you read through this assessment chapter.

(See p. 1111 for more information on L.M.)

Answers available at *http://evolve.elsevier.com/Lewis/medsurg.*

## Subjective Data

Information obtained from the patient can provide important clues as to the functioning of the endocrine system. You will need to obtain a thorough history from the patient and/or a caregiver if the patient's mental acuity is compromised.

### Important Health Information

***Past Health History.*** Patients with endocrine disorders often present with nonspecific complaints. The chief complaint may relate to not just one but a group of symptoms. The most common presenting problems include fatigue, weakness, menstrual irregularities, and weight changes. It is important to determine if the onset of symptoms has been gradual or sudden and what the patient has done about them.

Because some of the more general signs of dysfunction are the easiest to overlook, you must evaluate any reported or observed changes in weight, appetite, skin, libido, mental acuity, emotional stability, or energy levels.

***Medications.*** Ask about the use of all medications (both prescription and over-the-counter drugs), herbs, and dietary supplements. Ask about the reason for taking the drug, the dosage, and the length of time the drug has been taken. In particular, ask about the use of hormone replacements. Knowing that the patient is currently taking hormone replacements such as insulin, thyroid hormone, or corticosteroids (e.g., prednisone) alerts the nurse to potential adverse drug events. For example, corticosteroids may increase blood glucose levels and cause bone loss with long-term use. Thyroid preparations may cause tachycardia or dysrhythmias. Drug-to-drug interactions and adverse effects of nonhormonal medications can contribute to endocrine problems.

***Surgery or Other Treatments.*** Inquire about past medical, surgical, and obstetric history, including number of pregnancies and live births. Ask about traumatic events, birth weight, growth patterns, and stages of physical and emotional development. The depth of information required may vary depending on the presenting condition. For example, data regarding past radiation therapy to the head and neck are important when thyroid or pituitary dysfunction is suspected.

**Functional Health Patterns.** Key questions to ask the patient with an endocrine problem are summarized in Table 47-4.

***Health Perception–Health Management Pattern.*** Heredity often plays an important role in the development of endocrine dysfunction. Ask about first-degree relatives with diabetes mellitus, thyroid disease, or endocrine gland cancers, since these conditions have a familial tendency. A genetic assessment of family members may be appropriate.

## GENETIC RISK ALERT

**Pituitary**

- Nephrogenic diabetes insipidus can be inherited as a sex-linked or autosomal disorder.

**Thyroid**

- Genetics has a role in many cases of hypothyroid and hyperthyroid disorders.
- Hashimoto's thyroiditis, the most common cause of hypothyroidism, and Graves' disease, a cause of hyperthyroidism, are autoimmune disorders. Both likely result from a combination of genetic and environmental factors.[4]

**Multiple Endocrine Neoplasia**

- Multiple endocrine neoplasia (MEN) involves tumors in two or more different endocrine glands.
- There are several types of MEN. Mutations of *MEN1, RET,* and *CDKN1B* genes determine the type.
- The features of MEN are relatively consistent within any one family.
- A common tumor associated with MEN type 2 is medullary thyroid carcinoma.[4]

**Diabetes Mellitus**

- Genetics has a strong role in the development of type 2 diabetes and to a lesser extent in type 1 diabetes.

***Nutritional-Metabolic Pattern.*** Changes in appetite and weight can indicate endocrine dysfunction. Weight loss with increased appetite may indicate hyperthyroidism or diabetes mellitus. Weight gain may indicate hypothyroidism or hypocortisolism. Obese persons are more likely to develop type 2 diabetes.

Ask if there have been problems with nausea, vomiting, or diarrhea. Difficulty swallowing or a change in neck size may indicate an enlarged thyroid gland. Increased SNS activity, including nervousness, palpitations, sweating, and tremors, may indicate thyroid dysfunction or a rare tumor of the adrenal medulla *(pheochromocytoma).* Heat or cold intolerance may indicate hyperthyroidism or hypothyroidism, respectively.

Ask about changes in the patient's skin, particularly on the face, neck, hands, or body creases. Changes in skin texture and skin that seems thicker or drier may indicate endocrine dysfunction. A patient with hypothyroidism or excess GH may have skin that feels coarse or leathery. Ask if the patient has noticed any change in the distribution of hair anywhere on the body.

***Elimination Pattern.*** Because maintaining fluid balance is a major role of the endocrine system, questions related to fluid intake and elimination patterns may uncover endocrine dysfunction. For example, increased thirst and urination can indicate diabetes mellitus (pancreas disorder) or diabetes insipidus (pituitary disorder). Ask about the frequency and consistency of bowel movements. Frequent defecation may indicate hyperthyroidism or autonomic neuropathy of diabetes mellitus. Constipation occurs with hypothyroidism, hypoparathyroidism, and hypopituitarism.

***Activity-Exercise Pattern.*** Determine if there are any acute or gradual changes in energy level or persistent fatigue. Changes in

## TABLE 47-4 Health History

***Endocrine System***

**Health Perception–Health Management**
- What is your usual day like?
- Have you noticed any changes in your ability to perform your usual activities compared with last year? Five years ago?*

**Nutritional-Metabolic**
- What is your weight and height?
- How much do you want to weigh?
- Have there been any changes in your appetite or weight?*
- Have you noticed any changes in the distribution of the hair anywhere on your body?*
- Have you noticed any changes in the color of your skin, particularly on your face, neck, hands, or body creases?*
- Has the texture of your skin changed? For example, does it seem thicker and drier than it used to?*
- Have you noticed any difficulty swallowing, throat pain, or hoarseness? Is the top button on your shirt or blouse more difficult to button?*
- Do you feel more nervous than you used to? Do you notice your heart pounding or that you sweat when you do not think you should be sweating?
- Do you have difficulty holding things because of shakiness of your hands?*
- Do you feel that most rooms are too hot or too cold? Do you frequently have to put on a sweater, or feel as though you need to open windows when others in the room seem comfortable?*
- Do you have or have you had any wounds that were slow to heal?*

**Elimination**
- Do you have to get up at night to urinate? If so, how many times? Do you keep water by your bed at night?
- Have you ever had a kidney stone?*
- Describe your usual bowel pattern. Have you noted any bowel changes?*
- Do you use anything, such as laxatives, to help you move your bowels?*

**Activity-Exercise**
- What is your usual activity pattern during a typical day?
- Do you have a planned exercise program? If yes, what is it and have you had to make any changes in this routine lately? If so, why and what kinds of changes?
- Do you experience fatigue with or without activity?*
- Have you had any trouble with breathing?*

**Sleep-Rest**
- How many hours do you sleep at night? Do you feel rested on awakening?
- Are you ever awakened by sweating during the night?*
- Do you have nightmares?*

**Cognitive-Perceptual**
- How is your memory? Have you noticed any changes?*
- Have you experienced any blurring or double vision?*
- When was your last eye examination?

**Self-Perception–Self-Concept**
- Have you noticed any changes in your physical appearance or size?*
- Are you concerned about your weight?*
- Do you feel you are able to do what you think you should be capable of doing? If not, why not?
- Does your health problem affect how you feel about yourself?*

**Role-Relationship**
- Do you have a support system or partner? Are you married? Do you have any children? Do you think you are able to take care of your family and home? If not, why not?
- Where do you work? What kind of work do you do? Are you able to do what is expected of you and what you expect of yourself?
- Are you retired? What type of work did you do before you retired? How do you spend your time now that you have retired?

**Sexuality-Reproductive**

***Women***
- When did you start to menstruate? Was this earlier or later than other women in your family?
- When was your last menstrual period? Do you have scant, heavy, or irregular menstrual flows?
- How many children have you had? How much did they weigh at birth? Were you told you had diabetes during any pregnancy?*
- Are you menopausal? If so, for how long?
- Are you attempting to get pregnant but cannot?*
- Are you postmenopausal? If so, do you have any bleeding from your uterus?

***Men***
- Have you noticed any changes in your ability to get and maintain an erection?*
- Are you trying to have children but cannot?*

**Coping–Stress Tolerance**
- What kind of stressors do you have?
- How do you deal with stress or problems?
- What is your support system? To whom do you turn when you have a problem?

**Value-Belief**
- Do you think medicine should still be taken even though you feel okay?
- Do any of your prescribed therapies cause any conflict in your value-belief system?*

*If yes, describe.

activity level can identify a patient with chronic fatigue secondary to hypothyroidism, hypocortisolism, or diabetes mellitus.

***Sleep-Rest Pattern.*** Ask the patient how many hours he or she typically sleeps, and if he or she feels rested on awakening. Sleep disturbances can result from nocturia, nightmares, anxiety, depression, or insomnia that occurs with diabetes or thyroid dysfunction.

***Cognitive-Perceptual Pattern.*** Memory deficits are apparent in hypothyroidism and occur with changes in sodium levels. Hyponatremia can occur because of inappropriate secretion of antidiuretic hormone (SIADH) or pituitary tumors. These issues can occur gradually, so it is sometimes difficult for family members or care providers to identify changes in cognition. Gathering information from patient and family regarding memory, cognitive abilities, and balance can increase the chances of an earlier diagnosis.

***Self-Perception–Self-Concept Pattern.*** Many endocrine disorders may affect a patient's self-esteem because of associated changes in physical appearance. For example, weight gain associated with hypothyroidism or exophthalmos and goiter associated with hyperthyroidism can cause problems related to body image.

***Role-Relationship Pattern.*** Questions related to roles and relationships can highlight depression, chronic fatigue, and sleep disorders. With chronic fatigue, depression and anxiety, patients and their families will experience stressed relationships. Questions related to home life and the patient's ability to fulfill their role in the family will aid in the identification of these disorders.

***Sexuality-Reproductive Pattern.*** Growth hormone, prolactin, LH, FSH, testosterone, and estrogen are regulated by the endocrine system. Therefore menstrual dysfunction, hirsutism, infertility, and growth disorders can be a result of endocrine disorders. Some women experience hypothyroidism during or after menopause. Other patients begin to develop type 2 diabetes during middle age when sex hormones are changing. Document the presence of abnormal secondary sex characteristics, such as facial hair *(hirsutism)* in women. Obtain a detailed history of menstruation and pregnancy. Menstrual dysfunction can occur with disorders of the ovaries and pituitary, thyroid, and adrenal glands. A history of large-birth-weight babies may indicate gestational diabetes, which may put the patient at a higher risk of developing type 2 diabetes later in life. Male sexual dysfunction may take the form of impotence, decreased libido, infertility, or the lack of development of secondary sexual characteristics. Retrograde ejaculation can occur in diabetes mellitus.

***Coping–Stress Tolerance Pattern.*** Because stress exacerbates some endocrine conditions, ask patients about their stress level and usual coping patterns. Patients with adrenal insufficiency have difficulty dealing with stress. These patients are at risk for developing hypotension and fluid and electrolyte imbalance. Patients' perception of the impact of their condition and treatments on their lifestyle is significant.

***Value-Belief Pattern.*** Determining a patient's ability to make lifestyle changes is an important nursing function. Identify the patient's value-belief patterns so that you can help to determine appropriate treatment regimens. This is particularly important in a condition such as diabetes mellitus, which may require major lifestyle changes. Other disorders, such as hypothyroidism or hypocortisolism, may be managed with medications but require lifelong monitoring with an HCP.

## Objective Data

Most endocrine glands (with the exception of the thyroid and testes) are inaccessible to direct examination. Assessment can be accomplished using objective data, including physical examination and diagnostic tests. It is essential to understand the actions of hormones in order to assess the function of a gland by monitoring the target tissue.

**Physical Examination.** Specific clinical findings for the various endocrine problems are discussed in Chapters 48 and 49. Regardless of the type of endocrine dysfunction, use the following general examination.[5]

Take a full set of vital signs at the beginning of the examination. Variations in temperature, heart rate, and blood pressure can occur with a variety of endocrine-related problems.

Include a history of growth and development patterns, weight distribution and changes, and comparisons of these factors with normal findings. Calculate body mass index (BMI) to assess nutritional status.

Endocrine disorders may cause changes in mental and emotional status. Throughout the examination, assess the patient's orientation, alertness, memory, cognitive abilities, affect, personality, and anxiety and the appropriateness of his or her behavior.

### CASE STUDY—cont'd

#### *Subjective Data*

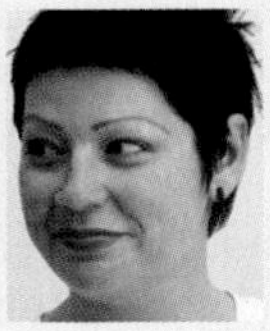
(©iStockphoto/Thinkstock)

A focused subjective assessment of L.M. revealed the following information:

- ***PMH:*** Denies any medical or surgical history. Has not seen an HCP for 8 yr.
- ***Medications:*** None.
- ***Health Perception–Health Management:*** L.M. works as a receptionist for a local law firm and states it is all she can do some days to make it through the work day. She states she frequently wakes up with a headache and goes to bed with the same headache, describing it as a dull, throbbing ache between her eyes. She definitely does not have the energy she had 5 yr ago or even 6 mo ago. She used to enjoy gardening and going out with friends but now can barely manage work and coming home.
- ***Nutritional-Metabolic:*** L.M. reports a steady weight gain over the past 6 mo, mainly in her abdominal area. She feels as if she looks pregnant but knows that is not possible. Her appetite has decreased, but she is not able to lose any weight. She says she feels "bloated." She complains of facial hair growth and notices she is bruising easily. L.M. denies difficulty with swallowing, hoarseness, palpitations, or tremors.
- ***Elimination:*** Denies any changes or difficulty with urination or bowel movements.
- ***Activity-Exercise:*** L.M. states that she has no ambition to exercise. She is just too tired at the end of the workday and has no energy on the weekends either. She complains of leg cramps with walking.
- ***Sleep-Rest:*** Sleeps 10+ hr at night but does not feel rested on awakening.
- ***Cognitive-Perceptual:*** L.M. is worried she is going crazy. She finds herself easily angered and irritable, frequently snapping at co-workers and her partner. She states this is not her usual self. At first, she thought it was because she was dealing with a constant, dull headache. Lately, she has noticed that her vision is blurry and that is making work and life even more difficult and stressful. When asked about her headache, she states it hurts between her eyes. She rates the pain as a 4 on a scale of 0 to 10 and states that ibuprofen does not ease the pain. The pain is typically worse on arising in the morning. It slowly decreases during the day.
- ***Self-Perception–Self-Concept:*** L.M. hates the way she looks. She says when she looks in the mirror, she can't believe what she sees. She feels as if she has aged 10 yr over the past 6 mo and has gained weight in her face, neck, and trunk. She is concerned that her scalp hair is thinning, and she is growing a beard. She states that she is beginning to wonder if she is "turning into a man"!
- ***Coping–Stress Tolerance:*** L.M. states that she is finding it more and more difficult to cope with the stresses of her job, her relationship with her partner, and life in general. She believes her emotions are very "raw and labile," totally different from the easy-going, smiling person she had once prided herself in being.

**Discussion Questions**

1. Which subjective assessment findings are of most concern to you?
2. Based on the subjective assessment findings, what should be included in the physical assessment? What would you be looking for?

You will learn more about the physical examination of the endocrine system in the next section.

(See p. 1112 for more information on L.M.)

Answers available at *http://evolve.elsevier.com/Lewis/medsurg.*

***Integument.*** Assess the color and texture of the skin, hair, and nails. Note the overall skin color as well as pigmentation and possible ecchymosis (bruise). Decreased skin pigmentation can occur in hypopituitarism, hypothyroidism, and hypoparathyroidism. Hyperpigmentation, or "bronzing" of the skin (particularly on knuckles, elbows, knees, genitalia, and palmar creases), is a classic finding in a form of adrenal insufficiency known as *Addison's disease.* Palpate the skin for texture and moisture. Examine hair distribution on the head, face, trunk, and extremities. Assess the hair's appearance and texture. Hair loss, excessive hair growth, or dull, brittle hair may indicate endocrine dysfunction. Assess for delayed wound healing.

***Head.*** Inspect the size and contour of the head. Facial features should be symmetric. Hyperreflexia and facial muscle contraction upon percussion of the facial nerve *(Chvostek's sign)* may occur in hypoparathyroidism. Inspect the eyes for position, symmetry, and shape. Large and protruding eyes (exophthalmos) are associated with hyperthyroidism. Assess visual acuity using a Snellen eye chart. Visual field loss may indicate a pituitary tumor. In the mouth, inspect the buccal mucosa, condition of teeth, and tongue size. Note hair distribution on the scalp and face. Hearing loss is common in acromegaly from excess GH.[6]

***Neck.*** The thyroid gland is not usually visible during inspection. A feature that distinguishes the thyroid from other masses in the neck is its upward movement on swallowing. Inspect the neck while the patient swallows a sip of water. The neck should appear symmetric without lumps or bulging.

Palpate the thyroid for its size, shape, symmetry, and tenderness and for any nodules. *Goiter*, an enlarged thyroid gland, can occur with hyper- or hypothyroidism. Be careful not to press too hard or massage an enlarged thyroid gland. This can cause a sudden release of thyroid hormone into an already overloaded system. An experienced clinician should perform palpation in patients with a known diagnosis of hyperthyroidism.

Perform palpation using a posterior or anterior approach. For *anterior palpation,* stand in front of the patient, with the patient's neck flexed. Place your thumb horizontally with the upper edge along the lower border of the cricoid cartilage. Then move your thumb over the isthmus as the patient swallows water. Place your fingers laterally to the anterior border of the sternocleidomastoid muscle, and palpate each lateral lobe before and while the patient swallows water.

For *posterior palpation,* stand behind the patient (Fig. 47-10). With the thumbs of both hands resting on the nape of the patient's neck, use your index and middle fingers of both hands to feel for the thyroid isthmus and for the anterior surfaces of the lateral lobes. To relax the neck muscles, ask the patient to flex the neck slightly forward and to the right. Displace the thyroid cartilage to the right with your left hand and fingers. Palpate with your right hand after placing the thumb deep and behind the sternocleidomastoid muscle with the index and middle fingers in front of it. Ask the patient to swallow water, and feel for the thyroid to move up. In a normal person, the thyroid is often not palpable. If palpable, it usually feels smooth with a firm consistency. It is not tender with gentle pressure. If nodules, enlargement, asymmetry, or hardness (abnormal findings) are present, refer the patient for further evaluation. Auscultate the lateral lobes of an enlarged thyroid gland with the stethoscope bell to identify a *bruit,* a soft swishing sound that may indicate a goiter or hyperthyroidism.

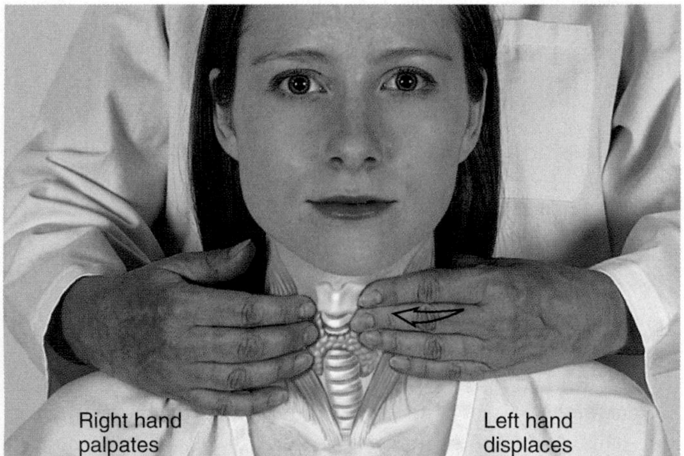


**FIG. 47-10** Posterior palpation of the thyroid gland. (From Jarvis C: *Physical examination and health assessment,* ed 6, St Louis, 2012, Saunders.)

***Thorax.*** Inspect the thorax for shape and characteristics of the skin. Note the presence of breast gynecomastia in men. Auscultate lung sounds and heart sounds. Note any adventitious lung sounds (wheezing, diminished sounds) or extra heart sounds. Signs of fluid overload or heart failure may be present in patients with secretion of inappropriate antidiuretic hormone or hypothyroidism (SIADH).

***Abdomen.*** Inspect the contour of the abdomen and note the symmetry and color. Cushing syndrome (hypercortisolism) causes the skin to be fragile, resulting in purple-blue striae across the abdomen. Note general obesity or truncal obesity. Auscultate bowel sounds.

***Extremities.*** Assess the size, shape, symmetry, and general proportion of hands and feet. Patients with acromegaly from pituitary tumors may have large hands and feet. Inspect the skin for changes in pigmentation, lesions, and edema. Evaluate muscle strength and deep tendon reflexes. In the upper extremities, assess for tremors by placing a piece of paper on the outstretched fingers, palm down. Muscular spasms of the hand elicited on application of an occlusive BP cuff for 3 minutes *(Trousseau's sign)* may occur in hypoparathyroidism.

***Genitalia.*** Inspect the genital hair distribution pattern, since it may be altered with hormone irregularities.

Assessment abnormalities related to the endocrine system are presented in Table 47-5. A focused assessment of the endocrine system is presented on p. 1114.

## CASE STUDY—cont'd

### *Objective Data: Physical Examination*

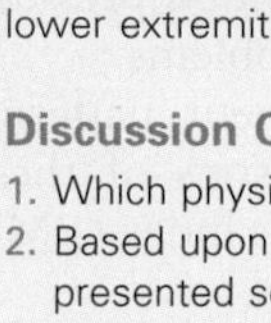

(©iStockphoto/ Thinkstock)

A focused assessment of L.M. reveals the following:

L.M. is sitting on the edge of the examination table. She appears somewhat anxious. Her BP is 190/80, heart rate 84, respiratory rate 20, temp 98.6° F (37° C). Her weight is 160 lb, and she is 5 ft 4 inches tall. L.M.'s face is reddened and puffy, and she appears to have a lump on the back of her neck and shoulders. She has some acne on her face, along with some hair growth on her upper lip and chin area. Her abdomen is protruding, but her arms and legs are thin. She has +1 edema in her ankles bilaterally. There are several ecchymotic areas on her upper and lower extremities, as well as purple stretch marks on her abdomen.

**Discussion Questions**

1. Which physical assessment findings are of most concern to you?
2. Based upon the subjective and objective assessment data presented so far, what are three priority nursing diagnoses?
3. What diagnostic studies would you expect to be ordered?

You will learn more about diagnostic studies related to the endocrine system in the next section.

(See p. 1118 for more information on L.M.)

Answers available at *http://evolve.elsevier.com/Lewis/medsurg.*

## TABLE 47-5 Assessment Abnormalities

### *Endocrine System*

| Finding | Description | Possible Etiology and Significance |
|---|---|---|
| **Integument** | | |
| **Hyperpigmentation** | Darkening of the skin, particularly in creases and skinfolds | Addison's disease caused by increased secretion of melanocyte-stimulating hormone, acanthosis nigricans |
| **Depigmentation (vitiligo)** | Patchy areas of light skin | May be a marker of autoimmune endocrine disorders |
| **Striae** | Purplish red marks below the skin surface. Usually seen on abdomen, breasts, and buttocks | Cushing syndrome |
| **Changes in skin texture** | Thick, cold, dry skin | Hypothyroidism |
| | Thick, leathery, oily skin | Growth hormone excess (acromegaly) |
| | Warm, smooth, moist skin | Hyperthyroidism |
| **Changes in hair distribution** | Hair loss | Hypothyroidism, hyperthyroidism, decreased pituitary secretion |
| | Diminished axillary and pubic hair | Cortisol deficiency |
| | Hirsutism (excessive facial hair on women) | Cushing syndrome, prolactinoma (a pituitary tumor) |
| **Skin ulceration** | Areas of ulcerated skin, most commonly found on legs and feet | Peripheral neuropathy and peripheral vascular disease, which are contributory factors in the development of diabetic foot ulcers |
| **Bruises easily** | Multiple bruises over various parts of body | Cushing syndrome |
| **Edema** | Generalized edema | Mucopolysaccharide accumulation in tissue in hypothyroidism |
| **Head and Neck** | | |
| **Visual changes** | Decreased visual acuity and/or decreased peripheral vision | Pituitary gland enlargement or tumor leading to pressure on optic nerve |
| **Exophthalmos** | Eyeball protrusion from orbits | Occurs in hyperthyroidism as a result of fluid accumulation in eye and retroorbital tissue |
| **Moon face** | Periorbital edema and facial fullness | Cushing syndrome as a result of increased cortisol secretion |
| **Myxedema** | Puffiness, periorbital edema, masklike affect | Hydrophilic mucopolysaccharides infiltrating dermis in patients with hypothyroidism |
| **Goiter** | Generalized enlargement of thyroid gland | Hyperthyroidism, hypothyroidism, iodine deficiency |
| **Thyroid nodule(s)** | Localized enlargement of thyroid gland | May be benign or malignant |
| **Cardiovascular** | | |
| **Chest pain** | Angina caused by increased metabolic demands, effusions | Hyperthyroidism, hypothyroidism |
| **Dysrhythmias** | Tachycardia, atrial fibrillation | Hypothyroidism or hyperthyroidism, hypoparathyroidism or hyperparathyroidism, pheochromocytoma |
| **Hypertension** | Elevated BP caused by increased metabolic demands and catecholamines | Hyperthyroidism, pheochromocytoma, Cushing syndrome |
| **Fluid overload or signs of heart failure** | Crackles in the lungs, peripheral edema, shortness of breath | Syndrome of inappropriate antidiuretic hormone, hypothyroidism, myxedema |
| **Musculoskeletal** | | |
| **Changes in muscular strength or muscle mass** | Generalized weakness and/or fatigue | Common symptoms associated with many endocrine problems, including pituitary, thyroid, parathyroid, and adrenal dysfunctions<br>Diabetes mellitus, diabetes insipidus |
| | Decreased muscle mass | Specifically seen in those with growth hormone deficiency and in Cushing syndrome secondary to protein wasting |
| **Enlargement of bones and cartilage** | Coarsening of facial features. Increases in size of hands and feet over a period of several years | Gradual enlargement and thickening of bony tissue occurring with growth hormone excess in adults as seen in acromegaly secondary to pituitary dysfunction |
| **Nutrition** | | |
| **Changes in weight** | Weight loss | Hyperthyroidism caused by increases in metabolism, type 1 diabetes mellitus, diabetic ketoacidosis |
| **Altered glucose levels** | Weight gain | Hypothyroidism, Cushing syndrome, type 2 diabetes mellitus |
| | Increased serum glucose | Diabetes mellitus, Cushing syndrome, growth hormone excess |
| **Neurologic** | | |
| **Lethargy** | State of mental sluggishness or somnolence | Hypothyroidism |
| **Tetany** | Intermittent involuntary muscle spasms usually involving the extremities | Severe hypocalcemia that can occur with hypoparathyroidism |
| **Seizure** | Sudden involuntary contraction of muscles | Consequence of a pituitary tumor<br>Hypervolemia and hyponatremia associated with syndrome of inappropriate antidiuretic hormone<br>Complications of diabetes mellitus, severe hypothyroidism |
| **Increased deep tendon reflexes** | Hyperreflexia | Hyperthyroidism, hypoparathyroidism |
| **Gastrointestinal** | | |
| **Constipation** | Passage of infrequent hard stools | Hypothyroidism, hyperparathyroidism |

## TABLE 47-5 Assessment Abnormalities
### *Endocrine System—cont'd*

| Finding | Description | Possible Etiology and Significance |
|---|---|---|
| **Reproductive** | | |
| **Changes in reproductive function** | Menstrual irregularities, decreased libido, decreased fertility, impotence | Pituitary hypofunction, growth hormone excess, thyroid dysfunction, adrenocortical dysfunction |
| **Other** | | |
| **Polyuria** | Excessive urine output | Diabetes mellitus (secondary to hyperglycemia) or diabetes insipidus (associated with decreased ADH) |
| **Polydipsia** | Excessive thirst | Extreme water losses in diabetes mellitus (with severe hyperglycemia), diabetes insipidus, dehydration |
| **Decreased urine output** | Decreased water reabsorption from kidney tubules | Syndrome of inappropriate antidiuretic hormone |
| **Thermoregulation** | Cold sensitivity | Hypothyroidism caused by a slowing of metabolic processes |
| | Heat intolerance | Hyperthyroidism caused by excessive metabolism |

## FOCUSED ASSESSMENT
### *Endocrine System*

*Use this checklist to ensure the key assessment steps have been done.*

**Subjective**

*Ask the patient about any of the following and note responses.*

| | | |
|---|---|---|
| Excessive or increased thirst | Y | N |
| Excessive or decreased urination | Y | N |
| Excessive hunger | Y | N |
| Intolerance to heat or cold | Y | N |
| Excessive sweating | Y | N |
| Recent weight gain or loss | Y | N |

**Objective: Diagnostic**

Check the following laboratory results for critical values.

| | |
|---|---|
| Potassium | ✓ |
| Glucose | ✓ |
| Sodium | ✓ |
| Glycosylated hemoglobin (A1C) | ✓ |
| Thyroid studies: TSH, $T_3$, $T_4$ | ✓ |
| Serum osmolality | ✓ |

**Objective: Physical Examination**

***Inspect/Measure***

| | |
|---|---|
| Body temperature | ✓ |
| Height and weight | ✓ |
| Alertness and emotional state | ✓ |
| Skin for changes in color and texture | ✓ |
| Hair for changes in color, texture, and distribution | ✓ |

***Auscultate***

| | |
|---|---|
| Heart rate, BP | ✓ |

***Palpate***

| | |
|---|---|
| Extremities for edema | ✓ |
| Skin for texture and temperature | ✓ |
| Neck for thyroid size, shape | ✓ |

*$T_3$*, Triiodothyronine; *$T_4$*, thyroxine; *TSH*, thyroid-stimulating hormone.

## DIAGNOSTIC STUDIES OF ENDOCRINE SYSTEM

Diagnostic studies of the endocrine system are presented in Table 47-6. Pertinent findings from the history and physical examination guide the selection of diagnostic studies. Imaging studies can identify pituitary tumors, thyroid nodules, or adrenal tumors. Laboratory studies may include direct measurement of the hormone level or involve an indirect indication of gland function by evaluating blood or urine components affected by the hormone such as glucose or electrolytes. It is also possible to measure the releasing or stimulating hormone. For example, TSH can be measured to evaluate thyroid function.

Hormones with constant basal levels, such as $T_4$, can be assessed with a single measurement. Note the time of the sample collection on the laboratory slip. Information about night shift work is important for hormones with circadian or sleep-related secretion (e.g., cortisol). Evaluation of other hormones may require multiple blood samplings, such as in suppression tests (e.g., dexamethasone) and stimulation tests (e.g., glucose tolerance). In these situations, it is often necessary to obtain IV access to administer the testing medication and fluids and to draw multiple blood samples.

Disorders associated with the pituitary gland can manifest in a wide variety of ways because of the number of hormones produced. Many diagnostic studies evaluate these hormones either directly or indirectly.

A number of tests are available to evaluate thyroid function. The most sensitive and accurate laboratory test is the measurement of TSH. Thus it is often the first diagnostic test done to evaluate thyroid function.[7] Common additional tests ordered in the presence of an abnormal TSH level include total $T_4$, free $T_4$, and total $T_3$. Free $T_4$ is the unbound thyroxine and is a more accurate reflection of thyroid function than total $T_4$.

The only hormone secreted by the parathyroid glands is PTH. Because PTH regulates serum calcium and phosphate levels, abnormalities in PTH secretion are reflected by these levels. For this reason, diagnostic tests for the parathyroid gland typically include PTH, serum calcium, and serum phosphate levels.

Tests associated with the adrenal cortex function focus on measuring blood plasma and urine levels of the three types of hormones secreted: glucocorticoids, mineralocorticoids, and androgens. Urine studies often require a 24-hour urine collection to eliminate the impact of short-term fluctuations in plasma hormone levels.

The tests used to evaluate glucose metabolism are important in the diagnosis and management of diabetes mellitus. See Chapter 48 for information regarding diagnostic studies for diabetes mellitus.

## TABLE 47-6 Diagnostic Studies
### *Endocrine System*

| Study | Purpose and Description | Nursing Responsibility |
|---|---|---|
| **Pituitary Studies** | | |
| ***Blood Studies*** | | |
| **Growth hormone (GH)** (somatotropin) | Evaluates GH secretion. Used to identify GH deficiency or GH excess. GH levels are affected by time of day, food intake, and stress. Difficult to interpret significance of isolated GH level. Further evaluation requires stimulation tests.<br>*Reference interval:*<br>*Men:* <4 ng/mL (<4.0 mcg/L), *Women:* <18 ng/mL (<18 mcg/L) | *Before:* Make sure that patient has been fasting. Emotional and physical stress may alter results. Indicate patient fasting status and recent activity level on the laboratory slip.<br>*After:* Send blood sample to laboratory immediately. |
| **Somatomedin C** (insulin-like growth factor 1 [IGF-1]) | Evaluates GH secretion. Provides a more accurate reflection of mean plasma concentration of GH because it is not subject to circadian rhythm and fluctuations. Low levels indicate GH deficiency. High levels indicate GH excess.<br>*Reference interval:* 42-110 ng/mL | *Before:* Overnight fasting is preferred but not necessary. |
| **Growth hormone (GH) stimulation** | ***Insulin tolerance test:*** Regular insulin given IV and blood drawn at –30, 0, 30, 45, 60, and 90 min for measurement of glucose and GH.<br>*Reference interval:* GH >5 mcg/L<br>***Arginine-GHRH test:*** GHRH bolus followed by 30-min infusion of arginine.<br>*Reference interval:* GH >4.1 mcg/L | *Before:* Patient is NPO after midnight. Water is permitted on morning of test. Establish IV access for medication administration and blood sampling.<br>*During:* Continually assess for hypoglycemia and hypotension. Keep 50% dextrose and 5% dextrose IV solution at the bedside in case severe hypoglycemia occurs. |
| **Gonadotropins**<br>• Follicle-stimulating hormone (FSH)<br>• Luteinizing hormone (LH) | Used to distinguish primary gonadal problems from pituitary insufficiency. In women, there are marked differences during menstrual cycle and in postmenopausal period. Levels are low in pituitary insufficiency and high in primary gonadal failure.<br>***FSH Reference intervals***<br>*Women:*<br>Follicular phase: 1.37-9.9 mU/mL<br>Ovulatory phase: 6.17-17.2 mU/mL<br>Luteal phase: 1.09-9.2 mU/mL<br>Postmenopause: 19.3-100.6 mU/mL<br>*Men:* 1.42-15.4 mU/mL<br>***LH Reference intervals***<br>*Women:*<br>Follicular phase: 1.68-15 IU/L<br>Ovulatory phase: 21.9-56.6 IU/L<br>Postmenopause: 14.2-52.3 IU/L<br>*Men:* 1.24-7.8 IU/L | *Before:* Explain procedure to patient.<br>*During:* Note on the laboratory slip time of menstrual cycle or whether woman is menopausal. |
| **Water deprivation (restriction)** (ADH stimulation) | Used to differentiate causes of diabetes insipidus (DI), including central DI, nephrogenic DI, and psychogenic polydipsia. ADH (vasopressin) is administered.<br>In patients with central DI, urine osmolality increases after ADH. In patients with nephrogenic DI, no or minimal response to ADH. | *Before:* Obtain baseline weight and urine and plasma osmolality. Should be performed only if serum sodium is normal and urine osmolality is <300 mOsm/kg.<br>*During:* Patient is NPO for test. Severe dehydration may occur with central or nephrogenic diabetes insipidus. Assess urine hourly for volume and specific gravity. Send hourly urine samples to laboratory for osmolality determination. Send blood samples for sodium and osmolality every 2 hr. Discontinue test and rehydrate if patient's weight drops >2 kg at any time.<br>*After:* Rehydrate with oral fluids. Check orthostatic BP and pulse to ensure adequate fluid volume. |
| ***Radiologic Studies*** | | |
| **Magnetic resonance imaging (MRI)** | Examination of choice for radiologic evaluation of the pituitary gland and hypothalamus. Used to identify tumors involving the hypothalamus or pituitary. | *Before:* Inform patient of the need to lie as still as possible during the test. Assess for contraindications, including pregnancy, presence of metal implants (e.g., pacemaker). |
| **Computed tomography (CT) scan** | Used to detect tumor and size of tumor. Oral and/or IV contrast medium may be used. | *Before:* Assess renal function before test. If IV contrast is used, check for iodine or shellfish allergy. Contrast medium may induce renal failure in at-risk patients. |

*Continued*

## TABLE 47-6 Diagnostic Studies
### *Endocrine System—cont'd*

| Study | Purpose and Description | Nursing Responsibility |
|---|---|---|
| **Thyroid Studies** | | |
| ***Blood Studies*** | | |
| **Thyroid-stimulating hormone (TSH) (thyrotropin)** | Measures TSH levels. Considered the most sensitive diagnostic test for evaluating thyroid dysfunction.<br>*Reference interval:* 0.4-4.2 μU/mL (0.4-4.2 mU/L) | *Before:* Explain blood draw procedure to the patient. No specific preparations are necessary. |
| **Triiodothyronine ($T_3$), total** | Measures serum levels of $T_3$. Used to diagnose hyperthyroidism if $T_4$ levels are normal.<br>*Reference interval: Ages 20-50:* 70-204 ng/dL (1.08-3.14 nmol/L)<br>*Ages >50:* 40-181 ng/dL (0.62-2.79 nmol/L) | See above. |
| **Thyroxine ($T_4$), total** | Measures total serum level of $T_4$. Used to evaluate thyroid function and monitor thyroid therapy.<br>*Reference interval:* 4.6-11.0 mcg/dL (59-142 nmol/L) | See above. |
| **Free thyroxine ($FT_4$)** | Measures active component of total $T_4$. Because level remains constant, considered better indicator of thyroid function than total $T_4$.<br>*Reference interval:* 0.8-2.7 ng/dL (10-35 pmol/L) | *Before:* Tell patient that $FT_4$ levels may be measured until symptoms of hyperthyroidism have abated and levels have returned to normal. |
| **Free triiodothyronine ($FT_3$)** | Measures active component of total $T_3$.<br>*Reference interval:* 260-480 pg/dL (4.0-7.4 pmol/L) | See above. |
| **$T_3$ uptake ($T_3$ resin uptake)** | Indirectly measures binding capacity of thyroid-binding globulin.<br>*Reference interval:* 24%-34% | See above. |
| **Thyroid antibodies (Ab)**<br>• Thyroid peroxidase (TPO) Ab<br>• Thyroglobulin Ab<br>• Thyroid-stimulating Ab | Measures levels of thyroid antibodies. Assists in the diagnosis of autoimmune thyroid disease and separates it from other forms of thyroiditis. One or more antibody tests may be ordered depending on symptoms. | See above. |
| **Thyroglobulin** | Identifies functioning thyroid tissue and thyroid cancer cells. Used primarily as a tumor marker for patients being treated for thyroid cancer.<br>*Reference interval:*<br>*Men:* 0.5-53 ng/mL<br>*Women:* 0.5-43 ng/mL | See above. |
| ***Radiologic Studies*** | | |
| **Ultrasound** | Evaluates thyroid nodule(s) to determine if it is a fluid-filled (cystic) or solid tumor and follows change over time. | *Before:* Explain that gel and a transducer will be used over the neck. The test lasts 15 min. No fasting or sedation required. |
| **Thyroid scan and uptake** | ***Scan:*** Used to evaluate nodules of thyroid. Radioactive isotopes are given orally or IV. Scanner passes over thyroid and makes graphic record of radiation emitted. Normal thyroid scan reveals homogeneous pattern with symmetric lobes. Benign nodules appear as warm spots because they take up radionuclide. Malignant tumors appear as cold spots because they tend not to take up radionuclide.<br>***Radioactive iodine uptake (RAIU):*** Provides direct measure of thyroid activity. Evaluates function of thyroid nodules. Patient is given radioactive iodine either orally or IV. The uptake by the thyroid gland is measured with a scanner at several time intervals such as 2-4 hr and at 24 hr. The values of RAIU are expressed in percentage of uptake.<br>*Reference interval:*<br>For 2-4 hr: 3%-19%<br>For 24 hr: 11%-30% | *Before:* Explain procedure to the patient. Reaction to iodine in allergic patients is rare because amount of iodine in preparation is minimal.<br>*After:* Tell patient to drink increased amount of fluids for 24-48 hr unless contraindicated. Radionuclide will be eliminated in 6-24 hr. |
| **Parathyroid Studies** | | |
| ***Blood Studies*** | | |
| **Parathyroid hormone (PTH)** | Measures PTH level in serum. Must be interpreted in terms of concurrently drawn serum calcium level.<br>*Reference interval:* 50-330 pg/mL (50-330 ng/L) | *Before:* Fasting specimen preferred. Inform patient that blood sample will be drawn.<br>*After:* Keep sample on ice. |
| **Calcium (total)** | Used to detect bone and parathyroid disorders. Hypercalcemia can indicate primary hyperparathyroidism. Hypocalcemia can indicate hypoparathyroidism.<br>*Reference interval:* 8.6-10.2 mg/dL (2.15-2.55 mmol/L) | See above. |

## TABLE 47-6 Diagnostic Studies

### *Endocrine System—cont'd*

| Study | Purpose and Description | Nursing Responsibility |
|---|---|---|
| **Calcium (ionized)** | Free form of calcium unaffected by variable serum albumin levels.<br>*Reference interval:* 4.64-5.28 mg/dL (1.16-1.32 mmol/L) | See above. |
| **Phosphate** | Measures inorganic phosphorus. High levels indicate primary hypoparathyroidism or secondary causes (e.g., renal failure). Low levels indicate hyperparathyroidism.<br>*Reference interval:* 2.4-4.4 mg/dL (0.78-1.42 mmol/L) | See above. |
| ***Radiologic Studies*** | | |
| **Parathyroid scan** | Assists in identifying the number and location of parathyroid glands. Uses radioactive isotopes that are taken up by cells in parathyroid glands to obtain an image of the glands and any abnormally active areas. | *Before:* Explain procedure to the patient. No specific preparations are necessary. |
| **Adrenal Studies** | | |
| ***Blood Studies*** | | |
| **Cortisol (total)** | Measures amount of total cortisol in serum and evaluates status of adrenal cortex function. Cortisol has diurnal variation; levels are higher in morning than in evening. Stress and excessive physical activity produce elevated results.<br>*Reference interval:*<br>At 8 AM: 5-23 mcg/dL (138-635 nmol/L)<br>At 4 PM: 3-16 mcg/dL (83-441 nmol/L) | *Before:* Sample should be drawn in morning. Note if patient does night shift work. Mark time of blood draw on laboratory slip. |
| **Aldosterone** | Used to assess for hyperaldosteronism.<br>*Reference interval:*<br>Upright posture: 7-30 ng/dL (0.19-0.83 nmol/L)<br>Supine position: 3-16 ng/dL (0.08-0.44 nmol/L) | *Before:* Usually morning blood sample is preferred. Inform patient that the required position (supine or sitting/standing) must be maintained for 2 hr before specimen is drawn. |
| **Adrenocorticotropic hormone (ACTH) (corticotropin)** | Measures plasma level of ACTH. Since ACTH controls adrenal cortex secretion, levels help determine if underproduction or overproduction of cortisol is caused by adrenal gland or pituitary gland dysfunction. Diurnal levels correspond with variation of cortisol levels. Levels are higher in morning, lower in evening.<br>*Reference interval:*<br>Morning: <120 pg/mL (<26 pmol/L)<br>Evening: <85 pg/mL (<19 pmol/L) | *Before:* Patient should be NPO after midnight. Do morning blood draw between 6-8 AM.<br>*During:* Use prechilled blood tube and place on ice.<br>*After:* Send to laboratory immediately. |
| **ACTH stimulation with cosyntropin** | Used to evaluate adrenal function. After baseline cortisol sample is drawn, give cosyntropin (synthetic ACTH) by IV bolus. Cortisol samples are drawn 30 and 60 min after bolus. Plasma cortisol at 60 min should increase by >7 mcg/dL from baseline. | *Before:* Obtain baseline cortisol level at beginning of cosyntropin infusion.<br>*During:* Inject cosyntropin with a plastic syringe and collect blood samples in plastic heparinized tubes. Administer test with continuous-infusion method. Monitor site and rate of IV infusion. Ensure sample collection at appropriate times. |
| **ACTH suppression** (dexamethasone suppression) | Assesses adrenal function. Especially helpful if hyperactivity (Cushing syndrome) is suspected.<br>*Overnight method:* Dexamethasone (Decadron) 1 mg (low dose) or 4 mg (high dose) is given at 11 PM to suppress secretion of corticotropin-releasing hormone. Plasma cortisol sample is drawn at 8 AM.<br>*Reference interval:* Cortisol level <3 mcg/dL (<0.08 μmol/L) for low dose and <50% of baseline in high dose indicates normal adrenal response. | *Before:* Obtain a fasting specimen. Ensure accurate timing of medication and sample collection. Inform patient that blood sample will be taken. Do not test acutely ill patients or those under stress. Stress-stimulated ACTH may override suppression. Screen patient for drugs such as estrogen and corticosteroids that may give false-positive results. |
| **Metanephrine** | Screens for pheochromocytoma. A more accurate test than urinary vanillylmandelic acid (VMA) and catecholamine measurements. | *Before:* Ask about recent history of vigorous exercise, high levels of stress, or starvation (may artificially ↑ levels). Use of caffeine, alcohol, levodopa, lithium, nitroglycerin, acetaminophen, and medications containing epinephrine or norepinephrine can alter test results. |
| ***Urine Studies*** | | |
| **17-Ketosteroids** | Measures androgen metabolites in urine and evaluates adrenocortical and gonadal function.<br>*Reference interval:*<br>*Men:* 6-20 mg/day (20-70 μmol/day)<br>*Women:* 6-17 mg/day (20-60 μmol/day) | *Before:* Explain the 24-hr urine collection. Tell patient that specimen must be kept refrigerated or iced during entire collection period. Determine whether preservative is required. |

*Continued*

## TABLE 47-6 Diagnostic Studies

### *Endocrine System—cont'd*

| Study | Purpose and Description | Nursing Responsibility |
|---|---|---|
| **Adrenal Studies—cont'd** | | |
| ***Urine Studies—cont'd*** | | |
| **Cortisol (free)** | Measures free (unbound) cortisol. Preferred test to evaluate hypercortisolism.<br>*Reference interval:* 20-90 mcg/24 hr (55-248 nmol/day) | *Before:* Explain the 24-hr urine collection and need to avoid stressful situations and excessive physical exercise. Assess for drug use (e.g., reserpine, diuretics, phenothiazines, insulin, amphetamines) that may alter results. |
| **Vanillylmandelic acid (VMA)** | Measures urinary excretion of catecholamine metabolite. Levels are increased in pheochromocytoma.<br>*Reference interval:* 1.4-6.5 mg/24 hr (7-33 μmol/day) | *Before:* Keep 24-hr urine collection at pH <3.0 with HCl acid as preservative. Keep on ice. Consult with laboratory or HCP about patient discontinuing any drugs 3 days before urine collection. |
| ***Radiologic Studies*** | | |
| **CT** | Abdominal CT is radiologic examination of choice for the adrenal gland. Used to detect tumor and size or metastatic spread. Oral and/or IV contrast medium may be used. | *Before:* Inform patient of procedure. Patient must lie still during the procedure. Assess renal function if IV contrast is used. Check for iodine or shellfish allergy. |
| **MRI** | Same as MRI above. | Same as MRI above. |
| **Pancreatic Studies** | | |
| ***Blood Studies*** | | |
| **Fasting blood glucose (FBG)** | Measures circulating glucose level.<br>*Reference interval:* 70-99 mg/dL (3.9-5.5 mmol/L). | *Before:* Patient should fast 8–12 hr. Water intake is permitted. Many medications may influence results. |
| **Oral glucose tolerance test (OGTT)** | Used to evaluate abnormal FBG levels that do not clearly indicate diabetes. Patient drinks 75 g of glucose, samples for glucose are drawn at baseline and at 30, 60, and 120 min. Test takes 2 hr to complete.<br>*Reference interval:* <100 mg/dL (5.5 mmol/L) at baseline, <200 mg/dL (11.1 mmol/L) at 30 and 60 min, and <140 mg/dL (7.8 mmol/L) at 120 min. Values >200 mg/dL (11.1 mmol/L) at 120 min are considered diagnostic for diabetes mellitus. | *Before:* Perform test on ambulatory patients after fasting 8-12 hr. Many drugs may influence results, including caffeine and smoking. Ensure that patient's diet 3 days before test includes 150-300 g of carbohydrate with intake of at least 1500 cal/day. |
| **Glycosylated hemoglobin (A1C)** | Indicates the amount of glucose linked to hemoglobin. Assesses long-term glycemic control during previous 3 mo.<br>*Reference interval:* 4.0%-6.0%<br>ADA treatment goal <7% | *Before:* Inform patient that fasting is not necessary and that blood sample will be drawn. |
| ***Urine Studies*** | | |
| **Glucose** | Estimate amount of glucose in urine by using an enzymatic method. Dip dipstick into urine and read for color changes after 1 min.<br>*Reference interval:* Negative | *Before:* Use freshly voided urine. Many drugs alter glucose readings. Follow directions exactly to avoid errors. |
| **Ketones** | Measures amount of acetone (a type of ketone) excreted in urine as result of incomplete fat metabolism. Tested with a dipstick as described above. Positive result can indicate lack of insulin and diabetic acidosis.<br>*Reference interval:* Negative | *Before:* Use freshly voided urine specimen. Test is often done with glucose test. Follow directions exactly. Certain drugs can produce false-positive or false-negative results. |
| ***Radiologic Studies*** | | |
| **CT** | Abdominal CT is the radiologic examination of choice for pancreas. Used to identify tumors or cysts. Oral and/or IV contrast medium may be ordered. | *Before:* Inform patient of procedure. Patient must lie still during the procedure. If IV contrast is used, check for iodine and shellfish allergy. Assess renal function if contrast is used. |

*ADA,* American Diabetes Association; *ADH,* antidiuretic hormone; *GHRH,* growth hormone–releasing hormone.

## CASE STUDY—cont'd

### *Objective Data: Diagnostic Studies*

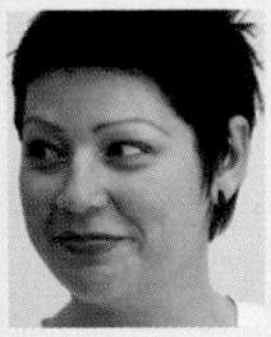

(©iStockphoto/Thinkstock)

The health care provider orders the following initial diagnostic studies to be drawn in the morning after an 8-hr fast:

- CBC, basic metabolic panel (electrolytes, BUN, creatinine)
- Fasting blood glucose (FBG)
- TSH, free $T_4$
- Plasma cortisol levels
- Plasma ACTH levels

CBC results reveal a WBC of 12,200/μL and a decreased lymphocyte count at 800 cells/μL. The rest of the CBC is within normal limits (WNL). The FBG is 130 mg/dL. The plasma cortisol and ACTH levels are elevated. Thyroid studies are WNL.

**Discussion Questions**

1. Which diagnostic study results are of most concern to you?
2. Do you anticipate any additional diagnostic studies being ordered for L.M.?
3. What are the interprofessional team's priorities for L.M. at this time?

Answers available at *http://evolve.elsevier.com/Lewis/medsurg.*

## BRIDGE TO NCLEX EXAMINATION

The number of the question corresponds to the same-numbered outcome at the beginning of the chapter.

1. A characteristic common to all hormones is that they
   - **a.** circulate in the blood bound to plasma proteins.
   - **b.** influence cellular activity of specific target tissues.
   - **c.** accelerate the metabolic processes of all body cells.
   - **d.** enter a cell to alter the cell's metabolism or gene expression.
2. A patient is receiving radiation therapy for cancer of the kidney. The nurse monitors the patient for signs and symptoms of damage to the
   - **a.** pancreas.
   - **b.** thyroid gland.
   - **c.** adrenal glands.
   - **d.** posterior pituitary gland.
3. A patient has a serum sodium level of 152 mEq/L (152 mmol/L). The normal hormonal response to this situation is
   - **a.** release of ADH.
   - **b.** release of ACTH.
   - **c.** secretion of aldosterone.
   - **d.** secretion of corticotropin-releasing hormone.
4. All cells in the body are believed to have intracellular receptors for
   - **a.** insulin.
   - **b.** glucagon.
   - **c.** growth hormone.
   - **d.** thyroid hormone.
5. When obtaining subjective data from a patient during assessment of the endocrine system, the nurse asks specifically about
   - **a.** energy level.
   - **b.** intake of vitamin C.
   - **c.** employment history.
   - **d.** frequency of sexual intercourse.
6. An appropriate technique to use during physical assessment of the thyroid gland is
   - **a.** asking the patient to hyperextend the neck during palpation.
   - **b.** percussing the neck for dullness to define the size of the thyroid.
   - **c.** having the patient swallow water during inspection and palpation of the gland.
   - **d.** using deep palpation to determine the extent of a visibly enlarged thyroid gland.
7. Endocrine disorders often go unrecognized in the older adult because
   - **a.** symptoms are often attributed to aging.
   - **b.** older adults rarely have identifiable symptoms.
   - **c.** endocrine disorders are relatively rare in the older adult.
   - **d.** older adults usually have subclinical endocrine disorders that minimize symptoms.
8. An abnormal finding by the nurse during an endocrine assessment would be *(select all that apply)*
   - **a.** blood pressure of 100/70 mm Hg.
   - **b.** excessive facial hair on a woman.
   - **c.** soft, formed stool every other day.
   - **d.** 3-lb weight gain over last 6 months.
   - **e.** hyperpigmented coloration in lower legs.
9. A patient has a total serum calcium level of 3 mg/dL (1.5 mEq/L). If this finding reflects hypoparathyroidism, the nurse would expect further diagnostic testing to reveal
   - **a.** decreased serum PTH.
   - **b.** increased serum ACTH.
   - **c.** increased serum glucose.
   - **d.** decreased serum cortisol levels.

1. b, 2. c, 3. a, 4. d, 5. a, 6. c, 7. a, 8. b, e, 9. a

For rationales to these answers and even more NCLEX review questions, visit *http://evolve.elsevier.com/Lewis/medsurg.*

## EVOLVE WEBSITE

http://evolve.elsevier.com/Lewis/medsurg

**NCLEX Review Questions (Online Only)**

**Key Points**

**Answer Keys for Questions**

- Rationales for Bridge to NCLEX Examination Questions
- Answer Guidelines for the Case Study on pp. 1109, 1111, 1112, and 1118

**Conceptual Care Map Creator**

**Audio Glossary**

**Supporting Media**

- Animations
  - Overview of the Endocrine System
  - Thyroid and Parathyroid Glands
  - Thyroid Secretion

**Supporting Media**

**Content Updates**

## REFERENCES

1. Huether SE, McCance KL: *Understanding pathophysiology*, ed 5, St Louis, 2014, Mosby.
*2. Gamble KL, Berry R, Frank SJ, et al: Circadian clock control of endocrine factors, *Nat Rev Endocrinol* 10:466, 2014.
3. McCance KL, Huether SE: *Pathophysiology: the biological basis for disease in adults & children*, ed 7, St Louis, 2014, Mosby.
4. Genetics Home Reference: Endocrine conditions. Retrieved from *http://ghr.nlm.nih.gov/conditionCategory/endocrine-system-hormones.*
5. Jarvis C: *Physical examination and health assessment*, ed 7, St Louis, 2015, Saunders.
*6. Aydin K, Ozturk B, Turkyilmaz MD, et al: Functional and structural evaluation of hearing loss in acromegaly, *Clin Endocrinol* 76:415, 2012.
7. Pagana K, Pagana T: *Mosby's manual of diagnostic and laboratory tests*, ed 5, St Louis, Mosby, 2014.

*Evidence-based information for clinical practice.

# 48

# Diabetes Mellitus

*Jane K. Dickinson*

*You don't have to let your life be destroyed by diabetes. You can reclaim your life.*

***Della Reese***

http://evolve.elsevier.com/Lewis/medsurg/

## LEARNING OUTCOMES

1. Describe the pathophysiology and clinical manifestations of diabetes mellitus.
2. Differentiate between type 1 and type 2 diabetes mellitus.
3. Describe the interprofessional care of a patient with diabetes mellitus.
4. Describe the role of nutrition and exercise in the management of diabetes mellitus.
5. Discuss the nursing management of a patient with newly diagnosed diabetes mellitus.
6. Describe the nursing management of a patient with diabetes mellitus in the ambulatory and home care settings.
7. Relate the pathophysiology of acute and chronic complications of diabetes mellitus to the clinical manifestations.
8. Explain the interprofessional care and nursing management of a patient with acute and chronic complications of diabetes mellitus.

## KEY TERMS



This chapter discusses the pathophysiology, clinical manifestations, complications, and interprofessional care of diabetes mellitus. To promote the patient's self-management of diabetes, you have a very important role in teaching both the patient and caregiver.

## DIABETES MELLITUS

**Diabetes mellitus (DM)** is a chronic multisystem disease characterized by hyperglycemia related to abnormal insulin production, impaired insulin utilization, or both. Diabetes mellitus is a serious health problem throughout the world, and its prevalence is rapidly increasing. Currently in the United States an estimated 29.1 million people, or 9.3% of the population, have diabetes mellitus, and 86 million more people have prediabetes.[1] Approximately 8.1 million people with diabetes mellitus have not been diagnosed and are unaware that they have the disease. Diabetes mellitus is the seventh leading cause of death in the United States, but it is likely to be underreported.[2]

The long-term complications associated with diabetes can make it a devastating disease. Diabetes is the leading cause of adult blindness, end-stage renal disease, and nontraumatic lower limb amputations. It is also a major contributing factor to heart disease and stroke. Adults with diabetes have heart disease death rates two to four times higher than adults without diabetes. The risk for stroke is also two to four times higher among people with diabetes. In addition, more than half of adults with diabetes have hypertension and high cholesterol levels.[2]

### Etiology and Pathophysiology

Current theories link the causes of diabetes, singly or in combination, to genetic, autoimmune, and environmental factors (e.g., virus, obesity). Regardless of its cause, diabetes is primarily a disorder of glucose metabolism related to absent or insufficient insulin supply and/or poor utilization of the insulin that is available.

The American Diabetes Association (ADA) recognizes four different classes of diabetes. The two most common are type 1 and type 2 diabetes mellitus (Table 48-1). The two other classes are gestational diabetes and other specific types of diabetes with various causes.

**Normal Glucose and Insulin Metabolism.** Insulin is a hormone produced by the β-cells in the islets of Langerhans of the pancreas. Under normal conditions, insulin is continuously released into the bloodstream in small increments, with increased release when food is ingested (Fig. 48-1). Insulin lowers blood glucose and facilitates a stable, normal glucose range of approximately 70 to 110 mg/dL (3.9 to 6.1 mmol/L). The average amount of

Reviewed by Cora Espina, RN, MN, ARNP, CWN, Nurse Practitioner, Inpatient Diabetes Consult Service and Diabetes Care Center, University of Washington Medical Center, Seattle, Washington; Carolyn Lyon, RN, MSN, Assistant Professor, Jefferson College of Health Science, Carilion Health System, Roanoke, Virginia; Lorraine Nowakowski-Grier, MSN, APRN, BC, CDE, Diabetes Nurse Practitioner, Christiana Care Health Services, Nursing Development and Education, Newark, Delaware; and Susan A. Sandstrom, RN, MSN, BC, CNE, Associate Professor in Nursing (retired), College of Saint Mary, Omaha, Nebraska.

**TABLE 48-1 Comparison of Type 1 and Type 2 Diabetes Mellitus**

| Factor | Type 1 Diabetes Mellitus | Type 2 Diabetes Mellitus |
|---|---|---|
| **Age at onset** | More common in young people but can occur at any age. | More common in adults but can occur at any age. Incidence is increasing in children. |
| **Type of onset** | Signs and symptoms usually abrupt, but disease process may be present for several years. | Insidious, may go undiagnosed for years. |
| **Prevalence** | Accounts for 5%-10% of all types of diabetes. | Accounts for 90%-95% of all types of diabetes. |
| **Environmental factors** | Virus, toxins. | Obesity, lack of exercise. |
| **Primary defect** | Absent or minimal insulin production. | Insulin resistance, decreased insulin production over time, and alterations in production of adipokines. |
| **Islet cell antibodies** | Often present at onset. | Absent. |
| **Endogenous insulin** | Absent. | Initially increased in response to insulin resistance. Secretion diminishes over time. |
| **Nutritional status** | Thin, normal, or obese. | Frequently overweight or obese. May be normal. |
| **Symptoms** | Polydipsia, polyuria, polyphagia, fatigue, weight loss without trying. | Frequently none. Fatigue, recurrent infections. May also experience polyuria, polydipsia, and polyphagia. |
| **Ketosis** | Prone at onset or during insulin deficiency. | Resistant except during infection or stress. |
| **Nutrition therapy** | Essential. | Essential. |
| **Insulin** | Required for all. | Required for some. Disease is progressive and insulin treatment may need to be added to treatment regimen. |
| **Vascular and neurologic complications** | Frequent. | Frequent. |

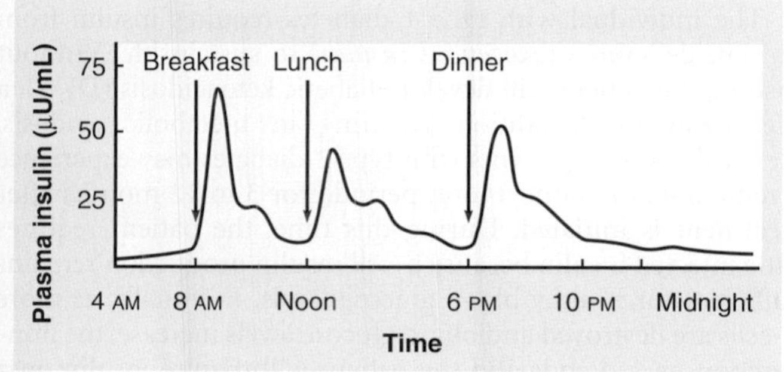


**FIG. 48-1** Normal endogenous insulin secretion. In the first hour or two after meals, insulin concentrations rise rapidly in blood and peak at about 1 hour. After meals, insulin concentrations promptly decline toward preprandial values as carbohydrate absorption from the gastrointestinal tract declines. After carbohydrate absorption from the gastrointestinal tract is complete and during the night, insulin concentrations are low and fairly constant, with a slight increase at dawn.

insulin secreted daily by an adult is approximately 40 to 50 U, or 0.6 U/kg of body weight.

Insulin promotes glucose transport from the bloodstream across the cell membrane to the cytoplasm of the cell (Fig. 48-2). Cells break down glucose to make energy, and liver and muscle cells store excess glucose as glycogen. The rise in plasma insulin after a meal inhibits gluconeogenesis, enhances fat deposition of adipose tissue, and increases protein synthesis. For this reason, insulin is an *anabolic*, or storage, hormone. The fall in insulin level during normal overnight fasting facilitates the release of stored glucose from the liver, protein from muscle, and fat from adipose tissue.

Skeletal muscle and adipose tissue have specific receptors for insulin and are considered insulin-dependent tissues. Insulin is required to "unlock" these receptor sites, allowing the transport of glucose into the cells to be used for energy. Other tissues (e.g., brain, liver, blood cells) do not directly depend on insulin for glucose transport but require an adequate glucose supply for normal function. Although liver cells are not considered insulin-dependent tissue, insulin receptor sites on the liver facilitate hepatic uptake of glucose and its conversion to glycogen.

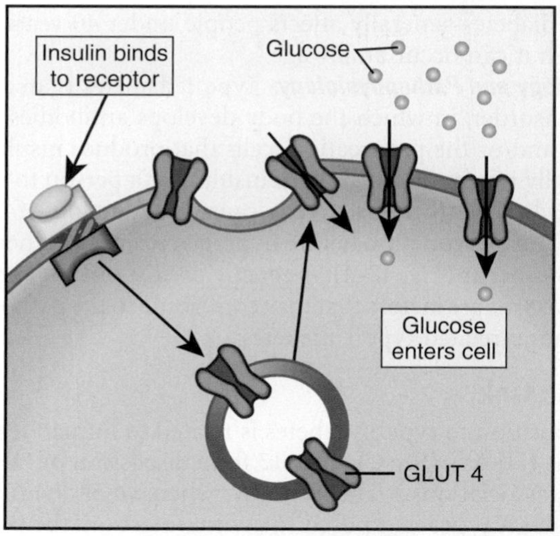


**FIG. 48-2** Normal glucose metabolism. Insulin binds to receptors along the cell walls of muscle, adipose, and liver cells. Glucose transport proteins (GLUT 4) then attach to the cell wall and allow glucose to enter the cell, where it is either stored or used to make energy.

Other hormones (glucagon, epinephrine, growth hormone, and cortisol) work to oppose the effects of insulin and are referred to as *counterregulatory hormones.* These hormones increase blood glucose levels by (1) stimulating glucose production and release by the liver and (2) decreasing the movement of glucose into the cells. The counterregulatory hormones and insulin usually maintain blood glucose levels within the normal range by regulating the release of glucose for energy during food intake and periods of fasting.

Insulin is synthesized from a precursor, proinsulin. Enzymes split proinsulin to form insulin and C-peptide, and then the two substances are released in equal amounts. Therefore measuring C-peptide in serum and urine is a useful clinical indicator of pancreatic β-cell function.

**Type 1 Diabetes Mellitus.** *Type 1 diabetes mellitus,* formerly known as *juvenile-onset diabetes* or *insulin-dependent diabetes,* accounts for about 5% to 10% of all people with diabetes.

## GENETICS IN CLINICAL PRACTICE

### *Types 1 and 2 Diabetes Mellitus and MODY*

| Type 1 Diabetes Mellitus | Type 2 Diabetes Mellitus | Maturity-Onset Diabetes of the Young (MODY) |
|---|---|---|
| **Genetic Basis** | | |
| • Increased susceptibility (40%-50%) when one has specific human leukocyte antigens (HLA-DR3, HLA-DR4).<br>• Polygenic (>40 genes influence susceptibility). | • Polygenic (>25 genes influence susceptibility). | • Autosomal dominant.<br>• Monogenic (single gene).<br>• Caused by mutations in any of six MODY genes (types 1-6).<br>• Mutations in genes lead to β-cell dysfunction. |
| **Risk to Offspring** | | |
| • Risk to offspring of mothers with diabetes is 1%-4%.<br>• Risk to offspring of fathers with diabetes is 5%-6%.<br>• When one identical twin has type 1 diabetes, the other gets the disease about 30%-40% of the time. | • Risk to offspring is 8%-14%.<br>• When one identical twin has type 2 diabetes, the other gets it about 60%-75% of the time. | • If one parent has MODY, a child has a 50% chance of developing disease.<br>• If one parent has MODY, a child has a 50% chance of being a carrier. |
| **Clinical Implications** | | |
| • Disease is a result of complex interaction of genetic, autoimmune, and environmental factors. | • Disease is a result of complex genetic interactions, which are modified by environmental factors such as body weight and exercise. | • MODY accounts for 1% to 5% of people with diabetes.<br>• Characterized by young age of onset (often before age 25).<br>• Not associated with obesity or hypertension.<br>• Treatment varies depending on the genetic mutation that caused MODY. |

Type 1 diabetes generally affects people under 40 years of age, although it can occur at any age.[3]

***Etiology and Pathophysiology.*** Type 1 diabetes is an autoimmune disorder, in which the body develops antibodies against insulin and/or the pancreatic β-cells that produce insulin. This eventually results in not enough insulin for a person to survive. Autoantibodies to the islet cells cause a reduction of 80% to 90% of normal function before hyperglycemia and other manifestations occur (Fig. 48-2). A genetic predisposition and exposure to a virus are factors that may contribute to the pathogenesis of immune-related type 1 diabetes.

#### Genetic Link

Predisposition to type 1 diabetes is related to human leukocyte antigens (HLAs). (See Chapter 13 for a discussion of HLAs and disease associations.) Theoretically, when an individual with certain HLA types is exposed to a viral infection, the β-cells of the pancreas are destroyed, either directly or through an autoimmune process. The HLA types associated with an increased risk for type 1 diabetes include HLA-DR3 and HLA-DR4 (Genetics in Clinical Practice box).

*Idiopathic diabetes* is a form of type 1 diabetes that is strongly inherited and not related to autoimmunity. It only occurs in a small number of people with type 1 diabetes, most often of Hispanic, African, or Asian ancestry.[3] *Latent autoimmune diabetes in adults* (LADA), a slowly progressing autoimmune form of type 1 diabetes, occurs in adults, and is often mistaken for type 2 diabetes.

***Onset of Disease.*** In type 1 diabetes, the islet cell autoantibodies responsible for β-cell destruction are present for months to years before the onset of symptoms. Manifestations of type 1 diabetes develop when the person's pancreas can no longer produce sufficient amounts of insulin to maintain normal glucose. Once this occurs, the onset of symptoms is usually rapid, and patients often are initially seen with impending or actual ketoacidosis. The patient usually has a history of recent and sudden weight loss and the classic symptoms of *polydipsia* (excessive thirst), *polyuria* (frequent urination), and *polyphagia* (excessive hunger).

The individual with type 1 diabetes requires insulin from an outside source *(exogenous insulin)* to sustain life. Without insulin, the patient will develop diabetic ketoacidosis (DKA), a life-threatening condition resulting in metabolic acidosis. Newly diagnosed patients with type 1 diabetes may experience a remission, or "honeymoon period," for 3 to 12 months after treatment is initiated. During this time, the patient requires little injected insulin because β-cell insulin production remains sufficient for healthy blood glucose levels. Eventually, as more β-cells are destroyed and blood glucose levels increase, the honeymoon period ends and the patient will require insulin on a permanent basis.

**Type 2 Diabetes Mellitus.** *Type 2 diabetes mellitus* was formerly known as *adult-onset diabetes (AODM)* or *non–insulin-dependent diabetes (NIDDM)*. Type 2 diabetes is, by far, the most prevalent type of diabetes, accounting for approximately 90% to 95% of patients with diabetes.[2] Many risk factors contribute to the development of type 2 diabetes, including being overweight or obese, being older, and having a family history of type 2 diabetes. Although the disease is seen less frequently in children, the incidence is increasing due to the increasing prevalence of childhood obesity. Type 2 diabetes is more prevalent in some ethnic populations. African Americans, Asian Americans, Hispanics, Native Hawaiians or other Pacific Islanders, and Native Americans have a higher rate of type 2 diabetes than whites.[4]

***Etiology and Pathophysiology.*** Type 2 diabetes is characterized by a combination of inadequate insulin secretion and insulin resistance. The pancreas usually produces some *endogenous* (self-made) insulin. However, the body either does not produce enough insulin or does not use it effectively, or both. The presence of endogenous insulin is a major distinction between type 1 and type 2 diabetes. (In type 1 diabetes, there is an absence of endogenous insulin.)

#### Genetic Link

Although the genetics of type 2 diabetes is not yet fully understood, it is likely multiple genes are involved. Genetic mutations that lead to insulin resistance and a higher risk for obesity have been found in many people with type 2 diabetes. Individuals

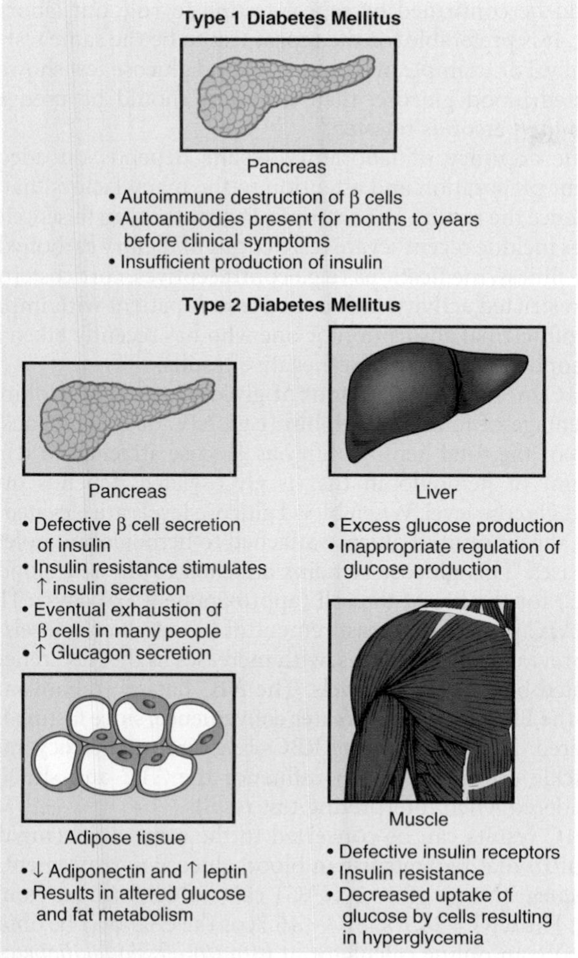


**FIG. 48-3** Altered mechanisms in type 1 and type 2 diabetes mellitus.

with a first-degree relative with the disease are 10 times more likely to develop type 2 diabetes.

Metabolic abnormalities have a role in the development of type 2 diabetes (Fig. 48-3). The first factor is **insulin resistance**, a condition in which body tissues do not respond to the action of insulin because insulin receptors are unresponsive, are insufficient in number, or both. Most insulin receptors are located on skeletal muscle, fat, and liver cells. When insulin is not properly used, the entry of glucose into the cell is impeded, resulting in hyperglycemia. In the early stages of insulin resistance, the pancreas responds to high blood glucose by producing greater amounts of insulin (if β-cell function is normal). This creates a temporary state of hyperinsulinemia that coexists with hyperglycemia.

A second factor in the development of type 2 diabetes is a marked decrease in the ability of the pancreas to produce insulin, as the β-cells become fatigued from the compensatory overproduction of insulin or when β-cell mass is lost. The underlying basis for the failure of β-cells to adapt is unknown. It may be linked to the adverse effects of chronic hyperglycemia or high circulating free fatty acids. In addition, the α-cells of the pancreas increase production of glucagon.

This leads to a third factor, which is inappropriate glucose production by the liver. Instead of properly regulating the release of glucose in response to blood levels, the liver does so in a haphazard way that does not correspond to the body's needs at the time.

A fourth factor is altered production of hormones and cytokines by adipose tissue *(adipokines)*. Adipokines secreted by adipose tissue appear to play a role in glucose and fat metabolism and are likely to contribute to the pathophysiology of type 2 diabetes.[5] Adipokines are thought to cause chronic inflammation, a factor involved in insulin resistance, type 2 diabetes, and cardiovascular disease (CVD). The two main adipokines believed to affect insulin sensitivity are adiponectin and leptin. Finally, the brain, kidneys, and gut also have roles in the development of type 2 diabetes, and scientists are continuously learning more about metabolic factors in the development of type 2 diabetes.[6]

Individuals with *metabolic syndrome* are at an increased risk for the development of type 2 diabetes. Metabolic syndrome has five components: elevated glucose levels, abdominal obesity, elevated BP, high levels of triglycerides, and decreased levels of high-density lipoproteins (HDLs) (see Table 41-10). An individual with three of the five components is considered to have metabolic syndrome.[7] Overweight individuals with metabolic syndrome can reduce their risk for diabetes through a program of weight loss and regular physical activity. (See Chapter 40 for a discussion of metabolic syndrome.)

***Onset of Disease.*** The disease onset in type 2 diabetes is usually gradual. The person may go for many years with undetected hyperglycemia that may produce few, if any, symptoms. Many people are diagnosed on routine laboratory testing or when they undergo treatment for other conditions, and elevated glucose or glycosylated hemoglobin (A1C) levels are found. The signs and symptoms of hyperglycemia develop when about 50% to 80% of β-cells are no longer secreting insulin. At the time of diagnosis, the average person has had type 2 diabetes for 6½ years.

**Prediabetes.** Individuals diagnosed with prediabetes are at increased risk for the development of type 2 diabetes. **Prediabetes** is defined as **impaired glucose tolerance (IGT)**, **impaired fasting glucose (IFG)**, or both. It is an intermediate stage between normal glucose homeostasis and diabetes, in which the blood glucose levels are elevated but not high enough to meet the diagnostic criteria for diabetes. A diagnosis of IGT is made if the 2-hour oral glucose tolerance test (OGTT) values are 140 to 199 mg/dL (7.8 to 11.0 mmol/L).[3] IFG is diagnosed when fasting blood glucose levels are 100 to 125 mg/dL (5.56 to 6.9 mmol/L).

Persons with prediabetes usually do not have symptoms. However, long-term damage to the body, especially the heart and blood vessels, may already be occurring. It is important for patients to undergo screening and to understand risk factors for diabetes. Patients with prediabetes can take action to prevent or delay the development of type 2 diabetes. Encourage those with prediabetes to have their blood glucose and A1C checked regularly and monitor for symptoms of diabetes, such as fatigue, frequent infections, or slow healing wounds. Maintaining a healthy weight, exercising regularly, and making healthy food choices have all been found to reduce the risk of developing overt type 2 diabetes in people with prediabetes.

**Gestational Diabetes.** *Gestational diabetes* develops during pregnancy and occurs in about 4.6% to 9.2% of pregnancies in the United States.[8] Women with gestational diabetes have a higher risk for cesarean delivery, and their babies have increased risk for perinatal death, birth injury, and neonatal complications. Women who are at high risk for gestational diabetes are screened at the first prenatal visit.[9] Those at high risk include women who are obese, are of advanced maternal age, or have a family history of diabetes. Women with an average risk for gestational diabetes are screened using an OGTT at 24 to 28 weeks of gestation. Most women with gestational diabetes have normal glucose levels within 6 weeks postpartum. Be aware that women with a history of gestational diabetes have up to a 63% chance of developing type 2 diabetes within 16 years.[10] Gestational diabetes and management of the pregnant patient with diabetes are specialized areas not covered in detail in this chapter. Consult an obstetric text for more information.

**Other Specific Types of Diabetes.** Diabetes occurs in some people because of another medical condition or treatment of a medical condition that causes abnormal blood glucose levels. Conditions that may cause diabetes can result from injury to, interference with, or destruction of the β-cell function in the pancreas. These include Cushing syndrome, hyperthyroidism, recurrent pancreatitis, cystic fibrosis, hemochromatosis, and parenteral nutrition. Commonly used medications that can induce diabetes in some people include corticosteroids (prednisone), thiazides, phenytoin (Dilantin), and atypical antipsychotics (e.g., clozapine [Clozaril]). Diabetes caused by medical conditions or medications can resolve when the underlying condition is treated or the medication discontinued.

## Clinical Manifestations

**Type 1 Diabetes Mellitus.** Because the onset of type 1 diabetes is rapid, the initial manifestations are usually acute. The classic symptoms are *polyuria, polydipsia,* and *polyphagia.* The osmotic effect of glucose produces the manifestations of polydipsia and polyuria. Polyphagia is a consequence of cellular malnourishment when insulin deficiency prevents utilization of glucose for energy. Weight loss may occur because the body cannot get glucose and turns to other energy sources, such as fat and protein. Weakness and fatigue may result because body cells lack needed energy from glucose. Ketoacidosis, a complication most common in those with untreated type 1 diabetes, is associated with additional clinical manifestations and is discussed later in this chapter.

**Type 2 Diabetes Mellitus.** The clinical manifestations of type 2 diabetes are often nonspecific, although it is possible that an individual with type 2 diabetes will experience some of the classic symptoms associated with type 1 diabetes, including polyuria, polydipsia, and polyphagia. Some of the more common manifestations associated with type 2 diabetes are fatigue, recurrent infections, recurrent vaginal yeast or candidal infections, prolonged wound healing, and visual changes.

## Diagnostic Studies

The diagnosis of diabetes mellitus is made using one of the following four methods.

1. A1C of 6.5% or higher.
2. Fasting plasma glucose (FPG) level greater than or equal to 126 mg/dL (7.0 mmol/L). *Fasting* is defined as no caloric intake for at least 8 hours.
3. Two-hour plasma glucose level greater than or equal to 200 mg/dL (11.1 mmol/L) during an OGTT, using a glucose load of 75 g.
4. In a patient with classic symptoms of hyperglycemia (polyuria, polydipsia, unexplained weight loss) or hyperglycemic crisis, a random plasma glucose greater than or equal to 200 mg/dL (11.1 mmol/L).

If a patient is seen with a hyperglycemic crisis or clear symptoms of hyperglycemia (polyuria, polydipsia, polyphagia) with a random plasma glucose greater than or equal to 200 mg/dL, repeat testing is not warranted. Otherwise, criteria 1 through 3 should be confirmed by repeat testing to rule out laboratory error. It is preferable for the repeat test to be the same test used initially. For example, if a random blood glucose test showed an elevated blood glucose, that same test should be used again when the person is retested.

The accuracy of laboratory results depends on adequate patient preparation and attention to the many factors that may influence the results. For example, factors that can falsely elevate values include recent severe restrictions of dietary carbohydrate, acute illness, medications (e.g., contraceptives, corticosteroids), and restricted activity such as bed rest. A patient with impaired gastrointestinal absorption or one who has recently taken acetaminophen may have false-negative results.

A1C measures the amount of glycosylated hemoglobin as a percentage of total hemoglobin (e.g., A1C of 6.5% means that 6.5% of the total hemoglobin has glucose attached to it). The amount of hemoglobin that is glycosylated depends on the blood glucose level. When blood glucose levels are elevated over time, the amount of glucose attached to hemoglobin molecules increases. This glucose remains attached to the red blood cell (RBC) for the life of the cell (approximately 120 days). Therefore A1C provides a measurement of blood glucose levels over the previous 2 to 3 months, with increases in the A1C reflecting elevated blood glucose levels. The A1C has several advantages over the FPG, including greater convenience, since fasting is not required. Diseases affecting RBCs (e.g., iron deficiency anemia or sickle cell anemia) can influence the A1C and should be considered when interpreting test results.

A1C results can be converted to the same units (mg/dL or mmol/L) that patients use in blood glucose measurements. An *estimated average glucose* (eAG) can be determined from the A1C. The $eAG = 28.7 \times A1C - 46.7$, or the eAG may be obtained by using an online calculator at *http://professional.diabetes.org/glucosecalculator.aspx.* For example, an A1C of 8.0% is equivalent to a glucose level of 183 mg/dL.

Teach patients with diabetes and prediabetes to have their A1C monitored regularly to determine the success of the current treatment plan and make changes in the plan if glycemic goals are not achieved. The ADA identifies an A1C goal for patients with diabetes of less than 7.0%. The American College of Endocrinology recommends an A1C of less than 6.5%. When the A1C is maintained at near-normal levels, the risk for the development of microvascular and macrovascular complications is greatly reduced. For individuals with prediabetes, monitoring the A1C can detect overt diabetes and provide feedback on efforts to prevent diabetes.

Fructosamine is another way to assess glucose levels. Fructosamine is formed by a chemical reaction of glucose with plasma protein. It reflects glycemia in the previous 1 to 3 weeks. Fructosamine levels may show a change in blood glucose levels before A1C does.

Islet cell autoantibody testing is primarily ordered to help distinguish between autoimmune type 1 diabetes and diabetes from other causes. Autoantibodies can develop to one or several of the autoantigens: GAD65, IA-2, or insulin.

## Interprofessional Care

The goals of diabetes management are to reduce symptoms, promote well-being, prevent acute complications related to hyper- and hypoglycemia, and prevent or delay the onset and progression of long-term complications. These goals are most likely to be met when the patient is able to maintain blood glucose levels as near to normal as possible. Diabetes is a chronic disease that requires daily decisions about food intake, blood glucose monitoring, medication, and exercise. Patient teaching, which enables the patient to become the most active participant in his or her own care, is essential to achieve glycemic goals. Nutritional therapy, drug therapy, exercise, and self-monitoring of blood glucose are the tools used in the management of diabetes (Table 48-2).

The three major types of glucose-lowering agents (GLAs) used in the treatment of diabetes are insulin, oral agents (OAs), and noninsulin injectable agents. All individuals with type 1 diabetes require insulin. For some people with type 2 diabetes, a healthy eating plan, regular physical activity, and maintenance of healthy body weight are sufficient to attain optimal blood glucose levels. However, eventually most people with type 2 diabetes will require medication management because diabetes is a progressive disease.

## Drug Therapy: Insulin

Exogenous (injected) insulin is needed when a patient has inadequate insulin to meet specific metabolic needs. People with type 1 diabetes require exogenous insulin to survive and often use multiple daily injections of insulin (often four or more) or continuous insulin infusion via an insulin pump to adequately manage blood glucose levels. People with type 2 diabetes may require exogenous insulin during periods of severe stress such as illness or surgery. In addition, since type 2 diabetes is a progressive disease, over time the combination of nutrition therapy, exercise, OAs, and noninsulin injectable agents may no longer adequately manage blood glucose levels. At that point, exogenous insulin would be added as part of the management plan. People with type 2 diabetes may also need up to four injections per day to adequately maintain their blood glucose levels. Insulin pumps can also be used for patients with type 2 diabetes.

**Types of Insulin.** Today people use only genetically engineered human insulin made in laboratories. The insulin is derived from common bacteria (e.g., *Escherichia coli*) or yeast cells using recombinant deoxyribonucleic acid (DNA) technology. In the past, insulin was extracted from beef and pork pancreases, but these forms of insulin are no longer available.

Insulins differ by their onset, peak action, and duration (Fig. 48-4) and are categorized as rapid-acting, short-acting, intermediate-acting, and long-acting insulin (Table 48-3).

**Insulin Regimens.** Examples of insulin regimens are presented in Table 48-4. The insulin regimen that most closely mimics endogenous insulin production is the basal-bolus regimen, which uses rapid- or short-acting (bolus) insulin before meals and intermediate- or long-acting (basal) background insulin once or twice a day. The basal-bolus regimen is **intensive or physiologic insulin therapy**, consisting of multiple daily insulin injections together with frequent self-monitoring of blood glucose. The goal is to achieve a glucose level of 80 to 130 mg/dL before meals.

Other, less intense regimens can also promote healthy blood glucose levels for some people. Ideally, the patient and the HCP will work together to select a plan. The criteria for selection are based on the desired and feasible blood glucose levels and the patient's lifestyle, food choices, and activity patterns. If a less intense regimen is not giving the person optimal results, the HCP may encourage a more intense approach.

**Mealtime Insulin (Bolus).** To manage postprandial blood glucose levels, the timing of rapid- and short-acting insulin in relation to meals is crucial. Rapid-acting synthetic insulin analogs, which include lispro (Humalog), aspart (NovoLog), and glulisine (Apidra), have an onset of action of approximately 15 minutes and should be injected within 15 minutes of mealtime. The rapid-acting analogs most closely mimic natural insulin secretion in response to a meal.

### TABLE 48-2 Interprofessional Care
### *Diabetes Mellitus*

**Diagnostic Assessment**
- History and physical examination
- Blood tests, including fasting blood glucose, postprandial blood glucose, A1C, fructosamine, lipid profile, blood urea nitrogen and serum creatinine, electrolytes, islet cell autoantibodies
- Urine for complete urinalysis, albuminuria, and acetone (if indicated)
- Blood pressure
- ECG (if indicated)
- Funduscopic examination (dilated eye examination)
- Dental examination
- Neurologic examination, including monofilament test for sensation to lower extremities
- Ankle-brachial index (ABI) (if indicated) (see Table 37-3)
- Foot (podiatric) examination
- Monitoring of weight

**Management**
- Patient and caregiver teaching and follow-up programs
- Nutrition therapy (Table 48-8)
- Exercise therapy (Tables 48-9 and 48-10)
- Self-monitoring of blood glucose (SMBG) (Table 48-11)

***Drug Therapy***
- Insulin (Fig. 48-3 and Tables 48-3 and 48-4)
- Oral and noninsulin injectable agents (Table 48-7)
- Enteric-coated aspirin (81-162 mg/day)
- Angiotensin-converting enzyme (ACE) inhibitors (see Table 32-7)
- Angiotensin II receptor blockers (ARBs) (see Table 32-7)
- Antihyperlipidemic drugs (see Table 33-5)

### TABLE 48-3 Drug Therapy
### *Types of Insulin*

| Classification | Examples* |
|---|---|
| **Rapid-acting insulin** | lispro (Humalog)<br>aspart (NovoLog)<br>glulisine (Apidra) |
| **Short-acting insulin** | regular (Humulin R, Novolin R) |
| **Intermediate-acting insulin** | NPH (Humulin N, Novolin N) |
| **Long-acting insulin** | glargine (Lantus)<br>detemir (Levemir)<br>degludec (Tresiba) |
| **Combination therapy (premixed)** | NPH/regular 70/30† (Humulin 70/30, Novolin 70/30)<br>NPH/regular 50/50† (Humulin 50/50)<br>lispro protamine/lispro 75/25† (Humalog Mix 75/25)<br>lispro protamine/lispro 50/50† (Humalog Mix 50/50)<br>aspart protamine/aspart 70/30† (NovoLog Mix 70/30)<br>degludec/aspart 70/30 (Ryzodeg) |
| **More concentrated insulin** | Toujeo U-300 (insulin glargine)<br>Humulin R U-500 |
| **Inhaled insulin** | Afrezza |

*Insulin preparations are clear solutions except for NPH and protamine-containing insulin, which are cloudy.
†These numbers refer to percentages of each type of insulin.

| INSULIN PREPARATION | ONSET, PEAK, DURATION | EXAMPLE |
|---|---|---|
| **Rapid acting**<br>lispro (Humalog)<br>aspart (NovoLog)<br>glulisine (Apidra) | *Onset:* 10-30 min<br>*Peak:* 30 min-3 hr<br>*Duration:* 3-5 hr | 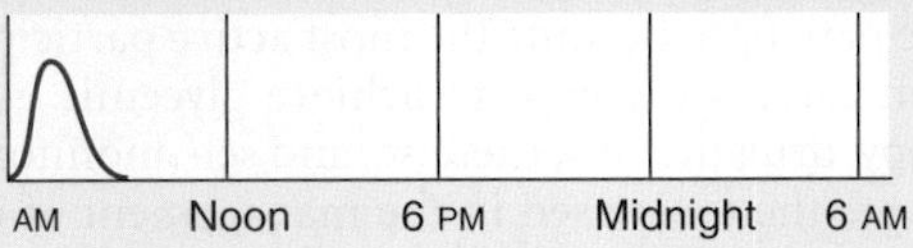 |
| **Short acting**<br>Regular (Humulin R, Novolin R) | *Onset:* 30 min-1 hr<br>*Peak:* 2-5 hr<br>*Duration:* 5-8 hr | 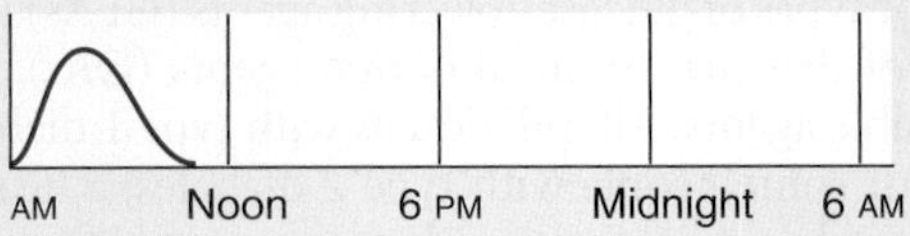 |
| **Intermediate acting**<br>NPH (Humulin N, Novolin N) | *Onset:* 1.5-4 hr<br>*Peak:* 4-12 hr<br>*Duration:* 12-18 hr | 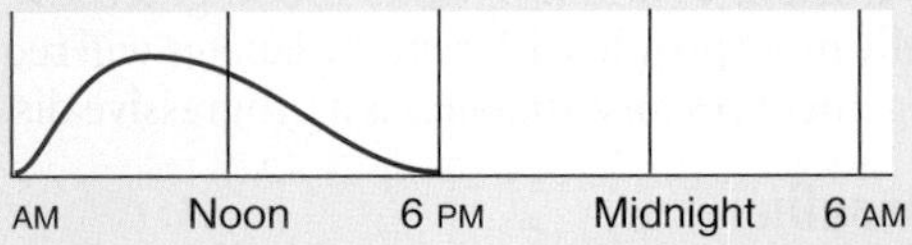 |
| **Long acting**<br>glargine (Lantus)<br>detemir (Levemir)<br>degludec (Tresiba) | *Onset:* 0.8-4 hr<br>*Peak:* Less defined or no pronounced peak<br>*Duration:* 16-24 hr | 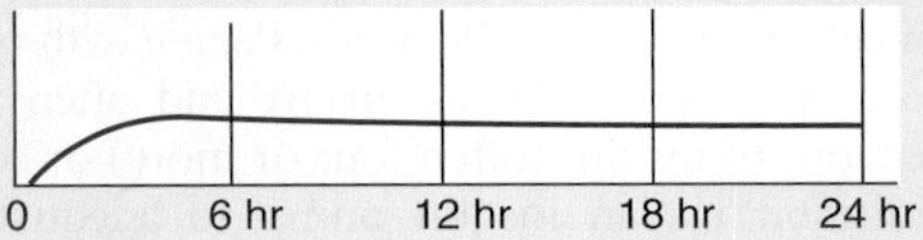 |
| **Inhaled insulin**<br>Afrezza | *Onset:* 12-15 min<br>*Peak:* 60 min<br>*Duration:* 2.5-3 hr | 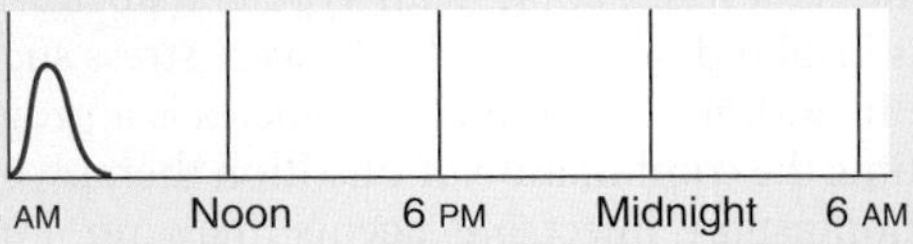 |

**FIG. 48-4** Commercially available insulin preparations showing onset, peak, and duration of action. Individual patient responses to each type of insulin are different and affected by many different factors.

Short-acting regular insulin has an onset of action of 30 to 60 minutes and is injected 30 to 45 minutes before a meal to ensure that the onset of action coincides with meal absorption. Because timing an injection 30 to 45 minutes before a meal is difficult for people to incorporate into their lifestyles, the flexibility that rapid-acting insulins offer is preferred by those taking insulin with their meals.[11] Short-acting insulin is also more likely to cause hypoglycemia because of a longer duration of action.

**Long- or Intermediate-Acting (Basal) Background Insulin.** In addition to mealtime insulin, people with type 1 diabetes use a long- or intermediate-acting basal (background) insulin to maintain blood glucose levels in between meals and overnight. Without 24-hour background insulin, people with type 1 diabetes are more prone to developing DKA. Many people with type 2 diabetes who use oral medications will also require insulin to adequately manage blood glucose levels.

The long-acting insulins include glargine (Lantus, Toujeo), detemir (Levemir), and degludec (Tresiba). This type of insulin is released steadily and continuously, and for many people does not have a peak of action. The action time for long-acting insulin varies (Fig. 48-4). Although they can be used for once-daily subcutaneous administration, detemir is often given twice daily. Because they lack peak action time, the risk for hypoglycemia from this type of insulin is greatly reduced. Glargine and detemir must not be diluted or mixed with any other insulin or solution in the same syringe. Ryzodeg 70/30 is a mixture of degludec and aspart (rapid-acting) insulin.

If oral agents and long-acting insulin are not adequate to achieve glycemic goals, mealtime insulin may also be added.

Intermediate-acting insulin (NPH) is also used as a basal insulin. It has a duration of 12 to 18 hours. The disadvantage of NPH is that it has a peak ranging from 4 to 12 hours, which can result in hypoglycemia. NPH can be mixed with short- and rapid-acting insulins. NPH insulin should never be given IV.

### CHECK YOUR PRACTICE

You are preparing your patient's order for NPH insulin. When you look at the vial, you notice that it is cloudy. You are thinking that you should throw away the vial because it must be contaminated.

- Before you take this action, what should you do?

NPH, lispro protamine, and aspart protamine are cloudy insulins because they contain protamine. This substance decreases solubility, and as a result these insulins must be gently agitated before administration.

**Combination Insulin Therapy.** For those who want to use only one or two injections per day, a short- or rapid-acting insulin is mixed with intermediate-acting insulin in the same syringe. This allows the patient to have both mealtime and basal coverage without having to administer two separate injections. Although this may be more appealing to the patient, most patients achieve more optimal blood glucose levels with basal-bolus therapy. Patients may mix the two types of insulin themselves or may use a commercially premixed formula or pen (Table 48-3). Premixed formulas offer convenience to patients, who do not have to draw up and mix insulin from two different vials. This is especially helpful to those who lack the visual, manual, or cognitive skills to mix insulin themselves. However, the convenience of these formulas limits the potential for optimal blood glucose levels because there is less opportunity for flexible dosing based on need.

## TABLE 48-4 Drug Therapy

### *Insulin Regimens*

| Regimen | Type of Insulin and Frequency | Action Profile | Comments |
|---|---|---|---|
| **Once a day**<br>Single dose | Intermediate (NPH)<br>*At bedtime* | 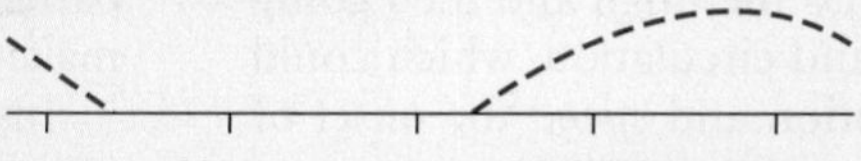 | One injection should provide nighttime coverage. |
| | OR<br>Long-acting (glargine [Lantus], detemir [Levemir])<br>*In AM or at bedtime* | 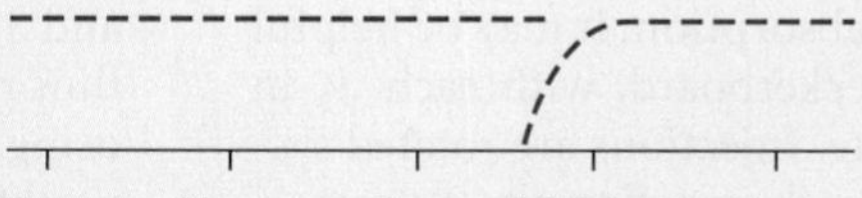 | One injection may last up to 24 hr with less defined peaks and less chance for hypoglycemia. Does not cover postprandial blood glucose levels. |
| **Twice a day**<br>Split-mixed dose | NPH and regular or rapid (both regular and rapid are shown on the diagram)<br>*Before breakfast and at dinner* | 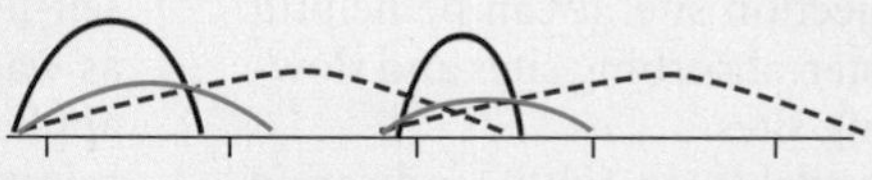 | Two injections provide coverage for 24 hr.<br>Patient must eat at certain times to avoid hypoglycemia. |
| **Three times a day**<br>Combination of mixed and single dose | NPH and regular or rapid (both regular and rapid are shown on the diagram)<br>*Before breakfast*<br>+<br>Regular or rapid<br>*Before dinner*<br>+<br>NPH<br>*At bedtime* | 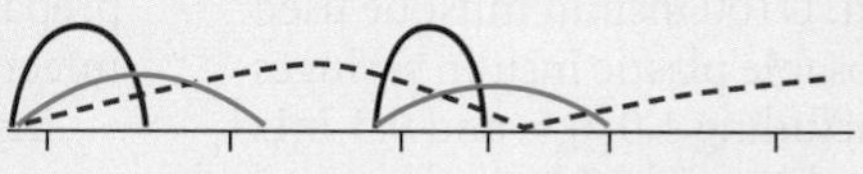 | Three injections provide coverage for 24 hr, particularly during early AM hours. Decreased potential for 2-3 AM hypoglycemia. |
| **Basal-bolus**<br>Multiple dose | Regular or rapid (both regular and rapid are shown on the diagram)<br>*Before breakfast, lunch, and dinner*<br>+<br>Long-acting (glargine or detemir)<br>*Once or twice a day*<br>OR<br>Regular or rapid (both regular and rapid are shown on the diagram)<br>*Before breakfast, lunch, and dinner*<br>+<br>NPH<br>*Twice a day* | 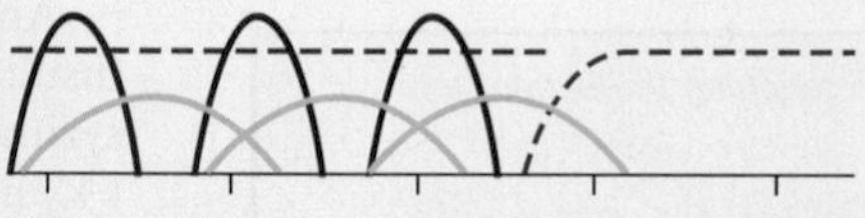<br>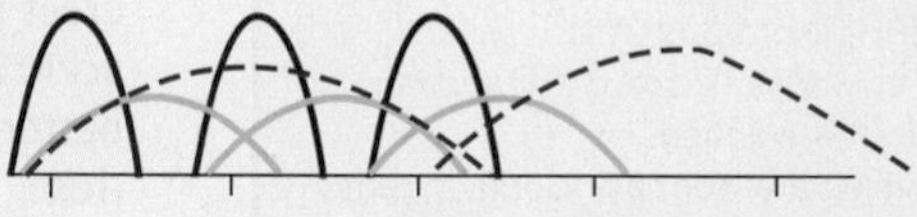 | More flexibility is allowed at mealtimes and for amount of food intake. Good postprandial coverage.<br>Preprandial blood glucose checks and establishing and following individualized algorithms are necessary. Patients with type 1 diabetes require basal insulin to cover 24 hr.<br>Most physiologic approach, except for pump. |

——— Rapid-acting (lispro, aspart, glulisine) insulin.
——— Short-acting (regular) insulin.
- - - - Intermediate-acting (NPH) or long-acting (glargine, detemir) insulin.

**Storage of Insulin.** As a protein, insulin requires special storage considerations. Heat and freezing alter the insulin molecule and can make it less effective. Insulin vials and insulin pens currently in use may be left at room temperature for up to 4 weeks unless the room temperature is higher than 86° F (30° C) or below freezing (less than 32° F [0° C]). Prolonged exposure to direct sunlight should be avoided. A patient who is traveling in hot climates may store insulin in a thermos or cooler to keep it cool (not frozen). Store unopened insulin vials and insulin pens in the refrigerator.

Patients who are traveling or caregivers of patients who are sight impaired or who lack the manual dexterity to fill their own syringes may prefill insulin syringes. Prefilled syringes containing two different insulins are stable for up to 1 week when stored in the refrigerator, whereas syringes containing only one type of insulin are stable up to 30 days.[12]

Teach patients to store syringes in a vertical position with the needle pointed up to avoid clumping of suspended insulin in the needle. Before injection, gently roll prefilled syringes between the palms 10 to 20 times to warm the insulin and resuspend the particles. Some insulin combinations are not appropriate for prefilling and storage because the mixture can alter the onset, action, and/or peak times of either of the types. Consult a pharmacy reference as needed when mixing and prefilling different types of insulin.

**Administration of Insulin.** Routine doses of insulin are administered by subcutaneous injection. Regular insulin can be given IV when immediate onset of action is desired. Insulin is not taken orally because it is inactivated by gastric fluids. Teach patients to avoid injecting insulin IM because rapid and unpredictable absorption could result in hypoglycemia.

***Insulin Injection.*** The steps in administering a subcutaneous insulin injection are outlined in Table 48-5. Teach this technique to new insulin users and review it periodically with long-term users. Never assume that because the patient already uses insulin, he or she knows and practices the correct insulin injection technique. The patient may not have understood prior instructions, or changes in eyesight may result in inaccurate preparation. The patient may not see air bubbles in the syringe or may improperly read the scale on the syringe. The patient receiving mixed insulins in the same syringe needs to learn the proper technique for combining them if commercially prepared premixed insulins are not used.

The speed with which peak serum concentrations are reached varies with the anatomic site for injection. The fastest subcutaneous absorption is from the abdomen, followed by the arm, thigh, and buttock. Although the abdomen is often the preferred injection site, other sites also work well (Fig. 48-5). Caution the patient about injecting into a site that is to be exercised. For example, injecting into the thigh and then going jogging could increase body heat and circulation, which could increase the rate of insulin absorption and speed the onset of action, thus resulting in hypoglycemia.

Teach patients to rotate the injection within and between sites. This allows for better insulin absorption. It may be helpful to think of the abdomen as a checkerboard, with each $\frac{1}{2}$-in square representing an injection site. Injections are rotated systematically across the board, with each injection site at least $\frac{1}{2}$ to 1 in away from the previous injection site. It can be helpful to inject fast-acting insulin into faster-absorbing sites and slow-acting insulin into slower-absorbing sites.

Most commercial insulin is available as U100, indicating that 1 mL contains 100 U of insulin. U100 insulin must be used with a U100-marked syringe. Disposable plastic insulin syringes are available in a variety of sizes, including 1.0, 0.5, and 0.3 mL. The 0.5-mL size may be used for doses of 50 U or less, and the 0.3-mL syringe can be used for doses of 30 U or less. The 0.5- and 0.3-mL syringes are in 1-U increments. This provides more accurate delivery when the dose is an odd number. The 1.0-mL syringe is necessary for patients who require more than 50 U of insulin. The 1.0-mL syringe is in 2-U increments. When patients change from a 0.3- or a 0.5-mL to a 1.0-mL syringe, make them aware of the dose increment difference.

Insulin syringe needles come in the following lengths: 6 mm ($\frac{1}{4}$ in), 8 mm ($\frac{5}{16}$ in), and 12.7 mm ($\frac{1}{2}$ in).[13] Needle gauges also vary among syringes. The needle gauges available are 28, 29, 30, and 31. The higher the gauge number, the smaller the diameter, thus resulting in a more comfortable injection. Only the person using the syringe should recap the needle; never recap a needle used for a patient. The use of an alcohol swab on the site before self-injection is no longer recommended. Routine hygiene such as washing with soap and rinsing with water is adequate. This applies primarily to patient self-injection technique. When injection occurs in a health care facility, policy may dictate site preparation with alcohol to prevent health care–associated infection (HAI).

Insulin injections are typically given at a 90-degree angle. For extremely thin or muscular patients in the hospital, perform injections at a 45-degree angle. At home, patients inject at a 90-degree angle using the shortest needle desired. Pinching up of the skin to avoid IM injection is no longer necessary because of the availability of short needles.

An insulin pen is a compact portable device loaded with an insulin cartridge that serves the same function as a needle and syringe (Fig. 48-6). Pen needles are available in lengths of 4 mm ($\frac{5}{32}$ in), 5 mm ($\frac{3}{16}$ in), 8 mm ($\frac{5}{16}$ in), and 12.7 mm ($\frac{1}{2}$ in) and in three gauges: 29, 31, and 32. Insulin pens offer convenience and flexibility. They are portable and compact, are more discreet than using a vial and syringe, and provide consistent and accurate dosing. For patients with poor vision, the pen is a better option, since they can hear the clicks of the pen as the dose is selected. Insulin pens come packaged with printed instructions, including pictures of the steps to take when using the pen. These instructions are helpful when teaching new users and reviewing technique with current users of a pen.

***Insulin Pump.*** An *insulin pump* delivers a continuous subcutaneous insulin infusion through a small device worn on the belt, in a pocket, or under clothing. Insulin pumps use rapid-acting insulin, which is loaded into a reservoir or cartridge and connected via plastic tubing to a catheter inserted into the subcutaneous tissue. Insulet Corporation has an insulin pump that is a tubing-free system (Fig. 48-7). All insulin pumps are programmed to deliver a continuous infusion of rapid-acting insulin 24 hours a day, known as the *basal rate.* Basal insulin can be temporarily increased or decreased based on carbohy-

## TABLE 48-5 Patient & Caregiver Teaching
### *Insulin Therapy*

*Include the following instructions when teaching the patient and caregiver about insulin therapy.*

1. Wash hands thoroughly.
2. Always inspect insulin bottle before using it. Make sure that it is the proper type and concentration, expiration date has not passed, and top of bottle is in perfect condition. Insulin solutions (except for intermediate-acting insulins [NPH, lispro/protamine, aspart/protamine]) should look clear and colorless. Discard if it appears discolored or if you see particles in the solution.
3. For intermediate-acting insulins (which are normally cloudy), gently roll the insulin bottle between the palms of hands to mix the insulin. (Clear insulins do not need to be agitated.)
4. Select proper injection site (Fig. 48-5).
5. Ensure that the site is clean and dry.
6. Push the needle straight into the skin (90-degree angle). If you are very thin, muscular, or using an 8- or 12-mm needle, you may need to pinch the skin and/or use a 45-degree angle.
7. Push the plunger all the way down, leave needle in place for 5 sec to ensure that all insulin has been injected, and then remove needle.
8. Destroy and dispose of single-use syringe safely.

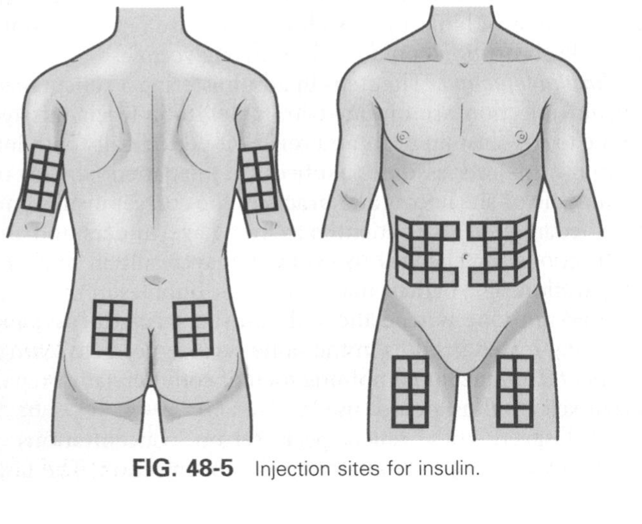

**FIG. 48-5** Injection sites for insulin.

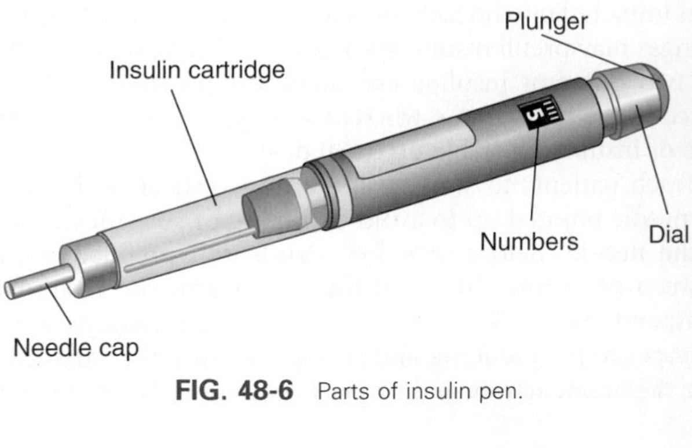


**FIG. 48-6** Parts of insulin pen.

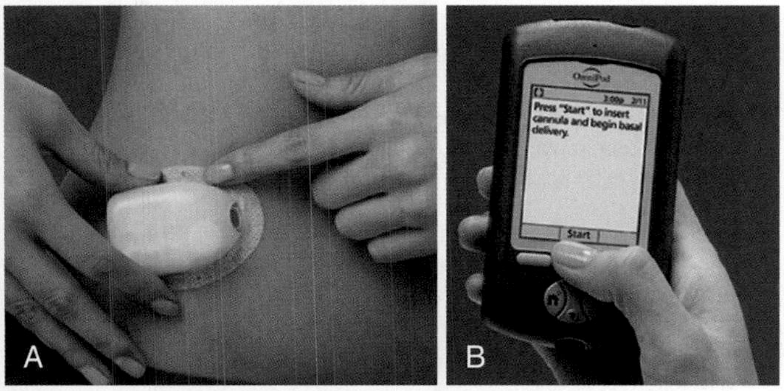


**FIG. 48-7** **A,** OmniPod Insulin Management System. The Pod holds and delivers insulin. **B,** The Personal Diabetes Manager (PDM) wirelessly programs insulin delivery via the Pod. The PDM has a built-in glucose meter. (Courtesy of Insulet Corporation.)

drate intake, activity changes, or illness. Many individuals require different basal rates at different times of the day.

At mealtime, the user programs the pump to deliver a bolus infusion of insulin appropriate to the amount of carbohydrate ingested and an additional amount, if needed, to bring down or "correct" high preprandial blood glucose. The infusion set is changed every 2 to 3 days and placed in a new site to avoid infection and to promote good insulin absorption. Insulin pump users check their blood glucose level at least four times per day. Monitoring eight times or more per day is common.

A major advantage of the insulin pump is the potential for keeping blood glucose levels in a tighter range. This is possible because insulin delivery is similar to the normal physiologic pattern. Pumps offer users more flexibility with meal and activity patterns. Potential challenges of insulin pump therapy include infection at the insertion site, an increased risk for DKA if the insulin infusion is disrupted, the increased cost of the pump and supplies, and being attached to a device.[14]

**Problems With Insulin Therapy.** Problems associated with insulin therapy include hypoglycemia, allergic reactions, lipodystrophy, and the Somogyi effect. Hypoglycemia is discussed in detail later in this chapter. (Guidelines for assessing patients treated with insulin and other GLAs are presented in Table 48-6.)

***Allergic Reactions.*** Local inflammatory reactions to insulin may occur, such as itching, erythema, and burning around the injection site. Local reactions may be self-limiting within 1 to 3 months or may improve with a low dose of antihistamine. A true insulin allergy, which is rare, is manifested by a systemic response with urticaria and possibly anaphylactic shock. Zinc or protamine used as a preservative in the insulin and the latex or rubber stoppers on the vials have been implicated in allergic reactions.

***Lipodystrophy.*** *Lipodystrophy* (atrophy or hypertrophy of subcutaneous tissue) may occur if the same injection sites are used frequently. The use of human insulin has significantly reduced the risk for lipodystrophy. *Atrophy* is the wasting of subcutaneous tissue and presents as indentations in injection sites. *Hypertrophy,* a thickening of the subcutaneous tissue, eventually regresses if the patient does not use the site for at least 6 months. The use of hypertrophied sites may result in erratic insulin absorption.

***Somogyi Effect and Dawn Phenomenon.*** Hyperglycemia in the morning may be due to the **Somogyi effect**. A high dose of insulin produces a decline in blood glucose levels during the night. As a result, counterregulatory hormones (e.g., glucagon, epinephrine, growth hormone, cortisol) are released, stimulating lipolysis, gluconeogenesis, and glycogenolysis, which in turn produce rebound hyperglycemia. The danger of this effect is that when blood glucose levels are measured in the morning, hyperglycemia is apparent and the patient (or the HCP) may increase the insulin dose.

If a patient is experiencing morning hyperglycemia, checking blood glucose levels between 2:00 and 4:00 AM for hypoglycemia will help determine if the cause is the Somogyi effect. The patient may report headaches on awakening and recall having night sweats or nightmares. A bedtime snack, a reduction in the dose of insulin, or both can help to prevent the Somogyi effect.

**TABLE 48-6 Assessing the Patient Treated With Glucose-Lowering Agents**

| Category | Assessment |
|---|---|
| **For Patient With Newly Diagnosed Diabetes or for Reevaluation of Drug Regimen** | |
| **Cognitive** | • Is patient or caregiver able to understand why insulin or OAs are being used as part of diabetes management?<br>• Is patient or caregiver able to understand concepts of asepsis, combining insulins, and side effects of medications?<br>• Is patient able to remember to take >1 dose/day?<br>• Does patient take medications at right times in relation to meals? |
| **Psychomotor** | • Is patient or caregiver physically able to prepare and administer accurate doses of the drugs? |
| **Affective** | • What emotions and attitudes are patient and caregiver displaying concerning diagnosis of diabetes and insulin or OA treatment? |
| **For Follow-up of Patients Taking GLAs** | |
| **Effectiveness of therapy** | • Is patient having symptoms of hyperglycemia?<br>• Does blood glucose record show blood glucose levels in or out of the target range?<br>• Is A1C in a healthy range and consistent with glucose records? |
| **Side effects of therapy** | • Is atrophy or hypertrophy present at injection sites?<br>• Has patient had hypoglycemia? If so, how often? What time of day? What were the symptoms of hypoglycemia?<br>• Are there complaints of nightmares, night sweats, or early morning headaches?<br>• Has patient had a skin rash or GI upset since taking OAs?<br>• Has patient gained or lost weight? |
| **Self-management behaviors** | • If patient is having hyperglycemia or hypoglycemia, how are those episodes managed?<br>• Has patient determined reason for hyperglycemia or hypoglycemia?<br>• How much insulin or OA is patient taking and at what time of day? Is patient adjusting insulin dose? Under what circumstances and by how much?<br>• Has exercise pattern changed?<br>• Is patient making healthy food choices? Are meals taken at times corresponding to peak insulin action? |

*A1C,* Glycosylated hemoglobin; *GLA,* glucose-lowering agent; *OA,* oral agent.

The **dawn phenomenon** is also characterized by hyperglycemia that is present on awakening. Two counterregulatory hormones (growth hormone and cortisol), which are excreted in increased amounts in the early morning hours, may be the cause of this phenomenon. The dawn phenomenon affects a majority of people with diabetes and tends to be most severe when growth hormone is at its peak in adolescence and young adulthood.

Careful assessment is required to document the Somogyi effect or dawn phenomenon because the treatment for each differs. The treatment for Somogyi effect is less insulin in the evening. The treatment for dawn phenomenon is an increase in insulin or an adjustment in administration time. Your assessment must include insulin dose, injection sites, and variability in the time of meals or insulin administration. Ask the patient to measure and document bedtime, nighttime (between 2:00 and 4:00 AM), and morning fasting blood glucose levels on several occasions. If the predawn levels are less than 60 mg/dL (3.3 mmol/L) and signs and symptoms of hypoglycemia are present, the insulin dosage should be reduced. If the 2:00 to 4:00 AM blood glucose is high, the insulin dosage should be increased. In addition, counsel the patient on appropriate bedtime snacks.

**Inhaled Insulin.** Afrezza, a rapid-acting inhaled insulin, is administered at the beginning of each meal or within 20 minutes after starting a meal. It is not a substitute for long-acting insulin. Afrezza must be used in combination with long-acting insulin in patients with type 1 diabetes. It is not recommended for the treatment of diabetic ketoacidosis or in patients who smoke. The most common adverse reactions are hypoglycemia, cough, and throat pain or irritation. Afrezza should not be used in patients with chronic lung disease, such as asthma or COPD, because bronchospasm can occur.

### Drug Therapy: Oral and Noninsulin Injectable Agents

OAs and noninsulin injectable agents work to improve the mechanisms by which the body produces and uses insulin and glucose. These drugs work on three defects of type 2 diabetes: (1) insulin resistance, (2) decreased insulin production, and (3) increased hepatic glucose production. These drugs may be used in combination with agents from other classes or with insulin to achieve blood glucose goals. Oral and noninsulin injectable agents are listed in Table 48-7.

**Biguanides.** The most widely used oral diabetes agent is metformin, the only medication in the biguanide class available in the United States. Metformin is the most effective first-line treatment for type 2 diabetes.[15] Forms of metformin include Glucophage (immediate release), Glucophage XR (extended release), Fortamet (extended release), and Riomet (liquid form of metformin). The primary action of metformin is to reduce glucose production by the liver. It also enhances insulin sensitivity at the tissue level and improves glucose transport into the cells. Additionally, it has beneficial effects on plasma lipids.

Because it may cause moderate weight loss, metformin may be useful for people with type 2 diabetes and prediabetes who are overweight or obese. It is also used in the prevention of type 2 diabetes in those with prediabetes who are less than age 60 and have risk factors such as hypertension or a history of gestational diabetes.

Patients who are undergoing surgery or any radiologic procedures that involve the use of a contrast medium are instructed to temporarily discontinue metformin before surgery or the procedure. They should not resume the metformin until 48 hours afterward, once their serum creatinine has been checked and is normal.

**DRUG ALERT Metformin**

- Do not use in patients with kidney disease, liver disease, or heart failure. Lactic acidosis is a rare complication of metformin accumulation.
- IV contrast media that contain iodine pose a risk of acute kidney injury, which could exacerbate metformin-induced lactic acidosis.
- To reduce risk of kidney injury, discontinue metformin a day or two before the procedure.
- May be resumed 48 hours after the procedure, assuming kidney function is normal.
- Do not use in people who drink excessive amounts of alcohol.
- Take with food to minimize GI side effects.

**Sulfonylureas.** Sulfonylureas include glipizide (Glucotrol, Glucotrol XL), glyburide (DiaBeta, Glynase), and glimepiride (Amaryl). The primary action of the sulfonylureas is to increase insulin production by the pancreas. Therefore hypoglycemia is the major side effect with sulfonylureas.

**Meglitinides.** Like the sulfonylureas, repaglinide (Prandin) and nateglinide (Starlix) increase insulin production by the pancreas. However, because they are more rapidly absorbed and eliminated than sulfonylureas, they are less likely to cause hypoglycemia. When they are taken just before meals, pancreatic insulin production increases during and after the meal, mimicking the normal response to eating. Instruct patients to take meglitinides any time from 30 minutes before each meal right up to the time of the meal. These drugs should not be taken if a meal is skipped.

**α-Glucosidase Inhibitors.** Also known as "starch blockers," these drugs work by slowing down the absorption of carbohydrate in the small intestine. Acarbose (Precose) and miglitol (Glyset) are the available drugs in this class. Taken with the first bite of each main meal, they are most effective in lowering postprandial blood glucose. Their effectiveness is measured by checking 2-hour postprandial glucose levels.

**Thiazolidinediones.** Sometimes referred to as "insulin sensitizers," these agents include pioglitazone (Actos) and rosiglitazone (Avandia). They are most effective for people who have insulin resistance. These agents improve insulin sensitivity, transport, and utilization at target tissues. Because they do not increase insulin production, thiazolidinediones do not cause hypoglycemia when used alone. However, these drugs are rarely used today because of their adverse effects. Rosiglitazone is associated with adverse cardiovascular events (e.g., myocardial infarction) and can be obtained only through restricted access programs. Pioglitazone can worsen heart failure and is associated with an increased risk of bladder cancer.

**Dipeptidyl Peptidase-4 (DPP-4) Inhibitors.** Incretin hormones are released by the intestines throughout the day, but levels increase in response to a meal. When glucose levels are normal or elevated, incretins increase insulin synthesis and release from the pancreas, as well as decrease hepatic glucose production. The incretin hormones are normally inactivated by dipeptidyl peptidase-4 (DPP-4).

DPP-4 inhibitors (also known as *gliptins*) come in pill form and include sitagliptin (Januvia), saxagliptin (Onglyza), linagliptin (Tradjenta), and alogliptin (Nesina). DPP-4 inhibitors block the action of the DPP-4 enzyme, which is responsible for inactivating incretin hormones (gastric inhibitory peptide [GIP] and glucagon-like peptide-1 [GLP-1]). The result is an increase in insulin release, decrease in glucagon secretion,

## TABLE 48-7 Drug Therapy

### Oral Agents and Noninsulin Injectable Agents

| Type | Mechanism of Action | Side Effects |
|---|---|---|
| **Oral Agents** | | |
| ***Biguanides*** | | |
| metformin (Glucophage, Glucophage XR, Riomet, Fortamet, Glumetza) | Decreases rate of hepatic glucose production. Augments glucose uptake by tissues, especially muscles. | Diarrhea, lactic acidosis. Must be held 1-2 days before IV contrast media given and for 48 hr after. |
| ***Sulfonylureas*** | | |
| glipizide (Glucotrol, Glucotrol XL)<br>glyburide (DiaBeta, Glynase)<br>glimepiride (Amaryl) | Stimulate release of insulin from pancreatic islets. Decrease glycogenolysis and gluconeogenesis. Enhance cellular sensitivity to insulin. | Weight gain, hypoglycemia. |
| ***Meglitinides*** | | |
| nateglinide (Starlix)<br>repaglinide (Prandin) | Stimulate a rapid and short-lived release of insulin from the pancreas. | Weight gain, hypoglycemia. |
| ***α-Glucosidase Inhibitors*** | | |
| acarbose (Precose)<br>miglitol (Glyset) | Delay absorption of complex carbohydrates (starches) from GI tract. | Gas, abdominal pain, diarrhea. |
| ***Thiazolidinediones*** | | |
| pioglitazone (Actos)<br>rosiglitazone (Avandia) | Increase glucose uptake in muscle. Decrease endogenous glucose production. | Weight gain, edema.<br>*pioglitazone:* may increase risk for bladder cancer and exacerbate heart failure.<br>*rosiglitazone:* may increase risk for cardiovascular events (e.g., myocardial infarction, stroke). |
| ***Dipeptidyl Peptidase-4 (DPP-4) Inhibitors*** | | |
| linagliptin (Tradjenta)<br>saxagliptin (Onglyza)<br>sitagliptin (Januvia)<br>alogliptin (Nesina) | Enhance activity of incretins. Stimulate release of insulin from pancreatic β-cells. Decrease hepatic glucose production. | Pancreatitis, allergic reactions. |
| ***Dopamine Receptor Agonists*** | | |
| bromocriptine (Cycloset) | Activates dopamine receptors in central nervous system. Unknown how it improves glycemic levels. | Orthostatic hypotension. |
| ***Sodium-Glucose Co-Transporter 2 (SGLT2) Inhibitors*** | | |
| canagliflozin (Invokana)<br>dapagliflozin (Farxiga)<br>empagliflozin (Jardiance) | Decreases renal glucose reabsorption and increases urinary glucose excretion | Increased risk of genital and urinary tract infections. Hypoglycemia. |
| ***Combination Oral Therapy*** | | |
| Glucovance | Same as for metformin and glyburide. | See side effects for individual drugs. |
| Duetact | Same as for pioglitazone and glimepiride. | Same as above. |
| Actoplus Met, Actoplus Met XR | Same as for metformin and pioglitazone. | Same as above. |
| Janumet, Janumet XR | Same as for metformin and sitagliptin. | Same as above. |
| Jentadueto | Same as for linagliptin and metformin. | Same as above. |
| PrandiMet | Same as for metformin and repaglinide. | Same as above. |
| Kombiglyze | Same as for saxagliptin and metformin. | Same as above. |
| Kazano | Same as for alogliptin and metformin. | Same as above. |
| Oseni | Same as for alogliptin and pioglitazone. | Same as above. |
| Glyxambi | Same as for empagliflozin and linagliptin. | Same as above. |
| Xigduo | Same as for dapagliflozin and metformin. | Same as above. |
| Synjardy | Same as metformin and empagliflozin. | Same as above. |
| **Noninsulin Injectable Agents** | | |
| ***Glucagon-Like Peptide-1 (GLP-1) Receptor Agonists**** | | |
| exenatide (Byetta)<br>exenatide extended-release (Bydureon)<br>liraglutide (Victoza)<br>albiglutide (Tanzeum)<br>dulaglutide (Trulicity)<br>lixisenatide (Adlyxin) | Stimulate release of insulin, decrease glucagon secretion, and slow gastric emptying. Increase satiety. | Nausea, vomiting, hypoglycemia, diarrhea, headache. |
| ***Amylin Analogs†*** | | |
| pramlintide (Symlin) | Slows gastric emptying, decreases glucagon secretion and endogenous glucose output from liver. Increases satiety. | Hypoglycemia, nausea, vomiting, decreased appetite, headache. |

*Administered subcutaneously.
†Administered subcutaneously only in abdomen or thigh.

and decrease in hepatic glucose production. Since the DPP-4 inhibitors are glucose dependent, they lower the potential for hypoglycemia. The main benefit of these drugs over other medications for diabetes with similar effects is the absence of weight gain as a side effect.

**Sodium-Glucose Co-Transporter 2 (SGLT2) Inhibitors.** Sodium-glucose co-transporter 2 (SGLT2) inhibitors work by blocking the reabsorption of glucose by the kidney, increasing glucose excretion, and lowering blood glucose levels. Drugs in this class include canagliflozin (Invokana), dapagliflozin (Farxiga), and empagliflozin (Jardiance).

**Dopamine Receptor Agonist.** Bromocriptine (Cycloset) is a dopamine receptor agonist that improves glycemic levels. The mechanism of action is unknown. Patients with type 2 diabetes are thought to have low levels of dopamine activity in the morning. These low levels of dopamine may interfere with the body's ability to control blood glucose. Bromocriptine increases dopamine receptor activity. It can be used alone or as an add-on to another type 2 diabetes treatment.

**Combination Oral Therapy.** Many combination drugs are currently available (Table 48-7). These drugs combine two different classes of medications to treat diabetes. One advantage of combination therapy is that the patient takes fewer pills, thus improving adherence to taking medications.

**Glucagon-Like Peptide-1 Receptor Agonists.** Exenatide (Byetta), exenatide extended-release (Bydureon), liraglutide (Victoza), albiglutide (Tanzeum), dulaglutide (Trulicity), and lixisenatide (Adlyxin) simulate GLP-1 (one of the incretin hormones), which is found to be decreased in people with type 2 diabetes. These drugs increase insulin synthesis and release from the pancreas, inhibit glucagon secretion, slow gastric emptying, and reduce food intake by increasing satiety.

These drugs may be used as monotherapy or adjunct therapy for patients with type 2 diabetes who have not achieved optimal glucose levels on OAs. These drugs are administered using a subcutaneous injection in a prefilled pen. In contrast to exenatide, which is given twice a day, and liraglutide, which is given once daily, dulaglutide, albiglutide, and Bydureon are given once every 7 days. The delayed gastric emptying that occurs with these medications may affect the absorption of oral medications. Advise patients to take fast-acting oral medications at least 1 hour before injecting a GLP-1 agonist drug.

**DRUG ALERT Exenatide (Byetta)**

- Acute pancreatitis and kidney problems have been associated with its use.

**DRUG ALERT Liraglutide (Victoza) and Dulaglutide (Trulicity)**

- Do not use in patients with a personal or family history of medullary thyroid cancer.
- Acute pancreatitis has been associated with its use.

**Amylin Analogs.** Pramlintide (Symlin) is the only available amylin analog. Amylin, a hormone secreted by the β-cells of the pancreas in response to food intake, slows gastric emptying, reduces glucagon secretion, and increases satiety.[12] Pramlintide is used in addition to mealtime insulin in patients with type 1 or type 2 diabetes who have elevated blood glucose levels on insulin therapy. It is only used concurrently with insulin and is not a replacement for insulin. Pramlintide is administered before major meals subcutaneously into the thigh or abdomen. It cannot be injected into the arm because absorption from this site is too variable. The drug cannot be mixed in the same syringe with insulin.

The concurrent use of pramlintide and insulin increases the risk of severe hypoglycemia during the 3 hours after injection, especially in patients with type 1 diabetes. Instruct patients to eat a meal with at least 250 calories and keep a form of fast-acting glucose on hand in the event that hypoglycemia develops. When pramlintide is used, the bolus dose of insulin should be reduced.

**DRUG ALERT Pramlintide (Symlin)**

- Can cause severe hypoglycemia when used with insulin.

**Other Drugs Affecting Blood Glucose Levels.** Both the patient and the HCP must be aware of drug interactions that can potentiate hypoglycemia and hyperglycemia effects. For example, β-adrenergic blockers can mask symptoms of hypoglycemia and prolong the hypoglycemic effects of insulin. Thiazide and loop diuretics can potentiate hyperglycemia by inducing potassium loss, although low-dose therapy with a thiazide is usually considered safe.

## Nutritional Therapy

Individualized nutrition therapy, consisting of counseling, education, and ongoing monitoring, is a cornerstone of care for people with diabetes and prediabetes.[16] Changing eating habits can be challenging for many people. Achieving nutrition goals requires a coordinated team effort that takes into account the person's behavioral, cognitive, socioeconomic, cultural, and religious backgrounds and preferences. Because of these complexities, it is recommended that a dietitian with expertise in diabetes management work with the person who has diabetes. The dietitian starts with a nutrition assessment and develops an individualized food plan. Additional team members may include nurses, certified diabetes educators, clinical nurse specialists, HCPs, and social workers.

Guidelines from the ADA indicate that, within the context of an overall healthy eating plan, a person with diabetes can eat the same foods as a person who does not have diabetes. This means that the same principles of healthy nutrition that apply to the general population also apply to the person with diabetes. Table 48-8 describes nutrition guidelines for patients with diabetes. According to the ADA, the overall goal of nutrition therapy is to assist people with diabetes in making healthy nutritional choices that will lead to achieving and/or maintaining safe and healthy blood glucose levels. Additional specific goals include the following:

- Maintain blood glucose levels as close to normal as safely possible to prevent or reduce the risk for complications of diabetes.
- Achieve lipid profiles and BP levels that reduce the risk for CVD.
- Prevent or slow the rate of development of chronic complications of diabetes by modifying nutrient intake and lifestyle.
- Address individual nutrition needs while taking into account personal and cultural preferences and respecting the individual's willingness or ability to change eating and dietary habits.
- Maintain the pleasure of eating by encouraging a variety of healthy food choices.

**Type 1 Diabetes Mellitus.** People with type 1 diabetes base their meal planning on usual food intake and preferences balanced with insulin and exercise patterns. The patient coordinates insulin dosing with eating habits and activity pattern in mind. Day-to-day consistency in timing and amount of food eaten makes it much easier to manage blood glucose levels, especially for those individuals using conventional, fixed insulin

**TABLE 48-8 Nutritional Therapy**

***Diabetes Mellitus***

| Component | Recommendations |
|---|---|
| **Total carbohydrate** | • Include carbohydrate from fruits, vegetables, grains, legumes, and low-fat milk.<br>• Monitor by carbohydrate counting, exchange lists, or use of appropriate proportions.<br>• Sucrose-containing food can be substituted for other carbohydrates in meal plan.<br>• Fiber intake at 25-30 g/day.<br>• Nonnutritive sweeteners are safe when consumed within FDA daily intake levels. |
| **Protein** | • Individualize goals.<br>• High-protein diets are not recommended for weight loss. |
| **Fat** | • Individualize goals.<br>• Minimize *trans* fat.<br>• Dietary cholesterol <200 mg/day.<br>• ≥2 servings of fish per week to provide polyunsaturated fatty acids. |
| **Alcohol** | • Limit to moderate amount (maximum 1 drink per day for women and 2 drinks per day for men).<br>• Consume alcohol with food to reduce risk of nocturnal hypoglycemia in those using insulin or insulin secretagogues.<br>• Moderate alcohol consumption has no acute effect on glucose and insulin concentrations, but carbohydrate taken with the alcohol (mixed drink) may raise blood glucose. |

Source: Evert AB, Boucher JL, Cypress M: Nutrition therapy recommendations for the management of adults with diabetes, *Diabetes Care* 36(11): 3821, 2013.

regimens. Patients using rapid-acting insulin can adjust the dose before each meal based on the current blood glucose level and the carbohydrate content of the meal. Intensified insulin therapy, such as multiple daily injections or the use of an insulin pump, allows considerable flexibility in food selection and can be adjusted for alterations from usual eating and exercise habits.

**Type 2 Diabetes Mellitus.** Nutrition therapy in type 2 diabetes emphasizes achieving glucose, lipid, and BP goals. Modest weight loss has been associated with improved insulin resistance. Therefore weight loss is recommended for all individuals with diabetes who are overweight or obese.[16]

No one proven strategy or method can be uniformly recommended. A nutritionally adequate meal plan with appropriate serving sizes, a reduction of saturated and *trans* fats, and low carbohydrates can decrease calorie consumption. Spacing meals is another strategy that spreads nutrient intake throughout the day. A weight loss of 5% to 7% of body weight often improves blood glucose levels, even if desirable body weight is not achieved. Weight loss is best attempted by a moderate decrease in calories and an increase in caloric expenditure. Regularly exercising and adopting new behaviors and attitudes can facilitate long-term lifestyle changes. Monitoring of blood glucose levels, A1C, lipids, and BP provides feedback on how well the goals of nutrition therapy are being met.

**Food Composition.** A healthy balance of nutrients is essential to maintain blood glucose levels and overall health. Energy from food intake can be balanced with the patient's energy output. Patients plan their individual meal plan with their lifestyle and health goals in mind. The following are general recommendations for nutrient balance.

***Carbohydrates.*** Carbohydrates include sugars, starches, and fiber. Carbohydrates provide important sources of energy, fiber, vitamins, and minerals and are therefore important to all people, including those with diabetes. Foods containing carbohydrates from whole grains, fruits, vegetables, and low-fat dairy are part of a healthy meal plan. The ADA recommends individualizing carbohydrate intake as there is no ideal number for all people with diabetes.

All individuals benefit from including dietary fiber as part of a healthy meal plan. The current recommendation for the general population is 25 to 30 g/day.[16]

Nutritive and nonnutritive sweeteners may be included in a healthy meal plan in moderation. Nonnutritive sweeteners include the sugar substitutes saccharine, aspartame, sucralose, neotame, and acesulfame-K.

***Fats.*** Dietary fat provides energy, carries fat-soluble vitamins, and provides essential fatty acids. The ADA recommends individualizing saturated fat intake. Less than 200 mg/day of cholesterol and limited *trans* fats are also recommended as part of a healthy meal plan. Decreasing fat and cholesterol intake assists in reducing the risk for CVD. Healthy fats are those that come from plants, such as olives, nuts, and avocados.

***Protein.*** The amount of daily protein in the diet for people with diabetes and normal renal function is the same as for the general population. The ADA recommends individualizing protein intake.

***Alcohol.*** Alcohol inhibits gluconeogenesis (breakdown of glycogen to glucose) by the liver. This can cause severe hypoglycemia in patients on insulin or oral hypoglycemic medications that increase insulin secretion. Create a trusting environment where patients feel comfortable being honest about their use of alcohol because its use can make blood glucose more difficult to manage.

Moderate alcohol consumption can be safely incorporated into the meal plan if the person is monitoring blood glucose levels and if the patient is not at risk for other alcohol-related problems. Moderate consumption is defined as one drink per day for women and two drinks per day for men. A patient can reduce the risk for alcohol-induced hypoglycemia by eating carbohydrates when drinking alcohol. On the other hand, mixed drinks often contain sweetened mixers and can lead to elevated blood glucose levels. To decrease the carbohydrate content, recommend using sugar-free mixes and drinking dry, light wines.

**Patient Teaching Related to Nutrition Therapy.** Most often the dietitian initially teaches the principles of nutrition management. Whenever possible, work with dietitians as part of an interprofessional diabetes care team. Some patients who have limited insurance coverage or live in remote areas do not have access to a dietitian. In these cases, you may need to assume responsibility for teaching basic nutrition principles to patients with diabetes.

*Carbohydrate counting* is a meal planning technique used to keep track of the amount of carbohydrates eaten with each meal and per day. Advise patients to keep carbohydrates within a healthy range. The amount of total carbohydrates per day depends on blood glucose levels, age, weight, activity level, patient preference, and prescribed medications. A serving size of carbohydrates is 15 g. A typical adult usually starts with 45 to 60 g of carbohydrate per meal. For some patients, insulin doses are tailored to the number of carbohydrates that a patient will consume at the meal, with a set number of units of insulin given per gram of carbohydrate (e.g., 1 U/15 g carbohydrate, 2 U/25 g carbohydrate). Teach the patient about the foods that contain carbohydrates, how to read food labels, and appropriate serving sizes.

*Diabetes exchange lists* are another method for meal planning. Instead of counting carbohydrates, the individual is given a meal plan with specific numbers of helpings from a list of exchanges for each meal and snack. The exchanges are starches, fruits, milk, meat, vegetables, fats, and free foods. The patient chooses foods from the various exchanges based on the prescribed meal plan. This method may be easier for some patients than carbohydrate counting. It also encourages a well-balanced meal plan. Another advantage is that this approach helps the patient limit portion sizes and overall food intake, an important component of weight management.

MyPlate was developed by the U.S. Department of Agriculture (USDA) to represent national nutrition guidelines for people with or without diabetes. This simple method helps the patient visualize the amount of vegetables, starch, and meat that fills a 9-in plate. The recommendation is that each meal has one half of the plate filled with nonstarchy vegetables, one fourth filled with a starch, and one fourth filled with a protein (*www.diabetes.org/food-and-fitness/food/planning-meals/create-your-plate*). An 8-ounce glass of nonfat milk and a small piece of fresh fruit complete the meal.[17]

Whenever possible, include family members and caregivers in nutrition education and counseling, particularly the person who cooks for the household. However, the responsibility for maintaining a healthy eating plan still belongs to the person with diabetes. Reliance on another person to make health decisions interferes with the patient's ability to develop self-care skills, which are essential in the management of diabetes. Foster independence, even in patients with visual or cognitive impairment. It is also important to discuss traditional foods with the patient. Individualize food choices to take into account the patient's preferences and foods that are culturally appropriate.

## Exercise

Regular, consistent exercise is an essential part of diabetes and prediabetes management.[18] The ADA recommends that people with diabetes engage in at least 150 min/wk (30 minutes, 5 days/week) of a moderate-intensity aerobic physical activity (Table 48-9). The ADA also encourages people with type 2 diabetes to perform resistance training three times a week in the absence of contraindications.[19]

Exercise decreases insulin resistance and can have a direct effect on lowering blood glucose levels. It also contributes to weight loss, which further decreases insulin resistance. The therapeutic benefits of regular physical activity may result in a decreased need for diabetes medications to reach target blood glucose goals in people with type 2 diabetes. Regular exercise may also help reduce triglyceride and low-density lipoprotein (LDL) cholesterol levels, increase high-density lipoprotein (HDL), reduce BP, and improve circulation.[7]

Any new exercise program for patients with diabetes can be started after medical clearance. Patients start slowly with gradual progression toward the desired goal. Patients who use insulin, sulfonylureas, or meglitinides are at increased risk for hypoglycemia when they increase physical activity, especially if they exercise at the time of peak drug action or eat too little to maintain adequate blood glucose levels. This can also occur if a normally sedentary patient with diabetes has an unusually active day.

The glucose-lowering effects of exercise can last up to 48 hours after the activity, so it is possible for hypoglycemia to occur long after the activity. It is recommended that patients who use medications that can cause hypoglycemia schedule exercise about 1 hour after a meal or that they have a 10- to 15-g carbohydrate snack and check their blood glucose before exercising. They can eat small carbohydrate snacks every 30 minutes during exercise to prevent hypoglycemia. Patients using medications that place them at risk for hypoglycemia should always carry a fast-acting source of carbohydrate, such as glucose tablets or hard candies, when exercising. Table 48-10 describes exercise guidelines for patients with diabetes.

Although exercise is generally beneficial to blood glucose levels, strenuous activity can be perceived by the body as a stress, causing a release of counterregulatory hormones and a temporary elevation of blood glucose. In a person with type 1 diabetes

**TABLE 48-9 Activities That Affect Caloric Expenditure**

| Light Activity (100-200 kcal/hr) | Moderate Activity (200-350 kcal/hr) | Vigorous Activity (400-900 kcal/hr) |
|---|---|---|
| • Fishing | • Active housework | • Aerobic exercise |
| • Light housework | • Bicycling (light) | • Bicycling (vigorous) |
| • Secretarial work | • Bowling | • Hard labor |
| • Teaching | • Dancing | • Ice skating |
| • Walking casually | • Gardening | • Outdoor sports |
| | • Golf | • Running |
| | • Roller skating | • Soccer |
| | • Walking briskly | • Tennis |
| | | • Wood chopping |

**TABLE 48-10 Patient & Caregiver Teaching**

***Exercise for Patients With Diabetes Mellitus***

*Include the following information in the exercise teaching plan for the patient and caregiver.*

1. Exercise does not have to be vigorous to be effective. The blood glucose–reducing effects of exercise can be attained with activity such as brisk walking.
2. The exercises selected should be enjoyable to foster regularity.
3. It is important to have properly fitting footwear.
4. The exercise session includes a warm-up period and a cool-down period. Start the exercise program gradually and increase slowly.
5. Exercise is best done after meals, when the blood glucose level is rising.
6. Exercise plans are individualized and monitored by the HCP.
7. It is important to self-monitor blood glucose levels before, during, and after exercise to determine the effect exercise has on blood glucose level at particular times of the day.
8. *Before exercise, if blood glucose ≤100 mg/dL,* eat a 15-g carbohydrate snack. After 15 to 30 min, recheck blood glucose levels. Delay exercise if <100 mg/dL.
9. *Before exercise, if blood glucose ≥250 mg/dL* in a person with type 1 diabetes and ketones are present, delay vigorous activity until ketones are gone. Drink fluids.
10. Exercise-induced hypoglycemia may occur several hours after the completion of exercise.
11. Taking a glucose-lowering medication does not mean that planned or spontaneous exercise cannot occur.
12. It is important to compensate for extensive planned and spontaneous activity by monitoring blood glucose levels to make adjustments in the insulin dose (if taken) and food intake.

who has hyperglycemia and ketones, exercise can worsen these conditions. Teach these patients to delay activity if the blood glucose level is over 250 mg/dL and ketones are present in the urine. If hyperglycemia is present without ketosis, it is not necessary to postpone exercise.[15]

## EVIDENCE-BASED PRACTICE

### Applying the Evidence

**Education: Text Messaging and Diabetes**

A.Y. is a 62-yr-old female recently diagnosed with type 2 diabetes. She understands the importance of maintaining blood glucose levels that are close to normal to reduce symptoms and prevent long-term complications. A.Y. tells you she wants to be an active participant in her care. You determine she is motivated and wants to learn the knowledge and skills necessary to manage her own care. You arrange for A.Y. to receive education text messages about diabetes as part of the teaching plan.

*Making Clinical Decisions*

***Best Available Evidence.*** The delivery of education related to diabetes self-management may include remote electronic messages transmitted by mobile or cell phone. Electronic education text messaging can significantly improve glycemic levels in patients with type 2 diabetes, resulting in an almost 50% reduction in Hb A1C (A1C) levels.

***Clinician Expertise.*** You know self-management diabetes education is effective in helping patients improve glycemic levels. You also know that education text messaging may be a useful method for delivering information to patients with chronic diseases who are managing their own care.

***Patient Preferences and Values.*** A.Y. indicates strong interest in receiving text education messages 4 times/week from diabetes clinic that emphasize the importance of physical activity, blood glucose monitoring, and healthy food choices.

*Implications for Nursing Practice*

1. How can you use text messaging for communication with A.Y. related to her self-monitoring of blood glucose levels?
2. As you empower A.Y. to initially manage her care, why is it important for you to frequently assess A.Y.'s knowledge and skills?
3. What parameters will you use to assess if she is able to manage her own care?

*Reference for Evidence*

Saffari M, Ghanizadeh G, Koenig H: Health education via mobile text messaging for glycemic control in adults with type 2 diabetes: a systematic review and meta-analysis, *Prim Care Diabetes* 8:275, 2014.

## Monitoring Blood Glucose

Self-monitoring of blood glucose (SMBG) is a critical part of diabetes management. By providing a current blood glucose reading, SMBG enables the patient to make decisions regarding food intake, activity patterns, and medication dosages. It also produces accurate records of daily glucose fluctuations and trends, and it alerts the patient to acute episodes of hyperglycemia and hypoglycemia. Furthermore, it provides patients with a tool for achieving and maintaining specific glycemic goals. SMBG is recommended for all patients who use insulin to manage their diabetes. Other patients with diabetes use SMBG to help achieve and maintain glycemic goals and monitor for acute fluctuations in blood glucose related to medications, food, and exercise.

The frequency of monitoring depends on several factors, including the patient's glycemic goals, type of diabetes, medication regimen, patient's ability to check blood glucose independently, and patient's willingness and ability to do so. The recommendation for patients who use multiple insulin injections or insulin pumps is to monitor their blood glucose four or more times each day. Patients using less frequent insulin injections, noninsulin therapy, or nutrition management will monitor as often as needed to achieve their glycemic goals.[12]

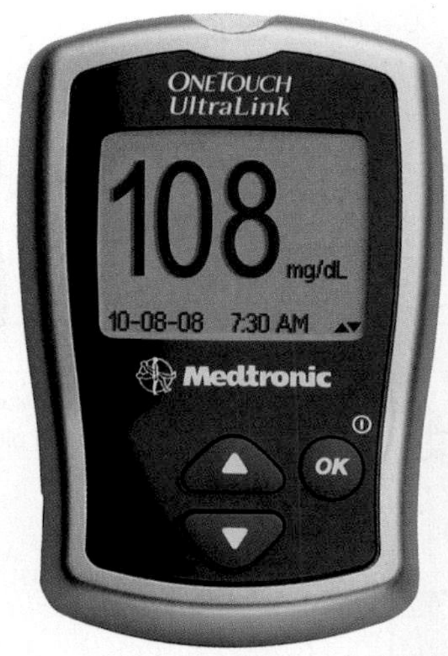


**FIG. 48-8** Blood glucose monitors are used to measure blood glucose levels. Bayer Contour Link glucose meter. (Courtesy of Bayer Diabetes.)

Patients who perform SMBG use portable blood glucose monitors. A wide variety of blood glucose monitors are available (Fig. 48-8). Disposable lancets are used to obtain a small drop of capillary blood (usually from a finger stick) that is placed in a reagent strip. After a specified time, the monitor displays a digital reading of the capillary blood glucose value. The technology of SMBG is rapidly changing, with newer and more convenient systems being introduced on an ongoing basis.

Some systems allow the user to collect blood from alternative sites such as the forearm or palm. Alternate site use is not recommended with rapidly changing blood glucose readings, during pregnancy, or when symptoms of low blood glucose are present (Fig. 48-9). The data from some glucose monitors can be uploaded to a computer and reviewed by HCPs, allowing for more frequent and efficient adjustment of the plan of care if needed.

Continuous glucose monitoring (CGM) systems provide another route for monitoring glucose. Insulin pumps can also be matched with CGM (Fig. 48-10).

Using a sensor inserted subcutaneously, the systems display glucose values that are updated every 1 to 5 minutes. CGM assesses interstitial glucose, which lags behind blood glucose by up to 20 minutes.[20] The patient inserts the sensor using an automatic insertion device. Data are sent from the sensor to a transmitter, which displays the glucose value on either an insulin pump or a pager-like receiver. The continuous glucose monitor can be used with or without an insulin pump.

CGMs assist the patient and HCP to identify trends and patterns in glucose levels. In addition, they are useful for the management of insulin therapy or when continuous blood glucose readings are clinically important. The patient is alerted to episodes of hypoglycemia and hyperglycemia, thus allowing corrective action to be quickly taken. These systems still require finger-stick measurements using a blood glucose monitor to calibrate the sensor and to make treatment decisions.

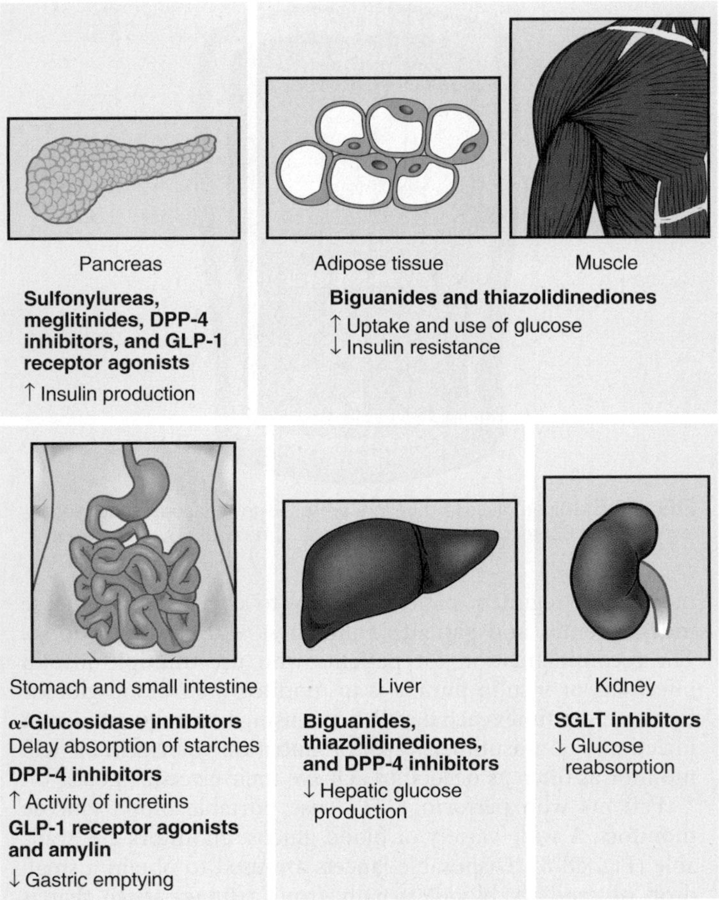


**FIG. 48-9** Sites and mechanisms of action of type 2 diabetes drugs. *DDP-4,* Dipeptidyl peptidase; *GLP-1,* glucagon-like peptide-1; *SGLT,* sodium-glucose co-tranporter.

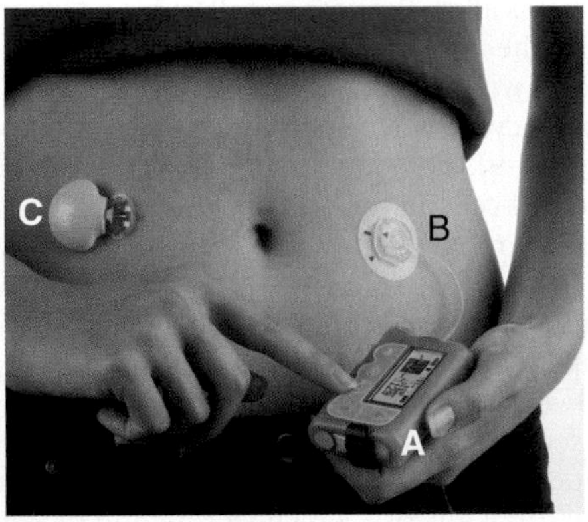


**FIG. 48-10** The MiniMed® 530/730G with Enlite *(A)* delivers insulin through a thin plastic tubing to an infusion set, which has a cannula *(B)* that sits under the skin. Continuous glucose monitoring occurs through a tiny sensor *(C)* inserted under the skin. Sensor data are sent continuously to the insulin pump through wireless technology giving a more complete picture of glucose levels, which can lead to better treatment decisions and improved health. (MiniMed® 530G with Enlite® manufactured by the diabetes division of Medtronic, Inc.)

The blood glucose level reported by a laboratory is sometimes higher than the patient's home glucose monitor or the hospital's portable monitor. This is because some home monitors give capillary blood glucose values from whole blood (via finger stick), whereas tests performed in laboratories provide plasma readings. Plasma samples, or venous samples, are approximately 10% to 12% higher. Most current monitors are automatically calibrated to give a "plasma" result (even though whole blood was used for the sample) so that the home readings can be more readily compared with laboratory values. It is important to read the literature accompanying a monitor to find out if it is displaying values as whole blood or plasma.

**TABLE 48-11 Patient & Caregiver Teaching**

***Self-Monitoring of Blood Glucose (SMBG)***

*Include the following instructions when teaching the patient and caregiver about SMBG.*

1. Wash hands in warm water. It is not necessary to clean the site with alcohol, and it may interfere with test results. Finger should be dry before puncturing it.
2. If it is difficult to obtain an adequate drop of blood for testing, warm the hands in warm water or let the arms hang dependently for a few minutes before the finger puncture is made.
3. A lancing device is usually used. Place the lancet in the device, following the instructions that come with it. If the puncture is made on the finger, use the side of the finger pad rather than near the center. Fewer nerve endings are along the side of the finger pad. If an alternative site is used (e.g., forearm), special equipment may be needed. Refer to manufacturer's instructions for alternative site use, except during hypoglycemic episodes.
4. Set lancing device to make a puncture just deep enough to obtain a sufficiently large drop of blood. Unnecessarily deep punctures may cause pain and bruising. Current meters require very small amounts of blood.
5. Follow instructions on monitor for checking the blood.
6. Record results. Compare with personal target blood glucose goals.

Because errors in monitoring technique can cause errors in management strategies, comprehensive patient teaching is essential. Initial instruction should be followed up with regular reassessment. Review the instructions that accompany each product. If a product has a control solution, teach patients to use and interpret control solutions. Control solution should be used when first using a blood glucose meter, when a new bottle of strips is used, or when there is a reason to believe that the readings are not correct. Table 48-11 lists the steps to include when teaching the patient how to perform SMBG.

People with type 1 diabetes often check their blood glucose before meals. This is because many patients use insulin pumps or multiple daily injections and base the insulin dose on the carbohydrates in a meal or make adjustments if the preprandial value is above or below target. Checking blood glucose 2 hours after the first bite of food helps a person determine if the bolus insulin dose was adequate for that meal.

Teach patients to monitor blood glucose whenever hypoglycemia is suspected so that immediate action can be taken. During times of illness, check blood glucose levels at 4-hour intervals to determine the effects of the illness on glucose levels. Teach the patient to monitor blood glucose before and after exercise to determine the effects of exercise on blood glucose levels. This is especially important in the patient with type 1 diabetes.

A patient who is visually impaired, cognitively impaired, or limited in manual dexterity needs careful evaluation of the degree to which SMBG can be performed independently. Nurses preparing patients for discharge from the hospital and nurses working in home health and outpatient settings may need to identify caregivers who can assume this responsibility. Adaptive devices are available to help patients with certain limitations. These include talking meters and other equipment for the visually impaired.

### Bariatric Surgery

*Bariatric surgery* may be considered for patients with type 2 diabetes, especially if the diabetes or associated co-morbidities are difficult to manage with lifestyle and drug therapy. Patients with type 2 diabetes who have undergone bariatric surgery need lifelong lifestyle support and monitoring. (Bariatric surgery is discussed in Chapter 40.)

### Pancreas Transplantation

Pancreas transplantation can be used as a treatment option for patients with type 1 diabetes. Usually it is done for patients who have end-stage renal disease and have had or plan to have a kidney transplant. Kidney and pancreas transplants are often performed together, or a pancreas may be transplanted after a kidney transplant. If renal failure is not present, the ADA recommends that pancreas transplantation be considered only for patients who exhibit the following three criteria: (1) a history of frequent, acute, and severe metabolic complications (e.g., hypoglycemia, hyperglycemia, ketoacidosis) requiring medical attention; (2) clinical and emotional problems with the use of exogenous insulin therapy that are so severe as to be incapacitating; and (3) consistent failure of insulin-based management to prevent acute complications.

Successful pancreas transplantation can improve quality of life for people with diabetes, primarily by eliminating the need for exogenous insulin, frequent blood glucose measurements, and the risks involved with hyper- and hypoglycemia. Transplantation can also eliminate the acute complications commonly experienced by patients with type 1 diabetes (e.g., hypoglycemia, hyperglycemia). However, pancreas transplantation is only partially successful in reversing the long-term renal and neurologic complications of diabetes. The patient will also require lifelong immunosuppression to prevent rejection of the organ. Complications can result from immunosuppressive therapy. (Immunosuppressive therapy is discussed in Chapter 13.)

Pancreatic islet cell transplantation is another potential treatment measure. During this procedure, the islets are harvested from the pancreas of a deceased organ donor. Most recipients require the use of two or more pancreases. The islets are infused via a catheter through the upper abdomen into the portal vein of the liver. With only the islets transplanted, pain and recovery time are diminished compared with whole pancreas transplants. Currently this procedure is experimental in the United States. Research is continuing to investigate the best ways to implant the islet cells and to prevent their rejection.

### Culturally Competent Care: Diabetes Mellitus

Because culture can have a strong influence on dietary preferences and meal preparation practices, culturally competent care has special relevance for the patient with diabetes. For example, certain ethnic and cultural groups, such as Hispanics, Native Americans, African Americans, and Asians and Pacific Islanders have a high incidence of diabetes. The increased prevalence can be attributed to genetic predisposition, environmental factors, and dietary choices.

Explore the influences of culture on food choices and meal planning with the patient as part of the health history. When giving diet instructions, consider the patient's cultural food preferences. Nutrition resources specifically designed for members of different cultural groups are available from the ADA.

**CULTURAL & ETHNIC HEALTH DISPARITIES**

***Diabetes Mellitus***

- The highest incidence of diabetes is among Native Americans and Alaska Natives (16.5% are being treated for diabetes).
- Pima Indians in Arizona have the highest rate of diabetes in the world (50% of adults have diabetes).
- The rates of diabetes are: non-Hispanic whites 7.1%, Asian Americans 8.4%, Hispanics 11.8%, and non-Hispanic blacks 12.6%.
- Diabetes is 1.5 times more likely to cause death in Hispanics and 2.2 times more likely to cause death in African Americans than in non-Hispanic whites.
- Complications from diabetes are a major cause of death among Native Americans. Native Americans have a six times higher rate of end-stage renal disease and a four times higher rate of amputation than other ethnicities with diabetes.

## NURSING MANAGEMENT: DIABETES MELLITUS

### Nursing Assessment

Table 48-12 provides initial subjective and objective data that you should obtain from a person with diabetes mellitus. After the initial assessment, perform periodic patient assessments on a regular basis.

### Nursing Diagnoses

Nursing diagnoses related to diabetes mellitus may include, but are not limited to, the following:

- Ineffective health management *related to* deficient knowledge of diabetes management and lack of understanding of diabetes management plan
- Risk for unstable blood glucose levels *related to* infrequent blood glucose monitoring and lack of following diabetes management plan
- Risk for injury *related to* decreased tactile sensation, episodes of hypoglycemia
- Risk for peripheral neurovascular dysfunction *related to* vascular effects of diabetes

Additional information on nursing diagnoses for the patient with diabetes is presented in eNursing Care Plan 48-1 available on the website.

### Planning

The overall goals are for the patient with diabetes mellitus to (1) engage in self-care behaviors to actively manage his or her diabetes, (2) experience few or no hyperglycemia or hypoglycemia emergencies, (3) maintain blood glucose levels at normal or near-normal levels, (4) prevent or minimize chronic complications related to diabetes, and (5) adjust lifestyle to accommodate the diabetes plan with a minimum of stress. The patient with diabetes needs to safely and effectively fit diabetes into life, rather than living life around diabetes.

### Nursing Implementation

**Health Promotion.** Your role in health promotion is to identify, monitor, and teach the patient at risk for diabetes. Obesity is the primary risk factor for type 2 diabetes. The findings from the Diabetes Prevention Program indicated that a modest

## TABLE 48-12 Nursing Assessment

### *Diabetes Mellitus*

**Subjective Data**

***Important Health Information***

*Past health history:* Mumps, rubella, coxsackievirus, or other viral infections. Recent trauma, infection, or stress. Pregnancy, gave birth to infant >9 lb. Chronic pancreatitis, Cushing syndrome, acromegaly, family history of type 1 or type 2 diabetes mellitus

*Medications:* Use of and adherence to regimen with insulin or OAs, corticosteroids, diuretics, phenytoin (Dilantin)

*Surgery or other treatments:* Any recent surgery

***Functional Health Patterns***

*Health perception–health management:* Positive family history, malaise

*Nutrition-metabolic:* Obesity, weight loss (type 1), weight gain (type 2). Thirst, hunger, nausea and vomiting. Poor healing (especially involving the feet), eating habits in patients with previously diagnosed diabetes

*Elimination:* Constipation or diarrhea, frequent urination, frequent bladder infections, nocturia, urinary incontinence

*Activity-exercise:* Muscle weakness, fatigue

*Cognitive-perceptual:* Abdominal pain, headache, blurred vision, numbness or tingling of extremities, pruritus

*Sexuality-reproductive:* Erectile dysfunction, frequent vaginal infections, decreased libido

*Coping–stress tolerance:* Depression, irritability, apathy

*Value-belief:* Commitment to lifestyle changes involving diet, medication, and activity patterns

**Objective Data**

***Eyes***

Soft, sunken eyeballs.* History of vitreal hemorrhages, cataracts

***Integumentary***

Dry, warm, inelastic skin. Pigmented lesions (on legs), ulcers (especially on feet), loss of hair on toes, acanthosis nigricans

***Respiratory***

Rapid, deep respirations (Kussmaul respirations)*

***Cardiovascular***

Hypotension.* Weak, rapid pulse*

***Gastrointestinal***

Dry mouth, vomiting.* Fruity breath*

***Neurologic***

Altered reflexes, restlessness, confusion, stupor, coma

***Musculoskeletal***

Muscle wasting

***Possible Findings***

Serum electrolyte abnormalities. Fasting blood glucose level ≥126 mg/dL. Oral glucose tolerance test >200 mg/dL, random glucose ≥200 mg/dL. Leukocytosis. ↑ Blood urea nitrogen, creatinine, triglycerides, cholesterol, LDL, VLDL. ↓ HDL. A1C >6.0% (A1C >7.0% in those with diagnosed diabetes), glycosuria, ketonuria, albuminuria. Acidosis

*A1C,* Glycosylated hemoglobin; *HDL,* high-density lipoprotein; *LDL,* low-density lipoprotein; *OAs,* oral agents; *VLDL,* very-low-density lipoprotein.
*Indicates manifestations of diabetic ketoacidosis (DKA).

## TABLE 48-13 Screening for Diabetes in Asymptomatic, Undiagnosed Individuals

**Who to Screen**

1. Consider screening all adults who are overweight (BMI >25 kg/m$^2$) and have additional risk factors:
   - First-degree relative with diabetes
   - Physically inactive
   - Members of a high-risk ethnic population (e.g., African American, Hispanic, Native American, Asian American,* Pacific Islander)
   - Women who delivered a baby weighing >9 lb or were diagnosed with gestational diabetes mellitus
   - Hypertensive (≥140/90 mm Hg) or on therapy for hypertension
   - HDL cholesterol level ≤35 mg/dL (0.90 mmol/L) and/or a triglyceride level ≥250 mg/dL (2.82 mmol/L)
   - Women with polycystic ovary syndrome
   - A1C ≥5.7%, IGT, or IFG on previous screening
   - Other clinical conditions associated with insulin resistance (e.g., obesity, acanthosis nigricans)
2. In the absence of the above criteria, screening for diabetes should begin at age 45 yr regardless of weight.
3. If results are normal, screening should be repeated at least at 3-yr intervals, with consideration of more frequent screening depending on initial results and risk status.

**What Measurements Are Used**

To screen for diabetes or to assess risk of future diabetes, A1C, FPG, or 2-hour OGTT is appropriate.

Source: American Diabetes Association: Standards of Medical Care in Diabetes, *Diabetes Care* 39 (Suppl 1):S1, 2016.
*A1C,* Glycosylated hemoglobin; *BMI,* body mass index; *FPG,* fasting plasma glucose; *HDL,* high-density lipoprotein; *IFG,* impaired fasting glucose; *IGT,* impaired glucose tolerance; *OGTT,* oral glucose tolerance test.
*Consider screening in Asian Americans with a BMI of 23 kg/m$^2$ or higher.

weight loss of 5% to 7% of body weight and regular exercise of 30 minutes five times a week lowered the risk of developing type 2 diabetes up to 58%.[21]

The ADA recommends routine screening for type 2 diabetes for all adults who are overweight or obese (BMI greater than or equal to 25 kg/m$^2$) or have one or more risk factors. For people who do not have risk factors for diabetes, screening should begin at age 45. Table 48-13 provides criteria to screen for prediabetes and diabetes. If results are normal, repeat screening at 3-year intervals.[3] Many factors put an individual at an increased risk for diabetes. These include age, ethnicity (being Native American, Hispanic, African American, Asian, Pacific Islander), obesity, having a baby that weighed more than 9 lb at birth, history of gestational diabetes, and a family history of diabetes. A diabetes risk test is available at *www.diabetes.org/risk-test.jsp.* The diabetes risk test determines if the person is at risk for prediabetes or diabetes based on the number of risk factors present.

## HEALTHY PEOPLE

### *Prevention and Early Detection of Diabetes Mellitus*

- Increase level of exercise because physical activity reduces the risk of type 2 diabetes.
- Maintain a healthy weight because obesity increases the risk of type 2 diabetes.
- If overweight, lose weight and participate in a regular exercise program to reduce the risk of diabetes.
- Choose foods that are low in fat content, total calories, and processed foods and high in whole grains, fruits, and vegetables.
- If overweight and over age 45, get screened for diabetes.

◆ **Acute Care.** Acute situations involving the patient with diabetes include hypoglycemia, DKA, and hyperosmolar hyperglycemic syndrome (HHS). Nursing management for these situations is discussed in more detail later in this chapter. Other areas of acute care relate to management during acute illness and surgery.

◆ ***Acute Illness and Surgery.*** Both emotional and physical stress can increase the blood glucose level and result in hyperglycemia. Because stress is unavoidable, certain situations may require more intense treatment, such as extra insulin and more frequent blood glucose monitoring, to maintain glycemic goals and avoid hyperglycemia.

Acute illness, injury, and surgery are situations that may evoke a counterregulatory hormone response, resulting in hyperglycemia. Even common illnesses such as a viral upper respiratory tract infection or the flu can cause this response. Encourage patients with diabetes to check blood glucose at least every 4 hours during times of illness. Acutely ill patients with type 1 diabetes with a blood glucose greater than 240 mg/dL (13.3 mmol/L) should also check urine for ketones every 3 to 4 hours.

Teach patients to report to the HCP when glucose levels are over 300 mg/dL twice in a row or urine ketone levels are moderate to high. A patient with type 1 diabetes may need an increase in insulin to prevent DKA. Elevated blood glucose levels can lead to poor healing and infection. Insulin therapy may be required for a patient with type 2 diabetes to prevent or treat hyperglycemia symptoms and avoid an acute hyperglycemia emergency. In critically ill patients, insulin therapy may be started if the blood glucose is persistently greater than 180 mg/dL. These patients have a higher targeted blood glucose goal, which is usually 140 to 180 mg/dL. Food intake is important during times of stress and illness, when the body requires extra energy. If patients are able to eat normally, they can continue with their regular meal plan while increasing the intake of noncaloric fluids, such as water, sugar-free gelatin, and other decaffeinated beverages, and continue taking OAs, noninsulin injectable agents, and insulin as prescribed. When illness causes patients to eat less than normal, they can continue to take OAs, noninsulin injectable agents, and/or insulin as prescribed while supplementing food intake with carbohydrate-containing fluids. Examples include low-sodium soups, juices, and regular, sugar-sweetened decaffeinated soft drinks. It is important to tell the patient to contact an HCP if he or she is unable to keep down food or fluid.

During the intraoperative period, adjustments in the diabetes regimen can be planned to ensure safe and healthy blood glucose levels. The patient is given IV fluids and insulin (if needed) immediately before, during, and after surgery when there is no oral intake. Explain to the patient with type 2 diabetes who has been on OAs that this is a temporary measure, not a sign of worsening diabetes.

When caring for an unconscious surgical patient receiving insulin, be alert for signs of hypoglycemia such as sweating, tachycardia, and tremors. Frequent monitoring of blood glucose can prevent episodes of severe hypoglycemia.

◆ **Ambulatory Care.** Successful management of diabetes involves ongoing interaction among the patient, caregiver, and interprofessional team. It is important that a certified diabetes educator (CDE) be involved in the care of the patient and family. Because diabetes is a complex chronic condition, a great deal of patient contact takes place in outpatient and home settings. The major goal of patient care in these settings is to enable the patient (with the help of a caregiver as needed) to reach an optimal level of independence in self-care activities. Unfortunately, many patients with diabetes face challenges in reaching these goals. Diabetes increases the risk for other chronic conditions that can affect self-care activities. These include visual impairment, lower-extremity problems that affect mobility, and other functional limitations related to a stroke.

An important nursing function is to assess the ability of patients and caregivers in performing activities such as SMBG and insulin injection. Assistive devices for self-administration of insulin include syringe magnifiers, vial stabilizers, and dosing aids for the visually impaired. In some cases, referrals are made to help the patient achieve the self-care goal. These may include an occupational therapist, a social worker, a home care nurse, a home health aide, or a dietitian.

A diagnosis of diabetes affects the patient in many profound ways. Self-management of the disease is demanding. Patients with diabetes continually face lifestyle choices that affect the foods they eat, their activities, and demands on their time and energy. The requirements of scheduled meals, SMBG, medication, and insulin management may interfere with the patient's other responsibilities. Any change in the daily routine can be difficult. In addition, they face the challenge of preventing or dealing with the devastating complications of diabetes.

Careful assessment of what it means to the patient to have diabetes is a good starting point for teaching. The goals of teaching are mutually determined by the patient and you, based on individual needs and therapeutic requirements. Identify the patient's support system, and include them in planning, teaching, and counseling. When family members and other individuals close to the patient are included, they can support the patient's self-care behaviors. Additionally, they can provide care if self-care is not possible. Encourage the family and caregivers to provide emotional support and encouragement as the patient deals with the reality of living with a chronic disease.

***Insulin Therapy.*** Nursing responsibilities for the patient receiving insulin include proper administration, assessment of the patient's response to insulin therapy, and teaching the patient about administration, storage, and side effects of insulin (Table 48-5). Table 48-6 lists guidelines for assessing a patient using glucose-lowering agents, including insulin and OAs.

Assessment of the patient who is a new user of insulin must include an evaluation of his or her ability to safely manage this therapy. This includes the ability to understand the interaction of insulin, food, and activity and to recognize and treat the symptoms of hypoglycemia appropriately. If the patient does not have the cognitive skills to do these things, identify and teach another responsible person. The patient or caregiver must have the cognitive and manual skills needed to prepare and inject insulin. Otherwise, additional resources will be needed to assist the patient. For patients with cognitive, physical, and other barriers, consider referral to a CDE because he or she has the specialized knowledge and skills to promote self-care behaviors for these patients.

Many patients are fearful when they first begin using insulin.[22] Some find it difficult to self-inject because they are afraid of needles or the pain associated with an injection. Others may think that the insulin is not necessary or that they will experience hypoglycemia after an injection. Explore the patient's underlying fears before beginning the teaching. Assessment of the patient's beliefs and concerns regarding starting insulin will guide the teaching, counseling, and plan of care. Having open discussion with patients, providing educational materials and programs, and working with a diabetes educator are all beneficial for patients starting insulin.

Follow-up assessment of the patient who has been using insulin therapy includes an inspection of injection sites for signs of lipodystrophy and other reactions, review of insulin preparation and injection technique, a history pertaining to the occurrence of hypoglycemia, and assessment of the patient's method for handling hypoglycemia. A review of the patient's recorded blood glucose readings is vital in assessing how the patient is doing and making any needed adjustments.

◆ ***Oral and Noninsulin Injectable Agents.*** Your responsibilities for the patient taking oral and noninsulin injectable agents are similar to those for the patient taking insulin. Proper administration of these drugs, assessment of the patient's use of and response to these drugs, and teaching the patient and family are all essential nursing actions.

Your assessment is valuable in determining the most appropriate drug for a patient. Factors such as the patient's mental status, eating habits, home environment, attitude toward diabetes, and medication history all play a significant role in determining the most appropriate drug. For example, frail older adults who live alone are at high risk for severe hypoglycemia because low blood glucose is frequently undetected or untreated in this population. This is especially true if the patient has cognitive impairment. In these cases, an OA that does not cause hypoglycemia, or a shorter-acting OA, would be most appropriate.

Patient teaching is essential. Some patients may assume that their diabetes is not a serious condition if they are only taking a pill to treat it. Instruct the patient that these agents will help manage blood glucose and help prevent serious long- and short-term complications of diabetes. Teach patients that OAs and noninsulin injectable agents are used in addition to food choices and activity as therapy for diabetes and the importance of following their meal and activity plans. Teach patients not to take extra pills if they have overeaten. If the patient uses sulfonylureas and metformin, instruct the patient about prevention, symptom recognition, and management of hypoglycemia.

◆ ***Personal Hygiene.*** The potential for infection requires diligent skin and dental hygiene practices. Because of the susceptibility to periodontal disease, encourage daily brushing and flossing in addition to regular visits to the dentist. When having dental work done, have the patient inform the dentist that he or she has diabetes.

Routine care includes regular bathing, with particular emphasis on foot care. Advise patients to inspect their feet daily, avoid going barefoot, and wear shoes that are supportive and comfortable. If cuts, scrapes, or burns occur, treat them promptly and monitor them carefully. Wash the area and apply a nonabrasive or nonirritating antiseptic ointment. Cover the area with a dry, sterile pad. Teach patients to notify the HCP immediately if the injury does not begin to heal within 24 hours or if signs of infection develop.

◆ ***Medical Identification and Travel.*** Instruct the patient to carry medical identification at all times indicating that he or she has diabetes. Police, paramedics, and many private citizens are aware of the need to look for this identification when working with sick or unconscious persons. Every person with diabetes is encouraged to wear a Medic Alert bracelet or necklace. An identification card (Fig. 48-11) can supply valuable information,

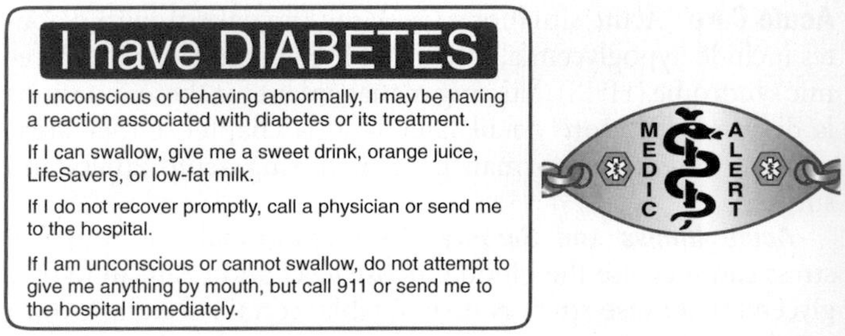


**FIG. 48-11** Medical alerts. A patient with diabetes should carry a card and wear a bracelet or necklace that indicates diabetes. If the patient with diabetes is unconscious, these measures will ensure prompt and appropriate attention.

such as the name of the HCP; the type of diabetes; and the type and dosage of insulin, noninsulin injectable agents, or OAs.

Travel for a patient with diabetes requires planning. Being sedentary for long periods may raise the person's glucose level. Encourage the patient to get up and walk at least every 2 hours to lower the risk for deep vein thrombosis and to prevent elevation of glucose levels. Teach the patient to have a full set of diabetes care supplies in the carry-on luggage when traveling by plane, train, or bus. This includes blood glucose monitoring equipment, insulin, noninsulin injectable agents, oral medications, and syringes or insulin pens.

When equipment such as syringes, lancing devices, insulin vials or pens, and insulin pumps are taken onto a commercial airliner, it is a good idea to have the professional printed pharmaceutical labels that accompany them. A letter from the prescribing HCP indicating medical necessity may prevent delays at security checkpoints. Notify screeners if an insulin pump is used so that they can inspect it while it is on the body, rather than removing it.

For patients who use insulin or OAs that can cause hypoglycemia, keep snack items and a quick-acting carbohydrate source for treating hypoglycemia in the carry-on luggage. Keep extra insulin available in case a bottle breaks or is lost. For longer trips, carry a full day's supply of food in the event of canceled flights, delayed meals, or closed restaurants. If the patient is planning a trip out of the country, it is wise to have a letter from the HCP explaining that the patient has diabetes and requires all the materials, particularly syringes, for ongoing health care.

When travel involves time changes, such as traveling coast to coast or across the International Date Line, the patient can contact the HCP to plan an appropriate insulin schedule. During travel, most patients find it helpful to keep watches set to the time of the city of origin until they reach their destination. The key to travel when taking insulin is to know the type of insulin being taken, its onset of action, the anticipated peak time, and mealtimes.

◆ ***Patient and Caregiver Teaching.*** The goals of diabetes self-management education are to match the level of self-management to the patient's individual ability so that he or she can become the most active participant possible. Patients who actively manage their diabetes care have better outcomes than those who do not. For this reason, an educational approach that facilitates informed decision making by the patient is advocated. Sometimes this is referred to as the *empowerment approach* to education.

Unfortunately, patients can encounter a variety of physical, psychologic, and emotional barriers when it comes to effectively managing their diabetes. These barriers may include feelings of

## COMPLEMENTARY & ALTERNATIVE THERAPIES

### *Herbs and Supplements That May Affect Blood Glucose*

**Scientific Evidence***

- Herbs and supplements that may lower blood glucose include aloe, α-lipoic acid, cinnamon, chromium, garlic, and ginseng.
- However, many studies have been small and not well designed. Further research is needed.

**Nursing Implications**

- Teach patients to use herbs and supplements with caution, since they may affect blood glucose.
- Patients with diabetes mellitus should consult their health care provider before using herbs or nutritional supplements.
- Patients who use herbs should monitor their blood glucose levels carefully and regularly.

*Based on a systematic review of scientific literature. Retrieved from *www.naturalstandard.com.*

## INFORMATICS IN PRACTICE

### *Patient Teaching Using Smart Phone Apps*

- Teaching is a critical part of nursing care for patients with diabetes. Put some fun into patient teaching by using smart phone applications.
- Introduce patients to a variety of smart phone apps for healthy living and managing diabetes.
- Sample apps include Moves, Glucose Buddy, Diabetes Companion, Diabetes App, and Calorie King.

Based on list provided by American Diabetes Association. Retrieved from *www.diabetesforecast.org/2014/Jan/app-happy.html.*

inadequacy about one's own abilities, unwillingness to make the necessary behavioral changes, ineffective coping strategies, and cognitive deficits. If the patient is not able to manage the disease, a family member may be able to assume part of this role. If the patient or caregiver cannot make decisions related to diabetes management, consider a referral to a CDE, social worker, or other resources within the community. These resources can assist the patient and family in outlining a feasible treatment program that meets their capabilities.

An assessment of the patient's knowledge of diabetes and lifestyle preferences is useful in planning a teaching program. Tables 48-14 and 48-15 present guidelines to use for patient and caregiver teaching. Assess the patient's knowledge base frequently so that gaps in knowledge or incorrect or inaccurate ideas can be corrected.

The ADA offers resources for patients in the form of pamphlets, booklets, books, and a monthly magazine called *Diabetes Forecast.* Affiliates of the ADA are located in all states, and most can be reached by dialing 1-800-DIABETES (800-342-2383). The ADA publishes materials and sponsors conferences for health care professionals concerned with diabetes education, research, and management of patients. The ADA website (*www.diabetes.org*) has extensive information for the public and health care professionals. This organization also recognizes education programs that meet the national standards of diabetes education and can provide a list of these programs. Drug companies manufacturing diabetes-related products also have free educational materials for patients and HCPs. It is critical that you stay current in your diabetes knowledge so that you can effectively teach and support patients with diabetes.

## TABLE 48-14 Patient & Caregiver Teaching

### *Management of Diabetes Mellitus*

*Include the following instructions when teaching the patient and caregiver how to manage diabetes mellitus.*

| Component | What to Teach |
|---|---|
| **Disease process** | • Include an introduction about the pancreas and the islets of Langerhans.<br>• Describe how insulin is made and what affects its production.<br>• Discuss the relationship of insulin and glucose.<br>• Explain the difference between type 1 and type 2 diabetes. |
| **Physical activity** | • Discuss the effect of regular exercise on the management of blood glucose, improvement of cardiovascular function, and general health. |
| **Menu planning** | • Stress the importance of a well-balanced diet as part of a diabetes management plan.<br>• Explain the impact of carbohydrates on blood glucose levels. |
| **Medication** | • Ensure that the patient understands the proper use of prescribed medication (e.g., insulin [Table 48-5], OAs, and noninsulin injectables).<br>• Account for a patient's physical limitations or inabilities for self-medication. If necessary, involve the family or caregiver in proper use of medication.<br>• Discuss all side effects and safety issues regarding medication. |
| **Monitoring blood glucose** | • Teach correct blood glucose monitoring.<br>• Include when to check blood glucose levels, how to record them, and how to adjust insulin levels if necessary. |
| **Risk reduction** | • Ensure that the patient understands and appropriately responds to the signs and symptoms of hypoglycemia and hyperglycemia (Table 48-16).<br>• Stress the importance of proper foot care (Table 48-21), regular eye examinations, and consistent glucose monitoring.<br>• Inform the patient about the effect that stress can have on blood glucose. |
| **Psychosocial** | • Help the patient identify resources that are available to facilitate the adjustment and answer questions about living with a chronic condition such as diabetes. |

*OAs,* Oral agents.

## ◆ Evaluation

The expected outcomes are that the patient with diabetes mellitus will

- Verbalize key elements of the therapeutic regimen, including knowledge of disease and treatment plan
- Describe self-care measures that may prevent or slow progression of chronic complications
- Maintain a balance of nutrition, activity, and insulin availability that results in stable, safe, and healthy blood glucose levels
- Experience no injury resulting from decreased sensation in feet
- Implement measures to increase peripheral circulation

Additional information on expected outcomes for the patient with diabetes is presented in eNursing Care Plan 48-1 available on the website for this chapter.

## TABLE 48-15 Patient & Caregiver Teaching

### Instructions for Patients With Diabetes Mellitus

*Include the following essential instructions for diabetes management for the patient and caregiver.*

**Blood Glucose**

- Monitor your blood glucose at home and record results in a log.
- Take your insulin, OA, and/or noninsulin injectable agent as prescribed.
- Take insulin consistently, especially when you are sick.
- Keep an adequate supply of insulin on hand at all times.
- Obtain A1C blood test every 3-6 mo as an indicator of your long-term blood glucose levels.
- Be aware of symptoms of hypoglycemia and hyperglycemia.
- Carry some form of rapid-acting glucose at all times so that you can treat hypoglycemia quickly.
- Instruct family members how and when to use glucagon if patient becomes unresponsive because of hypoglycemia.

**Exercise**

- Learn how exercise and food affect your blood glucose levels.
- Remember that exercise will usually lower your blood glucose level.
- Begin an exercise program after approval from HCP.

**Food**

- Work with a dietitian to create an individualized meal plan.
- Make healthy food choices most of the time and eat regular meals at regular times.
- Choose foods low in saturated and *trans* fat. Know your cholesterol level.
- Limit the amount of alcohol you drink.
- Be aware that excessive amounts of alcohol may lead to unpredictable low blood glucose reactions.
- Avoid fad diets.
- Limit regular soda and fruit juice.

**Other Guidelines**

- Obtain an annual eye examination by an ophthalmologist.
- Obtain annual urine monitoring for protein.
- Examine your feet at home.
- Wear comfortable, well-fitting shoes to help prevent foot injury. Break in new shoes gradually.
- Always carry identification that says you have diabetes.
- Have other medical problems treated, especially high BP and high cholesterol.
- Have a yearly influenza vaccination.
- Quit or never start smoking cigarettes or using nicotine products.
- Avoid applying heat or cold directly to your feet.
- Avoid going barefoot.
- Keep skin moisturized by applying cream to surfaces of feet, but not between toes.

*A1C*, Glycosylated hemoglobin; *OA*, oral agent.

# ACUTE COMPLICATIONS OF DIABETES MELLITUS

The acute complications of diabetes mellitus arise from events associated with hyperglycemia and hypoglycemia. Hyperglycemia occurs when there is not enough insulin working, and hypoglycemia occurs when there is too much insulin working. It is important for the HCP to distinguish between hyperglycemia and hypoglycemia because hypoglycemia worsens rapidly and is a serious threat if action is not immediately taken. Table 48-16 compares the manifestations, causes, management, and prevention of hyperglycemia and hypoglycemia.

## EVIDENCE-BASED PRACTICE

### Translating Research Into Practice

**Can Exercise Improve Blood Pressure Levels in Patients With Diabetes?**

***Clinical Question***

For adults with type 2 diabetes (P), what is the effect of structured exercise training (I) versus advice on physical activity (C) on blood pressure levels (O)?

***Synthesis of Best Available Evidence***

- Systematic review of randomized controlled trials (RCTs).
- 51 RCTs of patients ($n = 9540$) with type 2 diabetes receiving structured exercise training or physical activity advice only. Structured exercise was aerobic and/or resistance training. Activity advice was information provided on gradually increasing the frequency of moderate/vigorous activity up to 150 min/wk. Control groups received no exercise training or advice on activity. Outcome was BP level.

***Conclusion***

- All types of structured exercise training were associated with a reduction in both systolic and diastolic BP in patients with type 2 diabetes. Greatest decreases in BP occurred in structured exercise programs lasting >150 min/wk.
- Physical activity advice only is also associated with lowered BP levels.

***Implications for Nursing Practice***

1. Why is it important for patients with diabetes to seek nonpharmacological methods to decrease BP level?
2. What would you discuss with a patient who has an elevated BP and appears motivated to engage in a regular exercise program?
3. How will you facilitate the provision of physical activity information to patients with diabetes?

***Reference for Evidence***

Figueira F, Umpierre D, Cureau F, et al: Association between physical activity advice only or structured exercise training with blood pressure levels in patients with type 2 diabetes: a systematic review and meta-analysis, *Sports Med* 44:1557, 2014.

*P*, Patient population of interest; *I*, intervention or area of interest; *C*, comparison of interest or comparison group; *O*, outcomes of interest; *T*, timing (see p. 15).

# DIABETIC KETOACIDOSIS

## Etiology and Pathophysiology

**Diabetic ketoacidosis (DKA)** is caused by a profound deficiency of insulin and is characterized by hyperglycemia, ketosis, acidosis, and dehydration. It is most likely to occur in people with type 1 diabetes but may be seen in people with type 2 diabetes in conditions of severe illness or stress when the pancreas cannot meet the extra demand for insulin. Precipitating factors include illness and infection, inadequate insulin dosage, undiagnosed type 1 diabetes, poor self-management, and neglect.

When the circulating supply of insulin is insufficient, glucose cannot be properly used for energy. The body compensates by breaking down fat stores as a secondary source of fuel (Fig. 48-12). Ketones are acidic by-products of fat metabolism that can cause serious problems when they become excessive in the blood. Ketosis alters the pH balance, causing metabolic acidosis to develop. Ketonuria is a process that occurs when ketone bodies are excreted in the urine. During this process, electrolytes become depleted as cations are eliminated along with the anionic ketones in an attempt to maintain electrical neutrality.

**TABLE 48-16 Comparison of Hyperglycemia and Hypoglycemia**

| Hyperglycemia | Hypoglycemia |
|---|---|
| **Manifestations*** | |
| • Elevated blood glucose† <br>• Increase in urination <br>• Increase in appetite followed by lack of appetite <br>• Weakness, fatigue <br>• Blurred vision <br>• Headache <br>• Glycosuria <br>• Nausea and vomiting <br>• Abdominal cramps <br>• Progression to DKA or HHS | • Blood glucose <70 mg/dL (3.9 mmol/L) <br>• Cold, clammy skin <br>• Numbness of fingers, toes, mouth <br>• Rapid heartbeat <br>• Emotional changes <br>• Headache <br>• Nervousness, tremors <br>• Faintness, dizziness <br>• Unsteady gait, slurred speech <br>• Hunger <br>• Changes in vision <br>• Seizures, coma |
| **Causes** | |
| • Illness, infection <br>• Corticosteroids <br>• Too much food <br>• Too little or no diabetes medication <br>• Inactivity <br>• Emotional, physical stress <br>• Poor absorption of insulin | • Alcohol intake without food <br>• Too little food—delayed, omitted, inadequate intake <br>• Too much diabetes medication <br>• Too much exercise without adequate food intake <br>• Diabetes medication or food taken at wrong time <br>• Loss of weight without change in medication <br>• Use of β-adrenergic blockers interfering with recognition of symptoms |
| **Treatment** | |
| • Get medical care <br>• Continue diabetes medication as prescribed <br>• Check blood glucose frequently and check urine for ketones; record results <br>• Drink fluids at least on an hourly basis <br>• Contact HCP regarding ketonuria | • Follow the Rule of 15 (see pp. 1146-1147). <br>• See Table 48-19 for treatment of hypoglycemia. |
| **Preventive Measures** | |
| • Take prescribed dose of medication at proper time <br>• Accurately administer insulin, noninsulin injectables, OA <br>• Make healthy food choices <br>• Follow sick-day rules when ill <br>• Check blood glucose routinely <br>• Wear or carry diabetes identification | • Take prescribed dose of medication at proper time <br>• Accurately administer insulin, noninsulin injectables, OA <br>• Coordinate eating with medications <br>• Eat adequate food intake needed for calories for exercise <br>• Be able to recognize and know symptoms and treat them immediately <br>• Carry simple carbohydrates <br>• Teach family and caregiver about symptoms and treatment <br>• Check blood glucose routinely <br>• Wear or carry diabetes identification |

*DKA,* Diabetic ketoacidosis; *HHS,* hyperosmolar hyperglycemic syndrome; *OA,* oral agent.

*There is usually a gradual onset of symptoms in hyperglycemia and a more rapid onset in hypoglycemia. Many signs and symptoms of hyper- and hypoglycemia overlap. Signs and symptoms of hypoglycemia often change over time.

†Specific clinical manifestations related to elevated levels of blood glucose vary according to the patient.

**PATHOPHYSIOLOGY MAP**

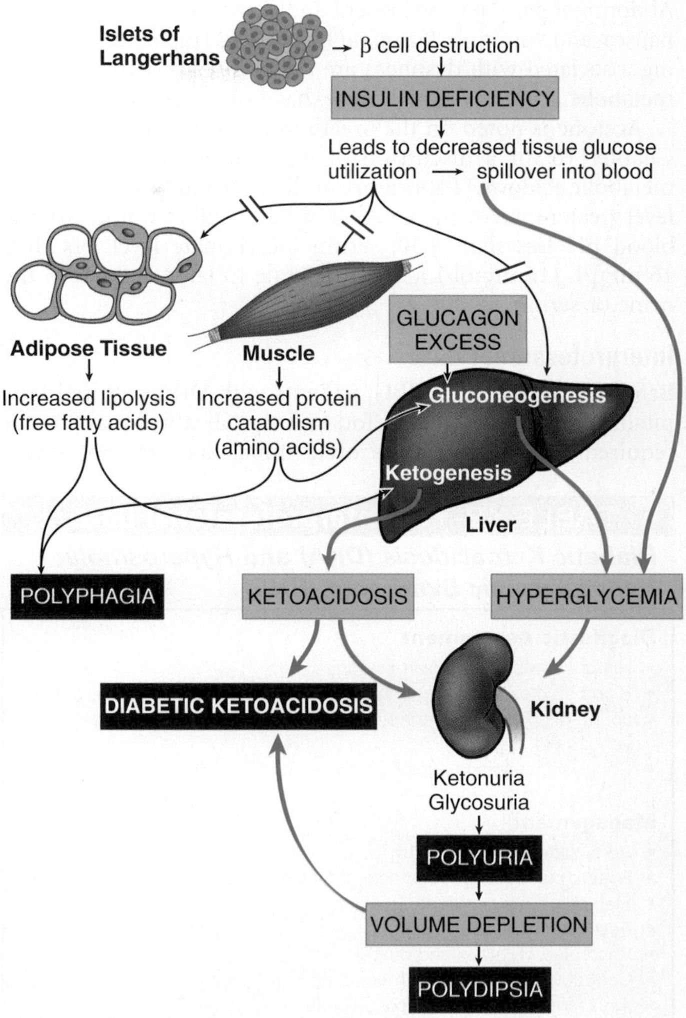


**FIG. 48-12** Metabolic events leading to diabetic ketoacidosis. (From Kumar V, Abbas AK, Aster JC, Fausto N: *Robbins and Cotran pathologic basis of disease,* ed 8, Philadelphia, 2010, Saunders.)

Insulin deficiency impairs protein synthesis and causes excessive protein degradation. This results in nitrogen losses from the tissues. Insulin deficiency also stimulates the production of glucose from amino acids (from proteins) in the liver and leads to further hyperglycemia. Because of the deficiency of insulin, the additional glucose cannot be used and the blood glucose level rises further, adding to the osmotic diuresis.

If not treated, the patient will develop severe depletion of sodium, potassium, chloride, magnesium, and phosphate. Vomiting caused by the acidosis results in more fluid and electrolyte losses. Eventually, hypovolemia followed by shock will ensue. Renal failure, which may eventually occur from hypovolemic shock, causes the retention of ketones and glucose, and the acidosis progresses. Untreated, the patient becomes comatose as a result of dehydration, electrolyte imbalance, and acidosis. If the condition is not treated, death is inevitable.

## Clinical Manifestations

Dehydration occurs in DKA with manifestations of poor skin turgor, dry mucous membranes, tachycardia, and orthostatic hypotension. Early symptoms may include lethargy and weakness. As the patient becomes severely dehydrated, the skin becomes dry and loose, and the eyes become soft and sunken. Abdominal pain may be present and accompanied by anorexia, nausea, and vomiting. *Kussmaul respirations* (rapid, deep breathing associated with dyspnea) are the body's attempt to reverse metabolic acidosis through the exhalation of excess $CO_2$.

Acetone is noted on the breath as a sweet, fruity odor. (See Chapter 16 for a discussion of respiratory compensation of metabolic acidosis.) Laboratory findings include a blood glucose level greater than or equal to 250 mg/dL (13.9 mmol/L), arterial blood pH less than 7.30, serum bicarbonate level less than 16 mEq/L (16 mmol/L), and moderate to large ketones in the urine or serum.

## Interprofessional Care

Before the advent of SMBG, patients with DKA required hospitalization for treatment. Today, hospitalization may not be required. If fluid and electrolyte imbalances are not severe and blood glucose levels can be safely monitored at home, DKA may be managed on an outpatient basis (Table 48-17). Other factors to consider when deciding where the patient is managed include the presence of fever, nausea, vomiting, and diarrhea; altered mental status; the cause of the ketoacidosis; and availability of frequent communication with the HCP (every few hours). Patients with DKA who have an illness such as pneumonia or a urinary tract infection are usually admitted to the hospital.

DKA is a serious condition that proceeds rapidly and must be treated promptly. Refer to Table 48-18 for the emergency management of a patient with DKA. Because fluid imbalance is potentially life threatening, the initial goal of therapy is to establish IV access and begin fluid and electrolyte replacement. Typically, an infusion of 0.45% or 0.9% NaCl at a rate to restore urine output to 30 to 60 mL/hr and to raise BP constitutes the initial fluid therapy regimen. When blood glucose levels approach 250 mg/dL (13.9 mmol/L), add 5% to 10% dextrose to the fluid regimen to prevent hypoglycemia and a sudden drop in glucose that can be associated with cerebral edema. Overzealous rehydration, especially with hypotonic IV solutions, can result in cerebral edema.

The aim of fluid and electrolyte therapy is to replace extracellular and intracellular water and to correct deficits of sodium, chloride, bicarbonate, potassium, phosphate, magnesium, and nitrogen. Monitor patients with renal or cardiac compromise for fluid overload. Obtain a serum potassium level before starting insulin. If the patient is hypokalemic, insulin administration will further decrease the potassium levels, making early potassium replacement essential. Although initial serum potassium may be normal or high, levels can rapidly decrease once therapy starts as insulin drives potassium into the cells, leading to life-threatening hypokalemia.

IV insulin administration therapy is directed toward correcting hyperglycemia and hyperketonemia. Insulin is immediately started at 0.1 U/kg/hr by a continuous infusion. It is important to prevent rapid drops in serum glucose to avoid cerebral edema. A blood glucose reduction of 36 to 54 mg/dL/hr (2 to 3 mmol/L/hr) will avoid complications. Insulin allows water and potassium to enter the cell along with glucose and can lead

### TABLE 48-17 Interprofessional Care

***Diabetic Ketoacidosis (DKA) and Hyperosmolar Hyperglycemic Syndrome (HHS)***

**Diagnostic Assessment**
- History and physical examination
- Blood studies, including immediate blood glucose, complete blood count, pH, ketones, electrolytes, blood urea nitrogen, arterial or venous blood gases
- Urinalysis, including specific gravity, glucose, acetone

**Management**
- Administration of IV fluids
- IV administration of short-acting insulin
- Electrolyte replacement
- Assessment of mental status
- Recording of intake and output
- Central venous pressure monitoring (if indicated)
- Assessment of blood glucose levels
- Assessment of blood and urine for ketones
- ECG monitoring
- Assessment of cardiovascular and respiratory status

### TABLE 48-18 Emergency Management

***Diabetic Ketoacidosis***

| Etiology | Assessment Findings | Interventions |
|---|---|---|
| • Undiagnosed diabetes mellitus<br>• Inadequate treatment of existing diabetes mellitus<br>• Insulin not taken as prescribed<br>• Infection<br>• Change in eating, insulin, or exercise plan<br>• Malfunction of insulin pump/ nondelivery of insulin | • Dry mouth<br>• Thirst<br>• Abdominal pain<br>• Nausea and vomiting<br>• Gradually increasing restlessness, confusion, lethargy<br>• Flushed, dry skin<br>• Eyes appearing sunken<br>• Breath odor of ketones<br>• Rapid, weak pulse<br>• Labored breathing (Kussmaul respirations)<br>• Fever<br>• Urinary frequency<br>• Serum glucose >250 mg/dL (13.9 mmol/L)<br>• Glucosuria and ketonuria | **Initial**<br>• Ensure patent airway.<br>• Administer $O_2$ via nasal cannula or non-rebreather mask.<br>• Establish IV access with large-bore catheter.<br>• Begin fluid resuscitation with 0.9% NaCl solution 1 L/hr until BP stabilized and urine output 30-60 mL/hr.<br>• Begin continuous regular insulin drip 0.1 U/kg/hr.<br>• Identify history of diabetes, time of last food, and time and amount of last insulin injection.<br>**Ongoing Monitoring**<br>• Monitor vital signs, level of consciousness, cardiac rhythm, $O_2$ saturation, and urine output.<br>• Assess breath sounds for fluid overload.<br>• Monitor serum glucose and serum potassium.<br>• Administer potassium to correct hypokalemia.<br>• Administer sodium bicarbonate if severe acidosis (pH < 7.0).<br>• Add dextrose to IV fluid for blood glucose <250 mg/dL. |

### CHECK YOUR PRACTICE

A 36-yr-old female patient was admitted to your unit with DKA. You are trying to regulate her IV rate. You know that too rapid administration of IV fluids and a rapid lowering of serum glucose can lead to cerebral edema. You also know that incorrect fluid replacement, especially with hypotonic fluids, can cause a sudden fall in serum sodium that can cause cerebral edema.

- What are the best clinical indicators of successful treatment of DKA?
- What is your role as a nurse in the care of this patient?

to a depletion of vascular volume and hypokalemia, so monitor the patient's fluid balance and potassium levels.

## HYPEROSMOLAR HYPERGLYCEMIC SYNDROME

**Hyperosmolar hyperglycemic syndrome (HHS)** is a life-threatening syndrome that can occur in the patient with diabetes who is able to produce enough insulin to prevent DKA, but not enough to prevent severe hyperglycemia, osmotic diuresis, and extracellular fluid depletion (Fig. 48-13). HHS is less common than DKA (Table 48-17). It often occurs in patients over 60 years of age with type 2 diabetes.

Common causes of HHS are urinary tract infections, pneumonia, sepsis, any acute illness, and newly diagnosed type 2 diabetes. HHS is often related to impaired thirst sensation and/or a functional inability to replace fluids. There is usually a history of inadequate fluid intake, increasing mental depression, and polyuria.

The main difference between HHS and DKA is that the patient with HHS usually has enough circulating insulin so that ketoacidosis does not occur. Because HHS produces fewer symptoms in the earlier stages, blood glucose levels can climb quite high before the problem is recognized. The higher blood glucose levels increase serum osmolality and produce more severe neurologic manifestations, such as somnolence, coma, seizures, hemiparesis, and aphasia. Since these manifestations resemble a stroke, immediate determination of the glucose level is critical for correct diagnosis and treatment.

Laboratory values in HHS include a blood glucose level greater than 600 mg/dL (33.33 mmol/L) and a marked increase in serum osmolality. Ketone bodies are absent or minimal in both blood and urine.

### Interprofessional Care

HHS is a medical emergency and has a high mortality rate. The management of DKA and HHS is similar and includes immediate IV administration of insulin and either 0.9% or 0.45% NaCl. HHS usually requires large volumes of fluid replacement. This should be accomplished slowly and carefully. Patients with HHS are commonly older and may have cardiac or renal compromise, requiring hemodynamic monitoring to avoid fluid overload during fluid replacement. When blood glucose levels fall to approximately 250 mg/dL (13.9 mmol/L), IV fluids containing dextrose are administered to prevent hypoglycemia.

Electrolytes are monitored and replaced as needed. Hypokalemia is not as significant in HHS as it is in DKA, although fluid losses may result in milder potassium deficits that require replacement. Assess vital signs, intake and output, tissue turgor, laboratory values, and cardiac monitoring to check the efficacy

### PATHOPHYSIOLOGY MAP

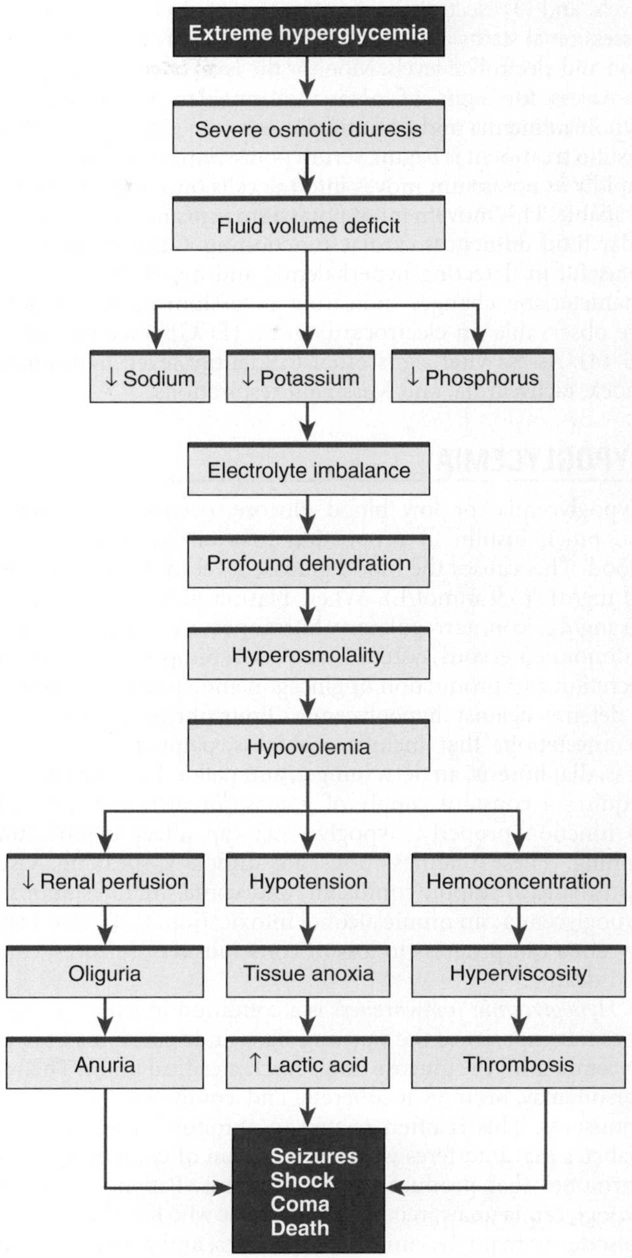


**FIG. 48-13** Pathophysiology of hyperosmolar hyperglycemic syndrome. (Modified from Urden LD, Stacy KM, Lough ME: *Critical care nursing: diagnosis and management,* ed 6, St Louis, 2010, Mosby.)

of fluid and electrolyte replacement. This includes monitoring serum osmolality and frequently assessing cardiac, renal, and mental status. Once the patient is stabilized, initiate attempts to detect and correct the underlying cause.

## ❖ NURSING MANAGEMENT: DIABETIC KETOACIDOSIS AND HYPEROSMOLAR HYPERGLYCEMIC SYNDROME

Closely monitor the hospitalized patient with appropriate blood and urine tests. You are responsible for monitoring blood glucose and urine for output and ketones and using laboratory data to determine appropriate patient care.

Monitor the administration of (1) IV fluids to correct dehydration, (2) insulin therapy to reduce blood glucose and serum ketone levels, and (3) electrolytes given to correct electrolyte imbalance. Assess renal status and cardiopulmonary status related to hydration and electrolyte levels. Monitor the level of consciousness.

Assess for signs of potassium imbalance resulting from hypoinsulinemia and osmotic diuresis (see Chapter 16). When insulin treatment is begun, serum potassium levels may decrease rapidly as potassium moves into the cells once insulin becomes available. This movement of potassium into and out of extracellular fluid influences cardiac functioning. Cardiac monitoring is useful in detecting hyperkalemia and hypokalemia because characteristic changes indicating potassium excess or deficit are observable on electrocardiogram (ECG) tracings (see Fig. 16-14). Assess vital signs often to identify fever, hypovolemic shock, tachycardia, and Kussmaul respirations.

## HYPOGLYCEMIA

Hypoglycemia, or low blood glucose, occurs when there is too much insulin in proportion to available glucose in the blood. This causes the blood glucose level to drop to less than 70 mg/dL (3.9 mmol/L). When plasma glucose drops below 70 mg/dL, counterregulatory hormones are released and the autonomic nervous system is activated. Suppression of insulin secretion and production of glucagon and epinephrine provide a defense against hypoglycemia. Epinephrine release causes manifestations that include shakiness, palpitations, nervousness, diaphoresis, anxiety, hunger, and pallor. Because the brain requires a constant supply of glucose in sufficient quantities to function properly, hypoglycemia can affect mental functioning. These manifestations are difficulty speaking, visual disturbances, stupor, confusion, and coma. Manifestations of hypoglycemia can mimic alcohol intoxication. Untreated hypoglycemia can progress to loss of consciousness, seizures, coma, and death.

*Hypoglycemia unawareness* is a condition in which a person does not experience the warning signs and symptoms of hypoglycemia until the glucose levels reach a critical point. Then the person may become incoherent and combative or lose consciousness. This is often related to autonomic neuropathy of diabetes that interferes with the secretion of counterregulatory hormones that produce these symptoms. Patients at risk for hypoglycemia unawareness include those who have had repeated episodes of hypoglycemia, older patients, and patients who use β-adrenergic blockers. Using intensive treatment to get tight blood glucose levels in patients who are at risk for hypoglycemia unawareness may not be an appropriate goal because a major drawback is hypoglycemia. These patients are usually managed with blood glucose goals that are somewhat higher than those of patients who are able to detect and manage the onset of hypoglycemia.

Causes of hypoglycemia are often related to a mismatch in the timing of food intake and the peak action of insulin or oral hypoglycemic agents that increase endogenous insulin secretion. The balance between blood glucose and insulin can be disrupted by administering too much insulin or medication, ingesting too little food, delaying the time of eating, and performing unusual amounts of exercise. Hypoglycemia can occur at any time, but most episodes occur when the OA or insulin is at its peak of action or when the patient's daily routine is disrupted without adequate adjustments in diet, medications, and activity. Although hypoglycemia is more common with insulin therapy, it can occur with noninsulin injectable agents and OAs, and it may be severe and persist for an extended time because of the longer duration of action of these drugs.

Symptoms of hypoglycemia may occur when a very high blood glucose level falls too rapidly (e.g., a blood glucose level of 300 mg/dL [16.7 mmol/L] falling quickly to 180 mg/dL [10 mmol/L]). Although the blood glucose level is above normal by definition and measurement, the sudden metabolic shift can evoke hypoglycemia symptoms. Too vigorous management of hyperglycemia with insulin can cause this type of situation.

## ❖ NURSING AND INTERPROFESSIONAL MANAGEMENT: HYPOGLYCEMIA

Hypoglycemia can usually be quickly reversed with effective treatment. At the first sign of hypoglycemia, check the blood glucose if possible. If it is less than 70 mg/dL (3.9 mmol/L), immediately begin treatment for hypoglycemia. If the blood glucose is greater than 70 mg/dL, investigate other possible causes of the signs and symptoms. If the patient has manifestations of hypoglycemia and monitoring equipment is not available or the patient has a history of fluctuating blood glucose levels, hypoglycemia should be assumed and treatment initiated.

Follow the "Rule of 15" to treat hypoglycemia (Table 48-19). A blood glucose less than 70 mg/dL is treated by ingesting 15 g of a simple (fast-acting) carbohydrate, such as 4 to 6 oz of fruit juice or a regular soft drink. Commercial products such as gels or tablets containing specific amounts of glucose are convenient for carrying in a purse or pocket to be used in such situations. Recheck the blood glucose 15 minutes later. If the value is still

### TABLE 48-19 Interprofessional Care
### *Hypoglycemia*

**Diagnostic Assessment**

- History of hypoglycemia and symptoms.
- Blood glucose—immediately.

**Management**

- Determine cause of hypoglycemia (after correction of condition).

***Conscious Patient***

- Have patient eat or drink 15 g of quick-acting carbohydrate (4-6 oz of regular soda, 5-8 LifeSavers, 1 Tbsp syrup or honey, 4 tsp jelly, 4-6 oz orange juice, commercial dextrose products [per label instructions]).
- Wait 15 min. Then check blood glucose again.
- If blood glucose is still <70 mg/dL, have patient repeat treatment of 15 g of carbohydrate.
- Once the glucose level is stable and the next meal is more than 1 hr away, give patient additional food of carbohydrate plus protein or fat (e.g., crackers with peanut butter or cheese) after symptoms subside. Give additional food if patient is engaged in physical activity regardless of time until next meal.
- Immediately notify HCP or emergency service (if patient outside hospital) if symptoms do not subside after two or three administrations of quick-acting carbohydrate.

***Worsening Symptoms or Unconscious Patient***

- Subcutaneous or IM injection of 1 mg glucagon. IV administration of 20-50 mL of 50% glucose.

less than 70 mg/dL, ingest 15 g more of carbohydrate and recheck the blood glucose in 15 minutes. If no significant improvement occurs after two or three doses of 15 g of simple carbohydrate, contact the HCP. After an acute episode of hypoglycemia, have the patient ingest a complex carbohydrate after recovery to prevent repeat hypoglycemia.

Avoid treatment with carbohydrates that contain fat, such as candy bars, cookies, whole milk, and ice cream. The fat in those foods will slow the absorption of the glucose and delay the response to treatment. Avoid overtreatment with large quantities of quick-acting carbohydrates so that a rapid fluctuation to hyperglycemia does not occur.

In an acute care setting, patients with hypoglycemia may be treated with 20 to 50 mL of 50% dextrose IV push. If the patient is not alert enough to swallow and no IV access is available, another option is to administer 1 mg of glucagon by IM or subcutaneous injection. An IM injection in a site such as the deltoid muscle will result in a quicker response. Glucagon stimulates a strong hepatic response to convert glycogen to glucose and therefore makes glucose rapidly available. Nausea is a common reaction after glucagon injection. Therefore, to prevent aspiration if vomiting occurs, turn the patient on the side until he or she becomes alert. Patients with minimal glycogen stores will not respond to glucagon. This includes patients with alcohol-related hepatic disease, starvation, and adrenal insufficiency. Teach family members and others likely to be present when severe hypoglycemia occurs when and how to inject glucagon.

Once the acute hypoglycemia has been reversed, explore with the patient the reasons why the situation developed. This assessment may indicate the need for additional teaching of the patient and the family to avoid future episodes of hypoglycemia.

# CHRONIC COMPLICATIONS OF DIABETES MELLITUS

## ANGIOPATHY

Chronic complications associated with diabetes are primarily those of end-organ disease from damage to blood vessels *(angiopathy)* secondary to chronic hyperglycemia (Fig. 48-14). Angiopathy is one of the leading causes of diabetes-related deaths, with about 68% of deaths caused by CVD and 16% caused by strokes for those ages 65 or older.[23] These chronic blood vessel dysfunctions are divided into two categories: macrovascular complications and microvascular complications.

Several theories exist as to how and why chronic hyperglycemia damages cells and tissues. Possible causes include (1) the accumulation of damaging by-products of glucose metabolism, such as sorbitol, which is associated with damage to nerve cells; (2) the formation of abnormal glucose molecules in the basement membrane of small blood vessels such as those that circulate to the eyes and kidneys; and (3) a derangement in red blood cell function that leads to a decrease in oxygenation to the tissues.

The Diabetes Control and Complications Trial (DCCT), a landmark study in diabetes management, demonstrated that in patients with type 1 diabetes the risk for microvascular complications could be significantly reduced by keeping blood glucose levels as near to normal as possible for as much of the time as

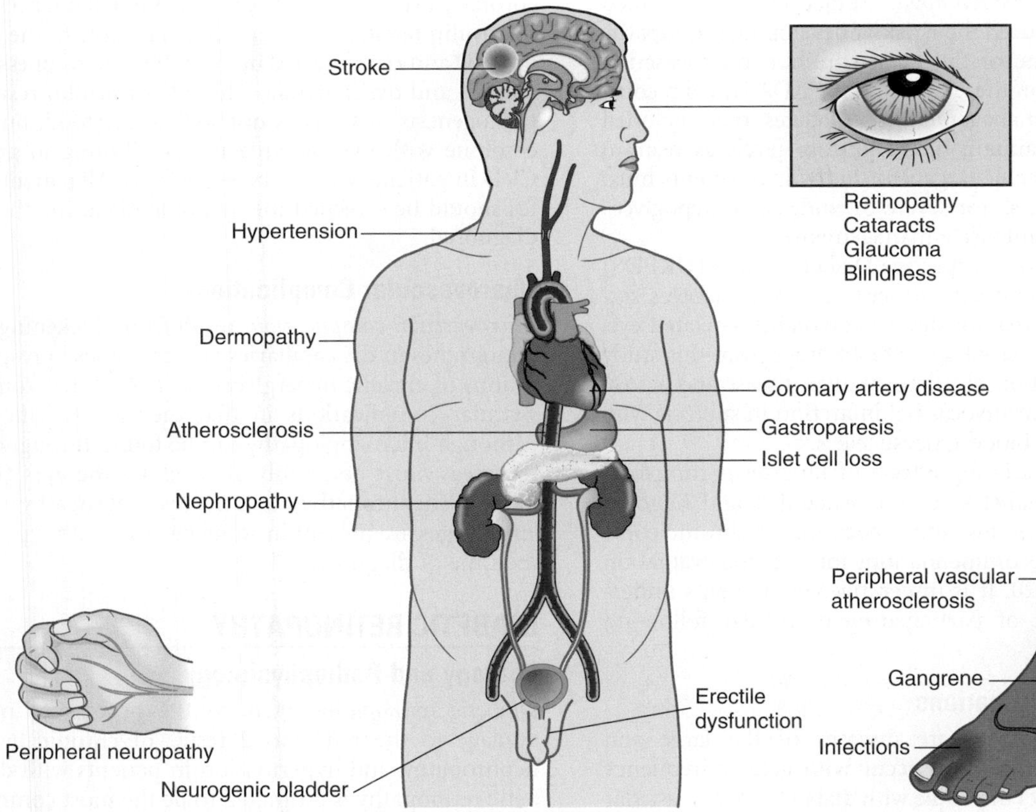


**FIG. 48-14** Long-term complications of diabetes mellitus. (From Kumar V, Abbas AK, Aster JC, Fausto N: *Robbins and Cotran pathologic basis of disease,* ed 8, Philadelphia, 2010, Saunders.)

**TABLE 48-20 Monitoring for Long-Term Complications of Diabetes Mellitus**

| Complication | Type of Examination | Frequency |
|---|---|---|
| **Retinopathy** | • Funduscopic: dilated eye examination | • Annually |
| | • Fundus photography | |
| **Nephropathy** | • Urine for albuminuria<br>• Serum creatinine | • Annually |
| **Neuropathy** (foot and lower extremities) | • Visual examination of foot | • Daily by patient<br>• Every visit to HCP |
| | • Comprehensive foot:<br>• Visual examination<br>• Sensory examination with monofilament and tuning fork<br>• Palpation (pulses, temperature, callus formation) | • Annually* |
| **Cardiovascular disease** | • Risk factor assessment: hypertension, dyslipidemia, smoking, family history of premature coronary artery disease, and presence of albuminuria or | • At least annually |
| | • Exercise stress testing (may include stress ECG, stress echocardiogram, stress nuclear imaging) | • As needed based on risk factors |

Source: American Diabetes Association: Standards of medical care in diabetes, *Diabetes Care* 39 (Suppl 1):S1, 2016.

*If patients have a history of foot ulcers, loss of sensation in their feet, or other foot abnormalities, the recommendation is to have a foot exam at every visit.

possible *(tight or intensive therapy)*.[24] Subjects who maintained tight glucose levels reduced their risk of developing retinopathy and nephropathy, some of the most common microvascular complications. Based on these findings, the ADA issued recommendations for the management of diabetes that included treatment goals to maintain blood glucose levels as near to normal as possible. Specific targets for individual patients must take into account the risk for severe or undetected hypoglycemia as a side effect of intensive management.

The United Kingdom Prospective Diabetes Study (UKPDS) demonstrated that intensive treatment of type 2 diabetes significantly lowered the risk for developing diabetes-related eye, kidney, and neurologic problems. The findings from this study included a 25% reduction of microvascular disease and a 16% reduction in the risk for myocardial infarction in subjects who maintained long-term blood glucose levels.[25]

Because of the devastating effects of long-term complications, patients with diabetes require scheduled and ongoing monitoring for the detection and prevention of chronic complications. The ADA recommendations for ongoing evaluation are listed in Table 48-20. It is imperative that patients understand the importance of participating in regular follow-up examinations.

### Macrovascular Complications

*Macrovascular complications* are diseases of the large and medium-size blood vessels that occur with greater frequency and with an earlier onset in people with diabetes. Macrovascular diseases include cerebrovascular, cardiovascular, and peripheral vascular disease. Women with diabetes have a four to six times increased risk for CVD, and men with diabetes have a two to three times increased risk for CVD compared with those without diabetes.[4] Patients with diabetes can decrease several risk factors associated with macrovascular complications, such as obesity, smoking, hypertension, high fat intake, and sedentary lifestyle. Smoking, which is detrimental to health in general, is especially injurious to people with diabetes and significantly increases their risk for blood vessel and cardiovascular disease, stroke, and lower extremity amputation. The ADA recommends yearly screening for CVD risk factors in people with diabetes.[12]

Optimizing BP control in patients with diabetes is significant for the prevention of cardiovascular and renal disease. Treating hypertension in those with diabetes results in a decrease in macrovascular and microvascular complications. Hypertension in people with diabetes causes an increase in mortality greater than for those with hypertension without diabetes.[2] A target BP of less than 140/90 mm Hg is recommended for most patients with diabetes.[15]

Patients with diabetes have an increase in lipid abnormalities. This contributes to the increase in CVD seen in this population. The ADA recognizes that diabetes alone is a CVD risk factor. Therefore it recommends that all adults with diabetes take a statin. Dosing is based on the presence of age and additional atherosclerotic CVD risk factors. The ADA advocates lifestyle interventions, including nutritional therapy, exercise, weight loss, and smoking cessation to treat hyperlipidemia.

The ADA recommends BP screening at every routine visit for people with diabetes. They also recommend lifestyle advisement for BP greater than 130/80 and treatment for BP greater than 140/90. (Hypertension is discussed in Chapter 32, and coronary artery disease is discussed in Chapter 33.)

Insulin resistance has an important role in the development of CVD and is implicated in the pathogenesis of essential hypertension and dyslipidemia. The role of insulin resistance in the pathogenesis of CVD is not well understood, but it seems to combine with dyslipidemia in contributing to greater risk of CVD in patients with diabetes mellitus. All patients with diabetes should be screened for dyslipidemia at the time diabetes is diagnosed.

### Microvascular Complications

*Microvascular complications* result from thickening of the vessel membranes in the capillaries and arterioles in response to conditions of chronic hyperglycemia. They differ from the macrovascular complications in that they are specific to diabetes. Although microangiopathy can be found throughout the body, the areas most noticeably affected are the eyes (retinopathy), kidneys (nephropathy), and nerves (neuropathy). Microvascular changes are present in some patients with type 2 diabetes at the time of diagnosis.

## DIABETIC RETINOPATHY

### Etiology and Pathophysiology

*Diabetic retinopathy* refers to the process of microvascular damage to the retina as a result of chronic hyperglycemia, nephropathy, and hypertension in patients with diabetes. Diabetic retinopathy is estimated to be the most common cause of new cases of adult blindness.[2]

Retinopathy can be classified as nonproliferative or proliferative. In *nonproliferative retinopathy,* the most common form, partial occlusion of the small blood vessels in the retina causes microaneurysms to develop in the capillary walls. The walls of these microaneurysms are so weak that capillary fluid leaks out, causing retinal edema and eventually hard exudates or intraretinal hemorrhages. This may cause mild to severe vision loss, depending on which parts of the retina are affected. If the center of the retina (macula) is affected, vision loss can be severe.

*Proliferative retinopathy,* the most severe form, involves the retina and vitreous. When retinal capillaries become occluded, the body compensates by forming new blood vessels to supply the retina with blood, a pathologic process known as *neovascularization.* These new vessels are extremely fragile and hemorrhage easily, producing vitreous contraction. Eventually light is prevented from reaching the retina as the vessels become torn and bleed into the vitreous cavity. The patient sees black or red spots or lines. If these new blood vessels pull the retina while the vitreous contracts, causing a tear, partial or complete retinal detachment will occur. If the macula is involved, vision is lost. Without treatment, more than half of patients with proliferative diabetic retinopathy will be blind.

Persons with diabetes are also prone to other visual problems. Glaucoma occurs as a result of the occlusion of the outflow channels secondary to neovascularization. This type of glaucoma is difficult to treat and often results in blindness. Cataracts develop at an earlier age and progress more rapidly in people with diabetes.

### Interprofessional Care

The earliest and most treatable stages of diabetic retinopathy often produce no changes in the vision. Therefore patients with type 2 diabetes should have a dilated eye examination by an ophthalmologist or a specially trained optometrist at the time of diagnosis and annually thereafter for early detection and treatment. A person with type 1 diabetes should have a dilated eye examination within 5 years after the onset of diabetes and then repeated annually.

The best approach to the management of diabetes-related eye disease is to prevent it by maintaining healthy blood glucose levels and managing hypertension. Laser photocoagulation therapy is indicated to reduce the risk of vision loss in patients with proliferative retinopathy or macular edema and in some cases of nonproliferative retinopathy. Laser photocoagulation destroys the ischemic areas of the retina that produce growth factors that encourage neovascularization. A patient who develops vitreous hemorrhage and retinal detachment of the macula may need to undergo vitrectomy. *Vitrectomy* is the aspiration of blood, membrane, and fibers from the inside of the eye through a small incision just behind the cornea. (Photocoagulation and vitrectomy are discussed in Chapter 21.)

Iluvien (fluocinolone acetonide intravitreal implant) is used to treat retinopathy. It is an injectable micro-insert that provides sustained treatment through continuous delivery of corticosteroid fluocinolone acetonide for 36 months. Iluvien is injected in the back of the patient's eye with an applicator that uses a 25-gauge needle, which allows for a self-sealing wound.

Recent research has identified the importance of vascular endothelial growth factor (VEGF) in the development of diabetic retinopathy. Drugs injected into the eye that block the action of VEGF and reduce inflammation are currently being studied for their effectiveness in treating retinopathy.[26]

## NEPHROPATHY

**Diabetic nephropathy** is a microvascular complication associated with damage to the small blood vessels that supply the glomeruli of the kidney. It is the leading cause of end-stage renal disease in the United States and is seen in 20% to 40% of people with diabetes. Risk factors for diabetes-related nephropathy include hypertension, genetic predisposition, smoking, and chronic hyperglycemia. Results of the DCCT and UKPDS research have demonstrated that kidney disease can be significantly reduced when near-normal blood glucose levels are maintained.[24,25]

Patients with diabetes are screened for nephropathy annually with a random spot urine collection to assess for albuminuria and measure the albumin-to-creatinine ratio. Serum creatinine is also measured to provide an estimation of the glomerular filtration rate and thus the degree of kidney function.

Patients with diabetes who have albuminuria receive either angiotensin-converting enzyme (ACE) inhibitor drugs (e.g., lisinopril [Prinivil, Zestril]) or angiotensin II receptor antagonists (e.g., losartan [Cozaar]). Both classifications of these drugs are used to treat hypertension and have been found to delay the progression of nephropathy in patients with diabetes.[12] Hypertension significantly accelerates the progression of nephropathy. Therefore aggressive BP management is indicated for all patients with diabetes. Keeping blood glucose levels in a healthy range is also critical in the prevention and delay of diabetes-related nephropathy. (See Chapter 32 for a discussion of hypertension and Chapter 46 for a discussion of renal failure.)

## NEUROPATHY

**Diabetic neuropathy** is nerve damage that occurs because of the metabolic derangements associated with diabetes mellitus. About 60% to 70% of patients with diabetes have some degree of neuropathy.[2] The most common type of neuropathy affecting persons with diabetes is sensory neuropathy. This can lead to the loss of protective sensation in the lower extremities, and, coupled with other factors, significantly increases the risk for complications that result in a lower limb amputation. More than 60% of nontraumatic amputations in the United States occur in people with diabetes.[2] Screening for neuropathy begins at the time of diagnosis in patients with type 2 diabetes and 5 years after diagnosis in patients with type 1 diabetes.[12]

### Etiology and Pathophysiology

The pathophysiologic processes of diabetes-related neuropathy are not well understood. Several theories exist, including metabolic, vascular, and autoimmune factors. The prevailing theory is that persistent hyperglycemia leads to an accumulation of sorbitol and fructose in the nerves that causes damage by an unknown mechanism. The result is reduced nerve conduction and demyelinization. Ischemic damage by chronic hyperglycemia in blood vessels that supply the peripheral nerves is also implicated in the development of diabetes-related neuropathy. Neuropathy can precede, accompany, or follow the diagnosis of diabetes.

### Classification

The two major categories of diabetes-related neuropathy are *sensory neuropathy,* which affects the peripheral nervous system, and *autonomic neuropathy.* Each of these types can take on several forms.

**Sensory Neuropathy.** The most common form of sensory neuropathy is distal symmetric polyneuropathy, which affects the hands and/or feet bilaterally. This is sometimes referred to as *stocking-glove neuropathy.* Characteristics of distal symmetric polyneuropathy include loss of sensation, abnormal sensations, pain, and paresthesias. The pain, which is often described as burning, cramping, crushing, or tearing, is usually worse at night and may occur only at that time. The paresthesias may be associated with tingling, burning, and itching sensations. The patient may report a feeling of walking on pillows or numb feet. At times the skin becomes so sensitive (hyperesthesia) that even light pressure from bed sheets cannot be tolerated. Complete or partial loss of sensitivity to touch and temperature is common. Foot injury and ulcerations can occur without the patient ever having pain (Fig. 48-15). Neuropathy can also cause atrophy of the small muscles of the hands and feet, causing deformity and limiting fine movement.

Managing blood glucose is the only treatment for diabetes-related neuropathy. It is effective in many, but not all, cases. Drug therapy may be used to treat neuropathic symptoms, particularly pain. Medications commonly used include topical creams (e.g., capsaicin [Zostrix]), tricyclic antidepressants (e.g., amitriptyline), selective serotonin and norepinephrine reuptake inhibitors (e.g., duloxetine [Cymbalta]), and antiseizure medications (e.g., gabapentin [Neurontin], pregabalin [Lyrica]). Capsaicin is a moderately effective topical cream made from chili peppers. It depletes the accumulation of pain-mediating chemicals in the peripheral sensory neurons. The cream is applied three or four times a day.

At the start of therapy, symptoms usually increase, followed by relief of pain in 2 to 3 weeks. Tricyclic antidepressants are moderately effective in treating the symptoms of diabetic neuropathy. They work by inhibiting the reuptake of norepinephrine and serotonin, which are neurotransmitters believed to play a role in the transmission of pain through the spinal cord. Duloxetine is thought to relieve pain by increasing the levels of serotonin and norepinephrine, which improves the body's ability to regulate pain. Antiseizure medications decrease the release of neurotransmitters that transmit pain.[27]

**Autonomic Neuropathy.** Autonomic neuropathy can affect nearly all body systems and lead to hypoglycemia unawareness, bowel incontinence and diarrhea, and urinary retention. *Gastroparesis* (delayed gastric emptying) is a complication of autonomic neuropathy that can produce anorexia, nausea, vomiting, gastroesophageal reflux, and persistent feelings of fullness. Gastroparesis can trigger hypoglycemia by delaying food absorption. Cardiovascular abnormalities associated with autonomic neuropathy are postural hypotension, resting tachycardia, and painless myocardial infarction. Assess patients with diabetes for postural hypotension to determine if they are at risk for falls. Instruct the patient with postural hypotension to change from a lying or sitting position slowly.

Diabetes can affect sexual function in men and women. Erectile dysfunction (ED) in men with diabetes is well recognized and common, often being the first manifestation of autonomic neuropathy. ED in diabetes is also associated with other factors, including vascular disease, elevated blood glucose levels, endocrine disorders, psychogenic factors, and medications. Decreased libido is a problem for some women with diabetes. Candidal and nonspecific vaginitis is also common. ED or sexual dysfunction requires sensitive therapeutic counseling for both the patient and the patient's partner. (See Chapter 55 for a further discussion of ED.)

A neurogenic bladder may develop as the sensation in the inner bladder wall decreases, causing urinary retention. A patient with retention has infrequent voiding, difficulty voiding, and a weak stream of urine. Emptying the bladder every 3 hours in a sitting position helps prevent stasis and subsequent infection. Tightening the abdominal muscles during voiding and using the Credé maneuver (mild massage downward over the lower abdomen and bladder) may also help with complete bladder emptying. Cholinergic agonist drugs such as bethanechol (Urecholine) may be used. The patient may also need to learn self-catheterization (see Chapter 45).

## COMPLICATIONS OF FEET AND LOWER EXTREMITIES

People with diabetes are at high risk for foot ulcerations and lower extremity amputations.[12] The development of diabetes-related foot complications can be the result of a combination of microvascular and macrovascular diseases that place the patient at risk for injury and serious infection (Fig. 48-16).

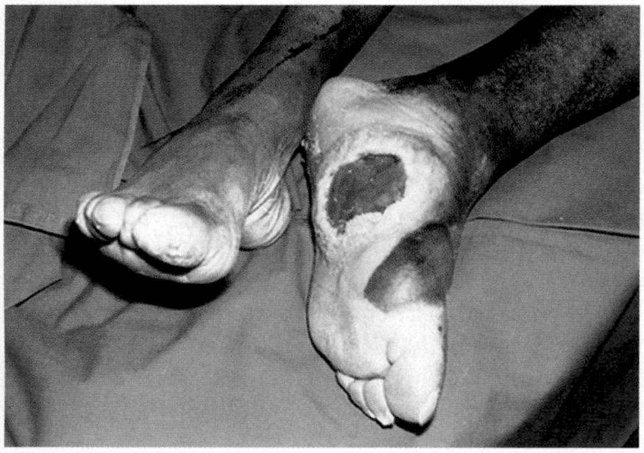

**FIG. 48-15** Neuropathy: neurotrophic ulceration.

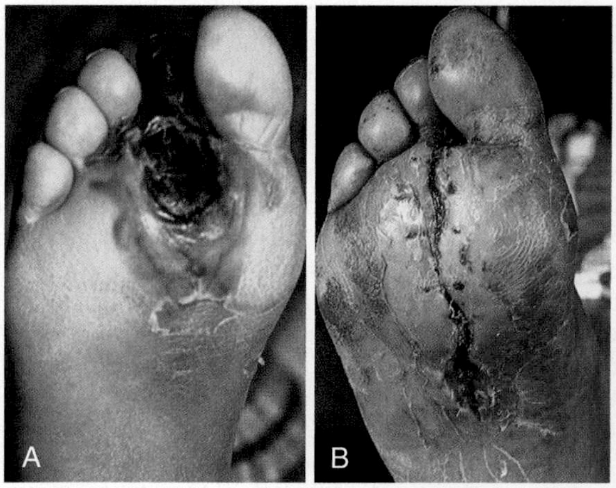


**FIG. 48-16** The necrotic toe developed as a complication of diabetes. **A,** Before amputation. **B,** After amputation. (From Chew SL, Leslie D: *Clinical endocrinology and diabetes: an illustrated colour text,* Edinburgh, 2006, Churchill Livingstone.)

Sensory neuropathy and peripheral artery disease (PAD) are risk factors for foot complications. In addition, clotting abnormalities, impaired immune function, and autonomic neuropathy also have a role. Smoking is deleterious to the health of lower extremity blood vessels and increases the risk for amputation.

*Sensory neuropathy* is a major risk factor for lower extremity amputation in the person with diabetes. *Loss of protective sensation* (LOPS) often prevents the patient from being aware that a foot injury has occurred. Improper footwear and injury from stepping on foreign objects while barefoot are common causes of undetected foot injury in the person with LOPS.[12] Because the primary risk factor for lower extremity amputation is LOPS, annual screening using a *monofilament* is important. This is done by applying a thin, flexible filament to several spots on the plantar surface of the foot and asking the patient to report if it is felt. Insensitivity to a monofilament has been shown to greatly increase the risk for foot ulcers that can lead to amputation.

PAD increases the risk for amputation by causing a reduction in blood flow to the lower extremities. When blood flow is decreased, oxygen, white blood cells, and vital nutrients are not available to the tissues. Wounds take longer to heal, and the risk for infection increases. Signs of PAD include intermittent claudication, pain at rest, cold feet, loss of hair, delayed capillary filling, and dependent rubor (redness of the skin that occurs when the extremity is in a dependent position). The disease is diagnosed by history, ankle-brachial index (ABI) (see Table 37-3), and angiography. Management includes reduction of risk factors, particularly smoking, cholesterol intake, and hypertension. Bypass or graft surgery is indicated in some patients. (PAD is discussed in Chapter 37.)

If the patient has LOPS or PAD, aggressive measures must be taken to teach the patient how to prevent foot ulcers. These measures include the selection of proper footwear, including protective shoes. Teach the patient to carefully avoid injury to the foot, practice diligent skin and nail care, inspect the foot thoroughly each day, and treat small problems promptly. Guidelines for patient teaching are listed in Table 48-21.

Proper care of a foot ulcer is critical for wound healing. Several forms of treatment can be used. Casting can be done to redistribute the weight on the plantar surface of the foot. Wound care for the ulcer can include debridement, dressings, advanced wound healing products (becaplermin [Regranex]), vacuum-assisted closure, ultrasound, hyperbaric oxygen, and skin grafting.

Neuropathic arthropathy, or *Charcot's foot,* results in ankle and foot changes that ultimately lead to joint dysfunction and footdrop. These changes occur gradually and promote an abnormal distribution of weight over the foot, further increasing the chances of developing a foot ulcer as new pressure points emerge. Foot deformity should be recognized early and proper footwear fitted before ulceration occurs.

## INTEGUMENTARY COMPLICATIONS

Up to two thirds of persons with diabetes develop skin problems.[12] Diabetes-related dermopathy, the most common diabetic skin lesion, is characterized by reddish brown, round or oval patches. They initially are scaly, then they flatten out and become indented. The lesions appear most frequently on the shins but can also be found on the front of the thighs, forearm, side of the foot, scalp, and trunk.

### TABLE 48-21 Patient & Caregiver Teaching*
**Foot Care**

*Include the following instructions when teaching the patient and caregiver about foot care.*

1. Wash feet daily with a mild soap and warm water. First test water temperature with elbow.
2. Pat feet dry gently, especially between toes.
3. Examine feet daily for cuts, blisters, swelling, and red, tender areas. Do not depend on feeling sores. If eyesight is poor, have others inspect feet.
4. Use lanolin on feet to prevent skin from drying and cracking. Do not apply between toes.
5. Use mild foot powder on sweaty feet.
6. Do not use commercial remedies to remove calluses or corns.
7. Cleanse cuts with warm water and mild soap, covering with clean dressing. Do not use iodine, rubbing alcohol, or strong adhesives.
8. Report skin infections or nonhealing sores to HCP immediately.
9. Cut toenails evenly with rounded contour of toes. Do not cut down corners. The best time to trim nails is after a shower or bath.
10. Separate overlapping toes with cotton or lamb's wool.
11. Avoid open-toe, open-heel, and high-heel shoes. Leather shoes are preferred to plastic ones. Wear slippers with soles. Do not go barefoot. Inspect socks and shoes for foreign objects before putting on.
12. Wear clean, absorbent (cotton or wool) socks or stockings that have not been mended. Colored socks must be colorfast.
13. Do not wear clothing that leaves impressions, hindering circulation.
14. Do not use hot water bottles or heating pads to warm feet. Wear socks for warmth.
15. Guard against frostbite.
16. Exercise feet daily either by walking or by flexing and extending feet in suspended position. Avoid prolonged sitting, standing, and crossing of legs.

*This teaching guide is also appropriate for patients with peripheral vascular problems.

*Acanthosis nigricans* is a manifestation of insulin resistance. It can appear as a velvety light brown to black skin thickening, predominantly seen on flexures, axillae, and the neck. *Necrobiosis lipoidica diabeticorum* usually appears as red-yellow lesions, with atrophic skin that becomes shiny and transparent revealing tiny blood vessels under the surface (Fig. 48-17). This condition is uncommon and occurs more frequently in young women. It may appear before other clinical signs or symptoms of diabetes. Because the thin skin is prone to injury, special care must be taken to protect affected areas from injury and ulceration.

## INFECTION

A person with diabetes is more susceptible to infections because of a defect in the mobilization of white blood cells and an impaired phagocytosis by neutrophils and monocytes. Recurring or persistent infections such as *Candida albicans,* as well as boils and furuncles, in the undiagnosed patient often lead the HCP to suspect diabetes. Loss of sensation (neuropathy) may delay the detection of an infection.

Persistent glycosuria may predispose patients to bladder infections, especially patients with a neurogenic bladder. Decreased circulation resulting from angiopathy can prevent or delay the immune response. Antibiotic therapy has prevented infection from being a major cause of death in patients with diabetes. The

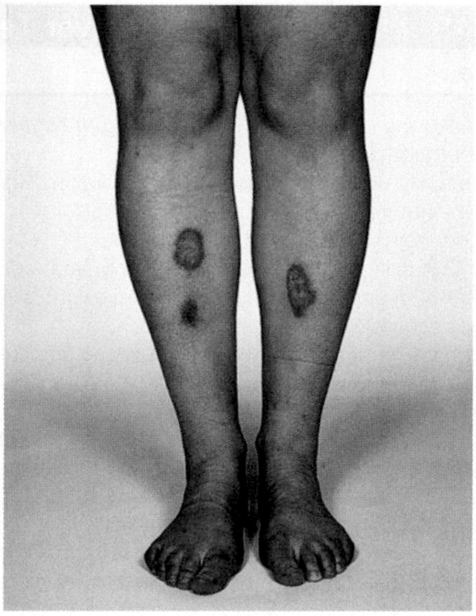

**FIG. 48-17** Necrobiosis lipoidica diabeticorum. (From Chew SL, Leslie D: *Clinical endocrinology and diabetes: an illustrated colour text,* Edinburgh, 2006, Churchill Livingstone.)

treatment of infections must be prompt and vigorous. Teach patients to prevent infection by practicing good hand hygiene, avoiding exposure to individuals who have a communicable illness, and getting an annual influenza vaccine and pneumococcal vaccine. (Guidelines for pneumococcal vaccine are presented in Table 27-5.)

## PSYCHOLOGIC CONSIDERATIONS

Patients with diabetes have high rates of depression, anxiety, and eating disorders. Depression contributes to diminished diabetes self-care, feelings of helplessness related to chronic illness, and poor outcomes.[12] Assess patients for manifestations of depression and/or diabetes distress.

Disordered eating behaviors (DEB) can occur in people with both type 1 and type 2 diabetes. DEBs include anorexia, bulimia, binge eating, excessive restriction of calories, and intense exercise. The greatest incidence of eating disorders is seen in females. Adolescent girls with diabetes are more than twice as likely to develop DEB than those who do not have diabetes.[28] Patients may intentionally decrease their dose of insulin or omit the dose. This is called "diabulimia" and leads to weight loss, hyperglycemia, and glycosuria because the food ingested cannot be used for energy without adequate insulin. Insulin omission and DEBs can have serious consequences, including retinopathy, neuropathy, lipid abnormalities, DKA, and death.[28]

Open communication is critical to identify these behaviors early. Patients with eating disorders need to be seen by a mental health professional with expertise in eating disorders and an understanding of diabetes management.

### Gerontologic Considerations: Diabetes Mellitus

Diabetes is present in more than 25% of persons over 65 years of age, with this age group being the fastest-growing segment of the population developing diabetes.[2] Older people with diabetes have higher rates of premature death, functional disability, and coexisting illnesses such as hypertension and stroke than those without diabetes. The prevalence of diabetes increases with age. A major reason for this is that the process of aging is associated with a reduction in β-cell function, decreased insulin sensitivity, and altered carbohydrate metabolism. Aging is also associated with a number of conditions that are more likely to be treated with medications that impair insulin action (e.g., corticosteroids, antihypertensives, phenothiazines). Undiagnosed and untreated diabetes is more common in older adults, partly because many of the normal physiologic changes of aging resemble those of diabetes, such as low energy levels, falls, dizziness, confusion, and chronic urinary tract infections.

Several factors are taken into account when determining glycemic goals for an older adult. One is that hypoglycemia unawareness is more common in older adults, making these patients more likely to suffer adverse consequences from blood glucose–lowering therapy. They may have delayed psychomotor function that could interfere with the ability to treat

## TEAMWORK & COLLABORATION

### *Caring for the Patient With Diabetes Mellitus*

Oral agents (OAs), noninsulin injectable agents, and insulin can be administered by licensed practical/vocational nurses (LPN/LVNs) (and in some states and settings by unlicensed assistive personnel [UAP]) to stable patients. In patients experiencing acute complications of diabetes mellitus (DM), actions such as insulin administration and infusion of IV fluids are done or directly supervised by a registered nurse (RN).

**Role of Nursing Personnel**

***Registered Nurse (RN)***

- Assess for risk factors for prediabetes and type 1 and type 2 DM.
- Teach the patient and caregiver about self-management of DM, including self-monitoring of blood glucose (SMBG), insulin, noninsulin injectables, OAs, nutrition, physical activity, and recognition and management of hypoglycemia.
- Develop a plan to avoid hypoglycemia or hyperglycemia in a patient with DM who is acutely ill or having surgery.
- Assess for acute complications and implement appropriate actions: hypoglycemia, diabetic ketoacidosis (DKA), and hyperosmolar hyperglycemic syndrome (HHS).
- Assess for chronic complications, including cardiovascular disease, retinopathy, nephropathy, neuropathy, and foot complications.
- Teach patient and caregiver about prevention and management of chronic complications related to diabetes.

***Licensed Practical/Vocational Nurse (LPN/LVN)***

- Administer OAs and routinely scheduled insulin regimens.
- Monitor the patient for symptoms of hypoglycemia, DKA, and HHS.
- In the ambulatory or home setting, monitor patient self-management of insulin, OAs, nutrition, and physical activity.
- Report concerns with patient self-management in the home setting to the RN.

***Unlicensed Assistive Personnel (UAP)***

- Check capillary blood glucose (CBG) levels (after being trained and evaluated in this procedure) and report values to the RN.
- Report changes in patient vital signs, urine output, behavior, or level of consciousness to the RN.
- In a community or home care setting, administer OAs and insulin to a stable patient (consider state nurse practice act and agency policy).

**Role of Other Team Members**

***Dietitian***

- Assess patient's knowledge of diabetes. Provide teaching about disease process as needed.
- Teach the patient and caregiver about nutrition and diet to self-manage DM and any complications (e.g., hypoglycemia).

## ETHICAL/LEGAL DILEMMAS

### *Durable Power of Attorney for Health Care*

**Situation**

G.V., a 64-yr-old woman, is admitted to the intensive care unit with heart failure. She has many complications from a long-term history of type 1 diabetes and hypertension, including a right leg above-the-knee amputation and blindness related to retinopathy. She severed ties with her family 30 yr ago. She has a life partner of 35 yr whom she designated as her proxy in her signed Durable Power of Attorney. She has stated many times that she would rather die than have renal dialysis. She has been sedated and intubated for 3 days. The physician plans to extubate her and resuscitate her so that dialysis can be initiated. Her brother shows up at the hospital and supports the physician's decision. Her partner disagrees with the decision. The physician refuses to recognize her partner as proxy because she is not a blood relative.

**Ethical/Legal Points for Consideration**

- The Patient Self-Determination Act (1990) requires all health care facilities receiving Medicare and Medicaid funding to make available advance directives allowing individuals to state their preferences or refusals of health care in the event that they are incapable of consenting for themselves.
- Durable Power of Attorney for health care is one type of advance directive in which people, when they are competent, identify someone else to make decisions for them, should they lose their decision-making ability in the future.
- The Living Will, another type of advance directive, permits individuals to state their own preferences and refusals.
- Many HCPs mistakenly think that proxies must be family members or blood relatives. Lesbian, gay, bisexual, and transgender (LGBT) individuals often have difficulty having their partnership recognized as valid, especially if the patient's family disputes their rights.
- Some families are deeply divided on decisions for their loved ones, and sometimes difficulties occur when money and property are also disputed. The passage of time may be an issue where the original documents were executed and then changes occurred (e.g., divorce, death or disability of the proxy, inability to contact the proxy, inability to find a valid original of the advance directive).
- Within your scope of nursing practice, you need to be informed as to decision-making laws and regulations in your own state and make advance directive documents available to patients. In addition, you need to (1) teach patients and their families about advance directives, (2) make sure that HCPs are aware of and follow advance directives, (3) assist the patient and family in communicating with the HCPs when a "No Code" order is requested, and (4) assist a conflicted family in obtaining appropriate counseling whenever necessary.*
- Counsel LGBT patients on the importance of having a health care proxy and a will to legally protect their end-of-life choices.

**Discussion Questions**

1. How would you handle a situation in which the family and surrogate decision maker disagree?
2. How can you assess the patient and family's understanding of durable power of attorney and assist them in understanding their role in decision making?
3. What should you do when a physician orders dialysis to be initiated when you know that this goes against the patient's advance directive?

*Advance directives are discussed in Table 9-6.

hypoglycemia. Other factors to consider in establishing glycemic goals for the older patient include the patient's own desire for treatment and coexisting medical problems such as cognitive impairment. Compounding the challenge, diabetes increases the rate of decline of cognitive function. Although it is generally agreed that treatment is indicated to prevent complications, intensive diabetes management may be difficult and dangerous to achieve, especially in older adults.

Meal planning and exercise are recommended as therapy for older adult patients with diabetes. This should take into account functional limitations that may interfere with physical activity and the ability to prepare meals. Because of the physiologic changes that occur with aging, the therapeutic outcome for the older adult with diabetes who receives OAs may be altered. Assess renal function and creatinine clearance in patients over 80 years of age taking metformin. Monitor those taking sulfonylurea drugs (e.g., glipizide) for hypoglycemia and renal and liver dysfunction. Insulin therapy may be instituted if OAs are not effective. However, it is important to recognize that older adults are more likely to have limitations in the manual dexterity and visual acuity necessary for accurate insulin administration. Insulin pens may be a safer alternative for older adults.

Patient education issues for the older patient include those related to altered vision, mobility, cognitive status, and functional ability. Plan patient teaching based on the individual's needs, using a slower pace with simple printed or audio materials in patients with cognitive and functional limitations. Include the family or caregivers in the teaching. Consider the patient's financial and social situation and the effect of multiple medications, eating habits, and quality-of-life issues.

## CASE STUDY

### Diabetic Ketoacidosis

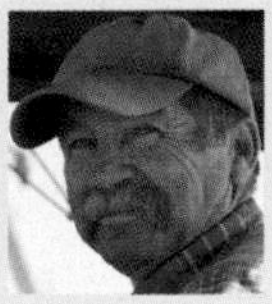

(©katrinaelena/ iStock/ Thinkstock)

**Patient Profile**

N.B., a 48-yr-old farmer, was admitted to the emergency department after he was found unconscious by his wife in their barn. They live 40 miles from the nearest health care facility.

**Subjective Data (Provided by Wife)**

- Was diagnosed with type 1 diabetes mellitus 15 years ago
- Was taking 50 U/day of insulin via insulin pump: 5 U of lispro insulin bolus with breakfast, 5 U bolus with lunch, and 10 U bolus with dinner plus 30 U of basal insulin
- Has history of gastroenteritis for 1 wk with vomiting and anorexia
- Stopped taking meal time boluses 2 days ago when he was unable to eat
- Has not changed his infusion set in 5 days

**Objective Data**

***Physical Examination***

- Breathing is deep and rapid
- Fruity acetone smell on breath
- Skin flushed and dry

***Diagnostic Studies***

- Blood glucose level 730 mg/dL (40.5 mmol/L)
- Blood pH 7.26

**Discussion Questions**

1. Briefly explain the pathophysiology of the development of diabetic ketoacidosis (DKA) in this patient.
2. What clinical manifestations of DKA does this patient exhibit?
3. What factors precipitated this patient's DKA?
4. ***Priority Decision:*** What is the priority nursing intervention for N.B.?
5. What distinguishes this case history from one of hyperosmolar hyperglycemic syndrome (HHS) or hypoglycemia?
6. ***Priority Decision:*** What is the priority teaching for this patient and his family?
7. What role should N.B.'s wife have in the management of his diabetes?
8. ***Priority Decision:*** Based on the assessment data presented, what are the priority nursing diagnoses? Are there any collaborative problems?
9. ***Evidence-Based Practice:*** N.B.'s wife asks you if she should have given her husband insulin when he got sick. How would you respond?
10. ***Teamwork and Collaboration:*** How can the interprofessional team be most effective in the care of N.B?
11. ***Quality Improvement:*** What outcomes would indicate that the interprofessional team was effective in the care of N.B.?

Answers and a corresponding concept map are available at *http://evolve.elsevier.com/Lewis/medsurg.*

## BRIDGE TO NCLEX EXAMINATION

The number of the question corresponds to the same-numbered outcome at the beginning of the chapter.

**1.** Polydipsia and polyuria related to diabetes mellitus are primarily due to
- **a.** the release of ketones from cells during fat metabolism.
- **b.** fluid shifts resulting from the osmotic effect of hyperglycemia.
- **c.** damage to the kidneys from exposure to high levels of glucose.
- **d.** changes in RBCs resulting from attachment of excessive glucose to hemoglobin.

**2.** Which statement would be correct for a patient with type 2 diabetes who was admitted to the hospital with pneumonia?
- **a.** The patient must receive insulin therapy to prevent ketoacidosis.
- **b.** The patient has islet cell antibodies that have destroyed the pancreas's ability to produce insulin.
- **c.** The patient has minimal or absent endogenous insulin secretion and requires daily insulin injections.
- **d.** The patient may have sufficient endogenous insulin to prevent ketosis but is at risk for hyperosmolar hyperglycemic syndrome.

**3.** Analyze the following diagnostic findings for your patient with type 2 diabetes. Which result will need further assessment?
- **a.** A1C 9%
- **b.** BP 126/80 mm Hg
- **c.** FBG 130 mg/dL (7.2 mmol/L)
- **d.** LDL cholesterol 100 mg/dL (2.6 mmol/L)

**4.** Which statement by the patient with type 2 diabetes is accurate?
- **a.** "I will limit my alcohol intake to one drink."
- **b.** "I am not allowed to eat any sweets because of my diabetes."
- **c.** "I cannot exercise because I take a blood glucose-lowering medication."
- **d.** "The amount of fat in my diet is not important. Only carbohydrates raise my blood sugar."

**5.** You are caring for a patient with newly diagnosed type 1 diabetes. What information is *essential* to include in your patient teaching before discharge from the hospital *(select all that apply)*?
- **a.** Insulin administration
- **b.** Elimination of sugar from diet
- **c.** Need to reduce physical activity
- **d.** Use of a portable blood glucose monitor
- **e.** Hypoglycemia prevention, symptoms, and treatment

**6.** What is the *priority* action for the nurse to take if the patient with type 2 diabetes complains of blurred vision and irritability?
- **a.** Call the physician.
- **b.** Administer insulin as ordered.
- **c.** Check the patient's blood glucose level.
- **d.** Assess for other neurologic symptoms.

**7.** A patient with diabetes has a serum glucose level of 824 mg/dL (45.7 mmol/L) and is unresponsive. After assessing the patient, the nurse suspects diabetic ketoacidosis rather than hyperosmolar hyperglycemic syndrome based on the finding of
- **a.** polyuria.
- **b.** severe dehydration.
- **c.** rapid, deep respirations.
- **d.** decreased serum potassium.

**8.** Which are appropriate therapies for patients with diabetes mellitus *(select all that apply)*?
- **a.** Use of statins to reduce CVD risk
- **b.** Use of diuretics to treat nephropathy
- **c.** Use of ACE inhibitors to treat nephropathy
- **d.** Use of serotonin agonists to decrease appetite
- **e.** Use of laser photocoagulation to treat retinopathy

1. b, 2. d, 3. a, 4. a, 5. a, d, e, 6. c, 7. c, 8. a, c, e

For rationales to these answers and even more NCLEX review questions, visit *http://evolve.elsevier.com/Lewis/medsurg.*

## EVOLVE WEBSITE

http://evolve.elsevier.com/Lewis/medsurg

**Review Questions (Online Only)**

**Key Points**

**Answer Keys for Questions**

- Rationales for Bridge to NCLEX Examination Questions
- Answer Guidelines for Case Study(ies) on p. 1153

**Student Case Studies**

- Patient With Type 1 Diabetes Mellitus and Diabetic Ketoacidosis
- Patient With Type 2 Diabetes Mellitus and Hyperosmolar Hyperglycemic Syndrome

**Nursing Care Plans**

- eNursing Care Plan 48-1: Patient With Diabetes Mellitus

**Conceptual Care Map Creator**

- Conceptual Care Map for Case Study on p. 1153

**Audio Glossary**

**Supporting Media**

- Animation
  - Insulin Function

**Content Updates**

## REFERENCES


1. American Diabetes Association: Statistics about diabetes. Retrieved from *www.diabetes.org/diabetes-basics/statistics*.
2. Centers for Disease Control and Prevention: 2014 National Diabetes Statistics Report. Retrieved from *www.cdc.gov/diabetes/data/statistics/2014StatisticsReport.html*.
3. American Diabetes Association: Diagnosis and classification of diabetes mellitus, *Diabetes Care* 39 (Suppl):S13, 2016.
4. Centers for Disease Control and Prevention: Diabetes public health resource: groups especially affected. Retrieved from *www.cdc.gov/diabetes*.
5. Dumore S, Brown J: The role of adipokines in β cell failure of type 2 diabetes, *J Endocrinol* 216:T37, 2013.
6. Bansal N: Prediabetes diagnosis and treatment: a review, *World J Diabetes* 6(2):296, 2015.
7. Ben-Shmuel S, Rostoker R, Scheinman EJ, et al: Metabolic syndrome, type 2 diabetes, and cancer: epidemiology and potential mechanisms, *Handb Exp Pharmacol* 233:355, 2016.
8. Centers for Disease Control and Prevention: Preventing chronic disease: prevalence estimates of gestational diabetes mellitus in the United States, pregnancy risk assessment monitoring system (PRAMS), 2014. Retrieved from *www.cdc.gov/pcd/issues/2014/13_0415.htm*.

*9. HAPO Study Cooperative Research Group: Hyperglycemia and adverse pregnancy outcomes, *N Engl J Med* 358:1991, 2008. (Classic)

*10. Schwartz N, Nachum Z, Green MS: The prevalence of gestational diabetes mellitus recurrence-effect of ethnicity and parity: a meta-analysis, *Am J Obstet Gynecol* 213:310, 2015.

11. Tran L, Zielinski A, Roach AH, et al: The pharmacologic treatment of type 2 diabetes: injectable medications, *Ann Pharmacother* 49:700, 2015.
12. American Association of Diabetes Educators: *The art and science of self-management education desk reference*, ed 3, Chicago, 2014, American Association of Diabetes Educators.
13. BD Diabetes: Syringe and needle sizes. Retrieved from *www.bd.com/us/products/category.asp*.
14. Joslin Diabetes Center: The advantages and disadvantages of an insulin pump, 2015. Retrieved from *www.joslin.org/info/the_advantages_and_disadvantages_of_an_insulin_pump.html*.
15. American Diabetes Association: Standards of medical care in diabetes, *Diabetes Care* 39 (Suppl 1):S1, 2016.
16. Evert AB, Boucher JL, Cypress M: Nutrition therapy recommendations for the management of adults with diabetes, *Diabetes Care* 36(11):3821, 2013.
17. American Diabetes Association: Food and fitness: create your plate. Retrieved from *www.diabetes.org/food-and-fitness/food*.
18. US Department of Health and Human Services: Physical activity guidelines advisory committee report. Retrieved from *www.cdc.gov/nccdphp/sgr/contents.htm*.
19. American Diabetes Association: Fitness, 2015. Retrieved from *www.diabetes.org/food-and-fitness/fitness*.
20. Cengiz E, Tamborlane W: A tale of two compartments: Interstitial versus blood glucose monitoring, *Diabetes Technol Ther* S-11, 2008. (Classic)
21. Ratner R: An update on the Diabetes Prevention Program, *Endocrine Pract* 12(Suppl 1):20, 2006. (Classic)
22. Kruger DF, LaRue S, Estepa P: Recognition of and steps to mitigate anxiety and fear of pain in injectable diabetes treatment, *Diabetes Metab Syndr Obes* 8:49, 2015.
23. Boucher J, Hurrell D: Cardiovascular disease and diabetes, *Diabetes Spectrum* 21:154, 2008. (Classic)

*24. Diabetes Control and Complications Trial Research Group: The effect of intensive treatment of diabetes on the development and progression of long-term complications in insulin-dependent diabetes mellitus, *N Engl J Med* 329:977, 1993. (Classic)

*25. UK Prospective Diabetes Study (UKPDS) Group: Intensive blood-glucose control with sulphonylureas or insulin compared with conventional treatment and risk of complications in patients with type 2 diabetes, *Lancet* 352:837, 1998. (Classic)

26. El-Shazly S, El-Bradey M, Tameesh M: Vascular endothelial growth factor gene polymorphism prevalence in patients with diabetic macular oedema and its correlation with anti-vascular endothelial growth factor treatment outcomes, *Clin Exp Opthalmol* 42:369, 2014.

*27. Javed S, Petropoulos N, Alam U, Malik, R: Treatment of painful diabetic neuropathy, *Ther Adv Chronic Dis* 6:15, 2015.

28. Pinhas-Hamiel O, Levy-Shraga Y: Eating disorders in adolescents with type 1 and type 2 diabetes, *Curr Diab Rep* 13:289, 2013.


*Evidence-based information for clinical practice.

# 49

# Endocrine Problems

*Katherine A. Kelly*

*The best way to cheer yourself up is to try to cheer somebody else up.*

*Mark Twain*

http://evolve.elsevier.com/Lewis/medsurg/

## LEARNING OUTCOMES

1. Explain the pathophysiology, clinical manifestations, interprofessional care, and nursing management of the patient with an imbalance of hormones produced by the anterior pituitary gland.
2. Describe the pathophysiology, clinical manifestations, interprofessional care, and nursing management of the patient with an imbalance of hormones produced by the posterior pituitary gland.
3. Explain the pathophysiology, clinical manifestations, interprofessional care, and nursing management of the patient with thyroid dysfunction.
4. Describe the pathophysiology, clinical manifestations, interprofessional care, and nursing management of the patient with an imbalance of the hormone produced by the parathyroid glands.
5. Identify the pathophysiology, clinical manifestations, interprofessional care, and nursing management of the patient with an imbalance of hormones produced by the adrenal cortex.
6. Describe the pathophysiology, clinical manifestations, interprofessional care, and nursing management of the patient with an excess of hormones produced by the adrenal medulla.
7. List the side effects of corticosteroid therapy.
8. Describe common nursing assessments, interventions, rationales, and expected outcomes related to patient teaching for management of chronic endocrine problems.

## KEY TERMS



The endocrine system is made up of a number of organs and glands that are involved in the synthesis and secretion of hormones that affect every body system. Because these hormones have such a wide range of action, endocrine problems are associated with a variety of clinical manifestations. An endocrine problem often affects many aspects of a person's life.

## DISORDERS OF ANTERIOR PITUITARY GLAND

The pituitary gland is considered the master gland of the endocrine system. The anterior pituitary gland secretes GH, prolactin, and the tropic hormones, ACTH, TSH, FSH, and LH. These hormones affect growth, sexual maturation, reproduction, metabolism, stress response, and fluid balance. As a result, pituitary gland disorders manifest in a variety of ways.

Tumors of the pituitary gland account for 5% to 20% of primary intracranial tumors.[1] The most common, the pituitary adenoma, is a slow-growing, benign tumor. It is generally found in adults between 40 and 60 years of age. Hypersecretory pituitary adenomas secrete an excess of a specific hormone causing manifestations related to the action of that hormone. The most common are prolactinomas and growth hormone and ACTH-secreting adenomas.[1]

## ACROMEGALY

**Acromegaly** is a rare condition characterized by an overproduction of growth hormone (GH). Around four out of every 1 million adults in the United States are diagnosed annually.[2] It affects both genders equally. The mean age at the time of diagnosis is 40 to 45 years old.

### Etiology and Pathophysiology

Acromegaly most often occurs because of a benign growth hormone–secreting pituitary adenoma. The excess GH results

Reviewed by Crystal Sheaves, RN, MSN, APRN, FNP-BC, Senior Lecturer, West Virginia University School of Nursing, Charleston, West Virginia; and Crystal R. Sherman, DNP, CNP, FNP-BC, APHN-BC, Assistant Professor of Nursing, Shawnee State University, Portsmouth, Ohio.

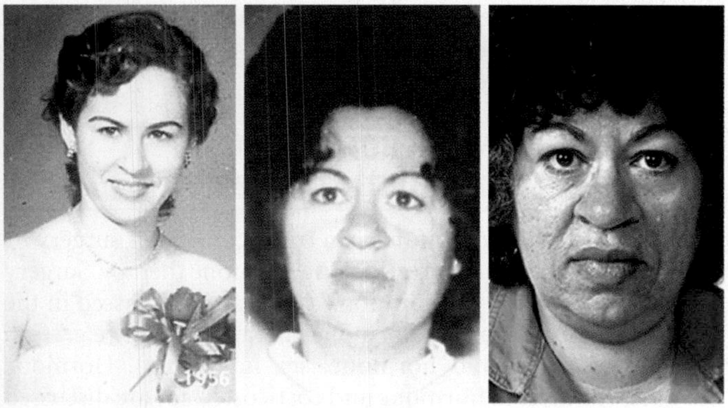


**FIG. 49-1** Progressive development of facial changes associated with acromegaly. (Courtesy Linda Haas, Seattle, Wash.)

in an overgrowth of soft tissues and bones in the hands, feet, and face. Because the problem develops after epiphyseal closure, the bones of the arms and legs do not grow longer.

### Clinical Manifestations

The changes resulting from excess GH in adults can occur slowly, over a number of years, and may go unnoticed by the person, family, and friends. Thickening and enlargement of the bony and soft tissues on the face, feet, and head occur (Fig. 49-1). Patients may experience proximal muscle weakness and joint pain that can range from mild to crippling. Carpal tunnel syndrome and peripheral neuropathy may be present.

Tongue enlargement results in dental problems and speech difficulties. The voice deepens because of hypertrophy of the vocal cords. Sleep apnea may occur because of upper airway narrowing and obstruction from increased amounts of pharyngeal soft tissues. The skin becomes thick, leathery, and oily with acne outbreaks.

Visual changes may occur due to pressure on the optic nerve from a pituitary adenoma. Headaches are common. Since GH antagonizes the action of insulin, glucose intolerance and manifestations of diabetes mellitus may occur, including *polydipsia* (increased thirst) and *polyuria* (increased urination).[3]

The life expectancy of those with acromegaly is reduced by 5 to 10 years. They are prone to cardiovascular disease, diabetes mellitus, and colorectal cancer.[4] Even if patients are cured or the disease is well controlled, manifestations such as joint pain and deformities often remain.

### Diagnostic Studies

In addition to the history and physical examination, a diagnosis requires evaluating plasma insulin-like growth factor (IGF-1) levels and GH response to an oral glucose tolerance test (OGTT). IGF-1 mediates the peripheral actions of GH. As GH levels rise, so do IGF-1 levels. However, GH is released in a pulsatile fashion, requiring several samples to obtain an accurate assessment. Serum IGF-1 levels are more constant, giving a more reliable diagnostic measure of acromegaly. During an OGTT, GH concentration normally falls because glucose inhibits GH secretion. In acromegaly GH levels do not fall, and in some cases GH levels rise.

MRI or high-resolution CT scan with contrast media can detect pituitary adenomas. A complete eye examination, including visual fields, is done because a tumor may cause pressure on the optic chiasm or optic nerves.

## ❖ NURSING AND INTERPROFESSIONAL MANAGEMENT: ACROMEGALY

The patient's prognosis depends on the age at onset, age when treatment started, and tumor size. The overall goal is to return the patient's GH levels to normal. Treatment consists of surgery, radiation therapy, drug therapy, or a combination of these therapies. With treatment, bone growth can be stopped and tissue hypertrophy reversed. However, sleep apnea, diabetes, and cardiac complications may persist.

Surgery (hypophysectomy) is the treatment of choice. It offers the best chance for a cure and optimal symptom management, especially for smaller pituitary adenomas.[5] Surgery produces an immediate reduction in GH levels followed by a drop in IGF-1 levels within a few weeks. Patients with larger tumors or those with GH levels greater than 45 ng/mL may require adjuvant radiation or drug therapy. Surgery and radiation therapy for pituitary tumors are discussed later in this chapter on p. 1158.

Drug therapy is an option for patients whose surgery did not result in a cure and/or in combination with radiation therapy. The primary drug used is octreotide (Sandostatin), a somatostatin analog. It reduces GH levels to normal in many patients. Octreotide is given by subcutaneous injection three times a week. Long-acting somatostatin analogs, octreotide (Sandostatin LAR), pasireotide (Signifor, Signifor LAR), and lanreotide SR (Somatuline Depot), are available as IM injections given every 4 weeks. GH levels are measured every 2 weeks to guide drug dosing and then every 6 months until the desired response is obtained.

Dopamine agonists (e.g., bromocriptine, cabergoline) may be given alone or with somatostatin analogs if complete remission has not been achieved after surgery. These drugs reduce the secretion of GH from the tumor.

GH antagonists (e.g., pegvisomant [Somavert]) reduce the effect of GH in the body by blocking the hepatic production of IGF-1. Most patients taking this drug achieve normal IGF-1 levels with symptom improvement.[4]

Serial photographs showing improvement in appearance may be helpful to the patient's recovery. Psychosocial effects of acromegaly include body image disturbances, sexual dysfunction, and depression. Fatigue and sleep disturbances may persist after surgery. Patients will need strategies for dealing with these symptoms. Referral to a support group may be helpful.

## EXCESSES OF OTHER TROPIC HORMONES

Excess secretion of prolactin or the tropic hormones (e.g., ACTH, TSH) by the anterior pituitary gland will cause other endocrine glands to overproduce certain hormones. An excess of these hormones (discussed later in the chapter) can cause significant disturbances in metabolism and general health.

A prolactin-secreting adenoma is known as a *prolactinoma*. Prolactinomas constitute about 40% of pituitary adenomas.[6] Women with prolactinomas frequently experience galactorrhea, anovulation, infertility, oligomenorrhea or amenorrhea, decreased libido, and hirsutism. In men, impotence, decreased sperm density, and libido may result. Compression of the optic chiasm can cause visual problems and signs of increased intracranial pressure, including headache, nausea, and vomiting.

Because prolactinomas do not typically progress in size, drug therapy is usually the first-line treatment. The dopamine agonists cabergoline and bromocriptine are used to treat prolactinomas. Surgery may be an option, depending on the extent and size of the tumor. Radiation therapy can reduce the risk of tumor recurrence for patients with large tumors.

## HYPOFUNCTION OF PITUITARY GLAND

**Hypopituitarism** is a rare disorder that involves a decrease in one or more of the pituitary hormones. A deficiency of only one pituitary hormone is referred to as *selective hypopituitarism.* Total failure of the pituitary gland results in deficiency of all pituitary hormones—a condition referred to as *panhypopituitarism.* The most common hormone deficiencies associated with hypopituitarism involve GH and gonadotropins (i.e., LH, FSH).

### Etiology and Pathophysiology

The usual cause of pituitary hypofunction is a pituitary tumor. Autoimmune disorders, infections, pituitary infarction (Sheehan syndrome), or destruction of the pituitary gland (from trauma, radiation, or surgical procedures) can also cause hypopituitarism. African Americans have a higher incidence of pituitary adenomas than other ethnic groups.[7]

Anterior pituitary hormone deficiencies can lead to end-organ failure. Deficiencies of TSH and ACTH are life threatening. ACTH deficiency can lead to acute adrenal insufficiency and hypovolemic shock from sodium and water depletion. (Acute adrenal insufficiency is discussed later in this chapter on pp. 1178-1179.)

### Clinical Manifestations and Diagnostic Studies

The manifestations of hypopituitarism vary with the type and degree of dysfunction. Early manifestations associated with a space-occupying lesion include headaches, visual changes (decreased visual acuity or decreased peripheral vision), loss of smell, nausea and vomiting, and seizures. Manifestations associated with hyposecretion of the target glands vary widely (Table 49-1).

In addition to a history and physical examination, diagnostic studies such as MRI and CT can identify a pituitary tumor. Laboratory tests vary widely but generally involve the direct measurement of pituitary hormones (e.g., TSH) or an indirect determination of the target organ hormones (e.g., triiodothyronine [$T_3$], thyroxine [$T_4$]). (See Chapter 47 for more information regarding diagnostic studies.)

**TABLE 49-1 Manifestations of Hypopituitarism**

| Hormone Deficiency | Manifestations |
|---|---|
| Growth hormone (GH) | Subtle, nonspecific findings: Truncal obesity, osteoporosis, decreased muscle mass and strength, weakness, fatigue, depression, or flat affect. |
| Follicle-stimulating hormone (FSH) and luteinizing hormone (LH) | *Women:* Menstrual irregularities, loss of libido, changes in secondary sex characteristics such as decreased breast size.<br>*Men:* Testicular atrophy, diminished spermatogenesis, loss of libido, impotence, decreased facial hair and muscle mass. |
| Thyroid-stimulating hormone (TSH) | Mild form of primary hypothyroidism: Fatigue, cold intolerance, constipation, lethargy, weight gain. |
| Adrenocorticotropic hormone (ACTH) | Involves cortisol deficiency: Weakness, fatigue, headache, dry and pale skin, diminished axillary and pubic hair, lowered resistance to infection, fasting hypoglycemia. |

## ❖ NURSING AND INTERPROFESSIONAL MANAGEMENT: HYPOPITUITARISM

The treatment for hypopituitarism often consists of surgery or radiation therapy followed by lifelong hormone therapy. Surgery and radiation therapy for pituitary tumors are discussed in the next section. Appropriate hormone therapy is used (e.g., GH, corticosteroids, thyroid hormone, sex hormones). Hormone therapies for thyroid hormone and corticosteroids are discussed later in this chapter on p. 1169 and pp. 1179-1180.

Somatropin (Omnitrope, Genotropin, Humatrope), which is recombinant human GH, is used for long-term hormone therapy in adults with GH deficiency. These patients respond well to GH replacement and experience increased energy, increased lean body mass, a feeling of well-being, and improved body image. Mild to moderate side effects of GH include fluid retention with swelling in the feet and hands, myalgia, joint pain, and headache. GH is given daily as a subcutaneous injection (preferably in the evening). The dosing is variable because it is adjusted based on symptoms, IGF-1 levels, and the development of adverse effects.

Although gonadal deficiency is not life threatening, hormone therapy will improve sexual function and general well-being. It is contraindicated in those with certain medical conditions, such as phlebitis, pulmonary embolism, breast cancer in women, and prostate cancer in men. Estrogen and progesterone replacement therapy may be indicated for hypogonadal women to treat hot flashes, vaginal dryness, and decreased libido. (Hormone therapy for women is discussed in Chapter 53.) Testosterone is used to treat men with gonadotropin deficiency. The benefits achieved with testosterone therapy include a return of male secondary sex characteristics; improved libido; and increased muscle mass, bone mass, and bone density. (Hormone therapy for men is discussed in Chapter 54.)

## PITUITARY SURGERY

A *hypophysectomy* is the surgical removal of the pituitary gland. It is the treatment of choice for tumors in the pituitary area, especially smaller pituitary adenomas. Most surgeries are done by an endoscopic *transsphenoidal* approach (Fig. 49-2). When the entire pituitary gland is removed, there is permanent loss of all pituitary hormones. The patient will require lifelong replacement therapy of thyroid hormone, sex hormones, and glucocorticoids.

Radiation therapy can reduce the size of a tumor before surgery. It is also used when surgery fails to produce a cure or when patients are poor candidates for surgery. Its full effects may not be noted for months to years. Radiation therapy may lead to hypopituitarism, which then requires lifelong hormone replacement therapy. Stereotactic radiosurgery (gamma knife surgery, proton beam, linear accelerator) is an option for small, surgically inaccessible pituitary tumors or in place of conventional radiation.

## ❖ NURSING MANAGEMENT: PITUITARY SURGERY

Postoperatively, assess the patient for the formation of a hematoma compressing the optic nerve or optic chiasma. Monitor

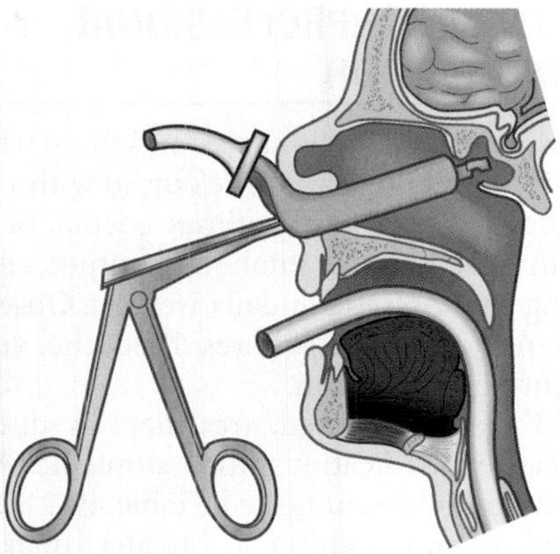

FIG. 49-2 Surgery on the pituitary gland is most commonly performed with the transsphenoidal approach. An incision is made in the inner aspect of the upper lip and gingiva. The sella turcica is entered through the floor of the nose and sphenoid sinuses.

## BECOMING A NURSE LEADER

### *Dealing With Conflict in the Workplace*

**Situation**

It is your first 7 PM to 7 AM shift on a general medical unit. You quickly observe that Debbie and Carrie do not get along. In fact, they loudly bicker with each other the entire shift, and they refuse to watch each other's patients for breaks. Their relationship seems to negatively affect other team members. In addition, your patients want to know what is going on and why the nurses are so loud in the hallways. You are very uncomfortable and don't want to rock the boat, but you approach the charge nurse and are told, "Oh, everyone knows Debbie and Carrie don't get along. It's always like this."

**Points for Consideration**

- Some people will go to extreme lengths to avoid conflict. They may have so little confidence in their own communication skills that they fear losing control of their emotions and making the situation worse.
- People often avoid dealing with conflict in the workplace because they fear confronting others:
  - Afraid confronting them will make the situation worse
  - Afraid confrontation will hurt the relationship
  - Concerned that the other party will "attack"
  - Fear retribution in some way
- Help resolve conflict by choosing your words carefully and avoiding labeling people. Establish a win-win approach to help those in conflict view each other as partners.
- Model good conflict management behaviors by remaining neutral and being an active listener. Define the issue in neutral terms by taking personalities out of the problem. Invite the conflicting parties to suggest ways to reach an agreement, while adding objectivity to the situation.

**Discussion Questions**

1. As a new nurse on this shift, what actions can you take to resolve the conflict?
2. Why is decreased patient satisfaction likely to be an issue on this shift? What can be done about it by you and/or the nurse manager?

peripheral vision, visual acuity, extraocular movements, and pupillary response. Report changes immediately because timely intervention may prevent visual deterioration from becoming permanent.

CSF leaks and epistaxis are other common postoperative complications.[8] The surgeon may place a petroleum jelly–coated ribbon of gauze or a balloon-tipped catheter (like an indwelling urinary catheter) in the sphenoid sinus. It is usually removed after 24 hours. It can be left in for 2 to 3 days if there is concern for bleeding or CSF leak. It is important that the patient does not blow the nose for at least 48 hours after surgery and avoid vigorous coughing, sneezing, and straining at stool (Valsalva maneuver).

Monitor the "moustache" dressing regularly for any drainage. Check any clear drainage with a urine dipstick for glucose and protein. If present, notify the HCP of a possible CSF leak. A sample can be sent to the laboratory. A glucose level greater than 30 mg/dL (1.67 mmol/L) indicates CSF leakage from an open connection with the brain. If this happens, the patient is at increased risk for meningitis.

Complaints of persistent and severe generalized or supraorbital headache may indicate CSF leakage into the sinuses. A CSF leak usually resolves within 72 hours when treated with head elevation and bed rest. If the leak persists, daily spinal taps may be done to reduce pressure to below-normal levels.

Other postoperative measures include elevating the head of the patient's bed at all times to a 30-degree angle. This elevation avoids pressure on the sella turcica and decreases headaches. Monitor the pupillary response, speech patterns, and extremity strength to detect neurologic complications. Gentle mouth care every 4 hours is essential to keep the surgical area clean and free of debris. Advise the patient to avoid tooth brushing for at least 10 days to protect the suture line.

Fluid and electrolyte disturbances can occur from the development of diabetes insipidus (DI).[8] Transient DI may occur because of the loss of antidiuretic hormone (ADH), which is stored in the posterior lobe of the pituitary gland, or cerebral edema related to manipulation of the pituitary during surgery. To assess for DI, closely monitor urine output and measure specific gravity. Report a urine output of >200 mL/hour for more than 3 consecutive hours or a specific gravity level of <1.005. Patients with DI will have an elevated serum sodium and extreme thirst. DI is treated by giving desmopressin acetate (DDAVP). Fluid replacement may be necessary to avoid hypovolemia related to high urine output.

Syndrome of inappropriate ADH secretion (SIADH) can occur after any intracranial surgery. SIADH typically occurs later than DI, usually around the fourth postoperative day. It may occur due to manipulation of the pituitary and other structures causing release of ADH. The fluid retention caused by circulating ADH leads to dilutional hyponatremia. Sodium levels of less than 125 mEq/L will exhibit as headache, vomiting, and decreased level of consciousness. The manifestations and treatment of DI and SIADH are discussed in the next section.

ADH, cortisol, and thyroid hormone replacement are needed after a hypophysectomy. Teach the patient about the need for lifelong therapy. Surgery may result in permanent loss or deficiencies in follicle-stimulating hormone (FSH) and luteinizing hormone (LH). This can lead to decreased fertility. Assist the patient in working through the grieving process associated with these losses.

## DISORDERS OF POSTERIOR PITUITARY GLAND

The hormones secreted by the posterior pituitary are antidiuretic hormone (ADH) and oxytocin. ADH, also referred to as *arginine vasopressin* (AVP) or vasopressin, plays a major role in the regulation of water balance and serum osmolarity (see Chapter 47). The two primary problems associated with ADH secretion are a result of either overproduction or underproduction of ADH. The overproduction of ADH results in a condition known as **syndrome of inappropriate antidiuretic hormone**

(SIADH). Underproduction of ADH results in a condition referred to as *diabetes insipidus* (DI).

## SYNDROME OF INAPPROPRIATE ANTIDIURETIC HORMONE

### Etiology and Pathophysiology

SIADH is the release of ADH despite normal or low plasma osmolarity (Fig. 49-3). ADH increases the permeability of the renal distal tubule and collecting duct, which leads to the reabsorption of water into the circulation. Extracellular fluid volume expands, plasma osmolality declines, glomerular filtration rate increases, and sodium levels decline (dilutional hyponatremia).[9] Thus the disorder is characterized by fluid retention, serum hypoosmolality, dilutional hyponatremia, hypochloremia, and concentrated urine in the presence of normal or increased intravascular volume.

This syndrome occurs more commonly in older adults. SIADH has various causes (Table 49-2). The most common cause is cancer, especially small cell lung cancer. Although SIADH tends to be self-limiting when caused by head trauma or drugs, it is chronic when associated with tumors or metabolic diseases.

### Clinical Manifestations and Diagnostic Studies

The patient with SIADH experiences low urine output and increased body weight. Initially, the patient displays thirst, dyspnea on exertion, and fatigue. Mild hyponatremia causes muscle cramping, irritability, and headache. As the serum sodium level falls (usually below 120 mEq/L [120 mmol/L]), manifestations become more severe and include vomiting, abdominal cramps, and muscle twitching. As plasma osmolality and serum sodium levels continue to decline, cerebral edema may occur, leading to lethargy, confusion, seizures, and coma.

The diagnosis of SIADH is made by simultaneous measurements of urine and serum osmolality. Dilutional hyponatremia is indicated by a serum sodium less than 134 mEq/L, serum osmolality less than 280 mOsm/kg (280 mmol/kg), and urine specific gravity greater than 1.025. A serum osmolality much lower than the urine osmolality indicates the body is inappropriately excreting concentrated urine in the presence of dilute serum.

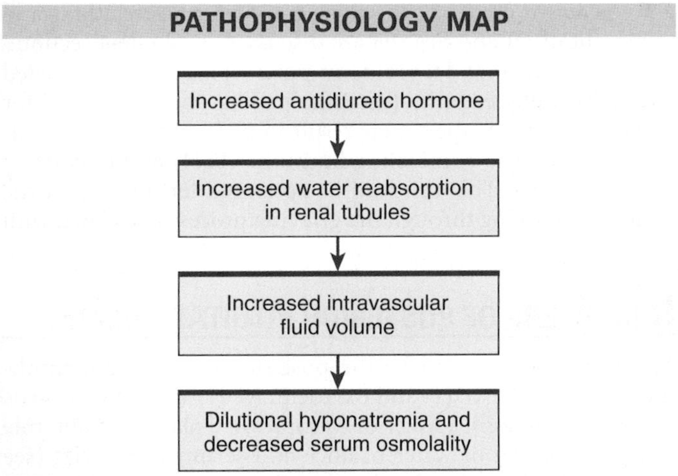


**FIG. 49-3** Pathophysiology of syndrome of inappropriate antidiuretic hormone (SIADH). (Modified from Urden LD, Stacy KM, Lough ME: *Critical care nursing: diagnosis and management,* ed 6, St Louis, 2010, Mosby.)

## ❖ NURSING AND INTERPROFESSIONAL MANAGEMENT: SIADH

In your assessment of persons at risk and those who have confirmed SIADH, be alert for low urine output with a high specific gravity, a sudden weight gain without edema, or a decreased serum sodium level. Monitor intake and output, vital signs, and heart and lung sounds. Obtain daily weights. Observe for signs of hyponatremia, including seizures, headache, vomiting, and decreased neurologic function.

Once SIADH is diagnosed, treatment is directed at the underlying cause. Medications that stimulate ADH release should be avoided or discontinued (Table 49-2). If symptoms are mild and serum sodium is greater than 125 mEq/L (125 mmol/L), the only treatment may be a fluid restriction of 800 to 1000 mL/day. This restriction should result in weight reduction and a gradual rise in serum sodium concentration and osmolality. An improvement in symptoms should accompany normalization of serum sodium and osmolality. Provide the patient with frequent oral care and distractions to decrease discomfort related to thirst from the fluid restriction.

A loop diuretic such as furosemide (Lasix) may be used to promote diuresis. The serum sodium must be at least 125 mEq/L (125 mmol/L) because it may promote further sodium loss. Because furosemide increases potassium, calcium, and magnesium losses, supplements may be needed. Demeclocycline may also be given. This drug blocks the effect of ADH on the renal tubules, resulting in more dilute urine.

Initiate seizure and fall precautions if the patient has an altered sensorium or is having seizures. Position the head of the bed flat or elevated no more than 10 degrees to enhance venous return to the heart and increase left atrial filling pressure, thereby reducing the release of ADH. Frequent turning, positioning, and range-of-motion exercises are important to maintain skin integrity and joint mobility.

**TABLE 49-2 Causes of SIADH**

**Malignant Tumors**
- Small cell lung cancer
- Pancreatic cancer
- Lymphoid cancers (Hodgkin's lymphoma, non-Hodgkin's lymphoma, lymphocytic leukemia)
- Thymus cancer
- Prostate cancer
- Colorectal cancer

**Central Nervous System Disorders**
- Head injury (skull fracture, subdural hematoma, subarachnoid hemorrhage)
- Stroke
- Brain tumors
- Infection (encephalitis, meningitis)
- Cerebral atrophy
- Guillain-Barré syndrome
- Systemic lupus erythematosus

**Drug Therapy**
- carbamazepine (Tegretol)
- chlorpropamide
- General anesthesia agents
- Opioids
- oxytocin
- Thiazide diuretics
- Selective serotonin reuptake inhibitor (SSRI) antidepressants
- Tricyclic antidepressants
- Chemotherapy drugs (vincristine, vinblastine, cyclophosphamide)

**Miscellaneous Conditions**
- Hypothyroidism
- Lung infection (pneumonia, tuberculosis, lung abscess)
- Chronic obstructive pulmonary disease
- Positive pressure mechanical ventilation
- HIV
- Adrenal insufficiency

*SIADH,* Syndrome of inappropriate antidiuretic hormone.

In cases of severe hyponatremia (less than 120 mEq/L), especially in the presence of neurologic manifestations such as seizures, small amounts of IV hypertonic saline solution (3% sodium chloride) may be slowly given. It is important to correct hyponatremia slowly. The level should not increase by more than 8 to 12 mEq/L in the first 24 hours. Quickly increasing levels can cause osmotic demyelination syndrome with permanent damage to nerve cells in the brain.[9] A fluid restriction of 500 mL/day may be indicated for those with severe hyponatremia.

Vasopressor receptor antagonists (drugs that block the activity of ADH) are used to treat euvolemic hyponatremia in hospitalized patients. Two drugs are FDA-approved: conivaptan (Vapriosol) and tolvaptan (Samsca). Conivaptan is given IV; tolvaptan is given orally. Neither should be given to patients with liver disease because they worsen liver function.

Assist the patient with chronic SIADH in self-managing the treatment regimen. In chronic SIADH, a fluid restriction of 800 to 1000 mL/day is recommended. The use of ice chips or sugarless chewing gum helps to decrease thirst. Have the patient weigh daily to monitor changes in fluid balance. Have the patient supplement the diet with sodium and potassium, especially if loop diuretics are prescribed. Teach the patient the symptoms of fluid and electrolyte imbalances, especially those involving sodium and potassium (see Chapter 16).

## DIABETES INSIPIDUS

### Etiology and Pathophysiology

**Diabetes insipidus (DI)** is caused by a deficiency of production or secretion of ADH or a decreased renal response to ADH. The decrease in ADH results in fluid and electrolyte imbalances caused by increased urine output and increased plasma osmolality (Fig. 49-4). Depending on the cause, DI may be transient or a chronic, lifelong condition.

There are several types of DI (Table 49-3). Central DI is the most common form.

### Clinical Manifestations

DI is characterized by polydipsia and polyuria. The primary characteristic of DI is the excretion of large quantities of urine (2 to 20 L/day) with a very low specific gravity (less than 1.005) and urine osmolality of less than 100 mOsm/kg (100 mmol/kg). Serum osmolality is elevated (usually greater than 295 mOsm/kg [295 mmol/kg]) because of hypernatremia (serum sodium greater than 145 mg/dL) caused by pure water loss in the kidneys. Most patients compensate for fluid loss by drinking large amounts of water so that serum osmolality remains normal or is moderately elevated. The patient may be tired from nocturia and experience generalized weakness. Uncorrected hypernatremia can cause brain shrinkage and intracranial bleeding.[9]

The onset of central DI is usually acute and accompanied by excessive fluid loss. After intracranial surgery, central DI has a triphasic pattern: the acute phase with an abrupt onset of polyuria, an interphase in which urine volume normalizes, and a third phase in which central DI may become permanent. The third phase occurs within 10 to 14 days postoperatively. Central DI that results from head trauma is often self-limiting and improves with treatment of the underlying problem. Although the clinical manifestations of nephrogenic DI are similar to those of central DI, the onset and amount of fluid loss are less dramatic.

Severe dehydration can result if oral fluid intake cannot keep up with urinary losses. The patient will have hypotension, tachycardia, and hypovolemic shock. Increasing serum osmolality and hypernatremia can cause central nervous system (CNS) manifestations, ranging from irritability and mental dullness to coma.

### Diagnostic Studies

Patients with DI excrete dilute urine at a rate greater than 200 mL/hr with a specific gravity of less than 1.005. Identification of central DI requires a water deprivation test. Before the test, body weight, and urine osmolality, volume, and specific gravity are measured. The patient is deprived of water for 8 to 12 hours and then given desmopressin acetate (DDAVP) subcutaneously or nasally. Patients with central DI exhibit a dramatic increase in urine osmolality (from 100 to 600 mOsm/kg) and a significant decrease in urine volume. The patient with nephrogenic DI will not be able to increase urine osmolality to greater than 300 mOsm/kg.

Another test to differentiate central DI from nephrogenic DI is to measure the level of ADH after an analog of ADH (e.g., desmopressin) is given. If the cause is central DI, the kidneys will respond to the hormone by concentrating urine. If the kidneys do not respond in this way, then the cause is nephrogenic.

PATHOPHYSIOLOGY MAP

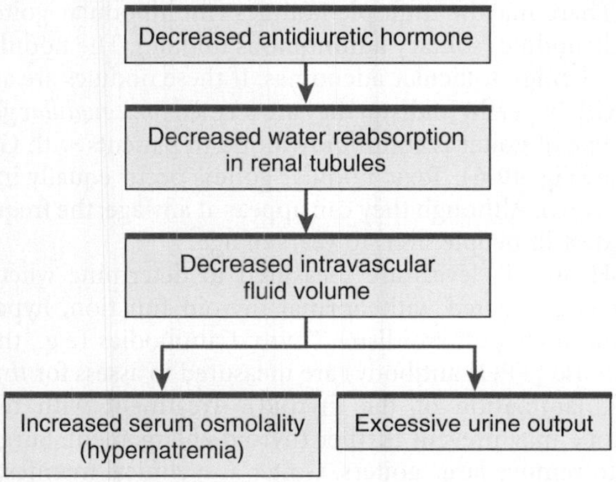


**FIG. 49-4** Pathophysiology of diabetes insipidus (DI).

**TABLE 49-3 Types of Diabetes Insipidus**

| Type | Etiology |
|---|---|
| **Central (neurogenic) DI** | Results from an interference with ADH synthesis, transport, or release<br>*Examples:* Brain tumor, head injury, brain surgery, CNS infections |
| **Nephrogenic DI** | Results from inadequate renal response to ADH despite presence of adequate ADH<br>*Examples:* Drug therapy (especially lithium), renal damage, hereditary renal disease |
| **Primary DI** | Results from excessive water intake<br>*Examples:* Structural lesion in thirst center, psychologic disorder |

## ❖ NURSING AND INTERPROFESSIONAL MANAGEMENT: DIABETES INSIPIDUS

Nursing management of the patient with DI includes early detection, maintaining adequate hydration, and patient teaching for long-term management. A therapeutic goal is maintaining fluid and electrolyte balance.

For central DI, fluid and hormone therapy is the cornerstone of treatment. Fluids are replaced orally or IV, depending on the patient's condition and ability to drink copious amounts of fluids. In acute DI, IV hypotonic saline or dextrose 5% in water ($D_5W$) is given and titrated to replace urine output. If IV glucose solutions are used, monitor serum glucose levels because hyperglycemia and glycosuria can lead to osmotic diuresis, which increases the fluid volume deficit. Monitoring BP, heart rate, urine output, level of consciousness, and specific gravity is essential and may be required hourly in the acutely ill patient. Assess for signs of acute dehydration. Maintain an accurate record of intake and output and daily weights to determine fluid volume status. Adjustments in fluid replacement should be made accordingly.

DDAVP, an analog of ADH, is the hormone replacement of choice for central DI. Another ADH replacement drug is aqueous vasopressin. DDAVP can be given orally, IV, subcutaneously, or as a nasal spray. Assess the response to DDAVP by monitoring pulse, BP, level of consciousness, intake and output, and specific gravity. Chlorpropamide and carbamazepine (Tegretol) are used to help decrease thirst associated with central DI.

Because the kidney is unable to respond to ADH in nephrogenic DI, hormone therapy has little effect. Instead, the treatment includes dietary measures (low-sodium diet) and thiazide diuretics (e.g., hydrochlorothiazide, chlorothiazide [Diuril]), which may reduce flow to the ADH-sensitive distal nephrons. Limiting sodium intake to no more than 3 g/day often helps decrease urine output. If a low-sodium diet and thiazide drugs are not effective, indomethacin (Indocin) may be prescribed. Indomethacin, a nonsteroidal antiinflammatory drug (NSAID), helps increase renal responsiveness to ADH.

## DISORDERS OF THYROID GLAND

Alterations in thyroid function are among the most common endocrine disorders. The thyroid hormones, thyroxine ($T_4$) and triiodothyronine ($T_3$), regulate energy metabolism and growth and development. Disorders of the thyroid gland include goiter, benign and malignant nodules, inflammatory conditions leading to hyperthyroidism, and hypothyroidism (Fig. 49-5).

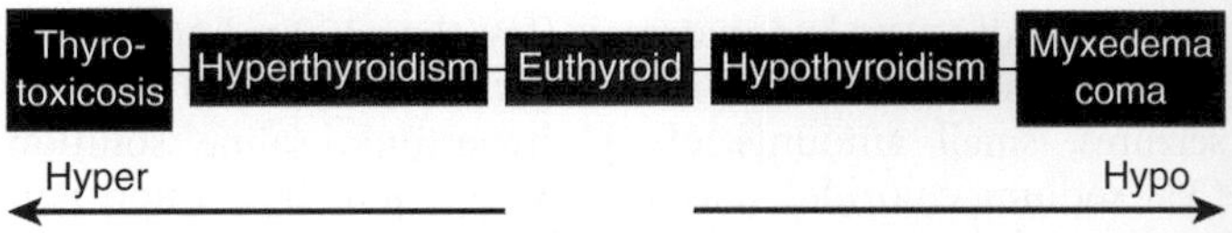


**FIG. 49-5** Continuum of thyroid dysfunction.

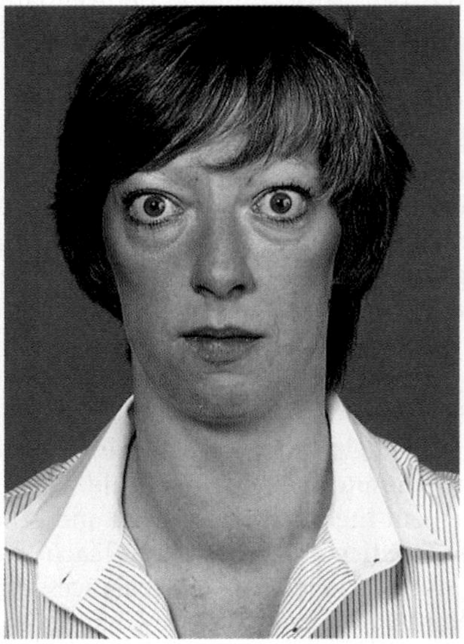

**FIG. 49-6** Exophthalmos and goiter of Graves' disease. (From Forbes CD, Jackson WF: *Colour atlas and text of clinical medicine,* ed 3, London, 2003, Mosby.)

**TABLE 49-4 Goitrogens**

| Thyroid Inhibitors | Select Foods |
|---|---|
| • propylthiouracil (PTU) | • Broccoli |
| • methimazole (Tapazole) | • Brussels sprouts |
| • Iodine in large doses | • Cabbage |
| | • Cauliflower |
| **Other Drugs** | • Kale |
| • Sulfonamides | • Mustard |
| • Salicylates | • Peanuts |
| • *p*-Aminosalicylic acid | • Strawberries |
| • lithium | • Turnips |
| • amiodarone (Cordarone) | |

## GOITER

A **goiter** is an enlarged thyroid gland. In a person with a goiter, the thyroid cells are stimulated to grow. This may result in an overactive thyroid (hyperthyroidism) or an underactive thyroid (hypothyroidism). The most common cause of goiter worldwide is a lack of iodine in the diet.[10] In the United States, where most people use iodized salt, goiter is more often due to the overproduction or underproduction of thyroid hormones or to nodules that develop in the gland itself. *Goitrogens* (foods or drugs that contain thyroid-inhibiting substances) can cause a goiter (Table 49-4).

A nontoxic goiter is a diffuse enlargement of the thyroid gland that does not result from a malignancy or inflammatory process. Normal levels of thyroid hormone are associated with this type of goiter. *Nodular goiters* are thyroid hormone–secreting nodules that function independent of TSH stimulation. There may be multiple nodules (multinodular goiter) or a single nodule (solitary autonomous nodule). The nodules are usually benign follicular adenomas. If these nodules are associated with hyperthyroidism, they are termed *toxic nodular goiters.* This type of goiter is commonly found in patients with Graves' disease (Fig. 49-6). Toxic nodular goiters occur equally in men and women. Although they can appear at any age, the frequency is greatest in people over 40 years of age.

TSH and $T_4$ levels are measured to determine whether a goiter is associated with normal thyroid function, hyperthyroidism, or hypothyroidism. Thyroid antibodies (e.g., thyroid peroxidase [TPO] antibody) are measured to assess for *thyroiditis* (inflammation of the thyroid). Treatment with thyroid hormone may prevent further thyroid enlargement. Surgery is used to remove large goiters. Goiter as a clinical manifestation of thyroid disorders is further discussed in the following sections.

## THYROIDITIS

**Thyroiditis**, an inflammation of the thyroid gland, encompasses several clinical disorders.[11] It is a frequent cause of goiter. *Subacute granulomatous thyroiditis* is thought to be caused by a viral infection. *Acute thyroiditis* is due to bacterial or fungal infection. Subacute and acute forms of thyroiditis have an abrupt onset. The patient complains of pain localized in the thyroid or radiating to the throat, ears, or jaw. Other systemic manifestations include fever, chills, sweats, and fatigue.

*Hashimoto's thyroiditis (chronic autoimmune thyroiditis)* is caused by the destruction of thyroid tissue by antibodies.[11] It is the most common cause of hypothyroid goiters in the United States. Factors placing a person at higher risk include female gender, a positive family history, older age, and white ethnicity. The goiter, which is the hallmark of Hashimoto's thyroiditis, may develop gradually or rapidly. If it enlarges rapidly, it may compress structures in the neck (e.g., trachea, laryngeal nerves), changing the voice and affecting breathing. As thyroid tissue is destroyed by antibodies, there may be a transient phase of hyperthyroidism due to leaking thyroid hormone from the damaged tissues.

*Silent, painless thyroiditis,* which may be early Hashimoto's thyroiditis, can occur in postpartum women. This condition, which is usually seen in the first 6 months after delivery, may be due to an autoimmune reaction to fetal cells in the mother's thyroid gland.

$T_4$ and $T_3$ levels are initially elevated in subacute, acute, and silent thyroiditis but become depressed with time. Suppression of radioactive iodine uptake (RAIU) is seen in subacute and silent thyroiditis. In Hashimoto's thyroiditis, thyroid hormone levels are usually low and the TSH level is high. Antithyroid antibodies are present in Hashimoto's thyroiditis.

Recovery from acute or subacute thyroiditis may be complete in weeks or months without any treatment. If the thyroiditis is bacterial in origin, treatment may include specific antibiotics or surgical drainage. In the subacute and acute forms, NSAIDs (aspirin or naproxen [Aleve]) are used to relieve symptoms. With more severe pain, corticosteroids (e.g., prednisone up to 40 mg/day) can relieve discomfort. Propranolol (Inderal) or atenolol (Tenormin) may be used to treat the cardiovascular symptoms related to a hyperthyroid condition. Thyroid hormone therapy is indicated if the patient is hypothyroid.

Nursing care of the patient with thyroiditis includes patient teaching regarding the disease process and course of treatment. Teach the patient not to discontinue medications abruptly. Instruct the patient to remain under close health care supervision so that progress can be monitored. Tell the patient to report to the HCP any change in symptoms, such as difficulty breathing or swallowing, swelling to face and extremities, or rapid weight gain or loss. Teach those receiving thyroid hormone about the expected side effects of these drugs and measures to manage them (see p. 1170).

The patient with Hashimoto's thyroiditis is at risk for other autoimmune diseases such as Addison's disease, pernicious anemia, or Graves' disease. Teach the patient the signs and symptoms of these disorders, particularly Addison's disease.

## HYPERTHYROIDISM

**Hyperthyroidism** is hyperactivity of the thyroid gland with sustained increase in synthesis and release of thyroid hormones. Hyperthyroidism occurs in women more than men, with the highest frequency in persons 20 to 40 years old. The most common form of hyperthyroidism is Graves' disease. Other causes include toxic nodular goiter, thyroiditis, excess iodine intake, pituitary tumors, and thyroid cancer. Since hyperthyroidism may be precipitated by iodinated contrast media used in CT scans and other radiological studies, those who are at-risk for hyperthyroidism should be monitored closely after iodinated contrast media exposure.[12]

### GENDER DIFFERENCES
#### *Endocrine Problems*

**Men**

- Ectopic ACTH production is more common in men.

**Women**

- Hyperthyroidism and hypothyroidism are more common in women than men.
- Graves' disease affects five times more women than men.
- Thyroid nodules and thyroid cancer affect up to four times as many women as men.
- Hyperparathyroidism affects twice as many women as men.
- Cushing disease and primary hyperaldosteronism are more common in women than men.

The term **thyrotoxicosis** refers to the physiologic effects or clinical syndrome of hypermetabolism resulting from excess circulating levels of $T_4$, $T_3$, or both.[13] Hyperthyroidism and thyrotoxicosis usually occur together. Subclinical hyperthyroidism occurs when the patient has a serum TSH level below 0.4 mU/L but normal $T_4$ and $T_3$ levels. Overt hyperthyroidism is defined by low or undetectable TSH and elevated $T_4$ and $T_3$ levels. The patient may or may not have symptoms of hyperthyroidism.

### Etiology and Pathophysiology

**Graves' Disease.** **Graves' disease** is an autoimmune disease of unknown etiology characterized by diffuse thyroid enlargement and excess thyroid hormone secretion. Graves' disease accounts for 75% of the cases of hyperthyroidism. Women are five times more likely than men to develop Graves' disease. Precipitating factors such as insufficient iodine supply, cigarette smoking, infection, and stressful life events may interact with genetic factors to cause Graves' disease.

In Graves' disease the patient develops antibodies to the TSH receptor. These antibodies attach to the receptors and stimulate the thyroid gland to release $T_3$, $T_4$, or both. The excess release of thyroid hormones leads to the clinical manifestations associated with thyrotoxicosis. The disease is characterized by remissions and exacerbations, with or without treatment. It may progress to destruction of the thyroid tissue, ultimately causing hypothyroidism. Graves' disease is associated with the presence of other autoimmune disorders, including rheumatoid arthritis, pernicious anemia, systemic lupus erythematosus (SLE), Addison's disease, celiac disease, and vitiligo.

### Clinical Manifestations

Clinical manifestations of hyperthyroidism are related to the effect of excess circulating thyroid hormone. It directly increases metabolism and tissue sensitivity to stimulation by the sympathetic nervous system.

Palpation of the thyroid gland may reveal a goiter. When the thyroid gland is excessively large, a goiter may be noted on inspection. Auscultating the thyroid gland may reveal bruits, a reflection of increased blood supply. Another common finding is *ophthalmopathy*, a term used to describe abnormal eye appearance or function. A classic finding in Graves' disease is **exophthalmos**, a protrusion of the eyeballs from the orbits that is usually bilateral (Fig. 49-6). Exophthalmos results from increased fat deposits and fluid (edema) in the orbital tissues and ocular muscles. The increased pressure forces the eyeballs outward. The upper lids are usually retracted and elevated, with the sclera visible above the iris. When the eyelids do not close completely, the exposed corneal surfaces become dry and irritated. Serious consequences, such as corneal ulcers and eventual loss of vision, can occur. The changes in the ocular muscles result in muscle weakness, causing diplopia.

Other manifestations of hyperthyroidism are summarized in Table 49-5. Abnormal laboratory findings are listed in Table 49-6. A patient in the early stages of hyperthyroidism may only exhibit weight loss and increased nervousness. *Acropachy* (clubbing of the digits) may occur with advanced disease (Fig. 49-7). Manifestations (e.g., palpitations, tremors, weight loss) in older adults with hyperthyroidism do not differ significantly from those of younger adults (Table 49-7). In older patients who are confused and agitated, dementia may be suspected and delay the diagnosis.

## Complications

*Acute thyrotoxicosis* (also called *thyrotoxic crisis* or *thyroid storm*) is an acute, severe, and rare condition that occurs when excessive amounts of thyroid hormones are released into the

**TABLE 49-6 Laboratory Results for Hyperthyroid and Hypothyroid Patients**

| | | HYPOTHYROID | |
|---|---|---|---|
| **Test** | **Hyperthyroid** | **Primary** | **Secondary** |
| Thyroid-stimulating hormone (TSH) | ↓ | ↑ | ↓ |
| $T_4$ (thyroxine) | ↑ | ↓ | ↓ |
| Total cholesterol | N | ↑ | ↑ |
| Low-density lipoproteins (LDLs) | ↓ | ↑ | ↑ |
| Triglycerides | N | ↑ | ↑ |
| Creatine kinase (CK) | N | ↑ | ↑ |
| Basal metabolic rate (BMR) | ↑ | ↓ | ↓ |
| Thyroid peroxidase (TPO) antibody | N | + (in autoimmune hypothyroidism) | N |

*N*, Normal; +, positive.

**TABLE 49-5 Manifestations of Thyroid Dysfunction**

| Hyperfunction | Hypofunction |
|---|---|
| **Cardiovascular System** | |
| • Systolic hypertension<br>• Increased rate and force of cardiac contractions<br>• Bounding, rapid pulse<br>• Increased cardiac output<br>• Cardiac hypertrophy<br>• Systolic murmurs<br>• Dysrhythmias<br>• Palpitations<br>• Angina | • Increased capillary fragility<br>• Decreased rate and force of contractions<br>• Varied changes in BP<br>• Cardiac hypertrophy<br>• Distant heart sounds<br>• Anemia<br>• Heart failure<br>• Angina |
| **Respiratory System** | |
| • Dyspnea on mild exertion<br>• Increased respiratory rate | • Dyspnea<br>• Decreased breathing capacity |
| **Gastrointestinal System** | |
| • Increased appetite, thirst<br>• Weight loss<br>• Increased peristalsis<br>• Diarrhea, frequent defecation<br>• Increased bowel sounds<br>• Splenomegaly<br>• Hepatomegaly | • Decreased appetite<br>• Weight gain<br>• Nausea and vomiting<br>• Constipation<br>• Distended abdomen<br>• Enlarged, scaly tongue<br>• Celiac disease |
| **Integumentary System** | |
| • Warm, smooth, moist skin<br>• Thin, brittle nails detached from nail bed (onycholysis)<br>• Hair loss (may be patchy)<br>• Clubbing of fingers (thyroid acropachy) (Fig. 49-7)<br>• Palmar erythema<br>• Fine, silky hair<br>• Premature graying (in men)<br>• Diaphoresis<br>• Vitiligo<br>• Pretibial myxedema (infiltrative dermopathy) | • Dry, thick, inelastic, cold skin<br>• Thick, brittle nails<br>• Dry, sparse, coarse hair<br>• Poor turgor of mucosa<br>• Generalized interstitial edema<br>• Puffy face<br>• Decreased sweating<br>• Pallor |
| **Musculoskeletal System** | |
| • Fatigue<br>• Weakness<br>• Proximal muscle wasting<br>• Dependent edema<br>• Osteoporosis | • Fatigue<br>• Weakness<br>• Muscular aches and pains<br>• Slow movements<br>• Arthralgia |
| **Nervous System** | |
| • Difficulty focusing eyes<br>• Nervousness<br>• Fine tremor of fingers and tongue<br>• Insomnia<br>• Lability of mood, delirium<br>• Restlessness<br>• Personality changes of irritability, agitation<br>• Exhaustion<br>• Hyperactive deep-tendon reflexes<br>• Depression, fatigue<br>• Lack of ability to concentrate<br>• Stupor, coma | • Apathy<br>• Lethargy<br>• Fatigue<br>• Forgetfulness<br>• Slowed mental processes<br>• Hoarseness<br>• Slow, slurred speech<br>• Prolonged relaxation of deep tendon reflexes<br>• Stupor, coma<br>• Paresthesias<br>• Anxiety, depression |
| **Reproductive System** | |
| • Menstrual irregularities<br>• Amenorrhea<br>• Decreased libido<br>• Impotence in men<br>• Gynecomastia in men<br>• Decreased fertility | • Prolonged menstrual periods or amenorrhea<br>• Decreased libido<br>• Infertility |
| **Other** | |
| • Intolerance to heat<br>• Elevated basal temperature<br>• Lid lag, stare<br>• Eyelid retraction<br>• Exophthalmos<br>• Goiter (Fig. 49-6)<br>• Rapid speech | • Intolerance to cold<br>• Increased susceptibility to infection<br>• Increased sensitivity to opioids, barbiturates, anesthesia<br>• Decreased hearing<br>• Goiter<br>• Sleepiness |

circulation. Although considered a life-threatening emergency, death is rare when treatment is initiated early. Acute thyroiditis is thought to result from stressors (e.g., infection, trauma, surgery) in a patient with preexisting hyperthyroidism. Patients having a thyroidectomy are at risk because manipulation of the hyperactive thyroid gland results in an increase in hormones released.[14]

In acute thyrotoxicosis, all the symptoms of hyperthyroidism are prominent and severe. Manifestations include severe tachycardia, heart failure, shock, hyperthermia (up to 106° F [41.1° C]), agitation, delirium, seizures, abdominal pain, vomiting, diarrhea, and coma.

## Diagnostic Studies

The two primary laboratory findings used to confirm the diagnosis of hyperthyroidism are low or undetectable TSH levels (<0.4 mU/L) and elevated free thyroxine (free $T_4$) levels. Total $T_3$ and $T_4$ levels may also be assessed, but they are not as definitive. Total $T_3$ and $T_4$ determine both free and bound (to protein) hormone levels. The free hormone is the only biologically active form of these hormones.

The RAIU test is used to differentiate Graves' disease from other forms of thyroiditis. The patient with Graves' disease shows a diffuse, homogeneous uptake of 35% to 95%, whereas the patient with thyroiditis shows an uptake of less than 2%.

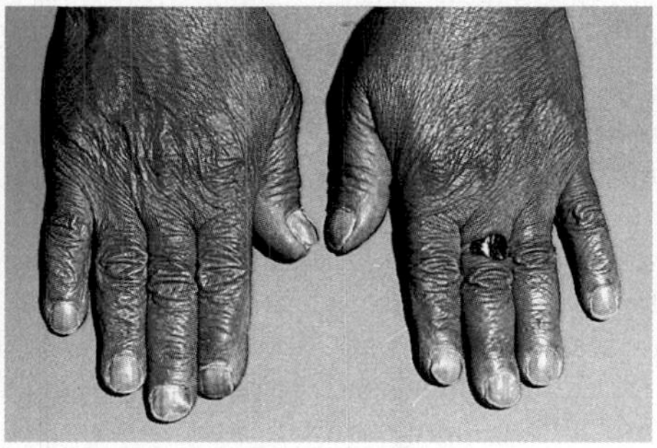

**FIG. 49-7** Thyroid acropachy. Digital clubbing and swelling of fingers. (From Chew SL, Leslie D: *Clinical endocrinology and diabetes: an illustrated colour text,* Edinburgh, 2006, Churchill Livingstone.)

**TABLE 49-7 Comparison of Hyperthyroidism in Younger and Older Adults**

| | Younger Adult | Older Adult |
|---|---|---|
| **Common causes** | Graves' disease in >90% of cases | Graves' disease or toxic nodular goiter |
| **Common symptoms** | Nervousness, irritability, weight loss, heat intolerance, warm moist skin | Anorexia, weight loss, apathy, lassitude, depression, confusion |
| **Goiter** | Present in >90% of cases | Present in about 50% of cases |
| **Ophthalmopathy** | Exophthalmos (Fig. 49-6) present in 20%-40% of cases | Exophthalmos less common |
| **Cardiac features** | Tachycardia and palpitations common, but without heart failure | Angina, dysrhythmia (especially atrial fibrillation with rapid ventricular response), heart failure may occur |

The person with a nodular goiter has an uptake in the high normal range.

## Interprofessional Care

The goal of management of hyperthyroidism is to block the adverse effects of excessive thyroid hormone, suppress oversecretion of thyroid hormone, and prevent complications. There are several treatment options, including antithyroid medications, radioactive iodine therapy, and surgical intervention (Table 49-8). Supportive therapy is directed at managing respiratory distress, reducing fever, replacing fluid, and eliminating or managing the initiating stressor(s).

The choice of treatment is influenced by the patient's age and preferences, coexistence of other diseases, and pregnancy status.

**Drug Therapy.** Drugs used in the treatment of hyperthyroidism include antithyroid drugs, iodine, and β-adrenergic blockers. These drugs are useful in treating thyrotoxic states, but they are not considered curative. Radiation therapy or surgery may ultimately be required.

***Antithyroid Drugs.*** The first-line antithyroid drugs are propylthiouracil and methimazole (Tapazole).[13] These drugs inhibit the synthesis of thyroid hormones. Indications for use include Graves' disease in the young patient, hyperthyroidism during pregnancy, and the need to achieve a euthyroid state before surgery or radiation therapy. Propylthiouracil is generally used for patients who are in the first trimester of pregnancy, had an adverse reaction to methimazole, or require a rapid reduction in symptoms. Propylthiouracil is considered first-line therapy in thyrotoxicosis, since it also blocks the peripheral conversion of $T_4$ to $T_3$. An advantage of propylthiouracil is that it achieves the therapeutic goal of being euthyroid more quickly. However, it must be taken three times per day. Methimazole is given in a single daily dose.

Improvement usually begins 1 to 2 weeks after the start of drug therapy. Good results are usually seen within 4 to 8 weeks. Therapy is usually continued for 6 to 15 months to allow for spontaneous remission, which occurs in 20% to 40% of patients. Emphasize to the patient the importance of adhering to the

**TABLE 49-8 Interprofessional Care**

***Hyperthyroidism***

| Diagnostic Assessment | Management |
|---|---|
| • History and physical examination<br>• Ophthalmologic examination<br>• ECG<br>• Laboratory tests<br>  • TSH levels, serum free $T_4$<br>  • Thyroid antibodies (e.g., thyroid peroxidase [TPO] antibody)<br>  • Total serum $T_3$ and $T_4$<br>• Radioactive iodine uptake (RAIU) | ***Drug Therapy***<br>• Antithyroid drugs<br>  • methimazole (Tapazole)<br>  • propylthiouracil<br>• Iodine (SSKI)<br>• β-Adrenergic receptor blockers<br>  • propranolol (Inderal)<br>  • atenolol (Tenormin) or metoprolol (Toprol)<br>***Radiation Therapy***<br>• Radioactive iodine<br>***Surgical Therapy***<br>• Subtotal thyroidectomy<br>***Nutritional Therapy***<br>• High-calorie, high-protein diet<br>• Frequent meals |

drug regimen. Abruptly discontinuing drug therapy can result in a return of hyperthyroidism.

***Iodine.*** Iodine is available as saturated solution of potassium iodine (SSKI) and Lugol's solution. Iodine is used with other antithyroid drugs to prepare the patient for thyroidectomy or for treatment of thyrotoxicosis. Rapidly giving large doses of iodine inhibits synthesis of $T_3$ and $T_4$ and blocks the release of these hormones into circulation. It also decreases the vascularity of the thyroid gland, making surgery safer and easier. The maximal effect is usually seen within 1 to 2 weeks. Because of a reduction in the therapeutic effect, long-term iodine therapy is not effective in controlling hyperthyroidism.

Iodine is mixed with water or juice, sipped through a straw, and given after meals. Assess the patient for signs of iodine toxicity, such as swelling of the buccal mucosa and other mucous membranes, excessive salivation, nausea and vomiting, and skin reactions. If toxicity occurs, discontinue iodine administration and notify the HCP.

***β-Adrenergic Blockers.*** β-Adrenergic blockers are used for symptomatic relief of thyrotoxicosis. These drugs block the effects of sympathetic nervous stimulation, thereby decreasing tachycardia, nervousness, irritability, and tremors. Propranolol is usually given with antithyroid agents. Atenolol is the preferred β-adrenergic blocker for use in the hyperthyroid patient with asthma or heart disease.

**Radioactive Iodine Therapy.** Radioactive iodine (RAI) therapy is the treatment of choice for most nonpregnant adults. RAI damages or destroys thyroid tissue, thus limiting thyroid hormone secretion. RAI has a delayed response. The maximum effect may not be seen for up to 3 months. For this reason, the patient is usually treated with antithyroid drugs and propranolol before and for 3 months after starting RAI until the effects of radiation become apparent. Although RAI is usually effective, 80% of patients have posttreatment hypothyroidism, resulting in the need for lifelong thyroid hormone therapy. Teach the patient the symptoms of hypothyroidism and to seek medical help if these symptoms occur.

RAI therapy is usually given on an outpatient basis. A pregnancy test is done before starting therapy for all women who experience menstrual cycles. Tell the patient that radiation thyroiditis and parotiditis are possible and may cause dryness and irritation of the mouth and throat. Relief may be obtained with frequent sips of water, ice chips, or a salt and soda gargle three or four times per day. This gargle is made by dissolving 1 tsp of salt and 1 tsp of baking soda in 2 cups of warm water. The discomfort should subside in 3 to 4 days. A mixture of antacid (Mylanta or Maalox), diphenhydramine, and viscous lidocaine can be used to swish and spit, increasing patient comfort when eating.

To limit radiation exposure to others, teach the patient receiving RAI home precautions, including (1) using private toilet facilities if possible and flushing two or three times after each use; (2) separately laundering towels, bed linens, and clothes daily at home; (3) not preparing food for others that requires prolonged handling with bare hands; and (4) avoiding being close to pregnant women and children for 7 days after therapy.

**Surgical Therapy.** Thyroidectomy is indicated for those who have (1) a large goiter causing tracheal compression, (2) a lack of response to antithyroid therapy, or (3) thyroid cancer (Fig. 49-8). Additionally, surgery may be done when a person is not a candidate for RAI. One advantage that thyroidectomy has over RAI is a more rapid reduction in $T_3$ and $T_4$ levels. A *subtotal thyroidectomy* is the preferred surgical procedure, which involves removing a significant portion (90%) of the thyroid gland.

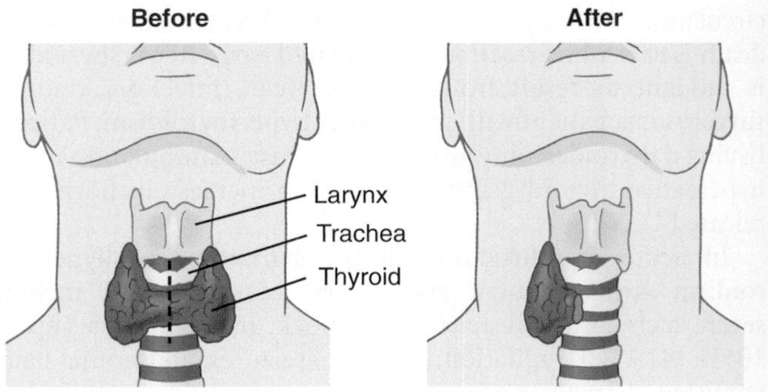


**FIG. 49-8** Subtotal thyroidectomy. Part of the thyroid gland is removed.

Some patients may undergo minimally invasive endoscopic or robotic thyroidectomy. Endoscopic thyroidectomy is an appropriate procedure for patients with small nodules (less than 3 cm) and no evidence of cancer. Robotic surgery is best for those who are not overweight and have small nodules on only one side of the gland. Advantages of endoscopic and robotic procedures over open thyroidectomy include less scarring, less pain, and a faster return to normal activity.

**Nutritional Therapy.** With the increased metabolic rate in hyperthyroid patients, there is a high potential for the patient to have a nutritional deficit. A high-calorie diet (4000 to 5000 cal/day) may be needed to satisfy hunger, prevent tissue breakdown, and decrease weight loss. This can be accomplished with six full meals a day and snacks high in protein, carbohydrates, minerals, and vitamins. The protein content should be 1 to 2 g/kg of ideal body weight. Increase carbohydrate intake to compensate for increased metabolism. Carbohydrates provide energy and decrease the use of body-stored protein. Teach the patient to avoid highly seasoned and high-fiber foods because these foods can further stimulate the already hyperactive GI tract. Have the patient avoid caffeine-containing liquids such as coffee, tea, and cola to decrease the restlessness and sleep disturbances associated with these fluids. Refer the patient to a dietitian for help in meeting individual nutritional needs.

## NURSING MANAGEMENT: HYPERTHYROIDISM

### Nursing Assessment

Subjective and objective data you should obtain from a person with hyperthyroidism are presented in Table 49-9.

### Nursing Diagnoses

Nursing diagnoses for the patient with hyperthyroidism include, but are not limited to, the following:

- Activity intolerance *related to* fatigue and heat intolerance
- Imbalanced nutrition: less than body requirements *related to* hypermetabolism and inadequate food intake

Additional information on nursing diagnoses is presented in eNursing Care Plan 49-1 for the patient with hyperthyroidism (available on the website for this chapter).

### Planning

The overall goals are that the patient with hyperthyroidism will (1) experience relief of symptoms, (2) have no serious complications related to the disease or treatment, (3) maintain nutritional balance, and (4) cooperate with the therapeutic plan.

## Nursing Implementation

**Acute Care.** Patients with hyperthyroidism are usually treated in an outpatient setting. However, those who develop acute thyrotoxicosis or undergo thyroidectomy require hospitalization and acute care.

**TABLE 49-9 Nursing Assessment**

***Hyperthyroidism***

**Subjective Data**

***Important Health Information***

*Past health history:* Preexisting goiter. Recent infection or trauma, immigration from iodine-deficient area, autoimmune disease

*Medications:* Thyroid hormones, herbal therapies that may contain thyroid hormone

***Functional Health Patterns***

*Health perception–health management:* Positive family history of thyroid or autoimmune disorders

*Nutritional-metabolic:* Iodine intake, weight loss, increased appetite, thirst, nausea, vomiting

*Elimination:* Diarrhea, polyuria, sweating

*Activity-exercise:* Dyspnea on exertion, palpitations, muscle weakness, fatigue

*Sleep-rest:* Insomnia

*Cognitive-perceptual:* Chest pain, nervousness, heat intolerance, pruritus

*Sexuality-reproductive:* Decreased libido, impotence, gynecomastia (in men), amenorrhea (in women)

*Coping–stress tolerance:* Emotional lability, irritability, restlessness, personality changes, delirium

**Objective Data**

***General Observation***

Agitation, rapid speech and body movements, anxiety, restlessness, hyperthermia, enlarged or nodular thyroid gland

***Eyes***

Exophthalmos, eyelid retraction, infrequent blinking

***Integumentary***

Warm, diaphoretic, velvety skin. Thin, loose nails. Fine, silky hair and hair loss. Palmar erythema, clubbing, white pigmentation of skin (vitiligo), diffuse edema of legs and feet

***Respiratory***

Tachypnea, dyspnea on exertion

***Cardiovascular***

Tachycardia, bounding pulse, systolic murmurs, dysrhythmias, hypertension, bruit over the thyroid gland

***Gastrointestinal***

Increased bowel sounds. Increased appetite, diarrhea, weight loss, hepatosplenomegaly

***Neurologic***

Hyperreflexia; diplopia. Fine tremors of hands, tongue, eyelids

***Musculoskeletal***

Muscle wasting

***Reproductive***

Menstrual irregularities, infertility, impotence, gynecomastia in men

***Possible Diagnostic Findings***

↑ $T_3$, ↑ $T_4$, ↑ $T_3$ resin uptake, ↓ or undetectable TSH. Chest x-ray showing enlarged heart. ECG findings of tachycardia, atrial fibrillation.

***Acute Thyrotoxicosis.*** Acute thyrotoxicosis is a systemic syndrome that requires aggressive treatment, often in an intensive care unit. Administer medications (previously discussed) that block thyroid hormone production and the sympathetic nervous system. Provide supportive therapy, including monitoring for cardiac dysrhythmias and decompensation, ensuring adequate oxygenation, and giving IV fluids to replace fluid and electrolyte losses. This is especially important in the patient who experiences fluid losses due to vomiting and diarrhea.

Ensuring adequate rest may be a challenge because of the patient's irritability and restlessness. Provide a calm, quiet room because increased metabolism and sensitivity of the sympathetic nervous system causes sleep disturbances. Other interventions may include (1) placing the patient in a cool room away from very ill patients and noisy, high-traffic areas; (2) using light bed coverings and changing the linen frequently if the patient is diaphoretic; and (3) encouraging and assisting with exercise involving large muscle groups (tremors can interfere with small-muscle coordination) to allow the release of nervous tension and restlessness. It is important to establish a supportive, trusting relationship to facilitate coping by a patient who is irritable, restless, and anxious.

If exophthalmos is present, there is a potential for corneal injury related to irritation and dryness. The patient may have orbital pain. To relieve eye discomfort and prevent corneal ulceration, apply artificial tears to soothe and moisten conjunctival membranes. Salt restriction may help reduce periorbital edema. Elevate the patient's head to promote fluid drainage from the periorbital area. The patient should sit upright as much as possible.

Dark glasses reduce glare and prevent irritation from smoke, air currents, dust, and dirt. If the eyelids cannot be closed, lightly tape them shut for sleep. To maintain flexibility, teach the patient to exercise the intraocular muscles several times a day by turning the eyes in the complete range of motion. Good grooming can help reduce the loss of self-esteem from an altered body image. If the exophthalmos is severe, treatment options include corticosteroids, radiation of retroorbital tissues, orbital decompression, or corrective lid or muscle surgery.

***Thyroid Surgery.*** When a subtotal thyroidectomy is the treatment of choice, the patient must be adequately prepared to avoid postoperative complications. Before surgery, antithyroid drugs, iodine, and β-adrenergic blockers may be given to achieve a euthyroid state. Iodine also reduces the vascularization of the thyroid gland, reducing the risk of hemorrhage.

Preoperatively, teach the patient about routine postoperative care and comfort and safety measures. Teach the patient the importance of performing leg exercises. Instruct the patient how to support the head manually while turning in bed, since this maneuver minimizes stress on the suture line after surgery. The patient should practice range-of-motion exercises of the neck. Tell the patient that talking is likely to be difficult for a short time after surgery.

***Postoperative Care.*** Postoperative complications include hypothyroidism, damage to or inadvertent removal of parathyroid glands, causing hypoparathyroidism and hypocalcemia, hemorrhage, injury to the recurrent or superior laryngeal nerve, thyrotoxicosis, and infection.[15] Recurrent laryngeal nerve damage leads to vocal cord paralysis. If both cords are paralyzed, spastic airway obstruction will occur, requiring an immediate tracheostomy.

**SAFETY ALERT Airway Obstruction**
- Although not common, airway obstruction after thyroid surgery is an emergency situation.
- $O_2$, suction equipment, and a tracheostomy tray should be readily available in the patient's room.

Respiration may become difficult because of excess swelling of the neck tissues, hemorrhage, and hematoma formation. *Laryngeal stridor* (harsh, vibratory sound) may occur during inspiration and expiration because of edema of the laryngeal nerve. Laryngeal stridor may also be related to tetany from hypocalcemia, which occurs if the parathyroid glands were removed or damaged during surgery. To treat tetany, IV calcium salts (e.g., calcium gluconate) should be available.

Important nursing interventions after a thyroidectomy include the following:
- Assess the patient every 2 hours for 24 hours for signs of hemorrhage or tracheal compression, such as irregular breathing, neck swelling, frequent swallowing, choking, blood on the dressings, and sensations of fullness at the incision site. Expect some hoarseness for 3 or 4 days after surgery because of edema.
- Place the patient in a semi-Fowler's position and support the patient's head with pillows. Avoid flexion of the neck and any tension on the suture lines.
- Monitor vital signs and calcium levels. Assess for signs of tetany secondary to hypoparathyroidism (e.g., tingling in toes, fingers, around the mouth; muscular twitching; apprehension) and any difficulty in speaking and hoarseness. Monitor Trousseau's sign and Chvostek's sign (see Fig. 16-15).
- Control postoperative pain by giving medication.

If postoperative recovery is uneventful, the patient ambulates within hours after surgery and is permitted fluids as soon as tolerated. A soft diet starts the day after surgery.

The appearance of the incision may be distressing to the patient. Reassure the patient that the scar will fade in color and eventually look like a normal neck wrinkle. A scarf, jewelry, a high collar, or other covering can effectively camouflage the scar.

◆ **Ambulatory Care.** The patient and caregiver must be aware that thyroid hormone balance should be monitored periodically. Most patients experience a period of relative hypothyroidism soon after surgery because of the substantial reduction in the size of the thyroid. However, the remaining tissue usually hypertrophies over time and recovers the capacity to produce hormones. The administration of thyroid hormone is avoided because the exogenous hormone inhibits pituitary production of TSH and delays or prevents the restoration of normal gland function and tissue regeneration.

To prevent weight gain, caloric intake must be substantially reduced below the amount that was required before surgery. Adequate iodine is necessary to promote thyroid function, but excesses can inhibit the thyroid gland. Seafood once or twice a week or normal use of iodized salt should provide sufficient iodine intake. Encourage regular exercise to stimulate the thyroid gland. Teach the patient to avoid high environmental temperatures because they inhibit thyroid regeneration.

Regular follow-up care is necessary. The patient should see the HCP biweekly for a month and then at least semiannually to assess thyroid function. Tell the patient who had a complete thyroidectomy about the need for lifelong thyroid hormone replacement. Teach the patient the signs and symptoms of thyroid failure and to seek medical care promptly if these develop.

### ◆ Evaluation

The expected outcomes are that the patient with hyperthyroidism will
- Experience relief of symptoms
- Have no serious complications related to the disease or treatment
- Cooperate with the therapeutic plan
- Maintain nutritional balance

Additional information on expected outcomes is presented in eNursing Care Plan 49-1 for the patient with hyperthyroidism (available on the website for this chapter).

## HYPOTHYROIDISM

**Hypothyroidism** is a deficiency of thyroid hormone that causes a general slowing of the metabolic rate. About 4% of the U.S. population has mild hypothyroidism, with about 0.3% having more severe disease. Hypothyroidism is more common in women than men. Subclinical hypothyroidism occurs when the TSH is greater than 4.5 mU/L, but the thyroxine ($T_4$) levels are normal. Up to 10% of women older than 60 years have subclinical hypothyroidism.[16] Patients with overt hypothyroidism have elevated TSH and decreased thyroxine levels. Critically ill patients may present with nonthyroidal illness syndrome (NTIS).[17] Those with NTIS have low $T_3$, $T_4$, and TSH levels.

### Etiology and Pathophysiology

Hypothyroidism can be classified as primary or secondary. *Primary hypothyroidism* is caused by destruction of thyroid tissue or defective hormone synthesis. *Secondary hypothyroidism* is caused by pituitary disease with decreased TSH secretion or hypothalamic dysfunction with decreased thyrotropin-releasing hormone (TRH) secretion. Hypothyroidism can be transient and related to thyroiditis or discontinuing thyroid hormone therapy.

Iodine deficiency is the most common cause of hypothyroidism worldwide. In the United States, the most common cause of primary hypothyroidism is atrophy of the thyroid gland. This atrophy is the end result of Hashimoto's thyroiditis or Graves' disease. These autoimmune diseases destroy the thyroid gland. Hypothyroidism may also develop after treatment for hyperthyroidism, specifically thyroidectomy or RAI therapy. Drugs such as amiodarone (Cordarone), which contains iodine, and lithium, which blocks hormone production, can cause hypothyroidism.

Hypothyroidism that develops in infancy *(cretinism)* is caused by thyroid hormone deficiencies during fetal or early neonatal life. All infants in the United States are screened for decreased thyroid function at birth.

### Clinical Manifestations

Regardless of the cause, hypothyroidism has common features. It has systemic effects characterized by a slowing of body processes. Manifestations vary, depending on the severity and the duration of thyroid deficiency as well as the patient's age at the onset of the deficiency. Symptoms may develop over months to years, unless hypothyroidism occurs after a thyroidectomy, after thyroid ablation, or during treatment with antithyroid drugs.

The patient is often fatigued, lethargic, and experiences personality and mental changes, including impaired memory, slowed speech, decreased initiative, and somnolence. Many appear depressed. Weight gain is most likely a result of a decreased metabolic rate.

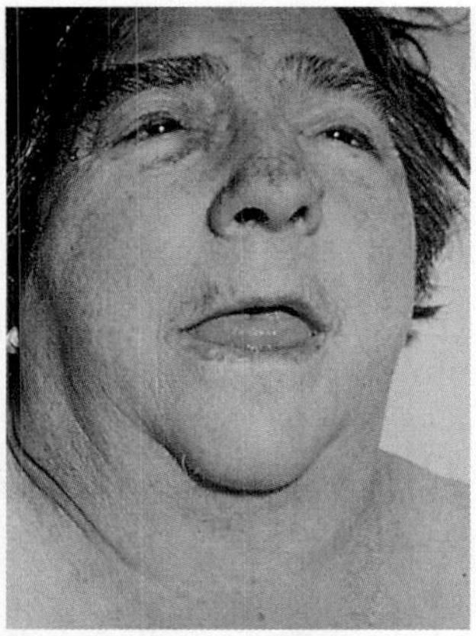

**FIG. 49-9** Common features of myxedema. Dull, puffy skin; coarse, sparse hair; periorbital edema; and prominent tongue. (Courtesy Paul W. Ladenson, MD, The Johns Hopkins University and Hospital, Baltimore, Md. From Seidel HM, Ball JW, Dains JE, et al, editors: *Mosby's guide to physical examination,* ed 6, St Louis, 2006, Mosby.)

Hypothyroidism may cause significant cardiovascular problems, especially in a person with previous cardiovascular disorders. It is associated with decreased cardiac contractility and decreased cardiac output. Thus the patient may experience low exercise tolerance and shortness of breath on exertion. Increased serum cholesterol and triglyceride levels and the accumulation of mucopolysaccharides in the intima of small blood vessels can result in coronary atherosclerosis. Anemia is common.

Patients with severe, long-standing hypothyroidism may display **myxedema**, which alters the physical appearance of the skin and subcutaneous tissues with puffiness, facial and periorbital edema, and a masklike affect. Myxedema occurs due to the accumulation of hydrophilic mucopolysaccharides in the dermis and other tissues (Fig. 49-9). People with hypothyroidism may describe an altered self-image related to their disabilities and altered appearance. Other manifestations of hypothyroidism are summarized in Table 49-5.

In the older adult, the typical manifestations of hypothyroidism (fatigue, cold and dry skin, hoarseness, hair loss, constipation, and cold intolerance) may be attributed to normal aging. For this reason, the patient's symptoms may not raise suspicion of an underlying condition. Older adults who have confusion, lethargy, and depression should be evaluated for thyroid disease.

## Complications

The mental sluggishness, drowsiness, and lethargy of hypothyroidism may progress gradually or suddenly to a notable impairment of consciousness or coma. This situation, termed *myxedema coma,* is a medical emergency. Myxedema coma can be precipitated by infection, drugs (especially opioids, tranquilizers, and barbiturates), exposure to cold, and trauma. It is characterized by subnormal temperature, hypotension, and hypoventilation. Cardiovascular collapse can result from hypoventilation, hyponatremia, hypoglycemia, and lactic acidosis. For the patient to survive myxedema coma, vital functions must be supported and IV thyroid hormone replacement administered.

## Diagnostic Studies

The most reliable laboratory tests for thyroid function are TSH and free $T_4$. These values, correlated with symptoms obtained from the history and physical examination, confirm the diagnosis of hypothyroidism. Serum TSH levels help determine the cause of hypothyroidism. Serum TSH is high when the defect is in the thyroid and low when it is in the pituitary or the hypothalamus. The presence of thyroid antibodies suggests an autoimmune origin. Other abnormal laboratory findings are elevated cholesterol and triglycerides, anemia, and increased creatine kinase (Table 49-6).

**TABLE 49-10 Interprofessional Care**
***Hypothyroidism***

| Diagnostic Assessment | Management |
|---|---|
| • History and physical examination<br>• Serum TSH and free $T_4$<br>• Total serum $T_3$ and $T_4$<br>• Thyroid peroxidase (TPO) antibodies | • Thyroid hormone replacement (e.g., levothyroxine)<br>• Monitor thyroid hormone levels and adjust dosage (if needed)<br>• Nutritional therapy to promote weight loss<br>• Patient and caregiver teaching (Table 49-11) |

## Interprofessional Care

The treatment goal for a patient with hypothyroidism is restoration of a euthyroid state as safely and rapidly as possible with hormone therapy (Table 49-10). A low-calorie diet is indicated to promote weight loss or prevent weight gain.

Levothyroxine (Synthroid) is the drug of choice to treat hypothyroidism. In the young and otherwise healthy patient, the maintenance replacement dosage is adjusted according to the patient's response and laboratory findings. When initiating thyroid hormone therapy, the initial dosages are low to avoid increases in resting heart rate and BP. In the patient with compromised cardiac status, careful monitoring is needed when starting and adjusting the dosage because the usual dose may increase myocardial $O_2$ demand.[16] This may cause angina and cardiac dysrhythmias.

**DRUG ALERT Levothyroxine (Synthroid)**
- Carefully monitor patients with cardiovascular disease who take this drug.
- Monitor heart rate and report pulse greater than 100 beats/min or an irregular heartbeat.
- Promptly report chest pain, weight loss, nervousness, tremors, and/or insomnia.

In a patient without side effects, the dose is increased at 4- to 6-week intervals as needed based on the TSH levels. It may take up to 8 weeks before the full effect of hormone therapy is seen. Levothyroxine has a peak of action of 1 to 3 weeks. It is important that the patient regularly take replacement medication. Lifelong thyroid therapy is usually required.

Liotrix is a synthetic mix of levothyroxine ($T_4$) and liothyronine ($T_3$) in a 4:1 combination. In contrast, liotrix has a faster onset of action with a peak of 2 to 3 days. Liotrix can be used in acutely ill patients with hypothyroidism.

# NURSING MANAGEMENT: HYPOTHYROIDISM

## Nursing Assessment

Careful assessment may reveal early and subtle changes in a patient suspected of having hypothyroidism. Note any previous history of hyperthyroidism and treatment with antithyroid medications, radioactive iodine, or surgery. Ask the patient about using iodine-containing medications (Table 49-4) and any changes in appetite, weight, activity level, speech, memory, and skin (e.g., increased dryness or thickening). Assess for cold intolerance, constipation, and signs of depression. Further assessment should focus on heart rate, tenderness over the thyroid gland, and edema in the extremities and face.

### ◆ Nursing Diagnoses

Nursing diagnoses for the patient with hypothyroidism may include, but are not limited to, the following:

- Activity intolerance *related to* weakness and fatigue
- Constipation *related to* GI hypomotility
- Impaired memory *related to* hypometabolism

Additional information on nursing diagnoses is presented in the eNursing Care Plan 49-2 for the patient with hypothyroidism (available on the website for this chapter).

### ◆ Planning

The overall goals are that the patient with hypothyroidism will (1) experience relief of symptoms, (2) maintain a euthyroid state, (3) maintain a positive self-image, and (4) comply with lifelong thyroid therapy.

### ◆ Nursing Implementation

◆ **Health Promotion.** Routine screening of thyroid function is not recommended in nonpregnant, asymptomatic adults. Risk factors for hypothyroidism include being female, white ethnicity, advancing age or having type 1 diabetes, Down syndrome, family history of thyroid disease, goiter, previous hyperthyroidism, and external beam radiation in the head and neck area.[18] High-risk populations should be screened for subclinical thyroid disease.

◆ **Acute Care.** Most people with hypothyroidism are treated on an outpatient basis. The person who develops myxedema coma requires acute nursing care, often in an intensive care setting. Mechanical respiratory support and cardiac monitoring are frequently necessary.

Give thyroid hormone therapy and all other medications IV because severe gastric hypomotility may prevent the absorption of oral preparations. Monitor the core temperature for hypothermia that often occurs in myxedema and myxedema coma. Use gentle soap and moisturize frequently to prevent skin breakdown. Frequent position changes and a low-pressure mattress assist in maintaining skin integrity.

Monitor the patient's progress by assessing vital signs, body weight, fluid intake and output, and edema. Cardiac assessment is especially important because the cardiovascular response to hormone therapy determines the medication regimen. Note energy level and mental alertness, which should improve within 2 to 14 days and continue a steady progression to normal levels. Neurologic status and TSH levels are used to determine continuing treatment.

◆ **Ambulatory Care.** Patient teaching regarding medication management and identification of complications is essential (Table 49-11). Initially the hypothyroid patient may have difficulty processing complex instructions. It is important to provide written instructions, repeat the information often, and assess the patient's comprehension level.

Stress the need for lifelong drug therapy and avoiding abrupt discontinuation of drugs. Caution patients against doubling up on doses for any reason. Some patients notice weight loss and are tempted to increase dosing to achieve a desired weight. Teach the patient the expected and unexpected side effects, including the signs and symptoms of hypothyroidism and hyperthyroidism

**TABLE 49-11 Patient & Caregiver Teaching**

***Hypothyroidism***

*Include the following instructions when teaching the patient and caregiver about management of hypothyroidism.*

1. Discuss the importance of thyroid hormone therapy.
   - Need for lifelong therapy
   - Taking thyroid hormone in the morning before food
   - Need for regular follow-up care
2. Caution the patient not to switch brands of the hormone unless prescribed, since the bioavailability of thyroid hormones may differ.
3. Emphasize the need for a comfortable, warm environment because of cold intolerance.
4. Teach measures to prevent skin breakdown. Soap should be used sparingly and lotion applied to skin.
5. Caution the patient, especially if an older adult, to avoid sedatives. If they must be used, suggest that the lowest dose be used. Caregiver should closely monitor mental status, level of consciousness, and respirations.
6. Discuss measures to minimize constipation, including
   - Gradual increase in activity and exercise
   - Increased fiber in diet
   - Use of stool softeners
   - Regular bowel elimination time
7. Tell patient to avoid using enemas because they produce vagal stimulation, which can be hazardous if cardiac disease is present.

(Table 49-5). The manifestations of overdose are the same as hyperthyroidism. Tell the patient to immediately contact an HCP if symptoms, such as orthopnea, dyspnea, rapid pulse, palpitations, chest pain, nervousness, or insomnia, are present.

The patient with diabetes mellitus should test his or her capillary blood glucose at least daily because the return to the euthyroid state frequently increases insulin requirements. Thyroid drugs potentiate the effects of anticoagulants and decrease the effect of digitalis compounds. Teach the patient the toxic signs and symptoms of these medications and the need to remain under close medical observation until stable. Medication interactions are an important reason for patients to consult their HCP before switching brands of thyroid replacement medication. Switching brands may alter bioavailability of the drug and physiologic response.

With treatment, striking transformations occur in both appearance and mental function. Most adults return to a normal state. Cardiovascular conditions and psychosis may persist despite corrections of the hormonal imbalance. Relapses occur if treatment is interrupted.

### ◆ Evaluation

The expected outcomes are that the patient with hypothyroidism will

- Have relief from symptoms
- Maintain a euthyroid state as evidenced by normal thyroid hormone and TSH levels
- Avoid complications of therapy
- Adhere to lifelong therapy

Additional information on expected outcomes is presented in the eNursing Care Plan 49-2 for the patient with hypothyroidism (available on the website for this chapter).

## THYROID NODULES AND CANCER

A *thyroid nodule* (growth in the thyroid gland) may be benign or malignant (thyroid cancer). More than 95% of all thyroid gland nodules are benign. Prevalence of thyroid nodule development increases with age. Benign nodules are usually not dangerous, but they can cause tracheal compression if they become too large.

**Thyroid cancer** is the most common type of cancer of the endocrine system. An estimated 62,450 new cases of thyroid cancer are diagnosed annually. The incidence of thyroid cancer has increased significantly in the past 25 years. It is the most rapidly increasing cancer in the United States. Thyroid cancer affects more women, and the incidence is higher in whites and Asian Americans.[19] Adults at risk include those who had head and neck radiation therapy during childhood, were exposed to radioactive fallout, or have a personal or family history of goiter.

### Types of Thyroid Cancer

The four main types of thyroid cancer are papillary, follicular, medullary, and anaplastic. *Papillary* thyroid cancer is the most common type, accounting for about 70% to 80% of all thyroid cancers. Papillary cancer tends to grow slowly and spreads initially to lymph nodes in the neck.

*Follicular* thyroid cancer makes up about 15% of all thyroid cancers. It tends to occur in older patients. Follicular cancer first metastasizes into the cervical lymph nodes and then spreads to the neck, lungs, and bones.

*Medullary* thyroid cancer, which accounts for up to 10% of all thyroid cancers, is more likely to occur in families and be associated with other endocrine problems. It is diagnosed by genetic testing for a proto-oncogene called *RET*. Medullary thyroid cancer is a type of multiple endocrine neoplasia. It is often poorly differentiated and associated with early metastasis.

*Anaplastic* thyroid cancer, which is found in less than 2% of patients with thyroid cancer, is the most advanced and aggressive thyroid cancer. It is the least likely to respond to treatment and has a poor prognosis.

### Clinical Manifestations and Diagnostic Studies

The primary manifestation of thyroid cancer is a painless, palpable nodule or nodules in an enlarged thyroid gland. Most nodules are found during routine palpation of the neck. The presence of firm, palpable, cervical masses suggests lymph node metastasis. Some patients may have difficulty swallowing or breathing because of tumor growth invading the trachea or esophagus. Hemoptysis and airway obstruction may occur if the trachea is involved. Patients with thyroid cancer generally are euthyroid.

Nodular enlargement of the thyroid gland or palpation of a mass requires further evaluation. Ultrasound is often the first test used. Follow-up testing may involve CT, MRI, positron emission tomography (PET), and ultrasound-guided fine-needle aspiration (FNA). FNA is indicated when a tissue sample for pathologic examination is necessary. A thyroid scan may be done. The scan shows whether nodules on the thyroid are "hot" or "cold." "Hot" tumors take up radioactive iodine and are nearly always benign. If the nodule does not take up the radioactive iodine, it appears as "cold" and has a higher risk of being malignant.

Elevations in serum calcitonin are associated with medullary thyroid cancer. In papillary and follicular cancers, serum thyroglobulin is elevated. In families with a history of medullary thyroid cancer, family members should be encouraged to get genetic testing done and have thyroid screening on a regular basis.

## ❖ NURSING AND INTERPROFESSIONAL MANAGEMENT: THYROID CANCER

Surgical removal of the tumor is the primary treatment for thyroid cancer.[19] Surgical procedures range from unilateral total lobectomy to near-total thyroidectomy with bilateral lobectomy. Lymph nodes in the neck may be removed to determine if the cancer has spread. RAI may be given to some patients to destroy any remaining cancer cells after surgery. RAI therapy has been shown to improve survival rates in patients with papillary and follicular thyroid cancer. External beam radiation may be given as palliative treatment for patients with metastatic thyroid cancer.

Many thyroid cancers are TSH dependent. Thyroid hormone therapy in high doses is often prescribed to inhibit pituitary secretion of TSH. Chemotherapy, including doxorubicin, may be used for advanced disease. Vandetanib (Caprelsa), lenvatinib (Lenvima), sorafenib tosylate (Nexavar), and cabozantinib (Cometriq) are targeted therapies used for metastatic thyroid cancer. These drugs inhibit tyrosine kinases, enzymes that are involved in growth of cancer cells.

Nursing care for the patient with thyroid cancer is similar to that of a patient undergoing thyroidectomy (see p. 1167). Because of the surgical site location and the potential for hypocalcemia, the patient requires frequent postoperative assessment. Assess the patient for airway obstruction, bleeding, and tetany, since the parathyroid gland may have been disturbed or removed during surgery.

## MULTIPLE ENDOCRINE NEOPLASIA

*Multiple endocrine neoplasia* is an inherited condition characterized by hormone-secreting tumors.[20] It is caused by the mutation of one of two genes, *MEN1* or *RET,* that normally control cell growth. Tumors may develop in childhood or later in life.

The two major types of multiple endocrine neoplasia are type 1 and type 2. Both types are commonly inherited as autosomal dominant disorders. Persons with type 1 commonly have parathyroid gland hyperactivity (hyperparathyroidism). Other signs may include hyperactivity of the pituitary gland (prolactinoma) and pancreas (gastrinomas). In most cases the tumors are initially benign. Some tumors later become malignant. Persons with type 2 neoplasia often have medullary thyroid carcinoma. They may also develop pheochromocytoma (tumor of the adrenal glands). (Pheochromocytoma is discussed later in this chapter on p. 1181.)

Treatment of the tumor(s) may include conservative management (watchful waiting), medication to block the effects of excess hormone, and surgical removal of the gland and/or tumor. It is important for patients to have regular screening visits with their HCP so that new tumors may be detected early and existing tumors carefully monitored.

# DISORDERS OF PARATHYROID GLANDS

## HYPERPARATHYROIDISM

### Etiology and Pathophysiology

**Hyperparathyroidism** is a condition involving an increased secretion of parathyroid hormone (PTH). PTH helps regulate

**TABLE 49-12 Manifestations of Parathyroid Dysfunction**

| Hyperfunction | Hypofunction |
|---|---|
| **Cardiovascular System** | |
| • Hypertension<br>• Angina<br>• Dysrhythmias<br>• Shortened ST segment<br>• Shortened QT interval<br>• Increased digitalis effect | • Hypotension<br>• Edema<br>• Dysrhythmias<br>• Elongation of ST segment<br>• Prolonged QT interval<br>• Decreased cardiac output |
| **Neurologic System** | |
| • Lethargy, weakness, fatigue<br>• Psychosis, depression<br>• Depressed reflexes<br>• Personality changes<br>• Irritability<br>• Memory impairment<br>• Delirium, confusion, coma<br>• Headache<br>• Poor coordination<br>• Gait abnormalities<br>• Psychomotor retardation<br>• Paresthesias | • Weakness, fatigue<br>• Depression<br>• Hyperreflexia, muscle cramps<br>• Personality changes<br>• Irritability<br>• Memory impairment<br>• Disorientation, confusion (in older adult)<br>• Headache, increased intracranial pressure<br>• Tetany, seizures<br>• Positive Chvostek's and Trousseau's sign<br>• Tremor<br>• Paresthesias of lips, hands, feet |
| **Renal/Urinary System** | |
| • Hypercalciuria<br>• Kidney stones (nephrolithiasis)<br>• Urinary tract infections<br>• Polyuria | • Urinary frequency<br>• Urinary incontinence |
| **Visual System** | |
| • Impaired vision<br>• Corneal calcification | • Eye changes, including lenticular opacities, cataracts, papilledema |
| **Gastrointestinal System** | |
| • Vague abdominal pain<br>• Anorexia<br>• Nausea and vomiting<br>• Constipation<br>• Pancreatitis<br>• Peptic ulcer disease<br>• Cholelithiasis<br>• Weight loss | • Abdominal cramps<br>• Fecal incontinence (in older adult)<br>• Malabsorption |
| **Integumentary System** | |
| • Skin necrosis<br>• Moist skin | • Dry, scaly skin<br>• Hair loss on scalp and body<br>• Brittle nails, transverse ridging<br>• Lack of tooth enamel |
| **Musculoskeletal System** | |
| • Weakness, fatigue<br>• Skeletal pain<br>• Backache<br>• Pain on weight bearing<br>• Osteoporosis<br>• Pathologic fractures of long bones<br>• Compression fractures of spine<br>• Decreased muscle tone, muscle atrophy | • Weakness, fatigue<br>• Painful muscle cramps<br>• Skeletal x-ray changes, osteosclerosis<br>• Soft tissue calcification<br>• Difficulty walking |

serum calcium and phosphate levels by stimulating bone resorption of calcium, renal tubular reabsorption of calcium, and activation of vitamin D. Thus oversecretion of PTH is associated with increased serum calcium levels. Primary hyperparathyroidism affects 25 of 100,000 persons per year.[21]

Hyperparathyroidism is classified as primary, secondary, or tertiary. *Primary hyperparathyroidism* is due to an increased secretion of PTH leading to disorders of calcium, phosphate, and bone metabolism. The most common cause is a benign tumor (adenoma) in the parathyroid gland. Patients who have previously undergone head and neck radiation have an increased risk of developing a parathyroid adenoma. Long-term lithium therapy is also associated with primary hyperparathyroidism. The peak incidence of primary hyperparathyroidism is in the 40s and 50s. Women are twice as likely to develop primary hyperparathyroidism as men.[21]

*Secondary hyperparathyroidism* is a compensatory response to conditions that induce or cause hypocalcemia, the main stimulus of PTH secretion. These conditions include vitamin D deficiencies, malabsorption, chronic kidney disease, and hyperphosphatemia.

*Tertiary hyperparathyroidism* occurs when there is hyperplasia of the parathyroid glands and a loss of negative feedback from circulating calcium levels. Thus there is autonomous secretion of PTH, even with normal calcium levels. This condition is seen in patients who have had a kidney transplant after a long period of dialysis treatment for chronic kidney disease (see Chapter 46).

Excess levels of circulating PTH usually lead to hypercalcemia and hypophosphatemia. Multiple body systems are affected (Table 49-12). Decreased bone density can occur because of the effect of PTH on osteoclastic (bone resorption) and osteoblastic (bone formation) activity. In the kidneys the excess calcium cannot be reabsorbed, leading to increased urinary calcium levels (hypercalciuria). This urinary calcium, along with a large amount of urinary phosphate, can lead to calculi formation.

## Clinical Manifestations and Complications

Clinical manifestations range from an asymptomatic person (diagnosed through testing for unrelated problems) to a patient with overt symptoms.[21] The manifestations are associated with hypercalcemia (Table 49-12). Loss of appetite, constipation, fatigue, emotional disorders, shortened attention span, and muscle weakness, particularly in the proximal muscles of the lower extremities, are often noted. Complications include osteoporosis, renal failure, kidney stones, pancreatitis, cardiac changes, and long bone, rib, and vertebral fractures.

## Diagnostic Studies

PTH levels are elevated in patients with hyperparathyroidism. Serum calcium levels usually exceed 10 mg/dL (2.50 mmol/L). Because of its inverse relation with calcium, the serum phosphorus level is usually less than 3 mg/dL (0.1 mmol/L). Hypercalcemia in asymptomatic cases is often identified through a routine chemistry panel.

Elevations in other laboratory tests include urine calcium, serum chloride, uric acid, creatinine, amylase (if pancreatitis is present), and alkaline phosphatase (in the presence of bone disease). Bone density measurements may be used to detect bone loss. Conversely, those found to have bone loss on a screening dual-energy x-ray absorptiometry (DEXA) scan should be tested for hypercalcemia. MRI, CT, and/or ultrasound can detect an adenoma.

### Interprofessional Care

The goal of treatment is to relieve symptoms and prevent complications caused by excess PTH. The choice of therapy depends on the urgency of the clinical situation, degree of hypercalcemia, and underlying cause of the disorder.

**Surgical Therapy.** The most effective treatment of primary and secondary hyperparathyroidism is surgical intervention. Surgery involves partial or complete removal of the parathyroid glands. The most commonly used procedure involves endoscopy and is done on an outpatient basis. Criteria for surgery include elevated serum calcium levels (more than 1 mg/dL above the upper limit of normal), hypercalciuria (greater than 400 mg/day), markedly reduced bone mineral density, overt symptoms (e.g., neuromuscular effects, nephrolithiasis), or those under age 50. Parathyroidectomy leads to a rapid reduction of high calcium levels.

Patients who have multiple parathyroid glands removed may undergo autotransplantation of normal parathyroid tissue in the forearm or near the sternocleidomastoid muscle. This allows PTH secretion to continue with normalization of calcium levels. If autotransplantation is not possible or if it fails, the patient will need to take calcium supplements for life.

**Nonsurgical Therapy.** A conservative approach is often used in patients who are asymptomatic or have mild symptoms of hyperparathyroidism. Ongoing care includes regular examination with measurements of serum PTH, calcium, phosphorus, alkaline phosphatase, creatinine and blood urea nitrogen (BUN) (to assess renal function), and urinary calcium excretion. Annual x-rays and DEXA scans are done to assess for metabolic bone loss. Continued ambulation and avoiding immobility are important. Dietary measures include high fluid and moderate calcium intake.

Severe hypercalcemia is managed with IV sodium chloride solution and loop diuretics such as furosemide to increase the urinary excretion of calcium. Several drugs help to lower calcium levels, but they do not treat the underlying problem. Bisphosphonates (e.g., alendronate [Fosamax]) inhibit osteoclastic bone resorption, normalizing serum calcium levels and improving bone mineral density. IV bisphosphonates (e.g., pamidronate [Aredia]) can rapidly lower serum calcium in patients with dangerously elevated levels. Phosphates are given if the patient has normal renal function and low serum phosphate levels.

Calcimimetic agents (e.g., cinacalcet [Sensipar]) increase the sensitivity of the calcium receptor on the parathyroid gland, resulting in decreased PTH secretion and calcium blood levels. They are useful in treating secondary hyperparathyroidism in those with chronic kidney disease on dialysis or in patients with parathyroid cancer.

## ❖ NURSING MANAGEMENT: HYPERPARATHYROIDISM

Nursing care for the patient after a parathyroidectomy is similar to that for a patient after thyroidectomy. The major postoperative complications are associated with hemorrhage and fluid and electrolyte disturbances. *Tetany,* a condition of neuromuscular hyperexcitability associated with sudden decrease in calcium levels, is another concern. It is usually apparent early in the postoperative period but may develop over several days. Mild tetany, characterized by unpleasant tingling of the hands and around the mouth, may be present but should decrease over time. If tetany becomes more severe (e.g., muscular spasms or laryngospasms), IV calcium may be given. IV calcium gluconate should be readily available for patients after parathyroidectomy in the event that acute tetany occurs.

Monitor intake and output to evaluate the patient's fluid status. Assess calcium, potassium, phosphate, and magnesium levels frequently, as well as Chvostek's and Trousseau's signs (see Fig. 16-15). Encourage mobility to promote bone calcification.

If surgery is not performed, treatment to relieve symptoms and prevent complications is initiated. Assist the patient with hyperparathyroidism to adapt the meal plan to his or her lifestyle. A referral to a dietitian may be useful. Because immobility can aggravate the bone loss, emphasize the importance of an exercise program. Encourage the patient to keep the regular follow-up appointments. Teach the patient the symptoms of hypocalcemia and hypercalcemia and to report them if they occur. Hypocalcemia and hypercalcemia are discussed in Chapter 16.

## HYPOPARATHYROIDISM

**Hypoparathyroidism** is an uncommon condition associated with inadequate circulating PTH. It is characterized by hypocalcemia due to a lack of PTH to maintain serum calcium levels. PTH resistance at the cellular level may also occur *(pseudohypoparathyroidism).* This is caused by a genetic defect resulting in hypocalcemia despite normal or high PTH levels. It is often associated with hypothyroidism and hypogonadism.

The most common cause of hypoparathyroidism is iatrogenic. This may include accidental removal of the parathyroid glands or damage to the vascular supply of the glands during neck surgery (e.g., thyroidectomy). Idiopathic hypoparathyroidism resulting from the absence, fatty replacement, or atrophy of the glands is a rare disease. It usually occurs early in life and may be associated with other endocrine disorders. Affected patients may have antiparathyroid antibodies. Severe hypomagnesemia (e.g., malnutrition, chronic alcoholism, renal failure) also leads to a suppression of PTH secretion. Other causes of parathyroid deficiency include tumors and heavy metal poisoning.

The clinical features of acute hypoparathyroidism are due to hypocalcemia (Table 49-12). Sudden decreases in calcium concentration cause tetany, characterized by tingling of the lips and stiffness in the extremities. Painful tonic spasms of smooth and skeletal muscles can cause dysphagia and laryngospasms, which compromise breathing. Lethargy, anxiety, and personality changes may occur. Abnormal laboratory findings include decreased serum calcium and PTH levels and increased serum phosphate levels.

## ❖ NURSING AND INTERPROFESSIONAL MANAGEMENT: HYPOPARATHYROIDISM

Treatment goals for the patient with hypoparathyroidism are to treat acute complications such as tetany, maintain normal serum calcium levels, and prevent long-term complications. Emergency treatment of tetany after surgery requires the administration of IV calcium.

Give IV calcium slowly. Use ECG monitoring during calcium administration because high serum calcium levels can cause hypotension, serious cardiac dysrhythmias, or cardiac arrest. The patient who takes digoxin is particularly vulnerable. It is important to assess IV patency before administration. Calcium chloride can cause venous irritation and inflammation, and extravasation may cause cellulitis, necrosis, and tissue sloughing.

Rebreathing may partially relieve acute neuromuscular symptoms associated with hypocalcemia such as generalized muscle cramps or mild tetany. Instruct the patient (if cooperative) to breathe in and out of a paper bag or breathing mask. This reduces $CO_2$ excretion from the lungs, increases carbonic acid levels in the blood, and lowers the pH. A lower pH (acidic environment) enhances calcium ionization, which causes more total body calcium to be available in the active form.

**CHECK YOUR PRACTICE**

You are caring for a 56-yr-old man admitted 18 hours ago to your clinical unit. He had a total thyroidectomy for papillary thyroid cancer. As you are preparing to administer oral pain medication, he tells you he hopes he "doesn't have any trouble" taking the medication because his lips feel "a little numb."

- What complication do you suspect could be occurring?
- What assessments do you need to make at this time?
- Describe the actions needed if this complication is occurring.

Teach the patient how to manage long-term drug and nutritional therapy. PTH replacement is not recommended because of the expense and need for parenteral administration. Most patients receive a regimen of oral calcium supplements (totaling 1.5 to 3 g/day in divided doses), magnesium supplements, and vitamin D.

Vitamin D is used to enhance intestinal calcium absorption. Vitamin D (e.g., dihydrotachysterol, 1,25-dihydroxycholecalciferol, or calcitriol [Rocaltrol]) increases calcium levels rapidly and is quickly metabolized. Rapid metabolism is desired because vitamin D is a fat-soluble vitamin and toxicity can cause irreversible renal impairment.

A high-calcium meal plan includes foods such as dark green vegetables, soybeans, and tofu. Tell the patient to avoid foods containing oxalic acid (e.g., spinach, rhubarb) because they inhibit the absorption of calcium. Teach the patient about the need for follow-up care, including monitoring of calcium levels three or four times a year.

# DISORDERS OF ADRENAL CORTEX

Adrenal cortex steroid hormones have three main classifications: glucocorticoids, mineralocorticoids, and androgens. Glucocorticoids regulate metabolism, increase blood glucose levels, and are critical in the physiologic stress response. The primary glucocorticoid is cortisol. Mineralocorticoids regulate sodium and potassium balance. The primary mineralocorticoid is aldosterone. Androgens contribute to growth and development in both genders and to sexual development in women. The term *corticosteroid* refers to any one of these three types of hormones produced by the adrenal cortex.

## CUSHING SYNDROME

### Etiology and Pathophysiology

**Cushing syndrome** is a clinical condition that results from chronic exposure to excess corticosteroids, particularly glucocorticoids.[22] Several conditions can cause Cushing syndrome. The most common cause is iatrogenic administration of exogenous corticosteroids (e.g., prednisone). About 85% of the cases of endogenous Cushing syndrome are due to an ACTH-secreting pituitary adenoma (Cushing disease). Less common causes include adrenal tumors and ectopic ACTH production by tumors (usually of the lung or pancreas) outside of the hypothalamic-pituitary-adrenal axis. Cushing disease and primary adrenal tumors are more common in women in the 20- to 40-year-old age group. Ectopic ACTH production is more common in men.

### Clinical Manifestations

Manifestations of Cushing syndrome occur in most body systems and are related to excess levels of corticosteroids (Table 49-13). Although signs of glucocorticoid excess usually predominate, symptoms of mineralocorticoid and androgen excess can occur.

Corticosteroid excess causes pronounced changes in physical appearance (Fig. 49-10). Weight gain, the most common feature, results from the accumulation of adipose tissue in the trunk (centripetal obesity), face ("moon face"), and cervical areas ("buffalo hump") (Fig. 49-11). Hyperglycemia occurs because of glucose intolerance (associated with cortisol-induced insulin resistance) and increased gluconeogenesis by the liver. Muscle wasting causes weakness, especially in the extremities. A loss of bone matrix leads to osteoporosis and back pain. The loss of collagen makes the skin weaker, thinner, and more easily bruised. Purplish red striae (usually depressed below the skin surface) appear on the abdomen, breast, or buttocks (Fig. 49-12). Catabolic processes lead to a delay in wound healing.

Mineralocorticoid excess may cause hypokalemia from potassium excretion and hypertension secondary to fluid retention. Adrenal androgen excess may cause severe acne, virilization in women, and feminization in men. Menstrual disorders and hirsutism in women and gynecomastia and impotence in men are seen more commonly in adrenal cancers.

### Diagnostic Studies

Diagnosing Cushing syndrome begins with confirming elevated plasma cortisol levels. Three tests are used: (1) midnight or late-night salivary cortisol, (2) low-dose dexamethasone suppression test, and (3) 24-hour urine cortisol.[23] Urine cortisol levels higher than the normal range of 80 to 120 mcg/24 hr

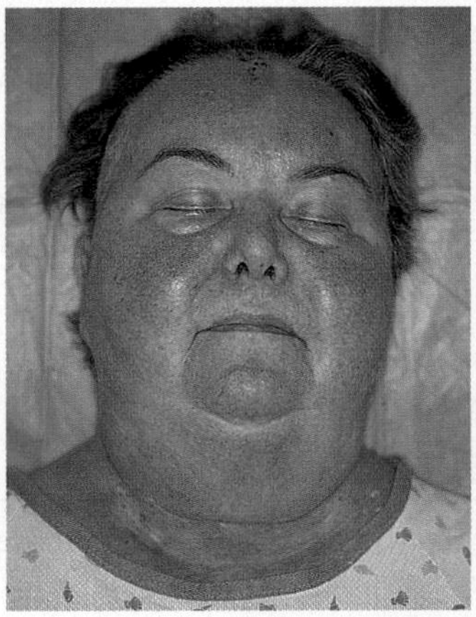

**FIG. 49-10** Cushing syndrome. Facies include a rounded face ("moon face") with thin, reddened skin. Hirsutism may also be present. (From Seidel HM, Ball JW, Dains JE, et al: *Mosby's guide to physical examination,* ed 6, St Louis, 2006, Mosby.)

**TABLE 49-13 Manifestations of Adrenocortical Dysfunction**

| System | Cushing Syndrome | Addison's Disease |
|---|---|---|
| **Glucocorticoids** | | |
| **General appearance** | Truncal obesity, thin extremities, rounding of face (moon face), fat deposits on back of neck and shoulders (buffalo hump) (Fig. 49-11). | Weight loss, emaciation. |
| **Integumentary** | Thin, fragile skin, purplish red striae (Fig. 49-12). Petechial hemorrhages, bruises. Florid cheeks (plethora), acne, poor wound healing. | Bronzed or smoky hyperpigmentation of face, neck, hands (especially creases) (Fig. 49-13), buccal membranes, nipples, genitalia, and scars (if pituitary function normal). Vitiligo, alopecia. |
| **Cardiovascular** | Hypervolemia, hypertension, edema of lower extremities. | Hypotension, tendency to develop refractory shock, vasodilation. |
| **Gastrointestinal** | Increase in secretion of pepsin and HCl acid, risk of peptic ulcer disease, anorexia. | Anorexia, nausea and vomiting, cramping abdominal pain, diarrhea. |
| **Renal/urinary** | Glycosuria, hypercalciuria, risk for kidney stones. | |
| **Musculoskeletal** | Muscle wasting in extremities, fatigue, osteoporosis, awkward gait, back pain, weakness, compression fractures. | Fatigue. |
| **Immune** | Inhibition of immune response, suppression of allergic response. | Tendency for coexisting autoimmune diseases. |
| **Metabolic** | Hyperglycemia, negative nitrogen balance, dyslipidemia. | Hyponatremia, insulin sensitivity, fever. |
| **Emotional** | Euphoria, irritability, depression, insomnia, anxiety. | Depression, exhaustion or irritability, confusion, delusions. |
| **Mineralocorticoids** | | |
| **Fluid and electrolytes** | Marked sodium and water retention, edema, marked hypokalemia, alkalosis. | Sodium loss, decreased volume of extracellular fluid, hyperkalemia, salt craving. |
| **Cardiovascular** | Hypertension, hypervolemia. | Hypovolemia, tendency toward shock, decreased cardiac output. |
| **Androgens** | | |
| **Integumentary** | Hirsutism, acne, hyperpigmentation. | Decreased axillary and pubic hair (in women). |
| **Reproductive** | *Women:* Menstrual irregularities and enlargement of clitoris<br>*Men:* Gynecomastia and testicular atrophy. | *Women:* Decreased libido in women<br>*Men:* No effect in men. |
| **Musculoskeletal** | Muscle wasting and weakness. | Decrease in muscle size and tone. |

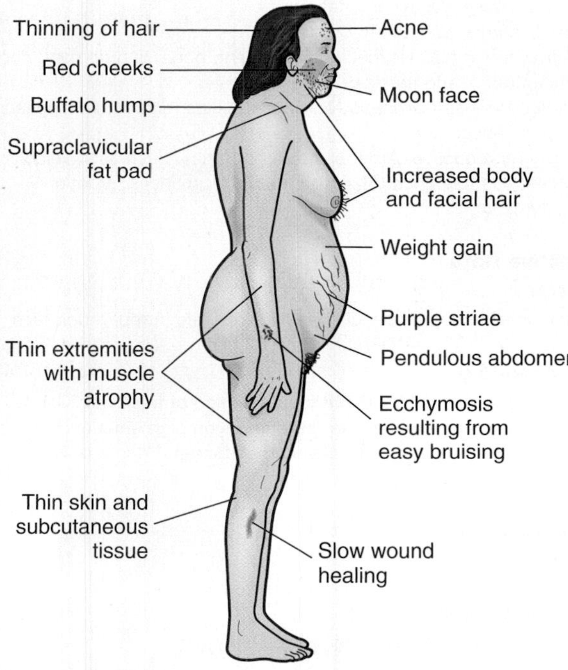


**FIG. 49-11** Common characteristics of Cushing syndrome.

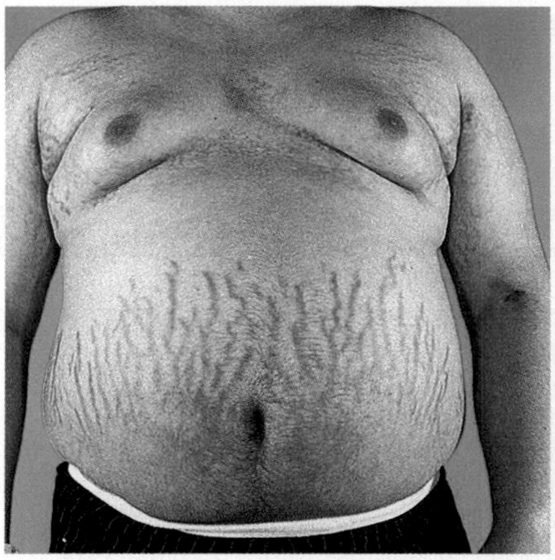

**FIG. 49-12** Cushing syndrome. Truncal obesity; broad, purple striae; and easy bruising (left antecubital fossa). (From Chew SL, Leslie D: *Clinical endocrinology and diabetes: an illustrated colour text,* Edinburgh, 2006, Churchill Livingstone.)

indicate Cushing syndrome. Urine levels of 17-ketosteroids may be elevated. A CT scan or MRI of the pituitary and adrenal glands can detect a tumor.

Plasma ACTH levels may be low, normal, or elevated, depending on the underlying cause of Cushing syndrome. High or normal ACTH levels indicate Cushing disease, whereas low or undetectable levels indicate an adrenal or medication etiology. Other findings on diagnostic tests associated with, but not diagnostic of, Cushing syndrome include leukocytosis, lymphopenia, eosinopenia, hyperglycemia, glycosuria, hypercalciuria, and osteoporosis. Hypokalemia and alkalosis are seen in ectopic ACTH syndrome and adrenal carcinoma.

## Interprofessional Care

The primary goal of treatment is to normalize hormone secretion. The specific treatment depends on the underlying cause (Table 49-14). If the underlying cause is a pituitary adenoma, the standard treatment is surgical removal of the pituitary tumor using the transsphenoidal approach.[23] (The transsphenoidal approach is discussed earlier in this chapter on p. 1158.) Radiation therapy is an option for patients who are not good surgical candidates.

Adrenalectomy is indicated for Cushing syndrome caused by adrenal tumors or hyperplasia. Occasionally, bilateral adrenalectomy is necessary. A laparoscopic approach is used unless a malignant adrenal tumor is suspected. An open surgical adrenalectomy is usually performed for adrenal cancer.

Patients with ectopic ACTH-secreting tumors are best managed by locating and removing the tumor (usually lung or pancreas). This is usually possible when the tumor is benign. When a tumor is malignant and it has already metastasized, surgical removal may not be possible or successful.

When the patient is a poor candidate for surgery or prior surgery has failed, then drug therapy may be attempted. The goal of drug therapy is to suppress the synthesis and secretion of cortisol from the adrenal gland *(medical adrenalectomy)*. Drugs used include ketoconazole, aminoglutethimide, and mitotane. These are used cautiously because they are often toxic at the dosages needed to reduce cortisol secretion. Hydrocortisone or prednisone may be needed to avoid adrenal insufficiency. Mifepristone (Korlym) may be used to control hyperglycemia in patients with endogenous Cushing syndrome who have type 2 diabetes.

If Cushing syndrome has developed during the course of prolonged administration of corticosteroids (e.g., prednisone), the following alternatives may be tried: (1) gradually discontinuing corticosteroid therapy, (2) reducing the corticosteroid dose, and (3) converting to an alternate-day regimen. Gradual tapering of the corticosteroids is necessary to avoid potentially life-threatening adrenal insufficiency. In an alternate-day regimen, twice the daily dosage of a shorter-acting corticosteroid is given every other morning to minimize hypothalamic-pituitary-adrenal suppression, growth suppression, and altered appearance. This regimen is not used when the corticosteroids are given as hormone therapy.

### TABLE 49-14 Interprofessional Care

**Cushing Syndrome**

**Diagnostic Assessment**

- History and physical examination
- Dexamethasone suppression test
- 24-hr urine for free cortisol and 17-ketosteroids
- Plasma and salivary cortisol levels
- Plasma ACTH levels
- Complete blood count (CBC) with WBC differential
- Blood chemistries for sodium, potassium, glucose
- CT scan, MRI

**Management**

***Pituitary Adenoma***

- Transsphenoidal resection
- Radiation therapy

***Adrenocortical Adenoma, Carcinoma, or Hyperplasia***

- Adrenalectomy (open or laparoscopic)
- Drug therapy (e.g., ketoconazole, aminoglutethimide, mitotane, mifepristone [Korlym])

***Ectopic ACTH-Secreting Tumor***

- Treatment of the tumor (surgical removal or radiation)

***Exogenous Corticosteroid Therapy***

- Discontinue or alter the dose of exogenous corticosteroids

## NURSING MANAGEMENT: CUSHING SYNDROME

### Nursing Assessment

Subjective and objective data that should be obtained from a patient with Cushing syndrome are presented in Table 49-15.

### Nursing Diagnoses

Nursing diagnoses for the patient with Cushing syndrome may include, but are not limited to, the following:

- Risk for infection *related to* lowered resistance to stress and suppression of immune system
- Risk for overweight *related to* increased appetite, high caloric content of foods, and inactivity

### TABLE 49-15 Nursing Assessment

**Cushing Syndrome**

**Subjective Data**

***Important Health Information***

*Past health history:* Pituitary tumor (Cushing disease). Adrenal, pancreatic, or pulmonary neoplasms. GI bleeding, frequent infections

*Medications:* Corticosteroids

***Functional Health Patterns***

*Health perception–health management:* Malaise

*Nutritional-metabolic:* Weight gain, anorexia. Prolonged wound healing, easy bruising

*Elimination:* Polyuria

*Activity-exercise:* Weakness, fatigue

*Sleep:* Insomnia, poor sleep quality

*Cognitive-perceptual:* Headache. Back, joint, bone, and rib pain. Poor concentration and memory

*Self-perception–self-concept:* Negative feelings regarding changes in personal appearance

*Sexuality-reproductive:* Amenorrhea, impotence, decreased libido

*Coping–stress tolerance:* Anxiety, mood disturbances, emotional lability, psychosis

**Objective Data**

***General***

Truncal obesity, supraclavicular fat pads, buffalo hump, moon face

***Integumentary***

Plethora. Hirsutism of body and face, thinning of head hair. Thin, friable skin. Acne, petechiae, purpura, hyperpigmentation. Purplish red striae on breasts, buttocks, and abdomen. Edema of lower extremities

***Cardiovascular***

Hypertension

***Musculoskeletal***

Muscle wasting, thin extremities, awkward gait

***Reproductive***

Gynecomastia, testicular atrophy (in men), enlarged clitoris (in women)

***Possible Diagnostic Findings***

Hypokalemia, hyperglycemia, dyslipidemia, polycythemia, granulocytosis, lymphocytopenia, eosinopenia. ↑ plasma cortisol, ↑ salivary cortisol. High, low, or normal ACTH levels. Abnormal dexamethasone suppression test. ↑ Urine free cortisol, 17-ketosteroids. Glycosuria, hypercalciuria. Osteoporosis on x-ray

- Disturbed body image *related to* change in appearance from disease process
- Impaired skin integrity *related to* excess corticosteroids, immobility, and altered skin fragility

Additional information on nursing diagnoses is presented in eNursing Care Plan 49-3 for the patient with Cushing syndrome (available on the website for this chapter).

## Planning

The overall goals are that the patient with Cushing syndrome will (1) experience relief of symptoms, (2) avoid serious complications, (3) maintain a positive self-image, and (4) actively participate in the therapeutic plan.

## Nursing Implementation

**Health Promotion.** Health promotion is focused on identifying patients at risk for Cushing syndrome. Patients receiving long-term, exogenous corticosteroids are at risk. Teaching related to using medications and monitoring side effects is an important preventive measure.

**Acute Care.** The patient with Cushing syndrome is seriously ill. Because the therapy has many side effects, assessment focuses on signs and symptoms of hormone and drug toxicity and complicating conditions (e.g., cardiovascular disease, diabetes mellitus, infection). Monitor vital signs, daily weight, and glucose. Assess for possible infections. Because signs and symptoms of inflammation (e.g., fever, redness) may be minimal or absent, assess for pain, loss of function, and purulent drainage. Monitor for signs and symptoms of thromboembolic events such as pulmonary emboli (e.g., sudden chest pain, dyspnea, tachypnea).

Another important focus of nursing care is emotional support. Changes in appearance, such as truncal obesity, multiple bruises, hirsutism in women, and gynecomastia in men, can be distressing. The patient may feel unattractive, repulsive, or unwanted. You can help by remaining sensitive to the patient's feelings and offering respect and unconditional acceptance. Reassure the patient that the physical changes and much of the emotional lability will resolve when hormone levels return to normal.

If treatment involves surgical removal of a pituitary adenoma, an adrenal tumor, or one or both adrenal glands, nursing care will include preoperative and postoperative care.

***Preoperative Care.*** Before surgery the patient should be brought to optimal physical condition. Hypertension and hyperglycemia must be controlled. Hypokalemia must be corrected with diet and potassium supplements. A high-protein diet helps correct the protein depletion. Preoperative teaching depends on the type of surgical approach planned (hypophysectomy or adrenalectomy) and should include information regarding the anticipated postoperative care.

***Postoperative Care.*** Surgery on the adrenal glands poses great risks. Because the adrenal glands are vascular, the risk of hemorrhage is increased. In the postoperative period for both laparoscopic and open adrenalectomy, the patient may have a nasogastric tube, a urinary catheter, IV therapy, central venous pressure monitoring, and leg sequential compression devices to prevent emboli.

Manipulating glandular tissue during surgery may release large amounts of hormones into the circulation, producing marked fluctuations in the metabolic processes affected by these hormones. Postoperatively, BP, fluid balance, and electrolyte levels may be unstable due to these hormone fluctuations.

High doses of corticosteroids (e.g., hydrocortisone [Solu-Cortef]) are given IV during surgery and for several days afterward to ensure adequate responses to the stress of the procedure. If large amounts of endogenous hormone were released into the systemic circulation during surgery, the patient is likely to develop hypertension, increasing the risk of hemorrhage. High corticosteroid levels cause problems with glycemic control, increase susceptibility to infection, and delay wound healing.

The critical period for circulatory instability ranges from 24 to 48 hours after surgery. During this time you must constantly be alert for signs of corticosteroid imbalance. Report any rapid or significant changes in BP, respirations, or heart rate. Monitor fluid intake and output carefully and assess for potential imbalances. IV corticosteroids are given, and the dosage and flow rate are adjusted to the patient's clinical manifestations and fluid and electrolyte balance. Oral doses are given as tolerated. After IV corticosteroids are withdrawn, keep the IV line open for quick administration of corticosteroids or vasopressors. Obtain morning urine samples at the same time each morning for cortisol measurement to evaluate the surgery's effectiveness.

If corticosteroid dosage is tapered too rapidly after surgery, acute adrenal insufficiency may develop. Vomiting, increased weakness, dehydration, and hypotension are signs of hypocortisolism. In addition, the patient may complain of painful joints, pruritus, or peeling skin and may experience severe emotional disturbances. Report these signs and symptoms so that drug doses can be adjusted as necessary.

The patient is usually maintained on bed rest until the BP stabilizes. Be alert for subtle signs of postoperative infection because the usual inflammatory responses are suppressed. To prevent infection, provide meticulous care when changing the dressing and during any other procedures that involve access to body cavities, circulation, or areas under the skin.

**Ambulatory Care.** Discharge instructions are based on the patient's lack of endogenous corticosteroids and resulting inability to react physiologically to stressors. Consider a home health nurse referral, especially for older adults, because of the need for ongoing evaluation and teaching. Instruct the patient to wear a Medic Alert bracelet at all times and carry medical identification and instructions in a wallet or purse. Teach the patient to avoid exposure to extreme temperatures, infections, and emotional disturbances. Stress may produce or precipitate acute adrenal insufficiency because the remaining adrenal tissue cannot meet an increased hormonal demand. Teach patients to adjust their corticosteroid replacement therapy in accordance with their stress levels. Consult with the patient's HCP to determine the parameters for dosage changes if this plan is feasible. If the patient cannot adjust his or her own medication or if weakness, fainting, fever, or nausea and vomiting occur, the patient should contact the HCP for a possible adjustment in corticosteroid dosage. Many patients require lifetime replacement therapy. However, patients should be prepared for it to take several months to adjust the hormone dose satisfactorily.

## Evaluation

The expected outcomes are that the patient with Cushing syndrome will

- Experience no signs or symptoms of infection
- Maintain weight appropriate for height
- Verbalize acceptance of appearance and treatment regimen
- Demonstrate healing of skin and maintenance of intact skin

Additional information on expected outcomes is presented in eNursing Care Plan 49-3 for the patient with Cushing syndrome (available on the website for this chapter).

## ADRENOCORTICAL INSUFFICIENCY

### Etiology and Pathophysiology

Adrenocortical insufficiency (hypofunction of the adrenal cortex) may be from a primary cause (**Addison's disease**) or a secondary cause (lack of pituitary ACTH secretion). In Addison's disease, all three classes of adrenal corticosteroids (glucocorticoids, mineralocorticoids, and androgens) are reduced. In secondary adrenocortical insufficiency, corticosteroids and androgens are deficient, but mineralocorticoids rarely are. ACTH deficiency may be caused by pituitary disease or suppression of the hypothalamic-pituitary axis because of the administration of exogenous corticosteroids.

Up to 80% of Addison's disease cases in the United States are caused by an autoimmune response.[24] Autoimmune adrenalitis causes the adrenal cortex to be destroyed by antibodies. This results in loss of glucocorticoid, mineralocorticoid, and adrenal androgen hormones. Addison's disease can be present along with other endocrine conditions. This is known as *autoimmune polyglandular syndrome*. It is most common in white females. Those with autoimmune adrenalitis often have other autoimmune disorders such as type 1 diabetes, autoimmune thyroid disease, pernicious anemia, and celiac disease.[25]

Although tuberculosis causes Addison's disease worldwide, it is now an uncommon cause in the United States. Other causes include amyloidosis, fungal infections (e.g., histoplasmosis), acquired immunodeficiency syndrome (AIDS), and metastatic cancer. Iatrogenic Addison's disease may be due to adrenal hemorrhage, often related to anticoagulant therapy, chemotherapy, ketoconazole therapy for AIDS, or bilateral adrenalectomy. Adrenal insufficiency most often occurs in adults younger than 60 years of age and affects both genders equally.

### Clinical Manifestations

Because manifestations do not tend to become evident until 90% of the adrenal cortex is destroyed, the disease is often advanced before it is diagnosed. The manifestations have a slow (insidious) onset and include anorexia, nausea, progressive weakness, fatigue, and weight loss. Increased ACTH causes the striking feature of a bronze-colored skin hyperpigmentation. It is seen primarily in sun-exposed areas of the body; at pressure points; over joints; and in the creases, especially palmar creases (Fig. 49-13). The changes in the skin are most likely due to increased secretion of β-lipotropin (which contains melanocyte-stimulating hormone [MSH]). This tropic hormone is increased because of decreased negative feedback and subsequent low corticosteroid levels. Other manifestations include abdominal pain, diarrhea, headache, orthostatic hypotension, salt craving, and joint pain. Irritability and depression may occur in primary adrenal hypofunction.

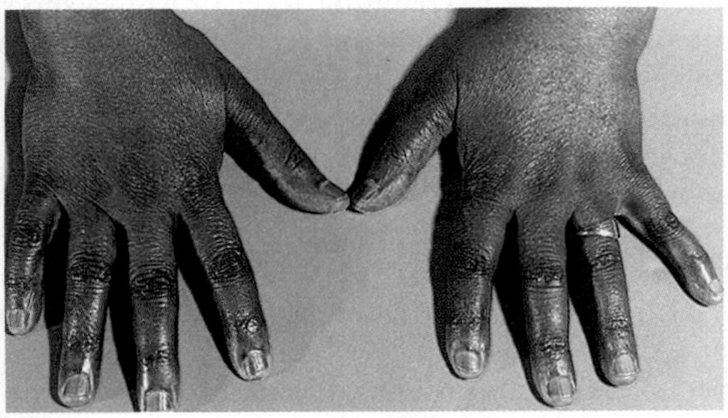

**FIG. 49-13** Hyperpigmentation typically seen in Addison's disease. (From Chew SL, Leslie D: *Clinical endocrinology and diabetes: an illustrated colour text*, Edinburgh, 2006, Churchill Livingstone.)

Patients with secondary adrenocortical hypofunction may have many signs and symptoms similar to those of patients with Addison's disease. However, they usually do not have hyperpigmented skin because ACTH levels are low.

### Complications

Patients with adrenocortical insufficiency are at risk for acute adrenal insufficiency *(addisonian crisis)*, a life-threatening emergency caused by insufficient adrenocortical hormones or a sudden sharp decrease in these hormones. Addisonian crisis is triggered by (1) stress (e.g., from infection, surgery, psychologic distress), (2) the sudden withdrawal of corticosteroid hormone therapy (which is often done by a patient who lacks knowledge of the importance of this therapy), (3) adrenal surgery, or (4) sudden pituitary gland destruction.

During acute adrenal insufficiency, the patient exhibits severe manifestations of glucocorticoid and mineralocorticoid deficiencies, including hypotension, tachycardia, dehydration, hyponatremia, hyperkalemia, hypoglycemia, fever, weakness, and confusion. Hypotension may lead to shock. Circulatory collapse associated with adrenal insufficiency is often unresponsive to the usual treatment (vasopressors and fluid replacement). GI manifestations include severe vomiting, diarrhea, and pain in the abdomen. Pain may occur in the lower back and legs.

### Diagnostic Studies

The ACTH stimulation test is a common test to diagnose adrenal insufficiency. Baseline cortisol and ACTH levels are measured, and the patient is given an IV injection of synthetic ACTH (cosyntropin). Cortisol and ACTH levels are rechecked after 30 and 60 minutes. The normal response is a rise in blood cortisol levels. People with Addison's disease have little or no increase in cortisol levels. Those with primary adrenal insufficiency have a high ACTH level.[24]

When the response to the ACTH test is abnormal, a corticotropin-releasing hormone (CRH) stimulation test may be done. The patient is given an IV injection of synthetic CRH, and blood is taken after 30 and 60 minutes. Those with Addison's disease have high ACTH levels but no cortisol. People with secondary adrenal insufficiency due to pituitary or hypothalamus problems do not produce ACTH or have a delayed response.[25]

Other abnormal laboratory findings may include hyperkalemia, hypochloremia, hyponatremia, hypoglycemia, anemia, and increased BUN levels.[25] An ECG may show low voltage and peaked T waves caused by hyperkalemia. CT scans and MRI can identify causes other than autoimmune, including tumors, fungal infections, tuberculosis, or adrenal calcification.

### Interprofessional Care

Treatment of adrenocortical insufficiency focuses on managing the underlying cause when possible. The mainstay is lifelong hormone therapy with glucocorticoids and mineralocorticoids (Table 49-16). Overall, patients who take their medications consistently can anticipate a normal life expectancy. Hydrocortisone,

**TABLE 49-16 Interprofessional Care**

***Addison's Disease***

**Diagnostic Assessment**

- History and physical examination
- ACTH stimulation test
- Serum cortisol and ACTH
- Urine cortisol and aldosterone
- CRH suppression test
- Serum electrolytes
- CT scan, MRI

**Management**

- Daily glucocorticoid (e.g., prednisone, hydrocortisone) replacement (two thirds on awakening in morning, one third in late afternoon)
- Daily mineralocorticoid (fludrocortisone) in morning
- Increased salt in the diet
- Androgen replacement with dehydroepiandrosterone (DHEA) for women
- Salt additives for excess heat or humidity
- Increased doses of glucocorticoid for stress situations (e.g., surgery, hospitalization)

**TABLE 49-17 Patient & Caregiver Teaching**

***Addison's Disease***

*Include the following information in the teaching plan for patient with Addison's disease and the caregiver.*

1. Names, dosages, and actions of drugs
2. Symptoms of overdosage and underdosage
3. Conditions requiring increased medication (e.g., trauma, infection, surgery, emotional crisis)
4. Course of action to take related to changes in medication
   - Increase in dose of corticosteroid
   - Administration of large dose of corticosteroid IM, including demonstration and return demonstration
   - Consultation with HCP
5. Prevention of infection and need for prompt and vigorous treatment of existing infections
6. Need for lifelong replacement therapy
7. Need for lifelong medical supervision
8. Need to carry medical identification
9. Prevention of falls
10. Adverse effects of corticosteroid therapy and prevention techniques
11. Special instruction for patients who are diabetics and management of blood glucose when taking corticosteroids

the most commonly used form of hormone therapy, has both glucocorticoid and mineralocorticoid properties. The dosage is increased in stressful situations to prevent addisonian crisis. Mineralocorticoids are replaced with fludrocortisone. Women need androgen replacement with dehydroepiandrosterone (DHEA) as their only source of androgen production is the adrenal glands.[25] Increased salt is added to the diet.

Addisonian crisis is a life-threatening emergency requiring aggressive management. Treatment is directed toward shock management and high-dose hydrocortisone replacement. Large volumes of 0.9% saline solution and 5% dextrose are given to reverse hypotension and electrolyte imbalances until BP returns to normal.

## NURSING MANAGEMENT: ADDISON'S DISEASE

### Nursing Implementation

**Acute Care.** When the patient with Addison's disease is hospitalized, nursing management focuses on monitoring the patient while correcting fluid and electrolyte balance. Assess vital signs and neurologic status. Monitor for signs of fluid volume deficit and electrolyte imbalance. Obtain a daily weight and keep an accurate intake and output record. Take a complete medication history to determine drugs that can potentially interact with corticosteroids. These drugs include oral hypoglycemics, cardiac glycosides, oral contraceptives, anticoagulants, and NSAIDs.

Note changes in BP, weight gain, weakness, or other manifestations of Cushing syndrome. Guard the patient against exposure to infection and assist with daily hygiene. Protect the patient from noise, light, and environmental temperature extremes. The patient cannot cope with these stresses because of the inability to produce corticosteroids.

**Ambulatory Care.** As a nurse, you have an important role in the long-term management of Addison's disease. The serious nature of the disease and the need for lifelong hormone therapy necessitate a comprehensive teaching plan. Table 49-17 outlines the major areas to include in a teaching plan.

Glucocorticoids are usually given in divided doses, two thirds in the morning and one third in the afternoon. Mineralocorticoids are given once daily, preferably in the morning. This schedule reflects normal circadian rhythm in endogenous hormone secretion and decreases the side effects associated with corticosteroid therapy. Teach patients using mineralocorticoid therapy (fludrocortisone) how to take their BP, increase salt intake, and report any significant changes to their HCP.

The patient with Addison's disease is unable to tolerate physical or emotional stress without additional exogenous corticosteroids. Long-term care revolves around recognizing the need for extra medication and techniques for stress management. Examples of situations requiring corticosteroid adjustment are fever, influenza, tooth extraction, and rigorous physical activity such as playing tennis on a hot day or distance running. Provide written and verbal instructions on when to change the dose. If vomiting or diarrhea occurs, as may happen with gastroenteritis, the patient should notify the HCP immediately, because electrolyte replacement and parenteral administration of cortisol may be necessary.

Teach patients the signs and symptoms of corticosteroid deficiency and excess (Cushing syndrome) and to report these signs to their HCP so that the drug dose can be adjusted. It is critical that the patient wear an identification bracelet (Medic Alert) and carry a wallet card stating the patient has Addison's disease so that appropriate therapy can be started in case of an emergency. The patient should carry an emergency kit at all times with 100 mg of IM hydrocortisone, syringes, and instructions for use. Teach the patient, caregiver, and significant others how to give an IM injection.

## CORTICOSTEROID THERAPY

Corticosteroids are effective in treating many diseases and disorders (Table 49-18). However, the long-term administration of corticosteroids at therapeutic doses often leads to serious complications and side effects (Table 49-19). For this reason, corticosteroid therapy is not recommended for minor chronic conditions. Therapy should be reserved for diseases that have a risk of death or permanent loss of function and for conditions in which short-term therapy is likely to produce remission or

**TABLE 49-18 Drug Therapy**

***Diseases/Disorders Treated With Corticosteroids***

**Hormone Therapy**
- Adrenal insufficiency
- Congenital adrenal hyperplasia

**Therapeutic Effect**

***Allergic Reactions***
- Anaphylaxis
- Bee stings
- Contact dermatitis
- Drug reactions
- Serum sickness
- Urticaria

***Connective Tissue Diseases***
- Mixed connective tissue disorders
- Polymyositis
- Polyarteritis nodosa
- Rheumatoid arthritis
- Systemic lupus erythematosus

***Neurologic Diseases***
- Prevention of cerebral edema and increased intracranial pressure
- Head trauma

***Gastrointestinal Diseases***
- Inflammatory bowel disease
- Celiac disease

***Endocrine Diseases***
- Hypercalcemia
- Hashimoto's thyroiditis
- Thyrotoxicosis

***Liver Diseases***
- Alcoholic hepatitis
- Autoimmune hepatitis

***Pulmonary Diseases***
- Aspiration pneumonia
- Asthma
- Chronic obstructive pulmonary disease

***Other Diseases or Disorders***
- Skin diseases
- Cancer, leukemia, lymphoma
- Immunosuppression
- Inflammation
- Nephrotic syndrome

**TABLE 49-19 Drug Therapy**

***Effects and Side Effects of Corticosteroids***

- Hypokalemia may develop.
- Patient is predisposed to peptic ulcer disease.
- Skeletal muscle atrophy and weakness occur.
- Mood and behavior changes may be observed.
- Glucose intolerance predisposes patient to diabetes mellitus.
- Fat from extremities is redistributed to trunk and face.
- Hypocalcemia related to anti–vitamin D effect may occur.
- Healing is delayed, with increased risk for wound dehiscence.
- Susceptibility to infection is increased. Infection develops more rapidly and spreads more widely.
- Manifestations of inflammation, including redness, tenderness, heat, swelling, and local edema, are suppressed.
- Pituitary ACTH synthesis is suppressed. Corticosteroid deficiency is likely if hormones are withdrawn abruptly. Taper corticosteroid doses.
- BP increases because of excess blood volume and potentiation of vasoconstrictor effects. Hypertension predisposes patient to heart failure.
- Protein depletion decreases bone formation, density, and strength, leading to predisposition to pathologic fractures, especially compression fractures of the vertebrae (osteoporosis).

**CHECK YOUR PRACTICE**

You are working in the outpatient clinic. Your 39-yr-old female patient is experiencing Cushing syndrome secondary to high doses of prednisone use for her severe systemic lupus erythematosus. At her office visit today, she tells you, "I looked in the mirror this morning and did not recognize the fat, ugly woman looking back at me."
- How would you respond to her?

recovery. The potential benefits of treatment must always be weighed against the risks.

A beneficial effect of corticosteroids in one situation may be a harmful one in another. For example, decreasing inflammation in arthritis is an important therapeutic effect, but increasing the risk for infection is a harmful effect. Suppressing inflammation and the immune response may help save lives in persons with anaphylaxis and in those receiving an organ transplant, but it can reactivate latent tuberculosis and greatly reduce resistance to other infections and cancers. The vasopressive effect of corticosteroids is critical in enabling a person to function in stressful situations but can produce hypertension when used for drug therapy.

**DRUG ALERT Corticosteroids**
- Teach the patient not to abruptly discontinue these drugs.
- Monitor the patient for signs of infection.
- Have patients with diabetes closely monitor blood glucose.

Patients receive corticosteroid therapy for many reasons. Detailed instruction is necessary to ensure patient adherence. When corticosteroids are used as nonreplacement therapies, they are taken once daily or once every other day. They should be taken early in the morning with food to decrease gastric irritation. Because exogenous corticosteroid administration may suppress endogenous ACTH and therefore endogenous cortisol (suppression is time and dose dependent), emphasize the danger of abruptly stopping corticosteroid therapy to patients and caregivers. Corticosteroids taken for longer than 1 week will suppress adrenal production, and oral corticosteroids must be tapered. Ensure that increased doses of corticosteroids are prescribed in acute care or home care settings in situations of physical or emotional stress.

Corticosteroid-induced osteoporosis is an important concern for patients who receive corticosteroid treatment for prolonged periods (longer than 3 months).[26] Therapies to reduce bone resorption may include increased calcium intake, vitamin D supplementation, bisphosphonates (e.g., alendronate), and a low-impact exercise program. Further instruction and interventions to minimize the side effects and complications of corticosteroid therapy are outlined in Table 49-20.

## HYPERALDOSTERONISM

**Hyperaldosteronism** (Conn's syndrome) is characterized by excessive aldosterone secretion. The main effects of aldosterone are (1) sodium retention and (2) potassium and hydrogen ion excretion. Thus the hallmark of this disease is hypertension with hypokalemic alkalosis. *Primary hyperaldosteronism* (PA) is most commonly caused by a small solitary adrenocortical adenoma. Occasionally multiple lesions are involved and are associated with bilateral adrenal hyperplasia.

PA affects women more than men and usually occurs between 30 and 50 years of age. A genetic link has been identified in some patients.[27] Up to 2% of all cases of hypertension are caused by PA. *Secondary hyperaldosteronism* occurs in response to a nonadrenal cause of elevated aldosterone levels such as renal artery stenosis, renin-secreting tumors, and chronic kidney disease.

Elevated aldosterone levels are associated with sodium retention and potassium excretion. Sodium retention leads to hypernatremia, hypertension, and headache. Edema does not usually occur because the rate of sodium excretion increases, which

**TABLE 49-20 Patient & Caregiver Teaching**

***Corticosteroid Therapy***

*Include the following instructions when teaching the patient and caregiver to manage corticosteroid therapy.*

1. Plan a diet high in protein, calcium (at least 1500 mg/day), and potassium and low in fat and concentrated simple carbohydrates, such as sugar, honey, syrups, and candy.
2. Identify measures to ensure adequate rest and sleep, such as daily naps and avoiding caffeine late in the day.
3. Develop and maintain an exercise program to help maintain bone integrity.
4. Recognize edema and ways to restrict sodium intake to <2000 mg/day if edema occurs.
5. Monitor glucose levels and recognize symptoms of hyperglycemia (e.g., polydipsia, polyuria, blurred vision). Report hyperglycemic symptoms or capillary glucose levels >120 mg/dL (10 mmol/L).
6. Notify HCP if experiencing heartburn after meals or epigastric pain that is not relieved by antacids.
7. See an eye specialist yearly to assess for cataracts.
8. Use safety measures such as getting up slowly from bed or a chair and use good lighting to avoid accidental injury.
9. Maintain good hygiene practices and avoid contact with persons with colds or other contagious illnesses to prevent infection.
10. Inform all HCPs about long-term corticosteroid use.
11. Recognize need for increased doses of corticosteroids in times of physical and emotional stress.
12. Never abruptly stop the corticosteroids because this could lead to addisonian crisis and possibly death.

prevents more severe sodium retention. Potassium wasting leads to hypokalemia, which causes generalized muscle weakness, fatigue, cardiac dysrhythmias, glucose intolerance, and metabolic alkalosis that may lead to tetany.

Hyperaldosteronism should be suspected in hypertensive patients with hypokalemia who are not being treated with diuretics. PA is associated with elevated plasma aldosterone levels, elevated sodium levels, decreased serum potassium levels, and decreased plasma renin activity. A CT scan or MRI can detect an adenoma.[27] If a tumor is not found, plasma 18-hydroxycorticosterone is measured after overnight bed rest. A level greater than 50 ng/dL indicates an adenoma.

## NURSING AND INTERPROFESSIONAL MANAGEMENT: PRIMARY HYPERALDOSTERONISM

The preferred treatment for PA is surgical removal of the adenoma (adrenalectomy). A laparoscopic approach is most often used. Before surgery, patients should be treated with potassium-sparing diuretics (spironolactone [Aldactone], eplerenone [Inspra]) and antihypertensive agents to normalize serum potassium levels and BP. Spironolactone and eplerenone block the binding of aldosterone to the mineralocorticoid receptor in the terminal distal tubules and collecting ducts of the kidney, thus increasing sodium and water excretion and potassium retention. Oral potassium supplements and sodium restrictions may be necessary. However, potassium supplementation and a potassium-sparing diuretic should not be started simultaneously because of the danger of hyperkalemia. Teach patients taking eplerenone to avoid grapefruit juice as it may increase potential for hyperkalemia.

Patients with bilateral adrenal hyperplasia are treated with a potassium-sparing diuretic (e.g., spironolactone) or aminoglutethimide, which blocks aldosterone synthesis. Calcium channel blockers may be used to control BP. Dexamethasone may be used to decrease adrenal hyperplasia.

Nursing care includes careful assessment of fluid and electrolyte balance (especially potassium) and cardiovascular status. Monitor BP frequently before and after surgery because unilateral adrenalectomy is successful in controlling hypertension in only 80% of patients with an adenoma. Tell patients receiving spironolactone about the possible side effects of gynecomastia, impotence, and menstrual disorders, as well as the signs and symptoms of hypokalemia and hyperkalemia. Teach patients how to monitor their own BP and the need for frequent monitoring. Stress the need for continued health supervision.

# DISORDERS OF ADRENAL MEDULLA

## PHEOCHROMOCYTOMA

**Pheochromocytoma** is a rare condition caused by a tumor in the adrenal medulla. It affects the chromaffin cells, resulting in an excess production of catecholamines (epinephrine, norepinephrine). The most dangerous immediate effect of the disease is severe hypertension. If left untreated, it may lead to encephalopathy, diabetes mellitus, cardiomyopathy, multiple organ failure, and death. It is most commonly seen in young to middle-aged adults. Pheochromocytoma may be inherited in persons with multiple endocrine neoplasia.[28]

The most striking clinical features of pheochromocytoma are severe, episodic hypertension accompanied by severe, pounding headache; tachycardia with palpitations; profuse sweating; and unexplained abdominal or chest pain. Attacks can be induced by direct trauma, mechanical pressure to the tumor, stress (e.g., surgery, exercise, defecation, sexual intercourse, alcohol consumption, smoking), or many medications, including antihypertensives, opioids, radiologic contrast media, and tricyclic antidepressants. Attacks can last from a few minutes to several hours.

The simplest and most reliable diagnostic test for pheochromocytoma is measurement of urinary fractionated metanephrines (catecholamine metabolites) and fractionated catecholamines and creatinine, usually done as a 24-hour urine collection. Values are elevated in at least 95% of persons with pheochromocytoma. Serum catecholamines may be elevated during an "attack." CT scans and MRI can detect tumors. Avoid palpating the abdomen of a patient with suspected pheochromocytoma, since it may cause the sudden release of catecholamines and severe hypertension.

## NURSING AND INTERPROFESSIONAL MANAGEMENT: PHEOCHROMOCYTOMA

The primary treatment is surgical removal of the tumor. Treatment with α- and β-adrenergic receptor blockers is required preoperatively to control BP and prevent an intraoperative hypertensive crisis. Therapy begins with an α-adrenergic receptor blocker (e.g., doxazosin, prazosin, phenoxybenzamine) 10 to 14 days preoperatively to reduce BP.[28] After adequate α-adrenergic blockade, β-adrenergic receptor blockers (e.g., propranolol) are used to decrease tachycardia and dysrhythmias. If β-blockers are started too early, unopposed α-adrenergic stimulation can precipitate a hypertensive crisis. Therapy can cause orthostatic hypotension. Advise the patient to make postural changes cautiously.

Surgery is usually done using a laparoscopic approach. Removing the adrenal tumor usually cures the hypertension, but hypertension persists in about 10% to 30% of patients. If surgery is not an option, metyrosine (Demser) is used to decrease catecholamine production by the tumor.

Case finding is an important nursing role. Although pheochromocytoma is associated with a number of symptoms, the diagnosis is often missed. Any patient with hypertension accompanied by symptoms of sympathoadrenal stimulation should be referred to an HCP for definitive diagnosis. Assess the patient for the classic triad of symptoms of pheochromocytoma: severe pounding headache, tachycardia, and profuse sweating. Monitor the BP immediately if the patient is experiencing an "attack."

Make the patient as comfortable as possible. Monitor blood glucose levels to assess for diabetes mellitus. Patients need rest, nourishing food, and emotional support during this period. Preoperative and postoperative care is similar to that for any patient undergoing adrenalectomy. Note that BP fluctuations from catecholamine excesses tend to be severe and must be carefully monitored. Emphasize the importance of follow-up and routine BP monitoring because hypertension may persist even when the tumor is removed.

## CASE STUDY

### *Graves' Disease*

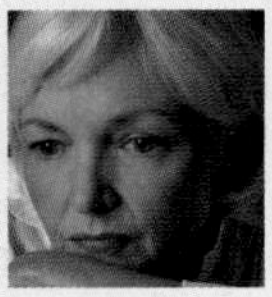

(©Hemera Technologies/ AbleStock.com/ Thinkstock)

#### Patient Profile

R.D., a 52-yr-old white woman, was admitted to the hospital with a high fever. Unable to find a source of infection, the HCP does an endocrine workup. R.D. is diagnosed with Graves' disease.

#### Subjective Data

- Reports recent job loss because she is no longer able to tolerate work-related stress
- Reports symptoms including fatigue, unintentional weight loss, insomnia, palpitations, and heat intolerance

#### Objective Data

***Physical Examination***

- Fever of 104°F (40°C)
- BP of 150/80 mm Hg, pulse of 116 beats/min, and respiratory rate of 26 breaths/min
- Hot, moist skin
- Fine tremors of the hands
- 4+ deep tendon reflexes and muscle strength of 1 to 2 out of 5

#### Interprofessional Care

- Subtotal thyroidectomy planned for 2 months later
- Started on methimazole and propranolol (Inderal LA)

#### Discussion Questions

1. What is the etiology of R.D.'s symptoms?
2. What diagnostic studies were probably ordered? What would the results have been to establish the diagnosis of Graves' disease?
3. Why was surgery delayed?
4. ***Teamwork and Collaboration:*** What is the interprofessional team's top priority at this time for R.D.?
5. ***Quality Care:*** What is the expected outcome associated with drug therapy?
6. ***Priority Decision:*** What are her priority teaching needs at this time?
7. ***Patient-Centered Care:*** What teaching will you provide after surgery so that R.D. can successfully self-manage her care?
8. ***Priority Decision:*** Based on the assessment data presented, what are the priority nursing diagnoses pertinent to this patient while hospitalized? Are there any collaborative problems?
9. ***Evidence-Based Practice:*** Why is R.D. counseled to give up her long-standing cigarette smoking habit?

Answers available at *http://evolve.elsevier.com/Lewis/medsurg.*

## BRIDGE TO NCLEX EXAMINATION

The number of the question corresponds to the same-numbered outcome at the beginning of the chapter.

1. After a hypophysectomy for acromegaly, immediate postoperative nursing care should focus on
   **a.** frequent monitoring of serum and urine osmolarity.
   **b.** parenteral administration of a GH-receptor antagonist.
   **c.** keeping the patient in a recumbent position at all times.
   **d.** patient teaching regarding the need for lifelong hormone therapy.
2. A patient with a head injury develops SIADH. Manifestations the nurse would expect to find include
   **a.** hypernatremia and edema.
   **b.** muscle spasticity and hypertension.
   **c.** low urine output and hyponatremia.
   **d.** weight gain and decreased glomerular filtration rate.
3. The health care provider prescribes levothyroxine for a patient with hypothyroidism. After teaching regarding this drug, the nurse determines that further instruction is needed when the patient says
   **a.** "I can expect the medication dose may need to be adjusted."
   **b.** "I only need to take this drug until my symptoms are improved."
   **c.** "I can expect to return to normal function with the use of this drug."
   **d.** "I will report any chest pain or difficulty breathing to the doctor right away."
4. After thyroid surgery, the nurse suspects damage or removal of the parathyroid glands when the patient develops
   **a.** muscle weakness and weight loss.
   **b.** hyperthermia and severe tachycardia.
   **c.** hypertension and difficulty swallowing.
   **d.** laryngospasms and tingling in the hands and feet.

5. Important nursing intervention(s) when caring for a patient with Cushing syndrome include *(select all that apply)*
   a. restricting protein intake.
   b. monitoring blood glucose levels.
   c. observing for signs of hypotension.
   d. administering medication in equal doses.
   e. protecting patient from exposure to infection.
6. An important preoperative nursing intervention before an adrenalectomy for hyperaldosteronism is to
   a. monitor blood glucose levels.
   b. restrict fluid and sodium intake.
   c. administer potassium-sparing diuretics.
   d. advise the patient to make postural changes slowly.
7. To control the side effects of corticosteroid therapy, the nurse teaches the patient who is taking corticosteroids to
   a. increase calcium intake to 1500 mg/day.
   b. perform glucose monitoring for hypoglycemia.
   c. obtain immunizations due to high risk of infections.
   d. avoid abrupt position changes because of orthostatic hypotension.
8. The nurse teaches the patient that the *best* time to take corticosteroids for replacement purposes is
   a. once a day at bedtime.
   b. every other day on awakening.
   c. on arising and in the late afternoon.
   d. at consistent intervals every 6 to 8 hours.

1. a, 2. c, 3. b, 4. d, 5. b, e, 6. c, 7. a, 8. c

For rationales to these answers and even more NCLEX review questions, visit *http://evolve.elsevier.com/Lewis/medsurg.*

## EVOLVE WEBSITE

http://evolve.elsevier.com/Lewis/medsurg

**Review Questions (Online Only)**

**Key Points**

**Answer Keys for Questions**

- Rationales for Bridge to NCLEX Examination Questions
- Answer Guidelines for Case Study(ies) on p. 1182

**Student Case Studies**

- Patient With Addison's Disease
- Patient With Cushing Syndrome
- Patient With Hyperthyroidism

**Nursing Care Plans**

- eNursing Care Plan 49-1: Patient With Hyperthyroidism
- eNursing Care Plan 49-2: Patient With Hypothyroidism
- eNursing Care Plan 49-3: Patient With Cushing Syndrome

**Conceptual Care Map Creator**

**Audio Glossary**

**Supporting Media**

- Animation
  - Hypophysectomy

**Content Updates**

## REFERENCES


1. Kopczak A, Ulrich R, Günter KS: Advances in understanding pituitary tumors, *F1000Prime Reports* 6:2014.
2. Acromegaly. Retrieved from *www.niddk.nih.gov/health-information/health-topics/endocrine/acromegaly/Pages/fact-sheet.aspx.*
3. American Diabetes Association: Diagnosis and classification of diabetes mellitus, *Diabetes Care* 37:S81, 2014.
4. About acromegaly. Retrieved from *http://acromegaly.org/en/about/about-acromegaly.*

*5. Sarkar S, Rajaratnam S, Chacko G, et al: Endocrinological outcomes following endoscopic and microscopic transsphenoidal surgery in 113 patients with acromegaly, *Clin Neurol Neurosurg* 126:190, 2014.

*6. Brandon A, Miller A, Ioachimescu N, et al: Contemporary indications for transsphenoidal pituitary surgery, *World Neurosurg* 82:S147, 2014.

*7. Gittleman H, Ostrom Q, Farah P, et al: Descriptive epidemiology of pituitary tumors in the United States 2004-2009, *J Neurosurg* 121:527, 2014.

*8. Thomas J, Gadgil N, Samson S, et al: Prospective trial of a short hospital stay protocol after endoscopic endonasal pituitary adenoma surgery, *World Neurosurg* 81:576, 2014.

9. Braun M, Barstow C, Pyzocha N: Diagnosis and management of sodium disorders: hyponatremia and hypernatremia, *Am Fam Physician* 91:299, 2015.

*10. Zimmermann M, Boelaert K: Iodine deficiency and thyroid disorders, *Lancet Diabetes Endocrinol* 3:286, 2015.

11. Sweeney L, Stewart C, Gaitonde D: Thyroiditis: an integrated approach, *Am Fam Physician* 90:389, 2014.

*12. Lee S, Chang D, He X, et al: Urinary iodine excretion and serum thyroid function in adults after iodinated contrast administration, *Thyroid* 25:471, 2015.

13. Vaidya B, Pearce SH: Diagnosis and management of thyrotoxicosis, *BMJ* 349:5128, 2014.

*14. Chiha M: Thyroid storm: an updated review, *J Intens Care Med* 30:131, 2015.

*15. Orosco RK, Lin HW, Bhattacharyya N: Ambulatory thyroidectomy: a multistate study of revisits and complications, *Otolaryngol Head Neck Surg* 152:1017, 2015.

16. Nygaard B: Primary hypothyroidism, *Am Fam Physician* 91:359, 2015.

*17. Fliers E, Bianco A, Langouche L, et al: Endocrine and metabolic considerations in critically ill patients: thyroid function in critically ill patients, *Lancet.* Online June 11, 2015.

*18. Screening for thyroid disease: systematic evidence review. Retrieved from *www.ahrq.gov/clinic.*

19. Thyroid cancer. Retrieved from *www.cancer.org.*

20. Multiple endocrine neoplasia. Retrieved from *ghr.nlm.nih.gov/condition/multiple-endocrine-neoplasia.*

21. Michels T, Kelly K: Parathyroid disorders, *Am Fam Physician* 88:249, 2013.

*22. Lacroix A, Feelders R, Stratakis C, et al: Cushing's syndrome, *Lancet* 386:913, 2015.

*23. Raff H, Carroll T: Cushing's syndrome: from physiological principles to diagnosis and clinical care, *J Physiol* 593:493, 2015.

24. Michels A, Michels N: Addison disease: early detection and treatment principles, *Am Fam Physician* 89:563, 2014.

25. Addison's disease: adrenal insufficiency. Retrieved from *www.niddk.nih.gov/health-information/health-topics/endocrine/adrenal-insufficiency-addisons-disease/Pages/fact-sheet.aspx.*

26. Treating corticosteroid-induced bone loss. Retrieved from *www.arthritis.org/living-with-arthritis/treatments/medication/drug-types/corticosteroids/osteoporosis-bone-loss.php.*

27. Galati SJ: Primary aldosteronism: challenges in diagnosis and management, *Endocrinol Metab Clin North Am* 44:355, 2015.

28. Ahmed I, Jepegnanam C: Recognition and management of pheochromocytoma, *Anaesth Intens Care* 15:465, 2014.


*Evidence-based information for clinical practice.

50

# Assessment of Reproductive System

*Kim K. Choma*

*Happiness is not being pained in body or troubled in mind.*

***Thomas Jefferson***

http://evolve.elsevier.com/Lewis/medsurg/

## LEARNING OUTCOMES

1. Describe the structures and functions of the male and female reproductive systems.
2. Summarize the functions of the major hormones essential for the functioning of the male and female reproductive systems.
3. Explain the physiologic changes during the stages of sexual response for both a man and a woman.
4. Link the age-related changes of the male and female reproductive systems to the differences in assessment findings.
5. Obtain significant subjective and objective data related to the male and female reproductive systems and information about sexual function from a patient.
6. Perform a physical assessment of the male and female reproductive systems using the appropriate techniques.
7. Differentiate normal from common abnormal findings of a physical assessment of the male and female reproductive systems.
8. Describe the purpose, significance of results, and nursing responsibilities related to diagnostic studies of the male and female reproductive systems.

## KEY TERMS

**amenorrhea, p. 1190**
**clitoris, p. 1187**
**ductus deferens, p. 1184**
**dyspareunia, p. 1194**
**epididymis, p. 1184**
**gonads, p. 1184**
**menarche, p. 1189**
**menopause, p. 1190**
**menstrual cycle, p. 1189**
**mons pubis, p. 1187**
**nulliparous, p. 1186**
**spermatogenesis, p. 1184**

## STRUCTURES AND FUNCTIONS OF MALE AND FEMALE REPRODUCTIVE SYSTEMS

The reproductive systems of males and females consist of primary (or essential) organs and secondary (or accessory) organs. The primary reproductive organs are referred to as **gonads**. The female gonads are the ovaries; the male gonads are the testes. The main purpose of the gonads is secretion of hormones and production of gametes (ova and sperm, sex cells that unite during fertilization to form a new cell called a *zygote*). Secondary (or accessory) organs begin their maturity at puberty under the influence of sex hormones and are responsible for (1) transporting and nourishing the ova (eggs) and sperm and (2) preserving and protecting the fertilized ova. Secondary (accessory) organs are discussed in the male and female reproductive portions of this chapter.

### Male Reproductive System

The three primary roles of the male reproductive system are (1) production and transportation of sperm, (2) deposition of sperm in the female reproductive tract, and (3) secretion of hormones. The primary male reproductive organs are the testes. Secondary reproductive organs include ducts (epididymis, ductus deferens, ejaculatory duct, and urethra), sex glands (prostate gland, Cowper's glands, and seminal vesicles), and the external genitalia (scrotum and penis)[1] (Fig. 50-1).

**Testes.** The paired testes are ovoid, smooth, firm organs measuring 1.4 to 2.2 in (3.5 to 5.6 cm) long and 0.8 to 1.2 in (2 to 3 cm) wide. They are within the scrotum, which is a loose protective sac composed of a thin outer layer of skin over a tough connective tissue layer. Within the testes, coiled structures known as seminiferous tubules form *spermatozoa* (immature sperm). The process of sperm production is called **spermatogenesis**. Interstitial cells of the testes lie between the seminiferous tubules and produce the male sex hormone testosterone.

**Ducts.** Sperm formed in the seminiferous tubules move through a series of ducts. These ducts transport sperm from the testes to the outside of the body. As sperm exit the testes, they enter and pass through the epididymis, ductus deferens, ejaculatory duct, and urethra.

The **epididymis** is a comma-shaped structure located on the posterosuperior aspect of each testis within the scrotum (see Figs. 50-1 and 50-2). It is a long, tightly coiled structure that measures about 20 ft in length.[1] The epididymis transports sperm as they mature. Sperm exit the epididymis through a long, thick tube known as the **ductus deferens**.

The ductus deferens (also known as the *vas deferens*) is continuous with the epididymis within the scrotal sac. It travels

Reviewed by Courtney Reinisch, RN, DNP, APN-BC, DCC, Clinical Associate Professor, Doctoral Candidate, School of Nursing, Rutgers University, Newark, New Jersey; and Crystal Sheaves, RN, MSN, APRN, FNP-BC, Senior Lecturer, West Virginia University School of Nursing, Charleston, West Virginia.

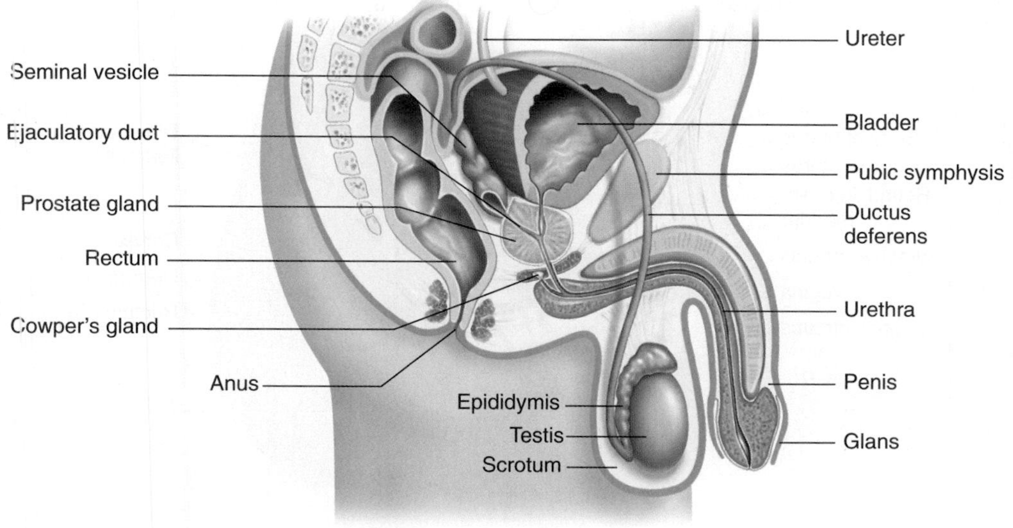


**FIG. 50-1** Male reproductive tract. (Modified from Patton KT, Thibodeau GA: *Anatomy and physiology,* ed 8, St Louis, 2013, Mosby.)

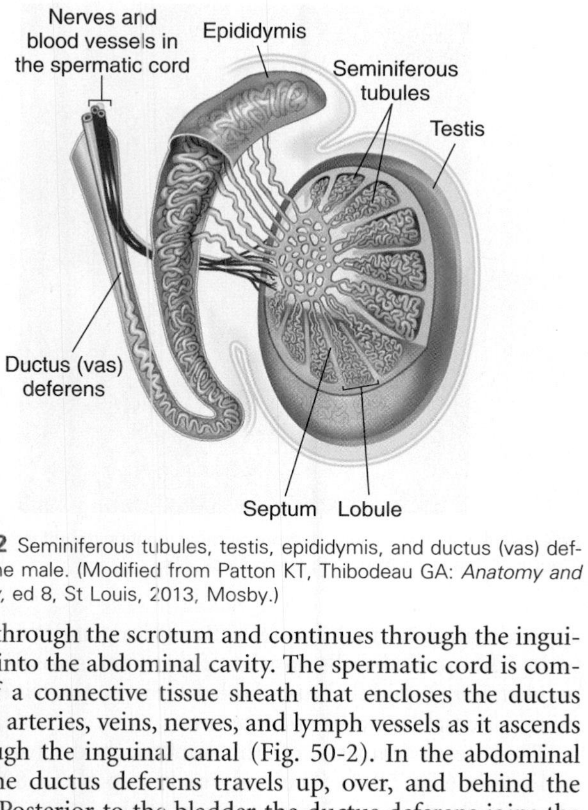


**FIG. 50-2** Seminiferous tubules, testis, epididymis, and ductus (vas) deferens in the male. (Modified from Patton KT, Thibodeau GA: *Anatomy and physiology,* ed 8, St Louis, 2013, Mosby.)

upward through the scrotum and continues through the inguinal ring into the abdominal cavity. The spermatic cord is composed of a connective tissue sheath that encloses the ductus deferens, arteries, veins, nerves, and lymph vessels as it ascends up through the inguinal canal (Fig. 50-2). In the abdominal cavity, the ductus deferens travels up, over, and behind the bladder. Posterior to the bladder the ductus deferens joins the seminal vesicle to form the ejaculatory duct (Fig. 50-1).

The ejaculatory duct passes downward through the prostate gland, connecting with the urethra. The urethra extends from the bladder, through the prostate, and ends in a slit-like opening (the meatus) on the ventral side of the *glans,* the tip of the penis. During the process of ejaculation, sperm travel through the urethra and out of the penis.

**Glands.** The seminal vesicles, prostate gland, and Cowper's (bulbourethral) glands are the accessory glands of the male reproductive system. These glands produce and secrete seminal fluid *(semen),* which surrounds the sperm and forms the *ejaculate.*

The seminal vesicles lie posterior to the bladder and between the rectum and bladder. The ducts of the seminal vesicles fuse with the ductus deferens to form the ejaculatory ducts that enter the prostate gland. The prostate gland lies beneath the bladder. Its posterior surface is in contact with the rectal wall. The prostate normally measures 0.8 in (2 cm) wide and 1.2 in (3 cm) long and is divided into the right and left lateral lobes and an anteroposterior median lobe. Cowper's glands lie on each side of the urethra and slightly posterior to it, just below the prostate. The ducts of these glands enter directly into the urethra.

Secretions from the seminal vesicles, prostate, and Cowper's glands make up most of the fluid in the ejaculate. These various secretions serve as a medium for the transport of sperm and create an alkaline, nutritious environment that promotes sperm motility and survival.

**External Genitalia.** The male external genitalia consist of the penis and scrotum. The penis consists of a shaft, and the tip is known as the *glans.* The glans is covered by a fold of skin, the prepuce (or foreskin), that forms at the junction of the glans and shaft of the penis. In circumcised males the prepuce has been removed. The shaft of the penis consists of erectile tissue composed of the corpus cavernosum, corpus spongiosum (fibrous sheath that encases the erectile tissue), and urethra. The skin covering the penis is thin, loose, and hairless.

## Female Reproductive System

The three primary roles of the female reproductive system are (1) production of ova, (2) secretion of hormones, and (3) protection and facilitation of the development of the fetus in a pregnant female. Like the male, the female has primary and secondary reproductive organs. The primary reproductive organs in the female are the paired ovaries. Secondary reproductive organs include the ducts (fallopian tubes), uterus, vagina, sex glands (Bartholin's glands and breasts), and external genitalia (vulva).

### Pelvic Organs

***Ovaries.*** The ovaries are located on either side of the uterus, just behind and below the fallopian tubes (Fig. 50-3). The almond-shaped ovaries are firm and solid, approximately 0.6 in

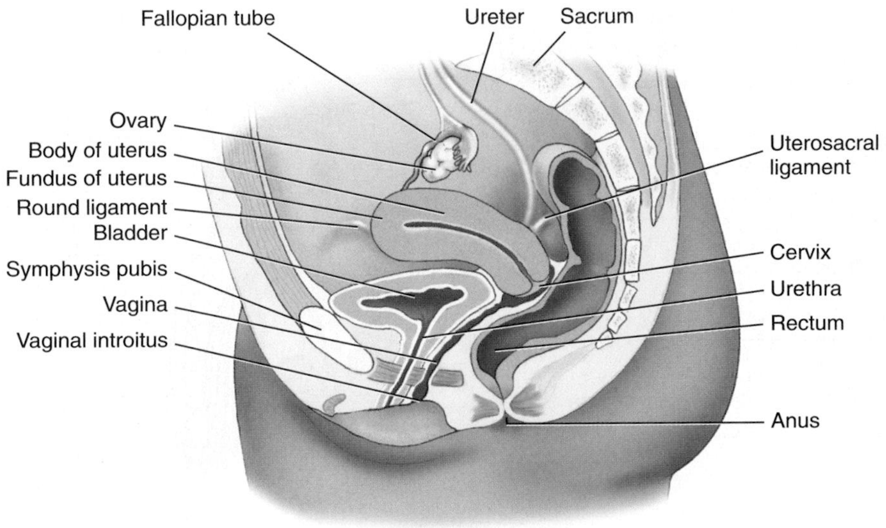


**FIG. 50-3** Female reproductive tract. (Modified from McKenry L, Tessier E, Hogan M: *Mosby's pharmacology in nursing,* St Louis, 2006, Mosby.)

(1.5 cm) wide and 1.2 in (3 cm) long. Their functions include ovulation and secretion of the two major reproductive hormones: estrogen and progesterone.

The outer zone of the ovary contains follicles with germ cells, or *oocytes.* Each follicle contains a primordial (immature) oocyte surrounded by granulosa and theca cells. These two layers protect and nourish the oocyte until the follicle reaches maturity and ovulation occurs. However, not all follicles reach maturity. In a process termed *atresia,* most of the primordial follicles become smaller and are reabsorbed by the body. Thus the number of follicles declines from 1 million at birth to approximately 400,000 at *menarche* (first menstruation). This is the female's lifetime supply of sex cells. In contrast, males produce spermatocytes throughout their reproductive life cycle. As a woman ages, both the number and quality of the oocytes decline, with fewer than 500 oocytes actually released by ovulation during the reproductive years of the normal healthy woman.[2]

***Fallopian Tubes.*** The fallopian tubes have two responsibilities: (1) transporting the ovum towards the uterus, allowing for fertilization, and (2) facilitating the passage of the ovum to the uterus for implantation. The tubes are uterine appendages that end by curling around the ovary. The distal ends of the fallopian tubes consist of fingerlike projections called *fimbriae,* which sweep the ovum from the ruptured ovarian follicle (ovulation) to the fallopian tube. The tubes, which average 4.8 in (12 cm) in length, extend from the fimbriae to the superior lateral borders of the uterus. Fertilization usually takes place within the outer one third of the fallopian tubes.[3]

Normally, each month during a woman's reproductive years, one ovarian follicle reaches maturity, and the ovum is ovulated, or expelled, from the ovary through the stimulus of the gonadotropic hormones: follicle-stimulating hormone (FSH) and luteinizing hormone (LH). The ovum then travels through a fallopian tube, where fertilization by sperm may occur (if sperm are present). An ovum can be fertilized up to 72 hours after its release.

***Uterus.*** The uterus is a pear-shaped, hollow, muscular organ located between the bladder and rectum (Fig. 50-3). In the mature **nulliparous** (never pregnant) woman, the uterus is approximately 2.4 to 3.2 in (6 to 8 cm) long and 1.6 in (4 cm) wide. The uterine walls consist of an outer serosal layer, the *perimetrium;* a middle muscular layer, the *myometrium;* and an inner mucosal layer, the *endometrium.*

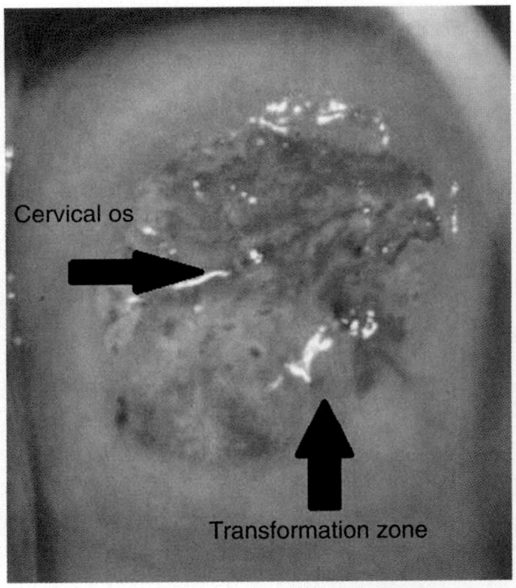


**FIG. 50-4** Cervical os and squamocolumnar junction (transformation zone). (Courtesy Candy Tedschi, NP, Great Neck, NY.)

The uterus consists of the fundus, body (or corpus), and cervix (Fig. 50-3). The body makes up about 80% of the uterus and connects with the cervix at the isthmus, or neck. The cervix is the lower portion of the uterus that projects into the anterior wall of the vaginal canal. It makes up about 15% to 20% of the uterus in the nulliparous female. The cervix consists of the *ectocervix,* the outer portion that protrudes into the vagina, and the *endocervix,* the canal in the opening of the cervix. The opening of the cervix is referred to as the *cervical os* (Fig. 50-4).

The ectocervix is covered with squamous epithelial cells, which give it a smooth, pinkish appearance. The endocervix contains a lining of columnar epithelial cells, which give it a rough, reddened appearance. The junction at which the two types of epithelial cells meet is termed the *squamocolumnar junction* or the *transformation zone* (Fig. 50-4). Cells sampled from the squamocolumnar junction are examined as part of a Papanicolaou (Pap) test, which is a critical component of cervical cancer screening.

The cervical canal is 0.8 to 1.6 in (2 to 4 cm) long and is relatively tightly closed. However, the cervix allows sperm to enter the uterus through the cervical os and also allows menses to be expelled. The columnar epithelium, under hormonal influence, provides elasticity during labor. The cervix is able to stretch to allow passage of a fetus during the birth process. The entrance of sperm into the uterus is facilitated by mucus produced by the cervix under the influence of estrogen. Under normal conditions, the cervical mucus becomes watery, stretchy, and more abundant at ovulation. The postovulatory cervical mucus, under the influence of progesterone, is thick and inhibits sperm passage.

***Vagina.*** The vagina is a tubular structure 3 to 4 in (7.6 to 10 cm) long that is lined with squamous epithelium. In reproductive-age women, the vagina has multiple transverse folds known as *rugae*. The secretions of the vagina consist of cervical mucus, desquamated epithelium, and, during sexual stimulation, a watery secretion. These fluids help protect against vaginal infection. The muscular and erectile tissue of the vaginal walls allows enough dilation and contraction to accommodate the passage of the fetus during labor, as well as penetration of the penis during intercourse. The anterior vaginal wall lies along the urethra and bladder. The posterior vaginal wall is adjacent to the rectum.

***Pelvis.*** The female pelvis consists of four bones (two pelvic bones, sacrum, coccyx) held together by several strong ligaments. The pelvis in the female has a larger diameter and is circular, whereas a male pelvis is more heart shaped. The wider female pelvis plays an important role in *parturition* (childbirth), as the fetal head adapts its position to the pelvic dimensions during labor and delivery through rotation and flexion to pass through the pelvic inlet.[4]

**External Genitalia.** The external portion of the female reproductive system (Fig. 50-5), commonly called the *vulva,* consists of the mons pubis, labia majora, labia minora, clitoris, urethral meatus, Skene's glands, vaginal introitus (opening), and Bartholin's glands.

The **mons pubis** is a fatty layer lying over the pubic bone. It is covered with coarse hair that lies in a triangular pattern. The labia majora are folds of adipose tissue that form the outer borders of the vulva. The hairless labia minora form the borders of the vaginal orifice and extend anteriorly to enclose the clitoris.

The *vestibule* is the space between the labia minora that is observed when they are held apart. It extends from the clitoris to the *posterior forchette* (a mucous membrane band that connects the posterior ends of the labia minora to the vagina). The perineum is the area between the vagina and anus. The vaginal introitus (vaginal opening) is surrounded by thin membranous tissue called the *hymen.* It is usually perforated and has many variations in shape. In the adult woman the hymen usually appears as folds or hymenal tags *(carunculae myrtiformes)* and separates the external genitalia from the vagina. At the posterior aspect of the vagina, a tense band of mucous membrane connecting the posterior ends of the labia minora is referred to as the *posterior fourchette.*

The **clitoris** is erectile tissue that becomes engorged during sexual excitation. It lies anterior to the urethral meatus and the vaginal orifice and is usually covered by the prepuce. Clitoral stimulation is an important part of sexual activity for many women.

Ducts of the Skene's glands lie alongside the urinary meatus and are thought to help lubricate the urinary meatus.[5] The Bartholin's glands, located at the posterior and lateral aspects of the vaginal orifice, secrete a thin, mucoid material believed to contribute slightly to lubrication during sexual intercourse. These glands are not usually palpable unless sebaceous-like cysts form or they are swollen in the presence of an infection, such as a sexually transmitted infection (STI).

**Breasts.** The breasts are a secondary sex characteristic that develops during puberty in response to estrogen and progesterone. Cyclic hormonal changes lead to regular changes in breast tissue to prepare it for lactation when fertilization and pregnancy occur.

The breasts extend from the second to the sixth ribs. The extension of breast tissue into the upper-outer quadrant into the axilla is an area referred to as the *tail of Spence* (Fig. 50-6). The fully mature breast is dome shaped and contains a

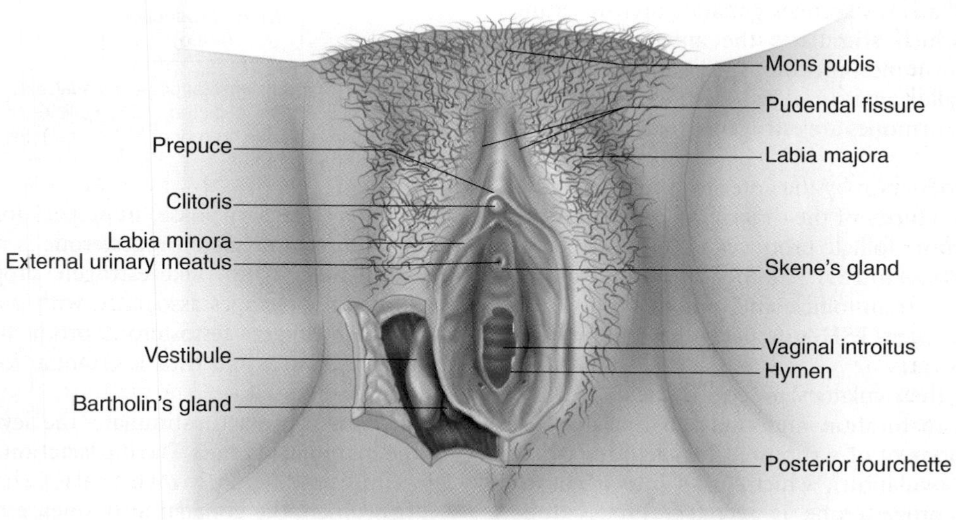


**FIG. 50-5** External female genitalia. (Modified from Patton KT, Thibodeau GA: *Anatomy and physiology,* ed 8, St Louis, 2013, Mosby.)

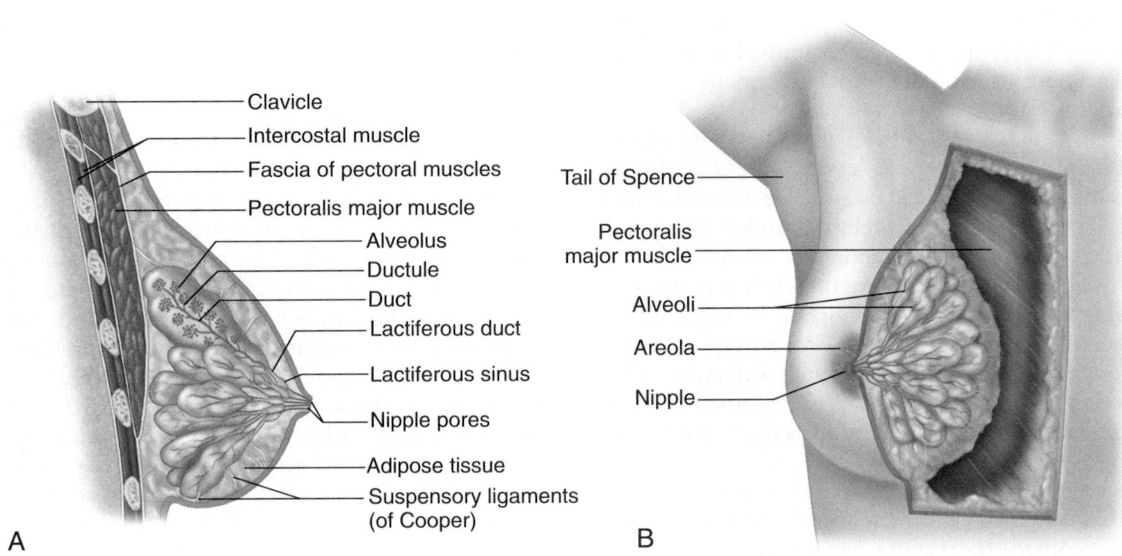


**FIG. 50-6** The lactating female breast. **A,** Glandular structures are anchored to the overlying skin and the pectoralis muscle by suspensory ligaments of Cooper. Each lobule of glandular tissue is drained by a lactiferous duct that eventually opens through the nipple. **B,** Anterior view of a lactating breast. In nonlactating breasts, glandular tissue is less evident, with adipose tissue comprising most of the breast. (Modified from Patton KT, Thibodeau GA: *Anatomy and physiology,* ed 8, St Louis, 2013, Mosby.)

pigmented center termed the *areola.* The areolar region contains Montgomery's tubercles, which are similar to sebaceous glands and assist in lubricating the nipple. During lactation, the alveoli secrete milk. The milk then flows into a ductal system and is transported to the lactiferous sinuses. The nipple contains 15 to 20 tiny openings through which the milk flows during breastfeeding. The fibrous and fatty tissue that supports and separates the channels of the mammary duct system is primarily responsible for the varying sizes and shapes of the breasts in different individuals.

## Neuroendocrine Regulation of Reproductive System

The hypothalamus, pituitary gland, and gonads secrete numerous hormones (Fig. 50-7). (Endocrine hormones are discussed in Chapter 47.) These hormones regulate the processes of ovulation, spermatogenesis (formation of sperm), and fertilization and the formation and function of the secondary sex characteristics. The hypothalamus secretes gonadotropin-releasing hormone (GnRH), which stimulates the anterior pituitary gland to secrete its hormones, including FSH and LH. LH in males is sometimes called *interstitial cell–stimulating hormone (ICSH).* The gonadal hormones are estrogen, progesterone, and testosterone.

In women, FSH production by the anterior pituitary stimulates the growth and maturity of the ovarian follicles necessary for ovulation. The mature follicle produces estrogen, which in turn suppresses the release of FSH. Another hormone, inhibin, is also secreted by the ovarian follicle and inhibits both GnRH and FSH secretion. In men, FSH stimulates the seminiferous tubules to produce sperm.

LH contributes to the ovulatory process because it causes follicles to complete maturation and undergo ovulation. It also affects the development of a ruptured follicle (area where ovum exited during ovulation), which turns into a corpus luteum from which progesterone is secreted. Progesterone plays a major role in the menstrual cycle, but most specifically in the secretory phase. It maintains the rich vascular state of

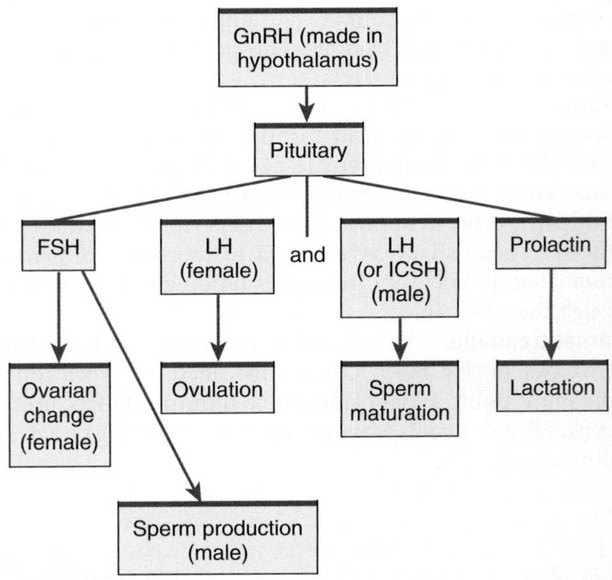


**FIG. 50-7** Hypothalamic-pituitary-gonadal axis. Only the major pituitary hormone actions are depicted. *FSH,* Follicle-stimulating hormone; *GnRH,* gonadotropin-releasing hormone; *ICSH,* interstitial cell–stimulating hormone; *LH,* luteinizing hormone.

the uterus (secretory phase) in preparation for fertilization and implantation. Adequate progesterone is necessary to maintain an implanted ovum. Like estrogen, progesterone is involved in the bodily changes associated with pregnancy. In men, LH (or ICSH) triggers testosterone production by the interstitial cells of the testes and thus is essential for the full maturation of sperm.

In women, prolactin stimulates the development and growth of the mammary glands. During lactation, it initiates and maintains milk production. In men, prolactin has no known function.

In women, the gonadal hormones, estrogen and progesterone, are produced by the ovaries. Small amounts of an estrogen precursor are also produced in the adrenal cortices. Estrogen is

**TABLE 50-1 Gonadal Feedback Mechanisms**

| |
|---|
| **Negative Feedback** |
| ***Female*** |
| ↓ Estrogen → ↑ GnRH (hypothalamus) → ↑ FSH (pituitary) → ↑ Estrogen (ovaries) |
| ***Male*** |
| ↓ Testosterone → ↑ GnRH (hypothalamus) → ↑ FSH and LH (or ICSH) (pituitary) → ↑ Testosterone (testes) |
| **Positive Feedback** |
| ↑ Estrogen → ↑ GnRH (hypothalamus) → ↑ LH (pituitary) |

*FSH,* Follicle-stimulating hormone; *GnRH,* gonadotropin-releasing hormone; *ICSH,* interstitial cell–stimulating hormone; *LH,* luteinizing hormone.

essential to the development and maintenance of the secondary sex characteristics, proliferative phase of the menstrual cycle immediately after menstruation, and uterine changes essential to pregnancy. In men, estrogen is produced predominantly in the adrenal cortices. The role and importance of estrogen in men are not well understood.

In men, the major gonadal hormone is testosterone, which is produced by the testes. Testosterone is responsible for the development and maintenance of secondary sex characteristics, as well as for adequate spermatogenesis. In women, androgens are produced in small amounts by the adrenal glands and ovaries.

The circulating levels of gonadal hormones are controlled primarily by a *negative feedback process.* Receptors within the hypothalamus and pituitary are sensitive to the circulating blood levels of the hormones (Table 50-1). Increased levels of hormones stimulate a hypothalamic response to decrease the high circulating levels. Likewise, low circulating levels provoke a hypothalamic response that increases the low circulating levels. For example, if the circulating level of testosterone in men is low, the hypothalamus is stimulated to secrete GnRH. This triggers the anterior pituitary to secrete greater amounts of FSH and LH, which in turn cause an increase in the production of testosterone. The high level of testosterone signals a decrease in the production of GnRH and thus of FSH and LH.

In women, however, there is a slight variation in the control of gonadal hormones. The circulating levels are controlled through a combination of both a negative and positive feedback system. A *negative feedback control* mechanism exists similar to that described above for men. When circulating estrogen levels are low, the hypothalamus is stimulated to increase its production of GnRH. GnRH stimulates the pituitary to secrete greater amounts of FSH and LH, resulting in higher levels of estrogen production by the ovaries. Reciprocally higher levels of circulating estrogen result in a decreasing secretion of GnRH and thus a decrease in the secretion of FSH by the pituitary.

Women also have a *positive feedback control* mechanism. Thus with increasing levels of circulating estrogen, a greater level of GnRH is produced, resulting in an increased level of LH from the pituitary. Likewise, lowered levels of estrogen result in a lowered level of LH.

## Menarche

**Menarche** is the first episode of menstrual bleeding, indicating that a girl has reached puberty. Menarche usually occurs at approximately 12 to 13 years of age but can occur as early as 10 years of age in some individuals. Menstrual cycles are often irregular for the first 1 to 2 years after menarche because of *anovulatory cycles* (cycles without ovulation).

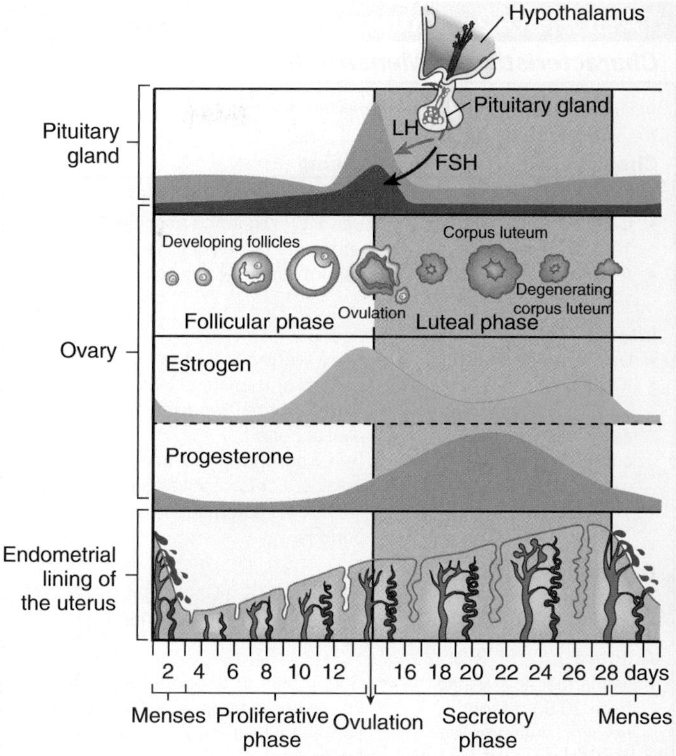


**FIG. 50-8** Events of the menstrual cycle. The lines depict the changes in blood hormone levels, the development of the follicles, and the changes in the endometrium during the cycle. *FSH,* Follicle-stimulating hormone; *LH,* luteinizing hormone. (Modified from Patton KT, Thibodeau GA: *Anatomy and physiology,* ed 8, St Louis, 2013, Mosby.)

## Menstrual Cycle

The major functions of the ovaries are ovulation and the secretion of hormones. These functions are accomplished during the normal **menstrual cycle**, a monthly process mediated by the hormonal activity of the hypothalamus, pituitary gland, and ovaries. Menstruation occurs during each month in which an ovum is not fertilized (Fig. 50-8). The endometrial cycle is divided into three phases labeled in relation to uterine and ovarian changes: (1) the *proliferative,* or *follicular, phase;* (2) the *secretory,* or *luteal, phase;* and (3) the *menstrual,* or *ischemic, phase.* The length of the menstrual cycle ranges from 21 to 35 days, with an average of 28 days.

The menstrual cycle begins on the first day of menstruation, which usually lasts 4 to 6 days. The first day of the menstrual cycle is charted as the *LMP,* or last menstrual period. Table 50-2 includes characteristics of the menstrual cycle and related teaching. During menstruation, estrogen and progesterone levels are low, but FSH levels begin to increase. During the follicular phase, a single follicle matures fully under the stimulation of FSH. (The mechanism that ensures that usually only one follicle reaches maturity is not known.) The mature follicle stimulates estrogen production, causing a negative feedback with resulting decreased FSH secretion.

Although the initial stage of follicular maturation is stimulated by FSH, complete maturation and ovulation occur only in the presence of LH. When estrogen levels peak on about the

TABLE 50-2 **Patient Teaching**

***Characteristics of Menstruation***

*Include the following information when teaching the patient about menstruation.*

| Characteristic | Teaching |
|---|---|
| **Menarche** | |
| • Occurs between ages 10 and 16 yr.<br>• Average age at onset is 12-13 yr. | • See HCP regarding possible endocrine or developmental abnormality when delayed. |
| **Interval** | |
| • Usually is 21-35 days.<br>• Regular cycles as short as 17 days or as long as 45 days are considered normal if pattern is consistent for individual. | • Keep written record to identify own pattern of menstrual cycle.<br>• Expect some irregularity in perimenopausal period.<br>• Be aware that drugs (phenothiazines, opioids, contraceptives) and stressful life events can result in missed periods. |
| **Duration** | |
| • Menstrual flow generally lasts 2-8 days. | • Realize that pattern is fairly constant but that wide variations do exist. |
| **Amount** | |
| • Menstrual flow varies from 20-80 mL per menses. Average is 30 mL.<br>• Amount varies among women and in same woman at different times.<br>• It is usually heaviest first 2 days. | • Count pads or tampons used per day.<br>• The average tampon or pad (when completely saturated) absorbs 20-30 mL.<br>• Very heavy flow is indicated by complete soaking of two pads in 1-2 hr.<br>• Flow increases and then gradually decreases in perimenopausal period.<br>• IUD or drugs such as anticoagulants and thiazides can produce heavy menses.<br>• Women with uterine fibroids may also experience increased or heavy menses. |
| **Composition** | |
| • Menstrual discharge is mixture of endometrium, blood, mucus, and vaginal cells.<br>• It is dark red and less viscous than blood and usually does not clot. | • Clots indicate heavy flow or vaginal pooling. |

*IUD,* Intrauterine device.

twelfth day of the cycle, there is a surge of LH, which triggers ovulation a day or two later. After ovulation (maturation and release of an ovum), LH promotes the development of the corpus luteum, a temporary functional cyst that forms with the ruptured follicle.

The fully developed corpus luteum continues to secrete estrogen and initiates progesterone secretion. If fertilization occurs, high levels of estrogen and progesterone continue to be secreted because of the continued activity of the corpus luteum from stimulation by human chorionic gonadotropin (hCG). If fertilization does not take place, menstruation occurs because of a decrease in estrogen production and progesterone withdrawal.

During the *follicular phase,* the endometrial lining of the uterus also undergoes change. As more estrogen is produced, the endometrial lining undergoes proliferative changes, including an increase in the length of blood vessels and glandular tissue.

With ovulation and the resulting increased levels of progesterone, the *luteal* (or *secretory*) *phase* begins. If the corpus luteum regresses (when fertilization does not occur) and estrogen and progesterone levels fall, the endometrial lining can no longer be supported. As a result, the blood vessels contract, and tissue begins to slough (fall away). This sloughing results in the menses and the start of the menstrual phase. Although most women have regular cycles, irregular cycles may occur and can be due to a variety of factors, including hormonal fluctuations, medications, or conditions such as uterine fibroids.

## Menopause

**Menopause** is the physiologic cessation of menses associated with declining ovarian function. It is usually considered complete after 1 year of **amenorrhea** (absence of menstruation). (Menopause is discussed in Chapter 53.)

## Phases of Sexual Response

The sexual response is a complex interplay of psychologic and physiologic phenomena and is influenced by a number of variables (e.g., stress, illness). The changes that occur during sexual excitement are similar for men and women. Masters and Johnson described the sexual response in terms of the excitement, plateau, orgasmic, and resolution phases.[6]

**Male Sexual Response.** The penis and urethra are essential to the transport of sperm into the vagina and cervix during intercourse. This transport is facilitated by penile erection in response to sexual stimulation during the *excitement phase.* Erection results from the filling of the large venous sinuses within the erectile tissue of the penis. In the flaccid state the sinuses hold only a small amount of blood, but during the erection stage they are congested with blood. Because the penis is richly endowed with sympathetic, parasympathetic, and pudendal nerve endings, it is readily stimulated to erection. The loose skin of the penis becomes taut as a result of the venous congestion. This erectile tautness allows for easy insertion into the vagina.

As the man reaches the *plateau phase,* the erection is maintained, and the penis increases in diameter as a result of a slight increase in vasocongestion. Testicle size also increases. Sometimes the glans penis becomes more reddish purple.

The subsequent contraction of the penile and urethral musculature during the *orgasmic phase* propels the sperm outward through the meatus. In this process, termed *ejaculation,* sperm are released into the ductus deferens during contractions. Sperm advance through the urethra, where fluids from the prostate and seminal vesicles are added to the ejaculate. The sperm continue their path through the urethra, receiving a small amount of fluid from the Cowper's glands, and are finally ejaculated through the urinary meatus. *Orgasm* is characterized by the rapid release of the vasocongestion and muscular tension (myotonia) that have developed. The rapid release of muscular tension (through rhythmic contractions) occurs primarily in the penis, prostate gland, and seminal vesicles. After ejaculation, a man enters the *resolution phase.* The penis undergoes involution, gradually returning to its unstimulated, flaccid state.

**Female Sexual Response.** The changes that occur in a woman during sexual excitation are similar to those in a man. In response to stimulation, the clitoris becomes congested and vaginal lubrication increases from secretions from the cervix, Bartholin's glands, and vaginal walls. This initial response is the excitation phase.

As excitation is maintained in the plateau phase, the vagina expands and the uterus is elevated. In the orgasmic phase, contractions occur in the uterus from the fundus to the lower uterine segment. There is a slight relaxation of the cervical os, which helps the entrance of the sperm, and rhythmic contractions of the vagina. Muscular tension is rapidly released through rhythmic contractions in the clitoris, vagina, and uterus. This phase is followed by a resolution phase, in which these organs return to their preexcitation state. However, women do not have to go through the resolution (refractory) recovery state before they can be orgasmic again. They can be multi-orgasmic without resolution between orgasms.

### Gerontologic Considerations: Effects of Aging on Reproductive Systems

With advancing age, changes occur in the male and female reproductive systems (Table 50-3). In women many of these changes are related to the altered estrogen production that is associated with menopause.[7] A reduction in circulating estrogen and other sex steroids in postmenopausal women is associated with breast and genital atrophy, reduction in bone mass, and increased rate of atherosclerosis. Vaginal dryness may occur, which can lead to urogenital atrophy and changes in the composition of vaginal *microbiome* (the aggregate of microorganisms and their genetic material in a particular environment).[8]

Testosterone levels decline in men as they age. Manifestations of hormonal decline are more gradual in men and can be physical, psychologic, or sexual. Some of the changes include an increase in prostate size and a decrease in testosterone level, sperm production, muscle tone of the scrotum, and size and firmness of the testicles. Erectile dysfunction and sexual dysfunction occur in some men as a result of these changes.

Gradual changes resulting from advancing age occur in the sexual responses of men and women. The cumulative effects of these changes, as well as the negative social attitude toward sexuality in older adults, can affect the sexual practices of older adults. Many factors affect sexuality in later life. Illness, disability, medicines, and surgeries can affect a person's ability to participate in sexual activities.

Nurses play an important role in providing accurate and unbiased information about sexuality and age. Emphasize the normalcy of sexual activity in older adults and refer them to resources that address such issues.

**TABLE 50-3 Gerontologic Assessment Differences**

***Reproductive Systems***

| Structure | Changes | Assessment Findings Abnormalities |
|---|---|---|
| **Male** | | |
| **Breasts** | Enlargement | Gynecomastia (abnormal enlargement). |
| **Penis** | Decreased subcutaneous fat | Easily retractable foreskin (if uncircumcised). Decrease in size. Fewer sustained erections. |
| **Prostate** | Benign hyperplasia | Enlargement, urinary obstruction, incontinence. |
| **Testes** | Decreased testosterone production | Decrease in size, firmness. |
| **Female** | | |
| **Breasts** | Decreased subcutaneous fat, increased fibrous tissue, decreased skin turgor | Less resilient, looser, more pendulous tissue. Decreased size. Duct around nipple may feel like stringy strand. |
| **Ovaries** | Decreased ovarian function | Nonpalpable ovaries normal postmenopause. |
| **Urethra** | Decreased muscle tone, mucosal thinning | Possible urinary tract infections, painful urination (dysuria), urgency, frequency, incontinence. |
| **Uterus** | Decreased thickness of myometrium | Uterine prolapse. |
| **Vagina** | Atrophy of tissue, decreased muscle tone, alkaline pH | Mucosa becomes pale, dry, smooth and thins. Vagina narrows and shortens. |
| **Vulva** | Decreased skin turgor | Atrophy. Decreased amount of pubic hair. Decreased size of clitoris and labia. |

## ASSESSMENT OF MALE AND FEMALE REPRODUCTIVE SYSTEMS

### Subjective Data

**Important Health Information.** In addition to general health information, elicit information specifically relating to the reproductive system. Reproduction and sexual issues are often considered extremely personal and private. Develop trust with the patient to elicit such information. A professional demeanor is important when taking a reproductive or sexual history. Be sensitive, use gender-neutral terms when asking about partners, and maintain an awareness of a patient's culture and beliefs. Begin with the least sensitive information (e.g., menstrual history) before asking questions about more sensitive issues such as sexual practices or STIs.

**CASE STUDY**

***Patient Introduction***

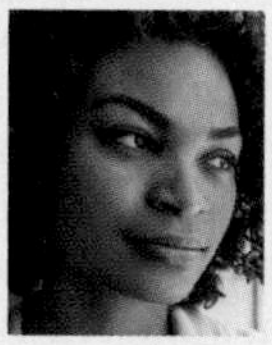

(©Benjamin A. Peterson/Mother Image/mother image/Fuse/Thinkstock)

A.K. is a 30-yr-old African American, divorced, single mother who is being evaluated for irregular and heavy menses with clots for the past several months. She has frequent migraine headaches. She takes the following medications: topiramate (Topamax) 100 mg orally once daily, sumitriptan (Imitrex) 100 mg orally PRN migraine, oral contraceptive pills orally once daily, consistent with use and timing.

**Discussion Questions**

1. What are the possible causes for A.K.'s irregular and heavy menstrual bleeding?
2. What type of assessment would you anticipate for A.K.: comprehensive? focused? emergency?

You will learn more about A.K. and her condition as you read through this assessment chapter.

(See p. 1195 for more information on A.K.)

Answers available at *http://evolve.elsevier.com/Lewis/medsurg.*

**GENDER DIFFERENCES**

***Effects of Aging on Sexual Function***

| Men | Women |
|---|---|
| • Increased stimulation necessary for erection | • Decreased vaginal lubrication |
| • Decreased force of ejaculation | • Decreased sensitivity with labia shrinking and more clitoris exposed |
| • Decreased ability to attain or sustain erection | • Difficulty in maintaining arousal |
| • Decreased size and rigidity of the penis at full erection | • Difficulty in achieving orgasm after stimulation |
| • Decreased libido and interest in sex | • Decreased libido and interest in sex |

***Past Health History.*** The past health history should include information about major illnesses, hospitalizations, immunizations, and surgeries. Inquire about any infections involving the reproductive system, including STIs. Also take a complete obstetric and gynecologic history from the female patient.

Common pediatric illnesses that affect reproductive function are mumps and rubella. The occurrence of mumps in young men has been associated with an increase in sterility. Bilateral testicular atrophy may occur secondary to mumps-related orchitis. In the health history ask male patients if they have had mumps, have been immunized with the mumps vaccine, or have any indications of sterility.

Rubella is of primary concern to women of childbearing age. If rubella occurs during the first 3 months of pregnancy, the possibility of congenital anomalies is increased. For this reason, you should encourage immunization for all women of childbearing age who have not been immunized for rubella or have not already had the disease. (Rubella immunity can be determined by antibody titers.) However, women should not be immunized if they are already pregnant.[9] Advise women to avoid becoming pregnant for 28 days after vaccination.

Question the patient regarding current health status and any acute or chronic health problems. Co-morbidities are often related to problems with the reproductive system. Chronic illnesses such as cardiovascular disease, respiratory disorders, anemia, cancer, and kidney and urinary tract disorders may affect the reproductive system and sexual functioning.

Ask questions relating to possible endocrine disorders, particularly diabetes mellitus (DM), hypothyroidism, and hyperthyroidism, because these disorders directly interfere with women's menstrual cycles and with sexual performance. Men who have DM may experience erectile dysfunction and retrograde ejaculation. In women with uncontrolled DM, pregnancy may pose significant health risks to both the woman and unborn fetus.

Determine if the patient has a history of a stroke. In men, strokes may cause physiologic or psychologic erectile dysfunction. Men who have suffered a myocardial infarction (MI) may experience erectile dysfunction because of fear that sexual activity could precipitate another MI. Post MI medication, such as β-blockers, may affect a man's ability to achieve an erection.[10] Although most patients have concerns about sexual activity after an MI, many are not comfortable expressing these fears to the nurse. Be sensitive to this concern.

***Medications.*** Document all prescription and over-the-counter medications that the patient is taking, including the reason for the medication, dosage, and length of time that the medication has been taken. Ask the patient about the use of herbal products and dietary or nutritional supplements.

Particularly relevant in the assessment of the reproductive system is the use of diuretics (sometimes prescribed for premenstrual edema), psychotropic agents (which may interfere with sexual performance), and antihypertensives (some of which may cause erectile dysfunction). Patients who use drugs such as amlodipine (Norvasc), lisinopril (Prinivil), propranolol (Inderal), and clonidine (Catapres) must be closely assessed for these problems. Also note the use of drugs such as alcohol, marijuana, barbiturates, amphetamines, or phencyclidine hydrochloride (PCP [also called "angel dust"]), which can have serious behavioral or physiologic effects on the reproductive system.

In women, document the use of hormonal contraceptives or other hormone therapy (HT). The long-term use of combined hormone therapy (specifically a combination of oral conjugated equine estrogen and a progestin called *medroxyprogesterone acetate*) appears to increase the risk of stroke, breast cancer, deep vein thrombosis, gallbladder disease, and urinary incontinence in postmenopausal women.[11] The short-term use of HT appears to be appropriate for women experiencing moderate to severe menopausal symptoms. Women who use tobacco have a much higher risk of clotting disorders. (HT is discussed in Chapter 53.)

A history of cholecystitis and hepatitis is important because these conditions may be contraindications for the use of oral contraceptives. Cholecystitis is often aggravated by oral contraceptives, and chronic active inflammation of the liver generally precludes the use of estrogen products because they are metabolized by the liver. Chronic obstructive pulmonary disease may be a contraindication to oral contraceptive use because progesterone thickens respiratory secretions.

***Surgery or Other Treatments.*** Note any surgical procedures in the health history. Examples of surgical procedures involving the female reproductive system are listed in Table 53-15. Also document any therapeutic or spontaneous abortions and type of intervention (e.g., medical versus surgical abortion).

**Functional Health Patterns.** The key questions to ask a patient with a reproductive problem are presented in Table 50-4.

***Health Perception–Health Management Pattern.*** Two of the primary focuses of a health pattern are the patient's perception of his or her own health and measures that the patient takes to maintain health. Specifically, ask about self-examination practices and screenings. Mammography (based on current guidelines [see Chapter 51]), Pap tests, and clinical breast examinations are integral to a woman's health.

Men are at risk for testicular and prostate cancer. However, controversy exists regarding the benefits of routine screening for these cancers.[12] Patients should discuss the benefits and risks of screening with their primary care provider.

**GENETIC RISK ALERT**

- Breast, ovarian, uterine, and prostate cancer have known genetic risk factors.
- Having a first-degree relative with any of these cancers significantly increases the risk of cancer for the patient.
- The risk increases if several family members have been affected with these cancers over succeeding generations.
- Individuals with a known hereditary predisposition to breast or ovarian cancer can use this information to make informed decisions about how to minimize their risks.

Family history is also an important component of this health pattern. Inquire about a history of cancer, particularly cancer of the reproductive organs. Determine if the patient has a familial tendency for diabetes mellitus, hypothyroidism, hyperthyroidism, hypertension, stroke, angina, MI, endocrine disorders, or anemia.

Assessment of the reproductive system is incomplete without knowledge of the patient's lifestyle choices. Determine whether a patient has smoked or is currently smoking, the amount (if any) of alcohol consumption, or if the patient uses illicit drugs. Risks associated with smoking include ectopic pregnancy, spontaneous abortion, an increased risk of perinatal mortality and morbidity, placental abnormalities, preterm delivery, and congenital facial defects of the fetus.[13] In addition, smoking increases the risk of morbidity and mortality in women who

## TABLE 50-4 Health History

***Reproductive System***

**Health Perception–Health Management**
- How would you describe your overall health?
- Describe the health of your family members. Any history of breast, uterine, ovarian, or prostate cancer?*

*Women*
- Do you perform self breast examination? Any concerns?
- What was the date of your last Pap test and the results?*
- Any prior abnormalities with your Pap tests?
- What was the date of your last mammogram and the results?*
- Any prior abnormalities with your mammograms?

*Men*
- Do you perform testicular self-examination? Any concerns?

**Nutritional-Metabolic**
- Describe what you usually eat and drink.
- Have you experienced any changes in weight?*
- How do you feel about your current weight?
- Do you take any nutritional supplements, such as calcium or vitamins?*
- Do you have any dietary restrictions?*

**Elimination**
- Do you experience problems with urination (e.g., pain, burning, dribbling, incontinence, frequency)?*
- Have you had bladder infections? If so, when? How often?
- Do you experience problems with bowel movements?*
- Do you experience any constipation, loose stools, or blood with stools?*
- Do you use laxatives?*

**Activity-Exercise**
- What activities do you typically do each day?
- Do you have enough energy for your desired activities?
- Can you dress yourself? Feed yourself? Walk without help?

**Sleep-Rest**
- How many hours do you typically sleep each night?
- Do you feel rested after sleep?
- Do you experience any problems associated with sleeping?*

**Cognitive-Perceptual**
- Are you able to read and write?
- Do you experience problems with dizziness?*
- Do you experience pain? If yes, where?
- Do you experience pain during sexual activity or intercourse?*

**Self-Perception–Self-Concept**
- How would you describe yourself?
- Have there been any recent changes that have made you feel differently about yourself?*
- Are you experiencing any problems that are affecting your sexuality?*

**Role-Relationship**
- Describe your living arrangements. With whom do you live?
- Do you have a significant other? If yes, is this relationship satisfying?
- Are you experiencing any role-related problems in your family?* At work?*
- What are the relationships among your family members?

**Sexuality-Reproductive**
- Are you sexually active? If so, how many partners do you have?
- What kind of sex do you engage in (e.g., oral, vaginal, anal)?
- How do you protect yourself against sexually transmitted infections and unwanted pregnancy?
- Are you satisfied with your present means of sexual expression? If not, explain.
- Have you experienced any recent changes in your sexual practices?*

*Women*
- How old were you when you had your first menstrual period? (Menarche)
- What was the first day of your last menstrual period?
- Describe your period. How many days does it last? How often does it come (for example, every 28 days)?
- Do you experience pain with your period? Do you pass clots?
- Do you feel your flow is heavy or excessive?
- How old were you when you went through menopause?
- Have you experienced any postmenopausal bleeding or spotting?*
- Pregnancy history: How many times have you been pregnant? How many living children do you have? Have you ever had any miscarriages or abortions? Did they require medical intervention?

*Men*
- Do you experience any difficulty with obtaining or sustaining an erection?

**Coping–Stress Tolerance**
- Have there been any major changes in your life within the past couple of years?*
- What is stressful in your life right now?
- How do you handle health problems when they occur?

**Value-Belief**
- What beliefs do you have about your health and illnesses?
- Do you use home remedies?*
- Is religion an important part of your life?*
- Do you think that any of your personal beliefs or values may be compromised because of your treatment?*

*If yes, describe.

use oral contraceptives. Smoking in women is also associated with early menopause.[8] Decreased sperm counts and erectile dysfunction are seen in male smokers. Finally, smoking is a known cofactor for persistence of *human papillomavirus* (HPV) infection and anogenital cancers among men and women.[14]

Document the patient's allergies, especially if the patient is allergic to sulfonamides, macrolides, cephalosporins, tetracyclines, penicillin, or latex. Sulfonamides, macrolides, cephalosporins, tetracyclines, and penicillin are used frequently in the treatment of reproductive and genitourinary problems such as STIs and urinary tract infections (UTIs). Silicone and latex are commonly used in diaphragms and condoms. An allergy to these substances precludes their use as contraceptive methods.

***Nutritional-Metabolic Pattern.*** Anemia is a common problem in women in their reproductive years, particularly during pregnancy and the postpartum period. Evaluate the adequacy of the diet with this condition in mind. Iron deficiency anemia is the most common cause of anemia in menstruating females.

Take a thorough nutritional and psychologic history to assess for the presence of an eating disorder. Anorexia nervosa can cause amenorrhea and subsequent problems, such as osteoporosis, that are related to menopause. Obesity can be related to polycystic ovarian syndrome and may be a precursor to type 2 DM.

From early adolescence, counsel women regarding adequate calcium and vitamin D intake to prevent osteoporosis. Estimate the patient's daily calcium intake to determine whether supplementation is needed. Evaluate folic acid intake for women in their reproductive years because a deficiency can result in spina bifida and other neural tube defects in the fetus.[15]

***Elimination Pattern.*** Many gynecologic problems can result in genitourinary problems. Urinary incontinence is common in older women. Factors associated with female incontinence include relaxation of the pelvic musculature caused by multiple births, advancing age, fibroid tumors, DM, obesity, and weight gain. Use of condoms, diaphragms, and spermicides is associated with an increased risk of UTIs. In addition, vaginal infections such as bacterial vaginosis (BV) can facilitate the growth of *Escherichia coli,* which causes the majority of UTIs.[16] Men may suffer from urethritis, an inflammation of the urethra, which may be caused by an STI. Urethritis can cause painful urination. Benign prostatic hyperplasia (BPH) is a common problem of older men. It can alter normal urination by causing retention or difficulty in initiating the urinary stream.

***Activity-Exercise Pattern.*** Record the amount, type, and intensity of activity and exercise. Lack of weight-bearing exercise is an important factor in the development of osteoporosis, especially in postmenopausal women. Adolescent females who engage in excessive leanness sports may experience *female athlete triad,* characterized by secondary amenorrhea, low energy availability, and osteoporosis.[17] Anemia can result in fatigue and activity intolerance and interfere with satisfactory performance of activities of daily living.

***Sleep-Rest Pattern.*** Sleep patterns for women may be affected during the postpartum period and also while raising young children. Hot flashes and sweating that are often present during perimenopause can cause serious sleep interruption when the woman awakens in a drenching sweat. The need to change her nightgown and bedding further disrupts her sleep. Insomnia is also a common complaint of perimenopausal women. Daytime fatigue often results from such sleep disruptions. In men, sleep disturbances may be caused by frequent urination at night associated with prostate enlargement or hormone therapy for prostate cancer.

***Cognitive-Perceptual Pattern.*** Pelvic pain is associated with various gynecologic disorders such as pelvic inflammatory disease, ovarian cysts, and endometriosis. **Dyspareunia** (painful intercourse) can be particularly problematic for women in the postmenopausal period. The pain associated with intercourse can create a reluctance to participate in sexual activity and strain relationships with sexual partners. Refer women with dyspareunia to their HCPs.

***Self-Perception–Self-Concept Pattern.*** Changes that occur with aging, such as pendulous breasts and vaginal dryness in women and decreased size of the penis in men, may lead to emotional distress. The subtle changes associated with sexuality and advancing age may alter the self-concept of many persons.

***Role-Relationship Pattern.*** Obtain information regarding the family structure and occupation. Question the patient regarding recent changes in work-related relationships or family conflict. Determine the patient's role in the family as a starting point to determine family dynamics.

Roles and relationships are affected by changes within the family. The addition of a new baby may change family dynamics. Role-relationship patterns change as children begin their careers and move away from home. Another change occurs when people lose their jobs at midlife or retire.

***Sexuality-Reproductive Pattern.*** The extent and depth of the interview about a patient's sexuality depend primarily on the interviewer's expertise and on the patient's needs and willingness to discuss the topic. Before taking a sexual history, assess your comfort with your own sexuality, because any discomfort in questioning becomes obvious to the patient. Carry out interviews in an environment that provides reassurance, confidentiality, and a nonjudgmental attitude. Begin with the least sensitive areas of questioning and then move to more sensitive areas.

For women, obtain a menstrual and a chronologic obstetric history. The menstrual history includes the first day of the last menstrual period, description of menstrual flow, age of menarche, and, if applicable, age at menopause. Menstrual history data are used in the detection of pregnancy, infertility, and numerous other gynecologic problems. Have the patient explicitly describe changes in her usual menstrual pattern to determine whether the change is transient and unimportant or connected with a more serious gynecologic problem. Terminology that describes abnormal uterine bleeding patterns is discussed in Chapter 53.

Identify changes in menstrual patterns associated with the use of contraceptive pills, intrauterine devices (IUDs), birth control patches, vaginal rings, progestin-only implants, or medroxyprogesterone injections. Contraceptive pills usually decrease the amount and duration of flow, whereas some intrauterine devices can increase menstrual flow.[18] Some IUDs may be used for both contraception as well as a nonsurgical treatment for heavy menstrual bleeding.

The obstetric history includes the number of pregnancies, full-term births, preterm births, stillbirths, living children, and abortions (including spontaneous [miscarriage], ectopic, or induced). Document the course of each pregnancy, including the duration of each pregnancy, date of delivery, problems that may have occurred with each pregnancy, and any medical or surgical interventions that were needed.

A sexual history should include information regarding sexual activity, beliefs, and practices. Explore the (1) gender of the patient's partners (does the patient have sex with men? women? both?), (2) frequency and type of sexual activity (penile-vaginal, penile-rectal, receptive rectal, oral), (3) number of partners and protective measures against STI, and (4) contraceptive methods (if applicable). Determine the patient's knowledge of safe sexual practices. A history of multiple sex partners and unprotected sex increases the risk of contracting an STI. For a woman, this can increase the risk of pelvic inflammatory disease, which can compromise her ability to become pregnant.

Table 50-5 outlines *The 5 Ps of Sexual Health* approach for taking a sexual history that was developed by the Centers for Disease Control and Prevention. Never make an assumption about a patient's sexual orientation. Ask both men and women about their general satisfaction with their sexuality. Question the patient about sexual beliefs and practices and whether orgasm is achieved. Explore any unexplained change in sexual practices or performance. Problems of the reproductive system can cause physiologic or psychologic problems that can lead to painful intercourse, erectile dysfunction, sexual dysfunction, or infertility.

***Coping–Stress Tolerance Pattern.*** The stress related to situations such as pregnancy or menopause increases dependence on support systems. Determine whom the support people are in

**TABLE 50-5 Sexual History Format**

***The Five Ps of Taking a Sexual History****

| The 5 *Ps* | Questions |
|---|---|
| **1. Partners** | Are you currently sexually active? (yes or no)<br>• Do you have sex with men, women, or both?<br>• In the past 2 months, with how many partners have you had sex?<br>• In the past 12 months, with how many partners have you had sex? |
| **2. Practices** | To understand your risk for STIs, I need to understand the kind of sex you have had recently.<br>• Genital (penis in the vagina)<br>• Anal (penis in the anus)<br>• Oral (mouth on penis, vagina, or anus) |
| **3. Protection from STIs** | Do you and your partner(s) use any protection against STIs?<br>• What kind?<br>• How often? |
| **4. Past history of STIs** | Have you ever been diagnosed with an STI?<br>• What type?<br>• When?<br>• How were you treated? |
| **5. Prevention of pregnancy** | Are you or your partner trying to get pregnant?<br>• If not, what are you doing to prevent pregnancy? |

*This guide may need to be modified to be culturally appropriate for some patients based on culture or gender dynamics.
Adapted from *www.cdc.gov/STI/treatment/sexualhistory.pdf*.

**CASE STUDY—cont'd**

***Subjective Data***

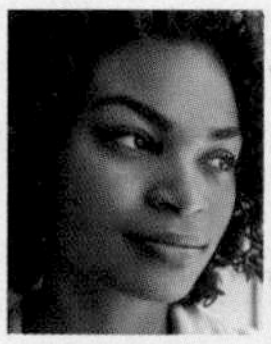

(©Benjamin A. Peterson/Mother Image/mother image/Fuse/Thinkstock)

A focused assessment of A.K. revealed the following information:

***Health Perception–Health Management:*** In good health. Last Pap smear 2 years ago was normal. Has not had any surgeries.

***Nutritional-Metabolic:*** 5′4″ 140 lb (BMI 24 kg/m$^2$)

***Elimination:*** Denies any changes with urination or bowel movements.

***Activity-Exercise:*** Exercises at gym three times a week.

***Cognitive-Perceptual:*** Denies dyspareunia.

***Self-Perception–Self Concept:*** Single mother of a 5-yr-old daughter.

***Role-Relationship:*** Divorced 3 years ago. Lives with daughter and partner. Works full time as a schoolteacher.

***Sexuality-Reproductive:*** Menarche at age 12. Last menstrual period 3 months ago. Menses every 28-30 days, lasting 5 days. Sexually active with men—four lifetime partners. In a mutually monogamous relationship of 2 years' duration. Practices vaginal and oral sex.

***Coping–Stress Tolerance:*** Denies stressors.

***Value-Belief:*** She was raised Baptist. She attends services at a local church periodically.

**Discussion Questions**

1. What assessment questions would you ask A.K.?
2. How would you individualize the assessment based on her age, ethnic/cultural background, and condition?
3. What should be included in the physical assessment?

You will learn more about physical examination of the reproductive system in the next section.

(See p. 1196 for more information on A.K.)

Answers available at *http://evolve.elsevier.com/Lewis/medsurg*.

the patient's life. The diagnosis of an STI can cause stress for the patient and partner. Explore ways to manage this stress with the patient by encouraging them to verbalize their fears and concerns.

***Value-Belief Pattern.*** Sexual and reproductive functioning is closely related to cultural, religious, moral, and ethical values. Be aware of your own beliefs in these areas, and recognize and sensitively react to the patient's personal beliefs associated with reproductive and sexuality issues.

## Objective Data

**Physical Examination: Male.** The examination of the male external genitalia by the nurse includes inspection and palpation of the pubis, penis, and scrotum. An examination may be performed with the patient lying or standing. The standing position is generally preferred. Sit in front of the standing patient. Use gloves during examination of the male genitalia.

If breast cancer is suspected or there is a strong family history of breast cancer in a male patient, a clinical breast examination is conducted in the same pattern for a male patient as a female breast examination (see Fig. 51-1).

***Pubis.*** Assess for hair distribution and presence of body lice. Normally, the hair is in a diamond-shaped pattern and coarser than scalp hair. The absence of hair is not a normal finding unless the man is shaving or waxing the pubic hair. Carefully assess the skin for irritation and inflammation.

***Penis and Scrotum.*** Inspect the penis for any lesions, bleeding, or swelling. Also note the location of the urethral meatus and the presence or absence of a foreskin. If present, the foreskin should be retracted to note any redness, discharge, irritation, lesions, or swelling from the meatus. Replace the foreskin over the glans after observation. Inspect the scrotum by lifting each testis to inspect all sides of the scrotal sac. Palpate the testes for tenderness or masses. The left testis usually hangs lower than the right. An undescended testis *(cryptorchidism)* is a major risk factor for testicular cancer and a potential cause of male infertility.[19]

***Anus.*** Note if the buttocks have any lesions, swelling, or inflammation. Spread the buttocks apart with both hands to expose the anus. Inspect the anal sphincter and perineal regions for fissures, lesions, masses, and hemorrhoids. The anus should be free from inflammation or skin changes.

**Physical Examination: Female.** With a chaperone present, physical examination of women often begins with inspection and palpation of the breasts and axillae and then proceeds to the abdomen and genitalia. Examination of the abdomen provides an opportunity to detect pain or any masses that may involve the genitourinary system. Abdominal examination is discussed in Chapter 38.

***Breasts.*** First examine the breasts by visual inspection. With the patient seated, observe the breasts for symmetry, size, shape, skin color, vascular patterns, dimpling, and unusual lesions. Ask the patient to put her arms at her sides, arms overhead, lean forward, and press hands on hips. Observe for any abnormalities during these maneuvers. Palpate the axillae and clavicular areas for enlarged lymph nodes.

After the patient assumes a supine position, place a pillow under her back on the side to be examined. Ask the patient to put her arm above and behind her head. These maneuvers flatten breast tissue and make palpation easier. Then palpate the breast in a systematic fashion, preferably using a vertical line (see Fig. 51-1). Use the distal finger pads of the index, middle, and ring fingers for palpation. Include the axillary tail of Spence in the examination. This area of the breast lies adjacent to the upper outer quadrant, which is where most breast malignancies develop (see Fig. 51-1). Finally, palpate the area around the areolae for masses. Document the color, consistency, and odor of any discharge.

***External Genitalia.*** The examination of a woman's genitalia by the nurse includes inspection and palpation of the mons pubis, vulva, and anus. Use gloves for the examination. Assess for hair distribution, presence of body lice, lesions, erythema, edema, or discharge. Many women remove hair from the genital region via shaving, waxing, or laser hair removal and may develop folliculitis (infection of the hair follicle). Separate the labia to fully inspect the clitoris, urethral meatus, and vaginal orifice. Spread the buttocks apart to inspect the anus for fissures, lesions, and hemorrhoids.

***Internal Pelvic Examination.*** This part of the examination is usually performed by clinicians with advanced or specialized training. During the speculum examination, the examiner observes the walls of the vagina and cervix for inflammation, discharge, polyps, and suspicious growths. If indicated, a Pap test and specimens for culture and microscopic examination are obtained. After the speculum examination, a bimanual examination is performed to assess the size, shape, and consistency of the uterus and ovaries. The tubes are not normally palpable.

Table 50-6 provides an example of a recording format for the physical assessment findings for the male and female reproductive systems. Tables 50-7 through 50-9 summarize assessment abnormalities of the breasts, female reproductive system, and male reproductive system, respectively.

A *focused assessment* is used to evaluate the status of previously identified reproductive problems and to monitor for signs of new problems (see Table 3-7). A focused assessment of the reproductive system is presented in the box on this page.

## CASE STUDY—cont'd

### *Objective Data: Physical Examination*

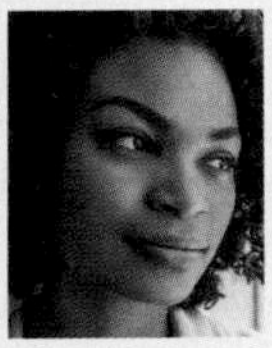

(©Benjamin A. Peterson/Mother Image/mother image/Fuse/Thinkstock)

Focused assessment of A.K. reveals the following:

BP is 118/76 mmHg; her pulse is 70 beats per minute and regular. Skin warm and dry without lesions. No cyanosis of lips, mucous membranes, or nail beds. Thyroid is not enlarged. Cardiac examination is normal. Abdomen soft and nontender. External genitalia examination is normal. Bimanual examination performed by the physician is negative for cervical motion tenderness, adnexal masses, or pain. Uterus is enlarged, approximately 14 weeks in size, and boggy.

**Discussion Questions**

1. Based on the subjective and objective assessment findings, what diagnostic tests would you anticipate being ordered for A.K.?

You will learn more about diagnostic studies related to the reproductive system in the next section.

(See p. 1202 for more information on A.K.)

Answers available at *http://evolve.elsevier.com/Lewis/medsurg.*

## DIAGNOSTIC STUDIES OF REPRODUCTIVE SYSTEMS

The most commonly used diagnostic studies in the assessment of the reproductive systems are summarized in Table 50-10. Diagnostic studies of the endocrine system may also be done in a person with a reproductive system problem (see Table 47-6).

*Text continued on p. 1202*

**TABLE 50-6 Normal Physical Assessment of Reproductive System**

| Male | Female |
|---|---|
| **Breasts** | |
| Nipples soft. No lumps, nodules, swelling, or enlarged tissue noted. | Symmetric without dimpling. Nipples soft. No drainage, retraction, or lesions noted. No masses or tenderness. No lymphadenopathy. |
| **External Genitalia** | |
| Diamond-shaped hair distribution. No penile lesions or discharge noted. Scrotum symmetric, no masses, descended testes. No inguinal hernia. | Triangular hair distribution. Genitalia dark pink, no lesions, redness, swelling, or inflammation in perineal region. No vaginal discharge noted. No tenderness with palpation of Skene's ducts and Bartholin's glands. |
| **Anus** | |
| No hemorrhoids, fissures, or lesions noted. | No hemorrhoids, fissures, or lesions noted. |

## FOCUSED ASSESSMENT

### *Reproductive System*

*Use this checklist to ensure the key assessment steps have been done.*

**Subjective**

*Ask the patient about any of the following and note responses.*

| | | |
|---|---|---|
| Vaginal or vulvar: discharge, lesions, itching, unusual bleeding, odor | Y | N |
| Penile pain, lesions, discharge | Y | N |
| Medications: oral contraceptives, antihypertensives, psychotropics, hormones | Y | N |
| Clinical examinations of reproductive systems (breast, pelvis, testicular, prostate) and results | Y | N |
| Pain: abdomen, pelvis, or genitalia | Y | N |

**Objective: Diagnostic**

*Check the following for results and critical values.*

| | |
|---|---|
| Serum hCG | ✓ |
| Serum PSA | ✓ |
| Culture and sensitivity | ✓ |
| Hormone studies (testosterone, progesterone, estrogen, FSH, LH) | ✓ |
| STI results (e.g., *Chlamydia*, gonorrhea) | ✓ |
| In office testing (e.g., wet mounts, pH assessment) | ✓ |
| Mammography and/or ultrasound of breasts | ✓ |
| Ultrasound: abdominal, pelvic, transvaginal, prostate | ✓ |

**Objective: Physical Examination**

***Inspect***

| | |
|---|---|
| External genitalia for erythema, swelling, discharge, lesions | ✓ |
| Breasts for swelling, dimpling, retraction, drainage, erythema, skin changes, masses, | ✓ |

***Palpate***

| | |
|---|---|
| Breast tissue for masses or tenderness | ✓ |
| External genitalia: tenderness, pain | ✓ |

*hCG,* Human chorionic gonadotropin; *PSA,* prostate-specific antigen; *STIs,* sexually transmitted infections.

## TABLE 50-7 Assessment Abnormalities

### *Breast*

| Finding | Description | Possible Etiology and Significance |
|---|---|---|
| **Nipple inversion or retraction** | Recent onset, erythematous, pain, unilateral. | Abscess, inflammation, cancer. |
| | Recent onset (usually within past year), unilateral presentation, lack of tenderness. | Neoplasm. |
| **Nipple secretions** | | |
| • Galactorrhea (female) | Milky, no relationship to lactation, unilateral or bilateral, intermittent or consistent presentation. | Drug therapy, particularly phenothiazines, tricyclic antidepressants, methyldopa. Hypofunction or hyperfunction of thyroid or adrenal glands. Tumors of hypothalamus or pituitary gland. Excessive estrogen. Prolonged suckling or breast foreplay. |
| • Galactorrhea (male) | Milky, bilateral presentation. | Chorioepithelioma of testes, manifestation of pituitary tumor. |
| • Purulent | Gray-green or yellow color. Frequent unilateral presentation. Association with pain, erythema, induration, nipple inversion. | Puerperal (after birth) mastitis (inflammatory condition of breast) or abscess. |
| | Same as above but usually without nipple inversion. | Infected sebaceous cyst. |
| • Serous discharge | Clear appearance, unilateral or bilateral, intermittent or consistent presentation. | Intraductal papilloma. |
| • Dark green or multicolored discharge | Thick, sticky, and frequently bilateral. | Ductal ectasia (dilation of mammary ducts). |
| • Serosanguineous or bloody drainage | Unilateral presentation. | Papillomatosis (widespread development of nipple-like growths), intraductal papilloma, carcinoma (male and female). |
| **Scaling or irritation of nipple** | Unilateral or bilateral presentation, crusting, possible ulceration. | Paget's disease, eczema, infection. |
| **Nodules, lumps, or masses** | Multiple, bilateral, well-delineated, soft or firm, mobile cysts. Pain. Premenstrual occurrence. | Fibrocystic changes. |
| | Rubbery consistency, fluid-filled interior, pain. | Ductal ectasia. |
| | Soft, mobile, well-delineated cyst, absence of pain. | Lipoma, fibroadenoma. |
| | Erythema, tenderness, induration. | Infected sebaceous cysts, abscesses. |
| | Usually singular, hard, irregularly shaped, poorly delineated, nonmobile. | Neoplasm. |
| **Dimpling of breast** | Unilateral, recent onset, no pain. | Neoplasm. |

## TABLE 50-8 Assessment Abnormalities

### *Female Reproductive System*

| Finding and Description | Possible Etiology and Significance |
|---|---|
| **Vulvar Discharge** | |
| White, thick, curdy, frequent itching and inflammation, lack of odor or yeast-like smell | Candidiasis (*Candida* or yeast infection), vaginitis |
| Thin gray or white, copious flow, malodorous or fishy, vulvar irritation | Bacterial vaginosis infection |
| Frothy green or yellow color; malodorous | *Trichomonas vaginalis* |
| Bloody discharge | *Chlamydia trachomatis* or *Neisseria gonorrhoeae* infection, menstruation, trauma, cancer |
| **Vulvar Erythema** | |
| Bright or beefy red color, itching | *Candida albicans*, allergy, chemical vaginitis |
| Reddened base, painful vesicles or ulcerations | Genital herpes |
| Macules or papules, itching | Chancroid, contact dermatitis, scabies, pediculosis |
| **Vulvar Growths** | |
| Soft, fleshy growth, nontender | Condyloma acuminatum |
| Flat and warty appearance, nontender | Condyloma latum |
| Same as either of above, possible pain | Neoplasm |
| Reddened base, vesicles, and small erosions; pain | Lymphogranuloma venereum, genital herpes, chancroid |
| Indurated, firm ulcers, no pain | Chancre (syphilis), granuloma inguinale |
| **Abdominal Pain or Tenderness** | |
| Intermittent or consistent tenderness in right or left lower quadrant | Salpingitis (infection of fallopian tube), ectopic pregnancy, ruptured ovarian cyst, PID, tubal or ovarian abscess |
| Periumbilical location, consistent occurrence | Cystitis, endometritis (inflammation of endometrium), ectopic pregnancy |

*PID,* Pelvic inflammatory disease.

## TABLE 50-9 Assessment Abnormalities

### *Male Reproductive System*

| Finding and Description | Possible Etiology and Significance |
|---|---|
| **Penile Growths or Masses** | |
| Indurated, smooth, disklike appearance. Absence of pain. Singular presentation | Chancre |
| Papular to irregularly shaped ulceration with pus, lack of induration | Chancroid |
| Ulceration with induration and nodularity | Cancer |
| Flat, wartlike nodule | Condyloma latum |
| Elevated, fleshy, moist, elongated projections with single or multiple projections | Condyloma acuminatum |
| Localized swelling with retracted, tight foreskin | Paraphimosis (inability to replace foreskin to its normal position after retraction), trauma |
| **Vesicles, Erosions, or Ulcers** | |
| Painful, erythematous base. Vesicular or small erosions | Genital herpes, balanitis (inflammation of glans penis), chancroid |
| Painless, singular, small erosion with eventual lymphadenopathy | Lymphogranuloma venereum, cancer |
| **Scrotal Masses** | |
| Localized swelling with tenderness, unilateral or bilateral presentation | Epididymitis (inflammation of epididymis), testicular torsion, orchitis (mumps) |
| Swelling, tenderness | Incarcerated hernia |
| Swelling without pain. Unilateral or bilateral presentation. Translucent, cordlike or wormlike appearance | Hydrocele (accumulation of fluid in outer covering of testes), spermatocele (firm, sperm-containing cyst of epididymis), varicocele (dilation of veins that drain testes), hematocele (accumulation of blood within scrotum) |
| Firm, nodular testes or epididymis. Frequent unilateral presentation | Tuberculosis, cancer |
| **Penile Discharge** | |
| Clear to purulent color, minimal to copious flow | Urethritis or gonorrhea, *Chlamydia trachomatis* infection, trauma |
| **Penile or Scrotal Erythema** | |
| Macules and papules | Scabies, pediculosis |
| **Inguinal Masses** | |
| Bulging unilateral presentation during straining | Inguinal hernia |
| 1- to 3-cm nodules | Lymphadenopathy |

## TABLE 50-10 Diagnostic Studies

### *Male and Female Reproductive Systems*

| Study | Description and Purpose | Nursing Responsibility |
|---|---|---|
| **Urine and Blood Studies** | | |
| **Anti-mullerian hormone (AMH)** | Measures ovarian function. Level reflects size of the remaining egg supply ("ovarian reserve"). May be done when a woman has manifestations of polycystic ovarian syndrome (PCOS). Used to monitor AMH-producing ovarian tumor.<br>Females with higher AMH have a better response to ovarian stimulation during fertility treatments.<br>Females 13-45 years: 0.9-9.5 ng/mL<br>Females >45 years: <1.0 ng/mL | *Before:* Inform patient that blood sample will be drawn.<br>*After:* Observe venipuncture site for bleeding or hematoma formation. |
| **Estradiol** | Measures ovarian function. Useful in assessing estrogen-secreting tumors and states of precocious female puberty. May be used to confirm perimenopausal status. Increased serum estradiol levels in men may be indicative of testicular tumors.<br>*Female:*<br>Follicular phase: 20-150 pg/mL (73-1285 pmol/L)<br>Luteal phase: 30-450 pg/mL (110-1652 pmol/L)<br>Postmenopause: ≤20 pg/mL (≤73 pmol/L)<br>*Male:* 10-50 pg/mL (37-184 pmol/L) | Same as above. |
| **Fluorescent treponemal antibody absorption (FTA-Abs)** | Detects antibodies to syphilis.<br>*Reference interval:* Negative or nonreactive. | Same as above. |

**TABLE 50-10 Diagnostic Studies**

***Male and Female Reproductive Systems—cont'd***

| Study | Description and Purpose | Nursing Responsibility |
|---|---|---|
| **Follicle-stimulating hormone (FSH)** | Assesses gonadal function and abnormal levels may indicate pituitary tumors or dysfunction. Increased in menopause. May be used to validate menopausal status.<br>In 24-hr urine samples:<br>*Female:*<br>Follicular phase: 2-15 U/24 hr<br>Midcycle: 8-60 U/24 hr<br>Luteal phase: 2-10 U/24 hr<br>Postmenopause: 35-100 U/24 hr<br>*Male:* 3-11 U/24 hr<br>In blood:<br>*Female:*<br>Follicular phase: 1.37-9.9 mU/mL<br>Ovulatory phase: 6.17-17.2 mU/mL<br>Luteal phase: 1.09-9.2 mU/mL<br>Postmenopause: 19.3-100.6 mU/mL<br>*Male:* 1.42-15.4 mU/mL | Same as above. |
| **Human chorionic gonadotropin (hCG)** | Detects pregnancy. Also detects hydatidiform mole and chorioepithelioma (in men and women). Can be done in urine or blood.<br>*Qualitative:* Negative<br>*Quantitative:* <5 mIU/mL (<5 IU/L) *(males and nonpregnant females)* | *Before:* Obtain menstrual history from patient, including birth control methods.<br>*During:* Urine tests can be purchased over the counter or used in HCP office. |
| **Luteinizing hormone (LH)** | Associated with ovulation in women and testosterone production in men. Particularly useful in women in the workup of infertility and menstrual irregularities.<br>*Female: Premenopause*: 5-25 IU/L<br>With higher peaks at ovulation<br>*Female: Postmenopause*: 14-52.3 IU/L<br>*Male:* 1.8-8.6 IU/L | *Before:* Inform patient that blood sample will be drawn.<br>*After:* Observe venipuncture site for bleeding or hematoma formation. |
| **Prolactin** | Detects pituitary dysfunction that can cause amenorrhea, decreased libido, and impotence.<br>*Female:* 3.8-23.2 ng/mL (3.8-23.2 mg/L)<br>*Male:* 3.0-14.7 ng/mL (3.0-14.7 mg/L) | Same as above. |
| **Progesterone** | Used to assess infertility, monitors success of drugs for infertility or the effect of treatment with progesterone, determines whether ovulation is occurring, and diagnoses problems with adrenal glands and some types of cancer.<br>*Female:*<br>Follicular phase: 15-70 ng/dL (0.5-2.2 nmol/L)<br>Luteal phase: 200-2500 ng/dL (6.4-79.5 nmol/L)<br>Postmenopause: <40 ng/dL (1.28 nmol/L)<br>*Male:* 13-97 ng/dL (0.4-3.1 nmol/L) | Same as above. |
| **Prostate-specific antigen (PSA)** | Detects prostate cancer. Also used to monitor response to therapy.<br>*Reference interval:* <4 ng/mL (<4 mcg/L) | Same as above. |
| **Rapid plasma reagin (RPR) (agglutination)** | Screening test for syphilis. Test is most sensitive during secondary stage.<br>*Reference interval:* Negative or nonreactive | Same as above. |
| **Testosterone** | Detects tumors and developmental anomalies of the testicles. Used to assess male infertility.<br>In 24-hr urine samples:<br>*Female:* 2-12 mcg/24 hr (6.9-41.6 nmol/24 hr)<br>*Male:* 40-135 mcg/24 hr (139-469 nmol/24 hr)<br>In blood:<br>*Female:* 15-70 ng/dL (0.52-2.43 nmol/L)<br>*Male:* 280-1100 ng/dL (10.4-38.17 nmol/L) | Same as above.<br>*Before:* Obtain health history to eliminate potential sources of inaccuracy of results (e.g., use of corticosteroids or barbiturates, hypo- or hyperthyroidism). In males, can also be measured in saliva. |
| **Cultures, Smears, and Nucleic Acid Amplification Tests** | | |
| **Dark-field microscopy** | Direct examination of specimen obtained from potential syphilitic lesion (chancre) is performed to detect *Treponema pallidum*. | *During:* Avoid direct skin contact with open lesion. |
| **Wet mounts** | Direct microscopic examination of specimen of vaginal discharge is performed immediately after collection. Determines presence or absence and number of *Trichomonas* organisms, bacteria, white and red blood cells, and candidal buds or hyphae. | *Before:* Explain procedure and purpose to patient. Instruct patient not to douche before examination.<br>*During:* Prepare for collection of specimens (glass slide, cover slips, 10%-20% potassium hydroxide [KOH] solution, sodium chloride [NaCl] solution, and applicators). |

*Continued*

**TABLE 50-10 Diagnostic Studies**

***Male and Female Reproductive Systems—cont'd***

| Study | Description and Purpose | Nursing Responsibility |
|---|---|---|
| **Cultures, Smears, and Nucleic Acid Amplification Tests—*cont'd*** | | |
| **Cultures** | Specimens from urine or vaginal, urethral, or cervical discharge are cultured to assess for gonorrhea or *Chlamydia* organisms. Rectal and throat cultures may also be taken, depending on data obtained from sexual history. | *Before:* Obtain specific contact and sexual history, including oral and rectal intercourse. *During:* Obtain urethral specimen from men before they void. |
| **Nucleic acid amplification test (NAAT)** | Nonculture test used to identify small amounts of DNA or RNA in test samples with sensitivity similar to culture tests. Uses ligase or polymerase chain reaction that amplifies the signal of the nucleic acids in the test sample so that they are easier to identify. Can be done on a wide variety of samples, including vaginal, endocervical, urethral, and urine specimens. Preferred method to test for gonorrhea, *Chlamydia,* and trichomoniasis. | *During:* Do not require special handling of specimens and are easier to perform than cell cultures. |
| **Gram stain** | Used for rapid detection of gonorrhea. Presence of gram-negative intracellular diplococci generally warrants treatment. Not highly accurate for women. Also a valid alternative for *Chlamydia* testing. | Same as culture. |
| **Cytologic Studies** | | |
| **Papanicolaou (Pap) test** | Microscopic study of exfoliated cervical cells to detect abnormal cells. *Conventional cytology* entails fixing cells directly to a slide at the time of collection and sending the slide to the laboratory for interpretation. In *liquid-based cytology* the specimen is sent to the laboratory in a liquid solution that preserves it and is processed for microscopic evaluation at the laboratory. Testing for human papillomavirus (HPV) may be done on specimen obtained for liquid-based Pap test (see Chapter 53). | *Before:* Obtain data about menstrual history and current hormone therapy use. Instruct women that best time to schedule examination is 10-14 days after the first day of LMP and to avoid vaginal medications, lubricants, contraceptives, or douches 2 days prior to test. |
| **Nipple discharge test** | Cytologic study of nipple discharge. | *Before:* Find out if patient is taking hormonal preparations or other drugs, is breastfeeding, or has a history of amenorrhea. Document this information. |
| **Radiologic Studies** | | |
| **Mammography** | X-ray image used to assess breast tissue. Detects benign and malignant masses. (Screening guidelines for mammography are discussed in Chapter 51.) | *Before:* Instruct patient to avoid use of deodorants, antiperspirants, powders, lotions, or creams under the arms or on breasts. Try to schedule test the week after menses when breasts are least likely to be tender. |
| **Ultrasound (US) (breast, pelvic, testicular, transvaginal [TV], rectal [TRUS])** | Measures and records high-frequency sound waves as they pass through tissues of variable density. Breast US useful in detecting fluid-filled masses and for follow-up screening after mammography in women with dense breast tissue. In women, pelvic and TV US useful to detect pelvic masses such as ectopic pregnancy, ovarian cysts, fibroids, and other pelvic masses. In men, US used to detect testicular masses and testicular torsion. Transrectal ultrasound (TRUS) is useful for diagnosing prostate tumors. | *Before:* Instruct patient that a full bladder is required for a pelvic ultrasound. |
| **Ultrasound-guided biopsy** | Use of ultrasound guidance while performing a biopsy. Ultrasound is used to direct the biopsy needle into the region of interest and obtain a sample of tissue. Removal of small tissue sample to diagnose infection, inflammation, or mass. | *Before:* Inform patient of purpose for this procedure. It is usually done as an outpatient procedure. *After:* Instruct patient to monitor for signs and symptoms of infection at biopsy site. |
| **CT scan of pelvis** | Detects tumors in the pelvis. | *Before:* Inform patient of procedure. *During:* Patient must lie still during the procedure. If IV contrast medium is used, check for iodine allergy. |
| **MRI** | Radio waves and magnetic field are used to assess soft tissue. Useful after an abnormal mammogram or in women with dense breast tissue. Breast MRI may be used in addition to mammography to detect breast cancer in women at high risk for breast cancer. Also used to diagnose abnormalities in female and male reproductive systems. | *Before:* Screen patient for metal parts and pacemaker. Inform patient the procedure is painless. Patient must lie still during the procedure. |
| **Invasive Procedures** | | |
| **Hysteroscopy** | Allows visualization of uterine lining through insertion of scope through cervix. Used mainly to diagnose and treat abnormal bleeding such as polyps and fibroids. Biopsy may be taken during procedure. May be used as part of infertility assessment. | *Before:* Explain purpose and method of procedure and that it may be done in the physician's office or an outpatient setting. Inform patient that mild cramping and slight bloody discharge after procedure is normal. |

**TABLE 50-10 Diagnostic Studies**
***Male and Female Reproductive Systems—cont'd***

| Study | Description and Purpose | Nursing Responsibility |
|---|---|---|
| **Hysterosalpingogram** | Involves instillation of contrast media through cervix into uterine cavity and subsequently through fallopian tubes. X-ray images taken to detect abnormalities of uterus and its adnexa (ovaries and tubes) as contrast progresses through them. Most useful in diagnostic assessment of fertility (e.g., to detect adhesions near ovary, abnormal uterine shape, blockage of tubal pathways). | *Before:* Inform patient about procedure and that it may be fairly uncomfortable. Contrast medium is used.<br>*After:* Inform patient she may experience slight vaginal bleeding and cramping. Monitor for foul-smelling vaginal discharge, severe pain, fever, or chills. |
| **Colposcopy** | Direct visualization of cervix with binocular microscope that allows magnification of cervix and study of cellular abnormalities. Used as follow-up for abnormal Pap test and for examination of women exposed to DES in utero. Biopsy(ies) of cervix may be taken during examination. Also used to assess for vaginal or vulvar dysplasia. | *Before:* Instruct patient about this procedure. Inform patient that this examination is similar to speculum examination. |
| **Conization** | Cone-shaped sample of squamocolumnar tissue of cervix is removed for direct study. | *Before:* Explain purpose and method of procedure and that it requires use of surgical facilities and anesthesia.<br>*After:* Instruct patient to avoid sexual intercourse and tampons for about 3-4 wk. Also discuss necessity for 3-wk follow-up. |
| **Loop electrosurgical excision procedure (LEEP)** | Excision of cervical tissue via an electrosurgical instrument. Diagnoses and treats cervical dysplasia. Minimal amount of tissue removed and preserves childbearing ability. | *Before:* Explain purpose and method of procedure and that it may be done in the physician's office. Patient may feel slight tingling or abdominal cramping during procedure.<br>*After:* Tell patient that discharge, bleeding, and cramping may occur for 1-3 days after procedure. |
| **Culdotomy, culdoscopy, and culdocentesis** | *Culdotomy* is an incision made through posterior fornix of cul-de-sac and allows visualization of peritoneal cavity (i.e., uterus, tubes, and ovaries). *Culdoscopy* can then be used to closely study these structures. This technique is valuable in fertility evaluations. Withdrawal of fluid *(culdocentesis)* allows examination of fluid. | *Before:* Explain purpose and method of procedure. Prepare patient for vaginal operation with preoperative instruction and sedation.<br>*After:* Perform assessment of bleeding and discomfort after surgery. |
| **Laparoscopy** | Allows visualization of pelvic structures via fiberoptic scopes inserted through small abdominal incisions. Instillation of $CO_2$ into cavity improves visualization. Used in diagnostic assessment of uterus, tubes, and ovaries (Fig. 50-9, on following page). Often used for tubal sterilization or part of infertility assessment. | *Before:* Instruct patient about procedure, prepare abdomen, and reassure patient about sedation. Inform patient of probability of referred shoulder pain secondary to residual air in the abdomen. |
| **Dilation and curettage (D&C)** | Operative procedure that dilates cervix and allows curetting of endometrial lining. Used in assessment of abnormal bleeding and cytologic evaluation of lining. | *Before:* Instruct patient about procedure and sedation.<br>*After:* Perform assessment of degree of bleeding (frequent pad check during first 24 hr). |
| **Fertility Studies** | | |
| **Semen analysis** | Semen is assessed for volume (2-5 mL), viscosity, sperm count (>20 million/mL), sperm motility (60% motile), and percent of abnormal sperm (60% with normal structure). | *Before:* Instruct patient that no more than 1 hr should elapse between collection and examination of sample. Do not have any sexual activity that causes ejaculation 2-3 days before the test. |
| **Basal body temperature assessment** | Measurement indirectly indicates whether ovulation has occurred. (Temperature rises at ovulation and remains elevated during secretory phase of normal menstrual cycle.) | *Before:* Instruct woman to take temperature using special basal temperature thermometer (calibrated in tenths of degrees) every morning before getting out of bed. Instruct to record temperature on graph. |
| **Hysterosalpingogram** | Same as operative procedures. | Same as operative procedures. |
| **Serum AMH, estradiol, FSH, progesterone** | Same as blood studies. | Same as blood studies. |
| **Urinary LH** | Over-the-counter "ovulation predictor kits." Identifies midcycle LH surge that precedes ovulation by 1 to 2 days. | Inform patient to follow directions carefully of specific test used. |

*DES,* Diethylstilbestrol; *IUD,* intrauterine device.

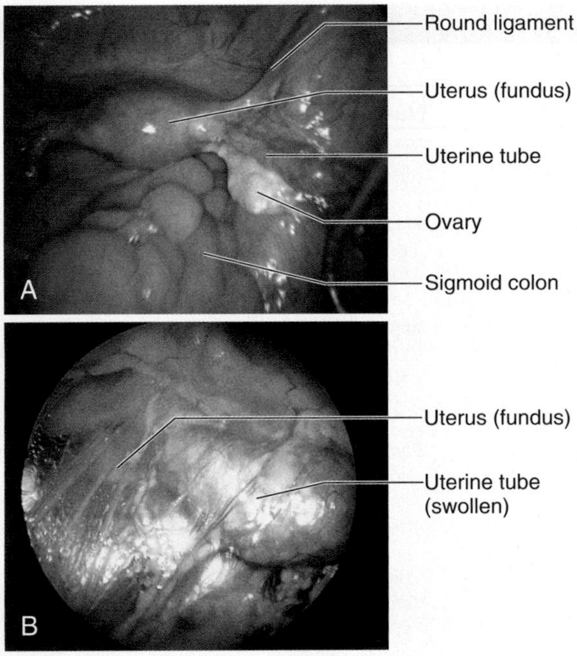


**FIG. 50-9** Laparoscopic views of the female pelvis. **A,** Normal image. **B,** Pelvic inflammatory disease. (Note reddish inflammatory membrane covering and fixing the ovary and uterus to the surrounding structures.) (*A,* From Abrahams P, Marks S, Hutching R: *McMinn's color atlas of human anatomy,* ed 5, Philadelphia, 2003, Saunders. *B,* From Symonds EM, MacPherson MB: *Color atlas of obstetrics and gynecology,* London, 1994, Mosby Wolfe.)

## CASE STUDY—cont'd

### *Objective Data: Diagnostic Studies*

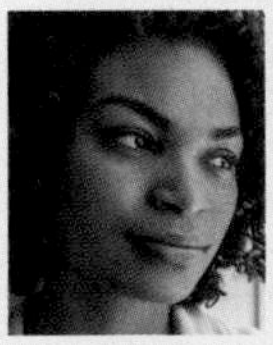

(©Benjamin A. Peterson/Mother Image/mother image/Fuse/Thinkstock)

The following laboratory and diagnostic tests are ordered for A.K.:

Urine pregnancy test, pelvic and transvaginal ultrasound, complete blood count (CBC), thyroid stimulating hormone (TSH), and iron studies.

Pregnancy test

CBC findings:

- Hemoglobin, 10.3 g/dL
- Hematocrit, 31%

Serum iron level, decreased

TSH, 2.3 IU/L

The pelvic and transvaginal ultrasound revealed a uterine fibroid. The patient is scheduled for a hysteroscopic myomectomy.

**Discussion Questions**

1. Which diagnostic and laboratory test results are of concern to you?
2. What additional patient teaching can you provide A.K. based on her diagnostic test results?

Answers available at *http://evolve.elsevier.com/Lewis/medsurg.*

## BRIDGE TO NCLEX EXAMINATION

The number of the question corresponds to the same-numbered outcome at the beginning of the chapter.

1. A normal male reproductive function that may be altered in a patient who undergoes a orchiectomy (removal of testes) is
   **a.** production of GnRH
   **b.** production of testosterone.
   **c.** production of progesterone.
   **d.** production of seminal fluid.
2. Luteinizing hormone (LH) secretion by the anterior pituitary (*select all that apply*)
   **a.** results in ovulation.
   **b.** causes follicles to complete maturation.
   **c.** affects development of ruptured follicles.
   **d.** directly inhibits both GnRH and FSH secretion.
   **e.** stimulates testosterone production by interstitial cells of testes.
3. Male orgasm is characterized by
   **a.** resolution.
   **b.** increased testicular size.
   **c.** vasodilation and dystonia.
   **d.** vasocongestion and myotonia.
4. An age-related finding during the assessment of the older woman's reproductive system is
   **a.** dyspareunia.
   **b.** vaginal atrophy.
   **c.** nipple enlargement.
   **d.** increased vulvar skin turgor.
5. Significant information about a person's health history related to the reproductive system should include *(select all that apply)*
   **a.** tobacco use.
   **b.** intellectual status.
   **c.** current pain level.
   **d.** previous history of shingles.
   **e.** previous sexually transmitted infections.
6. Cultures used in the diagnosis of STIs can be obtained from *(select all that apply)*
   **a.** urine.
   **b.** vagina.
   **c.** urethra.
   **d.** rectum.
   **e.** endocervix.
7. An abnormal finding noted during physical assessment of the male reproductive system is
   **a.** descended testes.
   **b.** symmetric scrotum.
   **c.** slight clear urethral discharge.
   **d.** the glans covered with prepuce.

8. The nurse is caring for a patient scheduled for an endometrial biopsy who is having difficulty becoming pregnant. The nurse explains to the woman that
   a. the outpatient procedure is usually done preovulation.
   b. bleeding and discharge is common 2 to 4 days after the procedure.
   c. a small sample of tissue is obtained to diagnose and treat cervical dysplasia.
   d. common changes in endometrial cells in relation to progesterone levels will be assessed.

1. b, 2. a, b, c, e, 3. d, 4. b, 5. a, c, e, 6. a, b, c, d, e, 7. c, 8. d

For rationales to these answers and even more NCLEX review questions, visit *http://evolve.elsevier.com/Lewis/medsurg.*

## ⓔ EVOLVE WEBSITE

http://evolve.elsevier.com/Lewis/medsurg

**Review Questions (Online Only)**

**Key Points**

**Answer Keys for Questions**

- Rationales for Bridge to NCLEX Examination Questions
- Answer Guidelines for the Case Study on pp. 1191, 1195, 1196, and 1202

**Conceptual Care Map Creator**

**Audio Glossary**

**Supporting Media**

- Animations
  - Ovulation
  - Reproductive System Overview
  - Spermatogenesis

**Content Updates**

## REFERENCES


1. Thibodeau GA, Patton KT: *Structure and function of the body*, ed 14, St Louis, 2012, Mosby.
2. Strauss J. Barbieri R, editors: *Yen and Jaffe's reproductive endocrinology: physiology, pathophysiology and clinical management*, ed 7, Philadelphia, 2014, Saunders.
3. Lentz GM, Lobo RA, Gerhenson DM, et al: *Comprehensive gynecology*, ed 6, Philadelphia, 2012, Saunders.
4. Singh V: *Textbook of anatomy abdomen and lower limb*, vol 2, ed 2, New Delhi, 2014, Elsevier.
5. Gynecologic cysts. Retrieved from *www.merckmanuals.com/home/womens_health_issues/noncancerous_gynecologic_abnormalities/gynecologic_cysts.html.*
6. Masters WH, Johnson E: *Human sexual response*, Boston, 1966, Little Brown. (Classic)
7. Menopause. Retrieved from *www.womenshealth.gov/menopause/index.html?from=AtoZ.*

*8. The North American Menopause Society (NAMS). *Menopause practice: a clinician's guide*, ed 5, Mayfield Heights, Ohio, 2014, NAMS.

*9. Centers for Disease Control and Prevention. Guidelines for vaccinating pregnant women. 2013. Retrieved from *www.cdc.gov/vaccines/pubs/downloads/b_preg_guide.pdf.*

10. Aging changes in the male reproductive system. Retrieved from *www.nlm.nih.gov/medlineplus/ency/article/004017.htm.*
11. The American College of Obstetricians and Gynecologists: Patient education fact sheet: hormone therapy. Retrieved from *www.acog.org/-/media/For-Patients/pfs003.pdf?dmc=1&ts=20141029T1921516354.*
12. American Cancer Society: Can prostate cancer be found early? 2014. Retrieved from *www.cancer.org/cancer/prostatecancer/detailedguide/prostate-cancer-detection.*
13. Centers for Disease Control and Prevention: 2014 Surgeon General's Report: The health consequences of smoking—50 years of progress. Retrieved from *www.surgeongeneral.gov/library/reports/50-years-of-progress/full-report.pdf.*
14. Moscicki AB, Schiffman M, Burchell A, et al: Updating the natural history of human papillomavirus and anogenital cancers, *Vaccine* 30:F24, 2012.
15. Centers for Disease Control and Prevention: Folic acid recommendations. Retrieved from *www.cdc.gov/ncbddd/folicacid/recommendations.html.*
16. Foxman B: Urinary tract infection syndromes: occurrence, recurrence, bacteriology, risk factors, and disease burden, *Infect Dis Clin North Am* 28:1, 2014.
17. Barrack MT, Ackerman KE, Gibbs JC: Update on the female athlete triad, *Curr Rev Musculoskelet Med* 6:195, 2013.
18. Hubacher D, Chen PL, Park S: Side effects from the copper IUD: Do they decrease over time? *Contraception* 79:356, 2010.
19. Viatori M: Testicular cancer, *Semin Oncol Nurs* 28:180, 2012.

*Evidence-based information for clinical practice.

51

# Breast Disorders

*Darcy Burbage*

*People grow through experience if they meet life honestly and courageously. This is how character is built.*

***Eleanor Roosevelt***

ⓔ http://evolve.elsevier.com/Lewis/medsurg/

## LEARNING OUTCOMES

1. Summarize screening guidelines for the early detection of breast cancer.
2. Describe accurate clinical breast examination techniques, including inspection and palpation.
3. Explain the types, causes, clinical manifestations, and nursing and interprofessional management of common benign breast disorders.
4. Assess the risk factors for breast cancer.
5. Describe the pathophysiology and clinical manifestations of breast cancer.
6. Describe the interprofessional care and nursing management of breast cancer.
7. Specify the physical and psychologic preoperative and postoperative aspects of nursing management for the patient undergoing breast cancer surgery.
8. Explain the indications for reconstructive breast surgery, types and complications of reconstructive breast surgery, and nursing management after reconstructive breast surgery.

## KEY TERMS

ductal ectasia, p. 1208
fibroadenoma, p. 1207
fibrocystic changes, p. 1207
galactorrhea, p. 1208
gynecomastia, p. 1208
intraductal papilloma, p. 1208
lumpectomy, p. 1213
lymphedema, p. 1214
mammoplasty, p. 1222
mastalgia, p. 1206
mastitis, p. 1206
Paget's disease, p. 1211

Breast disorders are a significant health concern for women. Whether the actual diagnosis is a benign condition or a malignancy, the initial discovery of a lump or change in the breast often triggers intense feelings of anxiety, fear, and denial.

The most frequently encountered breast disorders in women are fibrocystic changes, fibroadenoma, intraductal papilloma, ductal ectasia, and breast cancer. In a woman's lifetime, there is a 1 in 8 (12%) chance that she will be diagnosed with breast cancer.[1] Although rare, breast cancer does occur in men.

## ASSESSMENT OF BREAST DISORDERS

### Breast Cancer Screening Guidelines

Screening guidelines for the early detection of breast cancer vary depending on a woman's age and risk. For women at average risk for breast cancer, the following is recommended by the American Cancer Society:[2]

- Women should undergo regular screening mammography starting at age 45 years.
- Women aged 45 to 54 years should be screened annually.
- Women 55 years and older should transition to biennial screening or have the opportunity to continue screening annually.
- Women should continue screening mammography as long as their overall health is good and they have a life expectancy of 10 years or longer.
- The ACS does not recommend clinical breast examination for breast cancer screening among average-risk women at any age.

Women at increased risk of breast cancer (family history, genetic link, prior breast cancer, past history of thoracic radiation therapy, or certain atypical findings on a prior breast biopsy) should talk with their HCP about the benefits and limitations of starting mammography screening earlier, using breast magnetic resonance imaging (MRI), and having more frequent clinical breast examinations.[3]

Consistent breast self-examination (BSE) may facilitate breast self-awareness.[3] In recent years there has been some

Reviewed by Jane E. Lacovara, RN, MSN, CMSRN, Clinical Nurse Specialist-BC, Nursing Administration, University of Arizona Medical Center–University Campus, Tucson, Arizona; Karen Meneses, RN, PhD, FAAN, Professor and Associate Dean for Research, School of Nursing, University of Alabama at Birmingham, Birmingham, Alabama; Mary Schied, RN, MSN, OCN, CBCN, Breast Health Nurse, North Colorado Medical Center, Greeley, Colorado; Kathryn J. Trotter, DNP, CNM, FNP-C, Assistant Clinical Professor, Duke University Medical Center, Durham, North Carolina; and Deborah Kirk Walker, DNP, FNP-BC, NP-C, AOCN, Assistant Professor/Nurse Practitioner, Coordinator of Dual Adult–Gerontology Primary Care and Oncology Nurse Practitioner Specialty Track, University of Alabama at Birmingham School of Nursing, Birmingham, Alabama.

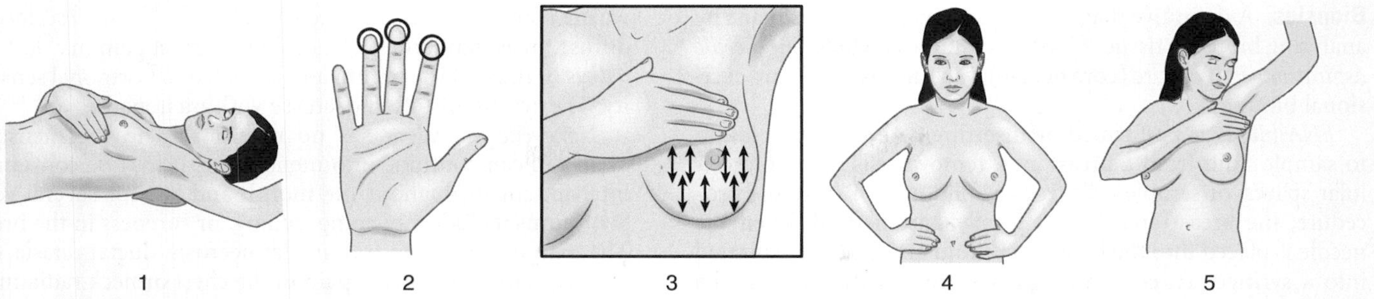


**FIG. 51-1** Breast self-examination and patient instruction. *1,* Lie down and place your left arm behind your head. Lying down spreads breast tissue evenly and thinly over the chest wall, making it easier to feel the tissue. *2,* Use finger pads of three middle fingers on your right hand to feel for lumps in left breast. Use overlapping dime-sized circular motions to feel the breast tissue. Use three different levels of pressure to feel the breast tissue: light pressure to feel tissue closest to the skin; medium pressure to feel a little deeper; and firm pressure to feel tissue closest to the chest and ribs. A firm ridge in the lower curve of each breast is normal. *3,* The up-and-down (vertical) pattern is recommended for examining the entire breast. Move around the breast in an up-and-down pattern starting at an imaginary line straight down your side from the underarm (including the tail of Spence, which is the triangular breast tissue projecting into the axilla), and moving across the breast to the middle of the sternum. Examine the entire breast going down until you feel only ribs and up to the neck or clavicle. Repeat procedure while examining your right breast. *4,* Stand in front of a mirror. Place your hands firmly on your hips, which will tighten the pectoralis muscles. Look at your breasts for size, shape, redness, scaliness, or dimpling of the breast skin or nipple. *5,* Examine each underarm while standing or sitting with arm slightly raised. Check for any lump, hard knot, or thickening of tissue. (Source: American Cancer Society: How to examine your breasts. Retrieved from *www.cancer.org/cancer/breastcancer/moreinformation/breastcancerearlydetection/breast-cancer-early-detection-acs-recs-bse.*)

controversy regarding the value of BSE and its role in reducing mortality rates from breast cancer in women. While the benefit of BSE in reducing breast cancer deaths continues to be reviewed, BSE remains a useful technique in helping women develop awareness of how their breasts normally look and feel. Teach women beginning at age 20 the benefits and limitations of BSE and the importance of reporting breast changes (e.g., nipple discharge, a lump) to their HCP.[3]

When teaching the woman about BSE, include information related to potential benefits, limitations, and harm (chance of a false-positive test result). Allow time for questions about the procedure and a return demonstration. At every periodic health examination, ask the woman who is performing BSE to demonstrate her technique. For women who choose to perform BSE, the technique is described in Fig. 51-1.

## Diagnostic Studies

**Radiologic Studies.** Several techniques can be used to screen for breast disorders or to help diagnose a suspicious physical finding. *Mammography* is a method used to visualize the breast's internal structure using x-rays (Fig. 51-2). This generally well-tolerated procedure can detect suspicious lumps that cannot be felt. Mammography has significantly improved the early and accurate detection of breast malignancies. Improved imaging technology has also reduced the radiation dose from mammography.

A comparison of current and prior mammograms may show early tissue changes. Because some tumors metastasize late, early detection by mammography allows for earlier treatment and the prevention of metastasis. In younger women, mammography is less sensitive because of the greater density of breast tissue, resulting in more false-negative results.

*Digital mammography* is a technique in which x-ray images are digitally coded and stored in a computer (Fig. 51-2). Digital mammograms are more accurate than traditional film mammography in younger women with dense breasts. The availability and associated costs of digital mammography are additional issues related to this technology.

*Three-dimensional (3D) mammography*, or tomosynthesis mammography, produces a 3D image of the breast. It provides a clearer view of overlapping breast tissue structures.

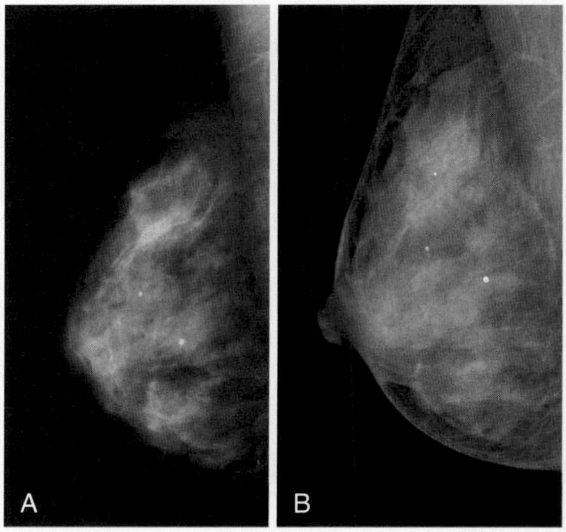


**FIG. 51-2** Screening mammogram showing dense breast tissue and benign, scattered microcalcifications of a 57-year-old. **A,** Using conventional x-rays. **B,** Using digital x-rays. (From Adam A, Dixon AK, Grainger RG, et al: *Grainger and Allison's diagnostic radiology,* ed 5, St Louis, 2008, Churchill Livingstone.)

Calcifications are the most easily recognized mammogram abnormality (Fig. 51-2). These deposits of calcium crystals form in the breast for many reasons, such as inflammation, trauma, and/or aging. Although most calcifications are benign, they may also be associated with breast cancer.

About 10% to 15% of all breast cancers cannot be seen on mammography. They can be detected by palpation or additional breast imaging studies, such as ultrasound and MRI. If the clinical findings are suspicious and the mammogram is normal, an ultrasound or MRI may be used. Based on these additional findings, a biopsy may be done.

Ultrasound is used in conjunction with mammography to differentiate a solid mass from a cystic mass, to evaluate a mass in a pregnant or lactating woman, and to locate and biopsy a suspicious lesion. MRI is recommended as a screening tool in addition to mammography for women who are at risk for breast cancer (e.g., first-degree relative with a *BRCA* mutation).[3]

**Biopsies.** A definitive diagnosis of a suspicious area is made by analyzing biopsied tissue. Biopsy techniques include *fine-needle aspiration* (FNA), core (core needle), vacuum-assisted, and excisional biopsies.

*FNA biopsy* is performed by inserting a needle into a lesion to sample fluid from a breast cyst, remove cells from intercellular spaces, or sample cells from a solid mass. Before the procedure, the breast area is first locally anesthetized. Then the needle is placed into the breast, and fluid and cells are aspirated into a syringe. Three or four passes are usually made. If the results are negative with a suspicious lesion, an additional biopsy may be necessary.

A *core (core needle) biopsy* involves removing small samples of breast tissue using a hollow "core" needle. For palpable lesions, this is accomplished by fixing the lesion with one hand and performing a needle biopsy with the other. In the case of nonpalpable lesions, *stereotactic mammography, ultrasound,* or MRI image guidance is used. Stereotactic mammography uses computers to pinpoint the exact location of a breast mass based on mammograms. With ultrasound, the radiologist or surgeon watches the needle on the ultrasound monitor to help guide it to the area of concern. Because a core biopsy removes more tissue than an FNA, it is more accurate.

*Vacuum-assisted biopsy* is a version of core biopsy that uses a vacuum technique to help collect the tissue sample. In core biopsy, several separate needle insertions are used to acquire multiple samples. During vacuum-assisted biopsy, the needle is inserted only once into the breast, and the needle can be rotated, which allows for multiple samples through a single needle insertion.

Minimally invasive breast biopsies have become the standard of care for diagnosing abnormalities found either on imaging studies or through clinical examination. However, in some cases an *excisional biopsy* is recommended. An excisional biopsy is performed in an operating room.

# BENIGN BREAST DISORDERS

## MASTALGIA

Mastalgia (breast pain) is the most common breast-related complaint in women. The most common form is *cyclic mastalgia,* which coincides with the menstrual cycle.[4] It is described as diffuse breast tenderness or heaviness. Breast pain may last 2 or 3 days or most of the month and is related to hormonal sensitivity. The symptoms often decrease with menopause.

*Noncyclic mastalgia* has no relationship to the menstrual cycle and can continue into menopause. It may be constant or intermittent throughout the month and last for several years. Symptoms include a burning, aching, or soreness in the breast. The pain may be from trauma, fat necrosis, ductal ectasia, costochrondritis, or arthritic pain in the chest or neck radiating to the breast.

For patients with mastalgia, mammography and targeted ultrasound are frequently done to exclude cancer and provide information on the etiology of mastalgia. Although evidence supporting treatments for benign breast pain have yielded conflicting results, some relief for cyclic pain may occur by reducing intake of caffeine and dietary fat; taking vitamins E, A, B complex, gamma-linolenic acid (evening primrose oil); and continually wearing a supportive bra. Compresses, ice, analgesics, and antiinflammatory drugs may also help. Prescription medication such as oral contraceptives and danazol may also be used. However, the androgenic side effects of danazol (acne, edema, hirsutism) may make this therapy unacceptable for many women.

## BREAST INFECTIONS

### Mastitis

Mastitis is an inflammatory condition of the breast that occurs most frequently in lactating women (Table 51-1). *Lactational mastitis* manifests as a localized area that is erythematous, painful, and tender to palpation. Fever is often present. The infection develops when organisms (usually staphylococci) gain access to the breast through a cracked nipple. In its early stages, mastitis can be cured with antibiotics. Breastfeeding should continue unless an abscess is forming or purulent drainage is noted. The mother may wish to use a nipple shield or to hand-express milk from the involved breast until the pain subsides. The woman should see her HCP promptly to begin a course of antibiotic therapy. Any breast that remains red, tender, and not responsive to antibiotics requires follow-up care and evaluation for inflammatory breast cancer.[5]

**TABLE 51-1 Benign Breast Disorders***

| Disorder | Risk Factors | Clinical Manifestations |
|---|---|---|
| **Lactational mastitis** | Occurs in up to 10% of postpartum lactating mothers (both primipara and multipara), usually 2-4 wk after birth. | • Warm to touch, indurated, painful, often unilateral.<br>• Most commonly caused by *Staphylococcus aureus.* |
| **Fibrocystic changes** | Most common between ages 35 and 50. | • Not usually discrete masses—nodularity instead.<br>• Usually accompanied by cyclic pain and tenderness.<br>• Mass(es) often cyclic in occurrence (movable, soft). |
| **Cysts** | Most common over age 35. Incidence decreases after menopause. Develop in 1 of every 14 women. | • Palpable fluid-filled mass (movable, soft).<br>• Multiple cysts can occur and recur.<br>• Rarely associated with breast cancer. |
| **Fibroadenoma** | Commonly occurs in 10% of all women ages 15-40. | • Palpable mass (firm, movable), usually 2-3 cm in size.<br>• Rarely associated with breast cancer. |
| **Fat necrosis** | Many women report previous history of trauma to breast. | • Usually a hard, tender, mobile, indurated mass with irregular borders. |
| **Ductal ectasia** | Perimenopausal woman—most common in women in their 50s, previous lactation, inverted nipples. | • Fixation of nipple, usually accompanied by nipple discharge of thick gray material.<br>• Often associated with breast pain. |

*This list is not inclusive; other benign breast disorders are discussed in the text.

### Lactational Breast Abscess

If lactational mastitis persists after several days of antibiotic therapy, a lactational breast abscess may have developed. In this condition, the skin may become red and edematous over the involved breast, often with a corresponding palpable mass, and the patient may have a fever. Antibiotics alone are insufficient treatment for a breast abscess. Ultrasound-guided drainage of the abscess or surgical incision and drainage are necessary. The drainage is cultured, sensitivities are obtained, and therapy with an appropriate antibiotic is begun. Breastfeeding can continue in most cases with ongoing treatment of the abscess.

## FIBROCYSTIC CHANGES

**Fibrocystic changes** in the breast are a benign condition characterized by changes in breast tissue[5,6] (Fig. 51-3). Fibrocystic changes are the most common breast disorder.

The changes include the development of excess fibrous tissue, hyperplasia of the epithelial lining of the mammary ducts, proliferation of mammary ducts, and cyst formation. Fibrocystic changes are thought to be due to a heightened responsiveness of breast tissue to circulating estrogen and progesterone. These changes produce pain related to nerve irritation (from edema in the connective tissue) and fibrosis (from pinching of the nerve).

The use of the term *fibrocystic disease* is incorrect because the cluster of problems is actually an exaggerated response to hormonal influence. The terms *fibrocystic condition* or *fibrocystic complex* are more accurate.

Fibrocystic changes alone are not associated with increased breast cancer risk. Masses or nodularities can appear in both breasts. They are often found in the upper, outer quadrants and usually occur bilaterally.

Fibrocystic changes occur most frequently in women between 35 and 50 years of age but often begin as early as 20 years of age. Pain and nodularity often increase over time but tend to subside after menopause unless high doses of estrogen replacement are used. Fibrocystic changes most commonly occur in women with premenstrual abnormalities, nulliparous women, women with a history of spontaneous abortion, nonusers of oral contraceptives, and women with early menarche and late menopause. Symptoms related to fibrocystic changes often worsen in the premenstrual phase and subside after menstruation.

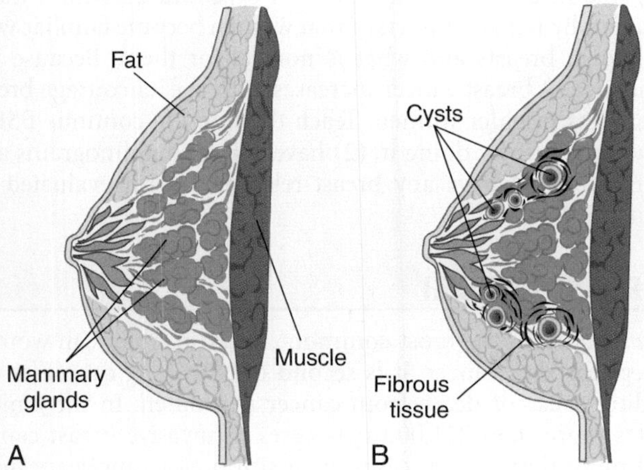


**FIG. 51-3** **A,** Normal breast tissue. **B,** Fibrocystic breast tissue.

Manifestations of fibrocystic breast changes include one or more palpable lumps that are often round, well delineated, and freely movable within the breast (Table 51-1). Discomfort ranging from tenderness to pain may also occur. The lump is usually observed to increase in size and perhaps in tenderness before menstruation. Cysts may enlarge or shrink rapidly. Nipple discharge associated with fibrocystic breasts is often milky, watery-milky, yellow, or green.

Mammography may be helpful in distinguishing fibrocystic changes from breast cancer. However, in some women the breast tissue is so dense that it is difficult to obtain a mammogram. In these situations, ultrasound may be more useful in differentiating a fluid-filled cyst from a solid mass.

## ❖ NURSING AND INTERPROFESSIONAL MANAGEMENT: FIBROCYSTIC CHANGES

With the initial discovery of a discrete mass in the breast by a woman or her HCP, aspiration or biopsy may be indicated. If the nodularity is recurrent, a wait of 7 to 10 days may be planned in order to note any changes that may be related to the menstrual cycle. With large or frequent cysts, an excisional biopsy may be preferred over repeated aspiration. An excisional biopsy may be done if (1) no fluid is found on aspiration, (2) the fluid that is found is hemorrhagic, or (3) a residual mass remains after fluid aspiration. The biopsy is usually performed in an outpatient surgery unit.

Severe fibrocystic changes may make palpation of the breast more difficult. Teach the woman with cystic changes to maintain regular follow-up care with her HCP and encourage breast self-awareness and to report any changes found so that they can be evaluated.

Treatment for a fibrocystic condition is similar to that described earlier for mastalgia. Teach the woman with fibrocystic breasts that she may expect a recurrence of the cysts in one or both breasts until menopause and that the cysts may enlarge or become painful just before menstruation. Additionally, reassure her that the cysts do not "turn into" cancer. Advise her that any new lump that does not respond in a cyclic manner over 1 to 2 weeks should be examined by her HCP.

## FIBROADENOMA

**Fibroadenoma** is a common cause of discrete benign breast lumps in young women. It generally occurs in women between 15 and 40 years of age. It is the most frequent cause of breast masses in women under 25 years of age.

The possible cause of fibroadenoma may be increased estrogen sensitivity in a localized area of the breast. Fibroadenomas are usually small (but can be large [2 to 3 cm]), painless, round, well delineated, and very mobile. They may be soft but are usually solid, firm, and rubbery in consistency. There is no accompanying retraction or nipple discharge. The fibroadenoma may appear as a single unilateral mass, although multiple bilateral fibroadenomas have been reported. Growth is slow and often ceases when the size reaches 2 to 3 cm. Size is not affected by menstruation. However, pregnancy can stimulate dramatic growth.

Fibroadenomas are easily detected by physical examination and may be visible on mammography and ultrasound. However, definitive diagnosis requires FNA, core, or excisional biopsy and tissue examination by a pathologist to exclude a malignancy.

Treatment of fibroadenomas can include observation with regular monitoring after a malignancy has been ruled out. In women over 35 years of age, all new lesions should be evaluated by breast ultrasound and possible biopsy.[3]

## NIPPLE DISCHARGE

Nipple discharge may occur spontaneously or as a result of nipple manipulation. A milky secretion is due to inappropriate lactation (termed **galactorrhea**) and may be a result of certain medications or endocrine or neurologic disorders. Nipple discharge may also be idiopathic (no known cause).

Secretions can also be serous, bloody, or brown to green. A cytology slide may be made of the secretion to determine the specific cause and recommended treatment. Disorders associated with nipple discharge include benign breast conditions such as fibrocystic changes, intraductal papilloma, or ductal ectasia. In most cases, nipple discharge is not related to malignancy.

### Intraductal Papilloma

An **intraductal papilloma** is a benign, soft, wartlike growth found in the mammary ducts. It is usually unilateral. Typically, the nipple has a bloody discharge that can be intermittent or spontaneous. Most intraductal papillomas are beneath the areola, and they may be difficult to palpate. They are usually found in women 40 to 60 years of age. A single duct or several ducts may be involved. Treatment includes excision of the papilloma and the involved duct or duct system. Papillomas are associated with a slightly increased risk (1.5 to 2 times) of developing breast cancer over the general population.[7]

### Ductal Ectasia

**Ductal ectasia** (duct dilation) is a benign breast disease of perimenopausal and postmenopausal women involving the ducts in the subareolar area. It usually involves several bilateral ducts. Multicolored, sticky nipple discharge is the primary symptom. Ductal ectasia is initially painless but may progress to burning, itching, and pain around the nipple, as well as swelling in the areolar area. Inflammatory signs are often present, the nipple may retract, and the discharge may become bloody in more advanced disease. Ductal ectasia is not associated with malignancy. If an abscess develops, warm compresses and antibiotics are usually effective treatments. Therapy consists of close follow-up examinations or surgical excision of the involved ducts.

## ATYPICAL HYPERPLASIA

Atypical hyperplasia is usually discovered after a biopsy is done to evaluate a suspicious area found on a mammogram or during a clinical breast examination. Atypical hyperplasia is found in either the ducts (atypical ductal hyperplasia) or in the lobules (atypical lobular hyperplasia). Both are associated with an increased risk of developing breast cancer. To follow up on a diagnosis of atypical hyperplasia an excisional biopsy or lumpectomy may be done to remove all of the affected tissue.[8]

## GYNECOMASTIA IN MEN

**Gynecomastia**, a transient, noninflammatory enlargement of one or both breasts, is the most common breast problem in men. The condition is usually temporary and benign. Gynecomastia in itself is not a risk factor for breast cancer. The most common cause of gynecomastia is a disturbance of the normal ratio of active androgen to estrogen in plasma or within the breast itself.[9]

Gynecomastia can also occur in puberty. During puberty, there is often a transient relative imbalance between estrogen and testosterone, leading to gynecomastia. This condition usually resolves by age 18 years when adult androgen/estrogen ratios are achieved. The treatment of pubertal gynecomastia is reassurance of the parent and teenager regarding the benign nature of the condition.

Gynecomastia may also be a manifestation of other problems. It may accompany diseases such as testicular tumors, adrenal cancer, pituitary adenomas, hyperthyroidism, and liver disease. Gynecomastia may occur as a side effect of drug therapy, particularly with estrogen and androgen, digitalis, isoniazid, ranitidine (Zantac), and spironolactone (Aldactone). The use of heroin and marijuana can also cause gynecomastia.

### Senescent Gynecomastia

*Senescent gynecomastia* occurs in many older men. A probable cause is the elevation in plasma estrogen in older adult men as the result of increased conversion of androgens to estrogens in peripheral circulation. Although initially unilateral, the tender, firm, centrally located enlargement may become bilateral. When gynecomastia is characterized by a discrete, circumscribed mass, it must be biopsied to differentiate it from the rarer breast cancer in males. Senescent hyperplasia requires no treatment and generally regresses within 6 to 12 months.

### Gerontologic Considerations: Age-Related Breast Changes

The loss of subcutaneous fat and structural support and the atrophy of mammary glands often result in pendulous breasts in the postmenopausal woman. Encourage older women to wear a well-fitting bra. Adequate support can improve physical appearance and reduce pain in the back, shoulders, and neck. It can also prevent *intertrigo* (dermatitis caused by friction between opposing surfaces of skin). Sagging breasts can be surgically lifted (mastopexy).

The decrease in glandular tissue in older women makes a breast mass easier to palpate. This decreased density is likely a result of age-related decreases in estrogen. Rib margins may be palpable in a thin woman and can be confused with a mass. That is why it is so important that women become familiar with their own breasts and what is normal for them. Because the incidence of breast cancer increases with age, encourage breast awareness in older women. Teach them to (1) continue BSE if they are routinely doing it, (2) have annual mammograms and CBEs, and (3) have any breast-related concern evaluated by their HCP.

## BREAST CANCER

*Breast cancer* is the most common cancer in American women except for skin cancer. It is second only to lung cancer as the leading cause of death from cancer in women. In the United States more than 231,000 new cases of invasive breast cancer and more than 60,000 cases of in situ breast cancer are diagnosed annually. An additional 2200 cases of breast cancer are diagnosed in men. Approximately 40,300 deaths occur each year related to breast cancer.[1]

The incidence of breast cancer is slowly decreasing, with a slight drop in the number of deaths related to breast cancer. This decline may be the result of the decreased use of hormone therapy after menopause. Breast cancer survivors are the largest group of any cancer survivors.[1] (Survivorship is discussed later in this chapter.)

## Etiology and Risk Factors

Although the etiology is not completely understood, a number of risk factors are related to breast cancer (Table 51-2). Risk factors appear to be cumulative and interacting. Therefore the presence of multiple risk factors may greatly increase the overall risk, especially for people with a positive family history.

**Risk Factors for Women.** The risk factors most associated with breast cancer include female gender and advancing age. Women are at far greater risk than men, with 99% of breast cancers occurring in women. Increasing age also increases the risk of developing breast cancer. The incidence of breast cancer in women under 25 years of age is very low and increases gradually until age 60. After age 60, the incidence increases dramatically.

Hormonal regulation of the breast is related to the development of breast cancer, but the mechanisms are poorly understood. The hormones estrogen and progesterone may act as tumor promoters to stimulate breast cancer growth if malignant changes in the cells have already occurred. The Women's Health Initiative study showed that the use of combined hormone therapy (estrogen plus progesterone) increases the risk of breast cancer. It also showed that there was a risk of having a larger, more advanced breast cancer at diagnosis. The use of estrogen therapy alone for longer than 10 years (for women with a prior hysterectomy) increases a woman's long-term risk for breast cancer.[10] A link may exist between oral contraceptive use and increased risk of breast cancer for younger women.[11]

Modifiable risk factors include excess weight gain during adulthood, sedentary lifestyle, smoking, dietary fat intake, obesity, and alcohol intake. Environmental factors such as radiation exposure may also play a role.

**TABLE 51-2 Risk Factors for Breast Cancer**

| Risk Factor | Comments |
|---|---|
| Female | Women account for 99% of breast cancer cases. |
| Age ≥50 yr | Majority of breast cancers are found in postmenopausal women. After age 60, increase in incidence. |
| Hormone use | Use of estrogen and/or progesterone as hormone therapy, especially in postmenopausal women. |
| Family history | Breast cancer in a first-degree relative, particularly when premenopausal or bilateral, increases risk. |
| Genetic factors | Gene mutations *(BRCA1, BRCA2, P53, PTEN, PALB2)* play a role in 5%-10% of breast cancer cases. |
| Personal history of breast cancer, colon cancer, endometrial cancer, ovarian cancer | Personal history significantly increases risk of breast cancer, risk of cancer in other breast, and recurrence. |
| Early menarche (before age 12), late menopause (after age 55) | A long menstrual history increases the risk of breast cancer. |
| First full-term pregnancy after age 30, nulliparity | Prolonged exposure to unopposed estrogen increases risk for breast cancer. |
| Benign breast disease with atypical epithelial hyperplasia, lobular carcinoma in situ | Atypical changes in breast biopsy increase the risk of breast cancer. |
| Weight gain and obesity after menopause | Fat cells store estrogen, which increases the likelihood of developing breast cancer. |
| Exposure to ionizing radiation | Radiation damages DNA (e.g., prior treatment for Hodgkin's lymphoma). |
| Alcohol consumption | Women who drink ≥1 alcoholic beverage per day may have an increased risk of breast cancer. |

## Genetic Link

Family history of breast cancer is an important risk factor, especially if the involved family member also had ovarian cancer, was premenopausal, had bilateral breast cancer, or is a first-degree relative (i.e., mother, father, sister, brother, daughter). Having any first-degree relative with breast cancer increases a woman's risk of breast cancer 1.5 to 3 times, depending on age.[12,13] A breast cancer risk assessment tool for HCPs is available *(www.cancer.gov/bcrisktool)*. Genetic counseling must be considered for an individual at high risk for breast cancer and appropriate referrals made.

About 5% to 10% of all breast cancers are hereditary. This means that specific genetic abnormalities that contribute to the development of breast cancer have been inherited (passed from parent to child). Most inherited cases of breast cancer are associated with mutations in two genes: *BRCA1* and *BRCA2* (*BRCA* stands for *BR*east *CA*ncer). Everyone has *BRCA* genes. The *BRCA1* gene, located on chromosome 17, is a tumor suppressor gene that inhibits tumor development when functioning normally. Women who have *BRCA1* mutations have a 40% to 80% lifetime chance of developing breast cancer. The *BRCA2* gene, located on chromosome 11, is another tumor suppressor gene. Women with a mutation of this gene have a similar risk of breast cancer.[12,13]

Mutations in *BRCA* genes may cause as many as 10% to 40% of all inherited breast cancers. As many as 1 in 200 to 400 women in the United States may be carriers for these genetic abnormalities. Women with *BRCA* mutations are also at higher risk for developing ovarian, colon, pancreatic, and uterine cancers.[12]

In addition to *BRCA* gene mutations, many other abnormal genes have been identified that increase a person's risk of developing breast cancer. These include the tumor suppressor genes *p53* and *PTEN* (which inhibit tumor development when functioning normally), *ATM* (which helps to repair damaged deoxyribonucleic acid [DNA]), *CHEK2* (which stops tumor growth), and *PALB2* (which partners with *BRCA* to suppress tumor growth).[14]

Most people who develop breast cancer do not have an abnormal breast cancer gene, nor do they have a family history of breast cancer. Ongoing research continues to investigate the role of genes in the development of breast cancer. (Genomics and genetics are discussed in Chapter 12.)

**Risk Factors for Men.** Predisposing risk factors for breast cancer in men include hyperestrogenism, a family history of breast cancer, and radiation exposure. A thorough examination of the

## GENETICS IN CLINICAL PRACTICE

### *Breast Cancer*

**Genetic Basis**
- Mutations occur in *BRCA1* and/or *BRCA2* genes.
- Normally these genes are tumor suppressor genes involved in DNA repair.
- Transmission is autosomal dominant.
- Additional genes (e.g., *ATM, CHEK-2, p53, PTEN, PALB2*) may increase the risk of breast cancer.

**Incidence**
- Approximately 5% to 10% of breast cancers are related to *BRCA1* and *BRCA2* gene mutations.
- Women with *BRCA1* and *BRCA2* gene mutations have a 40% to 80% lifetime risk of developing breast cancer.
- *BRCA1* and *BRCA2* gene mutations are associated with early-onset breast cancer that is more likely to involve both breasts.
- Men with mutations in *BRCA1* and *BRCA2* have an increased risk of breast cancer and prostate cancer.
- Family history of both breast and ovarian cancer increases the risk of having a *BRCA* mutation.

**Genetic Testing**
- DNA testing is available for *BRCA1* and *BRCA2* gene mutations.
- Newer genetic tests are available to analyze an entire panel of genes in specific breast cancer patient populations.

**Clinical Implications**
- Most breast cancers (about 90%-95%) are not inherited. They are associated with genetic changes that occur after a person is born (somatic mutations). There is no risk of passing on the mutated gene to children.
- Bilateral oophorectomy and/or bilateral mastectomy reduces the risk of breast cancer and ovarian cancer in women with *BRCA1* and *BRCA2* mutations.
- Mutations in the *BRCA1* and *BRCA2* genes increase the risk of ovarian cancer.
- Genetic counseling and testing for *BRCA* mutations should be considered for patients whose personal or family history puts them at high risk for a genetic predisposition to breast cancer.

*BRCA, BReast CAncer.*

male breast should be a routine part of a physical examination. Men in *BRCA*-positive families should consider genetic testing. Men who test positive for a *BRCA* gene mutation should receive BSE training starting at the age of 35, a CBE every 6 months starting at the age of 35, and a baseline mammogram beginning at the age of forty. These men should also begin prostate screening at the age of 40 as they also have an increased risk of developing prostate cancer.[13]

## CHECK YOUR PRACTICE

Your best female friend calls you on the phone and you can tell she has been crying. Her mother has just been diagnosed with Stage 3A breast cancer. Between sobs, she tells you that her grandmother died of breast cancer and her aunt (her mother's sister) is being treated with chemotherapy for breast cancer. She asks you, "Don't you think that I should just get mine whacked off? Then I would not have to worry anymore."
- How would you respond to her?

**Prophylactic Oophorectomy and Mastectomy.** In women with *BRCA1* or *BRCA2* mutations, prophylactic bilateral oophorectomy can decrease the risk of breast cancer as well as ovarian cancer. Removing the ovaries lowers the risk of breast cancer because the ovaries are the main source of estrogen in a premenopausal woman. Removing the ovaries does not reduce the risk of breast cancer in postmenopausal women because the ovaries are not the main producers of estrogen in these women. A woman who has a high risk of developing breast cancer (i.e., related to factors such as family history and prior tissue biopsies) may choose (in consultation with her physician and genetic counselor) to undergo prophylactic bilateral mastectomy.

Younger women with hereditary (non-*BRCA*) early-stage, estrogen receptor–negative breast cancer may have a higher risk of developing a secondary primary breast cancer in the unaffected (contralateral) breast.[14] These women may also choose to have the unaffected breast removed prophylactically at the time of initial surgery for breast cancer or at a later time.

## Pathophysiology

The main components of the breast are lobules (milk-producing glands) and ducts (milk passages that connect the lobules and the nipple). In general, breast cancer arises from the epithelial lining of the ducts *(ductal carcinoma)* or from the epithelium of the lobules *(lobular carcinoma)*. Breast cancers may be *in situ* (within the duct) or invasive (invading through the wall of the duct).

Metastatic breast cancer is breast cancer that has spread to other organs, with the most common sites being bone, liver, lung, and brain. Cancer growth rates can range from slow to rapid. Factors that affect cancer prognosis are tumor size, axillary node involvement (the more nodes involved, the worse the prognosis), tumor differentiation, estrogen and progesterone receptor status, and *human epidermal growth factor receptor 2* (HER-2) status. HER-2 is a protein that helps regulate cell growth.[15]

## Types of Breast Cancer

Breast cancer is not just one disease, but a group of diseases characterized by different pathologic findings and clinical behaviors. Breast cancer can be classified as (1) ductal or lobular or other or (2) noninvasive or invasive (Table 51-3). It can also be classified based on hormonal status and genetic subtypes.

**Noninvasive Breast Cancer.** An estimated 20% of breast cancers are noninvasive. These intraductal cancers include *ductal carcinoma in situ* (DCIS) and *lobular carcinoma in situ* (LCIS). DCIS tends to be unilateral and may progress to invasive breast cancer if left untreated.

To determine treatment options for DCIS, the Oncotype DX Assay (a genomic test) can be used to (1) predict the risk of local recurrence or invasive carcinoma and (2) guide personalized treatment based on tumor biology.[16] Treatment options include breast-conserving treatment (lumpectomy), total mastectomy with or without sentinel lymph node biopsy, radiation therapy, and/or hormone therapy (e.g., tamoxifen).

The term *lobular carcinoma in situ* is somewhat misleading. Although women with LCIS are more likely to develop invasive breast cancer than women without LCIS, it is not considered to be a premalignant lesion. No surgical or radiation treatment is indicated for LCIS. Hormone therapy may be used as a preventive measure to reduce breast cancer risk for some patients.

**Invasive Ductal Carcinoma.** *Invasive (infiltrating) ductal carcinoma* is the most common type of breast cancer accounting for approximately 80% of all invasive breast cancers. It starts in the milk ducts and then breaks through the walls of the duct, invading the surrounding tissue. From there it may metastasize to

**TABLE 51-3 Classification of Breast Cancer**

**Based on Tissue Type**
- Ductal carcinoma (affects milk ducts)
  - Medullary
  - Tubular
  - Colloid (mucinous)
- Lobular carcinoma (affects milk-producing glands)
- Other
  - Inflammatory
  - Paget's disease
  - Phyllodes tumor

**Based on Invasiveness**
***Noninvasive (In situ)***
- Ductal carcinoma in situ (DCIS)
- Lobular carcinoma in situ (LCIS)

***Invasive (Spreading to Other Locations)***
- Invasive ductal carcinoma
- Invasive lobular carcinoma

**Based on Hormone Receptor and Genetic Status**
***Estrogen and Progesterone Receptor Status***
- Estrogen receptor positive
- Estrogen receptor negative
- Progesterone receptor positive
- Progesterone receptor negative

***HER-2 Genetic Status***
- HER-2 positive
- HER-2 negative

*HER-2*, Human epidermal growth factor receptor 2.

other parts of the body. Subtypes of invasive ductal carcinoma include medullary carcinoma, tubular carcinoma, colloid (mucinous) carcinoma, papillary carcinoma, and metaplastic carcinoma.

**Invasive Lobular Carcinoma.** *Invasive (infiltrating) lobular carcinoma* begins in the lobules (milk-producing glands) of the breast and accounts for approximately 10% to 15% of invasive breast cancers. The cancer cells can break out of the lobule and have the potential to metastasize to other areas of the body. Invasive lobular carcinoma usually presents as a subtle thickening in the upper outer quadrant of the breast. It is a type of breast cancer that is generally not detected by mammography.

### Other Types of Breast Cancer

***Inflammatory Breast Cancer.*** *Inflammatory breast cancer* is an aggressive and fast-growing breast cancer with a high risk for metastasis accounting for approximately 1% to 3% of all breast cancers. In the early stages, it is often mistaken for mastitis. However, the inflammatory changes do not improve with antibiotics, as the lymph channels in the skin of the breast are blocked by cancer cells. Because of skin involvement, the breast looks red, feels warm, and has a thickened appearance that is often described as resembling an orange peel *(peau d'orange)*. Sometimes the breast develops ridges and small bumps that look like hives. A breast mass may not be present and changes may not show up on mammograms, thus making diagnosis difficult. Inflammatory breast cancer is associated with a worse prognosis as compared to invasive ductal and lobular breast cancer.[17]

***Paget's Disease.*** Paget's disease is a rare breast malignancy that starts in the breast ducts and spreads to the nipple and areola. It is rare, causing approximately 1% of all breast cancers (This is different from Paget's disease of the bone, which is discussed in Chapter 63.) Most women with Paget's disease have underlying ductal carcinoma. Only in rare cases is the cancer confined to the nipple.

Itching, burning, bloody nipple discharge with superficial skin erosion and ulceration may be present. Diagnosis of Paget's disease is confirmed by pathologic examination of the lesion. Nipple changes are often diagnosed as an infection or dermatitis, which can lead to treatment delays.

The treatment of Paget's disease is surgical removal of the involved tissue (central lumpectomy or mastectomy). Radiation therapy may also be used after surgery. The prognosis is good when the cancer is confined to the nipple.

***Phyllodes Tumor.*** A phyllodes tumor is a rare tumor that develops in the connective tissue (stroma) of the breast as compared with invasive ductal or lobular carcinomas. Treatment for this tumor is usually mastectomy and if needed, chemotherapy.

**Triple-Negative Breast Cancer.** A patient whose breast cancer tests negative for all three receptors (estrogen, progesterone, and HER-2) has *triple-negative breast cancer.* (Receptor testing is discussed on pp. 1212-1213.) The incidence of triple-negative breast cancer is higher in African Americans, Hispanics, premenopausal women, and those with a *BRCA1* mutation. These patients tend to have more aggressive tumors with a poorer prognosis because these tumors do not respond to treatment.

These cancers do not usually respond to hormone therapy or therapy for the human epidermal growth factor receptor 2 (HER-2). Chemotherapy appears to be the most successful method for treating triple-negative breast cancer.

## Clinical Manifestations

Breast cancer is usually detected as a lump or thickening in the breast or mammography abnormality. It occurs most often in the upper, outer quadrant of the breast, which is the location of most of the glandular tissue (Fig. 51-4). Breast cancers vary in their growth rate. If palpable, breast cancer is characteristically hard and may be irregularly shaped, poorly delineated, nonmobile, and nontender.

A small percentage of breast cancers cause nipple discharge. The discharge is usually unilateral and may be clear or bloody. Nipple retraction may occur. Peau d'orange may occur due to plugging of the dermal lymphatics. In large cancers, infiltration, induration, and dimpling (pulling in) of the overlying skin may also occur.

## Complications

The main complication of breast cancer is recurrence (Table 51-4). Recurrence may be *local* or *regional* (skin or soft tissue near the mastectomy site, axillary or internal mammary lymph nodes) or distant (most commonly involving bone, lung, brain, and liver). However, metastatic disease can be found in any site in the body.

Widely disseminated or metastatic disease involves the growth of cancerous breast cells in parts of the body distant from the breast. Metastases primarily occur through the lymphatics, usually those of the axilla (Fig. 51-5). However, the cancer can spread to other parts of the body.

## Diagnostic Studies

In addition to radiologic and biopsy studies used to diagnose breast cancer (see earlier discussion in this chapter on

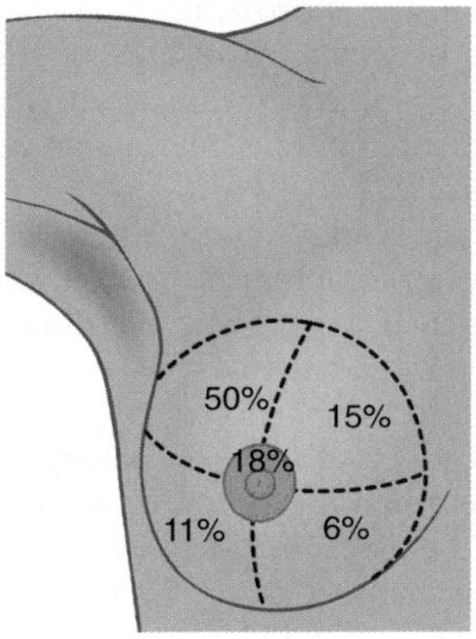


**FIG. 51-4** Distribution of where breast cancer occurs.

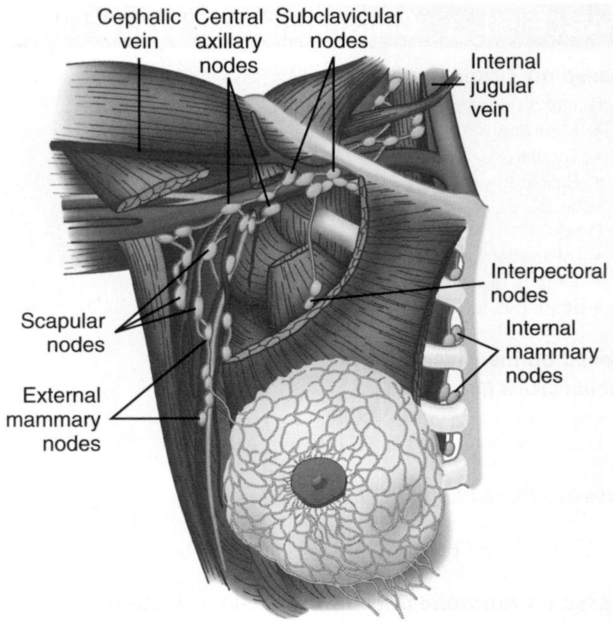


**FIG. 51-5** Lymph nodes and drainage in the axilla. The sentinel lymph node is usually found in the external mammary nodes. A complete axillary dissection would remove all nodes. (From Donegan WL, Spratt JS: *Cancer of the breast,* ed 3, Philadelphia, 1988, Saunders.)

**TABLE 51-4 Sites of Breast Cancer Recurrence and Metastasis**

| Site | Manifestations |
|---|---|
| **Local Recurrence** | |
| Skin, chest wall | Firm, discrete nodules. Occasionally pruritic, usually painless, commonly in or near a scar. |
| **Regional Recurrence** | |
| Lymph nodes | Enlarged nodes in axilla or supraclavicular area, usually nontender. |
| **Distant Metastasis** | |
| Skeletal | Localized pain of gradually increasing intensity, percussion tenderness at involved sites, pathologic fracture caused by involvement of bone cortex. |
| Spinal cord | Progressive back pain, localized and radiating. Change in bladder or bowel function. Loss of sensation in lower extremities. |
| Brain | Headache described as "different," unilateral sensory loss, focal muscular weakness, hemiparesis, incoordination (ataxia), nausea and vomiting unrelated to medication, cognitive changes. |
| Pulmonary (including lung nodules and pleural effusions) | Shortness of breath, tachypnea, nonproductive cough (not present in all patients). |
| Liver | Abdominal distention. Right lower quadrant abdominal pain sometimes radiating to scapular area. Nausea and vomiting, anorexia, weight loss. Weakness and fatigue. Hepatomegaly, ascites, jaundice. Peripheral edema. Elevated liver enzymes. |
| Bone marrow | Anemia, infection, increased bleeding, bruising, petechiae. Weakness, fatigue, mild confusion, light-headedness. Dyspnea. |

pp. 1205-1206), other tests are used to predict the risk of local or systemic recurrence. These tests include axillary lymph node analysis, tumor size, estrogen and progesterone receptor status, cell-proliferative indices, and genomic assays.

**Axillary Lymph Node Analysis.** Axillary lymph node involvement is one of the most important prognostic factors in breast cancer. *Axillary lymph nodes* are often examined to determine if cancer has spread to the axilla on the side of the breast cancer (Fig. 51-5). The more nodes involved, the greater the risk of recurrence.

A *sentinel lymph node biopsy* (SLNB) helps to identify the lymph node(s) that drain first from the tumor site *(sentinel node).* In SLNB a radioisotope and/or blue dye, which will travel the same route as the cancer, is injected into the affected breast. Then intraoperatively it is determined in which sentinel lymph nodes (SLNs) the radioisotope (using radioactive detector) or dye (visually see blue nodes) is located. A local incision is made in the axilla, and the surgeon dissects the blue-stained and/or radioactive SLNs. Generally, with a SLNB, one to four axillary lymph nodes are removed. The nodes are sent for pathologic analysis. If the SLNs are negative, no further axillary surgery is required.

If the SLNs are positive, a complete *axillary lymph node dissection* (ALND) may be done. In an ALND, the surgeon will typically remove 12 to 20 lymph nodes. SLNB is less invasive than ALND and is associated with lower morbidity rates and greater accuracy compared with ALND.

**Tumor Size.** *Tumor size* is a prognostic variable: the larger the tumor, the poorer the prognosis. The wide variety of biologic types of breast cancer explains the variability of disease behavior. In general, the more well differentiated (like the original cell type) the tumor, the less aggressive it is. The cells of poorly differentiated (unlike the original cell type) tumors appear morphologically disorganized, and they are more aggressive.

**Estrogen and Progesterone Receptor Status.** *Estrogen and progesterone receptor status* is another diagnostic test useful for decisions about both treatment and prognosis. Receptor-positive tumors (1) commonly show histologic evidence of being well differentiated, (2) frequently have a *diploid* (more normal) DNA content and low proliferative indices, (3) have a lower chance for recurrence, and (4) are frequently hormone dependent and responsive to hormone therapy. Receptor-negative tumors (1) are often poorly differentiated histologically, (2) have a high incidence of *aneuploidy* (abnormally high or low DNA content) and higher proliferative indices, (3) frequently recur, and (4) are usually unresponsive to hormone therapy. Ploidy status correlates with tumor aggressiveness. Diploid tumors have been shown to have a significantly lower risk of recurrence than aneuploid tumors.

**Cell-Proliferative Indices.** *Cell-proliferative indices* indirectly measure the rate of tumor cell proliferation. The percentage of tumor cells in the synthesis (S) phase of the cell cycle (see Chapter 15, Fig. 15-1) is another important prognostic indicator. Although cell-proliferative indices are not routinely performed as part of the breast cancer pathology evaluation, patients with cells that have high S-phase fractions have a higher risk for recurrence and earlier cancer death.

**Genomic Assay.** An important *genomic assay* is to determine HER-2, which is a prognostic indicator. Overexpression of this receptor has been associated with unusually aggressive tumor growth, a greater risk for recurrence, and a poorer prognosis in breast cancer.[15] HER-2 is overexpressed in about 10% to 20% of patients with breast cancer. The presence or absence of this marker assists in the selection and sequence of drug therapy and predicts the patient's response to treatment.

A *genomic* test uses a sample of the breast cancer tissue to analyze the activity of a group of genes that can affect how a cancer is likely to behave and respond to treatment. Knowing whether certain genes are present or absent, or overly active or not active enough, can provide information about the risk of recurrence and the likely benefit of chemotherapy or hormone therapy. The Oncotype DX test is the most commonly used genomic test. Other genomic tests are MammaPrint, Mammostrat, and Prosigna.

## Interprofessional Care

A wide range of treatment options is available to the patient and HCPs making critical decisions about how to treat breast cancer (Table 51-5). Prognostic factors are considered when treatment decisions are made. The therapeutic regimen is often determined by the clinical stage and biology of the cancer.

**Staging of Breast Cancer.** The most widely accepted staging method for breast cancer is the TNM system.[18] This system uses tumor size (T), nodal involvement (N), and presence of metastasis (M) to determine the stage of disease. The stage of a breast cancer describes its size and the extent to which it has spread (Table 51-6).

The stages range from 0 to IV, with stage 0 being in situ cancer with no lymph node involvement and no metastasis. Further classification within these stages depends on the tumor size and number of lymph nodes involved. Stage IV indicates metastatic spread, regardless of tumor size or lymph node involvement. The presence or absence of malignant cells in lymph nodes remains a powerful prognostic factor related to local recurrence or metastasis after primary therapy.

**Surgical Therapy.** Surgery is considered the primary treatment for breast cancer. Table 51-7 describes the most common surgical procedures used to treat breast cancer. The most common surgical options for operable breast cancer are (1) breast conservation surgery (lumpectomy [segmental mastectomy]) and (2) mastectomy with or without reconstruction. Most women diagnosed with early stage breast cancer (tumors smaller than 5 cm) are candidates for either treatment choice as the overall survival rate with lumpectomy and radiation is the same as that with mastectomy.[19]

### TABLE 51-5 Interprofessional Care

**Breast Cancer**

**Diagnostic Assessment**

***Prediagnosis***

- Health history, including risk factors
- Physical examination, including breast and lymph nodes
- Mammography
- Ultrasound (if indicated)
- Breast MRI (if indicated)
- Biopsy

***Postdiagnosis***

- Lymph node analysis
- Estrogen and progesterone receptor status
- Cell-proliferative indices
- HER-2 marker
- Genetic assays (e.g., MammaPrint or Oncotype DX)

**Staging**

- Complete blood count, platelet count
- Alkaline phosphatase
- Liver function tests
- Chest x-ray (if indicated)
- Bone scan (if indicated)
- CT scan of chest, abdomen, pelvis (if indicated)
- MRI (if indicated)
- PET/CT scan (if indicated)

**Management**

***Surgical Therapy***

- Breast-conserving surgery (lumpectomy) with SLNB and/or axillary lymph node dissection
- Simple (total) mastectomy with SLNB and/or axillary lymph node dissection
- Modified radical mastectomy
- Reconstructive surgery

***Radiation Therapy***

- External radiation
- Brachytherapy
- Palliative radiation therapy

***Drug Therapy*** (Table 51-8)

- Chemotherapy
- Hormone therapy
- Immunotherapy
- Targeted therapy

*SLNB,* Sentinel lymph node biopsy.

It is important to note that breast reconstruction is an option for any woman undergoing surgical treatment for breast cancer. For women undergoing mastectomy, breast reconstruction can be performed at the time of the mastectomy or delayed for months or even years. Women may opt to not have reconstruction and choose to use a breast prosthesis instead.

***Breast-Conserving Surgery.*** Breast-conserving surgery (also called lumpectomy) involves removal of the entire tumor along with a margin of normal surrounding tissue (Fig. 51-6, *A*). In some cases, it may take two to three additional surgeries to remove all the cancer from the margins. After surgery, radiation therapy is delivered to the entire breast, ending with a boost to the tumor bed. If the risk for recurrence is high, chemotherapy may be administered before radiation therapy.

Not everyone is a candidate for breast conservation surgery. Contraindications include breast size too small in relation to the tumor size to yield an acceptable cosmetic result, multifocal masses and calcifications, multicentric masses (in more than one quadrant), diffuse calcifications in more than one quadrant, or prior radiation therapy. In addition to these issues, the choice between mastectomy and breast conservation surgery depends on additional factors. Because of the time commitment (i.e., 6 to 7 weeks of daily radiation therapy treatments) and travel distances to access radiation therapy treatment facility, some patients may chose mastectomy over breast conservation surgery.

***Axillary Lymph Node Analysis.*** Sentinel lymph node biopsy (SLNB) is the preferred standard for axillary lymph node analysis and staging. It was described on p. 1212. However, if the sentinel lymph node cannot be identified, or if the node is positive for cancer, ALND may have to be performed.

**TABLE 51-6 Staging of Breast Cancer**

| Stage | Tumor Size | Lymph Node Involvement | Metastasis |
|---|---|---|---|
| **0** | TIS* | No | No |
| **I** | <2 cm | No | No |
| **II** | | | |
| A | No evidence of tumor ranging to 5 cm | No, or 1-3 axillary nodes and/or internal mammary nodes | No |
| B | Ranging from 2 to >5 cm | No, or 1-3 axillary nodes and/or internal mammary nodes | No |
| **III** | | | |
| A | No evidence of tumor ranging to >5 cm | Yes, 4-9 axillary nodes and/or internal mammary nodes | No |
| B | Any size with extension to chest wall or skin | Yes, 4-9 axillary nodes and/or internal mammary nodes | No |
| C | Any size | Yes, ≥10 axillary nodes, internal mammary nodes, or infraclavicular nodes | No |
| **IV** | Any size | Any type of nodal involvement | Yes |

Modified from American Joint Committee on Cancer: AJCC cancer staging manual, ed 7. Retrieved from *www.cancerstaging.org/staging/changes2010.*
**TIS,* Tumor in situ.

**Lymphedema.** Lymphedema (accumulation of lymph in soft tissue) can occur as a result of the lymph node sampling procedure or radiation therapy (Fig. 51-7). When the axillary nodes cannot return lymph fluid to the central circulation, the fluid accumulates in the arm, hand, or breast, causing obstructive pressure on the veins and venous return. The patient may experience heaviness, impaired motor function in the arm, and numbness and paresthesia of the fingers. Cellulitis and progressive fibrosis of the skin can result from untreated lymphedema. (See further discussion on lymphedema later in this chapter on p. 1220.)

***Mastectomy.*** A *total* or *simple mastectomy* removes the entire breast. A *modified radical mastectomy* includes removal of the breast and axillary lymph nodes, but it preserves the pectoralis major muscle (Fig. 51-6, *B*). In a *nipple-sparing mastectomy*, the nipple and/or areola are left in place while the breast tissue under them is removed. Women who have a small cancer near the outer part of the breast, with no signs of cancer in the skin or near the nipple, may be able to have nipple-sparing surgery.[16]

For women who have a mastectomy, breast reconstruction can be performed immediately or it can be delayed. If the woman chooses, it may not be done at all. There are two main types of breast reconstruction procedures: implant reconstruction or tissue flap procedures (Table 51-7). Breast reconstructive surgery is discussed on pp. 1222-1224.

**CHECK YOUR PRACTICE**

You are working in the breast clinic and doing a postoperative assessment on a 56-yr-old woman who had a right radical mastectomy 6 weeks ago. She is complaining of sharp, prickly feelings in her right arm. She tells you, "I also feel pain in the breast that was removed. Am I going crazy? That breast is not even attached to my body anymore!"

- How would you respond and what follow-up would you provide?

***Post–Breast Therapy Pain Syndrome.*** *Post–breast therapy pain syndrome* (PBTPS) occurs in some people who have undergone procedures for breast cancer. Most commonly it is caused by injury to nerves during surgery. However, it can also be due to chemotherapy and radiation therapy. The most common theory for the onset of this syndrome is injury to intercostobrachial nerves, which are sensory nerves that exit the chest wall muscles and provide sensation to the shoulder and upper arm.

Because of its multiple causes, PBTPS symptoms can range from mild to debilitating.[20] Common symptoms include chest

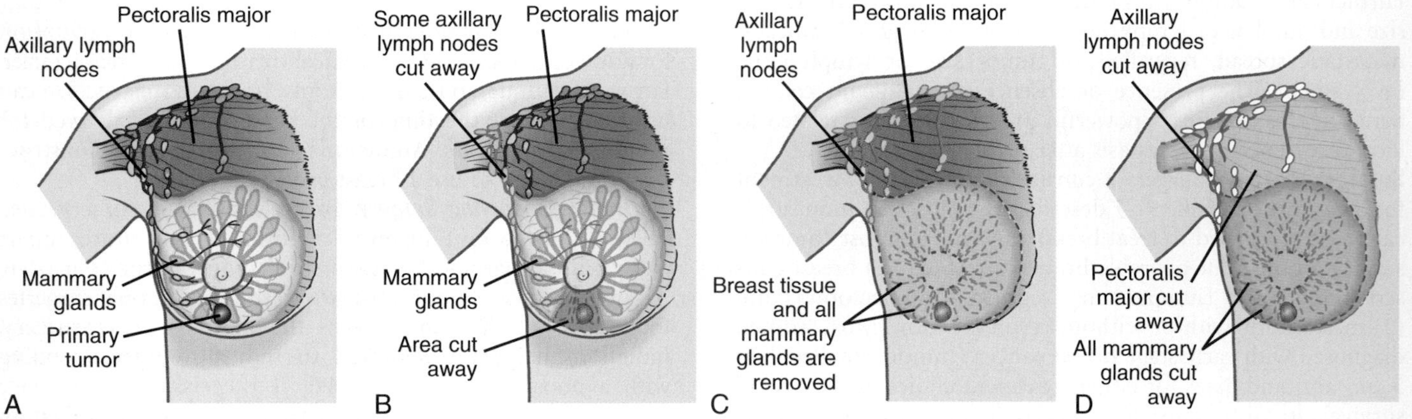


**FIG. 51-6** Breast cancer surgery. **A,** Preoperative. **B,** Lumpectomy. **C,** Simple mastectomy. **D,** Modified radical mastectomy.

**TABLE 51-7 Surgical Procedures for Breast Cancer**

| Procedure | Side Effects | Complications | Patient Issues |
|---|---|---|---|
| **Breast-Conserving Surgery (Lumpectomy) With Radiation Therapy** | | | |
| Wide excision of tumor, sentinel lymph node biopsy (SLNB) and/or axillary lymph node dissection (ALND)<br>Radiation therapy | • Breast soreness<br>• Breast edema<br>• Skin reactions<br>• Arm swelling<br>• Sensory changes in breast and arm | *Short-term:* Moist desquamation,* hematoma, seroma, infection<br>*Long-term:* Fibrosis, lymphedema,† myositis, pneumonitis,* rib fractures* | • Prolonged treatment*<br>• Impaired arm mobility†<br>• Change in texture and sensitivity of breast |
| **Mastectomy** | | | |
| **Simple Mastectomy**<br>Removal of breast, preservation of pectoralis muscle with SLNB<br>**Modified Radical Mastectomy**<br>Removal of breast and pectoralis muscle with ALND | • Chest wall tightness, scar<br>• Phantom breast sensations<br>• Lymphedema<br>• Sensory changes<br>• Impaired range of motion | *Short-term:* Skin flap necrosis, seroma, hematoma, infection<br>*Long-term:* Sensory loss, muscle weakness, lymphedema | • Loss of breast<br>• Incision<br>• Body image<br>• Need for prosthesis<br>• Impaired arm mobility |
| **Breast Implants and Tissue Expansion** | | | |
| Expander used to slowly stretch tissue. Saline gradually injected into reservoir over weeks to months<br>Insertion of implant under musculofascial layer of chest wall | • Discomfort<br>• Chest wall tightness | *Short-term:* Skin flap necrosis, wound separation, seroma, hematoma, infection<br>*Long-term:* Capsular contractions, displacement of implant | • Altered body image<br>• Prolonged physician visits to expand implants<br>• Potential additional surgeries for nipple construction, symmetry |
| **Breast Reconstruction Tissue Flap Procedures‡** | | | |
| ***Transverse Rectus Abdominis Musculocutaneous (TRAM) Flap*** | | | |
| Musculocutaneous flap (muscle, skin, fat, blood supply) is transposed from abdomen to the mastectomy site<br>May be done concurrently with mastectomy | • Pain related to two surgical sites and extensive surgery | *Short-term:* Delayed wound healing, infection, skin flap necrosis, abdominal hernia, hematoma | • Prolonged postoperative recovery |
| ***Deep Inferior Epigastric Artery Perforator (DIEP) Flap*** | | | |
| Free flap that transfers skin and fat from the abdomen to the chest. Differs from TRAM flap because no muscle is moved | • Requires more time in surgery than TRAM flap<br>• Pain related to two surgical sites | If procedure fails, tissue flap may die and have to be completely removed<br>If tissue dies, new reconstruction may not be done for 6-12 mo | • Patients may experience less pain and restriction of movement than with a TRAM flap. |

*Specific to radiation therapy.
†If ALND (less likely with SLNB).
‡This list is not inclusive as additional breast reconstruction options are available to patients.

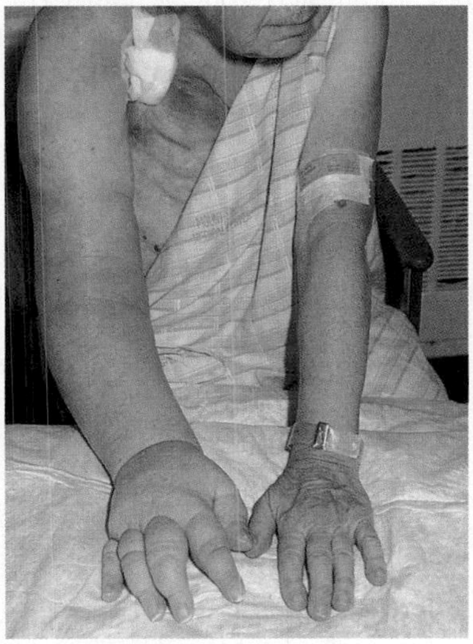

**FIG. 51-7** Lymphedema. Accumulation of fluid in the tissue after excision of lymph nodes. (From Swartz MH: *Textbook of physical diagnosis: history and examination,* ed 6, Philadelphia, 2010, Saunders.)

and upper arm pain, tingling down the arm, continuous aching and burning, numbness, edema, shooting or pricking pain, and unbearable itching that persists beyond the normal 3-month healing time.

Treatment includes nonsteroidal antiinflammatory drugs (NSAIDs), low-dose antidepressants, EMLA (local anesthetics: lidocaine and prilocaine), and antiseizure drugs (e.g., gabapentin [Neurontin]). Other possible treatment modalities include biofeedback, physical therapy to prevent "frozen shoulder" syndrome as a result of inadequate movement, guided imagery, and psychologic counseling with a therapist trained in the management of chronic pain syndromes.

***Phantom Breast Pain.*** *Phantom breast pain* is feeling pain in the breast after a mastectomy. Phantom breast pain can happen after the breast has been removed for the same reasons phantom limb sensation occurs after limb amputations. The brain continues to send signals to nerves in the breast area that were cut during surgery, even though the breast is no longer physically there.

**Radiation Therapy.** Radiation therapy is one form of *adjuvant (additional)* therapy that can be used after surgery. Radiation therapy may be used for breast cancer to (1) prevent local breast cancer recurrences after breast-conserving surgery; (2) prevent local and lymph node recurrences after mastectomy; or (3) relieve pain caused by local, regional, or distant spread of cancer.

***External Radiation Therapy.*** When radiation therapy is a primary treatment, it is usually performed after surgery for the breast cancer. The decision to use radiation therapy after mastectomy is based on the probability that local residual cancer cells are present. Radiation of the axilla and/or supraclavicular nodes may be indicated when lymph nodes are involved to decrease the risk of axillary recurrence. Radiating a localized area will not prevent distant metastasis.

In traditional whole breast (and regional lymph nodes in some cases) radiation treatment, the area is radiated 5 days per week over the course of about 5 to 7 weeks. An external beam of radiation is used to deliver 1.8 Gy to 2 Gy daily fractions to an approximate total dose of 45 to 50 Gy (4500 to 5000 cGy). In patients who have had breast-conserving surgery, a "boost" is a dose of radiation delivered to the area in which the original tumor was located. It is given by external beam and adds five to eight more treatments to the total number given.

For some breast cancer patients, accelerated external beam radiation may be used. With this type of radiation, a shortened schedule of radiation therapy is given daily for 3 to 4 weeks for a total dose of 42.5 Gy.[17]

Fatigue, skin changes, and breast edema may be temporary side effects of external radiation therapy. (Nursing management of the patient receiving radiation therapy is discussed in Chapter 15.)

***Brachytherapy.*** *Brachytherapy* (internal radiation) is used for partial-breast radiation as an alternative to traditional external radiation treatment for some patients with early stage breast cancer.[17] Radiation is delivered directly into the cavity left after a tumor is surgically removed by a lumpectomy. This approach is a minimally invasive way to deliver radiation. Because the radiation is concentrated and focused on the area with the highest risk for tumor recurrence, internal radiation only requires 5 days. Traditional external radiation treatments can take 5 to 7 weeks. Internal radiation therapy is primarily delivered using a multicatheter method or balloon-catheter system.

In the *multicatheter method* (e.g., SAVI) many very small catheters are placed in the breast at the site of the tumor. The SAVI is inserted through a small incision, and the catheter bundle expands uniformly. The ends of the catheters stick out through little holes in the skin. Small radioactive seeds are placed in the catheters. The seeds are left in place just long enough to deliver the radiation dose (e.g., 5 to 10 minutes). The tiny radioactive seeds are inserted only during treatment and then removed. The radiation does not remain in the body between treatments or after the final treatment is over.

In the *balloon-catheter system,* the balloon is placed where the tumor is located. The balloon is filled with fluid to keep it in place. Radioactive seeds are inserted (Fig. 51-8). Radiation is emitted by a tiny radioactive seed attached by a wire on the way to an afterloader, a computer-controlled machine. The seed travels through the MammoSite applicator into the inflated balloon. As with the multicatheter system, the radiation does not remain in the body between treatments or after the final treatment is over. Once the final session is completed, the balloon is deflated and the system is removed.

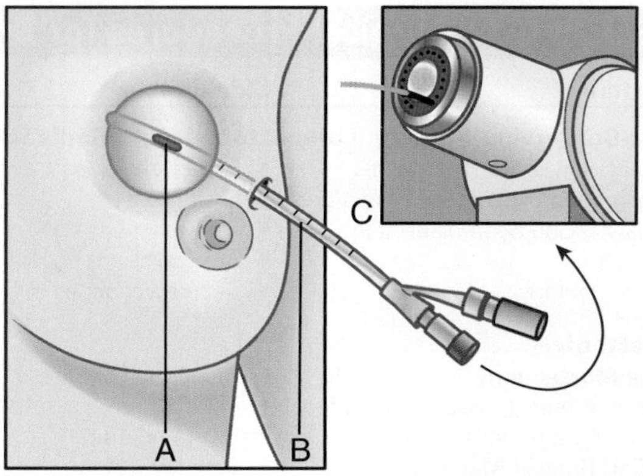


**FIG. 51-8** High-dose brachytherapy for breast cancer. The MammoSite system involves the insertion of a single small balloon catheter *(B)* at the time of the lumpectomy or shortly thereafter into the tumor resection cavity (the space that is left after the surgeon removes the tumor). A tiny radioactive seed *(A)* is inserted into the balloon, connected to a machine called an *afterloader (C),* and delivers the radiation therapy.

***Palliative Radiation Therapy.*** In addition to reducing the primary tumor mass with a resultant decrease in pain, radiation therapy is also used to treat symptomatic metastatic lesions in such sites as bone, soft tissue organs, brain, and chest. Radiation therapy often relieves pain and is successful in controlling recurrent or metastatic disease.

**Drug Therapy.** Drug therapy (systemic therapy) is treatment that travels through the bloodstream to all parts of the body, not just the cancer. Drug therapy includes chemotherapy, hormone therapy, immunotherapy, and targeted therapy.

When drug therapy is given before surgery, it is called *neoadjuvant therapy.* Neoadjuvant therapy is often used to shrink the size of the tumor enough to make surgical removal possible, or to allow for breast-conserving surgery in women who would have been recommended to have a mastectomy. Drug therapy after surgery is called *adjuvant therapy*. Drug therapy can decrease the rate of recurrence and increase the length of survival. Because of the risk for recurrent disease, nearly all patients with evidence of node involvement, particularly those who are hormone receptor negative, will have some type of drug therapy. Some patients, particularly those with a larger or more aggressive tumor, are known to be at higher risk for recurrent or metastatic disease. Drug therapy may be used for these patients even when there is no evidence of node involvement. Weighing the risks and benefits of drug therapy is a complex process.[17]

***Chemotherapy.*** Chemotherapy is the use of cytotoxic drugs to destroy cancer cells. A combination of drugs is usually superior to the use of a single drug. Combination treatment is beneficial because the drugs have different mechanisms of action and work at different parts of the cell cycle.

When used in the neoadjuvant and adjuvant setting, chemotherapy is usually given for 3 to 6 months. However, when a patient has metastasis, chemotherapy may be given for the rest of the patient's life.

Common combination-therapy protocols in the adjuvant and neoadjuvant setting are (1) CMF: cyclophosphamide, methotrexate, and 5-fluorouracil (5-FU); (2) AC: doxorubicin and cyclophosphamide, with or without the addition of a taxane such as paclitaxel (Taxol) or docetaxel (Taxotere); or (3) CEF or CAF: cyclophosphamide, epirubicin (Ellence) or doxorubicin, and 5-FU.

**DRUG ALERT Doxorubicin**

- Monitor for signs of cardiotoxicity and heart failure (e.g., new onset of shortness of breath, pedal edema, decreased activity tolerance, dysrhythmias, ECG changes).
- Instruct patient not to have immunizations without HCP's approval.
- Instruct patient to avoid contact with those who recently received live virus vaccine.

Because healthy cells are also affected by chemotherapy, a variety of side effects accompany this treatment modality. The incidence and severity of common side effects are related to specific drug combination, drug schedule, and dosage. The most common side effects involve rapidly dividing cells in the gastrointestinal tract (nausea, anorexia, weight loss), bone marrow (anemia), and hair follicles (alopecia [hair loss]).

Cognitive changes during and after treatment, especially with chemotherapy, can occur in patients with cancer. This phenomenon is called *"chemobrain."* These changes include difficulties in concentration, memory, focus, and attention. (Cognitive changes in cancer are discussed in Chapter 15 on p. 256.)

***Hormone Therapy.*** Estrogen can promote the growth of breast cancer cells if the cells are estrogen receptor positive. Hormone therapy can block the effect and source of estrogen, thus promoting tumor regression.

Both estrogen and progesterone receptor status assays have been developed to identify women whose breast cancers are likely to respond to hormone therapy. These assays predict whether hormone therapy is a treatment option. Chances of tumor regression are significantly greater in women whose tumors have estrogen and progesterone receptors.

Hormone therapy can (1) block estrogen receptors or (2) suppress estrogen synthesis by inhibiting aromatase, an enzyme needed for estrogen synthesis (Table 51-8). Premenopausal women with estrogen receptor (ER)–positive breast cancers may also benefit from the removal or suppression of their ovaries. Ovarian ablation can be accomplished surgically or by using luteinizing hormone releasing hormone (LHRH) analogs such as goserelin (Zoladex) or leuprolide (Lupron).

**Estrogen receptor blockers.** Estrogen receptor blockers include tamoxifen, toremifene (Fareston), and fulvestrant (Faslodex).

Tamoxifen has been the hormone therapy of choice in ER-positive women with all stages of breast cancer over the past 30 years. Tamoxifen may also be used in high-risk premenopausal and postmenopausal women to prevent breast cancer. The most common side effects of tamoxifen include hot flashes, mood swings, vaginal discharge and dryness, and other effects commonly associated with decreased estrogen. It also increases the risk of blood clots, cataracts, stroke, and endometrial cancer in postmenopausal women.

**DRUG ALERT Tamoxifen**

- Irregular vaginal bleeding or spotting may occur.
- Decreased visual acuity, corneal opacity, and retinopathy can occur in women receiving high doses (240-320 mg/day for >17 mo). These problems may be irreversible.
- Instruct patient to immediately report decreased visual acuity.
- Monitor for signs of deep vein thrombosis, pulmonary embolism, and stroke, including shortness of breath, leg cramps, and weakness.

**Aromatase inhibitors.** Aromatase inhibitor drugs interfere with the anastrozole enzyme aromatase, which is needed for the synthesis of estrogen. These drugs include anastrozole, letrozole (Femara), and exemestane (Aromasin). They are used in the treatment of breast cancer in postmenopausal women. Aromatase inhibitors do not block the production of estrogen by the ovaries. Thus they are of little benefit and may be harmful in premenopausal women.

Aromatase inhibitors have different side effects than tamoxifen. They rarely cause blood clots, and they do not cause

**TABLE 51-8 Drug Therapy**

***Breast Cancer***

| Drug Class | Mechanism of Action | Indications |
|---|---|---|
| **Hormone Therapy** | | |
| ***Estrogen Receptor Blockers*** | | |
| tamoxifen | Blocks estrogen receptors (ERs) | ER-positive breast cancer in premenopausal and postmenopausal women<br>Used as a preventive measure in high-risk premenopausal and postmenopausal women |
| toremifene (Fareston) | Blocks ERs | ER-positive breast cancer in postmenopausal women only |
| fulvestrant (Faslodex) | Blocks ERs | ER-positive breast cancer in postmenopausal women only |
| ***Aromatase Inhibitors*** | | |
| anastrozole (Arimidex)<br>letrozole (Femara)<br>exemestane (Aromasin) | Prevents production of estrogen by inhibiting aromatase | ER-positive breast cancer in postmenopausal women only |
| ***Estrogen Receptor Modulator*** | | |
| raloxifene (Evista) | In breast blocks the effect of estrogen<br>In bone promotes effect of estrogen and prevents bone loss | Postmenopausal women |
| **Immunotherapy and Targeted Therapy** | | |
| trastuzumab (Herceptin)<br>pertuzumab (Perjeta) | Blocks HER-2 receptor | HER-2-positive breast cancer |
| lapatinib (Tykerb) | Inhibits HER-2 tyrosine kinase and EGFR tyrosine kinase | HER-2-positive breast cancer |
| ado-trastuzumab emtansine (Kadcyla) | trastuzumab connected to a chemotherapy drug called DM1 | HER-2-positive breast cancer |
| everolimus (Afinitor) | Binds to mammalian target of rapamycin (mTOR), thereby suppressing T cell activation and proliferation | ER-positive, HER-2-negative breast cancer in postmenopausal women |
| palbociclib (Ibrance) | Kinase inhibitor | ER-positive, HER-2-negative breast cancer in postmenopausal women |

*EGFR,* Epidermal growth factor receptor; *HER-2,* human epidermal growth factor receptor 2.

endometrial cancer. Because they block the production of estrogen in postmenopausal women, osteoporosis and bone fractures may occur. These drugs have been associated with night sweats, nausea, arthralgias, and myalgias.

**Estrogen receptor modulator and others.** Raloxifene (Evista) is a selective estrogen receptor modulator that produces both estrogen-agonistic effects on bone and estrogen-antagonistic effects on breast tissue. (Raloxifene is discussed in the section on osteoporosis in Chapter 63.)

Additional drugs that may be used to suppress hormone-dependent breast tumors include megestrol acetate (Megace), diethylstilbestrol (DES), and fluoxymesterone (Halotestin).

**Immunotherapy and Targeted Therapy.** As more is known about the genetic changes in breast cancer, drugs have been developed to specifically target cells that have altered gene expression. One of these genetic changes is the overexpression of HER-2. Tumors that overexpress the HER-2 protein tend to be more aggressive and are more likely to recur.

Trastuzumab (Herceptin) is a monoclonal antibody to HER-2. After the antibody attaches to the antigen, it is taken into the cells and eventually kills them. It can be used alone or in combination with chemotherapy agents. The most common side effects are flu-like symptoms (fever, chills, myalgia). Another possible, but more serious side effect, is damage to the heart.

**DRUG ALERT Trastuzumab (Herceptin)**
- Use with caution in women with preexisting heart disease.
- Monitor for signs of ventricular dysfunction and heart failure.

Other drugs that target HER-2 include pertuzumab (Perjeta), ado-trastuzumab emtansine (Kadcyla), which is trastuzumab connected to a chemotherapy drug called DM1, and lapatinib (Tykerb), which works inside the cell by blocking the function of the HER-2 protein.

Drugs in other classes that are used to treat breast cancer include everolimus (Afinitor) and palbociclib (Ibrance). Everolimus works by blocking mTOR, a protein that normally promotes cell growth and division. Palbociclib is a kinase inhibitor that prevents cells from dividing, thus slowing cancer growth. (The use of immunotherapy and targeted therapy is discussed in Chapter 15.)

### Culturally Competent Care: Breast Cancer

Differences exist in the incidence, mortality rates, and care issues among diverse racial and ethnic groups related to breast cancer (see Cultural & Ethnic Health Disparities box on this page). In addition, cultural differences may involve gender roles, health beliefs, religion, family structure, socioeconomic factors (e.g., poverty) and lack of health insurance. In addition, the lack of education may influence disparities related to access to health care and the use of recommended surveillance examinations.[21]

Cultural values strongly influence how individuals respond to and cope with breast cancer and treatment. Health beliefs and behaviors are influenced by diverse cultural norms. Breast cancer screening, diagnosis, and treatment are affected by the cultural values and meanings (body image, sexuality, modesty, motherhood) associated with the breasts. Women may delay screening or treatment for varying reasons, including an acceptance of disease as inevitable fate or "God's will," a mistrust of Western medicine, lack of health care benefits, fear, or the stigma of a cancer diagnosis.

**CULTURAL & ETHNIC HEALTH DISPARITIES**

***Breast Cancer***

- White women have a higher incidence of breast cancer than other ethnic groups.
- African American women have lower survival rates from breast cancer than white women, even when diagnosed at an early stage.
- Triple-negative breast cancer (negative for estrogen, progesterone, and HER-2 receptors) has a higher incidence in African American and Hispanic women.
- Breast cancer incidence and mortality rates are lower among Hispanic and Asian/Pacific Islander women than among white and African American women.
- Breast cancer is the most commonly diagnosed cancer among Hispanic women.
- Hispanic women, especially Mexican Americans, have the lowest rate of breast cancer screening of any ethnic group.
- Hispanic and African American women are more likely to be diagnosed at a later stage of breast cancer than white women.

*HER-2,* Human epidermal growth factor receptor 2.

## NURSING MANAGEMENT: BREAST CANCER

### Nursing Assessment

Many factors must be considered when assessing a patient with a breast problem. The history of the breast disorder assists in establishing a diagnosis. Investigate the presence of nipple discharge, pain, rate of growth of the lump, breast asymmetry, and correlation with the menstrual cycle.

Carefully document the size and location of the lump or lumps. Assess the physical characteristics of the lesion, such as consistency, mobility, and shape. If nipple discharge is present, note the color and consistency and whether it occurs from one or both breasts.

Subjective and objective data that should be obtained from an individual suspected of having or diagnosed with breast cancer are presented in Table 51-9.

### Nursing Diagnoses

Nursing diagnoses related to the care of a patient diagnosed with breast cancer vary. After diagnosis and before a treatment plan has been selected, the following nursing diagnoses would apply:
- Decisional conflict *related to* lack of knowledge about treatment options and their effects
- Fear and/or anxiety *related to* diagnosis of breast cancer
- Disturbed body image *related to* physical and emotional effects of treatment modalities

If surgery is planned, the nursing diagnoses may include, but are not limited to, those presented in eNursing Care Plan 51-1 (available on the website for this chapter).

### Planning

The overall goals are that the patient with breast cancer will (1) actively participate in the decision-making process related to treatment, (2) adhere to the therapeutic plan, (3) communicate about and manage the side effects of adjuvant therapy, (4) access and benefit from the support provided by significant others and HCPs, and (5) comply with recommended follow-up and surveillance after treatment.

### Nursing Implementation

**Health Promotion.** Review the risk factors in Table 51-2. People can reduce their risk factors by maintaining a healthy weight,

**TABLE 51-9 Nursing Assessment**

***Breast Cancer***

**Subjective Data**

***Important Health Information***

*Past health history:* Benign breast disease with atypical changes. Previous unilateral breast cancer. Menstrual history (early menarche with late menopause), pregnancy history (nulliparity or first full-term pregnancy after age 30). Previous endometrial, ovarian, or colon cancer. Hyperestrogenism and testicular atrophy (in men)

*Medications:* Hormones, especially as postmenopausal hormone therapy and in oral contraceptives. Infertility treatments

*Surgery or other treatments:* Exposure to therapeutic radiation (e.g., Hodgkin's lymphoma or thyroid radiation)

***Functional Health Patterns***

*Health perception–health management:* Family history of breast cancer (young age at diagnosis). History of abnormal mammogram or atypical prior biopsy. Palpable change found on BSE. Known BRCA mutation carrier, first-degree relative of *BRCA* carrier (but untested)

*Nutritional-metabolic:* Obesity; unexplained severe weight loss (possible indicator of metastasis)

*Activity-exercise:* Level of usual activity

*Cognitive-perceptual:* Changes in cognition, headache, bone pain (possible indicators of metastasis)

*Sexuality-reproductive:* Unilateral nipple discharge (clear, milky, or bloody). Change in breast contour, size, or symmetry

*Coping–stress tolerance:* Psychologic stress

*Self-perception–self-concept:* Anxiety regarding threat to self-esteem

**Objective Data**

***General***

Axillary and supraclavicular lymphadenopathy

***Integumentary***

Hard, irregular, nonmobile breast lump most often in upper, outer sector, possibly fixated to fascia or chest wall. Thickening of breast. Nipple inversion or retraction, erosion. Edema ("peau d'orange"), erythema, induration, infiltration, or dimpling (in later stages). Firm, discrete nodules at mastectomy site (possible indicator of local recurrence). Peripheral edema (possible indicator of metastasis)

***Respiratory***

Pleural effusions (possible indicator of metastasis)

***Gastrointestinal***

Hepatomegaly, jaundice, ascites (possible indicators of liver metastasis)

***Possible Diagnostic Findings***

Finding of mass or change in tissue on breast examination. Abnormal mammogram, ultrasound, or breast MRI. Positive results of FNA or surgical biopsy or similar results with a needle biopsy

*BSE,* Breast self-examination; *FNA,* fine-needle aspiration.

exercising regularly, limiting alcohol, eating nutritious food, and never smoking (or quitting if currently smoking).

Encourage people to adhere to the breast cancer screening guidelines presented on pp. 1204-1205. If a person is at high risk, he or she needs to develop an individualized plan with the HCP. Early detection can decrease the morbidity and mortality associated with breast cancer.

Along with these lifestyle choices, there are other risk-reduction options for individuals at high risk. Genetic testing for *BRCA* gene mutations is available. People with a strong family history of breast cancer should talk with their HCP about the possibility of genetic testing. Routine screening for genetic abnormalities in women without evidence of a strong family history of breast cancer is not warranted.

In women with an abnormal *BRCA1* or *BRCA2* gene, prophylactic oophorectomy may reduce their risk of developing breast cancer and ovarian cancer. In deciding whether and when to undergo this surgical procedure, women should receive counseling about the risks and benefits of prophylactic oophorectomy, including fertility issues.

Prophylactic surgery decisions require a great deal of thought, patience, and discussion with the HCP, genetic counselor, and family. Patients need to consider these options and make decisions with which they feel comfortable. Removing both breasts and ovaries at a young age does not eliminate the risk of breast cancer. A small risk exists that cancer can develop in the areas where the breasts used to be. Close follow-up is necessary, even after prophylactic surgery.

◆ **Acute Care.** The times of waiting for the initial biopsy results and waiting for the HCP to make treatment recommendations are difficult for patients and their families. Even after the HCP has discussed treatment options, the patient often relies on you to clarify and expand on these options. During this stressful time, the patient may not be coping effectively. Appropriate nursing interventions are to explore the patient's usual decision-making processes, help to evaluate the advantages and disadvantages of the options, provide information relevant to the decision, clarify unresolved issues with the HCP, and support the patient and family once the decision is made.

Regardless of the surgery planned, provide the patient with sufficient information to ensure informed consent. Some patients seek extensive, detailed information to maintain a sense of control, whereas others avoid information to decrease anxiety and fear. Be sensitive to the individual's need for and preferred type of information. These include (1) preoperative instructions on pain control and what to expect after surgery (e.g., reporting of complications, dressing and drain care, turning, coughing, deep breathing); (2) a review of mobility restrictions and postoperative exercises; and (3) explanation of the recovery period from the time of surgery until the first postoperative visit.

The woman who has breast-conserving surgery usually has an uncomplicated postoperative course with variable pain intensity. Pain depends primarily on the extent of the lymph node sampling procedure performed. If an ALND has been done or if the patient had a mastectomy, drains are generally left in place, and patients are discharged home with them. Teach the patient and family, with a return demonstration, how to manage the drains at home.

Most patients are discharged from the hospital within 24 to 48 hours after a mastectomy, depending on if reconstructive surgery was performed. Restoring arm function on the affected side after breast cancer surgery is a key nursing goal. Postoperative arm and shoulder exercises, which are started gradually, may begin prior to discharge (Fig. 51-9). These exercises are designed to prevent contractures and muscle shortening, maintain muscle tone, and improve lymph and blood circulation. The difficulty and pain encountered in performing what used to be simple tasks may cause frustration and depression. The goal of all exercise is a gradual return to full range of motion.

## EVIDENCE-BASED PRACTICE

### Applying the Evidence

**Treatment for Breast Cancer**

C.P. is a 56-yr-old woman who was diagnosed with stage IIIA breast cancer. Her treatment plan is to receive neoadjuvant chemotherapy and then have surgery and radiation. C.P. tells you that she is anxious and will have surgery and radiation but does not want chemotherapy because she is afraid of the side effects.

*Making Clinical Decisions*

***Best Available Evidence.*** The use of chemotherapy before surgery reduces the size and extent of the tumor, thus making the surgery more likely to succeed. It also reduces the consequences of a more extensive treatment that would be required if the tumor were not reduced.

***Clinician Expertise.*** Neoadjuvant chemotherapy is usually recommended for stage IIIA breast cancer. The common side effects (e.g., nausea, vomiting, fatigue) can be managed with appropriate treatment.

***Patient Preferences and Values.*** C.P. does not want chemotherapy and prefers to take her chances. If the cancer comes back, she will have chemotherapy.

*Implications for Nursing Practice*

1. Why is it important to discuss with C.P. why chemotherapy is recommended?
2. What information would you share with her regarding possible treatment side effects and how they can be managed?
3. You note her spouse appears attentive and supportive. How will you involve him in C.P.'s care?

*Reference for Evidence*

National Comprehensive Cancer Network: NCCN guidelines for patients. Stage III breast cancer. Retrieved from *www.nccn.org/patients/guidelines/stage_iii_breast/index.html.*

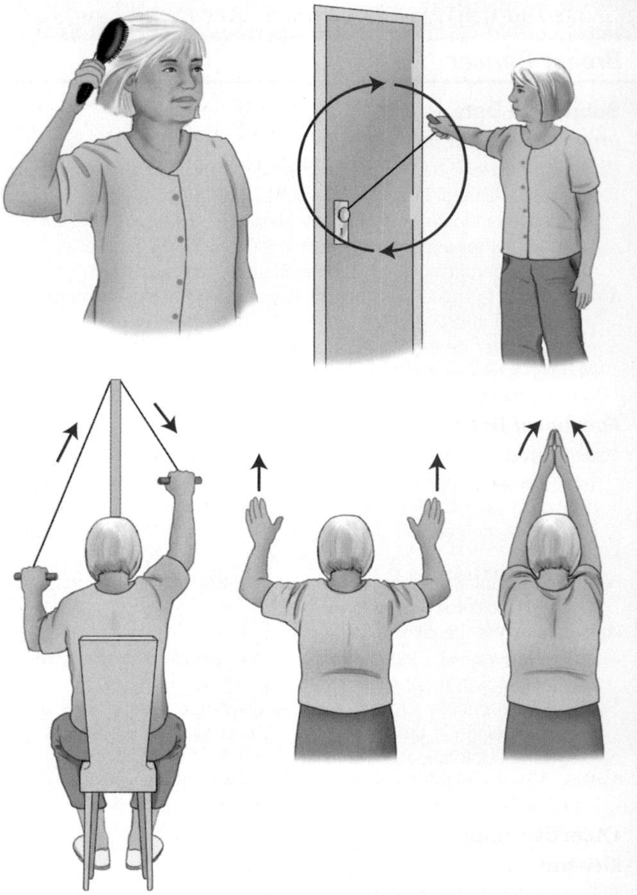

**FIG. 51-9** Postoperative exercises for the patient with a mastectomy or lumpectomy with axillary lymph node sampling and/or dissection.

Postoperative discomfort can be minimized by administering analgesics regularly when the patient is in pain and about 30 minutes before initiating exercises. When the patient is able to shower, the warm water on the involved shoulder often relaxes the muscle and reduces joint stiffness.

Upper extremity lymphedema can occur at any point after treatment for breast cancer. Teach the patient measures to prevent and reduce lymphedema, including no BP readings, venipunctures, or injections on the affected arm. The affected arm should not be dependent for long periods. Caution should be used to prevent infection, burns, or compromised circulation on the affected side.

If trauma to the arm occurs, the area should be washed thoroughly with soap and water and observed. A topical antibiotic ointment and a bandage or other sterile dressing may be applied.

When the patient's lymphedema is acute (Fig. 51-7), complete decongestive therapy will be recommended. This therapy is performed by specially trained professionals and consists of a massage-like technique to mobilize the subcutaneous accumulation of fluid. This may be followed by use of compression bandaging and an intermittent pneumatic compression sleeve. The sleeve applies mechanical massage to the arm and facilitates lymph drainage up toward the heart. Elevation of the arm so that it is level with the heart and isometric exercises may be used to reduce the fluid in the arm. To maintain maximum volume reduction, the patient may need to wear a fitted compression sleeve during waking hours and preventively during air travel.

◆ ***Psychosocial Support.*** Throughout history, the female breast has been regarded as a symbol of beauty, femininity, sexuality, and motherhood. The potential loss of a breast, or part of a breast, may be devastating for many women because of the significant psychologic, social, sexual, and body image implications associated with it. For men diagnosed with breast cancer, isolation and embarrassment related to the diagnosis can occur. You must be aware of resources for men *(www.malebreastcancer.org)*.

As difficult as it is to predict which patients will develop physical effects of treatment, it can be even more difficult to foresee the psychosocial effects of treatment. In some cases, psychosocial concerns may increase the physical effects of cancer, such as pain, fatigue, sleep disturbances, fear of recurrence, and cognitive changes.

Screening all cancer patients for psychosocial distress has been added to the Commission on Cancer accreditation requirements.[22] From the time of diagnosis through treatment, survivorship, or metastatic disease, the patient may exhibit signs of distress or tension (e.g., tachycardia, increased muscle tension, sleep disturbances, restlessness, changes in appetite or mood). Assess the patient's body language and affect during periods of high stress and indecision so that appropriate interventions, including referral to a mental health provider, can be initiated.

Remain sensitive to the complex psychologic impact that a diagnosis of cancer and subsequent breast surgery can have on patients and their families. With an accepting attitude and the offer of resources, you can help the patient cope with feelings of fear, anger, anxiety, and depression. You can help to:

- Provide a safe environment for the expression of feelings.
- Identify sources of support and strength, such as his or her partner, family, and spiritual or religious practices.
- Encourage the patient to identify and learn individual coping strengths.
- Promote communication between the patient and his or her family and friends.
- Provide accurate and complete answers to questions about the disease; treatment options; and reproductive, fertility, or lactation issues (if appropriate).
- Make resources available for mental health counseling.
- Offer information about local and national community resources. Referring patients to support resources, such as the Cancer Support Community, Breastcancer.org, or local breast cancer organizations, is invaluable. The American Cancer Society and National Cancer Institute can provide excellent materials to assist you in meeting the special needs of patients with breast cancer. In addition to in-person and online support programs, multiple free smart phone applications are available through national cancer organizations that provide reliable and current information for the patient and his or her family.

◆ **Ambulatory Care.** Explain the specific follow-up plan to the patient and emphasize the importance of ongoing monitoring and self-care. Immediately after surgery, advise the patient to report symptoms such as fever, inflammation at the surgical site, erythema, postoperative constipation, and unusual swelling. Other changes to report are new back pain, weakness, shortness of breath, and change in mental status, including confusion.

For women who have had a mastectomy without breast reconstruction, a variety of products are available. These include garments such as camisoles with soft breast prosthetic inserts or a fitted prosthesis with bra. Should the woman choose a breast prosthesis, a certified fitter can help her select a comfortable, more permanent weighted prosthesis and bra, generally at 4 to 8 weeks postoperatively. Your role is to present the choices and resources without judgment.

How the loss of part or all of the breast and cancer affect the patient's sexual identity, body image, and relationships can vary. If you are comfortable, initiate a discussion of sexuality by inviting questions about relationships or intimacy concerns. Often the patient's partner and/or family members need help dealing with their emotional reactions to the diagnosis and surgery before they can provide effective support for the patient. There are no physical reasons why a mastectomy would prevent sexual satisfaction. A woman taking hormone therapy may have a decreased sexual drive or vaginal dryness. She may need to use lubrication to prevent discomfort during intercourse. Concerns about sexuality are not well addressed by many HCPs. If difficulty in adjustment or other problems develop, individual or couples counseling may be necessary to deal with the emotional component of a diagnosis of cancer.

## COMPLEMENTARY & ALTERNATIVE THERAPIES

### Imagery

Imagery is the use of one's mind to generate images that have a calming effect on the body.

**Scientific Evidence***

- Good evidence for decreasing cancer pain and postoperative pain.
- Good evidence for treatment of migraine or tension headache in conjunction with standard medical care.

**Nursing Implications**

- Used by nurses to help patients promote relaxation, decrease stress, and manage pain.
- Should be used as a supplemental technique, not a replacement for medical care.

*Source: *www.naturalstandard.com.*

## EVIDENCE-BASED PRACTICE

### *Translating Research Into Practice*

**Are Integrative Therapies Helpful During Breast Cancer Treatment?**

***Clinical Question***

For women receiving breast cancer treatment (P), what is the effect of integrative therapy (I) versus usual care (C) on anxiety, depression, fatigue, and quality of life (O)?

***Synthesis of Best Available Evidence***

- Systematic review of randomized controlled trials (RCTs).
- 203 RCTs of patients receiving breast cancer treatments of surgery, chemotherapy, radiation therapy, and/or hormonal therapy. Intervention was the use of integrative therapies (complementary and alternative therapies) during treatment. Many therapies were examined including meditation, acupuncture, hypnosis, yoga, natural products (e.g., botanicals, minerals), relaxation with imagery, stress management, yoga, massage, music therapy, Tai Chi/qigong, and energy conservation. Outcomes included anxiety, stress reduction, pain, hot flashes, depression, fatigue, sleep, skin changes, and quality of life.
- *Strongest evidence:* Meditation, relaxation with imagery, and yoga decreased anxiety, depression, and fatigue and improved quality of life.
- *Moderate evidence:* Stress management, yoga, massage, music therapy, energy conservation, and meditation decreased stress, fatigue, anxiety, and depression and improved quality of life.

***Conclusions***

- Women use a variety of integrative therapies during breast cancer treatment.
- Meditation, yoga, relaxation with imagery, stress management, massage, music therapy, and energy conservation may be particularly helpful in managing symptoms and improving quality of life during treatment.

***Implications for Nursing Practice***

1. Why is it important for you to determine patient use of complementary and alternative therapies and document your findings?
2. How will you stay informed on evidence that supports or discourages the use of specific complementary and alternative therapies during breast cancer treatment?
3. How can you best help a patient who is exploring various complementary and alternative therapies to reduce treatment-related fatigue?
4. Why are patient preferences for complementary and alternative therapies an integral part of evidence-based practice?

***Reference for Evidence***

Greenlee H, Balneaves L, Carlson L, et al: Clinical practice guidelines on the use of integrative therapies as supportive care in patients treated for breast cancer, *J Natl Cancer Inst Monogr* 50: 346, 2014.

*P,* Patient population of interest; *I,* intervention or area of interest; *C,* comparison of interest or comparison group; *O,* outcomes of interest; *T,* timing (see p. 15).

Depression and anxiety may occur with the continued stress and uncertainty of a cancer diagnosis. A patient's self-esteem and identity may also be threatened. The support of family and friends and participation in a cancer support group and/or individual counseling are important aspects of care that may improve the patient's quality of life.

Almost 3 million breast cancer survivors are alive in the United States, making this population the largest group of cancer survivors. This number is expected to grow due to an aging population and improved methods for early detection and treatment. After treatment for breast cancer, the patient will have ongoing survivorship care.[22,23]

A history and physical examination is recommended one to four times per year as clinically appropriate for 5 years, then annually thereafter. In addition, advise breast cancer survivors to perform monthly BSE and chest wall self-examination, and report any changes to their HCP. Local recurrence of breast cancer is usually at the surgical site. Breast cancer survivors should have an annual mammogram. Other breast imaging studies such as a breast ultrasound or breast MRI should only be performed as an adjunct to mammography and not for annual routine surveillance. (Cancer survivorship is discussed in Chapter 15 on p. 266.)

### Evaluation

Expected outcomes are that the patient after breast cancer surgery will

- Identify activities that can reduce postoperative edema and improve mobility
- Use pain control measures appropriately
- Demonstrate effective use of coping strategies that provide reduction of anxiety
- Discuss feelings about and the meaning of changes in physical appearance
- Identify community and online resources, individual counseling resources, and support groups

Additional information on expected outcomes for the patient after breast cancer surgery is presented in eNursing Care Plan 51-1 (available on the website for this chapter).

### Gerontologic Considerations: Breast Cancer

A major risk for breast cancer is increasing age, and more than half of all breast cancers are diagnosed in women who are age 65 or older.[1] Older women are less likely to have mammograms. Screening and treatment decisions for breast cancer should be based on a woman's general health status rather than biologic age, since health status has a greater influence on tolerance to treatment and long-term prognosis. In addition to medical co-morbidities and life expectancy, treatment decisions for the older woman with breast cancer should be based on an assessment of nutritional and functional status; vision, gait, and balance; and the presence of delirium, dementia, or depression.

Breast cancer treatment is similar for older and younger patients, including the use of surgery, radiation therapy, and drug therapy. For healthy older women, breast cancer survival rates are similar to those of younger women when matched by cancer stage.

## BECOMING A NURSE LEADER

### *Protecting Patient Privacy*

#### Situation

During your clinical rotation on the oncology unit, Felicia, a fellow nursing student, asks you to take a photo of her with her patient, who is a famous TV newscaster. Felicia assures you that this photo will only be for her private collection. Later, you see the photo posted on Felicia's Facebook page with the caption: "Look who I took care of in the hospital today! Hope her treatments for breast cancer are successful."

#### Points for Consideration

- Privacy and confidentiality are basic rights in our society. As nurses, it is our ethical and legal obligation to safeguard those rights.
- *Privacy* is the right of individuals to keep information about themselves from being disclosed. *Confidentiality* is the principle that the information that a patient reveals to an HCP is private and has limits on how and when it can be disclosed to a third party.
- The Health Insurance Portability and Accountability Act (HIPAA) of 1996 privacy rule protects an individual's health information. This information includes the individual's past, present, or future physical or mental health or condition. If you violate HIPAA confidentiality laws by posting patient information online, you may be fired or lose your license.[1]
- The American Nurses Association Code of Ethics details that nurses promote, advocate for, and strive to protect the health, safety, and rights of patients.[2] This includes their right to privacy and confidentiality. The nurse has a duty to maintain confidentiality of all patient information. The patient's well-being could be jeopardized and the fundamental trust between patient and nurse destroyed.
- Our patients trust us with intimate details of their lives, and we should never post patient-related issues on any social media site.

#### Discussion Questions

1. What should you have done when asked to take a photo of the nursing student and her patient?
2. What consequences could happen to Felicia as a result of posting this photo and comment on Facebook?
3. What consequences could you face?

#### References


1. Tortorice J: What is right and wrong when it comes to posting medical pictures online? Retrieved from *www.ceufast.com/blog/julia-tortorice/what-is-right-and-wrong-when-it-comes-to-posting-medical-pictures-online.*
2. American Nurses Association: Code of ethics. Retrieved from *www.nursingworld.org/MainMenuCategories/EthicsStandards/CodeofEthicsforNurses/Code-of-Ethics.pdf.*


## MAMMOPLASTY

**Mammoplasty** is the surgical change in the size or shape of the breast. It may be done electively for cosmetic purposes to either enlarge or reduce the size of the breasts. It may also be done to reconstruct the breast after a mastectomy.

A professional, nonjudgmental attitude and clear information about surgical breast options are most useful for women engaged in decision making about mammoplasty. The desire to change the appearance of the breasts has special significance for each woman as she attempts to alter or recreate her body image. Be aware of the cultural value that the woman places on the breast. Help the patient set realistic expectations about what mammoplasty can accomplish and about possible complications (e.g., hematoma formation, hemorrhage, infection). If an implant is involved, capsular contracture and loss of the implant are possible.

### Breast Reconstruction

Breast reconstructive surgery is a type of surgery for women who have had all or part of a breast removed. It is done to

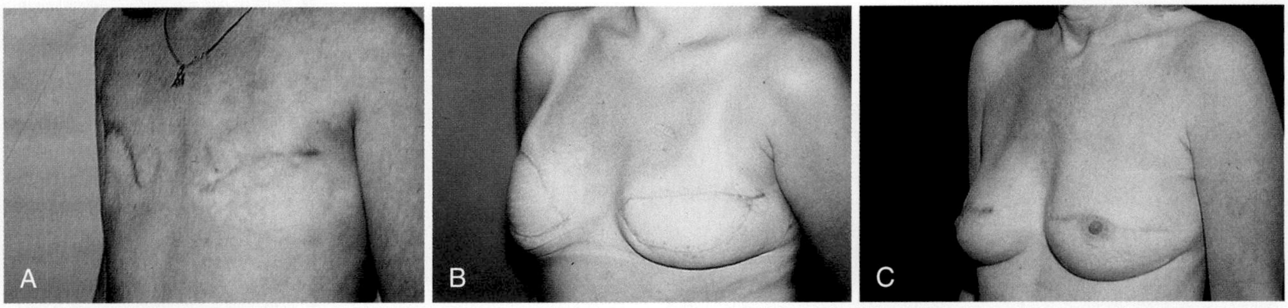


**FIG. 51-10** **A,** Appearance of chest after bilateral mastectomy. **B,** Postoperative breast reconstruction before nipple-areolar reconstruction. **C,** Postoperative breast reconstruction after nipple-areolar reconstruction. (Courtesy Brian Davies, MD. From Fortunato N, McCullough S: *Plastic and reconstructive surgery,* St Louis, 1998, Mosby.)

achieve symmetry and to restore or preserve body image. It may be done simultaneously with a mastectomy or some time afterward. The timing of reconstructive surgery is individualized based on the patient's physical and psychologic needs.[24]

**Indications.** The main indication for breast reconstruction is to improve a woman's self-image, regain a sense of normalcy, and assist in coping with the loss of the breast. The contour of the breast is restored without the use of an external prosthesis. Reconstruction techniques cannot restore lactation, nipple sensation, or erectility. Although the breast will not fully resemble its premastectomy appearance, the reconstructed appearance usually represents an improvement over the mastectomy scar (Fig. 51-10).

**Types of Reconstruction**

***Breast Implants and Tissue Expansion.*** Implants have a silicone shell filled with either silicone gel or saline.[25] Some newer types use a cohesive gel, which is a thicker silicone gel. Implant surgery can be done during one stage or two stages.

In the *one-stage procedure,* the implant is placed at the same time as the mastectomy. The implant is usually placed under the pectoralis muscle.

In the *two-stage procedure,* a tissue expander is inserted after the mastectomy. It is used to stretch the skin and muscle at the mastectomy site before inserting permanent implants (Fig. 51-11). The tissue expander is placed in a pocket under the pectoralis muscle, which protects the implant and provides soft tissue coverage. The tissue expander is minimally inflated and then gradually filled by weekly injections of sterile saline solution. This procedure stretches the skin and muscle and can be painful. A small magnet is embedded in most expanders to help locate the port where the fluid is injected. Therefore a woman should not have an MRI with a magnet in place.

The expander can be (1) surgically removed and a permanent implant is inserted or (2) remain in place to become the implant, thus eliminating the need for a second surgical procedure. Tissue expansion does not work well in individuals with extensive scar tissue from surgery or radiation therapy.

The body's natural response to the presence of a foreign substance is the formation of a fibrous capsule around the implant. If excessive capsular formation occurs as a result of infection, hematoma, trauma, or reaction to a foreign body, a contracture can develop, resulting in deformity. Although surgeons differ in their approaches to the prevention of contracture formation, gentle manual massage around the implant is

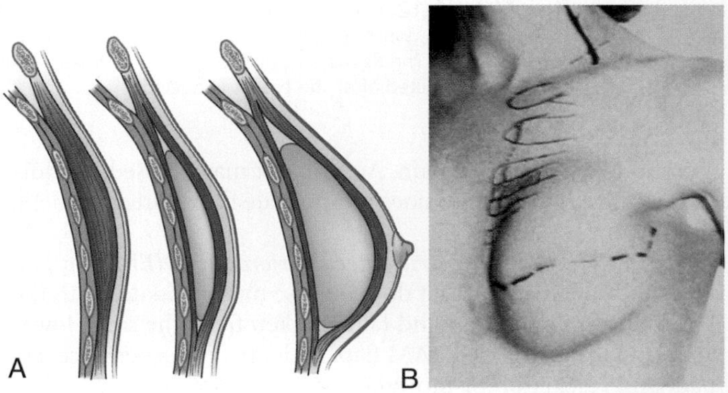


**FIG. 51-11** **A,** Tissue expander with gradual expansion. **B,** Tissue expander in place after mastectomy. (*A,* Modified from Cameron J: *Current surgical therapy,* ed 5, St Louis, 1995, Mosby. *B,* Courtesy Brian Davies, MD. From Fortunato N, McCullough S: *Plastic and reconstructive surgery,* St Louis, 1998, Mosby.)

routine. Other adverse outcomes include wrinkling, scarring, asymmetry, pain, and infection at the incision site.[22]

***Tissue Flap Procedures.*** Another type of breast reconstruction uses autologous (person's own) tissue to recreate a breast mound. In autologous breast reconstruction, tissue from the abdomen, back, thighs, or buttocks is used to create a reconstructed breast. The most common types of tissue flap procedures are *transverse rectus abdominis musculocutaneous (TRAM) flap, deep inferior epigastric artery perforator (DIEP) flap,* and *latissimus dorsi flap.*

The *transverse rectus abdominis musculocutaneous (TRAM) flap* is a frequently used flap operation. The rectus abdominis muscles are paired flat muscles running from the rib cage down to the pubic bone. Arteries running inside the muscles provide branches at many levels, and these branches supply the fat and skin across a large expanse of the abdomen.

There are two different types of TRAM: pedicle flap and free flap. In a pedicle flap, the tissue remains attached to the rectus muscle and is tunneled under the skin to the patient's chest (Fig. 51-12). In a free flap, the tissue is completely separated from the muscle and its blood supply and moved to the new place on the patient's chest.

The tissue is molded and fashioned to form a breast. The abdominal incision is closed, giving the patient a result that is similar to having an abdominoplasty ("tummy tuck"). This surgical procedure can last 6 to 8 hours with recovery taking 6 to 8 weeks. Some patients have reported pain and fatigue for up to 3 months. Complications include bleeding, seroma, hernia,

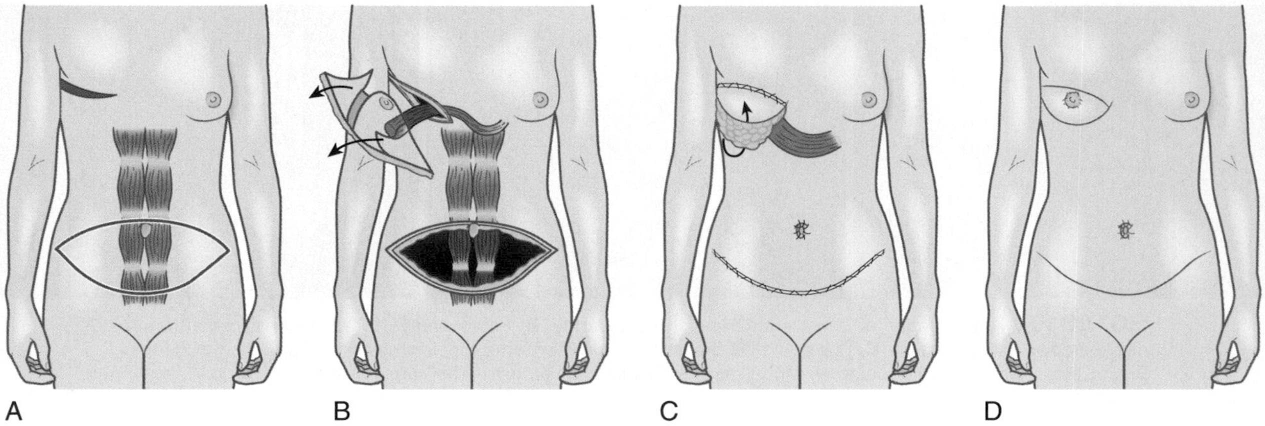


**FIG. 51-12** Transverse rectus abdominis musculocutaneous (TRAM) flap. **A,** TRAM flap is planned. **B,** The abdominal tissue, while attached to the rectus muscle, nerve, and blood supply, is tunneled through the abdomen to the chest. **C,** The flap is trimmed to shape the breast. The lower abdominal incision is closed. **D,** Nipple and areola are reconstructed after the breast is healed.

infection, and low back pain. An implant may be used in addition to the flap if the flap does not provide the desired cosmetic result alone.

A *deep inferior epigastric artery perforator (DIEP) flap* is a version of the free flap that does not use muscle tissue. With the DIEP flap, only the skin and fat are taken from the same lower abdominal area as the TRAM flap. Patients may experience less pain and restriction of movement with this procedure.

In a *latissimus dorsi flap*, a block of skin and muscle from the patient's back is used to replace tissue removed during mastectomy. A small implant may be needed beneath the flap to gain reasonable breast shape and size. A disadvantage of this technique is an additional scar on the back.

Other types of breast reconstruction include gluteal free flap (tissue is used from buttocks, including the gluteal muscle) and transverse upper gracilis flap or inner thigh flap (tissue is taken from the bottom fold of the buttock extending into the inner thigh.)

***Nipple-Areolar Reconstruction.*** Many patients undergoing breast reconstruction also have nipple-areolar reconstruction. Nipple reconstruction gives the reconstructed breast a much more natural appearance (Fig. 51-10, *C*). Nipple-areolar reconstruction is usually done a few months after breast reconstruction. Tissue to construct a nipple may be taken from the opposite breast or from a small flap of tissue on the reconstructed breast mound. The areola may be grafted from the labia, skin in the area of the groin, or lower abdominal skin. Tattooing may be done with a permanent pigmented dye. In some patients, a small implant may be placed under the completed nipple-areolar reconstruction to provide additional projection.

### Breast Augmentation

In *augmentation mammoplasty* (procedure to enlarge the breasts), an implant is placed in a surgically created pocket between the capsule of the breast and pectoral fascia, or ideally under the pectoralis muscle. (Implants are discussed on p. 1223.)

### Breast Reduction

For some women, large breasts can be a source of physical and psychologic discomfort. They can interfere with normal daily activities, such as walking, using a computer, and driving a car. The weight of large breasts can lead to back, shoulder, and neck problems, including degenerative nerve changes. Overly large breasts can interfere with self-esteem, self-image, and comfort in wearing some clothing. Reduction in the size of the breasts can have positive effects on the patient's psychologic and physical health.

Reduction mammoplasty is performed by resecting wedges of tissue from the upper and lower quadrants of the breast. The excess skin is removed, and the areola and nipple are relocated on the breast. Lactation can usually be accomplished if massive amounts of tissue are not removed and the nipples are left connected during surgery.

## ❖ NURSING MANAGEMENT: BREAST AUGMENTATION AND REDUCTION

Breast augmentation and breast reduction may be done in the outpatient surgical area or they may involve overnight hospitalization. General anesthesia is used. Drains are generally placed in the surgical site to prevent hematoma formation and then removed when drainage is under 20 to 30 mL/day. The drainage must be examined for color and odor to detect postoperative infection or hemorrhage. Also monitor the woman's temperature. Dressings should be changed as necessary using sterile technique.

After surgery, assure the woman that the breast's appearance will improve when healing is complete. Depending on physician preference, the patient may be instructed to wear a bra that provides good support continuously for 2 or 3 days after breast reduction or augmentation. Depending on the extent of the operation, most women resume normal activities within 2 to 3 weeks. Strenuous exercise may not be appropriate until several weeks later.

## CASE STUDY

### Breast Cancer

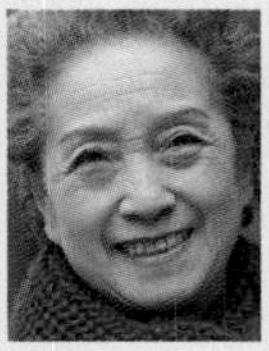

(©XiXinXing/ iStock/ Thinkstock)

**Patient Profile**

A.K., a 68-yr-old married Asian American woman, has been diagnosed with breast cancer. She is scheduled for surgery in the morning for a lumpectomy and sentinel lymph node biopsy with possible axillary node dissection.

**Interprofessional Care**

***Preoperative***

- When she is seen in the preoperative clinic 1 week before surgery, she is crying uncontrollably and says, "My husband does not want to look at me anymore. He is afraid of what I am going to look like with a flat chest."
- She says, "I cannot sleep and I just pace the floor at night."
- "My mother died of breast cancer when she was 60, and my sister got it when she was 40."
- Expresses concern that her two daughters (34 and 32) and their daughters are going to get "this horrible disease."

***Operative Procedure***

- A lumpectomy and sentinel lymph node biopsy are performed.
- A.K. has cancer cells in her sentinel lymph node.
- Axillary node dissection is then done, involving the removal of 12 nodes.

***Postoperative***

- Does not want to leave hospital. She wants to stay in bed.
- Swelling and restricted range of motion in right arm.
- Pain not controlled well with pain medication.

**Follow-Up Findings and Treatment**

- Two positive lymph nodes are found.
- Scheduled for outpatient chemotherapy followed by external radiation.

**Discussion Questions**

1. What in A.K.'s breast cancer experience with her family members may influence her coping response?
2. ***Patient-Centered Care:*** What information would you provide to A.K. about her surgery?
3. What complication did she develop after her surgery?
4. Which common postoperative exercises will A.K. need to practice after her surgery?
5. ***Teamwork and Collaboration:*** Which of the following personnel should provide this instruction to A.K.: registered nurse, licensed practical/vocational nurse, unlicensed assistive personnel?
6. What community resources are available to help A.K. and her family adjust to the change in her body and to cope with the diagnosis of cancer? How can you access these resources?
7. What information is important for you to provide to A.K. about her radiation treatment and chemotherapy?
8. ***Priority Decision:*** Based on the assessment data, what are the priority nursing diagnoses? Are there any collaborative problems?
9. What information is important for you to provide to A.K. and her daughters? What early detection measures are important for them to know?
10. ***Evidence-Based Practice:*** A.K. wants to know what the psychologic benefit may be for her daughters if they decide on a breast cancer genetic risk assessment.
11. ***Patient-Centered Care:*** How will you include cultural preferences in A.K.'s plan of care?
12. ***Teamwork and Collaboration:*** What types of referrals may be indicated for A.K.?
13. ***Safety:*** Describe specific nursing interventions aimed at minimizing risk of harm for A.K.
14. ***Quality Improvement:*** What outcomes would indicate nursing interventions were successful for A.K.?

Answers and a corresponding conceptual care map available at *http://evolve.elsevier.com/Lewis/medsurg.*

## BRIDGE TO NCLEX EXAMINATION

The number of the question corresponds to the same-numbered outcome at the beginning of the chapter.

1. You are a community health nurse planning a program on breast cancer screening guidelines for women in the neighborhood. To best promote the participants' learning and adherence, you would include *(select all that apply)*
   **a.** a short audiotape on the BSE procedure.
   **b.** a packet of articles from the medical literature.
   **c.** written guidelines for mammography and CBE.
   **d.** a discussion of the value of early breast cancer detection.
   **e.** community resources where they can obtain an ultrasound and MRI.
2. In teaching a patient who wants to perform BSE, you inform her that the technique involves both the palpation of the breast tissue and
   **a.** palpation of cervical lymph nodes.
   **b.** hard squeezing of the breast tissue.
   **c.** a mammogram to evaluate breast tissue.
   **d.** inspection of the breasts for any changes.
3. You are caring for a young woman who has painful fibrocystic breast changes. Management of this patient would include
   **a.** scheduling a biopsy to rule out malignant changes.
   **b.** teaching that symptoms will probably subside if she stops using oral contraceptives.
   **c.** preparing her for surgical removal of the lumps, since they will become larger and more painful.
   **d.** explaining that restrictions of coffee and chocolate and supplements of vitamin E may relieve some discomfort.
4. When discussing risk factors for breast cancer with a group of women, you emphasize that the greatest known risk factor for breast cancer is
   **a.** being a woman over age 60.
   **b.** experiencing menstruation for 30 years or more.
   **c.** using hormone therapy for 5 years for menopausal symptoms.
   **d.** having a paternal grandmother with postmenopausal breast cancer.

5. A patient with breast cancer has a lumpectomy with sentinel lymph node biopsy that is positive for cancer. You explain that, of the other tests done to determine the risk for cancer recurrence or spread, the results that support the more favorable prognosis are *(select all that apply)*
   **a.** well-differentiated tumor.
   **b.** estrogen receptor–positive tumor.
   **c.** overexpression of HER-2 cell marker.
   **d.** involvement of two to four axillary nodes.
   **e.** aneuploidy status from cell proliferation studies.
6. A simple mastectomy has been scheduled for your patient with breast cancer. Postoperatively, to restore arm function on the affected side, you would
   **a.** apply heating pads or blankets to increase circulation.
   **b.** place daily ice packs to minimize the risk of lymphedema.
   **c.** teach passive exercises with the affected arm in a dependent position.
   **d.** emphasize regular exercises for the affected shoulder to increase range of motion.
7. Preoperatively, to meet the psychologic needs of a woman scheduled for a simple mastectomy, you would
   **a.** discuss the limitations of breast reconstruction.
   **b.** include her significant other in all conversations.
   **c.** promote an environment for expression of feelings.
   **d.** explain the importance of regular follow-up screening.
8. To prevent capsular formation after breast reconstruction with implants, teach the patient to
   **a.** gently massage the area around the implant.
   **b.** bind the breasts tightly with elastic bandages.
   **c.** exercise the arm on the affected side to promote drainage.
   **d.** avoid strenuous exercise until the implant has healed.

1. c, d, 2. d, 3. d, 4. a, 5. a, b, 6. d, 7. c, 8. a

For rationales to these answers and even more NCLEX review questions, visit *http://evolve.elsevier.com/Lewis/medsurg.*

## EVOLVE WEBSITE

http://evolve.elsevier.com/Lewis/medsurg

**Review Questions (Online Only)**

**Key Points**

**Answer Keys for Questions**

- Rationales for Bridge to NCLEX Examination Questions
- Answer Guidelines for Case Study(ies) on p. 1225

**Student Case Study**

- Patient With Breast Cancer

**Nursing Care Plan**

- eNursing Care Plan 51-1: Patient After Breast Surgery

**Conceptual Care Map Creator**

- Conceptual Care Map for Case Study on p. 1225

**Audio Glossary**

**Content Updates**

## REFERENCES


1. American Cancer Society: Breast cancer facts and figures. Retrieved from *www.cancer.org/research/cancerfactsstatistics/breast-cancer-facts-figures.*
2. Oeffinger KC, Fontham ETH, Etzioni R, et al: Breast cancer screening for women at average risk : 2015 guideline update from the American Cancer Society, *JAMA* 314(15):1599, 2015.

*3. National Comprehensive Cancer Network (NCCN): NCCN Guidelines Version1.2014. Breast Cancer Screening and Diagnosis. Retrieved from *www.nccn.org/professionals/physician_gls/pdf/breast-screening.pdf.*

4. Mansel R: Management of breast pain. In Harris JR, Morrow M, Osborne CK, et al, editors: *Diseases of the breast*, ed 5, Philadelphia, 2014, Wolters Kluwer Health.
5. Twoon M, Ng NY, Thomson SE: Breast lumps, *BMJ* 349:g5275, 2014.
6. Collins LC, Schnitt S: Pathology of benign breast disorders. In Harris JR, Morrow M, Osborne CK, et al, editors: *Diseases of the breast*, ed 5, Philadelphia, 2014, Wolters Kluwer Health.
7. Fatemi Y, Hurley R, Grant C, et al: Challenges in the management of giant intraductal breast papilloma, *Clin Case Rep* 3(1):7, 2015.
8. Mayo Clinic: Atypical hyperplasia. Retrieved from *www.mayoclinic.org/diseases-conditions/atypical-hyperplasia/basics/definition/con-20032601.*
9. Braunstein G: Management of gynecomastia. In Harris JR, Morrow M, Osborne CK, et al, editors: *Diseases of the breast*, ed 5, Philadelphia, 2014, Wolters Kluwer Health.

*10. National Institutes of Health: Women's Health Initiative study. Retrieved from *www.nhlbi.nih.gov/whi.*

11. National Cancer Institute: Oral contraceptives and cancer risk. Retrieved from *www.cancer.gov/about-cancer/causes-prevention/risk/hormones/oral-contraceptives-fact-sheet.*
12. National Cancer Institute: BRCA1 and BRCA2: cancer risk and genetic testing. Retrieved from *www.cancer.gov/about-cancer/causes-prevention/genetics/brca-fact-sheet.*

*13. National Comprehensive Cancer Network (NCCN): NCCN Guidelines Version 2.2014. Genetic/Familial High-Risk Assessment: Breast and Ovarian. Retrieved from *www.nccn.org/professionals/physician_gls.pdf/genetics_screening.pdf.*

14. Breastcancer.org: Other abnormal gene testing. Retrieved from *www.breastcancer.org/symptoms/diagnosis/other-gene-testing.*
15. Zelnak AB, Wisinski KB: Management of patients with HER2-positive metastatic breast cancer: is there an optimal sequence of HER2-directed approaches? *Cancer* 121(1):17, 2015.
16. Oncotype testing for DCIS. Retrieved from *http://breast-cancer.oncotypedx.com/en-US/Patient-DCIS/WhatIsTheOncotypeDXCancerTest.aspx.*

*17. National Comprehensive Cancer Network (NCCN). NCCN Guidelines Version1.2015. Breast Cancer. Retrieved from *www.nccn.org/professionals/_gls.pdf/.pdf.*

18. Joint Committee on Cancer: AJCC cancer staging manual, ed 7. Retrieved from *www.cancerstaging.org.*
19. National Cancer Institute. Breast cancer treatment: Stage I, II, IIIA, and Operable Stage IIIC Breast Cancer. Retrieved from *www.cancer.gov/cancertopics/pdq/treatment/breast/healthprofessional.*
20. Post-breast therapy pain syndrome. Retrieved from *http://cancersupportivecare.com/neuropathicpain.php.org.*
21. Reeder-Hayes KE, Wheeler SB, Mayer DK: Health disparities across the breast cancer continuum, *Semin Oncol Nurs* 31(2):170, 2015.
22. American College of Surgeons Commission on Cancer (2012). Cancer Program Standards 2012, Version 1.1: Ensuring Survivor-Centered Care Manual, retrieved from *www.facs.org/cancer/coc/programstandards2012.html.*
23. Hulett JM, Armer JM, Stewart BR, et al: Perspectives of the breast cancer survivorship continuum: diagnosis through 30 months post-treatment, *J Pers Med* 5(2):174, 2015.
24. American Cancer Society: Types of reconstruction. Retrieved from *www.cancer.org/cancer/breastcancer/moreinformation/breastreconstructionaftermastectomy/breast-reconstruction-after-mastectomy-types-of-br-recon.*
25. Food and Drug Administration: Breast implants. Retrieved from *www.fda.gov/MedicalDevices/ProductsandMedicalProcedures/ImplantsandProsthetics/BreastImplants/default.htm.*

*Evidence-based information for clinical practice.

52

# Sexually Transmitted Infections

*Adena Bargad*

*They may forget your name, but they will never forget how you made them feel.*

***Maya Angelou***

http://evolve.elsevier.com/Lewis/medsurg/

## LEARNING OUTCOMES

1. Identify factors contributing to the high rates of sexually transmitted infections (STIs) in the United States.
2. Describe the etiology, clinical manifestations, complications, and diagnostic studies for chlamydia, gonorrhea, trichomoniasis, genital herpes, genital warts, and syphilis.
3. Compare and contrast primary genital herpes with recurrent genital herpes.
4. Explain the interprofessional care and drug therapy of chlamydia, gonorrhea, trichomoniasis, genital herpes, genital warts, and syphilis.
5. Integrate the nursing assessment and nursing diagnoses for patients who have an STI.
6. Describe the nursing management of patients with STIs, including the teaching and counseling appropriate for each STI.
7. Summarize the nursing role in the prevention and control of STIs.

## KEY TERMS

chlamydial infections, p. 1228
genital herpes, p. 1232
genital warts, p. 1234
gonorrhea, p. 1230
sexually transmitted infections (STIs), p. 1227
syphilis, p. 1235
trichomoniasis, p. 1231

**Sexually transmitted infections (STIs)** are infectious diseases that are spread through sexual contact with the penis, vagina, anus, mouth, or sexual fluids of an infected person. Mucosal tissues in the genitals (urethra in men, vagina in women), rectum, and mouth are especially susceptible to the bacteria and viruses that cause STIs. A list of common STIs is presented in Table 52-1.

Some STIs, such as genital human papillomavirus (HPV), may also be spread from direct skin-to-skin contact with an infected person. Other STIs, such as human immunodeficiency virus (HIV), may also be contracted via blood or blood products or be transmitted from mother to baby during pregnancy or labor and delivery. Some STIs may also be spread through *autoinoculation* (spread of infection by touching or scratching an infected area and transferring it to another part of the body). STIs cannot typically be transmitted from inanimate objects.

STIs are very common. It is estimated that nearly 20 million new infections occur in the United States each year. An estimated 110 million Americans are currently infected with one or more STIs.[1] Having one STI increases the risk of getting another. A person can have more than one STI at the same time.

All STIs have an incubation period, which refers to the time from initial infection to the time when symptoms first appear or screening tests for the infection are positive. This can lead to the transmission of disease from an asymptomatic (but infected) person to another person, even before any symptoms or signs begin.

In the United States, all cases of gonorrhea and syphilis, and, in most states, chlamydial infection must be reported to public health authorities for purposes of surveillance and partner notification. Surveillance and partner notification are a major part of the effort to prevent and control the spread of STIs. Nurses play an important role in STI reporting and are mandated to report these STIs to public health authorities. In spite of this requirement, many cases of these infections go unreported. Every year, only a small percentage of the estimated 20 million new STIs are reported.

## FACTORS AFFECTING INCIDENCE OF STIs

Many factors contribute to the high rate of STIs. Earlier reproductive maturity and increased longevity make for a longer sexual life span. Other factors include (1) greater sexual freedom, (2) inconsistent or incorrect use of barrier methods (e.g., condoms) during sexual activity, and (3) the media's increasing emphasis on sexuality without mentioning safer sex. Substance

Reviewed by Suzanne Jed, MSN, FNP-BC, Senior Clinical Technical Advisor, International Training and Education Center for Health (I-TECH) South Africa, University of Washington, Pretoria, South Africa; Crystal Sheaves, RN, MSN, APRN, FNP-BC, Senior Lecturer, West Virginia University School of Nursing, Charleston, West Virginia; and Whitney Starr, MSN, FNP-BC, Assistant Professor, Division of Infectious Diseases, University of Colorado, Denver, Colorado.

**TABLE 52-1 Causes of Sexually Transmitted Infections (STIs)**

| Sexually Transmitted Infection | Cause |
|---|---|
| **Bacterial Infections** | |
| Chlamydial | *Chlamydia trachomatis* |
| Gonorrhea | *Neisseria gonorrhoeae* |
| Syphilis | *Treponema pallidum* |
| **Viral Infections** | |
| Genital herpes | Herpes simplex virus (HSV 1 or 2) |
| Genital warts *(condylomata acuminata)* | Human papillomavirus (HPV) |
| Human immunodeficiency virus infection (HIV) | Human immunodeficiency virus (HIV) (see Chapter 14) |
| Acquired immunodeficiency syndrome (AIDS) | |
| Hepatitis B and C | Hepatitis B and C viruses (see Chapter 43) |
| Molluscum | *Molluscum contagiosum* |
| **Parasitic/Protozoan Infection** | |
| Trichomoniasis | *Trichomonas vaginalis* |

**TABLE 52-2 Risk Factors for STIs**

**High-Risk Populations**
- Women
- Men who have sex with men
- Adolescents and young adults (age <25)
- Men and women in correctional facilities
- Victims of sexual assault

**High-Risk Behaviors**
- Having new or multiple sexual partners
- Having more than one sexual partner
- Having sexual partners who have had multiple partners
- Sharing needles used to inject drugs
- Alcohol or drug dependence or abuse (inhibits judgment)
- Inconsistent or incorrect use of condoms or other barrier methods

**High-Risk Medical History**
- Not being vaccinated for STIs that have vaccines
- Having one STI is a risk factor for getting another

use and abuse can further contribute to unsafe sexual practices by impairing judgment. Risk factors for STIs are presented in Table 52-2.

Urbanization and easier national and international travel are some of the more global changes that may contribute to increased opportunities for exposure to all infectious diseases, including STIs. Finally, certain groups of people are disproportionately affected by STIs, including youth under age 25 and those who are socially and economically disadvantaged.[1]

The rate of STIs is also reflected in trends in methods of contraceptive use. For example, the male condom is considered to be the best form of protection (other than abstinence) against STIs. Although condom use has increased in the United States, condoms are not frequently used in the general population for contraception. Only a small percentage of women use condoms as their method of contraception. It is important to note that hormone contraceptives (oral contraceptive pills, patch, injectables) and long-acting reversible contraceptives (e.g., intrauterine devices or implantable devices) provide no barrier protection against STIs.[2]

**CULTURAL & ETHNIC HEALTH DISPARITIES**

***Sexually Transmitted Infections***

**Incidence of STIs**
- *Chlamydial infection:* African Americans represent 52% of cases.
- *Syphilis:* African Americans represent 47% of cases, a rate 60 times higher than that of whites.
- *Herpes simplex virus-2:* More common in African Americans (39%) than whites (12%).
- *Gonococcal infection:* African Americans represent 69% of reported cases.

**Factors Influencing Disparities**
- Social and economic disadvantages can make it difficult for individuals to care for their overall health, including their sexual health.
- People who cannot afford basic necessities may have trouble accessing and affording quality sexual health services.
- Fear and distrust of HCPs and institutions can negatively affect racial and ethnic minorities from seeking health care.
- In ethnic communities where there is a high prevalence of STIs, it may be difficult to reduce the risk of infection because with any sexual encounter, a person faces a higher chance of encountering an infected partner than in those communities with a lower prevalence.

# STIs CHARACTERIZED BY DISCHARGE, CERVICITIS, OR URETHRITIS

## CHLAMYDIAL INFECTIONS

Chlamydial infection is the most common STI in the United States, with an estimated nearly 3 million new cases per year.[1]

### Etiology and Pathophysiology

**Chlamydial infections** are caused by *Chlamydia trachomatis,* a gram-negative bacterium and intracellular pathogen. *Chlamydia* is transmitted through exposure to sexual fluids during vaginal, anal, or oral sex. Ejaculation does not have to occur for this infection to be transmitted. The incubation period for chlamydial infection is 1 to 3 weeks. Infection with *Chlamydia* does not confer immunity to future infection. This means that people who have been treated for chlamydial infection can be reinfected.

The most common site for infection in men is the urethra. Infections in the male urethra are called *urethritis.* The most common site for infection for women is the cervix. Infections in the female cervix are called *cervicitis.* Both men and women can get chlamydial infections of the rectum from anal sex. Because the vagina acts as a natural reservoir for infectious secretions, transmission of STIs is often more efficient from men to women than it is from women to men.

There are many strains of the *C. trachomatis* bacteria. Some of these strains can cause other sexually acquired infections, such as *nongonococcal urethritis* (NGU) or lymphogranuloma venereum (LGV).

### Clinical Manifestations

Persons with chlamydial infection may have no symptoms. However, if symptoms develop in men, they may experience pain with urination or a urethral discharge. Rarely, men can have pain or swelling of the testicles caused by infection of the epididymis (Fig. 52-1). Symptoms of cervicitis in women include

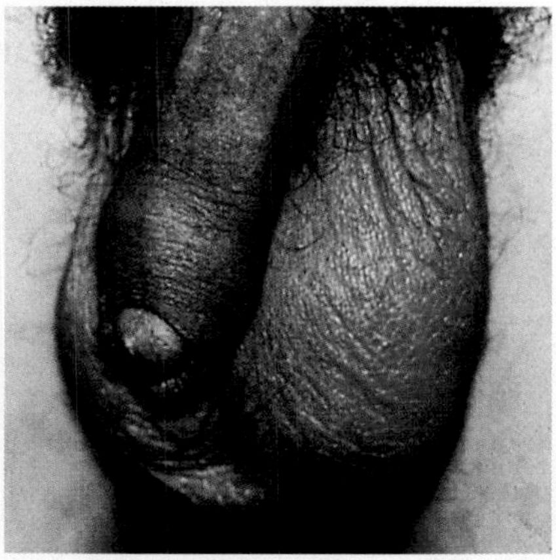

**FIG. 52-1** Chlamydial epididymitis. Red, swollen scrotum. (From Morse S, Moreland A, Holmes K, editors: *Atlas of sexually transmitted diseases and AIDS,* London, 1996, Mosby-Wolfe.)

### TABLE 52-3 Interprofessional Care

#### *Chlamydial Infections*

**Diagnostic Assessment**

- History and physical examination
- Nucleic acid amplification test (NAAT)
- Testing for other STIs (gonorrhea, HIV, syphilis)

**Management**

- azithromycin (Zithromax) or doxycycline (Vibramycin)
- Alternative regimen: erythromycin, ofloxacin, or levofloxacin (Levaquin)
- Instruction on abstinence from sexual intercourse for 7 days after completing treatment
- Treatment of all sexual partners

mucopurulent discharge (mucus with pus), bleeding, dysuria, and pain with intercourse. Symptoms of rectal chlamydial infection can include rectal pain, discharge, and bleeding.

## Complications

Complications often develop from poorly managed, inaccurately diagnosed, or undiagnosed chlamydial infections. Chlamydial infection is often not diagnosed until complications occur. While men rarely have long-term complications from chlamydial infection, epididymitis can result in male infertility. More commonly, chlamydial infections can affect a woman's reproductive tract, resulting in *pelvic inflammatory disease* (PID). PID can damage fallopian tubes and increases a woman's risk for an ectopic pregnancy (pregnancy outside of uterus), infertility, and chronic pelvic pain. The risk of developing PID increases with repeated chlamydial infection. The more episodes of PID, the more likely a woman will experience infertility.[3] Both men and women can develop a rare reactive arthritis, an autoimmune response to infection with *C. trachomatis.*

## Diagnostic Studies

The preferred method for diagnosing chlamydial infection is through nucleic acid amplification testing (NAAT) (Table 52-3). NAAT is used to identify small amounts of DNA or RNA in test samples.

NAAT can be performed on endocervical or vaginal swabs from women, urethral swabs from men, and urine from both men and women. NAATs are also the recommended test for

### EVIDENCE-BASED PRACTICE

#### *Translating Research Into Practice*

**Is Home-Based STI Testing Effective?**

***Clinical Question***

In females screened for sexually transmitted infections (P) what is the effectiveness of home-based self-sampling (I) versus clinic-based testing (C) on acceptability and specimen quality (O)?

***Synthesis of Best Available Evidence***

- Systematic review of randomized controlled trials (RCTs).
- 7 RCTs of females ($n$ = 4042) 14 to 50 years old. Intervention was sampling method used to screen for sexually transmitted infections (STIs) of *Chlamydia,* gonorrhea, and trichomoniasis. Outcome was uptake or nonuptake of screening, which is the number of females screened as a proportion of all those that should have been screened. Also measured were acceptability of sampling method and quality of specimen obtained.
- Home-based STI testing had greater uptake compared to clinic-based testing and was the preferred screening method.
- Specimen quality did not differ according to sampling method used.

***Conclusions***

- Home-based testing increased screening uptake for STIs with no compromise in specimen quality.
- Greater ease (acceptability) occurred when specimens are obtained at home.

***Implications for Nursing Practice***

1. Why is home-based sampling important for younger females who do not want to attend a screening clinic?
2. How will you provide teaching to older women with STI symptoms who refuse clinic testing because "only young people get STIs"?
3. Why is it important for HCPs to learn new strategies to improve STI screening rates?

***Reference for Evidence***

Odesanmi TY, Wasti SP, Odesanmi OS, et al: Comparative effectiveness and acceptability of home-based and clinic-based sampling methods for sexually transmissible infections screening in females aged 14-50 years: a systematic review and meta-analysis, *Sexual Health* 10:559, 2013.

*P,* Patient population of interest; *I,* intervention or area of interest; *C,* comparison of interest or comparison group; *O,* outcomes of interest; *T,* timing (see p. 15).

rectal and oropharyngeal screening and diagnosis in these extragenital sites.[4]

## Interprofessional Care

Because of the high prevalence of asymptomatic infections, regular screening for chlamydial infection in high-risk populations is recommended (Table 52-2). Anyone diagnosed and treated for chlamydial infection should be retested 3 months posttreatment to detect repeat infections.

**Drug Therapy.** The preferred treatment for chlamydial infection is a single dose of azithromycin or doxycycline for 7 days (Table 52-3). Instruct patients to abstain from sexual intercourse for 7 days after treatment and until all sexual partners have completed a full course of treatment. Advise patients to return if symptoms persist or recur.

**DRUG ALERT Doxycycline (Vibramycin)**

- Patients on this drug should avoid unnecessary exposure to sunlight.
- Do not take with antacids, iron products, or dairy products.
- Pregnant women should not take doxycycline.

Any sexual partner within the preceding 60 days of diagnosis or onset of symptoms needs to be treated. Teach patients to return for testing 3 months after treatment to be sure that they have not been reinfected. Encourage patients to use condoms or barrier methods consistently and correctly every time they have sex.

**CHECK YOUR PRACTICE**

You are working in a public health STI clinic. You are seeing a 28-yr-old woman for the second time in 2 months for recurrent vaginal discharge. The patient states she has not been with anyone else except her regular partner and she says, "I don't know why I have this again. The doctor gave me the pills and I took them."

- How would you respond?
- What do you think is causing her symptoms?

Unfortunately, there is a high rate of recurrence for chlamydial infections. This may be due to the fact that sexual partners of infected people may not be treated. This "ping-pong" effect (treatment, reexposure, and reinfection) can end only when infected partners are also treated. Because of this issue, the CDC recommends *Expedited Partner Therapy* (EPT). EPT means HCPs can provide medications or prescriptions to their patients with STIs to give to partners without actually examining the partner. The legality of EPT varies from state to state, but few states actually prohibit EPT. EPT is not routinely recommended for men who have sex with men (MSM) because of a higher risk for coexisting infections in partners of MSM, especially undiagnosed syphilis or HIV.[5]

## GONOCOCCAL INFECTIONS

In the United States, approximately 800,000 gonococcal infections occur per year, making it the second most common STI.[1]

### Etiology and Pathophysiology

Gonorrhea is caused by *Neisseria gonorrhoeae,* a gram-negative, diplococcus bacterium. Gonorrhea can be transmitted by exposure to sexual fluids during vaginal, anal, or oral sex, but ejaculation does not have to occur for gonorrhea to be transmitted. The incubation period is from a few days to 1 week. The infection confers no immunity to subsequent reinfection. The most common site for infection for men is the urethra and for women, the cervix. Both men and women can get gonorrheal infections of the rectum from anal sex or of the oropharynx from oral sex.

### Clinical Manifestations

The initial site of infection in men is usually the urethra. Many men with gonorrhea are asymptomatic, while many others do report symptoms. The most common symptoms of gonococcal urethritis among men are dysuria, purulent urethral discharge (Fig. 52-2), or epididymitis. Most women who contract gonorrhea are asymptomatic or have minor symptoms that are often overlooked. For women, common symptoms are increased vaginal discharge, dysuria, frequency of urination, or bleeding after sex. Often, redness and swelling can occur at the cervix or urethra along with a purulent exudate (Fig. 52-3).

Both men and women can contract rectal gonorrhea during anal intercourse and oropharyngeal gonorrhea during oral sex. Symptoms of rectal gonorrhea may include mucopurulent rectal discharge, bleeding, pain, pruritus, and painful bowel movements.

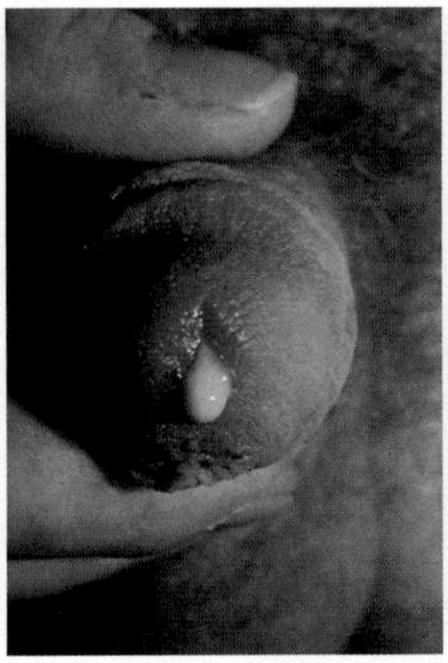

**FIG. 52-2** Profuse, purulent drainage in a patient with gonorrhea. (From Marx J, Walls R, Hockberger R: *Rosen's emergency medicine: concepts and clinical practice,* ed 7, St Louis, 2010, Mosby.)

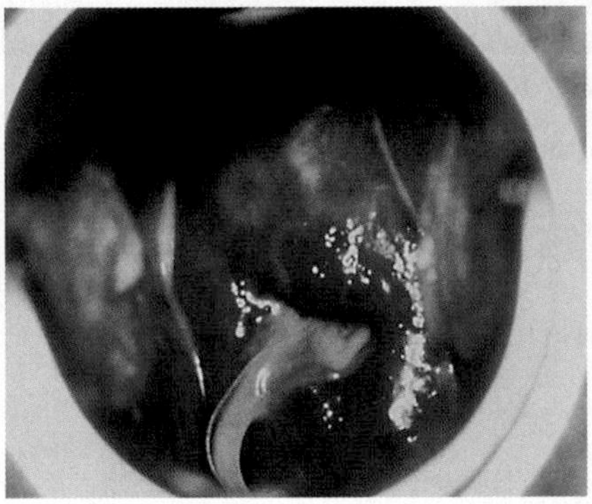

**FIG. 52-3** Endocervical gonorrhea. Cervical redness and edema with discharge. (From Morse S, Moreland A, Holmes K, editors: *Atlas of sexually transmitted diseases and AIDS,* London, 1996, Mosby-Wolfe.)

Most patients with gonorrheal infections in the throat have few if any symptoms. Some may complain of a sore throat.

### Complications

Because men are often symptomatic and seek treatment early in the course of gonorrhea infection, they are less likely to develop serious complications than women. The complication that can occur in men is epididymitis, which can result in infertility.

Because women who are asymptomatic seldom seek treatment, serious complications are more common for women and are usually the reason for seeking medical attention. Untreated gonorrhea can cause an infection in the Bartholin's glands (located internally on either side of the vaginal opening) and can also result in PID. PID increases risk for ectopic pregnancy, infertility, and chronic pelvic pain.

Although rare, both men and women can develop a disseminated gonococcal infection (DGI). DGI is associated with skin lesions, fever, arthralgia, arthritis, and/or endocarditis (Fig. 52-4).

Neonates can develop gonococcal conjunctivitis *(ophthalmia neonatorum)* from exposure to an infected mother during delivery that can result in permanent blindness. Almost all states have a law or a health department regulation requiring the use of a prophylactic treatment in the eyes of all newborns to prevent such infections. Because of both improved prenatal screening for gonorrhea and prophylactic treatment regimens, *ophthalmia neonatorum* caused by gonorrhea is relatively rare.

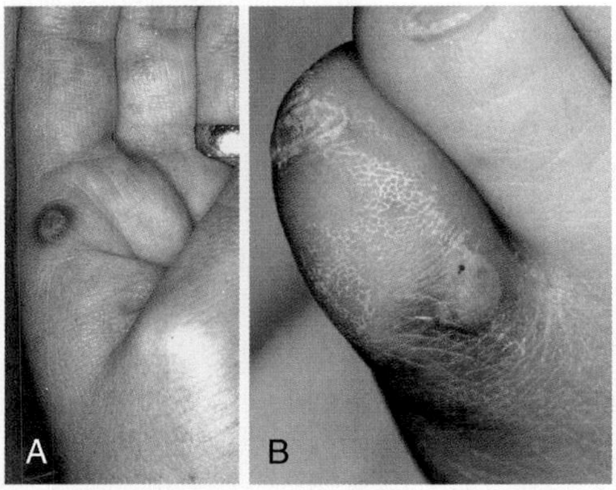


**FIG. 52-4** Skin lesions with disseminated gonococcal infection. **A,** On the hand. **B,** On the fifth toe. (*A,* From Cohen J, Powderly WG: *Infectious diseases,* ed 2, St Louis, 2004, Mosby. *B,* From Mandell GL, Bennett JE, Dolin R: *Mandell, Douglas, and Bennett's principles and practice of infectious diseases,* ed 7, Philadelphia, 2010, Churchill Livingstone.)

**GENDER DIFFERENCES**

***Sexually Transmitted Infections***

| Men | Women |
|---|---|
| • Syphilis more common, especially in men who have sex with men<br>• More likely to have symptoms<br>• Chlamydial infection results in few complications<br>• Easier to diagnose because of less complex anatomy<br>• Less likely to seek medical care | • Anatomy increases risk for STI<br>• Chlamydial infection three times more common<br>• Gonorrhea, trichomoniasis, and HSV-2 more common<br>• HPV is most common STI in women<br>• Have more frequent and serious complications related to STIs (e.g., PID, infertility, ectopic pregnancy, untreated syphilis in pregnant women can result in infant death) |

Adapted from Centers for Disease Control and Prevention: 10 Ways STDs impact women differently than men. Retrieved from *www.cdc.gov/nchhstp/newsroom/docs/STDs-Women-042011.pdf.*
*HSV-2,* Herpes simplex type 2; *PID,* pelvic inflammatory disease; *STIs,* sexually transmitted infections.

## Diagnostic Studies

Diagnosis of any STI requires an accurate sexual history, a physical exam, and appropriate laboratory tests specific to each infection. For men, a presumptive diagnosis of gonorrhea is made if there is a history of sexual contact with a new or infected partner followed within a few days by urethral discharge. For women, making a diagnosis of gonorrhea on the basis of symptoms is difficult. Most women are asymptomatic or have complaints that may be confused with other conditions, such as chlamydial or urinary tract infection.

As with chlamydial infection, NAATs are used for detecting gonorrhea. Culture may also be used to diagnose infection. Gram stains of urethral secretions may also be used, but the sensitivity of gram stain is not as good as other methods.

## Interprofessional Care

**Drug Therapy.** Because of a short incubation period and high rates of infectivity, treatment for gonorrhea is often given without waiting for positive test results. The first-line treatment for gonorrhea is dual therapy with ceftriaxone (Rocephin) given IM with oral azithromycin (Table 52-4). Over the years, *N. gonorrhoeae* has developed resistance to many classes of antibiotics, including fluoroquinolones (ciprofloxacin [Cipro], ofloxacin, levofloxacin [Levaquin]) and tetracyclines (doxycycline [Vibramycin]). Given the increasing rate of drug resistance, all patients with gonococcal infection must receive treatment with at least two antibiotics as a way of reducing or minimizing the chance of incomplete treatment to combat the potential for drug resistance. Patients treated with a preferred regimen but who have a persistently positive test 7 days after treatment need antibiotic sensitivity testing.

As with *C. trichomatis,* all sexual contacts of patients with gonorrhea should be evaluated and treated to prevent reinfection and further transmission. All sexual partners within 60 days of diagnosis should also be treated. Counsel patients to abstain from sexual intercourse during and one week after treatment. Review the ways to reduce risk of acquiring a repeat or new STI in the future.

**TABLE 52-4 Interprofessional Care**

***Gonococcal Infections***

**Diagnostic Assessment**
- History and physical examination
- Gram-stained smears of urethral or endocervical exudate
- Culture for *Neisseria gonorrhoeae*
- Nucleic acid amplification test (NAAT) to detect *N. gonorrhoeae*
- Testing for other STIs (syphilis, HIV, chlamydial infection)

**Management**
- Uncomplicated gonorrhea: ceftriaxone (Rocephin) IM with azithromycin (Zithromax)
- Treatment of sexual contacts
- Instruction on abstinence from sexual intercourse and alcohol during treatment
- Reexamination if symptoms persist or recur after completion of treatment

# TRICHOMONIASIS

**Trichomoniasis**, a type of STI caused by a protozoan, *Trichomonas vaginalis,* is one of the most common STIs in the world. Also known as "trich," this infection was often overlooked compared to other STIs. However, better testing methods have improved detection of trichomoniasis. Trichomoniasis is much more common among women than men, particularly among women with HIV.[6]

## Etiology and Pathophysiology

*Trichomonas vaginalis* is a flagellate protozoan parasite. *Trichomonas* can be transmitted by exposure to sexual fluids during vaginal, anal, or oral sex, even if ejaculation does not occur. The incubation period for trichomoniasis is approximately 1 week to 1 month but can be much longer. The infection confers no immunity to future reinfection.

The most common site for infection in men is the urethra, and in women, the cervix. It is uncommon for *Trichomonas* to infect the rectum, and it is not known to infect the oropharynx. Routine screening for *T. vaginalis* should be considered for women in high-risk populations, including HIV-positive women and women seeking care for vaginal discharge.

## Clinical Manifestations

The majority of people with trichomoniasis do not have symptoms. Men may report burning with urination or ejaculation or urethral discharge. Women with trichomoniasis may report painful urination, vaginal itching, painful intercourse, bleeding after sex, or a yellow-green discharge with a foul odor. On speculum exam, the cervix can have a "strawberry" appearance.

### Complications

The main complications of untreated trichomoniasis are related to the inflammation and irritation that the infection causes in the genital tract. This irritation makes an infected person more likely to acquire or transmit another STI, particularly HIV. While gonorrhea and chlamydial infection are responsible for the vast majority of PID, trichomoniasis infection is associated with PID in women with HIV.

### Diagnostic Studies

Diagnosis of trichomoniasis can be achieved by several methods. The preferred method is nucleic acid amplification testing (NAAT) of vaginal or endocervical secretions, or urine. Other methods include culture, point of care testing, or direct visualization of trichomonads under the microscope. Identification of motile trichomonads in the vaginal secretions confirms infection. Tests can be done on liquid-based cervical Pap samples. In men, NAAT testing is recommended.[7]

### Interprofessional Care

**Drug Therapy.** Patients and their partners should be treated with either metronidazole (Flagyl) or tinidazole (Tindamax). Instruct patients to abstain from sexual intercourse for 7 days after treatment and until all sexual partners have completed a full course of treatment. Advise patients to return if symptoms persist or recur. Any sexual partner within the preceding 60 days should be treated. Teach patients to use condoms or other barrier methods with every sexual contact. Because of a high rate of recurrence of trichomoniasis, repeat testing 3 months after treatment is recommended.

# STIs CHARACTERIZED BY GENITAL LESIONS OR ULCERS

## GENITAL HERPES INFECTIONS

Genital herpes infection is a lifelong, incurable infection that is very common. There are two strains of herpes that cause genital infections, herpes simplex virus type 1 (HSV-1) and herpes simplex virus type 2 (HSV-2). Although both forms of HSV may cause genital infection, HSV-1 is more commonly associated with oral lesions, and HSV-2 is more common in the genitals. However, an increasing proportion of genital herpes infections is caused by HSV-1.[8]

More than 24 million people in the United States have HSV-2. Nearly 800,000 new infections occur annually. Rates of new infections are high, partly due to the fact that an estimated 80% of those infected with genital HSV-2 have never received a clinical diagnosis and are unaware that they are capable of transmitting the virus.[1] The prevalence of new genital HSV-2 infections is twice as high among women compared to men.

### Etiology and Pathophysiology

HSV-1 and HSV-2 are strains of herpesvirus that cause genital herpes. Having one type does not confer immunity against getting the other type. The virus enters through the mucous membranes or breaks in the skin during contact with an infected person. The virus reproduces inside the cell and spreads to the surrounding cells. Then the virus enters the peripheral or autonomic nerve endings and ascends to the sensory or autonomic nerve ganglion near the infection site, where it often becomes dormant. Viral reactivation (recurrence) may occur when the virus descends to that initial site of infection, either the mucous membranes or skin.

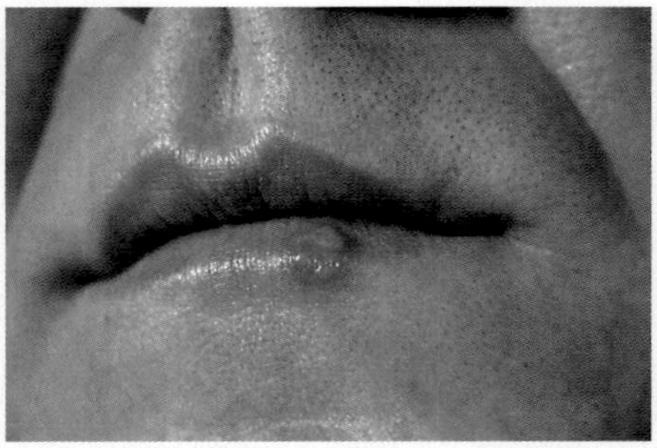

FIG. 52-5 Herpes simplex virus (HSV) to the lips. (From Centers for Disease Control and Prevention. Courtesy Dr. Hermann.)

When a person is infected with HSV-1 or HSV-2, the virus persists within the individual for life. Transmission of either strain of HSV occurs through direct contact with skin or mucous membranes when an infected individual is symptomatic. HSV-1 and HSV-2 can also be transmitted without any symptoms being apparent, called *asymptomatic shedding*. It is impossible to predict when asymptomatic shedding will occur.

HSV type 1 (HSV-1) was primarily associated with orolabial disease, commonly known as "cold sores" or "fever blisters" (Fig. 52-5) and HSV-2 with genital disease. However, there has been a shift in understanding that either HSV-1 or HSV-2 can cause genital or orolabial infections. In most cases, HSV-1 infections are more common "above the waist," involving the gingivae, dermis, upper respiratory tract, and, rarely the CNS. HSV-2 almost always infects sites "below the waist," the genital tract or perineum. It is important to understand that there is no absolute, single site for either virus. Among young women, HSV-1 is more commonly associated with genital infection than HSV-2.[9]

### Clinical Manifestations

**Primary Episode.** A *primary (initial) episode* of genital herpes has an incubation of 2 days to 2 weeks. The vast majority of people do not have any recognizable symptoms of primary HSV genital infection. If symptoms do occur, they follow a series of stages. During the *prodromal stage*, the period before lesions appear, the patient may have burning, itching, or tingling at the site of inoculation. In the *vesicular stage*, few to multiple small, often painful vesicles (blisters) may appear on the buttock, inner thigh, penis, scrotum, vulva, perineum, perianal region, vagina, or cervix. The vesicles contain large quantities of infectious viral particles.

Next in the *ulcerative stage*, the lesions rupture and form shallow, moist ulcerations. In the *final stage*, spontaneous crusting and epithelialization of the erosions occur (Fig. 52-6). Primary infections also tend to be associated with local inflammation and pain, regional (inguinal node) lymphadenopathy and systemic flu-like symptoms, including fever, headache, malaise, and myalgia. Urination may be painful from the urine touching active lesions. The whole process from prodrome to healing varies and can take approximately 3 weeks.

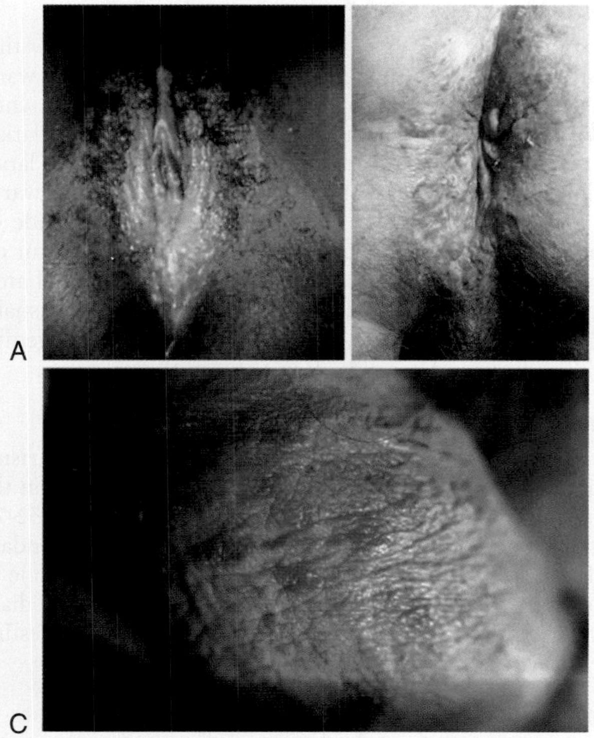


**FIG. 52-6** Unruptured vesicles of herpes simplex virus type 2 (HSV-2). **A,** Vulvar area. **B,** Perianal area. **C,** Penile herpes simplex, ulcerative stage. (*A* and *C,* From Centers for Disease Control and Prevention. Courtesy Susan Lindsley. *B,* From Morse S, Moreland A, Holmes K, editors: *Atlas of sexually transmitted diseases and AIDS,* London, 1996, Mosby-Wolfe.)

Autoinoculation can occur if active lesions are touched or scratched, causing additional and potentially recurrent infection at extragenital sites.

**Recurrent Episodes.** *Recurrent genital herpes* occurs in many individuals during the year following the primary episode. The symptoms of recurrent episodes are less severe, and the lesions usually heal more quickly. HSV-1 genital infections recur less frequently than HSV-2 genital infections, and over time, both decrease in frequency.

Common triggers of recurrence include stress, fatigue, sunburn, general illness, immunosuppression, and menses. Many patients can predict a recurrence by noticing the prodromal symptoms of tingling, burning, and itching at the site where the lesions will recur. The greatest risk for transmitting infection exists when active lesions are present. However, it is possible to transmit the virus when no visible lesions or symptoms are present. The majority of HSV transmission occurs during these asymptomatic periods.[8]

## Complications

Both HSV-1 and HSV-2 can cause rare but serious complications, such as blindness, encephalitis (inflammation of the brain), and aseptic meningitis (inflammation of the linings of the brain). Autoinoculation can result in the development of extragenital lesions in the buttocks, groin, thighs, fingers, and eyes. Genital ulcers increase the risk of acquiring HIV, and HSV lesions can be more severe and more persistent in HIV-infected patients.

Pregnant women with HSV can transmit the virus to the baby, most commonly if the virus is shed while the infant passes though the birth canal. Women with a primary episode of HSV near the time of delivery have the highest risk of transmitting genital herpes to the neonate. The virus can infect the neonate's skin, eyes, mouth, or the CNS or become disseminated and cause significant morbidity and mortality. An active genital lesion at the time of delivery is usually an indication for cesarean delivery.[10]

In addition to the physiologic complications associated with HSV infection, one of the most serious consequences for people diagnosed with genital herpes is the overall impact it can have on their psychologic well-being, their relationships, and their sexual lives. You can help teach patients to understand how to talk to sexual partners about HSV. Refer patients who need counseling. Teach patients with herpes that it is a manageable condition and help them to understand their treatment options.

## Diagnostic Studies

Diagnosis of genital herpes is often based on the patient's reported symptoms and then confirmation by visual exam. Culture from direct lesion samples can be used to diagnose HSV and differentiate between HSV-1 and HSV-2. Highly accurate blood tests for antibodies are available for HSV-1 and HSV-2. These antibodies usually appear by 12 weeks after exposure.

## Interprofessional Care

**Drug Therapy.** Although not a cure, antiviral medications can shorten the duration of HSV viral shedding, shorten the healing time of genital lesions, and reduce the frequency of outbreaks by 75%.[9] Treatment of HSV infection should be started before diagnostic results are available because early treatment reduces the duration of the ulcers and risk of transmission (Table 52-5).

Three antiviral agents are available for the treatment of HSV: acyclovir, valacyclovir, and famciclovir. These drugs inhibit herpetic viral replication and are prescribed for both primary and recurrent infections. These antiviral medications can also be used on a daily basis as suppressive therapy to decrease

### TABLE 52-5 Interprofessional Care
### *Genital Herpes*

**Diagnostic Assessment**
- History and physical examination
- Antibody assay for HSV type
- Viral isolation by tissue culture

**Management**

***Primary (Initial) Infection***
- acyclovir (Zovirax), famciclovir (Famvir), or valacyclovir (Valtrex)

***Recurrent Episodic Infection***
- acyclovir, famciclovir, or valacyclovir
- Identify triggering factors
- Abstinence from sexual contact while lesions are present
- Symptomatic care
- Confidential counseling and testing for HIV

***Suppressive Therapy***
- acyclovir, famciclovir, or valacyclovir

***Severe Infection***
- acyclovir IV until clinical improvement, followed by oral antiviral therapy

frequent recurrences. Teach patients with active outbreaks to maintain good genital hygiene and wear loose-fitting cotton undergarments.

The primary goal is to keep lesions clean and dry. Techniques to reduce pain on urination include pouring water onto the perineal area while voiding to dilute the urine or voiding in the shower. Pain may require a local anesthetic such as lidocaine gel or analgesics such as ibuprofen, acetaminophen, acetaminophen with codeine, or aspirin. Ice packs to the affected area can provide some relief.

IV acyclovir is reserved for severe or life-threatening infections in which hospitalization is required for the treatment of disseminated infections, central nervous system infections (meningitis), or pneumonitis.

## GENITAL WARTS

**Genital warts** *(condylomata acuminata)* are caused by the human papillomavirus (HPV). There are approximately 150 papillomavirus types. More than 40 types can be sexually transmitted. Some of these can cause warts on the skin, while others can cause cancers of the genital tract or oropharynx. Ninety percent of genital warts are caused by HPV types 6 and 11. About 360,000 people get genital warts each year. Most sexually active men and women will get some type of HPV at some point in their lives.[1] In most states, genital warts are not a reportable infection. (HPV infection of the cervix is discussed in Chapter 53.)

### Etiology and Pathophysiology

HPV is transmitted by skin-to-skin contact, most commonly during vaginal, anal, or oral sex, but it can be transmitted during nonpenetrative sexual activity. The basal epithelial cells infected with HPV undergo transformation and proliferation to form a warty growth (Fig. 52-7). The incubation period of the virus can range from weeks to months to years. Infection with one type of HPV does not prevent infection with another type.

In general, genital HPV infection is considered transient (virus is "cleared" or resolves spontaneously usually after 1 to 2 years). However, HPV infection can also persist even when the warts themselves are not visible after treatment. It is unclear whether removing visible genital warts helps a person to clear the virus, cure the virus, or reduces a person's ability to transmit the virus.[11]

### Clinical Manifestations

Most individuals who have HPV infection do not know that they are infected because they are asymptomatic. Genital warts are discrete single or multiple papillary growths that are white to gray and pink-flesh colored or can be brownish on darker skin types. They may grow and coalesce to form large, cauliflower-like masses. Most patients have 1 to 10 genital warts.

In men, warts occur on the penis and scrotum, inside or around the anus, or in the urethra. In women, warts occur on the inner thighs, vulva, vagina, or cervix, in the perianal area, including in the internal anal canal (Fig. 52-7). There are usually no other signs or symptoms. Itching may occur with anogenital warts. Bleeding on defecation may occur with anal warts.

### Diagnostic Studies

Most early lesions caused by HPV are undetectable by visual examination. A diagnosis of genital warts can be made on the basis of the characteristic appearance of the lesions (Fig. 52-7). Warts may be confused with *condylomata lata* of secondary syphilis, cancer, or benign growths. Testing should be done to rule out other conditions. At present, the only definitive diagnostic procedure is biopsy of any questionable growth. Testing for cervical HPV is discussed in Chapter 53.

### Complications

Genital warts have few long-term complications. Approximately 90% of warts are caused by noncancerous strains of HPV. However, certain strains of HPV (types 16 and 18) can lead to cancer of the cervix, vagina, vulva, penis, rectum, and throat or pharynx. For some individuals, HPV lesions can cause psychosocial burden due to the cosmetic appearance of lesions on the genitals or the need for long courses of HPV-related treatment. During pregnancy, genital warts tend to grow rapidly and increase in size.

### Interprofessional Care

**HPV Vaccines.** It may be possible to eradicate some of the oncogenic HPV types over the next few decades, particularly if both girls and boys are vaccinated.[11,12] Currently three vaccines are available to protect against HPV. A quadrivalent vaccine (Gardasil) protects against types 6, 11, 16, and 18; a bivalent vaccine (Cervarix) offers protection against HPV types 16 and 18; and a 9-valent vaccine (Gardasil 9) protects against HPV types 6, 11, 16, 18 and five other HPV types. These vaccines are

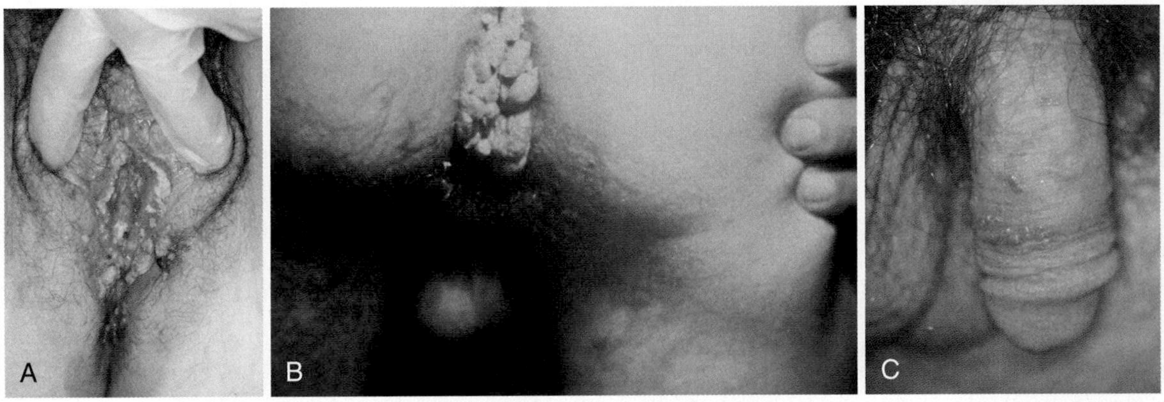


**FIG. 52-7** Genital warts. **A,** Severe vulvar warts. **B,** Perineal wart. **C,** Multiple genital warts of the glans penis. (*A,* From Centers for Disease Control and Prevention. Courtesy Joe Millar. *B,* From Centers for Disease Control and Prevention. Courtesy Dr. Wiesner. *C,* From Centers for Disease Control and Prevention. Courtesy Susan Lindsley.)

given in three IM doses over a 6-month period and have few side effects. The CDC recommends that all children, males and females, be vaccinated at age 11 to 12, but vaccination can be started as early as age 9. The bivalent and quadrivalent vaccines are approved for persons up to age 26. The 9-valent vaccine is approved for girls 9 to 26 and boys 9 to 15.

These vaccines do not treat active HPV infection. Ideally, individuals should receive the vaccine before the start of sexual activity, but even those who are infected with HPV can still get protection against HPV types not already acquired. The HPV vaccine reduces the risk of anal cancer and may also protect against oropharynx cancer.[11]

## EVIDENCE-BASED PRACTICE

### Applying the Evidence

**HPV Vaccine and Young Men**

T.N. is a 19-yr-old man who is being seen in the health care center for signs and symptoms of a urinary tract infection. After reviewing his health history, you learn he has not received the human papillomavirus (HPV) vaccine. When asked, he shares with you that he is sexually active and that he does not need to get the vaccine because his girlfriend already has.

***Making Clinical Decisions***

***Best Available Evidence.*** Males ages 9 to 26 can get vaccinated with Gardasil to reduce the incidence of anogenital HPV infections, which are caused by HPV types 6, 11, 16, or 18. Gardasil protects against the two HPV types (6 and 11) that cause 90% of genital warts.

***Clinician Expertise.*** You know younger men may be unaware of expanded recommendations for Gardasil, which was originally approved to prevent cervical, vulvar, and vaginal cancer in females ages 9 through 26.

***Patient Preferences and Values.*** T.N. states he never has unprotected sex and does not like injections.

***Implications for Nursing Practice***

1. Why is it important to discuss the risks and benefits of the vaccine with T.N.?
2. How would you respond to T.N., who has heard that if you are already sexually active the vaccine will not be effective?

***Reference for Evidence***

Centers for Disease Control: HPV vaccination. Retrieved from *www.cdc.gov/vaccines/vpd-vac/hpv* and Centers for Disease Control: HPV-associated cancers statistics. Retrieved from *www.cdc.gov/cancer/hpv/statistics/index.htm.*

**Drug Therapy.** Treatment of genital warts is hampered by the high proportion of asymptomatic infections and lack of curative treatment. The primary goal when treating visible genital warts is the removal of symptomatic warts.

Treatment consists of chemical or ablative (removal with laser or electrocautery) methods. One common treatment is the use of trichloroacetic acid (TCA) or bichloroacetic acid (BCA) applied directly to the wart surface. Petroleum jelly is applied to the surrounding normal skin to minimize irritation before a small amount of TCA or BCA is applied to the wart with a cotton swab. A sharp, stinging pain is often felt with initial acid contact, but this quickly subsides.

Patient-managed treatment is also an option. Podofilox liquid and gel are available by prescription (Condylox, Condylox Gel). The patient applies the solution or gel for 3 successive days. Treatment can be repeated for up to 4 weeks or until resolution of the lesions. Imiquimod (Aldara) cream is an immune response modifier that is applied at bedtime, three times a week for up to 16 weeks. Sinecatechin (Veregen) ointment (made from extract of green tea leaves) is applied three times weekly.

The removal of warts may or may not decrease infectivity. Genital warts are difficult to treat and often require multiple office visits. The therapy should be modified if a patient has not improved after three treatments or if the warts have not completely disappeared after six treatments.

If the warts do not regress with any of these therapies, treatments such as cryotherapy with liquid nitrogen, electrocautery, laser therapy, intralesional use of α-interferon, and surgical excision may be indicated. Because treatment does not destroy the virus, merely the infected tissue, recurrence and reinfection are possible, and careful long-term follow-up is advised.

## SYPHILIS

Syphilis is a sexually transmitted bacterial infection that can cause serious long-term complications if not treated effectively. Over 55,000 cases of syphilis are reported annually in the United States. There has been a shift in the population most affected by syphilis, with rates highest among young men 20 to 29 years old, with 75% of cases reported among MSM.[1]

### Etiology and Pathophysiology

Syphilis is caused by *Treponema pallidum,* a bacterial spirochete. It is transmitted via direct contact with a syphilitic lesion called a *chancre* that can occur externally on the genitals, anus, or lips, or internally in the vagina, rectum, or mouth or tongue (Fig. 52-8). The transmission of this bacterium occurs during vaginal, anal, or oral sex. The incubation period for syphilis can range from 10 to 90 days (average 21 days). Having the infection does not confer immunity to future infection, even after successful treatment. An infected pregnant woman can transmit syphilis to her fetus during her pregnancy and is at high risk for stillbirth or having babies who develop complications after birth, including seizures and death.

### Clinical Manifestations

Syphilis is called "*The Great Pretender*" because it can infect many organs in the body and present with a variety of signs and symptoms that can mimic a number of other diseases. Consequently, compared with other STIs, syphilis is more difficult to recognize. If it is not diagnosed and treated, specific clinical stages are characteristic of the progression of the disease (Table 52-6). It can take weeks to years to progress through all of the stages. At each stage, if no treatment is initiated, the disease will progress to the next stage.

### Complications

Complications of the disease occur mostly in late syphilis. The gummas of late syphilis may produce irreparable damage to skin, bone, or liver. In cardiovascular syphilis, the resulting aneurysm may press on structures such as the intercostal nerves, causing pain. The possibility of a rupture exists as the aneurysm increases in size. Scarring of the aortic valve results in aortic valve insufficiency and eventually heart failure. Neurosyphilis occurs when *T. pallidum* invades the central nervous system. It can occur at any of the stages of syphilis. Visual impairment, *tabes dorsalis* (progressive locomotor ataxia), and dementia are extreme manifestations and are rare.

TABLE 52-6 **Stages of Syphilis**

**Primary**
- *Infectivity:* Highly infectious
- Single or multiple chancres (painless indurated lesions) of penis, vulva, lips, mouth, vagina, and rectum) (Fig. 52-8). Occurs 10-90 days after inoculation
- Regional lymphadenopathy (draining of the microorganisms into the lymph nodes)
- Exudate and blood from chancre are highly infectious
- *Duration of stage:* 3-6 wk

**Secondary**
- *Infectivity:* Highly infectious
- Occurs a few weeks after primary chancre heals
- Flu-like symptoms: malaise, fever, sore throat, headaches, fatigue, arthralgia, generalized adenopathy
- Mucous patches in mouth (Fig. 52-9), tongue, or cervix
- Symmetric, nonpruritic rash bilaterally that appears on trunk, palms, and/or soles (Fig. 52-10)
- *Condylomata lata* (moist, weeping papules) in the anogenital area
- Weight loss, alopecia
- *Duration of stage:* 1-2 yr

**Latent**
- *Infectivity:* Early (<1 yr)–Infectious; Late (≥1 yr)–Noninfectious
- Absence of signs or symptoms
- Diagnosis based on positive specific treponemal antibody test together with normal CSF and absence of clinical manifestations
- *Duration of stage:* Throughout life or progression to late stage

**Late**
- *Infectivity:* Noninfectious
- Occurs 1-20 years after initial infection
- Gummas (chronic, destructive lesions affecting any organ of body, especially skin, bone, liver, mucous membranes) (Fig. 52-11)
- *Cardiovascular:* Aneurysms, heart valve insufficiency, heart failure, aortitis
- *Neurosyphilis*: Can occur at any stage of syphilis
- *General paresis*: Personality changes from minor to psychotic, tremors, physical and mental deterioration
- *Tabes dorsalis* (ataxia, areflexia, paresthesias, lightning pains, damaged joints)
- *Duration of stage:* Chronic (without treatment), possibly fatal

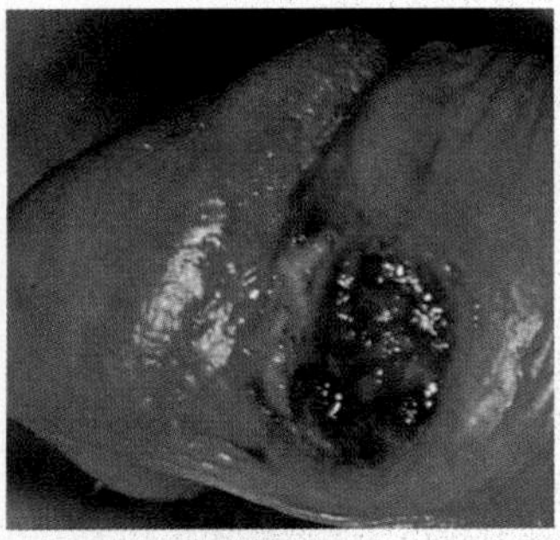

**FIG. 52-8** Primary syphilis chancre. (From Forbes CD, Jackson WF. *Color atlas and text of clinical medicine,* ed 3, London, 2003, Mosby.)

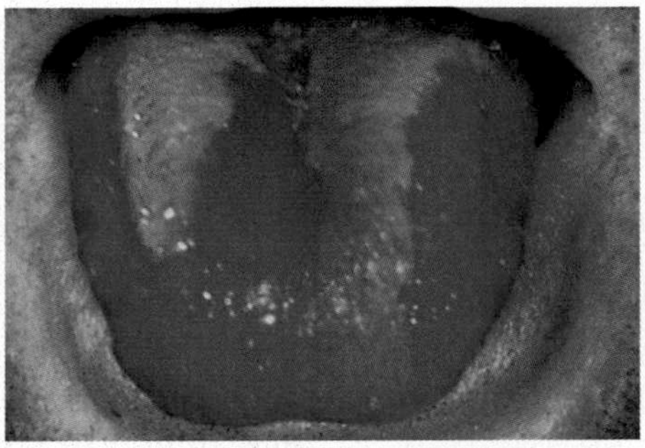

**FIG. 52-9** Secondary syphilis. Mucous patch in the mouth. (From Mandell GL, Bennett JE, Dolin R: *Mandell, Douglas, and Bennett's principles and practice of infectious diseases,* ed 7, Philadelphia, 2010, Churchill Livingstone.)

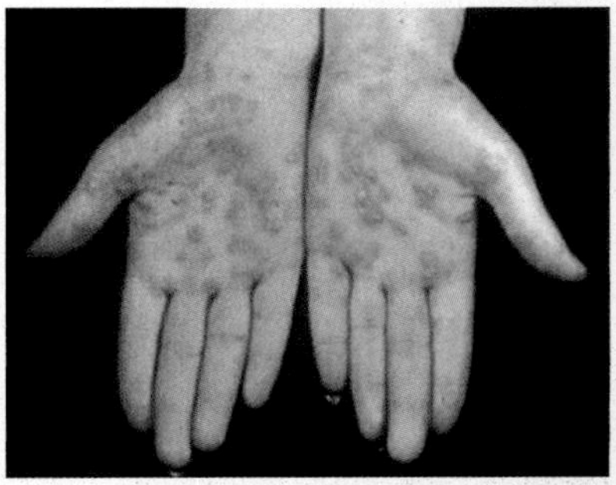

**FIG. 52-10** Secondary syphilis. Palmar rash. (From Centers for Disease Control and Prevention Public Health Image Library. Courtesy Robert Sumpter.)

Chancres on the genitalia enhance HIV transmission. Patients with HIV and syphilis appear to be at greatest risk for clinically significant CNS involvement and may require more intensive treatment than do other patients with syphilis.

## Diagnostic Studies

Syphilis is most commonly diagnosed by a blood test. Tests for syphilis are classified as those performed for screening and those performed for confirmation of a positive screening test. Nontreponemal tests used for screening detect antibodies that are not specific for syphilis. Nontreponemal tests include the Venereal Disease Research Laboratory (VDRL) test and the rapid plasma reagin (RPR) test. These screening tests usually become positive 10 to 14 days after the appearance of a chancre. The fluorescent treponemal antibody absorption (FTA-Abs) test and the *T. pallidum* particle agglutination (TP-PA) test are called *treponemal tests* because they specifically detect treponemal antibodies. These treponemal tests are used for confirming the diagnosis.[13]

False-negative and false-positive test results do occur with the nontreponemal tests (VDRL, RPR). A false-negative result may be obtained during primary syphilis if the test is done before the individual has had time to produce antibodies. A false-positive finding may occur if patients have various other diseases or conditions. Positive nontreponemal test results are always confirmed by more specific treponemal tests to rule out other causes. In the cerebrospinal fluid (CSF), changes such as an increased WBC count, increased total protein, and a positive treponemal antibody test are diagnostic of neurosyphilis.[13]

If treatment with antibiotics is initiated early in the course of the disease on the basis of the history and the symptoms, the serologic testing may not indicate syphilis. Once a person has tested positive for syphilis, these findings may remain positive for an indefinite period in spite of successful treatment.

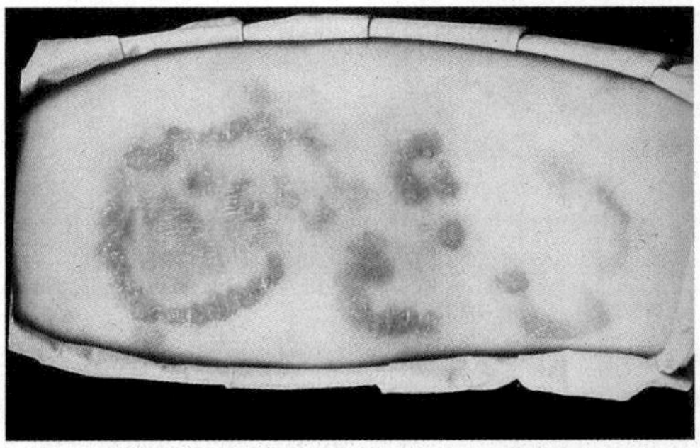

**FIG. 52-11** Destructive skin gummas associated with tertiary syphilis. (From Cohen J, Powderly WG: *Infectious diseases,* ed 2, St Louis, 2004, Mosby.)

## TABLE 52-7 Interprofessional Care

***Syphilis***

**Diagnostic Assessment**

- History and physical examination
- Dark-field microscopy
- Nontreponemal and/or treponemal serologic testing
- Testing for other STIs (HIV, gonorrhea, chlamydial infection)

**Management**

- Antibiotic therapy
  - penicillin G benzathine (Bicillin LA)
  - doxycycline (Vibramycin) or tetracycline (when penicillin is contraindicated)
- Confidential counseling and testing for HIV infection
- Surveillance
- Repeat of nontreponemal tests at 6 and 12 months
- Examination of cerebrospinal fluid at 1 yr*

*If treatment involves alternative antibiotics or treatment failure has occurred.

### Interprofessional Care

Because of the serious complications associated with untreated syphilis, screening programs for high-risk groups are important for reducing morbidity and mortality. The evaluation of all patients with syphilis should also include HIV testing, and the CDC recommends annual syphilis testing for HIV patients[13] (Table 52-7).

**Drug Therapy.** Management of syphilis is aimed at initiating treatment early and eradicating the syphilitic organisms. Penicillin G benzathine (Bicillin LA) is the recommended treatment for all stages (Table 52-7). When penicillin is contraindicated, doxycycline or tetracycline may be used. Aqueous procaine penicillin G is the treatment of choice for neurosyphilis. Treatment cannot reverse damage that is already present in the later stages of the disease. All sexual contacts from the preceding 90 days should be treated presumptively. Reexamination and follow-up testing are recommended every 6 months for up to 2 years.[13]

## NURSING MANAGEMENT: STIs

### Nursing Assessment

Subjective and objective data that should be obtained from a person with an STI are presented in Table 52-8. Assess the patient's risk for contracting an STI. Questions to ask include number of partners, types of partners ("Do you have sex with men, women, or both?"), type of birth control used (if applicable), use of condoms or other barrier methods, history of an STI, use of drugs and alcohol, exchange of sex for drugs or money, and risk for violence and personal safety. Plan teaching based on the responses to these questions.

Interpersonal skills necessary for this interview include respect, compassion, and a nonjudgmental attitude. Tailor your counseling to the individual. Do not assume that older people are not at risk: sex and sexuality are dynamic across the life cycle, and sexually active older individuals can be at risk for STIs.[14]

**CHECK YOUR PRACTICE**

You are working on the medicine unit caring for a 68-yr-old man admitted for IV penicillin for neurosyphilis. The nurse that you are working with says, "I can't believe a man that old could get a sexually transmitted infection."

- How would you respond?
- What should you discuss with your colleague?

## TABLE 52-8 Nursing Assessment

***Sexually Transmitted Infections***

**Subjective Data**

***Important Health Information***

*Sexual health history:* Sexual activity with individuals with STIs, past history of STIs, multiple sexual partners, unsafe sexual practices

*Medications:* Allergy to any antibiotics

***Functional Health Patterns***

*Health perception–health management:* Unsafe sexual practices, drug and/or alcohol use

*Nutritional-metabolic:* Nausea, vomiting, anorexia. Pharyngitis, oral lesions, chills. Alopecia

*Elimination:* Dysuria, urinary frequency, urethral discharge, pain with bowel movements

*Cognitive-perceptual:* Arthralgia, headache, painful, burning lesions, itching or irritation at infected site

*Sexuality-reproductive:* Dyspareunia, vaginal or penile discharge, bleeding with sex, genital or perianal lesions

**Objective Data**

***General***

Fever, lymphadenopathy (generalized or inguinal)

***Integumentary***

*Syphilis:* Primary: Painless, indurated genital, oral, or perianal lesions

Secondary: Bilateral, symmetric rash on palms, soles, or entire body. Mucous patches on mouth or tongue; alopecia

*Genital herpes:* Painful genital or anal vesicular lesions

*Genital warts:* Single or multiple gray or white genital or anal warts

***Gastrointestinal***

Rectal discharge, rectal lesions

***Urinary***

Urethral discharge, erythema

***Reproductive***

Cervical mucopurulent discharge, cervical erythema, cervical bleeding; penile purulent discharge, epididymitis, proctitis, genital lesions

***Possible Diagnostic Findings***

*Chlamydia:* Positive culture or NAAT cervical, urethral, anal, oropharyngeal, or urine samples

*Gonorrhea:* Positive cultures or NAAT from cervical, urethral, anal, oropharyngeal, or urine samples

*Genital herpes:* Positive HSV-1 or HSV-2 serum antibody test. Positive culture from active lesion indicating HSV-1 or HSV-2

*Syphilis:* Positive findings on VDRL and RPR, spirochetes on dark-field microscopy

*Trichomoniasis:* Positive increased pH and positive motile protozoa on wet prep of discharge. Positive FDA-approved rapid test or liquid-based Pap positive for trichomoniasis.

*HSV-1,* Herpes simplex virus type 1; *HSV-2,* herpes simplex virus type 2; *NAAT,* nucleic acid amplification test; *RPR,* rapid plasma reagin; *STIs,* sexually transmitted infections; *VDRL,* Venereal Disease Research Laboratory.

### Nursing Diagnoses

Nursing diagnoses for the patient with an STI include, but are not limited to, the following:

- Risk for infection *related to* lack of knowledge about modes of STI transmission, failure to practice safer sex, and engaging in other high-risk behaviors
- Anxiety *related to* impact of the condition on relationships, long-term effects of infection, and lack of knowledge regarding the infection

- Ineffective health maintenance *related to* lack of knowledge about disease process and transmission, inadequate follow-up measures, and possibility of reinfection

## ◆ Planning

The overall goals are that the patient with an STI will (1) demonstrate understanding of the mode of transmission of STIs and the risks associated with STIs, (2) complete treatment and return for appropriate follow-up, (3) notify or assist in notification of sexual contacts about their need for testing and treatment, (4) abstain from intercourse until infection is resolved, and (5) demonstrate knowledge of safer sex practices.

## ◆ Nursing Implementation

◆ **Health Promotion.** Many approaches to stopping the spread of STIs have been met with varying degrees of success. Be prepared to discuss "safer" sex practices with all patients, not only those who are perceived to be at risk. These practices include abstinence, monogamy, avoidance of high-risk sexual behaviors, and the correct use of condoms and other barriers with every sexual act. Sexual abstinence is the only certain method of avoiding all STIs, but few people consider this a feasible alternative to sexual expression. Limiting sexual contacts to a well-established, monogamous relationship in which both partners are tested regularly for STIs can reduce the risk of contracting an STI. Addressing issues related to drug and alcohol dependence or abuse is important for the promotion of healthy sexual behavior.

Be prepared to teach special populations, such as MSM, women who have sex with women (WSW), and transgender persons, about their particular risks (Table 52-9). A teaching guide for the patient with an STI is presented in Table 52-10.

◆ ***Measures to Prevent Infection.*** Encourage patients to take notice of a sexual partner's genitalia before sex, paying attention to any discharge, sores, blisters, or rashes. Help patients to be aware of specific signs and symptoms of infection. This can assist them to make good decisions about whether to continue a sexual interaction with safer-sex modifications or to elect not to have sexual relations at all. Remind patients that most STIs may have no symptoms but can still be transmitted. Also emphasize with patients that when they have sex, they are exposed to the infections of everyone with whom their partner has ever had sex.

Proper use of a condom provides a highly effective mechanical barrier to infection. Partners should openly discuss any objections to condom usage, such as interference with spontaneity and the presence of a barrier. Information about the mechanics of sexual arousal and incorporating a condom into sex can help in overcoming the individual's or partner's resistance to its use. Refusing sexual activity with any partner who will not use a condom is a safe and legitimate option.

The *female condom,* a lubricated polyurethane sheath designed for vaginal use, is another option for some individuals. Remind patients to avoid the spermicide nonoxynol 9 (N-9), which can be used alone to prevent pregnancy or as a condom lubricant. Nonoyxynol 9 is one of the least effective methods of birth control when used alone and can act as an irritant to the vagina and rectum, increasing the risk for acquiring an STI.

◆ ***Screening Programs.*** Screening programs are an effective means of identifying, treating, preventing, and controlling the spread of STIs. At present, there are CDC-recommended screening programs for certain populations, including young people, MSM, pregnant women, and anyone at increased risk for exposure to an STI (new partners, nonmonogamous relationships, not using condoms/barriers).[7]

◆ ***Case Finding.*** Interviewing and case finding are other methods used to control the spread of STIs. These activities are directed toward locating and examining all sexual contacts of patients with reportable STIs so that effective treatment can be initiated. Public health professionals, often nurses, are aware of the social implications of these diseases and the need for discretion in locating partners. Sexual contacts are not informed about the origin of the information naming them as a contact so that patient privacy mandates are ensured.

Partner notification and treatment impose a heavy burden on public health departments and, as a result, the notification often becomes the responsibility of the infected partner. The infected partner may choose not to inform sexual partners, and the partners may choose not to seek treatment.

◆ ***Educational and Research Programs.*** Actively encourage your community to provide better education about STIs for its citizens. High-risk populations (e.g., young people under age 25,

### TABLE 52-9 Understanding Risk for STIs in Special Populations

*When dealing with the following populations at risk for STIs, it is important to consider cultural, behavioral, and other risk factors that may place them at increased risk for STIs or not receiving appropriate screening.*

**Women Who Have Sex with Women (WSW)**

- WSW should not be presumed to be at low or no risk for STIs based on sexual orientation.
- Self-identified WSW report having had sex with men and indicate that they may continue this practice in the future.
- WSW are at risk for acquiring bacterial, viral, and protozoal infections from current and prior partners, both male and female.
- Practices involving digital-vaginal or digital-anal contact, particularly with shared penetrative sex items, present a possible means for transmission of infected cervicovaginal secretions.
- Female-to-female transmission of *Chlamydia,* trichomoniasis, HIV, HPV, HSV, and syphilis have all been reported.
- Report of same-sex behavior in women should not deter HCPs from screening for all STIs.

**Men Who Have Sex with Men (MSM)**

- MSM are at higher risk for HIV, syphilis, hepatitis C, and other viral and bacterial STIs compared to the general population.
- Rates of rectal gonorrhea infection are increasing in MSM, particularly in HIV-infected MSM.
- HCPs should assess risk for STIs among MSM patients and be comfortable asking questions about sexual practices, including anal sex.

**Transgender Individuals**

- Transgender man is a term used to describe a person born anatomically female but who identifies as male. Transgender woman is a term used to describe a person born anatomically male but who identifies as female.
- Rates of certain STIs, including HIV, are higher among transgender women, compared to the general population.
- Not all transgender persons have had genital reassignment surgery and may still have the genitals they were assigned at birth. Therefore these individuals should be screened for STIs based on both risk history and current anatomy. For example, a transgender man may still have a vagina and cervix.
- HCPs must remain aware of their patients' gender identity, current anatomy, and screen patients based on risk history and sexual behaviors.

Source: Centers for Disease Control, Sexually Transmitted Disease Treatment Guidelines, 2015, *www.cdc.gov/std/tg2015/specialpops.htm.*

**TABLE 52-10 Patient Teaching**

***Sexually Transmitted Infections***

*When teaching the patient with sexually transmitted infections:*

1. Explain precautions to take such as
   - Using condoms and other barrier methods with every sexual encounter
   - Being monogamous
   - Asking potential partners about sexual history
   - Asking potential partners if they have been tested for STIs
   - Avoiding sex with partners who use IV drugs or who have visible oral, inguinal, genital, perineal, or anal lesions
   - Voiding and washing genitalia and surrounding area after sex to flush out some organisms and potentially reduce exposure infection
2. Explain the importance of taking all antibiotics and/or antiviral agents as prescribed. Symptoms will improve after 1-2 days of therapy, but organisms may still be present.
3. Teach patients about the need for treatment of sexual partners to prevent transmission and reinfection.
4. Instruct patients to abstain from sexual intercourse during treatment and to use condoms or other barrier methods when sexual activity is resumed to prevent spread of infection and reinfection.
5. Explain the importance of follow-up examination and retesting at least once after treatment if appropriate to confirm complete cure and prevent relapse.
6. Allow patients and partners to verbalize concerns to clarify areas that need explanation.
7. Instruct patient about symptoms of complications and need to report problems to ensure proper follow-up and early treatment of reinfection.
8. Inform patient regarding state of infectivity to prevent a false sense of security, which may result in careless sexual practices and poor personal hygiene.
9. Inform patients about health department requirements for reporting certain STIs.

MSM) should be a prime target for such educational programs. STI rates are also rising in older adults.[14] Older adults are less likely to use condoms and often have a hard time initiating discussion of sexual health issues.

Knowledge and understanding can decrease the incidence of STIs. The HPV vaccine that protects against genital warts and cervical cancer should be encouraged for boys and girls before the start of sexual activity. Accurate and current information may help reduce parental fears related to the vaccine. Consider stressing the prevention of cancer as a reason for the vaccine, which may be more productive and less controversial, thus making the parent and adolescent more receptive.

### Acute Care

***Psychologic Support.*** The diagnosis of an STI may be met with a variety of emotions, such as shame, guilt, anger, and a desire for vengeance. Encourage the patient to verbalize feelings. Couples in marital or committed relationships are confronted with an added problem when an STI is diagnosed if they must face the implication of possible sexual activity outside the relationship. The STI raises other concerns about their relationship and may serve as an incentive for further problem solving. A referral for professional counseling to explore the ramifications of an STI in their relationship may be indicated.

A patient who has genital herpes is faced with the fact that repeated infections can occur and that no cure is available. This can be frustrating and disruptive to the patient's physical, emotional, social, and sexual life. Help the patient identify and avoid any factors that may precipitate the condition. Inform the patient that the frequency and severity of recurrences will decrease over time.

**ETHICAL/LEGAL DILEMMAS**

***Confidentiality and HIPAA***

**Situation**

P.H., a 22-yr-old woman, is informed of the positive results of a test for chlamydial infection. You advise her to tell her sexual partners that she has this disease. She refuses to tell her boyfriend because he will know that she has had sex with another partner. You later learn that the nursing student who was in the clinic for the day, who is a friend of the boyfriend, hinted to him that he should have STI testing.

**Ethical/Legal Points for Consideration**

- Each state has requirements for reporting communicable diseases and other health-related data. Inform the patient of the reporting requirements for communicable diseases.
- Nurses and other HCPs have both a legal and an ethical obligation to maintain confidentiality of patient information. The Health Insurance Portability and Accountability Act (HIPAA) ensures the privacy of personal health information.
- The duty to maintain confidentiality is not absolute and may be limited, as necessary, to protect the patient or other parties, or by law or regulation such as mandated reporting for safety or public health reasons.[1]
- Your primary obligation is to the patient seeking care. Patient teaching is one way to establish a partnership with this woman. Share information about the effects of the disease if it is not treated, the consequences of reinfection, and the effect of the disease on others who may not know that they are infected. Then encourage the patient to inform her partners of the diagnosis for the good of everyone, and discuss the option of expedited partner therapy (EPT) where applicable.*

**Discussion Questions**

1. What are your state's requirements for reportable conditions?
2. In your opinion, what is the best way to balance the needs of an individual patient with those of the general public?
3. What are the risks to the institution for the breach of confidentiality and HIPAA?

**Reference**

1. Code of Ethics for Nurses. *www.nursingworld.org/MainMenuCategories/EthicsStandards/Ethics-Position-Statements.*

*EPT is discussed on p. 1230.

Genital warts involve a prolonged course of treatment. The patient can become frustrated and distressed because of frequent office visits, associated costs, potential for unpleasant side effects as a result of treatment, and effects of the infection on future health and sexual relationships. Support and a willingness to listen to the patient's concerns are needed. Local or online support groups are available for almost all STIs. Help patients to connect with support groups.

***Follow-Up.*** If you work in public health facilities, clinics, or other outpatient settings, you are more likely to care for a patient with an STI than if you work in a hospital setting. Whatever the setting, as a nurse you are in a position to explain and interpret treatment measures such as the purpose and possible side effects of prescribed drugs and the need for follow-up care (Table 52-10).

Frequently, single-dose treatment for gonorrhea, chlamydial infection, and syphilis helps prevent the problems associated with nonadherence with drug therapy. Give special instructions to the patient requiring multiple-dose therapy to complete the prescribed regimen. Also inform the patient about problems resulting from nonadherence. All patients should return to the treatment center for a repeat culture from the infected sites or for serologic testing at designated times to determine the effectiveness of the treatment. Explaining to the patient that cures are not always obtained on the first treatment can reinforce the need for a follow-up visit. Also advise the patient to inform sexual partners of the need for testing and treatment, regardless of whether they are free of symptoms or experiencing symptoms.

◆ ***Hygiene Measures.*** Emphasize to the patient with an STI the importance of certain hygiene measures, such as frequent hand washing. Tell the patient not to itch or scratch infection sites in order to avoid autoinoculation of STIs that can be spread to other parts of the body that way. Washing with soap and water as well as voiding after sex may theoretically provide some benefit in decreasing the exposure to STIs but certainly does not provide adequate protection against transmission. Teach patients that douching after sex is never recommended, as it can push bacteria higher into the reproductive tract or undermine local immune responses.

◆ ***Sexual Activity.*** Sexual abstinence is indicated during the communicable phase of any STI, and long-term precautions must be taken with those STIs that are chronic or recurrent. Emphasize that even single-dose treatments can take up to 1 week to be effective and thus the patient is infectious during this period. Emphasize to the patient the importance of using condoms or other barrier methods to help prevent the spread of infection and reinfection. Also encourage condom or other barrier methods use after treatment to prevent future exposure to infection. Remind patients that complications can follow if unprotected sexual activity occurs before treatment completion. Patients need to discuss re-treatment or continued treatment with an HCP. During treatment, the patient can also choose to relate to a partner in an intimate way that avoids penetrative, oral-genital contact, or skin-to-skin contact.

◆ **Ambulatory Care.** Because many STIs are cured with a single dose or short course of antibiotic therapy, many patients are casual about the outcome of these infections. The consequences of this attitude can include delays in treatment, nonadherence with instructions, and subsequent development of complications. The complications are serious and costly and can include future infertility.

Surgery and prolonged therapy are indicated for many patients with infection-related complications. Major surgical procedures such as resection of an aneurysm or aortic valve replacement may be necessary to treat cardiovascular problems caused by syphilis. Pelvic surgery and procedures to correct fertility problems secondary to an STI may be necessary and, if not successful, patients may require assisted reproductive technologies to achieve future pregnancy. Because young people ages 15 to 24 represent about 50% of new STIs annually, it is important to know that almost every state and the District of Columbia have laws that allow minors to consent to STI services without parental involvement (the minimum age varies by state).[1]

### ◆ Evaluation

Expected outcomes for the patient with an STI are that the patient will

- Understand the course, modes of transmission, and treatment options for the STI
- Understand the potential long-term complications of the infection
- Demonstrate compliance with medication regimens and the follow-up protocol
- Understand the importance of partner notification and treatment
- Experience no reinfection and understand STI risk-reducing behaviors and practices

## CASE STUDY

### *Gonococcal and Chlamydial Infection*

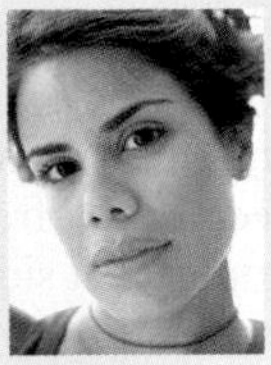

(©Eyecandy Images/ Thinkstock)

**Patient Profile**

C.R. is a 24-yr-old Hispanic woman who is seen at the outpatient clinic with complaints of increased yellow vaginal discharge and bleeding after sex for the past 2 weeks. She is sexually active with a new partner. She was treated in the past for chlamydial infection at age 20.

**Subjective Data**

- She and her partner use condoms "sometimes"
- Last menstrual period was 3 weeks ago and she does not use a birth control method
- Noticed her partner had some unusual discharge before they had sex
- Appears anxious and teary

**Objective Data**

- Cervix: erythematous
- Mucopurulent cervical discharge
- Urine pregnancy test is negative
- Nucleic acid amplification testing (NAAT) of the cervix is positive for both *Neisseria gonorrhoeae* and *Chlamydia trachomatis*

**Interprofessional Care**

- ceftriaxone 250 mg IM × 1 dose
- azithromycin 1 g PO × 1 dose

**Discussion Questions**

1. What were C.R.'s risk factors for acquiring gonorrhea and chlamydial infection?
2. What complications could occur if C.R.'s infections are not treated?
3. ***Priority Decision:*** What is the priority of care for C.R.?
4. ***Patient-Centered Care:*** What instructions should C.R. receive to ensure successful treatment? To prevent reinfection? To prevent further transmission of the infection?
5. ***Teamwork and Collaboration:*** Which nursing personnel should be responsible for teaching C.R. what she needs to know about other sexually transmitted infections (STIs): RN, LPN/LVN, UAP?
6. ***Patient-Centered Care:*** What impact is her diagnosis likely to have on C.R.'s self-image? On her relationship with her sexual partner?
7. ***Safety:*** C.R. tells you she is worried about how her partner will react when she discloses this information. What safety precautions should be considered?
8. ***Priority Decision:*** Based on the assessment data presented, what are the priority nursing diagnoses?
9. ***Evidence-Based Practice:*** C.R. mentions she is using the spermicide nonoxynol-9 (N-9) to protect herself against STIs. Would you advise her to continue to use it?

Answers available *at http://evolve.elsevier.com/Lewis/medsurg.*

## BRIDGE TO NCLEX EXAMINATION

The number of the question corresponds to the same-numbered outcome at the beginning of the chapter.

1. The individual with the lowest risk for sexually transmitted pelvic inflammatory disease is a woman who uses
   a. oral contraceptives.
   b. barrier methods of contraception.
   c. an intrauterine device for contraception.
   d. Norplant implant or injectable Depo-Provera for contraception.
2. The nurse is obtaining a subjective data assessment from a woman reported as a sexual contact of a man with chlamydial infection. The nurse understands that symptoms of chlamydial infection in women
   a. are frequently absent.
   b. are similar to those of genital herpes.
   c. include a macular palmar rash in the later stages.
   d. may involve chancres inside the vagina that are not visible.
3. A primary HSV infection differs from recurrent HSV episodes in that *(select all that apply)*
   a. only primary infections are sexually transmitted.
   b. symptoms are less severe during recurrent episodes.
   c. transmission of the virus to a fetus is less likely during primary infection.
   d. systemic manifestations such as fever and myalgia are more common in primary infection.
   e. lesions from recurrent HSV are more likely to transmit the virus than lesions from primary HSV.
4. Explain to the patient with gonorrhea that treatment will include both ceftriaxone and azithromycin because
   a. azithromycin helps prevent recurrent infections.
   b. some patients do not respond to oral drugs alone.
   c. coverage with more than one antibiotic will prevent reinfection.
   d. the increasing rates of drug resistance requires the use of at least two drugs.
5. In assessing patients for STIs, the nurse needs to know that many STIs can be asymptomatic. Which STIs can be asymptomatic *(select all that apply)*?
   a. Syphilis
   b. Gonorrhea
   c. Genital warts
   d. Genital herpes
   e. Chlamydial infection
6. To prevent the infection and transmission of STIs, the nurse's teaching plan would include an explanation of
   a. the appropriate use of oral contraceptives.
   b. sexual positions that can be used to avoid infection.
   c. the necessity of annual Pap tests for patients with HPV.
   d. sexual practices that are considered high-risk behaviors.
7. Provide emotional support to a patient with an STI by
   a. offering information on how safer sexual practices can prevent STIs.
   b. showing concern when listening to the patient who expresses negative feelings.
   c. reassuring the patient that the disease is highly curable with appropriate treatment.
   d. helping the patient who received an STI from his or her sexual partner in forgiving the partner.

1. b, 2. a, 3. b, d, 4. d, 5. a, b, c, d, e, 6. d, 7. b

For rationales to these answers and even more NCLEX review questions, visit *http://evolve.elsevier.com/Lewis/medsurg.*

## EVOLVE WEBSITE

http://evolve.elsevier.com/Lewis/medsurg

**Review Questions (Online Only)**
**Key Points**
**Answer Keys for Questions**
- Rationales for Bridge to NCLEX Examination Questions
- Answer Guidelines for Case Study on p. 1240

**Conceptual Care Map Creator**
**Audio Glossary**
**Content Updates**

## REFERENCES


1. Centers for Disease Control and Prevention: Sexually transmitted disease surveillance, 2013. Retrieved from *www.cdc.gov/std/stats13/default.htm.*
2. Daniels K, Daugherty J, Jones J: Current contraceptive status among women aged 15–44: United States, 2011–2013. *NCHS Data Brief,* No. 173, 2014. Retrieved from *www.cdc.gov/nchs/data/databriefs/db173.pdf.*
3. Centers for Disease Control and Prevention: STDs and infertility. Retrieved from *www.cdc.gov/std/infertility.*
4. Centers for Disease Control and Prevention: Recommendations for the laboratory-based detection of *Chlamydia trachomatis* and *Neisseria gonorrhoeae*—2014, *MMWR* 63(No. RR-2), 2014.
5. Centers for Disease Control and Prevention: Sexually transmitted diseases: expedited partner therapy 2015. Retrieved from *www.cdc.gov/std/ept/legal/default.htm.*
6. Lewis D: Trichomoniasis, *Medicine* 42:369, 2014.

*7. Centers for Disease Control and Prevention: Sexually transmitted diseases treatment guidelines 2015, *MMWR* 64(3):1, 2015.

8. Hofstetter AM: Current thinking on genital herpes, *Curr Opin Infect Dis* 27:75, 2014.
9. Garland S: Vulvovaginal disease: genital herpes, *Best Pract Res Clin Obstet Gynaecol* 26:1098, 2014.
10. James SH, Kimberlin DW: Neonatal herpes simplex virus infection: epidemiology and treatment, *Clin Perinatol* 42:47, 2015.
11. Centers for Disease Control and Prevention: HPV. Retrieved from *www.cdc.gov/std/hpv/default.htm*
12. Crossignani P, De Stefani A, Fara GM, et al: Towards eradication of HPV infection through universal specific vaccination, *BMC Public Health* 13:642, 2013.
13. Centers for Disease Control and Prevention: Syphilis. Retrieved from *www.cdc.gov/std/syphilis/stdfact-syphilis-detailed.htm.*
14. Poynten IM, Grulich AE, Templeton DJ: Sexually transmitted infections in older populations, *Curr Opin Infect Dis* 26:80, 2013.

*Evidence-based information for clinical practice.

53

# Female Reproductive and Genital Problems

*Amy McKeever, Kim K. Choma*

*A woman is the full circle. Within her is the power to create, nurture, and transform.*

***Diane Mariechild***

http://evolve.elsevier.com/Lewis/medsurg/

## LEARNING OUTCOMES

1. Summarize the etiologies of infertility and the strategies for diagnosis and treatment of the infertile woman.
2. Describe the etiology, clinical manifestations, interprofessional care, and nursing management of menstrual problems and abnormal uterine bleeding.
3. Identify the risk factors, clinical manifestations, and nursing and interprofessional management of ectopic pregnancy.
4. Describe the changes related to menopause and the interprofessional care and nursing management of the patient with menopausal symptoms.
5. Describe the assessment, interprofessional care, and nursing management of women with pelvic inflammatory disease and endometriosis.
6. Explain the clinical manifestations, diagnostic studies, interprofessional care, including surgical therapy for cervical, endometrial, ovarian, and vulvar cancers.
7. Summarize the preoperative and postoperative nursing management of the patient requiring surgery of the female reproductive system.
8. Differentiate among the common problems that occur with cystoceles, rectoceles, and fistulas and the related interprofessional care and nursing management.
9. Summarize the clinical manifestations of sexual assault and the appropriate nursing and interprofessional management of the patient who has been sexually assaulted.

## KEY TERMS



## INFERTILITY

**Infertility** is the inability to conceive after at least 1 year of regular unprotected intercourse. Approximately 15% of couples in North America are infertile.[1]

### Etiology and Pathophysiology

Infertility may be caused by either female or male or combined factors. (Conditions that cause male infertility are discussed in Chapter 54.) In some cases, the cause of infertility may not be identified.

Female infertility may be due to problems with ovulation, the fallopian tubes, or conditions that affect the uterus or cervix. In women, the risk for infertility begins around age 30. By the time a woman reaches the age of 40, the chances of conceiving are 10% or less. For both genders, chronic diseases, genital infections, and exposure to environmental toxins can affect fertility.

### Diagnostic Studies

Couples who are being evaluated for infertility usually have a detailed history and physical examination. Based on the findings from the history and physical examination, additional diagnostic testing may be ordered (Table 53-1). Formal evaluation of the infertile couple is usually conducted after 1 year of regular unprotected intercourse. Earlier evaluation may occur in women over age 35 or based on medical or physical findings, such as a history of irregular menstrual cycles or if the partner has a known fertility problem.

A comprehensive evaluation of the female reproductive system includes cervical, uterine, endometrial, tubal, peritoneal, and ovarian factors that may be the source of infertility. A

Reviewed by Adena Bargad, PhD, CNM, Assistant Professor, Columbia University Medical Center, Director, Sub-Specialty Program in Women's Health, Columbia University School of Nursing, New York, New York; Courtney Reinisch, RN, DNP, APN-BC, DCC, Clinical Associate Professor, School of Nursing, Rutgers University, Newark, New Jersey; and Crystal Sheaves, RN, MSN, APRN, FNP-BC, Senior Lecturer, West Virginia University School of Nursing, Charleston, West Virginia.

**TABLE 53-1 Interprofessional Care**

***Infertility***

**Diagnostic Assessment**

- History and physical examination of both partners, including psychosocial functioning
- Review of menstrual and gynecologic history
- Assessment of possible sexually transmitted infections
- Hormone levels
  - Serum hormone levels (e.g., FSH, LH, prolactin)
  - Urinary LH
- Pap test
- Ovulatory study
- Tubal patency study
  - Hysterosalpingogram
- Postcoital test
  - Cervical mucus
  - Sperm penetration assay
  - Semen analysis
- Pelvic ultrasound
- Genetic screening

**Management**

- Hormone therapy
- Drug therapy (Table 53-2)
- Intrauterine insemination
- Assisted reproductive technologies (ARTs)

*FSH,* Follicle-stimulating hormone; *LH,* luteinizing hormone.

semen sample is required to determine if the cause is related to the male partner.

## ❖ NURSING AND INTERPROFESSIONAL MANAGEMENT: INFERTILITY

Infertility management depends on the cause. If the cause is due to ovarian function, supplemental hormone therapy may be required. Table 53-2 provides a review of drugs commonly used for women experiencing infertility.

*Assisted reproductive technology* (ART) can be used to help women who are experiencing difficulty becoming pregnant. ART includes fertility medications, artificial insemination, and surrogacy. Different types of ART include (1) in vitro fertilization (IVF); (2) gamete intrafallopian transfer (GIFT); (3) zygote intrafallopian transfer (ZIFT); (4) donor gametes; and (5) freezing of ova. Some types of ART, such as IVF, are expensive and can be emotionally stressful. Assisting couples experiencing infertility is critical. You can provide teaching about the physiology of reproduction and an overview of infertility evaluation and treatments.

## EARLY PREGNANCY LOSS

*Early pregnancy loss* is a term used to describe the loss of a pregnancy before 20 weeks gestation.[2] **Abortion** is another term that is used to describe the loss of pregnancy. Abortions are classified as *spontaneous* (those occurring naturally [e.g., miscarriage]) or *induced* (those occurring as a result of medical intervention). *Miscarriage* is the common term for the unintended loss of a pregnancy.

### Spontaneous Abortion

*Spontaneous abortion* is the natural loss of pregnancy before 20 weeks of gestation (Table 53-3). Nearly 20% of pregnancies can result in miscarriage, a loss that can be devastating for both the mother and her partner. Fetal chromosomal abnormalities account for many miscarriages before 8 weeks of gestation. Other causes of spontaneous abortions include endocrine abnormalities, maternal infection, uterine abnormalities (e.g., uterine fibroids, endometriosis), immunologic factors, and environmental factors.

Treatment to prevent spontaneous abortion is limited. Although bed rest and avoidance of vaginal intercourse are often recommended, there is no evidence that these measures improve the outcome. Women are advised to report any bleeding to their HCP.

If the pregnancy is not viable, two types of management are considered: expectant management or medical management. *Expectant management* refers to monitoring the patient to see if the *products of conception* (POC) are expelled naturally without complications. *Medical management* may be indicated if the POCs do not pass completely or bleeding becomes

**TABLE 53-2 Drug Therapy**

***Infertility***

| Drug | Mechanism of Action |
|---|---|
| **Selective Estrogen Receptor Modulator** | |
| clomiphene (Clomid) | Stimulates hypothalamus to ↑ production of GnRH, which ↑ release of LH and FSH. End result is stimulation of ovulation. |
| **Menotropins (Human Menopausal Gonadotropin)** | |
| Pergonal<br>Repronex<br>Humegon | Product made of FSH and LH to promote the development and maturation of follicles in ovaries. |
| **Follicle-Stimulating Hormone Agonists** | |
| urofollitropin (Bravelle)<br>follitropin (Gonal-f) | Stimulate follicle growth and maturation by mimicking the body's natural FSH. |
| **GnRH Antagonists** | |
| cetrorelix (Cetrotide)<br>ganirelix | Prevent premature LH surges and premature ovulation in women undergoing ovarian stimulation. |
| **GnRH Agonists** | |
| leuprolide (Lupron)<br>nafarelin (Synarel) | Suppress release of LH and FSH with continuous use. May also be used in the treatment of endometriosis. |
| **Human Chorionic Gonadotropin (hCG)** | |
| Pregnyl<br>Profasi<br>Novarel | Induces ovulation by stimulating release of eggs from follicles. |

*FSH,* Follicle-stimulating hormone; *GnRH,* gonadotropin-releasing hormone; *LH,* luteinizing hormone.

**TABLE 53-3 Types of Spontaneous Abortion**

| Type | Description |
|---|---|
| **Complete abortion** | All products of conception (POC) are expelled |
| **Incomplete abortion** | Parts of POC are retained |
| **Inevitable abortion** | Cervix is open and pregnancy loss cannot be prevented |
| **Infected (septic) abortion** | Endometrium (uterine lining) and POC become infected |
| **Missed abortion** | Fetus has died but has not been expelled |
| **Threatened abortion** | Unexplained bleeding with or without pain. Suggests pregnancy loss may occur |

**TABLE 53-4 Methods for Inducing Abortions**

| Method | Length of Pregnancy | Description |
|---|---|---|
| **Medical vacuum aspiration** | Usually up to 2 wk after first missed period | Catheter is inserted through cervix into uterus, and suction is applied. Contents of uterus are aspirated. |
| **Suction aspiration (curettage)** | Up to 12 wk | Cervix is dilated, uterine aspirator is introduced, and suction is applied, removing contents of uterus. |
| **Dilation and evacuation (D&E)** | 10-16 wk (approximate) | Cervix is dilated and contents of uterus are removed by vacuum cannula and use of other instruments as needed. |
| **Mifepristone (Mifeprex) with misoprostol (Cytotec)** | Up to 49-63 days* | Mifepristone is administered orally, followed by misoprostol orally 48 hr later. |

*FDA recommends 49 days. The American Congress of Obstetricians and Gynecologists guidelines indicate it is safe to use up to 63 days.

excessive. This may involve a *dilation and curettage (D&C)* or the use of medications to expel the remaining contents from the uterus. The D&C involves surgically dilating the cervix and scraping the endometrium of the uterus to empty the contents of the uterus.

Women who experience moderate-to-heavy bleeding and the passage of clots during pregnancy may require emergency care at a hospital. Vital signs and blood loss are monitored along with an assessment of her psychologic well-being. Any heavy bleeding, severe pain, or fever that occurs after medical management should be reported to the HCP. Ovulation can occur as soon as 2 weeks after early pregnancy loss, and normal menses should return within 4 to 6 weeks.

Provide grief support as the couple deals with the psychologic distress of their loss. Encourage them to verbalize their feelings and refer them to a pregnancy loss support group.

### Induced Abortion

*Induced abortion* is an elective termination of a pregnancy.[3] Several methods can be used for induced abortions (Table 53-4). Deciding which method to use depends on the length of the pregnancy and the woman's condition.

Once the decision is made to have an abortion, the woman and her partner need support and acceptance. Prepare the patient for what to expect both emotionally and physically. Grief and sadness are normal emotions after an abortion. Nursing care for a women who terminates her pregnancy includes assessment of a woman's need for counseling and support, providing for privacy, maintaining her physical comfort, and monitoring her vital signs.

After the abortion, teach the patient the signs and symptoms of possible complications, such as abnormal vaginal bleeding, severe abdominal cramping, fever, and foul-smelling drainage. Also stress to the patient that as soon as 1 week after having an abortion she is able to become pregnant again. Normal menstruation returns in 4 to 6 weeks.

Instruct patients to refrain from intercourse and putting anything into the vagina for 1 week after the abortion. (The one exception is for women who use NuvaRing birth control.) Oral contraception can be started the day of the abortion or 1 to 2 weeks after the procedure, depending on the patient's needs and desires.

## PROBLEMS RELATED TO MENSTRUATION

The normal menstrual cycle is discussed in Chapter 50. After *menarche* (onset of menses), the menstrual cycle may be irregular during the first few years as well as the years preceding menopause. Although most women have a predictable menstrual cycle, considerable normal variation exists among women in cycle length and in duration, amount, and character of the menstrual flow (see Table 50-2). During the perimenopausal period as ovarian function begins to diminish, women may note a change in their menstrual patterns.

## PREMENSTRUAL SYNDROME

**Premenstrual syndrome (PMS)** refers to a group of symptoms that occur during a woman's menstrual cycle. Many women experience symptoms of PMS. The syndrome includes a variety of physical, psychologic, and somatic symptoms that may be severe enough to affect interpersonal relationships, professional responsibilities, academic performance, and social activities.

As many as 150 symptoms have been associated with PMS. *Premenstrual dysphoric disorder* (PMDD) is the term used to describe PMS associated with a severe mood disorder.

### Etiology and Pathophysiology

The cause of PMS is not well understood. PMS is probably due to a combination of biologic and psychosocial factors. Genetics, imbalances in hormones and neurotransmitters (e.g., serotonin), and nutritional deficiencies have all been thought to be causes of PMS.

### Clinical Manifestations

PMS is extremely variable in its clinical manifestations, frequency, and severity among women. Symptoms may also vary from one cycle to another. Common symptoms include breast discomfort, peripheral edema, abdominal bloating, sensation of weight gain, episodes of binge eating, headaches, anxiety, depression, irritability and moodiness, back pain, insomnia, menstrual cramps, fatigue, and generalized muscle pain.

### Diagnostic Studies and Interprofessional Care

A focused health history and physical examination are performed to identify any underlying conditions such as thyroid dysfunction, uterine fibroids, anemia, nutritional and vitamin deficiencies, autoimmune disorders, endometriosis, and/or depression that may account for the symptoms.

To accurately diagnose PMS or PMDD, four factors are critical: (1) consistency of the syndrome complex, (2) occurrence of the symptoms in the luteal phase and resolution after the beginning of menses, (3) documented ovulatory cycles, and (4) symptoms that disrupt the woman's life.

A holistic approach to managing PMS symptoms for women includes stress management, dietary changes, exercise, teaching, and cognitive behavioral therapy.

**Drug Therapy.** Selective serotonin reuptake inhibitors (SSRIs), such as sertraline (Zoloft) and fluoxetine (Prozac, Sarafem), have provided relief to women who suffer from symptoms of anxiety, irritability, and mood changes associated with PMS. Many women choose to take oral contraceptives and/or NSAIDs to reduce cramping and back pain. Vitamin $B_6$, calcium, and magnesium have been recommended for mood changes associated with PMS.

**CHECK YOUR PRACTICE**

You are working in the GYN outpatient clinic. Your patient is a 28-yr-old woman who is being seen for symptoms of PMS. She tells you, "My PMS has gotten so bad lately that I spend the entire day in bed due to pain. I am very anxious and overwhelmed. I can't function like this anymore."

- How would you respond?
- What are things she can do to relieve symptoms?

## NURSING MANAGEMENT: PREMENSTRUAL SYNDROME

Nursing care for the patient with PMS includes teaching her about the symptoms associated with PMS and how to manage them (Table 53-5). Acknowledging that she has PMS can be therapeutic and empowering. Teaching the woman's partner about the nature of PMS helps the partner better understand PMS and its effects. Provide the patient with support and reassure her that PMS is not an emotional disorder, but one that has a physiologic basis and one that can be managed.

## DYSMENORRHEA

**Dysmenorrhea** is painful menses with abdominal cramping. The two types of dysmenorrhea are *primary* (no pathologic condition exists) and *secondary* (pelvic disease is the underlying cause). Dysmenorrhea is one of the most common gynecologic problems.

### Etiology and Pathophysiology

*Primary dysmenorrhea* begins in the first few years after menarche, typically with the onset of regular menstrual cycles. It is usually related to elevated levels of prostaglandin, a hormone that is found in the endometrium. Stimulation of the endometrium by estrogen and progesterone results in a dramatic increase in prostaglandin production. Prostaglandin stimulates the uterus to contract. Uterine contractions and constriction of small endometrial blood vessels result in tissue ischemia and increased sensitization of the pain receptors. This results in painful menstrual cramps. As menstruation continues, prostaglandin levels decrease each day, and menstrual cramping lessens.

*Secondary dysmenorrhea* usually occurs after adolescence, most commonly at 30 to 40 years of age and worsens as a woman ages. Common pelvic conditions that cause secondary dysmenorrhea include endometriosis, chronic pelvic inflammatory disease, and uterine fibroids. Because secondary dysmenorrhea can be caused by many conditions, the clinical manifestations and severity vary. However, painful menses is the primary manifestation.

### Clinical Manifestations

Clinical manifestations of dysmenorrhea include menstrual pain that is most severe during the first few days of menses. Painful menstruation rarely lasts more than 2 days. Typical symptoms reported by women include lower, colicky abdominal pain, frequently radiating to the lower back and upper thighs. Nausea, diarrhea, fatigue, and headache may also occur.

Secondary dysmenorrhea usually occurs after the woman has little to no pain during the menstrual cycle. The pain, which may be unilateral, is generally more constant and continues longer than in primary dysmenorrhea. Depending on the cause, symptoms such as *dyspareunia* (painful intercourse), painful defecation, or irregular bleeding may occur at times other than menstruation.

### Diagnostic Studies

Evaluating a patient for dysmenorrhea begins with a complete health history and pelvic examination. A probable diagnosis of primary dysmenorrhea is given if the history reveals an onset shortly after menarche with symptoms that are associated only with menses. The pelvic examination is otherwise normal. If the HCP finds an underlying cause of dysmenorrhea, the diagnosis is secondary dysmenorrhea.

## NURSING AND INTERPROFESSIONAL MANAGEMENT: DYSMENORRHEA

Treatment for primary dysmenorrhea includes pharmacologic and nonpharmacologic therapy. Nonsteroidal antiinflammatory drugs (NSAIDs) (e.g., naproxen [Naprosyn]) inhibit prostaglandins. Oral contraceptives (OCPs) may also be used to decrease estrogen and progesterone. This results in lower prostaglandin levels, decreased monthly endometrial lining proliferation, and decreased menstrual flow.

Nonpharmacologic interventions include applying heat to the lower abdomen or back and physical exercise. Regular exercise helps to reduce prostaglandin production. Acupuncture and transcutaneous nerve stimulation may be used for women who have inadequate relief from drugs or who prefer not to take drugs.

Treatment of secondary dysmenorrhea depends on the etiology. Some individuals with secondary dysmenorrhea are helped by the approaches used for primary dysmenorrhea. However, if a gynecologic abnormality is the main cause of secondary dysmenorrhea, then treating the underlying gynecologic abnormality is the priority. For example, women with endometriosis who have secondary dysmenorrhea may benefit from taking OCPs. Nursing interventions include teaching women with dysmenorrhea about the cause, symptoms, and treatment. This will

**TABLE 53-5 Interprofessional Care**

***Premenstrual Syndrome (PMS)***

**Diagnostic Assessment**
- History and physical examination
- Symptom diary

**Management**
- Stress management
- Nutritional therapy
- Aerobic exercise

***Drug Therapy***
- Diuretics
- Prostaglandin inhibitors (e.g., ibuprofen)
- Selective serotonin reuptake inhibitors (e.g., sertraline [Zoloft])
- Combined oral contraceptives

provide women with a basis for coping with this common problem and increase feelings of self-control. Advise women that during acute pain, relief may be obtained by applying heat to the abdomen or back and taking NSAIDs. Also suggest noninvasive pain-relieving practices such as relaxation breathing and guided imagery, yoga, and meditation. Other measures to reduce the discomfort of dysmenorrhea include regular exercise and good nutrition.

## ABNORMAL UTERINE BLEEDING

**Abnormal uterine bleeding (AUB)** is any change in a woman's menstrual flow, including volume, duration, or cycle pattern. AUB can be classified based on the cause of bleeding (Fig. 53-1). *Heavy menstrual bleeding* (HMB) (instead of the term *menorrhagia*) describes excessive bleeding. *Intermenstrual bleeding* (instead of the term *metrorrhagia*) refers to bleeding between regular menstrual cycles.

*Chronic AUB* is classified as uterine bleeding that is abnormal in volume, timing, or regularity and has been present for most of the past 6 months. *Acute AUB* is an episode of heavy bleeding that requires immediate treatment.

In reproductive-age women, the causes of AUB may include uterine fibroids, polyps, ovulatory dysfunction, endometrial problems, or cancer. Other causes of AUB may include bleeding disorders (e.g., thrombocytopenia), leukemia, medications, eating disorders, or liver failure.[4] For postmenopausal women, endometrial cancer must be considered whenever bleeding or spotting is experienced after her menstrual bleeding has ceased for 1 year or longer.

*Anovulation* is the most common reason for missing menses. Ovulation is often erratic for several years after menarche and before menopause. Bleeding in between periods (spotting) is also common for women who start taking oral contraceptives. If spotting continues beyond the first few months on oral contraceptives, a different pill formulation may be prescribed. Spotting with long-acting progestin therapies (e.g., intrauterine devices [IUDs], Nexplanon implant, progestin-only pills [levonorgestrel, norethindrone], progesterone injections [medroxyprogesterone-Depo-Provera] is also common and not usually associated with any serious complications.

**Amenorrhea** is the absence or abnormal interruption of menstruation (Table 53-6). *Primary amenorrhea* refers to the failure of menstrual cycles to begin by 16 years of age. *Secondary amenorrhea* occurs when menstrual cycles stop for 3 to 6 months in menstruating women. Primary amenorrhea is often associated with chromosomal or congenital abnormalities. Many causes of secondary amenorrhea can be attributed to primary ovarian insufficiency, polycystic ovary syndrome (PCOS), hypothalamic disorders, and hyperprolactinemia.

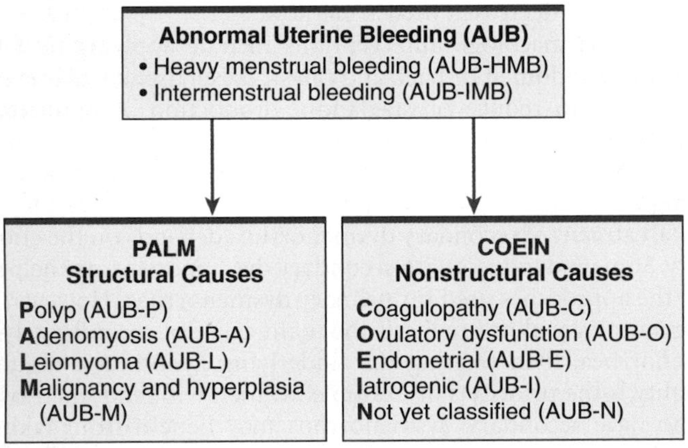


**FIG. 53-1** PALM-COIEN classification system for abnormal uterine bleeding. (Used with permission. The American College of Obstetricians and Gynecologists: *Practice Bulletin* 128:1, 2012.)

### Diagnostic Studies and Interprofessional Care

Once it is determined that a patient has AUB, the HCP will determine if the AUB is related to a structural cause or nonstructural cause. A comprehensive history and physical examination are done to determine the cause of AUB (Table 53-7). Laboratory evaluation and diagnostic procedures are based on findings from the history and physical examination. Treatment depends on the cause of the problem, degree of threat to the patient's health, her quality of life, and whether children are desired in the future.

**TABLE 53-6 Causes of Amenorrhea**

**Natural Amenorrhea**
- Pregnancy
- Breastfeeding
- Menopause

**Lifestyle**
- Stress
- Excessive exercise
- Low body weight
- Acute and chronic illness

**Hormonal Imbalance**
- Polycystic ovary syndrome (PCOS)
- Pituitary tumors
- Thyroid dysfunction

**Medications**
- Antipsychotics
- Antihypertensives
- Chemotherapy
- Antidepressants
- Hormone therapy (oral or injectable contraceptives, intrauterine devices)

**Structural Problems**
- Damage or scarring to reproductive organs from infection, trauma, radiation

**Genetic**
- Congenital absence of reproductive organ(s)
- Turner's syndrome

**TABLE 53-7 Interprofessional Care**

***Abnormal Uterine Bleeding***

**Diagnostic Assessment**
- History, including surgical history and medication history
- Pelvic examination
- Age of menarche/menopause
- Bleeding patterns and perceived severity of bleeding (clots, soaking through clothing)
- Evaluation for manifestations of obesity/hirsutism (suggestive of polycystic ovary syndrome)
- Pregnancy test
- Complete blood count (CBC)
- Thyroid-stimulating hormone (TSH)
- STI screening
- Screening for bleeding disorders (if indicated)
- Imaging studies and tissue sampling
  - Transvaginal/pelvic ultrasound
  - Saline infusion sonohysterography
  - MRI
  - Hysteroscopy
  - Endometrial biopsy

**Management**

Based on etiology of problem, may include:
- Oral contraceptives
- Hormonal therapy
- Nonsteroidal antiinflammatory drugs
- Mirena IUD

Combined oral contraceptives may be prescribed for a woman with amenorrhea to ensure regular shedding of the endometrium. Tranexamic acid (Lysteda) may be used to treat heavy menstrual bleeding. This drug stabilizes a protein that helps blood to clot. The use of tranexamic acid is contraindicated in women who use combined oral contraceptives.

Estradiol valerate/dienogest (Natazia) is the only combined oral contraceptive approved for treatment of heavy menstrual bleeding. It may be given to women who desire an oral contraceptive to prevent pregnancy. Other options for treatment of heavy menstrual bleeding include nonsteroidal antiinflammatory drugs (NSAIDs) and the Mirena IUD (progestin IUD).

## ❖ NURSING MANAGEMENT: ABNORMAL UTERINE BLEEDING

Teach women about the characteristics of the menstrual cycle to help them identify variations (see Table 50-2). This knowledge can decrease apprehension and dispel misconceptions about the menstrual cycle. Encourage the patient to report excessive bleeding, passing of clots, and unusually long duration of menstrual cycles.

Teach women to avoid the prolonged use of superabsorbent tampons that can increase the risk of toxic shock syndrome (TSS). TSS is an acute life-threatening condition caused by a toxin from *Staphylococcus aureus.* TSS causes high fever, vomiting, diarrhea, weakness, myalgia, and a sunburn-like rash.

## ECTOPIC PREGNANCY

An **ectopic pregnancy** is the implantation of the fertilized ovum anywhere outside the uterus. Almost all ectopic pregnancies occur within the fallopian tube. Approximately 3% of all pregnancies are ectopic (Fig. 53-2). Ectopic pregnancy is a life-threatening condition. Early detection can lead to successful management as well as reduced morbidity and mortality.

### Etiology and Pathophysiology

Ectopic pregnancy can be caused by blockage of the fallopian tube(s) or reduction of tubal peristalsis that impedes or delays the fertilized ovum from passing to the uterus. After the fertilized egg implants itself in the fallopian tube, the growth of the gestational sac expands the tubal wall and eventually the fallopian tube ruptures. This leads to manifestations of acute peritonitis 6 to 8 weeks after the last normal menstrual period. Often the woman presents to the HCP or the emergency department (ED) due to bleeding and/or pelvic pain or pressure.

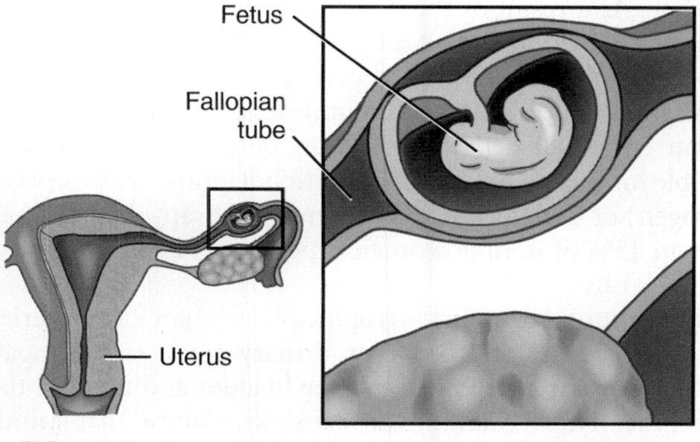


**FIG. 53-2** Ectopic pregnancy occurring in the fallopian tube.

Risk factors or causes for ectopic pregnancy include a history of pelvic inflammatory disease, prior ectopic pregnancy, current progestin-releasing IUD, and prior pelvic or tubal surgery. Additional risk factors include procedures used in infertility treatment (e.g., IVF, embryo transfer, ovulation induction).

### Clinical Manifestations

The classic manifestations of ectopic pregnancy are abdominal or pelvic pain, missed menses, and/or irregular vaginal bleeding. Other manifestations include morning sickness, breast tenderness, gastrointestinal disturbance, malaise, and syncope.

Pelvic and/or abdominal pain is almost always present and is caused by distention of the fallopian tube. The character of the pain varies among women and can be colicky or vague, unilateral or bilateral.

Symptom severity does not necessarily correlate with the extent of vaginal bleeding. The vaginal bleeding that may accompany ectopic pregnancy is usually described as spotting. However, bleeding may be heavier and can be confused with menses. If tubal rupture occurs, there is risk of hemorrhage and hypovolemic shock. This situation is an emergency.

### Diagnostic Studies

Diagnosing an ectopic pregnancy can be challenging because of the clinical manifestations. If an HCP suspects an ectopic pregnancy, a pelvic examination should be performed along with a serum pregnancy test (quantitative human chorionic gonadotropin β-hCG). If the patient is in stable condition, a combination of serial measurements of serum β-hCG and vaginal ultrasound is indicated to monitor the ectopic pregnancy.

**CHECK YOUR PRACTICE**

You are working in the ED. Your patient is a 29-yr-old woman who presented with acute abdominal pain. She has had in vitro fertilization. Her pain is 7 (on 0 to 10 pain scale). The HCP suspects an ectopic pregnancy. She is crying, "I am going to lose this baby, and we have been trying so hard to have one."

- As her nurse, what are your priorities?
- How would you respond to her?

## ❖ NURSING AND INTERPROFESSIONAL MANAGEMENT: ECTOPIC PREGNANCY

There are two ways to treat ectopic pregnancies: drug therapy or surgery.[5] Drug therapy is used (1) when an ectopic pregnancy is confirmed on ultrasound, (2) the woman is hemodynamically stable, (3) the woman is compliant with the required follow-up, and (4) the pregnancy is small and the fallopian tube has not ruptured.

Methotrexate therapy is the drug therapy of choice. Methotrexate stops the growth of rapidly dividing cells, such as embryonic, fetal, and early placenta cells. Methotrexate can be given as a single shot or as several injections. The most common side effect of methotrexate is cramping abdominal pain. It usually occurs during the first 2 to 3 days of treatment. Other side effects may include vaginal bleeding, nausea, vomiting, indigestion, or dizziness.

Serum β-hCG levels are determined on posttreatment days 4 and 7. A 15% reduction in β-hCG is expected. Weekly β-hCG are performed until negative. If at any time serum β-hCG levels plateau or increase, methotrexate may be repeated. If an ectopic

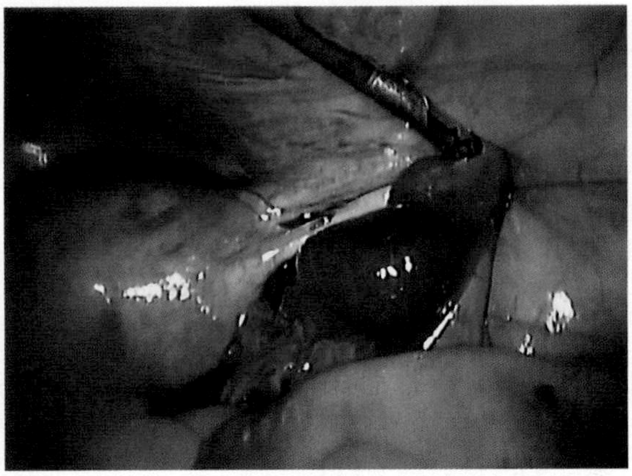

**FIG. 53-3** Laparoscopic treatment of ectopic pregnancy in the right fallopian tube. (From Katz V: *Comprehensive gynecology,* ed 5, St Louis, 2007, Mosby.)

pregnancy continues after 2 or 3 doses of methotrexate, surgical treatment is needed to remove the ectopic pregnancy.

If surgery is needed, a conservative approach that limits damage to the reproductive system is the goal. If the pregnancy is small, the pregnancy is removed laparoscopically (Fig. 53-3). If the tube ruptures, emergent surgery is required to stabilize the patient.

Nursing care includes closely monitoring vital signs and observing for signs of shock. Provide patient teaching to prepare her for the diagnostic procedures and drug therapy. Explain the side effects of methotrexate and tell her to avoid NSAIDs. Follow-up with weekly β-hCG measurements is required. If the patient requires laparoscopic surgery, provide patient teaching and emotional support.

**TABLE 53-8 Manifestations of Perimenopause and Postmenopause**

| Perimenopause | Postmenopause |
|---|---|
| • Irregular menstrual cycles<br>• Occasional vasomotor symptoms (e.g., hot flashes)<br>• Mood changes<br>• Sleep disturbances<br>• Vaginal dryness | • Cessation of menses<br>• Vasomotor instability (e.g., hot flashes and night sweats)<br>• Atrophy of genitourinary tissue (e.g., vaginal epithelium)<br>• Stress and urge incontinence<br>• Breast tenderness<br>• Atrophy of genitourinary tissue with decreased support<br>• Osteoporosis |

**TABLE 53-9 Manifestations of Estrogen Deficiency**

| | |
|---|---|
| **Vasomotor**<br>• Hot flashes<br>• Night sweats | **Musculoskeletal**<br>• Increased fracture rate, especially vertebral bodies but also humerus, distal radius, and upper femur |
| **Genitourinary**<br>• Atrophic vaginitis<br>• Dyspareunia secondary to poor lubrication<br>• Incontinence | **Cardiovascular**<br>• Decreased high-density lipoproteins (HDLs)<br>• Increased low-density lipoproteins (LDLs) |
| **Psychologic**<br>• Emotional lability<br>• Change in sleep pattern<br>• Decreased REM sleep | **Other**<br>• Diminished collagen content of skin<br>• Breast tissue changes |

*REM,* Rapid eye movement.

## PERIMENOPAUSE AND POSTMENOPAUSE

**Perimenopause** is a normal life transition for women that begins with the first signs of change in menstrual cycles and ends after cessation of menses. Menstrual changes can include shorter cycles, less frequent cycles, lighter cycles, or heavier cycles.

**Menopause** is a normal physiologic cessation of menses associated with declining ovarian function that ends in cessation of the menstrual cycle and ovulation. *Natural menopause* is diagnosed retrospectively after 12 months of no periods. The average age for a woman is 52 years, but the age can vary from 40 to 58 years.

*Induced menopause* occurs as a result of surgical intervention to remove the ovaries or from side effects of chemotherapy, radiation therapy, or other drugs. *Postmenopause* is a term that refers to the time in a woman's life after menopause.

### Clinical Manifestations

Clinical manifestations of perimenopause and menopause are presented in Table 53-8. Perimenopause is a time of erratic hormonal fluctuation and irregular menstrual cycles. With the decrease in function of the ovaries, estrogen levels drop and hot flashes and other symptoms begin. The signs and symptoms of diminished estrogen are listed in Table 53-9.

The loss of estrogen plays a significant role in the cause of age-related alterations. Changes most critical to a woman's well-being are the increased risks for coronary artery disease (CAD) and osteoporosis (secondary to bone density loss). Other changes include a redistribution of fat, a tendency to gain weight more easily, muscle and joint pain, loss of skin elasticity, changes in hair amount and distribution, and atrophy of external genitalia and breast tissue.

*Vasomotor instability* (hot flashes) and irregular menses are the two main clinical manifestations associated with menopause. A hot flash is a sudden sensation of intense heat along with perspiration and flushing. Other manifestations of menopause include atrophy of the vagina. Vaginal atrophy is due to decreased estrogen levels related to the loss of ovarian function. Decreased estrogen causes thinning of the vaginal mucosa and disappearance of rugae, which results in a decrease in vaginal secretions and causes the vaginal secretions to become more alkaline. As a result of these changes, the vagina is easily traumatized, the woman can experience more dyspareunia, and she can be more susceptible to infection.

Vaginal atrophy can lead to unnecessary and premature cessation of sexual activity. This can be corrected with water-soluble lubricants or, if needed, with hormonal creams (vaginal estrogen) or oral hormone replacement therapy. Approximately 20% to 45% of midlife women experience vaginal atrophy, but few seek care.

In addition to vaginal atrophy, the woman can experience atrophic changes in the lower urinary tract. In menopause, bladder capacity decreases, and the bladder and urethral tissue lose tone. These changes can cause symptoms that mimic a bladder infection (e.g., dysuria, urgency, frequency) when no infection is present. Decreasing blood serum estrogen levels can cause an array of physical and cognitive changes during menopause that include depression, irritability, insomnia, and memory loss.

## EVIDENCE-BASED PRACTICE

### *Translating Research Into Practice*

**Is Sleep Disturbance Associated With Menopausal Stage?**

***Clinical Question***

For women who are premenopausal, perimenopausal, or postmenopausal (P), what is the association between menopausal stage (I) and sleep disturbance (O)?

***Synthesis of Best Available Evidence***

- Systematic review and meta-analysis of cross-sectional, cohort, and experimental studies.
- Included 24 studies of community-dwelling midlife women ($n = 63{,}542$) in various stages of natural menopause, including premenopausal, perimenopausal, and postmenopausal stages. Also included women with surgical menopause. Women from ethnically diverse backgrounds included white, Asian (Chinese and Japanese), Iranian, and Hispanic.
- Significant association was found between perimenopausal and postmenopausal stages and higher rates of sleep disturbance.
- Surgical menopause had stronger link to sleep disturbance than natural menopause.
- Asian and white women had more increased sleep disturbance compared than other ethnic groups when comparing perimenopausal to premenopausal and postmenopausal to premenopausal stages.

***Conclusions***

- Sleep disturbance is associated with menopausal stage.
- Association between menopausal stage and sleep disturbance may be influenced by a women's ethnicity.

***Implications for Nursing Practice***

1. What would you advise a woman who is in the perimenopausal stage and asks if her sleep problems are "normal"?
2. Why is it important for health care professionals to be knowledgeable of menopausal attitudes and beliefs when caring for ethnically diverse women with sleep problems?

***Reference for Evidence***

Xu Q, Lang C: Examining the relationship between subjective sleep disturbance and menopause: a systematic review and meta-analysis, *Menopause* 21:1301, 2014.

*P*, Patient population of interest; *I*, intervention or area of interest; *C*, comparison of interest or comparison group; *O*, outcomes of interest; *T*, timing (see p. 15).

## Interprofessional Care

The diagnosis of menopause should be made only after careful consideration of other possible causes for a woman's symptoms. Follicle-stimulating hormone (FSH) levels may be done to confirm a diagnosis of menopause. (The FSH levels are increased in menopause.) Because of the hormonal fluctuations that occur before menopause, routine testing of the serum FSH level to establish a diagnosis is not indicated until the woman has stopped menstruating for 12 months.

**Drug Therapy.** Hormone replacement therapy (HRT) using estrogen, with or without progesterone, is prescribed for some women. Women may choose to use HRT for short-term symptom management and treatment for several years (4 to 5 years) of menopausal symptoms. The risks (e.g., increased risk of breast and endometrial cancer, risk for blood clots) and benefits (e.g., minimizes bone loss, hot flashes, vaginal atrophic changes) must be carefully considered for an individual woman.[6]

**Nonhormonal Therapy.** Because of the risks associated with HRT some women choose to use nonhormonal and nonpharmacologic interventions to manage their symptoms. If a woman does not want to use HRT but has significant menopausal symptoms, other nonhormonal pharmacologic agents may be used. For example, the SSRI antidepressants, paroxetine (Paxil, Brisdelle), fluoxetine, and venlafaxine (Effexor XR), are an effective alternative to HRT to reduce hot flashes.

Clonidine (Catapres), an antihypertensive drug, and gabapentin (Neurontin), an antiseizure drug, have also been shown to manage vasomotor symptoms during menopause. Selective estrogen receptor modulators (SERMs), such as raloxifene (Evista), are also used to manage menopausal symptoms. SERMs have positive benefits of estrogen, such as preventing bone loss, without the negative effects that include risk for endometrial hyperplasia.

**Nutritional Therapy.** Good nutrition can decrease the risk of cardiovascular disease and osteoporosis in addition to assisting with vasomotor symptoms. A decrease in metabolic rate and careless eating habits can cause the weight gain and fatigue often attributed to menopause. An adequate intake of calcium and vitamin D helps maintain healthy bones and counteracts loss of bone density.

Postmenopausal women not taking supplemental HRT should have a daily calcium intake of at least 1500 mg. Women taking estrogen replacement need at least 1000 mg/day. Calcium supplements are best absorbed when taken with meals. Either dietary calcium or calcium supplements may be used (see Table 63-14).

## COMPLEMENTARY & ALTERNATIVE THERAPIES

### *Herbs and Supplements for Menopause*

| Herb | Scientific Evidence | Nursing Implications |
|---|---|---|
| Black cohosh | Mixed evidence for use in the treatment of menopausal symptoms* | • Generally well tolerated in recommended doses for up to 6 mo.<br>• Should not be used in people with a liver disorder. |
| Soy | Mixed evidence for treatment of menopausal symptoms* | • Women with a history of breast, ovarian, or uterine cancer or endometriosis should consult with their HCP before using soy or soy products.<br>• Soy may interact with warfarin. Patients taking warfarin should consult with their HCP before using soy or soy products. |

Source: *www.nlm.nih.gov/medlineplus/herbalmedicine.html#summary.*
*In general, the evidence for use of these herbs as treatments for menopause symptoms is limited by a lack of well-designed, controlled trials.

## NURSING MANAGEMENT: PERIMENOPAUSE AND POSTMENOPAUSE

Menopause is a time of great transition for a woman both physically and psychologically. Many women experience symptoms for years during the perimenopausal period while others transition without any difficulty. In addition, menopause may be occurring simultaneously with role changes in the woman's personal and professional life. The combination of menopause and these changes can cause great emotional distress or a renewed sense of self and well-being.

Women in their perimenopausal and menopausal years need a lot of emotional support. Provide reassurance that symptoms can be treated and managed with either hormonal or nonhormonal therapies. It is also important to teach them about strategies to prevent or reduce the risk of cardiovascular disease and osteoporosis.

## INFECTIONS OF LOWER GENITAL TRACT

### Etiology and Pathophysiology

The female genital tract is susceptible to different types of infections, especially if the pH of the genital tract is altered. In most women, the vaginal pH is typically below 4.5, which helps prevent certain bacterial infections from occurring. The pH level of the vagina is maintained through a combination of sufficient levels of estrogen and *Lactobacillus,* a naturally occurring bacteria that colonizes the vagina.

Infection and inflammation of the vagina, cervix, and vulva commonly occur when estrogen levels decrease and/or the presence of *Lactobacillus* is disrupted. Aging, poor nutrition, and drugs (e.g., antibiotics, oral contraceptives, corticosteroids) can affect the bacterial flora or mucosa, leading to alterations in the pH balance of the genital tract. For example, *Candida albicans* may be present in small numbers in the vagina. However, some women who take an antibiotic for another type of infection may experience an overgrowth of *Candida albicans,* leading to a condition called *vulvovaginal candidiasis* (more commonly referred to as "yeast infection").

Organisms gain entrance to the lower genital tract through contaminated hands, clothing, douching, and intercourse. Most lower genital tract infections are related to sexual intercourse. Intercourse can transmit organisms, injure tissue, and alter the acid-base balance of the vagina.

Table 53-10 presents the causes, manifestations, and interprofessional care of common infections of the female lower genital tract.

### Clinical Manifestations

The clinical manifestations of lower genital tract infections depend on the type of infection. Abnormal vaginal discharge and reddened vulvar lesions are common clinical manifestations. Women with vulvovaginal candidiasis have a curd-like discharge accompanied with intense itching and pain with urination. Women who have bacterial vaginosis often produce vaginal discharge that has a fishy odor. Women with cervicitis may notice spotting (bleeding) after intercourse.

Common vulvar lesions include herpes infection and genital warts. Initial or primary herpes infections may be extremely painful. Herpes infections begin as a small vesicle followed by a superficial red, painful, ulcer. Genital warts, caused by the human papillomavirus (HPV), vary in appearance. Irregularly shaped "cauliflower" lesions are common. Genital warts are painless unless traumatized. (Herpes infection and genital warts are discussed in Chapter 52.)

Postmenopausal women may develop vulvar changes such as *lichen sclerosis.* This chronic inflammatory skin condition is associated with intense itching in the genital skin area (e.g., labia minora, clitoris). Although the lesions are white with a "tissue paper" appearance initially, scratching produces changes in the appearance. The cause is unknown.

### Interprofessional Care

Evaluation of genital problems includes a history, physical examination, and appropriate laboratory and diagnostic studies. Because many problems relate to sexual activity, a sexual history is essential. The nature of the problem determines the extent of the evaluation. When ulcerative lesions are present, an HCP will usually obtain a culture for herpes and a blood test for syphilis.

**TABLE 53-10 Infections of the Lower Genital Tract**

| Infection and Etiology | Manifestations | Drug Therapy |
|---|---|---|
| **Vulvovaginal Candidiasis** | | |
| *Candida albicans* (fungus) | Pruritus, thick white curd-like discharge. | Antifungal agents (e.g., miconazole [Monistat], clotrimazole [Gyne-Lotrimin, Mycelex] [available over the counter, in cream or suppository]).<br>Fluconazole (Diflucan). Terconazole (Terazol) vaginal creams and suppositories. |
| **Trichomonas Vaginitis** | | |
| *Trichomonas vaginalis* (protozoa) | Sexually transmitted. Pruritus, frothy greenish or gray discharge. Hemorrhagic spots on cervix or vaginal walls. | Metronidazole (Flagyl) or tinidazole (Tindamax) for patient and partner. |
| **Bacterial Vaginosis** | | |
| *Gardnerella vaginalis*<br>*Corynebacterium vaginale* | Watery discharge with fish-like odor. May or may not have other symptoms. | Oral or vaginal metronidazole (Flagyl), vaginal clindamycin (Clindesse), or oral tinidazole (Tindamax).<br>*Lactobacillus acidophilus* taken orally by diet (e.g., yogurt, fermented soy products) or supplements can decrease unwanted vaginal bacteria. |
| **Cervicitis** | | |
| *Chlamydia trachomatis* or *Neisseria gonorrhoeae* (most often) | Sexually transmitted. Mucopurulent discharge with postcoital spotting from cervical inflammation. | Based on cause. Common treatment includes azithromycin (Zithromax) and ceftriaxone (Rocephin). Treat patient and partner. |
| **Severe Recurrent Vaginitis (more than four episodes per year)** | | |
| *C. albicans* (most often) or non-*albicans* strains | May be indication of HIV infection. All women who are unresponsive to first-line treatment should be offered HIV testing. | Drug appropriate to opportunistic organism. |

*KOH,* Potassium hydroxide.

Genital warts are usually identified by their clinical appearance. Vulvar skin conditions may be examined by colposcopy and biopsy of the skin lesion.

Problems involving vaginal discharge are evaluated by examining the discharge under a microscope and obtaining cultures. To assess for cervicitis, specimens are obtained for chlamydial infection and gonorrhea. (Sexually transmitted infections [STIs] are discussed in Chapter 52.)

Drug therapy is based on the diagnosis (Table 53-10). Antibiotics taken as directed will cure bacterial infections. Teach patients how to properly take their medications and get follow-up care. Partners should be treated so that reinfection does not occur.

Women with vaginal conditions or cervical infection should abstain from intercourse for at least 1 week. Douching should be avoided. Sexual partners must be evaluated and treated if the patient is diagnosed with trichomoniasis, chlamydial infection, gonorrhea, syphilis, or HIV.

Treatment of vulvar skin conditions is symptomatic because no cures are available. Treatment involves controlling the itching and hence the scratching. High-potency topical corticosteroid ointment such as clobetasol (Temovate) helps relieve itching. Interrupting the "itch-scratch cycle" prevents further secondary damage to the skin.

## NURSING MANAGEMENT: INFECTIONS OF LOWER GENITAL TRACT

Teach women about common infections of the genital tract and how to reduce their risks for infection. Recognize symptoms that indicate a problem, and help women seek care in a timely manner. Discussing problems that concern the patient's genitalia or sexual intercourse is frequently difficult. Use a nonjudgmental attitude to make women feel more comfortable while empowering them to ask questions.

When a woman is diagnosed with a genital infection, ensure that she fully understands the treatment. Taking the full course of medication is especially important to decrease the chance of relapse. Because genitalia are such a private area, the use of graphs and models is especially helpful for patient teaching. When a woman is using a vaginal medication for the first time, show her the applicator and how to fill it. Also teach where and how the applicator should be inserted using visual aids or models. Vaginal creams should be inserted before going to bed so that the medication will remain in the vagina for a long period. Women using vaginal creams or suppositories may wish to use panty liners during the day when the residual medication may drain out.

## PELVIC INFLAMMATORY DISEASE (PID)

**Pelvic inflammatory disease (PID)** is an infectious condition of the pelvic cavity that may involve the fallopian tubes (salpingitis), ovaries (oophoritis), and pelvic peritoneum (peritonitis). A tubo-ovarian abscess may also form (Fig. 53-4).

### Etiology and Pathophysiology

PID is often the result of untreated cervical infection. The organism infecting the cervix can spread into the uterus, fallopian tubes, ovaries, and peritoneal cavity. *Chlamydia trachomatis* and *Neisseria gonorrhoeae* are the most common causative organisms of PID.[7] These organisms, as well as anaerobes, mycoplasma, streptococci, and enteric gram-negative rods, gain entrance during sexual intercourse or after pregnancy termination, pelvic surgery, or childbirth. It is important to remember that not all cases of PID are the result of an STI.

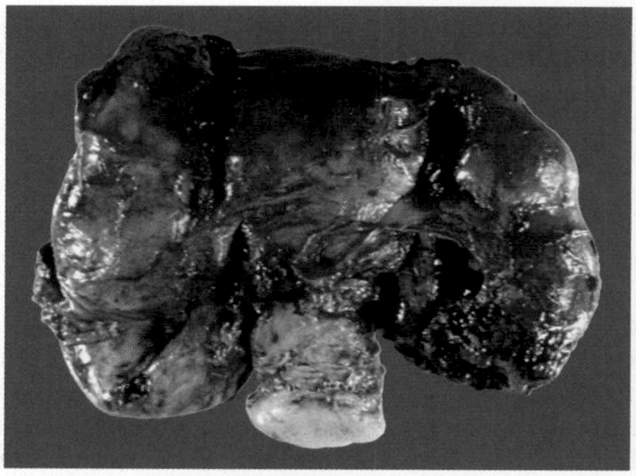

**FIG. 53-4** Pelvic inflammatory disease. Acute infection of the fallopian tubes and the ovaries. The tubes and the ovaries have become an inflamed mass attached to the uterus. A tubo-ovarian abscess is also present. (From Kumar V, Abbas AK, Aster JC, Fausto N: *Robbins and Cotran pathologic basis of disease,* ed 8, Philadelphia, 2010, Saunders.)

Women at increased risk for chlamydial infections (e.g., younger than 24 years of age, have multiple sex partners, have a new sex partner) should be routinely tested for *Chlamydia*. Chlamydial infections can be asymptomatic and unknowingly transmitted during intercourse.

### Clinical Manifestations

Lower abdominal pain is a common manifestation of PID. The pain typically starts gradually and then becomes constant. The intensity may vary from mild to severe. Movement such as walking can increase the pain. The pain is also frequently associated with intercourse. Spotting after intercourse and purulent cervical or vaginal discharge may also be noted. Fever and chills may be present.

Women with less acute symptoms often notice increased cramping pain with menses, irregular bleeding, and some pain with intercourse. Women who have mild symptoms may go untreated either because they did not seek care or the HCP misdiagnosed their complaints.

### Complications

Complications of PID may include septic shock, perihepatitis, tubo-ovarian abscess, peritonitis, and embolism. PID can cause adhesions and strictures in the fallopian tubes, which may lead to ectopic pregnancy. After one episode of PID, the risk of having an ectopic pregnancy increases nearly 10 times. Further damage can obstruct the fallopian tubes and cause infertility.

### Interprofessional Care

A pelvic examination assists in the diagnosis of PID. Women with PID have lower abdominal tenderness, adnexal tenderness, and positive cervical motion tenderness.

Diagnostic testing includes examination for *N. gonorrhoeae* and *C. trachomatis* and a pregnancy test to rule out an ectopic pregnancy. When the patient's pain or obesity compromises the pelvic examination, a vaginal ultrasound may be ordered.

PID is usually treated on an outpatient basis. The patient is given a combination of antibiotics to provide broad coverage against the causative organisms. With effective antibiotic therapy, the pain should subside. The patient should abstain from intercourse for 3 weeks. Her partner(s) must be examined and treated. An important part of care is physical rest and oral fluids. Reevaluation in 48 to 72 hours, even if symptoms are improving, is an essential part of outpatient care.

If outpatient treatment is unsuccessful or if the patient is acutely ill or in severe pain, admission to a hospital is indicated. If a tubo-ovarian abscess is present, hospitalization is also indicated. Maximum doses of IV antibiotics are given in the hospital. Corticosteroids may be added to the antibiotic regimen to reduce inflammation, allowing for faster recovery and optimizing the chances for subsequent fertility. Application of heat to the lower abdomen or sitz baths may improve circulation and decrease pain. Bed rest in a semi-Fowler's position promotes drainage of the pelvic cavity by gravity and may prevent the development of abscesses high in the abdomen. Analgesics to relieve pain and IV fluids to prevent dehydration are also used.

Surgery is indicated for abscesses that fail to resolve with IV antibiotics. The abscess may be drained by laparoscopy or laparotomy. In extreme cases of infection or severe chronic pelvic pain, a hysterectomy may be performed. When surgery is necessary, the capacity for childbearing is preserved whenever possible.

## ❖ NURSING MANAGEMENT: PELVIC INFLAMMATORY DISEASE

Subjective and objective data that should be obtained from the woman with PID are presented in Table 53-11. Prevention, early recognition, and prompt treatment of vaginal and cervical infections can help prevent PID and its serious complications. Provide accurate information about factors that place a woman at increased risk for PID. Urge women to seek medical attention for any unusual vaginal discharge or possible infection of their reproductive organs. Inform patients that not all vaginal discharge indicates infection, but early diagnosis and treatment of an infection, if present, can prevent serious complications. Teach patients methods to decrease the risk of getting STIs and to recognize the signs of infection in their partner(s).

The patient may feel guilty about having PID, especially if it is associated with an STI. She may also be concerned about the complications associated with PID, such as infertility, and the increased incidence of ectopic pregnancy. Discuss with the patient her feelings and concerns to help her cope with them more effectively.

For patients requiring hospitalization, you have an important role in implementing drug therapy, monitoring the patient's health status, and providing symptom relief and patient teaching. Record vital signs and the character, amount, color, and odor of the vaginal discharge. Explain the need for limiting activity, being in a semi-Fowler's position, and increasing fluid intake. Assess the degree of abdominal pain to determine the effectiveness of drug therapy.

### TABLE 53-11 Nursing Assessment
#### *Pelvic Inflammatory Disease*

**Subjective Data**

***Important Health Information***

*Past health history:* Use of IUD. Previous PID, gonorrhea, or chlamydial infection. Multiple sexual partners. Exposure to partner with urethritis. Infertility

*Medications:* Use of and allergy to any antibiotics

*Surgery or other treatments:* Recent abortion or pelvic surgery

***Functional Health Patterns***

*Health perception–health management:* Malaise

*Nutritional-metabolic:* Nausea, vomiting; chills, fever

*Elimination:* Urinary frequency, urgency

*Cognitive-perceptual:* Lower abdominal and pelvic pain, low back pain, onset of pain just after a menstrual cycle. Dysmenorrhea, dyspareunia, dysuria, vulvar pruritus

*Sexuality-reproductive:* Abnormal vaginal bleeding and menstrual irregularity. Vaginal discharge

**Objective Data**

***Reproductive***

Mucopurulent cervicitis, vulvar maceration, vaginal discharge (heavy and purulent to thin and mucoid), tenderness on motion of cervix and uterus. Presence of inflammatory masses on palpation

***Possible Diagnostic Findings***

Leukocytosis, ↑ erythrocyte sedimentation rate, positive culture of secretions or endocervical fluid, pelvic inflammation and positive endometrial biopsy on laparoscopic examination, abscess or inflammation on ultrasonography

*IUD,* Intrauterine device; *PID,* pelvic inflammatory disease.

## CHRONIC PELVIC PAIN

*Chronic pelvic pain* refers to pain in the pelvic region (below the umbilicus and between the hips) that lasts 6 months or longer. The cause of chronic pelvic pain is often hard to find. Many different conditions can cause pelvic pain. Gynecologic etiologies include PID, endometriosis, ovarian cysts, uterine fibroids, pelvic adhesions, and ectopic pregnancies. Abdominal etiologies include irritable bowel syndrome, interstitial cystitis, appendicitis, and colitis. Psychologic factors (e.g., depression, chronic stress, history of sexual or physical abuse) may increase the risk of developing chronic pelvic pain. Emotional distress makes pain worse, and living with chronic pain contributes to emotional distress.

Chronic pelvic pain has many different clinical manifestations, including severe and steady pain, intermittent pain, dull and achy pain, pelvic pressure or heaviness, and sharp pain or cramping. In addition, pain may occur during intercourse or while having a bowel movement.

Determining the cause of chronic pelvic pain often involves a process of elimination. In addition to a detailed history and physical examination (including a pelvic examination), the patient may be asked to keep a journal of the onset of symptoms and any precipitating factors.

Diagnostic tests may include cultures from the cervix or vagina (used to detect STIs), ultrasound, CT scan, or MRI to detect abnormal structures or growths. Laparoscopy may be used to visualize the pelvic organs. This procedure is especially useful in detecting endometriosis and chronic PID.

If the cause of chronic pelvic pain is found, treatment focuses on that cause. If no cause can be found, treatment involves managing the pain. Over-the-counter pain medications (e.g., aspirin, ibuprofen, acetaminophen) may provide some relief. Sometimes stronger pain drugs may be needed. Birth control pills or other hormonal medications may help relieve cyclic pelvic pain related to menstrual cycles. If an infection is the source of the problem, antibiotics are used.

Tricyclic antidepressants (e.g., amitriptyline, nortriptyline [Pamelor]) have pain-relieving and antidepressant effects.

These drugs may help improve chronic pelvic pain even in women who do not have depression. The patient may be encouraged to get counseling for any emotional issues.

Laparoscopic surgery may be used to remove pelvic adhesions or endometrial tissue. As a last resort, a hysterectomy may be done.

## ENDOMETRIOSIS

**Endometriosis** is a benign gynecologic condition in which endometrial tissue accumulates outside the endometrium. Endometriosis is a common gynecologic problem.

In endometriosis, the most frequent sites for endometrial tissue growth is in or near the ovaries, uterosacral ligaments, and uterovesical peritoneum (Fig. 53-5). The tissue responds to the hormones of the ovarian cycle and undergoes a "mini-menstrual cycle" similar to the uterine endometrium. Although it is not a life-threatening condition, endometriosis can cause considerable pain. Endometriosis can significantly affect a woman's quality of life and ability to conceive. It also increases the risk of ovarian cancer.

### Etiology and Pathophysiology

Although the etiology of endometriosis is poorly understood, many theories have been proposed. Some of the theories include the possibility that the disorder may be due to retrograde (backward) flow of endometrial tissue. Instead of flowing out the cervix, the endometrial tissue flows through the fallopian tubes, depositing endometrial tissue into the pelvis.

Other theories have suggested that endometrial tissue is spread to the pelvic area through the lymph system or bloodstream. Another theory suggests that there is an increased sensitivity and production of prostaglandins, which are released prior to onset of menses. Other proposed causes include a genetic predisposition and altered immune function.

### Clinical Manifestations

Patients with endometriosis have a wide range of clinical manifestations. The severity of symptoms does not always correlate with the degree of disease found. The most common manifestations are secondary dysmenorrhea, infertility, pelvic pain, painful intercourse, and irregular bleeding. Less common manifestations include backache, painful bowel movements, and pain with urination. With menopause, estrogen is no longer produced in the ovaries, and the symptoms may disappear.

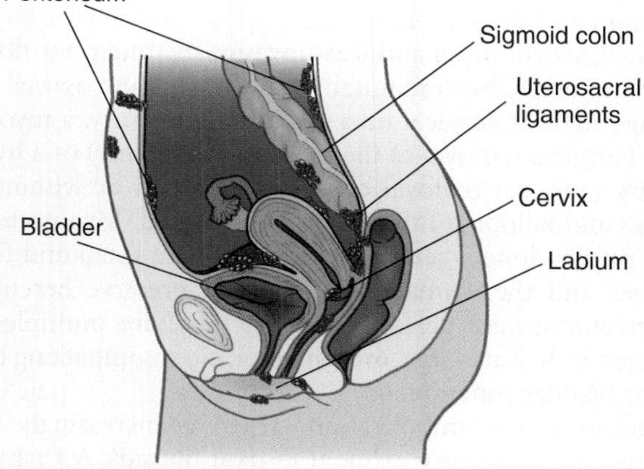


**FIG. 53-5** Common sites of endometriosis.

### Interprofessional Care

Endometriosis may be suspected based on a woman's history of the characteristic symptoms and the HCP's palpation of firm nodular lumps in the adnexa on bimanual examination. However, laparoscopy with a biopsy is necessary for a definitive diagnosis. MRI is now being used more frequently prior to surgery as a way to determine if the gynecologic symptoms the woman is experiencing are a result of endometriosis.

The treatment of endometriosis is influenced by the patient's age, desire for pregnancy, symptom severity, and extent and location of the disease. When symptoms are not disruptive, a "watch and wait" approach is used (Table 53-12). When endometriosis is identified as a probable cause of infertility, therapy proceeds more rapidly.

**Drug Therapy.** Drug therapy is used to reduce symptoms. Pain may be relieved with the use of NSAIDs such as ibuprofen, naproxen (Naprosyn), and diclofenac (Voltaren). The most common agent used to control symptoms and cause regression of endometrial tissue is combined oral contraceptives (OCPs). The continuous use of combined OCPs causes regression of endometrial tissue.

Another class of drugs used is GnRH agonists (e.g., leuprolide [Lupron], nafarelin [Synarel]). These drugs result in amenorrhea. Side effects are usually the same as those of menopause (hot flashes, vaginal dryness, emotional lability). Loss of bone density has also been reported in women who remain on the therapy longer than 6 months.

Endometriosis is controlled but not cured by drug therapy. Persistent lesions give rise to subsequent recurrences once the menstrual cycle is reestablished.

**DRUG ALERT Leuprolide (Lupron)**
- Assess patient for pregnancy before initiating therapy.
- Monitor patient for dysrhythmias, palpitations.
- Instruct patient to use nonhormonal contraceptive measures during therapy.

**Surgical Therapy.** The only cure for endometriosis is surgical removal of all endometrial tissue.[8] It involves removal or

**TABLE 53-12 Interprofessional Care**
***Endometriosis***

**Diagnostic Assessment**
- History and physical examination
- Pelvic examination
- Laparoscopy
- Pelvic ultrasound
- MRI

**Management**

***Conservative Therapy***
- Watch and wait

***Drug Therapy***
- Nonsteroidal antiinflammatory drugs (NSAIDs)
- Oral contraceptives
- danazol
- GnRH agonists (e.g., leuprolide [Lupron])

***Surgical Therapy***
- Laparotomy to remove implanted tissue and adhesions
- Total abdominal hysterectomy and bilateral salpingo-oophorectomy (TAH-BSO)

*GnRH,* Gonadotropin-releasing hormone.

destruction of endometrial tissue and excision of adhesions by means of laparoscopic laser surgery or laparotomy. Definitive surgery involves removal of the uterus, fallopian tubes, ovaries, and as many endometrial implants as possible. GnRH agonist therapy can be given for 4 to 6 months to reduce the size of the lesions before surgery.

For women wishing to get pregnant, conservative surgical therapy is used to remove implants blocking the fallopian tube. Adhesions are removed from the tubes, ovaries, and pelvic structures. Efforts are made to conserve all tissues necessary to maintain fertility.

Patients should be actively involved in making the decision about preserving part or all of their ovaries, if surgically possible. Explore the patient's feelings about maintaining her ovarian function. The HCP should assess the woman's risk for ovarian cancer and provide this information for her consideration.

## ❖ NURSING MANAGEMENT: ENDOMETRIOSIS

Nursing care for the woman with endometriosis includes reassurance that endometriosis is not life threatening and treatment options exist. When the symptoms are less severe, teach the patient about comfort measures that may be helpful. If pharmacologic therapy is required, then teach her about the action and side effects of the prescribed medication. Psychologic support may be needed for women experiencing severe disabling pain, sexual difficulties secondary to dyspareunia, and infertility.

# BENIGN TUMORS OF THE FEMALE REPRODUCTIVE SYSTEM

## LEIOMYOMAS

### Etiology and Pathophysiology

**Leiomyomas** (uterine fibroids) are benign smooth-muscle tumors (noncancerous) that occur during the childbearing years. Leiomyomas do not increase a woman's risk of endometrial cancer. They may be present inside the uterus within the endometrium, within the muscle of the uterus (myometrium), or outside on the surface of the uterus (subserosal). The size, shape, location, and number of leiomyomas vary among women. Some fibroids grow in spurts, while others slowly grow during the reproductive years (Fig. 53-6). Leiomyomas can occur at any age but are commonly found in women ages 30 to 40 years.

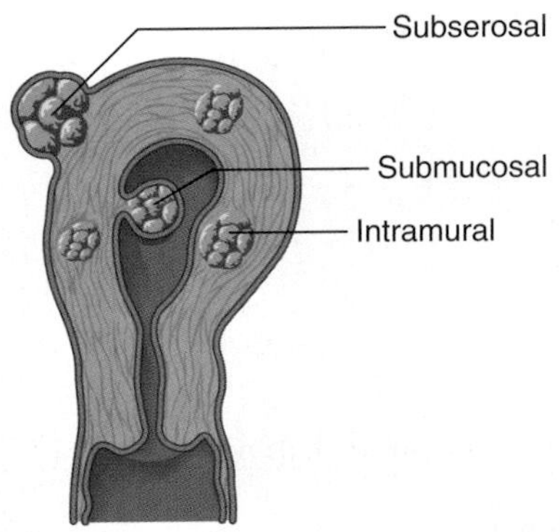


**FIG. 53-6** Leiomyomas. Uterine section showing whorl-like appearance and locations of leiomyomas. (From McCance KL, Huether SE: *Pathophysiology: the biologic basis for disease in adults and children,* ed 6, St Louis, 2010, Mosby.)

The etiology of leiomyomas is unknown. Their growth appears to depend on estrogen and progesterone because they grow during the reproductive years and undergo atrophy after menopause. In addition, leiomyomas contain more estrogen and progesterone receptors than normal uterine tissue. Thus they are more sensitive and grow in response to the release of these hormones.

In addition, genetics may play a role. Identical twins and women with mothers and sisters with leiomyomas have an increased risk. African American women seem to have increased incidence of leiomyomas and present with larger uterine fibroids and ones at an early age compared to other women. Other risk factors for fibroids include early age of menarche, alcohol use, and a diet high in red meat and low in green vegetables.

### Clinical Manifestations

The majority of women who have uterine fibroids do not report any symptoms. Those who report clinical manifestations may have abnormal uterine bleeding (AUB), abdominal and pelvic pain (i.e., dull, heaving and or achy pain and with pelvic pressure), painful sexual intercourse, pressure or pain during urination, or frequent urination. If leiomyomas are large, some women will report constipation and difficulty passing stool. AUB can manifest as increased duration, more frequent, or increased menstrual bleeding. The pain associated with a leiomyoma seems to be caused from uterine blood vessel compression as the fibroid grows or from the fibroid pressing on surrounding organs.

## ❖ NURSING AND INTERPROFESSIONAL MANAGEMENT: LEIOMYOMAS

Clinical diagnosis is based on the characteristic pelvic examination findings of an enlarged uterus distorted by nodular masses. Ultrasound can confirm the diagnosis. In some cases, small leiomyomas are found during a hysteroscopy, laparoscopy, or hysterosalpingogram when a woman is having a comprehensive workup for other gynecologic conditions, especially infertility.

The treatment of uterine fibroids depends on the patient's clinical manifestations, patient's age, a woman's desire to conceive, and the location and size of the fibroid.[9] If the symptoms are minimal, the HCP may elect to follow the patient closely for a period of time. Treatment may be required if a woman is seeking conception, is experiencing AUB, has pelvic pain and pressure, has anemia, or if she is experiencing difficulty with urination and defecation.

The most common and least invasive treatment for fibroids is the use of OCPs to maintain and slow growth as well as to manage AUB. If surgical intervention is necessary, a myomectomy (surgical removal of the uterine fibroid only) or a **hysterectomy** (surgical removal of the uterus with or without the ovaries and fallopian tubes) may be indicated. Myomectomies are typically done when the leiomyomas are small and few in number and the woman would like to preserve her uterus. Hysterectomies are performed when there are multiple leiomyomas, if they are large, or if their location is impacting bowel and or bladder function.

Uterine artery embolization (UAE) is increasingly being used as an alternative treatment to treat fibroids. A UAE is the process by which embolic material (small plastic or gelatin beads) is injected into the uterine artery. This process blocks blood flow to the uterus and shrinks the fibroid.

## OVARIAN CYSTS

*Ovarian cysts* are usually soft and surrounded by a thin capsule. Follicle and corpus luteum cysts are common ovarian cysts (Fig. 53-7). Multiple small ovarian follicles may occur in a condition called *polycystic ovary syndrome* (PCOS).

Ovarian cysts are often asymptomatic until they are large enough to cause pressure in the pelvis. Depending on the tumor's size and location, constipation, menstrual irregularities, urinary frequency, a full feeling in the abdomen, anorexia, an increase in abdominal girth, and peripheral edema may occur.

Pelvic pain may be present if the tumor is growing rapidly. Severe pain results when the cyst twists on its pedicle (ovarian torsion). In some cases, an ovarian cyst can rupture. A ruptured ovarian cyst is not only extremely painful, but it can lead to serious complications such as hemorrhage and infection.

Pelvic examination reveals a mass or an enlarged ovary. A pelvic ultrasound may be done to determine a diagnosis. In premenopausal women, ovarian cysts often resolve on their own. If the mass is cystic (does not appear cancerous) and smaller than 5 cm, the patient is asked to return for reexamination in 4 to 6 weeks. This is called "watchful waiting."

In postmenopausal women, watchful waiting may be an option depending on the results of the ultrasound. If the mass is cystic and greater than 5 cm or is solid, laparoscopic surgery or laparotomy is performed. Immediate surgery is necessary if ovarian torsion occurs, causing the ovary to rotate and cutting off circulation. Surgical techniques are used to save as much of the ovary as possible (if indicated).

### Polycystic Ovary Syndrome

*Polycystic ovary syndrome* (PCOS) is a disorder that includes ovulatory dysfunction, polycystic ovaries, and hyperandrogenism.[10] It most commonly occurs in women under 30 years old and is a cause of infertility.

The etiology of this disorder is unknown and the treatment is based on symptoms. PCOS is thought to be due to the ovaries producing estrogen and excess testosterone but not progesterone. As a result of this hormonal imbalance, ovulation fails and multiple fluid-filled cysts develop from mature ovarian follicles (Fig. 53-8). Classic manifestations of PCOS include irregular menstrual periods, amenorrhea, hirsutism, and obesity (80% of women). Of these manifestations, obesity in particular has been associated with severe symptoms such as excess androgens, oligomenorrhea, amenorrhea, and infertility. Many women start with normal menstrual periods, which become irregular after 1 to 2 years, and then the periods become infrequent. If PCOS is left untreated, cardiovascular disease and abnormal insulin resistance with type 2 diabetes mellitus may develop.

Pelvic ultrasound reveals enlarged ovaries with multiple small cysts. Successful management includes early diagnosis and treatment to improve quality of life and decrease the risk of complications. OCPs are useful in regulating menstrual cycles. Hirsutism may be treated with spironolactone. Hyperandrogenism can be treated with flutamide and a GnRH agonist such as leuprolide. Metformin (Glucophage) reduces hyperinsulinemia, improves hyperandrogenism, and restores ovulation. For women wishing to become pregnant, fertility drugs (e.g., clomiphene [Clomid]) may be used to induce ovulation. If all other treatments are unsuccessful, a hysterectomy with bilateral salpingectomy and oophorectomy may be performed.

Nursing management of a woman with PCOS includes teaching about the importance of weight management and exercise to decrease insulin resistance. Obesity exacerbates the problems related to PCOS. Monitor lipid profile and fasting glucose levels. Hirsutism is cosmetically distressing for many women. Support the patient as she explores measures to remove unwanted hair (e.g., depilating agents, electrolysis). Stress the importance of regular follow-up care to monitor the effectiveness of therapy and to detect any complications.

## CERVICAL POLYPS

*Cervical polyps* are benign pedunculated lesions that generally arise from the endocervical mucosa and are seen protruding through the cervical os during a speculum examination. Polyps are a characteristic bright cherry red and are soft and fragile. They are generally small, measuring less than 3 cm in length, and may be single or multiple. Their cause is unknown. Symptoms are usually not present, but intermenstrual bleeding after straining for a bowel movement and coitus can occur. Polyps are prone to infection.

When the polyp is small, it can be excised in an outpatient procedure. If the point of attachment of the polyp cannot be identified and is not accessible to cautery, a polypectomy is

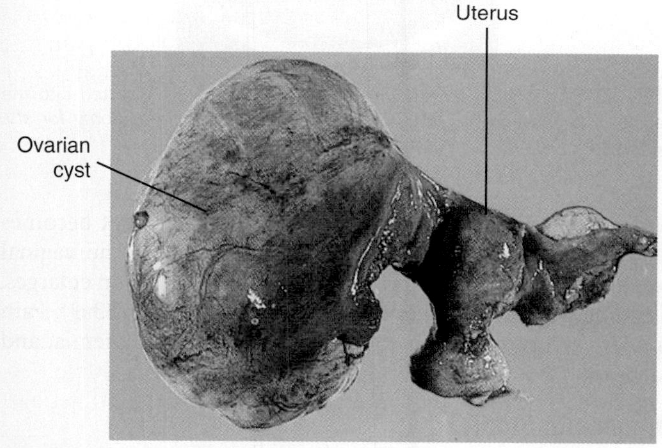


**FIG. 53-7** Large ovarian cyst. (From Symonds EM, McPherson MBA: *Colour atlas of obstetrics and gynecology,* London, 1994, Mosby.)

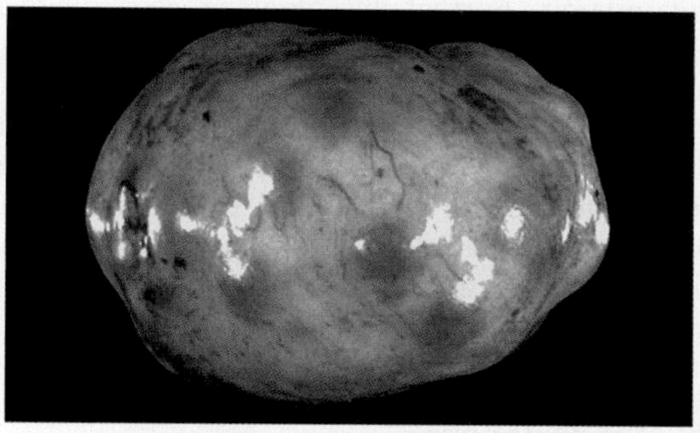

**FIG. 53-8** Polycystic ovary syndrome. Multiple fluid-filled cysts in the ovary. (From Kumar V, Abbas A, Fausto N: *Robbins and Cotran pathologic basis of disease,* ed 7, Philadelphia, 2005, Saunders.)

performed in an operating room. All tissue removed is sent for pathologic review because polyps occasionally undergo malignant changes.

# CANCERS OF THE FEMALE REPRODUCTIVE SYSTEM

## CERVICAL CANCER

Approximately 12,900 women in the United States are diagnosed with cervical cancer and approximately 4100 women will die from cervical cancer each year. While Hispanic women are the most likely to be diagnosed with cervical cancer, African American women have the highest mortality rate from cervical cancer.[11]

Cervical cancer was once the most frequent cause of cancer death in women. However, with early detection (using Pap test), the mortality rate from cervical cancer has significantly declined.

### CULTURAL & ETHNIC HEALTH DISPARITIES

***Cancers of the Female Reproductive System***

**Ovarian Cancer**

- Japanese women have a low incidence of ovarian cancer.
- However, second- and third-generation Japanese women in the United States have much higher rates, similar to those of white women born in the United States.

**Endometrial Cancer**

- Incidence is higher for white women and African American women than other ethnic groups.
- Mortality rate for African American women is nearly twice that of white women.

**Cervical Cancer**

- Incidence is higher among Hispanic, African American, and Native American women than among white women.
- Mortality rates are more than twice as high among African American women as among white women.

### Etiology and Pathophysiology

Risk factors for cervical cancer include (1) infection with high-risk strains of human papillomavirus (HPV) 16 and 18, (2) immunosuppression, (3) low socioeconomic status, (4) chlamydia infection, and (5) smoking.[12]

The cervix is the lower third of the uterus that projects into the vagina and comprises glandular cells that line the uterine cavity and endocervical canal. Squamous epithelium lines the vagina and outer portion of the cervix. These two cell types meet and undergo a normal physiologic process known as *squamous metaplasia,* the transformation of columnar epithelium into squamous epithelium, resulting in an area called the *transformation zone.* This process begins at puberty and continues throughout a women's reproductive life cycle, with the transformation zone moving in and out the endocervical canal, depending upon her hormonal status and other factors. While the entire anogenital tract can be infected by HPV, the transformation zone is an area that is particularly susceptible to HPV-associated carcinogenesis.

### Clinical Manifestations

Early cervical cancer generally has no symptoms. However, an unusual discharge, AUB, or postcoital bleeding eventually occurs. The discharge is usually thin and watery but becomes dark and foul smelling as the disease advances. The vaginal bleeding initially presents as spotting. As the tumor enlarges, bleeding becomes heavier and more frequent (Fig. 53-9). Pain is a late symptom and is followed by weight loss, anemia, and cachexia.

### EVIDENCE-BASED PRACTICE

***Applying the Evidence***

**Pap Test and Cervical Cancer**

E.V. is a 36-yr-old African American woman who had a tubal ligation in the outpatient surgery unit. As you prepare her for discharge, you remind her that she needs to have regular Pap tests to screen for cervical cancer. She expresses concern over the expense of this procedure. She tells you she does not know if her health care insurance pays for screening diagnostic testing, and she does not remember when she last had a Pap test done.

***Making Clinical Decisions***

***Best Available Evidence.*** For women between the ages of 30 and 65 yr old, the screening preference for cervical cancer is a Pap test and human papillomavirus (HPV) test every 5 years. A Pap test alone every 3 years is also within the recommended guidelines.

***Clinician Expertise.*** You know the incidence and death rate of cervical cancer is twice as high for African American as for white women.

***Patient Preferences and Values.*** E.V. is concerned about the costs related to her current procedure and future Pap tests. She adds that no one in her family has ever had cervical cancer.

***Implications for Nursing Practice***

1. How would you explain to her the current recommendations and her increased risk for cervical cancer?
2. Why is it important to encourage E.V. to learn more about her health care coverage?

***Reference for Evidence***

American Cancer Society: American Cancer Society guidelines for the early detection of cancer. Retrieved from *www.cancer.org/Healthy/FindCancerEarly/CancerScreeningGuidelines.*

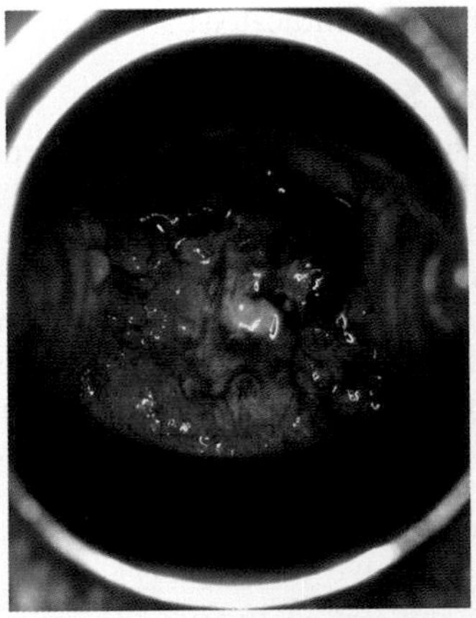

**FIG. 53-9** Cervical cancer. View through a speculum inserted into the vagina. (From Drake RL, Vogl W, Mitchell AWM: *Gray's anatomy for students,* ed 2, Edinburgh, 2010, Churchill Livingstone.)

### Diagnostic Studies

The two tests used for cervical cancer screening are the Papanicolaou (Pap) test and the HPV test. The Pap test identifies changes in cervical cells that may indicate precancerous changes. Cells are obtained from the cervix during a pelvic examination.

HPV testing can be used to identify the high-risk HPV types 16 and 18, which are associated with cervical cancer. To do the test, cervical scrapings are obtained and tested for viral DNA or RNA.

The use of these two tests to screen for cervical cancer may be referred to as cotesting. While the Pap test helps find cervical cell changes, the HPV test checks for the HPV virus that can cause these cell changes.

All women should begin cervical cancer screening at age 21. Women ages 21 to 29 years should get a Pap test every 3 years. Women between the ages of 30 and 65 should have a Pap test and HPV test every 5 years. This is the preferred approach, but the woman may choose to get a Pap test without an HPV test every 3 years.[13]

If both tests are negative, the risk for cervical cancer is very low and women can wait 5 years before another screening. HPV tests may also be used to provide more information when a Pap test has unclear results.

Women found to have an abnormal Pap test typically need a *colposcopy* (an examination of the cervical tissue under magnification). Typically a cervical biopsy is taken and sent for further analysis.

### Interprofessional Care

Vaccination against HPV provides for primary prevention of cervical cancer. Inform both parents and patients about the need to complete the HPV vaccination series prior to first sexual contact.

Currently three vaccines are available to protect against HPV: (1) Gardasil protects against types 6, 11, 16, and 18; (2) Cervarix offers protection against HPV types 16 and 18; and (3) Gardasil 9 protects against HPV types 6, 11, 16, 18 and five other HPV types. These vaccines are given in three IM doses over a 6-month period and have few side effects. The CDC recommends that all children, males and females, be vaccinated at age 11 to 12, but vaccination can be started as early as age 9. (More specific information about HPV vaccines is discussed on p. 1234 in Chapter 52.)

Women diagnosed with cervical cancer are typically referred to an oncologist for treatment recommendations. Treatment options can include surgery or a combination of chemotherapy and radiation (Table 53-13). For patients with advanced disease, bevacizumab (Avastin), a targeted therapy drug, may be used in addition to cisplatin-based chemotherapy. Bevacizumab is an angiogenesis inhibitor and works by interfering with the blood vessels that supply nutrients to cancer cells. (Chemotherapy, radiation therapy, and targeted therapy are discussed in Chapter 15.)

**TABLE 53-13 Staging and Treatment of Cervical Cancer**

| Stage | Extent | Treatment |
|---|---|---|
| 0 | In situ | Cervical conization, hysterectomy, cryosurgery, laser surgery |
| I | Confinement to cervix | Radiation, radical hysterectomy |
| II | Spread beyond cervix to upper two thirds of vagina but not to tissues around uterus | Radiation, cisplatin-based chemotherapy, radical hysterectomy |
| III | Spread to pelvic wall, involvement of lower third of vagina, and/or has caused kidney problems | Radiation, cisplatin-based chemotherapy |
| IV | Spread to other parts of the body such as bladder, rectum, liver, lungs, and bones | Radiation, surgery (e.g., pelvic exenteration), cisplatin-based chemotherapy |

Modified from National Cancer Institute: Cancer cervical treatment: stages of cervical cancer. Retrieved from *www.cancer.gov/cancertopics/pdq/treatment/cervical/Patient/page2*.

## ENDOMETRIAL CANCER

Endometrial cancer is the most common gynecologic malignancy. About 55,000 women are diagnosed each year with endometrial cancer, and 10,200 will die. If endometrial cancer is diagnosed in the early stage, it has a relatively low mortality rate, with survival rates over 95%.[11]

### Etiology and Pathophysiology

The major risk factor for the development of endometrial cancer is exposure to estrogen, especially unopposed estrogen. Obesity is a risk factor because adipose cells store estrogen, thus increasing the amount of circulating estrogen. Additional risk factors include increasing age, never being pregnant, early menarche, late menopause, smoking, diabetes mellitus, and a personal or family history of hereditary nonpolyposis colorectal cancer (HNPCC) (see the Genetics in Clinical Practice box for HNPCC in Chapter 42 on p. 954). Pregnancy, use of oral contraceptives and IUDs, and physical exercise are associated with reduced risk.

Endometrial cancer arises from the lining of the endometrium within the uterus and most tumors are adenocarcinomas. If endometrial cancer is not diagnosed in early stages, it can invade the myometrium (muscle of the uterus) and the regional lymph nodes.

If metastasis occurs, the common sites include the lung, liver, bone, and brain. Prognosis depends on tumor size, cell type, degree of invasion into the myometrium, and any metastasis.[14]

### Clinical Manifestations

Early clinical manifestations of endometrial cancer include abnormal uterine bleeding, especially in postmenopausal women. Later symptoms can include pain during urination or intercourse or in the pelvic area.

### Interprofessional Care

No routine screening test is available for endometrial cancer. Most cases are diagnosed at an early stage because of postmenopausal bleeding.

An endometrial biopsy is the primary diagnostic test for identifying endometrial cancer. This procedure is typically performed in the office. For women who have or are at risk of developing HNPCC, the American Cancer Society recommends annual screening with an endometrial biopsy beginning at 35 years of age.[11]

Treatment of endometrial cancer in the early stage is a total hysterectomy and bilateral salpingo-oophorectomy with lymph node biopsies. (Various types of hysterectomies are shown in Fig. 53-10.) Surgery may be followed by external radiation either to the pelvis or abdomen or internal radiation (brachytherapy) intravaginally if there is local or distant metastasis.

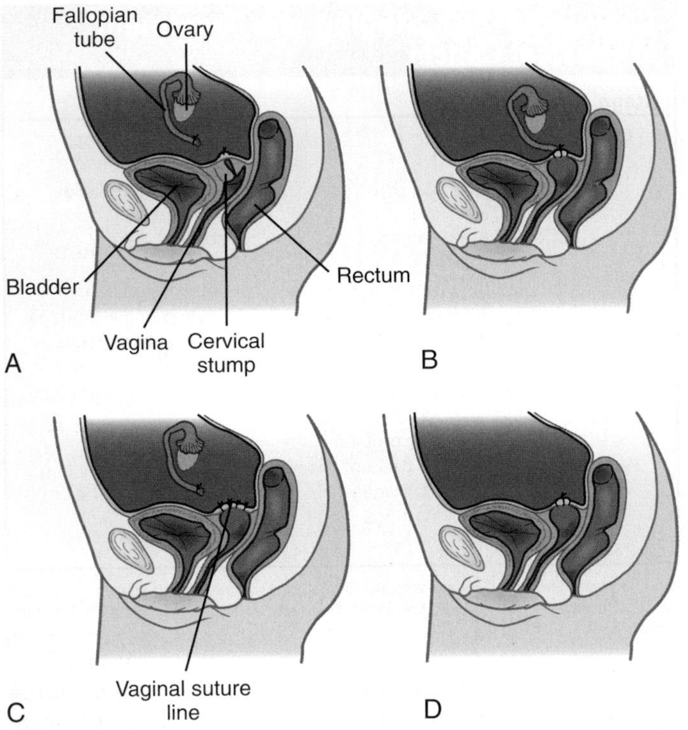


**FIG. 53-10** Hysterectomies. **A,** Cross section of subtotal hysterectomy. Note that cervical stump, fallopian tubes, and ovaries remain. **B,** Cross section of total hysterectomy. Note that fallopian tubes and ovaries remain. **C,** Cross section of vaginal hysterectomy. Note that fallopian tubes and ovaries remain. **D,** Total hysterectomy, salpingectomy, and oophorectomy. Note that uterus, fallopian tubes, and ovaries are completely removed.

If the woman has advanced or recurrent disease, chemotherapy and hormonal therapy may be indicated. The 5- and 10-year survival rates are 82% and 79%, respectively.[11]

## OVARIAN CANCER

Ovarian cancer is the most deadly gynecologic malignancy. Approximately 21,290 new cases of ovarian cancer are diagnosed each year, and about 14,200 women die. It is the fifth leading cause of cancer deaths in women in the United States. In most women, ovarian cancer is diagnosed when the disease is in the advanced stages.[11] It is most common in women between 55 and 65 years of age.

### Etiology and Pathophysiology

The cause of ovarian cancer is not known. The major risk factor for ovarian cancer is family history (one or more first-degree relatives). A family history of breast or colon cancer is also a risk factor. Other risk factors include a personal history of breast or colon cancer and HNPCC (see the Genetics in Clinical Practice box on HNPCC in Chapter 42 on p. 954).

**Genetic Link.** Women who have mutations of the *BRCA* genes have an increased susceptibility to ovarian cancer. The *BRCA* genes are tumor suppressor genes that inhibit tumor growth when functioning normally. When they mutate, they lose their tumor suppressor ability. This results in an increased risk for women to develop ovarian or breast cancer (see the Genetics in Clinical Practice box).

Women who have never been pregnant (nulliparity) are also at higher risk. Other risk factors include increasing age, high-fat diet, increased number of ovulatory cycles (usually associated

## GENETICS IN CLINICAL PRACTICE

### *Ovarian Cancer*

**Genetic Basis**
- Mutations in *BRCA1* and/or *BRCA2* genes.
- Normally these genes are tumor suppressor genes involved in DNA repair.
- Autosomal dominant transmission.
- Mutations passed down from either mother or father.

**Incidence**
- About 10% of cases of ovarian cancer are related to hereditary factors.
- Women with *BRCA1* mutations have a 25%-40% lifetime risk of developing ovarian cancer.
- Women with *BRCA2* mutations have a 10%-20% lifetime risk of developing ovarian cancer.
- Family history of both breast and ovarian cancer increases the risk of having a BRCA mutation.
- *BRCA* mutations occur in 10%-20% of patients with ovarian cancer who have no family history of breast or ovarian cancer.

**Genetic Testing**
- DNA testing is available for *BRCA1* and *BRCA2* genetic mutations.

**Clinical Implications**
- Bilateral oophorectomy reduces the risk of ovarian cancer in women with *BRCA1* and *BRCA2* mutations.
- Genetic counseling and testing for *BRCA* mutations should be considered for women whose personal or family history puts them at high risk for a genetic predisposition to ovarian cancer.

with early menarche and late menopause), HRT, and possibly the use of infertility drugs.

Breastfeeding, multiple pregnancies, oral contraceptive use (more than 5 years), and early age at first birth seem to reduce the risk of ovarian cancer. These factors may have a protective effect because they reduce the number of ovulatory cycles and thus reduce the exposure to estrogen.

About 90% of ovarian cancers are epithelial carcinomas that arise from malignant transformation of the surface epithelial cells. Germ cell tumors account for another 10%. Histologic grading is important to determine the prognosis of the disease. Tumor cells are graded according to the level of differentiation, ranging from well differentiated (grade I) to poorly differentiated (grade III) to undifferentiated (grade IV). Grade IV cells have a poorer prognosis than the other grades.

Intraperitoneal dissemination is a common characteristic of ovarian cancer. It metastasizes to the uterus, bladder, bowel, and omentum. In advanced disease, it can spread to the stomach, colon, liver, and other parts of the body.

### Clinical Manifestations

Early ovarian cancer usually has no obvious symptoms. Most clinical manifestations are vague and nonspecific. These include pelvic or abdominal pain, bloating, urinary urgency or frequency, and difficulty eating or feeling full quickly. Late stage disease typically presents with abdominal enlargement with ascites (fluid in the abdominal cavity), unexplained weight loss or gain, and menstrual changes.

### Diagnostic Studies

No accurate screening test exists for early detection of ovarian cancer. Since early ovarian cancer has vague symptoms, yearly

**TABLE 53-14 Interprofessional Care**

***Ovarian Cancer***

**Diagnostic Assessment**
- History and physical examination
- Pelvic examination
- Abdominal and transvaginal ultrasound
- CA-125 level
- Laparotomy for diagnostic staging

**Management**
- Surgery
  - Abdominal hysterectomy and bilateral salpingo-oophorectomy with pelvic lymph node biopsies
  - Debulking for advanced disease
- Chemotherapy
  - Adjuvant and palliative
- Radiation therapy
  - Adjuvant and palliative

bimanual pelvic examinations should be performed to identify an ovarian mass (Table 53-14). Postmenopausal women should not have palpable ovaries, so a mass of any size should be considered suspicious. An abdominal or a transvaginal ultrasound can be done to detect ovarian masses. An exploratory laparotomy may be used to establish the diagnosis and stage the disease.

For women at high risk for ovarian cancer, screening using a combination of the tumor marker CA-125 and ultrasound is often recommended in addition to a yearly pelvic examination. The CA-125 test is positive in 80% of women with epithelial ovarian cancer. CA-125 is also used to monitor the course of the disease and response to treatment. Of concern is that levels of CA-125 may be elevated with other malignancies (e.g., pancreatic cancer) or with benign gynecologic conditions such as fibroids or endometriosis.

### Interprofessional Care

Options for women identified as being at high risk based on family and health history include prophylactic removal of the ovaries and fallopian tubes and the use of OCPs.[15] Although oophorectomy significantly reduces the risk of ovarian cancer, it does not completely eliminate the possibility of the disease in the peritoneum.

The initial treatment for all stages of ovarian cancer is a total abdominal hysterectomy and bilateral salpingo-oophorectomy with omentectomy and removal of as much of the tumor as possible (i.e., tumor debulking). Depending on the differentiation of the cells and the stage of cancer, treatment options include intraperitoneal and systemic chemotherapy, intraperitoneal instillation of radioisotopes, and external abdominal and pelvic radiation therapy. The chemotherapy agents most commonly used are taxanes (paclitaxel or docetaxel) and platinum agents (carboplatin or cisplatin). (See Table 15-7 for a discussion of these drugs.)

Targeted therapy that is used to treat advanced ovarian cancer includes Bevacizumab (Avastin) (discussed on p. 1257) and olaparib (Lynparza). Olaparib is a poly ADP-ribose polymerase (PARP) inhibitor that blocks enzymes involved in repairing damaged DNA. It used for women with ovarian cancer that is associated with defective *BRCA* genes.

Overall the 5- and 10-year survival rates are 45% and 35%, respectively. The majority of patients with ovarian cancer are diagnosed when the disease is advanced, for which the 5-year survival rate is 27%.[11]

## VAGINAL CANCER

Vaginal cancers are rare, with about 4000 new cases reported annually.[11] They are usually found in women between ages 50 and 70. Vaginal tumors can be secondary sites or metastases of other gynecologic cancers, such as cervical or endometrial cancer. The most common type of vaginal cancer is squamous cell carcinoma. Intrauterine exposure to diethylstilbestrol (DES) places a woman at risk for clear cell adenocarcinoma of the vagina.

Treatment of vaginal cancer depends on the type of cells involved, stage of the disease, and the size and location of the tumor. Squamous cell carcinomas can be treated with both surgery and radiation.

## VULVAR CANCER

Vulvar cancer is relatively rare, with about 5150 new cases reported annually.[11] Preinvasive lesions referred to as *vulvar intraepithelial neoplasia (VIN)* precede invasive vulvar cancer. The invasive form occurs mainly in women over 60 years of age, with the highest incidence being in women in their 70s.

Patients with vulvar cancer may have symptoms of vulvar itching or burning, pain, bleeding, or discharge. Women who are immunosuppressed and/or have diabetes mellitus, hypertension, or chronic vulvar dystrophies are at a higher risk for developing vulvar cancers. HPV DNA have been identified in some but not all vulvar cancers.

Diagnosis of vulvar cancer is based on physical examination, colposcopy, and biopsy results of the suspicious lesion. VIN can be treated topically with imiquimod cream (Aldara) or laser surgery. Surgery is the most common treatment for vulvar cancer with the goal to remove all the cancer without any loss of the woman's sexual function. In some cases, surgery to remove the lesion is performed.

If a woman has extensive lesions, a vulvectomy is recommended. Various types of vulvectomies are presented in Table 53-15. As adjuvant measures, the patient may have chemotherapy or radiation therapy after surgery.

## NURSING AND INTERPROFESSIONAL MANAGEMENT: CANCERS OF FEMALE REPRODUCTIVE SYSTEM

### Nursing Assessment

Malignant tumors of the female reproductive system can be found in the cervix, endometrium, ovaries, vagina, and vulva. A patient with any of these malignant tumors may experience a variety of clinical manifestations, including leukorrhea, irregular vaginal bleeding, vaginal discharge, abdominal pain and pressure, bowel and bladder dysfunction, and vulvar itching and burning. Assessment for these signs and symptoms is an important nursing responsibility.

### Nursing Diagnoses

Nursing diagnoses for the female patient with cancer of the reproductive system include, but are not limited to, the following:

- Anxiety *related to* threat of a malignancy and lack of knowledge about the disease process and prognosis

**TABLE 53-15 Surgical Procedures Involving the Female Reproductive System**

| Type of Surgery | Description |
|---|---|
| **Hysterectomy** | |
| Total abdominal hysterectomy (TAH) | Uterus and cervix removed using abdominal incision (bikini cut). |
| Total abdominal hysterectomy and bilateral salpingo-oophorectomy (TAH-BSO) | Uterus, cervix, fallopian tubes, and ovaries removed using abdominal incision. |
| Radical hysterectomy | Panhysterectomy, partial vaginectomy, and dissection of lymph nodes in pelvis. |
| Vaginal hysterectomy | Uterus and cervix removed through a cut in the top of vagina. |
| Laparoscopic hysterectomy | Laparoscope (video camera and small surgical instruments). |
| • Laparoscopic-assisted vaginal hysterectomy (LAVH) | Incision made at top of vagina. Uterus and cervix removed through the vagina. Laparoscope inserted into abdomen to assist in the procedure. |
| • Laparoscopic supracervical hysterectomy | Uterus removed using only laparoscopic instruments. Cervix is left intact. |
| **Myomectomy** | Surgical removal of fibroid from the uterus, leaving the uterus in place. |
| **Vulvectomy** | Surgical procedure to remove part or all of the vulva. |
| • Skinning vulvectomy | Removal of top layer of vulvar skin where the cancer is found. Skin grafts from other parts of the body may be needed to cover the area. |
| • Simple vulvectomy | Entire vulva is removed. |
| • Radical vulvectomy | Entire vulva, including clitoris, labia majora and minora, and nearby tissue, is removed. Nearby lymph nodes may also be removed. |
| **Vaginectomy** | Removal of vagina. |
| **Pelvic exenteration** | Radical hysterectomy, total vaginectomy, removal of bladder with diversion of urinary system and resection of colon and rectum with colostomy. |
| **Dilation and curettage** | Dilation of cervix and scraping of endometrium. |

- Acute pain *related to* pressure secondary to an enlarging tumor
- Disturbed body image *related to* loss of body part and loss of good health
- Ineffective sexuality pattern *related to* physiologic limitations and fatigue
- Grieving *related to* poor prognosis of advanced disease

## ◆ Planning

The overall goals are that the patient with cancer of the female reproductive system will (1) actively participate in treatment decisions, (2) achieve satisfactory pain and symptom management, (3) recognize and report problems promptly, (4) maintain preferred lifestyle as long as possible, and (5) continue to practice cancer detection strategies.

## ◆ Nursing Implementation

◆ **Health Promotion.** Through your contact with women in a variety of settings, teach women the importance of routine screening for cancers of the reproductive system. Cancer can be prevented when screening reveals precancerous conditions of the vulva, cervix, endometrium, and, rarely, the ovaries. Also routine screening increases the chance that a cancer will be found in an early stage.

Teaching women about risk factors for cancers of the reproductive system is also important. Limiting sexual activity during adolescence, using condoms, having fewer sexual partners, and not smoking reduce the risk of cervical cancer. When high-risk behaviors are identified, assist women in modifying their lifestyles to decrease risk.

**CHECK YOUR PRACTICE**

You are working in the preoperative surgery holding unit. Your patient is a 42-yr-old woman who is scheduled for a total abdominal hysterectomy for endometrial cancer. When you ask her how she is doing, she tells you that she's worried because "life will never be the same."

- How would you approach this situation? What do you think are her major concerns?

◆ **Acute Intervention Related to Surgery.** Various types of surgery of the female reproductive tract are presented in Table 53-15 and Fig. 53-10. All patients experience a degree of anxiety when contemplating surgery, but the prospect of major gynecologic surgery increases these concerns. Some women are relieved by the thought of no longer having menstrual periods or becoming pregnant.

Some women may focus on the effect the surgery will have on their reproductive and sexual functions. The ability to bear children may be associated with her perception of womanhood. Grief from this loss is normal.

Elicit the woman's feelings and concerns about her surgery. Assess each patient individually. Be willing to listen, since this can provide considerable psychologic support.

Preoperatively, prepare the patient physically for surgery with the standard perineal or abdominal preparation. A vaginal douche and enema may be given (based on the surgeon's preference). The bladder should be emptied before the patient is sent to the operating room. An indwelling catheter is commonly inserted preoperatively.

◆ ***Hysterectomy.*** Following a hysterectomy, abdominal distention may develop from the sudden release of pressure on the intestines when a large tumor is removed or from paralytic ileus secondary to anesthesia and pressure on the bowel. Food and fluids may be restricted if the patient is nauseated. Ambulation will help relieve flatus.

Take special care to prevent the development of deep vein thrombosis (DVT). Frequent changes of position, avoidance of the high Fowler's position, and avoidance of pressure under the knees minimize stasis and pooling of blood. Pay special attention to patients with varicosities. Encourage leg exercises to promote circulation.

Teach the patient what to expect after surgery (e.g., she will not menstruate). Instructions should include specific activity restrictions. Intercourse should be avoided until the wound is healed (about 4 to 6 weeks). However, intercourse is not contraindicated once healing is complete.

If a vaginal hysterectomy is performed, inform the patient that she may have a temporary loss of vaginal sensation. Reassure her that the sensation will return in several months.

Physical restrictions are limited for a short time. Heavy lifting should be avoided for 2 months. Teach her to avoid activities that may increase pelvic congestion, such as dancing and walking swiftly, for several months. However, activities such as swimming may be both physically and mentally helpful. Assure her that once healing is complete, all previous activity can be resumed.

◆ ***Salpingectomy and Oophorectomy.*** Postoperative care of the woman who has undergone removal of a fallopian tube (salpingectomy) or an ovary (oophorectomy) is similar to that for any patient having abdominal surgery. However, if a large ovarian cyst is removed, she may have abdominal distention caused by the sudden release of pressure in the intestines. An abdominal binder may provide relief until the distention subsides.

When both ovaries are removed (bilateral oophorectomy), surgical menopause results. The symptoms are similar to those of regular menopause but may be more severe because of the sudden withdrawal of hormones.

◆ ***Vulvectomy.*** It is important to recognize the extent of the vulvectomy and the significant effect it is likely to have on the patient's life. Because the surgery causes mutilation of the perineal area and the healing process is slow, the patient is likely to become discouraged. Provide opportunities for the patient to express her feelings and concerns about the operation.

Special attention to bowel and bladder care is needed. A low-residue diet and stool softeners prevent straining and wound contamination. An indwelling catheter is used to provide urinary drainage. Be careful not to dislodge the catheter because extensive edema makes its reinsertion difficult. Heavy, taut sutures are often used to close the wounds, resulting in severe discomfort. In other instances, the wound may be allowed to heal by granulation. Analgesics may be required to control pain. Carefully position the patient using strategically placed pillows to provide comfort. Anticoagulant therapy to prevent DVTs is commonly used.

Teach the patient specific instructions in self-care before discharge. Instruct her to report any unusual odor, fresh bleeding, breakdown of incision, or perineal pain. Home care nursing can benefit the patient during her adjustment period.

Sexual function is often retained. Whether clitoral sensation is retained may be critical to some women, particularly if it was a primary source of orgasmic satisfaction. Discussing alternative methods of achieving sexual satisfaction may be indicated.

◆ ***Pelvic Exenteration.*** When other forms of therapy fail to control the spread of cancer and no metastases have been found outside of the pelvis, pelvic exenteration may be performed. This radical surgery usually involves removal of the uterus, ovaries, fallopian tubes, vagina, bladder, urethra, and pelvic lymph nodes (Fig. 53-11). In some situations, the descending colon, rectum, and anal canal may also be removed. Candidates for this procedure are selected on the basis of their likelihood

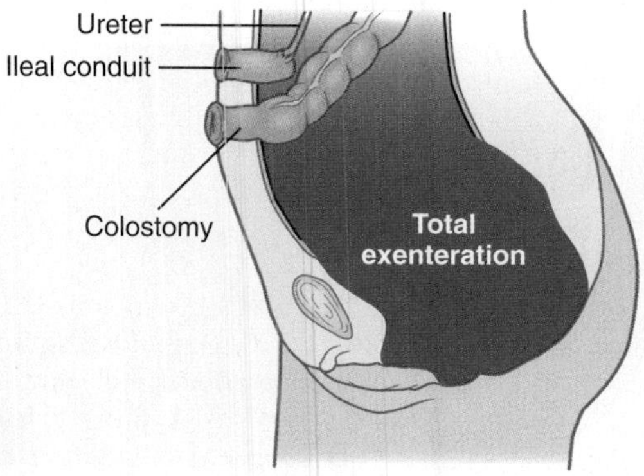


**FIG. 53-11** Total exenteration is removal of all pelvic organs with creation of an ileal conduit and a colostomy.

of surviving the surgery and their ability to adjust to and accept the resulting limitations.

Postoperative care is similar to that of a patient who has had a radical hysterectomy, an abdominal perineal resection, and an ileostomy or a colostomy. The physical, emotional, and social adjustments to life required by the woman and her family are great. There are urinary or fecal diversions in the abdominal wall, a reconstructed vagina, and the onset of menopausal symptoms.

Assess the patient's physical and emotional adjustment to the changes in body image produced by the surgery and her ability to carry out any treatment measures. The patient's rehabilitative process should keep pace with her acceptance of the situation. You need to provide understanding and support during a long recovery period. Gently encourage the patient to regain her independence. She needs to verbalize her feelings about her altered body structure. Include her caregiver and family in the plan of care. Careful follow-up monitoring is needed so that early recurrence of the cancer can be identified and treated.

◆ **Acute Intervention With Radiation Therapy.** Instruct the patient who is to receive external radiation to urinate immediately before the treatment to minimize radiation exposure to the bladder. Advise her about radiation side effects, including enteritis and cystitis. These are natural reactions to radiation therapy and do not indicate an overdose. Fully inform the patient of the possible side effects and measures that can be used to reduce their impact.

Nursing management of the patient receiving internal radiation therapy requires special considerations. Do not stay in the immediate area any longer than is necessary to give proper care and attention. (Radiation therapy is discussed in Chapter 15.)

### ◆ Evaluation

The expected outcomes are that the patient with cancer of the female reproductive system will

- Actively participate in treatment decisions
- Achieve satisfactory pain and symptom management
- Recognize and report problems promptly
- Maintain preferred lifestyle as long as possible
- Continue to practice cancer detection strategies

## PELVIC ORGAN PROLAPSE

The most common problems with pelvic support are uterine prolapse, cystocele, and rectocele. Although vaginal birth increases the risk for these problems, these conditions can occur in women who have never experienced childbirth. Obesity, chronic coughing, and straining during bowel movements can increase the likelihood of these problems. The decreased estrogen that normally accompanies perimenopause also decreases connective tissue support.

## UTERINE PROLAPSE

**Uterine prolapse** is the downward displacement of the uterus into the vaginal canal (Fig. 53-12). Prolapse is rated by degrees. In first-degree prolapse the cervix rests in the lower part of the vagina. Second-degree prolapse means the cervix is at the vaginal opening. Third-degree prolapse means the uterus protrudes through the introitus.

Symptoms vary with the degree of prolapse. The patient may describe a feeling of "something coming down." She may have

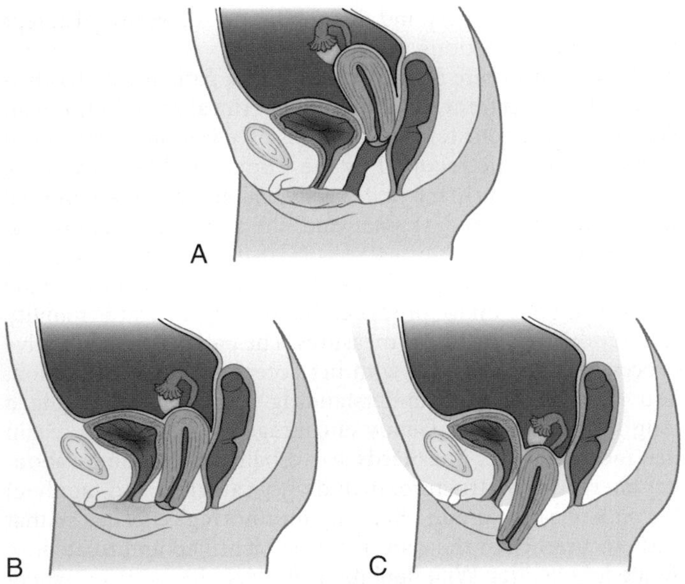


**FIG. 53-12** Uterine prolapse. **A,** First-degree prolapse. **B,** Second-degree prolapse. **C,** Third-degree prolapse.

dyspareunia, a dragging or heavy feeling in the pelvis, backache, and bowel or bladder problems if a cystocele or rectocele is also present. Stress incontinence is a common and troubling problem. When third-degree uterine prolapse occurs, the protruding cervix and vaginal walls are subjected to constant irritation, and tissue changes may occur.

Therapy depends on the degree of prolapse and how much the woman's daily activities have been affected.[16] Pelvic muscle strengthening exercises (Kegel exercises) may be effective for some women (see Table 45-18). If not, a pessary may be used. A *pessary* is a device that is placed in the vagina to help support the uterus.[17] A wide variety of shapes exist, including rings, arches, and balls. Most are made of plastic or wire coated with plastic. When a woman first receives a pessary, she needs instructions on how to clean it. Pessaries that are left in place for long periods are associated with erosion, fistulas, and vaginal carcinoma.

If more conservative measures are not successful, surgery is indicated. Surgery generally involves a vaginal hysterectomy with anterior and posterior repair of the vagina and the underlying fascia.

## CYSTOCELE AND RECTOCELE

Cystocele occurs when support between the vagina and bladder is weakened (Fig. 53-13). Similarly, a *rectocele* results from weakening between the vagina and rectum (Fig. 53-14). Cystocele and rectocele are common problems, and in many women they are asymptomatic.[18] With large cystoceles, complete emptying of the bladder can be difficult, predisposing women to bladder infections. A woman with a large rectocele may not be able to completely empty her rectum when defecating unless she helps push the stool out by putting her fingers in her vagina.

As with uterine prolapse, Kegel exercises (see Table 45-18) may be used to strengthen the weakened perineal muscles if the cystocele or rectocele is not too problematic. A pessary may be helpful for cystoceles.

Surgery designed to tighten the vaginal wall (colporrhaphy) is generally the method of treatment. A cystocele is corrected with a procedure called an *anterior colporrhaphy,* whereas a posterior colporrhaphy is done for a rectocele. If further surgery

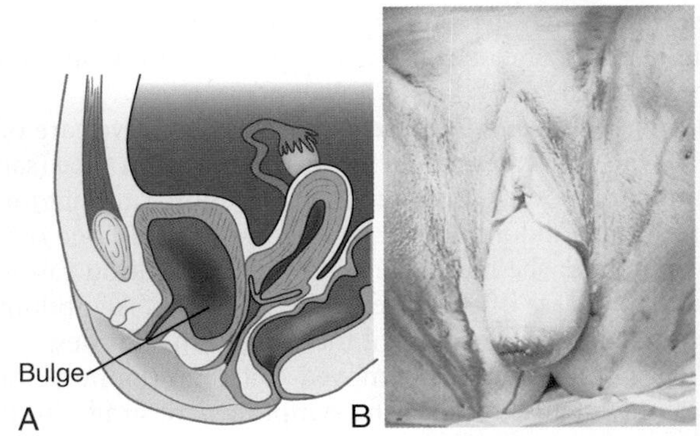


**FIG. 53-13** **A,** Cystocele. **B,** Bladder has prolapsed into the vagina, causing a uterine prolapse.

is needed to relieve stress incontinence, procedures to support the urethra and restore the proper angle between the urethra and the posterior bladder wall are used.

## NURSING AND INTERPROFESSIONAL MANAGEMENT: PELVIC ORGAN PROLAPSE

Assist women to avoid or decrease problems with pelvic support by teaching them how to do Kegel exercises.[19] Women of all ages may benefit from these exercises. Instruct the patient to pull in or contract her muscles as if she were trying to stop the flow of urine, control the passing of gas, or pinch off a stool (see Table 45-18).

If vaginal surgery is necessary, the preoperative preparation usually includes a cleansing douche the morning of surgery. A cleansing enema is usually given when a rectocele repair is scheduled. A perineal shave may be done.

In the postoperative period, the goals of care are to prevent wound infection and pressure on the vaginal suture line. Perineal care must be done at least twice a day and after each urination or defecation. Apply an ice pack locally to help relieve the initial perineal discomfort and swelling. A disposable glove filled with ice and covered with a cloth works well to create an ice pack. Later, sitz baths may be used.

After an anterior colporrhaphy, an indwelling catheter is usually left in the bladder for 4 days to allow the local edema to subside. The catheter keeps the bladder empty, preventing strain on the sutures. Twice-daily catheter care with an antiseptic is generally done. To prevent constipation after a posterior colporrhaphy, a high-fiber diet and stool softener may be used.

Review discharge instructions before the patient leaves the hospital. These include the (1) use of douches or a mild laxative

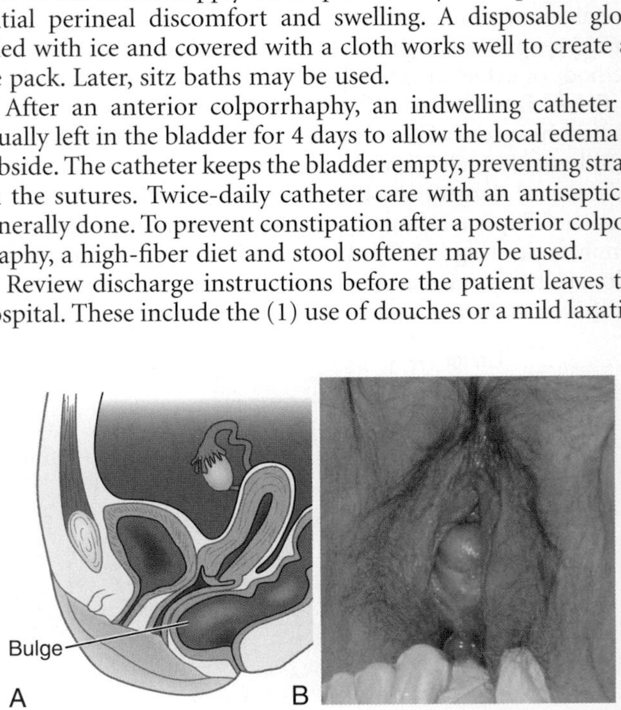


**FIG. 53-14** **A,** Rectocele. **B,** Rectum has prolapsed into the vagina. (*B,* From Townsend CM: *Sabiston textbook of surgery,* ed 18, St Louis, 2009, Mosby.)

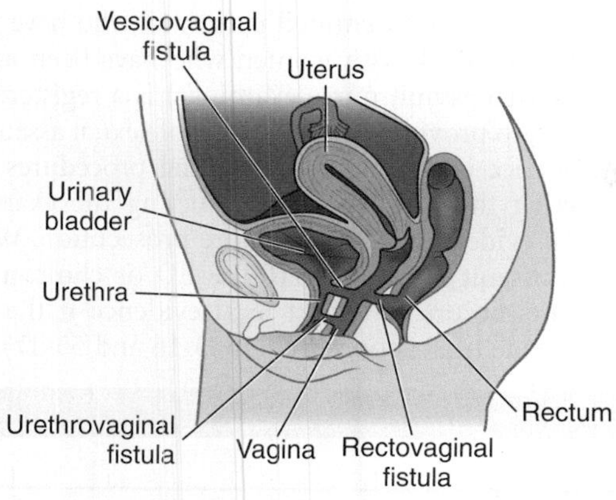


**FIG. 53-15** Common fistulas involving the vagina.

as needed; (2) restrictions on heavy lifting and prolonged standing, walking, or sitting; and (3) avoidance of intercourse until the HCP gives permission. There may be a temporary loss of vaginal sensation, which can last for several months.

## FISTULA

A *fistula* is an abnormal opening between internal organs or between an organ and the exterior of the body (Fig. 53-15). Gynecologic procedures cause most urinary tract fistulas. Other causes include injury during childbirth and disease processes, such as cancer. Fistulas may develop between the vagina and bladder, urethra, ureter, or rectum. When *vesicovaginal* fistulas (between the bladder and vagina) develop, some urine leaks into the vagina, whereas with *rectovaginal* fistulas (between the rectum and vagina), flatus and feces escape into the vagina. In both instances, excoriation and irritation of the vaginal and vulvar tissues occur and may lead to severe infections. In addition to wetness, offensive odors may develop, causing embarrassment and severely limiting socialization.

## ❖ NURSING AND INTERPROFESSIONAL MANAGEMENT: FISTULAS

Because small fistulas may heal spontaneously within a matter of months, treatment may not be needed. If the fistula does not heal, surgical repair is required. Inflammation and tissue edema must be eliminated before surgery is attempted, which may involve a wait of many months. The fistulectomy may result in the patient's having an ileal conduit or temporary colostomy. (See Chapter 45 for care of a patient with an ileal conduit and Chapter 42 for care of a patient with a colostomy.)

Surgical repair of fistulas is not always effective, even in the best conditions. Therefore supportive nursing care for the patient and her significant others is especially important.[20]

Perineal hygiene is of great importance both preoperatively and postoperatively. Cleanse the perineum every 4 hours. Warm sitz baths should be taken three times daily if possible. Change perineal pads frequently. Encourage the patient to maintain an adequate fluid intake.

Encouragement and reassurance are needed to help the patient cope with her problems. Postoperatively emphasize the avoidance of stress on the repaired areas and prevention of infection. Take care so that the indwelling catheter, usually in place for 7 to 10 days, is draining at all times. Urge oral fluids to provide for internal catheter irrigation. Use minimal pressure and strict asepsis if catheter irrigation becomes necessary.

The first stool after bowel surgery may be purposely delayed to prevent contamination of the wound. Later, give stool softeners or mild laxatives (as ordered).

## SEXUAL ASSAULT

**Sexual assault** is the forcible perpetration of a sexual act on a person without his or her consent. It is a crime of violence and aggression. It can include any of the following actions: sodomy (anal or oral copulation with a person of the same or opposite sex), forced vaginal intercourse, assault with a foreign object, unwanted kissing, touching, or fondling as well as serial battery and rape. The Federal Bureau of Investigation's (FBI) definition of *rape* includes female or male victims who have experienced sexual assault that includes oral or anal penetration.

Sexual assault may be committed by a stranger or by an intimate partner. *Intimate partner violence (IPV)* is a major health problem in the United States.[21] Sexual assault that is perpetrated by a family member is termed *incest. Statutory rape* is consensual sexual intercourse with someone younger than a specific age. This age usually varies state to state, but most states use the criteria of a person younger than 16 years of age. Most states consider that an adolescent who is 16 years of age or older can consent to consensual sexual intercourse.

The involvement of children 14 years of age or younger in sexual activity either consensual or forced is termed *child sexual abuse.* Child sexual abuse is defined as the employment, persuasion, inducement, or enticement or even coercion of a person younger than 14 years of age in any sexually explicit conduct or simulation of sexual conduct. It also includes behaviors that are forced onto the child for the purpose of production of video material as well as rape, molestation, prostitution, or other forms of exploitation of children involving any sexual behavior.

Approximately 1.3 million rape or rape-related assaults occur to women annually. Approximately 18% of women reported that they had been victims of an attempted or completed rape during their lifetime. Most (80%) reported that they were victimized before the age of 25. Survivors suffer an array of physical and psychologic health consequences.[21]

### Clinical Manifestations

**Physical.** Some female victims of assault experience more injuries than others. Factors that influence the severity of injury include the woman's age, if the perpetrator used a weapon, and if the victim knew the perpetrator. Physical injuries may include fractures, subdural hematomas, cerebral concussions, and intraabdominal injuries. In addition, sexual injuries may include bruising and lacerations of the perineum, hymen, vulva, vagina, cervix, and anus. Sexual assault also places women at risk for STIs and pregnancy.

**Psychologic.** Immediately after the assault, women may demonstrate signs of shock, numbness, denial, or withdrawal. Some women may seem unnaturally calm, while others may cry or express anger. Feelings of humiliation, degradation, embarrassment, anger, self-blame, and fear of another assault are commonly expressed.

These symptoms usually decrease after 2 weeks, and victims may appear to have adjusted. Yet any time from 2 to 3 weeks to months or years after the assault, symptoms may return and become more severe.

*Rape trauma syndrome* is a classification of posttraumatic stress disorder. Flashbacks, intrusive recall, sleep disturbances, gastrointestinal symptoms, and numbing of feelings are common initial symptoms. Women feel embarrassment, self-blame, and powerlessness. Later symptoms include mood swings, irritability, and anger. Feelings of despair, shame, and hopelessness may be internalized and lead to depression, and the risk of suicide may increase.[22]

## Interprofessional Care

The highest priority for the victim of assault is her emotional and physical safety. Table 53-16 outlines the emergency management of the patient who has been sexually assaulted. Most emergency departments (EDs) have identified personnel who have received special training to work with women who have been assaulted. The SANE (sexual assault nurse examiner) is a registered nurse who is certified to provide care to victims of sexual assault, while ensuring evidence is safeguarded.[23] Special procedures are followed in taking the history and conducting the examination to preserve all evidence in case of future prosecution. When the victim of an assault is admitted to the ED or clinic, a specific chain of events occurs to collect legal evidence if the woman chooses to pursue legal action (Tables 53-16 and 53-17).

### TABLE 53-16 Emergency Management

**Sexual Assault**

| Etiology | Assessment Findings | Interventions |
|---|---|---|
| • Sexual molestation<br>• Sodomy<br>• Assault involving genitalia (male or female) without consent | • Emotional or physical manifestations of shock<br>• Hysteria<br>• Crying<br>• Anger<br>• Silence<br>• Decreased level of consciousness<br>• Hyperventilation<br>• Oral, vaginal, and rectal injuries<br>• Extragenital injuries<br>• Pain in genital or extragenital area | **Initial**<br>• Treat shock and other urgent medical problems (e.g., head injury, hemorrhage, wounds, fractures).<br>• Assess emotional state.<br>• Contact support person (i.e., social worker, rape advocate, sexual assault nurse examiner).<br>• Do *not* clean the patient until all evidence is collected. Make sure the patient does not wash, douche, urinate, brush teeth, or gargle.<br>• Place sheet on floor. Then have patient stand on sheet to remove clothing. Place sheet with clothing in paper bag.<br>• Obtain forensic evidence per local protocol (e.g., body hair, nail scrapings, tissue, dried semen, vaginal washing, blood samples).<br>• Maintain chain of evidence for all legal specimens. Clearly label evidence and keep in locked cabinet until given to law enforcement agency.<br>• Obtain baseline HIV, syphilis, and other STI screening.<br>• Determine method of contraception, date of last menstrual period, and date of last tetanus immunization.<br>• Consider tetanus prophylaxis if lacerations contain soil or dirt.<br>• Vaccinate against hepatitis B if not already done.<br>**Ongoing Monitoring**<br>• Monitor vital signs and emotional status.<br>• Provide clothing as needed.<br>• Counsel patient regarding confidential HIV and STI testing. |

*HIV,* Human immunodeficiency virus; *STI,* sexually transmitted infection.

### TABLE 53-17 Evaluation of Alleged Sexual Assault

**1. Medicolegal**
- Valid written consent for examination, photographs, laboratory tests, release of information, and laboratory samples
- Appropriate "chain of evidence" documentation

**2. History**
- History of assault (who, what, when, where)
- Penetration, ejaculation, extragenital acts
- Activities since assault (e.g., changed clothes, bathed, douched)
- Inquire about safety
- Menstrual and contraceptive history
- Medical history
- Emotional status
- Current symptoms

**3. General Physical Examination**
- Vital signs and general appearance
- Extragenital trauma: mouth, breasts, neck
- Cuts, bruises, scratches (photographs taken)

**4. Pelvic Examination**
- Vulvar trauma, erythema. Hymen, anal, and rectal status
- Matted hairs or free hairs
- Vaginal examination with unlubricated speculum for discharge, blood, lacerations
- Uterine size
- Adnexa, especially hematomas

**5. Laboratory Samples**
- Vaginal vault content sampling
- Vaginal smears: microscope evaluation for trichomonads and semen
- Oral or rectal swabs and smears (if indicated)
- Blood samples: pregnancy test; serologic testing for syphilis, HIV, and hepatitis B infection
- Freeze serum sample for later testing
- Cultures: cervix and other areas (if indicated) for gonorrhea and chlamydial infection
- Fingernail scrapings
- Pubic hair scrapings
- Clipping of matted pubic hairs

**6. Treatment**
- Care of injuries and emotional trauma
- Prophylaxis for STIs, tetanus, and hepatitis B (see appropriate chapters)
- If appropriate, consider levonorgestrel (Plan-B One-Step) emergency contraceptive pill up to 72 hr after assault; follow-up for pregnancy test in 2-3 wk
- Testing for HIV, syphilis, and hepatitis B may be done at 6-8 wk
- Protection of legal rights
- Recommendation of continued follow-up and services of rape crisis center

The SANE nurse takes a comprehensive gynecologic and sexual history and an account of the assault (who, what, when, and where), as well as a general physical and pelvic examination. Laboratory tests are performed to identify sperm in the vagina and to screen for STIs or pregnancy. The patient is provided preventive treatment for pregnancy and STIs as well as treatment for injuries sustained in the assault.

Follow-up physical and psychologic care is recommended. Women should return weekly for the first month after the assault. This includes the time period when a woman's psychologic reactions may be the most severe.

## NURSING MANAGEMENT: SEXUAL ASSAULT

Nursing care for a sexual assault victim is complex. Provide emotional and nonjudgmental support. Obtain referrals as needed for follow-up care. Part of the role of the SANE nurse is to discuss the possibility of pregnancy and STIs, and offer the patient an emergency contraception pill as well as antibiotics (Table 53-18). A social worker or nurse case manager referral should be made by the primary nurse in the ED to assist the patient in follow-up with financial compensation to assist them in paying for emergency services as a result of the assault as well as for emotional injuries sustained from the assault and any missed work.

### TABLE 53-18 Patient Teaching

**Sexual Assault Prevention**

*Include the following instructions when teaching measures to prevent sexual assault.*

1. Be proactive and take a self-defense class.
2. Be aware of date-rape drugs (e.g., GHB, Rohypnol, ketamine). Never leave your beverage unattended when socializing.
3. Place and maintain lights at all entrances to your home.
4. Keep your doors locked and do not open them to a stranger. Ask for identification if a service person comes to the door.
5. Do not advertise that you live alone. List only your initials with your last name in the telephone directory or on the mailbox. Never reveal to a caller that you are home alone.
6. Avoid walking alone in deserted areas. Walk to the parking lot with a friend. Be sure you see each other leave.
7. Have your keys ready as you approach your car or home.
8. Keep all doors locked and the windows up when driving.
9. Never get on an elevator with a suspicious person. Pretend you have forgotten something and get off.
10. Say what you mean in social situations. Be sure your voice and body language reflect your response.
11. Proceed with caution in online correspondence.
12. Carry a loud whistle and use it when you think you are in danger.
13. Yell "Fire!" if you are attacked and run toward a lighted area.

## CASE STUDY

**Uterine Fibroids and Endometrial Cancer**

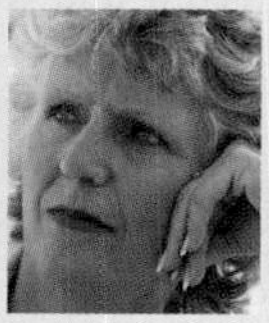

(©Wavebreak-media/iStock/Thinkstock)

### Patient Profile

T.J. is a 56-yr-old white woman who has lower pelvic discomfort and stress incontinence. She also has hypertension and type 2 diabetes. T.J. is the mother of four adult children. She has had abnormal uterine bleeding for 5 months. Large multiple uterine fibroids were diagnosed on ultrasound. She comes to the hospital for an abdominal hysterectomy.

### Subjective Data

- Was initially reluctant about surgery
- Concerned about her dyspareunia and her husband's reaction to the surgery
- States she has pelvic discomfort and stress incontinence

### Objective Data (Preoperative)

- BP 148/90 mm Hg, pulse 82 beats/min, respirations 14 breaths/min
- Height 5′6″ Weight 175 lb.

### Operative

- During surgery, abnormal-looking endometrial tissue was sent for pathologic analysis. The results were positive for endometrial cancer.
- Had total hysterectomy and bilateral salpingo-oophorectomy with lymph node biopsies. Five large fibroids were found in the uterus.

### Postoperative Status

- Returned to room with indwelling urinary catheter in place
- Abdominal incision
- Sequential compression devices on lower extremities
- Patient-controlled analgesia (PCA) pump for pain management

### Discussion Questions

1. Can the manifestations of uterine fibroids be differentiated from endometrial cancer?
2. ***Patient-Centered Care:*** Preoperatively T.J. asks you about the effect of the surgery on her sexuality. How would you respond, and what type of patient teaching would you do?
3. ***Patient-Centered Care:*** When she is told about the diagnosis of endometrial cancer, she is shocked. She cannot believe that was not discovered before surgery. How would you respond to her?
4. ***Priority Decision:*** What are priorities of care for T.J.?
5. ***Safety:*** When assessing T.J. after you got her out of bed, you note that her abdominal dressing is saturated with blood and she is complaining that she feels weak and dizzy. What would you do?
6. What other possible complications (including reasons for their development) can occur after an abdominal hysterectomy?
7. ***Teamwork and Collaboration:*** Which nursing personnel should be responsible for teaching T.J. related to her hypertension and diabetes: registered nurse, licensed practical/vocational nurse, unlicensed assistive personnel? What should she be taught?
8. ***Priority Decision:*** Based on the assessment data presented, what are the priority nursing diagnoses? Are there any collaborative problems?
9. ***Evidence-Based Practice:*** Her 37-yr-old daughter asks you if she is at risk for endometrial cancer. How would you respond?

Answers available at *http://evolve.elsevier.com/Lewis/medsurg.*

## BRIDGE TO NCLEX EXAMINATION

The number of the question corresponds to the same-numbered outcome at the beginning of the chapter.

1. In telling a patient with infertility what she and her partner can expect, the nurse explains that
   - **a.** ovulatory studies can help determine tube patency.
   - **b.** a hysterosalpingogram is a common diagnostic study.
   - **c.** the cause will remain unexplained for 40% of couples.
   - **d.** if postcoital studies are normal, infection tests will be done.
2. An appropriate question to ask the patient with painful menstruation to differentiate primary from secondary dysmenorrhea is
   - **a.** "Does your pain become worse with activity or overexertion?"
   - **b.** "Have you had a recent personal crisis or change in your lifestyle?"
   - **c.** "Is your pain relieved by nonsteroidal antiinflammatory medications?"
   - **d.** "When in your menstrual history did the pain with your period begin?"
3. The nurse should advise the woman recovering from surgical treatment of an ectopic pregnancy that
   - **a.** she has an increased risk for salpingitis.
   - **b.** bed rest must be maintained for 12 hours to assist in healing.
   - **c.** having one ectopic pregnancy increases her risk for another one.
   - **d.** intrauterine devices and infertility treatments should be avoided.
4. To prevent or decrease age-related changes that occur after menopause in a patient who chooses not to take hormone therapy, the *most* important self-care measure to teach is
   - **a.** maintaining usual sexual activity.
   - **b.** increasing the intake of dairy products.
   - **c.** performing regular aerobic, weight-bearing exercise.
   - **d.** taking vitamin E and B-complex vitamin supplements.
5. In caring for a patient with endometriosis, the nurse teaches the patient that interventions used to treat or cure this condition may include (*select all that apply*)
   - **a.** radiation.
   - **b.** antibiotic therapy.
   - **c.** oral contraceptives.
   - **d.** surgical removal of tissue.
   - **e.** total abdominal hysterectomy and salpingo-oophorectomy.
6. Nursing responsibilities related to the patient with endometrial cancer who has a total abdominal hysterectomy and salpingectomy and oophorectomy include
   - **a.** maintaining absolute bed rest.
   - **b.** keeping the patient in high Fowler's position.
   - **c.** need for supplemental estrogen after removal of ovaries.
   - **d.** encouraging movement and walking as much as tolerated.
7. Postoperative goals in caring for the patient who has undergone an abdominal hysterectomy include (*select all that apply*)
   - **a.** monitoring urine output.
   - **b.** changing position frequently.
   - **c.** restricting all food for 24 hours.
   - **d.** observing perineal pad for bleeding.
   - **e.** encouraging leg exercises to promote circulation.
8. Postoperative nursing care for the woman with a gynecologic fistula includes (*select all that apply*)
   - **a.** bed rest.
   - **b.** bladder training.
   - **c.** warm sitz baths.
   - **d.** perineal hygiene.
   - **e.** use of stool softeners.
9. The *first* nursing intervention for the patient who has been sexually assaulted is to
   - **a.** treat urgent medical problems.
   - **b.** contact support person for the patient.
   - **c.** provide supplies for the patient to cleanse self.
   - **d.** document bruises and lacerations of the perineum and the cervix.

1. b, 2. d, 3. c, 4. c, 5. c, d, e, 6. d, 7. a, b, e, 8. c, d, 9. a

For rationales to these answers and even more NCLEX review questions, visit *http://evolve.elsevier.com/Lewis/medsurg.*

## EVOLVE WEBSITE

http://evolve.elsevier.com/Lewis/medsurg

**Review Questions (Online Only)**

**Key Points**

**Answer Keys for Questions**

- Rationales for Bridge to NCLEX Examination Questions
- Answer Guidelines for Case Study on p. 1265

**Student Case Study**

- Patient With Endometrial Cancer

**Nursing Care Plan(s)**

- eNursing Care Plan 53-1: Patient Having Abdominal Hysterectomy

**Conceptual Care Map Creator**

**Audio Glossary**

**Content Updates**

## REFERENCES


1. American Society for Reproductive Medicine: Defining infertility. Retrieved from *www.asrm.org/FACTSHEET_Defining_Infertility.*
2. American Congress of Obstetricians & Gynecologists: Early pregnancy loss. Retrieved from *www.acog.org/~/media/For%20Patients/faq090.pdf.*
3. American Congress of Obstetricians & Gynecologists: Retrieved from *www.acog.org/-/media/For-Patients/faq043.pdf?dmc=1&ts=20150208T1033249676.*
4. Contraceptive technology update: classify the causes of abnormal uterine bleeding, 2014. Retrieved from *www.ctcfp.org/wp-content/uploads/Contraceptive-Technology-Update-1-2014.pdf.*
5. Tulundi T: Ectopic pregnancy: choosing a treatment and methotrexate therapy. Retrieved from *www.uptodate.com/contents/ectopic-pregnancy-choosing-a-treatment-and-methotrexate-therapy?source=search_result&search=ectopic+pregnancy&selectedTitle=2~150.*

*6. Shifren J, Gass L: The North American Menopause Society Recommendations for clinical care of midlife women, *Menopause* 21:1038, 2014.

7. CDC: Pelvic inflammatory disease (PID). Retrieved from *www.cdc.gov/std/pid/treatment.htm.*
8. Schenken R: Overview of the treatment of endometriosis. Retrieved from *www.uptodate.com/contents/overview-of-the-treatment-of-endometriosis?source=search_result&search=endometriosis&selectedTitle=1~150.*
9. Owen C, Armstrong A: Clinical management of leiomyoma, *Obstet Gynecol Clin North Am* 42:67, 2015.

*10. The Endocrine Society: Diagnosis and treatment of polycystic ovary syndrome: an endocrine society clinical practice guideline. Retrieved from *www.endocrine.org/~/media/endosociety/Files/Publications/Clinical%20Practice%20Guidelines/120513_PCOS_FinalA_2013.pdf.*
11. American Cancer Society: American Cancer Society: Cancer facts and figures 2015. Retrieved from *www.cancer.org/research/cancerfactsstatistics/allcancerfactsfigures/index.*
12. National Cancer Institute: A snapshot of cervical cancer: incidence and mortality. Retrieved from *www.cancer.gov/researchandfunding/snapshots/cervical.*
13. The American College of Obstetricians and Gynecologists: Cervical cancer screening. Retrieved from *www.acog.org/Patients/FAQs/Cervical-Cancer-Screening.*
14. American Cancer Society: Endometrial (uterine) cancer overview. Retrieved from *www.cancer.org/acs/groups/cid/documents/webcontent/003048-pdf.pdf.*
15. National Cancer Institute: Ovarian epithelial, fallopian tube, and primary peritoneal cancer treatment (PDQ). Retrieved from *www.cancer.gov/types/ovarian/patient/ovarian-epithelial-treatment-pdq.*
16. Anderson K, Davis K, Flynn B: Urinary incontinence and pelvic organ prolapse, *Med Clin North Am* 99:405, 2015.
17. Ding J, Chen C, Song X, et al: Successful use of ring pessary with support for advanced pelvic prolapse, *Int Urogynecol J* 26:1517, 2015.
18. Guzman Rojas R, Quintero C, Shek K, et al: Does childbirth play a role in the etiology of rectocele? *Int Urogynecol J* 26:737, 2015.
19. Alas A, Anger J: Management of apical pelvic organ prolapse, *Curr Urol Rep* 16:33-2015.
20. The Bowel and Bladder Foundation: Vaginal fistulas. Retrieved from *www.bladderandbowelfoundation.org/bladder/bladder-conditions-and-symptoms/vaginal-and-recto-vaginal-fistulas.*
21. Centers for Disease Control and Prevention: Intimate partner violence. Retrieved from *www.cdc.gov/violenceprevention/intimatepartnerviolence.*
22. American Congress of Obstetrics and Gynecologists: Sexual assault. Retrieved from *www.acog.org/Resources-And-Publications/Committee-Opinions/Committee-on-Health-Care-for-Underserved-Women/Sexual-Assault.*
23. Georgia Network to End Sexual Assault: Basic SANE training. Retrieved from *www.gnesa.org.*

*Evidence-based information for clinical practice.

# 54

# Male Reproductive and Genital Problems

*Susanne A. Quallich*

*Only those who risk going too far can possibly find out how far they can go.*

*T.S. Eliot*

http://evolve.elsevier.com/Lewis/medsurg/

## LEARNING OUTCOMES

1. Describe the pathophysiology, clinical manifestations, and interprofessional care of benign prostatic hyperplasia.
2. Describe the nursing management of benign prostatic hyperplasia.
3. Describe the pathophysiology, clinical manifestations, and interprofessional care of prostate cancer.
4. Explain the nursing management of prostate cancer.
5. Specify the pathophysiology, clinical manifestations, and nursing and interprofessional management of prostatitis and problems of the penis and scrotum.
6. Explain the clinical manifestations and interprofessional care of testicular cancer.
7. Describe the pathophysiology, clinical manifestations, and nursing and interprofessional management of problems related to male sexual function.
8. Summarize the psychologic and emotional implications related to male reproductive problems.

## KEY TERMS

benign prostatic hyperplasia (BPH), p. 1268
epididymitis, p. 1284
erectile dysfunction (ED), p. 1286
orchitis, p. 1284
paraphimosis, p. 1283
phimosis, p. 1283
prostate cancer, p. 1275
prostatitis, p. 1282
radical prostatectomy, p. 1278
testicular cancer, p. 1285
testicular torsion, p. 1285
transurethral resection of the prostate (TURP), p. 1272
vasectomy, p. 1286

This chapter discusses problems of the male reproductive system. These involve a variety of structures, including the prostate, penis, urethra, ejaculatory duct, scrotum, testes, epididymis, ductus (vas) deferens, and rectum (Fig. 54-1).

## PROBLEMS OF THE PROSTATE GLAND

## BENIGN PROSTATIC HYPERPLASIA

**Benign prostatic hyperplasia (BPH)** is a condition in which the prostate gland increases in size, leading to disruption of the outflow of urine from the bladder through the urethra. Almost half of the men with BPH will have bothersome lower urinary tract symptoms (LUTS), such as difficulty starting a urine stream, a decreased flow of urine, or urinary frequency.[1] Research is not clear about whether having BPH leads to an increased risk of developing prostate cancer.[2,3]

### Etiology and Pathophysiology

The etiology of BPH is not completely understood. However, hormonal changes associated with aging are believed to be contributing factors.[1] Dihydroxytestosterone (DHT), one of several sex hormones, stimulates prostate cell growth. Excess amounts of DHT can cause overgrowth of prostate tissue. As men age, they have a decrease in testosterone but continue to produce and accumulate high levels of DHT, resulting in prostate enlargement.

Another possible cause of BPH is an increased proportion of estrogen (as compared to testosterone). Throughout their lives, men produce both testosterone and small amounts of estrogen. As men age, the amount of active testosterone in the blood decreases, leaving a higher proportion of estrogen. A higher amount of estrogen within the prostate gland increases the activity of substances (including DHT) that promote prostate cell growth.

BPH usually develops in the inner part of the prostate. (Prostate cancer is most likely to develop in the outer part.) As the prostate enlarges, it gradually compresses the urethra, leading to partial or complete obstruction (Fig. 54-2). This compression of the urethra leads to the development of clinical manifestations. There is no direct relationship between prostate size and the severity of manifestations or degree of obstruction. The location of the enlargement is most significant in the development of obstructive symptoms (Fig. 54-3). For example, it is

Reviewed by Shari Gould, RN, MSN, Associate Professor of Nursing, Victoria College, Victoria, Texas; and Anthony R. Lutz, RN, MSN, A-GNP-C, Urology Nurse Practitioner, Carolinas Health Care System, Charlotte, North Carolina.

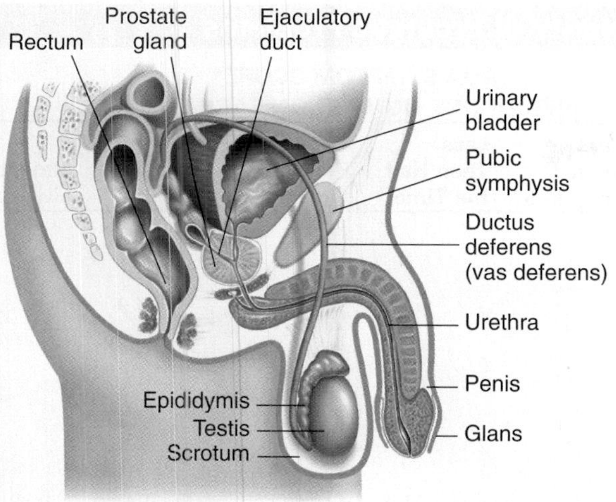


**FIG. 54-1** Areas of the male reproductive system in which problems are likely to develop.

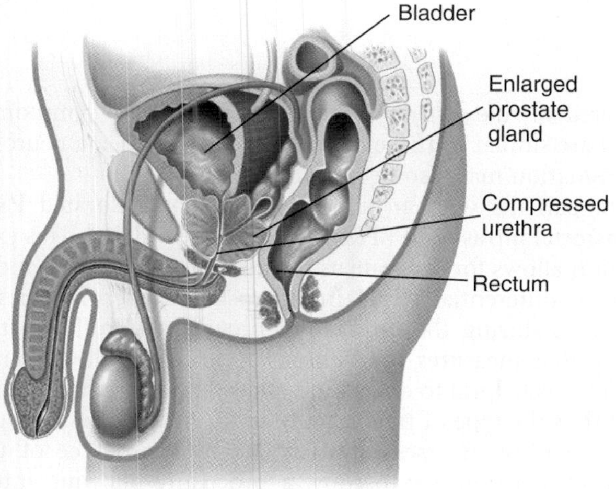


**FIG. 54-2** Benign prostatic hyperplasia. The enlarged prostate compresses the urethra.

possible for mild prostate enlargement to cause severe obstruction, or for extreme prostate enlargement to cause few obstructive symptoms.

Risk factors for BPH include aging, obesity (in particular increased waist circumference), lack of physical activity, alcohol consumption, erectile dysfunction, smoking, and diabetes.[4] A family history of BPH in a first-degree relative may also be a risk factor.

## Clinical Manifestations

Manifestations of BPH occur gradually and may not be noticed until prostate enlargement has been present for some time. Early symptoms may not cause significant problems because the bladder can compensate for a small amount of resistance to urine flow. As the severity of urethral obstruction increases, the symptoms gradually worsen.

Symptoms can be divided into two groups: irritative and obstructive. *Irritative symptoms* include nocturia, urinary frequency, urgency, dysuria, bladder pain, and incontinence. These symptoms are associated with inflammation or infection. Nocturia is often the first symptom that the patient notices. *Obstructive symptoms,* caused by prostate enlargement, include a decrease in the caliber and force of the urinary stream, difficulty in initiating a stream, intermittency (stopping and starting stream several times while voiding), and dribbling at the end of urination. These symptoms are due to the increased effort of the bladder as it tries to empty through the decreased diameter of the urethra. As a group, both irritative and obstructive symptoms are considered lower urinary tract symptoms (LUTS).

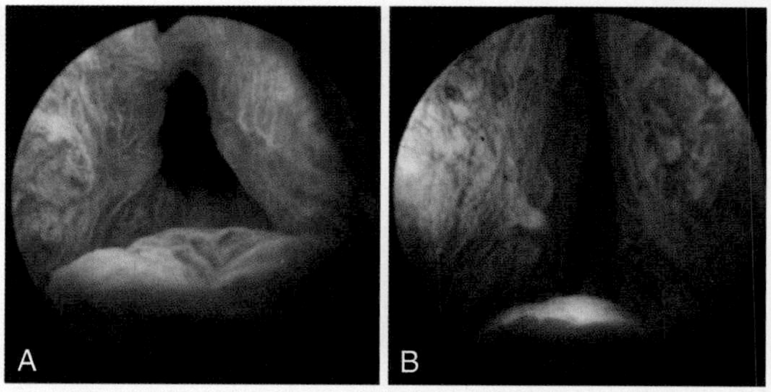


**FIG. 54-3** Views of the prostate by cystoscopy. **A,** Normal appearance. **B,** Moderate benign prostatic hyperplasia with urethral obstruction. (From Townsend CM, Beauchamp RD, Evers BM, et al: *Sabiston textbook of surgery,* ed 19, Philadelphia, 2012, Saunders.)

The American Urological Association (AUA) symptom index for BPH (Table 54-1) is a widely used tool to assess voiding symptoms associated with obstruction.[5] Although this tool is not diagnostic, it helps determine the extent of symptoms and provides guidelines for treatment.[6] Higher scores on this tool indicate greater symptom severity.

## Complications

Complications of BPH are relatively rare. However, some men may experience acute urinary retention. This complication is manifested by the sudden and painful inability to urinate. Treatment involves the insertion of a catheter to drain the bladder. Surgery may be indicated in severe situations.

Urinary tract infection (UTI) can also be a complication of BPH. Since the bladder is unable to empty completely, bacteria can grow and cause infection within the urinary tract. In more severe cases, sepsis may also develop. Bladder calculi (stones) may develop in the bladder because of the alkalinization of the residual urine. Although bladder stones are more common in men with BPH, the risk of kidney stones is not significantly increased.

Additional complications include renal failure caused by *hydronephrosis* (distention of pelvis and calyces of the kidney by urine that cannot flow through the ureter to the bladder), pyelonephritis, and bladder damage if treatment for acute urinary retention is delayed.

## Diagnostic Studies

A history and physical examination are important for diagnosis. (Diagnostic studies are outlined in Table 54-2.) A digital rectal examination (DRE) is done to estimate the prostate size, symmetry, and consistency. In BPH, the prostate is symmetrically enlarged, firm, and smooth.

Other diagnostic testing may include a urinalysis with culture to look for bacteria, white blood cells (WBCs), or microscopic hematuria, which indicate infection or inflammation.

A prostate-specific antigen (PSA) blood test may be done to screen for prostate cancer. However, PSA levels may be slightly elevated in patients with BPH. Serum creatinine levels may be

**TABLE 54-1 AUA Symptom Index to Determine Severity of Prostatic Problems**

| Questions | AUA SYMPTOM SCORE* (CIRCLE ONE NUMBER ON EACH LINE) Not At All | Less Than 1 Time in 5 | Less Than Half the Time | About Half the Time | More Than Half the Time | Almost Always |
|---|---|---|---|---|---|---|
| **Over the past month** | | | | | | |
| 1. How often do you have the sensation that your bladder is not completely empty after you finish urinating? | 0 | 1 | 2 | 3 | 4 | 5 |
| 2. How often do you have to urinate again, less than 2 hr after you finish urinating? | 0 | 1 | 2 | 3 | 4 | 5 |
| 3. How often do you stop and start again several times when you urinate? | 0 | 1 | 2 | 3 | 4 | 5 |
| 4. How often do you find it difficult to postpone urination? | 0 | 1 | 2 | 3 | 4 | 5 |
| 5. How often do you have a weak urinary stream? | 0 | 1 | 2 | 3 | 4 | 5 |
| 6. How often do you have to push or strain to begin urination? | 0 | 1 | 2 | 3 | 4 | 5 |
| 7. How many times do you usually get up to urinate from the time you go to bed at night until the time you get up in the morning? | 0 (None) | 1 (1 time) | 2 (2 times) | 3 (3 times) | 4 (4 times) | 5 (5 times or more) |
| **Sum of circled numbers (AUA Symptom Score): _____*** | | | | | | |

Source: Barry MJ, Fowler FJ, O'Leary MP, et al: The American Urological Association symptom index for benign prostatic hyperplasia, *J Urol* 148:1549, 1992. Used with permission.
*AUA,* American Urological Association.
*Score is interpreted as follows: 0-7, mild; 8-19, moderate; 20-35, severe.

**TABLE 54-2 Interprofessional Care**

***Benign Prostatic Hyperplasia***

**Diagnostic Assessment**
- History and physical examination
- Digital rectal examination (DRE)
- Urinalysis with culture
- Prostate-specific antigen (PSA)
- Serum creatinine
- Postvoid residual
- Transrectal ultrasound (TRUS)
- Uroflowmetry
- Cystoscopy

**Management**

***Active Surveillance***
- Annual PSA and DRE

***Drug Therapy***
- 5α-Reductase inhibitors (e.g., finasteride [Proscar], dutasteride [Avodart], dutasteride plus tamsulosin [Jalyn])
- α-Adrenergic receptor blockers (e.g., silodosin [Rapaflo], alfuzosin [Uroxatral], doxazosin [Cardura], prazosin [Minipress], terazosin, tamsulosin [Flomax])
- Erectogenic drugs (e.g., tadalafil [Cialis])

***Minimally Invasive Therapy****
- Transurethral microwave thermotherapy (TUMT)
- Transurethral needle ablation (TUNA)
- Laser prostatectomy
- Transurethral electrovaporization of the prostate (TUVP)

***Invasive (Surgery) Therapy****
- Transurethral resection of the prostate (TURP)
- Transurethral incision of the prostate (TUIP)
- Open prostatectomy

*See Table 54-3.

ordered to rule out renal insufficiency. Because symptoms of BPH are similar to those of a neurogenic bladder, a neurologic examination may also be performed.

In patients with an abnormal DRE and elevated PSA, a transrectal ultrasound (TRUS) is typically ordered. This examination allows for accurate assessment of prostate size and can help to differentiate BPH from prostate cancer. Biopsies can be taken during the ultrasound procedure. Uroflowmetry, a study that measures the volume of urine expelled from the bladder, is helpful to determine the extent of urethral blockage and thus the type of treatment needed. Postvoid residual urine volume is often assessed to determine the degree of urine flow obstruction. Cystoscopy, a procedure allowing internal visualization of the urethra and bladder, is performed if the diagnosis is unclear or to visualize the degree of prostatic enlargement.

## Interprofessional Care

The goals of interprofessional care are to (1) restore bladder drainage, (2) relieve the patient's symptoms, and (3) prevent or treat the complications of BPH. Treatment is generally based on the degree to which the symptoms bother the patient or the presence of complications, rather than the size of the prostate. Alternatives to surgical intervention for some patients include drug therapy and minimally invasive procedures.

The most conservative treatment that may be recommended for some patients with BPH is referred to as *active surveillance,* or watchful waiting. When the patient has mild symptoms (AUA symptom scores of 0 to 7), a wait-and-see approach is taken. Teaching patients to make lifestyle changes can help relieve early or mild symptoms. Making dietary changes (decreasing intake of caffeine, artificial sweeteners, and spicy or acidic foods), avoiding drugs such as decongestants and anticholinergics, and restricting evening fluid intake may improve symptoms.

In addition, a timed voiding schedule may reduce or eliminate symptoms, thus eliminating the need for further intervention. If the patient begins to have signs or symptoms that indicate an increase in obstruction, further treatment is indicated.

**Drug Therapy.** Two classes of drugs that are used to treat BPH include 5α-reductase inhibitors and α-adrenergic receptor blockers. Combination therapy using both types of drugs may be more effective in reducing symptoms than using one drug alone.

***5α-Reductase Inhibitors.*** 5α-Reductase inhibitors work by reducing the size of the prostate gland. Finasteride (Proscar) blocks the enzyme 5α-reductase, which is necessary for the conversion of testosterone to DHT (principal intraprostatic androgen). Prostate size is directly related to the amount of DHT. By blocking DHT, overly enlarged prostates can decrease in size. This class of medication is more effective for men with larger prostates who experience bothersome symptoms.

Finasteride is an appropriate treatment option for men who have a moderate to severe symptom score on the AUA symptom index (Table 54-1). Although most men who are treated with the drug have symptom improvement, it can take up to 6 months to be effective. These drugs must be taken on a regular basis to have an effect.

Serum PSA levels may be decreased by almost 50% when taking finasteride. Therefore to "correct" for the decrease caused by the finasteride, the HCP should double the PSA result. This allows for an accurate comparison to premedication levels to more accurately track trends in the PSA over time.

Dutasteride (Avodart) has the same effect on prostatic tissue as finasteride and is a dual inhibitor of 5α-reductase type 1 and 2 isoenzymes. (Finasteride inhibits only the type 2 isoenzyme.) The combination of a 5α-reductase inhibitor (dutasteride) and an α-adrenergic receptor blocker (tamsulosin) is available in a single oral medication (Jalyn).

In addition to decreasing the symptoms of BPH, finasteride, dutasteride, and Jalyn (finasteride plus tamsulosin) may also lower the risk of prostate cancer.[7] However, the use of these drugs in the prevention of prostate cancer has not been recommended. Patients with an increased PSA level while taking these medications should be referred to their HCP. Also encourage the patient to discuss the need for prostate cancer screening with the HCP.

**DRUG ALERT Finasteride (Proscar)**

- Women who may be or are pregnant should not handle tablets due to potential risk to male fetus (anomaly).

***α-Adrenergic Receptor Blockers.*** α-Adrenergic receptor blockers are another drug treatment option for BPH. These medications selectively block $\alpha_1$-adrenergic receptors, which are abundant in the prostate, and are increased in hyperplastic prostate tissue. Although nonspecific α-adrenergic blockers are more commonly used for the treatment of hypertension, these drugs promote smooth muscle relaxation in the prostate, thus facilitating urinary flow through the urethra.

Several α-adrenergic blockers are used, including silodosin (Rapaflo), alfuzosin (Uroxatral), doxazosin (Cardura), prazosin (Minipress), terazosin, and tamsulosin (Flomax). Although these drugs offer symptom relief of BPH by relaxing the smooth muscle of the prostate that surrounds the urethra, these medications do not decrease the overall size of the prostate.

***Erectogenic Drugs.*** Tadalafil (Cialis) has been used in men who have symptoms of BPH alone or in combination with erectile dysfunction (ED). The drug has shown to be effective in reducing symptoms for both of these conditions.[8]

***Herbal Therapy.*** Some patients take plant extracts such as saw palmetto *(Serenoa repens)*. However, research indicates that saw palmetto has no benefit over a placebo.[9,10] Advise patients to discuss herbal therapies with their HCP.

**Minimally Invasive Therapy.** Minimally invasive therapies are becoming more common as an alternative to watchful waiting and invasive treatment (Table 54-3). They generally do not require hospitalization or catheterization and are associated with few adverse events. Many minimally invasive therapies have outcomes comparable to those of invasive techniques.[11]

***Transurethral Microwave Thermotherapy.*** *Transurethral microwave thermotherapy* (TUMT) is an outpatient procedure that involves the delivery of microwaves directly to the prostate through a transurethral probe (probe inserted into the meatus and through the urethra). The microwaves increase the temperature of the prostate tissue to about 113° F (45° C). The heat causes death of tissue, thus relieving the obstruction. A rectal temperature probe is used during the procedure to ensure that the temperature in the rectum is kept below 110° F (43.5° C) to prevent rectal tissue damage. The procedure takes about 90 minutes.

Postoperative urinary retention is a common complication. Patients who have a TUMT are generally sent home with an indwelling catheter for 2 to 7 days to maintain urinary flow and to facilitate the passing of small clots or necrotic tissue. Antibiotics, pain medication, and bladder antispasmodic medications are used to treat and prevent postprocedure problems. The procedure is not appropriate for men with rectal problems. Anticoagulant therapy should be stopped 10 days before treatment. Mild side effects include occasional problems of bladder spasm, hematuria, dysuria, and retention.

***Transurethral Needle Ablation.*** *Transurethral needle ablation* (TUNA) is another procedure that increases the temperature of prostate tissue, thus causing localized necrosis. TUNA differs from TUMT in that low-wave radiofrequency is used to heat the prostate. Only prostate tissue in direct contact with the needle is affected, which allows for more precise removal of the target tissue. The majority of the patients undergoing TUNA have an improvement in symptoms.

**CHECK YOUR PRACTICE**

You are working in the preoperative unit and caring for a patient who is scheduled for a transurethral needle ablation for BPH. He appears anxious. He tells you, "I'm afraid of the pain after the procedure. They told me I might have to have a tube in my bladder. I don't know how I'll manage at home."

- What type of information and teaching would you provide him?

This procedure is performed in an outpatient unit or physician's office using local anesthesia and IV or oral sedation. The TUNA procedure lasts approximately 30 minutes. The patient typically experiences little pain with an early return to regular activities. Complications include urinary retention, UTI, and irritative voiding symptoms (e.g., frequency, urgency, dysuria). Some patients require a urinary catheter for a short time. Patients often have hematuria for up to a week, and irritative voiding symptoms may persist for several weeks.

***Laser Prostatectomy.*** The use of laser therapy through visual or ultrasound guidance is an effective alternative to transurethral resection of the prostate (TURP) in treating BPH. The laser beam is delivered transurethrally through a fiber instrument and is used for cutting, coagulation, and vaporization of prostatic tissue. There are a variety of laser procedures using different sources, wavelengths, and delivery systems. Retreatment rates are comparable to those of a TURP.[12]

**TABLE 54-3 Treatment for Benign Prostatic Hyperplasia**

| Description | Advantages | Disadvantages |
|---|---|---|
| **Minimally Invasive** | | |
| ***Transurethral Microwave Thermotherapy (TUMT)*** | | |
| Use of microwave radiating heat to produce coagulative necrosis of the prostate. | • Outpatient procedure<br>• Erectile dysfunction, urinary incontinence, and retrograde ejaculation are rare | • Potential for damage to surrounding tissue<br>• Urinary catheter needed after procedure |
| ***Transurethral Needle Ablation (TUNA)*** | | |
| Low-wave radiofrequency used to heat the prostate, causing necrosis. | • Outpatient procedure<br>• Erectile dysfunction, urinary incontinence, and retrograde ejaculation are rare<br>• Precise delivery of heat to desired area<br>• Very little pain experienced | • Urinary retention common<br>• Irritative voiding symptoms<br>• Hematuria |
| ***Laser Prostatectomy*** | | |
| Procedure uses a laser beam to cut or destroy part of the prostate. Different techniques are available:<br>• Visual laser ablation of prostate (VLAP)<br>• Contact laser<br>• Photovaporization of prostate (PVP)<br>• Interstitial laser coagulation (ILC) | • Short procedure<br>• Comparable results to TURP<br>• Minimal bleeding<br>• Fast recovery time<br>• Rapid symptom improvement<br>• Very effective | • Catheter (up to 7 days) needed after procedure due to edema and urinary retention<br>• Delayed sloughing of tissue<br>• Takes several weeks to reach optimal effect<br>• Retrograde ejaculation |
| ***Transurethral Electrovaporization of Prostate (TUVP)*** | | |
| Electrosurgical vaporization and desiccation are used together to destroy prostatic tissue. | • Minimal risks<br>• Minimal bleeding and sloughing | • Retrograde ejaculation<br>• Intermittent hematuria |
| **Invasive (Surgery)** | | |
| ***Transurethral Resection of Prostate (TURP)*** | | |
| Use of excision and cauterization to remove prostate tissue via cystoscope. Remains the standard for treatment of BPH. | • Erectile dysfunction unlikely | • Bleeding<br>• Retrograde ejaculation |
| ***Transurethral Incision of Prostate (TUIP)*** | | |
| Involves transurethral incisions into prostatic tissue to relieve obstruction. Effective for men with small to moderate prostates. | • Outpatient procedure<br>• Minimal complications<br>• Low occurrence of erectile dysfunction or retrograde ejaculation | • Urinary catheter needed after procedure |
| ***Open Prostatectomy*** | | |
| Surgery of choice for men with large prostates, bladder damage, or other complicating factors. Involves external incision with two possible approaches (see Fig. 54-6). | • Complete visualization of prostate and surrounding tissue | • Erectile dysfunction<br>• Bleeding<br>• Postoperative pain<br>• Risk of infection |

One common procedure is *visual laser ablation of the prostate* (VLAP), which uses the laser beam to produce deep coagulation necrosis. The affected prostate tissue gradually sloughs in the urinary stream. It takes several weeks before the patient reaches optimal results after this type of laser therapy. At the completion of VLAP, a urinary catheter is inserted to allow for drainage.

*Contact laser techniques* involve the direct contact of the laser with the prostate tissue, producing an immediate vaporization of the tissue. Blood vessels near the laser tip are immediately cauterized. Thus bleeding during the procedure is rare. A three-way catheter with slow-drip irrigation is placed immediately after the procedure for a short time. Typically the catheter is removed within 6 to 8 hours after the procedure. Advantages of this procedure over TURP include minimal bleeding both during and after the procedure, faster recovery time, and ability to perform the surgery on patients taking anticoagulants.

*Photovaporization of the prostate* (PVP) uses a high-power green laser light to vaporize prostate tissue. Improvements in urine flow and symptoms are almost immediate after the procedure. Bleeding is minimal, and a catheter is usually inserted for 24 to 48 hours afterward. PVP works well for larger prostate glands, but irritative voiding symptoms may persist for several weeks.

Another approach to laser prostatectomy is *interstitial laser coagulation* (ILC). The prostate is viewed through a cystoscope. A laser is used to quickly treat precise areas of the enlarged prostate by placement of interstitial light guides directly into the prostate tissue.

**Invasive (Surgery) Therapy.** Invasive treatment of symptomatic BPH involves surgery. The choice of the treatment approach depends on the size and location of the prostatic enlargement and patient factors such as age and surgical risk. Invasive treatments are summarized in Table 54-3.

Invasive therapy is indicated when a decrease in urine flow causes discomfort, persistent residual urine, acute urinary retention because of obstruction with no reversible precipitating cause, or hydronephrosis. Intermittent catheterization or insertion of an indwelling catheter can temporarily reduce symptoms and bypass the obstruction. However, avoid long-term catheter use because of the increased risk of infection.

***Transurethral Resection of the Prostate.*** Transurethral resection of the prostate (TURP) is a surgical procedure involving the removal of prostate tissue using a resectoscope inserted through the urethra. TURP has long been considered the gold standard for surgical treatments of obstructing BPH. Results of a TURP are superior but at the cost of a longer hospital stay. The number of TURP procedures done in recent years has declined due to the development of less invasive technologies.[6]

In TURP no external surgical incision is made. A resectoscope is inserted through the urethra to excise and cauterize obstructing prostatic tissue (Fig. 54-4). A large three-way

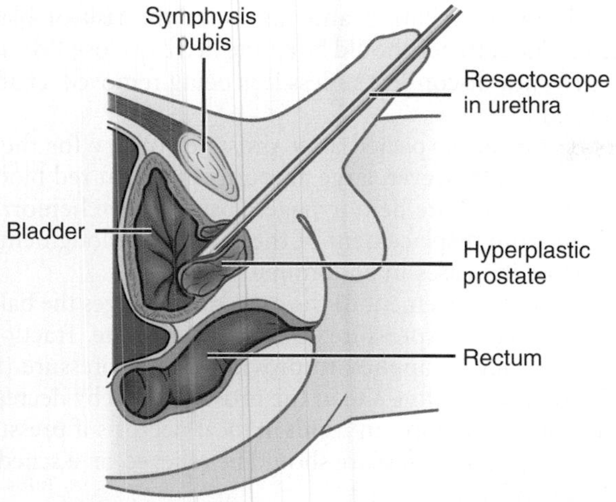


**FIG. 54-4** Transurethral resection of the prostate.

indwelling catheter with a 30-mL balloon is inserted into the bladder after the procedure to provide hemostasis and to facilitate urinary drainage. The bladder is irrigated, either continuously or intermittently, usually for the first 24 hours to prevent obstruction from mucus and blood clots.

The outcome for the majority of patients is excellent, with marked improvements in symptoms and urinary flow rates. TURP is a surgical procedure with a relatively low risk, but caregivers must be vigilant for signs or symptoms of transurethral resection syndrome (TUR or TURP syndrome). This condition is manifested by nausea, vomiting, confusion, bradycardia, and hypertension. TUR syndrome is the result of hyponatremia due to longer operative times and prolonged intraoperative bladder irrigation.

Other postoperative complications include bleeding and clot retention. Because bleeding is a common complication, patients taking aspirin, warfarin (Coumadin), or other anticoagulants must discontinue these medications several days before surgery. BPH medications are also stopped after this procedure.

***Transurethral Incision of the Prostate.*** Transurethral incision of the prostate (TUIP) is a surgical procedure done under local anesthesia for men with moderate to severe symptoms. Several small incisions are made into the prostate gland to expand the urethra, which relieves pressure on the urethra and improves urine flow. TUIP is an option for patients with a small or moderately enlarged prostate gland. TUIP has similar patient outcomes to TURP in relieving symptoms.

## NURSING MANAGEMENT: BENIGN PROSTATIC HYPERPLASIA

Because you will be most directly involved in care of patients with BPH having invasive therapies, the focus of nursing management in this section is on preoperative and postoperative care.

### Nursing Assessment

Subjective and objective data that should be obtained from a patient with BPH are presented in Table 54-4.

### Nursing Diagnoses

Nursing diagnoses for the patient with BPH preoperatively may include, but are not limited to, the following:

- Acute pain *related to* bladder distention secondary to enlarged prostate

**TABLE 54-4 Nursing Assessment**

***Benign Prostatic Hyperplasia***

**Subjective Data**

***Important Health Information***

*Medications:* Testosterone supplementation
*Surgery or other treatments:* Previous treatment for BPH

***Functional Health Patterns***

*Health perception–health management:* Knowledge of the condition
*Nutritional-metabolic:* Voluntary fluid restriction
*Elimination:* Urinary urgency, diminution in caliber and force of urinary stream. Hesitancy in initiating voiding. Postvoid dribbling, urinary retention, urinary incontinence
*Sleep-rest:* Nocturia
*Cognitive-perceptual:* Dysuria, sensation of incomplete voiding, bladder discomfort
*Sexuality-reproductive:* Anxiety about sexual dysfunction

**Objective Data**

***General***

Older adult male

***Urinary***

Distended bladder on palpation. Smooth, firm, elastic enlargement of prostate on rectal examination

***Possible Diagnostic Findings***

Enlarged prostate on ultrasonography, vesicle neck obstruction on cystoscopy, residual urine with postvoiding catheterization. White blood cells, bacteria, or microscopic hematuria with bladder infection. ↑ serum creatinine levels with renal involvement

- Risk for infection *related to* an indwelling catheter, urinary stasis, or environmental pathogens

Nursing diagnoses for the patient with BPH who has invasive therapy (surgery) are presented in eNursing Care Plan 54-1 (available on the website for this chapter).

### Planning

The overall preoperative goals for the patient having invasive procedures are to have (1) restoration of urinary drainage; (2) treatment of any UTI; and (3) understanding of the upcoming procedure, implications for sexual function and urinary control. The overall postoperative goals are to have (1) no complications, (2) restoration of urinary control, (3) complete bladder emptying, and (4) satisfying sexual expression.

### Nursing Implementation

**Health Promotion.** The cause of BPH is largely attributed to the aging process.[13] Health promotion focuses on early detection and treatment. The American Urological Association (AUA) currently recommends that men age 55 to 69 have the greatest potential benefit from PSA screening. The recommended screening interval is every 2 years.[14] When symptoms of prostatic hyperplasia are present, further diagnostic screening may be necessary (Table 54-2).

Some men find that consuming alcohol, caffeine, or other bladder irritants tends to increase prostatic symptoms because the diuretic effect increases bladder distention. Compounds found in common cough and cold remedies such as pseudoephedrine (in Sudafed) and phenylephrine (in Allerest PE and Coricidin D) often worsen the symptoms of BPH. These drugs are α-adrenergic agonists that cause smooth muscle contraction. If this occurs, the patient should avoid these drugs.

Teach patients with obstructive symptoms to urinate every 2 to 3 hours and when they first feel the urge. This will minimize urinary stasis and acute urinary retention. Instruct patients to maintain a normal level of fluid so that they do not become dehydrated. The patient may believe that if he restricts his fluid intake, symptoms will be less severe, but this only increases the chances of an infection while concentrating his urine.

◆ **Acute Care.** The following discussion focuses on preoperative and postoperative care for the patient undergoing a TURP.

◆ ***Preoperative Care.*** Antibiotics are usually administered before any invasive GU procedure. Any infection of the urinary tract must be treated before surgery. Restoring urinary drainage and encouraging a high fluid intake (2 to 3 L/day unless contraindicated) are helpful in managing the infection. Prostatic obstruction may result in acute retention or inability to void. Urinary drainage must be restored before surgery.

A urethral catheter such as a coudé (curved-tip) catheter may be needed to restore bladder drainage. In many health care settings, 10 mL of sterile 2% lidocaine gel is injected into the urethra before insertion of the catheter. The lidocaine gel not only acts as a lubricant but also provides local anesthesia and helps open the urethral lumen. If a sizable obstruction of the urethra exists, the urologist may insert a filiform catheter with sufficient rigidity to pass the obstruction. Aseptic technique is important at all times to avoid introducing bacteria into the bladder. (Urinary catheters are discussed in Chapter 45.)

Patients may be concerned about the impact of the impending surgery on sexual function. Provide an opportunity for the patient and his partner to express their concerns. Inform the patient that his ejaculate volume may be decreased or absent after the procedure. Most types of prostatic surgery results in some degree of *retrograde ejaculation*, a condition in which some semen travels back into the bladder during orgasm instead of traveling out of the penis. This may decrease orgasmic sensations felt during ejaculation. Retrograde ejaculation is not harmful, and the semen is voided during the next urination.

◆ ***Postoperative Care.*** The main complications after surgery are hemorrhage, bladder spasms, urinary incontinence, and infection. Adjust the plan of care to the type of surgery, reasons for surgery, and patient's response to surgery.

After surgery the patient will have a standard catheter or a triple-lumen catheter. Bladder irrigation is typically done to remove clotted blood from the bladder and ensure drainage of urine. The bladder is irrigated either manually on an intermittent basis or more commonly as continuous bladder irrigation (CBI) with sterile normal saline solution or another prescribed solution. If the bladder is manually irrigated (if ordered), instill 50 mL of irrigating solution and then withdraw with a syringe to remove clots that may be in the bladder and catheter. Painful bladder spasms often occur as a result of manual irrigation.

With CBI, irrigating solution is continuously infused and drained from the bladder. The rate of infusion is based on the color of drainage. Ideally the urine drainage should be light pink without clots. Continuously monitor the inflow and outflow of the irrigant. If outflow is less than inflow, assess the catheter patency for kinks or clots. If the outflow is blocked and patency cannot be reestablished by manual irrigation, stop the CBI and notify the physician.

Use careful aseptic technique when irrigating the bladder because bacteria can easily be introduced into the urinary tract. Secure the catheter to the leg with tape or a catheter strap to prevent urethral irritation and minimize the risk of bladder infection. The catheter should be connected to a closed-drainage system. Do not disconnect unless it is being removed, changed, or irrigated.

Blood clots are expected after prostate surgery for the first 24 to 36 hours. However, large amounts of bright red blood in the urine can indicate hemorrhage. Postoperative hemorrhage may occur from displacement of the catheter, dislodgment of a large clot, or increases in abdominal pressure.

Release or displacement of the catheter dislodges the balloon that provides counterpressure on the operative site. Traction on the catheter may be applied to provide counterpressure (tamponade) on the bleeding site in the prostate, thereby decreasing bleeding. Such traction can result in local necrosis if pressure is applied for too long. Pressure should be relieved on a scheduled basis by qualified personnel.

Activities that increase abdominal pressure should be avoided in the postoperative recovery period. These include sitting or walking for prolonged periods and straining to have a bowel movement (Valsalva maneuver).

Bladder spasms are a distressing complication for the patient after transurethral procedures. They occur as a result of irritation of the bladder mucosa from the insertion of the resectoscope, presence of a catheter, or clots leading to obstruction of the catheter. If bladder spasms develop, check the catheter for clots. If present, remove the clots by irrigation so that urine can

## TEAMWORK & COLLABORATION

### Patient Receiving Bladder Irrigation

Intermittent or continuous bladder irrigation (CBI) is usually required after invasive prostate surgery to prevent bladder obstruction by clots or mucus.

**Role of Nursing Personnel**

***Registered Nurse (RN)***

- Assess for bleeding and clots.
- Assess catheter patency by measuring intake and output and presence of bladder spasms.
- Manually irrigate catheter if bladder spasms or decreased outflow occurs.
- Discontinue CBI and notify physician if obstruction occurs.
- Teach patient Kegel exercises after catheter removal.
- Provide care instructions for patient discharged with indwelling catheter.

***Licensed Practical/Vocational Nurse (LPN/LVN)***

- Monitor catheter drainage for increased blood or clots.
- Increase flow of irrigating solution to maintain light pink color in outflow.
- Administer antispasmodics and analgesics as needed.

***Unlicensed Assistive Personnel (UAP)***

- Clean around catheter daily.
- Record intake and output.
- Notify RN if large amount of bright red blood is in urine.
- Report complaints of pain or bladder spasms to RN.

**Role of Other Team Members**

***Physician or Advanced Practice Clinician (Nurse Practitioner or Physician Assistant)***

- Assess for bleeding and clots.
- Assess and manage catheter if obstruction occurs.
- Order antispasmodics and analgesics as needed.

flow freely. Instruct the patient not to urinate around the catheter because this increases the likelihood of spasm. Belladonna and opium suppositories or other antispasmodics (e.g., oxybutynin [Ditropan XL]), along with relaxation techniques, are used to relieve the pain and decrease spasm.

The catheter is often removed 2 to 4 days after surgery. The patient should have a voiding trial after catheter removal. If he cannot urinate, he will have a catheter reinserted for a day or two or be taught to perform clean intermittent self-catheterization (see Chapter 45).

Sphincter tone may be poor immediately after catheter removal, resulting in urinary incontinence or dribbling. This is a common but distressing situation for the patient. Sphincter tone can be strengthened by having the patient practice Kegel exercises (pelvic floor muscle technique) 10 to 20 times per hour while awake. (Kegel exercises are discussed in Table 45-18.) Encourage the patient to practice starting and stopping the stream several times during urination. This helps the patient to target the correct pelvic floor muscles when performing Kegel exercises.

It can take several weeks to achieve urinary continence. In some instances, control of urine may never be fully regained. Continence can improve for up to 12 months. If continence has not been achieved by that time, the patient may be referred to a continence clinic. A variety of methods, including biofeedback, have been used to achieve positive results.

Teach the patient how to use a penile clamp, a condom catheter, or incontinence pads or briefs to avoid embarrassment from dribbling. In severe cases, an occlusive cuff that serves as an artificial sphincter can be surgically implanted to restore continence. Assist the patient in finding ways to manage the problem that allow him to continue socializing and interacting with others. (Urinary incontinence is discussed in Chapter 45.)

Observe the patient for signs of postoperative infection. If an external wound is present (from an open prostatectomy), assess the area for redness, heat, swelling, and purulent drainage. Special care must be taken if a perineal incision is present because of the proximity of the anus. Avoid rectal procedures, such as taking rectal temperatures and administering enemas. The insertion of well-lubricated belladonna and opium suppositories is acceptable.

Dietary intervention and stool softeners are important in the postoperative period to prevent the patient from straining while having bowel movements. Straining increases the intraabdominal pressure, which can lead to bleeding at the operative site. A diet high in fiber facilitates the passage of stool.

◆ **Ambulatory Care.** Discharge planning and home care issues are important aspects of care after prostate surgery. Patient teaching includes (1) caring for an indwelling catheter (if one is left in place); (2) managing urinary incontinence; (3) maintaining adequate oral fluid intake; (4) observing for signs and symptoms of urinary tract and wound infection; (5) preventing constipation; (6) avoiding heavy lifting (more than 10 lb [4.5 kg]); and (7) refraining from driving or intercourse after surgery as directed by the provider.

The patient may experience a change in sexual function after surgery. Many men experience retrograde ejaculation because of trauma to the internal urethral sphincter. Erectile dysfunction (ED) may occur if the nerves are cut or damaged during surgery. The patient may experience anxiety over the change because of a perceived loss of his sex role, self-esteem, or quality of sexual interaction with his partner. Discuss these changes with the patient and his partner and allow them to ask questions and express their concerns. Sexual counseling and treatment options may be necessary if ED becomes a chronic issue. (ED is discussed later in this chapter on pp. 1286-1288.)

Some patients experience concerns regarding change in sexual function, but this is not a universal concern. Recovery depends on the type of surgery performed and the interval of time between when symptoms first appeared and the date of surgery. It may take up to 1 year for complete sexual function to return.

The bladder may take up to 2 months to return to its normal capacity. Instruct the patient to drink at least 2 to 3 L of fluid per day and urinate every 2 to 3 hours to flush the urinary tract. Teach the patient to avoid or limit the amounts of bladder irritants such as caffeine products, citrus juices, and alcohol. Because the patient may experience incontinence or dribbling, he may incorrectly believe that decreasing fluid intake will relieve this problem.

Urethral strictures may result from instrumentation or catheterization. Treatment may include teaching the patient intermittent clean self-catheterization or having a urethral dilation.

Advise the patient to discuss the need for a yearly DRE with his HCP if he has had any procedure other than complete removal of the prostate. Hyperplasia or cancer can occur in the remaining prostatic tissue.

### ◆ Evaluation

The expected outcomes are that the patient with BPH who has surgery will

- Report satisfactory pain control
- Report improved urinary function with no pain or incontinence

Additional information on expected outcomes for the patient with BPH is presented in eNursing Care Plan 54-1.

## PROSTATE CANCER

**Prostate cancer** is a malignant tumor of the prostate gland. Prostate cancer is the most common cancer among men, excluding skin cancer, and is the second leading cause of cancer death in men (exceeded only by lung cancer). Annually 220,800 men are diagnosed and 27,580 die. Men have a 1 in 7 risk of developing prostate cancer. Almost 2.9 million men in the United States are survivors of prostate cancer.[15]

### Etiology and Pathophysiology

Prostate cancer is slow-growing, androgen-dependent cancer. It can spread by three routes: by direct extension, through the lymph system, or through the bloodstream. Spread by direct extension involves the seminal vesicles, urethral mucosa, bladder wall, and external sphincter. The cancer later spreads through the lymphatic system to the regional lymph nodes. The bloodstream seems to be the mode of spread to the axial skeleton: pelvic bones, head of the femur, lower lumbar spine, and finally liver and lungs.

Age, ethnicity, and family history are known risk factors for prostate cancer. (See the Cultural & Ethnic Health Disparities box.) The incidence of prostate cancer rises markedly after age 50 with a median age at diagnosis of 67 years old.[15] However, many cases occur in younger men who sometimes have a more aggressive type of cancer.

## CULTURAL & ETHNIC HEALTH DISPARITIES

### *Cancers of the Male Reproductive System*

**Prostate Cancer**

- African American men have the highest rate of prostate cancer in the world (except Jamaican men of African descent).
- African American men are diagnosed with prostate cancer at an earlier age, have more advanced disease at the time of diagnosis, and have a higher mortality rate than do white men.
- Although the mortality rate for prostate cancer among African American men is higher than that among whites, the mortality rate is declining.
- Asian American men have a lower incidence and lower mortality rates from prostate cancer than white men.

**Testicular Cancer**

- Testicular cancer occurs more frequently among whites than in other ethnic groups.

The incidence of prostate cancer is higher in African Americans than in any other ethnic group (except Jamaican men of African descent).[15] The reasons for the higher rate are unknown. African American men are likely to have more aggressive tumors at diagnosis and have higher mortality rates from prostate cancer. Differences in survival may be due to body composition, dietary factors, and endogenous hormones. It is not clear if smoking is a risk factor for prostate cancer. Neither is it clear if having BPH increases the risk of developing prostate cancer.[3]

Dietary factors and obesity may be associated with prostate cancer. A diet high in red and processed meat and high-fat dairy products along with a low intake of vegetables and fruits may increase the risk of prostate cancer.[15] Environment may also play a role, as there is an increased prevalence of prostate cancer in farmers and commercial pesticide applicators, possibly due to chemicals found in pesticides.[16]

## Genetic Link

Currently no known single gene causes prostate cancer. Some genes or gene mutations are more common in men with prostate cancer. From a genetics viewpoint, prostate cancer can be classified into three categories.

Most prostate cancers (about 75%) are considered *sporadic,* which means that damage to the genes occurs by chance after a person is born. Prostate cancer that runs in a family, called *familial prostate cancer,* is less common (about 20%). It occurs because of a combination of shared genes and shared environment or lifestyle factors. Familial prostate cancer is when two or more first-degree relatives (father, brother, son) are diagnosed with prostate cancer.

*Hereditary (inherited) prostate cancer* is rare (5% to 10%) and occurs when gene mutations are passed down in a family from one generation to the next. In hereditary prostate cancer, a family has any of the following characteristics: (1) three or more first-degree relatives with prostate cancer, (2) prostate cancer in three generations on the same side of the family, and (3) two or more close relatives (father, brother, son, grandfather, uncle, nephew) on the same side of the family diagnosed with prostate cancer before age 55.

Only genetic testing can determine whether a man has a genetic mutation. However, no genetic tests are available to determine if a man is predisposed to developing prostate cancer.

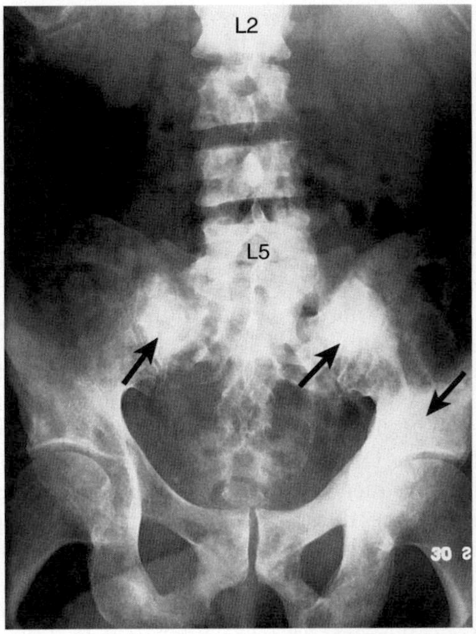


**FIG. 54-5** Metastasis of prostate cancer to the pelvis and lumbar spine indicated by *arrows.* (From Mettler F: *Essentials of radiology,* ed 2, Philadelphia, 2004, Saunders.)

Having a family history does not mean that a man will develop prostate cancer; it indicates that he has an increased risk. Men with a family history of prostate cancer should talk with their HCP about their concerns. It is important for the HCP to obtain a detailed family history, including a family pedigree (see Figs. 12-4 and 12-5). Depending on the findings of the family history, a referral to a genetic counselor may be appropriate.

Hereditary breast and ovarian cancer (HBOC) syndrome is associated with mutations in the *BRCA1* and/or *BRCA2* genes (BRCA stands for *BR*east *CA*ncer). HBOC is most commonly associated with an increased risk of breast and ovarian cancer in women. However, men with HBOC also have an increased risk of breast cancer and prostate cancer. Mutations in *BRCA1* and *BRCA2* cause only a small percentage of familial prostate cancers. Genetic testing may be appropriate for families with prostate cancer that also have HBOC.

## Clinical Manifestations and Complications

Prostate cancer may have no symptoms in the early stages. Eventually the patient may have LUTS similar to those of BPH. Pain in the lumbosacral area that radiates down to the hips or the legs, when combined with urinary symptoms, may indicate metastasis.

The tumor can spread to pelvic lymph nodes, bones, bladder, lungs, and liver. Once the tumor has spread to distant sites, the major problem becomes the management of pain. As the cancer spreads to the bones (common site of metastasis), pain can become severe, especially in the back and legs because of compression of the spinal cord and destruction of bone (Fig. 54-5).

## Diagnostic Studies

Most men in the United States with prostate cancer are diagnosed by PSA screening. As prostate cancer screening has become more widespread, smaller cancers are being found in older men. In most cases, slow-growing cancers probably do not need to be treated. Many men live and die *with* prostate cancer, but most will not die *from* it.

Men have a chance to make an informed decision with their HCP about whether to be screened for prostate cancer. Men should be informed about the potential risks (e.g., subsequent evaluation and treatment that may be unnecessary) and benefits (early detection of prostate cancer) of PSA screening before being tested. After this discussion with their HCP, men who want to be screened may have an annual PSA test and DRE. On DRE, an abnormal prostate may feel hard, nodular, and asymmetric.

The AUA believes that men age 55 to 69 have the greatest potential benefit from PSA screening and recommend screening every 2 years.[14] Men at higher risk (African American men, men with a first-degree relative with prostate cancer) will have an individualized schedule for screening.

The American Cancer Society recommends that men should have a discussion with their HCP about screening for prostate cancer (as mentioned earlier). Men should not be screened unless they have received this information. The discussion about screening should take place at:

- Age 50 for men who are at average risk of prostate cancer and are expected to live at least 10 more years.
- Age 45 for men at high risk of developing prostate cancer. This includes African Americans and men who have a first-degree relative (father, brother, or son) diagnosed with prostate cancer at an early age (younger than age 65).
- Age 40 for men at even higher risk (those with more than one first-degree relative who had prostate cancer at an early age).

Elevated levels of PSA (normal level, 0 to 4 ng/mL [0 to 4 mcg/L]), a glycoprotein produced by the prostate, do not necessarily indicate prostate cancer. Mild elevations in PSA may occur with aging, BPH, recent ejaculation, constipation, acute or chronic prostatitis, or after long bike rides. In addition, cystoscopy, indwelling urethral catheters, and prostate biopsies may also produce transient elevations in PSA levels.

Neither PSA nor DRE is a definitive diagnostic test for prostate cancer. If PSA levels are continually elevated or if the DRE is abnormal, a biopsy of the prostate tissue is usually indicated. Biopsy of prostate tissue is necessary to confirm the diagnosis of prostate cancer. The biopsy is typically done using a transrectal approach. In a transrectal ultrasound (TRUS) procedure, an ultrasound probe enables the urologist to visualize abnormalities where the biopsy needles are going to be placed into the prostate. When a suspicious area is located, biopsy needles are inserted through the wall of the rectum into the prostate to obtain tissue samples. A pathologic examination of the specimen is done to assess for malignant changes.

Another approach for biopsies is to use an MRI/ultrasound fusion biopsy. In this approach, MRIs are fused with real-time, three-dimensional ultrasound. This new technique is more accurate than the traditional approach. Men who are candidates for this procedure are those who have a history of a previous negative ultrasound-guided biopsy and increasing PSA. This approach may also be used for men who are on active surveillance.

PSA is used not only to detect prostate cancer but also to monitor the success of treatment. When treatment has been successful, PSA levels should fall to undetectable levels. The regular measurement of PSA levels after treatment is important to evaluate the effectiveness of treatment and possible recurrence of prostate cancer.[17]

An elevated level of prostatic isoenzyme of serum acid phosphatase (prostatic acid phosphatase [PAP]) is another indicator of prostate cancer, especially if the cancer has spread outside of the prostate. With advanced prostate cancer, serum alkaline phosphatase is increased as a result of bone metastasis.

Other tests used to determine the location and extent of the spread of the cancer may include bone scan, CT scan, and MRI using an endorectal probe.

### Interprofessional Care

Chemoprevention of prostate cancer is an active area of research. As discussed earlier in this chapter, finasteride and dutasteride used to treat BPH may reduce the chance of getting prostate cancer. Men who are concerned about prostate cancer should discuss with their HCP the potential risks and benefits of taking finasteride or dutasteride.

Early recognition and treatment are important to control tumor growth, prevent metastasis, and preserve quality of life. Most patients (93%) with prostate cancer are initially diagnosed when the cancer is at a local or regional stage.[15,18] The 5-year survival rate with an initial diagnosis at this stage is almost 100%.

The most common classification system for determining the extent of the prostate cancer is the tumor, node, and metastasis (TNM) system (Table 54-5). The tumor is graded on the basis of tumor histology using the Gleason scale.[19] The Gleason scale grades the tumor from 1 to 5 based on the degree of glandular differentiation. Grade 1 represents the most well-differentiated or lowest grade (most like the original cells), and grade 5 represents the most poorly differentiated (unlike the original cells) or highest grade. The two most commonly occurring patterns of cells are graded, and then the two scores are added together to create a Gleason score, which ranges from 2 to 10. The PSA level at diagnosis and the patient's Gleason score are used with the TNM system to determine the stage of the tumor, which is vital to determine treatment options.

The interprofessional care of the patient with prostate cancer depends on the stage of the cancer and the patient's overall health. None of these diagnostic options can predict the progression of prostate cancer, but at all stages, there is more than

**TABLE 54-5 Staging of Prostate Cancer**

| Stage | Tumor Size | Lymph Node Involvement | Metastasis | PSA Level | Gleason Score |
|---|---|---|---|---|---|
| I | Not felt on DRE. Not seen by visual imaging. | No | No | <10 | ≤6 |
| II | Felt on DRE. Seen by imaging. Tumor confined to prostate. | No | No | 10-20 | 6-7 |
| III | Cancer outside prostate. Possible spread to seminal vesicles. | No | No | Any level | Any score |
| IV | Any size. | Any nodal involvement. | Yes | Any level | Any score |

*DRE*, Digital rectal examination.
Adapted from American Cancer Society: How is prostate cancer staged? Retrieved from *www.cancer.org/Cancer/ProstateCancer/DetailedGuide/prostate-cancer-staging.*

## TABLE 54-6 Interprofessional Care

### *Prostate Cancer*

**Diagnostic Assessment**
- History and physical examination
- Digital rectal examination (DRE)
- Prostate-specific antigen (PSA)
- Prostatic acid phosphatase (PAP)
- Transrectal ultrasound (TRUS)
- Biopsy of prostate and lymph nodes
- CT scan, MRI
- Bone scan (to evaluate for metastatic disease)

**Management**

***Active Surveillance***
- Annual PSA and DRE

***Surgery***
- Radical prostatectomy
- Cryotherapy
- Orchiectomy (for metastatic disease)

***Radiation Therapy***
- External beam for primary, adjuvant, and recurrent disease
- Brachytherapy

***Drug Therapy***
- Androgen deprivation therapy (Table 54-7)
- Chemotherapy for metastatic disease

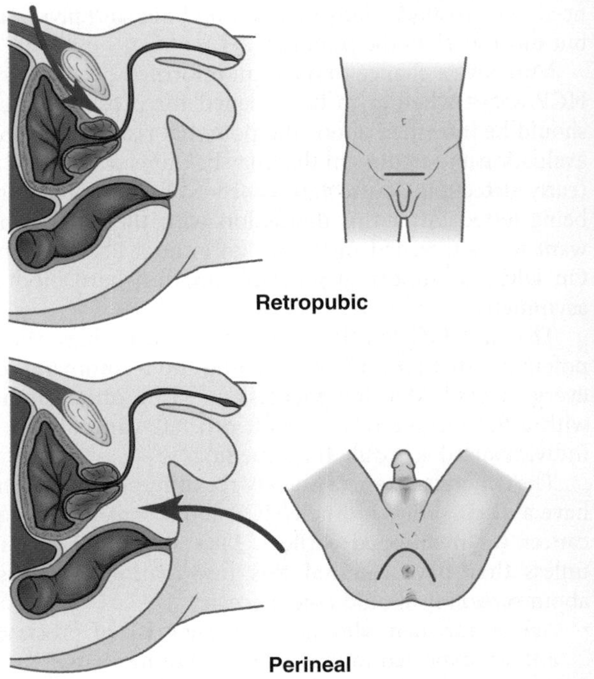


**FIG. 54-6** Common approaches used to perform a prostatectomy. **A,** Retropubic approach involves a midline abdominal incision. **B,** Perineal approach involves an incision between the scrotum and the anus.

one possible treatment option (Table 54-6), depending on the stage, Gleason score, and PSA. The decision of which treatment course to pursue should be made jointly by patients, their partners, and the interprofessional care team.[17,18]

**Active Surveillance.** Prostate cancer is relatively slow growing. Therefore a conservative approach to management of prostate cancer is active surveillance, or "watchful waiting." This strategy is appropriate when the patient has (1) a life expectancy of less than 10 years (low risk of dying of the disease); (2) a low-grade, low-stage tumor; and (3) serious coexisting medical conditions. With active surveillance, patients are typically followed with frequent PSA measurements and DRE to monitor the progress of the disease. Significant changes in the PSA level or the DRE, or the development of symptoms, warrant a reevaluation of treatment options.

**Surgical Therapy**

***Radical Prostatectomy.*** With radical prostatectomy, the entire prostate gland, seminal vesicles, and part of the bladder neck (ampulla) are removed. The entire prostate is removed because the cancer tends to be in many different locations within the gland. Retroperitoneal lymph node dissection is performed only on men with a high risk for metastatic disease. Surgery is usually not considered an option for advanced stage disease (except to relieve symptoms associated with obstruction) because metastasis has already occurred.

Traditional surgical approaches for a radical prostatectomy include retropubic and perineal resection (Fig. 54-6). With the *retropubic* approach, a low midline abdominal incision is made to access the prostate gland, and the pelvic lymph nodes can be dissected. With the *perineal* resection, an incision is made between the scrotum and anus.

A *robotic-assisted* (e.g., da Vinci system) prostatectomy is a type of surgery in which the surgeon sits at a computer console while controlling high-resolution cameras and microsurgical instruments. Robotics is being used more frequently since it allows for increased precision, visualization, and dexterity by the surgeon when removing the prostate gland. It results in less bleeding, less pain, and a faster recovery compared with other approaches.[20,21]

After surgery, the patient has a large indwelling catheter with a 30-mL balloon placed in the bladder via the urethra. A drain is left in the surgical site to aid in the removal of drainage from the area. This drain is typically removed after a couple of days. Because the perineal approach has a higher risk of postoperative infection (because of the location of the incision related to the anus), careful dressing changes and perineal care after each bowel movement are important for comfort and to prevent infection. Depending on the type of surgery, the length of hospital stay postoperatively ranges from 1 to 3 days.

Two major adverse outcomes after a radical prostatectomy are erectile dysfunction (ED) and urinary incontinence.[22] The incidence of ED depends on the patient's age, preoperative sexual function, whether nerve-sparing surgery was performed, and the surgeon's expertise. Sexual function after surgery tends to return gradually over at least 24 months or more, but phosphodiesterase type 5 (PDE5) medications may help improve sexual function.

Problems with urinary control may occur for the first few months after surgery because the bladder must be reattached to the urethra after the prostate is removed. Over time, the bladder adjusts and most men regain control.[22] Kegel exercises strengthen the urinary sphincter and may help improve continence. (Kegel exercises are presented in Table 45-18.) Other complications associated with surgery include hemorrhage, urinary retention, infection, wound dehiscence, deep vein thrombosis, and pulmonary emboli.

***Nerve-Sparing Procedure.*** Near the prostate gland are neurovascular bundles that maintain erectile functioning. The preservation of these bundles during a prostatectomy is possible while still removing all of the cancer. Nerve-sparing prostatectomy is not indicated for patients with cancer outside of the prostate gland. Although the risk of ED is reduced with this procedure, there is no guarantee that potency will be maintained.

***Cryotherapy.*** *Cryotherapy* (cryoablation) is a surgical technique for prostate cancer that destroys cancer cells by freezing the tissue. It has been used both as an initial treatment and as a second-line treatment after radiation therapy has failed. A TRUS probe is inserted to visualize the prostate gland. Probes containing liquid nitrogen are then inserted into the prostate. Liquid nitrogen delivers freezing temperatures, thus destroying the tissue. The treatment takes about 2 hours under general or spinal anesthesia and does not involve an abdominal incision.

Possible complications include damage to the urethra and, in rare cases, an urethrorectal fistula (an opening between the urethra and rectum) or a urethrocutaneous fistula (an opening between the urethra and skin). Tissue sloughing, ED, urinary incontinence, prostatitis, and hemorrhage can also occur.

**Radiation Therapy.** Radiation therapy is another common treatment option for prostate cancer. Radiation therapy may be the only treatment, or it may be used in combination with surgery or with hormone therapy. Salvage radiation therapy given for prostate cancer recurrence after a radical prostatectomy may improve survival in some men.

***External Beam Radiation.*** External beam radiation is the most widely used method of delivering radiation treatments for men with prostate cancer. This therapy can be used to treat patients with prostate cancer confined to the prostate and/or surrounding tissue. Patients are usually treated on an outpatient basis 5 days a week for 4 to 8 weeks; each treatment lasts only a few minutes.

Side effects from radiation can be acute (occurring during treatment or within 90 days that follow) or delayed (occurring months or years after treatment). The most common side effects involve changes to the skin (dryness, redness, irritation, pain), gastrointestinal tract (diarrhea, abdominal cramping, bleeding, radiation proctitis), urinary tract (dysuria, frequency, hesitancy, urgency, nocturia), and sexual function.[23,24] Fatigue may also occur. In patients with localized prostate cancer, cure rates with external beam radiation are comparable to those with radical prostatectomy.[15]

***Brachytherapy.*** *Brachytherapy* involves placing radioactive seed implants into the prostate gland, allowing higher radiation doses directly in the tissue while sparing the surrounding tissue (rectum and bladder). The radioactive seeds are placed in the prostate gland with a needle through a grid template guided by TRUS (Fig. 54-7) to ensure accurate placement of the seeds.

Because brachytherapy is a one-time outpatient procedure, many patients find this more convenient than external beam radiation treatment. Brachytherapy is best suited for patients with early stage disease. The most common side effect is the development of urinary irritative or obstructive problems. Some men may also experience ED. The AUA Symptom Index (Table 54-1) can be used to measure urinary function for patients undergoing brachytherapy and can be incorporated into postoperative nursing management. For those with more advanced tumors, brachytherapy may be offered in combination with external beam radiation treatment.[24] (Brachytherapy is further discussed in Chapter 15.)

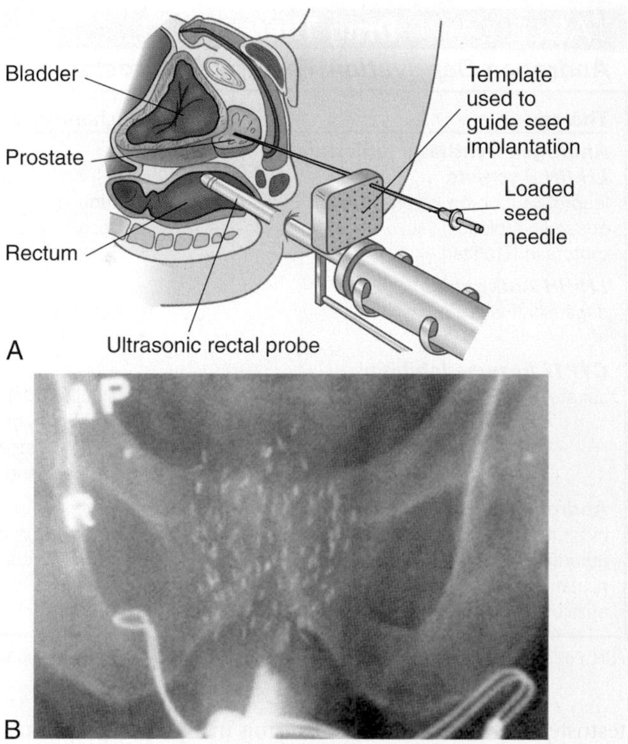


**FIG. 54-7** **A,** Prostate brachytherapy. Implantation of radioactive seeds with a needle guided by ultrasound and a template grid. **B,** Radioactive seeds. (*B,* From Abeloff MD, Armitage JO, Niederhuber JE, et al, editors: *Abeloff's clinical oncology,* ed 4, 2008, Churchill Livingstone.)

**Drug Therapy.** The forms of drug therapy available for the treatment of advanced or metastatic prostate cancer are androgen deprivation (hormone) therapy, chemotherapy, or a combination of both.

***Androgen Deprivation Therapy.*** Prostate cancer growth is largely dependent on the presence of androgens. *Androgen deprivation therapy* (ADT) reduces the levels of circulating androgens to reduce the tumor growth. Androgen deprivation can be produced by inhibiting androgen production or blocking androgen receptors (Table 54-7).

One of the biggest challenges with ADT is that almost all tumors treated become resistant to this therapy *(hormone refractory)* within a few years. An elevated PSA level is often the first sign that this therapy is no longer effective. Patients taking ADT have an increased risk of cardiovascular side effects, including elevated serum cholesterol and triglyceride levels and coronary artery disease.[25]

Osteoporosis and fractures may occur in prostate cancer patients receiving ADT. Drugs recommended to reduce bone mineral loss in these patients include zoledronic acid (Reclast) and raloxifene (Evista).[26] Denosumab (Prolia), a drug that slows the breakdown of bone, may also be used to increase bone mass in men with nonmetastatic prostate cancer.

**Androgen synthesis inhibitors.** The hypothalamus produces luteinizing hormone–releasing hormone (LH-RH), which stimulates the anterior pituitary to produce luteinizing hormone (LH) and follicle-stimulating hormone (FSH). LH stimulates the testicular Leydig cells to produce testosterone. *LH-RH agonists* super stimulate the pituitary, downregulating the LH-RH receptors, and leading to a refractory condition in which the anterior pituitary is unresponsive to LH-RH. These drugs cause an initial transient increase in LH and FSH;

TABLE 54-7 **Drug Therapy**

***Androgen Deprivation Therapy for Prostate Cancer***

| Therapy | Mechanism of Action | Side Effects |
|---|---|---|
| **Androgen Synthesis Inhibitors** | | |
| ***LH-RH Agonists*** | | |
| leuprolide (Lupron, Lupron Depot, Eligard)<br>goserelin (Zoladex)<br>triptorelin (Trelstar) | • Reduce secretion of LH and FSH<br>• Decrease testosterone production | • Hot flashes, gynecomastia, decreased libido, erectile dysfunction<br>• Depression and mood changes |
| ***LH-RH Antagonist*** | | |
| degarelix (Firmagon) | • Blocks LH receptors<br>• Immediate testosterone suppression | • Pain, redness, and swelling at injection site<br>• Elevated liver enzymes |
| ***CYP17 Enzyme Inhibitor*** | | |
| abiraterone (Zytiga) | • Inhibits CYP17, an enzyme needed for production of testosterone<br>• Inhibits testosterone synthesis from testes, adrenal glands, and prostate cancer cells | • Joint swelling, fluid retention<br>• Muscle discomfort<br>• Hot flashes<br>• Diarrhea |
| **Androgen Receptor Blockers** | | |
| bicalutamide (Casodex)<br>flutamide<br>nilutamide (Nilandron)<br>enzalutamide (Xtandi) | • Block action of testosterone by competing with receptor sites | • Loss of libido, erectile dysfunction, and hot flashes<br>• Breast pain and gynecomastia may also occur |

*FSH,* Follicle-stimulating hormone; *LH,* luteinizing hormone; *LH-RH,* luteinizing hormone–releasing hormone.

testosterone abruptly rises resulting in a *flare.* Symptoms may worsen during this time. However, with continued administration, LH and testosterone levels are decreased.

LH-RH agonists include leuprolide (Lupron, Lupron Depot, Eligard), goserelin (Zoladex), and triptorelin (Trelstar) (Table 54-7). These drugs essentially produce a chemical castration similar to the effects of an orchiectomy. These drugs are given by subcutaneous or IM injections on a regular basis. Viadur is an implant that is placed subcutaneously and delivers leuprolide continuously for 1 year.

Degarelix is an *LH-RH antagonist* that lowers testosterone levels to castration levels. Unlike the LH-RH agonists, degarelix does not cause a testosterone flare because it acts directly to block LH and FSH receptors. It is given as a subcutaneous injection, and results are seen in 3 days.

Abiraterone (Zytiga) works by inhibiting an enzyme, CYP17, which is needed for the production of testosterone. This drug is given orally to men with castration-resistant prostate cancer, and improves overall survival by 4 to 5 months.

**Androgen receptor blockers.** Androgen receptor blockers are another classification of antiandrogen drugs that compete with circulating androgens at the receptor sites. Flutamide, nilutamide (Nilandron), bicalutamide (Casodex), and enzalutamide (Xtandi) are androgen receptor blockers. They are taken daily as an oral medication and can be used in combination with an LH-RH agonist (e.g., goserelin, leuprolide). Combining an androgen receptor blocker with an LH-RH agonist results in combined androgen blockade.

***Chemotherapy.*** The use of chemotherapy has primarily been limited to treatment for those with hormone-refractory prostate cancer (HRPC) in late-stage disease. In HRPC the cancer is progressing despite treatment. This occurs in patients who have taken an antiandrogen for a certain period. The goal of chemotherapy is mainly palliative.

Some commonly used chemotherapy drugs for prostate cancer include docetaxel (Taxotere), cabazitaxel (Jevtana), paclitaxel (Abraxane), mitoxantrone, vinblastine, cyclophosphamide, and estramustine (Emcyt).

Men with advanced prostate cancer who have HRPC may receive a vaccine (sipuleucel-T [Provenge]). The vaccine stimulates the patient's system against the cancer and may prolong survival, although its exact mechanism is unknown. It prolongs survival by about 4 months but does not reduce tumor burden. It is individually prepared for each man by a process that combines his own white blood cells with granulocyte macrophage colony-stimulating factor (GMCSF), which then attacks the prostate tumor cells.

***Radiotherapy.*** Radium-223 dichloride (Xofigo) can be used in the treatment of patients with castration-resistant prostate cancer, symptomatic bone metastases, and no known visceral metastatic disease. It is an alpha particle–emitting radiotherapy drug that mimics calcium and forms complexes with hydroxyapatite at areas of increased bone turnover, such as bone metastases.

***Orchiectomy.*** A bilateral orchiectomy is the surgical removal of the testes that may be done alone or after prostatectomy. It is the gold standard for androgen deprivation, as there are no side effects to be managed, and it is very low cost when compared with other options. For advanced stages of prostate cancer, an orchiectomy is one treatment option for cancer control, with rapid relief of bone pain associated with advanced tumors.

Orchiectomy may also shrink the prostate, thus relieving urinary obstruction in the later stages of disease when surgery is not an option. After an orchiectomy, weight gain and loss of muscle mass can alter a man's physical appearance. These physical changes can affect self-esteem, leading to grief and depression. Because this procedure is permanent, many men prefer drug therapy over an orchiectomy. Currently orchiectomy is rarely performed.

## Culturally Competent Care: Prostate Cancer

Nurses need to be aware of ethnic and cultural considerations when providing information about the risk for prostate cancer and screening recommendations. Consider not only the ethnic differences in the incidence of prostate cancer but also differences in health promotion practices.

African American men have the highest mortality rates from prostate cancer, in part because their prostate cancer often is more advanced at the time of diagnosis. Despite the availability of screening measures (PSA and DRE), African American men and those in lower socioeconomic groups may not access these services. This is only partially related to knowledge levels about prostate cancer. In comparison to white men, African American men with prostate cancer report more problems with financial access to transportation and health care costs, and they indicate using more religious coping strategies. White men are also perceived as receiving more favorable treatment from their HCPs than African Americans.[27]

Although exposure to electronic and print media is successful in informing some men about prostate cancer, the effectiveness differs significantly based on demographic variables such as ethnicity, age, education level, and socioeconomic level. Ideally, all men should be aware of the risks associated with prostate cancer and the screening methods available. Consider the best method to communicate this information to men of all cultures and ethnicities, while being aware of the changing guidelines, to promote understanding and participation in prostate cancer screening for men in at risk groups.

## NURSING MANAGEMENT: PROSTATE CANCER

### Nursing Assessment

Subjective and objective data that should be obtained from a patient with prostate cancer are presented in Table 54-8.

**TABLE 54-8 Nursing Assessment**
***Prostate Cancer***

**Subjective Data**

***Important Health Information***

*Medications:* Testosterone supplements. Use of any medications affecting urinary tract such as morphine, anticholinergics, monoamine oxidase inhibitors, and tricyclic antidepressants

***Functional Health Patterns***

*Health perception–health management:* Positive family history. Increasing fatigue and malaise

*Nutritional-metabolic:* High-fat diet. Anorexia, weight loss (possible indicators of metastasis)

*Elimination:* Hesitancy or straining to start stream, urinary urgency, frequency, retention with dribbling, weak stream, hematuria

*Sleep-rest:* Nocturia

*Cognitive-perceptual:* Dysuria. Low back pain radiating to legs or pelvis, bone pain (possible indicators of metastasis). Pain level

*Self-perception–self-concept:* Anxiety regarding self-concept

**Objective Data**

***General***

Older adult male. Pelvic lymphadenopathy (late sign)

***Urinary***

Distended bladder on palpation. Unilaterally hard, enlarged, fixed prostate on rectal examination

***Musculoskeletal***

Pathologic fractures (metastasis)

***Possible Diagnostic Findings***

Serum PSA. ↑ serum PAP (metastasis). Nodular and irregular prostate on ultrasonography, positive biopsy results. Anemia

*PAP,* Prostatic acid phosphatase; *PSA,* prostate-specific antigen.

### Nursing Diagnoses

Nursing diagnoses for the patient with prostate cancer depend on the stage of the cancer. General nursing diagnoses may include, but are not limited to, the following.

- Decisional conflict *related to* numerous alternative treatment options
- Acute pain *related to* surgery, prostatic enlargement, bone metastasis, and bladder spasms
- Urinary retention and impaired urinary elimination *related to* obstruction of the urethra by the prostate and loss of bladder tone
- Sexual dysfunction *related to* effects of treatment
- Anxiety *related to* uncertain outcome of disease process on life and lifestyle and effect of treatment on sexual function

### Planning

The overall goals are that the patient with prostate cancer will (1) be an active participant in the treatment plan, (2) have satisfactory pain control, (3) follow the therapeutic plan, (4) understand the effect of the therapeutic plan on sexual function, and (5) find a satisfactory way to manage the impact on bladder and bowel function.

### Nursing Implementation

**Health Promotion.** One of the most important roles in relation to prostate cancer is to encourage patients, in consultation with their HCPs, to have annual prostate screening (PSA and DRE). (The age at which to begin screening is discussed on pp. 1276-1277.) Because of their increased risk of prostate cancer, African American men and other men at high risk, such as those with a family history of prostate cancer, should discuss the need for annual PSA and DRE beginning at age 45.[15]

**Acute Care.** Preoperative and postoperative phases of radical prostatectomy are similar to surgical procedures for BPH (see pp. 1273-1275). Nursing interventions for the patient who undergoes radiation therapy and chemotherapy are discussed in Chapter 15. An additional consideration is the patient's psychologic response to a diagnosis of cancer. Provide sensitive, caring support for the patient and his family to help them cope with the diagnosis. Prostate cancer support groups are available for men and their families to encourage them to be active, informed participants in their own care.

**Ambulatory Care.** Teach appropriate catheter care if the patient is discharged with an indwelling catheter in place. Instruct the patient to clean the urethral meatus with soap and water once a day; maintain a high fluid intake; keep the collecting bag lower than the bladder at all times; keep the catheter securely anchored to the inner thigh or abdomen; and report any signs of bladder infection, such as bladder spasms, fever, or hematuria.

If urinary incontinence is a problem, encourage the patient to practice pelvic floor muscle exercises (Kegel exercises) at every urination and throughout the day. Continuous practice during the 4- to 6-week healing process improves the success rate. Products used for incontinence specifically designed for men are available through home care product catalogs and retail stores. (Urinary incontinence is discussed in Chapter 45.)

Palliative and end-of-life care are often appropriate and beneficial to the patient with advanced disease and his family (see

Chapter 9). Common problems experienced by the patient with advanced prostate cancer include fatigue, bladder outlet obstruction and ureteral obstruction (caused by compression of the urethra and/or ureters from tumor mass or lymph node metastasis), severe bone pain and fractures (caused by bone metastasis), spinal cord compression (from spinal metastasis), and leg edema (caused by lymphedema, deep vein thrombosis, and other medical conditions). Nursing interventions must focus on all of these problems.

Pain management is one of the most important aspects of your care for these patients. Pain control involves ongoing pain assessment, administration of prescribed medications (both opioid and nonopioid agents), and nonpharmacologic methods of pain relief (e.g., relaxation breathing). (Pain management is further discussed in Chapter 8.)

### ◆ Evaluation

The outcomes are that the patient with prostate cancer will

- Be an active participant in the treatment plan
- Have satisfactory pain control
- Follow the therapeutic plan
- Understand the effect of the treatment on sexual function
- Find a satisfactory way to manage the impact on bladder or bowel function

## PROSTATITIS

### Etiology and Pathophysiology

**Prostatitis** is a broad term that describes a group of inflammatory and noninflammatory conditions affecting the prostate gland. Prostatitis is one of the most common urologic disorders. It is estimated that 12% of all men experience prostatitis in their lifetime.[28] Almost 2 million men are treated for prostatitis every year, and the most common type is nonbacterial.

The four categories of prostatitis syndromes are: (1) acute bacterial prostatitis, (2) chronic bacterial prostatitis, (3) chronic prostatitis/chronic pelvic pain syndrome, and (4) asymptomatic inflammatory prostatitis.

Both acute and chronic bacterial prostatitis generally result from organisms reaching the prostate gland by one of the following routes: ascending from the urethra, descending from the bladder, and invading via the bloodstream or the lymphatic channels. Common causative organisms are *Escherichia coli* (most common), *Klebsiella, Pseudomonas, Enterobacter, Proteus, Chlamydia trachomatis, Neisseria gonorrhoeae,* and group D streptococci.

Chronic bacterial prostatitis differs from acute prostatitis in that it involves recurrent episodes of infection. It is the most common reason for recurrent UTIs in adult men.

*Chronic prostatitis/chronic pelvic pain syndrome* describes a syndrome of prostate and urinary pain in the absence of an obvious infectious process. The etiology of this syndrome is not known. It may occur after a viral illness, or it may be associated with sexually transmitted infections (STIs), particularly in younger adults. A culture reveals no causative organisms, but leukocytes may be found in prostatic secretions.

*Asymptomatic inflammatory prostatitis* is usually diagnosed in individuals who have no symptoms but are found to have an inflammatory process in the prostate. These patients are usually diagnosed during the evaluation of other genitourinary tract problems. Leukocytes are present in the seminal fluid from the prostate, but the cause of this process is unclear.

### Clinical Manifestations and Complications

Common manifestations of acute prostatitis include fever, chills, back pain, and perineal pain. In addition, acute urinary symptoms such as dysuria, urinary frequency, urgency, and cloudy urine may occur. The patient may progress to acute urinary retention caused by prostatic swelling if he remains untreated. With DRE, the prostate is extremely swollen, extremely tender, and boggy.

The complications of prostatitis are epididymitis and cystitis. Sexual function may be affected as manifested by postejaculation pain, libido problems, and ED. Prostatic abscess is also a potential, but uncommon, complication.

In chronic bacterial prostatitis and chronic prostatitis/chronic pelvic pain syndrome, manifestations are similar but generally milder than those of acute bacterial prostatitis. These include irritative voiding symptoms (frequency, urgency, dysuria), backache, perineal and pelvic pain, and ejaculatory pain. Obstructive symptoms are uncommon unless there is coexisting BPH.[29] With DRE, the prostate feels enlarged and soft or boggy and can be slightly tender with palpation. Chronic prostatitis can predispose the patient to recurrent UTIs.

The clinical features of prostatitis can mimic those of a UTI. However, it is important to remember that acute cystitis is not common in men.

### Diagnostic Studies

Because patients with prostatitis have urinary symptoms, a urinalysis (UA) and urine culture are indicated. Often WBCs and bacteria are present. If the patient has a fever, WBC count and blood cultures are also indicated. The PSA test may be done to rule out prostate cancer. However, PSA levels are often elevated with prostatic inflammation. Thus it is not in itself considered diagnostic.

Microscopic evaluation and culture of expressed prostate secretion can be useful in the diagnosis of prostatitis. Expressed prostate secretion is obtained using a premassage and postmassage test.[29] The patient is asked to void into a specimen cup just before and just after a vigorous prostate massage. Prostatic massage (for expressed prostate secretion) should be avoided if acute bacterial prostatitis is suspected, since compression is extremely painful and can increase the risk of bacterial spread. TRUS has not been useful in the diagnosis of prostatitis. However, TRUS or MRI may be done to rule out an abscess in the prostate.

## ❖ NURSING AND INTERPROFESSIONAL MANAGEMENT: PROSTATITIS

Antibiotics commonly used for acute and chronic bacterial prostatitis include trimethoprim/sulfamethoxazole (Bactrim), ciprofloxacin (Cipro), ofloxacin, carbachol (Miostat), carbenicillin, cephalexin (Keflex), and doxycycline (Vibramycin) or tetracycline. Antibiotics are usually given orally for up to 4 weeks for acute bacterial prostatitis. However, if the patient has high fever or other signs of impending sepsis, he will be hospitalized and IV antibiotics given.

Men with chronic bacterial prostatitis may be given oral antibiotic therapy for 8 to 12 weeks. Antibiotics may be given for a lifetime if the patient is immunocompromised. A short course of oral antibiotics is usually prescribed for those with chronic prostatitis/chronic pelvic pain syndrome in case of bacterial infection. However, antibiotic therapy is often ineffective for patients whose prostatitis is not due to bacteria.

Although patients with acute and chronic bacterial prostatitis tend to experience a great amount of discomfort, the pain resolves as the infection is treated. However, they may have residual discomfort for several weeks after a course of antibiotics, as it takes time for the prostate to return to normal. Pain management for patients with chronic prostatitis/chronic pelvic pain syndrome is more difficult because the pain persists for weeks to months. No single approach has been shown to provide relief for everyone with this condition. Antiinflammatory agents (e.g., ibuprofen, indomethacin) may be used for pain control in prostatitis, but these drugs provide only moderate pain relief.

Warm sitz baths may help to relieve pain. Relaxation of muscle tissue in the prostate using α-adrenergic blockers (e.g., tamsulosin, alfuzosin) has been shown to be effective in reducing discomfort for some men.

Acute urinary retention can develop in acute prostatitis, requiring insertion of a urinary catheter. However, passage of a catheter through an inflamed urethra is contraindicated in acute prostatitis. The placement of a suprapubic catheter may then be indicated. Repetitive prostatic massage may be recommended as adjunct therapy for prostatitis for men. This potentially relieves congestion within the prostate by squeezing out excess prostatic secretions, providing pain relief. Similar to massage, measures to stimulate ejaculation (masturbation and intercourse) may help to drain the prostate and provide some relief.

Because the prostate can serve as a source of bacteria, fluid intake should be kept at a high level for all patients experiencing prostatitis. Encourage the patient to drink plenty of fluids, especially men with acute bacterial prostatitis because of the increased fluid needs associated with fever and infection. Management of fever is also an important nursing intervention.

## PROBLEMS OF THE PENIS

Health problems of the penis are rare if STIs are excluded (see Chapter 52). Problems of the penis may be classified as congenital, problems of the prepuce, problems with the erectile mechanism, and cancer.

### CONGENITAL PROBLEMS

*Hypospadias* is a urologic abnormality in which the urethral meatus is located on the ventral surface of the penis anywhere from the corona to the perineum. Possible causes are hormonal influences in utero, environmental factors, and genetic factors. Surgical repair of hypospadias, especially those that are closest to the scrotum or perineum, is usually done while the boy is young. Surgery may be necessary if it is associated with *chordee* (a painful downward curvature of the penis during erection) or if it prevents intercourse or normal urination. Surgery may be considered for cosmetic reasons or emotional well-being in older boys and adult men.

### PROBLEMS OF PREPUCE

Problems of the prepuce (foreskin) in the United States are not common because circumcision (surgical removal of the foreskin of the penis) has been a routine procedure for many male infants.

**Phimosis** is a tightness or constriction of the foreskin around the head of the penis, making retraction difficult (Fig. 54-8, *A*). It is caused by chronic inflammation of the foreskin, usually associated with poor hygiene techniques that allow bacterial and yeast organisms to become trapped under the foreskin. Topical corticosteroid cream, with or without an antifungal, applied two or three times daily to the exterior and interior of the tip of the foreskin may be effective in the initial treatment of any inflammation. Definitive treatment is either circumcision or a dorsal slit surgical procedure.

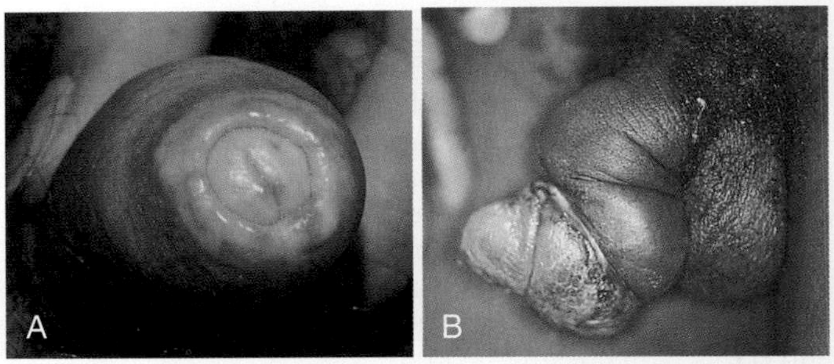


**FIG. 54-8** **A,** Phimosis: inability to retract the foreskin due to secondary lesions on the prepuce. **B,** Paraphimosis: ulcer with edema from foreskin remaining contracted over the prepuce (foreskin).

**Paraphimosis** is tightness of the foreskin resulting in the inability to pull it forward from a retracted position and preventing normal return over the glans. It is a urologic emergency, as a sufficiently tight retracted phimotic ring will compromise arterial flow to the glans. An ulcer can develop if the foreskin remains contracted (Fig. 54-8, *B*). Paraphimosis can occur when the foreskin is pulled back during bathing, use of urinary catheters, or intercourse and is not placed back in the forward position. Replacement of the foreskin after careful cleaning helps to prevent this condition. The goal of treatment is to return the foreskin to its natural position over the glans penis through manual reduction. One strategy involves pushing the glans back through the prepuce by applying constant thumb pressure while the index fingers pull the prepuce over the glans. Ice and/or hand compression on the foreskin, glans, and penis may be done before this technique to reduce edema. Treatment may include antibiotics or warm soaks. Definitive treatment is either circumcision or a dorsal slit.

### PROBLEMS OF ERECTILE MECHANISM

*Priapism* is a painful erection lasting longer than 6 hours that may constitute a medical emergency. Priapism is caused by complex vascular and neurologic factors that result in an obstruction of venous outflow in the penis. Conditions that may be associated with priapism include sickle cell disease, diabetes mellitus, trauma to the spinal cord, degenerative lesions of the spine, and drugs (e.g., cocaine, trazodone). Vasoactive drugs (e.g., alprostadil) injected into the corpora cavernosa for ED can also cause priapism. Complications include penile tissue necrosis caused by lack of blood flow or hydronephrosis from bladder distention. With immediate medical treatment, the risk of permanent ED is low.

Treatment varies depending on the cause. In patients with sickle cell disease, a blood exchange transfusion may be done, whereas other patients may be treated with sedatives, an injection of a smooth muscle relaxant directly into the penis, or aspiration and irrigation of the corpora cavernosa with a large-bore needle.

*Peyronie's disease* is caused by plaque formation in one of the corpora cavernosa of the penis that results in inelasticity during erection. The palpable, nontender, hard plaque formation may occur spontaneously or result from trauma to the penile shaft. The plaque prevents adequate blood flow into the spongy tissue, which results in a curvature during erection. The condition is not dangerous but can result in painful erections, ED, or embarrassment. Patients may improve slightly over time, stabilize, or need surgery. Collagenase clostridium histolyticum (Xiaflex) is a series of injections into the plaque that can reduce the curvature over the course of the injections and allows men to avoid surgery.

## CANCER OF PENIS

Cancer of the penis is rare in the United States. More than 95% are squamous cell carcinoma. It occurs more commonly in men who have human papillomavirus (HPV) infection and phimosis or uncircumcised men.[30] The tumor may appear as a superficial ulceration or a pimple-like nodule. Pain is not a usual complaint, and this contributes to a delay in seeking treatment. The nontender warty lesion may be mistaken for a genital wart. Treatment in the early stages is laser removal of the growth. A radical resection of the penis may be done if the cancer has spread. Surgery, radiation, or chemotherapy may be attempted, depending on the extent of the disease, lymph node involvement, or metastasis.

# PROBLEMS OF SCROTUM AND TESTES

It is important for the patient to see his HCP if he feels any scrotal lumps or painful areas in his scrotum or testes. He would be unable to distinguish normal variations from cancer when performing self-examination, and an incidental finding of a "scrotal lump" results in high anxiety for the patient.

## INFLAMMATORY AND INFECTIOUS PROBLEMS

### Skin Problems

The skin of the scrotum is susceptible to a number of common skin diseases. The most common are fungal infections, dermatitis (neurodermatitis, contact dermatitis, seborrheic dermatitis), and parasitic infections (scabies, lice). These conditions involve discomfort for the patient but are associated with few severe complications (see Chapter 23).

### Epididymitis

**Epididymitis** is an acute, painful inflammatory process of the epididymis (Fig. 54-9), which is often due to an infectious process, trauma, or urinary reflux down the ductus (vas) deferens. It is usually unilateral. Swelling may progress to the point that the epididymis and testis are indistinguishable. In men younger than 35 years of age, the most common cause is gonorrhea or chlamydial infection; in men greater than 35 the most common cause is *E. coli*. BPH and prostatitis are common contributors in older men.

The use of antibiotics is important for both partners if the transmission is through sexual contact. Encourage patients to refrain from sexual intercourse until treatment is complete. If they do engage in intercourse, a condom should be used. Conservative treatment consists of elevation of the scrotum, ice packs, and analgesics. Ambulation places the scrotum in a dependent position and increases pain. Acute tenderness subsides within 1 week, although some discomfort and swelling may last for weeks or months.

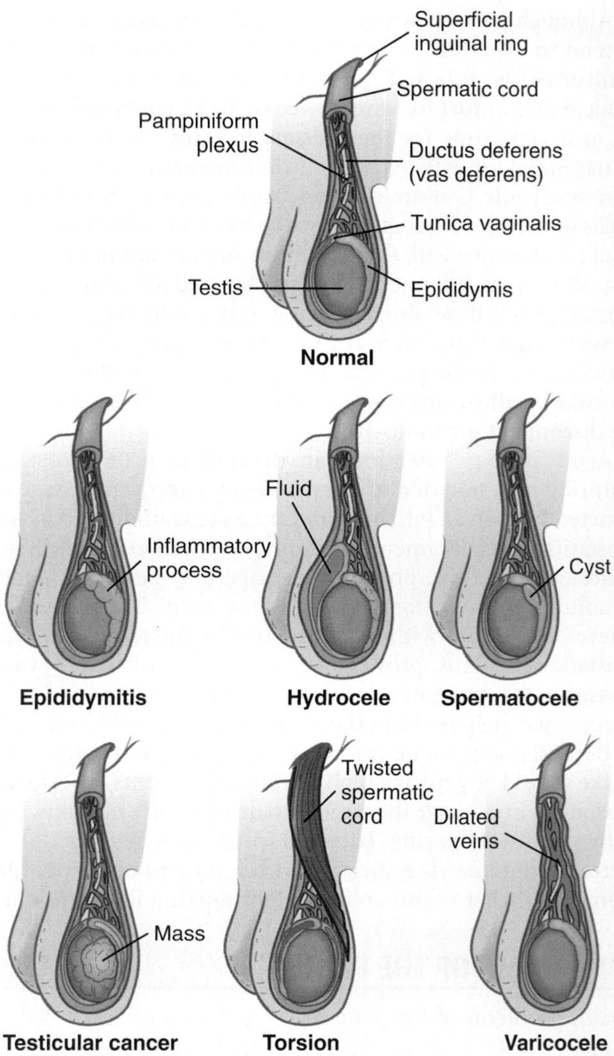


**FIG. 54-9** Scrotal masses.

### Orchitis

**Orchitis** refers to an acute inflammation of the testis. In orchitis, the testis is painful, tender, and swollen. It generally occurs after an episode of bacterial or viral infection such as mumps, pneumonia, tuberculosis, or syphilis. It can also be a side effect of epididymitis, trauma, infectious mononucleosis, influenza, catheterization, or complicated UTI. Mumps orchitis is a condition contributing to infertility that could be avoided by childhood vaccination against mumps. Treatment is similar to that for epididymitis.

## CONGENITAL PROBLEMS

*Cryptorchidism* (undescended testes) is failure of the testes to descend into the scrotal sac before birth. It is the most common congenital testicular condition and is more common on the right. It may occur bilaterally or unilaterally and may be a contributing factor to male infertility if corrective surgery is not done by 2 years of age. The incidence of testicular cancer is also higher if the condition is not corrected before puberty. Surgery is performed to locate and suture the testis or testes to the scrotum.

## ACQUIRED PROBLEMS

### Hydrocele

A *hydrocele* is a nontender, fluid-filled mass that results from interference with lymphatic drainage of the scrotum and swelling of the tunica vaginalis that surrounds the testis (Fig. 54-10; also Fig. 54-9). Diagnosis is aided by shining a flashlight through the scrotum (transillumination). No treatment is indicated unless the swelling becomes large and uncomfortable, in which case surgical repair of the hydrocele is performed. Hydrocele repair is avoided in men who have not started their family or seek to add to their family as repair can contribute to subfertility or infertility.

### Spermatocele

A *spermatocele* is a firm, sperm-containing cyst of the epididymis that may be visible with transillumination (Fig. 54-9). The cause is unknown, and these structures can become large, tense and painful, and their size can wax and wane with time. Spermatocele repair is also avoided in men who have not started their family or seek to add to their family as repair can contribute to subfertility or infertility.

### Varicocele

A *varicocele* is a dilation of the veins that drain the testes (Fig. 54-9). The scrotum can feel wormlike when palpated if the venous dilation is significant. However, this is dependent on the examiner's experience and skill. The cause of the problem is unknown.

A varicocele is usually located on the left side of the scrotum as a consequence of retrograde blood flow from the left renal vein. Surgery can be considered if the patient is infertile, as varicoceles are associated with 40% to 50% of cases of infertility. Sperm is thought to be damaged by varicoceles via an undetermined mechanism. Repair of the varicocele may be through injection of a sclerosing agent or by surgical ligation of the spermatic vein. Untreated varicoceles are not associated with any long-term health risk.

### Testicular Torsion

**Testicular torsion** involves a twisting of the spermatic cord that supplies blood to the testes and epididymis (Fig. 54-9). It is considered a surgical emergency. It is most commonly seen in males younger than age 20. It can occur spontaneously, as a result of trauma, or as a result of an anatomic abnormality. The patient experiences severe, sudden onset of scrotal pain, tenderness, swelling, nausea, and vomiting. Urinary symptoms, fever, and WBCs or bacteria in the urine are absent. The pain does not usually subside with rest or elevation of the scrotum.

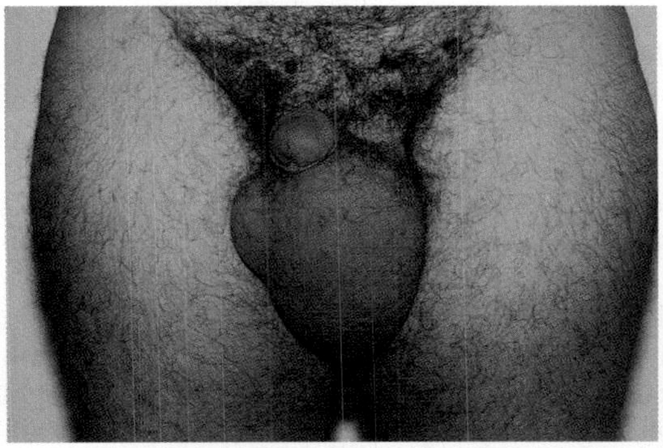

**FIG. 54-10** Hydrocele. (From Swartz MH: *Textbook of physical diagnosis*, ed 6, Philadelphia, 2010, Saunders.)

In testicular torsion, the cremasteric reflex is absent on the side of the swelling. Normal anatomic landmarks are lost due to tissue edema.

A nuclear scan of the testes or Doppler ultrasound is typically performed to assess blood flow within the testicle. Decreased or absent blood flow confirms the diagnosis. Torsion is an emergency if the blood supply to the affected testicle is not restored within 4 to 6 hours. Ischemia to the testis will occur, leading to necrosis. Unless the torsion resolves spontaneously, surgery to untwist the cord and restore the blood supply must be performed emergently.

## TESTICULAR CANCER

### Etiology and Pathophysiology

**Testicular cancer** is rare, accounting for less than 1% of all cancers found in males. It is the most common type of cancer in young men between 15 and 44 years of age. In the United States about 8430 new cases occur annually with a median age at diagnosis of 33 years old.[15,31]

Testicular tumors are more common in males who have had undescended testes (cryptorchidism) or a family history of testicular cancer or anomalies. Other predisposing factors include orchitis, human immunodeficiency virus (HIV) infection, maternal exposure to exogenous estrogen, and testicular cancer in the contralateral (other) testis.

Most testicular cancers develop from two types of embryonic germ cells: seminomas and nonseminomas. Although seminoma germ cell cancers are the most common, they are the least aggressive. Nonseminoma testicular germ cell tumors are rare but very aggressive. Non–germ cell tumors arise from other testicular tissue and include Leydig cell and Sertoli cell tumors. These account for less than 10% of testicular cancers.

### Clinical Manifestations and Complications

Testicular cancer may have a slow or rapid onset depending on the type of tumor (Fig. 54-9). The patient may notice a painless lump in his scrotum, scrotal swelling, and a feeling of heaviness. The scrotal mass usually is nontender and firm. Some patients complain of a dull ache or heavy sensation in the lower abdomen, perianal area, or scrotum. Acute pain is the initial symptom in about 10% of patients. Manifestations associated with advanced disease are varied and include lower back or chest pain, cough, and dyspnea.

### Diagnostic Studies

Palpation of the scrotal contents is the first step in diagnosing testicular cancer. A cancerous mass is firm and does not transilluminate. Ultrasound of the testes is indicated whenever testicular cancer is suspected (e.g., palpable mass) or when persistent or painful testicular swelling is present. If a testicular neoplasm is suspected, blood is obtained to determine the serum levels of α-fetoprotein (AFP), lactate dehydrogenase (LDH), and human chorionic gonadotropin (hCG).[32] (The tumor markers AFP and hCG are discussed in Chapter 15.)

A chest x-ray and CT scan of the abdomen and pelvis are done to detect metastasis. Anemia may be present, and liver function levels may be elevated in metastatic disease.

## ❖ NURSING AND INTERPROFESSIONAL MANAGEMENT: TESTICULAR CANCER

Testicular cancer is one of the most curable types of cancer. Interprofessional care generally involves a radical orchiectomy (surgical removal of the affected testis, spermatic cord, and regional lymph nodes). Some patients with early stage disease do not need further treatment after an orchiectomy. Retroperitoneal lymph node dissection and removal may also be done in early stage disease. These nodes are the primary route for metastasis.

Postorchiectomy treatment may also involve surveillance, radiation therapy, or chemotherapy, depending on the stage of the cancer. Radiation therapy is mainly used for patients with a seminoma, which is very sensitive to radiation. Radiation does not work well for nonseminomas.

Testicular germ cell tumors are more sensitive to systemic chemotherapy than any other adult solid tumor. Chemotherapy protocols use a combination of agents, including bleomycin, etoposide, ifosfamide (Ifex), and cisplatin. Retroperitoneal lymph node dissection may be done after chemotherapy as adjunct therapy in patients with advanced testicular cancer.[33]

### CHECK YOUR PRACTICE

You are working on the urologic oncology unit caring for a 24-yr-old man who recently underwent orchiectomy for testicular cancer. He appears quiet and nonengaged when you assess him. He says, "I'm never going to have a normal sex life."

- How would you respond? What kind of support or information would you provide?

The prognosis for patients with testicular cancer in recent years has greatly improved, and 95% of the patients obtain complete remission if the disease is detected in the early stages. As a result of treatment successes, a majority of men with testicular cancer are long-term survivors.

However, some of the drugs used to treat testicular cancer can cause serious long-term side effects. These include pulmonary toxicity, kidney damage, nerve damage (which can cause numbness and tingling), and hearing loss (from nerve damage). Secondary malignancies can occur as a result of chemotherapy (see Chapter 15).

All patients with testicular cancer, regardless of pathology or stage, require surveillance and regular physical examinations, chest x-rays, CT scans, and assessment of hCG and AFP. The goal is to detect relapse when the tumor burden is minimal.

Pretreatment subfertility or impaired fertility is identified at diagnosis. In treatment of testicular cancer, chemotherapy with cisplatin and/or pelvic radiation often damages the testicular germ cells.[33] However, spermatogenesis can return in some patients. Because of the high risk for infertility, the cryopreservation of sperm in a sperm bank before treatment begins should be sensitively discussed and recommended for the man with testicular cancer. Ejaculatory dysfunction may result from retroperitoneal lymph node dissection. These issues may be hard to discuss with the newly diagnosed patient. Men may think that the disease is a threat to their masculinity and self-worth.

# SEXUAL FUNCTION

## VASECTOMY

**Vasectomy** is the bilateral surgical ligation or resection of the ductus deferens performed for the purpose of sterilization (Fig. 54-11). The procedure requires only 15 to 30 minutes and is usually performed with the patient under local anesthesia on an outpatient basis. Although vasectomy is considered a permanent form of sterilization, successful vasectomy reversals *(vasovasotomy, vasoepididymostomy)* are common.

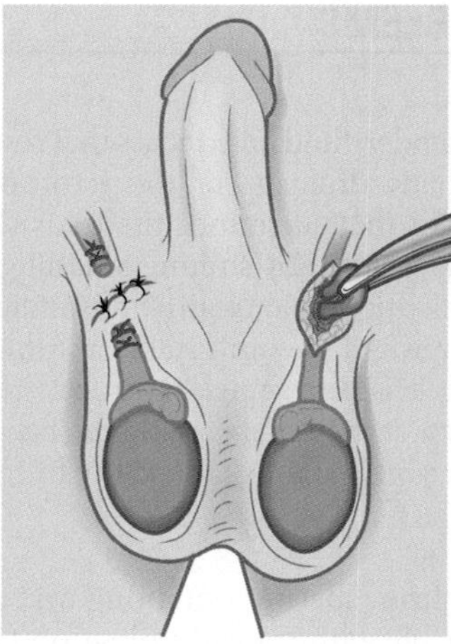

**FIG. 54-11** Vasectomy procedure. The ductus deferens is ligated or resected for the purpose of sterilization.

After vasectomy, the patient should not notice any difference in the look or feel of the ejaculate because its major components are seminal and prostatic fluid. The patient must use an alternative form of contraception until semen examination reveals no sperm. Sperm cells continue to be produced by the testes but are stored in the epididymis and reabsorbed by the body rather than being passed through the ductus deferens. Vasectomy does not affect the production of hormones, ability to ejaculate, or physiologic mechanisms related to erection or orgasm. Psychologic adjustment may be a problem after surgery. It may be difficult for the patient to separate vasectomy from castration at a subconscious level. Some men may develop psychogenic ED or may feel the need to become more sexually active than they were in the past to prove their masculinity.

## ERECTILE DYSFUNCTION

**Erectile dysfunction (ED)** is the inability to attain or maintain an erection that allows satisfactory sexual activity. Although sexual function is a topic that many individuals are uncomfortable discussing, health care professionals must be able and willing to address ED.

ED is a condition that is significant because of its prevalence, with more than 10 million men in the United States estimated to have ED. It can occur at any age, although the incidence increases with age. In fact, it is estimated that about 50% of all men between ages 40 and 70 have at least some degree of ED. Regardless of age, ED is increasing in all sexually active males. In younger men, the increase is attributed to substance abuse (e.g., recreational drugs, alcohol) or stress and anxiety. Middle-aged men are more likely to experience ED due to chronic medical conditions (e.g., diabetes, hypertension) or treatment for these conditions (e.g., antihypertensive drugs) that may cause ED.

### Etiology and Pathophysiology

ED can be due to many factors (Table 54-9). Common causes include diabetes, vascular disease, side effects from medications, result of surgery (e.g., prostatectomy), trauma, chronic illness, stress, difficulty in a relationship, or depression. Since ED results

**TABLE 54-9 Risk Factors for Erectile Dysfunction***

| Vascular | Genitourinary |
|---|---|
| • Atherosclerosis<br>• Hypertension<br>• Peripheral vascular disease | • Radical prostatectomy<br>• Renal failure |
| **Drug Induced** | **Neurologic** |
| • Alcohol<br>• Antiandrogens<br>• Antihypertensives<br>• Antilipidemic agents<br>• Major tranquilizers (diazepam [Valium], alprazolam [Xanax])<br>• Marijuana, cocaine<br>• Nicotine<br>• Tricyclic antidepressants (e.g., amitriptyline [Elavil]) | • Cerebrovascular disease<br>• Diabetes mellitus<br>• Parkinson's disease<br>• Trauma to the spinal cord<br>• Tumors or transection of spinal cord |
| | **Psychologic** |
| | • Anxiety<br>• Depression<br>• Stress |
| **Endocrine** | **Other** |
| • Diabetes mellitus<br>• Hypogonadism<br>• Obesity | • Aging |

*Table is not all-inclusive.

**TABLE 54-10 Interprofessional Care**

***Erectile Dysfunction***

| Diagnostic Assessment | Management |
|---|---|
| • History and physical examination<br>• Sexual history<br>• Serum glucose and lipid profile<br>• Testosterone, prolactin, and thyroid hormone levels<br>• Nocturnal penile tumescence and rigidity testing<br>• Vascular studies | • Modify reversible causes<br>• Sexual counseling<br><br>***Drug Therapy***<br>• sildenafil (Viagra)<br>• vardenafil (Levitra, Staxyn)<br>• tadalafil (Cialis)<br>• avanafil (Stendra)<br><br>***Devices and Implants***<br>• Vacuum erection device (VED)<br>• Intraurethral medication pellet<br>• Intracavernosal self-injection<br>• Penile implants |

from reduced blood flow to the penis, there is a potential association with cardiovascular disease (CVD) because the risk factors for both of these disorders are the same.

Normal physiologic age-related changes are associated with changes in erectile function and may be an underlying cause of ED for some men. Table 50-3 lists age-related changes in sexual function. Explain these age-related changes (if necessary) to reassure an anxious older man regarding normal changes in his sexual abilities. (The male sexual response is discussed in Chapter 50.)

## Clinical Manifestations and Complications

The typical symptom of ED is a patient's self-report of problems associated with erectile activity, describing an inability to attain or maintain an erection. The symptoms may occur only occasionally, may be continual with a gradual onset, or may occur with a sudden onset. A gradual onset of symptoms is usually associated with physiologic factors, whereas a sudden or rapid onset of symptoms may be associated with psychologic issues. It is not uncommon for younger men who seek care for ED to be diagnosed with diabetes, hypertension, depression, or cholesterol abnormalities during their evaluation for ED.

A man's inability to perform sexually can cause great distress in his interpersonal relationships and may interfere with his concept of himself as a man. It can also affect the relationship between the man and his partner. Problems with ED can lead to a number of personal issues, including anger, anxiety, and depression.

## Diagnostic Studies

The first step in diagnosis and management of ED begins with a thorough sexual, health, and psychosocial history. Self-administered assessment and treatment-related questionnaires have been developed and may prove useful as primary screening tools. For example, the International Index of Erectile Function (IIEF) identifies a man's response to five key areas of male sexual function: erectile function, orgasmic function, sexual desire, intercourse satisfaction, and overall satisfaction.[34]

Second, a physical examination should focus on secondary sexual characteristics, noting if secondary sexual characteristics reflect the individual's chronologic age (Tanner stage). A DRE should be done to assess prostate size, consistency, and presence of nodules. Assessment of BP with palpation and auscultation of the femoral arteries and peripheral pulses should also be included.

Further examination or diagnostic testing is typically based on findings from the history and physical examination. A serum glucose and lipid profile is recommended to rule out diabetes mellitus. Hormonal levels for testosterone, prolactin, LH, and thyroid hormones may help identify endocrine-related problems. PSA level and a complete blood count may help to identify other diseases.

Other diagnostic tests may be done to diagnose ED. Nocturnal penile tumescence and rigidity testing is a noninvasive method that involves the continuous measurement of penile circumference and axial rigidity during sleep. Such measurements are used to differentiate between physiologic or psychogenic causes of ED. Vascular studies, including penile arteriography, penile blood flow study, and duplex Doppler ultrasound studies, are used to assess penile blood inflow and outflow. These tests help to identify vascular problems interfering with erection.

## Interprofessional Care

The goal of ED therapy is for the patient and his partner to achieve a satisfactory sexual relationship. The treatment for ED can be based on the underlying cause, but generally men are moved directly into treatment without a costly workup. A variety of treatment options are available (Table 54-10). Advise patients that none of the options will restore ejaculation or tactile sensations if they were absent before treatment.

It is important to determine if ED is reversible before treatment is started. For example, if ED appears to be a side effect of prescribed drugs, alternative treatments can be explored. With an established diagnosis of testicular failure (hypogonadism), androgen replacement therapy may be part of the prescribed treatment.

For individuals who have ED that is psychologic in nature, counseling for the patient (with or without his partner) is recommended. This counseling should be carried out by a qualified sex therapist.

**Erectogenic Drugs.** Sildenafil (Viagra), tadalafil (Cialis), vardenafil (Levitra, Staxyn), and avanafil (Stendra) are erectogenic drugs.[35,36] These drugs are phosphodiesterase type 5 (PDE5) inhibitors that cause smooth muscle relaxation and increased blood flow into the corpus cavernosum, thus promoting penile erection. They are taken orally before sexual activity. These drugs have been found to be generally safe and effective for the treatment of most types of ED but are ineffective in the absence of arousal.

Side effects of these drugs include headaches, dyspepsia, flushing, and nasal congestion. Additional rare side effects are blurred or blue-green visual disturbances, sudden hearing loss, and an erection lasting more than 4 hours (priapism). Instruct the patient to seek immediate medical attention if any of these reactions occur. Because these drugs may potentiate the hypotensive effect of nitrates, they are contraindicated for individuals taking nitrates (e.g., nitroglycerin).

**DRUG ALERT Phosphodiesterase Type 5 (PDE5) Inhibitors**
- Should not be used with nitrates (nitroglycerin) in any form.
- Can potentiate hypotensive effects of nitrates.

**Vacuum Erection Devices.** Vacuum erection devices (VEDs) are suction devices that can be applied to the flaccid penis to produce an erection by pulling blood up into the corporeal bodies. A penile ring or constrictive band is placed around the base of the penis to retain venous blood, thereby preventing the erection from subsiding.

**Intraurethral Devices and Intracavernosal Injections.** Intraurethral devices include the use of vasoactive drugs administered as a topical gel or a medication pellet inserted into the urethra using a medicated urethral system for erection (MUSE) device. Intracavernosal self-injections may also be performed, which should be injected directly into the corpus cavernosum while taking care to avoid the corpus spongiosum.

Alprostadil (Caverject, Edex) is a vasoactive drug that enhances blood flow into the penile arteries. It can be given either by injection or as a transurethral pellet (suppository). When given as a suppository, the drug is placed into the opening at the tip of the penis. When injected, a needle and syringe is used to inject the drug directly into the penis. Trimix (a combination product) includes alprostadil, papaverine, and phentolamine.

**Penile Implants.** Implantation requires surgery but can sometimes be accomplished in an outpatient setting. The devices are implanted into the corporeal bodies to provide an erection firm enough for penetration. The inflatable implant consists of cylinders in the penis, a small pump in the scrotum, and a reservoir in the lower abdomen. The main complications associated with penile prostheses are infection, erosions, and rarely, mechanical failure.

**Sexual Counseling.** Sexual counseling can be recommended at any point during treatment for ED and may be most valuable in cases with a component of psychogenic ED. Counseling should address psychologic or interpersonal factors that may enhance sexual expression, as well as other factors that are of concern. Counseling can be effective for an individual patient, but it can include his partner, particularly if he is involved in a long-term relationship.[37]

## NURSING MANAGEMENT: ERECTILE DYSFUNCTION

The man experiencing ED requires a great deal of emotional support for both himself and his partner. Men often do not feel comfortable discussing their problems with others because of their perceptions of society's expectations of a man's sexual abilities. Reassure the patient that confidentiality will be maintained. The majority of men delay seeking medical assistance and may expect immediate solutions to their problems. The interprofessional care team should provide a support system and accurate information.

Conducting routine health assessments on men seeking any form of medical treatment places you in a unique position. It provides an opportunity to ask the patient questions pertaining to general health, as well as sexual health and function. Given the opportunity, men will be less hesitant to answer these questions when they know that someone cares and can address their concerns.

Be aware that increasing numbers of men are seeking alternate methods for obtaining medications to treat their ED. This can include compounding pharmacies and online pharmacies. Seeking alternate methods can be due to both the cost of these medications and lack of insurance coverage for ED.

## HYPOGONADISM

*Hypogonadism* is a gradual decline in androgen secretion that occurs in most men as they age. The primary male androgen that is reduced is testosterone (Fig. 54-12). This has also been called *late onset hypogonadism* or *hypogonadism of old age,* but it can begin as early as age 40. It is unclear what causes a decline in testosterone, but obesity has been identified as one contributing factor.

Manifestations associated with low testosterone include decreased libido, fatigue, ED, depression and mood swings, and sleep disturbances. Since many of these manifestations can be associated with aging, some patients may not mention this to their HCP, or the HCP may not recognize these manifestations as signs of low testosterone. Long-term effects of low testosterone include loss of muscle mass and strength, which may contribute to an increased risk of falls and fractures.

Hypogonadism is diagnosed with a blood test and a physical examination. Normal serum testosterone levels can range from 280 to 1100 ng/dL. Replacement testosterone therapy is considered once levels drop below 200 ng/dL.[38] Therapy may be started earlier depending on severity of symptoms. Testosterone replacement therapy (TRT) should not be started until the patient, in consultation with his HCP, considers the risks and benefits of therapy. Potential risks of TRT include lowered levels of high-density lipoprotein (HDL) cholesterol, increased hematocrit, and worsening sleep apnea, although these are uncommon. Since TRT may cause increased growth of prostate tissue, TRT is contraindicated in patients with unmanaged BPH

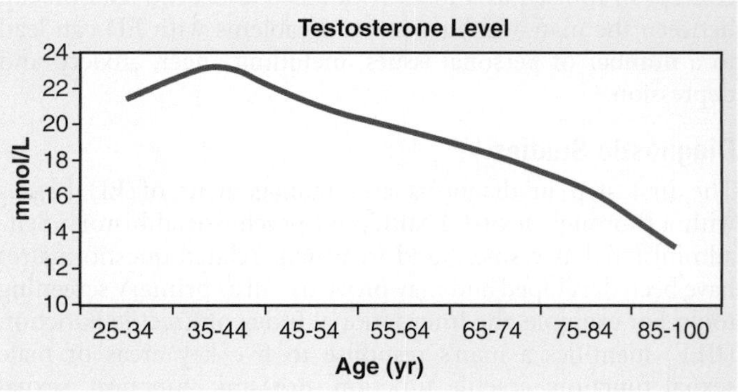


**FIG. 54-12** Changes in testosterone plasma level in men as they age.

or prostate cancer. Before treatment is initiated, a DRE and PSA test should be performed. Once TRT begins, patients should be closely monitored by their HCP.

Replacement therapy is available in different forms, including injection, transdermal, topical, buccal, or intranasal preparations. Oral TRT is not approved for use in the United States.[39] IM injections such as testosterone cypionate (Depo-Testosterone) and testosterone enanthate (Delatestryl) are available in varying doses. These drugs create a cyclic rise and fall in serum testosterone levels with the highest levels 2 or 3 days after the injection. Testosterone levels slowly decrease until the next injection. One of the side effects of this form of TRT is that men may complain of mood swings with these fluctuations.

Transdermal preparations, including patches and gels (e.g., Androderm, Testim), are more commonly prescribed. They are generally applied to the skin daily at product-specific sites, including the back, arm, and abdomen. Skin irritation is a common side effect. Testosterone may also be given as a buccal tablet (Striant) or intranasally (Natesto).

Emphasize to the patient the importance of hand washing with soap and water after applying testosterone preparations to the skin. Covering the area with clothing until the preparation has dried is recommended.

Women of childbearing age and children should avoid direct contact with testosterone products. Testosterone may cause early signs of puberty in young children and changes (virilization) in the external genitalia of a female fetus.

## INFERTILITY

*Infertility* in a couple is defined as the inability to conceive after 1 year of frequent unprotected intercourse. Infertility is a disorder of a couple, not of one individual. For this reason, both partners must be involved in determining the cause of infertility. In 20% to 30% of cases, infertility is caused primarily by factors involving the man.[40]

Male infertility can be caused by disorders of the hypothalamic-pituitary system, disorders of the testes, and abnormalities of the ejaculatory system. The physical causes of infertility can be divided into three categories: pretesticular, testicular, and posttesticular. The *pretesticular* or endocrine causes occur only in about 3% of the cases and can generally be treated with medication or surgery.

*Testicular problems* make up 50% of the cases. The most common cause of male infertility is a varicocele. Other factors that influence the testes include infection (e.g., mumps virus, STIs, bacterial infections), congenital anomalies, drugs, radiation, substance abuse (alcohol, nicotine, drugs), and environmental hazards.

*Posttesticular* causes account for approximately 5% to 7% of the cases, with obstruction, infection, and the result of a surgical procedure being the primary causes. The remaining 40% are classified as *idiopathic,* or of unknown causes.

A careful health history and examination may reveal the cause of a patient's infertility. Thus the history is a starting point for determining cause and treatment. The history should include age; occupation; past injury, surgery, or infections to the genital tract; lifestyle issues such as hot tubs, weight training, or wearing tight undergarments; sexual practices; frequency of intercourse; and emotional factors such as stress levels and the desire for children. Document the use of drugs, such as chemotherapeutic agents, anabolic steroids or testosterone, sulfasalazine (Azulfidine), cimetidine (Tagamet HB), and recreational drugs, since these drugs can reduce the sperm count. A physical examination may identify a varicocele, Peyronie's disease, or other physical findings.

The first test in the male infertility evaluation is a semen analysis to determine sperm concentration, motility, and morphology. Hormone studies are also helpful in determining the etiology, including plasma testosterone and serum LH and FSH measurements. Be tactful in dealing with the male patient undergoing infertility studies. Many cultures equate fertility and masculinity. Both male and female partners should undergo evaluation simultaneously to avoid potential treatment delays for the couple.

Treatment options for the man include drugs, conservative lifestyle changes (e.g., avoidance of scrotal heat, substance abuse, high stress), in vitro fertilization techniques, and corrective surgery. Infertility can seriously strain a relationship, and the couple may require counseling and discussion of alternatives if conception is not achieved. (Female infertility is discussed in Chapter 53.)

## CASE STUDY

### *Benign Prostatic Hyperplasia With Acute Urinary Retention*

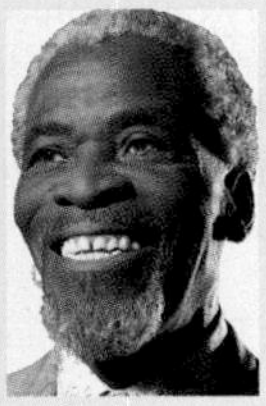

(©IPGGutenberg-UKLtd/iStock/Thinkstock)

**Patient Profile**

B.G., a 60-yr-old married African American man, comes to the ED because of an inability to void for the past 13 hours and pain in the lower abdomen.

**Subjective Data**

- Complains of the urge to void
- Is restless, anxious, and agitated

**Objective Data**

- Has prostate enlargement on digital rectal examination
- Has hematuria, bacteria, and WBCs in urine
- Has a tender and palpable bladder above the umbilicus
- PSA test: 5 ng/mL

**Interprofessional Care**

- Indwelling catheter inserted by a urology resident
- Admitted to the hospital for observation

**Discussion Questions**

1. What risk factors for prostate problems are present in B.G.?
2. Explain the etiology of the manifestations that B.G. exhibited.
3. What are possible reasons for B.G.'s elevated PSA level?
4. Discuss the drug and surgical options available to B.G.
5. ***Patient-Centered Care:*** B.G. asks you about the effect of the various surgical options on his ability to have sex. How would you respond and what type of teaching would you provide?
6. ***Priority Decision:*** Based on the assessment data, what are the priority nursing diagnoses? Are there any collaborative problems?
7. ***Priority Decision:*** What is the priority nursing intervention for B.G.?
8. ***Patient-Centered Care:*** On further assessment, you note that B.G. has a nursing diagnosis of decisional conflict. How would you help him resolve this conflict related to treatment options, and how would you teach him about these options?
9. ***Evidence-Based Practice:*** What information would you offer to B.G. when he asks if he should start taking saw palmetto to prevent future UTIs?

Answers available at *http://evolve.elsevier.com/Lewis/medsurg.*

## BRIDGE TO NCLEX EXAMINATION

The number of the question corresponds to the same-numbered outcome at the beginning of the chapter.

1. Symptoms of BPH are *primarily* caused by
   - **a.** obstruction of the urethra.
   - **b.** untreated chronic prostatitis.
   - **c.** decreased bladder compliance.
   - **d.** excessive secretion of testosterone.
2. Postoperatively, a patient who has had a laser prostatectomy has continuous bladder irrigation with a three-way urinary catheter with a 30-mL balloon. When he complains of bladder spasms with the catheter in place, the nurse should
   - **a.** deflate the balloon to 10 mL to decrease bulk in the bladder.
   - **b.** deflate the balloon and then reinflate to ensure that it is patent.
   - **c.** encourage the patient to try to have a bowel movement to relieve colon pressure.
   - **d.** explain that this feeling is normal and that he should not try to urinate around the catheter.
3. Which factors would place a patient at a higher risk for prostate cancer *(select all that apply)*?
   - **a.** Older than 65 years
   - **b.** Asian or Native American
   - **c.** Long-term use of an indwelling urethral catheter
   - **d.** Father diagnosed and treated for early stage prostate cancer
   - **e.** Previous history of undescended testicle and testicular cancer
4. A patient scheduled for a prostatectomy for prostate cancer expresses the fear that he will have erectile dysfunction. In responding to this patient, the nurse should keep in mind that
   - **a.** erectile dysfunction can occur even with a nerve-sparing procedure.
   - **b.** the most common complication of this surgery is postoperative bowel incontinence.
   - **c.** retrograde ejaculation affects sexual function more frequently than erectile dysfunction.
   - **d.** preoperative sexual function is the most important factor in determining postoperative erectile dysfunction.
5. The nurse explains to the patient with chronic bacterial prostatitis who is undergoing antibiotic therapy that *(select all that apply)*
   - **a.** all patients require hospitalization.
   - **b.** pain will lessen once treatment has ended.
   - **c.** course of treatment is generally 2 to 4 weeks.
   - **d.** long-term therapy may be indicated in immunocompromised patient.
   - **e.** if the condition is unresolved and untreated, he is at risk for prostate cancer.
6. In assessing a patient for testicular cancer, the nurse understands that the manifestations of this disease often include
   - **a.** acute back spasms and testicular pain.
   - **b.** rapid onset of scrotal swelling and fever.
   - **c.** fertility problems and bilateral scrotal tenderness.
   - **d.** painless mass and heaviness sensation in the scrotal area.
7. The nurse should explain to the patient who has erectile dysfunction (ED) that *(select all that apply)*
   - **a.** the most common cause is benign prostatic hypertrophy.
   - **b.** ED may be due to medications or conditions such as diabetes.
   - **c.** only men who are over 65 years or older benefit from PDE5 inhibitors.
   - **d.** there are medications and devices that can be used to help with erections.
   - **e.** this condition is primarily due to anxiety and best treated with psychotherapy.
8. To decrease the patient's discomfort related to discussing his reproductive organs, the nurse should
   - **a.** relate his sexual concerns to his sexual partner.
   - **b.** arrange to have male nurses care for the patient.
   - **c.** maintain a nonjudgmental attitude toward his sexual practices.
   - **d.** use technical terminology when discussing reproductive function.

1. a, 2. d, 3. a, d, 4. a, 5. b, d, 6. d, 7. b, d, 8. c

For rationales to these answers and even more NCLEX review questions, visit *http://evolve.elsevier.com/Lewis/medsurg.*

## EVOLVE WEBSITE

http://evolve.elsevier.com/Lewis/medsurg

**Review Questions (Online Only)**

**Key Points**

**Answer Keys for Questions**

- Rationales for Bridge to NCLEX Examination Questions
- Answer Guidelines for Case Study on p. 1289
- Answer Guidelines for Managing Care of Multiple Patients Case Study (Section 10) on p. 1292

**Student Case Study**

- Patient With Benign Prostatic Hyperplasia

**Nursing Care Plan**

- eNursing Care Plan 54-1: Patient Having Prostate Surgery

**Conceptual Care Map Creator**

**Audio Glossary**

**Supporting Media**

- Animations
  - Prostatectomy
  - Vasectomy

**Content Updates**

## REFERENCES


1. Rosenberg M, Witt E, Miner M, et al: A practical primary care approach to lower urinary tract symptoms caused by benign prostatic hyperplasia (BPH-LUTS), *Can J Urol* 21 (Suppl 2):12, 2014.
2. Weight C, Kim S, Jacobson D, et al: The effect of benign lower urinary tract symptoms on subsequent prostate cancer testing and diagnosis, *Eur Urol* 63:1021, 2013.
3. Ørsted D, Bojesen S: The link between benign prostatic hyperplasia and prostate cancer, *Nat Review Urol* 10:49, 2013.
4. American Urological Association Foundation: What is benign prostatic hyperplasia (BPH)? Retrieved from *www.urologyhealth.org/urologic-conditions/benign-prostatic-hyperplasia-(bph)*.
5. Barry M, Fowler F, O'Leary M, et al: The American Urologic Association symptom index for benign prostatic hyperplasia, *J Urol* 148:1549, 1992. (Classic)

*6. American Urological Association: American Urological Association Guideline: Management of benign prostatic hyperplasia (BPH). Retrieved from *www.auanet.org/education/guidelines/benign-prostatic-hyperplasia.cfm*.

7. National Cancer Institute: Prostate cancer prevention trial, National Institutes of Health. Retrieved from *www.cancer.gov*.

8. Brock G, McVary K, Roehrborn C, et al: Direct effects of tadalafil on lower urinary tract symptoms versus indirect effects mediated through erectile dysfunction symptom improvement: integrated data analyses from 4 placebo controlled clinical studies, *J Urol* 191:405, 2014.
9. Barry M, Cantor A, Roehrborn C, et al: Relationships among participant international prostate symptom score, benign prostatic hyperplasia impact index changes and global ratings of change in a trial of phytotherapy in men with lower urinary tract symptoms, *J Urol* 189:987, 2013.
10. Andriole G, McCullum-Hill C, Sandhu G, et al: The effect of increasing doses of saw palmetto fruit extract on serum prostate specific antigen: analysis of the CAMUS randomized trial, *J Urol* 189:486, 2013.
*11. Cornu J, Ahyai S, Bachmann A, et al: A systematic review and meta-analysis of functional outcomes and complications following transurethral procedures for lower urinary tract symptoms resulting from benign prostatic obstruction: an update, *Eur Urol* 67:1066, 2015.
12. Chughtai B, Simma-Chiang V, Lee R, et al: Trends and utilization of laser prostatectomy in ambulatory surgical procedures for the treatment of benign prostatic hyperplasia in New York State (2000-2011), *J Endourol* 29:700, 2015.
13. National Kidney and Urologic Diseases Information Clearinghouse: Prostate enlargement: benign prostatic hyperplasia, US Department of Health and Human Services. Retrieved from *www.niddk.nih.gov/health-information/health-topics/urologic-disease/benign-prostatic-hyperplasia-bph/pages/facts/aspx.*
*14. American Urological Association (2013). PSA Testing for the Pretreatment Staging and Posttreatment Management of Prostate Cancer: 2013 Revision of 2009 Best Practice Statement. Retrieved from *www.auanet.org/education/guidelines/prostate-specific-antigen.cfm.*
15. American Cancer Society: What are the key statistics about prostate cancer? Retrieved from *www.cancer.org/cancer/prostatecancer/detailedguide/prostate-cancer-key-statistics.*
16. Alavanja M, Ross M, Bonner M: Increased cancer burden among pesticide applicators and others due to pesticide exposure, *CA Cancer J Clin* 63:120, 2013.
*17. Skolarus T, Wolf A, Erb N, et al: American Cancer Society prostate cancer survivorship care guidelines, *CA Cancer J Clin* 64:225, 2014.
18. National Institutes of Health, National Cancer Institute: Treatment choices for men with early-stage prostate cancer. Retrieved from *www.cancer.gov/types/prostate/patient/prostate-treatment-pdq.*
19. Brimo F, Montironi R, Egevad L, et al: Contemporary grading for prostate cancer: implications for patient care, *Eur Urol* 63:892, 2013.
*20. Gandaglia G, Sammon J, Chang S, et al: Comparative effectiveness of robot-assisted and open radical prostatectomy in the postdissemination era, *J Clin Oncol* 32:1419, 2014.
*21. Sukumar S, Rogers C, Trinh Q, et al: Oncological outcomes after robot-assisted radical prostatectomy: long-term follow-up in 4803 patients, *BJU Int* 114:824, 2014.
22. Steineck G, Bjartell A, Hugosson J, et al: Degree of preservation of the neurovascular bundles during radical prostatectomy and urinary continence 1 year after surgery, *Eur Urol* 67:559, 2015.
23. Chen R, Chang P, Vetter R, et al: Recommended patient-reported core set of symptoms to measure in prostate cancer treatment trials, *J Natl Cancer Inst* 106:7, 2014.
*24. Smolska-Ciszewska B, Miszczyk L, Bialas B, et al: The effectiveness and side effects of conformal external beam radiotherapy combined with high-dose-rate brachytherapy boost compared to conformal external beam radiotherapy alone in patients with prostate cancer, *Radiat Oncol* 10:60, 2015.
*25. Gandaglia G, Sun M, Popa I, et al: The impact of androgen-deprivation therapy (ADT) on the risk of cardiovascular (CV) events in patients with non-metastatic prostate cancer: a population-based study, *BJU Int* 114:E82, 2014.
*26. Limburg C, Maxwell C, Mautner B: Prevention and treatment of bone loss in patients with nonmetastatic breast or prostate cancer who receive hormonal ablation therapy, *Clin J Oncol Nurs* 18:223, 2014.
*27. Dilori C, Steenland K, Goodman M, et al: Differences in treatment-based beliefs and coping between African American and white men with prostate cancer, *J Commun Health* 36:505, 2011.
28. National Institute of Diabetes and Digestive and Kidney Disorders Information Clearinghouse: Prostatitis: inflammation of the prostate. Retrieved from *www.niddk.nih.gov/healht-information/health-topics/urologic-disease/prostatitis-disorders-of-the-prostate/pages/facts.aspx.*
*29. Wagenlehner F, van Till J, Magri V, et al: National Institutes of Health chronic prostatitis symptoms index (NIH-CPSI) symptom evaluation in multinational cohorts of patients with chronic prostatitis/chronic pelvic pain syndrome, *Eur Urol* 63:953, 2013.
30. Inman B, Stewart S, Kattan M: Staging and risk stratification in penile cancer. In Spiess PE, editor: *Penile cancer*, New York, 2013, Humana Press.
31. Znaor A, Lortet-Tieulent J, Jemal A, et al: International variations and trends in testicular cancer incidence and mortality, *Eur Urol* 65:1095, 2014.
32. Hanna N, Einhorn L: Testicular cancer-discoveries and updates, *N Eng J Med* 371: 2005-16, 2014.
*33. Bujan L, Walschaerts M, Moinard N, et al: Impact of chemotherapy and radiotherapy for testicular germ cell tumors on spermatogenesis and sperm DNA: a multicenter prospective study from the CECOS network, *Fertil Steril* 100:673, 2013.
34. Rosen R, Riley A, Wagner G, et al. The International Index of Erectile Function (IIEF): a multidimensional scale for assessment of erectile dysfunction, *Urology* 49:822, 1997. (Classic)
35. Porst H, Burnett A, Brock G, et al: SOP conservative (medical and mechanical) treatment of erectile dysfunction, *J Sex Med* 10:130, 2013.
36. Smith W, McCaslin I, Gokce A, et al: PDE5 inhibitors: considerations for preference and long-term adherence, *Int J Clin Pract* 67:768, 2013.
*37. Schmidt H, Munder T, Gerger H, et al: Combination of psychological intervention and phosphodiesterase-5 inhibitors for erectile dysfunction: a narrative review and meta-analysis, *J Sex Med* 11:1376, 2014.
*38. Buvat J, Maggi M, Guay A, et al: Testosterone deficiency in men: systematic review and standard operating procedures for diagnosis and treatment, *J Sex Med* 10:245, 2013.
39. Basaria S: Male hypogonadism, *Lancet* 383:1250, 2014.
*40. American Urological Association (2011). The optimal evaluation of the infertile male: Best practice statement reviewed and validity confirmed 2011. Retrieved from *www.auanet.org/education/guidelines/male-infertility-d.cfm.*

*Evidence-based information for clinical practice.

## CASE STUDY

### *Managing Care of Multiple Patients*

You are working on the medical-surgical unit and have been assigned to care for the following six patients. You have one LPN and one UAP on your team to help you.

#### Patients

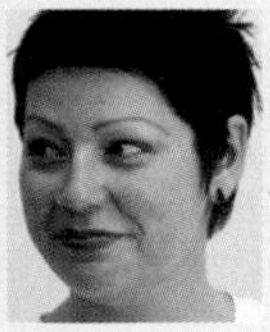

(©iStockphoto/Thinkstock)

L.M. is a 35-yr-old Hispanic woman who went to the clinic 3 days ago complaining of "just not feeling well." She was admitted to the hospital for treatment of hypertension caused by newly diagnosed Cushing syndrome. She has been depressed and crying because of her physical appearance. Her most recent BP was 164/94 mm Hg.

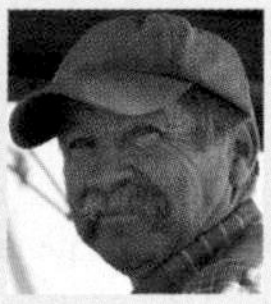

(©iStockphoto/Thinkstock)

N.B. is a 48-yr-old farmer admitted to the ICU 2 days ago with a diagnosis of diabetic ketoacidosis. He was transferred to the clinical unit yesterday evening. His fasting blood glucose level this morning is 296 mg/dL.

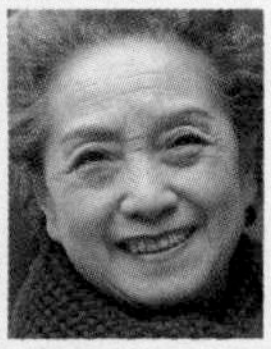

(©XiXinXing/iStock/Thinkstock)

A.K. is a 68-yr-old Asian American woman recently diagnosed with adenocarcinoma of her right breast. She had a lumpectomy and axillary node dissection yesterday. She has a Jackson-Pratt drain in her right chest. Her last pain medication was administered 1 hour ago, at which time she rated her pain as a 7 on a scale of 0-10.

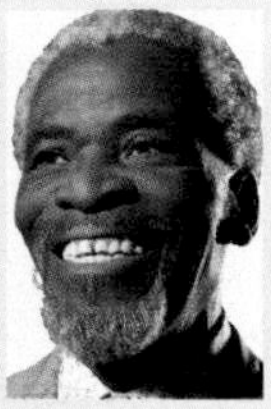

(©IPGGutenberg-UKLtd/iStock/Thinkstock)

B.G. is a 60-yr-old African American man who was admitted to the hospital because of an inability to void for 13 hours and pain in the lower abdomen. He has a urinary tract infection and prostatic enlargement. An indwelling catheter was inserted by a urology resident. B.G. is scheduled to undergo a transurethral resection of his prostate (TURP) this morning.

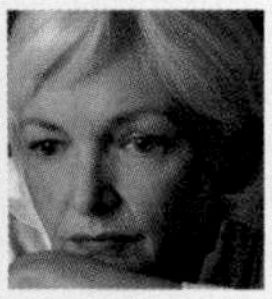

(©Jupiterimages/Photos.com/Thinkstock)

R.D. is a 52-yr-old white woman who was diagnosed with Graves' disease 2 months ago. She was treated with antithyroid medication for 2 months and underwent a subtotal thyroidectomy yesterday. In report it is noted that her voice has become slightly "hoarse" in the last hour.

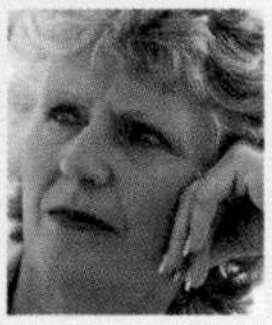

(©Wavebreakmedia/iStock/Thinkstock)

T.J. is a 56-yr-old white woman who underwent a total abdominal hysterectomy and bilateral salpingo-oophorectomy 1 day ago. She has a urinary catheter in place. Her vital signs are stable and she is not complaining of pain.

#### Discussion Questions

1. ***Priority Decision:*** After receiving report, which patient should you see first? Second? Provide a rationale.
2. ***Teamwork and Collaboration:*** Which tasks could you delegate to UAP *(select all that apply)?*
   a. Assist T.J. to ambulate in the hallway.
   b. Teach B.G. what to expect postoperatively.
   c. Take R.D.'s vital signs and report the results to you.
   d. Assess A.K.'s mastectomy incision for manifestations of infection.
   e. Listen to L.M. talk about her feelings while helping her with AM care.
3. ***Priority Decision and Teamwork and Collaboration:*** While you are assessing R.D., the LPN informs you that A.K.'s chest dressing is totally saturated with bloody drainage. Which *initial* action would be most appropriate?
   a. Ask the LPN to call the laboratory for a stat Hgb and Hct on A.K.
   b. Have the LPN reinforce the dressing with sterile 4 × 4 gauze pads.
   c. Have the LPN stay with R.D. while you assess the patency of A.K.'s Jackson-Pratt drain.
   d. Ask the LPN to stay with A.K. and the UAP to monitor R.D. while you call A.K.'s surgeon.

#### Case Study Progression

A.K.'s Jackson-Pratt drain was not functioning properly. You get it working and change the chest dressing. The incision is well approximated without signs of infection. When you leave the room, the Jackson-Pratt has a small amount of serosanguineous drainage in it. As you enter R.D.'s room you notice that the patient is having a carpal spasm on the same arm that the LPN is taking her BP on. You recognize this as a manifestation of hypocalcemia and notify the health care provider.

4. Which assessment findings would be *most* important to include in a discussion with the health care provider regarding R.D. *(select all that apply)?*
   a. Patient is anxious
   b. Hoarseness of voice
   c. Most recent Hgb and Hct
   d. Carpal spasm upon inflation of BP cuff
   e. Blood pressure of 138/76 and heart rate of 78
5. ***Priority Decision:*** Which intervention would be of *highest* priority in caring for L.M.?
   a. Assess her for fall risk.
   b. Assess her for signs and symptoms of hypoglycemia.
   c. Teach her the need for a high-carbohydrate, low-protein diet.
   d. Reassure her that her physical appearance will improve with treatment.
6. B.G. asks you what to expect when he returns from surgery. You explain that he will have a(n)
   a. dressing in his groin as well as a urinary catheter.
   b. 3-way urinary catheter connected to an irrigation system.
   c. patient-controlled analgesia (PCA) pump for pain control.
   d. abdominal and a perineal drain that will be recharged q4h.
7. ***Priority Decision and Management Decision:*** The LPN is assigned to administer medications to N.B., including his sliding scale Novolog insulin with breakfast. The UAP, who is also a senior nursing student, tells you that the LPN administered N.B.'s insulin at least 30 min after the patient ate his breakfast. What is your *best* initial action?
   a. Report the incident to the charge nurse for follow-up.
   b. Talk to the LPN about the importance of timely medication administration.
   c. Ask the LPN what time the insulin was given and when the patient ate breakfast.
   d. Ask the UAP to first discuss the concern with the LPN so as to follow proper channels of communication.

Answers available at *http://evolve.elsevier.com/Lewis/medsurg.*

# SECTION 11

# Problems Related to Movement and Coordination

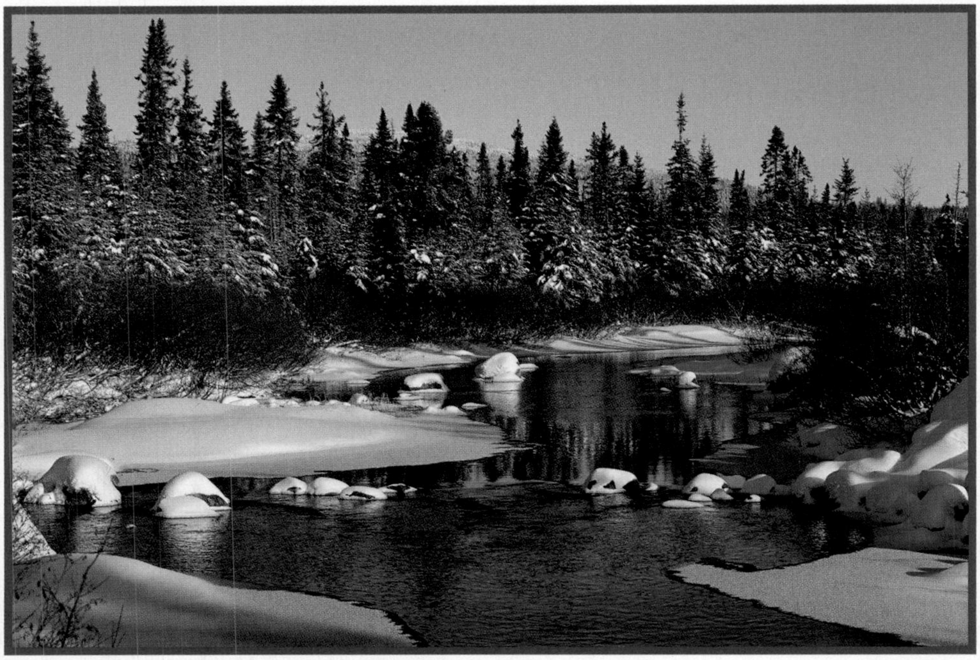

(©Stockbyte/Stockbyte/Thinkstock)

*The river has taught me to listen; you will learn from it, too.*
*The river knows everything; one can learn everything from it.*

**Hermann Hesse**

55

# Assessment of Nervous System

*Linda Littlejohns*

*It always seems impossible until it is done.*

***Nelson Mandela***

http://evolve.elsevier.com/Lewis/medsurg/

## LEARNING OUTCOMES

1. Differentiate between the functions of neurons and glial cells.
2. Explain the anatomic location and functions of the cerebrum, brainstem, cerebellum, spinal cord, peripheral nerves, and cerebrospinal fluid.
3. Identify the major arteries supplying the brain.
4. Describe the functions of the 12 cranial nerves.
5. Compare the functions of the two divisions of the autonomic nervous system.
6. Link the age-related changes in the neurologic system to the differences in assessment findings.
7. Obtain significant subjective and objective data related to the nervous system from a patient.
8. Perform a physical assessment of the nervous system using the appropriate techniques.
9. Differentiate normal from abnormal findings of a physical assessment of the nervous system.
10. Describe the purpose, significance of results, and nursing responsibilities related to diagnostic studies of the nervous system.

## KEY TERMS



## STRUCTURES AND FUNCTIONS OF NERVOUS SYSTEM

The nervous system is responsible for the control and integration of the body's many activities. It can be divided into the central nervous system and peripheral nervous system. The **central nervous system (CNS)** consists of the brain, spinal cord, and cranial nerves I and II. The **peripheral nervous system (PNS)** consists of cranial nerves III to XII, spinal nerves, and peripheral components of the **autonomic nervous system (ANS)**.

### Cells of Nervous System

The nervous system is made up of two types of cells: neurons and supportive glial cells.

**Neurons.** **Neurons** are the primary functional unit of the nervous system. Although neurons come in many shapes and sizes, they share three characteristics: (1) *excitability,* or the ability to generate a nerve impulse; (2) *conductivity,* or the ability to transmit an impulse; and (3) *influence,* or the ability to influence other neurons, muscle cells, or glandular cells.

A typical neuron consists of a cell body, multiple dendrites, and an axon (Fig. 55-1). The *cell body* containing the nucleus and cytoplasm is the metabolic center of the neuron. *Dendrites* are short processes extending from the cell body that receive impulses or signals from other neurons and conduct them toward the cell body. The *axon* projects varying distances from the cell body. The axon carries nerve impulses to other neurons or to end organs, such as smooth and striated muscles and glands.

Many axons in the CNS and PNS are covered by a *myelin sheath,* a white, lipid protein substance that acts as an insulator for the conduction of impulses. Axons may be myelinated or unmyelinated, as in the case of smaller fibers.

**Glial Cells.** **Glial cells** (glia or neuroglia) provide support, nourishment, and protection to neurons. Glial cells constitute almost half of the brain and spinal cord mass. Glial cells are divided into microglia and macroglia. *Microglia,* specialized macrophages capable of phagocytosis, protect the neurons. These cells are mobile within the brain and multiply when the brain is damaged.

Types of *macroglial cells* include the astrocytes, oligodendrocytes, and ependymal cells. *Astrocytes* are found primarily in

Reviewed by Tara Back, RN, MSN, Instructor, Goldfarb School of Nursing at Barnes Jewish College, St. Louis, Missouri; Julia R. Popp, RN, MSN, Professor of Nursing, Owens Community College, Toledo, Ohio; and Crystal R. Sherman, DNP, CNP, FNP-BC, APHN-BC, Assistant Professor of Nursing, Shawnee State University, Portsmouth, Ohio.

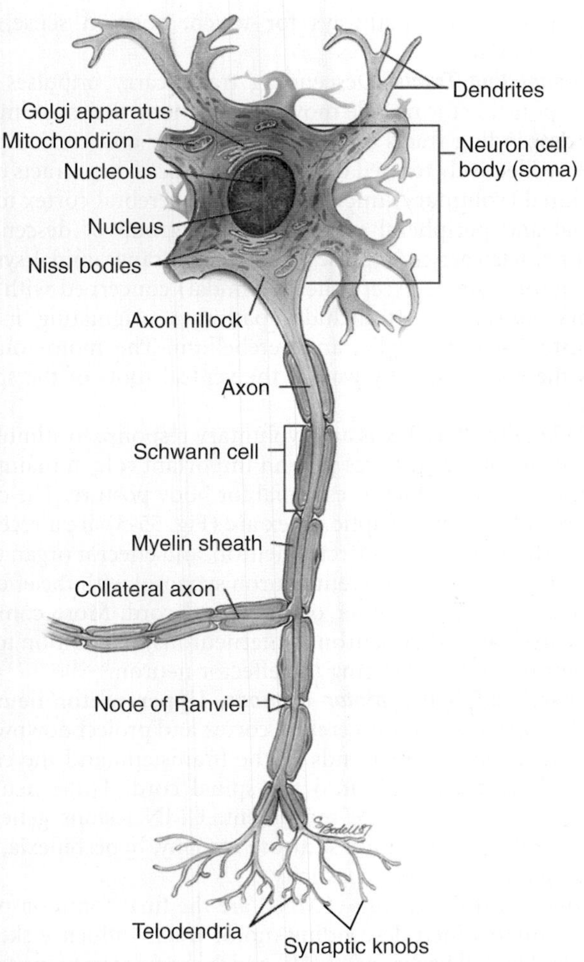


**FIG. 55-1** Structural features of neurons: dendrites, cell body, and axons. (Modified from Thibodeau GA, Patton KT: *Anatomy and physiology,* ed 8, St Louis, 2013, Mosby.)

gray matter and provide structural support to neurons. Their delicate processes form the *blood-brain barrier* with the endothelium of the blood vessels. They also play a role in *synaptic transmission* (conduction of impulses between neurons). When the brain is injured, astrocytes act as phagocytes for cleaning up neuronal debris. They help restore the neurochemical milieu and provide support for repair. Proliferation of astrocytes contributes to the formation of scar tissue *(gliosis)* in the CNS.

*Oligodendrocytes* are specialized cells that produce the myelin sheath of nerve fibers in the CNS and are found primarily in the white matter of the CNS. (*Schwann cells* myelinate the nerve fibers in the periphery.) *Ependymal cells* line the brain ventricles and aid in the secretion of cerebrospinal fluid (CSF).

Neuroglia are mitotic and can replicate. In general, when neurons are destroyed, the tissue is replaced by the proliferation of neuroglial cells. Most primary CNS tumors involve glial cells. Primary malignancies involving neurons are rare.

## Nerve Regeneration

If the axon of the nerve cell is damaged, the cell attempts to repair itself. Damaged nerve cells attempt to grow back to their original destinations by sprouting many branches from the damaged ends of their axons. Axons in the CNS are generally less successful than peripheral axons in regeneration.[1]

Injured nerve fibers in the PNS can regenerate by growing within the protective myelin sheath of the supporting Schwann cells if the cell body is intact and the environment is optimal.[1] The final result of nerve regeneration depends on the number of axon sprouts that join with the appropriate Schwann cell columns and reinnervate appropriate end organs.

Neurons have long been thought to be nonmitotic. That is, after being damaged, neurons could not be replaced. Although cell proliferation historically was not believed to be possible, recent evidence indicates a subset of glial cells (astrocytes) proliferate after certain injuries in the CNS, and neurogenesis may occur from stem cells.[2] These findings support the expectation that the patient will experience a certain amount of recovery after injury involving the neurons.

## Nerve Impulse

The purpose of a neuron is to initiate, receive, and process messages about events both within and outside the body. The initiation of a neuronal message *(nerve impulse)* involves the generation of an action potential. A series of action potentials travel along the axon. When the impulse reaches the end of the nerve fiber, it is transmitted across the junction *(synapse)* between nerve cells by a chemical interaction involving neurotransmitters. This chemical interaction generates another set of action potentials in the next neuron. These events are repeated until the nerve impulse reaches its destination.

Because of its insulating capacity, myelination of nerve axons facilitates the conduction of an action potential. Many peripheral nerve axons have *nodes of Ranvier* (gaps in the myelin sheath) that allow an action potential to travel much faster by jumping from node to node. This is called *saltatory* (hopping) conduction. In an unmyelinated fiber, the wave of depolarization travels the entire length of the axon, with each portion of the membrane becoming depolarized in turn.

**Synapse.** A synapse is the structural and functional junction between two neurons. It is the point at which the nerve impulse is transmitted from one neuron to another. The nerve impulse also can be transmitted from neurons to glands or muscles. The essential structures of synaptic transmission are a presynaptic terminal, synaptic cleft, and receptor site on the postsynaptic cell (Fig. 55-2).

**Neurotransmitters.** Neurotransmitters are chemicals that affect the transmission of impulses across the synaptic cleft. *Excitatory neurotransmitters* (e.g., epinephrine, norepinephrine, glutamate) activate postsynaptic receptors that increase the likelihood that an action potential will be generated. *Inhibitory neurotransmitters* (e.g., serotonin, GABA, dopamine) activate postsynaptic receptors to decrease the likelihood that an action potential will be generated. Endorphins block pain transmission while substance P makes nerves more sensitive to pain.

In general, the net effect (excitatory or inhibitory) depends on the number of presynaptic neurons releasing neurotransmitters on the postsynaptic cell. A presynaptic cell that releases an excitatory neurotransmitter does not always cause the postsynaptic cell to depolarize enough to generate an action potential.

Neurotransmitters can be affected by drugs and toxins, which can modify their function or block their attachment to receptor sites on the postsynaptic membrane. When many presynaptic cells release excitatory neurotransmitters on a single neuron, the sum of their input is enough to generate an action potential. Neurotransmitters continue to combine with the receptor sites at the postsynaptic membrane until they are

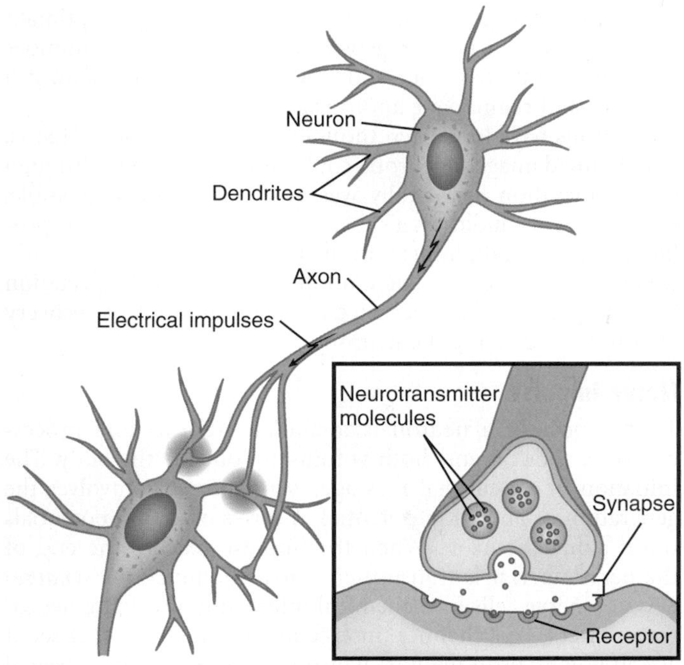


**FIG. 55-2** Impulse generation between neurons. Synapse shown with neurotransmitters and receptors.

inactivated by enzymes, are taken up by the presynaptic endings, or diffuse away from the synaptic region. (See Chapter 56 for information regarding the use of cerebral microdialysis for measuring neurotransmitter levels in the cerebral cortex.)

## Central Nervous System

The components of the CNS include the cerebrum (cerebral hemispheres), brainstem, cerebellum, and spinal cord.

**Spinal Cord.** The *spinal cord* is continuous with the brainstem and exits from the cranial cavity through the foramen magnum. A cross section of the spinal cord reveals gray matter that is centrally located in an H shape and surrounded by white matter. The gray matter contains the cell bodies of voluntary motor neurons, preganglionic autonomic motor neurons, and association neurons (interneurons). The white matter contains the axons of the ascending sensory and descending motor fibers. The myelin surrounding these fibers gives them their white appearance. The spinal pathways or tracts are named for the point of origin and the point of destination (e.g., spinocerebellar tract [ascending], corticospinal tract [descending]).

***Ascending Tracts.*** In general, the ascending tracts carry specific sensory information to higher levels of the CNS. This information comes from special sensory receptors in the skin, muscles and joints, viscera, and blood vessels and enters the spinal cord by way of the dorsal roots of the spinal nerves. The fasciculus gracilis and the fasciculus cuneatus (commonly called the *dorsal* or *posterior columns*) carry information concerned with touch, deep pressure, vibration, position sense, and kinesthesia (appreciation of movement, weight, and body parts). The *spinocerebellar tracts* carry information about muscle tension and body position to the cerebellum for coordination of movement. The *spinothalamic tracts* carry pain and temperature sensations. Thus the ascending tracts are organized by sensory modality, as well as by anatomy.

Although the functions of these pathways are generally accepted, other ascending tracts may also carry sensory modalities. The signs and symptoms of various neurologic diseases suggest additional pathways for touch, position sense, and vibration exist.

***Descending Tracts.*** Descending tracts carry impulses that are responsible for muscle movement. Among the most important descending tracts are the corticobulbar and corticospinal tracts, collectively termed the *pyramidal tract.* These tracts carry volitional (voluntary) impulses from the cerebral cortex to the cranial and peripheral nerves. Another group of descending motor tracts carries impulses from the extrapyramidal system (all motor systems except the pyramidal) concerned with voluntary movement. It includes pathways originating in the brainstem, basal ganglia, and cerebellum. The motor output exits the spinal cord by way of the ventral roots of the spinal nerves.

***Reflex Arc.*** A reflex is an involuntary response to stimuli. In the spinal cord, reflex arcs play an important role in maintaining muscle tone, which is essential for body posture. The components of a monosynaptic reflex arc (Fig. 55-3) are a receptor organ, afferent neuron, effector neuron, and effector organ (e.g., skeletal muscle). The afferent neuron synapses with the efferent neuron in the gray matter of the spinal cord. More complex reflex arcs have other neurons (interneurons) in addition to the afferent neuron influencing the effector neuron.

***Lower and Upper Motor Neurons.*** Upper motor neurons (UMNs) originate in the cerebral cortex and project downward. The corticobulbar tract ends in the brainstem, and the corticospinal tract descends into the spinal cord. These neurons influence skeletal muscle movement. UMN lesions generally cause weakness or paralysis, disuse atrophy, hyperreflexia, and increased muscle tone (spasticity).

Lower motor neurons (LMNs) are the final common pathway through which descending motor tracts influence skeletal muscle. The cell bodies of LMNs, which send axons to innervate the skeletal muscles of the arms, trunk, and legs, are located in the anterior horn of the corresponding segments of the spinal cord (e.g., cervical segments contain LMNs for the arms). LMNs for skeletal muscles of the eyes, face, mouth, and throat are located in the corresponding segments of the brainstem. These cell bodies and their axons make up the somatic motor components of the cranial nerves. LMN lesions generally cause weakness or paralysis, denervation atrophy, hyporeflexia or areflexia, and decreased muscle tone (flaccidity).

**Brain.** The *brain* has three major intracranial components: cerebrum, brainstem, and cerebellum.

***Cerebrum.*** The *cerebrum* is composed of the right and left cerebral hemispheres and divided into four lobes: frontal, temporal, parietal, and occipital (Fig. 55-4). The functions of the cerebrum are multiple and complex (Table 55-1). The *frontal lobe* controls higher cognitive function, memory retention, voluntary eye movements, voluntary motor movement, and motor functions involved in speech production *(Broca's area).* The *temporal lobe* integrates somatic, visual, and auditory data and contains *Wernicke's receptive speech area.* (Language and potential functional deficits are described further in the discussion of stroke in Chapter 57 [Table 57-4]).

The *parietal lobe* interprets spatial information and contains the sensory cortex. Processing of sight takes place in the *occipital lobe.*

The division of the cerebrum into lobes is useful to delineate portions of the neocortex (gray matter), which makes up the outer layer of the cerebral hemispheres. Neurons in specific parts of the neocortex are essential for various highly complex

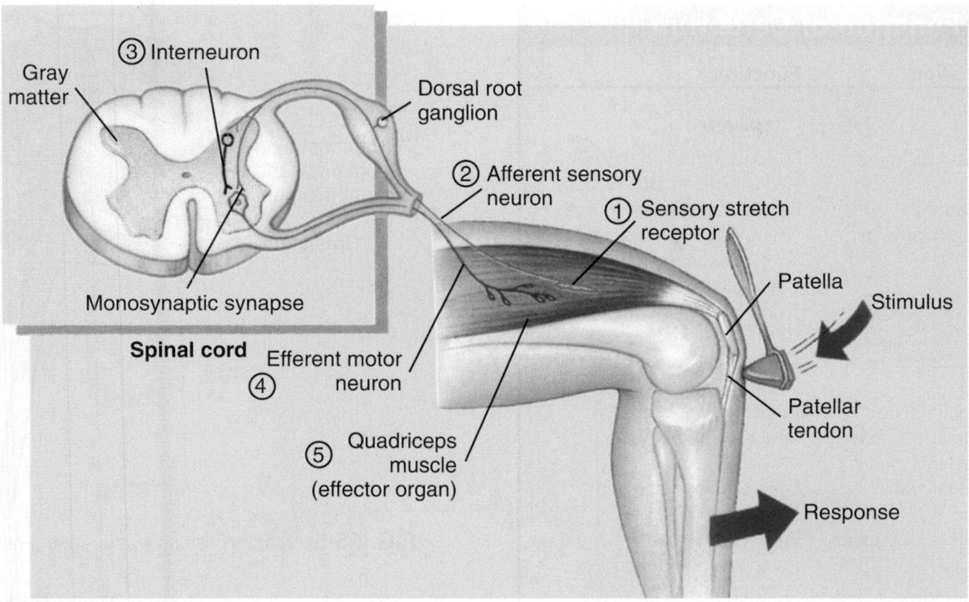


**FIG. 55-3** Basic diagram of the patellar "knee jerk" reflex arc, including the *(1)* sensory stretch receptor, *(2)* afferent sensory neuron, *(3)* interneuron, *(4)* efferent motor neuron, and *(5)* quadriceps muscle (effector organ). (Modified from Thibodeau GA, Patton KT: *Anatomy and physiology,* ed 6, St Louis, 2007, Mosby.)

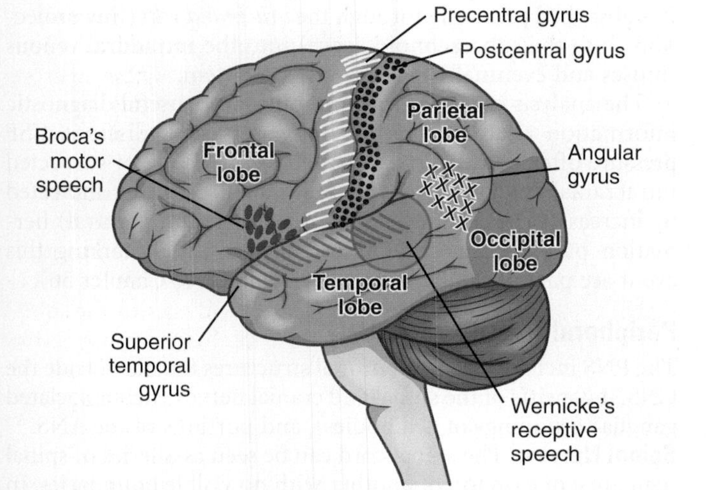


**FIG. 55-4** Left hemisphere of cerebrum, lateral surface, showing major lobes and areas of the brain.

and sophisticated functions, such as language, memory, and appreciation of visual-spatial relationships.

The basal ganglia, thalamus, hypothalamus, and limbic system are also located in the cerebrum. The *basal ganglia* are a group of structures located centrally in the cerebrum and midbrain. Most of them are on both sides of the thalamus. The function of the basal ganglia includes the initiation, execution, and completion of voluntary movements, learning, emotional response, and automatic movements associated with skeletal muscle activity (e.g., swallowing saliva, blinking, and swinging the arms while walking).

The *thalamus* lies directly above the brainstem (Fig. 55-5) and is the major relay center for sensory input from the body, face, retina, and cochlear and taste receptors. Motor relay nuclei in the thalamus connect the cerebellum and basal ganglia to the frontal cortex.

The *hypothalamus* is located just inferior to the thalamus and slightly in front of the midbrain. It exerts a direct influence on release of hormones from the anterior pituitary gland and has a rich capillary connection to this gland to assist in the transport of hormones. These hormones include thyroid-stimulating hormone, growth hormone, luteinizing hormone, and prolactin-releasing hormone, which play a role in regulating reproductive function. In contrast, the supraoptic and paraventricular neurons travel directly through the pituitary stalk to the posterior pituitary, where they release vasopressin and oxytocin. The hypothalamus contains the satiety center that regulates appetite. Subject to input from the limbic system, it also regulates body temperature, water balance (through influence on vasopressin secretion), circadian rhythm, and expression of emotion. The *limbic system* is located near the inner surfaces of the cerebral hemispheres and is concerned with emotion, aggression, feeding behavior, and sexual response.

***Brainstem.*** The *brainstem* includes the midbrain, pons, and medulla (Fig. 55-5). Ascending and descending fibers to and from the cerebrum and cerebellum pass through the brainstem. The nuclei of cranial nerves III through XII are in the brainstem. The vital centers concerned with respiratory, vasomotor, and cardiac function are located in the medulla.

Also located in the brainstem is the *reticular formation,* a diffusely arranged group of neurons and their axons that extends from the medulla to the thalamus and hypothalamus. The functions of the reticular formation include relaying sensory information, influencing excitatory and inhibitory control of spinal motor neurons, and controlling vasomotor and respiratory activity. The *reticular activating system* (RAS) is a complex system that requires communication among the brainstem, reticular formation, and cerebral cortex. The RAS is responsible for regulating arousal and sleep-wake transitions. The brainstem also contains the centers for sneezing, coughing, hiccuping, vomiting, sucking, and swallowing.

***Cerebellum.*** The *cerebellum* is located in the posterior cranial fossa inferior to the occipital lobe. The cerebellum coordinates voluntary movement and maintains trunk stability and equilibrium. The cerebellum receives information from the cerebral cortex, muscles, joints, and inner ear. It influences motor

**TABLE 55-1 Function of Cerebrum**

| Part | Location | Function |
|---|---|---|
| **Cortical Areas** | | |
| ***Motor*** | | |
| Primary | Precentral gyrus | Motor control and movement on opposite side of body |
| Supplemental | Anterior to precentral gyrus | Facilitates proximal muscle activity, including activity for stance and gait, and spontaneous movement and coordination |
| ***Sensory*** | | |
| Somatic | Postcentral gyrus | Sensory response from opposite side of body |
| Visual | Occipital lobe | Registers visual images |
| Auditory | Superior temporal gyrus | Registers auditory input |
| Association areas | Parietal lobe | Integrates somatic and sensory input |
| | Posterior temporal lobe | Integrates visual and auditory input for language comprehension |
| | Anterior temporal lobe | Integrates past experiences |
| | Anterior frontal lobe | Controls higher-order processes (e.g., judgment, reasoning) |
| ***Language*** | | |
| Comprehension | Wernicke's area in dominant posterior temporal lobe | Integrates auditory language (understanding of spoken words) |
| Expression | Broca's area in dominant frontal lobe | Regulates motor speech |
| **Basal Ganglia** | Near lateral ventricles of both cerebral hemispheres | Controls and refines learned and automatic movements |
| **Thalamus** | Below and slightly posterior to basal ganglia | Relays sensory and motor input to and from cerebrum |
| **Hypothalamus** | Below and anterior to thalamus | Regulates endocrine and autonomic functions |
| **Limbic System** | Lateral to hypothalamus | Influences emotional behavior and basic drives such as feeding and sexual behavior |

activity through axonal connections to the thalamus, motor cortex, and brainstem nuclei and their descending pathways.

***Ventricles and Cerebrospinal Fluid.*** The ventricles are four interconnected fluid-filled cavities. The lower portion of the fourth ventricle becomes the central canal in the lower part of the brainstem. The spinal canal extends centrally through the full length of the spinal cord.

**Cerebrospinal fluid (CSF)** is produced largely in the choroid plexuses of the brain within the ventricles. It circulates within the subarachnoid space that surrounds the brain, brainstem, and spinal cord, cushioning the brain and spinal cord. CSF flows from the cranial cavity to the spinal cavity, carrying nutrients through both passive diffusion and active transport. CSF is produced at an average rate of about 500 mL/day. The ventricles and central canal are filled with an average of 150 mL at any given time. Changes in the rate of CSF production or absorption can occur, leading to a change in the volume within the ventricles and central canal. Excessive buildup of CSF results in a condition known as *hydrocephalus*.

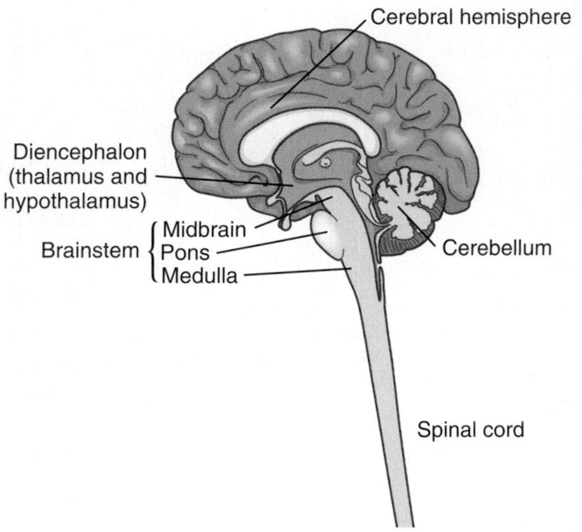


**FIG. 55-5** Major divisions of the central nervous system (CNS).

The CSF circulates throughout the ventricles and seeps into the subarachnoid space surrounding the brain and spinal cord. It is absorbed primarily through the *arachnoid villi* (tiny projections into the subarachnoid space) into the intradural venous sinuses and eventually into the venous system.

The analysis of CSF composition provides useful diagnostic information related to certain nervous system diseases. CSF pressure often is measured in patients with actual or suspected intracranial injury. Increased intracranial pressure, indicated by increased CSF pressure, can force downward (central) herniation of the brain and brainstem. The signs marking this event are part of the herniation syndrome (see Chapter 56).

## Peripheral Nervous System

The PNS includes all the neuronal structures that lie outside the CNS. It consists of the spinal and cranial nerves, their associated ganglia (groupings of cell bodies), and portions of the ANS.

**Spinal Nerves.** The spinal cord can be seen as a series of spinal segments, one on top of another with no visible boundaries. In addition to the cell bodies, each segment contains a pair of dorsal (afferent) sensory nerve fibers or roots and ventral (efferent) motor fibers or roots, which innervate a specific region of the body. This combined motor-sensory nerve is called a *spinal nerve* (Fig. 55-6). The cell bodies of the voluntary motor system are located in the anterior horn of the spinal cord gray matter. The cell bodies of the autonomic (involuntary) motor system are located in the anterolateral portion of the spinal cord gray matter. The cell bodies of sensory fibers are located in the dorsal root ganglia just outside the spinal cord. On exiting the spinal column, each spinal nerve divides into ventral and dorsal rami, a collection of motor and sensory fibers that eventually goes to peripheral structures (e.g., skin, muscles, viscera).

A **dermatome** is the area of skin innervated by the sensory fibers of a single dorsal root of a spinal nerve (Fig. 55-7). The dermatomes give a general picture of somatic sensory innervation by spinal segments. A *myotome* is a muscle group innervated by the primary motor neurons of a single ventral root. The dermatomes and myotomes of a given spinal segment overlap with those of adjacent segments because of the development of ascending and descending collateral branches of nerve fibers.

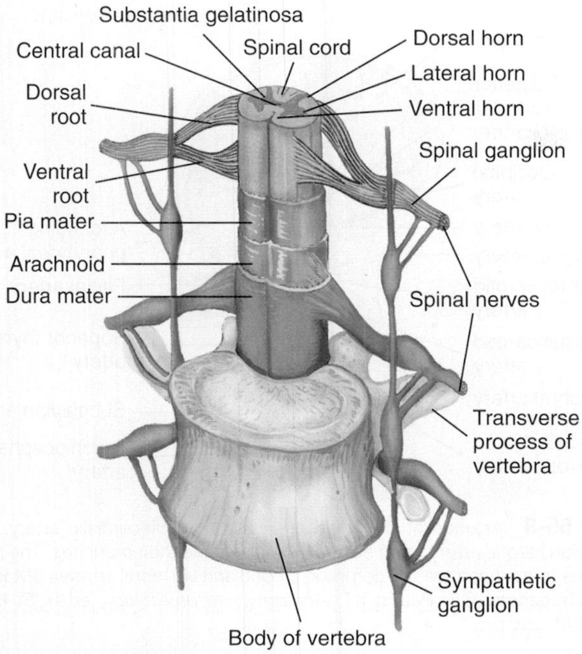


**FIG. 55-6** Cross section of spinal cord showing attachments of spinal nerves and coverings of the spinal cord.

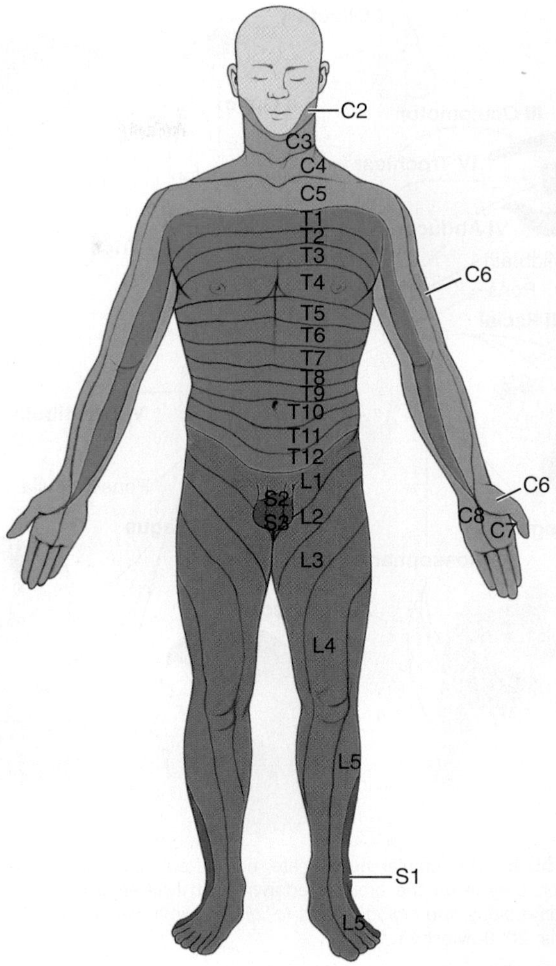


**FIG. 55-7** Dermatomes of the body. (From Herlihy B: *The human body in health and illness,* ed 4, St Louis, 2011, Saunders.)

**Cranial Nerves.** The cranial nerves (CNs) are the 12 paired nerves composed of cell bodies with fibers that exit from the cranial cavity. Unlike the spinal nerves, which always have both afferent sensory and efferent motor fibers, some CNs are only sensory, some only motor, and some both.

Table 55-4 (later in this chapter) summarizes the motor and sensory components of the CNs. Fig. 55-8 shows the position of the CNs in relation to the brain and spinal cord. Just as the cell bodies of the spinal nerves are located in specific segments of the spinal cord, so are the cell bodies (nuclei) of the CNs located in specific segments of the brainstem. Exceptions are the nuclei of the olfactory and optic nerves. The primary cell bodies of the olfactory nerve are located in the nasal epithelium, and those of the optic nerve are in the retina.

**Autonomic Nervous System.** The autonomic nervous system (ANS) is divided into the sympathetic and parasympathetic systems. The ANS governs involuntary functions of cardiac muscle, smooth muscle, and glands through both efferent and afferent pathways. The two systems function together to maintain a relatively balanced internal environment. The preganglionic cell bodies of the *sympathetic nervous system* (SNS) are located in spinal segments T1 through L2. The major neurotransmitter released by the postganglionic fibers of the SNS is norepinephrine, and the neurotransmitter released by the preganglionic fibers is acetylcholine.

The preganglionic cell bodies of the *parasympathetic nervous system* (PSNS) are located in the brainstem and sacral spinal segments (S2 through S4). Acetylcholine is the neurotransmitter released at both preganglionic and postganglionic nerve endings.

SNS stimulation activates the mechanisms required for the "fight-or-flight" response that occurs throughout the body. In contrast, the PSNS is geared to act in localized and discrete regions. It conserves and restores the body's energy stores. The ANS provides dual and often reciprocal innervation to many structures. For example, the SNS increases the rate and force of heart contraction, and the PSNS decreases the rate and force.

## Cerebral Circulation

Knowledge of the distribution of the brain's major arteries is essential for understanding and evaluating the signs and symptoms of cerebrovascular disease and trauma. The brain's blood supply arises from the internal carotid arteries (anterior circulation) and the vertebral arteries (posterior circulation), which are shown in Fig. 55-9.

The internal carotid arteries provide blood flow to the anterior and middle portions of the cerebrum. The vertebral arteries join to form the basilar artery and provide blood flow to the brainstem, cerebellum, and posterior cerebrum. The *Circle of Willis* is formed by communicating arteries that join the basilar and internal carotid arteries (Fig. 55-10). Although the Circle of Willis is considered a safety valve for blood flow, variations exist in 31% to 44% of patients.[3]

Superior to the Circle of Willis, three pairs of arteries supply blood to the left and right hemispheres. The anterior cerebral artery feeds the medial and anterior portions of the frontal lobes. The middle cerebral artery feeds the outer portions of the frontal, parietal, and superior temporal lobes. The posterior cerebral artery feeds the medial portions of the occipital and inferior temporal lobes. Venous blood drains from the brain through the dural sinuses, which form channels that drain into the two jugular veins.

**Blood-Brain Barrier.** The blood-brain barrier is a physiologic barrier between blood capillaries and brain tissue. This barrier

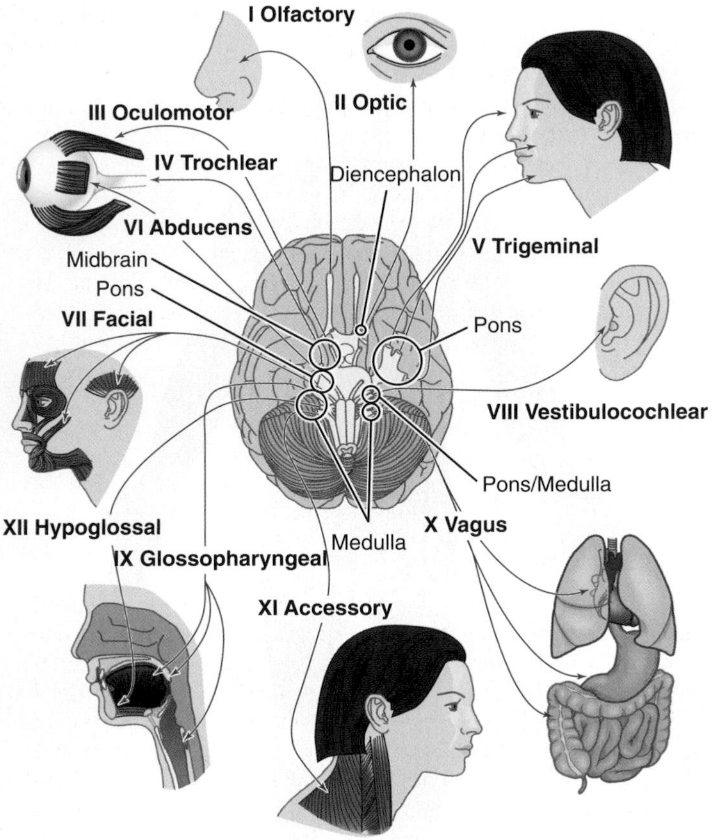


**FIG. 55-8** The cranial nerves are numbered according to the order in which they leave the brain. (Redrawn from McCance KL, Huether SE: *Pathophysiology: the biologic basis for disease in adults and children,* ed 6, St Louis, 2010, Mosby.)

protects the brain from harmful agents, while allowing nutrients and gases to enter. The structure of brain capillaries differs from that of other capillaries, so substances that normally pass into most tissues are prevented from entering brain tissue. Lipid-soluble compounds enter the brain easily, whereas water-soluble and ionized drugs enter the brain and the spinal cord slowly. Thus the blood-brain barrier affects the penetration of drugs. Only certain drugs can enter the CNS from the bloodstream.

## Protective Structures

**Meninges.** The meninges consist of three protective membranes that surround the brain and spinal cord: dura mater, arachnoid, and pia mater (Fig. 55-11). The thick *dura mater* forms the outermost layer. The *falx cerebri* is a fold of the dura that separates the two cerebral hemispheres and slows expansion of brain tissue in conditions such as a rapidly growing tumor or acute hemorrhage. The *tentorium cerebelli* is a fold of dura that separates the cerebral hemispheres from the posterior fossa (which contains the brainstem and cerebellum).

The *arachnoid* layer is a fragile, web-like membrane that lies between the dura mater and *pia mater* (the vascular innermost layer of the meninges). The area between the arachnoid layer and pia mater *(subarachnoid space)* is filled with CSF. Structures such as arteries, veins, and cranial nerves passing to and from the brain and skull must pass through the subarachnoid space. A larger subarachnoid space in the region of the third and fourth lumbar vertebrae is the area used to obtain CSF during a lumbar puncture.

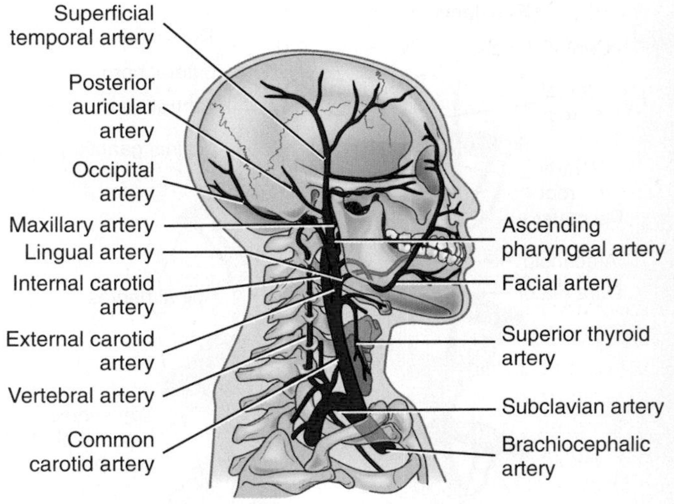


**FIG. 55-9** Arteries of the head and neck. Brachiocephalic artery, right common carotid artery, right subclavian artery, and their branches. The major arteries to the head are the common carotid and vertebral arteries. (Modified from Thibodeau GA, Patton KT: *Anatomy and physiology,* ed 8, St Louis, 2013, Mosby.)

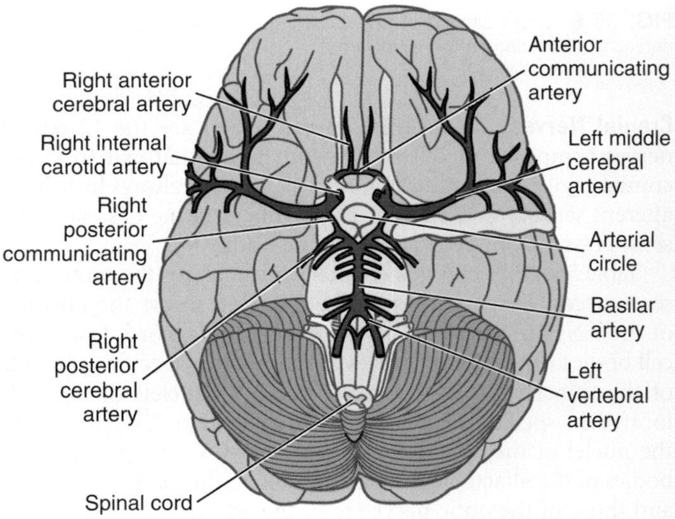


**FIG. 55-10** Arteries at the base of the brain. The arteries that compose the Circle of Willis are the two anterior cerebral arteries joined to each other by the anterior communicating cerebral artery and to the posterior cerebral arteries by the posterior communicating arteries. (Modified from Thibodeau GA, Patton KT: *Anatomy and physiology,* ed 8, St Louis, 2013, Mosby.)

**Skull.** The *skull* protects the brain from external trauma. It is composed of eight cranial bones and 14 facial bones. Although the top and sides of the inside of the skull are relatively smooth, the bottom surface is uneven. It has many ridges, prominences, and foramina (holes through which blood vessels and nerves enter the intracranial vault). The largest hole is the *foramen magnum,* through which the brainstem extends to the spinal cord. This foramen offers the only major space for the expansion of brain contents when increased intracranial pressure occurs.

**Vertebral Column.** The *vertebral column* protects the spinal cord, supports the head, and provides flexibility. The vertebral column is made up of 33 individual vertebrae: 7 cervical, 12 thoracic, 5 lumbar, 5 sacral (fused into one), and 4 coccygeal (fused into one). Each vertebra has a central opening through which the spinal cord passes. The vertebrae are held together by a series of ligaments. Intervertebral discs occupy the spaces between vertebrae, allowing movement of the column. Fig.

55-12 shows the natural curvature of the spinal column and its relation to the trunk.

### Gerontologic Considerations: Effects of Aging on Nervous System

Several parts of the nervous system are affected by aging. In the CNS the gradual loss of neurons in certain areas of the brainstem, cerebellum, and cerebral cortex begins in early adulthood. With loss of neurons, the ventricles widen or enlarge, brain weight decreases, cerebral blood flow decreases, and CSF production declines.[4,5]

In the PNS, degenerative changes in myelin cause a decrease in nerve conduction. Coordinated neuromuscular activity, such as the maintenance of BP in response to changing from a lying to a standing position, is altered with aging. As a result, older adults are more likely to experience orthostatic hypotension. Similarly, coordination of neuromuscular activity to maintain body temperature also becomes less efficient with aging. Older adults are less able to adapt to extremes in environmental temperature and are more vulnerable to both hypothermia and hyperthermia.

Additional relevant changes associated with aging include decreases in memory, vision, hearing, taste, smell, vibration, position sense, muscle strength, and reaction time. Sensory changes, including decreases in taste and smell perception, may result in decreased dietary intake in the older adult.[6] Reduced hearing and vision can result in perceptual confusion. Problems with balance and coordination can put the older adult at risk for falls and subsequent fractures.[7] Changes in assessment findings result from age-related alterations in the various components of the nervous system (Table 55-2). Changes should not be attributed to aging without considering other underlying causes.

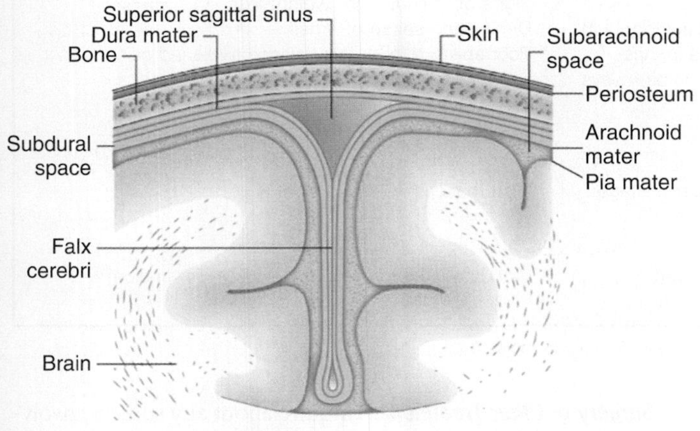


**FIG. 55-11** Meninges.

## ASSESSMENT OF NERVOUS SYSTEM

### Subjective Data

#### Important Health Information

***Past Health History.*** When performing a neurologic examination, first determine if an emergency exists. For example, does the patient demonstrate decreasing level of consciousness? The neurologic assessment is performed when an abnormality is identified during screening or can be expected based on patient history. Is the patient a reliable historian and able to provide detailed information? If not, interview someone with firsthand knowledge of the patient's history and current complaint. Avoid suggesting symptoms or asking leading questions.

Second, the mode of onset and course of the illness are especially important aspects of the history. Often the nature of a neurologic disease process can be described by these facts alone. Obtain all pertinent data in the history of the present illness, especially data related to the characteristics and progression of the symptoms. In some cases, the history may include

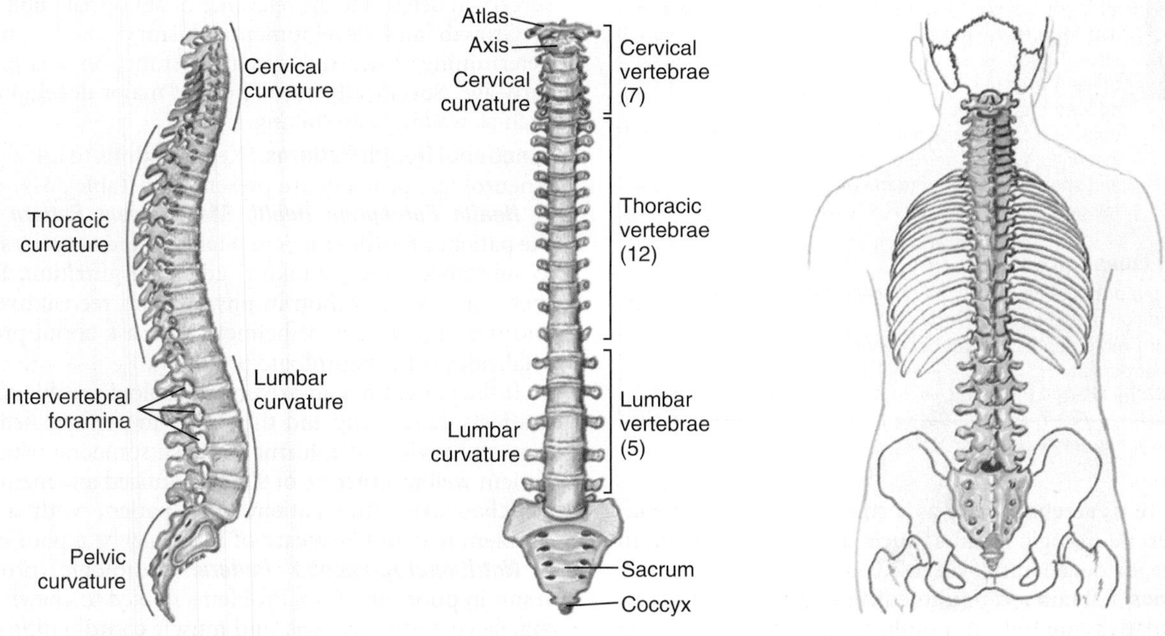


**FIG. 55-12** The vertebral column (three views). (Modified from Thibodeau GA, Patton KT: *Anatomy and physiology,* ed 8, St Louis, 2013, Mosby.)

## TABLE 55-2 Gerontologic Assessment Differences

### Nervous System

| Component | Changes | Differences in Assessment Findings |
|---|---|---|
| **Central Nervous System** | | |
| ***Brain*** | ↓ Cerebral blood flow and metabolism<br>↓ Efficiency of temperature-regulating mechanism<br>↓ Neurotransmitters, loss of neurons<br>↓ $O_2$ supply<br>Cerebral tissue atrophy and ↑ size of ventricles | Alterations in mental functioning.<br>Impaired ability to adapt to environmental temperature.<br>Slowed conduction of nerve impulses, with slowed response time.<br>Changes in gait and ambulation. Diminished kinesthetic sense.<br>Altered balance, vertigo, syncope. ↑ Postural hypotension. Proprioception diminished. ↓ Sensory input. |
| **Peripheral Nervous System** | | |
| ***Cranial and spinal nerves*** | Loss of myelin and ↓ conduction time<br>Cellular degeneration, death of neurons | ↓ Reaction time in specific nerves.<br>↓ Speed and intensity of neuronal reflexes. |
| **Functional Divisions** | | |
| ***Motor*** | ↓ Muscle bulk | Diminished strength and agility. |
| ***Sensory**** | ↓ Sensory receptors<br>↓ Electrical activity<br>Atrophy of taste buds<br>Degeneration and loss of fibers in olfactory bulb<br>Degenerative changes in nerve cells in inner ear, cerebellum, and proprioceptive pathways | Diminished sense of touch, pain, and temperature.<br>Slowing of or alteration in sensory reception.<br>Signs of malnutrition, weight loss.<br>Diminished sense of smell.<br>Poor ability to maintain balance, widened gait. |
| ***Reflexes*** | ↓ Deep tendon reflexes<br>↓ Sensory conduction velocity | Below-average reflex score.<br>Sluggish reflexes, slowed reaction time. |
| **Reticular Formation** | | |
| ***Reticular activating system*** | Modification of hypothalamic function, ↓ stage IV sleep | Disturbances in sleep patterns. |
| **Autonomic Nervous System** | | |
| ***Sympathetic nervous system and parasympathetic nervous system*** | Morphologic features of ganglia, slowed autonomic nervous system responses | Orthostatic hypotension, systolic hypertension. |

*Specific changes related to the eye are listed in Table 20-1, and specific changes related to the ear are listed in Table 20-7.

## CASE STUDY

### Patient Introduction

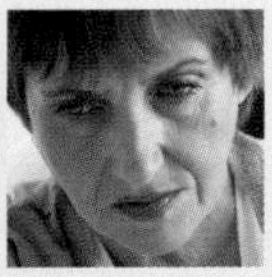

(©TatyanaGl/iStock/Thinkstock)

J.K. is a 57-yr-old white woman who went to see her HCP for severe, persistent headaches that she has had for a few weeks. She lives alone and has a very stressful job as an office manager in an engineering office. When her HCP did a neurologic examination, he noticed that she had a visual field deficit, especially in upper left quadrant of her visual field. During the examination, J.K. had a seizure in his office. 911 was called and she was admitted to the hospital. The on-call neurologist was notified.

**Discussion Questions**

1. What are the possible causes of J.K.'s headaches and seizure?
2. Is her condition stable or an emergency?

You will learn more about J.K. and her condition as you read through this assessment chapter.

(See p. 1304 for more information on J.K.)

Answers available at *http://evolve.elsevier.com/Lewis/medsurg.*

birth injury (e.g., cerebral palsy as a consequence of hypoxia) and/or other neurologic insults, such as a traumatic brain injury, stroke, or degenerative disease.

***Medications.*** Obtain a careful medication history, especially the use of sedatives, opioids, tranquilizers, and mood-elevating drugs. Many other drugs also can cause neurologic side effects. Additionally, ask the patient to describe the medication regimen to determine adherence to prescribed therapies.

***Surgery or Other Treatments.*** Inquire about any surgery involving any part of the nervous system, such as head, spine, or sensory organs. If a patient had surgery, determine the date, cause, procedure, recovery, and current status. Also note any history of eye surgery to determine the relevance of abnormal pupil assessment.

Growth and developmental history can be important in determining if nervous system dysfunction was present at an early age. Specifically inquire about major developmental tasks such as walking and talking.

**Functional Health Patterns.** Key questions to ask a patient with a neurologic problem are presented in Table 55-3.

***Health Perception–Health Management Pattern.*** Ask about the patient's health practices related to the nervous system, such as substance abuse, smoking, adequate nutrition, BP management, safe participation in physical and recreational activities, and use of seat belts or helmets. Also ask about previous hospitalizations for neurologic problems.

If the patient has an existing neurologic problem, assess how it affects daily living and the ability to perform self-care. After a careful review of information, ask someone who knows the patient well whether he or she has noticed any mental or physical changes in the patient. The patient with a neurologic problem may not be aware of it or may be a poor historian.

***Nutritional-Metabolic Pattern.*** Neurologic problems can result in poor nutrition. Problems related to chewing, swallowing, facial nerve paralysis, and muscle coordination could make it difficult for the patient to ingest adequate nutrients. Also, certain vitamins such as thiamine ($B_1$), niacin, and pyridoxine ($B_6$) are essential for the maintenance and health of the CNS.

## TABLE 55-3 Health History

### *Nervous System*

**Health Perception–Health Management**
- What are your usual daily activities?
- Do you use alcohol, tobacco, or recreational drugs?*
- What safety practices do you perform in a car? On a motorcycle? On a bicycle?
- Do you have hypertension? If so, how is it managed?
- Have you ever been hospitalized for a neurologic problem?*

**Nutritional-Metabolic**
- Are you able to feed yourself?
- Do you have any problems getting adequate nutrition because of chewing or swallowing difficulties, facial nerve paralysis, or poor muscle coordination?*
- Give a 24-hr dietary recall.

**Elimination**
- Do you have incontinence of your bowels or bladder?*
- Do you ever experience problems with urinary hesitancy, urgency, retention?*
- Do you postpone your bowel movements?*
- Do you take any medication to manage neurologic problems? If so, what?

**Activity-Exercise**
- Describe any problems you experience with usual activities and exercise as a result of a neurologic problem.
- Do you have weakness or lack of coordination?*
- Are you able to perform your personal hygiene needs independently?*

**Sleep-Rest**
- Describe your sleep pattern.
- When you have trouble sleeping, what do you do?

**Cognitive-Perceptual**
- Have you noticed any changes in your memory?*
- Do you experience dizziness, heat or cold sensitivity, numbness, or tingling?*
- Do you have chronic pain?*
- Do you have any difficulty with verbal or written communication?*
- Have you noticed any changes in vision or hearing?*

**Self-Perception–Self-Concept**
- How do you feel about yourself, about who you are?
- Describe your general emotional pattern.

**Role-Relationship**
- Have you experienced changes in roles such as spouse, parent, or breadwinner?*

**Sexuality-Reproductive**
- Are you dissatisfied with your sexual function?*
- Are problems related to your sexual function causing tension in an important relationship?*
- Do you feel the need for professional counseling related to your sexual function?*

**Coping–Stress Tolerance**
- Describe your usual coping pattern.
- Do you think your present coping pattern is adequate to meet the stressors of your life?*
- What needs are unmet by your current support system?

**Value-Belief**
- Describe any culturally specific beliefs and attitudes that may influence your care.

*If yes, describe.

## GENETIC RISK ALERT

- Huntington's disease is a genetically transmitted, autosomal dominant disorder.
- Major neurologic disorders that may have a genetic basis are multiple sclerosis, headaches, Parkinson's disease, and Alzheimer's disease. The presence of these problems in a family history increases the likelihood of similar problems occurring in the patient.
- A careful family history may determine if a neurologic problem has a genetic basis.

Deficiencies in one or more of these vitamins could result in such nonspecific complaints as depression, apathy, neuritis, weakness, mental confusion, and irritability. Cobalamin (vitamin $B_{12}$) deficiency can occur in older adults, who may have problems with vitamin absorption from supplements as well as natural food sources such as meat, fish, and poultry. Untreated, cobalamin deficiency can cause mental function decline. In the patient with brain injury, early nutritional support can markedly improve outcomes.[8]

***Elimination Pattern.*** Bowel and bladder problems often are associated with neurologic problems such as stroke, head injury, spinal cord injury, multiple sclerosis, and dementia. To plan appropriate interventions, determine if the bowel or bladder problem was present before or after the current neurologic event. Urinary retention and incontinence of urine and feces are the most common elimination problems associated with a neurologic problem or its treatment. For example, nerve root compression (as occurs in cauda equina conditions) leads to a sudden onset of incontinence. Document key details, such as number of episodes, accompanying sensations or lack of sensations, and measures to control the problem.

***Activity-Exercise Pattern.*** Many neurologic disorders can cause problems in the patient's mobility, strength, and coordination. Neurologic problems can result in changes in the patient's usual activity and exercise patterns. These problems can also result in falls.[7] Assess the person's activities of daily living because neurologic diseases can affect the ability to perform motor tasks, which increases the possibility of injury.

***Sleep-Rest Pattern.*** Sleep pattern alteration can be both a cause and a response to neurologic problems. Pain and reduced ability to change position because of muscle weakness and paralysis could interfere with sleep quality. Hallucinations resulting from dementia or drugs can also interrupt sleep. Carefully assess and document the patient's sleep pattern and bedtime routines.

***Cognitive-Perceptual Pattern.*** Because the nervous system controls cognition and sensory integration, many neurologic disorders affect these functions.[9] Consider culture, age, and education when assessing communication because they play a role in the interaction among people. Assess memory, language, calculation ability, problem-solving ability, insight, and judgment. Ask the patient hypothetical questions such as, "What is a reasonable price for a cup of coffee?" or "What would you do if you saw a car crash outside your house?" Often a structured mental status questionnaire is used to evaluate these functions and provide baseline data.

*Delirium* is an acute and transient disorder of cognition that can be seen at any time during a patient's illness. As discussed in Chapter 59, delirium is often an early indicator of various illnesses (see Table 59-17). The Confusion Assessment Method tool is used to assess for delirium (see Table 59-18).

Assess a person's ability to use and understand language. Appropriateness of responses is a useful indicator of cognitive and perceptual ability. Determine the patient's understanding and ability to carry out necessary treatments. Neurologic-related cognitive changes can interfere with the patient's understanding of the disease and adherence to related treatment.

Pain is commonly associated with many neurologic problems, and is often the reason a patient seeks care. Carefully assess the patient's pain. (Pain and pain assessment are discussed in Chapter 8.)

***Self-Perception–Self-Concept Pattern.*** Neurologic diseases can drastically alter a patient's control over life and create dependency on others for meeting daily needs. Also, the patient's physical appearance and emotional control can be affected. Sensitively inquire about the patient's evaluation of self-worth, perception of abilities, body image, and general emotional pattern.

***Role-Relationship Pattern.*** Physical impairments such as weakness and paralysis can alter or limit participation in usual roles and activities. Cognitive changes can permanently alter a person's ability to maintain previous roles. These changes can dramatically affect the patient, caregiver, and family. Ask the patient if a role change has occurred (e.g., spouse or breadwinner) as a result of neurologic problems and determine how long it has lasted. Family members or caregivers should participate in decision making when neurologic deficits preclude the patient from decisions that will affect the role.

***Sexuality-Reproductive Pattern.*** Assess the person's ability to participate in sexual activity because many neurologic disorders can affect sexual response. Cerebral lesions may inhibit the desire phase or the reflex responses of the excitement phase. The hypothalamus stimulates the pituitary gland to release hormones that influence sexual desire. Brainstem and spinal cord lesions may partially or completely interrupt the desire or ability to have intercourse. Neuropathies and spinal cord lesions may prevent reflex activities of the sexual response or affect sensation and decrease desire. Despite neurologically related changes in sexual function, many persons can achieve satisfying expression of intimacy and affection.

***Coping–Stress Tolerance Pattern.*** The physical sequelae of a neurologic problem can strain a patient's coping ability. Often the problem is chronic and requires the patient to learn new coping skills. Assess if the patient's coping skills are adequate to deal with the stress of this problem. Also assess the patient's support system.

***Value-Belief Pattern.*** Many neurologic problems have serious, long-term, life-changing effects. Determine what these effects are because they can strain the patient's belief system. Also determine if any religious or cultural beliefs could affect the planned treatment regimen.

## Objective Data

**Physical Examination.** The standard neurologic examination helps determine the presence, location, and nature of nervous system disease. The examination assesses six categories of function: mental status, cranial nerve function, motor function, sensory function, cerebellar function, and reflexes.[10] Develop a consistent pattern of completing the neurologic examination to remember to include each element for every patient examination.

### CASE STUDY—cont'd

#### Subjective Data

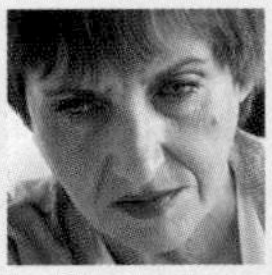

(©TatyanaGl/ iStock/ Thinkstock)

After her admission to the hospital, a subjective assessment of J.K. revealed the following information:

***PMH:*** No history of seizures, migraine, or other headache prior to the current headaches and seizure.

***Medications:*** lisinopril 10 mg PO daily.

***Health Perception–Health Management:*** Never smoked. Occasional social alcohol use. Reports good health other than mild hypertension.

***Nutritional-Metabolic:*** J.K. is 5 ft 5 in tall and weighs 145 lb.

***Activity-Exercise:*** Moderate activity. No formal exercise or participation in sports.

***Cognitive-Perceptual:*** States her headaches led her to get her eyes tested but only had minor decrease in visual acuity.

***Coping–Stress Tolerance:*** Is depressed and fearful. She is worried that something serious is wrong. Denies dizziness, change in hearing, or memory deficits.

**Discussion Questions**

1. What type of assessment would be most appropriate for J.K.: comprehensive, focused, or emergency? What would be your priority?
2. What assessment questions will you ask her?
3. Which subjective assessment findings are of most concern to you?
4. Based on these subjective assessment findings, what type of physical assessment should be performed?

You will learn more about the physical examination of the neurologic system in the next section.

(See p. 1307 for more information on J.K.)

Answers available at *http://evolve.elsevier.com/Lewis/medsurg.*

***Mental Status.*** Assessment of mental status (cerebral function) gives a general impression of how the patient is functioning. It involves determining complex and high-level cerebral functions governed by many areas of the cerebral cortex. Complete most of the mental status examination during your interaction with the patient. For example, assess language and memory when asking the patient for details of the illness and significant past events. Consider the patient's age, cultural background, and level of education when evaluating mental status.

The components of the mental status examination include:

- *General appearance and behavior:* This component includes level of consciousness (awake, asleep, comatose), motor activity, body posture, dress and hygiene, facial expression, and speech pattern. A patient who has deficits in self-care as evidenced by poor grooming is more likely to have other cognitive deficits.
- *Cognition:* Note orientation to time, place, person, and situation, as well as memory, general knowledge, insight, judgment, problem solving, and calculation. Common questions are "Who were the last three presidents?" "Does a rock float on water?" "How much money is a quarter, two dimes, and a nickel?" Consider if the patient's plans and goals match the physical and mental capabilities. Note the presence of factors affecting intellectual capacity, such as cognitive impairment, hallucinations, delusions, and dementia.
- *Mood and affect:* Note any agitation, anger, depression, or euphoria, and the appropriateness of these states. Use suitable questions to reveal the patient's feelings.

***Cranial Nerves.*** Testing each CN is an essential part of the neurologic examination (Table 55-4).

## TABLE 55-4 Cranial Nerves: Function and Assessment

| Nerve | Function | Assessment |
|---|---|---|
| **I Olfactory** | *Sensory:* from olfactory (smell) | Ask patient to close one nostril at a time and identify easily recognized odors (e.g., coffee). Any asymmetry in sense of smell is important. |
| **II Optic** | *Sensory:* from retina of eyes (vision) | Examine each eye independently.<br>*Visual fields:* Position yourself opposite the patient. Ask him or her to look directly at the bridge of your nose and indicate when an object (finger, pencil tip) presented from the periphery of each of the visual fields is seen (Fig. 55-13).<br>*Visual acuity:* Ask patient to read a Snellen chart. Record the number on the lowest line the patient can read with 50% accuracy. The patient who wears glasses should wear them during testing unless they are used only for close reading. If a Snellen chart is not available, ask the patient to read newsprint for gross assessment of acuity. Record the distance from patient to newsprint required for accurate reading. |
| **III Oculomotor** | *Motor:* to four eye movement muscles and levator palpebrae muscle<br>*Parasympathetic:* smooth muscle in eyeball | Ask the person to hold the head steady and to follow the movement of your finger, pen, or penlight only with the eyes. Hold the target back about 12 inches so that the person can focus on it comfortably. Move the target to each of the six positions (right and up, right, right and down, left and up, left, left and down), hold it momentarily, and then move back to center. Progress clockwise. A normal response is parallel tracking of the object with both eyes.<br>Check for pupillary constriction and *accommodation* (pupils constricting with near vision). To test pupillary constriction, shine a light into the pupil of one eye; look for ipsilateral constriction of the same pupil and contralateral (consensual) constriction of the opposite eye. Note the size and shape of the pupils. (The optic nerve must be intact for this reflex to occur.) |
| **IV Trochlear** | *Motor:* to one eye movement muscle, the superior oblique muscle | See testing for CN III. (Because the oculomotor [CN III], trochlear [CN IV], and abducens [CN VI] nerves help move the eye, they are tested together.) |
| **V Trigeminal** | | |
| • Ophthalmic branch | *Sensory:* from forehead, eye, superior nasal cavity | *Sensory:* Have patient close eyes and identify light touch (cotton wisp) and pinprick in each of the three divisions (ophthalmic, maxillary, and mandibular) of nerve on both sides of face. |
| • Maxillary branch | *Sensory:* from inferior nasal cavity, face, upper teeth, mucosa of superior mouth | *Motor:* Ask patient to clench teeth and then palpate masseter muscles just above the mandibular angle. Muscles should feel equally strong on both sides. |
| • Mandibular branch | *Sensory:* from surfaces of jaw, lower teeth, mucosa of lower mouth, and anterior tongue<br>*Motor:* to muscles of mastication | *Corneal (blink) reflex:* Evaluates CN V and CN VII simultaneously. (Sensory component of this reflex [corneal sensation] is innervated by the ophthalmic division of CN V. The motor component [eye blink] is innervated by the facial nerve [CN VII]). Have patient look up and away. Then from the other side, lightly touch the cornea with cotton wisp. Look for normal blink reaction of both eyes. Repeat on other side. |
| **VI Abducens** | *Motor:* to the lateral rectus muscle of the eye (one eye movement) | See testing for CN III. (Because the oculomotor [CN III], trochlear [CN IV], and abducens [CN VI] nerves help move the eye, they are tested together.) |
| **VII Facial** | *Motor:* to facial muscles of expression and cheek muscle<br>*Sensory:* taste from anterior two thirds of tongue | Ask patient to raise eyebrows, close eyes tightly, purse lips, draw back the corners of mouth in an exaggerated smile, and frown. Note any asymmetry in the facial movements because this can indicate damage to nerve. |
| **VIII Vestibulocochlear** | | |
| • Vestibular branch | *Sensory:* from equilibrium sensory organ (vestibular apparatus) | Not routinely tested unless the patient complains of dizziness, vertigo, or unsteadiness, or has auditory dysfunction. |
| • Cochlear branch | *Sensory:* from auditory sensory organ (cochlea), hearing | Have patient close eyes and indicate when he or she hears the rustling of your fingertips. For more precise assessment of hearing, perform the Weber and Rinne tests or use an audiometer (see Table 20-11). |
| **IX Glossopharyngeal** | *Sensory:* from pharynx and posterior tongue, including taste<br>*Motor:* to superior pharyngeal muscles | The glossopharyngeal and vagus nerves (CN IX and X) are tested together because both innervate the pharynx. To test the gag reflex, touch the sides of the posterior pharynx or soft palate with a tongue blade. If the reflex is weak or absent, the patient is in danger of aspirating food or secretions.<br>Another test for the awake, cooperative patient is to ask the patient to say "ah," and note the bilateral symmetry of elevation of the soft palate.<br>If a patient has an endotracheal tube, the cough reflex (elicited when the suction catheter contacts the *carina* of the respiratory tree) is a method of assessing the vagus nerve. |
| **X Vagus** | *Sensory:* from much of viscera of thorax and abdomen<br>*Motor:* to larynx and middle and inferior pharyngeal muscles<br>*Parasympathetic:* to heart, lungs, most of digestive system | See testing for CN IX. (The glossopharyngeal and vagus nerves [CN IX and X] are tested together because both innervate the pharynx.) |
| **XI Accessory** | *Motor:* to sternocleidomastoid and trapezius muscles | Ask patient to shrug the shoulders and to turn head to either side against resistance. Sternocleidomastoid and trapezius muscles should contract smoothly. Note symmetry, atrophy, or fasciculation of muscle. |
| **XII Hypoglossal** | *Motor:* to muscles of tongue | Ask to protrude tongue, which should protrude in midline. Next ask the patient to move the tongue up and down and side to side. Finally, the patient should also be able to push the tongue to either side against the resistance of a tongue blade. Note any asymmetry, atrophy, or fasciculation. |

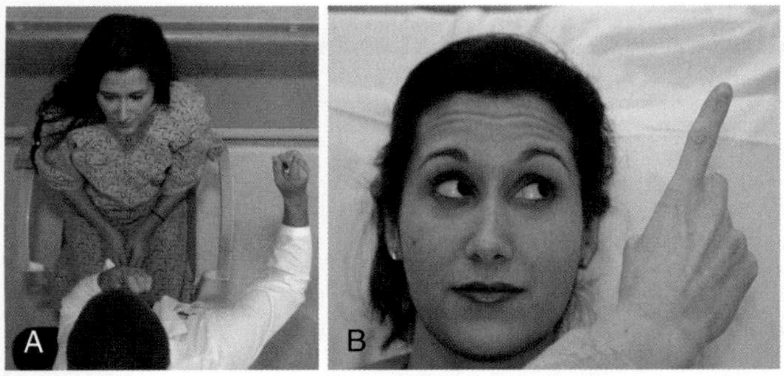

**FIG. 55-13** **A,** Nurse checking visual fields. **B,** Nurse checking extraocular movement (EOM). (Courtesy DaiWai Olson, RN, PhD, CCRN, Dallas, Tex.)

**Olfactory nerve.** Chronic rhinitis, sinusitis, and heavy smoking may decrease the sense of smell. Disturbance in ability to smell may be associated with a tumor involving the olfactory bulb or may be the result of a basilar skull fracture that has damaged the olfactory fibers as they pass through the delicate cribriform plate of the skull. *Anosmia* (loss of sense of smell) also has been identified as an early sign in Parkinson's disease and Lewy body dementia.[11]

**Optic nerve.** Visual field defects may arise from lesions of the optic nerve, optic chiasm, or tracts that extend through the temporal, parietal, or occipital lobes. Visual field changes resulting from brain lesions include *hemianopsia* (one half of the visual field is affected), *quadrantanopsia* (one fourth of the visual field is affected), *bitemporal hemianopsia* (bilateral peripheral vision is affected), or monocular vision. It may be difficult to test acuity if the patient does not read English or is aphasic.

**Oculomotor, trochlear, and abducens nerves.** Because the oculomotor (CN III), trochlear (CN IV), and abducens (CN VI) nerves help move the eye, they are tested together (Table 55-4). With weakness or paralysis of one of the eye muscles, the eyes do not move together, and the patient has a *disconjugate gaze.* The presence and direction of *nystagmus* (fine, rapid jerking movements of the eyes) are observed at this time, even though this condition most often indicates vestibulocerebellar problems.

Because the oculomotor nerve exits at the top of the brainstem at the tentorial notch, it can be compressed easily by expanding mass lesions. When this occurs, sympathetic input to the pupil is unopposed; the pupil changes shape and becomes dilated. The lack of pupillary constriction is an early sign of central herniation (see Chapter 56).

Two abbreviations commonly used to record the reaction of the pupils are *PERRL* (*P*upils are *E*qual [in size], *R*ound, and *R*eactive to *L*ight) and *PERRLA* (*P*upils are *E*qual, *R*ound, and *R*eactive to *L*ight and *A*ccommodation). The *PERRL* abbreviation is appropriate when accommodation cannot be assessed, as in an unconscious patient. Convergence and accommodation are tested by having the patient focus on the examiner's finger as it moves toward the patient's nose.

Another function of the oculomotor nerve is to keep the eyelid open. Damage to the nerve can cause *ptosis* (drooping eyelid), pupillary abnormalities, and eye muscle weakness.

***Motor System.*** The motor system examination includes assessment of strength, tone, coordination, and symmetry of the major muscle groups. Test muscle strength by asking the patient to push and pull against the resistance of your arm as it opposes flexion and extension of the patient's muscle. Ask the patient to offer resistance at the shoulders, elbows, wrists, hips, knees, and ankles. Mild weakness of the arm is demonstrated by downward drifting of the arm or pronation of the palm *(pronator drift).* The pronator drift test is particularly sensitive when the patient has a potential for vasospasm or increasing edema in one hemisphere of the cerebrum. Ask the patient to close the eyes and hold the arms out with palms facing up (as though he or she is holding a large pizza). The patient should hold this position for 30 seconds. Downward drift with palm pronation indicates a problem in the opposite motor cortex. Note any weakness or asymmetry of strength between the same muscle groups of the right and left sides.

Test muscle tone by passively moving the limbs through their range of motion. You should identify a slight resistance to these movements. Abnormal tone is described as *hypotonia* (flaccidity) or *hypertonia* (spasticity). Note any involuntary movements, such as tics, tremor, *myoclonus* (spasm of muscles), *athetosis* (slow, writhing, involuntary movements of extremities), *chorea* (involuntary, purposeless, rapid motions), and *dystonia* (impairment of muscle tone).

Test cerebellar function by assessing balance and coordination. A good screening test for both balance and muscle strength is to observe the patient's stature (posture while standing) and gait. Note the pace and rhythm of the gait, and observe for normal symmetric and oppositional arm swing. The patient's ability to ambulate helps to determine the level of nursing care required and the risk of falling.

The finger-to-nose test (having the patient alternately touch the nose, then touch the examiner's finger) and the heel-to-shin test (having the patient stroke the heel of one foot up and down the shin of the opposite leg) assess coordination and cerebellar function. Reposition your finger while the patient is touching the nose so that the patient must adjust to a new distance each time your finger is touched. These movements should be performed smoothly and accurately. Other tests include asking the patient to pronate and supinate both hands rapidly and to do a shallow knee bend, first on one leg and then on the other. Note dysarthria or slurred speech because it is a sign of incoordination of the speech muscles.

***Sensory System.*** In the somatic sensory examination, several modalities are tested. Each modality is carried by a specific ascending pathway in the spinal cord before it reaches the sensory cortex. As a rule, perform the examination with the patient's eyes closed and avoid providing the patient with clues. Ask "How does this feel?" rather than "Is this sharp?" In the routine neurologic examination, sensory testing of the anterior torso, posterior torso, and the four extremities is sufficient. However, if a disturbance is identified in sensory function of the skin, the boundaries of that dysfunction should be carefully delineated along the dermatome.

**Touch, pain, and temperature.** Light touch is usually tested first using a cotton wisp or light pinprick. Gently touch each of the four extremities and ask the patient to indicate when he or she feels the stimulus. Test pain by alternately touching the skin with the sharp and dull end of a pin. Tell the patient to respond "sharp" or "dull." Evaluate each limb separately.

*Extinction* is assessed by simultaneously touching both sides of the body symmetrically. Normally, the simultaneous stimuli are both perceived (sensed). An abnormal response occurs when the patient perceives the stimulus on only one side. The other stimulus is *extinguished.*

The sensation of temperature (only to be assessed when the response to deep pain is abnormal) can be tested by applying tubes of warm and cold water to the skin and asking the patient to identify the stimuli with the eyes closed. If pain sensation is intact, assessment of temperature sensation may be omitted because both sensations are carried by the same ascending pathways.

**Vibration sense.** Assess vibration sense by applying a vibrating tuning fork to the fingernails and bony prominences of the hands, legs, and feet. Ask the patient if the vibration or "buzz" is felt. Then ask the patient to indicate when the vibration ceases.

**Position sense.** Assess position sense *(proprioception)* by placing your thumb and forefinger on either side of the patient's forefinger or great toe and gently moving his or her digit up or down. Ask the patient to close the eyes and indicate the direction in which the digit is moved.

Another test of proprioception is the Romberg test. Ask the patient to stand with feet together and then close his or her eyes. If the patient is able to maintain balance with the eyes open but sways or falls with the eyes closed (i.e., a positive Romberg test), vestibulocochlear dysfunction or disease in the posterior columns of the spinal cord may be indicated. Be aware of patient safety during this test.

**Cortical sensory functions.** Several tests evaluate cortical integration of sensory perceptions (which occurs in the parietal lobes). Explain these tests to the patient before performing them, while his or her eyes are still open. Assess *two-point discrimination* by placing the two points of a calibrated compass on the tips of the fingers and toes. The minimum recognizable separation is 4 to 5 mm in the fingertips and a greater degree of separation elsewhere. This test is important in diagnosing diseases of the sensory cortex and PNS.

*Graphesthesia* (ability to feel writing on skin) is tested by having the patient identify numbers traced on the palm of the hands. *Stereognosis* (ability to perceive the form and nature of objects) is tested by having the patient close the eyes and identify the size and shape of easily recognized objects (e.g., coins, keys, safety pin) placed in the hands.

***Reflexes.*** Tendons have receptors that are sensitive to stretch. A reflex contraction of the skeletal muscle occurs when the tendon is stretched. In general, the biceps, triceps, brachioradialis, patellar, and Achilles tendon reflexes are tested. Initiate a simple muscle stretch reflex by briskly tapping the tendon of a stretched muscle, usually with a reflex hammer (Fig. 55-14). The response (muscle contraction of the corresponding muscle) is measured on a 0 to 5 scale as follows: 0 = absent reflex, 1 = weak response, seen only with reinforcement, 2 = normal response, 3 = brisk response, 4 = hyperreflexia with nonsustained clonus, and 5 = hyperreflexia with sustained clonus. *Clonus,* an abnormal response, is a continued rhythmic contraction of the muscle with continuous application of the stimulus.

Elicit the *biceps reflex,* with the patient's arm partially flexed and palm up, by placing your thumb over the biceps tendon in the antecubital space and striking the thumb with a hammer. The normal response is flexion of the arm at the elbow or contraction of the biceps muscle that can be felt by your thumb.

Elicit the *triceps reflex* by striking the triceps tendon above the elbow while the patient's arm is flexed. The normal response is extension of the arm or visible contraction of the triceps.

Elicit the *brachioradialis reflex* by striking the radius 3 to 5 cm above the wrist while the patient's arm is relaxed. The normal response is flexion and supination at the elbow or visible contraction of the brachioradialis muscle.

Elicit the *patellar reflex* by striking the patellar tendon just below the patella. The patient can be sitting or lying as long as the leg being tested hangs freely. The normal response is extension of the leg with contraction of the quadriceps.

Gently dorsiflex the patient's foot at the ankle. Elicit the *Achilles tendon reflex* by striking the Achilles tendon while the patient's leg is flexed at the knee. The normal response is plantar flexion at the ankle.

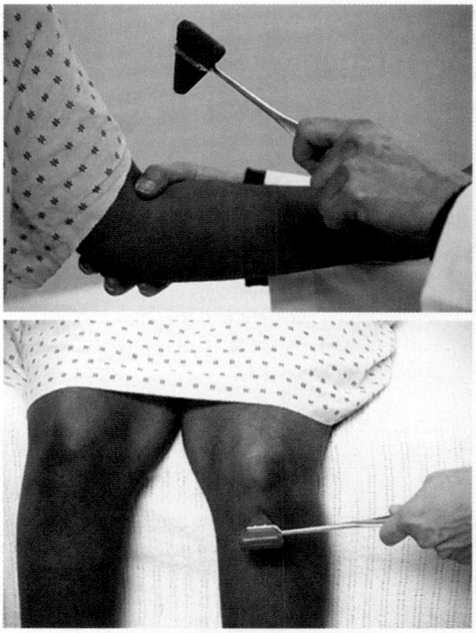
A
B

**FIG. 55-14** The examiner strikes a swift blow over a stretched tendon to elicit a stretch reflex. **A,** Biceps reflex. **B,** Patellar reflex.

## CASE STUDY—cont'd

### *Objective Data: Physical Examination*

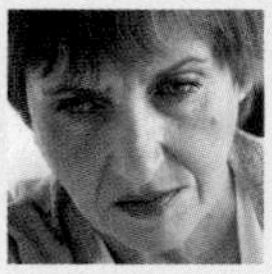
(©TatyanaGl/iStock/Thinkstock)

A physical assessment of J.K. reveals the following:
- BP 145/80, HR 78, RR 20, T 37°C
- Alert, oriented, and appropriate but anxious
- Strength 5/5 on all extremities
- Visual field deficits in upper left quadrant of visual field

**Discussion Question**
1. What should be included in the physical assessment? For what would you be looking?
2. Which physical assessment findings are of most concern to you?
3. Based on the results of the subjective and physical assessment, what diagnostic studies do you think may be ordered for J.K.?

You will learn more about diagnostic studies related to the neurologic system in the next section.

(See p. 1312 for more information on J.K.)

Answers available at *http://evolve.elsevier.com/Lewis/medsurg.*

A *focused assessment* is used to evaluate the status of previously identified neurologic problems and to monitor for signs of new problems (see Table 3-7). A focused assessment of the neurologic system is presented in the box.

Table 55-5 is an example of a normal neurologic physical assessment. Abnormal assessment findings of the neurologic system are presented in Table 55-6.

## DIAGNOSTIC STUDIES OF NERVOUS SYSTEM

Numerous diagnostic studies are available to assess the nervous system (Table 55-7). CSF analysis provides information about a variety of CNS diseases. Normal CSF is clear, colorless, odorless, and free of red blood cells. It contains little protein. Normal CSF values are listed in Table 55-8. CSF may be obtained through lumbar puncture (most common) or ventriculostomy.

## TABLE 55-5 Normal Physical Assessment of Nervous System*

| Parameter | Findings |
|---|---|
| **Mental status** | • Alert and oriented, orderly thought processes.<br>• Appropriate mood and affect. |
| **Cranial nerves†** | • Smell intact to soap or coffee.<br>• Visual fields full to confrontation.<br>• Intact extraocular movements.<br>• No nystagmus. Pupils equal, round, reactive to light and accommodation.<br>• Intact facial sensation to light touch and pinprick.<br>• Facial movements full.<br>• Hearing intact bilaterally.<br>• Intact gag and swallow reflexes. Symmetric smile. Midline protrusion of tongue.<br>• Full strength with head turning and shoulder shrugging. |
| **Motor system** | • Normal gait and station. Normal tandem walk. Negative Romberg test.<br>• Normal and symmetric muscle bulk, tone, and strength.<br>• Smooth performance of finger-nose, heel-shin movements. |
| **Sensory system** | • Intact sensation to light touch, position sense, pinprick, heat, and cold. |
| **Reflexes‡** | • Biceps, triceps, brachioradialis, patellar, and Achilles tendon reflexes 2/5 bilaterally.<br>• Toes pointed down with plantar stimulation. |

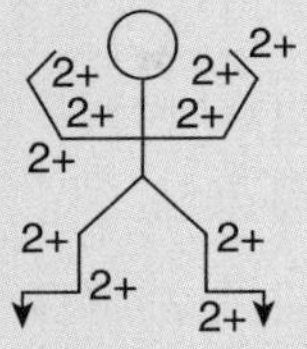


*If some portion of the neurologic examination was not done, this should be indicated (e.g., "Smell not tested").
†May also be recorded as "CN I to XII intact."
‡May also be recorded as drawing of stick figure indicating reflex strength at appropriate sites.

## FOCUSED ASSESSMENT
### Nervous System

Use this checklist to make sure the key assessment steps have been done.

**Subjective**

*Ask the patient about any of the following and note responses.*

| | | |
|---|---|---|
| Blackouts/loss of memory | Y | N |
| Weakness, numbness, tingling in arms or legs | Y | N |
| Headaches, especially new onset | Y | N |
| Loss of balance/coordination | Y | N |
| Orientation to person, place, time, and situation | Y | N |

**Objective: Diagnostic**

*Check the following diagnostic results for critical values.*

| | |
|---|---|
| Lumbar puncture | ✓ |
| CT or MRI of brain | ✓ |
| EEG | ✓ |

**Objective: Physical Examination**

***Inspect/Observe***

| | |
|---|---|
| General level of consciousness/orientation | ✓ |
| Oropharynx for gag reflex and soft palate movement | ✓ |
| Peripheral sensation of light touch and pinprick (face, hands, feet) | ✓ |
| Smell with coffee or soap | ✓ |
| Eyes for extraocular movements, PERRLA, peripheral vision, nystagmus | ✓ |
| Gait for smoothness and coordination | ✓ |

***Palpate***

| | |
|---|---|
| Strength of neck, shoulders, arms, and legs for fullness and symmetry | ✓ |

***Percuss***

| | |
|---|---|
| Reflexes | ✓ |

*CT,* Computed tomography; *EEG,* electroencephalogram; *MRI,* magnetic resonance imaging; *PERRLA,* pupils equal, round, and reactive to light and accommodation.

## TABLE 55-6 Assessment Abnormalities
### Nervous System

| Finding | Description | Possible Etiology and Significance |
|---|---|---|
| **Mental Status** | | |
| **Altered consciousness** | Stuporous, mute, diminished response to verbal cues or pain | Intracranial lesions, metabolic disorder, psychiatric disorders |
| **Anosognosia** | Inability to recognize bodily defect or disease | Lesions in right parietal cortex |
| **Speech** | | |
| **Aphasia, dysphasia** | Loss of or impaired language faculty (comprehension, expression, or both) | Left cerebral cortex lesion |
| **Dysarthria** | Lack of coordination in articulating speech | Cerebellar or cranial nerve lesion<br>Antiseizure drugs, sedatives, hypnotic drug toxicity (including alcohol) |
| **Eyes** | | |
| **Anisocoria** | Inequality of pupil size | Oculomotor nerve injury<br>Sympathetic pathway injury |
| **Diplopia** | Double vision | Lesions affecting nerves of extraocular muscles, cerebellar damage |
| **Homonymous hemianopsia** | Loss of vision in one side of visual field | Lesions in the contralateral occipital lobe |
| **Cranial Nerves** | | |
| **Dysphagia** | Difficulty in swallowing | Lesions involving motor pathways of CNs IX, X (including lower brainstem) |
| **Ophthalmoplegia** | Paralysis of eye muscles | Lesions in brainstem |
| **Papilledema** | "Choked disc," swelling of optic nerve head | Increased intracranial pressure |

## TABLE 55-6 Assessment Abnormalities

### *Nervous System—cont'd*

| Finding | Description | Possible Etiology and Significance |
|---|---|---|
| **Motor System** | | |
| **Apraxia** | Inability to perform learned movements despite having desire and physical ability to perform them | Cerebral cortex lesion |
| **Ataxia** | Lack of coordination of movement | Lesions of sensory or motor pathways, cerebellum<br>Antiseizure drugs, sedatives, hypnotic drug toxicity (including alcohol) |
| **Dyskinesia** | Impairment of voluntary movement, resulting in fragmentary or incomplete movements | Disorders of basal ganglia, idiosyncratic reaction to psychotropic drugs |
| **Hemiplegia** | Paralysis on one side | Stroke and other lesions involving contralateral motor cortex |
| **Nystagmus** | Jerking or bobbing of eyes as they track moving object | Lesions in cerebellum, brainstem, vestibular system<br>Antiseizure drugs, sedatives, hypnotic toxicity (including alcohol) |
| **Sensory System** | | |
| **Analgesia** | Loss of pain sensation | Lesion in spinothalamic tract or thalamus. Analgesic drugs |
| **Anesthesia** | Absence of sensation | Lesions in spinal cord, thalamus, sensory cortex, or peripheral sensory nerve. Anesthesia drugs |
| **Paresthesia** | Alteration in sensation | Lesions in the posterior column or sensory cortex |
| **Astereognosis** | Inability to recognize form of object by touch | Lesions in parietal cortex |
| **Reflexes** | | |
| **Extensor plantar response** | Toes pointing up with plantar stimulation | Suprasegmental or upper motor neuron lesion |
| **Deep tendon reflexes** | Diminished or absent motor response | Lower motor neuron lesions |
| **Spinal Cord** | | |
| **Bladder dysfunction** | | |
| • Atonic (autonomous) | Absence of muscle tone and contractility, enlargement of capacity, no sensation of discomfort, overflow with large residual, inability to voluntarily empty | Early stage of spinal cord injury |
| • Hypotonic | More ability than atonic bladder but less than normal | Interruption of afferent pathways from bladder |
| • Hypertonic | Increased muscle tone, diminished capacity, reflex emptying, dribbling, incontinence | Lesions in pyramidal tracts (efferent pathways) |
| **Paraplegia** | Paralysis of lower extremities | Spinal cord transection or mass lesion (thoracolumbar region) |
| **Tetraplegia (quadriplegia)** | Paralysis of all extremities | Spinal cord transection or mass lesion (cervical region) |

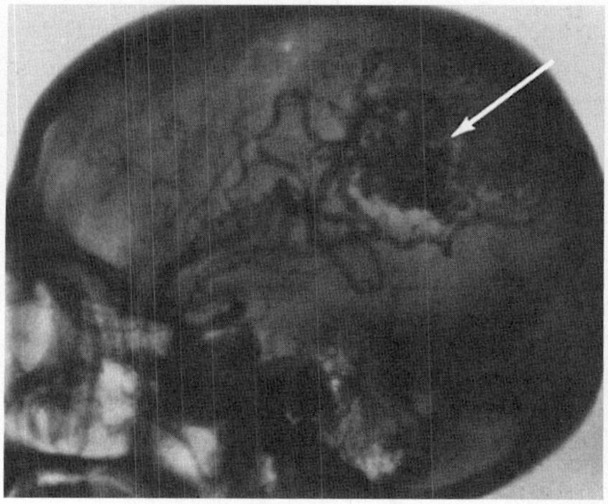

**FIG. 55-15** Cerebral angiogram illustrating an arteriovenous malformation *(arrow)*. (From Chipps E, Clanin N, Campbell V: *Neurologic disorders,* St Louis, 1992, Mosby.)

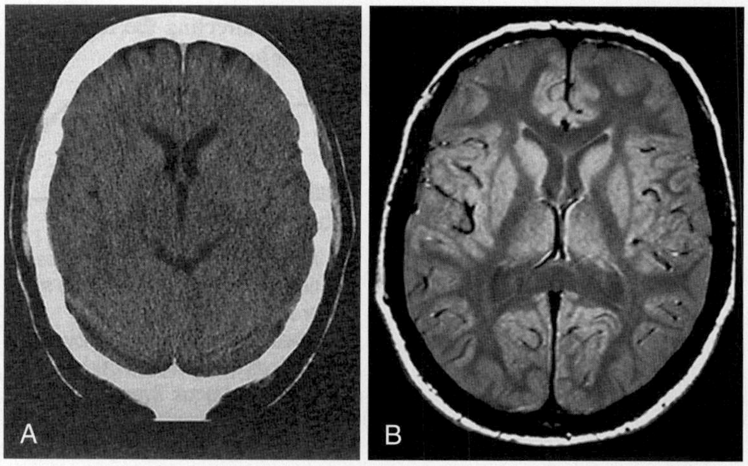


**FIG. 55-16** Normal images of the brain. **A,** Computed tomography scan. **B,** Magnetic resonance imaging. (From Fuller G, Manford M: *Neurology: an illustrated colour text,* ed 3, New York, 2010, Churchill Livingstone.)

## TABLE 55-7 Diagnostic Studies

***Nervous System***

| Study | Description and Purpose | Nursing Responsibility |
|---|---|---|
| **Cerebrospinal Fluid Analysis** | | |
| **Lumbar puncture** | CSF is aspirated by needle insertion in L3-4 or L4-5 interspace. Manometer is attached to needle to obtain CSF pressure. CSF is withdrawn in a series of tubes and sent for analysis (Table 55-8). Contraindicated in the presence of increased intracranial pressure (risk of downward herniation from CSF removal) or infection at site of puncture. | *Before:* Have patient void. Inform the patient that he or she may feel temporary, sharp pain or tingling radiating down the leg as a sterile needle is passed between 2 lumbar vertebrae.<br>*During:* Most commonly, the patient is side lying. Seated position may also be used. Ensure labeling of CSF specimens in proper sequence.<br>*After:* Encourage fluids. Monitor neurologic signs and VS. Monitor for headache intensity, meningeal irritation *(nuchal rigidity),* or signs and symptoms of local trauma (e.g., hematoma, pain). Administer analgesia as needed. |
| **Radiology** | | |
| **Skull and spine x-rays** | Simple x-ray of skull and spinal column is done to detect fractures, bone erosion, calcifications, abnormal vascularity. | *Before:* Explain that procedure is noninvasive. |
| **Cerebral angiography** | Serial x-ray visualization of intracranial and extracranial blood vessels performed to detect vascular lesions (aneurysms, hematomas, arteriovenous malformations) and tumors of brain (Fig. 55-15 on p. 1309). Catheter is inserted into the femoral (sometimes brachial) artery and passed through the aortic arch into the base of a carotid or a vertebral artery for injection of contrast medium. Timed-sequence radiographic images are obtained as contrast flows through arteries, smaller vessels, and veins. | *Before:* Assess patient for stroke risk before procedure because thrombi may be dislodged during procedure. Withhold preceding meal. Explain that patient will have hot flush of head and neck when contrast medium is injected. Explain need to be absolutely still during procedure.<br>*During:* Allergic (anaphylactic) reaction may occur from contrast medium. May require emergency resuscitation measures.<br>*After:* Monitor neurologic signs and VS every 15-30 min for first 2 hr, every hour for next 6 hr, then every 2 hr for 24 hr. Maintain bed rest for 6 hr (1 hr if a closure device is used) and monitor for bleeding. Report any neurologic status changes. |
| **CT scan** | Provides a rapid means of obtaining radiographic images of the brain (Fig. 55-16, *A*, on p. 1309). Computer-assisted x-ray of multiple cross sections of body parts to detect problems such as hemorrhage, tumor, cyst, edema, infarction, brain atrophy, and other abnormalities. Contrast medium may be used to enhance visualization of brain structures. | *Before:* Assess for contraindications to contrast media, including allergy to shellfish, iodine, or dye. Explain appearance of scanner. Instruct patient to remain still during procedure. |
| • CT angiography (CTA) | Noninvasive imaging of vascular system (e.g., aneurysms). Evaluates blood volume, flow, and mean transit time as a measure of perfusion. Has fewer complications than cerebral angiography and is less expensive. | Similar to CT (see above). |
| **MRI** | Imaging of brain, spinal cord, and spinal canal by means of magnetic energy (Fig. 55-16, *B*, on p. 1309). Used to detect strokes, multiple sclerosis, tumors, trauma, herniation, and seizures. Provides greater detail than CT and improved resolution (detail) of intracranial structures. Takes a longer time to complete and may not be appropriate in life-threatening emergencies.<br>Contrast medium may be used to enhance visualization. Advantage of MRI is that the contrast agent *gadolinium* has a lower incidence of allergy than iodine used in CT. | *Before:* Screen patient for metal parts and pacemaker in body. Instruct patient on need to lie very still for up to 1 hr. Sedation may be necessary if patient is claustrophobic. |
| • Magnetic resonance angiography (MRA) | Uses differential signal characteristics of flowing blood to evaluate extracranial and intracranial blood vessels. Provides both anatomic and hemodynamic information. Can be used in conjunction with contrast medium. | Similar to MRI (see above). |
| • Functional MRI (fMRI) | MRI technique that provides time-related (temporal) images that can be used to evaluate how the brain responds to various stimuli. Makes it possible to detect the brain areas that are involved in a task, process, or an emotion. | Similar to MRI (see above). |
| • MR spectroscopy (MRS) | Noninvasive test for measuring biochemical changes in the brain, especially the presence of tumors. Compares the chemical composition of normal brain tissue with abnormal tumor tissue. Can also be used to detect tissue changes in stroke and epilepsy. | Similar to MRI (see above). |

**TABLE 55-7 Diagnostic Studies**

***Nervous System—cont'd***

| Study | Description and Purpose | Nursing Responsibility |
|---|---|---|
| **Positron emission tomography (PET)** | Measures metabolic activity of brain to assess cell death or damage. Uses radioactive material that shows up as a bright spot on the image (see Fig. 15-7). Used for patients with stroke, Alzheimer's disease, seizure disorders, Parkinson's disease, and tumors. | *Before:* Explain procedure to patient. Explain that 2 IV lines will be inserted. Instruct patient not to take sedatives or tranquilizers. Have patient empty bladder before procedure.<br>*During:* Patient may be asked to perform different activities during test. |
| **Single-photon emission computed tomography (SPECT)** | Method of scanning similar to PET, but using more stable substances and different detectors. Radiolabeled compounds are injected, and their photon emissions can be detected. Resulting images are accumulation of labeled compound. Used to visualize blood flow or $O_2$ or glucose metabolism in the brain. Useful in diagnosing strokes, brain tumors, and seizure disorders. | Similar to PET (see above). |
| **Myelogram** | X-ray of spinal cord and vertebral column after injection of contrast medium into subarachnoid space. Used to detect spinal lesions (e.g., herniated or ruptured disc, spinal tumor). | *Before:* Administer sedative as ordered. Instruct patient to empty bladder. Inform patient that test is performed with patient on tilting table that is moved during test.<br>*After:* Patient should lie flat for a few hours. Encourage fluids. Monitor neurologic signs and VS. Headache, nausea, and vomiting may occur after procedure. |
| **Electrographic Studies** | | |
| **Electroencephalography (EEG)** | Electrical activity of brain is recorded using scalp electrodes to evaluate seizure disorders, cerebral disease, CNS effects of systemic diseases, brain injury, brain death. Specific tests may be done to evaluate brain's electrical response to lights and loud noises. | *Before:* Inform patient procedure is noninvasive and without danger of electric shock. Determine if any medications (e.g., tranquilizers, antiseizure drugs) should be withheld.<br>*After:* Resume medications and instruct patient to wash electrode paste out of hair after test. |
| **Magnetoencephalography (MEG)** | Uses a biomagnetometer to detect magnetic fields generated by neural activity. Can accurately pinpoint the part of the brain involved in a stroke, seizure, or other disorder or injury. Measures extracranial magnetic fields and scalp electric field (EEG). | *Before:* Explain procedure to patient. MEG, a passive sensor, does not make physical contact with patient. |
| **Electromyography (EMG)** | Recording of electrical activity associated with innervation of skeletal muscle. Needle electrodes are inserted into the muscle to record specific motor units. Normal muscle at rest shows no electrical activity. Electrical activity occurs only when the muscle contracts.<br>Activity may be altered in diseases of muscle itself (e.g., myopathic conditions) or in disorders of muscle innervation (e.g., segmental or LMN lesions, peripheral neuropathic conditions). | *Before:* Explain procedure and inform patient that pain and discomfort are associated with insertion of needles. |
| **Electroneurography (nerve conduction studies)** | Measures conduction velocity of peripheral nerves. Involves applying a brief electrical stimulus to a distal portion of a sensory nerve and recording the resulting wave of depolarization at a point proximal to the stimulation. The time between the stimulus onset and the initial wave of depolarization at the recording electrode is measured. This is termed *nerve conduction velocity.* Damaged nerves have slower conduction velocities. | *Before:* Explain procedure to patient. For example, a stimulus can be applied to the forefinger and a recording electrode placed over the median nerve at the wrist will detect the speed of the conduction. |
| **Evoked potentials** | Electrical activity associated with nerve conduction along sensory pathways is recorded by electrodes placed on skin and scalp. A stimulus generates the impulse. Increases in the normal time from stimulus onset to a given peak (latency) indicate slowed nerve conduction or nerve damage.<br>Used to diagnose disease (e.g., multiple sclerosis), locate nerve damage, and monitor function intraoperatively. Useful in diagnosing abnormalities of the visual or auditory systems because it indicates if a sensory impulse is reaching the appropriate part of brain. | *Before:* Explain procedure to patient and instruct to shampoo hair before test. |

*Continued*

**TABLE 55-7 Diagnostic Studies**
***Nervous System—cont'd***

| Study | Description and Purpose | Nursing Responsibility |
|---|---|---|
| **Ultrasound** | | |
| **Carotid artery duplex scan** | Noninvasive study that evaluates the degree of stenosis of carotid and vertebral arteries. Combines ultrasound and Doppler technology. Probe is placed over the carotid artery and slowly moved along the course of common carotid artery. Frequency of reflected ultrasound signal corresponds to blood velocity. Increased blood flow velocity can indicate stenosis of a vessel. | *Before:* Explain procedure to patient. |
| **Transcranial Doppler** | Same technology as carotid duplex but evaluates blood flow velocities of intracranial blood vessels. Probe is placed on skin at various "windows" in the skull (areas in the skull that have only a thin bony covering) to record velocities of the blood vessels. | *Before:* Explain procedure to patient. |
| **Biopsies (neurologic pathology tests)** | Biopsy of brain, nerve, muscle, and artery with a needle or through a small incision. Brain biopsy is done primarily using stereotactic procedure. Local anesthesia is used at the site for all types of biopsy. Indications include tumors, infectious disease, degenerative diseases, weakness, and temporal artery for arteritis. | *Before:* Explain procedure to patient.<br>*After:* Follow up with results of the biopsy and plans for surgery if needed. |

*CNS,* Central nervous system; *CSF,* cerebrospinal fluid; *ICP,* intracranial pressure; *LMN,* lower motor neuron.

**TABLE 55-8 Normal Cerebrospinal Fluid Values**

| Parameter | Normal Value |
|---|---|
| Specific gravity | 1.007 |
| pH | 7.35 |
| Appearance | Clear, colorless |
| Red blood cells (RBCs) | None |
| White blood cells (WBCs) | 0-5 cells/μL (0-5 × $10^6$ cells/L) |
| Protein | |
| • Lumbar | 15-45 mg/dL (0.15-0.45 g/L) |
| • Cisternal | 15-25 mg/dL (0.15-0.25 g/L) |
| • Ventricular | 5-15 mg/dL (0.05-0.15 g/L) |
| Glucose | 40-70 mg/dL (2.2-3.9 mmol/L) |
| Microorganisms | None |
| Pressure | 60-150 mm $H_2O$ |

## CASE STUDY—cont'd

### *Objective Data: Diagnostic Studies*

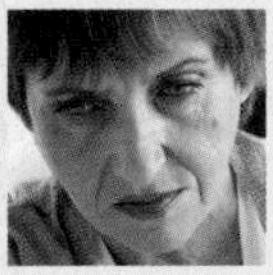
(©TatyanaGl/ iStock/ Thinkstock)

MRI/MRA results indicate a temporal-parietal glioblastoma that has extended into margins of the occipital lobes.

**Discussion Questions**

1. Are these the diagnostic studies that you expected to be ordered?
2. Why are these diagnostic study results of concern to you?

This case study is continued in Chapter 57 on p. 1366.

Answers available at *http://evolve.elsevier.com/Lewis/medsurg.*

## BRIDGE TO NCLEX EXAMINATION

The number of the question corresponds to the same-numbered outcome at the beginning of the chapter.

1. In a patient with a disease that affects the myelin sheath of nerves, such as multiple sclerosis, the glial cells affected are the
   - **a.** microglia.
   - **b.** astrocytes.
   - **c.** ependymal cells.
   - **d.** oligodendrocytes.
2. Drugs or diseases that impair the function of the extrapyramidal system may cause loss of
   - **a.** sensations of pain and temperature.
   - **b.** regulation of the autonomic nervous system.
   - **c.** integration of somatic and special sensory inputs.
   - **d.** automatic movements associated with skeletal muscle activity.
3. During the admitting neurologic examination, the nurse determines the patient has speech difficulties as well as weakness of the right arm and lower face. The nurse would expect a CT scan to show pathology in the distribution of the
   - **a.** basilar artery.
   - **b.** left middle cerebral artery.
   - **c.** right anterior cerebral artery.
   - **d.** left posterior communicating artery.
4. A patient is seen in the emergency department after diving into the pool and hitting the bottom with a blow to the face that hyperextended the neck and scraped the skin off the nose. The patient also described "having double vision" when looking down. During the neurologic exam, the nurse finds the patient is unable to abduct either eye. The nurse recognizes this finding is related to
   - **a.** a basal skull fracture.
   - **b.** a stretch injury to bilateral CN VI.
   - **c.** a stiff neck from the hyperextension injury.
   - **d.** facial swelling from the scrape on the bottom of the pool.
5. Stimulation of the parasympathetic nervous system results in *(select all that apply)*
   - **a.** constriction of the bronchi.
   - **b.** dilation of skin blood vessels.
   - **c.** increased secretion of insulin.
   - **d.** increased blood glucose levels.
   - **e.** relaxation of the urinary sphincters.

6. The nurse is assessing the muscle strength of an older adult patient. The nurse knows the findings cannot be compared with those of a younger adult because
   a. nutritional status is better in young adults.
   b. muscle bulk and strength decrease in older adults.
   c. muscle strength should be the same for all adults.
   d. most young adults exercise more than older adults.
7. A patient is admitted with a headache, fever, and general malaise. The HCP has asked that the patient be prepared for a lumbar puncture. What is a *priority* nursing action to avoid complications?
   a. Ensure that CT scan is performed prior to lumbar puncture.
   b. Assess laboratory results for changes in the white cell count.
   c. Provide acetaminophen for the headache and fever before the procedure.
   d. Administer antibiotics before the procedure to treat the potential meningitis.
8. During neurologic testing, the patient is able to perceive pain elicited by pinprick. Based on this finding, the nurse may omit testing for
   a. position sense.
   b. patellar reflexes.
   c. temperature perception.
   d. heel-to-shin movements.
9. A patient's eyes jerk while the patient looks to the left. The nurse will record this finding as
   a. nystagmus.
   b. CN VI palsy.
   c. ophthalmic dyskinesia.
   d. oculocephalic response.
10. The nurse is caring for a patient with peripheral neuropathy who is scheduled for EMG studies tomorrow morning. The nurse should
   a. ensure the patient has an empty bladder.
   b. instruct the patient about the risk of electric shock.
   c. ensure the patient has no metallic jewelry or metal fragments.
   d. instruct the patient that pain may be experienced during the study.

1. d, 2. d, 3. b, 4. b, 5. a, b, c, e, 6. b, 7. a, 8. c, 9. a, 10. d

For rationales to these answers and even more NCLEX review questions, visit *http://evolve.elsevier.com/Lewis/medsurg.*

## EVOLVE WEBSITE

http://evolve.elsevier.com/Lewis/medsurg

**Review Questions (Online Only)**
**Key Points**
**Answer Keys for Questions**
- Rationales for Bridge to NCLEX Examination Questions
- Answer Guidelines for Case Study on pp. 1302, 1304, 1307, and 1312

**Conceptual Care Map Creator**
**Audio Glossary**
**Supporting Media**
- Animations
  - Cervical Nerves
  - Overview of Nervous System
  - Parts of the Brain
  - Synaptic Transmission
  - The Synapse
  - Vertebral Column and Spinal Nerves

**Content Updates**

## REFERENCES


1. Arslantunali D, Dursun T, Yucel D, et al: Peripheral nerve conduits: technology update, *Med Devices (Auckl)* 2014:405, 2014.
2. Banerjee S, Bentley P, Hamady M, et al: Intra-arterial immunoselected CD34+ stem cells for acute ischemic stroke, *Stem Cells Trans Med* 3:1322, 2014.
3. Raghavendra R, Shirol VS, Daksha D, et al: Circle of Willis and its variations: morphometric study in adult human cadavers, *Int J Med Res Health Sci* 3:394, 2014.
4. Hafkemeijer A, Altmann-Schneider I, de Craen A, et al: Associations between age and gray matter volume in anatomical brain networks in middle-age to older adults, *Aging Cell* 13:1068, 2014.
5. Pedersen NL, Gerritsen L: Genetics of brain and cognitive aging: introduction to the special issue of neuropsychology review, *Neuropsychol Rev* 25(1):1, 2015.
6. NIH MedlinePlus: Aging changes in the senses. Retrieved from *www.nlm.nih.gov/medlineplus/ency/article/004013.htm.*
7. Quigley P, White S: Hospital-based fall program measurement and improvement in high reliability organizations, *Online J Issues Nurs* 18:2, 2013.
8. Gerber L, Chiu Y, Carney N, et al: Marked reduction in mortality of patients with severe traumatic brain injury, *J Neurosurg* 119:1583, 2013.
9. Saracoglu K: Patient safety and preoperative assessment of neurological status in neurosurgical patients, *Surg Curr Res* 4:e114, 2014.
10. Rank W: Performing a focused neurologic assessment, *Nursing* 43(12):37, 2013.
11. Donaghy P, McKeith I: The clinical characteristics of dementia with Lewy bodies and a consideration of prodromal diagnosis, *Alzheimers Res Ther* 6:46, 2014.

56

# Acute Intracranial Problems

*Linda Littlejohns*

*You can observe a lot by just watching.*

*Yogi Berra*

http://evolve.elsevier.com/Lewis/medsurg/

## LEARNING OUTCOMES

1. Explain the physiologic mechanisms that maintain normal intracranial pressure.
2. Describe the common etiologies, clinical manifestations, and interprofessional care of the patient with increased intracranial pressure.
3. Describe the interprofessional and nursing management of the patient with increased intracranial pressure.
4. Differentiate types of head injury by mechanism of injury and clinical manifestations.
5. Describe the interprofessional care and nursing management of the patient with a brain injury.
6. Compare the types, clinical manifestations, and interprofessional care of patients with brain tumors.
7. Discuss the nursing management of the patient with a brain tumor.
8. Describe the nursing management of the patient undergoing cranial surgery.
9. Differentiate among the primary causes, interprofessional care, and nursing management of brain abscess, meningitis, and encephalitis.

## KEY TERMS

brain abscess, p. 1338
cerebral edema, p. 1316
coma, p. 1317
concussion, p. 1327
contusion, p. 1328
diffuse axonal injury (DAI), p. 1327
encephalitis, p. 1341
epidural hematoma, p. 1328
Glasgow Coma Scale (GCS), p. 1323
head injury, p. 1326
intracerebral hematoma, p. 1329
intracranial pressure (ICP), p. 1314
meningitis, p. 1339
nuchal rigidity, p. 1339
subdural hematoma, p. 1329
unconsciousness, p. 1318

Acute intracranial problems include diseases and disorders that can increase intracranial pressure (ICP). This chapter discusses the mechanisms that maintain normal ICP and increase ICP. In addition, head injury, brain tumors, and cerebral inflammatory disorders are discussed.

## INTRACRANIAL PRESSURE

Understanding the dynamics associated with ICP is important in caring for patients with many different neurologic problems. The skull is an enclosed space with three essential volume components: brain tissue, blood, and cerebrospinal fluid (CSF) (Fig. 56-1). The intracellular and extracellular fluids of brain tissue make up approximately 78% of this volume. Blood in the arterial, venous, and capillary network makes up 12% of the volume, and the remaining 10% is the volume of the CSF.

Primary versus secondary injury is another important concept in understanding ICP. *Primary injury* occurs at the initial time of an injury (e.g., impact of car accident, blunt-force trauma) that results in displacement, bruising, or damage to any of the three components.

*Secondary injury* is the resulting hypoxia, ischemia, hypotension, edema, or increased ICP that follows the primary injury. Secondary injury, which could occur several hours to days after the initial injury, is a primary concern when managing brain injury. Nursing management of the patient with an acute intracranial problem must include management of secondary injury and thus increased ICP.

### Regulation and Maintenance of Intracranial Pressure

**Normal Intracranial Pressure.** **Intracranial pressure (ICP)** is the hydrostatic force measured in the brain CSF compartment. Under normal conditions in which intracranial volume remains relatively constant, the balance among the three components (brain tissue, blood, CSF) maintains the ICP. Factors that influence ICP under normal circumstances are changes in (1) arterial pressure; (2) venous pressure; (3) intraabdominal and intrathoracic pressure; (4) posture; (5) temperature; and

*Acknowledgment*: We would like to acknowledge the contributions of Meg Zomorodi, RN, PhD, CNL, University of North Carolina at Chapel Hill School of Nursing, Chapel Hill, North Carolina to this chapter over the past three editions of the book.
Reviewed by Molly McNett, RN, PhD, CNRN, Director, Nursing Research, The MetroHealth System, Cleveland, Ohio and Meg Zomorodi, RN, PhD, CNL, Clinical Associate Professor, University of North Carolina at Chapel Hill School of Nursing, Chapel Hill, North Carolina.

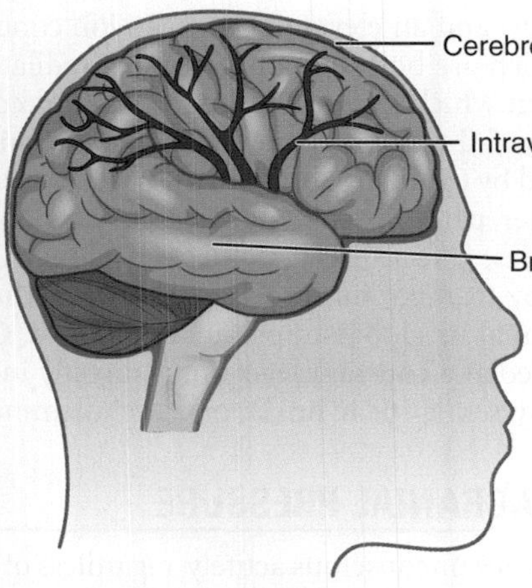


**FIG. 56-1** Components of the brain.

(6) blood gases, particularly $CO_2$ levels. The degree to which these factors increase or decrease the ICP depends on the brain's ability to adapt to changes.

The Monro-Kellie doctrine states that the three components must remain at a relatively constant volume within the closed skull structure. If the volume of any one of the three components increases within the cranial vault and the volume from another component is displaced, the total intracranial volume will not change.[1] This hypothesis is only applicable in situations in which the skull is closed. The hypothesis is not valid in persons with displaced skull fractures or hemicraniectomy.

ICP can be measured in the ventricles, subarachnoid space, subdural space, epidural space, or brain tissue using a pressure transducer.[2] Normal ICP ranges from 5 to 15 mm Hg. A sustained pressure greater than 20 mm Hg is considered abnormal and must be treated.

**Normal Compensatory Adaptations.** In applying the Monro-Kellie doctrine, the body can adapt to volume changes within the skull in three different ways to maintain a normal ICP. First, compensatory mechanisms can include changes in the CSF volume. The CSF volume can be changed by altering CSF absorption or production and by displacing CSF into the spinal subarachnoid space. Second, changes in intracranial blood volume can occur through the collapse of cerebral veins and dural sinuses, regional cerebral vasoconstriction or dilation, and changes in venous outflow. Third, brain tissue volume compensates through distention of the dura or compression of brain tissue.

Initially an increase in volume produces no increase in ICP as a result of these compensatory mechanisms. However, the ability to compensate for changes in volume is limited. As the volume increase continues, the ICP rises and decompensation ultimately occurs, resulting in compression and ischemia.

## Cerebral Blood Flow

*Cerebral blood flow* (CBF) is the amount of blood in milliliters passing through 100 g of brain tissue in 1 minute. The global CBF is approximately 50 mL/min/100 g of brain tissue. The maintenance of blood flow to the brain is critical because the brain requires a constant supply of $O_2$ and glucose. The brain uses 20% of the body's $O_2$ and 25% of its glucose.[3]

**Autoregulation of Cerebral Blood Flow.** The brain regulates its own blood flow in response to its metabolic needs despite wide fluctuations in systemic arterial pressure. *Autoregulation* is the automatic adjustment in the diameter of the cerebral blood vessels by the brain to maintain a constant blood flow during changes in arterial blood pressure (BP). The purpose of autoregulation is to ensure a consistent CBF to provide for the metabolic needs of brain tissue and to maintain cerebral perfusion pressure within normal limits.

**TABLE 56-1 Calculation of Cerebral Perfusion Pressure**

$$CPP = MAP - ICP$$

$$MAP = DBP + 1/3\,(SBP - DBP)$$

OR

$$MAP = \frac{SBP + 2\,(DBP)}{3}$$

*Example:* Systemic BP = 122/84 mm Hg
MAP = 97 mm Hg
ICP = 12 mm Hg
CPP = 85 mm Hg

*CPP,* Cerebral perfusion pressure; *DBP,* diastolic blood pressure; *ICP,* intracranial pressure; *MAP,* mean arterial pressure; *SBP,* systolic blood pressure.

The lower limit of systemic arterial pressure at which autoregulation is effective in a normotensive person is a mean arterial pressure (MAP) of 70 mm Hg. Below this, CBF decreases, and symptoms of cerebral ischemia, such as syncope and blurred vision, occur. The upper limit of systemic arterial pressure at which autoregulation is effective is a MAP of 150 mm Hg. When this pressure is exceeded, the vessels are maximally constricted, and further vasoconstrictor response is lost.

The *cerebral perfusion pressure* (CPP) is the pressure needed to ensure blood flow to the brain. CPP is equal to the MAP minus the ICP (CPP = MAP − ICP) (see the example in Table 56-1). This formula is clinically useful, although it does not consider the effect of cerebrovascular resistance. Cerebrovascular resistance, generated by the arterioles within the cranium, links CPP and blood flow as follows:

$$CPP = Flow \times Resistance$$

When cerebrovascular resistance is high, blood flow to brain tissue is impaired. Transcranial Doppler is a noninvasive technique used in intensive care units (ICUs) to monitor changes in cerebrovascular resistance.

As the CPP decreases, autoregulation fails and CBF decreases. Normal CPP is 60 to 100 mm Hg. A CPP of less than 50 mm Hg is associated with ischemia and neuronal death. A CPP of less than 30 mm Hg results in ischemia and is incompatible with life.

Normally, autoregulation maintains an adequate CBF and perfusion pressure primarily by adjusting the diameter of cerebral blood vessels and metabolic factors that affect ICP. It is critical to maintain MAP when ICP is elevated.

Remember that CPP may not reflect perfusion pressure in all parts of the brain. There may be local areas of swelling and compression limiting regional perfusion pressure. Thus a higher CPP may be needed for these patients to prevent localized tissue damage. For example, a patient with an acute stroke may require a higher BP, increasing MAP and CPP, in order to increase perfusion to the brain and prevent further tissue damage.

**Pressure Changes.** The relationship of pressure to volume is depicted in the pressure-volume curve (Fig. 56-2). The curve is affected by the brain's compliance. *Compliance* is the expandability of the brain. It is represented as the volume increase for

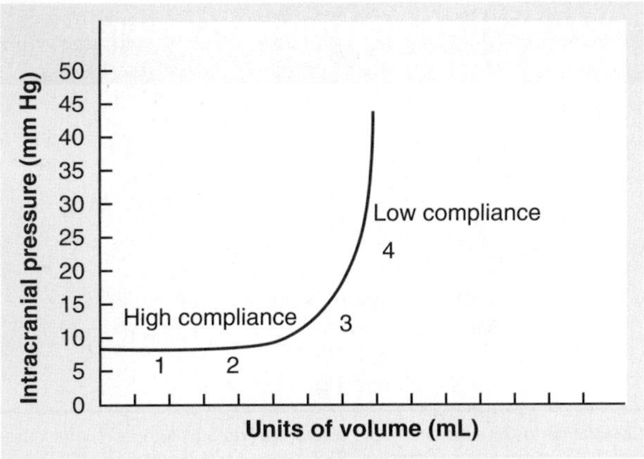


**FIG. 56-2** Intracranial pressure-volume curve. (See text for descriptions of *1, 2, 3,* and *4.*)

each unit increase in pressure. With low compliance, small changes in volume result in greater increases in pressure.

Compliance = Volume/Pressure

The concept of the pressure-volume curve can be used to represent the stages of increased ICP. At stage 1 on the curve, there is high compliance. The brain is in total compensation, with accommodation and autoregulation intact. An increase in volume (brain tissue, blood, or CSF) does not increase the ICP.

At stage 2, the compliance is beginning to decrease, and an increase in volume places the patient at risk of increased ICP and secondary injury. At stage 3, there is significant reduction in compliance. Any small addition of volume causes a great increase in ICP. Compensatory mechanisms fail, there is a loss of autoregulation, and the patient exhibits manifestations of increased ICP (e.g., headache, changes in level of consciousness or pupil responsiveness).

With a loss of autoregulation, the body attempts to maintain cerebral perfusion by increasing systolic BP. However, decompensation is imminent. The patient's response is characterized by systolic hypertension with a widening pulse pressure, bradycardia with a full and bounding pulse, and altered respirations. This is known as *Cushing's triad* and is a neurologic emergency.

As the patient enters stage 4, the ICP rises to lethal levels with little increase in volume. *Herniation* occurs as the brain tissue is forcibly shifted from the compartment of greater pressure to a compartment of lesser pressure. In this situation, intense pressure is placed on the brainstem, and if herniation continues, brainstem death is imminent.

**Factors Affecting Cerebral Blood Flow.** $CO_2$, $O_2$, and hydrogen ion concentration affect cerebral blood vessel tone. An increase in the partial pressure of $CO_2$ in arterial blood ($PaCO_2$) relaxes smooth muscle, dilates cerebral vessels, decreases cerebrovascular resistance, and increases CBF. A decrease in $PaCO_2$ constricts cerebral vessels, increases cerebrovascular resistance, and decreases CBF.

Cerebral $O_2$ tension of less than 50 mm Hg results in cerebrovascular dilation. This dilation decreases cerebrovascular resistance, increases CBF, and increases $O_2$ tension. However, if $O_2$ tension is not increased, anaerobic metabolism begins, resulting in an accumulation of lactic acid. As lactic acid increases and hydrogen ions accumulate, the environment becomes more acidic. Within this acidic environment, further vasodilation occurs in a continued attempt to increase blood flow. The combination of a severely low partial pressure of $O_2$ in arterial blood ($PaO_2$) and an elevated hydrogen ion concentration (acidosis), which are both potent cerebral vasodilators, may produce a state in which autoregulation is lost and compensatory mechanisms fail to meet tissue metabolic demands.

CBF can be affected by cardiac or respiratory arrest, systemic hemorrhage, and other pathophysiologic states (e.g., diabetic coma, encephalopathies, infections, toxicities). Regional CBF can also be affected by trauma, tumors, cerebral hemorrhage, or stroke. When regional or global autoregulation is lost, CBF is no longer maintained at a constant level but is directly influenced by changes in systemic BP, hypoxia, or catecholamines.

## INCREASED INTRACRANIAL PRESSURE

Any patient who becomes unconscious acutely, regardless of the cause, should be suspected of having increased ICP.

### Mechanisms of Increased Intracranial Pressure

Increased ICP is a potentially life-threatening situation that results from an increase in any or all of the three components (brain tissue, blood, CSF) within the skull. Elevated ICP is clinically significant because it diminishes CPP, increases risks of brain ischemia and infarction, and is associated with a poor prognosis.[4] Common causes of increased ICP include a mass (e.g., hematoma, contusion, abscess, tumor) and cerebral edema (associated with brain tumors, hydrocephalus, head injury, or brain inflammation).

These cerebral insults, which may result in hypercapnia, cerebral acidosis, impaired autoregulation, and systemic hypertension, increase the formation and spread of cerebral edema. This edema distorts brain tissue, further increasing the ICP, and leads to even more tissue hypoxia and acidosis. Fig. 56-3 illustrates the progression of increased ICP.

It is critical to maintain CBF to preserve tissue and thus minimize secondary injury. Sustained increases in ICP result in brainstem compression and herniation of the brain from one compartment to another.

Displacement and herniation of brain tissue can cause a potentially reversible process to become irreversible. Ischemia and edema are further increased, compounding the preexisting problem. Compression of the brainstem and cranial nerves may be fatal. (Fig. 56-4 illustrates types of herniation.) Herniation forces the cerebellum and brainstem downward through the foramen magnum. If compression of the brainstem is unrelieved, respiratory arrest will occur due to compression of the respiratory control center in the medulla.

### Cerebral Edema

As shown in Table 56-2, there are a variety of causes of **cerebral edema** (increased accumulation of fluid in the extravascular spaces of brain tissue). Regardless of the cause, cerebral edema results in an increase in tissue volume that can increase ICP. The extent and severity of the original insult are factors that determine the degree of cerebral edema.

There are three types of cerebral edema: vasogenic, cytotoxic, and interstitial. The same patient may have more than one type.

**Vasogenic Cerebral Edema.** *Vasogenic cerebral edema,* the most common type of cerebral edema, occurs mainly in the white matter and is characterized by leakage of large molecules from the capillaries into the surrounding extracellular space. This results in an osmotic gradient that favors the flow of fluid from the intravascular to extravascular space. A variety of insults,

### PATHOPHYSIOLOGY MAP

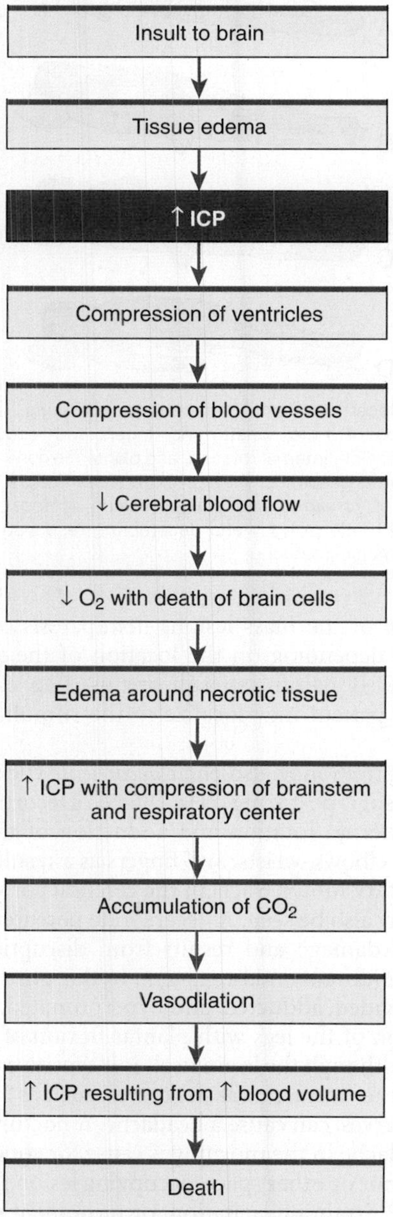


**FIG. 56-3** Progression of increased intracranial pressure *(ICP)*.

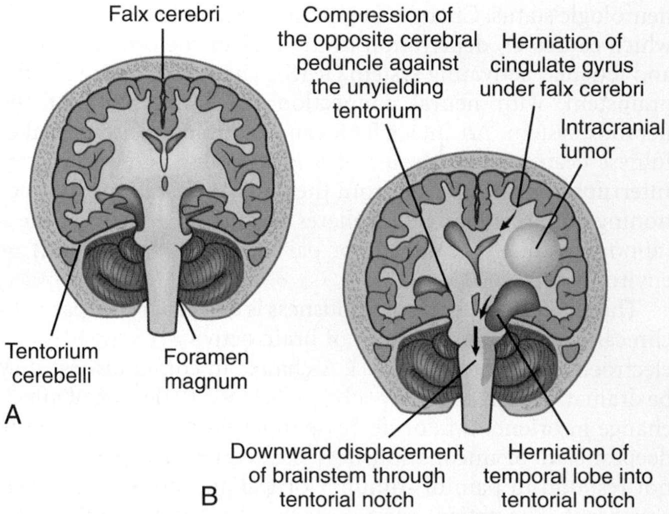


**FIG. 56-4** Herniation. **A,** Normal relationship of intracranial structures. **B,** Shift of intracranial structures. (Modified from McCance KL, Huether SE: *Pathophysiology: the biologic basis for disease in adults and children,* ed 6, St Louis, 2010, Mosby.)

**TABLE 56-2 Causes of Cerebral Edema**

| | |
|---|---|
| **Mass Lesions**<br>• Brain abscess<br>• Brain tumor (primary or metastatic)<br>• Hematoma (intracerebral, subdural, epidural)<br>• Hemorrhage (intracerebral, cerebellar, brainstem) | **Cerebral Infections**<br>• Encephalitis<br>• Meningitis |
| | **Vascular Insult**<br>• Anoxic and ischemic episodes<br>• Cerebral infarction (thrombotic or embolic)<br>• Venous sinus thrombosis |
| **Head Injuries and Brain Surgery**<br>• Contusion<br>• Hemorrhage<br>• Posttraumatic brain swelling | **Toxic or Metabolic Encephalopathic Conditions**<br>• Hepatic encephalopathy<br>• Lead or arsenic intoxication<br>• Uremia |

such as brain tumors, abscesses, and ingested toxins, may cause an increase in the permeability of the blood-brain barrier and produce an increase in the extracellular fluid volume. The speed and extent of the spread of the edema fluid are influenced by the systemic BP, site of the brain injury, and extent of the blood-brain barrier defect.

This edema may produce a continuum of symptoms ranging from headache to disturbances in consciousness, including **coma** (profound state of unconsciousness) and focal neurologic deficits.

It is important to recognize that although a headache may seem to be a benign symptom, in cases of cerebral edema it can quickly progress to coma and death. Therefore you must be vigilant in your assessment.

**Cytotoxic Cerebral Edema.** *Cytotoxic cerebral edema* results from disruption of the integrity of the cell membranes. It develops from destructive lesions or trauma to brain tissue, resulting in cerebral hypoxia or anoxia and syndrome of inappropriate antidiuretic hormone (SIADH) secretion. In this type of edema, the blood-brain barrier remains intact. Cerebral edema occurs as a result of a fluid and protein shift from the extracellular space directly into the cells, with subsequent swelling and loss of cellular function.

**Interstitial Cerebral Edema.** *Interstitial cerebral edema* is usually a result of hydrocephalus. *Hydrocephalus* is a buildup of fluid in the brain and is manifested by ventricular enlargement. It can be due to excess CSF production, obstruction of flow, or an inability to reabsorb the CSF. Hydrocephalus treatment usually consists of a ventriculostomy or ventriculoperitoneal shunt. (Management of hydrocephalus is discussed later in this chapter.)

## Clinical Manifestations

The clinical manifestations of increased ICP can take many forms, depending on the cause, location, and rate of increases in ICP.

**Change in Level of Consciousness.** The *level of consciousness* (LOC) is the most sensitive and reliable indicator of the patient's neurologic status. Changes in LOC are a result of impaired CBF, which causes $O_2$ deprivation to the cells of the cerebral cortex and reticular activating system (RAS). The RAS is located in the brainstem, with neural connections to many parts of the nervous system. An intact RAS can maintain a state of wakefulness even in the absence of a functioning cerebral cortex. Interruptions of impulses from the RAS or alterations in functioning of the cerebral hemispheres can cause **unconsciousness** (abnormal state of complete or partial unawareness of self or environment).

The patient's state of consciousness is defined by the patient's clinical responses and pattern of brain activity (recorded by an electroencephalogram [EEG]). A change in consciousness may be dramatic (as in coma) or subtle (such as a flattening of affect, change in orientation, or decrease in level of attention). In the deepest state of unconsciousness (i.e., coma), the patient does not respond to painful stimuli. Corneal and pupillary reflexes are absent. The patient cannot swallow or cough and is incontinent of urine and feces. The EEG pattern demonstrates suppressed or absent neuronal activity.

**Changes in Vital Signs.** Changes in vital signs are caused by increasing pressure on the thalamus, hypothalamus, pons, and medulla.

## CHECK YOUR PRACTICE

You are monitoring the vital signs of an 82-yr-old female who was admitted for a head injury after she fell while walking on the sidewalk. She hit her head on a fire hydrant. She was confused on admission, but vital signs were stable at BP 150/86, pulse 84, respirations 14/minute. Two hours after admission, her vital signs are now BP 166/74, pulse 54, respirations 10-16/minute.

- What is your interpretation of her vital signs?

Manifestations such as *Cushing's triad* (systolic hypertension with a widening pulse pressure, bradycardia with a full and bounding pulse, and irregular respirations) may be present but often do not appear until ICP has been increased for some time or is suddenly and markedly increased (e.g., head trauma). Always recognize Cushing's triad as a medical emergency, since this is a sign of brainstem compression and impending death. A change in body temperature may also occur because increased ICP affects the hypothalamus.

**Ocular Signs.** Compression of cranial nerve (CN) III, the oculomotor nerve, results in dilation of the pupil on the same side *(ipsilateral)* as the mass lesion, sluggish or no response to light, inability to move the eye upward and adduct, and ptosis of the eyelid. These signs can be the result of the brain shifting from midline, compressing the trunk of CN III, and paralyzing the muscles controlling pupillary size and shape. In this situation, a fixed, unilateral, dilated pupil is considered a neurologic emergency that indicates herniation of the brain.

Other cranial nerves may also be affected, such as the optic (CN II), trochlear (CN IV), and abducens (CN VI) nerves. Signs of dysfunction of these cranial nerves include blurred vision, diplopia, and changes in extraocular eye movements. *Central herniation* may initially manifest as sluggish but equal pupil response. *Uncal herniation* may cause a dilated unilateral pupil. *Papilledema* (an edematous optic disc seen on retinal examination) is also noted and is a nonspecific sign associated with persistent increases in ICP.

**Decrease in Motor Function.** As the ICP continues to rise, the patient manifests changes in motor ability. A *contralateral*

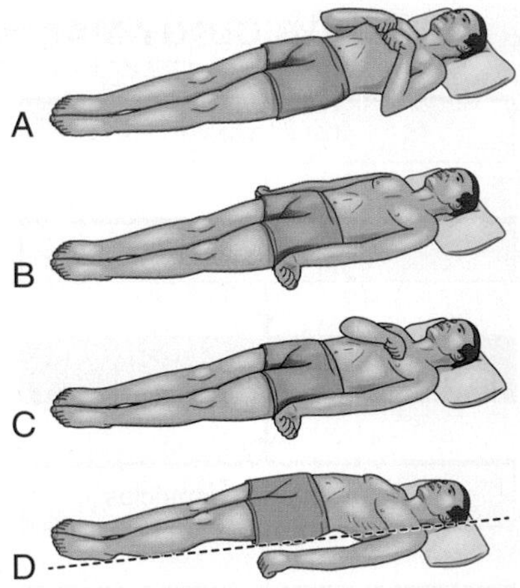


**FIG. 56-5** Decorticate and decerebrate posturing. **A,** Decorticate response. Flexion of arms, wrists, and fingers with adduction in upper extremities. Extension, internal rotation, and plantar flexion in lower extremities. **B,** Decerebrate response. All four extremities in rigid extension, with hyperpronation of forearms and plantar flexion of feet. **C,** Decorticate response on right side of body and decerebrate response on left side of body. **D,** Opisthotonic posturing.

(opposite side of the mass lesion) hemiparesis or hemiplegia may develop, depending on the location of the source of the increased ICP. If painful stimuli are used to elicit a motor response, the patient may localize to the stimuli or withdraw from it.

Noxious stimuli may also elicit *decorticate* (flexor) or *decerebrate* (extensor) posturing (Fig. 56-5). Decorticate posture consists of internal rotation and adduction of the arms with flexion of the elbows, wrists, and fingers as a result of interruption of voluntary motor tracts in the cerebral cortex. Extension of the legs may also be seen. A decerebrate posture may indicate more serious damage and results from disruption of motor fibers in the midbrain and brainstem. In this position, the arms are stiffly extended, adducted, and hyperpronated. There is also hyperextension of the legs with plantar flexion of the feet.

**Headache.** Although the brain itself is insensitive to pain, compression of other intracranial structures, such as arteries, veins, and cranial nerves, can cause a headache. A nocturnal headache and/or a headache in the morning is cause for concern and may indicate a tumor or other space-occupying lesion that is causing increased ICP. Straining, agitation, or movement may accentuate the pain.

**Vomiting.** Vomiting, usually not preceded by nausea, is often a nonspecific sign of increased ICP. This is called *unexpected vomiting* and is related to pressure changes in the cranium. Projectile vomiting may also occur and is related to increased ICP.

### Complications

The major complications of uncontrolled increased ICP are inadequate cerebral perfusion and cerebral herniation (Fig. 56-4). To better understand cerebral herniation, two important structures in the brain must be described. The *falx cerebri* is a thin wall of dura that folds down between the cortex, separating the two cerebral hemispheres. The *tentorium cerebelli* is a rigid fold of dura that separates the cerebral hemispheres from the cerebellum (Fig. 56-4). It is called the *tentorium* (meaning tent) because it forms a tentlike cover over the cerebellum.

*Tentorial herniation* (central herniation) occurs when a mass lesion in the cerebrum forces the brain to herniate downward through the opening created by the brainstem. *Uncal herniation* occurs when there is lateral and downward herniation. *Cingulate herniation* occurs when there is lateral displacement of brain tissue beneath the falx cerebri.

## Diagnostic Studies

Diagnostic studies can be used to identify the cause of increased ICP (Table 56-3). CT and MRI are used to differentiate the many conditions that can cause increased ICP and to assess the effect of treatment.

Additional tests include EEG, cerebral angiography, ICP measurement, brain tissue oxygenation measurement via the LICOX catheter (described later), transcranial Doppler studies, and evoked potential studies. Positron emission tomography (PET) is also used to diagnose the cause of increased ICP. In general, a lumbar puncture is not performed when increased ICP is suspected. The reason for this is that cerebral herniation could occur from the sudden release of the pressure in the skull from the area above the lumbar puncture.

In some institutions, a hand-held near-infrared scanner (Infrascanner) is used to detect life-threatening intracranial bleeding. The scanner directs a wavelength of light that can penetrate tissue and bone. Blood from intracranial hematomas absorbs the light differently than other areas of the brain.

**TABLE 56-3 Interprofessional Care**

***Increased Intracranial Pressure***

**Diagnostic Assessment**

- History and physical examination
- Vital signs, neurologic assessments, ICP measurements
- Skull, chest, and spinal x-ray studies
- CT scan, MRI, cerebral angiography, EEG, PET
- Transcranial Doppler studies
- Infrascanner
- ECG
- Evoked potential studies
- Laboratory studies, including CBC, coagulation profile, electrolytes, serum creatinine, ABGs, ammonia level, drug and toxicology screen, CSF analysis (for protein, WBC, and glucose)*

**Management**

- Elevation of head of bed to 30 degrees with head in a neutral position
- Intubation and mechanical ventilation
- ICP monitoring
- Cerebral oxygenation monitoring ($PbtO_2$, $SjvO_2$)
- Maintenance of $PaO_2$ ≥100 mm Hg
- Maintenance of fluid balance and assessment of osmolality
- Maintenance of systolic arterial pressure between 100 and 160 mm Hg
- Maintenance of CPP >60 mm Hg
- Reduction of cerebral metabolism (e.g., high-dose barbiturates)

***Drug Therapy***

- Osmotic diuretic (mannitol)
- Hypertonic saline
- Antiseizure drugs (e.g., phenytoin [Dilantin])
- Corticosteroids (dexamethasone) for brain tumors, bacterial meningitis
- Histamine ($H_2$)-receptor antagonist (e.g., cimetidine) or proton pump inhibitor (e.g., pantoprazole [Protonix]) to prevent GI ulcers and bleeding

*CPP,* Cerebral perfusion pressure; *ICP,* intracranial pressure; *$PaO_2$,* partial pressure of $O_2$ in arterial blood; *$PbtO_2$,* pressure of $O_2$ in brain tissue; *$SjvO_2$,* jugular venous $O_2$ saturation.

*A lumbar puncture to obtain CSF for analysis should not be done if there is a possibility of herniation.

## Monitoring ICP and Cerebral Oxygenation

**Indications for Intracranial Pressure Monitoring.** ICP monitoring is used to guide clinical care when the patient is at risk for or has elevations in ICP.[4] It may be used in patients with a variety of neurologic insults, including hemorrhage, stroke, tumor, infection, or traumatic brain injury. ICP should be monitored in patients admitted with a Glasgow Coma Scale (GCS) score of 8 or less and an abnormal CT scan or MRI. These results indicate that the patient may have bleeding, contusion, edema, or other problems. (The GCS is presented later in Table 56-5.)

**Methods of Measuring ICP.** Patients with conditions known to elevate ICP, except those with irreversible problems or advanced neurologic disease, usually undergo ICP monitoring in an ICU. Multiple methods and devices are available to monitor ICP in various sites (Fig. 56-6).

The gold standard for monitoring ICP is the *ventriculostomy,* in which a specialized catheter is inserted into the lateral ventricle and coupled to an external transducer (Figs. 56-7 and 56-8). This technique directly measures the pressure within the ventricles, facilitates removal and/or sampling of CSF, and allows for intraventricular drug administration. In this system the transducer is external, and it is important to ensure that the transducer of the ventriculostomy is level with the foramen of Monro (interventricular foramen). The ventriculostomy system must also be at the ideal height (Fig. 56-9, *A*). A reference point for this foramen is the tragus of the ear. Every time the patient is repositioned, the system must be assessed to ensure it is level.

The *fiberoptic catheter,* an alternative technology, uses a sensor transducer located within the catheter tip. The sensor tip is placed within the ventricle or the brain tissue and provides a direct measurement of brain pressure.

The *air pouch/pneumatic technology,* another system for monitoring ICP, has an air-filled pouch at the tip of the catheter that maintains a constant volume. The pressure changes within the cranium are transmitted through the changes exerted on this pouch to the monitor.

ICP is represented on the monitor as a mean pressure in mm Hg. If a CSF drainage device is in place, the drain must be closed for at least 6 minutes to ensure an accurate reading. Record the waveform strip along with other pressure monitoring waveforms. The normal ICP waveform has three phases (Fig. 56-7

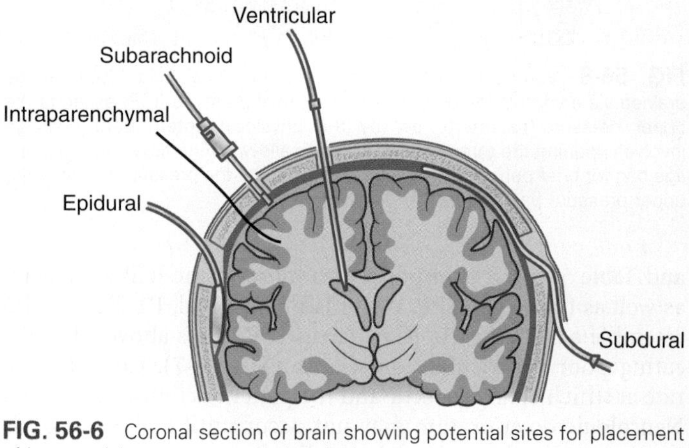


**FIG. 56-6** Coronal section of brain showing potential sites for placement of intracranial pressure monitoring devices.

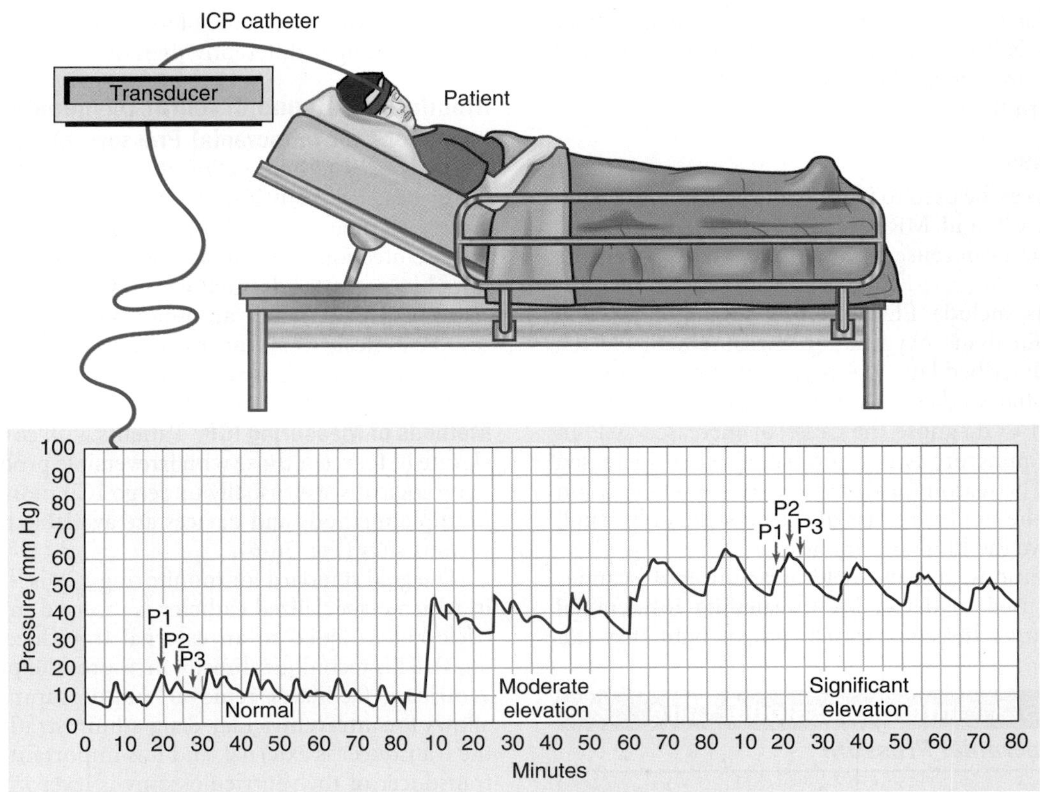


**FIG. 56-7** Intracranial pressure (ICP) monitoring can be used to continuously measure ICP. The ICP tracing shows normal, elevated, and plateau waves. At high ICP, the P2 peak is higher than the P1 peak, and the peaks become less distinct and plateau. (Modified from Copstead-Kirkhorn LC, Banasik JL: *Pathophysiology,* ed 5, St Louis, 2013, Mosby.)

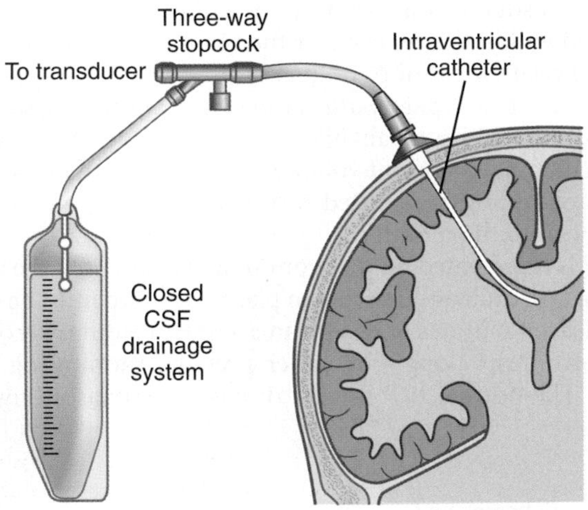


**FIG. 56-8** Ventriculostomy in place. Cerebrospinal fluid (CSF) can be drained via a ventriculostomy when intracranial pressure (ICP) exceeds the upper pressure parameter set by the physician. Intermittent drainage involves opening the three-way stopcock to allow CSF to flow into the drainage bag for brief periods (30 to 120 seconds) until the pressure is below the upper pressure parameters.

and Table 56-4). It is important to monitor the ICP waveform, as well as the mean CPP. When ICP is normal, P1, P2, and P3 resemble a staircase. As ICP increases, P2 rises above P1, indicating poor ventricular compliance (Fig. 56-7). Consider the rate at which changes occur and the patient's clinical condition. Neurologic deterioration may not occur until ICP elevation is pronounced and sustained. Immediately report to the HCP any ICP elevation, either as a mean increase in pressure or as an abnormal waveform configuration.

**TABLE 56-4 Normal Intracranial Pressure Waveforms***

| Waveform | Meaning |
|---|---|
| **P1** Percussion wave | Represents arterial pulsations. Normally the highest of the three waveforms. |
| **P2** Rebound wave or tidal wave | Reflects intracranial compliance or relative brain volume. When P2 is higher than P1, intracranial compliance is compromised. |
| **P3** Dicrotic wave | Follows dicrotic notch. Represents venous pulsations. Normally the lowest waveform. |

*See Fig. 56-7.

Inaccurate ICP readings can be caused by CSF leaks around the monitoring device, obstruction of the intraventricular catheter (from tissue or blood clot), a difference between the height of the catheter and the transducer, kinks in the tubing, and incorrect height of the drainage system relative to the patient's reference point. Bubbles or air in the tubing can also dampen the waveform.

Infection is a serious complication with ICP monitoring. Factors that contribute to the development of infection include ICP monitoring more than 5 days, use of a ventriculostomy, a CSF leak, and a concurrent systemic infection. Routinely assess the insertion site, use aseptic technique, and monitor the CSF for a change in drainage color or clarity.

**Cerebrospinal Fluid Drainage.** With the ventricular catheter, it is possible to control ICP by removing CSF (Fig. 56-8). The

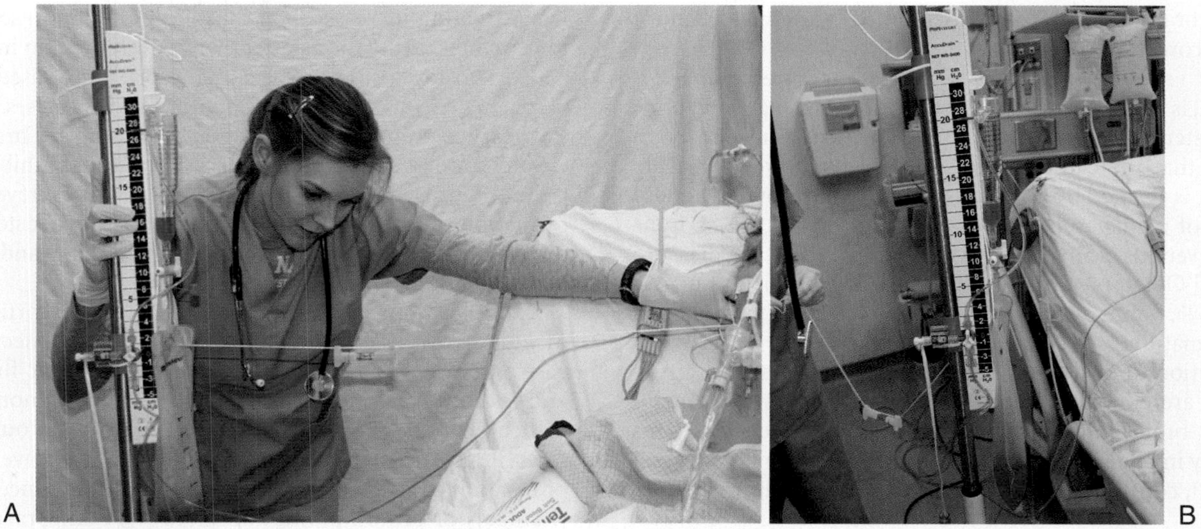


**FIG. 56-9** **A,** Leveling a ventriculostomy. **B,** Cerebrospinal fluid is drained into a drainage system. (Courtesy Meg Zomorodi, RN, PhD, CNL, Raleigh, N.C.)

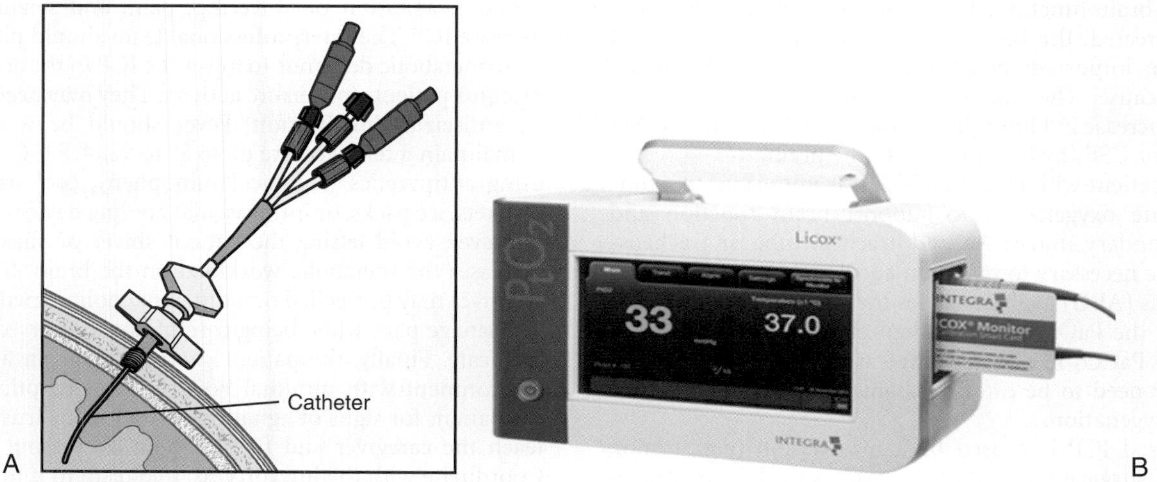


**FIG. 56-10** **A,** The LICOX brain tissue $O_2$ system involves insertion of a catheter. **B,** The system measures $O_2$ in the brain ($PbtO_2$), brain tissue temperature, and intracranial pressure. (*B,* Permission granted by Integra Life-Sciences Corporation, Plainsboro, N.J.)

HCP typically orders a specific level at which to initiate drainage (e.g., if ICP is greater than 20 mm Hg) and the frequency of drainage (intermittent or continuous). When the ICP is above the indicated level, the ventriculostomy system is opened by turning a stopcock and allowing the drainage of CSF, thus relieving pressure inside the cranial vault (Fig. 56-9, *B*).

The two options for CSF drainage are intermittent or continuous. If intermittent drainage is ordered, open the ventriculostomy system at the indicated ICP and allow CSF to drain for 2 to 3 minutes. Then close the stopcock to return the ventriculostomy to a closed system. If continuous ICP drainage is ordered, carefully monitor the volume of CSF drained. Keep in mind that normal CSF production is about 20 to 30 mL/hr, with a total CSF volume of about 150 mL within the ventricles and subarachnoid space. It is also recommended that a sign be posted above the patient's bed to notify anyone before turning, moving, or suctioning the patient to prevent the removal of too much CSF, which can result in other complications.

Strict aseptic technique during dressing changes or sampling of CSF is imperative to prevent infection. The system must remain intact to ensure that the ICP readings are accurate because treatment is initiated based on the pressures.

Complications of this type of drainage system include ventricular collapse, infection, and herniation or subdural hematoma formation from rapid decompression. Although it is generally recognized that CSF removal decreases ICP and improves CPP, guidelines for CSF removal are not universally accepted but are typically based on institution or HCP preference.[5]

**Cerebral Oxygenation Monitoring.** Technology is available to measure cerebral oxygenation and assess perfusion. Three intracranial devices used in ICU settings are the LICOX catheter, Neurovent catheter, and jugular venous bulb catheter.

The LICOX and Neurovent catheters are placed in viable (healthy) white matter of the brain (Fig. 56-10). These catheters can measure brain oxygenation and temperature. These systems provide continuous monitoring of the pressure of $O_2$ in brain tissue ($PbtO_2$). The normal range for $PbtO_2$ is 20 to 40 mm Hg. A lower-than-normal $PbtO_2$ level is indicative of ischemia.[6] These catheters can also measure brain temperature.

A cooler brain temperature (96.8° F [36° C]) may produce better outcomes.

*Jugular venous bulb oximetry,* which measures global $O_2$ extraction, is also used in some institutions. The jugular venous bulb catheter is placed in the internal jugular vein and positioned so that the catheter tip is located in the jugular bulb. Placement is verified by an x-ray. This catheter provides a measurement of jugular venous $O_2$ saturation ($SjvO_2$), which indicates total venous brain tissue extraction of $O_2$. This is a measure of cerebral $O_2$ supply and demand. The normal $SjvO_2$ range is 55% to 75%. Values less than 50% demonstrate impaired cerebral oxygenation.[7]

In addition to measuring ICP and brain oxygenation, many clinicians are now looking at multimodality monitoring in traumatic brain injury and intracranial hypertension. This technology includes brain microdialysis (measurement of small molecules), continuous EEG, and blood flow monitoring.

## Interprofessional Care

The goals of interprofessional care (Table 56-3) are to (1) identify and treat the underlying cause of increased ICP and (2) support brain function. The earlier the condition is recognized and treated, the better the patient outcome. A careful history is an important diagnostic aid in the search for the underlying cause. The underlying cause of increased ICP is usually an increase in blood (hemorrhage), brain tissue (tumor or edema), or CSF (hydrocephalus) in the brain.

For any patient with increased ICP, it is important to maintain adequate oxygenation to support brain function and prevent secondary injury. An endotracheal tube or tracheostomy may be necessary to maintain adequate ventilation. Arterial blood gas (ABG) analysis guides the $O_2$ therapy. The goal is to maintain the $PaO_2$ at greater than or equal to 100 mm Hg and to keep $PaCO_2$ in normal range at 35 to 45 mm Hg. The patient may need to be on a mechanical ventilator to ensure adequate oxygenation.

If increased ICP is caused by a mass lesion (e.g., tumor, hematoma), surgical removal of the mass is the best treatment (see the sections on brain tumors and cranial surgery later in this chapter). In aggressive situations, a craniectomy (removal of part of skull) may be performed to reduce ICP and prevent herniation (see head injury section for further details).

**Drug Therapy.** Drug therapy plays an important part in the management of increased ICP. Mannitol (Osmitrol) (25%) is an osmotic diuretic given IV. Mannitol decreases the ICP in two ways: plasma expansion and osmotic effect. The immediate plasma-expanding effect reduces the hematocrit and blood viscosity, thereby increasing CBF and cerebral $O_2$ delivery. A vascular osmotic gradient is created by mannitol. Thus fluid moves from the tissues into the blood vessels, reducing the ICP because of the decrease in the total brain fluid content. Monitor fluid and electrolyte status when osmotic diuretics are used. Mannitol may be contraindicated if renal disease is present and if serum osmolality is elevated.

Hypertonic saline solution is another drug treatment used to manage increased ICP. It produces massive movement of water out of edematous swollen brain cells and into blood vessels. This movement of water out of the brain can reduce swelling and improve cerebral blood flow. Hypertonic solution infusion requires frequent monitoring of BP and serum sodium levels because intravascular fluid volume excess can occur. Hypertonic saline infusion has been shown to be just as effective as mannitol when treating increased ICP, and both are often used concurrently when caring for a patient with a severe brain injury.[8]

Corticosteroids (e.g., dexamethasone) are used to treat vasogenic edema surrounding tumors and abscesses. However, these drugs are not recommended for traumatic brain injury. Corticosteroids stabilize the cell membrane and inhibit the synthesis of prostaglandins (see Fig. 11-2), thus preventing the formation of proinflammatory mediators. Corticosteroids also improve neuronal function by improving CBF and restoring autoregulation.

Complications associated with the use of corticosteroids include hyperglycemia, increased incidence of infections, and gastrointestinal (GI) bleeding. Regularly monitor fluid intake and sodium levels, and perform blood glucose monitoring at least every 6 hours until hyperglycemia is ruled out. Patients receiving corticosteroids should concurrently be given antacids or histamine ($H_2$)-receptor blockers (e.g., cimetidine, ranitidine [Zantac]) or proton pump inhibitors (e.g., omeprazole [Prilosec], pantoprazole [Protonix, Protonix IV]) to prevent GI ulcers and bleeding.

Metabolic demands such as fever (greater than 100.4° F [38° C]), agitation or shivering, pain, and seizures can also increase ICP. The interprofessional team should plan to reduce these metabolic demands to lower the ICP in the at-risk patient. Monitor patients for seizure activity. They may need prophylactic antiseizure medication. Fever should be well controlled to maintain a temperature of 96.8° to 98.6° F (36° to 37° C) by using antipyretics (e.g., acetaminophen), cool baths, cooling blankets, ice packs, or intravascular cooling devices as necessary. However, avoid letting the patient shiver or shake, since this increases the metabolic workload on the brain. If this occurs, sedatives may be needed or a different cooling method selected.

Manage pain while being careful not to oversedate or overmedicate. Finally, the patient should remain in a quiet, calm environment with minimal noise and interruptions. Observe the patient for signs of agitation, irritation, or frustration. Also teach the caregiver and family about decreasing stimulation. Coordinate with the interprofessional team to minimize procedures that may produce agitation.

Drug therapy for reducing cerebral metabolism may be an effective strategy to control ICP. Reducing the metabolic rate decreases the CBF and therefore the ICP. High doses of barbiturates (e.g., pentobarbital, thiopental) are used in patients with increased ICP refractory to other treatments. Barbiturates decrease cerebral metabolism, causing a decrease in ICP and a reduction in cerebral edema. When this treatment is used, monitor the patient's ICP, blood flow, and EEG. Barbiturate dosing is typically based on analysis of the bedside EEG tracing and the ICP. The HCP orders the barbiturate infusion at a rate that achieves a desired level of brain wave suppression as a means to control ICP. Total *burst suppression,* recognized by the absence of spikes showing brain activity on the EEG monitor, indicates that maximal therapeutic effect has been achieved.

**Nutritional Therapy.** Regardless of their state of consciousness, patients must have their nutritional needs met. Because malnutrition promotes continued cerebral edema, maintenance of optimal nutrition is imperative. The patient with increased ICP is in a hypermetabolic and hypercatabolic state that increases the need for glucose as fuel for metabolism of the injured brain. If the patient cannot maintain an adequate oral intake, other means of meeting the nutritional requirements, such as enteral feedings or parenteral nutrition, should be initiated.

Early feeding after brain injury may improve patient outcome.[9] Nutritional replacement should begin within 3 days after injury to reach full nutritional replacement within 7 days after the injury is sustained. (Nutritional therapy is discussed in Chapter 39.) Feedings or supplements should be guided by the patient's fluid and electrolyte status and metabolic needs. The patient should remain in a normovolemic fluid state. Continuously evaluate the patient based on clinical factors such as urine output, insensible fluid loss, serum and urine osmolality, and serum electrolytes.

IV 0.9% sodium chloride is the preferred solution for administration of piggyback medications. If 5% dextrose in water or 0.45% sodium chloride is used, serum osmolarity decreases and an increase in cerebral edema may occur.

## NURSING MANAGEMENT: INCREASED INTRACRANIAL PRESSURE

### Nursing Assessment

Subjective data about the patient with increased ICP can be obtained from the patient, caregiver, or family member who is familiar with the patient. Learn appropriate neurologic assessment techniques. Describe the LOC by noting the specific behaviors observed. Assess the LOC using the Glasgow Coma Scale (Table 56-5). Also assess body functions, especially circulation and respiration.

**Glasgow Coma Scale.** The Glasgow Coma Scale (GCS) is a quick, practical, and standardized system for assessing the LOC. The three areas assessed in the GCS are the patient's ability to (1) open the eyes when a verbal or painful stimulus is applied, (2) speak, and (3) obey commands. Specific assessments evaluate the patient's response to varying degrees of stimulus. Three indicators of response are evaluated: (1) opening of the eyes, (2) best verbal response, and (3) best motor response (Table 56-5).

Specific behaviors observed as responses to the testing stimulus are given a numeric value. Your responsibility is to elicit the best response on each of the scales: the higher the scores, the higher the level of brain functioning. The subscale scores are particularly important if a patient is untestable in one area. For example, severe periorbital edema may make eye opening impossible.

The total GCS score is the sum of the numeric values assigned to each of the three areas evaluated. The highest GCS score is 15 for a fully alert person, and the lowest possible score is 3. A GCS score of 8 or less generally indicates coma, and mechanical ventilation should be considered. Plot the results of the GCS scores on a graph, which can be used to determine whether the patient is stable, improving, or deteriorating.

The GCS offers several advantages in the assessment of the unconscious patient. It allows different health care professionals to arrive at the same conclusion regarding the patient's status and can be used to discriminate between different or changing states.

Although the GCS is the gold standard assessment tool for LOC, other scales such as the *Full Outline of Unresponsiveness (FOUR) scale* are also used in the clinical setting.[10] In cases of stroke or hemorrhage associated with increased ICP, use the NIH Stroke Scale (Table 57-10). Other components of the neurologic assessment include cranial nerve assessment and motor and sensory testing.

**Neurologic Assessment.** Compare the pupils with one another for size, shape, movement, and reactivity (Fig. 56-11). If the oculomotor nerve (CN III) is compressed, the pupil on the affected side *(ipsilateral)* becomes larger until it fully dilates. If ICP continues to increase, both pupils dilate.

**TABLE 56-5 Glasgow Coma Scale**

| Appropriate Stimulus | Response | Score |
|---|---|---|
| **Eyes Open** | | |
| • Approach to bedside<br>• Verbal command<br>• Pain | Spontaneous response. | 4 |
| | Opening of eyes to name or command. | 3 |
| | Lack of opening of eyes to previous stimuli but opening to pain. | 2 |
| | Lack of opening of eyes to any stimulus. | 1 |
| | Untestable.* | U |
| **Best Verbal Response** | | |
| • Verbal questioning with maximum arousal | Appropriate orientation, conversant. Correct identification of self, place, yr, and mo. | 5 |
| | Confusion. Conversant, but disorientation in one or more spheres. | 4 |
| | Inappropriate or disorganized use of words (e.g., cursing), lack of sustained conversation. | 3 |
| | Incomprehensible words, sounds (e.g., moaning). | 2 |
| | Lack of sound, even with painful stimuli. | 1 |
| | Untestable.* | U |
| **Best Motor Response** | | |
| • Verbal command (e.g., "raise your arm, hold up two fingers")<br>• Pain (pressure on proximal nail bed) | Obedience of command. | 6 |
| | Localization of pain, lack of obedience but presence of attempts to remove offending stimulus. | 5 |
| | Flexion withdrawal,* flexion of arm in response to pain without abnormal flexion posture. | 4 |
| | Abnormal flexion, flexing of arm at elbow and pronation, making a fist. | 3 |
| | Abnormal extension, extension of arm at elbow usually with adduction and internal rotation of arm at shoulder. | 2 |
| | Lack of response. | 1 |
| | Untestable.* | U |

Test pupillary reaction with a penlight. The normal reaction is brisk constriction when the light is shone directly into the eye. Also note a consensual response (slight constriction in the opposite pupil) at the same time. A sluggish reaction can indicate early pressure on CN III. A fixed pupil unresponsive to light stimulus usually indicates increased ICP. However, note that there are other causes of a fixed pupil, including direct injury to CN III, previous eye surgery, administration of atropine, and use of mydriatic eye drops.

In some hospitals, clinicians are using a handheld device *(pupillometer)* to measure the pupil reactivity and size. The device removes any subjectivity from the pupil evaluation.

Evaluation of other cranial nerves can be included in the neurologic assessment. (Cranial nerve assessment is presented in Table 55-4.)

Eye movements controlled by CN III, IV, and VI can be examined in the patient who is awake and able to follow

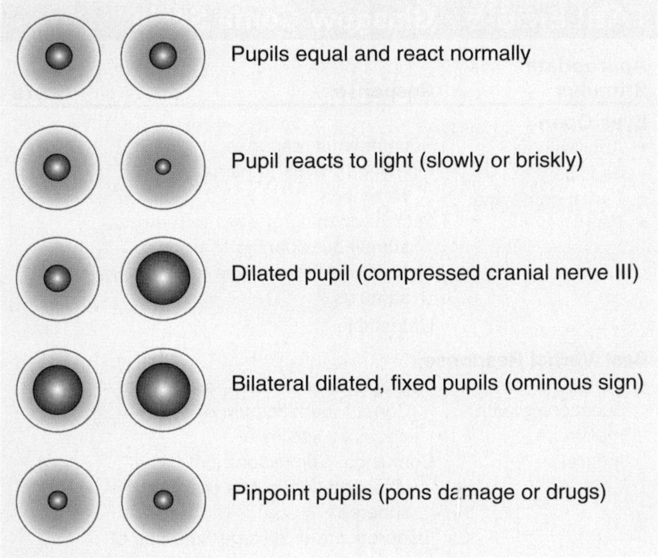


**FIG. 56-11** Pupillary check for size and response.

| Pattern | Location of Lesion | Description |
|---|---|---|
| 1. Cheyne-Stokes 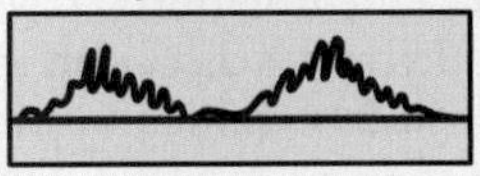 | Bilateral hemispheric disease or metabolic brain dysfunction | Cycles of hyperventilation and apnea |
| 2. Central neurogenic hyperventilation 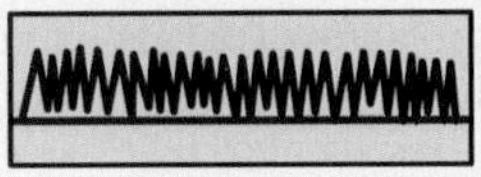 | Brainstem between lower midbrain and upper pons | Sustained, regular rapid and deep breathing |
| 3. Apneustic breathing 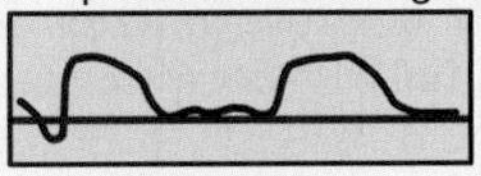 | Mid or lower pons | Prolonged inspiratory phase or pauses alternating with expiratory pauses |
| 4. Cluster breathing 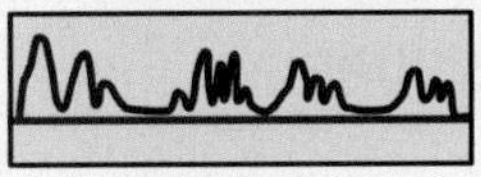 | Medulla or lower pons | Clusters of breaths follow each other with irregular pauses between |
| 5. Ataxic breathing 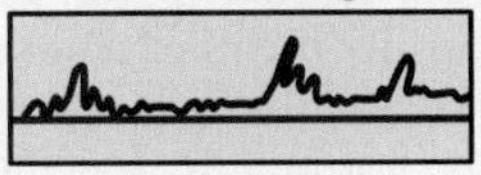 | Reticular formation of the medulla | Completely irregular with some breaths deep and some shallow. Random, irregular pauses, slow rate |

**FIG. 56-12** Common abnormal respiratory patterns associated with coma.

commands and can be used to assess the function of the brainstem. Testing the corneal reflex gives information about the functioning of CN V and VII. If this reflex is absent, initiate routine eye care to prevent corneal abrasion (see Chapter 21).

Eye movements of the uncooperative or unconscious patient can be elicited by reflex with the use of head movements (oculocephalic) and caloric stimulation (oculovestibular). To test the oculocephalic reflex (doll's eye reflex), turn the patient's head briskly to the left or right while holding the eyelids open. A normal response is movement of the eyes across the midline in the direction opposite that of the turning. Next, quickly flex and then extend the neck. Eye movement should be opposite to the direction of head movement—up when the neck is flexed and down when it is extended. Abnormal responses can help locate the intracranial lesion. This test should not be attempted if a cervical spine problem is suspected.

Test motor strength by asking the awake and cooperative patient to squeeze your hands to compare strength in the hands. The pronator drift test is an excellent measure of strength in the upper extremities. The patient raises the arms in front of the body with the palms facing upward and eyes closed. If there is any weakness in the upper extremity, the palmar surface turns downward and the arm drifts down. This would indicate a problem in the opposite motor cortex. Asking the patient to raise the foot from the bed or to bend the knees up in bed is a good assessment of lower extremity strength. Test all four extremities for strength and for any asymmetry in strength or movement.

Assess the motor response of the unconscious or uncooperative patient by observation of spontaneous movement. If no spontaneous movement is possible, apply a pain stimulus to the patient, and note the response. Resistance to movement during passive range-of-motion exercises is another measure of strength. Do not include hand squeezing as part of the assessment of motor movement in the unconscious or uncooperative patient, since this is a reflex action and can misrepresent the patient's status.

Also record the vital signs, including BP, pulse, respiratory rate, and temperature. Be aware of Cushing's triad, which indicates severely increased ICP. Besides recording respiratory rate, also note the respiratory pattern. Specific respiratory patterns are associated with severely increased ICP (Fig. 56-12).

## ◆ Nursing Diagnoses

Nursing diagnoses for the patient with increased ICP include, but are not limited to, the following:

- Decreased intracranial adaptive capacity *related to* decreased cerebral perfusion or increased ICP
- Risk for ineffective cerebral tissue perfusion *related to* reduction of venous and/or arterial blood flow and cerebral edema
- Risk for disuse syndrome *related to* altered LOC, immobility, and altered nutritional intake

Additional information on nursing diagnoses for patients with increased ICP is presented in eNursing Care Plan 56-1 (available on the website for this chapter).

## ◆ Planning

The overall goals for the patient with increased ICP are to (1) maintain a patent airway; (2) have ICP within normal limits; (3) have normal fluid, electrolyte, and nutritional balance; and (4) prevent complications secondary to immobility and decreased LOC.

## ◆ Nursing Implementation

### ◆ Acute Care

◆ ***Respiratory Function.*** Maintaining a patent airway is critical in the patient with increased ICP and is a primary nursing responsibility. As the LOC decreases, the patient is at an increased risk of airway obstruction from the tongue dropping back and occluding the airway or from accumulation of secretions.

**! SAFETY ALERT Altered Breathing**

- Be alert to altered breathing patterns in a patient with increased ICP.
- Snoring sounds indicate obstruction and require immediate intervention.

Remove accumulated secretions by suctioning as needed. An oral airway facilitates breathing and provides an easier suctioning route in the comatose patient. In general, any patient with a GCS of 8 or less or an altered LOC who is unable to maintain a patent airway or effective ventilation needs intubation and mechanical ventilation.

Prevent hypoxia and hypercapnia to minimize secondary injury. Proper positioning of the head is important. Elevation of the head of the bed to 30 degrees enhances respiratory exchange and aids in decreasing cerebral edema. Suctioning and coughing cause transient decreases in the $PaO_2$ and increases in the ICP. Keep suctioning to a minimum and less than 10 seconds in duration, with administration of 100% $O_2$ before and after to prevent decreases in the $PaO_2$. To avoid cumulative increases in the ICP with suctioning, limit suctioning to two passes per suction procedure, if possible. Patients with elevated ICP are at risk for lower CPP during suctioning.

Try to prevent abdominal distention, since it can interfere with respiratory function. Insertion of a nasogastric tube to aspirate the stomach contents can prevent distention, vomiting, and possible aspiration. However, in patients with facial and skull fractures, a nasogastric tube is contraindicated unless a basilar skull fracture (at base of skull) has been ruled out, and oral insertion of a gastric tube is preferred.

Pain, anxiety, and fear related to the primary injury, therapeutic procedures, or noxious stimuli can increase ICP and BP, thus complicating the management and recovery of the brain-injured patient. The appropriate choice or combination of sedatives, paralytics, and analgesics for symptom management presents a challenge to the ICU team. Administration of these agents may alter the neurologic state, thus masking true neurologic changes. It may be necessary to temporarily suspend drug therapy to appropriately assess neurologic status. The choice, dose, and combination of agents may vary depending on the patient's history, neurologic state, and overall clinical presentation.

Opioids, such as morphine sulfate and fentanyl (Sublimaze), are rapid-onset analgesics with minimal effect on CBF or $O_2$ metabolism. The IV anesthetic sedative propofol (Diprivan) is used in the management of anxiety and agitation in the ICU because of its rapid onset and short half-life. An accurate neurologic assessment can be performed soon after turning off the infusion of propofol. Dexmedetomidine (Precedex), an $\alpha_2$-adrenergic agonist, is used for continuous IV sedation of intubated and mechanically ventilated patients in the ICU setting for up to 24 hours. When using continuous IV sedatives, be aware of the side effects of these drugs, especially hypotension, since this can result in a lower CPP value.

Nondepolarizing neuromuscular blocking agents (e.g., vecuronium, cisatracurium besylate [Nimbex]) are useful for achieving complete ventilatory control in the treatment of refractory intracranial hypertension. Because these agents paralyze muscles without blocking pain or noxious stimuli, they are used in combination with sedatives, analgesics, or benzodiazepines.

Benzodiazepines, although useful for sedation, are usually avoided in the management of the patient with increased ICP because of the hypotensive effect and long half-life, unless they are used as an adjunct to neuromuscular blocking agents.

Frequently monitor and evaluate the ABG values, and take measures to maintain the levels within prescribed or acceptable parameters (see Chapter 25). The appropriate ventilatory support can be ordered on the basis of the $PaO_2$ and $PaCO_2$ values.

◆ ***Fluid and Electrolyte Balance.*** Fluid and electrolyte disturbances can have an adverse effect on ICP. Closely monitor IV fluids with the use of an accurate IV infusion control device or pump. Intake and output, with insensible losses and daily weights taken into account, are important parameters in the assessment of fluid balance.

Make electrolyte determinations daily, and discuss any abnormal values with the HCP. It is especially important to monitor serum glucose, sodium, potassium, magnesium, and osmolality.

Monitor urine output to detect problems related to diabetes insipidus and SIADH. Diabetes insipidus is caused by a decrease in antidiuretic hormone (ADH). It results in increased urine output and hypernatremia. The usual treatment of diabetes insipidus is fluid replacement, vasopressin, or desmopressin acetate (DDAVP) (see Chapter 49). If it is not treated, severe dehydration will occur.

SIADH is caused by an excess secretion of ADH. SIADH results in decreased urine output and dilutional hyponatremia. It may result in cerebral edema, changes in LOC, seizures, and coma. (Treatment of SIADH is described in Chapter 49.)

◆ ***Monitoring ICP.*** ICP monitoring is used in combination with other physiologic parameters to guide the care of the patient and assess the patient's response to treatment. Valsalva maneuver, coughing, sneezing, suctioning, hypoxemia, and arousal from sleep are factors that can increase ICP. Be alert to these factors and attempt to minimize them.

◆ ***Body Position.*** Maintain the patient with increased ICP in the head-up position. The head should be maintained in a midline position, avoiding extreme neck flexion. This position can cause venous obstruction and contribute to elevated ICP. Adjust the body position to decrease the ICP and improve the CPP. Elevation of the head of the bed promotes drainage from the head and decreases the vascular congestion that can produce cerebral edema. However, raising the head of the bed above 30 degrees may decrease the CPP by lowering systemic BP. Carefully evaluate the effects of elevation of the head of the bed on both the ICP and CPP. Position the bed so that it lowers the ICP while optimizing the CPP and other indices of cerebral oxygenation.

Take care to turn the patient with slow, gentle movements because rapid changes in position may increase the ICP. Prevent discomfort in turning and positioning the patient because pain or agitation also increases pressure. Increased intrathoracic pressure contributes to increased ICP by impeding the venous return. Thus coughing, straining, and the Valsalva maneuver should be avoided. Avoid extreme hip flexion to decrease the risk of raising the intraabdominal pressure, which increases ICP. Turn the patient at least every 2 hours.

Decorticate or decerebrate posturing is a reflex response in some patients with increased ICP. Turning, skin care, and even passive range of motion can elicit the posturing reflexes. Provide the physical care to minimize complications of immobility, such as atelectasis and contractures.

◆ ***Protection From Injury.*** The patient with increased ICP and decreased LOC needs protection from self-injury. Confusion, agitation, and the possibility of seizures increase the risk for injury. Use restraints judiciously in the agitated patient. If restraints are absolutely necessary to keep the patient from removing tubes or falling out of bed, they should be secure enough to be effective, and observe the skin area under the restraints regularly for irritation. Agitation may increase with the use of restraints, which indicates the need for other measures to protect the patient from injury. Light sedation with agents such as midazolam or lorazepam (Ativan) may be needed. Having a family member stay with the patient may have a calming effect.

For the patient with seizures or the patient at risk for such activity, institute seizure precautions. These include padded side rails, an airway at the bedside, suction readily available, accurate and timely administration of antiseizure drugs, and close observation. The use of prophylactic antiseizure drugs has been controversial as their use may not decrease seizures.[11]

The patient can benefit from a quiet, nonstimulating environment. Always use a calm, reassuring approach. Touch and talk to the patient, even one who is in a coma.

◆ ***Psychologic Considerations.*** In addition to carefully planned physical care, also be aware of the psychologic well-being of patients and their families. Anxiety over the diagnosis and the prognosis can be distressing to the patient, caregiver and family, and nursing staff. Your competent and assured manner in performing care is reassuring to everyone involved. Short, simple explanations are appropriate and allow the patient and caregiver to acquire the amount of information they desire. There is a need for support, information, and teaching of both patients and families. Assess the family members' desires to assist in providing care for the patient and allow for their participation as appropriate. Encourage interprofessional management (social work, chaplain, etc.) of the patient and family in decision making as much as possible.

### ◆ Evaluation

The expected outcomes are that the patient with increased ICP will

- Maintain ICP and cerebral perfusion within normal parameters
- Experience no serious increases in ICP during or after care activities
- Experience no complications of immobility

Additional expected outcomes for the patient with increased ICP are addressed in eNursing Care Plan 56-1 (available on the website for this chapter).

## HEAD INJURY

**Head injury** includes any injury or trauma to the scalp, skull, or brain. A serious form of head injury is *traumatic brain injury* (TBI). Statistics regarding the occurrence of head injuries are incomplete because many victims die at the injury scene or because the condition is considered minor and health care services are not sought. In U.S. hospital emergency departments, an estimated 1.7 million persons are treated and released with TBI. Fifty thousand people die and 275,000 persons are hospitalized with TBI. Of individuals hospitalized, 20% of the patients die.[12] At least 5.3 million Americans (2% of the U.S. population) currently live with disabilities resulting from TBI (*www.braintrauma.org*).

The most common causes of head injury are falls and motor vehicle accidents. Other causes of head injury include firearms, assaults, sports-related trauma, recreational injuries, and war-related injuries.[13] Males are twice as likely to sustain a TBI as females.

Head trauma has a high potential for a poor outcome. Deaths from head trauma occur at three points after injury: immediately after the injury, within 2 hours after injury, and approximately 3 weeks after injury.[13] The majority of deaths after a head injury occur immediately after the injury, either from the direct head trauma or from massive hemorrhage and shock. Deaths occurring within a few hours of the trauma are caused by progressive worsening of the brain injury or internal bleeding.[14]

Deaths occurring 3 weeks or more after the injury result from multisystem failure. Expert nursing care in the weeks after the injury is crucial in decreasing the mortality risk and in optimizing patient outcomes.[15]

### Types of Head Injuries

**Scalp Lacerations.** *Scalp lacerations* are an easily recognized type of external head trauma. Because the scalp contains many blood vessels with poor constrictive abilities, most scalp lacerations are associated with profuse bleeding. Even relatively small wounds can bleed significantly. The major complications associated with scalp laceration are blood loss and infection.

**Skull Fractures.** *Skull fractures* frequently occur with head trauma. Skull fractures can be described in several ways: (1) linear or depressed; (2) simple, comminuted, or compound; and (3) closed or open (Table 56-6). Fractures may be closed or open, depending on the presence of a scalp laceration or extension of the fracture into the air sinuses or dura. The type and severity of a skull fracture depend on the velocity, momentum, direction and shape (blunt or sharp) of the injuring agent, and site of impact.

The location of the fracture determines the clinical manifestations (Table 56-7). For example, a basilar skull fracture is a specialized type of linear fracture involving the base of the skull. Manifestations can evolve over the course of several hours; vary with the location and severity of fracture; and may include cranial nerve deficits, Battle's sign (postauricular ecchymosis), and periorbital ecchymosis (raccoon eyes) (Fig. 56-13). This fracture generally is associated with a tear in the dura and subsequent leakage of CSF.

*Rhinorrhea* (CSF leakage from the nose) or *otorrhea* (CSF leakage from the ear) generally confirms that the fracture has traversed the dura (Fig. 56-13). Rhinorrhea may also manifest as postnasal sinus drainage. The significance of rhinorrhea may be overlooked unless the patient is specifically assessed for this finding. The risk of meningitis is high with a CSF leak, and antibiotics should be administered as a preventive measure.

Two methods of testing can be used to determine whether the fluid leaking from the nose or ear is CSF. The first method

**TABLE 56-6 Types of Skull Fractures**

| Type | Description | Cause |
|---|---|---|
| **Linear** | Break in continuity of bone without alteration of relationship of parts | Low-velocity injuries |
| **Depressed** | Inward indentation of skull | Powerful blow |
| **Simple** | Linear or depressed skull fracture without fragmentation or communicating lacerations | Low to moderate impact |
| **Comminuted** | Multiple linear fractures with fragmentation of bone into many pieces | Direct, high-momentum impact |
| **Compound** | Depressed skull fracture and scalp laceration with communicating pathway to intracranial cavity | Severe head injury |

**TABLE 56-7 Manifestations of Skull Fractures**

| Location | Manifestations |
|---|---|
| **Frontal fracture** | Exposure of brain to contaminants through frontal air sinus, possible association with air in forehead tissue, CSF rhinorrhea, or pneumocranium (air between cranium and dura mater) |
| **Orbital fracture** | Periorbital ecchymosis (raccoon eyes), optic nerve injury |
| **Temporal fracture** | Boggy temporal muscle because of extravasation of blood, oval-shaped bruise behind ear in mastoid region (Battle's sign), CSF otorrhea, middle meningeal artery disruption, epidural hematoma |
| **Parietal fracture** | Deafness, CSF or brain otorrhea, bulging of tympanic membrane caused by blood or CSF, facial paralysis, loss of taste, Battle's sign |
| **Posterior fossa fracture** | Occipital bruising resulting in cortical blindness, visual field defects, rare appearance of ataxia or other cerebellar signs |
| **Basilar skull fracture** | CSF or brain otorrhea, bulging of tympanic membrane caused by blood or CSF, Battle's sign, tinnitus or hearing difficulty, rhinorrhea, facial paralysis, conjugate deviation of gaze, vertigo |

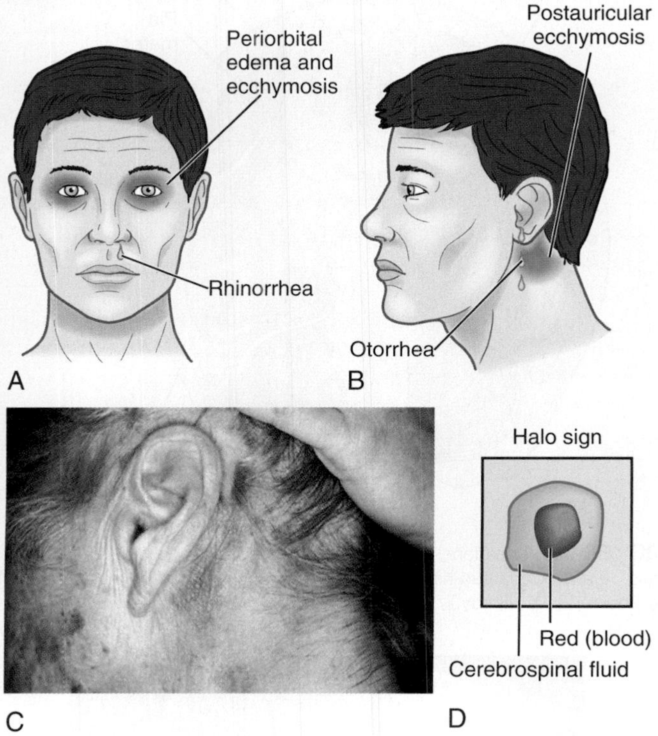


**FIG. 56-13** **A,** Raccoon eyes and rhinorrhea. **B,** Battle's sign (postauricular ecchymosis) with otorrhea. **C,** Battle's sign. **D,** Halo or ring sign (see text). (*C,* From Bingham BJG, Hawke M, Kwok P: *Clinical atlas of otolaryngology,* St Louis, 1992, Mosby.)

is to test the leaking fluid with a Dextrostix or Tes-Tape strip to determine whether glucose is present. CSF gives a positive reading for glucose. If blood is present in the fluid, testing for glucose is unreliable because blood also contains glucose. In this event, look for the *halo* or *ring* sign (Fig. 56-13, *D*). Allow the leaking fluid to drip onto a white gauze pad (4 × 4) or towel, and then observe the drainage. Within a few minutes, the blood coalesces into the center, and a yellowish ring encircles the blood if CSF is present. Note the color, appearance, and amount of leaking fluid because both tests can give false-positive results.

The major potential complications of skull fractures are intracranial infections, hematoma, and meningeal and brain tissue damage. Note that in cases where a basilar skull fracture is suspected, an orogastric tube should be inserted rather than a nasogastric tube.

**Head Trauma.** Brain injuries are categorized as diffuse (generalized) or focal (localized). In a *diffuse* injury (e.g., concussion, diffuse axonal injury), damage to the brain cannot be localized to one particular area. In a *focal injury* (e.g., contusion, hematoma), damage can be localized to a specific area of the brain. Brain injury can be classified as *minor* (GCS 13 to 15), *moderate* (GCS 9 to 12), and *severe* (GCS 3 to 8).

***Diffuse Injury.*** Concussion (a sudden transient mechanical head injury with disruption of neural activity and a change in the LOC) is considered a minor diffuse head injury. The patient may or may not lose total consciousness with this injury.

Typical signs of concussion include a brief disruption in LOC, amnesia regarding the event (retrograde amnesia), and headache. The manifestations are generally of short duration. If the patient has not lost consciousness, or if the loss of consciousness lasts less than 5 minutes, the patient is usually discharged from the care facility with instructions to notify the HCP if symptoms persist or if behavioral changes are noted.

*Postconcussion syndrome* may develop in some patients, usually anywhere from 2 weeks to 2 months after the injury. Manifestations include persistent headache, lethargy, personality and behavioral changes, shortened attention span, decreased short-term memory, and changes in intellectual ability. This syndrome can significantly affect the patient's abilities to perform activities of daily living.

Although concussion is generally considered benign and usually resolves spontaneously, the signs and symptoms may be the beginning of a more serious, progressive problem, especially in a patient with a history of prior concussion or head injury. At the time of discharge, it is important to give the patient and caregiver instructions for observation and accurate reporting of symptoms or changes in neurologic status.

**Diffuse axonal injury.** Diffuse axonal injury (DAI) is widespread axonal damage occurring after a mild, moderate, or severe TBI. The damage occurs primarily around axons in the subcortical white matter of the cerebral hemispheres, basal ganglia, thalamus, and brainstem.[16] Initially, DAI was believed to occur from the tensile forces of trauma that sheared axons, resulting in axonal disconnection. There is increasing evidence that axonal damage is not preceded by an immediate tearing of the axon from the traumatic impact, but rather the trauma changes the function of the axon, resulting in axon swelling and disconnection. This process takes approximately 12 to 24 hours to develop and may persist longer.

The clinical signs of DAI are varied but may include a decreased LOC, increased ICP, decortication or decerebration, and global cerebral edema. Approximately 90% of patients with DAI remain in a persistent vegetative state.[16] Patients with DAI who survive the initial event are rapidly triaged to an ICU, where they will be vigilantly watched for signs of increased ICP and treated accordingly (as previously discussed).

***Focal Injury.*** Focal injury can be minor to severe and can be localized to an area of injury. Focal injury consists of lacerations, contusions, hematomas, and cranial nerve injuries.

*Lacerations* involve actual tearing of the brain tissue and often occur in association with depressed and open fractures and penetrating injuries. Tissue damage is severe, and surgical repair of the laceration is impossible because of the nature of brain tissue. Medical management consists of antibiotics (until meningitis is ruled out) and prevention of secondary injury related to increased ICP. If bleeding is deep into the brain tissue, focal and generalized signs develop.

When major head trauma occurs, many delayed responses are seen, including hemorrhage, hematoma formation, seizures, and cerebral edema. Intracerebral hemorrhage is generally associated with cerebral laceration. This hemorrhage manifests as a space-occupying lesion accompanied by unconsciousness, hemiplegia on the contralateral side, and a dilated pupil on the ipsilateral side. As the hematoma expands, signs of increased ICP become more severe. Subarachnoid hemorrhage and intraventricular hemorrhage can also occur secondary to head trauma.

A **contusion** is bruising of the brain tissue within a focal area. It is usually associated with a closed head injury. A contusion may contain areas of hemorrhage, infarction, necrosis, and edema, and it frequently occurs at a fracture site.

With contusion, the phenomenon of *coup-contrecoup injury* is often noted (Fig. 56-14), and injuries can range from minor to severe. Damage from coup-contrecoup injury occurs when the brain moves inside the skull due to high-energy or high-impact injury mechanisms. Contusions or lacerations occur both at the site of the direct impact of the brain on the skull *(coup)* and at a second area of damage on the opposite side away from injury *(contrecoup)*, leading to multiple contused areas. *Contrecoup* injuries tend to be more severe, and overall patient prognosis depends on the amount of bleeding around the contusion site.

Contusions may continue to bleed or rebleed and appear to "blossom" on subsequent CT scans of the brain. Bleeding worsens the neurologic outcome. Neurologic assessment may demonstrate focal and generalized manifestation, depending on the contusion's size and location. Seizures can occur as a result of a brain contusion, particularly when the injury involves the frontal or temporal lobes. Anticoagulant use and coagulopathy are associated with increased hemorrhage, more severe head injury, and an increased mortality rate.[17] This is especially important when considering older individuals who are taking anticoagulants. If they fall, their contusion is likely to be more severe due to the use of anticoagulants. Risk for falls should be assessed in all patients taking anticoagulants (see Table 62-1).

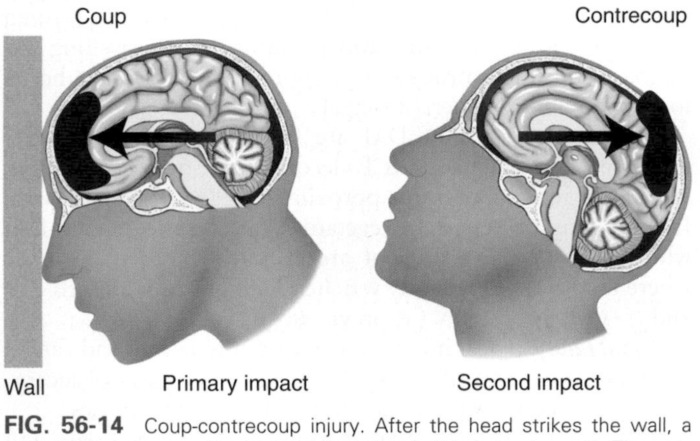


**FIG. 56-14** Coup-contrecoup injury. After the head strikes the wall, a coup injury occurs as the brain strikes the skull (primary impact). The contrecoup injury (the second impact) occurs when the brain strikes the skull surface opposite the site of the original impact.

## Complications

**Epidural Hematoma.** An **epidural hematoma** results from bleeding between the dura and inner surface of the skull (Figs. 56-15 and 56-16). An epidural hematoma is a neurologic emergency and is usually associated with a linear fracture crossing a major artery in the dura, causing a tear. It can have a venous or an arterial origin. Venous epidural hematomas are associated with a tear of the dural venous sinus and develop slowly. With arterial hematomas, the middle meningeal artery lying under the temporal bone is often torn. Hemorrhage occurs into the epidural space, which lies between the dura and inner surface of the skull (Fig. 56-15). Because this is an arterial hemorrhage, the hematoma develops rapidly.

Classic signs of an epidural hematoma include an initial period of unconsciousness at the scene, with a brief lucid interval followed by a decrease in LOC. Other manifestations may be a headache, nausea and vomiting, or focal findings. Rapid surgical intervention to evacuate the hematoma and prevent

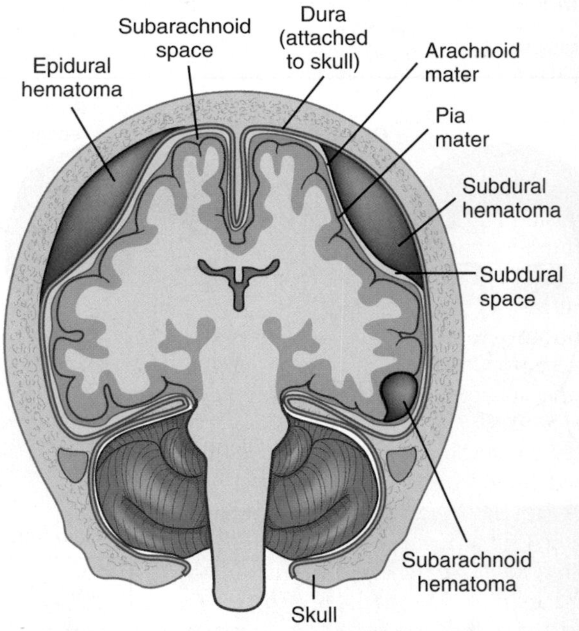


**FIG. 56-15** Locations of epidural, subdural, and subarachnoid hematomas. (From Copstead-Kirkhorn LC, Banasik JL: *Pathophysiology*, ed 4, St Louis, 2010, Mosby.)

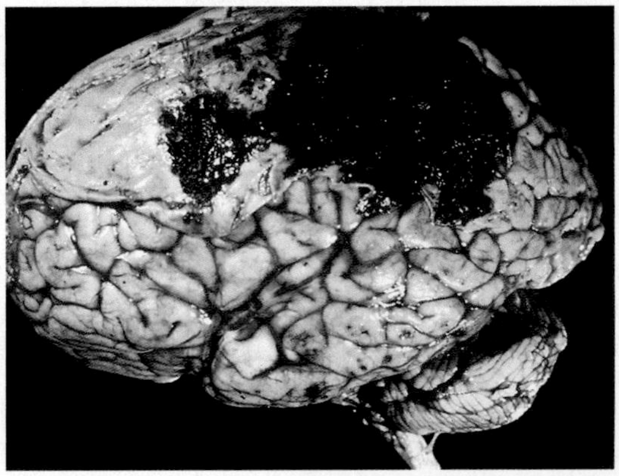

**FIG. 56-16** Epidural hematoma covering a portion of the dura. Multiple small contusions are seen in the temporal lobe. (From Kumar V, Abbas AK, Aster JC, Fausto N: *Robbins and Cotran pathologic basis of disease*, ed 8, Philadelphia, 2010, Saunders.)

**TABLE 56-8 Types of Subdural Hematomas**

| Occurrence After Injury | Progression of Symptoms | Treatment |
|---|---|---|
| **Acute** | | |
| 24-48 hr after severe trauma. | Immediate deterioration. | Craniotomy, evacuation, and decompression. |
| **Subacute** | | |
| 48 hr to 2 wk after severe trauma. | Alteration in mental status as hematoma develops. Progression dependent on size and location of hematoma. | Evacuation and decompression. |
| **Chronic** | | |
| Weeks or months, usually >20 days after injury. Often injury seemed trivial or was forgotten by patient. | Nonspecific, nonlocalizing progression. Progressive alteration in LOC. | Evacuation and decompression, membranectomy. |

*LOC,* Level of consciousness.

cerebral herniation, along with medical management for increasing ICP, can dramatically improve outcomes.

**Subdural Hematoma.** A **subdural hematoma** occurs from bleeding between the dura mater and arachnoid layer of the meninges (Fig. 56-15). A subdural hematoma usually results from injury to the brain tissue and its blood vessels. The veins that drain from the surface of the brain into the sagittal sinus are the source of most subdural hematomas. Because it is usually venous in origin, the subdural hematoma may be slower to develop. However, a subdural hematoma may be caused by an arterial hemorrhage, in which case it develops more rapidly. Subdural hematomas may be acute, subacute, or chronic (Table 56-8).

An *acute subdural hematoma* manifests within 24 to 48 hours of the injury.[18] The signs and symptoms are similar to those associated with brain tissue compression in increased ICP and include decreasing LOC and headache. The size of the hematoma determines the patient's clinical presentation and prognosis. The patient's appearance may range from drowsy and confused to unconscious. The ipsilateral pupil dilates and becomes fixed if ICP is significantly elevated. Blunt force injuries that produce acute subdural hematomas may also cause significant underlying brain injury, resulting in cerebral edema. The resulting increase in ICP from the cerebral edema can cause an increased morbidity and mortality risk despite surgical intervention to evacuate the hematoma.

A *subacute subdural hematoma* usually occurs within 2 to 14 days of the injury. After the initial bleeding, a subdural hematoma may appear to enlarge over time as the breakdown products of the blood draw fluid into the subdural space.

A *chronic subdural hematoma* develops over weeks or months after a seemingly minor head injury.[19] Chronic subdural hematomas are more common in older adults because of a potentially larger subdural space as a result of brain atrophy. With atrophy, the brain remains attached to the supportive structures, but tension is increased, and it is subject to tearing. Because the subdural space is larger, the presenting complaint is focal symptoms (specific to a certain area of the brain), rather than signs of increased ICP.[20] Chronic alcoholics are also prone to cerebral atrophy and subsequent development of subdural hematoma because of an increased incidence of falls.

**CHECK YOUR PRACTICE**

You are doing BP screenings in the senior center when you meet a 76-yr-old man and his wife. As you perform their BP screening, the wife tells you that her husband has been getting severe headaches, is dizzy, and sometimes has difficulty talking. Based on your advice, they go to an urgent care center, where a CT scan is done. The results indicate he has a chronic subdural hematoma.

When you find out the diagnosis, you are really puzzled about the diagnosis because you thought he was having a stroke and cannot understand how he got a subdural hematoma.

- If you had been the nurse, what would you have done differently when screening this man?

Diagnosis of a subdural hematoma in the older adult may be delayed because symptoms mimic other health problems in this age group, such as somnolence, confusion, lethargy, and memory loss. The manifestations of a subdural hematoma are often misinterpreted as vascular disease (stroke, transient ischemic attack [TIA]) or dementia.

**Intracerebral Hematoma.** **Intracerebral hematoma** occurs from bleeding within the brain tissue in approximately 16% of head injuries. It usually occurs within the frontal and temporal lobes, possibly from rupture of intracerebral vessels at the time of injury. The size and location of the hematoma are key determinants of the patient's outcome.

### Diagnostic Studies and Interprofessional Care

CT scan is the best diagnostic test to evaluate for head trauma because it allows for rapid diagnosis and intervention in the acute care setting. MRI, PET, and evoked potential studies may also be used in the diagnosis and differentiation of head injuries. An MRI scan is more sensitive than the CT scan in detecting small lesions. Transcranial Doppler studies allow for the measurement of cerebral blood flow (CBF) velocity. A cervical spine x-ray series, CT scan, or MRI of the spine may also be indicated, since cervical spine trauma often occurs at the same time as a head injury. In general, the diagnostic studies are similar to those used for a patient with increased ICP (Table 56-3).

Emergency management of the patient with a head injury is presented in Table 56-9. In addition to measures to prevent secondary injury by treating cerebral edema and managing increased ICP, the principal treatment of head injuries is timely diagnosis and surgery (if necessary). For the patient with concussion and contusion, observation and management of increased ICP are the primary management strategies.

The treatment of skull fractures is usually conservative. For depressed fractures and fractures with loose fragments, a craniotomy is necessary to elevate the depressed bone and remove the free fragments. If large amounts of bone are destroyed, the bone may be removed (craniectomy), and a cranioplasty will be needed later (see the section on cranial surgery later in this chapter).

In cases of large acute subdural and epidural hematomas or those associated with significant neurologic impairment, the blood must be removed through surgical evacuation. A craniotomy is generally performed to visualize and allow control of the bleeding vessels. Burr-hole openings may be used in an

**TABLE 56-9 Emergency Management**

***Head Injury***

| Etiology | Assessment Findings | Interventions |
|---|---|---|
| **Blunt**<br>• Motor vehicle collision<br>• Fall<br>• Assault<br>• Sports injury<br>**Penetrating**<br>• Gunshot wound<br>• Arrow | **Surface Findings**<br>• Scalp lacerations<br>• Fracture or depressions in skull<br>• Bruises or contusions on face, Battle's sign (bruising behind ears)<br>• Raccoon eyes (dependent bruising around eyes)<br>**Respiratory**<br>• Central neurogenic hyperventilation<br>• Cheyne-Stokes respirations<br>• Decreased $O_2$ saturation<br>• Pulmonary edema<br>**Central Nervous System**<br>• Unequal or dilated pupils, photophobia<br>• Asymmetric facial movements<br>• Garbled speech, abusive speech<br>• Confusion<br>• Decreased level of consciousness<br>• Combativeness<br>• Involuntary movements<br>• Seizures<br>• Bowel and bladder incontinence<br>• Flaccidity<br>• Depressed or hyperactive reflexes<br>• Decerebrate or decorticate posturing<br>• GCS score <12<br>• CSF leaking from ears or nose | **Initial**<br>• If unresponsive, assess circulation, airway, and breathing.<br>• If responsive, monitor airway, breathing, and circulation.<br>• Assume neck injury with head injury.<br>• Stabilize cervical spine.<br>• Administer $O_2$ via non-rebreather mask.<br>• Establish IV access with two large-bore catheters to infuse normal saline or lactated Ringer's solution.<br>• Intubate if GCS score <8.<br>• Control external bleeding with sterile pressure dressing.<br>• Remove patient's clothing.<br>**Ongoing Monitoring**<br>• Maintain normothermia using blankets, warm IV fluids, as necessary.<br>• Monitor vital signs, level of consciousness, $O_2$ saturation, cardiac rhythm, GCS score, pupil size and reactivity.<br>• Anticipate need for intubation if gag reflex is impaired or absent.<br>• Assess for rhinorrhea, otorrhea, scalp wounds.<br>• Administer fluids cautiously to prevent fluid overload and increasing ICP. |

*GCS,* Glasgow Coma Scale, *ICP,* intracranial pressure.

extreme emergency for a more rapid decompression, followed by a craniotomy. A drain may be placed postoperatively for several days to prevent reaccumulation of blood. In cases in which extreme swelling is expected (e.g., DAI, hemorrhage), a craniectomy may be performed, which involves removing a piece of skull to reduce the pressure inside the cranial vault, thus reducing the risk of herniation.

## NURSING MANAGEMENT: HEAD INJURY

### Nursing Assessment

A patient with a head injury always has the potential to develop increased ICP, which is associated with higher mortality rates and poorer functional outcomes. Objective data are obtained by applying the GCS (Table 56-5), assessing and monitoring the neurologic status, and determining whether a CSF leak has occurred. (Nursing assessment related to increased ICP is discussed on pp. 1323-1324.) Nursing assessment of the patient with a head injury is presented in Table 56-10.

### Nursing Diagnoses

Nursing diagnoses and a potential complication for the patient who has sustained a head injury may include, but are not limited to, the following:

- Risk for ineffective cerebral tissue perfusion *related to* interruption of CBF associated with cerebral hemorrhage, hematoma, and edema
- Hyperthermia *related to* increased metabolism, infection, and hypothalamic injury
- Impaired physical mobility *related to* decreased LOC
- Anxiety *related to* abrupt change in health status, hospital environment, and uncertain future
- Potential complication: increased ICP *related to* cerebral edema and hemorrhage

### Planning

The overall goals are that the patient with an acute head injury will (1) maintain adequate cerebral oxygenation and perfusion; (2) remain normothermic; (3) achieve control of pain and discomfort; (4) be free from infection; (5) have adequate nutrition; and (6) attain maximal cognitive, motor, and sensory function.

### Nursing Implementation

**Health Promotion.** One of the best ways to prevent head injuries is to prevent car and motorcycle accidents. The use of helmets by cyclists has led to fewer TBIs. The use of car seat belts and child car seats is also associated with reduced TBI mortality rates.

Be active in campaigns that promote driving safety, and speak to driver education classes regarding the dangers of unsafe driving and of driving after drinking alcohol and using drugs. Wearing seat belts in cars and helmets for riding on motorcycles is the most effective measure for increasing survival after crashes. Protective helmets should also be worn by lumberjacks, construction workers, athletes who play contact sports, miners, horseback riders, bicycle riders, snowboarders, skiers, and skydivers. Additionally, individuals who are at risk for falls (e.g., older adults) should be evaluated for safety in the home, since falls are the second leading cause of head injuries.

**Acute Care.** Management at the injury scene can have a significant impact on the outcome of the head injury. Emergency management of head injury is presented in Table 56-9. The general goal of nursing management of the head-injured patient

## TABLE 56-10 Nursing Assessment

### *Head Injury*

**Subjective Data**

***Important Health Information***

*Past health history:* Mechanism of injury: motor vehicle collision, sports injury, industrial incident, assault, falls

*Medications:* Anticoagulant medications

***Functional Health Patterns***

*Health perception–health management:* Alcohol or recreational drugs. Risk-taking behaviors

*Cognitive-perceptual:* Headache, mood or behavioral change, mentation changes, aphasia, dysphasia, impaired judgment

*Coping–stress tolerance:* Fear, denial, anger, aggression, depression

**Objective Data**

***General***

Altered mental status

***Integumentary***

Lacerations, contusions, abrasions, hematoma, Battle's sign, periorbital edema and ecchymosis, otorrhea, exposed brain matter

***Respiratory***

Rhinorrhea, impaired gag reflex, inability to maintain a patent airway. Impending herniation: altered/irregular respiratory rate and pattern

***Cardiovascular***

Impending herniation: Cushing's triad (systolic hypertension with widening pulse pressure, bradycardia with full and bounding pulse, irregular respirations)

***Gastrointestinal***

Vomiting, projectile vomiting, bowel incontinence

***Urinary***

Bladder incontinence

***Reproductive***

Uninhibited sexual expression

***Neurologic***

Altered level of consciousness, seizure activity, pupil dysfunction, cranial nerve deficit(s)

***Musculoskeletal***

Motor deficit/impairment, weakness, palmar drift, paralysis, spasticity, decorticate or decerebrate posturing, muscular rigidity or increased tone, flaccidity, ataxia

***Possible Diagnostic Findings***

Location and type of hematoma, edema, skull fracture, and/or foreign body on CT scan and/or MRI; abnormal EEG; positive toxicology screen or alcohol level, ↓ or ↑ blood glucose level; ↑ ICP

*ICP,* Intracranial pressure.

is to maintain cerebral oxygenation and perfusion and prevent secondary cerebral ischemia.

Surveillance or monitoring for changes in neurologic status is critically important because the patient's condition may deteriorate rapidly, necessitating emergency surgery. Appropriate preoperative and postoperative nursing interventions are initiated if surgery is anticipated. Because of the close association

## ETHICAL/LEGAL DILEMMAS

### *Brain Death*

**Situation**

The emergency nurse receives a radio call from emergency response system (ERS) personnel about R.G., a young man involved in a motorcycle crash. He was not wearing a helmet and has a large open skull fracture. Transport from the accident scene was delayed by 45 min as a result of a severe thunderstorm and traffic congestion. On the way to the hospital, R.G. exhibits fixed, dilated pupils and experiences cardiac arrest. Estimated arrival at the hospital is still an additional 45 min as a result of the severe weather. EMS personnel request permission to stop resuscitation efforts.

**Ethical/Legal Points for Consideration**

- Criteria for brain death include coma or unresponsiveness, absence of brainstem reflexes, and apnea (see Chapter 9).
- The definition of death has changed with the advent of new technology, monitoring devices, and interventions.
- A circumstance that influences the manner in which a state of death is determined is the customary practice or best practice for the specific situation.
- In a situation in which the professional responsible for determining a state of death is in remote contact with the patient, but the monitoring devices available provide virtual contact with the patient, a remote diagnosis of death may be legally acceptable.
- Brain death criteria do not address patients in a permanent vegetative state, since the brainstem activity in these patients is adequate to maintain heart and lung function.
- CPR is inappropriate when survival is not expected or if the patient is expected to survive without the ability to communicate. Quantitative futility implies that survival is not expected after CPR under given circumstances. In the absence of mitigating factors, prolonged resuscitative efforts are unlikely to be successful and can be discontinued if there is no return of spontaneous circulation at any time during 30 minutes of cumulative advanced life support.
- It is ethical for ED personnel to discontinue treatment initiated by ERS personnel in the prehospital setting, provided that there is valid, after-the-fact evidence that these interventions are now inappropriate.

**Discussion Questions**

1. What are your feelings about cessation of brain function vs. cessation of heart and lung function as the criteria for death of a patient?
2. What are your state's laws or practices about stopping cardiopulmonary resuscitation (CPR) efforts by ERS personnel in the field?
3. When brain death has occurred, what is your obligation for teaching the family or significant other regarding organ donation?

between hemodynamic status and cerebral perfusion, be aware of any coexisting injuries or conditions.

Explain the need for frequent neurologic assessments to both the patient and caregiver. Behavioral manifestations associated with head injury can result in a frightened, disoriented patient who is combative and resists help. Your approach should be calm and gentle. A family member may be available to stay with the patient and thus decrease anxiety and fear. One of the most important needs of the caregiver and family members in the acute injury phase is information about the patient's diagnosis, treatment plan, and rationale for the interventions. Other teaching points are presented in Table 56-11.

Perform neurologic assessments at intervals based on the patient's condition. The GCS is useful in assessing the LOC (Table 56-5). Report any indications of a deteriorating neurologic state, no matter how subtle, such as a decreasing LOC or

**TABLE 56-11 Patient & Caregiver Teaching**

***Head Injury***

*Include the following instructions when teaching the patient and caregiver about care during the first 2 or 3 days after a head injury.*

1. Notify your HCP immediately if experiencing signs and symptoms that may indicate complications. These include the following:
   - Increased drowsiness (e.g., difficulty arousing, confusion)
   - Nausea or vomiting
   - Worsening headache or stiff neck
   - Seizures
   - Vision difficulties (e.g., blurring) or sensitivity to light (photophobia)
   - Behavioral changes (e.g., irritability, anger)
   - Motor problems (e.g., clumsiness, difficulty walking, slurred speech, weakness in arms or legs)
   - Sensory disturbances (e.g., numbness)
   - A heart rate <60 beats/min
2. Have someone stay with you.
3. Abstain from alcohol.
4. Check with your HCP before taking drugs that may increase drowsiness, including muscle relaxants, tranquilizers, and opioid pain medications.
5. Avoid driving, using heavy machinery, playing contact sports, and taking hot baths.

decreasing motor strength, to the HCP. Monitor the patient's condition closely.

The major focus of nursing care for the brain-injured patient relates to increased ICP (see eNursing Care Plan 56-1). However, some problems may require specific nursing intervention.

Eye problems may include loss of the corneal reflex, periorbital ecchymosis and edema, and diplopia. Loss of the corneal reflex may necessitate administering lubricating eye drops or taping the eyes shut to prevent abrasion. Periorbital ecchymosis and edema decrease with time, but cold and, later, warm compresses provide comfort and hasten the process. Diplopia can be relieved by use of an eye patch. Consider a consult with an ophthalmologist.

Hyperthermia may occur from injury to or inflammation of the hypothalamus. Elevations in body temperature can result in increased CBF, cerebral blood volume, and ICP. Increased metabolism secondary to hyperthermia increases metabolic waste, which in turn produces further cerebral vasodilation. Avoid hyperthermia with a goal of a temperature of 96.8° to 98.6° F (36° to 37° C) as the standard of care. Use interventions to reduce temperature as previously discussed (see p. 1322) in conjunction with sedation as necessary to prevent shivering.

If CSF rhinorrhea or otorrhea occurs, inform the HCP immediately. The head of the bed may be raised to decrease the CSF pressure so that a tear can seal. A loose collection pad may be placed under the nose or over the ear. Do not place a dressing in the nasal or ear cavities and document the amount of drainage each shift. Instruct the patient not to sneeze or blow the nose. Do not use nasogastric tubes. Do not perform nasotracheal suctioning on these patients because of the high risk of meningitis.

Nursing measures specific to the care of the immobilized patient, such as those related to bladder and bowel function, skin care, and infection, are also indicated. Nausea and vomiting may be a problem and can be alleviated by antiemetic drugs. Headache can usually be controlled with acetaminophen or small doses of codeine.

If the patient's condition deteriorates, intracranial surgery may be necessary (see the section on cranial surgery later in this chapter). A burr-hole opening or craniotomy may be indicated, depending on the underlying injury that is causing the problems. The emergency nature of the surgery may hasten the usual preoperative preparation. Consult with the neurosurgeon to determine specific preoperative nursing measures.

The patient is often unconscious before surgery, making it necessary for a family member to sign the consent form for surgery. This is a difficult and frightening time for the patient's caregiver and family and requires sensitive nursing management. The suddenness of the situation makes it especially difficult for the family to cope. Use the interprofessional team, including social workers, to assist the patient and family throughout the hospitalization and recovery time.

◆ **Ambulatory Care.** Once the condition has stabilized, the patient is usually transferred for acute rehabilitation management. There may be chronic problems related to motor and sensory deficits, communication, memory, and intellectual functioning. Many of the principles of nursing management of the patient with a stroke are appropriate for these patients (see Chapter 57).

Conditions that may require nursing and interprofessional management include poor nutritional status, bowel and bladder management, spasticity, dysphagia, deep vein thrombosis, and hydrocephalus. The patient's outward appearance is not a good indicator of how well he or she will ultimately function in the home or work environment. The outward physical appearance does not necessarily reflect what has happened in the brain.

Seizure disorders may occur in patients with nonpenetrating head injury. Seizures may develop during the first week after the head injury, but some patients may not develop a seizure disorder until years later. Antiseizure drugs may be used prophylactically to manage posttraumatic seizure activity, but this practice is controversial as previously discussed on p. 1326.

The mental and emotional sequelae of brain trauma are often the most incapacitating problems. One of the consequences of TBI is that the person may not realize that a brain injury has occurred. Many of the patients with head injuries who have been comatose for more than 6 hours undergo some personality change. They may suffer loss of concentration and memory and defective memory processing. Personal drive may decrease. Apathy may increase. Euphoria and mood swings, along with a seeming lack of awareness of the seriousness of the injury, may occur. The patient's behavior may indicate a loss of social restraint, judgment, tact, and emotional control.

Progressive recovery may continue for years. Specific nursing management in the posttraumatic phase depends on specific residual deficits. Being able to return to work and maintaining employment is one of the challenges during the recovery period.[21]

In all cases, the family must be given special consideration. They need to understand what is happening and be taught appropriate interaction patterns. Provide guidance and referrals for financial aid, child care, and other personal needs. Assist the family in involving the patient in family activities whenever possible. Help the patient and family remain hopeful. The family often has unrealistic expectations of the patient as the coma begins to recede. The family expects full return to pretrauma status. In reality, the patient usually experiences a reduced awareness and ability to interpret environmental stimuli. Prepare the family for the patient's emergence from coma and explain that the process of awakening often takes several weeks. In addition, arrange for social work and chaplain consultations for the family.

When it is the time for discharge planning, the patient, caregiver, and family may benefit from specific posthospitalization instructions to avoid family-patient friction. Special "no" policies that may be appropriately suggested by the neurosurgeon, neuropsychologist, and nurse include no drinking of alcoholic beverages, no driving, no use of firearms, no working with hazardous implements and machinery, and no unsupervised smoking. Family members, particularly spouses, go through role transition as the role changes from that of spouse to that of caregiver. (The stresses and needs of family caregivers are discussed in Chapter 4.)

### ◆ Evaluation

The expected outcomes are that the patient with a head injury will

- Maintain normal CPP
- Achieve maximal cognitive, motor, and sensory function
- Experience no infection or hyperthermia

## BRAIN TUMORS

Annually there are an estimated 23,400 newly diagnosed people with brain tumors in the United States. The brain is also a frequent site for metastasis from other sites.[22] Males have a slightly higher incidence of brain tumors than females. Brain tumors are more commonly seen in middle-aged persons, but they may occur at any age.

**CULTURAL & ETHNIC HEALTH DISPARITIES**

***Brain Tumors***

- Whites have a higher incidence of malignant brain tumors than African Americans.
- White males have the highest incidence of malignant brain tumors.
- African Americans have a higher incidence of benign brain tumors (e.g., meningiomas) than whites.

### Types

Brain tumors can occur in any part of the brain or spinal cord. Tumors of the brain may be *primary,* arising from tissues within the brain, or *secondary,* resulting from a metastasis from a malignant neoplasm elsewhere in the body.[23] Metastatic brain tumors are the most common brain tumor. The cancers that most commonly metastasize to the brain are lung and breast.

Primary brain tumors are generally classified according to the tissue from which they arise (Table 56-12). Meningiomas are the most common primary brain tumor. Other common brain tumors are gliomas (e.g., astrocytoma, glioblastoma [most common form of glioma]).

More than half of brain tumors are malignant. They infiltrate the brain tissue and are not amenable to complete surgical removal. Other tumors may be histologically benign but are located such that complete removal is not possible.

Brain tumors rarely metastasize outside the central nervous system (CNS) because they are contained by structural (meninges) and physiologic (blood-brain) barriers. Table 56-12 compares the most common brain tumors. A glioblastoma and meningioma are shown in Fig. 56-17.

### Clinical Manifestations and Complications

The clinical manifestations of brain tumors depend mainly on their location and size (Table 56-13). The rate of growth and appearance of manifestations depend on the location, size, and mitotic rate of the cells of the tissue of origin. Fig. 56-18 illustrates the functional areas of the cerebral cortex and can be used as a guide to correlate the clinical manifestations with the location of the tumor, as indicated by an alteration in the function controlled by the affected area.

Wide ranges of possible clinical manifestations are associated with brain tumors. Headache is a common problem. Tumor-related headaches tend to be worse at night and may awaken the patient. The headaches are usually dull and constant but occasionally throbbing. Seizures are common in gliomas and brain metastases. Brain tumors can cause nausea and vomiting from increased ICP. Cognitive dysfunction, including memory problems and mood or personality changes, is another common manifestation, especially in patients with brain metastases. Muscle weakness, sensory losses, aphasia, and visual-spatial dysfunction are also manifestations of brain tumors.

If the tumor mass obstructs the ventricles or occludes the outlet, ventricular enlargement (hydrocephalus) can occur. As the brain tumor expands, it may also produce manifestations of increased ICP, cerebral edema, or obstruction of the CSF pathways. Unless treated, all brain tumors eventually cause death from increasing tumor volume leading to increased ICP.

**TABLE 56-12 Types of Brain Tumors**

| Type | Tissue of Origin | Characteristics |
|---|---|---|
| **Gliomas** | | |
| • Astrocytoma | Supportive tissue, glial cells, and astrocytes | Can range from low-grade to moderate-grade malignancy. |
| • Glioblastoma | Primitive stem cell (glioblast) | Highly malignant and invasive. Among the most devastating of primary brain tumors. |
| • Oligodendroglioma | Oligodendrocytes | Benign (encapsulation and calcification). |
| • Ependymoma | Ependymal epithelium | Range from benign to highly malignant. Most are benign and encapsulated. |
| • Medulloblastoma | Primitive neuroectodermal cell | Highly malignant and invasive. Metastatic to spinal cord and remote areas of brain. |
| **Meningioma** | Meninges | Can be benign or malignant. Most are benign. |
| **Acoustic neuroma (Schwannoma)** | Cells that form myelin sheath around nerves. Commonly affects cranial nerve VIII | Many grow on both sides of the brain. Usually benign or low-grade malignancy. |
| **Pituitary adenoma** | Pituitary gland | Usually benign. |
| **Hemangioblastoma** | Blood vessels of brain | Rare and benign. Surgery is curative. |
| **Primary central nervous system lymphoma** | Lymphocytes | Increased incidence in transplant recipients and acquired immunodeficiency syndrome (AIDS) patients. |
| **Metastatic tumors** | Lungs and breast (most common) | Malignant. |

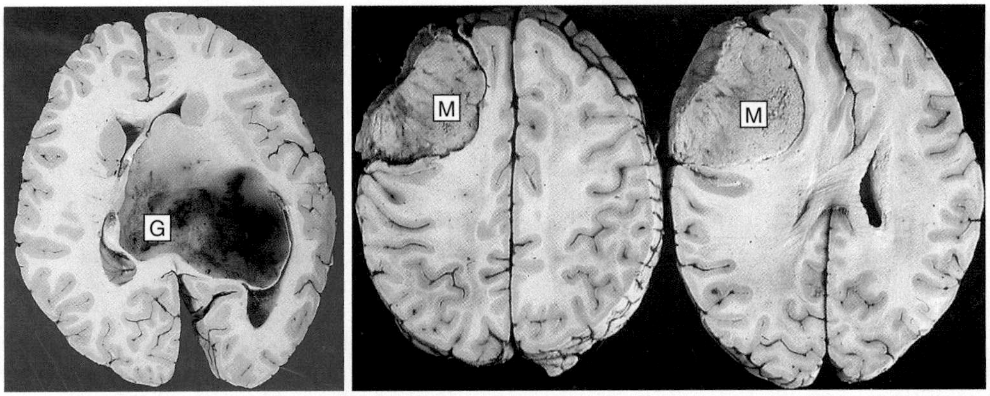


**FIG. 56-17** **A,** A large glioblastoma *(G)* arises from one cerebral hemisphere and has grown to fill the ventricular system. **B,** Meningioma. These two different sections from different levels in the same brain show a meningioma *(M)* compressing the frontal lobe and distorting underlying brain. (From Stevens A, Lowe J: *Pathology: illustrated review in colour,* ed 2, London, 2000, Mosby.)

**TABLE 56-13 Manifestations of Brain Tumors**

| Tumor Location | Manifestations |
|---|---|
| **Cerebral hemisphere** | |
| • Frontal lobe (unilateral) | Unilateral hemiplegia, seizures, memory deficit, personality and judgment changes, visual disturbances. |
| • Frontal lobe (bilateral) | Symptoms associated with unilateral frontal lobe tumors. Ataxic gait. |
| • Parietal lobe | Speech disturbance (if tumor is in the dominant hemisphere), inability to write, spatial disorders, unilateral neglect. |
| • Occipital lobe | Vision disturbances and seizures. |
| • Temporal lobe | Few symptoms. Seizures, dysphagia, hallucinations, auras. |
| **Subcortical** | Hemiplegia. Other symptoms may depend on area of infiltration. |
| **Meningeal tumors** | Symptoms associated with compression of the brain and depend on tumor location. |
| **Metastatic tumors** | Headache, nausea, or vomiting (occur from ↑ ICP). Other symptoms depend on tumor location. |
| **Thalamus and sellar tumors** | Headache, nausea, vision disturbances, papilledema, and nystagmus (occur from ↑ ICP). Diabetes insipidus may occur. |
| **Fourth ventricle and cerebellar tumors** | Headache, nausea, and papilledema (occur from ↑ ICP). Ataxic gait and changes in coordination. |
| **Cerebellopontine tumors** | Tinnitus and vertigo, deafness. |
| **Brainstem tumors** | Headache on awakening, drowsiness, vomiting, ataxic gait, facial muscle weakness, hearing loss, dysphagia, dysarthria, "crossed eyes" or other visual changes, hemiparesis. |

*ICP,* Intracranial pressure.

## Diagnostic Studies

An extensive history and a comprehensive neurologic examination must be done in the workup of a patient with a suspected brain tumor. A careful history and physical examination may provide data with respect to location. New onset of seizures or adult-onset migraines may be indicative of a brain tumor and should be investigated. Diagnostic studies are similar to those used for a patient with increased ICP (Table 56-3).

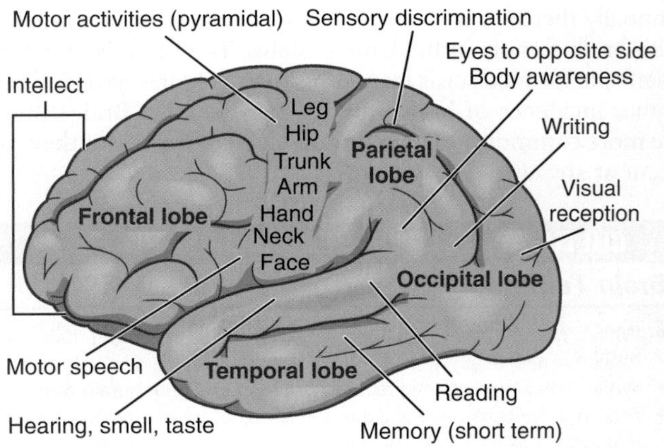


**FIG. 56-18** Each area of the brain controls a particular activity.

The sensitivity of techniques such as MRI and PET scans allows for detection of small tumors and may provide more reliable diagnostic information than a CT scan. CT with contrast and MRI are used to identify the lesion's location. Other tests include magnetic resonance spectroscopy, functional MRI, and single-photon emission computed tomography (SPECT). The EEG is useful for ruling out seizures but is of less importance. A lumbar puncture is seldom diagnostic and carries with it the risk of cerebral herniation. Cerebral angiography can be used to determine blood flow to the tumor and further localize the tumor. Other studies are done to rule out a primary lesion elsewhere in the body. Endocrine studies are helpful when a pituitary adenoma is suspected (see Chapter 49).

The correct diagnosis of a brain tumor can be made by obtaining tissue for histologic study. In most patients, tissue is obtained at the time of surgery. Computer-guided stereotactic biopsy is also an option. A smear or frozen section can be performed in the operating room for a preliminary interpretation of the histologic type. With this information, the neurosurgeon can make a better decision about the extent of surgery.

## Interprofessional Care

Treatment goals are aimed at (1) identifying the tumor type and location, (2) removing or decreasing tumor mass, and (3) preventing or managing increased ICP.

**Surgical Therapy.** Surgical removal is the preferred treatment for brain tumors (see the section on cranial surgery later in this chapter). Stereotactic surgical techniques are used with greater frequency to perform a biopsy and remove small brain tumors. The outcome of surgical therapy depends on the tumor's type, size, and location. Meningiomas and oligodendrogliomas can usually be completely removed, whereas the more invasive gliomas and medulloblastomas may only be partially removed. Computer-guided stereotactic biopsy, ultrasound, functional MRI, and cortical mapping can be used to localize brain tumors intraoperatively.

Complete surgical removal of brain tumors is not always possible because the tumor is not always accessible or may involve vital parts of the brain. Surgery can reduce tumor mass, which decreases ICP, provides relief of symptoms, and extends survival time.

**Ventricular Shunts.** Hydrocephalus due to a tumor obstructing the CSF flow can be treated with the placement of a ventricular shunt. A catheter with one-way valves is placed in the lateral ventricle and then tunneled under the skin to drain CSF into the peritoneal cavity. Rapid decompression of ICP can cause total body collapse and weakness, including a headache that may be prevented by gradually introducing the patient to the upright position.

Manifestations of shunt malfunction, which are related to increased ICP, include decreasing LOC, restlessness, headache, blurred vision, or vomiting. This may necessitate shunt revision or replacement. Infection may also occur, as exhibited by high fever, persistent headache, and stiff neck. Antibiotics are used to treat the infection. In some situations, the shunt must be replaced and CSF drainage managed with an extraventricular drainage system while the infection is treated.

**Radiation Therapy and Stereotactic Radiosurgery.** Radiation therapy may be used as a follow-up measure after surgery. Radiation seeds can also be implanted into the brain. Cerebral edema and rapidly increasing ICP may be a complication of radiation therapy, but these problems can be managed with high doses of corticosteroids (dexamethasone, prednisone, or methylprednisolone [Solu-Medrol]). (Radiation therapy is discussed in Chapter 15.)

Stereotactic radiosurgery is a method of delivering a highly concentrated dose of radiation to a precise location within the brain. Stereotactic radiosurgery may be used when conventional surgery has failed or is not an option because of the tumor location. (Radiosurgery is discussed on p. 1337.)

**Chemotherapy and Targeted Therapy.** The effectiveness of chemotherapy has been limited by the difficulty with getting drugs across the blood-brain barrier, tumor cell heterogeneity, and tumor cell drug resistance. Chemotherapy drugs called *nitrosoureas* (e.g., carmustine, lomustine) are used to treat brain tumors. Normally the blood-brain barrier prohibits the entry of most drugs into the brain. The most malignant tumors cause a breakdown of the blood-brain barrier in the area of the tumor, thus allowing chemotherapy agents to be used to treat the malignancy. Chemotherapy-laden biodegradable wafers (e.g., Gliadel wafer [polifeprosan with carmustine implant]) implanted at the time of surgery can deliver chemotherapy directly to the tumor site. Other drugs being used include methotrexate and procarbazine (Matulane). One method used to deliver chemotherapy drugs directly to the CNS is intrathecal administration via an Ommaya reservoir.

Temozolomide (Temodar) is an oral chemotherapy agent that can cross the blood-brain barrier. In contrast with many traditional chemotherapy drugs, which require metabolic activation to exert their effects, temozolomide can convert spontaneously to a reactive agent that directly interferes with tumor growth. It does not interact with other drugs commonly taken by patients with brain tumors, such as antiseizure medications, corticosteroids, and antiemetics.

**DRUG ALERT Temozolomide (Temodar)**

- Causes myelosuppression. Before using, it is recommended that absolute neutrophil count be ≥1500/μL and platelet count be ≥100,000/μL.
- To reduce nausea and vomiting, take on empty stomach.

Bevacizumab (Avastin) is used to treat patients with glioblastoma that continues to progress after standard therapy. Bevacizumab is a targeted therapy that inhibits the action of vascular endothelial growth factor, which helps form new blood vessels. These vessels can feed a tumor, helping it to grow, and can also provide a pathway for cancer cells to circulate in the body. (Targeted therapy is discussed in Chapter 15 and Table 15-13.)

**Other Therapies.** A medical device system, OpTune System, is used to treat glioblastoma that recurs or progresses after receiving chemotherapy and radiation therapy. With this system, electrodes are placed on the surface of the patient's scalp to deliver low-intensity, changing electrical fields called *tumor treatment fields* (TTFs) to the tumor site.

## NURSING MANAGEMENT: BRAIN TUMORS

### Nursing Assessment

Structure the initial assessment to provide baseline data of the patient's neurologic status. Use this information to design a realistic, individualized care plan. Assess the patient's LOC, motor abilities, sensory perception, integrated function (including bowel and bladder function), and balance and proprioception. In addition, assess the coping abilities of the patient, caregiver, and family. Watching a patient perform activities of daily living and listening to the patient's conversation can be part of the neurologic assessment. Having the patient or caregiver explain the problem can be helpful to determine the patient's limitations and obtain information about the patient's insight into the problems. Record all initial data to provide a baseline for comparison to determine whether the patient's condition is improving or deteriorating.

Interview data are as important as the actual physical assessment. Ask questions about the medical history, intellectual abilities and educational level, and history of nervous system infections and trauma. Determine the presence of seizures, syncope, nausea and vomiting, and headaches or other pain to help better plan care for the patient.

### Nursing Diagnoses

Nursing diagnoses and collaborative problems for the patient with a brain tumor may include, but are not limited to, the following:

- Risk for ineffective cerebral tissue perfusion *related to* cerebral edema
- Acute pain (headache) *related to* cerebral edema and increased ICP
- Anxiety *related to* diagnosis and treatment
- Potential complications: seizures *related to* abnormal electrical activity of the brain and increased ICP *related to* tumor and failure of normal compensatory mechanisms

### Planning

The overall goals are that the patient with a brain tumor will (1) maintain normal ICP, (2) maximize neurologic functioning, (3) achieve control of pain and discomfort, and (4) be aware of the long-term implications with respect to prognosis and cognitive and physical functioning.

### Nursing Implementation

A primary or metastatic tumor of the frontal lobe can cause behavioral and personality changes. Loss of emotional control, confusion, disorientation, memory loss, impulsivity, and depression may be signs of a frontal lobe lesion. These behavioral changes are often not perceived by the patient but can be disturbing and even frightening to the caregiver and family. These changes can also cause a distancing to occur between the family and patient. Assist the caregiver and family in understanding what is happening to the patient, and support the family.

The confused patient with behavioral instability can be a challenge. Protecting the patient from self-harm is an important part of nursing care. Essential techniques in the care of these patients include close supervision of activity, use of side rails, judicious use of restraints, appropriate sedative medications, padding of the rails and the area around the bed, and a calm, reassuring approach.

Perceptual problems associated with frontal and parietal lobe tumors contribute to a patient's disorientation and confusion. Minimize environmental stimuli, create a routine, and use reality orientation for the confused patient. Tumors in the temporal lobe can cause hallucinations, which may be confused with dementia or delirium in the hospitalized patient.

Seizures, which often occur with brain tumors, are managed with antiseizure drugs. Also use seizure precautions for the patient's protection. Some behavioral changes seen in the patient with a brain tumor are a result of seizure disorders and can improve with adequate seizure control. Patients at risk for seizures may be unable to drive, so be aware of the extra resources needed and collaborate with the social worker and family. (Seizure disorders are discussed in Chapter 58.)

Motor and sensory dysfunctions interfere with activities of daily living. Alterations in mobility must be managed. Encourage the patient to provide as much self-care as physically possible. Self-image often depends on the patient's ability to participate in care within the limitations of the physical deficits.

Language deficits can also occur in patients with brain tumors. Motor (expressive) or sensory (receptive) dysphasia may occur. The disturbance in communication can be frustrating for the patient and may interfere with your ability to meet the patient's needs. Make attempts to establish a communication system that can be used by both the patient and staff.

Nutritional intake may be decreased because of the patient's inability to eat, loss of appetite, or loss of desire to eat. Assess the patient's nutritional status, and ensure adequate nutritional intake. Encourage the patient to eat. Some patients may need enteral or parenteral nutrition (see Chapter 39). The patient with a brain tumor who undergoes cranial surgery requires complex nursing care (discussed in the next section).

Provide help and support during the adjustment phase and in long-range planning. Social work and home health nurses may be needed to assist the caregiver with discharge planning and to help the family adjust to role changes and psychosocial and socioeconomic factors. Issues related to palliative and end-of-life care must be discussed with both the patient and family (see Chapter 9).

### Evaluation

The expected outcomes are that the patient with a brain tumor will

- Achieve control of pain, vomiting, and other discomforts
- Maintain ICP within normal limits
- Demonstrate maximal neurologic function (cognitive, motor, sensory) given the location and extent of the tumor
- Maintain optimal nutritional status
- Accept the long-term consequences of the tumor and its treatment

## CRANIAL SURGERY

Indications for cranial surgery are related to brain tumors, CNS infection (e.g., abscess), vascular abnormalities, craniocerebral trauma, seizure disorder, or intractable pain (Table 56-14).

### Types

Various types of cranial surgical procedures are presented in Table 56-15.

**Craniotomy.** Depending on the location of the pathologic condition, a *craniotomy* may be frontal, parietal, occipital, temporal, suboccipital, or a combination of any of these. The surgeon drills a set of burr holes and uses a saw to connect the holes to remove the bone flap. Sometimes operating microscopes are used to magnify the site. After surgery, the bone flap is secured with small plates or wired shut. Sometimes drains are placed to remove fluid and blood. Patients are usually cared for in an ICU until stable.

**TABLE 56-14 Indications for Cranial Surgery**

| Indication | Cause | Surgical Procedure |
|---|---|---|
| **Brain abscess** | Bacteria that caused intracranial infection | Excision or drainage of abscess |
| **Hydrocephalus** | Overproduction of CSF, obstruction to flow, defective reabsorption | Placement of ventriculoperitoneal or (rarely) ventriculoatrial shunt |
| **Brain tumors** | Benign or malignant cell growth | Excision or partial resection of tumor |
| **Intracranial bleeding** | Rupture of cerebral vessels because of trauma or stroke | Surgical evacuation through burr holes or craniotomy |
| **Skull fractures** | Trauma to skull | Debridement of fragments and necrotic tissue, elevation and realignment of bone fragments |
| **Arteriovenous (AV) malformation** | Congenital tangle of arteries and veins (frequently in middle cerebral artery) | Excision of malformation |
| **Aneurysm repair** | Dilation of weak area in arterial wall (usually near anterior portion of circle of Willis) | Dissection and clipping or coiling of aneurysm |

*CSF,* Cerebrospinal fluid.

**TABLE 56-15 Types of Cranial Surgery**

| Type | Description |
|---|---|
| **Burr hole** | Opening into the cranium with a drill. Used to remove localized fluid and blood beneath the dura. |
| **Craniotomy** | Opening into cranium with removal of bone flap and opening the dura to remove a lesion, repair a damaged area, drain blood, or relieve ↑ ICP. |
| **Craniectomy** | Excision into the cranium to cut away bone flap. |
| **Cranioplasty** | Repair of cranial defect resulting from trauma, malformation, or previous surgical procedure. Artificial material used to replace damaged or lost bone. |
| **Stereotactic procedure** | Precise localization of a specific area of the brain using a frame or frameless system based on three-dimensional coordinates. Procedure is used for biopsy, radiosurgery, or dissection. |
| **Shunt procedures** | Alternate pathway to redirect cerebrospinal fluid from one area to another using a tube or implanted device. Examples include ventricular shunt and Ommaya reservoir. |

*ICP,* Intracranial pressure.

**Stereotactic Radiosurgery.** Stereotactic procedures use precision apparatus (often computer guided) to help the physician precisely target an area of the brain. Stereotactic biopsy can be performed to obtain tissue samples for histologic examination. CT scanning and MRI are used to image the targeted tissue. With the patient under general or local anesthesia, the surgeon drills a burr hole or creates a bone flap for an entry site and then introduces a probe and biopsy needle. Stereotactic procedures are used for removal of small brain tumors and abscesses, drainage of hematomas, ablative procedures for extrapyramidal diseases (e.g., Parkinson's disease), and repair of arteriovenous malformations. A major advantage of the stereotactic approach is a reduction in damage to surrounding tissue.

*Stereotactic radiosurgery* is not a form of surgery in the traditional sense. Instead, radiosurgery uses precisely focused radiation to destroy tumor cells and other abnormal growths in the brain. Computers create three-dimensional images of the brain, and these images are used to guide the focused radiation while the patient's head is held still in a stereotactic frame (Fig. 56-19). Radiosurgical techniques can use ionizing radiation generated by a linear accelerator, gamma knife, or CyberKnife. In these procedures, a high dose of cobalt radiation is delivered to precisely targeted tumor tissue. The dose of radiation is delivered in a single treatment lasting a few hours or in multiple sessions. Side effects of stereotactic radiosurgery may include fatigue, headache, and nausea.

In combination with stereotactic procedures to identify and localize tumor sites, surgical lasers can be used to destroy tumors. Three surgical lasers currently used are the carbon dioxide, argon, and neodymium:yttrium-aluminum-garnet (Nd:YAG) lasers. All three work by creating thermal energy, which destroys the tissue on which it is focused. Laser therapy also provides the benefit of reducing damage to surrounding tissue.

## NURSING MANAGEMENT: CRANIAL SURGERY

### Nursing Implementation

**Acute Care.** The general preoperative and postoperative nursing care for the patient undergoing cranial surgery is similar regardless of the cause. Nursing management is similar to that for the patient with increased ICP (presented in eNursing Care Plan 56-1). The patient (if conscious and coherent), caregiver, and family will be concerned about the potential physical and emotional problems that can result from surgery. The uncertainty regarding prognosis and outcome requires compassionate nursing care in the preoperative period.

Preoperative teaching is important in allaying the fears of the patient, caregiver, and family, and also in preparing them for the postoperative period. Provide general information concerning the type of operation that will be performed and what can be expected immediately after the operation. Explain that some hair may be shaved to allow for better exposure and to prevent contamination. The hair is usually removed in the operating room after induction of anesthesia. Also inform the family that the patient will be taken to an ICU or to a special care unit after surgery.

The primary goal of care after cranial surgery is prevention of increased ICP. (Nursing management of the patient with increased ICP is presented on pp. 1323-1326.) Frequent assessment of the patient's neurologic status is essential during the first 48 hours. In addition to the neurologic functions, closely monitor fluid and electrolyte levels and serum osmolality to detect changes in sodium regulation, the onset of diabetes insipidus, or severe hypovolemia. Turning and positioning the patient may depend on the site of the operation.

Monitor the patient for pain and nausea. Although the brain itself does not possess pain receptors, patients often report headache caused by edema or pain at the incision site. Control pain with short-acting opioids and monitor neurologic status. Nausea and vomiting are common after surgery and are usually treated with antiemetics. The use of promethazine is discouraged because it can increase somnolence, thus altering the accuracy of a neurologic assessment.

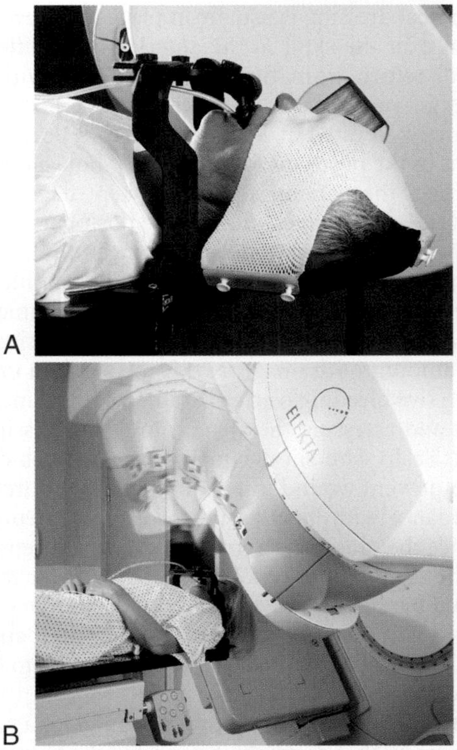


**FIG. 56-19** **A,** Patient in a stereotactic frame. **B,** Elekta's Fraxion head frame helps ensure accuracy and precision in stereotactic radiation therapy (SRT) of cancer targets in the brain and cranium. (Courtesy Elekta.)

The surgical dressing is usually in place for a few days. With an incision over the skull in the anterior or middle fossa, the patient will return from the operating room with the head elevated at an angle of 30 to 45 degrees. The head of the bed should remain elevated at least 30 degrees unless the surgical approach is in the posterior fossa or a burr hole has been made. In these cases, the patient is generally kept flat or at a slight elevation (10 to 15 degrees) during the postoperative phase.

If a bone flap has been removed (craniectomy), do not position the patient on the operative side. A sign should be placed at the head of the bed, alerting everyone of the craniectomy site and position of the surgical site. Observe the dressing for color, odor, and amount of drainage. Notify the surgeon immediately of any excessive bleeding or clear drainage. Checking drains for placement and assessing the area around the dressing are also important. Scalp care should include meticulous care of the incision to prevent wound infection. Cleanse the area and treat it in accordance with hospital protocol or the neurosurgeon's orders. Once the dressing is removed, use an antiseptic soap for washing the scalp. The psychologic impact of hair removal can be alleviated by the use of a wig, turban, scarves, or cap. For the patient who is receiving radiation, instruct the patient to use a sunblock and head covering if any exposure to the sun is anticipated.

◆ **Ambulatory Care.** The rehabilitative potential for a patient after cranial surgery depends on the reason for the surgery, postoperative course, and patient's general state of health. Base your nursing interventions on a realistic appraisal of these factors. An overall goal is to foster independence for as long as possible and to the highest degree possible.

Specific rehabilitation potential cannot be determined until cerebral edema and increased ICP subside postoperatively. Take care to maintain as much function as possible through measures such as careful positioning, meticulous skin and mouth care, regular range-of-motion exercises, bowel and bladder care, and adequate nutrition.

Referrals may be made to other specialists on the interprofessional team. For example, the speech therapist may be helpful to the patient who has a speech problem, or the physical therapist may provide an exercise plan to regain functional deficits. Address the needs and problems of each patient individually because many variables affect the plan. The patient's mental and physical deterioration, including seizures, personality disorganization, apathy, and wasting, is difficult for both family and health care professionals to watch. Cognitive and emotional residual deficits are often harder to accept than are motor and sensory losses.

## INFLAMMATORY CONDITIONS OF THE BRAIN

Brain abscesses, meningitis, and encephalitis are the most common inflammatory conditions of the brain and spinal cord (Table 56-16). Inflammation can be caused by bacteria, viruses, fungi, and chemicals (e.g., contrast media used in diagnostic tests, blood in the subarachnoid space). CNS infections may occur via the bloodstream, by extension from a primary site, or along cranial and spinal nerves.

The mortality rate for inflammatory conditions of the brain is approximately 10% to 30% in the general population, with higher rates in older patients. Up to 19% of those who recover can have long-term neurologic deficits, including hearing loss.[24]

### ETHICAL/LEGAL DILEMMAS

#### *Withholding Treatment*

**Situation**

C.J., a 26-yr-old patient in a permanent vegetative state, is diagnosed with her fifteenth bladder infection. As her home care nurse, you must determine whether to seek antibiotics for this infection. The family members have expressed a concern that no heroic measures be used to extend the biologic life of their daughter and sister. However, they have been unwilling to withdraw the existing treatment, which is enteral nutrition through a gastrostomy tube. Should antibiotics be withheld?

**Ethical/Legal Points for Consideration**

- Patients in a persistent vegetative state do not recover.
- The primary legal issue here is who has the legal right to refuse or consent to treatment for this incapacitated patient. You need to know if a guardian has been appointed by the court or if her parents retain a form of guardianship to make health care decisions for her.
- You also need to know when the vegetative state began; that is, did the patient ever have the right to consent having reached the age of majority as a competent adult, or did the vegetative state begin while she was a minor? If the patient did become a competent adult before the vegetative state, did she ever express any preference for quality-of-life and end-of-life decision making?
- The courts have widespread legal precedents for accepting the decision of the patient's guardian or parents or the patient's clearly expressed preferences for quality-of-life decision making.
- Life-sustaining treatment is any treatment that serves to prolong life without reversing the underlying medical condition. Life-sustaining treatment may include, but is not limited to, mechanical ventilation, renal dialysis, chemotherapy, antibiotics, and artificial nutrition and hydration.
- There is no ethical distinction between withdrawing and withholding life-sustaining treatment. If there is not adequate evidence of the incompetent patient's preferences and values, the decision should be based on the best interests of the patient (i.e., what outcome would most likely promote the patient's well-being).

**Discussion Questions**

1. How would you approach C.J.'s family?
2. What are your feelings about providing nutrition, hydration, and treatments that will prolong life in a patient for whom there is no hope of recovery?
3. What options are available to the family for the care of their daughter once a decision is made about withholding antibiotics?

## BRAIN ABSCESS

**Brain abscess** is an accumulation of pus within the brain tissue that can result from a local or systemic infection. Direct extension from an ear, tooth, mastoid, or sinus infection is the primary cause. Other causes for brain abscess formation include spread from a distant site (e.g., pulmonary infection, bacterial endocarditis), skull fracture, and prior brain trauma or surgery. Streptococci and *Staphylococcus aureus* are the primary infective organisms.

Manifestations of brain abscess, which are similar to those of meningitis and encephalitis, include headache, fever, and nausea and vomiting. Signs of increased ICP may include drowsiness, confusion, and seizures. Focal symptoms may reflect the local area of the abscess. For example, visual field defects or psychomotor seizures are common with a temporal lobe abscess, whereas an occipital abscess may be accompanied by visual impairment and hallucinations. CT and MRI are used to diagnose a brain abscess.

**TABLE 56-16 Comparison of Cerebral Inflammatory Conditions**

| | Meningitis | Encephalitis | Brain Abscess |
|---|---|---|---|
| **Cause** | Bacteria (*Streptococcus pneumoniae, Neisseria meningitidis*, group B streptococci, viruses, fungi) | Bacteria, fungi, parasites, herpes simplex virus (HSV), other viruses (e.g., West Nile virus) | Streptococci, staphylococci through bloodstream |
| **CSF (Reference Interval)** | | | |
| • Pressure (70-150 mm $H_2O$) | Increased<br>*Bacterial:* 200-500<br>*Viral:* ≤250 | Normal to slight increase | Increased |
| • WBC count (0-5 cells/μL) | *Bacterial:* >1000/μL (mainly neutrophils)<br>*Viral:* 25-500/μL (mainly lymphocytes) | 500/μL, neutrophils (early), lymphocytes (later) | 25-300/μL (neutrophils) |
| • Protein (15-45 mg/dL [0.15-0.45 g/L]) | *Bacterial:* >500 mg/dL<br>*Viral:* 50-500 mg/dL | Slight increase | Normal |
| • Glucose (40-70 mg/dL [2.2-3.9 mmol/L]) | *Bacterial:* Decreased 5-40<br>*Viral:* Normal or low >40 | Normal | Low or absent |
| • Appearance | *Bacterial:* Turbid, cloudy<br>*Viral:* Clear or cloudy | Clear | Clear |
| **Diagnostic Studies** | CT scan, Gram stain, smear, culture, PCR* | CT scan, EEG, MRI, PET, PCR, IgM antibodies to virus in serum or CSF | CT scan |
| **Treatment** | Antibiotics, dexamethasone, supportive care, prevention of ↑ ICP | Supportive care, prevention of ↑ ICP, acyclovir (Zovirax) for HSV | Antibiotics, incision and drainage<br>Supportive care |

*CSF*, Cerebrospinal fluid; *ICP*, intracranial pressure; *PCR*, polymerase chain reaction.
*PCR is used to detect viral RNA or DNA.

Antimicrobial therapy is the primary treatment for brain abscess. Other manifestations are treated symptomatically. If drug therapy is not effective, the abscess may have to be drained or removed if it is encapsulated.

Nursing measures are similar to those for management of meningitis or increased ICP. If surgical drainage or removal is the treatment of choice, nursing care is similar to that described under cranial surgery.

## BACTERIAL MENINGITIS

**Meningitis** is an acute inflammation of the meningeal tissues surrounding the brain and spinal cord. Meningitis usually occurs in fall, winter, or early spring and is often secondary to viral respiratory disease. Older adults and persons who are debilitated are affected more frequently than the general population. College students living in dormitories and individuals living in institutions (e.g., prisoners) have a high risk for contracting meningitis. Untreated bacterial meningitis has a mortality rate near 100%.[25]

### Etiology and Pathophysiology

*Streptococcus pneumoniae* and *Neisseria meningitidis* are the leading causes of bacterial meningitis. *Neisseria meningitides* has at least 13 different subtypes (serogroups) with five of them (A, B, C, Y, W) causing most cases. *Haemophilus influenzae* was once the most common cause of bacterial meningitis. However, the use of *H. influenzae* vaccine has resulted in a significant decrease in meningitis related to this organism.

The organisms usually gain entry to the CNS through the upper respiratory tract or bloodstream. However, they may enter by direct extension from penetrating wounds of the skull or through fractured sinuses in basilar skull fractures.

The inflammatory response to the infection tends to increase CSF production with a moderate increase in ICP. In bacterial meningitis the purulent secretions produced quickly spread to other areas of the brain through the CSF and cover the cranial nerves and other intracranial structures. If this process extends into the brain parenchyma or if concurrent encephalitis is present, cerebral edema and increased ICP become more of a problem. Closely observe all patients with meningitis for manifestations of increased ICP, which is thought to be a result of swelling around the dura and increased CSF volume.

### Clinical Manifestations

Fever, severe headache, nausea, vomiting, and **nuchal rigidity** (neck stiffness) are key signs of meningitis. Photophobia, a decreased LOC, and signs of increased ICP may also be present. Coma is associated with a poor prognosis and occurs in 5% to 10% of patients with bacterial meningitis. Seizures occur in one third of all cases. The headache becomes progressively worse and may be accompanied by vomiting and irritability.

If the infecting organism is a meningococcus, a skin rash is common, and petechiae may be seen on the trunk, lower extremities, and mucous membranes. A *Tumbler test* can be done by pressing the base of a drinking glass against the rash. The rash does not blanch or fade under pressure.

### Complications

The most common acute complication of bacterial meningitis is increased ICP. Most patients have increased ICP, and it is the major cause of an altered mental status. Another complication of bacterial meningitis is residual neurologic dysfunction.

Dysfunction often occurs involving many cranial nerves. Cranial nerve irritation can have serious sequelae. The optic nerve (CN II) is compressed by increased ICP. Papilledema is often present, and blindness may occur. When the oculomotor (CN III), trochlear (CN IV), and abducens (CN VI) nerves are irritated, ocular movements are affected. Ptosis, unequal pupils, and diplopia are common. Irritation of the trigeminal nerve (CN V) results in sensory losses and loss of the corneal reflex. Irritation of the facial nerve (CN VII) results in facial paresis. Irritation of the vestibulocochlear nerve (CN VIII) causes tinnitus, vertigo, and deafness. The dysfunction usually disappears within a few weeks. However, hearing loss may be permanent after bacterial meningitis.

Hemiparesis, dysphasia, and hemianopsia may also occur. These signs usually resolve over time. If they do not, a cerebral abscess, subdural empyema, subdural effusion, or persistent meningitis is suspected. Acute cerebral edema may cause seizures, CN III palsy, bradycardia, hypertensive coma, and death.

Headaches may occur for months after the diagnosis of meningitis until the irritation and inflammation have completely resolved. It is important to implement pain management for chronic headaches.

A noncommunicating hydrocephalus may occur if the exudate causes adhesions that prevent the normal flow of CSF from the ventricles. CSF reabsorption by the arachnoid villi may also be obstructed by the exudate. In this situation, surgical implantation of a shunt is the only treatment.

*Waterhouse-Friderichsen syndrome* is a complication of meningococcal meningitis. The syndrome is manifested by petechiae, disseminated intravascular coagulation (DIC), adrenal hemorrhage, and circulatory collapse. DIC and shock, which are some of the most serious complications of meningitis, are associated with meningococcemia. (DIC is discussed in detail in Chapter 30.)

### TABLE 56-17 Interprofessional Care

**Bacterial Meningitis**

| Diagnostic Assessment | Management |
|---|---|
| • History and physical examination<br>• Analysis of CSF (for protein, WBC, and glucose), Gram stain, and culture<br>• CBC, coagulation profile, electrolyte levels, glucose, platelet count<br>• Blood culture<br>• CT scan, MRI, PET scan<br>• Skull x-ray studies | • Rest<br>• IV fluids<br>• Hypothermia<br><br>***Drug Therapy***<br>• IV antibiotics<br>  • ampicillin, penicillin<br>  • cephalosporin (e.g., cefotaxime [Claforan], ceftriaxone [Rocephin])<br>• codeine for headache<br>• dexamethasone<br>• acetaminophen or aspirin for temperature >100.4° F (38° C)<br>• phenytoin IV<br>• mannitol (Osmitrol) IV for diuresis |

*CSF*, Cerebrospinal fluid; *PET*, positron emission tomography.

## Diagnostic Studies

When a patient has manifestations suggestive of bacterial meningitis, a blood culture and CT scan should be done. Diagnosis is usually verified by doing a lumbar puncture with analysis of the CSF. A lumbar puncture should be completed only after the CT scan has ruled out an obstruction in the foramen magnum in order to prevent a fluid shift resulting in herniation.

Specimens of the CSF, sputum, and nasopharyngeal secretions are taken for culture before the start of antibiotic therapy to identify the causative organism. A Gram stain is done to detect bacteria. The predominant white blood cell type in the CSF during bacterial meningitis is neutrophils (Table 56-16).

X-rays of the skull may demonstrate infected sinuses. CT scans and MRI may be normal in uncomplicated meningitis. In other cases, CT scans may reveal evidence of increased ICP or hydrocephalus.

## Interprofessional Care

Bacterial meningitis is a medical emergency. Rapid diagnosis based on history and physical examination is crucial because the patient is usually in a critical state when health care is sought. When meningitis is suspected, antibiotic therapy is begun after the collection of specimens for cultures, even before the diagnosis is confirmed (Table 56-17).

Ampicillin, penicillin, vancomycin, cefuroxime (Ceftin), cefotaxime (Claforan), ceftriaxone (Rocephin), ceftizoxime, and ceftazidime are some commonly prescribed drugs for treating bacterial meningitis. Dexamethasone (a corticosteroid) may also be prescribed before or with the first dose of antibiotics. Collaborate with the HCP to manage the headache, fever, and nuchal rigidity often associated with meningitis.

# NURSING MANAGEMENT: BACTERIAL MENINGITIS

## Nursing Assessment

Initial assessment should include vital signs, neurologic assessment, fluid intake and output, and evaluation of the lungs and skin.

## Nursing Diagnoses

Nursing diagnoses for the patient with bacterial meningitis may include, but are not limited to, the following:

- Decreased intracranial adaptive capacity *related to* decreased cerebral perfusion or increased ICP
- Risk for ineffective cerebral tissue perfusion *related to* reduction of blood flow and cerebral edema
- Hyperthermia *related to* infection
- Acute pain *related to* headache and muscle aches

Additional information on nursing diagnoses for the patient with bacterial meningitis is presented in eNursing Care Plan 56-2 (available on the website for this chapter).

## Planning

The overall goals for the patient with bacterial meningitis are to (1) return to maximal neurologic functioning, (2) resolve the infection, and (3) control pain and discomfort.

## Nursing Implementation

**Health Promotion.** Prevention of respiratory tract infections through vaccination programs for pneumococcal pneumonia and influenza is important. Meningococcal vaccines are available that protect against all serogroups of meningococcal disease that are most commonly seen in the United States, but they will not prevent all cases. Three kinds of meningococcal vaccines available in the United States include:

- Meningococcal conjugate vaccines (MCV4) (Menactra, MenHibrix, Menveo)
- Meningococcal polysaccharide vaccine (MPSV4) (Menomune)
- Serogroup B meningococcal vaccines (Bexsero and Trumenba)

Early and vigorous treatment of respiratory tract and ear infections is important. Persons who have close contact with anyone who has bacterial meningitis should be given prophylactic antibiotics.

**Acute Care.** The patient with bacterial meningitis is usually acutely ill. The fever is high, and head pain is severe. Irritation of the cerebral cortex may result in seizures. The changes in mental status and LOC depend on the degree of increased ICP.

Assess and record vital signs, neurologic status, fluid intake and output, skin, and lung fields at regular intervals based on the patient's condition.

Head and neck pain secondary to movement requires attention. Codeine provides some pain relief without undue sedation for most patients. Assist the patient to a position of comfort, often curled up with the head slightly extended. The head of the bed should be slightly elevated. A darkened room and a cool cloth over the eyes relieve the discomfort of photophobia.

For the patient with delirium, additional low lighting may be necessary to decrease hallucinations. All patients suffer some degree of mental distortion and hypersensitivity, and they may be frightened and misinterpret the environment. Make every attempt to minimize environmental stimuli and prevent injury. A familiar person at the bedside may have a calming effect. Be efficient with care but also convey an attitude of caring and of unhurried gentleness. The use of touch and a soothing voice to give simple explanations of activities is helpful. If seizures occur, make appropriate observations and take protective measures. Administer antiseizure drugs such as phenytoin (Dilantin) or levetiracetam (Keppra) as ordered. Problems associated with increased ICP must be managed (see the section on increased ICP earlier in this chapter).

Fever must be vigorously treated because it increases cerebral edema and the frequency of seizures. In addition, neurologic damage may result from an extremely high temperature over a prolonged time. Acetaminophen or aspirin may be used to reduce fever. However, if the fever is resistant to aspirin or acetaminophen, more vigorous means are necessary, such as a cooling blanket. Take care not to reduce the temperature too rapidly because shivering may result, causing a rebound effect and increasing the temperature. Wrap the extremities in soft towels or a blanket covered with a sheet to reduce shivering (which can raise ICP). If a cooling blanket is not available or desirable, tepid sponge baths with water may be effective in lowering the temperature. Protect the skin from excessive drying and injury and prevent breaks in the skin.

Because high fever greatly increases the metabolic rate and thus insensible fluid loss, assess the patient for dehydration and adequacy of fluid intake. Diaphoresis further increases fluid losses, which should be noted on the output record. Calculate replacement fluids as 800 mL/day for respiratory losses and 100 mL for each degree of temperature above 100.4° F (38° C). Supplemental feeding (e.g., enteral nutrition) to maintain adequate nutritional intake may be necessary. Follow the designated antibiotic schedule to maintain therapeutic blood levels.

Meningitis generally requires respiratory isolation until the cultures are negative. Meningococcal meningitis is highly contagious, whereas other causes of meningitis may pose minimal to no infection risk with patient contact. However, standard precautions are essential to protect the patient and nurse.

◆ **Ambulatory Care.** After the acute period has passed, the patient requires several weeks of convalescence before resuming normal activities. In this period, stress the importance of adequate nutrition, with an emphasis on a high-protein, high-calorie diet in small, frequent feedings.

Muscle rigidity may persist in the neck and backs of the legs. Progressive range-of-motion exercises and warm baths are useful. Have the patient gradually increase activity as tolerated, but encourage adequate rest and sleep.

Residual effects can result in sequelae such as dementia, seizures, deafness, hemiplegia, and hydrocephalus. Assess vision, hearing, cognitive skills, and motor and sensory abilities after recovery, with appropriate referrals as indicated. Throughout the acute and convalescent periods, be aware of the anxiety and stress experienced by the caregiver and other family members.

### ◆ Evaluation

The expected outcomes are that the patient with bacterial meningitis will

- Demonstrate appropriate cognitive function
- Be oriented to person, place, and time
- Maintain body temperature within normal range
- Report satisfaction with pain control

Additional information on expected outcomes for the patient with bacterial meningitis is provided in eNursing Care Plan 56-2.

## VIRAL MENINGITIS

The most common causes of viral meningitis are enteroviruses, arboviruses, human immunodeficiency virus, and herpes simplex virus (HSV). Enteroviruses are most often spread through direct contact with respiratory secretions. Viral meningitis usually manifests as a headache, fever, photophobia, and stiff neck.[24] The fever may be moderate or high.

The Xpert EV test is used to rapidly diagnose viral meningitis. A sample of CSF is used to determine if enterovirus is present, and results are available within hours of symptom onset.[26]

The CSF can be clear or cloudy, and the typical finding is lymphocytosis (Table 56-16). Organisms are not seen on Gram stain or acid-fast smears. Polymerase chain reaction (PCR) used to detect viral-specific deoxyribonucleic acid (DNA) or ribonucleic acid (RNA) is a highly sensitive method for diagnosing CNS viral infections.

Antibiotics should be administered after the lumbar puncture while awaiting the results of the CSF analysis. Antibiotics are the best defense for bacterial meningitis and can be easily discontinued if the meningitis is found to be viral.

Viral meningitis is managed symptomatically because the disease is self-limiting. Full recovery from viral meningitis is expected. Rare sequelae include persistent headaches, mild mental impairment, and incoordination.

## ENCEPHALITIS

**Encephalitis**, an acute inflammation of the brain, is a serious, and sometimes fatal, disease. In the United States, encephalitis is responsible for about 20,000 cases and 1400 deaths annually.[27]

Encephalitis is usually caused by a virus. Many different viruses have been implicated in encephalitis. Some of the viruses are associated with certain seasons of the year and endemic to certain geographic areas.

Ticks and mosquitoes transmit epidemic encephalitis. Examples include eastern equine encephalitis, La Crosse encephalitis, St. Louis encephalitis, West Nile encephalitis, and western equine encephalitis.[27] Nonepidemic encephalitis may occur as a complication of measles, chickenpox, or mumps. HSV encephalitis is the most common cause of acute nonepidemic viral encephalitis. Cytomegalovirus encephalitis is a common complication in patients with acquired immunodeficiency syndrome (AIDS).

### Clinical Manifestations and Diagnostic Studies

The onset of infection is typically nonspecific, with fever, headache, nausea, and vomiting. Encephalitis can be acute or subacute. Signs of encephalitis appear on day 2 or 3 and may vary from minimal alterations in mental status to coma. Virtually any CNS abnormality can occur, including hemiparesis, tremors, seizures, cranial nerve palsies, personality changes, memory impairment, amnesia, and dysphasia.

Early diagnosis and treatment of viral encephalitis are essential for favorable outcomes. Diagnostic findings related to viral encephalitis are shown in Table 56-16. Brain imaging techniques include CT, MRI, and PET. PCR tests allow for early detection of HSV and West Nile encephalitis. West Nile virus should be strongly considered in adults over 50 years old who develop encephalitis or meningitis in summer or early fall. The best diagnostic test for West Nile virus is a blood test that detects viral RNA. This test is also used in screening blood, organs, cells, and tissues that have been donated.

## ❖ NURSING AND INTERPROFESSIONAL MANAGEMENT: ENCEPHALITIS

Prevention of encephalitis requires mosquito control, including cleaning rain gutters, removing old tires, draining bird baths, and removing water where mosquitoes can breed. In addition, insect repellent should be used during mosquito season.

Interprofessional and nursing management of encephalitis, including West Nile virus infection, is symptomatic and supportive. In the initial stages of encephalitis, many patients require intensive care.

Acyclovir (Zovirax) and vidarabine (Vira-A) are used to treat encephalitis caused by HSV infection. Acyclovir has fewer side effects than vidarabine and is often the preferred treatment. Use of these antiviral agents has been shown to reduce mortality rates, although neurologic complications may not be reduced. For maximal benefit, antiviral agents should be started before the onset of coma. Treat seizure disorders with antiseizure drugs. Prophylactic treatment with antiseizure drugs may be used in severe cases of encephalitis. Treatment of cytomegalovirus encephalitis in AIDS patients is discussed in Chapter 14.

## CASE STUDY

### *Traumatic Brain Injury*

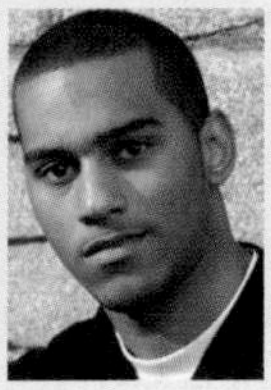

(©Comstock/ Thinkstock)

**Patient Profile**

C.G. is a 24-yr-old African American man who has just returned from a 15-month Army deployment to Afghanistan. He comes to the outpatient clinic with a report of chronic headaches (pain rating of 8 [0-10 point scale]) and difficulty sleeping. His wife has noticed some personality changes since his return from deployment and is concerned that he has posttraumatic stress disorder (PTSD).

**Subjective Data**

- Reports that he has been depressed lately but attributes it to headache and difficulty returning home.
- Headache is worse in the morning or when he lies down.
- Uses tobacco and drinks coffee throughout the day.
- Has difficulty sleeping.
- Reports "incidents" of heavy combat and blasts with a loss of consciousness. Cannot remember how many times. Unable to obtain a more through history as he becomes quite agitated.

**Objective Data**

- During your assessment, you note that C.G. is looking around the room and jumps when the phone rings next door.
- Loss of short-term memory (remembers one of three items).
- Heart rate ranges from 100 to 130 beats/min.
- ECG strip is shown below:

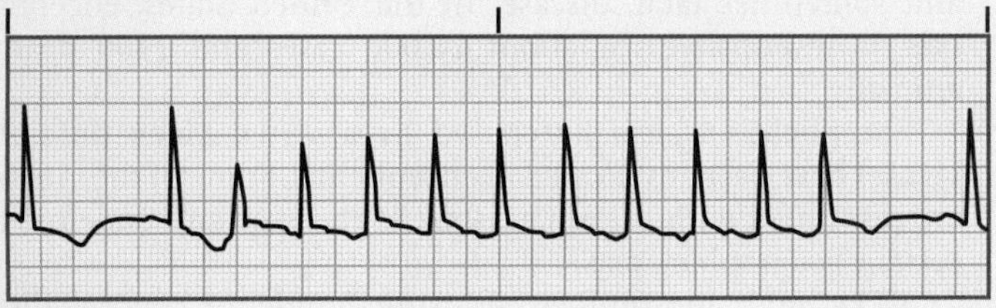

- Systolic BP ranges from 120 to 160 mm Hg.
- Right pupil, 3 mm sluggishly reactive; left pupil, 3 mm briskly reactive.

**Diagnostic Studies**

- CT of the head: negative for skull fracture, hematoma, or hemorrhage. Cerebral edema is noted with cingulate herniation on the right side.
- MRI performed following CT. Results indicate mild diffuse axonal injury.

**Discussion Questions**

1. What could be the cause of C.G.'s hypertension, tachycardia, and ECG rhythm?
2. In addition to PTSD, what do his clinical manifestations suggest?
3. ***Priority Decision:*** What are the priority nursing interventions that should be implemented?
4. ***Teamwork and Collaboration:*** How can the interprofessional team work together to meet his needs?
5. ***Safety:*** Are there any safety concerns for this patient or his wife?
6. ***Priority Decision:*** Based on the assessment data presented, what are the priority nursing diagnoses? Are there any collaborative problems?
7. ***Evidence-Based Practice:*** What interventions and support can help his wife?

Answers available at *http://evolve.elsevier.com/Lewis/medsurg.*

## BRIDGE TO NCLEX EXAMINATION

The number of the question corresponds to the same-numbered outcome at the beginning of the chapter.

1. Vasogenic cerebral edema increases intracranial pressure by
   a. shifting fluid in the gray matter.
   b. altering the endothelial lining of cerebral capillaries.
   c. leaking molecules from the intracellular fluid to the capillaries.
   d. altering the osmotic gradient flow into the intravascular component.
2. A patient with intracranial pressure monitoring has a pressure of 12 mm Hg. The nurse understands that this pressure reflects
   a. a severe decrease in cerebral perfusion pressure.
   b. an alteration in the production of cerebrospinal fluid.
   c. the loss of autoregulatory control of intracranial pressure.
   d. a normal balance between brain tissue, blood, and cerebrospinal fluid.
3. A nurse plans care for the patient with increased intracranial pressure with the knowledge that the *best* way to position the patient is to
   a. keep the head of the bed flat.
   b. elevate the head of the bed to 30 degrees.
   c. maintain patient on the left side with the head supported on a pillow.
   d. use a continuous-rotation bed to continuously change patient position.
4. The nurse is alerted to a possible acute subdural hematoma in the patient who
   a. has a linear skull fracture crossing a major artery.
   b. has focal symptoms of brain damage with no recollection of a head injury.
   c. develops decreased level of consciousness and a headache within 48 hours of a head injury.
   d. has an immediate loss of consciousness with a brief lucid interval followed by decreasing level of consciousness.
5. During admission of a patient with a severe head injury to the emergency department, the nurse places the *highest* priority on assessment for
   a. patency of airway.
   b. presence of a neck injury.
   c. neurologic status with the Glasgow Coma Scale.
   d. cerebrospinal fluid leakage from the ears or nose.
6. A patient is suspected of having a brain tumor. The signs and symptoms include memory deficits, visual disturbances, weakness of right upper and lower extremities, and personality changes. The nurse recognizes that the tumor is *most* likely located in the
   a. frontal lobe.
   b. parietal lobe.
   c. occipital lobe.
   d. temporal lobe.
7. Nursing management of a patient with a brain tumor includes *(select all that apply)*
   a. discussing with the patient methods to control inappropriate behavior.
   b. using diversion techniques to keep the patient stimulated and motivated.
   c. assisting and supporting the family in understanding any changes in behavior.
   d. limiting self-care activities until the patient has regained maximum physical functioning.
   e. planning for seizure precautions and teaching the patient and the caregiver about antiseizure drugs.
8. The nurse on the clinical unit is assigned to four patients. Which patient should she assess *first*?
   a. Patient with a skull fracture whose nose is bleeding
   b. Older patient with a stroke who is confused and whose daughter is present
   c. Patient with meningitis who is suddenly agitated and reporting a headache of 10 on a 0-to-10 scale
   d. Patient who had a craniotomy for a brain tumor and who is now 3 days postoperative and has had continued vomiting
9. A nursing measure that is indicated to reduce the potential for seizures and increased intracranial pressure in the patient with bacterial meningitis is
   a. administering codeine for relief of head and neck pain.
   b. controlling fever with prescribed drugs and cooling techniques.
   c. keeping the room dark and quiet to minimize environmental stimulation.
   d. maintaining the patient on strict bed rest with the head of the bed slightly elevated.

1. b, 2. d, 3. b, 4. c, 5. a, 6. a, 7. c, e, 8. c, 9. b

For rationales to these answers and even more NCLEX review questions, visit *http://evolve.elsevier.com/Lewis/medsurg.*

## EVOLVE WEBSITE

http://evolve.elsevier.com/Lewis/medsurg

**Review Questions (Online Only)**

**Key Points**

**Answer Keys for Questions**

- Rationales for Bridge to NCLEX Examination Questions
- Answer Guidelines for Case Study on p. 1342

**Student Case Studies**

- Patient With Head Injury
- Patient With Meningitis

**Nursing Care Plans**

- eNursing Care Plan 56-1: Patient With Increased Intracranial Pressure
- eNursing Care Plan 56-2: Patient With Meningitis

**Conceptual Care Map Creator**

**Audio Glossary**

**Supporting Media**

- Animation
  - Parts of the Brain Controlling Body Function

**Content Updates**

## REFERENCES


1. Cushing H: *Studies in intracranial physiology and surgery,* London, 1925, Oxford University Press. (Classic)
2. Miller C, Torbey M: *Neurocritical care monitoring,* New York, 2015, Demos Medical Publishing.
3. Seidman R: Cerebrovascular disease, Stonybrook University Medical Center. Retrieved from *www.stonybrookmedicalcenter.org/pathology/neuropathology/chapter2.*
4. Perez-Barcena J, Llompart-Pou JA, O'Phelan KH: Intracranial pressure monitoring and management of intracranial hypertension, *Crit Care Clin* 30(4):735, 2014.

*5. Olson D, Zomorodi M, Britz G, et al: Continuous cerebral spinal fluid drainage associated with complications in patients admitted with subarachnoid hemorrhage, *J Neurosurg* 119(4):974, 2013.

6. Oddo M, Le Roux P: Brain oxygen. In Le Roux P, Levine J, Kofke W, editors: *Monitoring in neurocritical care,* Philadelphia, 2013, Saunders.
7. Stochetti N, Magnoni S, Zanier E: My paper 20 years later: cerebral venous oxygen saturation studied with bilateral samples in the internal

jugular veins, Intensive Care Medicine. Retrieved from *www.ncbi.nlm.nih.gov/pubmed/25614058*.

*8. Surani S, Lockwood G, Macias M, et al: Hypertonic saline in elevated intracranial pressure: past, present, and future, *J Intens Care Med* 30:1, 2015.

9. Wang X, Dong Y, Han X, et al: Nutritional support for patients sustaining traumatic brain injury: A systematic review and meta-analysis of prospective studies, *PLoS One* 8(3): ee58838, 2013. Retrieved from *www.ncbi.nlm.nih.gov/pmc/articles/PMC3602547*.

*10. Jalali R, Rezaei M: A comparison of the Glasgow Coma Scale Score with Full Outline of Unresponsiveness Scale to predict patients' traumatic brain injury outcomes in intensive care units, *Crit Care Res Prac* 2014 Article ID 289803. Retrieved from *www.hindawi.com/journals/ccrp/2014/289803*.

*11. Bhullar I, Johnson D, Paul J, et al: More harm than good: Antiseizure prophylaxis after traumatic brain injury does not decrease seizure rates but may inhibit functional recovery, *J Trauma Acute Care Surgery* 76(1):54, 2014.

12. Faul M, Xu L, Wald M, et al: Traumatic brain injury in the United States: emergency department visits, hospitalizations, and deaths 2002-2006, Atlanta. Centers for Disease Control and Prevention, National Center for Injury Prevention and Control. Retrieved from *www.cdc.gov/traumaticbraininjury/pdf/blue_book.pdf*.

13. Centers for Disease Control and Prevention: Traumatic brain injury in the United States fact sheet. Retrieved from *www.cdc.gov/traumaticbraininjury/get_the_facts.html*.

14. American Association of Neurological Surgeons: Traumatic brain injury: fact sheets. Retrieved from *www.aans.org/patientinformation/conditionsandtreatments/traumaticbraininjury.aspx*.

15. Lump D: Managing patients with severe traumatic brain injury, *Nursing* 44(3):30, 2014.

16. Wasserman J, Koenigsberg RA: Diffuse axonal injury. Retrieved from *http://emedicine.medscape.com/article/339912-overview*.

17. Hyatt KS: Mild traumatic brain injury, *AJN* 114:36, 2014.

18. Phan N, Hemphill J: Management of acute severe traumatic brain injury. Retrieved from *www.uptodate.com/contents/management_of_acute_traumatic_brain_injury*.

19. Bauman M, McCourt TR: Assessing and managing patients with chronic subdural hematoma, *Am Nurse Today* 9:38, 2014.

20. Chronic subdural hematoma. Retrieved from *www.nlm.nih.gov/medlineplus/ency/article/000781.html*.

*21. Waljas M, Iverson G, Lange R, et al: Return to work following mild traumatic brain injury, *J Head Trauma Rehab* 29(5):443, 2014.

22. National Cancer Institute: Brain tumor, approved by the US National Institutes of Health. Retrieved from *www.cancer.gov/cancertopics/types/brain*.

23. University of Pittsburgh: Types of brain tumors. Retrieved from *www.neurosurgery.pitt.edu/neuro_oncology/brain/types.html*.

24. Centers for Disease Control and Prevention: Meningitis questions and answers. Retrieved from *www.cdc.gov/meningitis/about/fac/html*.

25. Miller A: Fire up to beat the threat of bacterial meningitis, *Nursing* 43(12):52, 2013.

26. Nordqvist C: Rapid test approved by FDA. Retrieved from *www.medicalnewstoday.com/articles/65448.php*.

27. Venkatesan A, Tunkel A, Bloch K, et al: Case definitions, diagnostic algorithms, and priorities in encephalitis: consensus statement of the international encephalitis consortium, *Clin Infect Dis* 57(8):1114, 2013.

*Evidence-based information for clinical practice.

57

# Stroke

*Meg Zomorodi*

*If I have the belief that I can do it, I shall surely acquire the capacity to do it even if I may not have it at the beginning.*

***Gandhi***

http://evolve.elsevier.com/Lewis/medsurg/

## LEARNING OUTCOMES

1. Describe the incidence of and risk factors for stroke.
2. Explain mechanisms that affect cerebral blood flow.
3. Compare and contrast the etiology and pathophysiology of ischemic and hemorrhagic strokes.
4. Correlate the clinical manifestations of stroke with the underlying pathophysiology.
5. Identify diagnostic studies performed for patients with strokes.
6. Differentiate among the interprofessional care, drug therapy, and surgical therapy for patients with ischemic strokes and hemorrhagic strokes.
7. Describe the acute nursing management of a patient with a stroke.
8. Describe the rehabilitative nursing management of a patient with a stroke.
9. Explain the psychosocial impact of a stroke on the patient, caregiver, and family.

## KEY TERMS

**aneurysm**, p. 1349
**aphasia**, p. 1351
**brain attack**, p. 1345
**cerebrovascular accident (CVA)**, p. 1345
**dysarthria**, p. 1351
**dysphasia**, p. 1351
**embolic stroke**, p. 1349
**hemorrhagic strokes**, p. 1349
**intracerebral hemorrhage**, p. 1349
**ischemic stroke**, p. 1348
**stroke**, p. 1345
**subarachnoid hemorrhage (SAH)**, p. 1349
**thrombotic stroke**, p. 1348
**transient ischemic attack (TIA)**, p. 1347

**Stroke** occurs when there is (1) *ischemia* (inadequate blood flow) to a part of the brain or (2) *hemorrhage* (bleeding) into the brain that results in death of brain cells. In a stroke, functions such as movement, sensation, thinking, talking, or emotions that were controlled by the affected area of the brain are lost or impaired. The severity of the loss of function varies according to the location and extent of the brain damage.

The terms **brain attack** and **cerebrovascular accident (CVA)** are also used to describe stroke. The term *brain attack* communicates the urgency of recognizing the warning signs of a stroke and treating it as a medical emergency, as would be done with a heart attack (Table 57-1). After the onset of a stroke, immediate medical attention is crucial to decrease disability and the risk of death.

Stroke is a major public health concern. An estimated 7 million people over the age of 20 in the United States have had a stroke.[1] With an aging population, a further increase in the incidence of stroke can be expected. However, stroke can occur at any age. About 34% of strokes occur in people younger than 65 years old.[2]

Stroke is currently the fifth most common cause of death in the United States. More than 137,000 deaths occur annually from stroke.[3] While death due to stroke has been reduced, stroke is the leading cause of serious long-term disability. About 800,000 people have a stroke each year, with 15% to 30% with permanent disability.[4]

Common long-term disabilities include *hemiparesis* (partial paralysis on one side), inability to walk, complete or partial dependence for activities of daily living (ADLs), *aphasia* (dysfunction in communication), and depression. In addition to the physical, cognitive, and emotional impact of the stroke on the stroke survivor, the stroke affects the lives of the stroke victim's caregiver and family.[5] A stroke is a lifelong change for both the stroke survivor and family. Be mindful of this impact when caring for patients who survive stroke.

Reviewed by Carol Annesser, RN, MSN, BC, CNE, Assistant Professor of Nursing, Mercy College of Ohio, Toledo, Ohio; Regina Gonzalez-Lama, RN, MS, Lecturer, College of Staten Island–CUNY, Staten Island, New York; Linda Littlejohns, RN, MSN, CNRN, FAAN, Neuroscience Clinical Nurse Consultant, San Juan Capistrano, California; Molly McClelland, RN, PhD, ACNS-BC, CMSRN, Associate Professor of Nursing, College of Health Professions, University of Detroit Mercy, Detroit, Michigan; and Kathy Morrison, RN, MSN, CNRN, SCRN, Stroke Program Manager, Neuroscience Institute, Penn State Hershey Medical Center, Hershey, Pennsylvania.

**TABLE 57-1 Patient & Caregiver Teaching**

***FAST for Warning Signs of Stroke***

FAST is an easy way to remember the signs of stroke. Include the following information in the teaching plan for a patient at risk for stroke and the patient's caregiver.

| | | |
|---|---|---|
| **F** | Face drooping | Does one side of the face droop or is it numb? Ask the person to smile. Is the smile uneven? |
| **A** | Arm weakness | Is one arm weak or numb? Ask the person to raise both arms. Does one arm drift downward? |
| **S** | Speech difficulties | Is speech slurred? Is the person unable to speak or hard to understand? Ask the person to repeat a simple sentence like "The sky is blue." Is the sentence repeatedly correctly? |
| **T** | Time | Time is CRITICAL! If someone shows any of these signs (even if they go away), call 911 and get the person to the hospital. Note the time when the signs first appeared. |

***In addition, the following should be reported:***

- Sudden trouble seeing in one or both eyes
- Sudden trouble walking, dizziness, loss of balance or coordination
- Sudden, severe headache with no known cause

Source: American Stroke Association: FAST. Retrieved from *www.strokeassociation.org/STROKEORG/WarningSigns/Stroke-Warning-Signs-and-Symptoms_UCM_308528_SubHomePage.jsp.*

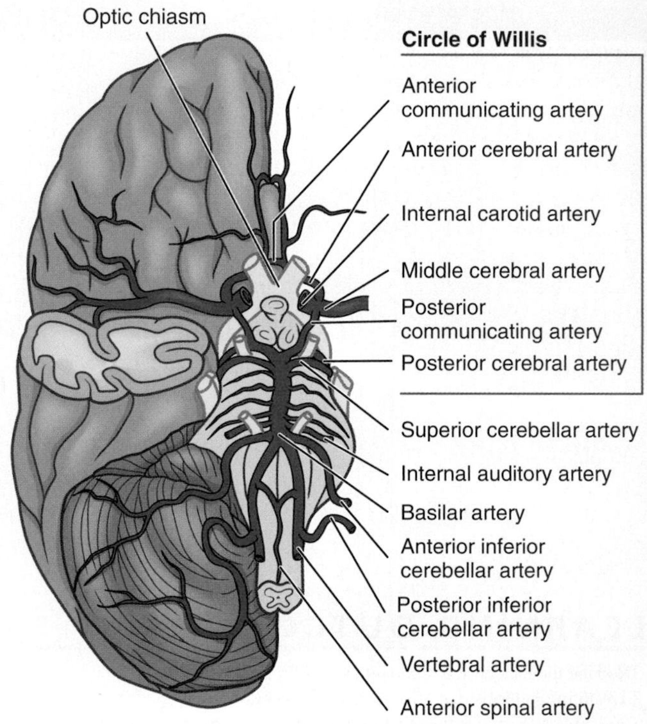


**FIG. 57-1** Cerebral arteries and the circle of Willis. The top of the temporal lobe has been removed to show the course of the middle cerebral artery.

## PATHOPHYSIOLOGY OF STROKE

### Anatomy of Cerebral Circulation

Blood is supplied to the brain by two major pairs of arteries: internal carotid arteries (anterior circulation) and vertebral arteries (posterior circulation). The carotid arteries branch to supply most of the (1) frontal, parietal, and temporal lobes; (2) basal ganglia; and (3) part of the diencephalon (thalamus and hypothalamus). The major branches of the carotid arteries are the middle cerebral and anterior cerebral arteries. The vertebral arteries join to form the basilar artery, which branches to supply the middle and lower parts of the temporal lobes, occipital lobes, cerebellum, brainstem, and part of the diencephalon. The main branch of the basilar artery is the posterior cerebral artery. The anterior and posterior cerebral circulation is connected at the *Circle of Willis* by the anterior and posterior communicating arteries (Fig. 57-1). (Fig. 55-10 illustrates the arteries at the base of the brain.) Genetic variations in this area are common, and all connecting vessels may not be present.

### Regulation of Cerebral Blood Flow

The brain requires a continuous supply of blood to provide the $O_2$ and glucose that neurons need to function. Blood flow must be maintained at 750 to 1000 mL/min (55 mL/100 g of brain tissue), or 20% of the cardiac output, for optimal brain functioning. If blood flow to the brain is totally interrupted (e.g., cardiac arrest), neurologic metabolism is altered in 30 seconds, metabolism stops in 2 minutes, and cellular death occurs in 5 minutes.

The brain is normally well protected from changes in mean systemic arterial BP over a range from 50 to 150 mm Hg by a mechanism known as *cerebral autoregulation.* This involves changes in the diameter of cerebral blood vessels in response to changes in pressure so that the blood flow to the brain stays constant. When cerebral ischemia occurs, cerebral autoregulation may be impaired, making the brain dependent on systemic BP. $CO_2$ is a potent cerebral vasodilator. Changes in arterial $CO_2$ levels have a dramatic effect on cerebral blood flow (increased $CO_2$ levels increase cerebral blood flow, and decreased $CO_2$ levels decrease cerebral blood flow). Very low arterial $O_2$ levels (partial pressure of arterial $O_2$ less than 50 mm Hg) or increases in hydrogen ion concentration also increase cerebral blood flow.

Factors that affect blood flow to the brain include systemic BP, cardiac output, and blood viscosity. During normal activity, $O_2$ requirements vary considerably, but changes in cardiac output, vasomotor tone, and distribution of blood flow normally maintain adequate blood flow to the brain. Cardiac output has to be reduced by one third before cerebral blood flow is reduced. Changes in blood viscosity affect cerebral blood flow, with decreased viscosity increasing blood flow.

Collateral circulation may develop over time to compensate for a decrease in cerebral blood flow. An area of the brain can potentially receive blood supply from another blood vessel even if blood supply from the original vessel has been cut off (e.g., because of thrombosis). In other words, the vessels in the brain make an "alternate route" for blood flow to reach damaged areas, thus preventing a stroke.

Intracranial pressure (ICP) also influences cerebral blood flow. Increased ICP causes brain compression and reduced cerebral blood flow. One of your major goals when caring for a stroke patient is to reduce secondary injury related to increased ICP (see Chapter 56).

## RISK FACTORS FOR STROKE

The most effective way to decrease the burden of stroke is prevention and teaching, especially about risk factors. Risk factors can be divided into nonmodifiable and modifiable. Stroke risk increases with multiple risk factors. Thus primary prevention of stroke, and reduction of these risk factors, can dramatically reduce the morbidity and mortality of stroke.[6]

## Nonmodifiable Risk Factors

*Nonmodifiable risk factors* include age, gender, ethnicity or race, and family history or heredity. Stroke risk increases with age, doubling each decade after 55 years of age. Two thirds of all strokes occur in individuals older than 65 years, but stroke can occur at any age. Strokes are more common in men, but more women die from stroke than men. Because women tend to live longer than men, they have more opportunity to suffer a stroke.[2]

African Americans have twice the incidence of stroke and a higher death rate from stroke compared to any other ethnic group. This may be related in part to a higher incidence of hypertension, obesity, and diabetes mellitus in African Americans.[2]

### CULTURAL & ETHNIC HEALTH DISPARITIES

***Stroke***

**African Americans**

- Have a higher incidence of strokes than whites.
- Have a rate of first strokes that is almost twice that of any other ethnic group.
- Are three times more likely than whites to have an ischemic stroke and four times more likely to have a hemorrhagic stroke.
- Experience increased rates of hypertension, diabetes mellitus, and sickle cell anemia, which may be related to their high incidence of strokes.
- Have a higher incidence of smoking and obesity than whites, which are two risk factors for stroke.
- Are twice as likely to die from a stroke as whites.

**Other Ethnicities**

- Hispanics, Native Americans, and Asian Americans have a higher incidence of strokes than whites.
- Diabetes (an important risk factor for strokes) has a high incidence among Hispanics.
- Native Americans are more likely than whites to have at least two risk factors for stroke.

Genetic risk factors are important in the development of all vascular diseases, including stroke. A person with a family history of stroke has an increased risk of having a stroke. Genes encoding products involved in lipid metabolism, thrombosis, and inflammation are believed to be potential genetic factors for stroke. Individuals who have at least two first-degree relatives with a history of subarachnoid hemorrhage or aneurysm should be screened to rule out anomalies in their cerebral vasculature.[7]

## Modifiable Risk Factors

*Modifiable risk factors* are those that can potentially be altered through lifestyle changes and medical treatment, thus reducing the risk of stroke. Ninety percent of strokes are a result of modifiable risk factors.[7] Modifiable risk factors include hypertension, heart disease, diabetes mellitus, smoking, obesity, sleep apnea, metabolic syndrome, lack of physical exercise, poor diet, and drug and alcohol abuse.

Hypertension is the single most important modifiable risk factor, but it is still often undetected and inadequately treated. Increases in systolic and diastolic BP independently increase the risk of stroke. Stroke risk can be reduced by up to 50% with appropriate treatment of hypertension. New recommendations by the American Heart Association include home BP monitoring with a goal of SBP less than 140 mm Hg.[4,7]

Heart disease, including atrial fibrillation, myocardial infarction, cardiomyopathy, cardiac valve abnormalities, and cardiac congenital defects, is also a risk factor for stroke. Atrial fibrillation is responsible for about 25% of all strokes.[8] The incidence of atrial fibrillation increases with age. Oral anticoagulants (e.g., warfarin, dabigatran [Pradaxa]) and adherence to these medications play an important role in the prevention of stroke.[4,7]

Diabetes mellitus is a significant risk factor for stroke. The risk for stroke in people with diabetes mellitus is five times higher than in the general population.[8]

Increased serum cholesterol and smoking are risk factors for stroke. Smoking nearly doubles the risk of ischemic stroke, and smokers are four times as likely to have a hemorrhagic stroke than nonsmokers.[6] The risk associated with smoking decreases substantially over time after the smoker quits. After 5 to 10 years of no tobacco use, former smokers have the same risk of stroke as nonsmokers.

The effect of alcohol on stroke risk appears to depend on the amount consumed. Women who drink more than one alcoholic drink per day and men who drink more than two alcoholic drinks per day are at higher risk for hypertension, which increases their chance of stroke. Illicit drug use, especially cocaine use, has been associated with stroke risk.[7]

A waist circumference to hip circumference ratio equal to or above the mid-value for the population increases the risk of ischemic stroke threefold. In addition, obesity is also associated with hypertension, high blood glucose, and elevated blood lipid levels, all of which increase the risk of stroke.[6] An association of physical inactivity and increased stroke risk is present in both men and women, regardless of ethnicity. Benefits of physical activity can occur with even light to moderate regular activity. The American Stroke Association recommends 40 minutes of exercise 3 to 4 days per week in order to reduce risk of stroke.[7] Nutrition teaching is important for the individual at risk for stroke, since a diet high in fat and low in fruits and vegetables may increase stroke risk.

The early forms of birth control pills that contained high levels of progestin and estrogen increased a woman's chance of experiencing a stroke, especially if the woman also smoked heavily. Newer, low-dose oral contraceptives have lower risks for stroke except in those individuals who have hypertension and smoke.

Women who experience migraine with aura are at an increased risk for stroke. The American Heart Association recommends smoking cessation and alternatives to estrogen oral contraceptives for these women to reduce the incidence of stroke.[4,7]

Other conditions that may increase the risk for strokes include inflammatory conditions (rheumatoid arthritis), sickle cell disease, lack of exercise, and obesity.[6]

### Transient Ischemic Attack

Another risk factor associated with stroke is a history of a **transient ischemic attack (TIA)**. A TIA is a transient episode of neurologic dysfunction caused by focal brain, spinal cord, or retinal ischemia, but without acute infarction of the brain. Clinical symptoms typically last less than 1 hour. In the past, TIAs were operationally defined as any focal cerebral ischemic event with symptoms lasting less than 24 hours.

However, it is important to teach the patient to seek treatment for any stroke symptoms, since there is no way to predict if a TIA will resolve or if it is in fact the development of a stroke. In general, one third of individuals who experience a TIA do not experience another event, one third have additional TIAs, and one third progress to stroke.[9]

TIAs may be due to microemboli that temporarily block the blood flow. TIAs are a warning sign of progressive cerebrovascular disease. The signs and symptoms of a TIA depend on the blood vessel that is involved and the area of the brain that is ischemic. If the carotid system is involved, patients may have a temporary loss of vision in one eye *(amaurosis fugax)*, transient hemiparesis, numbness or loss of sensation, or a sudden inability to speak. Signs of a TIA involving the vertebrobasilar system may include tinnitus, vertigo, darkened or blurred vision, diplopia, ptosis, dysarthria, dysphagia, ataxia, and unilateral or bilateral numbness or weakness.

### CHECK YOUR PRACTICE

You are talking with your uncle at your family reunion. He knows that you are a nurse and seems very eager to talk with you. He tells you that earlier this morning he was having problems talking, got dizzy, and then "blanked" out for a while. He found himself just lying on the floor in his room.

- He says, "I think it is just all the excitement of the reunion, but what do you think?"

A TIA should be treated as a medical emergency as it is usually a precursor to ischemic stroke.

Teach people at risk for TIAs to seek medical attention immediately with any stroke-like symptom and to identify the time of onset of symptoms.

## TYPES OF STROKE

Unlike a TIA, in which ischemia occurs without infarction, a stroke results in infarction (cell death). Strokes are classified as ischemic or hemorrhagic based on the cause and underlying pathophysiologic findings (Fig. 57-2 and Table 57-2).

### Ischemic Stroke

An **ischemic stroke** results from inadequate blood flow to the brain from partial or complete occlusion of an artery.[10] Ischemic strokes are further divided into thrombotic and embolic strokes.

**Thrombotic Stroke.** A **thrombotic stroke** occurs from injury to a blood vessel wall and formation of a blood clot (Fig. 57-2, *A*). The lumen of the blood vessel becomes narrowed and, if it becomes occluded, infarction occurs. Thrombosis develops readily where atherosclerotic plaques have already narrowed blood vessels. Thrombotic stroke, which is the result of thrombosis or narrowing of the blood vessel, is the most common cause of stroke, accounting for about 60% of strokes.[2] Thrombotic strokes are more common in older individuals, especially those with high cholesterol, atherosclerosis, or diabetes. A

**TABLE 57-2 Types of Stroke**

| Gender and Age | Warning and Onset | Prognosis |
|---|---|---|
| **Ischemic** | | |
| *Incidence:* Accounts for 87% of strokes | | |
| ***Thrombotic*** | | |
| Men more than women<br>Oldest median age | *Warning:* TIA (30%-50% of cases)<br>*Onset:* Often during or after sleep | Stepwise progression, signs and symptoms develop slowly, usually some improvement, recurrence in 20%-25% of survivors. |
| ***Embolic*** | | |
| Men more than women | *Warning:* TIA (uncommon)<br>*Onset:* Sudden onset, most likely to occur during activity | Single event, signs and symptoms develop quickly, usually some improvement, recurrence common without aggressive treatment of underlying disease. |
| **Hemorrhagic** | | |
| *Incidence:* Accounts for 13% of strokes | | |
| ***Intracerebral*** | | |
| Slightly higher in women | *Warning:* Headache (25% of cases)<br>*Onset:* Activity (often) | Progression over 24 hr. Poor prognosis, fatality more likely with presence of coma. |
| ***Subarachnoid*** | | |
| Slightly higher in women<br>Youngest median age | *Warning:* Headache (common)<br>*Onset:* Activity (often), sudden onset, most commonly related to head trauma | Usually single sudden event, fatality more likely with presence of coma. |

*TIA,* Transient ischemic attack.

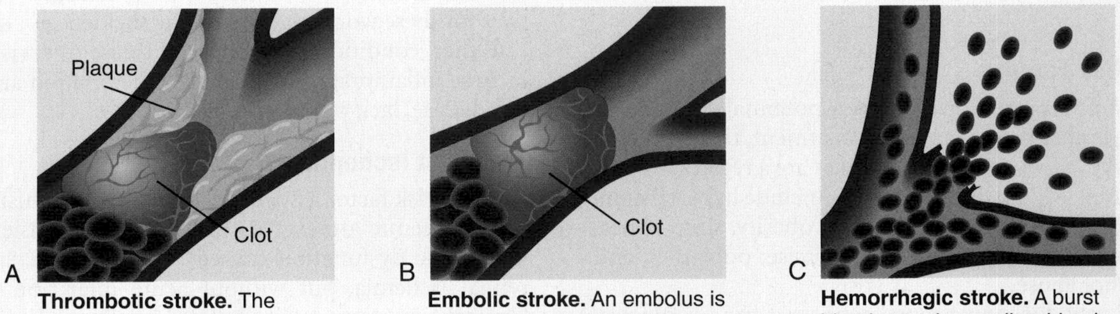


A **Thrombotic stroke.** The process of clot formation (thrombosis) results in a narrowing of the lumen, which blocks the passage of the blood through the artery.

B **Embolic stroke.** An embolus is a blood clot or other debris circulating in the blood. When it reaches an artery in the brain that is too narrow to pass through, it lodges there and blocks the flow of blood.

C **Hemorrhagic stroke.** A burst blood vessel may allow blood to seep into and damage brain tissues until clotting shuts off the leak.

**FIG. 57-2** Major types of stroke.

majority of thrombotic strokes are associated with hypertension or diabetes mellitus, both of which accelerate atherosclerosis. Many times thrombotic strokes are preceded by a TIA.[8]

The extent of the stroke depends on rapidity of onset, size of the damaged area, and presence of collateral circulation. Most patients with ischemic stroke do not have a decreased level of consciousness in the first 24 hours, unless it is due to a brainstem stroke or other conditions such as seizures, increased ICP, or hemorrhage. Manifestations of ischemic stroke may progress in the first 72 hours as infarction and cerebral edema increase.

**Embolic Stroke.** Embolic stroke occurs when an embolus lodges in and occludes a cerebral artery, resulting in infarction and edema of the area supplied by the involved vessel (Fig. 57-2, *B*). Embolism is the second most common cause of stroke.[2] Most emboli originate in the endocardial (inside) layer of the heart, with plaque breaking off from the endocardium and entering the circulation. The embolus travels upward to the cerebral circulation and lodges where a vessel narrows or bifurcates (splits). Heart conditions, which account for most of embolic ischemic strokes, include atrial fibrillation, myocardial infarction, infective endocarditis, rheumatic heart disease, valvular heart prostheses, and atrial septal defects.[2] Less common causes of emboli include air and fat from long bone (e.g., femur) fractures.

The patient with an embolic stroke commonly has severe clinical manifestations that occur suddenly. Embolic strokes can affect any age group. Rheumatic heart disease is a cause of embolic stroke in young to middle-aged adults. An embolus arising from an atherosclerotic plaque is more common in older adults.

Warning signs are less common with embolic than with thrombotic stroke. The embolic stroke often occurs rapidly, giving little time to accommodate to an obstructed blood vessel with the development of collateral circulation. The patient usually remains conscious, although he or she may have a headache. The effects of the emboli are initially characterized by severe neurologic deficits, which can be temporary if the clot breaks up and allows blood to flow. Smaller emboli then continue to obstruct smaller vessels, which in turn involve smaller portions of the brain with fewer deficits noted.

The prognosis is related to the amount of brain tissue deprived of its blood supply. Recurrence of embolic stroke is common unless the underlying cause is aggressively treated.

### Hemorrhagic Stroke

Hemorrhagic strokes result from bleeding into the brain tissue itself (intracerebral or intraparenchymal hemorrhage) or into the subarachnoid space or ventricles (subarachnoid hemorrhage or intraventricular hemorrhage).

**Intracerebral Hemorrhage.** Intracerebral hemorrhage is bleeding within the brain caused by a rupture of a vessel (usually in the basal ganglia) (Fig. 57-2, *C*). The prognosis of patients with intracerebral hemorrhage is poor, with the 30-day mortality rate at 40% to 80%. Fifty percent of the deaths occur within the first 48 hours.[2]

Hypertension is the most common cause of intracerebral hemorrhage (Fig. 57-3). Other causes include vascular malformations, coagulation disorders, anticoagulant and thrombolytic drugs, trauma, brain tumors, and ruptured aneurysms. Hemorrhage commonly occurs during periods of activity. Most often there is a sudden onset of symptoms, with progression over minutes to hours because of ongoing bleeding.

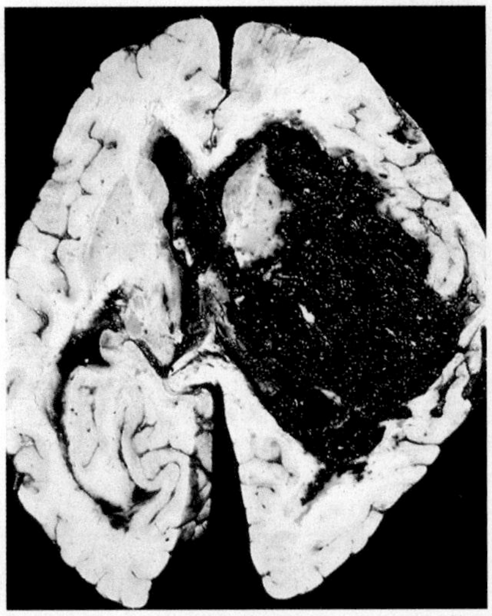

**FIG. 57-3** Massive hypertensive hemorrhage rupturing into a lateral ventricle of the brain. (From Kumar V, Abbas AK, Aster JC, et al: *Robbins and Cotran pathologic basis of disease,* ed 8, Philadelphia, 2010, Saunders.)

Manifestations include neurologic deficits, headache, nausea, vomiting, decreased level of consciousness, and hypertension. The extent of the symptoms varies depending on the amount, location, and duration of the bleeding. A blood clot within the closed skull can result in a mass that causes pressure on brain tissue, displaces brain tissue, and decreases cerebral blood flow, leading to ischemia and infarction.

Approximately half of intracerebral hemorrhages occur in the putamen and internal capsule, central white matter, thalamus, cerebellar hemispheres, and pons. Initially, patients experience a severe headache with nausea and vomiting. Clinical manifestations of putaminal and internal capsule bleeding include weakness of one side (including the face, arm, and leg), slurred speech, and deviation of the eyes. Progression of symptoms related to a severe hemorrhage includes hemiplegia, fixed and dilated pupils, abnormal body posturing, and coma. Thalamic hemorrhage results in hemiplegia with more sensory than motor loss. Bleeding into the subthalamic areas of the brain leads to problems with vision and eye movement. Cerebellar hemorrhages are characterized by severe headache, vomiting, loss of ability to walk, dysphagia, dysarthria, and eye movement disturbances.

Hemorrhage in the pons is the most serious because basic life functions (e.g., respiration) are rapidly affected. Hemorrhage in the pons can be characterized by hemiplegia leading to complete paralysis, coma, abnormal body posturing, fixed pupils (small in size), hyperthermia, and death.

**Subarachnoid Hemorrhage.** Subarachnoid hemorrhage (SAH) occurs when there is intracranial bleeding into the cerebrospinal fluid–filled space between the arachnoid and pia mater membranes on the surface of the brain. SAH is commonly caused by rupture of a cerebral aneurysm (congenital or acquired weakness and ballooning of vessels). Aneurysms may be saccular or berry aneurysms, ranging from a few millimeters to 20 to 30 mm in size, or fusiform atherosclerotic aneurysms. The majority of aneurysms are in the Circle of Willis. Other causes of SAH include trauma and illicit drug (cocaine) abuse. The incidence of SAH increases with age and is higher in women than men.

The patient may have warning signs and symptoms if the ballooning artery applies pressure to brain tissue, or minor warning symptoms may result from leaking of an aneurysm before major rupture. In general, cerebral aneurysms are viewed as a "silent killer," since individuals do not have warning signs or symptoms of an aneurysm until rupture has occurred.

**CHECK YOUR PRACTICE**

You are watching your husband's "for fun" soccer game. He leaves the game and is kneeling on the ground. When you try to assess what is going on he says, "I've got a terrible headache. It just started." Knowing that he sometimes gets headaches when he is stressed, you ask him if he is feeling stressed. He almost screams back at you, "NO! This is the worst headache of my life!"

- What should you do?

Loss of consciousness may or may not occur. The patient's level of consciousness may range from alert to comatose, depending on the severity of the bleed. Other manifestations include focal neurologic deficits (including cranial nerve deficits), nausea, vomiting, seizures, and stiff neck.

Complications of aneurysmal SAH include rebleeding before surgery or other therapy is initiated and cerebral vasospasm (narrowing of the blood vessels), which can result in cerebral infarction. Cerebral vasospasm is most likely due to an interaction between the metabolites of blood and the vascular smooth muscle. This occurs when the subarachnoid blood clots break down or dissolve, releasing metabolites that can cause endothelial damage and vasoconstriction. In addition, release of endothelin (a potent vasoconstrictor) may play a major role in the induction of cerebral vasospasm after SAH. Patients with SAH who are at risk for vasospasm are often kept in the intensive care unit (up to 14 days) until the threat of vasospasm is reduced. Peak time for vasospasm occurs 6 to 10 days after the initial bleed.

Despite improvements in surgical techniques and management, many patients with SAH die. Some die almost immediately when a rupture occurs. Others die from subsequent bleeding. Survivors may be left with significant morbidity, including cognitive difficulties.

## CLINICAL MANIFESTATIONS OF STROKE

Neurologic manifestations do not significantly differ between ischemic and hemorrhagic stroke. The reason for this is that destruction of neural tissue is the basis for neurologic dysfunction caused by both types of stroke. The clinical manifestations are related to the location of the stroke. Specific manifestations related to the type of stroke are discussed in the previous section. The general clinical manifestations of ischemic and hemorrhagic stroke are discussed together here.

A stroke can affect many body functions, including motor activity, bladder and bowel elimination, intellectual function, spatial-perceptual alterations, personality, affect, sensation, swallowing, and communication. The functions affected are directly related to the artery involved and area of the brain that it supplies (Table 57-3). Manifestations related to right- and left-brain damage differ somewhat and are shown in Fig. 57-4.

An additional assessment question that you need to ask is the time of the onset of symptoms. This is important for all types of stroke, especially ischemic strokes, since the time can affect treatment decisions.

### Motor Function

Motor deficits are the most obvious effect of stroke. Motor deficits include impairment of (1) mobility, (2) respiratory function, (3) swallowing and speech, (4) gag reflex, and (5) self-care abilities. Symptoms are caused by the destruction of motor neurons in the pyramidal pathway (nerve fibers from the brain that pass through the spinal cord to the motor cells). The characteristic motor deficits include loss of skilled voluntary movement *(akinesia)*, impairment of integration of movements, alterations in muscle tone, and alterations in reflexes. The initial *hyporeflexia* (depressed reflexes) progresses to *hyperreflexia* (hyperactive reflexes) for most patients.

Motor deficits after a stroke follow certain specific patterns. Because the pyramidal pathway crosses at the level of the medulla, a lesion on one side of the brain affects motor function

**TABLE 57-3 Stroke Manifestations Related to Artery Involvement**

| Artery | Manifestations |
|---|---|
| **Anterior cerebral** | Motor and/or sensory deficit (contralateral), sucking or rooting reflex, rigidity, gait problems, loss of proprioception and fine touch |
| **Middle cerebral** | *Dominant side:* Aphasia, motor and sensory deficit, hemianopsia<br>*Nondominant side:* Neglect, motor and sensory deficit, hemianopsia |
| **Posterior cerebral** | Hemianopsia, visual hallucination, spontaneous pain, motor deficit |
| **Vertebral** | Cranial nerve deficits, diplopia, dizziness, nausea, vomiting, dysarthria, dysphagia, and/or coma |

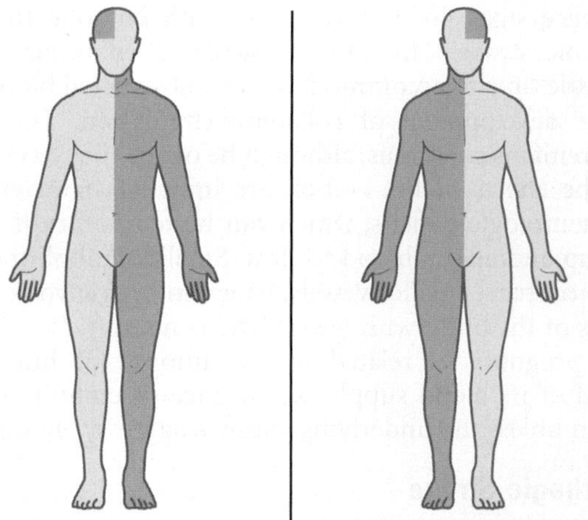

| Right-brain damage (stroke on right side of the brain) | Left-brain damage (stroke on left side of the brain) |
|---|---|
| • Paralyzed left side: hemiplegia<br>• Left-sided neglect<br>• Spatial-perceptual deficits<br>• Tends to deny or minimize problems<br>• Rapid performance, short attention span<br>• Impulsive, safety problems<br>• Impaired judgment<br>• Impaired time concepts | • Paralyzed right side: hemiplegia<br>• Impaired speech/language aphasias<br>• Impaired right/left discrimination<br>• Slow performance, cautious<br>• Aware of deficits: depression, anxiety<br>• Impaired comprehension related to language, math |

**FIG. 57-4** Manifestations of right-brain and left-brain stroke.

on the opposite side of the body (contralateral). The arms and legs of the affected side may be weakened or paralyzed to different degrees depending on which part of and to what extent the cerebral circulation was compromised. A stroke affecting the middle cerebral artery leads to a greater weakness in the upper extremity than the lower extremity. The affected shoulder tends to rotate internally, and the hip rotates externally. The affected foot is plantar flexed and inverted. An initial period of flaccidity may last from days to several weeks and is related to nerve damage. Spasticity of the muscles, which follows the flaccid stage, is related to interruption of upper motor neuron influence.

### Communication

The left hemisphere is dominant for language skills in right-handed persons and in most left-handed persons.[10] Language disorders involve expression and comprehension of written and spoken words. The patient may experience **aphasia**, which may be *receptive aphasia* (loss of comprehension), *expressive aphasia* (inability to produce language), or *global aphasia* (total inability to communicate). Aphasia occurs when a stroke damages the dominant hemisphere of the brain.

**Dysphasia** refers to impaired ability to communicate. However, in most settings the terms *aphasia* and *dysphasia* are used interchangeably, with aphasia often being the more common term used. (Dysphasia should not be confused with the similarly pronounced *dysphagia,* which is difficulty swallowing.)

Patterns of aphasia may differ, since the stroke affects different portions of the brain. Aphasia may be classified as *nonfluent* (minimal speech activity with slow speech that requires obvious effort) or *fluent* (speech is present but contains little meaningful communication) (Table 57-4). Most types of aphasia are mixed, with impairment in both expression and understanding. A massive stroke may result in global aphasia.

Many stroke patients also experience **dysarthria**, a disturbance in the muscular control of speech. Impairment may involve pronunciation, articulation, and phonation. Dysarthria does not affect the meaning of communication or the comprehension of language, but it does affect the mechanics of speech. Some patients experience a combination of aphasia and dysarthria.

### Affect

Patients who have had a stroke may have difficulty controlling their emotions. Emotional responses may be exaggerated or unpredictable. Depression and feelings associated with changes in body image and loss of function can make this worse.[11] Patients may also be frustrated by mobility and communication problems.

**CHECK YOUR PRACTICE**

You are working in the outpatient stroke clinic and counseling with the family of one of your favorite patients. He is a well-respected 65-yr-old business man who has returned home following a stroke. His family tells you that during meals he becomes frustrated and begins to cry because of the difficulty getting food into his mouth and chewing. They tell you that this is something that he was able to do easily before his stroke. His family cannot understand why a previously very competent man is so emotional.

- How should you counsel the family and what teaching is needed?

**TABLE 57-4 Types of Aphasia**

| Type | Characteristics |
|---|---|
| **Broca's** | • Type of nonfluent aphasia.<br>• Damage to frontal lobe of brain.<br>• Frequently speak in short phrases that make sense but are produced with great effort.<br>• Often omit small words such as "is," "and," and "the."<br>• May say, "Walk dog," meaning, "I will take the dog for a walk," or "book book two table," for "There are two books on the table."<br>• Typically understand speech of others fairly well.<br>• Often aware of their difficulties and can become easily frustrated. |
| **Wernicke's** | • Type of fluent aphasia.<br>• Damage occurs in left temporal lobe, although it can result from damage to right lobe.<br>• May speak in long sentences that have no meaning, add unnecessary words, and even create made-up words.<br>• May say, "You know that smoodle pinkered and that I want to get him round and take care of him like you want before."<br>• Often difficult to follow what person is trying to say.<br>• Usually have great difficulty understanding speech.<br>• Often unaware of their mistakes. |
| **Global** | • Type of nonfluent aphasia.<br>• Results from damage to extensive portions of language areas of brain.<br>• Have severe communication difficulties.<br>• May be extremely limited in ability to speak or comprehend language. |
| **Other** | • Results from damage to different language areas in brain.<br>• Some patients may have difficulty repeating words and sentences, even though they can speak and they understand the meaning of the word or sentence.<br>• Other patients may have difficulty naming objects, even though they know what the object is and what its use is. |

### Intellectual Function

Both memory and judgment may be impaired as a result of stroke. These impairments can occur with strokes affecting either side of the brain. A left-brain stroke is more likely to result in memory problems related to language. Patients with a left-brain stroke often are cautious in making judgments. The patient with a right-brain stroke tends to be impulsive and to move quickly.

An example of behavior in people with right-brain stroke is that they try to rise quickly from a wheelchair without locking the wheels or raising the footrests. On the other hand, people with a left-brain stroke would move slowly and cautiously from the wheelchair. Patients with either type of stroke may have difficulty making generalizations, which interferes with their ability to learn.

### Spatial-Perceptual Alterations

Individuals who have had a stroke on the right side of the brain are more likely to have problems with spatial-perceptual orientation. However, this can also occur in people with left-brain stroke.

Spatial-perceptual problems may be divided into four categories.

- The first is the result of damage of the parietal lobe and causes the patient to have an incorrect perception of self and illness. In this situation, patients may deny their illnesses or not recognize their own body parts.
- The second category occurs when the patient neglects all input from the affected side (erroneous perception of self in space). This may be worsened by *homonymous hemianopsia,* in which blindness occurs in the same half of the visual fields of both eyes. The patient also has difficulty with spatial orientation, such as judging distances.
- The third spatial-perceptual deficit is *agnosia,* the inability to recognize an object by sight, touch, or hearing.
- The fourth deficit is *apraxia,* the inability to carry out learned sequential movements on command. Because patients may or may not be aware of their spatial-perceptual alterations, you need to assess for this potential problem, since it will affect rehabilitation and recovery.

### Elimination

Most problems with urinary and bowel elimination occur initially and are temporary. When a stroke affects one hemisphere of the brain, the prognosis for normal bladder function is excellent. At least partial sensation for bladder filling remains, and voluntary urination is present. Initially, the patient may experience frequency, urgency, and incontinence. Although motor control of the bowel is usually not a problem, patients are frequently constipated. Constipation is associated with immobility, weak abdominal muscles, dehydration, and diminished response to the defecation reflex. Urinary and bowel elimination problems may also be related to inability to verbalize the need to eliminate and difficulty with managing clothing (resulting in incontinence). Scheduled toileting and clothes that are easily removed may encourage independence.

## DIAGNOSTIC STUDIES FOR STROKE

When manifestations of a stroke occur, diagnostic studies (Table 57-5) are done to (1) confirm that it is a stroke and not another type of brain lesion and (2) identify the likely cause of the stroke. Diagnostic study results also guide decisions about therapy.

Important diagnostic tools for patients who have experienced a stroke are an MRI or noncontrast CT scan.[12] These tests can rapidly distinguish between ischemic and hemorrhagic stroke and help determine the size and location of the stroke. Serial scans may be used to assess the effectiveness of treatment and to evaluate recovery. Once the individual suspected of TIA or stroke arrives in the emergency department, it is important to rapidly assess and diagnose the patient (usually through a noncontrast head CT or MRI). Rapid access to these diagnostic tools is important, since the results will determine treatment options for the patient. MRI is more effective in identifying ischemic stroke than CT scans. However, a CT scan is a rapid diagnostic tool to rule out hemorrhage.[12]

CT angiography (CTA) provides visualization of cerebral blood vessels. It can be performed after or at the same time as the noncontrast CT scan. CTA can provide an estimate of perfusion and detect filling defects in the cerebral arteries. Magnetic resonance angiography (MRA) can detect vascular lesions and blockages, similar to CTA. CT/MRI perfusion and diffusion imaging may also be done.

**TABLE 57-5 Diagnostic Studies**

***Stroke***

**Diagnosis of Stroke (Including Extent of Involvement)**
- CT scan
- CT angiography (CTA)
- MRI
- Magnetic resonance angiography (MRA)
- CT/MRI perfusion and diffusion imaging

**Cerebral Blood Flow**
- Cerebral angiography
- Carotid angiography
- Digital subtraction angiography
- Transcranial Doppler ultrasonography
- Carotid duplex scanning

**Cardiac Assessment**
- Electrocardiogram
- Chest x-ray
- Cardiac markers (troponin, creatine kinase-MB)
- Echocardiography (transthoracic, transesophageal)

**Additional Studies**
- Complete blood count (including platelets) and glucose
- Coagulation studies: prothrombin time, activated partial thromboplastin time
- Electrolytes, blood glucose
- Renal and hepatic studies
- Lipid profile
- Cerebrospinal fluid analysis*

*A lumbar puncture to obtain cerebrospinal fluid is avoided if increased intracranial pressure is suspected.

Cardiac imaging is also recommended because many strokes are caused by blood clots from the heart. Angiography can identify cervical and cerebrovascular occlusion, atherosclerotic plaques, and malformation of vessels. Cerebral angiography is a definitive study to identify the source of SAH. Risks of angiography include dislodging an embolus, causing vasospasm, inducing further hemorrhage, and provoking an allergic reaction to contrast media.

Intraarterial digital subtraction angiography (DSA) reduces the dose of contrast material, uses smaller catheters, and shortens the length of the procedure compared with conventional angiography. DSA involves the injection of a contrast agent to visualize blood vessels in the neck and the large vessels of the Circle of Willis. It is considered safer than cerebral angiography because less vascular manipulation is required.

Transcranial Doppler (TCD) ultrasonography is a noninvasive study that measures the velocity of blood flow in the major cerebral arteries. TCD is effective in detecting microemboli and vasospasm and is ideal for the patient suspected of having an SAH. Carotid duplex scanning is used not only to detect the cause of the stroke but also to stratify patients for either medical management or carotid intervention if they have carotid stenoses.

A lumbar puncture may be done to look for evidence of red blood cells in the cerebrospinal fluid if an SAH is suspected but the CT does not show hemorrhage. A lumbar puncture is avoided if the patient is suspected of having an obstruction in the foramen magnum or other signs of increased ICP because of the danger of herniation of the brain downward, leading to pressure on cardiac and respiratory centers in the brainstem and potentially death.

If the suspected cause of the stroke includes emboli from the heart, diagnostic cardiac tests should be done. Blood tests are also done to help identify conditions contributing to stroke and to guide treatment (Table 57-5).

The LICOX system may be used as a diagnostic tool to evaluate the progression of stroke. LICOX measures brain oxygenation and temperature (see discussion in Chapter 56 on pp. 1321-1322 and Fig. 56-10). Secondary brain injury adds significantly to mortality risk and poor functional outcome after a stroke.

## INTERPROFESSIONAL CARE FOR STROKE

### Preventive Therapy

Primary prevention is a priority for decreasing morbidity and mortality risk from stroke (Table 57-6). The goals of stroke prevention include health promotion for a healthy lifestyle and management of modifiable risk factors to prevent a stroke. Health promotion focuses on (1) healthy diet, (2) weight control, (3) regular exercise, (4) no smoking, (5) limiting alcohol consumption, (6) BP management, and (7) routine health assessments. Patients with known risk factors such as diabetes mellitus, hypertension, obesity, high serum lipids, or cardiac dysfunction require close management.

**HEALTHY PEOPLE**

***Prevention of Stroke***

- Reduce salt and sodium intake.
- Maintain a normal body weight.
- Maintain a normal BP.
- Increase level of physical exercise.
- Avoid cigarette smoking or tobacco products.
- Limit consumption of alcohol to moderate levels.
- Follow a diet that is low in saturated fat, total fat, and dietary cholesterol and high in fruits and vegetables (e.g., Mediterranean diet).

**Preventive Drug Therapy.** Measures to prevent the development of a thrombus or an embolus are used in patients with TIAs, since they are at high risk for stroke. Antiplatelet drugs are usually the chosen treatment to prevent stroke in patients who have had a TIA. Aspirin is the most frequently used antiplatelet agent, commonly at a dose of 81 to 325 mg/day. Other drugs include ticlopidine, clopidogrel (Plavix), dipyridamole (Persantine), and combined dipyridamole and aspirin (Aggrenox).

**DRUG ALERT Ticlopidine and Clopidogrel (Plavix)**

- All HCPs and dentists must be informed that the drug is being taken, especially before scheduling surgery or major dental procedures.
- Drug may have to be discontinued 10 to 14 days before surgery if antiplatelet effect is not desired.

For patients who have atrial fibrillation, oral anticoagulation can include warfarin (Coumadin) and the direct factor Xa inhibitors: rivaroxaban (Xarelto), dabigatran (Pradaxa), and apixaban (Eliquis). The primary advantage of direct factor Xa inhibitors (compared to warfarin) is that these drugs do not need close monitoring or dosage adjustments. Statins (simvastatin [Zocor], lovastatin) have also been shown to be effective in the prevention of stroke for individuals who have experienced a TIA in the past.[9]

**Left Atrial Appendage Occlusion.** The left atrial appendage (LAA) is a pouch that extends off the left atrium. The LAA is believed to be the source of a majority of stroke-causing emboli in patients with atrial fibrillation. LAA occlusion is a treatment strategy to prevent blood clot formation in patients who have atrial fibrillation. By removing or occluding the LAA, the incidence of strokes can be decreased.

A special stapler can be used to remove the LAA or sutures can be used to manually occlude the LAA. In addition, LAA occlusion devices (e.g., AtriClip, Watchman) are available. These devices are positioned around the LAA and then closed, similar to a clamp that is used to shut off the blood supply. This prevents blood from flowing into and out of the LAA. LAA occlusion can be used as an alternative for patients who cannot use oral anticoagulants such as warfarin. This procedure may reduce the risk of stroke, and patients may be able to stop taking anticoagulants.

**Surgical/Endovascular Therapy for TIA and Stroke Prevention.** Surgical interventions for the patient with TIAs due to carotid disease include carotid endarterectomy, transluminal angioplasty, and stenting. In a *carotid endarterectomy* (CEA), the atheromatous lesion is removed from the carotid artery to improve blood flow.[13]

*Transluminal angioplasty* is the insertion of a balloon to open a stenosed artery in the brain and improve blood flow. The balloon is threaded up to the carotid artery via a catheter inserted in the femoral artery.

*Stenting* involves intravascular placement of a stent in an attempt to maintain patency of the artery (Fig. 57-5). The stent can be inserted during an angioplasty. Once in place, the system can be used with a tiny filter that opens like an umbrella. The

**TABLE 57-6 Interprofessional Care**

***Stroke***

**Diagnostic Assessment**

- History and physical examination
- Diagnostic studies (Table 57-5)

**Management**

***Prevention***

- Control of hypertension
- Control of diabetes mellitus
- Treatment of underlying cardiac problem
- No smoking
- Limiting alcohol intake

*Drug Therapy*

- Platelet inhibitors (e.g., aspirin)
- Anticoagulation therapy for patients with atrial fibrillation

*Surgical Therapy*

- Carotid endarterectomy
- Stenting of carotid artery
- Transluminal angioplasty
- Surgical interventions for aneurysms at risk of bleeding

***Acute Care***

- Maintenance of airway
- Fluid therapy
- Treatment of cerebral edema
- Prevention of secondary injury

*Ischemic Stroke*

- Tissue plasminogen activator (tPA) IV or intraarterial
- Endovascular therapy

*Hemorrhagic Stroke*

- Surgical decompression if indicated
- Clipping or coiling of aneurysm

***Rehabilitation***

- Focus on helping patient achieve independence and functional recovery filter catches and removes the debris that is stirred up during the stenting procedure before it floats to the brain, where it can trigger a stroke. Stenting is a less invasive strategy for revascularization in patients unable to withstand the CEA because of coexisting medical conditions.

Postoperative nursing care for these patients consists of neurovascular assessment, BP management, assessment of stent occlusion or retroperitoneal hemorrhage as complications, and minimization of complications at the insertion site by keeping the patient's leg straight for the prescribed time.

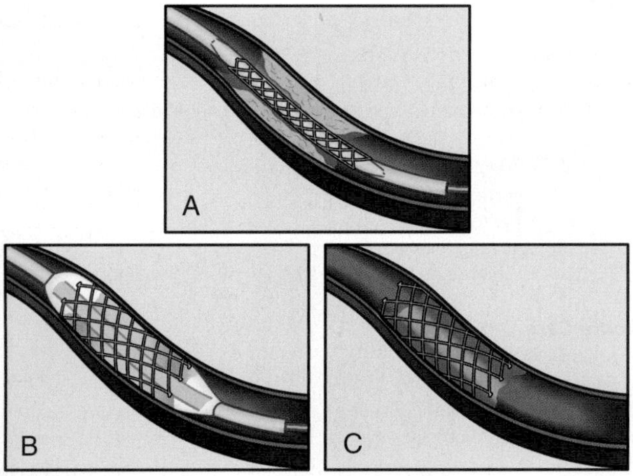


**FIG. 57-5** Brain stent used to treat blockages in cerebral blood flow. **A,** A balloon catheter is used to implant the stent into an artery of the brain. **B,** The balloon catheter is moved to the blocked area of the artery and then inflated. The stent expands due to inflation of the balloon. **C,** The balloon is deflated and withdrawn, leaving the stent permanently in place holding the artery open and improving the flow of blood.

### Acute Care for Ischemic Stroke

During initial evaluation, the single most important point in the patient's history is the time of onset of symptoms. Interprofessional goals during the acute phase are preserving life, preventing further brain damage, and reducing disability.

Table 57-7 outlines the emergency management of the patient with a stroke. In the unresponsive person, acute care begins with assessing circulation, airway, and breathing. Patients may have difficulty keeping an open and clear airway because of a decreased level of consciousness or decreased or absent gag and swallowing reflexes. Maintaining adequate oxygenation is important. $O_2$ administration, artificial airway insertion, intubation, and mechanical ventilation may be required. Baseline neurologic assessment is carried out, and patients are monitored closely for signs of increasing neurologic deficit. Many patients may worsen in the first 24 to 48 hours.

For emergency care, patients should be transported to the closest certified stroke center or, when such an institution is not available, the closest facility offering emergency stroke care. The American Heart Association recommends that acute care facilities have stroke teams in place. The stroke team generally consists of a registered nurse, neurologist, radiologist, and radiologic technician.[13]

Elevated BP is common immediately after a stroke and may be a protective response to maintain cerebral perfusion. However, it can also be detrimental. Immediately after an ischemic stroke in those patients who do not receive fibrinolytic therapy (discussed later), the use of drugs to lower BP is recommended only if BP is markedly increased (systolic BP greater than 220 mm Hg or diastolic greater than 120 mm Hg). In a patient who is going to have fibrinolytic therapy, the BP must be less than 185/110 mm Hg and then maintained at or below 180/105 mm Hg for at least 24 hours after fibrinolytic therapy. In an acute stroke, IV antihypertensives such as labetalol and

**TABLE 57-7 Emergency Management**

***Stroke***

| Etiology | Assessment Findings | Interventions |
|---|---|---|
| • Sudden vascular compromise causing disruption of blood flow to brain<br>• Thrombosis<br>• Trauma<br>• Aneurysm<br>• Embolism<br>• Hemorrhage<br>• Arteriovenous malformation | • Altered level of consciousness<br>• Weakness, numbness, or paralysis of portion of body<br>• Speech or visual disturbances<br>• Severe headache<br>• Heart rate ↑ or ↓<br>• Respiratory distress<br>• Unequal pupils<br>• Hypertension<br>• Facial drooping on affected side<br>• Difficulty swallowing<br>• Seizures<br>• Bladder or bowel incontinence<br>• Nausea and vomiting<br>• Vertigo | **Initial**<br>• If unresponsive, assess circulation, airway, and breathing.<br>• If responsive, monitor airway, breathing, and circulation.<br>• Call stroke code or stroke team.<br>• Remove dentures.<br>• Perform pulse oximetry.<br>• Maintain adequate oxygenation ($SaO_2$ >95%) with supplemental $O_2$, if necessary.<br>• Establish IV access with normal saline.<br>• Maintain BP according to guidelines (e.g., Cardiac Life Support).*<br>• Remove clothing.<br>• Obtain CT scan or MRI immediately.<br>• Perform baseline laboratory tests (including blood glucose) immediately, and treat if hypoglycemic.<br>• Position head in midline.<br>• Elevate head of bed 30 degrees if no symptoms of shock or injury.<br>• Institute seizure precautions.<br>• Anticipate thrombolytic therapy for ischemic stroke.<br>• Keep patient NPO until swallow reflex evaluated.<br>**Ongoing Monitoring**<br>• Monitor vital signs and neurologic status, including level of consciousness (NIH Stroke Scale), motor and sensory function, pupil size and reactivity, $SaO_2$, and cardiac rhythm.<br>• Reassure patient and family. |

*NIH,* National Institutes of Health; *$SaO_2$,* arterial $O_2$ saturation.
*See Appendix A.

nicardipine (Cardene) are preferred. Although low BP immediately after a stroke is uncommon, hypotension and hypovolemia should be corrected if present.

Fluid and electrolyte balance must be controlled carefully. Generally the goal is to keep the patient adequately hydrated to promote perfusion and decrease further brain injury. Overhydration may compromise perfusion by increasing cerebral edema. Adequate fluid intake during acute care via oral, IV, or tube feedings is a priority. Also monitor urine output to make sure the patient does not become dehydrated.

If secretion of antidiuretic hormone (ADH) increases in response to the stroke, urine output decreases and fluid is retained. Low serum sodium (hyponatremia) may occur. IV solutions with glucose and water are avoided because they are hypotonic and may further increase cerebral edema and ICP. Glycemic control should be maintained to avoid extreme hypo- or hyperglycemia. In general, decisions regarding individualized fluid and electrolyte replacement therapy are based on the extent of intracranial edema, manifestations of increased ICP, central venous pressure levels, electrolyte levels, and intake and output.

Increased ICP is more likely to occur with hemorrhagic strokes but can occur with ischemic strokes. Increased ICP from cerebral edema usually peaks in 72 hours and may cause brain herniation. Management of increased ICP includes practices that improve venous drainage, such as elevating the head of the bed, maintaining head and neck in alignment, and avoiding hip flexion. Additional measures for reducing ICP include management of hyperthermia (goal temperature of 96.8° to 98.6° F [36° to 37° C]), drug therapy to prevent seizures, pain management, avoidance of hypervolemia, and management of constipation. Cerebrospinal fluid drainage may be used in some patients to reduce ICP. (The specific management of increased ICP is discussed in Chapter 56.)

**Drug Therapy for Ischemic Stroke.** Fibrinolytic therapy should not be delayed. Recombinant tissue plasminogen activator (tPA) is used to produce localized fibrinolysis by binding to the fibrin in the thrombi. The fibrinolytic action of tPA occurs as the plasminogen is converted to plasmin, whose enzymatic action then digests fibrin and fibrinogen, thus breaking down the clot. Other fibrinolytic agents cannot be substituted for tPA. (Fibrinolytic [thrombolytic] therapy is discussed in Chapter 33.)

tPA is administered IV to reestablish blood flow through a blocked artery to prevent cell death in patients with the acute onset of ischemic stroke. tPA must be administered within 3 to 4½ hours of the onset of clinical signs of ischemic stroke.[9] Patients are screened carefully before tPA can be given. Screening includes a noncontrast CT scan or MRI to rule out hemorrhagic stroke; blood tests for glucose level and coagulation disorders; screening for recent history of gastrointestinal bleeding, stroke, or head trauma within the past 3 months; major surgery within 14 days; or recent active internal bleeding within 22 days.[14]

During infusion of the drug, closely monitor the patient's vital signs and neurologic status to assess for improvement or for potential deterioration related to intracerebral hemorrhage. Control of BP (SBP less than 185 mm Hg) is critical during treatment and for 24 hours following.

Intraarterial infusion of tPA may also be used for patients with an ischemic stroke when mechanical thrombectomy is not an option. To be effective, intraarterial tPA must be administered within 6 hours of the onset of stroke symptoms. In the intraarterial tPA procedure, the neurovascular specialist inserts a thin, flexible catheter into an artery (usually the femoral artery) and guides the catheter (using angiogram) to the area of the clot. The tPA is administered through the catheter and immediately targets the clot. Less tPA is needed when it is delivered directly to the clot, which can reduce the possibility of intracranial hemorrhage.[15]

The use of anticoagulants (e.g., heparin) in the emergency phase after an ischemic stroke is generally not recommended because of the risk for intracranial hemorrhage. Acetylsalicylic acid (aspirin) at a dose of 325 mg may be initiated within 24 to 48 hours after the onset of an ischemic stroke. Complications of aspirin (with higher doses) include gastrointestinal bleeding. Aspirin should be administered cautiously if the patient has a history of peptic ulcer disease.

After the patient has stabilized and to prevent further clot formation, patients with strokes caused by thrombi and emboli may be treated with anticoagulants and platelet inhibitors (see discussion on prevention of stroke on pp. 1353-1354). For patients who have atrial fibrillation, oral anticoagulants include warfarin and the direct factor Xa inhibitors: rivaroxaban (Xarelto), dabigatran (Pradaxa), and apixaban (Eliquis). Platelet inhibitors include aspirin, ticlopidine, clopidogrel, and dipyridamole. Additionally, the use of statins has been shown to be effective for the patient with an ischemic stroke.[7]

**Endovascular Therapy for Ischemic Stroke.** Stent retrievers (e.g., Solitaire FR) are a way of opening blocked arteries in the brain by using a removable stent system.[16] During the procedure, a catheter is used to guide the small stent from the femoral artery in the groin area to the affected artery in the brain. The stent is guided (using neuroimaging) into the part of the artery where a blood clot has formed. The stent expands the interior walls of the artery and allows blood to get to the patient's brain immediately to prevent as much brain damage as possible. The clot seeps into the mesh of the stent. Then, after a few minutes the stent and clot are removed together. Stent retrievers are becoming the most effective way of managing ischemic stroke.[16,17]

The ENROUTE device accesses the carotid arteries through the neck, rather than the groin. The ENROUTE uses a blood flow reversal system to capture pieces of the blockage dislodged during stenting procedures, while also maintaining blood flow to the brain.[18]

## Acute Care for Hemorrhagic Stroke

**Drug Therapy for Hemorrhagic Stroke.** Anticoagulants and platelet inhibitors are contraindicated in patients with hemorrhagic strokes. The main drug therapy for patients with hemorrhagic stroke is the management of hypertension. Oral and IV agents may be used to maintain BP within a normal to high-normal range (systolic BP less than 160 mm Hg). Seizure prophylaxis in the acute period after intracerebral and subarachnoid hemorrhages is situation specific and should be discussed with the interprofessional care team.[19]

**Surgical Therapy for Hemorrhagic Stroke.** Surgical interventions for hemorrhagic stroke include immediate evacuation of aneurysm-induced hematomas or cerebellar hematomas larger than 3 cm. Individuals who have an arteriovenous malformation (AVM) may experience a hemorrhagic stroke if the AVM ruptures. The treatment of AVM is surgical resection and/or radiosurgery (i.e., gamma knife). Both may be preceded by interventional neuroradiology to embolize the blood vessels that supply the AVM.

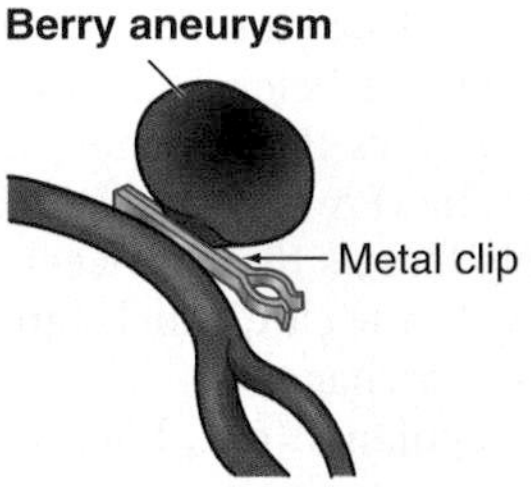


**FIG. 57-6** Clipping of aneurysms.

In a subarachnoid hemorrhage, bleeding from a damaged vessel causes blood to accumulate between the brain and skull. The leaked blood can irritate, damage, or destroy the surrounding brain cells. When blood enters the subarachnoid space, it mixes with the cerebrospinal fluid (CSF). This can block CSF circulation, thus causing increased pressure on the brain. The open spaces in the brain (ventricles) may enlarge, resulting in hydrocephalus. This further increases ICP (due to the large accumulation of blood) and can result in further brain injury. Insertion of a ventriculostomy for CSF drainage can dramatically improve these situations by reducing the ICP.[20] Goals for managing ICP are the same for patients with SAH as they are for patients dealing with acute stroke. (The management of ICP is discussed in Chapter 56.)

SAH is usually caused by a ruptured aneurysm. Patients may have multiple aneurysms. Treatment of an aneurysm involves clipping or coiling the aneurysm to prevent rebleeding (Figs. 57-6 and 57-7). In *clipping* the aneurysm, the neurosurgeon places a metallic clip on the neck of the aneurysm to block blood flow and prevent rupture. The clip remains in place for life.

In the procedure known as *coiling*, a hydrogel-coated platinum coil is inserted into the lumen of the aneurysm via interventional neuroradiology (Fig. 57-7). Guglielmi detachable coils (GDCs) provide immediate protection against hemorrhage by reducing the blood pulsations within the aneurysm. Eventually, a thrombus forms within the aneurysm. Then the aneurysm becomes sealed off from the parent vessel by the formation of an endothelialized layer of connective tissue.

After aneurysmal occlusion via clipping or coiling, hyperdynamic therapy (hemodilution-induced hypertension using vasoconstricting agents such as phenylephrine or dopamine and hypervolemia) may be instituted in an effort to increase the mean arterial pressure and increase cerebral perfusion. Volume expansion is achieved via crystalloid or colloid solution.

Interventions to treat cerebral vasospasm either before or after aneurysm clipping or coiling include administration of the calcium channel blocker nimodipine, which is given to patients with SAH to decrease the effects of vasospasm and minimize cerebral damage. Nimodipine restricts the influx of calcium ions into cells by reducing the number of open calcium channels. Although nimodipine is a calcium channel blocker, its exact mechanism of action in reducing vasospasm is not well understood.

**DRUG ALERT Nimodipine**
- Assess BP and apical pulses before administration.
- If pulse is ≤60 beats/min or systolic BP is <90 mm Hg, hold medication and contact physician.

## Rehabilitation Care

After the stroke patient has stabilized for 12 to 24 hours, interprofessional care shifts from preserving life to lessening disability and attaining optimal function. Many of the interventions discussed in the acute phase are maintained during this phase. The patient may be evaluated by a physiatrist (a physician who specializes in physical medicine and rehabilitation). Remember that some aspects of rehabilitation actually begin in the acute care phase as soon as the patient is stabilized. Specific measures related to rehabilitation are discussed in the section on Ambulatory Care on pp. 1362-1365.

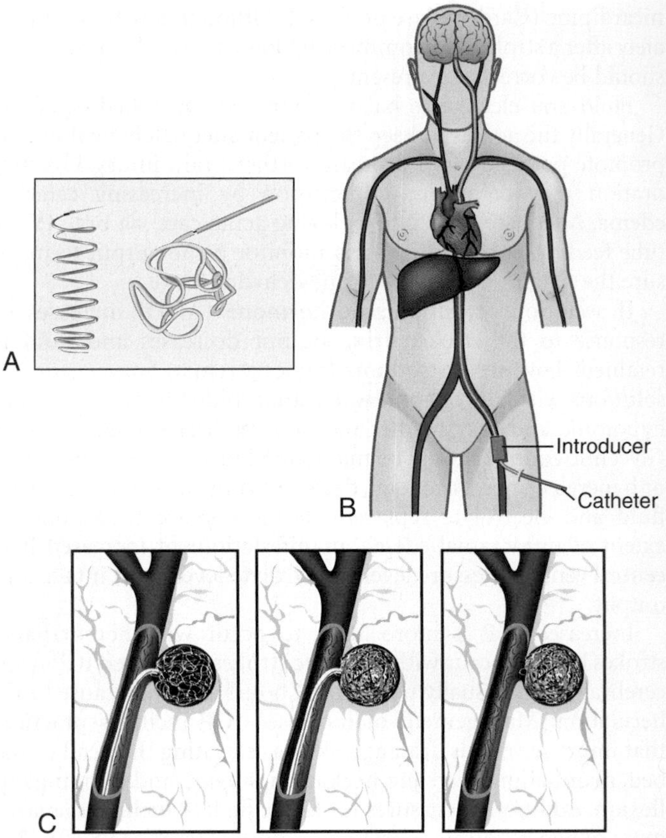


**FIG. 57-7** Guglielmi detachable coil (GDC). **A,** A coil is used to occlude an aneurysm. Coils are made of soft, springlike platinum. The softness of the platinum allows the coil to assume the shape of irregularly shaped aneurysms while posing little threat of rupture of the aneurysm. **B,** A catheter is inserted through an introducer (small tube) in an artery in the leg. The catheter is threaded up to the cerebral blood vessels. **C,** Platinum coils attached to a thin wire are inserted into the catheter and then placed in the aneurysm until the aneurysm is filled with coils. Packing the aneurysm with coils prevents the blood from circulating through the aneurysm, reducing the risk of rupture.

## Core Measures for Stroke

The stroke (STK) core measures (Table 57-8) were developed in partnership with the American Stroke Association (ASA) for use by primary stroke centers. These core measures are used by hospitals for accreditation and certification. Measures are implemented during the hospital admission and prior to discharge and align with guidelines supported by the AHA Get With The Guidelines (GWTG) stroke patient management tool and the Centers for Disease Control and Prevention (CDC) Paul Coverdell National Acute Stroke Registry (PCNASR).

# ❖ NURSING MANAGEMENT: STROKE

## ◆ Nursing Assessment

Subjective and objective data that should be obtained from a person who has had a stroke are presented in Table 57-9.

**TABLE 57-8 Stroke (STK) Core Measure Set**

| Measure | Topic |
|---|---|
| STK-1 | Venous thromboembolism (VTE) prophylaxis |
| STK-2 | Discharged on antithrombotic therapy |
| STK-3 | Anticoagulation therapy for atrial fibrillation/flutter |
| STK-4 | Thrombolytic therapy |
| STK-5 | Antithrombotic therapy by end of hospital day 2 |
| STK-6 | Discharged on statin medication |
| STK-8 | Stroke education |
| STK-10 | Assessed for rehabilitation |

Source: The Joint Commission. Stroke Core Measures. Retrieved from *www.jointcommission.org/stroke*.

Primary assessment focuses on cardiac and respiratory status and neurologic assessment. If the patient is stable, the nursing history is obtained as follows: (1) description of the current illness with attention to initial symptoms, particularly symptom onset and duration, nature (intermittent or continuous), and changes; (2) history of similar symptoms previously experienced; (3) current medications; (4) history of risk factors and other illnesses such as hypertension; and (5) family history of stroke, aneurysm, or cardiovascular diseases. This information is gained through an interview of the patient, caregiver, family members, and/or significant others.

Secondary assessment includes a comprehensive neurologic examination of the patient. This includes (1) level of consciousness, including assessment using the National Institutes of Health (NIH) Stroke Scale (NIHSS) (Table 57-10); (2) cognition; (3) motor abilities; (4) cranial nerve function; (5) sensation; (6) proprioception; (7) cerebellar function; and (8) deep tendon reflexes. Clear documentation of initial and ongoing neurologic examinations is essential to note changes in the patient's status.

## Nursing Diagnoses

Nursing diagnoses for the person with a stroke may include, but are not limited to

- Decreased intracranial adaptive capacity *related to* decreased cerebral perfusion pressure of ≤50 to 60 mm Hg and sustained increase in ICP secondary to thrombus, embolus, or hemorrhage
- Risk for aspiration *related to* decreased level of consciousness and decreased or absent gag and swallowing reflexes
- Impaired physical mobility *related to* neuromuscular and cognitive impairment and decreased muscle strength and control
- Impaired verbal communication *related to* aphasia
- Unilateral neglect *related to* visual field cut and loss on one side of body (hemianopsia) and brain injury from cerebrovascular problems
- Impaired swallowing *related to* weakness or paralysis of affected muscles
- Situational low self-esteem *related to* actual or perceived loss of function and altered body image

Additional information on nursing diagnoses are presented in eNursing Care Plan 57-1 (available on the website for this chapter).

## Planning

Establish the goals of nursing care together with the patient, caregiver, and family. Typical goals are that the patient will (1) maintain a stable or improved level of consciousness,

**TABLE 57-9 Nursing Assessment**

***Stroke***

**Subjective Data**

***Important Health Information***

*Past health history:* Hypertension. Previous stroke, TIA, aneurysm, cardiac disease (including recent myocardial infarction), dysrhythmias, heart failure, valvular heart disease, infective endocarditis. Hyperlipidemia, polycythemia, diabetes, gout. Previous head injury, family history of hypertension, diabetes, stroke, or coronary artery disease

*Family history:* Neurologic disorders, aneurysms, stroke, or transient ischemic attack (TIA)

*Medications:* Oral contraceptives; use of and compliance with antihypertensive and anticoagulant therapy; illegal substances and drug use (cocaine)

***Functional Health Patterns***

*Health perception–health management:* Positive family history of stroke. Alcohol abuse, smoking, drug abuse

*Nutritional-metabolic:* Anorexia, nausea, vomiting. Dysphagia, altered sense of taste and smell

*Elimination:* Change in bowel and bladder patterns

*Activity-exercise:* Loss of movement and sensation. Syncope, weakness on one side, generalized weakness, easy fatigability

*Cognitive-perceptual:* Numbness, tingling of one side of the body, loss of memory. Alteration in speech, language, problem-solving ability. Pain, headache (possibly sudden and severe) (hemorrhage). Visual disturbances. Denial of illness

**Objective Data**

***General***

Emotional lability, lethargy, apathy or combativeness, fever

***Respiratory***

Loss of cough reflex, labored or irregular respirations, tachypnea, wheezes (aspiration), airway occlusion (tongue), apnea, coughing when eating or delayed coughing

***Cardiovascular***

Hypertension, tachycardia, carotid bruit

***Gastrointestinal***

Loss of gag reflex, bowel incontinence, decreased or absent bowel sounds, constipation

***Urinary***

Frequency, urgency, incontinence

***Neurologic***

Contralateral motor and sensory deficits, including weakness, paresis, paralysis, anesthesia. Unequal pupils, hand grasps. Akinesia, aphasia (expressive, receptive, global), dysarthria (slurred speech), agnosias, apraxia, visual deficits, perceptual or spatial disturbances, altered level of consciousness (drowsiness to deep coma) and Babinski's sign, ↓ followed by ↑ deep tendon reflexes, flaccidity followed by spasticity, amnesia, ataxia, personality change, nuchal rigidity, seizures

***Possible Diagnostic Findings***

Positive CT, CTA, MRI, MRA, or other neuroimaging scans showing size, location, and type of lesion. Positive Doppler ultrasonography and angiography indicating stenosis

*CTA,* Computed tomographic angiography; *MRA,* magnetic resonance angiography; *TIA,* transient ischemic attack.

## TABLE 57-10 National Institutes of Health Stroke Scale (NIHSS)

**Description**

The National Institutes of Health Stroke Scale (NIHSS) is a 15-item neurologic examination used to evaluate the effect of an acute stroke. Total scores on the NIHSS range from 0-42, with higher values reflecting more severity.

**Procedure for Use**

A trained observer rates the patient's ability to answer questions and perform activities. Ratings for each item are scored and there is an allowance for untestable (UN) items. If an item is left untested, a detailed explanation must be clearly written on the form. Training can be completed free at *www.nihstrokescale.org.*

| Item | Scale Definition |
|---|---|
| **Level of consciousness** | 0 = Alert<br>1 = Not alert, but arousable by minor stimulation<br>2 = Not alert, requires repeated stimulation to get attention<br>3 = Responds only with reflex motor or autonomic effects or totally unresponsive, flaccid, areflexic |
| **Level of consciousness questions** | 0 = Answers both questions correctly<br>1 = Answers one question correctly<br>2 = Answers neither question correctly |
| **Level of consciousness commands** | 0 = Performs both tasks correctly<br>1 = Performs one task correctly<br>2 = Performs neither task correctly |
| **Best gaze** | 0 = Normal<br>1 = Partial gaze palsy<br>2 = Forced deviation, or total gaze paresis |
| **Visual** | 0 = No visual loss<br>1 = Partial hemianopsia<br>2 = Complete hemianopsia<br>3 = Bilateral hemianopsia or blind |
| **Facial palsy** | 0 = Normal symmetric movement<br>1 = Minor paralysis<br>2 = Partial paralysis<br>3 = Complete paralysis of one or both sides |
| **Motor and drift (for each extremity)** | 0 = No drift<br>1 = Drift<br>2 = Some effort against gravity<br>3 = No effort against gravity, limb falls<br>4 = No movement<br>UN = Amputation |
| **Limb ataxia** | 0 = Absent<br>1 = Present in one limb<br>2 = Present in two limbs |
| **Sensory** | 0 = Normal<br>1 = Mild to moderate sensory loss<br>2 = Severe to total sensory loss |
| **Best language** | 0 = No aphasia, normal<br>1 = Mild to moderate aphasia<br>2 = Severe aphasia<br>3 = Mute, no usable speech or auditory comprehension |
| **Dysarthria** | 0 = Normal<br>1 = Mild to moderate<br>2 = Severe<br>UN = Intubated or other physical barrier |
| **Extinction or inattention** | 0 = No abnormality<br>1 = Inattention or extinction to bilateral stimulation<br>2 = Does not recognize own hand |
| **Distal motor function** | 0 = Normal (no flexion after 5 sec)<br>1 = At least some extension but not fully extended<br>2 = No voluntary extension after 5 sec |

Source: American Stroke Association: NIH stroke scale, 2009. Retrieved from *www.ninds.nih.gov/doctors/NIH_Stroke_Scale.pdf.*

(2) attain maximum physical functioning, (3) attain maximum self-care abilities and skills, (4) maintain stable body functions (e.g., bladder control), (5) maximize communication abilities, (6) maintain adequate nutrition, (7) avoid complications of stroke, and (8) maintain effective personal and family coping.

## Nursing Implementation

**Health Promotion.** You have a major role in the promotion of a healthy lifestyle. Teaching should focus on stroke prevention, particularly for persons with known risk factors. As previously mentioned, most strokes are caused by modifiable risk factors. Nursing measures to reduce risk factors for stroke are similar to those for coronary artery disease (see Chapter 33, Table 33-2) and are discussed earlier in this chapter on pp. 1346-1348.

Uncontrolled or undiagnosed hypertension is the primary cause of stroke. Therefore you need to be involved in BP screening and ensuring that patients adhere to the use of their antihypertensive medications and home monitoring of BP. If a person is a diabetic, it is important that the diabetes is well controlled. If an individual has atrial fibrillation, an anticoagulant (see p. 1347) or aspirin may be used to reduce the risk of stroke. Because smoking is a major risk factor for stroke, you need to be actively involved in helping patients to stop smoking (see Chapter 10, Tables 10-4 to 10-6).

Another important aspect of health promotion is teaching patients and families about early symptoms associated with stroke or TIA. Table 57-1 presents information on when to seek health care for these symptoms.

### Acute Care

***Respiratory System.*** During the acute phase after a stroke, management of the respiratory system is a nursing priority.[21] Stroke patients are particularly vulnerable to respiratory problems. Advancing age and immobility increase the risk for atelectasis and pneumonia.

Risk for aspiration pneumonia is high because of impaired consciousness or dysphagia. Dysphagia after stroke is common. Airway obstruction can occur because of problems with chewing and swallowing, food pocketing (food remaining in the buccal cavity of the mouth), and the tongue falling back. Some stroke patients, especially those with brainstem or hemorrhagic stroke, may require endotracheal intubation and mechanical ventilation initially. Enteral tube feedings also place the patient at risk for aspiration pneumonia. All patients should be screened for their ability to swallow and kept on nothing-by-mouth (NPO) status until dysphagia has been ruled out.

Nursing interventions to support adequate respiratory function are individualized to meet the patient's needs. An oropharyngeal airway may be used in comatose patients to prevent the tongue from falling back and obstructing the airway and to provide access for suctioning. Alternatively, a nasopharyngeal airway may be used to provide airway protection and access. When an artificial airway is required for a prolonged time, a tracheostomy may be performed.

Nursing interventions include frequently assessing airway patency and function, providing oxygenation, suctioning, promoting patient mobility, positioning the patient to prevent aspiration, and encouraging deep breathing. In patients who are on mechanical ventilation, oral care at least every 2 hours reduces the occurrence of ventilator-assisted pneumonia.[21]

Patients who have an unclipped or uncoiled aneurysm may experience rebleeding and the possibility of increasing ICP further with coughing or suctioning, so nursing management is aimed at reducing these interventions while maintaining a proper airway.

Interventions related to maintenance of airway function are described in eNursing Care Plan 57-1.

***Neurologic System.*** The primary clinical assessment tool to evaluate and document neurologic status in acute stroke patients is the NIH Stroke Scale (NIHSS), which measures stroke severity[22] (Table 57-10). The NIHSS is a predictor of both short- and long-term outcomes of stroke patients. Additionally, it serves as a data collection tool for planning patient care and exchanging information among HCPs.

Additional neurologic assessment includes mental status, pupillary responses, and extremity movement and strength. Also closely monitor vital signs. A decreasing level of consciousness may indicate increasing ICP. Monitor ICP and cerebral perfusion pressure if the patient is in a critical care environment. Record your nursing assessment on flowsheets to communicate the patient's neurologic status to the stroke team.

***Cardiovascular System.*** Nursing goals for the cardiovascular system are aimed at maintaining homeostasis. Many patients with stroke have decreased cardiac reserves secondary to cardiac disease. Cardiac efficiency may be further compromised by fluid retention, overhydration, dehydration, or BP variations. Central venous pressure, pulmonary artery pressure, or hemodynamic monitoring may be used as indicators of fluid balance or cardiac function in the critical care unit.

Nursing interventions include (1) monitoring vital signs frequently; (2) monitoring cardiac rhythms; (3) calculating intake and output, noting imbalances; (4) regulating IV infusions; (5) adjusting fluid intake to individual patient needs; (6) monitoring lung sounds for crackles and wheezes, indicating pulmonary congestion; and (7) monitoring heart sounds for murmurs. Bedside monitors or telemetry may record cardiac rhythms.

Hypertension is sometimes seen after a stroke as the body attempts to increase cerebral blood flow. It is also important to monitor for orthostatic hypotension before ambulating the patient for the first time. Neurologic changes can occur with a sudden decrease in BP.

After a stroke, the patient is at risk for venous thromboembolism (VTE), especially in the weak or paralyzed lower extremity. VTE is related to immobility, loss of venous tone, and decreased muscle pumping activity in the leg. The most effective prevention is to keep the patient moving. Teach the patient active range-of-motion exercises if the patient has voluntary movement in the affected extremity. For the patient with hemiplegia, perform passive range-of-motion exercises several times a day. Additional measures to prevent VTE include positioning to minimize the effects of dependent edema and using sequential compression devices for bedridden patients. VTE prophylaxis may include low-molecular-weight heparin (e.g., enoxaparin [Lovenox]). The nursing assessment for VTE includes measuring the calf and thigh daily, observing for swelling of the lower extremities, noting unusual warmth of the leg, and asking the patient about pain in the calf.[23]

***Musculoskeletal System.*** The nursing goal for the musculoskeletal system is to maintain optimal function by preventing joint contractures and muscular atrophy. In the acute phase, range-of-motion exercises and positioning are important nursing interventions. Passive range-of-motion exercise is begun on the first day of hospitalization. Muscle atrophy secondary to lack of innervation and activity can develop after stroke, so exercise is an important intervention for rehabilitation and recovery.

The paralyzed or weak side requires special attention when the patient is positioned. Position each joint higher than the joint proximal to it to prevent dependent edema. Specific deformities on the weak or paralyzed side that may be present in patients with stroke include internal rotation of the shoulder; flexion contractures of the hand, wrist, and elbow; external rotation of the hip; and plantar flexion of the foot. Subluxation of the shoulder on the affected side is common. Careful positioning and moving of the affected arm may prevent development of a painful shoulder condition. Immobilization of the affected upper extremity may precipitate a painful shoulder-hand syndrome.

Nursing interventions to optimize musculoskeletal function include (1) trochanter roll at the hip to prevent external

## TEAMWORK & COLLABORATION

### *Caring for the Patient With an Acute Stroke*

During the first 48 hr after an acute stroke, some nursing activities may be delegated to licensed practical/vocational nurses (LPNs/LVNs) and unlicensed assistive personnel (UAP). The registered nurse (RN) should communicate frequently with these staff members to rapidly intervene based on changes in the patient status.

**Role of Nursing Personnel**

***Registered Nurse (RN)***

- Assess clinical manifestations of stroke and determine when clinical manifestations started.
- Screen patient for contraindications for tissue plasminogen activator (tPA) therapy.
- Infuse tPA for patients with ischemic stroke who meet the criteria for tPA administration.
- Assess respiratory status and initiate needed actions such as $O_2$, oropharyngeal or nasopharyngeal airways, suctioning, and patient positioning to prevent aspiration, obstruction, and atelectasis.
- Assess neurologic status, including intracranial pressure (ICP), if needed.
- Monitor cardiovascular status, including hemodynamic monitoring, if needed.
- Assess patient's ability to swallow (in conjunction with the speech therapist).

***Licensed Practical/Vocational Nurse (LPN/LVN)***

- Administer scheduled anticoagulant and antiplatelet medications.

***Unlicensed Assistive Personnel (UAP)***

- Obtain vital signs frequently and report these to RN.
- Measure and record urine output.
- Assist with positioning patient and turning patient at least every 2 hr (as directed by RN).
- Perform passive and active range-of-motion exercises (after being trained and evaluated in these procedures).
- Place equipment needed for seizure precautions in patient room.

**Role of Other Team Members**

***Speech Therapy***

- Assess swallowing reflex.
- Evaluate patient for communication defects (e.g., aphasia).

***Physical Therapy***

- Position patient in a functional position.
- Assess function and together with patient, plan a rehabilitation program.

rotation; (2) hand cones (not rolled washcloths) to prevent hand contractures; (3) arm supports with slings and lap boards to prevent shoulder displacement; (4) avoidance of pulling the patient by the arm to avoid shoulder displacement; (5) posterior leg splints, footboards, or high-top tennis shoes to prevent footdrop; and (6) hand splints to reduce spasticity.

Use of a footboard for the patient with spasticity is controversial. Rather than preventing plantar flexion (footdrop), the sensory stimulation of a footboard against the bottom of the foot increases plantar flexion. Likewise, experts disagree on whether hand splints facilitate or diminish spasticity. The decision regarding the use of footboards or hand splints is made on an individual patient basis.

◆ ***Integumentary System.*** The skin of the patient with stroke is particularly susceptible to breakdown related to loss of sensation, decreased circulation, and immobility. This is compounded by advanced age, poor nutrition, dehydration, edema, and incontinence.

The nursing plan for prevention of skin breakdown includes (1) pressure relief by position changes, special mattresses, or wheelchair cushions; (2) good skin hygiene; (3) emollients applied to dry skin; and (4) early mobility. An example of a position change schedule is side-back-side, with a maximum duration of 2 hours for any position. Position the patient on the weak or paralyzed side for only 30 minutes. If an area of redness develops and does not return to normal color within 15 minutes of pressure relief, the epidermis and dermis are damaged.

Do not massage the damaged area because this may cause additional damage. Control of pressure is the single most important factor in both the prevention and treatment of skin breakdown. Pillows can be used under lower extremities to reduce pressure on the heels. Vigilance and good nursing care are required to prevent pressure sores.

◆ ***Gastrointestinal System.*** The most common bowel problem for the stroke patient is constipation. Patients may be prophylactically placed on stool softeners and/or fiber (psyllium [Metamucil]). If a patient has liquid stools, check for stool impaction. Fluid and fiber intake goals should be discussed with the stroke team and are based on the patient's nutritional and fluid status.

Physical activity also promotes bowel function. Laxatives, suppositories, or additional stool softeners may be ordered if the patient does not respond to increased fluid and fiber. Enemas are used only if suppositories and digital stimulation are ineffective because they cause vagal stimulation and increase ICP.

Bowel retraining may be needed and continues into the rehabilitation phase. A bowel management program consists of placing the patient on the bedpan or bedside commode or taking the patient to the bathroom at a regular time daily to reestablish bowel regularity. A good time for the bowel program is 30 minutes after breakfast because eating stimulates the gastrocolic reflex and peristalsis, but timing may have to be adjusted, since individual bowel habits may vary.

◆ ***Urinary System.*** In the acute stage of stroke, the primary urinary problem is poor bladder control, resulting in incontinence. Take steps to promote normal bladder function and avoid the use of indwelling catheters. If an indwelling catheter must be used initially, remove it as soon as the patient is medically and neurologically stable. Long-term use of an indwelling catheter is associated with urinary tract infections and delayed bladder retraining.

Avoid bladder overdistention. An intermittent catheterization program may be used for patients with urinary retention because of the lower incidence of urinary infections. An alternative to intermittent catheterizations is the external catheter for male patients with urinary incontinence. External catheters do not alleviate the problem of urine retention.

Assist the patient with urinary difficulties or incontinence. Often the patient with stroke has functional incontinence, which is associated with communication difficulties, mobility problems, and dressing or undressing difficulties. A bladder retraining program consists of (1) adequate fluid intake with most of it given between 7:00 AM and 7:00 PM; (2) scheduled toileting every 2 hours using bedpan, commode, or bathroom while encouraging the usual position for urinating (standing for men and sitting for women); (3) observation for signs of restlessness, which may indicate the need for urination; and (4) assessment for bladder distention by palpation. Encourage patients to wear pants without drawstrings, buttons, or zippers, as these can be difficult to manage if motor or sensory deficits exist.

Assessment of postvoid residual volume is often done using bladder ultrasound. The ultrasound measures how much urine is in the bladder after voiding. If urine remains in the bladder, incomplete emptying is a problem and may cause urinary tract infections. A coordinated program by the entire nursing staff is needed to achieve urinary continence.

◆ ***Nutrition.*** The patient's nutritional needs require quick assessment and treatment. The patient may initially receive IV infusions to maintain fluid and electrolyte balance and to administer drugs. Patients with severe impairment may require enteral or parenteral nutrition support. Patients should have their nutritional needs addressed in the first 24 hours of admission to the hospital because nutrition is important for recovery and healing.[24]

**! SAFETY ALERT Oral Feeding After Stroke**

- The gag reflex may be impaired due to dysphagia and must be assessed.
- Therefore the first oral feeding should be carefully planned.

Speech therapists (if available) should perform a swallowing evaluation before a patient's oral intake is initiated. The majority of patients experience dysphagia after a stroke.[24] Before initiating feeding, assess the gag reflex by gently stimulating the back of the throat with a tongue blade. If a gag reflex is present, the patient will gag spontaneously. If it is absent, defer the feeding, and begin exercises to stimulate swallowing. The speech therapist or occupational therapist is usually responsible for designing this program. However, you may be involved in helping to develop the program in some clinical settings.

To assess swallowing ability, elevate the head of the bed to an upright position (unless contraindicated) and give the patient a small amount of crushed ice or ice water to swallow. If the gag reflex is present and the patient is able to swallow safely, you may proceed with feeding.

After careful assessment of swallowing, chewing, gag reflex, and pocketing, oral feedings can be initiated. Mouth care before feeding helps stimulate sensory awareness and salivation and can facilitate swallowing. The patient should remain in a high Fowler's position, preferably in a chair with the head flexed forward, for the feeding and for 30 minutes afterward.

The speech therapist may recommend various dietary items. Foods should be easy to swallow and provide enough texture,

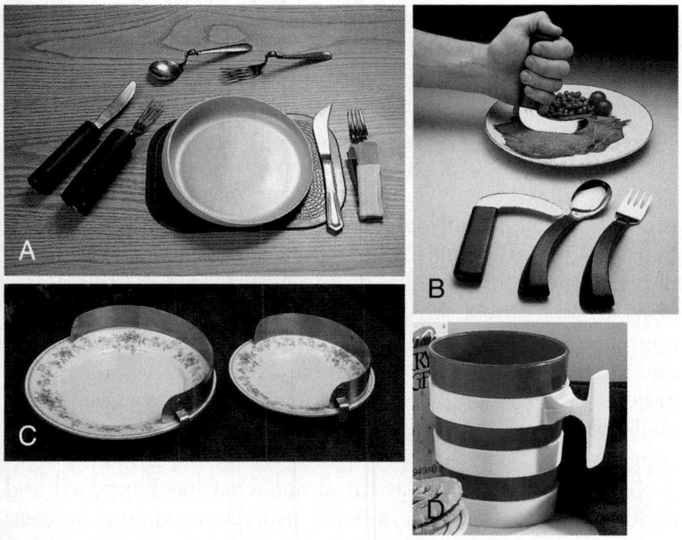


**FIG. 57-8** Assistive devices for eating. **A,** The curved fork fits over the hand. The rounded plate helps keep food on the plate. Special grips and swivel handles are helpful for some persons. **B,** Knives with rounded blades are rocked back and forth to cut food. The person does not need a fork in one hand and a knife in the other. **C,** Plate guards help keep food on the plate. **D,** Cup with special handle. (Courtesy Sammons Preston, Bolingbrook, Ill.)

temperature (warm or cold), and flavor to stimulate a swallow reflex. Crushed ice can be used as a stimulant. Instruct the patient to swallow and then swallow again. Pureed foods are not usually the best choice because they are often bland and too smooth. Thin liquids are often difficult to swallow and may promote coughing. Thin liquids can be thickened with a commercially available thickening agent (e.g., Thick-It). Avoid milk products because they tend to increase the viscosity of mucus and increase salivation.

Place food on the unaffected side of the mouth. Feedings must be followed by scrupulous oral hygiene because food may collect on the affected side of the mouth. During the acute and rehabilitation phase of the stroke, a dietitian can assist in determining the appropriate daily caloric intake based on the patient's size, weight, and activity level. If the patient is unable to take in an adequate oral diet and dysphagia persists, a percutaneous endoscopic gastrostomy (PEG) tube (see Chapter 39, Fig. 39-7) may be used for nutritional support. Most commercially prepared formulas provide about 1 cal/mL. (Enteral feedings are described in Chapter 39.)

The inability to feed oneself can be frustrating and may result in malnutrition and dehydration. Interventions to promote self-feeding include using the unaffected upper extremity to eat; employing assistive devices such as rocker knives, plate guards, and nonslip pads for dishes (Fig. 57-8); removing unnecessary items from the tray or table, which can reduce spills; and providing a calm environment (e.g., turn off the television) to decrease sensory overload and distraction. The effectiveness of the dietary program is evaluated in terms of maintenance of weight, adequate hydration, and patient satisfaction. Introduce these interventions in the acute care setting so that maximum rehabilitation can occur once the patient is discharged.

◆ ***Communication.*** During the acute stage of stroke, your role in meeting the patient's psychologic needs is primarily supportive. Speech, comprehension, and language deficits are the most difficult problems for the patient and caregiver. Assess the patient for both the ability to speak and the ability to understand. The patient's response to simple questions can guide you in structuring explanations and instructions. If the patient cannot understand words, use gestures to support verbal cues. Collaborate with the speech therapist to assess and formulate a plan of care to enhance communication.

**TABLE 57-11 Communication With a Patient With Aphasia**

*The following are guidelines for communicating with a patient with aphasia.*

1. Decrease environmental stimuli that may be distracting and disrupting to communication efforts.
2. Treat the patient as an adult.
3. Speak with normal volume and tone.
4. Present one thought or idea at a time.
5. Keep questions simple or ask questions that can be answered with "yes" or "no."
6. Let the person speak. Do not interrupt. Allow time for the individual to complete thoughts.
7. Make use of gestures or demonstration as an acceptable alternative form of communication. Encourage this by saying, "Show me ..." or "Point to what you want."
8. Do not pretend to understand the person if you do not. Calmly say you do not understand and encourage the use of nonverbal communication, or ask the person to write out what he or she wants.
9. Give the patient time to process information and generate a response before repeating a question or statement.
10. Allow body contact (e.g., clasp of a hand, touching) as much as possible. Realize that touching may be the only way the patient can express feelings.
11. Organize the patient's day by preparing and following a schedule (the more familiar the routine, the easier it will be).
12. Do not push communication if the person is tired or upset. Aphasia worsens with fatigue and anxiety.
13. Teach communication techniques to caregiver and family members.

Nursing interventions that support communication include (1) communicating frequently and meaningfully; (2) allowing time for the patient to comprehend and answer; (3) using simple, short sentences; (4) using visual cues; (5) structuring conversation so that it permits simple answers by the patient; and (6) praising the patient honestly for improvements with speech.[25]

An alert patient is usually anxious because of lack of understanding about what has happened and because of difficulty with communication or inability to communicate. The stroke patient with aphasia may easily be overwhelmed by verbal stimuli. Give the patient extra time to comprehend and respond to communication. (Guidelines for communicating with a patient who has aphasia are presented in Table 57-11.) A picture board may be helpful for communicating with the stroke patient. Further evaluation and treatment of language and communication deficits are often done by the speech therapist once the patient has stabilized. It is also important to teach the caregiver and family these communication strategies.

◆ ***Sensory-Perceptual Alterations.*** Patients who have had a stroke frequently have perceptual deficits. Patients with a stroke on the right side of the brain usually have difficulty judging position, distance, and rate of movement. These patients are often impulsive and impatient and tend to deny problems related to strokes. They may fail to correlate spatial-perceptual problems with the inability to perform activities, such as guiding a wheelchair through the doorway. The patient with a right-brain stroke (left hemiplegia) is at higher risk for injury because

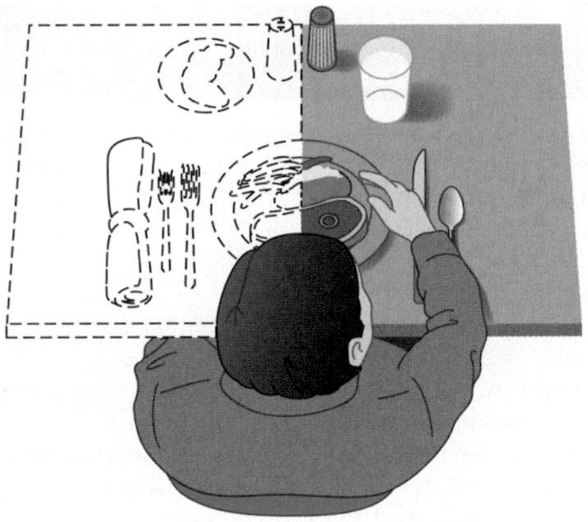

**FIG. 57-9** Spatial and perceptual deficits in stroke. Perception of a patient with homonymous hemianopsia shows that food on the left side is not seen and thus is ignored. (Modified from Hoeman SP: *Rehabilitation nursing,* ed 2, St Louis, 1995, Mosby.)

of mobility difficulties. Directions for activities are best given verbally for comprehension. Break the task down into simple steps for ease of understanding. Environmental control, such as removing clutter and obstacles and using good lighting, aids in concentration and safer mobility. Provide nonslip socks at all times. One-sided neglect is common for people with right-brain stroke, so you may assist or remind the patient to dress the weak or paralyzed side or shave the forgotten side of the face.

Patients with a left-brain stroke (right hemiplegia) commonly are slower in organization and performance of tasks. They tend to have impaired spatial discrimination. These patients usually admit to deficits and have a fearful, anxious response to a stroke. Their behaviors are slow and cautious. Nonverbal cues and instructions are helpful for comprehension with patients who have had a left-brain stroke.

*Homonymous hemianopsia* (blindness in the same half of each visual field) is a common problem after a stroke. Persistent disregard of objects in part of the visual field should alert you to this possibility. Initially, help the patient to compensate by arranging the environment within the patient's perceptual field, such as arranging the food tray so that all foods are on the right side or the left side to accommodate for field of vision (Fig. 57-9). Later, the patient learns to compensate for the visual defect by consciously attending or by scanning the neglected side. The weak or paralyzed extremities are carefully checked for adequacy of dressing, hygiene, and trauma.

In the clinical situation, it is often difficult to distinguish between a visual field cut and a neglect syndrome. Both problems may occur with strokes affecting either the right or the left side of the brain. A person may be unfortunate enough to have both homonymous hemianopsia and a neglect syndrome, which increases the inattention to the weak or paralyzed side. A neglect syndrome results in decreased safety awareness and places the patient at high risk for injury. Immediately after the stroke, anticipate safety hazards and provide protection from injury. Safety measures can include closely observing the patient, elevating side rails, lowering the height of the bed, and using video monitors. Avoid the use of restraints and soft vests because this may agitate the patient.

Other visual problems may include *diplopia* (double vision), loss of the corneal reflex, and *ptosis* (drooping eyelid), especially if the stroke is in the vertebrobasilar distribution. Diplopia is often treated with an eye patch. If the corneal reflex is absent, the patient is at risk for corneal abrasion and should be observed closely and protected against eye injuries. Corneal abrasion can be prevented with artificial tears or gel to keep the eyes moist and an eye shield (especially at night). Ptosis is generally not treated because it usually does not inhibit vision.

◆ ***Coping.*** A stroke is usually a sudden, extremely stressful event for the patient, caregiver, family, and significant others. A stroke is often a family disease, affecting the family emotionally, socially, and financially and changing roles and responsibilities within the family. The stroke patient and family may perceive the stroke as a threat to life and to accustomed lifestyle. Reactions to this threat vary considerably but may involve fear, apprehension, denial of the severity of stroke, depression, anger, and sorrow. During the acute phase of caring for the stroke patient, caregiver, and family, nursing interventions designed to facilitate coping involve providing information and emotional support.

Explanations to the patient about what has happened and about diagnostic and therapeutic procedures should be clear and understandable, with reinforcement as needed. Decision making and upholding the patient's wishes during this challenging time are of upmost importance. Advance directives should be honored, and family meetings or updates should be held daily about feeding tube placement or tracheostomy.

Give the caregiver and family a careful, detailed explanation of what has happened to the patient. However, if the family is extremely anxious and upset during the acute phase, explanations may have to be repeated at a later time. Because family members usually have not had time to prepare for the illness, they may need assistance in arranging care for family members or pets and for transportation and finances. A social services referral is often helpful.

It is particularly challenging to keep the patient with aphasia adequately informed. Use demeanor and touch to convey support. When communicating with a patient who has a communication deficit, speak in a normal volume and tone, keep questions simple, and present one thought or idea at a time. To decrease frustration, always let the patient speak without interruption and make use of gestures. Do not forget to use writing and communication boards.[25]

◆ **Ambulatory Care.** The patient is usually discharged from the acute care setting to home, an intermediate- or long-term care facility, or a rehabilitation facility. Ideally, discharge planning with the patient and caregiver starts early in the hospitalization and promotes a smooth transition from one care setting to another. The stroke team provides guidance for the appropriate care necessary after discharge. If the patient requires a short- or long-term health care facility, the team can make appropriate referrals that allow time to select and arrange for care. A critical factor in discharge planning is the patient's level of independence in performing ADLs.[26] If the patient is returning home, the team can make referrals for needed equipment and services in preparation for discharge.

You have an excellent opportunity to prepare the patient and caregiver for discharge through teaching, demonstration and return demonstration, practice, and evaluation of self-care skills. Total care is considered in discharge planning: medications, nutrition, mobility, exercises, hygiene, and toileting. Follow-up care is carefully planned to permit continuing nursing care; physical, occupational, and speech therapy; and medical care. Identify community resources to provide recreational activities, group support, spiritual assistance, respite care, adult day care, and home assistance based on the patient's needs.

**Rehabilitation.** *Rehabilitation* is the process of maximizing the patient's capabilities and resources to promote optimal functioning related to physical, mental, and social well-being. The goals of rehabilitation are to prevent deformity and maintain and improve function. Regardless of the care setting, ongoing rehabilitation is essential to maximize the patient's abilities. Most patients recover in the first 6 months following a stroke, with maximum benefit 1 year after a stroke.[1]

Rehabilitation requires a team approach so that the patient and caregiver can benefit from the combined, expert care of a stroke interprofessional team. The team must communicate and coordinate care to achieve the patient's goals. As a nurse, you are in a good position to facilitate this process and are often the key to successful rehabilitation efforts. The stroke interprofessional team is composed of many members, including nurses, physicians, psychiatrist, physical therapist, occupational therapist, speech therapist, registered dietitian, respiratory therapist, vocational therapist, recreational therapist, social worker, psychologist, pharmacist, and chaplain.

Physical therapy focuses on mobility, progressive ambulation, transfer techniques, and equipment needed for mobility. Occupational therapy emphasizes retraining for skills of daily living such as eating, dressing, hygiene, and cooking. Occupational therapists are also skilled in cognitive and perceptual evaluation and training. Speech therapy focuses on speech, communication, cognition, and eating abilities.

## INFORMATICS IN PRACTICE

### *Video Games for Stroke Recovery*

- Patients dealing with the effects of a stroke often have difficulty performing activities of daily living.
- Playing active video games, such as Nintendo Wii or Xbox Kinect, brings some fun into stroke recovery and may get patients to spend more time in therapy.
- Gaming helps patients regain lost strength, improve motor skills, and improve problem solving and short- and long-term memory.
- Patients can play with their families, including children, making gaming a way to involve others in rehabilitation.

Many of the nursing interventions outlined in eNursing Care Plan 57-1 for the patient with a stroke are initiated in the acute phase of care and continue throughout rehabilitation. Some of the interventions are independent nursing actions, whereas others involve the entire team.

The rehabilitation nurse assesses the patient, caregiver, and family with attention to the (1) patient's rehabilitation potential, (2) physical status of all body systems, (3) complications caused by the stroke or other chronic conditions, (4) patient's cognitive status, (5) family resources and support, and (6) expectations of the patient and caregiver related to the rehabilitation program.

**Musculoskeletal Function.** Initially emphasize the musculoskeletal functions of eating, toileting, and walking for rehabilitation of the patient. Initial assessment consists of determining the stage of recovery of muscle function. If the muscles are still flaccid several weeks after the stroke, the prognosis for regaining function is poor, and care focuses on preventing additional loss (Fig. 57-10).

Most patients begin to show signs of spasticity with exaggerated reflexes within 48 hours after the stroke. Spasticity at this phase of stroke denotes progress toward recovery. As improvement continues, small voluntary movements of the hip or shoulder may be accompanied by involuntary movements in the rest of the extremity *(synergy)*. The final stage of recovery occurs when the patient has voluntary control of isolated muscle groups.

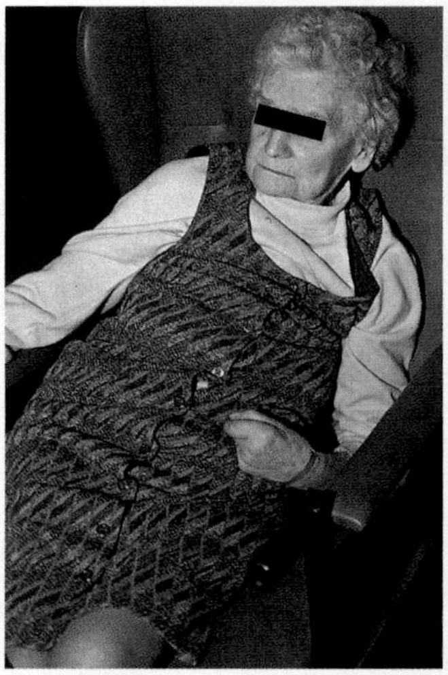

**FIG. 57-10** Loss of postural stability is common after stroke. When the nondominant hemisphere is involved, walking apraxia and loss of postural control are usually apparent. The patient is unable to sit upright and tends to fall sideways. Provide appropriate support with pillows or cushions. (From Forbes CD, Jackson WF: *Colour atlas and text of clinical medicine,* ed 3, London, 2003, Mosby.)

## EVIDENCE-BASED PRACTICE

### *Applying the Evidence*

**Virtual Reality and Stroke**

You are a nurse working in an outpatient rehabilitation facility with C.W., a 70-yr-old female who was diagnosed with a stroke 3 months ago. You note she has right-sided weakness, especially in her arm. She tells you that she cannot write very well or use a computer, and she misses e-mailing her friends and family since her stroke.

***Making Clinical Decisions***

***Best Available Evidence.*** Virtual reality and interactive video gaming may improve upper limb mobility and daily functioning in patients undergoing rehabilitation for stroke.

***Clinician Expertise.*** You know the therapeutic use of interactive video games in rehabilitation helps patients to move the unaffected hand with the assistance of virtual mirror feedback. You also note the benefit of virtual reality for practicing daily tasks that may currently be unsafe in the home, such as showering and dressing.

***Patient Preferences and Values.*** C.W. says, "It will be fun to play video games while I rehab."

***Implications for Nursing Practice***

1. What parameters will you use to assess C.W.'s progression with the virtual reality intervention?
2. Why is it important for you to determine with C.W. if virtual training translates into the actual performance of activities at home?
3. As you coordinate her rehabilitation care, how will you facilitate communication among interprofessional team members?

***Reference for Evidence***

Laver KE, George S, Thomas S, et al: Virtual reality for stroke rehabilitation, *Cochrane Database Syst Rev* 2:CD008349, 2015.

Interventions for the musculoskeletal system advance in a manner of progressive activity. Balance training is the initial step and begins with the patient sitting up in bed or dangling the legs over the edge of the bed. Evaluate tolerance by noting dizziness or syncope caused by vasomotor instability.

## EVIDENCE-BASED PRACTICE

### *Applying the Evidence*

#### Walking and Stroke

You are a nurse caring for S.F., a 68-yr-old male who had a stroke 7 months ago. S.F. is unhappy that he is not able to perform activities on his own because of difficulties with physical mobility. You note his gait remains unsteady when walking with assistance from his wife who is his caregiver. He tells you a physical therapist is coming to his home but not on a regular basis.

#### *Making Clinical Decisions*

***Best Available Evidence.*** In the chronic stage of stroke (>6 months after stroke), high-frequency walking training can increase walking capacity including speed and walking distance. Training frequency should be at least 24 sessions over 7 weeks for effective improvements in walking.

***Clinician Expertise.*** You know a consistent walking program is an important part of rehabilitation following stroke. You also know improvements in physical mobility reach their maximum potential in the first year following stroke.

***Patient Preferences and Values.*** S.F. has a goal of being able to walk independently in the next 6 months.

#### *Implications for Nursing Practice*

1. In what ways will you collaborate with physical therapy to monitor the progress of S.F. in meeting his goal?
2. How will you determine S.F.'s motivation to stay engaged in a consistent supervised walking program?
3. Why is it important to assess caregiver needs and coping at every patient visit, and how will you assist in providing caregiver resources?

#### *Reference for Evidence*

Peurala S, Karttunen A, Sjögren T, et al: Evidence for the effectiveness of walking training on walking and self-care after stroke: A systematic review and meta-analysis of randomized controlled trials, *J Rehabil Med* 46:387, 2014.

Also assess whether patients autocorrect their posture when sitting on the edge of the bed. If the patient can straighten his or her posture instead of leaning to the weaker side, the patient may be ready for the next step of transferring from bed to chair. Place the chair beside the bed so that the patient can lead with the stronger arm and leg. The patient sits on the side of the bed, stands, places the strong hand on the far wheelchair arm, and sits down. You may either supervise the transfer or provide minimal assistance by guiding the patient's strong hand to the wheelchair arm, standing in front of the patient while blocking the patient's knees with your knees to prevent knee buckling, and guiding the patient into a sitting position.

In some rehabilitation units, the Bobath method is used as an approach to mobility *(http://ibita.org)*. The goal of this approach is to help the patient gain control over patterns of spasticity by inhibiting abnormal reflex patterns. Therapists and nurses use the Bobath approach to encourage normal muscle tone, normal movement, and bilateral function of the body. An example is to have the patient transfer into the wheelchair using the weak or paralyzed side and the stronger side to facilitate more bilateral functioning.

Another approach to stroke rehabilitation is *constraint-induced movement therapy* (CIMT). CIMT encourages the patient to use the weakened extremity by restricting movement of the normal extremity. Complying with this approach can be challenging for patients and may limit its use. Movement training, skill acquisition, splinting, and exercise are additional therapies offered for rehabilitation of the stroke patient.[27]

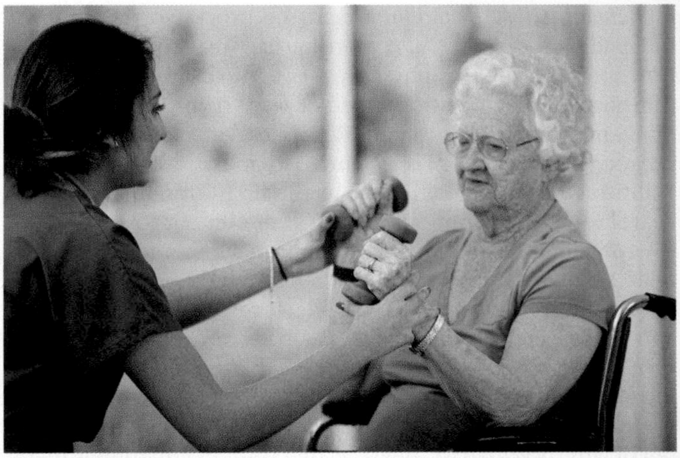

**FIG. 57-11** A patient who had a stroke works with a physical therapist to improve arm strength. (©Thinkstock 78783452)

Supportive or assistive equipment, such as canes, walkers, and leg braces, may be needed on a short- or long-term basis for mobility. The physical therapist usually selects the most appropriate supportive device(s) to meet individual needs and instructs the patient regarding use. Incorporate physical therapy activities into the patient's daily routine for additional practice and repetition of rehabilitation efforts (Fig. 57-11).

◆ ***Stroke Survivorship and Coping.*** Patients who have had strokes often exhibit emotional responses that are not appropriate or typical for the situation. Patients may appear apathetic, depressed, fearful, anxious, weepy, frustrated, and angry. Some patients, especially those with a stroke on the left side of the brain (right hemiplegia), have exaggerated mood swings. The patient may be unable to control emotions and may suddenly burst into tears or laughter. This behavior is out of context and often is unrelated to the patient's underlying emotional state. Nursing interventions for atypical emotional response are to (1) distract the patient who suddenly becomes emotional, (2) explain to the patient and family that emotional outbursts may occur after a stroke, (3) maintain a calm environment, and (4) avoid shaming or scolding the patient during emotional outbursts.

The patient with a stroke may experience many losses, including sensory, intellectual, communicative, functional, role behavior, emotional, social, and vocational losses. The patient, caregiver, and family often go through the process of grief and mourning associated with the losses. Some patients experience long-term depression with symptoms such as anxiety, weight loss, fatigue, poor appetite, and sleep disturbances. In addition, the time and energy required to perform previously simple tasks can result in anger and frustration.

The patient, caregiver, and family need help coping with the losses associated with stroke. Provide assistance by (1) supporting communication between the patient and family; (2) discussing lifestyle changes resulting from stroke deficits; (3) discussing changing roles and responsibilities within the family; (4) being an active listener to allow the expression of fear, frustration, and anxiety; (5) including the family and patient in short- and long-term goal planning and patient care; (6) supporting family conferences, and (7) identifying support groups and referrals as needed.

Maladjusted dependence with inadequate coping occurs when the patient does not maintain optimal functioning for self-care, family responsibilities, decision making, or socialization. This situation can cause resentment from both the patient and family with a negative cycle of interpersonal dependency and control. Caregivers and family members must cope with three aspects of the patient's behavior: (1) recognition of behavioral changes resulting from neurologic deficits that are not changeable, (2) responses to multiple losses by both the patient and family, and (3) behaviors that may have been reinforced during the early stages of stroke as continued dependency.

The patient, caregiver, and family may express guilt over not living healthy lifestyles or not seeking professional help sooner. Family therapy is a helpful adjunct to rehabilitation. Open communication, information regarding the total effects of stroke, teaching regarding stroke treatment, and therapy are helpful. Stroke support groups in rehabilitation facilities and in the community are helpful in terms of mutual sharing, education, coping skills, and understanding.

***Sexual Function.*** A patient who has had a stroke may be concerned about the loss of sexual function. Many patients are comfortable talking about their anxieties and fears regarding sexual function if you are comfortable and open to the topic. You may initiate a discussion about the topic with the patient and spouse or significant other. Common concerns regarding sexual activity are impotence and the occurrence of another stroke during sex. Nursing interventions for sexual activity include teaching about (1) optional positioning of partners, (2) timing for peak energy periods, and (3) patient and partner counseling.

***Community Integration.*** Traditionally, successful community integration after stroke has been difficult for the patient because of persistent problems with cognition, coping, physical deficits, and emotional changes that interfere with functioning. Older patients who have had a stroke often have more severe deficits and frequently experience multiple health problems. Failure to continue the rehabilitation regimen at home may result in deterioration and further complications.

Community resources can be an asset to patients and their families. The National Stroke Association provides information, resources, referral services, and quarterly newsletters on stroke. The American Stroke Association, a division of the American Heart Association, has information regarding stroke, hypertension, diet, exercise, and assistive devices. This association sponsors self-help groups in many areas. Easter Seals provides wheelchairs and other assistive devices for stroke patients. Local groups can offer more daily assistance such as meals and transportation. These resources can be identified by nurse case managers, home health nurses, discharge planners, and clinical nurse specialists.

## Gerontologic Considerations: Stroke

Stroke is a significant cause of death and disability. The majority (66%) of strokes that require hospitalization occur in adults over 65.[4] Stroke can result in a profound disruption in the life of an older person. The magnitude of disability and changes in total function can leave patients wondering if they can ever return to their "old self," and loss of independence may be a major concern. The ability to perform ADLs may require many adaptive changes because of physical, emotional, perceptual, and cognitive deficits. Home management may be a particular challenge if the patient has an older spouse caregiver who also has health problems. There may be limited family members (including adult children) living in close proximity to provide help.

The rehabilitative phase and helping the older patient deal with the residual deficits of stroke, as well as aging, can provide a challenging nursing experience. Patients may become fearful and depressed because they think they may have another stroke or die. The fear can become immobilizing and interfere with effective rehabilitation.

Changes may occur in the patient-spouse relationship. The dependency resulting from a stroke may threaten the relationship. The spouse may also have chronic medical problems that can affect the ability to take care of the stroke survivor. The patient may not want anyone other than the spouse to provide care, thus putting a significant burden on the spouse.

You have the opportunity to assist the patient and caregiver in the transition through acute hospitalization, rehabilitation, long-term care, and home care. The needs of the patient, caregiver, and family require ongoing nursing assessment and adaptation of interventions in response to changing needs to optimize quality of life for all of them.

## BECOMING A NURSE LEADER

### *Dealing With a Changing Environment*

**Situation**

You have just gotten your first job after nursing school. You are so excited to be working at a rehabilitation center that has just moved into a new building and has new ownership. On your first day of work, you meet Evelyn and Martha, two older nurses who have worked for the center for over 20 years. In your first conversation with them Evelyn tells you, "The new management requires specialized computer training for all nursing staff. We are not going to do it and we will fight them on this issue and all the other changes they want to make." Martha adds, "Not only that, but we will threaten to quit if they do not listen to us and they better listen as we have been here for many years."

**Points for Consideration**

- Change is inevitable. Health care is constantly adapting and changing to new policies, technology, and medical advances.
- Resistance to change may be due to a variety of reasons. Deal with resistance by identifying the underlying fears that are causing it. Manage resistance by recognizing the benefits that change will bring. Reassure others that training will be provided for adapting to the new changes.
- Traditional practices are challenged with a changing environment. Nurses are put in positions of needing to do things that they have little experience with or have never done before.
- Integrating technology into nursing practice can improve health care, prevent medical errors, and decrease paperwork. However, technology can be very intimidating for nurses who have no or limited experience with it.
- Being leaders and responding to change is the responsibility of every nurse. Recognize that people will respond better to change if they are involved in the change process. Support other nurses as they adapt to and accept the changes.

**Discussion Questions**

1. Why are Evelyn and Martha resistant to the changes at the rehabilitation center?
2. How would you respond to Evelyn and Martha? Is there anything that you can do or say that would change their attitude about change?
3. As a new nurse, how can you take a leadership role to pave the way for the new changes at the center?

## CASE STUDY

### *Stroke*

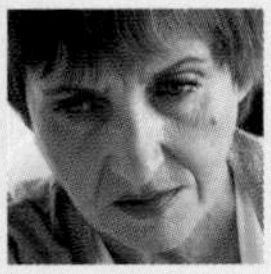

(©iStockphoto/ Thinkstock)

**Patient Profile**

J.K. is a 57-yr-old white woman who was is referred to the neurosurgery service for management of her temporal-parietal glioblastoma (see Assessment Case Study in Chapter 55 on pp. 1302, 1304, and 1307). She was diagnosed after presenting with persistent headaches, a seizure in her HCP's office, and left side upper visual field loss and neglect. Her MRI/MRA demonstrated a temporal-parietal glioblastoma that extends into the occipital lobes. She is scheduled for surgery to debulk the tumor. J.K. lives alone and holds a management position. She is concerned about her ability to return to work after her surgery.

J.K. returns from surgery to the neurosurgery unit drowsy but following commands. During the night J.K. is noted to have a pronator drift of the left arm, her pupils are equal and respond to light, but she has also developed left-sided weakness of both arm and leg and difficulty with answering questions.

*Medications:* dexamethasone 4 mg q6hr, famotidine, metoclopramide, ondansetron (Zofran), codeine, and levetiracetam (Keppra) since her admitting seizure

**Subjective Data**

- Left arm and leg are weak and feel numb
- She is trying to answer questions but looks confused and cannot follow commands

**Objective Data**

- BP 150/90 mm Hg
- Right gaze preference
- Left homonymous hemianopsia
- Left arm weakness (3/5) greater than leg weakness (4/5)
- Decreased sensation on both left arm and leg
- Has speech but not clear. Difficulty with word finding and following commands
- A diagnostic CT scan demonstrates a hemorrhagic stroke into the site of the tumor bed, and temporal-parietal and anterior occipital areas extending into the thalamus.

**Discussion Questions**

1. How does J.K.'s diagnosis (glioblastoma) put her at risk for a stroke?
2. ***Priority Decisions:*** What are the priority decisions that need to made regarding safety and self-care related to the left neglect and visual field cut?
3. ***Patient-Centered Care:*** What factors should you assess for related to rehabilitation for J.K.?
4. ***Priority Decisions:*** What are the priority nursing interventions for J.K.?
5. ***Priority Decisions:*** Based on the assessment data provided, what are the priority nursing diagnoses and are there any collaborative problems?
6. ***Teamwork and Collaboration:*** What nursing interventions for J.K. can the RN delegate to unlicensed assistive personnel ((UAP)?
7. ***Teamwork and Collaboration:*** How can you work together with the interprofessional team to develop and implement strategies to improve communication for J.K.?
8. ***Safety:*** How can you ensure safety for J.K. in light of her homonymous hemianopsia and left-sided neglect?
9. ***Patient-Centered Care:*** How can you address J.K.'s concerns about her finances and self-care?
10. ***Patient-Centered Care:*** J.K.'s family wants to know if her tumor surgery caused her hemorrhagic stroke and if so, what they should watch out for at home.

Answers available at *http://evolve.elsevier.com/Lewis/medsurg.*

## BRIDGE TO NCLEX EXAMINATION

The number of the question corresponds to the same-numbered outcome at the beginning of the chapter.

1. Of the following patients, the nurse recognizes that the one with the highest risk for a stroke is a(n)
   **a.** obese 45-yr-old Native American.
   **b.** 35-yr-old Asian American woman who smokes.
   **c.** 32-yr-old white woman taking oral contraceptives.
   **d.** 65-yr-old African American man with hypertension.
2. The factor related to cerebral blood flow that *most* often determines the extent of cerebral damage from a stroke is the
   **a.** amount of cardiac output.
   **b.** $O_2$ content of the blood.
   **c.** degree of collateral circulation.
   **d.** level of $CO_2$ in the blood.
3. Information provided by the patient that would help differentiate a hemorrhagic stroke from a thrombotic stroke includes
   **a.** sensory disturbance.
   **b.** a history of hypertension.
   **c.** presence of motor weakness.
   **d.** sudden onset of severe headache.
4. A patient is exhibiting word finding difficulty and weakness in his right arm. What area of the brain is *most* likely involved?
   **a.** brainstem.
   **b.** vertebral artery.
   **c.** left middle cerebral artery.
   **d.** right middle cerebral artery.
5. The nurse explains to the patient with a stroke who is scheduled for angiography that this test is used to determine the
   **a.** presence of increased ICP.
   **b.** site and size of the infarction.
   **c.** patency of the cerebral blood vessels.
   **d.** presence of blood in the cerebrospinal fluid.
6. A patient experiencing TIAs is scheduled for a carotid endarterectomy. The nurse explains that this procedure is done to
   **a.** decrease cerebral edema.
   **b.** reduce the brain damage that occurs during a stroke in evolution.
   **c.** prevent a stroke by removing atherosclerotic plaques blocking cerebral blood flow.
   **d.** provide a circulatory bypass around thrombotic plaques obstructing cranial circulation.
7. For a patient who is suspected of having a stroke, one of the *most* important pieces of information that the nurse can obtain is
   **a.** time of the patient's last meal.
   **b.** time at which stroke symptoms first appeared.
   **c.** patient's hypertension history and management.
   **d.** family history of stroke and other cardiovascular diseases.
8. Bladder training in a male patient who has urinary incontinence after a stroke includes
   **a.** limiting fluid intake.
   **b.** keeping a urinal in place at all times.
   **c.** assisting the patient to stand to void.
   **d.** catheterizing the patient every 4 hours.

9. Common psychosocial reactions of the stroke patient to the stroke include *(select all that apply)*
   a. depression.
   b. disassociation.
   c. intellectualization.
   d. sleep disturbances.
   e. denial of severity of stroke.

1. d, 2. c, 3. d, 4. c, 5. c, 6. c, 7. b, 8. c, 9. a, d, e

For rationales to these answers and even more NCLEX review questions, visit *http://evolve.elsevier.com/Lewis/medsurg.*

## EVOLVE WEBSITE

http://evolve.elsevier.com/Lewis/medsurg

**Review Questions (Online Only)**

**Key Points**

**Answer Keys for Questions**

- Rationales for Bridge to NCLEX Examination Questions
- Answer Guidelines for Case Study on p. 1366

**Student Case Studies**

- Patient With Hypertension and Stroke
- Patient With Stroke

**eNursing Care Plans**

- eNursing Care Plan 57-1: Patient With Stroke

**Conceptual Care Map Creator**

- Conceptual Care Map for Case Study on p. 1366

**Audio Glossary**

**Content Updates**

## REFERENCES


1. National Stroke Association: Stroke Survivors. Retrieved from *www.stroke.org/we-can-help/survivors.*
2. Center for Disease Control and Prevention: Stroke Facts. Retrieved from *www.cdc.gov/stroke/facts.htm.*
3. American Heart Association: Stroke falls to No. 5 Killer in US. Retrieved from *http://blog.heart.org/stroke-falls-no-5-killer-u-s.*
4. Vega C: Updated guidelines available for primary prevention of stroke CME/CE. Retrieved from *www.medscape.org/viewarticle/834329.*

*5. Kruithof W, Post M, Visser-Meily J: Measuring negative and positive caregiving experiences: A psychometric analysis of the Caregiver Strain Index Expanded, *Clin Rehabil* 29:1224, 2015.

*6. O'Donnell M and INTERSTROKE Study Team: Risk factors for ischaemic and intracerebral haemorrhagic stroke in 22 countries (the INTERSTROKE study): a case-control study, *Lancet Neurol* 376(9735):112, 2010.

7. Meschia J, Bushnel C, Boden-Albala B, et al: Guidelines for the primary prevention of stroke: A statement for healthcare professionals from the American Heart Association/American Stroke Association, *Stroke* 45(12):3754, 2014.
8. National Institute of Neurological Disorders and Stroke: Brain basics, preventing strokes. Retrieved from *www.ninds.nih.gov/disorders/stroke/preventing_stroke.htm#Risk%20Factors.*
9. American Heart Association/American Stroke Association: Transient ischemic attacks. Retrieved from *www.strokeassociation.org/STROKEORG/AboutStroke/TypesofStroke/TIA/TIA-Transient-Ischemic-Attack_UCM_310942_Article.jsp.*
10. American Heart Association/American Stroke Association: Ischemic Strokes (Clots). Retrieved from *www.strokeassociation.org/STROKEORG/AboutStroke/TypesofStroke/IschemicClots/Ischemic-Strokes-Clots_UCM_310939_Article.jsp.*

*11. Eriksen S, Gay C, Lerdal A: Acute phase factors associated with the course of depression during the first 18 months after first ever stroke, *Disability and Rehabilitation* 38:30, 2016.

*12. Schellinger P, Bryan R, Caplan L, et al: Evidence-based guideline: The role of diffusion and perfusion MRI for the diagnosis of acute ischemic stroke. Report of the Therapeutics and Technology Assessment Subcommittee of the American Academy of Neurology, *Neurology* 75(2):177, 2010.

13. Patel V, Gupta R, Horn C, et al: The neuro-critical care management of the endovascular stroke patient, *Curr Treat Options Neurol* 15(2):113, 2013.

*14. Hanselman C: Timing of tissue plasminogen activator for acute ischemic stroke: outcomes-based recommendations for practice, *J Neuroscience Nurs* 46(6): 314, 2014.

*15. Spiotta A, Chaudry M, Hui F, et al: Evolution of thrombectomy approaches and devices for acute stroke: A technical review, *J Neurointerv Surg* 7:12, 2015.

*16. Campbell BC, Mitchell PJ, Kleinig TJ, et al: Endovascular therapy for ischemic stroke with perfusion-imaging selection, *N Engl J Med* 372:1009, 2015.

17. Furlan AJ: Endovascular therapy for stroke—it's about time, *N Engl J Med* 2015; 150417035025009 DOI: 10.1056/NEJMe1503217.
18. U.S. Food and Drug Administration FDA: Clears system to reduce stroke during stent and angioplasty procedures. Retrieved from *www.fda.gov/NewsEvents/Newsroom/PressAnnouncements/ucm433482.htm?source=govdelivery&utm_medium=email&utm_source=govdelivery.*
19. Kirkman M, Citerio G, Smith M: The intensive care management of acute ischemic stroke: an overview, *Intens Care Med* 40(5):640, 2014.
20. Watson J: Subarachnoid hemorrhage surgery. Retrieved from *http://emedicine.medscape.com/article/247090-overview.*
21. Green T, Kelloway L, Davies-Schinkel C, et al: Nurses' accountability for stroke quality of care, part one: review of the literature on nursing-sensitive outcomes, *Can J Neurosci* 33(3):13, 2011.
22. American Stroke Association: NIH stroke scale international. Retrieved from *www.nihstrokescale.org.*

*23. CLOTS Trial Collaboration: Effect of intermittent pneumatic compression on disability, living circumstances, quality of life, and hospital costs after stroke: secondary analyses from CLOTS 3, *Lancet Neurol* 13(12):1186, 2014.

*24. Hutchinson E, Wilson N: Acute stroke, dysphagia, and nutritional support, *Br J Community Nurs* S26-29, 2013.

*25. Wallace S, Purdy M, Skidmore E: A multimodal communication program for aphasia during inpatient rehabilitation: a case study, *NeuroRehabilitation* 35(3):615, 2014.

*26. Van der Cruyssen K, Vereeck L, Saeys W, et al: Prognostic factors for discharge destinations after acute stroke: a comprehensive literature review, *Disabil Rehabil* 37:1214, 2015.

*27. Saunders DH, Sanderson M, Brazzelli M, et al: Physical fitness training for stroke patients, *Cochrane Database Syst Rev*, 2013. Issue 10. CD003316. DOI:10.1002/146518.CD003316.pub5.

*Evidence-based information for clinical practice.

# 58

# Chronic Neurologic Problems

*Dottie Roberts, Madona Plueger*

*If you don't like something, change it. If you can't change it, change your attitude.*

***Maya Angelou***

http://evolve.elsevier.com/Lewis/medsurg/

## LEARNING OUTCOMES

1. Compare and contrast the etiology, clinical manifestations, interprofessional care, and nursing management of tension-type, migraine, and cluster headaches.
2. Differentiate the etiology, clinical manifestations, diagnostic studies, interprofessional care, and nursing management of seizure disorders, multiple sclerosis, Parkinson's disease, and myasthenia gravis.
3. Describe the clinical manifestations and nursing and interprofessional management of restless legs syndrome, amyotrophic lateral sclerosis, and Huntington's disease.
4. Explain the potential impact of chronic neurologic disease on physical and psychologic well-being.
5. Outline the major goals of treatment for the patient with a chronic, progressive neurologic disease.

## KEY TERMS



This chapter discusses headaches, chronic neurologic disorders, and degenerative neurologic disorders. Chronic neurologic disorders include seizure disorders and restless legs syndrome. Degenerative neurologic disorders include multiple sclerosis, Parkinson's disease, myasthenia gravis, amyotrophic lateral sclerosis, and Huntington's disease.

## HEADACHES

**Headache** is probably the most common type of pain that humans experience. The majority of people have functional headaches, such as migraine or tension-type headaches. Others have organic headaches caused by intracranial or extracranial disease.

Pain-sensitive structures in the head include venous sinuses, dura, cranial blood vessels, three divisions of the trigeminal nerve (cranial nerve [CN] V), facial nerve (CN VII), glossopharyngeal nerve (CN IX), vagus nerve (CN X), and the first three cervical nerves. Because these nerves have both motor and sensory functions, increased pain intensity and symptoms can occur when a person moves.

Headaches are classified as primary or secondary headache. *Primary headache* classifications include tension-type, migraine, and cluster headaches. Primary headaches are not caused by a disease or another medical condition. The type of primary headache is determined using the International Headache Society (IHS) guidelines based on characteristics of the headache (Table 58-1). *Secondary headaches* are caused by another condition or disorder, such as sinus infection, neck injury, and brain tumor.

A patient may have more than one type of headache. The history and neurologic examination are diagnostic keys to determine the type of headache. The examination of a person with a headache is often normal. Unexplained abnormal findings require additional diagnostic studies to identify underlying causes and additional risk factors.

Reviewed by Sonya H. Blevins, RN, DNP, CMSRN, CNE, Assistant Professor of Nursing, Mary Black School of Nursing, University of South Carolina Upstate, Greenville, South Carolina; Regina Gonzalez-Lama, RN, MS, Lecturer, College of Staten Island–CUNY, Staten Island, New York; Linda Littlejohns, RN, MSN, CNRN, FAAN, Neuroscience Clinical Nursing Consultant, San Juan Capistrano, California; Pamela K. Newland, RN, PhD, CMSRN, Assistant Professor, Goldfarb School of Nursing at Barnes Jewish College, St. Louis, Missouri; and Daryle Wane, PhD, ARNP, FNP-BC, RN to BSN Coordinator, Professor of Nursing, Department of Health Occupations, Pasco-Hernando State College, New Port Richey, Florida.

## TABLE 58-1 Interprofessional Care

### *Headaches*

| Tension-Type Headaches | Migraine Headache | Cluster Headache |
|---|---|---|
| **Location** | | |
| Bilateral, band-like pressure at base of skull | Unilateral (in 60%), may switch sides, commonly anterior location | Unilateral, radiating up or down from one eye |
| **Quality** | | |
| Constant, squeezing tightness | Throbbing, synchronous with pulse | Severe, bone crushing |
| **Frequency** | | |
| Cycles for many years | Periodic, cycles of several months and years | May have months or years between attacks<br>Attacks occur in clusters over a period of 2-12 wk |
| **Duration** | | |
| 30 min-7 days | 4-72 hr | 5 min-3 hr |
| **Time and Mode of Onset** | | |
| Not related to time | May be preceded by premonitory symptoms or aura<br>Onset after awakening<br>Improves with sleep | Nocturnal, commonly awakens person from sleep |
| **Associated Symptoms** | | |
| Palpable neck and shoulder muscle tension<br>Stiff neck<br>Tenderness | Irritability, sweating<br>Nausea, vomiting<br>Photophobia<br>Phonophobia<br>Premonitory symptoms: sensory, motor, or psychic phenomena<br>Family history (in 65%) | Facial flushing or pallor<br>Unilateral lacrimation, ptosis, rhinitis |
| **Treatment: Abortive and Symptomatic Drugs** | | |
| Non-opioid analgesics: aspirin, acetaminophen, NSAIDS<br>Analgesic combinations<br>• butalbital/aspirin/caffeine (Fiorinal)<br>• butalbital/acetaminophen/caffeine<br>• dichloralphenazone/acetaminophen/ isomethepetene<br>Muscle relaxants | Non-opioid analgesics: aspirin, NSAIDs<br>Serotonin receptor agonists<br>• almotriptan (Axert)<br>• eletriptan (Relpax)<br>• frovatriptan (Frova)<br>• naratriptan (Amerge)<br>• rizatriptan (Maxalt)<br>• sumatriptan (Imitrex)<br>• zolmitriptan (Zomig)<br>• sumatriptan transdermal system (Zecuity)<br>Combination<br>• sumatriptan/naproxen (Treximet)<br>α-Adrenergic blockers<br>• ergotamine tartrate (Ergomar)<br>• dihydroergotamine nasal spray (Migranal)<br>Analgesic combinations<br>• acetaminophen/caffeine/aspirin<br>• acetaminophen/isometheptene/ dichloralphenazone<br>Corticosteroids<br>• dexamethasone | α-Adrenergic blockers<br>• ergotamine tartrate (Ergomar)<br>Serotonin receptor agonists<br>• almotriptan<br>• eletriptan<br>• frovatriptan<br>• naratriptan<br>• rizatiptan<br>• sumatriptan<br>• zolmitriptan<br>$O_2$ 100% inhalation via mask |
| **Treatment: Preventive** | | |
| Tricyclic antidepressants<br>• amitriptyline<br>• nortriptyline (Pamelor)<br>• doxepin<br>Selective serotonin reuptake inhibitors<br>• fluoxetine (Prozac)<br>• paroxetine (Paxil)<br>β-Adrenergic blocker:<br>• propranolol (Inderal)<br>Antiseizure drugs<br>• topiramate (Topamax)<br>• divalproex (Depakote)<br>Other drugs<br>• mirtazapine (Remeron)<br>Biofeedback<br>Psychotherapy<br>Muscle relaxation training | β-Adrenergic blocker<br>• propranolol<br>Antidepressants<br>• amitriptyline<br>• imipramine (Tofranil)<br>Antiseizure drugs<br>• valproic acid (Depakene)<br>• divalproex<br>• topiramate<br>• gabapentin (Neurontin)<br>Calcium channel blocker<br>• verapamil (Calan)<br>• nifedipine (Procardia)<br>Botulinum toxin A (Botox)<br>Biofeedback<br>Relaxation therapy<br>Cognitive-behavioral therapy | α-Adrenergic blockers<br>• ergotamine tartrate<br>Corticosteroid<br>• prednisone<br>Calcium channel blocker<br>• verapamil<br>Lithium<br>Biofeedback |

## TENSION-TYPE HEADACHE

**Tension-type headache**, also called *stress headache*, is the most common type of headache. These headaches are characterized by their bilateral location and pressing or tightening quality. Tension-type headaches are usually of mild or moderate intensity and can last from minutes to days. Tension-type headaches are divided by frequency into episodic and chronic types.[1]

### Etiology and Pathophysiology

The cause of tension-type headache is not fully understood, but it may have a neurobiologic basis similar to migraine headaches. For some, episodic headaches evolve to chronic headaches. Increased frequency does not necessarily produce increased headache intensity. However, chronic tension-type headache can cause diminished quality of life and severe disability.[1]

### Clinical Manifestations

Patients often have a bilateral frontal-occipital headache described as a constant, dull pressure, or band-like headache associated with neck pain and increased tone in the cervical and neck muscles. The headache may involve sensitivity to light *(photophobia)* or sound *(phonophobia)* but does not involve nausea or vomiting. There are no *premonitory symptoms* (warning symptoms of impending headache), and physical activity does not aggravate symptoms. The headaches may occur intermittently for weeks, months, or even years.

Many patients have a combination of migraine and tension-type headaches, with features of both occurring simultaneously. Patients with migraine headaches may experience tension-type headaches between migraine attacks. Fig. 58-1 shows the location of pain for common headache syndromes.

### Diagnostic Studies

Careful history taking may be the most important tool for diagnosing tension-type headache (Table 58-2). If tension-type headache is present during physical examination, increased resistance to passive movement of the head and tenderness of the head and neck may be noted. Electromyography (EMG) may reveal sustained contraction of neck, scalp, or facial muscles. However, the patient may not show increased muscle tension with this test, even when it is done during an actual headache.

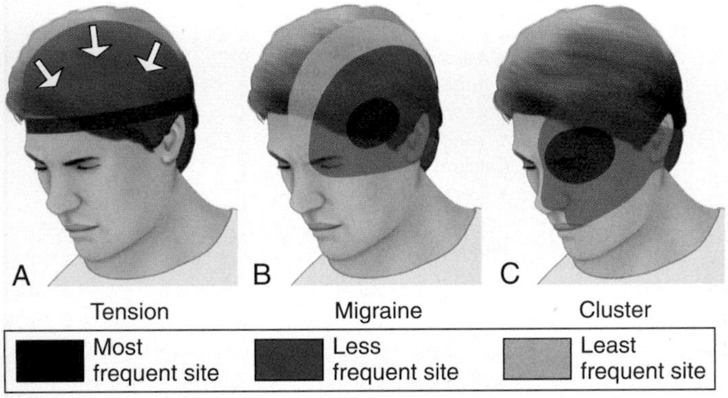


**FIG. 58-1** Location of pain for common headache syndromes. **A,** Tension headache is often described as feeling of a weight in or on the head or a band squeezing the head. **B,** Migraine headache is described as an intense throbbing or pounding pain that involves one temple. The pain usually is unilateral (on one side of the head), although it can be bilateral. **C,** Cluster headache pain is focused in and around one eye and is often described as sharp, penetrating, or burning.

## MIGRAINE HEADACHE

**Migraine headache** is a recurring headache characterized by unilateral throbbing pain. Light, sound, and smell sensitivity and other environmental factors may be either premonitory symptoms or triggers for the migraine headache.[2] Manifestations of migraine are associated with neurologic and autonomic nervous system dysfunction. The most common age for onset of migraine is between 20 and 30 years. Migraine affects as many as 18% of females and 6% of males in the United States.[3] Migraines are more common in women than men (see Gender Differences box). Risk factors for migraine include family history, low level of education, low socioeconomic status, high workload, and frequent tension-type headaches.

**GENDER DIFFERENCES**

***Headaches***

| Men | Women |
|---|---|
| • Cluster headaches are more common than in women (6:1).<br>• Exercise-induced headaches are more common than in women. | • Migraine headaches are more common than in men (3:1).<br>• Tension headaches are more common than in men. |

The IHS subdivides migraines into categories. *Migraine without aura* (formerly called *common migraine*) is the most common type. *Migraine with aura* (formerly called *classic migraine*) occurs in only 10% of migraine headache episodes.[1]

### Etiology and Pathophysiology

Although many theories have addressed the cause of migraine headaches, the exact etiology is not known. The current theory is that a complex series of neurovascular events initiates a migraine headache. People who have migraines have a state of neuronal hyperexcitability in the cerebral cortex, especially in the occipital cortex. Genetic factors may account for about 50% of an individual's risk for migraine headache.[3]

Migraine is associated with seizure disorders, ischemic stroke, asthma, depression, anxiety, myocardial infarction, Raynaud's syndrome, and irritable bowel syndrome. In many cases, migraine headaches have no known precipitating events. However, for some patients, specific factors may trigger a headache. These include foods, menstruation, head trauma, physical exertion,

**TABLE 58-2 Diagnostic Studies**

***Headaches***

**History and Physical Examination**
- Neurologic examination (often negative)
- Inspection for local infection
- Palpation of head for tenderness, bony swellings
- Auscultation for bruits over major arteries, especially neck

**Routine Laboratory Studies**
- Complete blood count (CBC) (may indicate anemia, infection)
- Electrolytes (may indicate dehydration, other illnesses)
- Urinalysis (may indicate infection, other medical diagnoses [e.g., diabetes])
- Other diagnostic studies to assess evidence of disease, deformity, or infection: angiography, EMG, EEG, MRA, MRI, lumbar puncture

*EEG*, Electroencephalography; *EMG*, electromyography; *MRA*, magnetic resonance angiography.

fatigue, stress, missed meals, weather, and drugs. Food triggers include chocolate, cheese, oranges, tomatoes, onions, monosodium glutamate, aspartame, and alcohol (particularly red wine).

### Clinical Manifestations

Premonitory symptoms and an *aura* may precede the headache phase by several hours or several days. Premonitory symptoms may include neurologic (e.g., photophobia), psychologic (e.g., hyperactivity, irritability), and other (e.g., food craving) manifestations. An **aura** is a complex of neurologic symptoms that occur before a headache for some patients. It may be characterized by visual symptoms, such as bright lights, scotomas (patchy blindness), visual distortions, or zigzag lines. Sensory (voices or sounds that do not exist, strange smells), and/or motor (e.g., weakness, paralysis, feeling that limbs are moving) phenomena may also be part of an aura.

A migraine headache may last 4 to 72 hours. The headache is described as a steady, throbbing pain that is synchronous with the pulse. Although the headache is usually unilateral, it may switch to the opposite side in another episode. During the headache phase, some patients with migraine may tend to seek shelter from noise, light, odors, people, and problems.

The presentation of migraine varies in severity. Not all migraine headaches are disabling, and many patients who have migraines do not seek treatment for them. In some patients, migraine symptoms may become worse over time.

### Diagnostic Studies

The diagnosis of migraine headache is usually based on the patient history. The neurologic and other diagnostic examinations are often normal (Table 58-2).

No specific laboratory or radiologic test can diagnose migraine headache. Neuroimaging techniques (e.g., head CT scan, with or without contrast, and MRI) are not recommended for routine evaluation of headache, unless the neurologic examination reveals abnormal findings. If atypical features are present, then additional testing is done to rule out a secondary headache.

## CLUSTER HEADACHE

**Cluster headaches** are the most severe form of primary headache. Repeated headaches occur in clusters, generally at the same time of day or night. Age at onset is typically 20 to 45 years, but they can start at any age. Men are affected three times more often than women.[4]

### Etiology and Pathophysiology

Neither the cause nor the pathophysiologic mechanism of cluster headache is fully known. The unilateral pain may occur with activation of neurons in the ophthalmic branch of the trigeminal nerve. Cluster headaches also involve the hypothalamus, with irregularities in melatonin and cortisol. This indicates a dysfunction of circadian rhythm. Imaging studies show hypothalamic activation at the onset of cluster headache.[5] Alcohol is a dietary trigger. Strong odors, weather changes, and napping are other triggers.

### Clinical Manifestations

The cluster headache is one of the most severe forms of headache, with intense pain lasting from a few minutes to 3 hours. In contrast to the pulsing pain of migraine headache, the pain of cluster headache is sharp and stabbing. The pain is generally located around the eye, radiating to the temple, forehead, cheek, nose, or gums. Other manifestations may include swelling around the eye, lacrimation (tearing), facial flushing or pallor, nasal congestion, and miosis (constriction of the pupil). During the headache, the patient is often agitated and restless, unable to sit still or relax. A majority of patients have at least three of these symptoms. In addition, an aura similar to migraine may occur in 14% of patients up to 60 minutes before an attack.[5]

Cluster headaches can occur every other day and as often as eight times a day. A cluster typically lasts 2 weeks to 3 months, and then the patient goes into remission for months to years. Typically, two cluster periods a year may be separated by months without symptoms. Because cluster periods often occur seasonally, headaches may be mistaken for symptoms of allergies.

### Diagnostic Studies

The diagnosis of cluster headache is based on the patient history according to IHS criteria. Asking patients to keep a headache diary can be useful. CT scan, MRI, or magnetic resonance angiography (MRA) may rule out an aneurysm, a tumor, or an infection. A lumbar puncture may rule out other disorders that may cause similar symptoms.

## OTHER TYPES OF HEADACHES

Although tension, migraine, and cluster headaches are by far the most common types of headaches, other types can occur. These headaches may be the first symptom of a more serious illness. Headache can accompany subarachnoid hemorrhage; brain tumors; other intracranial masses; vascular abnormalities; trigeminal neuralgia (tic douloureux); diseases of the eyes, nose, and teeth; and systemic illness (e.g., bacteremia, carbon monoxide poisoning, altitude sickness, polycythemia vera). Because of the varied causes of headache, clinical evaluation must be thorough. It should include assessment of personality, life adjustment, environment, and family situation, as well as a comprehensive evaluation of neurologic and physical status.

**INFORMATICS IN PRACTICE**

***Social Media Use for Patients With Migraine Headaches***

- Many patients with migraine headaches believe their pain and its impact on their quality of life are poorly understood by others.
- Encourage patients to participate in a social media outlet (e.g., Twitter) where people who have migraines share their experiences.
- Using social media allows patients to describe their physical and emotional pain and can help them cope better with their condition and improve their quality of life.

## INTERPROFESSIONAL CARE FOR HEADACHES

If no systemic underlying disease is the cause, the type of headache guides therapy. Table 58-2 outlines the general workup for a patient with headache to rule out any intracranial or extracranial disease. Table 58-1 summarizes current therapies for prevention and management of different types of headaches. These therapies include drugs, meditation, yoga, biofeedback, cognitive-behavioral therapy, and relaxation training.

Cognitive-behavioral therapy and relaxation therapy used alone or in conjunction with drug therapy may be beneficial to some patients. Biofeedback involves the use of physiologic monitoring equipment to give the patient information regarding muscle tension and peripheral blood flow (e.g., skin temperature of the fingers). The patient is trained to relax the muscles and raise the finger temperature and is given reinforcement (operant conditioning) in accomplishing these changes. Acupuncture, acupressure, and hypnosis also work well in some patients with headaches.

## Drug Therapy

**Tension-Type Headache.** Drug therapy for tension-type headache usually involves aspirin, acetaminophen (Tylenol), or nonsteroidal antiinflammatory drugs (NSAIDs) used alone or in combination with a sedative, muscle relaxant, or tranquilizer. However, many of these drugs have serious side effects. Caution the patient about the long-term use of aspirin and aspirin-containing drugs because they can cause upper gastrointestinal (GI) bleeding and coagulation abnormalities in susceptible patients. Drugs containing acetaminophen can cause kidney damage with chronic use and liver damage when taken in large doses or when combined with alcohol. To decrease the recurrence of tension-type headache, the patient may receive preventive therapy with a tricyclic antidepressant (e.g., amitriptyline, nortriptyline) or mirtazapine (Remeron), a nonadrenergic serotonergic antidepressant (NaSSA). Antiseizure medications such as topiramate (Topamax) or divalproex (Depakote) may also be used.

**Migraine Headache.** The aim of drug treatment of an acute migraine attack is terminating or decreasing the symptoms. Many people with mild or moderate migraine can obtain relief with NSAIDs, aspirin, or caffeine-containing combination analgesics. For moderate to severe headaches, the triptans have become the first line of therapy. Triptans (e.g., sumatriptan [Imitrex]) affect selected serotonin receptors, thus reducing neurogenic inflammation of the cerebral blood vessels and producing vasoconstriction (Table 58-1). They are most effective when taken at the onset of migraine headache or during the aura. Sumatriptan is available in various forms: oral, subcutaneous, nasal spray, transdermal.

Some patients respond better to one triptan than to others, so HCPs need to be knowledgeable about all of them. Because these drugs cause vasoconstriction, patients with a history of heart disease or stroke should avoid their use. The combination drug sumatriptan/naproxen (Treximet) combines a triptan with an antiinflammatory drug. However, risk of serious cardiovascular events such as myocardial infarction, thromboembolic events, and stroke may increase over time with this drug.

**DRUG ALERT Sumatriptan (Imitrex)**

- Should not be given to patients with the following:
  - History or manifestations of ischemic cardiac, cerebrovascular, or peripheral vascular problems.
  - Uncontrolled hypertension (may increase BP).
- Excess dosage may produce tremor and decrease respirations.

Zecuity (sumatriptan transdermal system) is the first skin patch indicated for the treatment of migraine headache and for intense nausea secondary to the headache itself. Zecuity is applied either to the upper arm or thigh. It should not be applied over red or irritated skin or over scars, tattoos, or broken skin. The patient pushes a button to deliver the drug through the skin over a course of 4 hours. Zecuity has similar contraindications to other triptans.[6] When triptans are contraindicated or ineffective, other drugs can be used (Table 58-1).

Preventive treatment is important in the management of migraine headaches. The decision to initiate preventive treatment is individually determined based on frequency, severity, and any disability related to headaches. Several different classes of medications are used.

Topiramate, an antiseizure drug, may be taken daily for migraine prevention. Common side effects include hypoglycemia, paresthesia, weight loss, and cognitive changes. Usually these side effects are mild to moderate and transient. Topiramate must be used for 2 to 3 months to determine its effectiveness. Not all patients become pain free on this medication. HCPs must offer thorough teaching regarding topiramate to promote patient adherence.

**DRUG ALERT Topiramate (Topamax)**

Instruct patient to do the following:

- Not abruptly discontinue because this may cause seizures.
- Avoid tasks that require alertness until response to drug is established.
- Take adequate fluids to decrease risk of renal stone development.

Botulinum toxin A (Botox) may be an effective prophylactic treatment for patients who have chronic migraines lasting for 4 hours or more at least 15 days each month, or migraines that do not respond to other medications. Botox is given by multiple injections around the head and neck. Effects last 2 to 4 months; the injections are repeated every 3 months. The most common adverse reactions are neck pain and headache. A slight risk exists for the toxin to migrate from the injection site to other areas of the face and neck, causing swallowing and breathing difficulties. Teach the patient to seek immediate medical attention if this occurs.

Gabapentin (Neurontin) is another antiseizure drug used for migraine prevention. Selective serotonin reuptake inhibitors (e.g., fluoxetine [Prozac]) may also be prescribed. Other drugs used for migraine headache prevention are listed in Table 58-1.

**Cluster Headache.** Triptans are a gold standard of treatment for occasional cluster headache. Either nasal administration or subcutaneous injection is appropriate. However, as noted in the discussion of migraine headache, triptans are vasoconstrictors. Thus they are contraindicated for patients with vascular risk factors.[5]

High-flow 100% $O_2$ by non-rebreather mask is well tolerated, safe, and effective as an alternative treatment. $O_2$ delivered at a rate of 6 to 8 L/min for 10 minutes may relieve headache by causing vasoconstriction and increasing synthesis of serotonin in the central nervous system. Treatment can be repeated after a 5-minute rest. However, a drawback to this treatment is that the patient must have continuous access to the $O_2$ supply.

For chronic cluster headache, preventive treatment is needed. High-dose verapamil is the first-choice drug. However, because of its effects on cardiac conduction, verapamil should be initiated only after careful consideration of the risks. Careful monitoring is needed during treatment. Other drug options may include lithium, ergotamine, antiseizure drugs (e.g., topiramate), and melatonin. Options for patients with refractory cluster headaches include invasive nerve blocks, deep brain stimulation, and ablative neurosurgical procedures (e.g., percutaneous radiofrequency).

**Other Headaches.** Patients with frequent headaches may overuse analgesics or other medications indicated for headache treatment. *Medication overuse headache* (MOH) is the term used to describe a new type of headache, or marked worsening of a preexisting headache condition. Drugs known to cause this problem are acetaminophen, aspirin, NSAIDs (e.g., ibuprofen), butalbital, triptans, ergotamine, and opioids.[1] Patients with daily headaches may complain of early awakening with decreased appetite, nausea, restlessness, decreased memory, and irritability. Treatment involves abrupt withdrawal of the offending drug (except for opioids, which must be tapered) and initiation of alternative drugs such as amitriptyline.

## NURSING MANAGEMENT: HEADACHES

### Nursing Assessment

Table 58-3 outlines subjective and objective data that you should obtain from a patient with headache. Because the history provides the key to assessment of headache, it should include specific details of the headache, such as the location and type of pain, onset, frequency, duration, relation to events (emotional, psychologic, physical), and time of day of the occurrence. Obtain information about previous illnesses, surgery, trauma, allergies, family history, and response to medication.

Suggest that the patient keep a diary of headache episodes with specific details. This record can be of great help in determining the type of headache and precipitating events. If the patient has a history of migraine, tension-type, or cluster headaches, ask the patient if the character, intensity, or location of the headache has changed. The answer may be an important clue about the cause of the headache.

### Nursing Diagnoses

Nursing diagnoses for the patient with headache may include, but are not limited to, the following:

- Acute pain *related to* headache
- Ineffective health management *related to* drug therapy and lifestyle adjustments

Additional information on nursing diagnoses is presented in eNursing Care Plan 58-1 for the patient with headache (available on the website for this chapter).

### Planning

The overall goals are that the patient with a headache will (1) have reduced or no pain, (2) demonstrate understanding of triggering events and treatment strategies, (3) use positive coping strategies to deal with pain, and (4) experience increased quality of life and decreased disability.

### Nursing Implementation

The patient with chronic headache presents a great challenge to HCPs. Because an inability to cope with daily stresses can cause headaches, an effective therapy may involve helping the patient examine the daily routine, recognize stressful situations, and develop more appropriate coping strategies. Help the patient identify precipitating factors and develop ways to avoid them. Encourage daily exercise, relaxation periods, and socialization because they can decrease the recurrence of headache. Suggest alternative ways to address headache pain through techniques, such as relaxation, meditation, and yoga.

In addition to using analgesics and analgesic combinations for symptomatic relief of headache, encourage the migraine sufferer to seek a quiet, dimly lit environment. Massage and moist hot packs to the neck and head can help a patient with tension-type headaches. The patient should learn about the drugs prescribed for preventive and abortive/symptomatic treatment of headache and should be able to describe the purpose, action, dosage, and side effects of the drugs. To prevent accidental overdose, the patient should make a written note of each dose of drug or headache remedy.

For the patient with headaches triggered by food, provide dietary counseling. Encourage the patient to eliminate foods that may provoke headaches, such as chocolate, cheese, oranges, tomatoes, onions, monosodium glutamate, aspartame, alcohol (particularly red wine), excessive caffeine, and fermented or

**TABLE 58-3 Nursing Assessment**

***Headaches***

**Subjective Data**

***Important Health Information***

*Past health history:* Seizures, cancer, recent fall or trauma, cranial infection, stroke. Asthma or allergies. Relationship of headache to overwork, stress, menstruation, exercise, food, sexual activity, travel, bright lights, or noxious environmental stimuli

*Medications:* Hydralazine, bromides, nitroglycerin, ergotamine (withdrawal), NSAIDs (in high daily doses), estrogen preparations, oral contraceptives, over-the-counter or prescription remedies

*Surgical interventions or other treatments:* Craniotomy, sinus surgery, facial surgery

***Functional Health Pattern***

*Health perception–health management:* Positive family history. Malaise

*Nutritional-metabolic:* Ingestion of alcohol, caffeine, cheese, chocolate, monosodium glutamate, aspartame, lunch meats (nitrites in cured meats), sausage, hot dogs, onions, avocados. History of anorexia, nausea, vomiting (migraine premonitory symptom); unilateral lacrimation (cluster)

*Activity, exercise:* Vertigo, fatigue, weakness, paralysis, fainting

*Sleep-rest:* Insomnia

*Cognitive-perceptual*

- *Migraine:* Aura. Unilateral, severe, throbbing headache (possible switching of side). Visual disturbances, photophobia, phonophobia, dizziness, tingling or burning sensations
- *Cluster:* Unilateral and severe, nocturnal headache. Nasal stuffiness
- *Tension type:* Bilateral, band-like, dull and persistent, base-of-skull headache, neck tenderness.

*Self-perception–self-concept:* Depression

*Coping–stress tolerance:* Stress, anxiety, irritability, withdrawal

**Objective Data**

***General***

Anxiety, apprehension

***Integumentary***

*Cluster:* Forehead diaphoresis, pallor, unilateral facial flushing with cheek edema, conjunctivitis

*Migraine:* Generalized edema (premonitory symptom) pallor, diaphoresis

***Neurologic***

Horner's syndrome, restlessness (cluster), hemiparesis (migraine)

***Musculoskeletal***

Resistance of head and neck movement, nuchal rigidity (meningeal, tension type), palpable neck and shoulder muscle tension (tension type)

***Possible Diagnostic Findings***

Evidence of disease, deformity, or infection on brain imaging (CT, MRI, MRA), cerebral angiogram, lumbar puncture, EEG, EMG

*EEG,* Electroencephalography; *EMG,* electromyography; *MRA,* magnetic resonance angiography.

**TABLE 58-4 Patient & Caregiver Teaching**
***Headaches***

*Include the following instructions when teaching the patient with a headache and the patient's caregiver.*

1. Keep a diary or calendar of headaches and possible precipitating events.
2. Avoid possible triggers for a headache:
   - Foods containing amines (cheese, chocolate), nitrites (meats such as hot dogs), vinegar, onions, monosodium glutamate
   - Fermented or marinated foods
   - Caffeine
   - Oranges
   - Tomatoes
   - Aspartame
   - Nicotine
   - Ice cream
   - Alcohol (particularly red wine)
   - Emotional stress
   - Fatigue
   - Drugs such as ergot-containing preparations (ergotamine tartrate [Ergomar]) and monoamine oxidase inhibitors (e.g., rasagiline [Azilect])
3. Learn the purpose, action, dosage, and side effects of drugs taken.
4. Self-administer sumatriptan (Imitrex) subcutaneously if prescribed.
5. Self-administer sumatriptan transdermal patch (Zecuity) (if prescribed) and describe appropriate disposal method for used patch.
6. Use stress management techniques (Chapter 6).
7. Participate in regular exercise.
8. Contact HCP if any of the following occur:
   - Symptoms become more severe, last longer than usual, or are resistant to medication
   - Nausea and vomiting (if severe or not typical), change in vision, or fever occurs with the headache
   - Problems occur with any drugs

marinated foods. Active challenge and provocative testing (designed specifically to provoke symptoms) with suspect foods may help determine specific causative agents. However, teach the patient that food triggers may change over time.

Teach patients to avoid smoking and exposure to triggers, such as strong perfumes, volatile solvents, and gasoline fumes. Cluster headaches may occur at high altitudes with low $O_2$ levels during air travel. Ergotamine, taken before the plane takes off, may decrease the likelihood of these attacks. See Table 58-4 for a teaching guide for the patient with a headache.

### ◆ Evaluation

Expected outcomes are that the patient with headache will
- Report satisfaction with pain management
- Use drug and nondrug measures appropriately to manage pain

Additional information on expected outcomes for the patient with headache is presented in eNursing Care Plan 58-1 (available on the website for this chapter).

# CHRONIC NEUROLOGIC DISORDERS

## EPILEPSY AND SEIZURE DISORDERS

**Epilepsy** is a disease marked by a continuing predisposition to seizures, with neurobiologic, cognitive, psychologic, and social consequences.[7] It is the fourth most common neurologic disorder, with only migraine, stroke, and Alzheimer's disease occurring more frequently. In the United States, approximately 2.2 million people have active epilepsy, with 150,000 new cases diagnosed each year.[8] The incidence of epilepsy is higher in young children and older adults.

New cases of epilepsy are more common in African Americans and in socially disadvantaged populations. Males are slightly more likely to develop epilepsy than females. People with Alzheimer's disease or who have had a stroke are at high risk for developing epilepsy. The risk is slightly increased in the child of a person who has epilepsy. However, most children will not inherit epilepsy from a parent.

**Seizure** is a transient, uncontrolled electrical discharge of neurons in the brain that interrupts normal function. Seizures may accompany a variety of disorders, or they may occur spontaneously without any apparent cause. Seizures resulting from systemic and metabolic disturbances are not considered epilepsy if the seizures cease when the underlying problem is corrected. Metabolic disturbances that cause seizures include acidosis, electrolyte imbalances, hypoglycemia, hypoxia, alcohol and barbiturate withdrawal, dehydration, and water intoxication. Extracranial disorders that can cause seizures are heart, lung, liver, or kidney diseases; systemic lupus erythematosus; diabetes mellitus; hypertension; and septicemia.

### Etiology and Pathophysiology

Seizure disorders have many possible causes, with the most common causes varying by age. The most common causes of seizure disorder during the first 6 months of life are severe birth injury, congenital defects involving the central nervous system (CNS), infections, and inborn errors of metabolism. In people between 2 and 20 years of age, primary causes are birth injury, infection, trauma, and genetic factors. In individuals between 20 and 30 years of age, seizure disorder usually occurs as the result of structural lesions, such as trauma, brain tumors, or vascular disease. After 50 years of age, the primary causes of seizure disorders are stroke and metastatic brain tumors. However, one third of all epilepsy cases are idiopathic, meaning they are not attributable to a specific cause. These cases are known as *idiopathic generalized epilepsy (IGE)*.

Epilepsy (recurring seizures) is caused by a group of abnormal neurons that seem to undergo spontaneous firing. This firing spreads by physiologic pathways to involve adjacent or distant areas of the brain. If this activity spreads to involve the whole brain, a generalized seizure occurs. The cause of this abnormal firing is not clear. Any stimulus that causes the neuron's cell membrane to depolarize induces a tendency for spontaneous firing. Localization of the *seizure focus* (the place where the seizure originates) is critical to the success of any anticipated surgical treatment.

Scar tissue *(gliosis)* is often found in the area of the brain from which the seizure activity arises. Scarring is believed to interfere with the normal chemical and structural environment of the brain neurons, making them more likely to fire abnormally.

In addition to neuronal alterations, changes in the function of astrocytes may play several key roles in recurring seizures. Activation of astrocytes by hyperactive neurons is one of the crucial factors that predisposes nearby neurons to generate an epileptic discharge.

### Genetic Link

Genetic abnormalities may be the most important factor contributing to IGE. Some types of epilepsy tend to run in families, suggesting a genetic influence. Other types of IGE are related to abnormalities in specific genes that control the flow of ions in and out of cells and regulate neuron signaling or are involved with protein and carbohydrate metabolism. Many genetic mutations associated with epilepsy appear to be acquired (occurring after birth) rather than inherited mutations.[9] (Genetics is discussed in Chapter 12.)

The role of genetics in the etiology of seizure disorders has been difficult to determine because of the problem of separating genetic from environmental or acquired influences. In some forms of epilepsy, families carry a predisposition to seizure disorders in the form of an inherently low threshold to seizure-producing stimuli, such as trauma, disease, and high fever.

Abnormal genes may influence the disorder in subtle ways. For example, a person with epilepsy may have an abnormally active version of a gene that increases resistance to drugs. This may help explain why antiseizure drugs do not work for some people.

## Clinical Manifestations

Specific clinical manifestations of a seizure are determined by the site of the electrical disturbance. The preferred method of classifying seizures is presented in Table 58-5. This system, which is based on the clinical and electroencephalographic manifestations of seizures, divides seizures into two major classes: *generalized* and *focal* (Fig. 58-2). Depending on the type, a seizure may occur in multiple phases: (1) *prodromal phase,* with sensations or behavior changes that precede a seizure; (2) *aural phase,* with a sensory warning that is similar each time a seizure occurs; (3) *ictal phase,* from first symptoms to the end of seizure activity; and (4) *postictal phase,* the recovery period after the seizure.

**Generalized Seizures.** Generalized seizures quickly involve both sides of the brain and are characterized by bilateral synchronous epileptic discharges in the brain from the onset of the seizure. In most cases, the patient loses consciousness for a few seconds to several minutes.

***Tonic-Clonic Seizures.*** The most common generalized seizure is the tonic-clonic seizure. Tonic-clonic seizure (formerly known as *grand mal*) is characterized by losing consciousness and falling to the ground if the patient is upright, followed by stiffening of the body (tonic phase) for 10 to 20 seconds and subsequent jerking of the extremities (clonic phase) for another 30 to 40 seconds. Cyanosis, excessive salivation, tongue or cheek biting, and incontinence may accompany the seizure.

In the postictal phase, the patient usually has muscle soreness, feels tired, and may sleep for several hours. Some patients may not feel normal for several hours or days after a seizure. The patient has no memory of the seizure.

***Typical Absence Seizures.*** Absence seizure (formerly called *petit mal*) usually occurs only in children and rarely continues beyond adolescence. This type of seizure may cease altogether as the child matures, or it may evolve into another type of seizure. The typical clinical manifestation of a simple absence seizure is a brief staring spell resembling "daydreaming" that lasts less than 10 seconds, so it often goes unnoticed. In complex absence seizures, the blank stare is accompanied by some type of movement (e.g., blinking, chewing, hand gestures) and can last up to 20 seconds. When untreated, seizures may occur up to 100 times a day. An electroencephalogram (EEG) demonstrates a 3-Hz (cycles per second) spike-and-wave pattern that

**TABLE 58-5 Classification of Seizure Disorders**

| Primary Generalized Seizures | Focal Seizures |
|---|---|
| (Involve both hemispheres of brain)<br>• Tonic-clonic seizures<br>• Absence seizures (simple or complex)<br>  • Typical<br>  • Atypical<br>  • Absence with special features<br>• Myoclonic seizures<br>• Tonic seizures<br>• Atonic seizures (akinetic)<br>• Clonic seizures | (Involve one hemisphere of brain)<br>• Simple focal seizures (no impairment of awareness/consciousness)<br>• Complex focal seizures (impairment of awareness/consciousness)<br>• Focal seizures evolving to secondary generalized seizures<br>**Unknown**<br>(Events not clearly diagnosed into categories above) |

Adapted from International League Against Epilepsy: ILAE revised terminology for organization of seizures and epilepsies 2011-2013. Retrieved from *www.ilae.org/visitors/centre/documents/OrganizationEpilepsy-overview.pdf.*

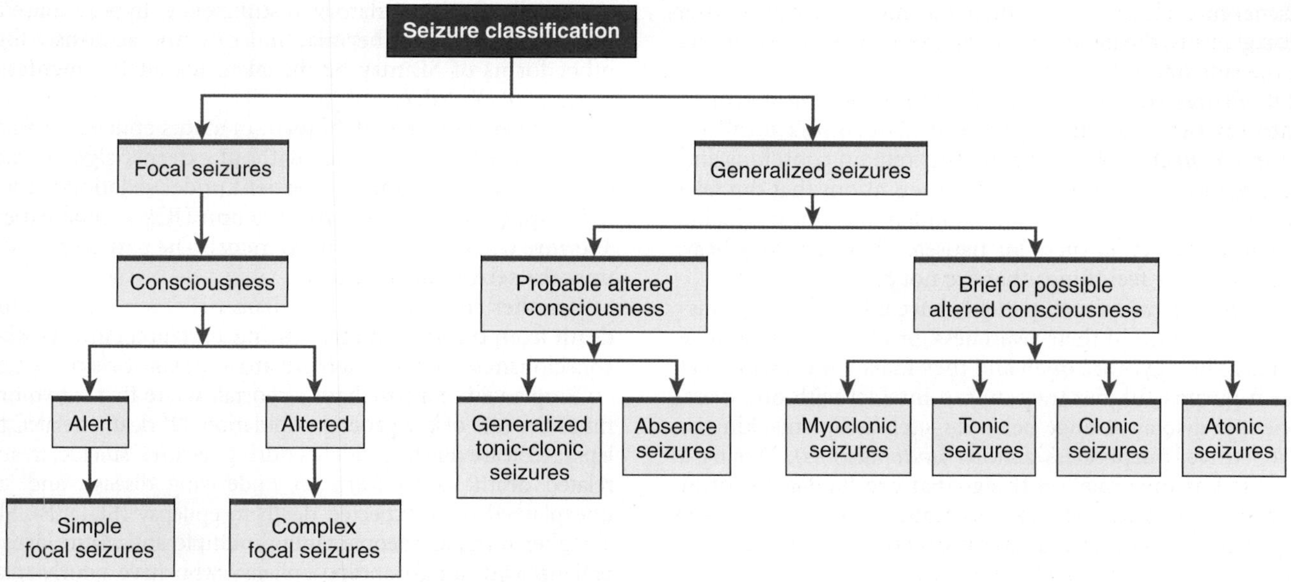


**FIG. 58-2** Algorithm for classification of seizures.

is unique to this type of seizure. Hyperventilation and flashing lights can precipitate absence seizures.

***Atypical Absence Seizures.*** In *atypical absence seizure,* the staring spell is accompanied by other signs and symptoms, such as eye blinking or jerking movements of the lips. The patient may be somewhat responsive during seizure activity. This type of seizure commonly lasts more than 10 seconds (as much as 30 seconds), with a gradual beginning and end. If the patient has cognitive impairment, seizure activity may be difficult to distinguish from usual behavior. Atypical absence seizures usually continue into adulthood. An EEG demonstrates atypical spike-and-wave patterns, usually greater or less than 3 Hz.

***Other Types of Generalized Seizures.*** Other generalized seizures are myoclonic, atonic, tonic, and clonic seizures. A *myoclonic seizure* is characterized by a sudden, excessive jerk or twitch of the body or extremities. The jerk represents a muscle contraction and may be forceful enough to hurl the person to the ground. These seizures last no more than a few seconds, but they may occur in clusters.

An *atonic seizure (akinetic seizure* or *drop attack)* involves either a tonic episode or a paroxysmal loss of muscle tone and begins suddenly with the person falling to the ground. Seizures typically last less than 15 seconds. The person usually remains conscious, and normal activity can be resumed immediately. Patients with this type of seizure are at a great risk of head injury and often have to wear protective helmets.

A tonic seizure involves a sudden onset of increased tone in the extensor muscles, contributing to sudden stiff movements. Tonic seizures most often occur in sleep and affect both sides of the body. Patients will fall if they are standing when the seizure occurs. Tonic seizures usually last less than 20 seconds. The patient usually remains conscious.

*Clonic seizures* begin with loss of consciousness and sudden loss of muscle tone, followed by rhythmic limb jerking that may or may not be symmetric. Clonic seizures are relatively rare.

**Focal Seizures.** *Focal seizures,* also called *partial* or *partial focal seizures,* are the other major class of seizures (Table 58-5). Focal seizures begin in one hemisphere of the brain in a specific region of the cortex, as indicated by the EEG. They produce sensory, motor, cognitive, or emotional manifestations based on the function of the involved area of the brain. For example, if the discharging focus is located in the medial aspect of the postcentral gyrus, the patient may experience paresthesia in the leg on the side opposite the focus.

Focal seizures are divided according to their clinical expression into (1) simple focal seizures and (2) complex focal seizures.[10] In a *simple focal seizure,* patients remain conscious and alert but experience unusual feelings or sensations that can take many forms. They may experience sudden and unexplainable feelings of joy, anger, sadness, or nausea. They also may hear, smell, taste, see, or feel things that are not real.

In a *complex focal seizure,* patients have a loss of consciousness or an alteration in their awareness, producing a dreamlike experience. Their eyes are open and they make movements that may seem purposeful, but they cannot interact with observers. Some people display strange behavior such as lip smacking or other repetitive, purposeless actions *(automatisms).* During a seizure, some people may do things that can be dangerous or embarrassing, such as walking into traffic or removing their clothes. These patients need to take precautions before a seizure occurs.

Patients may continue an activity started before the seizure, such as counting coins or choosing items from a grocery shelf, but after the seizure they do not remember the activity performed during the seizure. These seizures usually last between 30 seconds and 2 minutes. Patients may be tired or confused following the seizure and may not return to normal activity for hours.

Focal seizures may be confined to one side of the brain and remain focal (partial) in nature, or they may spread to involve the entire brain, culminating in a generalized tonic-clonic seizure. Any tonic-clonic seizure that is preceded by an aura or warning is a focal seizure that generalizes secondarily. Many tonic-clonic seizures that appear to be generalized from the outset may actually be secondary generalized seizures. However, the preceding partial component may be so brief that it is undetected by the patient or the observer, or even on the EEG. Unlike the primary generalized tonic-clonic seizure, the secondary generalized seizure may result in a transient residual neurologic deficit postictally. This is called *Todd's paralysis* (focal weakness), which resolves after varying lengths of time.

**Psychogenic Seizures.** Because they closely resemble epileptic seizures, psychogenic seizures may be misdiagnosed as epilepsy. Proper diagnosis usually requires video-EEG monitoring to identify associated events. If the diagnosis of epilepsy is excluded, history of emotional or physical abuse or a specific traumatic event often emerges. Some patients may have both psychogenic seizures and epilepsy. Care provided by a specialist in epilepsy is essential.

## Complications

**Physical.** Status epilepticus (SE) is a state of continuous seizure activity or a condition in which seizures recur in rapid succession without return to consciousness between seizures. It is defined as any seizure lasting longer than 5 minutes. The longer a seizure lasts, the less likely it is to stop without drug therapy.[11]

SE is a neurologic emergency that can occur with any type of seizure. The highest incidence occurs in children and older adults. During repeated seizures, the brain uses more energy than can be supplied. As neurons become exhausted and cease to function, permanent brain damage may result. *Convulsive status epilepticus* is the most dangerous type because it can cause potentially fatal ventilatory insufficiency, hypoxemia, cardiac dysrhythmias, hyperthermia, and systemic acidosis. However, other forms of SE may be mistaken for altered mentation or movement disorders.

*Subclinical seizures* are a form of status epilepticus in which a sedated patient seizes but without external signs because of sedative use. For example, a patient under sedation for ventilatory support in the intensive care unit (ICU) could experience a seizure without physical movements. The patient's HCP could miss the seizure occurrence.

Another complication of seizures is severe injury and even death from trauma suffered during a seizure. Patients who lose consciousness during a seizure are at greatest risk.

People with epilepsy have a mortality rate that is two or three times the rate of the general population. Of deaths related to epilepsy, 40% are due to accidents during seizures, suicide, treatment-related death, death from an underlying disease, and sudden unexplained or unexpected death in epilepsy (SUDEP). SUDEP is higher in males, people taking multiple antiseizure drugs, and patients with long-standing epilepsy who have poorly managed seizure activity. The direct cause of SUDEP is unknown but thought to be related to respiratory dysfunction, cardiac dysrhythmias, or cerebral depression.[12] Specific teaching about medication adherence and disease awareness is critical for at-risk people.

**Psychosocial.** Perhaps the most common complication of seizure disorders is its effect on a patient's lifestyle. Patients may develop ineffective coping methods because of psychosocial problems related to having a seizure disorder. In particular, an increased incidence of depression occurs in people who have seizures that are difficult to control. Antiseizure drugs and the continued need to manage a chronic disease also can contribute to depression.

Although attitudes have improved in recent years, a diagnosis of epilepsy still carries a social stigma. Patients with epilepsy may experience discrimination in employment and educational opportunities. Transportation may be difficult because of legal sanctions against driving. Screen patients frequently for depression, and encourage them to pursue available treatment options.

## Diagnostic Studies

A diagnosis of epilepsy or seizure disorder has many socioeconomic, physical, and psychologic consequences for the patient. Thus accurate diagnosis is crucial. The most useful diagnostic tool is an accurate, comprehensive description of seizures and the patient's health history (Table 58-6).

The EEG is a useful diagnostic adjuvant to the history, but only if it shows abnormalities. Abnormal findings help determine the type of seizure and pinpoint the seizure focus. Ideally, an EEG should be done within 24 hours of a suspected seizure. Unfortunately, only a small percentage of patients with seizure disorders have abnormal EEG findings the first time the test is done. Either repeated EEGs or continuous EEG monitoring may be needed to detect abnormalities. An EEG is not a definitive test because some patients without seizure disorders have abnormal patterns on their EEGs, while many patients with seizure disorders have normal EEG results between seizures. If abnormal discharges do not occur during the 30 to 40 minutes of sampling during EEG, the test may not indicate an abnormality. Magnetoencephalography may be done in conjunction with the EEG. This test has greater sensitivity in detecting small magnetic fields generated by neuronal activity.

A complete blood count, serum chemistries, studies of liver and kidney function, and a urinalysis should be done to rule out metabolic disorders. A CT scan or MRI should be done in any new-onset seizure to rule out a structural lesion. Cerebral angiography, single-photon emission computed tomography (SPECT), magnetic resonance spectroscopy (MRS), MRA, and positron emission tomography (PET) may be used in selected clinical situations.

The International League Against Epilepsy has developed specific diagnostic criteria for each type of seizure, including conditions that resolve over time (*www.ilae.org*). If a patient is diagnosed with a seizure disorder, the seizure type must be correctly identified (Fig. 58-2 and Table 58-6) to determine appropriate treatment.

**TABLE 58-6 Interprofessional Care**

***Epilepsy and Seizure Disorders***

| Diagnostic Assessment | Diagnostic Studies |
|---|---|
| ***History and Physical Examination*** | • CBC, urinalysis, electrolytes, creatinine, fasting blood glucose |
| • Birth and developmental history | • Lumbar puncture for CSF analysis |
| • Significant illnesses and injuries | • CT, MRI, MRA, MRS, PET scan |
| • Family history | • Electroencephalography (EEG) |
| • Febrile seizures | **Management** |
| • Comprehensive neurologic assessment | • Antiseizure drugs (Table 58-8) |
| ***Seizure History*** | • Surgery |
| • Precipitating factors | • Vagal nerve stimulation |
| • Antecedent events | • Psychosocial counseling |
| • Seizure description (including onset, duration, frequency, postictal state) | • Physical therapy |

*MRA,* Magnetic resonance angiography; *MRS,* magnetic resonance spectroscopy; *PET,* positron emission tomography.

## Interprofessional Care

Most seizures do not require emergency medical care because they are self-limiting and rarely cause bodily injury. However, if status epilepticus or significant bodily harm occurs, or if the event is a first-time seizure, medical care should be sought immediately. Table 58-6 outlines the diagnostic studies and interprofessional care of seizure disorders. Table 58-7 summarizes emergency care of the patient with a generalized tonic-clonic seizure, the seizure most likely to warrant emergency medical care.

**Drug Therapy.** The primary treatment for seizure disorders is antiseizure drugs (Table 58-8). Because a cure is not possible, the goal of therapy is to prevent seizures with minimal toxic side effects from drug therapy. Drugs generally act by stabilizing nerve cell membranes and preventing spread of the epileptic discharge. Drug therapy should begin with a single drug based on the patient's age and weight and type, frequency, and cause of seizure. Dosage should be increased until seizures are controlled or toxic side effects occur.

If seizure control is not achieved with a single drug, dosage or timing of administration may be changed or a second drug may be added. About one third of patients require a combination regimen for adequate control. Patients should discuss emerging treatments with their HCPs to provide the best control with the least amount of medication.

The therapeutic range for each drug indicates the serum level above which most patients experience toxic side effects and below which most continue to have seizures. However, therapeutic drug ranges are only guides for therapy. If the patient's seizures are well controlled with a subtherapeutic level, the drug dosage does not have to be increased. Likewise, if a drug level is above the therapeutic range and the patient has good seizure control without toxic side effects, the drug dosage does not have to be decreased. Serum drug levels are monitored if seizures continue to occur, seizure frequency increases, or drug adherence is questioned. Because they have a very large therapeutic range, many newer drugs do not require drug-level monitoring.

The primary drugs to treat generalized tonic-clonic and focal seizures are phenytoin (Dilantin), carbamazepine (Tegretol), phenobarbital, divalproex, and primidone (Mysoline). The drugs used to treat absence and myoclonic seizures include ethosuximide (Zarontin), divalproex, and clonazepam (Klonopin).

**TABLE 58-7 Emergency Management**

***Tonic-Clonic Seizures***

| Etiology | Assessment Findings | Interventions |
|---|---|---|
| **Head Trauma**<br>• Epidural hematoma<br>• Subdural hematoma<br>• Intracranial hematoma<br>• Cerebral contusion<br>• Traumatic birth injury<br>**Drug-Related Processes**<br>• Overdose<br>• Withdrawal of alcohol, opioids, antiseizure drugs<br>• Ingestion, inhalation<br>**Infectious Processes**<br>• Meningitis<br>• Septicemia<br>• Encephalitis<br>**Intracranial Events**<br>• Brain tumor<br>• Subarachnoid hemorrhage<br>• Stroke<br>• Hypertensive crisis<br>• Increased ICP secondary to clogged shunt<br>**Metabolic Imbalances**<br>• Fluid and electrolyte imbalance<br>• Hypoglycemia<br>**Medical Disorders**<br>• Heart, liver, lung, or kidney disease<br>• Systemic lupus erythematosus<br>**Idiopathic**<br>**Other**<br>• Cardiac arrest<br>• Psychiatric disorders<br>• High fever | **Aural Phase**<br>• Peculiar sensations that precede seizure<br>• Loss of consciousness<br>• Bowel and bladder incontinence<br>• Tachycardia<br>• Diaphoresis<br>• Warm skin<br>• Pallor, flushing, or cyanosis<br>**Tonic Phase**<br>• Continuous muscle contractions<br>**Hypertonic Phase**<br>• Extreme muscular rigidity lasting 5-15 sec<br>**Clonic Phase**<br>• Rigidity and relaxation alternating in rapid succession<br>**Postictal Phase**<br>• Lethargy, altered level of consciousness<br>• Confusion and headache<br>• Repeated tonic-clonic seizures for several min | **Initial**<br>Ensure patent airway.<br>Protect patient from injury during seizure. *Do not restrain.* Pad side rails.<br>Remove or loosen tight clothing.<br>Establish IV access.<br>Stay with patient until seizure has passed.<br>Anticipate administration of phenobarbital, phenytoin (Dilantin), or benzodiazepines (e.g., diazepam [Valium], midazolam [Versed], lorazepam [Ativan]) to attempt to abort seizures.<br>Suction as needed.<br>Assist ventilations if patient does not breathe spontaneously after seizure.<br>Anticipate need for intubation if gag reflex absent.<br>**Ongoing Monitoring**<br>Monitor vital signs, level of consciousness, $O_2$ saturation, Glasgow Coma Scale results, pupil size and reactivity.<br>Reassure and orient patient after seizure.<br>Never force an airway between patient's clenched teeth.<br>Give IV dextrose for hypoglycemia. |

*ICP,* Intracranial pressure.

**TABLE 58-8 Drug Therapy**

***Seizure Disorders***

| | |
|---|---|
| • brivaracetam (Briviact) | • levetiracetam (Keppra) |
| • carbamazepine (Tegretol) | • lorazepam (Ativan) |
| • clonazepam (Klonopin) | • oxcarbazepine (Trileptal) |
| • daclizumab (Zinbryta) | • perampanel (Fycompa) |
| • diazepam (Diastat) | • phenytoin (Dilantin) |
| • divalproex (Depakote) | • pregabalin (Lyrica) |
| • eslicarbazepine (Aptiom) | • primidone (Mysoline) |
| • ethosuximide (Zarontin) | • tiagabine (Gabitril) |
| • ezogabine (Potiga) | • topiramate (Topamax) |
| • felbamate (Felbatol) | • valproic acid (Depakene) |
| • gabapentin (Neurontin) | • vigabatrin (Sabril) |
| • lacosamide (Vimpat) | • zonisamide (Zonegran) |
| • lamotrigine (Lamictal) | |

**DRUG ALERT Carbamazepine (Tegretol)**
- Do not take with grapefruit juice.
- Instruct patient to report visual abnormalities.
- Abrupt withdrawal after long-term use may precipitate seizures.

Other antiseizure drugs include gabapentin, topiramate, lamotrigine (Lamictal), tiagabine (Gabitril), levetiracetam (Keppra), and zonisamide (Zonegran). Some of these drugs are broad spectrum and appear to be effective for multiple seizure types. Pregabalin (Lyrica) is used as an additional treatment for focal seizures not successfully controlled with a single medication.

Treatment of status epilepticus requires initiation of a rapid-acting IV antiseizure drug. The drugs most commonly used are lorazepam (Ativan) and diazepam (Valium). Because these are short-acting drugs, their administration is followed with long-acting drugs such as phenytoin or phenobarbital.

Because many of the antiseizure drugs (e.g., phenytoin, phenobarbital, ethosuximide, lamotrigine, topiramate) have a long half-life, they can be given in once- or twice-daily doses. This simplifies the drug regimen and increases the patient's adherence because the drug does not have to be taken at work or school. Unnecessary combination therapy should be avoided whenever possible. Medications should be reviewed routinely and the least effective medication discontinued by tapering.

**DRUG ALERT Antiseizure Drugs**
- Abrupt withdrawal after long-term use may precipitate seizures.
- If weaning is to occur, the patient must be seizure free for a prolonged period (e.g., 2 to 5 yr) and have a normal neurologic examination and EEG.

Side effects of antiseizure drugs involve the CNS and include diplopia, drowsiness, ataxia, and mental slowness. Neurologic assessment for dose-related toxicity involves testing the eyes for nystagmus and evaluating hand and gait coordination, cognitive functioning, and general alertness.

As a nurse, be knowledgeable about these side effects so that you can inform patients and institute proper treatment. Common side effects of phenytoin are gingival hyperplasia (excessive growth of gingival tissue) and hirsutism, especially in young adults. Good dental hygiene, including regular tooth brushing and flossing, can decrease gingival hyperplasia. If gingival hyperplasia is extensive, the hyperplastic tissue may have to be surgically removed (gingivectomy) and phenytoin replaced with another antiseizure drug.

Medication nonadherence can be a problem in people with a seizure disorder. Take measures to increase patient adherence to the prescribed drug regimens. If HCPs are aware of nonadherence issues, they can work with the patient to find an acceptable drug regimen. For example, using pregabalin as an adjunct medication in some cases may allow a decreased dose of the primary antiseizure drug, thus decreasing undesirable side effects.

### Gerontologic Considerations: Drug Therapy for Seizure Disorders

Many older adults experience a first single seizure, and a large percentage of them do not have another seizure. To be considered for antiseizure drug therapy, older adults should have recurrent seizures, an obvious structural predisposition for seizures, or onset of epilepsy presenting as status epilepticus. Older adults are more responsive to antiseizure drugs than younger adults, but they also are more likely to experience side effects at lower serum drug concentrations.

In considering antiseizure drug therapy for older adults, you should recall the relationship between drug action and normal changes that occur with aging. For example, phenytoin is widely used to treat seizure disorders. However, because the liver metabolizes phenytoin, its use should be avoided in older patients with compromised liver function. Age-related changes in liver enzymes decrease the liver's ability to metabolize drugs. Because phenobarbital, carbamazepine, and primidone have potential effects on cognitive function, their use may also be less desirable for older adults. Use of carbamazepine, phenytoin, phenobarbital, primidone, topiramate, and oxcarbazepine can increase the risk of osteopenia and osteoporosis in older adults.[13]

Several newer antiseizure drugs offer greater treatment benefit to older adults. Compared with older drugs, gabapentin, lamotrigine, oxcarbazepine, and levetiracetam may be safer, have fewer effects on cognitive function, and have fewer interactions with other drugs.

**Surgical Therapy.** Despite availability of newer drugs with fewer side effects, no solution has been found for *medically refractory epilepsy* (unresponsive to drug therapy). If a patient's seizures fail to respond to the first two prescribed antiseizure medications, the likelihood of achieving a seizure-free life with further medication changes is only 5% to 10%.[14] However, a substantial number of patients with uncontrolled epilepsy are candidates for surgical therapy to remove the epileptic focus or prevent spread of epileptic activity in the brain. The classic surgical intervention has been an anterior temporal lobe resection. However, the current goal of neurosurgery is a careful resection of a precisely localized area within a lobe of the brain. Approximately 70% to 80% of patients become seizure free after surgery, and 10% to 20% experience a marked reduction in seizure activity.[14]

Not all types of epilepsy benefit from surgery. An extensive preoperative evaluation is important, including continuous EEG monitoring and other specific tests to ensure precise localization of the focal point. Surgical candidates must meet three requirements: (1) a confirmed diagnosis of epilepsy, (2) an adequate trial with drug therapy without satisfactory results, and (3) a defined electroclinical syndrome (type of seizure disorder).

**Other Therapies.** *Vagal nerve stimulation*, a form of neuromodulation, is used as an adjunct to drugs when an accessible focal point cannot be identified for surgical removal. The exact mechanism of action is unknown, but it is thought to interrupt the synchronization of epileptic brain wave activity and stop excessive discharge of neurons. In vagal nerve stimulation, a surgically implanted electrode in the neck is programmed to deliver the electrical impulse to the vagus nerve, usually on the left side. The patient can activate it with a magnet when he or she senses a seizure is imminent. Vagal nerve stimulation can cause adverse effects such as coughing, hoarseness, dyspnea, and tingling in the neck. Battery life is 5 to 10 years, and surgical replacement is required. Benefits of this therapy can be seen within 24 months after implantation.

A *ketogenic diet* is a special high-fat, low-carbohydrate diet that has been used to control seizures in some people with epilepsy. When a person is on this diet, ketones are produced and pass into the brain and replace glucose as an energy source. Meals must be carefully planned because the amount of protein and carbohydrate in the diet must be restricted. Patients on this diet who use anticoagulants need close monitoring for bleeding. Although HCPs are more likely to recommend the diet for children than adults, the diet can work equally well in both age groups. However, long-term effects of the diet are not clear.[15]

Biofeedback to control seizures is aimed at teaching the patient to maintain a certain brain wave frequency that is refractory to seizure activity. Further trials are needed to assess the effectiveness of biofeedback for seizure control.

## NURSING MANAGEMENT: SEIZURE DISORDERS AND EPILEPSY

### Nursing Assessment

Subjective and objective data to obtain from a patient with a seizure disorder are presented in Table 58-9. Obtain data related to a specific seizure episode from a witness.

### Nursing Diagnoses

Nursing diagnoses for the patient with seizure disorders and epilepsy may include, but are not limited to, the following:

- Ineffective breathing pattern *related to* neuromuscular impairment
- Ineffective health management *related to* drug therapy and lifestyle adjustments
- Risk for injury *related to* loss of consciousness during seizure activity and postictal physical weakness

Additional information on nursing diagnoses for the patient with a seizure disorder is presented in eNursing Care Plan 58-2 (available on the website for this chapter).

### Planning

The overall goals are that the patient with seizures will (1) be free from injury during a seizure, (2) have optimal mental and physical functioning while taking antiseizure drugs, and (3) have satisfactory psychosocial functioning.

## TABLE 58-9 Nursing Assessment

### *Epilepsy and Seizure Disorders*

**Subjective Data**

***Important Health Information***

*Past health history:* Previous seizures, birth defects or injuries, anoxic episodes. CNS trauma, tumors, or infections. Stroke, metabolic disorders, alcoholism, exposure to metals and carbon monoxide, hepatic or renal failure, fever, pregnancy, systemic lupus erythematosus

*Medications:* Adherence to antiseizure medication regimen. Barbiturate or alcohol withdrawal. Use and overdose of cocaine, amphetamines, lidocaine, theophylline, penicillin, lithium, phenothiazines, tricyclic antidepressants, benzodiazepines

***Functional Health Patterns***

*Health perception–health management:* Positive family history

*Cognitive-perceptual:* Headaches, aura, mood or behavioral changes before seizure. Mentation changes. Abdominal pain, muscle pain (postictal)

*Self-perception–self-concept:* Anxiety, depression. Loss of self-esteem, social isolation

*Sexuality-reproductive:* Decreased sexual drive, erectile dysfunction. Increased sexual drive (postictal)

**Objective Data**

***General***

Precipitating factors, including severe metabolic acidosis or alkalosis, hyperkalemia, hypoglycemia, dehydration, or water intoxication

***Integumentary***

Bitten tongue, soft tissue damage, cyanosis, diaphoresis (postictal)

***Respiratory***

Abnormal respiratory rate, rhythm, or depth. Apnea (ictal). Absent or abnormal breath sounds, possible airway occlusion

***Cardiovascular***

Hypertension, tachycardia or bradycardia (ictal)

***Gastrointestinal***

Bowel incontinence, excessive salivation

***Urinary***

Incontinence

***Neurologic***

***Generalized***

*Tonic-clonic:* Loss of consciousness, muscle tightening, then jerking. Dilated pupils. Hyperventilation, then apnea. Postictal somnolence

*Absence:* Altered consciousness (5-30 sec), minor facial motor activity

***Focal***

*Simple:* Aura. Focal sensory, motor, cognitive, or emotional phenomena (focal motor). Unilateral "marching" motor seizure (jacksonian)

*Complex:* Altered consciousness with inappropriate behaviors, automatisms, amnesia of event

***Musculoskeletal***

Weakness, paralysis, ataxia (postictal)

***Possible Diagnostic Findings***

Positive toxicology screen or blood alcohol level. Altered serum electrolytes, acidosis or alkalosis, very low blood glucose, ↑ blood urea nitrogen or serum creatinine, abnormal liver function tests, ammonia; abnormal CT scan or MRI of head, abnormal findings from lumbar puncture. Abnormal discharges on EEG

## ◆ Nursing Implementation

◆ **Health Promotion.** Some seizure disorders can be prevented by promoting general safety measures, such as wearing helmets in situations involving risk of head injury. Improved perinatal, labor, and delivery care have reduced fetal trauma and hypoxia and thus have reduced brain damage leading to seizure disorders.

The patient with a seizure disorder should practice good general health habits (e.g., maintain proper diet, get adequate rest, exercise). Help the patient identify events or situations that precipitate the seizures and provide suggestions for avoiding them or handling them better. Teach the patient to avoid excessive alcohol intake, fatigue, and loss of sleep. Help the patient handle stress constructively.

◆ **Acute Care.** Nursing care for a hospitalized patient with a seizure disorder or a patient who has had seizures secondary to other factors involves observation and treatment of the seizure, patient and caregiver teaching, and psychosocial intervention.

**CHECK YOUR PRACTICE**

You are making your morning rounds and go to check your 34-yr-old male patient who was admitted the night before with increased seizure activity. When you go to his room, his roommate is yelling, "Help, help!" You notice that the patient is on the floor jerking and stiffening and does not respond to you.

- What should you do?

When a seizure occurs, carefully observe and record details of the event because the diagnosis and subsequent treatment often rest solely on the seizure description. Note all aspects of the seizure. What events preceded the seizure? When did the seizure occur? How long did each phase (aural [if any], ictal, postictal) last? What occurred during each phase?

Both subjective data (usually the only type of data in the aural phase) and objective data are important. Note the exact onset of the seizure (which body part was affected first and how); the course and nature of the seizure activity (loss of consciousness, tongue biting, automatisms, stiffening, jerking, total lack of muscle tone); body parts involved and their sequence of involvement; and autonomic signs, such as dilated pupils, excessive salivation, altered breathing, cyanosis, flushing, diaphoresis, or incontinence. Assessment of the postictal period should include a detailed description of the level of consciousness, vital signs, pupil size and position of the eyes, memory loss, muscle soreness, speech disorders (aphasia, dysarthria), weakness or paralysis, sleep period, and the duration of each sign or symptom.

**! SAFETY ALERT Seizure**

During a seizure, you should do the following:

- Maintain a patent airway for the patient.
- Protect the patient's head, turn the patient to the side, loosen constrictive clothing, ease patient to the floor (if seated).
- Do not restrain the patient.
- Do not place any objects in the patient's mouth.

After the seizure the patient may require repositioning (to open and maintain the airway), suctioning, and $O_2$. A seizure can be frightening for the patient and for others who witnessed it. Assess their level of understanding and provide information about how and why the event occurred. This is an excellent opportunity for you to dispel many common misconceptions about seizures.

## TEAMWORK & COLLABORATION

### *Caring for the Patient With a Seizure Disorder*

Because any nursing staff member may be present when a patient experiences a seizure, all staff members are responsible for maintaining patient safety.

**Role of Nursing Personnel**

***Registered Nurse (RN)***

- Teach patient about factors that increase risk for seizures, such as alcohol use, fatigue, inadequate sleep, and stress.
- Teach patient about prescribed antiseizure medications, including drug regimen, side effects, and required monitoring of drug levels.
- Assess and document details of seizure events, including events preceding the seizure; length of each phase of the seizure; course and nature of seizure activity; and level of consciousness, vital signs, and activity during the postictal period.
- Assess airway patency, and position patient to maintain airway during and after any seizures.
- Administer IV antiseizure medications to the patient experiencing status epilepticus.
- Make appropriate referrals to the Epilepsy Foundation and community agencies to assist patient with financial impact of the disorder, work training, employment, and living arrangements.
- Teach family members and caregivers about management of seizures and status epilepticus.
- In the ambulatory and home care setting, evaluate patient self-management of medications and lifestyle.

***Licensed Practical/Vocational Nurse (LPN/LVN)***

- Administer oral antiseizure medications as scheduled.
- In the ambulatory and home setting, monitor patient adherence to medications and lifestyle changes and report problems to the RN.

***Unlicensed Assistive Personnel (UAP)***

- Place suction equipment, bag valve mask, and $O_2$ at the patient's bedside.
- Remove potentially harmful objects from the bedside and pad side rails.
- Immediately report any seizure activity to the RN.
- Observe and report events of the seizure to the RN.
- Obtain vital signs during the postictal period.
- Provide oropharyngeal suctioning after a seizure (after being trained and evaluated in this procedure).

**Role of Other Team Members**

***Physical, Occupational, or Respiratory Therapist***

- Remove potentially harmful objects from the bedside and pad side rails.
- Assess airway patency and position patient to maintain airway during and after any seizures.
- Immediately report any seizure activity to the RN.
- Observe and report events of the seizure to the RN.

**Ambulatory Care.** Prevention of recurring seizures is the major goal in the treatment of epilepsy. For treatment to be effective, drugs must be taken regularly and continuously, often for a lifetime. Help the patient understand this and review details of the drug regimen and what to do if a dose is missed. Usually the dose is made up if the omission is remembered within 24 hours. Caution the patient not to adjust drug dosages without professional guidance because this can increase seizure frequency and even cause status epilepticus. Encourage the patient to report any medication side effects and to keep regular appointments with the HCP.

You have an important role in teaching the patient and caregiver. Review the guidelines for teaching presented in Table 58-10. Teach the caregiver, family members, and significant others the emergency management of tonic-clonic seizures (Table 58-7). Remind them that it is not necessary to call an ambulance or send a person to the hospital after a single seizure unless the seizure is prolonged, another seizure immediately follows, extensive injury has occurred, or if it is unknown if there was a first-time seizure.

Patients with a seizure disorder may experience concerns or fears related to recurrent seizures, incontinence, or loss of self-control. Support the patient through teaching and by helping him or her use effective coping mechanisms.

Perhaps the greatest challenge for a patient with a seizure disorder is adjusting to the personal and societal limitations imposed by the illness. Discrimination in employment is the most serious problem facing the person with a seizure disorder. For issues relating to job discrimination, refer patients to the state department of vocational rehabilitation or the U.S. Equal Employment Opportunity Commission (EEOC).

## TABLE 58-10 Patient & Caregiver Teaching

### *Seizure Disorders*

*Include the following information in the teaching plan for the patient with a seizure disorder.*

1. Take antiseizure medications as prescribed. Report any and all drug side effects to the HCP. When necessary, blood is drawn to ensure maintenance of therapeutic drug levels. Schedule regular communication with the HCP to explore additional treatment options.
2. Use nondrug techniques, such as relaxation therapy, to potentially reduce the number of seizures.
3. Be aware of community and online resources for education and help with tracking and explaining seizure activity.
4. Wear a medical alert bracelet or necklace, and carry an identification card.
5. Avoid excessive alcohol intake, fatigue, and loss of sleep.
6. Eat regular meals and snacks in between if feeling shaky, faint, or hungry.
7. Be knowledgeable as a woman of childbearing age regarding antiseizure medications and contraceptive use.

*Caregivers should receive the following information.*

**Focal Seizures**

1. Stay calm. Guide patient to safety to prevent injury but do not restrain.
2. Observe for asymmetry of activity and focus on specific actions, such as lip smacking and abnormal movements.
3. Assess patient's level of consciousness and ability to converse and respond appropriately
4. Observe the time the event started and stopped. Pay attention to the time of return to baseline.
5. Provide respect and explanation of occurrence.

**Generalized Tonic-Clonic Seizures**

1. When seizure occurs outside the hospital setting, activate ERS if (1) the duration is greater than 5 minutes; (2) events recur without the patient recovering to baseline; (3) the patient is unable to establish a normal breathing pattern, is injured or pregnant; or (4) you do not know if this is a first-time seizure event.
2. Maintain patient safety. Lower the patient to the floor or bed, remove glasses if on, and loosen restrictive clothing.
3. Do not place anything in the patient's mouth. Patient's teeth/dentures may be damaged, and caregiver may be bitten.
4. Position patient on side (if possible) to improve the patient's ability to release oral secretions.
5. Observe the time event started and stopped. Pay attention to the time of return to baseline.
6. Assess for possible injury or any lingering motor weakness.

Assist the patient in finding appropriate resources. If you believe that associating with others who have a seizure disorder would be beneficial, refer the patient to the local chapter of the Epilepsy Foundation (EF), a volunteer agency that offers varied services to patients with epilepsy *(www.epilepsy.com)*. Refer the patient who is an eligible veteran to a Department of Veterans Affairs medical center that provides comprehensive care. If intensive psychologic counseling is needed, refer the patient to a community mental health center.

Social workers and welfare agencies can help with financial implications and living arrangements. State agencies specializing in vocational rehabilitation services can provide vocational assessment, counseling, funding for training, and assistance with job placement for patients whose seizures are not well controlled. They can also offer financial assistance for transportation and medical costs related to vocational rehabilitation or job maintenance.

Driving laws for patients who have had a seizure vary from state to state. For example, some states require a 3-month seizure-free period before issuing or reissuing a driver's license, whereas others require up to 1 year. The EF provides current information on driving laws for each state.

Inform the patient that medical alert bracelets, necklaces, and identification cards are available through the EF, local pharmacies, or companies specializing in identification devices (e.g., Medic Alert). However, the use of these medical identification tags is optional. Some patients have found them beneficial, but others prefer not to be identified as having a seizure disorder.

Encourage the patient to learn more about epilepsy through self-education. The EF provides informational pamphlets, has an extensive website, and may facilitate support groups. Many agencies that offer services to patients with epilepsy also offer teaching aids and support.

### ◆ Evaluation

Expected outcomes are that the patient with seizures will

- Experience breathing pattern adequate to meet $O_2$ needs
- Experience no seizure-related injury
- Express acceptance of seizure disorder by admitting presence of epilepsy and adhering to recommended treatment regimen

Additional expected outcomes are presented in eNursing Care Plan 58-2 available on the website.

## RESTLESS LEGS SYNDROME

### Etiology and Pathophysiology

**Restless legs syndrome (RLS)**, also called *Willis-Ekbom disease,* is a relatively common condition characterized by unpleasant sensory (paresthesia) and motor abnormalities of one or both legs. Up to 10% of the U.S. population may have RLS.[16] However, the numbers may be higher because the condition is underdiagnosed. RLS is more common in older adults. It is also more common in women than men, and women may have an earlier age of onset.

Two distinct types of RLS have been identified: primary (idiopathic) and secondary. The majority of cases are primary, and many patients with this type of RLS report a positive family history. Secondary RLS can occur with metabolic abnormalities associated with iron deficiency, renal failure, hypertension, diabetes mellitus, spinal disorders, or rheumatoid arthritis. Conditions such as anemia or pregnancy and certain medications can cause or worsen symptoms.

Although the exact pathophysiology of the primary disorder is unknown, RLS is believed to be related to a dysfunction in the brain's basal ganglia circuits that use the neurotransmitter dopamine, which controls movements. In RLS, this dysfunction causes the urge to move the legs. Abnormal iron metabolism or brain iron deficiencies reflected by low serum ferritin may also play a role in RLS.[16]

### Clinical Manifestations

The severity of RLS sensory symptoms ranges from infrequent minor discomfort (paresthesia, including numbness, tingling, and "pins and needles" sensation) to severe pain. Sensory symptoms often appear first. Patients describe annoying and uncomfortable (but usually not painful) sensations in the legs. Some compare the sensations to bugs creeping or crawling on the legs. The leg pain is localized within the calf muscles. Patients can also experience pain in the upper extremities and trunk. The discomfort occurs when the patient is sedentary and is most common in the evening or at night.

The pain at night can disrupt sleep. Physical activity, such as walking, stretching, rocking, or kicking, often relieves the pain. In the most severe cases, patients sleep only a few hours at night, resulting in daytime fatigue and disruption of the daily routine. The motor abnormalities associated with RLS consist of voluntary restlessness and stereotyped, periodic, involuntary movements. The involuntary movements usually occur during sleep. Fatigue further aggravates symptoms. Over time, RLS advances to more frequent and severe episodes.

### Diagnostic Studies

RLS is a clinical diagnosis, based in large part on the patient's history or the report of the bed partner related to nighttime activities. The diagnosis of RLS can be made when the patient meets all five specific criteria: (1) urge to move the legs, often accompanied by uncomfortable or unpleasant sensations in the legs; (2) any uncomfortable sensations begin or worsen with periods of inactivity; (3) any uncomfortable sensations are partially or totally relieved by movement, as long as the activity continues; (4) urge to move the legs and any accompanying sensations become worse in the evening or night; and (5) occurrence of these features is not primary to another medical or behavioral condition.[17]

The patient may undergo polysomnography studies during sleep to distinguish RLS from other clinical conditions that can disturb sleep (e.g., sleep apnea). However, periodic leg movements in sleep are a common feature in RLS patients. Blood tests, such as a complete blood count, serum ferritin, and renal function tests (e.g., serum creatinine), may help exclude secondary causes of RLS. A patient's history of diabetes mellitus and its management may provide information to determine if paresthesia is caused by peripheral neuropathy related to diabetes or RLS.

## ❖ NURSING AND INTERPROFESSIONAL MANAGEMENT: RESTLESS LEGS SYNDROME

The goal of interprofessional management is to reduce patient discomfort and distress and to improve sleep quality. When RLS is secondary to renal failure or iron deficiency, treatment of these conditions will decrease symptoms. Nondrug approaches to RLS management include establishing regular sleep habits; exercising; avoiding activities that cause symptoms; and eliminating aggravating factors, such as alcohol, caffeine, and certain drugs (neuroleptics, lithium, antihistamines, antidepressants). Yoga has been found to improve mood, sleep, and function in RLS.[18]

If nondrug measures fail to provide symptom relief, drug therapy is an option. No single medication effectively manages RLS for all patients. The main drugs used in RLS include dopamine precursors (e.g., carbidopa/levodopa) and dopamine agonists (e.g., ropinirole [Requip], pramipexole [Mirapex]) to increase the amount of dopamine in the brain. The antiseizure drug gabapentin enacarbil (Horizant) is used to decrease the sensory sensations. If the patient has iron deficiency or low serum ferritin, iron supplementation is considered.

Other drugs may relieve some symptoms of RLS. These include opioids and benzodiazepines. Low doses of opioids (e.g., oxycodone) are usually reserved for patients with severe symptoms who fail to respond to other drug therapies. The main side effect of opioids is constipation, so patients may need to take a stool softener or laxative. Clonidine (Catapres) and propranolol (Inderal) are also effective in some patients.

Relaxis is a device that produces vibration and provides a counterstimulation that competes with and diminishes the RLS sensations. The patient places the legs on the Relaxis pad, which provides 30 minutes of uninterrupted vibration after being activated and then slowly winds down over an additional 5 minutes to complete a 35-minute therapy cycle. If needed, it may be restarted one more time. The patient chooses the vibration intensity based on symptoms.[19]

# DEGENERATIVE NEUROLOGIC DISORDERS

*Degenerative nerve diseases* lead to nerve damage that worsens as the diseases progress. These diseases affect many activities, including balance, movement, speech, and respiratory and heart function. Some diseases have no known cause, but many are known to have a genetic basis. Most degenerative nerve diseases have no cure. Treatment aims to reduce symptoms and help the patient maintain an optimal level of function.

Patients with these diseases have similar concerns and problems. They must deal with not only their disease but also the impact of the disease on their quality of life. Many patients have concerns regarding safety, mobility, self-care, and coping. Patients and their families often require psychosocial support, especially as the disease progresses and patients' disability gets worse.

## MULTIPLE SCLEROSIS

**Multiple sclerosis (MS)** is a chronic, progressive, degenerative disorder of the CNS characterized by disseminated demyelination of nerve fibers of the brain and spinal cord. MS can affect people of any age. The onset of MS is usually between 20 and 50 years of age, with symptoms first appearing at an average of 30 to 35 years of age. People who are diagnosed at 50 years of age or older generally have more progressive disease. Women are affected two to three times more often than men. An estimated 400,000 people in the United States have MS, with approximately 10,000 new cases diagnosed annually.[20]

MS is more prevalent in temperate climates (between 45 and 65 degrees of latitude), such as those found in the northern United States, Canada, and Europe, as compared with tropical regions. People who are born in an area of high risk but migrate to an area of low risk before age 15 assume the risk of their new home. Researchers thus suspect that exposure to some environmental agent before puberty may predispose a person to develop MS later in life. MS is less common in Hispanics, Asians, and people of African descent. It rarely occurs in some ethnic groups, including Alaskan Natives and Aborigines.

### Etiology and Pathophysiology

Although the cause of MS is unknown, it is unlikely to be related to a single cause. The disease develops in a genetically susceptible person as a result of environmental exposure, such as an infection. Multiple genes are believed to be involved in the inherited susceptibility to MS. Having a first-degree relative with MS increases a person's risk of developing the disease. Common genetic factors have also been found in families with more than one affected member.[21]

Possible precipitating factors include infection, smoking, physical injury, emotional stress, excessive fatigue, pregnancy, and a poor state of health. The role of precipitating factors such as exposure to pathogenic agents is controversial. More than a dozen viruses and bacteria have been investigated, but none has definitely been proven to cause MS.

Three pathologic processes characterize MS: chronic inflammation, demyelination, and gliosis in the CNS. The primary neuropathologic condition is an autoimmune process orchestrated by activated T cells. An unknown trigger in genetically susceptible individuals may initiate this process. The activated T cells in the systemic circulation migrate to the CNS, disrupting the blood-brain barrier. This is likely the initial event in the development of MS. Subsequent antigen-antibody reaction within the CNS activates the inflammatory response and leads to the demyelination of axons.

Initially, attacks on the myelin sheaths of the neurons in the brain and spinal cord result in damage to the myelin sheath (Fig. 58-3, *A* to *C*). However, the nerve fiber is not affected. Transmission of nerve impulses still occurs, but it is slowed. The patient may complain of a noticeable impairment of function (e.g., weakness). However, myelin can regenerate. When it does,

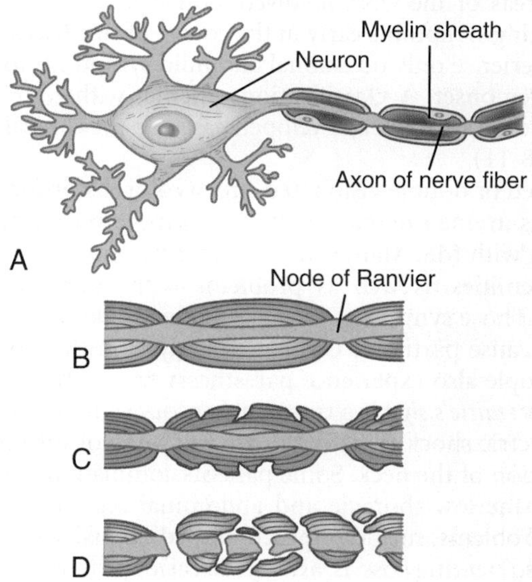


**FIG. 58-3** Pathogenesis of multiple sclerosis. **A,** Normal nerve cell with myelin sheath. **B,** Normal axon. **C,** Myelin breakdown. **D,** Myelin totally disrupted; axon not functioning.

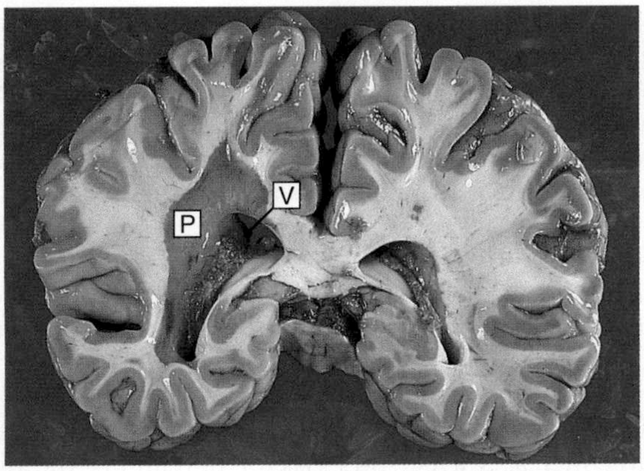


**FIG. 58-4** Chronic multiple sclerosis. Demyelination plaque *(P)* at gray-white junction and adjacent partially remyelinated shadow plaque *(V)*. (From Stevens A, Lowe J: *Pathology: illustrated review in colour,* ed 2, London, 2000, Mosby.)

symptoms disappear. At that point, the patient experiences a remission.

As ongoing inflammation occurs, nearby oligodendrocytes are affected, and myelin loses the ability to regenerate. Eventually damage occurs to the underlying axon. Nerve impulse transmission is disrupted, resulting in permanent loss of nerve function (Fig. 58-3, *D*). As inflammation subsides, glial scar tissue replaces damaged tissue, leading to formation of hard, sclerotic plaques (Fig. 58-4). These plaques are found throughout the white matter of the CNS.

## Clinical Manifestations

The onset of MS is often insidious and gradual, with vague symptoms occurring intermittently over months or years that do not prompt the patient to seek medical attention. Thus the disease may not be diagnosed until long after the onset of the first symptom. The disease is characterized by chronic, progressive deterioration in some patients, and remissions and exacerbations in others. With repeated exacerbations, the overall trend is progressive deterioration in neurologic function.

Because the disease process has a spotty distribution in the CNS, clinical manifestations vary with each patient according to the areas of the CNS involved. Some patients have severe, long-lasting symptoms early in the course of the disease. Others may experience only occasional and mild symptoms for several years after onset. A classification scheme, with four primary patterns of MS, has been developed based on the clinical course[22] (Table 58-11).

Blurred or double vision, red-green color distortion, or even blindness in one eye may be the first symptom experienced by a person with MS. Many patients describe muscle weakness in the extremities as well as problems with coordination and balance. Those symptoms may even affect walking or standing. MS can cause partial or complete paralysis in the worst cases. Most people also experience paresthesia or numbness and tingling. *Lhermitte's sign* is a transient sensory symptom described as an electric shock radiating down the spine or into the limbs with flexion of the neck. Some patients complain of pain, especially in the low thoracic and abdominal regions. Other frequent problems include speech impediments, tremors, and dizziness. Hearing loss is also an occasional finding. Possible cerebellar signs include nystagmus, ataxia, dysarthria, and dysphagia. Many patients have severe fatigue, sometimes with significant disability. The fatigue is aggravated by heat, humidity, deconditioning, and medication side effects.

**TABLE 58-11 Patterns of Multiple Sclerosis**

| Category | Characteristics |
|---|---|
| **Relapsing-remitting** | • Clearly defined attacks of worsening neurologic function *(relapses)* with partial or complete recovery *(remission)*.<br>• Approximately 85% of people are initially diagnosed with this type of MS. |
| **Primary-progressive** | • Steadily worsening neurologic function from the beginning with minor improvements but no distinct relapses or remissions.<br>• About 10% of people are diagnosed with this type of MS. |
| **Secondary-progressive** | • A relapsing-remitting initial course, followed by progression with or without occasional relapses, minor remissions, and plateaus.<br>• New treatments may slow progression.<br>• Most people initially diagnosed with relapsing-remitting MS eventually transition to this type. |
| **Progressive-relapsing** | • Progressive disease from onset, with clear acute relapses, with or without full recovery. Periods between relapses are characterized by continuing progression.<br>• Only 5% of people experience this type of MS. |

Bowel and bladder function can be affected if the sclerotic plaque is located in areas of the CNS that control elimination. Problems with defecation usually involve constipation rather than fecal incontinence. Urinary problems are variable. A common problem in patients with MS is a *spastic* (uninhibited) bladder. As a result, the bladder has a small capacity for urine, and its contractions are unchecked. The result is urinary urgency and frequency, often accompanied by dribbling or incontinence.

A *flaccid* (hypotonic) bladder indicates a lesion in the reflex arc controlling bladder function. A flaccid bladder has a large capacity for urine because there is no sensation or desire to void, no pressure, and no pain. Generally, the patient has urinary retention, but urgency and frequency may also occur with this type of lesion. Another urinary problem is a combination of the previous two. Urinary problems cannot be adequately diagnosed and treated without urodynamic studies.

Sexual dysfunction occurs in many people with MS. Physiologic erectile dysfunction may result from spinal cord involvement in men. Women may experience decreased libido, difficulty with orgasmic response, painful intercourse, and decreased vaginal lubrication. Diminished sensation can prevent a normal sexual response in both men and women. The emotional effects of chronic illness and the loss of self-esteem also contribute to loss of sexual response.

Some women with MS who become pregnant experience remission or an improvement in their symptoms during the gestation period. Hormonal changes associated with pregnancy appear to affect the immune system. However, during the postpartum period, women are at greater risk for exacerbation of the disease.

About half of people with MS experience some problems with cognitive function. For most people, the problems are difficulties with short-term memory, attention, information processing, planning, visual perception, and word finding. General intellect remains unchanged and intact, including long-term memory, conversational skills, and reading comprehension. Symptoms can be mild and thus easily overlooked. However, cognitive changes are so severe in about 5% to 10% of patients with MS that they significantly impair the person's ability to perform activities of daily living. Most of the time, cognitive difficulties occur later in the course of the disease. However, they can occur much earlier in the disease process, and occasionally they are present at the onset of MS.

People with MS may also experience emotional changes such as anger, depression, or euphoria. Physical and emotional trauma, fatigue, and infection may aggravate or trigger signs and symptoms.

The average life expectancy after the onset of symptoms is more than 25 years. Death usually occurs due to infectious complications of immobility (e.g., pneumonia) or because of an unrelated disease.

## Diagnostic Studies

Because there is no definitive diagnostic test for MS, factors considered are the history, clinical manifestations, and results of certain diagnostic tests (Table 58-12). An MRI of the brain and spinal cord may show plaques, inflammation, atrophy, and tissue breakdown and destruction. Cerebrospinal fluid (CSF) analysis may show an increase in immunoglobulin G and the presence of oligoclonal banding.[23] Evoked potential responses are often delayed in people with MS because of decreased nerve conduction from the eye and ear to the brain.

To be diagnosed with MS, the patient must have (1) evidence of at least two inflammatory demyelinating lesions in at least two different locations within the CNS, (2) damage or an attack occurring at different times (usually 1 month or more apart), and (3) all other possible diagnoses ruled out. If evidence exists for only one lesion, or only one clinical attack has occurred, the HCP will monitor the patient for another attack or for an attack at a different site in the CNS.[23]

## Interprofessional Care

**Drug Therapy.** Because no cure currently exists for MS, interprofessional care is aimed at treating the disease process and providing symptomatic relief (Table 58-12). Because no two cases of MS are alike, therapy is tailored specifically to the disease pattern and manifestations experienced by each patient (Table 58-13). Disease-modifying therapy has been found to be more effective when initiated early in the course of MS. Delays in treatment have been associated with poor outcomes.

Treatment of MS begins with use of immunomodulator drugs to modify the disease progression and prevent relapses. These drugs include (1) interferon β-1a (Rebif, Plegridy [given subcutaneously]) and interferon β-1a (Avonex) (given IM), (2) interferon β-1b (Betaseron, Extavia) (given subcutaneously), and (3) glatiramer acetate (Copaxone) (given subcutaneously).

**DRUG ALERT β-Interferon**
- Rotate injection sites with each dose.
- Assess for depression and suicidal ideation.
- Instruct patient to wear sunscreen and protective clothing while exposed to sun.
- Inform the patient that flu-like symptoms are common after initiation of therapy.

Teriflunomide (Aubagio) is an immunomodulatory agent with antiinflammatory properties. The exact mechanism of action is unknown but may involve a reduction in the number

### TABLE 58-12 Interprofessional Care
**Multiple Sclerosis**

| Diagnostic Assessment | Management |
|---|---|
| • History and physical examination | • Drug therapy (Table 58-13) |
| • CSF analysis | • Surgical therapy |
| • CT scan | • Thalamotomy (unmanageable tremor) |
| • MRI, MRS | • Neurectomy, rhizotomy, cordotomy (unmanageable spasticity) |
| • Evoked potential testing | • Physical therapy |
| • Somatosensory evoked potential (SSEP) | • Occupational therapy |
| • Auditory evoked potential (AEP) | |
| • Visual evoked potential (VEP) | |

*MRS,* Magnetic resonance spectroscopy.

### TABLE 58-13 Drug Therapy
**Multiple Sclerosis**

| Drug | Patient Teaching |
|---|---|
| **Disease-Modifying Drugs** | |
| ***Immunomodulators*** | |
| β-1a interferon (Rebif, Plegridy, Avonex) | • Perform self-injection techniques. • Report side effects. |
| β-1b interferon (Betaseron, Extavia) | • Treat flu-like symptoms with an NSAID or acetaminophen. |
| glatiramer acetate (Copaxone) | |
| teriflunomide (Aubagio) | • Because it may cause serious liver disease, monitor liver tests. • Avoid pregnancy. |
| ***Immunosuppressant*** | |
| mitoxantrone | • Report side effects. |
| dimethyl fumarate (Tecfidera) | • Avoid pregnancy. • Avoid contact with large crowds and people who have an infection. |
| ***Sphingosine 1-Phosphate Receptor Modulator*** | |
| fingolimod (Gilenya) | • Report side effects. • Monitor blood pressure regularly. • Avoid pregnancy. |
| ***Monoclonal Antibody*** | |
| natalizumab (Tysabri) | • Report side effects. |
| alemtuzumab (Lemtrada) | • Avoid pregnancy. |
| daclizumab (Zinbryta) | |
| **Drugs for Managing Exacerbations** | |
| ***Corticosteroids*** | |
| ACTH | • Restrict salt intake. |
| prednisone | • Do not abruptly stop therapy. |
| methylprednisolone | • Know drug interactions. |
| **Drugs for Symptom Management** | |
| ***Cholinergics*** | |
| bethanechol (Urecholine) | • Consult with HCP before using other drugs, including over-the-counter drugs. |
| neostigmine | |
| ***Anticholinergics*** | |
| propantheline | • Consult HCP before using other drugs, especially sleeping aids, antihistamines (possibly leading to potentiated effect). |
| oxybutynin (Ditropan XL) | |
| ***Muscle Relaxants*** | |
| diazepam (Valium) | • Avoid driving and similar activities because of sedative effects. |
| baclofen (Lioresal) | |
| dantrolene (Dantrium) | • Do not abruptly stop therapy. |
| tizanidine (Zanaflex) | • Avoid use with tranquilizers and alcohol. |
| ***Nerve Conduction Enhancer*** | |
| dalfampridine (Ampyra) | • Be aware that it may cause seizures, especially at higher doses. • Take the tablet whole. Do not take more than 2 in 24 hr. |

*ACTH,* Adrenocorticotropic hormone.

of activated lymphocytes in the CNS. Fingolimod (Gilenya) reduces MS disease activity by preventing lymphocytes from reaching the CNS and causing damage. Both drugs are specifically indicated for treatment of relapsing forms of MS.

For more active and aggressive forms of MS, natalizumab (Tysabri), alemtuzumab (Lemtrada), mitoxantrone, and dimethyl fumarate (Tecfidera) may be used. Natalizumab is given when patients have had an inadequate response to other drugs. An adverse effect of natalizumab is the increased risk of progressive multifocal leukoencephalopathy, a potentially fatal viral infection of the brain. Because of its safety profile, alemtuzumab is generally reserved for patients who have an inadequate response to two or more drugs indicated for the treatment of MS.[24]

Mitoxantrone, an antineoplastic medication, has serious effects, including cardiotoxicity, leukemia, and infertility. Dimethyl fumarate provides a new approach to treating MS by activating the Nrf2 pathway. This pathway provides a way for cells in the body to defend themselves against the inflammation and oxidative stress caused by MS.

Corticosteroids (e.g., methylprednisolone, prednisone) are most helpful to treat acute exacerbations of MS. They reduce edema and acute inflammation at the site of demyelination. However, these drugs do not affect the ultimate outcome or the degree of residual neurologic impairment from the exacerbation. Therapeutic plasma exchange *(plasmapheresis)* and IV immunoglobulin G may be considered when treatment with corticosteroids alone does not achieve symptom improvement.

Many other drugs are used to treat the various symptoms of MS, which may include fatigue, spasticity, tremor, vertigo or dizziness, depression, pain, bowel problems, bladder problems, sexual dysfunction, and cognitive changes. For example, muscle relaxants are used for spasticity. Amantadine and CNS stimulants (pemoline, methylphenidate [Ritalin], and modafinil [Provigil]) are used to treat fatigue. Anticholinergics are used to treat bladder symptoms. Tricyclic antidepressants and antiseizure drugs are used for chronic pain syndromes.

Dalfampridine (Ampyra) is used to improve walking speed in MS patients. It is a selective potassium channel blocker and improves nerve conduction in damaged nerve segments. It should not be used in patients with a history of seizure disorders or with moderate to severe kidney disease.

**Other Therapies.** Spasticity is treated primarily with muscle relaxants. However, surgery (e.g., neurectomy, rhizotomy, cordotomy), dorsal-column electrical stimulation, or intrathecal baclofen (Lioresal) delivered by pump may be required. Tremors that become unmanageable with drugs are sometimes treated by thalamotomy or deep brain stimulation.

Neurologic dysfunction sometimes improves with physical and speech therapies. Exercise improves the daily functioning for patients with MS not experiencing an exacerbation. Exercise decreases spasticity, increases coordination, and retrains unaffected muscles to substitute for impaired ones. An especially beneficial type of physical therapy is water exercise (Fig. 58-5). Water, which gives buoyancy to the body, allows the patient to have more control over the body and perform activities that would normally be impossible.

## NURSING MANAGEMENT: MULTIPLE SCLEROSIS

### Nursing Assessment

Subjective and objective data that should be obtained from a patient with MS are presented in Table 58-14.

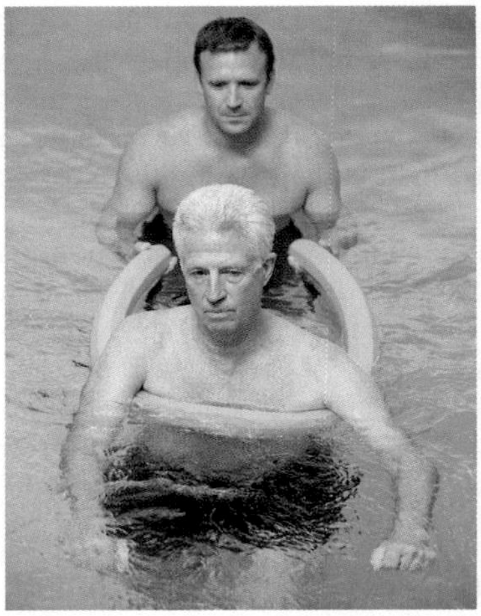

**FIG. 58-5** Water therapy provides exercise and recreation for the patient with a chronic neurologic disease. (©Photos.com/AbleStock.com/Thinkstock)

**TABLE 58-14 Nursing Assessment**
***Multiple Sclerosis***

**Subjective Data**

***Important Health Information***

*Past health history:* Recent or past viral infections or vaccinations, other recent infections, residence in cold or temperate climates, recent physical or emotional stress, pregnancy, exposure to extremes of heat and cold

*Medications:* Adherence to regimen of corticosteroids, immunomodulators, immunosuppressants, cholinergics, anticholinergics, antispasmodics

***Functional Health Patterns***

*Health perception–health management:* Positive family history; malaise

*Nutritional-metabolic:* Weight loss; difficulty in chewing, dysphagia

*Elimination:* Urinary frequency, urgency, dribbling or incontinence, retention; constipation

*Activity-exercise:* Generalized muscle weakness, muscle fatigue; tingling and numbness; ataxia (clumsiness)

*Cognitive-perceptual:* Eye, back, leg, joint pain; painful muscle spasms; vertigo; blurred or lost vision; diplopia; tinnitus

*Sexuality-reproductive:* Impotence, decreased libido

*Coping–stress tolerance:* Anger, depression, euphoria, social isolation

**Objective Data**

***General***

Apathy, inattentiveness

***Integumentary***

Pressure ulcers

***Neurologic***

Scanning speech, nystagmus, ataxia, tremor, spasticity, hyperreflexia, decreased hearing

***Musculoskeletal***

Muscle weakness, paresis, paralysis, spasms, foot dragging, dysarthria

***Possible Diagnostic Findings***

↓ T suppressor cells, demyelinating lesions on MRI or MRS scans, ↑ IgG or oligoclonal banding in cerebrospinal fluid, delayed evoked potential responses

*IgG,* Immunoglobulin G; *MRS,* magnetic resonance spectroscopy.

## ◆ Nursing Diagnoses

Nursing diagnoses for the patient with MS may include, but are not limited to, the following:

- Impaired physical mobility *related to* muscle weakness or paralysis and muscle spasticity
- Impaired urinary elimination *related to* sensorimotor deficits
- Ineffective health management *related to* knowledge deficit regarding management of MS

Additional information on nursing diagnoses for the patient with MS is presented in the eNursing Care Plan 58-3 (available on the website for this chapter).

## ◆ Planning

The overall goals are that the patient with MS will (1) maximize neuromuscular function, (2) maintain independence in activities of daily living for as long as possible, (3) manage disabling fatigue, (4) optimize psychosocial well-being, (5) adjust to the illness, and (6) reduce factors that precipitate exacerbations.

## ◆ Nursing Implementation

The patient with MS should be aware of triggers that may cause exacerbations or worsening of the disease. Exacerbations of MS are triggered by infection (especially upper respiratory and urinary tract infections), trauma, immunization, childbirth, stress, and change in climate. Each person responds differently to these triggers. Assist the patient in identifying triggers and developing ways to avoid them or minimize their effects.

During the diagnostic phase, the patient needs reassurance that certain diagnostic studies must be done to rule out other neurologic disorders, even though a tentative diagnosis of MS has been made. Assist the patient in dealing with anxiety caused by a diagnosis of a disabling illness. The patient with recently diagnosed MS may need assistance with the grieving process.

During an acute exacerbation, the patient may be immobile and confined to bed. The focus of nursing interventions at this phase is to prevent major complications of immobility, such as respiratory and urinary tract infections and pressure ulcers.

Focus patient teaching on building general resistance to illness, including avoiding fatigue, extremes of heat and cold, and exposure to infection. Encourage vigorous and early treatment of infection when it occurs. Teach the patient to achieve a good balance of exercise and rest; minimize caffeine intake; and eat nutritious, well-balanced meals. A diet high in fiber may help relieve constipation. The patient should know the treatment regimens, drug side effects, how to identify and manage side effects, and drug interactions with over-the-counter medications. The patient should consult an HCP before taking nonprescription drugs.

Bladder control is a major problem for many patients with MS. Although anticholinergics may be beneficial for some patients to decrease spasticity, you may need to teach others self-catheterization (discussed in Chapter 45 on p. 1050). Bowel problems, particularly constipation, frequently occur in patients with MS. Increasing dietary fiber intake may help some patients achieve regularity in bowel elimination.

The patient with MS and the caregiver need to make many emotional adjustments because of the unpredictability of the disease, need for lifestyle changes, and challenge of avoiding or decreasing precipitating factors. The National Multiple Sclerosis Society and its local chapters can offer a variety of services to meet the needs of patients with MS.

## ◆ Evaluation

The expected outcomes are that the patient with MS will

- Maintain or improve muscle strength and mobility
- Use assistive devices appropriately for ambulation and mobility
- Maintain urinary continence
- Make decisions about health and lifestyle modifications necessary for management of MS

Additional information on expected outcomes for the patient with MS are presented in eNursing Care Plan 58-3 (available on the website for this chapter).

# PARKINSON'S DISEASE

**Parkinson's disease (PD)** is a chronic, progressive neurodegenerative disorder characterized by slowness in the initiation and execution of movement *(bradykinesia),* increased muscle tone *(rigidity),* tremor at rest, and gait disturbance. It is the most common form of *parkinsonism* (a syndrome characterized by similar symptoms).

Up to 1 million Americans are believed to be living with PD, with approximately 60,000 diagnosed each year. Incidence of PD increases with age, but an estimated 4% of people with PD are diagnosed before 50 years of age. PD is more common in men by a ratio of 3:2.[25]

## Etiology and Pathophysiology

The exact cause of PD is unknown. Although PD is not considered a hereditary condition, genetic risk factors should be evaluated for their interplay with environmental factors. About 15% of patients with PD have a positive family history for the disease *(familial cases)* that may be caused by mutations in specific genes. In other people, risk for PD may be increased by well water, pesticides, herbicides, industrial chemicals, and wood pulp mills. Rural residence is also considered a risk factor.[26]

Many forms of secondary *(atypical)* parkinsonism exist other than PD. Symptoms of parkinsonism have occurred after exposure to a variety of chemicals, including carbon monoxide and manganese (among copper miners) and the product of meperidine analog synthesis, MPTP. Drug-induced parkinsonism can also follow therapy with metoclopramide (Reglan), reserpine, methyldopa, lithium, haloperidol (Haldol), and chlorpromazine. Parkinsonism can be seen after the use of illicit drugs, including amphetamine and methamphetamine. After stopping these drugs, symptoms of parkinsonism generally disappear; one notable exception is irreversible parkinsonism following MTPT exposure. Other causes of parkinsonism include hydrocephalus, other neurodegenerative disorders, hypoparathyroidism, infections, stroke, tumor, and trauma.[27]

Many changes found in the brains of people with PD may play a role in development of the disease, including a lack of dopamine (DA). The pathologic process of PD involves degeneration of the DA-producing neurons in the substantia nigra of the midbrain (Figs. 58-6 to 58-8), which in turn disrupts the normal balance between DA and acetylcholine (ACh) in the basal ganglia. The neurotransmitter DA is essential for normal functioning of the extrapyramidal motor system, including control of posture, support, and voluntary motion. Manifestations of PD do not occur until 80% of neurons in the substantia nigra are lost.

*Lewy bodies,* unusual clumps of protein, are found in the brains of patients with PD. It is not known what causes these bodies to form, but their presence indicates abnormal functioning of the brain. Lewy body dementia is discussed in Chapter 59.

## Genetic Link

Approximately 15% of patients with PD have a family history of PD. Many autosomal dominant and recessive genes have been linked to familial PD. The most common genetic contributor to PD is the *LRRK2* gene. Mutations in this gene also appear to have a role in sporadic, or noninherited, cases of PD. Other genes involved in familial PD are parkin *(PARK2, PARK7)*, *PINK1*, and SNCA. Mutations in these genes are often associated with a younger age of onset and have additional manifestations than those typically seen with age-related PD.[26] *PINK1* mutations are related to a rare, early-onset form of PD. It is not fully understood how genetic changes cause PD or influence the risk of developing the disorder.

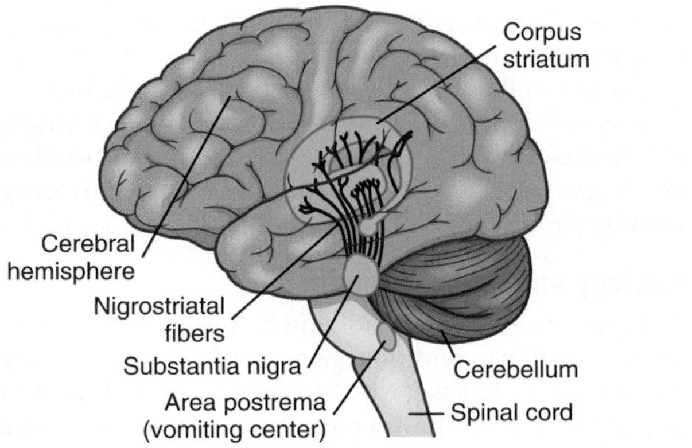


**FIG. 58-6** Nigrostriatal disorders produce parkinsonism. Left-sided view of the human brain showing the substantia nigra and the corpus striatum *(shaded area)* lying deep within the cerebral hemisphere. Nerve fibers extend upward from the substantia nigra, divide into many branches, and carry dopamine to all regions of the corpus striatum.

## Clinical Manifestations

The onset of PD is gradual and insidious, with an ongoing progression. Only one side of the body may be involved initially. Classic manifestations of PD are easily remembered by the mnemonic *TRAP* (**t**remor, **r**igidity, **a**kinesia, and **p**ostural instability).[26] In the beginning stages, only a mild tremor, a slight limp, or a decreased arm swing may be evident. Later in the disease, the patient may have a shuffling, propulsive gait with arms flexed, and show loss of postural reflexes. Up to 90% of patients also experience speech abnormalities *(hypokinetic dysarthria)* that can affect communication and quality of life.[28] None of these manifestations alone is sufficient evidence for a diagnosis of the disease.

**Tremor.** *Tremor* is often the first sign and may be minimal initially, so the patient is the only one who notices it. This tremor can affect handwriting, causing it to trail off, particularly toward the ends of words. Parkinsonian tremor is more prominent at rest and is aggravated by emotional stress or increased concentration. The hand tremor is described as "pill rolling"

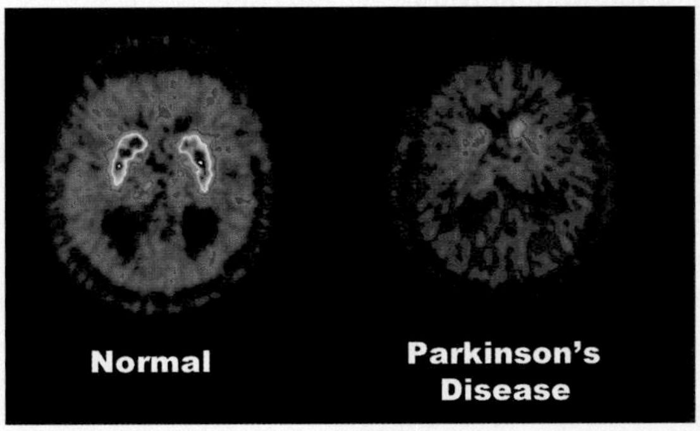


**FIG. 58-8** In Parkinson's disease, positron emission tomography (PET) scan showing reduced fluorodopa uptake in the basal ganglia *(right)* compared with a normal control *(left)*. (From Aminoff MJ, Daroff RB: *Encyclopedia of the neurological sciences,* Waltham, Mass, 2003, Academic Press.)

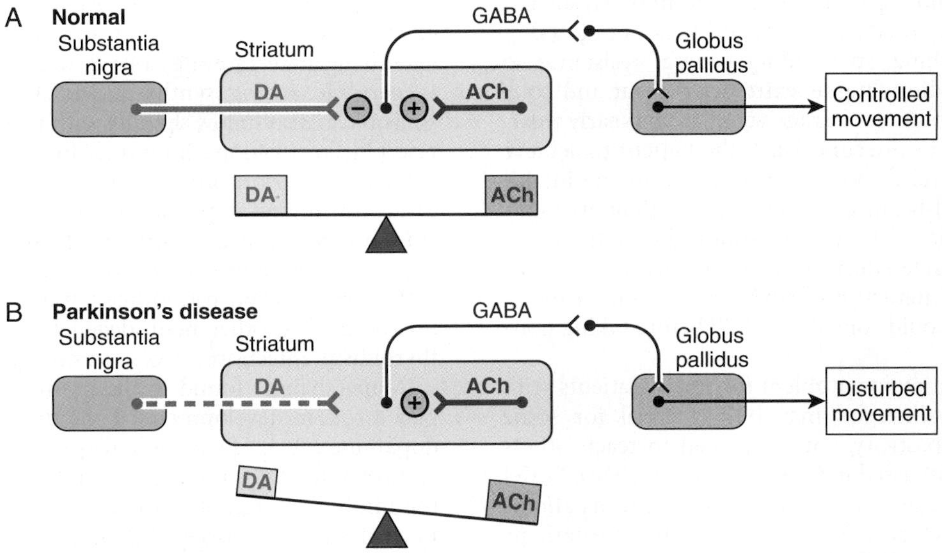


**FIG. 58-7** A deficit in dopamine (DA) exists in Parkinson's disease. This deficit creates an imbalance between dopamine and the excitatory neurotransmitter acetylcholine. **A,** In a healthy person, dopamine released from neurons originating in the substantia nigra inhibits the firing of neurons in the striatum that release γ-aminobutyric acid *(GABA)*. Conversely, neurons located within the striatum, which release acetylcholine *(ACh)*, excite the GABAergic neurons. Under normal conditions, inhibitory actions of DA are balanced by excitatory actions of ACh, and controlled movement results. **B,** In Parkinson's disease, neurons in the substantia nigra that supply DA to the striatum degenerate. When a deficit of DA occurs, excitatory effects of ACh go unopposed and disturbed movements (tremor, rigidity) result. (From Lehne RA: *Pharmacology for nursing care,* ed 8, St Louis, 2013, Saunders.)

because the thumb and forefinger appear to move in a rotary fashion as if rolling a pill, coin, or other small object. Tremor can also involve the diaphragm, tongue, lips, and jaw but rarely causes shaking of the head.

Unfortunately, in many people a benign *essential tremor* is mistakenly diagnosed as PD. Essential tremor occurs during voluntary movement, has a more rapid frequency than parkinsonian tremor, and is often familial.

**Rigidity.** *Rigidity* is the increased resistance to passive motion when the limbs are moved through their range of motion. Parkinsonian rigidity is typified by a jerky quality *(cogwheel rigidity)*, as if there were intermittent catches in the passive movement of a joint. Sustained muscle contraction causes the rigidity and consequently elicits complaints of muscle soreness; feeling tired and achy; or pain in the head, upper body, spine, or legs. Slowness of movement is another consequence of rigidity because it inhibits the alternating contraction and relaxation in opposing muscle groups (e.g., biceps and triceps).

**Akinesia.** *Akinesia* is the absence or loss of control of voluntary muscle movements. In PD *bradykinesia* (slowness of movement) is particularly evident in the loss of automatic movements. This occurs because of the physical and chemical alteration of the basal ganglia and related structures in the extrapyramidal portion of the CNS. In the unaffected patient, automatic movements are involuntary and occur subconsciously. They include blinking of the eyelids, swinging of the arms while walking, swallowing of saliva, using facial and hand movements for self-expression, and making minor movements for postural adjustment.

The patient with PD does not execute these movements and lacks spontaneous activity. This accounts for the stooped posture, masked face (deadpan expression), drooling of saliva, and shuffling gait *(festination)* that are characteristic of a person with this disease. The posture is that of a slowed "old man" image, with the head and trunk bent forward and the legs constantly flexed (Fig. 58-9).

**Postural Instability.** *Postural instability* is common. Patients may complain of being unable to stop themselves from going forward *(propulsion)* or backward *(retropulsion)*. Assessment of postural instability includes the "pull test." The examiner stands behind the patient and gives a tug backward on the shoulder, causing the patient to lose his or her balance and fall backward.

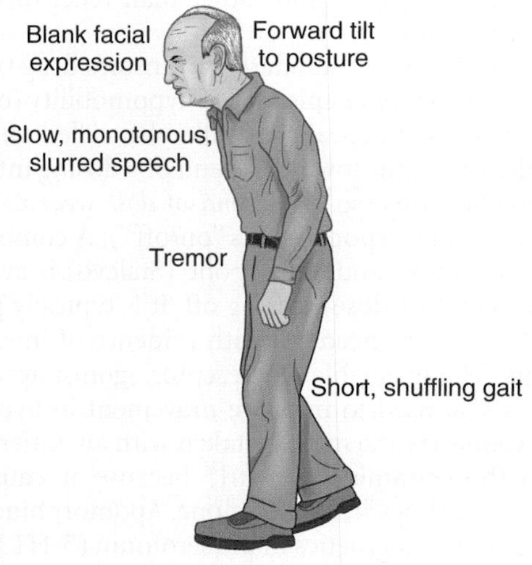


**FIG. 58-9** Characteristic appearance of a patient with Parkinson's disease.

In addition to the motor signs of PD, many nonmotor symptoms are common. They include depression, anxiety, apathy, fatigue, pain, urinary retention and constipation, erectile dysfunction, and memory changes. Sleep problems are common and include difficulty staying asleep at night, restless sleep, nightmares, and drowsiness or sudden sleep onset during the day. In particular, rapid eye movement (REM) behavior disorder is a preparkinsonian state that occurs in about one third of patients with PD. It is characterized by violent dreams and potentially dangerous motor activity during REM sleep.[26]

## Complications

As the disease progresses, complications increase. These include motor symptoms (e.g., dyskinesias [spontaneous, involuntary movements], weakness, neurologic problems (e.g., dementia), and neuropsychiatric problems (e.g., depression, hallucinations, psychosis). As PD progresses, it often results in dementia, which is associated with an increase in mortality.

As swallowing becomes more difficult (dysphagia), malnutrition or aspiration may result. General debilitation may lead to pneumonia, urinary tract infections, and skin breakdown. Orthostatic hypotension occurs commonly and, along with loss of postural reflexes, may result in falls or other injury. The patient's increased fall risk increases the need for the primary caregiver to be aware of environmental conditions that may also contribute to falls.

## Diagnostic Studies

Because no specific diagnostic test exists for PD, diagnosis is based on the patient's history and clinical features. Clinical diagnosis requires the presence of TRAP and asymmetric onset. Confirmation of PD is a positive response to antiparkinsonian drugs (levodopa or dopamine agonist). MRI and CT have a limited role in diagnosis of PD because they do not show a specific pathologic finding. However, they can rule out a stroke or brain tumor.

## Interprofessional Care

Because PD has no cure, interprofessional care focuses on symptom management (Table 58-15).

**Drug Therapy.** Drug therapy for PD is aimed at correcting the imbalance of neurotransmitters within the CNS. Antiparkinsonian drugs either enhance the release or the supply of DA (dopaminergic) or antagonize or block the effects of the overactive cholinergic neurons in the striatum (anticholinergic) (Fig. 58-7). Levodopa with carbidopa (Sinemet) is the primary treatment for symptomatic patients. Levodopa is a chemical

**TABLE 58-15 Interprofessional Care**

***Parkinson's Disease***

| Diagnostic Assessment | Management |
|---|---|
| • History and physical examination<br>• TRAP (tremor, rigidity, akinesia and postural instability)<br>• Positive response to antiparkinsonian drugs<br>• MRI<br>• Rule out side effects of phenothiazines, reserpine, benzodiazepines, haloperidol | • Antiparkinsonian drugs (Table 58-16)<br>• Surgical therapy<br>• Deep brain stimulation<br>• Ablation surgery<br>• Physical therapy<br>• Occupational therapy<br>• Dietitian consult for nutritional therapy |

## EVIDENCE-BASED PRACTICE

### Applying the Evidence

**Dancing and Parkinson's Disease**

You are a nurse working with T.K., a 77-yr-old male, who was diagnosed with Parkinson's disease 5 yr ago. You note he has a moderate tremor, shuffling gait, and decreased arm flexion. He asks you what types of physical activity he can do with his decreased mobility. He currently enjoys daily neighborhood walks but finds it hard to keep his balance.

***Making Clinical Decisions***

***Best Available Evidence.*** Patients with mild to moderately severe Parkinson's disease (PD) have improvements in balance, motor impairment, endurance, quality of life, and participation in social activities after engaging in dance classes at least twice/week.

***Clinician Expertise.*** You know it is important to promote and encourage patients with PD to engage in physical exercise to help maintain functional mobility. You are also aware that personal exercise programs should be designed around physical activities that the individual enjoys.

***Patient Preferences and Values.*** T.K. states that in years past he enjoyed dancing with his wife and would like to do so again.

***Implications for Nursing Practice***

1. What information will you provide to T.K. related to muscle atrophy and joint contractures and the importance of physical activity?
2. How will you assist T.K. and his wife in exploring community resources related to adaptive physical activities and in particular dance programs?

***Reference for Evidence***

Shanahan J, Morris ME, Bhriain O, et al: Dance for people with Parkinson disease: what is the evidence telling us? *Arch Phys Med Rehabil* 96:141, 2015.

precursor of DA and can cross the blood-brain barrier. It is converted to DA in the basal ganglia. Sinemet is the preferred drug because it also contains carbidopa, an agent that inhibits the enzyme dopa-decarboxylase in the peripheral tissues. Dopa-decarboxylase breaks down levodopa before it reaches the brain. The net result of the combination of levodopa and carbidopa is that more levodopa reaches the brain, and therefore less drug is needed. Levodopa has many side effects and drug interactions. Prolonged use often results in dyskinesias and "off/on" periods when the medication will unpredictably start or stop working.

**DRUG ALERT Carbidopa/Levodopa (Sinemet)**

- Monitor for signs of dyskinesia.
- Effects may be delayed for several weeks to months.
- Instruct patient or caregiver to report any uncontrolled movement of face, eyelids, mouth, tongue, arms, hands, or legs; mental changes; palpitations; severe nausea and vomiting; and difficulty urinating.

Many patients are given Sinemet early in the disease course for the management of motor symptoms. However, some HCPs believe that, after a few years of therapy, the effectiveness of Sinemet wears off. Therefore they prefer to start therapy with a DA receptor agonist, a drug that directly stimulates DA receptors. Ropinirole (Requip) and pramipexole (Mirapex) may be used alone or in combination with Sinemet. Bromocriptine (Parlodel) should not be used as first-line treatment because of possible serious side effects (e.g., high blood pressure, seizure, heart attack, stroke). Many of these medications are available in extended-release forms that improve patients' ability to adhere to treatment regimens. Rotigotine (Neupro), another DA receptor agonist, is available a transdermal patch applied once daily as an adjunctive therapy for patients taking Sinemet.

**DRUG ALERT Bromocriptine (Parlodel)**

- Patient may become dizzy or faint due to orthostatic hypotension, especially after the first dose.
- Notify physician immediately if a severe headache develops that does not improve or continues to get worse.

The antiviral agent amantadine is a weak antagonist of NMDA-type glutamate receptors, increases dopamine release, and blocks dopamine reuptake. Thus it provides only mild relief and is seldom used in early stages of PD.[29] In addition, withdrawal of amantadine even after extended therapy can worsen dyskinesia.

Anticholinergic drugs such as trihexyphenidyl and benztropine (Cogentin) are also used to manage PD. These drugs decrease the activity of ACh, thus providing balance between cholinergic and dopaminergic actions. Antihistamines (e.g., diphenhydramine) with anticholinergic properties may be used to manage tremors.

Selegiline (Eldepryl) and rasagiline (Azilect) are monoamine oxidase type B (MAO-B) inhibitors that may be used in combination with Sinemet. By inhibiting MAO-B, the degradative enzyme for DA, these agents increase the levels of DA and prolong the half-life of levodopa. Rasagiline can also be used alone as therapy in early PD. However, MAO-B inhibitors are less effective at treating motor symptoms than DA receptor agonists.

Entacapone (Comtan) and tolcapone (Tasmar) block the enzyme catechol *O*-methyltransferase (COMT), which breaks down levodopa in the peripheral circulation, and thus prolong the effect of Sinemet. These drugs are used only as adjuncts to levodopa; both drugs can exacerbate adverse effects of levodopa. Tolcapone is rarely prescribed because it has been associated with fatal hepatotoxicity.[26]

Rivastigmine (Exelon) or donepezil (Aricept) is used to treat dementia. Amitriptyline may be used to treat depression.

Table 58-16 summarizes the drugs commonly used in PD. The use of only one drug is preferred because fewer side effects occur and the drug dosage is easier to adjust than when several drugs are used. However, as the disease progresses, combination therapy is often required. Excessive amounts of dopaminergic drugs can lead to aggravation rather than relief of symptoms *(paradoxic intoxication)*.

Within 3 to 5 years of standard Parkinson's drug treatments, many patients experience episodes of hypomobility (e.g., inability to rise from chair, speak, or walk; also called *off episodes*). The episodes can occur toward the end of a dosing interval with standard medications (so-called *end-of-dose wearing off*) or at unpredictable times (spontaneous "on/off"). A combination of carbidopa, levodopa, and entacapone (Stalevo) is available for patients with end-of-dose wearing off. It is typically prescribed for patients with advanced PD with evidence of intense motor fluctuations. The injectable DA receptor agonist apomorphine (Apokyn) is also used to improve movement in hypomobility episodes. Apomorphine must be taken with an antiemetic drug (e.g., trimethobenzamide [Tigan]) because it causes severe nausea and vomiting when taken alone. Apomorphine must not be taken with the antiemetics in the serotonin (5-HT3) receptor

## TABLE 58-16 Drug Therapy
### *Parkinson's Disease*

| Drug | Mechanism of Action |
|---|---|
| **Dopaminergics** | |
| ***Dopamine Precursors*** | |
| levodopa (L-dopa)<br>levodopa/carbidopa (Sinemet) | Converted to dopamine in basal ganglia |
| ***Dopamine Receptor Agonists*** | |
| bromocriptine (Parlodel)<br>cabergoline<br>pramipexole (Mirapex)<br>ropinirole (Requip, Requip XL)<br>rotigotine (Neupro [transdermal patch]) | Stimulate dopamine receptors |
| ***Dopamine Agonists*** | |
| amantadine | Blocks NMDA-type glutamate receptors, increases dopamine release, and blocks dopamine reuptake |
| apomorphine (Apokyn) | Stimulates postsynaptic dopamine receptors |
| **Anticholinergics** | |
| trihexyphenidyl<br>benztropine (Cogentin) | Block cholinergic receptors, thus helping to balance cholinergic and dopaminergic activity |
| **Antihistamine** | |
| diphenhydramine | Has anticholinergic effect |
| **Monoamine Oxidase Inhibitors** | |
| selegiline (Eldepryl)<br>rasagiline (Azilect) | Block breakdown of dopamine |
| **Catechol *O*-Methyltransferase (COMT) Inhibitors** | |
| entacapone (Comtan)<br>tolcapone (Tasmar) | Block COMT and slow the breakdown of levodopa, thus prolonging the action of levodopa |

antagonist class (e.g., ondansetron [Zofran]) because this drug combination can lead to very low blood pressure and loss of consciousness.

**Surgical Therapy.** Surgical procedures aimed at relieving symptoms of PD are usually used in patients who are unresponsive to drug therapy or who have developed severe motor complications. Surgical procedures fall into three categories: deep brain stimulation (DBS), ablation (destruction), and transplantation. The most common surgical treatment is DBS, which involves placing an electrode in the thalamus, globus pallidus, or subthalamic nucleus and connecting it to a generator placed in the upper chest (similar to a pacemaker) (Fig. 58-10). The device is programmed to deliver a specific current to the targeted brain location. DBS is preferred to ablation procedures because it is reversible and programmable and can be safely performed bilaterally. DBS procedures reduce the increased neuronal activity produced by DA depletion. It has been shown to improve motor function and reduce dyskinesia and medication usage. DBS is most effective when candidates are carefully selected and screened.[30]

*Ablation surgery* involves locating, targeting, and destroying an area of the brain affected by PD. The goal is to destroy tissue that produces abnormal chemical or electrical impulses leading to tremors or other symptoms. Typical targets of ablation are

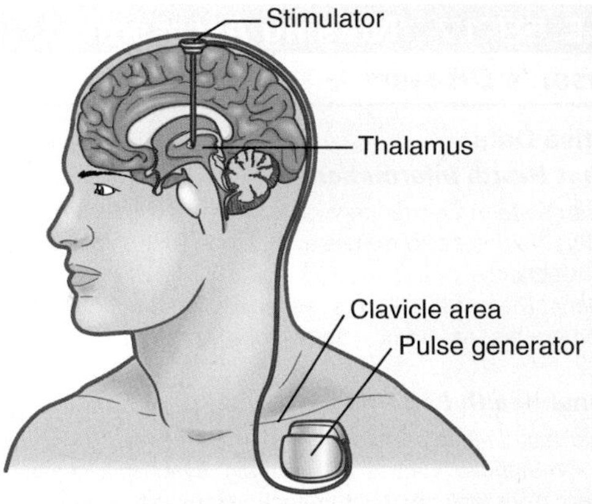


**FIG. 58-10** Deep brain stimulation (DBS) can be used to treat tremors and uncontrolled movements of Parkinson's disease. Electrodes are surgically placed in the brain and connected to a neurostimulator (pacemaker device) in the chest.

the thalamus *(thalamotomy)*, globus pallidus *(pallidotomy)*, and subthalamic nucleus *(subthalamic nucleotomy)*.

*Transplantation* of fetal neural tissue into the basal ganglia is designed to provide DA-producing cells in the brains of patients with PD. Research and clinical trials of this form of therapy are ongoing.

**Nutritional Therapy.** Diet is of major importance to patients with PD because malnutrition and constipation can be serious consequences of inadequate nutrition. Patients who have dysphagia and bradykinesia need appetizing foods that are easily chewed and swallowed. The diet should contain adequate fiber and fruit to avoid constipation. Cut food into bite-sized pieces before it is served, and serve it on a warmed plate to preserve its appeal.

Eating six small meals a day may be less exhausting than eating three large meals a day. Plan ample time for eating to avoid frustration. The absorption of levodopa can be impaired by protein ingestion and vitamin $B_6$. Therefore some patients are advised to limit their protein intake to the evening meal to decrease this problem. They also need to consult with their HCP regarding possible inclusion of vitamin $B_6$ in their multivitamins and fortified cereals.

## NURSING MANAGEMENT: PARKINSON'S DISEASE

### Nursing Assessment

Subjective and objective data that should be obtained from a patient with PD are presented in Table 58-17.

### Nursing Diagnoses

Nursing diagnoses for the patient with PD may include, but are not limited to, the following:

- Impaired physical mobility *related to* rigidity, bradykinesia, akinesia, and postural instability
- Imbalanced nutrition: less than body requirements *related to* inability to ingest food
- Impaired swallowing *related to* neuromuscular impairment (e.g., decreased or absent gag reflex)
- Impaired verbal communication *related to* dysarthria, tremor, and bradykinesia

Additional information on nursing diagnoses for the patient with PD is presented in eNursing Care Plan 58-4 (available on the website for this chapter).

**TABLE 58-17 Nursing Assessment**

***Parkinson's Disease***

**Subjective Data**

***Important Health Information***

*Past health history:* Central nervous system trauma, cerebrovascular disorders, exposure to metals and carbon monoxide, encephalitis or other infections

*Medications:* Major tranquilizers, especially haloperidol (Haldol), and phenothiazines, reserpine, methyldopa, amphetamines

***Functional Health Patterns***

*Health perception–health management:* Fatigue

*Nutritional-metabolic:* Excessive salivation, dysphagia, weight loss

*Elimination:* Constipation, incontinence, excessive sweating

*Activity-exercise:* Difficulty in initiating movements, frequent falls, loss of dexterity, micrographia (handwriting deterioration)

*Sleep-rest:* Insomnia, nightmares, daytime sleepiness

*Cognitive-perceptual:* Diffuse pain in head, shoulders, neck, back, legs, and hips. Muscle soreness and cramping

*Self-perception–self-concept:* Depression, mood swings, hallucinations

**Objective Data**

***General***

Blank (masked) facial expression, slow and monotonous speech, infrequent blinking

***Integumentary***

Seborrhea, dandruff; ankle edema

***Cardiovascular***

Postural hypotension

***Gastrointestinal***

Drooling

***Neurologic***

Tremor at rest, first in hands (pill rolling), later in legs, arms, face, and tongue. Aggravation of tremor with anxiety, absence in sleep. Poor coordination, cognitive impairment and dementia, impaired postural reflexes

***Musculoskeletal***

Cogwheel rigidity, dysarthria, bradykinesia, contractures, stooped posture, shuffling gait

***Possible Diagnostic Findings***

No specific tests. Diagnosis based on history and physical findings and ruling out of other diseases

## ◆ Planning

The overall goals are that the patient with PD will (1) maximize neurologic function, (2) maintain independence in activities of daily living for as long as possible, and (3) optimize psychosocial well-being.

## ◆ Nursing Implementation

Because PD is a chronic degenerative disorder with no acute exacerbations, teaching and nursing care are directed toward maintenance of good health, encouragement of independence, and avoidance of complications such as contractures and falls. Problems secondary to bradykinesia can be alleviated by relatively simple measures.

**CHECK YOUR PRACTICE**

You are working in a rehabilitation facility where one of your patients is a 78-yr-old man with Parkinson's disease. Six months ago he was also at your facility with a fractured hip after falling in his yard. The family has asked to talk with you about their fear of taking him for a walk in the hallways because he is so unstable.

- What advice would you provide to the family?

Promotion of physical exercise and a well-balanced diet are major concerns for nursing care. Exercise can limit the consequences of decreased mobility, such as muscle atrophy, contractures, and constipation. The American Parkinson Disease Association *(www.apdaparkinson.org)* publishes a series of booklets and videotapes with helpful exercises that can be used by family members and health care professionals.

A physical therapist may be consulted to design a personal exercise program aimed at strengthening and stretching specific muscles. Overall muscle tone and specific exercises to strengthen the muscles involved with speaking and swallowing should be included. Although exercise will not halt the progress of the disease, it will enhance the patient's functional ability. An occupational therapist can also assist the patient with strategies to increase self-care measures, including eating and dressing.

**SAFETY ALERT Preventing Falls**

Have patients who are at risk for falling and tend to "freeze" while walking do the following:

- Consciously think about stepping over imaginary or real lines on the floor.
- Drop rice kernels and step over them.
- Rock from side to side.
- Lift the toes when stepping.
- Take one step backward and two steps forward.

Work closely with the patient's caregiver and family in exploring creative adaptations that allow maximum independence and self-care. The patient can get out of a chair better by using an upright chair with arms and placing the back legs of the chair on small (2-inch) blocks. Encourage environmental alterations, such as removing rugs and excess furniture to avoid stumbling, using an elevated toilet seat to facilitate getting on and off the toilet, and elevating the legs on an ottoman to decrease dependent ankle edema. Clothing can be simplified by the use of slip-on shoes and Velcro hook-and-loop fasteners or zippers on clothing, instead of buttons and hooks.

Effective management of sleep problems can greatly improve the quality of life for patients with PD. Some patients find the use of satin nightwear or satin sheets beneficial. Information on teaching regarding sleep hygiene practices is presented in Chapter 7.

In the early stages of PD, many patients experience depression and anxiety. Patients need to adjust their lifestyle, including work and home responsibilities. As the disease progresses, the impact on the patient's psychologic well-being also increases. Assist the patient by listening, providing teaching, challenging distorted thoughts, and encouraging social interactions. Psychologic therapy and counseling can be helpful. Also ensure that patients with PD receives prescribed medications on time to avoid on-off effects.

In the early stage of the disease, the patient has subtle changes in cognitive function that can progress to dementia. This results in increased caregiver burden and the potential for long-term care placement. Information on care of the patient with dementia is provided in Chapter 59.

Family members (e.g., spouse, children) care for the majority of patients with PD. As the disease progresses, the caregiver burden increases, often while the caregiver's physical and mental health decline. Strategies to reduce caregiver burden are described in Chapter 4. Other interventions for patients with PD are presented in eNursing Care Plan 58-4 (available on the website for this chapter).

### Evaluation

The expected outcomes are that the patient with PD will

- Perform physical exercise to deter muscle atrophy and joint contractures
- Use assistive devices appropriately for ambulation and mobility
- Maintain nutritional intake adequate for metabolic needs
- Experience safe passage of fluids and/or solids from the mouth to the stomach
- Use methods of communication that meet needs for interaction with others

Additional information on expected outcomes for the patient with PD is presented in eNursing Care Plan 58-4 (available on the website).

## MYASTHENIA GRAVIS

**Myasthenia gravis (MG)** is an autoimmune disease of the neuromuscular junction characterized by the fluctuating weakness of certain skeletal muscle groups. This weakness increases with muscle use. MG occurs in either gender and in people of any ethnicity. The prevalence rate is approximately 20 per 100,000; currently an estimated 60,000 people have MG in the United States. The mean age at onset in women is 28 years; in men the mean age at onset of MG is 42 years. Women are affected more often than men (3:2). In older adults, both men and women are equally affected.[31]

### Etiology and Pathophysiology

MG is caused by an autoimmune process in which antibodies attack acetylcholine (ACh) receptors. This results in a decreased number of ACh receptor (AChR) sites at the neuromuscular junction. This prevents ACh molecules from attaching to receptors and stimulating muscle contraction. Anti-AChR antibodies are detectable in the serum of 90% of patients with generalized MG. In the 10% of patients who lack autoantibodies to AChR, their muscular weakness may be related to autoantibodies to muscle-specific tyrosine kinase or to other unknown antigens.[31] Thymic hyperplasia and tumors are common in patients with MG, suggesting autoantibody production occurs in the thymus.

### Clinical Manifestations and Complications

The primary feature of MG is fluctuating weakness of skeletal muscles. The condition usually affects multiple muscle groups, including muscles used to move the eyes and eyelids, chew, swallow, speak, and breathe. These muscles are generally strongest in the morning and become exhausted with continued activity. By the end of the day muscle weakness is prominent. A period of rest usually restores strength.

At onset, only the ocular muscles are involved for about 50% of patients; bilateral ptosis and constant or transient diplopia result (Fig. 58-11). The disease does not progress beyond the ocular muscles in about 20% of patients.[32] When facial muscles are affected, facial mobility and expression can be impaired. Patients may have difficulty chewing and swallowing food. Speech is affected, and the voice often fades after a long conversation. The muscles of the trunk and limbs are less often affected. Of these, the proximal muscles of the neck, shoulder, and hip are more often affected than the distal muscles. No other signs of neural disorder accompany MG. No sensory loss occurs, reflexes are normal, and muscle atrophy is rare.

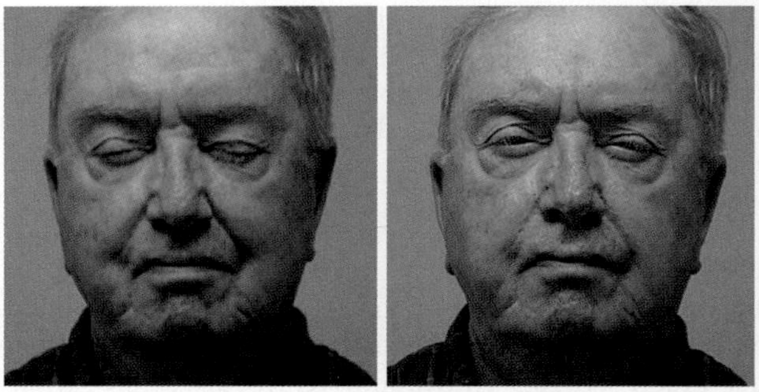

**FIG. 58-11** "Peek" sign in myasthenia gravis. During sustained forced eyelid closure he is unable to bury his eyelashes *(left)* and, after 30 sec, he is unable to keep the lids fully closed *(right)*. (From Sanders DB, Massey JM: Clinical features of myasthenia gravis. In AG Engel, editor: *Neuromuscular junction disorders: handbook of clinical neurology,* New York, 2008, Elsevier.)

The course of this disease is highly variable. Some patients may have short-term remissions, others may stabilize, and others may have severe, progressive involvement. Exacerbations of MG can be precipitated by emotional stress, pregnancy, menses, another illness, trauma, temperature extremes, and hypokalemia. Ingestion of drugs, including aminoglycoside antibiotics, β-adrenergic blockers, procainamide, quinidine, and phenytoin, can aggravate MG.[32] Psychotropic drugs (e.g., lithium carbonate, phenothiazines, benzodiazepines, tricyclic antidepressants) have also been associated with worsening of myasthenia, as have neuromuscular blocking agents (tubocurarine chloride, pancuronium, succinylcholine [Anectine]).

**Myasthenic crisis** is an acute exacerbation of muscle weakness triggered by respiratory infection, surgery, emotional distress, pregnancy, exposure to drugs that may increase myasthenic weakness, or beginning treatment with corticosteroids. The major complications of MG result from muscle weakness in areas that affect swallowing and breathing. This results in aspiration, respiratory insufficiency, and respiratory tract infection.

### Diagnostic Studies

The diagnosis of MG can be made based on history and physical examination. However, other tests may be used to confirm a diagnosis. EMG may show a decreased response to repeated stimulation of the hand muscles, indicative of muscle fatigue. Single-fiber EMG is sensitive in confirming the diagnosis of MG. Use of drugs may also aid in the diagnosis. In addition, serologic testing for specific antibodies is useful.

The Tensilon test in a patient with MG reveals improved muscle contractility after IV injection of edrophonium chloride (Tensilon), which is an anticholinesterase agent. (Anticholinesterase blocks the enzyme acetylcholinesterase.) This test also aids in the diagnosis of cholinergic crisis (secondary to overdose of anticholinesterase drug), which occurs due to excessive cholinesterase inhibition. Clinical features include muscle fasciculation, sweating, excessive salivation, and constricted pupils. In this condition, edrophonium does not improve muscle weakness but may actually increase it. Atropine, a cholinergic antagonist, should be readily available to counteract the effects of edrophonium when it is used diagnostically. In patients with a confirmed diagnosis of MG, a chest CT scan may be done to evaluate the thymus.

### Interprofessional Care

**Drug Therapy.** Drug therapy for MG includes anticholinesterase drugs, alternate-day corticosteroids, and immunosuppressants (Table 58-18). Anticholinesterase drugs are given to enhance transmission at the neuromuscular junction. Acetylcholinesterase is the enzyme that breaks down ACh. Thus inhibition of this enzyme by an anticholinesterase inhibitor will prolong the action of ACh and facilitate transmission of impulses at the neuromuscular junction. Pyridostigmine (Mestinon) is the most successful drug of this group in the long-term treatment of MG.

Tailoring the dose to avoid a myasthenic or cholinergic crisis often presents a clinical challenge. Corticosteroids (specifically prednisone) are used to suppress the immune response. Drugs such as azathioprine (Imuran), mycophenolate (CellCept), and cyclosporine (Sandimmune) may also be used for immunosuppression.

Many drugs are contraindicated or must be used with caution in patients with MG. Classes of drugs that should be cautiously evaluated before use include anesthetics, antidysrhythmics, antibiotics, quinine, antipsychotics, barbiturates and sedative-hypnotics, cathartics, diuretics, opioids, muscle relaxants, thyroid preparations, and tranquilizers.

**Surgical Therapy.** Because the presence of the thymus gland in the patient with MG appears to enhance the production of AChR antibodies, removal of the thymus gland results in improvement in a majority of patients. Thymectomy is indicated for almost all patients with thymoma, for patients with generalized MG between the ages of puberty and about 65 years, and for patients with purely ocular MG.

**Other Therapies.** Plasmapheresis and IV immunoglobulin G can yield short-term improvement in symptoms. They are indicated for patients in myasthenic crisis or in preparation for surgery when corticosteroids must be avoided. Plasmapheresis directly removes circulating AChR antibodies, leading to a decrease in symptoms. (Plasmapheresis is discussed in Chapter 13.) It is not certain how IV immunoglobulin works, but it is probably related to a decrease in antibody production.[32]

**TABLE 58-18 Interprofessional Care**

***Myasthenia Gravis***

| Diagnostic Assessment | Management |
|---|---|
| • History and physical examination | • Drug therapy |
| • Fatigability with prolonged upward gaze (2-3 min) | • Anticholinesterase agents |
| • Muscle weakness | • Corticosteroids |
| • EMG | • Immunosuppressive agents |
| • Tensilon test | • Surgery (thymectomy) |
| • Acetylcholine receptor antibodies | • Plasmapheresis |
| • Chest x-ray | • IV immunoglobulin G |

*EMG,* Electromyography.

## NURSING MANAGEMENT: MYASTHENIA GRAVIS

### Nursing Assessment

Assess the severity of MG by asking the patient about fatigability, what body parts are affected, and how severely they are affected. Some patients become so fatigued that they are no longer able to work or even walk. Assess the patient's coping abilities and strategies as well as understanding of the disorder.

Objective data should include respiratory rate and depth, $O_2$ saturation, arterial blood gas analyses, pulmonary function tests, and any evidence of respiratory distress in patients with acute myasthenic crisis. Assess muscle strength of all face and limb muscles, swallowing, speech (volume and clarity), and cough and gag reflexes.

### Nursing Diagnoses

Nursing diagnoses for the patient with MG may include, but are not limited to, the following:

- Ineffective airway clearance *related to* intercostal muscle weakness and impaired cough and gag reflex
- Impaired verbal communication *related to* weakness of the larynx, lips, mouth, pharynx, and jaw
- Activity intolerance *related to* muscle weakness and fatigability
- Disturbed body image *related to* inability to maintain usual lifestyle and role responsibilities

### Planning

The overall goals are that the patient with MG will (1) have a return of normal muscle endurance, (2) manage fatigue, (3) avoid complications, and (4) maintain a quality of life appropriate to the disease course.

### Nursing Implementation

The patient with MG who is admitted to the hospital usually has a respiratory tract infection or is in an acute myasthenic crisis. Nursing care is aimed at maintaining adequate ventilation, continuing drug therapy, and watching for side effects of therapy. Be able to distinguish cholinergic from myasthenic crisis (Table 58-19) because the causes and treatment of the two conditions differ greatly.

As with other chronic illnesses, focus care on the neurologic deficits and their impact on daily living. Teach the patient about a balanced diet that can easily be chewed and swallowed. Semisolid foods may be easier to eat than solids or liquids. Scheduling doses of drugs so that peak action is reached at mealtime may make eating less difficult. Arrange diversional activities that require little physical effort and match the patient's interests. Help the patient plan activities of daily living to avoid fatigue. Teaching should focus on adherence to the medical regimen, complications of the disease, potential adverse reactions to specific drugs, and complications of therapy (crisis conditions), and what to do about them. Explore community resources such as the Myasthenia Gravis Foundation of America and MG support groups.

### Evaluation

The expected outcomes are that the patient with MG will

- Maintain optimal muscle function
- Be free from side effects of drugs
- Not experience complications (myasthenic or cholinergic crises) from the disease
- Maintain a quality of life appropriate to the disease course

**TABLE 58-19 Comparison of Myasthenic and Cholinergic Crises**

| Myasthenic Crisis | Cholinergic Crisis |
|---|---|
| **Causes** | |
| Exacerbation of myasthenia following precipitating factors or failure to take drug as prescribed or drug dose too low | Overdose of anticholinesterase drugs resulting in increased ACh at the receptor sites, remission (spontaneous or after thymectomy) |
| **Differential Diagnosis** | |
| Improved strength after IV administration of anticholinesterase drugs | Weakness within 1 hr after ingestion of anticholinesterase drugs |
| Increased weakness of skeletal muscles manifesting as ptosis, bulbar signs (e.g., difficulty swallowing, difficulty articulating words), or dyspnea | Increased weakness of skeletal muscles manifesting as ptosis, bulbar signs, dyspnea<br>Effects on smooth muscle include pupillary miosis, salivation, diarrhea, nausea or vomiting, abdominal cramps, increased bronchial secretions, sweating, or lacrimation |

*ACh*, Acetylcholine.

## AMYOTROPHIC LATERAL SCLEROSIS

**Amyotrophic lateral sclerosis (ALS)** is a rare progressive neuromuscular disorder characterized by loss of motor neurons. ALS usually leads to death 2 to 5 years after diagnosis, but a few patients may survive for more than 10 years. This disease became known as *Lou Gehrig's disease* after the famous baseball player was stricken with it in 1939. Perhaps the best known patient with ALS is British theoretical physicist Stephen Hawking, diagnosed at age 21 years and now in his mid 70s. The typical onset is between 55 and 75 years of age. ALS is more common in men than women by a ratio of 2:1. Prevalence is approximately 3.9 cases of ALS per 100,000 people.[33,34]

In ALS, motor neurons in the brainstem and spinal cord gradually degenerate for unknown reasons. Dead motor neurons cannot produce or transport signals to muscles. Consequently, electrical and chemical messages originating in the brain do not reach the muscles to activate them.

Progressive muscle weakness, a classic sign of ALS, occurs in approximately 60% of diagnosed people. Early symptoms of weakness vary, but they often include tripping, dropping things, abnormal fatigue of the extremities, slurred speech, and muscle cramps and twitches. Muscle wasting and fasciculations result from the denervation of the muscles and lack of stimulation and use. Other symptoms include pain, sleep disorders, spasticity and hyperreflexia, drooling, emotional lability, constipation, and esophageal reflux. ALS does not affect a patient's intelligence, but affected people may experience depression and have alterations in decision making and memory. Death often results from respiratory tract infection secondary to compromised respiratory function.[34]

Unfortunately, there is no cure for ALS. Riluzole (Rilutek) slows the progression of ALS. This drug reduces damage to motor neurons by decreasing the release of glutamate (an excitatory neurotransmitter) in the brain.[34]

The illness trajectory for ALS is devastating because the patient remains cognitively intact while wasting away. Guide the patient in the use of moderate-intensity, endurance-type exercises for the trunk and limbs because this may help to reduce ALS spasticity. Nursing interventions include (1) facilitating communication, (2) reducing risk of aspiration, (3) facilitating early identification of respiratory insufficiency, (4) decreasing pain secondary to muscle weakness, (5) decreasing risk of injury related to falls, and (6) providing diversional activities such as reading and companionship.

Support the patient's cognitive and emotional functions. Help the patient and family manage the disease process, including grieving related to the loss of motor function and ultimately death. Discuss advance directives and artificial methods of ventilation with the patient and caregiver.

**INFORMATICS IN PRACTICE**

***Voice Banking Applications in Amyotrophic Lateral Sclerosis***

- For patients with amyotrophic lateral sclerosis (ALS), the loss of voice and the ability to communicate can be isolating.
- Speech pathologists encourage patients to participate in voice banking programs to record key words and phrases in their own voices.
- Voice banking is intended to be used as an alternative communication tool when patients may not be able to speak.

## HUNTINGTON'S DISEASE

**Huntington's disease (HD)** is a genetically transmitted, autosomal dominant disorder that affects men and women equally across races. The offspring of a person with this disease have a 50% risk of inheriting it (see Genetics in Clinical Practice box). The onset of HD is usually between 35 and 45 years of age. Often the diagnosis is made after the affected individual has had children. About 25,000 to 30,000 Americans are symptomatic and 150,000 or more are at risk for HD.[35]

The diagnostic process begins with a review of the family history and clinical symptoms. Genetic testing confirms the disease in a person with symptoms. People who are asymptomatic but who have a positive family history of HD face the dilemma of whether to be genetically tested. If the test is positive, the person will develop HD, but when and to what extent the disease develops cannot be determined.

Similar to PD, the pathologic process of HD involves the basal ganglia and the extrapyramidal motor system. However, instead of a deficiency of DA, HD involves a deficiency of the neurotransmitters ACh and $\gamma$-aminobutyric acid (GABA). The net effect is an excess of DA, which leads to symptoms that are the opposite of those of parkinsonism.

The clinical manifestations include a movement disorder and cognitive and psychiatric manifestations. The movement disorder is characterized by abnormal and excessive involuntary movements *(chorea)*. These are writhing, twisting movements of the face, limbs, and body. The movements get worse as the disease progresses. Because facial movements involving speech, chewing, and swallowing are affected, aspiration and malnutrition are likely. The gait deteriorates, and ambulation eventually becomes impossible.

Psychiatric symptoms are frequently present in the early stage of the disease, often before the onset of motor symptoms. Depression is common. Other psychiatric symptoms include anxiety, agitation, impulsivity, apathy, social withdrawal, and obsessiveness. Cognitive deterioration is more variable and

## GENETICS IN CLINICAL PRACTICE

### *Huntington's Disease (HD)*

**Genetic Basis**
- Autosomal dominant disorder.
- Caused by mutation in *HTT* gene located on chromosome 4.

**Incidence**
- 3 to 7 in 100,000 people of European ancestry.
- Less common in other populations, including people of Japanese, Chinese, and African descent.
- Offspring of a person with a pathogenic variant have a 50% chance of inheriting the disease-causing allele.

**Genetic Testing**
- DNA testing is available.
- DNA testing can be done on fetal cells obtained by amniocentesis or chorionic villus sampling.
- Preimplantation genetic diagnosis can be done on embryos before implantation and pregnancy.
- One copy of altered gene (heterozygous) is sufficient to cause HD.
- No test is available to predict when symptoms will develop.

**Clinical Implications**
- HD is a progressive, degenerative brain disorder.
- Onset of disease usually occurs at 30-50 yr of age. No cure is available.
- Drugs are available to control movements and behavioral problems.
- Genetic counseling may be considered if there is a family history of HD.
- Because HD is an autosomal dominant disorder, individuals who are at risk have a strong motivation to seek genetic testing.
- A positive result is not considered a diagnosis because it may be obtained decades before symptoms begin.
- A negative test means the individual does not carry the mutated gene and will not develop HD.

involves perception, memory, attention, and learning. Eventually all psychomotor processes, including the ability to eat and talk, are impaired.

Death usually occurs 10 to 20 years after the onset of symptoms.[36] The most common cause of death is pneumonia, followed by suicide. Other causes of death include injuries related to a fall and other complications.

Because HD has no cure, interprofessional care is palliative. Tetrabenazine (Xenazine) is used to treat the chorea by decreasing the amount of DA available at synapses in the brain and thus reducing the involuntary movements of chorea. If chorea is accompanied by other symptoms, tetrabenazine may not be the treatment of choice. For example, depression can be exacerbated by tetrabenazine, so aripripazole (Abilify) may be a better treatment option.[35]

Other medications used for the movement disorder include neuroleptics such as haloperidol and risperidone (Risperdal), benzodiazepines such as diazepam and clonazepam, and DA-depleting agents such as reserpine. Cognitive disorders are treated as needed with nondrug therapies (e.g., counseling, memory books). Psychiatric disorders can be treated with selective serotonin reuptake inhibitors such as sertraline (Zoloft) and paroxetine (Paxil). Antipsychotic medication, such as haloperidol or risperidone, may also be needed. HD presents a great challenge to health care professionals. The goal of nursing management is to provide the most comfortable environment possible for the patient and caregiver by maintaining physical safety, treating physical symptoms, and providing emotional and psychologic support.

Because of the choreic movements, caloric requirements are high. The patient may require as many as 4000 to 5000 cal/day to maintain body weight. As the disease progresses, meeting caloric needs becomes a greater challenge when the patient has difficulty swallowing and holding the head still. Depression and mental deterioration can also compromise nutritional intake. Alternative sources of nutrition may be indicated as the disease progresses.

End-of-life issues need to be discussed with the patient and caregiver. These include care in the home or long-term care facility, artificial methods of feeding, advance directives and cardiopulmonary resuscitation (CPR), use of antibiotics to treat infections, and guardianship. These topics should be addressed throughout the course of the disease as the patient and caregiver adapt to increasing disability.

## CASE STUDY

### *Epilepsy With Headache*

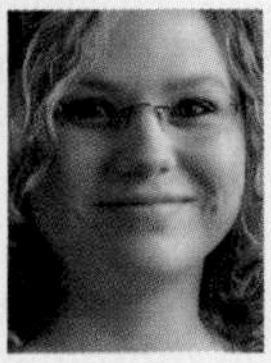
(©Purestock/ Thinkstock)

**Patient Profile**

J.P. is a 24-yr-old woman who was diagnosed with epilepsy at age 15. At that time, she had a tonic-clonic seizure and was given a prescription for valproate (Depakote). She had a second witnessed seizure 4 mo later but has since been seizure free. J.P. now has complaints of headaches and says she is afraid her seizures are going to return. She is single, lives alone, and describes her job as stressful.

**Subjective Data**
- Describes headache pain on the left side of her forehead as throbbing
- Has vomited with headache
- Describes changes in vision, including flashing lights
- Headache occurs nearly every month on a regular cycle

**Objective Data**
- Alert and oriented to person
- Neurologic examination negative
- Serum valproate levels within normal limits
- EEG normal
- CT of head normal

**Discussion Questions**
1. What is epilepsy?
2. What is the pathophysiology of epilepsy?
3. What is the significance of the laboratory and diagnostic findings?
4. Is the headache related to seizure activity?
5. ***Safety:*** To ensure J.P.'s safety, what nursing interventions are necessary?
6. ***Patient-Centered Care:*** What teaching will you include in the plan of care for J.P. regarding the course of the disease?
7. ***Priority Decision:*** Based on the assessment data, what are the priority nursing diagnoses?
8. ***Evidence-Based Practice:*** Based on current treatment guidelines, what medication may be effective in managing both J.P.'s epilepsy and her migraine headaches?

Answers available at *http://evolve.elsevier.com/Lewis/medsurg.*

## BRIDGE TO NCLEX EXAMINATION

The number of the question corresponds to the same-numbered outcome at the beginning of the chapter.

1. A 50-yr-old man complains of recurring headaches. He describes these as sharp, stabbing, and located around his left eye. He also reports that his left eye seems to swell and get teary when these headaches occur. Based on this history, you suspect that he has
   **a.** cluster headaches.
   **b.** tension headaches.
   **c.** migraine headaches.
   **d.** medication overuse headaches.
2. A 65-yr-old woman was just diagnosed with Parkinson's disease. The priority nursing intervention is
   **a.** searching the Internet for educational videos.
   **b.** evaluating the home for environmental safety.
   **c.** promoting physical exercise and a well-balanced diet.
   **d.** designing an exercise program to strengthen and stretch specific muscles.
3. The nurse finds an 87-yr-old woman with Alzheimer's disease is continually rubbing, flexing, and kicking her legs throughout the day. The night shift reports this same behavior escalates at night, preventing her from obtaining her required sleep. The next step the nurse should take is to
   **a.** ask the physician for a daytime sedative for the patient.
   **b.** request soft restraints to prevent her from falling out of her bed.
   **c.** ask the physician for a nighttime sleep medication for the patient.
   **d.** assess the patient more closely, suspecting a disorder such as restless legs syndrome.
4. Social effects of a chronic neurologic disease include *(select all that apply)*
   **a.** divorce.
   **b.** job loss.
   **c.** depression.
   **d.** role changes.
   **e.** loss of self-esteem.
5. The nurse is reinforcing teaching with a patient newly diagnosed with amyotrophic lateral sclerosis (ALS). Which statement would be appropriate to include in the teaching?
   **a.** "ALS results from an excess chemical in the brain, and the symptoms can be controlled with medication."
   **b.** "Even though the symptoms you are experiencing are severe, most people recover with treatment."
   **c.** "You need to consider advance directives now, because you will lose cognitive function as the disease progresses."
   **d.** "This is a progressing disease that eventually results in permanent paralysis, though you will not lose any cognitive function."

1. a, 2. c, 3. d, 4. a, b, c, d, e, 5. d

For rationales to these answers and even more NCLEX review questions, visit *http://evolve.elsevier.com/Lewis/medsurg.*

## EVOLVE WEBSITE

http://evolve.elsevier.com/Lewis/medsurg

**Review Questions (Online Only)**

**Key Points**

**Answer Keys for Questions**
- Rationales for Bridge to NCLEX Examination Questions
- Answer Guidelines for Case Study on p. 1396

**Student Case Studies**
- Patient With Parkinson's Disease and Hip Fracture
- Patient With Seizures

**Nursing Care Plans**
- eNursing Care Plan 58-1: Patient With Headache
- eNursing Care Plan 58-2: Patient With Seizure Disorder or Epilepsy
- eNursing Care Plan 58-3: Patient With Multiple Sclerosis
- eNursing Care Plan 58-4: Patient With Parkinson's Disease

**Conceptual Care Map Creator**
- Conceptual Care Map for Case Study on p. 1396

**Audio Glossary**

**Content Updates**

## REFERENCES


1. Headache Classification Committee of the International Headache Society. The international classification of headache disorders, ed 3, *Cephalgia* 33:629, 2013.
*2. Charles A: The evolution of a migraine attack: a review of recent evidence, *Headache* 53:413, 2013.
3. Lipton RB, Silberstein SD: Episodic and chronic migraine headache: breaking down barriers to optimal treatment and prevention, *Headache* 55:S2, 2015.
4. National Institute of Neurological Disorders and Stroke: Headache: hope through research. 2015. Retrieved from *www.ninds.nih.gov/disorders/headache/detail_headache.htm.*
5. Braine ME: Cluster headache, *Br J Neuro Nurs* 9:8, 2013.
6. Zecuity (package insert). North Wales, Penn, Teva Pharmaceuticals USA, Inc. 2014.
7. Fisher RS: International League Against Epilepsy announces epilepsy: a new definition. 2014. Retrieved from *www.epilepsy.com/article/2014/4/revised-definition-epilepsy.*
8. Epilepsy Foundation: Epilepsy statistics. 2014. Retrieved from *www.epilepsy.com/learn/epilepsy-statistics.*
9. National Institute of Neurological Disorders and Stroke: NIH-funded study discovers new genes for childhood epilepsies. 2013. Retrieved from *http://www.ninds.nih.gov/news_and_events/news_articles/pressrelease_childhood_epilepsy_genes_08112013.htm.*
10. Epilepsy Foundation: Types of seizures. 2013. Retrieved from *www.epilepsy.com/learn/types-seizures.*
11. Epilepsy Foundation: Status epilepticus. 2015. Retrieved from *www.epilepsy.com/information/professionals/about-epilepsy-seizures/classifying-seizures/status-epilepticus.*
12. Epilepsy Foundation: How SUDEP occurs. 2013. Retrieved from *http://www.epilepsy.com/learn/impact/mortality/sudep/how-sudep-occurs.*
13. Tatum WO, Sirven JI, Cascino GD: *Epilepsy case studies: pearls for patient care*, New York, 2014, Springer.
14. Schulze-Bonhage A, Zentner J: The preoperative evaluation and surgical treatment of epilepsy, *Dtsch Arztebl Int* 111:313, 2014.
15. Epilepsy Foundation: Ketogenic diet. 2014. Retrieved from *http://www.epilepsy.com/learn/treating-seizures-and-epilepsy/dietary-therapies/ketogenic-diet.*
16. National Institute of Neurological Disorders and Stroke: Restless legs syndrome fact sheet. Retrieved from *www.ninds.nih.gov/disorders/restless_legs/detail_restless_legs.htm.*
17. Allen RP, Picchietti D, Garcia-Borreguero D, et al: Restless legs syndrome/Willis-Ekbom disease diagnostic criteria: updated International Restless Legs Study Group (IRLSG) consensus criteria—history, rationale, description, and significance, *Sleep Med* 15:860, 2014.

*18. Innes KE, Selfe TK, Agarwal P, et al: Efficacy of an eight-week yoga intervention on symptoms of restless legs syndrome (RLS): a pilot study, *J Alt Comp Med* 19:527, 2013.
19. Sleep Review: FDA clears non-pharmacological device for restless legs syndrome. 2014. Retrieved from *www.sleepreviewmag.com/2014/05/fda-clears-non-pharmacological-device-restless-legs-syndrome.*
20. Multiplesclerosis.net: MS statistics. 2013. Retrieved from *http://multiplesclerosis.net/what-is-ms/statistics.*
21. National Multiple Sclerosis Society: What causes MS? Retrieved from *www.nationalmssociety.org/What-is-MS/What-Causes-MS.*
22. National Multiple Sclerosis Society: Types of MS. Retrieved from *www.nationalmssociety.org/What-is-MS/Types-of-MS.*
23. Polman CH, Reingold SC, Banwell B, et al: Diagnostic criteria for multiple sclerosis: 2010 revisions to the McDonald Criteria, *Ann Neurol* 69:292, 2011.
24. National Multiple Sclerosis Society: FDA approves Lemtrada (alemtuzumab) for relapsing MS—update. 2014. Retrieved from *www.nationalmssociety.org/About-the-Society/News/FDA-Approves-Lemtrada%E2%84%A2-%28alemtuzumab%29-for-Relapsing.*
25. Parkinson's Disease Foundation: Statistics on Parkinson's, 2015. Retrieved from *www.pdf.org/en/parkinson_statistics.*
26. Nolden LF, Tartavoulle T, Porche DJ: Parkinson's disease: assessment, diagnosis, and management, *J Nurs Pract* 10:500, 2014.
27. Merck Manual: Parkinson disease. 2013. Retrieved from *http://www.merckmanuals.com/professional/neurologic-disorders/movement-and-cerebellar-disorders/parkinson-disease.*
28. Sapir S: Multiple factors are involved in the dysarthria associated with Parkinson's disease: a review with implications for clinical practice and research, *J Speech Lang Hear Res* 57:1330, 2014.
29. National Parkinson Foundation: Amantadine (Symmetrel). 2015. Retrieved from *www.parkinson.org/Parkinson-s-Disease/Treatment/Medications-for-Motor-Symptoms-of-PD/Amantadine-%28Symmetrel%29.aspx.*
30. Shukla AW, Okun MS: Surgical treatment of Parkinson's disease: patients, targets, devices, and approaches, *Neurother* 11:47, 2014.
31. Schub T, Buckley L, Pravicoff D: Myasthenia gravis. *CINAHL Information Systems*, 2014.
32. Mestecky AM: Myasthenia gravis, *Br J Neuro Nurs* 9:110, 2013.
33. Mehta P, Antao V, Kaye W, et al: Prevalence of amyotrophic lateral sclerosis—United States, 2010-2011, *MMWR* 63:1, 2014.
34. National Institute of Neurological Disorders and Stroke: Amyotrophic lateral sclerosis (ALS) fact sheet. Retrieved from *www.ninds.nih.gov/disorders/amyotrophiclateralsclerosis/detail_ALS.htm.*
35. Frank S: Treatment of Huntington's disease, *Neurother* 11:153, 2014.
*36. Scerri R: Living with advanced stage Huntington's disease: an exploration of the experiences of Maltese family caregivers, *Br J Neuro Nurse* 11:20, 2015.

*Evidence-based information for clinical practice.

# 59

# Dementia and Delirium

*Sharon L. Lewis*

*I am going to make the rest of my life the best of my life.*
**Unknown**

http://evolve.elsevier.com/Lewis/medsurg/

## LEARNING OUTCOMES

1. Define dementia and describe its impact on society.
2. Compare and contrast different etiologies of dementia.
3. Describe the clinical manifestations, diagnostic studies, and interprofessional care of dementia.
4. Differentiate among neurodegenerative disorders associated with dementia, including dementia with Lewy bodies, frontotemporal lobar degeneration, and Down syndrome.
5. Describe the clinical manifestations of mild cognitive impairment.
6. Describe the clinical manifestations, diagnostic studies, and interprofessional care of Alzheimer's disease.
7. Describe the nursing management of the patient with Alzheimer's disease.
8. Describe the etiology, pathophysiology, clinical manifestations, diagnostic studies, and nursing and interprofessional management of delirium.

## KEY TERMS

Alzheimer's disease (AD), p. 1401
delirium, p. 1414
dementia, p. 1399
dementia with Lewy bodies (DLB), Table 59-3, p. 1401
familial Alzheimer's disease (FAD), p. 1402
frontotemporal lobar degeneration (FTLD), Table 59-3, p. 1401
mild cognitive impairment (MCI), p. 1405
mixed dementia, p. 1400
neurofibrillary tangles, p. 1403
normal pressure hydrocephalus, p. 1400
retrogenesis, p. 1403
sundowning, p. 1411
vascular dementia, p. 1400

This chapter discusses the cognitive disorders of dementia and delirium, with a focus on the nursing management of patients with Alzheimer's disease. The etiology and pathophysiology of dementia and delirium are differentiated, and interprofessional and nursing management of patients with these cognitive disorders are described.

The three most common cognitive problems in adults are dementia, delirium (acute confusion), and depression (Table 59-1). Although this chapter focuses on dementia and delirium, depression is often associated with these conditions.

Depression is often mistaken for dementia in older adults, and, conversely, dementia for depression. Manifestations of depression (especially in the older adult) include sadness, difficulty thinking and concentrating, fatigue, apathy, feelings of despair, and inactivity. When depression is severe, poor concentration and attention may result, causing memory and functional impairment. When dementia and depression occur together (as happens in many patients with dementia), the intellectual deterioration can be extreme. Depression, alone or in combination with dementia, is treatable. The challenge is to make an accurate and early assessment and diagnosis (Table 59-1).

## DEMENTIA

**Dementia** is a neurocognitive disorder characterized by dysfunction or loss of memory, orientation, attention, language, judgment, and reasoning. Personality changes and behavioral problems such as agitation, delusions, and hallucinations may occur. Ultimately, these problems result in alterations in the individual's ability to work, fulfill social and family responsibilities, and perform activities of daily living.

Fifteen percent of older Americans have dementia. As the average life span increases, the number of those affected with dementia is growing. There are about 100 causes of dementia, with about 60% to 80% of the patients with dementia having a diagnosis of Alzheimer's disease (AD) (Fig. 59-1). In the United States, about half of all patients in long-term care facilities have AD or a related dementia.[1]

### Etiology and Pathophysiology

Dementia is due to both treatable and untreatable conditions. Treatable causes may initially be reversible (Table 59-2). However, with prolonged exposure or disease, irreversible changes may occur.

Reviewed by Abimbola Farinde, PharmD, MS, Professor, Columbia Southern University, Orange Beach, Alabama; Shari Gould, RN, MSN, Associate Professor of Nursing, Victoria College, Victoria, Texas; and Linda Littlejohns, MSN, RN, CNRN, FAAN, Vice President of Clinical Development Integra LifeSciences, Irvine, California.

**TABLE 59-1 Comparison of Dementia, Delirium, and Depression**

| Feature | Dementia | Delirium | Depression |
|---|---|---|---|
| **Onset** | Usually insidious. | Abrupt, although initially can be subtle. | Often coincides with life changes. Often abrupt. |
| **Progression** | Slow. | Abrupt. Can fluctuate from day to day. | Variable, rapid to slow but may be uneven. |
| **Duration** | Years (average of 8 yr but can be much longer). | Hours to days to weeks. Can be prolonged in some. | Can be several months to years, especially if not treated. |
| **Thinking** | Difficulty with abstract thinking, impaired judgment, words difficult to find. | Disorganized, distorted. Slow or accelerated incoherent speech. | Intact but with apathy, fatigue. May be indecisive. Feels sense of hopelessness. May not want to live. |
| **Perception** | Misperceptions often present. Delusions and hallucinations. | Distorted. Delusions and hallucinations. | May deny or be unaware of depression. May have feelings of guilt. |
| **Psychomotor behavior** | May pace or be hyperactive. As disease progresses, may not be able to perform tasks or movements when asked. | Variable. Can be hyperactive or hypoactive, or mixed. | Often withdrawn and hypoactive. |
| **Sleep-wake cycle** | Sleeps during day. Frequent awakenings at night. Fragmented sleep. | Disturbed sleep. Reversed sleep-wake cycle. | Disturbed, often with early morning awakening. |

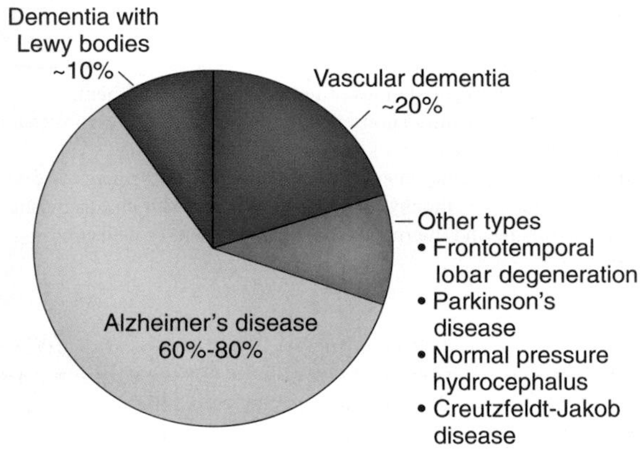


**FIG. 59-1** Causes of dementia.

The most common causes of dementia are neurodegenerative conditions, with the majority of cases being Alzheimer's disease (Table 59-3). Vascular conditions are the second most common cause of dementia.[1] **Vascular dementia**, also called *multiinfarct dementia,* is loss of cognitive function resulting from ischemic or hemorrhagic brain lesions caused by cardiovascular disease. This type of dementia is the result of decreased blood supply from narrowing and blocking of arteries that supply the brain. Vascular dementia may be caused by a single stroke (infarct) or by multiple strokes.

**Mixed dementia** occurs when two or more types of dementia are present at the same time. It is characterized by the hallmark abnormalities of Alzheimer's disease and another type of dementia. Usually the other type of dementia is vascular dementia, but it can be other types.

**Normal pressure hydrocephalus** is an uncommon disorder characterized by an obstruction in the flow of CSF, causing a buildup of CSF in the brain. Manifestations include dementia, urinary incontinence, and difficulty walking. Meningitis, encephalitis, or head injury may cause the condition. If diagnosed early, normal pressure hydrocephalus is treatable by surgery in which a shunt is inserted to divert the fluid away from the brain.

## Clinical Manifestations

Depending on the cause of the dementia, the onset of manifestations may be insidious and gradual or more abrupt. Often dementia associated with neurologic degeneration is gradual

**TABLE 59-2 Causes of Dementia**

| Type of Dementia | Cause |
|---|---|
| **Neurodegenerative disorders** | • Alzheimer's disease<br>• Dementia with Lewy bodies (DLB)<br>• Frontotemporal lobar degeneration (FTLD)<br>• Down syndrome<br>• Parkinson's disease<br>• Huntington's disease<br>• Amyotrophic lateral sclerosis (ALS) |
| **Vascular diseases** | • Vascular (multiinfarct) dementia<br>• Subarachnoid hemorrhage*<br>• Chronic subdural hematoma* |
| **Toxic, metabolic, or nutritional diseases** | • Alcoholism<br>• Thiamine (vitamin $B_1$) deficiency*<br>• Cobalamin (vitamin $B_{12}$) deficiency*<br>• Folate deficiency*<br>• Hyperthyroidism*<br>• Hypothyroidism* |
| **Immunologic diseases or infections** | • Multiple sclerosis<br>• Systemic exertion intolerance disease<br>• Infections (e.g., Creutzfeldt-Jakob disease)<br>• Acquired immunodeficiency syndrome (AIDS)<br>• Meningitis*<br>• Encephalitis*<br>• Neurosyphilis*<br>• Systemic lupus erythematosus* |
| **Systemic diseases** | • Uremic encephalopathy*<br>• Dialysis dementia*<br>• Hepatic encephalopathy*<br>• Wilson's disease |
| **Trauma** | • Head injury* |
| **Tumors** | • Brain tumors (primary)*<br>• Metastatic tumors* |
| **Ventricular disorders** | • Hydrocephalus* |
| **Drugs†** | • Anticholinergics<br>• phenytoin (Dilantin)<br>• Opioids<br>• Hypnotics<br>• Tranquilizers<br>• Antiparkinsonian drugs<br>• Cardiac drugs: digoxin, methyldopa<br>• Cocaine<br>• Heroin |

*Potentially reversible.
†These are examples of drugs that may cause cognitive impairment that is potentially reversible.

**TABLE 59-3 Neurodegenerative Causes of Dementia***

| Neurodegenerative Disorder | Characteristics | Management |
|---|---|---|
| **Dementia With Lewy Bodies (DLB)** | | |
| • Characterized by presence of Lewy bodies (abnormal deposits of protein α-synuclein) in brainstem and cortex<br>• Has features of both AD and Parkinson's disease.<br>• Imperative that a correct diagnosis is made | • Typically have manifestations of parkinsonism, hallucinations, short-term memory loss, unpredictable cognitive shifts, and sleep disturbances<br>• Diagnosis of LBD is based on clinical manifestations:<br>  • Extrapyramidal signs (bradykinesia, rigidity, and postural instability, but not always a tremor)<br>  • Fluctuating cognitive ability<br>  • Hallucinations<br>• Pneumonia is a common complication | • Drugs may include levodopa/carbidopa and acetylcholinesterase inhibitors.<br>• Manage dementia and problems related to dysphagia and immobility<br>• Swallowing problems can lead to impaired nutrition<br>• At risk for falls from impaired mobility and balance. |
| **Frontotemporal Lobar Degeneration (FTLD)** | | |
| • Associated with atrophy of frontal and temporal lobes of brain<br>• In Pick's disease, one type of FTLD, brain may have abnormal microscopic deposits called *Pick bodies*<br>• Often misdiagnosed as a psychiatric problem because of strange behaviors | • Characterized by disturbances in behavior, sleep, personality, and eventually memory<br>• Progresses relentlessly and may ultimately include language impairment, erratic behavior, and dementia.<br>• Tends to occur at a younger age than does AD, typically about age 60 | • No specific treatment<br>• Antidepressants and antipsychotics to treat behavioral manifestations |
| **Down Syndrome** | | |
| • Genetic disorder caused by presence of all or part of a third copy of chromosome 21 | • Typically associated with physical growth delays, characteristic facial features, and mild to moderate intellectual disability | • Much higher risk of developing dementia<br>• Estimated 80% will develop dementia |
| **Parkinson's Disease, Huntington's Disease, and Amyotrophic Lateral Sclerosis** | | |
| • Chronic, progressive, and incurable diseases | • Associated with development of dementia in the later stages of disease | See Chapter 58 |

*Alzheimer's disease is the most common neurodegenerative disorder causing dementia. It is the focus of this chapter.

and progressive over time. Causes of vascular dementia often result in symptoms that appear suddenly or progress in a stepwise pattern. However, it is difficult to distinguish the etiology of dementia (vascular versus neurodegenerative) based on symptom progression alone.

An acute (days to weeks) or subacute (weeks to months) pattern of change may be indicative of an infectious or metabolic cause of dementia, including encephalitis, meningitis, hypothyroidism, or drug-related dementia. The manifestations of different types of dementia overlap and can be further complicated by coexisting medical conditions.

Other clinical manifestations of dementia are discussed in the section on clinical manifestations of AD on pp. 1403-1404.

### Diagnostic Studies

The diagnosis of dementia is focused on determining the cause (e.g., reversible versus irreversible factors). An important first step is a thorough medical, neurologic, and psychologic history. A thorough physical examination is performed to rule out other potential medical conditions. Screening for cobalamin (vitamin $B_{12}$) deficiency and hypothyroidism is often performed. Based on patient history, testing for neurosyphilis (see Chapter 52) may be performed. Neuroimaging techniques (CT or MRI) may be used to rule out or confirm causes of dementia. (Diagnostic studies for Alzheimer's disease are discussed later in this chapter on pp. 1405-1408.)

## ❖ NURSING AND INTERPROFESSIONAL MANAGEMENT: DEMENTIA

In many ways, management of the patient with dementia is similar to management of the patient with AD (described later in this chapter). One form of dementia, vascular dementia, can often be prevented. Preventive measures include treatment of risk factors such as hypertension, diabetes, smoking, hypercholesterolemia, and cardiac dysrhythmias. (Stroke is discussed in Chapter 57.) Drugs that are used for patients with AD are also useful in patients with vascular dementia. Drug therapy is discussed on p. 1408 later in this chapter.

## ALZHEIMER'S DISEASE

**Alzheimer's disease (AD)** is a chronic, progressive, neurodegenerative disease of the brain. It is the most common form of dementia, accounting for 60% to 80% of all cases of dementia.[1] AD is named after Alois Alzheimer, a German physician who in 1906 described changes in the brain tissue of a 55-year-old woman who had died of an unusual mental illness.

Approximately 5.4 million Americans suffer from AD. It is estimated that 11% of people age 65 and older, and nearly one third of those over age 85, have AD. Ultimately the disease is fatal, with death typically occurring 4 to 8 years after diagnosis, although some patients live for 20 years. AD is the sixth leading cause of death in the United States.[1]

AD is the only cause of death among the top 10 in United States that cannot be prevented or cured, or its progression even slowed. The burden of care for the patient with AD on the family, caregivers, and society is staggering. AD has often been referred to as the "long good-bye" or "death in slow motion."

The incidence of AD is higher in African Americans and Hispanics than in whites. AD has been associated with lower socioeconomic status and education level and poor access to health care.[1] Women are more likely than men to develop AD, primarily because they live longer (see the Gender Differences box).

### Etiology

The exact etiology of AD is unknown but is likely a combination of multiple factors. These factors are discussed in this section.

## GENDER DIFFERENCES

### Alzheimer's Disease and Dementia

| Men | Women |
|---|---|
| • Men have a higher incidence of vascular dementia than women. | • Nearly two thirds of people with Alzheimer's disease are women.<br>• Women are more likely to develop Alzheimer's disease than men, primarily because they live longer.<br>• About twice as many women as men die each year from Alzheimer's disease. |

## CULTURAL & ETHNIC HEALTH DISPARITIES

### Alzheimer's Disease and Dementia

- Older African Americans are about twice as likely to have Alzheimer's and other dementias as older whites.
- Older Hispanics are about one and one-half times as likely to have Alzheimer's and other dementias as older whites.
- Variations in health, lifestyle, and socioeconomic risk factors across ethnic groups account for most of the differences in risk of Alzheimer's disease and other dementias.
- Health conditions such as cardiovascular disease and diabetes, which increase risk for Alzheimer's disease and other dementias, account for differences as they are more prevalent in African American and Hispanic people.
- Lower levels of education and other socioeconomic characteristics may also increase risk.

Source: Alzheimer's Association: 2015 Alzheimer's Association facts and figures report. Retrieved from *www.alz.org/facts/downloads/facts_figures_2015.pdf.*

**Aging.** The greatest risk factor for AD is age. Most people with AD are diagnosed at age 65 or older. While age is the greatest risk factor, AD is not a normal part of aging, and age alone is not sufficient to cause the disease.[1]

**Family History.** Family history is also an important risk factor, since those with a first-degree relative with dementia are more likely to develop the disease. Those who have more than one first-degree relative (parent, brother, sister) with dementia are even at higher risk of developing the disease. However, a family history is not necessary for an individual to develop AD.[1]

### Genetic Link

Only a small percentage of people younger than 60 years old develop AD. When AD develops in someone younger than 60 years old, it is referred to as *early-onset AD.* AD that becomes evident in individuals more than 60 years old is called *late-onset AD* (see the Genetics in Clinical Practice box).

Individuals with a clear pattern of inheritance within a family have **familial Alzheimer's disease (FAD)**. Other cases in which no familial connection can be made are termed *sporadic.* FAD is associated with an early onset (before 60 years of age) and a more rapid disease course. In both FAD and sporadic AD, the pathogenesis of AD is similar.

In patients with early-onset AD, three genes have been identified as important in the etiology (see the Genetics in Clinical Practice box). When the *presenilin-1, presenilin-2,* and *amyloid precursor protein* (*APP*) genes are mutated, they cause brain cells to overproduce β-amyloid.[2]

The first gene associated with AD was the *epsilon (E)-4* allele of the *apolipoprotein E (ApoE)* gene on chromosome 19. *ApoE* comes in several different alleles or forms, but three alleles occur

## GENETICS IN CLINICAL PRACTICE

### Alzheimer's Disease (AD)

**Genetic Basis**

***Early Onset (Familial) (<60 Yr Old at Onset)***

- Autosomal dominant disorder.
- Various mutations in the following genes:
  - Amyloid precursor protein *(APP)* gene on chromosome 21
  - Presenilin-1 *(PSEN1)* gene on chromosome 14
  - Presenilin-2 *(PSEN2)* gene on chromosome 1

***Late Onset (Sporadic) (>60 Yr Old at Onset)***

- Genetically more complex than early-onset form.
- Apolipoprotein E-4 *(ApoE-4)* allele on chromosome 19 increases the likelihood of developing AD.
- Presence of *ApoE-2* allele is associated with a lower risk of AD.

**Incidence**

***Early Onset***

- Rare form of AD, accounting for <5% of cases.
- Fifty percent risk of disease for children of affected parents.
- May occur in people as young as 30 yr old.

***Late Onset***

- *ApoE-4* is present in about 40% of people with late-onset AD. (It is present in 25%-30% of normal population.)
- Many *ApoE-4*-positive people do not develop AD, and many *ApoE-4*-negative people do.

**Genetic Testing**

***Early Onset***

- Genetic screening is available for mutations on chromosomes 1, 14, and 21.

***Late Onset***

- Blood test can identify which *ApoE* allele a person has but cannot predict who will develop disease.
- *ApoE* testing is mainly used in research to identify people who may have an increased risk of developing AD.*

**Clinical Implications**

- AD is the most common cause of dementia.
- Genetic testing and counseling for family members of patients with early-onset AD may be appropriate.
- If person tests positive for *ApoE-4,* it does not mean that the person will develop AD.

*ApoE testing is useful for studying AD risk in large groups of people, but not for determining an individual's specific risk.

most commonly. People inherit one allele (i.e., *ApoE-2, ApoE-3,* or *ApoE-4*) from each parent. *ApoE* contains the instructions to make a protein that helps to carry cholesterol and other types of fat in the bloodstream. *ApoE* may have a role in clearing amyloid plaques. Mutations in this gene result in greater amyloid deposition. The presence of *ApoE-4,* which is a risk-factor gene, increases the risk of a person developing late-onset AD. However, the presence of the gene alone is not adequate to account for AD, since many people with *ApoE-4* do not develop AD.

**Cardiovascular Factors.** The health of the brain is closely linked to the health of the heart and blood vessels. The functioning of the brain is dependent on a good blood supply and nutrients delivered to it by that blood supply.

Many factors increase the risk of cardiovascular disease. These include diabetes mellitus, hypertension, obesity, hypercholesterolemia, and smoking. Diabetes dramatically increases a person's risk of developing AD or other types of dementia. Diabetes can contribute to dementia in several ways. Chronic high levels of insulin and glucose may be directly toxic to brain cells. Insulin resistance, which causes high blood glucose and in some cases leads to type 2 diabetes, may interfere with the body's ability to break down amyloid, a protein that forms brain plaques in AD. In addition, high blood glucose along with high cholesterol has a role in atherosclerosis, which contributes to vascular dementia.[3,4]

Diabetes may contribute to poor memory and diminished mental function in various other ways. The disease causes microangiopathy, which damages small blood vessels throughout the body. Ongoing damage to blood vessels in the brain may be one reason why people with diabetes are at a higher risk of cognitive problems as they grow older. People with diabetes may lose brain volume (especially gray matter) as the disease progresses.[3,4]

**Head Trauma.** Head trauma is also a risk factor for dementia. Professional football players and military veterans who had traumatic brain injury or posttraumatic stress disorder have an increased risk for AD and other types of dementia.[5,6]

## Pathophysiology

Characteristic findings of AD relate to changes in the brain's structure and function: (1) amyloid plaques, (2) neurofibrillary tangles, (3) loss of connections between neurons, and (4) neuron death. Fig. 59-2 shows the pathologic changes in AD.

As part of aging, people develop some plaques in their brain tissue, but in AD more plaques appear in certain parts of the brain. These plaques consist of clusters of insoluble deposits of a protein called *β-amyloid,* other proteins, remnants of neurons, non-nerve cells such as microglia (cells that surround and digest damaged cells or foreign substances), and other cells such as astrocytes.

β-Amyloid is cleaved from amyloid precursor protein (APP), which is associated with the cell membrane (Fig. 59-3). The normal function of APP is unknown. Genetic factors may play a critical role in how the brain processes the β-amyloid protein. Overproduction of β-amyloid appears to be an important risk factor for AD. Abnormally high levels of β-amyloid cause cell damage either directly or by eliciting an inflammatory response and ultimately neuron death.

In AD, plaques develop first in areas of the brain used for memory and cognitive function, including the hippocampus (a structure that is important in forming and storing short-term memories). Eventually AD attacks the cerebral cortex, especially the areas responsible for language and reasoning.

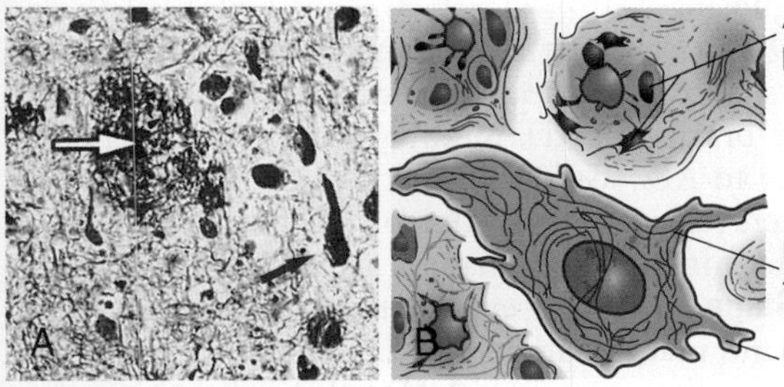


**FIG. 59-2** Pathologic changes in Alzheimer's disease **A,** Plaque with central amyloid core *(white arrow)* next to a neurofibrillary tangle *(red arrow)* on the histologic specimen from a brain autopsy. **B,** Schematic representation of amyloid plaque and neurofibrillary tangle.

**Neurofibrillary tangles** are abnormal collections of twisted protein threads inside nerve cells. The main component of these structures is a protein called *tau.* Tau proteins in the central nervous system (CNS) are involved in providing support for intracellular structure through their support of microtubules. Tau proteins hold the microtubules together like railroad ties hold railroad tracks together. In AD the tau protein is altered, and as a result, the microtubules twist together in a helical fashion (Fig. 59-3). This ultimately forms the neurofibrillary tangles found in the neurons of people with AD.

Plaques and neurofibrillary tangles are not unique to patients with AD or dementia. They are also found in the brains of individuals without evidence of cognitive impairment. However, they are more abundant in the brains of individuals with AD.

The other feature of AD is the loss of connections between neurons and neuron death. These processes result in structural damage. Affected parts of the brain begin to shrink in a process called brain atrophy. By the final stage of AD, brain tissue has shrunk significantly (Fig. 59-4).

## Clinical Manifestations

Pathologic changes often precede clinical manifestations of dementia by anywhere from 5 to 20 years. The Alzheimer's Association has developed a list of 10 warning signs that are common manifestations of AD (Table 59-4). The stages of AD can be categorized as mild, moderate, and severe (Table 59-5). The rate of progression from mild to severe is highly variable and ranges from 3 to 20 years.

The initial manifestations are usually related to changes in cognitive functioning. Patients may have complaints of memory loss, mild disorientation, or trouble with words and numbers. Often it is a family member, in particular the spouse, who reports the patient's declining memory to the HCP.

Normal age-related memory decline is characterized by mild changes that do not interfere with activities of daily living (Table 59-6). In AD the memory loss initially relates to recent events, with remote memories still intact. With time and progression of AD, memory loss includes both recent and remote memory and ultimately affects the ability to perform self-care.

As AD progresses, personal hygiene deteriorates, as does the ability to concentrate and maintain attention. Ongoing loss of neurons in AD can cause a person to act in altered or unpredictable ways. Behavioral manifestations of AD (e.g., agitation, aggression) result from changes that take place within the brain. They are neither intentional nor controllable by the individual with the disease. Some patients develop delusions and hallucinations.

With progression of AD, additional cognitive impairments are noted. These include *dysphasia* (difficulty comprehending language and oral communication), *apraxia* (inability to manipulate objects or perform purposeful acts), *visual agnosia* (inability to recognize objects by sight), and *dysgraphia* (difficulty communicating via writing). Eventually long-term memories cannot be recalled, and patients lose the ability to recognize family members and friends. Other problems include aggression and a tendency to wander.

Later in the disease, the ability to communicate and perform activities of daily living is lost. In the late stages of AD, the patient is unresponsive and incontinent and requires total care.

**Retrogenesis.** **Retrogenesis** is the process in AD patients in which degenerative changes occur in the reverse order in which

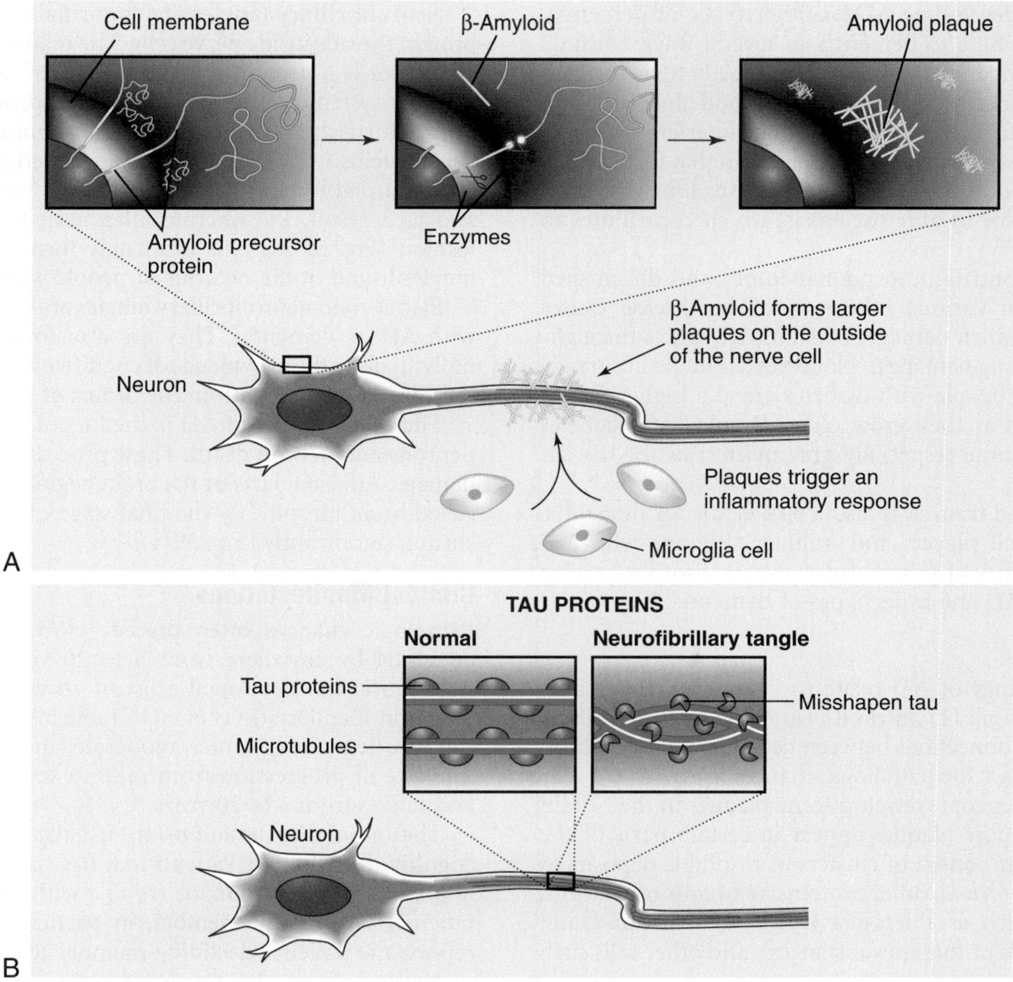


**FIG. 59-3** Current etiologic theories for the development of Alzheimer's disease. **A,** Abnormal amounts of β-amyloid are cleaved from the amyloid precursor protein *(APP)* and released into the circulation. The β-amyloid fragments come together in clumps to form plaques that attach to the neuron. Microglia react to the plaque, and an inflammatory response results. **B,** Tau proteins provide structural support for the neuron microtubules. Chemical changes in the neuron produce structural changes in tau proteins. This results in twisting and tangling (neurofibrillary tangles).

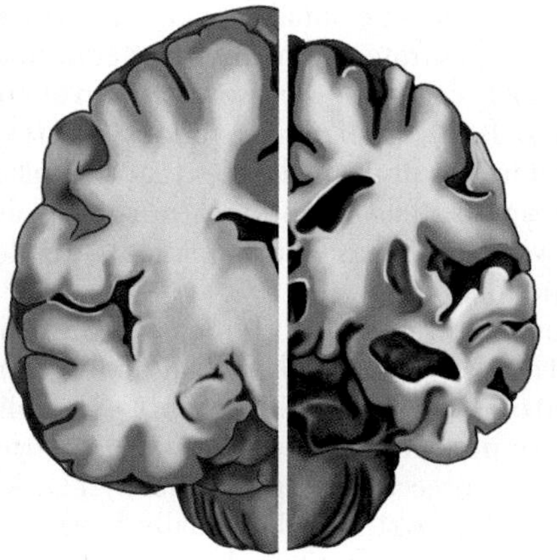

**FIG. 59-4** Effects of Alzheimer's disease on the brain. This figure compares a normal brain *(left)* with a brain that has been affected by Alzheimer's disease *(right).*

they were acquired.[7] This theory compares the developmental stages in children with the deterioration in AD patients. As seen in Fig. 59-5, a relationship exists between the developmental stage and deterioration of function. For example, it is appropriate for a person with AD in the moderate stage to feel good about putting together puzzles that belong to his 3-year-old grandson. In fact, they may play well together on the same task or project.

## Diagnostic Criteria for Alzheimer's Disease

AD may cause changes in the brain many years before symptoms appear. In addition, symptoms do not always directly relate to abnormal changes in the brain caused by AD. Based on these findings, in 2011 the National Institute on Aging and the Alzheimer's Association proposed revised criteria and guidelines for diagnosing AD.[8,9]

AD is now considered on a spectrum, where dementia marks the terminal stage of the disease (Table 59-7). The stages in this spectrum are preclinical AD, mild cognitive impairment, and dementia due to AD.[8] Guidelines address the use of imaging and biomarkers (discussed in section on diagnostic studies) that may help determine whether changes are due to AD.[9]

**Preclinical Stage.** A long lag exists between pathologic changes in the brain and manifestations of AD. The future goal would be to modify the disease process of AD before it becomes symptomatic. Once plaques and tangles have formed in sufficient quantity, it may be too late to intervene to prevent the disease or its progression. Although currently all attempts at modifying

**TABLE 59-4 Patient & Caregiver Teaching**

***Early Warning Signs of Alzheimer's Disease***

*Include the following information in the teaching plan for the patient with Alzheimer's disease.*

1. **Memory loss that affects job skills**
   - Frequent forgetfulness or unexplainable confusion at home or in the workplace may signal that something is wrong.
   - This type of memory loss goes beyond forgetting an assignment, colleague's name, deadline, or phone number.
2. **Difficulty performing familiar tasks**
   - It is normal for most people to become distracted and to forget something (e.g., leave something on the stove too long).
   - People with AD may cook a meal but then forget not only to serve it but also that they made it.
3. **Problems with language**
   - Most people have trouble finding the "right" word from time to time.
   - People with AD may forget simple words or substitute inappropriate words, making their speech difficult to understand.
4. **Disorientation to time and place**
   - Most individuals occasionally forget the day of the week or what they need from the store.
   - People with AD can become lost on their own street, not knowing where they are, how they got there, or how to get back home.
5. **Poor or decreased judgment**
   - Many individuals from time to time may choose not to dress appropriately for the weather (e.g., not bringing a coat or sweater on a cold evening).
   - The person with AD may dress inappropriately in more noticeable ways, such as wearing a bathrobe to the store or a sweater on a hot day.
6. **Problems with abstract thinking**
   - For the person with AD, this goes beyond challenges such as balancing a checkbook.
   - The person with AD may have difficulty recognizing numbers or doing even basic calculations.
7. **Misplacing things**
   - For many individuals, temporarily misplacing keys, purses, or wallets is a normal, albeit frustrating, event.
   - The person with AD may put items in inappropriate places (e.g., eating utensils in clothing drawers) but have no memory of how they got there.
8. **Changes in mood or behavior**
   - Most individuals experience mood changes.
   - The person with AD tends to exhibit more rapid mood swings for no apparent reason.
9. **Changes in personality**
   - As most individuals age, they may demonstrate some change in personality (e.g., become less tolerant).
   - The person with AD can change dramatically, either suddenly or over time. For example, someone who is generally easygoing may become angry, suspicious, or fearful.
10. **Loss of initiative**
    - The person with AD may become and remain uninterested and uninvolved in many or all of his or her usual pursuits.

Adapted from Alzheimer's Association: *Early warning signs*, Chicago, The Association. *www.alz.org/alzheimers_disease_know_the_10_signs.asp.*

the disease process have failed, research is ongoing. The model for early intervention is seen in other diseases, such as removing polyps to prevent colon cancer, controlling blood glucose in diabetes before the disease progresses to heart and kidney disease, and treating cardiac risk factors before a person has a myocardial infarction.

**Mild Cognitive Impairment.** Mild cognitive impairment (MCI), the second stage in the AD spectrum, is a state of cognitive function in which individuals have problems with memory, language, or another essential cognitive function that are severe enough to be noticeable to others and show up on tests. However, these manifestations may not be severe enough to interfere with activities of daily living. Because the problems do not interfere with daily activities, the person does not meet the criteria for being diagnosed with dementia.[10]

To the casual observer, an individual with MCI may seem fairly normal. However, the person with MCI is often aware of a significant change in memory, and family members may observe changes in the individual's abilities (Table 59-6).

Between 10% and 20% of people 65 years old and older have MCI and are at high risk of developing AD. Some individuals with MCI show no progression and do not go on to develop AD, but an estimated 15% of people with MCI eventually do.[1]

No drugs have been approved for the treatment of MCI. There is little evidence that medications used in AD (e.g., cholinesterase inhibitors) affect progression to dementia or cognitive test scores in people with MCI.[11]

Currently the primary treatment of MCI consists of ongoing monitoring. Recognize the importance of monitoring the patient with MCI for changes in memory and thinking skills that would indicate a worsening of symptoms or a progression to dementia. It is critical that you understand the 10 early warning signs of AD (Table 59-4).

## Diagnostic Studies

No definitive diagnostic test exists for AD. The diagnosis of AD is primarily a diagnosis of exclusion. In patients with cognitive impairment, there is increased emphasis on early and careful evaluation. As indicated earlier in this chapter, many conditions can cause manifestations of dementia, some of which are treatable or reversible (Table 59-2).

When all other possible conditions that can cause cognitive impairment have been ruled out, a clinical diagnosis of AD can be made. A comprehensive patient evaluation includes a complete health history, physical examination, neurologic and mental status assessments, and laboratory tests (Table 59-8). Brain imaging tests (e.g., CT or MRI) may show brain atrophy in the later stages of the disease, although this finding occurs in other diseases and can also be seen in people without cognitive impairment. Positron emission tomography (PET) scanning can be used to differentiate AD from other forms of dementia (Fig. 59-6). Neuroimaging techniques allow for detection of changes early in the disease and monitoring of treatment response. A definitive diagnosis of AD usually requires examination of brain tissue at autopsy and findings of neurofibrillary tangles and plaques.

The new criteria and guidelines identify two biomarker categories: (1) biomarkers showing the level of β-amyloid accumulation in the brain and (2) biomarkers showing that nerve cells in the brain are injured or actually degenerating. Biomarkers include (1) cerebrospinal fluid (CSF) neurochemical markers: β-amyloid and tau proteins and (2) imaging biomarkers: volumetric MRI and PET. The level of tau in the CSF is an indication of neurodegeneration. (Plasma levels of tau or β-amyloid are not of any value in diagnosing AD.) In AD, multiple brain structures atrophy and the volume of the brain correlates with neurodegeneration. PET determines brain metabolism using glucose tracers (Fig. 59-6). PET can also be used to detect amyloid.

Some imaging biomarkers are used in specialized clinical settings. CSF biomarkers are mainly used for research.

**TABLE 59-5 Stages of Alzheimer's Disease**

| Mild | Moderate | Severe |
|---|---|---|
| • Forgetfulness beyond what is seen in a normal person<br>• Short-term memory impairment, especially for new learning<br>• Loss of initiative and interests<br>• May forget recent events or the names of people or things<br>• Small personality changes<br>• May no longer be able to solve simple math problems<br>• Slowly loses the ability to plan and organize | • Memory loss and confusion become more obvious<br>• Has more trouble organizing, planning, and following directions<br>• May need help getting dressed<br>• May start having episodes of incontinence<br>• Trouble recognizing family members and friends<br>• Agitation, restlessness<br>• May lack judgment and begin to wander, gets lost<br>• May have trouble sleeping<br>• Delusions, hallucinations, paranoia<br>• Behavioral problems | • Severe impairment of all cognitive functions<br>• Little memory, unable to process new information<br>• Unable to perform self-care activities<br>• Often needs help with daily needs<br>• May not be able to talk<br>• Cannot understand words<br>• May have difficulty eating, swallowing<br>• May not be able to walk or sit up without help<br>• Immobility<br>• Incontinence |

**TABLE 59-6 Comparison of Normal Forgetfulness and Memory Loss**

| Normal Forgetfulness | Memory Loss in Mild Cognitive Impairment | Memory Loss in Alzheimer's Disease |
|---|---|---|
| • Sometimes misplaces keys, eyeglasses, or other items | • Frequently misplaces items | • Forgets what an item is used for or puts it in an inappropriate place |
| • Momentarily forgets an acquaintance's name | • Frequently forgets people's names and is slow to recall them | • May not remember knowing a person |
| • Occasionally has to search for a word | • Has increasing difficulty finding desired words | • Begins to lose language skills and may withdraw from social interaction |
| • Occasionally forgets to run an errand | • Begins to forget important events and appointments | • Loses sense of time, does not know what day it is |
| • May forget an event from the distant past | • May forget recent events or newly learned information | • Has seriously impaired recent memory and difficulty learning and remembering new information |
| • When driving, may momentarily forget where to turn, but quickly orients self | • Becomes temporarily lost more often, may have trouble understanding and following a map | • Becomes easily disoriented or lost in familiar places, sometimes for hours |
| • Jokes about memory loss | • Worries about memory loss, family and friends notice lapses | • May have little or no awareness of cognitive problems |

Adapted from Rabins P: Memory. In *The Johns Hopkins white papers,* Baltimore, 2007, Johns Hopkins University.

**TABLE 59-7 Diagnostic Criteria for Alzheimer's Disease***

| | Stage and Description | Recommendations for Biomarkers |
|---|---|---|
| **Preclinical Alzheimer's disease (AD)** | • Brain changes, including amyloid buildup and other early neuron changes, may already be in process<br>• At this point, significant clinical symptoms are not yet evident<br>• In some people, amyloid buildup can be detected with positron emission tomography (PET) scans and cerebrospinal fluid (CSF) analysis | • Use of imaging and biomarker tests at this stage are recommended only for research<br>• Biomarkers are still being developed and standardized, and are not used by clinicians in general practice |
| **Mild cognitive impairment (MCI) due to Alzheimer's disease** | • MCI stage is marked by symptoms of memory problems, enough to be noticed and measured, but not compromising a person's independence<br>• People with MCI may or may not progress to Alzheimer's dementia | • Used primarily by researchers<br>• May be used in specialized clinical settings to supplement standard clinical tests to help determine possible causes of MCI<br>• May help confirm that the person's impairment is related to AD |
| **Dementia due to Alzheimer's disease** | • Characterized by memory, thinking, and behavioral symptoms that impair a person's ability to function in daily life<br>• Dementia marks the terminal stage of AD<br>• Encompasses all stages presented in Table 59-5 | • May be used in some cases to increase the level of certainty about a diagnosis of AD<br>• Also may be used to distinguish AD from other dementias |

Source: Jack CR, Albert MS, Knopman DS, et al: Introduction to the recommendations from the National Institute on Aging–Alzheimer's Association workgroups on diagnostic guidelines for Alzheimer's disease, *Alzheimers Dement* 7:257, 2011.

*Note that these are recommended criteria and guidelines. More research is needed, especially biomarker research, before the new criteria and guidelines can be used in clinical settings.

| Stage | Alzheimer's Disease | Reisberg Stage* | Developmental Age | Diversion/Distraction Activities |
|---|---|---|---|---|
| Mild | No difficulty at all | 1 | | |
| | Some memory trouble begins to affect job/home. Forgets familiar names. | 2 | | |
| | Much difficulty maintaining job performance. Withdrawal from difficult situations. | 3 | 12+ yr | Can function with understanding. Enjoy things previously enjoyed—watch TV, play and listen to music, play games. |
| | Can no longer hold a job, plan and prepare meals, handle personal finances, etc. Driving becomes difficult although can drive to familiar places. | 4 | 8-12 yr | Can still enjoy simple games, watch TV and videos. Enjoys family photos and memories. |
| Moderate | Can no longer select proper clothing for occasion or season. Needs help to remain safe in home. Forgets to bathe. | 5 | 5-7 yr | Needs age appropriate toys and games. |
| | Requires assistance with dressing. | 6a | 4-5 yr | Enjoy many of the same activities as preschoolers. |
| | Requires assistance with bathing. | 6b | 4-5 yr | |
| | Can no longer use toilet without assistance. | 6c | 4 yr | |
| | Urinary incontinence | 6d | 3-4.5 yr | |
| | Fecal incontinence | 6e | 2-3 yr | |
| Severe | Speech now limited to about words per day. | 7a | 15 mo | Enjoys infant toys, mobiles, dangling ribbons. |
| | Speech now limited to one word per day. | 7b | 1 yr | |
| | Can no longer walk without assistance. | 7c | 1 yr | |
| | Can no longer sit up without assistance. | 7d | 6-10 mo | |
| | Can no longer smile. | 7e | 2-4 mo | |
| | Can no longer hold up head. | 7f | 1-3 mo | |

**FIG. 59-5** Retrogenesis (back to birth) in Alzheimer's disease. (*These stages are based on Functional Assessment Staging. Reisberg B: Functional assessment staging [FAST], *Psychopharmacol Bull* 24:653, 1988.)

## TABLE 59-8 Interprofessional Care

### *Alzheimer's Disease*

**Diagnostic Assessment**

- History and physical examination, including psychologic evaluation
- Neuropsychologic testing, including Mini-Cog (Table 59-9), Mini-Mental State Examination (Table 59-10)
- Brain imaging tests: CT, MRI, MRS, PET
- Complete blood count
- Electrocardiogram
- Serum glucose, creatinine, BUN
- Serum levels of vitamins $B_1$, $B_6$, $B_{12}$
- Thyroid function tests
- Liver function tests
- Screening for depression

**Management**

- Drug therapy for cognitive problems (Table 59-11)
- Behavioral modification
- Moderate exercise
- Assistance with functional independence
- Assistance and support for caregiver

*MRS,* Magnetic resonance spectroscopy; *PET,* positron emission tomography.

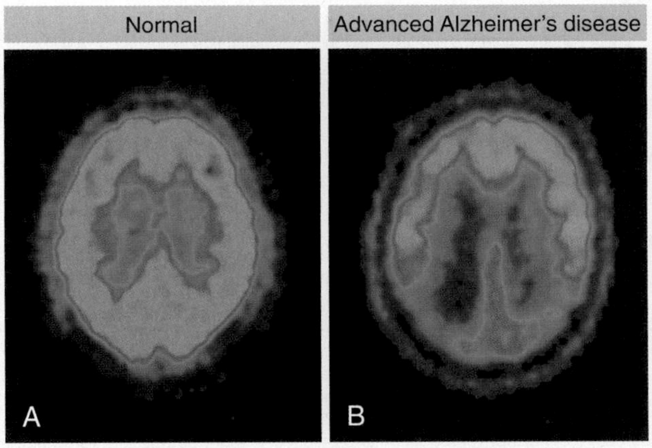


**FIG. 59-6** Positron emission tomography (PET) scan can be used to assist in the diagnosis of Alzheimer's disease (AD). Radioactive fluorine is applied to glucose (fluorodeoxyglucose), and the yellow areas indicate metabolically active cells. **A,** A normal brain. **B,** Advanced AD is recognized by hypometabolism in many areas of the brain. (From Roberts GS: *Neuropsychiatric disorders,* London, 1993, Mosby-Wolfe.)

### TABLE 59-9 The Mini-Cog

**Introduction**

The Mini-Cog is used as a brief assessment tool for cognitive impairment. It can be quickly administered and can guide the need for further evaluation.

**Administration**

1. Instruct the patient to listen carefully to and remember three unrelated words and then to repeat the words. *Example:* apple, table, penny. (This initial step is not scored.) The same three words may be repeated to the patient up to three tries to register all three words.
2. Instruct the patient to draw the face of a clock, either on a blank sheet of paper or on a sheet with the clock circle already drawn on the page. After the patient puts the numbers on the clock face, ask him or her to draw the hands of the clock to read a specific time (11:10). The test is considered normal if all numbers are present in the correct sequence and position, and the hands readably display the requested time.
3. Ask the patient to repeat the three previously stated words.

**Scoring (out of total of 5 points)**

Give 1 point for each recalled word after the clock drawing test.

- Patients recalling none of the three words are classified as cognitively impaired (score = 0).
- Patients recalling all three words are classified as not cognitively impaired (score = 3).
- Patients with intermediate word recall of one or two words are classified on the clock drawing test:
  The clock drawing test is scored 2 if normal and 0 if abnormal.
  Interpretation of results
  0-2: Positive screen for dementia
  3-5: Negative screen for dementia

Source: Borson S, Scanlan J, Brush M, et al: The Mini-Cog: a cognitive "vital signs" measure for dementia screening in multi-lingual elderly, *Intern J Geriatr Psychiatry* 15(11):1021, 2000.

### TABLE 59-10 Mini-Mental State Examination (MMSE)

***Sample Items***

**Orientation to Time**

"What is the date?"

**Registration**

"Listen carefully, I am going to say three words. You say them back after I stop. Ready? Here they are . . . HOUSE (pause), CAR (pause), LAKE (pause). Now repeat those words back to me." (Repeat up to five times, but score only the first trial.)

**Naming**

"What is this?" (Point to a pencil or pen.)

**Reading**

"Please read this and do what it says." (Show examinee the words CLOSE YOUR EYES on the stimulus form.)



Biomarkers may be used in some cases to increase the level of certainty about a diagnosis of Alzheimer's dementia and to distinguish Alzheimer's dementia from other dementias. However, more research is needed with biomarkers before they are used routinely in clinical practice.

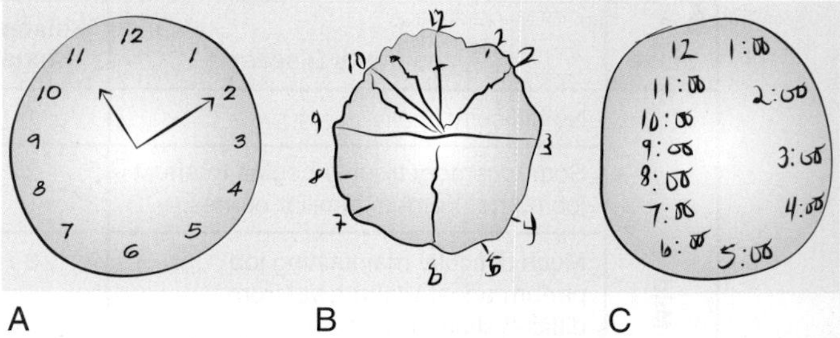


**FIG. 59-7** Clock drawing is a simple test that can be used as an assessment technique in dementia. The person undergoing testing is asked to draw a clock, put in all of the numbers, and set the hands at 10 past 11. **A,** Shows a clock drawn by a person with no dementia. **B** and **C** show clocks drawn by people with dementia. (Modified from Stern TA: *Massachusetts General Hospital comprehensive clinical psychiatry,* Philadelphia, 2008, Mosby.)

### TABLE 59-11 Drug Therapy

***Alzheimer's Disease***

| Problem | Drugs |
|---|---|
| **Decreased memory and cognition** | Cholinesterase inhibitors<br>• donepezil (Aricept)<br>• rivastigmine (Exelon)<br>• galantamine (Razadyne)<br>*N*-methyl-D-aspartate (NMDA) receptor antagonist<br>• memantine (Namenda) |
| **Depression** | Selective serotonin reuptake inhibitors (SSRIs)<br>• sertraline (Zoloft)<br>• fluvoxamine (Luvox)<br>• citalopram (Celexa)<br>• fluoxetine (Prozac)<br>Atypical antidepressants<br>• mirtazapine (Remeron)<br>• trazodone |
| **Behavioral problems** (e.g., agitation, physical aggression, disinhibition) | Antipsychotics*<br>• haloperidol (Haldol)<br>• risperidone (Risperdal)<br>• olanzapine (Zyprexa)<br>• quetiapine (Seroquel)<br>• aripiprazole (Abilify)<br>Benzodiazepines<br>• lorazepam (Ativan)<br>• clonazepam (Klonopin) |
| **Sleep disturbances** | • zolpidem (Ambien) |

*The use of these drugs in older patients with dementia is associated with an increased risk of death.

Neuropsychologic testing with tools such as the Mini-Cog (Table 59-9) and the Mini-Mental State Examination (Table 59-10) can help document the degree of cognitive impairment.[12] The clock drawing test can be used as part of the Mini-Cog or by itself to assess cognitive function (Fig. 59-7). Neuropsychologic testing is important not only for diagnostic purposes but also to establish a baseline for evaluating changes over time.

## Interprofessional Care

At this time there is no cure for AD. No treatment is available to stop the deterioration of brain cells in AD. Nothing stops or really slows the progression of the disease.

The interprofessional care of AD is aimed at (1) controlling the undesirable behavioral manifestations that the patient may exhibit and (2) providing support for the family caregiver.

**Drug Therapy.** Although drug therapy for AD is available (Table 59-11), these drugs do not cure or reverse the progression of the disease. Drugs help many people, but not for very long and

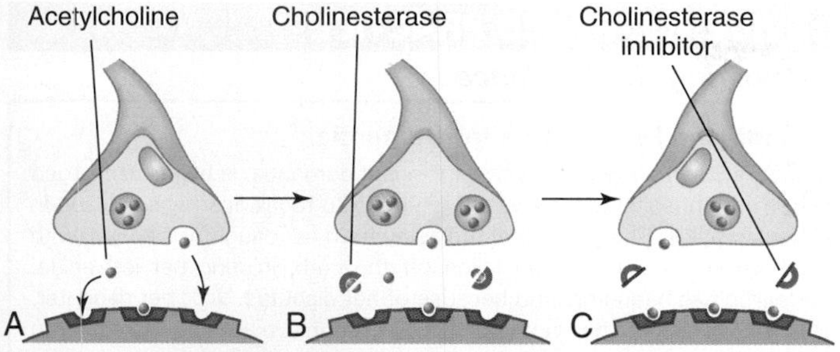


**FIG. 59-8** Mechanism of action of cholinesterase inhibitors. **A,** Acetylcholine is released from the nerve synapses and carries a message across the synapse. **B,** Cholinesterase breaks down acetylcholine. **C,** Cholinesterase inhibitors block cholinesterase, thus giving acetylcholine more time to transmit the message.

not very well. The use of drugs may lead to a modest decrease in the rate of decline of cognitive function. However, the drugs have no effect on overall disease progression.[1]

Cholinesterase inhibitors block cholinesterase, the enzyme responsible for the breakdown of acetylcholine in the synaptic cleft (Fig. 59-8). Cholinesterase inhibitors include donepezil (Aricept), rivastigmine (Exelon), and galantamine (Razadyne). Rivastigmine is available as a patch.

Memantine (Namenda) protects the brain's nerve cells against excess amounts of glutamate, which is released in large amounts by cells damaged by AD. The attachment of glutamate to *N*-methyl-D-aspartate (NMDA) receptors permits calcium to flow freely into the cell, which in turn may lead to cell degeneration. Memantine may prevent this destructive sequence by blocking the action of glutamate.

Treating the depression that is often associated with AD may improve cognitive ability. Depression is often treated with selective serotonin reuptake inhibitors, including fluoxetine (Prozac), sertraline (Zoloft), fluvoxamine (Luvox), and citalopram (Celexa). The antidepressant trazodone may help with problems related to sleep.

Although antipsychotic drugs are approved for treating psychotic conditions (e.g., schizophrenia), they have been used for the management of behavioral problems (e.g., agitation, aggressive behavior) that occur in patients with AD. However, these drugs have been shown to increase the risk of death in older dementia patients. The Food and Drug Administration (FDA) has warned that antipsychotics are not indicated for the treatment of dementia-related psychosis. However, the warning does not mean that the drugs cannot be used for these patients with dementia.[13]

## NURSING MANAGEMENT: ALZHEIMER'S DISEASE

### Nursing Assessment

Subjective and objective data that should be obtained from a person with AD are presented in Table 59-12. Useful questions for the patient and caregiver are, "When did you first notice the memory loss?" and "How has the memory loss progressed since then?"

### Nursing Diagnoses

Nursing diagnoses for AD may include, but are not limited to, the following:

- Impaired memory *related to* the effects of dementia
- Self-neglect *related to* memory deficit, cognitive impairment, and neuromuscular impairment

**TABLE 59-12 Nursing Assessment**
***Alzheimer's Disease***

**Subjective Data**

***Important Health Information***

*Past health history:* Repeated head trauma, stroke, previous CNS infection, family history of dementia
*Medications:* Use of any drug to decrease symptoms (e.g., tranquilizers, hypnotics, antidepressants, antipsychotics)

***Functional Health Patterns***

*Health perception–health management:* Positive family history. Emotional lability
*Nutritional-metabolic:* Anorexia, malnutrition, weight loss
*Elimination:* Incontinence
*Activity-exercise:* Poor personal hygiene, gait instability, weakness, inability to perform activities of daily living
*Sleep-rest:* Frequent nighttime awakening, daytime napping
*Cognitive-perceptual:* Forgetfulness, inability to cope with complex situations, difficulty with problem solving (early signs), depression, withdrawal, suicidal ideation (early)

**Objective Data**

***General***

Disheveled appearance, agitation

***Neurologic***

*Mild:* Loss of recent memory, disorientation to date and time, flat affect, lack of spontaneity. Impaired abstraction, cognition, and judgment
*Moderate:* Agitation, impaired ability to recognize close family and friends, loss of remote memory, confusion, apraxia, agnosia, alexia (inability to understand written language); aphasia, inability to do simple tasks
*Severe:* Inability to do self-care, incontinence, immobility, limb rigidity, flexor posturing

***Possible Diagnostic Findings***

Diagnosis by exclusion, cerebral cortical atrophy on CT scan, poor scores on mental status tests, hippocampal atrophy on MRI scan, abnormal changes on PET

- Risk for injury *related to* impaired judgment, gait instability, muscle weakness, and sensory/perceptual alteration
- Wandering *related to* cognitive impairment

Additional information on nursing diagnoses for the patient with AD is presented in eNursing Care Plan 59-1 (available on the website for this chapter).

### Planning

The overall goals are that the patient with AD will (1) maintain functional ability for as long as possible, (2) be maintained in a safe environment with a minimum of injuries, (3) have personal care needs met, and (4) have dignity maintained. The overall goals for the caregiver of a patient with AD are to (1) reduce caregiver stress; (2) maintain personal, emotional, and physical health; and (3) cope with the long-term effects of caregiving.

### Nursing Implementation

**Health Promotion.** Can AD be prevented? Although there is no known definitive way to prevent AD, there are several things that you can do to keep your brain healthy and modify your risks for developing dementia[14] (Table 59-13).

Early recognition and treatment of AD are important. You have a responsibility to inform patients and their families regarding the early signs of AD (Table 59-4).

**TABLE 59-13 Decreasing Risk of Cognitive Decline**

*The following are tips to reduce the risk of cognitive decline and dementia.*

1. **Avoid harmful substances**
   Excessive drinking and drug abuse can damage brain cells. Stop smoking because it increases the risk of cognitive decline.
2. **Challenge your mind**
   Read frequently, do crossword puzzles. Keep mentally active. Learn new skills. Go back to school. This strengthens the brain connections and promotes new ones.
3. **Exercise regularly**
   Even low to moderate level activity such as walking or gardening three to five times per week can make you feel better. Daily physical activity, even in older adults, can decrease the risk for cognitive decline.
4. **Stay socially active**
   Pursue social activities that have meaning to you. Family, friends, church, and a sense of community may all contribute to better brain health.
5. **Avoid trauma to the brain**
   Because traumatic brain injury may be a risk factor for developing AD, promote safety in physical activities and driving. Use the car seat belt. Wear a helmet when playing contact sports or riding a bike. Fall proof your home.
6. **Take care of mental health**
   Recognize and treat depression early. Depression may cause or worsen memory loss and other cognitive impairment.
7. **Treat diabetes.**
   Better blood glucose control can help to prevent the cognitive decline associated with diabetes.
8. **Take care of your heart**
   Risk factors for cardiovascular disease and stroke (hypertension, obesity) negatively affect your cognitive health. Heart health is linked to brain health.
9. **Get enough sleep**
   Not getting enough sleep may result in problems with memory and thinking.
10. **Get the right fuel**
   A healthy and balanced diet low in fats and high in vegetables and fruits helps to reduce the risk of cognitive decline.

Adapted from Alzheimer's Association: 10 Ways to love your brain. Retrieved from *www.alz.org/northcentraltexas/in_my_community_101405.asp;* and Baumgart M, Snyder HM, Carrillo MC, et al: Summary of evidence on modifiable risk factors for cognitive decline and dementia: a population-based perspective, *Alzheimers Dement* 11:718, 2015.

◆ **Acute Care.** The diagnosis of AD is traumatic for both the patient and family. It is not unusual for the patient to respond with depression, denial, anxiety, fear, withdrawal, and feelings of loss.[15] In the early stages of AD, patients are often aware that their memory is faulty and do things to cover up or mask the problem. *What Happens Next?* is a free booklet specifically for people dealing with the beginning stages of dementia (available at *www.alzheimers.nia.nih.gov*).

You are in an important position to assess for depression. Antidepressant drugs and counseling may be indicated. Family caregivers may also be in denial and may not seek medical attention early in the disease. Along with patient assessment, assess family caregivers and their ability to accept and cope with the diagnosis.

Although no current treatment is available for reversing AD, there is a need for ongoing monitoring of both the patient with AD and the patient's caregiver. An important nursing responsibility is to work collaboratively with the caregiver to manage clinical manifestations effectively as they change over time.[16] You are often responsible for teaching the caregiver to perform the many tasks that are required to manage the patient's care.

## EVIDENCE-BASED PRACTICE

### *Applying the Evidence*

**Modifying Risk Factors for Dementia**

G.C., a 63-yr-old woman with early-onset dementia, is being discharged from the hospital tomorrow after surgery to repair ligament damage in her left ankle. She had wandered away from her daughter's house (with whom she lives) and had fallen off the curb, injuring her left ankle. Healing has been impaired because of her diabetes. V.Z., her daughter, is very upset with her mother's declining cognitive abilities and asks you what she can do to help her mother. She also asks you what she personally can do to prevent getting this "awful" disease.

***Making Clinical Decisions***

***Best Available Evidence.*** Regular physical activity and management of cardiovascular risk factors (diabetes, obesity, smoking, and hypertension) reduce the risk of cognitive decline and may reduce the risk of dementia. A healthy diet and lifelong learning/cognitive training may also reduce the risk of cognitive decline.

***Clinician Expertise.*** Good nutrition and physical exercise can improve both a person's physical as well as emotional health. G.C. and V.Z. can exercise (e.g., walking) together, and that may also decrease G.C's wandering.

***Patient Preferences and Values.*** V.Z. recognizes that her meal planning for the family is very haphazard and they eat a lot of fast foods. She also recognizes that sitting in front of the TV has become a refuge and they get very little exercise.

***Implications for Nursing Practice***

1. How will you assess the risk factors for dementia and cognitive decline in both G.C. and V.Z.?
2. What strategies can you discuss with V.Z. that she can personally implement in her life to decrease her risk for dementia?
3. How can you engage G.C. in activities to prevent further cognitive decline?

***Reference for Evidence***

Baumgart M, Snyder HM, Carrillo MC, et al: Summary of evidence on modifiable risk factors for cognitive decline and dementia: a population-based perspective, *Alzheimers Dement* 11:718, 2015.

Consider both the patient with AD and the caregiver as patients with overlapping but unique problems.[17]

Patients with AD may be hospitalized for other health problems. Patients with AD have other illnesses (both acute and chronic) and may require surgical interventions. Their inability to communicate symptoms of health problems places the responsibility for assessment and diagnosis on caregivers and health care professionals. Hospitalization of the patient with AD can be a traumatic event for both the patient and caregiver and can precipitate a worsening of dementia or development of delirium. Patients with AD in the acute care setting need to be observed more closely because of concerns for safety, frequently oriented to place and time, and given reassurance. Anxiety or disruptive behavior may be reduced with using consistent nursing staff.

◆ **Ambulatory Care.** Currently, family members and friends care for most individuals with AD in their homes. Others with AD reside in various facilities, including long-term care and assisted living facilities. A facility that is good for one person may not be suitable for another. Also, what is helpful for a person at one point in the disease process may be completely different from what is best when the disease progresses.

Patients with AD move through the stages at variable rates. The nursing care required by the patient with AD changes as the disease progresses, which emphasizes the need for regular assessment and support. Regardless of the setting, the severity of the problems and amount of nursing care required intensify over time. The specific manifestations of the disease depend on the area of the brain involved. Nursing care focuses on decreasing clinical manifestations, preventing harm, and supporting the patient and caregiver throughout the disease process.

In the early stages of AD, memory aids (e.g., calendars) may be beneficial. Patients often develop depression during this phase. Depression may be related to the diagnosis of an incurable disorder and the impact of the disease on activities of daily living (e.g., driving, socializing with friends, participating in hobbies or recreational activities).

After the initial diagnosis, patients need to be aware that the progression of the disease is variable. Effective management of the disease may slow the progress of the disease and decrease the burden on the patient, caregiver, and family. However, decisions related to care should be made with the patient, family members, and interprofessional care team early in the disease. You have a role in advising the patient and caregiver to initiate health care decisions, including advance directives, while the patient has the capacity to do so. This can ease the burden for the caregiver as the disease progresses.

Adult day care is one of the options available to the person with AD. Although programs vary in size, structure, physical environment, and staff experience, the common goals of all day care programs are to provide respite for the family and a protective environment for the patient. During the early and moderate stages of AD, the person can still benefit from stimulating activities that encourage independence and decision making in a protective environment. The patient returns home tired, content, less frustrated, and ready to be with the family. The respite from the demands of care allows the caregiver to be more responsive to the patient's needs.

As the disease progresses, the demands on the caregiver eventually exceed the resources, and the person with AD may need to be placed in a long-term care facility. Special dementia units are becoming increasingly common. The dementia unit is designed with an emphasis on safety. For example, many facilities have designated areas that allow the patient to walk freely within the unit, while the unit is secured so that the patient cannot wander outside of it.

As the patient with AD progresses to the late stages (severe impairment) of AD, he or she has increased difficulty with the most basic functions, including walking and talking. Total care is required.

Specific problems relate to the care of the patient with AD in all phases of the disease. These problems are described below.

◆ ***Behavioral Problems.*** Behavioral problems occur in about 90% of patients with AD. These problems include repetitiveness (asking the same question repeatedly), delusions (false beliefs), hallucinations, agitation, aggression, altered sleeping patterns, wandering, hoarding, and resisting care. Many times these behaviors are unpredictable and may challenge caregivers. Caregivers must be aware that these behaviors are not intentional and are often difficult to control. Behavioral problems are often the reason that patients are placed in institutional care settings.

These behaviors are often the patient's way of responding to a precipitating factor (e.g., pain, frustration, temperature extremes, anxiety). When these behaviors become problematic, you must plan interventions carefully. Initially assess the patient's physical status. Check the patient for changes in vital signs, urinary and bowel patterns, and pain that could account for behavioral problems. Then assess the environment to identify factors that may trigger behavior disruptions. Extremes in temperature or excessive noise may lead to behavior changes. When a patient is agitated by the environment, either move the patient or remove the stimulus.

When a patient resists or pulls tubes or dressings, cover these items with stretch tube gauze or remove them from the visual field. Reassure the patient that you are present to keep him or her safe. Do not ask the confused or agitated patient challenging "why" questions. The person with AD cannot think logically. If the patient cannot verbalize distress, validate his or her mood. Rephrase the patient's statement to validate its meaning. Closely observe the patient's emotional state.

Nursing strategies that address difficult behavior include redirection, distraction, and reassurance. For the patient who is restless or agitated, redirecting involves changing the patient's focus (e.g., having the patient perform activities such as sweeping, raking, or dusting). Ways to distract the agitated patient may include providing snacks, taking a car ride, sitting on a porch swing or rocker, listening to favorite music, watching videotapes, looking at family photographs, or walking. Reassurance involves communicating to the patient that he or she will be protected from danger, harm, or embarrassment. Use of repetitive activities, songs, poems, music, massage, aromas, or a favorite object can be soothing to patients.

When dealing with the difficult patient, do not threaten to restrain the patient or call the HCP. A calming family member can be asked to stay with the patient until the patient becomes calmer. Monitor the patient frequently, and document all interventions. As verbal skills decline, you and the caregiver must rely more on the patient's body language to communicate care needs. The use of positive nurse actions can reduce the use of chemical (drug therapy) restraints.

Disruptive behaviors have been treated with antipsychotic drugs (Table 59-11). However, as discussed on p. 1409, these drugs have adverse side effects. Before these drugs are used, all other measures of treating behavioral issues should be exhausted.

### CHECK YOUR PRACTICE

You are working in a secure Alzheimer's unit. Today while making rounds at 4 PM you observe Dan, one of the assistants, screaming and yelling at an 84-yr-old man who has been a resident in the facility for 6 months. When you approach Dan and the resident, you ask what is going on. Dan responds, "Every day about this time he gets so agitated and starts yelling at me so I yell back."

- How would you handle the situation, and what teaching is needed for Dan?

A specific type of agitation, termed **sundowning**, is when the patient becomes more confused and agitated in the late afternoon or evening. Behaviors related to sundowning include agitation, aggressiveness, wandering, resistance to redirection, and increased verbal activity such as yelling. The cause of sundowning is unclear, but it may be due to a disruption of circadian rhythms. Other possible causes include fatigue, unfamiliar environment and noise (especially in an acute care setting), medications, reduced lighting, and sleep fragmentation.

When a patient has sundowning, remain calm and avoid confrontation. Assess the situation for possible causes of the agitation. Nursing interventions that may be helpful include (1) creating a quiet, calm environment; (2) maximizing exposure to daylight (open blinds and turn on lights during the day); (3) evaluating medications to determine if any could cause sleep disturbance; (4) limiting naps and caffeine; and

## TEAMWORK & COLLABORATION

### *Caring for the Patient With Alzheimer's Disease*

All staff members who care for a patient with Alzheimer's disease (AD) are responsible for ensuring the patient's physiologic and psychosocial safety. The registered nurse (RN) is responsible for ongoing assessments of the patient's level of function and for development of the plan of care. Since most patients with AD are cared for at home or in long-term care settings, many routine nursing activities are delegated to licensed practical/vocational nurses (LPN/LVNs), unlicensed assistive personnel (UAP), or family caregivers.

**Role of Nursing Personnel**

***Registered Nurse (RN)***

- Assess patient memory and level of function.
- Teach patient and caregivers memory enhancement aids (e.g., calendars, notes).
- Monitor for physiologic problems associated with AD, such as pain, swallowing difficulties, urinary tract infection, pneumonia, skin breakdown, and constipation.
- Assess patient's nutritional and fluid intake and develop a plan to ensure adequate intake.
- Evaluate patient's safety risk factors.
- Determine possible precipitating factors for behavioral changes and develop strategies to address difficult behavior.
- Assess the family caregiver's stress level and coping strategies.
- Make referrals for community services such as adult day care and respite care.

***Licensed Practical/Vocational Nurse (LPN/LVN)***

- Monitor for behavioral changes that may indicate physiologic problems.
- Check patient environment for potential safety hazards.
- Administer enteral feedings to patients who are unable to swallow (if ordered).
- Administer ordered drug therapy.

***Unlicensed Assistive Personnel (UAP)***

- Assist patient to use the toilet, commode, or bedpan at frequent intervals.
- Provide personal hygiene, skin care, oral care.
- Help patients with eating.
- Assist patients with daily activities.
- Use bed alarms and surveillance to decrease risk for falls.

(5) consulting with the HCP regarding drug therapy. Management of sundowning can be challenging for you, the patient, and the family.

***Safety.*** The person with AD is at risk for problems related to personal safety. Potential hazards include falling, ingesting dangerous substances, wandering, injuring others and self with sharp objects, being burned, and being unable to respond to crisis situations. These concerns require careful attention to the home environment to minimize risk. Supervision is also required. As the patient's cognitive function declines over time, the patient may have difficulty navigating physical spaces and interpreting environmental cues. Assist the caregiver in assessing the home environment for safety risks.

**SAFETY ALERT Preventing Falls**

Teach the caregiver to take the following steps:

- Have stairwells well lit.
- Make sure the patient can grasp the handrails.
- Tack down carpet edges.
- Remove throw rugs and extension cords.
- Use nonskid mats in tub or shower.
- Install handrails in the bath and by the commode.

Wandering is a major concern for caregivers. Wandering may be related to loss of memory or to side effects of drugs, or it may be an expression of a physical or emotional need, restlessness, curiosity, or stimuli that trigger memories of earlier routines. As with other behaviors, observe for factors or events that may precipitate wandering. For example, the patient may be sensitive to stress and tension in the environment. In such cases, wandering may reflect an attempt to leave.

When someone with AD is discovered missing, every second counts. To assist caregivers with locating them, the Alzheimer's Association and the MedicAlert Foundation have created an alliance called MedicAlert + Alzheimer's Association Safe Return.[18] This program includes identification products (e.g., bracelet, necklace, wallet cards), a national photo and information database, a 24-hour toll-free emergency crisis line, local chapter support, and wandering behavior education and training for caregivers and families.

Tracking devices such as a global positioning system (GPS) can also be used to detect and find people who wander. These devices can be placed in shoes, sewn into pockets, worn as a bracelet or pendant, or clipped to a belt.

***Pain Management.*** Because of difficulties with oral and written language, AD patients may have difficulty expressing physical complaints, including pain. You need to rely on other clues such as the patient's behavior. Pain can result in alterations in the patient's behavior, such as increased vocalization, agitation, withdrawal, and changes in function. Pain should be recognized and treated promptly and the patient's response monitored.

***Eating and Swallowing Difficulties.*** Undernutrition is a problem in the moderate and severe stages of AD. Loss of interest in food and decreased ability to self-feed *(feeding apraxia)*, as well as co-morbid conditions, can result in significant nutritional deficiencies in the patient with AD. In long-term care facilities, inadequate assistance with feeding may add to the problem.

Use pureed foods, thickened liquids, and nutritional supplements when chewing and swallowing become problematic for the patient. Patients may need reminders to chew their food and to swallow. Patients need a quiet and unhurried environment for eating. Avoid distractions at mealtimes, including the television. Low lighting, music, and simulated nature sounds may improve eating behaviors. Easy-grip eating utensils and finger foods may allow the patient to self-feed. Offer liquids frequently.

When oral feeding is not possible, explore alternative routes. Nasogastric (NG) feeding may be used for short periods. However, for the long term the NG tube is uncomfortable and may add to the patient's agitation. A percutaneous endoscopic gastrostomy (PEG) tube provides another option (see Fig. 39-7). However, PEG tubes can be problematic, since patients with AD are particularly vulnerable to aspiration of feeding formula and tube dislodgment. The potential positive outcomes to be gained from nutritional therapies are considered in light of overall outcome goals and potential adverse effects of the specific therapy. Nutritional support therapies are described in Chapter 39.

***Oral Care.*** In the late stages of AD, the patient is unable to perform oral self-care. With decreased tooth brushing and flossing, dental problems are likely to occur. Because of swallowing difficulties, patients may retain food in the mouth, adding to the potential for tooth decay. Dental caries and tooth abscess can add to patient discomfort or pain and subsequently may increase agitation. Inspect the mouth regularly and provide mouth care to those patients unable to do self-care.

◆ ***Infection Prevention.*** Urinary tract infection and pneumonia are the most common infections in patients with AD. Such infections are ultimately the cause of death in many patients with AD. Because of feeding and swallowing problems, the patient is at risk for aspiration pneumonia. Immobility can also predispose the patient to pneumonia.

Reduced fluid intake, prostate enlargement in men, poor hygiene, and urinary drainage devices (e.g., catheters) can predispose patients to bladder infection. Any manifestations of infection, such as a change in behavior, fever, cough (pneumonia), or pain on urination (bladder), need prompt evaluation and treatment.

◆ ***Skin Care.*** It is important to monitor the patient's skin over time. Note and treat rashes, areas of redness, and skin breakdown. In the late stages, incontinence along with immobility and undernutrition can place the patient at risk for skin breakdown. Keep the skin dry and clean, and change the patient's position regularly to avoid areas of pressure over bony prominences.

◆ ***Elimination Problems.*** During the moderate and severe stages of AD, urinary and fecal incontinence lead to increased need for nursing care. When possible, behavioral retraining of bladder and bowel function (e.g., scheduled toileting) may help decrease episodes of incontinence.

Another common elimination problem is constipation. Causes may relate to immobility, dietary intake (e.g., reduced fiber intake), and decreased fluid intake. Increased dietary fiber, fiber supplements, and stool softeners are the first lines of management. The combination of aging, other health problems, and swallowing difficulties may increase the risk of complications associated with the use of mineral oil, stimulants, osmotic agents, and enemas. Management of constipation is discussed in Chapter 42.

◆ ***Caregiver Support.*** More than 15 million Americans provide unpaid care for people with AD or other dementias.[1] The majority of these are family members providing care in the home (Fig. 59-9). AD is a disease that disrupts all aspects of personal and family life. Caregivers for people with AD describe it as very stressful (see Table 4-5). These caregivers also exhibit adverse consequences relating to their own emotional and physical health.

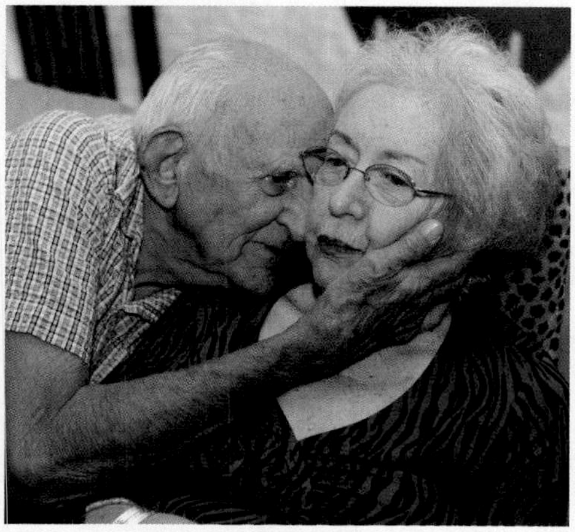

**FIG. 59-9** Caregivers of patients with dementia face an incredible challenge that often causes deterioration in their own physical and emotional health. (©iStock/Thinkstock)

The chronic and often severe stress associated with dementia caregiving increases the risk for the development of dementia in spouse caregivers.[19] One mechanism proposed is that the detrimental effects of the chronic stress of caregiving can affect the hippocampus, a region of the brain responsible for memory.

As the disease progresses, the relationship of the caregiver to the patient changes. Family roles may be altered or reversed (e.g., son caring for father). Decisions must be made, including when to tell the patient about the diagnosis, when to have the patient stop driving or doing activities that may be dangerous, when to ask for assistance, and when to place the patient in adult day care or a long-term care facility. With early-onset AD, the patient is affected during his or her most productive years in terms of career and family. The consequences can be devastating for the patient and family.

Sexual relations for couples are also seriously affected by AD. As the disease progresses, sexual interest may decline for both the patient and partner. A number of reasons account for this, including fatigue, memory impairment, and episodes of incontinence. The patient may also become sexually driven as the disease progresses and the patient becomes more uninhibited.

Work with the caregiver to assess stressors (see Table 4-4) and to identify coping strategies to reduce the burden of caregiving. For example, ask which behaviors are most disruptive to family life at a given time, while remembering that this is likely to change as the disease progresses. Determining what the caregiver views as most disruptive or distressful can help to establish priorities for care.

Safety of the patient is a high priority. It is also important to assess what the caregiver's expectations are regarding the patient's behavior. Are the expectations reasonable given the progression of the disease? A family and caregiver teaching guide based on the disease stages is provided in Table 59-14. Other tips for caregivers are listed in Table 59-15. A nursing care plan for the family caregiver (eNursing Care Plan 59-2) is available on the website for this chapter.

Support groups for caregivers and family members (Fig. 59-10) can provide an atmosphere of understanding and give current information about the disease itself and related topics such as safety, legal, ethical, and financial issues. The needs of family caregivers are discussed in Chapter 4 on pp. 49-50. Strategies related to stress management are discussed in Chapter 6.

The Alzheimer's Association has many educational and support systems available to help family caregivers (*www.alz.org*).

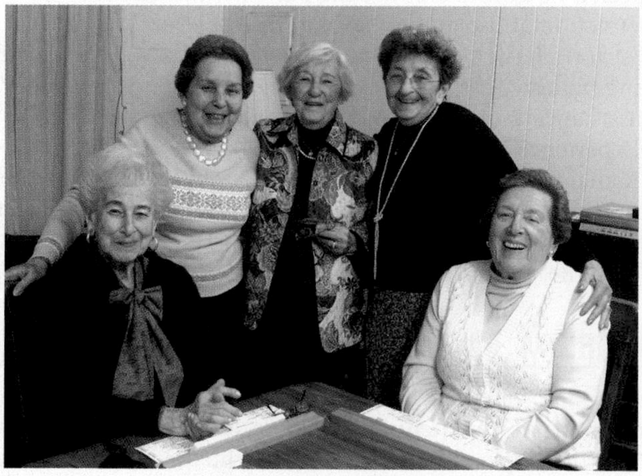

**FIG. 59-10** Support groups are an effective way to help caregivers cope. (©iStockphoto/Thinkstock)

### TABLE 59-14 Family & Caregiver Teaching

#### *Alzheimer's Disease*

*Include the following instructions when teaching families and caregivers the management of the patient with Alzheimer's disease.*

**Mild Stage**

- Many treatable (and potentially reversible) conditions can mimic dementia (Table 59-2). Try to get a definitive diagnosis.
- Get the person to stop driving. Confusion and poor judgment can impair driving skills and potentially put others at risk.
- Encourage activities such as visiting with friends and family, listening to music, participating in hobbies, and exercising.
- Provide cues in the home, establish a routine, and determine a specific location where essential items (e.g., glasses) must be kept.
- Do not correct misstatements or faulty memory.
- Register with MedicAlert + Alzheimer's Association Safe Return, a program established by the MedicAlert Foundation and the Alzheimer's Association to locate individuals who wander from their homes.
- Make plans for the future in terms of advance directives, care options, financial concerns, and personal preference for care.

**Moderate Stage**

- Install door locks for patient safety.
- Provide protective wear for urinary and fecal incontinence.
- Ensure that the home has good lighting, install handrails in stairways and bathroom, and remove area rugs.
- Label drawers and faucets (hot and cold) to ensure safety.
- Develop strategies such as distraction and diversion to cope with behavioral problems. Identify and reduce potential triggers (e.g., reduce stress, extremes in temperature) for disruptive behavior.
- Provide memory triggers, such as pictures of family and friends.

**Severe Stage**

- Provide a regular schedule for toileting to reduce incontinence.
- Provide care to meet needs, including oral care and skin care.
- Monitor diet and fluid intake to ensure their adequacy.
- Continue communication through talking and touching.
- Consider placement in a long-term care facility when providing total care becomes too difficult.

A booklet for caregivers, *Caring for a Person With Alzheimer's Disease,* is available at *www.nia.nih.gov/sites/default/files/caring_for_a_person_with_alzheimers_disease_0.pdf.*

## ◆ Evaluation

Expected outcomes are that the patient with AD will

- Function at the highest level of cognitive ability
- Perform basic personal care activities of daily living, including bathing, dressing, feeding, and toileting by self or with assistance as needed
- Experience no injury
- Remain in a restricted area during ambulation and activity

Additional information on the expected outcomes for the patient with AD is addressed in eNursing Care Plan 59-1 (available on the website for this chapter).

# DELIRIUM

**Delirium**, a state of temporary but acute mental confusion, is a common, life-threatening syndrome. Delirium affects as many as 50% of people older than 65 years who are hospitalized, and as many as 80% of patients in an ICU.[20,21] In many cases, delirium is preventable and/or reversible.

### TABLE 59-15 Guidelines for Dealing With Dementia Patients

**Do**

- Treat them like adults, with respect and dignity, even when their behavior is childlike.
- Use gentle touch and direct eye contact.
- Remain patient, flexible, calm, and understanding.
- Anticipate challenging behaviors, since the patient's ability to think logically has been affected.
- Give directions using gestures or pictures.
- Simplify tasks. Focus on one thing at a time.
- Avoid questions or topics that require extensive thought, memory, or words.
- Be flexible. If one approach does not work, try another.
- Use distraction, changing the subject, redirecting to another activity.
- Provide reassurance. Praise sincerely for success.

**Do Not**

- Criticize, correct, or argue.
- Rush or hurry the patient.
- Force participation in activities or events.
- Talk about the patient as if he or she is not there.
- Blame the person with AD. Instead, blame the disease.
- Take challenging behaviors personally. These behaviors are due to the patient's disease.
- Use condescending terms, such as "honey" or "sweetie."
- Use threatening gestures.
- Overreact to the person with AD.
- Try to explain "why" or rationalize.

### BECOMING A NURSE LEADER

#### *Elder Abuse*

**Situation**

While attending nursing school, you are working as a patient care technician in a long-term care facility. You are in charge of feeding five patients their dinner, including Mrs. Talbot, who is confused and has difficulty swallowing. You are approached by Joan, the LPN, who berates you for feeding Mrs. Talbot so slowly. Joan takes the spoon from your hand and feeds Mrs. Talbot a huge mouthful of food, which causes her to choke and cough. Joan then gives her a push and says, "Calm down." You are stunned and resume feeding Mrs. Talbot smaller bites. Joan then returns and says to you, "You will never get done at the rate you are going!"

**Points for Consideration**

- Elder abuse occurs in community settings, such as private homes as well as long-term care facilities.
- Types of abuse can include physical, sexual, emotional, neglect, self-neglect, and financial/exploitation.
- Elder mistreatment is often unrecognized, hidden, and underreported.
- People with dementia are at great risk of abuse.
- Health care professionals, including nurses, are frequently unaware of the various forms of elder abuse that take place and the proper course of action to pursue when mistreatment is suspected.

**Discussion Questions**

1. What responsibility do you have to Mrs. Talbot?
2. What should you say to Joan?
3. What role can you have to prevent this abuse from occurring again?

**Reference**

National Center on Elder Abuse. Administration on Aging: Retrieved from *www.ncea.aoa.gov.*

### Etiology and Pathophysiology

The pathophysiologic mechanism of delirium is poorly understood. A main contributing factor is impairment of cerebral oxidative metabolism (brain gets less oxygen and has problems using it). Multiple neurotransmitter abnormalities may also be involved. Cholinergic deficiency, excess release of dopamine, and both increased and decreased serotonergic activity may contribute to delirium. Proinflammatory cytokines, including interleukin-1, interleukin-2, interleukin-6, tumor necrosis factor–α (TNF-α), and interferon, appear to play a role.

Dementia is the leading risk factor for delirium. Furthermore, delirium is a risk factor for the subsequent development of dementia. Delirium may cause permanent neuronal damage and lead to dementia.[22]

Clinically, delirium is rarely caused by a single factor. Stress, surgery, and sleep deprivation have been linked to the onset of delirium. Pain and depression also contribute to delirium, especially in postoperative older patients.[21]

Delirium is often the result of the interaction of the patient's underlying condition with a precipitating event. Delirium can occur after a relatively minor insult in a vulnerable patient. For example, a patient with underlying health problems such as heart failure, cancer, cognitive impairment, or sensory limitations may develop delirium in response to a relatively minor change (e.g., use of a sleeping medication). In other less vulnerable patients, it may take a combination of factors (e.g., anesthesia, major surgery, mechanical ventilation, infection, prolonged sleep deprivation) to precipitate delirium. Delirium can also be a symptom of a serious medical illness such as bacterial meningitis.

Understanding factors that can lead to delirium can help in determining effective interventions. Several factors that can precipitate or cause delirium are listed in Tables 59-16 and 59-17. Many of these factors are more common in older patients. In addition, older patients have limited compensatory mechanisms to deal with physiologic insults such as hypoxia, hypoglycemia, and dehydration. Older adults are more susceptible to drug-induced delirium, in part because of their increased use of multiple drugs. Many medications, including sedative-hypnotics, opioids (especially meperidine [Demerol]), benzodiazepines, and drugs with anticholinergic properties, can cause or contribute to delirium, especially in older or vulnerable patients.[23]

### Clinical Manifestations

Patients with delirium can have a variety of manifestations ranging from hypoactivity and lethargy to hyperactivity, agitation, and hallucinations. Patients can also have mixed delirium, manifesting both hypoactive and hyperactive symptoms. Delirium can develop over the course of hours to days. In most patients, delirium usually develops over a 2- to 3-day period. The early manifestations often include inability to concentrate, disorganized thinking, irritability, insomnia, loss of appetite, restlessness, and confusion. Later manifestations may include agitation, misperception, misinterpretation, and hallucinations.

Delirium can last from 1 to 7 days. However, some delirium manifestations may persist up for months or years. Some patients do not completely recover.

Manifestations of delirium are sometimes confused with those of dementia. A key distinction between delirium and dementia is that the person who exhibits sudden cognitive impairment, disorientation, or clouded sensorium is more likely to have delirium rather than dementia. (A comparison of delirium and dementia is presented in Table 59-1.)

**TABLE 59-16 Factors That Precipitate Delirium**

**Demographic Characteristics**
- Age 65 yr or older
- Male gender

**Cognitive Status**
- Cognitive impairment
- Dementia
- Depression
- History of delirium

**Environmental**
- Admission to ICU
- Emotional stress
- Pain (especially untreated)
- Sleep deprivation
- Use of physical restraints

**Functional Status**
- Functional dependence
- History of falls
- Immobility

**Sensory**
- Sensory deprivation
- Sensory overload
- Visual or hearing impairment

**Decreased Oral Intake**
- Dehydration
- Malnutrition

**Drugs**
- Alcohol or drug abuse or withdrawal
- Aminoglycosides
- Anticholinergics
- Opioids
- Sedative-hypnotics
- Treatment with multiple drugs

**Coexisting Medical Conditions**
- Acute infection, sepsis, fever
- Chronic kidney or liver disease
- Electrolyte imbalances
- Fracture or trauma
- History of stroke
- Neurologic disease
- Severe acute illness
- Terminal illness

**Surgery**
- Cardiac surgery
- Noncardiac surgery
- Orthopedic surgery
- Prolonged cardiopulmonary bypass

**TABLE 59-17 Mnemonic for Causes of Delirium**

**D**ementia, dehydration
**E**lectrolyte imbalances, emotional stress
**L**ung, liver, heart, kidney, brain
**I**nfection, intensive care unit
**R**x drugs
**I**njury, immobility
**U**ntreated pain, unfamiliar environment
**M**etabolic disorders

### Diagnostic Studies

Diagnosing delirium is complicated because many critically ill patients cannot communicate their needs. A careful medical and psychologic history and physical examination are the first steps in diagnosing delirium. This includes careful attention to medications, both prescription and over-the-counter drugs. The Confusion Assessment Method (CAM) has been extensively studied and is a reliable tool for assessing delirium (Table 59-18). It is important to distinguish whether the delirium is part of an underlying problem of dementia.

Once delirium has been diagnosed, explore potential causes. Carefully review the patient's health history and medication record. Laboratory tests include complete blood count, serum electrolytes, blood urea nitrogen, and creatinine levels; ECG; urinalysis; liver and thyroid function tests; and oxygen saturation level. Drug and alcohol levels may be obtained. If unexplained fever or nuchal rigidity is present and meningitis or encephalitis is suspected, a lumbar puncture may be performed. CSF is examined for glucose, protein, and bacteria. If the

**TABLE 59-18 Confusion Assessment Method (CAM)**

*Delirium is diagnosed with the presence of features 1 and 2, and either 3 or 4.*

**Feature 1**
**Acute Onset and Fluctuating Course**
Data usually obtained from a family member or nurse.
Shown by positive responses to following questions:
- Is there evidence of an acute change in mental status from the patient's baseline?
- Did the (abnormal) behavior fluctuate during the day (i.e., tend to come and go, or increase and decrease in severity)?

**Feature 2**
**Inattention**
Shown by positive response to following question:
- Did the patient have difficulty focusing attention (e.g., being easily distractible, or having difficulty keeping track of what was being said)?

**Feature 3**
**Disorganized Thinking**
Shown by a positive response to following question:
- Was the patient's thinking disorganized or incoherent, such as rambling or irrelevant conversation, unclear or illogical flow of ideas, or unpredictable switching from subject to subject?

**Feature 4**
**Altered Level of Consciousness**
Shown by any answer other than "alert" to the following question:
- Overall, how would you rate this patient's level of consciousness (alert [normal], vigilant [hyperalert], lethargic [drowsy, easily aroused], stupor [difficult to arouse], or coma [unarousable])?

Adapted from Inouye S, van Dyck C, Alessi C, et al: Clarifying confusion: the Confusion Assessment Method, *Ann Intern Med* 113(12):941, 1990.

patient's history includes head injury, appropriate x-rays or scans may be ordered. In general, brain imaging studies such as CT and MRI are used only in situations in which head injury is known or suspected.

## NURSING AND INTERPROFESSIONAL MANAGEMENT: DELIRIUM

Treatment is important as many cases of delirium are potentially reversible. In caring for the patient with delirium, your roles include prevention, early recognition, and treatment. Prevention of delirium involves recognition of high-risk patients.[24] Patient groups at risk include those with neurologic disorders (e.g., dementia, stroke, CNS infection, Parkinson's disease), sensory impairment, and older age. Other risk factors, including surgery, hospitalization in an ICU, and untreated pain, are listed in Table 59-16.

Care of the patient with delirium focuses on eliminating precipitating factors. If it is drug induced, medications are discontinued. Keep in mind that delirium can also accompany drug and alcohol withdrawal. Depending on patient history, drug screening may be performed. Fluid and electrolyte imbalances and nutritional deficiencies (e.g., thiamine) are corrected if appropriate. If the problem is related to environmental conditions (e.g., an overstimulating or understimulating environment), changes should be made. If delirium is secondary to infection, appropriate antibiotic therapy is started. Similarly, if delirium is secondary to chronic illness such as chronic kidney disease or heart failure, treatment focuses on these conditions.

Care of the patient experiencing delirium includes protecting the patient from harm. Give priority to creating a calm and safe environment. This may include encouraging family members to stay at the bedside, providing familiar objects and family photos, transferring the patient to a private room or one closer to the nurses' station, and planning for consistent nursing staff if possible. Use reorientation and behavioral interventions in patients with delirium. Provide the patient with reassurance and reorienting information as to place, time, and procedures. Clocks, calendars, and lists of the patient's scheduled activities are also useful in reducing confusion. Reduce environmental stimuli, including noise and light levels.[25]

Personal contact through touch and verbal communication can be an important reorienting strategy. If the patient uses eyeglasses or a hearing aid, they should be readily available because sensory deprivation can precipitate delirium. Avoid the

### ETHICAL/LEGAL DILEMMAS
***Board of Nursing Disciplinary Action***

**Situation**

The State Board of Nursing has received multiple complaints about J.R., a registered nurse (RN) who works in a long-term care facility. J.R. has signed off on three controlled substances count sheets that have been determined to be inaccurate. During an investigation it was discovered that several members of the nursing staff knew about J.R.'s reported behavior, but they did not report their observations to the unit administrator. After the investigation, the board of nursing subpoenas J.R. to a meeting to discuss charges in preparation for a disciplinary hearing.

**Ethical/Legal Points for Consideration**

- Regulation of professional nursing practice is the right of each of the 50 states, most of which have separate regulatory agencies charged with writing regulations and rules to implement the State Nurse Practice Act. The regulations approved by these agencies carry the weight of law. Failure to behave accordingly places a nurse at risk for disciplinary action.
- The RN who is charged with unprofessional behavior has been charged with an offense and is entitled to the same legal rights as any other individual, including a fair and timely hearing, opportunity to confront the accusers, right to be represented by an attorney, and right to prepare a defense.
- Possible disciplinary actions include temporary suspension of the nursing license, revocation of the nursing license, mandatory rehabilitation for substance abuse, and mandated supervision and evaluation of practice. Sometimes the disciplinary action includes fines and requires reeducation. In addition, the State Board of Nursing may report the action to the state attorney general if evidence suggests that a crime has been committed. The RN who has been found guilty of unprofessional practice must report this action on all future applications for nursing positions.
- All RNs should be familiar with their state's nurse practice act and regulations, as well as the composition and actions of the State Board of Nursing. Nurses should pay particular attention to the regulation that lists examples of actionable behavior and disciplinary actions sanctioned by the state.
- RNs have a legal and ethical obligation to report suspected illegal behavior to their administrators and to continue reporting until the situation is resolved. By failing to report, the RN may be charged as an accessory to the act or aiding and abetting the behavior. This RN may be charged with unprofessional behavior and risks losing his or her nursing license. Shifting the obligation to someone else to report or failure to continue reporting each incident does not satisfy this duty.

**Discussion Questions**

1. How would you handle a situation where retaliation for reporting unprofessional behavior is likely?
2. What would you do if the nurse suspected of illegal behavior is related to someone in the administrative hierarchy?

## CHECK YOUR PRACTICE

You are working in the medical ICU. Your patient is an 82-yr-old man who had a hip replacement 4 days ago. He was doing well after surgery and then developed bilateral pneumonia. He was transferred to the ICU yesterday. When you walk into his room, you notice his daughter is staring out the window and does not respond to your greeting. When you approach her, you notice she is very upset. When you ask her what is wrong, she bursts out crying, "How can this be? My dad was always such a vibrant and brilliant man. Now look at him. He talks to himself. He screams at me. He thinks I am his wife. My mother died 5 years ago. What happened to him?"

- How would you assess the situation?
- What can you do to help the daughter?

use of restraints. Other interventions, including relaxation techniques, music therapy, and massage, may also be appropriate for some patients with delirium.

Comprehensive, multicomponent interventions to prevent delirium are the most effective and should be implemented by the interprofessional care team.[26] This team may also address issues related to polypharmacy, pain, nutritional status, and potential for incontinence. The patient experiencing delirium is also at risk for the adverse consequences of immobility, including skin breakdown. Give attention to increasing physical activity or providing range-of-motion exercises, when appropriate, and maintaining skin integrity.

Also focus on supporting the family and caregivers during episodes of delirium. Family members need to understand factors that may have precipitated the delirium, as well as the potential outcomes. Patient education materials are available at *www.ICUdelirium.org.*

### Drug Therapy

Drug therapy is reserved for patients with severe agitation, especially when it interferes with needed medical therapy (e.g., fluid replacement, intubation, dialysis). Agitation can put the patient at risk for falls and injury. Drug therapy is used cautiously because many of the drugs used to manage agitation have psychoactive properties. Drugs should be used only when nonpharmacologic interventions have failed.

Dexmedetomidine (Precedex), an α-adrenergic receptor agonist, has been used in ICU settings for sedation. In addition, low-dose antipsychotics (neuroleptics) may be used, such as haloperidol (Haldol), risperidone (Risperdal), olanzapine (Zyprexa), and quetiapine (Seroquel). Haloperidol can be administered IV, IM, or orally and will produce sedation. In addition to sedation, other side effects of antipsychotics include hypotension; extrapyramidal side effects, including *tardive dyskinesia* (involuntary muscle movements of face, trunk, and arms) and *athetosis* (involuntary writhing movements of the limbs); muscle tone changes; and anticholinergic effects. Carefully monitor older patients receiving antipsychotic agents.

Short-acting benzodiazepines (e.g., lorazepam [Ativan]) can be used to treat delirium associated with sedative and alcohol withdrawal or in conjunction with antipsychotics to reduce extrapyramidal side effects. However, these drugs may worsen delirium caused by other factors and must be used cautiously.

## CASE STUDY

### *Alzheimer's Disease*

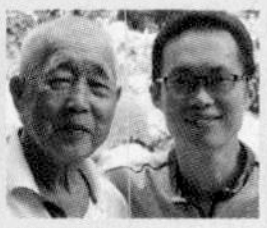

(©iStock/Thinkstock)

**Patient Profile**

M.Y., a 78-yr-old Asian American man, was diagnosed with Alzheimer's disease (AD) 3 yr ago shortly after his wife died. Today his 45-yr-old son brings him to the emergency department because he wandered from his son's home, fell, and injured his left hip.

**Subjective Data**

- Can state his name, confused as to place and time
- Denies memory of wandering or falling
- Agitated, trying to get up
- Denies pain

**Objective Data**

***Physical Examination***

- Left leg shorter than right leg
- Tense and anxious

***Diagnostic Studies***

- X-ray of left hip indicates a fracture
- Mini-Cog testing indicates cognitive impairment

**Discussion Questions**

1. What is the pathogenesis of AD?
2. What precipitating factors may have resulted in M.Y.'s fall?
3. ***Safety:*** What safety precautions need to be taken regarding the inpatient care of M.Y.?
4. ***Patient-Centered Care:*** What is the priority nursing intervention for M.Y.?
5. ***Patient-Centered Care:*** What teaching plan should you develop for M.Y. and his son?
6. Surgery is planned to repair his fractured hip. Why is he at risk for delirium?
7. ***Priority Decision:*** Based on the assessment data, what are the priority nursing diagnoses? Are there any collaborative problems?
8. ***Teamwork and Collaboration:*** What nursing activities can the RN delegate to unlicensed assistive personnel (UAP)?
9. ***Evidence-Based Practice:*** M.Y.'s son asks you if he should give his father ginkgo to help his memory. How would you respond?

Answers available at *http://evolve.elsevier.com/Lewis/medsurg.*

## BRIDGE TO NCLEX EXAMINATION

The number of the question corresponds to the same-numbered outcome at the beginning of the chapter.

1. Dementia is defined as a
   - **a.** syndrome that results only in memory loss.
   - **b.** disease associated with abrupt changes in behavior.
   - **c.** disease that is always due to reduced blood flow to the brain.
   - **d.** syndrome characterized by cognitive dysfunction and loss of memory.
2. Vascular dementia is associated with
   - **a.** transient ischemic attacks.
   - **b.** bacterial or viral infection of neuronal tissue.
   - **c.** cognitive changes secondary to cerebral ischemia.
   - **d.** abrupt changes in cognitive function that are irreversible.

3. The clinical diagnosis of dementia is based on
   a. CT or MRS.
   b. brain biopsy.
   c. electroencephalogram.
   d. patient history and cognitive assessment.
4. Dementia with Lewy bodies (DLB) is characterized by
   a. remissions and exacerbations over many years.
   b. memory impairment, muscle jerks, and blindness.
   c. parkinsonian symptoms, including muscle rigidity.
   d. increased intracranial pressure secondary to decreased CSF drainage.
5. Which statement(s) accurately describe(s) mild cognitive impairment *(select all that apply)*?
   a. Always progresses to AD
   b. Caused by variety of factors and may progress to AD
   c. Should be aggressively treated with acetylcholinesterase drugs
   d. Caused by vascular infarcts that, if treated, will delay progression to AD
   e. Patient is usually not aware that there is a problem with his or her memory
6. The early stage of AD is characterized by
   a. no noticeable change in behavior.
   b. memory problems and mild confusion.
   c. increased time spent sleeping or in bed.
   d. incontinence, agitation, and wandering behavior.
7. A *priority* goal of treatment for the patient with AD is to
   a. maintain patient safety.
   b. maintain or increase body weight.
   c. return to a higher level of self-care.
   d. enhance functional ability over time.
8. Which patient is *most* at risk for developing delirium?
   a. A 50-yr-old woman with cholecystitis
   b. A 19-yr-old man with a fractured femur
   c. A 42-yr-old woman having an elective hysterectomy
   d. A 78-yr-old man admitted to the medical unit with complications related to heart failure

1. d, 2. c, 3. d, 4. c, 5. b, 6. b, 7. a, 8. d

For rationales to these answers and even more NCLEX review questions, visit *http://evolve.elsevier.com/Lewis/medsurg.*

## EVOLVE WEBSITE

http://evolve.elsevier.com/Lewis/medsurg

**Review Questions (Online Only)**

**Key Points**

**Answer Keys for Questions**
- Rationales for Bridge to NCLEX Examination Questions
- Answer Guidelines for Case Study on p. 1417

**Student Case Study**
- Patient With Alzheimer's Disease

**eNursing Care Plans**
- eNursing Care Plan 59-1: Patient With Alzheimer's Disease
- eNursing Care Plan 59-2: Family Caregivers

**Conceptual Care Map Creator**

**Audio Glossary**

**Content Updates**

## REFERENCES


1. Alzheimer's Association: 2016 Alzheimer's Association facts and figures report. Retrieved from *www.alz.org/documents_custom/2016-facts-and-figures.pdf.*
2. Alzheimer's Disease Education and Referral Center: Alzheimer's disease genetics: facts sheet. Retrieved from *www.nia.nih.gov/alzheimers/publication/alzheimers-disease-genetics-fact-sheet.*
*3. Chiu WC, Ho WC, Liao DL, et al: Progress of diabetic severity and risk of dementia, *J Clin Endocrinol Metab* 100(8):2899, 2015.
*4. Bryan RN, Bilello M, Davatzikos C, et al. Effect of diabetes on brain structure: the action to control cardiovascular risk in diabetes MRI imaging baseline data, *Radiology* 272(1):210, 2014.
5. List J, Ott S, Bukowski M, et al: Cognitive function and brain structure after recurrent mild traumatic brain injuries in young-to-middle-aged adults, *Front Hum Neurosci* 9:228, 2015.
6. Barnes DE, Kaup A, Kirby KA, et al: Traumatic brain injury and risk of dementia in older veterans, *Neurology* 83(4):312, 2014.
*7. Reisberg B, Franssen EH, Souren LE, et al: Evidence and mechanisms of retrogenesis in Alzheimer's and other dementias: management and treatment import, *Am J Alzheimers Dis Other Demen* 17(4):202, 2002. (Classic)
*8. Jack CR, Albert MS, Knopman DS, et al: Introduction to the recommendations from the National Institute on Aging—Alzheimer's Association workgroups on diagnostic guidelines for Alzheimer's disease, *Alzheimers Dement* 7:257, 2011.
*9. McKhann GM, Knopman DS, Chertkow H, et al: The diagnosis of dementia due to Alzheimer's disease: recommendations from the National Institute on Aging and the Alzheimer's Association workgroup, *Alzheimers Dement* 7:263, 2011.
*10. Breitner JCS: Mild cognitive impairment and progression to dementia: new findings, *Neurology* 82:e34, 2014.
*11. Russ TC, Morling JR: Cholinesterase inhibitors for mild cognitive impairment, *Cochrane Database Syst Rev* 9:CD009132, 2012.
*12. Tsoi KK, Chan JY, Hirai HW, et al. Cognitive tests to detect dementia: a systematic review and meta-analysis, *JAMA Intern Med* 175(9):1450, 2015.
*13. Tan L, Tan L, Wang HF, et al: Efficacy and safety of atypical antipsychotic drug treatment for dementia: a systematic review and meta-analysis, *Alzheimers Res Ther* 7(1):20, 2015.
14. Baumgart M, Snyder HM, Carrillo MC, et al: Summary of evidence on modifiable risk factors for cognitive decline and dementia: a population-based perspective, *Alzheimers Dement* 11:718, 2015.
15. Volland J, Fisher A: Best practices for engaging patients with dementia, *Nursing* 44(11):44, 2014.
16. Brandon IL: Easing the burden on family caregivers, *Nursing* 43(8):36, 2013.
17. Beach PR, White BE: Applying the evidence to help caregivers torn in two, *Nursing* 45(6):30, 2015.
18. Alzheimer's Association: MedicAlert + Alzheimer's Association Safe Return. Retrieved from *www.alz.org/care/dementia-medic-alert-safe-return.asp.*
*19. Pertl MM, Lawlor BA, Robertson IH, et al: Risk of cognitive and functional impairment in spouses of people with dementia: evidence from the health and retirement study, *J Geriatr Psychiatry Neurol* 28(4):260, 2015.
20. Inouye SK, Westendorp RG, Saczynski JS: Delirium in elderly people, *Lancet* 83(9920):911, 2014.
21. Kosar CM, Tabloski PA, Travison TG, et al: Effect of preoperative pain and depressive symptoms on the development of postoperative delirium, *Lancet Psychiatry* 1(6):431, 2014.
22. Fong TG, Davis D, Growdon ME, et al: The interface between delirium and dementia in elderly adults, *Lancet Neurol* 14(8):823, 2015.
*23. American Geriatrics Society Expert Panel on Postoperative Delirium in Older Adults: Postoperative delirium in older adults: best practice statement from the American Geriatrics Society, *J Am Coll Surg* 220(2):136, 2015.
24. Delirium Prevention and Safety: Starting with the ABCDEF's. Retrieved from *www.icudelirium.org/medicalprofessionals.html.*
25. ICU Delirium and Cognitive Impairment Study Group: Delirium in the ICU. Retrieved from *www.icudelirium.org/docs/delirium_education_brochure.pdf*
*26. Hshieh TT, Yue J, Oh E, et al: Effectiveness of multicomponent nonpharmacological delirium interventions: a meta-analysis, *JAMA Intern Med* 175(4):512, 2015.

*Evidence-based information for clinical practice.

60

# Spinal Cord and Peripheral Nerve Problems

*Cindy M. Sullivan*

*I think a hero is an ordinary individual who finds strength to persevere and endure in spite of overwhelming obstacles.*

**Christopher Reeve**

http://evolve.elsevier.com/Lewis/medsurg/

## LEARNING OUTCOMES

1. Describe the classification of spinal cord injuries and associated clinical manifestations.
2. Describe the clinical manifestations, interprofessional care, and nursing management of neurogenic and spinal shock.
3. Relate the clinical manifestations of spinal cord injury to the level of disruption and rehabilitation potential.
4. Describe the nursing management of the major physical and psychologic problems of the patient with a spinal cord injury.
5. Describe the effects of spinal cord injury on the older adult.
6. Explain the types, clinical manifestations, interprofessional care, and nursing management of spinal cord tumors.
7. Explain the etiology, clinical manifestations, interprofessional care, and nursing management of trigeminal neuralgia and Bell's palsy.
8. Explain the etiology, clinical manifestations, interprofessional care, and nursing management of Guillain-Barré syndrome/acute inflammatory demyelinating polyneuropathy.
9. Explain the etiology, clinical manifestations, interprofessional care, and nursing management of chronic inflammatory demyelinating polyneuropathy.

## KEY TERMS

**acute inflammatory demyelinating polyneuropathy (AIDP), p. 1440**
**anterior cord syndrome, Table 60-1, p. 1422**
**autonomic hyperreflexia, p. 1431**
**Bell's palsy, p. 1439**
**botulism, p. 1442**
**Brown-Séquard syndrome, Table 60-1, p. 1422**
**cauda equina syndrome, Table 60-1, p. 1422**
**central cord syndrome, Table 60-1, p. 1422**
**chronic inflammatory demyelinating polyneuropathy (CIDP), p. 1441**
**conus medullaris syndrome, Table 60-1, p. 1422**
**Guillain-Barré syndrome (GBS), p. 1440**
**neurogenic bladder, p. 1423**
**neurogenic bowel, p. 1423**
**neurogenic shock, p. 1420**
**paraplegia, p. 1420**
**spinal cord injury (SCI), p. 1419**
**spinal shock, p. 1420**
**tetanus, p. 1442**
**tetraplegia, p. 1420**
**trigeminal neuralgia (TN), p. 1437**

This chapter discusses spinal cord and peripheral nerve problems, including spinal cord injuries, spinal cord tumors, cranial nerve disorders, and polyneuropathies. A focus of this chapter is the nursing management of the many problems encountered by the patient with a spinal cord injury.

## SPINAL CORD PROBLEMS

### SPINAL CORD INJURY

**Spinal cord injury (SCI)** is caused by trauma or damage to the spinal cord. It can result in temporary or permanent alteration in the function of the spinal cord. About 12,500 Americans experience SCI each year. Approximately 276,000 people in the United States are living with SCI. Young adult men ages 16 to 30 years have the greatest risk for SCI. With improved treatment strategies, even the very young patient with SCI can anticipate a long life.[1]

The number of older adults with SCI has increased. This increase is related to people with SCI living longer and older age at the time of injury.[1]

The potential for disruption of individual growth and development, altered family dynamics, economic loss in terms of employment, and the high cost of rehabilitation and long-term health care make SCI a major problem. Although many people with SCI can care for themselves independently, those with the highest level of injury may require around-the-clock care at home or in a long-term care facility.

Reviewed by Linda Littlejohns, RN, MSN, CNRN, FAAN, Neuroscience Clinical Nursing Consultant, San Juan Capistrano, California; Jessica Pastor, MSN, DNP(c), ACNP-BC, SANE-A, TNCC, Clinical Nursing Instructor, Wayne State University, Detroit, Michigan, and Nurse Practitioner, Infectious Diseases and Emergency Medicine, Troy Beaumont, Troy, Michigan; Crystal R. Sherman, DNP, CNP, FNP-BC, APHN-BC, Assistant Professor of Nursing, Shawnee State University, Portsmouth, Ohio; and Olga Van Dyke, RN, MSN, CAGS, Assistant Professor, School of Nursing, MCPHS University, Boston, Massachusetts.

## Etiology and Pathophysiology

SCI is usually a result of trauma. The most common causes are motor vehicle collisions (38%), falls (30%), violence (14%), sports injuries (9%), and other miscellaneous causes (9%).[1]

**Types of Injury.** The extent of neurologic damage caused by SCI results from primary injury (initial physical disruption of the spinal cord) and secondary injury (from processes such as ischemia, hypoxia, hemorrhage, and edema).

***Primary Injury.*** SCI can result from cord compression by bone displacement, interruption of blood supply to the cord, or traction from pulling on the cord. Penetrating trauma, such as gunshot and stab wounds, can cause tearing and transection. The initial mechanical disruption of axons as a result of stretch or laceration is referred to as the *primary injury.*

***Secondary Injury.*** *Secondary injury* refers to the ongoing, progressive damage that occurs after the primary injury. Several theories exist on what causes this ongoing damage. Possible causes include vascular changes due to hemorrhage, vasospasm, thrombosis, loss of autoregulation, breakdown of the blood-brain barrier, and infiltration of inflammatory cells that cause ischemia, edema, and cellular necrosis. Free radical formation, lipid peroxidation, release of glutamate, and disruption of the ionic balance of potassium, sodium, and calcium lead to neuronal cell death and reduced spinal cord blood flow. *Apoptosis* (programmed cell death) may continue for weeks after injury and contribute to postinjury demyelination.[2] These processes lead to scar tissue formation, irreversible nerve damage, and permanent neurologic deficit.

Fig. 60-1 illustrates the cascade of events causing secondary injury after traumatic SCI. The resulting hypoxia reduces $O_2$ levels below the metabolic needs of the spinal cord. Lactate metabolites accumulate, and an increase in vasoactive substances, including norepinephrine, serotonin, and dopamine occurs. High levels of these vasoactive substances cause vasospasms and hypoxia with subsequent necrosis. Unfortunately, the spinal cord has minimal ability to adapt to vasospasm.

Within 24 hours, permanent damage may occur because of edema. Edema secondary to the inflammatory response is particularly harmful because of limited space for tissue expansion. Thus compression of the spinal cord occurs. Edema extends above and below the injury, increasing ischemic damage. Because secondary injury progresses over time, the extent of the injury and prognosis for recovery are most accurately determined 72 hours or more after injury. Important signs of improvement include muscular strength and pinprick sensation below the level of injury. The greatest improvement occurs in the first 3 to 6 months following injury and can continue over years in 20% of cases.[3]

**Spinal and Neurogenic Shock.** **Spinal shock** may occur following acute SCI. This temporary shock is characterized by decreased reflexes, loss of sensation, absent thermoregulation, and flaccid paralysis below the level of injury. This syndrome lasts days to weeks and may mask postinjury neurologic function.

In contrast to spinal shock, **neurogenic shock** results from the loss of vasomotor tone caused by injury and is characterized by hypotension and bradycardia. Loss of sympathetic nervous system innervation causes peripheral vasodilation, venous pooling, and decreased cardiac output. These effects are generally associated with a cervical or high thoracic injury.[4]

**Classification of Spinal Cord Injury.** SCI is classified by the (1) mechanism of injury, (2) level of injury, and (3) degree of injury.

**PATHOPHYSIOLOGY MAP**

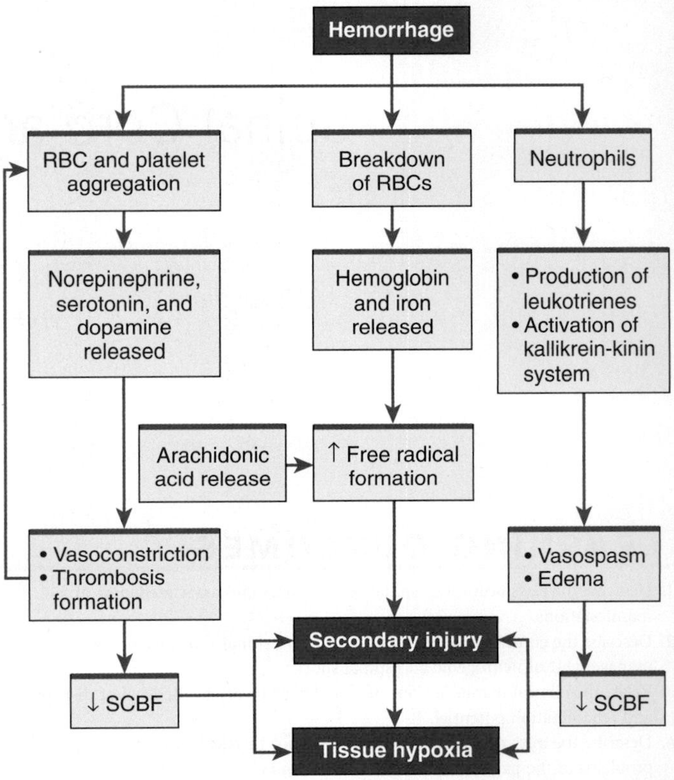


**FIG. 60-1** Cascade of metabolic and cellular events that leads to spinal cord ischemia and hypoxia of secondary injury. *RBCs,* Red blood cells; *SCBF,* spinal cord blood flow. (Modified from Marciano FF, Greene KA, Apostolides PJ, et al: Pharmacologic management of spinal cord injury: review of the literature, *BNI Q* 11[2]:11, 1995. In McCance KL, Huether SE, editors: *Pathophysiology: the biologic basis for disease in adults and children,* ed 5, St Louis, 2006, Mosby.)

***Mechanisms of Injury.*** The major mechanisms of injury are flexion, hyperextension, flexion-rotation, extension-rotation, and compression[5] (Fig. 60-2). The flexion-rotation injury is the most unstable because ligaments that stabilize the spine are torn. This injury most often contributes to severe neurologic deficits.

***Level of Injury.*** *Skeletal level of injury* is the vertebral level with the most damage to vertebral bones and ligaments. *Neurologic level* is the lowest segment of the spinal cord with normal sensory and motor function on both sides of the body. The level of injury may be cervical, thoracic, lumbar, or sacral. Cervical and lumbar injuries are most common because they are associated with the greatest flexibility and movement. If the cervical cord is involved, paralysis of all four extremities occurs, resulting in **tetraplegia** (formerly termed *quadriplegia*). The degree of impairment in the arms following cervical injury depends on the level of injury. The lower the level, the more function is retained in the arms.

If the thoracic, lumbar, or sacral spinal cord is damaged, the result is **paraplegia** (paralysis and loss of sensation in the legs). Fig. 60-3 shows affected structures and functions at different levels of cord injury.

***Degree of Injury.*** The degree of spinal cord involvement may be complete or incomplete (partial). *Complete cord involvement* results in total loss of sensory and motor function below the level of injury. *Incomplete cord involvement* results in a mixed

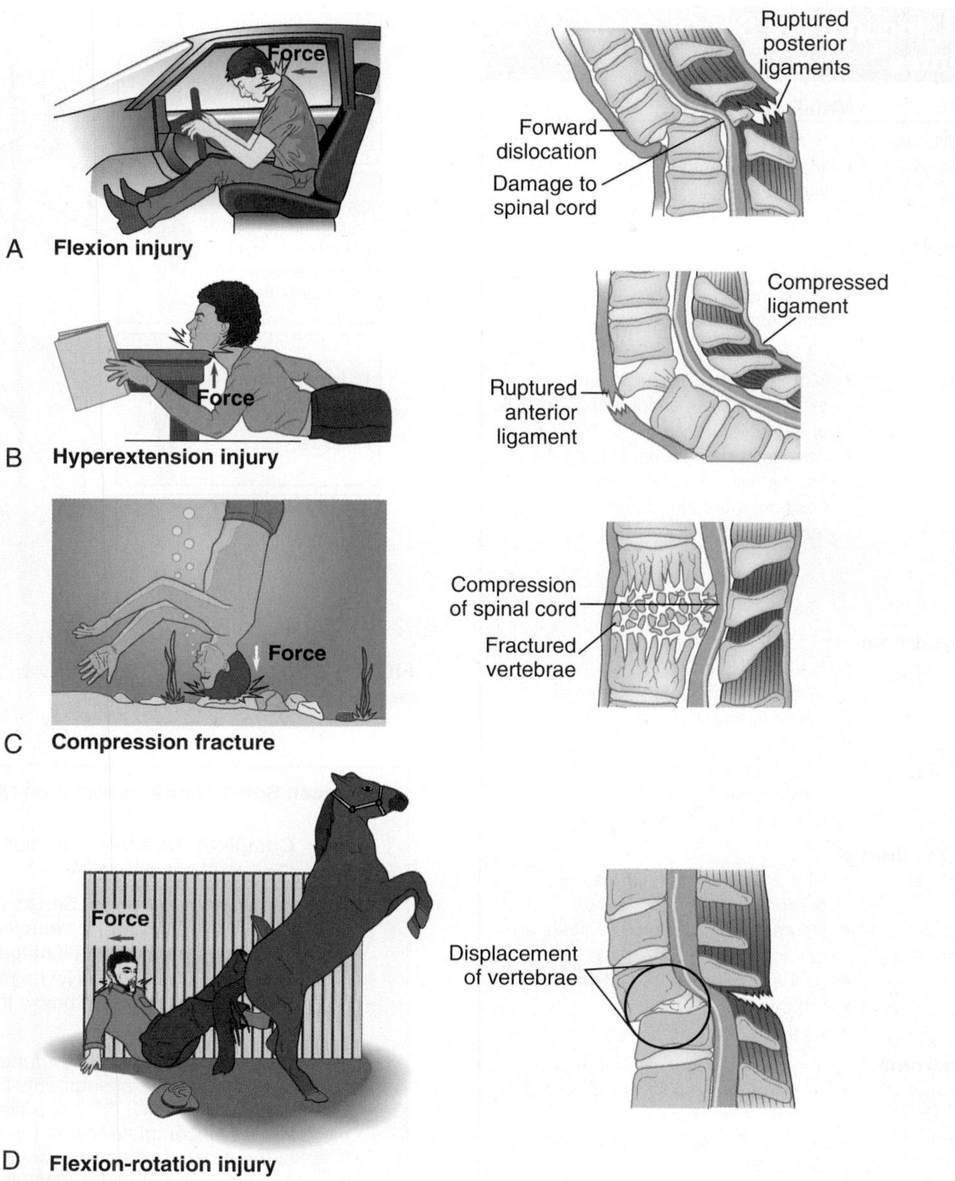


**FIG. 60-2** Examples of mechanisms of SCI. **A,** Flexion injury of the cervical spine ruptures the posterior ligaments. **B,** Hyperextension injury of the cervical spine ruptures the anterior ligaments. **C,** Compression fractures crush the vertebrae and force bony fragments into the spinal canal. **D,** Flexion-rotation injury of the cervical spine often results in tearing of ligamentous structures that normally stabilize the spine. (*A, B, C,* From Copstead-Kirkhorn LC, Banasik JL: *Pathophysiology,* ed 5, St Louis, 2014, Mosby.)

loss of voluntary motor activity and sensation and leaves some tracts intact. The degree of sensory and motor loss depends on the level of injury and reflects specific damaged nerve tracts.

Five major syndromes are associated with incomplete injuries: **central cord syndrome, anterior cord syndrome, Brown-Séquard syndrome, cauda equina syndrome**, and **conus medullaris syndrome** (Table 60-1).

## Clinical Manifestations

Manifestations of SCI are generally related to the direct result of trauma that causes cord compression, ischemia, edema, and possible cord transection. These manifestations are also related to the level and degree of injury. The patient with an incomplete injury may demonstrate a mixture of manifestations.

**Motor and Sensory Effects.** The American Spinal Injury Association (ASIA) Impairment Scale is recommended for classifying the severity of impairment from SCI. It combines assessments of motor and sensory function to determine neurologic level and completeness of injury[5] (Fig. 60-4).

The sensory regions are called *dermatomes,* with each segment of the spinal cord innervating a particular area of skin. Each dermatome has a specific point recommended for testing. A dermatome map is shown in Fig. 55-7 on p. 1299.

The ASIA Impairment Scale is useful for recording changes in neurologic status and identifying appropriate rehabilitation goals. Movement and rehabilitation potential related to specific locations of SCI are described in Table 60-2. In general, sensory function closely parallels motor function at all levels.

**Respiratory System.** Respiratory complications closely correspond to the level of injury. Cervical injuries above C4 present special problems because of the total loss of respiratory muscle function. Injury or fracture below C4 results in diaphragmatic

**TABLE 60-1 Incomplete Spinal Cord Injury Syndromes**

| Description | Manifestations |
|---|---|
| **Central Cord Syndrome** | |
| • Caused by damage to central spinal cord<br>• Occurs most commonly in cervical cord region<br>• More common in older adults | • Motor weakness and altered sensation present in upper extremities<br>• Lower extremities not usually affected<br>• Dysesthetic burning pain in upper extremities |
| **Anterior Cord Syndrome** | |
| • Caused by damage to anterior spinal artery<br>• Results in compromised blood flow to anterior spinal cord<br>• Typically results from acute compression of anterior portion of the spinal cord, often due to flexion injury | • Motor paralysis and loss of pain and temperature sensation below level of injury<br>• Because posterior cord tracts are not injured, sensations of touch, position, vibration, and motion remain intact |
| **Brown-Séquard Syndrome** | |
| • Results from damage to one half of the spinal cord<br>• Typically results from penetrating injury to spinal cord | • *Ipsilateral* (same side as injury): Loss of motor function and pressure, position, and vibratory sense<br>• *Contralateral* (opposite side of injury): Loss of light touch, pain, and temperature sensation below level of injury |
| **Conus Medullaris Syndrome** | |
| • Results from damage to the conus medullaris (lowest portion of spinal cord) | • Motor function in legs may be preserved, weak, or flaccid<br>• Decrease in or loss of sensation in perianal area<br>• Areflexic bowel and bladder<br>• Impotence<br>• Pain uncommon |
| **Cauda Equina Syndrome** | |
| • Results from damage to cauda equina (lumbar and sacral nerve roots) | • Asymmetric distal weakness, patchy sensation in lower extremities<br>• May cause flaccid paralysis of lower extremities<br>• Complete loss of sensation between legs and over buttocks, inner thighs, and backs of legs *(saddle area)*<br>• Areflexic (flaccid) bladder and bowel<br>• Severe, radicular, asymmetric pain |

breathing if the phrenic nerve is functioning. Even if the injury is below C4, spinal cord edema and hemorrhage can affect the function of the phrenic nerve and cause respiratory insufficiency. Hypoventilation and impairment of the intercostal muscles lead to a decrease in vital capacity and tidal volume.[6]

Cervical and thoracic injuries cause paralysis of abdominal muscles and often the intercostal muscles. Thus the patient cannot cough effectively enough to remove secretions, increasing the risk for aspiration, atelectasis, and pneumonia. Neurogenic pulmonary edema may occur secondary to a dramatic increase in sympathetic nervous system activity at the time of injury, which shunts blood to the lungs. In addition, pulmonary edema may occur in response to fluid overload. To improve respiratory function for patients with SCI, resistive inspiratory muscle training may be effective.[7]

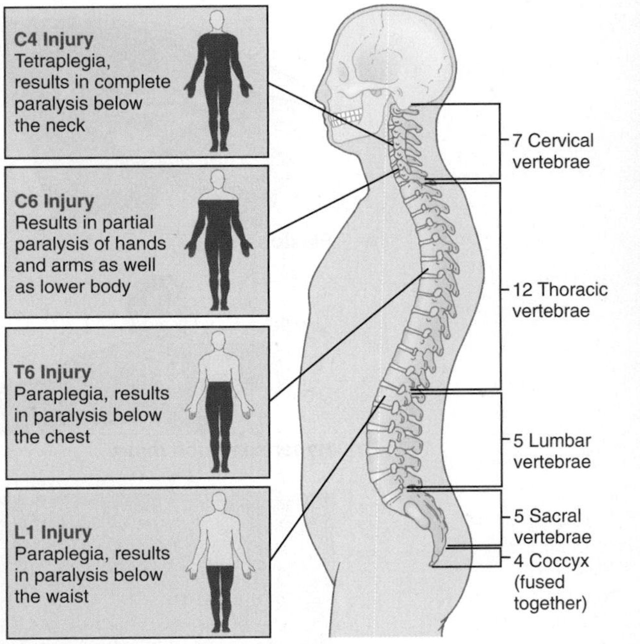


**FIG. 60-3** Symptoms, degree of paralysis, and potential for rehabilitation depend on level of spinal injury.

**American Spinal Injury Association (ASIA) Impairment Scale**

☐ A = **Complete.** No sensory or motor function is preserved in the sacral segments S4-5.

☐ B = **Sensory Incomplete.** Sensory but not motor function is preserved below the neurologic level and includes the sacral segments S4-5 (light touch or pin prick at S4-5 or deep anal pressure) AND no motor function is preserved more than three levels below the motor level on either side of the body.

☐ C = **Motor Incomplete.** Motor function is preserved at the most caudal sacral segments for voluntary anal contraction (VAC) OR the patient meets the criteria for sensory incomplete status (sensory function preserved at the most caudal sacral segments (S4-S5), and has some sparing of motor function more than three levels below the ipsilateral motor level on either side of the body.

☐ D = **Motor Incomplete.** Motor incomplete status as defined above, with at least half (half or more) of key muscle functions below the single neurologic level of injury (NLI) having a muscle grade ≥ 3.

☐ E = **Normal.** If sensation and motor function as tested with the ISNCSCI are graded as normal in all segments, and the patient had prior deficits, then the AIS grade is E. Someone without an initial SCI does not receive an AIS grade.

☐ ND = **Not Determined.** To document the sensory, motor, and NLI levels, the ASIA Impairment Scale grade, and/or the zone of partial preservation (ZPP) when they are unable to be determined based on the examination results.

**FIG. 60-4** The American Spinal Injury Association Impairment Scale. The worksheet for determining the classification is the International Standards for Neurologic Classification of Spinal Cord Injury (ISNCSCI) and is available at *www.asia-spinalinjury.org/elearning/isncsci_worksheet_2015_web.pdf.* (From American Spinal Injury Association.)

**TABLE 60-2 Level of Spinal Cord Injury and Rehabilitation Potential**

| Movement Remaining | Rehabilitation Potential |
|---|---|
| **Tetraplegia** | |
| ***C1-3*** | |
| • Often fatal injury<br>• Movement in neck and above, loss of innervation to diaphragm, absence of independent respiratory function | • Able to drive electric wheelchair equipped with portable ventilator by using chin control or mouth stick, headrest to stabilize head<br>• Able to use computer with mouth stick, head wand, or noise control<br>• Attendant care 24 hr/day. Able to instruct others |
| ***C4*** | |
| • Sensation and movement in neck and above<br>• May be able to breathe without a ventilator | • Same as C1-3 |
| ***C5*** | |
| • Full neck, partial shoulder, back, biceps<br>• Gross elbow, inability to roll over or use hands<br>• Decreased respiratory reserve | • Able to drive electric wheelchair with mobile hand supports<br>• Indoor mobility in manual wheelchair<br>• Able to feed self with setup and adaptive equipment<br>• Attendant care 10 hr/day |
| ***C6*** | |
| • Shoulder and upper back abduction and rotation at shoulder<br>• Full biceps to elbow flexion, wrist extension, weak grasp of thumb<br>• Decreased respiratory reserve | • Able to assist with transfer and perform some self-care<br>• Able to feed self with hand devices<br>• Able to push wheelchair on smooth, flat surface<br>• Able to drive adapted van from wheelchair<br>• Independent computer use with adaptive equipment<br>• Attendant care 6 hr/day |
| ***C7-8*** | |
| • All triceps to elbow extension, finger extensors and flexors<br>• Good grasp with some decreased strength<br>• Decreased respiratory reserve | • Able to transfer self to wheelchair<br>• Able to roll over and sit up in bed<br>• Able to push self on most surfaces<br>• Able to perform most self-care<br>• Independent use of wheelchair<br>• Able to drive car with powered hand controls (in some patients)<br>• Attendant care 0-6 hr/day |
| **Paraplegia** | |
| ***T1-6*** | |
| • Full innervation of upper extremities.<br>• Back, essential intrinsic muscles of hand. Full strength and dexterity of grasp.<br>• Decreased trunk stability, decreased respiratory reserve | • Full independence in self-care and in wheelchair<br>• Able to drive car with hand controls (in most patients)<br>• Independent standing in standing frame |
| ***T6-12*** | |
| • Full, stable thoracic muscles and upper back<br>• Functional intercostal muscles, resulting in increased respiratory reserve | • Full independent use of wheelchair<br>• Able to stand erect with full leg brace, ambulate on crutches with swing (although gait difficult)<br>• Unable to climb stairs |
| ***L1-2*** | |
| • Varying control of legs and pelvis<br>• Instability of lower back | • Good sitting balance<br>• Full use of wheelchair<br>• Able to ambulate with long leg braces |
| ***L3-4*** | |
| • Quadriceps and hip flexors<br>• Absence of hamstring function, flail ankles | • Completely independent ambulation with short leg braces and canes<br>• Unable to stand for long periods |

**Cardiovascular System.** Any cord injury above T6 leads to dysfunction of the sympathetic nervous system. The result may be bradycardia, peripheral vasodilation, and hypotension (neurogenic shock). Peripheral vasodilation causes a relative hypovolemia because of the increase in the capacity of the dilated veins. It also reduces venous return of blood to the heart. Cardiac output then decreases, leading to hypotension. Other injuries can also cause hemorrhagic shock and further reduce BP. It is important to identify all causes of hypotension in the person with SCI.

**Urinary System.** Urinary dysfunction occurs in the majority of patients following SCI. Neurogenic bladder describes any type of bladder dysfunction related to abnormal or absent bladder innervation. After spinal cord shock resolves, depending on the completeness of the SCI, patients usually have some degree of neurogenic bladder. Normal voiding requires nervous system coordination of urethral and pelvic floor relaxation, with simultaneous contraction of the detrusor muscle.

Depending on the injury, a neurogenic bladder may (1) have no reflex detrusor contractions *(flaccid, hypotonic)*, (2) have hyperactive reflex detrusor contractions *(spastic)*, or (3) lack coordination between detrusor contraction and urethral relaxation *(dyssynergia)*. Common problems with a neurogenic bladder include urgency, frequency, incontinence, inability to void, and high bladder pressures resulting in reflux of urine into the kidneys.[8]

Urinary retention is a common development in acute SCI and spinal shock. While the patient is in spinal shock, the bladder is atonic, becomes overdistended, and fails to empty. In the postacute phase of SCI, the bladder may become hyperirritable. A loss of inhibition from the brain results in reflex emptying and failure to store urine *(urinary incontinence)*.[9]

**Gastrointestinal System.** Decreased GI motor activity contributes to gastric distention and development of paralytic ileus. Gastric emptying may be delayed, especially in patients with higher level SCI. Excessive release of HCl acid in the stomach may cause stress ulcers. Dysphagia may also be present in patients who require mechanical ventilation, tracheostomy, and anterior spine surgery.

Intraabdominal bleeding may be difficult to diagnose because the person with SCI may not experience pain or tenderness. Continued hypotension and decreases in hemoglobin and hematocrit may indicate bleeding. Expanding abdominal girth may also be noted.

Loss of voluntary control of the bowel following SCI results in neurogenic bowel. SCI above the level of the conus medullaris causes the anal sphincter to remain tight, and the ability to sense a full rectum is lost. Bowel movement occurs on a reflex basis when the rectum is full *(incontinence)*. SCI at or below the conus medullaris causes the bowel to be *areflexic*. Peristalsis is impaired and stool propulsion is slow. The defecation reflex may be damaged and anal sphincter tone relaxed *(retention)*.

## ETHICAL/LEGAL DILEMMAS

### *Right to Refuse Treatment*

**Situation**

R.D., a 25-yr-old man, suffered a spinal cord injury (SCI) to C7-8 following a motorcycle accident. He was diagnosed with anterior cord syndrome and has motor paralysis, which may prevent him from riding motorcycles again. He has become extremely depressed and states he no longer wishes to live. Because of his emotional state, R.D. is now refusing to eat. Can he be forced to receive enteral nutrition (tube feeding)?

**Ethical/Legal Points for Consideration**

- Withholding treatment in a newly injured but otherwise healthy young adult may present an ethical dilemma for some nurses. They may consider it assisted suicide and believe that it violates the ethical principles of beneficence and nonmaleficence.
- A competent adult has the right to consent to or refuse medical treatment under the right to privacy, the Fourteenth Amendment of the Constitution, and case law.*
- Case law has also supported the concept that forced treatment constitutes battery (unlawful use of force). Furthermore, a mentally competent, physically incapacitated adult can refuse feeding by nasogastric tube and compel the health facility to follow the patient's wishes.†
- To be competent to participate in informed consent or refusal, an adult must be able to understand the information provided about the procedure or treatment, consider choices between alternatives available, and make a choice based on his values and preferences. Depression may not be a determinant in competency to make informed treatment choices.
- If, after adequate evaluation and treatment for pain, depression, or other medical conditions, the patient persists in his refusal, his wishes must be respected.
- Refusal to eat or drink has never been upheld as illegal, and the alternative—forced eating and drinking—is clearly a criminal act of battery and a violation of patient rights.

**Discussion Questions**

1. What are your feelings about requests to withhold treatment in a young person with a newly acquired disability?
2. What resources are available to help R.D., his family, and nursing staff deal with this emotionally charged and ethically complex situation?

* *Cruzan v. Director, Missouri Department of Health,* 497 U.S. 261, 1990. Retrieved from *http://supreme.justia.com/cases/federal/us/497/261.*

† *Bouvia v. Superior Court,* 1986. Retrieved from *http://law.justia.com/cases/california/calapp3d/179/1127.html.*

This leads to constipation, increased risk of incontinence, and possible impaction, ileus, or megacolon. Hemorrhoids can occur over time.

**Integumentary System.** The risk for skin breakdown over bony prominences in areas of decreased or absent sensation is a major consequence of immobility related to SCI. Pressure ulcers can occur quickly and lead to major infection and sepsis.

**Thermoregulation.** *Poikilothermism* is the adjustment of body temperature to room temperature. It occurs in SCI because interruption of the sympathetic nervous system prevents peripheral temperature sensations from reaching the hypothalamus. Spinal cord disruption is also marked by decreased ability to sweat or shiver below the level of injury, which affects the ability to regulate body temperature. The degree of poikilothermism depends on the level of injury. High cervical injuries are associated with a greater loss of ability to regulate temperature than are thoracic or lumbar injuries.

**Metabolic Needs.** Nasogastric suctioning may lead to metabolic alkalosis. It is especially important to monitor sodium and potassium until suctioning is discontinued and a normal diet is resumed.

The person with SCI has increased nutritional needs due to increased metabolism and more protein breakdown. Lean body mass is lost and muscle atrophy leads to weight loss. Nutritional support should focus on a diet that addresses the person's caloric and nitrogen needs.[10] Adequate nutrition helps to prevent skin breakdown, reduce infection, and decrease the rate of muscle atrophy.

**Peripheral Vascular Problems.** Venous thromboembolism (VTE) is a common problem accompanying SCI during the first 3 months.[11] Detecting deep venous thrombosis (DVT) may be difficult in a person with SCI because usual signs and symptoms, such as pain and tenderness, are not present. Pulmonary embolism is a leading cause of death in patients with SCI.[1]

**Pain.** Pain following SCI differs in type and severity, and is influenced by the patient's physical functioning and emotions. The pain can be nociceptive or neuropathic.

*Nociceptive pain* in SCI can develop from musculoskeletal, visceral, and/or other types of injury (e.g., skin ulceration, headache). Patients often describe musculoskeletal pain as dull or aching. It starts or worsens with movement. Visceral pain is located in the thorax, abdomen, and/or pelvis, and may be dull, tender, or cramping.

*Neuropathic pain* in SCI occurs from damage to the spinal cord or nerve roots. The pain can be located at or below the level of injury. Patients often identify neuropathic pain as hot, burning, tingling, pins and needles, cold, and/or shooting. They may be extremely sensitive to stimuli and even light touch can cause significant pain.[12] (Pain is discussed in Chapter 8.)

### Diagnostic Studies

CT scan is the preferred imaging study to diagnose the location and degree of injury as well as the degree of spinal canal compromise. Cervical x-rays are obtained when CT scan is not readily available. However, visualizing C7 and T1 on cervical x-rays is often difficult, and the ability to fully evaluate cervical spine injury is compromised.

MRI is used to assess soft tissue injury, neurologic changes, unexplained neurologic deficits, or worsening neurologic condition.[13] Perform a comprehensive neurologic examination with assessment of the head, chest, and abdomen for additional injuries or trauma. Patients with cervical injuries who demonstrate altered mental status may also need a CT angiogram to rule out vertebral artery damage. Duplex Doppler ultrasound, impedance plethysmography, venous occlusion plethysmography, venography, and clinical examination are used to diagnose DVT.

### Interprofessional Care

**Prehospital.** Immediate postinjury goals include maintaining a patent *airway*, adequate ventilation/*breathing*, and adequate *circulating* blood volume (ABCs) as well as preventing extension of spinal cord damage (secondary injury). Table 60-3 outlines emergency management of the patient with SCI. Recommended immobilization includes a combination of a rigid cervical collar and supportive blocks on a backboard with straps. Spinal immobilization with sandbags and tape is insufficient and is not recommended. Spinal immobilization in patients with penetrating trauma is also not recommended because of increased mortality. The concern during initial management of patients with potential cervical spinal injuries is impairment of neurologic function due to movement of the injured vertebrae.[14]

TABLE 60-3 **Emergency Management**

***Spinal Cord Injury***

| Etiology | Assessment Findings | Interventions |
|---|---|---|
| **Blunt Trauma**<br>• Compression, flexion, extension, or rotation injuries to spinal column<br>• Motor vehicle crash<br>• Pedestrian accidents<br>• Falls<br>• Diving<br>• Sports injuries<br>**Penetrating Trauma**<br>• Stretched, torn, crushed, or lacerated spinal cord<br>• Gunshot wounds<br>• Stab wounds | • Respiratory distress/difficulty breathing<br>• Neurogenic shock: hypotension, bradycardia, cool or warm dry skin<br>• Spinal shock<br>• Muscle weakness, paralysis, or flaccidity<br>• Alterations in sensation: temperature, light touch, deep pressure, proprioception<br>• Numbness, paresthesia<br>• Pain, tenderness, deformities, or muscle spasms adjacent to vertebral column<br>• Cuts; bruises; open wounds on head, face, neck, or back<br>• Bowel and bladder incontinence<br>• Urinary retention<br>• Priapism<br>• Diminished rectal sphincter tone | **Initial**<br>• Ensure patent airway and adequate respirations.<br>• Maintain $SaO_2$ > 90%: Administer $O_2$ via nasal cannula, non-rebreather mask, or endotracheal tube.<br>• Maintain SBP > 90 mm Hg.<br>• Establish IV access with two large-bore catheters to infuse normal saline or lactated Ringer's solution as appropriate.<br>• Immobilize and stabilize cervical spine.*<br>• Assess for other injuries.<br>• Control external bleeding.<br>• Obtain appropriate imaging.<br>**Ongoing Monitoring**<br>• Monitor vital signs, level of consciousness (neurologic status), $O_2$ saturation, cardiac rhythm, urine output.<br>• Anticipate need for intubation if in respiratory distress or gag reflex absent.<br>• Keep warm. |

*Spinal immobilization is not recommended in patients with penetrating trauma.

Systemic and neurogenic shock must be treated to maintain systolic BP greater than 90 mm Hg. Following cervical injury, all body systems must be maintained until the full extent of the damage can be evaluated. After stabilization at the injury scene, the person should be transferred by the most appropriate mode of transportation available to the nearest medical facility, preferably one that specializes in acute SCI care.[15] A thorough assessment allows evaluation of the degree of deficit and establishes the level and degree of injury.

**Acute Care.** Interprofessional care during the acute phase for a patient with a cervical injury is described in Table 60-4. Compared to cervical injury, patients with SCI of the thoracic and lumbar vertebrae require less intense support. At this level of injury, respiratory compromise is not as severe and bradycardia is usually not a problem. Other problems are treated symptomatically.

Obtain a history, with emphasis on how the incident occurred. Assess the extent of injury perceived by the patient or by the emergency response system (ERS) personnel immediately after the event. Initial assessment (which usually occurs in the emergency department) includes managing the person's ABCs and vital signs to ensure the airway is secure, oxygenation saturation ($SaO_2$) is greater than 90%, and SBP is greater than 90 mm Hg. Appropriate medical interventions and diagnostics are implemented to ensure the patient is hemodynamically stable.

A complete neurologic assessment is completed using the ASIA tool (Fig. 60-4). The International Standards for Neurologic Classification of Spinal Cord Injury is available at *www.asia-spinalinjury.org/elearning/isncsci_worksheet_2015_web.pdf.*

Muscle groups are tested with and against gravity, alone and against resistance, on both sides of the body. Ask the patient to move legs and then hands, spread fingers, extend wrists, and shrug shoulders. Record symmetry and spontaneous movement. After assessing motor status, complete a sensory examination, including touch and pain as tested by pinprick, starting at the toes and working upward toward the head. Assess rectal tone. Voluntary anal contraction indicates incomplete SCI. If time and conditions permit, also assess position sense and vibration.

Mechanisms of injury that cause spinal cord trauma, especially involving the cervical cord, may also result in brain injury and/or vertebral artery injury. Assess for a history of unconsciousness, signs of concussion, and increased intracranial pressure (see Chapter 56). In addition, perform a careful assessment for musculoskeletal injuries and trauma to internal organs. Because the patient has no muscle, bone, or visceral sensations, the only clue to internal trauma with hemorrhage may be a rapidly decreasing BP and increasing pulse. Examine urine for hematuria, which also indicates internal injuries.

Move the patient in alignment as a unit *(logroll)* during transfers and when repositioning to prevent further injury. Monitor respiratory, cardiac, urinary, and GI functions. The patient may go directly to surgery after initial immobilization or to the intensive care unit (ICU) for monitoring and management.

***Nonoperative Stabilization.*** Nonoperative treatments involve stabilization of the injured spinal segment and decompression, either through traction or realignment. Stabilization eliminates damaging motion at the injury site. It is intended to prevent secondary spinal cord damage caused by narrowing of the spinal canal, or continued contusion or compression of the spinal cord at the level of the injury. Early realignment of an unstable fracture-dislocation injury by closed reduction through craniocervical traction has been found to be effective and safe.

***Surgical Therapy.*** Surgical treatment is used following acute SCI to address the instability and decompress the spinal cord. The type of surgery depends on the severity and level of the injury, mechanism of injury, and location and degree of compression. Early spinal cord decompression may reduce secondary injury and thus improve the patient's outcome. Surgery within the first 24 hours after SCI is safe and associated with improved neurologic outcome.

Surgery to stabilize the spine can be performed from the back of the spine *(posterior approach)* or from the front of the spine *(anterior approach)*. In some cases, both approaches may be needed. Fusion involves attaching metal screws, plates, or other devices to the bones of the spine to keep them aligned. This procedure is usually done when two or more vertebrae have been injured. Small pieces of bone may also be attached to

**TABLE 60-4 Interprofessional Care**

***Cervical Cord Injury***

**Diagnostic Assessment**
- History and physical examination, including complete neurologic examination
- Arterial blood gases
- Electrolytes, serum glucose, coagulation profile, hemoglobin and hematocrit
- Urinalysis
- CT scan, MRI, EMG (measure evoked potentials)
- Anteroposterior, lateral, and odontoid spinal x-rays
- Serial bedside PFTs
- Duplex Doppler ultrasound, impedance plethysmography

**Management**

***Acute Care***
- Immobilization and stabilization of vertebral column
- ABCs (airway, breathing, circulation)
- $O_2$ by high-humidity mask ($PaO_2$ >60 mm Hg)
- Intubation (if indicated by ABGs and PFTs)
- Maintenance of heart rate (e.g., atropine) and BP (e.g., dopamine) (SBP >90 mm Hg, MAP >85)
- Administration of IV fluids
- Insertion of nasogastric tube and attach to suction.
- Assessment and management of nutrition
- Maintenance of normal body temperature *(normothermia)*
- Indwelling urinary catheter
- Pain management
- VTE prophylaxis
- Pressure ulcer prevention
- Stress ulcer prophylaxis
- Bowel and bladder care and training
- Mobilization once spine stabilized
- Physical, occupational, speech therapy and physiatrist consults

***Rehabilitation and Home Care***
- Physical therapy (ROM, mobility, strength, equipment)
- Occupational therapy (splints, ADLs training)
- Speech therapy (swallow and cognition)
- Pain management
- Spasticity management
- Bowel and bladder training
- Autonomic hyperreflexia prevention
- Pressure ulcer prevention
- Recreational therapy
- Patient and caregiver teaching

*ADL*, Activities of daily living; *PFT*, pulmonary function test; *VTE*, venous thromboembolism.

the injured bones to help them fuse into one solid piece. The bone used for this procedure can be obtained from the patient's spinal bone harvested during surgery, from another bone in the patient's body *(autologous)*, or from donor bone *(allograft)*. (Specific surgical and nursing interventions for these techniques are discussed in Chapter 63 on pp. 1506-1507.)

***Drug Therapy.*** Methylprednisolone (MP), which was used for many years to treat acute SCI, is no longer approved by the Food and Drug Administration (FDA) for this use. No evidence suggests clinical benefit of MP to treat acute SCI. High-dose MP is associated with harmful side effects, including immunosuppression with increased risk of infection, increased frequency of upper GI bleeding, sepsis, longer stays in the ICU, and even death.[16]

Low-molecular-weight heparin (e.g., enoxaparin [Lovenox]) is used to prevent VTE unless contraindicated. Contraindications include internal bleeding, abnormal kidney function, and recent surgery. Oral anticoagulation alone is not recommended as a prophylactic treatment strategy.

Vasopressor agents, such as phenylephrine or norepinephrine (Levophed), are used in the acute phase as adjuvants to treatment. These agents maintain the mean arterial pressure (MAP) at greater than 85 to 90 mm Hg to improve perfusion to the spinal cord. Use of vasopressors has significant risk of complications, including ventricular tachycardia, troponin elevation, metabolic acidosis, and atrial fibrillation. Dopamine has been shown to have more complications than phenylephrine in SCI.[17] Because drug metabolism is altered in patients with SCI, drug interactions may occur. Differences in drug metabolism correlate with level and completeness of injury, with greater change apparent following cervical cord injury than injury at lower spinal levels.

## NURSING MANAGEMENT: SPINAL CORD INJURY

### Nursing Assessment

Subjective and objective data that should be obtained from a patient with recent SCI are presented in Table 60-5.

### Nursing Diagnoses

Nursing diagnoses for the patient with SCI depend on the severity of the injury and level of dysfunction. Nursing diagnoses for a patient with SCI may include, but are not limited to, the following:
- Ineffective breathing pattern *related to* respiratory muscle fatigue, neuromuscular paralysis, and/or retained secretions
- Imbalanced nutrition: less than body requirements *related to* paralytic ileus and metabolic demands of body
- Ineffective peripheral tissue perfusion *related to* hypotension and lack of mobility
- Impaired skin integrity *related to* immobility and/or poor tissue perfusion
- Impaired urinary elimination *related to* spinal injury and/or limited fluid intake
- Constipation *related to* neurogenic bowel, inadequate fluid intake, and/or immobility
- Risk for autonomic hyperreflexia (dysreflexia) *related to* reflex stimulation of sympathetic nervous system

Additional information on nursing diagnoses for the patient with SCI is presented in eNursing Care Plan 60-1 (available on the website for this chapter). The care plan is for a patient with a complete cervical cord injury.

### Planning

Overall goals are that the patient with SCI will (1) maintain an optimal level of neurologic functioning; (2) have minimal or no complications of immobility; (3) learn new skills, gain new knowledge, and acquire new behaviors to be able to care for self or successfully direct others to do so; and (4) return home at an optimal level of functioning.

### Nursing Implementation

**Health Promotion.** Nursing interventions for prevention of SCI include identifying high-risk populations, counseling, and teaching. Support legislation to prohibit texting while driving and to mandate use of seat belts in cars, helmets for motorcyclists and bicyclists, and child safety seats. Also recommend tougher penalties for drunk-driving offenses.

Emphasize the importance of other health promotion and health screening following SCI. Health-promoting behaviors

## TABLE 60-5 Nursing Assessment
### Spinal Cord Injury

**Subjective Data**

***Important Health Information***

*Health history:* Motor vehicle crash, sports injury, industrial incident, gunshot or stabbing injury, falls

***Functional Health Patterns***

*Health perception–health management:* Use of alcohol or recreational drugs. Risk-taking behaviors
*Activity-exercise:* Loss of strength, movement, and sensation below level of injury. Dyspnea, inability to breathe adequately ("air hunger")
*Cognitive-perceptual:* Tenderness, pain at or above level of injury. Numbness, tingling, burning, twitching of extremities
*Coping–stress tolerance:* Fear, denial, anger, depression

**Objective Data**

***General***

Poikilothermism (unable to regulate body heat)

***Integumentary***

Warm, dry skin below level of injury (neurogenic shock)

***Respiratory***

*Injury at C1-3:* Apnea, inability to cough
*Injury at C4:* Poor cough, diaphragmatic breathing, hypoventilation
*Injury at C5-T6:* Decreased respiratory reserve

***Cardiovascular***

*Injury above T6:* Bradycardia, hypotension, postural hypotension, absence of vasomotor tone

***Gastrointestinal***

Decreased or absent bowel sounds (paralytic ileus in injuries above T5), abdominal distention, constipation, fecal incontinence, fecal impaction

***Urinary***

Retention (for injuries at T1-L2), flaccid bladder (acute stages), spasticity with reflex bladder emptying (later stages)

***Reproductive***

Priapism, altered sexual function

***Neurologic***

*Complete:* Areflexic, flaccid paralysis and anesthesia below level of injury resulting in tetraplegia (injuries above C8) or paraplegia (injuries below C8), hyperactive deep tendon reflexes and bilaterally positive Babinski test (after resolution of spinal shock)
*Incomplete:* Mixed loss of voluntary motor activity and sensation

***Musculoskeletal***

Muscle atony (in flaccid state), contractures (in spastic state)

***Pain***

Neuropathic, musculoskeletal, and/or visceral

***Possible Diagnostic Findings***

Location of level and type of bony involvement on spinal x-ray. Injury, edema, compression on CT scan and MRI; positive finding on myelogram

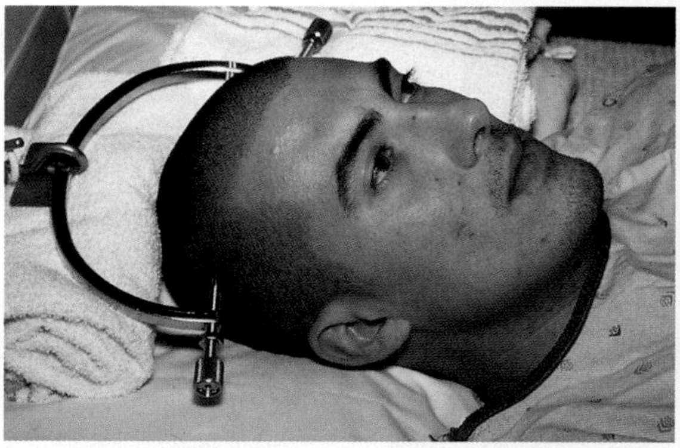

**FIG. 60-5** Cervical traction is attached to tongs inserted in the skull. (Courtesy Michael S. Clement, MD, Mesa, Ariz.)

after injury can have significant impact on the general health and well-being of the individual with SCI. Nursing interventions include (1) teaching and counseling; (2) referring to programs such as smoking cessation classes, recreation and exercise programs, and alcohol treatment programs; and (3) performing routine physical examinations for non-neurologic problems. Screening and prevention programs must be accessible to and accommodate people with SCI. Nurses in these clinical settings should advocate for wheelchair-accessible examination rooms, adjustable-height examination tables, and appointment scheduling that allows extra time if needed.

◆ **Acute Care.** High cervical cord injury caused by flexion-rotation is the most complex SCI and is discussed in this section. Interventions for this type of injury can be modified for patients with less severe injuries.

◆ ***Immobilization.*** Proper immobilization of the neck involves the maintenance of a neutral position.

**SAFETY ALERT Cervical Spine Injuries**
- Use a hard cervical collar and a backboard to stabilize the neck to prevent lateral rotation of the cervical spine.
- Always keep the patient's body in correct alignment.
- Turn the patient as a unit (logrolling) to prevent movement of the spine.

For cervical injuries, closed reduction with skeletal traction is used for early realignment *(reduction)* of the injury. Crutchfield (Fig. 60-5) or Gardner-Wells tongs or halo (halo ring) can provide this type of traction, using a rope that extends from the center of the device over a pulley to weights attached at the end. Traction must be maintained at all times. Possible displacement of the skull pins is a disadvantage of tongs. If displacement occurs, hold the head in a neutral position and get help. Immobilize the head while the surgeon reinserts the tongs.

No specific recommendations are available regarding maximum weight for traction. The surgeon may start with 10 pounds and add 5 pounds for each level to the injury. The goal is spinal reduction. Awake patients are monitored with x-ray as well as neurologic and pain assessment. Comatose patients require serial x-rays to evaluate the effects of traction.

The need for surgery is determined after the spine is reduced. After cervical fusion or other stabilization surgery, the patient may wear a hard cervical collar or sternal-occipital-mandibular immobilizer brace (Fig. 60-6).

When a patient can begin to mobilize after a stable injury (for which surgery is not needed), the halo frame can be attached to a special vest *(Halo vest)* (Fig. 60-7). This allows the patient to mobilize and ambulate while cervical bones fuse.

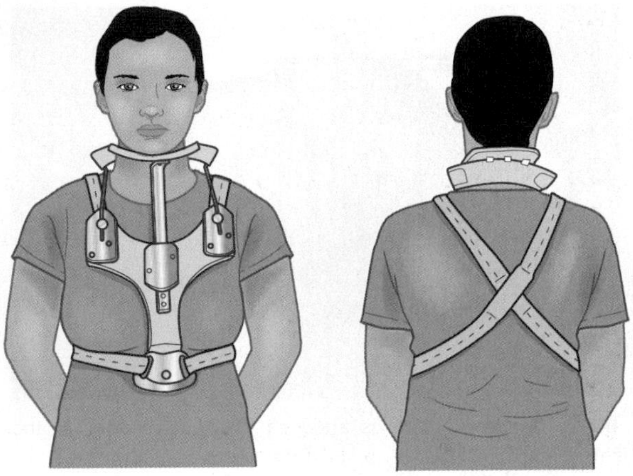

**FIG. 60-6** Sternal-occipital-mandibular immobilizer brace.

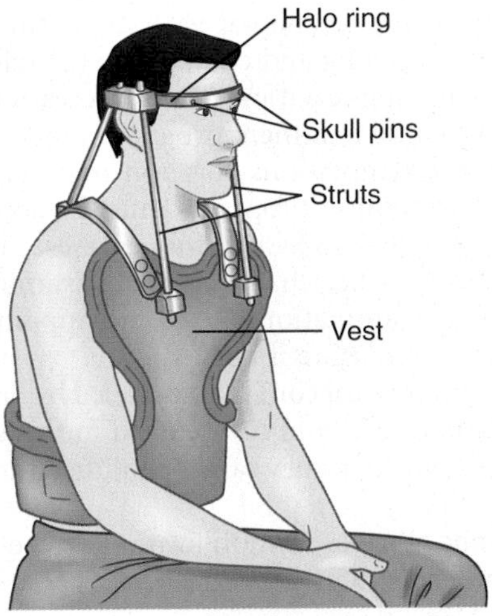


**FIG. 60-7** Halo vest. The halo traction brace immobilizes the cervical spine, which allows the patient to ambulate and participate in self-care. (Modified from Urden LD, Stacy KM, Lough ME: *Priorities in critical care nursing,* ed 6, St Louis, 2012, Mosby.)

However, the halo is not indicated if the patient has ligament instability from the injury. That patient will require surgery. Infection at the sites of tong or halo pin insertion is another potential problem. Preventive care is based on hospital protocol. A common protocol involves cleansing sites twice a day with half strength peroxide and normal saline solution and applying an antibiotic ointment to act as a mechanical barrier to the entrance of bacteria. Patient and caregiver teaching for a patient with a halo vest is presented in Table 60-6.

Special beds are often used in the management of the patient with SCI (Fig. 60-8). Kinetic therapy involves continuous side-to-side rotation of a patient to 40 degrees or more to help prevent pulmonary complications. This lateral rotation also redistributes pressure, helping prevent pressure ulcers.

Patients with stable thoracic or lumbar spine injuries may be immobilized with a custom thoracolumbar orthosis (TLSO or body jacket) to inhibit spinal flexion, extension, and rotation. Alternately, a Jewett brace may be used to restrict forward flexion. Unstable injuries may require surgical decompression and fusion in addition to the TLSO or lumbosacral orthotic (LSO).

Immobilization of the neck of the patient with SCI prevents further injury, but the effects of immobility are profound. Meticulous skin care is critical because decreased sensation and circulation make the patient more susceptible to skin breakdown. Remove the patient's backboard as soon as possible and replace it with other forms of immobilization to prevent skin breakdown in the coccygeal and occipital areas. Fit cervical collars properly. Inspect areas under the halo vest or jacket or under braces or orthoses to assess the skin.

## TABLE 60-6 Patient & Caregiver Teaching

### *Halo Vest Care*

*Include the following instructions when teaching the patient and caregiver management of a halo vest.*

1. Inspect the pins on the halo traction ring. Report to HCP if pins are loose or signs of infection are present, including redness, tenderness, swelling, or drainage at insertion sites.
2. Clean around pin sites carefully with half-strength hydrogen peroxide, water, or alcohol on a cotton swab as directed.
3. Apply antibiotic ointment as prescribed.
4. To receive skin care, have patient lie down with the head resting on a pillow to reduce pressure on the brace. Loosen one side of the vest. Gently wash the skin under the vest with soap and water, rinse area, and then dry it thoroughly. At the same time, check the skin for pressure points, redness, swelling, bruising, or chafing. Close the open side and repeat the procedure on the opposite side.
5. If the vest becomes wet or damp, carefully dry it with a blow dryer.
6. Encourage patient to use assistive device (e.g., cane, walker) to improve balance; encourage use of flat shoes.
7. Remind patient to turn the entire body, not just the head and neck, when trying to look sideways.
8. In case of an emergency, keep a set of wrenches close to the halo vest at all times.
9. Mark the vest strap to maintain consistent buckling and fit.
10. Avoid grabbing bars or vest to assist the patient.
11. Keep sheepskin pad under vest. Change and wash pad at least weekly.
12. If perspiration or itching is a problem, encourage patient to wear a cotton T shirt under the sheepskin. The T-shirt can be modified with a Velcro seam closure on one side.

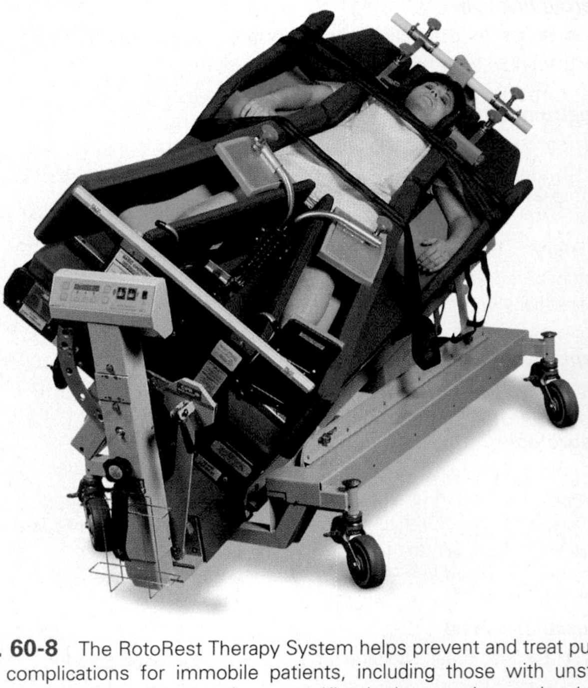

**FIG. 60-8** The RotoRest Therapy System helps prevent and treat pulmonary complications for immobile patients, including those with unstable cervical, thoracic, and lumbar fractures. Kinetic therapy, the continual side-to-side bilateral rotation of the patient, redistributes pulmonary blood flow and mobilizes secretions to improve ventilation and perfusion matching. The therapy system also helps to prevent pressure ulcers. (Courtesy Arjo Huntleigh, Addison, Ill.)

◆ ***Respiratory Dysfunction.*** Respiratory complications are the leading cause of death in people with SCI.[18] During the first 48 hours after injury, spinal cord edema may increase the level of dysfunction, and respiratory distress may occur. Patients with acute cervical SCI are initially managed in a monitored unit or ICU.[9] If the injury is at or above C4, the phrenic nerve leading to the diaphragm may be affected and breathing can stop. If the patient is exhausted from labored breathing or ABGs indicate inadequate oxygenation or ventilation, endotracheal intubation or tracheostomy and mechanical ventilation are needed. Monitor the patient carefully for respiratory compromise and be prepared for quick action if arrest occurs. Pneumonia and atelectasis may occur due to reduced vital capacity and loss of intercostal and abdominal muscle function, resulting in diaphragmatic breathing, pooled secretions, and ineffective cough.

Regularly assess (1) breath sounds, (2) ABGs, (3) tidal volume, (4) vital capacity, (5) skin color, (6) breathing patterns (especially use of accessory muscles), (7) subjective comments about the ability to breathe, and (8) amount and color of sputum. A $PaO_2$ (partial pressure of $O_2$ in arterial blood) greater than 60 mm Hg and a $PaCO_2$ (partial pressure of $CO_2$ in arterial blood) less than 45 mm Hg are acceptable values in a patient with uncomplicated tetraplegia. A patient who is unable to count to 10 aloud without taking a breath needs immediate attention.

In addition to ongoing assessment, intervene to maintain ventilation. Administer $O_2$ and provide ventilatory support until ABGs stabilize. Patients who experienced chest trauma or have difficulty weaning from the ventilator may require a tracheostomy for airway management.

Chest physiotherapy and assisted (augmented) coughing help to clear secretions. Assisted coughing simulates the action of the ineffective abdominal muscles during the expiratory phase of a cough. Place the heels of both hands just below the xiphoid process and exert firm upward pressure to the area timed with the patient's efforts to cough (see Fig. 67-7).

Perform tracheal suctioning if crackles or coarse breath sounds are present. Incentive spirometry can also be used to improve the patient's respiratory status. The older adult has more difficulty responding to hypoxia and hypercapnia. Thus aggressive chest physiotherapy, adequate oxygenation, and appropriate pain management are essential to maximize respiratory function and gas exchange. Other respiratory problems include nasal stuffiness and bronchospasm.

◆ ***Cardiovascular Instability.*** Because of unopposed vagal response, heart rate is slowed, often to less than 60 beats/minute. Any increase in vagal stimulation, as occurs with turning or suctioning, can cause cardiac arrest. Loss of sympathetic nervous system tone in peripheral vessels results in chronic low BP with potential postural hypotension. The lack of muscle tone to aid venous return can cause sluggish blood flow and predispose the patient to VTE. Dysrhythmias may also occur.

Frequently assess vital signs. If bradycardia is symptomatic, administer an anticholinergic drug such as atropine. A temporary or permanent pacemaker may be inserted. Maintain SBP greater than 90 mm Hg at all times and keep MAP between 85 and 90 mm Hg for the first 7 days following SCI. Manage hypotension with fluid replacement and a vasopressor agent, such as phenylephrine or norepinephrine.

If blood loss has occurred from other injuries, monitor hemoglobin and hematocrit and administer blood according to protocol. Also assess the patient for indications of hypovolemic shock secondary to hemorrhage.

Orthostatic hypotension is likely to occur in the patient with injury at T6 and above. The patient may complain of lightheadedness, dizziness, and nausea, and lose consciousness when moved from a bed to a chair. Assess orthostatic BP when mobilizing the patient. For symptomatic patients, use an abdominal binder and graduated compression stockings to promote venous return. Drugs used to increase intravascular volume include salt tablets and fludrocortisone. Midodrine may be given to promote blood vessel contraction and increase venous return.

Consider the effects of aging on the cardiovascular system of the older adult. The older patient is less able to manage the stress of traumatic injury because heart contractions weaken and cardiac output is reduced. Maximum heart rate is also reduced. In addition to the effects of aging, the older person may have cardiovascular disease.

Use low-molecular-weight heparin or low-dose heparin in combination, sequential compression devices (SCDs), or graduated compression stockings to promote venous return and prevent VTE.[11] Venous duplex studies may be performed before applying compression devices. Remove stockings every 8 hours for skin care. Also assess thighs and calves every shift for signs of DVT (e.g., deep reddish color, edema). Regularly perform range of motion (ROM) exercises and stretching. Continue VTE prophylaxis for 3 months following injury.

◆ ***Fluid and Nutritional Management.*** During the first 48 to 72 hours after the injury, the GI tract may stop functioning *(paralytic ileus)*. A nasogastric tube must be inserted if ileus occurs. Because the patient cannot have oral intake, carefully monitor fluid and electrolyte status.

Nutrition should be started within the first 72 hours following injury. Specific solutions and additives are ordered based on individual requirements. Due to severe catabolism, a high-protein, high-calorie diet is needed for energy and tissue repair. If the patient cannot be fed through the GI system, either orally or through a feeding tube placed into the duodenum, parenteral nutrition should be initiated to reduce nitrogen losses that occur during the hypermetabolic state.

Once bowel sounds are present or flatus is passed, and the patient is not receiving mechanical ventilation, a formal swallow evaluation should be done. If no risk of aspiration is identified, gradually introduce oral food and fluids. If the patient fails the swallow evaluation or is unable to eat due to an endotracheal tube or tracheostomy, a more secure feeding tube may be placed in the stomach or jejunum (see Chapter 39).

### CHECK YOUR PRACTICE

You are working in the spinal cord unit. Today your 28-yr-old male patient with SCI at T6 weighs 168 pounds. When he was admitted 3 weeks ago, he weighed 186 pounds. He asks you, "Well, what is my weight? Are you gonna make me eat now? You know you can't do that."

- What assessment data are important for you to obtain?
- What interventions would help him avoid further weight loss and regain lean body mass?

Patients may experience anorexia due to depression, boredom with institutional food, or discomfort at being fed (often by a hurried nurse). Some patients have a normally small appetite. Occasionally refusal to eat is a means of maintaining control over the environment because of diminished or absent body control. If the patient is not eating adequately, assess the cause.

Based on assessment findings, make a contract with the patient with mutual goal setting for the diet. This contract gives the patient increased control and often results in improved nutritional intake. General measures may also be effective, such as providing a pleasant eating environment, allowing adequate time to eat (including any self-feeding the patient can achieve), encouraging the family to bring in special foods, and planning social rewards for eating.

Keep a calorie count and record the patient's daily weight to evaluate progress. If feasible, the patient should participate in recording calorie intake. Dietary supplements may be needed to meet nutritional goals. Include increased dietary fiber to promote bowel function. Avoid allowing the patient's nutritional intake to become a basis for a power struggle.

◆ ***Bladder and Bowel Management.*** Immediately after the injury, urine is retained because of the loss of autonomic and reflex control of the bladder and sphincter *(neurogenic bladder).* Because there is no sensation of fullness, overdistention of the bladder can result in reflux into the kidney and cause renal failure. Bladder overdistention may even result in rupture of the bladder. Thus an indwelling catheter may be inserted as soon as possible after injury. Ensure patency of the catheter by frequent inspection and irrigation if necessary. In some institutions, an HCP's order is required for this procedure. Strict aseptic technique for catheter care is essential to prevent infection. During the period of indwelling catheterization, encourage a large fluid intake. Check the catheter to prevent kinking and ensure free flow of urine.

Catheter-acquired urinary tract infection (CAUTI) is a common problem. The best method for preventing UTI is regular and complete bladder drainage. After the patient is stabilized, assess the best means of managing long-term urinary function. Usually the patient is started on an intermittent catheterization program. (CAUTI and intermittent catheterization are discussed in Chapter 45.)

Intermittent catheterization should be done four to six times daily to prevent bacterial overgrowth from urinary stasis. Keep urine residuals under 500 mL to prevent bladder distention. If the urine is cloudy or has a strong, or if the patient develops symptoms of a UTI (e.g., chills, fever, malaise), send a specimen for culture.

Consider age-related changes in renal function. Older adults are more likely to develop renal calculi. Older men may have benign prostatic hyperplasia, which may interfere with urinary flow and complicate management of urinary problems.

Constipation is generally a problem during spinal shock because no voluntary or involuntary *(reflex)* evacuation of the bowel occurs *(neurogenic bowel).* Start a bowel program during acute care. This involves choosing a rectal stimulant (suppository or small-volume enema) to be inserted daily at a regular time, followed by gentle digital stimulation or manual evacuation until evacuation is complete. Initially the program may be done in bed with the patient in the side-lying position. However, as soon as the patient has resumed sitting, the patient should be in the upright position on a padded bedside commode chair. These programs typically require 30 to 60 minutes to complete. Constipation can be reduced with adequate fluid intake, a healthy diet of fiber and vegetables, and increased activity and exercise.[19]

◆ ***Temperature Control.*** Because the patient has no vasoconstriction, piloerection (erection of body hair), or heat loss through perspiration below the level of injury, temperature control is largely external. Monitor the environment closely to maintain an appropriate temperature. Also regularly monitor the patient's body temperature. Do not use excessive covers or unduly expose the patient (such as during bathing). If an infection with high fever develops, more aggressive methods for temperature control may be needed (e.g., a cooling blanket).

◆ ***Stress Ulcers.*** Stress ulcers can occur in the patient with SCI because of the physiologic response to severe trauma and psychologic stress. Peak incidence of stress ulcers is 6 to 14 days after injury. Test stool and gastric contents daily for blood, and monitor the hematocrit for a slow drop. Histamine ($H_2$)-receptor blockers (e.g., ranitidine [Zantac], famotidine [Pepcid]) or proton pump inhibitors (e.g., pantoprazole [Protonix], omeprazole [Prilosec]) may be given prophylactically to decrease the secretion of HCl acid and prevent ulcers during the initial phase.

◆ ***Sensory Deprivation.*** To prevent sensory deprivation, compensate for the patient's absent sensations by stimulating the patient above the level of injury. Conversation, music, and interesting foods can be part of the nursing care plan. If the head of the bed must remain flat, provide prism glasses to help the patient read and watch television.

Help the patient avoid withdrawing from the environment. Promote adequate rest and sleep and assess for changes in mood. Depression is a common problem (discussed later in chapter on p. 1435).

◆ ***Pain Management.*** Musculoskeletal nociceptive pain can develop secondary to injuries to bones, muscles, and ligaments. This pain is aggravated with movement or palpation. Antiinflammatory drugs such as ibuprofen may help with pain. Opioids may also be used to manage nociceptive pain.

Visceral nociceptive pain is a dull, tender, or cramping pain in the thorax, abdomen, or pelvis. This type of pain may result from the bladder and bowel. Assess the patient's bowel and bladder function to avoid bladder distention or constipation. Other causes of nociceptive pain include UTI and ureteral calculus. Notify the HCP if the patient experiences persistent pain despite treatment. Diagnostic imaging may be needed to fully evaluate its cause.

Neuropathic pain in the initial phase is usually at the level of SCI. It may occur on one or both sides of the body within the affected dermatome, and up to three levels below. The patient will complain of hot, burning, tingling, shooting, electric pain. Gabapentin (Neurontin) or pregabalin (Lyrica) may be used to reduce pain. Neuropathic pain can occur months or years after SCI and become chronic and permanent. The patient's mood can affect the pain, as can sudden noise, constipation, or infections. Teach the patient and caregiver about possible pain triggers and offer relaxation therapy. Other modes of treatment may include tricyclic antidepressants, intrathecal medication, antiseizure drugs, epidural stimulation, and destructive surgical intervention.

◆ ***Skin Care.*** Healthy skin requires adequate blood circulation. Constant pressure in one position can compress blood vessels and limit blood supply, causing cell death and pressure ulcers. The most common location of pressure ulcers, which occur in about 25% of all patients with SCI, is the sacrum.[20]

Pressure ulcers are preventable with diligent nursing care. Perform a comprehensive visual and tactile examination of the skin at least once daily, with special attention to areas over bony prominences. Areas most vulnerable to breakdown include the sacrum, ischia, trochanters, and heels. Assess surgical incisions for healing and integrity of the skin under collars and braces.

Carefully position and reposition the patient at least every 2 hours, with gradual increases in the times between turns if no redness over bony prominences is seen at the time of turning. While the patient is supine in bed, float the heels to reduce pressure. Move the patient carefully during turns and transfers to avoid stretching and folding of soft tissues *(shear)* or abrasion.

Specialty mattresses are used to reduce the incidence of pressure ulcers. When the patient is moved to a chair or wheelchair, use pressure-relieving cushions. Pressure relief should be performed every 15 to 20 minutes when the patient is in a chair and should last 30 to 60 seconds each time.

Regularly assess nutritional status. Both weight loss and gain can contribute to skin breakdown. Adequate intake of protein is essential for skin health. Evaluation of prealbumin, total protein, and albumin can help identify inadequate protein intake. Stress the importance of nutrition for skin health.

◆ ***Reflexes.*** Once spinal shock is resolved, return of reflexes may complicate rehabilitation. Lacking control from the higher brain centers, reflexes are often hyperactive and produce exaggerated responses. Penile erection can occur from a variety of stimuli, causing embarrassment and discomfort. Spasms ranging from mild twitches to convulsive movements below the level of injury may also occur. The patient or caregiver may interpret this reflex activity as a return of function. Tactfully explain the reason for the activity. Inform the patient of the positive use of these reflexes in sexual, bowel, and bladder retraining. Spasms may be controlled with the use of antispasmodic drugs such as baclofen, dantrolene (Dantrium), and tizanidine (Zanaflex). Botulism toxin injections may also be given to treat severe spasticity.

◆ ***Autonomic Hyperreflexia.*** The return of reflexes after the resolution of spinal shock means patients with injury at T6 or higher may develop autonomic hyperreflexia. **Autonomic hyperreflexia** (also known as *autonomic dysreflexia*) is a massive uncompensated cardiovascular reaction mediated by the sympathetic nervous system. It involves stimulation of sensory receptors below the level of the SCI. The intact sympathetic nervous system below the level of injury responds to the stimulation with a reflex arteriolar vasoconstriction that increases BP, but the parasympathetic nervous system is unable to directly counteract these responses via the injured spinal cord. Baroreceptors in the carotid sinus and aorta sense the hypertension and stimulate the parasympathetic system. This results in a decrease in heart rate, but visceral and peripheral vessels do not dilate because efferent impulses cannot pass through the injured spinal cord.

The most common precipitating cause of autonomic hyperreflexia is a distended bladder or rectum. However, autonomic hyperreflexia can be caused by any sensory stimulation, including contraction of the bladder or rectum, stimulation of the skin, or stimulation of pain receptors.

Manifestations include hypertension (up to 300 mm Hg SBP), throbbing headache, marked diaphoresis above the level of injury, bradycardia (30 to 40 beats/minute), piloerection as a result of pilomotor spasm, flushing of the skin above the level of injury, blurred vision or spots in the visual fields, nasal congestion, anxiety, and nausea. Measure BP when a patient with SCI complains of a headache.

Autonomic hyperreflexia is a life-threatening condition that requires immediate resolution. If uncorrected, it can lead to status epilepticus, stroke, myocardial infarction, and even death.

Nursing interventions in this serious emergency include elevating the head of the bed 45 degrees or sitting the patient upright, determining the cause, and notifying the HCP. The most common cause is bladder irritation. Immediate catheterization to relieve bladder distention may be necessary. Instill lidocaine jelly in the urethra before catheterization. If a catheter is already in place, check it for kinks or folds. If it is plugged, perform small-volume irrigation slowly and gently to open the catheter, or insert a new catheter.

Stool impaction can also cause autonomic hyperreflexia. Perform a digital rectal examination (if trained) only after application of an anesthetic ointment to decrease rectal stimulation and avoid increasing symptoms. Remove all skin stimuli, such as constrictive clothing and tight shoes. Monitor BP frequently during the episode. If symptoms persist after the source has been relieved, administer a rapid onset and short duration agent such as nitroglycerin, nitroprusside, or hydralazine. Continue careful monitoring until vital signs stabilize.

Teach the patient and caregiver to recognize causes and symptoms of autonomic hyperreflexia (Table 60-7). They must understand the life-threatening nature of this dysfunction, know how to relieve the cause, and activate the ERS if needed.

◆ **Rehabilitation and Home Care.** Rehabilitation of the person with SCI is complex. With physical and psychologic care and intensive and specialized rehabilitation, the patient with SCI can learn to function at the highest level of wellness. All patients with new SCI should receive comprehensive inpatient rehabilitation in a rehabilitation unit or center that specializes in spinal cord rehabilitation.

Many of the problems identified in the acute period become chronic and continue throughout life. Rehabilitation focuses on retraining physiologic processes as well as extensive patient, caregiver, and family teaching about how to manage the physiologic and life changes resulting from the injury (Fig. 60-9).

**TABLE 60-7 Patient & Caregiver Teaching**

***Autonomic Hyperreflexia***

*For a patient at risk for autonomic hyperreflexia, include the following information in the teaching plan for the patient and caregiver.*

1. Signs and symptoms
   - Sudden onset of acute headache
   - Elevation in BP and/or reduction in pulse rate
   - Flushed face and upper chest (above level of injury) and pale extremities (below level of injury)
   - Sweating above level of injury
   - Nasal congestion
   - Feeling of apprehension
2. Immediate interventions
   - Raise the person to a sitting position.
   - Remove the noxious stimulus (fecal impaction, kinked urinary catheter, tight clothing).
   - Call the HCP if above actions do not relieve the signs and symptoms.
3. Measures to decrease the incidence of autonomic hyperreflexia
   - Maintain regular bowel function.
   - Use a local anesthetic to prevent autonomic hyperreflexia if manual rectal stimulation is used to promote bowel function.
   - Monitor urine output.
   - Encourage the patient to wear a Medic Alert bracelet indicating a history of risk for autonomic hyperreflexia.

Rehabilitation is an interprofessional team effort. Team members include rehabilitation nurses, HCPs, physical therapists, occupational therapists, speech therapists, vocational counselors, psychologists, therapeutic recreation specialists, prosthetists, orthotists, case managers, social workers, and dietitians.

Rehabilitation care is organized around the patient's goals and needs. The patient is expected to be involved in therapies and learn self-care for several hours each day. Such intensive work at a time when the patient is dealing with the sudden change in health and function can be stressful. Progress may be slow. The rehabilitation nurse has a pivotal role in providing encouragement, specialized nursing care, and patient and caregiver teaching, and in helping to coordinate efforts of the rehabilitation team.

◆ ***Respiratory Rehabilitation.*** The patient with cervical injury above C3 requires mechanical ventilation because the phrenic nerve is not stimulated and thus the diaphragm is not functional. The patient will need around-the-clock caregivers who are knowledgeable about respiratory hygiene and tracheostomy care.[21] The rehabilitation nurse and respiratory therapist provide teaching on removing secretions through suctioning and assisted *(augmented)* coughing (see Fig. 67-7). The patient may also require chest percussion or postural drainage to manage secretions.

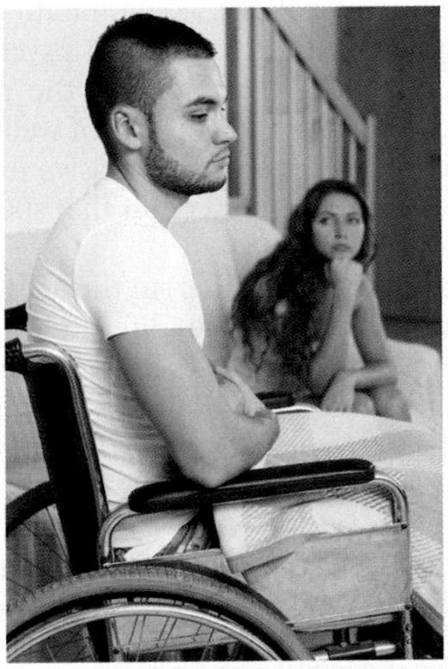

**FIG. 60-9** A spinal cord injury has a major effect on a person's physical, emotional, and psychologic health. (©JackF/iStock/Thinkstock)

Some patients with high cervical SCI may have greatly increased mobility with phrenic nerve stimulators or electronic diaphragmatic pacemakers. These devices are not appropriate for all ventilator-dependent patients but may be helpful for those with an intact phrenic nerve. Some ventilators are also portable, allowing ventilator-dependent patients with tetraplegia to be mobile and less dependent. Patients and caregivers should be taught home ventilator and tracheostomy care, with referrals to appropriate community agencies as needed.

If the patient was successfully weaned from the ventilator during hospitalization, downsizing (gradual decrease in size) and removal of the tracheostomy will be done during rehabilitation. Teach assisted coughing, regular use of incentive spirometry, and breathing exercises to the patient with cervical injury who is not ventilator dependent. Limit exposure to people with fever, cold, and cough. Adhere to swallowing precautions (e.g., proper positioning of head and neck) and diet recommendations to prevent aspiration.

◆ ***Neurogenic Bladder.*** Types of neurogenic bladder are presented in Table 60-8. Diagnostic and interprofessional care of neurogenic bladder is described in Table 60-9. The patient with SCI and a neurogenic bladder requires a comprehensive program to manage bladder function.

After the patient's overall condition is stable and assessment indicates return of neurologic reflexes, urodynamic testing (see Table 44-8) and a urine culture may be done. Many factors are considered when selecting a bladder management strategy. These include patient preference, upper extremity function, and availability of a caregiver. The type of bladder dysfunction (Table 60-8) also determines management options.

Various drugs can be used to treat the patient with a neurogenic bladder. Anticholinergic drugs (oxybutynin [Ditropan XL], tolterodine [Detrol]) may be used to suppress bladder contraction. α-Adrenergic blockers (e.g., terazosin, doxazosin [Cardura]) may be used to relax the urethral sphincter. Antispasmodic drugs (e.g., baclofen) may be used to decrease spasticity of pelvic floor muscles.

Numerous drainage methods are possible, including bladder reflex retraining if partial voiding control remains, indwelling catheter, intermittent catheterization, and external catheter (condom catheter). Evaluate long-term use of an indwelling catheter because of the associated high incidence of CAUTI, fistula formation, and diverticula. However, for some patients

**TABLE 60-8 Types of Neurogenic Bladder**

| Type | Characteristics | Causes | Manifestations |
|---|---|---|---|
| **Uninhibited bladder (reflexic)** | • No inhibitions influence time and place of voiding<br>• Bladder empties in response to stretching of bladder wall | • Results from lesions above the pons<br>• Observed in stroke, brain tumor, brain trauma | • Incontinence, frequency, urgency<br>• Voiding is unpredictable and incomplete |
| **Upper motor neuron bladder (mixed areflexic or hyperactive)** | • *Mixed A type* (most common):<br>  • Bladder is flaccid and external sphincter is spastic, leading to urinary retention<br>• *Mixed B type*:<br>  • Bladder is spastic with flaccid external sphincter leading to urinary incontinence. | • Results from lesions between pons and sacral spinal cord<br>• Observed in SCI or multiple sclerosis involving the cervicothoracic spinal cord | • Detrusor-sphincter dyssynergia<br>• Can lead to high bladder pressures and kidney damage from urinary reflex<br>• Sensory function impaired |
| **Lower motor neuron bladder (areflexic)** | • Bladder acts as if all motor functions were paralyzed<br>• Bladder fills without emptying | • Results from lower motor neuron injury caused by trauma involving S2-4<br>• Lesions of cauda equina, pelvic nerves | • If sensory function intact, patient feels bladder distention and hesitancy.<br>• No control of micturition, resulting in over distention of bladder, overflow incontinence, and UTI |

**TABLE 60-9 Interprofessional Care**

***Neurogenic Bladder***

**Diagnostic Assessment**
- History and physical examination, including neurologic examination
- Laboratory: Urinalysis, urine culture and sensitivity, blood urea nitrogen, serum creatinine, creatinine clearance
- Urodynamic testing (postvoid residual, cystometric testing, electromyography, urethral pressure profile)

**Management**
- Patient teaching
- Bladder retraining: time voiding, manual expression, intermittent catheterization
- Fluid schedule: intake of 1800-2000 mL/day
- Indwelling urinary catheter

***Drug Therapy***
- Tricyclic antidepressants
- Anticholinergic drugs
- α-Adrenergic blockers
- Antispasmodics
- Botulinum toxin injection into bladder wall

***Bladder and/or Urethral Surgical Therapy***
- Bladder augmentation
- Sphincter resection or removal *(sphincterotomy)*
- Electrode placement for electrical stimulation
- Urinary diversion
- Urethral stents and balloon dilation
- Artificial urinary sphincter

this may be the best option. Patients with indwelling catheters need to have adequate fluid intake (at least 3 to 4 L/day). Regularly check the patency of the indwelling catheter. Frequency of routine catheter changes ranges widely depending on the type of catheter used and agency policy.

Intermittent catheterization is the most commonly recommended method of bladder management (see Chapter 45). Nursing assessment is important in selecting the time interval between catheterizations. Initially, catheterization is done every 4 hours. Bladder volume can be assessed before catheterization using a portable bladder ultrasound machine. If less than 200 mL of urine is measured, the time interval until catheterization may be extended. If more than 500 mL of urine is measured, the time interval is shortened. Intermittent catheterization is usually done four to six times daily.

*Urinary diversion surgery* may be needed if the patient has repeated UTI with renal involvement or repeated stones, or if therapeutic interventions have been unsuccessful. Surgical treatment of neurogenic bladder includes bladder neck revision (sphincterotomy), bladder augmentation (augmentation cystoplasty), penile prosthesis, artificial sphincter, perineal ureterostomy, cystotomy, vesicotomy, and anterior urethral transplantation. (Urinary diversion procedures are discussed in Chapter 45.)

No matter which bladder management strategy is selected, teach the patient, caregiver, and family successful self-management. Inform them about the various management techniques, how to obtain necessary supplies, care of supplies and equipment, and when to seek health care.

◆ ***Neurogenic Bowel.*** Careful management of bowel evacuation is necessary in the patient with SCI because voluntary control of this function may be lost. Usual measures for

**TABLE 60-10 Patient & Caregiver Teaching**

***Bowel Management After Spinal Cord Injury***

*For the patient with a spinal cord injury, include the following information about bowel management in the teaching plan for the patient and caregiver.*

1. Optimal nutritional intake includes the following:
   - Three well-balanced meals each day
   - Two servings from the milk group
   - Two or more servings from the meat group, including beef, pork, poultry, eggs, fish
   - Four or more servings from the vegetable and fruit groups
   - Four or more servings from the bread and cereal group
2. Fiber intake should be approximately 20-30 g/day. Increase the amount of fiber eaten gradually over 1-2 wk.
3. At least 2 to 3 L of fluid should be consumed per day unless contraindicated. Water or fruit juices should be used (fluid softens hard stools). Caffeinated beverages such as coffee, tea, and cola should be limited (caffeine stimulates fluid loss through urination).
4. Avoid foods that produce gas (e.g., beans) or upper GI upset (e.g., spicy foods).
5. *Timing:* Establish a regular schedule for bowel evacuation. A good time is 30 min after the first meal of the day.
6. *Position:* If possible, an upright position with feet flat on the floor or on a step stool enhances bowel evacuation. Staying on the toilet, commode, or bedpan for longer than 20-30 min may cause skin breakdown. Based on stability, someone may need to stay with the patient.
7. *Activity:* Exercise is important for bowel function. In addition to improving muscle tone, it increases appetite and GI transit time. Exercise muscles, including stretching, ROM, position changing, and functional movement.
8. *Drug treatment:* Suppositories may be needed to stimulate a bowel movement. Manual stimulation of the rectum may also be helpful in initiating defecation. Use stool softeners as needed to regulate stool consistency. Use oral laxatives only if necessary.

preventing constipation include high-fiber diet and adequate fluid intake (see Table 42-7). Patient and caregiver teaching guidelines related to bowel management are presented in Table 60-10. However, these measures alone may not be adequate to stimulate evacuation. In addition, suppositories (bisacodyl or glycerin) or small-volume enemas and digital stimulation (performed 20 to 30 minutes after suppository insertion) by the nurse or patient may be needed. In the patient with an upper motor neuron injury, digital stimulation is needed to relax the external sphincter to promote defecation. A stool softener such as docusate sodium can be used to regulate stool consistency. Oral stimulant laxatives should be used only if absolutely necessary and not on a regular basis.

Valsalva maneuver and manual stimulation are useful in patients with lower motor neuron injuries. Because the Valsalva maneuver requires intact abdominal muscles, it is used in patients with injuries below T12. In general, a bowel movement every other day is considered adequate. However, consider preinjury patterns. Fecal incontinence can result from too much stool softener or a fecal impaction.

Record all bowel movements, including amount, time, and consistency. Timing of defecation may also be important. Planning bowel evacuation for 30 to 60 minutes after the first meal of the day may enhance success by taking advantage of the gastrocolic reflex induced by eating. This reflex may also be stimulated by drinking a warm beverage immediately after the meal. Patient, caregiver, and family teaching is required to promote successful independent bowel management. Timing of the bowel program should also be discussed among the interprofessional team so there are no interruptions when the patient is doing therapy (e.g., swimming pool therapy).

◆ ***Spasticity.*** Weeks after the initial SCI, the patient may start to have involuntary spasms of the muscles below the level of injury. This indicates resolution of the spinal shock or flaccid stage of SCI. Spasticity can be both beneficial and undesirable. It aids with mobility, especially for the patient with incomplete SCI. Spasticity improves circulation by promoting venous return and decreases orthostatic hypotension and the risk of VTE. Unfortunately, the patient with marked spasticity and tone may have difficulty with positioning and mobility secondary to the spasms. Spasms can cause significant pain and make activities of daily living (ADLs) difficult for the patient.

The Ashworth and modified Ashworth scales are used to evaluate spasticity *(www.scireproject.com/outcome-measures-new/ashworth-and-modified-ashworth-scale-mas).* Treatment strategies include ROM exercises to prevent muscle and joint tightness and reduce the risk of contracture. Antispasmodic medications such as baclofen or tizanidine may be administered. Botulinum toxin injection is useful for specific muscle involvement.

◆ ***Skin Care.*** Prevention of pressure ulcers is part of the lifelong treatment plan following SCI. Nurses in rehabilitation are responsible for teaching the patient and caregiver about daily skin care. A comprehensive visual and tactile examination should be performed daily with special attention to bony prominences. Teach the patient and caregiver to carefully move the patient to prevent injury and to reposition at least every 2 hours while in bed and every 15 to 20 minutes when in a chair or wheelchair. Also include information on the importance of adequate nutrition and how it affects the skin.

Protect the skin by avoiding thermal injury. Burns can be caused by hot food or liquids, bath or shower water that is too warm, radiators, heating pads, and uninsulated plumbing. Thermal injury also can result from extreme cold *(frostbite).* Injuries may not be noticed until severe damage has occurred. Anticipatory guidance about potential risks is essential. Patient and caregiver teaching related to skin care is provided in Table 60-11.

◆ ***Pain Management.*** The acute pain of the initial injury may persist during the first few weeks of rehabilitation. Assess, evaluate, and treat pain routinely. Use analgesics and interventions such as massage and repositioning to help the patient during therapy.

Chronic pain can also result from overuse of muscles in the shoulders and arms for movement and repositioning. Sleep may be disrupted due to pain. The patient may benefit from referral to an HCP who specializes in pain management.

◆ ***Sexuality.*** Sexuality is an important issue regardless of the patient's age or sex. To provide accurate and sensitive counseling and teaching about sexuality, be aware of your own sexuality and understand the human sexual responses. When discussing sexual potential, use scientific terminology rather than slang whenever possible. Knowledge of the level and completeness of injury is needed to understand the male patient's potential for orgasm, erection, and fertility, and the patient's capacity for sexual satisfaction.

Men normally have two types of erections: psychogenic and reflex. The process of *psychogenic erection* begins in the brain with sexual thoughts. Signals from the brain are sent through the nerves of the spinal cord to the T10-L2 levels. The signals are then relayed to the penis and trigger an erection. Men with low-level incomplete injuries are more likely to have psychogenic erection than men with higher-level incomplete injuries. Men with complete injuries are less likely to experience psychogenic erection.

A *reflex erection* occurs with direct physical contact to the penis or other erotic areas. A reflex erection is involuntary and can occur without sexually stimulating thoughts. These reflex erections are often short lived and uncontrolled and cannot be maintained or summoned at the time of coitus. The nerves that control a man's ability to have a reflex erection are located in the sacral nerves (S2-4) of the spinal cord. Most men with SCI are able to have a reflex erection with physical stimulation regardless of the extent of the injury if the S2-4 nerve pathways are not damaged.

Treatment for erectile dysfunction includes drugs, vacuum devices, and surgical procedures. Phosphodiesterase inhibitors such as sildenafil (Viagra) have become the first-line treatment in men with SCI. Sexual stimulation is required to get an erection after taking the medication. Penile injection of vasoactive substances (papaverine, prostaglandin E) is another medical treatment. Risks include prolonged penile erection *(priapism)* and scarring, so these substances should be considered only after failure of sildenafil. Vacuum suction devices use negative pressure to encourage blood flow into the penis. Erection is maintained by a constriction band placed at the base of the penis. The main surgical option is implantation of a penile prosthesis.[22] (Erectile dysfunction is discussed in Chapter 54.)

SCI affects male fertility, causing poor sperm quality and ejaculatory dysfunction. Recent advances in methods of sperm retrieval include penile vibratory stimulation and electroejaculation. Combined with ovulation induction and intrauterine insemination of the female partner, these techniques have changed the prognosis for men with SCI to father children from unlikely to a reasonable possibility of successful outcomes.

The effect of SCI on female sexual response is less clear. A woman of childbearing age with SCI usually remains fertile. The injury does not affect the ability to become pregnant or to deliver normally through the birth canal. Menses may cease for as long as 6 months after injury. If sexual activity is resumed, protection against unplanned pregnancy is needed. A normal pregnancy may be complicated by UTI, anemia, and autonomic

**TABLE 60-11 Patient & Caregiver Teaching**

***Skin Care After Spinal Cord Injury***

*To prevent skin breakdown in a patient with spinal cord injury, include the following instructions when teaching the patient and caregiver.*

**Change Position Frequently**

- If in a wheelchair, lift self and shift weight every 15-30 min.
- If in bed, change position with a regular turning schedule (at least every 2 hr) that includes sides, back, and abdomen.
- Use pressure-reducing mattresses and wheelchair cushions (not eggcrate).
- Use pillows to protect bony prominences when in bed.

**Monitor Skin Condition**

- Inspect skin frequently for areas of redness, swelling, and breakdown.
- Keep fingernails trimmed to avoid scratches and abrasions.
- If a wound develops, follow standard wound care procedures.

hyperreflexia. Because uterine contractions are not felt, precipitous delivery is always a danger.[23]

Care should be taken not to dislodge an indwelling catheter during sexual activity. If an external catheter is used, instruct the patient to refrain from fluids and remove the catheter before sexual activity. The bowel program should include evacuation the morning of sexual activity. Encourage the patient to inform the partner that incontinence is always possible. The woman may need a water-soluble lubricant to supplement diminished vaginal secretions and facilitate vaginal penetration.

Open discussion with the patient regarding sexual rehabilitation is essential. This important aspect of rehabilitation should be addressed by a professional trained in sexual counseling. A nurse or other rehabilitation professional with such expertise provides support for the patient and partner, with an emphasis on open communication. Alternative methods of obtaining sexual satisfaction, such as oral-genital sex (cunnilingus and fellatio), may be suggested. Explicit films may also be used, such as a film demonstrating the sexual activities of a patient with paraplegia and a nondisabled partner. Use graphics cautiously because they may focus too much on the mechanics of sex rather than on the relationship.

◆ ***Grief and Depression.*** Depression after SCI is common and disabling.[24] Patients with SCI may feel an overwhelming sense of loss. They may temporarily lose control over everyday activities as they depend on others for ADLs and for life-sustaining measures. Patients may believe they are useless and burdens to their families. At a life stage when independence is of great importance, they may be totally dependent on others.

Working through grief is a difficult, lifelong process for which the patient needs support and encouragement. Table 60-12 summarizes the grief response to SCI and appropriate nursing interventions. With recent advances in rehabilitation, the patient is often independent physically and discharged from the rehabilitation center before completing the grief process.

The goal of recovery is related more to adjustment than to acceptance. *Adjustment* implies the ability to go on with living with certain limitations. Although the patient who is cooperative and accepting is easier to treat, expect a wide fluctuation of emotions from a patient with SCI. Your role in grief work is to allow mourning as part of the rehabilitation process. Maintaining hope is important during the grieving process and should not be interpreted as denial.

When the patient is depressed, sympathy is not helpful. Treat the patient as an adult and encourage participation in care planning. A primary nurse relationship is helpful. Staff planning and sessions in which staff members can express their feelings help to provide consistency of care. To adjust, the patient needs continual support throughout the rehabilitation process in the form of acceptance, affection, and caring. Be attentive when the patient needs to talk and sensitive to needs at various stages of the grief process.

Although depression during the grief process usually lasts days to weeks, some individuals may become clinically depressed and require treatment for depression. Evaluation by a psychiatric nurse or psychiatrist is recommended. Treatment may include drugs and therapy. Treatment is maximized when the patient's personal preferences are identified and care is tailored to individual needs.

The patient's caregiver and family also require counseling to avoid promoting dependency in the patient through guilt or misplaced sympathy. The family also experiences intense grieving. A support group of family members and friends of patients with SCI can help family members increase their participation and knowledge of the grieving process, physical difficulties, rehabilitation plan, and meaning of the disability.

**TABLE 60-12 Grief Response in Spinal Cord Injury**

| Patient Behavior | Nursing Intervention |
|---|---|
| **Shock and Denial** | |
| Struggle for survival, complete dependence, excessive sleep, withdrawal, fantasies, unrealistic expectations | • Provide honest information.<br>• Use simple diagrams to explain injury.<br>• Encourage patient to begin road to recovery.<br>• Establish agreement to use and improve all current abilities while not denying the possibility of future improvement. |
| **Anger** | |
| Refusal to discuss paralysis, decreased self-esteem, manipulation, hostile and abusive language | • Coordinate care with patient and encourage self-care.<br>• Support family members.<br>• Use humor appropriately.<br>• Allow patient outbursts of emotions.<br>• Do not allow fixation on injury. |
| **Depression** | |
| Sadness, pessimism, anorexia, nightmares, insomnia, agitation, "blues," suicidal preoccupation, refusal to participate in any self-care activities | • Encourage family involvement and use of community resources.<br>• Plan graded steps in rehabilitation to give success with minimal opportunity for frustration.<br>• Give cheerful and willing assistance with ADLs.<br>• Avoid sympathy.<br>• Use firm kindness. |
| **Adjustment and Acceptance** | |
| Planning for future, actively participating in therapy, finding personal meaning in experience and continuation of growth, returning to premorbid personality. | • Remember patients have unique personalities.<br>• Balance support systems to encourage independence.<br>• Set goals with patient input.<br>• Emphasize potential. |

## ◆ Evaluation

Expected outcomes are that the patient with SCI will:

- Maintain adequate ventilation and have no signs of respiratory distress
- Maintain adequate circulation and BP
- Maintain intact skin over bony prominences
- Maintain adequate nutrition
- Establish a bowel management program based on neurologic function and personal preference
- Establish a bladder management program based on neurologic function, caregiver status, and lifestyle choices
- Experience no episodes of autonomic hyperreflexia

Additional information on expected outcomes for the patient with SCI is addressed in eNursing Care Plan 60-1 available on the website for this chapter.

## Gerontologic Considerations: Spinal Cord Injury

Because of the aging population and increased work and recreational activities among older adults, more of them experience SCI (Fig. 60-10). Falls are the leading cause of SCI for people age 65 years and older. Older adults with traumatic injuries experience more complications than younger patients, are hospitalized longer, and have higher mortality rates.

Demographics of people living with SCI are changing. Given their longer life spans, an increasing number of older adults are now living with SCI. Chronic illnesses associated with aging can also have a serious impact on these older adults. As patients with SCI age, both individual aging changes and length of time since injury can affect functional ability. For example, bowel and bladder dysfunction can increase with the duration and severity of SCI.

Health promotion and screening are important for the older patient with SCI. Daily skin inspections and UTI prevention measures are critical. Regular breast examinations for women and prostate cancer screening for men are recommended. Cardiovascular disease is the most common cause of morbidity and mortality among older adults with SCI. The lack of sensation, including chest pain, in people with high-level injuries may mask acute myocardial ischemia. Altered autonomic nervous system function and decreases in physical activity can place patients at risk for cardiovascular problems, including hypertension.

To decrease the risk of injury, instruct patients and caregivers on fall prevention strategies. For example, remove loose rugs from the floor, use a step stool or a long-handled reacher to access high shelves, and install handrails on stairs.

Rehabilitation for the older person with SCI may take longer because of preexisting conditions and poorer health status at the time of initial injury. An interprofessional team approach to rehabilitation is essential in preventing secondary complications associated with SCI, especially in older adults.

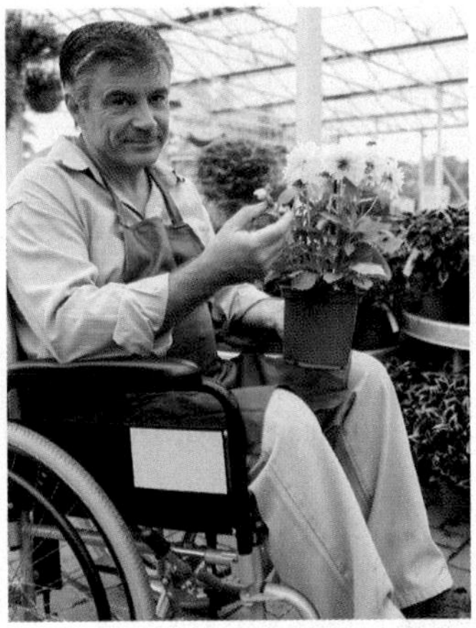

**FIG. 60-10** An increasing number of older adults are living with a chronic spinal cord injury. (©WavebreakmediaLtd/WavebreakMedia/Thinkstock)

## SPINAL CORD TUMORS

Spinal cord tumors can have a devastating impact due to spinal compression and neurologic dysfunction. Tumors are classified as *primary* (arising from some component of spinal cord, dura, nerves, or vessels) or *secondary* (from primary growths in other places in the body that have metastasized to the spinal cord).[25,26]

### Etiology and Pathophysiology

Spinal cord tumors are further classified as *extradural* (outside the dura), *intradural extramedullary* (between the spinal cord and dura), and *intramedullary* (within the substance of spinal cord itself) (Fig. 60-11, Table 60-13).

Extradural tumors account for about 60% of all spinal tumors. They include metastatic cancer and benign schwannomas. Many patients with cancer have metastasis to the spine.[27] These metastatic lesions can invade intradurally and compress the spinal cord. Tumors that commonly metastasize to the spinal epidural space are those that spread to bone, such as prostate, breast, lung, and kidney cancer.

Because many spinal cord tumors are slow growing, their symptoms are due to the mechanical effects of slow compression

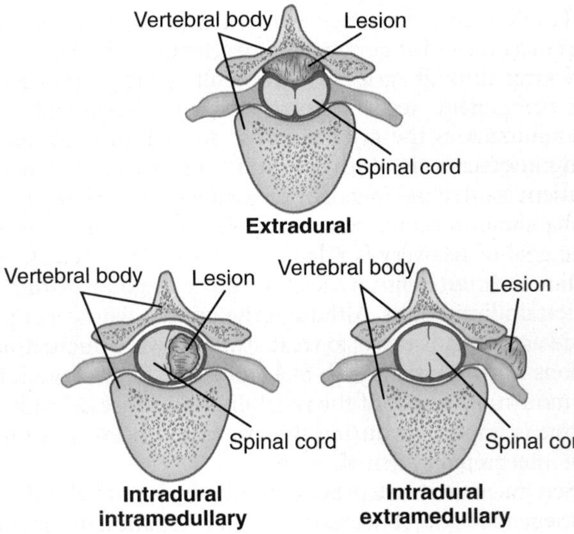


**FIG. 60-11** Types of spinal cord tumors.

**TABLE 60-13 Classification of Spinal Cord Tumors**

| Type | Incidence | Treatment | Prognosis |
|---|---|---|---|
| **Extradural** | | | |
| Outside spinal cord in extradural space | Metastatic lesions and benign schwannomas | Relief of cord pressure by surgical laminectomy, radiation, chemotherapy, or combination approach. | *Benign:* Excellent with resection. *Metastatic:* Poor. Treatment usually palliative. |
| **Intradural Extramedullary** | | | |
| Within dura mater but outside spinal cord | Mostly benign. Meningiomas, neurofibromas, and schwannomas | Complete surgical removal of tumor (if possible). Partial removal followed by radiation. | Usually very good if no damage to cord from compression. |
| **Intramedullary** | | | |
| Within spinal cord | Mostly benign Astrocytomas, ependymomas | Complete surgical removal of tumor (if possible). Partial removal followed by radiation. | Usually very good if no damage to cord from compression. Complete surgical resection of astrocytomas difficult. |

and irritation of nerve roots, displacement of the spinal cord, or gradual obstruction of the vascular supply. The slowness of growth does not cause autodestruction (secondary injury) as in traumatic SCI. Thus complete functional restoration may be possible when the tumor is removed.

### Clinical Manifestations

Both sensory and motor problems may result, with the location and extent of the tumor determining the severity and extent of the problem. The most common early symptom of a spinal cord tumor is back pain or pain radiating along the compressed nerve route. Location of the pain depends on the level of compression. Pain may worsen with activity, coughing, straining, and/or lying down. Motor disturbance may also occur as slowly increasing clumsiness, weakness, and spasticity. Paralysis can develop. Sensory disruption is later marked by coldness, numbness, and tingling in one or more extremities. Bladder disturbances are marked by urgency with difficulty in starting the flow, progressing to retention with overflow incontinence.

## NURSING AND INTERPROFESSIONAL MANAGEMENT: SPINAL CORD TUMORS

Extradural tumors can be seen on routine spinal x-rays, whereas intradural extramedullary and intramedullary tumors require MRI, CT scan, or CT myelogram for detection. Cerebrospinal fluid (CSF) analysis may reveal tumor cells. Patients with tumors suspicious for metastatic disease will require an oncology referral and further diagnostic testing to identify the primary cancer.

Compression of the spinal cord is an emergency. Relief of ischemia related to compression is the goal of therapy. Corticosteroids are generally prescribed immediately to relieve tumor-related edema. Dexamethasone, often in large doses, may also be administered to treat edema.

Indications for surgery depend on the type of tumor and neurologic deficit. Emergency surgery may be needed to decompress the spinal cord, obtain tissue for pathology, and help to determine appropriate adjunctive treatment.[28] Primary spinal tumors may be removed with the goal of cure. In patients with metastatic tumors, treatment is primarily palliative, with the goal of restoring or preserving neurologic function, stabilizing the spine, and alleviating pain. Radiation and/or chemotherapy may be used to treat the tumor.

Relieving pain and maximizing neurologic function are the ultimate goals of treatment. Assess the patient's neurologic status before and after treatment. Administering analgesia as needed is an important nursing responsibility. Depending on the amount of neurologic dysfunction, care of the patient may be similar to that of a patient recovering from SCI.

## CRANIAL NERVE DISORDERS

Cranial nerve disorders are commonly classified as peripheral neuropathies. The 12 pairs of cranial nerves are considered the peripheral nerves of the brain. The disorders usually involve the motor and/or sensory branches of a single nerve *(mononeuropathies)*. Causes of cranial nerve problems include tumors, trauma, infection, inflammatory processes, and unknown *(idiopathic)* causes. Two cranial nerve disorders discussed in this chapter are trigeminal neuralgia and Bell's palsy.

## TRIGEMINAL NEURALGIA

**Trigeminal neuralgia (TN)** *(tic douloureux)* is characterized by sudden, usually unilateral, severe, brief, stabbing, recurrent episodes of pain in the distribution of the trigeminal nerve. It is diagnosed in about 12 per 100,000 Americans each year and occurs approximately twice as often in women as in men. More than 90% of cases are diagnosed in people over the age of 50 years.[29]

TN is classified as *classic* (TN 1) or *atypical* (TN 2). Patients may experience both types. Although this condition is considered benign, pain intensity and lifestyle disruption can cause marked physical and psychologic dysfunction (even suicide).

### Etiology and Pathophysiology

The trigeminal nerve (CN V) has both motor and sensory branches. The sensory (afferent) branches of the second and third division (maxillary and mandibular branches) of CN V are most often affected in TN[30] (Fig. 60-12).

The majority of cases result from vascular compression of the trigeminal nerve root by an abnormal loop of the superior cerebellar artery. This artery compresses the nerve as it exits the brainstem. Constant compression of the blood vessel appears to lead to chronic injury, causing demyelination of the nerve and impairment of the nociceptive system.[31] In some cases, TN may be secondary to underlying pathology, such as multiple sclerosis, shingles, or masses in the cerebellum or brainstem.

### Clinical Manifestations

The first episode of TN is sudden with a memorable onset. Diagnosis is based almost entirely on history. In TN 1, the patient experiences an abrupt onset of paroxysms of excruciating pain described as a burning, knifelike, or lightning-like

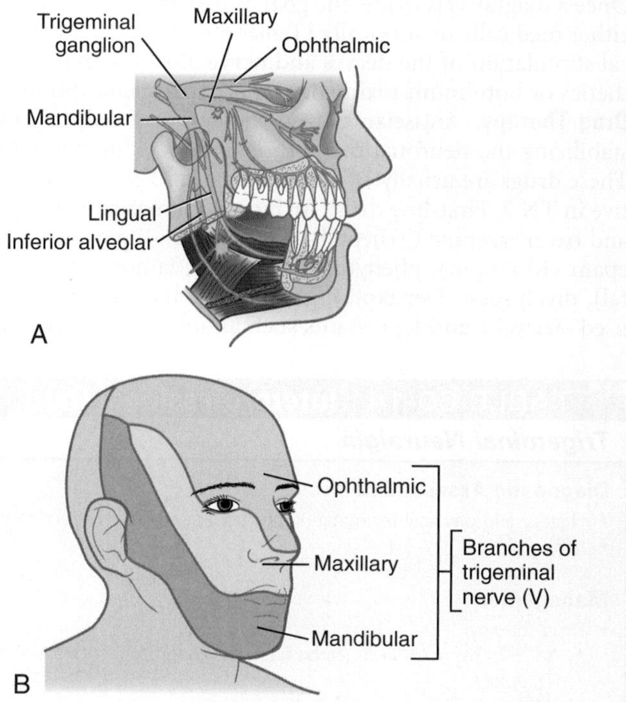


**FIG. 60-12** **A,** Trigeminal nerve (CNV) and its three main divisions: ophthalmic, maxillary, and mandibular nerves. **B,** Cutaneous innervation of the head. (Modified from Patton KT, Thibodeau GA: *Anatomy and physiology,* ed 8, St Louis, 2013, Mosby.)

shock in the lips, upper or lower gums, cheek, forehead, or side of the nose. Intense pain, facial twitching, grimacing, and frequent blinking and tearing of the eye occur during the acute attack (giving rise to the term *tic douloureux*). Some patients may also experience facial sensory loss. Attacks are usually brief, lasting only seconds to 2 or 3 minutes, and are unilateral.

Recurrences are unpredictable and may occur several times a day, or weeks or months apart. After the pain-free *(refractory)* period, a phenomenon known as *clustering* can occur. Clustering is characterized by a cycle of pain and refractoriness that continues for hours.

Painful episodes are usually initiated by a triggering mechanism of light touch at a specific point *(trigger zone)* along the distribution of the nerve branches. Precipitating stimuli include chewing, brushing the teeth, feeling a hot or cold blast of air on the face, washing the face, yawning, or even talking. As a result, the patient may eat improperly, neglect hygienic practices, wear a cloth over the face, and withdraw from interaction with others. The patient may sleep excessively as a means of coping with pain.

TN 2 is distinguished by constant aching, burning, crushing, or stabbing pain. The pain has a lower intensity and does not subside completely. The distinct attacks associated with TN 1 do not occur in TN 2.

### Diagnostic Studies

MRI with or without contrast is used to rule out other causes of pain, such as sinusitis, extracranial and cavernous sinus masses, cancer, multiple sclerosis, brain lesions in the thalamus or brainstem, or masses in the cerebellopontine angle.[32] A complete neurologic assessment is done, including audiologic evaluation. Results are usually normal.

### Interprofessional Care

Once a diagnosis is made, the goal of treatment is relief of pain either medically or surgically (Tables 60-14 and 60-15). Electrical stimulation of the nerves and nerve blocks with local anesthetics or botulinum toxin (Botox) are treatment options.

**Drug Therapy.** Antiseizure drug therapy may reduce pain by stabilizing the neuronal membrane and blocking nerve firing. These drugs are usually effective in treating TN 1 but less effective in TN 2. First-line drugs include carbamazepine (Tegretol) and oxcarbazepine (Trileptal). Topiramate (Topamax), clonazepam (Klonopin), phenytoin (Dilantin), lamotrigine (Lamictal), divalproex (Depakote), gabapentin, and baclofen may be used. Tricyclic antidepressants such as amitriptyline (Elavil) or nortriptyline (Pamelor) can be used to treat constant burning or aching pain. Analgesics or opioids are usually not effective in controlling pain in TN1 but may help with pain in TN2.

**Surgical Therapy.** If a conservative approach is ineffective or the patient is unable to tolerate adverse effects of medications, surgical therapy is available (Table 60-15). In percutaneous procedures, affected nerve fibers are damaged to eliminate pain. Although most patients are pain free after any of the procedures, pain relief lasts longer with microvascular decompression. Recurrence rates are about 50% at 1 year.[30-32]

## NURSING MANAGEMENT: TRIGEMINAL NEURALGIA

The patient with trigeminal neuralgia is primarily treated as an outpatient. Assess the attacks in detail, including triggering factors, characteristics, frequency, and pain management techniques. This information helps you to plan patient care. Include

**TABLE 60-14 Interprofessional Care**

***Trigeminal Neuralgia***

**Diagnostic Assessment**
- History and physical examination (including neurologic examination)
- MRI

**Management**
- Drug therapy
  - Antiseizure drugs (e.g., carbamazepine [Tegretol], oxcarbazepine [Trileptal])
  - gabapentin (Neurontin)
  - Tricyclic antidepressants (e.g., amitriptyline)
- Local nerve block
- Surgical therapy (Table 60-15)

**TABLE 60-15 Surgical Therapy for Trigeminal Neuralgia**

| Procedure | Description |
|---|---|
| **Percutaneous Procedures** | |
| Glycerol rhizotomy (injection into one or more branches of trigeminal nerve) (Fig. 60-13) | • Thin needle inserted through puncture in cheek and guided through natural opening in base of skull.<br>• Glycerol injected into trigeminal ganglion.<br>• Procedure can be repeated multiple times. |
| Percutaneous radiofrequency rhizotomy | • Needle passed through cheek thorough a natural opening in base of skull.<br>• Patient is awakened and a small electric current is passed through the needled causing tingling.<br>• When the needle is positioned so the tingling occurs in the same area of pain, patient is sedated again and radiofrequency current is used to destroy part of the nerve.<br>• Can result in facial numbness (although some degree of sensation may be retained), corneal anesthesia, and trigeminal motor weakness |
| Balloon compression | • Cannula is inserted through cheek and guided to a natural opening in the base of skull.<br>• Soft catheter with a balloon tip is threaded through cannula.<br>• Balloon is inflated and mechanical compression damages trigeminal nerve |
| **Surgical Procedures** | |
| Microvascular decompression (open surgery) | • Small craniotomy is first performed behind the ear (suboccipital craniotomy).<br>• Blood vessels that appear to be compressing the nerve at the root entry zone where it exits the pons are then displaced and repositioned. |
| Gamma knife radiosurgery | • Uses stereotactic localization to focus high doses of radiation to area where trigeminal nerve exits the brainstem.<br>• Radiation causes slow formation of a lesion on nerve and disrupts transmission of pain signals to brain.<br>• Pain relief from this procedure may take several months. (Radiosurgery is discussed in Chapter 56.) |

A

B

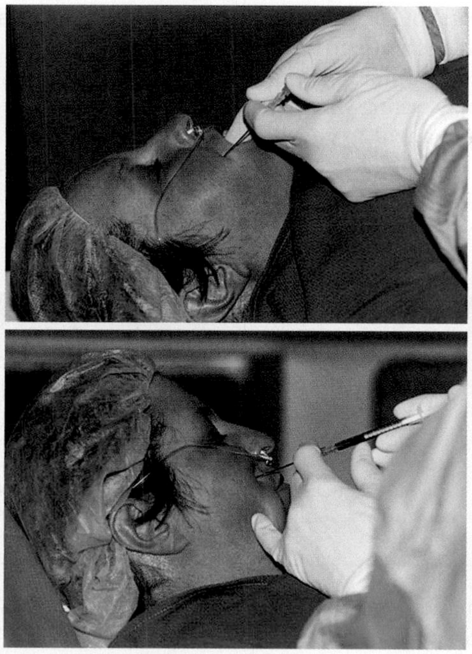

**FIG. 60-13** Glycerol rhizotomy for the treatment of trigeminal neuralgia. **A,** Patient with trigeminal neuralgia having needle placed. **B,** Physician injecting glycerol. (Courtesy Joe Rothrock, Media, Pa.)

the patient's nutritional status, hygiene (especially oral), and behavior (including withdrawal). Evaluate the degree of pain and its effects on the patient's lifestyle, drug use, emotional state, and suicidal tendencies.

Monitor the patient's response to drug therapy and note any side effects. Discuss alternative pain management measures, such as acupuncture, biofeedback, and yoga. Environmental assessment is essential during an acute period to decrease triggering stimuli. The room should be kept at an even, moderate temperature and free of drafts. The patient may prefer to complete all self-care activities, fearing someone else will inadvertently cause injury.

Teach the patient about the importance of nutrition, hygiene, and oral care, and convey understanding if previous oral neglect is apparent. A small, soft-bristled toothbrush or a warm mouthwash assists in promoting oral care. Hygiene activities are best performed when analgesia is at its peak.

Encourage food that is high in protein and calories and easy to chew. It should be served lukewarm and offered frequently. If oral intake is sharply reduced and the patient's nutritional status is compromised, a nasogastric tube can be inserted on the unaffected side for enteral feedings.

Appropriate teaching related to surgical procedures depends on the type of procedure planned (e.g., percutaneous). The patient needs to know he or she will be awake during local procedures in order to cooperate when corneal and ciliary reflexes and facial sensations are checked. After the procedure, compare the patient's pain with the preoperative intensity. Evaluate the corneal reflex, extraocular muscles, hearing, sensation, and facial nerve function frequently (see Chapter 55). If the corneal reflex is impaired, take special care to protect the eyes. This includes using artificial tears or eye shields.

After a percutaneous radiofrequency procedure, apply an ice pack to the jaw on the operative side for 3 to 5 hours. To avoid injuring the mouth, the patient should not chew on the operative side until sensation has returned.

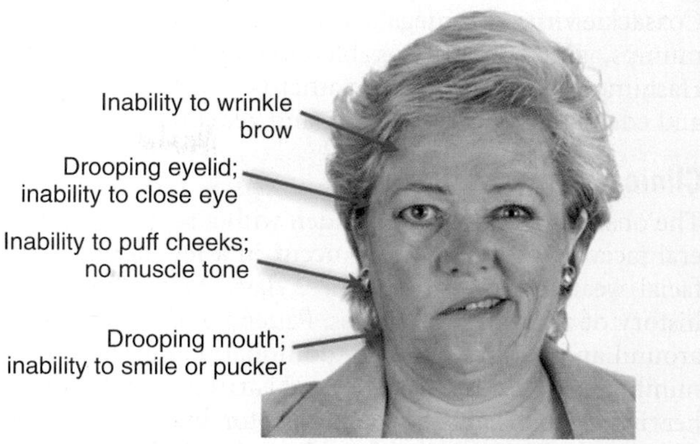


**FIG. 60-14** Facial characteristics of a person with Bell's palsy. (©Jo Ann Snover/123RF Stock Photo/123rf.com)

If intracranial surgery is performed, general postoperative nursing care after a craniotomy is appropriate. (Nursing care related to craniotomy is discussed in Chapter 56 on pp. 1337-1338.)

Plan for regular follow-up care, and instruct the patient on the dosage and side effects of medications. Although pain may be relieved, encourage the patient to keep environmental stimuli to a moderate level and to use stress management techniques. Long-term management after surgical intervention depends on residual effects of the procedure. If anesthesia is present or the corneal reflex is altered, teach the patient to (1) chew on the unaffected side; (2) avoid hot foods or beverages, which can burn the mucous membranes; (3) check the oral cavity after meals to remove food particles; (4) practice meticulous oral hygiene and continue with semiannual dental visits; (5) protect the face against extremes of temperature; (6) use an electric razor; (7) wear a protective eye shield and avoid rubbing eyes; and (8) examine eye regularly for symptoms of infection or irritation.

## BELL'S PALSY

**Bell's palsy** is an acute peripheral facial paresis of unknown cause. As the most common facial nerve disorder, it is characterized by inflammation of the facial nerve (CN VII) on one side of the face in the absence of any other disease (e.g., stroke).

Each year about 40,000 Americans are diagnosed with Bell's palsy. It is evenly distributed between men and women and can affect any age group, with peak incidence usually between ages 15 and 50 years.[33] Susceptible groups include women in the third trimester of pregnancy and early postpartum, older adults, and people with diabetes or hypothyroidism.

Bell's palsy is considered benign, and most patients recover spontaneously within 3 weeks to 9 months. One third of patients may have residual effects of facial weakness, involuntary movements, and persistent tearing of the eye on the affected side.[34]

### Etiology and Pathophysiology

Although the exact etiology is not known, several theories exist as to the underlying cause. One suggested mechanism is acute demyelination similar to Guillain-Barré disease. The most strongly supported cause is reactivation of herpes simplex virus isoform (HSV-1) and/or herpes zoster virus (HZV). The viral infection causes inflammation, leading to nerve compression and clinical features such as facial paralysis (Fig. 60-14). Other known documented infectious causes include adenovirus,

Coxsackie virus, cytomegalovirus, Epstein-Barr virus, influenza, mumps, and rubella. Possible noninfectious causes include Hashimoto's encephalopathy, atherosclerosis (causing ischemia and edema of the facial nerve), and genetic factors.

### Clinical Manifestations

The onset of Bell's palsy is sudden with a rapid onset of unilateral facial weakness that can occur in a few hours. Maximum facial weakness is seen within 2 days. Many patients have a history of a recent viral illness. Patients may complain of pain around and behind the ear. Additional manifestations include numbness of the face, tongue, and ear; tinnitus; headache; and hearing deficit. Paralysis of the motor branches of the facial nerve typically results in flaccidity of the affected side of the face, with drooping of the mouth accompanied by drooling.

*Bell's phenomenon*, an inability to close the eyelid with an upward movement of the eyeball when closure is attempted, is a hallmark sign of Bell's palsy. Other manifestations include a widened *palpebral fissure* (opening between the eyelids); flattening of the nasolabial fold; and inability to smile, frown, or whistle. Unilateral loss of taste is common. Decreased muscle movement may alter chewing ability. Although some patients experience a loss of tearing, many patients complain of excessive tearing. Muscle weakness causes the lower lid to turn out, allowing overflow of normal tear production. Pain may occur behind the ear on the affected side, especially before onset of paralysis.

Complications include psychologic withdrawal because of changes in appearance, malnutrition, dehydration, mucous membrane trauma, corneal abrasions, muscle stretching, and facial spasms and contractures.

### Diagnostic Studies

Diagnosis of Bell's palsy is by exclusion. No definitive diagnostic test exists. The diagnosis and prognosis are indicated by observing the typical pattern of onset and signs, and testing percutaneous nerve excitability by electromyography (EMG). MRI and CT can eliminate other causes for facial paralysis. Blood tests can be used to diagnose infections or other diseases. Patients should be referred to a neurologist or otolaryngologist as soon as possible to exclude other neurologic conditions.

### Interprofessional Care

Treatment of Bell's palsy includes moist heat, gentle massage, electrical stimulation of the nerve, and prescribed exercises. Stimulation may maintain muscle tone and prevent atrophy. Care is primarily focused on relief of symptoms, prevention of complications, and protection of the eye on the affected side.

Corticosteroids are started immediately, with best results if they are initiated before paralysis is complete. When the patient improves to the point that corticosteroids are no longer necessary, the drug should be tapered over a 2-week period. Treatment with antivirals, such as acyclovir (Zovirax), valacyclovir (Valtrex), and famciclovir (Famvir), has not been effective in the management of Bell's palsy. Surgical decompression of the facial nerve remains controversial and is considered in refractory cases.

## NURSING MANAGEMENT: BELL'S PALSY

The patient with Bell's palsy is treated as an outpatient. Mild analgesics can relieve pain. Hot wet packs can reduce the discomfort of herpetic lesions, aid circulation, and relieve pain. Tell the patient to protect the face from cold and drafts because trigeminal *hyperesthesia* (extreme sensitivity to pain or touch) may occur. Maintenance of good nutrition is important. Teach the patient to chew on the unaffected side of the mouth to avoid trapping food and to enjoy the taste of food. Thorough oral hygiene must be performed after each meal to prevent parotitis, caries, and periodontal disease from accumulated residual food.

#### CHECK YOUR PRACTICE

You are working in the outpatient neurology clinic. Your patient is a 68-yr-old woman who has been diagnosed with Bell's palsy. Her primary complaint today is dry eyes. When you are doing an assessment, she tells you, "I hate the way I look. I cannot go anywhere and I am afraid to leave the house. I am ugly and scary looking."

- How can you help her cope with her disorder?
- What will you suggest to decrease moisture loss in the eye on the affected side?

The patient may wear dark glasses for protective and cosmetic reasons. Artificial tears (methylcellulose) should be instilled frequently during the day to prevent drying of the cornea. Ointment and an impermeable eye shield can be used at night to retain moisture. Taping the lids closed at night may be needed to provide protection. Instruct the patient to report ocular pain, drainage, or discharge.

A facial sling may be helpful to support affected muscles, improve lip alignment, and facilitate eating. The facial sling is usually made and fitted by a physical or occupational therapist. When function begins to return, active facial muscle exercises should be performed several times a day.

The change in physical appearance as a result of Bell's palsy can be devastating. Reassure the patient that a stroke did not occur and that chances for a full recovery are good. Enlisting support from family and friends is important. Tell the patient most people recover within 3 to 6 months after onset of symptoms.

# POLYNEUROPATHIES

## GUILLAIN-BARRÉ SYNDROME

**Guillain-Barré syndrome (GBS)** is characterized by an autoimmune process that occurs a few days or weeks following a viral or bacterial infection.[35] GBS is a collection of clinical syndromes that manifest as acute inflammatory polyneuropathy. The most common type of GBS diagnosed in the United States is **acute inflammatory demyelinating polyneuropathy (AIDP)**. GBS is rare, affecting approximately 1 person in every 100,000.[36,37]

The main features of GBS include acute, ascending, rapidly progressive, symmetric weakness of the limbs. Maximal weakness is reached in 4 weeks. Reflexes in the affected limbs are weak or absent. Respiratory muscles may also be affected and some patients require mechanical ventilation.

### Etiology and Pathophysiology

The etiology of this syndrome is unknown. Both cellular and humoral immune mechanisms play a role in the immune reaction directed at the nerves. The result is segmental loss of myelin with edema and inflammation of affected nerves. As demyelination occurs, transmission of nerve impulses is stopped or slowed. Muscles innervated by the damaged peripheral nerves undergo denervation and atrophy. In the recovery phase, remyelination occurs slowly, and neurologic function returns in a proximal-to-distal pattern.

Most cases of GBS follow viral or bacterial infection of the gastrointestinal or upper respiratory tract. Cytomegalovirus is the most common viral cause. *Campylobacter jejuni* gastroenteritis is the most common bacterial cause. Surgery and trauma may also trigger GBS.

### Clinical Manifestations and Complications

GBS is a heterogeneous condition with manifestations ranging from mild to severe. The first symptoms are pain, *paresthesia* (numbness and tingling) and *hypotonia* (reduced muscle tone) of the limbs. *Areflexia* (lack of reflexes), and weakness or paralysis of the limbs usually peak within 4 weeks. Autonomic nervous system dysfunction results, with manifestations of orthostatic hypotension, hypertension, and abnormal vagal responses (bradycardia, heart block, asystole).

Other autonomic dysfunctions include bowel and bladder dysfunction, facial flushing, and diaphoresis. Cranial nerve involvement is manifested as facial weakness and paresthesia, extraocular eye movement difficulties, and dysphagia.

Pain is a common symptom in the patient with GBS. It can include paresthesia, muscular aches and cramps, and hyperesthesia, and appears to be worse at night. Pain may contribute to decreased appetite and may interfere with sleep.

The most serious complication of GBS is respiratory failure, which occurs as the paralysis progresses to nerves that innervate the thoracic area. Assess the respiratory system frequently by checking respiratory rate and depth to determine the need for immediate intervention, including intubation and mechanical ventilation. Respiratory infection or UTI may occur. Immobility from paralysis can cause paralytic ileus, muscle atrophy, VTE, pressure ulcers, orthostatic hypotension, and nutritional deficiencies.

### Diagnostic Studies

Diagnosis is based primarily on the patient's history and clinical signs. Clinical features required for diagnosis include progressive weakness of more than one limb and diminished or absent reflexes. CSF analysis is helpful in excluding other causes. In GBS, the CSF has more protein than normal. EMG and nerve conduction studies are used to confirm the diagnosis.

## NURSING AND PROFESSIONAL MANAGEMENT: GUILLAIN-BARRÉ SYNDROME

Management of GBS is interprofessional and is aimed at supportive care. Ventilatory support is critical during the acute phase, as 30% of GBS cases progress to respiratory failure.[35] Patients are admitted to ICU for hemodynamic monitoring.

Immunomodulating treatments such as plasma exchange *(plasmapheresis)* or high-dose IV immunoglobulin *(IV Ig)* are most effective if administered to patients within the first 2 weeks of symptom onset. They are equally effective. Plasmapheresis removes antibodies and other immune factors. It is used five times either daily or every other day in the first 2 weeks. (Plasmapheresis is discussed in Chapter 13.) IV Ig interferes with antigen presentation and is given over 5 days. Because it is more readily available, it has replaced plasmapheresis as the preferred treatment in many centers.[37] Beyond 4 weeks after disease onset, plasmapheresis and IV Ig therapies have little value. Corticosteroids appear to have little effect on the prognosis or duration of the disease.

Assessment of the patient is the most important aspect of nursing care during the acute phase. During the neurologic assessment, evaluate motor and sensory function. Report changes in motor function (e.g., ascending paralysis), reflexes, cranial nerve function (e.g., gag, cornea, swallow), and level of consciousness.

Carefully assess respiratory and cardiac function. Monitor arterial blood gases (ABGs) and vital capacity. Closely monitor BP and cardiac rate and rhythm during the acute phase because dysrhythmias may occur. Autonomic dysfunction commonly occurs, including tachycardia, bradycardia, hypertension, hypotension, abnormal sweating, and paralytic ileus.[37] Orthostatic hypotension secondary to muscle atony may occur in severe cases. Vasopressor agents and volume expanders may be needed to treat low BP. If fever develops, obtain sputum and blood cultures to identify the pathogen. Appropriate antibiotic therapy is then initiated.

Nutritional needs must be met in spite of possible problems associated with delayed gastric emptying, paralytic ileus, and potential for aspiration if the gag reflex is lost. In addition to testing for the gag reflex, note drooling and other difficulties with secretions that may indicate an inadequate gag reflex. Initially, enteral or parenteral nutrition may be used to ensure adequate caloric intake. Because of delayed gastric emptying, assess residual volumes of the feedings at regular intervals or before feedings (see Chapter 39).

Throughout the course of the illness, provide support and encouragement to the patient, caregiver, and family. Early referral should be made to physical, occupational, and speech therapists. Counseling may help the patient adjust to the sudden disabling syndrome and dependence on others.

Most patients with GBS will start to recover spontaneously at about 28 days. Although 80% of patients almost completely recover, the process is slow and takes months or years. About 65% of patients have minor residual signs or symptoms.[35] Older age, rapid onset, and mechanical ventilation are associated with poor prognosis.

## CHRONIC INFLAMMATORY DEMYELINATING POLYNEUROPATHY (CIDP)

**Chronic inflammatory demyelinating polyneuropathy (CIDP)** is a motor and sensory neuropathy. CIDP is a rare autoimmune disorder with a prevalence of 1.5 to 3.6 in a million people.[38] Similar to GBS, there are different types of CIDP. It occurs more than twice as often in men as is women and develops primarily when people are in their 60s and 70s.[39]

CIDP differs from GBS as the symptoms gradually occur over 8 weeks and there is not an acute onset. Also unlike GBS, CIDP is not self-limiting (with an end to the acute phase). If untreated, 30% of CIDP patients will progress to wheelchair dependence.[38] Early recognition and treatment can help the patient avoid significant disability.

### Etiology and Pathophysiology

The cause of CIDP is unclear. Although it is considered an autoimmune disease, no causative antigens have been found. It is unclear if CIDP is associated with a previous illness. It may be associated with infection, HIV, hepatitis C, Sjögren's syndrome, inflammatory bowel disease, melanoma, lymphoma, diabetes mellitus, and types of monoclonal gammopathy.

### Clinical Manifestations and Diagnostic Studies

Patients with CIDP have a similar clinical presentation to GBS, with symmetric weakness in the arms and legs, impaired sensation, paresthesia, and absent or diminished reflexes. However, development of CIDP symptoms occurs gradually over a period of at least 8 weeks. This is an important difference as patients may be diagnosed with GBS and the confusion may lead to incorrect or delayed treatment. Unlike GBS, CIDP does not automatically resolve. Most patients with GBS can walk without help within three months. Patients with CIDP require maintenance therapy to prevent relapse.[40]

CIDP assessment and diagnosis are similar to GBD. CSF demonstrates elevated protein levels. MRI may show changes. Key identifying features of CIDP include nerve conduction block and slowed conduction velocity, suggestive of demyelination.[41] Nerve biopsy shows unequivocal evidence of demyelination or remyelination.

## ❖ NURSING AND INTERPROFESSIONAL MANAGEMENT: CIDP

Early recognition and diagnosis of the syndrome are key to reducing permanent disability. The goal of treatment is to halt the immune response and stop nerve inflammation and demyelination. Unlike GBS, corticosteroids are recommended for all patients with CIDP and considered standard therapy. Additionally, IV Ig or plasmapheresis may be used. They have been shown to be equally effective, so the treatment decision is based on personal preference, cost, and availability.[37] Chemotherapy and immunosuppressive agents have also been used to treat CIDP.

Regardless of the treatment, patients continue on therapy until maximum clinical improvement is achieved or until they reach a clinical plateau. Patients will require maintenance therapy to prevent relapse or progression.[41] Appropriate referrals to rehabilitation should be made early to promote maximum recovery.

## TETANUS

**Tetanus** (lockjaw) is a severe infection of the nervous system affecting spinal and cranial nerves. It results from the effects of a potent neurotoxin released by the anaerobic bacillus *Clostridium tetani.* The spores of the bacillus are present in soil, garden mold, and manure. *C. tetani* enters the body through a wound that provides an appropriate low-$O_2$ environment for organisms to mature and produce toxin. Examples of possible wounds include IV drug use injection sites, human and animal bites, cuts from stepping on nails, gardening injuries, burns, frostbite, open fractures, and gunshot wounds.

Initial manifestations of tetanus include stiffness in the jaw *(trismus)* and neck and signs of infection (e.g., fever). As the disease progresses, the neck muscles, back, abdomen, and extremities become progressively rigid. In severe forms, continuous tonic seizures may occur with *opisthotonos* (extreme arching of the back and retraction of the head). Laryngeal and respiratory spasms cause apnea and anoxia. The slightest noise, jarring motion, or bright light can cause a seizure. These seizures are agonizingly painful. Mortality rate is almost 100% in the severe form.[42]

Tetanus prevention and immunizations, which are the most important factors influencing the incidence of this disease, are summarized in Table 68-6. Adults should receive a tetanus and diphtheria toxoid booster every 10 years. Teach the patient that immediate, thorough cleansing of all wounds with soap and water is important to prevent tetanus. If an open wound occurs and the patient has not been immunized within 5 years, the HCP should be contacted so that a tetanus booster can be given.

The management of tetanus includes administration of a tetanus toxoid, diphtheria toxoid, and pertussis (Tdap) booster and tetanus immune globulin (TIG) in different sites before the onset of symptoms to neutralize circulating toxins (see Table 68-6). A much larger dose of TIG is administered to patients with clinical manifestations of tetanus.

Control of spasms is essential and is managed by sedation and skeletal muscle relaxation, usually with diazepam (Valium), barbiturates, and, in severe cases, neuromuscular blocking agents that act to paralyze skeletal muscles. Opioid analgesics such as morphine or fentanyl are also indicated for pain management. A 10-14 day course of penicillin, metronidazole, tetracycline, or doxycycline is recommended to inhibit further growth of *C. tetani.*

Because of laryngospasm and the potential need for neuromuscular-blocking drugs, a tracheostomy is usually performed early and the patient is maintained on mechanical ventilation. Sedative agents and opioid analgesics are given concomitantly to all patients who are pharmacologically paralyzed. Any recognized wound should be debrided or an abscess drained. Antibiotics may be given to prevent secondary infections.

## BOTULISM

**Botulism** is rare but the most serious type of food poisoning. It is caused by gastrointestinal (GI) absorption of the neurotoxin produced by *Clostridium botulinum.* This organism is found in the soil, and the spores are difficult to destroy. It can grow in any food contaminated with the spores.

Improper home canning of foods is often the cause. It is thought that the neurotoxin destroys or inhibits the neurotransmission of acetylcholine at the myoneural junction, resulting in disturbed muscle innervation.

Neurologic manifestations can develop rapidly or evolve over several days. They include a descending paralysis with muscle incoordination and weakness, difficulty swallowing, seizures, and respiratory muscle weakness that can rapidly deteriorate to respiratory and/or cardiac arrest.

The clinical manifestations, prevention, and treatment are presented in Table 41-24. Patient and caregiving teaching related to food poisoning is presented in Table 41-25. Nursing care during the acute illness is similar to that for GBS. Supportive nursing interventions include rest, activities to maintain respiratory function, adequate nutrition, and prevention of loss of muscle mass.

## CASE STUDY

### *Spinal Cord Injury*

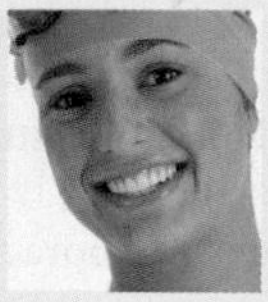

(©Comstock-Images/Stockbyte/Thinkstock)

**Patient Profile**

***Acute Phase***

S.W., an 18-yr-old white woman, is admitted to the emergency department with the diagnosis of a cervical SCI. S.W. was swimming at a neighbor's backyard pool. She dove into the shallow end, striking her head on the bottom of the pool. Her friends noticed she did not resurface. They rescued her and brought her to the side of the pool. They maintained neck immobilization until rescue crews arrived.

**Subjective Data**

- Awake and alert
- Complaining of neck pain
- Anxious and asking why she cannot move her legs
- Asking to see her family

**Objective Data**

***Physical Examination***

- Weak biceps movement bilaterally
- No triceps movement bilaterally
- Gross elbow movement present bilaterally
- No movement in bilateral lower extremities
- Decreased sensation from the shoulders down
- No bladder or bowel control
- BP 85/50 mm Hg; pulse 56 beats/min; respirations 32 breaths/min and labored

***Diagnostic Studies***

- CT C-spine shows C5 subluxation and compression fracture
- MRI C-spine shows severe spinal cord compression at C5-6

**Interprofessional Care**

- Intubated in the emergency department
- Started on mechanical ventilation
- Placed in tongs and traction on arrival to the ICU

**Discussion Questions (Acute Phase)**

1. ***Priority Decision:*** What nursing activities would be a priority on S.W.'s arrival in the ICU?
2. What physiologic problems are causing S.W. to have hypotension and bradycardia?
3. What would be the initial treatment for S.W.'s hypotension and bradycardia?
4. ***Safety:*** What signs and symptoms would indicate respiratory distress? What physiologic problem would cause respiratory distress in S.W.'s injury state?
5. ***Teamwork and Collaboration:*** What can the interprofessional team do to decrease S.W.'s anxiety?
6. ***Priority Decision:*** Based on the assessment data provided, what are the priority nursing diagnoses? What are the collaborative problems?
7. ***Teamwork and Collaboration:*** Identify activities that can be delegated to unlicensed assistive personnel (UAP).

**Patient Profile**

***Rehabilitation Phase***

S.W. is now 1 month postinjury and has been admitted to a local inpatient SCI rehabilitation facility. She has been extubated and uses a wheelchair to mobilize. She eats three meals a day with assistance and is on a strict bowel and bladder program.

**Subjective Data**

- Awake and alert but anxious
- Complaining of severe headache, blurred vision, and nausea

**Objective Data**

***Physical Examination***

- Flushed and diaphoretic above the level of injury
- No bowel movement for 2 days
- BP 235/106 mm Hg, pulse 32 beats/min, respirations 30 breaths/min and labored

**Discussion Questions (Rehabilitation Phase)**

1. ***Priority Decision:*** What initial priority nursing interventions would be appropriate?
2. What physiologic problem is causing S.W.'s hypertension and bradycardia?
3. Once the HCP has been notified, what other interventions would be appropriate?
4. ***Quality Improvement:*** What outcomes would indicate that nursing interventions were successful?
5. ***Priority Decision:*** Based on the assessment data provided, what are the priority nursing diagnoses?
6. ***Patient-Centered Care:*** Patient and family involvement in the rehabilitation process is vital. What teaching will you provide about bowel management?
7. ***Evidence-Based Practice:*** S.W. and her family are concerned about the risk of autonomic hyperreflexia. What effective strategies to prevent autonomic hyperreflexia would you discuss with the patient and family?

Answers available at *http://evolve.elsevier.com/Lewis/medsurg.*

## BRIDGE TO NCLEX EXAMINATION

The number of the question corresponds to the same-numbered outcome at the beginning of the chapter.

**1.** During rehabilitation, a patient with spinal cord injury begins to ambulate with long leg braces. Which level of injury does the nurse associate with this degree of recovery?
   **a.** L1-2
   **b.** T6-7
   **c.** T1-2
   **d.** C7-8

**2.** A patient with a T4 spinal cord injury experiences neurogenic shock as a result of sympathetic nervous system dysfunction. What would the nurse recognize as characteristic of this condition?
   **a.** Tachycardia
   **b.** Hypotension
   **c.** Increased cardiac output
   **d.** Peripheral vasoconstriction

**3.** A patient with spinal cord injury is experiencing severe neurologic deficits. What is the *most* likely mechanism of injury for this patient?
   **a.** Compression
   **b.** Hyperextension
   **c.** Flexion-rotation
   **d.** Extension-rotation

4. A patient with a C7 spinal cord injury undergoing rehabilitation tells the nurse he must have the flu because he has a bad headache and nausea. The nurse's *first priority* is to
   - **a.** call the HCP.
   - **b.** check the patient's temperature.
   - **c.** take the patient's blood pressure.
   - **d.** elevate the head of the bed to 90 degrees.
5. For a 65-year-old woman who has lived with a T1 spinal cord injury for 20 years, which health teaching instructions should the nurse emphasize?
   - **a.** A mammogram is needed every year.
   - **b.** Bladder function tends to improve with age.
   - **c.** Heart disease is not common in people with spinal cord injury.
   - **d.** As a person ages, the need to change body position is less important.
6. The most common early symptom of a spinal cord tumor is
   - **a.** urinary incontinence.
   - **b.** back pain that worsens with activity.
   - **c.** paralysis below the level of involvement.
   - **d.** impaired sensation of pain, temperature, and light touch.
7. During assessment of the patient with trigeminal neuralgia, the nurse should *(select all that apply)*
   - **a.** inspect all aspects of the mouth and teeth.
   - **b.** assess the gag reflex and respiratory rate and depth.
   - **c.** lightly palpate the affected side of the face for edema.
   - **d.** test for temperature and sensation perception on the face.
   - **e.** ask the patient to describe factors that initiate an episode.
8. During routine assessment of a patient with Guillain-Barré syndrome, the nurse finds the patient is short of breath. The patient's respiratory distress is caused by
   - **a.** elevated protein in the CSF.
   - **b.** immobility resulting from ascending paralysis.
   - **c.** degeneration of motor neurons in the brainstem and spinal cord.
   - **d.** paralysis ascending to the nerves that stimulate the thoracic area.
9. A nurse is caring for a patient newly diagnosed with chronic inflammatory demyelinating polyneuropathy (CIDP). Which statement can the nurse accurately use to teach the patient about CIDP?
   - **a.** "Corticosteroids have little effect on this disease."
   - **b.** "Maintenance therapy will be needed to prevent relapse."
   - **c.** "You will go into remission in approximately eight weeks."
   - **d.** "You should be able to walk without help within three months."

1. a, 2. b, 3. c, 4. c, 5. a, 6. b, 7. a, d, e, 8. d, 9. b.

For rationales to these answers and even more NCLEX review questions, visit *http://evolve.elsevier.com/Lewis/medsurg.*

## EVOLVE WEBSITE

http://evolve.elsevier.com/Lewis/medsurg

**Review Questions (Online Only)**

**Key Points**

**Answer Keys for Questions**

- Rationales for Bridge to NCLEX Examination Questions
- Answer Guidelines for Case Study on p. 1443

**Student Case Study**

- Patient With Spinal Cord Injury

**Nursing Care Plan**

- eNursing Care Plan 60-1: Patient With a Spinal Cord Injury

**Conceptual Care Map Creator**

**Audio Glossary**

**Content Updates**

## REFERENCES

1. The National SCI Statistical Center: Spinal cord injury (SCI) facts and figures at a glance. Retrieved from *www.nscisc.uab.edu/PublicDocuments/fact_figures_docs/Facts%202015.pdf.*
2. Silva NA, Sousa N, Reis RL, et al: From basics to clinical: a comprehensive review on spinal cord injury, *Prog Neurobiol* 114:25, 2014.
3. Grafman J, Salazar A: Traumatic Brain Injury, Part I. In Aminoff MJ, Boller F, Swaab DF: *Handbook of clinical neurology*, St Louis, 2015, Elsevier.
4. Fox A: Assessment and treatment of spinal cord injuries and neurogenic shock. *JEMS* Retrieved from *http://www.jems.com/articles/print/volume-39/issue-11/patient-care/assessment-and-treatment-spinal-cord-inj.html*, 2014.
5. International Standards for Neurologic Classification of Spinal Cord Injury (ISNCSCI). Retrieved from *www.asia-spinalinjury.org/elearning/isncsci_worksheet_2015_web.pdf.*
6. Vazquez RG, Sedes PR, Farina MM, et al: Respiratory management in the patient with spinal cord injury, *BioMed Res Internat* 2013:168757, 2013.

*7. Postma K, Haisma JA, Hopman MTE, et al: Resistive inspiratory muscle training in people with spinal cord injury during inpatient rehabilitation: a randomized controlled trial, *Phys Ther* 94:1709, 2014.

8. Merck Manual: Neurogenic bladder. Retrieved from *www.merckmanuals.com/professional/genitourinary-disorders/voiding-disorders/neurogenic-bladder.*
9. Christopher & Dana Reeve Foundation Paralysis Resource Center: Bladder management. Retrieved from *http://www.christopherreeve.org/atf/cf/%7B173bca02-3665-49ab-9378-be009c58a5d3%7D/BLADDERMGMT713.PDF.*
10. Dhall SS, Hadley MN, Bizhan A, et al: Nutritional support after spinal cord injury, *Neurosurg* 72(suppl 2):255, 2013.
11. Dhall SS, Hadley MN, Bizhan A, et al: Deep venous thrombosis and thromboembolism in patients with cervical spinal cord injuries, *Neurosurg* 72(suppl 2):244, 2013.
12. Widerstrom-Noga E, Biering-Sroensen F, Bryce TN, et al: The international spinal cord injury pain basic data set (version 2.0), *Spinal Cord* 52:282, 2014.
13. Ryken TC, Hadley MN, Walters BC, et al: Radiographic assessment. *Neurosurg* 72(suppl):3, 2013.
14. Theodore N, Hadley MN, Aarabi B, et al: Prehospital cervical spinal immobilization after trauma, *Neurosurg* 72(suppl):3, 2013.
15. Theodore N, Aarabi B, Dhall SS, et al: Transportation of patients with acute traumatic cervical spine injuries, *Neurosurg* 72(suppl):3, 2013.
16. Hurlbert RJ, Hadley MN, Walters B, et al: Pharmacological therapy for acute spinal cord injury, *Neurosurg* 72(suppl):93, 2013.
17. Inoue T, Manley GT, Patel N, et al: Medical and surgical management after spinal cord injury: vasopressor usage, early surgeries, and complications, *J Neurotraum* 31:284, 2014.
18. National Institute of Neurological Disorders and Stroke: Spinal cord injury hope through research. Retrieved from *www.ninds.nih.gov/disorders/sci/detail_sci.htm.*
19. Christopher & Dana Reeve Foundation Paralysis Resource Center: Bowel management. Retrieved from *www.christopherreeve.org/atf/cf/%7B173bca02-3665-49ab-9378-be009c58a5d3%7D/Bowel914.pdf.*

20. Saulino MF, Goldstein JA: Rehabilitation of persons with spinal cord injuries. Retrieved from *http://emedicine.Medscape.com/article/1265209-overview*, 2014.
21. Christopher & Dana Reeve Foundation Paralysis Resource Center: Respirator, ventilator, and trach resources. Retrieved from *www.christopherreeve.org/atf/cf/%7B173bca02-3665-49ab-9378-be009c58a5d3%7D/VENT-TRACH%20_RESPIRATORY_%208-10.PDF.*
22. Sexual function in men with SCI. Retrieved from *http://images.main.uab.edu/spinalcord/SCI%20Infosheets%20in%20PDF/Sexual%20Function%20for%20Men%20with%20SCI.pdf.*
23. Sexuality for women with spinal cord injury. Retrieved from *http://images.main.uab.edu/spinalcord/SCI%20Infosheets%20in%20PDF/Sexuality%20for%20Women%20with%20SCI.pdf.*
24. Fann JR, Crane DA, Graves DE, et al: Depression treatment preferences after acute traumatic spinal cord injury, *Arch Phys Med Rehab* 94:2389, 2013.
25. Huff JS, Brenner BE: Spinal cord neoplasms: epidemiology. Retrieved from *http://emedicine.medscape.com/article/779872-overview#a6.*
26. Mechtler LL: Spinal cord tumors: new views and future directions, *Neuro Clinic* 31:241, 2013.
27. American Association of Neurological Surgeons: Spinal tumors. Retrieved from *www.aans.org/Patient%20Information/conditions%20and%20Treatments/Spinal%20Tumor.aspx.*
*28. Sharma M, Sonig A, Ambekar S, et al: Discharge dispositions, complications, and costs of hospitalization in spinal cord tumor surgery: analysis of data from the United States nationwide inpatient sample, 2003-2010, *J Neurosurg Spine* 20:125, 2014.
29. Trigeminal neuralgia fact sheet. Retrieved from *www.ninds.nih.gov/disorders/trigeminal_neuralgia/detail_trigeminal_neuralgia.htm.*
30. Trigeminal neuralgia. Retrieved from *http://ihs-classification.org/en/02_klassifikation/04_teil3/13.01.01_facialpain.html.*
31. Zakrzewska JM, Linskey JE: Trigeminal neuralgia, *BMJ* 348:g474, 2014.
32. Lettmair S: Radiosurgery in trigeminal neuralgia, *Phys Med* 30:592, 2014.
33. National Institute of Neurological Disorders and Stroke: Bell's palsy fact sheet. Retrieved from *www.ninds.nih.gov/disorders/bells/detail_bells.htm.*
34. Zandian A, Osiro S, Hudson R, et al: The neurologist's dilemma: a comprehensive clinical review of Bell's palsy, with emphasis on current management trends, *Med Sci Mon* 20:83, 2014.
35. Dimachkie MM, Barohn RJ: Guillain-Barré syndrome, *Curr Treat Options Neurol* 15:338, 2013.
36. Van Doorn PA: Diagnosis, treatment, and prognosis of Guillain-Barré syndrome (GBS), *Presse Med* 42(6 Pt 2):e193, 2013.
37. Eldar AH, Chapman J: Guillain Barré syndrome and other immune mediated neuropathies: diagnosis and classification, *Autoimmune Rev* 13:525, 2014.
38. GBS/CIDP Foundation International: All about CIDP. Retrieved from *www.gbs-cidp.org/cidp/all-about-cidp.*
39. American Association of Neuromuscular and Electrodiagnostic Medicine: Chronic inflammatory demyelinating polyneuropathy. Retrieved from *http://aanem.org/Education/Patient-Resources/Disorders/Chronic-Inflammatory-Demyelinating-Polyradiculoneu.aspx.*
40. Sung JY, Tani J, Park SB, et al: Early identification of acute-onset chronic inflammatory demyelinating polyneuropathy, *Brain* 137:2155, 2014.
41. Taylor T: Chronic inflammatory demyelinating polyradiculoneuropathy: in a remote northern Ontario hospital, *Can Fam Phys* 59:368, 2013.
42. Centers for Disease Control and Prevention: Make sure your family is fully immunized. Retrieved from *www.cdc.gov/Features/Tetanus.*

*Evidence-based information for clinical practice.

61

# Assessment of Musculoskeletal System

*Michael E. Zychowicz*

*I think self-discipline is something, it's like a muscle. The more you exercise it, the stronger it gets.*

***Daniel Goldstein***

http://evolve.elsevier.com/Lewis/medsurg/

## LEARNING OUTCOMES

1. Describe the gross and microscopic anatomy of bone.
2. Explain the classification system for joints and movements at synovial joints.
3. Compare and contrast the types and structure of muscle tissue.
4. Describe the functions of cartilage, muscles, ligaments, tendons, fascia, and bursae.
5. Link age-related changes in the musculoskeletal system to the differences in assessment findings.
6. Obtain significant subjective and objective assessment data related to the musculoskeletal system from a patient.
7. Perform a physical assessment of the musculoskeletal system using appropriate techniques.
8. Differentiate normal from abnormal findings of a physical assessment of the musculoskeletal system.
9. Describe the purpose, significance of results, and nursing responsibilities related to diagnostic studies of the musculoskeletal system.

## KEY TERMS

ankylosis, Table 61-6, p. 1456
arthrocentesis, Table 61-7, p. 1459
arthroscopy, Table 61-7, p. 1458
atrophy, Table 61-6, p. 1456
contracture, Table 61-6, p. 1456
crepitation, Table 61-6, p. 1456
isometric contractions, p. 1449
isotonic contractions, p. 1449
kyphosis, Table 61-6, p. 1456
lordosis, Table 61-6, p. 1456
osteons, p. 1446
range of motion, p. 1454
scoliosis, p. 1455
x-ray, p. 1455

This chapter provides a review of the structure and function of the musculoskeletal system to facilitate nursing assessment and evaluation of the assessment findings for this system. The musculoskeletal system is composed of voluntary muscle and six types of connective tissue: bone, cartilage, ligaments, tendons, fascia, and bursae. The purpose of the musculoskeletal system is to protect body organs, provide support and stability for the body, and allow coordinated movement.

## STRUCTURES AND FUNCTIONS OF MUSCULOSKELETAL SYSTEM

### Bone

**Function.** The main functions of bone are support, protection of internal organs, voluntary movement, blood cell production, and mineral storage.[1] Bones provide the supporting framework that keeps the body from collapsing and also allows the body to bear weight. Bones also protect underlying vital organs and tissues. For example, the skull encloses the brain, vertebrae surround the spinal cord, and rib cage protects the lungs and heart.

Bones serve as a point of attachment for muscles, which are connected to bones by tendons. Bones act as a lever for muscles, and movement occurs as a result of muscle contractions applied to these levers. Bones also serve as a point of attachment for ligaments, which provide stability to joints. Bones contain hematopoietic tissue for the production of red and white blood cells. Bones also serve as a storage site for inorganic minerals such as calcium and phosphorus.

Bone is a dynamic tissue that continuously changes form and composition. It contains both organic material (collagen) and inorganic material (calcium, phosphate). The internal and external growth and remodeling of bone are ongoing processes.

**Microscopic Structure.** Bone is classified according to structure as *cortical* (compact and dense) or *cancellous* (spongy). In *cortical bone,* cylindrical structural units called **osteons** *(Haversian systems)* fit closely together, creating a dense bone structure (Fig. 61-1, *A*). Within the systems, the Haversian canals run parallel to the bone's long axis and contain the blood vessels that travel to the bone's interior from the periosteum. Surrounding each osteon are concentric rings known as *lamellae,*

Reviewed by Judy Carlyle, RN, MNSc, ARNEC Faculty, Clinical Liaison, Arkansas Rural Education Consortium, Nashville, Arkansas; and Colleen R. Walsh, RN, DNP, ONC, ONP-C, CNS, ACNP-BC, Contract Clinical Assistant Professor, Graduate Nursing, University of Southern Indiana, College of Nursing and Health Professions, Evansville, Indiana.

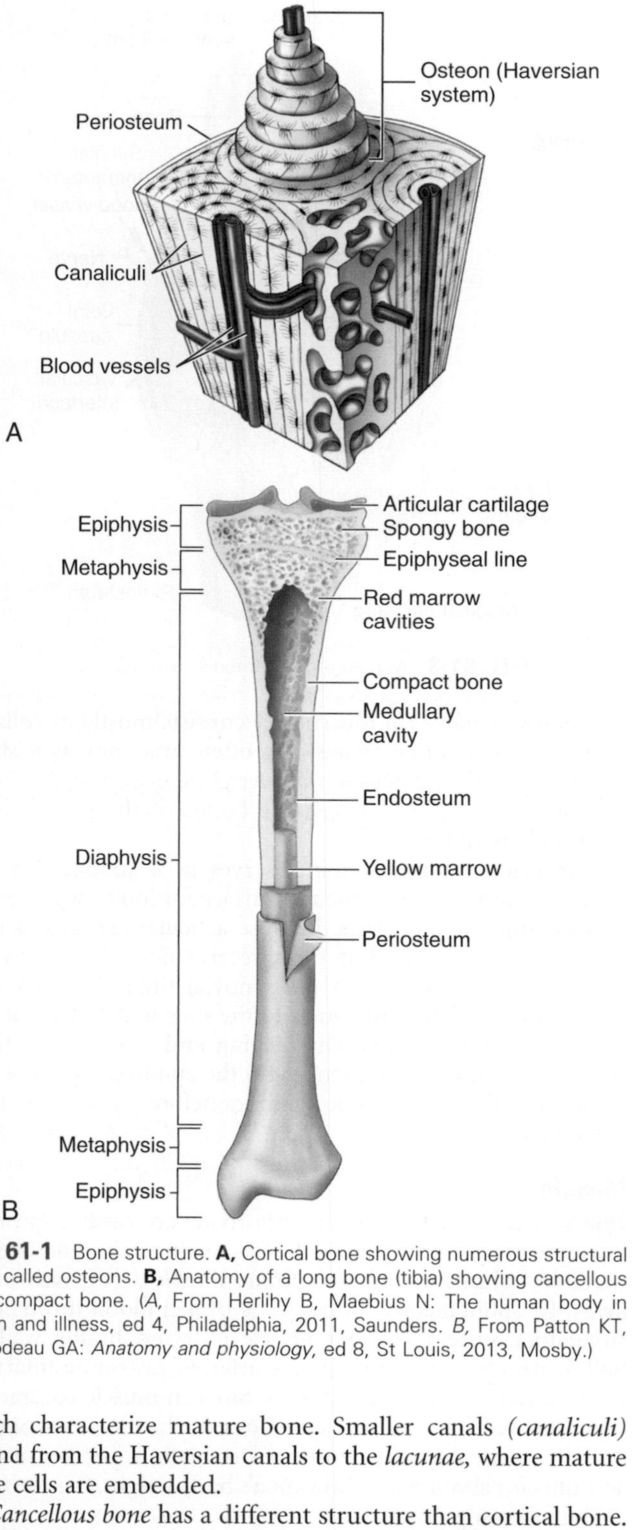


**FIG. 61-1** Bone structure. **A,** Cortical bone showing numerous structural units called osteons. **B,** Anatomy of a long bone (tibia) showing cancellous and compact bone. (*A,* From Herlihy B, Maebius N: The human body in health and illness, ed 4, Philadelphia, 2011, Saunders. *B,* From Patton KT, Thibodeau GA: *Anatomy and physiology,* ed 8, St Louis, 2013, Mosby.)

which characterize mature bone. Smaller canals *(canaliculi)* extend from the Haversian canals to the *lacunae,* where mature bone cells are embedded.

*Cancellous bone* has a different structure than cortical bone. The lamellae are not arranged in concentric rings but rather along the lines of maximum stress placed on the bone. Cancellous bone is filled with red or yellow marrow, and blood reaches the bone cells by passing through spaces in the marrow.

The three types of bone cells are osteoblasts, osteocytes, and osteoclasts.[2] *Osteoblasts* synthesize organic bone matrix (collagen) and are the basic bone-forming cells. *Osteocytes* are mature bone cells. *Osteoclasts* participate in bone remodeling by assisting in the breakdown of bone tissue. *Bone remodeling* is the removal of old bone by osteoclasts *(resorption)* and the deposition of new bone by osteoblasts *(ossification).* The inner layer of bone is composed primarily of osteoblasts with a few osteoclasts.

**Gross Structure.** The anatomic structure of bone is best represented by a typical long bone such as the tibia (Fig. 61-1, *B*). Each long bone consists of the epiphysis, diaphysis, and metaphysis. The *epiphysis,* the widened area at each end of a long bone, is composed primarily of cancellous bone. The wide epiphysis allows for greater weight distribution and provides stability for the joint. The epiphysis is also a primary location of muscle attachment. Articular cartilage covers the ends of the epiphysis to provide a smooth, low-friction surface for joint movement.

The *diaphysis* is the main shaft of the long bone. It provides structural support and is composed of cortical bone. The tubular structure of the diaphysis allows it to more easily withstand bending and twisting forces.

The *metaphysis* is the flared area between the epiphysis and diaphysis. Like the epiphysis, it is composed of cancellous bone.

The *epiphyseal plate* (physis or growth plate) is the cartilaginous area between the epiphysis and metaphysis. In skeletally immature children who still have open growth plates, the epiphyseal plate actively produces chondrocytes that become mature bone. Division of the chondrocytes causes longitudinal bone growth in children. Injury to the epiphyseal plate in a growing child can cause cessation of new bone formation at the growth plate. This leads to a shorter extremity and may contribute to significant functional problems. In the adult, the metaphysis and epiphysis become joined when chondrocyte formation at the growth plate ceases and the plate becomes fully ossified.

The *periosteum* is composed of fibrous connective tissue that covers the bone. Tiny blood vessels penetrate the periosteum to provide nutrition to underlying bone. Musculotendinous fibers attach to the outer layer of the periosteum. The inner layer of the periosteum is attached to the bone by collagen bundles. No periosteum exists on the articular surfaces of long bones. These bone ends are covered by articular cartilage.

The medullary *(marrow)* cavity in the center of the diaphysis contains either red or yellow bone marrow.[3] In the growing child, red bone marrow is actively involved in blood cell production (hematopoiesis). In the adult, the medullary cavity of long bones contains yellow bone marrow, which is mainly adipose tissue. Yellow marrow is involved in hematopoiesis only in times of great blood cell need. In adults, red marrow is found mainly in the *flat bones,* such as the pelvis, skull, sternum, cranium, ribs, vertebrae, and scapulae, and in the *cancellous* ("spongy") bone at the epiphyseal ends of long bones such as the femur and humerus.

**Types.** The skeleton consists of 206 bones, which are classified according to shape as long, short, flat, or irregular.

*Long bones* are characterized by a central shaft *(diaphysis)* and two widened ends *(epiphyses)* (Fig. 61-1, *B*). Examples include the femur, humerus, and tibia. *Short bones* are composed of cancellous bone covered by a thin layer of compact bone. Examples include the carpals in the hand and tarsals in the foot.

*Flat bones* have two layers of compact bone separated by a layer of cancellous bone. Examples include the ribs, skull, scapula, and sternum. The spaces in the cancellous bone contain bone marrow. *Irregular bones* appear in a variety of shapes

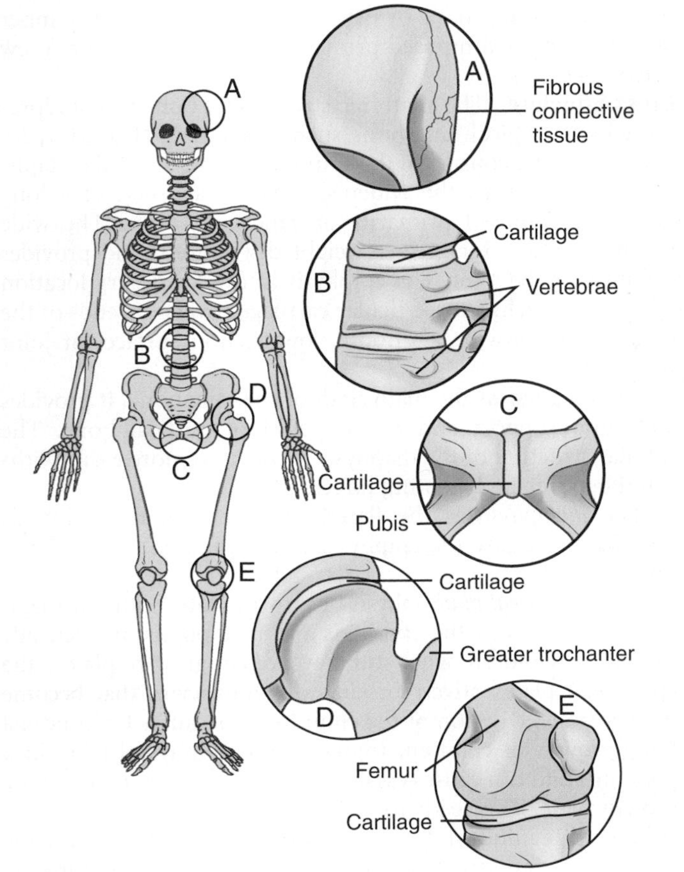


**FIG. 61-2** Classification of joints. **A** to **C,** Synarthrotic (immovable) and amphiarthrotic (slightly movable) joints. **D** and **E,** Diarthrodial (*freely* movable) joints.

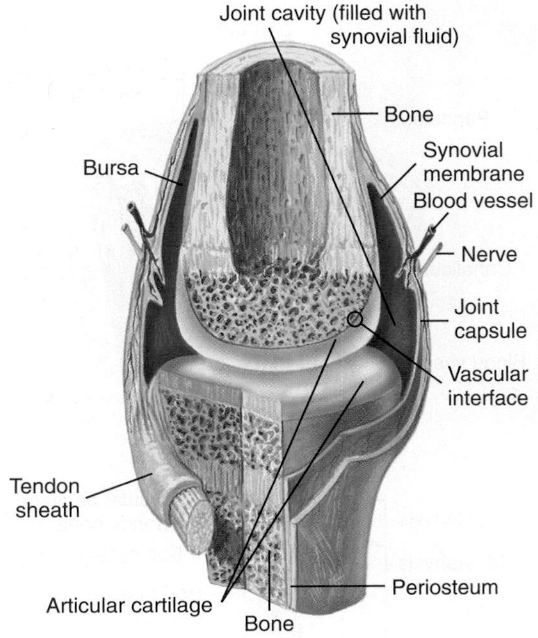


**FIG. 61-3** Structure of diarthrodial (synovial) joint.

and sizes. Examples include the sacrum, mandible, and ear ossicles.

## Joints

A *joint* (articulation) is a place where the ends of two bones are in proximity and move in relation to each other. Joints are classified by the degree of movement that they allow (Fig. 61-2).

The most common joint is the freely movable *diarthrodial* (synovial) type. Each joint is enclosed in a capsule of fibrous connective tissue, which joins the two bones together to form a cavity (Fig. 61-3). The capsule is lined by a synovial membrane, which secretes thick synovial fluid to lubricate the joint, reduce friction, and allow opposing surfaces to slide smoothly over each other. The end of each bone is covered with articular (hyaline) cartilage. Supporting structures (e.g., ligaments, tendons) reinforce the joint capsule and provide limits and stability to joint movement. Types of diarthrodial joints are shown in Fig. 61-4.

## Cartilage

The three types of *cartilage* are hyaline, elastic, and fibrous. *Hyaline cartilage,* the most common, contains a moderate amount of collagen fibers. It is found in the trachea, bronchi, nose, epiphyseal plate, and articular surfaces of bones.

*Elastic cartilage,* which contains both collagen and elastic fibers, is more flexible than hyaline cartilage. It is found in the ear, epiglottis, and larynx.

*Fibrous cartilage* (fibrocartilage) consists mostly of collagen fibers and is a tough tissue that often functions as a shock absorber. It is found between the vertebral discs and also forms a protective cushion between the bones of the pelvic girdle, knee, and shoulder.

Cartilage in synovial joints serves as a support for soft tissue and provides the articular surface for joint movement. It protects underlying tissues. Because articular cartilage is considered to be avascular, it must receive nourishment by the diffusion of material from the synovial fluid. The lack of a direct blood supply contributes to the slow metabolism of cartilage cells and explains why healing and repair of cartilage tissue occur slowly. The cartilage in the epiphyseal plate is also involved in the growth of long bones before physical maturity is reached.

## Muscle

**Types.** The three types of muscle tissue are cardiac (striated, involuntary), smooth (nonstriated, involuntary), and skeletal (striated, voluntary) muscle. *Cardiac muscle* occurs only in the heart. Its spontaneous contractions propel blood through the circulatory system. *Smooth muscle* is found in the walls of hollow structures such as airways, arteries, gastrointestinal (GI) tract, urinary bladder, and uterus. Smooth muscle contraction is modulated by neuronal and hormonal influences. *Skeletal muscle,* which requires neuronal stimulation for contraction, accounts for about half of a human's body weight. It is the focus of the following discussion.

**Structure.** The skeletal muscle is enclosed by the *epimysium,* a continuous layer of deep fascia. The epimysium helps muscles slide over nearby structures. Connective tissue surrounding and extending into the muscle can be subdivided into fiber bundles, or *fasciculi.* These bundles are covered by *perimysium* and an innermost connective tissue layer called the *endomysium* that surrounds each fiber (Fig. 61-5).

The structural unit of skeletal muscle is the muscle cell or muscle fiber, which is highly specialized for contraction. Skeletal muscle fibers are long, multinucleated cylinders that contain

| Joint | Movement | Examples | Illustration |
|---|---|---|---|
| **Hinge joint** | Flexion, extension | Elbow joint (shown), interphalangeal joints, knee joint | 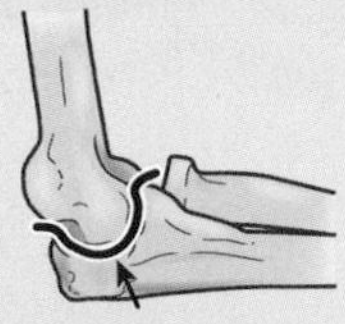 |
| **Ball and socket (spheroidal)** | Flexion, extension; adduction, abduction; circumduction | Shoulder (shown), hip | 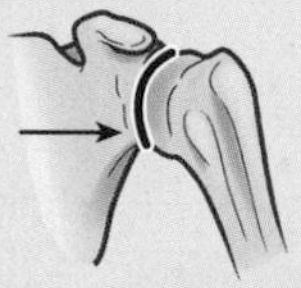 |
| **Pivot (rotary)** | Rotation | Atlas-axis, proximal radioulnar joint (shown) | 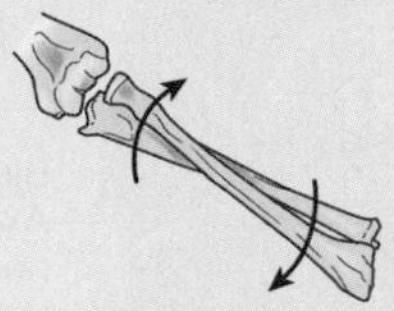 |
| **Condyloid** | Flexion, extension; abduction, adduction; circumduction | Wrist joint (between radial and carpals) (shown) | 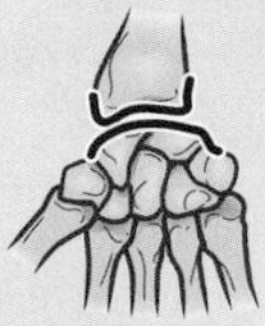 |
| **Saddle** | Flexion, extension; abduction, adduction; circumduction, thumb-finger opposition | Carpometacarpal joint of thumb (shown) | 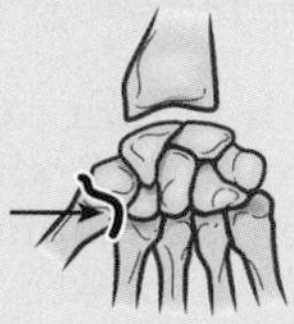 |
| **Gliding** | One surface moves over another surface | Between tarsal bones, sacroiliac joint, between articular processes of vertebrae, between carpal bones (shown) | 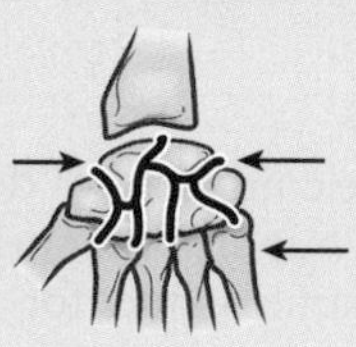 |

**FIG. 61-4** Types of diarthrodial (synovial) joints.

many mitochondria to support their high metabolic activity. Muscle fibers are composed of myofibrils, which in turn are made up of protein contractile filaments. The *sarcomere* is the contractile unit of the myofibrils. Each sarcomere consists of *myosin* (thick) filaments and *actin* (thin) filaments. The arrangement of the thin and thick filaments accounts for the characteristic banding of muscle when it is seen under a microscope. Muscle contraction occurs as thick and thin filaments slide past each other, causing the sarcomeres to shorten.

**Contractions.** Skeletal muscle contractions allow posture maintenance, body movement, and facial expressions. Isometric contractions increase the tension within a muscle but do not produce movement. Isotonic contractions shorten a muscle to produce movement. Most contractions are a combination of tension generation *(isometric)* and shortening *(isotonic)*. Repeated isometric and/or isotonic contractions provide stress to stimulate muscle growth. Muscular *atrophy* (decrease in size) occurs with the absence of contraction that results from immobility or decreased neuronal stimulation. Increased muscular activity leads to *hypertrophy* (increase in size).

Skeletal muscle fibers are divided into two groups based on the type of activity they demonstrate. *Slow-twitch muscle fibers* support prolonged muscle activity such as marathon running. Because they also support the body against gravity, they assist in posture maintenance. *Fast-twitch muscle fibers* are used for rapid muscle contraction required for activities such as blinking the eye, jumping, or sprinting. Fast-twitch fibers tend to tire more quickly than slow-twitch fibers.

**Neuromuscular Junction.** Skeletal muscle fibers require a nerve impulse to contract. A nerve fiber and the skeletal muscle fibers it stimulates are called a *motor endplate.* The junction between the axon of the nerve cell and the adjacent muscle cell is called the *myoneural* or *neuromuscular junction* (Fig. 61-6).

Acetylcholine is released from the presynaptic neuron and diffuses across the neuromuscular junction to bind with receptors on the motor endplate of the muscle. In response to this stimulation, the sarcoplasmic reticulum releases calcium ions into the cytoplasm. The presence of calcium triggers the contraction in the myofibrils. When calcium is low, *tetany* (involuntary contractions of skeletal muscle) can occur.

**Energy Source.** The direct energy source for muscle fiber contractions is adenosine triphosphate (ATP). ATP is synthesized by cellular oxidative metabolism in numerous mitochondria located close to the myofibrils. It is rapidly depleted through conversion to adenosine diphosphate (ADP) and must be rephosphorylated. Phosphocreatine provides a rapid source for

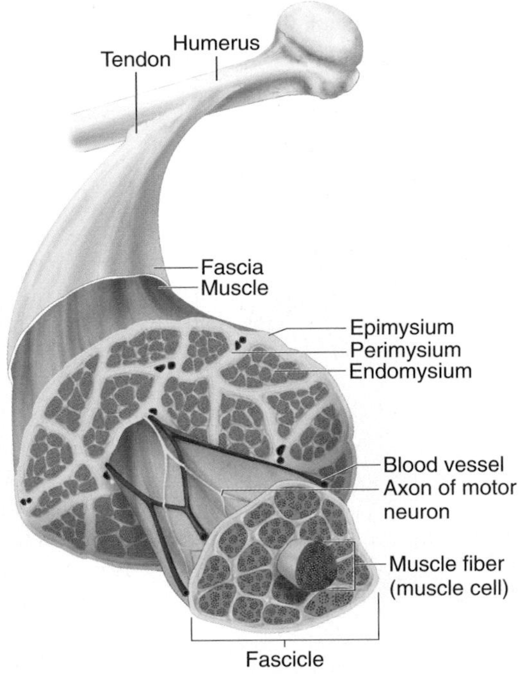


**FIG. 61-5** Structure of a muscle. (From Patton KT, Thibodeau GA, Douglas M: *Essentials of anatomy and physiology,* St Louis, 2012, Mosby.)

the resynthesis of ATP, but it is in turn converted to creatine. Glycolysis can serve as a source of ATP when the $O_2$ supply is inadequate for metabolic needs of the muscle tissue. In this process, one glucose molecule is broken down to two ATP molecules.

## Ligaments and Tendons

Ligaments and tendons are composed of dense, fibrous connective tissue that contains bundles of closely packed collagen fibers arranged in the same plane for additional strength. *Tendons* attach muscles to bones as an extension of the muscle sheath that adheres to the periosteum. *Ligaments* connect bones to bones (e.g., tibia to femur at knee joint). They have a higher elastic content than tendons.[4] Ligaments provide stability while permitting controlled movement at joints.

Ligaments and tendons have a relatively poor blood supply, usually making tissue repair a slow process after injury. For example, the stretching or tearing of ligaments that occurs with a sprain may require a long time to mend.

## Fascia

*Fascia* refers to layers of connective tissue with intermeshed fibers that can withstand limited stretching. Superficial fascia lies immediately under the skin. Deep fascia is a dense, fibrous tissue that surrounds muscle bundles, nerves, and blood vessels. It also encloses individual muscles, allowing them to act independently and to glide over each other during contraction. In addition, fascia provides strength to muscle tissues.

## Bursae

*Bursae* are small sacs of connective tissue lined with synovial membrane and containing viscous synovial fluid. They are typically located at bony prominences or joints to relieve pressure and decrease friction between moving parts.[5] For example, bursae are found between the (1) patella and skin (prepatellar bursae), (2) olecranon process of the elbow and skin (olecranon

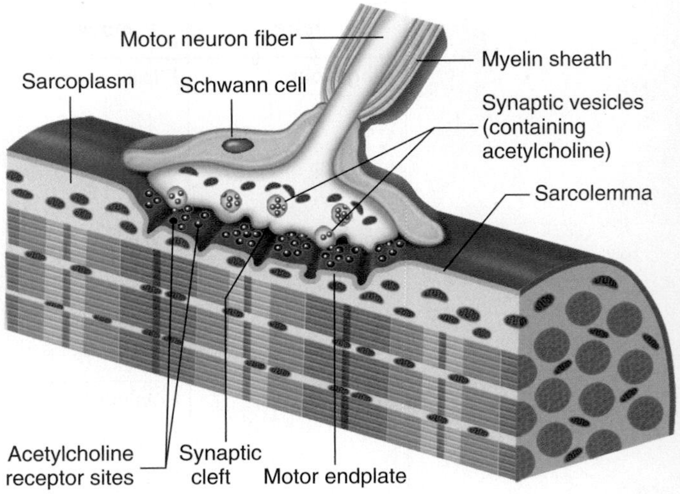


**FIG. 61-6** Neuromuscular junction. (From Patton KT, Thibodeau GA: *Anatomy and physiology,* ed 8, St Louis, 2013, Mosby.)

bursae), (3) head of the humerus and acromion process of the scapula (subacromial bursae), and (4) greater trochanter of the proximal femur and skin (trochanteric bursae). *Bursitis* is an inflammation of a bursa sac. The inflammation may be acute or chronic.

## Gerontologic Considerations: Effects of Aging on Musculoskeletal System

Many functional problems experienced by the older adult are related to changes of the musculoskeletal system. Although some changes begin in early adulthood, obvious signs of musculoskeletal impairment may not appear until later adult years. Alterations may affect the older adult's ability to complete self-care tasks and pursue other usual activities. Effects of musculoskeletal changes may range from mild discomfort and decreased ability to perform ADLs to severe, chronic pain and immobility.

The risk for falls also increases in the older adult due in part to a loss of strength. Aging can also bring changes in the patient's balance, thus making the person unsteady, and *proprioception* (awareness of self in relation to the environment) may be altered.

The bone remodeling process is altered in the aging adult. Increased bone resorption and decreased bone formation cause a loss of bone density, contributing to the development of osteopenia and osteoporosis (see Chapter 63). Muscle mass and strength also decrease with aging. Almost 30% of muscle mass is lost by age 70. A loss of motor neurons can cause additional problems with skeletal muscle movement. Tendons and ligaments become less flexible, and movement becomes more rigid. Joints in the aging adult are also more likely to be affected by osteoarthritis[6] (see Chapter 64).

Perform a musculoskeletal assessment with particular emphasis on exercise practices. Obtain information on the type of exercise performed, including frequency and warm-up activities. Determine the impact of age-related changes of the musculoskeletal system on the older adult's functional status. Specifically inquire about changes in self-care habits and ability to be self-sufficient in the home environment.

Identify any musculoskeletal changes that increase the patient's risk for falls, and discuss fall prevention strategies. Functional limitations that are accepted by the older adult as a

### TABLE 61-1 Gerontologic Assessment Differences

***Musculoskeletal System***

| Changes | Differences in Assessment Findings |
|---|---|
| **Muscle** | |
| • Decreased number and diameter of muscle cells. Replacement of muscle cells by fibrous connective tissue.<br>• Loss of elasticity and deterioration of cartilage.<br>• Reduced ability to store glycogen. Decreased ability to release glycogen as quick energy during stress.<br>• Decreased basal metabolic rate. | • Decreased muscle strength and mass. Abdominal protrusion.<br>• Increased rigidity in neck, shoulders, back, hips, and knees.<br>• Decreased fine motor dexterity, decreased agility.<br>• Slowed reaction times and reflexes as a result of slowed conduction of nerve impulses along motor units. Earlier fatigue with activity. |
| **Joints** | |
| • Increased risk for cartilage erosion that leads to direct contact between bone ends and overgrowth of bone around joint margins.<br>• Loss of water from discs between vertebrae, decreased height of intervertebral spaces. | • Joint stiffness, decreased mobility, limited ROM, possible crepitation on movement.<br>• Pain with motion and/or weight bearing.<br>• Loss of height and shortening of trunk from disc compression. Posture change. |
| **Bone** | |
| • Decreased bone density and strength.<br>• Slowed remodeling process. | • Loss of height and deformity such as dowager's hump (kyphosis) from vertebral compression and degeneration.<br>• Back pain, stiffness.<br>• Bony prominences more pronounced.<br>• Increased risk of osteopenia and osteoporosis. |

normal part of aging can often be halted or reversed with appropriate preventive strategies (see Table 62-1).

Diseases such as osteoarthritis and osteoporosis are not a normal part of growing older. These metabolic bone diseases involve the deterioration of bone tissue (osteoporosis) and destruction of cartilage (osteoarthritis). Carefully differentiate between expected changes and the effects of disease in the aging adult. Symptoms of disease can be treated in many cases, helping the older adult to return to a higher functional level. Age-related changes in the musculoskeletal system and differences in assessment findings are presented in Table 61-1.

## ASSESSMENT OF MUSCULOSKELETAL SYSTEM

### Subjective Data

**Important Health Information.** The most common manifestations of musculoskeletal impairment include pain, weakness, deformity, limitation of movement, stiffness, and joint crepitation (crackling sound). Ask the patient about changes in sensation or in the size of a muscle.

***Past Health History.*** Because certain illnesses are known to affect the musculoskeletal system directly or indirectly, question the patient about past medical problems, including tuberculosis, poliomyelitis, diabetes mellitus, parathyroid problems, hemophilia, rickets, soft tissue infection, and neuromuscular

## CASE STUDY

***Patient Introduction***

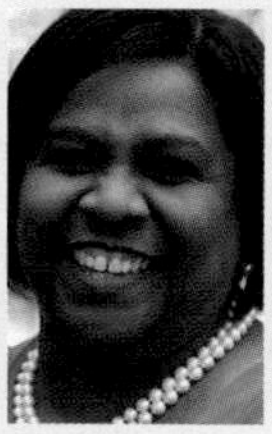

(©pixelhead-photo/iStock/Thinkstock)

G.A. is a 58-yr-old African-American woman who comes to the emergency department after waking with a sudden onset of excruciating pain in her left great toe. Her husband drove her to the ED this morning. She denies any injury to her foot and states she has never had this type of pain before.

**Discussion Questions**

1. What is the most likely cause for G.A.'s acute pain in her great toe?
2. Is this condition stable or an emergency?

You will learn more about how to assess G.A.'s condition as you read through this chapter.

See p. 1454 for more information on G.A.

Answers available at *http://evolve.elsevier.com/Lewis/medsurg.*

disability. In addition, past or developing musculoskeletal problems can affect the patient's overall health. Trauma to the musculoskeletal system is a common reason for seeking medical evaluation.

Questions should also focus on symptoms of arthritic and connective tissue diseases (e.g., gout, psoriatic arthritis, systemic lupus erythematosus), osteomalacia, osteomyelitis, and fungal infection of bones or joints. Ask the patient about possible sources of a secondary bacterial infection, such as ears, tonsils, teeth, sinuses, lungs, or genitourinary tract. These infections can enter the bones, resulting in osteomyelitis or joint destruction. Obtain a detailed account of the course and treatment of any of these problems.

***Medications.*** Question the patient regarding prescription and over-the-counter drugs, herbal products, and nutritional supplements (see the Complementary & Alternative Therapies box in Chapter 3 on p. 38). Obtain detailed information about each treatment, including its name, the dose and frequency, length of time it was taken, reason for use, and any possible side effects. Inquire about the use of skeletal muscle relaxants, opioids, nonsteroidal antiinflammatory drugs, and systemic and topical corticosteroids. Question the patient who has taken antiinflammatory drugs about GI distress or signs of bleeding.

In addition to drugs taken for treatment of a musculoskeletal problem, ask the patient about drugs that can have detrimental effects on the musculoskeletal system. Some of these drugs and their potential side effects include antiseizure drugs (osteomalacia), phenothiazines (gait disturbances), corticosteroids (avascular necrosis, decreased bone and muscle mass), and potassium-depleting diuretics (muscle cramps and weakness). Question women about their menstrual history. Episodes of premenopausal amenorrhea can contribute to the development of osteoporosis.[7] Ask postmenopausal women about their use of hormone therapy. Inquire about calcium and vitamin D supplements for women and men.

***Surgery or Other Treatments.*** Obtain information about past hospitalizations related to a musculoskeletal problem. Document the reason for hospitalization; the date and duration; and the treatment, including ongoing rehabilitation. Also record details of emergency treatment for musculoskeletal injuries. Obtain specific information regarding any surgical procedure, postoperative course, and complications. If the patient experienced a period of prolonged immobilization, consider the possible development of osteoporosis and muscle atrophy.

## TABLE 61-2 Health History

### Musculoskeletal System

**Health Perception–Health Management Pattern**
- Describe your usual daily activities.
- Do you experience any difficulties performing these activities?* Describe what you do if you experience difficulty in dressing, preparing meals and feeding yourself, performing basic hygiene, writing or using the phone, or maintaining your home.
- Do you have to lift heavy objects? Do your work or exercise habits require repetitive motion or joint stress? Describe any specialized equipment you use or wear when you work or exercise that helps protect you from injury.
- Do you take any drugs or herbal products to manage your musculoskeletal problem? If so, what are their names and what are the expected effects?

**Nutritional-Metabolic Pattern**
- What is your usual daily intake of food and snacks?
- Do you have difficulties preparing your food?
- What dietary supplements do you take? (Ask specifically about calcium, vitamin D supplements, and herbal products.)
- What is your weight? Describe any recent weight loss or gain.

**Elimination Pattern**
- Does your musculoskeletal problem make it difficult for you to reach the toilet in time?*
- Do you need any assistive devices or equipment to achieve satisfactory toileting?*
- Do you experience constipation related to decreased mobility or drugs taken for your musculoskeletal problem?*

**Activity-Exercise Pattern**
- Do you require assistance in completing your usual daily activities because of a musculoskeletal problem?*
- Describe your usual exercise pattern. Do you experience musculoskeletal symptoms before, during, or after exercising?*
- Are you able to move all your joints comfortably through full range of motion?
- Do you use any prosthetic or orthotic devices?*

**Sleep-Rest Pattern**
- Do you experience any difficulty sleeping because of a musculoskeletal problem?*
- Do you require frequent position changes at night?*
- Do you wake up at night because of musculoskeletal pain?*
- Do you use complementary and alternative therapies to help you sleep at night?*

**Cognitive-Perceptual Pattern**
- Describe any musculoskeletal pain you experience. How do you manage your pain? (Ask specifically about adjunctive therapies such as heat and cold or complementary and alternative therapies such as acupuncture.)

**Self-Perception–Self-Concept Pattern**
- Describe how changes in your musculoskeletal system (posture, walking, muscle strength) and decreased ability to do certain things may affect how you feel about yourself.
- Have these changes affected your lifestyle?*

**Role-Relationship Pattern**
- Do you live alone?
- Describe how family, friends, or others assist you with your musculoskeletal problem.
- Describe the effect of your musculoskeletal problem on your work and on your social relationships.

**Sexuality-Reproductive Pattern**
- Describe any sexual concerns related to your musculoskeletal problem.

**Coping–Stress Tolerance Pattern**
- Describe how you deal with problems such as pain, weakness, or immobility that have resulted from your musculoskeletal problem.

**Value-Belief Pattern**
- Describe any cultural practices or religious beliefs that may influence the treatment of your musculoskeletal problem.

*If yes, describe.

**Functional Health Patterns.** The use of functional health patterns assists in organizing assessment data. Table 61-2 summarizes specific questions to ask in relation to functional health patterns.

***Health Perception–Health Management Pattern.*** Ask about the patient's health practices related to the musculoskeletal system, such as maintenance of normal body weight, avoidance of excessive stress on muscles and joints, and use of proper body mechanics when lifting objects. Question the patient specifically about tetanus and polio immunizations. Obtain the most current date and reaction to a tuberculin skin test.

The patient who is a good historian can recount numerous minor and major injuries of the musculoskeletal system. Record information chronologically and include the following:
- Mechanism and circumstances of the injury (e.g., twist, crush, stretch)
- Methods and duration of treatment
- Current status related to the injury
- Need for assistive devices
- Interference with activities of daily living

Safety practices can affect the patient's predisposition for certain injuries and illnesses. Therefore ask the patient about safety practices related to the work environment, home life, recreation, and exercise. For example, if the patient is a computer programmer, ask about ergonomic adaptations in the office that decrease the risk of carpal tunnel syndrome or low back pain. Identification of problems in this area will direct your plan for patient teaching.

Obtain a family history related to rheumatoid arthritis, systemic lupus erythematosus, ankylosing spondylitis, osteoarthritis, gout, osteoporosis, and scoliosis because a patient may have a genetic predisposition to these or other musculoskeletal disorders.

***Nutritional-Metabolic Pattern.*** The patient's description of a typical day's diet provides clues to areas of nutritional concern that can affect the musculoskeletal system. Adequate intake of vitamins C and D, calcium, and protein is essential for a healthy, intact musculoskeletal system. Abnormal nutritional patterns can predispose individuals to problems such as osteomalacia and osteoporosis. In addition, maintenance of normal weight is an important nutritional goal. Obesity places additional stress on weight-bearing joints such as the knees, hips, and spine, predisposing individuals to cartilage deterioration and ligament instability.

***Elimination Pattern.*** Questions about the patient's mobility may reveal difficulty with ambulating to the toilet. Ask the

## GENETIC RISK ALERT

**Autoimmune Diseases**

- Many autoimmune diseases of the musculoskeletal system have a genetic basis involving human leukocyte antigens (HLAs).
- These diseases include ankylosing spondylitis, rheumatoid arthritis, and systemic lupus erythematosus.

**Osteoporosis**

- Genetic factors contribute to osteoporosis by influencing not only bone mineral density but also bone size, bone quality, and bone turnover.

**Osteoarthritis, Gout, and Scoliosis**

- A genetic predisposition is a contributing risk factor in all these diseases.

**Muscular Dystrophy**

- The most common types of muscular dystrophy are X-linked recessive disorders.

patient if an assistive device such as an elevated toilet seat or a grab bar is necessary to accomplish toileting. Decreased mobility secondary to a musculoskeletal problem can lead to constipation. In addition, musculoskeletal problems can contribute to bowel or bladder incontinence when ambulation is a problem.

***Activity-Exercise Pattern.*** Obtain a detailed account of the type, duration, and frequency of exercise and recreational activities. Compare daily, weekend, and seasonal patterns because occasional or sporadic exercise can be more problematic than regular exercise. Many musculoskeletal problems can affect the patient's activity-exercise pattern. Question the patient about clumsiness or limitations in movement, pain, weakness, crepitus, or any change in bones or joints that interferes with daily activities.

Extremes of activity related to occupation can also affect the musculoskeletal system. A sedentary occupation can negatively affect muscle flexibility and strength. Jobs that require extreme effort through heavy lifting or pushing can lead to damage of joints and supporting structures. Specifically question the patient about work-related injuries to the musculoskeletal system, including treatment and time lost from work.

***Sleep-Rest Pattern.*** The discomfort caused by musculoskeletal disorders can interfere with the patient's normal sleep pattern. Ask the patient about possible alterations in sleep patterns. If the patient describes sleep interference related to a musculoskeletal problem, inquire further about the type of bedding and pillows used, bedtime routine, sleeping partner, and sleeping positions.

***Cognitive-Perceptual Pattern.*** Fully explore and document any pain experienced by the patient as a result of a musculoskeletal problem. To provide a baseline for later reassessment, ask the patient to describe the intensity of the pain on a numeric scale from 0 to 10 (0 = no pain, 10 = most severe pain imaginable).[8] Reassessments over time assist in determining the effectiveness of any treatment plan. Question the patient about measures used at home for managing pain. Ask about related problems such as joint swelling or muscle weakness and any accommodations that help with the problem. (Pain is discussed in Chapter 8.)

***Self-Perception–Self-Concept Pattern.*** Many chronic musculoskeletal problems lead to deformities and a reduction in activities that can have a serious negative impact on the patient's body image and sense of personal worth. Assess the patient's feelings about these changes and the effect they may have on interactions with family and friends.

***Role-Relationship Pattern.*** Impaired mobility and chronic pain from musculoskeletal problems can negatively affect the patient's ability to perform in roles of spouse, parent, and/or employee. The ability to pursue and maintain meaningful social and personal relationships can also be affected by musculoskeletal problems. Carefully question the patient about role performance and relationships.

If the patient lives alone, the current musculoskeletal problem and rehabilitation may make it difficult or impossible to continue this arrangement. Determine the degree of assistance available from family, friends, and other caregivers. Find out if additional resources are needed such as physical therapy and home health care.

***Sexuality-Reproductive Pattern.*** The pain of musculoskeletal problems can impede the patient's ability to obtain sexual satisfaction. Explore this area with a sensitive and nonjudgmental attitude. Help the patient feel comfortable discussing any sexual problems related to pain, movement, and positioning. Additional information on obtaining patient data in this area is presented in Chapter 50.

***Coping–Stress Tolerance Pattern.*** Mobility limitations and pain (acute or chronic) are serious potential stressors that challenge the patient's coping resources. Recognize the potential for ineffective coping in the patient and family or significant other. Additional questioning will help to determine if a musculoskeletal problem is causing difficulties in coping and adjusting.

***Value-Belief Pattern.*** Ask the patient about cultural or religious beliefs that may influence the patient's acceptance of treatment for the musculoskeletal problem. These may include recommendations for diet, exercise, medication, and lifestyle modifications.

### Objective Data

**Physical Examination.** The basic musculoskeletal physical examination involves inspection, palpation, range of motion, strength testing, reflexes, and neurovascular assessment. Other special tests can be used to further assess for specific conditions. Conduct a general overview. While obtaining a careful health history, choose areas to concentrate on during the local examination. Take specific measurements as indicated by the local examination.

***Inspection.*** A systematic inspection is performed starting at the head and neck and proceeding to the upper extremities, lower extremities, and trunk. The regular use of a systematic approach is important to avoid missing important aspects of the examination. Inspect the skin for general color, scars, or other overt signs of previous injury or surgery. Certain cutaneous lesions require additional investigation because they can indicate underlying disorders. For example, butterfly rash over the cheeks and nose is characteristic of systemic lupus erythematosus.

Note the patient's general posture and body build, muscle size and symmetry, and symmetry and contour of joints. Observe for any swelling, deformity, nodules or masses, and discrepancies in limb length or muscle size. Use the patient's opposite body part for comparison when an abnormality is suspected.

***Palpation.*** As with inspection, palpation usually proceeds in a head to toe fashion, examining the neck, shoulders, elbows,

## CASE STUDY—cont'd

### *Subjective Data*

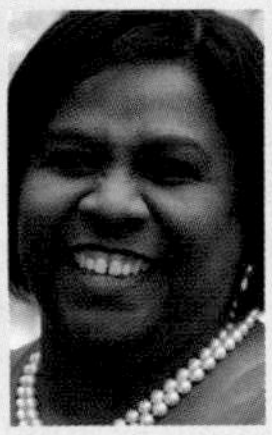

(©pixelhead-photo/iStock/Thinkstock)

A focused subjective assessment of G.A. revealed the following information:

***PMH:*** Hypertension for 6 years. Type 2 diabetes for 11 yr. 40-pack-yr smoking history.

***Medications:*** Metformin (Glucophage) 500 mg PO bid; glyburide (DiaBeta) 5 mg/day PO; hydrochlorothiazide 50 mg PO bid.

***Health Perception–Health Management:*** Currently smokes 1 pack of cigarettes per day. Is trying to quit but finding it difficult. Drinks alcohol at night.

***Nutritional-Metabolic:*** G.A. is 5 ft 2 in tall and weighs 160 lb (BMI 29.3 kg/m$^2$). Does not take any nutritional supplements and avoids milk and other dairy products because they make her "gassy."

***Activity-Exercise:*** Leads a very sedentary lifestyle. Able to perform ADLs without assistance. Denies any history of musculoskeletal problems.

***Cognitive-Perceptual:*** Rates toe pain at 8 on a scale of 0-10. Describes sharp, burning pain that increases in intensity with any movement.

***Coping–Stress Tolerance:*** Is asking for pain medicine "as strong as you can give me."

#### Discussion Questions

1. What type of assessment would be most appropriate for G.A.: comprehensive, focused, or emergency? On what basis would you make that decision?
2. What assessment questions will you ask G.A.?
3. How will you individualize the assessment based on her age, ethnic/cultural background, and condition?
4. What subjective assessment findings are of most concern to you?
5. Is this an appropriate time to talk with G.A. about her weight?
6. Based on these subjective findings, what type of physical assessment should be performed?

You will learn more about the physical assessment of the musculoskeletal system in the next section.

See p. 1457 for more information on G.A.

Answers available at *http://evolve.elsevier.com/Lewis/medsurg.*

wrists, hands, back, hips, knees, ankles, and feet. Warm your hands to prevent muscle spasm, which can interfere with identification of essential landmarks or soft tissue structures. Carefully palpate any specific areas of concern because of a subjective complaint or abnormal appearance on inspection.

Both superficial and deep palpation are usually performed consecutively. Consider the underlying anatomy structures and landmarks that are being palpated. Purposefully palpate both muscles and joints to allow evaluation of skin temperature, local tenderness, swelling, and crepitation. Establish the relationship of adjacent structures, and evaluate the general contour, abnormal prominences, and local landmarks. Make note of the specific anatomic location of any abnormal findings.

***Motion.*** When assessing the patient's joint mobility, carefully evaluate active and passive **range of motion** (full movement potential of a joint). Measurements should be similar for both active and passive maneuvers. *Active range of motion* means the patient takes his or her own joints through all movements without assistance. *Passive range of motion* occurs when someone else moves the patient's joints without his or her assistance through the full range of motion. Be careful in performing passive range of motion because of the risk of injury to underlying structures. If pain or resistance is encountered, stop manipulation immediately.

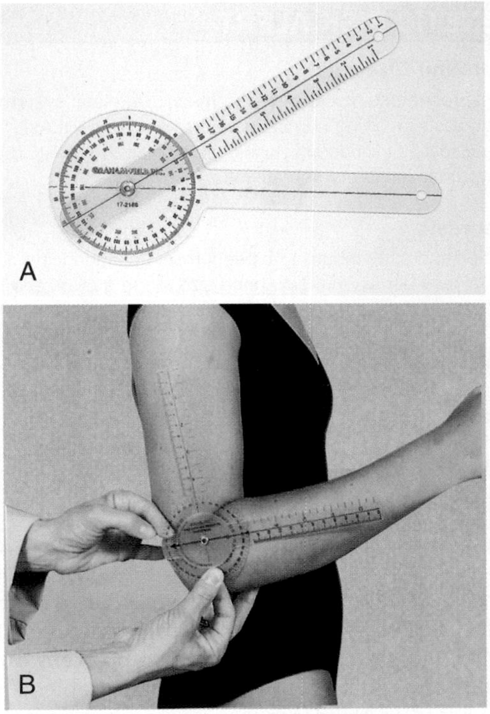


**FIG. 61-7 A,** Goniometer. **B,** Measurement of joint range of motion using a goniometer. (*A,* From Wilson SF, Giddens JF: *Health assessment for nursing practice,* ed 5, St Louis, 2013, Mosby. *B,* From Barkauskas V, Baumann L, Stoltenberg-Allen K, et al: *Health and physical assessment,* ed 2, St Louis, 1998, Mosby.)

If you note deficits in active or passive range of motion, also assess functional range of motion to determine if performance of ADLs has been affected by joint changes. This is done by asking the patient if activities such as eating, grooming, dressing, and bathing must be performed with assistance or cannot be done at all.

Range of motion is most accurately assessed with a goniometer, which measures the angle of the joint (Fig. 61-7). Specific degrees of range of motion of all joints are usually not measured. If a specific musculoskeletal problem has been identified, measure range of motion of the affected joint. A less exact but valuable assessment method is simply to compare the range of motion of one extremity with that on the opposite side. Common movements that occur at the synovial joints, including *abduction, adduction, flexion,* and *extension,* are described in Table 61-3.

***Muscle-Strength Testing.*** Grade the strength of individual muscles or groups of muscles during contraction on a 5-point scale (Table 61-4). Grade normal muscle strength with full resistance to opposition as a 5/5 bilaterally. To test resistance to opposition, have the patient apply resistance against a force you are exerting. For example, have the patient try to extend the elbow while you attempt to flex it. Compare muscle strength with the strength of the opposite extremity. Note any subtle variations in muscle strength when comparing the patient's dominant and nondominant sides. Variations in strength also exist when comparing individuals.

***Measurement.*** When limb length discrepancies or subjective problems are noted, obtain limb length and circumferential muscle mass measurements. For example, when gait disorders are observed, measure leg length between the anterosuperior iliac crest and the bottom of the medial malleolus. Then compare it with the similar measurement of the opposite extremity. Measure muscle mass circumferentially at the largest area of the muscle. When recording measurements, document the exact location at which the measurements were obtained (e.g., the left quadriceps muscle was measured 15 cm above the patella). This informs the next examiner of the exact area to measure and ensures consistency during reassessment.

***Other.*** Note the patient's use of an assistive device such as a walker or cane. Assess the patient for proper fit while reviewing the safe and correct technique for using these devices. Regularly review with the patient the use of the assistive device to ensure it remains appropriate and safe.[9]

If the patient is able to move independently, assess posture and gait by watching the patient walk, stand, and sit. Musculoskeletal and neurologic problems can result in abnormal gait patterns.

**Scoliosis** is a lateral S-shaped curvature of the thoracic and lumbar spine. Unequal shoulder and scapula height is usually noted when the patient is observed from the back (Fig. 61-8). Ask the patient to place the hands together above the head as if diving into a swimming pool and slowly bend forward at the waist, allowing for assessment of thoracic rib prominence or paravertebral muscle prominence in the lumbar spine. Lung and cardiac function may be impaired with advancing scoliosis deformity.

**TABLE 61-3 Synovial Joint Movements**

| Movement | Description |
|---|---|
| Abduction | Movement of part away from midline of body |
| Adduction | Movement of part toward midline of body |
| Circumduction | Circular motion of a body part resulting from a combination of flexion, abduction, extension, and adduction |
| Dorsiflexion | Flexion of the ankle and toes toward the shin |
| Eversion | Turning of sole outward away from midline of body |
| Extension | Straightening of joint that increases angle between two bones |
| External rotation | Movement along longitudinal axis away from midline of body |
| Flexion | Bending of joint as a result of muscle contraction that causes decreased angle between two bones |
| Hyperextension | Extension in which angle exceeds 180 degrees |
| Internal rotation | Movement along longitudinal axis toward midline of body |
| Inversion | Turning of sole inward toward midline of body |
| Opposition | Moving the first and fifth metacarpals anteriorly from a flattened palm ("cupping position"); makes it possible to hold objects between the thumb and fingers |
| Plantar flexion | Flexion of the ankle and toes toward the plantar surface of the foot ("toes pointed") |
| Pronation | Turning of palm downward |
| Supination | Turning of palm upward |

**TABLE 61-4 Muscle Strength Scale**

| | |
|---|---|
| 0/5 | No detection of muscular contraction |
| 1/5 | A barely detectable flicker or trace of contraction with observation or palpation |
| 2/5 | Active movement of body part with elimination of gravity |
| 3/5 | Active movement against gravity only and not against resistance |
| 4/5 | Active movement against gravity and some resistance |
| 5/5 | Active movement against full resistance without evident fatigue (normal muscle strength) |

The *straight-leg-raising test* is performed on the supine patient with sciatica or leg pain. Passively raise the patient's leg 60 degrees or less. The test is positive if the patient complains of pain along the distribution of the sciatic nerve. A positive test indicates nerve root irritation from intervertebral disc prolapse and herniation, particularly at the level of L4-5 or L5-S1.

Assessment of reflexes is discussed in Chapter 55. Table 61-5 is an example of how to record a normal physical assessment of the musculoskeletal system. Abnormal assessment findings of the musculoskeletal system are presented in Table 61-6.

A *focused assessment* is used to evaluate the status of previously identified musculoskeletal problems and to monitor for signs of new problems (see Table 3-7). A focused assessment of the musculoskeletal system is presented in the box.

## DIAGNOSTIC STUDIES OF MUSCULOSKELETAL SYSTEM

Numerous diagnostic studies are available to assess the musculoskeletal system. Table 61-7 presents the most common studies, and select studies are described in more detail below.

The use of studies such as x-rays, MRI, and bone scans has greatly improved orthopedic care. The **x-ray** is the most common diagnostic study used to assess musculoskeletal problems and to monitor the effectiveness of treatment. Because bones are denser than other tissues and contain calcium, most x-rays are absorbed by the bone tissue and do not penetrate it. Dense areas

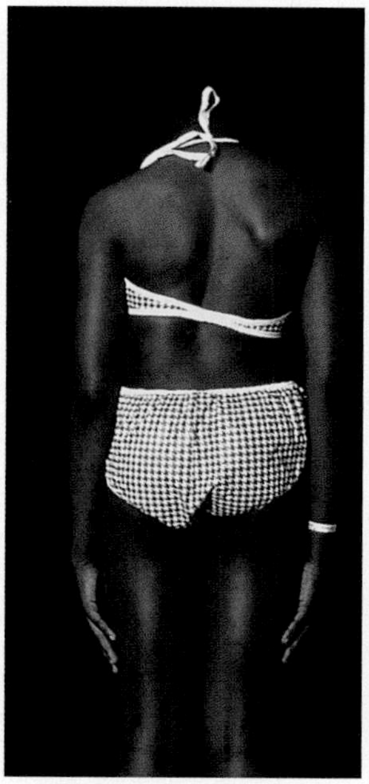

**FIG. 61-8** Scoliosis in a standing erect posture. (From Zitelli BJ, McIntire SC, Nowalk AJ: *Zitelli and Davis' atlas of pediatric physical diagnosis,* ed 6, St Louis, 2012, Mosby.)

**TABLE 61-5 Normal Physical Assessment of the Musculoskeletal System**

- Normal spinal curvatures
- No muscle atrophy or asymmetry
- No joint swelling, deformity, or crepitation
- No tenderness on palpation of spine, joints, or muscles
- Full range of motion of all joints without pain or laxity
- Muscle strength of 5/5

## TABLE 61-6 Assessment Abnormalities

### *Musculoskeletal System*

| Finding | Description | Possible Etiology and Significance |
|---|---|---|
| **Achilles tendonitis** | Pain in ankle and posterior calf, initially when running or walking. Can progress to pain at rest. | Cumulative stress on Achilles tendon resulting in inflammation. |
| **Ankylosis** | Stiffness and fixation of a joint. | Chronic joint inflammation and destruction (e.g., rheumatoid arthritis). |
| **Antalgic gait** | Shortened stride with minimal weight bearing on the affected side, resulting in a limp. | Pain or discomfort in the lower extremity on weight bearing. Can be related to trauma or other disorders. |
| **Ataxic gait** | Staggering, uncoordinated gait often with sway. | Neurogenic disorders (e.g., spinal cord lesion). |
| **Atrophy** | Decreased size and strength of muscle leading to decreased function and tone. | Muscle denervation, contracture, prolonged disuse as a result of immobilization. |
| **Boutonnière deformity** | Finger abnormality, flexion of proximal interphalangeal (PIP) joint and hyperextension of the distal interphalangeal (DIP) joint of the fingers (see Fig. 64-4, *B*). | Typical deformity of rheumatoid and psoriatic arthritis caused by disruption of extensor tendons over the fingers. |
| **Contracture** | Resistance of movement of muscle or joint as a result of fibrosis of supporting soft tissues. | Shortening of muscle or ligaments, tightness of soft tissue, incorrect positioning of immobilized extremity. |
| **Crepitation (crepitus)** | Frequent, audible crackling sound with palpable grating that accompanies movement. | Fracture, dislocation, temporomandibular joint dysfunction, osteoarthritis. |
| **Dislocation** | Separation of two bones from their normal position within a joint. | Trauma, disorders of surrounding soft tissues. |
| **Festinating gait** | While walking, neck, trunk, and knees flex and the body is rigid. Delayed start with short, quick, shuffling steps. Speed may increase as if patient is unable to stop (festination). | Neurogenic disorders (e.g., Parkinson's disease). |
| **Ganglion cyst** | Small fluid-filled mass over a tendon sheath or joint, usually on dorsal surface of wrist or foot. | Inflammation of tissues around a joint, which can increase in size or disappear. |
| **Kyphosis (dowager's hump)** | Exaggerated thoracic curvature. | Poor posture, tuberculosis, arthritis, osteoporosis, growth disturbance of vertebral epiphyses. |
| **Lateral epicondylitis (tennis elbow)** | Dull ache along outer aspect of elbow, worsens with twisting and grasping motions. | Injury, inflammation, and/or partial tearing of tendon at its insertion on epicondyle. |
| **Limited range of motion (ROM)** | Joint does not achieve expected degrees of motion. | Injury, inflammation, contracture. |
| **Lordosis (swayback)** | Exaggerated lumbar curvature. | Secondary to other spinal deformities, muscular dystrophy, obesity, flexion contracture of hip, congenital dislocation of hip. |
| **Muscle spasticity** | Increased muscle tone (rigidity) with sustained muscle contractions (spasms); stiffness or tightness may interfere with gait, movement, speech. | Neuromuscular disorders such as multiple sclerosis (MS) or cerebral palsy. |
| **Myalgia** | General muscle tenderness and pain. | Chronic pain syndromes (e.g., fibromyalgia). Overuse, injury, or strain. |
| **Paresthesia** | Numbness and tingling, often described as a "pins and needles" sensation. | Compromised sensory nerves, often due to edema in a closed space such as a cast or bulky dressing. May also result from spinal stenosis. |
| **Pes planus (flatfoot)** | Abnormal flatness of the sole and arch of the foot. | Hereditary, muscle paralysis, mild cerebral palsy, early muscular dystrophy, injury to posterior tibial tendon. |
| **Plantar fasciitis** | Burning, sharp pain on heel and sole of foot. Worse in the morning with first step out of bed. | Chronic degenerative/reparative cycle resulting in inflammation. |
| **Scoliosis** | Asymmetric elevation of shoulders, scapulae, and iliac crests with lateral spine curvature (Fig. 61-8). | Idiopathic or congenital condition, fracture or dislocation, osteomalacia. |
| **Short-leg gait** | A limp, unless corrective footwear used. | Leg length discrepancy ≥1 in, generally of structural origin (arthritis, fracture). |
| **Spastic gait** | Short steps with dragging of foot. Jerky, uncoordinated, cross-knee (scissor) movement. | Neurogenic (e.g., cerebral palsy, hemiplegia). |
| **Steppage gait** | Increased hip and knee flexion to clear the foot from the floor. Footdrop is evident, foot slaps down and along walking surface. | Neurogenic disorders (e.g., peroneal nerve injury, paralyzed dorsiflexor muscles). |
| **Subluxation** | Partial dislocation of joint. | Instability of joint capsule and supporting ligaments (e.g., trauma, arthritis). |
| **Swan neck deformity** | Hyperextension of the PIP joint with flexion of the metacarpophalangeal (MCP) and DIP joints of the fingers (see Fig. 64-4, *D*). | Typical deformity of rheumatoid and psoriatic arthritis caused by contracture of muscles and tendons. |
| **Swelling** | Enlargement, often of a joint due to fluid collection. Generally leads to pain, stiffness. | Trauma or inflammation. |
| **Tenosynovitis** | Superficial swelling, pain, and tenderness along a tendon sheath. | Inflammation that often occurs with infection, injury, or overuse. |
| **Torticollis (wryneck)** | Neck is rotated and laterally bent in unusual position to one side. | Prolonged contraction of neck muscles (congenital or acquired). |
| **Ulnar deviation (ulnar drift)** | Fingers drift to ulnar side of forearm (see Fig. 64-4, *A*). | Typical deformity of rheumatoid arthritis due to tendon contracture. |
| **Valgum deformity (knock-knees)** | When knees are together and there is >1 in (2.5 cm) between the medial malleoli. | Poliomyelitis, congenital deformity, arthritis. |
| **Varum deformity (bowlegs)** | When knees are apart and the medial malleoli are together, a space of >1 in (2.5 cm) exists. | Arthritis, congenital deformity. |

show as white on the standard x-ray. X-rays provide information about bone deformity, joint congruity, bone density, and calcification in soft tissue. X-rays are useful for diagnosing fractures and evaluating genetic, developmental, infectious, inflammatory, neoplastic, metabolic, and degenerative disorders.

Visualization and analysis of aspirated synovial fluid allows assessment of volume, color, clarity, viscosity, and mucin clot formation. Normal synovial fluid is transparent and colorless or straw colored. It should be scant in amount and of low viscosity. Fluid from an infected joint may be purulent and thick or gray and thin. In gout, the fluid may be whitish yellow. Blood may be aspirated if there is hemarthrosis due to injury or a bleeding disorder.

## CASE STUDY–cont'd

### Objective Data: Physical Examination

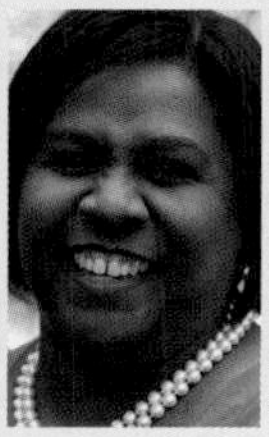
(©pixelhead-photo/iStock/Thinkstock)

A focused assessment of G.A. reveals the following: BP 128/94, heart rate 88, respiratory rate 26, temp 96.8° F, $O_2$ saturation 98%. Alert and oriented × 3. Lungs are clear bilaterally. Left great toe is red and swollen. No open wounds. Tremendous pain on palpation and with any movement of the left great toe. +1 Pedal pulses bilaterally.

**Discussion Questions**

1. What should be included in the physical assessment? What findings would be of most concern to you?
2. Based on results of the subjective and physical assessment, what diagnostic studies might you expect to be included for G.A.?

You will learn more about diagnostic studies related to the musculoskeletal system in the next section.

See p. 1460 for more information on G.A.

Answers available at *http://evolve.elsevier.com/Lewis/medsurg.*

The mucin clot test indicates the character of the protein portion of the synovial fluid. Normally a white, ropelike mucin clot is formed. In the presence of inflammation, the clot fragments easily. The fluid is examined grossly for floating fat globules, which indicate bone injury. In septic arthritis, protein content is elevated and glucose is considerably decreased. Presence of uric acid crystals suggests a diagnosis of gout. A Gram stain and culture may also be done to assess for the presence and type of infection.

## FOCUSED ASSESSMENT

### Musculoskeletal System

*Use this checklist to be sure key assessment steps have been done.*

**Subjective**

*Ask the patient about any of the following and note responses.*

| | | |
|---|---|---|
| Joint pain or stiffness | Y | N |
| Muscle weakness | Y | N |
| Bone pain | Y | N |

**Objective: Diagnostic**

*Check the results of the following diagnostic studies.*

| | |
|---|---|
| X-ray | ✓ |
| MRI or CT scan | ✓ |
| Bone scan | ✓ |

**Objective: Physical Examination**

***Inspect and Palpate***

| | |
|---|---|
| Spine and extremities (compare sides) for alignment, contour, symmetry, size, gross deformities | ✓ |
| Joints for range of motion, tenderness or pain, heat, crepitus, swelling | ✓ |
| Muscles (compare sides) for size, symmetry, tone, tenderness or pain | ✓ |
| Bones for tenderness or pain | ✓ |

## TABLE 61-7 Diagnostic Studies

### Musculoskeletal System

| Study | Description and Purpose | Nursing Responsibility |
|---|---|---|
| **Radiologic Studies** | | |
| **Standard x-ray** | Evaluates structural or functional changes of bones and joints. Can give a general impression of bone density. In anteroposterior view, x-ray beam passes from front to back, allowing one-dimensional view. Lateral position provides two-dimensional view. | *Before:* Remove any radiopaque objects that can interfere with results. Explain procedure to patient.<br>*During:* Avoid excessive exposure of patient and self. |
| **Diskogram** | X-ray of cervical or lumbar intervertebral disc is done after injection of contrast media into nucleus pulposus. Permits visualization of intervertebral disc abnormalities. | *Before:* Assess patient for possible allergy to contrast medium. Explain procedure. |
| **Computed tomography (CT) scan** | X-ray beam used with a computer to provide a 3D picture. Used to identify soft tissue abnormalities, bony abnormalities, and various types of musculoskeletal trauma. | *Before:* Inform patient that procedure is painless. Inform patient of importance of remaining still during procedure. If contrast medium is being used, verify that patient does not have shellfish allergy. |
| **Myelogram with or without CT** | Involves injecting a radiographic contrast medium into sac around nerve roots. CT scan may follow to show how the bone is affecting the nerve roots. Sensitive test for nerve impingement and can detect subtle lesions and injuries. | *Before:* Inform patient that headache may occur after procedure but should resolve in 1-2 days with rest and fluids, but should be reported to HCP. |
| **MRI** | Radio waves and magnetic field are used to view soft tissue. Especially useful in the diagnosis of avascular necrosis, disc disease, tumors, osteomyelitis, ligament tears, and cartilage tears. Patient is placed inside scanning chamber.<br>Gadolinium may be injected IV to enhance visualization of structures.<br>Open MRI (patient not placed in chamber) may be indicated for obese patient or patient with large chest and abdominal girth or severe claustrophobia. Contraindicated in patient with aneurysm clips, metallic implants, pacemakers, electronic devices, hearing aids, and shrapnel. | *Before:* Inform patient that procedure is painless. Explain that the machine will make loud tapping noises intermittently and there is no cause for alarm. Ear plugs can be requested or music to listen to. Ensure that patient has no metal on clothing (e.g., snaps, zippers), jewelry, credit cards. Inform patient to remain still throughout procedure.<br>Inform patients who are claustrophobic that they may experience symptoms during examination. Administer antianxiety agent if indicated and ordered. |

*Continued*

## TABLE 61-7 Diagnostic Studies

***Musculoskeletal System—cont'd***

| Study | Description and Purpose | Nursing Responsibility |
|---|---|---|
| **Bone Mineral Density (BMD) Measurements** | | |
| **Dual energy x-ray absorptiometry (DXA)** | Measures bone mineral density of spine, femur, forearm, and total body. Allows assessment of bone density with minimal radiation exposure. Used to diagnose metabolic bone disease (e.g., osteoporosis) and monitor changes in bone density with treatment. | *Before:* Inform patient that procedure is painless. |
| **Quantitative ultrasound (QUS)** | Evaluates density, elasticity, and strength of bone using ultrasound rather than radiation. Common area assessed is calcaneus (heel). | Same as above. |
| **Radioisotope Studies** | | |
| **Bone scan** | Involves injection of radioisotope (usually technetium [Tc]-99m) that is taken up by bone. Uniform uptake of the isotope is normal. Increased uptake is seen in osteomyelitis, primary and metastatic cancer of bone, and certain fractures. Decreased uptake is seen in areas of avascular necrosis. | *Before:* Explain that radioisotope is given 2 hr before procedure. Ensure that bladder is emptied before scan. Inform patient that procedure requires 1 hr while patient lies supine and that no pain or harm will result from isotopes.<br>*After:* Increase fluids after scan. |
| **Endoscopy** | | |
| **Arthroscopy** | Involves insertion of arthroscope into joint for visualization of interior of joint cavity. Can be used for surgery (removal of loose bodies, biopsy); repair of joint structures; and diagnosis of abnormalities of meniscus, articular cartilage, ligaments, or joint capsule. Structures that can be visualized through an arthroscope include knee, shoulder, elbow, wrist, jaw, hip, and ankle (Fig. 61-9). | *Before:* Inform patient that procedure can be performed in outpatient setting and that local or general anesthesia may be used.<br>*After:* Cover wound with sterile dressing. Explain any postprocedure activity restrictions. |
| **Mineral Metabolism** | | |
| **Alkaline phosphatase** | This enzyme is produced by osteoblasts and is needed for mineralization of organic bone matrix. Elevated levels are found in healing fractures, bone cancers, osteoporosis, osteomalacia, and Paget's disease.<br>*Reference interval:* 38-126 U/L (0.65-2.14 μkat/L) | *During:* Obtain blood samples by venipuncture. Observe venipuncture site for bleeding or hematoma formation. Inform patient that procedure does not require fasting. |
| **Calcium** | Bone is primary organ for calcium storage. Calcium provides bone with rigid structure. Decreased serum level is found in osteomalacia, kidney disease, and hypoparathyroidism.<br>Increased level is found in hyperparathyroidism and some bone tumors.<br>*Reference interval:* 8.6-10.2 mg/dL (2.20-2.55 mmol/L) | Same as above. |
| **Phosphorus** | Amount present is indirectly related to calcium metabolism. Decreased level is found in osteomalacia. Increased level is found in chronic kidney disease, healing fractures, and osteolytic metastatic tumor.<br>*Reference interval:* 2.4-4.4 mg/dL (0.78-1.42 mmol/L) | Same as above. |
| **Serologic Studies** | | |
| **Rheumatoid factor (RF)** | Assesses presence of autoantibody (rheumatoid factor) in serum. Factor is not specific for rheumatoid arthritis and is seen in other connective tissue diseases and in a small percentage of normal population.<br>*Reference interval:* Negative or titer <1:17 | Same as above. |
| **Anticyclic citrullinated peptide (anti-CCP)** | Assesses presence of CCP antibodies. More specific for rheumatoid arthritis than rheumatoid factor. Positive result indicates high likelihood of RA.<br>*Reference interval*: Negative or <20.0 U | Same as above. |
| **Antinuclear antibody (ANA)** | Assesses presence of antibodies capable of destroying nucleus of body's tissue cells. Finding is positive in 95% of patients with systemic lupus erythematosus and may also be positive in individuals with scleroderma or rheumatoid arthritis and in a small percentage of normal population.<br>*Reference interval:* Negative at 1:40 dilution | Same as above. |
| **Anti-DNA antibody** | Detects serum antibodies that react with DNA. Most specific test for systemic lupus erythematosus.<br>*Reference interval:* <70 IU/mL | Same as above. |

## TABLE 61-7 Diagnostic Studies
### *Musculoskeletal System—cont'd*

| Study | Description and Purpose | Nursing Responsibility |
|---|---|---|
| **Complement, total hemolytic ($CH_{50}$)** | Complement, a normal body protein, is essential to immune and inflammatory reactions. Complement components used in these reactions are depleted. Complement depletions may be found in patients with rheumatoid arthritis or systemic lupus erythematosus.<br>*Reference interval:* 75-160 U/mL (75-160 kU/L) | Same as above. |
| **Uric acid** | End product of purine metabolism normally excreted in urine. Although not specific, levels are usually elevated in gout.<br>*Male:* 4.4-7.6 mg/dL (262-452 µmol/L)<br>*Female:* 2.3-6.6 mg/dL (137-393 µmol/L) | Same as above. |
| **C-reactive protein (CRP)** | Used to diagnose inflammatory diseases, infections, and active widespread malignancy. Synthesized by the liver and is present in large amounts in serum 18-24 hr after onset of tissue damage.<br>*Reference interval:* 6.8-820 mcg/dL (68-8200 mcg/L) | Same as above. |
| **Human leukocyte antigen (HLA)–B27** | Antigen often present in autoimmune disorders such as ankylosing spondylitis and rheumatoid arthritis. | Same as above. |
| **Markers of Muscle Injury** | | |
| **Creatine kinase (CK)** | Highest concentration found in skeletal muscle. Increased serum CK found in progressive muscular dystrophy, polymyositis, and traumatic injuries.<br>*Male:* 20-200 U/L<br>*Female:* 20-180 U/L | Same as above. |
| **Potassium** | Increased in muscle trauma as cell destruction releases this electrolyte into serum. Cardiac dysrhythmias can be caused by hyperkalemia or hypokalemia.<br>*Reference interval:* 3.5-5.0 mEq/L (3.5-5.0 mmol/L) | Same as above. |
| **Aldolase** | Useful in monitoring muscular dystrophy and dermatomyositis.<br>*Reference interval:* 1.5-8.1 U/L | Same as above. |
| **Invasive Procedures** | | |
| **Arthrocentesis** | Incision or puncture of joint capsule to obtain samples of synovial fluid or to remove excess fluid. Local anesthesia and aseptic preparation are used before needle is inserted into joint and fluid aspirated. Useful in diagnosis of joint inflammation, infection, meniscal tears, and subtle fractures. | *Before:* Inform patient that procedure is usually done at bedside or in examination room.<br>*After:* Send samples of synovial fluid to laboratory for examination (if indicated). Apply compression dressing. Observe for leakage of blood or fluid on dressing. |
| **Electromyogram (EMG)** | Evaluates electrical potential associated with skeletal muscle contraction. Small-gauge needles are inserted into certain muscles. Needle probes are attached to leads that send information to EMG machine. Recordings of electrical activity of muscle are traced on audio transmitter and on oscilloscope and recording paper. Useful in providing information related to lower motor neuron dysfunction and primary muscle disease. | *Before:* Inform patient that procedure is usually done in EMG laboratory while patient lies supine on special table. Inform patient that procedure involves some discomfort from needle insertion. Avoid stimulants, including caffeine, and sedatives 24 hr before procedure. |
| **Miscellaneous** | | |
| **Duplex venous Doppler** | Ultrasound of the veins, usually of the lower extremities, to detect blood flow abnormalities that could indicate DVT. | *Before:* Inform patient that procedure is painless and noninvasive. |
| **Thermography** | Uses infrared detector to measure degree of heat radiating from skin surface. Useful in investigating cause of inflamed joint and in determining patient response to antiinflammatory drug therapy. | Same as above. |
| **Plethysmography** | Records variations in volume and pressure of blood passing through tissues. Test is nonspecific. | Same as above. |
| **Somatosensory evoked potential (SSEP)** | Evaluates evoked potential of muscle contractions. Electrodes are placed on skin and provide recordings of electrical activity of muscle. Useful in identifying subtle dysfunction of lower motor neuron and primary muscle disease. Measures nerve conduction along pathways not accessible by EMG. Transcutaneous or percutaneous electrodes are applied to the skin to help identify neuropathy and myopathy. Often used during spinal surgery for scoliosis to detect neurologic compromise when patient is under anesthesia. | *Before:* Inform patient that procedure is similar to EMG but does not involve needles. Electrodes are applied to the skin. |

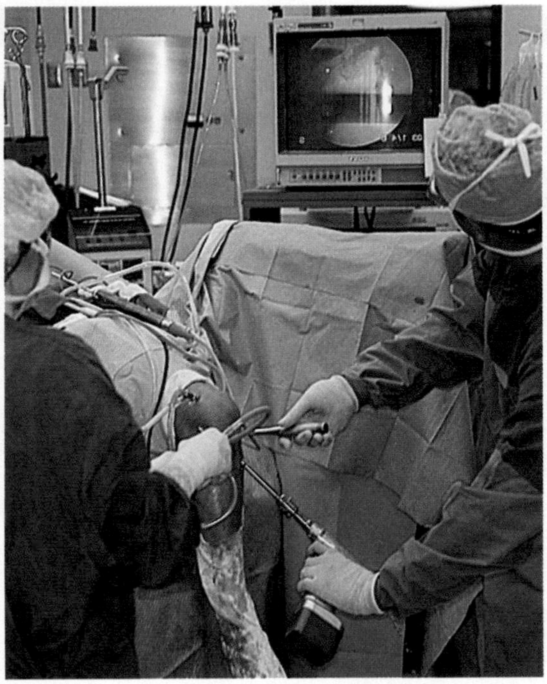

**FIG. 61-9** Knee arthroscopy in progress. Notice the monitor in the background. (From Miller MD, Howard RF, Plancher KD: *Surgical atlas of sports medicine*, Philadelphia, 2003, Saunders.)

## CASE STUDY–cont'd

### *Objective Data: Diagnostic Studies*

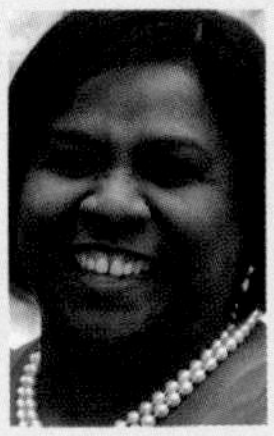

(©pixelhead-photo/iStock/Thinkstock)

The HCP in the ED immediately orders the following diagnostic studies:

- X-ray of left foot
- CBC, electrolytes
- Aspiration of the great toe

The x-ray of the foot reveals minor soft tissue swelling but no evidence of fracture. Very mild arthritis is noted at the interphalangeal joint of the great toe. CBC and electrolytes are within normal limits.

Aspiration of the interphalangeal joint shows clear synovial fluid. Protein and glucose are within normal limits. Microscopic analysis of the synovial fluid shows urate crystals.

#### Discussion Questions

1. Which diagnostic results are abnormal?
2. What diagnostic study results are of most concern to you?

Answers available at *http://evolve.elsevier.com/Lewis/medsurg.*

## BRIDGE TO NCLEX EXAMINATION

The number of the question corresponds to the same-numbered outcome at the beginning of the chapter.

1. The bone cells that function in the resorption of bone tissue are called
   - **a.** osteoids.
   - **b.** osteocytes.
   - **c.** osteoclasts.
   - **d.** osteoblasts.
2. While performing passive range of motion for a patient, the nurse puts the ankle joint through the movements of *(select all that apply)*
   - **a.** flexion and extension.
   - **b.** inversion and eversion.
   - **c.** pronation and supination.
   - **d.** flexion, extension, abduction, and adduction.
   - **e.** pronation, supination, rotation, and circumduction.
3. To prevent muscle atrophy, the nurse teaches the patient with a leg immobilized in traction to perform *(select all that apply)*
   - **a.** flexion contractions.
   - **b.** tetanic contractions.
   - **c.** isotonic contractions.
   - **d.** isometric contractions.
   - **e.** extension contractions.
4. A patient with tendonitis asks what the tendon does. The nurse's response is based on the knowledge that tendons
   - **a.** connect bone to muscle.
   - **b.** provide strength to muscle.
   - **c.** lubricate joints with synovial fluid.
   - **d.** relieve friction between moving parts.
5. The increased risk for falls in the older adult is *most* likely due to
   - **a.** changes in balance.
   - **b.** decrease in bone mass.
   - **c.** loss of ligament elasticity.
   - **d.** erosion of articular cartilage.
6. While obtaining subjective assessment data related to the musculoskeletal system, the nurse must ask a patient about other medical problems such as
   - **a.** hypertension.
   - **b.** thyroid problems.
   - **c.** diabetes mellitus.
   - **d.** chronic bronchitis.
7. When grading muscle strength, the nurse records a score of 3/5, which indicates
   - **a.** no detection of muscular contraction.
   - **b.** a barely detectable flicker of contraction.
   - **c.** active movement against full resistance without fatigue.
   - **d.** active movement against gravity but not against resistance.
8. A normal assessment finding of the musculoskeletal system is
   - **a.** no deformity or crepitation.
   - **b.** muscle and bone strength of 4.
   - **c.** ulnar deviation and subluxation.
   - **d.** angulation of bone toward midline.
9. A patient is scheduled for an electromyogram (EMG). The nurse explains that this diagnostic test involves
   - **a.** incision or puncture of the joint capsule.
   - **b.** insertion of small needles into certain muscles.
   - **c.** administration of a radioisotope before the procedure.
   - **d.** placement of skin electrodes to record muscle activity.
10. What would the nurse recognize as a possible difference in the assessment of a gerontologic patient?
    - **a.** Slowed reaction time
    - **b.** Quicker reflex response
    - **c.** Decreased joint stiffness
    - **d.** Increased fine motor dexterity

1. c, 2. a, b, 3. d, 4. a, 5. a, 6. c, 7. d, 8. a, 9. b, 10. a

For rationales to these answers and even more NCLEX review questions, visit *http://evolve.elsevier.com/Lewis/medsurg.*

## EVOLVE WEBSITE

http://evolve.elsevier.com/Lewis/medsurg

**Review Questions (Online Only)**

**Key Points**

**Answer Keys for Questions**

- Rationales for Bridge to NCLEX Examination Questions
- Answer Guidelines for Case Study on pp. 1451, 1454, 1457, and 1460

**Conceptual Care Map Creator**

**Audio Glossary**

**Supporting Media**

- Animation
  - Overview of the Musculoskeletal System

**Content Updates**

## REFERENCES

1. Moore KL, Anne MR, Dailey AF: *Essential clinical anatomy*, ed 5, Philadelphia, 2015, Wolters Kluwer Health.
2. Crowther-Radulewicz CL: The musculoskeletal system. In McCance KL, Heuther SE, editors: *Pathophysiology: the biologic basis for disease in adults and children*, ed 7, St Louis, 2014, Mosby.
3. Martini FH, Nath JL, Bartholomew EF: *Fundamentals of anatomy and physiology*, ed 10, New York, 2014, Pearson.
4. Patton KT, Thibodeau GA: *Anatomy & physiology*, ed 8, St Louis, 2013, Mosby.
5. Zychowicz ME, Ballard PC: Musculoskeletal system. In Estes MEZ, editor: *Health assessment & physical examination*, ed 5, Clifton Park, NY, 2014, Cengage.
6. Stoppiello LA, Mapp PI, Wilson D, et al: Structural associations of symptomatic knee osteoarthritis, *Arthr Rheum* 66:3018, 2014.
7. Zychowicz ME, South T, Martin-Plank L, et al: Musculoskeletal problems. In Dunphy LM, Winland-Brown JE, Porter BO, et al, editors: *Primary care: the art and science of advanced practice nursing*, ed 4, Philadelphia, 2015, FA Davis.
8. Ward CW: Procedure-specific postoperative pain management, *MEDSURG* 23:107, 2014.

*9. Fischer J, Nüesch C, Göpfert B, et al: Forearm pressure distribution during ambulation with elbow crutches: a cross-sectional study, *J Neuroeng Rehab* 11:61, 2014.

*Evidence-based information for clinical practice.

# 62

# Musculoskeletal Trauma and Orthopedic Surgery

*Mary K. Wollan*

*With the new day comes new strength and new thoughts.*

***Eleanor Roosevelt***

http://evolve.elsevier.com/Lewis/medsurg/

## LEARNING OUTCOMES

1. Differentiate among the etiology, pathophysiology, clinical manifestations, and interprofessional care of soft tissue injuries, including strains, sprains, dislocations, subluxations, bursitis, repetitive strain injury, carpal tunnel syndrome, and injuries to the rotator cuff, meniscus, and anterior cruciate ligament.
2. Relate the sequential events involved in fracture healing.
3. Compare closed reduction, cast immobilization, open reduction, and traction in terms of purpose, complications, and nursing management.
4. Assess the neurovascular condition of an injured extremity.
5. Explain common complications associated with a fracture and fracture healing.
6. Describe the interprofessional care and nursing management of patients with various kinds of fractures.
7. Describe indications for and interprofessional care and nursing management of the patient with an amputation.
8. Describe types of joint replacement surgery for arthritis and other disorders.
9. Prioritize preoperative and postoperative management of the patient having joint replacement surgery.

## KEY TERMS

**amputation, p. 1487**
**arthrodesis, p. 1492**
**arthroplasty, p. 1491**
**bursitis, p. 1468**
**carpal tunnel syndrome (CTS), p. 1465**
**compartment syndrome, p. 1479**
**debridement, p. 1491**
**dislocation, p. 1464**
**fat embolism syndrome (FES), p. 1480**
**fracture, p. 1468**
**osteotomy, p. 1490**
**phantom limb sensation, p. 1488**
**repetitive strain injury (RSI), p. 1465**
**sprain, p. 1463**
**strain, p. 1463**
**subluxation, p. 1464**
**synovectomy, p. 1490**
**traction, p. 1470**

Musculoskeletal problems resulting from trauma and common orthopedic surgical procedures are discussed in this chapter. The nurse's role in prevention of complications and promotion of function in patients with fractures and orthopedic surgery is emphasized.

The most common cause of musculoskeletal injury is a traumatic event resulting in fracture, dislocation, and/or soft tissue injury. Although most of these injuries are not fatal, the cost in terms of pain, disability, medical expense, and lost wages is enormous. Accidents are one of the top three causes of death for persons ages 1 to 64 years. Accidental injuries (e.g., motor vehicle collisions, drowning, burns) are the leading cause of death in children and young adults in the United States.[1]

Teaching the public about basic principles of safety and accident prevention is important. The morbidity associated with accidents can be significantly reduced if people are aware of environmental hazards, use appropriate safety equipment, and apply safety and traffic rules. In the occupational and industrial setting, teach employees and employers about use of proper safety equipment and avoidance of hazardous working situations.

**! SAFETY ALERT Falls**
- Falls account for many musculoskeletal injuries in the home.
- Provide preventive teaching to high-risk individuals (e.g., people with gait instability, visual or cognitive impairment).
- Stress the importance of wearing shoes with functional, stable soles and heels; avoiding wet or slippery surfaces; and removing throw rugs in the home.

Ways to prevent common musculoskeletal problems in the older adult are listed in Table 62-1.

## SOFT TISSUE INJURIES

*Soft tissue injuries,* including sprains, strains, dislocations, and subluxations, usually result from trauma. The increasing number of people involved in a fitness program or participating in sports has contributed to the increased incidence of soft

Reviewed by Judy Carlyle, RN, MNSc, Faculty/Clinical Liaison, Arkansas Rural Nursing Education Consortium (ARNEC), Nashville, Arkansas; Roberta Goff, RN, MSN Ed, ACNS-BC, RN-BC, ONC, Clinical Nurse Specialist, Munson Medical Center, Traverse City, Michigan; Matthew C. Price, RN, MSN, CNP, ONP-C, RNFA, Manager, Orthopedic Advanced Practice Providers, Riverside Methodist Hospital, Columbus, Ohio; and Laura C. Williams, RN, MSN, CNS, ONC, CCNS, Orthopedic Clinical Nurse Specialist, Orlando Health, Orlando, Florida.

tissue injuries. Common sports-related injuries are summarized in Table 62-2. The most common sports injuries that result in a visit to the emergency department for younger patients are sprains and strains, growth plate injuries, and repetitive motion injuries.[2]

## SPRAINS AND STRAINS

Sprains and strains commonly occur during vigorous activities from abnormal stretching or twisting forces. These injuries tend to occur around joints and in the spinal musculature.

A **sprain** is an injury to the ligaments surrounding a joint, usually caused by a wrenching or twisting motion. Most sprains occur in the ankle, wrist, and knee joints.[3] A sprain is classified according to the degree of ligament damage. A *first-degree (mild) sprain* involves tears in only a few fibers, resulting in mild tenderness and minimal swelling. A *second-degree (moderate) sprain* is partial disruption of the involved tissue with more swelling and tenderness. A *third-degree (severe) sprain* is complete tearing of the ligament in association with moderate to severe swelling. A gap in the muscle may be apparent or palpated through the skin if the muscle is torn. Because areas around joints are rich in nerve endings, the injury can be extremely painful.

A **strain** is an excessive stretching of a muscle, its fascial sheath, or a tendon. Most strains occur in the large muscle groups, including the lower back, calf, and hamstrings. Strains may also be classified as first degree (mild or slightly pulled muscle), second degree (moderate or moderately torn muscle), and third degree (severely torn or ruptured muscle).

Clinical manifestations of sprains and strains are similar and include pain, edema, decreased function, and contusion. Pain aggravated by continued use of the joint, tendon, or ligament is common. Edema develops in the injured area because of the local inflammatory response.

Mild sprains and strains are usually self-limiting, with full function returning within 3 to 6 weeks. X-rays of the affected part may be taken to rule out a fracture. A severe sprain can result in a concomitant *avulsion fracture,* in which the ligament pulls loose a fragment of bone. Alternatively, the joint structure may become unstable and result in subluxation or dislocation. At the time of injury, *hemarthrosis* (bleeding into a joint space or cavity) or disruption of the synovial lining may occur. Severe strains may require surgical repair of the muscle, tendon, or surrounding fascia.[4]

**TABLE 62-1 Patient & Caregiver Teaching**

***Prevention of Musculoskeletal Problems in Older Adults***

*To prevent musculoskeletal problems, include the following instructions when teaching older adults and their caregivers.*

1. Use ramps in buildings and at street corners instead of steps to prevent falls.
2. Eliminate scatter rugs in the home.
3. Treat pain and discomfort from osteoarthritis.
   - Rest in positions that decrease discomfort.
   - Use medication as prescribed for pain.
4. Use a walker or cane to help prevent falls.
5. Eat the amount and kind of foods needed to prevent excessive weight gain. Obesity adds stress to joints, which may predispose to osteoarthritis.
6. Get regular and frequent exercise.
   - Activities of daily living provide range-of-motion exercises. Tai Chi may also be helpful.
   - Hobbies (e.g., jigsaw puzzles, needlework, model building) exercise finger joints and prevent stiffness.
   - Weight-bearing exercise (e.g., walking) should be done on a daily basis to improve bone health.
7. Use shoes with good support for safety and comfort.
8. Avoid sudden change in position. Rise slowly to a standing position to prevent dizziness, falls, and fractures.
9. Avoid walking on uneven surfaces and wet floors.

## NURSING MANAGEMENT: SPRAINS AND STRAINS

### Nursing Implementation

**Health Promotion.** Warming up muscles before exercising and vigorous activity, followed by stretching, may significantly reduce the risk of sprains and strains. Strength, balance, and endurance exercises are also important. Strengthening exercises

**TABLE 62-2 Sports-Related Injuries**

| Injury | Description | Treatment |
|---|---|---|
| **Impingement syndrome** | Entrapment of soft tissues and nerves under coracoacromial arch of shoulder. | NSAIDs. Rest until symptoms decrease and then gradual ROM and strengthening exercises. |
| **Rotator cuff tear** | Tear within muscle, tendons, or ligaments around shoulder. | *If minor tear:* Rest, NSAIDs, and gradual mobilization with ROM and strengthening exercises.<br>*If major tear:* Surgical repair. |
| **Shin splints** | Inflammation of periosteal bone *(periostitis)* along anterior calf caused by improper shoes, overuse, or running on hard pavement. | Rest, ice, NSAIDs, proper shoes. Gradual increase in activity.<br>If pain persists, x-ray to rule out tibial stress fracture. |
| **Tendonitis** | Inflammation of tendon as a result of overuse or incorrect use. | Rest, ice, NSAIDs. Gradual return to sport activity. Protective brace *(orthosis)* may be necessary if symptoms recur. |
| **Ligament injury** | Tearing or stretching of ligament. Usually occurs as a result of inversion, eversion, shearing, or torque applied to a joint. Characterized by sudden pain, swelling, and instability. | Rest, ice, elevation of extremity if possible, NSAIDs. Protect affected extremity by use of brace. If symptoms persist, surgical repair may be needed. |
| **Meniscus injury** | Injury to fibrocartilage discs in knee characterized by popping, clicking, tearing sensation, effusion, and/or swelling. | Rest, ice, elevation of extremity if possible, NSAIDs. Gradual return to regular activities.<br>If symptoms persist, MRI to assess meniscus injury. Possible arthroscopic surgery. |
| **Anterior cruciate ligament tear** | Tearing of ligament by deceleration forces with pivoting or odd positions of the knee or leg. | Physical therapy with rehabilitation, knee brace.<br>If knee instability or additional injury, reconstructive surgery may be done. |

that involve working against resistance build muscle strength and bone density. Balance exercises, which may overlap with some strengthening exercises, help to prevent falls. Endurance exercises should start at a low level of effort and progress gradually to a moderate level.

### HEALTHY PEOPLE

***Health Impact of Regular Physical Activity***

- Assists in weight management.
- Helps maintain and improve bone mass.
- Helps prevent high BP.
- Increases lean muscle and decreases body fat.
- Increases muscle strength, flexibility, and endurance.
- Appears to reduce symptoms of depression and anxiety.
- Reduces the risk of heart disease, diabetes, and colon cancer.
- Enhances sense of well-being and may reduce risk of depression.

◆ **Acute Care.** If an injury occurs, immediate care focuses on (1) stopping the activity and limiting movement, (2) applying ice packs to the injured area, (3) compressing the involved area, (4) elevating the extremity, and (5) providing analgesia as needed (Table 62-3).

*RICE* (*R*est, *I*ce, *C*ompression, *E*levation) may decrease local inflammation and pain for most musculoskeletal injuries. Movement should be restricted and the extremity rested as soon as pain is felt. Unless the injury is severe, prolonged rest is usually not indicated.

Cold *(cryotherapy)* in several forms can be used to produce hypothermia in the involved part. The cold induces physiologic changes in soft tissue, including vasoconstriction and a reduction in the transmission and perception of nerve pain impulses. In addition to pain relief, these changes reduce muscle spasms, inflammation, and edema. Cold is most useful when applied immediately after the injury has occurred. Apply ice no more than 20 to 30 minutes at a time; avoid applying ice directly to the skin.

An elastic compression bandage can be wrapped around the injured part. To prevent edema and encourage fluid return, wrap the bandage starting distally (at the point farthest from the trunk of the body) and progress proximally (toward the trunk of the body). The bandage is too tight if numbness or tingling is felt below the area of compression or additional pain or swelling occurs beyond the edge of the bandage. Leave the bandage in place for 30 minutes and then remove it for 15 minutes. However, some elastic wraps are left on during training, athletic, and occupational activities.

Elevate the injured part above heart level, even during sleep, to help mobilize excess fluid from the area and prevent further edema. Mild analgesics and nonsteroidal antiinflammatory drugs (NSAIDs) may be used to manage patient discomfort.

After the acute phase (usually 24 to 48 hours), apply warm, moist heat to the affected part to reduce swelling and provide comfort. Heat applications should not exceed 20 to 30 minutes, allowing a "cool-down" time between applications. Encourage the patient to use the limb if the joint is protected by means of casting, bracing, taping, or splinting. Joint movement maintains nutrition to the cartilage, and muscle contraction improves circulation and resolution of contusion and swelling.

◆ **Ambulatory Care.** Most sprains and strains are treated in the outpatient setting. Instruct the patient to use ice and elevate for 24 to 48 hours after the injury to reduce edema. Encourage the use of mild analgesics to promote comfort. Use of an elastic wrap may provide additional support during activity. Emphasize to the patient the importance of strengthening and conditioning exercises to prevent reinjury.[5]

The physical therapist may help provide pain relief by modalities such as ultrasound. The therapist may also teach the patient exercises to improve flexibility and strength.

## DISLOCATION AND SUBLUXATION

A **dislocation** is the complete displacement or separation of the articular surfaces of the joint. It results from severe injury of the ligaments surrounding the joint. A **subluxation** is a partial or incomplete displacement of the joint surface. The clinical manifestations of a subluxation are similar to those of a dislocation but are less severe.

Dislocations characteristically result from forces transmitted to the joint that disrupt the soft tissue support structures

### TABLE 62-3 Emergency Management

***Acute Soft Tissue Injury***

| Etiology | Assessment Findings | Interventions |
|---|---|---|
| • Falls<br>• Direct blows<br>• Crush injury<br>• Motor vehicle crashes<br>• Sports injuries | • Edema<br>• Bruising (contusion)<br>• Pain, tenderness<br>• Decreased sensation with severe edema<br>• Decreased pulse, coolness, capillary refill >2 sec<br>• Decreased movement<br>• Pallor<br>• Shortening or rotation of extremity<br>• Inability to bear weight with lower extremity involvement<br>• Limited or decreased function with upper extremity involvement<br>• Muscle spasms | **Initial**<br>• Ensure airway, breathing, and circulation.<br>• Perform neurovascular assessment of involved limb.<br>• Elevate involved limb.<br>• Apply compression bandage unless dislocation present.<br>• Apply ice packs to affected area.<br>• Immobilize affected extremity in the position found. Do *not* attempt to realign or reinsert protruding bones.<br>• Anticipate x-rays of injured extremity.<br>• Give analgesia as necessary.<br>• Administer tetanus and diphtheria prophylaxis if there is an open fracture.<br>• Administer antibiotic prophylaxis for open fracture, large tissue defects, or mangled extremity injury.<br>**Ongoing Monitoring**<br>• Monitor for changes in neurovascular condition.<br>• Implement weight-bearing restrictions as ordered for lower extremity involvement.<br>• Anticipate compartment pressure monitoring if neurovascular assessment changes and compartment syndrome suspected. |

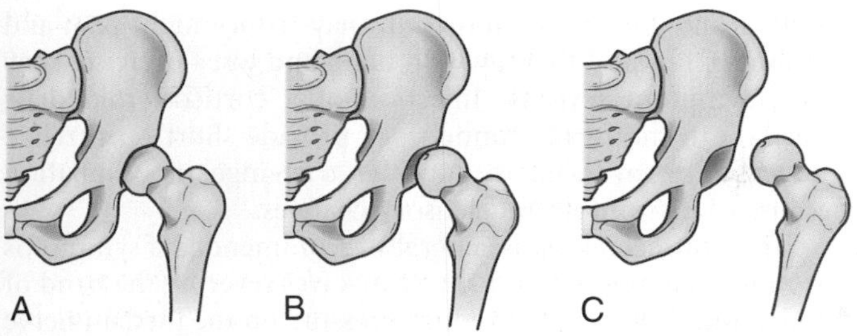


**FIG. 62-1** Soft tissue injury of the hip. **A,** Normal. **B,** Subluxation (partial dislocation). **C,** Dislocation.

surrounding it. The joints most frequently dislocated in the upper extremity include the thumb, elbow, and shoulder. In the lower extremity, the hip is vulnerable to dislocation as a result of severe trauma, often associated with motor vehicle crashes (Fig. 62-1). The kneecap *(patella)* may dislocate because of a sharp, direct blow or after a sudden twisting inward motion while the planted foot is pointed outward.[6]

The most obvious clinical manifestation of a dislocation is deformity. For example, if a hip is dislocated in a posterior (or backward) direction, the affected limb may be shorter and internally rotated. Additional manifestations include local pain, tenderness, loss of function of the injured part, and swelling of soft tissues near the joint. Major complications of a dislocated joint are open joint injuries, fractures within the joint *(intraarticular), avascular necrosis* (bone cell death due to inadequate blood supply), and damage to adjacent nerves and blood vessels.

X-rays are performed to determine the extent of displacement. The joint may also be aspirated to assess for hemarthrosis or fat cells. Fat cells in the aspirate indicate a probable intraarticular fracture.

## ❖ NURSING AND INTERPROFESSIONAL MANAGEMENT: DISLOCATION

A dislocation requires prompt attention. It is often considered an orthopedic emergency because it may be associated with significant vascular injury. The longer the joint remains unreduced, the greater the possibility of avascular necrosis. The femoral head of the hip joint is particularly susceptible to avascular necrosis. Compartment syndrome (discussed on p. 1479) may also occur after dislocation due to vascular injury and resulting ischemia. Neurovascular assessment is critical (see pp. 1474-1475).

The first goal of management of a dislocation is to realign the dislocated portion of the joint to its original anatomic position. Closed reduction (no incision) may be performed under local or general anesthesia or IV moderate to deep sedation (formerly called conscious sedation). Anesthesia is often needed to relax the muscle so that the bones can be manipulated. In some situations, open reduction (joint visualized through surgical incision) may be needed. After reduction, the extremity is immobilized by a brace, splint, or sling, or by taping to allow torn ligaments and surrounding tissue to heal.

Nursing management of subluxation or dislocation is directed toward pain management and support and protection of the injured joint. After the joint has been reduced and immobilized, motion is usually restricted. A carefully monitored rehabilitation program can prevent fracture instability and joint dysfunction. Gentle range-of-motion (ROM) exercises may be recommended if the joint is stable and well supported. An exercise program slowly restores the joint to its original ROM without causing another dislocation. The patient should gradually return to normal activities.

A patient who has dislocated a joint may be at greater risk for repeated dislocations because of loose ligaments. Activity restrictions may be imposed on the affected joint to decrease the risk of repeated dislocations.

## REPETITIVE STRAIN INJURY

**Repetitive strain injury (RSI)** and *cumulative trauma disorder* are terms used to describe injuries resulting from prolonged force or repetitive movements and awkward postures. RSI is also referred to as *repetitive trauma disorder, nontraumatic musculoskeletal injury, overuse syndrome* (sports medicine), *regional musculoskeletal disorder,* and *work-related musculoskeletal disorder.* Repeated movements strain the tendons, ligaments, and muscles, causing tiny tears that become inflamed. The exact cause of these disorders is unknown. No specific diagnostic tests exist, and diagnosis is often difficult.

Persons at risk for RSI include musicians, dancers, butchers, grocery clerks, vibratory tool workers, and those who frequently use a computer mouse and keyboard. Competitive athletes and poorly trained athletes may also develop RSI. Swimming, overhead throwing (e.g., baseball), weight lifting, gymnastics, tennis, skiing, and kicking sports (e.g., soccer) require repetitive motion. Overtraining compounds the effects of RSI.

In addition to repetitive movements, other factors related to RSI include poor posture and positioning, poor workspace ergonomics, badly designed workplace equipment (e.g., computer keyboard), and repetitive lifting of heavy objects without sufficient muscle rest. Inflammation, swelling, and pain in the muscles, tendons, and nerves of the neck, spine, shoulder, forearm, and hand may result. Symptoms of RSI include pain, weakness, numbness, or impaired motor function.

RSI can be prevented through education and *ergonomics* (the science that promotes efficiency and safety in the interaction of humans and their work environment). Ergonomic considerations for persons who work at a desk and use a computer include keeping the hips and knees flexed to 90 degrees with the feet flat, keeping the wrist straight to type, having the top of the computer monitor even with the forehead, and taking at least hourly stretch breaks.

Once RSI is diagnosed, treatment consists of (1) identification of the precipitating activity, (2) modification of equipment or activity, (3) pain management, including heat or cold application and NSAIDs, (4) rest, (5) physical therapy for strengthening and conditioning exercises, and (6) lifestyle changes.

## CARPAL TUNNEL SYNDROME

**Carpal tunnel syndrome (CTS)** is caused by compression of the median nerve, which enters the hand at the wrist through the narrow carpal tunnel (Fig. 62-2). The carpal tunnel is formed by ligaments and bones. CTS is the most common compression neuropathy in the upper extremity. It is associated with hobbies or occupations that require continuous wrist movement (e.g., musicians, carpenters, computer operators).

This condition is often caused by pressure from trauma or edema (secondary to inflammation of a tendon *[tenosynovitis]*), neoplasm, rheumatoid arthritis, or soft tissue masses such as

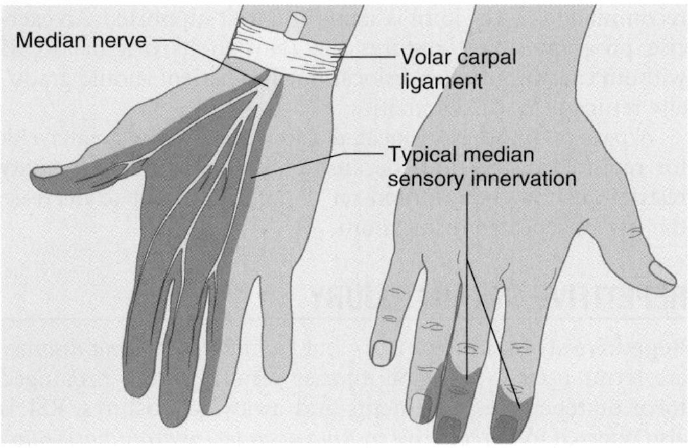


**FIG. 62-2** Wrist structures involved in carpal tunnel syndrome. Median nerve distribution. Shaded areas depict the locations of pain in carpal tunnel syndrome. (From Buttaravoli P: *Minor emergencies,* ed 3, Philadelphia, Saunders, 2012.)

ganglia. Hormones may be involved because initial manifestations of CTS often occur during the premenstrual period, pregnancy, and menopause. Persons with diabetes mellitus, peripheral vascular disease, and rheumatoid arthritis have a higher incidence of CTS because of swelling that changes blood flow to the nerve and narrows the carpal tunnel.[7] Women are more likely than men to develop CTS, possibly because of a smaller carpal tunnel.

Clinical manifestations of CTS are weakness, pain, numbness, or impaired sensation in the distribution of the median nerve (Fig. 62-2). Numbness and tingling may awaken the patient at night. Shaking the hands often relieves these symptoms. Clumsiness in performing fine hand movements is also common.

Manifestations of CTS include a positive Tinel's sign and Phalen's sign. *Tinel's sign* can be elicited by tapping over the median nerve as it passes through the carpal tunnel in the wrist. A positive response is a sensation of tingling in the distribution of the median nerve over the hand. *Phalen's sign* can be elicited by allowing the wrists to fall freely into maximum flexion and maintain the position for longer than 60 seconds. A positive response is a sensation of tingling in the distribution of the median nerve over the hand. In late stages, atrophy of the thenar muscles around the base of the thumb results in recurrent pain and eventual dysfunction of the hand.

## ❖ NURSING AND INTERPROFESSIONAL MANAGEMENT: CARPAL TUNNEL SYNDROME

To prevent CTS, teach employees and employers to identify risk factors. Adaptive devices such as wrist splints may be worn to hold the wrist in a slight extension and relieve pressure on the median nerve. Special keyboard pads and computer mice that help prevent repetitive pressure on the median nerve are available for computer users. Other ergonomic changes include workstation modifications, change in body positions, and frequent breaks from work-related activities.

Interprofessional care of the patient with CTS is directed toward relieving the underlying cause of the nerve compression. Early symptoms of CTS can usually be relieved by stopping the aggravating movement and by resting the hand and wrist by immobilization in a hand splint. Splints worn at night help keep the wrist in a neutral position and may reduce night pain and numbness. Physical therapy with hand and wrist exercises may lessen symptom severity. Injection of a corticosteroid drug directly into the carpal tunnel may provide short-term relief. The patient may need to consider a change in occupation because of discomfort and sensory changes.

Carpal tunnel release is generally recommended if symptoms last more than 6 months. Surgery involves severing the band of tissue around the wrist to reduce pressure on the median nerve (Fig. 62-2). Surgery is performed in the outpatient setting using local anesthesia. The types of carpal tunnel release surgery include open release and endoscopic surgery. In *open release surgery*, an incision is made in the wrist and then the carpal ligament is cut to enlarge the carpal tunnel. *Endoscopic carpal tunnel release* is performed through one or more small puncture incisions in the wrist and palm. A camera is attached to a tube, and the carpal ligament is cut. The endoscopic approach may allow a faster recovery and cause less postoperative discomfort than traditional open release surgery.

Although symptoms may be relieved immediately after surgery, full recovery may take months. After surgery, assess the hand's neurovascular status. Instruct the patient about wound care and appropriate assessments to perform at home.

## ROTATOR CUFF INJURY

The rotator cuff is a complex of four muscles in the shoulder: the supraspinatus, infraspinatus, teres minor, and subscapularis muscles. These muscles stabilize the humeral head in the glenoid fossa while assisting with ROM of the shoulder joint and rotation of the humerus.

A tear in the rotator cuff may occur as a gradual, degenerative process due to aging, repetitive stress (especially overhead arm motions), or injury to the shoulder while falling. The rotator cuff can also tear as a result of sudden adduction forces applied to the cuff while the arm is held in abduction. In sports, repetitive overhead motions, such as in swimming, weight lifting, and swinging a racquet (tennis, racquetball), often cause injury. Other causes include (1) falling onto an outstretched arm and hand, (2) a blow to the upper arm, (3) heavy lifting, or (4) repetitive work motions.

Manifestations of rotator cuff injury include shoulder weakness, pain, and decreased ROM. The patient usually experiences severe pain when the arm is abducted between 60 and 120 degrees (the painful arc). A positive *drop arm test* is another sign of rotator cuff injury. In this test, the arm is abducted 90 degrees, and the patient is asked to slowly lower the arm to the side. If the arm falls suddenly, rotator cuff injury is suspected. An x-ray alone is not beneficial in the diagnosis. A tear can usually be confirmed by MRI.

The patient with a partial tear or cuff inflammation may be treated conservatively with rest, ice and heat, NSAIDs, corticosteroid injections into the joint, ultrasound, and physical therapy.[8] If the patient does not respond to conservative treatment or if a complete tear is present, surgical repair may be needed. Most surgical repairs are performed as outpatient procedures through an arthroscope (Fig. 62-3). If the tear is extensive, part of the acromion may be surgically removed *(acromioplasty)* to relieve compression of the rotator cuff during movement. A sling and swathe or a shoulder immobilizer may be used immediately after surgery to limit shoulder movement. However, the shoulder should not be immobilized for too long

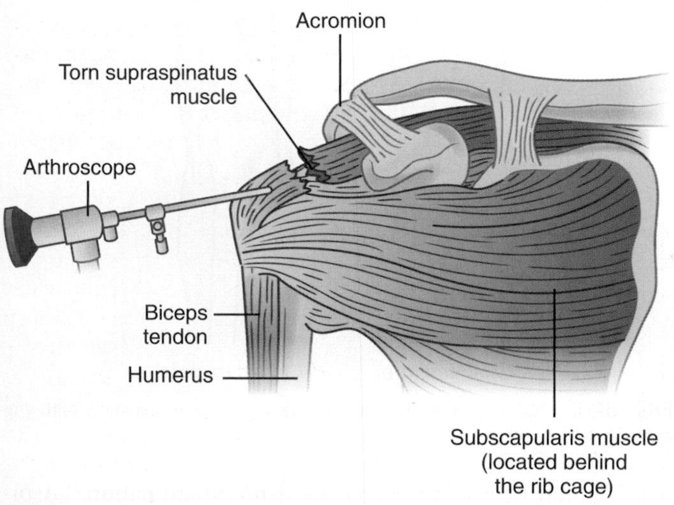


**FIG. 62-3** A torn rotator cuff is repaired using arthroscopic surgery.

because "frozen" shoulder *(arthrofibrosis)* may occur. Pendulum exercises and physical therapy begin the first postoperative day. Weight restrictions for lifting are usually given. Full recovery often takes up to 6 months.

## MENISCUS INJURY

The menisci are crescent-shaped pieces of fibrocartilage in the knee. Menisci are also found in other joints, including the acromioclavicular (AC), sternoclavicular, and temporomandibular joints. Meniscus injuries are closely associated with ligament sprains common among athletes in sports such as basketball, football, soccer, and hockey. These activities produce rotational stress when the knee is in varying degrees of flexion and the foot is planted or fixed. A blow to the knee can cause shearing of the meniscus between the femoral condyles and tibial plateau, resulting in a torn meniscus. Older patients and people who work in occupations that require squatting or kneeling may be at risk for degenerative tears.

Meniscus injuries alone do not usually cause significant edema because most of the cartilage is avascular. However, an acutely torn meniscus may be suspected when localized tenderness, pain, and effusion occur (Fig. 62-4). Pain is elicited by flexion, internal rotation, and then extension of the knee (*McMurray's test*). The patient may feel that the knee is unstable and often reports that the knee "clicks," "pops," "locks," or "gives way." Quadriceps atrophy is usually evident if the injury has been present for some time. Traumatic arthritis may occur from repeated meniscus injury and chronic inflammation.

MRI is beneficial in confirming the diagnosis before arthroscopy. The degree of knee pain and dysfunction, occupation, sport activities, and age may affect the patient's decision to have or postpone surgery.

## NURSING AND INTERPROFESSIONAL MANAGEMENT: MENISCUS INJURY

Because meniscus injuries are commonly caused by sports-related activity, teach athletes to do warm-up exercises. The acutely injured knee should be examined within 24 hours of injury. Initial care of this injury involves ice application, immobilization, and use of crutches with weight bearing as tolerated. Most meniscus injuries are treated in an outpatient setting.

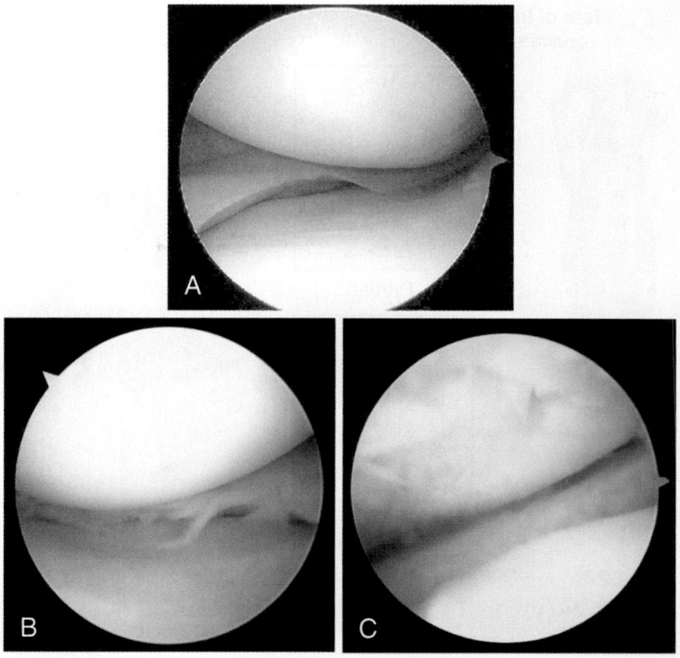


**FIG. 62-4** Arthroscopic views of the meniscus. **A,** Normal meniscus. **B,** Torn meniscus. **C,** Surgically repaired meniscus. (*A,* From David Lintner, MD, Houston, Tex., *www.drlintner.com. B* and *C,* Courtesy Peter Bonner, Placitas, N. Mex.)

Using a knee brace or immobilizer during the first few days after the injury protects the knee and offers some pain relief.

After acute pain has decreased, physical therapy can help the patient regain knee flexion and muscle strength to assist in returning to full function. In older adults with degenerative meniscus tears, progressive exercise therapy may improve neuromuscular function and muscle strength.[9]

Surgical repair or excision of part of the meniscus *(meniscectomy)* may be necessary (Fig. 62-4). Meniscal surgery is performed by arthroscopy. Pain relief may include NSAIDs or other analgesics. Rehabilitation starts soon after surgery, including quadriceps and hamstring strengthening exercises and ROM. When the patient's strength is back to its preinjury level, normal activities may be resumed.

## ANTERIOR CRUCIATE LIGAMENT INJURY

Knee injuries account for more than 50% of all sport injuries.[10] The most commonly injured knee ligament is the anterior cruciate ligament (ACL). ACL injuries are usually noncontact injuries that occur when the athlete pivots, lands from a jump, or slows down when running. Patients often report coming down on the knee, twisting, and hearing a pop, followed by acute knee pain and swelling. Athletes usually cannot continue playing, and the knee may feel unstable. Injury to the ACL can result in a partial tear, a complete tear, or an *avulsion* (tearing away) from the bones that form the knee (Fig. 62-5).

During examination of the affected knee, a positive *Lachman's test* will suggest an ACL tear.[10] This test is performed by flexing the knee 15 to 30 degrees and pulling the tibia forward while the femur is stabilized. The test is considered positive for an ACL tear if forward motion of the tibia occurs with the feeling of a soft or indistinct endpoint. MRI is often used to diagnose an ACL tear and coexisting conditions, including a fracture, meniscus tearing, and collateral ligament injuries.

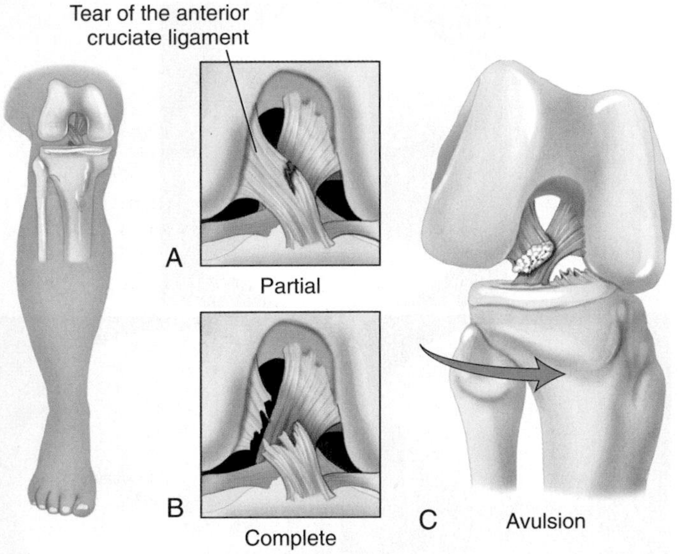


**FIG. 62-5** Anterior cruciate ligament (ACL) injury. **A,** Partial tear. **B,** Complete tear. **C,** Avulsion.

## ❖ NURSING AND INTERPROFESSIONAL MANAGEMENT: ANTERIOR CRUCIATE LIGAMENT INJURY

Prevention programs have been shown to significantly reduce ACL injuries in athletes. Conservative treatment for an intact ACL injury includes rest, ice, NSAIDs, elevation, and ambulation as tolerated with crutches. If present, a tight, painful effusion may be aspirated. A knee immobilizer or hinged knee brace may provide support. Physical therapy often assists the patient in maintaining knee joint motion and muscle tone.

Reconstructive surgery is usually recommended for physically active patients who have sustained severe injury to the ACL and meniscus. In reconstruction, the torn ACL tissue is removed and replaced with autologous or allograft tissue. ROM is encouraged soon after surgery, and the knee is placed in a brace or immobilizer. Rehabilitation with physical therapy is critical, with progressive weight bearing determined by the degree of surgical repair. A safe return to the patient's prior level of physical functioning may take 6 to 8 months.

## BURSITIS

Bursae are closed sacs that are lined with synovial membrane and contain a small amount of synovial fluid. They are located at sites of friction, such as between tendons and bones and near the joints. **Bursitis** (inflammation of the bursa) results from repeated or excessive trauma or friction, gout, rheumatoid arthritis, or infection.

Clinical manifestations of bursitis are warmth, pain, swelling, and limited ROM in the affected part. Common sites of bursitis include the hands, elbows, shoulders, knees, and greater trochanters of the hip. Improper body mechanics, repetitive kneeling (carpet layers, coal miners, and gardeners), jogging in worn-out shoes, and prolonged sitting with crossed legs are common precipitating activities.

Try to determine and correct the cause of the bursitis. Rest is often the only treatment needed. The affected part may be immobilized in a compression dressing or splint. Ice and NSAIDs may be used to reduce pain and inflammation.[11] Aspiration of the bursal fluid and intraarticular corticosteroid injection may be needed. If the bursal wall has become thickened and continues to interfere with normal joint function, surgical excision *(bursectomy)* is often done. Septic bursae usually require surgical incision and drainage.

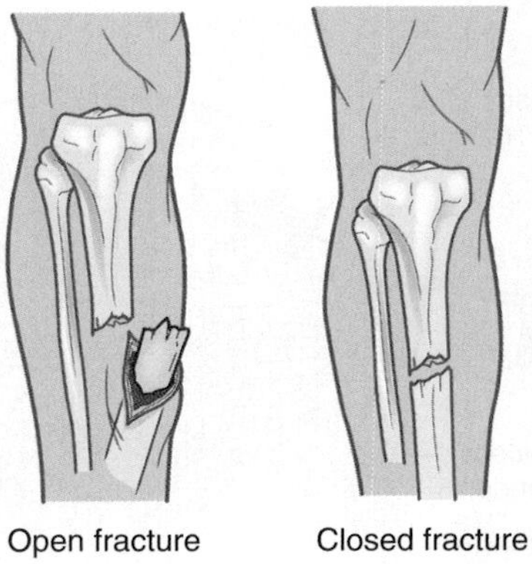


**FIG. 62-6** Fracture classification according to communication with the external environment.

## FRACTURES

### Classification

A **fracture** is a disruption or break in the continuity of bone. Although traumatic injuries account for the majority of fractures, some fractures are secondary to a disease process such as cancer or osteoporosis *(pathologic fracture).*

Fractures can be classified as *open* or *closed* based on possible communication with the external environment (Fig. 62-6). In an *open fracture,* the skin is broken and bone exposed, causing soft tissue injury. In a *closed fracture,* the skin remains intact.

Fractures can also be classified as complete or incomplete. A fracture is termed *complete* if the break goes completely through the bone. An *incomplete* fracture occurs partly across a bone shaft but the bone is still intact. An incomplete fracture is often the result of bending or crushing forces applied to a bone.

Fractures are also identified according to the direction of the fracture line. Types include linear, oblique, transverse, longitudinal, and spiral fractures (Fig. 62-7).

Fractures can be classified as displaced or nondisplaced. In a *displaced* fracture, the two ends of the broken bone are separated from one another and out of their normal positions. Displaced fractures are often *comminuted* (more than two fragments) or *oblique* (Fig. 62-7). In a *nondisplaced* fracture, the periosteum is intact across the fracture and the bone fragments are still in alignment. Nondisplaced fractures are usually transverse, spiral, or greenstick (Fig. 62-7).

### Clinical Manifestations

Clinical manifestations of fracture include immediate localized pain, decreased function, and inability to bear weight or use the affected part (Table 62-4). The patient guards and protects the extremity against movement. Obvious bone deformity may not be present. If a fracture is suspected, the extremity is immobilized in the position in which it is found. Unnecessary movement increases soft tissue damage. It may also convert a closed fracture to an open fracture or create further injury to adjacent nerves and blood vessels.

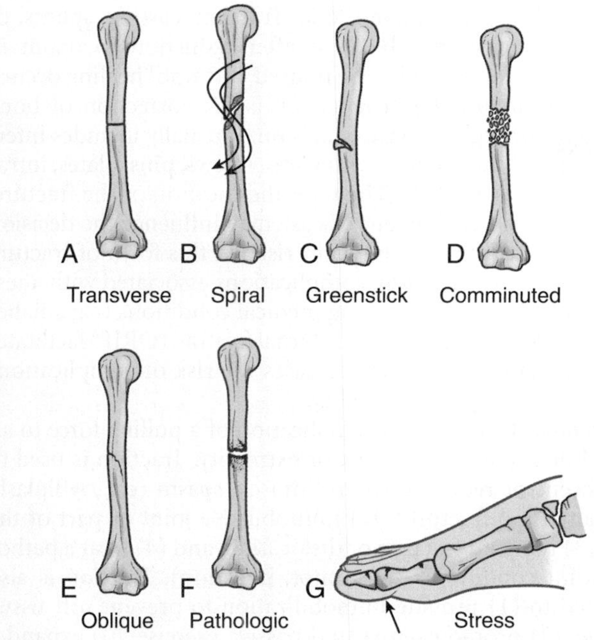


**FIG. 62-7** Types of fractures. **A,** Transverse fracture: the line of the fracture extends across the bone shaft at a right angle to the longitudinal axis. **B,** Spiral fracture: the line of the fracture extends in a spiral direction along the bone shaft. **C,** Greenstick fracture: an incomplete fracture with one side splintered and the other side bent. **D,** Comminuted fracture: a fracture with more than two fragments. The smaller fragments appear to be floating. **E,** Oblique fracture: the line of the fracture extends across and down the bone. **F,** Pathologic fracture: a spontaneous fracture at the site of a diseased bone. **G,** Stress fracture: occurs in normal or abnormal bone that is subject to repeated stress, such as from jogging or running.

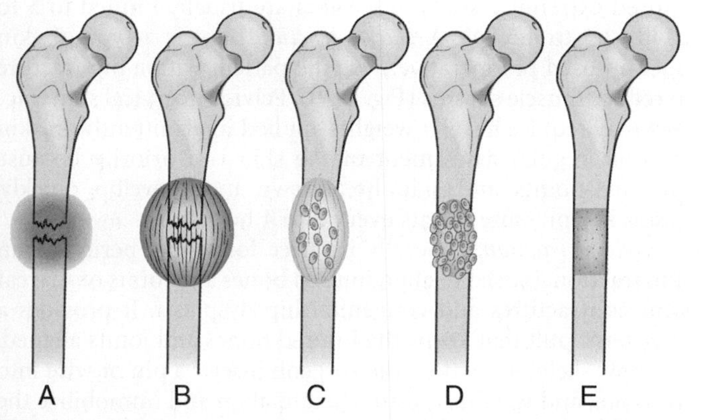


**FIG. 62-8** Bone healing (schematic representation). **A,** Bleeding at fractured ends of the bone with subsequent hematoma formation. **B,** Organization of hematoma into fibrous network. **C,** Invasion of osteoblasts, lengthening of collagen strands, and deposition of calcium. **D,** Callus formation: new bone is built up as osteoclasts destroy dead bone. **E,** Remodeling is accomplished as excess callus is resorbed and trabecular bone is laid down.

## Fracture Healing

Knowledge of the stages of fracture healing (Fig. 62-8) is needed to provide appropriate interventions. Bone goes through a complex multistage healing process *(union)* that occurs in the following stages[12]:

1. *Fracture hematoma:* When a fracture occurs, bleeding creates a hematoma that surrounds the ends of the bone fragments. The hematoma is extravasated blood that changes from a liquid to a semisolid clot. This occurs in the first 72 hours after injury.

**TABLE 62-4 Manifestations of Fracture**

| Manifestation | Significance |
|---|---|
| **Edema and Swelling** | |
| Disruption or penetration of skin or soft tissues by bone fragments, or bleeding into surrounding tissues. | Unchecked bleeding and swelling in closed space can occlude blood vessels and damage nerves (e.g., increased risk of compartment syndrome). |
| **Pain and Tenderness** | |
| Muscle spasm due to involuntary reflex action of muscle, direct tissue trauma, increased pressure on nerves, movement of fracture fragments. | Pain and tenderness encourage the patient to splint muscle around fracture and reduce motion of injured area. |
| **Muscle Spasm** | |
| Irritation of tissues and protective response to injury and fracture. | Muscle spasms may displace nondisplaced fracture or prevent it from reducing spontaneously. |
| **Deformity** | |
| Abnormal position of extremity or part as result of original forces of injury and action of muscles pulling fragment into abnormal position. Seen as a loss of normal bony contours. | Deformity is cardinal sign of fracture. If uncorrected, it may result in problems with bony union and restoration of function of injured part. |
| **Contusion** | |
| Discoloration of skin (bruising) as a result of extravasation of blood in subcutaneous tissues. | Bruising may appear immediately after injury and may appear distal to injury. Reassure patient that process is normal and discoloration will eventually resolve. |
| **Loss of Function** | |
| Disruption of bone or joint, preventing functional use of limb or part. | Fracture must be managed properly to ensure restoration of function to limb or part. |
| **Crepitation** | |
| Grating or crunching of bony fragments, producing palpable or audible crunching or popping sensation. | Crepitation may increase chance for nonunion if bone ends are allowed to move excessively. Micromovement of fragments (postfracture) assists in osteogenesis (new bone growth). |

2. *Granulation tissue:* During this stage, active phagocytosis absorbs the products of local necrosis. The hematoma converts to granulation tissue. Granulation tissue (consisting of new blood vessels, fibroblasts, and osteoblasts) forms the basis for new bone substance *(osteoid)* during days 3 to 14 after injury.
3. *Callus formation:* As minerals (calcium, phosphorus, and magnesium) and new bone matrix are deposited in the osteoid, an unorganized network of bone is formed and woven about the fracture parts. *Callus* is primarily composed of cartilage, osteoblasts, calcium, and phosphorus. It usually appears by the end of the second week after injury. Evidence of callus formation can be verified by x-ray.
4. *Ossification:* Ossification of the callus occurs from 3 weeks to 6 months after the fracture and continues until the fracture has healed. Callus ossification is sufficient to prevent

movement at the fracture site when the bones are gently stressed. However, the fracture is still evident on x-ray. During this stage of *clinical union,* the patient may be allowed limited mobility or the cast may be removed.
5. *Consolidation:* As callus continues to develop, the distance between bone fragments decreases and eventually closes. Ossification continues and can be equated with *radiologic union,* which occurs when an x-ray shows complete bony union. This phase can occur up to 1 year after injury.
6. *Remodeling:* Excess bone tissue is resorbed in the final stage of bone healing, and union is complete. Gradual return of the injured bone to its preinjury structural strength and shape occurs. Bone remodels in response to physical loading stress (Wolff's law). Initially, stress is provided through exercise. Weight bearing is gradually introduced. New bone is deposited in sites subjected to stress and resorbed at areas of little stress.

Many factors influence the time required for complete fracture healing, including displacement and site of the fracture, blood supply to the area, immobilization, and use of internal fixation devices (e.g., screws, pins). The ossification process may be slowed or even stopped by inadequate reduction and immobilization, excessive movement of fracture fragments, infection, poor nutrition, and systemic disease. Healing time for fractures increases with age. For example, an uncomplicated midshaft femur fracture heals in 3 weeks in a newborn and in 20 weeks in an adult. Smoking also increases fracture healing time. Fracture healing may not occur in the expected time *(delayed union)* or may not occur at all *(nonunion).* Table 62-5 summarizes complications of fracture healing.

## Interprofessional Care

The overall goals of fracture treatment are (1) anatomic realignment of bone fragments through reduction, (2) immobilization to maintain realignment, and (3) restoration of normal or near-normal function of the injured part. Table 62-6 summarizes the interprofessional care of fractures.

### Fracture Reduction

***Closed Reduction.*** *Closed reduction* is nonsurgical, manual realignment of bone fragments to their previous anatomic position. Traction and countertraction are manually applied to the bone fragments to restore position, length, and alignment. Closed reduction is usually performed while the patient is under local or general anesthesia. Traction, casting, splints, or orthoses (braces) may be used after reduction to maintain alignment and immobilize the injured part until healing occurs.

***Open Reduction.*** *Open reduction* is the correction of bone alignment through a surgical incision. It usually includes internal fixation of the fracture with wires, screws, pins, plates, intramedullary rods, or nails. The type and location of the fracture, patient age, and concurrent disease may influence the decision to use open reduction. The main risks of this form of fracture management are infection, complications associated with anesthesia, and effect of preexisting medical conditions (e.g., diabetes). However, open reduction internal fixation (ORIF) facilitates early ambulation and thus decreases the risk of complications related to prolonged immobility.

***Traction.*** Traction is the application of a pulling force to an injured or diseased body part or extremity. Traction is used to (1) prevent or reduce pain and muscle spasm (e.g., whiplash, unrepaired hip fracture), (2) immobilize a joint or part of the body, (3) reduce a fracture or dislocation, and (4) treat a pathologic joint condition (e.g., tumor, infection). Traction is also indicated to (1) provide immobilization to prevent soft tissue damage, (2) promote active and passive exercise, (3) expand a joint space during arthroscopic procedures, and (4) expand a joint space before major joint reconstruction.

Traction devices apply a pulling force on a fractured extremity to attain realignment while *countertraction* pulls in the opposite direction. The most common types of traction are skin traction and skeletal traction. *Skin traction* is generally used for short-term treatment (48 to 72 hours) until skeletal traction or surgery is possible. Tape, boots, or splints are applied directly to the skin, primarily to help diminish muscle spasms in the injured extremity. Traction weights are usually limited to 5 to 10 lb (2.3 to 4.5 kg). A *Buck's traction* boot is a type of skin traction used preoperatively for the patient with a hip fracture to reduce muscle spasms (Fig. 62-9). Pelvic or cervical skin traction may require heavier weights applied intermittently. In skin traction, regular assessment of the skin is a priority because pressure points and skin breakdown may develop quickly. Assess key pressure points every 2 to 4 hours.

*Skeletal traction,* generally in place for longer periods than skin traction, is used to align injured bones and joints or to treat joint contractures and congenital hip dysplasia. It provides a long-term pull that keeps the injured bones and joints aligned. To apply skeletal traction, the surgeon inserts a pin or wire into the bone, and weights are attached to align and immobilize the injured body part. Weight for skeletal traction ranges from 5 to

**TABLE 62-5 Complications of Fracture Healing**

| Complication | Description |
|---|---|
| **Delayed union** | Fracture healing progresses more slowly than expected. Healing eventually occurs. |
| **Nonunion** | Fracture fails to heal despite treatment. No x-ray evidence of callus formation. |
| **Malunion** | Fracture heals in expected time but in unsatisfactory position, possibly resulting in deformity or dysfunction. |
| **Angulation** | Fracture heals in abnormal position in relation to midline of structure (type of malunion). |
| **Pseudoarthrosis** | Type of nonunion occurring at fracture site in which a false joint is formed with abnormal movement at site. |
| **Refracture** | New fracture occurs at original fracture site. |
| **Myositis ossificans** | Deposition of calcium in muscle tissue at site of significant blunt muscle trauma or repeated muscle injury. |

**TABLE 62-6 Interprofessional Care**

***Fractures***

**Diagnostic Assessment**
- History and physical examination
- X-ray
- CT scan, MRI

**Management**

***Fracture Reduction***
- Manual traction
- Closed reduction
- Skeletal traction
- Open reduction

***Fracture Immobilization***
- Casting or splinting
- Skeletal traction
- External fixation
- Internal fixation

***Open Fractures***
- Surgical debridement and irrigation
- Tetanus and diphtheria immunization
- Prophylactic antibiotic therapy
- Immobilization

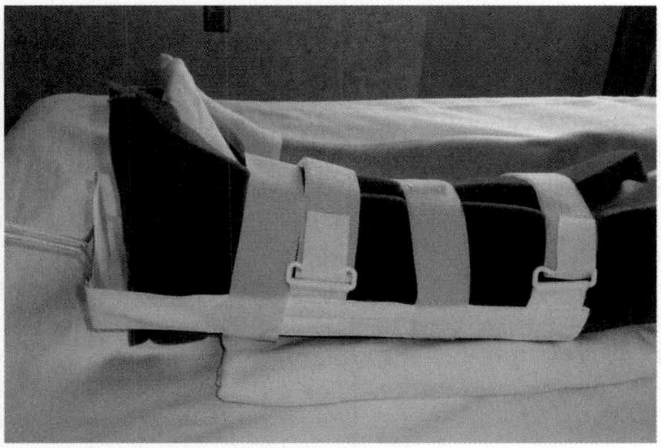

**FIG. 62-9** Buck's traction is most commonly used for fractures of the hip and femur. (Courtesy Mary Wollan, RN, BAN, ONC, Spring Park, Minn.)

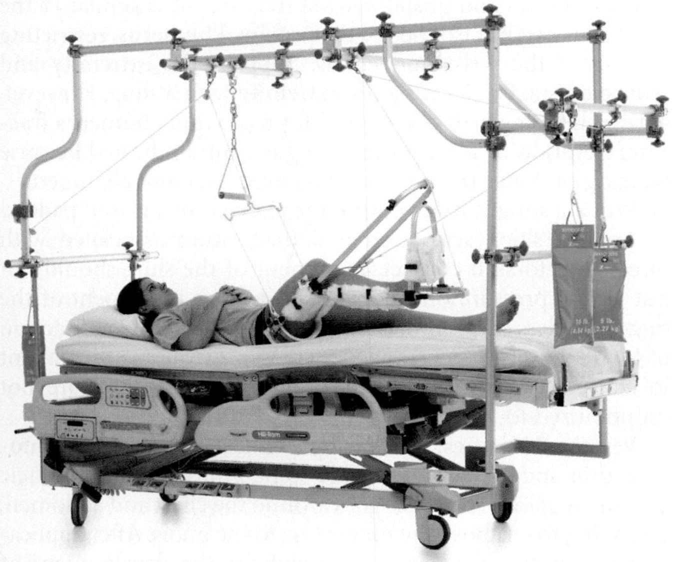

**FIG. 62-10** Balanced suspension skeletal traction. Most commonly used for fractures of the femur, hip, and lower leg. (Courtesy Zimmer, Inc.)

## TEAMWORK & COLLABORATION

### *Caring for the Patient With a Cast or Traction*

**Role of Nursing Personnel**

***Registered Nurse (RN)***

- Perform neurovascular assessment on the affected extremity.
- Assess for manifestations of compartment syndrome.
- Monitor cast during drying for denting or flattening.
- Teach patient and caregiver about cast care and complications of casting.
- Determine correct body alignment to enhance traction.
- Instruct patient and caregiver about traction and correct body positioning.
- Teach patient and caregiver ROM exercises.
- Assess for complications associated with immobility or fracture (e.g., wound infection, constipation, VTE, renal calculi, atelectasis).
- Develop plan to minimize complications associated with immobility or fracture.

***Licensed Practical/Vocational Nurse (LPN/LVN)***

- Check color, temperature, capillary refill, and pulses distal to the cast.
- Mark circumference of any drainage on the cast.
- Monitor skin integrity around cast and at traction pin sites.
- Pad cast edges and traction connections to prevent skin irritation.
- Monitor pain intensity and administer prescribed analgesics.
- Notify RN of changes in pain or if pain persists after prescribed analgesics are administered.

***Unlicensed Assistive Personnel (UAP)***

- Position casted extremity above heart level as directed by RN.
- Apply ice to cast as directed by RN.
- Maintain body position and integrity of traction (after being trained and evaluated in this procedure).
- Assist patient with passive and active ROM exercises.
- Notify RN about patient complaints of pain, tingling, or decreased sensation in the affected extremity.

**Role of Other Team Members**

***Physical Therapist***

- Assess patient's current mobility and need for assistance.
- Teach safe ambulation with assistive device based on patient's weight-bearing restrictions.
- Establish exercise regimen and teach patient to perform exercises safely.
- Coordinate physical therapy with RN so that patient can receive timely analgesia.
- Discuss home environment with patient and identify possible modifications to facilitate recovery (e.g., stair training if allowed by patient's weight-bearing restrictions, bed placement on first level to avoid stairs).

***Occupational Therapist***

- Assess impact of patient's condition on ability to perform ADLs.
- Instruct patient in use of assistive devices (e.g., long-handled reacher, shoe donner) to facilitate self-care while maintaining activity restrictions.
- Discuss home environment with patient and identify possible modifications to facilitate recovery (e.g., bed placement on first level for access to bathroom).

45 lb (2.3 to 20.4 kg). The use of too much weight can result in delayed union or nonunion. The major complications of skeletal traction are infection at the pin insertion site and the effects of prolonged immobility.[13]

When traction is used to treat fractures, the forces are usually exerted on the distal bone fragment to align it with the proximal fragment. Several types of traction are used for this purpose. One of the more common types of skeletal traction is balanced suspension traction (Fig. 62-10). Fracture alignment depends on the correct positioning and alignment of the patient while the traction forces remain constant. For extremity traction to be effective, forces must be pulling in the opposite direction *(countertraction)*. Countertraction is commonly supplied by the patient's body weight or by weights pulling in the opposite direction, and it may be augmented by elevating the end of the bed. Traction must be maintained continuously. Keep the weights off the floor and moving freely through the pulleys.

**Fracture Immobilization.** Fracture immobilization can be done using casts, braces, splints, immobilizers, and external and internal fixation devices.

***Casts.*** A *cast* is a temporary circumferential immobilization device. Casting is a common treatment following closed reduction. It allows the patient to perform many normal activities of daily living while providing sufficient immobilization to ensure stability. Cast materials are natural (plaster of Paris), synthetic acrylic, fiberglass-free, latex-free polymer, or a hybrid of materials. Synthetic casting materials are commonly used because they are lighter and dry more quickly than plaster of Paris. Plaster of Paris is now used primarily for contact casting in the treatment of diabetic foot ulcers.[14] A cast generally incorporates the joints above and below a fracture. Immobilization above and below a joint restricts tendon and ligament movement, thus assisting with joint stabilization while the fracture heals.

To apply a cast on an extremity, first cover the affected part with stockinette that is cut longer than the extremity. Then place cotton padding over the stockinette, with extra padding for bony prominences. If plaster of Paris casting material is used, immerse it in warm water and then wrap and mold it around the affected part. The number of layers of plaster bandage and the technique of application determine the strength of the cast. The plaster sets within 15 minutes, so the patient may move around without difficulty. However, it is not strong enough for weight bearing until about 24 to 72 hours after application. The final decision about the patient's weight bearing is made by the surgeon.

A fresh plaster cast should never be covered because air cannot circulate. Heat then builds up in the cast and may cause a burn, and drying is delayed. Avoid direct pressure on the cast during the drying period. Handle the cast gently with an open palm to avoid denting the cast. Once the cast is thoroughly dry, the rough edges may be *petaled* to minimize skin irritation. Petaling also prevents plaster of Paris debris from falling into the cast and causing irritation or pressure necrosis. Place several strips (petals) of tape over the rough areas to ensure a smooth cast edge.

Casts made of synthetic materials are used more than plaster because they are lightweight, stronger, and relatively waterproof and provide for early weight bearing. The synthetic casting materials (thermolabile plastic, thermoplastic resins, polyurethane, fiberglass) are activated by submersion in cool or tepid water. Then they are molded to fit the torso or extremity.

**Upper extremity injuries.** Immobilization of an acute fracture or soft tissue injury of the upper extremity is often accomplished by use of a (1) sugar-tong splint, (2) posterior splint, (3) short arm cast, or (4) long arm cast (Fig. 62-11). The *sugar-tong splint* is typically used for acute wrist injuries or injuries

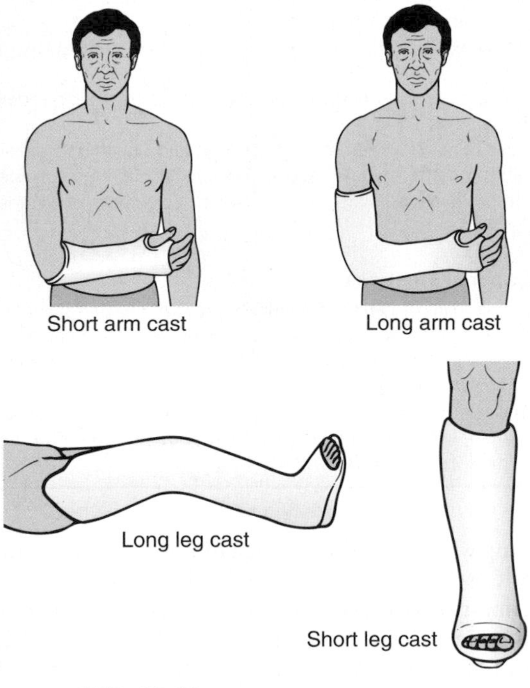


**FIG. 62-11** Common types of casts.

that may result in significant swelling. Splints are applied over a well-padded forearm, beginning at the phalangeal joints of the hand, extending up the dorsal aspect of the forearm around the distal humerus and then down the volar aspect of the forearm to the distal palmar crease. The splinting material is wrapped with either elastic bandage or bias stockinette. The sugar-tong posterior splint accommodates early swelling in the fractured extremity.

The *short arm cast* is often used for the treatment of stable wrist or metacarpal fractures. An aluminum finger splint can be incorporated into the short arm cast for concurrent treatment of phalangeal injuries. The short arm cast is a circular cast extending from the distal palmar crease to the proximal forearm. This cast provides wrist immobilization and permits unrestricted elbow motion.

The *long arm cast* is commonly used for stable forearm or elbow fractures and unstable wrist fractures. It is similar to the short arm cast but extends to the proximal humerus, restricting motion at the wrist and elbow. Support the extremity and reduce edema by elevating the extremity with a sling. However, when a hanging arm cast is used for a proximal humerus fracture, elevation or a supportive sling is contraindicated because hanging provides traction and maintains fracture alignment.

When a sling is used, ensure the axillary area is well padded to prevent skin excoriation and maceration associated with direct skin-to-skin contact. Placement of the sling should not put undue pressure on the neck. Encourage movement of the fingers (unless contraindicated) to enhance the pumping action of blood vessels to decrease edema. Also encourage the patient to actively move joints of the upper extremity that are not immobilized to prevent stiffness and contractures.

**Vertebral injuries.** The *body jacket brace* is used for immobilization and support for stable spine injuries of the thoracic or lumbar spine. The brace goes around the chest and abdomen, extending from above the nipple line to the pubis. After application of the brace, assess the patient for the development of superior mesenteric artery syndrome *(cast syndrome)*. This condition occurs if the brace is applied too tightly, compressing the superior mesenteric artery against the duodenum. The patient generally complains of abdominal pain, abdominal pressure, nausea, and vomiting. Assess the abdomen for decreased bowel sounds (a window in the brace may be left over the umbilicus). Treatment of cast syndrome includes gastric decompression with a nasogastric (NG) tube and suction. Also assess respiratory status, bowel and bladder function, and areas of pressure over the bony prominences, especially the iliac crest. The brace may have to be adjusted or removed if any complications occur.

**Lower extremity injuries.** Injuries to the lower extremity are often immobilized by long leg cast, short leg cast, cylinder cast, or prefabricated splint or immobilizer. The usual indications for a long leg cast are an unstable ankle fracture, soft tissue injuries, a fractured tibia, and knee injuries. The cast usually extends from the base of the toes to the groin and gluteal crease. The short leg cast is used primarily for stable ankle and foot injuries. A cylinder cast, which is used for knee injuries or fractures, extends from the groin to the malleoli of the ankle. A Robert Jones dressing may be used temporarily to limit mobility of a joint. It is composed of soft padding materials (absorption dressing and cotton sheet wadding), splints, and an elastic wrap or bias-cut stockinette.

After application of a lower extremity cast or dressing, the extremity should be elevated on pillows above heart level for the first 24 hours. After the initial phase, a casted extremity should not be placed in a dependent position because of the possibility of excessive edema. After cast application, observe for signs of compartment syndrome (discussed on p. 1479) and increased pressure, especially in the heel, anterior tibia, head of the fibula, and malleoli. This increased pressure is manifested by pain or a burning feeling in these areas.

Prefabricated knee and ankle splints and immobilizers are used in many settings. This type of immobilization is easy to apply and remove, which permits close observation of the affected joint for swelling and skin breakdown (Fig. 62-12). Depending on the injury, removal of the splint or immobilizer facilitates ROM of the affected joint and faster return to function.

The *hip spica cast* is now mainly used for femur fractures in children to immobilize the affected extremity and trunk. It extends from above the nipple line to the base of the foot (single spica) and may include the opposite extremity up to an area above the knee (spica and a half) or both extremities (double spica). Assess the patient with a hip spica cast for the same problems associated with the body jacket brace.

***External Fixation.*** An *external fixator* is a device composed of metal pins that are inserted into the bone and attached to external rods to stabilize the fracture while it heals. It can be used to apply traction or to compress fracture fragments and immobilize reduced fragments when the use of a cast or other traction is not appropriate. The external device holds fracture fragments in place similar to a surgically implanted internal device. The external fixator is attached directly to the bones by percutaneous transfixing pins or wires (Fig. 62-13). External fixation is indicated primarily for complex fractures with extensive soft tissue damage, correction of congenital bony defects, nonunion or malunion, and limb lengthening.

External fixation is often used in an attempt to salvage extremities that otherwise may require amputation. Because the use of an external device is a long-term process, ongoing assessment for pin loosening and infection is critical. Infection (indicated by exudate, erythema, tenderness, and pain) may require removal of the device. Instruct the patient and caregiver about meticulous pin care. Although each surgeon has a protocol for pin care cleaning, chlorhexidine 2 mg/mL is often used.[15] Hydrogen peroxide may be cytotoxic to osteoblasts and may not be bactericidal.

***Internal Fixation.*** Internal fixation devices (pins, plates, intramedullary rods, metal and bioabsorbable screws) are surgically inserted to realign and maintain position of bony fragments (Fig. 62-14). These metal devices are biologically inert and made from stainless steel, vitallium, or titanium. Proper alignment and bone healing are evaluated regularly by x-rays.

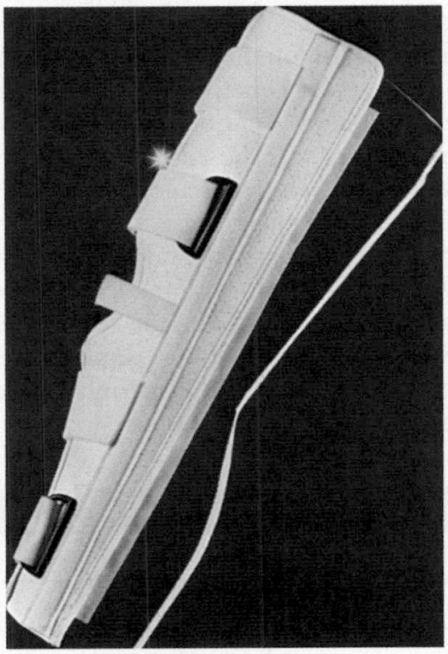

**FIG. 62-12** Knee immobilizer. (From Maher AB, Salmond SW, Pellino T, editors: *Orthopaedic nursing,* ed 3, Philadelphia, 2002, Saunders.)

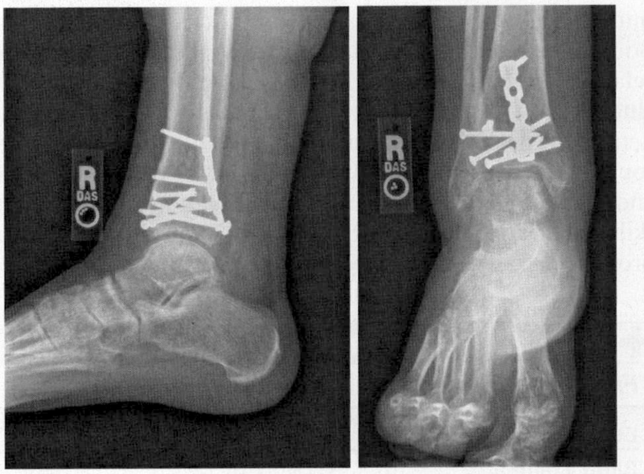


**FIG. 62-14** Views of internal fixation devices to stabilize a fractured tibia and fibula. (From Jeremy Lewis, MD, Albuquerque, N. Mex.)

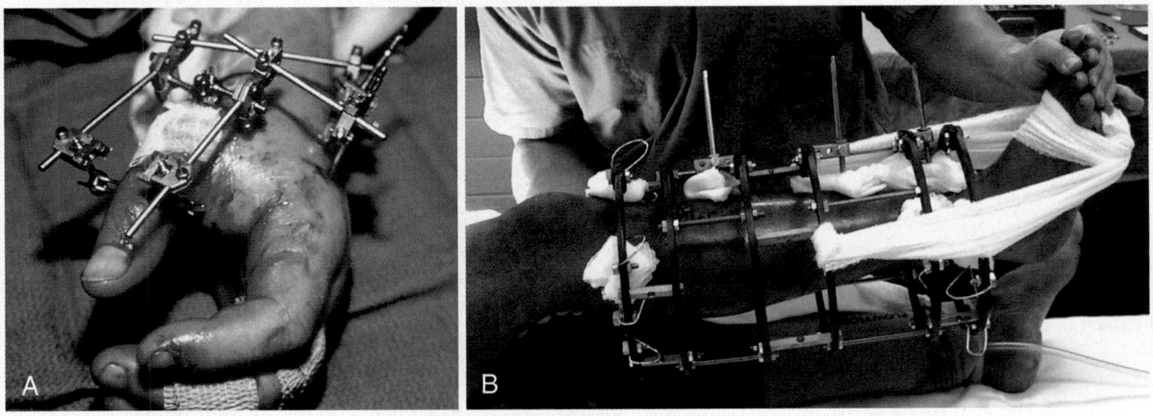


**FIG. 62-13** External fixators. **A,** Stabilization of hand injury. **B,** Stabilization of a tibial fracture. (*A,* Courtesy Howmedica, Inc, Allendale, Pa. *B,* From Canale ST, Beaty JH: *Campbell's operative orthopaedics,* ed 12, Philadelphia, 2013, Mosby.)

**Electrical Bone Growth Stimulation.** Electrical bone growth stimulation is used to facilitate the healing process, especially for fracture nonunion or delayed union. The mechanism of action of electrical bone growth stimulation may include (1) increasing the calcium uptake of bone, (2) activating intracellular calcium stores, and (3) increasing the production of bone growth factors (e.g., bone morphogenic protein).

Noninvasive, semi-invasive, and invasive methods of electrical bone growth stimulation are used. Noninvasive stimulators use direct current or pulsed electromagnetic fields (PEMFs) to generate a weak electrical current. Electrodes are typically in a band applied over the patient's skin or cast and worn 10 to 12 hours each day, usually while the patient is sleeping. Semi-invasive or percutaneous bone growth stimulators use an external power supply and electrodes that are inserted through the skin and into the bone. Invasive stimulators require surgical implantation of a current generator in an IM or subcutaneous space. An electrode is implanted in the bone fragments.

**Drug Therapy.** Patients with fractures experience varying degrees of pain associated with muscle spasms. Central and peripheral muscle relaxants, such as carisoprodol (Soma), cyclobenzaprine, or methocarbamol (Robaxin), may be prescribed for management of pain associated with muscle spasms.[16]

The threat of tetanus from an open fracture can be reduced by administering tetanus and diphtheria toxoid or tetanus immunoglobulin for the patient who has not been previously immunized or whose immunization is expired (see Table 68-6). Bone-penetrating antibiotics, such as a cephalosporin (e.g., cefazolin [Kefzol]), are used prophylactically before surgery.

**Nutritional Therapy.** Proper nutrition is an essential component of the healing process in injured tissue. An adequate energy source is needed to promote muscle strength and tone, build endurance, and provide energy for ambulation and gait-training skills. The patient's dietary requirements must include adequate protein (e.g., 1 g/kg of body weight), vitamins (especially B, C, and D), calcium, phosphorus, and magnesium to ensure optimal soft tissue and bone healing. Low serum protein and vitamin C deficiencies interfere with tissue healing. Immobility and bone healing increase calcium needs.

Three well-balanced meals a day usually provide the necessary nutrients. A well-balanced diet should be supplemented by fluid intake of 2000 to 3000 mL/day to promote optimal bladder and bowel function. Adequate fluid and a high-fiber diet with fruits and vegetables prevent constipation. If immobilized in bed with skeletal traction or in a body jacket brace, the patient should eat six small meals to avoid overeating that can contribute to abdominal pressure and cramping.

## ❖ NURSING MANAGEMENT: FRACTURES

### ◆ Nursing Assessment

A brief history of the traumatic episode, mechanism of injury, and position in which the victim was found can be obtained from the patient or witnesses. As soon as possible, the patient should be transported to an emergency department, where thorough assessment can be performed and treatment initiated (Table 62-7). Subjective and objective data that should be obtained from an individual with a fracture are presented in Table 62-8.

Place special emphasis on the region distal to the site of injury. Document clinical findings before fracture treatment to avoid doubts about if a problem identified later was missed during the original examination or was caused by the treatment.

◆ **Neurovascular Assessment.** Musculoskeletal injuries may cause changes in the neurovascular status of an injured extremity. Application of a cast or constrictive dressing, poor positioning, and physiologic responses to the traumatic injury can cause nerve or vascular damage, usually distal to the injury. The neurovascular assessment should consist of *peripheral vascular assessment* (color, temperature, capillary refill, peripheral pulses, edema) and *peripheral neurologic assessment* (sensation, motor function,

**TABLE 62-7 Emergency Management**

***Fractured Extremity***

| Etiology | Assessment Findings | Interventions |
|---|---|---|
| **Blunt Trauma**<br>• Motor vehicle crash<br>• Pedestrian event<br>• Fall<br>• Direct blow<br>• Forced flexion or hyperextension<br>• Twisting force<br>**Penetrating Trauma**<br>• Gunshot<br>• Blast<br>**Other**<br>• Pathologic condition<br>• Violent muscle contraction (seizures)<br>• Crush injury | • Deformity (loss of normal bony contours) or unnatural position of affected limb<br>• Edema, contusion<br>• Muscle spasm<br>• Tenderness, pain<br>• Warmth at site<br>• Loss of function<br>• Numbness, tingling, decreased distal pulses<br>• Grating (crepitus)<br>• Open wound over injured site, exposure of bone | **Initial**<br>• Treat life-threatening injuries first.<br>• If unresponsive, assess circulation, airway, and breathing.<br>• If responsive, monitor airway, breathing, and circulation.<br>• Control external bleeding with direct pressure or sterile pressure dressing and elevation of the extremity.<br>• Assess neurovascular condition distal to injury before and after splinting.<br>• Elevate injured limb if possible.<br>• Do *not* attempt to straighten fractured or dislocated joints.<br>• Do *not* manipulate protruding bone ends.<br>• Apply ice packs to affected area.<br>• Obtain x-rays of affected limb.<br>• Administer tetanus and diphtheria prophylaxis if there is a break in skin integrity.<br>• Mark location of pulses to facilitate repeat assessment.<br>• Splint fracture site, including joints above and below fracture site.<br>**Ongoing Monitoring**<br>• Assess vital signs, level of consciousness, $O_2$ saturation, neurovascular condition, pain.<br>• Assess for compartment syndrome characterized by excessive pain, pain with passive stretch of the affected extremity muscles, pallor, paresthesia (with late signs of paralysis and pulselessness).<br>• Assess for fat embolism (dyspnea, chest pain, temperature elevation). |

**TABLE 62-8 Nursing Assessment**

***Fracture***

**Subjective Data**

***Important Health Information***

*Past health history:* Traumatic injury, long-term repetitive forces (stress fracture), bone or systemic diseases, prolonged immobility, osteopenia, osteoporosis

*Medications:* Corticosteroids (osteoporotic fractures); analgesics

*Surgery or other treatments:* First aid treatment of fracture, previous musculoskeletal surgeries

***Functional Health Patterns***

*Health perception–health management:* Calcium and vitamin D supplementation

*Activity-exercise:* Loss of motion or weakness of affected part, muscle spasms

*Cognitive-perceptual:* Sudden and severe pain in affected area; numbness, tingling, loss of sensation distal to injury; ongoing pain that increases with activity (stress fracture)

**Objective Data**

***General***

Apprehension, guarding of injured site

***Integumentary***

Skin lacerations, pallor and cool skin or bluish and warm skin distal to injury; bruising, edema at fracture site

***Cardiovascular***

Reduced or absent pulse distal to injury, ↓ skin temperature, delayed capillary refill

***Neurovascular***

Paresthesia, absent or ↓ sensation, hypersensation

***Musculoskeletal***

Restricted or lost function of affected part; local bony deformities, abnormal angulation; shortening, rotation, or crepitation of affected part; muscle weakness

***Possible Diagnostic Findings***

Identification and extent of fracture on x-ray, bone scan, CT scan, or MRI

pain). Throughout the neurovascular assessment, compare both extremities to obtain an accurate assessment.

Assess an extremity's color (pink, pale, cyanotic) and temperature (hot, warm, cool, cold) in the area of the injury. Pallor or a cool-to-cold extremity below the injury could indicate arterial insufficiency. A warm, cyanotic extremity could indicate poor venous return. Next assess capillary refill (blanching of the nail bed). A compressed nail bed should return to its original color within 3 seconds.

Compare pulses on the unaffected and injured extremity to identify differences in rate or quality. This contralateral evaluation is critical. Pulses are described as strong, diminished, audible by Doppler, or absent. A diminished or absent pulse distal to the injury can indicate vascular dysfunction and insufficiency. Also assess peripheral edema. Pitting edema may be present with severe injury.

Assess ulnar, median, and radial nerve function to evaluate sensation and motor innervation in the upper extremity. Assess motor function by asking the patient to (1) abduct the fingers (ulnar nerve), (2) oppose the thumb and small finger (median nerve), and (3) flex and extend the wrist (or the fingers, if in a cast) (radial nerve). In the lower extremity, assess the patient's ability to perform dorsiflexion (peroneal nerve) and plantar flexion (tibial nerve). Evaluate sensory function of the peroneal nerve by touching the web space between the great and second toes. Stroke the plantar surface (sole) of the foot to assess sensory function of the tibial nerve.[17]

*Paresthesia* (abnormal sensation [e.g., numbness, tingling]) and hypersensation or hyperesthesia may be reported by the patient. Partial or full loss of sensation (paresis or paralysis) may be a late sign of neurovascular damage. Instruct patients to immediately report any changes in sensation or the ability to move the digits in the affected extremity.

## ◆ Nursing Diagnoses

Nursing diagnoses for the patient with a fracture may include, but are not limited to, the following:

- Impaired physical mobility *related to* loss of integrity of bone structures, movement of bone fragments, and prescribed movement restrictions
- Risk for peripheral neurovascular dysfunction *related to* vascular insufficiency and nerve compression secondary to edema and/or mechanical compression by traction, splints, or casts
- Acute pain *related to* edema, movement of bone fragments, and muscle spasms
- Readiness for enhanced self–health management

Additional information on nursing diagnoses for the patient with a fracture is presented in eNursing Care Plan 62-1 (on the website for this chapter).

## ◆ Planning

The overall goals are that the patient with a fracture will (1) have healing with no associated complications, (2) obtain satisfactory pain relief, and (3) achieve maximal rehabilitation potential.

## ◆ Nursing Implementation

◆ **Health Promotion.** Teach people in the community to take appropriate safety precautions to prevent injuries while at home or work, when driving, or when participating in sports. Be an advocate for personal actions known to reduce injuries, such as (1) regularly using seat belts, (2) driving within posted speed limits, (3) avoiding distracted driving (e.g., not texting on a cell phone) or driving under the influence of alcohol or drugs (prescribed or illicit) that may affect response times, (4) warming up muscles before exercise, (5) using protective athletic equipment (helmets and knee, wrist, and elbow pads), and (6) using safety equipment at work.

Encourage individuals, especially older adults, to participate in moderate exercise to help maintain muscle strength and balance. To reduce risk for falls, also urge them to wear nonskid, hard-soled footwear and assess their living environment for safety risks (e.g., remove scatter rugs, ensure adequate lighting, maintain clear paths to the bathroom for nighttime use) (Table 62-1). Also stress the importance of adequate calcium and vitamin D intake for bone health.

◆ **Acute Care.** Patients with fractures may be treated in an emergency department or a physician's office and released to home care, or they may require hospitalization for varying amounts of time. Specific nursing measures depend on the setting and type of treatment.

## EVIDENCE-BASED PRACTICE

### *Translating Research Into Practice*

**Do Physical Activity Exercises Decrease Sport Injuries?**

***Clinical Question***

Among physically active adults and adolescents (P), what is the effect of stretching, strength training, and proprioception exercises (I) versus control group (C) on acute and overuse sport injuries (O)?

***Synthesis of Best Available Evidence***

- Systematic review and meta-analysis of randomized controlled trials (RCTs).
- 25 RCTs of adults and adolescents (*n* = 26,610) with acute and overuse sport injuries (*n* = 3464). Intervention was physical activity exercises including strength training, stretching, and/or proprioception exercises that improve joint mobility.
- Sport injuries were not prevented by stretching before or after the sport activity.
- Strength training and/or proprioception exercises showed a positive effect in reducing sport injuries.
- Strength training reduced sports injuries by 30% with overuse injuries decreased by almost 50%.
- A trend was noted for strength training to have a greater preventive effect against injury compared to proprioception training.

***Conclusion***

- Participation in strength training and/or proprioception exercises decreases the incidence of acute and overuse sport injuries.

***Implications for Nursing Practice***

1. What would you advise a person who participates in sports and solely commits to stretching for physical activity exercise?
2. Why is it important for you to discuss the benefits of adherence to strength training when persons are involved in multiple extensive physical activity programs?

***Reference for Evidence***

Lauersen JB, Bertelsen DM, Andersen LB: The effectiveness of exercise interventions to prevent sports injuries: a systematic review and meta-analysis of randomised controlled trials, *Br J Sports Med* 48:871, 2014.

*P*, Patient population of interest; *I*, intervention or area of interest; *C*, comparison of interest or comparison group; *O*, outcomes of interest; *T*, timing (see p. 15).

◆ ***Preoperative Care.*** If surgical intervention is required to treat a fracture, patients need preoperative preparation. In addition to the usual preoperative nursing measures (see Chapter 17), inform patients of the type of immobilization and assistive devices that will be used and the expected activity limitations after surgery. Assure patients that nursing staff will help meet their personal needs until they can resume self-care. Remind patients that pain medication will be available if needed.

◆ ***Postoperative Care.*** In general, postoperative nursing care and management are directed toward monitoring vital signs and applying general principles of postoperative nursing care (see Chapter 19). Frequent neurovascular assessment of the affected extremity is necessary to detect early and subtle changes. Closely monitor any limitations related to turning, positioning, and extremity support. Minimize pain and discomfort through proper alignment and positioning. Carefully observe dressings or casts for any signs of bleeding or drainage. Report a significant increase in size of the drainage area. If a wound drainage system is in place, regularly measure the volume of drainage and assess its character (e.g., bloody, purulent). Report increased or purulent drainage immediately to the surgeon. Also assess the patency of the drainage system, using aseptic technique to avoid contamination.

Additional nursing responsibilities depend on the type of immobilization used. A blood salvage and reinfusion system may be used to allow recovery and reinfusion of the patient's own blood. The blood is retrieved from a joint space or cavity, and the patient receives this blood in the form of an autotransfusion. (Autotransfusion is discussed in Chapter 30.) Additional nursing measures for the patient who has had orthopedic surgery are discussed in eNursing Care Plan 62-2 (on the website for this chapter).

◆ ***Other Measures.*** Patients often have reduced mobility as a result of a fracture. Plan care to decrease risk for the many complications associated with immobility. Prevent constipation by increasing patient activity and maintaining high fluid intake (more than 2500 mL/day unless contraindicated by the patient's health status) and a diet high in bulk and roughage (fresh fruits and vegetables). If these measures are not effective in maintaining the patient's normal bowel elimination pattern, administer stool softeners, laxatives, or suppositories. Maintain a regular time for elimination to promote bowel regularity.

Renal calculi can develop from bone demineralization related to reduced mobility. Hypercalcemia from demineralization causes a rise in urine pH and stone formation from the precipitation of calcium. Unless contraindicated, fluid intake of 2500 mL/day is recommended to decrease the risk of calculi formation. (Renal calculi are discussed in Chapter 45.)

Rapid deconditioning of the cardiopulmonary system can occur as a result of prolonged bed rest, resulting in orthostatic hypotension and decreased lung capacity. Unless contraindicated, these effects can be diminished by having the patient sit on the side of the bed, allowing the patient's lower limbs to dangle over the bedside, and having the patient perform standing transfers. When the patient is allowed to increase activity, assess for orthostatic hypotension. Also assess patients for venous thromboembolism (VTE) (VTE is discussed in Chapter 37.)

◆ ***Traction.*** When slings are used with traction, regularly inspect exposed skin areas. Pressure over a bony prominence created by wrinkled sheets or blankets may cause pressure necrosis. Persistent skin pressure may impair blood flow and cause injury to peripheral nerves and blood vessels. Observe skeletal traction or external fixation pin sites for signs of infection. Pin site care may vary but often includes regularly cleansing with chlorhexidine, rinsing pin sites with sterile saline, and drying the area with sterile gauze.

External rotation of the affected extremity is a classic assessment finding for a patient with unrepaired hip fracture. If skin traction is ordered preoperatively, apply traction without attempting to reposition or realign the extremity. Movement of fracture fragments can occur during repositioning, causing increased pain and possible nerve impingement. Keep the patient in the center of the bed in a supine position to provide adequate countertraction.

To offset possible problems associated with prolonged immobility, discuss specific patient activity with the HCP. If exercise is permitted, encourage patient participation in a simple exercise regimen based on activity restrictions. Encourage the patient to participate in frequent position changes, ROM exercises of unaffected joints, deep-breathing exercises, isometric exercises, and use of the trapeze bar (if permitted) to raise the body off the bed for linen changes and placement of the bedpan. These activities should be performed several times

**INFORMATICS IN PRACTICE**

***Web-Based Knee and Hip Replacement Community***

- Many hospitals provide preoperative classes for patients undergoing joint replacement surgery, but fewer resources are available for postdischarge support.
- With careful research, the patient can locate online knee and hip replacement communities to share experiences and receive social support. The patient is likely to feel relieved knowing that others have similar experiences.
- Encourage patients to validate any advice with their surgeons before taking action.

each day. Encourage and help the hospitalized patient to stay connected with friends and family by telephone or through social media resources (see Informatics in Practice box).

## ◆ Ambulatory Care

◆ ***Cast Care.*** Because uncomplicated fractures are treated in an outpatient setting, the patient may require only a short hospitalization or none at all. Regardless of the type of cast material, a cast can interfere with circulation and nerve function if it is applied too tightly or excessive edema occurs after application. Frequent neurovascular assessment of the immobilized extremity is critical. Teach the patient to recognize and promptly report the signs of cast complications. Explain the importance of elevating the extremity above heart level to promote venous return and applying ice to control or prevent edema during the initial phase. However, if compartment syndrome is suspected, do not elevate the extremity above the heart.

Instruct the patient to exercise joints above and below the cast. Instruct the patient to avoid scratching or placing foreign objects inside the cast because this may cause skin breakdown and infection. For itching, suggest the use of a hair dryer on a cool setting to be directed under the cast.

Patient and caregiver teaching is important to prevent complications. In addition to specific instructions for cast care and recognition of complications, encourage the patient to contact the HCP with any questions. Table 62-9 summarizes patient and caregiver instructions for cast care. Validate the patient's and caregiver's understanding of these instructions before discharge. A follow-up phone call is appropriate. Home care nursing visits may be warranted, especially for the patient with a body jacket brace.

The cast is typically removed in the outpatient setting. Patients often fear being cut by the oscillating blade of the cast saw. Reassure the patient that damage to the skin is unlikely.[18] Teach the patient about possible alterations in the appearance of the extremity beneath the cast (e.g., dry, wrinkled skin; atrophied muscle). The patient may also have anxiety related to using the injured extremity after cast removal.

◆ ***Psychosocial Problems.*** Short-term rehabilitative goals address the transition from dependence to independence in performing simple ADLs and preserving or increasing strength and endurance. Long-term rehabilitative goals are aimed at preventing problems associated with musculoskeletal injury (Table 62-10). During the rehabilitative phase, help the patient adjust to any problems caused by the injury (e.g., separation from family, financial impact of medical care, loss of income from inability to work, potential for lifetime disability). Offer support and encouragement while actively listening to the patient's and caregiver's concerns.

**TABLE 62-9 Patient & Caregiver Teaching**

***Cast Care***

*After a cast is applied, include the following instructions when teaching the patient and the caregiver.*

**Do**

1. Apply ice directly over fracture site for first 24 hr (avoid getting cast wet by keeping ice in plastic bag and protecting cast with cloth).
2. Check with HCP before getting fiberglass cast wet.
3. Dry cast thoroughly if inadvertently exposed to water.
   - Blot dry with towel.
   - Use hair dryer on low setting until cast is thoroughly dry.
4. Elevate extremity above level of heart for first 48 hr.
5. Regularly move joints above and below cast.
6. Use hair dryer on cool setting for itching inside the cast.
7. Report signs of possible problems to HCP:
   - Increasing pain despite elevation, ice, analgesia.
   - Swelling associated with pain and discoloration of toes or fingers.
   - Pain during movement.
   - Burning or tingling under cast.
   - Sores or foul odor under cast.
8. Keep appointment to have fracture and cast checked.

**Do Not**

1. Get cast wet.
2. Remove any padding.
3. Insert any objects inside cast.
4. Bear weight on new cast for 48 hr (not all casts are made for weight bearing; check with HCP when unsure).
5. Cover cast with plastic for prolonged periods.

◆ ***Ambulation.*** Know the overall goals of physical therapy in relation to the patient's abilities, needs, and tolerance. Mobility training and instruction in the use of assistive aids (cane, crutches, walker) are major areas of responsibility for the physical therapist. Reinforce these instructions to the patient. The patient with lower extremity dysfunction usually starts mobility training when able to sit in bed and dangle the feet over the side. Collaborate with the physical therapist to administer analgesia before a physical therapy session.

When the patient begins to ambulate, know the patient's weight-bearing status and the correct technique if the patient is using an assistive device. Ambulation occurs in different degrees of weight-bearing: (1) non–weight bearing (no weight on the involved extremity), (2) touch-down/toe-touch weight bearing (contact with floor for balance but no weight borne), (3) partial–weight-bearing ambulation (25% to 50% of patient's weight borne), (4) weight bearing as tolerated (based on patient's pain and tolerance), and (5) full–weight-bearing ambulation (no limitations).

◆ ***Assistive Devices.*** Devices for ambulation range from a cane (can relieve up to 40% of the weight normally borne by a lower limb) to a walker or crutches (may allow for complete non–weight-bearing ambulation). The HCP decides which device is appropriate, balancing the need for maximum stability and safety with the need for maneuverabiliy in small spaces such as bathrooms. Discuss with the patient his or her lifestyle requirements and select a device that allows each patient to feel most secure and independent. The technique for using assistive ambulation devices varies. The involved limb is usually advanced at the same time or immediately after advance of the device. The uninvolved limb is advanced last. In almost all cases, canes are held in the hand opposite the involved extremity.

TABLE 62-10 **Problems Associated With Musculoskeletal Injuries**

| Problem | Description | Nursing Considerations |
|---|---|---|
| **Muscle atrophy** | • Decreased muscle mass occurs as a result of disuse after prolonged immobilization.<br>• Loss of nerve function can precipitate muscle atrophy. | • Isometric muscle-strengthening exercises as able with immobilization device assists in reducing amount of atrophy.<br>• Muscle atrophy interferes with and prolongs rehabilitation process. |
| **Contracture** | • Abnormal condition of joint characterized by flexion and fixation.<br>• Caused by atrophy and shortening of muscle fibers and ligaments, or by loss of normal elasticity of skin over joint. | • Can be prevented by frequent position change, correct body alignment, active-passive ROM exercises several times a day.<br>• Intervention requires gradual progressive stretching of muscles or ligaments in region of joint. |
| **Footdrop** | • Plantar-flexed position of the foot occurs when Achilles tendon in ankle shortens because it has been allowed to assume an unsupported position.<br>• Peroneal nerve palsy (a compression neuropathy) can cause footdrop and spinal nerve compression. | • For patient with long-term injuries, support foot in neutral position to decrease risk of footdrop.<br>• Once footdrop has developed, ambulation and gait training may be significantly hindered.<br>• May require splint to keep feet in neutral position.<br>• High-top athletic shoes may also help. Apply at scheduled times to keep feet in neutral position. |
| **Pain** | • Frequently associated with fractures, edema, muscle spasm.<br>• Pain may be mild to severe and is described as aching, dull, burning, throbbing, sharp, or deep. | • Causes of pain include incorrect positioning and alignment of extremity, incorrect support of extremity, sudden movement of extremity, immobilization device that is applied too tightly or incorrectly, constrictive dressings, motion at fracture site.<br>• Determine causes of pain so that corrective action can be taken. |
| **Muscle spasms** | • Caused by involuntary muscle contraction after fracture, muscle strain, or nerve injury.<br>• May last several weeks.<br>• Pain associated with muscle spasms is often intense and can last from several seconds to several minutes. | • Measures to reduce intensity of muscle spasms are similar to actions for pain management.<br>• Do not massage muscle spasms. Massage may stimulate muscle tissue contraction that increases spasm and pain.<br>• Thermotherapy, especially heat, may reduce muscle spasm. |

Place a transfer belt (gait belt) around the patient's waist to provide stability while he or she is learning to use an assistive device. Discourage the patient from reaching for furniture or relying on another person for support. If the patient has inadequate upper limb strength or poorly fitted crutches, he or she bears weight at the axilla rather than at the hands, endangering the neurovascular bundle that passes across the axilla. If verbal coaching does not correct the problem, instruct the patient in another form of ambulation (e.g., walker) until strength is adequate.

Patients who must ambulate without weight bearing require sufficient upper limb strength to lift their own weight at each step. Because the muscles of the shoulder girdle and upper arm may not be accustomed to this work, patients require vigorous and diligent training for this task. Push-ups, pull-ups using the overhead trapeze bar, and weight lifting develop the triceps and biceps muscles. Straight-leg raises and quadriceps-setting exercises strengthen the quadriceps muscles.

◆ ***Counseling and Referrals.*** During the rehabilitative process, the patient's caregiver assumes an important role in the provision of long-term care. Instruct the caregiver in strength and endurance exercises, assistance with mobility training, and promotion of activities that enhance the quality of daily living. Also evaluate patients for posttraumatic stress disorder. This is especially important if significant injury to others or fatalities were associated with the patient's injuries.

### ◆ Evaluation

The expected outcomes are that the patient with a fracture will

- Report satisfactory pain management
- Demonstrate appropriate care of cast or immobilizer
- Experience no peripheral neurovascular dysfunction
- Experience uncomplicated bone healing

## COMPLICATIONS OF FRACTURES

The majority of fractures heal without complications. Death after a fracture is usually the result of damage to underlying organs and vascular structures or from complications of the fracture or immobility. Complications of fractures may be direct or indirect. *Direct complications* include problems with bone infection, bone union, and avascular necrosis. *Indirect complications* are associated with blood vessel and nerve damage resulting in conditions such as compartment syndrome, VTE, fat embolism syndrome (FES), breakdown of skeletal muscle *(rhabdomyolysis),* and hypovolemic shock. Most musculoskeletal injuries are not life threatening. However, open fractures, fractures accompanied by severe blood loss, and fractures that damage vital organs (e.g., lung, heart) are medical emergencies requiring immediate attention.

### Infection

Open fractures and soft tissue injuries have a high incidence of infection. An open fracture usually results from severe external forces. Massive or blunt soft tissue injury often has more serious consequences than the fracture. Devitalized and contaminated tissue is an ideal medium for many common pathogens, including gas-forming (anaerobic) bacilli such as *Clostridium tetani.* Treatment of infection is costly in terms of extended nursing and medical care, time for treatment, and loss of patient income. Delayed or ineffective treatment can lead to the development of chronic osteomyelitis[19] (see Chapter 63).

Open fractures require aggressive surgical debridement. The wound is initially cleaned by pulsating saline lavage in the operating room. Gross contaminants are irrigated and mechanically removed. Contused, contaminated, and devitalized tissue (muscle, subcutaneous fat, skin, and bone fragments) are surgically excised *(debridement).* The extent of soft tissue damage determines if the wound is closed at the time of surgery and if it requires repeat debridement, closed suction drainage, and/or skin grafting. Depending on the location and extent of the fracture, reduction may be maintained by external fixation or traction. During surgery, the open wound may be irrigated with antibiotic solution. Antibiotic-impregnated beads may also be placed in the surgical site. The patient may have antibiotics administered IV for 3 to 7 days during the postoperative phase of care. In conjunction with aggressive surgical management, antibiotics have greatly reduced the occurrence of infection.

## Compartment Syndrome

**Compartment syndrome** is a condition in which swelling causes increased pressure within a limited space (muscle compartment). Because the fascia surrounding the muscle has limited ability to stretch, continued swelling can cause pressure that compromises the function of blood vessels and nerves in the compartment. Capillary perfusion is reduced below a level needed for tissue viability. Compartment syndrome usually involves the leg but can also occur in any muscle group (e.g., arm, shoulder, buttock, abdomen).

Thirty-eight compartments are located in the upper and lower extremities. Two basic causes of compartment syndrome are (1) decreased compartment size resulting from restrictive dressings, splints, casts, excessive traction, or premature closure of fascia; and (2) increased compartment contents related to bleeding, inflammation, edema, or IV infiltration.

Edema can create sufficient pressure to obstruct circulation and cause venous occlusion, which further increases edema. Arterial flow is eventually compromised, causing ischemia in the extremity. As ischemia continues, muscle and nerve cells are destroyed. Fibrotic tissue eventually replaces healthy tissue. Contracture, disability, and loss of function can occur. Delays in diagnosis and treatment result in irreversible muscle and nerve ischemia. The extremity may become functionally useless or severely impaired.

Compartment syndrome is usually associated with trauma, fractures (especially of long bones), extensive soft tissue damage, and crush injury. Fractures of the distal humerus and proximal tibia are the most common fractures associated with compartment syndrome. Compartment injury can also occur after knee or leg surgery. Prolonged pressure on a muscle compartment may result when someone is trapped under a heavy object or a person's limb is trapped beneath the body because of response to drugs or alcohol.

### CHECK YOUR PRACTICE

Your 32-yr-old male patient had a skiing injury. He returned from surgery 8 hours ago with a long leg cast placed for open fractures of the femur and tibia. He continually complains of pain and IV morphine does not seem to help.

- How will you assess his neurovascular condition? What signs and symptoms would suggest the development of compartment syndrome?
- What is the most likely intervention if compartment syndrome is developing?

**Clinical Manifestations.** Compartment syndrome may occur initially from the body's physiologic response to the injury, or it may be delayed for several days after the original insult or injury. Ischemia can occur within 4 to 8 hours after the onset of compartment syndrome.

One or more of the following six *P*s are characteristic of compartment syndrome: (1) *pain* out of proportion to the injury that is not managed by opioid analgesics, and *pain* on passive stretch of muscle traveling through the compartment; (2) increasing *pressure* in the compartment; (3) *paresthesia* (numbness and tingling); (4) *pallor,* coolness, and loss of normal color of the extremity; (5) *paralysis* or loss of function; and (6) *pulselessness* (diminished or absent peripheral pulses).

**Interprofessional Care.** Prompt, accurate diagnosis of compartment syndrome is critical.[20] Perform and document regular neurovascular assessment on all patients with fractures, especially those with injury of the extremities or soft tissue in these areas. Early recognition and effective treatment of compartment syndrome are essential to avoid permanent damage to muscles and nerves.

Carefully assess the location, quality, and intensity of the pain (see Chapter 8). Evaluate the patient's level of pain on a scale of 0 to 10. Pain unrelieved by drugs and out of proportion to the level of injury is one of the *first* indications of impending compartment syndrome. Paresthesia is also an early sign. Notify the HCP immediately of these changes in the patient's condition. If the source of pressure is relieved (e.g., cast is cut [bivalve] or dressing loosened by order of the HCP), pain and paresthesia typically decrease and compartment syndrome is avoided. Reducing traction weight may also decrease external pressures on the extremity. Pulselessness and paralysis are later signs of compartment syndrome. Do not wait until these late signs occur to contact the HCP, as the limb may require amputation if pressure progresses to this state.

Because of the possibility of muscle damage, assess urine output. Myoglobin released from damaged muscle cells precipitates and causes obstruction in renal tubules. This condition results in acute tubular necrosis and acute kidney injury (AKI). Common signs are dark reddish brown urine and clinical manifestations associated with AKI (see Chapter 46).

Elevation of the extremity may lower venous pressure and slow arterial perfusion. With suspected compartment syndrome, the extremity should not be elevated above the heart level. Similarly, application of cold compresses should be avoided because they may cause vasoconstriction and exacerbate compartment syndrome.

Surgical decompression (e.g., fasciotomy) of the involved compartment may be necessary (Fig. 62-15). The fasciotomy site is left open for several days to ensure adequate soft tissue decompression. Infection resulting from delayed wound closure is a potential problem after fasciotomy. In severe cases of compartment syndrome, amputation may be required.

## Venous Thromboembolism

Veins of the lower extremities and pelvis are highly susceptible to thrombus formation after a fracture, especially a hip fracture. VTE may also occur after total hip or total knee replacement surgery. In patients with limited mobility, venous stasis is aggravated by inactivity of muscles that normally assist in pumping venous blood from the extremities to the heart.

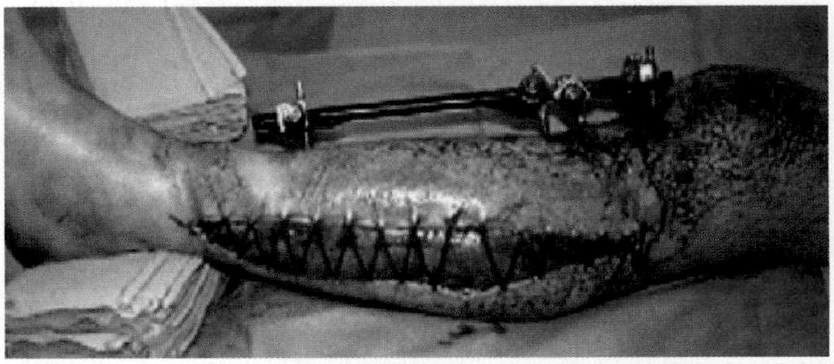

**FIG. 62-15** Fasciotomy associated with compartment syndrome. Stabilization of fracture with external fixator. (From Browner BD, Jupiter JB, Levine AM, Trafton P: *Skeletal trauma: fractures, dislocations, ligamentous injuries,* ed 4, Philadelphia, 2009, Saunders.)

Because of the high risk of VTE in the orthopedic surgical patient, prophylactic anticoagulant drugs may be ordered: (1) warfarin (Coumadin), (2) low-molecular-weight heparin (LMWH) (e.g., enoxaparin [Lovenox], dalteparin [Fragmin]), or (3) a factor Xa inhibitor (fondaparinux [Arixtra], rivaroxaban [Xarelto], apixaban [Eliquis]). In addition to wearing compression gradient stockings (antiembolism hose) or using sequential compression devices, the patient should dorsiflex and plantar flex the ankle of an affected lower extremity against resistance and perform ROM exercises on the unaffected leg. For upper extremity injuries, the patient should flex and extend the wrist if not immobilized by a cast or splint and perform ROM exercises on the unaffected arm. (Assessment and management of VTE are discussed in Chapter 37.)

**SAFETY ALERT Anticoagulant Therapy**

- Monitor for signs of external bleeding (e.g., nosebleeds) or internal bleeding (e.g., tea-colored urine).
- Teach patient about signs of bleeding and what to do if excessive bleeding occurs (i.e., apply pressure for 10 minutes, seek medical attention if bleeding does not stop).
- Teach patient safe self-injection if taking an injectable anticoagulant after discharge.
- Encourage patient to keep all follow-up appointments for laboratory testing to monitor effects of warfarin (if prescribed).

### Fat Embolism Syndrome

Fat embolism syndrome (FES) is characterized by systemic fat globules from fractures that are distributed into tissues, lungs, and other organs after a traumatic skeletal injury. FES is a contributory factor in mortality associated with fractures. The fractures that most often are associated with FES include those of the long bones, ribs, tibia, and pelvis. FES can also occur after total joint replacement, spinal fusion, liposuction, crush injuries, and bone marrow transplantation.

Two theories about FES exist. According to the mechanical theory, fat emboli may originate from fat released from the marrow of injured bone. The fat then enters systemic circulation, where it embolizes to other organs such as the brain.[21] As fat droplets lodge in small blood vessels, local ischemia and inflammation occur. The biochemical theory suggests hormonal changes caused by trauma or sepsis stimulate the systemic release of free fatty acids (e.g., chylomicrons) that form the fat emboli.

**Clinical Manifestations.** Early recognition of FES is crucial to prevent a potentially lethal course. Most patients manifest symptoms within 24 to 48 hours after injury. Severe forms have occurred within hours of injury. Fat emboli in the lungs cause a hemorrhagic interstitial pneumonitis with signs and symptoms of acute respiratory distress syndrome (ARDS), such as chest pain, tachypnea, cyanosis, dyspnea, apprehension, tachycardia, and decreased partial pressure of arterial $O_2$ ($PaO_2$). These symptoms are caused by poor oxygen exchange. Changes in mental status (a result of hypoxemia) are also part of the classic triad of signs and symptoms. Investigate memory loss, restlessness, confusion, elevated temperature, and headache so that central nervous system involvement is not mistaken for alcohol withdrawal or acute head injury. Petechiae located on the neck, anterior chest wall, axilla, buccal membrane, and conjunctiva of the eye may help distinguish fat emboli from other problems. They may appear due to intravascular thromboses caused by decreased oxygenation. However, petechiae are only seen in 25% to 50% of cases of FES and may fade before noticed.[21]

The clinical course of a fat embolus may be rapid and acute. Frequently the patient expresses a feeling of impending disaster. In a short time, skin color changes from pallor to cyanosis, and the patient may become comatose. No specific laboratory examinations are available to aid in the diagnosis. However, certain abnormalities may be present. These include fat cells in blood, urine, or sputum; a decrease of $PaO_2$ to less than 60 mm Hg; ST segment and T-wave changes on ECG; a decrease in the platelet count and hematocrit; and an elevated erythrocyte sedimentation rate (ESR). A chest x-ray may show bilateral pulmonary infiltrates.

**CHECK YOUR PRACTICE**

You are caring for a 24-yr-old male patient who had a femur fracture in a motorcycle accident last night. He is scheduled for ORIF later today. While doing your assessment, you notice that he seems very restless. You also observe some axillary petechiae.

- What complication would you suspect is occurring?
- Why is this patient particularly at risk for this complication?
- What is the most important intervention for a patient with this complication?

**Interprofessional Care.** Treatment of fat embolism is directed at prevention. Careful immobilization and handling of a long bone fracture are probably the most important factors in prevention of fat embolism. Reposition the patient as little as possible before fracture immobilization or stabilization because of the danger of dislodging fat droplets into the general circulation. Management of FES is mostly supportive and related to management of symptoms. Treatment includes fluid resuscitation to prevent hypovolemic shock, correction of acidosis, and blood transfusion. Use of corticosteroids to prevent or treat fat embolism is controversial.

Encourage coughing and deep breathing. Administer $O_2$ to treat hypoxia. Intubation or intermittent positive pressure ventilation may be considered if satisfactory $PaO_2$ cannot be obtained with supplemental oxygen alone. Some patients may develop pulmonary edema and/or ARDS leading to increased mortality. Most persons survive FES with few sequelae.

## TYPES OF FRACTURES

### COLLES' FRACTURE

A *Colles' fracture* is a fracture of the distal radius and is one of the most common fractures in adults (Fig. 62-16). The styloid process of the ulna may be involved as well. The injury usually occurs when the patient falls on an outstretched arm and hand. This type of fracture most often occurs in patients over 50 years old whose bones are osteoporotic *(fragility fracture)*. A younger person with a Colles' fracture caused by a low-energy force should be referred for an osteoporosis evaluation.

Clinical manifestations of Colles' fracture are pain in the immediate area of injury, pronounced swelling, and dorsal displacement of the distal fragment (silver-fork deformity). This displacement appears as an obvious deformity of the wrist. The major complication associated with a Colles' fracture is vascular insufficiency secondary to edema. Carpal tunnel syndrome can be a later complication.

A Colles' fracture is usually managed with closed reduction of the fracture and immobilization by a splint or cast. If displaced, the fracture is typically managed with open reduction

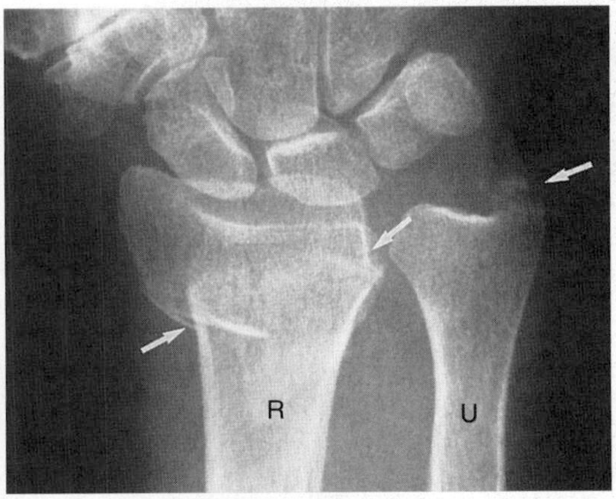


**FIG. 62-16** Colles' fracture. Fracture of the distal radius *(R)* and ulnar *(U)* styloid from patient falling on the outstretched hand. (From Mettler FA: *Essentials of radiology,* ed 2, Philadelphia, 2005, Saunders.)

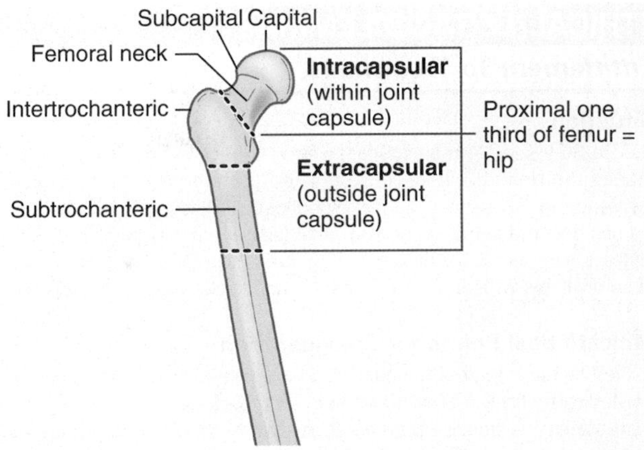


**FIG. 62-17** Femur with location of various types of fracture.

and internal or external fixation. Nursing management includes frequent neurovascular assessment and measures to reduce edema. Provide support and protect the extremity. Encourage active movement of the thumb and fingers to reduce edema and increase venous return. Also instruct the patient to perform active movements of the shoulder to prevent stiffness or contracture.

## HUMERAL SHAFT FRACTURE

Fractures involving the shaft of the humerus are common among young and middle-aged adults. The most common clinical manifestations are an obvious displacement of the humeral shaft, shortened extremity, abnormal mobility, and pain. Major complications associated with a humeral shaft fracture are radial nerve injury and injury to the brachial artery as a result of laceration, transection, or muscle spasm.

The treatment for a humeral shaft fracture depends on the location and displacement of the fracture. Nonoperative treatment may include a hanging arm cast; shoulder immobilizer; or sling and swathe (a type of immobilizer that prevents glenohumeral movement). The swathe encircles the trunk and humerus as an additional binder. It is often used after surgical repairs (e.g., rotator cuff repair) and shoulder dislocation.

When these devices are used, elevate the head of the bed to assist gravity in reducing the fracture. Allow the arm to hang freely when the patient is sitting or standing. Include measures to protect the axilla and prevent skin breakdown. Carefully place absorbable composite dressing pads (i.e., ABD pads) in the axilla and change them twice daily or as needed. Skin or skeletal traction may be used for reduction and immobilization.

During the rehabilitative phase, an exercise program to improve strength and motion of the injured extremity is extremely important. Exercises should include assisted motion of the hand and fingers. The shoulder can also be exercised if the fracture is stable. This helps prevent stiffness secondary to frozen shoulder or fibrosis of the shoulder capsule.

## PELVIC FRACTURE

Pelvic fractures range from relatively minor to life threatening, depending on the mechanism of injury and associated vascular damage. Although only a small percentage of all fractures are pelvic fractures, this type of injury is associated with a high mortality rate. Preoccupation with more obvious injuries at the time of a traumatic event may result in oversight of pelvic injuries.

Pelvic fractures may cause serious intraabdominal injury, including laceration and hemorrhage of the urethra, bladder, or colon. Pelvic fractures can cause acute pelvic compartment syndrome. Paralytic ileus may also occur following pelvic fracture. Patients may survive the initial pelvic injury, only to die from sepsis, FES, or VTE.

Physical examination of the abdomen may identify local swelling, tenderness, deformity, unusual pelvic movement, and ecchymosis. Assess the neurovascular condition of the lower extremities and determine associated injuries. Pelvic fractures are diagnosed by x-ray and CT scan.

Treatment of a pelvic fracture depends on the severity of the injury. Stable, nondisplaced fractures require limited intervention. Bed rest, sometimes with the use of a pelvic sling, is typically maintained for a few days. Progressive ambulation with guarded weight bearing is then encouraged. Complex or displaced fractures (e.g., open book fracture) require external fixation alone or combined with ORIF, often performed emergently. Use extreme care in handling or moving the patient to prevent additional injury. Turn the patient only when ordered by the HCP. Because a pelvic fracture can damage other organs, assess bowel and urinary elimination. Regularly perform distal neurovascular assessment. Provide back care while the patient is raised from the bed by independent use of the trapeze or with adequate assistance.

## HIP FRACTURE

Hip fractures are common in older adults, with 95% of these fractures resulting from a fall.[22] More than 320,000 patients are admitted to hospitals annually because of a hip fracture. By age 90, approximately 33% of all women and 17% of all men will have sustained a hip fracture. In adults more than 65 years old, hip fracture occurs more frequently in women than in men because of osteoporosis. Many older adults with a hip fracture develop disabilities that require long-term care. One in five people experiencing a hip fracture will die within 1 year of injury.[23]

Hip fracture (Fig. 62-17) refers to a fracture of the proximal (upper) third of the femur, which extends 5 cm below the lesser trochanter. Fractures that occur within the hip joint capsule are called *intracapsular fractures.* Intracapsular fractures are further identified by their specific locations: (1) *capital* (fracture of the

## ETHICAL/LEGAL DILEMMAS

### *Entitlement to Treatment*

**Situation**

H.Z., a 35-yr-old German tourist, was in a hang-gliding accident while touring the United States. He was taken to the regional trauma center for treatment of internal injuries, blood loss, and severe pelvic fractures. He has become septic, is now in renal failure, and has acute respiratory distress syndrome. He has no health insurance. Despite a poor chance of survival, his wife and parents want all possible measures to be taken.

**Ethical/Legal Points for Consideration**

- Federal law requires hospitals receiving federal funds through Medicare and Medicaid to provide emergency evaluation and treatment to stabilize patients (Emergency Medical Treatment and Active Labor Act [EMTALA]). They are under no obligation to continue treatment and may transfer the patient to another facility.
- In addition, the Hill-Burton Act requires states to have sufficient hospitals to provide necessary services for those unable to pay.
- Discussions with the family must occur to clarify treatment goals (e.g., recovery, survival, continued biologic existence, nonabandonment of the patient) and what they mean by wanting "everything done." There is no legal or ethical obligation to continue medical treatment when treatment goals cannot be met.
- Contact with the German consulate may result in collaboration to stabilize the patient and transport him to Germany.
- Neither HCPs nor hospitals are required to provide medically futile care (care that provides no benefit to the patient).
- Although his home country (Germany) offers universal health care, H.Z. assumed the risk when engaging in a potentially dangerous activity and did not obtain international health insurance coverage for his visit to a foreign country,

**Discussion Questions**

1. How can the nurse facilitate discussions with the family regarding treatment goals for H.Z.? Are family members able to verbalize H.Z.'s wishes for his own care in such a situation?
2. If a person engages in risky behavior, is withholding treatment an option because of the behavior?

## CHECK YOUR PRACTICE

You are taking care of an 83-yr-old patient who fell down the steps outside her house while getting her mail. She was diagnosed with a femoral neck fracture and Colles' fracture. She is returning to the clinical unit following surgery. She had an ORIF of the femoral neck fracture and closed reduction of the Colles' fracture.

- Based on these injuries, what do you think are possible complications?
- How will the interprofessional team mobilize a patient with these injuries?
- What are your postdischarge concerns for this patient?

head of the femur), (2) *subcapital* (fracture just below the head of the femur), and (3) *transcervical* (fracture of the femoral neck). These fractures are often associated with osteoporosis and minor trauma and are identified as *fragility fractures.*

*Extracapsular fractures* occur outside the joint capsule. They are termed (1) *intertrochanteric* (in a region between the greater and lesser trochanter) or (2) *subtrochanteric* (below the lesser trochanter). Extracapsular fractures are usually caused by severe direct trauma or a fall.

### Clinical Manifestations

Clinical manifestations of hip fractures are external rotation, muscle spasm, shortening of the affected extremity, and severe pain and tenderness around the fracture site. Displaced femoral neck fractures may cause serious disruption of blood supply to the femoral head, which can result in avascular necrosis of the femoral head.

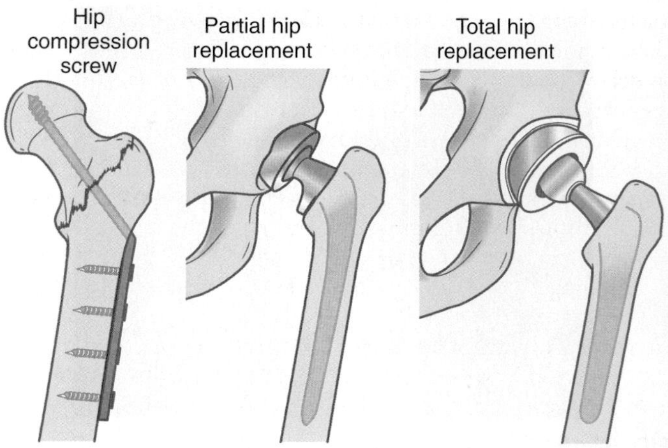


**FIG. 62-18** Types of surgical repair for a hip fracture.

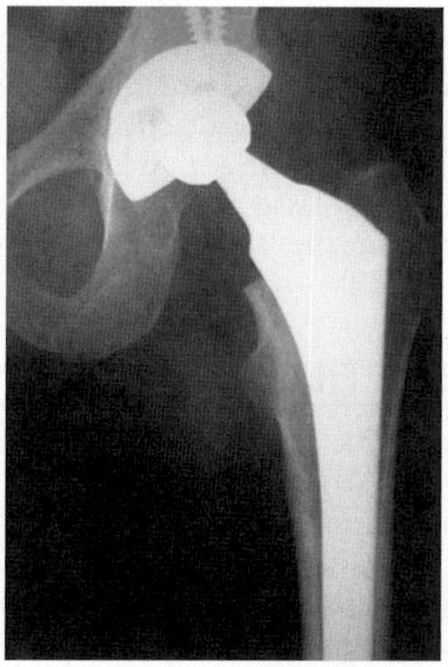

**FIG. 62-19** Total hip replacement (arthroplasty) with cementless femoral prosthesis of metal alloy with plastic acetabular socket.

### Interprofessional Care

Initially the affected extremity may be temporarily immobilized by Buck's traction (Fig. 62-9) until the patient's physical condition is stabilized and surgery can be performed. Buck's traction relieves painful muscle spasms and can be used for 24 to 48 hours.

Surgical treatment of hip fractures permits early mobilization and decreases the risk of major complications. The type of surgery depends on the location and severity of the fracture and the person's age. Surgical options include (1) repair with internal fixation devices (e.g., hip compression screw, intramedullary devices) (Fig. 62-18), (2) replacement of the femoral head with a prosthesis (partial hip replacement or *hemiarthroplasty*, often used for fracture of the femoral neck) (Fig. 62-18), and (3) total hip replacement (involves both the femur and acetabulum) (Figs. 62-18 and 62-19).

## NURSING MANAGEMENT: HIP FRACTURE

### Nursing Implementation

**Preoperative Care.** The majority of people who have hip fractures are older adults. When planning treatment of the hip fracture, consider the patient's chronic health problems (e.g., diabetes mellitus, cardiac and pulmonary disease). Surgery may be delayed for a brief time until the patient's general health is stabilized, but better outcomes are associated with surgery performed within 24 hours of injury.[24]

Before surgery, severe muscle spasms can increase pain. Appropriate analgesics or muscle relaxants, comfortable positioning (unless contraindicated), and properly applied traction (if used) can help to manage the spasms.

Teaching is often done in the emergency department because quick surgical intervention is the standard of care. Most patients are medically stable and thus do not have an overnight preoperative period in which to receive instructions. The patient also may not have the cognitive ability to retain this important patient teaching.

When possible, teach the patient the method for exercising the unaffected leg and both arms. Plans for discharge begin as soon as the patient enters the hospital because the length of stay postoperatively will only be a few days.

◆ **Postoperative Care.** Similar principles of patient care apply to any of the surgical procedures for hip fractures. In the initial postoperative period, assess vital signs, intake, and output; monitor respiratory function and encourage deep breathing and coughing; administer pain medication; and observe the dressing and incision for signs of bleeding. (eNursing Care Plan 62-2 for the orthopedic surgical patient is presented on the website for this chapter.)

Neurovascular impairment is possible. Assess the patient's extremity for (1) color, (2) temperature, (3) capillary refill, (4) distal pulses, (5) edema, (6) sensation, (7) motor function, and (8) pain. Edema is alleviated by elevating the leg when the patient is in bed or in a chair. The pain resulting from surgical repair of the affected extremity can be reduced by maintaining limb alignment with pillows between the patient's knees when turning the patient to the nonoperative side.

Encourage the patient to use the overhead trapeze bar and the opposite side rail to assist in changing positions. Avoid turning the patient to the affected side unless approved by the surgeon. A physical therapist can teach the patient how to perform out-of-bed and chair transfers.

If the hip fracture has been repaired with hemiarthroplasty or total joint replacement by a *posterior approach* (incision posterior to the midline of the greater trochanter down the femoral shaft), measures to prevent dislocation must be used (Table 62-11). Inform the patient and caregiver about positions and activities that place the patient at risk for dislocation (more than 90 degrees of flexion, adduction across the midline [crossing of legs and ankles], internal rotation of hip). Many daily activities may reproduce these positions: (1) putting on shoes and socks, (2) crossing the legs or feet while seated, (3) assuming the side-lying position incorrectly, (4) standing up or sitting down while the hip is flexed more than 90 degrees relative to the chair, and (5) sitting on low seats, especially low toilet seats. Teach the patient to avoid these activities until the soft tissue capsule around the hip has healed enough to stabilize the prosthesis (usually at least 6 weeks).

Elevated toilet seats and chair alterations (e.g., raising the seat with a folded blanket, maintaining a straight back) are necessary. Avoid placing a soft pillow in the patient's seat because sitting on it can cause internal rotation. If a foam abduction wedge is ordered to prevent joint dislocation, place it between the patient's legs (Fig. 62-20). Apply the top straps above the knee to avoid placing pressure on the peroneal nerve at the lateral tibial tubercle. Some HCPs prefer that the patient keep the abductor wedge in place except when bathing or walking.

If the hip fracture has been repaired with hemiarthroplasty or total joint replacement by an *anterior approach* (incision is made in the front of the hip with patient lying on the back), the hip muscles are left intact. This approach generally results in a more stable hip in the postoperative period with a lower rate of complications. Patient precautions related to motion and weight bearing are few but typically include instructions to avoid hyperextension.

Weight bearing on the involved extremity varies. Limited weight bearing is typically the only restriction for the patient who had ORIF of the hip fracture. Complete weight bearing following ORIF is generally restricted until x-ray examination indicates adequate healing, usually 6 to 12 weeks. Inform the caregiver about the patient's weight-bearing status after surgery.

Taking a tub bath and driving a car are not allowed for 4 to 6 weeks. An occupational therapist may teach the patient to use

## TABLE 62-11 Patient & Caregiver Teaching

### *Hip Replacement**

*After a hip replacement by posterior surgical approach, include the following instructions when teaching a patient and caregiver.*

**Do**

- Use an elevated toilet seat.
- Place chair inside shower or tub and remain seated while washing.
- Use pillow between legs for first 6 wk after surgery when lying on nonoperative side or when supine.
- Keep hip in neutral, straight position when sitting, walking, or lying.
- Notify surgeon immediately if severe pain, deformity, or loss of function occurs.
- Discuss personal risk factors for prosthetic joint infection with surgeon and dentist before dental work.

**Do Not**

- Flex hip greater than 90 degrees (e.g., sitting in low chairs or toilet seats).
- Adduct hip (i.e., bring legs together at knees).
- Internally rotate hip (i.e., turn toward planted foot on affected side).
- Cross legs at knees or ankles.
- Put on own shoes or stockings without adaptive device (e.g., long-handled shoehorn or stocking-helper) until 4-6 wk after surgery.
- Sit on chairs without arms. The arms of chairs will help the patient rise to a standing position.

*For patients having surgery by a posterior approach.

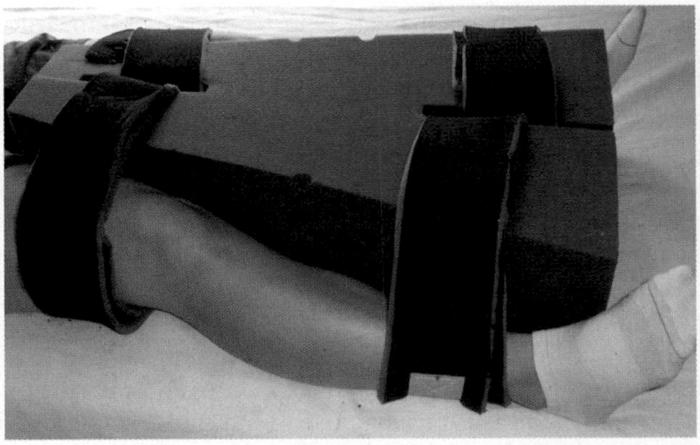

**FIG. 62-20** Maintaining postoperative abduction following total hip replacement. (Courtesy Mary Wollan, RN, BAN, ONC, Spring Park, Minn.)

assistive devices such as reachers or grabbers to avoid bending over to pick up something on the floor, long-handled shoehorns, or sock assists. The knees must be kept apart. Instruct the patient to never cross the legs or twist to reach behind.

The physical therapist usually supervises exercises for the affected extremity and ambulation when the surgeon permits it. The patient is usually out of bed by the first postoperative day. In collaboration with the physical therapist, monitor the patient's ambulation for proper use of crutches or a walker. To be discharged home, the patient must demonstrate the proper use of crutches or a walker over a functional distance (approximately 150 feet), and the ability to transfer to and from a chair and bed and to go up and down stairs.

Complications associated with femoral neck fracture include nonunion, avascular necrosis, dislocation, and osteoarthritis (OA). The affected leg may be shortened if the patient had an intertrochanteric fracture. A cane or shoe lift may be required for safe ambulation.

Sudden severe pain, a lump in the buttock, limb shortening, and external rotation indicate prosthesis dislocation. This requires a closed reduction with moderate to deep sedation or open reduction under general anesthesia to realign the femoral head in the acetabulum. If any of these manifestations occur, (regardless of the setting), keep the patient NPO in anticipation of surgical intervention.

Assist the patient and caregiver in adjusting to restrictions and dependence imposed by the hip fracture. Anxiety and depression can easily occur, but creative nursing care and awareness of potential problems can help to prevent them. Inform the patient and caregiver about community services that can help with rehabilitation after hospital discharge.

◆ **Ambulatory Care.** Hospitalization averages 3 or 4 days. Older adults or patients who live alone may require care in a subacute rehabilitation unit, at a skilled nursing facility, or in an acute rehabilitation facility for a few weeks before returning home. If the patient has skilled nursing needs or is homebound for physical therapy after discharge from post-acute care, the HCP may order follow-up home health care.

Home care considerations include ongoing assessment of pain management, monitoring for infection, and prevention of VTE. The incision is typically closed with metal staples, which are removed at the surgeon's office. If warfarin is used to decrease the high risk for VTE, inform the patient and caregiver of required testing for the international normalized ratio (INR), which is the standardized system of reporting prothrombin times. Adjust anticoagulation based on HCP order. Alternatives to warfarin include LMWH or factor Xa inhibitors. These newer anticoagulants require less monitoring than warfarin. Teach the patient who is receiving an anticoagulant to immediately report signs of bleeding to the HCP (see Chapter 37).

Exercises designed to restore strength and tone in the quadriceps and muscles around the hip are essential to improve function and ROM. These include quadriceps setting (e.g., pressing the kneecap down), gluteal muscle setting (e.g., tightening the buttocks), leg raises in supine and prone positions, and abduction exercises from the supine and standing positions (e.g., swinging the leg out but never crossing midline). The patient continues these exercises for many months after discharge. Teach the exercise program to the caregiver who will be encouraging the patient at home.

A physical therapist assesses ROM, ambulation, and adherence to the exercise program. The patient gradually increases the number of repetitions of exercises and may add ankle weights. Swimming and stationary cycling may also tone quadriceps and improve cardiovascular fitness. Instruct the patient to avoid high-impact exercises and sports, such as jogging and tennis, because they may loosen the implant. A physical therapist may also perform a home assessment to identify hazards that may cause the patient to fall again.

### ◆ Evaluation

The expected outcomes are that the patient with a hip fracture will

- Report satisfactory pain management
- Participate in exercise therapy
- Understand prescribed treatment plan

### Gerontologic Considerations: Hip Fracture

Factors that increase the risk of a hip fracture in older adults include (1) a tendency to fall due to an altered center of gravity and the inability to correct a postural imbalance, (2) decreased fat and muscle to act as local tissue shock absorbers, and (3) reduced skeletal strength. Other factors that increase the older adult's risk of falling include (1) gait and balance problems, (2) altered vision and hearing, (3) slowed reflexes, (4) orthostatic hypotension, and (5) medication use. Homes can be made safer by (1) eliminating tripping hazards (e.g., loose rugs, uneven surfaces), (2) adding grab bars inside and outside the tub or shower, and beside the toilet, (3) adding railings on both sides of the stairs, and (4) installing better lighting.[25]

Many falls are associated with getting in or out of a chair or bed. Falls to the side, the most common type seen in frail older adults, are more likely to result in a hip fracture than a forward fall. External hip protectors may help prevent hip fractures in the frail older patient.[26] Older adults may have low bone density *(osteopenia)* or osteoporosis, which increases their risk of fragility fractures.

Calcium and vitamin D supplementation is indicated for anyone with osteopenia or osteoporosis. A bisphosphonate drug (e.g., alendronate [Fosamax]) or teriparatide (Forteo, a form of parathyroid hormone) may also be prescribed to decrease bone loss or increase bone density and thus reduce the likelihood of fracture. (Osteoporosis is discussed in Chapter 63.)

## FEMORAL SHAFT FRACTURE

Because the femur can bend slightly to absorb stress, femoral shaft fracture occurs from a severe direct force. The force exerted to cause the fracture (e.g., from a motor vehicle crash or gunshot wound) frequently also damages the adjacent soft tissue. These injuries may be more serious than the bone injury. Young adults have a higher incidence of this type of fracture.

Displacement of fracture fragments often causes increased soft tissue damage. Considerable blood loss (1 to 1.5 L) can occur. The most common types of femoral shaft fracture include transverse, spiral, comminuted, oblique, and open (Figs. 62-6 and 62-7).

Clinical manifestations of a femoral shaft fracture are usually obvious. They include pain, marked deformity and angulation, shortening of the extremity, and inability to move the hip or knee. Common complications associated with femoral shaft fracture include FES; nerve and vascular injury; and problems associated with bone union, open fracture, and soft tissue damage.

Initial management of a femoral shaft fracture is directed toward stabilization of the patient and immobilization of the fracture. Traction may be used as a temporary measure before surgical treatment or in the patient unable to undergo surgery. Placement of an *intramedullary rod* is the most common surgical treatment for femoral shaft fracture. A metal rod is placed into the marrow canal of the femur. The rod passes across the fracture to keep it in position. Plates and screws may also be used. Internal fixation is preferred because it reduces the hospital stay and complications associated with prolonged bed rest. External fixation would be used for an open fracture.

After surgery, gluteal and quadriceps isometric exercises will promote and maintain strength in the affected extremity. Encourage the patient to perform ROM and strengthening exercises for all uninvolved extremities in preparation for ambulation. The patient may be allowed to begin non–weight-bearing activities with an ambulatory assistive device (e.g., walker, crutches). Full weight bearing is usually restricted until x-rays show union of fracture fragments. Teach the patient to carefully follow the HCP's instructions for weight bearing.

## TIBIAL FRACTURE

Although the tibia is vulnerable to injury because it lacks a covering of anterior muscle, strong force is required to cause a tibial fracture. As a result, soft tissue damage, devascularization, and open fracture are frequent. The tibia is a common site for stress fracture. Complications associated with tibial fracture are compartment syndrome, FES, delayed union or nonunion, and possible infection with an open fracture.

The recommended management for closed tibial fracture is closed reduction followed by immobilization in a long leg cast. ORIF with intramedullary rods, plate fixation, or external fixation is indicated for complex tibial fractures and those with extensive soft tissue damage. Locking plates (screw and plate system) may also be used for surgical repair. Emphasis for either type of reduction is on maintaining quadriceps strength.

Assess the neurovascular condition of the affected extremity at least every 2 hours during the first 48 hours. Instruct patients to perform active ROM exercises with the uninvolved leg and the upper extremities to build the strength required for crutch walking. When the HCP has determined the patient is ready for gait training, reinforce the principles of crutch walking introduced by the physical therapist. The patient may be non–weight bearing for 6 to 12 weeks, depending on healing. Home nursing visits may be initiated to monitor the patient's progress if the patient is homebound.

## STABLE VERTEBRAL FRACTURE

Stable fractures of the vertebral column are usually caused by motor vehicle crashes, falls, diving, or sports injuries. Patients with osteoporosis experience more than 700,000 vertebral compression fractures annually, many of which are stable. In a stable fracture, the fracture fragments are unlikely to move or cause spinal cord damage. This type of injury is frequently confined to the vertebral body (anterior element of the spinal column) in the lumbar region and less frequently involves the cervical and thoracic regions. Vertebral bodies are usually protected from displacement by intact spinal ligaments.

Most patients with stable spinal fractures experience only brief periods of disability. However, if spinal ligaments are significantly disrupted, dislocation of the vertebrae may occur. Instability and injury to the spinal cord may result (unstable fracture). These injuries generally require surgery. The most serious complication of vertebral fractures is fracture displacement, which can cause damage to the spinal cord (see Chapter 60). Although stable vertebral fractures are not associated with abnormal spinal cord pathology, all spinal injuries should be considered unstable and potentially serious until diagnostic tests determine the fracture to be stable.

The patient usually complains of pain and tenderness in the affected region of the spine. Sudden loss of function below the fracture indicates spinal cord impingement and paraplegia. Stable compression fractures are associated with a kyphotic deformity (flexion angulation of thoracic vertebrae) known as a *dowager's hump.* This deformity is readily identified during the physical examination (see Fig. 63-9). *Lordosis* (extreme inward curve of lumbar spine) and cervical spine involvement are also possible. Bowel and bladder dysfunction may indicate an interruption of the autonomic nervous system nerves or injury to the spinal cord.

The overall goal in management of stable vertebral fractures is to keep the spine in good alignment until union has been accomplished. Many nursing interventions are aimed at assessing for the possibility of spinal cord trauma. Regularly evaluate vital signs and bowel and bladder function. Also monitor the motor and sensory function of peripheral nerves distal to the injured region. Promptly report any deterioration in the patient's neurovascular condition.

Treatment includes pain medication followed by early mobilization and bracing. The patient's mattress should offer firm support to support the spinal column, relax muscles, decrease edema, and prevent potential compression on nerve roots. Teach the patient to keep the spine straight when turning by moving the shoulders and pelvis together. The patient will need nursing assistance to learn the technique of logrolling. Several days after the initial injury, the HCP may apply a specially constructed orthotic device (e.g., thoracolumbar sacral orthosis [TLSO]), a jacket cast, or a removable corset if there is no evidence of neurologic deficit. The device provides extra support during healing and is used for a short period of time.

Lightweight bracing (e.g., Jewett or Bähler-Vogt brace) may be used for patients with stable vertebral compression fractures due to osteoporosis. Patients with osteoporosis may also be treated with two outpatient procedures: vertebroplasty or balloon kyphoplasty. *Vertebroplasty* uses radioimaging to guide the injection of bone cement into a fractured vertebral body. When hardened, the cement stabilizes the vertebra and prevents further compression. *Balloon kyphoplasty* involves first inserting a balloon into the vertebral body and then inflating it. This creates a cavity that is filled with bone cement under low pressure to restore the height of the vertebral body. Kyphoplasty is now the surgical treatment of choice for compression fractures. This is due largely to the decreased incidence of bone cement leakage into nearby structures (e.g., colon, lung) compared to vertebroplasty. Patients experience decreased pain almost immediately with these procedures. However, later compression fractures of adjacent vertebrae are a risk.

If the fracture is in the cervical spine, the patient may wear a hard cervical collar. Some cervical fractures are immobilized by use of a halo vest (see Fig. 60-7). This consists of a plastic jacket or cast fitted about the chest and attached to a halo that is held in place by skeletal pins inserted into the cranium. These devices immobilize the spine in the fracture area but allow the patient to ambulate.

The patient with a stable vertebral fracture is discharged after (1) demonstrating safe ambulation, (2) learning care of the cast or orthotic device, and (3) verbalizing strategies to address safety and security concerns related to the injury and treatment. Unstable vertebral fractures and spinal cord injuries are discussed in Chapter 60.

## FACIAL FRACTURE

Any bone of the face can be fractured as a result of trauma, such as a motor vehicle crash, an assault, or a fall.[27] It is critically important after facial injury to establish and maintain a patent airway and provide adequate ventilation. Suctioning may be needed to remove foreign material and blood. A surgically created airway *(tracheostomy)* may be needed if a patent airway cannot be maintained.

Facial fractures and cervical spine injuries commonly occur together. All patients with facial injuries should be treated as if they have a cervical injury until proven otherwise by examination and CT scan or x-ray. Table 62-12 describes clinical manifestations of common facial fractures.

Related soft tissue injury often makes assessment of facial injury difficult. Perform oral and facial examinations after any life-threatening situations have been treated. Carefully assess ocular muscles and cranial nerves III, IV, and VI.[28] X-rays are used to determine the extent of the injury. CT scanning helps differentiate between bone and soft tissue.

Suspect injury to the eye when facial injury occurs, particularly if the injury is near the orbit. If an eye-globe rupture is suspected, stop the examination and place a protective shield over the eye. Signs of rupture include vitreous humor forced out of the eye, or brown tissue (iris or ciliary body) on the surface of the globe or penetrating through a laceration with an off-center or teardrop-shaped pupil.

Specific treatment depends on the site and extent of the facial fracture and associated soft tissue injury. Immobilization or surgical stabilization may be necessary. Maintain a patent airway and adequate nutrition throughout the recovery period.

Be sensitive about alterations in appearance that may occur after facial fracture. Changes in appearance may be drastic. Edema and discoloration subside with time, but concurrent soft tissue injuries may result in permanent scarring.

### Mandibular Fracture

Mandibular fracture may result from trauma to the face or jaw. Maxillary fractures may also occur, but they are less common than mandibular fractures. The mandibular fracture may be simple, with no bone displacement, or may involve loss of tissue and bone. The fracture may require immediate treatment to ensure the patient's survival. Long-term treatment is sometimes needed to restore satisfactory appearance and function.

Mandibular fractures may also be therapeutically performed to correct an underlying alignment problem *(malocclusion)* that cannot be adjusted by orthodontics alone. The mandible is resected during surgery and manipulated forward or backward to correct the occlusion problem.

Surgery for a mandibular fracture includes immobilization, usually by wiring the jaws *(intermaxillary fixation)*. Internal fixation may be done with screws and plates. In a simple fracture with no loss of teeth, the lower jaw is wired to the upper jaw. Wires are placed around the teeth, and then cross-wires or rubber bands are used to hold the lower jaw tight against the upper jaw (Fig. 62-21). Arch bars may be placed on the maxillary and mandibular arches of the teeth. Vertical wires are placed between the arch bars, holding the jaws together. If teeth are missing or bone is displaced, other forms of fixation may be needed (e.g., metal arch bars in the mouth or insertion of a pin in the bone). Bone grafting may also be required. Immobilization is usually necessary for only 4 to 6 weeks because the fractures often heal rapidly.

**TABLE 62-12 Manifestations of Facial Fractures**

| Fracture | Manifestation |
|---|---|
| **Frontal bone** | Rapid edema that may mask underlying fractures |
| **Periorbital bone** | Possible frontal sinus involvement, entrapment of ocular muscles |
| **Nasal bone** | Displacement of nasal bones, nosebleed *(epistaxis)* |
| **Zygomatic arch** | Depression of cheek bone *(zygomatic arch)* and entrapment of ocular muscles |
| **Maxilla** | Segmental motion (instability) of maxilla and tooth fracture at socket |
| **Mandible** | Tooth fractures, bleeding, limited motion of mandible |

## ❖ NURSING MANAGEMENT: MANDIBULAR FRACTURE

Inform the patient preoperatively about what is involved in the surgical procedure, how the face will look afterward, and alterations caused by the surgery. Reassure the patient about the ability to breathe normally, speak, and swallow liquids. Hospitalization for respiratory monitoring is brief unless there are other injuries or problems.

Postoperative care focuses on a patent airway, oral hygiene, communication, pain management, and adequate nutrition. Two potential problems in the immediate postoperative period are airway obstruction and aspiration of vomitus. Because the patient cannot open the jaws, an airway must be maintained. Observe for signs of respiratory distress (e.g., dyspnea; alterations in rate, quality, and depth of respirations). After surgery place the patient on the side with the head slightly elevated immediately.

Tape a wire cutter or scissors (for rubber bands) to the head of the bed and send it with the patient to all appointments and examinations away from the bedside. The wire cutter or scissors

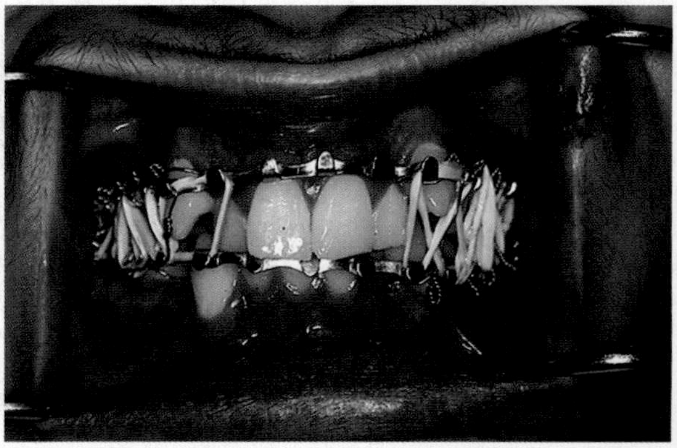

**FIG. 62-21** Intermaxillary fixation. (Courtesy R.A. Weinstein, Denver, Colo.)

may be used to cut the wires or elastic bands in case of an emergency requiring access to the pharynx or lungs (e.g., cardiac arrest or respiratory distress). In the care plan include a picture with the appropriate wires to cut in an emergency. In some cases, cutting the wires may cause the entire facial and upper jaw structure to shift or collapse and worsen the problem. A tracheostomy or endotracheal tray should always be available.

If the patient begins to vomit or choke, try to clear the mouth and airway. Suctioning may be done by the nasopharyngeal or oral route, depending on the extent of injury and type of repair. An NG tube may be used for decompression to remove fluids and gas from the stomach to help prevent aspiration. An NG tube also helps prevent vomiting. Antiemetics may also be used. The NG tube can later be used as a feeding tube. Teach the patient to clear secretions and vomitus.

Oral hygiene is extremely important. Teach the patient to remove food debris by rinsing the mouth often, particularly after meals and snacks. Warm normal saline solution, water, or alkaline mouthwashes may be used. A syringe and soft irrigation catheter or a Water Pik may be effective for thorough oral cleansing. Inspect the mouth several times a day to see that it is clean. Use a tongue depressor to retract the cheeks. Keep the lips, corners of the mouth, and buccal mucosa moist. Cover any sharp edges of the wires with dental wax to prevent irritation of the buccal mucosa.

Communication may be a problem, particularly in the early postoperative period. Establish an effective way of communicating preoperatively (e.g., use of dry erase board, pad and pencil). Usually the patient can speak well enough to be understood, especially a few days after surgery.

Intake of adequate nutrients poses a challenge because the diet must be liquid. The patient easily tires of sucking through a straw or laboriously using a spoon. Work with the dietitian and patient to plan a diet with adequate calories, protein, and fluids. Liquid protein supplements may help the patient improve the nutritional status. A low-bulk, high-carbohydrate diet and intake of air through the straw contribute to constipation and gas. Ambulation, prune juice, and bulk-forming laxatives may help relieve these problems.

The patient is usually discharged with the wires in place. Encourage the patient to verbalize feelings about the altered appearance. Discharge teaching should include oral care, diet, techniques for handling secretions, how and when to use wire cutters or scissors, and when to notify the HCP about concerns and problems.

## AMPUTATION

An **amputation** is the removal of a body extremity by trauma or surgery. About 2 million people in the United States are living with limb loss.[29] Older people have the highest incidence of amputation due to peripheral vascular disease (PVD), atherosclerosis, and vascular changes related to diabetes mellitus. Amputation in young people is usually secondary to trauma (e.g., motor vehicle crashes, land mines, farm-related injury). More than 1700 American military personnel have undergone a service-related amputation as part of the U.S. combat mission in Iraq.[30]

### Clinical Indications

Most amputations are performed due to PVD, especially in older patients with diabetes mellitus. These patients often experience peripheral neuropathy that progresses to trophic ulcers and gangrene. Other common reasons for amputation are trauma, thermal injuries, tumors, osteomyelitis, and congenital limb disorders. Although pain is often present, it is not usually the primary reason for amputation.

**TABLE 62-13 Interprofessional Care**

***Amputation***

| Diagnostic Assessment | Management |
|---|---|
| • History and physical examination<br>• Physical appearance of soft tissues<br>• Skin temperature<br>• Sensory function<br>• Quality of peripheral pulses<br>• Arteriography<br>• Venography<br>• Plethysmography<br>• Transcutaneous ultrasonic Doppler recordings | ***Medical***<br>• Appropriate management of underlying disease<br>• Stabilization of trauma victim<br>***Surgical***<br>• Residual limb management<br>• Immediate or delayed prosthesis fitting<br>***Rehabilitation***<br>• Coordination of prosthesis-fitting and gait-training activities<br>• Coordination of muscle-strengthening and physical therapy regimens |

### Diagnostic Studies

Diagnostic studies depend on the underlying problem that makes the amputation necessary (Table 62-13). An elevated white blood cell (WBC) count with abnormal differential may indicate infection. Vascular tests such as arteriography, Doppler studies, and venography provide information about the circulation of the extremity.

### Interprofessional Care

If amputation is planned or elective, as for the patient with PVD, carefully assess the patient's general health. Chronic illnesses and infection must be managed before an amputation is performed. Help the patient and caregiver understand the need for the amputation and assure them that rehabilitation can help with postoperative quality of life. If the amputation is performed emergently after trauma, patient management is physically and emotionally more complicated.

The goal of surgery is to preserve the greatest extremity length and function while removing all infected, pathologic, or ischemic tissue. (Levels of amputation of upper and lower extremities are illustrated in Fig. 62-22.) The type of amputation depends on the reason for the surgery. A closed amputation is performed to create a weight-bearing *residual limb* (or stump). An anterior skin flap with dissected soft tissue padding covers the bony part of the residual limb. The skin flap is sutured posteriorly so that the suture line will not be in a weight-bearing area. Special care is needed to prevent accumulation of drainage, which can produce pressure and harbor bacteria that may cause infection.

*Disarticulation* is an amputation performed through a joint. A *Syme's amputation* is a form of disarticulation at the ankle. After an open amputation *(guillotine amputation),* the surface of the residual limb is left uncovered with skin. This type of surgery is generally indicated to control actual or potential infection. The wound is usually closed later by a second surgical procedure or closed by skin traction surrounding the residual limb.

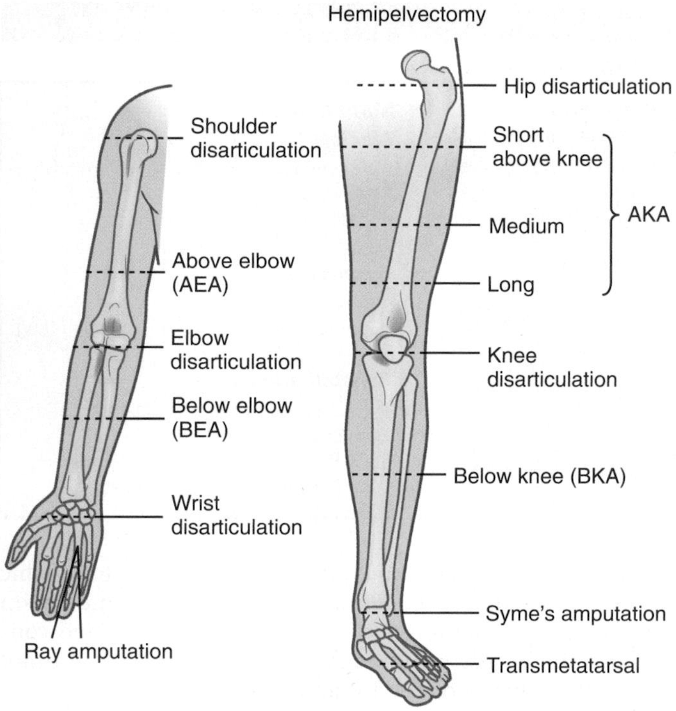


**FIG. 62-22** Location and description of amputation sites of the upper and lower extremities. *AKA,* Above-the-knee amputation.

## NURSING MANAGEMENT: AMPUTATION

### Nursing Assessment

Assess any preexisting illnesses. Because most amputations are performed for vascular problems, assessment of vascular and neurologic condition is especially important (see Chapters 31 and 55).

### Nursing Diagnoses

Nursing diagnoses for the patient with an amputation may include, but are not limited to, the following:

- Disturbed body image *related to* loss of body part and impaired mobility
- Impaired skin integrity *related to* immobility and improperly fitted prosthesis
- Chronic pain *related to* phantom limb sensation or residual limb pain
- Impaired physical mobility *related to* amputation of lower limb

### Planning

The overall goals are that the patient with an amputation will (1) have adequate relief from the underlying health problem, (2) have satisfactory pain management, (3) reach maximum rehabilitation potential (with the use of a prosthesis, if indicated), (4) cope with the body image changes, and (5) make satisfying lifestyle adjustments.

### Nursing Implementation

**Health Promotion.** Control of causative illnesses such as PVD, diabetes mellitus, chronic osteomyelitis, and pressure ulcers can eliminate or delay the need for amputation. Teach patients with these problems to carefully examine their lower extremities daily for signs of infection or skin breakdown. If the patient cannot do this, the caregiver should help. Instruct the patient and caregiver to report changes in the feet or toes to the HCP, including changes in skin color or temperature, decreased or absent sensation, tingling, burning pain, cuts, or abrasions.

Instruct people in safety precautions for recreational activities and potentially hazardous work. This responsibility is especially critical for the occupational health nurse.

**Acute Care.** Reasons for amputation and the rehabilitation potential depend on a person's age, diagnosis, occupation, personality, resources, and support system. Be aware of the tremendous psychologic and social implications of amputation. The disruption in body image caused by amputation often causes a patient to go through the grieving process. Use therapeutic communication to assist the patient and caregiver through this process to develop a realistic attitude about the future.

***Preoperative Care.*** Before surgery, reinforce information that the patient and caregiver have received about reasons for the amputation, proposed prosthesis, and mobility-training program. To meet the patient's educational needs, know the level of amputation, type of postsurgical dressings to be applied, and type of prosthesis to be used. Teach the patient to perform upper extremity exercises such as push-ups in bed or the wheelchair to promote arm strength essential for crutch walking and gait training. Discuss general postoperative nursing care, including positioning, support, and residual limb care. If a compression bandage is to be used after surgery, instruct the patient about its purpose and how it will be applied. If immediate prosthesis use is planned, discuss general ambulation expectations.

Tell the patient that the amputated limb may feel like it is still present after surgery. This phenomenon, termed **phantom limb sensation**, occurs in many amputees. (Nursing management of phantom limb sensation is discussed in the next section.)

***Postoperative Care.*** General postoperative care for the patient who has had an amputation depends largely on the patient's age and general state of health, and the reason for the amputation. Monitor individuals who undergo amputation as a result of a traumatic injury for posttraumatic stress disorder because they have had no time to prepare or perhaps even to participate in the decision to have a limb amputated.

Prevention and detection of complications are important after surgery. Carefully monitor the patient's vital signs. Assess dressings for hemorrhage in the operative area. Use sterile technique during dressing changes to reduce the risk for wound infection.

If an *immediate* postoperative prosthesis has been applied, carefully observe the surgical site. If excessive bleeding occurs, notify the surgeon immediately. A surgical tourniquet must always be available for emergency use.

The *delayed* prosthetic fitting may be the best choice for patients who have had amputations above the knee or below the elbow, older adults, and those with infection (Fig. 62-23). Appropriate timing for the use of a prosthesis depends on satisfactory healing of the residual limb and the patient's general condition. A temporary prosthesis may be used for partial weight bearing after sutures are removed. If there are no problems, the patient can bear full weight on a permanent prosthesis approximately 3 months after amputation.

Not all patients are candidates for prostheses. The seriously ill or debilitated patient may not have the upper body strength and energy needed to use a lower extremity prosthesis. Mobility with a wheelchair may be the most realistic goal for this patient.

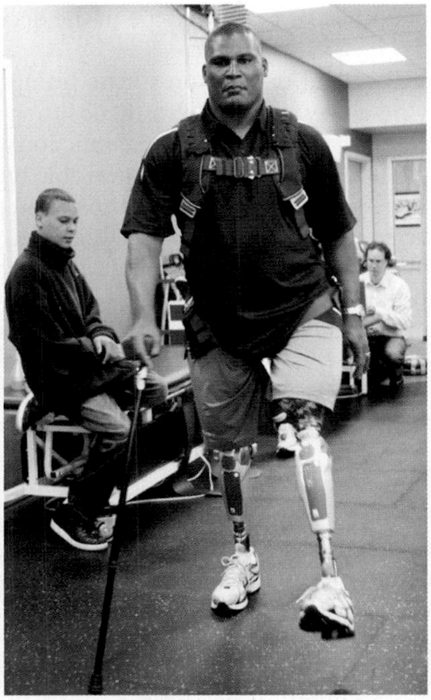

FIG. 62-23 A double amputee fitted with prostheses. (Photo courtesy U.S. Army.)

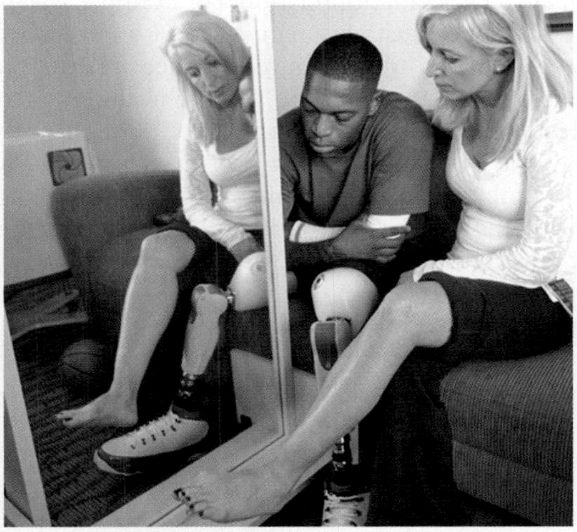

FIG. 62-24 Mirror therapy, a type of treatment that may reduce phantom limb sensation and pain. (U.S. Navy photo courtesy Mass Communication Specialist Seaman Joseph A. Boomhower.)

Patients are often extremely worried about phantom limb sensation because they still perceive pain in the missing portion of the limb. As recovery and ambulation progress, phantom limb sensation and pain usually subside. However, the pain may become chronic. The patient may complain of shooting, burning, or crushing pain as well as feelings of coldness, heaviness, and cramping,

Mirror therapy reduces phantom limb sensation and pain in some patients[31] (Fig. 62-24). The mirror is thought to provide visual information to the brain, replacing sensory feedback expected from the missing limb. However, it is unknown why looking in the mirror at the remaining limb would decrease phantom limb sensation and pain. Mirror therapy may also improve patient functioning after a stroke.

Success of the rehabilitation program depends on the patient's physical and emotional health. Chronic illness and

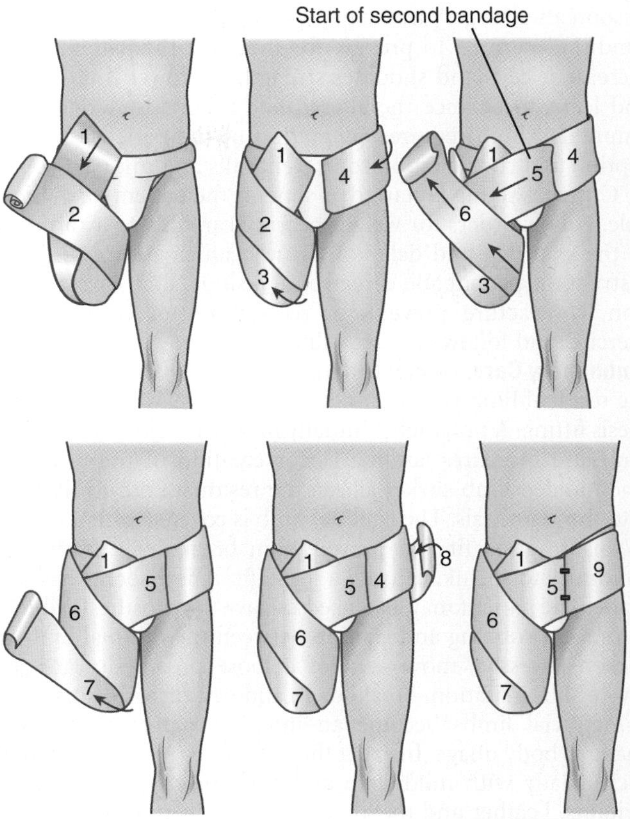


FIG. 62-25 Bandaging for the above-the-knee amputation residual limb. Figure-eight style covers progressive areas of the residual limb. Two elastic wraps are required.

deconditioning can complicate rehabilitation. Physical and occupational therapy must be an integral component of the patient's overall plan of care.

Flexion contractures may delay rehabilitation. The most common and debilitating contracture is hip flexion. Hip adduction contracture is rare. To prevent flexion contractures, have patients avoid sitting in a chair for more than 1 hour with hips flexed or having pillows under the surgical extremity. Unless specifically contraindicated, patients should lie on their abdomen for 30 minutes three or four times each day and position the hip in extension while prone.

Proper bandaging ensures the residual limb is shaped and molded for eventual prosthesis fitting (Fig. 62-25). The surgeon usually orders a compression bandage to be applied immediately after surgery to support soft tissues, reduce edema, hasten healing, minimize pain, and promote residual limb shrinkage and maturation. This bandage may be an elastic roll applied to the residual limb or a residual limb shrinker, which is an elastic stocking that fits tightly over the residual limb.

The patient initially wears the compression bandage at all times except during physical therapy and bathing. Remove and reapply the bandage several times daily. Take care to apply it snugly but not so tight as to interfere with circulation. Wash and change shrinker bandages daily. After the residual limb is healed, bandage it only when the patient is not wearing the prosthesis. Instruct the patient to avoid dangling the residual limb over the bedside to decrease edema.

As the patient's overall condition improves, the HCP and physical therapist generally start and supervise an exercise regimen. Active ROM exercises for all joints should be started as soon after surgery as the patient's pain intensity and medical condition permit. To prepare for mobility, the patient should increase triceps and shoulder strength for lower limb support and learn to balance the altered body. The lost weight of an amputated limb requires adaptation of the patient's proprioception and coordination to prevent falls and injury.

Crutch walking is started as soon as the patient is physically able. Follow orders for weight bearing carefully to avoid injury to the skin flap and delay of tissue healing. Before discharge, instruct the patient and caregiver in residual limb care, ambulation, contracture prevention, recognition of complications, exercise, and follow-up care (Table 62-14).

◆ **Ambulatory Care.** When healing has occurred satisfactorily and the residual limb is well molded, the patient is ready for prosthesis fitting. A prosthetist initially makes a mold of the residual limb and measures landmarks for creation of the prosthesis. The molded limb socket allows the residual limb to fit snugly into the prosthesis. The residual limb is covered with a stocking to ensure good fit and prevent skin breakdown. If the limb continues to shrink, causing a loose fit, a new socket has to be made. The patient may also need to have the prosthesis adjusted to prevent rubbing and friction between the residual limb and socket. Excessive movement of a loose prosthesis can cause severe skin irritation, breakdown, and gait disturbances.

Artificial limbs become an integral part of the patient's changed body image. Instruct the patient to clean the prosthesis socket daily with mild soap and rinse thoroughly to remove irritants. Leather and metal parts of the prosthesis should not get wet. Encourage the patient to have regular maintenance on the prosthesis. Also consider the condition of the patient's shoe. A badly worn shoe alters the gait and may damage the prosthesis.

◆ **Special Considerations in Upper Limb Amputation.** Emotional implications of an upper limb amputation are often more devastating than for lower limb amputation. The enforced dependency due to one-handedness may be depressing and frustrating to the patient. Because most upper extremity amputations result from trauma, the patient has likely had little time to adjust psychologically or to participate in the decision-making process.

Both immediate and delayed prosthetic fittings are possible for the below-the-elbow amputee. Prosthetic fitting is delayed for the above-the-elbow amputee. The usual functional prosthesis is the arm and hook. A cosmetic hand is available but has limited functional value. As with the lower limb prosthesis, patient motivation and perseverance are major factors contributing to a satisfactory outcome. Recent technologic advances in upper extremity prostheses have led to increased functionality, with movements and capabilities that are closer to the natural arm.[32]

**TABLE 62-14 Patient & Caregiver Teaching**

***Following Lower Extremity Amputation***

*After lower extremity amputation, include the following instructions when teaching the patient and caregiver.*

1. Inspect the residual limb daily for signs of skin irritation, especially redness, abrasion, and odor. Pay particular attention to areas prone to pressure.
2. Discontinue use of the prosthesis if irritation develops. Have the area checked before resuming use of the prosthesis.
3. Wash the residual limb thoroughly each night with warm water and bacteriostatic soap. Rinse thoroughly and dry gently. Expose the residual limb to air for 20 min.
4. Do not use lotions, alcohol, powders, or oil on residual limb unless prescribed by the HCP.
5. Wear only a residual limb sock in good condition and supplied by the prosthetist.
6. Change residual limb sock daily. Launder in mild soap, squeeze, lay flat to dry.
7. Use prescribed pain management techniques.
8. Perform ROM to all joints daily. Perform general strengthening exercises (including for upper extremities) daily.
9. Do not elevate residual limb on a pillow.
10. Lay prone with hip in extension for 30 min three or four times daily.

### ◆ Evaluation

The expected outcomes are that the patient with an amputation will

- Accept changed body image and integrate changes into lifestyle
- Have no evidence of skin breakdown
- Have reduction or absence of pain
- Become mobile within limitations imposed by amputation

### Gerontologic Considerations: Amputation

If a lower limb amputation has been performed on an older adult, the patient's previous ability to ambulate may affect the extent of recovery. Use of a prosthesis requires significant strength and energy for ambulation. For example, walking with a below-the-knee prosthesis requires 40% more energy than walking on two legs, and an above-the-knee prosthesis requires 60% more. Older adults whose general health is altered and weakened by disorders such as cardiac or pulmonary dysfunction may not be candidates for prosthesis use. The patient's ability to ambulate may be limited. If possible, discuss these issues with the patient and caregiver before surgery so that realistic expectations can be set.

# COMMON JOINT SURGICAL PROCEDURES

Surgery plays an important role in the treatment and rehabilitation of patients with various types of joint disease. Surgery is aimed at relieving chronic pain, improving joint motion, correcting deformity and misalignment, and removing diseased cartilage. If the joint problem is not corrected, contraction with permanent limitation of motion may occur. Limited joint motion can be demonstrated on physical examination. Joint-space narrowing is also apparent on x-rays.

## TYPES OF JOINT SURGERIES

### Synovectomy

**Synovectomy** (removal of synovial membrane) is performed to remove inflamed tissue that is causing unacceptable pain or limiting ROM in rheumatoid arthritis (RA). A synovectomy is best performed early in the disease process when there is minimal bone or cartilage destruction. Removal of the thickened synovium does not cure the disease but may relieve symptoms temporarily. Common sites for this surgery include the elbow, wrist, and fingers. Synovectomy in the knee is done less frequently because knee joint replacement is usually performed.

### Osteotomy

An **osteotomy** involves removing a wedge or slice of bone to restore alignment (joint and vertebral) and to shift weight bearing, thus relieving pain. Cervical osteotomy may be used to correct a kyphotic deformity in some patients with ankylosing spondylitis. Halo vests and body jacket braces are worn until fusion occurs (3 to 4 months). Osteotomy has proven ineffective in patients with inflammatory joint disease. However, femoral osteotomy may provide some pain relief and improve motion in selected patients with hip osteoarthritis (OA). Tibial osteotomy also provides pain relief in selected patients, but a majority of patients require later knee replacement surgery.

Care of a patient who has undergone osteotomy is similar to that of a patient with ORIF of a fracture at a comparable site (see pp. 1474-1478). Internal wires, screws and plates, bone grafts, or an external fixator usually fixes the bone in place.

## Debridement

**Debridement** is the removal of degenerative debris such as pieces of bone or cartilage *(loose bodies)* or osteophytes from a joint using a fiberoptic arthroscope. This procedure is usually performed on an outpatient basis on the knee or shoulder. A compression dressing is applied postoperatively. Weight bearing is permitted following knee arthroscopy. Patient teaching includes monitoring for signs of infection, managing pain, and restricting excessive activity for 24 to 48 hours.

## Arthroplasty

**Arthroplasty** is the reconstruction or replacement of a joint to relieve pain, improve or maintain ROM, and correct deformity. Arthroplasty is most commonly performed on patients with OA, RA, avascular necrosis, congenital deformities or dislocations, and other systemic problems. There are several types of arthroplasty, including surgical reshaping of the bones of the joints, replacement of part of a joint (hemiarthroplasty), and total joint replacement. Replacement arthroplasty is available for elbows, shoulders, phalangeal joints of the fingers, wrists, hips, knees, ankles, and feet. More than 1 million Americans have knee and hip replacement surgery annually.[33]

**Total Hip Arthroplasty.** Total hip arthroplasty (THA) (total hip replacement) provides significant relief of pain and improved function for patients with joint deterioration from OA, RA, and other conditions. Partial and total hip replacements are also used to treat hip fractures.

In THA, the prosthesis (implant) replaces the ball-and-socket joint and upper shaft of the femur (Fig. 62-19). The socket can be cemented in place with polymethyl methacrylate, which bonds to the bone. The socket may also be inserted without cement (cementless). Cementless THA may provide longer-term prosthesis stability by enabling biologic ingrowth of new bone tissue into the porous surface coating of the prosthesis. Cementless devices are most often recommended for younger, more active patients and patients with good bone quality so that bone ingrowth into the components can be readily achieved.

The nursing care for a patient who has THA is discussed in the section on nursing management of a patient with a hip fracture on pp. 1482-1484.

**Hip Resurfacing Arthroplasty.** An alternative to hip replacement is hip resurfacing arthroplasty, which allows the femoral head (ball) to be preserved and reshaped rather than replaced as in THA. The resurfaced femoral head is then capped by a metal prosthesis. Hip resurfacing is a more favorable option for patients younger than age 60 with larger frames. A small percentage of patients will experience femoral neck fracture after hip resurfacing; this is not possible with THA. In addition, metal ions may be released into the bloodstream from the prosthesis. Patients may develop sensitivity or allergy to these particles.[34] Patients receiving a smaller femoral head (including many women) have a higher failure rate with a resurfaced implant when compared with patients receiving THA.

**Knee Arthroplasty.** Unremitting pain and instability as a result of severe deterioration of the knee joint are the main indications for total knee arthroplasty (TKA). Partial *(unicompartmental)* arthroplasty can be performed on a patient with osteoarthritis limited to one part (compartment) of the knee.

Immediately after knee arthroplasty a compression dressing may be used to immobilize the knee in extension. This dressing is removed before discharge. If the patient is unable to perform a straight leg raise, a knee immobilizer or posterior plastic shell to maintain extension may be used during ambulation and at rest for about 4 weeks.

After surgery, an emphasis is placed on pain management and physical therapy. Because postoperative pain can significantly reduce the patient's ability to participate in therapy, effective pain management is a primary nursing care goal.[35] Physical therapy begins early with isometric quadriceps setting. Therapy progresses to straight-leg raises and gentle ROM to increase muscle strength and obtain 90-degree knee flexion. Active flexion exercises or passive flexion exercises with a continuous passive motion (CPM) machine may promote joint mobility. Ambulation is also begun early and typically progresses to full weight bearing before discharge. An active home exercise program involves progressive ROM with muscle strengthening and flexibility exercises.

Adequate analgesia should be ordered at discharge to allow the patient to continue with the exercise program. Effective pain management is key to achieving positive rehabilitation outcomes. After TKA, many older patients with advanced OA show significant improvement in mobility, motor function tests, and ability to complete daily tasks.

**Finger Joint Arthroplasty.** A silicone rubber arthroplastic device is used to restore function in the fingers of the patient with RA. Ulnar deviation often causes severe functional limitations of the hand. The goal of hand surgery is primarily to restore function related to grasp, pinch, stability, and strength rather than to correct cosmetic deformity. Before surgery the patient is instructed in hand exercises, including flexion, extension, abduction, and adduction of the fingers.

Postoperatively, a bulk dressing is placed and the hand is kept elevated. Perform regular neurovascular assessment and monitor for signs of infection. Success of the surgery depends largely on the postoperative treatment plan, which is usually implemented by an occupational therapist. After the dressing is removed, a guided splinting program is initiated. The patient is discharged with splints to use while sleeping and hand exercises to perform at least three or four times a day for 10 to 12 weeks. Instruct the patient to avoid lifting heavy objects.

**Elbow and Shoulder Arthroplasty.** Although available, total replacement of elbow and shoulder joints is not as common as other forms of arthroplasty. Shoulder replacements are performed in patients with severe pain because of RA, OA, avascular necrosis, or previous trauma. The shoulder replacement is usually considered if the patient has adequate surrounding muscle strength and bone density. If joint replacement is needed for both elbow and shoulder, the elbow is usually done first because a severely painful elbow interferes with the shoulder rehabilitation program.

Significant pain relief has been achieved after elbow and shoulder arthroplasty, with most patients having no pain at rest or minimal pain with activity. Functional improvements have also contributed to better hygiene and increased ability to perform activities of daily living. However, rehabilitation is longer and more difficult than with other joint surgeries.

**Ankle Arthroplasty.** Total ankle arthroplasty (TAA) is indicated for RA, OA, trauma, and avascular necrosis. Although use of TAA is not widespread, it is a viable alternative to fusion for treatment of severe ankle arthritis in certain patients. Available devices include several fixed-bearing devices and a mobile-bearing cementless prosthesis. This device more closely imitates natural ankle function.

Ankle fusion is often selected over arthroplasty because the result is more durable. However, the patient is left with a stiff foot and the inability to change heel height. TAA achieves a more normal gait pattern. Postoperatively, the patient may not bear weight for 6 weeks. Teach the patient to elevate the extremity to reduce and prevent edema, take steps to prevent postoperative infection, and maintain immobilization as directed by the surgeon.

### Arthrodesis

Arthrodesis is the surgical fusion of a joint. This procedure is indicated only if articular surfaces are too severely damaged or infected to allow joint replacement or if reconstructive surgery fails. Arthrodesis relieves pain and provides a stable but immobile joint. The fusion is usually accomplished by removing the articular hyaline cartilage and adding bone grafts across the joint surface. The affected joint must be immobilized until bone healing has occurred. Common areas of fusion are wrist, ankle, cervical spine, lumbar spine, and metatarsophalangeal (MTP) joint of the great toe.

### Complications of Joint Surgery

Infection is a serious complication of joint surgery, particularly joint replacement surgery. The most common causative organisms are gram-positive aerobic streptococci and staphylococci. Infection may lead to pain and loosening of the prosthesis, generally requiring additional surgery. Efforts to reduce the incidence of infection include the use of specially designed self-contained operating suites, operating rooms with laminar airflow, and prophylactic antibiotic administration.

VTE is another potentially serious complication after joint surgeries, particularly those involving the lower extremities. Prophylactic measures such as anticoagulant medications, sequential compression devices, and early ambulation are usually instituted. Patients may be assessed postoperatively with venous Doppler ultrasound to detect DVT, the source of most pulmonary emboli.

### Interprofessional Care

**Preoperative Management.** The primary goal of preoperative assessment is to identify risk factors for postoperative complications so nursing strategies can be implemented to promote optimal outcomes. A careful history includes (1) previous medical diagnoses and complications such as diabetes and VTE, (2) pain tolerance and management preferences, (3) current functional level and expectations following surgery, (4) current social support, and (5) home care needs after discharge. The patient should be free from infection and acute joint inflammation.

If lower extremity surgery is planned, assess upper extremity muscle strength and joint function to determine the type of assistive devices needed postoperatively for ambulation and ADL performance. Preoperative teaching about the expected hospital course and postoperative management at home is important for the patient and caregiver. Discuss ways to maximize the usefulness and longevity of the prosthesis. Patients also need to realize that recovery does not occur rapidly. Talking with other people who have had total joint arthroplasty may help the patient better understand the reality of rehabilitation.

**Postoperative Management.** Postoperatively, regularly perform neurovascular assessment. Administer anticoagulant medication, analgesia, and parenteral antibiotics. Pain management strategies may include epidural or intrathecal analgesia, femoral nerve block, patient-controlled IV analgesia, and oral opioids or NSAIDs. Assess patient comfort frequently during the postoperative period.

In general, the affected joint is exercised and ambulation is encouraged as early as possible to prevent complications of immobility. Specific protocols vary according to the patient, type of prosthesis, and surgeon preference. Depending upon the surgical approach, an abduction pillow may be used after THA. CPM machines may be used after TKA.

The hospital stay after arthroplasty is 3 to 5 days depending on the patient's course and need for physical therapy. Some patients are discharged in 1 to 2 days. Physical therapy and ambulation enhance mobility, build muscle strength, and reduce the risk of VTE. If the patient is taking warfarin, therapy starts on the day of surgery and the INR and prothrombin times are measured daily. With LMWH (e.g., enoxaparin), therapy starts 12 to 24 hours after surgery and continues for 7 to 10 days postoperatively. Fondaparinux is started no earlier than 6 hours after surgery, with the usual duration of therapy 5 to 9 days. Apixaban is generally taken for 12 days. Daily monitoring of the patient's coagulation status is not necessary when the patient is taking LMWH or a factor Xa inhibitor.

## ❖ NURSING MANAGEMENT: JOINT SURGERY

The nursing management of the patient undergoing joint surgery begins with preoperative teaching and realistic goal setting. Help the patient understand and accept limitations of the proposed surgery and realize surgery may not remove or cure the underlying disease. Explain postoperative procedures such as turning, deep breathing, use of bedpan and bedside commode, and use of an abductor pillow. Reassure the patient that analgesia will be available. A preoperative visit from a physical therapist allows practice of postoperative exercises and measurement for crutches or other assistive devices. Provide opportunities for practice with assistive devices.

Discharge planning begins immediately. Discuss the duration of the hospital stay and the expected postoperative events so that the patient and caregiver can prepare. Teach them to assess the home environment for safety (e.g., scatter rugs, electric cords) and accessibility. Are the bathroom and bedroom on the first floor? Are door frames wide enough to accommodate a walker? Assess the patient's social support. Is a friend or family member available to assist the patient in the home? Will the patient require homemaker or meal services? The older patient may need to be discharged to a subacute or extended care facility for a few weeks to progressively regain independent living skills. Nursing interventions for the patient having orthopedic surgery are presented in eNursing Care Plan 62-2 (on the website for this chapter).

Instruct the patient on reporting complications, including infection (e.g., fever, increased pain, drainage) and dislocation of the prosthesis (e.g., pain, loss of function, shortening or malalignment of an extremity). Act as the liaison between the patient and surgeon, while monitoring for postoperative complications. Also assess the patient's comfort level and ROM at regular intervals to facilitate the goal of improved functional performance.

## CASE STUDY

### *Periprosthetic Hip Fracture and Revision Arthroplasty*

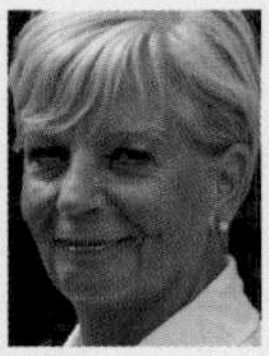

(©iStockphoto/ Thinkstock)

#### Patient Profile

M.C. is a 58-yr-old white woman who has had both hips replaced (left 10 yr ago, right 5 yr ago). She had a total hysterectomy 3 yr ago and stopping taking hormone replacement therapy at that time. She also has a history of hypothyroidism. She was admitted to emergency department after tripping over a short retaining wall in her backyard while gardening. She landed on her right side.

#### Subjective Data

- Acute, severe pain in right hip, unable to bear weight on right leg
- Taking levothyroxine (Synthroid) 125 mcg every morning
- Taking cholecalciferol (vitamin $D_3$) 1000 IU every day without calcium supplement. States calcium upsets her stomach
- Reports loss of approximately 30 lb in the last year through diet and exercise. Continues to exercise three times a week
- Lives in multilevel house with her husband. Bedrooms are on the second level
- Nonsmoker, identifies herself as "a very light social drinker"

#### Objective Data

- 5 ft 6 in tall, 155 lb

*Diagnostic Studies*

- X-rays reveal periprosthetic right femoral fracture at the greater trochanter with resulting loss of fixation in the femoral component of the right total hip replacement
- Normal CBC, chest x-ray
- Serum calcium 8.1 mg/dL

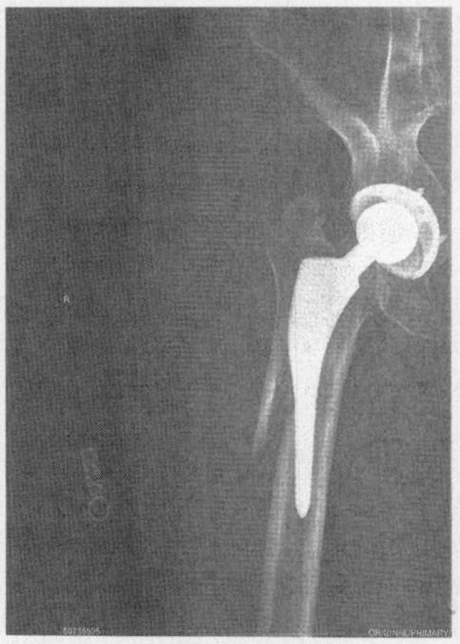

#### Interprofessional Care

- Revision of femoral component of her right total hip replacement with open reduction of the femoral fracture and fixation with three wires
- Pain management, transitioning from IV hydromorphone (Dilaudid) to oral oxycodone (Roxicodone) as tolerated
- Cefazolin 1 g IV every 8 hours for 24 hours
- Enoxaparin (Lovenox) 40 mg subcutaneous every day for 4 weeks
- Calcium citrate (Citracal) 600 mg plus 800 IU vitamin D PO every day with food
- Physical therapy for transfers, gait, and stair training
- Occupational therapy for ADL training

Discharge planning based on mobility limitations and need for continued PT and OT

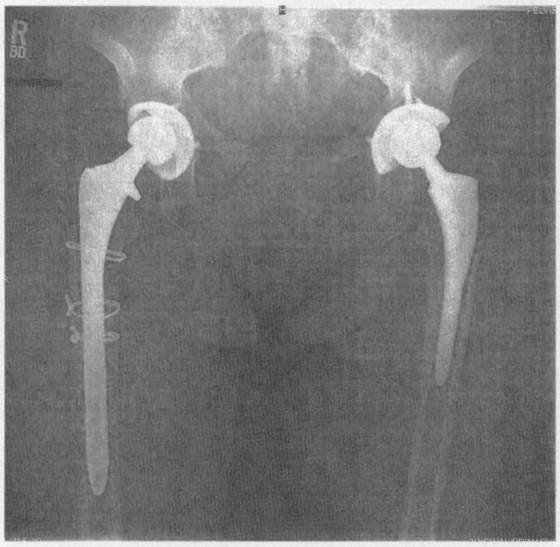

#### Discussion Questions

1. ***Patient-Centered Care:*** How do M.C.'s previous total joint surgeries affect her recovery following this surgery?
2. ***Priority Decision:*** As you plan care for M.C., what are the perioperative priority nursing interventions?
3. What are the most likely postoperative complications M.C. could develop?
4. In considering M.C.'s patient profile, what issues can you identify that may affect her bone healing?
5. ***Priority Decision:*** What are the priority assessments that should be done prior to discharge?
6. ***Teamwork and Collaboration:*** What is the interprofessional team's top priority at this time for M.C.?
7. ***Quality Improvement:*** What outcomes would indicate interprofessional care was effective?
8. ***Safety:*** What safety precautions should be considered for M.C.?
9. ***Evidence-Based Practice:*** Why is satisfactory pain management an important postoperative nursing goal for M.C.?

Answers available at *http://evolve.elsevier.com/Lewis/medsurg.*

## BRIDGE TO NCLEX EXAMINATION

The number of the question corresponds to the same-numbered outcome at the beginning of the chapter.

1. The nurse suspects an ankle sprain when a patient at the urgent care center describes
   - **a.** being hit by another soccer player during a game.
   - **b.** having ankle pain after sprinting around the track.
   - **c.** dropping a 10-lb weight on his lower leg at the health club.
   - **d.** twisting his ankle while running bases during a baseball game.
2. A patient with a humeral fracture is returning for a 4-week checkup. The nurse explains that initial evidence of healing on x-ray is indicated by
   - **a.** formation of callus.
   - **b.** complete bony union.
   - **c.** hematoma at the fracture site.
   - **d.** presence of granulation tissue.
3. A patient with a comminuted fracture of the tibia is to have an open reduction with internal fixation (ORIF) of the fracture. The nurse explains that ORIF is indicated when
   - **a.** the patient is unable to tolerate prolonged immobilization.
   - **b.** the patient cannot tolerate the surgery for a closed reduction.
   - **c.** a temporary cast would be too unstable to provide normal mobility.
   - **d.** adequate alignment cannot be obtained by other nonsurgical methods.
4. The nurse suspects a neurovascular problem based on assessment of
   - **a.** exaggerated strength with movement.
   - **b.** increased redness and heat below the injury.
   - **c.** decreased sensation distal to the fracture site.
   - **d.** purulent drainage at the site of an open fracture.
5. A patient with a stable, closed humeral fracture has a temporary splint with bulky padding applied with an elastic bandage. The nurse notifies the surgeon of possible early compartment syndrome when the patient experiences
   - **a.** increasing edema of the limb.
   - **b.** muscle spasms of the lower arm.
   - **c.** bounding pulse at the fracture site.
   - **d.** pain when passively extending the fingers.
6. A patient with a pelvic fracture should be monitored for
   - **a.** changes in urine output.
   - **b.** petechiae on the abdomen.
   - **c.** a palpable lump in the buttock.
   - **d.** sudden increase in blood pressure.
7. The nurse instructs the patient with an above-the-knee amputation that the residual limb should not be routinely elevated because this position promotes
   - **a.** hip flexion contracture.
   - **b.** clot formation at the incision.
   - **c.** skin irritation and breakdown.
   - **d.** increased risk of wound dehiscence.
8. A patient with osteoarthritis is scheduled for a total hip arthroplasty. The nurse explains the purpose of this procedure is to *(select all that apply)*
   - **a.** fuse the joint.
   - **b.** replace the joint.
   - **c.** prevent further damage.
   - **d.** improve or maintain ROM.
   - **e.** decrease the amount of destruction in the joint.
9. A patient is scheduled for total ankle replacement. The nurse should tell the patient that after surgery he should avoid
   - **a.** lifting heavy objects.
   - **b.** sleeping on the back.
   - **c.** abduction exercises of the affected ankle.
   - **d.** bearing weight on the affected leg for 6 weeks.

1. d, 2. a, 3. d, 4. c, 5. d, 6. a, 7. a, 8. b, d, 9. d

For rationales to these answers and even more NCLEX review questions, visit *http://evolve.elsevier.com/Lewis/medsurg.*

## EVOLVE WEBSITE

http://evolve.elsevier.com/Lewis/medsurg

**Review Questions (Online Only)**

**Key Points**

**Answer Keys for Questions**
- Rationales for Bridge to NCLEX Examination Questions
- Answer Guidelines for Case Study on p. 1493

**Student Case Studies**
- Patient With Musculoskeletal Trauma
- Patient With Parkinson's Disease and Hip Fracture

**Nursing Care Plans**
- eNursing Care Plan 62-1: Patient With a Fracture
- eNursing Care Plan 62-2: Patient Having Orthopedic Surgery

**Concept Map Creator**

**Audio Glossary**

**Supporting Media**
- Animations
  - ORIF Ankle
  - Total Knee Replacement

**Content Updates**

## REFERENCES


1. Centers for Disease Control and Prevention: Death in the United States, 2011. Retrieved from *http://www.cdc.gov/nchs/data/databriefs/db115.htm.*
2. National Institute of Arthritis and Musculoskeletal and Skin Diseases: Preventing sports injuries in youth: a guide for parents. Retrieved from *www.niams.nih.gov/Health_Info/Sports_Injuries/child_sports_injuries.asp.*
3. American Academy of Orthopaedic Surgeons: Sprains, strains, and other soft-tissue injuries. Retrieved from *www.orthoinfo.org/topic.cfm?topic=A00111.*
4. Myrick K: Clinical assessment and management of ankle sprains, *Orthop Nurs* 33:244, 2014.

*5. Lewis J: A systematic literature review of the relationship between stretching and athletic injury prevention, *Orthop Nurs* 33:321, 2014.

6. American Academy of Orthopaedic Surgeons: Common knee injuries. Retrieved from *http://orthoinfo.aaos.org/topic.cfm?topic=A00325.*
7. Mayo Clinic: Carpal tunnel syndrome. Retrieved from *www.mayoclinic.org/diseases-conditions/carpal-tunnel-syndrome/basics/definition/con-20030332.*

8. Agency for Healthcare Research and Quality: Comparative effectiveness of interventions for rotator cuff tears in adults: clinician guide. Retrieved from *http://effectivehealthcare.ahrq.gov/ehc/index.cfm/search-for-guides-reviews-and-reports/?pageAction=displayProduct&productID=544*.
9. National Institute of Arthritis and Musculoskeletal and Skin Diseases: Spotlight on research: Physical therapy to treat torn meniscus comparable to surgery for many patients. Retrieved from *www.niams.nih.gov/News_and_Events/Spotlight_on_Research/2013/pt_surgery_meniscus.asp*.
10. Atkinson Smith M, Smith WT: Anterior cruciate ligament tears reconstruction and rehabilitation, *Orthop Nurs* 33:25, 2015.
11. Mayo Clinic: Bursitis. Retrieved from *www.mayoclinic.org/diseases-conditions/bursitis/basics/definition/con-20015102*.
12. McDevitt KA: Orthopaedic trauma. In Schoenly L, editor: *Core curriculum for orthopaedic nursing*, ed 7, Chicago, 2013, National Association of Orthopaedic Nurses.
*13. Austin D, Donegan D, Mehta S: Low complication rates associated with the application of lower extremity traction pins, *J Orthop Trauma* 29:e259, 2015.
14. American Orthopaedic Foot and Ankle Society: Foot ulcers and the total contact cast. Retrieved from *www.aofas.org/footcaremd/conditions/diabetic-foot/Pages/Foot-Ulcers-and-the-Total-Contact-Cast.aspx*.
15. Royal College of Nursing: Guidance on pin site care. Retrieved from *www.rcn.org.uk/__data/assets/pdf_file/0009/413982/004137.pdf*.
16. *Saunders nursing drug handbook*, St Louis, 2016, Elsevier.
17. The Royal Children's Hospital Melbourne: Neurovascular observations. Retrieved from *www.rch.org.au/rchcpg/hospital_clinical_guideline_index/Neurovascular_observations*.
18. Abu-Ghanem Y, Abu-Ghanem N, Albagly A, et al: Limb position significantly affects safety distance during cast removal, *Orthop Nurs* 34:110, 2015.
19. Greene LR: Orthopaedic infections. In Schoenly L, editor: *Core curriculum for orthopaedic nursing*, ed 7, Chicago, 2013, National Association of Orthopaedic Nurses.
20. Azar F: Traumatic disorders. In Canale S, Beaty J, editors: *Canale and Beaty: Campbell's operative orthopaedics*, ed 12, St Louis, 2013, Mosby.
21. Parker R: Orthopaedic complications. In Schoenly L, editor: *Core curriculum for orthopaedic nursing*, ed 7, Chicago, 2013, National Association of Orthopaedic Nurses.
22. Centers for Disease Control and Prevention: Hip fractures among older adults. Retrieved from *www.cdc.gov/HomeandRecreationalSafety/Falls/adulthipfx.html*.
23. Abel LE: Metabolic bone conditions. In Schoenly L, editor: *Core curriculum for orthopaedic nursing*, ed 7, Chicago, 2013, National Association of Orthopaedic Nurses.
24. Kahn-Kastell B: The hip, femur, and pelvis. In Schoenly L, editor: *Core curriculum for orthopaedic nursing*, ed 7, Chicago, 2013, National Association of Orthopaedic Nurses.
25. Center for Disease Control and Prevention: Preventing falls among older adults. Retrieved from *www.cdc.gov/Features/OlderAmericans*.
*26. Santesso N, Carrasco-Labra A, Brignardello-Petersen R: Hip protectors for preventing hip fracture in older people. Retrieved from *www.cochrane.org/CD001255/MUSKINJ_hip-protectors-for-preventing-hip-fractures-in-older-people*.
*27. Motamedi MHK, Dadgar E, Ebrahimi A, et al: Pattern of maxillofacial fractures: a 5-year analysis of 8,818 patients, *J Trauma Acute Care Surg* 77:630, 2014.
28. Anthony A, Ranzer M, Cohen M: Assessment of the trauma patient. In Taub P, Patel P, Buchman S, et al, editors: *Ferraro's fundamentals of maxillofacial surgery*, New York, 2015, Springer.
29. Amputee Coalition: Limb loss statistics. Retrieved from *www.amputee-coalition.org/limb-loss-resource-center/resources-by-topic/limb-loss-statistics/limb-loss-statistics*.
30. Fischer H: U.S. military casualty statistics: Operation New Dawn, Operation Iraqi Freedom, and Operation Enduring Freedom. Retrieved from *http://journalistsresource.org/wp-content/uploads/2013/02/RS22452.pdf*.
*31. Kiabi FS, Habibi MR, Soleimani A, et al: Mirror therapy as an alternative treatment for phantom limb pain: a short literature review, *Korean J Pain* 26:309, 2013.
32. Gonzalez-Fernandez M: Development of upper limb prostheses: current progress and areas for growth, *Arch Phys Med and Rehab* 95:1013, 2014.
33. National Institute of Arthritis and Musculoskeletal and Skin Diseases: Joint replacement surgery: health information basics for you and your family. Retrieved from *www.niams.nih.gov/health_info/joint_replacement/#4*.
34. American Academy of Orthopaedic Surgeons: Hip resurfacing. Retrieved from *http://orthoinfo.aaos.org/topic.cfm?topic=A00586*.
*35. Wittig-Wells D, Shapiro S, Higgins M: Patients' experience of pain in the 48 hours following total knee arthroplasty, *Orthop Nurs* 32:39, 2013.

*Evidence-based information for clinical practice.

63

# Musculoskeletal Problems

*Matthew C. Price*

*Toughness is in the soul and spirit, not in muscles.*

*Alex Karras*

http://evolve.elsevier.com/Lewis/medsurg/

## LEARNING OUTCOMES

1. Describe the pathophysiology, clinical manifestations, interprofessional care, and nursing management of osteomyelitis.
2. Differentiate among the types, pathophysiology, clinical manifestations, and interprofessional care of bone cancer.
3. Differentiate between the causes and characteristics of acute and chronic low back pain.
4. Explain the conservative and surgical treatment of intervertebral disc damage.
5. Describe the postoperative nursing management of a patient who has undergone vertebral disc surgery.
6. Specify the etiology and nursing management of common foot disorders.
7. Describe the etiology, pathophysiology, clinical manifestations, and nursing and interprofessional management of osteomalacia, osteoporosis, and Paget's disease.

## KEY TERMS

degenerative disc disease (DDD), p. 1504
hallux valgus, p. 1508
herniated disc, p. 1505
low back pain, p. 1502
muscular dystrophy (MD), p. 1501
osteochondroma, p. 1500
osteomalacia, p. 1510
osteomyelitis, p. 1496
osteopenia, p. 1511
osteoporosis, p. 1510
osteosarcoma, p. 1500
Paget's disease, p. 1514
sarcoma, p. 1500

Acute and chronic musculoskeletal problems are a common source of pain and disability. A variety of problems unrelated to trauma that affect the musculoskeletal system are presented in this chapter, including osteomyelitis, bone cancer, muscular dystrophy, foot disorders, and metabolic bone diseases. Management of the patient with acute and chronic low back pain is addressed, and spinal vertebral disc surgery is discussed. The nurse's role in prevention of injury and maintenance of mobility is emphasized.

## OSTEOMYELITIS

### Etiology and Pathophysiology

**Osteomyelitis** is a severe infection of the bone, bone marrow, and surrounding soft tissue. Although *Staphylococcus aureus* is a common cause of infection, a variety of microorganisms may cause osteomyelitis[1] (Table 63-1).

Infecting microorganisms can invade by indirect or direct entry. *Indirect entry* (hematogenous) of microorganisms most frequently affects growing bone in boys younger than 12 years old and is associated with their higher incidence of blunt trauma. Adults with genitourinary and respiratory tract infections or disorders marked by vascular insufficiency (e.g., diabetes mellitus) are at high risk for the spread of a primary infection via the blood to the bone. As highly vascular bones, the pelvis, tibia, and vertebrae are the most common sites of infection.

*Direct entry* osteomyelitis can occur at any age when an open wound (e.g., penetrating wounds, fractures) allows microorganisms to enter the body. Osteomyelitis may also be related to a foreign body such as an implant or an orthopedic prosthetic device (e.g., plate, total joint prosthesis).

After gaining entry into the blood, microorganisms grow and pressure increases because of the nonexpanding nature of most bone. This increasing pressure eventually leads to ischemia and vascular compromise of the periosteum. The infection spreads through the bone cortex and marrow cavity, causing cortical devascularization and necrosis.

Bone death occurs as a result of ischemia. The area of dead bone eventually separates from the surrounding living bone, forming *sequestra.* The part of the periosteum that continues to have a blood supply forms new bone called *involucrum* (Fig. 63-1). Antibiotics or white blood cells (WBCs) have difficulty

Reviewed by Judy Carlyle, RN, MNSc, ARNEC Faculty/Clinical Liaison, Arkansas Rural Nursing Education Consortium (ARNEC), Nashville, Arkansas; Monica L. Johnson, RN, MSN, MBA-HCM, CMSRN, ONC, LNC, Acute Care Division Clinical Educator, East Jefferson General Hospital, and Adjunct Clinical Faculty, Delgado Community College Charity School of Nursing, New Orleans, Louisiana; Rebecca Liebert, RN, MSN, FNP-C, ONP-C, Nurse Practitioner, Tomah Memorial Hospital and Specialty Clinic/Orthopedics, Tomah, Wisconsin; and Laura C. Williams, RN, MSN, CNS, ONC, CCNS, Orthopedic Clinical Nurse Specialist, Orlando Health, Orlando, Florida.

**TABLE 63-1 Organisms Causing Osteomyelitis**

| Organism | Predisposing Problem |
|---|---|
| *Staphylococcus aureus* | Pressure ulcer, penetrating wound, open fracture, orthopedic surgery, disorders with vascular insufficiency (e.g., diabetes, atherosclerosis) |
| *Staphylococcus epidermidis* | Indwelling prosthetic devices (e.g., joint replacements, fracture fixation devices) |
| *Streptococcus viridans* | Abscessed tooth, gingival disease |
| *Escherichia coli* | Urinary tract infection |
| *Mycobacterium tuberculosis* | Tuberculosis |
| *Neisseria gonorrhoeae* | Gonorrhea |
| *Pseudomonas* | Puncture wounds, IV drug use |
| *Salmonella* | Sickle cell disease |
| Fungi, mycobacteria | Immunocompromised host |

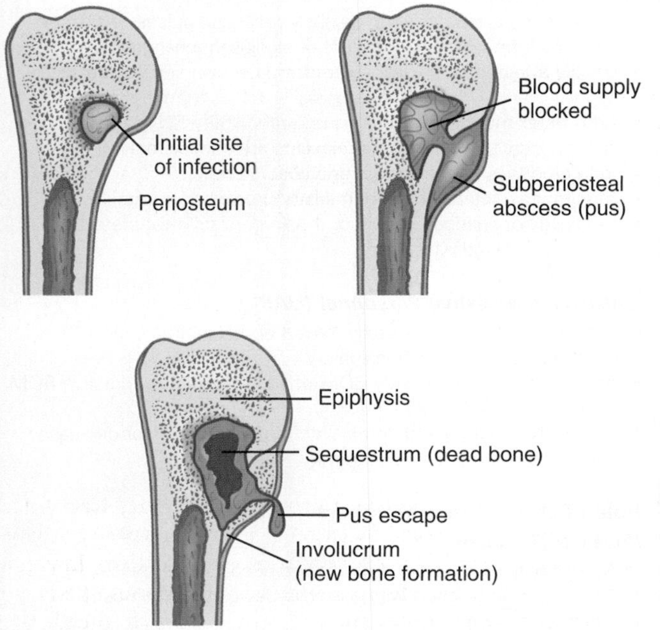


**FIG. 63-1** Development of osteomyelitis infection with involucrum and sequestrum.

reaching the sequestrum through the blood. Thus sequestrum may become a reservoir for microorganisms that spread to other sites, including the lungs and brain. If the sequestrum does not resolve or is not debrided surgically, a sinus tract may develop. Chronic, purulent cutaneous drainage from the tract results.

## Clinical Manifestations and Complications

*Acute osteomyelitis* refers to the initial infection or an infection of less than 1 month in duration. Clinical manifestations of acute osteomyelitis are local and systemic. Local manifestations include constant bone pain that worsens with activity and is unrelieved by rest; swelling, tenderness, and warmth at the infection site; and restricted movement of the affected part. Systemic manifestations include fever, night sweats, chills, restlessness, nausea, and malaise. Later signs include drainage from cutaneous sinus tracts or the fracture site.

*Chronic osteomyelitis* refers to a bone infection that lasts longer than 1 month or an infection that has failed to respond to initial antibiotic treatment. Chronic osteomyelitis may be a continuous, persistent problem (a result of inadequate acute treatment) or a process of exacerbations and remissions (Fig. 63-2). Systemic manifestations may be reduced. Local signs of infection become more common, including constant bone pain as well as swelling and warmth at the infection site. Over time, granulation tissue turns to scar tissue. The avascular scar tissue provides an ideal site for continued microorganism growth because it cannot be penetrated by antibiotics.

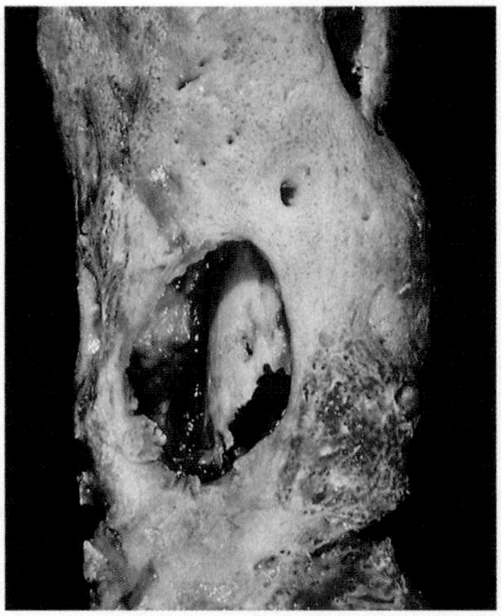

**FIG. 63-2** Resection of femur due to osteomyelitis. (From Thibodeau GA, Patton KT: *The human body in health and disease,* ed 5, St Louis, 2010, Mosby.)

Long-term and mostly rare complications of osteomyelitis include septicemia, septic arthritis, pathologic fractures, and amyloidosis.

## Diagnostic Studies

Bone or soft tissue biopsy is the definitive way to identify the causative microorganism. The patient's blood and wound cultures are frequently positive for microorganisms.[2] Elevated WBC count and erythrocyte sedimentation rate (ESR) may also be found. While elevated ESR is usually seen in chronic infective processes, elevated C-reactive protein (CRP) may also suggest acute infection. Signs of osteomyelitis usually do not appear on x-rays until 10 days to weeks after the initial clinical symptoms. By this time, the disease will have progressed. Compared to x-rays, CT scan may be more helpful in assessing the extent of infection. Especially in the acute phase, MRI may be more sensitive than CT in detecting bone marrow edema, which is an early indication of osteomyelitis.[3] Radionuclide bone scans (gallium and indium) are helpful in diagnosis and are usually positive in the area of infection.

## Interprofessional Care

Aggressive, prolonged IV antibiotic therapy is the treatment of choice for acute osteomyelitis if bone ischemia has not yet occurred. Cultures or a bone biopsy should be done if possible before initiating drug therapy. If antibiotic therapy is delayed, surgical debridement and decompression are often needed.

Patients are often discharged to home care or a skilled nursing facility with IV antibiotics delivered via a central venous access device (CVAD). These include centrally inserted catheters, peripherally inserted central catheters (PICCs), and implanted ports. (CVADs are discussed in Chapter 16.) IV antibiotic therapy may be started in the hospital and continued at home for 4 to 6 weeks or as long as 3 to 6 months. A variety of antibiotics may be prescribed depending on the microorganism. These drugs include penicillin, nafcillin, neomycin, vancomycin, cephalexin, cefazolin, cefoxitin, gentamicin, and tobramycin.

**DRUG ALERT Gentamicin**

- Assess patient for dehydration before starting therapy.
- Ensure renal function testing is done before starting therapy, especially in older patients.
- Monitor peak and trough blood levels to achieve therapeutic effect and minimize renal and inner ear toxicity.[4]
- Instruct patient to notify HCP if any visual, hearing, or urinary problems develop.

In adults with chronic osteomyelitis, oral therapy with a fluoroquinolone (e.g., ciprofloxacin [Cipro]) for 6 to 8 weeks may be prescribed instead of IV antibiotics. Oral antibiotics may also be given after acute IV therapy is completed to ensure the infection is resolved. The patient's response to drug therapy is monitored through bone scans and ESR testing.

Treatment of chronic osteomyelitis includes (1) surgical removal of the poorly perfused tissue and dead bone and (2) extended use of antibiotics.[5] Acrylic bead chains containing antibiotics may also be implanted to help combat the infection. After debridement of the dead, infected tissue, a suction irrigation system may be inserted and the wound closed. Intermittent or constant irrigation of the area with antibiotics may also be initiated. The limb or the surgical site is often protected with casts or braces. Postoperatively, negative-pressure wound therapy may be used (discussed in Chapter 11 on pp. 169-170).

Hyperbaric $O_2$ may be given as an adjunct therapy in refractory cases of chronic osteomyelitis. It stimulates new blood growth and healing in the infected tissue (see p. 170 in Chapter 11).

If orthopedic prosthetic devices are a source of chronic infection, they must be removed. Muscle flaps or skin grafts provide wound coverage over the dead space (cavity) in the bone. Bone grafts may help to restore blood flow. However, flaps or grafts should never be placed in the presence of active or suspected infection.

Amputation of the extremity may be needed if bone destruction is extensive. Amputation should improve quality of life and may save the patient's life if systemic complications are developing.

## NURSING MANAGEMENT: OSTEOMYELITIS

### Nursing Assessment

Subjective and objective data that should be obtained from an individual with osteomyelitis are presented in Table 63-2.

### Nursing Diagnoses

Nursing diagnoses for the patient with osteomyelitis may include, but are not limited to, the following:

- Acute pain *related to* inflammatory process secondary to infection
- Ineffective health maintenance *related to* lack of knowledge regarding long-term management of osteomyelitis
- Impaired physical mobility *related to* pain, immobilization devices, and weight-bearing limitations

Additional information on nursing diagnoses for the patient with osteomyelitis is available in eNursing Care Plan 63-1 (on the website for this chapter).

**TEAMWORK & COLLABORATION**

***Caring for the Patient With Osteomyelitis***

**Role of Nursing Personnel**

***Registered Nurse (RN)***

- Administer IV antibiotics as ordered.
- Assess wound for signs of worsening infection.
- Teach patient and caregiver about antibiotic side effects and length of treatment, signs and symptoms of worsening infection, and use of hyperbaric $O_2$ if ordered.
- Assess for muscle spasms and administer muscle relaxant as ordered.
- Assess pain intensity and administer analgesics as ordered. Assess patient response.
- Handle affected limb carefully to decrease pain and additional injury.
- Assess neurovascular condition of affected limb and immediately inform HCP of significant changes.

***Licensed Practical/Vocational Nurse (LPN/LVN)***

- Monitor color, temperature, capillary refill, and pulses of affected limb and immediately inform RN of significant changes.
- Handle affected limb carefully to decrease pain and additional injury.
- Administer muscle relaxants as ordered. Notify RN if muscle spasms persist after muscle relaxants are administered.
- Reinforce teaching related to antibiotic therapy.
- Monitor pain intensity and administer prescribed analgesics.
- Notify RN of changes in pain or if pain persists after prescribed analgesics are administered.

***Unlicensed Assistive Personnel (UAP)***

- Handle affected limb carefully (based on RN instruction) to decrease pain and additional injury.
- Assist patient with passive ROM of adjacent joints and active ROM exercises of unaffected limb.
- Notify RN about patient complaints of pain, tingling, or decreased sensation in the affected extremity.

**Role of Other Team Members**

***Physical Therapist***

- Assess patient's current mobility and need for assistance.
- Teach safe ambulation with assistive device based on patient's weight-bearing restrictions.
- Establish exercise regimen and teach patient to perform exercises safely.
- Coordinate PT with RN so that patient can receive timely analgesia.
- Discuss home environment with patient and identify possible modifications to facilitate recovery (e.g., stair training if allowed by patient's weight-bearing restrictions, bed placement on first level to avoid stairs).

***Occupational Therapist***

- Assess impact of patient's condition on ability to perform activities of daily living.
- Instruct patient in use of assistive devices (e.g., long-handled reacher, shoe donner) to facilitate self-care while maintaining activity restrictions.
- Discuss home environment with patient and identify possible modifications to facilitate recovery (e.g., bed placement on first level for access to bathroom).

### Planning

The overall goals are that the patient with osteomyelitis will (1) have satisfactory pain and fever management, (2) not experience any complications associated with osteomyelitis, (3) adhere to the treatment plan, and (4) maintain a positive outlook on the outcome of the disease.

**TABLE 63-2 Nursing Assessment**

***Osteomyelitis***

**Subjective Data**

***Important Health Information***

*Past health history:* Bone trauma, open fracture, open or puncture wounds, other infections (e.g., streptococcal sore throat, bacterial pneumonia, sinusitis, skin or tooth infection, chronic urinary tract infection)

*Medications:* Analgesics or antibiotics

*Surgery or other treatments:* Bone surgery

***Functional Health Patterns***

*Health perception–health management:* IV drug and alcohol abuse. Malaise

*Nutritional-metabolic:* Anorexia, weight loss. Chills

*Activity-exercise:* Weakness, paralysis, muscle spasms around affected area

*Cognitive-perceptual:* Local tenderness over affected area, increased pain with movement of affected area

*Coping–stress tolerance:* Irritability, withdrawal, dependency, anger

**Objective Data**

***General***

Restlessness. High, spiking temperature. Night sweats

***Integumentary***

Diaphoresis. Erythema, warmth, edema at site of infection

***Musculoskeletal***

Restricted movement; wound drainage. Spontaneous fracture

***Possible Diagnostic Findings***

Leukocytosis, positive blood and/or wound cultures, ↑ erythrocyte sedimentation rate. Presence of sequestrum and involucrum on x-rays, radionuclide bone scans, CT, and MRI

## ◆ Nursing Implementation

◆ **Health Promotion.** Control of other current infections (e.g., urinary or respiratory tract, pressure ulcers) is important in preventing osteomyelitis. Persons especially at risk for osteomyelitis are those who are immunocompromised, or who have diabetes, orthopedic prosthetic devices, or vascular insufficiency. Instruct the at-risk patient about the local and systemic signs of osteomyelitis. Encourage the patient to immediately tell the HCP about bone pain, fever, swelling, and restricted limb movement so that treatment can be started. Also teach family members about their role in monitoring the patient's health.

◆ **Acute Care.** Some immobilization of the affected limb (e.g., splint, traction) is usually needed to decrease pain and reduce risk of additional injury. Carefully handle the limb and avoid undue manipulation, which may increase pain and cause a pathologic fracture. Assess the patient's pain. Muscle spasms may cause minor to severe pain. Nonsteroidal antiinflammatory drugs (NSAIDs), opioid analgesics, and muscle relaxants may be prescribed for patient comfort. Encourage nondrug approaches to pain management (e.g., guided imagery, relaxation breathing) (see Chapter 6).

Dressings are used to absorb drainage from wounds and debride dead tissue from the wound bed. These include dry, sterile dressings; dressings saturated in saline or antibiotic solution; wet-to-dry dressings; and dressings applied with negative-pressure wound therapy. Sterile technique is essential when changing the dressing. Handle soiled dressings carefully to prevent transfer of bacteria to other areas of the wound. Discard dressings appropriately to prevent spread of infection to other patients. The patient is frequently placed on bed rest in the early stages of acute infection. Good body alignment and frequent position changes promote comfort and prevent complications related to immobility. Flexion contracture of the affected lower extremity is common as the patient frequently positions the leg in a flexed position to promote comfort. Footdrop can develop quickly due to Achilles tendon contracture if the foot is not correctly supported in a neutral position by a splint or boot. A tight splint or dressing may also compress and injure the peroneal nerve.

Teach the patient the possible adverse and toxic reactions associated with prolonged high-dose antibiotic therapy (e.g., tobramycin, neomycin). These reactions include hearing deficit, impaired renal function, and neurotoxicity (e.g., limb weakness or numbness, cognitive changes or loss of memory, vision changes, headache, behavioral problems). Reactions associated with cephalosporins (e.g., cefazolin) include hives, severe or watery diarrhea, blood in stools, and throat or mouth sores.

Tendonitis or tendon rupture (especially the Achilles tendon) can occur with use of fluoroquinolones (e.g., ciprofloxacin, levofloxacin [Levaquin]). Peak and trough blood levels of most antibiotics should be monitored to avoid adverse effects. Lengthy antibiotic therapy can also cause an overgrowth of *Candida albicans* and *Clostridium difficile* in the genitourinary and gastrointestinal (GI) tracts, especially in immunosuppressed and older patients. Instruct the patient to report any changes in the oral cavity (e.g., whitish yellow, curdlike lesions) or the genitourinary cavity (e.g., perianal itching or diarrhea).

**CHECK YOUR PRACTICE**

Your patient on the orthopedic unit is a 22-yr-old man who was involved in an all-terrain vehicle accident in a remote area 4 days ago. He was airlifted to your hospital because he was unconscious when he was found. He is now slowly recovering from his head injury and surgical repair of an open fracture of the femur. Yesterday he was diagnosed with acute osteomyelitis. He is very angry and at times disoriented. When you try to assess his leg, he yells at you, "It hurts. Leave it alone!"

- What are your priorities of care?
- What signs and symptoms would suggest the patient's condition is worsening?

The patient, caregiver, and family may be anxious and discouraged because of the serious nature of osteomyelitis, the uncertainty of the outcome, and the long, costly treatment. Continued psychologic and emotional support is an integral part of nursing management. A nursing care plan for the patient with osteomyelitis (eNursing Care Plan 63-1) is available on the website for this chapter.

◆ **Ambulatory Care.** IV antibiotics can be administered to the patient in a skilled nursing facility or home setting. If at home, instruct the patient and caregiver how to manage the CVAD. Also teach them how to administer the antibiotic when scheduled and reinforce the need for follow-up laboratory testing. Stress the importance of continuing to take antibiotics after symptoms have improved.

Dressing changes are often required if the patient has an open wound. The patient and caregiver may need supplies and instruction for completing the dressing change. If the osteomyelitis becomes chronic, the patient needs continued physical and psychologic support.

### ◆ Evaluation

The expected outcomes are that the patient with osteomyelitis will:

- Have satisfactory pain management
- Adhere to the recommended treatment regimen
- Verbalize confidence in ability to implement treatment regimen at home
- Demonstrate a consistent increase in mobility and range of motion

# BONE TUMORS

Primary bone tumors, both benign and malignant, are relatively rare in adults. They account for only about 3% of all tumors. Metastatic bone cancer in which cancer has spread from another site is a more common problem.

## BENIGN BONE TUMORS

Bone tumors are relatively rare when compared to other types of tumors. However, benign bone tumors are more common than primary malignant tumors. The main types of benign bone tumors are osteochondroma, osteoclastoma, and enchondroma (Table 63-3). These types of tumors are often removed by surgery.

### Osteochondroma

**Osteochondroma** is the most common primary benign bone tumor. It is characterized by an overgrowth of cartilage and bone near the end of the bone at the growth plate. It is more commonly found in the pelvis, scapula, or long bones of the leg.

Clinical manifestations include a painless, hard, immobile mass; lower-than-normal height for age; soreness of muscles close to the tumor; one leg or arm longer than the other; and pressure or irritation with exercise. Patients may also be asymptomatic. Diagnosis is confirmed using x-ray, CT scan, and MRI.

No treatment is necessary for asymptomatic osteochondroma. If the tumor is causing pain or neurologic manifestations because of compression, surgical removal is usually done. Patients should have regular screening examinations to detect progression to malignancy as soon as possible.

## MALIGNANT BONE TUMORS

A **sarcoma** is a malignant tumor that develops in bone, muscle, fat, nerve, or cartilage. The most common types of malignant bone tumors are osteosarcoma, chondrosarcoma, and Ewing's sarcoma (Table 63-3). About 2970 new cases of bone and joint cancer occur annually in the United States, with an estimated 1500 deaths.[6] Primary malignant tumors occur most often during childhood and young adulthood. They are characterized by their rapid metastasis and bone destruction.

### Osteosarcoma

**Osteosarcoma** is an extremely aggressive primary malignant bone tumor that rapidly spreads to distant sites. It usually occurs in the pelvis or metaphyseal region of the long bones of extremities, particularly in the distal femur, proximal tibia, and proximal humerus (Fig. 63-3, *A*). Osteosarcoma is the most common malignant bone tumor affecting children and young adults. It can also occur in older adults, but not as commonly.

**TABLE 63-3 Types of Primary Bone Tumors**

| Types | Description |
|---|---|
| **Benign** | |
| **Osteochondroma** | • Most common benign bone tumor<br>• Frequently located in pelvis, scapula, or metaphyseal portion of long bones<br>• Occurs most often in people ages 10-25 years<br>• May transform to malignancy (chondrosarcoma) |
| **Osteoclastoma** (giant cell tumor) | • Arises in cancellous ends of arm and leg bones<br>• About 10% are locally aggressive and may spread to lungs<br>• High rate of local recurrence after surgery and chemotherapy |
| **Enchondroma** | • Intramedullary cartilage tumor usually found in cavity of a single hand or foot bone<br>• Rarely transforms to malignancy<br>• If tumor becomes painful, surgical resection is done<br>• Peak incidence in people ages 10-20 |
| **Malignant** | |
| **Osteosarcoma** | • Most common primary bone cancer<br>• Occurs mostly in males ages 10-25<br>• Most often in pelvis or bones of arms, legs (Fig. 63-3, *A*) |
| **Chondrosarcoma** | • Occurs in cartilage most commonly in arm, leg, and pelvic bones of adults ages 50-70<br>• Can also arise from benign bone tumors (osteochondromas)<br>• Wide surgical resection is typically done as tumor rarely responds to radiation and chemotherapy<br>• Survival rate depends on stage, size, and grade of tumor (Fig. 63-3, *B*) |
| **Ewing's sarcoma** | • Develops in medullary cavity of pelvis and long bones, especially femur, humerus, and tibia<br>• Usually occurs in children and teenagers<br>• Use of wide surgical resection, radiation, and chemotherapy has improved 5-yr survival rate to 60% |

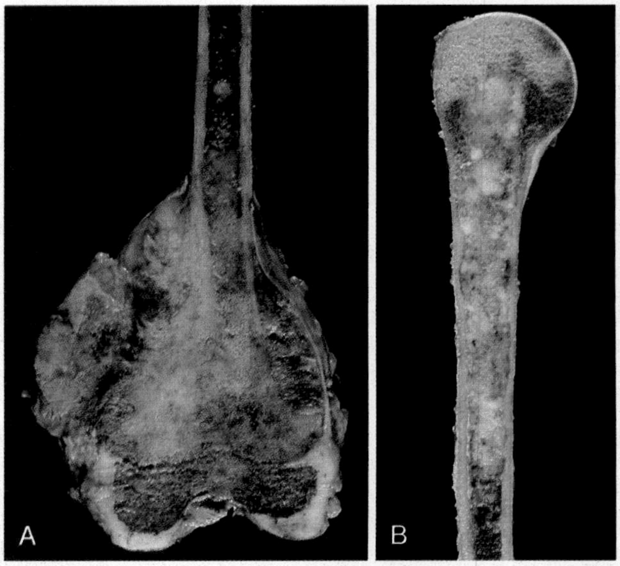


**FIG. 63-3** **A,** Osteosarcoma. **B,** Chondrosarcoma. (From Damjanov I, Linder J: *Anderson's pathology,* ed 10, St Louis, 1996, Mosby.)

It is most often associated with Paget's disease (discussed on p. 1514) and prior radiation.

Clinical manifestations of osteosarcoma are usually associated with the gradual onset of pain and swelling, especially around the knee. A minor injury does not cause the neoplasm but may bring the preexisting condition to medical attention. Metastasis is present in 10% to 20% of individuals when they are diagnosed with osteosarcoma.

Diagnosis is confirmed from tissue biopsy, elevation of serum alkaline phosphatase and calcium, x-ray, CT or positron emission tomography (PET) scans, and MRI.

Preoperative (neoadjuvant) chemotherapy may be used to decrease tumor size before surgery. Limb salvage procedures are usually considered if a clear (no cancer present) 6- to 7-cm margin surrounds the lesion. Limb salvage is usually contraindicated if the patient has major neurovascular involvement, pathologic fracture, infection, or extensive muscle involvement.

The use of adjunct chemotherapy after amputation or limb salvage has increased the 5-year survival rate to 70% in people without metastasis. Chemotherapy includes methotrexate, doxorubicin, cisplatin, cyclophosphamide, and etoposide.[7]

### Metastatic Bone Cancer

The most common type of malignant bone tumor occurs as a result of spread *(metastasis)* from a primary tumor at another site. Common primary sites include breast, prostate, lungs, kidney, and thyroid. Metastatic cancer cells travel from the primary tumor to the bone via the lymph and blood supply. Metastatic bone lesions are commonly found in vertebrae, pelvis, femur, humerus, or ribs.[8] Pathologic fractures at the site of metastasis are common because the bone has weakened. High serum calcium occurs as calcium is released from damaged bones.

Once a primary lesion has been identified, radionuclide bone scans are often done to detect metastatic lesions before they are visible on x-ray. Metastatic bone lesions may occur at any time (even years later) following diagnosis and treatment of the primary tumor. Metastasis to the bone should be suspected in any patient who has local bone pain and a past history of cancer. Surgical stabilization of the bone may be indicated for fracture or to prevent fracture in a high-risk patient. Prognosis depends on the primary type of cancer and any other sites of metastasis. Possible palliative treatment consists of radiation and pain management (see Chapter 15).

## ❖ NURSING MANAGEMENT: BONE CANCER

Assess the patient with bone cancer for the location and severity of pain. Also note weakness caused by anemia and decreased mobility. Monitor the tumor site for swelling; changes in circulation; and decreased movement, sensation, or joint function.

Nursing care of the patient with a malignant bone tumor does not differ significantly from the care provided to the patient with cancer of any other body system (see Chapter 15). However, use special care to prevent pathologic fractures or reduce the complications associated with them. Prevent fractures by careful handling and support of the affected extremity and logrolling for the patient on bed rest.

Treatment for hypercalcemia may be initiated if bone decalcification occurs (see Table 15-19, p. 263). The patient may be unwilling to participate in exercise or therapeutic activities because of weakness from the disease and treatment, fear of falling and fracturing a bone, and fear of pain. Provide regular rest periods between activities.

The pain associated with bone cancer can be severe. It is often caused by the tumor pressing against nerves and other organs near the bone. New onset or changes in severity of pain may also indicate pathologic fracture. Carefully assess the patient's pain and ensure adequate pain medication is provided. Sometimes radiation therapy is used as a palliative therapy to shrink the tumor and decrease pain.

Assist the patient and caregiver in accepting the poor prognosis associated with bone malignancy. General principles related to cancer nursing are applicable (see Chapter 15). Special attention is needed for problems of pain and disability, side effects of chemotherapy, and postoperative care (e.g., after spinal cord decompression or amputation). As with all types of cancer, stress the importance of follow-up examinations.

## MUSCULAR DYSTROPHY

**Muscular dystrophy** (MD) is a group of genetic diseases characterized by progressive symmetric wasting of skeletal muscles without evidence of neurologic involvement. A gradual loss of strength with increasing disability and deformity occurs with all forms of MD. The types of MD differ in the groups of muscles affected, age of onset, rate of progression, and mode of genetic inheritance (Table 63-4). Duchenne MD is the most common type.

**TABLE 63-4 Types of Muscular Dystrophy**

| Type* | Genetic Basis | Manifestations |
|---|---|---|
| **Duchenne** | • X-linked<br>• Mutation of dystrophin gene | • Most common form of MD<br>• Primarily affects boys<br>• Onset before age 5<br>• Progressive weakness of pelvic and shoulder muscles<br>• Unable to walk by age 12<br>• Cardiomyopathy<br>• Respiratory failure in 20s<br>• Mental impairment |
| **Becker** | • X-linked<br>• Mutation of dystrophin gene | • Very similar but less severe than Duchenne MD<br>• Onset ages 5-15<br>• Slower course of pelvic and shoulder muscle wasting than Duchenne<br>• Cardiomyopathy<br>• Respiratory failure<br>• May survive into 40s |
| **Facioscapulohumeral** | • Autosomal dominant<br>• Deletion of chromosome *4q35* | • Onset before age 20<br>• Slowly progressive weakness of face, shoulder muscles, and upper arms and lower legs<br>• Can affect vision and hearing |
| **Limb-girdle** | • Autosomal recessive or autosomal dominant<br>• Mutation in any of at least 15 genes affecting proteins needed for muscle function | • Group of disorders affecting voluntary muscles, especially those of hips and shoulders<br>• Onset ranges from early childhood to early adulthood or later<br>• Slow progressive weakness of hip and shoulder muscles |

*List is not all-inclusive.

### Genetic Link

Duchenne and Becker MD are X-linked recessive disorders usually seen only in males. (X-linked recessive disorders are discussed in Chapter 12.) These disorders are characterized by a mutation of the dystrophin *(DMD)* gene. Dystrophin is a protein that helps keep skeletal muscle fibers intact. Abnormal dystrophin can cause defects in the muscle fiber and results in muscle fiber degeneration.

A family history can be used to obtain a family pedigree. Family pedigrees for X-linked recessive disorders are shown in Figs. 12-4 and 12-5.

Diagnostic studies for MD include muscle serum enzymes (especially creatine kinase), electromyogram (EMG) testing, muscle fiber biopsy, and electrocardiogram for abnormalities that suggest cardiomyopathy. Muscle biopsy confirms the diagnosis with classic findings of fat and connective tissue deposits, muscle fiber degeneration and necrosis, and a deficiency of dystrophin.

No definitive therapy is available to stop the progressive wasting of MD. Primary treatment goals are to preserve mobility and independence through exercise, physical therapy, and use of assistive devices. Progressive muscle weakening around the trunk can cause spinal collapse. The patient may be fitted early with an orthotic jacket to provide stability and prevent further deformity or injury.

Cardiomyopathy often occurs and causes heart failure. Dysrhythmias are a frequent cause of death.[9] Gradual decreases in respiratory function often lead to the use of continuous positive airway pressure (CPAP). Eventually tracheostomy and mechanical ventilation are needed to support respiratory function. Corticosteroid therapy may slow disease progression for up to 2 years.[10]

Encourage communication between the patient and family to cope with the emotional and physical demands of MD. Teach the patient and caregiver range-of-motion (ROM) exercises, principles of good nutrition, and signs of disease progression. Genetic testing and counseling may be recommended for persons with a family history of MD.

Focus care on keeping the patient active as long as possible. Prolonged bed rest should be avoided because immobility can cause more muscle wasting. As the disease progresses, teach the patient to limit sedentary periods to prevent skin breakdown and respiratory complications. Ongoing medical and nursing care is required throughout the patient's life. The Muscular Dystrophy Association *(www.mda.org)* is an important resource and provides information on support services for the patient, caregiver, and family.

**SAFETY ALERT Muscular Dystrophy**

- Support respiratory function as needed.
- Fit patient with an orthotic jacket or brace to prevent deformity or injury.
- Teach patient, caregiver, and family the signs of disease progression.

## GENETICS IN CLINICAL PRACTICE

### *Duchenne and Becker Muscular Dystrophy (MD)*

**Genetic Basis**

- Caused by mutations in the dystrophin *(DMD)* gene. Many mutations have been identified.
- Gene provides instructions for making dystrophin (protein that helps to keep muscle cells intact) located primarily in skeletal and cardiac muscle.
- Inherited in an X-linked recessive pattern.

**Incidence**

- Between 400 and 600 boys are born with MD each year in the United States.
- Together these disorders affect 1 in 3500 to 5000 newborn males worldwide.
- Females in these families have a 50% chance of inheriting and passing the defective gene to their children.

**Genetic Testing**

- DNA testing for mutations in dystrophin gene is available.
- Genetic testing and counseling should be considered in individuals with a family history of MD.

**Clinical Implications**

- Muscular dystrophies are a group of genetic conditions characterized by progressive muscle weakness and atrophy.
- These conditions differ in their severity, age of onset, and rate of progression (Table 63-4).
- Males with Duchenne MD typically live into their 20s, whereas those with Becker MD may live into their 40s or beyond.
- Because there are many types of MD with different genetic bases, establishing the type of MD is important to determine treatment and possible genetic counseling recommendations.

## LOW BACK PAIN

**Low back pain** is most often due to a musculoskeletal problem. It may be experienced as localized or diffuse. In *localized pain,* patients feel soreness or discomfort when a specific area of the lower back is palpated or pressed. *Diffuse pain* occurs over a larger area and comes from deep tissue.

Low back pain may be radicular or referred. *Radicular pain* is caused by irritation of a nerve root. Radicular pain is not typically isolated to a single location but instead radiates or moves along a nerve distribution. Sciatica is an example of radicular pain. *Referred pain* is felt in the lower back, but the source of the pain is another location (e.g., kidneys, lower abdomen).

Low back pain has affected about 80% of adults in the United States at least once during their lives. Backache is second only to headache as the most common pain complaint. Low back pain is the leading cause of job-related disability and a major contributor to missed work days.[11]

Low back pain is a common problem because the lumbar region (1) bears most of the weight of the body, (2) is the most flexible region of the spinal column, (3) contains nerve roots that are at risk for injury or disease, and (4) has a naturally poor biomechanical structure. Risk factors associated with low back pain include lack of muscle tone, excess body weight, stress, poor posture, cigarette smoking, pregnancy, prior compression fracture of the spine, spinal problems since birth, and a family history of back pain. Jobs that require repetitive heavy lifting, vibration (such as a jackhammer operator), and extended periods of sitting are also associated with low back pain.

The causes of low back pain of musculoskeletal origin include (1) acute lumbosacral strain, (2) instability of the lumbosacral bony mechanism, (3) osteoarthritis of the lumbosacral vertebrae, (4) degenerative disc disease, and (5) herniation of an intervertebral disc.

Health care personnel who perform direct patient care activities are at high risk for development of low back pain.[12] Lifting and moving patients, excessive bending or leaning forward, and frequent twisting can result in low back pain that causes lost time and productivity and disability.

## ACUTE LOW BACK PAIN

*Acute low back pain* lasts 4 weeks or less. Most acute low back pain is caused by trauma or an activity that produces undue stress (often hyperflexion) on the lower back. Examples of trauma or activity that could cause acute back pain are heavy lifting, overuse of back muscles during yard work, a sports injury, or a sudden jolt as in a motor vehicle crash.

Often symptoms do not appear at the time of injury. They develop later (usually within 24 hours) because of a gradual increase in pressure on the nerve from an intervertebral disc and/or associated edema. Symptoms may range from muscle ache to shooting or stabbing pain, limited flexibility or ROM, or an inability to stand upright.

Few definitive diagnostic abnormalities are present with nerve irritation and muscle strain. One test is the straight-leg–raising test (see Chapter 61, p. 1455). MRI and CT scans are generally not done unless trauma or systemic disease (e.g., cancer, spinal infection) is suspected. MRI findings may also be limited in the acute phase of an injury due to increased edema near the injury.

## NURSING AND INTERPROFESSIONAL MANAGEMENT: ACUTE LOW BACK PAIN

### Nursing Assessment

Subjective and objective data that should be obtained from the patient with low back pain are summarized in Table 63-5.

### TABLE 63-5 Nursing Assessment
#### *Low Back Pain*

**Subjective Data**

***Important Health Information***

*Past health history:* Acute or chronic lumbosacral strain/trauma, osteoarthritis, degenerative disc disease, obesity

*Medications:* Opioid analgesics and NSAIDs, muscle relaxants, corticosteroids, over-the-counter remedies (e.g., topical ointments, patches)

*Surgery or other treatments:* Previous back surgery, epidural corticosteroid injections

***Functional Health Patterns***

*Health perception–health management:* Smoking, lack of exercise

*Nutritional-metabolic:* Obesity

*Activity-exercise:* Poor posture, muscle spasms, activity intolerance

*Elimination:* Constipation

*Sleep-rest:* Interrupted sleep

*Cognitive-perceptual:* Pain in back, buttocks, or leg associated with walking, turning, straining, coughing, leg raising. Numbness or tingling of legs, feet, toes

*Role-relationship:* Occupations requiring heavy lifting, vibrations, or extended driving. Change in role within family structure due to inability to work and provide income

**Objective Data**

***General***

Guarded movement

***Neurologic***

Depressed or absent Achilles tendon reflex or patellar tendon reflex. Positive straight-leg-raising test, positive crossover straight-leg-raising test, positive Trendelenburg test

***Musculoskeletal***

Tense, tight paravertebral muscles on palpation, ↓ range of motion in spine

***Possible Diagnostic Findings***

Localization of site of lesion or disorder on myelogram, CT scan, or MRI. Determination of nerve root impingement on electromyography (EMG)

### Nursing Implementation

**Health Promotion.** Use proper body mechanics at all times to serve as a role model. This includes increasing the patient's bed height, bending at the knees, asking for help in lifting and moving patients, and using lifting devices.

Assess the patient's use of body mechanics and offer advice when the person does activities that could produce back strain (Table 63-6). Some HCPs refer patients with back pain to a program called "Back School." This formal program is usually taught by health care professionals such as HCPs, nurses, and physical therapists. It is designed to teach the patient how to minimize back pain and avoid repeat episodes of low back pain. Tips for prevention of back injury are listed in Table 63-6. Referral to a physical therapist or personal trainer to address posture as well as core and abdomen strength may also be appropriate. Recommend flat shoes or shoes with low heels and shock-absorbing shoe inserts for women.

Advise patients to maintain a healthy body weight. Excess body weight places additional stress on the lower back. It also weakens abdominal muscles that support the lower back. The position assumed while sleeping is also important in preventing low back pain. Advise patients to avoid sleeping in a prone position because it produces excessive lumbar lordosis, placing excessive stress on the lower back. Encourage the patient to sleep in a supine or side-lying position with knees and hips flexed to prevent unnecessary pressure on support muscles, ligaments, and lumbosacral joints. Recommend use of a firm mattress.

Teach patients the importance of smoking cessation. Tobacco use impairs circulation to the intervertebral discs and may contribute to low back pain.

**Acute Care.** If acute muscle spasms and accompanying pain are not severe and unbearable, the patient may be treated as an outpatient with NSAIDs and muscle relaxants (e.g., cyclobenzaprine). Massage and back manipulation, acupuncture, and the application of cold and hot compresses may help some patients.[13] Severe pain may require a brief course of corticosteroids or opioid analgesics.

Some people may need a brief period (1 to 2 days) of rest at home but should avoid prolonged bed rest.[14] Most patients do better if they continue their regular activities. Patients should refrain from activities that increase the pain, including lifting, bending, twisting, and prolonged sitting. Symptoms of acute low back pain generally improve within 2 weeks and often resolve without treatment.

Teach the patient about the cause of the pain and ways to prevent additional episodes. Muscle stretching and strengthening exercises may be part of the management plan. Although

**TABLE 63-6 Patient & Caregiver Teaching**

***Low Back Problems***

*Include the following instructions when teaching the patient and caregiver how to manage low back problems.*

**Do**

- Maintain healthy body weight.
- Maintain a neutral pelvic position if standing. Place one foot on a low stool if standing for long periods.
- Choose a seat with good lower back support, armrests, and a swivel base. Place a pillow at the lumbar spine to maintain normal curvature. Keep knees and hips level.
- Sleep in a side-lying position with knees and hips bent, and a pillow between the knees for support.
- Sleep on back with a lift under knees and legs or on back with 10-in–high pillow under knees to flex hips and knees.
- Use proper body mechanics when lifting heavy objects. Bend at the knees, not at the waist, and stand up slowly while holding object close to your body.
- Participate in regular strength and flexibility training and low-impact aerobic exercise.
- Use local heat and cold application to relieve muscle tension.

**Do Not**

- Lean forward without bending knees.
- Lift anything above level of elbows.
- Stand unmoving for prolonged time.
- Sleep on abdomen or on back or side with legs out straight.
- Exercise without consulting HCP if having severe pain.
- Exceed prescribed amount and type of exercises without consulting HCP.
- Smoke or use tobacco products.

exercises are often taught by a physical therapist, reinforce the type and frequency of prescribed exercise and the rationale for the program.

Other nursing interventions for the patient with low back pain are summarized in eNursing Care Plan 63-2 (on the website for this chapter).

◆ **Ambulatory Care.** The goal of management is to make an episode of acute low back pain an isolated incident. If the lumbosacral area is unstable, repeated episodes are likely. Obesity, poor posture, poor muscle support, older age, or trauma may weaken the lumbosacral spine, so it is unable to meet the demands placed on it without strain. Exercise is aimed at strengthening the supporting muscles (see earlier).

Persistent use of poor body mechanics may also result in repeated episodes of low back pain. If the strain is work related, occupational counseling may be needed. Low back pain can cause frustration, pain, and disability. Provide emotional support and understanding care of the patient.

## CHRONIC LOW BACK PAIN

*Chronic low back pain* lasts more than 3 months or involves a repeated incapacitating episode. It is often progressive, and the cause can be difficult to determine. Causes include (1) degenerative conditions such as arthritis or disc disease; (2) osteoporosis or other metabolic bone diseases; (3) weakness from the scar tissue of prior injury; (4) chronic strain on lower back muscles from obesity, pregnancy, or stressful postures on the job; and (5) congenital spine problems.

### Spinal Stenosis

*Spinal stenosis* is a narrowing of the spinal canal (contains the spinal cord). Stenosis in the lumbar spine is a common cause of chronic low back pain. Spinal stenosis can be caused by acquired or inherited conditions. A common acquired cause is osteoarthritis. Arthritic changes (bone spurs, calcification of spinal ligaments, disc degeneration) narrow the space around the spinal canal and nerve roots, eventually leading to compression. Inflammation caused by the compression results in pain, weakness, and numbness.

Other acquired conditions that may cause spinal stenosis include rheumatoid arthritis, spinal tumors, Paget's disease, and traumatic damage to the vertebral column. Inherited conditions that lead to spinal stenosis include congenital spinal stenosis and scoliosis.

The pain associated with lumbar spinal stenosis often starts in the lower back and then radiates to the buttock and leg. It is worse with walking or prolonged standing. Numbness, tingling, weakness, and heaviness in the legs and buttocks may also be present. History of decreased pain when the patient bends forward or sits is often a sign of spinal stenosis. In most cases, stenosis slowly progresses.

## ❖ NURSING AND INTERPROFESSIONAL MANAGEMENT: CHRONIC LOW BACK PAIN

Nursing management and treatment of chronic low back pain are similar to acute low back pain. Manage the patient's pain and stiffness with mild analgesics, such as NSAIDs, for daily comfort. Antidepressants (e.g., duloxetine [Cymbalta]) may help with pain management and sleep problems. The antiseizure drug gabapentin (Neurontin) may improve walking and relieve leg symptoms.

Weight reduction, sufficient rest periods, local heat or cold application, physical therapy, and exercise and activity throughout the day assist in keeping the muscles and joints mobilized. Cold, damp weather aggravates the back pain, which can be decreased with rest and local heat application. Complementary and alternative therapies such as biofeedback, acupuncture, and yoga may also help reduce the pain. "Back School" (discussed on p. 1503) can significantly reduce pain and improve body posture.[15]

Minimally invasive treatments, such as epidural corticosteroid injections and implanted devices that deliver pain medication, may be used for patients with chronic low back pain that fails to respond to the usual therapeutic options. Surgical intervention may be indicated in patients with severe chronic low back pain who receive no benefit from conservative care and/or have continued neurologic deficits. (Surgery for low back pain is discussed on p. 1506.)

## INTERVERTEBRAL DISC DISEASE

Intervertebral discs separate the vertebrae and help absorb shock for the spine. *Intervertebral disc disease* involves the deterioration, herniation, or other dysfunction of the intervertebral discs. Disc disorders can affect the cervical, thoracic, and lumbar spine.

### Etiology and Pathophysiology

**Degenerative disc disease (DDD)** results from loss of fluid in the intervertebral discs with aging. The discs lose their elasticity, flexibility, and shock-absorbing abilities. Unless it is accompanied by pain, this condition is a normal process.[16] The discs become thinner as the *nucleus pulposus* (gelatinous center of the disc) starts to dry out and shrink. This change limits the disc's ability to distribute pressure between vertebrae. The pressure is then transferred to the *annulus fibrosus* (strong outside portion of the disc), causing progressive destruction. When the disc is damaged, the nucleus pulposus may seep through a torn or stretched annulus. This is called a **herniated disc** *(slipped disc),* a condition in which a spinal disc bulges outward between the vertebrae (Fig. 63-4).

A herniated disc can result from degeneration with age or repeated stress and trauma to the spine. The most common sites of herniation are the lumbosacral discs, specifically L4-5 and L5-S1. Disc herniation may also occur at C5-6 and C6-7. Disc herniation may be the result of spinal stenosis, in which narrowing of the spinal canal forces the intervertebral disc to bulge.

The spinal nerves emerge from the spinal column through an opening *(intervertebral foramen)* between adjacent vertebrae. Herniated discs can press against these nerves ("pinched nerve") causing *radiculopathy* (radiating pain, numbness, tingling, and diminished strength and/or range of motion).

Osteoarthritis (OA) of the spine is associated with DDD and the stresses placed on the vertebrae. As the poorly lubricated joints rub against each other, the protective cartilage is damaged and painful bone spurs occur as one of the changes found in OA.

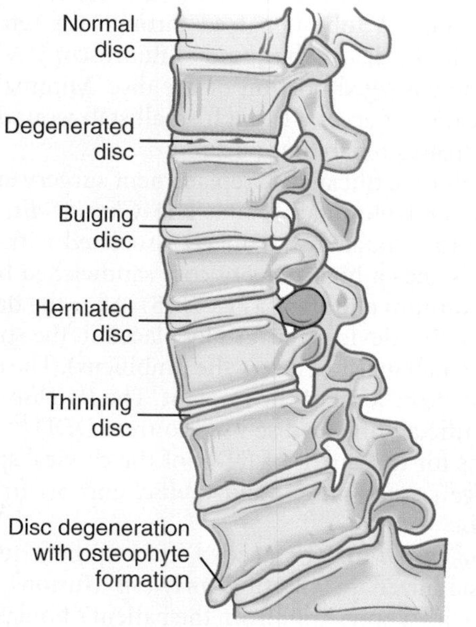


**FIG. 63-4** Common causes of degenerative disc damage.

## Clinical Manifestations

In *lumbar disc disease*, the most common manifestation is low back pain. Radicular pain that radiates down the buttock and below the knee, along the distribution of the sciatic nerve, generally indicates disc herniation. (Specific manifestations of lumbar disc herniation are summarized in Table 63-7.) A positive straight-leg-raising test may indicate nerve root irritation (see Chapter 61, p. 1455). Back or leg pain may be reproduced by raising the leg.

Low back pain from other causes may not be accompanied by leg pain. Reflexes may be depressed or absent, depending on the spinal nerve root involved. Numbness and tingling *(paresthesia)* or muscle weakness in the legs, feet, or toes may occur.

Multiple nerve root compressions *(cauda equina syndrome)* from a herniated disc, tumor, or an epidural abscess may be marked by (1) severe low back pain, (2) progressive weakness, (3) increased pain, and (4) bowel and bladder incontinence.[17] This condition is a medical emergency that requires surgical decompression to reduce pressure on the nerves.

In *cervical disc disease,* pain radiates into the arms and hands, following the pattern of the involved nerve. Similar to lumbar disc disease, reflexes may or may not be present. The handgrip is often weak. Because manifestations of cervical disc disease may include shoulder pain and dysfunction, the HCP must rule out shoulder disorders as part of the diagnosis.

## Diagnostic Studies

X-rays are done to detect any structural defects. A myelogram, MRI, or CT scan is helpful in localizing the damaged site. An epidural venogram or diskogram may be needed if other diagnostic studies are inconclusive. An EMG of the extremities can be performed to determine the severity of nerve irritation or to rule out other conditions such as peripheral neuropathy.

## Interprofessional Care

The patient with suspected disc damage is usually managed with conservative therapy (Table 63-8). This includes limitation of extremes of spinal movement (brace, corset, or belt), local heat or ice, ultrasound and massage, traction, and transcutaneous electrical nerve stimulation (TENS). Drug therapy to manage pain includes NSAIDs, short-term use of oral corticosteroids, opioid analgesics, muscle relaxants, antiseizure drugs, and antidepressants.[18] Epidural corticosteroid injections may reduce inflammation and relieve acute pain. However, if the underlying cause remains, pain tends to recur.

When symptoms subside, the patient should begin back-strengthening exercises twice a day and continue for life. Teach the patient the principles of good body mechanics. Discourage extremes of flexion and torsion. With a conservative treatment plan, most patients heal after 6 months.

**TABLE 63-7 Manifestations of Lumbar Disc Herniation***

| Intervertebral Level | Pain | Affected Reflex | Motor Function | Sensation |
|---|---|---|---|---|
| L3-4 | Back to buttocks to posterior thigh to inner calf | Patellar | Quadriceps, anterior tibialis | Inner aspect of lower leg, anterior part of thigh |
| L4-5 | Back to buttocks to dorsum of foot and big toe | None | Anterior tibialis, extensor hallucis longus, gluteus medius | Dorsum of foot and big toe |
| L5-S1 | Back to buttocks to sole of foot and heel | Achilles | Gastrocnemius, hamstring, gluteus maximus | Heel and lateral foot |

*A disc herniation can involve pressure on more than one nerve root.

**TABLE 63-8 Interprofessional Care**

***Intervertebral Disc Disease***

**Diagnostic Assessment**
- History and physical examination
- X-ray
- CT scan
- MRI
- Myelogram
- Diskogram
- Electromyogram (EMG)

**Management**

***Conservative Therapy***
- Restricted activity for several days, limited total bed rest
- Local ice or heat
- Physical therapy
- Analgesics (e.g., tramadol [Ultram])
- Nonsteroidal antiinflammatory drugs
- Muscle relaxants (e.g., cyclobenzaprine)
- Antiseizure drugs (e.g., gabapentin)
- Antidepressants (e.g., pregabalin [Lyrica])
- Epidural corticosteroid injections

***Surgical Therapy***
- Intradiscal electrothermoplasty (IDET)
- Radiofrequency discal nucleoplasty
- Interspinous process decompression system (X-Stop)
- Laminectomy with or without spinal fusion
- Discectomy
- Percutaneous laser discectomy
- Artificial disc replacement (e.g., Charité disc)
- Spinal fusion with instrumentation (e.g., plates, screws) or without instrumentation

**Surgical Therapy.** If conservative treatment is unsuccessful, radiculopathy becomes worse, or loss of bowel or bladder control (cauda equina syndrome) occurs, surgery may be considered. Surgery for a damaged disc is generally performed if the patient is in constant pain and/or has a persistent neurologic deficit.

*Intradiscal electrothermoplasty* (IDET) is a minimally invasive outpatient procedure for treatment of back and sciatic pain. A needle is inserted into the affected disc with x-ray guidance. A wire is then threaded through the needle and into the disc. As the wire is heated, small nerve fibers that have invaded the degenerating disc are destroyed. The heat also partially melts the annulus fibrosus. This causes the body to generate new reinforcing proteins in the fibers of the annulus.

Another outpatient technique is *radiofrequency discal nucleoplasty* (coblation nucleoplasty). A needle is inserted into the disc similar to IDET. Instead of a heated wire, a special radiofrequency probe is used. The probe generates energy that breaks the molecular bonds of the gel in the nucleus pulposus. Up to 20% of the nucleus is removed. This decompresses the disc and reduces pressure on the disc and surrounding nerve roots. Subsequent pain relief varies.

A third procedure involves use of an *interspinous process decompression system* (X-Stop). This titanium device fits onto a mount that is placed on vertebrae in the lower back. The X-Stop is used in patients with pain due to lumbar spinal stenosis. The device works by lifting vertebrae off the pinched nerve.

*Laminectomy* is a common, traditional surgical procedure for lumbar disc disease. It involves surgical excision of part of the vertebra (referred to as the *lamina*) to access and remove

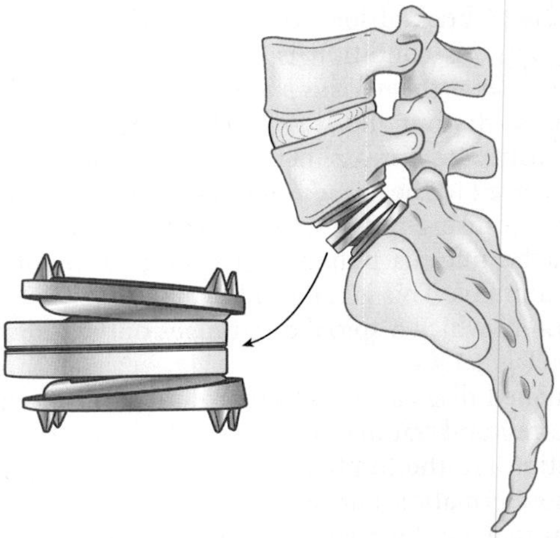

FIG. 63-5 The Charité artificial disc, used to replace a damaged intervertebral disc in degenerative disc disease of the lumbar spine. A movable high-density plastic core is sandwiched between two cobalt-chromium alloy endplates. The disc's design helps realign the spine and preserve movement.

the protruding disc. Laminectomy is often performed as an outpatient procedure, but a hospital stay of 1 to 3 days is not uncommon.

*Discectomy* can also be performed to decompress the nerve root.[11] Microsurgical discectomy is a version of the standard procedure. The surgeon uses a microscope for better visualization of the disc and disc space to aid in removal of the damaged portion. This helps maintain bony stability of the spine.

*Percutaneous discectomy* is a safe and effective outpatient surgical procedure. A tube is passed through the retroperitoneal soft tissues to the disc with the aid of fluoroscopy. A laser is then used on the damaged portion of the disc. Minimal blood loss occurs because of access through small stab wounds. The procedure decreases rehabilitation time.

The goals of artificial disc replacement surgery are to restore movement and eliminate pain. The *Charité disc* is used in patients with lumbar disc damage associated with DDD. This artificial disc has a high-density core sandwiched between two cobalt-chromium endplates (Fig. 63-5). After the damaged disc is removed, this device is surgically placed in the spine (usually through a small incision below the umbilicus). The disc restores movement at the level of the implant. The *ProDisc-L* is another type of artificial lumbar disc used to treat DDD.[19]

Options for treatment of DDD of the cervical spine include the *Prestige cervical disc, Mobi-C disc,* and *Secure-C artificial cervical disc.*

A *spinal fusion* may be needed if the spine is unstable. The spine is stabilized by creating *ankylosis* (fusion) of adjacent vertebrae with a bone graft from the patient's fibula or iliac crest *(autograft)* or from donated cadaver bone *(allograft)*. Metal fixation with rods, plates, or screws may also be placed at the time of spinal surgery to provide more stability and decrease vertebral motion. A posterior lumbar fusion may be performed in patients to provide extra support for bone grafting or a prosthetic device.

Bone morphogenetic protein (BMP), a genetically engineered protein, may be used to stimulate bone growth of the graft in spinal fusions.[20] A dissolvable sponge soaked with BMP is implanted into the spine. The protein on the sponge stimulates the body's cells to become active and produce bone. BMP begins the process of fusion, which continues after the protein and sponge dissolve to leave living bone behind.

## NURSING MANAGEMENT: VERTEBRAL DISC SURGERY

After vertebral disc surgery, postoperative nursing interventions mainly focus on maintaining proper alignment of the spine until it has healed. Depending on the type and extent of surgery and the surgeon's preference, the patient may be able to dangle the legs at the side of the bed, stand, or even ambulate the day of surgery.

After lumbar fusion, place pillows under the patient's thighs when supine and between the legs when in the side-lying position to provide comfort and ensure alignment. The patient often fears turning or any movement that may increase pain by stressing the surgical area. Reassure the patient that proper technique is being used to maintain body alignment. Enough staff should be available to move the patient without undue pain or strain for the patient or staff.

Postoperatively, most patients require opioids such as morphine IV for 24 to 48 hours. Patient-controlled analgesia (PCA) allows maintenance of optimal analgesic levels and is the preferred method of continuous pain management. Once the patient receives oral fluids, oral drugs such as acetaminophen with codeine, hydrocodone, or oxycodone (Percocet) may be used. Diazepam (Valium) may be prescribed for muscle relaxation. Assess and document pain intensity and pain management effectiveness.

Because the spinal canal may be entered during surgery, cerebrospinal fluid (CSF) leakage is possible. Immediately report leakage of CSF on the dressing or if the patient complains of severe headache. CSF appears as clear or slightly yellow drainage on the dressing. It has a high glucose concentration and is positive for glucose when tested with a dipstick. Note the amount, color, and characteristics of drainage.

Frequently assess the patient's peripheral neurologic condition after spinal surgery. Movement of the arms and legs and assessment of sensation should at least equal the preoperative status. Repeat these assessments every 2 to 4 hours during the first 48 hours after surgery and compare with the preoperative assessment. Paresthesia may not be relieved immediately after surgery. Report any new muscle weakness or paresthesia immediately to the surgeon and document this finding in the patient's medical record. Assess extremity circulation using skin temperature, capillary refill, and pulses.

Paralytic ileus and interference with bowel function may occur for several days and may manifest as nausea, abdominal distention, and constipation. Opioids can also slow bowel elimination. Assess if the patient is passing gas, has bowel sounds in all quadrants, and has a flat, soft abdomen. Stool softeners (e.g., docusate [Colace]) and laxatives may prevent and relieve constipation.

Emptying the bladder may be difficult due to activity restrictions, opioids, or anesthesia. Encourage men to dangle the legs over the side of the bed or stand to urinate if allowed by the surgeon. Urge patients to use a bedside commode or ambulate to the bathroom when allowed to promote bladder emptying. Ensure that privacy is maintained. Intermittent catheterization or an indwelling urinary catheter may be needed by patients who have difficulty urinating.

Loss of sphincter tone or bladder tone may indicate nerve damage. Monitor for incontinence or difficulty with bowel or bladder elimination, and immediately report problems to the surgeon.

In addition to nursing care appropriate for a patient who had a laminectomy, other nursing activities are indicated if the patient has also had a spinal fusion. Because a bone graft is usually involved, the postoperative healing time is prolonged compared with a laminectomy. Activity limitations may be needed for an extended time. A rigid orthosis (thoracic-lumbar-sacral orthosis [TLSO] or chairback brace) is often used during this period. Some surgeons want patients to be taught to apply and remove the brace by logrolling in bed. Others allow their patients to apply the brace in a sitting or standing position. Verify the surgeon's preferred method before starting this activity.

If surgery is done on the cervical spine, be alert for indications of spinal cord edema such as respiratory distress and a worsening neurologic condition of the upper extremities. After surgery, the patient's neck may be immobilized in a soft or hard cervical collar.

In addition to the primary surgical site, regularly assess the bone graft donor site. The posterior iliac crest is the most commonly used donor site, although the fibula may also be used. The donor site usually causes greater pain than the spinal fusion area. The donor site is bandaged with a pressure dressing to prevent excessive bleeding. If the donor site is the fibula, frequent neurovascular assessment of the extremity is a postoperative nursing responsibility.

After spinal fusion, the patient may experience some immobility of the spine at the fusion site. Instruct the patient to use proper body mechanics and avoid sitting or standing for prolonged periods. Encourage activities that include walking, lying down, and shifting weight from one foot to the other when standing. Instruct the patient on any lifting restrictions after spinal surgery. Encourage the patient to think through an activity before starting any potentially injurious task such as bending or stooping. Any twisting movement of the spine is contraindicated. Teach the patient to use the thighs and knees, rather than the back, to absorb the shock of activity and movement. A firm mattress or bed board is essential.

## NECK PAIN

Neck pain occurs almost as frequently as low back pain, affecting up to 10% of adults at any point in time. Neck pain may result from many different conditions, including benign (e.g., poor posture) and serious (e.g., herniated cervical disc)[21] (Table 63-9).

Cervical neck sprains and strains occur from hyperflexion and hyperextension injuries. Patients complain of stiffness and neck pain with possible radicular pain into the arm and hand. Pain may also radiate to the head, anterior chest, thoracic spine region, and shoulders. Weakness or paresthesia of the arm and hand may suggest cervical nerve root compression from stenosis, DDD, or herniation.

The cause of neck pain is diagnosed by history, physical examination, x-ray, MRI, CT scan, and myelogram. An EMG of the upper extremities may diagnose cervical radiculopathy.

**TABLE 63-9 Causes of Neck Pain**

| | |
|---|---|
| • Poor posture | • Spondylosis |
| • Strain or sprain | • Rheumatoid arthritis |
| • Degenerative disc disease, including herniation | • Tumor |
| • Trauma (e.g., fractures, subluxation) | • Osteoporosis |
| | • Osteomyelitis |
| | • Meningitis |

**TABLE 63-10 Patient & Caregiver Teaching**

***Neck Exercises***

*When teaching the patient exercises for neck pain, include the following instructions for the patient and caregiver.*

- Bend your head backward until you are looking up at the ceiling. Repeat slowly five times. Stop if experiencing dizziness.
- Bring your head forward so that your chin touches your chest and your face is looking down at the floor. Repeat slowly five times.
- With your head facing forward, bend your ear down toward one shoulder. Alternate this movement with your other ear. Repeat slowly five times on each side.
- Turn your head slowly around to one side as far as it will go. Repeat toward the other side. Repeat exercise five times on each side.

Conservative treatment for neck pain in patients without an underlying disorder includes head support using a soft cervical collar, gentle traction, heat and ice applications, massage, rest until symptoms subside, ultrasound, and NSAIDs. Therapeutic neck exercises and acupuncture may also be used for pain relief.[22] Most neck pain resolves without surgical intervention.

Preventing neck pain that occurs with everyday activities such as prolonged sitting at a computer or television, sleeping in nonaligned spinal positions, or making jarring movements during exercise is important. Encourage patients to practice good posture and maintain neck flexibility (Table 63-10).

## FOOT DISORDERS

The foot is the platform that supports the weight of the body and absorbs shock when the person ambulates. It is a complicated structure composed of bony structures, muscles, tendons, and ligaments that can be affected by (1) congenital conditions, (2) structural weakness, (3) traumatic and stress injuries, and (4) systemic conditions such as diabetes mellitus and rheumatoid arthritis. A great deal of the pain, deformity, and disability of foot disorders can be directly attributed to or worsened by poorly fitting shoes. Shoes may cause crowding and angulation of the toes and inhibit normal movement of foot muscles.

Footwear is used to (1) provide support, foot stability, protection, shock absorption, and a foundation for orthoses; (2) increase friction with the walking surface; and (3) treat foot abnormalities. (Table 63-11 summarizes common foot disorders.)

## NURSING MANAGEMENT: FOOT DISORDERS

### Nursing Implementation

**Health Promotion.** Well-made and properly fitted shoes are essential for healthy, pain-free feet. Women's footwear is often influenced by current styles instead of comfort and support. Stress the importance of having a shoe that conforms to the foot rather than to fashion trends. The shoe must be long enough and wide enough to avoid crowding the toes and forcing the great toe into a position of **hallux valgus** (Fig. 63-6). At the metatarsal head, the shoe should be wide enough to allow foot muscles to move freely and toes to bend. The shank (narrow part of sole under the instep) of the shoe should be rigid enough to give good support. The height of the heel should be realistic in relation to the shoe's purpose. Ideally, the heel of the shoe should not rise more than 1 inch higher than the forefoot support. Wearing higher-heeled shoes with a narrow toe box will cause hammertoes and corns over time.

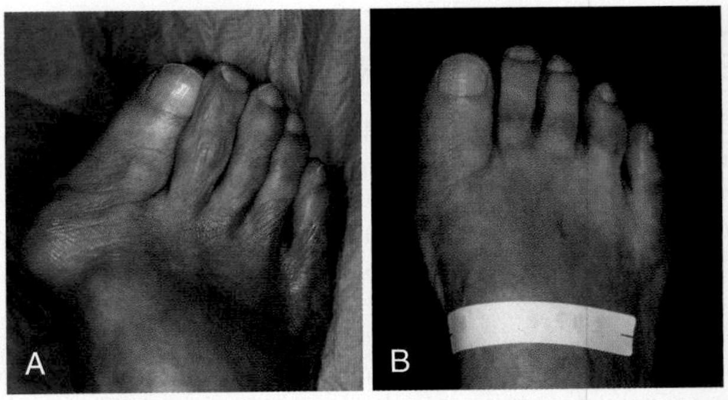

**FIG. 63-6** **A,** Severe hallux valgus with bursa formation. **B,** Postoperative correction. (From Canale ST, Beaty JH: *Campbell's operative orthopaedics,* ed 12, Philadelphia, 2013, Mosby.)

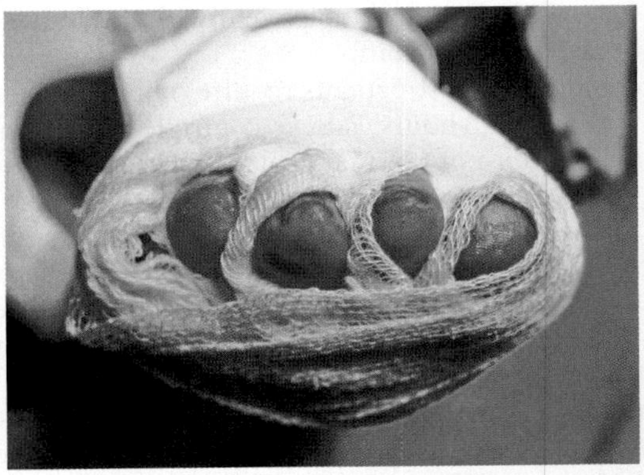

**FIG. 63-7** Postoperative supportive dressing for treatment of moderate forefoot deformity. Dressing must be conforming and binding enough to hold toe in exact position. (From Canale ST, Beaty JH: *Campbell's operative orthopaedics,* ed 12, Philadelphia, 2013, Mosby.)

Prolonged use of this type of footwear can also result in a *Morton's neuroma* (compression of an intermetatarsal plantar nerve, usually between the third and fourth toes, resulting in paresthesia). Initially, patients with Morton's neuroma may complain of feeling as if a sock is rolled up under their toes.[23]

**Acute Care.** Many foot problems require referral to a podiatrist. Depending on the problem, conservative therapies are tried first (Table 63-11). These therapies include NSAIDs, shock-wave therapy, ice, physical therapy, footwear alterations, stretching, warm soaks, orthotics, ultrasound, and corticosteroid injections. If these methods do not help, surgery may be recommended.

Depending on the type of surgery, pins or wires may extend through the toes, or a protective splint may be placed over the end of the foot. Postoperatively, the foot is usually immobilized by a bulky dressing (Fig. 63-7), short leg cast, slipper (plaster)

**CHECK YOUR PRACTICE**

A 52-yr-old woman is scheduled for surgical correction of a bunion after a diagnosis of hallux valgus. You are doing her preoperative assessment. She asks you, "Do you think I caused this problem? I have been so vain all my life and had to wear only fancy shoes. Now I have to wear an ugly bunion shoe. I am not sure I can handle taking care of myself after surgery."

- How will you respond when the patient asks about the cause of this disorder?
- What teaching will you provide her about her postoperative care?

**TABLE 63-11 Common Foot Disorders**

| Disorder | Description | Treatment |
|---|---|---|
| **Forefoot** | | |
| **Hallux valgus** (bunion) | Painful deformity of great toe with lateral angulation of great toe toward second toe, bony enlargement of medial side of first metatarsal head, swelling of bursa and formation of callus over bony enlargement (Fig. 63-6). | • Conservative treatment includes wearing shoes with wide forefoot or "bunion pocket" and use of bunion pads to relieve pressure on bursal sac.<br>• Surgical treatment involves removal of bursal sac and bony enlargement and correction of lateral angulation of great toe.<br>• May include temporary or permanent internal fixation. |
| **Hallux rigidus** | Painful stiffness of first MTP joint caused by osteoarthritis or local trauma. | • Conservative treatment includes intraarticular corticosteroids and passive manual stretching of first MTP joint.<br>• Shoe with a stiff sole decreases pain in the joint during walking.<br>• Surgical treatment is joint fusion or arthroplasty with silicone rubber implant. |
| **Hammer and claw toes** | Hammer toe is a deformity of PIP joint on 2nd to 5th toes causing toe to be permanently bent, resembling a hammer. Mallet toe is a similar condition affecting the DIP joint. Claw toe is a similar deformity with dorsiflexion of the proximal phalanx on the MTP joint combined with flexion of both PIP and DIP joints. Complaints include burning on bottom of foot and pain and difficulty walking when wearing shoes. | • Conservative treatment includes passive manual stretching of PIP joint and use of metatarsal arch support.<br>• Surgical correction consists of resection of base of middle phalanx and head of proximal phalanx, bringing raw bone ends together.<br>• Kirschner wire maintains straight position. |
| **Morton's neuroma** (Morton's toe or plantar neuroma) | Neuroma in web space between third and fourth metatarsal heads, causing sharp, sudden attacks of pain and burning sensations. | • Surgical excision is the usual treatment. |
| **Midfoot** | | |
| **Pes planus** (flatfoot) | Loss of metatarsal arch causing pain in foot or leg. | • Symptoms are relieved by use of resilient longitudinal arch supports.<br>• Surgical treatment consists of triple arthrodesis or fusion of subtalar joint. |
| **Pes cavus** | Elevation of longitudinal arch of foot resulting from contracture of plantar fascia or bony deformity of arch. | • Surgical correction is needed if condition interferes with ambulation. |
| **Hindfoot** | | |
| **Painful heels** | Complaint of heel pain with weight bearing. Common causes are plantar bursitis, plantar fasciitis, or bone spur. | • Corticosteroids are injected locally into inflamed bursa, and sponge-rubber heel cup is used.<br>• Surgical excision of bursa or spur is performed.<br>• Stretching exercises, ice, shoe heel cup, shock-wave therapy, NSAIDs, and corticosteroids are used for plantar fasciitis. |
| **Calcaneus stress fracture** | Complaint of heel pain after moderate walking. Common causes are overtraining, running on hard surfaces, or osteoporosis. | • Rest, ice, shoe heel pad, and NSAIDs are used.<br>• See HCP to assess for osteoporosis. |
| **Other Problems** | | |
| **Corn** | Localized thickening of skin caused by continual pressure over bony prominences, especially metatarsal head, frequently causing localized pain. | • Corn is softened with warm water or preparations containing salicylic acid and trimmed with razor blade or scalpel.<br>• Pressure on bony prominences caused by shoes is relieved. |
| **Soft corn** | Painful lesion caused by bony prominence of one toe pressing against adjacent toe. Usual location is web space between toes. Softness caused by secretions keeping web space relatively moist. | • Pain is relieved by placing cotton or spacers between toes to separate them.<br>• Surgical treatment is excision of projecting bone spur (if present). |
| **Callus** | Similar formation to corn but covering wider area and usually located on weight-bearing part of foot. | • Same as for corn. |
| **Plantar wart** | Painful papillomatous growth caused by virus that may occur on any part of skin on sole of foot. Warts tend to cluster on pressure points. | • Remedies containing salicylic acid (e.g., Compound W), excision with electrocoagulation, or surgical removal.<br>• Laser treatments may also be used.<br>• May disappear without treatment. |

*DIP*, Distal interphalangeal; *MTP*, metatarsophalangeal; *PIP*, proximal interphalangeal.

cast, or a platform shoe that fits over the dressing and has a rigid sole (also known as a *bunion shoe*).

Elevate the foot with the heel off the bed to reduce discomfort and prevent edema. Assess neurovascular condition frequently during the immediate postoperative period. Inserted devices may interfere with assessment for movement. Also be aware that evaluating sensation may be difficult because the patient may be unable to differentiate surgical pain from pain caused by nerve pressure or circulatory impairment.

The type and extent of surgery determine the orders for ambulation. Crutches, a walker, or a cane may be needed. The patient may experience pain or a throbbing sensation when lowering the affected leg. Reinforce instructions from the physical therapist. Remind the patient of the importance of walking with an erect posture with proper weight distribution. Report gait problems or continued pain to the surgeon. Instruct the patient about the importance of frequent rest periods with the foot elevated.

◆ **Ambulatory Care.** Instruct the patient to perform daily hygienic foot care and wear clean stockings. Stockings should be long enough to avoid wrinkling and causing pressure areas. Trimming toenails straight across helps prevent ingrown toenails and reduces the risk of infection. Provide detailed instruction to patients with impaired circulation or diabetes mellitus to prevent serious complications from blisters, pressure areas, and infection. (See Table 48-21 for guidelines on foot care.)

### Gerontologic Considerations: Foot Problems

The older adult is prone to foot problems because of poor circulation, atherosclerosis, and decreased sensation in the lower extremities. This is especially true for older patients with diabetes mellitus.[24] A patient may develop an open wound but not feel it because of altered sensation from peripheral vascular disease or diabetic neuropathy. Instruct older adults to inspect their feet daily and report any open wounds or breaks in the skin to their HCP.[25]

Untreated wounds may become infected, lead to osteomyelitis, and require surgical debridement. If the infection becomes widespread, lower limb amputation may be necessary. Teach the caregiver of the older adult who needs assistance with hygiene practices the importance of carefully assessing the feet at regular intervals.

## METABOLIC BONE DISEASES

Normal bone metabolism is affected by hormones, nutrition, and genetics. When dysfunction occurs in any of these factors, generalized reduction in bone mass and strength may result. Metabolic bone diseases include osteomalacia, osteoporosis, and Paget's disease.

## OSTEOMALACIA

**Osteomalacia** is caused by a vitamin D deficiency that causes bone to lose calcium and become soft. The disease is uncommon in the United States. It is the same disorder as rickets in children, except the epiphyseal growth plates are closed in adults. Vitamin D is required for the absorption of calcium from the intestine. Insufficient vitamin D intake can interfere with normal bone mineralization; with little or no calcification, bones become soft.

Causes of osteomalacia include limited sun exposure (ultraviolet rays needed for vitamin D synthesis), GI malabsorption, extensive burns, chronic diarrhea, pregnancy, kidney disease, and use of drugs such as phenytoin (Dilantin). Residents of long-term care settings may have inadequate sun exposure and thus poor synthesis of vitamin D. Persons with dark skin also do not synthesize vitamin D as easily as persons with fair skin. Obese persons are at higher risk for osteomalacia because of decreased physical activity and poor diet (i.e., inadequate calcium and vitamin D intake). Chronic diseases of the liver, kidneys, and small intestine may also contribute to vitamin D deficiency. Long-term use of antiseizure drugs, phosphate-binding antacids (e.g., Maalox), sedatives, and muscle relaxants may decrease calcium and vitamin D absorption.[26]

Common manifestations of osteomalacia are bone pain and difficulty walking or rising from a chair.[27] Other manifestations include muscle weakness, especially in the pelvic girdle, weight loss, and progressive deformity of weight-bearing bones (e.g., spine, extremities). Fractures are common and indicate delayed bone healing.

Laboratory findings commonly include decreased serum calcium or phosphorus, decreased serum 25-hydroxyvitamin D, and elevated serum alkaline phosphatase. X-rays may show effects of generalized bone demineralization, especially loss of calcium in the bones of the pelvis and associated bone deformity. *Looser's transformation zones* (ribbons of decalcification in bone found on x-ray) are diagnostic of osteomalacia. However, significant osteomalacia may exist without changes on x-ray.

Interprofessional care of osteomalacia is directed toward correction of vitamin D deficiency. The patient often shows a dramatic response when vitamin $D_3$ (cholecalciferol) and vitamin $D_2$ (ergocalciferol) supplements are used. Calcium or phosphorus supplements may also be prescribed. Encourage dietary intake of eggs, meat, and oily fish (e.g., salmon, tuna). Milk and breakfast cereals fortified with calcium and vitamin D should also be included in the diet. Exposure to sunlight and weight-bearing exercise are valuable as well.

Patients who have bariatric surgery to treat obesity should be assessed for osteomalacia. Any vitamin D deficiencies should be corrected before surgery.[26]

## OSTEOPOROSIS

**Osteoporosis** is a chronic, progressive metabolic bone disease marked by low bone mass and deterioration of bone tissue, leading to increased bone fragility (Fig. 63-8). More than 54 million persons in the United States have decreased bone density or osteoporosis.[28] One in two women and one in four men over age 50 will sustain an osteoporosis-related fracture during their lifetime. Osteoporosis is known as the "silent thief" because it slowly robs the skeleton of its banked resources. Bones eventually become so fragile that they cannot withstand normal mechanical stress.

Osteoporosis is more common in women than in men for several reasons: (1) women tend to have lower calcium intake than men throughout their lives (men between 15 and 50 years of age consume twice as much calcium as women); (2) women have less bone mass because of their generally smaller frames; (3) bone resorption begins at an earlier age in women and becomes more rapid at menopause; (4) pregnancy and breast-feeding deplete a woman's skeletal reserve unless calcium intake is adequate; and (5) longevity increases the likelihood of osteoporosis.

Current guidelines recommend an initial bone density test in all women over age 65 years. Women who are younger than

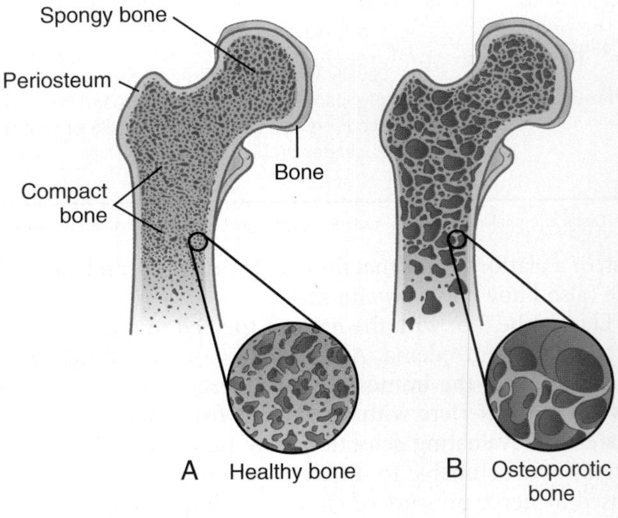


**FIG. 63-8** **A,** Normal bone. **B,** Osteoporotic bone.

65 and at high risk (e.g., low body weight, smoker, prior fractures) should also have a bone density test. If results are normal and the person is at low risk for osteoporosis, another test is not needed for 15 years. Testing should start earlier and be done more frequently if a person is at high risk for fractures. Currently there is not sufficient evidence to demonstrate significant benefit for osteoporosis screening in men.[29]

### CULTURAL & ETHNIC HEALTH DISPARITIES

#### Osteoporosis

- White and Asian American women have a higher incidence of osteoporosis than Native American, Hispanic, and African American women.
- African American women begin menopause with more bone mass and have a lower rate of bone loss after menopause than non–African American women.
- Risk of fracture in white women is higher than in nonwhite women of the same age.

## Etiology and Pathophysiology

Risk factors for osteoporosis are listed in Table 63-12. Decreased risk is associated with regular weight-bearing exercise and adequate intake of fluoride, calcium, and vitamin D. Low testosterone is a major risk factor in men.

Peak bone mass (maximum bone tissue) is typically achieved before age 20. It is largely determined by four factors: heredity, nutrition, exercise, and hormone function. Heredity may be responsible for up to 70% of a person's peak bone mass. Bone loss from midlife (ages 35 to 40 years) onward is inevitable, but the rate of loss varies. At menopause, women experience rapid bone loss when the decline in estrogen production is the greatest. The rate of loss then slows and eventually matches the rate of bone lost by men ages 65 to 70 years. Genetic factors influence not only bone mineral density but also bone size, quality, and turnover.

Bone is continuously being deposited by osteoblasts and resorbed by osteoclasts, a process called *remodeling.* Rates of bone deposition and resorption are normally equal, so total bone mass remains constant.[30] In osteoporosis, bone resorption exceeds bone deposition.

Specific diseases associated with osteoporosis include inflammatory bowel disease, intestinal malabsorption, kidney disease, rheumatoid arthritis, hyperthyroidism, alcoholism, cirrhosis of the liver, hypogonadism, and diabetes mellitus. Many drugs can interfere with bone metabolism, including corticosteroids, antiseizure drugs (e.g., divalproex sodium [Depakote], phenytoin), aluminum-containing antacids, heparin, some chemotherapy drugs, and excessive thyroid hormones. When one of these drugs is prescribed, inform the patient of this possible side effect. Long-term corticosteroid use is a major contributor to osteoporosis.

### TABLE 63-12 Risk Factors for Osteoporosis

- Advancing age (>65 yr)
- Female gender
- Low body weight
- White or Asian ethnicity
- Current cigarette smoking
- Sedentary lifestyle
- Estrogen deficiency in women (surgical or age-related menopause)
- Family history of osteoporosis
- Diet low in calcium or vitamin D deficiency
- Excessive use of alcohol (>2 drinks/day)
- Low testosterone in men
- Long-term use of corticosteroids, thyroid replacement, heparin, long-acting sedatives, or antiseizure drugs

### GENDER DIFFERENCES

#### Osteoporosis

| Men | Women |
|---|---|
| • Men are underdiagnosed and undertreated for osteoporosis as compared to women. | • Osteoporosis is eight times more common in women than in men. |
| • One in four men over age 50 will have an osteoporosis-related fracture in his lifetime. | • One in two women over age 50 years will have an osteoporosis-related fracture in her lifetime. |

## Clinical Manifestations

Osteoporosis occurs most commonly in bones of the spine, hips, and wrists. Typical early manifestations are back pain or spontaneous fractures. The loss of bone mass causes the bone to become mechanically weaker and prone to spontaneous fractures or fractures from minimal trauma. A person who has one vertebral fracture due to osteoporosis has an increased risk of having a second vertebral fracture within 1 year. Over time, vertebral fractures and wedging cause gradual loss of height and a humped thoracic spine (*kyphosis,* or "dowager's hump") (Fig. 63-9).

## Diagnostic Studies

Osteoporosis often goes unnoticed because it cannot be detected by conventional x-ray until 25% to 40% of calcium in the bone is lost. Serum calcium, phosphorus, and alkaline phosphatase levels usually are normal, although alkaline phosphatase may be elevated after a fracture.

Bone mineral density (BMD) measurements are typically expressed as grams of mineral per unit volume.[31] BMD is determined by peak bone mass and amount of bone loss. (Procedures for BMD measurement are presented in Table 61-7.) BMD may be measured by quantitative ultrasound (QUS) and dual-energy x-ray absorptiometry (DXA). QUS uses sound waves to measure bone density in the heel, kneecap, or shin. DXA (considered the gold standard of BMD studies by the World Health Organization) measures bone density in the spine, hips, and forearm. These represent the most common sites of fragility fractures from osteoporosis. DXA studies are also useful to evaluate changes in bone density over time and assess effectiveness of osteoporosis treatment.

The BMD test results are compared to the ideal or peak bone mineral density of a healthy 30-year-old adult, and reported as T-scores. A T-score of 0 means the BMD is equal to the norm for a healthy young adult. Differences between the BMD and that of the healthy young adult norm are measured in units called *standard deviations (SDs).* The more standard deviations below 0 (indicated as negative numbers), the lower the BMD and the higher the risk of fracture.

A T-score between +1 and −1 is considered normal. A T-score between −1 and −2.5 indicates **osteopenia** (bone loss that is more than normal, but not yet at the level for a diagnosis of osteoporosis). A T-score of −2.5 or lower indicates osteoporosis. The greater the negative number, the more severe the osteoporosis.

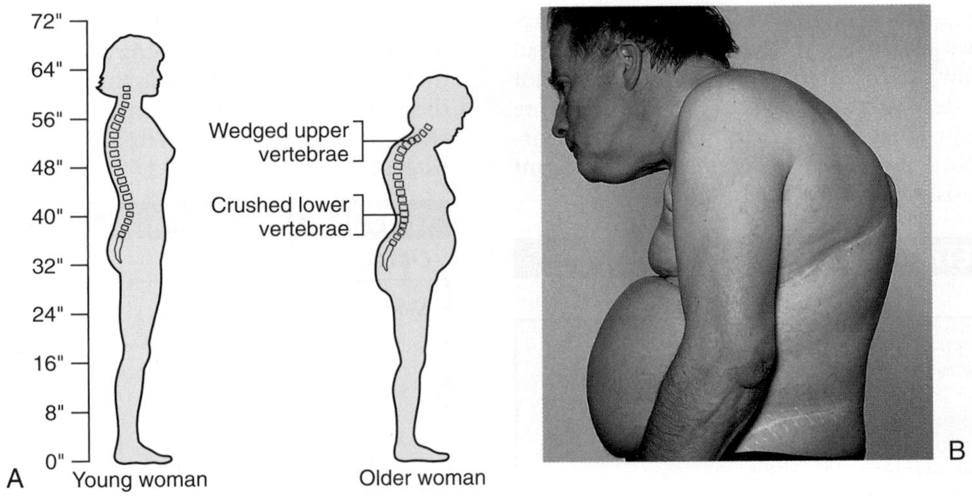


**FIG. 63-9** The effects of osteoporosis. **A,** Comparison of young woman with an older woman. **B,** Severe fixed kyphosis producing a question-mark appearance. (*A,* From Phillips N: *Berry & Kohn's operating room technique,* ed 12, St Louis, 2013, Mosby. *B,* Courtesy MA Mir. In Kanski JJ: *Clinical diagnosis in ophthalmology,* St Louis, 2006, Mosby.)

Sometimes the HCP asks for a Z-score instead of a T-score. In this case, a person is compared with someone his or her own age, gender, and/or ethnic group instead of a healthy 30-year-old. Among older adults, Z-scores can be misleading because decreased bone density is common. If the Z-score is −2 or lower, it may suggest that something other than aging is causing abnormal bone loss.

## NURSING AND INTERPROFESSIONAL MANAGEMENT: OSTEOPOROSIS

Interprofessional care for osteoporosis focuses on proper nutrition, calcium supplementation, exercise, prevention of falls and fractures, and drugs (Table 63-13). The National Osteoporosis Foundation *(www.nof.org)* recommends treatment for osteoporosis for postmenopausal women with (1) a T-score of less than −2.5, (2) a T-score between −1 and −2.5 with additional risk factors (Table 63-12), or (3) prior history of a hip or vertebral fracture.

A patient's risk of fracture from osteoporosis can also be calculated with the Fracture Risk Assessment (FRAX) tool *(www.shef.ac.uk/FRAX)*. The FRAX takes into account BMD and additional clinical factors when assessing fracture risk.[32]

Prevention and treatment of osteoporosis focus on adequate calcium intake (1000 mg/day for women ages 19 to 50 years and men ages 19 to 70 years; 1200 mg/day in women age 51 years or older and men 71 years or older). Foods high in calcium include milk, yogurt, turnip greens, cottage cheese, ice cream, sardines, and spinach (Table 63-14). If dietary intake of calcium is inadequate, supplemental calcium may be recommended.

Calcium is difficult to absorb in single doses greater than 500 mg.[33] Teach the patient the importance of taking calcium supplements as divided doses to increase absorption. The amount of elemental calcium varies in different calcium preparations. Calcium carbonate has 40% elemental calcium. It should be taken with meals because stomach acid is needed to dissolve and absorb this supplement. Calcium citrate offers about 20% elemental calcium but is less dependent on stomach acid for absorption. It is also better absorbed by patients taking a proton pump inhibitor (e.g., esomeprazole [Nexium]) or histamine receptor blocker (e.g., cimetidine) for acid reflux.[33]

### TABLE 63-13 Interprofessional Care

### *Osteoporosis*

**Diagnostic Assessment**
- History and physical examination
- Serum calcium, phosphorus, alkaline phosphatase, vitamin D
- Bone mineral densitometry
- Dual-energy x-ray absorptiometry (DXA)

**Management**
- Adequate dietary calcium (Table 63-14)
- Calcium supplements
- Sun exposure or vitamin D supplements
- Exercise program

***Drug Therapy***
- Bisphosphonates
  - alendronate (Fosamax, Binosto)
  - etidronate (Didronel)
  - ibandronate (Boniva)
  - pamidronate (Aredia)
  - risedronate (Actonel)
  - zoledronic acid (Reclast)
- Salmon calcitonin
- Selective estrogen receptor modulator (e.g., raloxifene [Evista])
- Recombinant parathyroid hormone (e.g., teriparatide [Forteo])
- Monoclonal antibody (e.g., denosumab [Prolia])

***Minimally Invasive Procedures***
- Vertebroplasty
- Kyphoplasty

Calcium lactate and calcium gluconate are not recommended because they have small amounts of elemental calcium.

Vitamin D is important in calcium absorption and function and may also have a role in bone formation. Most people get enough vitamin D from their diet or naturally through synthesis in the skin from exposure to sunlight. Being in the sun for 20 minutes a day is generally enough. However, supplemental vitamin D (800 IU) is recommended for postmenopausal women, older men, persons who are homebound or in long-term care settings, and those in northern climates due to decreased sun exposure.

**TABLE 63-14 Nutritional Therapy**

***Sources of Calcium***

| Food | Calcium (mg) | Food | Calcium (mg) |
|---|---|---|---|
| **Good Sources** | | **Good Sources—cont'd** | |
| 1 cup milk | | 3 oz seafood | |
| • Whole | 279 | • Salmon | 181 |
| • Skim | 299 | • Sardines | 325 |
| 6 oz calcium-fortified orange juice | 261 | 1 cup almonds | 304 |
| 1 oz cheese | | **Poor Sources** | |
| • Mozzarella | 222 | Egg | 28 |
| • Cheddar | 214 | 3 oz beef, pork, poultry | 10 |
| • Cottage | 138 | Apple, banana | 10 |
| 8 oz yogurt | 313-384 | 1 med potato | 14 |
| • Soft serve frozen | 206 | 1 med carrot | 14 |
| 1 cup ice cream | 168 | ¼ head lettuce | 27 |

Regular physical activity is important to build and maintain bone mass.[34] Exercise also increases muscle strength, coordination, and balance. The best exercises are weight-bearing exercises that force an individual to work against gravity. These exercises include walking, hiking, weight training, stair climbing, tennis, and dancing. Walking is preferred to high-impact aerobics or running, both of which may put too much stress on the bones and may cause stress fractures. Encourage patients to walk 30 minutes three times a week. Instruct patients to quit smoking and decrease alcohol intake to minimize negative effects on bone mass.

Although loss of bone cannot be significantly reversed, further loss can be prevented if the patient follows a regimen of calcium and vitamin D supplementation, exercise, and drugs (Table 63-13) as indicated. Encourage patients with osteoporosis to remain ambulatory to prevent further loss of bone density due to immobility.

Treatment may also involve the use of a gait aid to walk safely and protect areas of potential pathologic fractures. For example, a thoracolumbar sacral orthosis (TLSO) may be used to maintain the spine in proper alignment after fracture or treatment of a vertebral fracture. (Fractures are discussed in Chapter 62.)

*Vertebroplasty* and *kyphoplasty* are minimally invasive procedures used to treat osteoporotic vertebral fractures[35] (see Chapter 62). In vertebroplasty, bone cement is injected into the collapsed vertebra to stabilize the spine and improve the patient's pain. However, this procedure does not restore vertebral height or correct deformity. In kyphoplasty, a small balloon is inserted into the collapsed vertebra and inflated to restore vertebral body height before injection of bone cement. Kyphoplasty is now the preferred surgical treatment for vertebral compression fractures.

## Drug Therapy

Estrogen replacement therapy and estrogen with progesterone are no longer routinely given after menopause to prevent osteoporosis because they are associated with increased risk of heart disease as well as breast and uterine cancer. If a woman is taking short-term estrogen therapy to treat menopausal symptoms such as hot flashes, she may also receive some protection against bone loss and fractures of the hip and vertebrae.[36] Estrogen is believed to inhibit osteoclast activity, leading to decreased bone resorption and preventing loss of cortical and trabecular bone.

Bisphosphonates inhibit osteoclast-mediated bone resorption and slow the cycle of bone remodeling. Although a modest increase in BMD is typical, bone remodeling may be suppressed to the extent that normal bone formation is impaired and fracture risk increases. These drugs are widely used in the prevention and treatment of osteoporosis[37] (Table 63-13). Common side effects are anorexia, weight loss, and gastritis. Teach the patient to take the medication correctly to improve its absorption (see Drug Alert). These precautions have also been shown to decrease GI side effects (especially esophageal irritation). A rare and serious side effect of bisphosphonates is *osteonecrosis* (bone death) of the jaw. Its etiology is unknown. However, patients with dental disease, cancer, Paget's disease, or renal disease are most at risk for this complication. Patients should be evaluated by a dentist before beginning treatment and then annually to ensure good oral health.

**DRUG ALERT Bisphosphonates**

Instruct patient to:
- Take with full glass of water.
- Take 30 min before food or other medications.
- Remain upright for at least 30 min after taking.

Alendronate (Fosamax) is available as a daily or weekly oral tablet. Ibandronate (Boniva) is available as a once-per-month oral tablet or can be given every 3 months by IV infusion. The immediate-release form of risedronate (Actonel) is given daily, weekly, or monthly based on the dose. Zoledronic acid (Reclast) is approved as a once-yearly IV infusion to treat osteoporosis, or is given every 2 years to prevent the disease. Renal function tests and serum calcium must be assessed before administration of the drug. Other bisphosphonates are identified in Table 63-13.

Calcitonin is secreted by the thyroid gland and inhibits bone resorption by directly interacting with active osteoclasts. Salmon calcitonin is available in IM, subcutaneous, and intranasal forms. Administration of the IM or subcutaneous form of the drug at night has been shown to decrease associated side effects of nausea and facial flushing. Nausea does not occur with the nasal spray. If patients are using the nasal form, teach them to alternate nostrils daily. Nasal dryness and irritation are the most frequent side effects. Calcium supplementation is needed to prevent secondary hyperparathyroidism.

Raloxifene (Evista) is a selective estrogen receptor modulator (SERM). This drug mimics the effect of estrogen on bone by reducing bone resorption without stimulating the tissues of the breast or uterus. Raloxifene in postmenopausal women significantly increases BMD. Side effects included leg cramps, hot flashes, and blood clots. Raloxifene may decrease breast cancer risk. Similar to tamoxifen, it blocks the estrogen receptor sites.

Teriparatide (Forteo) is a recombinant form of human parathyroid hormone (PTH) that increases the action of osteoblasts. This drug is used to treat osteoporosis in men and postmenopausal women at high risk for fractures, including risk related to long-term corticosteroid use. Side effects include leg cramps and dizziness. Teriparatide is the first drug approved to stimulate new bone formation in osteoporosis; most drugs only prevent further bone loss. It is self-administered daily by subcutaneous injection from a preloaded pen.

Denosumab (Prolia) may be used for postmenopausal women with osteoporosis who are at high risk for fractures. It is a monoclonal antibody that binds to a protein (RANKL) involved in the formation and function of osteoclasts. Denosumab is given by a health care professional as a subcutaneous injection every 6 months.

Medical management of patients receiving corticosteroids includes prescribing the lowest effective dose for the shortest possible time. Ensure an adequate intake of calcium and vitamin D, including supplementation when osteoporosis drugs are prescribed. If osteopenia is evident on bone densitometry in people who are taking corticosteroids, treatment with bisphosphonates may be considered.

## PAGET'S DISEASE

**Paget's disease** *(osteitis deformans)* is a chronic skeletal bone disorder in which excessive bone resorption is followed by replacement of normal marrow by vascular, fibrous connective tissue. The new bone is larger, disorganized, and weaker. Commonly affected areas of the skeleton include pelvis, long bones, spine, ribs, sternum, and cranium. Up to 5% of adults in the United States are affected by Paget's disease.[38] The etiology is unknown, although a viral cause has been proposed. Up to 40% of all patients with Paget's disease have at least one relative with the disorder. Men are affected twice as often as women.

In milder forms of Paget's disease, patients may remain free of symptoms. The disease may be discovered incidentally through x-ray or serum chemistry findings of high alkaline phosphatase.[39] Bone pain may develop gradually and progress to severe intractable pain. Other early manifestations include fatigue and progressive development of a waddling gait. Patients may complain they are becoming shorter or their heads are becoming larger. Headaches, dementia, visual deficits, and loss of hearing can result from an enlarged, thickened skull. Increased bone volume in the spine can cause spinal cord or nerve root compression.

Pathologic fracture is the most common complication and may be the first indication of Paget's disease. Other complications include osteosarcoma, fibrosarcoma, and osteoclastoma (giant cell) tumors.

Serum alkaline phosphatase is markedly elevated in advanced disease, indicating high bone turnover.[40] X-rays may show curvature of an affected bone. The bone cortex becomes thicker and irregular, especially in weight-bearing bones and the cranium. Bone scans using a radiolabeled bisphosphonate demonstrate increased uptake in the affected skeletal areas.

Interprofessional care of Paget's disease is usually limited to symptomatic and supportive care with correction of secondary deformities by surgical intervention or braces. Bisphosphonate drugs (Table 63-13) are used to retard bone resorption. Zoledronic acid may be given specifically to build bone. Calcium and vitamin D are often given to decrease hypocalcemia, a common side effect with these drugs. Monitor drug effectiveness by regular assessment of serum alkaline phosphatase.

Calcitonin is recommended for patients who cannot tolerate bisphosphonates. Human calcitonin inhibits osteoclastic activity, prevents bone resorption, relieves acute symptoms, and lowers serum alkaline phosphatase. This drug is available as a subcutaneous injection. Salmon calcitonin can also be used to treat Paget's disease. It has a longer half-life and greater milligram potency than human calcitonin. Response to calcitonin therapy is not permanent and often stops when therapy is discontinued.

Pain is usually managed by NSAIDs. Orthopedic surgery for fractures, hip and knee replacement, and knee realignment may be needed.

A firm mattress should be used to provide back support and relieve pain. The patient may need to wear a corset or light brace to relieve back pain and provide support when upright. Teach the patient to correctly apply the device and regularly examine the skin for friction damage. Discourage lifting and twisting. Good body mechanics are essential. Physical therapy may increase muscle strength. A well-balanced diet is important in management of metabolic bone disorders. Vitamin D, calcium, and protein are especially important to ensure available components for bone formation. To decrease risk for falls and related fractures, teach the patient to use an assistive device and make environmental changes (e.g., eliminate throw rugs).

**! SAFETY ALERT Paget's Disease**

To reduce the risk of patient harm from falls:

- Evaluate environmental fall risk factors.
- Identify personal risk factors for falls, including drugs and uncorrected vision.
- Take action to address any identified risks.

### Gerontologic Considerations: Metabolic Bone Diseases

Osteoporosis and Paget's disease are common in older adults. Instruct patients in proper nutrition to decrease risk for further bone loss. Keep the patient as active as possible to slow demineralization of bone from disuse or extended immobilization.

Because metabolic bone disorders increase the possibility of pathologic fractures, use extreme caution when turning or moving the patient. Hip fractures in particular may decrease quality of life and lead to admission to a long-term care facility. A supervised exercise program is essential to osteoporosis treatment. Encourage ambulation if the patient's condition permits.

## CASE STUDY

### *Metastatic Bone Tumor/Pathologic Fracture*

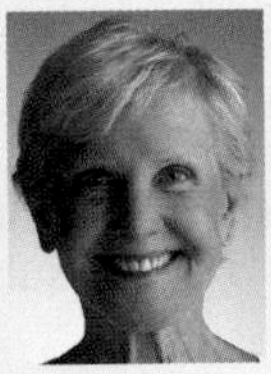

(©Christopher-Robbins/ Photodisc/ Thinkstock)

**Patient Profile**

L.R. is a 60-yr-old white woman with a history of hypertension, hypothyroidism, and osteoporosis. Four years ago she was diagnosed with Stage 3a breast cancer and treated with surgery, radiation therapy, and chemotherapy. Today she was admitted to the emergency department after a fall down two stairs.

**Subjective Data**

- Denies hitting her head or loss of consciousness
- States she was able to bear weight on her lower extremities but complains of significant left thigh pain after the fall
- Describes recent insidious onset of generalized weakness and fatigue
- Denies alcohol or tobacco use
- Takes levothyroxine (Synthroid) and atenolol (Tenormin) every morning. Takes ibandronate (Boniva) once a month

**Objective Data**

- Left lower extremity slightly shorter and externally rotated compared to right lower extremity
- Moderate edema with associated ecchymosis on left thigh
- Thigh soft, compressible to palpation
- Complains of pain with axial loading and internal/external rotation of left lower extremity
- Palpable dorsalis pedis and posterior tibialis pulses bilaterally
- Gross motor/sensation intact in all distributions in distal affected extremity

## CASE STUDY

### *Metastatic Bone Tumor/Pathologic Fracture—cont'd*

**Diagnostic Studies**

- X-ray reveals oblique mid-shaft left femur fracture with lytic lesion in the femoral neck
- Normal CBC and blood chemistry results, slightly elevated liver function tests
- CT scans of the chest, abdomen, and pelvis demonstrate multiple bony metastases throughout the pelvis as well as lesions of the liver and spleen, widespread abdominal cancer, compression fractures with lesions of T11 vertebral body, and bilateral rib fractures with associated lesions.
- Whole body bone scan consistent with findings from x-ray and CT
- CT-guided biopsy of femur fracture site showed poorly differentiated cells consistent with breast cancer

**Interprofessional Care**

- Diagnosed with stage IV breast cancer
- Intramedullary (IM) nail for femur fracture
- Pain management
- Postoperative chemotherapy and hormone therapy
- High-protein, high-calcium, nutrient-rich diet
- Depression assessment and management
- Ambulation evaluation with gait aids as needed

**Discussion Questions**

1. Why did a relatively low-energy injury cause L.R's fracture?
2. ***Patient-Centered Care:*** What factors could result in inadequate caloric intake postoperatively? How could you help L.R. increase her intake of protein and calcium?
3. What factors increase L.R.'s risk for delayed union or nonunion of the fracture?
4. ***Priority Decision:*** What are the priority teaching needs for L.R.?
5. ***Teamwork and Collaboration:*** Which personnel on the interprofessional team should be responsible for L.R.'s postoperative home care instructions? Who should be responsible for ambulation and home safety teaching and assessments? Who should assist L.R. with transfers and ambulation during her hospital stay?
6. ***Priority Decision:*** Based on the assessment data, what are the priority nursing diagnoses?
7. ***Quality Improvement:*** What outcomes would indicate that interprofessional care was effective?
8. ***Safety:*** What safety precautions should be considered for this patient?
9. ***Evidence-Based Practice:*** L.R asks why it is important for her to have daily injections of enoxaparin after surgery. How do you respond?

Answers available at *http://evolve.elsevier.com/Lewis/medsurg.*

## BRIDGE TO NCLEX EXAMINATION

The number of the question corresponds to the same-numbered outcome at the beginning of the chapter.

1. A patient with osteomyelitis undergoes surgical debridement with implantation of antibiotic beads. When the patient asks why the beads are used, the nurse answers *(select all that apply)*
   - **a.** "Oral or IV antibiotics are not effective in most cases of bone infection."
   - **b.** "The beads are an adjunct to debridement and antibiotics for deep infections."
   - **c.** "The beads are used to deliver antibiotics directly to the site of the infection."
   - **d.** "This is the safest method to deliver long-term antibiotic therapy for bone infection."
   - **e.** "Ischemia and bone death related to osteomyelitis are impenetrable to IV antibiotics."
2. A patient diagnosed with osteosarcoma of the humerus demonstrates understanding of his treatment options when he states
   - **a.** "I accept that I have to lose my arm with surgery."
   - **b.** "The chemotherapy before surgery will shrink the tumor."
   - **c.** "This tumor is related to the melanoma I had 3 years ago."
   - **d.** "I'm glad they can take out the cancer with such a small scar."
3. Which individuals would be at high risk for low back pain *(select all that apply)*?
   - **a.** A 63-year-old man who is a long-distance truck driver
   - **b.** A 36-year-old construction worker who is 6 ft 2 in and weighs 260 lb
   - **c.** A 44-year-old female chef with prior compression fracture of the spine
   - **d.** A 30-year-old nurse who works on an orthopedic unit and smokes
   - **e.** A 28-year-old female yoga instructor who is 5 ft 6 in and weighs 130 lb
4. A patient with suspected disc herniation is experiencing acute pain and muscle spasms. The nurse's responsibility is to
   - **a.** encourage total bed rest for several days.
   - **b.** teach principles of back strengthening exercises.
   - **c.** stress the importance of straight-leg raises to decrease pain.
   - **d.** promote use of cold and hot compresses and pain medication.
5. In caring for a patient after a spinal fusion, the nurse would immediately report which of the following to the surgeon?
   - **a.** The patient experiences a single episode of emesis.
   - **b.** The patient is unable to move the lower extremities.
   - **c.** The patient is nauseated and has not voided in 4 hours.
   - **d.** The patient complains of pain at the bone graft donor site.
6. A patient who has had surgical correction of bilateral hallux valgus is being discharged from the same-day surgery unit. The nurse will instruct the patient to
   - **a.** expect continued pain in the feet.
   - **b.** rest frequently with the feet elevated.
   - **c.** soak the feet in warm water several times a day.
   - **d.** expect the feet to be numb for the next few days.
7. What is important to include in the teaching plan for a patient with osteopenia?
   - **a.** Lose weight.
   - **b.** Stop smoking.
   - **c.** Eat a high-protein diet.
   - **d.** Start swimming for exercise.

1. b, c, 2. b, 3. a, b, c, d, 4. d, 5. b, 6. b, 7. b

For rationales to these answers and even more NCLEX review questions, visit *http://evolve.elsevier.com/Lewis/medsurg.*

## EVOLVE WEBSITE

http://evolve.elsevier.com/Lewis/medsurg

**Review Questions (Online Only)**

**Key Points**

**Answer Keys for Questions**

- Rationales for Bridge to NCLEX Examination Questions
- Answer Guidelines for Case Study on pp. 1514-1515

**Student Case Study**

- Patient With Osteoporosis

**Nursing Care Plans**

- eNursing Care Plan 63-1: Patient With Osteomyelitis
- eNursing Care Plan 63-2: Patient With Low Back Pain

**Conceptual Care Map Creator**

**Audio Glossary**

**Supporting Media**

- Animations
    - Diskectomy
    - Kyphoplasty

**Content Updates**

## REFERENCES


1. Huether S, McCance K: *Understanding pathophysiology*, ed 5, St Louis, 2012, Mosby.
2. Beck-Broichsitter BE, Smeets R, Heiland M: Current concepts in pathogenesis of acute and chronic osteomyelitis, *Curr Opin Infect Dis* 28(3):240, 2015.
3. Schmitt S: Osteomyelitis. Retrieved from *www.merckmanuals.com/professional/musculoskeletal-and-connective-tissue-disorders/infections-of-joints-and-bones/osteomyelitis#.*
4. Lehne R: *Pharmacology for nursing care*, ed 8, St Louis, 2013, Saunders.
5. Lima ALL, Oliveira PR, Carvalho VC, et al: Recommendations for the treatment of osteomyelitis, *Braz J Infect Dis* 18:526, 2014.
6. Siegel R, Naishadham D, Jemal A: Cancer statistics, *CA Cancer J Clin* 63:11, 2013.
7. Luetke A, Meyers PA, Lewis I, et al: Osteosarcoma treatment—Where do we stand? A state of the art review, *Canc Treat Rev* 40:523, 2014.
8. American Cancer Society: What is metastasis? Retrieved from *www.cancer.org/treatment/understandingyourdiagnosis/bonemetastasis/bone-metastasis-what-is-bone-mets.*
9. Leung DG, Herzka DA, Thompson WR, et al: Sildenafil does not improve cardiomyopathy in Duchenne/Becker muscular dystrophy, *Ann Neur* 76:541, 2014.
10. Ruegg UT: Pharmacological prospects in the treatment of Duchenne muscular dystrophy, *Curr Op Neur* 26:577, 2013.
11. National Institute of Neurological Disorders and Stroke: Low back pain fact sheet. Retrieved from *www.ninds.nih.gov/disorders/backpain/detail_backpain.htm.*
12. Lee S-J, Faucett J, Gillen M, et al: Musculoskeletal pain among critical-care nurses by availability and use of patient lifting equipment: an analysis of cross-sectional survey data, *Internat J Nurs Stud* 50:1648, 2013.
13. Knight CL, Deyo RA, Staiger TO, et al: Treatment of acute low back pain. Retrieved from *www.uptodate.com/contents/treatment-of-acute-low-back-pain?source=search_result&search=acute+back+pain&selectedTitle=2~145.*
14. Becker JA, Stumbo JR: Back pain in adults, *Prim Care Clin Office Pract* 40:271, 2013.
15. Webster LR, Markman J: Medical management of chronic low back pain: efficacy and outcomes, *Neuromodulation* 17(Suppl 2):18, 2014.
16. Cleveland Clinic: Degenerative back conditions. Retrieved from *http://my.clevelandclinic.org/services/orthopaedics-rheumatology/diseases-conditions/degenerative-back-conditions.*
17. American Academy of Orthopaedic Surgeons: Cauda equina syndrome. Retrieved from *http://orthoinfo.aaos.org/topic.cfm?topic=A00362&grpwebid=20DEEB.*
18. Mayo Clinic: Herniated disc: Treatment and drugs. Retrieved from *www.mayoclinic.org/diseases-conditions/herniated-disk/basics/treatment/con-20029957.*

*19. Phillips FM, Lee JYB, Geisler FH, et al: A prospective, randomized, controlled clinical investigation comparing PCM cervical disc arthroplasty with anterior cervical discectomy and fusion: 2-year results from the US FDA IDE Clinical Trial, *Spine* 38:E907, 2013.

20. Bae HW, Rajaee SS, Kanim LE: Nationwide trends in the surgical management of lumbar spinal stenosis, *Spine* 38:916, 2013.
21. Isaac Z: Evaluation of the patient with neck pain and cervical spine disorders. Retrieved from *www.uptodate.com/contents/evaluation-of-the-patient-with-neck-pain-and-cervical-spine-disorders?source=search_result&search=neck+pain&selectedTitle=1~150.*

*22. Gross A, Kay TM, Paquin JP, et al: Exercises for mechanical neck disorders, Cochrane Library Pub No. 10.1002/14651858.CD004250.pub5, 2015.

23. Fields KB: Evaluation and diagnosis of common causes of foot pain in adults. Retrieved from *www.uptodate.com/contents/evaluation-and-diagnosis-of-common-causes-of-foot-pain-in-adults?source=search_result&search=hammer+toe&selectedTitle=1~8.*
24. Edmonds ME, Foster AVM: *Managing the diabetic foot*, West Sussex, UK, 2014, Wiley Blackwell.
25. Stolt M, Suhonen R, Puukka P et al: Nurses' foot care activities in home health care, *Geriatric Nurs* 34:491, 2013.
26. Liu C, Wu D, Zhang J-F, et al: Changes in bone metabolism in morbidly obese patients after bariatric surgery: a meta-analysis, *Obes Surg* 26(1):91, 2016.
27. Blann A: An update on vitamin D deficiency and at risk groups, *J Fam Health* 25(3):16, 2015.
28. National Osteoporosis Foundation: Debunking the myths. Retrieved from *http://nof.org/OPmyths.*

*29. US Preventive Services Task Force: Screening for osteoporosis: systematic review to update the 2002 US Preventive Services Task Force recommendations. Retrieved from *www.ncbi.nlm.nih.gov/books/NBK45201.*

30. Cleveland Clinic: Osteoporosis. Retrieved from *http://my.clevelandclinic.org/health/diseases_conditions/hic_Osteoporosis.*
31. Adams JE: Advances in bone imaging for osteoporosis, *Nat Rev Endocrinol* 9:28, 2013.
32. Lewiecki EM: Osteoporotic fracture risk assessment. Retrieved from *www.uptodate.com/contents/osteoporotic-fracture-risk-assessment?source=machineLearning&search=frax&selectedTitle=1~19&sectionRank=3&anchor=H17#.*
33. Florence R, Allen S, Benedict L, et al: Diagnosis and treatment of osteoporosis. Retrieved from *www.guideline.gov/content.aspx?id=47543&search=osteoporosis.*
34. Golob AL, Laya MB: Osteoporosis: screening, prevention, and management, *Med Clin North Am* 99(3):587, 2015.
35. Wong CC, McGirt MJ: Vertebral compression fractures: a review of current management and multimodal therapy, *J Multidisc Health* 6:205, 2013.
36. Schmidt P: The 2012 hormone therapy position statement of the North American Menopause Society, *Menopause* 19:257, 2012.
37. Gatti D, Adami S, Viapiana O, et al: The use of bisphosphonates in women: when to use and when to stop, *Expert Opin Pharmacother* 11:1, 2015.
38. Ralston SH: Paget's disease of bone, *NEJM* 368:644, 2013.
39. White G, Rushbrook J: Paget's disease of bone, *Orthop Trauma* 27:254, 2013.
40. Pagana KD, Pagana TJ: *Mosby's manual of diagnostic and laboratory tests*, ed 5, St Louis, 2014, Mosby.

*Evidence-based information for clinical practice.

64

# Arthritis and Connective Tissue Diseases

Dottie Roberts

*Failure will never overtake me if my determination to succeed is strong enough.*

*Og Mandino*

http://evolve.elsevier.com/Lewis/medsurg/

## LEARNING OUTCOMES

1. Compare and contrast the sequence of events leading to joint destruction in osteoarthritis and rheumatoid arthritis.
2. Detail the clinical manifestations, interprofessional care, and nursing management of osteoarthritis and rheumatoid arthritis.
3. Describe the pathophysiology, clinical manifestations, and interprofessional care of gout, Lyme disease, and septic arthritis.
4. Summarize the pathophysiology, clinical manifestations, interprofessional care, and nursing management of ankylosing spondylitis, psoriatic arthritis, and reactive arthritis.
5. Differentiate the pathophysiology, clinical manifestations, interprofessional care, and nursing management of systemic lupus erythematosus, scleroderma, polymyositis, dermatomyositis, and Sjögren's syndrome.
6. Explain the drug therapy and related nursing management associated with arthritis and connective tissue diseases.
7. Compare and contrast possible etiologies, clinical manifestations, and interprofessional and nursing management of fibromyalgia and systemic exertion tolerance disease.

## KEY TERMS



This chapter discusses *rheumatic diseases,* which primarily affect body joints, tendons, ligaments, muscles, and bones. These diseases are often characterized by inflammation and loss of function in one or more of the body's connecting or supporting structures. More than 100 kinds of rheumatic diseases have been identified.[1] An estimated 52.5 million people in the United States have rheumatic conditions.[2]

## ARTHRITIS

**Arthritis**, a type of rheumatic disease, involves inflammation of a joint or joints. Most forms of arthritis affect women more frequently than men in every age group.[2] Osteoarthritis is the most common form of joint disease in the world.[3] Other forms that occur often include rheumatoid arthritis, fibromyalgia, systemic lupus erythematosus, and gout.

## OSTEOARTHRITIS

**Osteoarthritis (OA)** is a slowly progressive noninflammatory disorder of the diarthrodial *(synovial)* joints. Currently 27 million Americans are affected by OA, with the numbers expected to greatly increase as the population ages.[4]

### Etiology and Pathophysiology

OA involves the gradual loss of articular cartilage with formation of bony outgrowths *(osteophytes)* at the joint margins.[3] OA is not considered a normal part of the aging process, but aging is one risk factor for disease development.[4] Cartilage destruction may actually begin between ages 20 and 30, and the majority of adults are affected by age 40. Few patients experience symptoms until after age 50 or 60, but more than half of those over age 65 have x-ray evidence of OA in at least

Reviewed by Judy Carlyle, RN, MNSc, Faculty/Clinical Liaison, Arkansas Rural Nursing Education Consortium (ARNEC), Nashville, Arkansas; Kim Clevenger, RN, EdD, BC, Associate Professor of Nursing and BSN Program Coordinator, Morehead State University, Morehead, Kentucky; Michele M. Hughes, RN, MSN, ACNP, ONP-C, Nurse Practitioner, Bon Secours Memorial Regional Medical Center, Mechanicsville, Virginia; and Diane Ryzner, MSN, APN, CNS, OCNS-C, Advanced Practice Nurse, Northwest Community Hospital, Arlington Heights, Illinois.

**TABLE 64-1 Causes of Osteoarthritis**

| Cause | Effects on Joint Cartilage |
|---|---|
| Trauma | Dislocations or fractures may lead to avascular necrosis or uneven stress on cartilage. |
| Mechanical stress | Repetitive physical activities (e.g., sports) cause cartilage deterioration. |
| Inflammation | Release of enzymes in response to local inflammation can affect cartilage health. |
| Joint instability | Damage to supporting structures causes instability, placing uneven stress on joint cartilage. |
| Neurologic disorders | Pain and loss of reflexes from neurologic disorders, such as diabetic neuropathy and Charcot joint, cause abnormal movements that contribute to cartilage deterioration. |
| Skeletal deformities | Congenital or acquired conditions such as Legg-Calvé-Perthes disease or dislocated hip contribute to cartilage deterioration. |
| Hematologic or endocrine disorders | Chronic hemarthrosis (e.g., from hemophilia) contributes to cartilage deterioration. |
| Drugs | Drugs such as indomethacin (Indocin), colchicine, and corticosteroids can stimulate collagen-digesting enzymes in joint synovium. |

one joint. After age 50 years, women are affected by OA more often than men.[5]

OA may be caused by a known event or condition that directly damages cartilage or causes joint instability (Table 64-1). However, many persons with OA cannot identify a single cause. In these situations, subtle congenital or genetic cartilage defects may be present.

Decreased estrogen at menopause may contribute to the increased incidence of OA in aging women. Obesity is a modifiable risk factor that contributes to hip and knee OA by increasing the mechanical stress on the joints. Regular moderate exercise, which also helps with weight management, decreases the risk for disease development and progression. Anterior cruciate ligament injury from quick stops and pivoting, as in football and soccer, has been linked to an increased risk for knee OA.[6] Occupations that require frequent kneeling and stooping also increase the risk for knee OA.

The development of OA is complex. Genetic, metabolic, and local factors interact to cause cartilage deterioration from damage at the level of the chondrocytes (Fig. 64-1). The normally smooth, white, translucent articular cartilage becomes dull, yellow, and granular as the disease progresses. Affected cartilage steadily becomes softer and less elastic. It is less able to resist wear with heavy use.

The body's attempts at cartilage repair cannot keep up with the destruction of OA. As the collagen structure of the cartilage changes, articular surfaces become cracked and worn. While central cartilage becomes thinner, cartilage at the joint edges becomes thicker and osteophytes form. Joint surfaces become uneven, affecting the distribution of stress across the joint and causing reduced motion.

Although inflammation is not typical of OA, secondary synovitis may occur when phagocytes try to rid the joint of small pieces of cartilage torn from the joint surface. These changes cause the early pain and stiffness of OA. Pain in later disease occurs when articular cartilage is lost and bony joint surfaces rub on each other.

**GENDER DIFFERENCES**

***Osteoarthritis (OA)***

**Men**

- Except for traumatic arthritis, men do not experience OA as often as women until age 70 or 80 years.
- Hip OA is more common in men than in women.

**Women**

- Women are affected more often than men.
- Hand OA (interphalangeal joints and thumb base) is more common in women than in men.
- Knee OA is more common in women than in men, especially after menopause, and is likely to be more severe.

### Clinical Manifestations

**Systemic.** Fatigue, fever, and organ involvement are not present in OA. This is an important distinction between OA and inflammatory joint disorders such as rheumatoid arthritis.

**Joints.** Manifestations of OA range from mild discomfort to significant disability. Joint pain is the primary symptom and the typical reason the patient seeks medical attention. Pain generally gets worse with joint use. In early stages of OA, joint pain is relieved by rest. However, the patient with advanced disease may complain of pain at rest or have trouble sleeping due to increased joint pain. Pain may also worsen as the barometric pressure falls before the onset of severe weather.

As OA progresses, increasing pain can contribute greatly to disability and loss of function. The pain of OA may be referred to the groin, buttock, or the outside of the thigh or knee. Sitting down becomes difficult, as does rising from a chair when the hips are lower than the knees. As OA develops in the intervertebral *(apophyseal)* joints of the spine, local pain and stiffness are common.

Unlike pain, which typically worsens with activity, joint stiffness occurs after periods of rest or an unchanged position. Early morning stiffness is common but generally resolves within 30 minutes. This factor distinguishes OA from inflammatory arthritic disorders such as rheumatoid arthritis. Overactivity can cause a mild joint swelling that temporarily increases stiffness. *Crepitation,* a grating sensation caused by loose cartilage particles in the joint cavity, can also cause stiffness. Crepitation is common in patients with knee OA.

OA usually affects joints on one side of the body *(asymmetrically)* rather than in pairs. For example, the left knee may be affected and the right knee unchanged. The distal interphalangeal (DIP) and proximal interphalangeal (PIP) joints of the fingers, and the metacarpophalangeal (MCP) joint of the thumb are often affected. Weight-bearing joints (hips, knees), the metatarsophalangeal (MTP) joint of the foot, and the cervical and lower lumbar vertebrae are also commonly involved (Fig. 64-2).

**Deformity.** Deformity or instability associated with OA is specific to the involved joint. For example, *Heberden's nodes* occur on the DIP joints due to osteophyte formation and loss of joint space (Fig. 64-1, *D*). They can appear as early as age 40 and tend to be seen in family members. *Bouchard's nodes* on the PIP joints indicate similar disease involvement. Heberden's and Bouchard's nodes are often red, swollen, and tender. Although they usually do not cause significant loss of function, the patient may be bothered by the visible deformity.

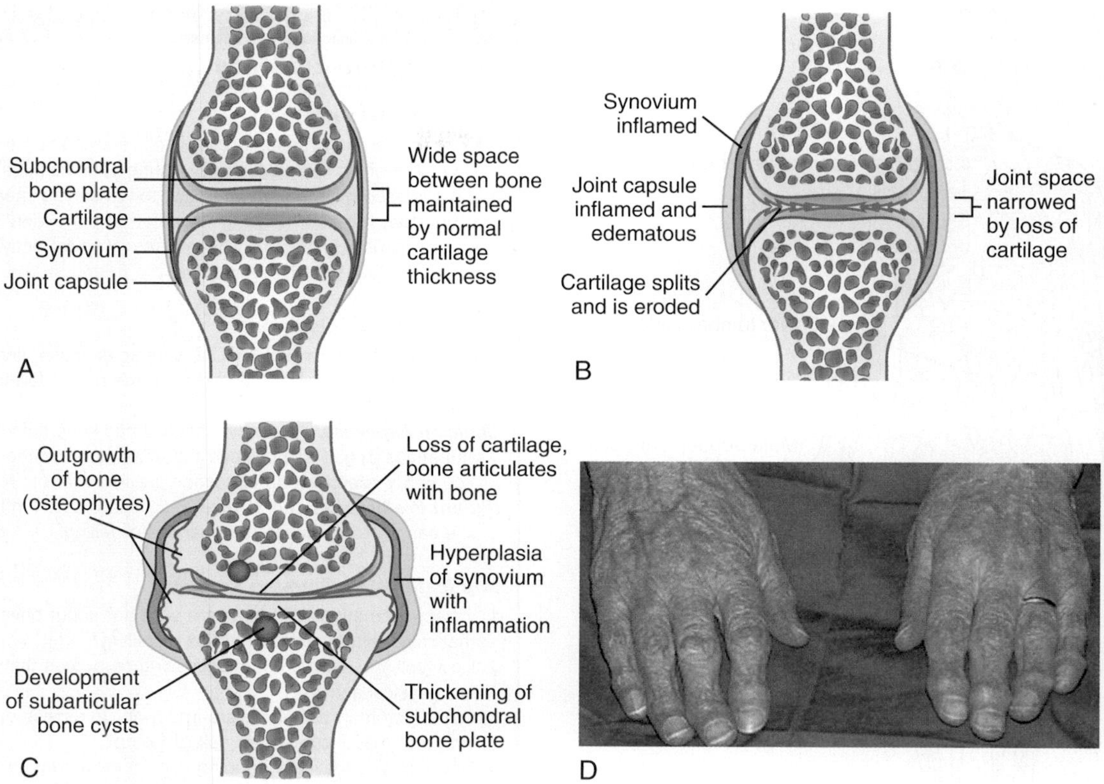


**FIG. 64-1** Pathologic changes in osteoarthritis. **A,** Normal synovial joint. **B,** Early change in osteoarthritis is destruction of articular cartilage and narrowing of the joint space. There is inflammation and thickening of the joint capsule and synovium. **C,** With time, thickening of subarticular bone occurs, caused by constant friction of the two bone surfaces. Osteophytes form around the periphery of the joint by irregular overgrowths of bone. **D,** In osteoarthritis of the hands, osteophytes on the distal interphalangeal joints of the fingers, termed *Heberden's nodes,* appear as small nodules. (*D,* From Forbes CD, Jackson WF: *Color atlas and text of clinical medicine,* ed 3, London, 2003, Mosby.)

Knee OA often leads to obvious joint deformity as a result of cartilage loss in one joint compartment. For example, the patient becomes bowlegged *(varus deformity)* in response to medial joint arthritis. Lateral joint arthritis causes a knock-kneed appearance *(valgus deformity)*. In advanced hip OA, one of the patient's legs may become shorter as the joint space narrows.

## Diagnostic Studies

A bone scan, CT scan, or MRI may be used to diagnose OA. These tests are able to detect early joint changes. X-rays are helpful in confirming disease and staging joint damage. As OA progresses, x-rays often show joint space narrowing and increasingly dense bone. Osteophytes are also visible. However, these changes do not always reflect the degree of pain the patient experiences. Despite strong x-ray evidence of disease, the patient may be relatively free of symptoms. On the other hand, another patient may have severe pain with only slight x-ray changes.

No laboratory tests or biomarkers can be used to diagnose OA. The erythrocyte sedimentation rate (ESR) is normal except during acute inflammation, when slight elevations may be seen. Other routine blood tests (e.g., complete blood count [CBC], renal and liver function tests) are useful only in screening for related conditions or for establishing baseline values before starting treatment. Synovial fluid analysis helps distinguish between OA and types of inflammatory arthritis. In OA, the fluid remains clear yellow with little or no sign of inflammation.

## Interprofessional Care

Because OA has no cure, interprofessional care focuses on managing pain and inflammation, preventing disability, and maintaining and improving joint function (Table 64-2). Nondrug interventions are the basis for OA management. They should be maintained throughout the patient's treatment. Drug therapy supplements nondrug treatments.

**Rest and Joint Protection.** Teach the patient with OA to balance rest and activity. Rest the affected joint during any periods of acute inflammation. Keep it in a functional position with splints or braces if needed. However, avoid immobilization of more than 1 week because of the risk of joint stiffness with inactivity. Modify usual activities to decrease stress on affected joints. Teach the patient with knee OA to avoid standing, kneeling, or squatting for long periods of time. Using an assistive device such as a cane, walker, or crutches can also decrease joint stress.

**Heat and Cold Applications.** Apply heat and cold to help reduce pain and stiffness. Ice is not used as often as heat in OA treatment, but it can be helpful if the patient has acute inflammation. Heat therapy is especially useful for stiffness. Treatments include hot packs, whirlpool baths, ultrasound, and paraffin wax baths.

**Nutritional Therapy and Exercise.** If the patient is overweight, a weight-reduction program is a critical part of the treatment plan. Help the patient evaluate the current diet to make needed changes. (Chapter 40 discusses ways to assist the patient in attaining and maintaining a healthy body weight.) Because

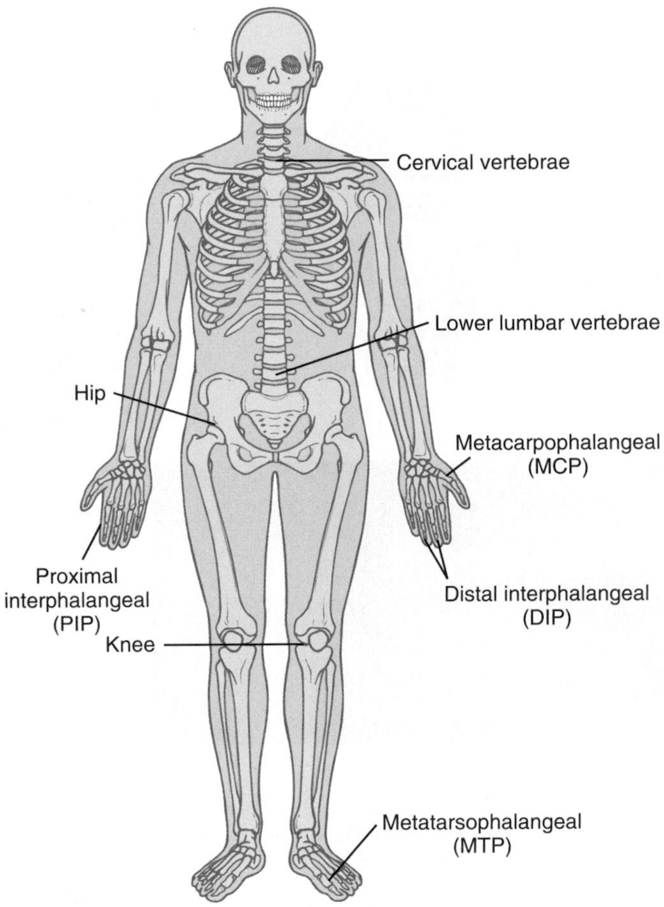


**FIG. 64-2** Joints most frequently involved in osteoarthritis.

## TABLE 64-2 Interprofessional Care

### *Osteoarthritis*

**Diagnostic Assessment**

- History and physical examination
- Radiologic studies of involved joints (e.g., x-ray, CT scan, MRI, bone scan)
- Synovial fluid analysis

**Management**

- Nutritional and weight management counseling
- Rest and joint protection, use of assistive devices
- Therapeutic exercise
- Heat and cold applications
- Complementary and alternative therapies
  - Herbs and nutritional supplements (e.g., fish oil, ginger, Sam-e)
  - Movement therapies (e.g., yoga, Tai Chi)
  - Acupuncture
  - Massage
- Transcutaneous electrical nerve stimulation (TENS)
- Reconstructive joint surgery

***Drug Therapy*** *(Table 64-3)*

- acetaminophen
- Nonsteroidal antiinflammatory drugs
- Intraarticular corticosteroids

loading and mobilizing the joint are needed to preserve articular cartilage health, exercise is an important part of OA management.[7] Aerobic conditioning, range-of-motion (ROM) exercises, and programs for quadriceps strengthening have been helpful for many patients with knee OA.

## EVIDENCE-BASED PRACTICE

### *Applying the Evidence*

**Falls and Osteoarthritis**

You are a community health nurse who is starting home visits with R.F., a 68-yr-old woman with OA. Today during your visit she states that her mobility is becoming more limited due to worsening knee pain. R.F. also tells you that her pain is being "somewhat controlled" by acetaminophen and capsaicin cream. She misses physical activity and is now concerned about falling in her home.

***Making Clinical Decisions***

***Best Available Evidence.*** Tai Chi, aerobic exercise, and strength training improve balance and reduce the risk of falling in older adults with knee OA.

***Clinician Expertise.*** You know that arthritic knee pain can cause alterations in gait and balance that may increase the risk of falling. You know exercise and education are important in reducing falls.

***Patient Preferences and Values.*** R.F. is interested in learning what she can do to decrease her chances of falling.

***Implications for Nursing Practice***

1. What information will you share with her about physical activities that may help to reduce her risk of falling?
2. How will you assist R.F. in accessing resources that will increase her physical activity?
3. What factors in the home are important to assess on your initial visit that may increase her risk of falling?
4. How will you facilitate ongoing communication with R.F's HCP to ensure satisfactory pain relief?

***References for Evidence***

Mat S, Tan M, Kamaruzzaman SB, et al: Physical therapies for improving balance and reducing falls risk in osteoarthritis of the knee: a systematic review, *Age Ageing* 44:16, 2015.

National Arthritis Foundation: Retrieved from *www.arthritistoday.org/about-arthritis/types-of-arthritis/osteoarthritis/daily-life/osteoarthritis-and-falls.php*.

**Complementary and Alternative Therapies.** Complementary and alternative therapies for OA symptom management are popular with patients who have not found relief through traditional medical care. Teach the patient to carefully research any alternative therapies and avoid replacing conventional OA treatments with unproven complementary approaches.[8] Acupuncture may reduce arthritis pain and improve joint mobility. Massage and Tai Chi may also reduce pain and improve function. Some nutritional supplements may have antiinflammatory effects (e.g., fish oil, ginger, Sam-e). However, results of studies on glucosamine and chondroitin are mixed. The American College of Rheumatology conditionally recommends that patients do not use glucosamine or chondroitin sulfate[7] (see the Complementary & Alternative Therapies boxes). Instruct patients to discuss any supplement use with their HCPs to identify possible interactions with prescribed medications.

**Drug Therapy.** Drug therapy is based on the severity of the patient's symptoms (Table 64-3). The patient with mild to moderate joint pain may get relief from acetaminophen (Tylenol).

A topical agent such as capsaicin cream may also be helpful, alone or with acetaminophen. It blocks pain by locally interfering with substance P, which is responsible for the transmission of pain impulses. A concentrated product is available by prescription, but creams of 0.025% to 0.075% capsaicin are available over the counter (OTC). Other OTC products that contain camphor, eucalyptus oil, and menthol (e.g., Bengay, Arthricare) may also provide temporary pain relief. Topical salicylates (e.g.,

**TABLE 64-3 Drug Therapy**

***Arthritis and Connective Tissue Diseases***

| Drug | Mechanism of Action | Nursing Considerations |
|---|---|---|
| **Salicylate** | | |
| aspirin, salicylate (salsalate) | Antiinflammatory<br>Analgesic<br>Fever reducer (antipyretic)<br>Act by inhibiting prostaglandin synthesis | Administer with food, milk, antacids (as prescribed), or full glass of water. May use enteric-coated aspirin. Report signs of bleeding (e.g., tarry stools, bruising, petechiae, nosebleeds). |
| **Nonsteroidal Antiinflammatory Drugs (NSAIDs)** | | |
| ibuprofen (Advil)<br>naproxen (Aleve)<br>ketoprofen<br>piroxicam (Feldene)<br>indomethacin (Indocin)<br>sulindac<br>tolmetin<br>diclofenac<br>meclofenamate<br>nabumetone<br>oxaprozin (Daypro)<br>meloxicam (Mobic)<br>celecoxib (Celebrex) | Antiinflammatory<br>Analgesic<br>Fever reducer (antipyretic)<br>Act by inhibiting prostaglandin synthesis | Administer drug with food, milk, or antacids (as prescribed).<br>Report signs of bleeding (e.g., tarry stools, bruising, petechiae, nosebleeds), edema, skin rashes, persistent headaches, visual disturbances.<br>Monitor BP for elevations related to fluid retention. Must be used regularly for maximal effect. |
| **Antibiotics** | | |
| doxycycline (Vibramycin) | Decreases action of enzymes on cartilage degradation | Possible treatment alternative for mild disease. |
| minocycline (Minocin) | Antirheumatic effect possibly related to immunomodulatory/antiinflammatory properties | |
| **Topical Analgesics** | | |
| capsaicin cream | Depletes substance P from nerve endings, interrupting pain signals to the brain | Must be used at regular intervals for maximal effect.<br>Aloe vera cream may decrease burning sensation.<br>Advise patient not to use cream with external heat source (heating pad) because of risk of burns. Available in OTC and prescriptive strengths. |
| diclofenac sodium (Voltaren gel) | Antiinflammatory<br>Analgesic | Advise patient to avoid sun and ultraviolet (UV) light exposure. Should not be used in combination with other oral NSAIDs or aspirin due to potential for increased side effects. |
| **Corticosteroids** | | |
| ***Intraarticular Injections*** | | |
| methylprednisolone acetate (Depo-Medrol)<br>triamcinolone (Aristospan) | Antiinflammatory<br>Analgesic<br>Act by inhibiting synthesis and/or release of inflammatory mediators | Use strict aseptic technique for corticosteroid injection. Inform patient that joint may temporarily feel worse right after injection. Advise patient to avoid overusing affected joint immediately after injection. Inform patient improvement lasts weeks to months after injection. |
| ***Systemic*** | | |
| hydrocortisone (Solu-Cortef)<br>methylprednisolone (Solu-Medrol)<br>dexamethasone<br>prednisone<br>triamcinolone | Antiinflammatory<br>Analgesic<br>Act by inhibiting synthesis and/or release of inflammatory mediators | Use only in life-threatening exacerbation or when symptoms persist after treatment with less potent antiinflammatory drugs. Administer for limited time only, tapering dose slowly. Be aware that exacerbation of symptoms occurs with abrupt withdrawal of drug. Monitor BP, weight, CBC, and serum potassium. Limit sodium intake. Report signs of infection. |
| **Disease-Modifying Antirheumatic Drugs (DMARDs)** | | |
| methotrexate (Trexall) | Antimetabolite<br>Inhibits DNA, RNA, protein synthesis | Monitor CBC and hepatic and renal function. Advise patient to report signs of anemia (fatigue, weakness). Keep patient well hydrated. Due to teratogenic effects, instruct female patient to use effective contraception during and 3 mo after treatment. |
| sulfasalazine (Azulfidine) | Sulfonamide<br>Antiinflammatory<br>Blocks prostaglandin synthesis | Advise patient drug may cause orange-yellow discoloration of urine or skin. Space doses evenly around the clock, taking drug after food with 8 oz water. Treatment may be continued even after symptoms are relieved. Monitor CBC. |
| leflunomide (Arava) | Antiinflammatory<br>Immunomodulatory agent that inhibits proliferation of lymphocytes | Monitor hepatic function. Assess for decreased pain, swelling, stiffness, and increase in joint mobility. Advise women of childbearing age to avoid pregnancy. |

*Continued*

## TABLE 64-3 Drug Therapy

***Arthritis and Connective Tissue Diseases—cont'd***

| Drug | Mechanism of Action | Nursing Considerations |
|---|---|---|
| **Disease-Modifying Antirheumatic Drugs (DMARDs)—*cont'd*** | | |
| penicillamine (Cuprimine, Depen) | Antiinflammatory<br>Exact mechanism unknown but may suppress cell-mediated immune response | Monitor WBC count, platelets, urinalysis. Advise patient to take medication 1 hr before or 2 hr after meals, and at least 1 hr away from any other drug, food, or milk. |
| ***Gold Compounds*** | | |
| *Parenteral:* gold sodium thiomalate, aurothioglucose<br>*Oral:* auranofin (Ridaura) | Alter immune responses, suppressing synovitis of active RA | Rule out pregnancy before beginning treatment. Monitor CBC, urinalysis, and hepatic and renal function. Advise patient therapeutic response may not occur for 3-6 mo. Advise patient to immediately report pruritus, rash, sore mouth, indigestion, or metallic taste. |
| ***Antimalarial*** | | |
| hydroxychloroquine (Plaquenil) | Exact mechanism unknown but may suppress formation of antigens | Monitor CBC and hepatic function. Advise patient therapeutic response may not occur for up to 6 mo. Advise patient to immediately report visual difficulties, muscular weakness, and decreased hearing or tinnitus. |
| ***Immunosuppressants*** | | |
| azathioprine (Imuran)<br>cyclophosphamide | Inhibit DNA, RNA, protein synthesis | Assess for decreased pain, swelling, stiffness, and increase in joint mobility. Advise patient to immediately report unusual bleeding or bruising. Advise patient therapeutic response may take up to 12 wk. Advise women of childbearing age to avoid pregnancy. Encourage increased fluid intake to decrease risk of hemorrhagic cystitis. |
| mycophenolate mofetil (CellCept) | Inhibits DNA synthesis | Monitor blood count and liver function tests every 2-4 wk for first 3 mo of treatment, thereafter every 1-3 mo.<br>Inform patient of increased infection risk. Instruct patients not to take antacids at same time because they may interfere with drug absorption. |
| ***JAK (Janus Kinase) Inhibitor*** | | |
| tofacitinib (Xeljanz) | Inhibits action of JAK enzymes, signaling pathways inside the cell with an important role in inflammation of RA | Inform patient of increased infection risk, including opportunistic infections. Monitor patient for any sign or symptom of infection for early treatment. |
| **Biologic Response Modifiers (Biologics, Immunotherapy)** | | |
| ***Tumor Necrosis Factor (TNF) Inhibitors*** | | |
| etanercept (Enbrel)<br>infliximab (Remicade)<br>adalimumab (Humira)<br>certolizumab (Cimzia)<br>golimumab (Simponi) | Bind to TNF, thus blocking its interaction with cell surface receptors. Decrease inflammatory and immune responses | Assess for decreased pain, swelling, stiffness, and increase in joint mobility. Advise patient of increased risk for tuberculosis. Instruct patient to have yearly PPD. Monitor for infection, bleeding, and emergence of malignancies. Advise patient injection site reaction generally occurs in first month of treatment and decreases with continued therapy. Advise patient to not receive live virus vaccines during treatment. |
| ***Interleukin-1 Receptor Antagonist*** | | |
| anakinra (Kineret) | Blocks the action of interleukin-1, decreasing inflammatory response | Assess for decreased pain, swelling, stiffness, and increase in joint mobility. Advise patient injection site reaction generally occurs in first month of treatment and decreases with continued therapy. Evaluate renal function. Monitor for infection. Inform patient to not take drug with TNF inhibitors. |
| ***Interleukin-6 Receptor Antagonist*** | | |
| tocilizumab (Actemra) | Blocks action of interleukin-6, thus decreasing inflammatory response | Given to patients with RA for whom other therapies have failed. Monitor BP and for infection. Advise patient of GI effects (e.g., perforation). Monitor liver enzyme and serum low-density lipoprotein (LDL). |
| ***T Cell Activation Inhibitor*** | | |
| abatacept (Orencia) | Inhibits T cell activation, thus suppressing immune response | Not recommended for concomitant use with TNF inhibitors. Assess for decreased pain, swelling, stiffness, and increase in joint mobility. |
| ***B Cell Depleting Agent*** | | |
| rituximab (Rituxan) | Monoclonal antibody that binds to CD20, an antigen on B cells, destroying B cells and suppressing immune response | Monitor for infection and bleeding. Advise patient to not receive live virus vaccines with treatment. Monitor for low BP if also taking BP medication. Advise patient fatigue is common with this medication. |

## COMPLEMENTARY & ALTERNATIVE THERAPIES

### Acupuncture

Acupuncture is a traditional Chinese medical practice of inserting very fine needles into the skin to stimulate specific anatomic points in the body (called *acupoints*) for therapeutic purposes.

**Scientific Evidence***

Acupuncture is associated with significant reduction in OA pain intensity, improved functional ability, and improved health-related quality of life.

**Nursing Implications**

- Research supports the use of acupuncture as an alternative for traditional analgesics in patients with OA.
- Refer interested patients to a practitioner who is appropriately trained and licensed.

*Source: Manyanga T, Froese M, Zarychanski R, et al: Pain management with acupuncture in osteoarthritis: a systematic review and meta-analysis, *BMC Comp Altern Med* 14:312, 2014.

## COMPLEMENTARY & ALTERNATIVE THERAPIES

### Glucosamine and Chondroitin

**Scientific Evidence***

- Combination of glucosamine plus chondroitin sulfate did not provide significant relief from OA pain among all participants.
- However, a smaller subgroup of study participants with moderate-to-severe pain showed significant relief with the combined supplements.
- Pain outcomes over 2 yr were similar to those of patients taking celecoxib (Celebrex) or placebo.
- Adverse reactions were mild. Serious adverse reactions were rare.

**Nursing Implications**

- Can be suggested to patients who are unable to take celecoxib or other NSAIDs.
- Discontinue if no effects after consistent use over 90-120 days.
- May decrease effectiveness of insulin or other drugs used to manage blood glucose.
- May increase the risk of bleeding.

*Source: National Center for Complementary and Alternative Medicine: Glucosamine/Chondroitin Arthritis Intervention Trial (GAIT): primary and ancillary study results. Retrieved from *https://nccih.nih.gov/research/results/gait*.

Aspercreme) may be an option for patients who are not able to take aspirin-containing medication. Several applications may be needed daily because topical agents have short-acting effects.

If a patient does not get adequate pain management with acetaminophen or has moderate to severe OA pain or signs of joint inflammation, a nonsteroidal antiinflammatory drug (NSAID) may be more effective. NSAID therapy typically is initiated in low-dose OTC strengths (e.g., ibuprofen) 200 mg up to four times daily). The dose may be increased if needed. If the patient is at risk for or develops gastrointestinal (GI) side effects with an NSAID, additional treatment with a protective agent such as misoprostol (Cytotec) may be needed. Arthrotec, a combination of misoprostol and the NSAID diclofenac, is also available. Diclofenac gel may be applied to the affected joint.

Because traditional NSAIDs block the production of prostaglandins from arachidonic acid by inhibiting the production of cyclooxygenase-1 (COX-1) and cyclooxygenase-2 (COX-2) (see Fig. 11-2), the risk for GI erosion and bleeding is increased. Traditional NSAIDs affect platelet aggregation, leading to a prolonged bleeding time. Patients taking an anticoagulant (e.g., warfarin [Coumadin]) and an NSAID are at high risk for bleeding. Long-term NSAID treatment may also affect cartilage metabolism, especially in older patients who may have poor cartilage integrity. As an alternative to traditional NSAIDs, the COX-2 inhibitor celecoxib (Celebrex) may be considered in selected patients. However, all NSAIDs carry the same risk for GI effects.[9]

## HEALTHY PEOPLE

### Prevention of Osteoarthritis

- Avoid cigarette smoking.
- Promptly treat any joint injury.
- Maintain healthy weight and eat a balanced diet.
- Use safety measures to protect and decrease risk of joint injury.
- Exercise regularly, including strength and endurance training.

When given in equivalent doses, all NSAIDs are comparably effective but vary widely in cost. Individual responses to the NSAIDs also vary. Some patients still prefer aspirin, but it is no longer a common treatment. It should be used cautiously with NSAIDs because both inhibit platelet function and prolong bleeding time. Intraarticular injections of corticosteroids may be suitable for the patient with local inflammation and swelling. Four or more injections without relief suggest the need for additional intervention. Systemic use of corticosteroids is not needed and may actually hasten the disease process.

Injection of hyaluronic acid *(viscosupplementation)* has been a common treatment for knee OA. However, its effectiveness in treating arthritis is not clear. Neither the American College of Rheumatology nor the American Academy of Orthopaedic Surgeons recommends using viscosupplementation with hyaluronates.[7,10] Research on the long-term effects of viscosupplementation continues.

Medications thought to slow the progression of OA or support joint healing are known as *disease-modifying osteoarthritis drugs (DMOADs)*. To date, no drugs have been approved to modify OA progression despite numerous clinical trials. Strontium ranelate is being evaluated in a variety of studies. Because of its potential ability to stimulate cartilage matrix, it may be helpful in OA treatment.[11]

**Surgical Therapy.** Symptoms of disease are often managed conservatively for many years. However, the patient's loss of joint function, unmanaged pain, and decreased independence in self-care may prompt a recommendation for surgery. Arthroscopy has been commonly performed for patients with knee OA. For most patients, however, this procedure provides no additional benefit over physical therapy and medical treatment.[12] Reconstructive surgical procedures (e.g., hip and knee replacements) are discussed in Chapter 62.

## NURSING MANAGEMENT: OSTEOARTHRITIS

### Nursing Assessment

Carefully assess and document the type, location, severity, frequency, and duration of the patient's joint pain and stiffness. Determine what makes the pain better or worse. Also ask the patient how these symptoms affect the ability to perform activities of daily living (ADLs). Identify the patient's pain management practices, and ask about success of each treatment.

Assess tenderness, swelling, limitation of movement, and crepitation of affected joints. Compare an involved joint with the opposite joint if it is not affected.

## ◆ Nursing Diagnoses

Nursing diagnoses for the patient with OA may include, but are not limited to, the following:

- Acute and chronic pain *related to* physical activity and lack of knowledge of pain self-management techniques
- Impaired physical mobility *related to* weakness, stiffness, or pain with ambulation
- Overweight or obesity *related to* intake in excess of energy output
- Depression *related to* chronic pain, changing physical appearance, and impaired social and work roles

## ◆ Planning

Overall goals are that the patient with OA will (1) maintain or improve joint function through a balance of rest and activity, (2) use joint protection measures (Table 64-4) to improve activity tolerance, (3) achieve independence in self-care and maintain optimal role function, and (4) use drug and nondrug strategies to manage pain satisfactorily.

## ◆ Nursing Implementation

◆ **Health Promotion.** Prevention of OA is possible in many cases. Focus community education on altering modifiable risk factors. For example, encourage the patient to lose weight and reduce occupational or recreational hazards. For athletic instruction and physical fitness programs, include safety measures that protect and reduce trauma to the joints. Traumatic joint injuries should be treated promptly to decrease the risk of OA.

◆ **Acute Care.** The person with OA most often complains of pain, stiffness, and limitation of function. In addition, the patient may experience daily frustration in coping with these physical difficulties. The older adult may believe OA is an inevitable part of aging and nothing can be done to decrease the discomfort and related disability.

The patient with OA is usually treated as an outpatient by an interprofessional team that may include an internal medicine physician or family HCP, a rheumatologist, a nurse, an occupational therapist, and a physical therapist. Health assessment questionnaires are often used to pinpoint areas of decreased function. Questionnaires are completed at regular intervals to document disease and treatment progression. Treatment goals can be based on data from the questionnaires and physical examination, with specific interventions for identified problems. The patient is usually hospitalized only if joint surgery is planned (see Chapter 62).

Drugs are administered for the treatment of pain and inflammation. Nondrug strategies to decrease pain and disability may include massage, use of heat (thermal packs) or cold (ice packs), meditation, and yoga.[13] Splints may be prescribed to rest and stabilize painful or inflamed joints.

Once an acute flare has subsided, a physical therapist can provide valuable assistance in planning an exercise program. The therapist may recommend Tai Chi as a low-impact form of exercise. Tai Chi can be performed by patients of all ages and may be done in a wheelchair. Stress the importance of warming up before any exercise to decrease risk for injury.

Patient and caregiver teaching related to OA is an important nursing responsibility. Provide information about the nature and treatment of the disease, pain management, body mechanics, correct use of assistive devices (e.g., cane, walker), principles of joint protection and energy conservation (Table 64-4), nutritional choices, weight and stress management, and an exercise program.

Assure the patient that OA is a localized disease and severe deforming arthritis is not the usual course. The patient can also gain support and understanding of the disease process through community resources such as the Arthritis Foundation's self-help course *(www.arthritis.org)*.

◆ **Ambulatory Care.** Adjust home management goals to meet the patient's needs. Include the caregiver, family members, and significant others in goal setting and teaching. Discuss home and work environment modification for patient safety, accessibility, and self-care. Measures include removing scatter rugs, providing rails at the stairs and bathtub, using night-lights, and wearing well-fitting supportive shoes. Assistive devices such as canes, walkers, elevated toilet seats, and grab bars also reduce the load on an affected joint and promote safety. Urge the patient to continue all prescribed therapies at home and be open to new approaches to symptom management.

Sexual counseling may help the patient and significant other to enjoy physical closeness by introducing the idea of alternate positions and timing for sexual activity. Discussion also increases awareness of each partner's needs. Encourage the patient to take analgesics or a warm bath to decrease joint stiffness before sexual activity.

## ◆ Evaluation

The expected outcomes are that the patient with OA will

- Experience adequate rest and activity
- Achieve satisfactory pain management
- Maintain joint flexibility and muscle strength through joint protection and therapeutic exercise
- Verbalize acceptance of OA as a chronic disease, collaborating with HCPs in disease management

### TABLE 64-4 Patient & Caregiver Teaching

***Joint Protection and Energy Conservation***

*Include the following instructions when teaching patients with arthritis to protect joints and conserve energy.*

- Maintain healthy weight.
- Use assistive devices, if indicated.
- Avoid forceful repetitive movements.
- Avoid awkward positions that stress joints.
- Use good posture and body mechanics.
- Seek help with needed tasks that may cause pain.
- Organize routine tasks and pace yourself to decrease fatigue and joint pain.
- Modify home and work environment to perform tasks in less stressful ways.

### CHECK YOUR PRACTICE

A 54-yr-old woman is diagnosed with osteoarthritis of the left knee. X-rays show joint space narrowing in the medial compartment with several bone spurs. She receives an intraarticular corticosteroid injection in the left knee. She also receives a prescription for physical therapy.

- What information will you provide about diclofenac to ensure the patient's safe, effective use?
- What type of exercises will be appropriate for this patient?
- The patient asks about complementary and alternative therapies for osteoarthritis. What will you tell her?

## RHEUMATOID ARTHRITIS

Rheumatoid arthritis (RA) is a chronic, systemic autoimmune disease characterized by inflammation of connective tissue in the diarthrodial (synovial) joints. RA is typically marked by periods of remission and exacerbation. RA often has extraarticular manifestations.

RA occurs globally, affecting all ethnic groups. It can occur at any time of life. However, incidence increases with age, peaking between ages 30 and 50 years. An estimated 1.5 million adult Americans are affected by RA. Almost three times as many women have the disease as men.[14]

### Etiology and Pathophysiology

The exact cause of RA is unknown. However, it probably results from a combination of genetics and environmental triggers. An autoimmune etiology is currently the most widely accepted theory, suggesting changes of RA begin when a genetically susceptible person has an initial immune response to an antigen. Although a bacterium or virus has been proposed as a possible antigen, no infection or organism has been identified to date.

The antigen, which is probably not the same in all patients, triggers formation of an abnormal immunoglobulin G (IgG). RA is marked by autoantibodies to this abnormal IgG. The autoantibodies are known as *rheumatoid factor (RF).* They combine with IgG to form immune complexes that initially deposit on synovial membranes or superficial articular cartilage in the joints. Immune complex formation leads to the activation of complement and an inflammatory response results. (Complement activation is discussed in Chapter 11, and immune complex formation is discussed in Chapter 13.)

Neutrophils are attracted to the site of inflammation, where they release proteolytic enzymes that damage articular cartilage and cause the synovial lining to thicken (Fig. 64-3). Other inflammatory cells include T helper (CD4) cells, which stimulate cell-mediated immune responses. Activated CD4 cells cause

**CULTURAL & ETHNIC HEALTH DISPARITIES**

***Arthritis and Connective Tissue Disorders***

- Arthritis is more common in whites and African Americans than in Hispanics.
- Hispanics and African Americans have a higher incidence of arthritis-related activity limitations than other ethnic groups.
- Some Native Americans (e.g., Pima, Chippewa, Yakima) have a higher incidence of RA than other ethnic groups in North America.
- Ankylosing spondylitis is more common in whites and certain Native American groups than in nonwhite groups.
- Systemic lupus erythematosus is more common and disease presentation is more severe among African American, Hispanic, Asian American, and Native American women than white women.
- African American and Hispanic women are at greater risk than white women for developing scleroderma.

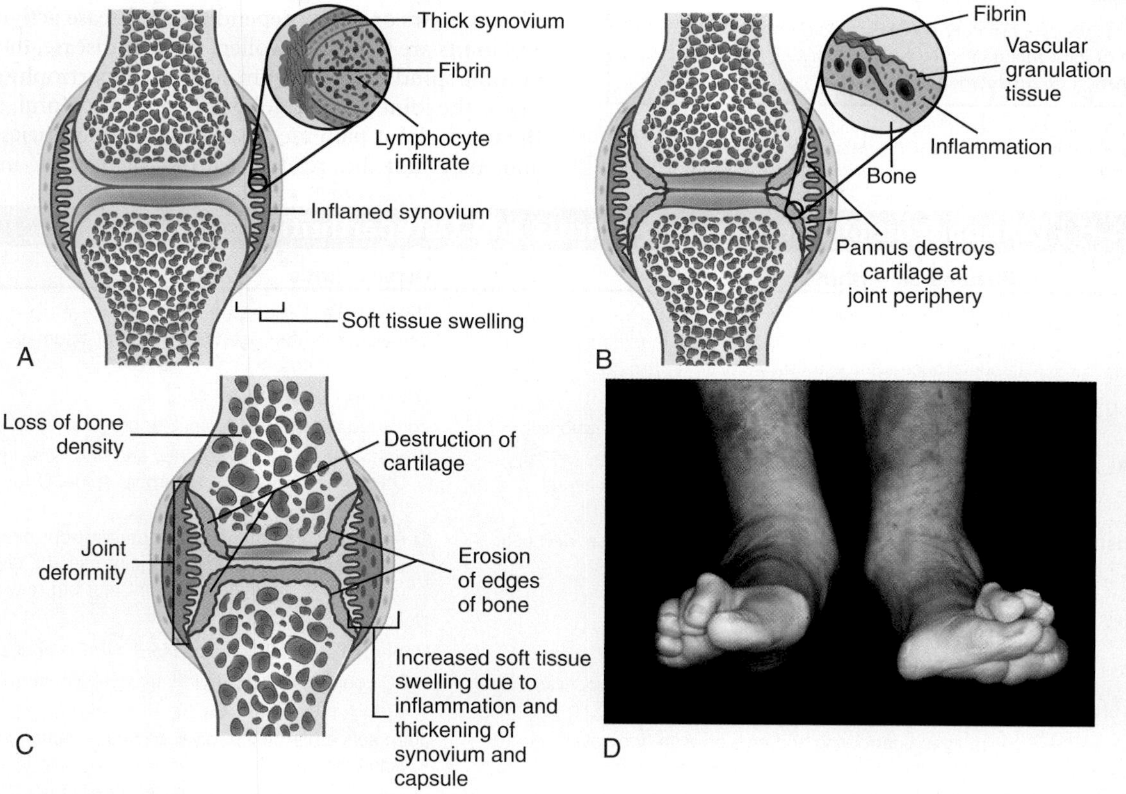


**FIG. 64-3** Rheumatoid arthritis. **A,** Early pathologic change is rheumatoid synovitis. Synovium becomes inflamed. Lymphocytes and plasma cells increase greatly. **B,** Over time, articular cartilage destruction occurs and vascular granulation tissue grows across the cartilage surface (pannus) from the edges of the joint. Joint surface shows loss of cartilage beneath the extending pannus, most marked at joint margins. **C,** Inflammatory pannus causes focal destruction of bone. Osteolytic destruction of bone occurs at joint edges, causing erosions seen on x-rays. This phase is associated with joint deformity. **D,** Multiple deformities of the foot from rheumatoid arthritis. (*D,* From Canale ST, Beaty JH: *Campbell's operative orthopaedics,* ed 12, Philadelphia, 2013, Mosby.)

monocytes, macrophages, and synovial fibroblasts to secrete the proinflammatory cytokines interleukin-1 (IL-1), interleukin-6 (IL-6), and tumor necrosis factor (TNF). These cytokines drive the inflammatory response in RA.

Without adequate treatment, more than 60% of patients with RA may develop marked functional impairment within 20 years of diagnosis.[15] This includes the need for mobility aids, loss of self-care ability, and need for joint reconstruction. By end-stage disease, patients experience loss of independence and require daily care (Table 64-5).

**TABLE 64-5 Stages of Rheumatoid Arthritis**

| Stage | Characteristics |
|---|---|
| I | • Synovitis marked by:<br>• Synovial membrane swelling with excess blood<br>• Membrane containing small areas of lymphocyte infiltration<br>• High WBC counts in synovial fluid (5000-60,000/μL)<br>• X-ray results: soft tissue swelling, possible osteoporosis, but no evidence of joint destruction |
| II | • Increased joint inflammation, spreading across cartilage into joint cavity<br>• Signs of gradual destruction in joint cartilage<br>• Narrowing joint space from loss of cartilage |
| III | • Formation of synovial pannus<br>• Joint cartilage becomes eroded, bone exposed<br>• X-ray results: extensive cartilage loss, erosion at joint margins, possible deformity |
| IV | • End-stage: inflammatory process subsides<br>• Loss of joint function<br>• Formation of subcutaneous nodules |

Source: Rheumatoid Arthritis.net: a Health Union Community: Understanding RA stages and progressions. Retrieved from *http://rheumatoidarthritis.net/what-is-ra/stages-and-progression.*

### Genetic Link

Genetic predisposition is important in the development of RA. The strongest evidence for a genetic influence is the role of human leukocyte antigens (HLA), especially the HLA-DR4 and HLA-DR1 antigens. (HLA is discussed in Chapter 13.) Smoking increases the risk of RA for persons who are genetically predisposed to the disease and may interfere with treatment for diagnosed persons.[16]

### Clinical Manifestations

**Joints.** The onset of RA is typically insidious. Nonspecific manifestations such as fatigue, anorexia, weight loss, and generalized stiffness may precede the onset of joint symptoms. Stiffness becomes more localized in the following weeks to months. Some patients report a precipitating stressful event such as infection, work stress, physical exertion, childbirth, surgery, or emotional upset. However, research has been unable to directly correlate such events with RA onset.

Specific joint involvement is marked by pain, stiffness, limited motion, and signs of inflammation (e.g., heat, swelling, tenderness). Joint symptoms occur symmetrically and often affect the small joints of the hands (PIP and MCP) and feet (MTP). Larger peripheral joints such as wrists, elbows, shoulders, knees, hips, ankles, and jaw may also be involved. The cervical spine may be affected, but the axial skeleton (spine and bones connected to it) is generally spared. Table 64-6 compares RA and OA.

The patient typically experiences joint stiffness after periods of inactivity. Morning stiffness may last from 60 minutes to several hours or more, depending on disease activity. MCP and PIP joints are typically swollen. In early disease, the fingers may become spindle shaped from synovial hypertrophy and thickening of the joint capsule. Joints are tender, painful, and warm to the touch. Joint pain increases with motion, varies in intensity, and may not be related to the degree of inflammation.

**TABLE 64-6 Comparison of Rheumatoid Arthritis and Osteoarthritis**

| Parameter | Rheumatoid Arthritis | Osteoarthritis |
|---|---|---|
| **Age at onset** | Young to middle age. | Usually >40 yr. |
| **Gender** | Female/male ratio is 2:1 or 3:1. Less marked sex difference after age 60. | Females 2:1 after age 60; except for traumatic arthritis, men less affected until age 70 or 80. |
| **Weight** | Lost or maintained weight. | Often overweight or obese. |
| **Disease** | Systemic disease with exacerbations and remissions. | Localized disease with variable, progressive course. |
| **Affected joints** | Small joints typically affected first (PIPs, MCPs, MTPs), wrists, elbows, shoulders, knees. Usually bilateral, symmetric joint involvement. | Weight-bearing joints of knees and hips, small joints (MCPs, DIPs, PIPs), cervical and lumbar spine. Often asymmetric. |
| **Pain characteristics** | Stiffness lasts 1 hr to all day and may decrease with use. Pain is variable, may disrupt sleep. | Stiffness occurs on arising but usually subsides after 30 min. Pain gradually worsens with joint use and disease progression, relieved with joint rest but may disrupt sleep. |
| **Effusions** | Common. | Uncommon. |
| **Nodules** | Present, especially on extensor surfaces. | Heberden's (DIPs) and Bouchard's (PIPs) nodes. |
| **Synovial fluid** | WBC count 5000-60,000/μL with mostly neutrophils; decreased viscosity. | WBC count <2000/μL (mild leukocytosis); normal viscosity. |
| **X-rays** | Joint space narrowing and erosion with bony overgrowths, subluxation with advanced disease. Osteoporosis related to decreased activity, corticosteroid use. | Joint space narrowing, osteophytes, subchondral cysts, sclerosis. |
| **Laboratory findings** | RF positive in 70%-90% of patients; negative titers in early disease for about 25% of patients.<br>ANA positive in 20%-30% of patients<br>Positive anti-CCP in more than 80% of patients<br>Elevated ESR, CRP indicative of active inflammation. | RF negative.<br>ANA negative.<br>Anti-CCP negative.<br>Transient elevation in ESR related to synovitis. |

*ANA,* Antinuclear antibodies; *anti-CCP,* anti-citrullinated peptide; *CRP,* C-reactive protein; *DIPs,* distal interphalangeal; *ESR,* erythrocyte sedimentation rate; *MCPs,* metacarpophalangeals; *MTPs,* metatarsophalangeals; *PIPs,* proximal interphalangeals; *RF,* rheumatoid factor.

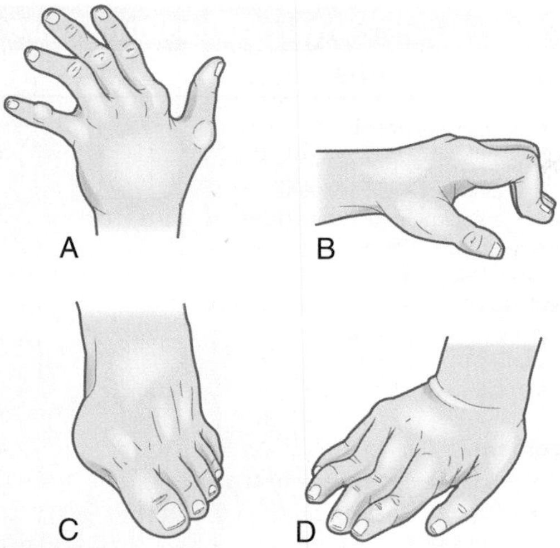


**FIG. 64-4** Typical deformities of RA. **A,** Ulnar drift. **B,** Boutonnière deformity. **C,** Hallux valgus. **D,** Swan neck deformity.

Tenosynovitis frequently affects the extensor and flexor tendons around the wrists, producing symptoms of carpal tunnel syndrome and making it difficult for the patient to grasp objects.

As the disease progresses, inflammation and fibrosis of the joint capsule and supporting structures may cause deformity and disability. Muscle atrophy and tendon destruction cause one joint surface to slip past the other *(subluxation)*. Metatarsal head dislocation and subluxation in the feet may cause pain and walking disability (Fig. 64-3, *D*). Ulnar drift ("zig-zag deformity"), swan neck, and boutonnière deformities are common in the hands (Fig. 64-4).

**Extraarticular Manifestations.** RA can affect nearly every body system (Fig. 64-5). Extraarticular manifestations are more likely to occur in the person with high levels of biomarkers such as RF.

*Rheumatoid nodules* develop in about half the patients with RA.[17] Rheumatoid nodules appear subcutaneously as firm, nontender, granuloma-type masses. They are often located on bony areas exposed to pressure, such as the fingers and elbows. Nodules at the base of the spine and back of the head are common in older adults. Treatment is usually not needed. However, these nodules can break down, similar to pressure ulcers. Cataracts and vision loss can result from scleral nodules. Nodular myositis and muscle fiber degeneration can cause pain similar to that of vascular insufficiency. In later disease, nodules in the heart and lungs can cause pleurisy, pleural effusion, pericarditis, pericardial effusion, and cardiomyopathy.

*Sjögren's syndrome* can occur by itself or in conjunction with other arthritic disorders, such as RA and SLE. Affected patients have diminished lacrimal and salivary gland secretion, leading to a dry mouth; burning, itchy eyes with decreased tearing; and photosensitivity. (Sjögren's syndrome is discussed later in this chapter on p. 1546.)

*Felty syndrome* is rare but can occur in patients with longstanding RA. It is characterized by an enlarged spleen and low white blood cell (WBC) count. Patients with Felty syndrome are at increased risk of infection and lymphoma.

Flexion contractures and hand deformities cause diminished grasp strength and affect the patient's ability to perform self-care tasks. Depression also may occur. However, it is unclear if the patient becomes depressed from struggling with chronic pain and disability, or if depression is part of the autoimmune disease process.[18]

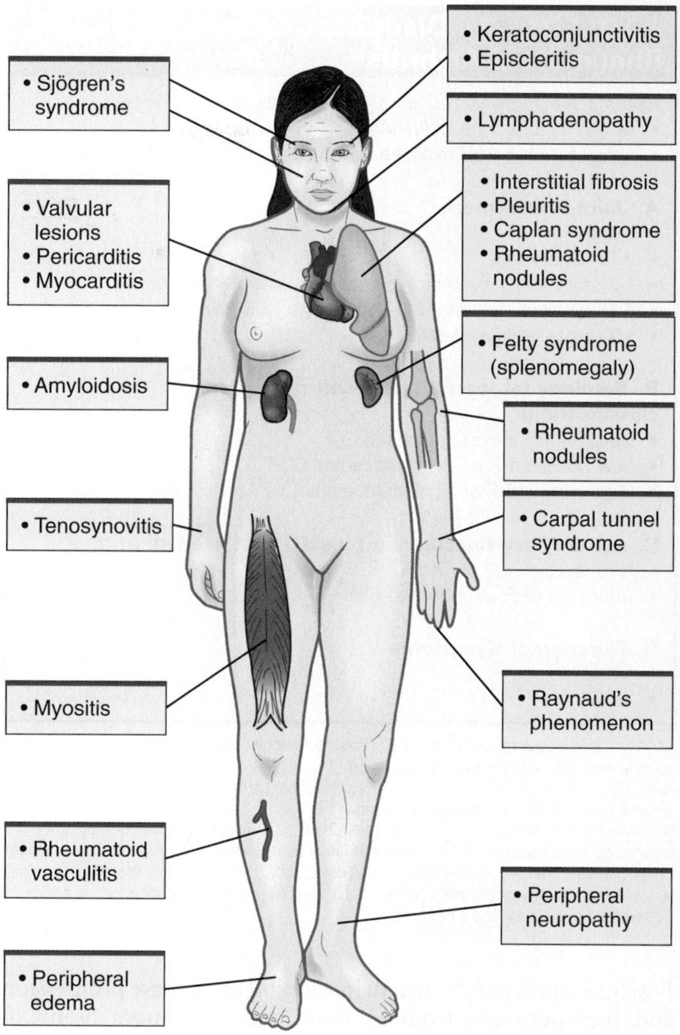


**FIG. 64-5** Extraarticular manifestations of RA.

## Diagnostic Studies

Accurate diagnosis is needed to start appropriate treatment and decrease the risk of disability. A diagnosis is often made based on history and physical findings. Some laboratory tests are also useful to confirm diagnosis and monitor disease progression (Tables 64-7 and 64-8).

Positive RF occurs in approximately 80% of adults with RA, and titers rise during active disease. ESR and C-reactive protein (CRP) are general indicators of active inflammation. An increase in antinuclear antibody (ANA) titers is also seen in 20% to 30% of patients with RA.[3] Testing for the antibodies to citrullinated peptide (anti-CCP) is also important in the diagnosis of RA. Levels of anti-CCP are more specific than RF for RA. In some cases, testing may allow an early, accurate diagnosis.[3]

Synovial fluid analysis in early disease often shows slightly cloudy, straw-colored fluid with many fibrin flecks. The enzyme MMP-3 is increased in the synovial fluid of the patient with RA, and it may be a marker of progressive joint damage. The WBC count of synovial fluid is elevated. Tissue biopsy can confirm inflammatory changes in the synovial membrane.

X-rays alone are not diagnostic of RA. They may show only soft tissue swelling and possible bone demineralization in early disease. A narrowed joint space, articular cartilage destruction, erosion, subluxation, and deformity are seen in later disease. Malalignment and ankylosis may be noted in advanced disease.

**TABLE 64-7 Diagnostic Criteria for Rheumatoid Arthritis***

| Patients should be tested for RA who initially are seen with: | |
|---|---|
| • At least 1 joint with definite clinical synovitis | |
| • Synovitis not better explained by another disease | |
| **A. Joint Involvement** | **Score** |
| • 1 large joint | 0 |
| • 2-10 large joints | 1 |
| • 1-3 small joints (with or without large joint involvement) | 2 |
| • 4-10 small joints (with or without large joint involvement) | 3 |
| • >10 joints (at least 1 small joint) | 5 |
| **B. Serology (at least 1 test result needed for classification)** | |
| • Negative RF *and* negative anti-CCP | 0 |
| • Low-positive RF *or* low-positive anti-CCP | 2 |
| • High-positive RF *or* high-positive anti-CCP | 3 |
| **C. Acute Phase Reactants (at least 1 test needed)** | |
| • Normal CRP *and* normal ESR | 0 |
| • Abnormal CRP *or* abnormal ESR | 1 |
| **D. Duration of Symptoms** | |
| • <6 wk | 0 |
| • ≥6 wk | 1 |

SCORING: Add score of categories A-D. Possible scores range from 0-10. A score of ≥6 indicates the definitive presence of RA.
*Anti-CCP,* Anti-citrullinated peptide; *CRP,* C-reactive protein; *ESR,* erythrocyte sedimentation rate; *RF,* rheumatoid factor.
From Aletaha D, Neogi T, Silman AJ, et al: 2010 Rheumatoid arthritis classification criteria: an American College of Rheumatology/European League Against Rheumatism Collaborative Initiative, *Arthr Rheum* 62:2569, 2010. Retrieved from *http://www.rheumatology.org/Portals/0/Files/2010_revised_criteria_classification_ra.pdf.*
*Used for newly diagnosed patients.

Baseline x-rays may be useful in monitoring disease progression and treatment effectiveness. Bone scans are more useful in detecting early joint changes and confirming diagnosis so that RA treatment can be initiated.

Criteria for diagnosis of RA in a newly presenting patient are described in Table 64-7.

## Interprofessional Care

Care of the patient with RA begins with a thorough program of education and drug therapy. Include information on correct administration, the need to report side effects, and medical and laboratory follow-up visits. Teach the patient and caregiver about the disease process and home management strategies. The physical therapist helps the patient maintain joint motion and muscle strength. An occupational therapist helps the patient maintain upper extremity function and encourages use of splints or other assistive devices for joint protection. A balance of rest and activity is also encouraged.

An individualized treatment plan considers disease activity, joint function, age, sex, family and social roles, and response to previous treatment (Table 64-8). A caring, long-term relationship with an interprofessional health care team can promote the patient's self-esteem and positive coping.

### Drug Therapy

***Disease-Modifying Antirheumatic Drugs.*** Drugs are the cornerstone of RA treatment (Table 64-3). Because irreversible joint changes can occur as early as the first year of RA, HCPs aggressively prescribe disease-modifying antirheumatic drugs (DMARDs). These drugs may slow disease progression and decrease risk of joint erosion and deformity. The choice of drug is based on disease activity; the patient's functional level; and lifestyle considerations, such as the wish to become pregnant.

**TABLE 64-8 Interprofessional Care**

***Rheumatoid Arthritis***

**Diagnostic Assessment**
- History and physical examination
- Complete blood cell (CBC) count
- Erythrocyte sedimentation rate (ESR)
- C-reactive protein (CRP)
- Rheumatoid factor (RF)
- Antibody to citrullinated peptide (anti-CCP)
- Antinuclear antibody (ANA)
- X-ray studies of involved joints
- Synovial fluid analysis

**Management**
- Nutritional and weight management counseling
- Therapeutic exercise
- Psychologic support
- Rest and joint protection, use of assistive devices
- Heat and cold applications
- Complementary and alternative therapies
  - Herbal products and nutritional supplements
  - Acupuncture
- Reconstructive surgery

***Drug Therapy*** *(Table 64-3)*
- Disease-modifying antirheumatic drugs (DMARDs)
- Intraarticular or systemic corticosteroids
- Nonsteroidal antiinflammatory drugs (NSAIDs)
- Biologic response modifiers (BRMs)

Methotrexate is preferred for early treatment of patients diagnosed with RA. It has a lower risk of toxicity than other drugs. Rare but serious side effects include bone marrow suppression and hepatotoxicity. The patient begins to experience therapeutic effects within 4 to 6 weeks. Methotrexate therapy requires frequent laboratory monitoring, including CBC and blood chemistry.

Sulfasalazine (Azulfidine) and the antimalarial drug hydroxychloroquine (Plaquenil) may be effective DMARDs for mild to moderate disease. They are rapidly absorbed, relatively safe, and well-tolerated medications. A baseline eye exam with yearly follow up is recommended for the patient taking hydroxychloroquine because of the risk of vision loss.

The synthetic DMARD leflunomide (Arava) blocks immune cell overproduction. Its efficacy and side effects are similar to those of methotrexate and sulfasalazine. Because the drug is teratogenic, the possibility of pregnancy in women of childbearing age must be excluded before therapy is initiated. Adequate contraception is needed during treatment.

Tofacitinib (Xeljanz), a JAK (Janus kinase) inhibitor, is used to treat moderate-to-severe active RA. The drug interferes with JAK enzymes that contribute to joint inflammation in RA.

***Biologic Response Modifiers.*** *Biologic response modifiers (BRMs)* (also called *biologics* or *immunotherapy*) are also used to slow disease progression in RA. These drugs are classified based on their mechanism of action (Table 64-3). They can be used to treat patients with moderate-to-severe who have not responded to DMARDs. They can also be used alone or in combination therapy with a DMARD such as methotrexate.

## TEAMWORK & COLLABORATION

### Caring for the Patient With Rheumatoid Arthritis

**Role of Nursing Personnel**

***Registered Nurse (RN)***

- Administer drug therapy as ordered.
- Teach patient and caregiver about medications, including increased risk of infection with disease-modifying agents.
- Assess disease impact on quality of life and joint function.
- Assess pain intensity and administer analgesics as ordered. Assess patient response.
- Develop program for rehabilitation and education with the interprofessional team.
- Teach patient about need for balance of rest and activity, with use of joint protective strategies.

***Licensed Practical/Vocational Nurse (LPN/LVN)***

- Reinforce teaching related to medication use and disease management strategies.
- Monitor pain intensity and administer prescribed analgesics.
- Notify RN of changes in pain or if pain persists after prescribed analgesics are administered.

***Unlicensed Assistive Personnel (UAP)***

- Assist patient with passive ROM of affected joints.
- Notify RN about patient complaints of pain.
- Assist patient with self-care needs.

**Role of Other Team Members**

***Physical Therapist***

- Assess patient's current mobility and need for assistance.
- Establish exercise regimen and teach patient to perform exercises safely.
- Coordinate PT with RN so that patient can receive timely analgesia.
- Discuss home environment with patient and identify possible modifications to facilitate disease management (e.g., bathroom on first level to avoid stairs).

***Occupational Therapist***

- Assess impact of patient's condition on ability to perform ADLs.
- Instruct patient in use of assistive devices (e.g., long-handled reacher, long-handled shoe horn) to facilitate self-care without increasing stress on joints.
- Discuss home environment with patient and identify possible modifications to facilitate role performance (e.g., kitchen modifications for meal preparation).

***Social Worker***

- Assess need for durable medical equipment (e.g., walker).
- Assess psychosocial and financial impact of disease. Arrange vocational retraining if needed.

TNF inhibitors include etanercept (Enbrel), infliximab (Remicade), adalimumab (Humira), certolizumab (Cimzia), and golimumab (Simponi). Etanercept is a biologically engineered copy of the TNF cell receptor. It binds to TNF in circulation before TNF can bind to the cell surface receptor. Thus etanercept inhibits the inflammatory response. This drug is given as a subcutaneous injection.

Infliximab and adalimumab are monoclonal antibodies that also bind to TNF, preventing it from binding to TNF receptors on cells. Infliximab is given IV in combination with methotrexate. Adalimumab is given subcutaneously.

Certolizumab and golimumab are TNF inhibitors that improve symptoms in patients with moderate-to-severe RA. Both drugs are given in combination with methotrexate.

**DRUG ALERT Tumor Necrosis Factor Inhibitors**

- Administer tuberculin test and perform chest x-ray before starting therapy.
- Monitor for signs of infection. Stop drug temporarily and notify HCP if acute infection develops.
- Instruct patients to avoid live vaccination while taking drug.
- Report bruising, bleeding, or persistent fever and other signs of infection.

Anakinra (Kineret) is an IL-1 receptor antagonist (IL-1Ra) created from new combinations of genetic material. It blocks the biologic activity of IL-1 by competitively inhibiting its ability to bind to the IL-1 receptor. Anakinra is given as a subcutaneous injection. It is used to reduce pain and swelling of moderate-to-severe RA. It can be used in combination with DMARDs but not with TNF inhibitors. Using these agents together can cause serious infection and neutropenia.

Tocilizumab (Actemra) blocks the action of IL-6, a cytokine that contributes to inflammation. It is used to treat patients with moderate-to-severe RA who have not adequately responded to or cannot tolerate other drugs for the disease.

Abatacept (Orencia) blocks T cell activation. It is recommended for patients who have inadequate response to DMARDs or TNF inhibitors. It is given IV. Similar to anakinra, it should not be used with TNF inhibitors.

Rituximab (Rituxan) is a monoclonal antibody that targets B cells (see Fig. 15-16). It may be used in combination with methotrexate for patients with moderate to severe RA not responding to TNF inhibitors. It is given IV.

***Other Drug Therapy.*** Other medications for treating RA include antibiotics (minocycline [Minocin]), immunosuppressants (azathioprine [Imuran]), penicillamine (Cuprimine), and gold preparations (auranofin [Ridaura], gold sodium thiomalate [Myochrysine]). However, these medications are not commonly used.

Corticosteroid therapy can be used to manage symptoms during disease flares. Intraarticular injections may temporarily reduce acute pain and inflammation. Low-dose oral corticosteroids may be used for a limited time to decrease disease activity until the effects of DMARD therapy are seen. However, they are inadequate as a sole therapy, and their long-term use should not be a mainstay of RA treatment. Possible complications include osteoporosis and avascular necrosis.

Various NSAIDs and salicylates are used to treat arthritic pain and inflammation. Aspirin may be used in dosages of 3 to 4 g/day in three to four doses. Blood salicylate levels should be monitored in a patient taking more than 3600 mg daily.[19] NSAIDs have antiinflammatory and analgesic effects. Some relief may be noted within days of starting treatment with NSAIDs, but full effect may take 2 to 3 weeks. NSAIDs may be used when the patient cannot tolerate aspirin. The patient may be able to better follow the treatment regimen if using an antiinflammatory drug that can be taken only once or twice a day (Table 64-3). Celecoxib (Celebrex), the only available COX-2 inhibitor, is effective in RA as well as OA.

**Nutritional Therapy.** Although no special diet is needed for RA, balanced nutrition is important. Fatigue, pain, and depression may cause a loss of appetite. In addition, limited endurance and mobility deficits may interfere with the patient's ability to shop for and prepare food. Weight loss may result. The occupational therapist may help the patient modify the home environment and use assistive devices for easier food preparation.

Corticosteroid therapy or decreased mobility due to pain may cause unwanted weight gain. Corticosteroids increase the appetite, leading to higher caloric intake. A sensible weight loss program with balanced nutrition and exercise reduces stress on affected joints. In addition, the patient taking corticosteroids may become distressed as signs and symptoms of Cushing syndrome (e.g., moon face, redistribution of fatty tissue to the trunk) change the physical appearance. Encourage the patient not to change the dose or stop therapy abruptly. Weight will return to normal several months after treatment ends. Remind the patient to continue to eat a balanced diet.

**Surgical Therapy.** Surgery may be needed to relieve severe pain and improve the function of severely deformed joints. Removal of the joint lining *(synovectomy)* is one type of surgery. Total joint replacement *(arthroplasty)* can be done for many different joints in the body. Joint surgery is discussed in Chapter 62.

## NURSING MANAGEMENT: RHEUMATOID ARTHRITIS

### Nursing Assessment

Subjective and objective data that should be obtained from the patient with RA are presented in Table 64-9.

**TABLE 64-9 Nursing Assessment**
***Rheumatoid Arthritis***

**Subjective Data**

***Important Health Information***

*Past health history:* Recent infections. Precipitating factors such as emotional upset, infections, overwork, childbirth, surgery. Pattern of remissions and exacerbations

*Medications:* Aspirin, NSAIDs, corticosteroids, DMARDs, BRMs

*Surgery or other treatments:* Any joint surgery

***Functional Health Patterns***

*Health perception–health management:* Positive family history for rheumatoid arthritis or other autoimmune disorders. Malaise, ability to participate in therapeutic regimen. Impact of disease on functional ability

*Nutritional-metabolic:* Anorexia, weight loss, dry mucous membranes of mouth and pharynx

*Activity-exercise:* Stiffness and joint swelling, muscle weakness, difficulty walking, fatigue

*Cognitive-perceptual:* Paresthesia of hands and feet, loss of sensation; symmetric joint pain and aching that increases with motion or stress on joint, may interfere with rest

**Objective Data**

***General***

Lymphadenopathy, fever

***Integumentary***

Scleritis, uveitis, Sjögren's syndrome. Subcutaneous rheumatoid nodules on forearms, elbows. Skin ulcers. Shiny, taut skin over involved joints. Peripheral edema

***Cardiovascular***

Symmetric pallor and cyanosis of fingers (Raynaud's phenomenon). Distant heart sounds, murmurs, dysrhythmias

***Respiratory***

Bronchiectasis, pleural effusion, tuberculosis, interstitial lung disease

***Gastrointestinal***

Splenomegaly (Felty syndrome)

***Musculoskeletal***

Symmetric joint involvement with swelling, erythema, heat, tenderness. Deformities (with later disease). Enlargement of PIP and MCP joints. Limitation of joint movement, muscle contractures, muscle atrophy

***Possible Diagnostic Findings***

Positive RF, ANA, Anti-CCP. ↑ ESR; anemia. ↑ WBCs in synovial fluid. On x-ray evidence of joint space narrowing, bony erosion, deformity, possible osteoporosis

*ANA,* Antinuclear antibody; *anti-CCP,* anti-citrullinated peptide; *BRMs,* biologic response modifiers; *DMARDs,* disease-modifying antirheumatic drugs; *ESR,* erythrocyte sedimentation rate; *MCP,* metacarpophalangeal; *NSAIDs,* nonsteroidal antiinflammatory drugs; *PIP,* proximal interphalangeal; *RF,* rheumatoid factor.

### Nursing Diagnoses

Nursing diagnoses for the patient with RA may include, but are not limited to, the following:

- Impaired physical mobility *related to* joint pain, stiffness, and deformity
- Chronic pain *related to* joint inflammation, overuse of joints, and ineffective pain and/or comfort measures
- Disturbed body image *related to* chronic disease activity, long-term treatment, deformities, stiffness, and inability to perform usual activities

Additional information on nursing diagnoses for the patient with RA is provided in eNursing Care Plan 64-1 (on the website for this chapter).

### Planning

The overall goals are that the patient with RA will (1) have satisfactory pain management, (2) have minimal loss of function of affected joints, (3) participate in planning and implementing the therapeutic regimen, (4) maintain a positive self-image, and (5) perform self-care to the maximum amount possible.

### Nursing Implementation

**Health Promotion.** Prevention of RA is not possible at this time. However, early treatment can help prevent further joint damage. Community education programs should focus on symptom recognition to promote early diagnosis and treatment. The Arthritis Foundation offers many publications, classes, and support activities to help persons with RA.

**Acute Care.** Primary goals in RA management are reduction of inflammation, management of pain, maintenance of joint function, and prevention or minimization of joint deformity. Goals may be met through a broad program of drug therapy, balance of rest and activity with joint protection, use of heat and cold applications, exercise, and patient and caregiver teaching. Work closely with the HCP, physical and occupational therapists, and social worker to help the patient regain function and adjust to chronic illness.

The patient newly diagnosed with RA is usually treated on an outpatient basis. Hospitalization may be needed for the patient who has systemic complications or requires surgery for disabling deformities.

Intervention begins with a careful physical assessment (e.g., joint pain, swelling, ROM, general health status). Also evaluate psychosocial needs (e.g., family support, sexual satisfaction, emotional stress, financial constraints, vocational and career limitations) and environmental concerns (e.g., transportation, home or work modifications). After identifying the patient's problems, carefully plan a program for rehabilitation and education with the interprofessional care team.

Inflammation may be effectively treated through administration of NSAIDs, DMARDs, and BRMs. Careful timing of drug administration is critical to maintain a therapeutic drug level and reduce early morning stiffness. Discuss the action and side effects of each prescribed drug and the importance of laboratory monitoring. Many patients with RA take several different drugs, so make the drug regimen as understandable as possible. Encourage patients to develop a way to remember to take their medications (e.g., pill containers).

Nondrug management may include the use of therapeutic heat and cold, rest, relaxation techniques, joint protection (Tables 64-4 and 64-10), biofeedback, transcutaneous electrical nerve stimulation (see Chapter 8), and hypnosis. Allow the patient and caregiver to choose therapies that promote optimal comfort and fit their lifestyle.

Lightweight splints may be prescribed to rest an inflamed joint and prevent deformity from muscle spasms and contractures. Remove the splints regularly to assess skin and perform ROM exercises. After assessment and supportive care, reapply splints as prescribed. The occupational therapist may identify additional self-help devices for ADLs.

Plan care and procedures around the patient's morning stiffness. Sitting or standing in a warm shower, sitting in a tub with warm towels around the shoulders, or simply soaking the hands in a basin of warm water may relieve joint stiffness and allow the patient to perform ADLs more comfortably.

### ◆ Ambulatory Care

◆ ***Rest.*** Alternating scheduled rest periods with activity throughout the day helps relieve fatigue and pain. The amount of rest needed varies based on disease severity and the patient's limitations. The patient should rest before becoming exhausted. Total bed rest is rarely necessary and should be avoided to prevent stiffness and other effects of immobility. However, even a patient with mild disease may require daytime rest in addition to 8 to 10 hours of sleep at night. Help the patient identify ways to modify daily activities to avoid overexertion and fatigue, which can worsen disease activity. For example, the patient may be able to prepare meals more easily while sitting on a high stool in front of the sink.

Teach the patient to maintain good body alignment during rest through use of a firm mattress or bed board. Encourage positions of extension, and teach the patient to avoid positions of flexion. To decrease the risk of joint contracture, never place pillows under the knees. Use a small, flat pillow under the head and shoulders if needed.

◆ ***Joint Protection.*** Protecting joints from stress is important. Help the patient identify ways to alter routine tasks to put less stress on joints (Table 64-10). Energy conservation requires careful planning. The emphasis is on work simplification. Work for short periods with scheduled rest breaks to avoid fatigue (pacing). Organize activities to avoid going up and down stairs repeatedly. Use carts to carry supplies, or store frequently used materials in a convenient, easy-to-reach area. Use joint-protective devices (e.g., electric can opener) whenever possible. Also teach patients to delegate tasks to other family members.

Occupational therapy training may increase patient independence with assistive devices that simplify tasks (e.g., built-up utensils, buttonhooks, modified drawer handles, lightweight plastic dishes, raised toilet seats). Encourage the patient to make dressing easier by wearing shoes with Velcro fasteners and clothing with buttons or a zipper in the front instead of the back. Use a cane or a walker for support and decreased pain when walking.

◆ ***Heat and Cold Therapy and Exercise.*** Heat and cold applications can help relieve stiffness, pain, and muscle spasm. Ice is especially helpful during periods of increased disease activity, while moist heat seems to offer better relief for chronic stiffness. Heating pads, moist hot packs, paraffin baths, and warm baths or showers can relieve stiffness to allow the patient to participate in therapeutic exercise. Plastic bags of small frozen vegetables (peas or kernel corn) can easily mold around the shoulder, wrists, or knees to be an effective home treatment. The patient can also use ice cubes or small paper cups of frozen water to massage areas on either side of a painful joint. Heat and cold can be used several times a day as needed. However, heat application should not exceed 20 minutes at one time. Cold application should not exceed 10 to 15 minutes at one time. Alert the patient to the risk of a burn and the need to avoid using a heat-producing cream (e.g., capsaicin) with an external heat device.

Individualized exercise is an important part of the treatment plan. A physical therapist may develop a therapeutic exercise program to improve flexibility and strength of affected joints and increase the patient's endurance. Encourage program participation and reinforce correct performance of the exercises. Progressive joint immobility and muscle weakness can occur if the patient does not move the joints. Overaggressive exercise can cause increased pain, inflammation, and joint damage. Emphasize that participating in a recreational exercise program (e.g., walking, swimming) or performing usual daily activities does not take the place of therapeutic exercise to maintain adequate joint motion.

Gentle ROM exercises are usually done daily to keep joints functional. The patient should practice exercises with supervision. Aquatic exercises in warm water (78° to 86° F [25° to 30° C]) allow easier joint movement because of the buoyancy and warmth of the water. Although movement seems easier, water also provides two-way resistance that makes muscles

**TABLE 64-10 Patient & Caregiver Teaching**

***Protection of Small Joints***

*Include the following instructions when teaching the patient with arthritis how to protect small joints.*

1. Maintain joint in neutral position to minimize deformity.
   - Press water from a sponge instead of wringing.
2. Use strongest joint available for any task.
   - When rising from chair, push with palms rather than fingers.
   - Carry laundry basket in both arms rather than with fingers.
3. Distribute weight over many joints instead of stressing a few.
   - Slide objects instead of lifting them.
   - Hold packages close to body for support.
4. Change positions frequently.
   - Do not hold book or grip steering wheel for long periods without resting.
   - Avoid grasping pencil or cutting vegetables with knife for extended periods.
5. Avoid repetitious movements.
   - Do not knit or sew for long periods.
   - Rest between rooms when vacuuming.
   - Modify home environment to include faucets and doorknobs that are pushed rather than turned.
6. Modify chores to avoid stress on joints.
   - Avoid heavy lifting.
   - Sit on stool instead of standing during meal preparation.

work harder than they would on land. During acute inflammation, limit exercise to one or two repetitions.

◆ ***Psychologic Support.*** For effective self-management and adherence to an individualized home treatment program, help the patient understand the nature and course of RA and the goals of therapy. Also consider the patient's value system and perception of the disease.

The patient is challenged constantly by problems of limited function and fatigue, loss of self-esteem, altered body image, and fear of disability and deformity. Discuss alterations in sexuality. Chronic pain or loss of function may make the patient vulnerable to claims of false advertising about unproven or even dangerous remedies. Help the patient recognize fears and concerns faced by all people who live with chronic illness.

Evaluate the family support system. Financial planning may be necessary. Consider community resources such as a home care nurse, homemaker services, and vocational rehabilitation. Self-help groups are helpful for some patients.

Living with chronic pain may lead to depression. To decrease depressive symptoms, suggest activities such as listening to music, reading, exercising, and counseling. Hypnosis and biofeedback may also be useful.

### Gerontologic Considerations: Arthritis

The prevalence of arthritis in older adults is high. The disease is also accompanied by problems unique to this age group. Areas of concern for older adults include the following:

- The high incidence of OA in older adults often keeps the HCP from considering other types of arthritis.
- Age alone causes changes in blood testing, making interpretation of laboratory values such as RF and ESR more difficult. Drugs taken for co-morbid conditions can also affect laboratory values.
- Polypharmacy in older adults can also cause arthritis.
- Musculoskeletal pain syndromes and weakness may have no physical cause. Instead, they may be related to depression and physical inactivity.
- Diseases such as SLE, which commonly occurs in younger adults, can develop in a milder form in older adults.

Physical and metabolic changes of aging may increase the older patient's sensitivity to both therapeutic and toxic effects of some drugs. The older adult who takes NSAIDs has an increased risk for side effects, especially GI bleeding and renal toxicity. Using NSAIDs with a shorter half-life may require more frequent dosing but may also produce fewer side effects in the older patient with altered drug metabolism.

The common occurrence of polypharmacy in the older adult is a concern. Use of additional drugs in RA treatment may increase the likelihood of unexpected drug interactions. The drug regimen should be as simple as possible to increase adherence (e.g., limited number of drugs with decreased frequency of administration). This is especially important for the patient who lacks regular assistance.

Osteopenia from corticosteroid use can worsen the problem of decreased bone density from aging and inactivity. The risk of pathologic fractures is increased, especially vertebral compression fractures. Myopathy related to corticosteroid use can be minimized or prevented by an age-appropriate exercise program. An adequate support system for the older adult is critical to the ability to follow a treatment regimen that includes nutritional planning, exercise, general health maintenance, and appropriate therapy.

## GOUT

**Gout** is a type of acute arthritis characterized by elevation of uric acid *(hyperuricemia)* and the deposit of uric acid crystals in one or more joints. Sodium urate crystals may be found in articular, periarticular, and subcutaneous tissues. Unlike chronic forms of arthritis, gout is marked by painful flares lasting days to weeks followed by long periods without symptoms. More than 8 million Americans are affected by gout, with men affected three times as often as women. The incidence among African American men is nearly twice that of white men.[20]

Hyperuricemia may be classified as primary or secondary.[21] In *primary hyperuricemia,* a hereditary error of purine metabolism leads to the overproduction or retention of uric acid. *Secondary hyperuricemia* may be related to another acquired disorder (Table 64-11) or may be caused by drugs known to inhibit uric acid excretion (e.g., thiazide diuretics, β-blockers, angiotensin-converting enzyme [ACE] inhibitors). Postmenopausal women and organ transplant recipients receiving immunosuppressive agents are also at risk for hyperuricemia.

### Etiology and Pathophysiology

Uric acid is the major end product of purine catabolism and is primarily excreted by the kidneys. Gout is caused by (1) an increase in uric acid production; (2) reduced excretion of uric acid by the kidneys; or (3) increased intake of foods containing purines (e.g., red and organ meat, shellfish, fructose drinks), which are metabolized to uric acid by the body. Increased uric acid production is most commonly linked to obesity. Excessive alcohol consumption is also a risk factor.

High dietary intake of purine alone has relatively little effect on uric acid. Hyperuricemia may result from prolonged fasting or excessive alcohol drinking because of the increased production of keto acids, which then inhibit uric acid excretion. Reduced uric acid excretion can occur with chronic kidney disease or metabolic syndrome.

### Clinical Manifestations and Complications

Gouty arthritis may occur acutely in one or more joints but usually less than four. Affected joints may appear dusky or cyanotic and are extremely tender. Inflammation of the great toe *(podagra)* is the most common initial problem. Other affected joints may include wrists, knees, ankles, and the midfoot. Olecranon bursae may also be involved. Acute gouty arthritis is usually triggered by events such as trauma, surgery, alcohol ingestion, or systemic infection. Symptom onset typically occurs at night with sudden swelling and severe pain peaking within several hours. Patients often indicate the painful

**TABLE 64-11 Causes of Hyperuricemia**

| | |
|---|---|
| • Acidosis or ketosis | • Malignant disease |
| • Alcohol use | • Myeloproliferative disorders |
| • Atherosclerosis | • Obesity or starvation |
| • Chemotherapy drugs | • Renal insufficiency |
| • Diabetes mellitus | • Sickle cell anemia |
| • Drug-induced renal impairment | • Use of certain common drugs (aspirin, thiazide, diuretics, niacin) |
| • Exposure to lead | |
| • Hyperlipidemia | |
| • Hypertension | |

area is highly sensitive to light touch. Low-grade fever is common.

Individual attacks usually end in 2 to 10 days with or without treatment. The affected joint returns to normal and patients have no symptoms between attacks.

Chronic gout is characterized by multiple joint involvement and visible deposits of sodium urate crystals *(tophi)*. These are typically seen in the synovium, subchondral bone, olecranon bursae, and vertebrae; along tendons; and in the skin and cartilage (Fig. 64-6). Tophi are generally only noted many years after the onset of disease.

The severity of gouty arthritis varies. The clinical course may involve infrequent mild attacks or multiple severe episodes (up to 12 per year) marked by slowly progressive disability. In general, tophi appear earlier and the patient is prone to more frequent, severe episodes of gout if serum uric acid remains high. Chronic inflammation may cause joint deformity, and cartilage destruction may lead to secondary OA. Large urate crystal deposits may pierce overlying skin, producing draining sinuses that often become infected.

Excessive uric acid excretion may lead to stone formation in the kidneys or urinary tract. Pyelonephritis related to sodium urate deposits and obstruction may contribute to kidney disease.

## Diagnostic Studies

In gout, serum uric acid is usually elevated above 6 mg/dL. However, hyperuricemia is not specifically diagnostic of gout because values may be normal during an acute gouty attack.[22] Increased uric acid may also be related to various drugs or may exist as an asymptomatic abnormality in the general population. Specimens may be obtained for 24-hour urine uric acid to determine if the disease is caused by decreased renal excretion or overproduction of uric acid.

### GENDER DIFFERENCES

***Gout***

**Men**

- Occurs three times more often in men than in women until age 60.
- Occurs predominantly in men ages 30 to 50.

**Women**

- Low occurrence in premenopausal women.

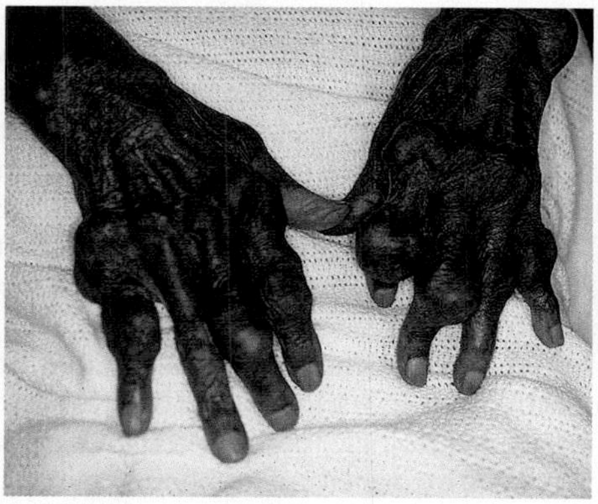

**FIG. 64-6** Tophi associated with chronic gout. Painless nodules are filled with uric acid crystals. (Courtesy John Cook, MD. From Goldstein BG, Goldstein AE: *Practical dermatology,* ed 2, St Louis, 1997, Mosby.)

The gold standard for diagnosis of gout is synovial fluid aspiration. Affected fluid characteristically contains needle-like monosodium urate crystals. This procedure is done in only about 11% of patients because diagnosis can typically be made on clinical symptoms alone.[21]

However, it is the only reliable way to distinguish gout from septic arthritis or *pseudogout* (calcium phosphate crystal formation). Aspiration also may have therapeutic value by decompressing a swollen joint capsule.

X-rays appear normal in the early stages of gout. In chronic disease, tophi may appear as eroded areas in the bone.

## Interprofessional Care

Goals for the care of the patient with gout (Table 64-12) include ending an acute attack with an antiinflammatory agent such as colchicine. Drug therapy is the primary way to treat acute and chronic gout. Also recommend weight reduction as needed and possible avoidance of alcohol and foods high in purine.

**Drug Therapy.** Acute gout is treated with colchicine and NSAIDs. Because colchicine has antiinflammatory effects but is not an analgesic, an NSAID is added for pain management. Oral administration of colchicine generally produces dramatic pain relief when given within 12 to 24 hours of an attack.[23] Colchicine also helps in diagnosis because good response to this drug is further evidence of gout.

Future attacks of gout are prevented in part by a maintenance dose of a drug that lowers urate such as a xanthine oxidase inhibitor (allopurinol [Zyloprim, Aloprim]), or a drug that increases the excretion of uric acid in the urine *(uricosuric)* (probenecid). Febuxostat (Uloric), a selective inhibitor of xanthine oxidase, is used for long-term management of hyperuricemia in people with chronic gout.

Patients who cannot take or do not respond to drugs that lower serum uric acid may be given pegloticase (Krystexxa).

### TABLE 64-12 Interprofessional Care

***Gout***

**Diagnostic Asessment**

- History and physical examination
- Family history of gout
- Sodium urate crystals in synovial fluid
- Elevated serum uric acid
- Elevated 24-hr urine for uric acid
- X-ray of affected joints

**Management**

- Joint immobilization
- Local application of heat and cold
- Joint aspiration and intraarticular corticosteroids
- Avoidance of food and fluids with high purine content (e.g., anchovies, liver, wine, beer)

***Drug Therapy***

- colchicine
- Nonsteroidal antiinflammatory drugs (e.g., naproxen [Naprosyn])
- allopurinol (Zyloprim)
- probenecid
- febuxostat (Uloric)
- pegloticase (Krystexxa)
- Corticosteroids (prednisone)
- Intraarticular corticosteroids (methylprednisolone)
- Adrenocorticotropic hormone (ACTH)

This drug is an enzyme that metabolizes uric acid into a harmless chemical excreted in the urine. The drug is given IV. Corticosteroids given orally or by intraarticular injection also can be helpful in treating acute attacks of gout. Systemic corticosteroids may be used only if routine therapies are contraindicated or ineffective. In addition, adrenocorticotropic hormone (ACTH) may be used for treating acute gout.

For many years, the standard therapy for hyperuricemia caused by decreased urate excretion has been uricosuric drugs such as probenecid. These drugs inhibit renal tubular reabsorption of urates. However, they are ineffective when creatinine clearance is reduced, as can occur in patients over age 60 years or with renal impairment. Aspirin inactivates the effect of these drugs, resulting in urate retention, and should be avoided during treatment. Acetaminophen can be used safely if analgesia is required.

Adequate urine volume with normal renal function (2 to 3 L/day) must be maintained to prevent precipitation of uric acid in the renal tubules. Allopurinol, which blocks the production of uric acid, is especially useful for patients with uric acid stones or renal impairment. Uricosuric drugs may be ineffective or dangerous for these patients. For patients who cannot tolerate allopurinol because of side effects, oxypurinol can be prescribed. Oxypurinol is the active metabolite of allopurinol. The angiotensin II receptor antagonist losartan (Cozaar) may be effective for treatment of older patients with gout and hypertension. Losartan promotes urate diuresis and may normalize serum urate. Combination therapy with losartan and allopurinol may also be used. Whatever drugs are prescribed, serum uric acid must be checked regularly to monitor treatment effectiveness.

**Nutritional Therapy.** Dietary restrictions that limit alcohol and foods high in purine help minimize uric acid production (see Table 45-12). Instruct obese patients in a carefully planned weight-reduction program.

## NURSING MANAGEMENT: GOUT

Nursing interventions for the patient with acute gout include supportive care of the inflamed joints. Avoid causing pain by careless handling of an inflamed joint. Bed rest may be appropriate to immobilize affected joints as needed. Use a cradle or footboard to protect a painful lower extremity from the weight of bed linens. Assess limitation of motion and degree of pain. Document treatment effectiveness.

Hyperuricemia and gout are chronic problems that can be controlled with effective patient education and careful adherence to a treatment program.[22] Explain the importance of drug therapy and the need for regular assessment of serum uric acid. Teach the patient about factors that may cause an attack: (1) excessive caloric intake or overindulgence in purine-containing foods and alcohol, (2) starvation (fasting), (3) drug use (e.g., diuretics), and (4) major medical events (e.g., surgery, myocardial infarction).

## LYME DISEASE

**Lyme disease** is an infection caused by the spirochete *Borrelia burgdorferi* and transmitted by the bite of an infected deer tick. It was first identified in 1975 in Lyme, Connecticut, after an unusual occurrence of arthritis in children. It is the most common vector-borne disease in the United States. The tick typically feeds on mice, dogs, cats, cows, horses, deer, and humans. Wild animals do not exhibit the illness, but clinical Lyme disease does occur in domestic animals. Person-to-person transmission does not occur.

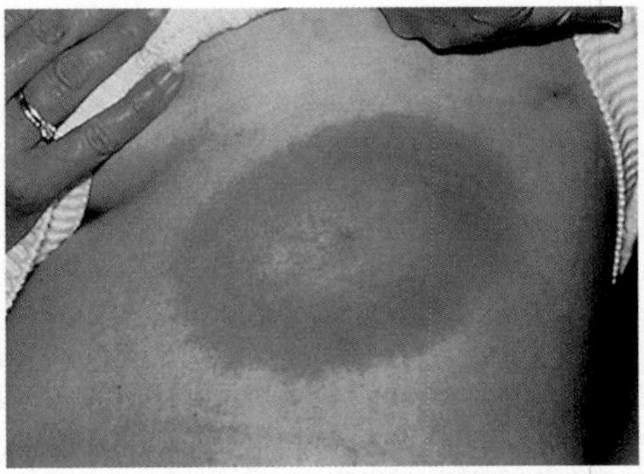

**FIG. 64-7** Erythema migrans. Typical skin lesion of Lyme disease occurs at the site of tick bite. (From Marx J, Hockberger R, Walls R: *Rosen's emergency medicine,* ed 7, Philadelphia, 2009, Mosby.)

### CHECK YOUR PRACTICE

A patient is admitted to the medical unit with acute gout. The right great toe is swollen, red, and painful. He is prescribed colchicine.

- What nursing interventions will you use to protect the right foot and decrease pain?
- What information will you provide about the patient's medication?
- How will you explain the role of hyperuricemia in development of acute gout?
- What will you discuss with the patient concerning possible dietary changes to decrease risk of future attacks?

The summer months are the peak season for human infection. Most U.S. cases occur in three areas: along the northeastern states from Virginia to Maine, in the Midwestern states of Wisconsin and Minnesota, and along the northwestern coast of California and Oregon. More than 30,000 cases are reported annually in the United States.[24] Reinfection is not uncommon.

Symptoms of Lyme disease can mimic those of other diseases such as multiple sclerosis, mononucleosis, and meningitis. The most characteristic clinical symptom of early localized disease is *erythema migrans* (EM). This "bull's eye rash" occurs in 70% to 80% of infected persons at the site of the tick bite within 3 to 30 days after exposure (Fig. 64-7). It may also appear anywhere else on the body as the disease progresses. The EM lesion begins as a central red macule or papule that slowly expands to include a red outer ring of up to 12 in, resembling a bull's eye. It may be warm to the touch but is not itchy or painful. The rash often occurs with acute flu-like symptoms: (1) low-grade fever, (2) chills, (3) headache, (4) stiff neck, (5) fatigue, (6) swollen lymph nodes, and (7) migratory joint and muscle pain. Loss of tone in facial muscles can appear as Bell's palsy. Symptoms usually occur in a week but may be delayed up to 30 days. Flu-like symptoms generally resolve over weeks or months, even if untreated.

If not treated, the spirochete can disseminate within several weeks or months to the heart, joints, and central nervous system (CNS). Chronic neurologic complaints include short-term memory loss, cognitive impairment, shooting pains, and numbness and tingling in the feet. Cardiac symptoms such as heart block and myocarditis may require hospitalization.[24] About 60% of persons with untreated infection develop chronic arthritic pain and swelling in the large joints, primarily the knee.

Diagnosis of Lyme disease is often based on clinical manifestations, in particular EM, and a history of exposure in one of the at-risk areas. CBC and ESR are usually normal. A two-step laboratory testing process is recommended by the Centers for Disease Control and Prevention (CDC) to confirm the diagnosis.[25] The first step is the enzyme immunoassay (EIA), which will have positive results for most people with Lyme disease. If the EIA is positive or inconclusive, a Western blot test is done. Results are diagnostic of Lyme disease only if both tests are positive. The CDC does not recommend completing the Western blot test alone as false-positive results lead to incorrect diagnosis and treatment. In individuals with neurologic involvement, cerebrospinal fluid should also be examined.

Active lesions can be treated with oral antibiotics. Doxycycline (Vibramycin), cefuroxime (Ceftin), and amoxicillin are often effective in treating early stage infection and preventing later stages of the disease. Doxycycline is preferred because it treats both Lyme disease and human granulocytic anaplasmosis, which can be transmitted as a co-infection with a single tick bite. Short-term therapy of 14 days is usually effective for solitary EM, but patients with neurologic or cardiac complications may require IV therapy with ceftriaxone (Rocephin) or penicillin G for 2 to 4 weeks.

Approximately 10% to 20% of persons treated with antibiotics for Lyme disease may experience lingering fatigue or joint and muscle pain. The International Lyme and Associated Diseases Society supports a definition of chronic Lyme disease in these cases, rather than posttreatment Lyme disease syndrome, and recommends extended antibiotic treatment until the patient shows subjective improvement.[25]

Reducing exposure to ticks is the best way to prevent Lyme disease. Patient and caregiver teaching for people living in endemic areas is outlined in Table 64-13. No vaccine is available for Lyme disease.

**TABLE 64-13 Patient & Caregiver Teaching**

***Prevention and Early Treatment of Lyme Disease***

*Include the following instructions when teaching patients how to prevent Lyme disease.*

- Avoid walking through tall grasses and low brush, and sitting on logs.
- Mow grass. Remove brush around paths, buildings, and campsites to create tick-safe zones.
- Move woodpiles and bird feeders away from house. Discourage deer (main source of food for adult ticks) from being in the area.
- Wear long pants or nylon tights of tightly woven, light-colored fabric so that ticks can be easily seen.
- Tuck pants into boots or long socks, wear long-sleeved shirts tucked into pants, and wear closed shoes when hiking.
- Check often for ticks crawling from pant legs to open skin.
- Thoroughly inspect and wash clothes. Placing clothing in dryer on high heat kills ticks.
- Spray insect repellent containing DEET sparingly on skin or clothing, or apply permethrin to clothing and camping gear; protects for several hours.
- Have pets wear tick collars, inspect them often, and do not allow pets on furniture or beds.

*Include the following instructions when teaching patients and caregivers living in endemic areas.*

- Remove attached ticks with fine-tipped tweezers (not fingers). Grasp tick's mouth parts as close to skin as possible and pull straight out with steady, even pressure. Do not twist or jerk. Avoid folk solutions such as painting the tick with nail polish or petroleum jelly.
- Save the tick in a bottle of alcohol (if you need it later for identification). Never crush a tick with your fingers.
- Wash bitten area with soap and water, iodine scrub, or rubbing alcohol. Apply antiseptic. Wash hands.
- See an HCP immediately if flu-like symptoms or a bull's-eye rash appears within 2-30 days after removal of tick.

Adapted from Centers for Disease Control and Prevention: Prevent Lyme disease. Retrieved from *www.cdc.gov/features/lymedisease*; and Centers for Disease Control and Prevention: Tick removal. Retrieved from *www.cdc.gov/lyme/removal/index.html*.
*DEET, N,N*-diethyl-m-toluamide.

## SEPTIC ARTHRITIS

**Septic arthritis** (infectious or bacterial arthritis) is caused by microorganisms invading the joint cavity. Bacteria can travel through the bloodstream from another site of active infection, resulting in hematogenous seeding of the joint. Organisms can also be introduced directly through trauma or surgical incision.

Any bacteria can cause the infection—even nonpathogenic bacteria in the immunocompromised patient. *Staphylococcus aureus* is the most common causative organism. Gonococcal infection was a common cause of septic arthritis in young sexually active adults, but its incidence is decreasing.[26] Factors that increase the risk of infection include (1) diseases with decreased host resistance (e.g., leukemia, diabetes mellitus), (2) treatment with corticosteroids or immunosuppressive drugs, and (3) debilitating chronic illness.

In septic arthritis, large joints such as the knee and hip are most frequently involved. Inflammation of the joint cavity causes severe pain, redness, and swelling. Septic arthritis of the hip can contribute to development of avascular necrosis. Because infection has often spread from a primary site elsewhere in the body, fever or shaking chills often accompany joint complaints. Diagnosis may be made by joint aspiration *(arthrocentesis)* and synovial fluid culture. WBC counts may be low early in the infectious process, especially in persons who are immunosuppressed, so diagnosis is not possible solely based on WBC counts. Blood cultures for aerobic and anaerobic organisms should also be obtained.

Septic arthritis is an emergency that requires prompt treatment to prevent joint destruction and bone loss.[26] Broad-spectrum antibiotics against gram-negative organisms, pneumococci, and staphylococci are often started before the causative organism is identified. Once the organism is identified, specific treatment can be determined. Infections may respond to treatment within 2 weeks or may take as long as 4 to 6 weeks, depending on the causative organism.

Local aspiration or surgical drainage may be needed. If diagnosis and treatment are delayed, articular cartilage can be destroyed and loss of joint function occur. Chronic infection can also develop.

Assess and monitor joint inflammation, pain, and fever. To manage pain, use resting splints or traction to immobilize affected joints. Local hot compresses can also decrease pain. Initiate gentle ROM exercises as soon as tolerated to prevent muscle atrophy and joint contractures. Explain the need for antibiotics and the importance of their continued use until the infection is resolved. Offer support to the patient who requires joint drainage. Use strict aseptic technique when assisting with joint aspiration.

## SPONDYLOARTHROPATHIES

The **spondyloarthropathies** are a group of multisystem inflammatory disorders that affect the spine, peripheral joints, and periarticular structures. These disorders are all negative for rheumatoid factor (RF) and thus are often referred to as *seronegative arthropathies.*

Inheritance of HLA-B27 is strongly associated with these diseases. Both genetic and environmental factors play a role in the development of this group of diseases, which includes ankylosing spondylitis, psoriatic arthritis, and reactive arthritis. (HLAs and their relationship to autoimmune diseases are discussed in Chapter 13.)

The spondyloarthropathies share clinical and laboratory characteristics that may make it difficult to distinguish among them in early disease. These characteristics include absence of antibodies in the serum, peripheral joint involvement predominantly of the lower extremities, low back pain *(sacroiliitis),* pain, and redness of the eyes *(uveitis),* intestinal inflammation, and skin lesions.[27]

## ANKYLOSING SPONDYLITIS

**Ankylosing spondylitis** (AS) is a chronic inflammatory disease that primarily affects the axial skeleton, including the sacroiliac joints, intervertebral disc spaces, and costovertebral articulations. HLA-B27 antigen is found in 90% to 95% of people with AS.[3] Onset of AS is usually in the third decade of life, but onset in adolescence is fairly common. Men are three times more likely to develop AS than women. The disease also may go undetected in women because of a milder course.

### Etiology and Pathophysiology

Genetic predisposition appears to play an important role in the pathogenesis of AS. However, the precise cause of the disease is unknown. Inflammation in the joints and adjacent tissue causes the formation of granulation tissue *(pannus)* and dense fibrous scars that can lead to joint fusions. Inflammation can affect the eyes, lungs, heart, kidneys, and peripheral nervous system.

### Clinical Manifestations and Complications

AS is characterized by symmetric sacroiliitis and progressive inflammatory arthritis of the axial skeleton. Symptoms of inflammatory spine pain are the first clues to diagnosis of AS. The patient typically complains of low back pain, stiffness, and limitation of motion that is worse during the night and in the morning but improves with mild activity. In women, early symptoms may include pain and stiffness in the neck rather than the lower back. General symptoms such as fever, fatigue, anorexia, and weight loss are rarely present. Uveitis is the most common non-skeletal symptom. It can appear as an initial presentation of the disease years before arthritic symptoms develop. Patients with AS may also experience distressing chest pain and sternal/costal cartilage tenderness.

Severe postural abnormalities and deformity can cause significant disability for the patient with AS (Fig. 64-8). Impaired spinal ROM and fusion contribute to altered vision, raising concerns about safe ambulation. Aortic insufficiency and pulmonary fibrosis are frequent complications. Cauda equina syndrome (compression of the nerves at the end of the spinal cord) can also result, contributing to lower-extremity weakness and bladder dysfunction. In addition, the patient is at risk for spinal fracture because of associated osteoporosis.

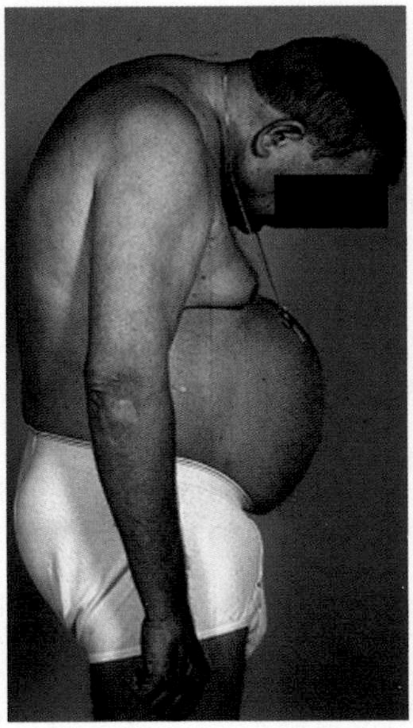

**FIG. 64-8** Advanced ankylosing spondylitis. Kyphotic posture causes many patients to have a bulging abdomen due to pulmonary restriction. (From Kim DH, Henn J, Vaccaro AR, Dickman C: *Surgical anatomy and techniques to the spine,* Philadelphia, 2006, Saunders.)

## GENETICS IN CLINICAL PRACTICE

### *Ankylosing Spondylitis*

**Genetic Basis**

- Inheritance of human leukocyte antigen (HLA)-B27 increases susceptibility to development of ankylosing spondylitis (AS). It is not known how HLA-B27 increases the risk of AS.

**Incidence**

- About 90% to 95% of people with AS have HLA-B27 antigen.
- Inheriting HLA-B27 does not mean a person will develop AS. Of children who inherit HLA-B27 from a parent with AS, 80% do not develop the disease.
- AS is three times more common in men than in women. The disease may go undetected in women because of a milder course.
- It occurs more often in whites than in other ethnic groups.

**Genetic Testing**

- Testing for HLA-B27 antigen is available.

**Clinical Implications**

- Diagnosis of AS usually occurs in the third decade of life, but adolescents can also be affected.
- Multiple genetic and environmental factors play a role in pathogenesis of disease.
- Inflammation can affect the eyes, lungs, heart, kidneys, and peripheral nervous system.
- Severe postural abnormalities and deformity can cause significant disability for the patient with AS.

### Diagnostic Studies

X-rays are the most important radiographic technique for the diagnosis and follow up of AS. However, x-rays are limited in detecting early sacroiliitis or subtle changes in posterior vertebrae. MRI is useful in assessing early cartilage abnormalities, while CT scan is appropriate in specific situations (e.g., cases with subtle x-ray changes). Changes on later spinal films include the appearance of "bamboo spine," the result of calcifications *(syndesmophytes)* that bridge from one vertebra to another.

Laboratory testing is not specific, but an elevated ESR and mild anemia may be seen. When the suspicion of AS is high, the presence of the HLA-B27 antigen improves the likelihood of this diagnosis.

### Interprofessional Care

Prevention of AS is not possible. However, families with other diagnosed HLA-B27-positive rheumatic diseases (e.g., psoriatic arthritis, juvenile spondyloarthritis) should be alert to signs of low back pain for early identification and treatment of AS.

Care of the patient with AS is aimed at maintaining maximal skeletal mobility while decreasing pain and inflammation. Heat applications can help relieve local symptoms. NSAIDs and salicylates are commonly prescribed. DMARDs such as sulfasalazine or methotrexate have little effect on spinal disease but may help with peripheral joint disease. Local corticosteroid injections may be helpful in relieving symptoms.

TNF, which promotes inflammation, is elevated in the blood and certain tissues of patients with AS. Etanercept, a BRM, binds TNF and inhibits its action. Etanercept reduces active inflammation and improves spinal mobility. Additional anti-TNF inhibitors (infliximab, adalimumab, golimumab) may also be effective.

Once pain and stiffness are managed, exercise is essential. Good posture is important to minimize spinal deformity. The exercise regimen should include back, neck, and chest stretches. Hydrotherapy (e.g., sauna, steam bath) has also been shown to decrease pain and facilitate spinal extension. Surgery may be needed for severe deformity and mobility impairment. Spinal osteotomy and total joint replacement are the most commonly performed procedures (see Chapter 62).

## NURSING MANAGEMENT: ANKYLOSING SPONDYLITIS

A key nursing responsibility is to teach the patient with AS about the disease and principles of therapy. The home management program should include regular exercise and attention to posture, local moist heat applications, and knowledgeable use of drugs.

Baseline ROM assessment includes chest expansion (using breathing exercises). Encourage smoking cessation to decrease the risk for lung complications in persons with reduced chest expansion. Ongoing physical therapy includes gentle, graded stretching and strengthening exercises to preserve ROM and improve thoracolumbar flexion and extension.

Discourage excessive physical exertion during periods of increased disease activity. Proper positioning at rest is essential. Encourage the patient to use a firm mattress and sleep on the back with a flat pillow, avoiding positions that encourage flexion deformity. Postural training emphasizes avoiding spinal flexion (e.g., leaning over a desk); heavy lifting; and prolonged walking, standing, or sitting. Encourage sports that facilitate natural stretching, such as swimming and racquet games. Family counseling and vocational rehabilitation are important.

## PSORIATIC ARTHRITIS

**Psoriatic arthritis (PsA)** is a progressive inflammatory disease that affects about 30% people with psoriasis.[28] *Psoriasis* is a common, benign, inflammatory skin disorder characterized by red, irritated, and scaly patches. Both PsA and psoriasis appear to have a genetic link with the HLA antigens in many patients. Although the exact cause of PsA is unknown, a combination of immune, genetic, and environmental factors is suspected. Most people develop psoriasis first and later are diagnosed with PsA.

PsA can occur in different forms. *Distal arthritis* primarily involves the ends of the fingers and toes, with pitting and color changes in the fingernails and toenails. *Asymmetric arthritis* involves different joints between the extremities. *Symmetric psoriatic arthritis* resembles RA and affects joints on both sides of the body at the same time. It accounts for about 50% of cases. *Psoriatic spondylitis* is marked by pain and stiffness in the spine and neck. *Arthritis mutilans* is the most severe form of the disease, affecting only 5% of people with psoriatic arthritis but causing complete destruction of small joints.[28]

On x-ray, the cartilage loss and erosion are similar to RA. Advanced cases of PsA often reveal widened joint spaces. A "pencil in cup" deformity is common in the DIP joints as a result of thinning, weakened bone. In this deformity, the narrowed ends of the metacarpals or phalanges insert into the expanded end of the other bone sharing the joint. Elevated ESR, mild anemia, and elevated serum uric acid can be seen in some patients. Thus the diagnosis of gout must be excluded.

Treatment includes splinting, joint protection, and physical therapy. NSAIDs given early in the course of the disease may help with inflammation. Drug therapy also includes the DMARDs such as methotrexate, which is effective for both articular and cutaneous manifestations. Sulfasalazine, cyclosporine, and BRMs (e.g., etanercept, golimumab, adalimumab, infliximab) may also be used. Apremilast (Otezla), an inhibitor of the enzyme phosphodiesterase-4, can also be used to decrease inflammation.

## REACTIVE ARTHRITIS

*Reactive arthritis (Reiter's syndrome)* occurs more commonly in young men than in young women. It is associated with a symptom complex that includes urethritis, conjunctivitis, and mucocutaneous lesions. Although the exact etiology is unknown, reactive arthritis appears to be a reaction triggered in the body after exposure to specific genitourinary or GI tract infections. *Chlamydia trachomatis* is most often implicated in sexually transmitted reactive arthritis.[3] Reactive arthritis is also associated with GI infections from *Shigella*, *Salmonella*, *Campylobacter*, or *Yersinia* species and other microorganisms.

Individuals who are positive for HLA-B27 are at increased risk of developing reactive arthritis after sexual contact or exposure to certain enteric pathogens. This finding supports the suggestion of genetic predisposition.

Urethritis develops within 1 to 2 weeks after sexual contact or GI infection. In women, symptoms include cervicitis. Low-grade fever, conjunctivitis, and arthritis may occur over the next several weeks. This type of arthritis tends to be asymmetric, frequently involving the large joints of the lower extremities and toes. Lower back pain may occur with severe disease. Lesions involving the skin and mucous membranes commonly occur as small, painless, superficial ulcerations on the tongue, oral mucosa, and glans penis. Soft tissue manifestations commonly include Achilles tendinitis or plantar fasciitis. Few laboratory abnormalities occur, although the ESR may be elevated.

Most patients recover in 2 to 16 weeks. Because reactive arthritis is often associated with *C. trachomatis* infection, treatment with doxycycline is widely recommended for patients and their sexual partners. Antibiotics have no effect on arthritis or other symptoms. Topical ophthalmic corticosteroids may be prescribed for treatment of uveitis, but conjunctivitis and lesions generally require no treatment. Drug therapy may also include NSAIDs and DMARDs (e.g., methotrexate, sulfasalazine). Physical therapy may be helpful during recovery.

Most patients have complete remission with return of full joint function. About 20% of patients may develop chronic arthritis, but the condition is often mild.[3] X-ray changes in chronic reactive arthritis closely resemble those of AS. Treatment is based on symptoms.

## SYSTEMIC LUPUS ERYTHEMATOSUS

**Systemic lupus erythematosus (SLE)** is a multisystem inflammatory autoimmune disease. It is a complex disorder of multifactorial origin resulting from interactions among genetic, hormonal, environmental, and immunologic factors. SLE typically affects the skin, joints, and serous membranes (pleura, pericardium), along with the renal, hematologic, and neurologic systems. SLE is marked by a chronic unpredictable course with alternating periods of remission and exacerbation.

About 250,000 people in the United States have SLE. Most cases occur in women in their childbearing years. Women are 6 to 10 times more likely than men to develop SLE. African Americans, Asian Americans, Hispanics, and Native Americans are more likely than whites to develop the disease.[3]

### Etiology and Pathophysiology

The etiology of the abnormal immune response in SLE is unknown. Based on the high prevalence of SLE among family members, a genetic influence is suspected. Multiple genes from the HLA complex, including *HLA-DR2* and *HLA-DR3,* show associations with SLE.

Hormones are also known to play a role in the etiology of SLE. Onset or worsening of disease symptoms sometimes occurs after the start of menses, with the use of oral contraceptives, and during and after pregnancy. The disease also tends to become worse in the immediate postpartum period.

Environmental factors are believed to contribute to the occurrence of SLE. These include sun or ultraviolet light exposure, stress, and exposure to some chemicals and toxins. Infectious agents such as viruses also may stimulate immune hyperactivity. In addition, at least 40 medications currently in use may trigger SLE. The most frequently identified drugs include procainamide, hydralazine, and quinidine. Drug-induced SLE should not be confused with medication side effects, which typically occur within a few hours or days of short-term drug use. SLE generally occurs months to years after continuous therapy with a causative drug.[29]

In SLE, varied autoantibodies are produced against nucleic acids (e.g., single- and double-stranded DNA), erythrocytes, coagulation proteins, lymphocytes, platelets, and many other self-proteins. Autoimmune reactions (antinuclear antibodies [ANA]) are typically directed against constituents of the cell nucleus, especially DNA.

Circulating immune complexes with antibody against DNA are deposited in the basement membranes of capillaries in the kidneys, heart, skin, brain, and joints. These complexes trigger inflammation that causes tissue destruction. Overaggressive autoimmune responses are also related to activation of B and T cells. Specific disease effects depend on the involved cell types or organs. (SLE is a type III hypersensitivity response [see Chapter 13].)

### Clinical Manifestations and Complications

Severity of SLE is extremely variable. It ranges from a relatively mild disorder to a rapidly progressive disease affecting many body systems (Fig. 64-9). No characteristic pattern occurs in the progressive involvement of SLE. Any organ can be affected by the circulating immune complexes. The most commonly affected tissues are the skin and muscle, lining of the lungs, heart, nervous tissue, and kidneys. General complaints such as fever, weight loss, joint pain *(arthralgia),* and excessive fatigue may precede worsened disease activity.

**Dermatologic Problems.** Vascular skin lesions can appear anywhere but are most likely to develop on sun-exposed areas. Severe skin reactions can occur in people who are sensitive to sunlight *(photosensitivity).* The classic butterfly rash over the cheeks and bridge of the nose occurs in 55% to 85% of patients at some time during the disease[3] (Fig. 64-10). About 20% of patients have *discoid* (round, coin-shaped) lesions. A small number of patients have persistent lesions, photosensitivity, and mild systemic disease in a syndrome known as *subacute cutaneous lupus.*

Oral or nasopharyngeal ulcers occur in up to one third of patients with SLE. Alopecia is also common, with or without related scalp lesions. The hair may grow back during remission, but hair loss may be permanent over lesions. The scalp becomes dry, scaly, and atrophied.

**Musculoskeletal Problems.** Arthritis occurs in about 95% of patients with SLE.[3] Pain in multiple joints *(polyarthralgia)* with morning stiffness is often the first complaint. It may precede the onset of multisystem disease by many years. Diffuse swelling occurs with joint and muscle pain and some stiffness. Lupus-related arthritis is generally nonerosive but may cause deformities (e.g., swan neck deformity of the fingers [Fig. 64-4, *D*], ulnar deviation, subluxation with joint laxity). Patients with SLE also have increased risk of bone loss and fracture.

**Cardiopulmonary Problems.** Tachypnea and cough in patients with SLE suggest presence of lung disease. Pleurisy is also possible. Cardiac involvement may include dysrhythmias due to fibrosis of the sinoatrial and atrioventricular nodes. This indicates advanced disease, contributing greatly to the morbidity and mortality of SLE. Pericarditis can also occur. Clinical factors such as hypertension and hypercholesterolemia require aggressive treatment and careful monitoring. In addition, people with SLE are at risk for secondary *antiphospholipid syndrome.* This disorder of coagulation leads to clots in the arteries and veins with related risk of stroke, gangrene, and heart attack.

**Renal Problems.** About 75% of persons with SLE experience kidney damage. Renal involvement is usually evident within the first 2 years after diagnosis.[3] Manifestations of renal involvement vary from mild proteinuria to rapidly progressive glomerulonephritis. Scarring and permanent damage can lead to end-stage renal disease (ESRD).

The primary goal is to slow the progression of nephropathy and preserve renal function by managing the underlying disease. The importance of obtaining a renal biopsy is controversial, but findings can help guide treatment. Although renal failure is the leading cause of death for patients with SLE, effective

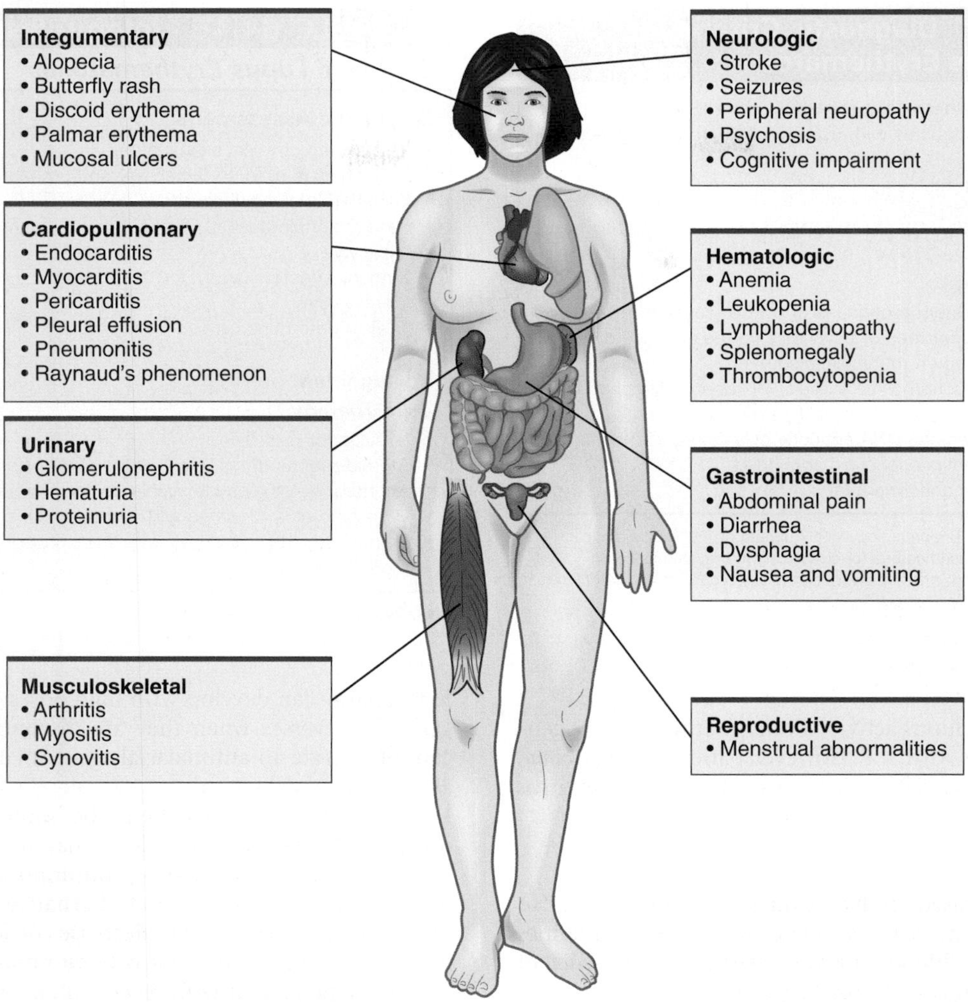


**FIG. 64-9** Multisystem involvement in systemic lupus erythematosus.

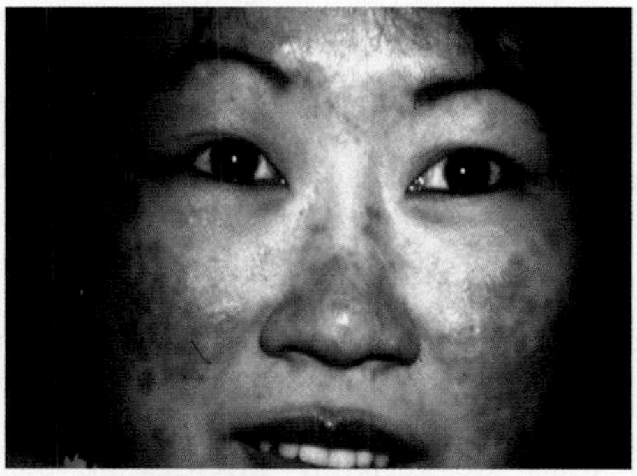

**FIG. 64-10** Butterfly rash of systemic lupus erythematosus. (From Firestein GS, Budd RC, Gabriel SE, McInnes IB: *Kelley's textbook of rheumatology*, ed 9, Philadelphia, 2012, Saunders.)

treatments are available. These typically include corticosteroids, cytotoxic agents (cyclophosphamide), and immunosuppressive agents (azathioprine, cyclosporine, mycophenolate mofetil [CellCept]). Rituximab and eculizumab (Soliris) are being studied as possible treatments.[30] Oral prednisone or pulsed IV methylprednisolone may also be used, especially in the initial treatment period when cytotoxic agents have not yet taken effect.

**Nervous System Problems.** Along with renal involvement, neuropsychiatric manifestations are prevalent in SLE. Generalized or focal seizures of the CNS occur in as many as 15% of patients with SLE by the time of diagnosis. Seizures are generally controlled by corticosteroids or antiseizure drugs. Peripheral neuropathy can also occur, leading to sensory and motor deficits.

Cognitive dysfunction may result from the deposit of immune complexes within the brain. It is marked by disordered thinking, disorientation, and memory deficits. Various psychiatric disorders are reported in SLE, including depression, mood disorders, anxiety, and psychosis. However, they may be related to the stress of having a major illness or to associated drug therapies. Occasionally SLE may cause a stroke or aseptic meningitis. Headaches are also common and can become severe during a disease flare.

**Hematologic Problems.** Abnormal blood conditions are common in SLE due to formation of antibodies against blood cells. Anemia, leukopenia, thrombocytopenia, and coagulation disorders (excessive bleeding or clotting) are often present.[31] Many patients with SLE benefit from high-intensity treatment with warfarin.

**Infection.** Patients with SLE appear to have increased susceptibility to infection. Risk may be due to impaired ability to phagocytize invading bacteria, deficient production of antibodies, and immunosuppressive effects of many antiinflammatory drugs. Infection is a major cause of death, and pneumonia is the most common infection. Fever may indicate an underlying

**TABLE 64-14 Diagnostic Criteria for Systemic Lupus Erythematosus***

- *Malar rash:* fixed erythema, flat or raised (butterfly rash)
- *Discoid rash:* raised patches with scaling follicular plugging; scarring in older lesions
- *Photosensitivity:* skin rash as unusual reaction to light
- *Oral ulcers:* usually painless
- *Nonerosive arthritis:* two or more peripheral joints with tenderness, swelling, effusion
- Pleuritis or pericarditis
- *Renal disorder:* persistent proteinuria or cellular casts in urine
- *Neurologic disorder:* seizures or psychosis (in the absence of causative drugs or known metabolic disorders)
- *Hematologic disorder:* hemolytic anemia, leukopenia, lymphopenia, or thrombocytopenia
- *Immunologic disorder:* anti-DNA antibody or antibody to Sm nuclear antigen or positive antiphospholipid antibodies
- *Antinuclear antibody:* abnormal titer

Source: American College of Rheumatology: 1997 update of the 1982 American College of Rheumatology revised criteria for classification of systemic lupus erythematosus. Retrieved from *http://www.rheumatology.org/Portals/0/Files/1997%20Update%20of%201982%20Revised.pdf.*
*Sm,* Smith.
*A person is classified as having SLE if four or more of the criteria are present, serially or simultaneously, during any interval of observation.

**TABLE 64-15 Interprofessional Care**

***Systemic Lupus Erythematosus***

**Diagnostic Assessment**

- History and physical examination
- Antibodies (e.g., ANA, anti-DNA, anti-Sm, antiphospholipid)
- Complete blood cell count
- Serum complement
- Urinalysis
- X-ray of affected joints
- Chest x-ray
- ECG to determine cardiac involvement

**Management**

***Drug Therapy***

- NSAIDs for mild disease
- Steroid-sparing drugs (e.g., methotrexate)
- Antimalarials (e.g., hydroxychloroquine [Plaquenil])
- Corticosteroids for flares and severe disease
- Immunosuppressive drugs (e.g., cyclophosphamide, mycophenolate mofetil [CellCept])

*ANA,* Antinuclear antibody; *anti-Sm,* Smith.

infection rather than lupus activity alone. Vaccinations are generally safe for patients with SLE. However, patients being treated with corticosteroids or cytotoxic drugs must avoid live virus vaccines.

## Diagnostic Studies

Diagnosis of SLE is based on distinct criteria (Table 64-14). No specific test is diagnostic for SLE, but a variety of abnormalities may be present in the blood. SLE is marked by the presence of ANA in 97% of persons with the disease.[32]

Anti-DNA antibodies are found in half the persons with SLE, but lupus can still be present if these antibodies are not identified. The anti-Smith (Sm) antibodies are found in 30% to 40% of persons with lupus and are almost always considered diagnostic. Nearly 30% of people with lupus will have antiphospholipid antibodies. Antibodies to histone are most often seen in people with drug-induced SLE. Elevated ESR and CRP are not diagnostic of SLE but may be used to monitor disease activity and effectiveness of therapy.

## Interprofessional Care

A major challenge in the treatment of SLE is managing active disease while preventing complications of treatment. Survival is influenced by several factors, including age, race, sex, socioeconomic status, co-morbid conditions, and disease severity. Prognosis can be improved with early diagnosis, ongoing assessment and prompt recognition of serious organ involvement, and effective therapeutic regimens.

**Drug Therapy.** NSAIDs continue to be an important intervention, especially for patients with mild arthralgia or arthritis. Careful patient monitoring during long-term NSAID use must include potential GI and renal effects.

Antimalarial agents such as hydroxychloroquine and chloroquine are often used to treat fatigue and skin and joint problems. They modulate the immune system but do not cause immunosuppression. These drugs may also reduce occurrence of flares. Patients taking hydroxychloroquine should have eye examinations by an ophthalmologist every 6 to 12 months. Retinopathy can develop with high doses of these drugs, but it generally reverses when they are discontinued. If the patient cannot tolerate an antimalarial agent, an antileprosy drug such as dapsone may be used.

Use of corticosteroids should be limited. However, tapering doses of IV methylprednisolone may manage severe flares of polyarthritis. Steroid-sparing immunosuppressants such as methotrexate can serve as an alternative treatment. They are prescribed with folic acid to decrease corticosteroid side effects. However, high doses of corticosteroids may be especially appropriate for the patient with severe cutaneous SLE.

Immunosuppressive drugs such as azathioprine and cyclophosphamide may be used to reduce the need for long-term corticosteroid therapy. Either drug is also an appropriate treatment for severe organ-system disease, especially renal problems. Close monitoring is needed to decrease the risk of drug toxicity and side effects. Because blood clots can be a life-threatening complication of SLE, anticoagulants such as warfarin may be prescribed.

Topical immunomodulators can be used instead of corticosteroids to treat serious skin conditions. Tacrolimus (Protopic, Prograf) and pimecrolimus (Elidel) suppress immune activity in the skin, affecting the butterfly rash and possibly discoid lesions.

Clinical trials are currently investigating the effect of various medications on SLE management. These include agents that interfere with the immune response such as abatacept, and hormones (prasterone) to combat corticosteroid-induced osteoporosis. Lenalidomide, a chemical derivative of thalidomide, can improve cutaneous lupus without adverse neurologic effects.

When teaching patients about their prescribed drugs, include indications for use, proper administration, and possible side effects. Help patients understand that abruptly stopping a medication may worsen disease activity.

Disease management is most appropriately monitored by serial anti-DNA titers and serum complement (Table 64-15). Simpler, less costly tests such as ESR or CRP may also be helpful.

## NURSING MANAGEMENT: SYSTEMIC LUPUS ERYTHEMATOSUS

### Nursing Assessment

Subjective and objective data that should be obtained from the patient with SLE are presented in Table 64-16. In particular, evaluate the effect of pain and fatigue on ability to perform ADLs.

### Nursing Diagnoses

Nursing diagnoses for the patient with SLE may include, but are not limited to, the following:

- Fatigue *related to* chronic inflammation and altered immunity
- Impaired skin integrity *related to* photosensitivity, skin rash, and alopecia
- Impaired comfort *related to* symptoms of illness, treatment side effects, and potential variable and unpredictable disease progression

Additional information on nursing diagnoses for the patient with SLE is presented in eNursing Care Plan 64-2 (on the website for this chapter).

### Planning

Overall goals are that the patient with SLE will (1) have satisfactory pain management, (2) adhere to the therapeutic regimen to achieve maximum symptom management, (3) demonstrate awareness of and avoid activities that worsen the disease, and (4) maintain optimal role function and positive self-image.

### Nursing Implementation

**Health Promotion.** Prevention of SLE is not currently possible. Education for health professionals and the community should create a clear understanding of the disease and the need for early diagnosis and treatment.

**Acute Care.** As in most rheumatic diseases, the unpredictable nature of SLE presents many challenges for the patient and caregiver. Physical, psychologic, and sociocultural problems linked to long-term management of SLE require varied approaches and skills from an interprofessional health care team.

During a disease flare, the patient may quickly become very ill. Nursing interventions include accurately recording the severity of symptoms and documenting the response to therapy. Specifically assess fever pattern, joint inflammation, limitation of motion, location and degree of discomfort, and fatigue. Monitor the patient's weight and fluid intake and output. This is especially important if corticosteroids are prescribed because of related fluid retention and possible renal failure. Collect 24-hour urine samples for protein and creatinine clearance as ordered. Observe for signs of bleeding due to drug therapy (e.g., pallor, skin bruising, petechiae, tarry stools).

Carefully assess neurologic function. Observe for vision problems, headaches, personality changes, seizures, and memory loss. Psychosis may result from CNS disease or be an effect of corticosteroid therapy. Nerve irritation of the extremities *(peripheral neuropathy)* may cause numbness, tingling, and weakness of the hands and feet.

Explain the nature of the disease, types of therapy, and all diagnostic procedures. Provide emotional support for the patient and family, especially during a disease flare.

**TABLE 64-16 Nursing Assessment**
***Systemic Lupus Erythematosus***

**Subjective Data**

***Important Health Information***

*Past health history:* Exposure to ultraviolet light, drugs, chemicals, viral infections. Physical or psychologic stress. States of increased estrogen activity, including early onset of menses, pregnancy, and postpartum period. Pattern of remissions and flares

*Medications:* Oral contraceptives, procainamide (Pronestyl), hydralazine, isoniazid, antiseizure drugs, antibiotics (possibly causing symptoms of SLE), corticosteroids, NSAIDs

***Functional Health Patterns***

*Health perception–health management:* Family history of autoimmune disorders, frequent infections, malaise, impact of disease on functional ability

*Nutritional-metabolic:* Weight loss, oral and nasal ulcers, nausea and vomiting, dry mouth *(xerostomia)*, dysphagia, photosensitivity with rash, frequent infections

*Elimination:* Decreased urine output, diarrhea or constipation

*Activity-exercise:* Morning stiffness, joint swelling and deformity, shortness of breath *(dyspnea)*, excessive fatigue

*Sleep-rest:* Insomnia

*Cognitive-perceptual:* Vision problems, vertigo, headache, arthralgia, chest pain (pericardial, pleuritic), abdominal pain. Painful, throbbing, cold fingers with numbness and tingling

*Sexuality-reproductive:* Amenorrhea, irregular menstrual periods

*Coping–stress tolerance:* Depression, withdrawal

**Objective Data**

***General***

Fever, lymphadenopathy, periorbital edema

***Integumentary***

Alopecia. Dry, scaly scalp. Keratoconjunctivitis, malar butterfly rash, palmar or discoid erythema, hives (urticaria), erythema at fingernails or toenails, purpura, or petechiae. Leg ulcers

***Respiratory***

Pleural friction rub, decreased breath sounds

***Cardiovascular***

Vasculitis, pericardial friction rub, hypertension, edema, dysrhythmias, murmurs. Bilateral, symmetric pallor and cyanosis of fingers (Raynaud's phenomenon)

***Gastrointestinal***

Oral and pharyngeal ulcers; splenomegaly

***Neurologic***

Facial weakness, peripheral neuropathies, papilledema, dysarthria, confusion, hallucination, disorientation, psychosis, seizures, aphasia, hemiparesis

***Musculoskeletal***

Myopathy, myositis, arthritis

***Urinary***

Proteinuria

***Possible Diagnostic Findings***

Presence of anti-DNA, anti-Sm, and antinuclear antibodies. Anemia, leukopenia, thrombocytopenia. ↑ Erythrocyte sedimentation rate (ESR), ↑ serum creatinine. Microscopic hematuria, cellular casts in urine. Pericarditis or pleural effusion on chest x-ray

*Sm,* Smith.

**TABLE 64-17 Patient & Caregiver Teaching**

***Systemic Lupus Erythematosus***

*Include the following information in the teaching plan for a patient with systemic lupus erythematosus and the caregiver.*

- Disease process
- Names of drugs, actions, side effects, dosage, administration
- Pain management strategies
- Energy conservation and pacing techniques
- Therapeutic exercise, use of heat therapy (for arthralgia)
- Relaxation therapy
- Avoidance of physical and emotional stress
- Avoidance of exposure to individuals with infection
- Avoidance of drying soaps, powders, household chemicals
- Use of sunscreen protection (at least SPF 15) and protective clothing, with minimal sun exposure from 11:00 AM to 3:00 PM
- Regular medical and laboratory follow-up
- Marital and pregnancy counseling as needed
- Community resources and health care agencies

*SPF,* Sun protection factor.

◆ **Ambulatory Care.** Emphasize the importance of patient involvement for successful home management. Help the patient understand that even strong adherence to the treatment plan is no guarantee against flares due to the unpredictable disease course. Various factors may increase disease activity, such as fatigue, sun exposure, emotional stress, infection, drugs, and surgery. Help the patient and caregiver eliminate or reduce exposure to such factors (Table 64-17).

◆ ***Lupus and Pregnancy.*** Because SLE is most common in women of childbearing age, treatment during pregnancy must be considered. The woman's primary HCP (or rheumatologist) and obstetrician should thoroughly discuss with the woman her desire to become pregnant. Infertility may have resulted from renal involvement and previous use of high-dose corticosteroid and immunosuppressive drugs. The patient should understand spontaneous abortion, stillbirth, and intrauterine growth retardation are common problems with pregnancy. They occur because immune complexes are deposited in the placenta and inflammation occurs in placental blood vessels.

Renal, cardiovascular, pulmonary, and central nervous systems may be affected during pregnancy. Women who already show serious effects in these systems should be counseled against pregnancy. For the best outcome, pregnancy should be planned when disease activity is minimal. Flares are common during the postpartum period. Therapeutic abortion offers the same risk of postdelivery exacerbation as carrying the fetus to term.

◆ ***Psychosocial Issues.*** The patient with SLE faces many psychosocial issues.[33] Disease onset and symptoms may be vague, and SLE may be undiagnosed for a long time. Supportive therapies may be as important as medical treatment in helping the patient cope with the disease. Inform the patient and caregiver that SLE has a good prognosis for most people.

Stress the importance of planning both recreational and occupational activities. The young adult may find sun restrictions and physical limitations difficult to follow. Help the patient develop and accomplish reasonable goals for improving or maintaining mobility, energy, and self-esteem.

Families worry about hereditary aspects and want to know if their children will also have SLE. Many couples require pregnancy and sexual counseling. Individuals making decisions about marriage and careers worry how SLE will interfere with their plans. Teach teachers, employers, and co-workers as needed about the impact of SLE.

### ◆ Evaluation

The expected outcomes are that the patient with SLE will

- Use energy-conservation techniques
- Adapt lifestyle to current energy
- Maintain skin integrity with use of topical treatments
- Prevent disease flare with use of sunscreens and limited sun exposure

Additional information on expected outcomes for the patient with SLE is presented in eNursing Care Plan 64-2 (on the website for this chapter).

## SCLERODERMA

**Scleroderma** *(systemic sclerosis)* is a disorder of connective tissue characterized by fibrotic, degenerative, and occasionally inflammatory changes in the skin, blood vessels, synovium, skeletal muscle, and internal organs.

Scleroderma occurs in all ethnic groups but is more common in African Americans than whites. Native Americans and persons of Japanese descent may also be at higher risk than whites. Although symptoms may begin at any time, the usual age at onset is between 30 and 50 years. Scleroderma is relatively rare, with approximately 20 adults per 1 million in the United States affected. Incidence in women is four times more common than in men.[3]

Two types of disease exist: *localized scleroderma,* which is the more common form, and *diffuse systemic scleroderma.* Skin changes of localized disease are usually limited to the face, fingers, and distal extremities without involvement of the trunk or internal organs. The prognosis of patients with limited disease is generally better than for those with diffuse disease. Skin changes are rapidly progressive during the first months of diffuse scleroderma, which is associated with internal organ involvement.

### Etiology and Pathophysiology

The exact cause of scleroderma is unknown. Immunologic dysfunction and vascular abnormalities are believed to play a role in the development of widespread systemic disease. Other risk factors for skin thickening include environmental or occupational exposure to coal, plastics, and silica dust.

In scleroderma, collagen (protein that gives normal skin its strength and elasticity) is overproduced (Fig. 64-11). This leads to progressive tissue fibrosis and occlusion of blood vessels. Proliferation of collagen also disrupts normal function of internal organs, such as the lungs, kidney, heart, and GI tract.

Vascular alterations, which primarily involve the small arteries and arterioles, are almost always present. These changes are some of the earliest changes in scleroderma.

### Clinical Manifestations

Manifestations of scleroderma range from diffuse cutaneous thickening with rapidly progressive and widespread organ involvement to the more benign limited cutaneous form. Localized disease is often marked by the **CREST syndrome**:

Calcinosis: painful deposits of calcium in skin of fingers, forearms, pressure points

Raynaud's phenomenon: intermittent vasospasm of fingertips in response to cold or stress

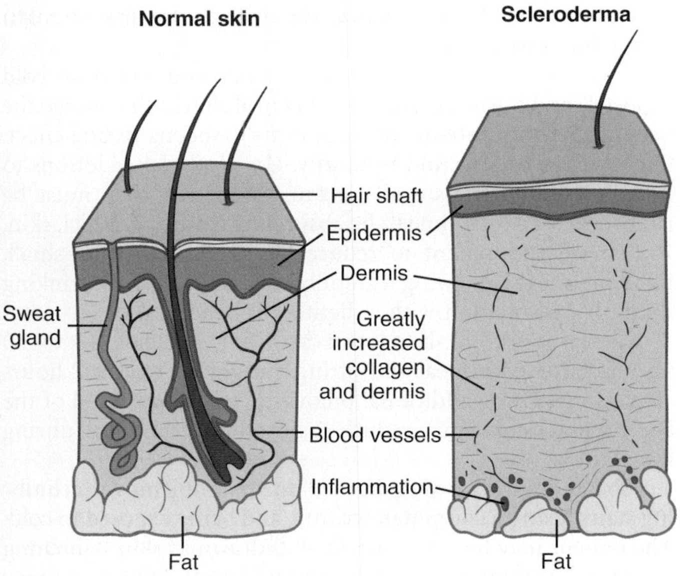


**FIG. 64-11** Skin changes in scleroderma.

Esophageal dysfunction: difficulty swallowing due to internal scarring
Sclerodactyly: tightening of skin on fingers and toes
Telangiectasia: red spots on hands, forearms, palms, face, and lips from capillary dilation

**Raynaud's Phenomenon.** Raynaud's phenomenon (sudden vasospasm of the digits) is the most common initial complaint in localized scleroderma. Patients have diminished blood flow to the fingers and toes on exposure to cold *(blanching or white phase),* followed by cyanosis as hemoglobin releases $O_2$ to the tissues *(blue phase),* and then erythema during rewarming *(red phase).* Color changes often occur with numbness and tingling. Raynaud's phenomenon may precede the onset of systemic disease by months, years, or even decades. (Raynaud's phenomenon is described in more detail in Chapter 37.)

**Skin and Joint Changes.** Symmetric painless swelling or thickening of the skin of the fingers and hands may progress to diffuse scleroderma of the trunk. In localized disease, skin thickening generally does not extend above the elbow or knee, although the face may be affected. In diffuse disease, the skin loses elasticity and becomes taut and shiny. This produces the typical expressionless face with tightly pursed lips. Skin changes in the face may also contribute to reduced ROM in the temporomandibular joint. The fingers may remain in a semi-flexed position *(sclerodactyly),* with tightened skin to the wrist (Fig. 64-12). Reduced peripheral joint function may occur as an early symptom of arthritis.

**Internal Organ Involvement.** About 20% of people with scleroderma develop secondary Sjögren's syndrome, a condition associated with dry eyes and dry mouth. Dysphagia, gum disease, and dental decay can result. Frequent reflux of gastric acid can also occur due to esophageal fibrosis. If swallowing becomes difficult, the patient is likely to decrease food intake and lose weight. Additional GI effects include constipation from colonic hypomotility and diarrhea due to malabsorption from bacterial overgrowth.

Lung involvement includes pleural thickening, pulmonary fibrosis, and abnormal pulmonary function. The patient develops a cough and dyspnea. Pulmonary arterial hypertension and interstitial lung disease may occur. (These disorders are

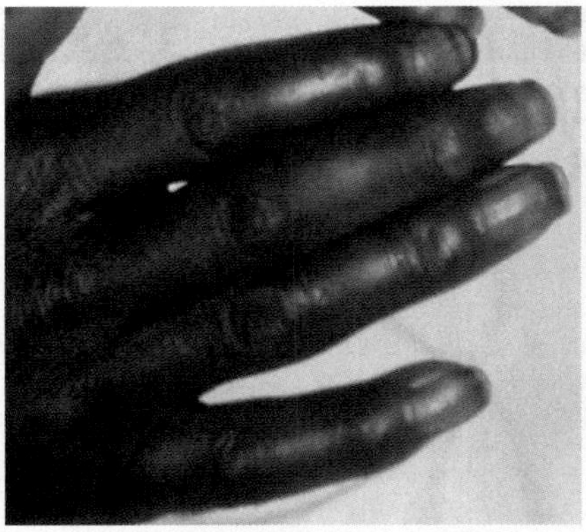

**FIG. 64-12** Sclerodactyly in the hand of a patient with scleroderma. (From Zitelli BJ, Davis HW: *Atlas of pediatric physical diagnosis,* ed 4, St Louis, 2002, Mosby.)

discussed in Chapter 27.) Lung disease is the main cause of death in scleroderma.

Primary heart disease consists of pericarditis, pericardial effusion, and dysrhythmias. Heart failure from myocardial fibrosis occurs most often in patients with diffuse disease.

Renal disease was previously a major cause of death in diffuse scleroderma. Because malignant hypertension associated with rapidly progressive, irreversible renal insufficiency can occur, early recognition of renal involvement and initiation of therapy are critical. Recent improvements in dialysis, bilateral nephrectomy in patients with uncontrollable hypertension, and kidney transplant have offered hope to patients with renal failure. In particular, use of angiotensin-converting enzyme (ACE) inhibitors (e.g., lisinopril [Prinivil]) has had a marked effect on the ability to treat renal disease.

## Diagnostic Studies

Laboratory results in scleroderma are relatively normal. Blood studies may reveal mild hemolytic anemia as a result of RBC damage in diseased small vessels. Anticentromere antibodies related to CREST syndrome are found in about 60% to 80% of people with localized scleroderma. Antibodies to topoisomerase-1 are present in about 30% of people with diffuse disease. Presence of either antibody is highly specific for diagnosis. If renal involvement is present, urinalysis may show proteinuria, microscopic hematuria, and casts. Serum creatinine may be elevated. X-ray evidence of subcutaneous calcification, distal esophageal hypomotility, or bibasilar pulmonary fibrosis is diagnostic of scleroderma. Pulmonary function studies reveal decreased vital capacity and lung compliance.

## Interprofessional Care

Interprofessional care of scleroderma (Table 64-18) offers no specific treatment. Supportive care is directed toward preventing or treating secondary complications of involved organs. Physical therapy helps to maintain joint mobility and preserve muscle strength. Occupational therapy assists the patient in maintaining functional abilities.

**Drug Therapy.** No specific drug or combination of drugs has proven effective for treatment of scleroderma. Vasoactive agents are often prescribed in early disease. Calcium channel blockers (nifedipine [Procardia], diltiazem [Cardizem]) and the angiotensin II blocker losartan are common treatments for Raynaud's phenomenon. Reserpine, an α-adrenergic blocking agent, increases blood flow to the fingers. Bosentan (Tracleer), an

**TABLE 64-18 Interprofessional Care**

***Scleroderma***

**Diagnostic Assessment**
- History and physical examination
- Antibodies to topoisomerase-1
- Anticentromere antibody
- Nail bed capillary microscopy
- Chest x-ray
- Skin or organ biopsy
- Urinalysis (proteinuria, hematuria, casts)
- Pulmonary function tests
- ECG

**Management**
- Physical therapy
- Occupational therapy

***Drug Therapy***
- *Vasoactive agents:* reserpine, bosentan, epoprostenol
- *Calcium channel blockers:* diltiazem, nifedipine
- *Angiotensin-converting enzyme inhibitors:* lisinopril (Prinivil)
- *Immunosuppressive drugs:* cyclophosphamide, mycophenolate mofetil (CellCept)

endothelin-receptor antagonist, and the vasodilator epoprostenol (Flolan) may help prevent and treat digital ulcers. They also improve exercise capacity and heart and lung dynamics.

Corticosteroids may have little effect on scleroderma and may actually cause a renal crisis. Topical agents may provide some relief from joint pain. Capsaicin cream may be useful, not only as a local analgesic but also as a vasodilator. Other therapies prescribed to treat specific systemic problems include (1) tetracycline for diarrhea caused by bacterial overgrowth, (2) histamine ($H_2$) receptor blockers (e.g., cimetidine) and proton pump inhibitors (e.g., omeprazole [Prilosec]) for esophageal symptoms, (3) antihypertensive agent (e.g., captopril, propranolol [Inderal], methyldopa) for hypertension with renal involvement, and (4) immunosuppressive drugs (e.g., cyclophosphamide, mycophenolate mofetil).

## NURSING MANAGEMENT: SCLERODERMA

Prevention of scleroderma is not possible. Nursing interventions often begin during a hospitalization for diagnosis. Assess vital signs, weight, intake and output, respiratory and bowel function, and joint ROM regularly as indicated by specific symptoms to plan appropriate care. Emotional stress and cold ambient temperatures may aggravate Raynaud's phenomenon. Instruct patients with scleroderma to avoid finger-stick blood testing because of compromised circulation and poor healing of the fingers.

Teaching is an important nursing intervention as the patient and family begin to live with this disease. Obvious changes in the face and hands often lead to poor self-image and loss of mobility and function. The patient must regularly participate in therapeutic exercises at home to prevent skin retraction and promote vascularization. Mouth excursion (yawning with an open mouth) is a good exercise to help with temporomandibular joint function. Isometric exercises are best if the patient has arthropathy because no joint movement occurs. Encourage the use of moist heat applications or paraffin baths to promote skin flexibility in the hands and feet. Teach the patient to use assistive devices as needed and organize activities to preserve strength and reduce disability.

Teach the patient to protect the hands and feet from cold exposure and burns or cuts that may heal slowly. Encourage the patient to avoid smoking because of its vasoconstricting effect. Report signs of infection promptly. Use alcohol-free lotions to improve skin dryness and cracking. However, they must be rubbed in for a long time to be absorbed through the thick skin.

Remind the patient to reduce dysphagia by eating small, frequent meals; chewing carefully and slowly; and drinking fluids. A consultation with a dietitian is beneficial.

Decrease risk for heartburn by using antacids 45 to 60 minutes after each meal and sitting upright for at least 2 hours after eating. Using additional pillows or raising the head of the bed on blocks also may reduce gastroesophageal reflux during the night.

Job alterations are often needed due to problems with climbing stairs, using a computer, writing, and being exposed to cold. The patient may become socially withdrawn as skin tightening changes the appearance of the face and hands. Dining out may become socially embarrassing because of the patient's small mouth, swallowing difficulty, and reflux. Some persons with scleroderma wear gloves to protect fingertip ulcers and provide extra warmth. Emphasize daily oral hygiene because neglect may lead to increased tooth and gum problems. The patient needs a dentist who is familiar with scleroderma and able to adapt care to a small mouth.

Psychologic support, biofeedback training, and relaxation can reduce stress and improve sleeping habits. Sexual dysfunction from body changes, pain, muscular weakness, limited mobility, decreased self-esteem, erectile dysfunction, and decreased vaginal secretions may require sensitive counseling.

**CHECK YOUR PRACTICE**

A 34-yr-old woman hospitalized for aspiration pneumonia also has a 5-year history of scleroderma.
- How could scleroderma have contributed to the aspiration pneumonia?
- What strategies will you suggest to decrease the risk of pneumonia recurrence?
- What other self-care strategies will you reinforce with this patient?

## POLYMYOSITIS AND DERMATOMYOSITIS

**Polymyositis (PM)** is diffuse, idiopathic, inflammatory myopathy of striated muscle that produces bilateral weakness, usually most severe in the proximal or limb girdle muscles. When muscle changes associated with PM are accompanied by distinctive skin changes, the disorder is called **dermatomyositis (DM)**.

These relatively rare disorders can be similar in signs, symptoms, and treatment, but they are two distinct diseases. They typically affect adults ages 40 to 60 years. Both PM and DM occur twice as often in women as in men. Patients with PM generally have more severe disease than those with DM.

### Etiology and Pathophysiology

The exact cause of PM and DM is unknown, but evidence suggests an autoimmune origin involving HLA immune response genes.[34] Environmental factors are also likely, including viral and bacterial infection; certain drugs, supplements, and vaccines; medical implants; and occupational exposures.

### Clinical Manifestations and Complications

**Muscular.** The patient with PM and DM experiences weight loss and increasing fatigue, with a gradually developing weakness of muscles that leads to difficulty performing routine activities. The most commonly affected muscles are in the shoulders, legs, arms, and pelvic girdle. The patient may have difficulty rising from a chair or bathtub, climbing stairs, combing hair, or reaching into a high cupboard. Repetitive movements are more likely to cause trouble than a single strength exercise. The patient may also be unable to raise the head from a pillow as neck muscles weaken. Muscle discomfort or tenderness is uncommon. Muscle examination reveals an inability to move against resistance or even gravity. Weak pharyngeal muscles may produce dysphagia and dysphonia (nasal or hoarse voice).

**Dermal.** Skin changes of DM include a classic red or purple symmetric rash *(heliotrope)* with edema around the eyelids. The typical skin rash is not commonly found with other disorders. An additional scaly, smooth, or raised rash may be seen on the knuckles and sides of the hands *(Gottron's papules)* (Fig. 64-13).

These skin changes usually prompt earlier recognition of DM than PM, which has no rash. Reddened, smooth, or scaly patches appear with the same symmetric distribution but sparing the interphalangeal spaces *(Gottron's sign)*. The rash can be confused with psoriasis or seborrheic dermatitis. A red, scaling rash *(poikiloderma)* may develop as a late finding on the back, buttocks, and a V-shaped area of the anterior neck and chest. Hyperemia and telangiectasia are often present at the nail beds. Calcium nodules *(calcinosis cutis)* can develop throughout the skin and are especially common in long-standing DM.

**Other Manifestations.** Joint redness, pain, and inflammation often occur and contribute to limited joint ROM in PM and DM. Contractures and muscle atrophy may occur with advanced disease. Weakened pharyngeal muscles can lead to poor cough effort, difficulty swallowing, and increased risk for aspiration pneumonia in both disorders. Interstitial lung disease is a frequent complication. All patients with PM or DM should be evaluated routinely with a chest x-ray and pulmonary function tests. People with DM also have an increased risk of cancer and should receive age- and gender-appropriate screenings. PM and DM may be associated with other connective tissue disorders (e.g., scleroderma).

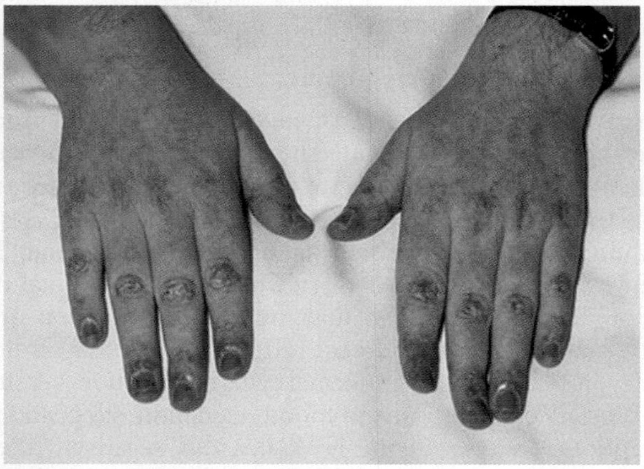

**FIG. 64-13** Dermatomyositis skin changes indicating Gottron's papules. (From Firestein GS, Budd RC, Gabriel SE, McInnes IB: *Kelley's textbook of rheumatology,* ed 9, Philadelphia, 2012, Saunders.)

### Diagnostic Studies

Biopsy is the gold standard for diagnosis of PM or DM after other neuromuscular diseases have been excluded. Muscle biopsy reveals necrosis, degeneration, regeneration, and fibrosis with pathologic findings distinct for DM or PM. MRI can be used to identify areas of inflammation and guide the biopsy site selection. Laboratory tests are helpful, but not diagnostic of either disease. Increased muscle enzymes (e.g., creatine kinase, myoglobin) reflect muscle damage but will decrease to normal or near normal with treatment. An electromyogram (EMG) suggestive of PM shows bizarre high-frequency discharges and spontaneous fibrillation, with positive spikes at rest. Elevation of the ESR or CRP occurs with active disease.

## NURSING AND INTERPROFESSIONAL MANAGEMENT: POLYMYOSITIS AND DERMATOMYOSITIS

PM and DM are treated initially with high-dose oral corticosteroids. Improvement generally occurs if corticosteroid therapy is instituted promptly. Dosage can be reduced as the patient improves until the lowest possible dose associated with symptom management is reached. Long-term corticosteroid therapy may be required because relapses are common when the drug is withdrawn.

For patients who do not respond to corticosteroids, immunosuppressive drugs (methotrexate, azathioprine, tacrolimus, cyclophosphamide) may be used. IV immunoglobulin (IV Ig) may also be administered with corticosteroids or immunosuppressants, but it is not a first-line treatment.

**DRUG ALERT IV Immunoglobulin (IV Ig)**

- Administer by slow infusion to decrease risk of thromboembolic complications.
- Hydrate patient well during infusion to decrease risk of renal failure.
- Treat transient adverse effects such as headache.

The role of newer drugs such as TNF inhibitors remains unclear. The most promising BRM for treatment of PM and DM is rituximab.[35]

Physical therapy can be helpful and should be tailored to disease activity. Massage and passive movement are appropriate during active disease. Delay more aggressive exercises until disease activity is minimal, as evidenced by low serum muscle enzymes.

Teach the patient about the disease, prescribed therapies, diagnostic tests, and the need for regular medical care. Help the patient understand that the benefits of therapy are often delayed. For example, weakness may increase during the first few weeks of corticosteroid therapy. Pay special attention to patient safety. Encourage the use of assistive devices to decrease risk of falls. To prevent aspiration, encourage the patient to rest before meals, maintain an upright position when eating, and choose easily swallowed foods.

Assist the patient to organize activities and use pacing techniques to conserve energy. Encourage daily ROM exercises to prevent contractures. When inflammation is decreased, start muscle-strengthening (repetitive) exercises. Home care and bed rest may be needed during acute PM because the patient may not be able to complete ADLs because of profound muscle weakness.

## MIXED CONNECTIVE TISSUE DISEASE

Patients having a combination of clinical features of several rheumatic diseases are described as having *mixed connective tissue disease.* The term describes a disorder with features primarily of SLE, scleroderma, and PM. This disease occurs most often in women in their 20s and 30s.

About 25% of persons with a connective tissue disease develop another related disease over the course of several years, which is known as *overlap syndrome.*[36]

## SJÖGREN'S SYNDROME

**Sjögren's syndrome** is a relatively common autoimmune disease that targets the moisture-producing exocrine glands, which leads to *xerostomia* (dry mouth) and *keratoconjunctivitis sicca* (dry eyes).[37] The nose, throat, airways, and skin can also become dry. The disease may affect other glands as well, including those in the stomach, pancreas, and intestines (extraglandular involvement). The disease is usually diagnosed in people over age 40 but can be found in all age groups. Women are 10 times more likely than men to have Sjögren's syndrome.

In primary Sjögren's syndrome, symptoms can be traced to problems with lacrimal and salivary glands. About half the cases of Sjögren's syndrome develop alone as primary disease.[37] The patient with secondary Sjögren's syndrome typically had another autoimmune disease (e.g., RA, SLE) before Sjögren's developed.

Sjögren's syndrome appears to be caused by genetic and environmental factors. Several genes seem to be involved. One gene predisposes whites to the disease, whereas other genes are linked to the disease in people of Japanese, Chinese, and African-American heritage. The trigger may be a viral or bacterial infection that adversely stimulates the immune system. In Sjögren's syndrome, lymphocytes attack and damage the lacrimal and salivary glands.

Decreased tearing causes dry eyes, which leads to a gritty sensation in the eyes, burning, blurred vision, and photosensitivity. Dry mouth produces buccal membrane fissures, altered sense of taste, dysphagia, and increased mouth infection or dental decay. Dry skin and rashes, joint and muscle pain, and thyroid problems may be present. Other exocrine glands can also be affected. For example, vaginal dryness may lead to painful intercourse *(dyspareunia).*

Autoimmune thyroid disorders, including Graves' disease and Hashimoto's thyroiditis, are common with Sjögren's syndrome. Histologic study reveals lymphocyte infiltration of salivary and lacrimal glands. The disease may become more generalized and involve the lymph nodes, bone marrow, and visceral organs (pseudolymphoma). Persons with Sjögren's syndrome have an increased risk of developing non-Hodgkin's lymphoma.[38]

Ophthalmologic examination (Schirmer's test for tear production), measures of salivary gland function, and lower lip biopsy of minor salivary glands aid in diagnosis. The treatment of Sjögren's syndrome is symptomatic, including (1) instillation of preservative-free artificial tears or ophthalmic antiinflammatory drops (e.g., cyclosporine [Restasis]) as needed for adequate hydration and lubrication, (2) surgical punctal occlusion, and (3) increased fluids with meals. Dental hygiene is important.

Pilocarpine (Salagen) and cevimeline (Evoxac) can be used to treat symptoms of dry mouth. Increased humidity at home may reduce respiratory tract infections. Vaginal lubrication with a water-soluble product such as K-Y jelly may increase comfort during intercourse.

**! SAFETY ALERT Sjögren's Syndrome**

To help with chewing and swallowing:

- Moisten food with mayonnaise, sauces, gravy, or yogurt.
- Thin foods with skim milk or broth.
- Use a food processor or blender to finely chop or liquefy foods.
- Try soft, creamy foods (e.g., mashed potatoes, macaroni and cheese).
- Drink high-calorie cold liquids (e.g., breakfast drinks).
- Avoid salty, acidic, or spicy foods.

## MYOFASCIAL PAIN SYNDROME

**Myofascial pain syndrome** is a chronic form of muscle pain. It is marked by musculoskeletal pain and tenderness, typically in the chest, neck, shoulders, hips, and lower back. Referred pain from these muscle groups can also travel to the buttocks, hands, and head, causing severe headaches. Temporomandibular joint pain may also originate in myofascial pain. Regions of pain are often within the connective tissue *(fascia)* that covers skeletal muscles. Trigger or tender points are thought to activate a characteristic pattern of pain that worsens with activity or stress.

Myofascial pain syndrome occurs more often in middle-aged adults and in women rather than men. Patients complain of deep, aching pain accompanied by a sensation of burning, stinging, and stiffness.

Physical therapy is one treatment used for myofascial pain syndrome. A typical treatment is the "spray and stretch" method, in which the painful area is iced or sprayed with a coolant such as ethyl chloride and then stretched. Positive results have been seen with topical patches and injection of the trigger points with a local anesthetic (e.g., 1% lidocaine). Massage, acupuncture, biofeedback, and ultrasound therapy have also benefited some patients.[39]

## FIBROMYALGIA

**Fibromyalgia** is a chronic central pain syndrome marked by widespread, nonarticular musculoskeletal pain and fatigue with multiple tender points. People with fibromyalgia may also experience nonrestorative sleep, morning stiffness, irritable bowel syndrome, and anxiety. Fibromyalgia is a commonly diagnosed musculoskeletal disorder and a major cause of disability. It affects an estimated 2% of the general U.S. population. The disease is 4 to 10 times more common in women than men.[3] Fibromyalgia and systemic exertion intolerance disease (SEID) (formerly called chronic fatigue syndrome) share many common features (Table 64-19).

### Etiology and Pathophysiology

Fibromyalgia is a disorder involving abnormal central processing of nociceptive pain input. The increased pain experienced by the affected patient is due to abnormal sensory processing in the CNS.

Multiple physiologic abnormalities have been found. They include (1) increased levels of substance P in the spinal fluid, (2) low blood flow to the thalamus, (3) dysfunction of the hypothalamic-pituitary-adrenal (HPA) axis, (4) low serotonin and tryptophan, and (5) abnormal cytokine function. Serotonin and substance P play a role in mood regulation, sleep, and pain perception. Changes in the HPA axis can negatively affect a person's physical and mental health. An increased incidence of depression and decreased response to stress occur. Genetic factors also contribute to the development of fibromyalgia, as

**TABLE 64-19 Common Features of Fibromyalgia and Systemic Exertion Intolerance Disease (SEID)**

| |
|---|
| **Occurrence**<br>Previously healthy, young and middle-aged women. |
| **Etiology (theories)**<br>Infectious trigger, dysfunction in HPA axis, alteration in CNS. |
| **Clinical Manifestations**<br>Generalized musculoskeletal pain, malaise and fatigue, cognitive dysfunction, headaches, sleep disturbances, depression, anxiety, fever. |
| **Disease Course**<br>Variable intensity of symptoms, fluctuates over time. |
| **Diagnosis**<br>No definitive laboratory tests or joint and muscle examinations. Mainly a diagnosis of exclusion. |
| **Management**<br>Symptomatic treatment may include antidepressant drugs such as amitriptyline and fluoxetine (Prozac). Other measures are heat, massage, regular stretching, biofeedback, stress management, and relaxation training. Patient and caregiver teaching is essential. |

*HPA,* Hypothalamic-pituitary-adrenal.

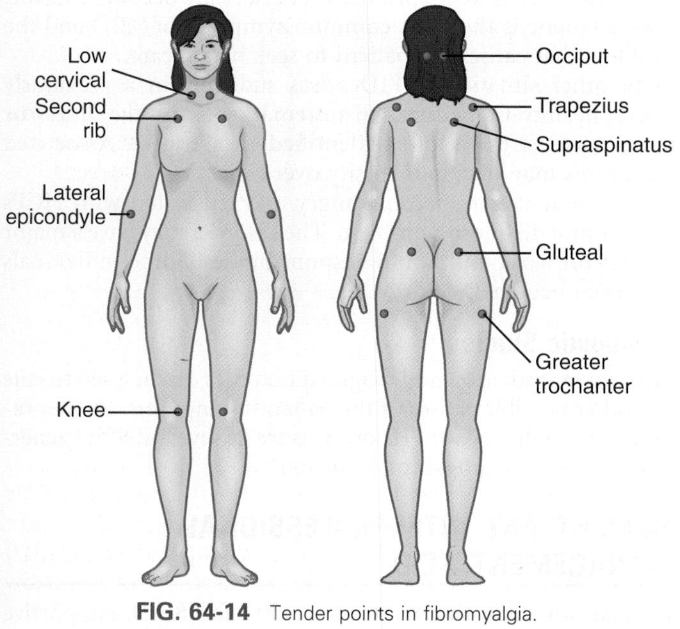


**FIG. 64-14** Tender points in fibromyalgia.

a familial tendency exists. Recent illness or trauma may be a trigger in susceptible people.

## Clinical Manifestations and Complications

The patient complains of a widespread burning pain that worsens and improves through the course of a day. The patient often has trouble determining if pain occurs in the muscles, joints, or soft tissues. Head or facial pain often results from stiff or painful neck and shoulder muscles. The pain can accompany temporomandibular joint dysfunction, which affects an estimated one third of patients with fibromyalgia.

Physical examination typically reveals point tenderness at 11 or more of 18 identified sites (Fig. 64-14). Patients with fibromyalgia are sensitive to painful stimuli throughout the body, not just at the identified tender sites. They may also experience pain in response to a stimulus that does not typically cause pain *(allodynia)*. In addition, point tenderness can vary from day to day. Sometimes, the patient may respond to fewer than 11 tender points. At other times, palpation of all sites may cause pain.

Cognitive effects range from difficulty concentrating to memory lapses and a feeling of being overwhelmed when dealing with multiple tasks. Many individuals report migraine headaches. Depression and anxiety often occur and may require drug therapy. Stiffness, nonrefreshing sleep, fatigue, and numbness or tingling in the hands or feet often accompany fibromyalgia. Restless legs syndrome is also typical, with patients describing an irresistible urge to move the legs when at rest or lying down.

Irritable bowel syndrome with manifestations of constipation and/or diarrhea, abdominal pain, and bloating is common. Patients may also experience difficulty swallowing, perhaps because of problems in esophageal smooth muscle function. Increased frequency of urination and urinary urgency, in the absence of a bladder infection, are typical complaints. Women with fibromyalgia may experience more difficult menstruation with a worsening of disease symptoms during this time.

## Diagnostic Studies

A definitive diagnosis of fibromyalgia is often difficult to establish. Lack of knowledge about the disease and its manifestations among HCPs may also cause delays in diagnosis and treatment.

Laboratory results in most cases help rule out other suspected disorders. Muscle biopsy may reveal a nonspecific moth-eaten appearance or fiber atrophy.

The American College of Rheumatology (ACR) classifies an individual as having fibromyalgia if two criteria are met: (1) pain is experienced in 11 of the 18 tender points on palpation (Fig. 64-14) and (2) a history of widespread pain is noted for at least 3 months.[40] Widespread pain is defined as pain that occurs on both sides of the body and above and below the waist. In addition, fatigue, cognitive symptoms, and extensive somatic symptoms are considered in establishing a diagnosis.

A subsequent classification by the ACR used non–tender point diagnostic criteria as an alternative method of diagnosis, using a symptom severity scale and a widespread pain index to identify disease characteristics.[41] It is suggested this classification be used with the previous ACR criteria.

## Interprofessional Care

Treatment of fibromyalgia is symptomatic and requires a high level of patient motivation. Teach the patient to be an active participant in the therapeutic regimen. Rest can help the pain, aching, and tenderness.

Drug therapy for the chronic widespread pain associated with fibromyalgia includes pregabalin (Lyrica), duloxetine (Cymbalta), and milnacipran (Savella). Low-dose tricyclic antidepressants, selective serotonin reuptake inhibitors (SSRIs), or benzodiazepines (e.g., diazepam [Valium]) may also be prescribed. If the tricyclic antidepressant amitriptyline is not well tolerated, similar drugs can be substituted (e.g., doxepin, imipramine [Tofranil], trazodone). SSRI antidepressants (e.g., sertraline [Zoloft] or paroxetine [Paxil]) tend to be reserved for patients who also have depression. SSRIs may have to be prescribed at higher doses than when used to treat depression. Both antidepressants and muscle relaxants (e.g., baclofen [Lioresal]) have sedative effects that can improve nighttime rest for the patient with fibromyalgia.

Long-acting opioids generally are not recommended unless other therapies are unsuccessful. In some patients, pain may be managed with OTC analgesics such as acetaminophen, ibuprofen, or naproxen (Aleve) used in combination with a TCA. Nonopioids such as tramadol (Ultram) may also be used. In addition, zolpidem (Ambien) or trazodone is sometimes prescribed for short-term intervention in patients with severe sleep problems.

## ❖ NURSING MANAGEMENT: FIBROMYALGIA

Because of the chronic nature of fibromyalgia, the patient needs consistent support from interprofessional team members. Massage is often combined with ultrasound or the application of alternating heat and cold packs to soothe tense, sore muscles and increase blood circulation. Gentle stretching to relieve muscle tension and spasm can be performed by a physical therapist or practiced by the patient at home. Yoga and Tai Chi are often helpful. Low-impact aerobic exercise, such as walking, can help prevent muscle atrophy.

Patients with fibromyalgia may consider limiting the consumption of sugar, caffeine, and alcohol because these substances may be muscle irritants. Vitamin and mineral supplements may help combat stress, correct deficiencies, and support the immune system. However, unproven miracle diets or supplements should be carefully investigated by the patient and discussed with the HCP before using them. Inform the patient that some foods and supplements can cause serious or even dangerous side effects when mixed with certain drugs.

Pain and the related symptoms of fibromyalgia can cause significant stress. Patients with fibromyalgia may not cope well with stress. Effective relaxation strategies include biofeedback, imagery, meditation, and cognitive behavioral therapy. Patients need to receive initial training for these interventions, but they can then continue to practice in their own homes. (Stress management is discussed in Chapter 6.) Psychologic counseling (individual or group) and a support group may also be beneficial for the patient with fibromyalgia.

## SYSTEMIC EXERTION INTOLERANCE DISEASE (SEID)

**Systemic exertion intolerance disease (SEID)**, formerly called *chronic fatigue syndrome,* is a serious, complex, multisystem disease in which exertion of any sort (physical, emotional, cognitive) can adversely affect multiple organs in a person.[42] SEID is a poorly understood condition that can have a devastating impact on the lives of patients and their families.

SEID affects 83,000 to 2.5 million people in the United States. Women are affected more often than men. SEID occurs in all ethnic and socioeconomic groups. The true prevalence of SEID is unknown because many people with the disease have not been diagnosed.[42]

### Etiology and Pathophysiology

Despite efforts to determine the etiology and pathology of SEID, precise mechanisms remain unknown. However, many theories exist about the cause of SEID. Neuroendocrine abnormalities have been implicated involving a hypofunction of the HPA axis and hypothalamic-pituitary-gonadal (HPG) axis, which together regulate the stress response and reproductive hormone levels. Several microorganisms have been investigated as causative agents, including herpes viruses (e.g., Epstein-Barr virus [EBV], cytomegalovirus [CMV]), retroviruses, enteroviruses, *Candida albicans,* and mycoplasma. Because many patients have cognitive deficits (e.g., decreased memory, attention, concentration), changes in the CNS have been suggested as the cause of SEID.

### Clinical Manifestations

Diagnosis of SEID requires that the patient have the following three symptoms:

1. Profound fatigue lasting at least 6 months
2. Postexertional malaise: total exhaustion after even minor physical or mental exertion that the patient sometimes describes as a "crash"
3. Unrefreshing sleep

At least one of the following manifestations is also required:

1. Cognitive impairment ("brain fog")
2. Worsening of symptoms upon standing *(orthostatic intolerance)*

SEID is often difficult to distinguish from fibromyalgia because many clinical features are similar (Table 64-19). In about half the cases, SEID develops insidiously, or the patient may have intermittent episodes that gradually become chronic. Severe fatigue is the most common symptom of SEID and the problem that causes the patient to seek health care.

In other situations, SEID arises suddenly in a previously active, healthy individual. An unremarkable flu-like illness or other acute stress is often identified as a trigger. Associated symptoms may vary in intensity over time.

The patient may become angry and frustrated with HCPs who cannot diagnose a problem. The disorder may have a major impact on work and family responsibilities. Some individuals may even need help with ADLs.

### Diagnostic Studies

Physical examination and diagnostic studies can be used to rule out other possible causes of the patient's symptoms. No laboratory test can diagnose SEID or measure its severity. SEID generally remains a diagnosis of exclusion.

## NURSING AND INTERPROFESSIONAL MANAGEMENT: SEID

Because no definitive treatment exists for SEID, supportive management is essential. Tell the patient what is known about the disease. Take all complaints seriously.

NSAIDs can be used to treat headaches, muscle and joint aches, and fever. Because many patients with SEID also have allergies and sinusitis, antihistamines and decongestants can be used to treat allergic symptoms. Tricyclic antidepressants (e.g., doxepin, amitriptyline) and SSRIs (e.g., fluoxetine, paroxetine) can improve mood and sleep problems. Clonazepam (Klonopin) can also be used to treat sleep disturbances and panic disorders. Use of low-dose hydrocortisone to decrease fatigue and disability is being studied.

Advise the patient to avoid total rest because it can contribute to the self-image of the patient as an invalid. On the other hand, strenuous exertion can exacerbate the exhaustion. Urge the patient to plan a carefully graduated exercise program. Also encourage a well-balanced diet, including fiber and fresh dark-colored fruits and vegetables for antioxidant action. Behavioral therapy may be used to promote a positive outlook and improve overall disability, fatigue, and other symptoms.

One of the major problems facing many patients with SEID is loss of livelihood and economic security. When the illness strikes, they cannot work or must decrease the amount of time working. Loss of a job often leads to loss of medical insurance. Obtaining disability benefits can be frustrating because of the difficulty of establishing a definitive diagnosis of SEID. Patients with SEID may experience substantial occupational and psychosocial loss, including the social pressure and isolation from being characterized as lazy or crazy.

SEID does not appear to progress. Although most patients recover or at least gradually improve, some do not show substantial improvement. Recovery is more common in persons with a sudden onset of SEID.

## EVIDENCE-BASED PRACTICE

### *Translating Research Into Practice*

#### Does Exercise Reduce Fatigue in Chronic Fatigue Syndrome?*

***Clinical Question***

For individuals with chronic fatigue syndrome (P), what is the effect of exercise therapy (I) versus control group (C) on fatigue, sleep, physical function, and self-perceived health (O) after 12 to 26 weeks of therapy (T)?

***Synthesis of Best Available Evidence***

- Systematic review of randomized controlled trials (RCTs).
- 8 RCTs of individuals ($n$ = 1518) with chronic fatigue syndrome (CFS). Intervention was anaerobic and aerobic exercise including cycling, dancing, and walking. Length of exercise therapy was 12 to 26 weeks. Control groups included usual, relaxation, cognitive behavior therapy (CBT), supportive listening, and pharmacologic treatment. Outcomes were fatigue, sleep, physical function, self-perceived health, quality of life, depression, anxiety, and pain.
- Reduction in fatigue following exercise therapy.
- Positive effects of exercise on sleep, physical function, and self-perceived changes in health.
- Unable to determine effect of exercise on pain, quality of life, anxiety, and depression.
- CBT appeared equally effective as exercise in reducing fatigue.

***Conclusions***

- Reductions in fatigue occurred following exercise therapy.
- Sleep, physical function, and self-reported health also improved with exercise.

***Implications for Nursing Practice***

1. Why is it important to discuss positive effects of exercise for patients with CFS who are sedentary and experience sleep difficulties?
2. What would you advise a patient who is interested in learning about CBT to improve physical functioning? How would you help this person access resources?

***Reference for Evidence***

Larun L, Brurberg KG, Odgaard-Jensen J, et al: Exercise therapy for chronic fatigue syndrome. *Cochrane Database Syst Rev* 2:CD003200, 2015.

*P*, Patient population of interest; *I*, intervention or area of interest; *C*, comparison of interest or comparison group; *O*, outcomes of interest; *T*, timing (see p. 15).
*Chronic fatigue syndrome is now referred to as systemic exertion intolerance disease.

## CASE STUDY

### *Rheumatoid Arthritis*

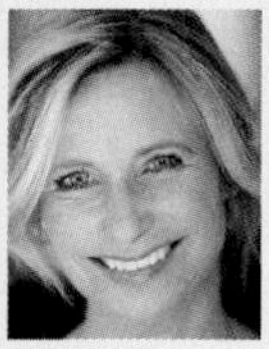

(©iStockphoto/Thinkstock)

#### Patient Profile

K.R., a 42-yr-old married white woman, is seen at the rheumatology clinic with complaints of tenderness and pain in the small joints of her hands.

#### Subjective Data

- Complains of tenderness, joint pain, and stiffness in her hands for the last 3 mo
- Experiencing fatigue, anorexia, and morning stiffness
- Mother diagnosed with ankylosing spondylitis 8 yr ago
- Expresses doubt about her ability to manage disease

#### Objective Data

***Physical Examination***

- Swelling, warmth, and tenderness of third and fourth metacarpophalangeal joints of both hands
- Mild pain with neck motion
- Tenosynovitis

***Diagnostic Studies***

- Positive ESR, RF, and anti-CCP
- Mild bone demineralization evident bilaterally in hand x-rays

#### Interprofessional Care

- Diagnosed with RA
- Started on methotrexate 7.5 mg PO once per week, etanercept (Enbrel) 50 mg subcutaneously once per week, prednisone 10 mg/day

#### Discussion Questions

1. How will you explain the pathophysiology of RA to K.R.?
2. K.R. asks you if genetic factors are related to a diagnosis of RA. How will you respond?
3. ***Safety:*** What are some home and work modifications you can suggest to K.R. to reduce her symptoms?
4. ***Patient-Centered Care:*** What suggestions can you make to K.R. about coping with fatigue?
5. ***Teamwork and Collaboration:*** What referrals may be needed for K.R.?
6. ***Priority Decision:*** Based on the assessment data presented, what are the priority nursing diagnoses? Are there any interprofessional problems?
7. ***Quality Improvement***: What outcomes would indicate interprofessional care was effective?
8. ***Evidence-Based Practice:*** Why is an exercise program important in the treatment plan for K.R.?

Answers and a corresponding conceptual care map are available at *http://evolve.elsevier.com/Lewis/medsurg*.

## BRIDGE TO NCLEX EXAMINATION

The number of the question corresponds to the same-numbered outcome at the beginning of the chapter.

1. In assessing the joints of a patient with osteoarthritis, the nurse understands that Bouchard's nodes
   - **a.** are often red, swollen, and tender.
   - **b.** indicate osteophyte formation at the PIP joints.
   - **c.** are the result of pannus formation at the DIP joints.
   - **d.** occur from deterioration of cartilage by proteolytic enzymes.
2. A patient with rheumatoid arthritis is experiencing articular involvement. The nurse recognizes these characteristic changes include *(select all that apply)*
   - **a.** bamboo-shaped fingers.
   - **b.** metatarsal head dislocation in feet.
   - **c.** noninflammatory pain in large joints.
   - **d.** asymmetric involvement of small joints.
   - **e.** morning stiffness lasting 60 minutes or more.
3. When administering medications to the patient with chronic gout, the nurse would recognize which drug is used as a treatment for this disease?
   - **a.** Colchicine
   - **b.** Febuxostat
   - **c.** Sulfasalazine
   - **d.** Cyclosporine
4. The nurse should teach the patient with ankylosing spondylitis the importance of
   - **a.** regularly exercising and maintaining proper posture.
   - **b.** avoiding extremes in environmental temperatures.
   - **c.** maintaining patient's usual physical activity during flares.
   - **d.** applying hot and cool compresses for relief of local symptoms.
5. In teaching a patient with SLE about the disorder, the nurse knows the pathophysiology of SLE includes
   - **a.** circulating immune complexes formed from IgG autoantibodies reacting with IgG.
   - **b.** an autoimmune T-cell reaction that results in destruction of the deep dermal skin layer.
   - **c.** immunologic dysfunction leading to chronic inflammation in the cartilage and muscles.
   - **d.** the production of a variety of autoantibodies directed against components of the cell nucleus.
6. In teaching a patient with Sjögren's syndrome about drug therapy for this disorder, the nurse includes instruction on use of which drug?
   - **a.** Pregabalin (Lyrica)
   - **b.** Etanercept (Enbrel)
   - **c.** Cyclosporine (Restasis)
   - **d.** Cyclobenzaprine (Flexeril)
7. Teach the patient with fibromyalgia the importance of limiting intake of which foods *(select all that apply)*?
   - **a.** Sugar
   - **b.** Alcohol
   - **c.** Caffeine
   - **d.** Red meat
   - **e.** Root vegetables

1. b, 2. b, e, 3. b, 4. a, 5. d, 6. c, 7. a, b, c

For rationales to these answers and even more NCLEX review questions, visit *http://evolve.elsevier.com/Lewis/medsurg*.

## EVOLVE WEBSITE

http://evolve.elsevier.com/Lewis/medsurg

**Review Questions (Online Only)**

**Key Points**

**Answer Keys for Questions**

- Rationales for Bridge to NCLEX Examination Questions
- Answer Guidelines for Case Study on p. 1549
- Answer Guidelines for Managing Care of Multiple Patients Case Study (Section 11 on p. 1552)

**Students Case Studies**

- Patient With Obesity and Osteoarthritis
- Patient With Rheumatoid Arthritis
- Patient With Systemic Lupus Erythematosus

**Nursing Care Plans**

- eNursing Care Plan 64-1: Patient With Rheumatoid Arthritis
- eNursing Care Plan 64-2: Patient With Systemic Lupus Erythematosus

**Conceptual Care Map Creator**

- Conceptual Care Map for Case Study on p. 1549

**Audio Glossary**

**Content Updates**

## REFERENCES


1. National Institute of Arthritis and Musculoskeletal and Skin Disease: Arthritis and rheumatic diseases. Retrieved from *www.niams.nih.gov/health_info/Arthritis/arthritis_rheumatic.asp*.
2. Centers for Disease Control and Prevention: Arthritis: meeting the challenge of living well. Retrieved from *www.cdc.gov/chronicdisease/resources/publications/aag/pdf/2014/arthritis-aag-2014.pdf*.
3. Roberts D: Arthritis and connective tissue disorders. In Schoenly L, editor: *NAON core curriculum for orthopaedic nursing*, ed 7, Chicago, 2013, National Association of Orthopaedic Nurses.
4. Arthritis Foundation: What is osteoarthritis? Retrieved from *www.arthritis.org/about-arthritis/types/osteoarthritis/what-is-osteoarthritis.php*.
5. Centers for Disease Control and Prevention: Osteoarthritis. Retrieved from *www.cdc.gov/arthritis/basics/osteoarthritis.htm*.

*6. Barenius B, Ponzer S, Shalabi A, et al: Increased risk of osteoarthritis after anterior cruciate ligament reconstruction: a 14-year follow-up study of a randomized controlled trial, *Am J Sports Med* 42:1049, 2014.

*7. *www.tylenol.com/safety-dosing/usage/dosage-for-adults*.

8. National Center for Complementary and Integrative Health: Osteoarthritis and complementary health approaches. Retrieved from *https://nccih.nih.gov/health/arthritis/osteoarthritis*.
9. RxList: Celebrex. Retrieved from *www.rxlist.com/celebrex-drug/warnings-precautions.htm*.
10. American Academy of Orthopaedic Surgeons: Viscosupplementation treatment for knee arthritis. Retrieved from *http://orthoinfo.aaos.org/topic.cfm?topic=A00217*.

*11. Reginster JY, Badurski J, Bellamy N, et al: Efficacy and safety of strontium ranelate in the treatment of knee osteoarthritis: results of a double-blind, randomized placebo-controlled trial, *Ann Rheum Dis* 72:179, 2013.

12. Arthritis Foundation: Arthroscopic knee surgery little help for arthritis. Retrieved from *www.arthritis.org/living-with-arthritis/treatments/joint-surgery/types/knee/arthroscopic-knee-surgery.php*.
13. Arthritis Foundation: Other natural therapies for osteoarthritis. Retrieved from *www.arthritis.org/living-with-arthritis/treatments/natural/other-therapies*.

14. Arthritis Foundation: What is rheumatoid arthritis? Retrieved from *www.arthritis.org/about-arthritis/types/rheumatoid-arthritis/what-is-rheumatoid-arthritis.php*.
15. Health Union: Understanding RA changes and progression. Retrieved from *http://rheumatoidarthritis.net/what-is-ra/stages-and-progression*.
16. Harrison P: Rheumatoid arthritis: smoking exacerbates disease activity. Retrieved from *http://www.medscape.com/viewarticle/821446*.
17. Arthritis Foundation: More than just joints: how rheumatoid arthritis affects the rest of your body. Retrieved from *www.arthritis.org/about-arthritis/types/rheumatoid-arthritis/articles/rheumatoid-arthritis-affects-body.php*.
18. Arthritis Foundation: Depression common in rheumatoid arthritis. Retrieved from *www.arthritis.org/living-with-arthritis/comorbidities/depression-and-arthritis/depression-rheumatoid-arthritis.php*.
19. Arthritis Foundation: Arthritis Today drug guide. Retrieved from *www.arthritis.org/living-with-arthritis/treatments/medication/drug-guide*.
20. Centers for Disease Control and Prevention: Gout. Retrieved from *www.cdc.gov/arthritis/basics/gout.html*.
21. Burbage G: Gout: clinical presentation and management, *Nurs Standard* 29:50, 2014.
22. Finney D: Managing gout: not a trivial matter, *Practice Nurs* 24;179, 2013.
23. Rees F, Doherty M: Patient with gout can be cured in primary care, *Practitioner* 258:15, 2014.
24. Moore KS: Lyme disease: diagnosis, treatment guidelines, and controversy, *J Nurse Pract* 11:64, 2015.
25. Centers for Disease Control and Prevention: Two-step laboratory testing process. Retrieved from *www.cdc.gov/lyme/diagnosistesting/labtest/twostep/index.html*.
26. Sharff KA, Richards EP, Townes JM: Clinical management of septic arthritis, *Curr Rheum Rep* 15:332, 2013.
27. Arthritis Foundation: Spondyloarthritis. Retrieved from *www.arthritis.org/about-arthritis/types/spondyloarthritis*.
28. Arthritis Foundation: What is psoriatic arthritis? Retrieved from *www.arthritis.org/about-arthritis/types/psoriatic-arthritis/what-is-psoriatic-arthritis.php*.
29. Lupus Foundation of America: Which medications cause drug-induced lupus? Retrieved from *www.lupus.org/answers/entry/which-medications-cause-drug-induced-lupus*.
30. Lupus Foundation of America: How does lupus affect the renal (kidney) system? Retrieved from *www.lupus.org/answers/entry/lupus-and-kidneys*.
31. Arthritis Foundation: Lupus symptoms. Retrieved from *www.arthritis.org/about-arthritis/types/lupus/symptoms.php*.
32. Lupus Foundation of America: What are the laboratory tests for lupus? Retrieved from *www.lupus.org/answers/entry/lupus-tests*.
*33. Sutanto B, Singh-Grewal D, McNeil HP, et al: Experiences and perspectives of adults living with systemic lupus erythematosus: thematic synthesis of qualitative studies, *Arthr Care Res* 65:1752, 2013.
34. Hylland TL, Doerner J: Polymyositis: essential information for primary care providers, *J Nurse Pract* 10:560, 2014.
35. Lundberg IE, Vencovsky J, Alexanderson H: Therapy of myositis: biological and physical, *Curr Opin Rheum* 26:704, 2014.
36. Cleveland Clinic: Mixed connective tissue disease. Retrieved from *http://my.clevelandclinic.org/health/diseases_conditions/hic_Mixed_Connective_Tissue_Disease*.
37. Catanzaro J, Dinkel S: Sjögren's syndrome: the hidden disease, *MED SURG Nurs* 23:219, 2014.
38. Arthritis Foundation: Sjögren's syndrome and lymphoma risk. Retrieved from *www.arthritis.org/about-arthritis/types/sjogrens-syndrome/articles/lymphoma-risk-and-sjogrens-syndrome-230.php*.
39. Mayo Clinic: Myofascial pain syndrome. Retrieved from *www.mayoclinic.org/diseases-conditions/myofascial-pain-syndrome/basics/treatment/con-20033195*.
40. Wolfe F, Smythe HA, Yunus MB, et al: The American College of Rheumatology 1990 criteria for the classification of fibromyalgia, *Arthr Rheum* 33:160, 1990. (Classic)
41. Wolfe F, Clauw DJ, Fitzcharles M-A, et al: The American College of Rheumatology preliminary diagnostic criteria for fibromyalgia and measurement of symptom severity, *Arthr Care Res* 62:600, 2010. (Classic)
42. Institute of Medicine: Beyond myalgic encephalopathy/chronic fatigue syndrome: redefining an illness. Retrieved from *http://iom.nationalacademies.org/~/media/Files/Report%20Files/2015/MECFS/MECFScliniciansguide.pdf*.

*Evidence-based information for clinical practice.

## CASE STUDY

### *Managing Care of Multiple Patients*

You are working on the medical-surgical unit and have been assigned to care for the following five patients. You have one LPN/LVN and one UAP on your team to help you.

#### Patients

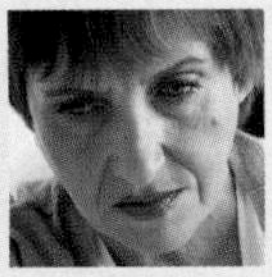

(©iStockphoto/Thinkstock)

J.K. is a 57-yr-old white woman who had debulking surgery for a temporal-parietal glioblastoma. She was diagnosed after presenting with persistent headaches, a seizure in her HCP's office, and left side upper visual field loss. Her MRI/MRA demonstrated a temporal-parietal glioblastoma that extended into the occipital lobes. Four days ago she developed a hemorrhagic stroke into the site of the tumor bed extending into the thalamus. She now has left homonymous hemianopsia and left-sided weakness.

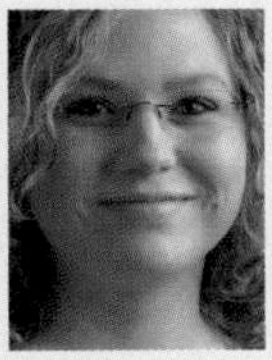

(©Purestock/Thinkstock)

J.P. is a 24-yr-old woman who fell and hit her head after experiencing a tonic-clonic seizure. Her boyfriend found her lying semiconscious on the floor of her apartment. She had an emergency evacuation of a subdural hematoma and was initially admitted to the ICU. She was transferred to the medical-surgical unit yesterday and is scheduled for a rehabilitation evaluation. She is oriented to person only and is somewhat restless. A safety sitter is at the bedside at all times.

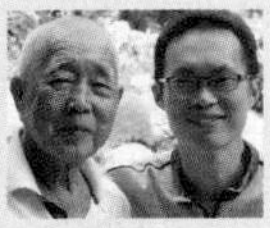

(©iStockphoto/Thinkstock)

M.Y., an 78-yr-old Asian American man, had an ORIF 2 days ago for a fractured left hip. He has a 3-yr history of Alzheimer's disease and is confused to place and time. Although he has a history of agitation, he has been pleasant and cooperative. He has a personal alarm and bed alarm on for safety. His hip dressing is dry and intact and the drainage in the Hemovac drain is minimal.

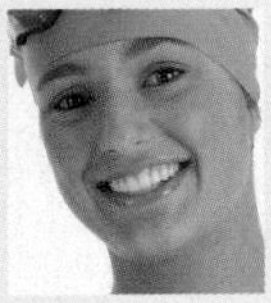

(©iStockphoto/Thinkstock)

S.W., an 18-yr-old woman, sustained a C5 cervical spinal cord injury when she dove into the shallow end of a neighbor's backyard pool and struck her head on the bottom. She was initially placed in cervical traction, intubated, and mechanically ventilated. She has since undergone surgical stabilization and the traction was removed. After spending 1 week in an inpatient SCI rehabilitation facility, she was transferred to the medical-surgical unit this morning with severe headache, blurred vision, and nausea.

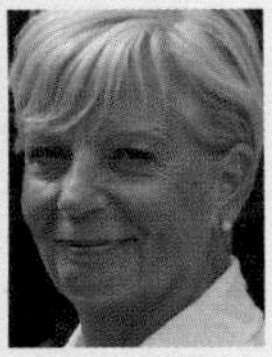

(©iStockphoto/Thinkstock)

M.C. is a 58-yr-old white woman who suffered a right femoral fracture of the greater trochanter after falling over a wall while gardening. She previously has had both hips replaced. She had surgery 4 days ago to repair the femoral component of her right total hip replacement. She is planning to be discharged home today.

#### Discussion Questions

1. ***Priority Decision:*** After receiving report, which patient should you see first? Provide a rationale.
2. **Teamwork and Collaboration:** Which tasks could you delegate to UAP *(select all that apply)*?
   a. Explain discharge instructions to M.C.
   b. Change the dressing on M.Y.'s left hip.
   c. Obtain vital signs on M.C. before discharge.
   d. Sit with J.P. while the safety sitter takes a break.
   e. Assess J.K.'s ability to swallow before feeding her breakfast.
3. ***Priority and Teamwork and Collaboration:*** When you enter the room to assess S.W., you find her diaphoretic with a flushed face and pale extremities. Her BP is 200/102 mm Hg. Which two initial actions would be *most* appropriate?
   a. Ask the UAP to obtain a stat bladder scan.
   b. Have the LPN administer her oral antihypertensive meds stat.
   c. Elevate the head of the bed while assessing for any noxious stimuli.
   d. Ask the LPN to stay with S.W. while you call S.W.'s health care provider.
   e. Insert rectal suppository after applying lidocaine to the area around the rectum.

#### Case Study Progression

S.W.'s bladder scan revealed 700 mL of urine. After you have the LPN catheterize her using a local anesthetic gel, her symptoms subside. You take this time to further teach S.W. about the clinical manifestations of autonomic dysreflexia and the need to report any symptom as soon as it appears. You also take the time to discuss bladder training strategies and how to avoid bladder distention in the future. S.W. is grateful for the information and your caring attitude. Just as you are finishing, the UAP informs you that M.Y. has pulled out his Hemovac drain.

4. What should be your *initial* intervention for M.Y.?
   a. Reinsert the Hemovac drain.
   b. Assess the incision site for a hematoma.
   c. Notify M.Y.'s surgeon that the drain was removed.
   d. Apply pressure to the incisional site where the drain had been placed.
5. Which intervention would be *most* appropriate in caring for J.K.?
   a. Place her left arm in a sling for support.
   b. Arrange the food tray so that all foods are on the right side.
   c. Position her left leg so that the ankle is lower than the knee to prevent contractures.
   d. Call the health care provider to get an order of warfarin to prevent deep vein thrombosis.
6. When teaching J.P.'s boyfriend about what to expect during recovery from a head injury, which statement is *most* accurate?
   a. "You can tell by how great she looks physically that she will ultimately function well at the home."
   b. "One good thing that will come out of this injury is that her seizures should occur less frequently."
   c. "Most patients are transferred out of the hospital for acute rehabilitation management to prepare them for going home."
   d. "She can expect a full recovery without any chronic problems, but it may take a few months to achieve that goal."
7. ***Priority and Management Decision:*** As you enter M.C.'s room to discuss her discharge plans, you find her all packed up and ready to go. She tells you the UAP already told her what she needed to do. What is your *best* initial action?
   a. Ask M.C. if she has any further questions.
   b. Call the UAP to M.C's room to find out what she told her.
   c. Review discharge instructions with M.C. to ascertain correct understanding.
   d. Give M.C. a telephone number to call in case she has any concerns when she gets home.

Answers and rationales available at *http://evolve.elsevier.com/Lewis/medsurg.*

# Nursing Care in Critical Care Settings

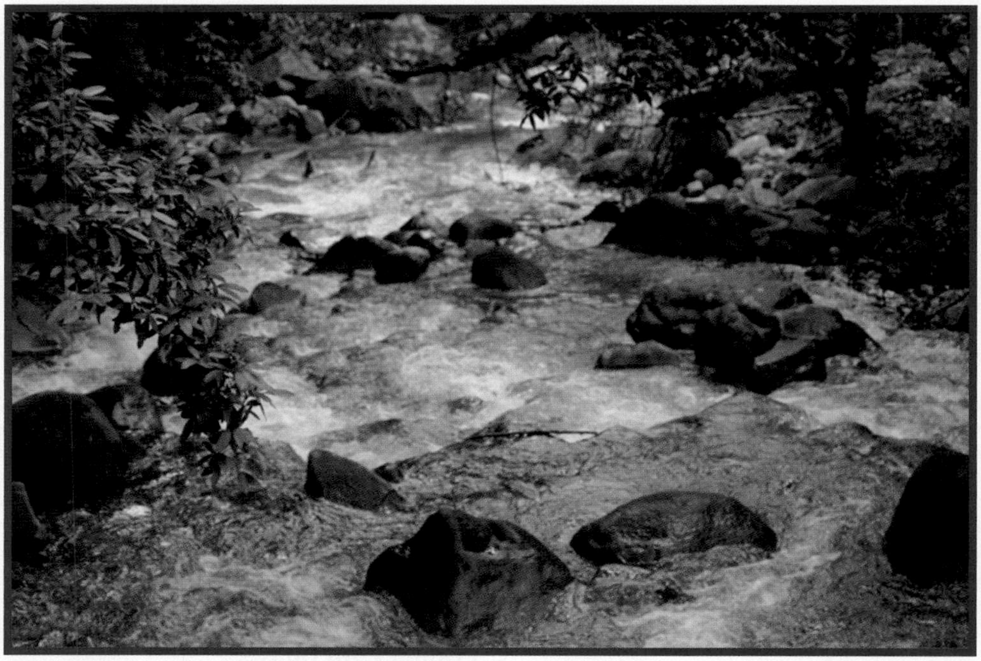

Peter Bonner

*Rivers have what man most respects and longs for in his own life—a capacity for renewal and replenishment, continual energy, creativity, cleansing.*

***John Kaufman***

65

# Critical Care

*Maureen A. Seckel, Linda Bucher*

*Health is not valued till sickness comes.*

***Thomas Fuller***

http://evolve.elsevier.com/Lewis/medsurg/

## LEARNING OUTCOMES

1. Differentiate the various certification opportunities for critical care nurses.
2. Select appropriate nursing interventions to manage common problems and needs of critically ill patients.
3. Develop strategies to manage issues related to caregivers of critically ill patients.
4. Apply the principles of hemodynamic monitoring to the nursing and interprofessional management of patients receiving this intervention.
5. Differentiate the purpose of, indications for, and function of circulatory assist devices and related nursing and interprofessional management.
6. Differentiate the indications for and modes of mechanical ventilation.
7. Select appropriate nursing interventions related to the care of an intubated patient.
8. Relate the principles of mechanical ventilation to the nursing and interprofessional management of patients receiving this intervention.

## KEY TERMS

**arterial pressure–based cardiac output (APCO), p. 1562**
**assist-control ventilation (ACV), p. 1575**
**circulatory assist devices (CADs), p. 1566**
**continuous positive airway pressure (CPAP), p. 1577**
**endotracheal (ET) intubation, p. 1569**
**hemodynamic monitoring, p. 1558**
**high-frequency oscillatory ventilation (HFOV), p. 1578**
**intraaortic balloon pump (IABP), p. 1566**
**mechanical ventilation, p. 1574**
**negative pressure ventilation, p. 1574**
**positive end-expiratory pressure (PEEP), p. 1577**
**positive pressure ventilation (PPV), p. 1574**
**pressure support ventilation (PSV), p. 1576**
**ventricular assist device (VAD), p. 1568**
**volume ventilation, p. 1574**
**weaning, p. 1582**

This chapter focuses on the role of the critical care nurse in the management of critically ill patients in an intensive care setting. The chapter reviews the concepts related to cardiovascular and respiratory dynamics. It emphasizes the interprofessional care and nursing management of patients needing aspects of critical care not addressed in other chapters. These include hemodynamic monitoring, circulatory assist devices, artificial airways, and mechanical ventilation.

## CRITICAL CARE NURSING

The American Association of Critical-Care Nurses (AACN) defines *critical care nursing* as that specialty dealing with human responses to life-threatening problems.[1] Critical care nurses care for patients with acute and unstable physiologic problems and their caregivers. This involves assessing life-threatening conditions, starting appropriate interventions, evaluating the outcomes of the interventions, and providing teaching and emotional support to caregivers.

### Critical Care Units

*Critical care units* (CCUs) or *intensive care units* (ICUs) are designed to meet the special needs of acutely and critically ill patients. In many hospitals, the concept of ICU care has expanded from delivering care in a standard unit to bringing ICU care to patients wherever they may be. For example, the *electronic* or *teleICU* assists the bedside ICU team by monitoring the patient from a remote location (Fig. 65-1).

Similarly, the development of *rapid response teams* (RRTs) provides for the delivery of advanced care by an interprofessional team usually composed of a critical care nurse, respiratory therapist, and critical care physician or an advanced practice registered nurse (APRN). RRTs bring rapid and immediate care to unstable patients in noncritical care settings. Patients often exhibit early and subtle signs of deterioration (e.g., mild confusion, tachypnea) 6 to 8 hours before cardiac or respiratory arrest. Early critical care intervention has made significant contributions to reducing mortality rates in these patients.[2]

Reviewed by Donna C. Bond, RN, DNP, CCNS, AE-C, CTTS, Pulmonary Clinical Nursing Specialist, Carilion Clinic, Roanoke, Virginia; Melissa Hutchinson, RN, MN, CCNS, CCRN, Clinical Nurse Specialist, MICU/CU VA Puget Sound Health Care System, Seattle, Washington; Patricia Lea, RN, DNP, CCRN, Assistant Professor, University of Texas Medical Branch School of Nursing, Galveston, Texas; and Eugene E. Mondor, RN, MN, CNCC(C), Clinical Nurse Educator, Adult Critical Care, Royal Alexandra Hospital, Edmonton, Alberta, Canada.

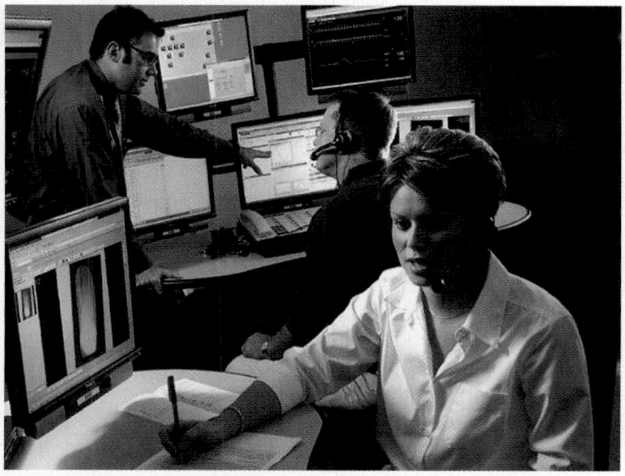

**FIG. 65-1** Tele-intensive care unit control room. (From Avera Health, Sioux Falls, S. Dak.)

The technology available in the ICU is extensive and always evolving. It is possible to continuously monitor the electrocardiogram (ECG), BP, $O_2$ saturation, cardiac output (CO), intracranial pressure, and temperature. More advanced monitoring devices measure cardiac index (CI), stroke volume (SV), stroke volume variation (SVV), ejection fraction (EF), end-tidal carbon dioxide ($CO_2$), and tissue $O_2$ consumption. Patients may receive ongoing support from mechanical ventilators, intraaortic balloon pumps (IABPs), circulatory assist devices (CADs), or dialysis machines.

*Progressive care units* (PCUs), also called *intermediate care* or *step-down units,* provide a transition between the ICU and the general care unit or discharge. Generally, PCU patients are at risk for serious complications, but their risk is lower than that of ICU patients. Examples of patients in PCUs include those scheduled for interventional cardiac procedures (e.g., stent placement), awaiting heart transplant, receiving stable doses of vasoactive IV drugs (e.g., diltiazem [Cardizem]), or being weaned from prolonged mechanical ventilation. Monitoring capabilities in these units may include continuous ECG, arterial BP, $O_2$ saturation, and end-tidal $CO_2$. The use of PCUs provides critical care nursing for an at-risk patient population in a more cost-effective environment.

## Critical Care Nurse

A critical care nurse has in-depth knowledge of anatomy, physiology, pathophysiology, pharmacology, and advanced assessment skills, as well as the ability to use advanced technology. As a critical care nurse, you perform frequent assessments to monitor trends (patterns) in the patient's physiologic parameters (e.g., BP, ECG). This allows you to rapidly recognize and manage complications while aiding healing and recovery. You must also provide psychologic support to the patient and caregiver. To be effective, you must be able to communicate and collaborate with all interprofessional team members (e.g., physician, dietitian, social worker, respiratory therapist, APRN).

As a critical care nurse, you will face ethical dilemmas related to the care of your patients. Moral distress over perceived issues of delivering futile or nonbeneficial care can lead to emotional exhaustion or burnout. Consequently, it is important that all members of the interprofessional care team coexist in a healthy work environment.

Specialization in critical care nursing requires formal education combined with a preceptored clinical orientation, often over several months. The AACN Certification Corporation offers (1) critical care certification (CCRN) in direct care adult, pediatric, and neonatal critical care nursing; (2) critical care certification knowledge (CCRN-K) for adult, pediatric, and neonatal critical care nurses who do not provide direct care but affect acute and critically ill patients and families in their role; (3) progressive care certification (PCCN); and (4) teleICU certification (CCRN-E). Additional certifications are available in cardiac medicine (CMC) and cardiac surgery (CSC). Certification requires registered nurse (RN) licensure, practice experience in the related area, and successful completion of a written test. It validates basic knowledge of critical or progressive care nursing. Certification is not the same as advanced practice.

APRNs have a graduate (master's or doctorate) degree.[3] These nurses function in a variety of roles: patient and staff educators, consultants, administrators, researchers, or expert practitioners. The APRN who is a clinical nurse specialist (CNS) typically provides advanced nursing care to meet the needs of adult-gerontology, pediatric, or neonatal patient populations. Certification for the CNS in acute and critical care (ACCNS) is available through the AACN.

Another APRN role is the acute care nurse practitioner (ACNP). This APRN provides comprehensive care to select critically ill patients and their caregivers. The ACNP conducts comprehensive assessments, orders and interprets diagnostic tests, manages health problems and disease-related symptoms, prescribes treatments, and coordinates care during transitions in settings. Certification as an ACNP in adult gerontology (ACNPC-AG) is available through the AACN. Prescriptive authority and licensure regulations for APRNs vary by state.

## Critical Care Patient

AACN defines a *critically ill patient* as one who is at high risk for actual or potential life-threatening health problems and who requires intense and vigilant nursing care.[1] A patient is generally admitted to the ICU for one of three reasons. First, the patient may be physiologically unstable, requiring advanced clinical judgments by you and the HCP. Second, the patient may be at risk for serious complications and need frequent assessments and often invasive interventions. Third, the patient may need intensive and complicated nursing support related to the use of IV polypharmacy (e.g., sedation, thrombolytics, drugs requiring titration [e.g., vasopressors]) and advanced technology (e.g., mechanical ventilation, intracranial pressure monitoring, continuous renal replacement therapy, hemodynamic monitoring).

ICU patients can be clustered by disease condition (e.g., neurology, pulmonary) or age-group (e.g., neonatal, pediatrics). ICU patients are sometimes clustered by acuity (e.g., acute and unstable versus chronic but technology dependent and stable). Patients commonly treated in the ICU include those with respiratory distress, myocardial infarction, or acute neurologic impairment or those receiving care after heart surgery or other major surgical procedures (e.g., organ transplantation). Trauma and burn ICUs care for critically injured patients. Patients with medical emergencies (e.g., sepsis, diabetic ketoacidosis, drug overdoses, thyroid crisis) are treated in a medical ICU. Fig. 65-2 shows a typical ICU.

The patient who is not expected to recover from an illness is usually not admitted to an ICU. For example, the ICU is not

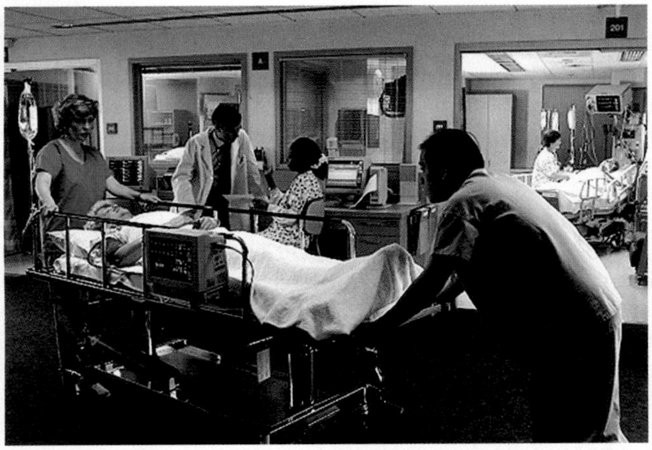

**FIG. 65-2** Typical intensive care unit. (Courtesy Spacelabs Medical, Snoquaime, Wash.)

used to manage the patient in a persistent, vegetative state or to prolong the natural process of death.

Despite the emphasis on caring for patients who are expected to survive, the incidence of death is higher in ICU patients than in non-ICU patients. In general, nonsurvivors are older, have co-morbidities (e.g., liver disease, obesity), and experience longer ICU stays.[4] Consequently, it is important that you are skilled in palliative and end-of-life care (see Chapter 9).

**Common Problems of Critical Care Patients.** The patient admitted to the ICU is at risk for numerous complications and special problems. Critically ill patients are often intubated and mechanically ventilated, immobile, and at high risk for skin problems (see Chapter 23) and venous thromboembolism (see Chapter 37). The use of multiple, invasive devices predisposes the patient to health care–associated infections (HAIs). Sepsis and multiple organ dysfunction syndrome (MODS) may follow (see Chapter 66). Other special problems relate to anxiety, pain, impaired communication, sensory-perceptual problems, sleep, and nutrition.

***Anxiety.*** Anxiety is a common problem for ICU patients. The primary sources of anxiety include the perceived or anticipated threat to health or life, loss of control of body functions, and an environment that is foreign. Many patients and caregivers feel uncomfortable in the ICU with its complex equipment, high noise and light levels, and intense pace of activity. Pain, impaired communication, sleeplessness, immobilization, and loss of control all enhance anxiety.

To help reduce anxiety, teach patients and caregivers to express concerns, ask questions, and state their needs. Include the patient and caregiver in all conversations and explain the purpose of equipment and procedures. Be sure to structure the patient's environment in a way that decreases anxiety. For example, encourage caregivers to bring in photographs and personal items. Appropriate use of antianxiety drugs (e.g., lorazepam [Ativan]) and relaxation techniques (e.g., music therapy) may reduce the stress response that can be triggered by anxiety.[5]

***Pain.*** The control of pain in the ICU patient is very important. As many as 70% of ICU patients report moderate to severe unrelieved pain.[6] Inadequate pain control is often linked with agitation and anxiety and is known to add to the stress response. ICU patients at high risk for pain include those who (1) have medical conditions that include ischemic, infectious, or inflammatory processes; (2) are immobilized; (3) have invasive monitoring devices, including endotracheal tubes; and (4) require invasive or noninvasive procedures.

For many critically ill patients (e.g., those intubated), continuous IV sedation (e.g., propofol [Diprivan]) and an analgesic agent (e.g., fentanyl [Sublimaze]) are used for sedation and pain control. However, patients getting deep sedation are often unresponsive. This prevents you and other HCPs from fully assessing the patient's neurologic status. To address this issue, guidelines should include a daily, scheduled interruption of sedation, or "sedation holiday" for select patients. These daily interruptions allow you to awaken the patient to conduct a neurologic examination.[6] (Pain management is discussed in Chapter 8.)

***Impaired Communication.*** Inability to communicate is distressing for patients who cannot speak because of the use of sedative and paralyzing drugs or an endotracheal tube. As part of every procedure, explain what will happen or is happening to the patient. When the patient cannot speak, explore other methods of communication, such as picture boards, notepads, magic slates, or computer keyboards. When speaking with the patient, look directly at the patient and use hand gestures when appropriate. For patients and caregivers who do not speak English, an approved interpreter or interpreter phone service must be provided (see Chapter 2).

Nonverbal communication is important. High levels of procedure-related touch and lower levels of comfort-related touch often characterize the ICU environment. Patients have different levels of tolerance for being touched, usually related to culture and personal history. If appropriate, use comforting touch with ongoing evaluation of the patient's response. Similarly, encourage caregivers to touch and talk with the patient even if the patient is unresponsive.

***Sleep.*** Nearly all ICU patients have sleep disturbances. Patients may have difficulty falling asleep or have disrupted sleep because of noise, anxiety, pain, frequent monitoring, or treatment procedures. Sleep disturbance has been associated with delirium and delayed recovery.[6]

Arrange the environment to promote the patient's sleep-wake cycle. Strategies include scheduling rest periods, dimming lights at nighttime, providing eye masks/ear plugs, opening curtains during the daytime, getting physiologic measurements without disturbing the patient, limiting noise, and providing comfort measures (e.g., massage).[7] If necessary, use benzodiazepines (e.g., temazepam [Restoril]) and benzodiazepine-like drugs (e.g., zolpidem [Ambien]) to aid and maintain sleep. (Sleep and sleep disorders are discussed in Chapter 7.)

## INFORMATICS IN PRACTICE

### *Smart Infusion Pumps*

- Smart infusion pumps, with preprogrammed drug libraries and wireless technology, calculate drug dose and delivery rates to help prevent IV drug errors and reduce the risk of patient harm.
- Smart pumps provide information used in driving safe practices, such as the total number of infusions programmed using the drug library, how many times pumps were manually overridden, or how often an alert resulted in reprogramming an infusion.
- Remember, if you make an error and enter incorrect data, you will get incorrect results. Some high-risk drugs (e.g., insulin, heparin) require that a second nurse confirm the pump settings.
- Always use your best nursing judgment when using smart infusion pumps and follow agency policy.

***Sensory-Perceptual Problems.*** Acute and reversible sensory-perceptual changes are common in ICU patients. The combination of alterations in mentation (e.g., delusions, short attention span, loss of recent memory), psychomotor behavior (e.g., restlessness, lethargy), and sleep-wake cycle (e.g., daytime sleepiness, nighttime agitation) has been inappropriately called *ICU psychosis.* The patient experiencing these changes is not psychotic but is suffering from *delirium.* It is estimated that the prevalence of delirium in ICU patients is as high as 80%.[8]

Significant risk factors for delirium include preexisting dementia, history of baseline hypertension or alcohol abuse, and severe illness on admission. Environmental factors that can contribute to delirium include sleep deprivation, anxiety, sensory overload, and immobilization. Physical conditions such as hemodynamic instability, hypoxemia, hypercarbia, electrolyte disturbances, and severe infections can lead to delirium. Last, certain drugs (e.g., sedatives [benzodiazepines], analgesics [opioids], and antimicrobials [aminoglycosides]) have been linked with the development of delirium.[8] (Chapter 59 discusses delirium.)

Monitor all ICU patients for delirium. Assessment tools include the Confusion Assessment Method (see Table 59-15) and the Intensive Care Delirium Screening Checklist[7] (both available at *www.icudelirium.org/delirium/monitoring.html*). It is critical to address physiologic factors (e.g., correction of oxygenation, perfusion, and electrolyte problems). The use of clocks and calendars can help orient the patient. If the patient has hyperactivity, insomnia, or delusions, treatment with sedative drugs with anxiolytic effects (e.g., dexmedetomidine [Precedex]) can be used.[8] In addition, the presence of a caregiver may help orient the patient and reduce agitation. Last, the introduction of early mobility protocols has also helped to reduce agitation and delirium in ICU patients.[9]

Sensory overload can also result in patient distress and anxiety. Environmental noise levels are particularly high in the ICU. You can limit noise and assist the patient in understanding noises that cannot be prevented. Conversation is a particularly stressful noise, especially when the discussion concerns the patient and is held in the presence of, but without participation from, the patient.[7] Reduce this source of stress by finding suitable places for patient-related discussions. Whenever possible, include the patient and caregiver in the discussion.

You can also limit noise levels by muting phones, setting alarms based on the patient's condition, and reducing unnecessary alarms. For example, silence the BP alarm when handling invasive lines and then reset the alarm when done. Similarly, silence ventilator alarms when suctioning. Last, limit overhead paging and all unnecessary noise in patient care areas.

***Nutrition.*** Patients often arrive at ICUs with conditions that result in either hypermetabolic states (e.g., burns, sepsis) or catabolic states (e.g., acute kidney injury). Other times, patients are in severely malnourished states (e.g., chronic heart, pulmonary, or liver disease). In general, inadequate nutrition is linked to increased mortality and morbidity rates. One contributing factor to underfeeding patients is the frequent interruptions in enteral feedings to give drugs and for tests and procedures. Determining whom to feed, what to feed, when to feed, and how to feed (e.g., route of administration) is crucial when caring for critically ill patients.[10] Collaborate with the HCP and dietitian to determine how best to meet the nutritional needs of ICU patients.

The primary goal of nutritional support is to prevent or correct nutritional deficiencies. This is usually done by the early provision of enteral nutrition (i.e., delivery of calories via the gastrointestinal [GI] tract) or parenteral nutrition (i.e., IV delivery of calories). Enteral nutrition preserves the structure and function of the gut mucosa and stops the movement of gut bacteria across the intestinal wall and into the bloodstream. In addition, early enteral nutrition is associated with fewer complications and shorter hospital stays and is less expensive than parenteral nutrition.[10] (Enteral and parenteral nutrition are discussed in Chapter 39.)

Parenteral nutrition is used when the enteral route cannot provide adequate nutrition or is contraindicated.[10] Examples of these conditions are paralytic ileus, diffuse peritonitis, intestinal obstruction, pancreatitis, GI ischemia, abdominal trauma or surgery, and severe diarrhea.

## Issues Related to Caregivers

When someone becomes critically ill, care extends beyond the patient to the patient's caregivers. Caregivers play a valuable role in the patient's recovery and are members of the interprofessional care team. They contribute to the patient's well-being by

- Advising the patient in health care decisions or serving as the decision maker when the patient cannot
- Helping with activities of daily living (e.g., bathing, oral care)
- Providing positive, loving, and caring support
- Providing a link to the patient's personal life (e.g., news of family, job)

To be effective in caring for their loved one, caregivers need your guidance and support. The experience of having a friend or relative in the ICU is physically and emotionally difficult, often to the point of exhaustion. Anxiety and concerns regarding the patient's condition, prognosis, and pain are some of the issues that caregivers have. In addition, caregivers commonly experience anxiety over the financial issues related to the provision of care during a critical illness. Consulting with the case manager or social worker is helpful in these instances.

Caregivers often disrupt their daily routines to support the patient. They may be far from their own home, friends, and relatives. Ultimately, caregivers of the critically ill are in crisis, and family-centered care is essential.[11] To provide family-centered care effectively, you must be skilled in crisis intervention. Conduct a family assessment and intervene as necessary. Strategies include active listening, reduction of anxiety, and support of those who become upset or angry. Recognize the caregivers' feelings, listen to them openly and without being judgmental, and acknowledge their decisions. Consult other team members (e.g., chaplains, psychologists, patient representatives) as necessary to help caregivers cope.

The major needs of caregivers of critically ill patients include information, reassurance, and access.[12] Lack of information is a major source of anxiety for the caregivers. Assess the caregiver's understanding of the patient's status, treatment plan, and prognosis and provide information as appropriate. Identify a spokesperson for the family to help coordinate information exchange between the interprofessional care team and family.

The caregiver needs reassurance regarding the way in which the patient's care is managed and decisions are made. Invite the caregiver to meet the interprofessional care team. Evaluate the appropriateness of including caregivers in rounds and patient care conferences. It helps caregivers accept and cope with problems when they see that the team is caring and competent, decisions are deliberate, and their input is valued. If the patient has an advance directive, the caregiver needs to see that the patient's wishes are followed. If the patient has a durable power of attorney for health care, this person must be involved in the patient's plan of care.

Caregivers of critically ill patients need access to the patient. Limiting visitation does not protect the patient from adverse physiologic consequences. AACN strongly recommends less restrictive, individualized visiting policies. This is accomplished by assessing the patient's and caregiver's needs and preferences and incorporating these into the plan of care.[13]

## ETHICAL/LEGAL DILEMMAS

### *Family Presence and Visitation in the Adult ICU*

**Situation**

B.W., a new nurse, is undergoing orientation in the surgical intensive care unit (ICU). He asks his preceptor why the patients' families are permitted on the unit throughout the day and even the night. B.W. states that, in his last position, visiting hours in the ICU were 10 AM to noon and 4 to 6 PM. He adds that families make him nervous when they watch what he is doing and ask him multiple questions. B.W. states that he intends to tell the visitors to leave the patient's room when he is providing care.

**Ethical/Legal Points for Consideration**

- The majority of nurses in adult ICUs prefer unrestricted visiting policies, but most ICU policies limit visitation.
- Family visitation was thought to cause the patient physiologic stress and interfere with care. Additionally, it was believed that family visitation was mentally exhausting to patients and families and even contributed to increased infection rates. Evidence does not support any of these beliefs.[1,2]
- Evidence suggests several positive benefits of flexible family visitation for the patient: decreases in anxiety, confusion, and agitation; reductions in cardiovascular complications; decreases in length of ICU stay; and reports that patients feel more secure and satisfied with care.[1]
- Similar evidence exists for the benefits of flexible visitation for family members: increases in satisfaction, decreases in anxiety, promotion of better communication, and increases in opportunities for patient and family teaching as the family becomes more involved in care.[1]
- Some conditions may require restricting visitation: a legal reason is documented in the chart; visitor behavior presents a risk to the patient, family, staff, or others; visitor behavior disrupts the functioning of the unit; visitor has a contagious illness or has been exposed to a contagious disease that could endanger the patient's health; or the patient requests fewer or no visitors.

**Discussion Questions**

1. How should the preceptor respond to B.W.'s statement of his intentions?
2. Does B.W. have an ethical or legal obligation to permit family visitation regardless of his personal concerns? Defend your position.

**References**

1. American Association of Critical-Care Nurses: AACN practice alert: family presence: visitation in the adult ICU. Retrieved from *www.aacn.org/WD/practice/docs/practicealerts/family-visitation-adult-icu-practicealert.pdf*.
2. American Association of Critical-Care Nurses: AACN practice alert: family presence during resuscitation and invasive procedures. Retrieved from *www.aacn.org/wd/practice/docs/practicealerts/family-presence-during-resuscitation-invasive-procedures.pdf*.

The first time that caregivers visit it is important for you to prepare them for the experience. Briefly describe the patient's appearance and physical environment (e.g., equipment, noise).[14] Join caregivers as they enter the room. Observe the responses of the patient and caregivers. Invite the caregivers to participate in the patient's care if they desire. In some ICUs, visitation includes animal-assisted therapy or pet visitation. The positive benefits of these interventions (e.g., decreases in BP and anxiety) far outweigh the risks (e.g., transmission of infection from animal to patient). They should be a part of the visitation policy.

In addition to traditional visiting, caregivers of patients undergoing invasive procedures (e.g., central line insertion) and cardiopulmonary resuscitation (CPR) want the option of being present at the bedside during these events. Even when the outcomes are not favorable, being present helps caregivers to (1) overcome doubts about the patient's condition, (2) reduce their anxiety and fear, (3) meet their need to be together with and to support their loved one, and (4) begin the grief process if death occurs. AACN encourages critical care nurses to develop policies and procedures that provide for the option of family presence during invasive procedures and CPR.[15]

### Culturally Competent Care: Critical Care Patients

Providing culturally competent care to critically ill patients and caregivers is challenging. Often, meeting the patient's physiologic needs is a priority and overshadows the influence of the patient's culture on the illness experience. It remains important to consider the cultural aspects of the meaning of sickness and health, pain, dying and death, and grief when caring for critically ill patients and their caregivers (see Chapter 2).

Cultural perspectives on dying and death are complex. Telling some patients that they are dying as a way of letting them prepare for death may impose on the family's role. Others view a discussion about advance directives as a legal way to withhold, withdraw, or deny care.

Customs surrounding dying and death vary. Caregiver requests may range from asking you to leave a window open so that the spirit of the deceased can leave, to providing the final bath for the deceased. Ask the caregivers about their cultural traditions when caring for the dying patient.

Several variables influence the expressions of grief that follow the loss of a loved one. These include the relationship between the grieving person and the deceased, whether the loss is sudden or anticipated, the support systems available to the grieving person, past experiences with loss, and the person's religious and cultural beliefs. Proceed cautiously when approaching patients facing death and their caregivers. Asking patients, "What do you want to know?" and "Who do you want with you when discussing options?" are good starting points.[16] (Chapter 9 provides additional information about end-of-life care.)

## HEMODYNAMIC MONITORING

**Hemodynamic monitoring** is the measurement of pressure, flow, and oxygenation within the cardiovascular system. The purpose of hemodynamic monitoring is to assess heart function, fluid balance, and the effects of fluids and drugs on CO. Both invasive (internally placed devices) and noninvasive (external devices) hemodynamic parameters (values) are obtained. These include systemic and pulmonary arterial pressures, central venous pressure (CVP), pulmonary artery wedge pressure

(PAWP) (also known as *pulmonary artery occlusive pressure [PAOP]*), CO/CI, SV/SV index [SVI], SVV, $O_2$ saturation of the hemoglobin of arterial blood ($SaO_2$), and mixed venous $O_2$ saturation ($SvO_2$).

From these measurements you can calculate several values, including the resistance of the systemic and pulmonary arterial vasculature and $O_2$ content, delivery, and consumption. When you combine these data, you get a picture of the patient's hemodynamic status and the effect of therapy over time (trends). Make all measurements with attention to accuracy. Inaccurate data can result in unnecessary or inappropriate treatment.

## Hemodynamic Terminology

**Cardiac Output and Cardiac Index.** *Cardiac output* (CO) is the volume of blood in liters pumped by the heart in 1 minute. *Cardiac index* (CI) is the measurement of the CO adjusted for body surface area (BSA). It is a more precise measurement of the efficiency of the heart's pumping action. Although minor beat-to-beat variations may occur, the left and right ventricles pump the same volume. The volume ejected with each heartbeat is the *stroke volume* (SV). Like CI, *stroke volume index* (SVI) is the measurement of SV adjusted for BSA.

CO and the forces opposing blood flow determine BP. *Systemic vascular resistance* (SVR) (opposition encountered by the left ventricle) or *pulmonary vascular resistance* (PVR) (opposition encountered by the right ventricle) is the resistance to blood flow by the vessels. Preload, afterload, and contractility (see Chapter 31) determine SV (and thus CO and BP). It is essential that you understand these concepts and relationships. In addition, you must understand the physiologic effects of manipulating each of these variables. Table 65-1 presents the formulas and values for common hemodynamic parameters.

**Preload.** *Preload* is the volume within the ventricle at the end of diastole. Unfortunately, chamber volume measurements are difficult to obtain. Instead, various pressures are used to estimate the volume. Left ventricular preload is called *left ventricular end-diastolic pressure.* PAWP, a measurement of pulmonary capillary pressure, reflects left ventricular end-diastolic pressure under normal conditions (i.e., when there is no mitral valve dysfunction, intracardiac defect, or dysrhythmia). CVP,

**TABLE 65-1 Resting Hemodynamic Parameters**

| Indicators | Normal Range |
|---|---|
| **Preload** | |
| Right atrial pressure (RAP) or central venous pressure (CVP) | 2-8 mm Hg |
| Pulmonary artery wedge pressure (PAWP) or left atrial pressure (LAP) | 6-12 mm Hg |
| Pulmonary artery diastolic pressure (PADP) | 4-12 mm Hg |
| Right ventricular end-diastolic volume (RVEDV) $= \frac{\text{Stroke volume (SV)}}{\text{Right ventricular ejection fraction (RVEF)}}$ | 100-160 mL |
| **Afterload** | |
| Pulmonary vascular resistance (PVR) $= \frac{\text{(Pulmonary artery mean pressure [PAMP]} - \text{PAWP)} \times 80}{\text{Cardiac output (CO)}}$ | <250 dynes/sec/cm$^{-5}$ |
| Pulmonary vascular resistance index (PVRI) $= \frac{(\text{PAMP} - \text{PAWP}) \times 80}{\text{Cardiac index (CI)}}$ | 160-380 dynes/sec/cm$^{-5}$/m$^2$ |
| Systemic vascular resistance (SVR) $= \frac{\text{(Mean arterial pressure [MAP]} - \text{CVP)} \times 80}{\text{CO}}$ | 800-1200 dynes/sec/cm$^{-5}$ |
| Systemic vascular resistance index (SVRI) $= \frac{(\text{MAP} - \text{CVP}) \times 80}{\text{CI}}$ | 1970-2390 dynes/sec/cm$^{-5}$/m$^2$ |
| $\text{MAP} = \frac{\text{Systolic blood pressure} + 2\ \text{(Diastolic blood pressure)}}{3^*}$ | 70-105 mm Hg |
| $\text{PAMP} = \frac{\text{Pulmonary artery systolic pressure (PASP)} + 2\ \text{PADP}}{3^*}$ | 10-20 mm Hg |
| **Other** | |
| Stroke volume $= \frac{\text{CO}}{\text{Heart rate}}$ | 60-150 mL/beat |
| Stroke volume index (SVI) $= \frac{\text{CI}}{\text{Heart rate}}$ | 30-65 mL/beat/m$^2$ |
| Stroke volume variation (SVV) $= \frac{SV_{max} - SV_{min}}{SV_{mean}}$ | <13% |
| Heart rate (HR) | 60-100 beats/min |
| $\text{CO} = \text{SV} \times \text{HR}$ | 4-8 L/min |
| $\text{CI} = \frac{\text{CO}}{\text{Body surface area (BSA)}}$ | 2.2-4 L/min/m$^2$ |
| $\text{RVEF} = \frac{\text{SV}}{\text{RVEDV} \times 100}$ | 40%-60% |
| Arterial hemoglobin $O_2$ saturation | 95%-100% |
| Mixed venous hemoglobin $O_2$ saturation | 60%-80% |
| Venous hemoglobin $O_2$ saturation | 70% |

*This formula is an approximation because it does not take into consideration the heart rate. The monitor looks at the area under the pressure curve, as well as the heart rate, to calculate MAP and PAMP.

measured in the right atrium or in the vena cava close to the heart, is the right ventricular preload or right ventricular end-diastolic pressure when there is no tricuspid valve dysfunction, intracardiac defect, or dysrhythmia.

*Frank-Starling's law* explains the effects of preload. It states that the more a myocardial fiber is stretched during filling, the more it shortens during systole and the greater the force of the contraction. As preload increases, force generated in the subsequent contraction increases, and thus SV and CO increase. The greater the preload, the greater the myocardial stretch and the greater the $O_2$ requirement of the myocardium. Thus increases in CO via increased preload require increased delivery of $O_2$ to the myocardium. However, the clinical measurement made is not a direct measurement of the muscle length. The measurement is of the pressure at the time of the peak stretch (end diastole) (Table 65-1). This pressure indirectly indicates the amount of stretch and the volume. This pressure is also important because it indicates pressure in the blood vessels of the lungs or in the blood returning to the heart. Diuresis and vasodilation decrease preload, and fluid administration increases preload.

**Afterload.** *Afterload* refers to the forces opposing ventricular ejection. These forces include systemic arterial pressure, the resistance offered by the aortic valve, and the mass and density of the blood to be moved. Clinically, although the measures fail to include all the components of afterload, SVR and arterial pressure are indices of left ventricular afterload. Similarly, PVR and pulmonary arterial pressure are indices of right ventricular afterload. Increased afterload often results in a decreased CO and increased $O_2$ demand. CO can be restored and myocardial $O_2$ needs reduced by decreasing afterload (i.e., decreasing forces opposing contraction). For example, vasodilator drug therapy (e.g., milrinone) can reduce afterload.

**Vascular Resistance.** *Systemic vascular resistance* (SVR) is the resistance of the systemic vascular bed. *Pulmonary vascular resistance* (PVR) is the resistance of the pulmonary vascular bed. Both these measures reflect afterload as described earlier and can be adjusted for body size (Table 65-1).

**Contractility.** *Contractility* describes the strength of contraction. Contractility is said to increase when preload is unchanged yet the heart contracts more forcefully. Epinephrine, norepinephrine (Levophed), isoproterenol (Isuprel), dopamine, dobutamine, digitalis-like drugs, calcium, and milrinone increase or improve contractility. These drugs are termed *positive inotropes.* Contractility is reduced by *negative inotropes.* Examples include certain drugs (e.g., calcium channel blockers, β-adrenergic blockers [β-blockers]) and clinical conditions (e.g., acidosis). Increased contractility results in increased SV and increased myocardial $O_2$ requirements.

There are no direct clinical measures of cardiac contractility. Measuring the patient's preload (PAWP) and CO and graphing the results indirectly indicate contractility. If preload, heart rate (HR), and afterload remain constant yet CO changes, contractility is changed. Contractility is reduced in the failing heart.

## Principles of Invasive Pressure Monitoring

Invasive lines are used in the ICU to measure systemic and pulmonary BPs. Fig. 65-3 shows the components of a typical invasive arterial BP monitoring system. The catheter, pressure tubing, flush system, and transducer are disposable.

Pressure monitoring equipment is referenced and zero balanced to the environment and dynamic response characteristics

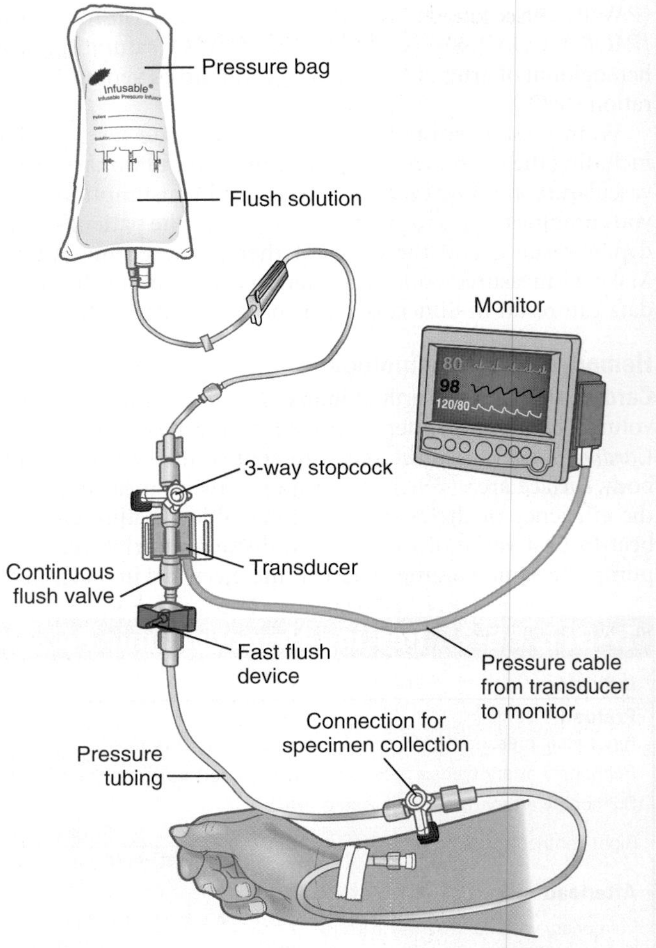


**FIG. 65-3** Components of a pressure monitoring system. The cannula, shown entering the radial artery, is connected via pressure (nondistensible) tubing to the transducer. The transducer converts the pressure wave into an electronic signal. The transducer is wired to the electronic monitoring system, which amplifies, conditions, displays, and records the signal. Stopcocks are inserted into the line for specimen withdrawal and for referencing and zero-balancing procedures. A flush system, consisting of a pressurized bag of IV fluid, tubing, and a flush device, is connected to the system. The flush system provides continuous slow (approximately 3 mL/hr) flushing and provides a mechanism for fast flushing of lines.

optimized for accuracy. *Referencing* means placing the transducer so that the zero reference point is at the level of the atria of the heart. The stopcock nearest the transducer is used for the zero reference. To place this level with the atria, use an external landmark, the phlebostatic axis. To identify the *phlebostatic axis,* draw two imaginary lines with the patient supine (Fig. 65-4, *A*). Draw a horizontal line down from the axilla, midway between the anterior and posterior chest walls. Draw a vertical line laterally through the fourth intercostal space along the chest wall. The phlebostatic axis is the intersection of the two imaginary lines. Mark this location on the patient's chest with a permanent marker. Position the port of the stopcock nearest the transducer level at the phlebostatic axis. Tape the transducer to the patient's chest at the phlebostatic axis or mount it on a bedside pole (Fig. 65-4, *B*).

*Zeroing* confirms that when pressure within the system is zero, the monitor reads zero. To do this, open the reference stopcock to room air (off to the patient) and observe the monitor for a reading of zero. This allows the monitor to use the atmospheric pressure as a reference for zero. Zero the transducer

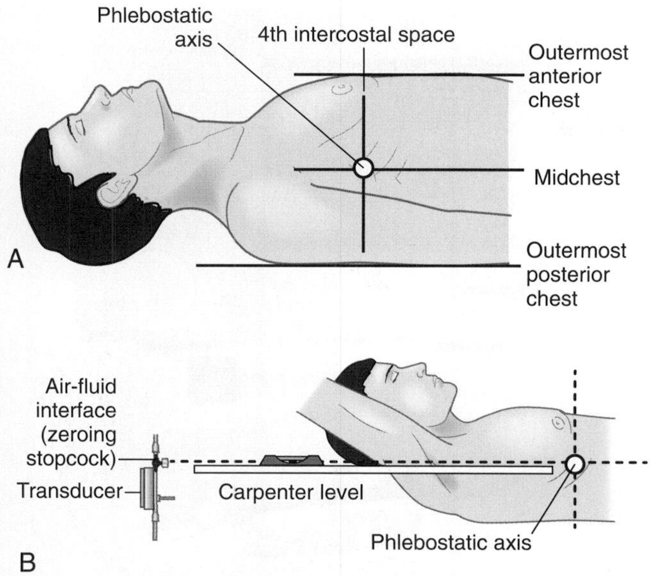


**FIG. 65-4** Identification of the phlebostatic axis. **A,** Phlebostatic axis is an external landmark used to identify the level of the atria in the supine patient. It is defined as the intersection of two imaginary lines: one drawn horizontally from the axilla, midway between the anterior and posterior chest walls, and the other drawn vertically through the fourth intercostal space along the lateral chest wall. **B,** Air-fluid interface (zeroing the stopcock) is level with the phlebostatic axis using a carpenter's or laser level.

**TABLE 65-2 Invasive Arterial Blood Pressure Measurement**

1. Explain the procedure to the patient.
2. Position the patient supine and flat or (if appropriate) with the head of the bed less than 45 degrees or prone.
3. Confirm that the zero reference (port of the stopcock nearest the transducer) is placed at the level of the phlebostatic axis (Fig. 65-4). If the reference stopcock is not taped to the patient's chest, use a leveling device to position the stopcock on a bedside pole at the point level with the phlebostatic axis.
4. Observe the monitor tracing and assess the quality of the tracing. Perform a dynamic response test (Fig. 65-5).
5. Obtain an analog printout (if available) and measure the systolic and diastolic pressures at end expiration (Fig. 65-6). If no printout is available, freeze the tracing on the oscilloscope screen and use the cursor to measure the pressures at end expiration.
6. Record the pressure measurements promptly, including (if available) the printout marked to identify the points read.

during the initial setup, immediately after insertion of the arterial line, when the transducer has been disconnected from the pressure cable or the pressure cable has been disconnected from the monitor, and when the accuracy of the measurements is questioned. Always follow the manufacturer's guidelines.

Optimizing dynamic response characteristics involves checking that the equipment reproduces, without distortion, a signal that changes rapidly. Perform a *dynamic response test (square wave test)* every 8 to 12 hours and when the system is opened to air or the accuracy of the measurements is questioned. It involves activating the fast flush and checking that the equipment reproduces a distortion-free signal (Fig. 65-5).

Table 65-2 outlines the steps in obtaining BP measurements with an invasive line. Obtain measurements from both digital and printed analog outputs. Readings from a printed pressure tracing at the end of expiration (to limit the effect of the respiratory cycle on arterial BP) are most accurate. Position the

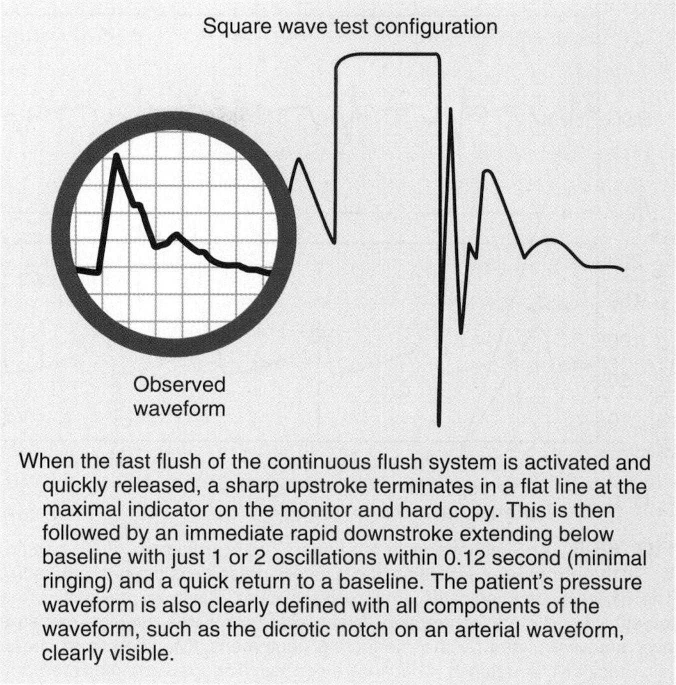


**FIG. 65-5** Optimally damped system. Dynamic response test (square wave test) using the fast flush system: normal response. No adjustment in the monitoring system is required. (From Darovic GO, Vanriper S, Vanriper J: Fluid-filled monitoring systems. In Darovic GO: *Hemodynamic monitoring,* ed 2, Philadelphia, 1995, Saunders.)

patient supine for initial readings. Values with head of bed (HOB) elevation (up to 45 degrees) are generally equal to measurements with the patient supine, unless the patient's BP is extremely sensitive to orthostatic changes. Additionally, readings in the prone position are generally accurate. However, there is little support for the accuracy of readings in the lateral positions.[17] It is not necessary to reposition the patient for each pressure reading. However, it is important to keep the zero reference stopcock level with the phlebostatic axis.

**! SAFETY ALERT Positioning the Zero Reference Stopcock**

- Mark the location of the phlebostatic axis on the patient's chest with a permanent marker.
- Recheck the leveling of the zero reference stopcock to the phlebostatic axis with any change in the patient's position before obtaining a reading.
- Transducers placed higher than the phlebostatic axis will produce falsely low BP readings.
- Transducers placed lower than the phlebostatic axis will produce falsely high BP readings.

## Types of Invasive Pressure Monitoring

**Arterial Blood Pressure.** Continuous arterial BP monitoring is indicated for patients in many situations, including acute hypertension and hypotension, respiratory failure, shock, neurologic injury, coronary interventional procedures, continuous infusion of vasoactive drugs (e.g., sodium nitroprusside), and frequent arterial blood gas (ABG) sampling. A nontapered Teflon catheter is typically used to cannulate an artery (e.g., radial, femoral) using a percutaneous approach. After insertion, the catheter is usually sutured in place. You must immobilize the insertion site to prevent dislodging or kinking the catheter line.

***Measurements.*** Use the arterial line to obtain systolic, diastolic, and mean arterial pressure (MAP) (Fig. 65-6). The

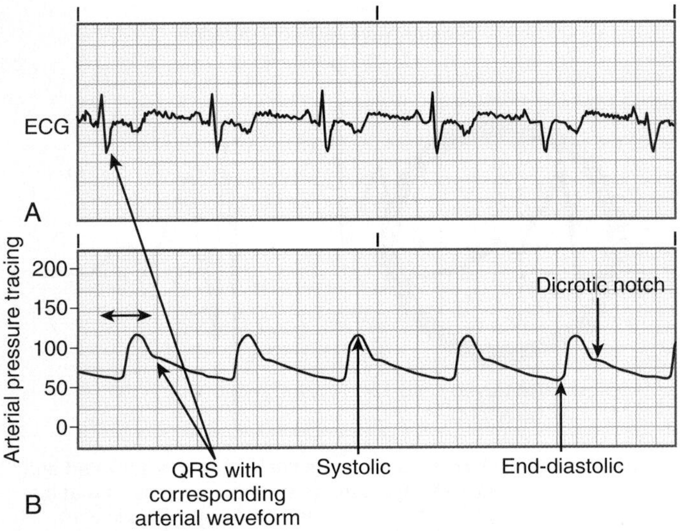


**FIG. 65-6** **A,** Simultaneously recorded electrocardiogram (ECG) tracing. **B,** Systemic arterial pressure tracing. Systolic pressure is the peak pressure. The *dicrotic notch* indicates aortic valve closure. Diastolic pressure is the lowest value before contraction. Mean pressure is the average pressure over time calculated by the monitoring equipment. (Modified from Urden LD, Stacy KM, Lough ME: *Critical care nursing: diagnosis and management,* ed 6, St Louis, 2010, Mosby.)

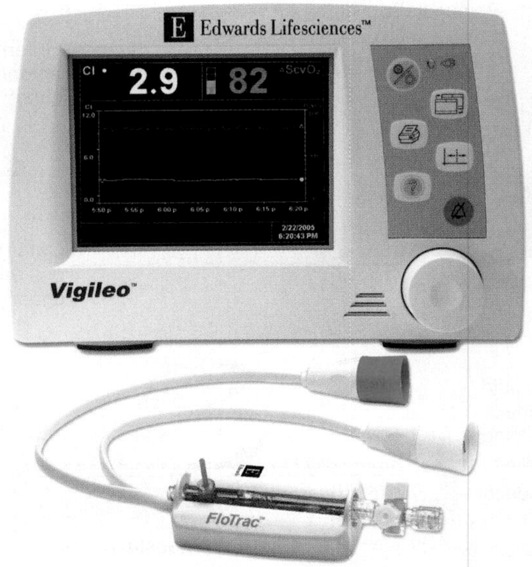


**FIG. 65-7** FloTrac sensor and Vigileo monitor. (Courtesy Edwards Lifesciences, Irvine, Calif.)

high- and low-pressure alarms are set based on the patient's current status and then activated. Various patient conditions will change the pressure tracings. In heart failure, the systolic upstroke may be slower. In volume depletion, systolic pressure varies greatly with mechanical ventilation, decreasing during inspiration. Observe simultaneous ECG and pressure tracings with dysrhythmias. Dysrhythmias that significantly diminish arterial BP are more urgent than those that cause only a slight decrease in systolic amplitude.

***Complications.*** Arterial lines carry the risk of hemorrhage, infection, thrombus formation, neurovascular impairment, and loss of limb. Hemorrhage is most likely to occur when the catheter dislodges or the line disconnects. To avoid this serious complication, use Luer-Lok connections, always check the arterial waveform, and activate alarms. If the pressure in the line falls (e.g., when the line is disconnected), the low-pressure alarm sounds immediately, allowing you to promptly correct the problem.

Infection is a risk with any invasive line. To limit the risk of catheter-related infection, inspect the insertion site for local signs of inflammation and monitor the patient for signs of systemic infection. Change the pressure tubing, flush bag, and transducer every 96 hours or according to agency policy. If infection is suspected, notify the HCP, remove the catheter, and replace the equipment.

Circulatory impairment can result from formation of a thrombus around the catheter, release of an embolus, spasm, or occlusion of the circulation by the catheter. Before inserting a line into the radial artery, perform an *Allen test* to confirm that ulnar circulation to the hand is adequate. In this test, apply pressure to the radial and ulnar arteries simultaneously. Ask the patient to open and close the hand repeatedly. The hand should blanch. Release the pressure on the ulnar artery while maintaining pressure on the radial artery. If pinkness fails to return within 6 seconds, the ulnar artery is inadequate and you should not use the radial artery for line insertion.

To maintain line patency and limit thrombus formation, assess the flush system every 1 to 4 hours to determine that the (1) pressure bag is inflated to 300 mm Hg, (2) flush bag contains fluid, and (3) system is delivering a continuous slow (approximately 3 mL/hr) flush. Because of the risk of heparin-induced thrombocytopenia (HIT), use normal saline for the flush solution.[17] (HIT is discussed in Chapter 30.)

Once the catheter is inserted, evaluate the neurovascular status distal to the arterial insertion site hourly. The limb with compromised arterial flow will be cool and pale, with capillary refill time longer than 3 seconds. The patient may have symptoms of neurologic impairment (e.g., paresthesia, pain, paralysis). Neurovascular impairment, which can result in the loss of a limb, is an emergency and must be reported to the HCP immediately.

**Arterial Pressure–Based Cardiac Output.** Arterial pressure–based cardiac output (APCO) monitoring is a minimally invasive technique to determine *continuous CO* (CCO)/*continuous CI* (CCI). In addition to measuring CCO, APCO is used to assess a patient's ability to respond to fluids by increasing SV *(preload responsiveness)*. This is determined by using *stroke volume variation* (SVV) or by measuring the percent increase in SV after a fluid bolus[18] (Table 65-1). This technology uses a specialized sensor that attaches to a standard arterial pressure line and a monitor (Fig. 65-7).

SVV is the variation of the arterial pulsation caused by the heart-lung interaction. It is a sensitive indicator of preload responsiveness when used on select patients. SVV helps predict whether or not a patient would benefit from an IV fluid challenge that may help optimize hemodynamic status. SVV is only used for patients on controlled mechanical ventilation with a fixed respiratory rate and a tidal volume ($V_T$) greater than 8 mL/kg. Also, the APCO monitor may not be able to filter certain dysrhythmias, specifically atrial fibrillation, thus limiting the use of SVV in these patients.[18] These limitations only apply to SVV, not to the use of APCO for CO monitoring.

***Measurements.*** *Arterial pressure* is the force generated by the ejection of blood from the left ventricle into the arterial circulation. Pulsatile pressure waves are produced by the heart's contractions (systole). The specialized sensor measures the arterial pulse pressure, which is proportional to SV. APCO monitoring uses the arterial waveform characteristics along with patient demographic data (i.e., gender, age, height, and weight) to calculate SV and pulse rate (PR) to calculate CCO/CCI and SV/SVI every 20 seconds. CO is calculated by multiplying the PR and calculated SV and is displayed on a continuous basis.[19]

APCO monitoring is frequently used in conjunction with a central venous oximetry catheter. Together, these allow for continuous monitoring of central venous $O_2$ saturation ($ScvO_2$) and SVR that is derived from the CVP. APCO is indicated only in adult patients and cannot be used in patients who are on IABP therapy.[19]

**Pulmonary Artery Flow-Directed Catheter.** Pulmonary artery (PA) pressure monitoring guides the management of patients with select complicated heart and lung problems (Table 65-3). PA diastolic (PAD) pressure and PAWP are sensitive indicators of heart function and fluid volume status. PAD pressure and PAWP increase in heart failure and fluid volume overload. They decrease with volume depletion. Fluid therapy based on PA pressures can restore fluid balance while limiting overcorrection or undercorrection of the problem. Monitoring PA pressures permits precise therapeutic manipulation of preload. This allows CO to be maintained without placing the patient at risk for pulmonary edema.

A PA flow-directed catheter (e.g., Swan-Ganz) is used to measure PA pressures, including PAWP. The standard PA catheter has multiple lumens (Fig. 65-8). When properly positioned, the distal lumen port (catheter tip) is within the PA. This port is used to monitor PA pressures and sample mixed venous blood (e.g., to evaluate $O_2$ saturation).

A balloon connected to an external valve surrounds the distal lumen port. Balloon inflation has two purposes: (1) to allow blood to "float" the catheter forward and (2) to allow PAWP measurement. The catheter has one or two proximal lumens, with exit ports in the right atrium or right atrium and right ventricle (if two). The right atrium port is used for measurement of CVP, injection of fluid for CO determination, and withdrawal of blood specimens. The second proximal port (if available) is used for infusion of fluids and drugs or blood sampling. A thermistor (temperature sensor) is located near the distal tip and is wired to an external connector. This is used to monitor core temperature and for the thermodilution method of measuring CO.[20]

In addition to providing most of the same functions as the standard PA catheter, the advanced technology PA catheter

## TABLE 65-3 Indications and Contraindications for Pulmonary Artery Catheterization*

**Indications**

- Assessment of response to therapy in patients with pulmonary hypertension and mixed types of shock
- Cardiogenic shock
- Differential diagnosis of pulmonary hypertension
- Myocardial infarction with complications (e.g., heart failure, cardiogenic shock)
- Potentially reversible systolic heart failure (e.g., fulminant myocarditis)
- Severe chronic heart failure requiring inotropic, vasopressor, and vasodilator therapy
- Transplantation work-up

**Contraindications**

- Coagulopathy (may be overlooked in emergency situations)
- Endocardial pacemaker
- Endocarditis
- Right heart mass (e.g., thrombus, tumor)
- Mechanical tricuspid or pulmonic valve

*List is not all-inclusive.

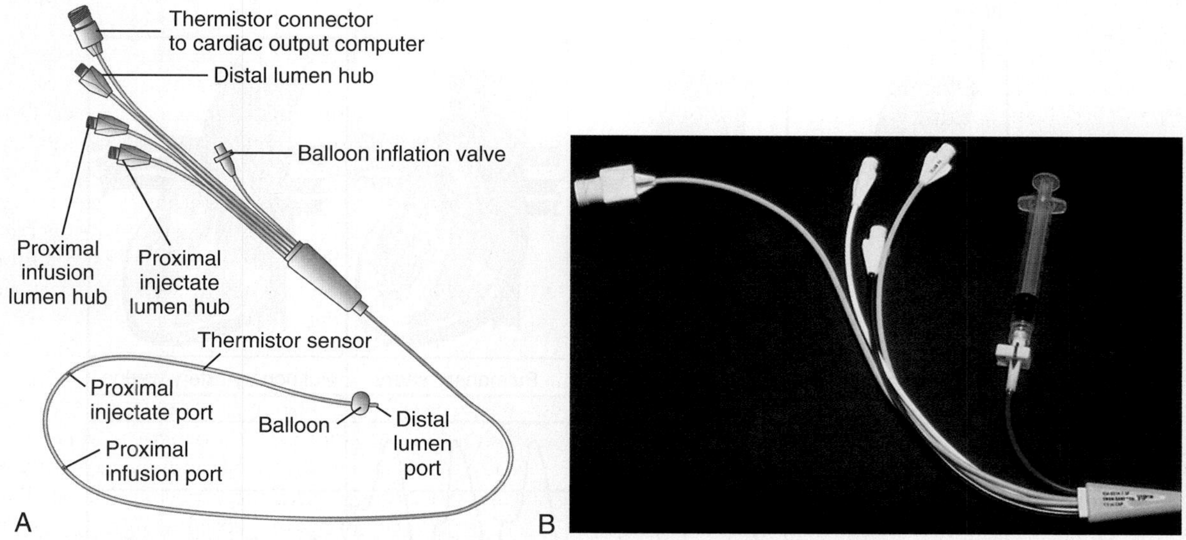


**FIG. 65-8** Pulmonary artery (PA) catheter. **A,** Illustrated catheter has five lumens. When properly positioned, the distal lumen exit port is in the PA and the proximal lumen ports are in the right atrium and right ventricle. The distal and one of the proximal ports are used to measure PA and central venous pressures, respectively. A balloon surrounds the catheter near the distal end. The balloon inflation valve is used to inflate the balloon with air to allow reading of the pulmonary artery wedge pressure. A thermistor located near the distal tip senses PA temperature and is used to measure thermodilution cardiac output when solution cooler than body temperature is injected into a proximal port. **B,** Photo of an actual catheter. (*B,* Courtesy Edwards Critical Care Division, Baxter Healthcare Corporation, Santa Ana, Calif.)

can continuously monitor the patient's $SvO_2$. This provides a global indicator of the balance between $O_2$ delivery and $O_2$ consumption. CCO and right ventricular EF (RVEF) also can be measured using advanced thermodilution technology. RVEF provides information regarding RV function and helps to assess right heart contractility. RV end-diastolic volume is continuously measured by dividing SV by RVEF (Table 65-1). This serves as a key indicator of preload.

***Pulmonary Artery Catheter Insertion.*** Before PA catheter insertion, note the patient's electrolyte, acid-base, oxygenation, and coagulation status. Imbalances such as hypokalemia, hypomagnesemia, hypoxemia, or acidosis can make the heart more irritable. This can increase the risk of ventricular dysrhythmia during catheter insertion. Coagulopathy increases the risk of hemorrhage. Preparation for the procedure includes arranging the monitor, cables, and infusion and pressurized flush solutions. The system is leveled and zero referenced to the phlebostatic axis.

The HCP explains the procedure to the patient and obtains informed consent. The patient is positioned supine and flat. The PA catheter is inserted percutaneously through a sheath (introducer) into the internal jugular, subclavian, antecubital, or femoral vein using surgical asepsis. Most catheters have a plastic "sleeve" connected to the sheath. This allows the catheter to be advanced or pulled back while maintaining sterility. Most catheters also have a side port that serves as a large-bore IV line. Venous cut-down is rarely needed. The catheter is advanced through the venous system to the right side of the heart. The HCP (e.g., ACNP) usually positions the PA catheter, but this practice varies by agency and state.

Continuously observe the characteristic waveforms on the monitor as the catheter is moved through the heart to the PA (Fig. 65-9). When the tip reaches the right atrium, the balloon is inflated. Inflation of the balloon should not exceed the balloon's capacity (1.5 mL of air). The catheter is then "floated" through the tricuspid valve into the right ventricle and then through the pulmonic valve to the PA. Monitor the ECG continuously during insertion because of the risk for dysrhythmias, particularly when the catheter reaches the right ventricle. Once a typical PAWP tracing is observed, the balloon is deflated, and the PA waveform should return on the monitor.

After insertion and before the PA catheter is used, a chest x-ray must confirm the catheter's position. To maintain the catheter in its proper place, secure it at the point of entry into the skin. Note and record the measurement at the exit point. Finally, apply an occlusive dressing and change it according to agency policy.

Recently, the use of PA pressure monitoring has decreased dramatically. This is due, in part, to risks associated with this invasive technology (e.g., dysrhythmias, infection) and the development of less invasive techniques (e.g., APCO monitoring, bedside echocardiography).

**Central Venous or Right Atrial Pressure Measurement.** CVP is a measurement of right ventricular preload and reflects fluid volume status. It is most often measured with a central venous catheter placed in the internal jugular or subclavian vein. It can be measured with a PA catheter using the proximal lumen located in the right atrium. CVP waveforms (Fig. 65-10) are similar to PAWP waveforms. CVP is measured as a mean pressure at the end of expiration. An elevated CVP indicates right ventricular failure or volume overload. A low CVP indicates hypovolemia.

**Venous Oxygen Saturation Monitoring.** In critically ill patients, measurement of the $O_2$ saturation of hemoglobin in venous blood helps to determine the adequacy of tissue oxygenation. The $O_2$ saturation of venous blood from the CVP catheter is termed *central venous $O_2$ saturation* ($ScvO_2$). Similarly, the $O_2$ saturation of blood from the PA catheter is termed *mixed venous*

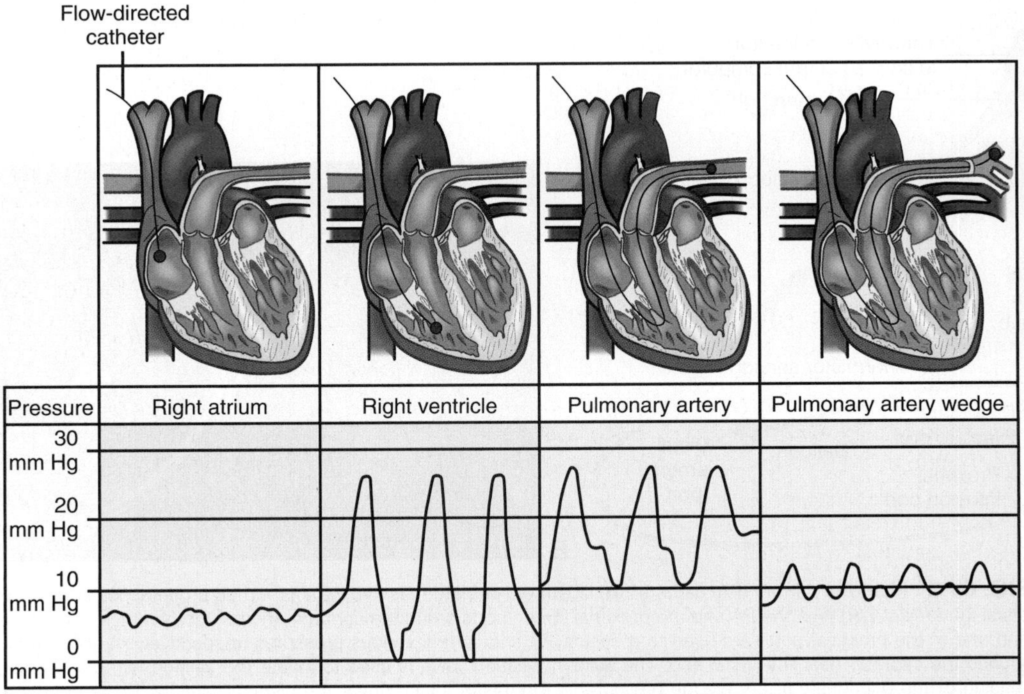


**FIG. 65-9** Position of the pulmonary artery flow-directed catheter during progressive stages of insertion with corresponding pressure waveforms. (Modified from Urden LD, Stacy KM, Lough ME: *Critical care nursing: diagnosis and management,* ed 6, St Louis, 2010, Mosby.)

**TABLE 65-4 Interpreting $ScvO_2$ and $SvO_2$* Measurements**

| $ScvO_2$ and $SvO_2$ Measurement | Physiologic Basis for Change in $ScvO_2$ or $SvO_2$ | Clinical Diagnosis and Rationale |
|---|---|---|
| **High $ScvO_2$ or $SvO_2$** (80%-95%) | Increased $O_2$ supply<br>Decreased $O_2$ demand | • Patient receiving more $O_2$ than required by clinical condition<br>• Anesthesia, which causes sedation and decreased muscle movement<br>• Hypothermia, which lowers metabolic demand (e.g., with cardiopulmonary bypass)<br>• Sepsis caused by decreased ability of tissues to use $O_2$ at the cellular level<br>• False high positive because pulmonary artery catheter is wedged in a pulmonary capillary ($SvO_2$ only) |
| **Normal $ScvO_2$ or $SvO_2$** (60%-80%) | Normal $O_2$ supply and metabolic demand | • Balanced $O_2$ supply and demand |
| **Low $ScvO_2$ or $SvO_2$** (<60%) | Decreased $O_2$ supply caused by<br>• Low hemoglobin<br>• Low arterial saturation ($SaO_2$)<br>• Low cardiac output<br>• Increased $O_2$ demand | • Anemia or bleeding with compromised cardiopulmonary system<br>• Hypoxemia resulting from decreased $O_2$ supply or lung disease<br>• Cardiogenic shock caused by left ventricular pump failure<br>• Metabolic demand exceeds $O_2$ supply in conditions that increase muscle movement and metabolic rate. These include physiologic states such as shivering, seizures, and hyperthermia and nursing interventions such as being weighed on a bedside scale and turning |

*$ScvO_2$ values are generally slightly higher than $SvO_2$ values.
Source: Urden LD, Lough ME, Stacy KM: *Critical care nursing: diagnosis and management,* ed 6, St Louis, 2010, Mosby.

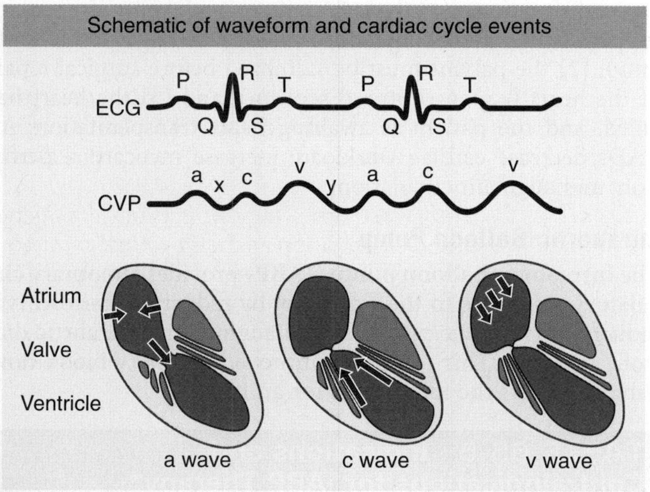


**FIG. 65-10** Cardiac events that produce the central venous pressure (CVP) waveform with *a, c,* and *v* waves. The *a* wave represents atrial contraction. The *x* descent represents atrial relaxation. The *c* wave represents the bulging of the closed tricuspid valve into the right atrium during ventricular systole. The *v* wave represents atrial filling. The *y* descent represents opening of the tricuspid valve and filling of the ventricle. (Modified from Urden LD, Stacy KM, Lough ME: *Critical care nursing: diagnosis and management,* ed 6, St Louis, 2010, Mosby.)

*oxygen saturation* ($SvO_2$). The measurements of $ScvO_2$ and $SvO_2$ reflect the balance among oxygenation of the arterial blood, tissue perfusion, and tissue $O_2$ consumption. $ScvO_2$ and $SvO_2$ are useful in assessing hemodynamic status and response to treatments or activities when considered in conjunction with arterial $O_2$ saturation (Table 65-4). Normal $ScvO_2$ or $SvO_2$ at rest is 60% to 80%.

Carefully review sustained decreases and increases in $ScvO_2$ or $SvO_2$. Decreased $ScvO_2$ or $SvO_2$ may indicate decreased arterial oxygenation, low CO, low hemoglobin level, or increased $O_2$ consumption or extraction. If the $ScvO_2$ or $SvO_2$ falls below 60%, determine which of these factors has changed. Observe for changes in arterial oxygenation (e.g., monitor pulse oximetry or ABGs) and indirectly assess CO and tissue perfusion. This is done by noting any changes in mental status, strength and quality of peripheral pulses, capillary refill, urine output, and skin color and temperature. If arterial oxygenation, CO, and hemoglobin level are unchanged, a fall in $ScvO_2$ or $SvO_2$ indicates increased $O_2$ consumption or extraction. This could represent an increased metabolic rate, pain, movement, or fever. If $O_2$ consumption increases without a comparable increase in $O_2$ delivery, more $O_2$ is extracted from the blood, and $ScvO_2$ and $SvO_2$ will continue to fall.[21]

Increased $ScvO_2$ or $SvO_2$ is also clinically significant. It may indicate a clinical improvement (e.g., increased arterial $O_2$ saturation, improved perfusion, decreased metabolic rate) or problem (e.g., sepsis). In sepsis, $O_2$ is not extracted properly at the tissue level, resulting in increased $ScvO_2$ or $SvO_2$.

Your interventions are guided by changes in $ScvO_2$ or $SvO_2$. For example, you may note that the patient's HR increased slightly during repositioning but that the $ScvO_2$ or $SvO_2$ remained stable. In this case, you would conclude that the patient tolerated the position change. If the $ScvO_2$ or $SvO_2$ dropped, this would be a sign to stop the activity until the $ScvO_2$ or $SvO_2$ returns to baseline.

In many cases, as activity or metabolism increases, HR and CO increase, and $ScvO_2$ or $SvO_2$ remains constant or varies slightly. However, critically ill patients often have conditions (e.g., heart failure, shock) that prevent substantial increases in CO. In these cases, $ScvO_2$ or $SvO_2$ can be a useful indicator of the balance between $O_2$ delivery and consumption.

**CHECK YOUR PRACTICE**

You are caring for a 38-yr-old woman admitted with sepsis secondary to a ruptured ectopic pregnancy. She has CVP and $ScvO_2$ monitoring in place. Trends in $ScvO_2$ have shown a slow, steady decline with the most recent reading being 55%.

- What additional assessment data would you explore to explain this drop in readings?

### Noninvasive Arterial Oxygenation Monitoring

*Pulse oximetry* is a noninvasive and continuous method of determining the $O_2$ saturation of hemoglobin ($SpO_2$). Monitoring $SpO_2$ may reduce the frequency of ABG sampling (see Chapter 25). $SpO_2$ is normally 95% to 100%. Accurate $SpO_2$ measurements may be difficult to obtain on patients who are hypothermic, receiving IV vasopressor therapy (e.g., norepinephrine), or experiencing hypoperfusion and vasoconstriction (e.g., shock). Consider alternative locations for placement of the pulse oximetry probe (e.g., forehead, earlobe).

A common use for pulse oximetry is to evaluate the effectiveness of $O_2$ therapy. Decreased $SpO_2$ indicates inadequate oxygenation of the blood in the pulmonary capillaries. You can correct this by increasing the fraction of inspired $O_2$ ($FIO_2$) and evaluating the patient's response. Similarly, use $SpO_2$ to monitor how the patient tolerates decreases in $FIO_2$ and responds to interventions. For example, if $SpO_2$ falls when you position the patient in a left lateral recumbent position, plan position changes that pose less risk for the patient.

### Noninvasive Hemodynamic Monitoring: Impedance Cardiography

*Impedance cardiography* (ICG) is a continuous or intermittent, noninvasive method of obtaining CO and assessing thoracic fluid status. Based on the concepts of *impedance* (the resistance to the flow of electric current [Ω]), ICG uses four sets of external electrodes to deliver a high-frequency, low-amplitude current that is similar to that used in apnea monitors. Blood is an excellent conductor of electricity (lower impedance), and pulsatile blood flow generates electrical impedance changes. ICG measures the change in impedance (dΩ) in the ascending aorta and left ventricle over time (dt) and is represented as dΩ/dt. Ωo is the measurement of the average impedance of the fluid in the thorax. Impedance-based hemodynamic parameters (CO, SV, and SVR) are calculated from Ωo, dΩ/dt, mean arterial pressure (MAP), CVP, and ECG.

Major indications for ICG include (1) early signs and symptoms of pulmonary or cardiac dysfunction, (2) differentiation of cardiac or pulmonary cause of shortness of breath, (3) evaluation of etiology and management of hypotension, (4) monitoring after discontinuing a PA catheter or justification for insertion of a PA catheter, (5) evaluation of drug therapy, and (6) diagnosis of rejection after heart transplantation. ICG is not recommended in patients who have generalized edema or third spacing because the excess volume interferes with accurate signals.

## ❖ NURSING AND INTERPROFESSIONAL MANAGEMENT: HEMODYNAMIC MONITORING

Assessment of hemodynamic status requires integrating data from many sources and trending these data over time. Comprehensive nursing observations provide important clues about the patient's hemodynamic status.

Begin by obtaining baseline data regarding the patient's general appearance, level of consciousness, skin color and temperature, vital signs, peripheral pulses, capillary refill, and urine output. Does the patient appear tired, weak, exhausted? There may be too little cardiac reserve to sustain even minimum activity. Pallor, cool skin, and diminished pulses may indicate decreased CO. Changes in mental status may reflect problems with cerebral perfusion or oxygenation. Monitor urine output to determine the adequacy of perfusion to the kidneys. The patient with diminished perfusion to the GI tract may develop hypoactive or absent bowel sounds. If the patient is bleeding and developing shock, BP may initially be relatively stable, yet the patient may become increasingly pale and cool from peripheral vasoconstriction. Conversely, the patient experiencing septic shock may remain warm and pink yet develop tachycardia and BP instability. Elevated HRs are common in stressed, compromised, critically ill patients. However, sustained tachycardia increases myocardial $O_2$ demand and can result in decreased CO.

Always correlate observational data with data obtained from technology (e.g., ECG, arterial and PA pressures, $ScvO_2$ or $SvO_2$). Single hemodynamic values are rarely helpful. You must monitor trends in these values over time and evaluate the whole clinical picture with the goals of recognizing early clues and intervening before problems escalate.

## CIRCULATORY ASSIST DEVICES

Mechanical **circulatory assist devices (CADs)** are used to decrease cardiac work and improve organ perfusion in patients with heart failure when conventional drug therapy is no longer adequate. CADs include intraaortic balloon pump (IABP) and left or right ventricular assist device (VAD).

The type of device used depends on the extent and nature of the heart problem. CADs provide interim support in three types of situations: (1) the left, right, or both ventricles require support while recovering from acute injury (e.g., postcardiotomy); (2) the patient must be stabilized before surgical repair of the heart (e.g., a ruptured septum); and (3) the heart has failed, and the patient is awaiting heart transplantation. All CADs decrease cardiac workload, increase myocardial perfusion, and augment circulation.

### Intraaortic Balloon Pump

The **intraaortic balloon pump (IABP)** provides temporary circulatory assistance to the sick heart by reducing afterload (via reduction in systolic pressure) and augmenting the aortic diastolic pressure. This results in improved coronary blood flow. Table 65-5 lists the indications for an IABP.

**TABLE 65-5 Indications and Contraindications for IABP Therapy***

**Indications**

- Refractory unstable angina (when drugs have failed)
- Short-term bridge to heart transplantation
- Acute myocardial infarction with any of the following:†
  - Ventricular aneurysm accompanied by ventricular dysrhythmias
  - Acute ventricular septal defect
  - Acute mitral valve dysfunction
  - Cardiogenic shock
  - Refractory chest pain with or without ventricular dysrhythmias
- Preoperative, intraoperative, and postoperative cardiac surgery (e.g., prophylaxis before surgery, failure to wean from cardiopulmonary bypass, left ventricular failure after cardiopulmonary bypass)
- High-risk interventional cardiology procedures

**Contraindications**

- Irreversible brain damage
- Major coagulopathy (e.g., disseminated intravascular coagulation [DIC])
- Terminal or untreatable diseases of any major organ system
- Abdominal aortic and thoracic aneurysms
- Moderate to severe aortic insufficiency
- Generalized peripheral vascular disease (e.g., aortoiliac disease)‡

*List is not all-inclusive.
†Allows time for emergent angiography and corrective heart surgery to be done.
‡May inhibit placement of balloon and is considered a relative contraindication; sheathless insertion may be used.

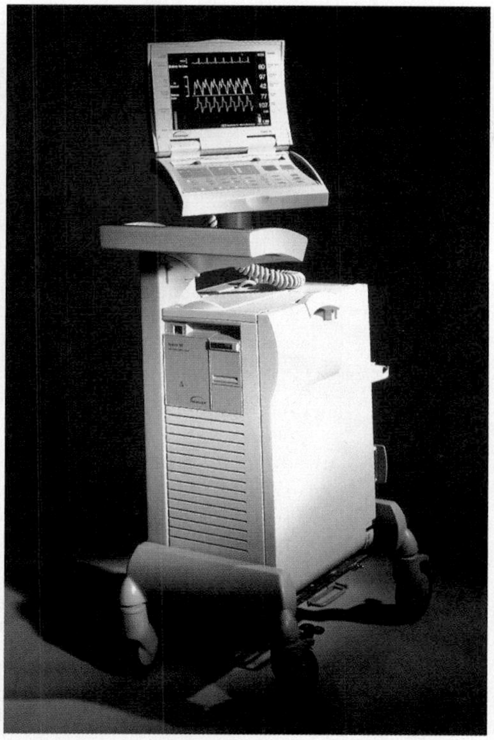

**FIG. 65-11** Intraaortic balloon pump machine. (Courtesy Datascope Corp, Fairfield, NJ.)

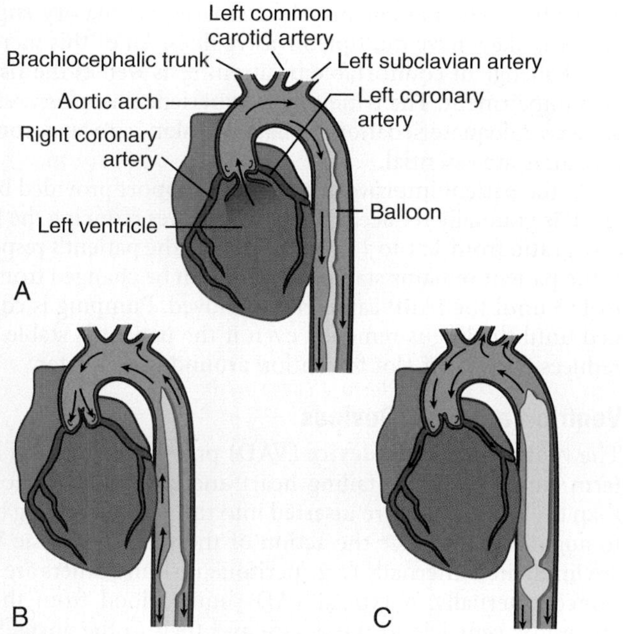


**FIG. 65-12** Intraaortic balloon pump. **A,** During systole the balloon is deflated, which facilitates ejection of blood into the periphery. **B,** In early diastole, the balloon begins to inflate. **C,** In late diastole, the balloon is totally inflated, which augments aortic pressure and increases the coronary perfusion pressure with the end result of increased coronary and cerebral blood flow.

The IABP consists of a sausage-shaped balloon, a pump that inflates and deflates the balloon, a control panel for synchronizing the balloon inflation to the cardiac cycle, and fail-safe features (Fig. 65-11). The balloon is inserted percutaneously or surgically into the femoral artery. It is moved toward the heart and placed in the descending thoracic aorta just below the left subclavian artery and above the renal arteries (Fig. 65-12). After placement, an x-ray confirms the position.

A pneumatic device fills the balloon with helium at the start of diastole (immediately after aortic valve closure) and deflates it just before the next systole. The ECG is the trigger used to start the deflation on the upstroke of the R wave (of the QRS) and inflation on the T wave. The dicrotic notch of the arterial pressure tracing is used to refine timing.

IABP therapy is known as *counterpulsation* because the timing of balloon inflation is opposite to ventricular contraction. The IABP assist ratio is 1:1 in the acute phase of treatment, meaning that one IABP cycle of inflation and deflation occurs for every heartbeat.

**TABLE 65-6 Hemodynamic Effects of Counterpulsation**

**Effects of Inflation During Diastole**
- Increased diastolic pressure (may exceed systolic pressure)
- Increased pressure in the aortic root during diastole
- Increased coronary artery perfusion pressure
- Improved $O_2$ delivery to the myocardium
  - Decreased angina
  - Decreased ECG evidence of ischemia
  - Decreased ventricular ectopy

**Effects of Deflation During Systole**
- Decreased afterload
- Decreased peak systolic pressure
- Decreased myocardial $O_2$ consumption
- Increased stroke volume, possibly associated with
  - Improved mentation
  - Warm skin
  - Increased urine output
  - Decreased heart rate
- Increased forward flow of blood, decreasing preload
  - Decreased PA pressures, including PAWP
  - Decreased crackles

*PA,* Pulmonary artery; *PAWP,* PA wedge pressure.

**Effects of Counterpulsation.** In late diastole when the balloon is totally inflated, blood is forcibly displaced distal to the extremities and proximal to the coronary arteries and main branches of the aortic arch. Diastolic arterial pressure rises (diastolic augmentation), increasing coronary artery perfusion pressure and perfusion of vital organs. The rise in coronary artery perfusion pressure causes an increase in blood flow to the myocardium. The balloon is rapidly deflated just before systole. This creates a vacuum that causes aortic pressure to drop. When aortic resistance to left ventricular ejection is reduced (reduced afterload), the left ventricle empties more easily and completely. As with other types of afterload reduction, the SV increases, yet the myocardial $O_2$ consumption decreases. Table 65-6 summarizes the hemodynamic effects of IABP therapy.

**Complications With IABP Therapy.** Vascular injuries such as dislodgment of plaque, aortic dissection, and compromised distal circulation are common with IABP therapy. Thrombus and embolus formation add to the risk of circulatory compromise to the extremity. The action of the IABP can also destroy platelets and cause thrombocytopenia. Movement of the balloon can block the left subclavian, renal, or mesenteric arteries. This can result in a weak or absent radial pulse, decreased urine output, and reduced or absent bowel sounds. Patients receiving IABP therapy are prone to infection. Local or systemic

## TABLE 65-7 Managing Complications of IABP Therapy

| Potential Complications | Nursing Interventions |
|---|---|
| Site infection from invasive lines | • Use strict aseptic technique for insertion and dressing changes for all lines.<br>• Cover all insertion sites with occlusive dressings.<br>• Give prescribed prophylactic antibiotic for entire course of therapy. |
| Issues related to immobilization (e.g., pressure ulcers, pneumonia) | • Reposition patient at least q2hr, being careful not to displace balloon.<br>• If patient requires chest physiotherapy, avoid introducing ECG artifact. |
| Arterial trauma caused by insertion or displacement of balloon | • Evaluate and mark peripheral pulses before insertion of balloon to use as baseline for assessing pulses after insertion.<br>• After insertion of balloon, evaluate perfusion to both upper and lower extremities at least every hour.<br>• Measure urine output at least every hour (occlusion of renal arteries causes severe decrease in urine output).<br>• Observe arterial waveforms for sudden changes.<br>• Keep head of bed no higher than 45 degrees.<br>• Do not flex cannulated leg at the hip.<br>• Immobilize cannulated leg to prevent flexion using a draw sheet tucked under the mattress, soft ankle restraint, or knee immobilizer. |
| Thromboembolism caused by trauma, balloon obstruction of blood flow distal to catheter | • Give prophylactic heparin therapy (if ordered).<br>• Evaluate pulses, urine output, and level of consciousness at least every hour.<br>• Check circulation, sensation, and movement in both legs at least every hour. |
| Hematologic complications caused by platelet aggregation along the balloon (e.g., thrombocytopenia) | • Monitor coagulation profiles, hematocrit, and platelet count. |
| Hemorrhage from insertion site | • Check site for bleeding at least every hour.<br>• Monitor vital signs for signs of hypovolemia with each check. |
| Balloon leak or rupture | • Prepare for emergent removal and possible reinsertion. |

signs of infection require catheter removal.[22] To reduce these complications, perform cardiovascular, neurovascular, and hemodynamic assessments every 15 to 60 minutes, depending on the patient's status (Table 65-7).

Mechanical complications from IABP are rare but can occur. Improper timing of balloon inflation may cause increased afterload, decreased CO, myocardial ischemia, and increased myocardial $O_2$ demand. These complications must be recognized immediately and reported to the HCP. If the balloon develops a leak, the pump will automatically stop. The catheter is promptly removed to avoid an embolus. Signs of a leak include less effective augmentation, repeated alarms for gas loss, and blood backing up into the catheter. A malfunction of the balloon or console triggers fail-safe alarms and automatically shuts down the unit.

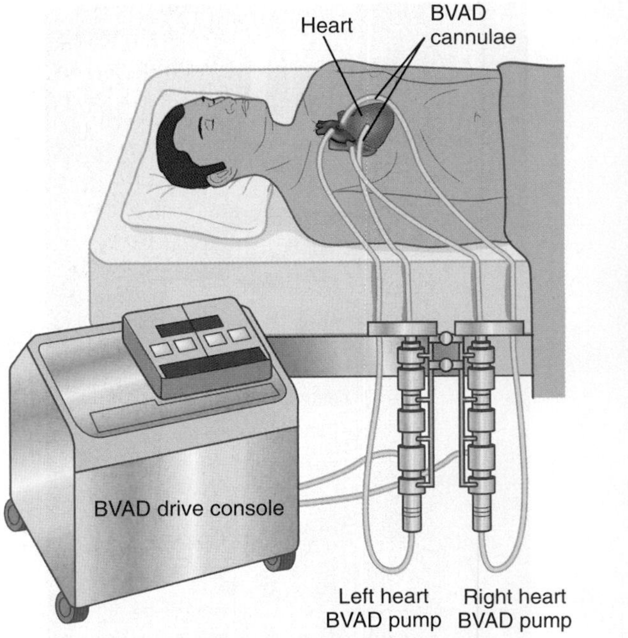


**FIG. 65-13** Schematic diagram of a biventricular assist device (BVAD).

The patient with an IABP is relatively immobile, limited to side-lying or supine positions with the HOB elevated less than 45 degrees. The patient may be receiving ventilatory support and will likely have multiple invasive lines. All of this increases the challenge of comfortable positioning as well as the risk for skin impairment. The patient may experience sleeplessness and anxiety. Adequate sedation, pain relief, skin care, and comfort measures are essential.

As the patient improves, circulatory support provided by the IABP is gradually reduced. Weaning involves reducing the IABP assist ratio from 1:1 to 1:2 and assessing the patient's response. If the patient remains stable, the ratio can be changed from 1:2 to 1:3 until the IABP catheter is removed. Pumping is continued until the line is removed even if the patient is stable. This reduces the risk of clot formation around the catheter.

### Ventricular Assist Devices

The **ventricular assist device (VAD)** provides short- and long-term support for the failing heart and allows more mobility than the IABP. VADs are inserted into the path of flowing blood to augment or replace the action of the ventricle. Some VADs are implanted internally (e.g., peritoneum), and others are positioned externally. A typical VAD shunts blood from the left atrium or ventricle to the device and then to the aorta. Some VADs provide right or biventricular support (Fig. 65-13).

Failure to wean from cardiopulmonary bypass (CPB) after surgery is a primary indicator for VAD support. VADs are also used to support patients with heart failure caused by myocardial infarction and patients awaiting heart transplantation. A VAD is a temporary device that can partially or totally support circulation until the heart recovers or a donor heart is found.

Appropriate patient selection for VAD therapy is critical. Indications include (1) failure to wean from CPB or postcardiotomy cardiogenic shock, (2) a bridge to recovery or heart transplantation, and (3) patients with New York Heart Association Class IV heart disease (see Table 34-3) who have failed medical therapy. Relative contraindications for VAD therapy include (1) body surface area (BSA) less than manufacturer's limit (e.g., 1.3 $m^2$), (2) renal or liver failure unrelated to a cardiac event, and (3) co-morbidities that would limit life expectancy to less than 3 years.[23]

### Implantable Artificial Heart

Every year about 2200 patients receive heart transplants, yet the demand for donor hearts far exceeds the supply. Research on mechanical CADs has led to the development of a fully implantable artificial heart that can sustain the body's circulatory system. This device is used to replace the hearts of patients who are not eligible for a transplant and have no other treatment options. One major advantage of the artificial heart compared with heart transplantation is decreased costs for implantation and drug therapies. Patients do not require immunosuppression therapy and thus do not experience its inevitable, long-term effects. However, patients do require lifelong anticoagulation.[24]

## NURSING AND INTERPROFESSIONAL MANAGEMENT: CIRCULATORY ASSIST DEVICES

The patient with an IABP requires highly skilled care. Perform frequent and thorough cardiovascular assessments. These include measurement of hemodynamic parameters (e.g., arterial BP, CO/CI, SVR), auscultation of the heart and lungs, and evaluation of the ECG (e.g., rate, rhythm). Assess for adequate tissue perfusion (e.g., skin color and temperature, mental status, capillary refill, peripheral pulses, urine output, bowel sounds) at regular intervals. It is expected that IABP therapy will improve these findings.

Nursing care of the patient with a VAD is similar to that of the patient with an IABP. Observe the patient for bleeding, cardiac tamponade, ventricular failure, infection, dysrhythmias, renal failure, hemolysis, and thromboembolism. Unlike the patient with an IABP, who must remain in bed with limited position change, the patient with VAD may be mobile and require an activity plan. In some cases, patients with VADs may go home. Preparation for discharge is complex and requires in-depth teaching about the device and support equipment (e.g., battery chargers). A competent caregiver must be present at all times.

Ideally, patients with CADs will recover, undergo heart transplantation, or receive an artificial heart. However, many patients die, or the decision to terminate the device is made and death follows. Both the patient and caregiver require emotional support. Consult other team members, such as social workers or clergy, as appropriate.

## ARTIFICIAL AIRWAYS

Patients in the ICU often need mechanical assistance to maintain airway patency. Inserting a tube into the trachea, bypassing upper airway and laryngeal structures, creates an artificial airway. The tube is placed into the trachea via the mouth or nose past the larynx (**endotracheal [ET] intubation**) or through a stoma in the neck *(tracheostomy)*. ET intubation is more common in ICU patients than a tracheostomy. It is performed quickly and safely at the bedside. Indications for ET intubation include (1) upper airway obstruction (e.g., secondary to burns, tumor, bleeding), (2) apnea, (3) high risk for aspiration, (4) ineffective clearance of secretions, and (5) respiratory distress. Fig. 65-14 shows the parts of an ET tube.

A *tracheotomy* is a surgical procedure that is performed when the need for an artificial airway is expected to be long term. There is ongoing debate regarding the timing of a tracheotomy in the patient requiring an ET tube. Research suggests that early tracheotomy (2 to 10 days) may have advantages over delayed tracheotomy, particularly when mechanical ventilation is predicted to be needed for longer than 10 to 14 days.[25] The situation varies with the patient, HCP, and agency. Chapter 26 discusses tracheostomy tubes and related nursing management.

### Endotracheal Tubes

In *oral intubation,* the ET tube is passed through the mouth and vocal cords and into the trachea with the aid of a laryngoscope or a bronchoscope. In *nasal ET intubation,* the ET is placed blindly (i.e., without seeing the larynx) through the nose,

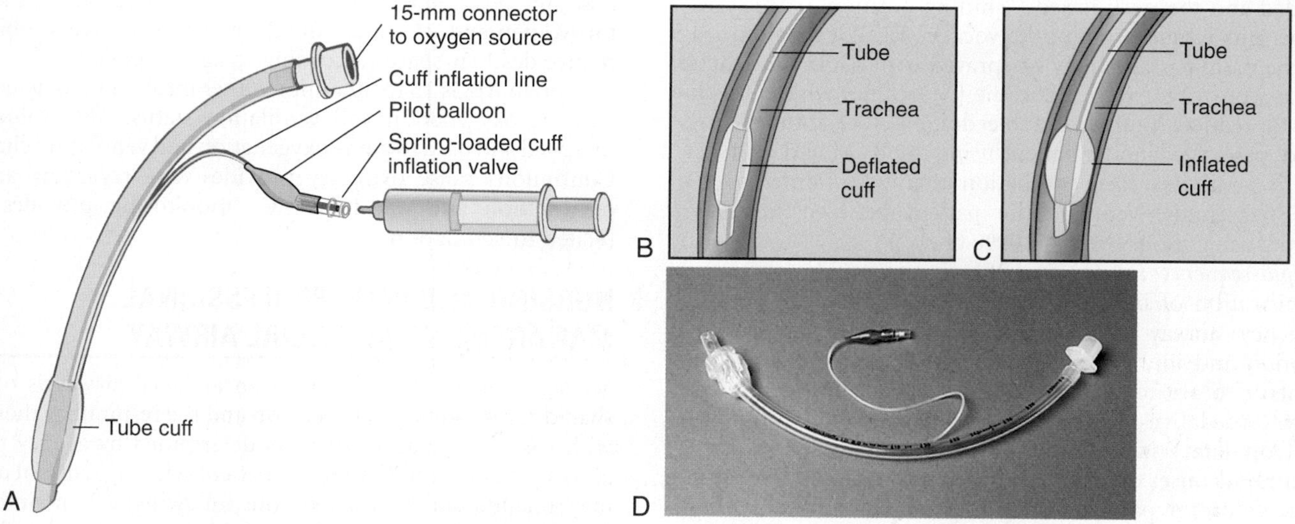


**FIG. 65-14** Endotracheal tube. **A,** Parts of an endotracheal tube. **B,** Tube in place with cuff deflated. **C,** Tube in place with the cuff inflated. **D,** Photo of tube before placement. (*A,* From Beare PG, Myers JL: *Adult health nursing,* ed 3, St Louis, 1998, Mosby.)

nasopharynx, and vocal cords. Oral ET intubation is preferred for most emergencies because the airway can be secured rapidly and a larger-diameter tube is used. A larger-bore ET tube reduces the *work of breathing* (WOB) because of less airway resistance. It is easier to remove secretions and perform bronchoscopy if needed. Nasal ET intubation is rarely used but may be needed when oral intubation is not possible (e.g., unstable cervical spine injury, dental abscess, epiglottitis).

There are risks associated with oral ET intubation. It is difficult to place an oral tube if head and neck mobility are limited (e.g., suspected spinal cord injury). Teeth can be chipped or accidentally removed during the procedure. Salivation is increased and swallowing is difficult. Patients can obstruct the ET tube by biting down on it. Sedation along with a bite block or oropharyngeal airway may be used to prevent this. The ET tube and bite block (if used) should be secured (separately) to the face. Mouth care is a challenge because of limited space in the oral cavity. Manage this by using smaller or pediatric-sized oral products for tooth brushing, cleaning, and suctioning.

### Endotracheal Intubation Procedure

Unless ET intubation is emergent, consent for the procedure is obtained. Tell the patient and caregiver the reason for ET intubation, steps in the procedure, and patient's role in the procedure (if indicated). Also explain that, while intubated, the patient will not be able to speak, but that you will provide other means of communication. Tell them that the patient's hands may have removable mitts placed to remind him or her not to touch the airway.

Have a self-inflating *bag-valve-mask* (BVM) (e.g., *Ambu bag*) attached to $O_2$, suctioning equipment ready at the bedside, and IV access. The BVM contains a reservoir that is filled with $O_2$ so that concentrations of 90% to 95% are delivered. The slower the bag is deflated and inflated, the higher the $O_2$ concentration that is delivered. Assemble and check the equipment to be used, remove the patient's dentures or partial plates (for oral intubation), and give drugs as ordered. Premedication varies depending on the patient's level of consciousness (e.g., awake, obtunded), nature of the procedure (e.g., emergent, nonemergent), and the HCP's preferences.

For oral intubation, place the patient supine with the head extended and the neck flexed ("sniffing position"). This position permits visualization of the vocal cords. For nasal intubation, the nasal passages may be sprayed with a local anesthetic and vasoconstrictor (e.g., lidocaine [Xylocaine] with epinephrine) to reduce trauma and bleeding. Before intubation is started, preoxygenate the patient using the BVM and 100% $O_2$ for 3 to 5 minutes. Each intubation attempt is limited to less than 30 seconds. Ventilate the patient between successive attempts using the BVM and 100% $O_2$.

*Rapid-sequence intubation* (RSI) is the rapid, concurrent administration of both a sedative and paralytic drug during emergency airway management to decrease the risks of aspiration and injury to the patient. RSI is not indicated in patients who are in cardiac arrest or have a known difficult airway.[26] A sedative-hypnotic-amnesic (e.g., midazolam, etomidate [Amidate]) is used to induce unconsciousness, along with a rapid-onset opioid (e.g., fentanyl) to blunt the pain of the procedure. A paralytic drug (e.g., succinylcholine [Anectine]) is then given to produce skeletal muscle paralysis. Monitor the patient's $O_2$ status during the procedure with pulse oximetry.

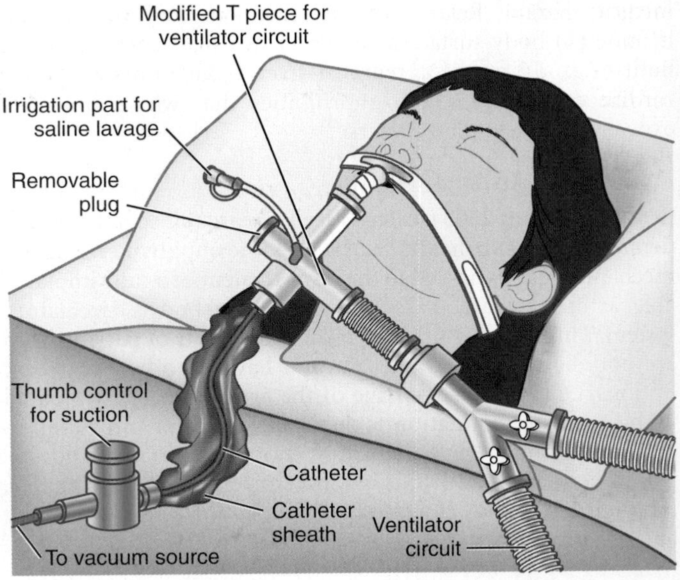


**FIG. 65-15** Closed tracheal suction system.

After intubation, inflate the cuff and confirm the placement of the ET tube while the patient is manually ventilated using the BVM with 100% $O_2$. Use an end-tidal $CO_2$ detector to confirm proper placement by noting the presence of exhaled $CO_2$ from the lungs. Place the detector between the BVM and ET tube and look for a color change (indicating the presence of $CO_2$) or a number. If no $CO_2$ is detected, the tube is in the esophagus and must be reinserted.[27] Auscultate the lungs for bilateral breath sounds and the epigastrium for the absence of air sounds. Observe the chest for symmetric chest wall movement. In addition, $SpO_2$ should be stable or improved.

If the findings support proper ET tube placement, connect the tube to a mechanical ventilator and secure per agency policy (Fig. 65-15). Suction the ET tube and pharynx, and insert a bite block if needed. Obtain a chest x-ray immediately to confirm tube location (2 to 6 cm above the carina in the adult). This position allows the patient to move the neck without moving the tube or causing it to enter the right mainstem bronchus. Once proper positioning is confirmed with x-ray, record and mark the position of the tube at the lip or teeth (usually 21 cm for women and 23 cm for men) or nose. Cut excess tubing to reduce dead air space (according to agency policy).

Obtain ABGs 15 to 30 minutes after intubation to determine baseline oxygenation and ventilation status. ABG values are reviewed and used to guide oxygenation and ventilation changes. Continuous pulse oximetry provides data regarding arterial oxygenation and end-tidal $CO_2$ monitoring provides data related to ventilation.

## ❖ NURSING AND INTERPROFESSIONAL MANAGEMENT: ARTIFICIAL AIRWAY

Management of a patient with an artificial airway is often a shared responsibility between you and the respiratory therapist, with specific management tasks determined by agency policy. Nursing responsibilities for the patient with an artificial airway may include some or all of the following: (1) maintaining correct tube placement, (2) maintaining proper cuff inflation, (3) monitoring oxygenation and ventilation, (4) maintaining tube patency, (5) providing oral care and maintaining skin integrity, (6) fostering comfort and communication, and (7) assessing for complications. eNursing Care Plan 65-1 for the patient on a mechanical ventilator is available on the website for this chapter.

## Maintaining Correct Tube Placement

Continuously monitor the patient with an ET tube for proper placement. If the tube moves or is dislodged, it could end up in the pharynx or enter the esophagus or the right mainstem bronchus (thus ventilating only the right lung).

**SAFETY ALERT Endotracheal Tube Placement**

- Maintain proper ET tube position by placing an "exit mark" on the tube.
- Confirm that the mark remains constant while at rest and during patient care, repositioning, and transport.

Observe for symmetric chest wall movement and auscultate to confirm bilateral breath sounds. If the ET tube is not positioned properly, it is an airway emergency. Stay with the patient, maintain the airway, support ventilation with a BVM and 100% $O_2$, and call for the appropriate help to immediately reposition the tube. If a dislodged tube is not repositioned, minimal or no $O_2$ is delivered to the lungs or the entire $V_T$ is delivered to one lung. This places the patient at risk for pneumothorax.

## Maintaining Proper Cuff Inflation

The cuff is an inflatable, pliable sleeve encircling the lower, outer wall of the ET tube (Fig. 65-14). The high-volume, low-pressure cuff stabilizes and "seals" the ET tube within the trachea and prevents escape of ventilating gases. However, excess volume in the cuff can damage the tracheal mucosa. To prevent this, inflate the cuff with air, and measure and monitor the cuff pressure. To ensure adequate tracheal perfusion, maintain cuff pressure at 20 to 25 cm $H_2O$.[28] Measure and record cuff pressure after intubation and on a routine basis (e.g., every 8 hours) using the *minimal occluding volume* (MOV) *technique* or *the minimal leak technique* (MLT).

The steps in the MOV technique for cuff inflation are as follows: (1) for the mechanically ventilated patient, place a stethoscope over the trachea and inflate the cuff to MOV by adding air until no air leak is heard at peak inspiratory pressure (end of ventilator inspiration); (2) for the spontaneously breathing intubated patient, inflate until no sound is heard after a deep breath or after inhalation with a BVM; (3) use a manometer to verify that cuff pressure is between 20 and 25 cm $H_2O$; and (4) record cuff pressure in the chart. If adequate cuff pressure cannot be maintained or larger volumes of air are needed to keep the cuff inflated, there could be a leak in the cuff or tracheal dilation at the cuff site. In these situations, notify the HCP.

The procedure for MLT is similar with one exception. Remove a small amount of air from the cuff until a slight air leak is auscultated at peak inflation. Both techniques aim to prevent the risks of tracheal damage from high cuff pressures.

## Monitoring Oxygenation and Ventilation

Closely monitor the patient with an ET tube for adequate oxygenation by assessing clinical findings, ABGs, $SpO_2$, and, if available, $ScvO_2$ or $SvO_2$. Assess for signs of hypoxemia such as a change in mental status (e.g., confusion), anxiety, dusky skin, and dysrhythmias. Periodic ABGs and continuous $SpO_2$ provide objective data regarding oxygenation. Lower $PaO_2$ values are expected in patients with some disease states, such as chronic obstructive pulmonary disease (COPD). CVP or PA catheters with $ScvO_2$ or $SvO_2$ capability provide an indirect indication of the patient's tissue oxygenation status (Table 65-4).

Indicators of ventilation include clinical findings, $PaCO_2$, and continuous partial pressure of end-tidal $CO_2$ ($PETCO_2$). Assess the patient's respirations for rate, rhythm, and use of accessory muscles. The patient who is hyperventilating will be breathing rapidly and deeply and may experience circumoral and peripheral numbness and tingling. The patient who is hypoventilating will be breathing shallowly or slowly and may appear dusky. $PaCO_2$ is the best indicator of alveolar hyperventilation (e.g., decreased $PaCO_2$, increased pH indicate respiratory alkalosis) or hypoventilation (e.g., increased $PaCO_2$, decreased pH indicate respiratory acidosis).

$PETCO_2$ monitoring *(capnography)* is done by analyzing exhaled gas directly at the patient-ventilator circuit *(mainstream sampling)* or by transporting a sample of gas via a small-bore tubing to a bedside monitor *(sidestream sampling)*. Continuous $PETCO_2$ monitoring can assess the patency of the airway and presence of breathing. In addition, gradual changes in $PETCO_2$ values may accompany an increase in $CO_2$ production (e.g., sepsis, hypoventilation, neuromuscular blockade) or a decrease in $CO_2$ production (e.g., hypothermia, decreased CO, metabolic acidosis). In patients with normal ventilation-to-perfusion ratios (see Chapter 67), $PETCO_2$ can be used as an estimate of $PaCO_2$, with $PETCO_2$ generally 1 to 5 mm Hg lower than $PaCO_2$. However, in patients with unusually large dead air space or serious mismatch between ventilation and perfusion, $PETCO_2$ is not a reliable estimate of $PaCO_2$.[27]

## Maintaining Tube Patency

Do not routinely suction a patient. Regularly assess the patient to determine if suctioning is needed. Indications for suctioning include (1) visible secretions in the ET tube, (2) sudden onset of respiratory distress, (3) suspected aspiration of secretions, (4) increase in respiratory rate with or without sustained coughing, and (5) sudden decrease in $SpO_2$. Other signs that may indicate the patient needs suctioning include an increase in peak airway pressure and auscultation of adventitious breath sounds over the trachea or bronchi.

Table 65-8 describes two recommended suctioning methods, the *closed-suction technique* (CST) and the *open-suction technique* (OST). The CST uses a suction catheter that is enclosed in a plastic sleeve connected directly to the patient-ventilator circuit (Fig. 65-15). With the CST, oxygenation and ventilation are maintained during suctioning, and exposure to the patient's secretions and possible infection is reduced for the patient's and HCP's safety. The CST should be used for patients who (1) require high levels of positive end-expiratory pressure (PEEP) (greater than 10 cm $H_2O$), (2) have high levels of $FIO_2$, (3) have bloody or infected pulmonary secretions, (4) require frequent suctioning, and (5) experience clinical instability with the OST.[29]

Potential complications associated with suctioning include hypoxemia, bronchospasm, increased intracranial pressure, dysrhythmias, hypertension, hypotension, mucosal damage, pulmonary bleeding, pain, and infection. Closely assess the patient before, during, and after the suctioning procedure. If the patient does not tolerate suctioning (e.g., decreased $SpO_2$, increased or decreased BP, sustained coughing, development of dysrhythmias), immediately stop the procedure. Hyperoxygenate the patient. Continue to reassess the patient

**TABLE 65-8 Suctioning Procedures for Patient on Mechanical Ventilator**

**General Measures for Open- and Closed-Suction Techniques**

1. Gather all equipment.
2. Wash hands and don personal protective equipment.
3. Explain procedure and patient's role in assisting with secretion removal by coughing.
4. Monitor patient's cardiopulmonary status (e.g., vital signs, $SpO_2$, $SvO_2$ or $ScvO_2$, ECG, level of consciousness) before, during, and after the procedure.
5. Turn on suction and set vacuum to 100-120 mm Hg.
6. Pause ventilator alarms.

**Open-Suction Technique**

7. Open sterile catheter package using the inside of the package as a sterile field. NOTE: Suction catheter should be no wider than half the diameter of the ET tube (e.g., for a 7-mm ET tube, select a 10F suction catheter).
8. Fill the sterile solution container with sterile normal saline or water.
9. Don sterile gloves.
10. Pick up sterile suction catheter with dominant hand. Using nondominant hand, secure the connecting tube (to suction) to the suction catheter.
11. Check equipment for proper functioning by suctioning a small volume of sterile saline solution from the container. **(Go to step 13.)**

**Closed-Suction Technique**

12. Connect the suction tubing to the closed suction port.
13. Hyperoxygenate the patient for 30 sec using one of the following methods:
    - Activate the suction hyperoxygenation setting on the ventilator using nondominant hand.
    - Increase $FIO_2$ to 100%. NOTE: Remember to return $FIO_2$ to baseline level at the completion of the procedure if not done automatically after preset time by ventilator.
    - Disconnect the ventilator tubing from the ET tube and manually ventilate the patient with 100% $O_2$ using a BVM device.* Administer five or six breaths over 30 sec. NOTE: Use of a second person to deliver the manual breaths significantly increases the $V_T$ delivered.
14. With suction off, gently and quickly insert the catheter using the dominant hand. When you meet resistance, pull back ½ in.
15. Apply continuous or intermittent suction using the nondominant thumb. Withdraw the catheter over 10 sec or less.
16. Hyperoxygenate for 30 sec as described in step 13.
17. If secretions remain and the patient has tolerated the procedure, perform two or three suction passes as described in steps 14 and 15. NOTE: Rinse the suction catheter with sterile saline solution between suctioning passes as needed.
18. Reconnect patient to ventilator (open-suction technique).
19. At the completion of ET tube suctioning, rinse the catheter and connecting tubing with the sterile saline solution.
20. Suction oral pharynx. NOTE: Use a separate catheter for this step when using the closed-suction technique.
21. Discard the suction catheter and rinse the connecting tubing with the sterile saline solution (open-suction technique).
22. Reset $FIO_2$ (if necessary) and ventilator alarms.
23. Reassess patient for signs of effective suctioning.

*BVM*, Bag-valve-mask; *ECG*, electrocardiogram; *ET*, endotracheal; *$FIO_2$*, fraction of inspired $O_2$; *PEEP*, positive end-expiratory pressure; *$V_T$*, tidal volume.
*Attach a PEEP valve to the BVM for patients on >5 cm $H_2O$ PEEP.
Adapted from Seckel MA: Suctioning: endotracheal or tracheostomy tube. In Wiegand DL-M, editor: *AACN procedure manual for critical care*, ed 7, St Louis, 2017, Elsevier. (in press)

until hemodynamic stability is achieved, the patient recovers, and/or the situation resolves before attempting another suction pass. Prevent hypoxemia by hyperoxygenating the patient before and after each suctioning pass and limiting each pass to 10 seconds or less (Table 65-8). Assess both the ECG and $SpO_2$ before, during, and after the suctioning procedure.

Causes of dysrhythmias during suctioning include (1) hypoxemia resulting in myocardial ischemia; (2) vagal stimulation caused by tracheal irritation; and (3) sympathetic nervous system stimulation caused by anxiety, discomfort, or pain. Dysrhythmias include tachydysrhythmias and bradydysrhythmias, premature beats, and asystole. Stop suctioning if any new dysrhythmias develop. Avoid excessive suctioning in patients with severe hypoxemia or bradycardia.

Tracheal mucosal damage may occur due to excessive suction pressures (greater than 120 mm Hg), overly vigorous catheter insertion, and the suction catheter itself. Blood streaks or tissue shreds in aspirated secretions may indicate mucosal damage. This increases the risk of infection and bleeding, particularly if the patient is receiving anticoagulants.[29] Trauma to the mucosa can be prevented by following the steps described in Table 65-8.

Secretions may be thick and difficult to suction because of inadequate hydration or humidification, infection, or inaccessibility of the lower airways. Adequately hydrate the patient (e.g., oral or IV fluids) and provide supplemental humidification of inspired gases to help thin secretions. Do not instill normal saline into the ET tube as it may be harmful. If infection is the cause of thick secretions, give the patient appropriate antibiotics. Mobilize and turn the patient (e.g., every 2 hours) to help move secretions into larger airways.

## ◆ Providing Oral Care and Maintaining Skin Integrity

When an oral ET tube is in place, the patient's mouth is always open. Moisten the lips, tongue, and gums with saline or water swabs to prevent mucosal drying. Proper oral care provides comfort and prevents injury to the gums and plaque formation (Table 65-9).

**TABLE 65-9 Oral Care for Patient on Mechanical Ventilator**

**General Measures**

1. Gather all equipment.
2. Wash hands and don personal protective equipment.
3. Explain procedure to the patient and caregiver (if present).
4. Perform oral care using pediatric or adult soft toothbrushes at least twice a day by gently brushing to clean and remove plaque.
5. Use oral swabs with a 1.5% hydrogen peroxide solution every 2-4 hr.
6. Use 0.12% chlorhexidine oral rinse twice daily.
7. Apply a mouth moisturizer to oral mucosa and lips with each cleaning.
8. Suction oral cavity and pharynx frequently. Fig. 65-16 is an example of an endotracheal tube that can provide continuous or intermittent subglottic suctioning.

NOTE:
- Change all oral suction equipment and suction tubing every 24 hr.
- Rinse nondisposable oral suction apparatus with sterile normal saline after each use and place on a dry paper towel.

Adapted from Vollman KM, Sole ML: Endotracheal tube and oral care. In Wiegand DL-M, editor: *AACN procedure manual for critical care*, ed 6, St Louis, 2011, Saunders; and Institute for Healthcare Improvement: How-to guide: prevent ventilator-associated pneumonia. Retrieved from *www.ihi.org/resources/Pages/Tools/HowtoGuidePreventVAP.aspx*.

Frequent assessment and meticulous care are required to prevent skin breakdown on the face, lips, tongue, and nares because of pressure from the ET tube or bite block or the method used to secure the ET tube to the patient's face. Reposition and retape the ET tube (per agency policy) and as needed to prevent skin breakdown.

For the nasally intubated patient, remove the old tape and clean the skin around the ET tube with saline-soaked gauze or cotton swabs. For the orally intubated patient, remove the bite block (if present) and the old tape. Provide oral hygiene and then reposition the ET tube to the opposite side of the mouth. Replace the bite block (if appropriate) and reconfirm proper cuff inflation and tube placement. Secure the ET tube again (per agency policy).

Commercial ET holders are often used. These may increase the risk for skin breakdown compared to tape.[30] If a commercial ET holder is used, follow the manufacturer's directions for maintaining tube position, providing skin care, and preventing skin breakdown.

Ongoing assessment is shared between nursing and respiratory therapy. Repositioning the ET tube may be limited to respiratory therapy. Two staff members should always perform the repositioning procedure to prevent accidental ET tube dislodgment. Monitor the patient for any signs of respiratory distress throughout the procedure.

## ◆ Fostering Comfort and Communication

Intubation is a major stressor for the patient.[31] The intubated patient may experience anxiety from not being able to talk or not knowing what to expect. Communicating with the intubated patient can be frustrating for the patient, caregiver, and interprofessional care team. To communicate more effectively, use a variety of methods.[32] (See Common Problems of Critical Care Patients earlier in this chapter on pp. 1556-1557.)

The physical discomfort associated with ET intubation and mechanical ventilation often requires sedating the patient and giving an analgesic until the ET tube is no longer needed. The patient may need fentanyl, midazolam, propofol, or other sedatives to blunt the anxiety and discomfort related to intubation. Evaluate the drugs' effectiveness in achieving an acceptable level of patient comfort by using a valid pain scale, sedation scale (e.g., Ramsey Sedation Scale), and/or delirium scale.[6] In addition, consider using relaxation techniques (e.g., music therapy) to complement drug therapy.

## ◆ Complications of Endotracheal Intubation

Two major complications of ET intubation are unplanned extubation and aspiration. Unplanned *extubation* (i.e., removal of the ET tube from the trachea) can be a catastrophic event and may complicate the patient's recovery. Unplanned extubations can be due to patient removal of the ET tube or accidental removal during movement or a procedure. Usually the unplanned extubation is obvious (i.e., the patient is holding the ET tube). Other times, the tip of the ET tube is in the hypopharynx or esophagus, and the extubation is not so obvious.

**! SAFETY ALERT Unplanned Extubation**

Observe for signs of unplanned extubation, which can be a life-threatening event:
- Patient talking
- Activation of the low-pressure ventilator alarm
- Diminished or absent breath sounds
- Respiratory distress

You are responsible for preventing unplanned extubation by ensuring that the ET tube is secured and observing and supporting the ET tube during repositioning, procedures, and patient transfers. Additionally, giving adequate sedation and analgesia and using standardized weaning protocols decrease the incidence of self-extubation.[33]

The use of soft wrist restraints to immobilize the patient's hands is not an absolute deterrent to self-extubation.[34] Be sure to explain to the patient and caregiver when you use short-term restraints for patient safety and discuss the use of alternatives. Reassess for the continued need of restraints (per agency policy).

Should an unplanned extubation occur, stay with the patient and call for help. Interventions are aimed at maintaining the patient's airway, supporting ventilation (e.g., manually ventilating the patient with a BVM and 100% $O_2$), securing the appropriate assistance to immediately reintubate the patient (if necessary), and providing psychologic support to the patient.

*Aspiration* is another potential hazard for the patient with an ET tube. The ET tube passes through the epiglottis, splinting it in an open position. Thus the intubated patient cannot protect the airway from aspiration. The high-volume, low-pressure ET or tracheal cuff cannot totally prevent the trickle of oral or gastric secretions into the trachea. Further, secretions collect above the cuff. When the cuff is deflated, those secretions can move into the lungs. Some ET tubes provide continuous suctioning of secretions above the cuff (Fig. 65-16).

Oral intubation increases salivation, yet swallowing is difficult, so suction the patient's mouth frequently. Use a Yankauer (tonsil-tip) suction catheter or a sterile single-use catheter. Other factors contributing to aspiration include improper cuff inflation, patient positioning, and decreased gastric mobility and bowel function if receiving tube feedings. The patient with an ET tube is at risk for aspiration of gastric contents. Even when the cuff is properly inflated, take precautions to prevent vomiting, which can lead to aspiration.[35]

Often, a nasogastric (NG) or an orogastric (OG) tube is inserted and connected to low, intermittent suction when a patient is first intubated. An OG tube is preferred over an NG tube to reduce the risk of sinusitis. All patients who are intubated or receiving enteral feedings must have the HOB elevated a minimum of 30 to 45 degrees unless medically contraindicated.

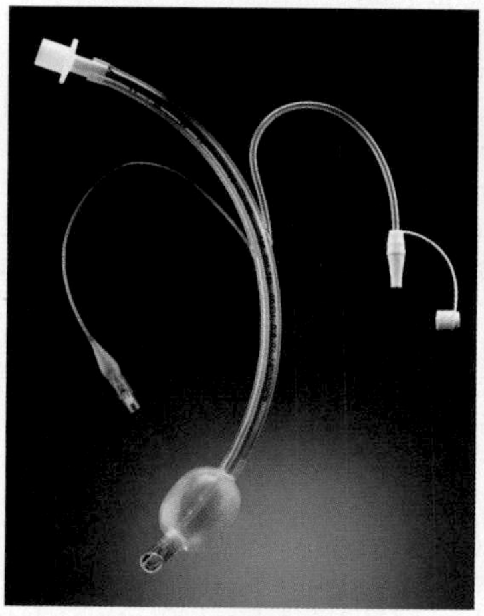

**FIG. 65-16** Continuous subglottal suctioning can be provided by the Hi Lo Evac Tube. A dorsal lumen above the cuff allows for suctioning of secretions from the subglottic area. (Reprinted by permission of Nellcor Puritan Bennett Inc, Pleasanton, Calif.)

## MECHANICAL VENTILATION

Mechanical ventilation is the process by which the $FIO_2$ (21% [room air] or more) is moved in and out of the lungs by a mechanical ventilator. Mechanical ventilation is not curative. It is a means of supporting patients until they recover the ability to breathe independently. It can also serve as a bridge to long-term mechanical ventilation, or until a decision is made to withdraw ventilatory support.

Indications for mechanical ventilation include (1) apnea or impending inability to breathe or protect the airway, (2) acute respiratory failure (see Chapter 67), (3) severe hypoxia, and (4) respiratory muscle fatigue.[36] Patients with chronic pulmonary disease and their caregivers should be given the opportunity to discuss mechanical ventilation before end-stage respiratory disease develops. Encourage all patients, particularly those with chronic illnesses, to discuss the subject with their families and HCPs. They should record and place the results of these discussions in an advance directive.

The decision to use, withhold, or withdraw mechanical ventilation must be made carefully, respecting the wishes of the patient and caregiver. When the interprofessional care team, patient, and/or caregiver disagree over the treatment plan, family conferences are essential to keep the lines of communication open and discuss options. You may need to consult the agency's ethics committee for assistance.

### Types of Mechanical Ventilation

The two major types of mechanical ventilation are negative pressure and positive pressure ventilation.

**Negative Pressure Ventilation.** Negative pressure ventilation involves the use of chambers that encase the chest or body and surround it with intermittent subatmospheric (or negative) pressure. The "iron lung" was the first form of negative pressure ventilation, developed during the polio epidemic. Intermittent negative pressure around the chest wall causes the chest to be pulled outward, reducing intrathoracic pressure. Air rushes in via the upper airway, which is outside the sealed chamber. Expiration is passive. The machine cycles off, allowing chest retraction. This type of ventilation is similar to normal ventilation in that decreased intrathoracic pressures produce inspiration, and expiration is passive. Negative pressure ventilation is delivered by noninvasive ventilation and does not require an artificial airway.

Several portable negative pressure ventilators are available for home use for patients with neuromuscular diseases, central nervous system disorders, diseases and injuries of the spinal cord, and severe COPD (Fig. 65-17). Negative pressure ventilators are not routinely used for acutely ill patients.

**Positive Pressure Ventilation.** Positive pressure ventilation (PPV) is the primary method used with acutely ill patients (Fig. 65-18). During inspiration the ventilator pushes air into the lungs under positive pressure. Unlike spontaneous ventilation, intrathoracic pressure is raised during lung inflation rather than lowered. Expiration occurs passively as in normal expiration. Modes of PPV are categorized into two groups: volume and pressure ventilation.[36]

***Volume Ventilation.*** With volume ventilation a predetermined tidal volume ($V_T$) is delivered with each inspiration, and the amount of pressure needed to deliver the breath varies based on compliance and resistance factors of the patient-ventilator system. Consequently, the $V_T$ is consistent from breath to breath, but airway pressures vary.

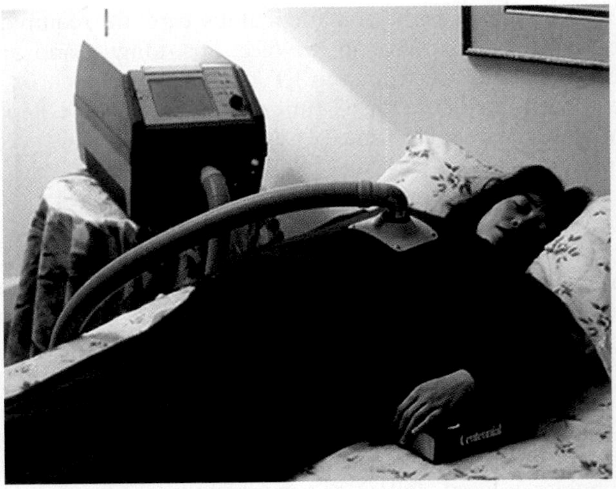

**FIG. 65-17** Negative pressure ventilator. (Courtesy Lifecare, Westminster, Colo.)

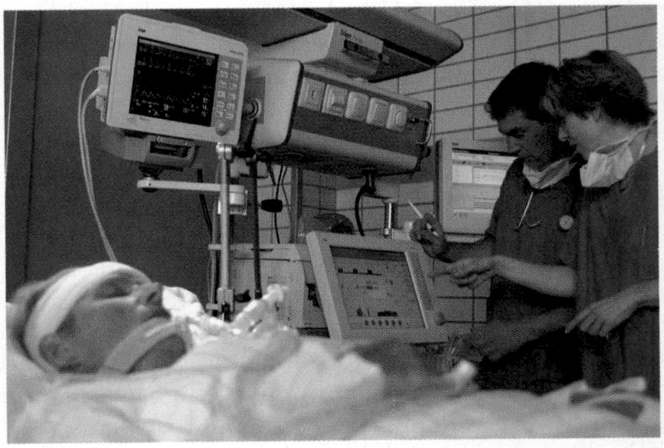

**FIG. 65-18** Patient receiving mechanical ventilation. (Courtesy Draeger Medical.)

***Pressure Ventilation.*** With *pressure ventilation* the peak inspiratory pressure is predetermined, and the $V_T$ delivered to the patient varies based on the selected pressure and compliance and resistance factors of the patient-ventilator system. With this understanding, careful attention must be given to the $V_T$ to prevent unplanned hyperventilation or hypoventilation. For example, when the patient breathes out of synchrony with the ventilator, the pressure limit may be reached quickly, and the volume of gas delivered may be small. Initially, pressure ventilation was used only in stable patients being weaned from the ventilator. Today, pressure ventilation is frequently used to treat critically ill patients.

### Settings of Mechanical Ventilators

Mechanical ventilator settings regulate rate, $V_T$, $O_2$ concentration, and other characteristics of ventilation (Table 65-10). Settings are based on the patient's status (e.g., ABGs, ideal body weight, current physiologic state, level of consciousness, respiratory muscle strength). Settings are evaluated and adjusted until oxygenation and ventilation targets have been reached.

**TABLE 65-10 Settings of Mechanical Ventilation**

| Parameter | Description |
|---|---|
| **Respiratory rate (f)** | Number of breaths the ventilator delivers per minute.<br>*Usual setting:* 6-20 breaths/min |
| **Tidal volume ($V_T$)** | Volume of gas delivered to patient during each ventilator breath.<br>*Usual volume:* 6-10 mL/kg |
| **$O_2$ concentration ($FIO_2$)** | Fraction of inspired $O_2$ ($FIO_2$) delivered to patient. May be set between 21% (essentially room air) and 100%.<br>*Usually adjusted* to maintain $PaO_2$ level >60 mm Hg or $SpO_2$ level >90% |
| **Positive end-expiratory pressure (PEEP)** | Positive pressure applied at the end of expiration of ventilator breaths.<br>*Usual setting:* 5 cm $H_2O$ |
| **Pressure support** | Positive pressure used to augment patient's inspiratory pressure.<br>*Usual setting:* 6-18 cm $H_2O$ |
| **I:E ratio** | Duration of inspiration (I) to duration of expiration (E).<br>*Usual setting:* 1:2 to 1:1.5 unless IRV is desired |
| **Inspiratory flow rate and time** | Speed with which the $V_T$ is delivered.<br>*Usual setting:* 40-80 L/min and time is 0.8-1.2 sec |
| **Sensitivity** | Determines the amount of effort the patient must generate to initiate a ventilator breath. It may be set for pressure triggering or flow triggering.<br>*Usual setting:* A pressure trigger is set 0.5-1.5 cm $H_2O$ below baseline pressure and a flow trigger is set 1-3 L/min below baseline flow |
| **High-pressure limit** | Regulates the maximal pressure the ventilator can generate to deliver the $V_T$. When the pressure limit is reached, the ventilator terminates the breath and spills the undelivered volume into the atmosphere.<br>*Usual setting:* 10-20 cm $H_2O$ above peak inspiratory pressure |

*IRV,* Inverse ratio ventilation.
Adapted from Urden LD, Lough ME, Stacy KM: *Critical care nursing: diagnosis and management,* ed 6, St Louis, 2010, Mosby.

It is important that you check that all ventilator alarms are always on. Alarms alert the staff to potentially dangerous situations such as mechanical malfunction, apnea, unplanned extubation, or patient asynchrony with the ventilator[37] (Table 65-11). On many ventilators the alarms can be temporarily suspended or silenced for up to 2 minutes for suctioning or testing while a staff member is in the room. After that time, the alarm system automatically turns back on.

**! SAFETY ALERT Alarm Fatigue**

- Alarm fatigue can develop in those who are exposed to an excessive number of alarms and results in sensory overload.
- This can cause a delayed response to alarms or dismissing them altogether and can lead to serious adverse events (e.g., patient death).
- One alarm management strategy to reduce alarm fatigue includes customizing alarm parameters based on individual patient needs.[37]

**TABLE 65-11 Mechanical Ventilation Alarms**

| Alarm | Possible Causes |
|---|---|
| **High-pressure limit** | • Secretions, coughing, or gagging<br>• Patient fighting ventilator (ventilator asynchrony)<br>• Condensate (water) in tubing<br>• Kinked or compressed tubing (e.g., patient biting on endotracheal tube [ET] tube)<br>• Increased resistance (e.g., bronchospasm)<br>• Decreased compliance (e.g., pulmonary edema, pneumothorax) |
| **Low-pressure limit** | • Total or partial ventilator disconnect<br>• Loss of airway (e.g., total or partial extubation)<br>• ET tube or tracheotomy cuff leak (e.g., patient speaking, grunting) |
| **Apnea** | • Respiratory arrest<br>• Oversedation<br>• Change in patient condition<br>• Loss of airway (e.g., total or partial extubation) |
| **High $V_T$, minute ventilation, or respiratory rate** | • Pain, anxiety<br>• Change in patient condition<br>• Excess condensate in tubing (i.e., false reading) |
| **Low $V_T$ or minute ventilation** | • Change in patient's breathing efforts (e.g., rate and volume)<br>• Patient disconnection, loose connection, or leak in circuit<br>• ET tube or tracheotomy cuff leak (e.g., patient speaking, grunting)<br>• Insufficient gas flow |
| **Ventilator inoperative or low battery** | • Machine malfunction<br>• Unplugged, power failure, or internal battery not charged |

*$V_T$,* Tidal volume.
Adapted from Pierce LN: *Management of the mechanically ventilated patient,* ed 2, St Louis, 2007, Saunders.

## Modes of Volume Ventilation

The methods by which the patient and ventilator interact to deliver effective ventilation are called *ventilator modes.* The selected ventilator mode is based on how much WOB the patient should or can perform. WOB refers to inspiratory effort needed to overcome the elasticity and viscosity of the lungs along with the airway resistance. The mode is determined by the patient's ventilatory status, respiratory drive, and ABGs. Generally, ventilator modes are controlled or assisted.

With controlled ventilatory support, the ventilator does all of the WOB. With assisted ventilatory support, the ventilator and patient share the WOB. Historically, volume modes such as controlled mandatory ventilation (CMV), assist-control ventilation (ACV), and synchronized intermittent mandatory ventilation (SIMV) have been used to treat critically ill patients. Currently, pressure modes such as pressure support ventilation (PSV), pressure-control ventilation (PCV), and inverse ratio ventilation (PC-IRV) are more common.[36] Table 65-12 describes these ventilator modes.

**Assist-Control Ventilation.** With **assist-control ventilation (ACV)**, the ventilator delivers a preset $V_T$ at a preset frequency. When the patient initiates a spontaneous breath, the ventilator senses a decrease in intrathoracic pressure and then delivers the

**TABLE 65-12 Modes of Mechanical Ventilation**

**Volume Modes**

***Assist-Control (AC) or Assisted Mandatory Ventilation (AMV)***

- Requires that rate, $V_T$, inspiratory time, and PEEP be set for the patient.
- The ventilator sensitivity is also set, and when the patient initiates a spontaneous breath, a full-volume breath is delivered.

***Intermittent Mandatory Ventilation (IMV) and Synchronized Intermittent Mandatory Ventilation (SIMV)***

- Requires that rate, $V_T$, inspiratory time, sensitivity, and PEEP are set for the patient.
- In between "mandatory breaths," patients spontaneously breathe at their own rates and $V_T$. With SIMV, the ventilator synchronizes the mandatory breaths with the patient's own inspirations.

**Pressure Modes**

***Pressure Support Ventilation (PSV)***

- Provides an augmented inspiration to a spontaneously breathing patient.
- The clinician selects an inspiratory pressure level, PEEP, and sensitivity.
- When the patient initiates a breath, a high flow of gas is delivered to the preselected pressure level, and pressure is maintained throughout inspiration.
- The patient determines the parameters of $V_T$, rate, and inspiratory time.

***Pressure-Control Inverse Ratio Ventilation (PC-IRV)***

- Combines pressure-limited ventilation with an inverse ratio of inspiration to expiration.
- The clinician selects the pressure level, rate, inspiratory time (1 : 1, 2 : 1, 3 : 1, 4 : 1), and the PEEP level.
- With the prolonged inspiratory times, auto-PEEP may result.
- The auto-PEEP may be a desirable outcome of the inverse ratios.
- Some clinicians use PC without IRV.
- Conventional inspiratory times are used and rate, pressure level, and PEEP are selected.

***Airway Pressure Release Ventilation (APRV)***

- Provides two levels of continuous positive airway pressure (CPAP) with timed releases, and permits spontaneous breathing throughout the respiratory cycle.
- The clinician selects both pressure high and pressure low along with time high and time low. $V_T$ is not a set variable and depends on the CPAP level, the patient's compliance and resistance, and spontaneous breathing effort.

**Positive End-Expiratory Pressure (PEEP) and Continuous Positive Airway Pressure (CPAP)**

***PEEP***

- Creates positive pressure at end exhalation and restores functional residual capacity (FRC).
- The term *PEEP* is used when end-expiratory pressure is provided during ventilator positive pressure breaths.

***CPAP***

- Similar to PEEP, CPAP restores FRC.
- This pressure is continuous during spontaneous breathing; no positive pressure breaths are present.

Modified from Burns SM: Invasive mechanical ventilation (through an artificial airway) volume and pressure modes. In Wiegand DL-M, editor: *AACN procedure manual for critical care,* ed 6, St Louis, 2011, Saunders.

preset $V_T$. The patient can breathe faster than the preset rate but not slower. This mode has the advantage of allowing the patient some control over ventilation while providing some assistance. ACV is used in patients with a variety of conditions, including neuromuscular disorders (e.g., Guillain-Barré syndrome), pulmonary edema, and acute respiratory failure.

In the ACV mode, the patient has the potential for hyperventilation. The spontaneously breathing patient can easily be overventilated, resulting in hyperventilation. If the volume or minimum rate is set too low and the patient is apneic or weak, the patient can be hypoventilated. Thus these patients require vigilant assessment and monitoring of ventilatory status, including respiratory rate, ABGs, $SpO_2$, and $ScvO_2$ or $SvO_2$. It is also important that the sensitivity or amount of negative pressure required to start a breath is appropriate to the patient's condition. For example, if it is too difficult for the patient to begin a breath, the WOB is increased and the patient may tire (i.e., the patient "rides" the ventilator) or develop ventilator asynchrony (i.e., the patient "fights" the ventilator).

**Synchronized Intermittent Mandatory Ventilation.** With *synchronized intermittent mandatory ventilation* (SIMV), the ventilator delivers a preset $V_T$ at a preset frequency in synchrony with the patient's spontaneous breathing. Between ventilator-delivered breaths, the patient is able to breathe spontaneously through the ventilator circuit. Thus the patient receives the preset $FIO_2$ during the spontaneous breaths but self-regulates the rate and $V_T$ of those breaths. This mode of ventilation differs from ACV, in which all breaths are of the same preset volume. It is used during continuous ventilation and during weaning from the ventilator. SIMV may also be combined with PSV (described later). Potential benefits of SIMV include improved patient-ventilator synchrony, lower mean airway pressure, and prevention of muscle atrophy as the patient takes on more of the WOB.

SIMV also has disadvantages. If spontaneous breathing decreases when the preset rate is low, ventilation may not be adequately supported. Only patients with regular, spontaneous breathing should use low-rate SIMV. Weaning with SIMV demands close monitoring and may take longer because the rate of breathing is gradually reduced. Patients being weaned with SIMV may also have increased muscle fatigue associated with spontaneous breathing efforts.

## Modes of Pressure Ventilation

**Pressure Support Ventilation.** With pressure support ventilation (PSV), positive pressure is applied to the airway only during inspiration and is used with the patient's spontaneous respirations. The patient must be able to initiate a breath in this modality. The level of positive airway pressure is preset so that the gas flow rate is greater than the patient's inspiratory flow rate. As the patient starts a breath, the machine senses the spontaneous effort and supplies a rapid flow of gas at the initiation of the breath and variable flow throughout the breath. With PSV the patient determines inspiratory length, $V_T$, and respiratory rate. $V_T$ depends on the pressure level and airway compliance.

PSV is used with continuous ventilation and during weaning. PSV may also be used with SIMV during weaning. PSV is not often used as ventilatory support during acute respiratory failure because of the risk of hypoventilation and apnea. Advantages of PSV include increased patient comfort, decreased WOB (because inspiratory efforts are augmented), decreased $O_2$ consumption (because inspiratory work is reduced), and increased endurance conditioning (because the patient is exercising respiratory muscles).

**Pressure-Control and Pressure-Control Inverse Ratio Ventilation.** *Pressure-control ventilation* (PCV) provides a pressure-limited breath delivered at a set rate and may permit spontaneous breathing. The $V_T$ is not set. It is determined by the pressure limit set. *Pressure-control inverse ratio ventilation* (PC-IRV) combines pressure-limited ventilation with an inverse ratio of inspiration (I) to expiration (E). Some HCPs use PC without IRV.

The *I/E ratio* is the ratio of duration of inspiration to the duration of expiration. This ratio is normally 1:2 or 1:3. With IRV, the I/E ratio begins at 1:1 and may progress to 4:1. Prolonged positive pressure is applied, increasing inspiratory time. IRV gradually expands collapsed alveoli. The short expiratory time has a PEEP-like effect, preventing alveolar collapse. Because IRV imposes a nonphysiologic breathing pattern, the patient needs sedation and often paralysis.

PC-IRV is indicated for patients with acute respiratory distress syndrome (ARDS) who continue to have refractory hypoxemia despite high levels of PEEP. Not all patients with poor oxygenation respond to PC-IRV.

**Airway Pressure Release Ventilation.** *Airway pressure release ventilation* (APRV) permits spontaneous breathing at any point during the respiratory cycle with a preset continuous positive airway pressure (CPAP) with short timed pressure releases. The CPAP level (pressure high, pressure low) is adjusted to keep oxygenation goals while the timed releases (time high, time low) are increased or decreased to meet ventilation goals. $V_T$ is not a set variable and depends on the CPAP level, the patient's compliance and resistance, and spontaneous breathing effort. The mode is designed for patients who need high pressure levels for alveolar recruitment (open collapsed alveoli). One advantage of this mode is the ability to permit spontaneous respirations. This may reduce the need for deep sedation or paralytics.

**Other Modes.** Advances in ventilator technology have led to the development of additional pressure modes. However, because of the nonstandardization of these options, the names and features are manufacturer specific. The superiority of these modes has not been established. Some examples include *volume-assured pressure ventilation* and *adaptive support ventilation.*

### Other Ventilatory Maneuvers

**Positive End-Expiratory Pressure.** Positive end-expiratory pressure (PEEP) is a ventilatory maneuver in which positive pressure is applied to the airway during exhalation. Normally during exhalation, airway pressure drops to near zero, and exhalation occurs passively. With PEEP, exhalation remains passive, but pressure falls to a preset level, often 3 to 20 cm $H_2O$. Lung volume during expiration and between breaths is greater than normal with PEEP. This increases functional residual capacity (FRC) and often improves oxygenation with restoration of lung volume that normally remains at the end of passive exhalation. The mechanisms by which PEEP increases FRC and oxygenation include increased aeration of patent alveoli, aeration of previously collapsed alveoli, and prevention of alveolar collapse throughout the respiratory cycle.

PEEP is titrated to the point that oxygenation improves without compromising hemodynamics. This is termed *optimal PEEP.* Often 5 cm $H_2O$ PEEP (referred to as *physiologic PEEP*) is used prophylactically to replace the glottic mechanism, help maintain a normal FRC, and prevent alveolar collapse. PEEP of 5 cm $H_2O$ is also used for patients with a history of alveolar collapse during weaning. PEEP improves gas exchange, vital capacity, and inspiratory force when used during weaning.

In contrast, *auto-PEEP* is not purposely set on the ventilator but is a result of inadequate exhalation time. Auto-PEEP is additional PEEP over what is set by the HCP. This additional PEEP may result in increased WOB, barotrauma, and hemodynamic instability. Interventions to limit auto-PEEP include sedation and analgesia, large-diameter ET tube, bronchodilators, short inspiratory times, and decreased respiratory rates. Reducing water accumulation in the ventilator circuit by frequent emptying or use of heated circuits also limits auto-PEEP. In patients with short exhalation times and early airway closure (e.g., asthma), setting PEEP above auto-PEEP can offset auto-PEEP effects by splinting the airway open during exhalation and preventing "air trapping."

In general, the major purpose of PEEP is to maintain or improve oxygenation while limiting risk of $O_2$ toxicity. $FIO_2$ can often be reduced when PEEP is used. PEEP is generally indicated in all patients who are mechanically ventilated. The classic indication for PEEP therapy is ARDS (see Chapter 67). PEEP is used with caution in patients with increased intracranial pressure, low cardiac output, and hypovolemia. In these cases the adverse effects of PEEP may outweigh any benefits.

**CHECK YOUR PRACTICE**

You are caring for a 75-yr-old woman who was orally intubated yesterday for respiratory distress secondary to pneumonia and placed on ACV. Her ventilator settings are: $FIO_2$ 40%, $V_T$ 400, RR 14 (set), PEEP 5. You respond to the ventilator alarm sounding and note that she is speaking. The alarm panel shows "low exhaled tidal volume." She appears confused with the following vital signs: HR 102, RR 24, and $SpO_2$ 89%.

- What would be your next steps?

**Continuous Positive Airway Pressure.** Continuous positive airway pressure (CPAP) restores FRC and is similar to PEEP. However, the pressure in CPAP is delivered continuously during spontaneous breathing, thus preventing the patient's airway pressure from falling to zero. For example, if CPAP is 5 cm $H_2O$, airway pressure during expiration is 5 cm $H_2O$. During inspiration, 1 to 2 cm $H_2O$ of negative pressure is generated, thus reducing airway pressure to 3 or 4 cm $H_2O$. CPAP is commonly used in the treatment of obstructive sleep apnea.[36] CPAP can be administered with a tight-fitting mask or an ET or tracheal tube. CPAP increases WOB because the patient must forcibly exhale against the CPAP. Therefore it must be used with caution in patients with myocardial compromise.

**Automatic Tube Compensation.** *Automatic tube compensation* (ATC) is an adjunct designed to overcome WOB through an artificial airway. It is currently available on many ventilators. ATC is increased during inspiration and decreased during expiration. It is set by entering the internal diameter of the patient's airway along with the desired percentage of compensation. ATC may become less effective in patients with excessive secretions and who require longer-term ventilation.[38]

**Bilevel Positive Airway Pressure.** In addition to $O_2$, *bilevel positive airway pressure* (BiPAP) provides two levels of positive pressure support: higher inspiratory positive airway pressure and lower expiratory positive airway pressure. It is a noninvasive modality and is delivered through a tight-fitting face mask, nasal mask, or nasal pillows. The patient must be able to spontaneously breathe and cooperate with this treatment.[36]

BiPAP is used for COPD patients with heart failure and acute respiratory failure and for patients with sleep apnea. BiPAP may also be used after extubation to prevent reintubation. Patients with shock, altered mental status, or increased airway secretions are not candidates for BiPAP because of the risk of aspiration and the inability to remove the mask.

**High-Frequency Oscillatory Ventilation.** High-frequency oscillatory ventilation (HFOV) involves delivery of a small $V_T$ (usually 1 to 5 mL/kg of body weight) at rapid respiratory rates (100 to 300 breaths/minute) in an effort to recruit and maintain lung volume and reduce intrapulmonary shunting. While HFOV may be a useful mode for patients with life-threatening hypoxia, it has not improved survival or provided lung protection in patients with ARDS.[39] Patients receiving HFOV must be sedated and may be paralyzed to suppress spontaneous respiration. All patients must receive concurrent sedation and analgesia if using a paralytic drug (see Chapter 67).

**Nitric Oxide.** *Nitric oxide* (NO) is a gaseous molecule that is made intravascularly and participates in the regulation of pulmonary vascular tone. Inhibition of NO production results in pulmonary vasoconstriction, and administration of continuous inhaled NO results in pulmonary vasodilation. NO may be administered via an ET tube, a tracheostomy, or a face mask. Currently, NO is used as a diagnostic screening tool for pulmonary hypertension and to improve oxygenation during mechanical ventilation in this patient population. Although the use of NO does not reduce mortality in patients with ARDS, it may be used in patients with life-threatening hypoxia.[40]

**Prone Positioning.** *Prone positioning* is the repositioning of a patient from a supine or lateral position to a prone (on the stomach, face down) position. This repositioning improves lung recruitment (i.e., alveolar expansion) through various mechanisms. Gravity reverses the effects of fluid in the dependent parts of the lungs as the patient is moved from supine to prone. The heart rests on the sternum, away from the lungs, contributing to an overall uniformity of pleural pressures. The prone position is a relatively safe (although nurse-intensive), supportive therapy used in critically ill patients with severe ARDS to improve oxygenation.[41]

**Extracorporeal Membrane Oxygenation.** *Extracorporeal membrane oxygenation* (ECMO) is an alternative form of pulmonary support for the patient with severe respiratory failure. It is used more frequently in the pediatric and neonatal populations but is increasingly being used in adults. ECMO is a modification of cardiac bypass and involves partially removing blood from a patient with large-bore catheters, infusing $O_2$, removing $CO_2$, and returning the blood to the patient. This intensive therapy requires systemic anticoagulation and is a time-limited intervention. A skilled team of specialists, including a perfusionist, is required continuously at the bedside.[42]

## INFORMATICS IN PRACTICE

### *Importing Monitor and Ventilator Data*

- In many ICUs, the monitor data (e.g., vital signs, hemodynamic pressures, core temperature, pulse oximetry) are directly imported into the electronic health record (EHR). Ventilator data may also be sent to the EHR.
- Depending on the agency's information technology system, this connectivity of monitoring devices and ventilators can help drive evidence-based practice. Trends can be readily noted and prompts can link the user to protocols.
- Some systems have the capability of sending alarms or notifications to the HCP from the EHR.
- Always verify that accurate patient data are imported when documenting. Check to ensure that artifact or false data are deleted and confirm the procedure according to your agency's policy.

## Complications of Positive Pressure Ventilation

Although PPV may be essential to maintain ventilation and oxygenation, it can cause adverse effects. It is often difficult to distinguish complications of mechanical ventilation from the underlying disease.

**Cardiovascular System.** PPV can affect circulation because of the transmission of increased mean airway pressure to various structures in the thorax. With increased intrathoracic pressure, thoracic vessels are compressed. The compression causes decreased venous return to the heart, left ventricular end-diastolic volume (preload), and CO, and results in hypotension. Mean airway pressure is further increased if PEEP is being titrated (greater than 5 cm $H_2O$) to improve oxygenation.

If the lungs are noncompliant (e.g., ARDS), airway pressures are not as easily transmitted to the heart and blood vessels. Thus effects of PPV on CO are reduced. Conversely, with compliant lungs (e.g., COPD), there is increased danger of transmission of high airway pressures and negative effects on hemodynamics.

Compromised venous return by PPV is worsened by hypovolemia (e.g., hemorrhage) and decreased venous tone (e.g., sepsis, spinal shock). Restoration and maintenance of the circulating blood volume are important in minimizing cardiovascular complications.

**Pulmonary System**

***Barotrauma.*** As lung inflation pressures increase, risk of *barotrauma* increases. Patients with compliant lungs (e.g., COPD) are at greater risk for barotrauma. This results when the increased airway pressure distends the lungs and possibly ruptures fragile alveoli or emphysematous blebs. Patients with stiff lungs (e.g., ARDS) who are given high inspiratory pressures and high levels of PEEP (greater than 5 cm $H_2O$) and patients with lung abscesses resulting from necrotizing organisms (e.g., staphylococci) are also susceptible to barotrauma.

Air can escape into the pleural space from alveoli or interstitium and become trapped. Pleural pressure increases and collapses the lung, causing pneumothorax. (Chapter 27 discusses the clinical manifestations of pneumothorax.) The lungs receive air during inspiration but cannot expel it during expiration. Respiratory bronchioles are larger on inspiration than expiration. They may close on expiration, and air becomes trapped. With PPV, a simple pneumothorax can become a life-threatening tension pneumothorax. The mediastinum and contralateral lung are compressed, reducing CO. Immediate treatment of the pneumothorax is required.

*Pneumomediastinum* usually begins with rupture of alveoli into the lung interstitium. Progressive air movement occurs into the mediastinum and subcutaneous neck tissue, and a pneumothorax often follows. New, unexplained subcutaneous emphysema is an indication for immediate chest x-ray. Pneumomediastinum and subcutaneous emphysema may be too small to detect on x-ray or clinically before the development of a pneumothorax.

***Volutrauma.*** The concept of *volutrauma* in PPV relates to the lung injury that occurs when a large $V_T$ is used to ventilate noncompliant lungs. Volutrauma results in alveolar fractures and movement of fluids and proteins into the alveolar spaces. Low-volume ventilation rather than pressure ventilation should be used in ARDS patients to protect the lungs.

***Alveolar Hypoventilation.*** *Alveolar hypoventilation* can be caused by inappropriate ventilator settings, leakage of air from the ventilator tubing or around the ET tube or tracheostomy cuff, lung secretions or obstruction, and low ventilation/perfusion ratio. A low $V_T$ or respiratory rate decreases minute ventilation. This results in hypoventilation, atelectasis, and respiratory acidosis. A leaking cuff or tubing that is not secured may cause air leakage and lower $V_T$. Lung secretions can cause hypoventilation. Mobilizing the patient, turning the patient at least every 2 hours, encouraging deep breathing and coughing, and suctioning (as needed) may limit this. Increasing the $V_T$, adding small increments of PEEP, and adding a preset number of *sighs* to the ventilator settings (i.e., a deeper than normal breath incorporated into the respiratory cycle) can help reduce the risk of atelectasis.

***Alveolar Hyperventilation.*** Respiratory alkalosis can occur if the respiratory rate or $V_T$ is set too high *(mechanical overventilation)* or if the patient receiving assisted ventilation is *hyperventilating.* It is easy to overventilate a patient on PPV. Particularly at risk are patients with chronic alveolar hypoventilation and $CO_2$ retention. For example, the patient with COPD may have a chronic $PaCO_2$ elevation (acidosis) and compensatory bicarbonate retention by the kidneys. When the patient is ventilated, the patient's "normal baseline" rather than the standard normal values is the therapeutic goal. If the COPD patient is returned to a standard normal $PaCO_2$, the patient will develop alkalosis because of the retained bicarbonate. Such a patient could move from compensated respiratory acidosis to serious metabolic alkalosis.

The presence of alkalosis makes weaning from the ventilator difficult. Alkalosis, especially if the onset is abrupt, can have additional serious consequences, including hypokalemia, hypocalcemia, and dysrhythmias. Usually the patient with COPD who is supported on the ventilator does better with a short inspiratory and longer expiratory time.

If hyperventilation is spontaneous, it is important to determine the cause and treat it. Possible causes include hypoxemia, pain, fear, anxiety, or compensation for metabolic acidosis. Patients who fight the ventilator or breathe out of synchrony may be anxious or in pain. If the patient is anxious and fearful, sitting with the patient and verbally coaching the patient to breathe with the ventilator may help. If these measures fail, manually ventilating the patient slowly with a BVM and 100% $O_2$ may slow breathing enough to bring it in synchrony with the ventilator.

***Ventilator-Associated Pneumonia.*** The risk for health care–associated pneumonia is highest in patients requiring mechanical ventilation because the ET or tracheostomy tube bypasses normal upper airway defenses. In addition, a poor nutritional state, immobility, and the underlying disease process (e.g., immunosuppression, organ failure) make the patient more prone to infection. *Ventilator-associated pneumonia* (VAP) is pneumonia that occurs 48 hours or more after ET intubation.[43] It occurs in as many as 27% of all intubated patients, with half of the cases developing within the first 4 days of mechanical ventilation. In addition, patients who develop VAP have significantly longer hospital stays and higher mortality rates than those who do not.

In patients with early VAP (within 96 hours of mechanical ventilation), sputum cultures often grow gram-negative bacteria (e.g., *Escherichia coli, Klebsiella, Streptococcus pneumoniae, Haemophilus influenzae*). Organisms associated with late VAP include antibiotic-resistant organisms such as *Pseudomonas aeruginosa* and oxacillin-resistant *Staphylococcus aureus.* These organisms are abundant in the hospital environment and the patient's GI tract. They can spread in a number of ways, including contaminated respiratory equipment, inadequate hand washing, adverse environmental factors such as poor room ventilation and high traffic flow, and decreased patient ability to cough and clear secretions. Colonization of the oropharynx tract by gram-negative organisms predisposes the patient to gram-negative pneumonia.

Clinical evidence suggesting VAP includes fever, elevated white blood cell count, purulent or odorous sputum, crackles or wheezes on auscultation, and pulmonary infiltrates noted on chest x-ray. The patient is given antibiotics after appropriate cultures are taken by tracheal suctioning or bronchoscopy and when infection is evident.

Guidelines on VAP prevention include (1) minimizing sedation including daily spontaneous awakening trials (SATs) and daily spontaneous breathing trials (SBTs), (2) early exercise and mobilization, (3) use of ET tubes with subglottic secretion drainage ports for patients likely to be intubated greater than 48 to 72 hours, (4) HOB elevation at a minimum of 30 to 45 degrees unless medically contraindicated, and (5) no routine changes of the patient's ventilator circuit tubing[44] (Fig. 65-16).

Prevention also includes strict hand washing before and after suctioning, whenever ventilator equipment is touched, and after contact with any respiratory secretions (see Nursing Management: Artificial Airway earlier in this chapter). Always wear gloves when in contact with the patient and change gloves between activities (e.g., emptying urinary catheter drainage, hanging an IV drug). Last, always drain the water that collects in the ventilator tubing away from the patient as it collects.

**DRUG ALERT Oxygen**

- $O_2$ is considered a drug and overexposure can lead to $O_2$ toxicity.
- Mechanically ventilated patients receiving high levels of $FIO_2$ for prolonged periods of time (e.g., 40% $FIO_2$ for >24 hours) are at risk for $O_2$ toxicity.
- Target $FIO_2$ levels are to maintain $SpO_2$ >90% and $PaO_2$ between 60 and 90 mm Hg.
- Assess ABGs for evidence of excess $O_2$.
- Monitor patient for signs of $O_2$ toxicity: uncontrolled coughing, chest pain, and dyspnea.

**Sodium and Water Imbalance.** Progressive fluid retention often occurs after 48 to 72 hours of PPV, especially PPV with PEEP. Fluid retention is associated with decreased urine output and increased sodium retention. Fluid balance changes may be due to decreased CO, which in turn results in diminished renal perfusion. Consequently, renin release is stimulated with subsequent production of angiotensin and aldosterone (see Chapter 44, Fig. 44-4). This results in sodium and water retention. It is also possible that pressure changes within the thorax are associated with decreased release of atrial natriuretic peptide, which also causes sodium retention. Mild water retention is also associated with PPV. Less insensible water loss occurs via the airway because ventilated delivered gases are humidified with body-temperature water. In addition, as a part of the stress response, release of antidiuretic hormone and cortisol contributes to sodium and water retention.

**Neurologic System.** In patients with head injury, PPV (especially with PEEP) can impair cerebral blood flow. The increased intrathoracic positive pressure impedes venous drainage from the head. This results in jugular venous distention. The patient may have increases in intracranial pressure due to the impaired venous return and subsequent increase in cerebral volume.

Elevating the HOB and keeping the patient's head in alignment may reduce the harmful effects of PPV on intracranial pressure.

**Gastrointestinal System.** Patients receiving PPV are stressed because of the serious illness, immobility, or discomforts associated with the ventilator. This places the ventilated patient at risk for developing stress ulcers and GI bleeding. Patients with a preexisting ulcer or those receiving corticosteroids are at an increased risk. Any kind of circulatory compromise, including reduction of CO caused by PPV, may contribute to ischemia of the gastric and intestinal mucosa and possibly increase the risk of translocation of GI bacteria.

Stress ulcer prophylaxis includes giving histamine ($H_2$)-receptor blockers (e.g., ranitidine [Zantac]), proton pump inhibitors (PPIs) (e.g., esomeprazole [Nexium]), or enteral nutrition to decrease gastric acidity and reduce the risk of stress ulcer and hemorrhage. The use of PPIs may be linked to an increase in the development of *Clostridium difficile*–associated diarrhea.[45] (This is discussed in Chapter 41 on p. 902.)

Gastric and bowel dilation may occur because of gas accumulation in the GI tract from swallowed air. The irritation of an artificial airway may cause excessive air swallowing and subsequent gastric dilation. Gastric or bowel dilation may put pressure on the vena cava, decrease CO, and prohibit adequate diaphragmatic excursion during spontaneous breathing. Elevation of the diaphragm as a result of paralytic ileus or bowel dilation leads to compression of the lower lobes of the lungs. This may cause atelectasis and compromise respiratory function. Decompression of the stomach is done by inserting an OG or NG tube.[46]

Immobility, sedation, circulatory impairment, decreased oral intake, use of opioid pain medications, and stress contribute to decreased peristalsis. The patient's inability to exhale against a closed glottis may make defecation difficult. As a result, the ventilated patient is at risk for constipation, and a bowel regimen should be started.

**Musculoskeletal System.** Maintenance of muscle strength and prevention of the problems linked with immobility are important. Adequate analgesia and nutrition can enhance exercise tolerance. Plan for early and progressive mobility of appropriate patients receiving PPV.[9,47] In collaboration with physical and occupational therapy, perform passive and active exercises to maintain muscle tone in the upper and lower extremities. Simple maneuvers such as leg lifts, knee bends, quadriceps setting, or arm circles are appropriate. Prevent contractures, pressure ulcers, foot drop, and external rotation of the hip and legs by proper positioning and the use of specialized mattresses or beds. Use a portable ventilator or manually ventilate the patient with a BVM and 100% $O_2$ when ambulating.

**Psychosocial Needs.** The patient receiving mechanical ventilation often experiences physical and emotional stress. In addition to the problems related to critical care patients discussed at the beginning of this chapter, the patient supported by a mechanical ventilator is unable to speak, eat, move, or breathe normally. Tubes and machines cause pain, fear, and anxiety. Usual activities of daily living such as eating, elimination, and coughing are extremely complicated.

Feeling safe is an overpowering need of patients on mechanical ventilation. In addition, four related needs include the need to know (information), the need to regain control, the need to hope, and the need to trust. When patients' needs are met, they feel safe. Work to strengthen the various factors that affect feeling safe. Encourage hope, as appropriate, and build trusting relationships with both the patient and caregiver. Involve patients and caregivers in decision making as much as possible.[14,15]

Patients receiving PPV may require sedation (e.g., propofol) and/or analgesia (e.g., fentanyl) to facilitate optimal ventilation. Before starting sedation or analgesia in the mechanically ventilated patient who is agitated or anxious, identify the cause of distress. Common problems that can result in patient agitation or anxiety include PPV, nutritional deficits, pain, hypoxemia, hypercapnia, drugs, and environmental stressors (e.g., sleep deprivation).

Delirium is an acute change in mental status. It is a marker of cerebral insufficiency and associated with longer hospital stays and higher mortality rates. ICU patients are particularly vulnerable to delirium. Assess for delirium using a valid tool, initiate prevention strategies, and recognize and treat delirium when it occurs.[6,8]

At times, the decision is made to paralyze the patient with a neuromuscular blocking agent (e.g., cisatracurium [Nimbex]) to provide more effective synchrony with the ventilator and improve oxygenation. Remember that the paralyzed patient can hear, see, and feel. It is essential to give IV sedation and analgesia concurrently when the patient is paralyzed. Monitoring patients receiving these drugs is challenging. Assess the patient using train-of-four (TOF) peripheral nerve stimulation, physiologic signs of pain or anxiety (e.g., changes in HR and BP), and ventilator synchrony. The TOF assessment involves using a peripheral nerve stimulator to deliver four successive stimulating currents to elicit muscle twitches (Fig. 65-19). The number of twitches varies with the percentage of neuromuscular blockade. The usual goal is one or two twitches out of four.

Noninvasive electroencephalogram technology (e.g., bispectral index monitoring [BIS]) may be useful and can help guide sedative and analgesic therapy in these patients.[6] Excessive administration of neuromuscular blocking agents may predispose the patient to prolonged paralysis and muscle weakness even after these agents are stopped.

Many patients have few memories of their time in the ICU, whereas others remember vivid details. Although appearing to be asleep, sedated, or paralyzed, patients may be aware of their

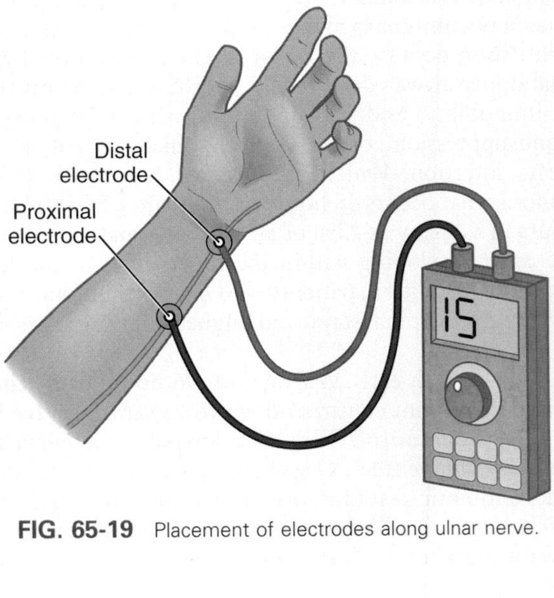


**FIG. 65-19** Placement of electrodes along ulnar nerve.

surroundings, and you should always address them as if they were awake and alert.[48]

**Ventilator Disconnection or Malfunction.** Mechanical ventilators may become disconnected or malfunction. When turned on and operative, alarms alert you to problems (Table 65-11). Most deaths from accidental ventilator disconnection occur while the alarm is off. Most accidental disconnections in critical care settings are discovered by low-pressure alarms. The most frequent site for disconnection is between the tracheal tube and the adapter. Push connections together and then twist to secure more tightly. Be certain that alarms are set and activated at all times, and chart that this is the case. You can pause alarms (not inactivate) during suctioning or removal from the ventilator, but you must reactivate them before leaving the patient's bedside.

Ventilator malfunction may also occur due to several factors. Although most agencies have emergency generators in the event of a power failure and newer ventilators may have battery backup, power failure is always a possibility. Have a plan for manually ventilating all patients who depend on a ventilator. If, at any time, you determine that the ventilator is malfunctioning (e.g., failure of $O_2$ supply), disconnect the patient from the machine and manually ventilate with a BVM and 100% $O_2$ until the ventilator is fixed or replaced.

### Nutritional Therapy: Patient Receiving Positive Pressure Ventilation

PPV and the hypermetabolism associated with critical illness can contribute to inadequate nutrition. The presence of an ET tube eliminates the normal route for eating. Patients with a long-term tracheostomy may be able to eat normally once the stoma heals. Swallowing studies and a consultation with a speech therapist are done to assess the patient's readiness. When eating with a tracheostomy tube in place, the patient should tilt the head slightly forward to facilitate swallowing and to prevent aspiration. Diet may be restricted to soft foods (e.g., puddings, ice cream) and thickened liquids.

Patients unlikely to be able to eat for 3 to 5 days should have a nutritional assessment and enteral feeding started within 24 to 48 hours of admission.[10,49] Inadequate nutrition makes the patient receiving prolonged mechanical ventilation prone to poor $O_2$ transport secondary to anemia and to poor tolerance of minimal exercise. Critically ill patients have frequent interruptions of enteral feedings because of problems with residuals, transportation to and during tests, and routine nursing care. Poor nutrition and the disuse of respiratory muscles contribute to decreased respiratory muscle strength. In addition, critical illness, trauma, and surgery are associated with

## TEAMWORK & COLLABORATION

### *Caring for the Patient Requiring Mechanical Ventilation*

In the critically ill patient who requires mechanical ventilation the registered nurse (RN) and respiratory therapist provide most of the care. Some patients who require chronic mechanical ventilation may be in long-term care settings or at home. In these settings, the RN and respiratory therapist assess the patient and plan and evaluate care, but implementation of some activities may be delegated.

#### Role of Nursing Personnel

***Registered Nurse (RN)***

- Develop plan for communication with the patient who has a tracheostomy or an ET tube.
- Give sedatives, analgesics, and paralytic drugs as needed.
- Teach patient and caregiver about mechanical ventilation and weaning procedures.
- Auscultate breath sounds and respiratory effort, assessing for decreased ventilation or adventitious sounds.
- Monitor ventilator settings and alarms.
- Determine need for ET tube suctioning and suction patients as needed.
- Reposition and secure ET tube (based on agency policy).
- Monitor oxygenation level and signs of respiratory fatigue during weaning procedure.

***Licensed Practical/Vocational Nurse (LPN/LVN)***

- Suction tracheostomy or ET tube for stable patients as directed by RN.
- Give routinely scheduled drugs (based on state Nurse Practice Act and agency policy).
- Assist RN or respiratory therapist with repositioning and securing ET tube.
- Administer enteral nutrition to stable patients as directed by RN.

***Unlicensed Assistive Personnel (UAP)***

- Obtain vital signs and report these to the RN.
- Perform bedside glucose testing, if needed and according to agency policy.
- Provide personal hygiene, skin care, and oral care, as directed by RN.
- Assist with frequent position changes, including ambulation, as directed by the RN.
- Help to perform passive or active range-of-motion exercises.
- Measure urine output and report information to RN.

#### Role of Other Team Members

***Respiratory Therapist****

- Auscultate breath sounds and respiratory effort, assessing for decreased ventilation or adventitious sounds.
- Monitor ventilator settings and alarms.
- Change ventilator settings as needed or ordered.
- Maintain appropriate cuff inflation on ET tube.
- Determine need for ET tube suctioning and suction patients as needed.
- Reposition and secure ET tube (based on agency policy).
- Monitor oxygenation level and signs of respiratory fatigue during weaning procedure.

***Physical/Occupational Therapist***

- Assist with range of motion exercises.
- Assist with early and progressive ambulation as directed by the RN.

***Dietitian***

- Assess and monitor patient's nutritional status.
- Recommend formulations for enteral and/or parenteral nutrition as needed.

***Speech Therapist***

- Perform swallowing studies as appropriate.
- Provide teaching for patient with a long-term tracheostomy.

*Some of these activities are often shared by RNs.

hypermetabolism, anxiety, pain, and increased WOB, which greatly increase caloric expenditure. Serum protein levels (e.g., albumin, prealbumin, transferrin, total protein) are usually decreased. Inadequate nutrition can delay weaning, decrease resistance to infection, and slow down recovery. Enteral gastric or small bowel feeding is the preferred method to meet caloric needs of ventilated patients (see Chapter 39 for discussion of enteral feeding).

Verification of feeding tube placement includes (1) x-ray confirmation before initial use, (2) marking and ongoing assessment of the tube's exit site, and (3) ongoing review of routine x-rays and aspirate.[46] The auscultatory method of assessment (i.e., listening for air after injection) is not a reliable method for verifying the placement of feeding tubes.

A concern regarding the nutritional support of patients receiving PPV is the carbohydrate content of the diet. Metabolism of carbohydrates may increase the serum $CO_2$ levels. This can result in a higher required minute ventilation and increased WOB. Limiting carbohydrate content in the diet may lower $CO_2$ production.[10] Consult the dietitian to determine the caloric and nutrient needs of these patients.

## Weaning From Positive Pressure Ventilation and Extubation

**Weaning** is the process of reducing ventilator support and resuming spontaneous breathing. The weaning process differs for patients requiring short-term ventilation (up to 3 days) versus long-term ventilation (longer than 3 days). Patients requiring short-term ventilation (e.g., after heart surgery) experience a linear weaning process. Patients likely to require prolonged PPV (e.g., patients with COPD who develop respiratory failure) often experience a weaning process that consists of alternating gains and losses. Preparation for weaning begins when PPV is started and involves a team approach (e.g., nurse, HCP, patient, caregiver, dietitian, respiratory therapist).

Weaning generally consists of three phases: the *preweaning phase,* the *weaning process,* and the *outcome phase.* The preweaning or assessment phase determines the patient's ability to breathe spontaneously. Assessment in this phase depends on a combination of respiratory (Table 65-13) and nonrespiratory factors. Note the resolution of the primary problem that prompted patient admission to the ICU. In addition, the patient's lungs should be reasonably clear on auscultation and chest x-ray. Weaning assessment parameters should include criteria to assess muscle strength (negative inspiratory force) and endurance (spontaneous $V_T$, vital capacity, minute ventilation, and rapid shallow breathing index).

Nonrespiratory factors include the patient's neurologic status; hemodynamics; fluid, electrolytes, and acid-base balance; nutrition; and hemoglobin. It is important to have an alert, well-rested, and well-informed patient relatively free from pain and anxiety who can cooperate with the weaning plan. This does not mean complete withdrawal from sedatives or analgesics. Instead, drugs should be titrated to achieve comfort without causing excessive drowsiness.

A *spontaneous awakening trial* (SAT) and a *spontaneous breathing trial* (SBT) are recommended in patients who meet a daily safety screen. This is part of what is known as the *Awakening and Breathing Trial Coordination, Daily Delirium Monitoring and Management, and Early Exercise and Mobility (ABCDE) bundle* for ventilator management.[50] An SAT should be done by stopping all sedatives and, in patients without active pain, all opioids. Sedation should be restarted at 50% the previous dose in patients who "fail" the SAT and remain off in patients who "pass."

An SBT should last at least 30 minutes but no more than 120 minutes. It may be done with low levels of CPAP, low levels of PSV, or a T piece. Tolerance of the trial may lead to extubation. Failure to tolerate an SBT should prompt a search for reversible or complicating factors and a return to a nonfatiguing ventilator modality for the patient. The SBT should be reattempted the next day.

The use of a weaning protocol decreases ventilator days. The ventilator settings are not as important as the use of a daily protocol to prevent delays in weaning. The patient receiving SIMV can have the ventilator breaths gradually reduced as his or her ventilatory status permits. CPAP or PSV can be added to SIMV. PSV is thought to provide gentle, slow respiratory muscle conditioning. It may be especially beneficial for patients who are deconditioned or have heart problems. Some patients may be weaned by simply providing humidified $O_2$ (T-piece or flow-by method).

Weaning may be tried at any time of day, although it is usually done during the day, with the patient ventilated at night in a rest mode. The rest mode should be a stable, nonfatiguing, and comfortable form of support for the patient. Regardless of the weaning mode selected, all health care team members should be familiar with the weaning plan. Additionally, it is important to permit the patient's respiratory muscles to rest between weaning trials. Once the respiratory muscles become fatigued, they may require 12 to 24 hours to recover.

The patient being weaned and the caregiver need ongoing emotional support. Explain the weaning process to them and keep them informed of progress. Place the patient in a comfortable sitting or semirecumbent position. Obtain baseline vital signs and respiratory parameters. During the weaning trial, closely monitor the patient for signs and symptoms that may signal a need to end the trial (e.g., tachypnea, dyspnea, tachycardia, dysrhythmias, sustained desaturation [$SpO_2$ less than 90%], hypertension or hypotension, agitation, diaphoresis, anxiety, sustained $V_T$ less than 5 mL/kg, changes in mentation). Record the patient's tolerance throughout the weaning process and include statements regarding the patient's and the caregiver's perceptions.

The weaning outcome phase is the period when the patient is extubated or weaning is stopped because no further progress is being made. The patient who is ready for extubation should receive hyperoxygenation and suctioning (e.g., oropharynx, ET tube). Loosen the ET tapes or commercial holder or the tracheostomy ties. Instruct the patient to take a deep breath, and at the peak of inspiration, deflate the cuff and remove the tube in one motion. After removal, encourage the patient to deep breathe and cough, and suction the oropharynx as needed. Give supplemental $O_2$ and provide naso-oral care. Carefully monitor the patient's vital signs, respiratory status, and oxygenation immediately after extubation, within 1 hour, and per agency policy. If the patient does not tolerate extubation (e.g., decreased level of consciousness, tachycardia, tachypnea or bradypnea, decrease in $PaO_2$, increase in $PaCO_2$, decreased $SpO_2$ levels), immediate reintubation or a trial of noninvasive ventilation may be needed.

## Chronic Mechanical Ventilation

Mechanical ventilators are no longer limited to the ICU but are now a part of long-term and home care. In some instances, terminally ill, ventilated patients may be discharged to hospice.

**TABLE 65-13 Indicators for Weaning**

**Weaning Readiness**

Patients receiving mechanical ventilation for respiratory failure should undergo a formal assessment of weaning potential if the following are satisfied:*

1. Reversal of the underlying cause of respiratory failure
2. Adequate oxygenation
   - $PaO_2/FIO_2$ >150-200
   - $SpO_2$ ≥90%
   - PEEP ≤5-8 cm $H_2O$
   - $FIO_2$ ≤40%-50%
   - pH ≥7.25
3. Hemodynamic stability
   - Absence of myocardial ischemia
   - Absence of clinically significant hypotension (no vasopressor therapy or low dose)
4. Patient ability to initiate an inspiratory effort
5. Optional criteria
   - Hemoglobin ≥7-10 g/dL
   - Core temperature ≤100.4°F (38°C) to 101.3°F (38.5°C)
   - Mental status awake and alert or easily arousable

**WEANING ASSESSMENT**

| Measurement | Significance | Normal Values | Indices for Weaning |
|---|---|---|---|
| **Spontaneous respiratory rate (f)** | Respiratory rate/frequency over 1 min. | 12-20 min | <35 min |
| **Spontaneous tidal volume ($V_T$)** | Amount of air exchanged during normal breathing at rest. Measure of muscle endurance. | 7-9 mL/kg | ≥5 mL/kg |
| **Minute ventilation ($V_E$)** | $V_T$ multiplied by respiratory rate over 1 min. *For example:* 0.350 ($V_T$) × 28 (f) = 9.8 L/min | 5-10 L/min | ≤10 L/min |
| **Negative inspiratory force or pressure (NIF, NIP)** | Amount of negative pressure that a patient is able to generate to initiate spontaneous respirations. *Measured by clinician*: After complete occlusion of inspiratory valve, a pressure manometer is attached to airway or mouth for 10-20 sec while negative inspiratory efforts are noted. | −75 to −100 cm $H_2O$ | >−20 cm $H_2O$ The more negative the number, the better indication for weaning. |
| **Positive expiratory pressure (PEP)** | Measure of expiratory muscle strength and ability to cough. *Measured by clinician*: After complete occlusion of expiratory valve, a pressure manometer is attached to the airway or mouth for 10-20 sec while positive expiratory efforts are noted. | 60-85 cm $H_2O$ | ≥30 cm $H_2O$ |
| **Compliance, rate, oxygenation, and pressure (CROP) index** | Combined index that is complex to calculate. $C_{Dyn}$ × NIF × ($PaO_2/PAO_2$)/f $C_{Dyn}$ = Compliance $PaO_2/PAO_2$ = Oxygenation ratio of arterial $O_2$/alveolar $O_2$ | Not applicable | >13 |
| **Rapid shallow breathing index (f/$V_T$)** | Spontaneous respiratory rate over 1 min divided by $V_T$ (in liters). *For example:* 30 (f)/0.400 ($V_T$) = 75/L | 60-105/L | <105/L |
| **Vital capacity (VC)** | Maximum inspiration and then measurement of air during maximal forced expiration. Measure of respiratory muscle endurance or reserve or both. Requires patient cooperation. | 65-75 mL/kg | ≥10-15 mL/kg |
| **Spontaneous breathing trial (SBT)** | If patient passes daily weaning screen, assess patient during spontaneous breathing with little or no ventilator assistance. Trial should be at least 30 min to a maximum of 120 min. | | Successful completion of trial is based on an integrated patient assessment. |

*The decision to use these criteria must be individualized to the patient.

Adapted from A Collective Task Force Facilitated by the American College of Chest Physicians, the American Association for Respiratory Care, and the American College of Critical Care Medicine: Evidence-based guidelines for weaning and discontinuing ventilatory support, *Resp Care* 47:69, 2002; and Burns SM: Weaning process. In Wiegand DL-M, editor: *AACN procedure manual for critical care,* ed 6, St Louis, 2011, Saunders.

The emphasis on controlling hospital costs has increased the early discharge of patients and the need to provide highly technical care such as mechanical ventilation in home settings. The success of home mechanical ventilation depends, in part, on careful predischarge assessment and planning for both the patient and caregivers.

Both negative pressure and positive pressure ventilators are used in the home. Negative pressure ventilators do not require an artificial airway and are less complicated to use. Several types of small, portable (battery-powered) positive pressure ventilators are available and can be attached to a wheelchair or placed on a bedside table. Settings and alarms on these ventilators are simpler to use than on the standard ICU ventilators.

Home mechanical ventilation has advantages and disadvantages. Having the patient in the home eliminates the strain that the hospital setting imposes on family dynamics. Caregivers may feel helpless when they first hear about the necessity for long-term mechanical ventilation. However, these feelings are frequently balanced by the opportunity to participate in the patient's care in the home setting. At home the patient may be able to take part in more activities of daily living around an individualized schedule and, because of the smaller size of the home ventilator, be more mobile. Another advantage of home mechanical ventilation is the reduced risk of HAIs.

Disadvantages of home mechanical ventilation include problems related to equipment, reimbursement, caregiver stress and fatigue, and the patient's complex needs. Ventilated patients are usually dependent, requiring extensive nursing care, at least initially. Disposable products may not be reimbursable. Financial resources must be carefully assessed when arranging home mechanical ventilation. Schedule a meeting with the interprofessional care team (e.g., social worker, home health care nurse, respiratory therapist) before starting a discharge teaching plan.

Another disadvantage of home mechanical ventilation is its potential impact on the family. Caregivers may seem enthusiastic about caring for their loved one in the home but may be motivated by numerous, complex factors. They may not understand the sacrifices they may have to make financially and in personal time and commitment. Encourage caregivers to consider respite care to periodically relieve their stress and fatigue.

## ❖ NURSING MANAGEMENT: MECHANICAL VENTILATION

eNursing Care Plan 65-1 for the patient receiving mechanical ventilation is available on the website for this chapter.

## OTHER CRITICAL CARE CONTENT

Table 65-14 lists additional critical care content presented in other chapters of this book.

**TABLE 65-14 Cross-References to Critical Care Content**

| Topic | Discussed in Chapter | Topic | Discussed in Chapter |
|---|---|---|---|
| Acute coronary syndrome (ACS) | 33 | Enteral nutrition (EN) | 39 |
| Acute heart failure | 34 | Head injury, including ICP monitoring | 56 |
| Acute respiratory distress syndrome (ARDS) | 67 | Multiple organ dysfunction syndrome (MODS) | 66 |
| Acute respiratory failure | 67 | Myocardial infarction (MI) | 33 |
| Basic life support and CPR | Appendix A | Oxygen delivery | 28 |
| Burns | 24 | Pain management | 8 |
| Cardiac dysrhythmias | 35 | Parenteral nutrition (PN) | 39 |
| Cardiac pacemakers | 35 | Pulmonary edema | 34 |
| Cardiac surgery | 33 | Renal dialysis | 46 |
| Central venous access device (CVAD) | 16 | Shock | 66 |
| Continuous renal replacement therapy (CRRT) | 46 | Stroke | 57 |
| Delirium | 59 | Systemic inflammatory response syndrome (SIRS) | 66 |
| Emergencies | 68 | Tracheostomy | 26 |
| End-of-life (EOL) care | 9 | Trauma | 68 |

*CPR,* Cardiopulmonary resuscitation; *ICP,* intracranial pressure.

## CASE STUDY

### *Critical Care and Mechanical Ventilation*

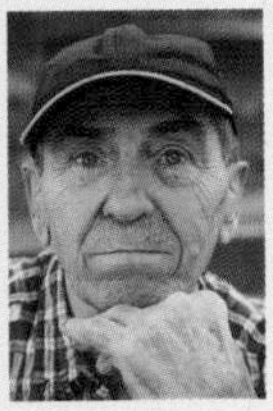
(©Thinkstock)

**Patient Profile**

R.K. is a 72-yr-old white man who collapsed in his home. He was found by his daughter, and she activated the emergency response system. He was unresponsive on admission to the emergency department and remains unresponsive on arrival to the ICU. He has an oral ET tube in place and is receiving mechanical ventilation. A large-bore, peripheral IV has been placed and fluids are infusing.

**Subjective Data**

None. Patient is unresponsive to painful stimuli.

**Objective Data**

***Physical Examination***

- Noninvasive BP 100/75 mm Hg; apical-radial heart rate 128; temperature 102°F (38.8°C); $SpO_2$ is 98%
- ECG: atrial fibrillation with a rapid ventricular response
- Purulent secretions suctioned from ET tube
- Breath sounds: coarse crackles bilaterally, decreased breath sounds on the right
- Weight: 168 lb (76 kg)

***Diagnostic Studies***

- Chest x-ray reveals right lower lung consolidation
- ABGs: pH 7.48; $PaO_2$ 94 mm Hg; $PaCO_2$ 30 mm Hg; $HCO_3$ 34 mEq/L
- CT scan is positive for a hemorrhagic stroke

**Interprofessional Care**

- Positive pressure ventilation settings: assist-control mode
- Settings: $FIO_2$ 70%, $V_T$ 700 mL, respiratory rate 16 breaths/min, PEEP 5 cm $H_2O$
- Orogastric tube to low, intermittent suction
- Enteral feeding at 25 mL/hr to start on day 2
- External condom catheter for urinary drainage and measurement
- HOB elevated at 40 degrees
- Reposition at least every 2 hr
- Azithromycin (Zithromax) 500 mg IV q24hr
- Cefotaxime (Claforan) 2 g IV q6hr
- NS with KCl 20 mEq/L at 100 mL/hr

**Discussion Questions**

1. Identify two reasons for intubating and providing mechanical ventilation for R.K.
2. What do R.K.'s ABGs indicate, and which ventilator setting(s) should be changed?
3. What is his $PaO_2/FIO_2$ ratio, and what does it indicate?
4. R.K.'s BP drops to 80 mm Hg. Despite increasing doses of vasopressors and fluid challenges, his BP remains low. A central venous catheter and an arterial line are inserted. APCO monitoring is started. What would be the purpose of hemodynamic monitoring in this patient?
5. ***Priority Decision:*** What are two priority nursing considerations for a patient with invasive monitoring?
6. R.K.'s pulmonary condition deteriorates. $PaO_2$ drops to 70 mm Hg, and $SpO_2$ is 89%. PEEP is increased to 7.5 cm $H_2O$. What implications does this have for R.K. given his hemodynamic status?
7. ***Priority Decision:*** Based on the data presented, what are the priority nursing diagnoses? Are there any collaborative problems?
8. ***Teamwork and Collaboration:*** What patient care activities can you delegate to unlicensed assistive personnel?
9. ***Evidence-Based Practice:*** R.K.'s family wants to know why he is to receive tube feedings. What would you tell the family? What is the evidence to support the use of tube feedings?
10. ***Patient-Centered Care:*** After 4 days, R.K. remains unresponsive and has developed renal failure. The HCP believes the patient will not recover from his neurologic injury and wishes to discuss goals of care with the patient's caregiver. What would be your role in this meeting?

Answers available at *http://evolve.elsevier.com/Lewis/medsurg.*

## BRIDGE TO NCLEX EXAMINATION

The number of the question corresponds to the same-numbered outcome at the beginning of the chapter.

1. Certification in critical care nursing (CCRN) by the American Association of Critical-Care Nurses indicates that the nurse
   a. is an advanced practice nurse who cares for acutely and critically ill patients.
   b. may practice independently to provide symptom management for the critically ill.
   c. has earned a master's degree in the field of advanced acute and critical care nursing.
   d. has practiced in critical care and successfully completed a test of critical care knowledge.
2. What are the appropriate nursing interventions for the patient with delirium in the ICU *(select all that apply)*?
   a. Use clocks and calendars to maintain orientation.
   b. Encourage round-the-clock presence of caregivers at the bedside.
   c. Silence all alarms, reduce overhead paging, and avoid conversations around the patient.
   d. Sedate the patient with appropriate drugs to protect the patient from harmful behaviors.
   e. Identify physiologic factors that may be contributing to the patient's confusion and irritability.
3. The critical care nurse recognizes that an ideal plan for caregiver involvement includes
   a. a caregiver at the bedside at all times.
   b. allowing caregivers at the bedside at preset, brief intervals.
   c. an individually devised plan to involve caregivers with care and comfort measures.
   d. restriction of visiting in the ICU because the environment is overwhelming to caregivers.
4. To establish hemodynamic monitoring for a patient, the nurse zeros the
   a. cardiac output monitoring system to the level of the left ventricle.
   b. pressure monitoring system to the level of the catheter tip located in the patient.
   c. pressure monitoring system to the level of the atrium, identified as the phlebostatic axis.
   d. pressure monitoring system to the level of the atrium, identified as the midclavicular line.
5. The hemodynamic changes the nurse expects to find after successful initiation of intraaortic balloon pump therapy in a patient with cardiogenic shock include *(select all that apply)*
   a. decreased SV.
   b. decreased SVR.
   c. decreased PAWP.
   d. increased diastolic BP.
   e. decreased myocardial $O_2$ consumption.
6. The purpose of adding PEEP to positive pressure ventilation is to
   a. increase functional residual capacity and improve oxygenation.
   b. increase $FIO_2$ in an attempt to wean the patient and avoid $O_2$ toxicity.
   c. determine if the patient is in synchrony with the ventilator or needs to be paralyzed.
   d. determine if the patient is able to be weaned and avoid the risk of pneumomediastinum.
7. The nursing management of a patient with an artificial airway includes
   a. maintaining ET tube cuff pressure at 30 cm $H_2O$.
   b. routine suctioning of the tube at least every 2 hours.
   c. observing for cardiac dysrhythmias during suctioning.
   d. preventing tube dislodgment by limiting mouth care to lubrication of the lips.
8. The nurse monitors the patient with positive pressure mechanical ventilation for
   a. paralytic ileus because pressure on the abdominal contents affects bowel motility.
   b. diuresis and sodium depletion because of increased release of atrial natriuretic peptide.
   c. signs of cardiovascular insufficiency because pressure in the chest impedes venous return.
   d. respiratory acidosis in a patient with COPD because of alveolar hyperventilation and increased $PaO_2$ levels.

1. d, 2. a, d, e, 3. c, 4. c, 5. b, c, d, e, 6. a, 7. c, 8. c

For rationales to these answers and even more NCLEX review questions, visit *http://evolve.elsevier.com/Lewis/medsurg.*

## EVOLVE WEBSITE

http://evolve.elsevier.com/Lewis/medsurg

**Review Questions (Online Only)**

**Key Points**

**Answer Keys to Questions**

- Rationales for Bridge to NCLEX Examination Questions
- Answer Guidelines for Case Study on p. 1584

**Student Case Study**

- Patient With Pulmonary Embolism and Respiratory Failure

**Nursing Care Plan**

- eNursing Care Plan 65-1: Patient on Mechanical Ventilation

**Conceptual Care Map Creator**

**Audio Glossary**

**Supporting Media**

- Animation
  - Endotracheal Intubation

**Content Updates**

## REFERENCES


1. American Association of Critical-Care Nurses: About critical care nursing. Retrieved from *www.aacn.org/wd/publishing/content/pressroom/aboutcriticalcarenursing.pcms?menu=*.

*2. Maharaj R, Raffaele I, Wendon J: Rapid response systems: a systematic review and meta-analysis, *Crit Care* 19:254, 2015.

3. American Association of Critical-Care Nurses: Frequently asked questions about APRN Consensus Model—for nurse practitioners. Retrieved from *www.aacn.org/wd/certifications/content/aprn-nurses-np-faqs.pcms?menu=certification.*

4. Society of Critical Care Medicine: Critical care statistics. Retrieved from *www.sccm.org/Communications/Pages/CriticalCareStats.aspx.*

*5. Woods S: Spiritual and complementary therapies to promote healing and reduce stress. In Molter NC, editor: *Protocols for practice: creating healing environments*, ed 2, Sudbury, Mass, 2007, Jones & Bartlett. (Classic)

*6. Barr J, Fraser GL, Puntillo K, et al: Clinical practice guidelines for the management of pain, agitation, and delirium in adult patients in the intensive care unit, *Crit Care Med* 41:263, 2013.
7. Stafford A, Haverland A, Bridges E: Noise in the ICU—what we know and what we can do about it, *AJN* 114:57, 2014.
*8. American Association of Critical-Care Nurses: Delirium assessment and management. Retrieved from *www.aacn.org/wd/practice/content/practicealerts/delirium-practice-alert.pcms?menu=practice.*
*9. American Association of Critical-Care Nurses: ABCDE tool kit, AACN PEARL: early progressive mobility protocol. Retrieved from *www.aacn.org/wd/practice/docs/tool%20kits/early-progressive-mobility-protocol.pdf.*
*10. McClave SA, Taylor BE, Martindale RG, et al: Guidelines for the provision and assessment of nutrition support therapy in the adult critically ill patient: Society of Critical Care Medicine (SCCM) and American Society for Parenteral and Enteral Nutrition (A.S.P.E.N.), *J Parenter Enteral Nutr* 40:159, 2016.
11. Bell L: Patient care page: patient-centered care, *Am J Crit Care* 23:325, 2014.
*12. Leske JS, Pasquale MA: Family needs, interventions and presence. In Molter NC, editor: *Protocols for practice: creating healing environments*, ed 2, Sudbury, Mass, 2007, Jones & Bartlett. (Classic)
*13. American Association of Critical-Care Nurses: AACN practice alert: family presence: visitation in the adult ICU. Retrieved from *www.aacn.org/wd/practice/content/practicealerts/family-visitation-icu-practice-alert.pcms?menu=practice.*
14. Society of Critical Care Medicine: Patient and family resources: ICU issues and answers brochures. Retrieved from *http://store.sccm.org/SearchResults.aspx?Category=BROC.*
*15. American Association of Critical-Care Nurses: AACN practice alert: family presence during CPR and invasive procedures. Retrieved from *www.aacn.org/wd/practice/docs/practicealerts/family-presence-during-resuscitation-invasive-procedures.pdf.*
*16. Medina J, Puntillo K, editors: *AACN protocols for practice: palliative care and end-of-life issues in critical care*, Sudbury, Mass, 2006, Jones & Bartlett. (Classic)
*17. Shaffer RB: Arterial catheter insertion (assist). In Wiegand DL-M, editor: *AACN procedure manual for critical care*, ed 6, St Louis, 2011, Saunders.
18. Edwards Lifesciences: Advanced hemodynamic monitoring. Retrieved from *www.edwards.com/products/mininvasive/Pages/strokevolumevariationwp.aspx.*
*19. Kern ME: Arterial pressure-based cardiac output monitoring. In Wiegand DL-M, editor: *AACN procedure manual for critical care*, ed 6, St Louis, 2011, Saunders.
*20. Klein DG: Cardiac output measurement techniques (invasive). In Wiegand DL-M, editor: *AACN procedure manual for critical care*, ed 6, St Louis, 2011, Saunders.
*21. Headley JM, Giuliano KK: Continuous venous oxygenation monitoring. In Wiegand DL-M, editor: *AACN procedure manual for critical care*, ed 6, St Louis, 2011, Saunders.
*22. Castelluci D: Intraaortic balloon pump management. In Wiegand DL-M, editor: *AACN procedure manual for critical care*, ed 6, St Louis, 2011, Saunders.
*23. Puhlman M, Hargraves J: Ventricular assist devices. In Wiegand DL-M, editor: *AACN procedure manual for critical care*, ed 6, St Louis, 2011, Saunders.
24. Abiomed: Frequently asked questions. Retrieved from *www.abiomed.com/assets/2010/11/AbioCor-FAQ-FINAL.pdf.*
25. Villwock JA, Jones K: Outcomes of early versus late tracheostomy: 2008-2010, *Laryngoscope* 124:1801, 2014.
26. Stollings JL, Diedrich DA, Oyen LJ, et al: Rapid-sequence intubation: a review of the process and considerations when choosing medications, *Ann Pharmacother* 48:62, 2014.
27. Walsh BK, Crotwell DN, Restrepo RD: Capnography/capnometry during mechanical ventilation, *Respir Care* 56:503, 2011.
*28. American Association of Respiratory Care: AARC clinical practice guidelines: endotracheal suctioning of mechanically ventilated patients with artificial airways, *Respir Care* 55:758, 2010.
*29. Seckel MA: Suctioning: endotracheal or tracheostomy tube. In Wiegand DL-M, editor: *AACN procedure manual for critical care*, ed 7, St Louis, 2017, Elsevier. *(in press)*
*30. Fisher DF, Chenelle CT, Marchese AD, et al: Comparison of commercial and noncommercial endotracheal tube-securing devices, *Respir Care* 59:1315, 2014.
*31. Wade D, Hardy R, Howell D, et al: Identifying clinical and acute psychological risk factors for PTSD after critical care: a systematic review, *Minerva Anestesiol* 79:944, 2013.
*32. Happ MB: Communicating with mechanically ventilated patients: state of the science, *AACN Clin Issues* 12:247, 2001. (Classic)
33. Jarachovic M, Mason M, Kerber K, et al: The role of standardized protocols in unplanned extubations in a medical intensive care unit, *Am J Crit Care* 20:304, 2011.
*34. Chang L, Wang KK, Yann-Fen C: Influence of physical restraint of unplanned extubation of adult intensive care patient: a case control study, *Am J Crit Care* 17:408, 2008. (Classic)
*35. American Association of Critical-Care Nurses: AACN practice alert: prevention of aspiration. Retrieved from *www.aacn.org/wd/practice/docs/practicealerts/prevention-aspiration-practice-alert.pdf?menu=aboutus.*
*36. Gallagher J: Mechanical ventilation (through an artificial airway): volume and pressure modes. In Wiegand DL-M, editor: *AACN procedure manual for critical care*, ed 7, St Louis, 2017, Elsevier. *(in press)*
*37. American Association of Critical-Care Nurses: Alarm management. Retrieved from *www.aacn.org/wd/practice/content/practicealerts/alarm-management-practice-alert.pcms?menu=practice.*
38. Oto J, Imanaka H, Nakataki E, et al: Potential inadequacy of automatic tube compensation to decrease inspiratory work load after at least 48 hours of endotracheal tube use in the clinical setting, *Respir Care* 57:697, 2012.
*39. Huang C, Lin H, Ruan S, et al: Efficacy and adverse events of high-frequency oscillatory ventilation in adult patients with acute respiratory distress syndrome: a meta-analysis, *Crit Care* 18:R102, 2014.
*40. Adhikari NK, Dellinger RP, Lundin S, et al: Inhaled nitric oxide does not reduce mortality in patients with acute respiratory distress syndrome regardless of severity: systematic review and meta-analysis, *Crit Care Med* 42:404, 2013.
*41. Lee JM, Bae W, Lee YJ, et al: The efficacy and safety of prone positional ventilation in acute respiratory distress syndrome: updated study-level meta-analysis of 11 randomized controlled trials, *Crit Care Med* 42:1252, 2014.
*42. Combes A, Brodie D, Bartlett R, et al: Position paper for the organization of extracorporeal membrane oxygenation programs for acute respiratory failure in adult patients, *Am J Respir Crit Care Med* 190:488, 2014.
43. Kalanuria AA, Zai W, Mirski M: Ventilator-associated pneumonia in the ICU, *Crit Care* 18:208, 2014.
*44. Klompas M, Branson R, Eichenwald EC, et al: Strategies to prevent ventilator-associated pneumonia in acute care hospitals: a 2014 update, *Infect Cont Hosp Epidemiol* 35:915, 2014.
*45. Dubberke ER, Carling P, Carrico R, et al: Strategies to prevent *Clostridium difficile* infections in acute care hospitals: 2014 update, *Infect Cont Hosp Epidemiol* 35:628, 2014.
*46. American Association of Critical-Care Nurses: AACN practice alert: verification of feeding tube placement. Retrieved from *www.aacn.org/WD/Practice/Docs/Verification_of_Feeding_Tube_Placement_05-2005.pdf*
47. Campbell MR, Fisher J, Anderson L, et al: Implementation of early exercise and mobility–steps to success, *Crit Care Nurs* 35:82, 2015.
48. Desai SV, Law TJ, Needham DM: Long-term complications of critical care, *Crit Care Med* 39:371, 2011.
49. Casaer MP, Van den Berghe G: Nutrition in the acute phase of critical illness, *NEJM* 370:1227, 2014.
50. Balas MC, Vasilevskis EE, Burke WJ, et al: Critical care nurses' role in implementing the "ABCDE bundle" into practice, *Crit Care Nurs* 32:35, 2012.

*Evidence-based information for clinical practice.

# Shock, Sepsis, and Multiple Organ Dysfunction Syndrome

Maureen A. Seckel

*In order for you to shine, you have to get through the darkness.*

*Mario Tomasello*

http://evolve.elsevier.com/Lewis/medsurg/

## LEARNING OUTCOMES

1. Relate the pathophysiology to the clinical manifestations of the different types of shock: cardiogenic, hypovolemic, distributive, and obstructive.
2. Compare the effects of shock, systemic inflammatory response syndrome, sepsis, and multiple organ dysfunction syndrome on the major body systems.
3. Compare the interprofessional care, drug therapy, and nursing management of patients experiencing different types of shock.
4. Describe the interprofessional care and nursing management of a patient experiencing multiple organ dysfunction syndrome.

## KEY TERMS

anaphylactic shock, p. 1590
cardiogenic shock, p. 1587
hypovolemic shock, p. 1589
multiple organ dysfunction syndrome (MODS), p. 1605
neurogenic shock, p. 1590
obstructive shock, p. 1593
sepsis, p. 1592
septic shock, p. 1592
shock, p. 1587
systemic inflammatory response syndrome (SIRS), p. 1604

Shock, systemic inflammatory response syndrome (SIRS), sepsis, and multiple organ dysfunction syndrome (MODS) are serious and interrelated problems (Fig. 66-1). This chapter provides an overview of the different types of shock, SIRS, sepsis, and MODS, and the related management of each.

## SHOCK

**Shock** is a syndrome characterized by decreased tissue perfusion and impaired cellular metabolism. This results in an imbalance between the supply of and demand for $O_2$ and nutrients. The exchange of $O_2$ and nutrients at the cellular level is essential to life. When cells experience hypoperfusion, the demand for $O_2$ and nutrients exceeds the supply at the microcirculatory level.

### Classification of Shock

The four main categories of shock are cardiogenic, hypovolemic, distributive, and obstructive[1,2] (Table 66-1). Although the cause, initial presentation, and management strategies vary for each type of shock, the physiologic responses of the cells to hypoperfusion are similar.

**Cardiogenic Shock.** **Cardiogenic shock** occurs when either systolic or diastolic dysfunction of the heart's pumping action results in reduced cardiac output (CO). Causes of cardiogenic shock are listed in Table 66-1. Mortality rates for patients with cardiogenic shock approach 60%.[3] Decreased filling of the heart results in decreased stroke volume (SV).

The heart's inability to pump the blood forward is called *systolic dysfunction.* Systolic dysfunction primarily affects the left ventricle, since systolic pressure is greater on the left side of the heart. When systolic dysfunction affects the right side of the heart, blood flow through the pulmonary circulation is reduced. The most common cause of systolic dysfunction is acute myocardial infarction (MI). Cardiogenic shock is the leading cause of death from acute MI.[4] Causes of diastolic dysfunction are listed in Table 66-1.

Fig. 66-2 describes the pathophysiology of cardiogenic shock. Whether the first event is myocardial ischemia, a structural problem (e.g., valvular disorder, ventricular septal rupture), or dysrhythmias, the physiologic responses are similar: the patient experiences impaired tissue perfusion and cellular metabolism.

The early clinical presentation of a patient with cardiogenic shock is similar to that of a patient with acute decompensated heart failure (see Chapter 34). The patient may have tachycardia and hypotension. Pulse pressure may be narrowed due to the heart's inability to pump blood forward during systole and increased volume during diastole. An increase in systemic vascular resistance (SVR) increases the workload of the heart, thus

Reviewed by Carla V. Hannon, MS, APRN, CCRN, CCNS, Clinical Nurse Specialist, Medical Intensive Care Unit, Yale–New Haven Hospital, New Haven, Connecticut; Patricia Lea, RN, DNP, CCRN, Assistant Professor, University of Texas Medical Branch School of Nursing, Galveston, Texas; and Anna P. Moore, RN, MS, Associate Professor, School of Nursing and Allied Health, J. Sargeant Reynolds Community College, Richmond, Virginia.

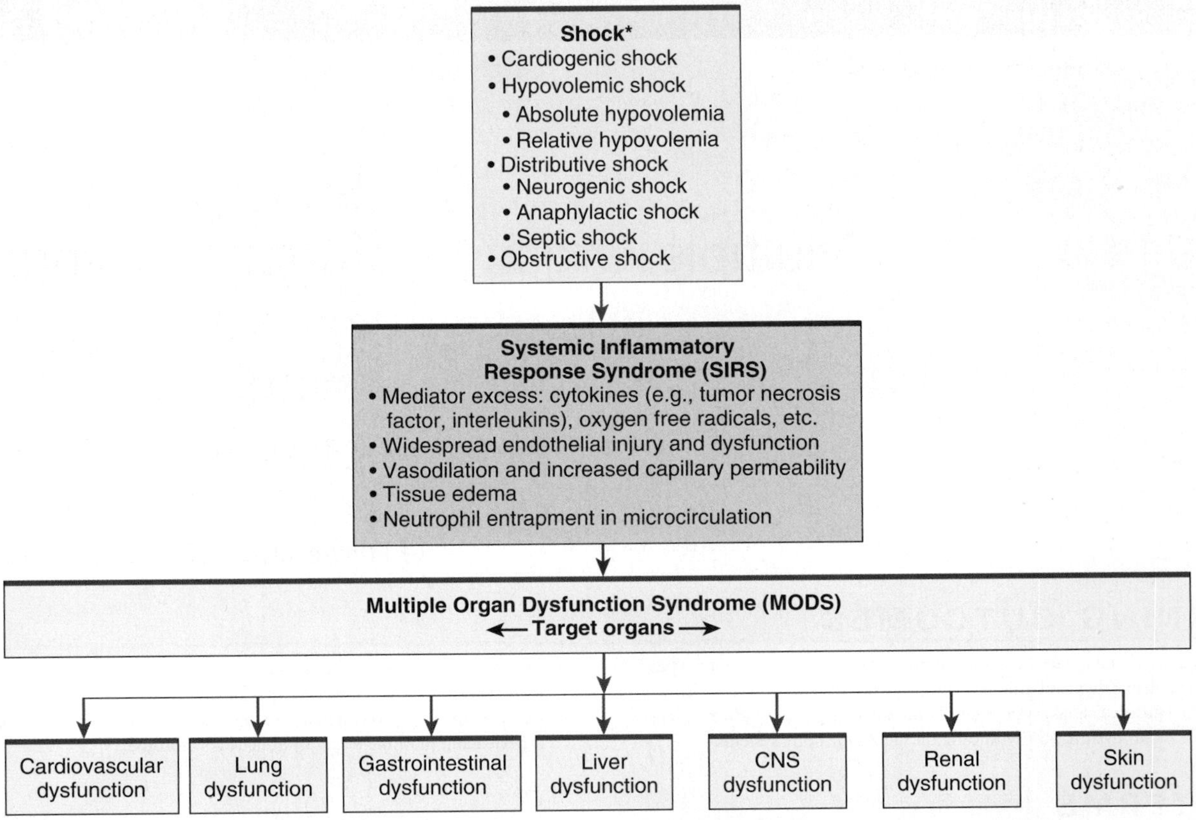


**FIG. 66-1** Relationship of shock, systemic inflammatory response syndrome, and multiple organ dysfunction syndrome. *CNS*, Central nervous system. (*See Table 66-1 for causes of shock states.)

## TABLE 66-1 Classification of Shock States

| Types and Causes | Examples |
|---|---|
| **Cardiogenic Shock** | |
| • Systolic dysfunction: inability of the heart to pump blood forward | Myocardial infarction, cardiomyopathy, blunt cardiac injury, severe systemic or pulmonary hypertension, myocardial depression from metabolic problems |
| • Diastolic dysfunction: inability of the heart to fill | Cardiac tamponade, ventricular hypertrophy, cardiomyopathy |
| • Dysrhythmias | Bradydysrhythmias, tachydysrhythmias |
| • Structural factors | Valvular stenosis or regurgitation, ventricular septal rupture, tension pneumothorax |
| **Hypovolemic Shock** | |
| ***Absolute Hypovolemia*** | |
| • External loss of whole blood | Hemorrhage from trauma, surgery, GI bleeding |
| • Loss of other body fluids | Vomiting, diarrhea, excessive diuresis, diabetes insipidus, diabetes mellitus |
| ***Relative Hypovolemia*** | |
| • Pooling of blood or fluids | Bowel obstruction |
| • Fluid shifts | Burn injuries, ascites |
| • Internal bleeding | Fracture of long bones, ruptured spleen, hemothorax, severe pancreatitis |
| • Massive vasodilation | Sepsis |
| **Distributive Shock** | |
| ***Neurogenic Shock*** | |
| • Hemodynamic consequence of spinal cord injury and/or disease at or above T5 | Severe pain, drugs, hypoglycemia, injury |
| • Spinal anesthesia | |
| • Vasomotor center depression | |
| ***Anaphylactic Shock*** | |
| • Hypersensitivity (allergic) reaction to a sensitizing substance | Contrast media, blood or blood products, drugs, insect bites, anesthetic agents, food or food additives, vaccines, environmental agents, latex |
| ***Septic Shock*** | |
| • Infection | Pneumonia, peritonitis, urinary tract, invasive procedures, indwelling lines and catheters |
| • At-risk patients | Older adults, patients with chronic diseases (e.g., diabetes mellitus, chronic kidney disease, heart failure), patients receiving immunosuppressive therapy or who are malnourished or debilitated |
| **Obstructive Shock** | |
| • Physical obstruction impeding the filling or outflow of blood resulting in reduced cardiac output | Cardiac tamponade, tension pneumothorax, superior vena cava syndrome, abdominal compartment syndrome, pulmonary embolism |

PATHOPHYSIOLOGY MAP

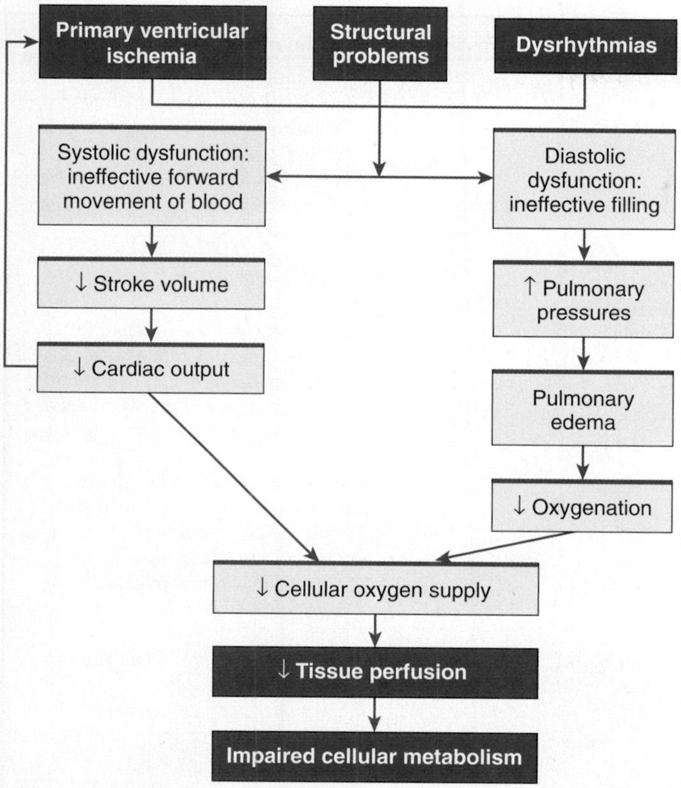


**FIG. 66-2** The pathophysiology of cardiogenic shock. (Modified from Urden LD, Stacy KM, Lough ME: *Critical care nursing: diagnosis and management,* ed 6, St Louis, 2010, Mosby.)

PATHOPHYSIOLOGY MAP

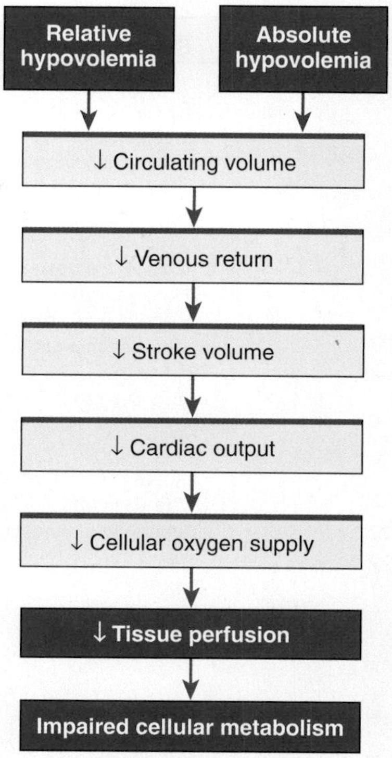


**FIG. 66-3** The pathophysiology of hypovolemic shock. (Modified from Urden LD, Stacy KM, Lough ME: *Critical care nursing: diagnosis and management,* ed 6, St Louis, 2010, Mosby.)

increasing the myocardial $O_2$ consumption. The heart's inability to pump blood forward also results in a low CO (less than 4 L/minute) and *cardiac index* (less than 2.5 L/minute/$m^2$).

On assessment, the patient is tachypneic and has crackles on auscultation of breath sounds because of pulmonary congestion. The hemodynamic profile demonstrates an increase in the pulmonary artery wedge pressure (PAWP), stroke volume variation (SVV), and pulmonary vascular resistance.

Signs of peripheral hypoperfusion (e.g., cyanosis, pallor, diaphoresis, weak peripheral pulses, cool and clammy skin, delayed capillary refill) are seen. Decreased renal blood flow results in sodium and water retention and decreased urine output. Anxiety, confusion, and agitation may develop as cerebral perfusion is impaired. Tables 66-2 and 66-3 describe the laboratory findings and clinical presentation of a patient with cardiogenic shock.

**Hypovolemic Shock.** Hypovolemic shock occurs after a loss of intravascular fluid volume (Table 66-1). The volume is inadequate to fill the vascular space. The volume loss may be either an absolute or a relative volume loss. *Absolute hypovolemia* results when fluid is lost through hemorrhage, gastrointestinal (GI) loss (e.g., vomiting, diarrhea), fistula drainage, diabetes insipidus, or diuresis. In *relative hypovolemia,* fluid volume moves out of the vascular space into the extravascular space (e.g., intracavitary space). This type of fluid shift is called *third spacing.* One example of relative volume loss is leakage of fluid from the vascular space to the interstitial space from increased capillary permeability, as seen in burns (see Chapter 24).

In hypovolemic shock the size of the vascular compartment remains unchanged while the volume of blood or plasma decreases. Whether the loss of intravascular volume is absolute or relative, the physiologic consequences are similar. A reduction in intravascular volume results in a decreased venous return to the heart, decreased preload, decreased SV, and decreased CO. A cascade of events results in decreased tissue perfusion and impaired cellular metabolism, the hallmarks of shock (Fig. 66-3).

The patient's response to acute volume loss depends on a number of factors, including extent of injury, age, and general state of health. However, the clinical presentation of hypovolemic shock is consistent (Table 66-3). An overall assessment of physiologic reserves may indicate the patient's ability to compensate. A patient may compensate for a loss of up to 15% of the total blood volume (approximately 750 mL). Further loss of volume (15% to 30%) results in a sympathetic nervous system (SNS)–mediated response. This response results in an increase in heart rate, CO, and respiratory rate and depth. The SV, central venous pressure (CVP), and PAWP are decreased because of the decreased circulating blood volume.

The patient may appear anxious, and urine output begins to decrease. If hypovolemia is corrected by crystalloid fluid replacement at this time, tissue dysfunction is generally reversible. If volume loss is greater than 30%, compensatory mechanisms may fail and immediate replacement with blood products should be started. Loss of autoregulation in the microcirculation and irreversible tissue destruction occur with loss of more than 40% of the total blood volume.[5] Common laboratory studies and assessments that are done include serial measurements of hemoglobin and hematocrit levels, electrolytes, lactate, blood gases, mixed central venous $O_2$ saturation ($SvO_2$), and hourly urine outputs (Table 66-2).

**TABLE 66-2 Diagnostic Studies**

***Shock***

| Study | Finding | Significance of Finding |
|---|---|---|
| **Red blood cells** | | |
| RBC count, hematocrit, hemoglobin | Normal | Remains within normal limits in shock because of relative hypovolemia and pump failure and in hemorrhagic shock before fluid resuscitation. |
| | ↓ | Hemorrhagic shock after fluid resuscitation when fluids other than blood are used. |
| | ↑ | Nonhemorrhagic shock caused by actual hypovolemia and hemoconcentration. |
| **White blood cells** | | |
| WBC count, presence of bands | ↑, ↓ | Infection, septic shock. |
| **DIC screen** | | Acute DIC can develop within hours to days after an initial assault on the body (e.g., shock). |
| • Fibrin split products (FSP) | ↑ | |
| • Fibrinogen level | ↓ | |
| • Platelet count | ↓ | |
| • PTT and PT | ↑ | |
| • INR | ↑ | |
| • Thrombin time | ↑ | |
| • D-dimer | ↑ | |
| **Creatine kinase** | ↑ | Trauma, myocardial infarction in response to cellular damage and/or hypoxia. |
| **Troponin** | ↑ | Increases in myocardial infarction. |
| **BUN** | ↑ | Indicates impaired kidney function caused by hypoperfusion as a result of severe vasoconstriction, or occurs secondary to catabolism of cells (e.g., trauma, infection). |
| **Creatinine** | ↑ | Indicates impaired kidney function caused by hypoperfusion as a result of severe vasoconstriction. Is more sensitive indicator of renal function than BUN. |
| **Procalcitonin (PCT)** | ↑ | Biomarker that is released in response to bacterial infections. |
| **Glucose** | ↑ | Found in early shock because of release of liver glycogen stores in response to sympathetic nervous system stimulation and cortisol. Insulin insensitivity develops. |
| | ↓ | Occurs because of depleted glycogen stores with liver dysfunction possible as shock progresses. |
| **Serum electrolytes** | | |
| • Sodium | ↑ | Found in early shock because of increased secretion of aldosterone, causing renal retention of sodium. |
| | ↓ | May occur iatrogenically when excess hypotonic fluid is administered after fluid loss. |
| • Potassium | ↑ | Results when dead cells release potassium. Also occurs in acute kidney injury and acidosis. |
| | ↓ | Found in early shock because of increased secretion of aldosterone, causing renal excretion of potassium. |
| **Arterial blood gases** | Respiratory alkalosis | Found in early shock secondary to hyperventilation. |
| | Metabolic acidosis | Occurs later in shock when lactate accumulates in blood from anaerobic metabolism. |
| **Base deficit** | >–6 | Indicates acid production secondary to hypoxia. |
| **Blood cultures** | Growth of organisms | May grow organisms in patients who are in septic shock. |
| **Lactate level** | ↑ | Usually increases once significant hypoperfusion and impaired $O_2$ utilization at the cellular level have occurred. By-product of anaerobic metabolism. |
| **Liver enzymes (ALT, AST, GGT)** | ↑ | Elevations indicate liver cell destruction in progressive stage of shock. |

*ALT,* Alanine aminotransferase; *AST,* aspartate aminotransferase; *BUN,* blood urea nitrogen; *DIC,* disseminated intravascular coagulation; *GGT,* γ-glutamyl transferase; *INR,* international normalized ratio; *PT,* prothrombin time; *PTT,* partial thromboplastin time.

### Distributive Shock

***Neurogenic Shock.*** Neurogenic shock is a hemodynamic phenomenon that can occur within 30 minutes of a spinal cord injury and can last up to 6 weeks. Neurogenic shock related to spinal cord injuries is generally associated with a cervical or high thoracic injury. The injury results in a massive vasodilation without compensation because of the loss of SNS vasoconstrictor tone. This massive vasodilation leads to a pooling of blood in the blood vessels, tissue hypoperfusion, and ultimately impaired cellular metabolism (Fig. 66-4).

In addition to spinal cord injury, spinal anesthesia can block transmission of impulses from the SNS. Depression of the vasomotor center of the medulla from drugs (e.g., opioids, benzodiazepines) also can decrease the vasoconstrictor tone of the peripheral blood vessels, resulting in neurogenic shock (Table 66-1).

The most important clinical manifestations in neurogenic shock are hypotension (from the massive vasodilation) and bradycardia (from unopposed parasympathetic stimulation).[6] The patient may not be able to regulate body temperature. Combined with massive vasodilation, the inability to regulate temperature promotes heat loss. Initially, the patient's skin is warm due to the massive vasodilation. As the heat disperses, the patient is at risk for hypothermia. Later, the patient's skin may be cool or warm depending on the ambient temperature (*poikilothermia,* taking on the temperature of the environment). In either case, the skin is usually dry. Tables 66-2 and 66-3 further describe the laboratory findings and clinical presentation of a patient with neurogenic shock.

Although spinal shock and neurogenic shock often occur in the same patient, they are not the same disorder. *Spinal shock* is a transient condition that is present after an acute spinal cord injury (see Chapter 60). The patient with spinal shock experiences the absence of all voluntary and reflex neurologic activity below the level of the injury.

***Anaphylactic Shock.*** Anaphylactic shock is an acute, life-threatening hypersensitivity (allergic) reaction to a sensitizing substance (e.g., drug, chemical, vaccine, food, insect venom). The reaction quickly causes massive vasodilation, release of vasoactive mediators, and an increase in capillary permeability.

**TABLE 66-3 Clinical Presentation of Types of Shock**

| | | DISTRIBUTIVE SHOCK | | | |
|---|---|---|---|---|---|
| **Cardiogenic Shock** | **Hypovolemic Shock** | **Neurogenic Shock** | **Anaphylactic Shock** | **Septic Shock** | **Obstructive Shock** |
| **Cardiovascular System** | | | | | |
| Tachycardia<br>↓ BP<br>↓ Capillary refill<br>Chest pain may or may not be present | ↓ Preload<br>↓ Stroke volume<br>↓ Capillary refill | ↓ BP<br>↓/↑ Temperature<br>Bradycardia | Chest pain<br>Third spacing of fluid | ↓/↑ Temperature<br>Myocardial dysfunction<br>Biventricular dilation<br>↓ Ejection fraction | ↓ BP<br>↓ Preload |
| **Respiratory System** | | | | | |
| Tachypnea<br>Crackles<br>Cyanosis | Tachypnea → bradypnea (late) | Dysfunction related to level of injury | Shortness of breath<br>Edema of larynx and epiglottis<br>Wheezing<br>Stridor<br>Rhinitis | Hyperventilation<br>Crackles<br>Respiratory alkalosis → respiratory acidosis<br>Hypoxemia<br>Respiratory failure<br>ARDS<br>Pulmonary hypertension | Tachypnea → bradypnea (late)<br>Shortness of breath |
| **Renal System** | | | | | |
| ↑ $Na^+$ and $H_2O$ retention<br>↓ Renal blood flow<br>↓ Urine output | ↓ Urine output | Bladder dysfunction | Incontinence | ↓ Urine output | ↓ Urine output |
| **Skin** | | | | | |
| Pallor<br>Cool, clammy | Pallor<br>Cool, clammy | ↓ Skin perfusion<br>Cool or warm<br>Dry | Flushing<br>Pruritus<br>Urticaria<br>Angioedema | Warm and flushed → cool and mottled (late) | Pallor<br>Cool, clammy |
| **Neurologic System** | | | | | |
| ↓ Cerebral perfusion:<br>• Anxiety<br>• Confusion<br>• Agitation | ↓ Cerebral perfusion:<br>• Anxiety<br>• Confusion<br>• Agitation | Flaccid paralysis below the level of the lesion<br>Loss of reflex activity | Anxiety<br>Feeling of impending doom<br>Confusion<br>↓ LOC<br>Metallic taste | Alteration in mental status (e.g., confusion)<br>Agitation<br>Coma (late) | ↓ Cerebral perfusion:<br>• Anxiety<br>• Confusion<br>• Agitation |
| **Gastrointestinal System** | | | | | |
| ↓ Bowel sounds<br>Nausea, vomiting | Absent bowel sounds | Bowel dysfunction | Cramping<br>Abdominal pain<br>Nausea<br>Vomiting<br>Diarrhea | GI bleeding<br>Paralytic ileus | ↓ to absent bowel sounds |
| **Diagnostic Findings*** | | | | | |
| ↑ Cardiac biomarkers<br>↑ b-Type natriuretic peptide (BNP)<br>↑ Blood glucose<br>↑ BUN<br>ECG (e.g., dysrhythmias)<br>Echocardiogram (e.g., left ventricular dysfunction)<br>Chest x-ray (e.g., pulmonary infiltrates) | ↓ Hematocrit<br>↓ Hemoglobin<br>↑ Lactate<br>↑ Urine specific gravity<br>Changes in electrolytes | | Sudden onset<br>History of allergies<br>Exposure to contrast media | ↑/↓ WBC<br>↓ Platelets<br>↑ Lactate<br>↑ Blood glucose<br>↑ Procalcitonin<br>↑ Urine specific gravity<br>↓ Urine $Na^+$<br>Positive blood cultures | Specific to cause of obstruction |

*ARDS*, Acute respiratory distress syndrome; *BUN*, blood urea nitrogen; *LOC*, level of consciousness.
*Also see Table 66-2.

As capillary permeability increases, fluid leaks from the vascular space into the interstitial space.

Anaphylactic shock can lead to respiratory distress due to laryngeal edema or severe bronchospasm, and circulatory failure from the massive vasodilation.[7,8] The patient has a sudden onset of symptoms, including dizziness, chest pain, incontinence, swelling of the lips and tongue, wheezing, and stridor. Skin changes include flushing, pruritus, urticaria, and angioedema. In addition, the patient may be anxious and confused and have a sense of impending doom.

A patient can have a severe allergic reaction, possibly leading to anaphylactic shock, after contact, inhalation, ingestion, or injection with an antigen (allergen) to which the individual has previously been sensitized (Table 66-1). Parenteral administration of the antigen (allergen) is the route most likely to cause anaphylaxis. However, oral, topical, and inhalation routes can also cause anaphylactic reactions. Tables 66-2 and 66-3 describe the laboratory findings and clinical presentation of a patient in anaphylactic shock. Quick and decisive action is critical to prevent the progression of an

**PATHOPHYSIOLOGY MAP**

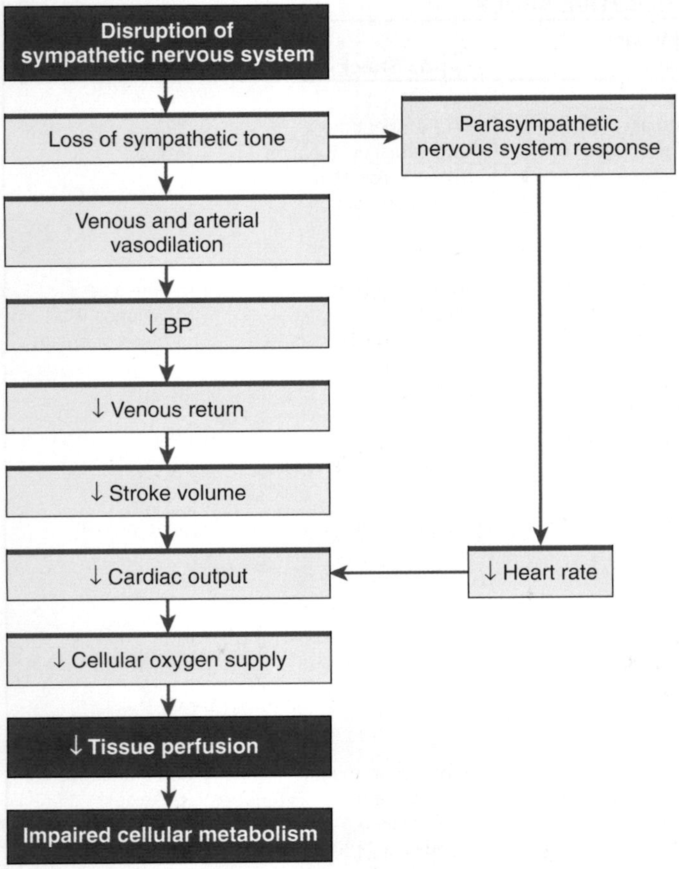


**FIG. 66-4** The pathophysiology of neurogenic shock. (Modified from Urden LD, Stacy KM, Lough ME: *Critical care nursing: diagnosis and management,* ed 6, St Louis, 2010, Mosby.)

**TABLE 66-4 Diagnostic Criteria for Sepsis**

Infection, documented or suspected, and some of the following:

**General Variables**
- Fever (temperature >100.9° F [38.3° C])
- Hypothermia (core temperature <97.0° F [36° C])
- Heart rate >90 beats/min
- Tachypnea (respiratory rate ≥ 22/min)
- SBP ≤ 100 mm Hg
- Altered mental status
- Significant edema or positive fluid balance (>20 mL/kg over 24 hr)
- Hyperglycemia (blood glucose >140 mg/dL) in the absence of diabetes

**Inflammatory Variables**
- Leukocytosis (WBC count >12,000/μL)
- Leukopenia (WBC count <4000/μL)
- Normal WBC count with >10% immature forms (bands)
- Elevated C-reactive protein
- Elevated procalcitonin

**Hemodynamic Variables**
- Arterial hypotension (SBP <90 mm Hg, MAP <70 mm Hg, or a decrease in SBP >40 mm Hg)

**Organ Dysfunction Variables**
- Arterial hypoxemia ($PaO_2/FIO_2$ <300)
- Acute oliguria (urine output <0.5 mL/kg/hr for at least 2 hr despite adequate fluid resuscitation)
- Serum creatinine increase >0.5 mg/dL
- Coagulation abnormalities (INR >1.5 or PTT >60 sec)
- Ileus (absent bowel sounds)
- Thrombocytopenia (platelet count <100,000/μL)
- Hyperbilirubinemia (total bilirubin >4 mg/dL)

**Tissue Perfusion Variables**
- Hyperlactatemia (>1 mmol/L)
- Decreased capillary refill or mottling

Sources: Dellinger RP, Levy MM, Rhodes A, et al: Surviving sepsis campaign: international guidelines for management of severe sepsis and septic shock: 2012, *Crit Care Med* 41:580, 2013; and Singer M, Deutschman CS, Seymour CW, et al: The third international consensus definitions for sepsis and septic shock (Sepsis-3), *JAMA* 315:801, 2016..

*$FIO_2$,* Fraction of inspired $O_2$; *INR,* international normalized ratio; *MAP,* mean arterial pressure; *$PaO_2$,* partial pressure of arterial $O_2$; *PTT,* partial thromboplastin time; *SBP,* systolic blood pressure.

allergic reaction to anaphylactic shock. (Anaphylaxis is discussed in Chapter 13.)

***Septic Shock.*** Sepsis is defined as a constellation of symptoms or syndrome in response to an infection. It is characterized by a dysregulated patient response along with new organ dysfunction related to the infection[9] (Table 66-4). In as many as 10% to 30% of patients with sepsis, the causative organism is not identified. Sepsis and septic shock have a high incidence worldwide with a mortality rate of 25% or higher.[10]

Septic shock is a subset of sepsis with an increased mortality risk due to profound circulatory, cellular, and metabolic abnormalities. Septic shock is characterized by persistent hypotension despite adequate fluid resuscitation requiring vasopressors, along with inadequate tissue perfusion resulting in tissue hypoxia.[9] The main organisms that cause sepsis are gram-negative and gram-positive bacteria. Parasites, fungi, and viruses can also cause sepsis and septic shock.[9] Fig. 66-5 presents the pathophysiology of septic shock.

When a microorganism enters the body, the normal immune or inflammatory responses are triggered. However, in sepsis and septic shock the body's response to the microorganism is exaggerated. Both proinflammatory and antiinflammatory responses are activated, coagulation increases, and fibrinolysis decreases.[9] Endotoxins from the microorganism cell wall stimulate the release of cytokines, including tumor necrosis factor (TNF), interleukin-1 (IL-1), and other proinflammatory mediators that act through secondary mediators such as platelet-activating factor, IL-6, and IL-8.[9] (See Chapter 11 for discussion of the inflammatory response.) The release of platelet-activating factor results in the formation of microthrombi and obstruction of the microvasculature. The combined effects of the mediators result in damage to the endothelium, vasodilation, increased capillary permeability, and neutrophil and platelet aggregation and adhesion to the endothelium.

Septic shock has three major pathophysiologic effects: vasodilation, maldistribution of blood flow, and myocardial depression. Patients may be euvolemic, but because of acute vasodilation, relative hypovolemia and hypotension occur. In addition, blood flow in the microcirculation is decreased, causing poor $O_2$ delivery and tissue hypoxia. The combination of TNF and IL-1 is thought to have a role in sepsis-induced myocardial dysfunction. The ejection fraction is decreased for the first few days after the initial insult. Because of a decreased ejection fraction, the ventricles dilate to maintain the SV. The ejection fraction typically improves, and ventricular dilation

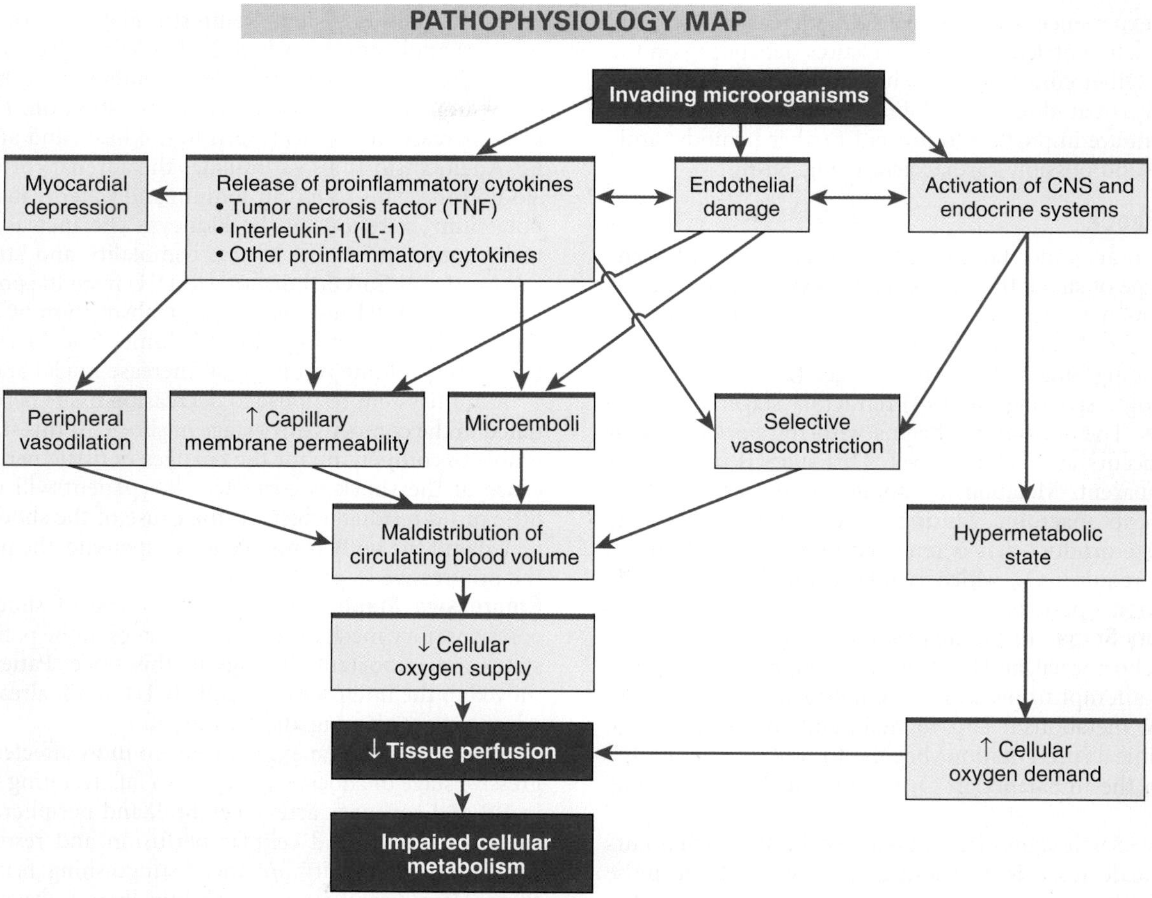


**FIG. 66-5** The pathophysiology of septic shock. *CNS,* Central nervous system. (Modified from Urden LD, Stacy KM, Lough ME: *Critical care nursing: diagnosis and management,* ed 6, St Louis, 2010, Mosby.)

resolves over 7 to 10 days. Persistence of a high CO and a low SVR beyond 24 hours is an ominous finding and is often associated with an increased development of hypotension and MODS. Coronary artery perfusion and myocardial $O_2$ metabolism are not primarily altered in septic shock.

In addition to the cardiovascular dysfunction that accompanies sepsis, respiratory failure is common. The patient initially hyperventilates as a compensatory mechanism, resulting in respiratory alkalosis. Once the patient can no longer compensate, respiratory acidosis develops. Respiratory failure develops in 85% of patients with sepsis, and 40% develop acute respiratory distress syndrome (ARDS) (see Chapter 67). These patients may need to be intubated and mechanically ventilated.

Other clinical signs of septic shock include alteration in neurologic status; decreased urine output; and GI dysfunction, such as GI bleeding and paralytic ileus. Table 66-3 gives the clinical presentation of a patient with septic shock.

**Obstructive Shock.** Obstructive shock develops when a physical obstruction to blood flow occurs with a decreased CO (Fig. 66-6). This can be caused by restricted diastolic filling of the right ventricle from compression (e.g., cardiac tamponade, tension pneumothorax, superior vena cava syndrome). Other causes include *abdominal compartment syndrome,* in which increased abdominal pressures compress the inferior vena cava, thus decreasing venous return to the heart (see Chapter 42). Pulmonary embolism and right ventricular thrombi cause an outflow obstruction as blood leaves the right ventricle through the pulmonary artery. This leads to decreased blood flow to the lungs and decreased blood return to the left atrium.

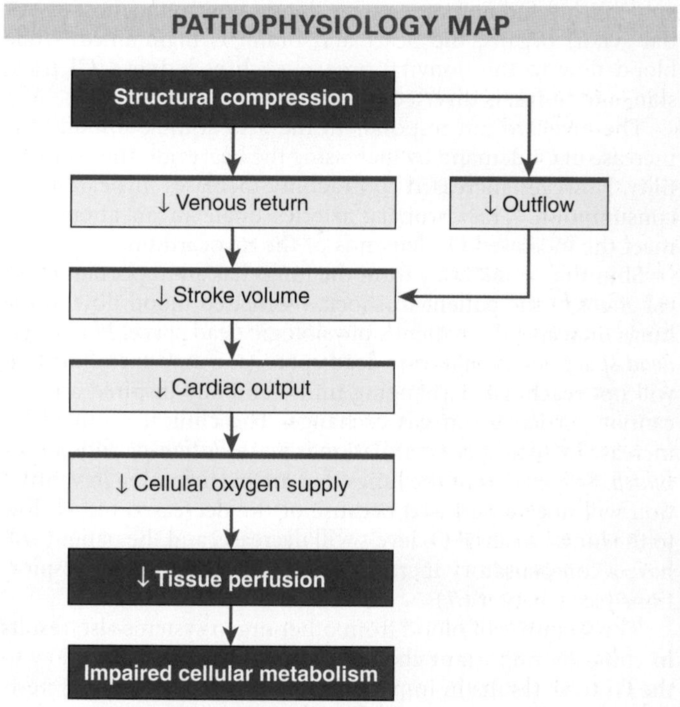


**FIG. 66-6** The pathophysiology of obstructive shock.

Patients experience a decreased CO, increased afterload, and variable left ventricular filling pressures depending on the obstruction. Other clinical signs include jugular venous distention and pulsus paradoxus (see Table 36-5). Rapid assessment and treatment are important to prevent further hemodynamic compromise and possibly cardiac arrest (Fig. 66-6).

### Stages of Shock

In addition to an understanding of the underlying pathogenesis of the type of shock that the patient is experiencing, monitoring and management are guided by knowing where the patient is on the shock "continuum." Shock is categorized into four overlapping stages: (1) initial stage, (2) compensatory stage, (3) progressive stage, and (4) refractory stage.[11]

**Initial Stage.** The continuum begins with the *initial stage* of shock that occurs at a cellular level. This stage is usually not clinically apparent. Metabolism changes at the cellular level from aerobic to anaerobic, causing lactic acid buildup. Lactic acid is a waste product that is removed by the liver. However, this process requires $O_2$, which is unavailable because of the decrease in tissue perfusion.

**Compensatory Stage.** In the *compensatory stage* the body activates neural, hormonal, and biochemical compensatory mechanisms in an attempt to overcome the increasing consequences of anaerobic metabolism and to maintain homeostasis. The patient's clinical presentation begins to reflect the body's responses to the imbalance in $O_2$ supply and demand (Table 66-5).

One of the classic signs of shock is a drop in BP, which occurs because of a decrease in CO and a narrowing of the pulse pressure. The baroreceptors in the carotid and aortic bodies immediately respond by activating the SNS. The SNS stimulates vasoconstriction and the release of the potent vasoconstrictors epinephrine and norepinephrine. Blood flow to the most essential (vital) organs, the heart and brain, is maintained, while blood flow to the nonvital organs, such as kidneys, GI tract, skin, and lungs, is diverted or shunted.

The myocardium responds to the SNS stimulation and the increase in $O_2$ demand by increasing the heart rate and contractility. However, increased contractility increases myocardial $O_2$ consumption. The coronary arteries dilate in an attempt to meet the increased $O_2$ demands of the myocardium.

Shunting blood away from the lungs has an important clinical effect in the patient in shock. Decreased blood flow to the lungs increases the patient's physiologic dead space. *Physiologic dead space* is the anatomic dead space (the amount of air that will not reach gas-exchanging units) and any inspired air that cannot participate in gas exchange. The clinical result of an increase in dead space ventilation is a *ventilation-perfusion mismatch.* Some areas of the lungs that are participating in ventilation will not be perfused because of the decreased blood flow to the lungs. Arterial $O_2$ levels will decrease, and the patient will have a compensatory increase in the rate and depth of respirations (see Chapter 67).

The shunting of blood from other organ systems also results in clinically important changes. The decrease in blood flow to the GI tract results in impaired motility and a slowing of peristalsis. This increases the risk for the development of a paralytic ileus.

Decreased blood flow to the skin results in the patient feeling cool and clammy. The exception is the patient in early septic shock who may feel warm and flushed because of a hyperdynamic state. Decreased blood flow to the kidneys activates the renin-angiotensin system. Renin stimulates angiotensinogen to produce angiotensin I, which is then converted to angiotensin II (see Fig. 44-4). Angiotensin II is a potent vasoconstrictor that causes both arterial and venous vasoconstriction. The net result is an increase in venous return to the heart and an increase in BP. Angiotensin II also stimulates the adrenal cortex to release aldosterone. This results in sodium and water reabsorption and potassium excretion by the kidneys. The increase in sodium reabsorption raises the serum osmolality and stimulates the release of antidiuretic hormone (ADH) from the posterior pituitary gland. ADH increases water reabsorption by the kidneys, thus further increasing blood volume. The increase in total circulating volume results in an increase in CO and BP.

A multisystem response to decreasing tissue perfusion is initiated in the compensatory stage of shock. At this stage the body is able to compensate for the changes in tissue perfusion. If the cause of the shock is corrected, the patient will recover with little or no residual effects. If the cause of the shock is not corrected and the body is unable to compensate, the patient enters the progressive stage of shock.

**Progressive Stage.** The *progressive stage* of shock begins as compensatory mechanisms fail. Changes in the patient's mental status are important findings in this stage. Patients must be moved to the intensive care unit (ICU), if not already there, for advanced monitoring and treatment.

The cardiovascular system is profoundly affected in the progressive stage of shock. CO begins to fall, resulting in a decrease in BP and coronary artery, cerebral, and peripheral perfusion. Continued decreased cellular perfusion and resulting altered capillary permeability are the distinguishing features of this stage. Altered capillary permeability allows leakage of fluid and protein out of the vascular space into the surrounding interstitial space. In addition to the decrease in circulating volume, there is an increase in systemic interstitial edema. The patient may have *anasarca* (diffuse profound edema). Fluid leakage from the vascular space also affects the solid organs (e.g., liver, spleen, GI tract, lungs) and peripheral tissues by further decreasing perfusion.

Sustained hypoperfusion results in weak peripheral pulses, and ischemia of the distal extremities eventually occurs. Myocardial dysfunction from decreased perfusion results in dysrhythmias, myocardial ischemia, and possibly MI. The end result is a complete deterioration of the cardiovascular system.

The pulmonary system is often the first system to display signs of critical dysfunction. During the compensatory stage, blood flow to the lungs is already reduced. In response to the decreased blood flow and the SNS stimulation, the pulmonary arterioles constrict, resulting in increased pulmonary artery (PA) pressure. As the pressure within the pulmonary vasculature increases, blood flow to the pulmonary capillaries decreases and ventilation-perfusion mismatch worsens.

Another key response in the lungs is the movement of fluid from the pulmonary vasculature into the interstitial space. As capillary permeability increases, the movement of fluid to the interstitial spaces results in interstitial edema, bronchoconstriction, and a decrease in functional residual capacity. With further increases in capillary permeability, the fluid moves to the alveoli, with resultant alveolar edema and a decrease in surfactant production. The combined effects of pulmonary vasoconstriction and bronchoconstriction are impaired gas exchange, decreased compliance, and worsening ventilation-perfusion mismatch. Clinically, the patient has tachypnea, crackles, and an overall increased work of breathing.

**TABLE 66-5 Manifestations of Stages of Shock***

| Compensatory Stage | Progressive Stage | Refractory Stage |
|---|---|---|
| **Neurologic System** | | |
| Oriented to person, place, time<br>Restless, apprehensive, confused<br>Change in level of consciousness | ↓ Cerebral perfusion pressure<br>↓ Cerebral blood flow<br>↓ Responsiveness to stimuli<br>Delirium | Unresponsive<br>Areflexia (loss of reflexes)<br>Pupils nonreactive and dilated |
| **Cardiovascular System** | | |
| Sympathetic nervous system response:<br>• Release of epinephrine/norepinephrine (vasoconstriction)<br>• ↑ $MVO_2$<br>• ↑ Contractility<br>• ↑ HR<br>Coronary artery dilation<br>Narrowed pulse pressure<br>↓ BP | ↑ Capillary permeability → systemic interstitial edema<br>↓ Cardiac output → ↓ BP and ↑ HR<br>MAP <60 mm Hg (or 40 mm Hg drop in BP from baseline)<br>↓ Coronary perfusion → dysrhythmias, myocardial ischemia, myocardial infarction<br>↓ Peripheral perfusion → ischemia of distal extremities, diminished pulses, ↓ capillary refill | Profound hypotension<br>↓ Cardiac output<br>Bradycardia, irregular rhythm<br>↓ BP inadequate to perfuse vital organs |
| **Respiratory System** | | |
| ↓ Blood flow to the lungs:<br>• ↑ Physiologic dead space<br>• ↑ Ventilation-perfusion mismatch<br>• Hyperventilation<br>• ↑ Minute ventilation ($V_E$)<br>• Tachypnea | Acute respiratory distress syndrome (ARDS):<br>• ↑ Capillary permeability<br>• Pulmonary vasoconstriction<br>• Pulmonary interstitial edema<br>• Alveolar edema<br>• Diffuse infiltrates<br>• Tachypnea<br>• ↓ Compliance<br>• Moist crackles | Severe refractory hypoxemia<br>Respiratory failure |
| **Gastrointestinal System** | | |
| ↓ Blood supply<br>↓ GI motility<br>Hypoactive bowel sounds<br>↑ Risk for paralytic ileus | Vasoconstriction and ↓ perfusion → ischemic gut (e.g., stomach, small and large intestines, gallbladder, pancreas)<br>• Erosive ulcers<br>• GI bleeding<br>• Translocation of GI bacteria<br>• Impaired absorption of nutrients | Ischemic gut |
| **Renal System** | | |
| ↓ Renal blood flow<br>↑ Renin resulting in release of angiotensin (vasoconstrictor)<br>↑ Aldosterone resulting in $Na^+$ and $H_2O$ reabsorption<br>↑ Antidiuretic hormone resulting in $H_2O$ reabsorption | Renal tubules become ischemic → acute tubular necrosis<br>↓ Urine output<br>↑ BUN/creatinine ratio<br>↑ Urine sodium<br>↓ Urine osmolality and specific gravity<br>↓ Urine potassium<br>Metabolic acidosis | Anuria |
| **Hepatic System** | | |
| | Failure to metabolize drugs and waste products<br>Cell death (↑ liver enzymes)<br>Jaundice (decreased clearance of bilirubin)<br>↑ $NH_3$ and lactate | Metabolic changes from accumulation of waste products (e.g., $NH_3$, lactate, $CO_2$) |
| **Hematologic System** | | |
| | DIC<br>• Thrombin clots in microcirculation<br>• Consumption of platelets and clotting factors | DIC progresses |
| **Temperature** | | |
| Normal or abnormal | Hypothermia or hyperthermia | Hypothermia |
| **Skin** | | |
| Pale and cool<br>Warm and flushed | Cold and clammy | Mottled, cyanotic |

*DIC*, Disseminated intravascular coagulation; *MAP*, mean arterial pressure; *$MVO_2$*, myocardial $O_2$ consumption; *$NH_3$*, ammonia.
*The shock continuum begins with the *initial stage* of shock. This stage occurs at the cellular level and is usually not clinically apparent. Also see Table 66-2 and Table 66-3.

The GI system is also affected by prolonged decreased tissue perfusion. As the blood supply to the GI tract is decreased, the normally protective mucosal barrier becomes ischemic. This ischemia predisposes the patient to ulcers and GI bleeding (see Chapter 41). It also increases the risk of bacterial migration from the GI tract to the blood. The decreased perfusion to the GI tract also leads to a decreased ability to absorb nutrients.

The effect of prolonged hypoperfusion on the kidneys is renal tubular ischemia. The resulting acute tubular necrosis may lead to acute kidney injury. This can be worsened by nephrotoxic drugs (e.g., certain antibiotics, anesthetics, diuretics) (see

Chapter 46). The patient has decreased urine output and elevated blood urea nitrogen (BUN) and serum creatinine. Metabolic acidosis occurs from the kidneys' inability to excrete acids (especially lactic acid) and reabsorb bicarbonate.

Other organ systems are also affected by the sustained hypoperfusion in the progressive stage of shock. The loss of the functional ability of the liver leads to a failure of the liver to metabolize drugs and waste products (e.g., lactate, ammonia). Jaundice results from an accumulation of bilirubin. As the liver cells die, enzymes become elevated (e.g., alanine aminotransferase [ALT], aspartate aminotransferase [AST], γ-glutamyl transferase [GGT]). The liver also loses its ability to function as an immune organ. Bacteria that may move from the GI tract are no longer destroyed by the Kupffer cells. Instead, they are released into the bloodstream, thus increasing the possibility of bacteremia.

Dysfunction of the hematologic system adds to the complexity of the clinical picture. The patient is at risk for disseminated intravascular coagulation (DIC). The consumption of the platelets and clotting factors with secondary fibrinolysis results in clinically significant bleeding from many orifices. These include, but are not limited to, the GI tract, lungs, and puncture sites (see Chapter 30). Altered laboratory values in DIC are presented in Table 66-3.

In this stage, aggressive interventions are necessary to prevent the development of MODS.

**Refractory Stage.** In the final stage of shock, the *refractory stage,* decreased perfusion from peripheral vasoconstriction and decreased CO exacerbate anaerobic metabolism. The accumulation of lactic acid contributes to increased capillary permeability and dilation. Increased capillary permeability allows fluid and plasma proteins to leave the vascular space and move to the interstitial space. Blood pools in the capillary beds secondary to the constricted venules and dilated arterioles. The loss of intravascular volume worsens hypotension and tachycardia and decreases coronary blood flow. Decreased coronary blood flow leads to worsening myocardial depression and a further decline in CO. Cerebral blood flow cannot be maintained and cerebral ischemia results.

The patient in this stage of shock demonstrates profound hypotension and hypoxemia. The failure of the liver, lungs, and kidneys results in an accumulation of waste products, such as lactate, urea, ammonia, and $CO_2$. The failure of one organ system affects several other organ systems. Recovery is unlikely in this stage. The organs are in failure and the body's compensatory mechanisms are overwhelmed (Table 66-5).

## Diagnostic Studies

There is no single diagnostic study to determine whether a patient is in shock. The diagnosis starts with a history and physical examination. Obtaining a thorough medical and surgical history, and a history of recent events (e.g., surgery, chest pain, trauma), provides valuable data.

Decreased tissue perfusion in shock leads to an elevation of lactate and a base deficit (the amount needed to bring the pH back to normal). These laboratory changes may reflect an increase in anaerobic metabolism. Table 66-2 summarizes other laboratory findings seen in shock.

Additional diagnostic studies include a 12-lead electrocardiogram (ECG), continuous ECG monitoring, chest x-ray, continuous pulse oximetry, and invasive and noninvasive hemodynamic monitoring. (Chapter 65 discusses hemodynamic monitoring.)

## Interprofessional Care: General Measures

Critical factors in the successful management of a patient experiencing shock relate to the early recognition and treatment of the shock state. Prompt intervention in the early stages of shock may prevent the decline to the progressive or irreversible stage. Successful management of the patient in shock includes the following:

1. Identification of patients at risk for developing shock
2. Integration of the patient's history, physical examination, and clinical findings to establish a diagnosis
3. Interventions to control or eliminate the cause of the decreased perfusion
4. Protection of target and distal organs from dysfunction
5. Provision of multisystem supportive care

Table 66-6 provides an overview of the initial assessment findings and interventions for the emergency care of patients in shock.[12] General management strategies begin with ensuring that the patient is responsive and has a patent airway. Once the airway is established, either naturally or with an endotracheal tube, $O_2$ delivery must be optimized. Supplemental $O_2$ and mechanical ventilation may be necessary to maintain an arterial $O_2$ saturation of 90% or more ($PaO_2$ greater than 60 mm Hg) to avoid hypoxemia (see Chapter 65). The mean arterial pressure (MAP) and circulating blood volume are optimized with fluid replacement and drug therapy.

**Oxygen and Ventilation.** $O_2$ delivery depends on CO, available hemoglobin, and arterial $O_2$ saturation ($SaO_2$). Methods to optimize $O_2$ delivery are directed at increasing supply and decreasing demand. Supply is increased by (1) optimizing the CO with fluid replacement or drug therapy, (2) increasing the hemoglobin through transfusion of whole blood or packed red blood cells (RBCs), and/or (3) increasing the arterial $O_2$ saturation with supplemental $O_2$ and mechanical ventilation.

Plan care to avoid disrupting the balance of $O_2$ supply and demand. Space activities that increase $O_2$ consumption (e.g., endotracheal suctioning, position changes) appropriately for $O_2$ conservation. Intermittent or continuous monitoring of $ScvO_2$ by a central venous catheter or mixed venous $O_2$ saturation ($SvO_2$) may be helpful. Both reflect the dynamic balance between $O_2$ supply and demand. Assess these values along with related hemodynamic measures (e.g., arterial pressure–based cardiac output [APCO], $O_2$ consumption, hemoglobin) to evaluate the patient's response to treatments or activities (see Chapter 65).

**Fluid Resuscitation.** The cornerstone of therapy for septic, hypovolemic, and anaphylactic shock is volume expansion with administration of the appropriate fluid. Fluid resuscitation should start using one or two large-bore (e.g., 14- to 16-gauge) IV catheters; an intraosseous (IO) access device; or a central venous catheter. Both crystalloids (e.g., normal saline, lactated Ringer's) and colloids (e.g., albumin) have a role in fluid resuscitation (Table 66-7; see Table 16-17).

**! SAFETY ALERT Intraosseous (IO) Access**

- Use an IO access device for emergency resuscitation when IV access cannot be obtained.
- Insertion sites include sternum, proximal and distal tibia, and proximal and distal humerus.
- Remove IO devices within 24 hours of insertion or as soon as possible after peripheral or central IV access is obtained.
- Monitor for complications: extravasation of drugs and fluids into the soft tissue, fractures caused during insertion, and osteomyelitis.

## TABLE 66-6 Emergency Management

### Shock

| Etiology* | Assessment Findings | Interventions |
|---|---|---|
| **Surgical**<br>• Postoperative bleeding<br>• Ruptured organ or vessel<br>• Gastrointestinal bleeding<br>• Aortic dissection<br>• Vaginal bleeding<br>• Ruptured ectopic pregnancy or ovarian cyst<br>**Medical**<br>• Myocardial infarction<br>• Dehydration<br>• Addisonian crisis<br>• Diabetes insipidus<br>• Sepsis<br>• Diabetes mellitus<br>• Pulmonary embolus<br>**Trauma**<br>• Ruptured or lacerated vessel or organ (e.g., spleen)<br>• Fractures, spinal injury<br>• Multiorgan injury | • Restlessness<br>• Confusion<br>• Anxiety<br>• Feeling of impending doom<br>• Decreased level of consciousness<br>• Weakness<br>• Rapid, weak, thready pulses<br>• Dysrhythmias<br>• Hypotension<br>• Narrowed pulse pressure<br>• Cool, clammy skin (warm skin in early onset of septic and neurogenic shock)<br>• Tachypnea, dyspnea, or shallow, irregular respirations<br>• Decreased $O_2$ saturation<br>• Extreme thirst<br>• Nausea and vomiting<br>• Chills<br>• Pallor<br>• Cyanosis<br>• Obvious hemorrhage or injury<br>• Temperature dysregulation | **Initial**<br>• If unresponsive, assess circulation, airway, and breathing (CAB).<br>• If responsive, monitor airway, breathing, and circulation (ABC).<br>• Stabilize cervical spine as appropriate.<br>• Control any external bleeding with direct pressure or pressure dressing.<br>• Give high-flow $O_2$ (100%) by non-rebreather mask or bag-valve-mask.<br>• Anticipate need for intubation and mechanical ventilation.<br>• Establish IV access with two large-bore catheters (14- to 16-gauge) or an intraosseous access device, or assist with insertion of central line.<br>• Begin fluid resuscitation with crystalloids (e.g., 30 mL/kg repeated until hemodynamic improvement is noted).<br>• Draw blood for laboratory studies (e.g., blood cultures, lactate, WBC).<br>• Assess for life-threatening injuries (e.g., cardiac tamponade, liver laceration, tension pneumothorax).<br>• Consider vasopressor therapy if hypotension persists after fluid resuscitation.<br>• Insert an indwelling urinary catheter and nasogastric tube.<br>• Start antibiotic therapy after blood cultures if sepsis is suspected.<br>• Obtain 12-lead ECG and treat dysrhythmias.<br>**Ongoing Monitoring**<br>• ABCs<br>• Level of consciousness<br>• Vital signs, including pulse oximetry; peripheral pulses, capillary refill, skin color and temperature<br>• Respiratory status<br>• Heart rate and rhythm<br>• Urine output |

*See Table 66-1 for additional causes of shock.

## TABLE 66-7 Fluid Therapy in Shock

| Fluid Type | Mechanism of Action | Type of Shock | Nursing Implications |
|---|---|---|---|
| **Crystalloids** | | | |
| ***Isotonic*** | | | |
| • 0.9% NaCl (NSS)<br>• Lactated Ringer's (LR) | Fluid primarily remains in the intravascular space, increasing intravascular volume. | Used for initial volume replacement in most types of shock. | Monitor patient closely for circulatory overload. Do not use LR in patients with liver failure. LR may be used if hyperchloremic acidosis develops from use of NSS in fluid resuscitation. |
| ***Hypertonic*** | | | |
| • 1.8%, 3%, 5% NaCl | Fluid remains in the intravascular space, increases serum osmolarity, shifts fluid volume from intracellular space to extracellular space to intravascular space. | May be used for initial volume expansion in hypovolemic shock. | Monitor patient closely for signs of hypernatremia (e.g., disorientation, convulsions).<br>Central line preferred for infusing saline solutions ≥3%, since these may damage veins. |
| **Blood or Blood Products** | | | |
| Packed red blood cells | Replaces blood loss, increases $O_2$-carrying capability. | All types of shock. | Same precautions as any blood administration (see Chapter 30). |
| Fresh frozen plasma | Replaces coagulation factors. | | |
| Platelets | Helps control bleeding caused by thrombocytopenia. | | |
| **Colloids** | | | |
| Human serum albumin (5% or 25%) | Can increase plasma colloid osmotic pressure. Rapid volume expansion. | All types of shock except cardiogenic and neurogenic shock. | Use 5% solution in hypovolemic patients. Use 25% solution in patients with fluid and sodium restrictions.<br>Monitor for circulatory overload. Mild side effects of chills, fever, and urticaria may develop.<br>More expensive than crystalloids. |
| dextran (dextran 40) | Hyperosmotic glucose polymer. | Limited use because of side effects, including reducing platelet adhesion, diluting clotting factors. | Increases risk of bleeding.<br>Important to monitor patient for allergic reactions and acute kidney injury.<br>Has maximum volume recommendations per manufacturer. |

*NSS,* Normal saline solution.

The ideal choice of fluid for resuscitation remains controversial. Currently, normal saline is most often used in the initial resuscitation of shock. While large volume resuscitation with normal saline can lead to hyperchloremic metabolic acidosis, lactated Ringer's solution may also cause serum lactate levels to increase because the failing liver cannot convert lactate to bicarbonate.[13] In some cases, hypertonic saline may be considered to expand plasma volume.

Colloids (4% to 5%) are effective volume expanders because the size of their molecules keeps them in the vascular space for a longer time. However, colloids are costly. Studies have shown that they are safe to use, but none have shown that using colloids versus crystalloids for resuscitation improves patient outcomes.[14]

The choice of resuscitation fluid is also based on the type and volume of fluid lost and the patient's clinical status. *Fluid responsiveness* is determined by clinical assessment. This includes vital signs, cerebral and abdominal perfusion pressures, capillary refill, skin temperature and urine output. Hemodynamic parameters, such as SVV or CO, are also used.[15] Monitor trends in BP with an automatic BP cuff or an arterial catheter to assess the patient's response. Use an indwelling urinary catheter to monitor urine output during resuscitation.

When large amounts of fluids are required, you must protect the patient against two major complications: hypothermia and coagulopathy. If the patient has persistent hypotension after adequate fluid resuscitation, a vasopressor (e.g., norepinephrine [Levophed], dopamine) and/or an inotrope (e.g., dobutamine) may be added. The goal for fluid resuscitation is restoration of tissue perfusion. Thus decisions on which drug to use should be based on the physiologic goal. Although BP helps determine whether the patient's CO is adequate, an assessment of end-organ perfusion (e.g., urine output, neurologic function, peripheral pulses) provides more relevant data.

**! SAFETY ALERT Fluid Resuscitation**

- Warm crystalloid and colloid solutions during massive fluid resuscitation.
- When administering large volumes of packed RBCs, remember that they do not contain clotting factors. Replace these factors based on the clinical situation and laboratory studies.

**Drug Therapy.** The primary goal of drug therapy for shock is the correction of decreased tissue perfusion. Drugs used to improve perfusion in shock are given IV via an infusion pump and central venous line. Many of these drugs have vasoconstrictor properties that are harmful if the drug extravasates while being infused peripherally (Table 66-8).

***Sympathomimetic Drugs.*** Many of the drugs used in the treatment of shock have an effect on the SNS. Drugs that mimic the action of the SNS are termed *sympathomimetic.* The effects of these drugs are mediated through their binding to $\alpha$- or $\beta$-adrenergic receptors. The various drugs differ in their relative $\alpha$- and $\beta$-adrenergic effects. (See Chapter 32 and Table 32-7.)

Many of the sympathomimetic drugs cause peripheral vasoconstriction and are called *vasopressor drugs* (e.g., norepinephrine, dopamine, phenylephrine). These drugs can cause severe peripheral vasoconstriction and an increase in SVR, further risking tissue perfusion. The increased SVR increases the workload of the heart and can harm a patient in cardiogenic shock by causing further myocardial damage. Use of vasopressor drugs is limited to patients who do not respond to fluid resuscitation. Adequate fluid resuscitation must be achieved before starting vasopressors because the vasoconstrictor effects in patients with low blood volume will cause further reduction in tissue perfusion.

The goal of vasopressor therapy is to achieve and maintain a MAP of greater than 65 mm Hg.[10] Continuously monitor end-organ perfusion (e.g., urine output, level of consciousness) and serum lactate levels (e.g., every 3 hours for the first 6 hours) to ensure that tissue perfusion is adequate.

***Vasodilator Drugs.*** Patients in cardiogenic shock have decreased myocardial contractility, and vasodilators may be needed to decrease afterload. This reduces myocardial workload and $O_2$ requirements. Although generalized sympathetic vasoconstriction is a useful compensatory mechanism for maintaining BP, excessive constriction can reduce tissue blood flow and increase the workload of the heart. The rationale for using vasodilator therapy for a patient in shock is to break the harmful cycle of widespread vasoconstriction causing a decrease in CO and BP, resulting in further sympathetic-induced vasoconstriction.

The goal of vasodilator therapy, as in vasopressor therapy, is to maintain the MAP greater than 65 mm Hg. Monitor hemodynamic parameters (e.g., CVP, CO, $ScvO_2/SvO_2$, SV, PA pressures) along with physical assessment so that fluids can be increased or vasodilator therapy decreased if a serious fall in CO or BP occurs. The vasodilator agent most often used for the patient in cardiogenic shock is nitroglycerin. Vasodilation may be enhanced with nitroprusside or nitroglycerin in noncardiogenic shock.

**Nutritional Therapy.** Protein-calorie malnutrition is one of the main manifestations of hypermetabolism in shock. Nutrition is vital to reducing mortality. Enteral nutrition should be started within the first 24 hours. However, full calorie replacement is not recommended for previously well-nourished adults early on in critical illness.[16] Generally, parenteral nutrition is used only if enteral feedings are contraindicated. (Chapter 39 discusses parenteral and enteral nutrition.)

Start the patient on a *trophic feeding.* This is defined as a slow drip of small amounts of enteral nutrition (e.g., 10 mL/hr). Early enteral feedings enhance the perfusion of the GI tract and help maintain the integrity of the gut mucosa. Advance feedings as tolerated and as prescribed.

Weigh the patient daily on the same scale (usually the bed scale) at the same time of day. If the patient has a significant weight loss, rule out dehydration before adding more calories. Large weight gains are common because of third spacing of fluids. Therefore daily weights serve as a better indicator of fluid status than caloric needs. Serum protein, total albumin, prealbumin, BUN, serum glucose, and serum electrolytes are all used to assess nutritional status.

## Interprofessional Care: Specific Measures

**Cardiogenic Shock.** For a patient in cardiogenic shock, the overall goal is to restore blood flow to the myocardium by restoring the balance between $O_2$ supply and demand. Cardiac catheterization is performed as soon as possible after the initial insult. Specific measures to restore blood flow include angioplasty with stenting, emergency revascularization, and valve replacement (see Chapter 33). Until these interventions are done, the heart must be supported to optimize SV and CO to achieve optimal perfusion (Tables 66-8 and 66-9).

Hemodynamic management of a patient in cardiogenic shock aims to reduce the workload of the heart through drug

## TABLE 66-8 Drug Therapy

### Shock

| Drug* | Mechanism of Action | Type of Shock | Nursing Implications |
|---|---|---|---|
| dobutamine | ↑ Myocardial contractility<br>↓ Ventricular filling pressures<br>↓ SVR, PAWP<br>↑ CO, stroke volume, CVP<br>↑/↓ HR | Used in cardiogenic shock with severe systolic dysfunction<br>Used in septic shock to increase $O_2$ delivery and raise $ScvO_2$ or $SvO_2$ to 70% if Hgb >7 g/dL or Hct ≥30% | Administration via central line is recommended (infiltration leads to tissue sloughing).<br>Do not administer in same line with $NaHCO_3$.<br>Monitor HR, BP (hypotension may worsen, requiring addition of a vasopressor).<br>Stop infusion if tachydysrhythmias develop. |
| dopamine | Positive inotropic effects:<br>↑ Myocardial contractility<br>↑ Automaticity<br>↑ Atrioventricular conduction<br>↑ HR, CO<br>↑ BP, ↑ MAP<br>↑ $MVO_2$<br>Can cause progressive vasoconstriction at high doses | Cardiogenic shock | Administration via central line is recommended (infiltration leads to tissue sloughing).<br>Do not give in same line with $NaHCO_3$.<br>Monitor for tachydysrhythmias.<br>Monitor for peripheral vasoconstriction (e.g., paresthesias, coldness in extremities) at moderate to high doses. |
| epinephrine (Adrenalin) | *Low doses:* β-Adrenergic agonist (cardiac stimulation, bronchodilation, peripheral vasodilation)<br>↑ HR, contractility, CO<br>↓ SVR<br>*High doses:* α-Adrenergic agonist (peripheral vasoconstriction)<br>↑ Stroke volume, SVR<br>↑ Systolic/↓ diastolic BP, widened pulse pressure<br>↑ CVP, PAWP | Cardiogenic shock<br>Anaphylactic shock<br>Septic shock requiring additional agent after norepinephrine<br>Cardiac arrest, pulseless ventricular tachycardia, ventricular fibrillation, asystole | Monitor for HR >110 beats/min.<br>Monitor for dyspnea, pulmonary edema.<br>Monitor for chest pain, dysrhythmias secondary to ↑ $MVO_2$.<br>Monitor for renal failure secondary to ischemia. |
| hydrocortisone (Solu-Cortef) | Decreases inflammation, reverses increased capillary permeability<br>↑ BP, HR | Septic shock requiring vasopressor therapy (despite fluid resuscitation) to maintain adequate BP<br>Anaphylactic shock if hypotension persists after initial therapy | Monitor for hypokalemia, hyperglycemia.<br>Consider use as continuous infusion. |
| norepinephrine (Levophed) | $\beta_1$-Adrenergic agonist (cardiac stimulation)<br>α-Adrenergic agonist (peripheral vasoconstriction)<br>Renal and splanchnic vasoconstriction<br>↑ BP, MAP, CVP, PAWP, SVR<br>↑/↓ CO | Cardiogenic shock after myocardial infarction<br>Septic shock—first drug of choice for BP unresponsive to adequate fluid resuscitation | Administration via central line is required (infiltration leads to tissue sloughing).<br>Monitor for dysrhythmias secondary to ↑ $MVO_2$ requirements. |
| phenylephrine | α-Adrenergic agonist (peripheral vasoconstriction)<br>Renal, mesenteric, splanchnic, cutaneous, and pulmonary blood vessel constriction<br>↑ HR, BP, SVR<br>↑/↓ CO | Neurogenic shock | Monitor for reflex bradycardia, headache, restlessness.<br>Monitor for renal failure secondary to ↓ renal blood flow.<br>Administration via central line is recommended (infiltration leads to tissue sloughing). |
| nitroglycerin | Venodilation<br>Dilates coronary arteries<br>↓ Preload, $MVO_2$, SVR, BP | Cardiogenic shock | Continuously monitor BP and HR, since reflex tachycardia may occur.<br>Glass bottle recommended for infusion. |
| sodium nitroprusside | Arterial and venous vasodilation<br>↓ Preload, afterload<br>↓ CVP, PAWP<br>↑/↓ CO<br>↓ BP | Cardiogenic shock with ↑ SVR | Continuously monitor BP.<br>Protect solution from light. Wrap infusion bottle with opaque covering.<br>Give with $D_5W$ only.<br>Monitor serum cyanide levels and for signs of cyanide toxicity (e.g., metabolic acidosis, tachycardia, altered level of consciousness, seizures, coma, almond smell on breath). |
| vasopressin | Antidiuretic hormone<br>Nonadrenergic vasoconstrictor<br>↑ MAP<br>↑ Urine output | Shock states (most commonly septic shock) refractory to other vasopressors | Administered with norepinephrine and in low doses.<br>Infusions are not titrated.<br>Monitor hemodynamic pressures and urine output. |

*CO,* Cardiac output; *CVP,* central venous pressure; *MAP,* mean arterial pressure; *$MVO_2$,* myocardial $O_2$ consumption; *PAWP,* pulmonary artery wedge pressure; *PT,* prothrombin time; *PTT,* partial thromboplastin time; *SVR,* systemic vascular resistance.

*Consult agency guidelines, pharmacist, pharmacology references, and drug manufacturer's administration materials for additional information and dosing recommendations.

## TABLE 66-9 Interprofessional Care

### *Shock*

| Oxygenation | Circulation | Drug Therapies | Supportive Therapies |
|---|---|---|---|
| **Cardiogenic Shock** | | | |
| • Provide supplemental $O_2$ (e.g., nasal cannula, non-rebreather mask)<br>• Intubation and mechanical ventilation, if necessary<br>• Monitor $ScvO_2$ or $SvO_2$ | • Restore blood flow with thrombolytics, angioplasty with stenting, emergent coronary revascularization<br>• Reduce workload of heart with circulatory assist devices: IABP, VAD | • Nitrates (e.g., nitroglycerin)<br>• Inotropes (e.g., dobutamine)<br>• Diuretics (e.g., furosemide)<br>• β-Adrenergic blockers (contraindicated with ↓ ejection fraction) | • Treat dysrhythmias |
| **Hypovolemic Shock** | | | |
| • Provide supplemental $O_2$<br>• Monitor $ScvO_2$ or $ScvO_2$ | • Rapid fluid replacement using two large-bore (14-16 gauge) peripheral IV lines, an intraosseous access device, or central venous catheter<br>• Restore fluid volume (e.g., blood or blood products, crystalloids)<br>• End points of fluid resuscitation:<br>  • CVP 15 mm Hg<br>  • PAWP 10-12 mm Hg | • No specific drug therapy | • Correct the cause (e.g., stop bleeding, GI losses)<br>• Use warmed IV fluids, including blood products (if appropriate) |
| **Septic Shock** | | | |
| • Provide supplemental $O_2$<br>• Intubation and mechanical ventilation, if necessary<br>• Monitor $ScvO_2$ or $SvO_2$ | • Aggressive fluid resuscitation (e.g., 30 mL/kg of crystalloids repeated as long as hemodynamic improvement is noted)<br>• End points of fluid resuscitation are based on:<br>1. Focused physical examination including vital signs, cardiopulmonary assessment, capillary refill, peripheral pulses, and skin or any 2 of the following:<br>  • $ScvO_2$ >70 or $SvO_2$ >65<br>  • CVP 8-12 mm Hg<br>  • Cardiovascular ultrasound<br>2. Assessment of fluid responsiveness with passive leg raise or fluid challenge | • Antibiotics as ordered<br>• Vasopressors (e.g., norepinephrine)<br>• Inotropes (e.g., dobutamine)<br>• Anticoagulants (e.g., low-molecular-weight heparin) | • Obtain cultures (e.g., blood, wound) before beginning antibiotics<br>• Monitor temperature<br>• Control blood glucose<br>• Stress ulcer prophylaxis |
| **Neurogenic Shock** | | | |
| • Maintain patent airway<br>• Provide supplemental $O_2$<br>• Intubation and mechanical ventilation (if necessary) | • Cautious administration of fluids | • Vasopressors (e.g., phenylephrine)<br>• Atropine (for bradycardia) | • Minimize spinal cord trauma with stabilization<br>• Monitor temperature |
| **Anaphylactic Shock** | | | |
| • Maintain patent airway<br>• Optimize oxygenation with supplemental $O_2$<br>• Intubation and mechanical ventilation, if necessary | • Aggressive fluid resuscitation with colloids | • Epinephrine (IM or IV)<br>• Antihistamines (e.g., diphenhydramine)<br>• Histamine ($H_2$)-receptor blockers (e.g., ranitidine [Zantac])<br>• Bronchodilators: nebulized (e.g., albuterol)<br>• Corticosteroids (if hypotension persists) | • Identify and remove offending cause<br>• Prevent via avoidance of known allergens<br>• Premedicate with history of prior sensitivity (e.g., contrast media) |
| **Obstructive Shock** | | | |
| • Maintain patent airway<br>• Provide supplemental $O_2$<br>• Intubation and mechanical ventilation, if necessary | • Restore circulation by treating cause of obstruction<br>• Fluid resuscitation may provide temporary improvement in CO and BP | • No specific drug therapy | • Treat cause of obstruction (e.g., pericardiocentesis for cardiac tamponade, needle decompression or chest tube insertion for tension pneumothorax, embolectomy for pulmonary embolism) |

*CO,* Cardiac output; *CVP,* central venous pressure; *IABP,* intraaortic balloon pump; *PAWP,* pulmonary artery wedge pressure; *VAD,* ventricular assist device.

therapy and/or mechanical interventions. Drug selection is based on the clinical goal and a thorough understanding of each drug's mechanism of action. Drugs can be used to decrease the workload of the heart by dilating coronary arteries (e.g., nitrates), reducing preload (e.g., diuretics), reducing afterload (e.g., vasodilators), and reducing heart rate and contractility (e.g., β-adrenergic blockers).

The patient may also benefit from a circulatory assist device (e.g., intraaortic balloon pump, ventricular assist device [VAD])[4,17] (see Chapter 65). The goals of this intervention are to decrease the SVR and the left ventricular workload so that the heart can heal. A VAD may be used as a temporary measure for the patient in cardiogenic shock who is awaiting heart transplantation. Heart transplantation is an option for a small, select group of patients with cardiogenic shock.

**Hypovolemic Shock.** The underlying principles of managing patients with hypovolemic shock focus on stopping the loss of fluid and restoring the circulating volume. Fluid resuscitation in hypovolemic shock initially is calculated using a 3:1 rule (3 mL of isotonic crystalloid for every 1 mL of estimated blood loss). Table 66-7 delineates the different types of fluid used for volume resuscitation, the mechanisms of action, and specific nursing implications for each fluid type.

**Septic Shock.** Patients in septic shock require large amounts of fluid replacement. Volume resuscitation of 30 to 50 mL/kg is usually done with isotonic crystalloids to achieve adequate fluid resuscitation. Albumin 4% to 5% may be added when patients require substantial volumes.

A fluid challenge technique (e.g., to achieve a minimum of 30 mL/kg of crystalloids) is used and repeated until hemodynamic improvement (e.g., increase in MAP and/or CVP, change in SVV) is noted.[18] Table 66-9 presents predetermined end points of fluid resuscitation along with methods to reassess volume status.

One of these methods is a *passive leg raise* (PLR) challenge along with hemodynamic measures to monitor response.[15] A PLR challenge provides a transient increase in fluid volume of 150 to 500 mL by placing the patient supine and raising the legs to 45 degrees. Response is monitored within 1 to 2 minutes by measuring CO, CI, SV, SVV, or other parameters for improvement. If the response is positive, then the patient is fluid responsive and should receive additional fluids. To optimize and evaluate large-volume fluid resuscitation, hemodynamic monitoring with various noninvasive or invasive monitors is necessary. The overall goal of fluid resuscitation is to restore the intravascular volume and organ perfusion.

If the patient remains hypotensive after initial volume resuscitation with minimally 30 mL/kg and the patient is no longer fluid responsive, vasopressors may be added. The first drug of choice is norepinephrine. Vasodilation and low CO, or vasodilation alone, can cause low BP in spite of adequate fluid resuscitation. Vasopressin may be added for patients refractory to initial vasopressor therapy. Exogenous vasopressin is used to replace the stores of physiologic vasopressin that are often depleted in septic shock.

**DRUG ALERT Vasopressin**

- Given along with norepinephrine.
- Infuse at low doses (e.g., 0.03 U/min) using an IV pump.
- Do not titrate infusion.
- Use cautiously in patients with coronary artery disease.

Vasopressor drugs may increase BP but may also decrease SV. An inotropic agent (e.g., dobutamine) may be added to offset the decrease in SV and increase tissue perfusion (Table 66-8). IV corticosteroids may be considered for patients in septic shock who cannot maintain an adequate BP with vasopressor therapy despite fluid resuscitation. In an attempt to meet the increasing tissue demands coupled with a low SVR, the patient initially demonstrates a normal or high CO. If the patient is unable to achieve and maintain an adequate CO and has unmet tissue $O_2$ demands, the CO may have to be increased using drug therapy (e.g., dopamine). $ScvO_2$ or $SvO_2$ monitoring is used to assess the balance between $O_2$ delivery and consumption, and the adequacy of the CO (see Chapter 65). If balance is maintained, the tissue demands will be met.

Antibiotics are an important and early component of therapy. They should be started within the first hour of severe sepsis or septic shock. Every hour delay has shown to significantly decrease survival.[19] Obtain cultures (e.g., blood, wound exudate, urine, stool, sputum) before antibiotics are started. However, this should not delay the start of antibiotics within the first hour. Broad-spectrum antibiotics are given first. More specific antibiotics may be ordered once the organism has been identified.

Glucose levels should be maintained below 180 mg/dL (10.0 mmol/L) for patients in shock. Intensive glucose control (81 to 108 mg/dL) actually increases mortality.[20] Monitor glucose levels in all patients in septic shock according to agency policy.

Stress ulcer prophylaxis with proton pump inhibitors (e.g., pantoprazole) for patients with bleeding risk factors and venous thromboembolism prophylaxis (e.g., heparin, enoxaparin [Lovenox]) are also recommended for these patients.[10]

**Neurogenic Shock.** The specific treatment of neurogenic shock is based on the cause. If the cause is spinal cord injury, general measures to promote spinal stability (e.g., spinal precautions, cervical stabilization with a collar) are initially used. Once the spine is stabilized, definitive treatment of the hypotension and bradycardia is essential to prevent further spinal cord damage. Hypotension, which occurs as a result of a loss of sympathetic tone, is associated with peripheral vasodilation and decreased venous return. Treatment involves the use of vasopressors (e.g., phenylephrine) to maintain BP and organ perfusion (Table 66-8). Bradycardia may be treated with atropine. Infuse fluids cautiously as the cause of the hypotension is not related to fluid loss.

The patient with a spinal cord injury also needs to be monitored for hypothermia caused by hypothalamic dysfunction (Table 66-9). Corticosteroids do not have an effect in neurogenic shock, and current guidelines no longer recommend the use of methylprednisolone (Solu-Medrol) for patients with a spinal cord injury.[21] (see Chapter 60).

**Anaphylactic Shock.** The first strategy in managing patients at risk for anaphylactic shock is prevention. A thorough history is key to avoiding the risk factors for anaphylaxis (Table 66-1). The clinical presentation of anaphylactic shock is dramatic, and immediate intervention is required. IM epinephrine is the first drug of choice to treat anaphylactic shock.[7,8] It causes peripheral vasoconstriction and bronchodilation and opposes the effect of histamine. Diphenhydramine and ranitidine (Zantac) are given as adjunctive therapies to block the ongoing release of histamine from the allergic reaction.

Maintaining a patent airway is important because the patient can quickly develop airway compromise from laryngeal edema or bronchoconstriction. Nebulized bronchodilators are highly effective. Aerosolized epinephrine can also be used to treat laryngeal edema. Endotracheal intubation or cricothyroidotomy may be necessary to secure and maintain a patent airway.

Hypotension results from leakage of fluid out of the intravascular space into the interstitial space as a result of increased vascular permeability and vasodilation. Aggressive fluid resuscitation, usually with crystalloids, is necessary. IV corticosteroids may be helpful in anaphylactic shock if significant hypotension persists after 1 to 2 hours of aggressive therapy (Tables 66-8 and 66-9).

**Obstructive Shock.** The primary strategy in treating obstructive shock is early recognition and treatment to relieve or manage the obstruction (Table 66-1). Mechanical decompression for pericardial tamponade, tension pneumothorax, and hemopneumothorax may be done by needle or tube insertion. Obstructive shock from a pulmonary embolism may require thrombolytic therapy. Superior vena cava syndrome, a compression or obstruction of the outflow tract of the mediastinum, may be treated by radiation, debulking, or removal of the mass or cause. A decompressive laparotomy may be indicated for abdominal compartment syndrome for patients with high intraabdominal pressures and hemodynamic instability.

## NURSING MANAGEMENT: SHOCK

### Nursing Assessment

Your role is vital in caring for patients who are at risk for developing shock or are in a state of shock. Focus your assessment on the ABCs: airway, breathing, and circulation. Next, assess for tissue perfusion. This includes evaluating vital signs, level of consciousness, peripheral pulses, capillary refill, skin (e.g., temperature, color, moisture), and urine output. As shock progresses, the patient's neurologic status declines, urine output decreases, skin becomes cooler and mottled, and peripheral pulses diminish.

To understand the complexity of the patient's clinical status, integrate all of the assessment data. It is essential to obtain a brief history from the patient or caregiver, including a description of the events leading to the shock condition, time of onset and duration of symptoms, and a health history (e.g., medications, allergies, date of last tetanus vaccination, recent travel). In addition, obtain details regarding any care that the patient received before hospitalization.

### Nursing Diagnoses

Nursing diagnoses for the patient in shock may include, but are not limited to, the following:

- Ineffective peripheral tissue perfusion and risk for decreased cardiac tissue perfusion, ineffective cerebral tissue perfusion, ineffective renal perfusion, impaired liver function, and ineffective GI perfusion *related to* low blood flow or maldistribution of blood
- Anxiety *related to* severity of condition and hypoxemia

Additional information on nursing diagnoses for the patient with shock is presented in eNursing Care Plan 66-1 (available on the website for this chapter).

### Planning

The overall goals for a patient in shock include (1) evidence of adequate tissue perfusion, (2) restoration of normal or baseline BP, (3) recovery of organ function, (4) avoidance of complications from prolonged states of hypoperfusion, and (5) prevention of health care–associated complications of disease management and care.

### Nursing Implementation

**Health Promotion.** You have an important role in the prevention of shock, beginning with the identification of patients at risk. In general, patients who are older, are immunocompromised, or have chronic illnesses are at an increased risk. Any person who has surgery or trauma is at risk for shock resulting from hemorrhage, spinal cord injury, sepsis, and other conditions (Table 66-1).

Planning is essential to help prevent shock after you identify an at-risk person. For example, a person with an acute anterior wall MI is at high risk for cardiogenic shock.[22] The primary goal for this patient is to limit the infarct size. This is done by restoring coronary blood flow through percutaneous coronary intervention, thrombolytic therapy, or surgical revascularization. Rest, analgesics, and sedation can reduce the myocardial demand for $O_2$. Modify the ICU environment to provide care at intervals that will not increase the patient's $O_2$ demand. For example, if the patient becomes tired with bathing, perform this care at a time that does not interfere with tests or other activities that may also increase $O_2$ demand.

A person with a severe allergy to things such as drugs, shellfish, insect bites, and latex is at increased risk for anaphylactic shock. This risk can be decreased if the patient is carefully questioned about allergies.

**SAFETY ALERT Preventing Allergic Reactions**

- Always confirm the patient's allergies before giving drugs or starting diagnostic procedures (e.g., CT scan with contrast media).
- Premedicate (e.g., diphenhydramine, methylprednisolone) patients who need a drug to which they are at high risk for an allergic reaction (e.g., contrast media).
- Encourage patients with allergies to obtain and wear a medical alert device and report their allergies to their HCPs.
- Tell patients about the availability of kits that contain equipment and drugs (e.g., epinephrine [EpiPen]) for the treatment of acute allergic reactions.

Careful monitoring of fluid balance can help prevent hypovolemic shock. Ongoing monitoring of intake and output and daily weights is important. In addition, monitoring the patient's clinical status is essential because trends in clinical findings are more meaningful than any one piece of clinical information.

Carefully monitor all patients for the development of infection. Progression from an infection to sepsis and septic shock depends on the patient's defense mechanisms. Patients who are immunocompromised are at high risk for opportunistic infections. Strategies to decrease the risk of health care–associated infections (HAIs) include decreasing the number of invasive catheters (e.g., central lines, bladder catheters), using aseptic technique during invasive procedures, and paying strict attention to hand washing. In addition, all equipment must be changed per agency policy and thoroughly cleaned or discarded (if disposable) between patient use.

Evidence-based guidelines are available to reduce the risk of HAIs (e.g., ventilator-associated pneumonia, central line infections, catheter-associated urinary tract infections). These guidelines, called *care bundles,* outline key interventions aimed at reducing infections (see *http://www.ihi.org/topics/Bundles/Pages/default.aspx*).

**Acute Care.** Your role in shock involves (1) monitoring the patient's ongoing physical and emotional status, (2) identifying trends to detect changes in the patient's condition, (3) planning and implementing nursing interventions and therapy, (4) evaluating the patient's response to therapy, (5) providing emotional support to the patient and caregiver, and (6) collaborating with other members of the interprofessional team to coordinate care (see Chapter 65).

◆ ***Neurologic Status.*** Assess the patient's neurologic status, including orientation and level of consciousness using a valid tool, at least every 1 to 2 hours. The patient's neurologic status is the best indicator of cerebral blood flow. Be aware of the clinical manifestations of neurologic involvement (e.g., changes in behavior, restlessness, hyperalertness, blurred vision, confusion, paresthesias). Note and report any subtle changes in the patient's mental status (e.g., mild agitation).

Orient the patient to person, place, time, and events on a regular basis. Orientation to the ICU environment is particularly important. Reduce noise and light levels to control sensory input. Keep a day-night cycle of activity and rest as much as possible. Sensory overload and disruption of the patient's diurnal cycle may contribute to delirium (see Chapter 65).

◆ ***Cardiovascular Status.*** Most of the therapy for shock is based on information about the patient's cardiovascular status. If the patient is unstable, continuously assess heart rate and rhythm, BP, CVP, and PA pressures, including CO, SVR, SV, and SVV (if available). (Chapter 65 discusses hemodynamic monitoring.) Monitoring trends in hemodynamic parameters provides more important information than single values. Integration of hemodynamic data with physical assessment data is essential in planning strategies to manage the patient with shock.

Patients in shock often have hypotension. The Trendelenburg (head-down) position should not be used to treat hypotension. Patients in this position may experience compromised pulmonary function and increased intracranial pressure.[23]

Continuously monitor the patient's ECG to detect dysrhythmias that may result from the cardiovascular and metabolic abnormalities associated with shock. Assess heart sounds for an $S_3$ or $S_4$ sound or new murmurs. An $S_3$ sound usually indicates heart failure.

In addition to monitoring the patient's cardiovascular status, give the prescribed therapy to correct the dysfunctions of the cardiovascular system. Assess the patient's response to fluid and drug administration as often as every 10 to 15 minutes. Make appropriate adjustments (e.g., drug titration) as needed. Once tissue perfusion is restored and the patient is stabilized, you can decrease the frequency of monitoring and slowly wean the patient off drugs to support BP and tissue perfusion.

### CHECK YOUR PRACTICE

A 69-yr-old male patient has just been transferred to the ICU from the emergency department with a diagnosis of sepsis. Your assessment indicates that he is confused with weak peripheral pulses and a BP of 84/50.

- What fluids would you expect to be ordered and what volume (amount) would you expect to be initially infused to improve his BP?
- In spite of aggressive fluid resuscitation, the patient remains hypotensive. What drug would you expect to be ordered to improve tissue perfusion?

◆ ***Respiratory Status.*** Frequently assess the respiratory status of the patient in shock to ensure adequate oxygenation, detect complications early, and provide data regarding the patient's acid-base status. Initially monitor the rate, depth, and rhythm of respirations as frequently as every 15 to 30 minutes. Increased rate and depth provide information regarding the patient's attempts to correct metabolic acidosis. Assess breath sounds every 1 to 2 hours and as needed for any changes that may indicate fluid overload or accumulation of secretions.

Use pulse oximetry to continuously monitor $O_2$ saturation. Pulse oximetry using a patient's finger may not be accurate in a shock state because of poor peripheral circulation. Instead, attach the probe to the ear, nose, or forehead (according to the manufacturer's guidelines). Arterial blood gases (ABGs) provide definitive information on ventilation and oxygenation status and acid-base balance. Initial interpretation of ABGs is often your responsibility. A $PaO_2$ below 60 mm Hg (in the absence of chronic lung disease) indicates hypoxemia and the need for higher $O_2$ concentrations or for a different mode of $O_2$ administration. Low $PaCO_2$ with a low pH and low bicarbonate level may indicate that the patient is attempting to compensate for metabolic acidosis from increasing lactate levels.

A rising $PaCO_2$ with a persistently low pH and $PaO_2$ indicates the need for advanced pulmonary management. Many patients in shock are intubated and on mechanical ventilation. Maintaining a patent airway and monitoring for ventilator-related complications are critical. (Chapter 65 discusses artificial airways and mechanical ventilation.)

◆ ***Renal Status.*** Initially, measure urine output every 1 to 2 hours to assess the adequacy of renal perfusion. Inserting an indwelling urinary catheter facilitates measurements during resuscitation. Urine output below 0.5 mL/kg/hr may indicate inadequate perfusion of the kidneys. Also use trends in serum creatinine values to assess renal function. Serum creatinine is a better indicator of renal function than BUN levels, since BUN is affected by the patient's catabolic state.

◆ ***Body Temperature and Skin Changes.*** Monitor temperature every 4 hours if normal. In the presence of an elevated or subnormal temperature, obtain hourly core temperatures (e.g., urinary, esophageal, or PA catheter). Use light covers and control the room temperature to keep the patient comfortably warm. If the patient's temperature rises above 101.5°F (38.6°C) and the patient becomes uncomfortable or experiences cardiovascular compromise, treat the fever with antipyretic drugs (e.g., ibuprofen, acetaminophen [Tylenol]) and remove some of the patient's covers. Consider a cooling device if fever persists despite treatment.

Monitor the patient's skin (e.g., upper and lower extremities) for signs of adequate perfusion. Changes in temperature, pallor, flushing, cyanosis, diaphoresis, and piloerection may indicate hypoperfusion.

◆ ***Gastrointestinal Status.*** Auscultate bowel sounds at least every 4 hours, and monitor for abdominal distention. If a nasogastric tube is present, measure drainage and check for occult blood. Similarly, check all stools for occult blood.

◆ ***Personal Hygiene.*** Hygiene is especially important for the patient in shock because impaired tissue perfusion predisposes the patient to skin breakdown and infection. Perform bathing and other nursing measures carefully because a patient in shock is experiencing problems with $O_2$ delivery to tissues. The increased $O_2$ demand that occurs during bathing and repositioning of patients with limited $O_2$ reserves makes the prevention of health care–associated pressure ulcers challenging. Turn the patient at least every 1 to 2 hours and maintain good body alignment to help prevent pressure ulcers. Use a pressure-relieving or pressure-reducing mattress or a specialty bed as needed.

Oral care for the patient in shock is essential because mucous membranes may become dry and fragile in the volume-depleted patient. In addition, the intubated patient usually has difficulty swallowing, resulting in pooled secretions in the mouth. Apply a water-soluble lubricant to the lips to prevent drying and cracking. Brush the patient's teeth or gums with a soft toothbrush every 12 hours, and swab the lips and oral mucosa with a moisturizing solution every 2 to 4 hours.[24] Perform passive range of motion three or four times a day to maintain joint mobility. Use good clinical judgment in determining priorities of care to limit the demands for increased $O_2$. Monitor trends in $O_2$ consumption (e.g., $SpO_2$, $ScvO_2/SvO_2$) during all nursing interventions to assess the patient's tolerance of activity.

◆ ***Emotional Support and Comfort.*** Do not underestimate the effects of fear and anxiety when the patient and caregiver are faced with a critical, life-threatening situation (see Chapter 65). Fear, anxiety, and pain may aggravate respiratory distress and increase the release of catecholamines. When implementing care, monitor the patient's mental state and level of pain using valid assessment tools. Provide drugs to decrease anxiety and pain as appropriate. Continuous infusions of a benzodiazepine (e.g., lorazepam [Ativan]) and an opioid or sedative (e.g., morphine, propofol [Diprivan]) are extremely helpful in decreasing anxiety and pain.

Talk to the patient and encourage the caregiver to talk to the patient, even if the patient is intubated, is sedated, or appears comatose. Hearing is often the last sense to decrease. Even if the patient cannot respond, he or she may still be able to hear. If the intubated patient is capable of writing, provide a "magic slate" or a pencil and paper. Alphabet boards or signboards with common requests (e.g., turn, fan, lights) are also useful.

Give the patient simple explanations of all procedures before you carry them out, as well as information regarding the current plan of care. If the patient or caregiver asks questions about progress and prognosis, provide simple and honest answers.

Do not overlook the patient's spiritual needs. Patients may desire a visit from a chaplain, priest, rabbi, or minister. One way to provide support is to offer to call a member of the clergy rather than wait for the patient or caregiver to express a wish for spiritual counseling.

Caregivers can have a therapeutic effect on the patient by providing support and comfort. Caregivers (1) link the patient to the outside world; (2) facilitate decision making and advise the patient; (3) assist with activities of daily living; (4) act as liaisons to advise the health care team of the patient's wishes for care; and (5) provide safe, caring, familiar relationships for the patient.[25,26]

Most important, caregivers wish to be kept informed of the patient's condition. If possible, the same nurses should continually care for the patient to decrease anxiety, limit conflicting information, and increase trust. If the prognosis becomes grave, support the patient's caregiver when making difficult decisions such as withdrawing life support. The interprofessional care team must promote realistic expectations and outcomes. Remember, compassion is as essential as scientific and technical expertise in the total care of the patient and caregiver.

Ensure that the caregiver is able to spend time with the patient, provided the patient perceives this time as comforting. Explain in simple terms the purpose of any tubes and equipment attached to or surrounding the patient. Inform the caregivers of what they may and may not touch. If possible, place the patient's hands and arms outside the sheets to encourage therapeutic touch. Encourage caregivers to perform simple comfort measures if desired. Provide privacy as much as possible, but assure the patient and caregiver that assistance is readily available should it be needed. Position the call bell in reach of the patient or caregiver at all times.

> **CHECK YOUR PRACTICE**
>
> Your patient is a 74-yr-old man recovering from septic shock secondary to a perforated diverticulum. He has been in the ICU for 7 days, and his condition has finally stabilized. His wife has been at his bedside for the duration of his ICU stay. While caring for him, you suggest that she could take a brief walk and get some coffee. She bursts out with tears, "I can't leave him. You know that he almost died."
>
> • How can you support this caregiver?

◆ **Ambulatory Care.** Rehabilitation of the patient who has experienced critical illness requires (1) correction of the precipitating cause, (2) prevention or early treatment of complications, and (3) teaching focused on disease management or prevention of recurrence based on the initial cause of shock. Continue to monitor the patient for indications of complications throughout the recovery period. These may include decreased range of motion, muscle weakness, decreased physical endurance, acute kidney injury (acute tubular necrosis) (see Chapter 46), and fibrotic lung disease (from ARDS) (see Chapter 67). Patients recovering from shock often require diverse services after discharge. These can include admission to transitional care units (e.g., for mechanical ventilation weaning), rehabilitation centers (inpatient or outpatient), or home health care agencies. Start planning for a safe transition from hospital to home as soon as the patient is admitted to the hospital.

### ◆ Evaluation

The expected outcomes are that the patient who experiences shock will have:

- Adequate tissue perfusion with restoration of normal or baseline BP
- Normal organ function with no complications from hypoperfusion
- Decreased fear and anxiety and increased psychologic comfort

Additional information on expected outcomes for the patient with shock is presented in eNursing Care Plan 66-1 (available on the website for this chapter).

## SYSTEMIC INFLAMMATORY RESPONSE SYNDROME AND MULTIPLE ORGAN DYSFUNCTION SYNDROME

### Etiology and Pathophysiology

**Systemic inflammatory response syndrome (SIRS)** is a systemic inflammatory response to a variety of insults, including infection (referred to as *sepsis*), ischemia, infarction, and injury (Table 66-4). Generalized inflammation in organs remote from the initial insult characterizes SIRS.[10] A systemic inflammatory response can be triggered by many different mechanisms, including the following:

- Mechanical tissue trauma: Burns, crush injuries, surgical procedures
- Abscess formation: Intraabdominal, extremities
- Ischemic or necrotic tissue: Pancreatitis, vascular disease, MI

- Microbial invasion: Bacteria, viruses, fungi, parasites
- Endotoxin release: Gram-negative and gram-positive bacteria
- Global perfusion deficits: Postcardiac resuscitation, shock states
- Regional perfusion deficits: Distal perfusion deficits

**Multiple organ dysfunction syndrome (MODS)** is the failure of two or more organ systems in an acutely ill patient such that homeostasis cannot be maintained without intervention. MODS results from SIRS. These two syndromes represent the ends of a continuum. Transition from SIRS to MODS does not occur in a clear-cut manner[10] (Fig. 66-1).

**Organ and Metabolic Dysfunction.** When the inflammatory response is activated, consequences include the release of mediators, direct damage to the endothelium, and hypermetabolism. In addition, vascular permeability increases. This allows mediators and protein to leak out of the endothelium and into the interstitial space. White blood cells begin to digest the foreign debris, and the coagulation cascade is activated (see Chapter 29). Hypotension, decreased perfusion, microemboli, and redistributed or shunted blood flow eventually compromise organ perfusion.

The respiratory system is often the first system to show signs of dysfunction in SIRS and MODS.[10] Inflammatory mediators have a direct effect on the pulmonary vasculature. The endothelial damage from the release of inflammatory mediators causes increased capillary permeability. This causes movement of fluid from the pulmonary vasculature into the pulmonary interstitial spaces. The fluid then moves to the alveoli, causing alveolar edema. Type I pneumocytes (alveolar cells) are destroyed. Type II pneumocytes are damaged, and surfactant production is decreased. The alveoli collapse. This creates an increase in *shunt* (blood flow to the lungs that does not participate in gas exchange) and worsening ventilation-perfusion mismatch. The end result is ARDS. Patients with ARDS need aggressive pulmonary management with mechanical ventilation. (See Chapter 67 for a complete discussion of ARDS.)

Cardiovascular changes include myocardial depression and massive vasodilation in response to increasing tissue demands. Vasodilation results in decreased SVR and BP. The baroreceptor reflex causes release of *inotropic* (increasing force of contraction) and *chronotropic* (increasing heart rate) factors that enhance CO. To compensate for hypotension, CO increases by an increase in heart rate and SV. Increases in capillary permeability cause a shift of albumin and fluid out of the vascular space, further reducing venous return and thus preload. The patient becomes warm and tachycardic with a high CO and a low SVR. Other signs include decreased capillary refill, skin mottling, increased CVP and PAWP, and dysrhythmias. $ScvO_2$ or $SvO_2$ may be abnormally high because the patient is perfusing areas not consuming much $O_2$ (e.g., skin, nonworking muscle) while other areas may have blood shunted away from them. Eventually, either perfusion of vital organs becomes insufficient or the cells are unable to use $O_2$ and their function is further compromised.

Neurologic dysfunction commonly presents as mental status changes with SIRS and MODS. These acute changes can be an early sign of SIRS or MODS. The patient may become confused and agitated, combative, disoriented, lethargic, or comatose. These mental status changes may be due to hypoxemia, the effects of inflammatory mediators, or impaired perfusion.

Acute kidney injury (AKI) is frequently seen in SIRS and MODS. Hypoperfusion and the effects of the mediators can cause AKI. Decreased perfusion to the kidneys activates the SNS and the renin-angiotensin system. The stimulation of the renin-angiotensin system results in systemic vasoconstriction and aldosterone-mediated sodium and water reabsorption. Another risk factor for the development of AKI is the use of nephrotoxic drugs. Antibiotics commonly used to treat gram-negative bacteria (e.g., aminoglycosides) can be nephrotoxic. Careful monitoring of drug levels is essential to avoid the nephrotoxic effects.

The GI tract also plays a key role in the development of MODS. GI motility is often decreased in critical illness, causing abdominal distention and paralytic ileus. In the early stages of SIRS and MODS, blood is also shunted away from the GI mucosa, making it highly vulnerable to ischemic injury. Decreased perfusion leads to a breakdown of this normally protective mucosal barrier, thus increasing the risk for ulceration, GI bleeding, and bacterial movement from the GI tract into circulation.

Metabolic changes are pronounced in SIRS and MODS. Both syndromes trigger a hypermetabolic response. Glycogen stores are rapidly converted to glucose (glycogenolysis). Once glycogen is depleted, amino acids are converted to glucose (gluconeogenesis), reducing protein stores. Fatty acids are mobilized for fuel. Catecholamines and glucocorticoids are released and result in hyperglycemia and insulin resistance. The net result is a catabolic state, and lean body mass (muscle) is lost.

The hypermetabolism associated with SIRS and MODS may last for several days and results in liver dysfunction. Liver dysfunction in MODS may begin long before clinical evidence of it is present. Protein synthesis is impaired. The liver cannot make albumin, one of the key proteins in maintaining plasma oncotic pressure. Consequently, plasma oncotic pressure is altered, and fluid and protein leak from the vascular spaces to the interstitial space. Administration of albumin does not normalize oncotic pressure in these patients at this point.

As the state of hypermetabolism persists, the patient cannot convert lactate to glucose, and lactate accumulates (lactic acidosis). Despite increases in glycogenolysis and gluconeogenesis, eventually the liver is unable to maintain an adequate glucose level and the patient becomes hypoglycemic. Hypoglycemia can also develop due to acute adrenal insufficiency.

DIC may result from dysfunction of the coagulation system. DIC causes simultaneous microvascular clotting and bleeding because of the depletion of clotting factors and platelets in addition to excessive fibrinolysis. (Chapter 30 discusses DIC.)

Electrolyte imbalances are common and result from the hormonal and metabolic changes and fluid shifts. These changes worsen mental status changes, neuromuscular dysfunction, and dysrhythmias. The release of ADH and aldosterone results in sodium and water retention. Aldosterone increases urinary potassium loss, and catecholamines cause potassium to move into the cell, resulting in hypokalemia. Hypokalemia is associated with dysrhythmias and muscle weakness. Metabolic acidosis results from impaired tissue perfusion, hypoxia, and a shift to anaerobic metabolism with a resultant increase in lactate levels. Progressive renal dysfunction also contributes to metabolic acidosis. Hypocalcemia, hypomagnesemia, and hypophosphatemia are common.

## Clinical Manifestations of SIRS and MODS

The clinical manifestations of SIRS and MODS are presented in Table 66-10.

**TABLE 66-10 Manifestations and Management of SIRS and MODS**

| Manifestations | Management |
|---|---|
| **Respiratory System** | |
| Development of ARDS (see Chapter 67):<br>• Severe dyspnea<br>• Tachypnea<br>• $PaO_2/FIO_2$ ratio <200<br>• Bilateral fluffy infiltrates on chest x-ray<br>• PAWP <18 mm Hg<br>• Ventilation-perfusion (V/Q) mismatch<br>• Pulmonary hypertension<br>• Increased minute ventilation<br>• Decreased compliance<br>• Refractory hypoxemia | Prevention<br>Optimize $O_2$ delivery and minimize $O_2$ consumption<br>Mechanical ventilation (see Chapter 65)<br>• Positive end-expiratory pressure<br>• Lung protective modes (e.g., pressure-control inverse ratio ventilation, low tidal volumes)<br>• Permissive hypercapnia<br>• Positioning (e.g., continuous lateral rotation therapy, prone positioning) |
| **Cardiovascular System** | |
| Myocardial depression<br>Massive vasodilation<br>↓ SVR, BP<br>↓ MAP<br>↑ HR, stroke volume<br>↑ CO<br>Systolic, diastolic dysfunction<br>Biventricular failure | Volume management<br>• Central venous or PA catheter for hemodynamic monitoring<br>• Minimally invasive hemodynamic monitoring<br>• ↑ Preload via volume replacement<br>• Arterial pressure monitoring<br>• Maintain MAP >65 mm Hg<br>Vasopressors<br>Intermittent or continuous $ScvO_2$ or $SvO_2$ monitoring<br>Balance $O_2$ supply and demand<br>Continuous ECG monitoring<br>Circulatory assist devices<br>Venous thromboembolism prophylaxis |
| **Central Nervous System** | |
| Acute change in neurologic status<br>Fever<br>Hepatic encephalopathy<br>Seizures<br>Confusion, disorientation, delirium<br>Failure to wean, prolonged rehabilitation | Evaluate for hepatic or metabolic encephalopathy<br>Optimize cerebral blood flow<br>↓ Cerebral $O_2$ requirements<br>Prevent secondary tissue ischemia<br>Calcium channel blockers (reduce cerebral vasospasm) |
| **Endocrine System** | |
| Hyperglycemia → hypoglycemia | Provide continuous infusion of insulin and glucose to maintain blood glucose 140-180 mg/dL (7.77-10.0 mmol/L) |
| **Renal System** | |
| *Prerenal:* Renal hypoperfusion<br>• BUN/creatinine ratio >20 : 1<br>• ↓ Urine $Na^+$ <20 mEq/L<br>• ↑ Urine specific gravity >1.020<br>• ↑ Urine osmolality<br>*Intrarenal:* Acute tubular necrosis<br>• BUN/creatinine ratio <10 : 1-15 : 1<br>• ↑ Urine $Na^+$ >20 mEq/L<br>• ↓ Urine osmolality<br>• Urine specific gravity ~1.010 | Diuretics<br>• Loop diuretics (e.g., furosemide [Lasix])<br>• May need to increase dosage due to ↓ glomerular filtration rate<br>Continuous renal replacement therapy (see Chapter 46) |
| **Gastrointestinal System** | |
| Mucosal ischemia<br>• ↓ Intramucosal pH<br>• Potential translocation of gut bacteria<br>• Potential abdominal compartment syndrome<br>Hypoperfusion → ↓ peristalsis, paralytic ileus<br>Mucosal ulceration on endoscopy<br>GI bleeding | Stress ulcer prophylaxis<br>• Antacids (e.g., Maalox)<br>• Proton pump inhibitors (e.g., omeprazole [Prilosec])<br>• sucralfate (Carafate)<br>• Monitor abdominal distention, intraabdominal pressures<br>• Dietary consultation<br>• Enteral feedings<br>• Stimulate mucosal activity<br>• Provide essential nutrients and optimal calories |
| **Hepatic System** | |
| Bilirubin >2 mg/dL (34 μmol/L)<br>↑ Liver enzymes (ALT, AST, GGT)<br>↑ Serum $NH_3$<br>↓ Serum albumin, prealbumin, transferrin<br>Jaundice<br>Hepatic encephalopathy | Maintain adequate tissue perfusion<br>Provide nutritional support (e.g., enteral feedings)<br>Careful use of drugs metabolized by liver |
| **Hematologic System** | |
| ↑ Bleeding times, ↑ PT, ↑ PTT<br>↓ Platelet count (thrombocytopenia)<br>↑ Fibrin split products<br>↑ D-dimer | Observe for bleeding from obvious and/or occult sites<br>Replace factors being lost (e.g., platelets)<br>Minimize traumatic interventions (e.g., IM injections, multiple venipunctures) |

*ALT,* Alanine aminotransferase; *APCO,* arterial pressure–based cardiac output; *ARDS,* acute respiratory distress syndrome; *AST,* aspartate aminotransferase; *BUN,* blood urea nitrogen; *CO,* cardiac output; *GGT,* γ-glutamyl transferase; *MAP,* mean arterial pressure; *$NH_3$,* ammonia; *PA,* pulmonary artery; *PAWP,* pulmonary artery wedge pressure; *PT,* prothrombin time; *PTT,* partial thromboplastin time; *$ScvO_2$,* $O_2$ saturation in venous blood; *$SvO_2$,* $O_2$ saturation in mixed venous blood; *SVR,* systemic vascular resistance.

## NURSING AND INTERPROFESSIONAL MANAGEMENT: SIRS AND MODS

The prognosis for the patient with MODS is poor, with mortality rates of 70% to 80% when three or more organ systems fail.[10] The most common cause of death continues to be sepsis. Survival improves with *early, goal-directed therapy.*[10] Therefore the most important goal is to prevent the progression of SIRS to MODS.

A critical part of your role is vigilant assessment and ongoing monitoring to detect early signs of deterioration or organ dysfunction. Interprofessional care for patients with SIRS and MODS focuses on (1) prevention and treatment of infection, (2) maintenance of tissue oxygenation, (3) nutritional and metabolic support, and (4) appropriate support of individual failing organs. Table 66-10 summarizes the management for patients with SIRS and MODS.

### Prevention and Treatment of Infection

Aggressive infection control strategies are essential to decrease the risk for HAIs. Early, aggressive surgery is recommended to remove necrotic tissue (e.g., early debridement of burn tissue) that can provide a culture medium for microorganisms. Aggressive pulmonary management, including early mobilization, can reduce the risk of infection. Strict asepsis can decrease infections related to intraarterial lines, endotracheal tubes, indwelling urinary catheters, IV lines, and other invasive devices or procedures. Daily assessment of the ongoing need for invasive lines and other devices is an important strategy to prevent or limit HAIs.

Despite aggressive strategies, infection may develop. Once an infection is suspected, begin interventions to treat the cause. Send appropriate cultures and start broad-spectrum antibiotic therapy, as ordered. Adjust therapy based on the culture results, if needed.

## Maintenance of Tissue Oxygenation

Hypoxemia frequently occurs in patients with SIRS and MODS. These patients have greater $O_2$ needs and decreased $O_2$ supply to the tissues. Interventions that decrease $O_2$ demand and increase $O_2$ delivery are essential. Sedation, mechanical ventilation, analgesia, and rest may decrease $O_2$ demand and should be considered. $O_2$ delivery may be optimized by using individualized tidal volumes with positive end-expiratory pressure, increasing preload (e.g., fluids) or myocardial contractility to enhance CO, or reducing afterload to increase CO.

## Nutritional and Metabolic Needs

Hypermetabolism in SIRS or MODS can result in profound weight loss, cachexia, and further organ failure. Protein-calorie malnutrition is one of the primary signs of hypermetabolism in SIRS and MODS. Total energy expenditure is often increased 1.5 to 2.0 times the normal metabolic rate. Because of their relatively short half-life, monitor plasma transferrin and prealbumin levels to assess hepatic protein synthesis.

The goal of nutritional support is to preserve organ function. Providing early and optimal nutrition decreases morbidity and mortality rates in patients with SIRS and MODS. The enteral route is preferred. If it cannot be used, parenteral nutrition should be considered.[16] (Chapter 39 discusses enteral and parenteral nutrition.) Provide glycemic control with a goal of 140 to 180 mg/dL with insulin infusions in these patients.[10,16]

## Support of Failing Organs

Support of any failing organ is a primary goal of therapy. For example, the patient with ARDS requires aggressive $O_2$ therapy and mechanical ventilation (see Chapter 67). DIC should be treated appropriately (e.g., blood products) (see Chapter 30). Renal failure may require dialysis. Continuous renal replacement therapy is better tolerated than hemodialysis, especially in a patient with hemodynamic instability (see Chapter 46).

A final consideration may be that further interventions are futile. It is important to maintain communication between the health care team and the patient's caregiver regarding realistic goals and likely outcomes for the patient with MODS. Withdrawal of life support and starting end-of-life care may be the best options for the patient.

## CASE STUDY

### *Shock*

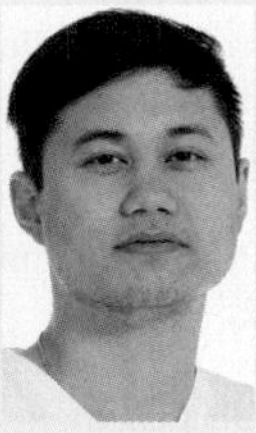
(©Thinkstock)

**Patient Profile**

K.L., a 25-yr-old Korean American, was not wearing his seat belt when he was the driver involved in a motor vehicle crash. The windshield was broken and K.L. was found 10 ft from his car. He was face down, conscious, and moaning. His wife and daughter were found in the car with their seat belts on. They sustained minor injuries and were very frightened and upset. All passengers were taken to the emergency department (ED). The following information pertains to K.L.

**Subjective Data**

- States, "I can't breathe"
- Cries out when abdomen is palpated

**Objective Data**

***Physical Examination***

- *Cardiovascular:* BP 80/56 mm Hg; apical pulse 138 but no palpable radial or pedal pulses; carotid pulse present but weak
  - ECG as follows:

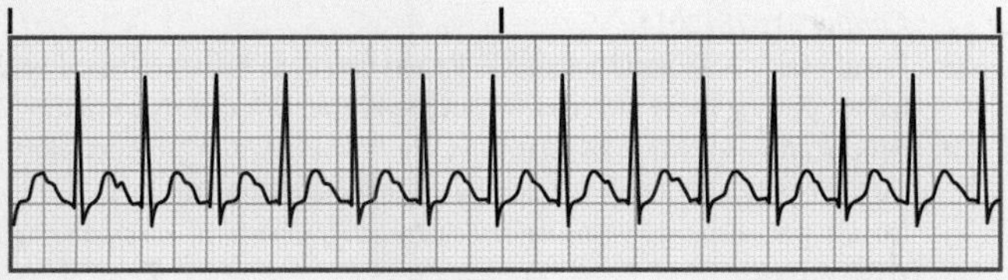

- *Respiratory:* respiratory rate 35 breaths/minute; labored breathing with shallow respirations; asymmetric chest wall movement; absence of breath sounds on left side
  - Trachea deviated slightly to the right
- *Abdomen:* slightly distended and left upper quadrant painful on palpation
- *Musculoskeletal:* open compound fracture of the lower left leg

***Diagnostic Studies***

- Chest x-ray: Hemothorax and six rib fractures on left side
- Hematocrit: 28%

**Interprofessional Care (in the ED)**

- Intraosseous access in right proximal tibia placed prehospital
- Left chest tube placed, draining bright red blood
- Fluid resuscitation started with crystalloids
- High-flow $O_2$ via non-rebreather mask

**Emergency Surgical Procedures**

- Splenectomy
- Repair of torn intercostal artery
- Repair of compound fracture

**Discussion Questions**

1. What types of shock is K.L. experiencing? What clinical manifestations did he display that support your answer?
2. What were the causes of K.L.'s shock states? What are other causes of these types of shock?
3. ***Priority Decision:*** What are the priority nursing responsibilities for K.L.?
4. ***Priority Decision:*** What ongoing nursing assessment parameters are essential for this patient?
5. What are his potential complications?
6. ***Patient-Centered Care:*** K.L.'s parents arrive. English is their second language. They are very anxious and asking about their son. What can you do to provide culturally competent family-centered care?
7. ***Priority Decision:*** Based on the assessment data presented, what are the priority nursing diagnoses?
8. ***Teamwork and Collaboration:*** Identify the tasks that could be delegated to unlicensed assistive personnel (UAP).
9. ***Evidence-Based Practice:*** You are orienting a new graduate RN. He asks you why crystalloids are used instead of colloids for fluid resuscitation. What is your response?

Answers available at *http://evolve.elsevier.com/Lewis/medsurg.*

## BRIDGE TO NCLEX EXAMINATION

The number of the question corresponds to the same-numbered outcome at the beginning of the chapter.

1. A patient has a spinal cord injury at T4. Vital signs include falling blood pressure with bradycardia. The nurse recognizes that the patient is experiencing
   **a.** a relative hypervolemia.
   **b.** an absolute hypovolemia.
   **c.** neurogenic shock from low blood flow.
   **d.** neurogenic shock from massive vasodilation.
2. A 78-yr-old man has confusion and temperature of 104° F (40° C). He is a diabetic with purulent drainage from his right heel. After an infusion of 3 L of normal saline solution, his assessment findings are BP 84/40 mm Hg; heart rate 110; respiratory rate 42 and shallow; CO 8 L/minute; and PAWP 4 mm Hg. This patient's symptoms are *most* likely indicative of
   **a.** sepsis.
   **b.** septic shock.
   **c.** multiple organ dysfunction syndrome.
   **d.** systemic inflammatory response syndrome.
3. Appropriate treatment modalities for the management of cardiogenic shock include *(select all that apply)*
   **a.** dobutamine to increase myocardial contractility.
   **b.** vasopressors to increase systemic vascular resistance.
   **c.** circulatory assist devices such as an intraaortic balloon pump.
   **d.** corticosteroids to stabilize the cell wall in the infarcted myocardium.
   **e.** Trendelenburg positioning to facilitate venous return and increase preload.
4. The *most* accurate assessment parameters for the nurse to use to determine adequate tissue perfusion in the patient with MODS are
   **a.** blood pressure, pulse, and respirations.
   **b.** breath sounds, blood pressure, and body temperature.
   **c.** pulse pressure, level of consciousness, and pupillary response.
   **d.** level of consciousness, urine output, and skin color and temperature.

1. d, 2. b, 3. a, c, 4. d

For rationales to these answers and even more NCLEX review questions, visit *http://evolve.elsevier.com/Lewis/medsurg.*

## EVOLVE WEBSITE

http://evolve.elsevier.com/Lewis/medsurg

**Review Questions (Online Only)**
**Key Points**
**Answer Keys to Questions**
- Rationales for Bridge to NCLEX Examination Questions
- Answer Guidelines for Case Study on p. 1607

**Student Case Studies**
- Patient With Acute Pancreatitis and Septic Shock
- Patient With Cardiogenic Shock
- Patient With Sepsis

**Nursing Care Plan**
- eNursing Care Plan 66-1: Patient in Shock

**Conceptual Care Map Creator**
**Audio Glossary**
**Content Updates**

## REFERENCES


1. Dries D, Sarani B: Diagnosis and management of shock. In Dries DJ, editor: *Guide for fundamental critical care support*, ed 5, Mount Pleasant, Ill, 2012, Society of Critical Care Medicine.
2. Galeski DF: Definition, classification, etiology, and pathophysiology of shock in adults. 2015. Retrieved from *www.uptodate.com+definition-classification-etiology-and-pathophysiology-of-shock-in-adults.*
3. Patel AK, Hollenberg SM: Cardiovascular failure and cardiogenic shock, *Semin Respir Crit Care Med* 22:598, 2011.
4. Shabana A, Moustafa M, El-Menyar A, et al: Cardiogenic shock complicating myocardial infarction: an updated review, *Br J Med Res* 3:622, 2013.
5. Mandel J, Palevsky PM: Treatment of severe hypovolemia or hypovolemic shock in adults, 2015. Retrieved from *www.uptodate.com/contents/treatment-of-severe-hypovolemia-or-hypovolemic-shock-in-adults.*

*6. Casha S, Christie S: A systematic review of intensive cardiopulmonary management after spinal cord injury, *J Neurotrauma* 28:1479, 2011.

*7. Simons FF, Ardusso LR, Dimov V, et al: World Allergy Organization Anaphylaxis Guidelines: 2013 update of the evidence base, *Int Arch Allergy Immunol* 162:193, 2013.

8. Zilberstein J, McCurdy MT, Winters ME: Anaphylaxis, *J Emerg Med* 47:182, 2014.

*9. Singer M, Deutschman CS, Seymour CW, et al: The third international consensus definitions for sepsis and septic shock (Sepsis-3), *JAMA* 315:801, 2016.

*10. Dellinger RP, Levy MM, Rhodes A, et al: Surviving sepsis campaign: international guidelines for management of severe sepsis and septic shock: 2012, *Crit Care Med* 41:50, 2013.

11. Leeper B: Cardiovascular system. In Burns S, editor: *AACN essentials of critical care nursing*, ed 3, New York, 2014, McGraw-Hill Education.
12. Strickler J: Halt the downward spiral of traumatic hypovolemic shock, *Nurs Crit Care* 7:42, 2012.
13. Finfer SR, Vincent JL: Resuscitation fluids, *N Engl J Med* 369:1243, 2013.

*14. Patel A, Laffan MA, Waheed U, et al: Randomized trials of albumin for adults with sepsis: systematic review and meta-analysis with trial sequential analysis of all-cause mortality, *BMJ* 349:g4561, 2014.

15. Marik PE, Monnet X, Teboul J: Hemodynamic parameters to guide fluid therapy, *Ann Intensive Care* 1:1, 2011.
16. Casaer MP, Van den Berghe G: Nutrition in the acute phase of critical illness, *N Engl J Med* 370:1227, 2014.
17. Myers TJ: Temporary ventricular assist devices in the intensive care unit as a bridge to decision, *AACN Adv Crit Care* 23:55, 2012.

*18. Surviving Sepsis Campaign: Updated bundles in response to new evidence, 2015. Retrieved from *www.survivingsepsis.org/SiteCollectionDocuments/SSC_Bundle.pdf.*

*19. Ferrer R, Martin-Loeches I, Phillips G, et al: Empiric antibiotic treatment reduces mortality in severe sepsis and septic shock from the first hour: results from a guideline-based performance improvement program, *Crit Care Med* 42:1749, 2014.

*20. Finfer S, Blair D, Bellomo R, et al: Intensive versus conventional glucose control in critically ill patients, *N Engl J Med* 360:1283, 2009. (Classic)

21. Hurlbert RJ, Hadley MN, Walters BC, et al: Pharmacological therapy for acute spinal cord injury, *Neurosurgery* 72:93, 2013.

*22. O'Gara PT, Kushner FG, Ascheim DD, et al: 2013 ACCF/AHA guideline for the management of ST-elevation myocardial infarction, *J Am Coll Cardiol* 61e:78, 2013.

23. Flynn Makic MB, VonRueden KT, Rauen CA, et al: Evidence-based practice habits: putting more sacred cows out to pasture, *Crit Care Nurse* 31:31, 2011.

*24. American Association of Critical-Care Nurses: AACN practice alert: oral care for patients at risk for ventilator-associated pneumonia. Retrieved from *www.aacn.org/wd/practice/docs/practicealerts/oral-care-patients-at-risk-vap.pdf.*

*25. American Association of Critical-Care Nurses: AACN practice alert: family presence during resuscitation and invasive procedures. Retrieved from *www.aacn.org/wd/practice/docs/practicealerts/family-presence-during-resuscitation-invasive-procedures.pdf.*

*26. American Association of Critical-Care Nurses: AACN practice alert: family presence: visitation in the adult ICU. Retrieved from *www.aacn.org/WD/practice/docs/practicealerts/family-visitation-adult-icu-practicealert.pdf*


*Evidence-based information for clinical practice.

67

# Acute Respiratory Failure and Acute Respiratory Distress Syndrome

*Richard Arbour*

*Hope lies in dreams, in imagination, and in the courage of those who dare to make dreams into reality.*

***Jonas Salk***

http://evolve.elsevier.com/Lewis/medsurg/

## LEARNING OUTCOMES

1. Compare the pathophysiologic mechanisms and clinical manifestations that result in hypoxemic and hypercapnic respiratory failure.
2. Differentiate between the nursing and interprofessional management of the patient with hypoxemic or hypercapnic respiratory failure.
3. Relate the pathophysiologic mechanisms and clinical manifestations associated with acute respiratory failure and acute respiratory distress syndrome (ARDS).
4. Select appropriate nursing and interprofessional interventions for the patient with ARDS.
5. Prioritize measures to prevent or reverse complications that can result from acute respiratory failure or ARDS.

## KEY TERMS

acute respiratory distress syndrome (ARDS), p. 1620
acute respiratory failure, p. 1609
alveolar hypoventilation, p. 1612
hypercapnia, p. 1609
hypercapnic respiratory failure, p. 1610
hypoxemia, p. 1609
hypoxemic respiratory failure, p. 1609
hypoxia, p. 1613
refractory hypoxemia, p. 1621
shunt, p. 1611
work of breathing (WOB), p. 1613

This chapter discusses the etiology, pathophysiology, and clinical manifestations of acute respiratory failure and acute respiratory distress syndrome (ARDS). Nursing and interprofessional management of patients with acute respiratory failure and ARDS focus on interventions to promote adequate oxygenation and ventilation while addressing the underlying causes.

## ACUTE RESPIRATORY FAILURE

The major function of the respiratory system is gas exchange. This involves the transfer of $O_2$ and $CO_2$ between atmospheric air and circulating blood within the pulmonary capillary bed (Fig. 67-1). **Acute respiratory failure** results when one or both of these gas-exchanging functions are inadequate (e.g., insufficient $O_2$ is transferred to the blood or inadequate $CO_2$ is removed from the lungs).

Conditions that interfere with adequate $O_2$ transfer result in **hypoxemia.** This causes a decrease in arterial $O_2$ ($PaO_2$) and saturation ($SaO_2$). Insufficient $CO_2$ removal results in **hypercapnia.** This causes an increase in arterial $CO_2$ ($PaCO_2$).[1] Arterial blood gases (ABGs) are used to assess changes in pH, $PaO_2$, $PaCO_2$, bicarbonate, and $SaO_2$. Pulse oximetry is used intermittently or continuously to assess arterial $O_2$ saturation ($SpO_2$).

Acute respiratory failure is not a disease but a symptom of underlying pathology affecting lung function. When respiratory function is insufficient, $O_2$ delivery, cardiac output (CO), clinical assessment findings, and/or baseline metabolic state may exhibit abnormalities specific to the affected body system(s). It is a condition that occurs because of one or more disorders involving the lungs or other body systems (Table 67-1).

Respiratory failure is classified as hypoxemic or hypercapnic (Fig. 67-2). Hypoxemic respiratory failure is also referred to as *oxygenation failure* because the primary problem is inadequate $O_2$ transfer between the alveoli and pulmonary capillaries. Although no universal definition exists, **hypoxemic respiratory failure** is commonly defined as a $PaO_2$ less than 60 mm Hg when the patient is receiving an inspired $O_2$ concentration of 60% or more. This definition incorporates two important concepts: (1) the $PaO_2$ level indicates inadequate $O_2$ saturation of

Reviewed by Susan J. Eisel, RN, MSEd, Associate Professor of Nursing, Mercy College of Ohio, Toledo, Ohio; Eugene E. Mondor, RN, MN, CNCC(C), Clinical Nurse Educator, Royal Alexandra Hospital, Edmonton, Alberta, Canada; and Julie Rogan, RN, MSN, ACCNS-AG, AOCNS, CCRN, Clinical Nurse Specialist, Medical Intensive Care Unit, Thomas Jefferson University Hospital, Philadelphia, Pennsylvania.

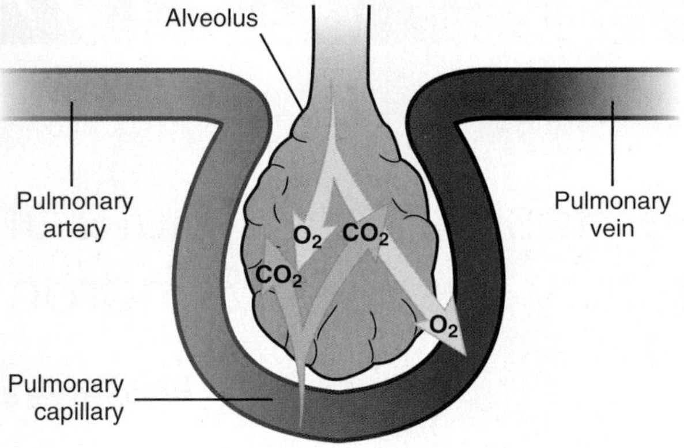


**FIG. 67-1** Normal gas exchange unit in the lung.

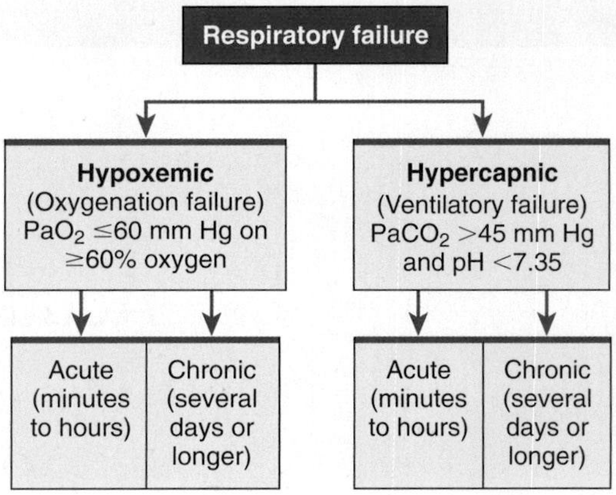


**FIG. 67-2** Classification of respiratory failure.

**TABLE 67-1 Causes of Hypoxemic and Hypercapnic Respiratory Failure***

| Hypoxemic Respiratory Failure | Hypercapnic Respiratory Failure |
|---|---|
| **Respiratory System**<br>• Acute respiratory distress syndrome (ARDS)<br>• Pneumonia<br>• Toxic inhalation (e.g., smoke inhalation)<br>• Hepatopulmonary syndrome (e.g., low-resistance flow state, V/Q mismatch)<br>• Massive pulmonary embolism (e.g., thrombus emboli, fat emboli)<br>• Pulmonary artery laceration and hemorrhage<br>• Inflammatory state and related alveolar injury | **Respiratory System**<br>• Asthma<br>• COPD<br>• Cystic fibrosis<br>**Central Nervous System**<br>• Brainstem injury or infarction<br>• Sedative and opioid overdose<br>• Spinal cord injury<br>• Severe head injury<br>**Chest Wall**<br>• Thoracic trauma (e.g., flail chest)<br>• Kyphoscoliosis<br>• Pain<br>• Severe obesity |
| **Cardiac System**<br>• Anatomic shunt (e.g., ventricular septal defect)<br>• Cardiogenic pulmonary edema<br>• Shock (decreasing blood flow through pulmonary vasculature)<br>• High cardiac output states: diffusion limitation | **Neuromuscular System**<br>• Myasthenia gravis<br>• Critical illness polyneuropathy<br>• Acute myopathy<br>• Toxin exposure or ingestion (e.g., tree tobacco, acetylcholinesterase inhibitors, carbamate or organophosphate poisoning)<br>• Amyotrophic lateral sclerosis<br>• Phrenic nerve injury<br>• Guillain-Barré syndrome<br>• Poliomyelitis<br>• Muscular dystrophy<br>• Multiple sclerosis |

*List is not all-inclusive.

hemoglobin and (2) this $PaO_2$ level exists despite giving supplemental $O_2$ at a percentage (60%) that is about three times that in room air (21%).

Hypercapnic respiratory failure is also referred to as *ventilatory failure* because the primary problem is insufficient $CO_2$ removal. **Hypercapnic respiratory failure** is commonly defined as a $PaCO_2$ greater than 45 mm Hg in combination with acidemia (arterial pH less than 7.35). This definition incorporates three important concepts: (1) the $PaCO_2$ is higher than normal, (2) there is evidence of the body's inability to compensate for this increase (acidemia), and (3) the pH is at a level where a further decrease may lead to severe acid-base imbalance. (See Chapter 16 for a discussion of acid-base balance.) Numerous disorders can compromise lung ventilation and subsequent $CO_2$ removal[2] (Table 67-1).

Patients may experience both hypoxemic and hypercapnic respiratory failure at the same time.[3] For example, a patient with chronic obstructive pulmonary disease (COPD) who develops pulmonary edema could be experiencing both acute and chronic respiratory failure. Always interpret patient-specific data within the context of your assessment findings and the patient's baseline (when known). A person with COPD who develops pneumonia may have a higher baseline $PaCO_2$. This information should be used for interpreting ABGs and other patient data.

## Etiology and Pathophysiology

**Hypoxemic Respiratory Failure.** Four physiologic mechanisms may cause hypoxemia and subsequent hypoxemic respiratory failure: (1) mismatch between ventilation (V) and perfusion (Q), commonly referred to as V/Q mismatch; (2) shunt; (3) diffusion limitation; and (4) alveolar hypoventilation. The most common causes are V/Q mismatch and shunt.

***Ventilation-Perfusion Mismatch.*** In normal lungs the volume of blood perfusing the lungs each minute (4 to 5 L) is approximately equal to the amount of gas that reaches the alveoli each minute (4 to 5 L). In a perfectly matched system, each portion of the lung would receive 1 mL of air (ventilation) for each 1 mL of blood flow (perfusion). This match of ventilation and perfusion would result in a V/Q ratio of 1 : 1, which is expressed as V/Q = 1. When the match is not 1 : 1, a *V/Q mismatch* occurs.

Although this example implies that ventilation and perfusion are ideally matched in all areas of the lung, this situation does not normally exist. In reality, some regional mismatch occurs. At the lung apex, V/Q ratios are greater than 1 (more ventilation than perfusion). At the lung base, V/Q ratios are less than 1 (less ventilation than perfusion). Because changes at the lung apex balance changes at the base, the net effect is a close overall match (Fig. 67-3).

Many diseases and conditions cause V/Q mismatch (Fig. 67-4). The most common are those in which increased secretions are present in the airways (e.g., COPD) or alveoli (e.g., pneumonia), and in which bronchospasm is present (e.g., asthma).[2] V/Q mismatch may also result from alveolar collapse (*atelectasis*) or as a result of pain.

Pain interferes with chest and abdominal wall movement, increases muscle tension, and produces generalized muscle rigidity. This often compromises ventilation. Pain also activates

| V/Q | $PaO_2$ | $PaCO_2$ |
|---|---|---|
| 3.3 | 132 | 28 |
| 1.0 | 108 | 39 |
| 0.63 | 89 | 42 |

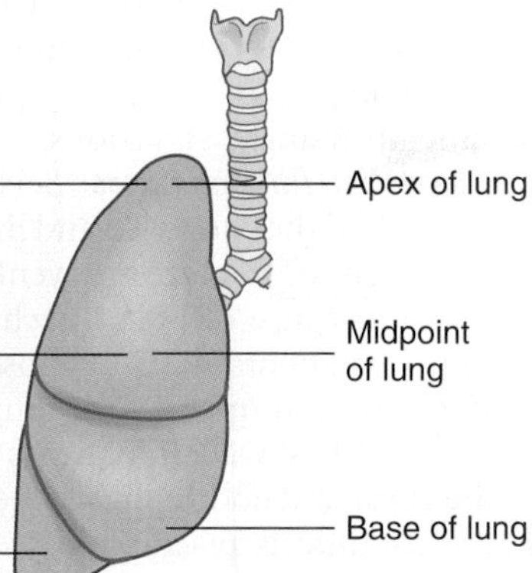


**FIG. 67-3** Regional V/Q differences in the normal lung. This difference causes the $PaO_2$ to be higher at the apex of the lung and lower at the base. Values for $PaCO_2$ are the opposite (i.e., lower at the apex and higher at the base). Blood that exits the lung is a mixture of these values.

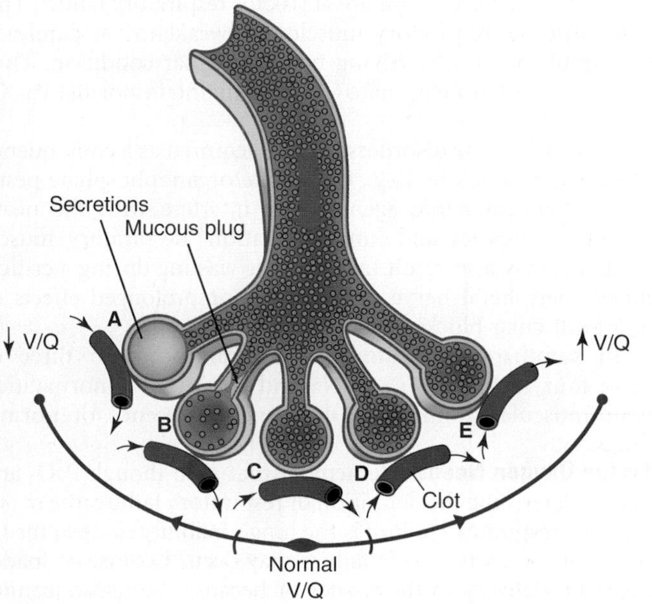


**FIG. 67-4** Range of ventilation-to-perfusion (V/Q) relationships. *A*, Absolute shunt, no ventilation because of fluid filling the alveoli. *B*, V/Q mismatch, ventilation partially compromised by secretions in the airway. *C*, Normal lung unit. *D*, V/Q mismatch, perfusion partially compromised by emboli obstructing blood flow. *E*, Dead space, no perfusion because of obstruction of the pulmonary capillary.

the stress response, increasing baseline metabolic state. It may increase $O_2$ consumption and $CO_2$ production.[4] With a significant increase in metabolic rate, $O_2$ is consumed and $CO_2$ (as a by-product of cell/tissue metabolism) is increased. In this case, increased $O_2$ demand and $CO_2$ production may increase ventilation demands. All these conditions result in limited airflow *(ventilation)* to alveoli but have no effect on blood flow *(perfusion)* to the gas exchange units (Fig. 67-1). The consequence of the imbalance is V/Q mismatch.

A pulmonary embolus affects the perfusion portion of the V/Q relationship. The embolus limits blood flow distal to the occlusion. When a pulmonary embolus occurs, areas of normal lung ventilation remain but have significantly decreased perfusion resulting from the vessel occlusion. This results in a V/Q

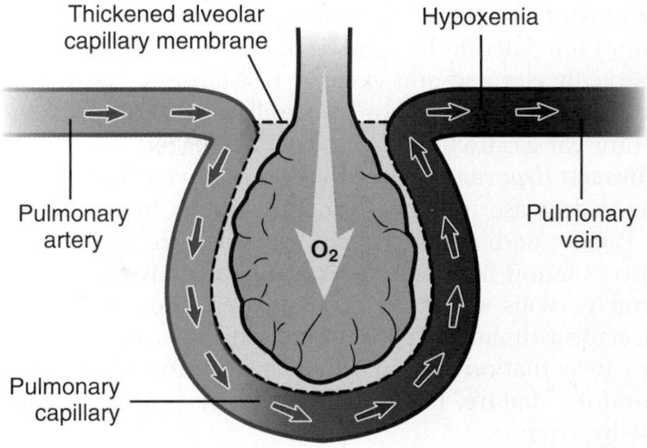


**FIG. 67-5** Diffusion limitation. Exchange of $CO_2$ and $O_2$ cannot occur because of the thickened alveolar-capillary membrane.

mismatch[5] (Fig. 67-4). If large enough, the embolus can cause hemodynamic compromise due to the blockage of a large pulmonary artery.

$O_2$ therapy is an appropriate first step to reverse hypoxemia caused by V/Q mismatch, even though not all gas exchange units are affected equally. $O_2$ therapy increases the $PaO_2$ in blood leaving normal gas exchange units, thus causing a higher-than-normal $PaO_2$. The well-oxygenated blood mixes with poorly oxygenated blood, raising the overall $PaO_2$ of blood leaving the lungs. The best approach to treat hypoxemia caused by a V/Q mismatch is aimed at the cause.

***Shunt.*** A **shunt** occurs when blood exits the heart without having participated in gas exchange. A shunt can be viewed as an extreme V/Q mismatch (Fig. 67-4). There are two types of shunt: anatomic and intrapulmonary. An *anatomic shunt* occurs when blood passes through an anatomic channel in the heart (e.g., a ventricular septal defect) and bypasses the lungs. An *intrapulmonary shunt* occurs when blood flows through the pulmonary capillaries without participating in gas exchange. An intrapulmonary shunt is seen in conditions in which the alveoli fill with fluid (e.g., acute respiratory distress syndrome [ARDS], pneumonia) and gas exchange is limited at the alveolar-capillary membrane.

$O_2$ therapy alone is often ineffective at increasing the $PaO_2$ if hypoxemia is due to a shunt. Patients with a shunt are usually more hypoxemic than patients with V/Q mismatch. They often require mechanical ventilation and a high fraction of inspired $O_2$ ($FIO_2$) to improve gas exchange.

***Diffusion Limitation.*** *Diffusion limitation* occurs when gas exchange across the alveolar-capillary membrane is compromised by a process that thickens, damages, or destroys the alveolar membrane or affects blood flow through the pulmonary capillaries (Fig. 67-5). Diffusion limitation is worsened by disease states affecting the pulmonary vascular bed, such as severe COPD or recurrent pulmonary emboli. Some disease states cause the alveolar-capillary membrane to become thicker (fibrotic), which slows gas transport. These include pulmonary fibrosis, interstitial lung disease, and ARDS.

The classic sign of diffusion limitation is hypoxemia that is present during exercise but not at rest. During exercise, blood moves more rapidly through the lungs. This decreases the time for diffusion of $O_2$ across the alveolar-capillary membrane. Diffusion limitation may also occur in a high CO state (e.g., hepatopulmonary syndrome) or other disease states (e.g., inflammatory response seen with pancreatitis or severe brain trauma) unrelated to lung tissue damage. In this situation, CO is markedly elevated and vascular resistance is low. Blood circulates through the pulmonary capillary bed rapidly, allowing less time for gas exchange to occur.[6]

***Alveolar Hypoventilation.*** Alveolar hypoventilation is a generalized decrease in ventilation that results in an increase in the $PaCO_2$ and a consequent decrease in $PaO_2$. Alveolar hypoventilation may be the result of restrictive lung diseases, central nervous system (CNS) diseases, chest wall dysfunction, acute asthma, or neuromuscular diseases. Although alveolar hypoventilation is primarily a mechanism of hypercapnic respiratory failure, it is mentioned here because it can also cause hypoxemia.

***Interrelationship of Mechanisms.*** Frequently, hypoxemic respiratory failure is caused by a combination of two or more of the following: V/Q mismatch, shunt, diffusion limitation, and alveolar hypoventilation. For example, the patient with acute respiratory failure secondary to pneumonia may have a combination of V/Q mismatch and shunt. In this case, inflammation, edema, and hypersecretion of exudate within the bronchioles and gas exchange units obstruct the airways (V/Q mismatch) and fill the alveoli with exudate (shunt). Additional contributing factors to hypoxemic respiratory failure include increases in $O_2$ demand such as with anxiety or agitation and unrelieved pain.

**Hypercapnic Respiratory Failure.** Hypercapnic respiratory failure is sometimes called *ventilatory failure.* When $CO_2$ levels cannot be maintained within normal limits by the respiratory system, one of two primary problems exists: (1) an increase in $CO_2$ production or (2) a decrease in alveolar ventilation. Hypercapnic respiratory failure may also be acute or chronic in nature. For example, a patient who experiences sudden onset of decreased level of consciousness due to drug overdose may not ventilate appropriately, producing an acute increase in $CO_2$ levels. Overall, hypercapnia often reflects substantial lung dysfunction.

Many different conditions can cause a limitation in ventilatory supply (Table 67-1). These can be grouped into four categories: (1) abnormalities of the airways and alveoli, (2) abnormalities of the CNS, (3) abnormalities of the chest wall, and (4) neuromuscular conditions.

***Airway and Alveoli Abnormalities.*** Patients with asthma, COPD, and cystic fibrosis are at high risk for hypercapnic respiratory failure because the underlying pathophysiology of these conditions results in airflow obstruction and air trapping. Ultimately respiratory muscle fatigue and ventilatory failure occur due to the additional work needed to inspire adequate tidal volumes against increased airway resistance and air trapped within the alveoli.[7]

***Central Nervous System Abnormalities.*** A variety of CNS problems may suppress the drive to breathe. A common example is an overdose of a respiratory depressant drug (e.g., opioids, benzodiazepines). In a dose-related manner, CNS depressants decrease $CO_2$ reactivity in the brainstem. This allows arterial $CO_2$ levels to rise. A brainstem infarction or severe head injury may also interfere with normal function of the respiratory center in the medulla. Patients with these conditions are at risk for respiratory failure because the medulla does not alter the respiratory rate in response to a change in $PaCO_2$.

CNS dysfunction may also include high-level spinal cord injuries that limit nerve supply to the respiratory muscles of the chest wall and diaphragm. Apart from direct brainstem dysfunction, metabolic or structural brain injury resulting in decreased or loss of consciousness may interfere with the patient's ability to adequately protect his or her own airway, breathe, or manage secretions.

***Chest Wall Abnormalities.*** Several conditions prevent normal movement of the chest wall and limit lung expansion. In patients with flail chest, fractures prevent the rib cage from expanding normally because of pain, mechanical restriction, and muscle spasm. In patients with kyphoscoliosis, the change in spinal configuration compresses the lungs and prevents normal expansion of the chest wall. In patients with severe obesity, the weight of the chest and abdominal contents may limit lung expansion. These conditions place patients at risk for respiratory failure because they limit lung expansion or diaphragmatic movement and consequently gas exchange.

***Neuromuscular Conditions.*** Various types of neuromuscular diseases may result in respiratory muscle weakness or paralysis (Table 67-1). For example, patients with Guillain-Barré syndrome, muscular dystrophy, myasthenia gravis (acute exacerbation), or multiple sclerosis are at risk for respiratory failure. This is because the respiratory muscles are weakened or paralyzed as a result of the underlying neuromuscular condition. Thus they are unable to eliminate $CO_2$ and maintain normal $PaCO_2$ levels.[8]

Neuromuscular disorders may be acquired as a consequence of exposure to toxins (e.g., carbamate/organophosphate pesticides, chemical nerve agents) that interfere with the nerve supply to muscles and lung ventilation. Respiratory muscle weakness may also result from muscle wasting during a critical illness, peripheral nerve damage, and/or prolonged effects of neuromuscular blocking agents.

In summary, respiratory failure can occur in three of these four categories (i.e., CNS and chest wall abnormalities, neuromuscular conditions) despite the presence of normal lungs.

**Tissue Oxygen Needs.** Remember that even though $PaO_2$ and $PaCO_2$ determine the definition of respiratory failure, the major cause of respiratory failure is the lung's inability to meet the $O_2$ needs of the tissues. This failure may occur because of inadequate $O_2$ delivery to the tissues or because the tissues cannot use the $O_2$ delivered to them. It may also occur as a result of the stress response and a demand for $O_2$ greater than what can be supplied to the tissues. Tissue $O_2$ delivery is determined by cardiac output and the amount of $O_2$ carried in hemoglobin. Therefore respiratory failure places the patient at greater risk if there are coexisting heart problems or anemia.

In some conditions, such as septic shock, adequate $O_2$ may be delivered to the tissues, but impaired $O_2$ extraction or diffusion limitation exists at the cellular level. The result is an abnormally high amount of $O_2$ returning in the venous blood because it is not used at the tissue level. (Chapter 66 discusses shock.) Acid-base alterations (e.g., alkalosis, acidosis) may also interfere with $O_2$ delivery to peripheral tissues (see Chapter 16).

## Clinical Manifestations

Respiratory failure may develop suddenly (minutes or hours) or gradually (several days or longer). A sudden decrease in $PaO_2$ or a rapid rise in $PaCO_2$ implies a serious condition, which can rapidly become a life-threatening emergency. An example is the patient with asthma who develops severe bronchospasm and a marked decrease in airflow, resulting in rapid respiratory muscle fatigue, acidemia, and acute respiratory failure.

Change in $PaCO_2$ is better tolerated over time because compensation can occur. An example is the patient with COPD who develops a progressive increase in $PaCO_2$ over several days after an acute respiratory tract infection. Because the change occurred over several days, there is time for renal compensation (e.g., retention of bicarbonate). This minimizes the change in arterial pH. (See Chapter 16 for a discussion of renal compensation for acid-base disorders.)

Signs of respiratory failure are related to the extent of change in $PaO_2$ or $PaCO_2$, the speed of change (acute versus chronic), and the patient's ability to compensate for this change. When the patient's compensatory mechanisms fail, respiratory failure occurs. Because clinical signs vary, it is important to watch trends in ABGs, pulse oximetry, and assessment findings to fully evaluate the extent of change. Frequently, the first sign of respiratory failure is a change in the patient's mental status. Mental status changes often occur early before ABG results are obtained. This is because the brain is very sensitive to variations in $O_2$ and $CO_2$ levels and acid-base balance.

Restlessness, confusion, agitation, and combative behavior suggest inadequate $O_2$ delivery to the brain and should be fully investigated. Conversely, morning headache, a slower respiratory rate, and a decreased level of consciousness may indicate issues with $CO_2$ removal. Tachycardia, tachypnea, and mild hypertension can be early signs of acute respiratory failure. Such changes can indicate an attempt by the heart and lungs to compensate for decreased $O_2$ delivery and rising $CO_2$ levels.

Cyanosis is an unreliable indicator of hypoxemia. It is a late sign of respiratory failure as it often does not occur until hypoxemia is severe ($PaO_2$ 45 mm Hg or less). You must identify the physiologic changes that can occur as a result of hypoxemia or hypercarbia. Your ability to detect the onset of acute respiratory failure and evaluate progression or resolution in response to treatment is essential (Table 67-2).

**Consequences of Hypoxemia and Hypoxia.** *Hypoxemia* occurs when the amount of $O_2$ in arterial blood is less than the normal value (normal $PaO_2$ is 80 to 100 mm Hg). **Hypoxia** occurs when the $PaO_2$ falls sufficiently to cause signs and symptoms of inadequate oxygenation (Table 67-2). Hypoxemia can lead to hypoxia if not corrected. If hypoxia or hypoxemia is severe, the cells shift from aerobic to anaerobic metabolism. Anaerobic metabolism uses more fuel, produces less energy, and is less efficient than aerobic metabolism. The waste product of anaerobic metabolism is lactic acid. This is more difficult to remove from the body than $CO_2$ because it has to be buffered with sodium bicarbonate. When the body does not have enough sodium bicarbonate to buffer the lactic acid produced by anaerobic metabolism, metabolic acidosis, tissue and cellular dysfunction, and cell death may occur. BP and CO can fall. Vasoactive or inotropic drugs may be needed for cardiovascular support. These drugs may be less effective in the presence of a severe acidotic environment.

Permanent brain damage may occur if the hypoxia is severe and prolonged. Renal function may also be impaired. Sodium retention, edema, acute tubular necrosis, and uremia may occur. Gastrointestinal (GI) system alterations include tissue ischemia, increased permeability of the intestinal wall, and possible migration of bacteria from the GI tract into circulation.

**TABLE 67-2 Manifestations of Hypoxemia and Hypercapnia***

| Specific | Nonspecific |
|---|---|
| **Hypoxemia** | |
| ***Respiratory*** | ***Central Nervous*** |
| Dyspnea | Agitation |
| Tachypnea | Disorientation |
| Prolonged expiration (I : E = 1 : 3, 1 : 4) | Restless, combative behavior |
| Nasal flaring | Delirium |
| Intercostal muscle retraction | Confusion |
| Use of accessory muscles in respiration | ↓ Level of consciousness |
| ↓ $SpO_2$ (<80%) | Coma (late) |
| Paradoxic chest or abdominal wall movement with respiratory cycle (late) | ***Cardiovascular*** |
| Cyanosis (late) | Tachycardia |
| | Hypertension |
| | Skin cool, clammy, and diaphoretic |
| | Dysrhythmias (late) |
| | Hypotension (late) |
| | ***Other*** |
| | Fatigue |
| | Inability to speak in complete sentences without pausing to breathe |
| **Hypercapnia** | |
| ***Respiratory*** | ***Central Nervous*** |
| Dyspnea | Morning headache |
| Use of tripod position | Disorientation, confusion |
| Pursed-lip breathing | Agitation |
| ↓ Respiratory rate or rapid rate with shallow respirations | Progressive somnolence |
| ↓ Tidal volume | Elevated intracranial pressure (if monitored) |
| ↓ Minute ventilation | Coma (late) |
| | ***Cardiovascular*** |
| | Dysrhythmias |
| | Hypertension |
| | Tachycardia |
| | Bounding pulse |
| | ***Neuromuscular*** |
| | Muscle weakness |
| | ↓ Deep tendon reflexes |
| | Tremors, seizures (late) |

*I : E*, Inspiratory : expiratory ratio.
*List is not all-inclusive.

**Specific Clinical Manifestations.** The patient in respiratory failure may have a rapid, shallow breathing pattern or a respiratory rate that is slower than normal. Both changes predispose the patient to insufficient $CO_2$ removal. The patient may increase the respiratory rate in an effort to blow off accumulated $CO_2$. This breathing pattern requires a substantial amount of work and can lead to respiratory muscle fatigue. A change from a rapid rate to a slower rate in a patient in acute respiratory distress such as that seen with acute asthma suggests extreme progression of respiratory muscle fatigue and increased probability of respiratory arrest.

The patient's position is an indication of the effort associated with the **work of breathing (WOB)**, or the effort used for muscle contraction during inhalation to accomplish lung ventilation. The patient may be able to lie down (mild distress), be able to lie down but prefer to sit (moderate distress), or be unable to breathe unless sitting upright (severe distress). A common position used by patients with moderate to severe COPD is to sit with the arms propped on the overbed table or

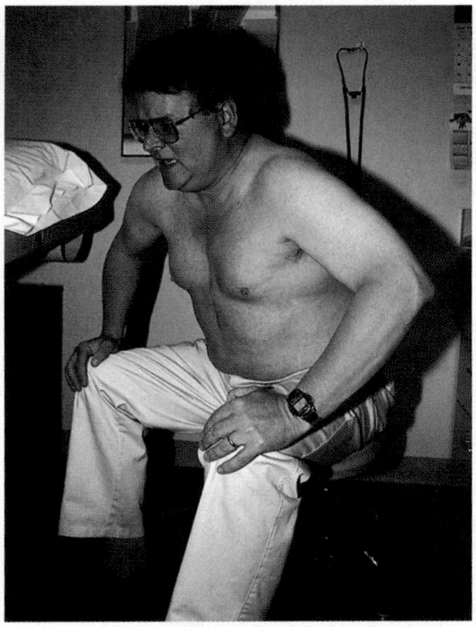

**FIG. 67-6** Tripod positioning is used to increase chest and lung expansion and decrease work of breathing for patients with COPD or asthma. (From Wilson SF, Giddens JF: *Health assessment for nursing practice,* ed 4, St Louis, 2009, Mosby.)

on the knees. This so-called *tripod position* helps decrease the WOB, since propping the arms increases the anteroposterior diameter of the chest and changes pressure in the thorax (Fig. 67-6).

The person who is experiencing dyspnea is working hard to breathe. You may see patients using pursed-lip breathing (see Table 28-13). This technique increases $SaO_2$ by slowing respirations, allowing more time for expiration, and preventing small bronchioles from collapsing. Similarly, the dyspneic patient may be able to speak only a few words at a time between breaths. The patient's ability to speak often indicates the severity of dyspnea. The patient may have "two-word" or "three word" dyspnea. This means that only two or three words can be spoken before pausing to breathe. These are important observations that can help you identify the onset of acute respiratory failure.

You may observe *retraction* (inward movement) of the intercostal spaces or supraclavicular area and use of the accessory muscles (e.g., sternocleidomastoid) during inspiration or expiration. Use of the accessory muscles signifies moderate distress. Paradoxic breathing indicates severe distress. Normally, the thorax and abdomen move outward on inspiration and inward on exhalation.

During *paradoxic breathing,* the abdomen and chest move in the opposite manner—outward during exhalation and inward during inspiration. Paradoxic breathing results from maximal use of the accessory muscles of respiration. The patient may also be diaphoretic from the WOB.

Perform auscultation to assess the patient's baseline breath sounds and any changes from baseline. Note and document the presence and location of any abnormal breath sounds. Crackles (generally heard on inspiration) may indicate pulmonary edema. Loud crackles heard on expiration indicate additional lung secretions and may be symptomatic of pneumonia or COPD. Absent or diminished breath sounds may indicate atelectasis, pleural effusion, or impaired inspiratory effort and hypoventilation. Bronchial breath sounds over the lung periphery often indicate lung consolidation from pneumonia. A pleural friction rub may also be heard in the presence of pneumonia that involves the pleura.

A thorough assessment may result in early detection of respiratory insufficiency, allowing interventions to be started sooner and preventing respiratory failure. Patients with end-stage chronic lung disease may have low $PaO_2$ or high $PaCO_2$ levels and crackles as their "normal" baseline. It is important to monitor specific and nonspecific signs of respiratory failure in patients with COPD because a small change can cause significant decompensation (Table 67-2). Immediately report any change in mental status (e.g., agitation, confusion, decreased level of consciousness). This may indicate the onset of rapid deterioration in clinical status and the need for mechanical ventilation. Obtain vital signs as clinically indicated. Changes in vital signs (especially respiratory rate) are often an early sign of respiratory failure.

### Diagnostic Studies

After physical assessment, the most common diagnostic studies used to evaluate acute respiratory failure are chest x-ray and ABG analysis. A chest x-ray helps to identify possible causes of respiratory failure (e.g., atelectasis, pneumonia). ABGs determine the levels of $PaCO_2$, $PaO_2$, bicarbonate, and pH. In respiratory failure, ABGs are used to evaluate oxygenation ($PaO_2$) and ventilation ($PaCO_2$) status and acid-base balance. Pulse oximetry monitors oxygenation status but reveals little about lung ventilation.

Other diagnostic studies that may be done include a complete blood cell count, serum electrolytes, urinalysis, and ECG. Blood and sputum cultures are obtained as necessary to determine sources of possible infection. If pulmonary embolus is suspected, a CT scan or V/Q lung scan may be done. For the patient in severe respiratory failure requiring endotracheal intubation, end-tidal $CO_2$ ($ETCO_2$) is used to help confirm correct tube placement within the airway immediately after intubation. (Chapter 65 discusses intubation.) $ETCO_2$ monitoring *(capnography)* and transcutaneous $CO_2$ monitoring may also be used during ventilator management to assess trends in lung ventilation.[9]

In severe respiratory failure, central venous or PA pressure monitoring or arterial pressure–based CO monitoring is used to measure hemodynamic parameters (e.g., central venous pressure, PA pressures, CO, stroke volume variation, central or mixed venous $O_2$ saturation [$ScvO_2$ or $SvO_2$]). These data help to determine the adequacy of tissue perfusion and the patient's response to treatment measures. Hemodynamic monitoring can also determine whether the accumulation of fluid in the lungs is the result of heart or lung problems. It can also provide feedback on the physiologic effects of mechanical ventilation on hemodynamic status.[10] (Chapter 65 discusses hemodynamic monitoring in detail.)

## NURSING AND INTERPROFESSIONAL MANAGEMENT: ACUTE RESPIRATORY FAILURE

Because many different problems cause respiratory failure, specific care of these patients varies. This section discusses general assessment and interventions that apply to patients with acute respiratory failure. In acute care settings, collaboration between nursing and other interprofessional care team members (e.g., respiratory therapists) is essential.

## ◆ Nursing Assessment

Table 67-3 presents subjective and objective data that should be obtained from the patient with acute respiratory failure.

## ◆ Nursing Diagnoses

Nursing diagnoses for the patient with acute respiratory failure may include, but are not limited to, the following:

- Impaired gas exchange *related to* alveolar hypoventilation, intrapulmonary shunting, V/Q mismatch, and diffusion impairment
- Ineffective airway clearance *related to* excessive secretions, decreased level of consciousness, presence of an artificial airway, neuromuscular dysfunction, and pain
- Ineffective breathing pattern *related to* neuromuscular impairment of respirations, pain, anxiety, decreased level of consciousness, respiratory muscle fatigue, and bronchospasm

Additional information on nursing diagnoses for the patient with acute respiratory failure is presented in eNursing Care Plan 67-1 (available on the website for this chapter).

## ◆ Planning

The overall goals for the patient with acute respiratory failure include (1) independent maintenance of the airway, (2) effective cough and ability to clear secretions, (3) normal ABG values or values within the patient's baseline, (4) absence of dyspnea or recovery to baseline breathing patterns for patient, and (5) breath sounds within the patient's baseline.

## ◆ Prevention

As part of the plan of care for any patient who may be at risk for respiratory failure, prevention and early recognition of respiratory distress are important. Prevention involves a thorough history and physical assessment to identify the patient at risk for respiratory failure and then the start of appropriate interventions. These include teaching the patient about deep breathing and coughing, use of incentive spirometry, and ambulation.

Prevention of atelectasis, pneumonia, and complications of immobility, as well as optimizing hydration and nutrition, can potentially decrease the risk of respiratory failure in acutely or critically ill patients. It is also important to consider age-related and acuity-related changes in physiology when assessing risk of acute respiratory failure. Patients at higher risk of acute respiratory failure should be assessed more frequently with additional attention to preventive measures.

## ◆ Respiratory Therapy

The major goals of care for acute respiratory failure include maintaining adequate oxygenation and ventilation. Interventions include $O_2$ therapy, mobilization of secretions, and positive pressure ventilation (PPV) (Table 67-4).

**◆ Oxygen Therapy.** The primary goal of $O_2$ therapy is to correct hypoxemia. The patient with acute respiratory failure must be able to tolerate the type of $O_2$ delivery system chosen. For example, a face mask may cause anxiety from feelings of claustrophobia. The anxiety can cause dyspnea, increase $O_2$ consumption and $CO_2$ production, and cause the patient to remove the $O_2$ device. The selected $O_2$ delivery system must also maintain $PaO_2$ at 55 to 60 mm Hg or higher and $SaO_2$ at 90% or higher at the lowest $O_2$ concentration possible.

Several methods are available to provide $O_2$ to patients in acute respiratory failure. (Chapter 28 and Table 28-20 discuss

### TABLE 67-3 Nursing Assessment
### *Acute Respiratory Failure*

**Subjective Data**

***Important Health Information***

*Past health history:* Chronic lung disease, potential occupational exposures to lung toxins, tobacco use (pack-years), alcohol or drug use, previous hospitalizations related to lung disease, thoracic or spinal cord trauma, severe obesity, altered consciousness, age (physiologic and chronologic)

*Medications:* Use of home $O_2$, inhalers (bronchodilators), home nebulization, over-the-counter drugs; immunosuppressant (e.g., corticosteroid) therapy, CNS depressants

*Surgery or other treatments:* Previous intubation and mechanical ventilation, recent thoracic or abdominal surgery

***Functional Health Patterns***

*Health perception–health management:* Exercise, self-care activities, immunizations (flu, pneumonia, hepatitis)

*Nutritional-metabolic:* Eating habits, bloating, indigestion; weight gain or loss, change in appetite. Use of vitamins or herbal supplements

*Activity-exercise:* Fatigue, dizziness, dyspnea at rest or with activity, wheezing, cough (productive or nonproductive), sputum (volume, color, viscosity), palpitations, swollen feet, change in exercise tolerance

*Sleep-rest:* Changes in sleep pattern, use of CPAP

*Cognitive-perceptual:* Headache, chest pain or tightness, chronic pain

*Coping–stress tolerance:* Anxiety, depression, hopelessness. Risk of drug, alcohol, or nicotine withdrawal

**Objective Data**

***General***

Restlessness, agitation

***Integumentary***

Pale, cool, clammy skin or warm, flushed skin. Peripheral and central cyanosis. Peripheral dependent edema

***Respiratory***

Shallow, increased respiratory rate progressing to decreased rate. Use of accessory muscles with evidence of retractions, increased diaphragmatic excursion or asymmetric chest expansion, paradoxic chest and abdominal wall movement. Tactile fremitus, crepitus, or deviated trachea on palpation. Absent, diminished, or adventitious breath sounds. Pleural friction rub. Bronchial or bronchovesicular sounds heard in other than normal location, inspiratory stridor

***Cardiovascular***

Tachycardia progressing to bradycardia, dysrhythmias, extra heart sounds ($S_3$, $S_4$). Bounding pulse. Hypertension progressing to hypotension. Pulsus paradoxus, jugular venous distention, pedal edema

***Gastrointestinal***

Abdominal distention, ascites, epigastric tenderness, hepatojugular reflex

***Neurologic***

Somnolence, confusion, slurred speech, restlessness, delirium, agitation, tremors, seizures, coma; asterixis, decreased deep tendon reflexes, papilledema

***Possible Diagnostic Findings***

↓/↑ pH, ↑/↓ $PaCO_2$, ↑/↓ bicarbonate, ↓ $PaO_2$, ↓ $SaO_2$, abnormal serum electrolytes, hemoglobin, hematocrit, and white blood cell count. Abnormal findings on chest x-ray. Abnormal central venous or pulmonary artery pressures. Initially cardiac output may be increased due to the stress response. As hypoxemia, hypercapnia, and acidosis become more severe, cardiac output will decrease.

*CPAP,* Continuous positive airway pressure.

## TABLE 67-4 Interprofessional Care

### Acute Respiratory Failure

**Diagnostic Assessment**

- Vital signs
- History and physical examination
- Arterial blood gases
- Pulse oximetry
- Chest x-ray
- CBC
- Serum electrolytes and urinalysis
- ECG
- Blood and sputum cultures (if indicated)
- Hemodynamic parameters: CVP, SVV, PAWP

**Management**

***Respiratory Therapy***

- $O_2$ therapy
- Mobilization of secretions
  - Effective coughing
  - Incentive spirometry
  - Hydration and humidification
  - Chest physiotherapy
  - Airway suctioning
  - Ambulation
  - Positioning: head of bed elevated to assist lung ventilation; tripod positioning for optimal comfort and efficiency during breathing
- Positive pressure ventilation
  - Noninvasive positive pressure ventilation
  - Intubation with positive pressure ventilation

***Drug Therapy***

- Relief of bronchospasm (e.g., albuterol)
- Reduction of airway inflammation (e.g., corticosteroids)
- Reduction of pulmonary congestion (e.g., furosemide [Lasix], morphine)
- Treatment of pulmonary infections (e.g., antibiotics)
- Reduction of severe anxiety, pain, and agitation (e.g., lorazepam [Ativan], fentanyl [Sublimaze], morphine)

***Medical Supportive Therapy***

- Management of the underlying cause of respiratory failure
- Maintenance of adequate cardiac output
- Maintenance of adequate hemoglobin concentration

***Nutritional Therapy***

- Enteral nutrition support
- Parenteral nutrition support

***Physical Therapy***

- Ambulation
- Muscle conditioning

*CVP*, Central venous pressure; *PAWP*, pulmonary artery wedge pressure; *SVV*, stroke volume variation.

$O_2$ delivery devices.) If hypoxemia is secondary to V/Q mismatch, one method is to give supplemental $O_2$ at 1 to 3 L/minute by nasal cannula. Another method is to give 24% to 32% $O_2$ by face mask or Venturi mask. This should improve the $PaO_2$ and $SaO_2$.

Hypoxemia secondary to an intrapulmonary shunt is usually not responsive to high $O_2$ concentrations. In this case, the patient usually needs $O_2$ given by invasive or noninvasive positive pressure ventilation (NIPPV). PPV provides $O_2$ therapy and humidification, decreases WOB, and reduces respiratory muscle fatigue. In addition, it assists in opening collapsed airways and decreasing shunt.[11] If respiratory status worsens despite NIPPV, PPV using an endotracheal tube is used and higher $O_2$ concentrations are given. (Chapter 65 discusses mechanical ventilation.)

High $O_2$ concentrations replace the nitrogen gas normally present in the alveoli, thus causing instability and atelectasis. In intubated patients, exposure to 60% or higher $FIO_2$ for longer than 48 hours poses a significant risk for *$O_2$ toxicity.* In nonintubated patients the risk is less clear. The effects of prolonged exposure to high levels of $O_2$ include increased pulmonary capillary permeability, decreased surfactant production and surfactant inactivation, and fibrotic changes in the alveoli. (Chapter 28 and Table 28-20 discuss $O_2$ delivery devices.)

Another possible risk of $O_2$ therapy is specific to patients with chronic hypercapnia (e.g., patients with COPD). Chronic hypercapnia blunts the response of chemoreceptors to elevated $CO_2$ levels as a respiratory stimulant. In this case, hypoxia stimulates respiration. Initial $O_2$ therapy may be provided to patients with chronic hypercapnia through a low-flow device such as a nasal cannula at 1 to 2 L/minute or a Venturi mask at 24% to 28%. $O_2$ should be given with careful titration and at the lowest possible dose needed to keep $SpO_2$ and $PaO_2$ within patient-specific clinical goals. Closely monitor patients for changes in mental status, respiratory rate, and ABGs until their $PaO_2$ level has reached their baseline normal value.

◆ **Mobilization of Secretions.** Retained pulmonary secretions may cause or exacerbate acute respiratory failure. This occurs because the movement of $O_2$ into the alveoli and removal of $CO_2$ are blocked. Secretions can be mobilized by effective coughing, adequate hydration and humidification, chest physiotherapy (physical therapy), airway suctioning, patient positioning, and ambulation when possible.

◆ ***Effective Coughing and Positioning.*** If secretions are obstructing the airway, encourage the patient to cough. The patient with a neuromuscular weakness from a disease or exhaustion may not be able to generate sufficient airway pressures to produce an effective cough. *Augmented coughing (quad coughing)* may benefit these patients. Perform augmented coughing by placing one or both hands at the anterolateral base of the patient's lungs (Fig. 67-7). As the patient ends a deep inspiration and begins the expiration, move your hands forcefully upward, increasing abdominal pressure and facilitating the cough. This measure helps increase expiratory flow and thereby facilitates secretion clearance.

Some patients may benefit from therapeutic cough techniques. *Huff coughing* is a series of coughs performed while saying the word "huff" (see Table 28-23). This technique prevents the glottis from closing during the cough. Patients with COPD generate higher flow rates with a huff cough than is possible with a normal cough. The huff cough is effective in clearing only the central airways, but it may assist in moving secretions upward.

The staged cough also assists in mobilizing secretions. To perform the *staged cough,* the patient assumes a sitting position, breathes three or four times in and out through the mouth, and coughs while bending forward and pressing a pillow inward against the diaphragm.

Positioning the patient upright, either by elevating the head of the bed at least 30 degrees or by using a reclining chair or chair bed, helps maximize thoracic expansion, thereby decreasing dyspnea and improving secretion mobilization. A sitting

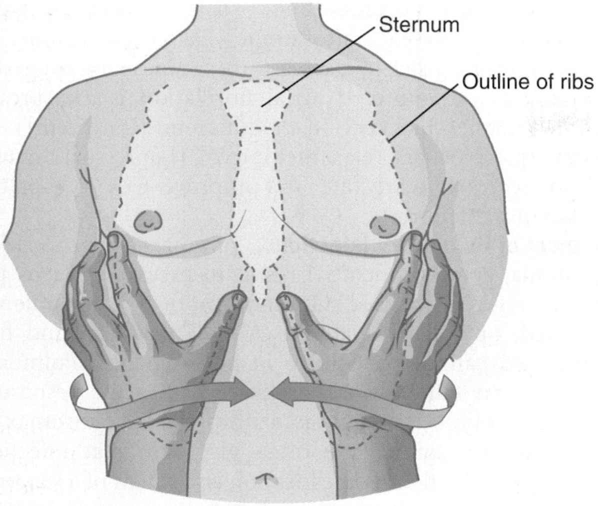


**FIG. 67-7** Augmented coughing is performed by placing one or both hands on the anterolateral base of the lungs. After the patient takes a deep inspiration and at the beginning of expiration, move the hand(s) forcefully upward. This increases abdominal pressure and aids in producing a forceful cough. (From American Association of Critical Care Nurses: *AACN advanced critical care nursing,* St Louis, 2009, Mosby.)

position improves pulmonary function and assists in venous pooling in dependent body areas such as the lower extremities. When lungs are upright, ventilation and perfusion are best in the lung bases.

For patients with a unilateral lung disorder such as right-sided pneumonia, lateral or side-lying positioning may be used. This position, termed *good lung down,* allows for improved V/Q matching in the affected lung. Pulmonary blood flow and ventilation are optimal in dependent lung areas. This position also allows secretions to drain out of the affected lung to the point where they may be removed by suctioning. For example, position patients with significant right-sided pneumonia on their left side to maximize ventilation and perfusion in the "good" lung and aid secretion removal from the affected lung (postural drainage). Patients with acute respiratory failure often have pathology affecting both lungs and may require repositioning at intervals on both sides to optimize air movement and drainage of secretions.

All patients should be side lying if there is any possibility that the tongue will obstruct the airway or that aspiration may occur. Airway control with endotracheal intubation and PPV is indicated when patients cannot maintain their airway and lung ventilation.

◆ ***Hydration.*** Thick and viscous secretions are difficult to expel. Adequate fluid intake (2 to 3 L/day) keeps secretions thin and easier to remove. If the patient is unable to take sufficient fluids orally, IV hydration is used. Thoroughly assess the patient's cardiac and renal status to determine whether he or she can tolerate the IV fluid volume and avoid heart failure and pulmonary edema. Regularly assess for signs of fluid overload by clinical evaluation (e.g., crackles, dyspnea) and invasive monitoring (e.g., increased central venous pressure).

◆ ***Humidification.*** An appropriate humidification device is an adjunct in secretion management. Aerosols of sterile normal saline, given with a nebulizer, may be used to liquefy secretions. $O_2$ may also be given by aerosol mask to thin secretions and facilitate their removal. Aerosol therapy may induce bronchospasm and severe coughing, causing a decreased $PaO_2$. Frequent assessment of the patient's tolerance to therapy is critical. Mucolytic drugs such as nebulized acetylcysteine mixed with a bronchodilator may be used to thin secretions. A side effect of these drugs is bronchospasm. Therefore during their use, closely monitor the patient's respiratory status.

◆ ***Chest Physiotherapy.*** Chest physiotherapy is indicated in patients who produce more than 30 mL of sputum per day or have evidence of severe atelectasis or pulmonary infiltrates. Postural drainage, percussion, and vibration to the affected lung segments assist in moving secretions to the larger airways, where they are removed by coughing or suctioning. Positioning affects oxygenation. Patients may not tolerate head-down or lateral positioning because of extreme dyspnea or hypoxemia caused by V/Q mismatch. (Chest physiotherapy is discussed in Chapter 28.)

◆ ***Airway Suctioning.*** Nasopharyngeal, oropharyngeal, or nasotracheal suctioning (blind suctioning without a tracheal tube in place) is done if the patient is unable to expectorate secretions. Suctioning through an artificial airway (e.g., endotracheal tube) is also done as needed (see Chapters 26 and 65).

At all times, deep airway suctioning should be done cautiously and the patient should be closely monitored for complications. These could include hypoxia, increased ICP, dysrhythmias, bradycardia, vasovagal response, hypotension from sudden elevation in intrathoracic pressure, and hypertension and tachycardia from noxious stimulation.

**CHECK YOUR PRACTICE**

You are caring for a 72-yr-old male patient admitted to the critical care unit with a diagnosis of acute respiratory failure. He has a history of COPD. A chest x-ray reveals a left-sided pneumonia. Your patient is awake but mildly confused and has a productive cough.

- What respiratory interventions would you expect to be ordered for this patient?

◆ **Positive Pressure Ventilation.** If initial measures fail to improve ventilation and oxygenation and the patient continues to show signs of acute respiratory failure, ventilatory assistance is needed. Invasive or NIPPV may be considered.[12] NIPPV is used for patients with acute or chronic respiratory failure. During NIPPV, a mask is placed tightly over the patient's nose or nose and mouth and the patient breathes spontaneously while PPV is delivered. With NIPPV, it is possible to decrease the WOB without the need for endotracheal intubation.

Bilevel positive airway pressure (BiPAP) is a form of NIPPV in which different positive pressure levels are set for inspiration and expiration (Fig. 67-8). Continuous positive airway pressure (CPAP) is another form of NIPPV, in which a constant positive pressure is delivered to the airway during inspiration and expiration.[12]

NIPPV is most useful in managing chronic respiratory failure in patients with chest wall and neuromuscular disease (Table 67-1). NIPPV may also be used for patients who refuse endotracheal intubation but still want some palliative ventilatory support (e.g., patients with end-stage COPD).[13] NIPPV is not appropriate for patients who have excessive secretions, decreased level of consciousness, high $O_2$ requirements, facial trauma, or hemodynamic instability. NIPPV is also used postextubation to avoid reintubation. (Chapter 65 discusses artificial airways, PPV, BiPAP, and CPAP in detail.)

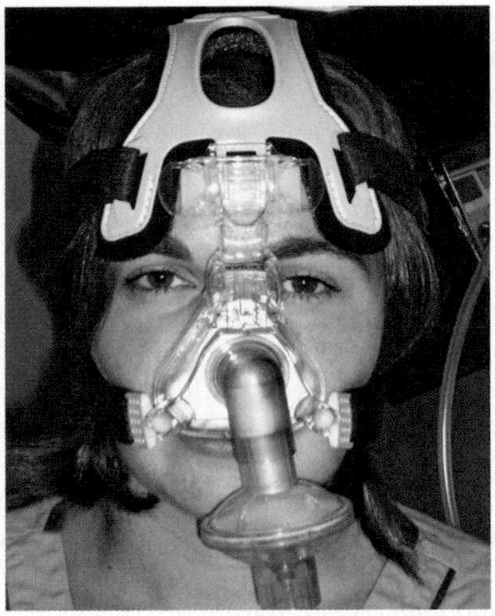

FIG. 67-8 Noninvasive bilevel positive airway pressure ventilation. A mask is placed over the nose or nose and mouth. Positive pressure from a mechanical ventilator assists the patient's breathing efforts, decreasing the work of breathing. (Courtesy Richard Arbour, RN, MSN, CCRN, CNRN, CCNS, FAAN and Anna Kirk, RN, MSN.)

## ◆ Drug Therapy

Goals of drug therapy for patients in acute respiratory failure include (1) relief of bronchospasm; (2) reduction of airway inflammation and pulmonary congestion; (3) treatment of pulmonary infection; and (4) reduction of severe pain, anxiety, and restlessness.

◆ **Relief of Bronchospasm.** Relief of bronchospasm increases alveolar ventilation. Short-acting bronchodilators, such as metaproterenol and albuterol, reverse bronchospasm. In acute bronchospasm these drugs may be given at 15- to 30-minute intervals until a response occurs. Side effects of these β-adrenergic agonists include tachycardia and hypertension. Prolonged use can increase the risk of dysrhythmias and cardiac ischemia. Monitor ECG and vital signs for any changes when giving these drugs.

The bronchodilator effects of these drugs can sometimes worsen hypoxemia by redistributing the inspired gas to areas of decreased perfusion. Giving the bronchodilator with an $O_2$-enriched gas mixture usually reduces this effect. (Chapter 28 discusses nursing management related to bronchodilators.) Give these drugs using a hand-held nebulizer or a metered-dose inhaler with a spacer.

◆ **Reduction of Airway Inflammation.** Corticosteroids (e.g., methylprednisolone [Solu-Medrol]) may be used with bronchodilating drugs for bronchospasm and inflammation. When given IV for conditions such as COPD exacerbation or acute asthma, corticosteroids aid resolution of airway inflammation and edema. Clinical effects may require several hours before onset. Inhaled corticosteroids require 4 to 5 days for optimum therapeutic effects and are not used for acute respiratory failure.

**DRUG ALERT IV Corticosteroids**

- Monitor potassium levels, since corticosteroids exacerbate hypokalemia caused by diuretics.
- Prolonged use causes adrenal insufficiency.

◆ **Reduction of Pulmonary Congestion.** Pulmonary interstitial fluid can accumulate because of direct or indirect injury to the alveolar capillary membrane (e.g., ARDS) or from heart failure. The result is decreased alveolar ventilation and hypoxemia. IV diuretics (e.g., furosemide [Lasix]), morphine, and nitroglycerin are used to decrease the pulmonary congestion caused by heart failure. If atrial fibrillation is also present, calcium channel blockers (e.g., diltiazem [Cardizem]) and β-adrenergic blockers (e.g., metoprolol [Lopressor]) may be used to decrease heart rate and improve CO. (Chapter 34 discusses heart failure.)

◆ **Treatment of Pulmonary Infections.** Pulmonary infections (e.g., pneumonia, acute bronchitis) result in excessive mucus production; fever; increased $O_2$ consumption; and inflamed, fluid-filled, or collapsed alveoli. Alveoli that are fluid filled or collapsed cannot participate in gas exchange. Pulmonary infections can either cause or exacerbate acute respiratory failure. IV antibiotics, such as azithromycin (Zithromax) or ceftriaxone (Rocephin), are often given to treat infections. Chest x-rays help identify the location and extent of a suspected infection. Sputum cultures help identify the type of organisms causing the infection and their sensitivity to antimicrobial drugs.

◆ **Reduction of Anxiety, Pain, and Agitation.** Anxiety, restlessness, and agitation result from hypoxia. In addition, fear caused by the inability to breathe and a sense of loss of control may increase anxiety. Anxiety, pain, and agitation increase $O_2$ consumption and $CO_2$ production from an elevated metabolic rate and increased WOB. This may cause asynchrony with mechanical ventilation and risk unplanned extubation. Several strategies can assist the patient in reducing anxiety and pain.

Sedation and analgesia with drug therapy such as propofol (Diprivan) (used for mechanically ventilated patients), benzodiazepines (e.g., lorazepam [Ativan], midazolam), and opioids (e.g., morphine, fentanyl [Sublimaze]) are used to decrease anxiety, agitation, and pain. Patients receiving these drugs are best managed by following an evidence-based and goal-directed protocol that uses the lowest possible drug dosing and duration of therapy needed to meet patient-specific goals. Some protocols include a regular *"sedation holiday"* (periodically decreasing sedative/hypnotic dosing) for ongoing assessment in patients who are intubated and mechanically ventilated. (Sedation holiday is discussed in Chapter 65.)

**! SAFETY ALERT Managing Agitation, Pain, and Sedation**

- Agitation is often caused by pain, hypoxemia, electrolyte imbalance, brain injury, and adverse drug reactions.
- Assess and aggressively treat all reversible causes of agitation.
- Monitor patients closely for cardiopulmonary depression when giving sedative and/or analgesic drugs.
- Sedative and analgesic drugs may have a prolonged effect in critically ill patients, delay weaning from mechanical ventilation, and contribute to increased length of stay.

Address treatable causes of agitation (e.g., hypoxemia, pain, hypercapnia) as part of a comprehensive plan of care. Frequently, agitation and mental status changes may be initial consequences of hypoxemia or ventilator asynchrony. You should address these causes and not depend solely on the use of sedatives.

Patients who breathe asynchronously with mechanical ventilation may also benefit from adjustment of ventilator flow rates and other settings. Patients who remain asynchronous with mechanical ventilation despite aggressive sedative and analgesic dosing may require neuromuscular blockade (paralysis) with agents such as vecuronium or cisatracurium (Nimbex). These drugs relax skeletal muscles by interfering with neuromuscular transmission and, ultimately, promote synchrony with mechanical ventilation. Remember that a patient receiving neuromuscular blockade can appear to be asleep but still possibly be awake and in pain. For this reason, deep sedation and analgesia are essential.

**SAFETY ALERT Neuromuscular Blockade**

- Provide concurrent sedation and analgesia to the point of unconsciousness for patients receiving neuromuscular blockade. This eliminates patient awareness, ensures patient comfort, and avoids the terrifying experience of being awake and in pain while paralyzed.
- Use neuromuscular blockade for the shortest duration and at the lowest dose possible to avoid complications (e.g., myopathy).

Monitoring levels of sedation in patients receiving neuromuscular blockade is challenging. Noninvasive electroencephalogram (EEG)–based technology may help guide sedative and analgesic therapy in these patients.[14] Levels of drug paralysis are monitored primarily by clinical assessment of ventilation and whether goals of care are being met. A frequent adjunct to monitoring paralysis is the use of a peripheral nerve stimulator (see Fig. 65-19). Clinical assessment is essential to determine the adequacy of sedation, analgesia, and neuromuscular blockade in critically ill patients.

### Medical Supportive Therapy

Goals and related interventions to maximize $O_2$ delivery are essential to improve the patient's oxygenation and ventilation status. The primary goal is to treat the underlying cause of the respiratory failure. Other supportive goals include maintaining an adequate CO and hemoglobin concentration.

**Treating the Underlying Cause.** Interventions are directed toward reversing the disease process that caused the acute respiratory failure. Patients with hypoventilation need to be diagnosed and treated rapidly. Patients with V/Q mismatch, shunting, or diffusion limitation are managed differently depending on the underlying cause. In all patient situations, monitoring treatment effects, including trends in ABGs and changes in respiratory status, is an ongoing process.

**Maintaining Adequate Cardiac Output.** CO reflects the blood flow reaching the tissues. BP and mean arterial pressure (MAP) are important indicators of the adequacy of CO. Always interpret BP and MAP readings within the context of the physical assessment to determine adequacy of CO and tissue perfusion. Usually a systolic BP of 90 mm Hg or more or a MAP greater than 60 mm Hg is adequate to maintain perfusion to the vital organs. At these levels, changes in mental status may be attributed to the level of $O_2$ and $CO_2$ rather than decreased cerebral perfusion. In a patient with chronic hypertension, a systolic BP of 90 to 100 mm Hg may be inadequate to maintain systemic and cerebral perfusion. Cerebral perfusion may require a higher BP and MAP to prevent episodes of brain ischemia or hypoperfusion to other organs.

Decreased CO is treated by giving IV fluids, drugs, or both. (Chapter 66 discusses drugs used to treat decreased CO and shock.) CO can also be decreased by changes in intrathoracic or intrapulmonary pressures from PPV. Patients experiencing exacerbation of COPD or asthma and those receiving PPV are at risk of alveolar hyperinflation, increased right ventricular afterload, and excessive intrathoracic pressures. These changes can limit blood flow from the right side of the heart through the pulmonary vasculature to the left side of the heart and cause hemodynamic compromise (e.g., decreased CO). Blood return from the systemic circulation to the right side of the heart may be impaired, decreasing preload and CO. Closely monitor BP and clinical indicators of adequate CO and tissue perfusion with the start of or changes in mechanical ventilation as these patients are always at risk for hemodynamic compromise.

**Maintaining Adequate Hemoglobin Concentration.** Hemoglobin is the primary carrier of $O_2$ to the tissues. Delivery of $O_2$ to the tissues is compromised in anemic patients. A hemoglobin of 7 g/dL (70 g/L) or higher typically ensures adequate $O_2$ saturation of the hemoglobin for tissue oxygenation.[15] Monitor the patient for signs of blood loss (e.g., hypotension, melena). Transfusion with packed red blood cells may be used if an adequate hemoglobin level is not maintained and the patient is symptomatic.

### Nutritional Therapy

Maintenance of protein and energy stores is especially important in patients with acute respiratory failure. The hypermetabolic state in critical illness increases the caloric requirements needed to maintain body weight and muscle mass. Thus nutritional depletion causes a loss of muscle mass, including the respiratory muscles, and may prolong recovery.

The dietitian, in collaboration with the interprofessional care team, determines the optimal method of feeding and optimal caloric and fluid requirements. During the acute manifestations of respiratory failure, the risk of aspiration typically prevents oral intake. Ideally, enteral or parenteral nutrition should be started within 24 to 48 hours. When acute manifestations subside, the patient may resume oral intake as able.

### Evaluation

The expected outcomes are that the patient with respiratory failure will

- Maintain a patent airway with effective removal of secretions
- Achieve normal or baseline respiratory rate and rhythm and breath sounds
- Maintain adequate oxygenation as indicated by normal or baseline ABGs
- Experience normal hemodynamic status

Additional outcomes are presented in eNursing Care Plan 67-1 (available on the website for this chapter).

### Gerontologic Considerations: Respiratory Failure

Older adults are the fastest-growing age-group in the United States, a trend that is increasingly reflected within the patient populations in acute and critical care settings. Multiple factors contribute to an increased risk of respiratory failure in older adults. The reduction in ventilatory capacity that accompanies aging places the older adult at risk for respiratory failure. Physiologic aging of the lung includes alveolar dilation, larger air spaces, and loss of surface area for gas exchange. Diminished elastic recoil within the airways, decreased chest wall compliance, and decreased respiratory muscle strength also occur.

In older adults, the $PaO_2$ falls further and the $PaCO_2$ rises to a higher level before the respiratory system is stimulated to alter the rate and depth of breathing. This delayed response can contribute to the development of respiratory failure. In addition, a history of tobacco use is a risk factor that can accelerate age-related respiratory changes. Poor nutritional status and l ess available physiologic reserve in the cardiopulmonary and autonomic nervous systems increase the risk of additional disease states such as pneumonia and heart disease. These may further compromise respiratory function and lead to respiratory failure.

Older adults are more vulnerable to delirium, health care–associated infections (HAIs), and the adverse effects of polypharmacy. Delirium is an independent risk factor for increased mortality and morbidity rates in critically ill patients. It can complicate ventilator management and weaning by interfering with patient cooperation. Delirium associated with agitation increases $CO_2$ elimination and $O_2$ consumption, increases the risk for unplanned extubation and device removal, and extends length of hospital stay and ventilator days.[16] (Delirium is discussed in Chapters 59 and 65.)

## ACUTE RESPIRATORY DISTRESS SYNDROME

**Acute respiratory distress syndrome (ARDS)** is a sudden and progressive form of acute respiratory failure in which the alveolar-capillary membrane becomes damaged and more permeable to intravascular fluid (Fig. 67-9). ARDS exists on a continuum. One way to assess the degree of impairment in gas exchange is to measure the $PaO_2/FIO_2$ (P/F) ratio. Under normal circumstances (e.g., $PaO_2$ 85 to 100 mm Hg; $FIO_2$ 0.21 [room air]), the P/F ratio would be greater than 400 (e.g., 95/0.21 = 452). With the onset and progression of lung injury and impairment in $O_2$ delivery through the alveolar-capillary membrane, the $PaO_2$ may remain lower than expected despite increased $FIO_2$. The PF ratio differentiates between mild, moderate, and severe ARDS[17] (Table 67-5).

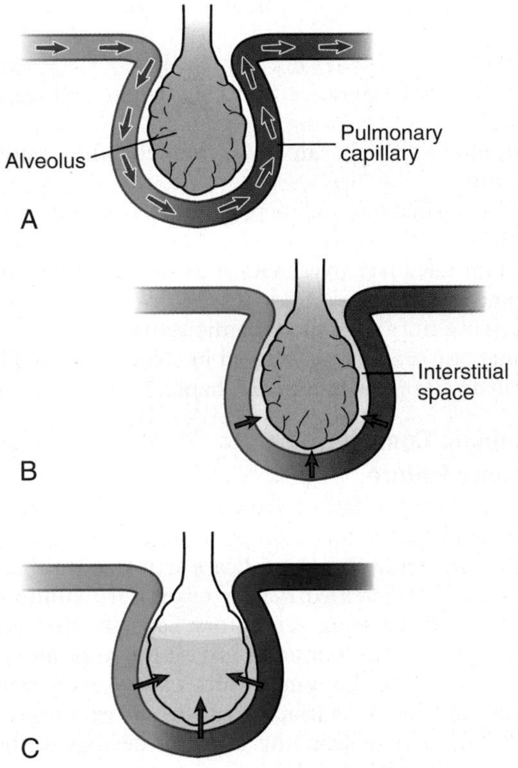


**FIG. 67-9** Stages of edema formation in acute respiratory distress syndrome. **A,** Normal alveolus and pulmonary capillary. **B,** Interstitial edema occurs with increased flow of fluid into the interstitial space. **C,** Alveolar edema occurs when the fluid crosses the alveolar-capillary membrane.

The incidence of ARDS in the United States is estimated at more than 150,000 cases annually. Despite supportive therapy, the mortality rate from ARDS is approximately 50%. Patients who have both gram-negative septic shock and ARDS have a mortality rate of 70% to 90%.

### Etiology and Pathophysiology

Table 67-6 lists conditions that predispose patients to the development of ARDS. Patients with multiple risk factors are three or four times more likely to develop ARDS.

The most common cause of ARDS is sepsis. Direct lung injury may cause ARDS (Fig. 67-10), or ARDS may develop because of the systemic inflammatory response syndrome (SIRS) (see Fig. 66-1). This is characterized by widespread inflammation or clinical responses to inflammation after a variety of

**TABLE 67-5 Diagnostic Findings in ARDS**

| | |
|---|---|
| **Timing** | Within 1 week of a known clinical insult or new or worsening respiratory symptoms |
| **Chest X-ray** | Bilateral opacities: not fully explained by effusions, lobar/lung collapse, or nodules |
| **Oxygenation** | *Mild ARDS:* $PaO_2/FIO_2$ ratio >200 to ≤300 with PEEP or CPAP ≥5 cm $H_2O$<br>*Moderate ARDS:* $PaO_2/FIO_2$ ratio 100 to ≤200 with PEEP or CPAP ≥5 cm $H_2O$<br>*Severe ARDS:* $PaO_2/FIO_2$ ratio <100 with PEEP or CPAP ≥5 cm $H_2O$ |

Modified from Pneumatikos L, Papaloannou VE: The new Berlin definition: what is, finally, the ARDS? *Pneumon* 25(4):365, 2012.

**TABLE 67-6 Predisposing Conditions to ARDS**

| Direct Lung Injury | Indirect Lung Injury |
|---|---|
| **Common Causes** | |
| • Aspiration of gastric contents or other substances | • Sepsis (especially gram-negative infection) |
| • Viral or bacterial pneumonia | • Severe massive trauma |
| • Sepsis | |
| **Less Common Causes** | |
| • Chest trauma | • Acute pancreatitis |
| • Embolism: fat, air, amniotic fluid, thrombus | • Cardiopulmonary bypass |
| • Inhalation of toxic substances | • Disseminated intravascular coagulation |
| • Near-drowning | • Opioid drug overdose (e.g., heroin) |
| • $O_2$ toxicity | • Severe head injury |
| • Radiation pneumonitis | • Shock states |
| | • Transfusion-related acute lung injury (e.g., multiple blood transfusions) |

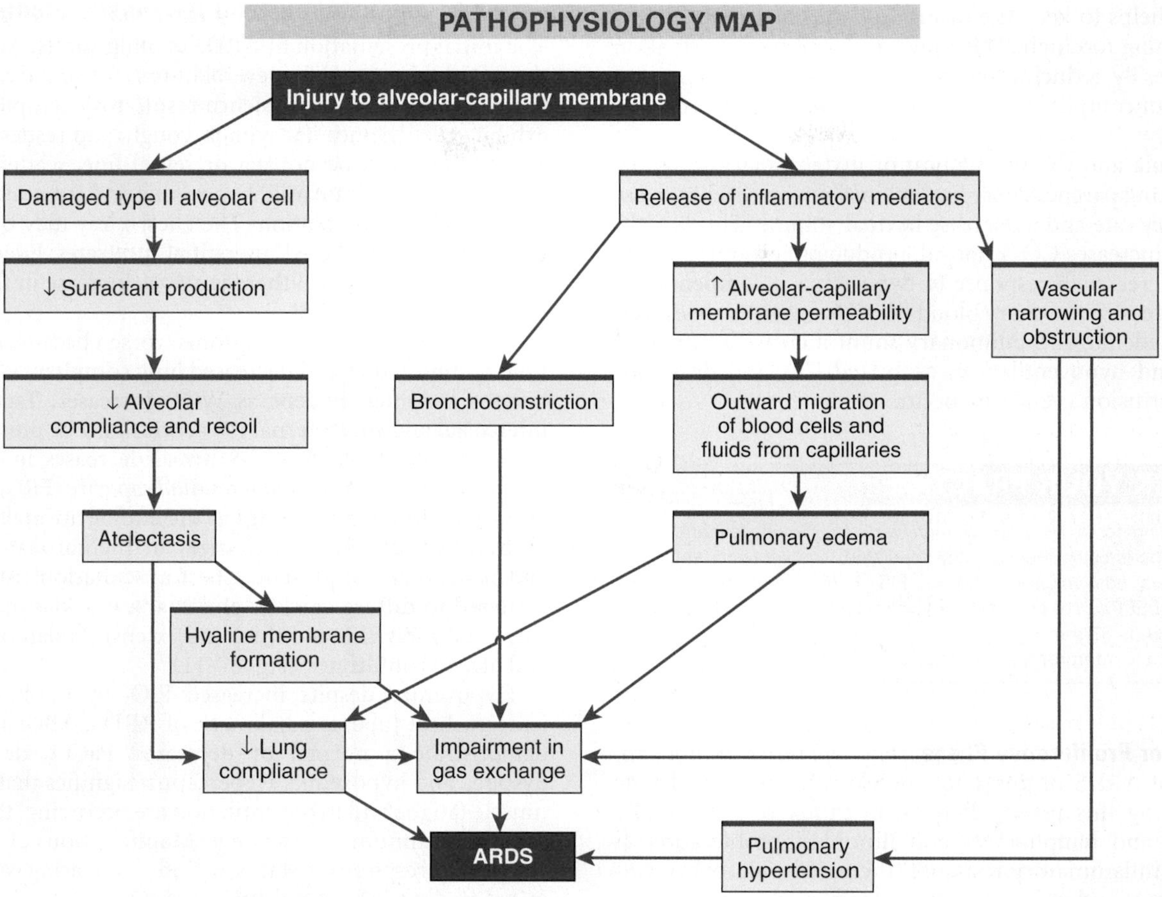


**FIG. 67-10** Pathophysiology of acute respiratory distress syndrome (ARDS).

physiologic insults, including severe trauma, gut ischemia, and lung injury. ARDS may also develop as a consequence of multiple organ dysfunction syndrome (MODS). MODS results from organ system dysfunction that progressively increases in severity and ultimately results in failure of one or more body systems. (Chapter 66 discusses SIRS, sepsis, and MODS.)

An exact cause for the damage to the alveolar-capillary membrane is not known. It is thought to be caused by stimulation of the inflammatory and immune systems. This causes an attraction of neutrophils to the pulmonary interstitium. The neutrophils release biochemical, humoral, and cellular mediators that produce changes in the lung. These include increased pulmonary capillary membrane permeability, destruction of elastin and collagen, formation of pulmonary microemboli, and pulmonary artery vasoconstriction (Fig. 67-10). (Chapters 11 and 13 discuss these mediators.)

The pathophysiologic changes in ARDS are divided into three phases: (1) injury or exudative phase, (2) reparative or proliferative phase, and (3) fibrotic phase.

**Injury or Exudative Phase.** The *injury or exudative phase* occurs approximately 1 to 7 days (usually 24 to 48 hours) after the initial direct lung injury or host insult. Initially, engorgement of the peribronchial and perivascular interstitial space produces interstitial edema. Next, fluid from the interstitial space crosses the alveolar membrane and enters the alveolar space. Intrapulmonary shunt develops because the alveoli fill with fluid, and blood passing through them cannot be oxygenated (Figs. 67-4 and 67-9).

Alveolar type I and II cells (which produce surfactant) are damaged by the changes caused by ARDS. This damage, in addition to further fluid and protein accumulation, results in surfactant dysfunction. The function of *surfactant* is to maintain alveolar stability by decreasing alveolar surface tension and preventing alveolar collapse. Decreased synthesis of surfactant and inactivation of existing surfactant cause the alveoli to become unstable and collapse *(atelectasis)*. Widespread atelectasis further decreases lung compliance, compromises gas exchange, and contributes to hypoxemia.

In addition, during this stage, necrotic cells, protein, and fibrin form hyaline membranes that line the alveoli. Hyaline membranes contribute to the development of fibrosis and atelectasis, leading to a decrease in gas exchange capability and lung compliance.

The primary pathophysiologic changes that describe the *injury or exudative phase* of ARDS are interstitial and alveolar edema and atelectasis. Severe V/Q mismatch and shunting of pulmonary capillary blood result in hypoxemia unresponsive to increasing concentrations of $O_2$ (termed **refractory hypoxemia**). Diffusion limitation, caused by hyaline membrane formation, worsens the hypoxemia. As the lungs become less compliant because of decreased surfactant, pulmonary edema, and atelectasis, the patient must generate higher airway pressures to inflate "stiff" lungs. Reduced lung compliance greatly increases the patient's WOB.

At this stage, ventilator management often includes a pressure-control type of ventilation. Pressure control ventilation helps to keep the inspiratory and plateau pressures from becoming too high. This prevents alveolar overdistention and rupture. By reducing the amount of pressure going into the stiff, noncompliant lungs, further lung injury may be prevented.[18]

Hypoxemia and the stimulation of juxtacapillary receptors in the stiff lung parenchyma *(J reflex)* initially cause an increase in respiratory rate and a decrease in tidal volume. This breathing pattern increases $CO_2$ removal, producing respiratory alkalosis. CO increases in response to hypoxemia, a compensatory effort to increase pulmonary blood flow. However, as atelectasis, pulmonary edema, and pulmonary shunt increase, compensation fails and hypoventilation, decreased CO, and decreased tissue $O_2$ perfusion eventually occur.

**CHECK YOUR PRACTICE**

You are caring for a 26-yr-old woman with ARDS who experienced drowning. She is being mechanically ventilated. The ventilator settings are as follows: tidal volume = 350 mL, $FIO_2$ = 70%, respiratory rate = 10/minute, PEEP = 10 cm $H_2O$, pressure limit = 35 cm $H_2O$. The patient's $PaO_2$ is 83 mm Hg.

- Calculate and interpret the P/F ratio.

**Reparative or Proliferative Phase.** The *reparative or proliferative phase* of ARDS begins 1 to 2 weeks after the initial lung injury. During this phase, there is an influx of neutrophils, monocytes, and lymphocytes and fibroblast proliferation as part of the inflammatory response. Increased pulmonary vascular resistance and pulmonary hypertension may occur in this stage because fibroblasts and inflammatory cells destroy the pulmonary vasculature. Lung compliance continues to decrease as a result of interstitial fibrosis. Hypoxemia worsens because of the thickened alveolar membrane, causing diffusion limitation and shunting. The proliferative phase is complete when the diseased lung is characterized by dense, fibrous tissue. If the reparative phase persists, widespread fibrosis results. If the reparative phase is stopped, the lesions will resolve.

**Fibrotic Phase.** The *fibrotic phase* of ARDS occurs approximately 2 to 3 weeks after the initial lung injury. This phase is also called the *chronic* or *late phase* of ARDS. By this time, the lung is completely remodeled by collagenous and fibrous tissues. The diffuse scarring and fibrosis result in decreased lung compliance. In addition, the surface area for gas exchange is significantly reduced because the interstitium is fibrotic, and therefore hypoxemia continues. Pulmonary hypertension results from pulmonary vascular destruction and fibrosis.

### Clinical Progression

Progression of ARDS varies among patients. Some survive the acute phase of lung injury. Pulmonary edema resolves, and complete recovery occurs in a few days. The chance for survival is poor in those who enter the fibrotic (chronic or late) stage, which requires long-term mechanical ventilation. It is not known why injured lungs repair and recover in some patients, and in others ARDS progresses. Several factors seem to be important in determining the course of ARDS. These include the nature of the initial injury, extent and severity of comorbidities, and pulmonary complications (e.g., pneumothorax).

### Clinical Manifestations and Diagnostic Studies

The initial presentation of ARDS is often subtle. At the time of the initial injury, and for several hours to 1 or 2 days afterward, the patient may not experience respiratory symptoms or may exhibit only dyspnea, tachypnea, cough, and restlessness. Chest auscultation may be normal or reveal fine, scattered crackles. ABGs usually indicate mild hypoxemia and respiratory alkalosis caused by hyperventilation. The chest x-ray may be normal or reveal minimal scattered interstitial infiltrates. Edema may not show on the x-ray until there is a 30% increase in fluid content in the lung (Table 67-5).

As ARDS progresses, symptoms worsen because of increased fluid accumulation and decreased lung compliance. Respiratory distress becomes evident as WOB increases. Tachypnea and intercostal and suprasternal retractions may be present. Pulmonary function tests in ARDS reveal decreases in compliance, lung volumes, and *functional residual capacity* (FRC, the amount of air remaining in the lungs at the end of normal expiration). Tachycardia, diaphoresis, changes in mental status, cyanosis, and pallor may be present. Chest auscultation usually reveals scattered to diffuse crackles and coarse crackles on expiration. The chest x-ray shows diffuse and extensive bilateral interstitial and alveolar infiltrates (Fig. 67-11).

Hypoxemia, despite increased $FIO_2$ by mask, cannula, or endotracheal tube, is a hallmark of ARDS. ABGs may initially demonstrate a normal or decreased $PaCO_2$ despite severe dyspnea and hypoxemia. Hypercapnia signifies that respiratory muscle fatigue and hypoventilation are occurring, thus interfering with optimum gas exchange. Manifestations of the patient's worsening respiratory status include increasing WOB despite initial findings of normal $PaO_2$ or $SaO_2$.

As ARDS progresses, it is associated with profound respiratory distress requiring endotracheal intubation and PPV. The chest x-ray is often termed *whiteout* or *white lung* because consolidation and infiltrates are widespread throughout the lungs, leaving few recognizable air spaces (Fig. 67-11). Pleural effusions may also be present. Severe hypoxemia, hypercapnia,

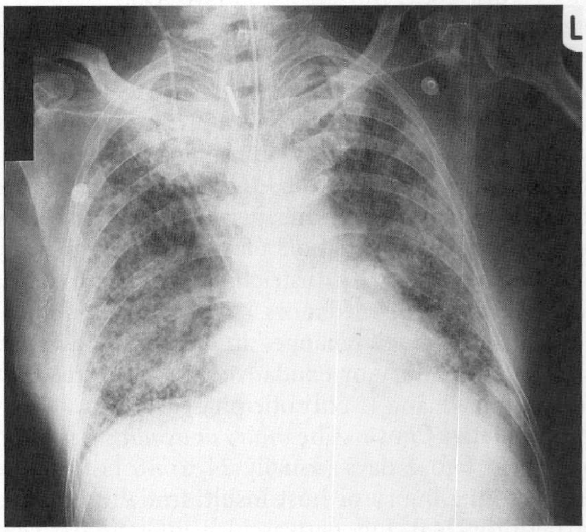


**FIG. 67-11** Chest x-ray of a patient with acute respiratory distress syndrome (ARDS). The x-ray shows new, bilateral, diffuse, homogeneous pulmonary infiltrates without cardiac failure, fluid overload, chest infection, or chronic lung disease. (From Cohen J, Powderly WG: *Infectious diseases*, ed 2, St Louis, 2004, Mosby.)

**TABLE 67-7 Complications Associated With ARDS**

| | |
|---|---|
| **Infection**<br>• Catheter-related infection (e.g., central and peripheral IV catheters, urinary catheters)<br>• Sepsis | **Renal**<br>• Acute kidney injury<br>**Cardiac**<br>• Decreased cardiac output<br>• Dysrhythmias |
| **Respiratory**<br>• $O_2$ toxicity<br>• Pulmonary barotrauma (e.g., pneumothorax, pneumomediastinum, subcutaneous emphysema)<br>• Pulmonary emboli<br>• Pulmonary fibrosis<br>• Ventilator-associated pneumonia | **Hematologic**<br>• Anemia<br>• Disseminated intravascular coagulation<br>• Thrombocytopenia<br>• Venous thromboembolism<br>**Endotracheal Tube**<br>• Laryngeal ulceration<br>• Tracheal malacia<br>• Tracheal stenosis<br>• Tracheal ulceration |
| **Gastrointestinal**<br>• Hypermetabolic state, dramatically increased nutrition requirements<br>• Paralytic ileus<br>• Pneumoperitoneum<br>• Stress ulceration and hemorrhage | **Central Nervous System and Psychologic**<br>• Delirium<br>• Posttraumatic stress disorder<br>• Sleep deprivation |

**TABLE 67-8 Components of a Ventilator Bundle**

- Elevation of head of the bed 30 to 45 degrees
- Daily "sedation holidays" and assessment of readiness for extubation (see Chapter 65)
- Peptic ulcer disease prophylaxis (see Chapter 41)
- Venous thromboembolism prophylaxis (see Chapter 37)
- Daily oral care with chlorhexidine (0.12%) solution (see Table 65-9)

Source: Institute for Healthcare Improvement: How-to guide: prevent ventilator-associated pneumonia. Retrieved from *www.ihi.org/resources/Pages/Tools/HowtoGuidePreventVAP.aspx.*

metabolic acidosis, and manifestations of specific organ dysfunction may develop if therapy is not promptly started.

## Complications

Complications may develop as a result of ARDS itself or its treatment (Table 67-7). The primary cause of death in ARDS is MODS, often accompanied by sepsis. The vital organs most commonly involved are the kidneys, liver, and heart.

**Ventilator-Associated Pneumonia.** A frequent complication of ARDS is ventilator-associated pneumonia (VAP). VAP occurs in as many as 68% of patients with ARDS. Risk factors include impaired host defenses, contaminated equipment, invasive monitoring devices, aspiration of GI contents (especially in patients receiving enteral feedings), and prolonged mechanical ventilation. Strategies to prevent VAP include strict infection control measures (e.g., strict hand washing, sterile technique during endotracheal suctioning, frequent mouth care and oral hygiene) and a ventilator bundle protocol[19] (Table 67-8). (Chapter 27 discusses pneumonia, and Chapter 65 discusses VAP.)

**Barotrauma.** *Barotrauma* may result from rupture of overdistended alveoli during mechanical ventilation. The high peak airway pressures required may predispose patients with ARDS to this complication. Barotrauma results in alveolar air escaping from ruptured alveoli. This can lead to pulmonary interstitial emphysema, pneumothorax, subcutaneous emphysema, pneumoperitoneum, pneumomediastinum, pneumopericardium, and tension pneumothorax.[20] (Chapter 27 discusses pneumothorax.)

To avoid barotrauma and minimize the risk associated with elevated plateau and peak inspiratory pressures, the patient with ARDS is often ventilated with smaller tidal volumes (e.g., 6 mL/kg) and varying amounts of positive end-expiratory pressure (PEEP) to minimize $O_2$ requirements and intrathoracic pressures. This approach, called the *Acute Respiratory Distress Syndrome Clinical Network (ARDSNet) protocol,* reduces mortality rate and the number of ventilator days for these patients. Unfortunately, one result of this protocol is an elevation in $PaCO_2$. This is termed *permissive hypercapnia* because the $PaCO_2$ is allowed to rise slowly above normal limits. It is generally well tolerated as long as the rise in $PaCO_2$ is gradual to allow systemic and brain circulation to compensate, the pH is 7.2 or higher, and the patient does not have preexisting ICP elevation.[21]

**Volutrauma.** *Volutrauma* occurs in patients with ARDS or other clinical states requiring mechanical ventilation and large tidal volumes (e.g., 10 to 15 mL/kg) to ventilate noncompliant lungs. Volutrauma results in *alveolar fractures* (damage or tears in the alveoli) and movement of fluids and proteins into the alveolar spaces. To limit this complication, smaller tidal volumes or pressure-control ventilation is now the standard in patients with ARDS (see Chapter 65).

**Stress Ulcers.** Critically ill patients with acute respiratory failure are at high risk for stress ulcers. Bleeding from stress ulcers occurs in 30% of patients with ARDS who require PPV, a higher incidence than other causes of acute respiratory failure. Management strategies include correction of predisposing conditions such as hypotension, shock, and acidosis. Prophylactic management includes antiulcer drugs such as proton pump inhibitors (e.g., pantoprazole [Protonix]) and mucosal-protecting drugs (e.g., sucralfate [Carafate]). Early initiation of enteral nutrition also helps prevent mucosal damage (see Chapters 39 and 65).

**Renal Failure.** Renal failure can occur from decreased renal perfusion and subsequent decreased delivery of $O_2$ to the kidneys. This can result from hypotension, hypoxemia, or hypercapnia. Renal failure may also result from nephrotoxic drugs (e.g., vancomycin [Vancocin]) used to treat ARDS-related infections.

## ❖ NURSING AND INTERPROFESSIONAL MANAGEMENT: ACUTE RESPIRATORY DISTRESS SYNDROME

The management of a patient with acute respiratory failure (Table 67-4) and the nursing care plan for acute respiratory failure (eNursing Care Plan 67-1, available on the website for this chapter) apply to patients with ARDS. The following section discusses additional interprofessional care for the patient with ARDS (Table 67-9).

**TABLE 67-9 Interprofessional Care**
***Acute Respiratory Distress Syndrome***

**Diagnostic Assessment**
See Table 67-5.

**Management**
***Respiratory Therapy***
- $O_2$ administration
- Positive pressure ventilation with PEEP
- Permissive hypercapnia
- Alternative modes of mechanical ventilation: pressure-control inverse ratio ventilation, airway pressure release ventilation, high-frequency ventilation (see Chapter 65)
- Positioning strategies
  - Prone positioning
  - Lateral rotation therapy
  - Kinetic therapy

***Supportive Therapy***
- Identification and treatment of underlying cause
- Hemodynamic monitoring
- Nutritional therapy

***Drug Therapy***
- Inotropic and vasopressor drugs
  - dopamine
  - dobutamine
  - norepinephrine (Levophed)
- Diuretics
- IV fluid administration
- Sedation/analgesia
- Neuromuscular blockade

*PEEP,* Positive end-expiratory pressure.

## ◆ Nursing Assessment

Because ARDS causes acute respiratory failure, the subjective and objective data that you should obtain from someone with ARDS are the same as those for acute respiratory failure (Table 67-3). Some patient information may not be possible to obtain initially due to management priorities of oxygenation and ventilation.

## ◆ Nursing Diagnoses

Nursing diagnoses for the patient with ARDS may include, but are not limited to, those described for acute respiratory failure (see p. 1615).

## ◆ Planning

Patients with moderate to severe ARDS are cared for in critical care units. With appropriate therapy, overall goals include a $PaO_2$ of 60 mm Hg or higher and adequate lung ventilation to maintain normal pH. Specific goals for a patient with ARDS include (1) $PaO_2$ within normal limits for age or at baseline on room air, (2) $SaO_2$ greater than 90%, (3) resolution of the precipitating factor(s) for ARDS, and (4) clear lungs on auscultation.

◆ **Oxygen Administration.** The primary goal of $O_2$ therapy is to correct hypoxemia. Initially use a nasal cannula or face mask with high-flow systems that deliver higher $O_2$ concentrations to maximize $O_2$ delivery. Continuously monitor $SpO_2$ to assess the effectiveness of $O_2$ therapy. Patients with moderate to severe ARDS and refractory hypoxemia need intubation with mechanical ventilation to maintain the $PaO_2$ at acceptable levels.

◆ **Positive Pressure Ventilation.** Endotracheal intubation and PPV provide additional respiratory support. However, even with these interventions it may be necessary to maintain the $FIO_2$ at 60% or higher to maintain a $PaO_2$ of at least 60 mm Hg. During PPV, it is common to apply PEEP at 5 cm $H_2O$ to compensate for loss of glottic function caused by the endotracheal tube. In patients with ARDS, higher levels of PEEP (e.g., 10 to 20 cm $H_2O$) may be used. PEEP increases FRC and opens up collapsed alveoli. PEEP is typically applied in 3- to 5-cm $H_2O$ increments until oxygenation is adequate with $FIO_2$ less than or equal to 60%. PEEP may improve V/Q in respiratory units that collapse at low airway pressures, thus allowing the $FIO_2$ to be lowered.

However, PEEP is not a benign therapy. The additional intrathoracic and intrapulmonic pressures can compromise venous return to the right side of the heart, thereby decreasing preload, CO, and BP. High levels of PEEP cause hyperinflation of the alveoli, compression of the pulmonary capillary bed, reduction in blood return to the left side of the heart, and a dramatic reduction in BP. In addition, high levels of PEEP or excessive inspiratory pressures can result in barotrauma and volutrauma.

If hypoxemic respiratory failure persists in spite of high levels of PEEP, alternative modes of mechanical ventilation and respiratory therapies may be used. These include airway pressure release ventilation, pressure-control inverse ratio ventilation, high-frequency ventilation, and permissive hypercapnia (low tidal volumes that allow $PaCO_2$ to increase slowly).[20] (Chapter 65 provides additional information on mechanical ventilation and PEEP.)

Extracorporeal membrane oxygenation (ECMO) and extracorporeal $CO_2$ removal ($ECCO_2R$) are external devices cannulated within large blood vessels. This allows blood to pass across a gas-exchanging membrane outside the body and then return oxygenated blood back to the body. $ECCO_2R$ with PPV allows the lungs to heal while lung function is inadequate to maintain adequate oxygenation and $CO_2$ removal.[22]

◆ ***Positioning Strategies.*** In the early phases of ARDS, fluid moves freely throughout the lung. Because of gravity, this fluid pools in dependent regions of the lung. As a result, some alveoli are fluid filled (dependent areas), whereas others are air filled (nondependent areas). In addition, when the patient is supine, the heart and mediastinal contents place more pressure on the lungs than in the prone position. Thus the supine position changes pleural pressure and predisposes the patient to atelectasis.

If you turn the patient from supine to prone, air-filled, alveoli in the ventral (anterior) portion of the lung become dependent. Perfusion may be better matched to ventilation.

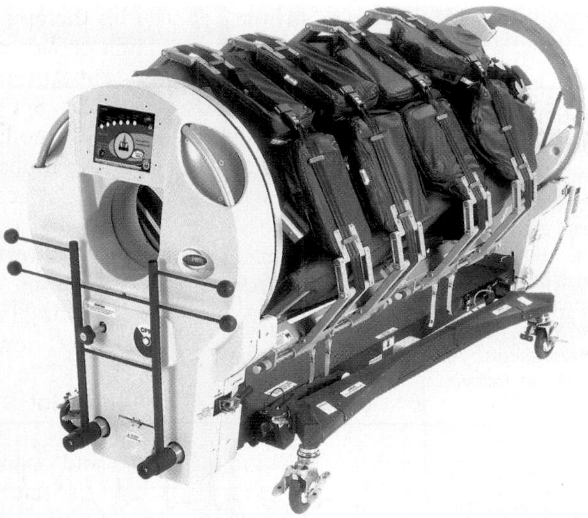

**FIG. 67-12** RotoProne bed. (ArjoHuntleigh. Reprinted with permission.) Note: The RotoProne Delta Therapy System allows clinicians to place patients in the prone position, safely and effectively. This product is not specifically indicated for the treatment of ARDS or VAP.

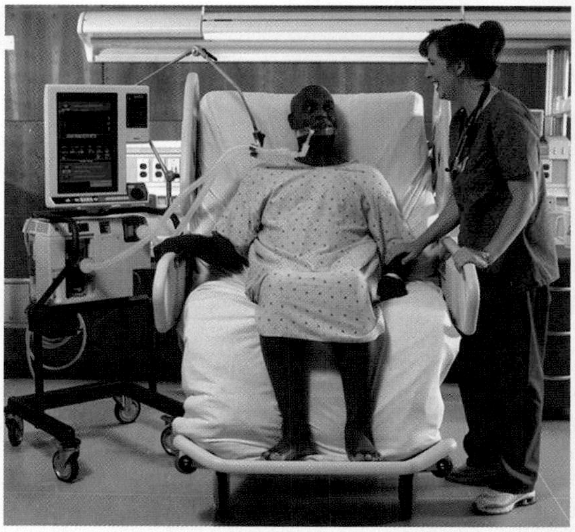

**FIG. 67-13** TotalCare SpO2RT Bed System offers continuous lateral rotation therapy and percussion and vibration therapies. Patients can easily and quickly be repositioned. (Copyright 2006 Hill-Rom Services, Inc. Reprinted with permission. All rights reserved.)

Prone positioning may be considered for patients with refractory hypoxemia who do not respond to other strategies to increase $PaO_2$ (Fig. 67-12). Some patients will have a marked improvement in $PaO_2$ when prone (e.g., $PaO_2$ 70 mm Hg supine, $PaO_2$ 90 mm Hg prone) with no change in $FIO_2$.[23]

Prone positioning helps to improve ventilation of better-perfused lung areas. This may be sufficient to allow a reduction in $FIO_2$ or PEEP. You may observe BP instability owing to fluid shifts and additional need for airway suctioning as secretions are mobilized by gravity.

Currently, there is no reliable way of predicting who will or will not respond to prone positioning.[23] When placing a patient in the prone position, pay special attention to the patient's skin to avoid the development of pressure ulcers.[24]

Other positioning strategies to consider for patients with ARDS include continuous lateral rotation therapy (CLRT) and kinetic therapy. CLRT provides continuous, slow, side-to-side turning of the patient by rotating the actual bed frame less than 40 degrees. The bed's lateral movement is maintained for 18 of every 24 hours to simulate postural drainage and to help mobilize pulmonary secretions. In addition, the bed may also contain a vibrator pack that provides chest physiotherapy. This feature assists with secretion mobilization and removal (Fig. 67-13). Kinetic therapy is similar to CLRT in that patients are rotated side-to-side 40 degrees or more. It is important to obtain baseline assessments of the patient's pulmonary status (e.g., respiratory rate and rhythm, breath sounds, ABGs, $SpO_2$) and continue to monitor the patient throughout the therapy.

## ◆ Medical Supportive Therapy

◆ **Maintenance of Cardiac Output and Tissue Perfusion.** Patients on PPV and PEEP frequently experience decreased CO. One cause is decreased venous return from the PEEP-induced increase in intrathoracic pressure. Impaired contractility and decreased preload can also decrease CO. Hemodynamic monitoring (e.g., CVP, CO, $ScvO_2$, $SvO_2$) via central venous or pulmonary artery pressure or arterial pressure-based CO monitoring is essential. This allows you to see trends, detect changes, and adjust therapy as needed. An arterial catheter also provides continuous monitoring of BP and sampling of blood for ABGs. If the CO falls, it may be necessary to administer crystalloid fluids or colloid solutions or to lower PEEP. Use of inotropic drugs such as dobutamine or dopamine may also be necessary. (Chapter 65 discusses hemodynamic monitoring.)

Packed red blood cells are used to increase hemoglobin and thus the $O_2$-carrying capacity of the blood. Controversy exists regarding the optimal hemoglobin level. Some advocate keeping the level around 9 g/dL (90 g/L) with an $SpO_2$ of 90% or more (when $PaO_2$ is greater than 60 mm Hg). Others recommend hemoglobin levels greater than 7 g/dL (70 g/L).[15]

◆ **Maintenance of Nutrition and Fluid Balance.** Maintenance of nutrition and fluid balance is challenging in the patient with ARDS. Consult with a dietitian to determine optimal caloric needs. Enteral or parenteral feedings are started to meet the high energy requirements of these patients.

Increasing pulmonary capillary permeability results in fluid in the lungs and causes pulmonary edema. At the same time, the patient may be volume depleted and thus at risk for hypotension and decreased CO from mechanical ventilation and PEEP. Monitor hemodynamic parameters (e.g., CVP, stroke volume variation), daily weights, and intake and output to assess the patient's fluid status. The patient is often placed on fluid restriction, and diuretics are used as necessary.

## ◆ Evaluation

The expected outcomes for the patient with ARDS are similar to those for a patient with acute respiratory failure (see p. 1619).

## CASE STUDY

### *Acute Respiratory Distress Syndrome*

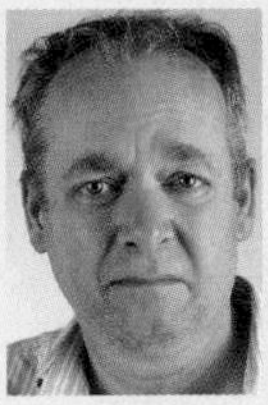
(©Thinkstock)

**Patient Profile**

J.N. is a 58-yr-old white man who was admitted 12 hr ago to a surgical ICU after emergent surgery for an acute ischemic bowel.

***Past Medical History***

- Lumbar spine surgery 5 yr ago
- Chronic back pain controlled with oxycodone (OxyContin) 15 mg PO tid

***Operative Procedure***

- Surgical procedure involved extensive abdominal surgery to repair a perforated colon, irrigate the abdominal cavity, and provide hemostasis
- During surgery his systolic BP dropped to 70 mm Hg
- Six units of packed red blood cells and 4 L of 0.9% saline were infused
- He is receiving 60% $O_2$ via an aerosol face mask

***Postoperative Orders***

- Continuous ECG and pulse oximetry monitoring
- Give 0.9% saline at 125 mL/hr via a central venous IV catheter
- Monitor hourly urine output via indwelling bladder catheter
- Pain management via a continuous IV infusion of morphine

***Immediate Postoperative Status***

- J.N.'s pulmonary status worsens. He requires progressively higher $FIO_2$ via high-flow face mask and a short trial of noninvasive positive pressure ventilation (NIPPV).
- J.N. continues to experience declining $SaO_2$ levels and increased WOB as well as worsening hemodynamic status. Emergent endotracheal intubation and PPV are needed.
- Sedation, analgesia, and neuromuscular blockade are started to achieve anxiolysis, pain control, and ventilator synchrony.
- Postintubation chest x-ray reveals 50% right-sided pneumothorax, requiring the emergent chest tube placement. Immediately after chest tube placement, his $SpO_2$ decreased significantly below baseline to 80% to 82%.
- No significant changes were evident in ventilation or lung compliance, and he remains synchronous with mechanical ventilation.
- ABGs shows $PaCO_2$ increased to 52 mm Hg and $PaO_2$ decreased to 44 mm Hg.
- J.N. is tachycardic during and immediately after chest tube insertion. A 10-mg bolus of morphine is given followed by an increase in the continuous infusion.
- After 30 min, his $O_2$ saturation improves to 90% to 91% and ABGs shows improved oxygenation ($PaO_2$ 63 mm Hg) and ventilation ($PaCO_2$ 45 mm Hg).

***Postoperative Day 1***

- J.N.'s lung function continues to worsen and his hypoxemia is refractory to 100% $FIO_2$ and high levels of PEEP.
- He experiences kidney and liver failure. There is little hope of weaning him from mechanical ventilation.
- He has an advance directive that indicates he does not want to be kept alive by artificial means.

**Subjective Data**

- Patient is sedated, paralyzed, and unable to communicate.
- His wife and two adult children are at the bedside and voicing concerns and questions regarding his progress.

**Objective Data**

***Physical Examination***

- *General:* Sedated, paralyzed; head of bed elevated 45 degrees; skin cool with moderate diaphoresis
- *Respiratory:* Endotracheal tube in place with PPV. No accessory muscle use, retractions, or paradoxic breathing; respiratory rate 18 breaths/min and in phase with ventilator; $SpO_2$ 85%, bilateral crackles at lung bases. Ventilator settings: tidal volume 350 mL, $FIO_2$ 100%, respiratory rate 10/minute, PEEP 10 cm $H_2O$, pressure limit 35 cm $H_2O$.
- *Cardiovascular:* Apical-radial pulse equal, BP 100/60 mm Hg
  - ECG as follows:

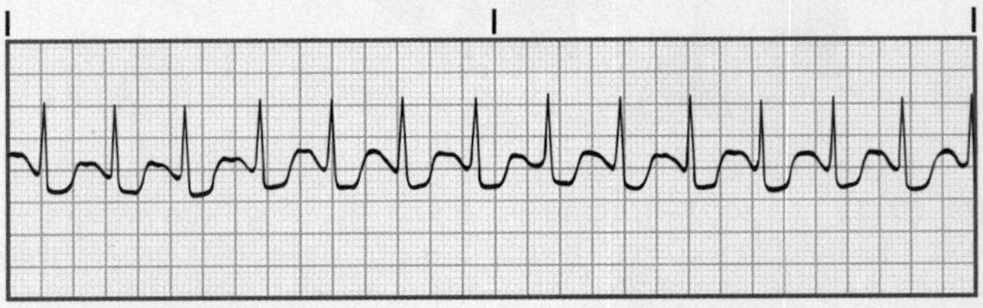

  - Weak peripheral pulses; temperature 101° F (38.3° C) rectally
- *Gastrointestinal:* Surgical dressing dry and intact; colostomy draining serosanguineous drainage
- *Urologic:* Indwelling bladder catheter draining concentrated urine less than 30 mL/hr

***Diagnostic Findings***

- ABGs obtained 4 hours following intubation and start of PPV: pH 7.15, $PaO_2$ 59 mm Hg, $PaCO_2$ 57 mm Hg, $HCO_3$ 16 mEq/L, $O_2$ saturation 86%.
- $PaO_2/FIO_2$ ratio 59
- Chest x-ray: new bilateral, scattered interstitial infiltrates compatible with an ARDS pattern as interpreted by the radiologist

**Discussion Questions**

1. How does the pathophysiology of ARDS predispose this patient to refractory hypoxemia?
2. What clinical manifestations does J.N. exhibit that support a diagnosis of ARDS?
3. What are the possible causes of ARDS in J.N.?
4. What are the possible complications that J.N. is at risk for developing secondary to ARDS?
5. What are possible reasons for J.N.'s sudden decline in pulmonary status during and immediately after chest tube insertion?
6. ***Evidence-Based Practice:*** You are orienting a new nurse who asks you why you offered J.N.'s family the opportunity to stay at the bedside while the chest tube was placed. How would you respond?
7. What are possible reasons for improved oxygenation and $CO_2$ levels after administration of additional opioid analgesia?
8. ***Priority Decision:*** What priority interventions should be implemented to improve J.N.'s respiratory status and hypoxemia?
9. ***Priority Decision:*** Based on the assessment data presented, what are the priority nursing diagnoses?
10. ***Teamwork and Collaboration:*** When developing the plan of care for J.N., what tasks can you delegate to unlicensed assistive personnel (UAP)?
11. ***Patient-Centered Care:*** What information should you provide to J.N.'s caregiver(s) given his decline in cardiopulmonary function?
12. ***Patient-Centered Care:*** Given the guidelines in the patient's advance directive, what ethical/legal issues could you encounter in this patient scenario?

Answers available at *http://evolve.elsevier.com/Lewis/medsurg.*

## BRIDGE TO NCLEX EXAMINATION

The number of the question corresponds to the same-numbered outcome at the beginning of the chapter.

1. Which signs and symptoms differentiate hypoxemic respiratory failure from hypercapnic respiratory failure *(select all that apply)*?
   **a.** Cyanosis
   **b.** Tachypnea
   **c.** Morning headache
   **d.** Paradoxic breathing
   **e.** Use of pursed-lip breathing
2. The $O_2$ delivery system chosen for the patient in acute respiratory failure should
   **a.** always be a low-flow device, such as a nasal cannula or face mask.
   **b.** administer continuous positive airway pressure ventilation to prevent $CO_2$ narcosis.
   **c.** correct the $PaO_2$ to a normal level as quickly as possible using mechanical ventilation.
   **d.** maintain the $PaO_2$ at greater than or equal to 60 mm Hg at the lowest $O_2$ concentration possible.
3. The *most* common early clinical manifestations of ARDS that the nurse may observe are
   **a.** dyspnea and tachypnea.
   **b.** cyanosis and apprehension.
   **c.** hypotension and tachycardia.
   **d.** respiratory distress and frothy sputum.
4. Maintenance of fluid balance in the patient with ARDS involves
   **a.** hydration using colloids.
   **b.** administration of surfactant.
   **c.** fluid restriction and diuretics as necessary.
   **d.** keeping the hemoglobin at levels above 9 g/dL (90 g/L).
5. Which intervention is *most* likely to prevent or limit barotrauma in the patient with ARDS who is mechanically ventilated?
   **a.** Decreasing PEEP
   **b.** Increasing the tidal volume
   **c.** Use of permissive hypercapnia
   **d.** Use of positive pressure ventilation

1. a, b, d; 2. d; 3. a; 4. c; 5. c

For rationales to these answers and even more NCLEX review questions, visit *http://evolve.elsevier.com/Lewis/medsurg.*

## EVOLVE WEBSITE

http://evolve.elsevier.com/Lewis/medsurg

**Review Questions (Online Only)**

**Key Points**

**Answer Keys to Questions**

- Rationales for Bridge to NCLEX Examination Questions
- Answer Guidelines for Case Study on p. 1626

**Student Case Studies**

- Patient With Acute Respiratory Failure and Ventilatory Management
- Patient With Pulmonary Embolism and Respiratory Failure

**Nursing Care Plans**

- eNursing Care Plan 67-1: Patient With Acute Respiratory Failure

**Conceptual Care Map Creator**

**Audio Glossary**

**Content Updates**

## REFERENCES


1. Kaynar AM: Respiratory failure: overview. 2015. Retrieved from *http://emedicine.medscape.com/article/167981-overview.*
*2. Chung KF, Wenzel SE, Brozek JL, et al: International ERS/ATS guidelines on definition, evaluation and treatment of severe asthma, *Eur Respir J* 43:343, 2014.
3. Taffet GE, Donahue JF, Altman PR: Considerations for managing chronic obstructive pulmonary disease in the elderly, *Clin Interv Aging* 9:23, 2014.
*4. Barr J, Fraser GL, Puntillo K, et al: Clinical practice guidelines for the management of pain, agitation, and delirium in adult patients in the intensive care unit, *Crit Care Med* 41(1):263, 2013.
5. Ouellette DR: Pulmonary embolism: overview. 2015. Retrieved from *http://emedicine.medscape.com/article/300901-overview.*
6. Cartin-Ceba R, Iyer VN, Krowka MJ: Hepatopulmonary syndrome and portopulmonary hypertension. In Cataldo D, editor: *Contemporary liver transplantation*, Switzerland, 2015, Springer International.
7. Laveneziana P, Webb KA, O'Donnell DE: Static and dynamic hyperinflation in chronic obstructive pulmonary disease. In Aliverti A, Pedotti A, editors: *Mechanics of breathing*, New York, 2014, Springer.
8. Fayyaz J: Hypoventilation syndromes: overview. 2015. Retrieved from *http://emedicine.medscape.com/article/304381-overview.*
9. Huttmann SE, Windisch W, Storre JH: Techniques for the measurement and monitoring of carbon dioxide in the blood, *Ann Am Thorac Soc* 11(4):645, 2014.
10. Terzano C, Romani S, Gaudio C, et al: Right heart functional changes in the acute, hypercapnic exacerbations of COPD, *BioMed Res Int* 2014:596051, 2014.
11. Schnell D, Timsit JF, Darmon M, et al: Noninvasive mechanical ventilation in acute respiratory failure: trends in use and outcomes, *Intens Care Med* 40(4):582, 2014.
12. Kelly CR, Higgins AR, Chandra S: Noninvasive positive-pressure ventilation, *N Engl J Med* 372:e30, 2015.
13. Bumbaeca D, Filip N, Valcu C, et al: Outcome of non-invasive ventilation in acute hypercapnic respiratory failure in the elderly, *Eur Respir J* 44(Suppl 58):P2958, 2014.
*14. Arbour R: Bispectral index monitoring. In Wiegand DL-M, editor: *AACN procedure manual for critical care*, ed 6, St Louis, 2011, Saunders.
*15. Shah A, Stanworth SJ, McKechnie S: Evidence and triggers for the transfusion of blood and blood products, *Anesth* 70(Suppl 1):10, 2015.
16. Inouye SK, Westendorp RGJ, Saczynski JS: Delirium in elderly people, *Lancet* 383(9920):911, 2014.
17. Ferguson ND, Fan E, Camporota L, et al: The Berlin definition of ARDS: an expanded rationale, justification, and supplementary material, *Intens Care Med* 38(10):1573, 2012.
18. Wilson JG, Matthay MA: Mechanical ventilation in acute hypoxemic respiratory failure: a review of new strategies for the practicing hospitalist, *J Hosp Med* 9(7):469, 2014.
19. Kalanuris AA, Zai W, Mirski M: Ventilator-associated pneumonia in the ICU, *Crit Care* 18(208):1, 2014.
20. Terzi E, Zarogoulidis K, Kougioumtzi I, et al: Acute respiratory distress syndrome and pneumothorax, *J Thorac Dis* 6(Suppl 4):S435, 2014.
21. Beitler JR, Schoenfeld DA, Thompson BT: Preventing ARDS: progress, promise and pitfalls, *Chest* 146(4):1102, 2014.
*22. Combes A, Brodie D, Bartlett R, et al: Position paper for the organization of extracorporeal membrane oxygenation programs for acute respiratory failure in adult patients, *Am J Respir Crit Care Med* 190(5):488, 2014.
*23. Beitler JR, Shaefi S, Montesi SB, et al: Prone positioning reduces mortality from acute respiratory distress syndrome in the low tidal volume era: a meta-analysis, *Intens Care Med* 40(3):332, 2014.
*24. Girard R, Baboi L, Ayzac L, et al: The impact of patient positioning on pressure ulcers in patients with severe ARDS: results from a multicentre randomized controlled trial on prone positioning, *Intens Care Med* 40:397, 2014.

*Evidence-based information for clinical practice.

68

# Emergency and Disaster Nursing

*Linda Bucher*

*One of the tests of leadership is the ability to recognize a problem before it becomes an emergency.*

***Arnold H. Glasow***

http://evolve.elsevier.com/Lewis/medsurg/

## LEARNING OUTCOMES

1. Apply the steps in triage, the primary survey, and the secondary survey to a patient experiencing a medical, surgical, or traumatic emergency.
2. Relate the pathophysiology to the assessment and interprofessional care of select environmental emergencies (e.g., hyperthermia, hypothermia, submersion injury, bites).
3. Relate the pathophysiology to the assessment and interprofessional care of select toxicologic emergencies.
4. Select appropriate nursing interventions for victims of violence.
5. Differentiate among the responsibilities of health care providers, the community, and select federal agencies in emergency and mass casualty incident preparedness.

## KEY TERMS

drowning, p. 1639
emergency, p. 1645
family presence (FP), p. 1632
frostbite, p. 1637
heat cramps, p. 1637
heat exhaustion, p. 1637
heatstroke, p. 1637
hypothermia, p. 1638
jaw-thrust maneuver, p. 1630
mass casualty incident (MCI), p. 1645
primary survey, p. 1630
secondary survey, p. 1632
submersion injury, p. 1639
terrorism, p. 1645
triage, p. 1628

This chapter presents an overview of triage and care of select emergency patients. Common emergency situations discussed include heat- and cold-related emergencies, submersion injuries, bites and stings, and various types of poisonings. The chapter concludes with a discussion of terrorism, followed by a description of a mass casualty incident, and the methods of responding to the incident.

The emergency management of various medical, surgical, and traumatic emergencies is discussed throughout the textbook. Tables summarize emergency management of specific problems. Table 68-1 lists the emergency management tables by title, chapter number, and page.

Patients with life-threatening or potentially life-threatening problems as well as less urgent problems come to the hospital through the emergency department (ED). Every year more than 136 million people visit EDs.[1] This number is increasing for a variety of reasons, including (1) the inability to see an HCP, (2) an aging population, (3) shorter hospital stays resulting in frequent readmissions, (4) acute mental health crises, (5) ED closures, and (6) lack of or inadequate health insurance or an HCP. These factors result in chronic overcrowding and long wait times.[2]

Emergency nurses care for patients of all ages and with a variety of problems. However, some EDs specialize in certain patient populations or conditions, such as pediatric ED or trauma ED. The Emergency Nurses Association (ENA) is the specialty organization aimed at advancing emergency nursing practice. The ENA provides standards of care for nurses working in the ED, and a certification process that allows nurses to become certified emergency nurses (CENs).[3]

## CARE OF EMERGENCY PATIENT

Recognition of life-threatening illness or injury is one of the most important goals of emergency nursing. Initiation of interventions to reverse or prevent a crisis is often a priority before a medical diagnosis is made. This process begins with your first contact with a patient. Prompt identification of patients requiring immediate treatment and determination of appropriate interventions are essential nurse competencies.

### Triage

**Triage**, a French word meaning "to sort," refers to the process of rapidly determining patient acuity.[4] It is one of the most

Reviewed by Rebecca Personett, RN, PhD, NEA-BC, Professor of Nursing, North Central Texas College, Gainesville, Texas and Brookhaven College, Dallas, Texas; and Matthew Soos, RN, BSN, BA, EMT, Interventional Radiology/Emergency Department Staff Nurse, AtlantiCare Regional Medical Center, Atlantic City, New Jersey.

important assessment skills needed by emergency nurses. Most often you will confront multiple patients who have a variety of problems. The triage process works on the premise that patients who have a threat to life must be treated before other patients.

A *triage system* identifies and categorizes patients so that the most critical are treated first. The ENA and American College of Emergency Physicians support the use of a five-level triage system.[5] The *Emergency Severity Index* (ESI) is a five-level triage system that incorporates concepts of illness severity and resource utilization (e.g., electrocardiogram [ECG], laboratory tests, radiology studies, IV fluids) to determine who should be treated first (Table 68-2). The ESI includes a triage algorithm that directs you to assign an ESI level to patients coming into the ED. The triage algorithm can be found in the ESI Implementation Handbook.[5]

First, assess the patient for any threats to life (ESI-1) (e.g., Is the patient dying?) or presence of a high-risk situation (ESI-2) (e.g., Is this a high-risk patient who should not wait to be seen?). Next, evaluate patients who do not meet the criteria for ESI-1 or ESI-2 for the number of anticipated resources that they may need. Assign patients to ESI-3, ESI-4, or ESI-5 based on this determination. Normal vital signs are required for patients assigned to ESI-3. Patients with abnormal vital signs may be reassigned to ESI-2.[5]

**TABLE 68-1 Emergency Management**

***Emergency Management Tables***

| Title | Chapter | Page |
|---|---|---|
| Abdominal Trauma | 42 | 942 |
| Acute Abdominal Pain | 42 | 939 |
| Acute Soft Tissue Injury | 62 | 1464 |
| Anaphylactic Shock | 13 | 202 |
| Chemical Burns | 24 | 436 |
| Chest Pain | 33 | 723 |
| Chest Trauma | 27 | 519 |
| Depressant Toxicity | 10 | 152 |
| Diabetic Ketoacidosis | 48 | 1144 |
| Dysrhythmias | 35 | 763 |
| Electrical Burns | 24 | 435 |
| Eye Injury | 21 | 371 |
| Fractured Extremity | 62 | 1474 |
| Head Injury | 56 | 1330 |
| Hyperthermia | 68 | 1636 |
| Hypothermia | 68 | 1639 |
| Inhalation Injury | 24 | 435 |
| Sexual Assault | 53 | 1264 |
| Shock | 66 | 1597 |
| Spinal Cord Injury | 60 | 1425 |
| Stimulant Toxicity | 10 | 151 |
| Stroke | 57 | 1354 |
| Submersion Injuries | 68 | 1641 |
| Thermal Burns | 24 | 434 |
| Thoracic Injuries | 27 | 520 |
| Tonic-Clonic Seizures | 58 | 1378 |

**CHECK YOUR PRACTICE**

You are working in the ED with your preceptor, who is a triage nurse. A 24-yr-old male arrives and states, "I think I have food poisoning. I've been vomiting all night and now I have diarrhea." The patient reports abdominal cramping that he rates as 6/10. He denies fever or chills. Vital signs: T = 97.8° F (36.6° C), HR = 94, RR = 16, BP = 121/74 mm Hg.

- Assign a triage acuity rating using the ESI (Table 68-2).

After you complete the initial focused assessment to determine the presence of actual or potential threats to life, proceed with a more detailed assessment. A systematic approach to this assessment decreases the time needed to identify potential threats to life and limits the risk of overlooking a life-threatening condition. A primary and secondary survey is the approach used for all trauma patients. For nontrauma patients, the

**TABLE 68-2 Five-Level Emergency Severity Index (ESI)**

| | LEVEL | | | | |
|---|---|---|---|---|---|
| **Definition** | **ESI-1** | **ESI-2** | **ESI-3** | **ESI-4** | **ESI-5** |
| **Stability of vital functions (ABCs)** | Unstable | Threatened | Stable | Stable | Stable |
| **Life threat or organ threat** | Obvious | Likely but not always obvious | Unlikely but possible | No | No |
| **How soon patient should be seen by HCP** | Immediately | Within 10 min | Up to 1 hr | Could be delayed | Could be delayed |
| **Expected resource intensity** | High resource intensity<br>Staff at bedside continuously<br>Often mobilization of team response | High resource intensity<br>Multiple, often complex diagnostic studies<br>Frequent consultation<br>Continuous monitoring | Medium to high resource intensity<br>Multiple diagnostic studies (e.g., multiple laboratory studies, x-rays) or brief observation<br>Complex procedure (e.g., IV fluids, drugs) | Low resource intensity<br>One simple diagnostic study (e.g., x-ray) or simple procedure (e.g., sutures) | Low resource intensity<br>Examination only |
| **Examples** | Cardiac arrest, intubated trauma patient, overdose with bradypnea, severe respiratory distress | Chest pain probably resulting from ischemia, multiple trauma unless responsive | Abdominal pain or gynecologic disorders unless in severe distress, hip fracture in older patient | Closed extremity trauma, simple laceration, cystitis | Cold symptoms, minor burn, recheck (e.g., wound), prescription refill |

*ABCs,* Airway, breathing, circulation.

Modified and reprinted with permission. Copyright 1999, Richard C. Wuerz, MD, and David R. Eitel, MD.

primary survey is followed by a focused assessment. (Focused assessments are discussed in Chapter 3.)

## Primary Survey

The **primary survey** (Table 68-3) focuses on airway, breathing, circulation (ABC), disability, exposure, facilitation of adjuncts and family, and other resuscitation aids. If uncontrolled external hemorrhage is noted, the usual ABC assessment format may be reprioritized to <C>ABC for hemorrhage control. The <C> stands for catastrophic hemorrhage and, if present, must be controlled first.[6] Apply direct pressure with a sterile dressing followed by a pressure dressing to any obvious bleeding sites.

The primary survey aims to identify life-threatening conditions so that appropriate interventions can be started. You may identify life-threatening conditions related to ABCs (Table 68-4) at any point during the primary survey. When this occurs, start interventions immediately, before moving to the next step of the survey.

**A = Alertness and Airway.** The alertness level of the patient can be an important factor for selecting appropriate airway interventions. Determine level of consciousness (LOC) by assessing the patient's response to verbal and/or painful stimuli. A simple mnemonic to remember is *AVPU: A* = alert, *V* = responsive to voice, *P* = responsive to pain, and *U* = unresponsive.[6]

Nearly all immediate trauma deaths occur because of airway obstruction. Saliva, bloody secretions, vomitus, laryngeal trauma, dentures, facial trauma, fractures, and the tongue can obstruct the airway. Patients at risk for airway compromise include those who drown or have seizures, anaphylaxis, foreign body obstruction, or cardiopulmonary arrest. If an airway is not maintained, obstruction of airflow, hypoxia, and death will result.

Primary signs and symptoms in a patient with a compromised airway include dyspnea, inability to speak, gasping (agonal) breaths, foreign body in the airway, and trauma to the face or neck. Airway maintenance should progress rapidly from the least to the most invasive method. Treatment includes opening the airway using the **jaw-thrust maneuver** (avoiding hyperextension of the neck) (Fig. 68-1), suctioning and/or removal of foreign body, insertion of a nasopharyngeal or an oropharyngeal airway (in unconscious patients only), and endotracheal intubation. If intubation is impossible because of airway obstruction, an emergency cricothyroidotomy or tracheotomy is performed (see Chapter 26). Ventilate patients with 100% $O_2$ using a bag-valve-mask (BVM) device before intubation or cricothyroidotomy.[7]

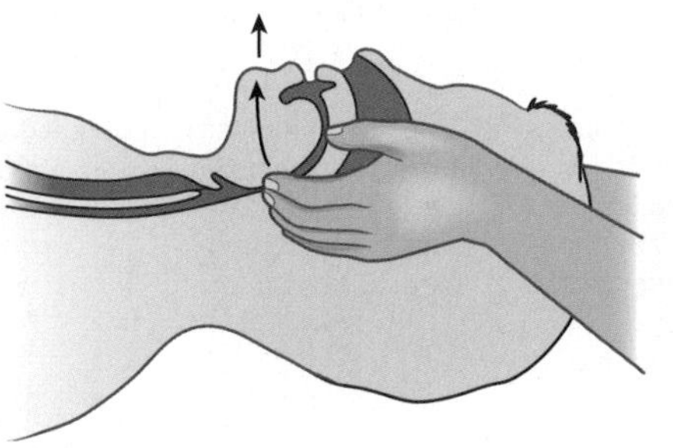

**FIG. 68-1** Jaw-thrust maneuver is the recommended procedure for opening the airway of an unconscious patient with a possible neck or spinal injury. With the patient lying supine, kneel at the top of the head. Place one hand on each side of the patient's head, resting your elbows on the surface. Grasp the angles of the patient's lower jaw and lift the jaw forward with both hands without tilting the head.

*Rapid-sequence intubation* is the preferred procedure for securing an unprotected airway in the ED. It involves the use of sedation (e.g., midazolam) or anesthesia (e.g., etomidate [Amidate]) and paralysis (e.g., succinylcholine [Anectine]). These drugs aid intubation and reduce the risk of aspiration and airway trauma. (See Chapter 65 for more information on intubation.)

Suspect cervical spine trauma in any patient with face, head, or neck trauma and/or significant upper chest injuries. Stabilize the cervical spine (head maintained in a neutral position) and/or immobilize during assessment of the airway. At the scene of the injury, the cervical spine is immobilized with a rigid *cervical collar* (C-collar) and a *cervical immobilization device* (CID) (also known as "head blocks"). Finally, secure the patient's forehead to the backboard. Do not use sandbags because the weight of the bags could move the head if the patient is logrolled.

**B = Breathing.** Adequate airflow through the upper airway does not ensure adequate ventilation. Many conditions cause breathing changes. These include fractured ribs, pneumothorax, penetrating injury, allergic reactions, pulmonary emboli, and asthma attacks. Patients with these conditions may have a variety of signs and symptoms, including dyspnea (e.g., pulmonary emboli), paradoxic or asymmetric chest wall movement (e.g., flail chest), decreased or absent breath sounds on the affected side (e.g., pneumothorax), visible wound to the chest wall (e.g., penetrating injury), cyanosis (e.g., asthma), tachycardia, and hypotension.

Every critically injured or ill patient has an increased metabolic and $O_2$ demand and should have supplemental $O_2$. Give high-flow $O_2$ (100%) via a non-rebreather mask and monitor the patient's response. Life-threatening conditions (e.g., flail chest, tension pneumothorax) can severely and quickly compromise ventilation. Interventions may include BVM ventilation with 100% $O_2$, needle decompression, intubation, and treatment of the underlying cause.

**C = Circulation.** An effective circulatory system includes the heart, intact blood vessels, and adequate blood volume. Uncontrolled internal or external bleeding places an individual at risk for hemorrhagic shock (see Chapter 66). Check a central pulse (e.g., carotid) because peripheral pulses may be absent due to direct injury or vasoconstriction. If you feel a pulse, assess the quality and rate. Assess the skin for color, temperature, and moisture. Altered mental status and delayed capillary refill (longer than 3 seconds) are common signs of shock. When evaluating capillary refill in cold environments, remember that a cold temperature delays refill.

Insert IV lines into veins in the upper extremities unless contraindicated, such as in a massive fracture or an injury that affects limb circulation. Insert two large-bore (14- to 16-gauge) IV catheters and start aggressive fluid resuscitation using normal saline or lactated Ringer's solution. Consider intraosseous or central venous access if unable to rapidly obtain venous access. (See Chapter 66 for more information on hypovolemic shock and fluid resuscitation.)

Give type-specific packed red blood cells if needed. In an emergency (life-threatening) situation, give uncrossmatched blood (e.g., O negative) if immediate transfusion is warranted. Pelvic splints or belts for pelvic fracture may be used for bleeding with hypotension.

## TABLE 68-3 Emergency Assessment: Primary Survey

| Assessment | Interventions |
|---|---|
| **Alertness and Airway With Cervical Spine Stabilization and/or Immobilization** | |
| • Assess for catastrophic external bleeding<br>• Assess alertness (e.g., AVPU)<br>• Assess for respiratory distress<br>• Assess airway for patency<br>• Check for loose teeth or foreign bodies<br>• Assess for bleeding, vomitus, or edema | • Control bleeding with direct pressure and pressure dressings<br>• Open airway<br>• Use jaw-thrust maneuver<br>• Remove or suction any foreign bodies<br>• Insert oropharyngeal or nasopharyngeal airway, cricothyroidotomy<br>• Rapid sequence intubation<br>• Immobilize cervical spine using rigid cervical collar and cervical immobilization device. Secure forehead to backboard |
| **Breathing** | |
| • Assess ventilation<br>• Scan chest for signs of breathing<br>• Look for paradoxic movement of the chest wall during inspiration and expiration<br>• Note use of accessory muscles or abdominal muscles<br>• Observe and count respiratory rate<br>• Note color of nail beds, mucous membranes, skin<br>• Auscultate lungs<br>• Assess for jugular venous distention and position of trachea | • Give supplemental $O_2$ via appropriate delivery system (e.g., non-rebreather mask)<br>• Ventilate with bag-valve-mask with 100% $O_2$ if respirations are inadequate or absent<br>• Prepare to intubate if severe respiratory distress (e.g., agonal breaths) or arrest<br>• Have suction available<br>• If absent breath sounds, prepare for needle thoracostomy and chest tube insertion |
| **Circulation** | |
| • Check carotid or femoral pulse<br>• Palpate pulse for quality and rate<br>• Assess skin color, temperature, and moisture<br>• Check capillary refill | • If absent pulse, initiate cardiopulmonary resuscitation and advanced life support measures<br>• If shock symptoms or hypotensive, start two large-bore (14- to 16-gauge) IVs and start infusions of normal saline or lactated Ringer's solution<br>• Consider intraosseous or central venous access if IV access cannot be rapidly obtained<br>• Administer blood products if ordered<br>• Consider autotransfusion if isolated chest trauma<br>• Consider use of pelvic splint or belt in the presence of pelvic fracture with hypotension |
| **Disability** | |
| • Assess level of consciousness by determining response to verbal and/or painful stimuli (e.g., Glasgow Coma Scale)<br>• Assess pupils for size, shape, equality, and reactivity | • Periodically reassess level of consciousness, mental status, and pupil size and reactivity |
| **Exposure and Environmental Control** | |
| • Assess full body for determination of additional or related injuries<br>• Assess environment | • Remove clothing for adequate examination<br>• Stabilize any impaled objects<br>• Keep patient warm with blankets, warmed IV fluids, overhead lights to prevent heat loss, if appropriate<br>• Maintain privacy |
| **Facilitate Adjuncts and Family** | |
| • Assess vital signs including pulse oximetry<br>• Determine caregiver's desire to be present during invasive procedures and/or cardiopulmonary resuscitation | • Obtain bilateral blood pressures if patient has sustained or is suspected of having sustained chest trauma, or if the BP is abnormally high or low<br>• Assign health team member to support caregiver(s) |
| **Get Resuscitation Adjuncts** | |
| • Determine need for additional adjunct measures for monitoring the patient's condition | • Facilitate laboratory tests (e.g., type and crossmatch, complete blood count and metabolic panel, blood alcohol, toxicology screening, arterial blood gases [ABGs], coagulation profile, cardiac biomarkers, pregnancy [urine])<br>• Continuously monitor ECG for heart rate and rhythm<br>• Insert nasogastric tube; insert orogastric tube in a patient with significant head or facial trauma<br>• Monitor oxygenation and ventilation (e.g., continuous pulse oximetry, capnography)<br>• Manage pain with pharmacologic (e.g., nonsteroidal antiinflammatory drugs, IV opioids) and nonpharmacologic (e.g., distraction, positioning, music) pain management strategies<br>• Provide emotional support to patient and caregiver<br>• Provide additional comfort measures as appropriate (e.g., ice, position of comfort, warm blanket) |

*AVPU, A* = alert, *V* = responsive to voice, *P* = responsive to pain, and *U* = unresponsive.

**TABLE 68-4 Potential Life-Threatening Conditions Found During Primary Survey***

**Airway**
- Inhalation injury (e.g., fire victim)
- Obstruction (partial or complete) from foreign bodies, debris (e.g., vomitus), or tongue
- Penetrating wounds and/or blunt trauma to upper airway structures

**Breathing**
- Anaphylaxis
- Flail chest with pulmonary contusion
- Hemothorax
- Pneumothorax (e.g., open, tension)

**Circulation**
- Direct cardiac injury (e.g., myocardial infarction, trauma)
- Pericardial tamponade
- Shock (e.g., massive burns, hypovolemia)
- Uncontrolled external hemorrhage
- Hypothermia

**Disability**
- Head injury
- Stroke

*List is not all-inclusive.

**D = Disability.** Conduct a brief neurologic examination as part of the primary survey. The patient's LOC is a measure of the degree of disability. Use the Glasgow Coma Scale (GCS) to determine the LOC (see Table 56-5). Although the GCS is not accurate for intubated or aphasic patients, it is a standardized tool. This allows for consistent communication among the interprofessional care team. Finally, assess the pupils for size, shape, equality, and reactivity.

**E = Exposure and Environmental Control.** Remove all trauma patients' clothing to perform a thorough physical assessment. This often requires cutting off the patient's clothing. Be careful not to cut through any area that may provide forensic evidence (e.g., bullet hole). Do not remove any impaled objects (e.g., knife). Removing these could result in serious bleeding and further injury. Once the patient is exposed, use warming blankets, overhead warmers, and warmed IV fluids to limit heat loss, prevent hypothermia, and maintain privacy.

**F = Facilitate Adjuncts and Family.** Obtain a full set of vital signs, including BP, heart rate, respiratory rate, $O_2$ saturation, and temperature after the patient is exposed. If the patient has sustained or is suspected of having sustained chest trauma, or if the BP is abnormally high or low, obtain the BP in both arms.

Facilitate family presence (FP). Research supports the benefits for patients, caregivers, and staff of allowing FP during resuscitation and invasive procedures.[8] Patients report that caregivers provide comfort, serve as advocates for them, and help remind the interprofessional care team of their "personhood." Caregivers who wish to be present during invasive procedures and resuscitation view themselves as active participants in the care process. They also believe that they comfort the patient and that it is their right to be with the patient.[8] Nurses report that family members serve as "patient helpers" (e.g., provide support) and "staff helpers" (e.g., act as a translator). It is essential to assign a member of the interprofessional care team to explain care delivered and answer questions should a caregiver request FP during resuscitation or invasive procedures.

**G = Get Resuscitation Adjuncts.** Start additional adjunct measures for monitoring the patient's condition, if not already done. Use the mnemonic "LMNOP" to remember these resuscitation aids:

*L:* Laboratory tests (e.g., type and crossmatch, complete blood count and metabolic panel, blood alcohol, toxicology screening, arterial blood gases [ABGs], coagulation profile, cardiac biomarkers, pregnancy [urine]).
*M:* Monitor ECG for heart rate and rhythm.
*N:* Nasogastric tube to decompress and empty the stomach, reduce the risk of aspiration, and test the contents for blood. Place an orogastric tube in a patient with significant head or facial trauma, since a nasogastric tube could enter the brain.
*O:* Oxygenation and ventilation assessment. Continuously monitor $O_2$ saturation and end-tidal $CO_2$ (if appropriate) (see Chapter 65).
*P:* Pain assessment and management

Pain is the primary complaint of most patients who come to the ED.[9] Provision of comfort measures is critical when caring for patients in the ED. Many EDs have developed pain management protocols for nurses to treat pain early, beginning at triage.

Pain management strategies should include a combination of pharmacologic (e.g., nonsteroidal antiinflammatory drugs, IV opioids) and nonpharmacologic (e.g., distraction, positioning, music) measures. You play a key role in ongoing pain management because of your frequent contact with patients.

General comfort measures such as providing verbal reassurance, listening, reducing stimuli (e.g., dimming lights, warm blankets), and developing a trusting relationship with the patient and caregiver should be provided to all patients in the ED. Additional measures include splinting, elevating, and icing injured extremities as appropriate.

### Secondary Survey

The secondary survey begins after addressing each step of the primary survey and starting any lifesaving interventions. The secondary survey is a brief, systematic process that aims to identify *all* injuries[7] (Table 68-5).

**H = History and Head-to-Toe Assessment.** The history and mechanism of the injury or illness provides clues to the cause of the crisis (e.g., Were the injuries self-inflicted or a result of abuse?) and suggests specific assessment and interventions. The patient may not be able to give a history. However, caregivers, friends, bystanders, and prehospital personnel can often provide necessary information. Prehospital information focuses on the mechanism and pattern of injury, injuries suspected, vital signs, treatments initiated, and patient responses.

Details of the incident are extremely important because the mechanism of injury and injury patterns can predict specific injuries.[7] For example, a restrained front-seat passenger may have a head injury or knee, femur, or hip fractures from hitting the dashboard and an abdominal injury from the seat belt. If there were deaths at the scene, the patient is at high risk for significant injury.

Patients who jump from buildings or bridges may have bilateral calcaneal (heel) fractures, bilateral wrist fractures, and lumbar spine compression fractures. They are also at risk for aortic tears. Older patients who have fallen may have had a stroke or heart attack that led to the fall.

Prehospital personnel provide a detailed description of the patient's general condition, level of consciousness, and apparent injuries.[7] If the patient is emergently ill, obtain a thorough history from caregivers or friends after the patient is taken to

**TABLE 68-5 Emergency Assessment: Secondary Survey**

| Assessment | Interventions |
|---|---|
| **History and Head-to-Toe Assessment** | |
| ***History*** | • Obtain details of the incident/illness, mechanism and pattern of injury, length of time since incident occurred, injuries suspected, treatment provided and patient's response, level of consciousness.<br>• Use the mnemonic **SAMPLE** to determine **S**ymptoms associated with injury or illness; **A**llergies, including tetanus status; **M**edication history; **P**ast health history (e.g., preexisting medical/psychiatric conditions, last menstrual period); **L**ast meal/oral intake; and **E**vents/Environment preceding illness or injury. |
| ***Head, Neck, and Face*** | • Note general appearance, including skin color.<br>• Examine face and scalp for lacerations, bone or soft tissue deformity, tenderness, bleeding, and foreign bodies.<br>• Inspect eyes, ears, nose, and mouth for bleeding, foreign bodies, drainage, pain, deformity, ecchymosis, lacerations.<br>• Palpate head for depressions of cranial or facial bones, contusions, hematomas, areas of softness, bony crepitus.<br>• Examine neck for stiffness, pain in cervical vertebrae, tracheal deviation, distended neck veins, bleeding, edema, difficulty swallowing, bruising, subcutaneous emphysema, bony crepitus. |
| ***Chest*** | • Observe rate, depth, and effort of breathing, including chest wall movement and use of accessory muscles.<br>• Palpate for bony crepitus, subcutaneous emphysema.<br>• Auscultate breath sounds.<br>• Obtain 12-lead ECG and chest x-ray.<br>• Inspect for external signs of injury: petechiae, bleeding, cyanosis, bruises, abrasions, lacerations, old scars. |
| ***Abdomen and Flanks*** | • Look for symmetry of abdominal wall and bony structures.<br>• Inspect for external signs of injury: bruises, abrasions, lacerations, punctures, old scars.<br>• Auscultate for bowel sounds.<br>• Palpate for masses, guarding, femoral pulses.<br>• Note type and location of pain, rigidity, or distention of abdomen. |
| ***Pelvis and Perineum*** | • Gently palpate pelvis.<br>• Assess genitalia for blood at the meatus, priapism, ecchymosis, rectal bleeding, anal sphincter tone.<br>• Determine ability to void. |
| ***Extremities*** | • Inspect for signs of external injury: deformity, ecchymosis, abrasions, lacerations, swelling.<br>• Observe skin color and palpate skin for pain, tenderness, temperature, and crepitus.<br>• Evaluate movement, strength, and sensation in arms and legs.<br>• Assess quality and symmetry of peripheral pulses. |
| **Inspect Posterior Surfaces** | • Logroll and inspect and palpate back for deformity, bleeding, lacerations, bruises while maintaining cervical spine immobilization, if appropriate. |

the treatment area. The mnemonic *SAMPLE* is a memory aid that prompts you to ask about the following[6]:

*S:* Symptoms associated with the injury or illness
*A:* Allergies (e.g., drugs, food, latex, environment) and tetanus status
*M:* Medication history
*P:* Past health history (e.g., preexisting medical or psychiatric conditions, previous surgeries, smoking history, recent use of drugs or alcohol, last menstrual period, baseline mental status)
*L:* Last meal/oral intake
*E:* Events or environmental factors leading to the illness or injury

***Head, Neck, and Face.*** Assess the patient for general appearance, skin color, and temperature. Check the eyes for extraocular movements. A disconjugate gaze is an indication of neurologic damage. Battle's sign, or bruising directly behind the ear(s), may indicate a fracture of the base of the posterior portion of the skull. "Raccoon eyes," or periorbital ecchymosis, is usually an indication of a fracture of the base of the frontal portion of the skull. Check the ears for blood and cerebrospinal fluid (see Chapter 56 and Fig. 56-13). Do not block clear drainage from the ear or nose.

Assess the airway for foreign bodies, bleeding, edema, and loose or missing teeth. Check for the ability to open the mouth and swallow. Inspect the neck for bruising, edema, bleeding, or distended neck veins. Palpate the trachea to determine whether it is midline. A deviated trachea may signal a life-threatening tension pneumothorax. Subcutaneous emphysema may indicate laryngotracheal disruption. A stiff or painful neck may signify a fracture of one or more cervical vertebrae. Protect the cervical spine using a C-collar and supine positioning if indicated.

***Chest.*** Inspect the chest for paradoxic chest movements and large sucking chest wounds. Palpate the sternum, clavicles, and ribs for deformity, point tenderness, and crepitus. Auscultate breath sounds and heart sounds. In addition to tension pneumothorax and open pneumothorax, evaluate the patient for rib fractures, pulmonary contusion, blunt cardiac injury, and hemothorax. Obtain a chest x-ray and 12-lead ECG, particularly on patients with known or suspected heart disease. The ECG can help detect dysrhythmias and signs of myocardial ischemia or infarction.

***Abdomen and Flanks.*** The abdomen and flanks are more difficult to assess. Frequent evaluation for subtle changes in the abdomen is essential. Motor vehicle crashes and assaults can cause blunt trauma. Penetrating trauma tends to injure specific, solid organs (e.g., spleen) based on their trajectory. Stabilize any impaled objects. They must be removed in a controlled environment such as an operating room.

Inspect the abdomen for bruising, petechiae, and ecchymosis. Auscultate for bowel sounds. Decreased bowel sounds may indicate a temporary paralytic ileus. Bowel sounds in the chest may indicate a diaphragmatic rupture. Percuss the abdomen for distention (e.g., tympany [excessive air] and dullness [excessive fluid]) and palpate for tenderness.

If you suspect intraabdominal hemorrhage, a *focused abdominal sonography for trauma* (FAST) to identify blood in the peritoneal space (hemoperitoneum) is preferred. This procedure is noninvasive and performed quickly at the bedside. However, a FAST cannot rule out a retroperitoneal bleed. If one is suspected, a CT scan is usually ordered.

***Pelvis and Perineum.*** Gently palpate the pelvis to determine stability. Do not rock the pelvis. Pain may indicate a pelvic fracture and the need for an x-ray. Inspect the genitalia for bleeding, priapism, and obvious injuries. Assess for bladder distention, hematuria, dysuria, or inability to void. The HCP may perform a rectal examination to check for blood, a high-riding prostate gland (e.g., urethral injury), and loss of sphincter tone (e.g., spinal cord injury).

***Extremities.*** Assess the upper and lower extremities for point tenderness, crepitus, and deformities. Splint injured extremities above and below the injury to decrease further soft tissue injury and pain if not done prehospital. Grossly deformed, pulseless extremities should be realigned by the HCP and then splinted. Check pulses before and after movement or splinting of an extremity. A pulseless extremity is a time-critical emergency. Immobilize and elevate injured extremities, and apply ice packs. Prophylactic antibiotics are ordered for open fractures.

Also, assess extremities for *compartment syndrome.* This occurs as pressure and swelling increase inside a section of an extremity (e.g., anterior compartment of lower leg) over several hours. This compromises the viability of the muscles, nerves, and arteries. Potential causes of compartment syndrome include crush injuries, fractures, edema (e.g., burns), and hemorrhage.

**I = Inspect Posterior Surfaces.** The trauma patient should always be logrolled (while maintaining cervical spine immobilization) to inspect the patient's posterior surfaces and whenever movement is needed. This often needs three to four or more people with one person supporting the head. Inspect the back for ecchymosis, abrasions, puncture wounds, cuts, and obvious deformities. Palpate the entire spine for deformity and pain.

## Acute Care and Evaluation

Once the secondary survey is complete, record all findings. Provide tetanus prophylaxis based on vaccination history and the condition of any wounds[10] (Table 68-6).

Regardless of the patient's chief complaint, ongoing monitoring and evaluation of interventions are critical. Provide appropriate care and assess the patient's response. The evaluation of airway patency and the effectiveness of breathing will always be the highest priority. Monitor respiratory rate and rhythm, $O_2$ saturation, and ABGs (if ordered) to evaluate the patient's respiratory status. Obtain a portable chest x-ray to confirm exact placement of tubes (e.g., endotracheal, gastric).

Closely monitor the LOC; vital signs; quality of peripheral pulses; and skin temperature, color, and moisture for key information about circulation and perfusion. Insert an indwelling catheter to decompress the bladder, monitor urine output, and check for hematuria. Do not insert an indwelling catheter if blood is present at the urinary meatus (e.g., urethral tear) or if scrotal hematoma or perineal ecchymosis is present. Men with a high-riding prostate gland on rectal examination are at risk for a urethral injury. The HCP may order a retrograde urethrogram before inserting a catheter.

Depending on the patient's injuries or illness, the patient may be (1) transported for diagnostic tests (e.g., CT scan, angiography) or to the operating room for immediate surgery; (2) admitted to an intensive care, telemetry, or general unit; or (3) transferred to another facility. You may go with critically ill patients on transports. You are responsible for monitoring the patient during transport, notifying the interprofessional care team should the patient's condition become unstable, and starting basic and advanced life-support measures as needed.

**TABLE 68-6 Tetanus Vaccines and TIG for Wound Management**

| | TYPE OF WOUND | |
|---|---|---|
| **Vaccination History** | **Clean, Minor Wounds** | **All Other Wounds** |
| **Age 11 and Older*** | | |
| Unknown or <3 doses of tetanus toxoid–containing vaccine | Tdap and recommend catch-up vaccination | Tdap and recommend catch-up vaccination TIG |
| ≥3 doses of tetanus toxoid–containing vaccine *and* <5 yr since last dose | No indication | No indication |
| ≥3 doses of tetanus toxoid–containing vaccine *and* 5–10 yr since last dose | No indication | Tdap preferred (if not yet received) or Td |
| ≥3 doses of tetanus toxoid–containing vaccine *and* >10 yr since last dose | Tdap preferred (if not yet received) or Td | Tdap preferred (if not yet received) or Td |

Source: Centers for Disease Control and Prevention: Disaster information: tetanus prevention after a disaster. Retrieved from *www.bt.cdc.gov/disasters/disease/tetanus.asp.*

*Td,* Tetanus-diphtheria toxoid absorbed; *Tdap,* tetanus toxoid, reduced diphtheria toxoid, and acellular pertussis vaccine; *TIG,* tetanus immune globulin (human).

*Pregnant women: As part of standard wound management care to prevent tetanus, a tetanus toxoid–containing vaccine might be recommended for wound management in a pregnant woman if ≥5 yr have elapsed since previous Td booster. If a Td booster is indicated for a pregnant woman, Tdap should be given.

## Cardiac Arrest and Therapeutic Hypothermia

Many patients arrive at the ED in cardiac arrest. Patients with nontraumatic, out-of-hospital cardiac arrest benefit from a combination of good chest compressions and rapid defibrillation (see Appendix A), therapeutic hypothermia, and supportive care. Mechanical chest compression devices are often used to provide chest compressions both prehospital and in the ED (Fig. 68-2).

*Therapeutic hypothermia* for 24 hours after the *return of spontaneous circulation* (ROSC) decreases mortality rates and improves neurologic outcomes in many patients.[11] It is recommended for all patients who are comatose or who do not follow commands after ROSC.[12]

Therapeutic hypothermia, also called *Targeted Temperature Management,* involves three phases: induction, maintenance, and rewarming. The induction phase begins in the ED. The goal core temperature is 89.6° to 93.2° F (32° to 34° C). Recent research has suggested that cooling to a target core temperature of 96.8° F (36° C) results in similar outcomes.[13]

A variety of methods are used to cool patients. These include cold saline infusions and cooling devices (e.g., Arctic Sun). Patients require intubation and mechanical ventilation, invasive monitoring (e.g., arterial and central pressures), and continuous assessment during this therapy. Protocols are used to direct

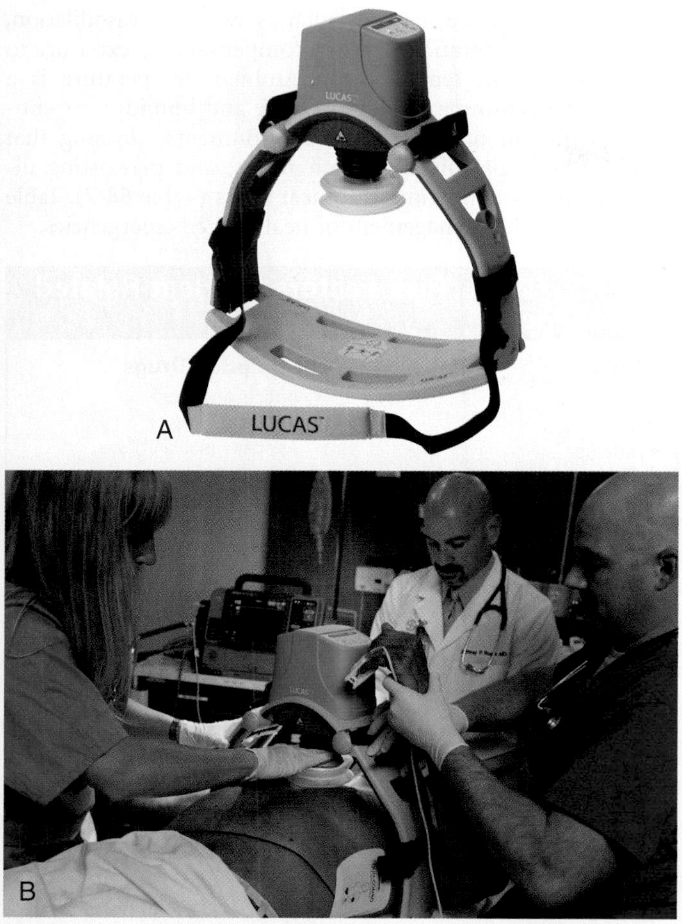


**FIG. 68-2** **A,** LUCAS 2 Mechanical Chest Compression Device. **B,** Application of the LUCAS 2 device on a patient during cardiopulmonary resuscitation. (Reprinted with permission from Physio-Control.)

the care of these patients. (Sample protocols are available at *www.med.upenn.edu/resuscitation/hypothermia/protocols.shtml.*)

## Death in the Emergency Department

Unfortunately, a number of patients will not benefit from the skill, expertise, and technology available in the ED. It is important for you to deal with your feelings about sudden death so that you can help caregivers begin the grieving process (see Chapter 9).

Recognize the importance of certain hospital rituals to help caregivers grieve. These can include collecting the personal belongings, viewing the body, and making mortuary arrangements. The death must seem real so that the caregivers can begin to accept the death. You play a significant role in providing comfort to the surviving loved ones after a death in the ED. Whenever possible, provide an area for privacy and, if appropriate, arrange for a visit from a chaplain.[14]

At times, you may need to contact the medical examiner or coroner. Autopsies may have to be arranged at the family's request or in the case of death within 24 hours of ED admission, or from suspected trauma or violence (e.g., gunshot wound).

Many patients who die in the ED could potentially be candidates for *non–heart-beating donation*. Certain tissues and organs (e.g., corneas, heart valves, skin, bone, kidneys) can be harvested from patients after death. *Organ procurement organizations* (OPOs) assist in the process of screening potential donors, counseling donor families, obtaining informed consent,

## EVIDENCE-BASED PRACTICE

### *Translating Research Into Practice*

**Does Prehospital Therapeutic Hypothermia Improve Outcomes in Cardiac Arrest?**

In patients following treatment for cardiac arrest (P), what is the effect of prehospital therapeutic hypothermia (I) versus in-hospital hypothermia or no hypothermia (C) on hospital admission body temperature, survival, and neurologic outcome to hospital discharge and re-arrest (O)?

***Synthesis of Best Available Evidence***

- Systematic review of randomized controlled trials (RCTs).
- Five RCTs of patients ($n$ = 633) with out-of-hospital cardiac arrest receiving prehospital therapeutic hypothermia, in-hospital hypothermia, or no hypothermia. Outcomes were temperature on hospital admission, survival to hospital discharge, favorable neurologic outcome at hospital discharge, and re-arrest.
- Therapeutic hypothermia helps reduce cerebral metabolism, inhibits excitatory amino acid release, and decreases brain edema and immune response during reperfusion.
- Temperatures on hospital admission for patients with prehospital therapeutic hypothermia were significantly lower compared to out-of-hospital hypothermia or no hypothermia.
- No differences were found related to timing or occurrence of hypothermia for survivor to discharge rates, neurologic outcomes at discharge, or re-arrest.

***Conclusion***

- After cardiac arrest, prehospital therapeutic hypothermia resulted in decreased patient temperature on hospital admission.

***Implications for Nursing Practice***

1. What information will you provide to other health team members regarding optimal timing for therapeutic hypothermia?
2. How will you respond to a family member who questions why prehospital therapeutic hypothermia is being done?
3. How would you critically evaluate the strength of evidence for these patients as you consider a change in best practice guidelines?

***Reference for Evidence***

Diao M, Huang F, Guan J, et al: Prehospital therapeutic hypothermia after cardiac arrest: a systematic review and meta-analysis of randomized controlled trials, *Resuscitation* 84:1021, 2013.

*P,* Patient population of interest; *I,* intervention or area of interest; *C,* comparison of interest or comparison group; *O,* outcomes of interest; *T,* timing (see p. 15).

and harvesting organs from patients who are on life support or who die in the ED.[15] Approaching caregivers about donation after an unexpected death can be distressing to both the staff and caregivers. However, for many individuals the act of donation may be the first positive step in the grieving process.

## Gerontologic Considerations: Emergency Care

The proportion of the population over age 65 is growing, with most leading active lives. Overall, people older than 65 account for 43% of all ED visits.[16] Regardless of a patient's age, aggressive interventions are warranted for all injuries or illnesses unless the patient has a preexisting terminal illness, an extremely low chance of survival, or an advance directive indicating a different course of action.

The older population is at high risk for injury because of many of the anatomic and physiologic changes that occur with aging (e.g., reduced visual acuity, limited neck rotation, slower gait, reduced reaction time). Of the injury-related admissions for people over 65 years old, most are for fractures, with many of these resulting from falls.[16]

The most common causes of falls in older adults are generalized weakness, environmental hazards (e.g., loose mats, furniture), cardiovascular syncope (e.g., dysrhythmias), and orthostatic hypotension (e.g., side effect of drugs, dehydration). When assessing a patient who has fallen, determine whether the physical findings may have caused the fall or may be due to the fall itself. For example, a patient may come to the ED with acute confusion. The confusion may be due to a heart attack or stroke that caused the patient to fall, or the patient may have suffered a head injury as a result of a fall from tripping on a rug.

Understanding the physiologic and psychosocial aspects of aging will improve the care delivered to older adults in the ED (see Chapter 5). Unfortunately, many older adults dismiss their symptoms as simply "normal for their age." It is important to fully explore any complaint by an older adult.

## ENVIRONMENTAL EMERGENCIES

Increased interest in outdoor activities such as running, hiking, cycling, skiing, and swimming has increased the number of environmental emergencies seen in the ED. Illness or injury may be caused by the activity, exposure to weather, or attack from various animals or humans. Specific environmental emergencies discussed in this section include heat-related emergencies, cold-related emergencies, submersion injuries, bites, and stings.

### HEAT-RELATED EMERGENCIES

Brief exposure to intense heat or prolonged exposure to less intense heat leads to heat stress. This occurs when thermoregulatory mechanisms such as sweating, vasodilation, and increased respirations cannot compensate for exposure to increased ambient temperatures. Ambient temperature is a product of environmental temperature and humidity. Strenuous activities in hot or humid environments, clothing that interferes with perspiration, high fevers, and preexisting illnesses predispose individuals to heat stress (Table 68-7). Table 68-8 presents the management of heat-related emergencies.

**TABLE 68-7 Risk Factors for Heat-Related Emergencies**

| | |
|---|---|
| **Alcohol**<br><br>**Age**<br>• Infants<br>• Older adults<br><br>**Environmental Conditions**<br>• High environmental temperatures<br>• High relative humidity<br><br>**Preexisting Illness**<br>• Cardiovascular disease<br>• Cystic fibrosis<br>• Dehydration<br>• Diabetes mellitus<br>• Obesity<br>• Previous stroke or other central nervous system lesion<br>• Skin disorders (e.g., large burn scars) | **Prescription Drugs**<br>• Anticholinergics<br>• Antihistamines<br>• Antiparkinsonian drugs<br>• Antispasmodics<br>• β-Adrenergic blockers<br>• Butyrophenones<br>• Diuretics<br>• Phenothiazines<br>• Tricyclic antidepressants<br><br>**Street Drugs**<br>• Amphetamines<br>• Jimson weed<br>• Lysergic acid diethylamide (LSD)<br>• Phencyclidine (PCP)<br>• 3,4-Methylenedioxymethamphetamine (MDMA, Ecstasy) |

Adapted from Howard PK, Steinmann RA, editors: *Sheehy's emergency nursing*, ed 6, St Louis, 2010, Mosby.

**TABLE 68-8 Emergency Management**

***Hyperthermia***

| Etiology | Assessment Findings | Interventions |
|---|---|---|
| **Environmental**<br>• Lack of acclimatization<br>• Physical exertion, especially during hot weather<br>• Prolonged exposure to extreme temperatures<br>**Trauma**<br>• Head injury<br>• Spinal cord injury<br>**Metabolic**<br>• Dehydration<br>• Diabetes<br>• Thyrotoxicosis<br>**Drugs**<br>• Amphetamines<br>• Antihistamines<br>• β-Adrenergic blockers<br>• Diuretics<br>• Phenothiazines<br>• Tricyclic antidepressants<br>**Other**<br>• Alcohol<br>• Cardiovascular disease<br>• CNS disorders | **Heat Cramps**<br>• Severe muscle contractions in exerted muscles<br>• Thirst<br>**Heat Exhaustion**<br>• Pale, ashen skin<br>• Fatigue, weakness<br>• Profuse sweating<br>• Extreme thirst<br>• Altered mental status (e.g., anxiety)<br>• Hypotension<br>• Tachycardia<br>• Weak, thready pulse<br>• Temperature (99.6° to 105.8° F [37.5° to 41° C])<br>**Heatstroke**<br>• Hot, dry skin<br>• Altered mental status (e.g., ranging from confusion to coma)<br>• Hypotension<br>• Tachycardia<br>• Weakness<br>• Temperature >105.8° F (41° C) | **Initial**<br>• Manage and maintain ABCs.<br>• Provide high-flow $O_2$ via non-rebreather mask or BVM.<br>• Establish IV access and begin fluid replacement for significant heat injury.<br>• Place patient in a cool environment.<br>• For patient with heatstroke, initiate rapid cooling measures: remove patient's clothing, place wet sheets over patient, and place in front of fan; immerse in a cool water bath; administer cool IV fluids or lavage with cool fluids.<br>• Obtain 12-lead ECG.<br>• Obtain blood for electrolytes and CBC.<br>• Insert urinary catheter.<br>**Ongoing Monitoring**<br>• Monitor ABCs, temperature and vital signs, level of consciousness.<br>• Monitor heart rhythm, $O_2$ saturation, and urine output.<br>• Replace electrolytes as needed.<br>• Monitor urine for development of myoglobinuria.<br>• Monitor clotting studies for development of disseminated intravascular coagulation. |

*ABCs,* Airway, breathing, circulation; *BVM,* bag-valve-mask.

### Heat Cramps

**Heat cramps** are severe cramps in large muscle groups fatigued by heavy work. Cramps are brief and intense and tend to occur during rest after exercise or heavy labor. Nausea, tachycardia, pallor, weakness, and profuse diaphoresis are often present. The condition is seen most often in healthy, acclimated athletes with inadequate fluid intake. Cramps resolve rapidly with rest and oral or parenteral replacement of sodium and water. Elevation, gentle massage, and analgesia minimize pain associated with heat cramps. Instruct the patient to avoid strenuous activity for at least 12 hours. Discharge teaching should emphasize salt replacement during strenuous exercise in hot, humid environments. You can also recommend the use of commercially prepared electrolyte solutions (e.g., sports drinks).

### Heat Exhaustion

Prolonged exposure to heat over hours or days leads to **heat exhaustion**. This is a clinical syndrome characterized by fatigue, nausea, vomiting, extreme thirst, and feelings of anxiety (Table 68-8). Hypotension, tachycardia, elevated body temperature, dilated pupils, mild confusion, ashen color, and profuse diaphoresis are also present. Hypotension and mild to severe temperature elevation (99.6° to 105.8°F [37.5° to 41°C]) are caused by dehydration. Heat exhaustion usually occurs in individuals engaged in strenuous activity in hot, humid weather, but it also occurs in sedentary individuals.

Begin treatment by placing the patient in a cool area and removing constrictive clothing. Monitor the patient for ABCs, including heart dysrhythmias (caused by electrolyte imbalances). Start oral fluid and electrolyte replacement unless the patient is nauseated. Do not use salt tablets because of potential gastric irritation and hypernatremia. Start a 0.9% normal saline IV solution if oral solutions are not tolerated. An initial fluid bolus may be needed to correct hypotension. Always correlate fluid replacement to clinical and laboratory findings. Place a moist sheet over the patient to decrease core temperature through evaporative heat loss. Consider hospital admission for older adults, the chronically ill, or those who do not improve within 3 to 4 hours.

### Heatstroke

**Heatstroke**, the most serious form of heat stress, results from failure of the hypothalamic thermoregulatory processes. It is a medical emergency. Increased sweating, vasodilation, and increased respiratory rate (the body's attempt to lower temperature) deplete fluids and electrolytes, specifically sodium. Eventually, sweat glands stop functioning, and core temperature increases rapidly, within 10 to 15 minutes. The patient has a core temperature greater than 105.8°F (41°C), altered mental status, absence of perspiration, and circulatory collapse. The skin is hot, dry, and ashen. A range of neurologic symptoms occur (e.g., hallucinations, loss of muscle coordination, combativeness) because the brain is extremely sensitive to thermal injuries. Cerebral edema and hemorrhage may occur as a result of direct thermal injury to the brain and decreased cerebral blood flow.

Death from heatstroke is directly related to the amount of time that the patient's body temperature remains elevated.[7] Prognosis is related to age, baseline health status, and length of exposure. Older adults and those with diabetes mellitus, chronic kidney disease, cardiovascular disease, pulmonary disease, or other physiologic compromise are particularly vulnerable.

**Interprofessional Care.** Treatment of heatstroke focuses on stabilizing the patient's ABCs and rapidly reducing the core temperature. Give 100% $O_2$ to compensate for the patient's hypermetabolic state. Ventilation with a BVM or intubation and mechanical ventilation may be needed. Correct fluid and electrolyte imbalances and start continuous ECG monitoring for dysrhythmias.

Various cooling methods are available. These include (1) removing clothing, covering with wet sheets, and placing the patient in front of a large fan (evaporative cooling); (2) immersing the patient in a cool water bath (conductive cooling); (3) applying ice packs to the groins and axillae; and, in refractory cases, (4) peritoneal lavaging with iced fluids.

Whatever method is selected, closely monitor the patient's temperature and control shivering. Shivering increases core temperature due to the heat generated by muscle activity. This complicates cooling efforts. Give chlorpromazine IV to control shivering. Antipyretics are not effective in this situation because the elevated temperature is not related to infection.

Monitor the patient for signs of *rhabdomyolysis* (a serious syndrome caused by the breakdown of skeletal muscle). The muscle breakdown leads to myoglobinuria. This places the kidneys at risk for acute kidney injury. Carefully monitor the urine for color (e.g., tea colored), amount, pH, and myoglobin. Finally, obtain clotting studies to monitor the patient for signs of disseminated intravascular coagulation (see Chapter 30).

Patient and caregiver teaching focuses on how to avoid future problems. Provide essential information regarding proper hydration during hot weather and physical exercise. Instruct patients on the early signs of and interventions for heat-related stress.

## COLD-RELATED EMERGENCIES

Cold injuries may be localized (frostbite) or systemic (hypothermia). Contributing factors include age, duration of exposure, environmental temperature, homelessness, preexisting conditions (e.g., diabetes mellitus, peripheral vascular disease), drugs that suppress shivering (e.g., opioids, psychotropic agents, antiemetics), and alcohol intoxication. Alcohol causes peripheral vasodilation, increases sensation of warmth, and depresses shivering. Smokers have an increased risk of cold-related injury because of the vasoconstrictive effects of nicotine.

### Frostbite

**Frostbite** is true tissue freezing that results in the formation of ice crystals in the tissues and cells.[7] Peripheral vasoconstriction is the initial response to cold stress and results in a decrease in blood flow and vascular stasis. As cellular temperature decreases and ice crystals form in intracellular spaces, the organelles are damaged and the cell membrane destroyed. This results in edema.

Depth of frostbite depends on ambient temperature, length of exposure, type and condition (wet or dry) of clothing, and contact with metal surfaces. Other factors that affect severity include skin color (dark-skinned people are more prone to frostbite), lack of acclimatization, previous episodes, exhaustion, and poor peripheral vascular status.

*Superficial frostbite* involves skin and subcutaneous tissue, usually the ears, nose, fingers, and toes. The skin appearance ranges from waxy pale yellow to blue to mottled, and the skin feels crunchy and frozen. The patient may complain of tingling,

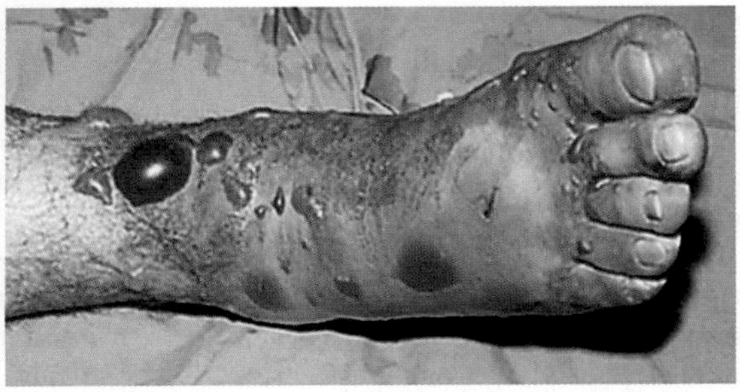

**FIG. 68-3** Edema and blister formation 24 hours after frostbite injury occurring in an area covered by a tightly fitted boot. (Courtesy Cameron Bangs, MD. From Auerbach PS, Donner HJ, Weiss EA: *Field guide to wilderness medicine,* ed 2, St Louis, 2003, Mosby.)

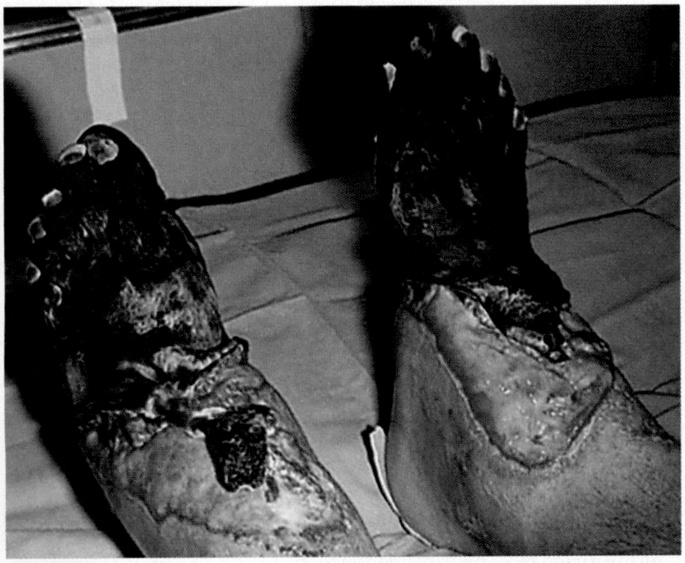

**FIG. 68-4** Gangrenous necrosis 6 weeks after the frostbite injury shown in Fig. 68-3. Courtesy Cameron Bangs, MD. (From Auerbach PS, Donner HJ, Weiss EA: *Field guide to wilderness medicine,* ed 2, St Louis, 2003, Mosby.)

numbness, or a burning sensation. Handle the area carefully and never squeeze, massage, or scrub the injured tissue because it is easily damaged. Remove clothing and jewelry because they may constrict the extremity and decrease circulation.

Immerse the affected area in circulating water that is temperature controlled (98.6° to 104° F) [37° to 40° C]). Use warm soaks for the face. The patient often experiences a warm, stinging sensation as tissue thaws. Blisters form within a few hours (Fig. 68-3). The blisters should be debrided and a sterile dressing applied. Avoid heavy blankets and clothing because friction and weight can lead to sloughing of damaged tissue. Rewarming is extremely painful. Residual pain may last weeks or even years. Give analgesia and tetanus prophylaxis as appropriate (Table 68-6). Evaluate the patient with superficial frostbite for systemic hypothermia.

*Deep frostbite* involves muscle, bone, and tendon. The skin is white, hard, and insensitive to touch. The area has the appearance of deep thermal injury with mottling gradually progressing to gangrene (Fig. 68-4). Immerse the affected extremity in a temperature controlled, circulating water bath (98.6° to 104° F [37° to 40° C]) until flushing occurs distal to the injured area.

After rewarming, the extremity should be elevated to reduce edema. Significant edema may begin within 3 hours, with blistering in 6 hours to days. IV analgesia is needed in severe frostbite because of the pain associated with tissue thawing. Give tetanus prophylaxis and evaluate the patient for systemic hypothermia.

Amputation may be required if the injured area is untreated or treatment is unsuccessful. It may take as long as 90 days for the final demarcation of the necrotic area.[7] The patient may be admitted to the hospital for observation with bed rest, elevation of the injured part, and prophylactic antibiotics if the wound is at risk for infection.

## Hypothermia

**Hypothermia**, defined as a core temperature below 95° F (35° C), occurs when heat produced by the body cannot compensate for heat lost to the environment.[7] Most body heat is lost as radiant energy, with the greatest loss from the head, thorax, and lungs (with each breath). Wet clothing increases evaporative heat loss to five times greater than normal; immersion in cold water (e.g., drowning) increases evaporative heat loss to 25 times greater than normal. Environmental exposure to freezing temperatures, cold winds, and wet terrain plus physical exhaustion, inadequate clothing, and inexperience predisposes individuals to hypothermia. Older adults are more prone to hypothermia because of decreased body fat, diminished energy reserves, decreased basal metabolic rate, decreased shivering response, decreased sensory perception, chronic medical conditions, and drugs that alter body defenses.[7]

Hypothermia mimics cerebral or metabolic disturbances causing ataxia, confusion, and withdrawal, so the patient may be misdiagnosed. Peripheral vasoconstriction is the body's first attempt to conserve heat. As cold temperatures persist, shivering and movement are the body's only mechanisms for producing heat.

Assessment findings in hypothermia are variable and depend on core temperature (Table 68-9). Patients with *mild hypothermia* (93.2° to 96.8° F [34° to 36° C]) have shivering, lethargy, confusion, rational to irrational behavior, and minor heart rate changes. *Moderate hypothermia* (89.6° to 93.2° F [32° to 34° C]) causes rigidity, bradycardia, slowed respiratory rate, BP obtainable only by Doppler, metabolic and respiratory acidosis, and hypovolemia. Shivering diminishes or disappears at core temperatures of 89.6° F (32° C).[7]

As core temperature drops, metabolic rate decreases two or three times. The cold myocardium is extremely irritable, making it vulnerable to dysrhythmias (e.g., atrial and ventricular fibrillation). Decreased renal blood flow decreases glomerular filtration rate, which impairs water reabsorption and leads to dehydration. The hematocrit increases as intravascular volume decreases. Cold blood becomes thick and acts as a thrombus, placing the patient at risk for stroke, myocardial infarction, pulmonary emboli, and renal failure. Decreased blood flow leads to hypoxia, anaerobic metabolism, lactic acid accumulation, and metabolic acidosis.

*Severe hypothermia* (below 89.6° F [32° C]) makes the person appear dead and is a potentially life-threatening situation. Metabolic rate, heart rate, and respirations are so slow that they may be difficult to detect. Reflexes are absent, and the pupils fixed and dilated. Profound bradycardia, ventricular fibrillation, or asystole may be present. Every effort is made to warm the patient to at least 86° F (30° C) before the person is pronounced dead. The cause of death is usually refractory ventricular fibrillation.

**TABLE 68-9 Emergency Management**

***Hypothermia***

| Etiology | Assessment Findings | Interventions |
|---|---|---|
| **Environmental**<br>• Inadequate clothing for environmental temperature<br>• Prolonged exposure to cold<br>• Prolonged immersion or drowning<br>**Metabolic**<br>• Hypoglycemia<br>• Hypothyroidism<br>**Health Care–Associated**<br>• Administration of neuromuscular blocking agents<br>• Blood administration<br>• Cold IV fluids<br>• Inadequate warming or rewarming in the ED or operating room<br>**Other**<br>• Alcohol<br>• Barbiturates<br>• Phenothiazines<br>• Shock<br>• Trauma | • Core body temperature:<br>  • *Mild hypothermia:* 93.2°-96.8° F (34°-36° C)<br>  • *Moderate hypothermia:* 89.6°-93.2° F (32°-34° C)<br>  • *Severe hypothermia:* ≤89.6° F (32° C)<br>• Shivering, diminished or absent at core body temperatures ≤89.6° F (32° C).<br>• Hypoventilation<br>• Hypotension<br>• Altered mental status (ranging from confusion to coma)<br>• Areflexia (absence of reflexes)<br>• Pale, cyanotic skin<br>• Blue, white, or frozen extremities<br>• Dysrhythmias: bradycardia, atrial fibrillation, ventricular fibrillation, asystole<br>• Fixed, dilated pupils | **Initial**<br>• Remove patient from cold environment.<br>• Manage and maintain ABCs.<br>• Provide high-flow $O_2$ via non-rebreather mask or BVM.<br>• Anticipate intubation for diminished or absent gag reflex.*<br>• Establish IV access with two large-bore catheters for fluid resuscitation<br>• Rewarm patient:<br>  • *Passive:* Remove wet clothing, apply dry clothing and warm blankets, use radiant lights.<br>  • *Active external:* Apply heating devices (e.g., air or fluid-filled warming blankets), use warm water immersion.<br>  • *Active internal:* Provide warmed IV fluids; heated, humidified $O_2$. Peritoneal lavage with warmed fluids. Extracorporeal circulation (e.g., cardiopulmonary bypass, rapid fluid infuser, hemodialysis).<br>• Obtain 12-lead ECG.<br>• Anticipate need for defibrillation.*<br>• Warm central trunk first in patients with severe hypothermia to limit rewarming shock.<br>• Assess for other injuries.<br>• Keep patient's head covered with warm, dry towels or stocking cap to limit loss of heat.<br>• Treat patient gently to avoid increased cardiac irritability.<br>**Ongoing Monitoring**<br>• Monitor ABCs, temperature, level of consciousness, vital signs.<br>• Monitor $O_2$ saturation, heart rate and rhythm.<br>• Monitor electrolytes, glucose. |

*ABCs,* Airway, breathing, circulation; *BVM,* bag-valve-mask.
*NOTE: Medications and defibrillation may not be effective with core temperatures <86° F (30° C).

**Interprofessional Care.** Treatment of hypothermia focuses on managing and maintaining ABCs, rewarming the patient, correcting dehydration and acidosis, and treating cardiac dysrhythmias (Table 68-9). Use passive or active external rewarming for mild hypothermia. *Passive* or *spontaneous rewarming* involves moving the patient to a warm, dry place; removing damp clothing; using radiant lights; and placing warm blankets on the patient. *Active external* or *surface rewarming* involves fluid- or air-filled warming blankets, or warm (98.6° to 104° F [37° to 40° C]) water immersion. Closely monitor the patient for marked vasodilation and hypotension during rewarming.

Use *active internal* or *core rewarming* for moderate to severe hypothermia. This refers to the application of heat directly to the core. Techniques include (1) heated (up to 111.2° F [44° C]), humidified $O_2$; (2) warmed IV fluids (up to 98.6° F [37° C]); (3) peritoneal lavage with warmed fluids (up to 113° F [45° C]); and (4) extracorporeal circulation with cardiopulmonary bypass, rapid fluid infuser, or hemodialysis.

Gentle handling is essential to prevent stimulation of the cold myocardium. Carefully monitor core temperature during rewarming procedures. Rewarming places the patient at risk for *afterdrop,* a further drop in core temperature. This occurs when cold peripheral blood returns to the central circulation. Rewarming shock can produce hypotension and dysrhythmias. Thus patients with moderate to severe hypothermia should have the core warmed before the extremities. Discontinue active rewarming once the core temperature reaches 89.6° to 93.2° F (32° to 34° C).

Patient teaching focuses on how to avoid future cold-related problems. Essential information includes dressing in layers for cold weather, covering the head, carrying high-carbohydrate foods for extra calories, and developing a plan for survival should an injury occur when in an extreme environment.

**CHECK YOUR PRACTICE**

You and your preceptor are working in the ED when the paramedics arrive with a patient who was found lying on the sidewalk outside the downtown bus station. He is wearing only a lightweight shirt and pants. The outdoor temperature is 12° F (-11.1° C). The patient is unresponsive. Initial vital signs are as follows: rectal temperature = 89.5° F (31.9° C), HR = 38, RR = 8, BP (by Doppler) = 86 mm Hg.

- What are your priority interventions for this patient?

## SUBMERSION INJURIES

**Submersion injury** results when a person becomes hypoxic as the result of submersion in a liquid, usually water.[7] More than 50,000 submersion events and approximately 4000 deaths from drowning occur each year in the United States. Most of the victims are children younger than 5 years of age or boys and men between ages 15 and 25. The primary risk factors for submersion injury include inability to swim, use of alcohol or drugs, trauma, seizures, hypothermia, stroke, and child neglect.

**Drowning** is the process of experiencing respiratory impairment after submersion in water or other fluid. Submersion in cold water (below 32° F [0° C]) may slow the progression of hypoxic brain injury.

Most drowning victims do not aspirate any liquid due to laryngospasm. If liquid is aspirated, it is in small amounts (e.g., 4 mL/kg). Drowning victims who do aspirate water develop

PATHOPHYSIOLOGY MAP

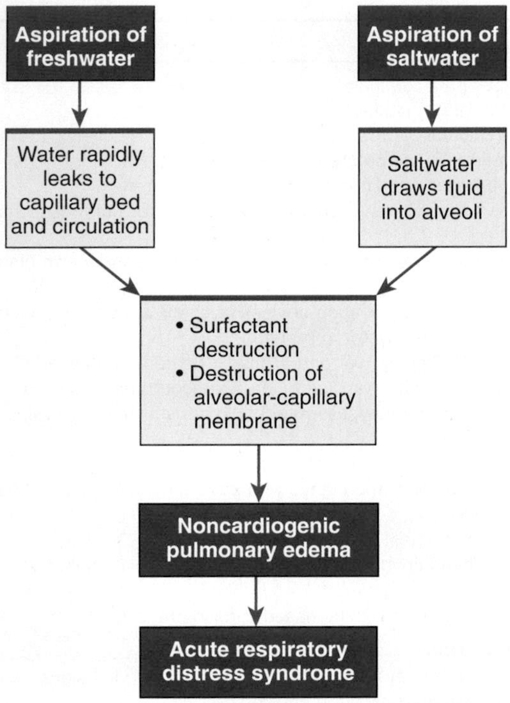


**FIG. 68-5** Pathophysiology of submersion injury.

pulmonary edema (Fig. 68-5). Regardless of what type of fluid is aspirated, the end result can be acute respiratory distress syndrome (see Chapter 67).

The osmotic gradient caused by aspirated fluid leads to fluid imbalances in the body. Hypotonic fresh water is rapidly absorbed into the circulatory system through the alveoli. Fresh water is often contaminated with chlorine, mud, or algae. This causes the breakdown of lung surfactant, fluid seepage, and pulmonary edema.

Hypertonic saltwater draws fluid from the vascular space into the alveoli, impairing alveolar ventilation and resulting in hypoxia. The body attempts to compensate for hypoxia by shunting blood to the lungs. This results in increased pulmonary pressures and deteriorating respiratory status. More and more blood is shunted through the alveoli. However, the blood is not adequately oxygenated, and hypoxemia worsens. This can result in cerebral injury, edema, and brain death.

Table 68-10 lists the assessment findings of a patient with a submersion injury. Aggressive resuscitation efforts (e.g., airway and ventilation management), especially in the prehospital phase, improve survival of drowning victims.

### Interprofessional Care

Treatment of submersion injuries focuses on correcting hypoxia and fluid imbalances, supporting basic physiologic functions, and rewarming when hypothermia is present. Initial evaluation involves assessment of airway, cervical spine, breathing, and circulation. Table 68-10 lists other interventions.

Mechanical ventilation with positive end-expiratory pressure or continuous positive airway pressure is used to improve gas exchange across the alveolar-capillary membrane when significant pulmonary edema is present. Ventilation and oxygenation are the primary techniques for treating respiratory failure (see Chapters 65 and 67). Mannitol (Osmitrol) or furosemide (Lasix) is used to treat cerebral edema or decrease free water.

Deterioration in neurologic status suggests cerebral edema, worsening hypoxia, or profound acidosis. Drowning victims may also have head and neck injuries that cause prolonged alterations in the LOC. Complications can develop in patients who are essentially free of symptoms immediately after the drowning episode. Consequently, observe all victims of drowning in a hospital for a minimum of 23 hours.[7] Additional observation is needed for patients who have co-morbidities (e.g., heart disease).

Patient teaching focuses on water safety and how to reduce the risks for drowning. Remind patients and caregivers to lock all swimming pool gates; use life jackets on all watercrafts, including inner tubes and rafts; and learn water survival skills (e.g., swimming lessons). Emphasize the dangers of combining alcohol and drugs with swimming and other water sports.

## STINGS AND BITES

Animals, spiders, snakes, and insects cause injury and even death by biting or stinging. Morbidity is a result of either direct tissue damage or lethal toxins. Direct tissue damage is a product of animal size, characteristics of the animal's teeth, and strength of the jaw. Tissue is lacerated, crushed, or chewed, while teeth, fangs, stingers, spines, or tentacles release toxins that have local or systemic effects. Death associated with animal bites is due to blood loss, allergic reactions, or lethal toxins. Injuries caused by select insects, ticks, animals (e.g., dogs, cats), and humans are described here.

### Hymenopteran Stings

The *Hymenoptera* family includes bees, yellow jackets, hornets, wasps, and fire ants. Stings can cause mild discomfort or life-threatening anaphylaxis (see Chapter 66). Venom may be cytotoxic, hemolytic, allergenic, or vasoactive. Symptoms may begin immediately or be delayed up to 48 hours. Reactions are more severe with multiple stings. Most hymenopterans sting repeatedly. However, the domestic honey bee stings only once, usually leaving a barbed stinger with an attached venom sac in the skin so that release of venom continues.

African honey bees (killer bees), which look like domestic bees, have migrated into North America. If threatened, these bees aggressively swarm and can repeatedly sting their victims (e.g., humans, animals). These attacks can be fatal.

**! SAFETY ALERT Hymenopteran Stings**
- Remove the stinger using a scraping motion with a fingernail, knife, or needle.
- Avoid using tweezers because they may squeeze the stinger and release more venom.
- Remove rings, watches, or any restrictive clothing around the sting site.

Manifestations vary from stinging, burning, swelling, and itching to edema, headache, fever, syncope, malaise, nausea, vomiting, wheezing, bronchospasm, laryngeal edema, and hypotension. Treatment depends on the severity of the reaction. Treat mild reactions with elevation, cool compresses, antipruritic lotions, and oral antihistamines. More severe reactions require IM or IV antihistamines (e.g., diphenhydramine), subcutaneous epinephrine, and corticosteroids (e.g., dexamethasone). Chapter 13 discusses allergic reactions and related patient teaching.

**TABLE 68-10 Emergency Management**

***Submersion Injuries***

| Etiology | Assessment Findings | Interventions |
|---|---|---|
| • Inability to swim or exhaustion while swimming<br>• Entrapment or entanglement with objects in water<br>• Loss of ability to move secondary to trauma, stroke, hypothermia, myocardial infarction (MI)<br>• Poor judgment due to alcohol or drugs<br>• Seizure while in water | **Respiratory**<br>• Ineffective breathing<br>• Dyspnea<br>• Respiratory distress<br>• Respiratory arrest<br>• Crackles, rhonchi<br>• Cough with pink-frothy sputum<br>• Cyanosis<br>**Cardiac**<br>• Tachycardia<br>• Bradycardia<br>• Dysrhythmia<br>• Hypotension<br>• Cardiac arrest<br>**Other**<br>• Panic<br>• Exhaustion<br>• Coma<br>• Coexisting illness (e.g., MI) or injury (e.g., cervical spine injury)<br>• Core temperature slightly elevated or below normal depending on water temperature and length of submersion | **Initial**<br>• Manage and maintain ABCs.<br>• Assume cervical spine injury in all drowning victims and stabilize or immobilize cervical spine.<br>• Provide 100% $O_2$ via non-rebreather mask or BVM.<br>• Anticipate need for intubation and mechanical ventilation if airway is compromised (e.g., absent gag reflex).<br>• Establish IV access with two large-bore catheters for fluid resuscitation and infuse warmed fluids if appropriate.<br>• Obtain 12-lead ECG.<br>• Assess for other injuries.<br>• Remove wet clothing and cover with warm blankets.<br>• Obtain temperature and begin rewarming if needed.<br>• Obtain cervical spine and chest x-rays.<br>• Insert gastric tube and urinary catheter.<br>**Ongoing Monitoring**<br>• Monitor ABCs, vital signs, level of consciousness.<br>• Monitor $O_2$ saturation, heart rate and rhythm.<br>• Monitor temperature and maintain normothermia.<br>• Monitor for signs of acute respiratory failure. |

*ABCs,* Airway, breathing, circulation; *BVM,* bag-valve-mask.

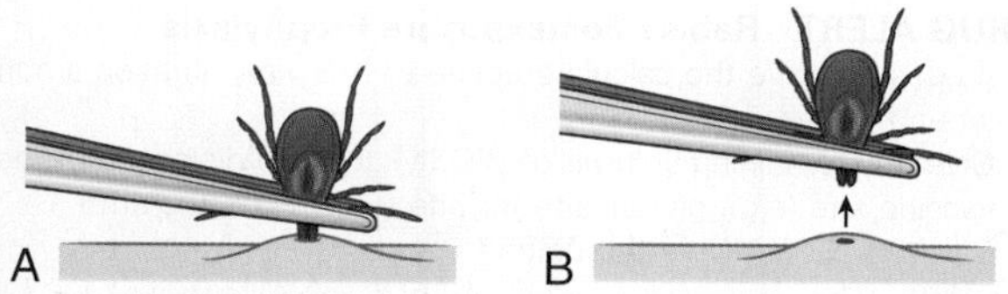


**FIG. 68-6** Tick removal. **A,** Use tweezers to grasp the tick close to the skin. **B,** With a steady motion, pull the tick's body up and away from the skin. Do not be alarmed if the tick's mouthparts remain in the skin. Once the mouthparts are removed from the rest of the tick, it can no longer transmit disease.

## Tick Bites

Ticks live throughout the United States but are most common in the northwestern, Rocky Mountain, and northeastern regions. Conditions associated with tick bites include Lyme disease, Rocky Mountain spotted fever, and tick paralysis. The infected tick or the release of neurotoxin causes the disease. Ticks release neurotoxic venom as long as the tick head attaches to the body. Therefore safe removal of the tick is essential for effective treatment.

Use forceps or tweezers to grasp the tick close to the point of attachment and pull upward in a steady motion (Fig. 68-6). After you remove the tick, clean the skin with soap and water. Do not use a hot match, petroleum jelly, nail polish, or other products to remove the tick, since these measures may cause a tick to salivate, thus increasing the risk for infection.[17]

Lyme disease is the most common tick-borne disease in the United States. Symptoms appear within days of a bite from the Ixodid (hard) tick that has been attached for at least 48 hours. Exposure to the spirochete *Borrelia burgdorferi* that lives on the tick causes the illness. The first stage of this disease begins with flu-like symptoms (e.g., headache, stiff neck, fatigue). Some patients may develop a characteristic bull's-eye rash (i.e., a circular area of redness 5 cm or more in diameter). Treatment at this stage includes doxycycline (Vibramycin). The rash, if it develops, will disappear even if the patient is not treated.

Monoarticular arthritis, meningitis, and neuropathies occur days or weeks after the initial manifestations. Recommended treatment includes ceftriaxone (Rocephin). Chronic arthritis, peripheral radiculoneuropathy, and heart disease characterize the later stage of the disease. These illnesses can last several months to years after the initial skin lesion. (Chapter 64 discusses Lyme disease.)

Rocky Mountain spotted fever is caused by *Rickettsia rickettsii,* a bacterium that is spread to humans by the Ixodid tick. It has an incubation period of 2 to 14 days. A pink, macular rash appears on the palms, wrists, soles, feet, and ankles within 10 days of exposure. Other symptoms include fever, chills, malaise, myalgias, and headache. Diagnosis is often difficult in the early stages, and without treatment the disease can be fatal. Antibiotic therapy with doxycycline is the treatment of choice.

Tick paralysis occurs 5 to 7 days after exposure to a neurotoxin introduced by a wood tick or dog tick. Classic manifestations are flaccid ascending paralysis, which develops over 1 to 2 days. Without tick removal, the patient dies as respiratory muscles become paralyzed. Tick removal leads to return of muscle movement, usually within 48 to 72 hours.

## Animal and Human Bites

Every year more than 5 million animal bites are reported in the United States. Children are at greatest risk. The most significant problems associated with animal bites are infection and mechanical destruction of skin, muscle, tendons, blood vessels, and bone. The bite may cause a simple laceration or be associated with crush injury, puncture wound, or tearing of multiple layers of tissue. The severity of injury depends on animal size, victim size, and anatomic location of the bite. Animal bites from

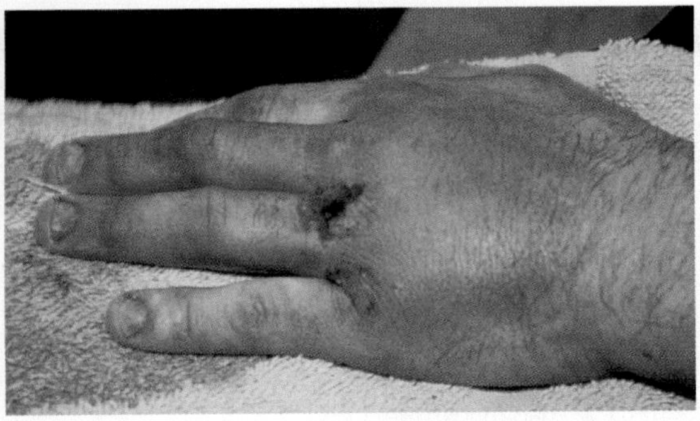

**FIG. 68-7** Probable human bite injury, although denied by patient. Human bites cause extensor tendon injuries, fractures, and joint capsule injuries and can harbor foreign bodies. (From Roberts JR, Hedges JR: *Clinical procedures in emergency medicine,* ed 5, Philadelphia, 2009, Saunders.)

dogs and cats are most common, with wild or domestic rodents (e.g., squirrels, hamsters) following as the third most frequently reported offenders.

Dog bites usually occur on the extremities. However, facial bites are common in small children. Most victims own the dogs that bite them. Dog bites may involve significant tissue damage with deaths reported, usually in children. A plastic surgeon should evaluate all disfiguring wounds of the face.

Cat bites cause deep puncture wounds that can involve tendons and joint capsules and result in a greater incidence of infection than with dog bites. Septic arthritis, osteomyelitis, and tenosynovitis can occur as a result of cat bites. The most common causative organisms of infections from dog and cat bites are from the *Pasteurella* species (e.g., *Pasteurella multocida*). Most healthy cats and dogs carry this organism in their mouths.

Human bites also cause puncture wounds or lacerations (Fig. 68-7). These carry a high risk of infection from oral bacterial flora, most commonly *Staphylococcus aureus, Streptococcus* organisms, and hepatitis virus. Hands, fingers, ears, nose, vagina, and penis are the most common sites of human bites and are frequently a result of violence or sexual activity.

Patients with Boxer's fracture (fracture of the fourth or fifth metacarpal) often have concurrent open wounds on the knuckles from striking teeth. The human jaw has great crushing ability, causing laceration, puncture, crush injury, soft tissue tearing, and even amputation. Infection rates are as high as 50% when victims do not seek medical care within 24 hours of injury.

**Interprofessional Care.** Initial treatment for animal and human bites includes cleaning with copious irrigation, debridement, tetanus prophylaxis, and analgesics as needed. Prophylactic antibiotics are used for animal and human bites at risk for infection, such as wounds over joints, those greater than 6 to 12 hours old, puncture wounds, and bites of the hand or foot. People at greatest risk of infection are infants, older adults, immunosuppressed patients, alcoholics, diabetics, and people taking corticosteroids.

Leave puncture wounds open. Splint wounds over joints. Lacerations are loosely sutured. However, initial closure is used for facial wounds. The patient is admitted for IV antibiotic therapy when an infection is present. These patients have an increased incidence of cellulitis, osteomyelitis, and septic arthritis. Report animal and human bites to the police as required.

Consider *rabies postexposure prophylaxis* in the management of all animal bites. Rabies is generally transmitted via saliva from the bite of an infected animal. It can also be spread by scratches and by contact with infected secretions through mucous membranes. Any warm-blooded mammal (e.g., dogs, raccoons, bats) can carry rabies.

A neurotoxic virus found in the saliva of infected mammals causes rabies. The virus spreads through the CNS via peripheral nerves. After a minimum 2-week incubation period, patients experience flu-like symptoms, pain, paresthesias, or numbness. Rabies prophylaxis must be started before symptoms appear. Otherwise, the disease will progress (e.g., agitation, hypersalivation, dysarthria, hallucinations, nuchal rigidity, seizures, coma) and is fatal. Death results from respiratory and cardiovascular collapse within a few days after the onset of coma.

Consider rabies exposure if an animal attack was not provoked, involves a wild animal, or involves a domestic animal not immunized against rabies. Always provide rabies postexposure prophylaxis when the animal is not found or a wild animal causes the bite. Start the regimen with an initial, weight-based dosage of rabies immune globulin (RIG [HyperRab S/D]) to provide passive immunity. Follow this with a series of four injections of human diploid cell vaccine (HDCV [Imovax Rabies]) on days 0, 3, 7, and 14 to provide active immunity.[18]

Since rabies is nearly always fatal, management efforts are directed at preventing the transmission and onset of the disease. Although death from rabies is significant worldwide, only one to three people die annually in the United States. Rabies vaccine is encouraged for persons who travel globally, since it remains a serious world health concern.

**DRUG ALERT Rabies Postexposure Prophylaxis**

- If possible, give the calculated dose of RIG via infiltration around the wound edges.
- Give any remaining volume of RIG IM at a site distant from the vaccine site (e.g., gluteal site for bite wounds on the arm).
- Give the HDCV IM in the deltoid.

## POISONINGS

A poison is any chemical that harms the body. More than 5 million cases of human poisonings occur each year in the United States. Poisonings can be accidental, occupational, recreational, or intentional. Natural or manufactured toxins can be ingested, inhaled, injected, splashed in the eye, or absorbed through the skin. Table 68-11 presents common poisons. Chapter 10 discusses other poisonings related to the use of illegal drugs such as amphetamines, opioids, and hallucinogens. Poisoning may also be due to toxic plants or contaminated foods. (Chapter 41 discusses food poisoning.)

Severity of the poisoning depends on type, concentration, and route of exposure. Toxins can affect every tissue of the body, so symptoms can be seen in any body system. Specific management of toxins involves decreasing absorption, enhancing elimination, and implementing toxin-specific interventions. Consult the local poison control center 24 hours a day (e.g., 800-222-1222) for the most current treatment protocols for specific poisons.[19]

Options for decreasing absorption of poisons include activated charcoal, dermal cleansing, eye irrigation, and gastric lavage. Gastric lavage involves oral insertion of a large-diameter (36F to 42F) gastric tube for irrigation of copious amounts of saline. Elevate the head of the bed or place the patient on the side to prevent aspiration. Patients with an altered LOC or diminished gag reflex are intubated before lavage. Patients who ingest caustic agents, co-ingest sharp objects, or ingest nontoxic

TABLE 68-11 **Common Poisons**

| Poison | Manifestations | Treatment |
|---|---|---|
| **Acetaminophen** (Tylenol) | *Phase 1* (within 24 hr of ingestion): Malaise, diaphoresis, nausea and vomiting<br>*Phase 2* (24-28 hr after ingestion): Right upper quadrant pain, decreased urine output, diminished nausea, increase in LFTs<br>*Phase 3* (72-96 hr after ingestion): Nausea and vomiting, malaise, jaundice, hypoglycemia, enlarged liver, possible coagulopathies, including DIC<br>*Phase 4* (7-8 days after ingestion): Recovery, resolution of symptoms or permanent liver damage, LFT results remain high | Activated charcoal, *N*-acetylcysteine (oral form may cause vomiting, IV form can be used) |
| **Acids and alkalis** | | |
| • *Acids:* Toilet bowl cleaners, antirust compounds<br>• *Alkalis:* Drain cleaners, dishwashing detergents, ammonia | Excess salivation, dysphagia, epigastric pain, pneumonitis; burns of mouth, esophagus, and stomach | Immediate dilution (water, milk), corticosteroids (for alkali burns), induced vomiting is contraindicated |
| • Aspirin and aspirin-containing drugs | Tachypnea, tachycardia, hyperthermia, seizures, pulmonary edema, occult bleeding or hemorrhage, metabolic acidosis | Activated charcoal, gastric lavage, urine alkalinization, hemodialysis for severe acute ingestion, intubation and mechanical ventilation, supportive care |
| **Bleaches** | Irritation of lips, mouth, and eyes, superficial injury to esophagus; chemical pneumonia and pulmonary edema | Washing of exposed skin and eyes, dilution with water and milk, gastric lavage, prevention of vomiting and aspiration |
| **Carbon monoxide** | Dyspnea, headache, tachypnea, confusion, impaired judgment, cyanosis, respiratory depression | Removal from source, administration of 100% $O_2$ via non-rebreather mask, BVM, or intubation and mechanical ventilation; consider hyperbaric $O_2$ therapy |
| **Cyanide** | Almond odor to breath, headache, dizziness, nausea, confusion, hypertension, bradycardia followed by hypotension and tachycardia, tachypnea followed by bradypnea and respiratory arrest | Amyl nitrate (nasally), IV sodium nitrate, IV sodium thiosulfate, supportive care |
| **Ethylene glycol** | Sweet aromatic odor to breath, nausea and vomiting, slurred speech, ataxia, lethargy, respiratory depression | Activated charcoal, gastric lavage, supportive care |
| **Iron** | Vomiting (often bloody), diarrhea (often bloody), fever, hyperglycemia, lethargy, hypotension, seizures, coma | Gastric lavage, chelation therapy (deferoxamine [Desferal]) |
| **Nonsteroidal antiinflammatory drugs** | Gastroenteritis, abdominal pain, drowsiness, nystagmus, hepatic and renal damage | Activated charcoal, gastric lavage, supportive care |
| **Tricyclic antidepressants** (e.g., amitriptyline) | *In low doses:* Anticholinergic effects, agitation, hypertension, tachycardia<br>*In high doses:* Central nervous system depression, dysrhythmias, hypotension, respiratory depression | Multidose activated charcoal, gastric lavage, serum alkalinization with sodium bicarbonate, intubation and mechanical ventilation, supportive care; never induce vomiting |
| **Alcohol, barbiturates, benzodiazepines, cocaine, hallucinogens, stimulants** | See Chapter 10 | See Chapter 10 |

*BVM,* Bag-valve-mask; *DIC,* disseminated intravascular coagulation; *LFT,* liver function test.

substances should not receive lavage. To be effective, perform gastric lavage within 1 hour of ingestion of most poisons. Problems associated with lavage include esophageal perforation and aspiration.

The most common and effective intervention for management of poisonings is administration of activated charcoal orally or via a gastric tube within 1 hour of poison ingestion. Many toxins adhere to charcoal and pass through the gastrointestinal (GI) tract rather than being absorbed into the circulation. Activated charcoal does not absorb ethanol, hydrocarbons, alkali, iron, boric acid, lithium, methanol, or cyanide.[20] Adults receive 50 to 100 g of charcoal. For some toxins (e.g., phenobarbital, digoxin) multiple-dose charcoal may be needed. Contraindications to charcoal administration include diminished bowel sounds, paralytic ileus, and ingestion of a substance poorly absorbed by charcoal. Charcoal can absorb and neutralize antidotes (e.g., *N*-acetylcysteine for acetaminophen toxicity). Do not give these immediately before, with, or shortly after charcoal.

Skin and ocular decontamination involves removal of toxins from skin and eyes using copious amounts of water or saline. Most toxins, with the exception of mustard gas, can be safely removed with water or saline. Water mixes with mustard gas and releases chlorine gas.

As a rule, brush dry substances from the skin and clothing before using water. Do not remove powdered lime with water. It should just be brushed off. Wear *personal protective equipment (PPE)* (e.g., gloves, gowns, goggles, respirators) for decontamination to prevent secondary exposure. Decontamination procedures are usually done by those specially trained in hazardous material decontamination before the patient arrives at the hospital and again at the hospital, if necessary. Decontamination takes priority over all interventions except those needed for basic life support.

Giving cathartics, whole-bowel irrigation, hemodialysis, urine alkalinization, chelating agents, and antidotes increases the elimination of poisons. Cathartics, such as sorbitol, are given together with the first dose of activated charcoal to stimulate intestinal motility and increase elimination.[20] Avoid multiple doses of cathartics because of potentially fatal electrolyte abnormalities. Whole-bowel irrigation is controversial and involves giving a nonabsorbable bowel evacuant solution (e.g., GoLYTELY). Give the solution every 4 to 6 hours until stools are clear. This process can be effective for swallowed objects, such as cocaine-filled balloons or condoms, and heavy metals such as lead and mercury. There is a high risk of electrolyte imbalance caused by fluid and electrolyte losses with this approach.

Hemodialysis is reserved for patients who develop severe acidosis from ingestion of toxic substances (e.g., aspirin). Other interventions include alkalinization and chelation therapy. Sodium bicarbonate administration increases the pH (greater than 7.5), which is particularly effective for phenobarbital and salicylate poisoning. Vitamin C is added to IV fluids to enhance excretion of amphetamines and quinidine. Chelation therapy is considered for heavy metal poisoning (e.g., edetate calcium disodium [calcium EDTA] for lead poisoning). A limited number of true antidotes are available, and many of these agents are themselves toxic.[20]

Focus patient teaching for toxic emergencies on how the poisoning occurred. Arrange for an evaluation and follow-up by a mental health professional for all patients who experience poisoning because of a suicide attempt or substance abuse.

Many health care workers (e.g., nurses, housekeepers) are at risk for exposure to hazardous materials (e.g., antineoplastic drugs, cleaning agents). Always consult the Material Safety Data Sheet (required by the Occupational Health and Safety Administration [OSHA]) for specific information regarding hazardous agents in the workplace. OSHA should evaluate all poisoning related to a workplace hazard.[21]

## VIOLENCE

*Violence* is the acting out of the emotions of fear and/or anger to cause harm to someone or something. It may be the result of organic disease (e.g., temporal lobe epilepsy), psychosis (e.g., schizophrenia), or criminal behavior (e.g., assault, murder). The patient cared for in the ED may be the victim or the perpetrator of violence. Violence can take place in a variety of settings, including the home, community, and workplace.

EDs have been identified as high-risk areas for *workplace violence.*[22] Measures to protect staff include the use of onsite security personnel and police officers, metal detectors, surveillance cameras, self-defense training, and locked access doors. The ENA supports comprehensive workplace violence prevention plans and recommends that they be implemented and evaluated in every ED.[22]

*Family and intimate partner violence* (IPV) is a pattern of coercive behavior in a relationship that involves fear; humiliation; intimidation; neglect; or intentional physical, emotional, financial, or sexual injury (see Chapter 53 for information on sexual assault). The ENA encourages ED nurses to become certified *sexual assault nurse examiners* (SANEs). These nurses provide expert emergency care, collect and document evidence, participate in staff and community education, and advocate for sexual assault and rape victims.[23]

### BECOMING A NURSE LEADER

#### *Patient and Visitor Violence/Abuse*

**Situation**

Since it has always been your desire to be an emergency department (ED) nurse, you are excited when you get to rotate to a busy metropolitan ED during your senior year of nursing school. While in the ED, you witness an intoxicated patient physically attacking and his family verbally abusing the nurses. You are pleased to see the rapid response by the staff and security to deal with the situation. However, you are still frightened and wonder if you should ever work in an ED.

**Points for Consideration**

- Workplace violence against nurses has become a problem affecting nurses in all settings. It is a serious problem, especially in EDs, mental health facilities, and long-term care facilities.
- Workplace violence can instantly transform nurses from being health care professionals to patients with physical and psychologic trauma caused when patients or visitors attack them.
- You can be a leader in promoting awareness of workplace violence and providing training and education to avoid situations for potential violence. These activities include:[1]
    - Helping to establish policies aimed at preventing workplace violence.
    - Making sure that you are not working alone, especially in certain areas such as the ED.
    - Being aware of your patient's history. Identify in some way the patients' charts if they have past incidents involving violence.
    - Avoiding being physically trapped in a room. Keeping yourself between the patient and the door.
    - Helping to plan work designs that provide for lockable areas for staff only (lounges, lockers rooms, bathrooms) and adequate lighting both inside and outside of the facility.

**Discussion Questions**

1. What can you do to protect yourself in situations where you are at risk for violence?
2. Describe how the following factors may be related to increased violence in the ED:
    - Prolonged wait times
    - Delays in providing pain medication
    - Influx of patients with mental health issues
    - Workplace design

**Reference**

1. Emergency Nurses Association: Toolkit—workplace violence. Retrieved from *www.ena.org/practice-research/practice/violencetoolkit/Documents/toolkitpg1.htm.*

IPV is found in all professions, cultures, socioeconomic groups, age groups, and genders. Although men can be victims of family violence and IPV, most victims are women, children, and older adults. Each year, more than 5 million women and 3 million men are treated in EDs for *battery* (assault) by spouses, caregivers, or individuals known to them. Many battered women are pregnant at the time of the assault.[23]

In the ED, you need to screen for family violence and IPV (e.g., Do you feel safe at home? Is anyone hurting you?). Routine screening for this risk factor is required.[23] Barriers to conducting effective screening include limited privacy in the ED, lack of time, and lack of knowledge about how to ask about family violence and IPV. The development and implementation of policies, procedures, and staff education programs improve screening practices.[22]

Start appropriate interventions for patients who you suspect or find are victims of abuse. These include making referrals, notifying appropriate agencies (i.e., as required by law), providing emotional support, and informing victims about their options (e.g., safe house, legal rights).[24]

## AGENTS OF TERRORISM

The threat of terrorism is an ongoing concern. Terrorism involves overt actions such as the dispensing of nuclear, biologic, or chemical (NBC) agents as weapons for the express purpose of causing harm. Prompt recognition and identification of potential health hazards are essential in the preparedness of health care professionals.

Biologic agents most commonly used in terrorist attacks include anthrax, smallpox, botulism, plague, tularemia, and hemorrhagic fever. Anthrax, plague, and tularemia are treated effectively with antibiotics if sufficient supplies are available and the organisms are not resistant.

Anthrax vaccine protects against cutaneous and inhalation anthrax. The vaccine is approved by the Food and Drug Administration for at-risk adults (e.g., military personnel) before exposure to anthrax.[25] Smallpox can be prevented or the incidence reduced by vaccination, even when given after exposure. Although botulism is treated with antitoxin, several vaccines are being studied. Vaccines for some hemorrhagic fevers (e.g., yellow fever, Argentine hemorrhagic fever) exist, and others are being investigated (e.g., Ebola).[26]

Chemicals are also used as agents of terrorism and are categorized according to their target organ or effect. For example, sarin is a highly toxic nerve gas that can cause death within minutes of exposure. It enters the body through the eyes and skin and acts by paralyzing the respiratory muscles. Antidotes for nerve agent poisoning include atropine and pralidoxime chloride (2-PAM chloride). Multiple doses may be needed to reverse the effects of the nerve agents.[27]

Phosgene is a colorless gas normally used in chemical manufacturing. If inhaled at high concentrations for a long enough period, it causes severe respiratory distress, pulmonary edema, and death. Mustard gas is yellow to brown and has a garlic-like odor. The gas irritates the eyes and causes skin burns and blisters. Protocols to treat victims of chemical exposure vary and relate to the specific agent.[28]

Radiologic or nuclear agents represent another category of agents of terrorism. *Radiologic dispersal devices* (RDDs), also known as "dirty bombs," consist of a mix of explosives and radioactive material (e.g., pellets). When the device is detonated, the blast scatters radioactive dust, smoke, and other material into the surrounding environment, resulting in radioactive contamination.[29]

The main danger from an RDD results from the explosion, which can cause serious injuries to the victims. The radioactive materials used in an RDD (e.g., uranium, iodine-131) do not usually generate enough radiation to cause immediate serious illness, except to those victims who are in close proximity to the explosion. However, the radioactive dust and smoke can spread and cause illness if inhaled. Since radiation cannot be seen, smelled, felt, or tasted, you should start measures to limit contamination (e.g., covering the patient's nose and mouth) and provide for decontamination (e.g., shower).[29,30]

*Ionizing radiation,* such as that from a nuclear bomb or damage to a nuclear reactor, represents a serious threat to the safety of victims and the environment. Exposure to ionizing radiation may or may not include skin contamination with radioactive material. Initiate decontamination procedures immediately if external radioactive contaminants are present. *Acute radiation syndrome* (ARS) develops after a substantial exposure to ionizing radiation and follows a predictable pattern.[31] (For additional information on ARS, see *www.bt.cdc.gov/radiation/arsphysicianfactsheet.asp.*)

Explosive devices (e.g., TNT, dynamite) that are used as agents of terrorism result in one or more of the following types of injuries: blast, crush, or penetrating. Blast injuries result from the supersonic overpressurization shock wave caused by the explosion. This shock wave primarily damages the lungs, GI tract, and middle ear. Crush injuries (i.e., blunt trauma) often result from explosions in confined spaces causing structural collapse (e.g., falling debris). Some explosive devices contain materials that are projected during the explosion (e.g., shrapnel), leading to penetrating injuries.

## EMERGENCY AND MASS CASUALTY INCIDENT PREPAREDNESS

The term emergency usually refers to any extraordinary event (e.g., multi-vehicle crash) that requires a rapid and skilled response and that the community's existing resources can manage. An emergency is differentiated from a mass casualty incident (MCI) in that an MCI is a man-made (e.g., involving NBC agents) or natural (e.g., hurricane) event or disaster that overwhelms a community's ability to respond with existing resources. MCIs usually involve large numbers of victims, physical and emotional suffering, and permanent changes within a community. In addition, MCIs always require assistance from resources outside the affected community (e.g., American Red Cross, Federal Emergency Management Agency [FEMA]) (Fig. 68-8).

When an emergency or an MCI occurs, first responders (e.g., police, emergency medical personnel) are sent to the scene. Triage of victims of an emergency or an MCI differs from the usual

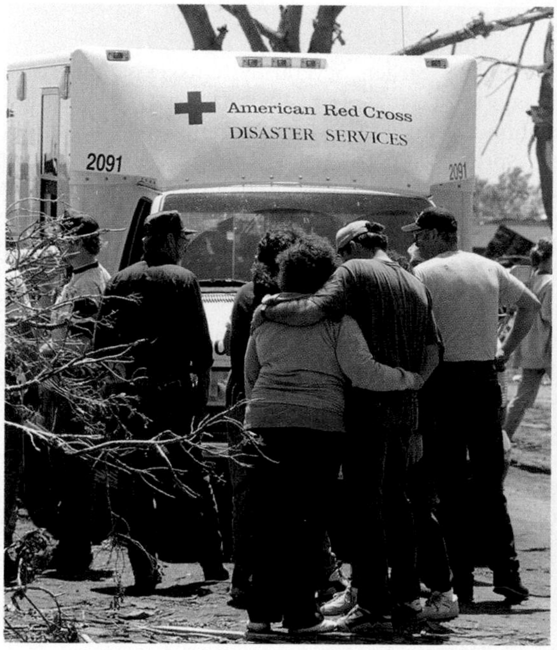


**FIG. 68-8** American Red Cross. (Photo used with the permission of the American Red Cross.)

## ETHICAL/LEGAL DILEMMAS

### *Good Samaritan*

**Situation**

You are a registered nurse, employed as a charge nurse at a subacute rehabilitation facility. It is midnight and you are driving home from work when you see a motor vehicle crash with a person at the side of the road waving and yelling for help. You stop and call 911 to report the incident. What do you do next?

**Ethical/Legal Points for Consideration**

- As a licensed health care professional, you are under no legal obligation to stop and render aid.
- If you do stop, you assume an obligation not to leave the scene until sufficiently trained first responders arrive and assume control.
- Between 50 and 75 yr ago, many states moved to encourage health care professionals to stop and render aid by passing "Good Samaritan" statutes. These statutes, which vary somewhat from state to state, offer immunity from lawsuit for bystanders who offer aid in emergencies except in the case of gross negligence.
- A Good Samaritan must not be in the place of employment or under employment conditions.
- An example of gross negligence may be refusing to assist someone who obviously had a serious hemorrhage in favor of a person with a minor injury because the bleeding person looked old or disheveled.
- Immunity covers only the scene of the accident and not subsequent care under the supervision of HCPs.
- If there is a national disaster, an act of terrorism, or a major emergent need for HCPs, you may be required to go to an assigned site to offer aid. You would not be covered by the Good Samaritan Act under these circumstances.

**Discussion Questions**

1. What factors do you think contribute to a health care professional's decision whether to stop to provide aid?
2. What basic aid would you feel comfortable providing if you do not have an emergency or trauma background?
3. Would your professional liability (malpractice) insurance cover you if someone claimed that you acted negligently while providing assistance?

triage described earlier. Several systems exist, and many use colored tags to designate both the seriousness of the injury and the likelihood of survival. One system uses green for minor injuries (e.g., sprains) and yellow for urgent, but not life-threatening injuries (e.g., open fractures). Red indicates a life-threatening injury requiring immediate intervention (e.g., shock). Blue indicates those who are expected to die (e.g., massive head trauma), and black identifies the dead.[32]

Triage of victims of an emergency or an MCI must be conducted in less than 15 seconds. In general, two thirds of victims are tagged green or yellow. The remaining are tagged red, blue, or black. Victims need to be treated and stabilized and, if there is known or suspected contamination, decontaminated at the scene. After this, they are moved to hospitals. Many other victims arrive at hospitals on their own (i.e., walking wounded). The total number of victims a hospital can expect is estimated by doubling the number of victims who arrive in the first hour. Generally, 30% of victims require admission to the hospital, and half of these need surgery within 8 hours.

In addition to the services provided by first responders, many communities have developed *community emergency response teams* (CERTs). CERTs are recognized by FEMA as important partners in emergency preparedness. The CERT training helps citizens understand their personal responsibility in preparing for a natural or man-made disaster. In addition, participants are taught what to expect after a disaster and how to safely help themselves, their family, and their neighbors. Training includes lifesaving skills with emphasis on decision making and rescuer safety. CERTs are an extension of the first responder services. They can offer immediate help to victims and organize untrained volunteers to assist until professional services arrive.[33]

All HCPs have a role in emergency and MCI preparedness. Knowledge of the hospital's *emergency response plan* is essential. This includes individual roles and responsibilities of the members of the response team plus participation in emergency/MCI preparedness drills on a regular basis. Several types of drills can assess a hospital's level of emergency preparedness. These include hospital disaster drills, computer simulations, and tabletop exercises. Drills allow HCPs to become familiar with the emergency response procedures.[34]

Response to MCIs often requires the aid of a federal agency. The National Incident Management System (NIMS) is a section within the U.S. Department of Homeland Security. NIMS is responsible for coordinating federal, state, and local government efforts to respond to and manage domestic MCIs. One important aspect of NIMS is the development of the *Incident Command System* (ICS). This standardized organizational structure provides for the management of all incidents. NIMS requires that all emergency services–related disciplines (e.g., hospitals, HCPs, emergency response services) wishing to participate in the emergency management of disasters must be NIMS and ICS trained. You can take courses online and at no cost *(http://training.fema.gov/is/nims.aspx)*.

The National Disaster Medical System (NDMS) is a part of the U.S. Department of Health and Human Services, Office of Preparedness and Response. The NDMS expands the nation's medical response capability by organizing and training volunteer disaster medical assistance teams (DMATs). Each DMAT consists of members with a variety of health or medical skills and those with specialized support skills (e.g., communications, logistics, security). DMATs are sent to disaster sites with enough supplies and equipment to remain self-sufficient for 72 hours while providing medical care. DMAT personnel are deployed for a period of 2 weeks.[35]

All disasters result in psychologic stress to the individuals involved. This stress can persist for an extended period and is influenced, in part, by the nature of the event, the individual's age, preexisting coping mechanisms, role in the event, and medical and psychologic history. Many hospitals and DMATs have a *critical incident stress management unit.* This unit arranges group discussions to allow participants to share and validate their feelings and emotions about the experience. This is important for emotional recovery.

## CASE STUDY

### *Trauma*

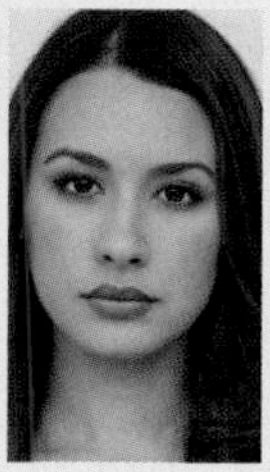

(©Thinkstock)

**Patient Profile**

D.F., a 20-yr-old Hispanic female trauma victim, is brought to the ED in an ambulance. She was the driver in a motor vehicle crash and was not wearing a seat belt. Two unrestrained children in the car were pronounced dead at the scene. The paramedics stated that there was significant damage to the car on the driver's side.

**Subjective Data**

- Patient asks, "What happened? Where am I?"
- Complains of shortness of breath and leg pain

**Objective Data**

***Physical Examination***

- Vital signs: BP = 85/40 mm Hg, HR = 140 beats/minute, RR = 36 breaths/minute; $O_2$ saturation = 85% with 100% non-rebreather mask
- Decreased breath sounds on left side of chest
- Asymmetric chest wall movement
- Glasgow Coma Score = 14; pupils slightly unequal
- Badly deformed left lower leg with significant swelling and a pedal pulse by Doppler only
- 4-cm head laceration, bleeding controlled

**Discussion Questions**

1. What are D.F.'s most likely life-threatening injuries?
2. ***Priority Decision:*** What is the priority of care for D.F.?
3. ***Priority Decision:*** What interventions does this patient need immediately?
4. What other interventions should you consider?
5. ***Teamwork and Collaboration:*** What activities could you delegate to unlicensed assistive personnel (UAP)?
6. ***Patient-Centered Care:*** Several family members have arrived in the ED, including the mother of one of the children who died. The second child who died was the patient's child. How should you approach the family?
7. ***Priority Decision:*** Based on assessment data presented, what are the priority nursing diagnoses? Are there any collaborative problems?
8. ***Evidence-Based Practice:*** What are the best practice guidelines for fluid resuscitation in patients who are experiencing hypovolemic shock?

Answers available at *http://evolve.elsevier.com/Lewis/medsurg.*

## BRIDGE TO NCLEX EXAMINATION

The number of the question corresponds to the same-numbered outcome at the beginning of the chapter.

**1.** An older man arrives in triage disoriented and dyspneic. His skin is hot and dry. His wife states that he was fine earlier today. The nurse's next *priority* would be to
- **a.** assess his vital signs.
- **b.** obtain a brief medical history from his wife.
- **c.** start supplemental $O_2$ and have the ED physician see him.
- **d.** determine the kind of insurance he has before treating him.

**2.** A patient has a core temperature of 90° F (32.2° C). The *most* appropriate rewarming technique would be
- **a.** passive rewarming with warm blankets.
- **b.** active internal rewarming using warmed IV fluids.
- **c.** passive rewarming using air-filled warming blankets.
- **d.** active external rewarming by submersing in a warm bath.

**3.** What are effective interventions to decrease absorption or increase elimination of an ingested poison *(select all that apply)*?
- **a.** Hemodialysis
- **b.** Milk dilution
- **c.** Eye irrigation
- **d.** Gastric lavage
- **e.** Activated charcoal

**4.** An older woman arrives in the ED complaining of severe pain in her right shoulder. The nurse notes that her clothes are soiled with urine and feces. She tells the nurse that she lives with her son and that she "fell." She is tearful and asks you if she can be admitted. What possibility should the nurse consider?
- **a.** Dementia
- **b.** Possible cancer
- **c.** Family violence
- **d.** Orthostatic hypotension

**5.** A chemical explosion occurs at a nearby industrial site. The first responders report that victims are being decontaminated at the scene and approximately 125 workers will need medical evaluation and care. The nurse receiving this report should know that this will *first* require activation of
- **a.** a code blue alert.
- **b.** a disaster medical assistance team.
- **c.** the local police and fire departments.
- **d.** the hospital's emergency response plan.

1. a, 2. b, 3. a, d, e, 4. c, 5. d

For rationales to these answers and even more NCLEX review questions, visit *http://evolve.elsevier.com/Lewis/medsurg.*

## EVOLVE WEBSITE

http://evolve.elsevier.com/Lewis/medsurg

**Review Questions (Online Only)**

**Key Points**

**Answer Keys for Questions**
- Rationales for Bridge to NCLEX Examination Questions
- Answer Guidelines for Case Study on p. 1647
- Answer Guidelines for Managing Care of Multiple Patients Case Study (Section 12) on p. 1649

**Student Case Study**
- Patient With Musculoskeletal Trauma

**Conceptual Care Map Creator**

**Audio Glossary**

**Content Updates**

## REFERENCES


1. Centers for Disease Control and Prevention: Emergency department visits. Retrieved from *www.cdc.gov/nchs/fastats/emergency-department.htm.*
2. American College of Emergency Physicians: Emergency department wait times, crowding and access fact sheet. Retrieved from *http://newsroom.acep.org/index.php?s=20301&item=29937.*
3. Board of Certification for Emergency Nurses: Get certified – CEN. Retrieved from *www.bcencertifications.org/Get-Certified/CEN.aspx.*
4. Rund DA, Rausch TS: *Triage*, St Louis, 1981, Mosby. (Classic)
5. Gilboy N, Tanabe P, Travers DA, et al: Emergency Severity Index (ESI): a triage tool for emergency department, version 4: Implementation handbook 2012 edition, AHRQ Pub No. 12-0014. Retrieved from *www.ahrq.gov/professionals/systems/hospital/esi/esihandbk.pdf.*
6. Emergency Nurses Association: Initial assessment. In *TNCC trauma nursing core course provider manual*, ed 7, Des Plaines, Ill, 2014, Emergency Nurses Association.
7. Hammond BB, Zimmermann PG, editors: *Sheehy's manual of emergency care*, ed 7, St Louis, 2013, Mosby.

*8. Emergency Nurses Association: Clinical practice guideline: family presence during invasive procedures and resuscitation. Retrieved from *www.ena.org/practice-research/research/CPG/Documents/FamilyPresenceCPG.pdf.*

*9. American College of Emergency Physicians: Optimizing the treatment of pain in patients with acute presentations. Retrieved from *www.acep.org/MobileArticle.aspx?id=48089&parentid=.*

10. Centers for Disease Control and Prevention: Tetanus: prevention. Retrieved from *www.cdc.gov/tetanus/about/prevention.html.*

*11. Diao M, Huang F, Guan J, et al: Prehospital therapeutic hypothermia after cardiac arrest: a systematic review and meta-analysis of randomized controlled trials, *Resuscitation* 84:1021, 2013.

*12. O'Gara P, Kushner FG, Ascheim DD, et al: 2013 ACCF/AHA guideline for the management of ST-elevation myocardial infarction, *J Am Coll Cardiol* 61:e78, 2013.

13. Bernard S: Inducing hypothermia after out of hospital cardiac arrest, *BMJ* 348:g2735, 2014.

*14. Emergency Nurses Association: Position statement: palliative and end-of-life care in the emergency department. Retrieved from *www.ena.org/SiteCollectionDocuments/Position%20Statements/PalliativeEndOfLifeCare.pdf.*

15. United Network for Organ Sharing: What every patient needs to know. Retrieved from *www.unos.org/wp-content/uploads/unos/WEPNTK.pdf.*

*16. American College of Emergency Physicians, the American Geriatrics Society, Emergency Nurses Association, and the Society for Academic Emergency Medicine: Geriatric emergency department guidelines. Retrieved from *www.acep.org/geriEDguidelines/.*

17. Centers for Disease Control and Prevention: Tick removal. Retrieved from *www.cdc.gov/ticks/removing_a_tick.html.*
18. Centers for Disease Control and Prevention: Rabies. Retrieved from *www.cdc.gov/rabies/medical_care.*
19. National Capital Poison Control Center: Act fast. Retrieved from *www.poison.org.*
20. Edmunds MW, Mayhew MS: *Pharmacology for the primary care provider*, ed 4, St Louis, 2014, Elsevier.
21. Occupational Health and Safety Administration: Reporting and recording occupational injuries and illness. Retrieved from *www.osha.gov/pls/oshaweb/owastand.display_standard_group?p_toc_level=1&p_part_number=1904.*

*22. Emergency Nurses Association: Position statement: violence in the emergency care setting. Retrieved from *www.ena.org/SiteCollectionDocuments/Position%20Statements/ViolenceintheEmergencyCareSetting.pdf.*

*23. Emergency Nurses Association: Position statement: intimate partner and family violence, maltreatment, and neglect. Retrieved from *http://ncdsv.org/images/ENA_IPVandFamilyViolenceMaltreatmentNeglect_2006.pdf.*

24. Dudgeon A, Evanson TA: Intimate partner violence in rural U.S. areas: what every nurse should know, *AJN* 114:26, 2014.
25. Centers for Disease Control and Prevention: Anthrax. Retrieved from *http://www.cdc.gov/anthrax/medical-care/prevention.html.*
26. Centers for Disease Control and Prevention: Viral hemorrhagic fevers. Retrieved from *www.cdc.gov/ncidod/dvrd/spb/mnpages/dispages/Fact_Sheets/Viral_Hemorrhagic_Fevers_Fact_Sheet.pdf.*
27. Agency for Toxic Substances and Disease Registry: Medical management guidelines for nerve agents: Tabun (GA), Sarin (GB), Soman (GD), and VX. Retrieved from *www.atsdr.cdc.gov/mmg/mmg.asp?id=523&tid=93.*
28. Agency for Toxic Substances and Disease Registry: Medical management guidelines for phosgene. Retrieved from *www.atsdr.cdc.gov/mmg/mmg.asp?id=1201&tid=182.*
29. Centers for Disease Control and Prevention: Frequently asked questions about dirty bombs. Retrieved from *http://emergency.cdc.gov/radiation/dirtybombs.asp.*

*30. Emergency Nurses Association: Position statement: hazardous material exposure. Retrieved from *www.ena.org/SiteCollectionDocuments/Position%20Statements/Archived/Hazardous_Material_Exposure_-_ENA_PS.pdf.*

*31. Military Medical Operations Armed Forces Radiobiology Research Institute: Medical management of radiological casualties. Retrieved from *www.orau.org/PTP/PTP%20Library/library/dod/radiologicalhandbooksp99-2.pdf.*

*32. Lerner EB, Schwartz RB, Coule PL, et al: Mass casualty triage: an evaluation of the data and development of a proposed national guideline, *Disaster Med Public Health Prep* 2:S25, 2008. (Classic)

33. Federal Emergency Management Agency: About community emergency response team. Retrieved from *www.fema.gov/community-emergency-response-teams/about-community-emergency-response-team.*

*34. Agency for Healthcare Research and Quality: Evidence report/technology assessment number 95: training of hospital staff to respond to a mass casualty incident. Retrieved from *http://archive.ahrq.gov/downloads/pub/evidence/pdf/hospmci/hospmci.pdf.*

35. US Department of Health and Human Services: Disaster medical assistance teams. Retrieved from *www.phe.gov/preparedness/responders/ndms/teams/pages/dmat.aspx.*


*Evidence-based information for clinical practice.

## CASE STUDY

### *Managing Care of Multiple Patients*

You are working in a 12-bed ICU and have been assigned to care for the following two patients. There is one UAP available to help as needed.

**Patients**

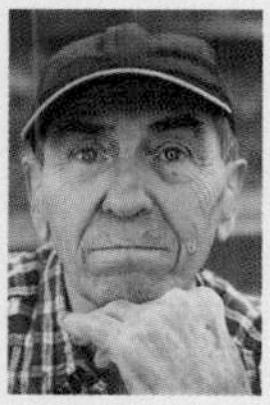

(©Thinkstock)

R.K. is a 72-yr-old white man who was admitted with a massive stroke after collapsing at his home. He is unresponsive, even to painful stimuli. He has an oral endotracheal (ET) tube in place and is receiving mechanical ventilation (assist-control mode, $FIO_2$ 70%, $V_T$ 700 mL, respiratory rate 16 breaths/minute, PEEP 7.5 cm $H_2O$). His chest x-ray reveals right lower lung consolidation. A subclavian central line was placed to monitor central venous pressure (CVP) and administer fluids and IV antibiotics. His cardiac rhythm on admission was atrial fibrillation with a rapid ventricular response. He is receiving IV diltiazem (Cardizem), and his ventricular response has slowed to 84 bpm. His temperature is elevated despite receiving acetaminophen (Tylenol) q4hr. Additionally, enteral feedings are running at 25 mL/hr via orogastric feeding tube and R.K. has a catheter for urinary drainage.

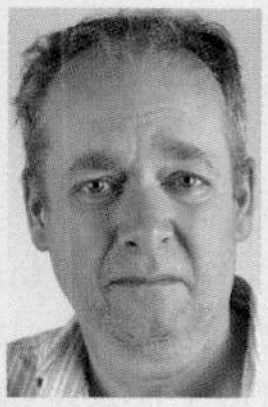

(©Thinkstock)

J.N. is a 58-yr-old white man who was admitted 24 hr ago after emergent surgery for an acutely ischemic bowel. The surgical procedure involved extensive abdominal surgery to repair a perforated colon, irrigate the abdominal cavity, and provide hemostasis. During surgery his systolic BP dropped to 70 mm Hg and remains in the low 90s. He is in sinus tachycardia at a rate of 128 bpm. Six units of packed RBCs and 4 L of 0.9% normal saline were infused. His pulmonary status worsened within 12 hr of admission to the ICU, requiring emergent ET intubation. He developed a right-sided pneumothorax after intubation, and a chest tube was placed at that time. His hypoxemia has rapidly progressed and is now refractory to 100% $FIO_2$ and high levels of PEEP. His laboratory tests indicate kidney and liver failure. He has an advance directive that indicates he does not want to be kept alive by artificial means, but he currently is full code status. He is sedated, paralyzed, and unable to communicate. His urinary catheter is draining concentrated urine <30 mL/hr and he has a central line in place with 0.9% saline running at 125 mL/hr. His most recent ABGs are as follows: pH 7.12, $PaO_2$ 50 mm Hg, $PaCO_2$ 62 mm Hg, $HCO_3^-$ 17 mEq/L, and $O_2$ saturation 84%. His $PaO_2/FIO_2$ ratio is 59, and his chest x-ray shows worsening bilateral interstitial infiltrates compatible with an ARDS pattern.

**Discussion Questions**

1. ***Priority Decision:*** After receiving report, which patient should you see first? Provide rationale.
2. ***Teamwork and Collaboration:*** Which tasks could you delegate to the UAP *(select all that apply)*?
   a. Record vital signs on R.K. and J.N.
   b. Drain the water from J.N.'s ventilator tubing as needed
   c. Change suction tubing on R.K.'s ET tubes as needed.
   d. Titrate the diltiazem IV drip based on R.K.'s heart rate.
   e. Talk to J.N.'s family regarding his advance directive and current code status.
3. ***Priority Decision and Teamwork and Collaboration:*** As you are assessing J.N., the UAP informs you that R.K. just vomited all over his bed. Which *initial* action would be *most* appropriate?
   a. Ask the UAP to give R.K. a bath while you finish assessing J.N.
   b. Turn off the enteral tube feeding on R.K. and auscultate his lungs.
   c. Ask the UAP to inform the HCP about J.N.'s ABG results while you assess R.K.
   d. Finish assessing R.K. and then suction R.K.'s endotracheal tube to remove any aspirated emesis.

**Case Study Progression**

R.K.'s lungs are clear to auscultation. Evaluation of his GI status reveals minimal bowel sounds and a gastric residual of 200 mL even after his emesis. You elevate the head of his bed to 60 degrees, hold the tube feeding, and notify his HCP.

4. Which intervention would you expect the HCP to order for R.K.?
   a. Morphine sulfate 2 mg IV stat
   b. Metoclopramide (Reglan) 10 mg IV q6hr
   c. Restart enteral tube feeding while maintaining HOB elevation at 90 degrees
   d. Hold enteral tube feeding for 1 hour and restart with half-strength fluids at same rate
5. J.N.'s ABG results reflect a worsening of his ARDS. You correctly identify that these results demonstrate
   a. uncompensated respiratory acidosis.
   b. uncompensated respiratory alkalosis.
   c. partially compensated respiratory acidosis.
   d. partially compensated respiratory alkalosis.
6. ***Management Decision:*** You walk into J.N.'s room and find his wife whispering in his ear with her hand on the ventilator tubing, appearing to be ready to disconnect him from life support. What is your *best* initial action?
   a. Ask J.N.'s wife to leave the room immediately.
   b. Report the incident to the charge nurse and security immediately.
   c. Ask J.N.'s wife if you could talk to her about her husband's condition.
   d. Report the incident to J.N.'s health care provider to address J.N.'s code status.

Answers and rationales available at *http://evolve.elsevier.com/Lewis/medsurg*.

# Basic Life Support for Health Care Professionals

*Linda Bucher*

*Basic life support* (BLS) for health care professionals consists of a series of actions and skills performed by the rescuer(s) based on assessment findings. The first action the rescuer performs on finding an adult victim is to assess for responsiveness. This is done by tapping or shaking the victim's shoulder and asking, "Are you all right?" If the victim does not respond, simultaneously scan the victim's chest for signs of breathing and perform a pulse check (described below).

If the rescuer is alone, the rescuer shouts for help. If someone responds, the rescuer asks him or her to activate the *emergency response system* (ERS) (e.g., through the use of a mobile phone) and get an *automatic external defibrillator* (AED) (if available). If no one responds and the rescuer does not have a mobile phone, the rescuer should leave to activate the ERS, get an AED (if available), and return to the victim before beginning *cardiopulmonary resuscitation* (CPR) and defibrillation if necessary.[1]

## CARDIOPULMONARY RESUSCITATION

*Cardiac arrest* is characterized by the absence of a pulse and breathing in an unconscious victim. The current approach for CPR is the chest *compressions-airway-breathing* (CAB) sequence.[1]

The first step in CPR is to perform a pulse check by palpating the carotid pulse for at least 5 but no more than 10 seconds. While maintaining a head-tilt position with one hand on the victim's forehead, locate the victim's trachea using two or three fingers of your other hand. Slide these fingers into the groove between the trachea and neck muscles where the carotid pulse can be felt. The technique is more easily performed on the side nearest you.

If a pulse is felt, give one rescue breath every 5 to 6 seconds (10 to 12 breaths/minute) and recheck the pulse every 2 minutes (Fig. A-1). If no pulse is felt, start CAB.[1,2]

### Chest Compressions

The proper technique for providing chest compressions is shown in Fig. A-2. Chest compression technique consists of fast and deep applications of pressure on the lower half of the sternum. The victim must be in the supine position when the compressions are performed. The victim must be lying on a flat, hard surface, such as a CPR board (specially designed for use in CPR), a headboard from a unit bed, or, if necessary, the floor. Position yourself close to the side of the victim's chest. More frequently, mechanical chest compression devices (see Fig. 68-2) are being used to provide chest compressions both prehospital and in the emergency department.

Chest compressions are combined with rescue breathing for an effective resuscitation effort of the adult victim of cardiac arrest. The compression-ventilation ratio for one- or two-rescuer CPR is 30 compressions to 2 breaths (Table A-1). However, if the patient has an advanced airway (e.g.,

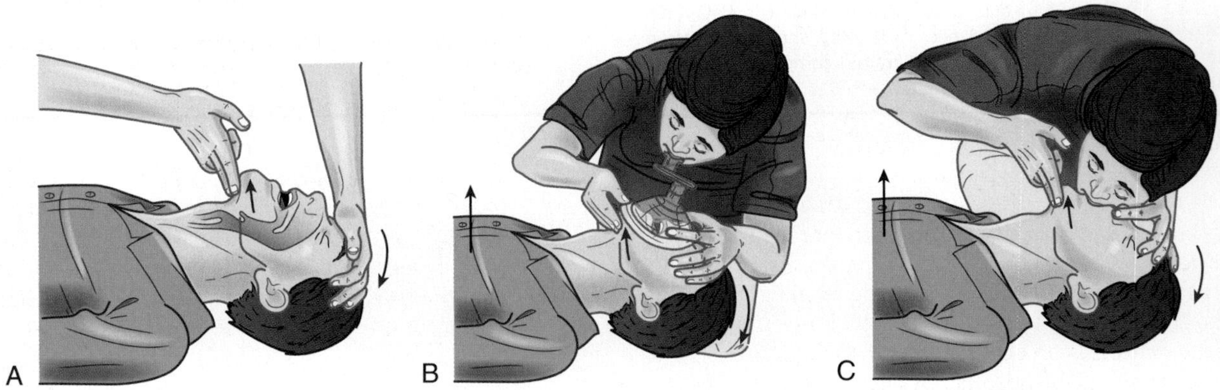


**FIG. A-1** The head tilt–chin lift maneuver is used to open the victim's airway to give rescue breaths. **A,** Rescuer places one hand on the victim's forehead and applies firm, backward pressure with the palm to tilt the head back. The chin is lifted and brought forward with the fingers of the other hand. **B,** Mouth-to-barrier device: Rescuer places the device tightly over the victim's mouth and nose and delivers a regular breath. **C,** Mouth-to-mouth technique: Rescuer pinches the victim's nostrils, tightly seals mouth over victim's mouth, and delivers a regular breath. NOTE: Rescuer should observe for a rise in the victim's chest *(black arrows).*

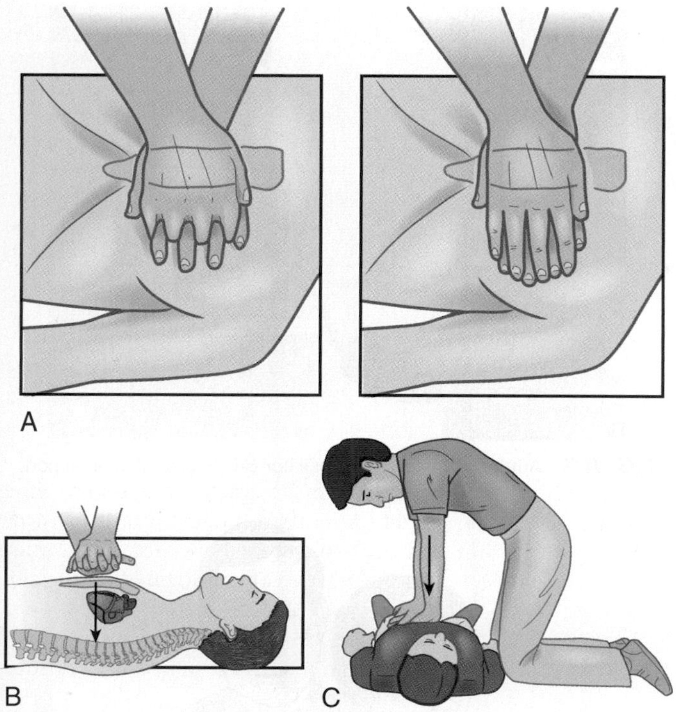


**FIG. A-2** Cardiopulmonary resuscitation. **A,** Position of the hands on the lower half of the sternum during chest compressions. **B,** When pressure is applied, the sternum is displaced posteriorly with the heel of the hand. **C,** Arms are kept straight and the rescuer pushes deep (at least 2 in [5 cm]) and fast (a rate of 100-120 compressions per minute).

endotracheal tube, laryngeal mask airway), do not pause between compressions for breaths and deliver 1 breath every 6 seconds (10 breaths/minute).[1]

If a mechanical chest compression device is not used, then it is preferable to have two persons performing CPR. One rescuer, positioned at the victim's side, performs chest compressions while the second rescuer, positioned at the victim's head, maintains an open airway and performs ventilations. To maintain the quality and rate of compressions, rescuers should change roles every 2 minutes.[2] Interruptions in CPR should be limited.

## Defibrillation

When the AED or advanced cardiovascular life support (ACLS) team arrives, assess the victim's rhythm. If the victim has a shockable rhythm (e.g., ventricular tachycardia, ventricular fibrillation), deliver one shock and immediately resume CPR for about 2 minutes before checking the rhythm again. If the rhythm is not a shockable rhythm, immediately resume CPR and recheck the rhythm after 2 minutes. CPR should continue between rhythm checks and shocks and until the ACLS team arrives or the victim shows signs of movement.[1]

The American Heart Association includes training in the use of AEDs with instruction of HCPs and laypersons in BLS. Survival from cardiac arrest is the highest when immediate CPR is provided and defibrillation occurs within 3 to 5 minutes.[2] AEDs are found in many out-of-hospital, public settings (Fig. A-3).

## Airway and Breathing

If a victim has a pulse but is gasping (e.g., agonal breathing) or not breathing, establish an open airway and begin rescue breathing. Open an adult's airway by hyperextending the head (Fig. A-1). Use the *head tilt–chin lift maneuver.* This involves tilting the head back with one hand and lifting the chin forward with the fingers of the other hand. Use the *jaw-thrust maneuver* if you suspect a cervical spine injury (see Fig. 68-1). Attempt to ventilate the victim using a mouth-to-barrier (recommended) device (e.g., face mask or bag-valve-mask) or mouth-to-mouth resuscitation[2] (Fig. A-1, *B, C*).

For mouth-to-mouth resuscitation give ventilations with the victim's nostrils pinched. Take a regular (not deep) breath and tightly seal your lips around the victim's mouth. Give one breath and watch for a rise in the victim's chest. Continue rescue breaths at a rate of 10 to 12 per minute. When the victim has a tracheostomy, give ventilations through the stoma.

### TABLE A-1 Adult One- and Two-Rescuer Basic Life Support With Automatic External Defibrillator (AED)

**Assess**

- Determine unresponsiveness: tap or shake victim's shoulder; shout, "Are you all right?"
- Check for no breathing or abnormal breathing (e.g., gasping) while simultaneously performing a pulse check (5-10 sec).

**Activate Emergency Response System (ERS)**

- Activate ERS (e.g., call 911) and get the AED (if available) (outside of hospital).
- Call a code and ask for the AED or crash cart (in hospital).

**Begin High-Quality CPR**

- If victim has a pulse but is not breathing or not breathing adequately, begin rescue breathing at a rate of 1 breath every 5-6 sec (Fig. A-1) and recheck the pulse every 2 minutes.*
- If there is no pulse, expose the victim's chest and immediately begin chest compressions (Fig. A-2).
- Deliver compressions at a rate of 100-120/minute.
- Compress the chest at least 2 inches (5 cm) but not greater than 2.4 inches (6 cm).
- Allow for complete chest recoil after each compression.
- Deliver a compression-ventilation ratio of 30 compressions to 2 breaths.†
- Minimize interruptions in compressions by delivering the 2 breaths in <10 sec.

**Deliver Effective Breaths**

- Open airway adequately (Fig. A-1, *A*).
- Deliver breath to produce a visible chest rise (Fig. A-1, *B, C*).
- Avoid excessive ventilation.

**Integrate Prompt Use of the AED**

- Use AED as soon as possible.
- If rhythm is shockable, deliver one shock and then resume chest compressions immediately after delivery of shock.
- If the rhythm is not shockable, resume CPR and recheck rhythm every five cycles.

**Continue CPR**

- Continue CPR between rhythm checks and shocks, and until ACLS providers arrive or the victim shows signs of movement.

*If possible opioid overdose, give naloxone if available and per protocol.
†For patients with ongoing CPR and an advanced airway in place, a ventilation rate of 1 breath every 6 seconds (10 breaths per minute) with no interruption in compressions is recommended.
*ACLS,* Advanced cardiovascular life support; *CPR,* cardiopulmonary resuscitation.
Sources: American Heart Association: *Highlights of the 2015 American Heart Association guidelines update for CPR and ECC,* Dallas, 2015, The Association and American Heart Association: *BLS for healthcare providers—student manual,* Dallas, 2011, The Association.

**TABLE A-2 Management of the Adult Choking Victim**

**Conscious Adult Choking Victim**

***Assess Victim for Severe Airway Obstruction***

Look for any of the following signs:

- Poor or no air exchange
- Clutching the neck with the hands, making the universal choking sign
- Weak, ineffective cough or no cough at all
- High-pitched noise while inhaling or no noise at all
- Increased respiratory difficulty
- Possible cyanosis

Ask the victim if he or she is choking. If the victim nods yes and cannot talk or has any of the symptoms noted above, severe airway obstruction is present and you must take immediate action.

***Abdominal Thrusts (Heimlich Maneuver) With Standing or Sitting Victim*** *(Fig. A-4)*

1. Stand or kneel behind victim and wrap arms around the victim's waist.
2. Make fist with one hand.
3. Place thumb side of fist against victim's abdomen. Position fist midline, slightly above navel and well below breastbone.
4. Grasp fist with other hand and press fist into victim's abdomen with a quick, forceful upward thrust.
5. Give each new thrust with a separate, distinct movement to relieve the obstruction. CAUTION: If victim is pregnant or obese, give chest thrusts instead of abdominal thrusts. Position hands (as described) over lower portion of the breastbone and apply quick backward thrusts.
6. Repeat thrusts until object is expelled or victim becomes unresponsive.

**Unconscious Adult Choking Victim**

If you see a choking victim collapse and become unresponsive:

1. Activate the emergency response system.
2. Lower the victim to the ground and begin CPR, starting with compressions (do not check for a pulse).
3. Open the victim's mouth wide each time you prepare to give breaths. Look for the object. If you see the object and can easily remove it, do so with your fingers. If you do not see the object, continue with CPR using the chest compression–airway-breathing sequence (Table A-1).
4. If efforts to ventilate are unsuccessful, continue with CPR.

Source: American Heart Association: *BLS for healthcare providers—student manual*, Dallas, 2011, The Association.

If the victim cannot be ventilated, proceed with CPR. When providing the next rescue breaths, look for any objects in the victim's mouth. If any objects are visible, remove them (Table A-2).

## HANDS-ONLY CPR

*Hands-only CPR* can be used to help adult victims who suddenly collapse from cardiac arrest outside of a health care setting. If you witness this event (as a bystander), you can choose to provide chest compressions only (push fast and deep in the center of the chest) or conventional CPR (described previously). Both methods are effective when done in the first few minutes of an out-of-hospital cardiac arrest.[3]

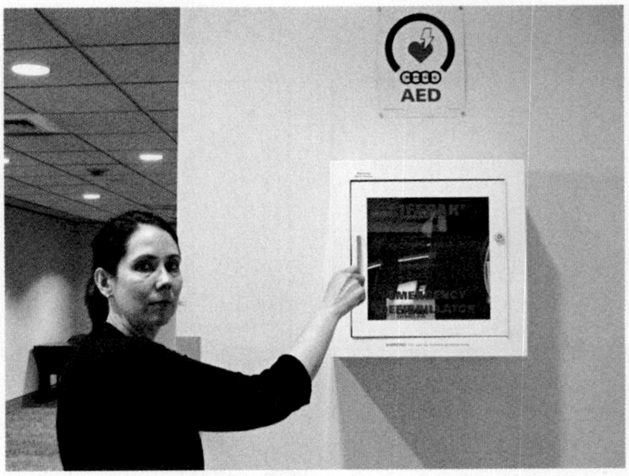


**FIG. A-3** Automatic external defibrillator (AED) located in an airport.

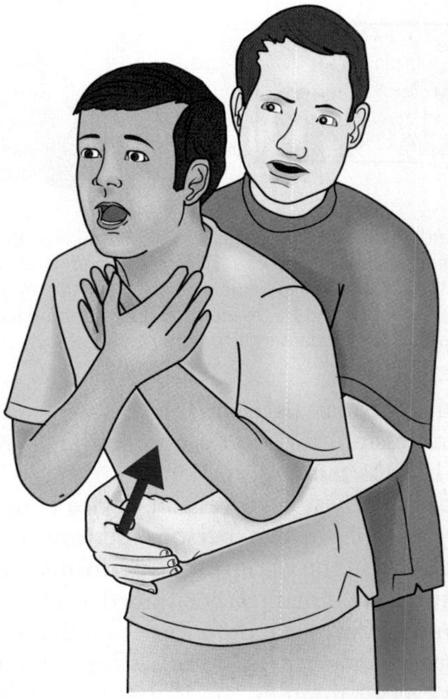

**FIG. A-4** Abdominal thrusts (Heimlich maneuver) administered to a conscious (standing) choking victim.

## REFERENCES*

1. American Heart Association: *Highlights of the 2015 American Heart Association guidelines update for CPR and ECC*, Dallas, 2015, The Association.
2. American Heart Association: *BLS for healthcare providers—student manual*, Dallas, 2011, The Association.
3. American Heart Association: Two steps to staying alive with hands-only CPR. Retrieved from *http://www.heart.org/HEARTORG/CPRAndECC/HandsOnlyCPR/Hands-Only-CPR_UCM_440559_SubHomePage.jsp*.

*The CPR guidelines will be updated on an ongoing basis and available at *https://eccguidelines.heart.org/index.php/circulation/cpr-ecc-guidelines-2*.

# Nursing Diagnoses

Activity Intolerance
Activity Intolerance, Risk for
Activity Planning, Ineffective
Activity Planning, Risk for Ineffective
Adaptive Capacity, Decreased Intracranial
Airway Clearance, Ineffective
Allergy Response, Risk for
Anxiety
Aspiration, Risk for
Attachment, Risk for Impaired
Autonomic Dysreflexia
Autonomic Dysreflexia, Risk for
Behavior, Disorganized Infant
Behavior, Readiness for Enhanced Organized Infant
Behavior, Risk for Disorganized Infant
Bleeding, Risk for
Blood Glucose Level, Risk for Unstable
Body Image, Disturbed
Body Temperature, Risk for Imbalanced
Breast Milk, Insufficient
Breastfeeding, Ineffective
Breastfeeding, Interrupted
Breastfeeding, Readiness for Enhanced
Breathing Pattern, Ineffective
Cardiac Output, Decreased
Cardiac Output, Risk for Decreased
Cardiovascular Function, Risk for Impaired
Childbearing Process, Ineffective
Childbearing Process, Readiness for Enhanced
Childbearing Process, Risk for Ineffective
Comfort, Impaired
Comfort, Readiness for Enhanced
Communication, Readiness for Enhanced
Confusion, Acute
Confusion, Chronic
Confusion, Risk for Acute
Constipation
Constipation, Chronic Functional
Constipation, Perceived
Constipation, Risk for
Constipation, Risk for Chronic Functional
Contamination
Contamination, Risk for
Coping, Compromised Family
Coping, Defensive
Coping, Disabled Family
Coping, Ineffective
Coping, Ineffective Community
Coping, Readiness for Enhanced
Coping, Readiness for Enhanced Community
Coping, Readiness for Enhanced Family
Death Anxiety
Decision Making, Readiness for Enhanced
Decisional Conflict
Denial, Ineffective
Dentition, Impaired
Development, Risk for Delayed
Diarrhea
Disuse Syndrome, Risk for
Diversional Activity, Deficient
Dry Eye, Risk for
Electrolyte Imbalance, Risk for
Elimination, Impaired Urinary
Elimination, Readiness for Enhanced Urinary
Emancipated Decision Making, Impaired
Emancipated Decision Making, Readiness for Enhanced
Emancipated Decision Making, Risk for Impaired
Emotional Control, Labile
Falls, Risk for
Family Processes, Dysfunctional
Family Processes, Interrupted
Family Processes, Readiness for Enhanced
Fatigue
Fear
Feeding Pattern, Ineffective Infant
Fluid Balance, Readiness for Enhanced
Fluid Volume, Deficient
Fluid Volume, Excess
Fluid Volume, Risk for Deficient
Fluid Volume, Risk for Imbalanced
Frail Elderly Syndrome
Frail Elderly Syndrome, Risk for
Gas Exchange, Impaired
Gastrointestinal Motility, Dysfunctional
Gastrointestinal Motility, Risk for Dysfunctional
Gastrointestinal Perfusion, Risk for Ineffective
Grieving
Grieving, Complicated
Grieving, Risk for Complicated
Growth, Risk for Disproportionate
Health, Deficient Community
Health Behavior, Risk-Prone
Health Maintenance, Ineffective
Health Management, Ineffective
Health Management, Ineffective Family
Health Management, Readiness for Enhanced
Home Maintenance, Impaired
Hope, Readiness for Enhanced
Hopelessness
Human Dignity, Risk for Compromised
Hyperthermia
Hypothermia
Hypothermia, Risk for
Hypothermia, Risk for Perioperative
Impulse Control, Ineffective
Incontinence, Bowel
Incontinence, Functional Urinary
Incontinence, Overflow Urinary

Incontinence, Reflex Urinary
Incontinence, Risk for Urge Urinary
Incontinence, Stress Urinary
Incontinence, Urge Urinary
Infection, Risk for
Injury, Risk for
Injury, Risk for Corneal
Injury, Risk for Perioperative Positioning
Injury, Risk for Thermal
Injury, Risk for Urinary Tract
Insomnia
Jaundice, Neonatal
Jaundice, Risk for Neonatal
Knowledge, Deficient
Knowledge, Readiness for Enhanced
Latex Allergy Response
Latex Allergy Response, Risk for
Lifestyle, Sedentary
Liver Function, Risk for Impaired
Loneliness, Risk for
Maternal/Fetal Dyad, Risk for Disturbed
Memory, Impaired
Mobility, Impaired Bed
Mobility, Impaired Physical
Mobility, Impaired Wheelchair
Mood Regulation, Impaired
Moral Distress
Nausea
Noncompliance
Nutrition, Imbalanced: Less Than Body Requirements
Nutrition, Readiness for Enhanced
Obesity
Oral Mucous Membrane, Impaired
Oral Mucous Membrane, Risk for Impaired
Other-Directed Violence, Risk for
Overweight
Overweight, Risk for
Pain, Acute
Pain, Chronic
Pain, Labor
Parenting, Impaired
Parenting, Readiness for Enhanced
Parenting, Risk for Impaired
Peripheral Neurovascular Dysfunction, Risk for
Personal Identity, Disturbed
Personal Identity, Risk for Disturbed
Poisoning, Risk for
Post-Trauma Syndrome
Post-Trauma Syndrome, Risk for
Power, Readiness for Enhanced
Powerlessness
Powerlessness, Risk for
Pressure Ulcer, Risk for
Protection, Ineffective
Rape-Trauma Syndrome
Reaction to Iodinated Contrast Media, Risk for
Relationship, Ineffective
Relationship, Readiness for Enhanced
Relationship, Risk for Ineffective
Religiosity, Impaired
Religiosity, Readiness for Enhanced
Religiosity, Risk for Impaired
Relocation Stress Syndrome
Relocation Stress Syndrome, Risk for
Renal Perfusion, Risk for Ineffective
Resilience, Impaired
Resilience, Readiness for Enhanced
Resilience, Risk for Impaired
Role Conflict, Parental
Role Performance, Ineffective
Role Strain, Caregiver
Role Strain, Risk for Caregiver
Self-Care, Readiness for Enhanced
Self-Care Deficit, Bathing
Self-Care Deficit, Dressing
Self-Care Deficit, Feeding
Self-Care Deficit, Toileting
Self-Concept, Readiness for Enhanced
Self-Directed Violence, Risk for
Self-Esteem, Chronic Low
Self-Esteem, Risk for Chronic Low
Self-Esteem, Situational Low
Self-Esteem, Risk for Situational Low
Self-Mutilation
Self-Mutilation, Risk for
Self-Neglect
Sexual Dysfunction
Sexuality Pattern, Ineffective
Shock, Risk for
Sitting, Impaired
Skin Integrity, Impaired
Skin Integrity, Risk for Impaired
Sleep, Readiness for Enhanced
Sleep Deprivation
Sleep Pattern, Disturbed
Social Interaction, Impaired
Social Isolation
Sorrow, Chronic
Spiritual Distress
Spiritual Distress, Risk for
Spiritual Well-Being, Readiness for Enhanced
Spontaneous Ventilation, Impaired
Standing, Impaired
Stress Overload
Sudden Infant Death Syndrome, Risk for
Suffocation, Risk for
Suicide, Risk for
Surgical Recovery, Delayed
Surgical Recovery, Risk for Delayed
Swallowing, Impaired
Thermoregulation, Ineffective
Tissue Integrity, Impaired
Tissue Integrity, Risk for Impaired
Tissue Perfusion, Ineffective Peripheral
Tissue Perfusion, Risk for Decreased Cardiac
Tissue Perfusion, Risk for Ineffective Cerebral
Tissue Perfusion, Risk for Ineffective Peripheral
Transfer Ability, Impaired
Trauma, Risk for
Unilateral Neglect
Urinary Retention
Ventilatory Weaning Response, Dysfunctional
Verbal Communication, Impaired
Walking, Impaired
Wandering

# Laboratory Reference Intervals

The tables in this appendix list some of the most common tests, their reference intervals (formally referred to as *normal values*), and possible etiologies of abnormal results. Laboratory results may vary depending on different techniques or different laboratories. Possible etiologies are presented in alphabetic order. Abbreviations appearing in the tables are defined as follows:

mEq = milliequivalent
mm Hg = millimeter of mercury
mm = millimeter
mOsm = milliosmole
L = liter
dL = deciliter ($10^{-1}$ liter)
mL = milliliter ($10^{-3}$ liter)
μL = microliter ($10^{-6}$ liter, $10^{-3}$ milliliter)
fL = femtoliter ($10^{-15}$ liter, $10^{-12}$ milliliter)
g = gram
mg = milligram ($10^{-3}$ gram)
mcg = microgram ($10^{-6}$ gram)
ng = nanogram ($10^{-9}$ gram)
pg = picogram ($10^{-12}$ gram)
U = unit
μU = microunit
IU = international unit
mmol = millimole ($10^{-3}$ mole)
μmol = micromole ($10^{-6}$ mole)
nmol = nanomole ($10^{-9}$ mole)
pmol = picomole ($10^{-12}$ mole)
kPa = kilopascal
μkat = microkatal

Source: Burtis CA, Ashwood ER, Bruns DE: *Tietz textbook of clinical chemistry and molecular diagnostics,* ed 5, St Louis, 2013, Elsevier.

## TABLE C-1 Serum, Plasma, and Whole Blood Chemistries

| | REFERENCE INTERVALS | | POSSIBLE ETIOLOGY | |
|---|---|---|---|---|
| **Test** | **Conventional Units** | **SI Units** | **Higher** | **Lower** |
| Acetone | | | Diabetic ketoacidosis, high-fat diet, low-carbohydrate diet, starvation | |
| • Quantitative | <2.0 mg/dL | <344 μmol/L | | |
| • Qualitative | Negative | Negative | | |
| Albumin | 3.5-5.0 g/dL | 35-50 g/L | Dehydration | Chronic liver disease, malabsorption, malnutrition, nephrotic syndrome |
| Aldolase | 1.5-8.1 U/L | 1.5-8.1 U/L | Skeletal muscle disease | Renal disease |
| $\alpha_1$-Antitrypsin | 78-200 mg/dL | 0.78-2.0 g/L | Acute and chronic inflammation, arthritis | Chronic lung disease (early onset), malnutrition, nephrotic syndrome |
| $\alpha_1$-Fetoprotein | <10 ng/mL | <10 mcg/L | Cancer of testes, ovaries, and liver | |
| Ammonia | 15-45 mcg N/dL | 11-32 μmol N/L | Severe liver disease | |
| Amylase | 30-122 U/L (method dependent) | 0.51-2.07 μkat/L | Acute and chronic pancreatitis, mumps (salivary gland disease), perforated ulcers | Acute alcoholism, cirrhosis of liver, extensive destruction of pancreas |
| Bicarbonate | 22-26 mEq/L | 22-26 mmol/L | Compensated respiratory acidosis, metabolic alkalosis | Compensated respiratory alkalosis, metabolic acidosis |
| b-Type natriuretic peptide (BNP) | <100 pg/mL | <100 pmol/L | Heart failure | |
| Bilirubin | | | Biliary obstruction, impaired liver function, hemolytic anemia, pernicious anemia | |
| • Total | 0.2-1.2 mg/dL | 3-21 μmol/L | | |
| • Indirect | 0.1-1.0 mg/dL | 1.7-17.0 μmol/L | | |
| • Direct | 0.1-0.3 mg/dL | 1.7-5.1 μmol/L | | |

*Continued*

## TABLE C-1 Serum, Plasma, and Whole Blood Chemistries—cont'd

| | REFERENCE INTERVALS | | POSSIBLE ETIOLOGY | |
|---|---|---|---|---|
| **Test** | **Conventional Units** | **SI Units** | **Higher** | **Lower** |
| Blood gases* | | | | |
| • Arterial pH | 7.35-7.45 | 7.35-7.45 | Alkalosis | Acidosis |
| • Venous pH | 7.32-7.43 | 7.32-7.43 | | |
| • $PaCO_2$ | 35-45 mm Hg | 4.66-5.98 kPa | Compensated metabolic alkalosis | Compensated metabolic acidosis |
| • $PvCO_2$ | 38-55 mm Hg | 5.06-7.32 kPa | Respiratory acidosis | Respiratory alkalosis |
| • $PaO_2$ | 80-100 mm Hg | 10.6-13.33 kPa | Administration of high concentration of oxygen | Chronic lung disease, decreased cardiac output |
| • $PvO_2$ | 38-42 mm Hg | 5.04-5.57 kPa | | |
| Calcium (total) | 8.6-10.2 mg/dL | 2.15-2.55 mmol/L | Acute osteoporosis, hyperparathyroidism, vitamin D intoxication, multiple myeloma | Acute pancreatitis, hypoparathyroidism, liver disease, malabsorption syndrome, renal failure, vitamin D deficiency |
| Calcium (ionized) | 4.64-5.28 mg/dL | 1.16-1.32 mmol/L | | |
| $CO_2$ | 23-29 mEq/L | 23-29 mmol/L | Same as bicarbonate | |
| Carotene | 10-85 mcg/dL | 0.19-1.58 µmol/L | Cystic fibrosis, hypothyroidism, pancreatic insufficiency | Dietary deficiency, malabsorption disorders |
| Chloride | 96-106 mEq/L | 96-106 mmol/L | Metabolic acidosis, respiratory alkalosis, corticosteroid therapy, uremia | Addison's disease, diarrhea, metabolic alkalosis, respiratory acidosis, vomiting |
| Cholesterol | <200 mg/dL | <5.2 mmol/L | Biliary obstruction, hypothyroidism, idiopathic hypercholesterolemia, renal disease, uncontrolled diabetes | Extensive liver disease, hyperthyroidism, malnutrition, corticosteroid therapy |
| • High-density lipoproteins (HDLs) | *Male:* >40 mg/dL<br>*Female:* >50 mg/dL | >1.04 mmol/L<br>>1.3 mmol/L | | |
| • Low-density lipoproteins (LDLs) | *Recommended:* <100 mg/dL<br>*Near optimal:* 100-129 mg/dL (2.6-3.34 mmol/L)<br>*Moderate risk for CAD:* 130-159 mg/dL (3.37-4.12 mmol/L)<br>*High risk for CAD:* >160 mg/dL (>4.14 mmol/L) | *Recommended:* <2.6 mmol/L<br>*Near optimal:* 2.6-3.34 mmol/L<br>*Moderate risk for CAD:* 3.37-4.12 mmol/L<br>*High risk for CAD:* >4.14 mmol/L | | |
| Copper | 80-155 mcg/dL | 12.6-24.3 µmol/L | Cirrhosis | Wilson's disease |
| Cortisol | 8 AM: 5-23 mcg/dL<br>8 PM: <10 mcg/dL | 0.14-0.63 µmol/L<br><0.28 µmol/L | Cushing syndrome, pancreatitis | Adrenal insufficiency, panhypopituitary states |
| Creatine | 0.2-1.0 mg/dL | 15.3-76.3 µmol/L | Active rheumatoid arthritis, biliary obstruction, hyperthyroidism, renal disorders, severe muscle disease | Diabetes mellitus |
| Creatine kinase (CK) | *Male:* 20-200 U/L<br>*Female:* 20-180 U/L | *Male:* 20-200 U/L<br>*Female:* 20-180 U/L | Musculoskeletal injury or disease, myocardial infarction, severe myocarditis, exercise, numerous IM injections | |
| • CK-MB | <4%-6% of total CK | <0.4-0.6 | Acute myocardial infarction | |
| Creatinine | 0.6-1.3 mg/dL | 53-115 µmol/L | Severe renal disease | |
| Ferritin | 10-250 ng/mL | 10-250 mcg/L | Sideroblastic anemia, anemia of chronic disease (infection, inflammation, liver disease) | Iron-deficiency anemia |
| Folate (folic acid) | 3-16 ng/mL | 7-36 nmol/L | Hypothyroidism | Alcoholism, hemolytic anemia, inadequate diet, malabsorption syndrome, megaloblastic anemia |
| Gamma glutamyl transferase (GGT) | 0-30 U/L | 0-0.5 µkat/L | Liver disease, infectious mononucleosis, pancreatitis, hyperthyroidism | Hypothyroidism |
| Glucose (fasting) | 70-99 mg/dL | 3.9-5.5 mmol/L | Acute stress, Cushing disease, diabetes mellitus, hyperthyroidism, pancreatic insufficiency | Addison's disease, hepatic disease, hypothyroidism, insulin overdosage, pancreatic tumor, pituitary hypofunction |

*$PaCO_2$*, Partial pressure of $CO_2$ in arterial blood; *$PaO_2$*, partial pressure of oxygen in arterial blood; *$PvCO_2$*, partial pressure of $CO_2$ in venous blood; *$PvO_2$*, partial pressure of oxygen in venous blood.

*Because arterial blood gases are influenced by altitude, the value for $PaO_2$ decreases as altitude increases. The lower value is normal for an altitude of 1 mile.

**TABLE C-1 Serum, Plasma, and Whole Blood Chemistries—cont'd**

| | REFERENCE INTERVALS | | POSSIBLE ETIOLOGY | |
|---|---|---|---|---|
| **Test** | **Conventional Units** | **SI Units** | **Higher** | **Lower** |
| Haptoglobin | 26-185 mg/dL | 260-1850 mg/L | Infectious and inflammatory processes, cancer | Hemolytic anemia, mononucleosis, toxoplasmosis, chronic liver disease |
| Insulin (fasting) | 4-24 μU/mL | 29-172 pmol/L | Acromegaly, adenoma of pancreatic islet cells, untreated mild case of type 2 diabetes | Inadequately treated type 1 diabetes mellitus |
| Iron, total | 50-175 mcg/dL | 9.0-31.3 μmol/L | Excessive RBC destruction | Iron-deficiency anemia, anemia of chronic disease |
| Iron-binding capacity | 250-425 mcg/dL | 44.8-76.1 μmol/L | Iron-deficient state, polycythemia | Cancer, chronic infections, pernicious anemia |
| Lactic acid (L-Lactate) | 6.3-22.5 mcg/dL | 0.7-2.5 mmol/L | Acidosis, heart failure, shock | |
| Lactic dehydrogenase (LDH) | 140-280 U/L | 0.83-2.5 μkat/L | Heart failure, hemolytic disorders, hepatitis, metastatic cancer of liver, myocardial infarction, pernicious anemia, pulmonary embolus, skeletal muscle damage | |
| Lactic dehydrogenase isoenzymes | | | | |
| • $LDH_1$ | 18%-33% | 0.18-0.33 | Myocardial infarction, pernicious anemia | |
| • $LDH_2$ | 28%-40% | 0.28-0.40 | Pulmonary embolus, sickle cell crisis | |
| • $LDH_3$ | 18%-30% | 0.18-0.30 | Malignant lymphoma, pulmonary embolus | |
| • $LDH_4$ | 6%-16% | 0.06-0.16 | Systemic lupus erythematosus, pulmonary infarction | |
| • $LDH_5$ | 2%-13% | 0.02-0.13 | Heart failure, hepatitis, pulmonary embolus and infarction, skeletal muscle damage | |
| Lipase | 31-186 U/L | 0.5-3.2 μkat/L | Acute pancreatitis, hepatic disorders, perforated peptic ulcer | |
| Magnesium | 1.5-2.5 mEq/L | 0.75-1.25 mmol/L | Addison's disease, hypothyroidism, renal failure | Chronic alcoholism, severe malabsorption |
| Osmolality | 275-295 mOsm/kg | 275-295 mmol/kg | Chronic renal disease, diabetes mellitus | Addison's disease, diuretic therapy |
| $O_2$ saturation (arterial) ($SaO_2$) | >95% | >0.95 | Polycythemia | Anemia, cardiac decompensation, respiratory disorders |
| pH | See Blood gases | | | |
| Phenylalanine | 0.8-1.8 mg/dL | 48-109 μmol/L | Phenylketonuria | |
| Phosphatase, acid | 0-0.6 U/L | 0-90 μkat/L | Advanced Paget's disease, cancer of prostate, hyperparathyroidism | |
| Phosphatase, alkaline | 38-126 U/L | 0.65-2.14 μkat/L | Bone diseases, marked hyperparathyroidism, obstruction of biliary system, rickets | Excessive vitamin D ingestion, hypothyroidism |
| Phosphorus (phosphate) | 2.4-4.4 mg/dL | 0.78-1.42 mmol/L | Healing fractures, hypoparathyroidism, renal disease, vitamin D intoxication | Diabetes mellitus, hyperparathyroidism, vitamin D deficiency |
| Potassium | 3.5-5.0 mEq/L | 3.5-5.0 mmol/L | Addison's disease, diabetic ketosis, massive tissue destruction, renal failure | Cushing syndrome, diarrhea (severe), diuretic therapy, gastrointestinal fistula, pyloric obstruction, starvation, vomiting |
| Progesterone (female) | | | | |
| • Follicular phase | 15-70 ng/dL | 0.5-2.2 nmol/L | Adrenal hyperplasia, choriocarcinoma of ovary, pregnancy, cysts of ovary | Threatened abortion, hypogonadism, amenorrhea, ovarian tumor |
| • Luteal phase | 200-2500 ng/dL | 6.4-79.5 nmol/L | | |
| • Postmenopause | <40 ng/dL | 1.28 nmol/L | | |

*RBC*, red blood cell; *$SaO_2$*, arterial oxygen saturation.

*Continued*

## TABLE C-1 Serum, Plasma, and Whole Blood Chemistries—cont'd

| | REFERENCE INTERVALS | | POSSIBLE ETIOLOGY | |
|---|---|---|---|---|
| **Test** | **Conventional Units** | **SI Units** | **Higher** | **Lower** |
| Prostate-specific antigen (PSA) | <4 ng/mL | <4 mcg/L | Prostate cancer | |
| Proteins | | | Burns, cirrhosis (globulin fraction), dehydration | Liver disease, malabsorption |
| • Total | 6.4-8.3 g/dL | 64-83 g/L | | |
| • Albumin | 3.5-5.0 g/dL | 35-50 g/L | | |
| • Globulin | 2.0-3.5 g/dL | 20-35 g/L | | |
| • Albumin/globulin ratio | 1.5:1-2.5:1 | 1.5:1-2.5:1 | Multiple myeloma (globulin fraction), shock, vomiting | Malnutrition, nephrotic syndrome, proteinuria, renal disease, severe burns |
| Sodium | 135-145 mEq/L | 135-145 mmol/L | Dehydration, impaired renal function, primary aldosteronism, corticosteroid therapy | Addison's disease, diabetic ketoacidosis, diuretic therapy, excessive loss from GI tract, excessive perspiration, water intoxication |
| Testosterone | *Male:* 280-1100 ng/dL | *Male:* 10.4-38.17 nmol/L | | Hypofunction of testes, hypogonadism |
| | *Female:* 15-70 ng/dL | *Female:* 0.52-2.43 nmol/L | Polycystic ovary, virilizing tumors | |
| $T_4$ (thyroxine), total | 4.6-11.0 mcg/dL | 59-142 nmol/L | Hyperthyroidism, thyroiditis | Cretinism, hypothyroidism, myxedema |
| $T_4$ (thyroxine), free | 0.8-2.7 ng/dL | 10-35 pmol/L | | |
| $T_3$ uptake | 24%-34% | 0.24-0.34 | Hyperthyroidism | Hypothyroidism |
| $T_3$ (triiodothyronine), total | *Age 20-50:* 70-204 ng/dL<br>*Age >50:* 40-181 ng/dL | 1.08-3.14 nmol/L<br>0.62-2.79 nmol/L | Hyperthyroidism | Hypothyroidism |
| Thyroid-stimulating hormone (TSH) | 0.4-4.2 μU/mL | 0.4-4.2 mU/L | Myxedema, primary hypothyroidism, Graves' disease | Secondary hypothyroidism |
| Transaminases | | | | |
| • Aspartate aminotransferase (AST) | 10-30 U/L | 0.17-0.51 μkat/L | Liver disease, myocardial infarction, pulmonary infarction, acute hepatitis | |
| • Alanine aminotransferase (ALT) | 10-40 U/L | 0.17-0.68 μkat/L | Liver disease, shock | |
| Transferrin | 190-380 mg/dL | 1.9-3.8 g/L | | |
| Transferrin saturation (%) | 15%-50% | 15%-50% | | |
| Triglycerides | <150 mg/dL | <1.7 mmol/L | Diabetes mellitus, hyperlipidemia, hypothyroidism, liver disease | Malnutrition |
| Troponins (cardiac) | | | Myocardial infarction | |
| • Troponin T (cTnT) | <0.1 ng/mL (<0.5 mcg/L) | | | |
| • Troponin I (cTnI) | <0.5 ng/mL (<0.1 mcg/L) | | | |
| Urea nitrogen (BUN) | 6-20 mg/dL | 2.1-7.1 mmol/L | Increase in protein catabolism (fever, stress), renal disease, urinary tract infection | Malnutrition, severe liver damage |
| Uric acid | *Male:* 4.4-7.6 mg/dL<br>*Female:* 2.3-6.6 mg/dL | *Male:* 262-452 μmol/L<br>*Female:* 137-393 μmol/L | Gout, gross tissue destruction, high-protein weight reduction diet, leukemia, renal failure | Administration of uricosuric drugs |
| Vitamin A (retinol) | 30-80 mcg/dL | 1.05-2.80 μmol/L | Excess ingestion of vitamin A | Vitamin A deficiency |
| Vitamin $B_{12}$ (cobalamin) | 200-835 pg/mL | 148-616 pmol/L | Chronic myeloid leukemia | Strict vegetarianism, malabsorption syndrome, pernicious anemia, total or partial gastrectomy |
| Vitamin C (ascorbic acid) | 0.4-2.0 mg/dL | 23-114 μmol/L | Excessive ingestion of vitamin C | Connective tissue disorders, hepatic disease, renal disease, rheumatic fever, vitamin C deficiency |
| Zinc | 70-120 mcg/dL | 10.7-120 μmol/L | | Alcoholic cirrhosis |

## TABLE C-2 Hematology

| | REFERENCE INTERVALS | | POSSIBLE ETIOLOGY | |
|---|---|---|---|---|
| **Test** | **Conventional Units** | **SI Units** | **Higher** | **Lower** |
| Bleeding time | 2-7 min | 120-420 sec | Defective platelet function, thrombocytopenia, von Willebrand disease, aspirin ingestion, vascular disease | |
| Activated partial thromboplastin time (aPTT) | 25-35 sec* | 25-35 sec* | Deficiency factors I, II, V, VIII, IX, X, XI, XII; hemophilia, liver disease; heparin therapy | |
| Prothrombin time (Protime, PT) | 11-16 sec* | 11-16 sec* | Warfarin therapy; deficiency of factors I, II, V, VII, and X; vitamin K deficiency; liver disease | |
| Fibrinogen | 200-400 mg/dL | 2-4 g/L | Burns (after first 36 hr), inflammatory disease | Burns (during first 36 hr), DIC, severe liver disease |
| Fibrin split (degradation) products | <10 mcg/mL | <10 mg/L | Acute DIC, massive hemorrhage, primary fibrinolysis | |
| D-Dimer | <250 ng/mL | <250 mcg/L | DIC, myocardial infarction, deep vein thrombosis, unstable angina | |
| Erythrocyte count† (altitude dependent) | *Male:* 4.3-5.7 × $10^6$/μL<br>*Female:* 3.8-5.1 × $10^6$/μL | *Male:* 4.3-5.7 × $10^{12}$/L<br>*Female:* 3.8-5.1 × $10^{12}$/L | Dehydration, high altitudes, polycythemia vera | Anemia, leukemia, posthemorrhage |
| Red blood indices | | | | |
| • Mean corpuscular volume (MCV) | 80-100 fL | 80-100 fL | Macrocytic anemia | Microcytic anemia |
| • Mean corpuscular hemoglobin (MCH) | 27-34 pg | 27-34 pg | Macrocytic anemia | Microcytic anemia |
| • Mean corpuscular hemoglobin concentration (MCHC) | 32%-37% | 0.32-0.37 | Spherocytosis | Hypochromic anemia |
| Erythrocyte sedimentation rate (ESR) | <30 mm/hr (some gender variation) | <30 mm/hr (some gender variation) | *Moderate increase:* acute hepatitis, myocardial infarction; rheumatoid arthritis<br>*Marked increase:* acute and severe bacterial infections, cancer, pelvic inflammatory disease | Malaria, severe liver disease, sickle cell anemia |
| Hematocrit† (altitude dependent) | *Male:* 39%-50%<br>*Female:* 35%-47% | *Male:* 0.39-0.50<br>*Female:* 0.35-0.47 | Dehydration, high altitudes, polycythemia | Anemia, hemorrhage, overhydration |
| Hemoglobin† (altitude dependent) | *Male:* 13.2-17.3 g/dL<br>*Female:* 11.7-15.5 g/dL | *Male:* 132-173 g/L<br>*Female:* 117-155 g/L | COPD, high altitudes, polycythemia | Anemia, hemorrhage |
| Hemoglobin, glycosylated (A1C) | 4.0%-6.0% | 4.0%-6.0% | Poorly controlled diabetes mellitus | Sickle cell anemia, chronic renal failure, pregnancy |
| Platelets (thrombocytes) | 150-400 × $10^3$/μL | 150-400 × $10^9$/L | Acute infections, chronic granulocytic leukemia, chronic pancreatitis, cirrhosis, collagen disorders, polycythemia, postsplenectomy | Acute leukemia, DIC, thrombocytopenic purpura |
| Reticulocyte count | 0.5%-1.5% of RBC | 0.5%-1.5% of RBC | Hemolytic anemia, polycythemia vera | Hypoproliferative anemia, macrocytic anemia, microcytic anemia |
| White blood cell count† | 4.0-11.0 × $10^3$/μL | 4.0-11.0 × $10^9$/L | Inflammatory and infectious processes, leukemia | Aplastic anemia, side effects of chemotherapy and irradiation |
| WBC differential | | | | |
| • Segmented neutrophils | 50%-70% | 0.50-0.70 | Bacterial infections, connective tissue diseases, Hodgkin's lymphoma | Aplastic anemia, viral infections |
| • Band neutrophils | 0-8% | 0-0.08 | Acute infections | |
| • Lymphocytes | 20%-40% | 0.20-0.40 | Chronic infections, lymphocytic leukemia, mononucleosis, viral infections | Corticosteroid therapy, whole body irradiation |
| • Monocytes | 4%-8% | 0.04-0.08 | Chronic inflammatory disorders, malaria, monocytic leukemia, acute infections, Hodgkin's lymphoma | |
| • Eosinophils | 0-4% | 0-0.04 | Allergic reactions, eosinophilic and chronic granulocytic leukemia, parasitic disorders, Hodgkin's lymphoma | Corticosteroid therapy |
| • Basophils | 0-2% | 0-0.02 | Hypothyroidism, ulcerative colitis, myeloproliferative diseases | Hyperthyroidism, stress |

*COPD,* Chronic obstructive pulmonary disease; *DIC,* disseminated intravascular coagulation.
*Values depend on reagent and instrumentation used.
†Components of complete blood count (CBC).

TABLE C-3 **Serology-Immunology**

| | REFERENCE INTERVALS | | POSSIBLE ETIOLOGY | |
|---|---|---|---|---|
| **Test** | **Conventional Units** | **SI Units** | **Higher** | **Lower** |
| Antinuclear antibody (ANA) | Negative at 1:40 dilution | Negative at 1:40 dilution | Chronic hepatitis, rheumatoid arthritis, scleroderma, systemic lupus erythematosus | |
| Anti-DNA antibody | <70 IU/mL | <70 IU/mL | Systemic lupus erythematosus | |
| Anti-Sm (Smith) | Negative | Negative | Systemic lupus erythematosus | |
| C-reactive protein (CRP) | 6.8-820 mcg/dL | 68-8200 mcg/L | Acute infections, any inflammatory condition, widespread cancer | |
| Carcinoembryonic antigen (CEA) | *Nonsmoker:* <3 ng/mL<br>*Smoker:* <5 ng/mL | *Nonsmoker:* <3 mcg/L<br>*Smoker:* <5 mcg/L | Carcinoma of colon, liver, pancreas; chronic cigarette smoking; inflammatory bowel disease; other cancers | |
| Complement, total hemolytic ($CH_{50}$) | 75-160 U/mL | 75-160 kU/L | | Acute glomerulonephritis, systemic lupus erythematosus, rheumatoid arthritis, subacute bacterial endocarditis |
| Direct Coombs or direct antihuman globulin test (DAT) | Negative | Negative | Acquired hemolytic anemia, drug reactions, transfusion reactions | |
| Fluorescent treponemal antibody absorption (FTA-Abs) | Negative or nonreactive | Negative or nonreactive | Syphilis | |
| Hepatitis A antibody | Negative | Negative | Hepatitis A | |
| Hepatitis B surface antigen ($HB_sAg$) | Negative | Negative | Hepatitis B | |
| Hepatitis C antibody | Negative | Negative | Hepatitis C | |
| Monospot or monotest | Negative | Negative | Infectious mononucleosis | |
| Rheumatoid factor (RF) | Negative or titer <1:17 | Negative or titer <1:17 | Rheumatoid arthritis, Sjögren's syndrome, systemic lupus erythematosus | |
| RPR | Negative or nonreactive | Negative or nonreactive | Syphilis, systemic lupus erythematosus, rheumatoid arthritis, leprosy, malaria, febrile diseases, IV drug abuse | |
| VDRL | Negative or nonreactive | Negative or nonreactive | Syphilis | |

*RPR*, Rapid plasma reagin test; *VDRL*, Venereal Disease Research Laboratory.

## TABLE C-4 Urine Chemistry

| | | REFERENCE INTERVALS | | POSSIBLE ETIOLOGY | |
|---|---|---|---|---|---|
| **Test** | **Specimen** | **Units** | **SI Units** | **Higher** | **Lower** |
| Acetone | Random | Negative | Negative | Diabetes mellitus, high-fat and low-carbohydrate diets, starvation | |
| Aldosterone | 24 hr | 3-30 mcg/day (low-sodium diet increases threefold to fivefold) | 0.08-0.83 nmol/day | *Primary aldosteronism:* adrenocortical tumors<br>*Secondary aldosteronism:* cardiac failure, cirrhosis, large dose of ACTH, salt depletion | ACTH deficiency, Addison's disease, corticosteroid therapy |
| Amylase | 24 hr | 1-17 U/hr | 1-17 U/hr | Acute pancreatitis | |
| Bence Jones protein | Random | Negative | Negative | Multiple myeloma | |
| Bilirubin | Random | Negative | Negative | Liver disorders | |
| Calcium | 24 hr | 100-250 mg/day | 2.5-6.3 mmol/day | Bone tumor, hyperparathyroidism | Hypoparathyroidism, malabsorption of calcium and vitamin D |
| Catecholamines | 24 hr | | | Pheochromocytoma, progressive muscular dystrophy, heart failure | |
| • Epinephrine | | <20 mcg/day | <109 nmol/day | | |
| • Norepinephrine | | 15-80 mcg/day | 89-473 nmol/day | | |
| Creatine | 24 hr | <100 mg/day | <763 μmol/day | Liver cancer, hyperthyroidism, diabetes, Addison's disease, infections, burns, muscular dystrophy, skeletal muscle atrophy | Hypothyroidism |
| Creatinine | 24 hr | 0.6-2.0 g/day | 5.3-17.7 mmol/day | Anemia, leukemia, muscular atrophy | Renal disease |
| Creatinine clearance | 24 hr | 59-137 mL/min/1.73 $m^2$ | 0.59-1.37 mL/sec/$m^2$ | | Renal disease |
| Estrogens | 24 hr | | | | |
| • Female | | | | Gonadal or adrenal tumor | Endocrine disturbance, ovarian dysfunction, menopause |
| • Premenopause | | 15-80 mcg/day | 15-80 mcg/day | | |
| • Postmenopause | | <20 mcg/day | <20 mcg/day | | |
| • Male | | 15-40 mcg/day | 15-40 mcg/day | | |
| Glucose | Random | Negative | Negative | Diabetes mellitus, pituitary disorders | |
| Hemoglobin | Random | Negative | Negative | Extensive burns, glomerulonephritis, hemolytic anemias, hemolytic transfusion reaction | |
| 5-Hydroxyindole acetic acid (5-HIAA) | 24 hr | 2-7 mg/day | 10.5-36.6 μmol/day | Malignant carcinoid syndrome | |
| Ketone bodies | 24 hr | 20-50 mg/day | 0.34-0.86 mmol/day | Diabetes mellitus, starvation, dehydration | |
| Metanephrine | 24 hr | 92-934 mcg/day | 500-5100 nmol/day | Pheochromocytoma | |
| Myoglobin | Random | Negative | Negative | Crushing injuries, electric injuries, extreme physical exertion | |
| Osmolality | Random | 300-1300 mOsm/kg | 300-1300 mmol/kg | Dehydration, tubular dysfunction (kidney lost ability to dilute urine) | Tubular dysfunction (kidney lost ability to concentrate urine) |
| pH | Random | 4.0-8.0 | 4.0-8.0 | Urinary tract infection, urine allowed to stand at room temperature | Respiratory or metabolic acidosis |
| Protein (dipstick) | Random | 0-trace | 0-trace | Acute and chronic renal disease, especially involving glomeruli; heart failure | |
| Protein (quantitative) | 24 hr | <150 mg/day | <0.15 g/day | Cardiac failure, inflammatory processes of urinary tract, nephritis, nephrosis, strenuous exercise | |
| Sodium | 24 hr | 40-220 mEq/day | 40-220 mmol/day | Acute tubular necrosis | Hyponatremia |
| Specific gravity | Random | 1.003-1.030 | Same as conventional units | Albuminuria, dehydration, glycosuria | Diabetes insipidus |
| Uric acid | 24 hr | 250-750 mg/day | 1.5-4.5 mmol/day | Gout, leukemia | Nephritis |
| Urobilinogen | 24 hr | 0.5-4.0 mg/day | 0.8-6.8 μmol/day | Hemolytic disease, hepatic parenchymal cell damage, liver disease | Complete obstruction of bile duct |
| Vanillylmandelic acid | 24 hr | 1.4-6.5 mg/day | 7-33 μmol/day | Pheochromocytoma | |

*ACTH,* Adrenocorticotropic hormone.

**TABLE C-5 Fecal Analysis**

| | REFERENCE INTERVALS | | POSSIBLE ETIOLOGY |
|---|---|---|---|
| **Test** | **Conventional Units** | **SI Units** | **Higher** |
| Fecal fat | <6 g/24 hr | Same as conventional units | Chronic pancreatic disease, obstruction of common bile duct, malabsorption syndrome |
| Mucus | Negative | Negative | Mucous colitis, spastic constipation |
| Pus | Negative | Negative | Chronic bacillary dysentery, chronic ulcerative colitis, localized abscesses |
| Blood* | Negative | Negative | Anal fissures, hemorrhoids, malignant tumor, peptic ulcer, inflammatory bowel disease |
| Color | | | |
| • Brown | | | Various color depending on diet |
| • Clay | | | Biliary obstruction or presence of barium sulfate |
| • Tarry | | | More than 100 mL of blood in gastrointestinal tract |
| • Red | | | Blood in large intestine |
| • Black | | | Blood in upper gastrointestinal tract or iron medication |

*Ingestion of meat may produce false-positive results. Patient may be placed on a meat-free diet for 3 days before the test.

**TABLE C-6 Cerebrospinal Fluid Analysis**

| | REFERENCE INTERVALS | | POSSIBLE ETIOLOGY | |
|---|---|---|---|---|
| **Test** | **Conventional Units** | **SI Units** | **Higher** | **Lower** |
| Pressure | 60-150 mm $H_2O$ | 60-150 mm $H_2O$ | Hemorrhage, intracranial tumor, meningitis | Head injury, spinal tumor, subdural hematoma |
| Blood | Negative | Negative | Intracranial hemorrhage | |
| Cell count (age dependent) | | | Inflammation or infections of CNS | |
| • WBC | 0-5 cells/μL | 0-5 × $10^6$ cells/L | | |
| • RBC | Negative | Negative | | |
| Chloride | 118-132 mEq/L | 118-132 mmol/L | Uremia | Bacterial infections of CNS (meningitis, encephalitis) |
| Glucose | 40-70 mg/dL | 2.2-3.9 mmol/L | Diabetes mellitus, viral infections of CNS | Bacterial infections and tuberculosis of CNS |
| Protein | | | | |
| • Lumbar | 15-45 mg/dL | 0.15-0.45 g/L | Guillain-Barré syndrome, poliomyelitis, trauma | |
| • Cisternal | 15-25 mg/dL | 0.15-0.25 g/L | Syphilis of CNS | |
| • Ventricular | 5-15 mg/dL | 0.05-0.15 g/L | Acute meningitis, brain tumor, chronic CNS infections, multiple sclerosis | |

*CNS,* Central nervous system.

## A

**acromegaly** a condition caused by excessive secretion of growth hormone characterized by an overgrowth of the bones and soft tissues.

**actinic keratosis** a slowly developing, localized thickening and scaling of the outer layers of the skin consisting of hyperkeratotic papules and plaques as a result of chronic, prolonged exposure to the sun; also known as *solar keratosis.*

**acute bronchitis** an inflammation of the lower respiratory tract that is usually due to infection.

**acute kidney injury (AKI)** clinical syndrome characterized by a rise in serum creatinine and/or a reduction in urine output.

**acute pancreatitis** an acute inflammatory process of the pancreas caused by autodigestion and marked by symptoms of an acute condition of the abdomen and spillage of pancreatic enzymes into surrounding pancreatic tissues.

**acute respiratory distress syndrome (ARDS)** a sudden and progressive form of acute respiratory failure in which the alveolar-capillary membrane becomes damaged and more permeable to intravascular fluid.

**acute tubular necrosis (ATN)** a type of intrarenal acute injury of the kidney that affects the renal tubules, caused by renal ischemia and nephrotoxic injury.

**adhesion** a band of scar tissue between or around organs.

**adventitious sounds** extra breath sounds that are not normally heard, such as crackles, wheezes, and pleural friction rubs.

**afterload** the peripheral resistance against which the left ventricle must pump.

**allergic rhinitis** the reaction of the nasal mucosa to a specific allergen.

**alopecia** partial or complete lack of hair resulting from normal aging, endocrine disorder, drug reaction, chemotherapy, or skin disease.

**Alzheimer's disease (AD)** a chronic, progressive, neurodegenerative disease of the brain.

**amyotrophic lateral sclerosis (ALS)** a rare progressive neuromuscular disorder characterized by loss of motor neurons and by weakness and atrophy of the muscles of the hands, forearms, and legs, spreading to involve most of the body and face.

**anaphylactic shock** an acute and life-threatening hypersensitivity (allergic) reaction to a sensitizing substance, such as a drug, chemical, vaccine, food, or insect venom.

**aneurysm** congenital or acquired weakness of the arterial wall resulting in dilation and ballooning of the vessel.

**angina** chest pain that is a clinical manifestation of reversible myocardial ischemia.

**ankylosing spondylitis** a chronic inflammatory disease that primarily affects the axial skeleton, including the sacroiliac joints, intervertebral disc spaces, and costovertebral articulations.

**ankylosis** stiffness or fixation of a joint usually resulting from destruction of articular cartilage and subchondral bone.

**aortic dissection** the result of a tear in the intimal (innermost) lining of the arterial wall that allows blood to enter between the intima and media, thus creating a false lumen.

**aphasia** an abnormal neurologic condition in which language function is disordered or absent because of an injury to certain areas of the cerebral cortex.

**aplastic anemia** a disease with a deficiency of all of the formed elements of blood (specifically red blood cells, white blood cells, and platelets), representing a failure of the cell-generating capacity of bone marrow.

**appendicitis** an inflammation of the appendix that, if undiagnosed, leads rapidly to perforation and peritonitis.

**arterial blood pressure** a measure of the pressure exerted by blood against the walls of the arterial system.

**arteriovenous fistula (AVF)** type of vascular access created most commonly in the forearm with an anastomosis between an artery (usually radial or ulnar) and a vein (usually cephalic).

**arteriovenous grafts (AVGs)** fistula made of synthetic materials that forms a "bridge" between the arterial and venous blood supplies.

**arthritis** inflammation of a joint; most prevalent types are osteoarthritis, rheumatoid arthritis, and gout.

**arthrocentesis** incision or puncture of joint capsule to obtain samples of synovial fluid from within joint cavity or to remove excess fluid.

**arthrodesis** the surgical fusion of a joint.

**arthroplasty** surgical reconstruction or replacement of a joint.

**arthroscopy** insertion of an arthroscope into a joint for visualization or surgery.

**ascites** an abnormal intraperitoneal accumulation of a fluid containing large amounts of protein and electrolytes as a result of portal hypertension.

**asterixis** flapping tremor commonly affecting the arms and hands that is a manifestation of hepatic encephalopathy.

**asthma** a chronic inflammatory lung disease that results in airflow obstruction; characterized by recurring episodes of paroxysmal dyspnea, wheezing on expiration and/or inspiration caused by constriction of the bronchi, coughing, and viscous mucoid bronchial secretions.

**asystole** represents the total absence of ventricular electrical activity.

**atherosclerosis** formation of focal deposits of cholesterol and lipids known as *atheromas* or *plaque,* primarily within the intimal wall of arteries, that obstruct circulation.

**atrial fibrillation** a cardiac dysrhythmia characterized by a total disorganization of atrial electrical activity without effective atrial contraction.

**atrial flutter** an atrial tachydysrhythmia identified by recurring, regular, sawtooth-shaped flutter waves.

**atrophy** wasting of muscle, characterized by decreased circumference and flabby appearance leading to decreased function and tone.

**aura** a sensation of light or warmth or other perception that may be a warning of an attack of a migraine or an epileptic seizure.

**auscultation** the act of listening for sounds within the body to evaluate the condition of the heart, blood vessels, lungs, pleura, intestines, or other organs.

**autoimmunity** an inappropriate immune reaction to self-proteins.

**azotemia** an accumulation of nitrogenous waste products such as blood urea nitrogen (BUN) and creatinine.

## B

**bariatric surgery** a surgical procedure on the stomach and/or intestines to help a person with extreme obesity lose weight.

**Barrett's esophagus** a precancerous esophageal disorder characterized by metaplastic cell changes.

**basal cell carcinoma** a malignant epithelial cell tumor arising from epidermal basal cells that begins as a papule and enlarges peripherally, developing a central crater that erodes, crusts, and bleeds.

**Bell's palsy** a disorder characterized by a disruption of the motor branches of the facial nerve (cranial nerve [CN] VII) on one side of the face in the absence of any other disease such as a stroke.

**benign prostatic hyperplasia (BPH)** a nonmalignant, noninflammatory enlargement of the prostate gland caused by an increase in the number of epithelial cells and stromal tissue.

**biologic therapy** treatment using biologic agents such as interferons, interleukins, monoclonal antibodies, and growth factors to modify the relationship between the host and tumor.

**borborygmi** audible abdominal sounds produced by hyperactive intestinal peristalsis.

**botulism** a rare but serious food poisoning caused by GI absorption of the neurotoxin produced by *Clostridium botulinum,* which results in disturbed muscle innervation.

**brachytherapy** radiation delivery system that means "closed" treatment and consists of the implantation or insertion of radioactive materials directly into the tumor or in close proximity to the tumor.

**brain attack** a stroke.

**bursitis** inflammation of the bursa.

## C

**calculus** an abnormal stone formed in body tissues by an accumulation of mineral salts.

**carcinogens** agents capable of producing cellular alterations leading to the development or increasing the incidence of neoplastic growth.

**carcinoma in situ** a lesion with all the histologic features of cancer except invasion.

**cardiac index (CI)** a measure of the cardiac output of a patient per square meter of body surface area.
**cardiac output (CO)** the amount of blood pumped by each ventricle in 1 minute.
**cardiac pacemaker** an electronic device used to increase the heart rate in severe bradycardia by electrically stimulating the heart muscle.
**cardiac reserve** the ability to respond to demands (exercise, stress, hypovolemia) by altering cardiac output threefold or fourfold.
**cardiac tamponade** compression of the heart produced by fluid accumulation in the pericardial sac.
**cardiogenic shock** shock occurring when either systolic or diastolic dysfunction of the myocardium results in compromised cardiac output.
**cardiomyopathy** a group of diseases that directly affect the structural or functional ability of the myocardium.
**carpal tunnel syndrome** a condition caused by compression of the median nerve beneath the transverse carpal ligament within the narrow confines of the carpal tunnel located in the wrist.
**cataract** an abnormal progressive condition of the lens of the eye characterized by an opacity within the lens.
**celiac disease** an inborn error of metabolism characterized by the inability to hydrolyze peptides contained in gluten.
**cell-mediated immunity** immunity that is initiated through specific antigen recognition by T lymphocytes, monocytes/macrophages, and natural killer cells.
**cellulitis** a diffuse, acute bacterial infection of the skin and subcutaneous tissue characterized most commonly by local heat, redness, pain, and swelling.
**central cord syndrome** damage to the central spinal cord characterized by microscopic hemorrhage, edema of the central spinal cord, and compression on anterior horn cells.
**cerebral edema** increased accumulation of fluid in the extravascular spaces of brain tissue that can lead to increased intracranial pressure.
**cheilosis** a disorder of the lips and mouth characterized by bilateral scales and fissures, resulting from a deficiency of riboflavin in the diet.
**chemotherapy** the treatment of disease with chemical agents.
**Cheyne-Stokes respiration** an abnormal breathing pattern characterized by alternating periods of apnea and deep, rapid breathing; usually seen as a person nears death.
**cholecystitis** inflammation of the gallbladder.
**cholelithiasis** stones in the gallbladder.
**chronic kidney disease (CKD)** progressive, irreversible loss of kidney function with either the presence of kidney damage or decreased glomerular filtration rate for at least 3 months.
**chronic kidney disease (CKD) mineral and bone disorder** a systemic disorder of mineral and bone metabolism due to progressive deterioration in kidney function.
**chronic pancreatitis** progressive destruction of the pancreas with fibrotic replacement of pancreatic tissue.
**chronic stable angina** chest pain that occurs intermittently over a long period with the same pattern of onset, duration, and intensity of symptoms.
**cirrhosis** end-stage liver disease characterized by extensive degeneration and destruction of the liver parenchymal cells.
**cluster headaches** repeated headaches that can occur as clusters, generally at the same time of day or night and followed by periods of remission.
**collateral circulation** development of arterial branching that occurs within the coronary circulation when occlusion of the coronary arteries occurs slowly over a long period.
**coma** a profound state of unconsciousness.
**community-acquired pneumonia (CAP)** a lower respiratory tract infection of the lung parenchyma with onset in the community or during the first 2 days of hospitalization.
**compartment syndrome** a condition in which elevated intracompartmental pressure within a confined myofascial compartment compromises the neurovascular function of tissues within that space.
**complete heart block** third-degree atrioventricular heart block in which no impulses from the atria are conducted to the ventricles.
**concussion** a sudden transient mechanical head injury, such as a blow or explosion, with disruption of neural activity and a change in the level of consciousness.
**continuous renal replacement therapy (CRRT)** provides a means by which uremic toxins and fluids can be removed slowly and continuously in the hemodynamically unstable patient.
**contracture** an abnormal, usually permanent condition of a joint, characterized by flexion and fixation.
**contusion** the bruising of the brain tissue within a focal area without altering the integrity of the pia mater and arachnoid layers.
**coronary artery disease (CAD)** an abnormal condition that may affect the heart's arteries and produce various pathologic effects, especially the reduced flow of oxygen and nutrients to the myocardium.
**cor pulmonale** hypertrophy of the right side of the heart, with or without heart failure, resulting from pulmonary hypertension.
**crackle** short, low-pitched sound consisting of discontinuous bubbling caused by air passing through the airway intermittently occluded by mucus, an unstable bronchial wall, or a fold of mucosa.
**crepitation** crackling sound or grating sensation as a result of friction between bones.
**cryosurgery** the use of subfreezing temperatures to perform surgery.
**curettage** scraping of material from the wall of a cavity or other surface; performed to remove tumors or other abnormal tissue or to obtain tissue.
**Cushing syndrome** a metabolic disorder resulting from the chronic and excessive production of cortisol by the adrenal cortex or by the administration of glucocorticoids in large doses for several weeks or longer.
**cystic fibrosis (CF)** an autosomal recessive, multisystem disease characterized by altered function of the exocrine glands involving primarily the lungs, pancreas, and sweat glands.
**cystitis** an inflammatory condition of the urinary bladder characterized by pain, urgency, frequency of urination, and hematuria.
**cystocele** herniation or protrusion of the urinary bladder through the wall of the vagina, resulting from weakened connective tissue support between the vagina and bladder.

## D

**death rattle** a sound produced by air moving through mucus that has accumulated in the throat of a dying person who has lost the cough reflex.
**debridement** removal of dirt, foreign objects, damaged tissue, and cellular debris from a wound or a burn to prevent infection and promote healing.
**deep vein thrombosis (DVT)** a disorder involving a thrombus in a deep vein; most commonly the iliac and femoral veins.
**degenerative disc disease (DDD)** progressive degeneration that is a normal process of aging; results in the intervertebral discs losing their elasticity, flexibility, and shock-absorbing capabilities.
**dehiscence** the separation and disruption of previously joined wound edges, typically an abdominal incision.
**delirium** a state of temporary but acute mental confusion.
**dementia** a neurocognitive disorder caused by brain disease, evidenced by chronic personality disintegration, confusion, memory impairment, and deterioration of intellectual capacity and function.
**dermatomyositis** a disease of the connective tissues characterized by pruritic or eczematous inflammation of the skin and tenderness of the muscles.
**diabetes insipidus (DI)** a group of conditions associated with deficient production or secretion of antidiuretic hormone (ADH), or a decreased renal response to ADH caused by injury of the neurohypophyseal system.
**diabetes mellitus (DM)** a multisystem disease related to abnormal insulin production, impaired insulin utilization, or both.
**diabetic ketoacidosis (DKA)** an acute metabolic complication of diabetes occurring when fats are metabolized in the absence of insulin resulting in formation of acid by-products, such as ketones.
**diabetic nephropathy** a microvascular complication of diabetes mellitus associated with damage to the small blood vessels that supply the glomeruli of the kidney.
**diabetic neuropathy** nerve damage caused by the metabolic derangements associated with diabetes mellitus.
**dialysis** technique in which substances move from the blood through a semipermeable membrane and into a dialysis solution.
**dislocation** a severe injury of the ligamentous structures that surround a joint resulting in

the complete displacement or separation of the articular surfaces of the joint.

**disseminated intravascular coagulation (DIC)** a grave coagulopathy resulting from the overstimulation of clotting and anticlotting processes in response to disease or injury.

**diverticulitis** inflammation of one or more diverticula, resulting in perforation into the peritoneum.

**dysarthria** a disturbance in the muscular control of speech resulting from interference in the control and execution over the muscles of speech.

**dysmenorrhea** abdominal cramping pain or discomfort associated with menstrual flow.

**dyspareunia** abnormal pain during sexual intercourse.

**dysphagia** difficulty swallowing.

**dysphasia** difficulty related to the comprehension or use of language.

**dysplastic nevi** nevi that are larger than usual with irregular borders and various shades of color; also known as *atypical moles.*

**dyspnea** shortness of breath; difficulty breathing that may be caused by certain heart or lung conditions, strenuous exercise, or anxiety.

## E

**ecchymoses** bruising.

**ectopic pregnancy** the implantation of a fertilized ovum anywhere outside the uterine cavity.

**embolic stroke** a stroke that occurs when an embolus lodges in and occludes a cerebral artery, resulting in infarction and edema of the area supplied by the involved vessel.

**emergence delirium** a neurologic alteration in recovery from anesthesia that can include behaviors such as restlessness, agitation, disorientation, thrashing, and shouting.

**empyema** an accumulation of purulent exudates in a body cavity, especially the pleural space, that results from bacterial infection, such as pleurisy or tuberculosis.

**encephalitis** an acute inflammation of the brain that usually caused by a virus.

**endometriosis** the presence of normal endometrial tissue in sites outside the endometrial cavity.

**endotracheal intubation** artificial airway created by inserting a tube into the trachea through the mouth or nose, past the larynx, and bypassing the upper airway and laryngeal structures.

**enteral nutrition (EN)** the administration of a nutritionally balanced, liquefied food or formula through a tube inserted into the stomach, duodenum, or jejunum.

**epididymitis** acute or chronic inflammation of the epididymis, usually secondary to an infectious process, trauma, or urinary reflux down the vas deferens.

**epidural block** injection of a local anesthetic into the epidural (extradural) space by either a thoracic or lumbar approach.

**epidural hematoma** collection of blood between the dura and inner surface of the skull, producing compression of the dura mater and thus of the brain.

**epilepsy** a condition in which a person has spontaneously recurring seizures caused by a chronic underlying condition.

**epistaxis** nosebleed.

**erectile dysfunction (ED)** the inability to attain or maintain an erection that allows satisfactory sexual activity.

**erythema** redness or inflammation of the skin or mucous membranes that results from dilation and congestion of superficial capillaries.

**escharotomy** incisions into necrotic tissue from a severe burn performed when eschar formation compromises circulation.

**esophageal diverticulum** saclike outpouching of one or more layers of the esophagus.

**esophageal varices** distended, tortuous, fragile veins at the lower end of the esophagus that result from portal hypertension.

**evisceration** the separation and disruption of previously joined wound edges to the extent that an internal organ, typically intestinal contents, protrudes through the wound.

**excision and grafting** procedure during which eschar is removed down to the subcutaneous tissue or fascia, depending on the degree of injury; a graft is then placed on clean, viable tissue to achieve good adherence.

**exophthalmos** protrusion of the eyeballs from the orbits caused by increased fat deposits and fluid in the retroorbital tissues.

**external otitis** inflammation or infection of the epithelium of the auricle and ear canal.

**extreme obesity** the classification used to describe individuals with body mass index values >40 $kg/m^2$.

## F

**fat embolism syndrome (FES)** embolization of fat globules that occurs in a small percentage of patients with fractures.

**fibroadenoma** a small, painless, round, well-delineated, mobile benign breast tumor commonly found in young women.

**fibrocystic changes** a benign condition of the breasts characterized by development of excess fibrous tissue, hyperplasia of the epithelial lining of the mammary ducts, proliferation of mammary ducts, and cyst formation.

**fibromyalgia** a chronic disorder characterized by widespread, nonarticular musculoskeletal pain and fatigue with multiple tender points.

**flail chest** instability of the chest wall resulting from multiple rib fractures.

**focal seizures** seizures that begin in a specific region of the cortex and may be confined to one side of the brain and remain partial or focal in nature, or they may spread to involve the entire brain.

**fracture** a disruption or break in the continuity of the structure of bone.

**fremitus** vibration of the chest wall produced by vocalization.

**frontotemporal lobar degeneration (FTLD)** a rare disorder caused by shrinking frontal and temporal lobes of the brain; characterized by disturbances in behavior, sleep, personality, and eventually memory.

**frostbite** freezing that results in the formation of ice crystals in the tissues and cells.

**full-thickness burn** destruction of all skin elements and subcutaneous tissues with possible involvement of muscles, tendons, and bones.

## G

**galactorrhea** a milky secretion from the nipple caused by inappropriate lactation.

**gastritis** inflammation of the gastric mucosa.

**gastroenteritis** an inflammation of the mucosa of the stomach and small intestine.

**gastroesophageal reflux disease (GERD)** any clinically significant symptomatic condition or histopathologic alteration presumed to be secondary to reflux of gastric contents into the lower esophagus.

**generalized seizures** seizures characterized by bilateral synchronous epileptic discharge in the brain with loss of consciousness for a few seconds to several minutes.

**genital herpes** a sexually transmitted infection caused by the herpes simplex virus type 2 (HSV-2), resulting in painful genital or anal vesicular lesions.

**Glasgow Coma Scale** assessment tool for altered states of consciousness that evaluates motor responses, verbal responses, and eye opening.

**glaucoma** a group of disorders characterized by (1) increased intraocular pressure and the consequences of elevated pressure, (2) optic nerve atrophy, and (3) peripheral visual field loss.

**glial cells** cells in the central nervous system that provide support, nourishment, and protection to neurons.

**glomerular filtration rate (GFR)** the amount of blood filtered by the glomeruli in a given time.

**glomerulonephritis** an immune-related inflammation of the glomeruli characterized by proteinuria, hematuria, decreased urine production, and edema.

**goiter** enlargement of the thyroid gland that may be associated with hyperthyroidism, hypothyroidism, or normal thyroid function.

**gonorrhea** infection of the genitalia, the rectum, and/or the oropharynx by *Neisseria gonorrhoeae,* which, if left untreated, leads to the formation of fibrous tissue and adhesions.

**Goodpasture syndrome** an example of cytotoxic autoimmune disease characterized by the presence of circulating antibodies against the glomerular basement membrane and alveolar basement membrane.

**gout** recurrent attacks of acute arthritis associated with increased levels of serum uric acid.

**Guillain-Barré syndrome** an acute, rapidly progressing, and potentially fatal form of polyneuritis possibly caused by a cell-mediated immunologic reaction directed at the peripheral nerves.

**gynecomastia** a transient enlargement of one or both breasts in men.

## H

**heat cramps** severe cramps in large muscle groups caused by depletion of both water and salt; usually follow vigorous exertion in an extremely hot environment.

**heat exhaustion** a clinical syndrome characterized by fatigue, light-headedness, nausea, vomiting, diarrhea, and feelings of impending doom precipitated by prolonged exposure to heat over hours or days.

**heatstroke** the most serious form of heat stress; results from failure of the central thermoregulatory mechanisms and is considered a medical emergency.

**heaves** sustained lifts of the chest wall in the precordial area that can be seen or palpated.

**hematemesis** vomiting of blood that indicates bleeding in the upper GI tract.

**hemochromatosis** an autosomal recessive disease characterized by increased intestinal iron absorption and, as a result, increased tissue iron deposition.

**hemodialysis (HD)** dialysis that uses an artificial membrane as the semipermeable membrane through which the patient's blood circulates.

**hemolytic anemia** an anemia caused by destruction of RBCs at a rate that exceeds production.

**hemophilia** hereditary bleeding disorders caused by defective or deficient clotting factors.

**hemorrhagic stroke** a stroke that results from bleeding into the brain tissue itself or into the subarachnoid space or ventricles.

**hemorrhoids** varicosities in the lower rectum or anus caused by congestion in the veins of the hemorrhoidal plexus.

**hemothorax** accumulation of blood in the pleural space.

**hepatic encephalopathy** changes in neurologic and mental function resulting from high levels of ammonia in the blood that a damaged liver cannot detoxify.

**hepatitis** inflammation of the liver.

**hepatorenal syndrome** type of renal failure in which the kidneys have no structural abnormality and characterized by azotemia, oliguria, and intractable ascites.

**hernia** a protrusion of a viscus through an abnormal opening or a weakened area in the wall of the cavity in which it is normally contained.

**herniated disc** herniation of nuclear material from the intervertebral disc that may compress or place tension on a cervical, lumbar, or sacral spinal nerve root.

**hiatal hernia** herniation of a portion of the stomach into the esophagus through an opening, or hiatus, in the diaphragm.

**histologic grading** a categorization of tumors in which the appearance of cells and the degree of differentiation are evaluated pathologically.

**Hodgkin's lymphoma** a malignant condition characterized by proliferation of abnormal giant, multinucleated cells, called *Reed-Sternberg cells,* which are located in lymph nodes.

**hordeolum** an infection of the sebaceous glands in the eyelid margin; commonly known as a *sty.*

**hospice** a concept of care that provides compassion, concern, and support for persons in the last phases of a terminal disease.

**hospital-acquired pneumonia (HAP)** pneumonia occurring 48 hours or longer after hospital admission and not incubating at the time of hospitalization.

**human immunodeficiency virus (HIV)** a retrovirus that causes HIV infection and acquired immunodeficiency syndrome.

**human leukocyte antigens (HLAs)** a system consisting of a series of linked genes that occur together on the sixth chromosome in humans and that is used to assess tissue compatibility.

**humoral immunity** antibody-mediated immunity.

**Huntington's disease** a genetically transmitted, autosomal dominant disorder that affects both men and women of all races and is characterized by chronic, devastating loss of all neurologic function, resulting in dementia.

**hydronephrosis** dilation or enlargement of the renal pelvis and calyces resulting from obstruction in the lower urinary tract with backflow of urine to the kidney.

**hydroureter** dilation of the renal pelvis due to backflow of urine.

**hyperaldosteronism** excessive aldosterone secretion caused by an adenoma of the adrenal zona glomerulosa or bilateral adrenal hyperplasia.

**hypercapnia** greater than normal amounts of carbon dioxide in the blood; also called *hypercarbia.*

**hypercapnic respiratory failure** a condition in which the $PaCO_2$ is above normal in combination with acidemia.

**hyperopia** farsightedness or the inability of the eye to focus on nearby objects.

**hyperosmolar hyperglycemic syndrome (HHS)** a life-threatening syndrome that can occur in the patient with diabetes who is able to produce enough insulin to prevent diabetic ketoacidosis but not enough to prevent severe hyperglycemia, osmotic diuresis, and extracellular fluid depletion.

**hyperparathyroidism** a condition involving increased secretion of parathyroid hormone resulting in increased serum calcium levels.

**hypertension** a common disorder characterized by sustained elevation of blood pressure.

**hypertensive crisis** a severe and abrupt elevation in blood pressure.

**hyperthyroidism** a clinical syndrome in which there is a sustained increase in the synthesis and release of thyroid hormones by the thyroid gland.

**hypertrophic scar** an inappropriately large, red, raised, and hard scar that occurs when the body produces excess collagen tissue.

**hypoparathyroidism** a condition of insufficient secretion of the parathyroid glands.

**hypopituitarism** a rare disorder that involves a decrease in one or more of the pituitary hormones and is marked by excessive deposits of fat and persistence or acquisition of adolescent characteristics.

**hypothermia** a core temperature <95° F (35° C) that occurs when heat produced by the body cannot compensate for heat lost to the environment.

**hypothyroidism** insufficient circulation of thyroid hormones resulting in a hypometabolic state.

**hypoxemia** low oxygen tension in the blood characterized by a variety of nonspecific clinical signs and symptoms.

**hypoxemic respiratory failure** a condition in which the $PaO_2$ is 60 mm Hg or less when the patient is receiving an inspired oxygen concentration of 60% or greater.

**hypoxia** the state in which the $PaO_2$ has fallen sufficiently to cause signs and symptoms of inadequate oxygenation.

## I

**ileal conduit** urinary diversion procedure in which ureters are implanted into a part of the ileum or colon that has been resected from the intestinal tract and an abdominal stoma is created.

**impaired fasting glucose (IFG)** an intermediate stage between normal glucose homeostasis and diabetes.

**impaired glucose tolerance (IGT)** an intermediate stage between normal glucose homeostasis and diabetes in which the blood glucose level is 140 mg/dL (7.8 mmol/L) to 199 mg/dL (11 mmol/L) 2 hours after a meal.

**infective endocarditis** an infection of the endocardial surface of the heart.

**infertility** the inability to achieve a pregnancy after at least 1 year of regular intercourse without contraception.

**inflammatory bowel disease (IBD)** chronic, recurrent inflammatory diseases of the intestinal tract that include ulcerative colitis and Crohn's disease.

**insulin resistance** a condition in which body tissues do not respond to the action of insulin.

**intensive insulin therapy** multiple daily insulin injections together with frequent self-monitoring of blood glucose.

**intermittent claudication** ischemic muscle ache or pain precipitated by a consistent level of exercise, resolves within 10 minutes or less with rest, and is reproducible.

**interstitial cystitis** chronic, painful inflammatory disease of the bladder probably associated with an autoimmune or allergic response.

**intraaortic balloon pump (IABP)** a temporary circulatory assist device used to enhance the function of a compromised heart by reducing afterload and augmenting the aortic diastolic pressure.

**intracerebral hematoma** collection of blood within the parenchyma of the brain, possibly from the rupture of an intracerebral vessel at the time of a head injury.

**intracranial pressure** the hydrostatic force measured in the brain cerebrospinal fluid compartment.

**iron-deficiency anemia** a microcytic hypochromic anemia caused by inadequate supplies of iron needed to synthesize hemoglobin; characterized by pallor, fatigue, and weakness.

**irritable bowel syndrome (IBS)** a disorder characterized by chronic abdominal pain or discomfort and alteration of bowel patterns (diarrhea or constipation).

**ischemic stroke** a stroke that results from inadequate blood flow to the brain due to partial or complete occlusion of an artery.

**isometric contractions** muscular contraction that increases tension but does not produce movement.

**isotonic contractions** muscular contraction with shortening that produces movement.

## J

**jaundice** a symptom of yellowish discoloration of body tissues that results from an increased concentration of bilirubin in the blood.

**jaw-thrust maneuver** a technique used to maintain an open airway that should be used in emergency situations.

## K

**keloid** an overgrowth of collagenous scar tissue at the site of a skin injury, particularly a wound or a surgical incision; the new tissue is elevated, rounded, and firm.

**keratinocytes** cells synthesized from epidermal cells in the basal layer; the cells produce a specialized protein (keratin) that is vital to the protective barrier function of the skin.

**keratitis** an inflammation or infection of the cornea; may be caused by a variety of microorganisms or by other factors.

**Korotkoff sounds** sounds heard during the taking of a blood pressure reading using a sphygmomanometer and stethoscope.

**Kupffer cells** a type of macrophage found in the liver that removes bacteria and toxins from the blood.

**kyphosis** anterior-posterior or forward bending of spine with convexity of curve in posterior direction.

## L

**leiomyoma** a benign smooth muscle tumor that occurs most commonly within the uterus, stomach, esophagus, or small intestine; uterine fibroid.

**leukemia** a broad term given to a group of malignant diseases characterized by diffuse replacement of bone marrow with proliferating leukocyte precursors.

**leukopenia** an abnormal decrease in the number of total white blood cells to <4000/μL.

**lichenification** the thickening of the skin as a result of proliferation of keratinocytes with accentuation of the normal markings of the skin often caused by repeated scratching of a pruritic lesion.

**lithotripsy** the use of sound waves to break renal stones into small particles that can be eliminated from the urinary tract.

**lordosis** lumbar spinal deformity resulting in anterior-posterior curvature with concavity in posterior direction.

**lumpectomy** breast-conserving surgery that involves the removal of the entire tumor along with a margin of normal tissue.

**Lyme disease** a spirochetal infection caused by *Borrelia burgdorferi* and transmitted by the bite of an infected deer tick; characterized by fever, chills, headache, stiff neck, and migratory joint and muscle pain.

**lymphedema** accumulation of lymph in soft tissue with swelling resulting from inflammation, obstruction, or removal of lymph channels and nodes.

**lymphomas** malignant neoplasms originating in the bone marrow and lymphatic structures resulting in the proliferation of lymphocytes.

## M

**malabsorption syndrome** a complex of symptoms resulting from disorders in the intestinal absorption of nutrients, characterized by anorexia, weight loss, abdominal bloating, muscle cramps, bone pain, and steatorrhea.

**malignant hyperthermia** a rare genetic metabolic disease characterized by hyperthermia with rigidity of skeletal muscles that can result in death.

**malignant melanoma** a tumor arising in cells producing melanin, usually the melanocytes of the skin.

**malignant neoplasm** a tumor that tends to grow, invade, and metastasize; usually has an irregular shape and is composed of poorly differentiated cells.

**Mallory-Weiss tear** a tear that occurs in the esophageal mucosa at the junction of the esophagus and stomach, caused by severe retching and vomiting and results in severe bleeding.

**mammoplasty** a change in the size or shape of the breast due to surgery.

**mass casualty incident** a human-caused (e.g., biologic warfare) or natural (e.g., hurricane) event or disaster that overwhelms a community's ability to respond with existing resources.

**mastalgia** breast pain; can be caused by congestion or "caking" during lactation, an infection, or fibrocystic disease, especially during or before menstruation, or in advanced cancer.

**mastitis** an inflammatory condition of the breast that occurs most frequently in lactating women, caused by streptococcal or staphylococcal infection.

**mean arterial pressure (MAP)** a calculated average of systolic and diastolic blood pressures; calculated by adding the diastolic pressure to one third of the pulse pressure.

**megaloblastic anemias** a group of disorders caused by impaired DNA synthesis and characterized by the presence of large red blood cells.

**melena** black, tarry stools that indicate slow bleeding from an upper GI source.

**menarche** the first episode of menstrual bleeding; indicates female has reached puberty.

**Ménière's disease** a disease characterized by symptoms caused by inner ear disease, including episodic vertigo, tinnitus, fluctuating sensorineural hearing loss, and aural fullness.

**meningitis** an acute inflammation of the pia mater and the arachnoid membrane surrounding the brain and the spinal cord.

**menopause** the physiologic cessation of menses associated with declining ovarian function.

**metabolic equivalent (MET)** a unit of measurement of heat production by the body; used to determine the energy costs of various exercises.

**metabolic syndrome** a group of metabolic risk factors that increase an individual's chance of developing cardiovascular disease and diabetes mellitus.

**metastasis** the spread of the cancer from the initial or primary site to a distant site.

**migraine headache** a recurring headache characterized by unilateral or bilateral throbbing pain and a triggering event or factor; can occur with and without an aura.

**mild cognitive impairment (MCI)** a state of cognition and functional ability between normal aging and early Alzheimer's disease.

**mitral valve prolapse (MVP)** a structural abnormality of the mitral valve leaflets and the papillary muscles or chordae that allows the leaflets to prolapse, or buckle, back into the left atrium during ventricular systole.

**mixed dementia** presentation of two or more types of dementia simultaneously.

**multiple myeloma** a condition in which malignant neoplastic plasma cells infiltrate the bone marrow and destroy bone.

**multiple organ dysfunction syndrome (MODS)** the failure of more than one organ system in an acutely ill patient such that homeostasis cannot be maintained without intervention.

**multiple sclerosis (MS)** a chronic, progressive, degenerative disorder of the central nervous system characterized by disseminated demyelination of nerve fibers of the brain and spinal cord.

**murmur** a gentle blowing, fluttering, or humming sound heard on auscultation and produced by turbulent blood flow through the heart or the walls of large arteries.

**muscular dystrophy (MD)** a group of genetically transmitted diseases characterized by progressive symmetric wasting of skeletal muscle without evidence of neurologic involvement.

**myasthenia gravis (MG)** an autoimmune disease of the neuromuscular junction characterized by the fluctuating weakness of certain skeletal muscle groups.

**myasthenic crisis** an acute exacerbation of myasthenia gravis triggered by infection, surgery, emotional distress, or overdose or inadequate medication.

**myelodysplastic syndrome (MDS)** a group of related hematologic disorders characterized by a change in the quantity and quality of bone marrow elements.

**myocardial infarction (MI)** an irreversible cardiac cellular death caused by sustained myocardial ischemia.

**myocarditis** a focal or diffuse inflammation of the myocardium.

**myopia** nearsightedness or the inability of the eye to focus on objects far away.

**myxedema** the progression of the mental sluggishness, drowsiness, and lethargy of hypothyroidism to a notable impairment of consciousness or coma, which is a medical emergency.

## N

**nadir** the lowest point, such as the blood cell count after it has been depressed by chemotherapy.

**nasal polyps** benign mucous membrane masses that form slowly in response to repeated inflammation of the sinus or nasal mucosa and project into the nasal cavity.

**nephrolithiasis** the formation of stones in the urinary tract.

**nephrosclerosis** a vascular disease of the kidney characterized by sclerosis of the small arteries and arterioles of the kidney, resulting in renal tissue necrosis.

**nephrotic syndrome** an abnormal condition of the kidney characterized by peripheral edema, massive proteinuria, hyperlipidemia, and hypoalbuminemia.

**neurofibrillary tangles** tangled bundles of fibers seen in the cytoplasm of abnormal neurons in those areas of the brain most affected by Alzheimer's disease.

**neurogenic bladder** any type of bladder dysfunction related to abnormal or absent bladder innervation caused by a lesion of the nervous system.

**neurogenic bowel** loss of voluntary neurologic control over the bowel.

**neurogenic shock** neurologic syndrome caused by the loss of vasomotor tone caused by spinal cord injury and characterized by hypotension, bradycardia, and warm, dry extremities.
**neuropathic pain** pain caused by damage to nerve cells or changes in spinal cord processing of nervous system input.
**neutropenia** an abnormal reduction of the neutrophil count to $<1000/\mu L$.
**nonalcoholic fatty liver disease (NAFLD)** a group of disorders characterized by hepatic *steatosis* (accumulation of fat in the liver) and is not associated with other causes such as hepatitis, autoimmune disease, or consumption of alcohol.
**normal pressure hydrocephalus** an uncommon disorder characterized by an obstruction in the flow of cerebrospinal fluid; causes a buildup of this fluid in the brain.
**nuchal rigidity** resistance to flexion of the neck.
**nulliparous** never having given birth.
**nystagmus** an abnormal, involuntary, repetitive movement of the eyes.

## O

**$O_2$ toxicity** a condition of $O_2$ overdosage caused by prolonged exposure to a high level of $O_2$.
**obese** the classification used to describe individuals with body mass index values $\geq 30$ kg/m$^2$.
**obstructive sleep apnea (OSA)** a condition characterized by partial or complete upper airway obstruction during sleep.
**oliguria** producing <400 mL of urine in 24 hours.
**oncogenes** potentially cancer-inducing genes.
**oncotic pressure** the osmotic pressure of a colloid in solution.
**orchitis** an acute inflammation of the testis.
**orthostatic hypotension** abnormally low blood pressure occurring when an individual suddenly assumes a standing position.
**osteoarthritis** a slowly progressive, noninflammatory disorder of the diarthrodial (synovial) joints.
**osteochondroma** primary benign bone tumor characterized by an overgrowth of cartilage and bone near the end of the bone at the growth plate.
**osteomalacia** a rare condition of adult bones associated with vitamin D deficiency, resulting in decalcification and softening of bone.
**osteomyelitis** a severe infection of the bone, bone marrow, and surrounding soft tissue.
**osteon** cylindrical structural units that fit closely together in compact bone, creating a dense bone structure.
**osteopenia** bone loss that is more than normal (a T-score between −1 and −2.5), but not yet at the level for a diagnosis of osteoporosis.
**osteoporosis** a metabolic bone disease characterized by low bone mass and structural deterioration of bone tissue, leading to increased bone fragility and pathologic fractures.
**osteosarcoma** a primary bone tumor that is extremely aggressive and rapidly metastasizes to distant sites; usually occurs in the metaphyseal region of the long bones of the extremities.
**osteotomy** removing or adding a wedge or slice of bone to change its alignment and shift weight bearing, thereby correcting deformity and relieving pain.
**ostomy** a surgical procedure in which an opening is made to allow the passage of urine from the bladder or intestinal contents from the bowel through an incision or stoma surgically created in the wall of the abdomen.
**otosclerosis** a hereditary condition in which irregular ossification occurring on the footplate of the stapes in the oval window results in decreased hearing acuity.

## P

**Paget's disease of the bone** a skeletal bone disorder in which there is excessive bone resorption followed by replacement of normal marrow by vascular, fibrous connective tissue and new bone that is larger, disorganized, and weaker.
**Paget's disease of the breast** a breast malignancy characterized by a persistent lesion of the nipple and areola with or without a palpable mass.
**palliative care** an approach that improves the quality of life of patients and their families who face problems associated with serious life-limiting illness.
**palpation** a physical examination technique in which the examiner feels the texture, size, consistency, and location of certain body parts with the hands.
**pancytopenia** a marked decrease in the number of red blood cells, white blood cells, and platelets.
**paralytic ileus** the lack of intestinal peristalsis.
**paraplegia** paralysis characterized by motor and/or sensory loss in the lower limbs and trunk.
**parasomnias** unusual and often undesirable behaviors that occur with sleep or during arousal from sleep, such as enuresis (bed-wetting), hallucinations, and eating.
**parenteral nutrition (PN)** the administration of nutrients by a route (e.g., bloodstream) other than the GI tract.
**Parkinson's disease (PD)** a disease of the basal ganglia characterized by a slowing down in the initiation and execution of movement, increased muscle tone tremor at rest, and impaired postural reflexes.
**paroxysmal nocturnal dyspnea (PND)** sudden attacks of respiratory distress that awaken the sleeper, usually after several hours of sleep in a reclining position.
**partial-thickness burn** varying degrees of epidermal and dermal skin injury in which some skin elements remain viable for regeneration.
**pelvic inflammatory disease (PID)** an infectious condition of the pelvic cavity that may involve infection of the fallopian tubes, ovaries, and pelvic peritoneum.
**peptic ulcer disease (PUD)** erosion of the GI mucosa that results from the digestive action of HCl acid and pepsin.
**percussion** a physical examination technique in which the examiner taps the body with the fingertips or fist.
**percutaneous coronary intervention (PCI)** a common intervention for coronary artery disease in which a catheter equipped with an inflatable balloon tip is inserted into a narrowed coronary artery and the balloon is inflated.
**pericardiocentesis** a procedure in which a 16- to 18-gauge needle is inserted into the pericardial space to remove fluid for analysis and to relieve cardiac pressure.
**pericarditis** a condition caused by inflammation of the pericardial sac.
**perimenopause** a normal life transition that begins with the first signs of change in menstrual cycles and ends after cessation of menses.
**peripheral artery disease (PAD)** the progressive narrowing and degeneration of the arteries of the neck, abdomen, and extremities.
**peripheral stem cell transplantation** the transplantation of stem cells obtained from the peripheral blood in an outpatient procedure; often takes more than one procedure to obtain enough stem cells.
**peritoneal dialysis (PD)** dialysis using the peritoneal membrane as the semipermeable membrane.
**peritonitis** the inflammation of the peritoneum.
**pernicious anemia** a progressive megaloblastic macrocytic anemia resulting from inadequate gastric secretion of intrinsic factor necessary for absorption of cobalamin.
**pertussis** a highly contagious infection of the lower respiratory tract with a gram-negative bacillus, *Bordetella pertussis.*
**petechiae** small purplish lesions.
**phantom limb sensation** the perception of sensations or pain in an amputated limb.
**pharmacogenetics** the study of variability of responses to drugs due to variations in single genes.
**pharmacogenomics** the study of variability of responses to drugs due to variations in and interactions of multiple genes.
**pheochromocytoma** a rare condition characterized by a tumor of the adrenal medulla that produces excessive catecholamines causing persistent or intermittent hypertension.
**phimosis** a constriction of the uncircumcised foreskin around the head of the penis, making retraction difficult.
**pleural effusion** an abnormal accumulation of fluid in the intrapleural spaces of the lungs.
**pleural friction rub** a creaking or grating sound from roughened, inflamed surfaces of the pleura rubbing together, evident during inspiration, expiration, or both.
**pleurisy (pleuritis)** inflammation of the pleura.
**pneumoconiosis** a general term for lung diseases caused by inhalation and retention of dust particles.
**pneumonia** an acute inflammation of the lungs, often caused by inhaled pneumococci of the species *Streptococcus pneumoniae.*
**pneumothorax** a collection of air or gas in the pleural space causing the lung to collapse.
**point of maximal impulse (PMI)** the site on the chest wall where the thrust or pulsation of the left ventricle is most prominent.
**polycystic kidney disease (PKD)** a genetic kidney disorder in which the cortex and medulla are filled with thin-walled cysts that enlarge and destroy surrounding tissue.

**polycythemia** an abnormal condition with excessive levels of red blood cells.

**polymyositis** diffuse, idiopathic, inflammatory myopathies of striated muscle, producing bilateral weakness usually most severe in the proximal or limb-girdle muscles; some forms of polymyositis are associated with malignancy.

**portal hypertension** increased venous pressure in the portal circulation caused by compression and destruction of the portal and hepatic veins and sinusoids.

**positive end-expiratory pressure (PEEP)** a ventilatory maneuver in which positive pressure is applied to the airway during exhalation.

**postural drainage** the use of various positions to promote gravity drainage of bronchial secretions.

**prediabetes** impaired glucose tolerance; occurs when a 2-hour plasma glucose level is higher than normal but lower than that considered diagnostic for diabetes.

**prehypertension** a disorder characterized by a systolic blood pressure of 120 to 139 mm Hg and a diastolic blood pressure of 80 to 89 mm Hg.

**preload** the volume of blood in the ventricles at the end of diastole before the next contraction.

**premature atrial contraction (PAC)** contraction originating from an ectopic focus in the atrium in a location other than the sinus node.

**premature ventricular contraction (PVC)** a contraction originating in an ectopic focus in the ventricles.

**premenstrual syndrome (PMS)** a common disorder in women in which a group of physical and psychologic symptoms occur during the last few days of the menstrual cycle and before the onset of menstruation.

**presbycusis** hearing loss associated with aging.

**presbyopia** a hyperopic shift to farsightedness resulting from a loss of elasticity of the lens of the eye.

**pressure ulcer** a localized area of tissue necrosis caused by unrelieved pressure that occludes blood flow to the tissues.

**primary hypertension** an elevated systemic arterial pressure for which no cause can be found and which is often the only significant clinical finding.

**Prinzmetal's angina** a variant angina; occurs at rest, usually in response to reversible, severe spasm of a major coronary artery.

**prostatitis** an acute or chronic inflammation of the prostate gland, usually as a result of infection.

**pruritus** itching.

**psoriasis** an autoimmune skin disorder characterized by circumscribed red patches covered by thick, dry, silvery, adherent scales.

**pulmonary edema** an acute, life-threatening situation in which the lung alveoli become filled with serous or serosanguineous fluid, caused most commonly by heart failure.

**pulmonary embolism** a thromboembolic occlusion of the pulmonary vasculature resulting from thrombi in the venous circulation or right side of the heart that travel as emboli until lodging in the pulmonary vessels.

**pulmonary hypertension** elevated pulmonary pressure resulting from an increase in pulmonary vascular resistance to blood flow through small arteries and arterioles.

**pulse pressure** the difference between the systolic and diastolic pressures.

**pursed-lip breathing** a technique of exhaling against pursed lips to prolong exhalation, preventing bronchiolar collapse and air trapping.

**pyelonephritis** a diffuse pyogenic infection of the renal parenchyma and collecting system.

**pyrosis** a burning sensation in the epigastric or substernal area; heartburn.

## R

**radical prostatectomy** the surgical removal of the entire prostate gland, seminal vesicles, and part of the bladder neck (ampulla).

**Raynaud's phenomenon** an episodic vasospastic disorder of small cutaneous arteries, most frequently involving the fingers and toes.

**refractive error** a defect in the ability of the lens of the eye to focus an image accurately on the retina, as occurs in nearsightedness and farsightedness.

**renal artery stenosis** a partial occlusion of one or both renal arteries and their major branches; is a major cause of abrupt-onset hypertension.

**repetitive strain injury (RSI)** a cumulative trauma disorder resulting from prolonged, forceful, or awkward movements resulting in strain of tendons, ligaments, and muscles, causing tiny tears that become inflamed.

**restless legs syndrome (RLS)** the unpleasant sensory and motor abnormalities of one or both legs; characterized by an irritating sensation of uneasiness, tiredness, and itching deep within the muscles of the leg.

**retinal detachment** a separation of the retina from the retinal pigment epithelium in the back of the eye, allowing the vitreous humor to leak between the two layers.

**retinopathy** the process of microvascular damage of the retina; may develop slowly or rapidly.

**rheumatic fever** an inflammatory disease of the heart that potentially involves all layers.

**rheumatic heart disease (RHD)** the resulting damage to the heart muscle and heart valves from rheumatic fever, a chronic condition characterized by scarring and deformity of the heart valves.

**rheumatoid arthritis (RA)** a chronic, systemic autoimmune disease characterized by inflammation of connective tissue in the diarthrodial (synovial) joints, typically with periods of remission and exacerbation.

**rhinoplasty** the surgical reconstruction of the nose.

## S

**sarcoma** a malignant tumor that originates from embryonal mesoderm that becomes connective tissue, muscle, bone, and fat.

**scleroderma** a disorder of connective tissue characterized by fibrotic, degenerative, and occasionally inflammatory changes in the skin, blood vessels, synovium, skeletal muscle, and internal organs.

**scoliosis** a lateral S-shaped curvature of the thoracic and lumbar spine.

**secondary hypertension** elevated blood pressure associated with any of several primary diseases, such as renal, pulmonary, endocrine, and vascular diseases.

**seizure** a paroxysmal, uncontrolled electrical discharge of neurons in the brain that interrupts normal function leading to a sudden, violent involuntary series of contractions of a group of muscles.

**sepsis** a systemic inflammatory response to infection.

**septic arthritis** infectious or bacterial arthritis caused by invasion of the joint cavity with microorganisms; bacterial inflammation of a joint may be caused by the spread of bacteria through the bloodstream from an infection elsewhere in the body or by contamination of a joint during trauma or surgery.

**septic shock** the presence of sepsis with hypotension despite adequate fluid resuscitation along with the presence of tissue perfusion abnormalities.

**sexually transmitted infections (STIs)** infectious diseases transmitted most commonly through sexual intercourse or genital contact.

**shock** a syndrome characterized by decreased tissue perfusion and impaired cellular metabolism resulting in an imbalance between the supply of and demand for oxygen and nutrients.

**sickle cell disease (SCD)** a group of inherited, autosomal recessive disorders characterized by the presence of an abnormal form of hemoglobin in the erythrocyte.

**silent ischemia** an asymptomatic ischemia that may damage the heart.

**Sjögren's syndrome** an autoimmune disease that targets moisture-producing glands, leading to the common symptoms of xerostomia (dry mouth) and keratoconjunctivitis sicca (dry eyes).

**Somogyi effect** a condition in which an excessive dose of insulin causes blood glucose levels to decline during sleep, triggering the release of counterregulatory hormones that increase the blood glucose levels, resulting in high blood glucose levels at morning testing; indicates a need for reduced dose of insulin.

**spermatogenesis** the formation of sperm.

**spider angiomas** small, dilated blood vessels with a bright red center point the size of a pinhead from which small blood vessels radiate.

**spinal shock** the immediate failure of all spinal cord function at the time of injury below the level of cord damage, resulting in flaccid paralysis, loss of reflexes, and loss of sympathetic innervation.

**spondyloarthropathies** a group of interrelated multisystem inflammatory disorders that affect the spine, peripheral joints, and periarticular structures.

**status epilepticus** a state of continuous seizure activity or a condition in which seizures recur in rapid succession without return to consciousness between seizures.

**steatorrhea** a greater than normal amount of fat in the feces.

**stenosis** a constriction or narrowing.

**stent** an expandable meshlike structure designed to maintain vessel patency by compressing the arterial walls and resisting vasoconstriction.

**stricture** an abnormal temporary or permanent narrowing of the lumen of a hollow organ.

**stroke** the death of brain cells that occurs when there is ischemia to a part of the brain or hemorrhage into the brain.

**subarachnoid hemorrhage** a stroke resulting from intracranial bleeding into the cerebrospinal fluid–filled space between the arachnoid and pia mater membranes on the surface of the brain.

**subdural hematoma** a collection of blood between the dura mater and the arachnoid layer of the meninges of the brain that is generally of venous origin, usually caused by injury.

**sudden cardiac death (SCD)** unexpected death from cardiac causes.

**sundowning** a condition in which the individual becomes more confused and agitated in the late afternoon or evening.

**surfactant** a lipoprotein that lowers the surface tension in the alveoli, reduces the amount of pressure needed to inflate the alveoli, and decreases the tendency of the alveoli to collapse.

**syndrome of inappropriate antidiuretic hormone (SIADH)** a condition associated with overproduction or oversecretion of ADH.

**synovectomy** the surgical removal of synovial membrane.

**syphilis** the infection of organs and tissues of the body by *Treponema pallidum.*

**systemic exertion intolerance disease (SEID)** was formerly called *chronic fatigue syndrome.* Is a serious, complex, multisystem disease in which exertion of any sort (physical, emotional, cognitive) can adversely affect multiple organs.

**systemic inflammatory response syndrome (SIRS)** a systemic inflammatory response to a variety of insults, including infection, ischemia, infarct, and injury.

**systemic lupus erythematosus (SLE)** a chronic multisystem inflammatory disorder associated with abnormalities of the immune system.

## T

**teletherapy** radiation therapy administered by a machine positioned at some distance from the patient; the most common form of radiation therapy treatment.

**tenesmus** the painful spasmodic contraction of the anal sphincter and a persistent desire to empty the bowel.

**tension pneumothorax** a rapid accumulation of air in the pleural space causing severely high intrapleural pressures with resultant tension on the heart and great vessels.

**tension-type headache** a headache characterized by a bilateral feeling of pressure around the head.

**tetanus** lockjaw; an extremely severe polyradiculitis and polyneuritis affecting spinal and cranial nerves that results from the effects of a potent neurotoxin released by the anaerobic bacillus *Clostridium tetani.*

**tetraplegia** the paralysis of the arms, legs, and trunk occurring with spinal cord damage at C8 or above.

**thalassemia** an autosomal recessive genetic disorder of inadequate production of normal hemoglobin.

**thoracentesis** a surgical procedure done to remove fluid from the pleural space.

**thoracotomy** a surgical opening into the thoracic cavity.

**thrombocytopenia** a reduction of the platelet count.

**thrombocytosis** a condition marked by excessive platelets; a disorder that occurs with inflammation and some malignant disorders.

**thrombotic stroke** a stroke resulting from thrombosis or narrowing of the blood vessel.

**thyroiditis** an inflammatory process in the thyroid gland.

**thyrotoxicosis** (also called *thyrotoxic crisis* or *thyroid storm*) a hypermetabolic state caused by excessive circulating levels of $T_4$, $T_3$, or both.

**tinnitus** a subjective noise sensation, often described as ringing, heard in one or both ears.

**tonic-clonic seizure** a seizure characterized by loss of consciousness and falling to the ground, followed by stiffening of the body for 10 to 20 seconds and subsequent jerking of the extremities for another 30 to 40 seconds.

**tracheostomy** a surgical opening into the trachea through which an indwelling tube may be inserted.

**traction** the application of a pulling force to an injured or diseased part of the body or an extremity while countertraction pulls in the opposite direction.

**transurethral resection of the prostate (TURP)** a surgical procedure involving the removal of prostate tissue with the use of a resectoscope inserted through the urethra.

**triage** a system that identifies and categorizes patients so that the most critical are treated first.

**trigeminal neuralgia** a neurologic condition of the trigeminal facial nerve characterized by paroxysms of flashing, stablike pain radiating along the course of a branch of the nerve from the angle of the jaw.

**trigger point** a circumscribed hypersensitive area within a tight band of muscle that is caused by acute or chronic muscle strain.

**tuberculosis (TB)** an infectious disease caused by *Mycobacterium tuberculosis;* usually involves the lungs but also occurs in the larynx, kidneys, bones, adrenal glands, lymph nodes, and meninges and can be disseminated throughout the body.

**tumor angiogenesis** the process of the formation of blood vessels within the tumor itself.

## U

**ulcerative colitis** a chronic inflammatory bowel disease that causes ulceration of the colon and rectum.

**unstable angina (UA)** an angina that is new in onset, occurs at rest, or has a worsening pattern.

**uremia** the presence of excessive amounts of urea and other nitrogenous waste products in the blood; renal function declines to the point that symptoms develop in multiple body systems.

**urethritis** inflammation of the urethra.

**urinary incontinence (UI)** an uncontrolled leakage of urine; can be caused by anything that interferes with bladder or urethral sphincter control, including confusion or depression, infection, atrophic vaginitis, urinary retention, restricted mobility, fecal impaction, or drugs.

**urinary retention** the inability to empty the bladder despite micturition, or the accumulation of urine in the bladder because of an inability to urinate.

**urosepsis** a urinary tract infection that has spread into the systemic circulation; life-threatening condition requiring emergency treatment.

**uterine prolapse** the downward displacement of the uterus into the vaginal canal as a result of impaired pelvic support.

## V

**Valsalva maneuver** a maneuver that involves contraction of the chest muscles on a closed glottis with simultaneous contraction of the abdominal muscles.

**varicose veins** the dilated, tortuous subcutaneous veins most frequently found in the saphenous system.

**vascular dementia** the loss of cognitive function resulting from ischemic, ischemic-hypoxic, or hemorrhagic brain lesions caused by cardiovascular disease.

**vasectomy** the bilateral surgical ligation or resection of the vas deferens performed for the purpose of sterilization.

**ventricular assist device (VAD)** a device that is applied externally or internally into the path of flowing blood to augment or replace the action of the ventricle of the heart.

**ventricular fibrillation** a severe derangement of the heart rhythm characterized on electrocardiogram (ECG) by irregular undulations of varying contour and amplitude.

**ventricular tachycardia (VT)** a condition that occurs when an ectopic focus or foci fire repetitively and the ventricle takes control as the pacemaker.

**vertigo** a sensation that a person or objects around the person are moving or spinning; usually stimulated by movement of the head.

**vesicants** agents that when accidentally infiltrated into the skin cause severe local tissue breakdown and necrosis.

**viral load** the quantity of viral particles in a biologic sample.

**Virchow's triad** three important factors in the etiology of venous thrombosis: (1) venous stasis, (2) damage of the endothelium (inner lining of the vein), and (3) hypercoagulability of the blood.

## W

**wheezes** a form of rhonchus characterized by a continuous high-pitched squeaking sound caused by rapid vibration of bronchial walls.

**window period** a time period of 3 weeks after HIV infection during which an infected individual will not test positive for HIV antibody.

# INDEX



NOTE: Disorder names and key terms are in **boldface**. Page numbers in **boldface** indicate main discussions. Page numbers followed by *f*, *t*, or *b* indicate figures, tables, or boxes, respectively.

## I

## J

## M

## O

## P

## T

## V

| | |
|---|---|
| ABG | arterial blood gas |
| ACE | angiotensin-converting enzyme |
| ACLS | advanced cardiac life support |
| ACS | acute coronary syndrome |
| ACTH | adrenocorticotropic hormone |
| ADH | antidiuretic hormone |
| AED | automatic external defibrillator |
| AIDS | acquired immunodeficiency syndrome |
| AKA | above-knee amputation |
| AKI | acute kidney injury |
| ALI | acute lung injury |
| ALL | acute lymphocytic leukemia |
| ALS | amyotrophic lateral sclerosis |
| AMI | acute myocardial infarction |
| ANA | antinuclear antibody |
| ANS | autonomic nervous system |
| AORN | Association of periOperative Room Nurses |
| APD | automated peritoneal dialysis |
| aPTT | activated partial thromboplastin time |
| ARDS | acute respiratory distress syndrome |
| ATN | acute tubular necrosis |
| BCLS | basic cardiac life support |
| BKA | below-knee amputation |
| BMI | body mass index |
| BMR | basal metabolic rate |
| BMT | bone marrow transplantation |
| BPH | benign prostatic hyperplasia |
| BSE | breast self-examination |
| BUN | blood urea nitrogen |
| CABG | coronary artery bypass graft |
| CAD | coronary artery disease; circulatory assist device |
| CAPD | continuous ambulatory peritoneal dialysis |
| CAVH | continuous arteriovenous hemofiltration |
| CBC | complete blood count |
| CCU | coronary care unit; critical care unit |
| CDC | Centers for Disease Control and Prevention |
| CIS | carcinoma in situ |
| CKD | chronic kidney disease |
| CLL | chronic lymphocytic leukemia |
| CML | chronic myelocytic leukemia |
| CMP | cardiomyopathy |
| CN | cranial nerve |
| CNS | central nervous system |
| CO | cardiac output |
| COPD | chronic obstructive pulmonary disease |
| CPAP | continuous positive airway pressure |
| CPR | cardiopulmonary resuscitation |
| CRRT | continuous renal replacement therapy |
| CRNA | certified registered nurse anesthetist |
| CSF | cerebrospinal fluid |
| CT | computed tomography |
| CVA | cerebrovascular accident; costovertebral angle |
| CVAD | central venous access device |
| CVI | chronic venous insufficiency |
| CVP | central venous pressure |
| D&C | dilation and curettage |
| DDD | degenerative disk disease |
| DI | diabetes insipidus |
| DIC | disseminated intravascular coagulation |
| DJD | degenerative joint disease |
| DKA | diabetic ketoacidosis |
| DM | diabetes mellitus; diastolic murmur |
| DRE | digital rectal examination |
| DVT | deep vein thrombosis |
| ECF | extracellular fluid |
| ECG | electrocardiogram |
| ED | emergency department; erectile dysfunction |
| EEG | electroencephalogram |
| EMG | electromyogram |
| EMS | emergency medical services |
| ENT | ear, nose, and throat |
| ERCP | endoscopic retrograde cholangiopancreatography |
| ERT | estrogen replacement therapy |
| ESKD | end-stage kidney disease |
| ESR | erythrocyte sedimentation rate |
| ET | endotracheal |
| FEV | forced expiratory volume |
| FRC | functional residual capacity |
| FUO | fever of unknown origin |
| GCS | Glasgow Coma Scale |
| GERD | gastroesophageal reflux disease |
| GFR | glomerular filtration rate |
| GH | growth hormone |
| GI | glycemic index |
| GTT | glucose tolerance test |
| GU | genitourinary |
| GYN, Gyn | gynecologic |
| HAI | health care–associated infection |
| HAV | hepatitis A virus |
| Hb, Hgb | hemoglobin |
| HBV | hepatitis B virus |
| Hct | hematocrit |
| HCV | hepatitis C virus |
| HD | hemodialysis, Huntington's disease |
| HDL | high-density lipoprotein |
| HF | heart failure |
| HIV | human immunodeficiency virus |
| H&P | history and physical examination |
| HPV | human papillomavirus |
| HSCT | hematopoietic stem cell transplantation |
| IABP | intraaortic balloon pump |
| IBS | irritable bowel syndrome |
| ICP | intracranial pressure |
| I&D | incision and drainage |
| IE | infective endocarditis |
| IFG | impaired fasting glucose |
| IGT | impaired glucose tolerance |
| INR | international normalized ratio |
| IOP | intraocular pressure |
| IPPB | intermittent positive-pressure breathing |
| ITP | idiopathic thrombocytopenic purpura |
| IUD | intrauterine device |
| IV | intravenous |
| IVP | intravenous push; intravenous pyelogram |
| JVD | jugular venous distention |
| KS | Kaposi sarcoma |
| KUB | kidney, ureters, and bladder (x-ray) |
| KVO | keep vein open |
| LAD | left anterior descending |
| LDL | low-density lipoprotein |